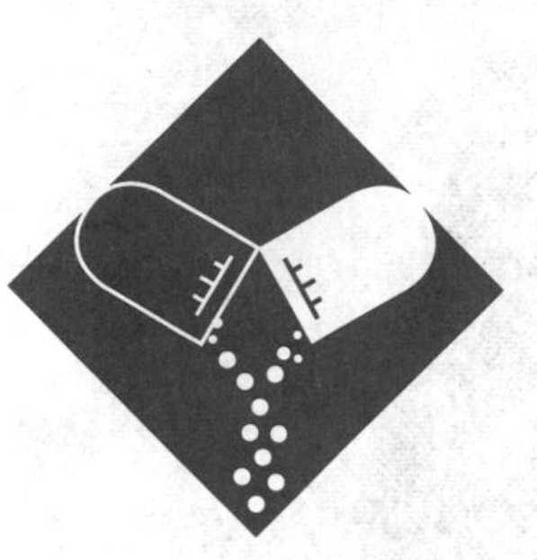

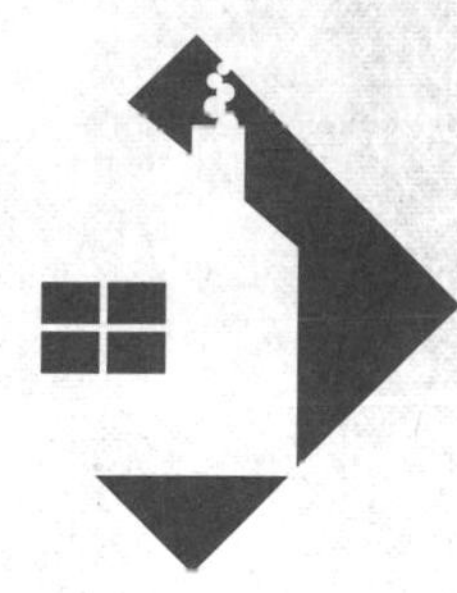

Ellenhorn's Medical Toxicology:

Diagnosis and Treatment of Human Poisoning

Second Edition

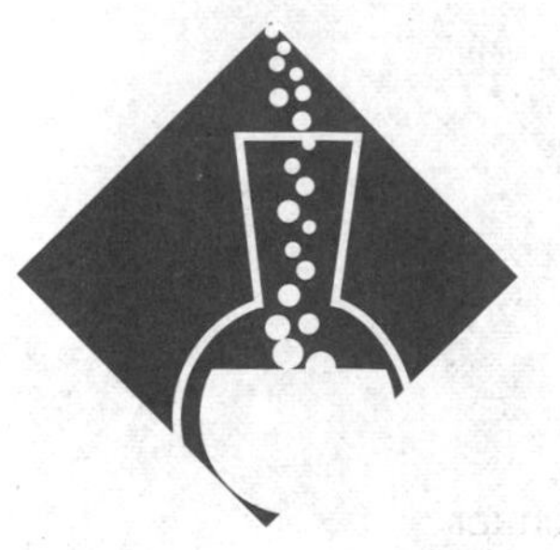

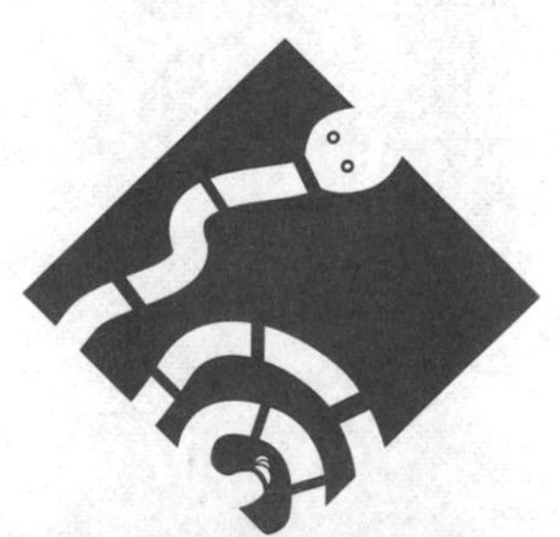

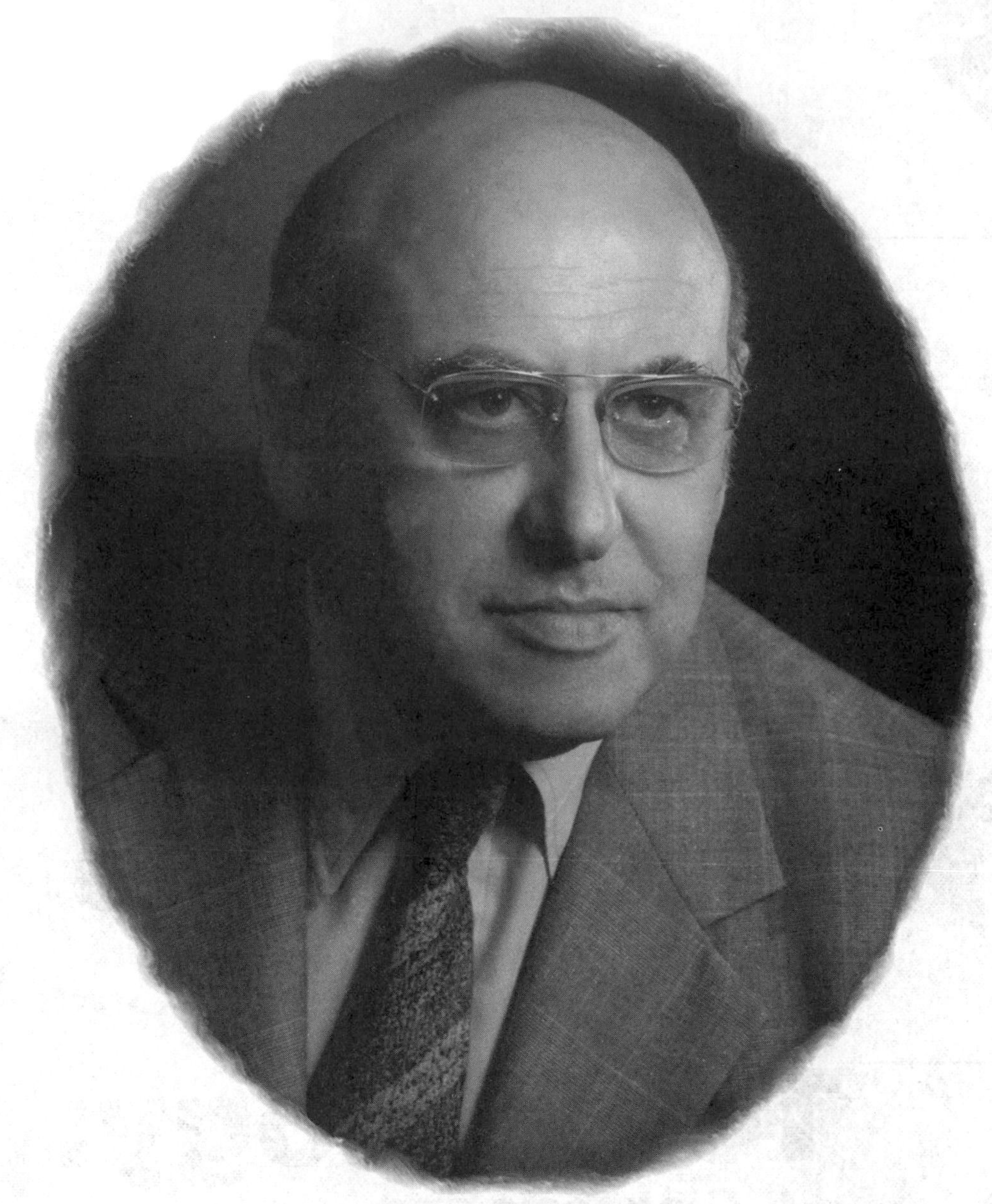

MATTHEW J. ELLENHORN, M.D.

He loved us, supported us and encouraged us to emulate his lifelong search for excellence. We proudly pass his legacy to our children.

Leah Ellenhorn Stromberg, M.S.W., L.C.S.W.
Naomi Ellenhorn Davis, M.D., F.A.C.S.
Joshua David Israel Ellenhorn, M.D., F.A.C.S.

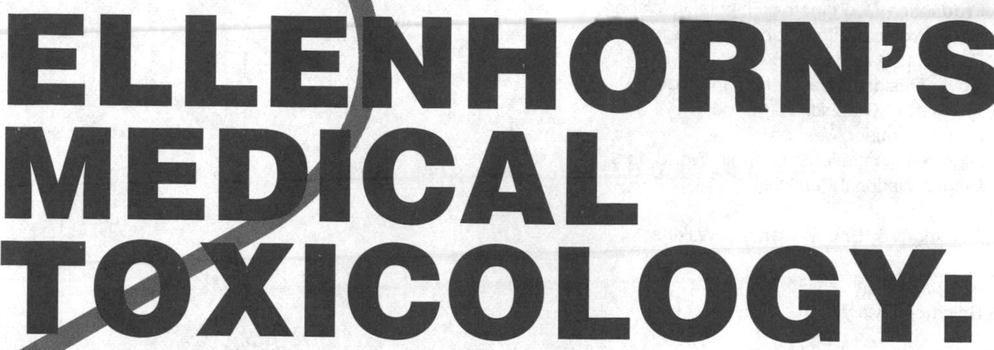

ELLENHORN'S MEDICAL TOXICOLOGY:

Diagnosis and Treatment of Human Poisoning

Second Edition

Matthew J. Ellenhorn, MD
Clinical Professor of Medical Toxicology
Drew/UCLA School of Medicine
Los Angeles, California
King/Drew Medical Center
Consultant Toxicologist, Los Angeles Regional Poison Information Center

Consulting Editors

Seth Schonwald, MD, FACEP
Instructor in Medicine, Emergency Medicine
Harvard Medical School
Mount Auburn Hospital, Cambridge, MA

Gary Ordog, MD, FACEP
Assistant Professor, Emergency Medicine
Charles R. Drew University of Medicine & Science
UCLA School of Medicine, Los Angeles, CA

Jonathan Wasserberger, MD, FACEP
Professor, Emergency Medicine
Charles R. Drew University of Medicine & Science
UCLA School of Medicine, Los Angeles, CA

TECHNICAL ASSOCIATE

Sylvia Syma Ellenhorn, B.A.

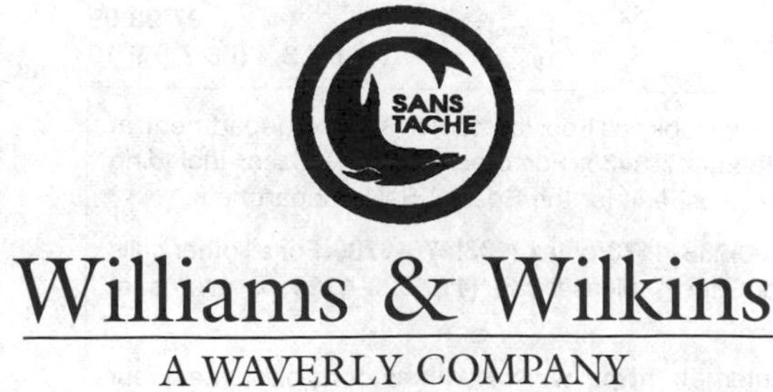

Williams & Wilkins

A WAVERLY COMPANY

BALTIMORE • PHILADELPHIA • LONDON • PARIS • BANGKOK
BUENOS AIRES • HONG KONG • MUNICH • SYDNEY • TOKYO • WROCLAW

Executive Editor: Darlene Barela Cooke
Senior Managing Editor: Sharon R. Zinner
Production Coordinator: Felecia R. Weber
Book Project Editor: Robert D. Magee
Designer: Nancy Hagan Abbott
Cover Designer: Nancy Hagan Abbott
Typesetter: Graphic World, Inc.
Printer: Courier Westford
Digitized Illustrations: Graphic World, Inc.
Binder: National Publishing

351 West Camden Street
Baltimore, Maryland 21201-2436 USA

Rose Tree Corporate Center
1400 North Providence Road
Building II, Suite 5025
Media, Pennsylvania 19063-2043 USA

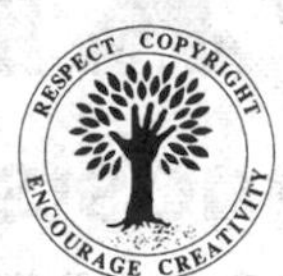

The first edition of MEDICAL TOXICOLOGY by Matthew J. Ellenhorn and Donald G. Barceloux was published by Elsevier Science Publishing Company in 1988, New York.

Accurate indications, adverse reactions, and dosage schedules for drugs are provided in this book, but it is possible that they may change. The reader is urged to review the package information data of the manufacturers of the medications mentioned.

Printed in the United States of America

Second Edition,

Library of Congress Cataloging-in-Publication Data

Ellenhorn's Medical toxicology : diagnosis and treatment of human poisoning / Matthew J. Ellenhorn ; consulting editors, Gary Ordog, Seth Schonwald, Jonathan Wasserberger ; technical associate, Sylvia Syma Ellenhorn.—2nd ed.
p. cm.
Rev. ed. of: Medical toxicology / Matthew J. Ellenhorn, Donald G. Barceloux. c1988.
Includes bibliographical references and index.
ISBN 0-683-30387-2
1. Toxicological emergencies. 2. Poisons. I. Ellenhorn, Matthew J. II. Barceloux, Donald G. III. Ellenhorn, Matthew J. Medical toxicology.
[DNLM: 1. Poisoning—diagnosis. 2. Poisoning—therapy. QV 600 M489 1997]
RA1224.5.M437 1997
615.9—dc20
DNLM/DLC
for Library of Congress 96-12738
CIP

The publishers have made every effort to trace the copyright holders for borrowed material. If they have inadvertently overlooked any, they will be pleased to make the necessary arrangements at the first opportunity.

97 98 99
1 2 3 4 5 6 7 8 9 10

To my four grandchildren:

Eliana Rose, Gideon Samuel, Amiad Yisrael, and Jacob Abraham, who will carry into the next century our hopes for a bright future.

To my children:

Leah and husband, Jeffrey; Dr. Naomi and husband, Avi; and Dr. Joshua and wife, Edith.

To the memory of my teacher,

Professor Clinton Thienes.

To all who care for the poisoned patient.

To my wife:

mother, grandmother, companion, advisor, indefatigable coworker on this volume.

He who saves one life is as one who has saved a whole world.

Talmud

Preface

SINCE THE FIRST EDITION

The past 8 years have witnessed an enormous expansion in the field of medical toxicology: organizations devoted to the study and improvement of the treatment of poisoning worldwide, new journals, electronic data systems, symposia, and postgraduate courses for practicing clinicians and poison control health professionals.

Many approaches to treatment that were used during this period are no longer considered to be supported by good clinical evidence. New treatments have gone through the usual process for most ideas: formulation, oversimplification, anarchy, and, hopefully, a conclusion. The clinician is not immune to the latest "fad." The pendulum continues to swing in patient management.

This volume reflects a synthesis of this knowledge filtered through the author's experiences in patient care, in consultations with clinicians, in teaching residents in training, and as consultant to a poison center. The book has been targeted to both a United States and an international audience and hopefully will find use throughout the world.

Reviews of the first edition of this book suggested additional areas of interest to health professionals. Since that time many others have suggested inclusion of additional subjects. These comments formed a matrix for the many new topics in the present volume, including chapters on AIDS drugs, antiviral drugs, bone drug toxicology, blood transfusions and citrate intoxication, cytokines, plasma volume expanders, ticlopidine, vasodilators, lipid-lowering drugs, endocrine drugs, gastrointestinal tract drugs, immunotoxicology, respiratory tract drugs, antimuscarinics, dopamine receptor drugs, serotonin receptor agents, certain unclassified drugs, anesthetic agents, antiseptics and disinfectants, chemical disasters, chemical warfare agents, contrast media, cytotoxic agents, explosives, hobbies, arts and crafts, plastics and plasticizers, radiation poisoning, veterinary product poisoning in man, and indigenous toxicology: folk medicine.

SCOPE

The book is organized into five major sections: I. Principles of Poison Management, II. Drugs, III. The Home, IV. Chemicals, and V. Natural Toxins throughout each area of the world.

THE MEDICAL LITERATURE: PROBLEMS

The published literature is replete with studies weakened by missed case reports, poor definition of terms, variable exclusion criteria, absence of control groups, failure to account for the influence of concurrent disease, nutritional status, smoking, alcohol use, hormone levels, diurnal variation in drug disposition or sensitivity, and environmental factors that induce or inhibit drug metabolism. The author has been cognizant of these factors and has remembered the advice of a beloved professor: "Don't draw long conclusions from short data." References quoted are as up to date as possible.

The author is indebted to Dr. A.T. Proudfoot for reference to the following gem of wisdom:

> The spectrum of man's diseases is complex, and his environment labyrinthine. Their interaction forms a thicket that is made only more dense by the addition of biochemical and other laboratory markers of exposure and/or disease. The imaginative investigator looks for patterns in this thicket, as others look for pictures in clouds. Investigators' own ambitions, as well as the demands of the systems in which we work, have led to widespread belief that on perceiving a pattern in the thicket it is better to report it, even if it turns out to be only a bunch of leaves, than fail to report a pattern that someone else later discovers to be a pheasant. (McMahon B: Pesticide residues and breast cancer? J Natl Cancer Inst 1994;86:572–573.)

FIGURES AND TABLES

I have included figures and tables with which I agree clinically for ease of subject presentation, to avoid textual redundancies (textual "padding") and to conserve space. They contain useful summaries and quick-to-learn facts.

ANECDOTAL REPORTS

Anecdotal reports have usually been cited if more than one similar observation indicates a significant clinical trend.

ANIMAL STUDIES

I have consciously avoided the temptation of extrapolating animal data to clinical experience. Animal studies are cited to enhance an understanding of the mechanism of action of toxic effects. The major part of the text depends on clinical observations for conclusions relating to human poisoning.

OCCUPATIONAL MEDICINE

Occupational medicine problems are addressed in a number of chapters (e.g., see Chapter 56—Anesthetics, Chapter 57—Antiseptics, and Chapter 60—Cytotoxic Drugs). Chapters 63 through 70 relate to common problems encountered in the practice of occupational medicine.

USE

This volume was written to be used by poison center health professionals, hospital emergency department physicians, critical care physicians and support staff, occupational physicians, industrial hygienists, governmental institutions, students in the health professions, practicing clinicians, and the medicolegal community. My goal has been to make a useful contribution to the current state-of-the-art in patient care.

M. J. Ellenhorn

Acknowledgments

The author acknowledges those health professionals who, knowingly or unknowingly, have provided the author with valuable insights into the practice of medical toxicology. To them and to the many academicians, medical educators, practicing clinicians, and to my students who devote their lives and energies to better patient care in this area of medical science, I owe a debt of gratitude. In the last analysis, responsibility for thc content of the book, both good and not so good, must be placed at the feet of the author.

Individual Acknowledgments

Yona Amitai, MD
Jerusalem, Israel

Syama Atluri, MD
Los Angeles, California

Jim Baumol, PhD
Los Angeles, California

Yedidia Bentur, MD
Haifa, Israel

Timothy Erickson, MD
Chicago, Illinois

Susan S. Fish, PharmD, MPH
Boston, Massachusetts

Leon Gussow, MD
Chicago, Illinois

J.A. Haines, PhD
Geneva, Switzerland

John A. Henry, MD
London, United Kingdom

Dag Jacobsen, MD, PhD
Oslo, Norway

A. Jaeger, MD
Strasbourg, France

Claus Koppel, MD
Berlin, Germany

Edward P. Krenzelok, PharmD
Pittsburgh, Pennsylvania

Jerrold B. Leikin, MD
Chicago, Illinois

Michael McCann PhD
New York, New York

Margaret McCarron, MD
Los Angeles, California

Michael A. McGuigan, MD
Toronto, Canada

Timothy Meredith, MD
Nashville, Tennessee

Gary Oderda, PharmD
Salt Lake City, Utah

Gary Ordog, MD, ABMT
Los Angeles, California

Hans Persson, MD
Stockholm, Sweden

Susan M. Pond, MD
Brisbane, Australia

Robert Ricks, PhD
Oak Ridge, Tennessee

William Shoemaker, MD
Los Angeles, California

Frederick R. Sidell, MD
Aberdeen Proving Ground, Maryland

Struan K. Sutherland, MD
Melbourne, Victoria, Australia

Uri Taitelman, MD
Haifa, Israel

Milton Tenenbein, MD
Winnipeg, Manitoba, Canada

J. Allister Vale, MD
Birmingham, United Kingdom

David Warrell, MD
Oxford, United Kingdom

Julian White, MD
North Adelaide, Australia

Frances Weindler, PIS
Los Angeles, California

Willis Wingert, MD
Los Angeles, California

Members of the Los Angeles Regional Poison Information Center

Anne Dillibe, Director Library Services,
City of Hope, National Medical Center, Duarte, California

Ivor Geft, MD
Los Angeles, California

Susan Koscielski, Assistant Librarian
City of Hope, National Medical Center, Duarte, California

Rose Ann G. Soloway, RN, MSEd, ABAT,
Administrator, American Association of Poison Control Centers, Inc.

Special Thanks

My special thanks to the support group who have been available to me at all times through thick and thin and through the many vicissitudes of temperament exhibited by the author:

My wife, Sylvia Syma Ellenhorn, without whom this book could not have been written.

Glenn Sato, Librarian, UCLA, Los Angeles, California, who dug out so many original papers for me and for a multitude of other clerical functions.

Josephine Della Peruta, Copy Editor, San Diego, California

Yale Altman, Harvard, Massachusetts

Phyllis Lanz, Production Editor, Boca Raton, Florida

and the staff of Williams & Wilkins: Darlene Barela Cooke, Executive Editor.

Contents

Section IV
CHEMICALS

Section V
NATURAL TOXINS

Wenn Sie eine Vergiftung behandeln, vergessen Sie nicht, das Ihr Patient schon vergiftet ist.

When you are managing a poisoning, do not forget that your patient has already been poisoned.

K. Bucher

PLATE I
Representative American Pit Vipers (CROTALIDAE)

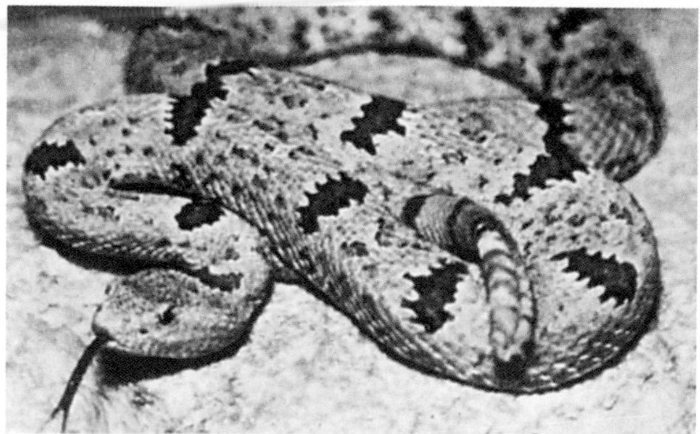

Figure 1. Rock Rattlesnake, *Crotalus lepidus.* Photo by Hal B. Harrison: National Audubon.

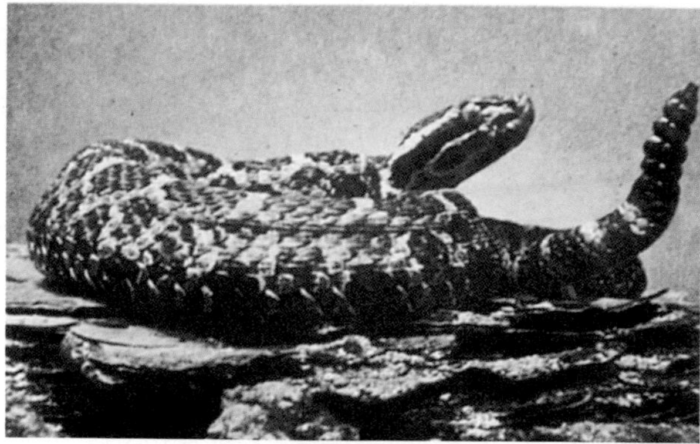

Figure 2. Massasauga, *Sistrurus catenatus*. Photo by Charles Hackenbrock and Staten Island Zoo.

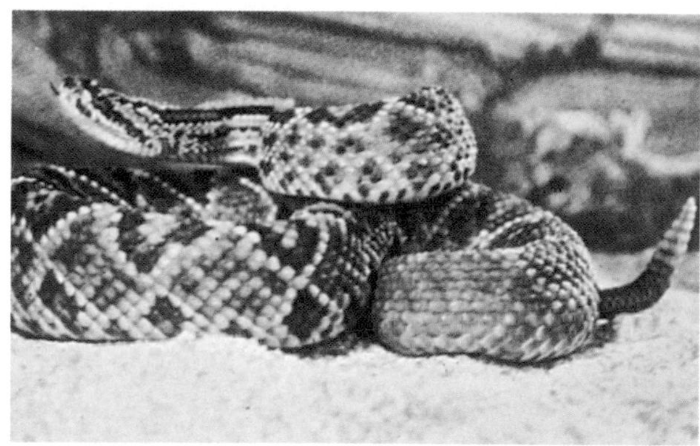

Figure 3. Cascabel, *Crotalus durissus.* Photo by Roy Pinney and Staten Island Zoo,

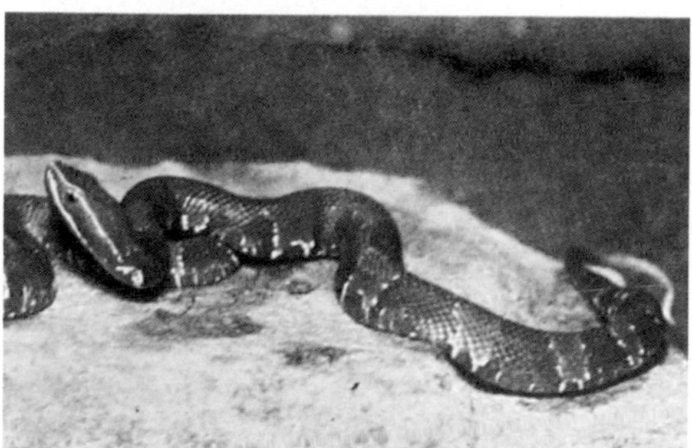

Figure 4. Cantil, *Agkistrodon bilineatus.* Photo by Hal B. Harrison: National Audubon.

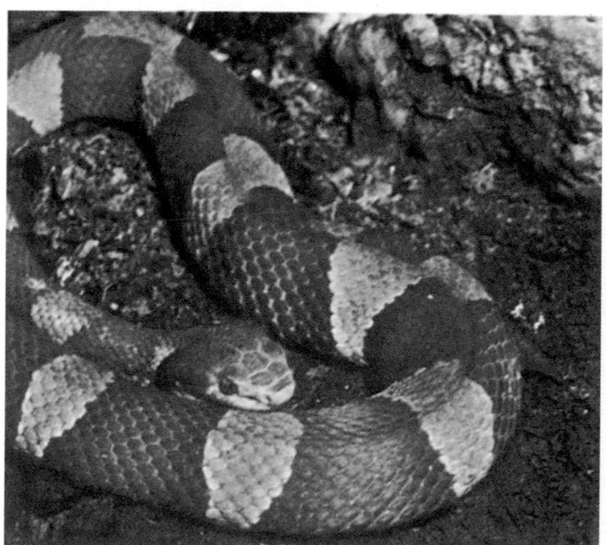

Figure 5. Broad-banded American Copperhead, *Agkistrodon contortrix* subspecies *laticinctus.* Photo by J. Markham.

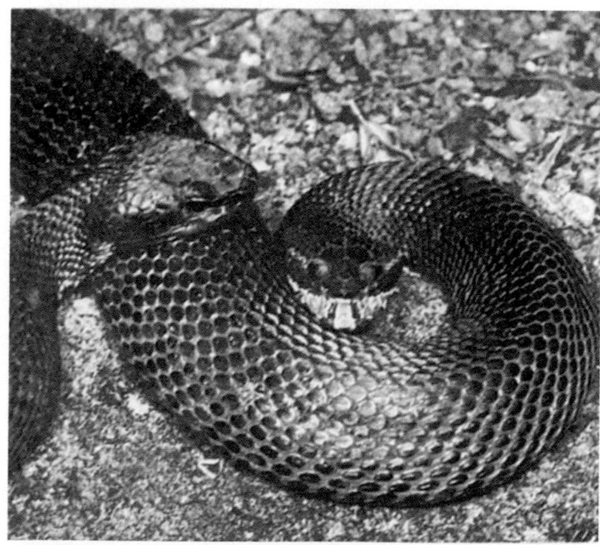

Figure 6. Cottonmouth, *Agkistrodon piscivorus.* Photo by J. Markham.

Plates I through VIII adapted from Poisonous snakes of the world—a manual for use by U.S. Amphibious Forces. Navmed P-5099. Department of the Navy. Bureau of Medicine and Surgery, Washington, DC: Superintendent of Documents. US Government Printing Office, 1990.

PLATE II
Representatives of Some Poisonous Snake Families

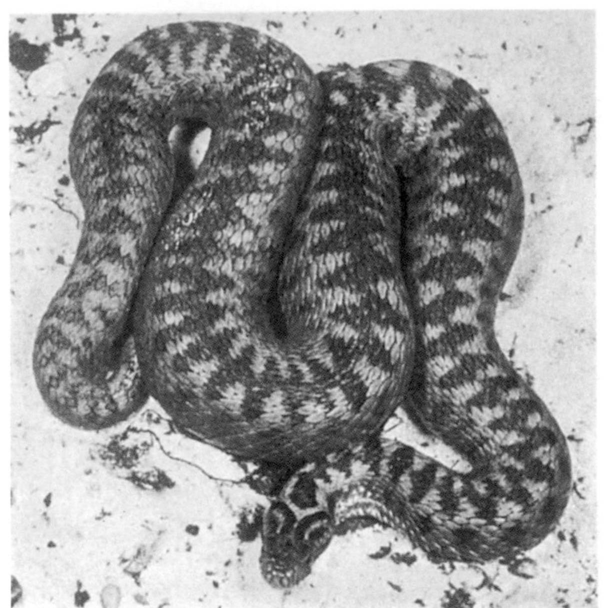

Figure 1. European Viper, *Vipera berus* (VIPERIDAE). Photo by J. Markham.

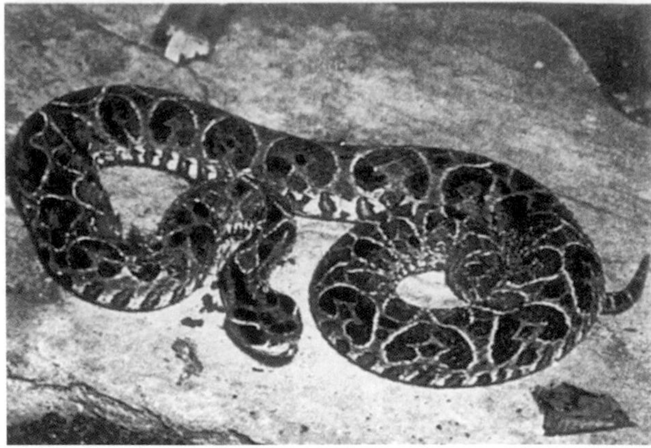

Figure 2. Urutu, *Bothrops alternatus* (CROTALIDAE). Photo by J. Markham.

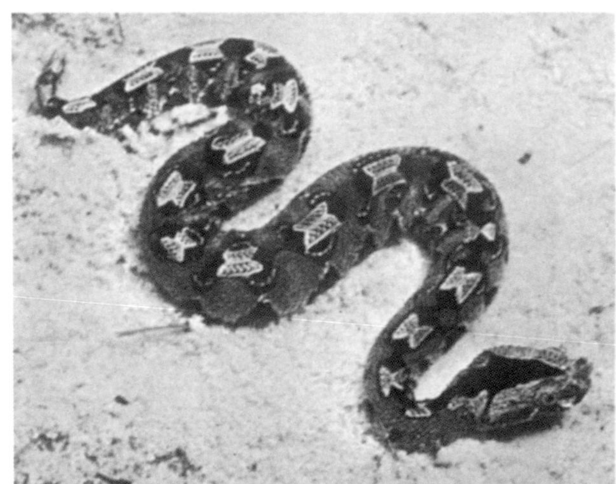

Figure 3. River Jack, *Bitis nasicornis* (VIPERIDAE). Photo by J. Markham.

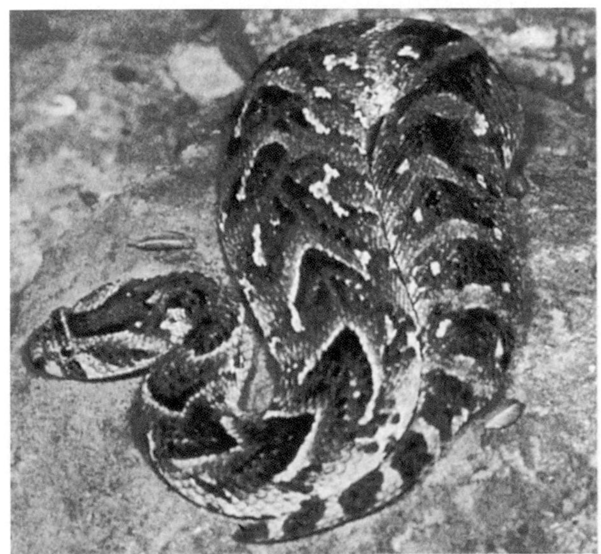

Figure 4. Puff Adder, *Bitis arietans* (VIPERIDAE). Photo by J. Markham.

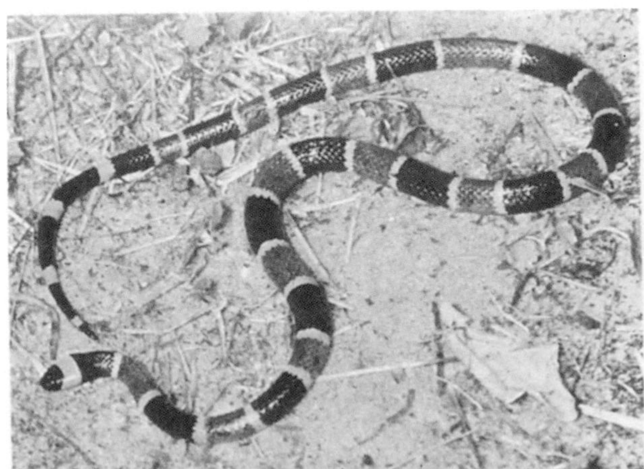

Figure 5. Eastern Coral Snake, *Micrurus fulvius* (ELAPIDAE). Photo by Allan D. Cruickshank: National Audubon.

PLATE III
Representatives of Some Poisonous Snake Families

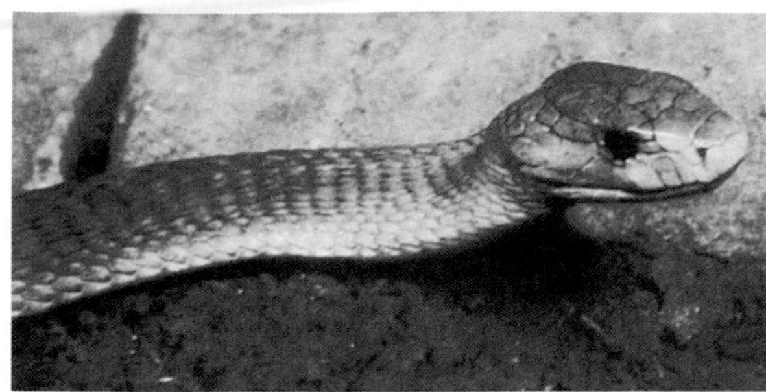

Figure 1. Black Mamba, *Dendroaspis polylepis* (ELAPIDAE). Photo by J. Markham.

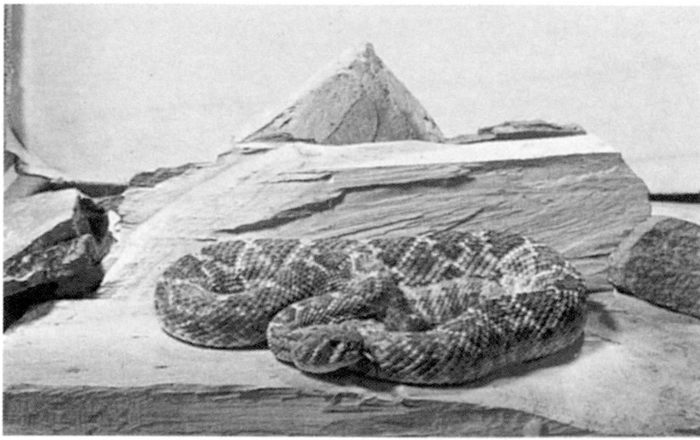

Figure 2. Western Diamondback Rattlesnake, *Crotalus atrox* (CROTALIDAE). Navy photo, courtesy U.S. National Zoological Park.

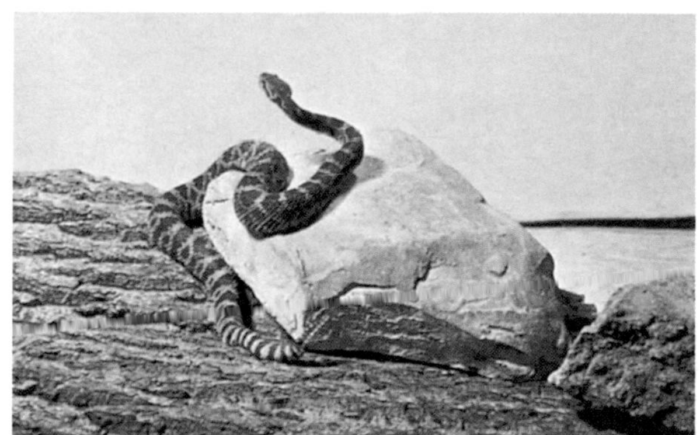

Figure 3. Prairie Rattlesnake, *Crotalus v. viridis* (CROTALIDAE). Navy photo, courtesy U.S. National Zoological Park.

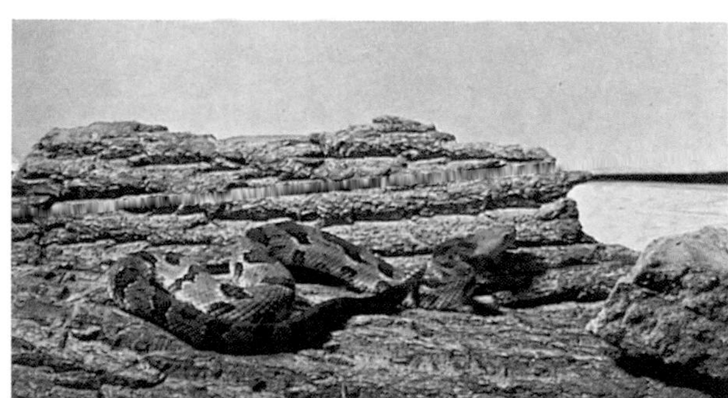

Figure 4. Timber Rattlesnake, *Crotalus horridus* (CROTALIDAE). Navy photo, courtesy U.S. National Zoological Park.

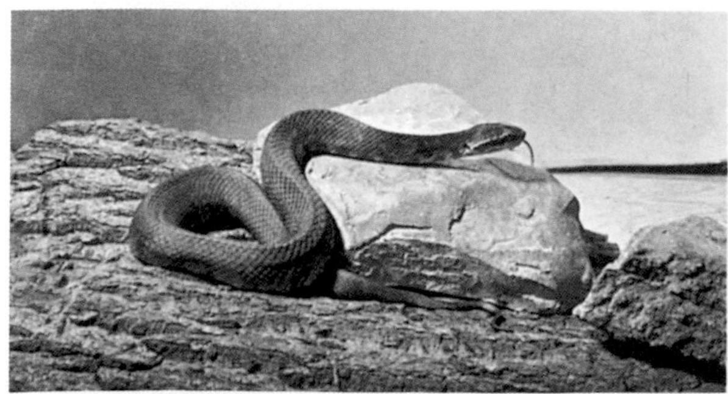

Figure 5. Cottonmouth, *Agkistrodon piscivorus* (CROTALIDAE). Navy photo, courtesy U.S. National Zoological Park.

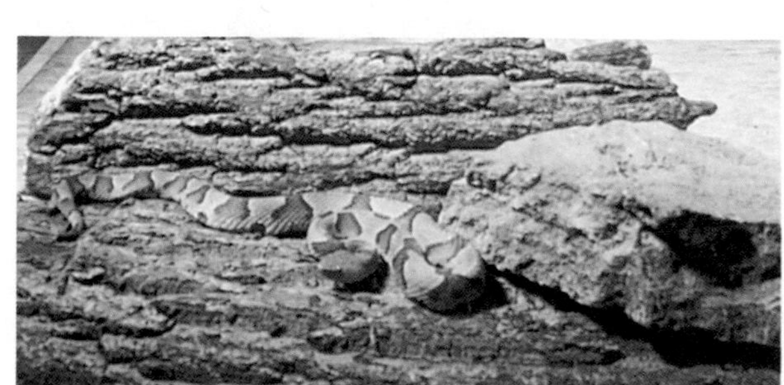

Figure 6. American Copperhead, *Agkistrodon contortrix* (CROTALIDAE). Navy photo, courtesy U.S. National Zoological Park.

PLATE IV
Representative Pit Vipers (CROTALIDAE)

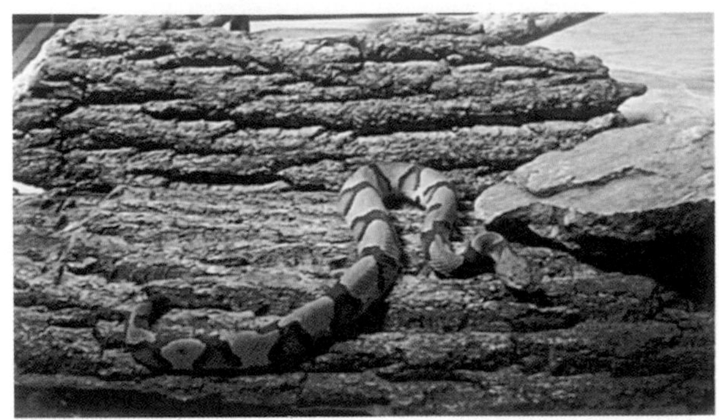

Figure 1. American Copperhead, *Agkistrodon contortrix,* south-eastern U.S. Navy photo, courtesy U.S. National Zoological Park.

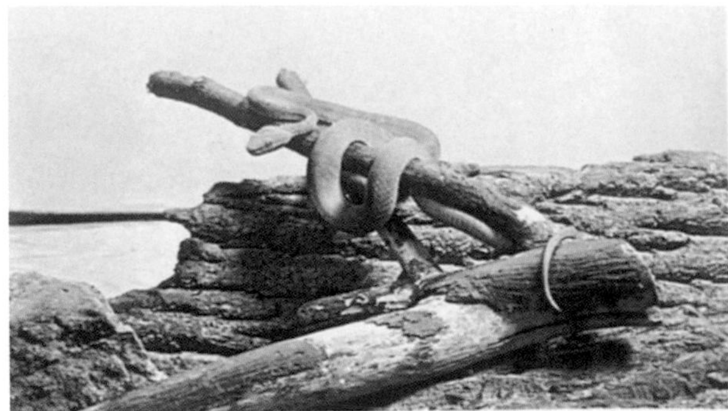

Figure 2. Chinese Green Tree Viper, *Trimeresurus stejnegeri.* Navy photo, courtesy U.S. National Zoological Park.

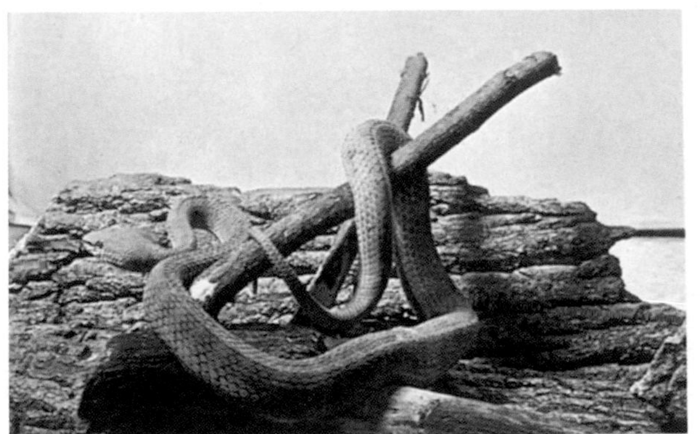

Figure 3. Green Tree Viper, *Trimeresurus* sp. Navy photo, courtesy U.S. National Zoological Park.

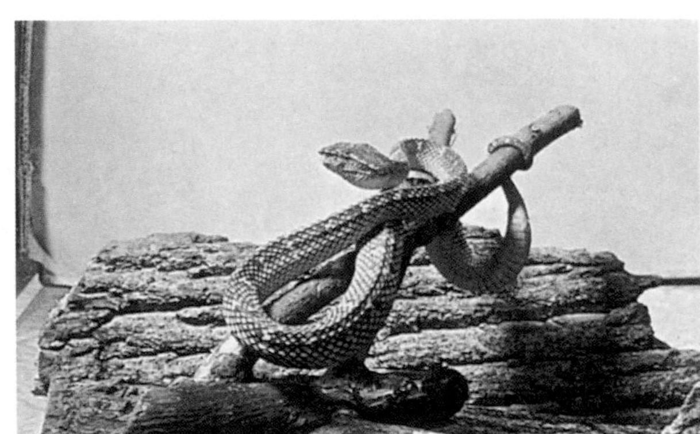

Figure 4. Wagler's Pit Viper, *Trimeresurus wagleri.* Navy photo, courtesy U.S. National Zoological Park.

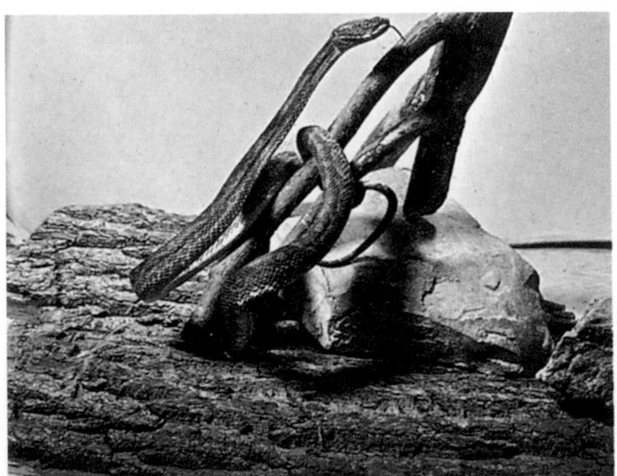

Figure 5. Okinawa Habu, *Trimeresurus flavoviridis.* Navy photo, courtesy U.S. National Zoological Park.

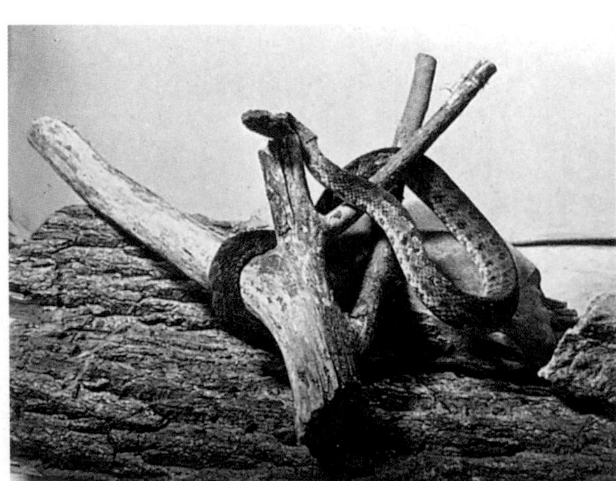

Figure 6. Sakishima Habu, *Trimeresurus elegans.* Navy photo, courtesy U.S. National Zoological Park.

PLATE V
Some Poisonous Snakes of Asia

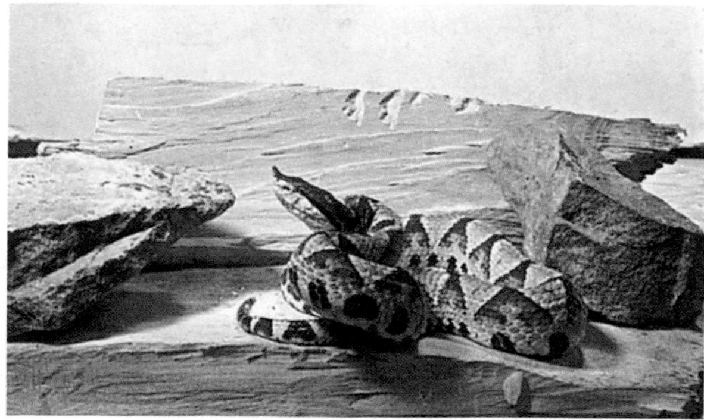

Figure 1. Sharp-nosed Pit Viper, *Agkistrodon acutus* (CROTALIDAE). Navy photo, courtesy U.S. National Zoological Park.

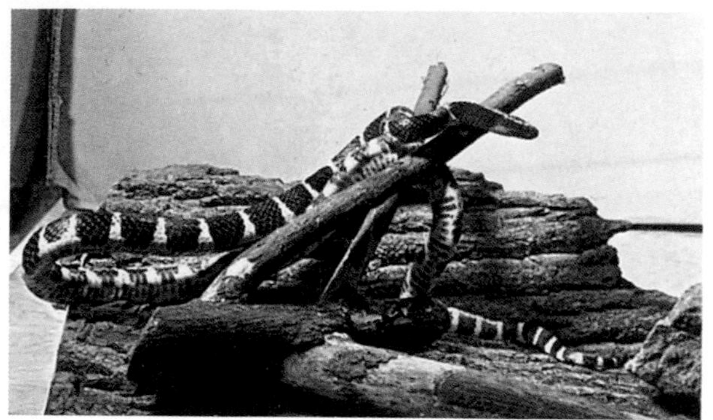

Figure 2. Many-banded Krait, *Bungarus multicinctus* (ELAPIDAE). Navy photo, courtesy U.S. National Zoological Park.

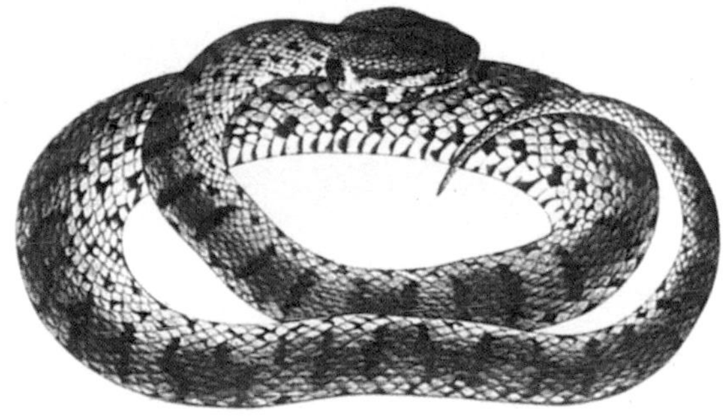

Figure 3. Chinese Mountain Viper, *Trimeresurus monticola* (CROTALIDAE). From a painting.

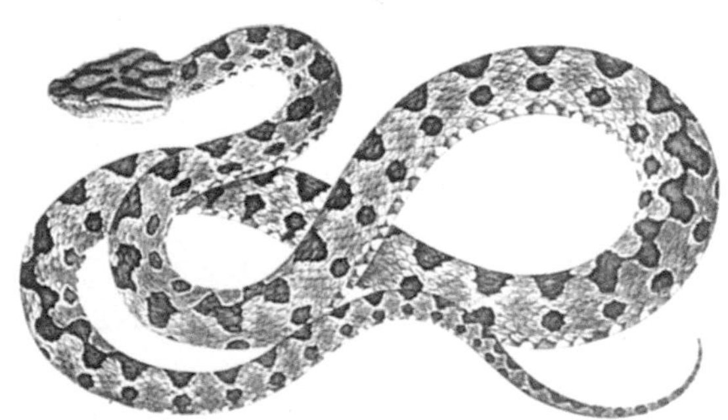

Figure 4. Chinese Habu, *Trimeresurus mucrosquamatus* (CROTALIDAE). From a painting.

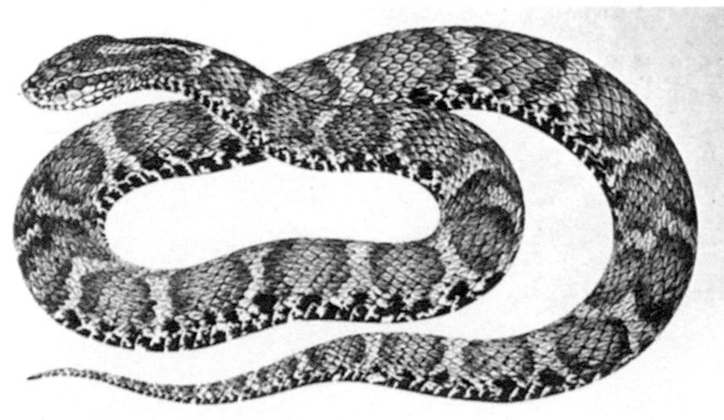

Figure 5. Japanese Mamushi, *Agkistrodon halys blomhoffi* (CROTALIDAE). From a painting.

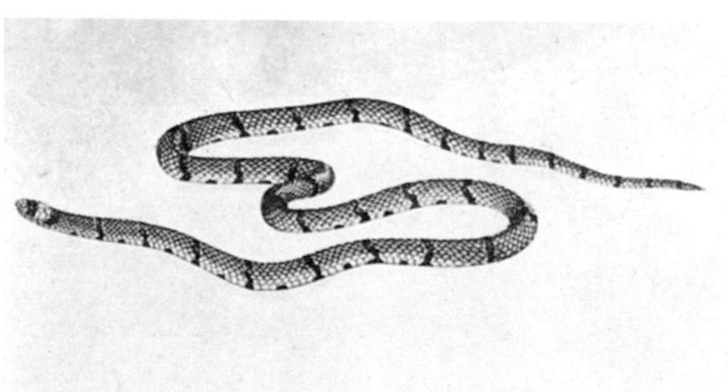

Figure 6. MacClelland's Coral Snake, *Calliophis macclellandii* (ELAPIDAE). From a painting.

PLATE VI
Some Poisonous Snakes of Asia

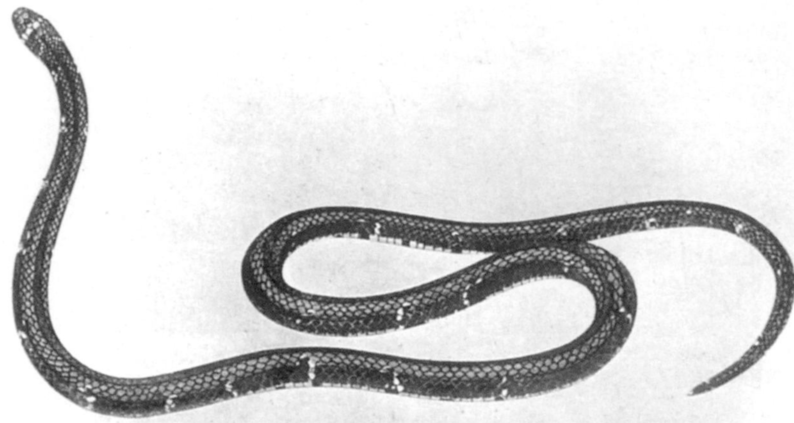

Figure 1. Asian Coral Snake, *Calliophis sauteri* (ELAPIDAE). From a painting.

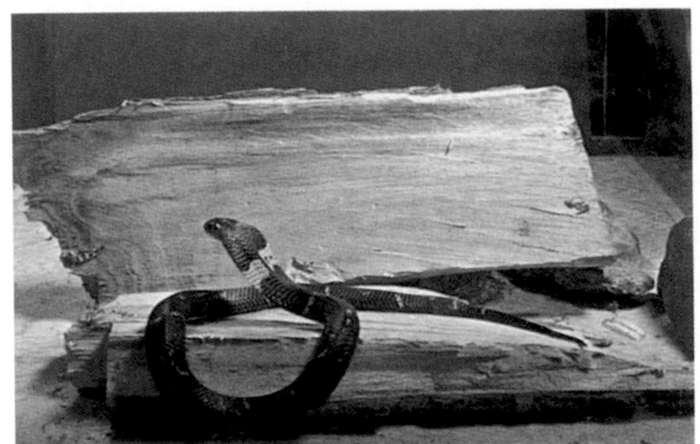

Figure 2. Chinese Cobra, *Naja naja atra* (ELAPIDAE). Navy photo, courtesy U.S. National Zoological Park.

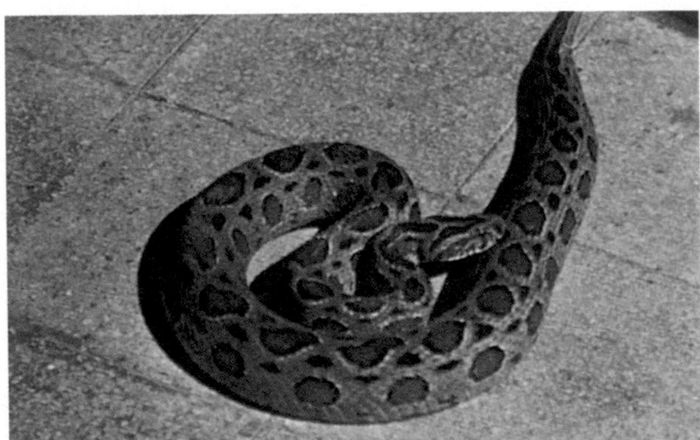

Figure 3. Russell's Viper, *Vipera russelii* (VIPERIDAE). Navy photo.

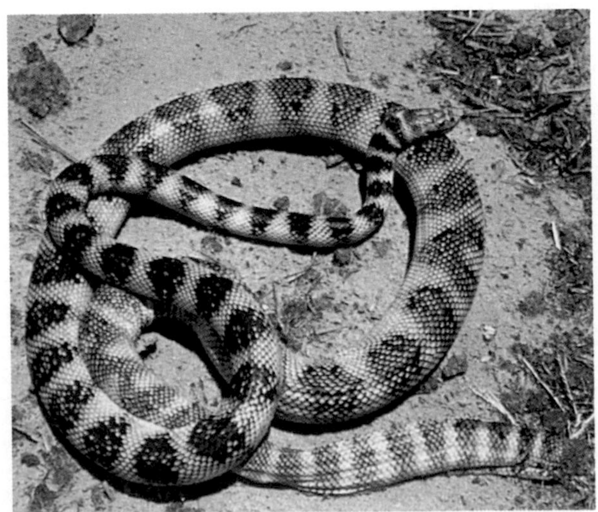

Figure 4. Annulated Sea Snake, *Hydrophis cyanocinctus* (HYDROPHIDAE). Photo by Sherman A. Minton.

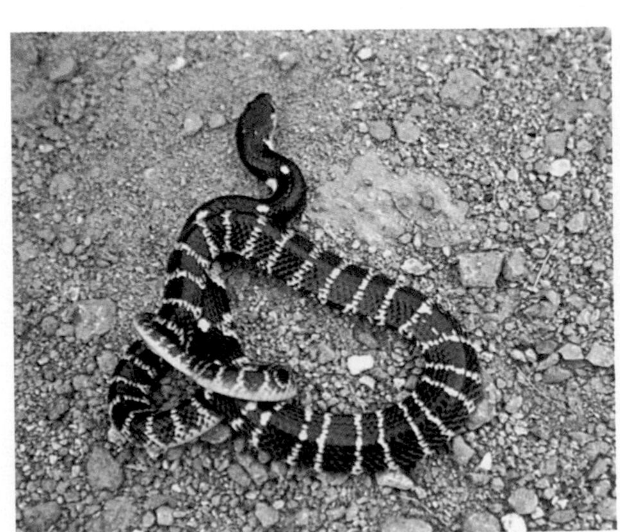

Figure 5. Indian Krait, *Bungarus caeruleus* (ELAPIDAE). Photo by Sherman A. Minton.

PLATE VII. Some Poisonous Snakes of Africa (From Pitman's *Snakes of Uganda*)

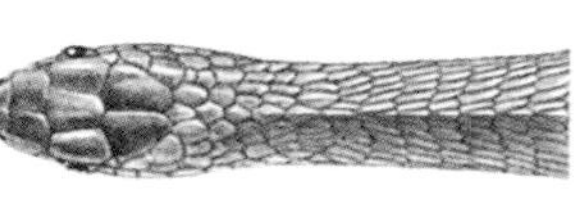
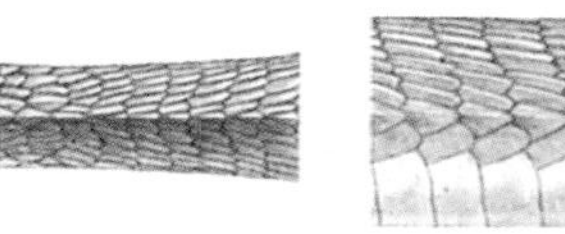

Figure 1. Boomslang, *Dispholidus typus* (COLUBRIDAE). Brown coloration. Note lack of distinct pattern. (See p. 90)

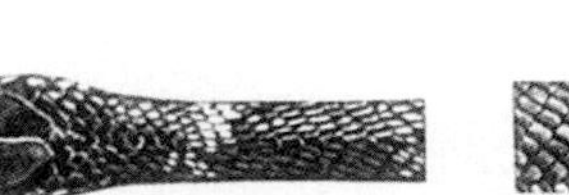
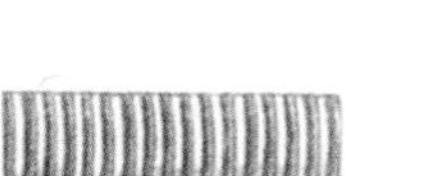

Figure 2. Gold's Tree Cobra, *Pseudohaje goldii* (ELAPIDAE). The very glossy appearance of scales is not well shown here.

Figure 3. Forest Cobra. *Naja melanoleuca* (ELAPIDAE). Juvenile coloration.

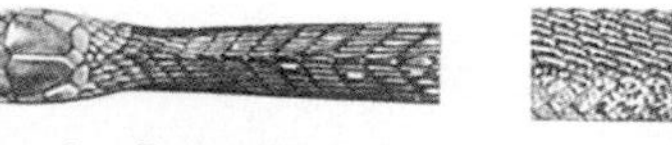
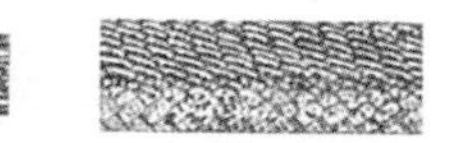
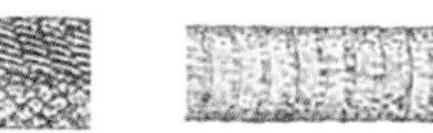

Figure 4. Boomslang, *Dispholidus typus* (COLUBRIDAE). Juvenile coloration.

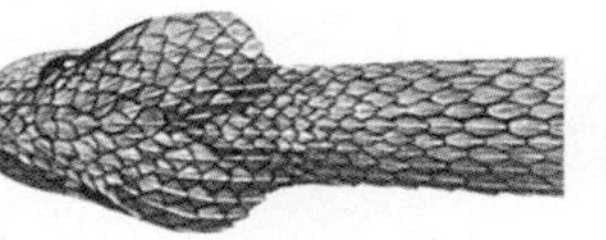
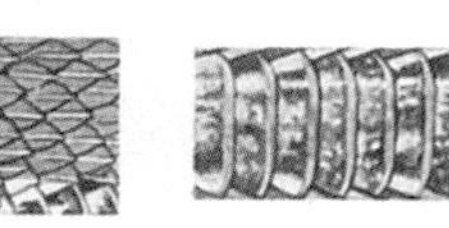
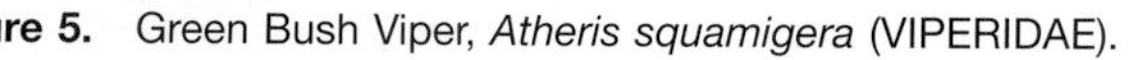

Figure 5. Green Bush Viper, *Atheris squamigera* (VIPERIDAE).

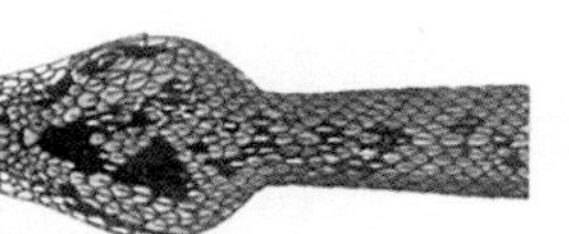
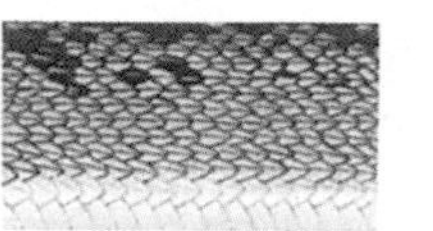
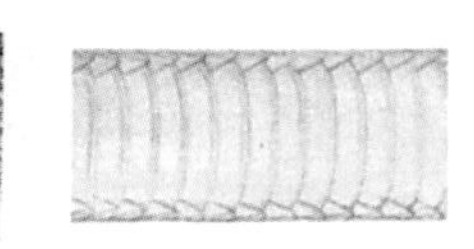

Figure 6. Sedge Viper, *Atheris nitschei* (VIPERIDAE).

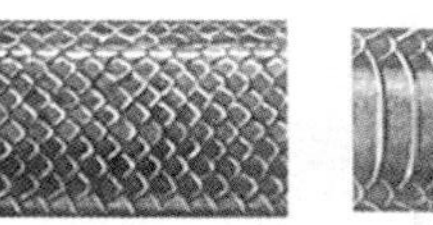
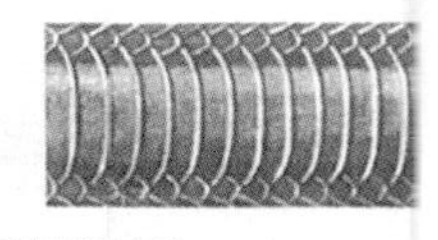

Figure 7. Black Mole Viper, *Atractaspis irregularis* (VIPERIDAE).

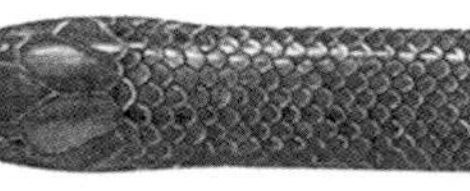
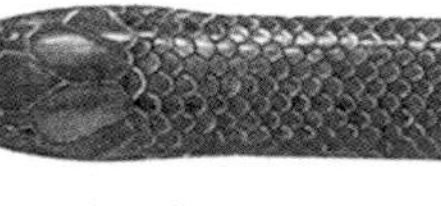
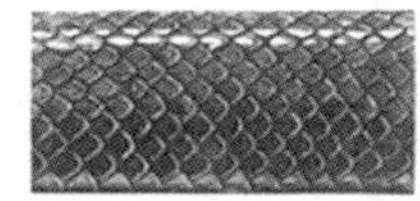
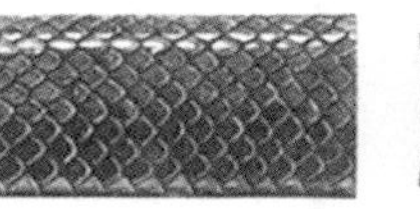
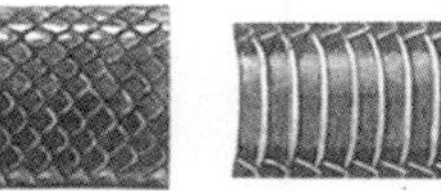

Figure 8. Günther's Mole Viper, *Atractaspis aterrima* (VIPERIDAE).

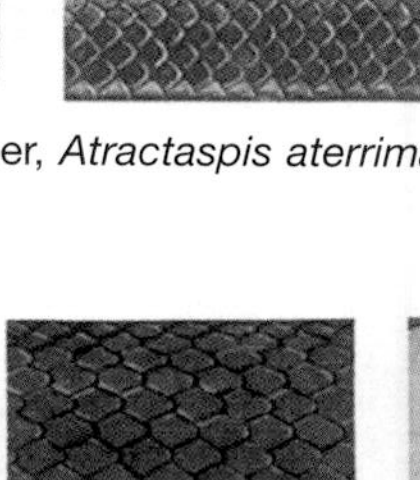
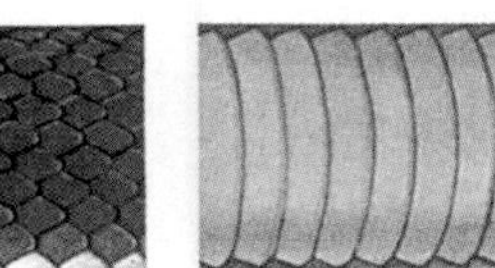
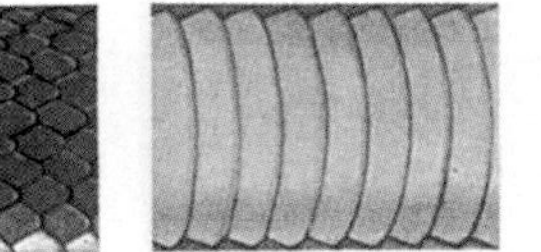

Figure 9. Banded Water Cobra, *Boulengerina annulata* (ELAPIDAE). This eastern subspecies is unicolor over most of body.

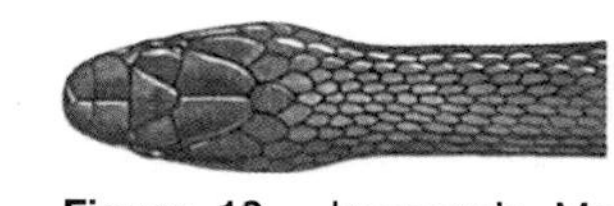
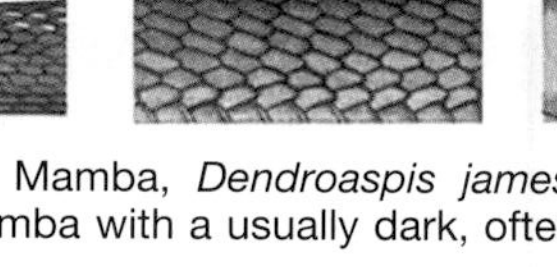

Figure 10. Jameson's Mamba, *Dendroaspis jamesoni* (ELAPIDAE). Widespread arboreal mamba with a usually dark, often black, tail.

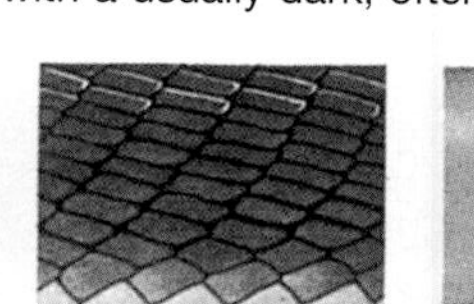
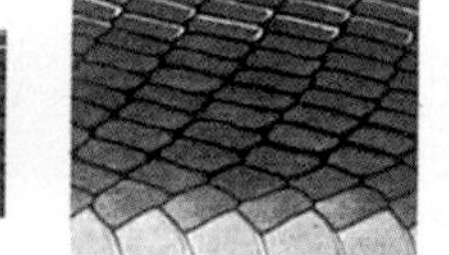
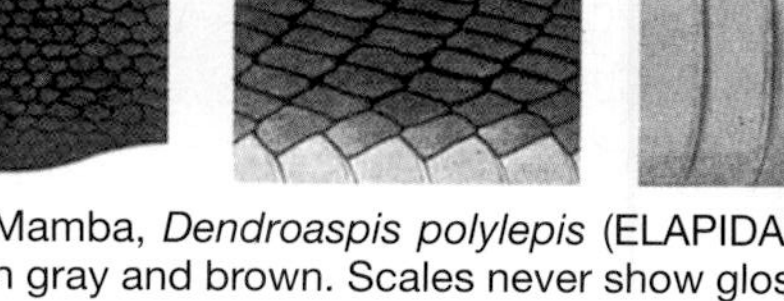

Figure 11. Black Mamba, *Dendroaspis polylepis* (ELAPIDAE). Ground color varies between gray and brown. Scales never show gloss that they do in some cobras.

PLATE VIII. Some Poisonous Snakes of Africa (From Pitman's *Snakes of Uganda*)

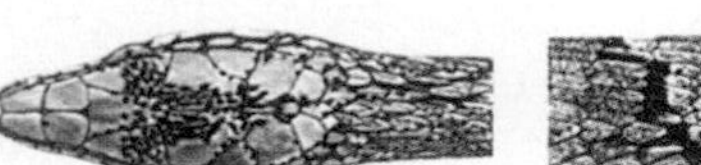
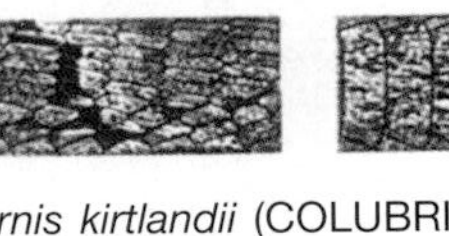

Figure 1. Bird Snake, *Thelotornis kirtlandii* (COLUBRIDAE). Note narrow pointed head, oblique dorsals, and lichen-like color pattern.

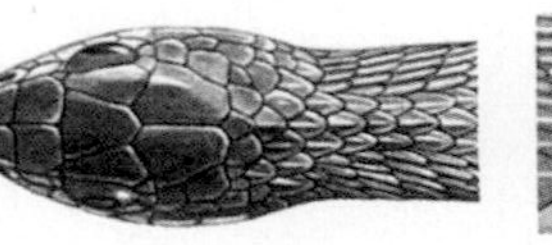
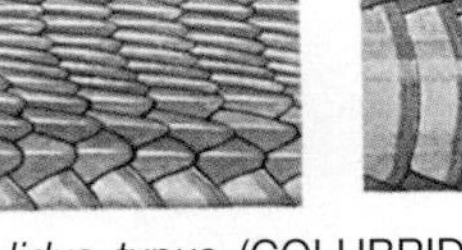

Figure 2. Boomslang, *Dispholidus typus* (COLUBRIDAE). Green coloration. Note distinctly oblique dorsals and absence of distinct color pattern.

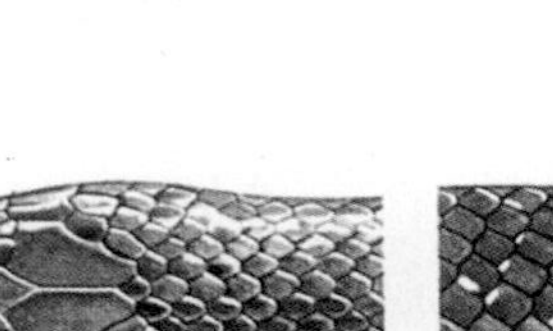
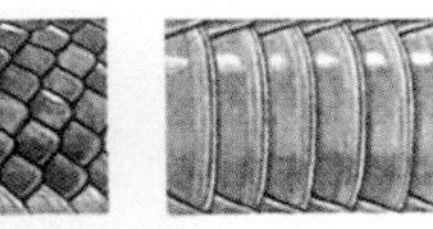
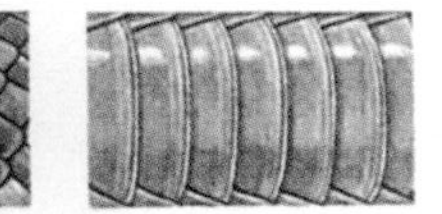

Figure 3. African Garter Snake, *Elapsoidea sundevallii* (ELAPIDAE).

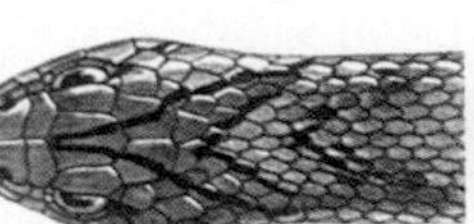
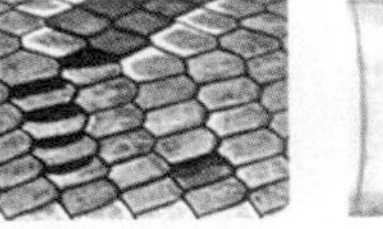
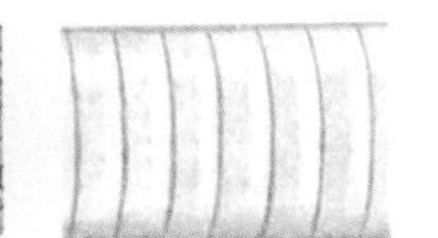
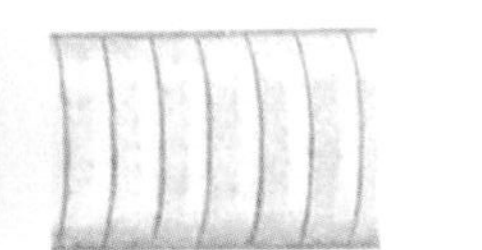

Figure 4. Rhombic Night Adder, *Causus rhombeatus* (VIPERIDAE). Chevron-shaped head marking is distinctive.

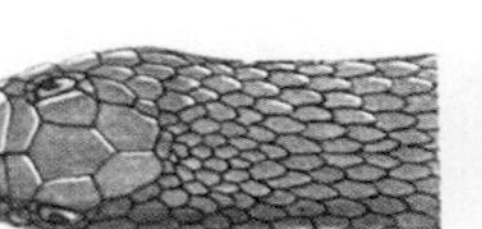
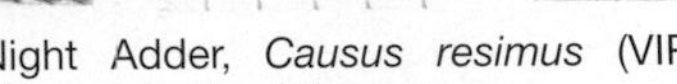

Figure 5. Green Night Adder, *Causus resimus* (VIPERIDAE). Oblique dorsals are characteristic of the genus.

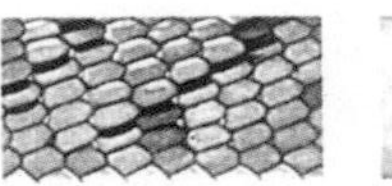
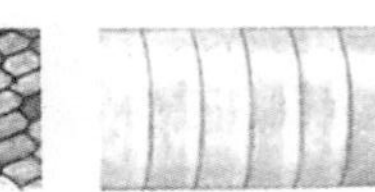

Figure 6. Lichtenstein's Night Adder, *Causus lichtensteinii* (VIPERIDAE).

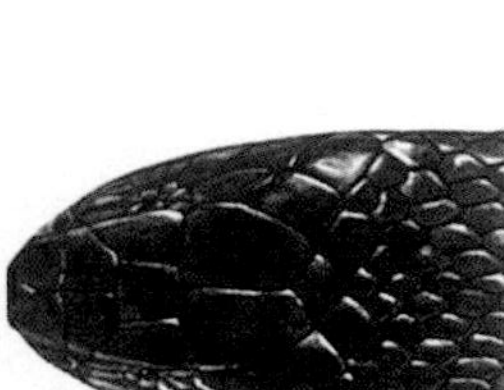
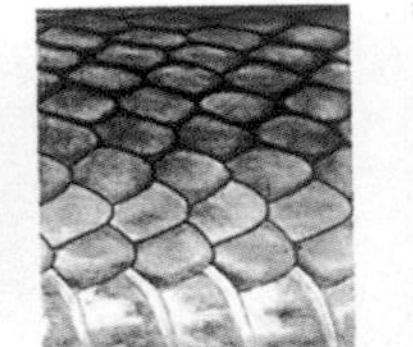
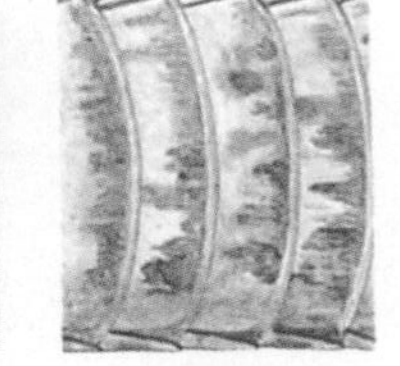

Figure 7. Egyptian Cobra, *Naja haje* (ELAPIDAE). Distinguished from other cobras by a row of subocular scales.

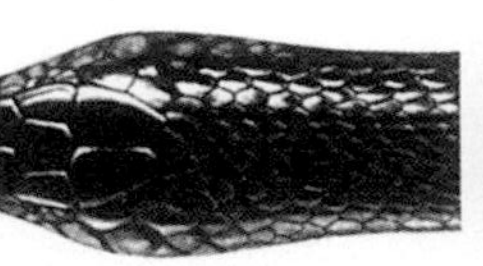
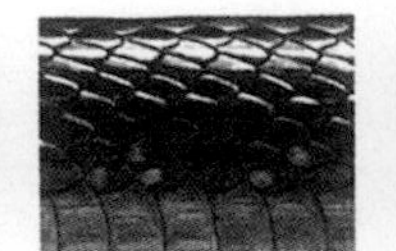

Figure 8. Forest Cobra, *Naja melanoleuca* (ELAPIDAE). Adult coloration. Note highly polished appearance of scales.

Figure 9. Spitting Cobra, *Naja nigricollis* (ELAPIDAE). Highly variable coloration; scales not as glossy as those of forest cobra.

Section I
PRINCIPLES OF POISON MANAGEMENT

Chapter 1 The Clinical Approach

SOURCES OF INFORMATION: PROBLEMS

Much of the accumulated knowledge of medical toxicology has been based on case reports of single acute overdoses, chronic overexposure, epidemiologic studies, and animal experiments. Case reports demonstrate a temporal but not necessarily a causative relationship between exposure and health effects. This information is often confounded by the inability to exclude other causes of illness.

THE MEDICAL TOXICOLOGIST

Appropriate medical qualification, training, knowledge, and clinical experience are paramount to the medical toxicologist. Vale summarized areas of knowledge and areas of toxicology that are central to the work of the medical toxicologist[1] (Figs. 1–1, 1–2). For those poison units that contain both treatment capability and information sources, the West Midlands Poisons Unit (in Birmingham) provides a model:

1. *Dedicated beds for the management of poisoned patients.* The unit acts as a focus for the provision of expert medical, psychiatric, and social care. The unit is staffed by physicians with a special interest in, and experience with, medical toxicology. A consultant psychiatrist with a specific commitment to the poisons unit provides psychosocial assessment on a daily basis.
2. *A poisons information service.* Information is given to medical practitioners and nursing staff and, occasionally, to veterinary practitioners (but not to members of the public) on the ingredients and toxicity of the many drugs, chemicals, household products, and plants available in present-day society. This service is available 24 hours a day, 365 days a year, and at all times physicians with extensive training in medical toxicology are available to provide expert advice to inquirers.
3. *Expert clinical advice to physicians on the management of specific cases of poisoning.* In such cases all the available information—circumstantial, clinical, laboratory, and from other sources—has to be assessed in relationship to the substances and circumstances of

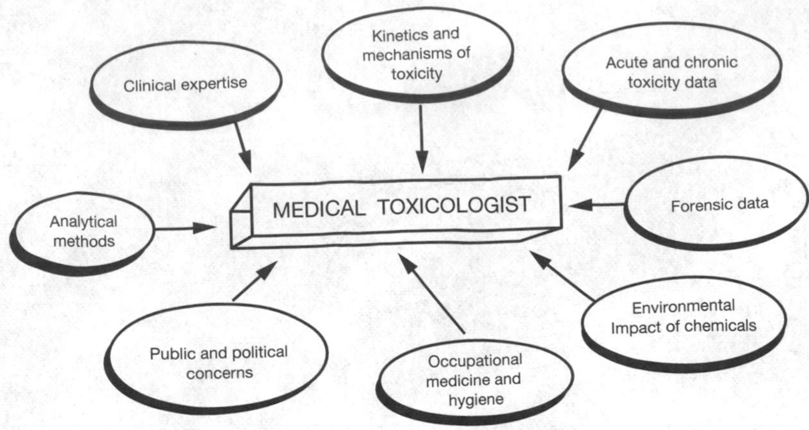

Figure 1–1 Areas of knowledge and influences that guide the medical toxicologist.

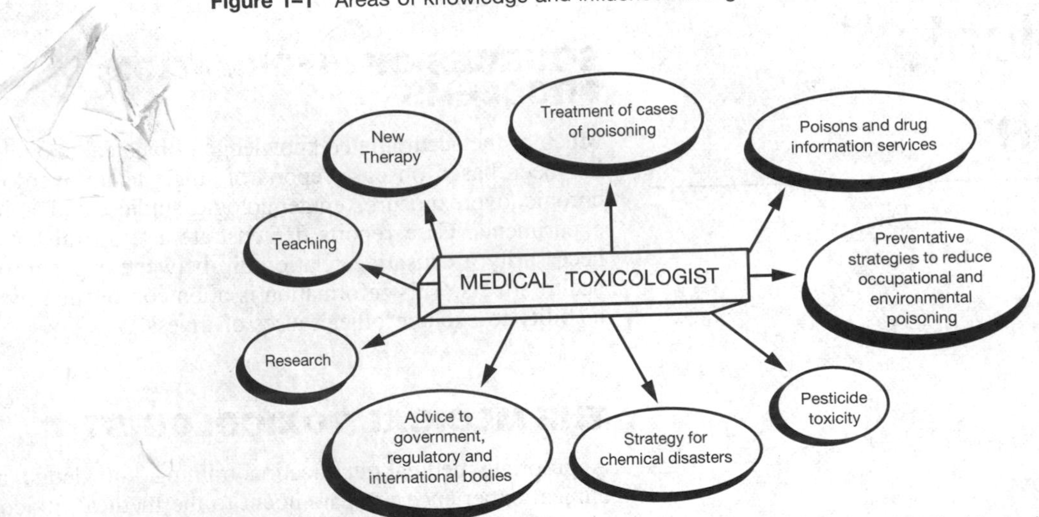

Figure 1–2 Areas of toxicology that are the concern of the medical toxicologist. (From Vale JA. Medical toxicology: Clinical aspects. Arch Toxicol 1991; suppl. 15:12–13.)

Table 1–1
Common Causes of Poisoning

	Western Europe	North America	Developing Countries
Childhood poisoning	Household products Pharmaceuticals	Household products Pharmaceuticals	Paraffin, traditional medicine Snake bites, insect stings
Childhood deaths	Carbon monoxide	Carbon monoxide	
Adolescent poisoning	Volatile substance abuse	Volatile substance abuse	
Adult poisoning (hospital admissions)	Analgesics Psychotropics Less barbiturates and nonbarbiturate hypnotics	Analgesics Psychotropics Less barbiturates and nonbarbiturate hypnotics	
Adult deaths (outside hospitals)	Carbon monoxide increasing	Carbon monoxide Petroleum distillate Pesticides Cleaning and polishing agents	Accidental and deliberate pesticide poisoning (agrochemicals)

From Meredith TJ. Epidemiology of poisoning. Pharmacol Ther 1993;59:251–256.

exposure to determine a detailed plan for clinical management that will maximize the chances of the victim surviving and minimize the risk of short- and long-term sequelae. This expert advice must be supplemented by a comprehensive collection of reference works and original papers. If necessary and appropriate, severely poisoned patients are transferred from other hospitals for more intensive and specialized treatment that cannot be provided locally even after advice from the unit.

4. *An outpatient advisory service.* The unit has for some years offered an advisory service particularly on chronic medical problems that are alleged to have a toxicologic basis; many of these have an occupational origin.
5. *Analytical support both for the unit and the surrounding region.* A close working relationship exists between the medical and analytical toxicologists which strengthens and improves the quality of the overall service even further.

EPIDEMIOLOGY OF POISONING

Common causes of poisoning in Western Europe, North America, and the developing countries are summarized in Table 1–1.

EXPOSURE TO TOXIC SUBSTANCES

There are, overall, about 4 to 5 million cases of poisoning per year in the United States. About 2 million exposures are reported each year to the American Association of Poison Centers Toxic Exposure Surveillance System (AAPCC TESS). Many cases of recognized poisoning go unreported and many cases of poisoning are never reported. Occupational and medical examiner data are often unreported.

TOXIC EXPOSURE SURVEILLANCE SYSTEM (TESS)

The average child presents to a health care facility about 1.5 hours after exposure. The average adult presents to a health care facility about 3.5 hours after exposure.

FATALITIES

Children less than 17 years of age account for most poisoning exposures but account for only about 10% of fatalities. Fatalities in children under the age of 6 are uncommon, representing about 4% of fatalities. Common toxins lethal to children and adults are listed in Table 1–2.

Childhood poisoning is usually accidental and is usually associated with a low morbidity and mortality. In adults, self-poisoning is usually deliberate (suicide or parasuicide) and has a higher morbidity and mortality rate.[2]

A total of 764 fatalities were reported in 1991 versus 545 in 1988 (United States). Eleven children died following the accidental ingestion of iron supplements, more than twice the number of pediatric fatalities from iron poisoning reported to the database in 1990. Pediatric deaths from hydrocarbons (gasoline, kerosene, lamp oil, charcoal lighter fluid) were also increased in 1991. In adults and teenagers, an increased frequency of deaths caused by ethylene glycol, toilet bowl cleaners, monoamine oxidase inhibitors, and isoniazid was noted in 1991. Fatal exposure associated with cocaine appeared constant from 1988 to 1991.

Figure 1–3 shows that from 1980 through 1986, the rate of mortality from unintentional poisoning in the United States increased from 1.9 to 2.3 deaths per 100,000 population. This 7-year trend appears to be explained by a 49% increase in the rate of deaths from drug poisoning. In 1986, the leading causes of fatal unintentional drug poisoning were

Table 1–2
Common Lethal Toxins (Toxic Exposure Surveillance System)

Children	Adult
Gases/fumes/vapors such as carbon monoxide	Same
Toxic alcohols	
Analgesics	Antidepressants
Iron	Drugs of abuse
Antidepressants	Cardiovascular toxins
Cleaning substances (through aspiration)	Analgesics
Cardiovascular toxins	Theophylline

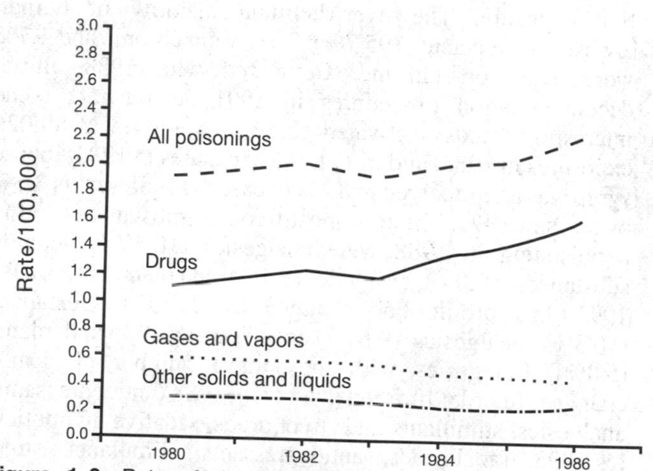

Figure 1–3 Rate of death from unintentional poisonings per 100,000 persons in the United States, 1980–1986. (From Centers for Disease Control and Prevention. Unintentional poisoning mortality: United States, 1980–1986. MMWR 1989; 38:153–158.)

opiates and related narcotics and local anesthetics including cocaine. Most fatal poisonings caused by other solids and liquids were due to alcohol ingestion.[3]

CHILDHOOD POISONING

Poisoning in Infants

In 1988, infants under 12 months accounted for 15% of all cases of poisoning under 6 years of age reported to the AAPCC. Poisoning peaked at 10 months and between 2 and 4 years. Most cases (>80%) occurred in the home: 61% occurred in the kitchen, 24% in the bedroom, 10% in the living room, and 8% in the bathroom.[4] The next most frequent place appears to be the homes of grandparents.

A major portion (30.1%) of pediatric ingestions reported to poison centers in the United States involve children with a prior history of a poisoning episode. Children tend to repeat with the same type of substance.[5] The mother was the caretaker in 70% of cases. The infant was often placed near the substance by the caretaker (43%). The infant was usually playing alone (66%) and the substance was within easy reach (78% on the floor or edge of tub or changing table).[6]

Woolf and Lovejoy suggest that impaired impulse suppression, hyperactivity, inability to discriminate safe from unsafe activities, living in a hazardous environment, and inadequate parental vigilance are all possible behavioral/

developmental determinants of childhood overdose.[7] Family stress also creates supervisory lapses conducive to childhood poisoning. Up to 30% of early childhood poisonings involve children whose parents can recall a history of prior poison exposure.

Data Collection System

The American Association of Poison Control Centers Data Collection System has collected experiences with pediatric poisoning exposures (Table 1–3).[8,9] Changes in human exposures from 1988 to 1991[4,10] are summarized in Table 1–4.

Ingestion accounted for 75.0% of exposure routes, followed in frequency by dermal exposure, inhalation, ocular exposure, bites and stings, parenteral exposure, and aspiration exposure. The overwhelming majority of human exposures were acute (95.7%); 2.1% were chronic and 1.7% were acute on chronic. Compared with 1988, initial decontamination procedures in 1991 demonstrate some interesting trends. Activated charcoal was used in 89,026 exposures in 1988, and in 114,563 exposures in 1993. Ipecac syrup was administered in 8.4% of cases in 1988 versus 3.7% of cases in 1991. The four most frequent substances used in a poisoning in 1988 were analgesics (10.5%), cleaning substances (10.0%), cosmetics (8.1%), and plants (6.9%). By 1993, this profile had changed to cleaning substances (10.3%), analgesics (9.6%), cosmetics (8.2%), and plants (5.4%). Categories with the largest number of deaths changed (in order of frequency) from 1988 (antidepressants, analgesics, stimulants and street drugs, sedative–hypnotics) to 1993, (analgesics, antidepressants, stimulants, street drugs, and sedative–hypnotics).

A survey for the AAPCC of childhood poisoning between 1985 and 1989 revealed that the three most commonly implicated substance categories, accounting for 30.4% of reported exposures, were cosmetics and personal care products, cleaning substances, and plants. Data summarized by the AAPCC between 1985 and 1989 indicate that the three most commonly implicated substances or categories leading to a life-threatening effect, residual disability or death, were cosmetics and personal care products, cleaning substances, and plants. Yet the hazard factor (sum of number of major effects and deaths divided by number of reported exposures) for these groups was low. Iron supplements were the single most frequent cause of pediatric unintentional ingestion fatalities. Antidepressants, cardiovascular medications, methyl salicylates, hydrocarbons, pesticides, and selenious acid-containing gun bluing, followed in frequency by carbon monoxide and hydrogen sulfide, posed the greatest hazards. In the past several decades the decline in the number of pediatric poisoning deaths can be attributed to child-resistant closures, product reformulations, heightened parental awareness and vigilance, and more sophisticated intervention by poisoning centers and health care professionals.[11]

Limitations of the AAPCC data include (1) underreporting of chronic pediatric poisonings with respect to environmental source; (2) important poisonings requiring hospitalization in which clinicians feel they are competent and do not require the assistance of a poison center; (3) death occurring in a community, out-of-hospital fatalities about which a poison center is not notified; and (4) applicability of a national data set to regional or local policy levels.[12]

Poisoning Severity Score

A guide for scoring poisoning severity has been proposed by members of the European Association of Clinical Poison Centers and Clinical Toxicologists. Preliminary studies suggest that this scoring system is an effective tool for comparing data from poison centers (Table 1–5).[13] A similar

Table 1–3
Toxic Effects of Pediatric Poisoning Exposures

	<6 years old		6–12 years old		13–17 years old	
	No.	%	No.	%	No.	%
None or presumed nontoxic	388,537	21.1	21,437	1.2	15,171	0.8
Minor effect	144,567	8.0	29,288	1.6	30,151	1.7
Moderate effect	5,645	0.3	1,704	0.1	3,920	0.2
Major effect	548	0.0	105	0.0	426	0.0
Death	44	0.0	4	0.0	48	0.0
Total	1,100,068	59.9	102,700	5.6	82,515	4.5

Adapted from Litovitz TL, Holm KC, Bailey KM, Schmitz BF. 1991 Annual report of the American Association of Poison Control Centers National Data Collection System. Am J Emerg Med 1992;10:452–505.

Table 1–4
Human Exposures, 1988–1991

Year	Number of Participating Poison Centers	Population Served (million)	Human Exposures Reported	Cases per Million
1988	64	155.7	1,368,748	8791
1991	73	200.7	1,837,939	9200

Data taken from Litovitz et al.[9] and Klein-Schwartz et al.[10]

Table 1-5
Guide for the Use of Poisoning Severity Score

Instructions

Poisoning Severity Score is a classification scheme for cases of poisoning in adults and children reported to poison information centers. This scheme should be used for the classification of *acute* poisonings regardless of the type and number of agents involved; however, modified schemes may eventually be required for certain poisonings and this scheme may then serve as a model.

Severity grading should take into account the overall clinical course and be applied according to the most severe signs and symptoms. Therefore it is a *retrospective* process, requiring follow-up of cases. If the grading is undertaken at any other time (e.g., on admission) this must be clearly stated when the data are presented.

Severity grading should take into account only the real clinical symptoms and signs and it should not estimate risks or hazards on the basis of parameters such as amounts ingested and serum/plasma concentrations.

Treatment measures employed are not graded themselves, but the type of symptomatic and/or supportive treatment applied (e.g., assisted ventilation, inotropic support, hemodialysis for renal failure) may help in the evaluation of severity. Preventive use of antidotes should not influence the grading, however, but should instead be mentioned when the data are presented.

Although the scheme is in principle intended for grading of acute stages of poisoning, if disabling sequelae and disfigurement occur, they would justify a high severity grade.

If a patient's past medical history is considered to influence the severity of poisoning, please comment on this.

Lethal cases and occurrence of sequelae should always be commented on separately when data are presented.

Severity Grades

None (0) No symptoms or signs; vague symptoms judged not to be related to poisoning
Minor (1) Mild, transient, and spontaneously resolving symptoms
Moderate (2) Pronounced or prolonged symptoms
Severe (3) Severe or life-threatening symptoms

Please note that the signs and symptoms given for each grade serve as *examples* to assist in grading severity. Numerical values given refer to adults.

In minor poisoning, symptomatic and supportive treatment is generally not required, whereas this normally is the case for moderate poisoning. In severe poisoning, advanced symptomatic and supportive treatment is always necessary.

The scheme must be used with flexibility as in some cases one single feature may determine the "level" at which the patient is graded, whereas in the majority of cases an overall evaluation of signs and symptoms is necessary for defining the seriousness of the case. In a simple system like this it is not possible to insist on strict criteria and the evaluation, therefore, largely depends on the judgment and experience of the professionals concerned.

Organ	None 0 No Symptoms or Signs	Minor 1 Mild, Transient, and Spontaneously Resolving Symptoms or Signs	Moderate 2 Pronounced or Prolonged Symptoms or Signs	Severe 3 Severe or Life-threatening Symptoms or Signs
Muscular system		Mild pain, tenderness	Pain, rigidity, cramping, and fasciculations	Intense pain, extreme rigidity, extensive cramping, and fasciculations
		Creatine phosphokinase (CPK) ~250–1500 IU/L	Rhabdomyolysis, CPK ~1500–10,000 IU/L	Rhabdomyolysis with complications, CPK ≥10,000 IU/L Compartment syndrome
Local effects on skin		Irritation, first-degree burns (reddening) or second-degree burns on <10% of body surface area	Second-degree burns on 10–50% of body surface (children: 10–30%) or third-degree burns on <2% of body surface area	Second-degree burns on >50% of body surface (children: >30%) or third-degree burns on >2% body surface area
Local effects on eye		Irritation, redness, lacrimation, mild palpebral edema	Intense irritation, corneal abrasion	
			Minor (punctate) corneal ulcers	Corneal ulcers (other than punctate), perforation Permanent damage
Local effects from bites and stings		Local swelling, itching	Regional swelling involving the whole extremity	Extensive swelling involving the whole extremity and significant parts of adjacent areas Critical localization of swelling threatening airways
Cardiovascular system		Mild pain	Moderate pain Sinus bradycardia (heart rate [HR] ~40–50) Sinus tachycardia (HR ~140–180)	Extreme pain Severe sinus bradycardia (HR ~<40) Severe sinus tachycardia (HR ~>180)

From Michell L-J, Dexter EM, Bradberry SM, et al. Assessment of IPCS/CEC/EAPCTT. Dexter EM, Michell L-J, Casey PB. The role and value of phonetoxscore in cases of poisoning. Phonetoxscore by staff of the PNPIS (Birmingham Centre). In: Proceedings, XVIth International Congress of the European Association of Poison Centres and Clinical Toxicologists, Vienna, April 12, 1994: Abstracts 0.83 and 0.84.

(continued)

Table 1-5 *(Continued)*

Organ	None 0 No Symptoms or Signs	Minor 1 Mild, Transient, and Spontaneously Resolving Symptoms or Signs	Moderate 2 Pronounced or Prolonged Symptoms or Signs	Severe 3 Severe or Life-threatening Symptoms or Signs
Cardiovascular system—cont'd		Isolated extrasystoles	Frequent extrasystoles, atrial fibrillation/flutter, atrioventricular block I–II, prolonged QRS and QT_c time, repolarization abnormalities	Life-threatening ventricular dysrhythmias, atrioventricular block III, asystole
			Myocardial ischemia	Myocardial infarction
		Mild and transient hypo/hypertension	Hypo/hypertension	Shock, hypertensive crisis
Metabolic balance		Mild acid–base disturbances (HCO_3 ~ 15–20 or 30–40 mmol/L, pH ~ 7.25–7.32 or 7.50–7.59)	Acid–base disturbances (HCO_3 ~ 10–14 or >40 mmol/L, pH ~ 7.15–7.24 or 7.60–7.69)	Severe acid–base disturbances HCO_3 ≤10 mmol/L, pH, ≤7.15 or >7.7)
		Mild electrolyte and fluid disturbances (K^+ 3.0–3.4 or 5.2–5.9 mmol/L)	Electrolyte and fluid disturbances (K^+ 2.5–2.9 or 6.0–6.9 mmol/L)	Severe electrolyte and fluid disturbances (K^+ <2.5 or >7.0 mmol/L)
		Mild hypoglycemia (~50–70 mg/dL or 2.8–3.9 mmol/L)	Hypoglycemia (~30–50 mg/dL or 1.7–2.8 mmol/L)	Severe hypoglycemia (≤30 mg/dL or 1.7 mmol/L)
		Hyperthermia of short duration	Hyperthermia of longer duration	Dangerous hypo/hyperthermia
Liver		Minimal rise in serum enzymes (aspartate transaminase [ASAT], alanine, transaminase [ALAT] ~ 2–5 × normal)	Rise in serum enzymes (ASAT, ALAT ~5–50 × normal) but no diagnostic biochemical (eg, ammonia, clotting factors) or clinical evidence of liver dysfunction	Rise in serum enzymes (≥50 × normal) or biochemical (e.g., ammonia, clotting factors) or clinical evidence of liver failure
Kidney		Minimal proteinuria/hematuria	Massive proteinuria/hematuria	
			Renal dysfunction (eg, oliguria, polyuria, serum creatinine ~200–500 µmol/L)	Renal failure (e.g., anuria, serum creatinine >500 µmol/L)
Blood		Mild hemolysis	Hemolysis	Massive hemolysis
		Mild methemoglobinemia (metHb ~ 10–30%)	Methemoglobinemia (metHb ~ 30–50%)	Severe methemoglobinemia (metHb >50%)
			Coagulation disturbances without bleeding	Coagulation disturbances with bleeding
			Anemia, leukopenia, thrombocytopenia	Severe anemia, leukopenia, thrombocytopenia
Gastrointestinal tract		Vomiting, diarrhea, pain	Pronounced or prolonged vomiting, diarrhea, pain	Massive hemorrhage, perforation
		Irritation, first-degree burns, minimal ulcerations in the mouth	First-degree burns of critical localization or second- and third-degree burns in restricted areas	More widespread second- and third-degree burns
			Dysphagia	Severe dysphagia
		Endoscopy: erythema, edema	Endoscopy: ulcerative transmucosal lesions	Endoscopy: ulcerative transmural lesions, circumferential lesions, perforation
Respiratory system		Irritation, coughing, breathlessness, mild dyspnea, mild bronchospasm	Prolonged coughing, bronchospasm, dyspnea, stridor, hypoxemia requiring extra oxygen	Manifest respiratory insufficient (due to severe bronchospasm, airway obstruction, edema, pulmonary edema, adult respiratory distress syndrome, pneumonitis, pneumonia, pneumothorax)

Table 1–5 *(Continued)*

Organ	None 0 No Symptoms or Signs	Minor 1 Mild, Transient, and Spontaneously Resolving Symptoms or Signs	Moderate 2 Pronounced or Prolonged Symptoms or Signs	Severe 3 Severe or Life-threatening Symptoms or Signs
Respiratory system—cont'd		Chest x-ray: abnormal with minor or no symptoms	Chest x-ray: abnormal with moderate symptoms	Chest x-ray: abnormal with severe symptoms
Nervous system		Drowsiness, vertigo, tinnitus, ataxia	Unconsciousness with appropriate response to pain	Deep coma with inappropriate response to or unresponsive to pain
			Brief apnea, bradypnea	Respiratory depression with insufficiency
		Restlessness	Confusion, agitation, hallucinations, delirium	Extreme agitation
			Infrequent, generalized or local seizures	Frequent, generalized seizures, status epilepticus, opisthotonus
		Mild extrapyramidal symptoms	Pronounced extrapyramidal symptoms	
		Mild cholinergic/anticholinergic symptoms	Pronounced cholinergic/anticholinergic symptoms	
		Paresthesia	Localized paralysis not affecting vital functions	Generalized paralysis or paralysis affecting functions
		Mild visual or auditory disturbances	Visual and auditory disturbances	Blindness, deafness

Table 1–6
Severity Grading of Childhood Poisoning

	Score = 1 (Mild Poisoning)	Score = 2 (Moderate Poisoning)
Gastrointestinal system	Nausea; non-induced vomiting and/or diarrhea ≤2×; dysphagia; salivation; oral burning	Vomiting and/or diarrhea >2×; persistent abdominal pain
Central nervous system	Headache; tiredness; vertigo; ataxia; anxiety/agitation	Lethargy; somnolence; coma responsive to pain; severe agitation; hallucinosis; isolated seizures; extrapyramidal reactions
Peripheral nervous system	Tremor; paresthesia	Muscular twitching; autonomic disturbances: anticholinergic, cholinergic, adrenergic, etc. (not requiring treatment or easily treated)
Respiratory system	Irritative coughing; mild cyanosis	Bronchospasm; dyspnea; brief apnea; cyanosis
Circulatory system	Mild tachycardia (75th–95th percentile)	Pronounced tachycardia (>95th percentile) or bradycardia (<5th percentile); isolated extrasystole; significant hypertension; first-degree AV block
Kidney		Proteinuria (150–300 mg/24 h); microhematuria; volume 0.5–1.0 mL/kg/h; serum creatinine (100–179 μmol/L; creatinine clearance 51–80 mL/min/1.73 m^2
Liver		S-ALT, S-AST <300 U/L; coagulation tests abnormal without clinical signs
Skin	Pallor; redness; edema/ecchymosis	
Other	Metabolic acidosis BE –5 or less; MetHb <10%; blood ethanol <22 mmol/L; serum salicylate "mild" by Done nomogram	Hypothermia < 35°C; hyperthermia 38–40°C; metabolic acidosis BE –6 to –15; serum potassium < 3 mmol/L or > 6 mmol/L; blood ethanol ≥22 mmol/L; MetHb 10–30%; serum salicylate "moderate" by Done nomogram
Caustics		
Skin	First-degree burns	Second-degree burns <10% of body surface (< 5% of infants); third-degree burns < 2% of body surface
Mucous membranes	Oral hyperemia; GI endoscopy: first-degree lesion	Oral erosions, ulcers (small and rare); GI endoscopy; second-degree lesions
Eye	Conjunctival hyperemia; corneal erosion	Initial necrosis (reversible ischemia)

(continued)

Table 1–6 ***(Continued)***

	Score = 3 (Severe Poisoning)	Score = 4 (Very Severe Poisoning)
Central nervous system	Coma without response to pain; delirium; repeated seizures; prolonged, severe dystonic reactions	Coma with respiratory depression; cerebral edema; status epilepticus;
Respiratory system	Pulmonary edema; pneumonia; bradypnea	Respiratory insufficiency requiring artificial ventilation; ARDS
Circulatory system	Hypotension with clinical signs; severe hypertension; ECG; serious arrhythmias (e.g., frequent, multifocal VEA), wide ECG complexes; second-degree AV block	Circulatory failure; shock; malignant arrhythmias (ventricular tachycardia, ventricular fibrillation, asystole)
Kidney	Proteinuria >300 mg/24 h; macrohematuria; volume <0.5 mL/kg/24 h; serum creatinine 180–910 μmol/L; creatinine clearance 10–50 mL/min/1.73 m^2	Renal failure (need of dialysis); anuria; serum creatinine >910 μmol/L; creatinine clearance <10 mL/min/1.73 m^2
Liver	S-ALT, S-AST 300–3000 U/L; moderately elevated bilirubin; coagulopathy with minimal bleeding (no anemia)	S-ALT, S-AST >3000 U/L; liver failure; hepatic encephalopathy; coagulopathy with severe bleeding and anemia
Other	Metabolic acidosis BE −16 to −25; serum potassium <2.5 mmol/L or >7.0 mmol/L; hyperthermia >40°C; MetHb 31–70%; blood ethanol 22–66 mm/L; rhabdomyolysis; serum salicylate "severe" by Done nomogram	Hyperthermia >41°C; MetHb >70%; metabolic acidosis BE over −26; serum potassium <2.0 mmol/L or >8.0 mmol/L
Caustics		
Skin	Second-degree burns: 10–20% of body surface (5–10% in infants); third-degree burns: 2–10% of body surface (<2% in infants)	Second-degree burns: >20% of body surface (>10% in infants); third-degree burns: >10% of body surface (>2% in infants)
Mucous membrane	Deep and wide oral ulcers; GI endoscopy: third-degree lesions	Perforation of esophagus or stomach; necrosis of GI walls with loss of normal mucosal aspects
Eye	Total necrosis; irreversible ischemia	Perforation

MetHb, methemoglobin; GI, gastrointestinal; S-ALT, serum alanine transaminase; S-AST, serum aspartate transaminase; AV, atrioventricular; ECG, electrocardiogram; ARDS, adult respiratory distress syndrome; BE, base excess; VEA, Ventricular Ectopic Activity.
(From March AG, Bet N, Persino MG, et al. Severity grading of childhood poisoning: The Matti Center study of poisoning children (MPXC) scare. Clin Toxicol 1995;33:223–231.)

grading of childhood poisoning has been suggested by March and associates[14] (Table 1–6).

Pediatric Fatalities

Koren reviewed data from the AAPCC National Data Collection System between 1983 and 1989. These data suggest that few drugs (eg, camphor, chloroquine, tricyclic antidepressants, phenothiazines, quinine, methyl salicylate, and theophylline) are fatal to toddlers (10 kg or 2 years of age or younger) after ingestion of one commercially available dose unit (Table 1–7).[15] Pediatric pharmaceutical and nonpharmaceutical fatalities between 1983 and 1990 are listed in Table 1–8.

Regional Poison Control Centers

Since 1978, AAPCC has maintained standards for staffing, staff qualifications, data resources, and service provisions required to achieve designation as an AAPCC Regional Poison Control Center (Table 1–9).[16] Regional centers surpass nonregional centers in population served, call volume and call volume per capita, center staffing, medical direction, staff orientation, and center follow-up protocols.

Child-Resistant Packaging

Childhood poisoning from prescription drugs has dropped since a federal regulation requiring child-resistant packaging was passed in 1974. Still, the Consumer Products Safety Commission found that 17% of drugs involved in childhood poisoning were in no container at all, but were found loose by the child. Almost one-third of all medicines that were in a prescription container at the time of the accident were not in child-resistant packaging.[17]

Table 1–7
Acute Drug Ingestion Fatalities in Infants and Toddlers (< 2 years) in the United States, 1983–1989

Drug	Number of Fatalities
Iron supplements	7
Desipramine and imipramine	6
Theophylline	2
Chloroquine	2
Dibucaine local anesthetic ointment	2
Methyl salicylate	1
Phenytoin	1
Chloramphenicol	1
Propoxyphene	1
Methadone	1
Amitriptyline	1
Verapamil	1

From Koren G. Medications which can kill a toddler with one tablet or teaspoonful. Clin Toxicol 1993;31:407–413.

Toxicity Gradations in Childhood Poisoning

Sibert and Routledge have suggested a gradation of the toxicity of substances taken in accidental child poisoning

Table 1-8
Pediatric Pharmaceutical and Nonpharmaceutical Ingestion Fatalities: 1983 Through 1990

Pharmaceutical

Age of Patient	Year of Poisoning	Substance Ingested
Anticonvulsants		
2 y	1986	Carbamazepine
2 y	1989	Carbamazepine
3 y	1986	Phenytoin
Antidepressants		
17 mo	1987	Amitriptyline
5 y	1988	Amitriptyline
10 mo	1990	Desipramine
15 mo	1988	Desipramine
18 mo	1989	Desipramine
20 mo	1989	Desipramine
<1 y	1983	Imipramine
13 mo	1987	Imipramine
18 mo	1985	Imipramine
11 mo	1990	Trazodone
Cardiovascular Drug		
4 y	1986	Digoxin
1 y	1984	Digoxin, quinidine
1 y	1985	Nifedipine
2 y	1984	Quinidine
2 y	1984	Verapamil
4 y	1988	Verapamil
4 y	1989	Verapamil, dextromethorphan, pseudoephedrine, chloropheniramine
Iron		
10 mo	1987	Ferrous sulfate
10 mo	1990	Ferrous sulfate
11 mo	1990	Ferrous sulfate
1 y	1984	Iron tablets
14 mo	1990	Iron tablets
15 mo	1988	Ferrous sulfate
15 mo	1989	Ferrous sulfate
15 mo	1990	Iron tablets
16 mo	1983	Iron tablets
16 mo	1990	Ferrous sulfate
17 mo	1983	Ferrous sulfate
17 mo	1988	Iron tablets
17 mo	1988	Ferrous sulfate (in prenatal vitamins)
18 mo	1986	Ferrous sulfate
22 mo	1989	Iron tablets
3 y	1985	Ferrous sulfate
Miscellaneous Agents		
1 y	1986	Caffeine
12 mo	1986	Chloroquine
2 y	1987	Chloroquine
9 mo	1985	Chlorpromazine
17 mo	1988	Dibucaine ointment
2 y	1987	Dibucaine ointment
11 mo	1990	Diphenhydramine
15 mo	1988	Diphenhydramine
14 mo	1989	Diphenoxylate/atropine
18 mo	1990	Morphine, levorphanol, and diphenoxylate/atropine
20 mo	1989	Propoxyphene
Salicylates		
3 y	1988	Aspirin
18 mo	1983	Methyl salicylate
2 y	1984	Methyl salicylate
18 mo	1988	Methyl salicylate and isopropanol
2 y	1990	Oil of wintergreen
3 y	1988	Salicylate

Nonpharmaceutical

Age of Patient	Year of Poisoning	Substance Ingested
Alcohols and Glycols		
3 y	1988	Ethanol (rum)
2 y	1985	Ethanol (tequila)
6 mo	1989	Ethylene glycol antifreeze and acetone
2 y	1985	Isopropanol and acetone (nail polish remover)
15 mo	1989	Methanol (brake line antifreeze)
6 mo	1989	Methanol (windshield washer)
18 mo	1984	Methanol (windshield washer)
Chemicals		
13 mo	1990	Cyanide
2 y	1990	Hydrogen peroxide (35%)
20 mo	1988	Methylene iodide
Cleaning Substances		
2 y	1988	Drain opener
8 mo	1989	Liquid detergent (3% ammonium chloride)
1 y	1984	Pine oil disinfectant
Cosmetics and Personal Care Products		
16 mo	1987	Acetonitrile (sculptured nail remover)
4 y	1987	Mouthwash (ethanol)
Hydrocarbons		
2 y	1990	Charcoal lighter fluid
2 y	1984	Fuel for stove
20 mo	1984	Hydrocarbon wood cleaner
13 mo	1990	Kerosene
18 mo	1988	Lamp oil (kerosene)
12 mo	1985	Lamp oil (kerosene)
12 mo	1990	Lamp oil (mineral and vegetable oil)
2 y	1990	Lamp oil
16 mo	1984	Lamp oil
1 y	1984	Mineral spirits
13 mo	1986	Mineral spirits
18 mo	1988	Saddle dressing (aliphatic hydrocarbon)
Pesticides		
18 mo	1989	Arsenic rodenticide
2 y	1986	Aldicarb
4 y	1984	Diazinon
15 mo	1985	Fonofos
18 mo	1988	Insecticide (for fire ants)
22 mo	1984	Methylparathion
26 mo	1985	Organophosphate
<5 y	1983	Organophosphate
2 y	1985	Pesticide (unknown type)
13 mo	1986	Sodium fluoride roach powder
18 mo	1990	Terbufos
2 y	1984	Trithion
Plants		
5 y	1985	*Conium maculatum* (poison hemlock)
Gun Bluing		
2 y	1989	Gun bluing
15 mo	1985	Gun bluing
2 y	1985	Gun bluing
2 y	1984	Gun bluing

From Litovitz T, Manoquerra A. Comparison of pediatric poisoning hazards: An analysis of 3.8 million exposure incidents: A report from the American Association of Poison Control Centers. Pediatrics 1992;89:999–1005.

Table 1–9
Criteria for Designation as a Regional Poison Control Center

- Region
  - Geographically defined
  - Population base 1,000,000 to 10,000,000
- Regional poison information service
  - Continuous availability
  - Comprehensive information
  - Written protocols
  - Qualified staff
- Regional treatment capabilities
  - Knowledge of medical facilities within region
  - Region has comprehensive analytical toxicology services
  - Regional patient transport facilities
- Regional data collection
  - Medical records
  - Participation in large-scale data collection programs
  - Regional tabulation of experience
- Education programs
  - For health professionals
  - For lay public

From Geller RJ, Fisher JG III, Leeper JD, Ranganathon S. American Poison Control Centers: Still not all the same? Ann Emerg Med 1988;17:599–603.

Table 1–10
Guide to Toxicity of Substances Taken in Accidental Child Poisoning

Low Toxicity

Medicines

Antibiotics (except ciprofloxacin, sulfasalazine, and chloramphenicol)
Antacids
Calamine
Oral contraceptives
Vitamin preparations that do not contain iron
Zinc oxide creams

Household Products

Chalks and crayons
Emulsion paints and water paints
Fabric softeners
Plant foods and fertilizers
Silica gel
Toothpaste
Wallpaper paste
Washing powder (except dishwasher powder)

Plants

Begonia
Cacti
Cotoneaster
Cyclamen
Honeysuckle
Mahonia
Rowan
Pyracantha
Spider plant
Sweet pea

Intermediate Toxicity

Medicines

Antihistamines (most)
Cough medicines (most)
Fluoride
Ibuprofen
Laxatives
Lignocaine gel
Paracetamol elixir
Thyroxine
Salbutamol

Household Products

Alcohol containing colognes, aftershaves, and perfumes
Bleach
Detergents
Disinfectants (most)
Mercury thermometers
Nail varnish remover
Paints (oil based)
Pyrethrins
Talc (if not inhaled)
Rat or mouse poison
Window cleaners

Plants

Berberis
Fuchsia
Holly
Philodendron
Mistletoe
Dieffenbachia (dumb cane)

Potentially Very Toxic Substances

Medicines

Barbiturates
Benzodiazepines
Carbamazepine
Clonidine
Digoxin
Diphenoxylate (Lomotil)
Iron
Lithium
Mefenamic acid (Ponstan)
Metoclopramide
Mianserin (Bulvidon)
Paracetamol tablets
Phenothiazines
Phenytoin
Quinine
Opiates (including codeine and cough medicines containing codeine)
Salicylates
Hyoscine
Tricylic antidepressants (including doxepin and amitriptyline) and monoamine oxidase inhibitors
Theophyllines

Household Products

Alcoholic beverages
Acids
Alkalis (including dishwasher powder and denture cleaner)
Camphor and camphorated oil
Cetrimide
Carbon monoxide
Disc batteries
Bottle sterilizing tablets
Ethylene glycol (antifreeze)
Essential oils (e.g., real turpentine, pine oil, citronella, and eucalyptus)
Methanol
Methylene chloride (paint stripper)
Organochloride insecticides
Organophosphate and carbonate insecticides
Paradichlorobenzene moth balls
Petroleum distillates (white spirit, kerosene, or turpentine substitute)
Paraquat and other weedkillers (phenoxyacetic acids)
Phenolic compounds
Slug pellets (metaldehyde)

Plants

Arum lily
Deadly nightshade
Laburnum
Yew

Adapted from Sibert R, Routledge PA. Accidental poisoning in children: Can we admit fewer children with safety. Arch Dis Child 1991;66:263–266.

Table 1–11
General Approach to the Poisoned Child

Initial Life Support Phase	
Airway	Emphasis on protective reflexes
Breathing	Adequate tidal volume?
	ABG?
Circulation	Early IV access
Disability	Level of consciousness
	Pupillary size, reactivity
Drugs	Dextrose (± rapid bedside test)
	Oxygen
	Naloxone
	Other ALS medications, as needed
Decontamination	Ocular
	Copious saline lavage
	Skin
	Copious water then soap and water
	GI
	Consider options
Evaluation and Detoxification Phase	
History: Brief, Focused	
Known toxin	Estimate amount
	Elapsed time
	Early symptoms
	Home treatment
	Significant past medical history
Suspected but unknown toxin—consider if:	
Patient	Acute onset
	Age 1–5 years
	Past history of pica ingestions
	Current household "stress"
	Multiorgan system dysfunction
	Altered mental status
	Puzzling clinical picture
Family:	Medications at home
	Recent illness (under treatment)
Social:	Grandparents visiting
	Holiday parties, etc.
Physical Examination	
Vital signs (include core temperature)	
Level of consciousness, neuromuscular status	
Eyes	Pupils, extraocular movements, fundi
Mouth	Corrosive lesions, odors, hydration of mucous membranes
Cardiovascular	Rate, rhythm, perfusion
Respiratory	Rate, chest excursion, air entry, auscultory signs
GI	Motility, corrosive effects
Skin	Color, bullae or burns, autonomic signs
Odors	Breath, clothing
Laboratory (individualize)	
CBC, cooximetry	
ABG, serum osmolarity	
ECG/cardiac monitor	
Chest x-ray, abdominal x-ray	
Electrolytes, BUN/creatinine, glucose, calcium, liver function tests	
Rapid overdose toxicologic screen	
Quantitative toxicology tests (especially acetaminophen)	
Assessment of Severity/Diagnosis	
Clinical findings	
Laboratory abnormalities (anion, osmolal gaps?)	
Toxidromes	
Specific Detoxification	
Reassess ABCDs	
Institute GI decontamination (if not already underway)	
Antidotal therapy, if indicated	
Consider excretion enhancement	
Supportive care	

ALS, advanced life support; ABG, arterial blood gas; CBC, complete blood count; ECG, electrocardiogram; BUN, blood urea nitrogen; GI, gastrointestinal. (From Henretig FM. Special considerations in the poisoned pediatric patient. Emerg Med Clin North Am 1994;12:552.)

(Table 1–10).[17] Henretig has suggested a general approach to the poisoned child (Table 1–11).[18]

MEDICATION ERRORS

Medication errors in and out of the hospital may result in unintentional poisoning. Such errors can be committed by both experienced and inexperienced staff, including pharmacists, physicians, nurses, supportive personnel (eg, pharmacy technicians, students, clerical staff [ward clerks], administrators, pharmaceutical manufacturers, patients and their caregivers).[19,20]

DISCONTINUED DRUGS

A number of drugs have been discontinued because of safety problems (Table 1–12). There are inherent risks, both known and unknown, associated with the therapeutic use of drugs (prescription and nonprescription) and other pharmaceutical agents. The incidents or hazards that result from such risks have been defined as drug misadventures and include adverse drug reactions and medication errors. Medication errors follow inappropriate prescribing, patient noncompliance, dispensing errors, and medication administration errors. The rate of medication errors in neonatal and pediatric intensive care admissions was as high as 1 per 6.8 admissions (14.7%) in one study. Prescribing errors with potential for "severe" or "serious" adverse consequences were recently reviewed in a tertiary care teaching hospital, where 57.7% of prescribing errors were rated as having the potential to produce adverse consequences (Table 1–13).[21–33]

Some look-alike or sound-alike medication pairs have been listed by Janda (Table 1–14).[34] Types of medication errors are summarized in Table 1–15.[19] Many adults and elderly patients are potential poisoning victims because of their inability to read and comprehend label instructions.[34,35]

Ten-Times-Higher Errors

One of every four doses computed by 95 registered nurses in one study contained an error that would result in the administration of an amount that was 10 times higher or lower than the dose ordered. Eleven pediatricians given the same test made errors at the rate of one of every 26 computations attempted.[36,37] A prospective study subsequently confirmed a 10-fold error rate in administration of drug doses.[38] Suggested solutions to this problem include (1) banning the decimal point[39] and (2) preparing a "Code Med" card that can be placed at the bedside or prominently in the chart.[40] Each institution, if it chooses, needs to prepare this type of card according to the local practice and available stock solutions. Additional suggestions include written tests for certification of all personnel involved in drug dosage preparation and administration and routine double-checking of medications with a narrow therapeutic index before their administration.[41]

Drug Donations: Dangers

To avoid unnecessary toxic effects in recipients, Hoen and colleagues suggest that drug donations to nations in need

Table 1–12
New Chemical Entities (NCEs) and New Biological Entities (NBEs) Approved and Subsequently Discontinued in Light of a Safety Question in the United Kingdom, the United States, or Spain, 1974 through 1993

Drug	Trade Name(s)*	Country	Therapeutic Class	Safety Issue
Azaribine	Triazure	U.S.	Antipsoriatic	Thromboembolism
Bendazac	Bendalina	Spain	Antiinflammatory, for prevention of cataracts	Liver damage
Benoxaprofen	Opren, Oraflex, Bexopron	U.K., U.S., Spain	Antiinflammatory	Liver damage, serious skin reactions
Cianidanol	Catergen	Spain	Hepatoprotector	Hemolytic anemia
Cinepazide	Vasolande, Arteripax	Spain	Vasodilator	Agranulocytosis
Dilevalol	Unicarde	U.K.	Beta-blocker, vasodilator	Liver damage
Encainide	Enkaid	U.K., U.S.	Antiarrhythmic	Proarrhythmic effect
Fenclofenac	Flenac	U.K.	Antiinflammatory	Serious skin reactions, carcinogenicity in animals
Feprazone	Methrazone	U.K.†	Antiinflammatory	Serious skin reactions, multiple problems
Flosequinan	Manoplax	U.K., U.S.	Vasodilator	Increased mortality
Gangliosides	Nevrotal	Spain	"Neurotrophic," treatment of neuritis, etc.	Acute polyneuropathy
Indoprofen	Flosint, Flosin	U.K., Spain	Antiinflammatory	Carcinogenicity in animals, multiple problems
Isoxicam	Pacyl	Spain	Antiinflammatory	Serious skin reactions
Nebacumab	Centoxin	U.K., Spain	Monoclonal antibody for treatment of septic shock	Increased mortality in patient subgroup
Nomifensine	Merital, Alival	U.K., U.S., Spain	Antidepressant	Hemolytic anemia
Perhexiline	Pexid	U.K., Spain	Vasodilator, antianginal	Peripheral neuropathy, liver damage
Pirprofen	Rengasil	Spain	Antiinflammatory	Gastrointestinal toxicity, liver damage
Polidexide	Secholex	U.K.	Hypolipidemic	Toxic impurities
Remoxipride	Roxiam	U.K.	Antipsychotic	Aplastic anemia
Somatropin	Crescormone, Asellacrin	U.K., U.S., Spain	Natural growth hormone	Creutzfeld–Jacob disease
Suloctidyl	Loctidon	Spain	Vasodilator	Liver damage
Suprofen	Suprol, Supranol	U.K., U.S., Spain	Antiinflammatory	Renal toxicity, lumbar pain
Temafloxin	Teflox	U.K., U.S.	Antibiotic	Multiorgan reactions
Terodiline	Terolin, Micturin, Uromictrol	U.K., Spain	Anticholinergic, calcium antagonist for urinary incontinence	Cardiac arrhythmias
Ticrynafen (tienilic acid)	Selacryn	U.S.	Diuretic	Liver damage
Triazolam	Halcion	U.K.‡	Hypnotic, anxiolytic	Amnesia, various psychiatric reactions
L-Tryptophan	Optimax, Pacitron	U.K.	Antidepressant	Eosinophilia–myalgia syndrome
Zimeldine	Zelmid	U.K.	Antidepressant	Neuropathy, convulsions, liver damage
Zomepirac	Zomax	U.K., U.S., Spain	Analgesic, antiinflammatory	Anaphylactic shock, renal failure

*Only originator's and/or principal licencee's trade name shown.
†Still marketed in Spain; not approved in the United States.
‡Still marketed in the United States and Spain. (From Bakke OM, Manoccho AM, de Abajos S, et al. Drug Safety discontinuations in the United Kingdom, the United States, and Spain from 1974 through 1995: A regulatory perspective. Clin Pharmacol Ther 1995;58:108–117.)

Table 1–13
Sound-Alike (Often Look-Alike) Drugs

acetohexamide/acetazolamide
Apronal label for acetaminophen/aprolidine
azathioprine/azidothymidine
chlorpropamide/chlorpromazine/clomipramine/clomiphene
desipramine/disopyramide
Diamox/Diabinese
Lanoxin (digoxin)/Levoxine (brand of levothyroxine sodium)
Lasix/Losec (now known as Prilosec)
norfloxacin (abbreviated norflox)/Norflex
quinidine/quinine
Stelazine/selegiline
tolazamide/tolmetin

Data taken from References 21–32.

should be based on a proper assessment of need; should consist only of drugs included in a national drug list, if it exists, or on the World Health Organization (WHO) essential drug list; should always be labeled by generic or international nonproprietary names; should be accompanied by product information in the local language; and should have a shelf life of at least 1 year.[42]

DEVELOPING COUNTRIES

The International Program on Chemical Safety (Dr. J. A. Haines, WHO, Geneva) has prepared a *Handbook on Poisoning for Developing Countries.* Joubert and Mathibe have reviewed some aspects of poisoning in developing

Table 1–14
Look-Alike or Sound-Alike Medication Pairs

Medication Pair	Reason for Potential Error
amiodarone/amrinone	Used in the cardiac setting, look alike when written
carboplatin/cisplatin	Both are chemotherapeutic agents, sound alike
Clonidine/Klonopin	Look and sound alike
Coumadin/Cardizem	Used in the cardiac setting, look alike when written
glipizide/glyburide	Used for diabetes, look and sound alike, similar strengths
Hismanal/Ismelin	Similar strengths, sound alike
Lasix/KCl	Similar strengths, often ordered in conjunction with one another
Loniten/Lotensin	Look alike when written, both used for hypertension
Mazicon/Mivacron	Both used in the anesthesia setting, sound alike. (Because of this similarity, Roche has changed the name of Mazicon to Romazicon)
Norvasc/Navane	Similar strengths, look alike when written
Paxil/paclitaxel (Taxol)	Sound alike
Platinol/Paraplatin	Both are chemotherapeutic agents, sound alike
rifabutin/rifampin	Similar drug names, same strengths
rimantadine/ranitidine	Similar drug names
Seldane/Feldene	Sound alike
sulfadiazine/sulfasalazine	Look alike when written
terbinafine/terfenadine	Look alike, sound alike
Xanax/Zantac	Look and sound alike

From Janda SM. Look-alike and sound-alike medication pairs. Vet Hum Toxicol 1994;36:256.
*Source: References 21–32.

countries (paraffin–kerosene, copper sulfate, pesticides, cantharidin, plant poisoning).[43]

BASIC APPROACH TO THE POISONED PATIENT

See Chapter 6.

PATIENT DECONTAMINATION

Eye Contamination

Immediately irrigate copiously for at least 15 to 20 minutes with neutralizing solution (eg, normal saline or water). Do not use acid or alkaline irrigating solution. Alkali corneal burns are ophthalmologic emergencies requiring immediate consultation from an ophthalmologist.

Skin Contamination

Cutaneous absorption is a common occurrence, as one in four industrial substances represents an appreciable hazard for skin absorption. Cutaneous absorption depends on several factors such as lipid solubility, skin condition, location, caustic effect, physical conditions, and the presence of certain vehicles (dimethyl sulfoxide, methanol, defatting agents). Serious toxicity has resulted from cutaneous absorption, and health personnel should be cautious about both continuing contamination and cross-contamination with such toxic substances as parathion and other organophosphates, organic metal compounds (eg, lead), aniline, phenol, hydrocyanic acid, and ethylene dibromide.

TREATMENT

1. Irrigate the area covered by a corrosive substance copiously with water or saline as soon as possible after exposure, and continue irrigating at least 15 minutes.
2. Do not use neutralizing substances.
3. Be sure to remove all contaminated clothes (eg, diaper in bleach ingestion), because damage is related both to concentration and to duration of exposure.
4. For potentially toxic substances subject to skin absorption, health personnel should wear impermeable gloves and gowns.
5. Exposed persons should rinse with cold water and then wash thoroughly (including skin folds, nail beds, and hair) with a nongermicidal soap. Green soap is highly effective but often not available. Repeat the rinse with cold water.
6. The process should be repeated twice more.
7. Some chemical exposures require special treatment. Lime (calcium oxide) and cement exposures are treated like alkali burns. In burns by flammable metals (eg, lithium, sodium), large particles are removed and the exposed surface is covered with mineral oil. Application of polyethylene decreases tissue penetration in burns caused by phenols (cresols). Copper sulfate solution improves debridement and reduces toxicity of white phosphorus burns. For hydrofluoric acid burns, use of intradermal or intraarterial calcium gluconate decreases tissue necrosis.
8. Chemical spills should be handled by specially trained teams (eg, HAZMAT teams) when available. In contrast to human skin decontamination, water is no longer used to neutralize and wash away a spill. Priorities of cleanup have shifted to containment, absorption, and dilution.

TOXIC SYNDROMES

Kulig has summarized the most common toxic poisoning syndrome groups likely to be encountered in an emergency department (Table 1–16).[44]

The Central Nervous System

Coma Scales

The Glasgow Coma Scale and Pediatric Glasgow Coma Scale are found in Tables 1–17 and 1–18.[45] Additional coma scales for use in pediatric practice have been suggested.[46]

The European Association of Poison Centers and Clinical Toxicologists has organized a working party to evaluate the usefulness of such scales. They came to the following conclusions:

Table 1–15
Types of Medication Errors*

Type	Definition
Prescribing error	Inappropriate drug selection (based on indications, contraindications, known allergies, existing drug therapy, and other factors), dose, dosage form, quantity, route, concentration, rate of administration, or instructions for use of a drug product ordered or authorized by physician (or other legitimate prescriber)
Omission error†	Failure to administer an ordered dose to a patient
Unauthorized drug error‡	Administration to the patient of a dose of medication not authorized by a legitimate prescriber for the patient
Extra dose error	Administration of duplicate doses to a patient, ie, one or more dosage units in addition to those that were ordered
Wrong dose error§	Administration to the patient of a dose that is greater than or less than the amount ordered by the prescriber
Wrong route error‖	Administration to the patient of a drug by a route other than that ordered by the physician
Wrong rate error	Incorrect rate of administration of a drug product to the patient
Wrong dosage form error#	Administration to the patient of a drug product in a different dosage form than was ordered by the prescriber
Wrong time error	Failure to administer a medication dose within a predefined interval from its scheduled administration time (this interval should be established by each individual health care facility)
Wrong drug preparation error¶	Drug product incorrectly formulated or manipulated before administration
Wrong administration technique error	Inappropriate procedure or improper technique in the administration of a drug
Deteriorated drug error**	Administration of a drug for which the physical or chemical dosage form integrity has been compromised.
Monitoring error	Failure to review a prescribed regimen for appropriateness, or failure to use appropriate clinical or laboratory data for adequate assessment of patient response to prescribed therapy
Potential error	Mistake in prescribing, dispensing, or planned medication administration that is detected and corrected through intervention (by another health care provider or patient) before actual medication administration
Compliance error	Inappropriate patient behavior regarding adherence to a prescribed medication regimen
Other medication error	Any medication error that does not fall into one of the above predefined categories

*The categories may not be mutually exclusive because of the multidisciplinary and multifactorial nature of medication errors.
†Assumes no prescribing error. Exclusions would include patient refusal to take the medication and failure to administer the dose because of recognized contraindications.
‡This would include, for example, a dose given to the wrong patient, unordered drugs, and doses given outside a stated set of clinical parameters or protocols.
§Exclusions would include (1) allowable deviations based on preset ranges established by individual health care organizations in consideration of measuring devices routinely provided to those who administer drugs to patients, or other factors such as conversion of doses expressed in the apothecary system to the metric system, and (2) topical dosage forms for which medication orders are not expressed quantitatively.
‖This would also include doses administered via the correct route but at the wrong site (eg, left eye instead of right eye).
#Exclusions would include accepted protocols (established by the pharmacy and therapeutics committee or its equivalent) that authorize pharmacists to dispense alternate dosage forms for patients with special needs (eg, liquid formulations for patients with tube feedings or those who have difficulty swallowing), as allowed by state regulations.
¶This would include, for example, incorrect dilution or reconstitution, mixing drugs that are physically or chemically incompatible, and inadequate product packaging.
**This would include, for example, use of expired drugs and improperly stored drugs.
(From ASHP Council on Professional Affairs. ASHP reports medication errors. Am J Hosp Pharm 1992;49:640–648.)

Table 1–16
The Most Common Toxic Syndromes

Anticholinergic Syndromes	
Common signs	Delirium with mumbling speech, tachycardia, dry, flushed skin, dilated pupils, myoclonus, slightly elevated temperature, urinary retention, and decreased bowel sounds. Seizures and dysrhythmias may occur in severe cases.
Common causes	Antihistamines, antiparkinsonian medication, atropine, scopolamine, amantadine, antipsychotic agents, antidepressant agents, antispasmodic agents, mydriatic agents, skeletal muscle relaxants, and many plants (notably jimson weed and *Amanita muscaria*).
Sympathomimetic Syndromes	
Common signs	Delusions, paranoia, tachycardia (or bradycardia if the drug is a pure alpha-adrenergic agonist), hypertension, hyperpyrexia, diaphoresis, piloerection, mydriasis, and hyperreflexia. Seizures, hypotension, and dysrhythmias may occur in severe cases.
Common causes	Cocaine, amphetamine, methamphetamine (and its derivatives 3,4-methylenedioxyamphetamine, 3,4-methylenedioxymethamphetamine, 3,4-methylenedioxyethamphetamine, and 2,5-dimethoxy-4-bromoamphetamine), and over-the-counter decongestants (phenylpropanolamine, ephedrine, and pseudoephedrine). In caffeine and theophylline overdoses, similar findings, except for the organic psychiatric signs, result from catecholamine release.
Opiate, Sedative, or Ethanol Intoxication	
Common signs	Coma, respiratory depression, miosis, hypotension, bradycardia, hypothermia, pulmonary edema, decreased bowel sounds, hyporeflexia, and needlemarks. Seizures may occur after overdoses of some narcotics, notably propoxyphene.
Common causes	Narcotics, barbiturates, benzodiazepines, ethchlorvynol, glutethimide, methyprylon, methaqualone, meprobamate, ethanol, clonidine, and guanabenz.
Cholinergic Syndromes	
Common signs	Confusion, central nervous system depression, weakness, salivation, lacrimation, urinary and fecal incontinence, gastrointestinal cramping, emesis, diaphoresis, muscle fasciculations, pulmonary edema, miosis, bradycardia or tachycardia, and seizures.
Common causes	Organophosphate and carbamate insecticides, physostigmine, edrophonium, and some mushrooms.

From Kulig K. Initial management of ingestions of toxic substances. N Engl J Med 1992;326:1678.

1. There is no merit in attempting to define individual symptoms and signs.
2. No single grading system is adequate for all situations in clinical toxicology, but this does not invalidate the benefits of a generally applicable severity grading scheme.
3. Parameters for data collection from telephone calls cannot be the same as the requirements in intensive care units. Therefore, two grading schemes are necessary–one simple and one detailed—but both using the same systematic basis.
4. The grading criteria require modification for application to pediatric cases.
5. Any scale that is adopted must be applicable over longer periods than the first 24 hours.
6. Severity scales based on therapeutic intervention have inherent problems which make them less satisfactory than those based on no intervention.
7. Severity should be graded according to the consequences that develop rather than those that might have occurred in the absence of treatment.
8. The Glasgow Coma Scale developed for trauma patients is inappropriate for acute poisoning. A new scale to encompass all types of impaired consciousness and disturbed behavior is required.
9. Inclusion of chronic health points in a scale for grading the severity of poisoning is irrelevant.
10. Analytical data should be used to identify cases in which specific treatment prevented the development of serious toxicity.

The predictive value of these scales in overdose remains to be determined.

Other proposed scales include the Reaction Level Scale (RLS85)[47]; Comprehensive Level of Consciousness Scale (CLOCS)[48]; Clinical Neurological Assessment Tool (CNA)[49]; Coma Recovery Scale[50]; Glasgow–Liege Scale (GLS)[51]; Innsbruck Coma Scale (ICS)[52]; and Glasgow Outcome Scale (GOS).[53] Details of these tests and scoring scales have been summarized by Segatore and Way.[54]

Table 1–17
Glasgow Coma Scale

Eyes		
Open	Spontaneously	4
	To verbal command	3
	To pain	2
No response		1
Best Motor Response		
To verbal command	Obeys	6
To painful stimulus	Localizes pain	5
	Flexion—withdrawal	4
	Flexion—abnormal (decorticate rigidity)	3
	Extension (decerebrate rigidity)	2
	No response	1
Best Verbal Response		
	Orlented and converses	5
	Disoriented and converses	4
	Inappropriate words	3
	Incomprehensible sounds	2
	No response	1
Total		3–15

From Teasdale G, Jennett B. Assessment of coma impaired consciousness. Lancet 1974;2:83.

Table 1–18
Pediatric Glasgow Coma Scale

		>1 Year	<1 Year
Eye opening	4	Spontaneously	Spontaneously
	3	To verbal command	To shout
	2	To pain	To pain
	1	No response	No response
Best motor response	5	Obeys commands	
	4	Localizes pain	Localizes pain
	3	Flexion to pain	Flexion to pain
	2	Extension to pain	Extension to pain
	1	No response	No response

		>5 Years	2–5 Years	0–2 Years
Best verbal response	5	Oriented and converses	Appropriate words and phrases	Smiles and cries appropriately
	4	Disoriented and converses	Inappropriate words	Cries
	3	Inappropriate words	Cries	Inappropriate crying
	2	Incomprehensible sounds	Grunting	Grunting
	1	No response	No response	No response
		Normal Aggregate Score		
		<6 months	12	
		6–12 months	12	
		1–2 years	13	
		2–5 years	14	
		>5 years	14	

From Lloyd-Thomas AP. Paediatric Glasgow Coma Scale. Br Med J 1990;301:382.

Table 1–19
Coma Due to Exogenous Toxins: Mechanisms

I. Hypoxia
  A. Displacement of oxygen in blood and tissues
    1. Carbon monoxide (carboxyhemoglobin)
    2. Methemoglobinemia (ferrous [2+] iron of hemoglobin is oxidized to ferric [3+] iron and cannot carry oxygen), eg, acetanilid, aniline dyes, chlorates, dinitrophenol, nitrites (At least 96 products may cause methemoglobinemia.)
  B. Displacement of oxygen in the atmosphere: carbon dioxide, butane, propane, methane

II. Depression of the central nervous system
  A. Alcohols—aliphatic, eg, ethanol, isopropanol, methanol
  B. Benzodiazepines, eg, diazepam (Valium)
  C. Anticholinergic drugs (rarely produce coma, usually delirium), eg, atropine
  D. Anticonvulsants, eg, phenytoin
  E. Antidepressants
    1. Monoamine oxidase inhibitors, eg, tranylcypromine (Parnate)
    2. Tricyclic antidepressants, eg, imipramine (Tofranil)
  F. Antihistamines, eg, diphenhydramine (Benadryl)
  G. Barbiturates
  H. Bromides
  I. Opiate narcotics
  J. Tranquilizers
    1. Major: phenothiazine (Thorazine), rauwolfia (Serpasil), lithium, butyrophenone (Haldol)
    2. Minor
      a. Chloral hydrate and derivatives: ethchlorvynol (Placidyl), methaqualone (Quaalude), paraldehyde
      b. Piperidinendiones: glutethimide (Doriden), methyprylon (Noludar)

III. Acidosis
  A. Ethylene glycol (glycolic acid metabolite) antifreeze
  B. Isopropanol (acetic acid, formic acid)
  C. Methanol (formic acid)
  D. Paraldehyde (acetic acid)
  E. Salicylate (salicylic acid)

IV. Hypoglycemic agents
  A. Alcohol: ethanol
  B. Exogenous insulin
  C. Hypoglycemic drugs: sulfonylureas
  D. Isoniazid
  E. Salicylates

V. Enzyme inhibitors
  A. Heavy metals: arsenic, cadmium, lead, mercury, thallium
  B. Organophosphate insecticides: parathion
  C. Salicylates
  D. Cyanide

VI. Postictal
  A. Amphetamines
  B. Boric acid
  C. Camphor
  D. Cocaine
  E. Chlorinated hydrocarbons: DDT and derivatives
  F. Hallucinogens: LSD, phencyclidine inhalants
  G. Opiate narcotics: codeine, meperidine (Demerol), propoxyphene (Darvon)
  H. Lead
  I. Plants: yellow jessamine *(Gelsemium sempervirens)*
  J. Phenothiazines
  K. Tricyclic antidepressants
  L. Withdrawal from alcohol, sedatives, minor tranquilizers

VII. Other causes
  A. Spider bites: black widow, scorpion
  B. Shellfish poisoning
  C. Snake bites
  D. Food poisoning: botulism
  E. Mushrooms
  F. Organophosphate insecticides

Drug-Induced Signs and Symptoms: A Systemic Review

Coma. Coma caused by exogenous toxins are listed in Table 1–19. Coma in narcotic users may be due to associated clinical problems (Table 1–20). The common pupillary abnormalities in coma are listed in Table 1–21. Skin changes in coma are summarized in Table 1–22.

Table 1–20
Clinical Problems in Narcotic Users Associated With Coma

Overdose: pure (rare); mixed and sedatives
Hypoxia: pulmonary edema, aspiration pneumonitis, pneumonia
Hypoglycemia
Postanoxic encephalopathy
Trauma
Seizure disorders
Sepsis
Hepatic encephalopathy

Table 1–21
The Pupil in Coma

Miosis	
Narcotics	Propoxyphene
Phenothiazine	Pentazocine
Ethanol	Oxycodone
Barbiturates	Organophosphates
Mydriasis	Clonidine
Usual; if deep coma, cardiorespiratory depression, cerebral hypoxia	
Sublethal coma	
Atropine	Alcohol
Glutethimide	Diphenhydramine
Imipramine	Anticholinergics
Cocaine	Scopolamine
LSD	
Normal	
Barbiturates (In stage II or III coma)	
Alcohol	
Nystagmus	
Barbiturates	
Phenytoin	
Phencyclidine	

Table 1–22
The Skin in Coma

Belladonna, datura, atropine	Dry, hot flushed face Low blood pressure, low temperature, high pulse
Organosphosphates, arsenic, salicylates, LSD	Heavy perspiration
Bromides	Brown skin, acne
Carbon monoxide	Pink, often pale
Cyanide	Deep cyanosis, but good pulmonary ventilation
Heroin, phencyclidine, barbiturates, morphine, codeine, methadone	Needle marks
Barbiturates, CO, methadone, meprobamate, imipramine, glutethimide, nitrazepam	Bullae

Mouth findings in coma are listed in Table 1–23. Drugs that cause coma with pulmonary edema are listed in Table 1–24. Diagnostic and therapeutic actions in coma patients are presented in Table 1–25.

Seizures. Common causes of drug-induced seizures include drug withdrawal (ethanol, barbiturates, benzodiazepines) and noncompliance with prescribed and convulsant therapy by epileptic patients (Table 1–26). In one survey the leading causes of seizure associated with poisoning were, in descending order, tricyclic antidepressants, cocaine, isoniazid, theophylline, and amphetamines.[55]

Status Epilepticus. Initial (emergent) diagnostic evaluation should include determination of antiepileptic drug levels; serum chemistry studies including glucose, sodium, calcium, and magnesium; and blood urea nitrogen determination. Urine and blood samples should be obtained for toxicologic screening. Oxygenation should be confirmed by oximetry or periodic arterial blood gas determinations. Lumbar puncture should be performed unless contraindicated by severe intracranial hypertension, suspected cerebral mass lesion, or obstructed cerebrospinal fluid flow (eg, hydrocephalus). Brain imaging by computed tomography scan or magnetic resonance imaging scan is usually performed before a lumbar puncture in adults. Brain imaging is usually and eventually necessary in adults with new-onset seizures, children with nonfebrile status epilepticus, and all patients with uncontrolled epilepsy.[56] Meningitis is relatively rare in patients with status epilepticus. A second phase of diagnostic studies begins when the seizures have stopped or occur only intermittently and the patient's cardiovascular function has stabilized.[57]

Peripheral Nervous System Toxicity. See Table 1–27.[58,59]

Axonopathy manifests as axon degeneration, myelin degeneration, partial recovery, and "dying-back" neuropathy. Examples of agents that may be involved are acrylamide (sensory, motor); hexacarbons (*n*-hexane, methyl-*n*-butyl [stocking and glove sensory motor and autonomic neurop-

Table 1–23
The Mouth in Coma

Increased salivation
- Organophosphates
- Arsenic
- Strychnine
- Some mushrooms

Dry mouth
- Atropine
- Belladonna
- Anticholinergics
- Narcotics

Table 1–24
Drugs That Cause Coma and Pulmonary Edema

Heroin
Methadone
Meperidine
Toxic fumes (eg, polyvinyl chloride)
Barbiturates
Glutethimide

Table 1–25
Diagnostic and Therapeutic Actions in Coma Patients

Immediate Need	Drug/Cause	Diagnostic Test	Treatment
Hypoxia	Carbon monoxide	Blood—pink	Oxygen
	Methemoglobinemia	Blood—chocolate	Methylene blue
	Cyanide	History	Sodium nitrite Sodium thiosulfate
Narcotics	See Chapter 25	Naloxone trial	Naloxone
Drug Withdrawal	Narcotic	Methadone trial	Methadone
	Barbiturate	Nembutal trial	Nembutal
	Alcohol	Valium trial	Valium
Cholinergics	Organophosphates Insecticides	Atropine	Atropine and pralidoxime
	Anticholinesterase drugs Parasympathomimetic agents, mushrooms, and plants	Atropine	Atropine
Food poisoning	Botulism	History	Antitoxin
Spider bite	Black widow, scorpion	History	Antivenin
Snake bite	Pit viper	History	Antivenin
Uncouplers of oxidative phosphorylation	Aspirin	Ferric chloride	Pharmacologic
Anticholinergic agents	See Table 1–16	Physostigmine trial	Physostigmine
Metals	Arsenic, mercury	X-ray of abdomen	Bronchoalveolar lavage, penicillamine
	Thallium	History	Dithiocarb
	Iron	X-ray of abdomen	Deferoxamine
Sedative drugs	See Table 1–16	Drug screen	Pharmacologic
	Methanol	History and drug screen	Ethanol
Sympathomimetic and stimulant drugs	See Table 1–16	Drug screen	Pharmacologic
Shellfish poisoning	Red tide	History	Pharmacologic

Table 1–26
Drug-Induced Seizures

- Antidepressants and lithium salts
  - Tricyclic antidepressants (frequent), including classic and "newer" antidepressants (mianserin, maprotiline, amoxapine)
  - Monoamine oxidase inhibitors
- Antipsychotics
  - Phenothiazines
  - Butyrophenones (less frequent)
  - Antihistamines (H_1-receptor antagonist), more frequent in children
  - Antiepileptic drugs and their paradoxical proconvulsant activity
- Central nervous system stimulants
  - Cortical stimulants
  - Theophylline
  - Cocaine (hyperthermia and cardiac arrhythmias are factors); (body packer's ruptured cocaine-filled condoms)
  - Amphetamine (in high-dose "binge" users)
- Brainstem stimulants
  - Pentatetrazol, picrotoxin (rarely used)
  - Spinal stimulants: strychnine
  - Nonprescription stimulants: caffeine, phenylpropanolamine, ephedrine)
- General anesthetics
  - Inhalation anesthetics
    - Enflurane
    - Isoflurane
  - Intravenous and nonnarcotic anesthetics
    - Ketamine
    - Etomidate
    - Methohexital
- Local anesthetics
  - Lidocaine (at high doses)
- Antiarrhythmic drugs (including lidocaine)
  - Mexiletine
  - Tocainide
  - Ajmaline
  - Disopyramide (severe hypoglycemia)
  - Quinidine
  - Quinine (adulteration of street drugs)
  - Propranolol (after high doses)
- Opioids and other narcotic analgesics
  - Morphine (at high doses in neonates and infants)
  - Meperidine (normeperidine)
  - Dextropropoxyphene
  - Fentanyl and sufentanyl
  - Partazone
- Nonnarcotic analgesics and nonsteroidal antiinflammatory drugs (NSAIDs)
  - Aspirin and salicylates (poisoning—depletion of brain glucose?)
  - Mefenamic acid (in overdose)
- Antimicrobial agents
  - Beta-lactam antibiotics
  - Penicillin
  - Cephalosporins (rare)
  - Imipenem/cilastatin
- Antitubercular drugs
  - Isoniazid (overdose or therapeutic dose)
  - Cycloserine
- Antifungal agents
  - Amphotericin B, miconazole (rare)
- Antimalarial drugs
  - Chloroquine, pyrimethamine (both in overdoses)
- Antineoplastic drugs (infrequent)
  - Alkylating agents: chlorambucil, bisulfate, mechlorethamine
  - Antimetabolites: high-dose methotrexate, cytarabine
  - Vinca alkaloids: vincristine
  - Others: cisplatin, carmustine, asparaginase (infrequent)
- Immunosuppressive drugs
  - Cyclosporine (10% neurologic side effects)
  - Glucocorticoids (occasionally, more often when used with cyclosporine)
- Radiologic contrast agents

Data taken from Zaccara et al.[57]

Table 1–27
Drugs Reported to Cause Peripheral Neuropathy

Drug Group	Predominantly Sensory Neuropathy	Mixed Sensorimotor Neuropathy	Predominantly Motor Neuropathy
Antimicrobial agents	Chloramphenicol Colistin Ethionamide Nalidixic acid Thiamphenicol	Chloroquine Ethambutol Isoniazid Metronidazole Nitrofurantoin Streptomycin	Amphotericin B Dapsone Sulfonamides
Anticonvulsants	Sulthiame	Phenytoin	
Antidepressants	Phenelzine	Amitriptyline	Amitriptyline Imipramine
Antimigraine drugs	Ergotamine Methysergide		
Antirheumatic drugs		Chloroquine Colchicine Penicillamine Gold Indomethacin Phenylbutazone	Gold
Cardiovascular drugs	Hydralazine	Amiodarone Clofibrate Disopyramide	
Cytotoxic drugs	Cytarabine Procarbazine Vincristine	Chlorambucil Vinblastine	
Gastrointestinal drugs		Chlorpropamide	Cimetidine
Oral hypoglycemics		Tolbutamide	Antitetanus toxin

From Morrow JI, Routledge BA. Drug-induced neurological disorders. Adverse Drug React Acute Poison Rev 1988;3:105–133.

athy]); carbon disulfide (sensory motor); tri-*o*-cresyl phosphate (motor paralysis); metals (thallium, arsenic, mercury, and platinum [motor]); colchicine, podophyllum; vincristine; taxol; ethanol; vacor; disulfiram; isoniazid; nitrous oxide; metronidazole; and dapsone.

In myelinopathies, the axon is spared, and myelin is destroyed. Proprioception, touch, and vibration are impaired (large fibers). Pain, temperature, and autonomic responses are intact, there is areflexia, and healing is rapid. Responsible agents include lead (motor neuropathy, wrist drop); buckthorn (ascending paralysis); diphtheria toxins; hexachlorophene; amiodarone; and trichlorethylene.

Neuronopathy may be caused by doxorubicin (dorsal root ganglia, autonomic ganglia, muscle necrosis intact) and pyridoxine (sensory loss, ataxia).

Toxins affecting nerve function without nerve injury include: botulism, tetanus, strychnine, elapid venom, and black widow spider venoms. Necrosis of the basal ganglia is caused by methanol, disulfiram, carbon monoxide, and 1-methyl-4-phenyl-1,2,3,6-tetrahydropyridine (MPTP) (designer drugs).

Cognitive Impairment

Conditions predisposing to drug-induced cognitive impairment include age, brain disease, and addiction to alcohol and/or drugs. The elderly are at particular risk because of multiple diseases, multiple drug use, and age-associated alterations in drug-induced cognitive impairment. These impairments are especially evident following the use of benzodiazepines, centrally acting sympathetic antihypertensive agents, sedating antipsychotic drugs, opioids, digitalis, antiparkinsonian drugs, antidepressants, and corticosteroids.[60]

Dementias

Toxic disorders associated with reversible dementias are listed in Table 1–28.

Stroke

Stroke can be caused by sympathomimetic drugs (oxymetazoline, phenoxazoline, phenylpropanolamine, amphetamine, methamphetamine, ephedrine, pseudoephedrine and cocaine).[61]

Impairment Of Consciousness

Impairment of consciousness is associated with use of amphetamines, barbiturates, benzodiazepines, insulin, opiates, phenothiazines, and tricyclic antidepressants. Signs and symptoms relative to each drug are described in Table 1–29.

Table 1–28
Drugs and Chemicals Associated With Reversible Dementias

Drug/Chemical	Clinical Characteristics	Treatment
Major tranquilizers	Chronic confusional state, parkinsonism	Lower dose or discontinue medication
Antidepressants	Chronic confusional state; tremors; anticholinergic effects	Lower dose or discontinue medication
Sedative–hypnotics	Lethargy, confusional state; withdrawal syndromes	Lower dose or discontinue medication (taper dose)
Narcotics	Pupillary constriction; constipation; respiratory depression; sensitivity to low doses in elderly	Lower dose or discontinue; give naloxone HCl for acute condition
Anticholinergic agents	Memory loss; confusional state; psychosis; dilated pupils; dry skin; tachycardia; wide variety of medications involved	Discontinue medication; give physostigmine in acute state
Antihypertensive agents	Psychomotor slowing, depression; use of methyldopa, reserpine, clonidine, propranolol	Switch to other agents for blood pressure control
Anticonvulsants	Sedation from barbiturates; possibly cerebellar signs with phenytoin use; toxic levels	Switch to another drug
Digoxin	Gastrointestinal and cardiac side effects; confusional state	Adjust dose
Antiparkinsonian agents	Use of levodopa, amantadine, bromocriptine; confusional state; psychosis	Reduce medication dose
Antibiotics	Use of penicillin, chloramphenicol; high doses, often decreased clearance in elderly	Adjust dose
Gastrointestinal agents	Chronic confusional state; cimetidine use; possibly extrapyramidal syndrome with metoclopramide	Adjust or discontinue medication
Antineoplastic agents	Asparaginase; intrathecal administration of methotrexate	Discontinue medication
Lead	Encephalopathy; motor neuropathy; headache; seizures; anemia; lead lines	Institute edetate chelation; eliminate exposure
Arsenic	Somnolence; sensory neuropathy; gastrointestinal symptoms; Mees' lines	Institute chelation; eliminate exposure
Organic solvents	Headache; lethargy; poor concentration; peripheral neuropathy	Eliminate exposure
Insecticides	Irritability; forgetfulness; organophosphates	Avoid exposure

From Mahler ME, Cummings JL, Benson DI. Treatable dementias. West J Med 1987;146:705–712.

Table 1–29
Clinical Features of Impairment of Consciousness Caused by Drugs

Drug	Clinical State	Physical Signs
Amphetamines	Agitation Aggression Paranoia Hallucinations	Pyrexia Hypertension Tachycardia Arrhythmias Dilated pupils Tremor Convulsions
Barbiturates	Stupor Coma	Hypothermia Hypotension Pupils reactive Oculocephalic reflex absent Apnea Bullous lesions
Benzodiazepines	Stupor, rarely unarousable	Little respiratory depression
Insulin	Stupor Coma	Pallor and sweating Tachycardia Dilated pupils Hyperreflexia and extensor plantar responses
Opiates	Stupor Coma	Hypotension Depressed respiration Pulmonary edema Skin cool and moist Pin point pupils (but reactive) Fasciculation
Phenothiazines	Drowsiness Coma	Hypotension Arrhythmias Dystonia
Tricyclic antidepressants	Drowsiness Delirium Coma	Hypotension Arrhythmias Dilated pupils Warm, dry skin Hyperreflexia and extensor plantar responses Urinary retention Paralytic ileus

From Morrow JI, Routledge BA. Drug-induced neurological disorders. Adverse Drug React Acute Poison Rev 1988;3:105–133.

Benign Intracranial Hypertension

Drugs most often associated with pseudotumor cerebri (benign intracranial hypertension) include tetracycline, minocycline, nifedipine, nalidixic acid, vitamin A and retinoid analogs, cotrimexazole, cimetidine, atenolol, and glyceryl trinitrate. This condition is characterized by a rise in cerebrospinal fluid pressure in the absence of a space-occupying lesion and with cerebral ventricles of normal or even reduced size. There may be diffuse cerebral edema. There are no localizing neurologic signs. In most cases the disorder is of unknown cause, but intracranial thrombosis and drugs are believed to be the most common precipitating factors.[62]

Headache

During Drug Use: Amyl nitrate, atenolol, captopril, cimetidine, cocaine, diclofenac, dipyridamole, griseofulvin, indomethacin, isosorbide dinitrate, isotretinoin, metoprolol, nalidixic acid, nifedipine, nitroglycerin, piroxicam, ranitidine, and trimethoprim–sulfamethoxazole.

Table 1–30
Odors Occasionally Helpful in Diagnosis of Poisoning

Garlic	Arsenic, parathion, organosphosphate
Acetone	Alcohol, salicylates
Carbon monoxide	Coal gas, petroleum exhaust
Methyl salicylate	Wintergreen
Chloral hydrate	Pear
Camphor	Camphor
Pesticides with parathion or organophosphates	Xylene or kerosene
Ethchlorvynol (Placidyl), paraldehyde	Pungent odor, aromatic
Solvent sniffing	Solvent

After Drug Withdrawal: Analgesics, caffeine, ergotamine, methysergide.

Depression

Drugs that cause depression include beta blockers, corticosteroids, fenfluramine, interferon-alfa, levodopa, methyldopa, methylphenidate, oral contraceptives, pemoline, and phenylpropanolamine. Additional anecdotes suggest an association with benzodiazepines, cimetidine, diltiazem, metoclopramide, nifedipine, ranitidine, and verapamil.[63]

Odors

Odors are not often helpful in the diagnosis of poisoning. Some anecdotal reports are summarized in Table 1–30.

Eye

Nystagmus: phencyclidine, phenytoin. Downbeat nystagmus: lithium, alcohol, toluene, felbamate.

Aggression

Drugs that may induce or aggravate aggression include alcohol, amitriptyline, amphetamines, barbiturates, benzodiazepines, hallucinogens, opiates, phencyclidine, and propranolol.[64]

Mania

Drug-induced mania is most often associated with steroids, levodopa and other dopaminergic agents, iproniazid, sympathomimetic amines, triazolobenzodiazepines, and hallucinogens.[65,66]

Violence

Violence is behavior characterized by an aggressive assault or combativeness. It may be precipitated by a mental disease, situational frustration, or organic disease. Drugs inducing violent reactions include ethanol (intoxication, intolerance, and withdrawal), amphetamines, anticholinergics, aromatic hydrocarbons, cocaine, corticosteroids, LSD (lysergic acid diethylamide), phencyclidine, and sedative–hypnotics (intoxication or withdrawal). Factors contributing to violent behavior may include anemia, dementia, electrolytic abnormalities, endocrinopathies, head trauma, hypoglycemia, hypoxia, postictal states, and vitamin deficiencies.[67]

Hyperthermia: Drug Induced Fever

Mechanisms of drug-induced fever and for drug-induced hyperthermic syndrome are summarized in Tables 1–31 and 1–32. In patients experiencing drug-induced fever, temperatures typically range from 39 to 40.6°C, and patients may appear inappropriately well. Drug-induced fever can be associated with low-grade eosinophilia and maculopapular rash. Fever usually normalizes within 48 to 72 hours of discontinuation of the offending drug, although it may persist for several days to weeks if the maculopapular rash presents as a component of the drug reaction. Dobutamine should be considered as a cause of fever in patients being treated for heart failure.[68] In the patient with drug-induced hyperthermia think of intoxication with phenothiazines,

Table 1–31
Drugs That May Cause Fever, Grouped by Postulated Mechanism*

Postulated Mechanism	Commonly Cause Fever	Occasionally Cause Fever
Hypersensitivity reaction	Methyldopa (Aldomet) Penicillins Procainamide (Procamide, Procan, Pronestyl) Quinidine Sulfonamides	Allopurinol (Lopurin, Zyloprim) Azathioprine (Imuran) Cephalosporins Hydralazine HCl (Apresoline) Iodides Isoniazid (Nydrazid) Nitrofurantoin (Furadantin) Aminosalicylate sodium Rifampin (Rifadin, Rimactane) Streptomycin sulfate
Idiosyncratic reaction	Halothane Quinine sulfate (Quinamm, Quine, Quinite) Sulfonamides Quinidine Primaquine phosphate	
Administration-related reaction	Amphotericin B (Fungizone) Bleomycin sulfate (Blenoxane)	Streptokinase (Kabikinase, Streptase) Vancomycin (Vancocin, Vancoled) Cephalosporins Pentazocine (Talwin) Paraldehyde
Pharmacologic action	Antineoplastics Antibiotics†	
Altered thermoregulation	Cocaine (abuse) Amphetamines (abuse) Atropine sulfate Antihistamines Levothyroxine sodium (Levothroid, Synthroid)	Cimetidine (Tagamet) Amphetamines (therapeutic)
Unknown	Phenytoin sodium (Dilantin) Salicylates Barbiturates	

*Some drugs may cause fever by more than one mechanism.
†During treatment of spirochetal disease.
Adapted from Lipsky BA, Hirschmann JW. Drug fever. JAMA 1981;245:851–854.

Table 1–32
Drug-Induced Central Hyperthermic Syndromes*

Condition (and Mechanism)	Common Drug Causes	Frequent Symptoms	Possible Treatment†	Clinical Course
Hyperthermia (↓ heat dissipation) (↑ heat production)	Atropine, lidocaine, meperidine Nonsteroidal antiinflammatory drug toxicity, pheochromocytoma, thyrotoxicosis	Hyperthermia, diaphoresis, malaise	Acetaminophen per rectum (325 mg every 4 h), diazepam PO or per rectum (5 mg every 8 h) for febrile seizures	Benign, febrile seizures in children

*Boldface indicates features that may be used to distinguish one syndrome from another.
(continued)
†Gastric lavage and supportive measures, including cooling, are required in most cases.
‡Oxygen consumption increases by 7% for every 1°F up in body temperature.
§Has been associated with idiosyncratic hepatocellular injury, as well as severe hypotension in one case.
(From Theoharides TC, Harris RS, Weckstein D. Neuroleptic malignant-like syndrome due to cyclobenzaprine. J Clin Psychopharmacol 1995;15:79–81. Letter.)

Table 1–32 *(Continued)*

Condition (and Mechanism)	Common Drug Causes	Frequent Symptoms	Possible Treatment†	Clinical Course
Malignant hyperthermia (↑ heat production)	Neuromuscular junction blockers (succinylcholine), halothane (1:50,000)	Hyperthermia, **muscle rigidity, arrhythmias,** ischemia,‡ hypotension, **rhabdomyolysis,** disseminated intravascular coagulation	Dantrolene sodium (1–2 mg/kg/min IV infusion)§	Familial, 10% mortality if untreated
Tricyclic overdose (↑ heat production)	Tricyclic antidepressants, cocaine	Hyperthermia, confusion, visual hallucinations, agitation, **hyperreflexia, muscle relaxation, anticholinergic effects** (dry skin, pupil dilation), arrhythmias	**Sodium bicarbonate** (1 mEq/kg IV bolus) if arrhythmias are present, physostigmine (1–3 mg IV) with cardiac monitoring	Fatalities have occurred if untreated
Autonomic hyperreflexia (↑ heat production)	Central nervous system stimulants (amphetamines)	Hyperthermia excitement, **hyperreflexia**	Trimethaphan (0.3–7 mg/min IV infusion)	Reversible
Lethal catatonia (↓ heat dissipation)	Lead poisoning	Hyperthermia, intense anxiety, **destructive behavior, psychosis**	Lorazepam (1–2 mg IV every 4 h), antipsychotics may be contraindicated	High mortality if untreated
Neuroleptic malignant syndrome (mixed: hypothalamic, ↑ heat dissipation, ↑ heat production)	Antipsychotics (neuroleptics), α-methyldopamine, reserpine	Hyperthermia, **muscle rigidity, diaphoresis (60%), leukocytosis, delirium, rhabdomyolysis, elevated creatine phosphokinase,** autonomic deregulation, **extrapyramidal symptoms**	**Bromocriptine** (2–10 mg **every 8 h PO or by nasogastric tube),** lisuride (0.02–0.1 mg/h IV infusion), Sinemet (carbidopa/levodopa [25/100] PO every 8 h), dantrolene sodium (0.3–1 mg/kg IV every 6 h)	Rapid onset, 20% mortality if untreated

*Boldface indicates features that may be used to distinguish one syndrome from another.
†Gastric lavage and supportive measures, including cooling, are required in most cases.
‡Oxygen consumption increases by 7% for every 1°F up in body temperature.
§Has been associated with idiosyncratic hepatocellular injury, as well as severe hypotension in one case.
(From Theoharides TC, Harris RS, Weckstein D. Neuroleptic malignant-like syndrome due to cyclobenzaprine. J Clin Psychopharmacol 1995;15:79–81. Letter.)

butyrophenones, haloperidol, cocaine, and amphetamines; alcohol abuse and alcohol withdrawal; and, uncommonly, salicylate intoxication.

Hypothermia

See Chapter 6.

Psychotic States

Psychotic states are induced by amphetamines, cocaine, and phencyclidine, although other psychotropic agents, therapeutic drugs, and occupational chemicals may be involved. Many patients who are violent may be paranoid schizophrenics.

Cardiovascular System

See Table 1–33.

Hypertension

Hypertension may be caused by sympathomimetics (eg, cocaine, amphetamines, phenylpropanolamine), anticholinergics, phencyclidine, scorpion venoms, and spider venoms. Other drugs associated with hypertension are listed in Tables 1–34 and 1–35.[69] An overview of the effects of drugs and chemical toxins on the cardiovascular system is presented in Tables 1–36 and 1–37.[70,71]

Cardiac Dysrhythmias

Antiarrhythmic drugs (tricyclic antidepressants, phenothiazines, sedative–hypnotics [eg, chloral hydrate]), include stimulants, hydrocarbons, phosphorus, carbon monoxide, and scorpion and spider stings (Table 1–37).

Hypersensitivity Myocarditis

The diagnosis of hypersensitivity myocarditis should be considered when new electrocardiographic changes, mildly elevated enzyme levels, cardiomegaly, or unexplained tachycardia is noted in a patient who has an ongoing allergic reaction to a drug, usually with evidence of eosinophilia.[72]

Torsade de Pointes

Antiarrhythmic agents (eg, quinidine, disopyramide, procainamide, lidocaine, amiodarone); psychotropics (eg, phenothiazines, tricyclic antidepressants, tetracyclic antidepressants, maprotiline); and organophosphates are associated with torsade de pointes (see Chapter 32).

Complete Heart Block

Class I antiarrhythmic agents (procainamide, quinidine), calcium channel blockers, beta blockers, digitalis, organophosphates, cocaine, clonidine, phenytoin, neuroleptic

Table 1–33
Summary of Adverse Effects of Drugs on the Cardiovascular System

Drugs Used to Treat Primarily Cardiovascular Diseases	
Drug	**Adverse Effect**
Digitalis glycosides	Various cardiac arrhythmias
Quinidine	Prolonged QT interval Intraventricular conduction disturbances Hypotension Quinidine syncope
Procainamide	Hypotension Intraventricular conduction disturbances Drug-induced lupus syndrome
Phenytoin (diphenylhydantoin)	Hypotension Arrhythmias Drug-induced lupus syndrome
Propranolol	Congestive heart failure Bradyarrhythmias Hypotension (rare) Rebound angina (abrupt withdrawal in severe ischemic heart disease)
Sympathomimetic amines	Tachycardia Myocardial ischemia
Diazoxide and hydralazine (parenterally)	Tachycardia Myocardial ischemia
Prazosin	Postural hypotension (excessive first dose or rapid dose increment)
Clofibrate	Various cardiac arrhythmias Elevation of serum glutamic–oxaloacetic transaminase, serum glutamic–pyruvic transaminase, and creatine phosphokinase levels Synergistic action with anticoagulants

Drugs Used to Treat Primarily Noncardiac Problems	
Drug	**Adverse Effect**
Oral contraceptives	Thromboembolism Hypertension
Doxorubicin and daunorubicin (Adriamycin and daunomycin)	Nonspecific ST segment, T wave abnormalities Drug-induced cardiomyopathy Endocardial fibrosis
Cyclophosphamide	Myocardial necrosis (in extremely high doses)
Lithium carbonate	Various arrhythmias
Phenothiazines	Cardiac arrhythmias Nonspecific ECG abnormalities Hypotension
Corticosteroids	Delayed healing of infarcted myocardium
Methylsergide	Endocardial fibrosis
Potassium penicillin	Hyperkalemia
Carbenicillin	Hypokalemia
Lincomycin	Bradycardia, cardiac arrest (rapid infusion of large doses)

Adapted from Deglin SM, Deglin JM, Chung SK. Drug-induced cardiovascular diseases. Drugs 1977;14:29–40.

Table 1–34
Chemically Induced Hypertension

Ingredient	Common Use/Abuse	Notes
Steroids		
Glucocorticoids	Replacement therapy and symptomatic treatment of various diseases	Dose-dependent, sustained increase mainly in systolic BP
Mineralocorticoids		
Black licorice	Candy, chewing gum, liquor	Dose-dependent, sustained increase in BP mimicking primary hyperaldosteronism characterized by hypokalemia, metabolic alkalosis, and suppressed plasma renin activity and aldosterone levels
Carbenoxolone	Ulcer medication	
9-α-fluoroprednisolone	Skin ointments, antihemorrhoid cream	
9-α-fluorocortisol	Ophthalmic drops and nasal sprays	
Ketoconazole	Antimycotic agent	
Estrogen	Contraception, replacement therapy, prostatic cancer	Mild, sustained BP elevation, more common in premenopausal women; severe HT has been reported
Progesterone	Contraception, replacement therapy	
Androgens	Anabolic effect (abuse in athletes)	Mild, dose-dependent sustained increase in systolic BP
Danazol (semisynthetic androgen)	Endometriosis, hereditary angioedema	
Anesthetics and Narcotics		
Cocaine	Local anesthetics; street drug	Transient severe increase in BP, especially when used with propranolol
Ketamine hydrochloride	Anesthetic agent	Transient severe increase in BP
Fentanyl citrate	Narcotic analgesic and anesthetic agent	—
Scopolamine	Preanesthetic medication, motion sickness	—
Naloxone hydrochloride	Opioid overdose	Transient BP evaluation

BP, blood pressure; HT, hypertension.
(From Grossman E, Messerli IH. High blood pressure: A side effect of drugs, poisons, and food. Arch Intern Med 1995;155:450–460.)

(continued)

Table 1–34 ***(Continued)***

Ingredient	Common Use/Abuse	Notes
Drugs Affecting the Sympathetic Nervous System		
Phenylephrine hydrochloride	Upper respiratory decongestant; ophthalmic drops	Dose-dependent, sustained increase in BP
Dipivalyladrenaline hydrochloride	Ophthalmic drops	Severe HT has been reported; may precipitate myocardial event and therefore should be used with caution in patients with coronary disease
Epinephrine (with β-blocker)	Local anesthetic, anaphylactic reaction, bronchodilation, decongestant, antihemorrhoidal treatment	—
Phenylpropanolamine	Anorexic/decongestant	—
Pseudoephedrine hydrochloride	Decongestant	—
Tetrahydrozoline hydrochloride	Ophthalmic vasoconstrictor drops; ophthalmic vasoconstrictor and nasal decongestant drops	—
Oxymetazoline hydrochloride	Decongestant drops	—
Caffeine	Analgesia, vascular headache, beverages	Acute transient increase in BP
Metoclopramide	Antiemetic	Transient increase in BP in association with cancer chemotherapy
Alizapride	Antiemetic	
Prochlorperazine	Antiemetic	
Yohimbine hydrochloride	Impotence	Acute, dose-dependent increase in BP
Glucagon	Bowel spasm	Only in patients with pheochromocytoma
Physostigmine	Reverse anticholinergic syndrome	—
Ritodrine hydrochloride	Inhibition of preterm labor	Hypertensive crisis has been reported
Monoamine oxidase inhibitors	Antidepressive agents	Mainly with sympathomimetic amines and with certain foods containing tyramine
Tricyclic antidepressants	Antidepressive	More common in patients with panic disorders
Buspirone	Anxiolytic	Mild dose-dependent increase in BP
Fluoxetine	Antidepressive	In combination with selegiline
Thioridazine hydrochloride	Psychotic and depressive disorders	Massive overdose may cause severe HT
Ions		
Sodium chloride	Food and drugs	In salt-sensitive subjects
Lithium	Manic–depressive illness	Acute intoxication can cause severe HT
Calcium	Food and drugs	—
Lead	Industry, paint	—
Cadmium	Industry	—
Mixed or Unknown Mechanism		
Cyclosporine	Immunosuppressive agent	Dose-dependent mild-to-moderate increase in BP; severe HT has been reported
Alkylating agents	Neoplastic disorders	—
Recombinant human erythropoietin	Anemia or renal failure	Dose-related mild increase in BP; hypertensive crisis with encephalopathy has been reported
Bromocriptine mesylate	Suppression of lactation and prolactinoma	Severe HT with stroke has been reported after use for suppression of lactation
Disulfiram	Alcoholism	Slight increase in BP; severe HT may occur in alcoholic-induced liver disease
Alcohol	Various	Dose-dependent, sustained increase in BP
Nicotine	Cigarette smoking	Acute transient increase in BP
Nonsteroidal antiinflammatory drugs	Analgesic antiinflammatory drugs	Mild, dose-dependent increase in BP

BP, blood pressure; HT, hypertension.
(From Grossman E, Messerli IH. High blood pressure: A side effect of drugs, poisons, and food. Arch Intern Med 1995;155:450–460.)

Table 1–35
Drugs Associated with Hyper/Hypotension

Hypertension and tachycardia	Amphetamines, cocaine, phencyclidine
Hypotension with bradycardia	Phenelzine, tranylcypromine, monoamine oxidase inhibitors, levodopa, bretylium, organophosphate insecticides, tricyclic antidepressants
Hypertension with normal or slowed pulse	Phenylpropanolamine
Malignant hypertension with intracranial hemorrhage	Amphetamine, cocaine, phencyclidine, phenylpropanolamine
Hypotension and tachycardia	Hypovolemia, shock, theophylline, cyanide, carbon monoxide poisoning
Tachycardia, little change in blood pressure	Lomotil (atropine and diphenoxylate), marijuana, thyroxine, theophylline (chronic)
Muscarinic syndrome	Organophosphate insecticides, bethanechol, pilocarpine
Clinical	Miosis, bradycardia, bronchorrhea, wheezing, hyperperistalsis, sweating

Table 1–36
Chemical Toxins and Cardiovascular Disease

Atherosclerotic ischemic heart disease	Arrhythmias
Carbon disulfide (1)*	Halogenated hydrocarbons (1)
Carbon monoxide (3)	Organophosphates (1)
Combustion products (3)	Antimony (2)
Arsenic (3)	Arsenic (2)
Nonatheromatous ischemic heart disease	Arsine (1)
Organic nitrates (1)	Hypertension
Myocardial asphyxiants	Lead (2)
Carbon monoxide (1)	Cadmium (3)
Cyanide (1)	Carbon disulfide (2)
Hydrogen sulfide (1)	Organic solvents (3)
Direct myocardial injury	Peripheral arterial occlusive disease
Cobalt (3)	Arsenic (2)
Arsenic (1)	Lead (2)
Arsine (1)	Carbon disulfide (2)
Lead (3)	
Antimony (2)	
Organic solvents (3)	

*Probability of causation: (1) definite, (2) probable, (3) possible.
(Adapted from Kristensen TS. Cardiovascular diseases and the work environment: A critical review of the epidemiologic literature on chemical factors. Scand J Work Environ Health 1989;15:245–264.)

Table 1–37
Drug- or Toxin-Induced Arrhythmias

Rhythm Disturbance	Possible Cause
Sinus bradycardia or atrioventricular block	Beta blockers, calcium antagonists, cyclic antidepressants, digoxin and other cardiac glycosides, organophosphate and carbamate insecticides, phenylpropanolamine and other alpha-adrenergic stimulants
Sinus tachycardia	Cocaine, amphetamines, phencyclidine, antihistamines, anticholinergics, cyclic antidepressants, phenothiazines, theophylline, ethanol or sedative–hypnotic withdrawal, carbon monoxide
Prolongation of QRS interval	Cyclic antidepressants, quinidine, procainamide, disopyramide, encainide, flecainide, beta blockers, calcium antagonists, diphenhydramine (massive doses), phenothiazines (especially thioridazine)
Prolongation of QT interval (including Torsade de pointes)	Cyclic antidepressants, quinidine, procainamide, disopyramide, encainide, flecainide, beta blockers, calcium antagonists, lithium, antihistamines (diphenhydramine, terfenadine, astemizole), phenothiazines, arsenic, organophosphates
Ventricular tachyarrhythmias	Cocaine, amphetamines, chloral hydrate and chlorinated hydrocarbons, theophylline, digoxin and other cardiac glycosides, tricyclic antidepressants

From Olson KR, Pentel RR, Kelley MT. Physical assessment and differential diagnosis of the poisoned patient. Med Toxicol 1987;2:52–81.

agents, and cyclic antidepressants may cause complete heart block.[73]

The Skin

Intravenous medications known to cause skin necrosis are listed in Table 1–38.[74] Compounds known to cause hypopigmentation are listed in Table 1–39. Chemical groups known to cause allergic contact dermatitis are listed in Table 1–40.

Toxic epidermal necrolysis has been associated with butazones, hydantoins, sulfonamides, barbiturates, and antibiotics.[75] Pemphigus may be secondary to penicillamine, captopril, pyritinol, thiopronin, penicillin, rifampin, pyrazolone compounds, beta blockers, progesterone, heroin, piroxicam, levodopa, lysine acetyl salicylate, gold, phenobarbital, cephalexin, enalapril, pentachlorophenol, phosphatide, and hydantoin/barbiturate. Most of these drugs induce pemphigus rarely, considering their widespread use.[76]

Systemic Lupus Erythematosus

As many as 10% of cases of systemic lupus erythematosus (SLE) are drug related.[77,78] Procainamide and hydralazine are the drugs most commonly implicated. A definite association has also been shown for isoniazid, methyldopa,

Table 1–38
Intravenous Drugs Known to Cause Skin Necrosis

Solutions and Electrolytes	**Chemotherapeutic Agents**
Dextrose 10%	Bleomycin
Mannitol	Dacabazine
Sodium bicarbonate	Vincalkaloids
Calcium salts	Doxorubicin
Potassium salts	Daunorubicin
Nafcillin	Dactinomycin
Vasopressors	Mitomycin
Norepinephrine	Fluorouracil
Dopamine	Streptozocin
Miscellaneous Drugs	Chlorozotocin
Radiologic dyes	Nitrogen mustard
Methylene blue	

Adapted from Dufresne RG. Skin necrosis from intravenously infused materials. Cutis 1987;39:197–198.

Table 1–39
Compounds Known to Cause Hypopigmentation

o-Benzylchlorophenol (antiseptic)
p-Butylphenol (used in the manufacture of varnish and lacquer resins, as an antioxidant in soaps, and as a motor oil additive)
p-Cresol (disinfectant)
Hydroquinone and its monoethyl and monobenzyl ethers (used in black-and-white photoprocessing, in skin lighteners, and as antioxidants in synthetic rubbers)
o-Phenylphenol (used as an agricultural fungicide, disinfectant, and in the rubber industry)
Pyrocatechol (topical antiseptic)
p-Tertiary butylcatechol (astringent)

Adapted from Hall AH, Hogan DJ. Skin lesions and environmental exposures: Rash decisions. Case Studies in Environmental Medicine, No. 28. Atlanta: ATSDR; May 1993.

Table 1–40
Common Causes of Allergic Contact Dermatitis

Germicides and Biocides
Formaldehyde-releasing compounds
Parabens
Quaternary ammonium compounds

Grains
Barley
Oat
Rye
Wheat

Foods/Spice

Cardamon	Lettuce
Carrot	Potato
Chicory	Radish
Coconut	Tamarind
Coffee	Tumeric
Endive	Vanilla

Medication/product Ingredients
Preservatives
- Lanolin
- Thimerosal

Fragrances and perfumes
- Balsam of Peru
- Benzyl alcohol
- Cinnamic acid derivatives
- Citronella derivatives

Metals
Chromium
Cobalt
Nickel

Organic Dyes
p-Aminoazobenzene
p-Phenylenediamine

Plastic Resins
Epoxies
Formaldehyde-based acrylics
Phenolics

Rhus* Plants
Poison ivy
Poison oak
Poison sumac

Rubber Products
Antioxidants
Polymerization accelerators

Topical Medications
Benzocaine
Neomycin

*For a more complete listing of plants that cause dermatitis see Adams RM. *Occupational Skin Disease.* 2nd ed. Philadelphia: WB Saunders; 1990:507–509. (From Hall AH, Hogan DJ. Skin lesions and environmental exposures: Rash decisions. Case Studies in Environmental Medicine, No. 28. Atlanta: ATSDR; May 1993.)

Table 1–41
Agents Most Often Associated with Vasculitis, Serum Sickness, and Reactions Resembling Serum Sickness

Vasculitis
Allopurinol
Penicillin
Aminopenicillins
Sulfonamides
Thiazides
Pyrazolones
Hydantoins
Propylthiouracil

Raynaud's Disease or Digital Necrosis
Beta-blockers
Ergot alkaloids
Bleomycin

Serum Sickness
Serum preparations
Vaccines

Reactions Resembling Serum Sickness
Beta blockers
Streptokinase
Beta-lactam antibiotics

From Roujeau JC, Stern RS. Severe adverse cutaneous reactions to drugs. N Engl J Med 1994;331:1272–1285.

quinidine, and chlorpromazine. Drugs less frequently implicated include many of the anticonvulsants, beta blockers, sulfasalazine, penicillamine, lithium, and antithyroid drugs. Drug-induced SLE usually occurs after long-term (6–12 months) high-dose therapy with the suspected drug. Clinical manifestations include arthralgias, arthritis, fever, skin rash, adenopathy, myalgias, pericarditis, pleuritis, pleural effusion, hepatosplenomegaly, and renal and central nervous system involvement. The antinuclear antibody (ANA) test is positive. Rapid remission (unlike retinopathy in SLE) follows discontinuation of the drug. The ANA test may remain positive up to 2 years.[79]

Scleroderma

Scleroderma may follow use of carbidopa, mazindol, L-5-hydroxytryptophan, diethylpropion, pentazocine hydrochloride, local anesthetics, bromocriptine, phytonadione, cocaine, and appetite suppressants.

The Hypersensitivity Syndrome

The aromatic antiepileptic agents (phenytoin, carbamazepine, and phenobarbital) and sulfonamides are the most frequent causes of the hypersensitivity syndrome.[80] Other drugs, especially allopurinol, gold salts, and dapsone, are also associated with the syndrome. The syndrome typically develops 2 to 6 weeks after a drug is first used, later than most other serious skin reactions. With antiepileptic drugs, fever and rash are the most frequent presenting symptoms (in 87% of cases). Lymphadenopathy (in about 75%) is frequent and usually due to benign lymphoid hyperplasia. Atypical lymphoid hyperplasia and pseudolymphoma occasionally occur. Some of these cases resolve with withdrawal of the drug, but in some cases lymphoma eventually develops. Hepatitis, interstitial nephritis, and hematologic abnormalities, especially eosinophilia and mononucleosis-like atypical lymphocytosis, are also common.

Agents most often associated with vasculitis, serum sickness, and reactions resembling serum sickness are listed in Table 1–41.

Hair

Hair loss evident 2 to 4 months after beginning treatment can be caused by anticoagulants, retinol and its derivatives, interferons, and antihyperlipidemic drugs. Such loss is usually reversible on the interruption of treatment. Hirsutism may follow use of testosterone, danazol, corticotropin, metyrapone, anabolic steroids, and glucocorticoids. Hypertrichosis is observed after use of cyclosporine, minoxidil, and diazoxide.[81]

Ototoxicity

Diuretics and antiinflammatory agents (eg, salicylates) are associated with acute and transient impairment of hearing or tinnitus. Some antineoplastic agents and aminoglycoside antibiotics are associated with delayed and often irreversible loss of hearing. Lesions in the organ of Corti include destruction of auditory sensory cells.[82] Drug-associated causes of tinnitus and deafness occurring in the same patient can include erythromycin, aspirin, gentamicin, cisplatin, metronidazole, and naproxen. Deafness alone is occasion-

Table 1–42
Drug-Induced Rhabdomyolysis

Syndrome	Primary Target	Pathogenetics	Clinical Features	Predisposing Factors	Typical Rise in Creatine Kinase (U/L)	Therapy	Drugs
Primary toxin-induced rhabdomyolysis	Striated muscle	Damage to membranes, metabolism	Generalized myonecrosis	Dehydration	10,000–100,000	Symptomatic	Heroin, doxylamine
Rhabdomyolysis secondary to: muscle ischemia in drug overdose Chronic intake of drugs including hypokalemia	Microcirculation, muscle perfusion, and/or metabolism	Muscle ischemia	Local or generalized myonecrosis	Hypokalemia, hypophosphatemia, dehydration	Wide range	Symptomatic	Barbiturates Laxatives, thiazides, emetics
Malignant hyperthermia	Sarcoplasmic reticulum of striated muscle		Extreme hyperthermia, hypercapnia, muscular hypertonicity	Genetic (50%)	100,000	Dantrolene	Succinylcholine, halothane, caffeine
Neuroleptic malignant syndrome	Central nervous system		Rigor hyperthermia	Dehydration, psychiatric disease	10,000	Dantrolene (physostigmine has no effect)	Butyrophenones, phenothiazines, antipsychotics, cocaine, diphenhydramine
Central anticholinergic syndrome	Central nervous system		Rigor hyperthermia	Dehydration	<10,000	Physostigmine	
Drug-induced polymyositis/dermatomyositis	Vessels of striated muscle	Vasculitis	Pain, diffuse swelling of musculature		<10,000	Abstinence from the incriminated drug, steroids	Penicillamine, phenytoin, phenylbutazone, quinidine

From Koppel C. Clinical features, pathogenesis and management of drug-induced rhabdomyolysis. Med Toxicol Adverse Drug Experience 1989;4:108–126.

ally observed after use of erythromycin, gentamicin, cisplatin, furosemide, metronidazole, and azithromycin. Tinnitus is more common with aspirin, quinine, indomethacin, sulindac, metoprolol, naproxen, and procaine penicillin.[83]

Rhabdomyolysis

Drugs

Koppel distinguishes a primary toxin-induced rhabdomyolysis (muscle disease caused by a direct myotoxic effect of a drug or toxin) (Table 1–42) from rhabdomyolysis secondary to muscle ischemia in drug overdose, which may be caused by local muscle compression in coma, prolonged seizures and myoclonus, and chronic intake of drugs that cause hypokalemia.[84,85] Factors predisposing to the development of rhabdomyolysis are listed in Table 1–43. Table 1–44 proposes a differential diagnosis of rhabdomyolysis. Etiologies of drug- and toxin-induced rhabdomyolysis have been reviewed by Curry and colleagues (Table 1–45).[86]

Table 1–43
Factors Predisposing to the Development of Rhabdomyolysis

Dehydration
Hypokalemia, hypophosphatemia, malnutrition
Psychiatric disease
Agitation, confusion, delirium
Endocrinopathies (eg, hypothyroidism, diabetic ketoacidosis)
Shock, hypotension
Hypoxia, acidosis

Adapted from Koppel C. Clinical features, pathogenesis and management of drug-induced rhabdomyolysis. Med Toxicol Adverse Drug Experience 1989; 4:108–126.

Myoglobin

Myoglobin is a 17,500-Da globular heme protein with a heme group identical to that of hemoglobin and the cytochromes. Myoglobin binds only one oxygen molecule and acts as an oxygen store, used when muscle is deprived

Table 1–44
Differential Diagnosis of Rhabdomyolysis

Drug-Induced Rhabdomyolysis
Toxin-induced rhabdomyolysis
Rhabdomyolysis secondary to muscle ischemia in drug overdose
Malignant hyperthermia
Neuroleptic malignant syndrome
Central anticholinergic syndrome
Drug-induced polymyositis dermatomyositis

Muscle Ischemia
Crush, compartment syndrome, tourniquet shock
Sickle cell trait
Shock and coma
Occlusive arterial disease

Excessive Muscular Stress
Marathon runners, military training
Status epilepticus, prolonged myoclonus or dystonia
Agitation, delirium

Physical Damage
Heat stroke
Burns

Infections
Viral (Coxsackie, herpes, echo, influenza)
Bacterial (Clostridia, Legionella, typhoid, staphylococci)

Electrolyte and Water Imbalances
Hypokalemia, hypernatremia, hypophosphatemia
Hyperosmolar states
Endocrine dysfunction

Genetic Defects
Deficiencies of glycolytic enzymes
Carnitine palmitoyl transferase deficiency

Neuropathy
Polyneuropathy
Motor neuron disease

Adapted from Koppel C. Clinical features, pathogenesis and management of drug-induced rhabdomyolysis. Med Toxicol Adverse Drug Experience 1989;4:108–126.

Table 1–45
Etiologies of Drug- and Toxin-Induced Rhabdomyolysis

ε-Aminocaproic acid
p-Aminosalicylate
Amitriptyline
Amoxapine
Amphetamines
Amphotericin B
Anticholinergics
Antidepressants
Antihistamines
Antimalarials
Antipyrine
5-Azacytidine
Barbiturates
Bee stings
Benzodiazepines
Benztropine*
Betamethasone
Bezafibrate
Butyrophenones
Carbenoxolone
Carbon monoxide
Carbromal
Cathine
Centipede
Chloral hydrate*
Chlorazepate*
Chlordiazepoxide
Chlorinated hydrocarbon insecticides
Chlormethiazole base
Chlorphenoxy herbicides
Chlorpromazine
Chlorthalidone
Clofibrate
Codeine
Colchicine
Copper sulfate
Corticosteroids
Cortisone
Cocaine
Cyanide
Dexamethasone
Dextromoramide
Diaminobenzene
Diazepam
Diazinon*
2,4-Dichlorophenoxyacetic acid
Diphenhydramine
Diquat
Diuretics
Doxepin*
Doxylamine
Emetine
Enflurane
Ethanol
Ethchlorvynol
Ethylene glycol
Etretinate
Fenfluramine
Fluoroacetate
9α-Fluoroprednisolone
Gasoline sniffing
General anesthetics
Glutethimide
Haff's disease
Haloperidol
Hallucinogens
Heroin
Hornet stings
Hydrocarbons
Hydrocortisone
Hydrogen sulfide
Hydroxyzine*
Iodoacetate
Isoflurane
Isoniazid
Isopropyl alcohol
Isotretinoin
Licorice
Lindane
Lithium
Lorazepam
Lovastatin
Loxapine
LSD
Marijuana
p-Mentha-1,8-diene*
Meperidine*
Mercuric chloride
Mescaline
Metabolic poisons
Methadone
Methamphetamine
Methanol
Methaqualone*
3,4-Methylenedioxyamphetamine
Methylparathion*
Mineralocorticoids
Molindone
Monoamine oxidase inhibitors
Morphine
Moxalactam
Muscle relaxants
Narcotics
Neuroleptics
Nitrazepam
Orphenadrine*
Oxyprenolol
Palfium
Paraquat
Parathion*
Peanut oil
Pemoline
Pentamidine
Perphenazine
Phenazone
Phenazopyridine
Phencyclidine
Phenelzine
Phenformin
Phenmetrazine
Phenobarbital
Phenothiazines
Phenylpropanolamine
Phenytoin
Phosphorus
Phosphine

(continued)

Table 1–45 *(Continued)*

Plasmocid	Selenium	Triazolam
Procainamide	Snake bite	2,4,5-Trichlorophenoxyacetic acid
Promethazone	Strychnine	Triethylene tetramine dihydrochloride
Propoxyphene	Succinylcholine	Trimethoprim–sulfamethoxazole
Protriptyline	Sympathomimetics	Toluene
Quail meat†	Tetraethyl lead	Vasopressin
Quinindine	Theophylline	Vitamin A derivatives
Quinine*	Thiopental	Water hemlock
Salicylate	Thiothixine	
Sedatives	Toxaphene	

*Personally observed by the authors, but not found in review of literature.
†Quail were thought to have eaten hemlock, causing rhabdomyolysis in those who feasted on quail meat.
(Adapted from Curry SC, Chang D, Connor D. Drug- and toxin-induced rhabdomyolysis. Ann Emerg Med 1989;18:1068–1084.)

of bloodborne oxygen. The normal level of myoglobin in serum is 3 to 80 μg/L. It has a volume of distribution of about 0.4 L/kg. Myoglobin in the circulation is bound to an α_2-globulin. It has a half-life of about 1 to 3 hours. In rhabdomyolysis and in myocardial infarction, a rise in serum myoglobulin precedes an increase in creatine kinase. Myoglobin serum levels greater than 2000 μg/L are associated with renal complications. When urine is highly concentrated, particularly when the urine pH is low, acute renal failure after infusions of myoglobin are consistently demonstrated. At or below pH 5.6, myoglobin dissociates into ferrihemate and globulin. The ferrihemate causes a deterioration in renal function and is excreted in the urine. At high myoglobin urine concentrations (>1000 μg/mL), red discoloration of the urine or plasma is observed. Myoglobin can be detected in the urine with a dipstick for blood (hemoglobin) with a detection limit as low as 5 to 10 μg/mL. A negative test for blood using a urine dipstick does not rule out rhabdomyolysis. Pink plasma with an orthotoluidine-positive urine indicates hemolysis and at least some hemoglobinemia is present. Urine that is orthotoluidine positive for blood in the absence of pink plasma is due to myoglobinuria (in the absence of large numbers of red blood cells in the urine from bleeding into the urinary tract).[87]

Movement Disorders

Drug-induced movement disorders occur during the early phase of neuroleptic (antipsychotic, major tranquilizer) administration. Parkinsonism is clinically indistinguishable from idiopathic Parkinson's disease; it appears within the first 3 months, more often in the elderly (Table 1–46).

Akathisia

Cyclic antidepressants, monoamine oxidase inhibitors, fluoxetine, lithium, buspirone, and levodopa are the principal causes.[88]

Dystonias

Dystonias are associated principally with phenothiazines, butyrophenones, metoclopramide, and tricyclic antidepressants; with phenytoin, carbamazepine, and propranolol in high doses; and with antiemetics, cocaine, chloroquine, and hydroxychloroquine.

Table 1–46
Agents That Induce Movement Disorders

Compound	Manifestation
Amoxapine	Parkinsonism
Amphetamines	Hyperkinetic movements
Anthistamines	Orofacial dystonia Myoclonic jerking
Black widow spider bite	Rigidity
Butyrophenones	Parkinsonism Orofacial dystonia Opisthotonus, trismus
Caffeine	Myoclonic jerking
Carbamazepine	Orofacial dystonia
Carbon monoxide	Parkinsonism
Chloroquine	Tongue protrusion
Cocaine	Jerking, tremor
Ethylene glycol	Myoclonic jerking
Fluoride	Generalized twitching
Ketamine	Tongue protrusion
Lead (tetraethyl)	Jerking, facial grimacing
Levodopa	Facial grimacing, dystonia Head tossing, flinging extremities
Lithium	Hypertonicity, tongue dystonia, lip smacking, tremor
Metaldehyde	Twitching, hyperreflexia
Methaqualone	Rigidity, hypertonicity
Methylphenidate	Motor and verbal tics
Metoclopramide	Parkinsonism
Monoamine oxidase inhibitors	Rigidity, opisthotonus
1-Methyl-4-phenyl-1,2,3,6-tetrahydropyridine (MPTP)	Parkinsonism
Narcotics (sufentanil)	Chest wall rigidity
Nicotine	Fasciculations → flaccid
Organophosphates	Fasciculations → flaccid
Pethidine (meperidine)	Tremor, muscle jerking
Phencyclidine	Generalized rigidity, trismus, orofacial dystonias, twitching, athetosis
Phenothiazines	Orofacial and other dystonias
Phenytoin	Choreoathetosis
Strychnine	Rigidity, opisthotonus, trismus
Toluene (chronic)	Ataxia, jerking eye movements
Tricyclic antidepressants	Twitching, myoclonic jerking

Chorea

Chorea is most commonly associated with the anticonvulsant drugs, especially phenytoin. Chorea has also been observed with anabolic steroids, benzhexane, amphetamines, methylphenidate, pemoline, cimetidine, levodopa and dopamine, as well as ethanol, toluene, manganese, and cocaine.

Tardive Dyskinesia

Phenothiazines constitute the principal group of drugs associated with the disorder. Metoclopramide has also been suspect.

Tremor. Resting tremor is most pronounced at rest; it decreases with activity. Think of any cause of toxin-induced parkinsonism (Table 1–47).

Postural tremor is most pronounced with an outstretched hand. Think of all beta agonists, phenytoin, valproic acid, cyclic antidepressants, monosodium glutamate, lithium, arsenic, and alcohol withdrawal.

Kinetic tremor is most pronounced with motion. Think of alcoholic cerebellar degeneration, mercury, lithium, sedative–hypnotic intoxication.

Chorea tremor consists of repetitive dancelike movements. Think of anticonvulsants (phenytoin, carbamazepine), anticholinergics, dopamine agonists (amantadine, bromocriptine), ethanol, toluene, manganese, and sympathomimetics (amphetamine, cocaine).

Dystonic tremor consists of muscle group spasms (oculogyric crises, torticollis, tortipelos, opisthotonus). Think of neuroleptics, antiemetics, cocaine, chloroquine, and hydroxychloroquine.

Myasthenic Crisis. Drug-induced myasthenic crisis may be associated with the aminoglycosides, polymyxin, penicillamine, tetracycline, quinidine, lidocaine, quinine, morphine, meperidine, curare, succinylcholine, and procainamide.[89] Recovery may occur within a few weeks of withdrawal of the toxic offender.

Myopathies. Drug-induced myopathies result from a direct toxic effect, which may be local when the drug is injected into a muscle or more diffuse when the drug is taken systematically. These myopathies also follow electrolyte disturbances, muscle compression, ischemia, and the development of an immunologic reaction directed against muscle.[90] Repeated injections of antibiotics or drugs of addiction often lead to severe muscle fibrosis and contractures. Clofibrate and ϵ-aminocaproic acid cause an acute or subacute painful necrotizing myopathy with myoglobinuria and acute renal failure. Other drugs that induce toxic myopathies are the lipid-lowering agents, succinylcholine, halothane, corticosteroids, and chloroquine. Drugs that cause a hypokalemic myopathy include the thiazide diuretics, amphotericin, carbenoxolone, emetine, and alcohol. Inflammatory myopathies have followed use of D-penicillamine, procainamide, hydralazine, phenytoin, and penicillin. Environmental agents associated with myositis include foods (adulterated rapeseed oil, L-trypotophan, ciguatera toxin), occupational exposures (silica), and medical devices (collagen and silicone implants).[91]

Table 1–47
Agents Reported to be Associated with Parkinsonism

Agent	Source
1-Methyl-4-phenyl-1,2,3,6-tetrahydropyridine (MPTP)	Intravenous drug abuse, occupational
Tranquilizers (flunarazine, conarazine, haloperidol, chlorpromazine, etc.)	Psychiatric medication
Antidepressants	Psychiatric medication
Lithium	Psychiatric medication
Phenothiazines	Antiemetic
Reserpine	Antihypertensive, psychiatric
Carbon monoxide	Occupational, environmental
Hydrogen cyanide	Occupational
Postanoxic injury	Environmental
Postencephalitic	Arthopodborne infection
Carbon disulfide	Occupational (viscose rayon)
Paraquat	Herbicide
Manganese	Occupational (welding)
Mercury	Occupational
Cycad	Dietary, folk medicine (Asia)
Lathyrus	Dietary (Asia, Africa, WWII)
Rural environment: well water?	Environmental
Suspected Protective Factors	
Cigarette smoking	Lifestyle
Hydrazine	Lifestyle, occupational
Measles	Environmental

From Goldsmith JR, Herishanu Y, Abarband JM, Weinbaum Z. Clustering of Parkinson's disease points to environmental neurotoxins. Arch Environ Health 1990;45:88–94.

Parkinsonism

Table 1–47 lists reported exposures associated with parkinsonism.[90] Drugs and toxins that induce parkinsonism include clebopride, MPTP (designer drug), disulfiram, lithium, organophosphates, metoclopramide, phenylpropanolamine, and antihistamines.[92] The most frequent causes are the phenothiazine or butyrophenone groups and the major tranquilizers.

Motor Neuron Disease

Excitatory amino acid neurotransmitters such as glutamate have been implicated in the pathogenesis of certain neurodegenerative disorders. Glutamate analogs such as β-methylaminoalanine, β-*N*-oxalylamino-L-alanine, and domoic acid are neurotoxic and have been linked to neurologic disorders in humans. Glutamate and its analogs act at N-methyl-D-aspartate (NMDA) receptors or neurons. Glycine, an inhibitory neurotransmitter, may also enhance NMDA-mediated neurotoxicity[93,94] (Table 1–48).

The Kidney

Abuelo has extensively reviewed potentially nephrotoxic chemicals, foods, plants, and animal venoms. Inhaled, cutaneously absorbed, and ingested nephrotoxic chemicals are listed in Tables 1–49 and 1–50.[108] Nephrotoxic foods and plants and animals, carrying potentially nephrotoxic venoms are listed in Tables 1–51, 1–52, and 1–53.[109] Drugs that when given in excessive dose by the physician or misused by the patient have resulted in damage to the kidney are summarized in Table 1–54.[108] Drugs that have been associated with a hemolytic uremic syndrome include cyclosporine, anticancer drugs (eg, mitomycin), ticlopidine, and quinine.[110]

Table 1–48
Motor Neuron Disorders

Lathyrism[96]
Disorder of corticospinal tract: weakness, spasticity, muscle cramps, usually in legs
Chickling pea, *Lathyrus* sativa, seeds
Africa and Asia; endemic in Mysore and Central India
Neurotoxin: β-*N*-oxalylanine-L-alanine (BOAA)

Parkinsonism, Dementia–Amyotrophic Lateral Sclerosis Complex[97,98]
Seeds of false sago palm, *Cycas circinalis*
Chamorros of Guam
Neurotoxin: β-*N*-methylamino-L-alanine (BMAA)
Delay in onset? (unconfirmed association)[99,100]

Parkinsonism in Drug Abusers[98]
Synthetic opiates contaminated with 1-methyl-4-phenyl-1,2,3,6-tetrahydropyridine
Selectively active against dopaminergic neurons in the substantia nigra

Mantakassa[98]
Spastic paresis
Northern Mozambique, 1981
Intake of cyanogenic glycosides from inadequate preparation of cassava

Motoneuron Disease in Leather Workers[101]
Leather workers in United Kingdom
Solvents?

Konzo[102]
Spastic paraparesis
East Africa
Cassava *(Manihot esculenta)* insufficiently processed
Toxin: cyanogen (cyanohydrin) plus insufficient sulfur intake

Amyotrophic lateral sclerosis
Early overexposure to lead, mercury, manganese, selenium[103,104]
Doubtful association[102–106]
Anecdotal reports[107]

Table 1–49
Inhaled or Cutaneously Absorbed Nephrotoxins

Probable Renal Lesion	Chemical
Chronic interstitial nephritis	Mineral spirits
Glomerulonephritis	Hydrocarbons or silicon
Hemoglobinuric acute tubular necrosis	Arsine gas
Myoglobinuric acute tubular necrosis	Carbon monoxide
Pseudoazotemia	Acetone (contaminating acetylene)
Nephrotoxic acute renal failure	Boric acid, cadmium, carbon tetrachloride, chromium, diethylene glycol, 1,2-dichloropropane, diesel fuel, dioxane, dynamite, ethylene dibromide, gasoline, Lysol (British), methylchloride or bromide gas, methylene chloride, phenol, polyethylene glycol, povidone–iodine, tetrachloroethylene, toluene, trichloroethylene

From Abuelo JG. Renal failure caused by chemicals, foods, plants, animal venoms and misuse of drugs. Arch Intern Med 1990;150:505–510.

Table 1–50
Ingested Nephrotoxic Chemicals

Probable Renal Lesion	Chemical
Chronic tubulointerstitial nephritis	Cadmium, fluoride, lead
Hemoglobinuric tubular necrosis	Aniline, chlorate compounds, copper sulfate, cresol, ethylene glycol dinitrate, Lysol (British), naphthalene, *p*-phenylenediamine, potassium or sodium bromate, propylene glycol
Myoglobinuric tubular necrosis	Copper sulfate, lindane, mercuric chloride, *p*-phenylenediamine, zinc phosphide
Nephrotoxic tubular necrosis	Arsenic salts, barium chloride, carbon tetrachloride, chlordane, chloroform, 2,4-dichlorophenoxyacetic and methylchlorophenoxyacetic acids, chromium compounds, diquat, ethylene dichloride, ethylene dibromide, germanium compounds, mercury salts, methylene chloride, oxalic acid, paraquat, tartaric acid, thallium, tetrachloroethylene, trichloroethylene, turpentine, yellow phosphorus
Oxalosis	Diethylene glycol, ethylene glycol, ethylene glycol butyl ether
Pseudoazotemia	Isopropyl alcohol

From Abuelo JG. Renal failure caused by chemicals, foods, plants, animal venoms and misuse of drugs. Arch Intern Med 1990;150:505–510.

Table 1–51
Nephrotoxic Foods

Probable Renal Lesion	Food	Toxic Component
Chronic interstitial nephritis	Vichy water	Fluoride
	Worcestershire sauce	Unknown
Hypercalcemia (milk–alkali syndrome)	Milk	Calcium
Hemoglobinuric tubular necrosis	Fava or broad beans (*Vicia faba* L)	Divicine and isouramil
Myoglobinuric tubular necrosis	Licorice	Glycyrrhizic acid (hypokalemia)
	Wild birds (chaffinch, quail, or european robin)	? Cicutoxin
Nephrotoxic tubular necrosis	Djenkol beans *(Pithecolabium lobatum)*	? Djenkolic acid
	Bile of the grass carp *(Clenopharyngodon idellus)*	? Cyprinol
Oxalosis	Rhubarb *(Rheum rhaponticum)*	Oxalic acid

From Abuelo JG. Renal failure caused by chemicals, foods, plants, animal venoms and misuse of drugs. Arch Intern Med 1990;150:505–510.

Table 1–52
Nephrotoxic Plants

Plant	Scientific Name	Toxic Compound
Autumn crocus	*Colchicum autumnale*	Colchicine
Castor bean	*Ricinus communis*	Ricin and recinine
Daphne	*Daphne mezereum*	Daphnin, vesicant resin, and mezerenic acid anhydride
Herbal remedies	Exact plants unknown	Unknown
Impila	*Callilepsis laureola*	Atractyloside
Marking-nut tree	*Semecarpus anacardium*	Phenolic constituents
Poison mushrooms	*Amanita phalloides* and *Cortinarius* species	Amatoxin cyclopeptides
Rosary pea	*Abrus precatorius*	Abrin and abric acid
?	*Securidaca longipedunculata*	Methyl salicylate, saponius, tanins, and gaultherin
Water hemlock	*Cicuta maculata*	Cicutoxin

From Abuelo JG. Renal failure caused by chemicals, foods, plants, animal venoms and misuse of drugs. Arch Intern Med 1990;150:505–510.

Incontinence

Medications that have the potential to cause incontinence are reviewed in Table 1–55.[111]

Gastrointestinal Tract

Tongue

"Glossitis" and tongue ulceration have followed use of trimethoprim–sulfamethoxazole, diclofenac, naproxen, metronidazole, sulindac, amoxicillin, erythromycin, captopril, and piroxicam[112] (Table 1–56).

Pancreas

Drugs can cause acute pancreatitis, but with the exception of ethanol, drugs rarely cause chronic pancreatitis. Reports of acute pancreatitis are generally anecdotal.[108] Definite, probable, and questionable associations of drugs with pancreatitis are listed in Table 1–57.[109]

Esophagus

Pill-induced esophageal injury may follow use of tetracycline, doxycycline, ipratropium bromide, slow-release potassium chloride, acetylsalicylic acid, nonsteroidal antiinflammatory drugs, and quinidine (Table 1–58). Symptoms of sudden onset of dysphagia, often accompanied by substernal chest pain and odynophagia, typically occur 4 to 12 hours after ingestion but may be delayed up to several weeks in quinidine-induced cases.[113] Iredale and George have summarized causes of drug-induced gastrointestinal obstruction (Table 1–59).[114]

Liver

Think drugs in the presence of raised aminotransferase activities, unexplained jaundice, acute hepatitis, chronic acute hepatitis, cryptogenic cirrhosis, "primary biliary cirrhosis" in the absence of antimitochondrial antibody, unexplained hepatic tumors, especially those not associated with cirrhosis, and liver disease of obscure cause.[115]

Hanson has proposed the following criteria for diagnosing drug-induced hepatitis[116]: (1) clinical and laboratory evidence of hepatocellular injury; (2) onset of symptoms related in time to drug therapy; (3) lack of serologic evidence for current infection with hepatitis A or B, cytomegalovirus,

Table 1–53
Animals With Potentially Nephrotoxic Venom

Common Name	Scientific Name	Location
Arthropods—arachnids		
Scorpion	*Buthus sauloci*	Iran
Brown recluse spider	*Loxosceles reclusa*	Western hemisphere
South American house spider	*Loxosceles lacta*	Western hemisphere
Arthropods—Hymenoptera		
Bees		
Africanized bee	*Apis mellifera scutellata*	Africa and Western hemisphere
Wax bee	*Apis mellificus*	Worldwide
Wasps		
Indian hornet	*Vespa affinis*	Asia
Oriental hornet	*Vespa orientalis*	Asia
Yellow jacket	*Vespula germanica*	Europe
Coelenterates		
Portuguese man-of-war	*Pysalia physalis*	North Carolina
Snakes		
Australian brown snake	*Pseudonaja textilis textilis*	Australia
Black mamba	*Dendroaspis polylepis*	Southern Africa
Boomslang	*Dispholidus typus*	Southern Africa
Small-eyed black snake	*Cryptophis nigrescens*	Australia
Dugite	*Demansia nuchalis affinis*	Australia
Gwardar	*Demansia nuchalis nuchalis*	Australia
Palestinian viper	*Vipera palestinae*	Israel
Pit vipers		
Copperhead	*Agkistrodon contortix*	Western hemisphere
Jaraca	*Bothrops jararaca*	South America
Mamushi	*Agkistrodon halys*	Japan
Rattlesnake	*Crotalus terrificus* and others	Western hemisphere
Water moccasin (cotton mouth)	*Agkistrodon piscivorus*	Western hemisphere
Pit viper	*Agkistrodon hypnale*	Sri Lanka
Puff adder	*Bitis arietans*	Africa
Rough-scaled snake	*Tropidechis carinatus*	Australia
Russel's viper	*Vipera russelli*	Asia
Saw-scaled sand viper	*Echis carinatus*	Africa, India, Middle East
Seasnake	*Enhydrina schistosa*	Asian waters
Small African snake	*Atracepaspis microlapidata*	Africa
Tiger snake	*Notechis scutatus*	Australia

From Abuelo JG. Renal failure caused by chemicals, foods, plants, animal venoms and misuse of drugs. Arch Intern Med 1990;150:505–510.

Table 1–54
Nephrotoxicity Resulting From Drugs Given in Excessive Dose by the Physician or Misused by the Patient

Renal Lesion	Drug	Circumstance of Administration
Acute interstitial nephritis	Chlorprothixene	Suicide
Acute tubular necrosis	Acetaminophen	Suicide
	Aspirin	Suicide
	Boric acid	Diaper rash
	Bismuth salts	Taken for warts
	Colchicine	Suicide
	Lead	Inadvertently self-injected with opium
	Nomifensine	Suicide
	Pennyroyal oil	Attempted abortion
	Paraldehyde	Drug overdose
	Triamterene	Suicide
	Uranium	Clinical investigation
Chronic glomerulonephritis (heroin nephropathy)	Heroin	Narcotic addiction
	Pentazocine	Narcotic addiction
Chronic interstitial nephritis (analgesic nephropathy)	Acetaminophen	Analgesic abuse
	Nonsteroidal anti-inflammatory drugs	Analgesic abuse
Hypercalcemia	Vitamin A	Acne treatment
	Vitamin D	Hypoparathyroidism* and metabolic bone disease*
Myoglobinuric tubular necrosis	Amoxapine	Suicide
	Amphetamines	Drug overdose
	Barbiturates	Drug overdose
	Cocaine	Drug overdose
	Diazepam	Drug overdose
	Doxepin hydrochloride or nitrazepam	Suicide
	Alcohol	Alcoholism
	Glutethimide	Drug overdose
	Heroin	Drug overdose
	Methadone	Drug overdose
	Phencyclidine hydrochloride	Drug overdose
	Phenylpropanolamine hydrochloride	Weight loss, drug overdose
	Strychnine	Mistaken for cocaine
Necrotizing vasculitis	Methamphetamine	Drug overdose
Obstruction (stones)	Magnesium antacid	Antacid abuse
Osmotic nephrosis	Mannitol	Excessive dose*
Oxalosis	Intravenous vitamin C	Excessive dose*

*Prescribed by a physician. (From Abuelo JG. Renal failure caused by chemicals, foods, plants, animal venoms and misuse of drugs. Arch Intern Med 1990;150:505–510.)

or Epstein–Barr virus; (4) absence of an acute hepatic insult such as septic shock; (5) lack of evidence of chronic liver disease; and (6) absence of other concomitantly administered drugs, especially any known hepatotoxins. The presence of fever, rash, eosinophilias, or lymphadenopathy is supportive but not essential.

Table 1–55
Drugs With the Potential to Cause Incontinence

Sedatives
Valium, Dalmane, other benzodiazepine drugs
Alcohol

Diuretics
Lasix, Bumex, Edecrin

Drugs With Potential to Weaken Bladder Contraction (Anticholinergics)
Thorazine, Stelazine, and related antipsychotic medications
Elavil, Sinequan, Tofranil, and related tricyclic antidepressants
Bentyl, Pro-Banthine, Donnatal, and other antispasmodics
Benadryl, Chlor-Trimeton, Contac, Phenergan, and other antihistamines or preparations containing them
Morphine, Codeine, Demerol, Methadone, and other opiates
Artane, Cogentin, and related drugs used for Parkinson's disease (not L-dopa or deprenyl)
Sominex, Unisom, and other over-the-counter insomnia medication
Eyedrops containing atropine, cyclopentolate, or tropicamide (used mainly for glaucoma)

Drugs Affecting Sympathetic Nerves
Minipress, Catapres, Aldomet, Regitine, Yohimex and other antagonists for sympathetic action
Allerest, Actifed, Sudafed, Contac, Sinutab, and other preparations (including nosedrops) containing phenylpropanolamine, pseudoephedrine, or other decongestants

From Urinary incontinence. Harvard Med School Health Lett 1990;15(10):10.

Table 1–56
Drug Effects on the Mouth

Dental discoloration	Fluorides, tetracycline antibiotics, chlorhexidine, liquid iron preparations
Gingival hyperplasia	Phenytoin, sodium valproate, phenobarbital, cyclosporine, nifedipine, diltiazem, verapamil, nitrendipine
Stomatitis	Cytotoxic drugs: nitrogen mustards, methotrexate, 5-fluorouracil, 6-mercaptopurine, chlorambucil, doxorubicin, daunorubicin, bleomycin; penicillamine, gold salts, locally applied aspirin, contents of chloral hydrate and valproic acid capsules, Gentian violet dye
Xerostomia	Centrally acting antihypertensive agents, diuretics, antipsychotics, tricyclic antidepressants, antihistamines, anticholinergics, anticonvulsants, laxatives, muscle relaxants, narcotics, hypnotics
Sialorrhea	Pilocarpine, neostigmine, iodides
Sialadenitis	Phenylbutazone, isoproterenol, nitrofurantoin, iodine
Parotitis	Bretylium, methyldopa, clonidine, guanethidine, phenylbutazone, oxyphenbutazone, thioridazine
Erythema multiforme	Penicillins, tetracyclines, clindamycin, sulfonamides, anticonvulsants
Systemic lupus erythematosus	Procainamide, hydralazine (see page 27)
Pigmentation	Cisplatin, oral contraceptives, minocycline, antimalarial agents, doxorubicin
Dental caries	Drugs inhibiting flow of saliva (xerostomia), preparation with high sucrose content: vitamin syrup, antibiotics and anticonvulsant suspensions, cough syrup

Data taken from Kane M, Zacharczenko N. Oral side effects of drugs. Oral Health 1993;83:29–35; and Thompson DF. Drug-induced parotitis. J Clin Pharm Ther 1993;18:255–258.

Table 1–57
Agents Associated with Acute Pancreatitis*

Definite Association	Questionable Association
Asparaginase	Acetaminophen
Azathioprine	Amiodarone
Didanosine	Ampicillin
Estrogens	Anticholinesterases
Furosemide	Carbamazepine
Mercaptopurine	Cisplatin
Pentamidine	Colchicine
Sulfonamides	Cyclosporine
Sulindac	Cytarabine
Tetracyclines	Diazoxide
Thiazides	Diphenoxylate
Valproic acid	Enalapril
Probable Association	Ergotamine
Bumetanide	Erythromycin
Chlorthalidone	Gold compounds
Cimetidine	Interleukin-2
Clozapine	Isotretinoin
Corticosteroids	Ketoprofen
Corticotropin	Lisinopril
ERCP† media	Mefenamic acid
Ethacrynic acid	Metolazone
Methyldopa	Nitrofurantoin
Metronidazole	Octreotide
Salicylates	Oxyphenbutazone
Sulfasalazine	Phenformin
Zalcitabine	Phenolphthalein
	Piroxicam
	Potassium permanganate
	Procainamide
	Ranitidine
	Roxithromycin
	Tryptophan

*Association is considered definite if pancreatitis developed during exposure to the agent, disappeared after withdrawal, and recurred after rechallenge. Association is considered probable if an association is thought to exist but the three criteria above were not all met. Association is considered questionable if published evidence is inadequate or contradictory.
†Endoscopic retrograde cholangiopancreatography.
(From Underwood TW, Frye CB. Drug-induced pancreatitis. Clin Pharm 1993;14:440–448.)

Table 1–58
Drugs That Induce Esophageal Injury

Lower Esophageal Sphincter Tone	Irritate Esophageal Mucosa
Alpha-adrenergic antagonists	Captopril
Phentolamine	Chlorazepate
Anticholinergic agents	Clindamycin
Atropine, belladonna tincture, dicyclomine, flavoxate, methantheline, oxybutynin, propantheline	Digoxin
	Ferrous sulfate
	Lincomycin
	Nonsteroidal antiinflammatory drugs
Benzodiazepines	
Diazepam	Aspirin, ibuprofen, indomethacin, ketoprofen, phenylbutazone, piroxicam
Beta-adrenergic agonists	
Caffeine, carbuterol, isoproterenol	
	Penicillin
Calcium channel blocking agents	Potassium chloride
	Quinidine
Nifedipine, verapamil	Tetracyclines
Dopamine	Doxycycline, tetracycline
Ethanol	Trimethoprim–sulfamethoxazole
Glucagon	Vitamin C
Narcotic analgesics	
Meperidine, morphine	
Prostaglandins E_1, E_2, A_2	
Theophylline	

From Lee M, Sharfi R. Oxybutynin-induced reflux esophagitis. DICP Ann Pharmacother 1990;34:583–585.

Primary Biliary Cirrhosis. Primary biliary cirrhosis has been associated with use of acetaminophen, chlorpromazine, phenylbutazone, tolbutamide, thiabendazole, benoxaprofen, and a compound containing glycyrrhizin, cysteine, and glycine.[117]

Colon

Cappell and Simon have presented a comprehensive review of drug-associated colonic toxicity (Table 1–60).[118]

Metabolic Disorders

Some drug-induced metabolic disorders are listed in Table 1–61.[119]

The Lungs

Noncardiogenic Pulmonary Edema

Many drugs have been associated with noncardiogenic pulmonary edema (NCPE).[120] NCPE is characterized by the simultaneous presence of severe hypoxemia, bilateral infiltrates on the chest roentgenogram, and normal pulmonary capillary wedge pressure with exclusion of other risk factors for NCPE. Agents known to cause pulmonary disease are noted in Table 1–62.[121] Agents associated with pleural effusion are listed in Table 1–63, and those associated with acute-onset pulmonary insufficiency in Table 1–64. Henry has suggested blockade of an oxygen cascade due to poisoning (Table 1–65).[122]

Asthma

Drugs causing or exacerbating asthma are listed in Table 1–66.[123] Nonsteroidal antiinflammatory drugs account for more than two thirds of drug-induced asthmatic reactions, with aspirin accounting for more than half of these. Beta blockers, cholinergic agonists, cholinomimetic alkaloids, chemotherapeutic agents, antibiotics, radiographic contrast agents, muscle relaxants, and intravenous anesthetic agents have also caused bronchospasm associated with systemic reactions.[123]

Endocrine System

It may be difficult to distinguish drug-induced sexual dysfunction from the effects of depression or disease, but most of the time, sexual dysfunction is reversed when drug use is stopped. Frequent offenders include antihypertensive agents, antipsychotic drugs, and antidepressants[124] (Table 1–67). Hyperprolactinemia may be associated with neuroleptic agents (phenothiazines, butyrophenones), monoamine oxidase inhibitors, tricyclic antidepressants, reserpine, methyldopa, metoclopramide, amoxapine, verapamil, and cocaine (Table 1–68).[125,126]

Table 1–59
Drug-Induced Gastrointestinal Obstruction

Site	Drugs
In the lumen without predisposing lesion	Barium sulfate, cholestyramine, potassium supplements, bulk laxatives, aluminum hydroxide suspension
In the lumen with predisposing lesion	Iron preparations in patients with Crohn's disease; bulk laxatives or bran in patients with renal failure, colon carcinoma, or diabetes mellitus
Within the gut wall	
Physical damage	Anticoagulants, nonsteroidal antiinflammatory drugs, penicillamine, methylene blue in utero, alprostadil (prostaglandin E_1) infusion in neonates
Dysmotility of smooth muscle	H_1 antagonists, opiates, clonidine, calcium antagonists, dantrolene, corticosteroid withdrawal, magnesium sulfate exposure in utero, erythromycin stearate
Interference with autonomic nerve transmission	Autonomic ganglion blockers, muscarinic antagonists (e.g., atropine), anticholinergics, phenothiazines, antiparkinsonian drugs, tricyclic antidepressants, disopyramide, vincristine
Outside the gut wall	
Vascular obstruction	Oral contraceptives, corticosteroids, vasopressors, cocaine abusers
Peritoneal fibrosis	Practolol, irradiation of abdomen or pelvis, intraperitoneal antineoplastic therapy
Meconium ileus-type lesion in cystic fibrosis	Cimetidine, ipratropium bromide

From Iredale JP, George CF. Drugs causing gastrointestinal obstruction. Adverse Drug React Toxicol Rev 1993;12:163–175.

Table 1–60
Drug-Induced Colon Toxicity

Toxic Effect	Drugs
Colonic ischemia	Cocaine, ergotamine, estrogen, amphetamines, digitalis, methysergide, vasopressin
Colonic pseudobstruction	Narcotics, phenothiazines, vincristine, atropine or other anticholinergics, ganglionic blocking agents, tricyclic antidepressants
Infectious or necrotizing enterocolitis	Antibiotics associated with pseudomembranous colitis, deferoxamine associated with *Yersinia* enterocolitis, chemotherapy associated with neutropenic colitis, hyperosmolar formulas in children
Allergic, inflammatory cytotoxic colitis	Gold compounds, nonsteroidal antiinflammatory drugs, α-methyldopa, flucytosine, methotrexate, salicylates, sulfasalazine
Intestinal ulcers	Slow-release (wax matrices) potassium chloride
Colonic hypomotility and abdominal distension	Chronic cathartic use
Colonic structure due to retroperitoneal fibrosis	Methysergide
Toxic colitis for intrarectally administered compound	Acids, bases, other corrosives
Colitis in patients with colonic obstruction	Enemas using hypertonic radiographic contrast agents

From Cappell MS, Simon T. Colonic toxicity of administered medications and chemicals. Am J Gastroenterol 1993;88:1684–1697.

Table 1–61
Drug-Induced Metabolic Disorders and Management in the Critical Care Setting

Disorder	Offending Agents	Intervention
Fluid overload	Large carbohydrate and Na loads; IV fluids	Monitor intake/output; maximally concentrate all fluids; restrict Na
Hyperkalemia	K-sparing diuretics; oversupplementation; acidosis	Conservatively diurese with loop diuretics; monitor serum and urine K; sodium polystyrene sulfonate may be necessary
Hypernatremia	Drugs with high Na content; blood products	Conservatively diurese with "free water" replacement; avoid drugs high in Na content; restrict Na and dextrose; monitor serum and urine Na
Hypocalcemia	Citrate loads from blood products; aggressive phosphate replacement	Replace Ca according to serum concentration; keep Ca • phosphate <70
Hypokalemia	Amphotericin B; corticosteroids; diuretics; alkalosis	Replace urine K losses; monitor serum and urine K
Hypomagnesemia	Cisplatin therapy; cyclosporine therapy; diuretics	Replace Mg according to serum concentration; monitor urine losses if necessary
Hyponatremia	Diuretics; nasogastric losses	Replace urine and nasogastric losses; monitor serum, urine, and nasogastric Na
Hypophosphatemia	Aluminum-containing antacids; corticosteroids; high serum insulin; aggressive calcium replacement	Replace phosphate according to serum concentration; ≤0.96 mM/kg/24 h; keep the product of Ca • phosphate <70
Metabolic acidosis	Amphotericin B; aminoglycosides	Estimate acid deficit; monitor arterial blood gases and replace deficit with acetate salts
Metabolic alkalosis	Diuretics; mineralocorticosteroids; large nasogastric losses with low pH; ≥140 mEq of citrate from blood products	Estimate base deficit; monitor arterial blood gases and replace deficit using chloride salts and/or HCl; use an H_2 antagonist for large nasogastric losses with low gastric pH

From Driscoll DF. Drug-induced metabolic disorders and parenteral nutrition in the intensive care unit: A pharmaceutical and metabolic perspective. DICP Ann Pharmacother 1989;23:363–371.

Table 1–62
Agents Known to Cause Pulmonary Disease

Chemotherapeutic Agents	**Analgesics**
Cytotoxic	Heroin*
Azathioprine	Methadone*
Bleomycin*	Naloxone*
Busulfan	Ethchlorvynol*
Chlorambucil	Propoxyphene*
Cyclophosphamide	Salicylates*
Etoposide	**Cardiovascular Agents**
Melphalan	Amiodarone*
Mitomycin*	Angiotensin-converting enzyme inhibitors
Nitrosoureas	Anticoagulants
Procarbazine	Beta blockers*
Vinblastine	Dipyridamole
Ifosfamide	Fibrinolytic agents*
Noncytotoxic	Protamine*
Methotrexate*	Tocainide
Cytosine arabinoside*	**Inhalants**
Bleomycin*	Aspirated oil
Procarbazine*	Oxygen*
Antibiotics	**Intravenous Agents**
Amphotericin B*	Blood*
Nitrofurantoin	Ethanolamine oleate (sodium morrhuate)*
Sulfasalazine	Ethiodized oil (lymphangiogram)
Sulfonamides	Talc
Pentamidine	Fat emulsion
Antiinflammation Agents	**Miscellaneous Agents**
Acetylsalicylic acid*	Bromocriptine
Gold	Dantrolene
Methotrexate	Hydrochlorothiazide*
Nonsteroidal antiinflammatory agents	Methysergide
Penicillamine*	Oral contraceptives
Immunosuppressive Agent	Tocolytic agents*
Cyclosporine	Tricyclics*
Interleukin-2*	L-Tryptophan
	Radiation
	Systemic lupus erythematosus (drug-induced)*
	Complement-mediated leukostasis*

*Typically cause acute or subacute respiratory insufficiency.
(From Rosenow EC III, Myers JL, Swenson SJ, Pisani RJ. Drug-induced pulmonary disease: An update. Chest 1992;102:239–250.)

Table 1–63
Agents Associated With Pleural Effusion

Chemotherapeutic agents
Nitrofurantoin (acute)
Bromocriptine
Dantrolene
Methysergide
L-Tryptophan
Drug-inducing systemic lupus erythematosus
Tocolytics
Amiodarone
Esophageal variceal sclerotherapy agents
Interleukin-2

From Rosenow EC III, Myers JL, Swenson SJ, Pisani RJ. Drug-induced pulmonary disease: An update. Chest 1992;102:239–250.

Table 1–64
Agents Associated With Acute-Onset Pulmonary Insufficiency*

Bleomycin plus O_2	Fibrinolytic agents
Mitomycin	Protamine
Bleomycin†	Blood products‡
Procarbazine†	Fat emulsion
Methotrexate†	Hydrochlorothiazide‡
Amphotericin B	Complement-mediated leukostasis
Nitrofurantoin (acute)‡	Hyskon (dextran-70)‡
Acetylsalicylic acid‡	Tumor necrosis factor‡
Interleukin-2‡	Intrathecal methotrexate
Heroin and other narcotics‡	Tricyclic antidepressants‡
Epinephrine‡	Amiodarone plus O_2
Ethchlorvynol‡	Naloxone

*Onset at less than 48 hours.
†Associated with hypersensitivity with eosinophilia.
‡Usually reversible within 48–72 hours, implying noncardiac pulmonary edema rather than inflammatory interstitial pneumonitis.
(From Rosenow EC III, Myers JL, Swenson SJ, Pisani RJ. Drug-induced pulmonary disease: An update. Chest 1992;102:239–250.)

Blood

Agranulocytosis has followed exposure to analgesic antiinflammatory drugs, antiarrhythmics, anticonvulsants, antidepressants, antihypertensive agents, antimicrobial agents, antipsychotic drugs, antithyroid drugs, diuretics, and other drugs (Table 1–69).[127] Some drugs and chemicals can induce a hemolytic anemia in persons with glucose-6-phosphate dehydrogenase deficiency (Table 1–70).[128]

Hemolysis

Hemolysis may follow exposure to arsine and stibine. It is also caused by direct erythrocyte binding (penicillin, cephalothin, streptomycin); binding to plasma protein (quinine, quinidine, sulfonylurea derivatives); and undetermined mechanisms (methyldopa, levodopa, mefenamic acid).

Drugs such as chloramphenicol may be associated with aplastic anemia. Drugs, foods, spices, and vitamins may cause abnormalities of platelet function (Table 1–71).[129]

Anaphylactic Reaction

Agents responsible for acute anaphylactic reactions are delineated in Table 1–72.[130–132]

Electrolyte Disturbances

Drug-induced hyperkalemia may follow inhibition of potassium entry into cells (inhibition of Na^+/K^+ ATPase activity) observed with digitalis, β_2-adrenoceptor antagonists, and drugs that cause acidosis. Reduced potassium excretion is observed with potassium-sparing diuretics, angiotensin-converting enzyme inhibitors, nonsteroidal antiinflammatory drugs, and agents that impair renal tubular function. Hyperkalemia follows renal Na^+ channel blockade (amiloride). Hyperkalemia is associated with abdominal pain, diarrhea, muscle pain and weakness, electrocardiographic changes (tall peaked T waves, ST-segment depression, prolonged PR interval, QRS prolongation), and cardiac arrhythmias (ventricular tachycardia, ventricular fibrillation).[133]

Table 1–65
Examples of Blockade of the Oxygen Cascade Due to Poisoning

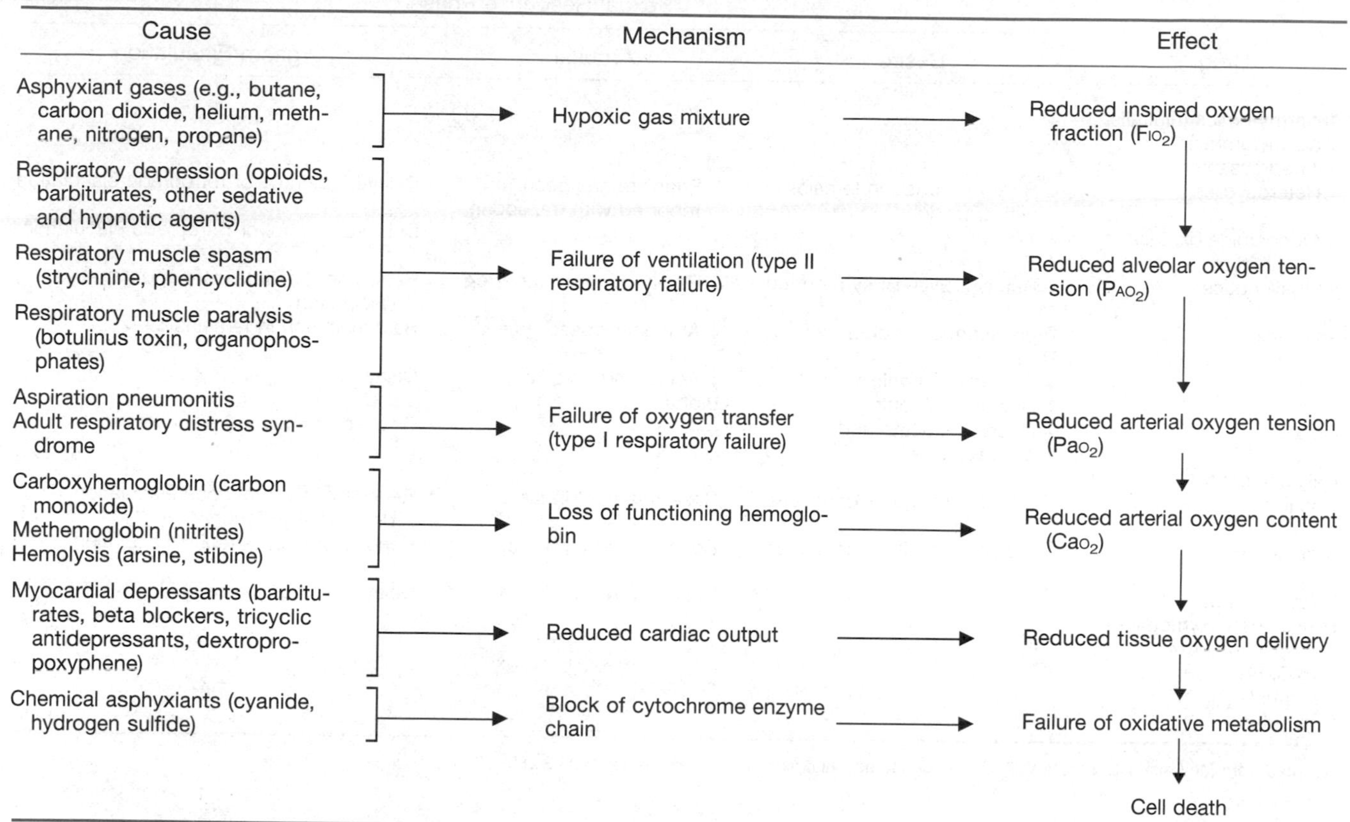

From Henry JA. Resuscitation from poisoning. In: Baskett PJF, ed. *Cardiopulmonary Resuscitation.* Amsterdam: Elsevier; 1989:231–257.

Table 1–66
Drugs That Cause or Exacerbate Asthma

Types of Drugs That Cause Asthma
Nonsteroidal antiinflammatory drugs
Antibiotics (nitrofurantoin, penicillins, cephalosporins, tetracycline)
Beta-adrenergic blocking agents (topical or systemic)
Cholinergic agonists (methacholine, carbachol, bethanechol, echothiophate iodide) and cholinomimetic alkaloids (pilocarpine, muscarine)
Corticosteroids (IV hydrocortisone in acetylsalicylic acid-sensitive asthma)
Diuretics (triamterene/hydrochlorothiazide)
Chemotherapeutic agents (bleomycin, podophyllotoxins, Zinostatin, methotrexate, vinca alkaloids in combination with mitomycin-C)

Unusual Causes of Drug-Induced Asthma
Agents encountered by airborne exposure in pharmaceutical manufacturing or in the hospital or laboratory workplace
Propellants or additives to inhalant medications
Metabisulfites
Agents inducing bronchospasm via non-IgE mast cell activation (radiographic contrast media, opiates, polymyxin, colistin)
Intravenous anesthetic agents and muscle relaxants
Agents aggravating bronchospasm via local irritant effect
Drugs causing or exacerbating gastroenteric reflex

Agents That Mimic Asthma Angiotensin-Converting Enzyme Inhibitors

Adapted from Hunt LW, Rosenow EC III. Asthma-producing drugs. Ann Allergy 1992;68:453–462.

Table 1–67
Summary of Effects of Drugs on Sexual Performance

	Sexual Response Phase		
Drug	Desire	Arousal	Orgasm/Ejaculation
Diuretics		↓	Rare delay
Spironolactone	↓	↓	
Methyldopa	↓	↓	Retrograde ejaculation
Guanethidine	↓	↓	Retrograde ejaculation
Reserpine	↓	↓	
Beta blockers	↓	↓	Rare
Clonidine	↓	↓	Retrograde, delayed or absence of ejaculation
Alpha blockers			Emission failure, retrograde ejaculation
Vasodilators		Rare ↓	
Hypolipidemics	↓	↓	

Adapted from McWaine DE, Procci WR. Drug-induced sexual dysfunction. Med Toxicol 1988;3:289–306.
(continued)

Table 1–67 *(Continued)*

Drug	Sexual Response Phase		
	Desire	Arousal	Orgasm/Ejaculation
Antiarrhythmics (digitalis, disopyramide)	↓	↓	
Antidepressants			
Heterocyclics	↓ Rarely reported in females, with trazodone	↓ Priapism has been reported with trazodone	Delayed, painful, or retrograde ejaculation
Monoamine oxidase inhibitors	↓	↓↓	Delayed, painful or retrograde ejaculation
Antipsychotics	↓ Rarely Kluver–Bucy reported	↓ Rarely priapism reported	Retrograde, painful, rare spontaneous ejaculation
Anxiolytics	Biphasic dose-related	↓ At higher doses	Rare inhibition in females
Lithium	Rare ↓		
Alcohol	↓ Biphasic, chronic	↓ Acute and chronic	Delay
Marijuana	↓ Biphasic, chronic	Biphasic	
Opiates	↓ Decrease, acute and chronic	↓	Delayed or inhibited ejaculation
Hallucinogens	↓	↓	↓
Cocaine	↑ Initially but with ↓ continued ingestion	Dose-related, biphasic	Reports of spontaneous ejaculation, delayed ejaculation
Amphetamines	↑ Initially but with ↓ continued ingestion	Dose-related biphasic	Reports of spontaneous ejaculation
Volatile nitrites	↑	Dose-related ↓	Delayed versus intensity
Methylenedioxymethyl-amphetamine (MDMA)	↑	↑	
Yohimbine		↑	
Cigarettes		Rare	

Adapted from McWaine DE, Procci WR. Drug-induced sexual dysfunction. Med Toxicol 1988;3:289–306.

Table 1–68
Drugs That Have Been Associated With Symptoms of Hyper- or Hypoprolactinemia

Drugs With a Higher Incidence of Chemical Symptoms of Hyper-prolactinemia
Antipsychotics (benperidol, butaparazine, chlorpromazine, flupenthixol, fluphenazine, flutroline, haloperidol, loxapine, molindone, penfluridol, perphenazine, pimozide, prochlorperazine, sulpiride, sultopride, thiethylperazine, thioridazine, thiotixene, tiapride, trifluoperazine, zetidoline)
Monoamine oxidase inhibitors (clorgilline, paragyline, selegiline)
Estrogens (ethinylestradiol, 2-hydroxyestradiol, estradiol valerate, estriols, polyestradiol phosphate, quinestrol, stilbestrol)
Morphine
Synthetic morphine analogs (buprenorphine, DAMME, dermorphine, methadone, nalorphine)
Mescaline
Fenfluramine
Amoxapine
Dibenzepine
α-Methyldopa
Reserpine
Benserazide
Carbidopa
Anesthetics (spinal, epidural, general)

Drugs With Lower Incidence of Hyperprolactinemia or With Less Well-Defined Affect
Oral contraceptives
Conjugated estrogens
Gestagens (medroxyprogesterone acetate, megestrol acetate, progesterone)
Human chorionic gonadotropin
Human calcitonin
Parathyroid hormone
Thyrotropin-releasing hormone
Luteinizing hormone/follicle-stimulating hormone
Dinoprost
Labetolol, tolamolol
Methyl-*p*-thyrosine
Verapamil
Fluoxetine
Buspirone
Cimetidine, ranitidine
5-Hydroxytryptophan
Clozapine, promazine
Clomipramine

Prolactin-Inhibiting Drugs That Are Highly Effective
Dopamine
Ipopamine
Levodopa
Methysergide
Nomifensine
Methylergometrine
Bromocriptine
Ergocriptine
Ergometrine
Lergotrile
Lisuride
Pergolide

Prolactin-Inhibiting Drugs With Minor or Not Well-Defined Effects
Corticotropin
Dexamethasone
Salmon calcitonin
17β-Estradiol
Antiestrogens (clomiphene, cyclofenil, hydrotestolactone, tamoxifen)
Testosterone propionate
Danazol
Alprostadil
Clonidine
Guanfacine
Cyproheptadine
Cysteamine
Piribedil
Pyridoxin
Calcitriol
Dexchlorpheniramine
Dihydroergocristine
Promethazine
Chlormethiazol
Valproic acid
Trazodone

From Hell K, Wemze H. Drug-induced changes in prolactin secretion: Clinical implications. Med Toxicol 1988;3:463–498.

Table 1–69
Drugs Associated With Agranulocytosis

Analgesic/Antiinflammatory Drugs
Amidopyrine (aminopyrine)
Antipyrine (phenazone)
Aspirin
Benoxaprofen
Colchicine
Fenoprofen
Gold salts
Ibuprofen
Indomethacin
Naproxen
Oxyphenbutazone
Paracetamol (acetaminophen)
Pentazocine
Phenylbutazone
Zomepirac

Antiarrhythmic Drugs
Ajmaline
Aprindine
Disopyramide
Procainamide
Propafenone
Propranolol
Quinidine
Tocainide

Anticonvulsant Drugs
Carbamazepine
Ethosuximide
Mephenytoin
Phenytoin
Primidone
Sodium valproate
Trimethadione

Antidepressant Drugs
Amoxapine
Clomipramine
Desipramine
Imipramine
Maprotiline
Mianserin

Antihypertensive Drugs
Captopril
Diazoxide
Hydralazine
Methyldopa
Nifedipine
Propranolol

Antimicrobial Drugs
Aminosalicylic acid
Amodiaquine
Ampicillin
Carbenicillin
Cephalexin
Cephalothin
Cephradine
Chloramphenicol
Clindamycin
Cloxacillin
Co-trimoxazole
Dapsone
Doxycycline
Flucytosine
Fumagillin
Gentamicin
Griseofulvin
Hydroxychloroquine
Isoniazid
Lincomycin
Methicillin
Metronidazole
Mezlocillin
Nafcillin
Nitrofurantoin
Novobiocin
Oxacillin
Oxophenarsine
Penicillin
Pyrimethamine
Quinine
Rifampicin (rifampin)
Ristocetin
Streptomycin
Sulfadiazine
Sulfamethoxypyridazine
Sulfapyridine
Sulfaselazine (salicylazosulphapyridine)
Sulfathazole
Thiacetazone
Ticarcillin

Antipsychotic Drugs
Chlorpromazine
Clozapine
Fluphenazine
Mepazine
Methylpromazine
Perazine
Prochlorperazine
Promazine
Thioridazine
Trimeprazine

Antithyroid Drugs
Carbimazole
Methimazole
Methylthiouracil
Propylthiouracil
Thiouracil

Diuretics
Acetazolamide
Bumetanide
Chlorthalidone
Chlorothiazide
Ethacryric acid
Hydrochlorothiazide
Mercurials
Methozolamide

Other Drugs
Allopurinol
Brompheniramine
Chlordiazepoxide
Chlorpropamide
Cimetidine
Diazepam
Levamisole
Levodopa
Mebendazole
Meprobamate
Methydroline
Metiamide
Penicillamine
Phenindione
Promethazine
Ranitidine
Thenalidine
Ticlopidine
Tolbutamide

From Heimpel H. Drug-induced agranulocytosis. Med Toxicol 1988;3:449–462.

Table 1–70
Drugs and Chemicals That Can Induce Hemolytic Anemia in Persons With Glucose-6-phosphate Dehydrogenase Deficiency

Acetanilid	Niridazole
Doxorubicin	Nitrofurantoin
Furazolidone	Phenazopyridine
Methylene blue	Primaquine
Nalidixic acid	Sulfamethoxazole

From Beutler E. Glucose-6-phosphate dehydrogenase deficiency. N Engl J Med 1991;324:169–174.

Treat with glucose, insulin infusions, sodium bicarbonate, and calcium gluconate. Exchange resins and hemodialysis may be required.

Drug-induced hypokalemia follows enhanced potassium entry into cells (increased Na^+/K^+ ATPase activity induced by β_2 agonists, theophylline, insulin), competitive blockade of potassium channels (chloroquine, barium), gastrointestinal losses, and drug-induced metabolic alkalosis. Hypokalemia results in generalized muscle weakness, paralytic ileus, electrocardiographic changes (flat or inverted T waves, prominent U waves, ST-segment depression), and cardiac arrhythmias (atrial tachycardia heart block, atrioventricular dissociation, ventricular tachycardia, ventricular fibrillation).[133] If the serum potassium level is greater than 3

Table 1–71
Drugs, Foods, Spices, and Vitamins That May Cause Abnormalities of Platelet Function

Agent*	Abnormality†
Nonsteroidal Antiinflammatory Drugs	
Meclofenamic acid, mefenamic acid, phenylbutazone, sulfinpyrazone	Abnormal platelet aggregation in vitro
Diflunisal, piroxicam, sulindac	Abnormal platelet aggregation
Tolmetin, zompirac	Abnormal bleeding time
Indomethacin, naproxen	Abnormal platelet aggregation and bleeding time
Aspirin	Abnormal platelet aggregation and bleeding time; clinical bleeding
Diclofenac	Abnormal bleeding time; clinical bleeding
Ibuprofen	Abnormal platelet aggregation in vitro; abnormal bleeding time
Beta-lactam Antibiotics	
Penicillins	
Carbenicillin, mezlocillin, piperacillin, ticarcillin	Abnormal platelet aggregation and bleeding time; clinical bleeding
Apalcillin, methicillin	Abnormal platelet aggregation
Ampicillin, penicillin G	Abnormal platelet aggregation and bleeding time
Sulbenicillin	Abnormal platelet aggregation in vitro
Azlocillin	Abnormal bleeding time
Nafcillin	Abnormal bleeding time; clinical bleeding
Cephalosporins	
Cephalothin	Abnormal platelet aggregation
Cefoperazone	Abnormal bleeding time
Cefotaxime	Abnormal bleeding time; clinical bleeding
Moxalactam	Abnormal platelet aggregation and bleeding time; clinical bleeding
Cardiovascular Drugs	
Dipyridamole‡	
Diltiazem, isosorbide dinitrate, isosorbide mononitrate, nimodipine, propranolol, sodium nitroprusside, verapamil	Abnormal platelet aggregation
Nifedipine, nitroglycerin	Abnormal platelet aggregation and bleeding time
Quinidine	Abnormal bleeding time; clinical bleeding
Anticoagulant, Fibrinolytic, and Antifibrinolytic Drugs	
Aminocaproic acid, heparin	Abnormal platelet aggregation and bleeding time
Protamine sulfate	Abnormal platelet aggregation in vitro
Alteplase	Abnormal bleeding time; clinical bleeding
Psychotropic Drugs	
Amitriptyline, fluphenazine, haloperidol, imipramine, nortriptyline, promazine, trifluoperazine	Abnormal platelet aggregation in vitro
Chlorpromazine	Abnormal platelet aggregation
Anesthetics and Narcotics	
Benoxinate, benzocaine, butacaine, cocaine, cyclaine, dibucaine, hydroxychloroquine, lidocaine, piperocaine, proparacaine, procaine, tetracaine	Abnormal platelet aggregation in vitro
Halothane, heroin	Abnormal platelet aggregation and bleeding time
Chemotherapeutic Agents	
Asparaginase, combination chemotherapy (cisplatin, cyclophosphamide, and either carmustine or melphalan), vincristine	Abnormal platelet aggregation
Carmustine, daunorubicin	Abnormal platelet aggregation in vitro
Plicamycin	Abnormal platelet aggregation and bleeding time; clinical bleeding
Antihistamines	
Chlorpheniramine, diphenhydramine, pyrilamine	Abnormal platelet aggregation in vitro
Radiographic Contrast Agents	
Iopamidol, iothalamate, ioxaglate	Abnormal platelet aggregation in vitro
Meglumine diatrizoate (Renografin-76), meglumine diatrizoate and sodium diatrizoate (Renovist II, Urografin)	Abnormal platelet aggregation
Other Drugs	
Clofibrate, guaifenesin, ketanserin	Abnormal platelet aggregation
Dextran, epoprostenol, nitrofurantoin	Abnormal platelet aggregation and bleeding time
Iloprost	Abnormal platelet aggregation in vitro
Ticlopidine	Abnormal platelet aggregation and bleeding time; clinical bleeding
Foods, Spices, and Vitamins	
Ginger, onion, vitamin C, vitamin E	Abnormal platelet aggregation
Cumin, turmeric, cloves	Abnormal platelet aggregation in vitro
Alcohol, *n*-3 fatty acids	Abnormal platelet aggregation and bleeding time
Chinese black tree fungus (mo-er), garlic	Abnormal platelet aggregation; clinical bleeding

*With the exception of studies demonstrating a significantly greater frequency of bleeding with aspirin, all are anecdotal observations in one or a few patients.
†"Abnormal platelet aggregation in vitro" indicates an abnormality when the agent is added to platelet-rich plasma. "Abnormal platelet aggregation" indicates an abnormality after administration of the agent to humans.
‡This drug has not been demonstrated to cause abnormal platelet function, but it has been used extensively as an antithrombotic agent.
(From George JM, Shattil SJ. The clinical importance of acquired abnormalities of platelet function. N Engl J Med 1991;324:27–40.)

Table 1–72
Mechanisms and Agents Responsible for Systemic Anaphylactic Reactions

Mechanism	Agent	Example
IgE-mediated reaction against native proteins	Venoms	Hymenoptera, fire ant, snake
	Airborne allergens	Pollens, molds, danders
	Foods	Peanuts, milk, egg, seafood, grains
	Enzymes	Trypsin, streptokinase, chymopapain
	Heterologous serum	Tetanus antitoxin, antilymphocyte globulin
	Human proteins	Insulin, corticotropin, vasopressin, serum and seminal proteins
	Others	Protamine, latex
IgE-mediated reaction against protein–hapten conjugates	Antibiotics	Penicillins, cephalosporins, sulfonamides
	Disinfectants	Ethylene oxide
Complement activation and generation of anaphylatoxins	Human proteins	Gamma globulins, other blood products
	Dialysis	Contact of blood with some dialysis membranes
Direct activation of mediator release from mast cells, basophils, or both	Hypertonic solutions	Radiocontrast medium, mannitol
	Drugs	Opiates, curare, *d*-tubocurarine, vancomycin
	Others	Dextran, fluorescein for angiography
Unknown	Nonsteroidal antiinflammatory drugs	Aspirin, indomethacin
	Anesthetics	Lidocaine, thiopental
	Preservatives	Metabisulfites, benzoates
	Steroids	Progesterone, hydrocortisone
	Exercise	—
	Exercise and food	—
	Idiopathic anaphylaxis	—

From Bochner BS, Lichtenstein LM. Anaphylaxis. N Engl J Med 1991;324:1785–1790.

Table 1–73
Drugs Commonly Associated With Orthostatic Hypotension in the Elderly

Antihypertensive Drugs	Drugs Producing Hypertension as an Adverse Effect
Diuretics	Nitrates
Calcium antagonists	Antiparkinsonian drugs (levodopa + decarboxylase inhibitors, bromocriptine, selegiline, anticholinergics)
Beta blockers	Antidepressants
Angiotensin-converting enzyme inhibitors	Antipsychotics (phenothiazine butyrophenones)
Miscellaneous (prazosin, clonidine, guanfacine)	

From Mets TF. Drug-induced orthostatic hypotension in older patients. Drugs and Aging 1995;6:219–228.

mmol/L, use oral potassium. If the serum potassium is below 3 mmol/L, replace with intravenous potassium.

Drug-induced hypernatremia follows excessive intake of sodium, salt emetics, enemas, intravenous saline solutions, excessive water loss, and drugs causing diabetes insipidus including lithium, phenytoin, and alcohol. Treatment comprises water restriction with or without loop diuretics.

Drug-induced hyponatremia follows excessive water intake and impaired water excretion by the kidney due to increased activity of antidiuretic hormone resulting from carbamazepine, chlorpropamide, and nonsteroidal antiinflammatory drug intoxication. Treatment comprises water restriction with or without loop diuretics. If the serum sodium level is less than 120 mmol/L and cerebral symptoms are present, use hypertonic saline cautiously. Watch for central pontine myelinosis and cerebral edema.

Hypoglycemia

Browning and colleagues suggest that administration of 50% glucose should be reserved for those patients in whom hypoglycemia is demonstrated. Preliminary animal and human evidence suggests that glucose-containing intravenous solutions should be avoided in patients at risk for cerebral ischemia, such as those with acute stroke, impending cardiac arrest, or severe hypotension or those receiving cardiopulmonary resuscitation.[134]

The Elderly

Elderly patients are particularly less tolerant of drugs that act on the central nervous system. This is compounded by multiple-drug therapy and reductions in lean body mass, renal blood flow, gastric motility, and synthesis of albumin[135] (see also Chapter 7).

Drug overdose in the elderly is usually due to suicidal thoughts, loneliness, chronic illness, poor eyesight, chaos in the medicine cabinet, noncompliance, suggestibility and erroneous interpretation, advertisements, gossip, poor interpretation of physician instructions, or confusion. Drugs commonly associated with orthostatic hypotension in the elderly are listed in Table 1–73.[136]

REFERENCES

1. Vale JA. Medical toxicology: Clinical aspects. Arch Toxicol 1991;suppl. 15:12–13.
2. Meredith TJ. Epidemiology of poisoning. Pharmacol Ther 1993;49:251–256.
3. Centers for Disease Control and Prevention. Unintentional poisoning mortality: United States, 1980–1986. MMWR 1989;38:153–158.
4. Centers for Disease Control and Prevention. Unintentional ingestion of prescription drugs in children under five years old. MMWR 1987;36:124–132.

5. Litovitz TL, Flagler SL, Manoguerra AS, et al. Recurrent poisoning among pediatric poisoning victims. Med Toxicol Adverse Drug Experience 1989;4:381–386.
6. Herrington LF, Geller RJ, Lopez GP, Garrettson LK. Poisoning in infants under 12 months. Who, which, when, where and why. Vet Hum Toxicol 1990;32:34.
7. Woolf AD, Lovejoy FH Jr: Epidemiology of drug overdose in children. Drug Saf 1993;9:291–304.
8. Litovitz TL, Clark LR, Soloway RA. 1993 Annual report of the American Association of Poison Control Centers Toxic Exposure Surveillance System. Am J Emerg Med 1994; 12:546–583.
9. Litovitz TL, Schmitz BF, Holm KC. 1988 Annual report of the American Association of Poison Control Centers National Data Collection System. Am J Emerg Med 1989;7:495–545.
10. Klein-Schwartz W, Oderda GM, Booze L. Poisoning in the elderly. J Am Geriatr Soc 1983;31:195–199.
11. Litovitz T, Manoguerra A. Comparison of pediatric poisoning hazards: An analysis of 3.8 million exposure incidents: A report from the American Association of Poison Control Centers. Pediatrics 1992;89:999–1005.
12. Woolf A, Liebett Z, Lovejoy FH Jr: Pediatric poisoning hazards. Pediatrics 1993;91:1017.
13. Michell L-J, Dexter EM, Bradberry SM, et al. Assessment of IPCS/CEC/EAPCTT. Dexter EM, Michell L-J, Casey PB: The role and value of phonetoxscore in cases of poisoning. Phonetoxscore by staff of the PNPIS (Birmingham Centre). In: Proceedings, XVIth International Congress of the European Association of Poison Centres and Clinical Toxicologists, Vienna, April 12, 1994:Abstracts 0.83 and 0.84.
14. March AG, Bet N, Persino MG, et al. Severity grading of childhood poisoning: The Matti Center study of poisoning children (MPXC) scare. Clin Toxicol 1995;33:223–231.
15. Koren G. Medications which can kill a toddler with one tablet or teaspoonful. Clin Toxicol 1993;31:407–413.
16. Geller RJ, Fisher JG III, Leeper JD, Ranganathon S. American Poison Control Centers: Still not all the same? Ann Emerg Med 1988;17:599–603.
17. Sibert R, Routledge PA. Accidental poisoning in children: Can we admit fewer children with safety? Arch Dis Child 1991;66:263–266.
18. Henretig FM. Special considerations in the poisoned pediatric patient. Emerg Med Clin North Am 1994;12:552.
19. Haslam R. Drug safety and medication systems in hospitals. Adverse Drug React Acute Poison Rev 1988;3:133–146.
20. Vitillo JA, Lesar TS. Preventing medication prescribing errors. DICP Ann Pharmacother 1991;25:1388–1394.
21. Mayer GA. Chlorpropamide or chlorpromazine? Can Med Assoc J 1991;144:119.
22. Hoffman JP. More on Losec or Lasix? N Engl J Med 1990; 323:1428.
23. Landis SJ. Azathioprine or azidothyridine. Can Med Assoc J 1990;143:611.
24. Olsen LA, Miller DR, Goswani A, McAskill AC, Newman WP. Inadvertent administration of acetohexamide instead of acetazolamide. DICP Ann Pharmacother 1991;25:100.
25. Pincus JM, Ike PW. Norflox or Norflex? N Engl J Med 1992; 326:1030.
26. Garvey CW. Desipramine sent when it's disopyramide. JAMA 1989;262:210.
27. Brierton D, Nunn-Thompson CW. Warning: Acetaminophen and aprolidine both labeled Apronal. DICP Ann Pharmacother 1990;24: 1232.
28. Hooper PL, Tello RJ, Burstein PJ, Abrams RS. Pseudoinsulinoma: The Diamox–Diabinese switch. N Engl J Med 1990; 1323:488.
29. Fallis G. Quinine or quinidine? Can Med Assoc J 1991;144: 540–541.
30. Kurth MC, Langston JW, Tetrud WW. "Stelazine" versus "selegiline": A hazard in prescription writing. N Engl J Med 1990;1323:1776.
31. Ahlquist DA, Nelson RL, Callaway CW. Pseudoinsulinoma syndrome from inadvertent tolazamide ingestion. Ann Intern Med 1980;93:281–282.
32. Kramer JM. More on drug name confusion. N Engl J Med 1995;332:753–754.
33. Lesar TS, Briceland LL, Delcoure K, et al. Medical prescribing errors in a teaching hospital. JAMA 1990;263:2329–2334.
34. Janda SM. Look-alike and sound-alike medication pairs. Vet Hum Toxicol 1994;36:256.
35. Mrvos R, Dean BS, Krenzelok EP. Illiteracy: A contributing factor to poisoning. Vet Hum Toxicol 1993;35:466–468.
36. Perlstein PH, Callison C, White M, et al. Errors in drug computations during newborn intensive care. Am J Dis Child 1979;133:376–379.
37. Bleyer WA, Koup JR. Medication errors during intensive care. Am J Dis Child 1979;133:366–367.
38. Koren G, Barzilay Z, Greenwald M. Tenfold errors in administration of drug doses: A neglected iatrogenic disease in pediatrics. Pediatrics 1986;77: 848–849.
39. Bury G. Errors in drug administration. Pediatrics 1987;79: 170.
40. Lamont JH. Errors in drug administration. Pediatrics 1987; 79:171–177.
41. Rieder WJ, Goldstein D, Zinman H, Koren G. Tenfold errors in drug dosage. Can Med Assoc J 1988;139:12–13.
42. Hoen E, Hodgkin C, Milkevicius D. Harmful use of donated veterinary drugs. Lancet 1993;342:308–309.
43. Joubert PH, Mathibe L. Acute poisoning in developing countries. Adverse Drug React Acute Poisoning Rev 1989; 8:165–178.
44. Kulig K. Initial management of ingestions of toxic substances. N Engl J Med 1992;326:1678.
45. Lloyd-Thomas AP. Paediatric Glasgow Coma Scale. Br Med J 1990;301:382.
46. Yaeger JY, Johnston B, Sesshia SS. Coma scales in pediatric practice. Am J Dis Child 1990;144:1088–1091.
47. Stanmark J-E, Stalhammer D, Holmgren E. The reaction level scale (RLS85): Manual and guidelines. Acta Neurochir 1988; 91:12–20.
48. Stanczak DE, White JG, Gouview W, et al. Assessment of level of consciousness following severe neurological insult. J Neurosurg 1984;60:955–961.
49. Crosby L, Parsons LC. Clinical neurologic assessment tool: Development and testing of an instrument to index neurologic status. Heart Lung 1989;18:121–129.
50. Giacino JT, Kezmarsky MA, De Luca J, Cicerone KD. Monitoring rate of recovery to predict outcome in minimally responsive patients. Arch Phys Med Rehabil 1991;72:897–901.
51. Born JD. The Glasgow–Liege Scale. Acta Neurochir (Wien) 1988;91:1–11.
52. Benzer A, Mittershiffthaler G, Marosi M, et al. Pediatric measures of non-survival after trauma: Innsbruck Coma Scale. Lancet 1991;338:977–978.
53. Jennett B, Bond M. Assessment of outcome after severe brain damage. Lancet 1975;1:484–485.
54. Segatore M, Way C. The Glasgow Coma Scale: Time for change. Heart Lung 1992;21:548–555.
55. Olson KR, Kerney TE, Dyer JE, Benowitz HL. Seizures associated with poisoning and drug overdose: Changing patterns of causes and poison center consultations. Vet Hum Toxicol 1990;32:361.
56. Working Group on Status Epilepticus. Treatment of convulsive status epilepticus: Recommendations of the Epilepsy Foundation of America Working Group on Status Epilepticus. JAMA 1993;270:854–859.
57. Zaccara G, Muscas GC, Messori A. Clinical features, pathogenesis and management of drug-induced seizures. Drug Saf 1990;5:109–151.
58. Hoffman R. Nervous system toxicity. Personal presentation, American College of Medical Toxicology, Board Examination Review Course, September 1994.
59. Morrow JI, Routledge BA. Drug-induced neurological disorders. Adverse Drug React Acute Poison Rev 1988;3: 105–133.
60. Francis J, Kapoor WN. Delirium in hospitalized elderly. J Gen Intern Med 1990;5:65–79.
61. Bruno A, Nolte KB, Chapinj J. Stroke associated with ephedrine use. Neurology 1993;43:1313–1316.
62. Griffen JP. A review of the literature on benign intracranial hypertension associated with medication. Adverse Drug React Toxicol Rev 1992;11:41–58.

63. Patter SB, Love EJ. Drug-induced depression: Incidence, avoidance and management. Drug Saf 1994;10:203–219.
64. Turnor P. Clinical pharmacology in criminal cases: Discussion paper. J R Soc Med 1987;8:438–439.
65. Sulter DL, Cummings JL. Drug-induced mania-causative agents, clinical characteristics and management: A retrospective analysis of the literature. Med Toxicol Adverse Drug Experience 1989;4:127–143.
66. Evans L. Psychological effects caused by drugs in overdose. Drugs 1980;19:220–242.
67. Mofenson HC, Caraccio TR. The agitated, violent or acutely psychotic patient. PP/T Review. Nassau County Medical Center Regional Poison Control Center. 1992;11(5): 301–306.
68. Chapman SA, Stephan T, Lake KD, et al. Fever induced by dobutamine infusion. Am J Cardiol 1994;74:517.
69. Thomas SHL. Drug-induced systemic hypertension. Adverse Drug React Bull 1993;5:559–562.
70. Kristensen TS. Cardiovascular diseases and the work environment: A critical review of the epidemiologic literature on chemical factors. Scand J Work Environ Health 1989;15: 245–264.
71. Benowitz NL. Cardiotoxicity in the workplace. Occup Med 1992;7(3):468–478.
72. Talieraco CP, Olney BA, Lie JT. Myocarditis related to drug hypersensitivity. Mayo Clin Proc 1985;60:463–468.
73. Hoff JS, Syverrud SA, Tucci MA. Case conference: Complete heart block in a young man. Acad Emerg Med 1995; 2:751–756.
74. Dufresne RG. Skin necrosis from intravenously infused materials. Cutis 1987;39:197–198.
75. Dolan PA, Flowers FP, Aranjo OE, Shuertz EF. Toxic epidermal necrolysis. J Emerg Med 1989;7:65–69.
76. Mutasim DF, Pelc NJ, Anhalt GJ. Drug induced pemphigus. Dermatol Clin 1993;11:463–471.
77. Krop LC. Drug-induced systemic lupus erythematosus. DICP Ann Pharmacokinet 1991;25:212–213.
78. Kale SA: Drug-induced systemic lupus erythematosus: Differentiating it from the real thing. Interstate Postgrad Med Assoc 1985;77:231–242.
79. Cohen MG, Prowse MV. Drug-induced rheumatic symptoms: Diagnosis, clinical features and management. Med Toxicol Adverse Drug Experience 1989;4:199–218.
80. Roujeau JC, Stern RS. Severe adverse cutaneous reactions to drugs. N Engl J Med 1994;331:1272–1285.
81. Tosti A, Misciali C, Piraccini BM, et al. Drug induced hair loss and hair growth: Incidence, management and avoidance. Drug Saf 1994;10:317–318.
82. Huang MY, Schacht J. Drug induced ototoxicity: Pathogenesis and prevention. Med Toxicol Adverse Drug Experience 1989;4:452–467.
83. Drug-induced hearing disorders. Aust Adverse Drug React Bull 1995;10(1):2.
84. Prendergast BD, George CP. Drug-induced rhabdomyolysis: Mechanisms and management. Postgrad Med J 1993; 66:333–336.
85. Koppel C. Clinical features, pathogenesis and management of drug-induced rhabdomyolysis. Med Toxicol Adverse Drug Experience 1989;4:108–126.
86. Curry SC, Chang D, Connor D. Drug- and toxin-induced rhabdomyolysis. Ann Emerg Med 1989;18:1068–1084.
87. Stone MJ, Willerson JT, Gomez-Sanchez CE, et al. Radioimmunoassay of myoglobin in human serum: Results in patients with acute myocardial infarction. J Clin Invest 1975; 56:1334–1339.
88. Sabaawi M, Holmes TF, Fragala MR. Drug-induced akathisias: Subjective experience and objective findings. Milit Med 1994;159:286–291.
89. Godley PJ, Morton TA, Karboski JA, Tani JA. Procainamide-induced myasthenic crisis. Ther Drug Monit 1990;12: 411–414.
90. Mastaglia FL. Adverse effects of drugs on muscle. Drugs 1982;24:304–321.
91. Plotz PH, Rider LG, Targoff IN, et al. Myositis: Immunologic contributions to understanding cause, pathogenesis, and therapy. Ann Intern Med 1995;122:715–725.
92. Goldsmith JR, Herishanu Y, Abarband JM, Weinbaum Z. Clustering of Parkinson's disease points to environmental etiology. Arch Environ Health 1990;45:88–94.
93. Ross RT. Drug-induced parkinsonism and other movement disorders. Can J Neurol Sci 1990;17:155–162.
94. Martyn CN. Neurological clues from environmental neurotoxins. Br Med J 1987;295:346–347.
95. Lane RJM, Dick JPR, de Belleroche J. Glycine and neurodegenerative disease. Lancet 1991;337:732–733.
96. Feldman RG, Mayer RM, Taub A. Evidence for peripheral neurotoxic effects of trichlorethylene. Neurology 1970; 20:599.
97. Spencer PS, Nunn PB, Hugon J, et al. Guam amyotrophic lateral sclerosis–parkinsonism–dementia linked to a plant excitant neurotoxin. Science 1987;237:517–522.
98. Spencer PS. Guam ALS/parkinsonism-dementia: A long-lasting neurotoxic disorder caused by "slow toxin(s)" in food? Can J Neurol Sci 1987;14:347–357.
99. Boothby JA, de Jesus PV, Rowland LP. Reversible form of motor neuron disease: Lead "neuritis." Arch Neurol 1974;31: 18–25.
100. Stober T, Stelte W, Kunze K. Lead concentrations in blood, plasma, erythrocytes and cerebrospinal fluid in amyotrophic lateral sclerosis. J Neurol Sci 1983;61:21–26.
101. Hawkes CH, Cavanagh JB, Fox AJ. Motoneuron disease: A disorder secondary to solvent exposure? Lancet 1989; 1:73–76.
102. Tylleskar T, Banea M, Bikangi N, et al. Cassava cyanogens and konzo, an upper motoneuron disease found in Africa. Lancet 1992;339:208–211.
103. Roelofs-Ivenson RA, Mulder DW, Elveback LP, et al. ALS and heavy metals: A pilot case–control study. Neurology 1984; 34:393–395.
104. Conradi S, Ronnevi L-O, Nise G, Vesterberg O. Long-time penicillamine treatment in amyotrophic lateral sclerosis with parallel determination of lead in blood, plasma and urine. Acta Neurol Scand 1982;65:203–211.
105. Yanagihara R. Heavy metals and essential minerals in motor neuron disease. In: Rowland LP, ed. *Human Motor Neuron Disease.* New York: Raven Press;1982:233–247.
106. Garruto RM, Yanagihara R, Gajdusek DC. Cycads and amyotrophic lateral sclerosis/parkinsonism dementia. Lancet 1988; 2:1079.
107. Duncan MW, Steele JC, Kopin IJ, Markey SP. 2-Amino 3 (methylamino)-propanoic acid (BMAA) in cycad flow: An unlikely cause of amyotrophic lateral sclerosis and parkinsonism–dementia of Guam. Neurology 1990;40:767–772.
108. Abuelo JG. Renal failure caused by chemicals, foods, plants, animal venoms and misuse of drugs. Arch Intern Med 1990; 150:505–510.
109. Underwood TW, Frye CB. Drug-induced pancreatitis. Clin Pharm 1993;14:440–448.
110. Nelid GH. Haemolytic syndrome in practice. Lancet 1994; 334:338–340.
111. Urinary incontinence. Harvard Med School Health Lett 1990; 15(10):10.
112. Oral drug effects. Aust Adverse Drug React Bull 1992;11(4).
113. Klegan KL, Young TL. Pill-induced esophageal injury. J Tenn Med Assoc 1992;85:417–418.
114. Iredale JP, George CF. Drugs causing gastrointestinal obstruction. Adverse Drug React Toxicol Rev 1993;12:163–175.
115. Committee on Safety of Medicines UK. CSM update: Adverse drug reactions and the liver. Br Med J 1985;291:46.
116. Hanson JS. Propylthiouracil and hepatitis: Two cases and a review of the literature. Arch Intern Med 1984;144:994–996.
117. Ishii M, Miyazaki Y, Yamamoto T, et al. A case of drug-induced ductopenia resulting in fatal biliary cirrhosis. Liver 1993;13:227–231.
118. Cappell MS, Simon T. Colonic toxicity of administered medications and chemicals. Am J Gastroenterol 1993;88:1684–1697.
119. Driscoll DF. Drug-induced metabolic disorders and parenteral nutrition in the intensive care unit: A pharmaceutical and metabolic perspective. DICP Ann Pharmacother 1989; 23:363–371.
120. Reed CR, Glauser FL. Drug-induced noncardiogenic pulmonary edema. Chest 1991;100:1120–1124.

121. Rosenow EC III, Myers JL, Swenson SJ, Pisani RJ. Drug-induced pulmonary disease: An update. Chest 1992;102: 239–250.
122. Henry JA. Resuscitation from poisoning. In Baskett PJF, ed. *Cardiopulmonary Resuscitation.* Amsterdam: Elsevier;1989: 231–257.
123. Hunt LW, Rosenow EC III. Asthma-producing drugs. Ann Allergy 1992;68:453–462.
124. McWaine DE, Procci WR. Drug-induced sexual dysfunction. Med Toxicol 1988;3:289–306.
125. Molitch ME, Russell EJ. The pituitary "incidentaloma." Ann Intern Med 1990;112:925–931.
126. Hell K, Wernze H. Drug-induced changes in prolactin secretion: Clinical implications. Med Toxicol 1988;3:463–498.
127. Heimpel H. Drug-induced agranulocytosis. Med Toxicol 1988;3:449–462.
128. Beutler E. Glucose-6-phosphate dehydrogenase deficiency. N Engl J Med 1991;324:169–174.
129. George JM, Shattil SJ. The clinical importance of acquired abnormalities of platelet function. N Engl J Med 1991; 324:27–40.
130. Bochner BS, Lichtenstein LM. Anaphylaxis. N Engl J Med 1991;324:1785–1790.
131. DeJarnett AC, Grant JA. Basic mechanisms of anaphylaxis and anaphylactoid reactions. Immunol Allergy Clin North Am 1992;12:501–515.
132. Lee M, Sharfi R. Oxybutynin-induced reflux esophagitis. DICP Ann Pharmacother 1990;34:583–585.
133. Bradberry SM, Vale JA. Disturbances of potassium homeostasis in poisoning. Clin Toxicol 1995;33:295–310.
134. Browning RG, Olson DW, Stueven HA, Mateer JR. 50% dextrose: Antidote or toxin? Ann Emerg Med 1990;19:683–687.
135. Ghose K. Prescribing CNS drugs for elderly patients. Drugs Aging 1994;4:275–284.
136. Mets TF. Drug-induced orthostatic hypotension in older patients. Drugs Aging 1995;6:219–228.

Chapter 2 Diagnostic Procedures

INTRODUCTION

Snyder and Vlasses have suggested a mnemonic (PROMISE) for potential indications for analytical (laboratory) toxicologic assistance including the following[1]: determination of **p**rognosis; collection of **r**esearch data; response to **o**rder of court, medical examiner, or law enforcement official; **m**onitoring of treatment; **i**dentification of a substance to establish a diagnosis; assessment of **s**everity of poisoning; and **e**xclusion (or confirmation) of toxic exposure (see also Appendix).

LABORATORY AND CLINICAL DISCORDANCE

The cornerstone of the management of overdose patients—aggressive support of ventilatory, cardiovascular, metabolic, and neurologic functions—is mostly independent of the drugs implicated in the overdose.[2,3] Discrepancies between the clinical impression and laboratory results may be due to unreliable histories given by patients and friends (the finding of an empty medicine container does not necessarily imply recent ingestion of that agent),[2] the time interval between ingestion of a drug and collection of a specimen, and the toxicokinetics of the drug. Also, the threshold concentration required for detection may influence the performance of the laboratory. Errors in toxicology have been documented in both false-positive and false-negative directions. The laboratory is not always the absolute "gold standard."

Brett found that potentially important unsuspected drugs are found in only a small minority of patients; clinical characteristics of patients with unsuspected drug identifications are not significantly different from those of other patients; and unexpected laboratory results rarely lead to changes in patient management and probably never affect the outcome.

Laboratory discovery of an unsuspected drug often does not appear as a marker for severity of illness and does not, in itself, identify patients requiring closer observation or having a poorer prognosis. "Objective" results may falsely provide reassurance to the physician, even if clinical management is unlikely to be affected. The ultimate value of reassurance must be weighed against the economic impact of performance of such tests in many patients who do not require them.

The health care professional should ascertain whether the local hospital laboratory is capable of performing tests in a timely manner for those drugs whose concentrations exhibit a useful correlation with the clinical status of the patient. Laboratories with specialized capabilities should be easily available.

THE LARGE HOSPITAL LABORATORY

In large hospitals, laboratories are usually isolated from the clinical environment and are often largely ignored by the doctors. Analytical service for drug analysis is less than optimally useful because dosage adjustments are often made on the basis of clinical judgment. In one large hospital most analyses were performed for theophylline, cyclosporine, phenytoin, digoxin, carbamazepine, valproate, and phenobarbital in descending order. Service to inpatients works well, but for outpatients the service is often inadequate largely because of the delay in delivering samples to the laboratory.[3]

ANION GAP

Drugs associated with a non-anion gap metabolic acidosis include acetazolamide, amphotericin B, amiloride, spironolactone, and toluene.[4,5]

The anion gap may be normal in the early stages of methanol and ethylene glycol poisonings when ethanol coingestion prevents formation of their metabolites.

LACTIC ACIDOSIS

The anion gap calculation (12 ± 4 mmol/L) may not signal the presence of all cases of clinically important lactic acidosis.[6,7] Hyperlactatemia is a reflection of ineffective tissue oxygenation and carries a poor prognosis in critically ill patients. Lactic acidosis may be defined as a pH less than 7.4 and a blood lactate greater than 2.5 mmol/L. Lactate elevations are considered high (usually 100% mortality) when levels are more than 10 mmol/L, moderate (usually 75% mortality) between 5 and 9.9 mmol/L, and mild (approximately 35% mortality) between 2.5 and 4.9 mmol/L. When the lactate level is very high the anion gap will be at the upper limits of normal or elevated; however, the anion gap may not be elevated in 50% of patients with a moderate lactate elevation and up to 80% of those with mild elevation.[8] Hyperlactatemia should be included in the differential diagnosis of non-anion gap acidosis as well. As a normal anion gap does not rule out an elevated blood lactate level, and the pH may be altered toward normal by manipulating ventilation settings or infusing bicarbonate, the only alternative is to measure blood lactate directly.

The limitations of the anion gap are summarized in Table 2–1.

Table 2–1
Limitations of the Anion Gap

1. Nearly one third of patients with anion gaps between 20 and 30 mEq/L do not have a demonstrable organic acidosis.[9]
2. Increases in the concentration of ketoanions and lactate are insufficient to explain the entire anion gap increment in organic acidosis.[10]
3. Patients with otherwise classic uncomplicated diabetic ketoacidosis may present with[10] or later show a metabolic acidosis with a normal anion gap.[11]
4. After resolution of lactic acidosis, an "overshoot" alkalosis may develop[7] because "excess" lactate typically exceeds the decrement in bicarbonate.[12]
5. The exact relationship between the increment in the anion gap and the decrement in bicarbonate in a high-anion-gap acidosis is not readily predictable.[12]

THE FALL OF THE SERUM ANION GAP

The currently used reference range for the anion gap, 12 ± 4 mmol/L, was developed with technology available in the

Table 2–2
Anion Gap Technology

	1970s	1990s
Sodium	Flame photometry	Ion-selective electrode
Chloride	Mercuric nitrate thiocyanate colorimetric reaction	Colorimetric titration or ion-selective electrode*
Total CO_2 content	Acidification Colorimetric titration	Rate of pH change as detected by a pH electrode
Normal individuals may exhibit the following:		
Sodium 140 mmol/L		136–143
Chloride 103 mmol/L		102–111
Bicarbonate 25 mmol/L		23–30
Anion gap		3–11

*ASTRA instrumentation (**A**utomated **Sta**t/**R**outine **A**nalyzer).

Table 2–3
Processes That Affect the Anion Gap

High Anion Gap
Metabolic acidosis*
Dehydration or loss of fluid with relatively little unmeasured anions
Infusions of salts of organic acids (lactate, acetate, citrate, penicillin, carbenicillin)
Reduced unmeasured cations (potassium, calcium, magnesium)
Alkalemia*
Systematic underestimation of serum chloride (in azotemic patients receiving allopurinol)†
Random laboratory error*

Low Anion Gap
Volume expansion with free water or fluid containing relatively little unmeasured anion
Systematic underestimation of serum sodium (hypernatremia, hyperviscosity, hyperlipidemia)*,†
Systematic overestimation of serum chloride (bromism,[13] iodide intoxication, hyperlipidemia)*
Raised unmeasured cations (potassium, calcium, magnesium, immunoglobulin G, lithium, polymyxins)*
Reduced unmeasured anions (hypoalbuminemia)*
Acidemia from a respiratory or hyperchloremic metabolic acidosis‡
Random laboratory error*

*Realistic clinical situations in which the anion gap may exceed 6 mEq/L.
†Systematic errors critically depend on laboratory methods used to measure particular ions under described conditions.
‡The acidemia usually associated with a high-anion-gap acidosis tends to reduce the increment in anion gap caused by the higher concentration of unmeasured anions.
Adapted from Di Nubile MJ. The increment in the anion gap: Overextension of a concept? Lancet 1988;2:951–953.

1970s. The majority of clinical laboratories are now using current technology (Table 2–2).[13]

Consultation with the clinical or hospital laboratory will provide guidance for the clinician and may avoid misinterpretations of the calculated anion gap.

Factors that contribute to a low anion gap are listed in Table 2–3.[4] The relationship between the rise in the anion gap and the fall in bicarbonate has been characterized by Wrenn with a numerical value, the delta gap: delta gap = rise in anion gap – decrement in HCO_3. If the delta gap is greater than +6, a metabolic acidosis is usually present. If the delta gap is less than –6, a hyperchloremic acidosis is usually present.[14]

OSMOLAL GAP

The osmolal gap (Table 2–4) reflects the difference between the measured osmolarity (by the freezing point depression method and $2Na^+ + \frac{glucose}{18} + \frac{BUN}{2.8}$). A mnemonic for causative factors is ME DIE (**m**ethanol, **e**thanol, **d**iuretics [mannitol, sorbitol, glycerine], **i**sopropanol, or **e**thylene glycol). The degree to which any chemical substance contributes to the osmolality of a solution is simply based on the number of molecules present. One millimole of substance will contribute 1 mOsm to the measured osmolality. One ethanol molecule (molecular weight 46) has the same osmotic activity as one molecule of albumin (molecular weight 66,500). Thus, for any given concentration, small-molecular-weight substances are significantly more osmotically active than an equivalent concentration of larger molecules. Glycol ethers and their metabolites are osmotically active; however, given their relatively large molecular weights compared with ethanol and other smaller alcohols, small concentrations of these substances do not exert a significant osmotic effect. The osmolal gap may be normal in the late stages when methanol and ethylene glycol are completely metabolized.[15–19]

Table 2–4
Osmolal Gap

- If $M - C$ is greater than 10 mOsm/kg H_2O, look for (1) laboratory error, (2) decreased serum water content, (3) low molecular-weight substances not used in equation for calculated osmolality.
- If M is normal and C is low, look for a decrease in serum water associated with hyperproteinemias and hyperlipidemias.
- If M is high and C is normal or low, gap = unmeasured osmoles.

Sorbitol	Ethanol
Mannitol	Methanol
Glycerin	Ethylene glycol
Diatrizoate sodium	Acetone
Isoniazid	Ether
Trichloroethane	

M = measured osmolality
C = calculated osmolality

Anion Gap Metabolic Acidosis
Normal Osmolar Gap

Iron	Abdominal pain, hematemesis, diarrhea, radiopaque
Toluene	Glue sniffing, odor, hypokalemia due to RTA
Phenformin	Hypoglycemia
Lactic acidosis	Cardiopulmonary distress, seizures, iron, etc.
Paraldehyde	Odor
Salicylates	Positive serum assay, respiratory alkalosis
Uremia	High serum creatine
Ketoacidosis	High ketone levels

ETHANOL

If the measured ethanol level is less than that predicted by the osmolal gap, the presence of another osmotically active substance, such as methanol, ethylene glycol, isopropyl alcohol, or acetone, is suggested. The finding of both an osmolal and an anion gap, in the absence of detectable ethanol, is considered strong evidence for poisoning by methanol or ethylene glycol. If the excess anion gap is not explained by an elevated lactate level, the diagnosis of methanol or ethylene glycol poisoning is almost certain because these substances produce nonlactate organic acids. The osmolal gap provides an accurate estimation of alcohol levels.

Frequently, an excess osmolal gap is not accounted for by the level of ethanol. Dehydration and rehydration may affect the accuracy of formulas used to calculate the osmolal gap. Most formulas are based on the assumption that serum is about 93% water; however, this numeric "constant" may change as the hydration state changes. A dehydrated patient may have a fraction as low as 0.89 or as high as 0.94 when rehydrated. Pathologic processes associated with alcoholism may contribute to the osmolal gap. Alcoholic ketoacidosis with an unexplained osmolal gap and a large anion gap could mimic ethylene glycol or methanol poisoning. Unmeasured osmoles may be generated in pathologic states. Osmolal gap excess may be secondary to metabolites of the toxin, differences in the formulas used to calculate the osmolar gap, and the nonconstancy of the fixed terms used in these formulas.

A suggested mnemonic for the causes of an anion gap acidosis is I Love Chocolate Raspberry Truffle MUDPIES.[20]

I	Iron, isoniazid (INH), ibuprofen
L	Lithium, lactate
C	Carbon monoxide, cyanide, caffeine
R	Respiratory dysfunction, beta-adrenergic agents, benzyl alcohol
T	Toluene
M	Methanol, metabolic dysfunction
U	Uremia, hepatorenal dysfunction
D	Diabetic ketoacidosis
P	Paraldehyde, phenformin
I	Idiopathic, iron, INH, ibuprofen
E	Ethanol, ethylene glycol
S	Salicylates, hydrogen sulfide, strychnine, seizures, starvation, sympathomimetic amines

When ethanol is included in the formula for calculating osmolality, the formula becomes

$$2[Na^+] + \frac{glucose}{18} + \frac{serum\ urea\ nitrogen}{2.8} + \frac{ethanol}{4.6}$$

The mean is usually –2 more or less than 6 mOsm/L. The use of either formula (see above) yields similar values for calculated osmolality.

Many alcohols (eg, methanol, ethanol, isopropyl alcohol) have boiling points less than that of water. As these volatile alcohols may remain in the vapor phase instead of condensing with the serum, the osmolality determined by vapor pressure measurement may be falsely normal. The freezing point depression method does not pose this problem and is

Table 2–5
Summary of the Emergency Drug/Poison "Screen" Offered by the Poisons Unit, Guy's Hospital*

Test 1: Acidic Drugs (blood)
BARBITURATES   CAFFEINE
CHLORMEZANONE   CHLORPROPAMIDE
GLUTETHIMIDE   IBUPROFEN
MEFENAMIC ACID   MEPROBAMATE
METHAQUALONE   METHYPRYLONE
PHENAZONE   THEOPHYLLINE

Test 2: Anticonvulsant Drugs (blood)
CARBAMAZEPINE   ETHOSUXIMIDE
METHSUXIMIDE   PHENOBARBITONE
PHENYTOIN   PRIMIDONE
THIOPENTONE   VALPROATE

Test 3: Nonsteroidal Antiinflammatory Drugs (blood)
DIFLUNISAL   FENOPROFEN
IBUPROFEN   INDOMETHACIN
KETOPROFEN   MEFENAMIC ACID
NAPROXEN   PIROXICAM

Test 4: Volatile Hypnotic Drugs (Blood)
CHLORMETHIAZOLE   TRICHLOROETHANOL
CHLORAL HYDRATE AND DICHLORALPHENAZONE AS TRICHLOROETHANOL

Test 5: Benzodiazepines (blood)
ALPRAZOLAM   BROMAZEPAM
CHLORDIAZEPOXIDE   CLOBAZAM
CLONAZEPAM   DIAZEPAM
FLUNITRAZEPAM   FLURAZEPAM
LORAZEPAM   LORMETAZEPAM
MIDAZOLAM   NITRAZEPAM
NORDIAZEPAM   OXAZEPAM
PRAZEPAM   TEMAZEPAM
TRIAZOLAM

Test 6: Alcohols (blood, urine, or fluids)
ACETONE   ETHANOL
ISOPROPANOL   METHANOL

Test 7: Glycols (blood, urine, or fluids)
ETHYLENE GLYCOL   OTHER GLYCOLS

Test 8: Solvent Screen (blood)
ALCOHOLS   BUTANE
HALONS   KETONES
TOLUENE   CHLORINATED HYDROCARBONS

Test 9: (blood or urine)
PARACETAMOL

Test 10: (blood or urine)
SALICYLATES

Test 11: Bipyridilium Herbicides (blood, urine, or fluids)
PARAQUAT   DIQUAT

Test 12: Chlorinated Phenoxy and Other Herbicides (blood, urine or fluids)
2,4-D   2,4,5-T   BROMOXYNIL
DICHLORPROP   IOXYNIL   MCPA
MECORPROP

Test 13: Basic Drugs (urine or gastric contents)
AMPHETAMINE-TYPE STIMULANTS   ANTICHOLINERGICS
CAFFEINE   CHLORMETHIAZOLE   CHLOROQUINE
DISOPYRAMIDE   LIGNOCAINE   METOCLOPRAMIDE
NARCOTIC ANALGESICS (EXCLUDING HEROIN AND MORPHINE)
METRONIDAZOLE   NICOTINE   ORPHENADRINE
PROCAINAMIDE   PROCYCLIDINE   TRANYLCYPROMINE
TRICYCLIC ANTIDE-PRESSANTS   TRIMETHOPRIM   VERAPAMIL

Test 14: Basic and Neutral Drugs (urine or gastric contents—20 mL)
Those in Test 13 plus:
BARBITURATES   BETA BLOCKERS   CIMETIDINE
HEROIN   MEFENAMIC ACID   MORPHINE
PHENOTHIAZINES   QUININE   RANITIDINE
STRYCHNINE   THEOPHYLLINE   TRAZODONE

Test 15: Test for Opiates (urine)
CODEINE   DIHYDROCODEINE   HEROIN
MORPHINE

Test 16: Basic Drugs (blood)
CHLORPROMAZINE   CODEINE   DIHYDROCODEINE
METHADONE   NEFOPAM   ORPHENADRINE
PETHIDINE   PROCYCLIDINE
TRICYCLIC ANTIDEPRESSANTS

Test 17: Test for Cannabis (urine)
CANNABINOIDS

Test 18: Test for Cocaine (urine)
BENZOYLECGONINE (COCAINE METABOLITE)

Test 19: Laxatives (urine or stool)
ANTHRAQUINONES   BISACODYL   PHENOLPTHALEIN

Test 20: Diuretics (urine)
LOOP   THIAZIDES

*Compounds in capital letters are usually measured in plasma/serum; the other compounds are normally reported qualitatively.
(From Flanagan RJ, Widdop B, Ramsey JD, Loveland M. Analytical toxicology. Hum Toxicol 1988;7:489–502.)

a preferred method for alcohol ingestions. Potentially serious alcohol poisoning may be missed.[21] The routine use of osmolal gaps to diagnose toxic alcohol ingestion is likely to produce many false-positive and false-negative results.[22]

ALCOHOLIC KETOACIDOSIS

An increased osmolal gap found in alcoholic ketoacidosis is only partially explained by the osmolal concentration of ethyl alcohol. Elevation of endogenous glycerol, acetone, and acetone metabolite levels is also a significant cause of an increased osmolal gap in an alcoholic patient. Both increased anion gap metabolic acidosis and an increased osmolal gap are increased in alcoholic acidosis in addition to the similar observation made after ingestion of methanol and ethylene glycol. Hence, alcoholic acidosis and lactic acidosis should first be excluded before alcohol therapy and/or hemodialysis is instituted in such patients.[15,21]

INCREASES IN BOTH THE ANION GAP AND OSMOLAL GAP

The anion gap may be normal in the early stages of methanol and ethylene glycol poisonings when ethanol coingestion prevents formation of their acid metabolism. The osmolal gap may be normal in late stages when methanol and ethylene glycol are completely metabolized. Elevation of both the anion gap and the osmolal gap strongly supports the diagnosis of ethylene or ethylene glycol poisoning. Treatment with bicarbonate and ethanol (or 4-methylpyrazole) should be initiated while considering the indications for hemodialysis treatment.[23]

THE "TOX SCREEN"

Drug screening is a useful tool in patients with altered mental status or coma of unclear etiology (Table 2–5). In known overdose cases, comprehensive toxicology screening contributes little when patients are responsive to verbal stimuli and have no seizures, hypoventilation, or cardiac abnormalities other than sinus tachycardia after several hours of observation. It seems reasonable to obtain general toxicology screens in the more seriously ill patients in whom antidotes, dialysis, or hemoperfusion may be beneficial (e.g., phenobarbital, ethanol, ethylene glycol, isopropyl alcohol, lithium, methanol, paraquat, salicylate, and theophylline) (Table 2–6).[24] Clinical judgment must ultimately guide decisions regarding the use of the laboratory.[25] A drug screen may be indicated when the history is unreliable, with a multiple-drug ingestion, with a patient in delirium or coma, for the identification of specific drugs, to indicate when antagonists may be used, and to aid in the estimation of prognosis. A drug screen should be obtained in the presence of coma, cardiotoxicity (unexplained), acidosis (unexplained), head trauma with neurologic signs and symptoms, suspected history, and seizures with an undetermined history.

LIMITATIONS

Few potentially important unsuspected drugs are found in most poisoned patients. Discovery of a clinically unsuspected drug does not serve as a marker of the severity of illness. The most common drugs found in patients determined to have ingested drugs include volatiles (ethanol, methanol, isopropyl alcohol), benzodiazepines, acetaminophen, sympathomimetics, antidepressants, barbiturates, opiates, phenothiazine, *d*-propoxyphene, meperidine, and cocaine. The toxicology screen will change management based on the clinical history in overdose with acetaminophen, salicylates, lithium, theophylline, methanol, ethylene glycol, and digoxin. A positive urine for drugs of abuse does not indicate that an individual was clinically affected when the specimen was collected, the frequency of use, the pattern of use, and addiction. Water-soluble drugs appear in the urine shortly after use and are excreted in a few days (alcohol, barbiturate, stimulants, and opiates). Lipid-soluble drugs are excreted slowly (marijuana, phencyclidine). The most common drugs found in a toxicology screen at death include carbon monoxide, ethanol, benzodiazepines, antidepressants, *d*-propoxyphene, acetamin-

Table 2–6
Some Poisons for Which Plasma Concentration Data May Influence Treatment

Treatment	Poison	Plasma Concentration Associated with Serious Toxicity
Protective therapy		
Acetylcysteine or methionine	Paracetamol (Acetaminophen)	200 mg/L at 4 h, 30 mg/L at 15 h
Ethanol	Methanol	0.5 g/L
	Ethylene glycol	0.5 g/L
Prussian blue	Thallium	200 µg/L (urine)
Chelation therapy		
Deferoxamine	Iron	5 mg/L (serum)
	Aluminum	200 µg/L (serum)
DTA/DMSA*	Lead	600 µg/L (blood)
	Cadmium	40 µg/L (blood)
DMSA/DMPS	Mercury	100 µg/L (blood)
	Arsenic	200 µg/L (blood)
Active elimination		
Alkaline diuresis	Salicylates	900 mg/L at 6 h, 450 mg/L at 24 h
	Phenobarbital	100 mg/L
	2,4-D	200 mg/L combined
	2,4,5-T	
	MCPA	
Peritoneal or hemodialysis	Ethanol	5 g/L
	Methanol	0.5 g/L
	Ethylene glycol	0.5 g/L
	Lithium	2.0 mmol/L
	Phenobarbital	100 mg/L
	Salicylates	900 mg/L at 6 h, 450 mg/L at 24 h
Charcoal hemoperfusion	Phenobarbital	100 mg/L
	Other barbiturates	50 mg/L
	Trichloroethanol	100 mg/L
	Theophylline	60 mg/L

DTA, ethylenediaminetetracetic acid; DMSA, dimercaptosuccinic acid; DMPS, dimercaptopropanesulfonic acid; 2,4-D, 2,4-dichlorophenoxyacetic acid; 2,4,5-T, 2,4,5-trichlorophenoxyacetic acid; MCPA, 2-methyl-4-chlorophenoxyacetic acid.
From Flanagan RJ, Widdop B, Ramsey JD, Loveland M. Analytical toxicology. Hum Toxicol 1988;7:489–502.

ophen, salicylates, opiates, barbiturates, meperidine, and cocaine.

Drug-specific therapy may be available for some poisonings which are corroborated by laboratory studies (methanol, isopropyl alcohol, ethylene glycol, salicylates, acetaminophen, opiates, iron, lead, arsenic, mercury, calcium, potassium, lithium, organophosphates).

Urine sample spot tests are available for salicylates, acetaminophen, ethychlorvynol, phenothiazines, glucose, ketone bodies, opiates, barbiturates, benzodiazepines, benzoylecgonine, phencyclidine, and tetrahydrocannabinol. Many such tests have not been subject to clinically controlled studies.

The toxicology screen may confirm a clinical impression (benzodiazepines, neuroleptics, hallucinogens, phencyclidine, amphetamines, cocaine, and phenylpropanolamine).

TREATMENT AND THE TOXICOLOGIC EVALUATION

Mahoney and associates have categorized treatment of an overdose into four groups with respect to a toxicologic evaluation[25]:

1. Toxicity can be predicted based on serum levels, and a drug-specific therapy can be instituted when dictated by serum levels (eg, acetaminophen, salicylates, lithium, methanol, ethylene glycol, digoxin, theophylline).
2. Toxicity closely correlates with serum level, but only nonspecific care is required (eg, ethanol, barbiturates, phenytoin).
3. Toxicity and requirement for drug-specific therapy are dependent on clinical parameters, and toxicologic testing serves only to confirm the clinical impression (eg, tricyclic antidepressants, narcotics, cyanide, organophosphates).
4. Toxicity poorly correlates with serum level, and only nonspecific care is required as dictated by clinical parameters (eg, benzodiazepines, neuroleptics, hallucinogens, phencyclidine, amphetamines, cocaine, phenylpropanolamine).[25]

Table 2–7
Examples of Compounds Not Commonly Detected in the Standard Toxicology Screen

1. Hemoglobins
   Carboxyhemoglobin, sulfhemoglobin, methemoglobin
2. Inorganic compounds
   Metals: arsenic, bismuth, mercury, lead, selenium, lithium
   Diuretics: mercurial and ammonia compounds
   Halogens: bromides, fluorides
3. Solvents
4. Pesticides
5. Radioactive compounds
6. Antibiotics
7. Vitamins
8. Nonsteroidal antiinflammatory agents (except aspirin and acetaminophen)
9. Calcium channel blockers
10. Beta blockers

From Gaudreault P, Timberlake S. Toxic compounds quantification: Type of samples and proper timing. Toxic screens, Part I. Clin Toxicol Rev 1989; 12(2):32.

Many drugs are often not detected by a toxicology screen (Table 2–7).[26] Some representative analytical techniques used for toxicologic evaluation of serum samples are found in Table 2–8.[24] Measurements valuable in industrial toxi-

Table 2–8
Analytical Techniques Used for Toxicologic Evaluation of Serum Samples

Analytical System	Representative Drugs Detected*	Detection Limits*
GC	Volatiles (eg, ethanol, methanol, isopropanol)	50 mg/L
$HPLC_1$	Acetaminophen	50 mg/L
	Salicylates	50 mg/L
	Xanthines	0.5 mg/L
$HPLC_2$	Tricyclic antidepressants, phenothiazines	50 μg/L
$HPLC_3$	Benzodiazepines	200 μg/L
Acid GC/mass spectroscopy	Barbiturates, anticonvulsants	0.2 mg/L
Basic GC/mass spectroscopy	Sedative–hypnotics	0.2 mg/L

GC, gas chromatography; HPLC, high-performance liquid chromatography.
*Drugs and detection limits listed are representative, and not a complete list, of all drugs detectable by this system.
From Mahoney JD, Gross PL, Stern TA, et al. Quantitative serum toxic screening in the management of suspected drug overdose. Am J Emerg Med 1990;8:16–22.

Table 2–9
Some Measurements Valuable in Industrial Toxicology

Compound (fluid)	Indicator of Exposure to
5-Aminolevuline acid (urine)	Lead
Arsenic (urine)	—
Bromide (blood and urine)	Methyl bromide
Carboxyhemoglobin	Carbon monoxide/ dichloromethane
Cadmium (blood and urine)	—
Cholinesterase (plasma and red cell)	Cholinesterase inhibitors
Chromium (blood and urine)	—
Cobalt (urine)	—
Dieldrin (blood)	—
Fluoride (urine	—
Hemoglobin (blood)	Lead
Hippuric acid (urine)	Toluene
Lead (blood)	—
Lindane (blood)	—
Mandelic acid (urine)	Styrene
Mercury (blood and urine)	—
Methylenebis(2-chloroaniline) (MbOCA) (urine)	—
Methylenedianiline acid (urine)	Xylene
4.4′-Methylenedianiline (MDA) (urine)	—
Pentachlorophenol (urine and plasma)	—
Polychlorinated biphenyls (blood)	—
Solvents (blood)	—
2-Thiothiazolidine-4-carboxylic acid (urine)	Carbon disulfide
Trichloroacetic acid (urine)	Chlorinated solvents
Zinc protoporphyrin (blood)	Lead

From Flanagan RJ, Widdop B, Ramsey JD, Loveland M. Analytical toxicology. Hum Toxicol 1988;7:489–502.

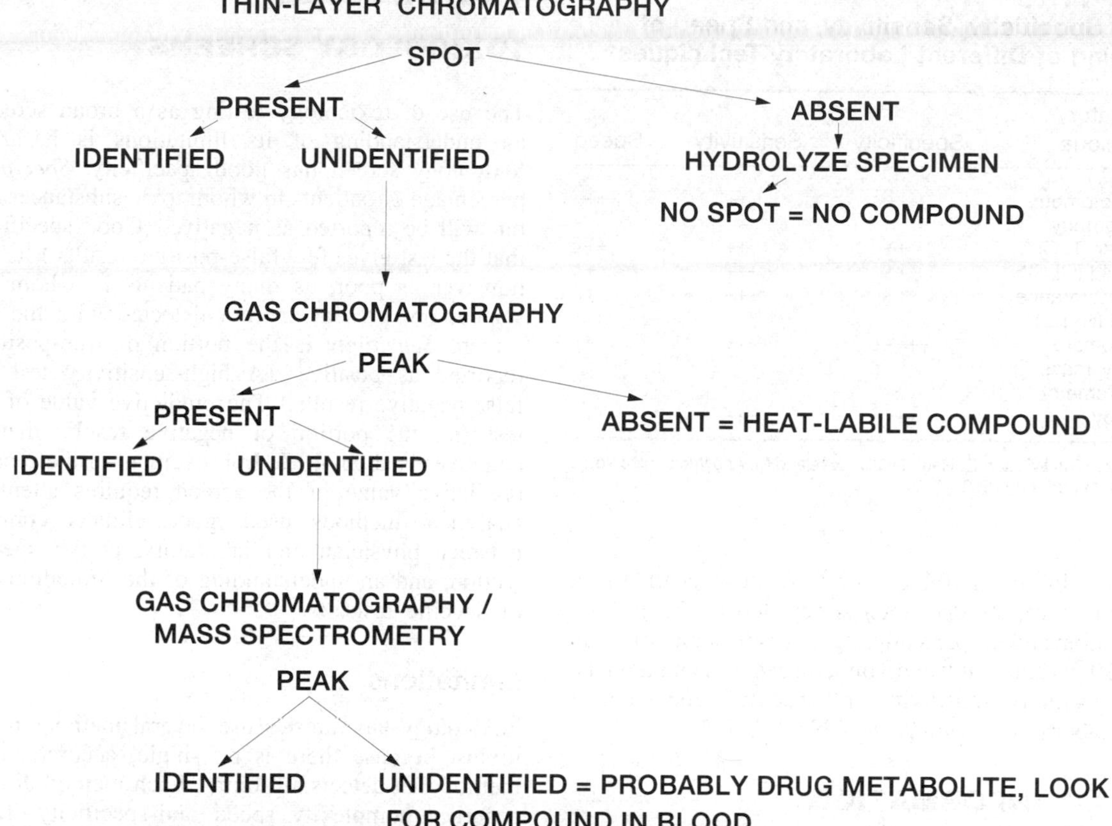

Figure 2–1 Flow chart for a toxicologic screening specimen. (From Gaudreault P, Timberlake S. Toxic compounds quantification: Type of samples and proper timing. Toxic screens, Part I. Clin Toxicol Rev 1989;12(2):32.)

Table 2–10
Toxic Compound Quantification

Substance	Sampling: Type	Sampling: Time (postingestion)	Commentary
Acetaminophen	Serum	4 h*	Hepatotoxicity >200 µg/mL
Alcohols	Serum	1–2 h	Ethanol >80–100 mg/dL Ethylene glycol >20 mg/dL Isopropranol >50–75 mg/dL Methanol >20 mg/dL
Carboxyhemoglobin	Blood	Stat	Intoxication >15%
Carbamazepine	Serum	Stat	Intoxication >12 µg/mL
Digitalis	Serum	6–8 h*	Intoxication >2.0 ng/mL
Iron	Serum	2–4 h	Intoxication >300 µg/dL
Lead	Serum	Stat	Intoxication >25 µg/dL
Lithium	Serum	6–8 h*	Intoxication >2.0 mEq/L
Methemoglobinemia	Blood	Stat	Intoxication >30%
Paraquat	Plasma	8 h*	Intoxication >1.0 µg/mL
Phenobarbital	Serum	Stat	Intoxication >30 µg/mL
Phenytoin	Serum	Stat	Intoxication >20 µg/mL
Primidone	Serum	Stat	Intoxication >12 µg/mL
Salicylate	Serum	>6 h*	Intoxication >30 mg/dL
Theophylline	Serum	Stat	Intoxication >20 µg/mL

*For these compounds measure the serum concentration twice, as soon as the patient arrives at the emergency room and a second time at the time noted in the table. These two measurements are recommended at the time because primarily the distribution phase of certain drugs (e.g., digitalis, lithium) is long and serum concentration does not reflect tissue concentration until 6 to 8 hours have elapsed. Second, the interpretation of serum concentration of other drugs based on nomogram (eg, salicylate, acetaminophen) can be carried out only after a certain amount of time has elapsed.
From Flanagan RJ, Widdop B, Ramsey JD, Loveland M. Analytical toxicology. Hum Toxicol 1988;7:489–502.

Table 2-11
Relative Specificity, Sensitivity, and Speed of Processing of Different Laboratory Techniques

Laboratory Technique	Specificity	Sensitivity	Speed
Spectrophotometry	+	++	+++
Chromatography			
Thin-layer (TLC)	++	++	++
Gas–liquid (GLC)*	+++	+++	+
High-performance liquid (HPLC)	+++	+++	+
Gas chromatography–mass spectrometry	++++	++++	+
Immunology	+++	+++	++++

From Flanagan RJ, Widdop B, Ramsey JD, Loveland M. Analytical toxicology. Hum Toxicol 1988;7:489–502.

cology are listed in Table 2–9.[24] A flow chart for a toxicologic screening specimen is depicted in Figure 2–1. Quantification and proper sampling times are summarized in Table 2–10.[26] Gaudreault and Timberlake have compared the relative specificity, sensitivity, and speed of processing of different laboratory techniques (Table 2–11).[26]

CLINICAL INFORMATION

The clinician should provide patient information to the clinical laboratory as follows:

1. Be specific.
2. List all possible drugs and medications.
3. Give patient information: vital signs, loss of consciousness, behavioral abnormalities.
4. Provide laboratory results already available.
5. List medications used chronically or used in the emergency care of the patient.

Optimal times for a toxicology screen are on arrival and again in several hours. The emergency department physician will benefit from meeting with laboratory personnel and learning which tests to order, when results are needed, how soon they can be available, whether the test should be quantitative or qualitative, when the specimen should be obtained, what type of specimen should be sent, and the nature and sensitivity of the methodology employed. Immunoassays are employed in screening urine for drugs of abuse (Table 2–12).[24]

DIFFICULTIES

Some compounds may be active in low quantities. A toxicology screen does not detect some that are heat labile and break apart before detection (LSD, psilocybin); some that are distributed to a compartment other than the one being tested (pesticides, LSD); some that evaporate in the extraction or concentration phase (solvents); and some that are inorganic, too polar, and are missed in analysis (Hg, P). Many drugs are quickly metabolized and only the metabolites are detected, and some are difficult to detect (haloperidol, oxycodone).

TECHNIQUES

TOXICOLOGY SCREENS

The use of toxicology testing as a broad screen without an understanding of its limitations is hazardous. The toxicology screen has good specificity. *Specificity* is the percentage of patients in whom toxic substances are present but will be reported as negative. (Good specificity means that the test gives few false-positive results.) Its sensitivity, however, is poor, as many patients in whom toxic substances are present are not detected with the toxicology screen. *Sensitivity* is the portion of true-positive results reported as positive. (A high-sensitivity test gives few false-negative results.) The predictive value of a negative test (ie, the portion of negative results that are truly negative) is about 40%. Improvement of the sensitivity and predictive value of the screen requires attention to the analytical methods used, good clinical communication between physician and laboratory, proper specimen collection, and an understanding of the limitations and value of specific tests.[27]

Limitations

Toxicology laboratories use several methods to screen for toxins, because there is no single, accurate, inexpensive method that detects all toxins. Each method differs in cost, accuracy, complexity, speed, and specificity (Table 2–12). Individual test reliability depends on expertise of the analyst, equipment, method, and number of requests processed. Problems arise from the changes that occur in the storage of biologic fluids, the transfer of drugs from tube to tube, and the standards used to test drugs. Deterioration of gas–liquid chromatograph columns produces unknown residues, and ionization of gases may cause the breakdown of chemicals. In addition, labile metabolites undergo chemical changes depending on the analytical technique employed. Hence, familiarity with specific laboratory requirements, processes, and limitations is critical to the proper utilization of the laboratory. To interpret toxicology screen results, the following questions are important:

1. For each drug category, which method is used and what is its specificity?
2. What chemicals are detected by the toxicology screen, and what varieties of screens are available (eg, coma panel, drugs of abuse, seizure panel)?
3. What information is required on the request form?
4. Which samples are best for each specific analysis?
5. Which tests are qualitative, which are quantitative, and how quickly are the results returned?

Comparison of Analytical Screening Methods

Chromatography, the most frequently used analytical technique, involves a separation method based on the flow of a mobile liquid or gas over a solid or stationary phase containing the unknown. Immunoassays (enzyme multiple immunoassay technique, radioimmunoassay) are sensitive techniques less specific than chromatographic or mass spectrometry methods.

Table 2–12
Some Immunoassays Employed in Screening for Drugs of Abuse in Urine

Technique	Manufacturer	Drug/Drug Group	Limit of Sensitivity* (mg/L)
Agglutination inhibition	Roche Agglutex	LSD	0.0005
Enzyme-multiplied (mediated) immunoassay technique	Syva EMIT-dau	Opiates	0.3
		Amphetamine	0.3
		Barbiturates	0.3
		Benzodiazepines	0.3 (diazepam)
		Cannabinoids	0.02–0.1†
		Cocaine‡	0.3
		Dextropropoxyphene	1.0
		Methadone	0.3
		Methaqualone	0.3
		Opiates	0.5
		Phencyclidine	0.075
Fluorescence polarization immunoassay	Abbot TDx	Amphetamine	0.3
		Barbiturates	0.5
		Benzodiazepines	0.2 (nordiazepam)
		Cannabinoids	0.025†
		Cocaine‡	0.3
		Opiates	0.2
		Phencyclidine	0.075
	Perkin-Elmer	Amphetamine	1.0
		Barbiturates	2.0
		Benzodiazepines	1.0 (diazepam)
		Cocaine‡	1.0
		Methadone	1.5
		Morphine	1.0
		Opiates	1.0
Hemagglutination inhibition	Boehringer Technam	Opiates	0.05
		Cocaine‡	0.1
		Methadone	0.25
		Opiates	0.2
Radioimmunoassay	Diagnostic Products	Amphetamine	0.25
		Barbiturates	0.1
		Buprenorphine	0.001
		Cannabinoids	0.1
		Cocaine‡	0.1
		Methadone	0.005–0.5
		Morphine	0.005
		Opiates	0.05
		Phencyclidine	0.001–0.25
	Janssen	Alfentanil	0.0001
		Carfentanil	0.0001
		Fentanyl	0.0001
	Roche Abuscreen	Amphetamine	1.0
		Barbiturates	0.2
		Benzodiazepines	0.1
		Cannabinoids	0.1
		Cocaine‡	0.3
		LSD	0.00025
		Methaqualone	0.75
		Opiates	0.3
		Phencyclidine	0.025

*As suggested by the manufacturers but can be varied especially with radioimmunoassay.
†As 11-nor-δ-8-tetrahydrocannabinol-9-carboxylic acid.
‡As benzoylecgonine.
From Flanagan, Widdop B, Ramsey JD, Loveland M. Analytical toxicology. Hum Toxicol 1988;7:489–502.

Thin-Layer Chromatography

A simple, inexpensive technique effective for qualitative screening, but not for quantitative measurements, is thin-layer chromatography (TLC). Separation results from absorption or partition as the mobile solvent moves across the stationary sorbent phase (usually silicic acid or aluminum oxide). For each substance a characteristic amount of migration occurs after the test specimen is applied to the base with the liquid solvent system. Tests take 2 hours and must be interpreted carefully by experienced technicians.

There are commercially available thin-layer chromatographic systems that chromatographically screen for drugs with less performance expertise than required for standard thin-layer chromatography.

Ultraviolet Spectrophotometry

Ultraviolet spectrophotometry (UVS) is an easy, economical, and quantitative test that can detect toxic blood acetaminophen and salicylate levels as well as elevated urine phenothiazine levels. Interference by multiple-drug ingestion, however, seriously impairs its accuracy and currently restricts its use.

Gas–Liquid Chromatography

Gas–liquid chromatography (GLC) is a sophisticated but somewhat slow method that is highly accurate and specific. Liquid or dissolved solid specimens are injected into the column and vaporized by heat. Inert gases carry the specimen out of the column where chemical detectors record the emergence of the specimen as a function of time. The comparison of retention times and peak areas with known standards allows identification and quantitation. This method is effective for quantitation of blood levels of volatile liquids (methanol, ethanol, ethylene glycol).

High-Pressure (High-Performance) Liquid Chromatography

High-pressure (high-performance) liquid chromatography (HPLC) is similar in speed, specificity, and expense to gas–liquid chromatography, but is not restricted to volatile compounds. Complex compounds, including conjugated metabolites, are well separated by facilitating the movement of specimens with high pressures (1000–6000 psi).

Radioimmunoassay

Radioimmunoassay is the slowest, most expensive method, but it has good accuracy. Mixing known quantities of drug-specific antibody and known amounts of radioactively labeled drug allows analysis of the precipitate with a gamma counter. The amount of emittance inversely correlates with the presence of assayed drug. This test is excellent for detection of drugs in extremely low blood concentrations (cannabis, lysergic acid diethylamide [LSD], digoxin, paraquat).

Enzyme-Mediated Immunoassay

A fast, expensive, and simple method with intermediate accuracy and specificity, the enzyme-mediated immunoassay (EMIT) system, works on the basis that the amount of drug present is proportional to the inhibition of an enzyme–substrate reaction. A known quantity of drug is labeled by chemical attachment to an enzyme. Drug-specific antibodies added to the specimen bind the drug–enzyme complex, thereby reducing enzyme activity. Free drug in the specimen competes with enzyme-labeled drug and limits the antibody-induced enzyme inactivation. Enzyme activity correlates with drug concentration in the specimen as measured by absorbance changes resulting from the enzyme's catalytic action on a substrate. EMIT is preferred over other radioimmunoassay methods in the emergency situation because of its simplicity and speed in providing information on toxic drug concentrations. EMIT eliminates the complex separation phase necessary in radioimmunoassays. The two systems are EMIT-st (single test), consisting of a compact spectrophotometer, for small laboratories, and EMIT-dau (drugs of abuse) for larger hospitals. Negative tests do not exclude the ingestion of a drug that may be present in undetectable quantities.

Antibody cross-reactions that can produce false-positive screens include the following[28]:

- Narcotics
  - Poppy seeds
  - Dextromethorphan
  - Chlorpromazine
  - Diphenoxylate
- Amphetamines
  - Ephedrine
  - Phenylephrine
  - Pseudoephedrine
  - *N*-Acetylprocainamide
  - Chloroquine
  - Procainamide
- Phencyclidine
  - Dextromethorphan
  - Diphenhydramine
  - Chlorpromazine
  - Doxylamine
  - Thioridazine

The most common cause of a genuinely false-positive result is antibody cross-reactivity with a substance bearing some structural similarity to the drug including poppy seeds, which may contain opium congeners, resulting in a drug screen that is positive for opiates. Also common is the ability of nasal decongestants such as ephedrine and phenylpropanolamine to produce a urine drug screen that is positive for amphetamines. Cross-reactivity may occur; phenmetrazine and L-ephedrine may produce such a positive result.

Causes of False Negative Screen

The reasons for a false-negative test can be divided into three general categories: technologic shortcomings, toxicokinetic characteristics, and intentional specimen alteration or adulteration, and are as follows:

Technological shortcomings
- Drug screen does not seek the drug
- Structural dissimilarity from drug class prototype, e.g., fentanyl
- Poor laboratory quality assurance

Toxicokinetic characteristics
- Large volume of distribution
- Short elimination half-life

Intentional specimen alteration or adulteration
- Use of a colleague's "clean" urine
- Use of a fluid other than urine
- Drinking excessive fluids
- Use of a diuretic
- Addition of bleach, caustics, golden seal tea, lemon juice, salt, soap, or vinegar to urine

Atomic Absorption Spectrophotometry

Atomic absorption spectrophotometry is the usual method for detecting inorganic agents (eg, lead, mercury, thallium, cadmium), but is not suitable as a screening technique. Hence most toxicology screens do not detect heavy metals. Inductively coupled plasma atomic emission spectroscopy (ICP-AES) is a new method that allows simultaneous multielement analysis useful for the industrial workplace. ICP-AES quantitatively measures 17 elements (aluminum, barium, cadmium, chromium, copper, iron, lanthanum, lead, manganese, molybdenum, nickel, platinum, silver, strontium, tin, titanium, zinc) from a single sample.[29]

Gas Chromatography–Mass Spectrometry

Probably the best technique with which to determine the presence of a chemical is gas chromatography–mass spectrometry (GC-MS), but the high capital equipment and operating costs limit its use to reference centers.

QUANTITATIVE BLOOD LEVELS

Drugs whose blood levels may be useful in the management of poisoning include acetaminophen, salicylates, carboxyhemoglobin, methemoglobin, methanol, ethylene glycol, lithium, iron, paraquat, digoxin, theophylline, and organophosphates. Specific use is discussed in this text.

URINE LEVELS

Urine samples are preferred when the blood concentration of the compound is too low for detection by conventional means. Such drugs usually either are rapidly eliminated or have large volumes of distribution. Examples are phenothiazines, barbiturates, benzodiazepines, sedative–hypnotic agents, tricyclic antidepressants, and antihistamines.

URINE COLOR

The differential diagnosis of substances that color the urine is given in Figure 2–2.

RADIOGRAPHS

Nelson and colleagues used an in vitro model to show that preparations found to be consistently radiopaque were matrix tablet preparations containing brompheniramine or chlorpheniramine and any preparation containing ferrous sulfate or potassium chloride (Table 2–13). A number of enteric-coated and sustained-release preparations previously thought to be radiopaque were negative in this study (eg, Ecotrin, Theo-Dur). Several others were unexpectedly positive (Donnatal Extentabs, Entex-LA, Procan SR, Proventil Repetabs, Quinidex Extentabs, Trinalin Repetabs, and Tussionex); all of these were matrix dissolution tablet formulations with the exception of Procan SR (matrix diffusion tablet) and Tussionex (ion-exchange tablet). Most modified release medications and transdermal patches are not radiopaque.[32] Chewable Pepto-Bismol tablets contain bismuth subsalicylate and may be radiopaque.[33] Medications known to form bezoars and their opacities are listed in Table 2–14.

ULTRASOUND

Diphenhydramine, theophylline, propoxyphene, and phenobarbital (substances previously shown to be poorly visualized on plain radiography) are easily detected by ultrasound. Ferrous sulfate, enteric-coated aspirin, and chloral hydrate are also detected. Preliminary data suggest that ultrasound may be useful in confirming suspected ingestions of certain nonradiopaque substances; determining success of attempts at gastric decontamination of such substances; assessing the number of pills ingested; and assessing toxic ingestions in situations where radiography may be contraindicated (eg, pregnant women). Further studies are required to determine the potential clinical application of ultrasound.[34,35]

HYPOCALCEMIA

Hypocalcemia is more frequently observed after poisoning with hydrogen fluoride, oxalates, ethylene glycol, and organic tin compounds and is often observed in critically ill patients in association with cardiovascular or neuromuscular insufficiency.

CRYSTALLURIA

Crystalluria may follow poisoning with sulfonamide, carbon tetrachloride, primidone, and ampicillin. Massive crystalluria is most commonly associated with the ingestion of oxalates or ethylene glycol.

LABORATORY PERSONNEL

Drugs involved in common poisonings of laboratory and health care personnel include barbiturates, carbon monoxide, cyanide, sodium azide, and methemoglobin-inducing chemicals. Diagnosis of such poisoning is summarized in Table 2–15.[36]

NEUROBEHAVIORAL TESTING

Neurobehavioral test batteries are often used to evaluate the central nervous system effects of known or suspected neurotoxins in groups of subjects who have been exposed to occupational and environmental chemicals. Application to specific patients is often difficult. For many of the tests, controlled studies on which to base sensitivity and specificity are not available. Some tests of possible encephalopathy secondary to exposure to toxic chemicals are summarized in Table 2–16.[37]

Such testing must be complemented by a detailed medical history, personal history, occupational history, complete physical and neurologic examinations, and specific tests for suspected neurotoxicants.

HAIR

Reports on detection of drugs of abuse in human hair have appeared for opiates, cocaine, benzoylecgonine, morphine, phencyclidine, methadone, methamphetamine, caffeine, nicotine, phenobarbital, haloperidol, digoxin, antidepressants, chloroquine, and desethylchloroquine (Table 2–17).[38]

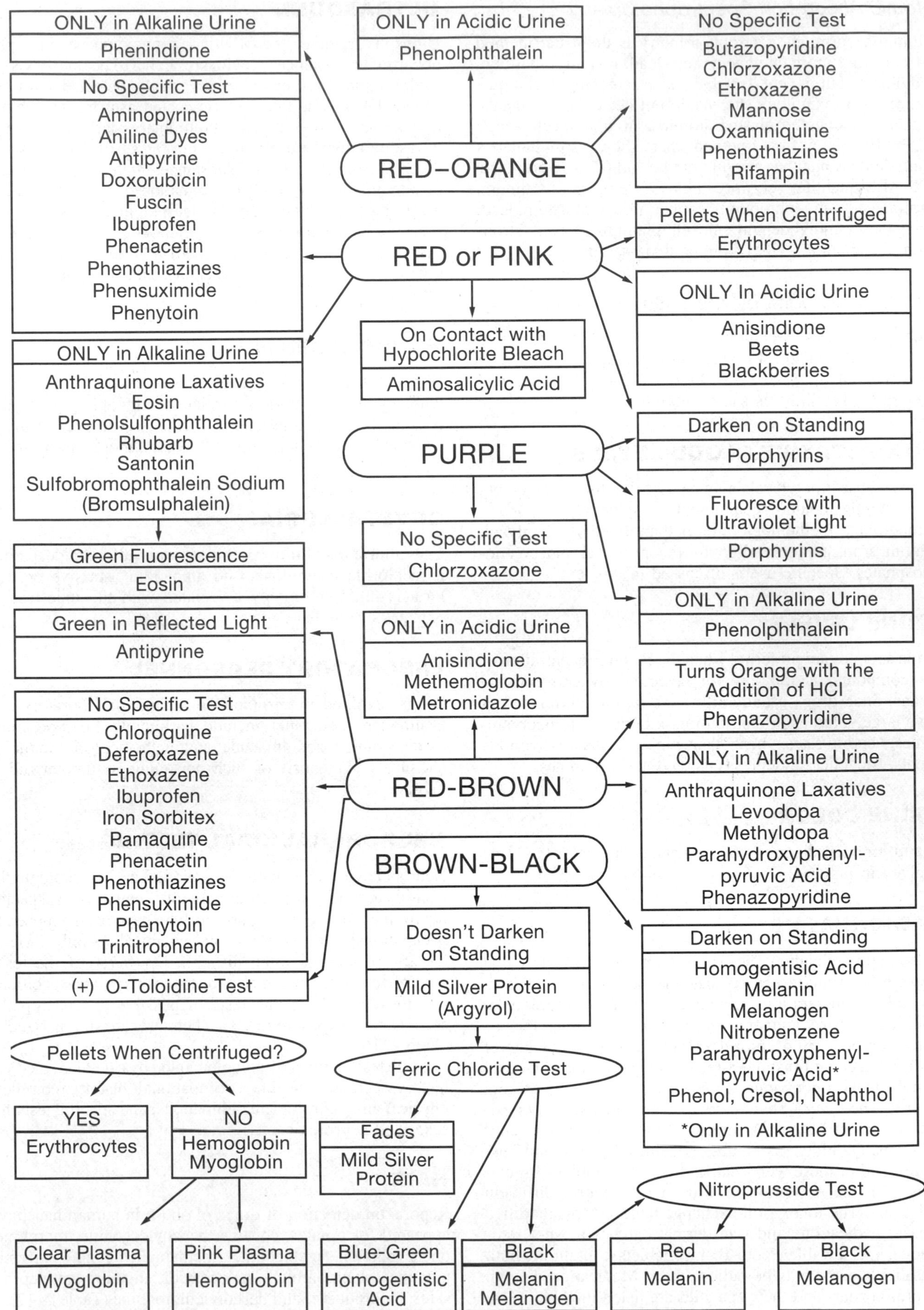

Figure 2–2 Algorithm for differential diagnosis of colored urine. (From Raymond JR, Yarger WE. South Med J 1988;81:837–841.)

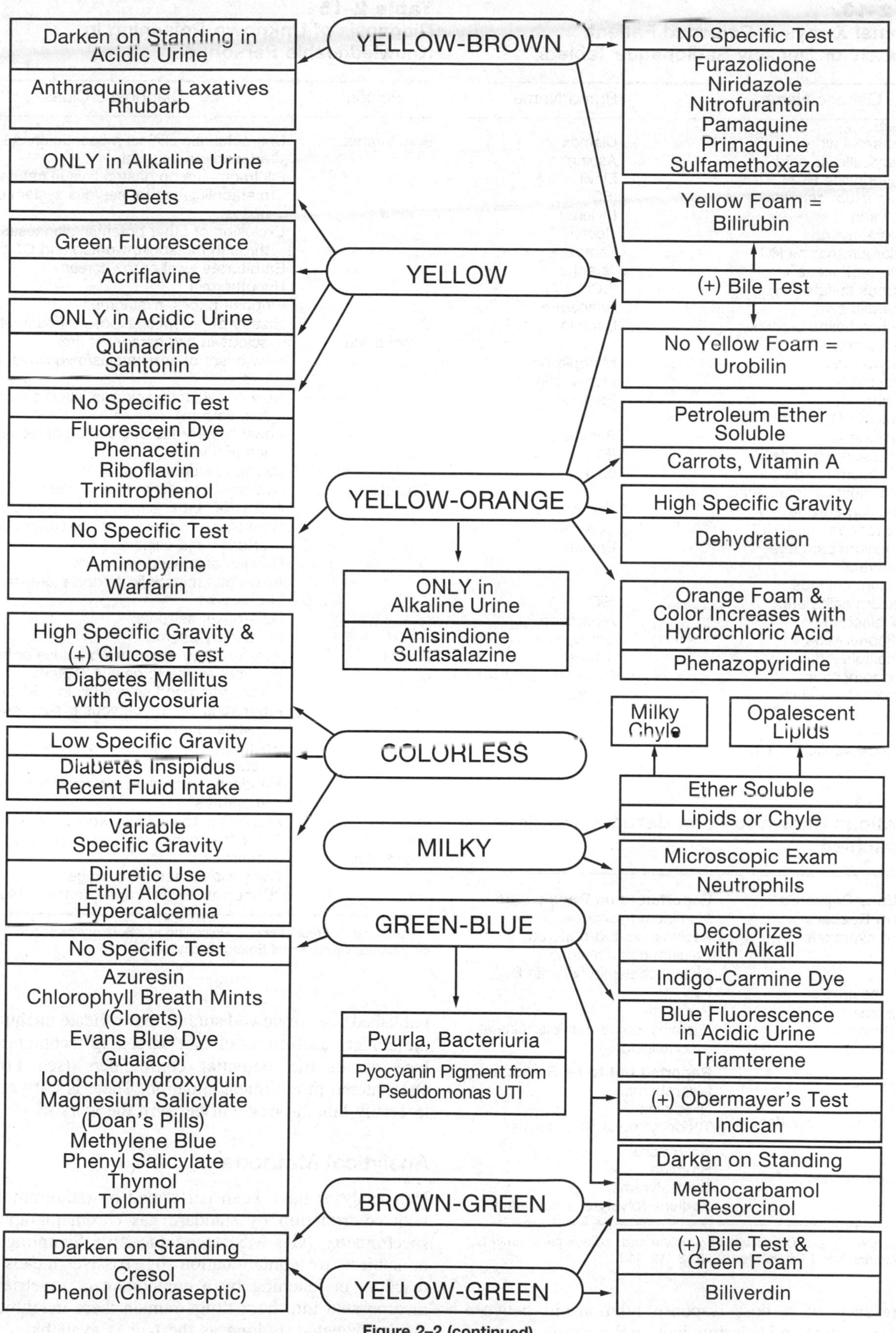

Figure 2–2 (continued)

Table 2–13
Abdominal X-rays in Poisoned Patient: Moderately or Densely Radiopaque Tablets*

Generic Name	Brand Name
Acetazolamide	Diamox
Acetylsalicylic acid	Aspirin
Amitriptyline HCl	Elavil
Ammonium chloride	(EC)
Busulfan	Myleran
Chloral hydrate	Noctec
Chloropromazine HCl	Thorazine
Chlorprothixene	Taractan
Ferrous sulfate	(EC)
Iopanoic acid	Telepaque
Methantheline bromide	Banthine
Methotrexate	
Metyrapone	Metopirone
Mystatin	Mycostatin
Pancreatin	Panteric
Penicillin G	
Penicillin K	PenVee K
Potassium chloride	(EC)
Potassium iodide	(EC)
Potassium permanganate	
Prochlorperazine	Compazine
Pseudoephedrine HCl	Sudafed
Pyrvinium pamoate	Provan
Quadrinal	
Sodium chloride	
Sodium salicylate	(EC)
Spirolactone	Aldactone
Trifluoperazine	Stelazine
Trihexiphenidyl	Artane
Triiodothyronine	Cytomel
Vitamins—Multiple	Sigtab
Vitamins—Prenatal	

*See also References 30 and 31.

Table 2–14
Medications Known to Form Bezoars and Their Radiopacities

Medications Reported to Form Bezoars	
Aluminum hydroxide	**Reported to be Radiopaque**
Aspirin	Aluminum hydroxide
Bromide	Aspirins, coated/buffered
Calcium phosphate	Calcium combinations
Cholestyramine	Cyanocobalamin (vitamin B_{12})
Cyanocobalamin (vitamin B_{12})	Iron
Iron	Sucralfate
Meprobamate	Vitamins, some multiple/mineral-containing
Nifedipine	**Reported not to be Radiopaque**
Sodium polystyrene sulfonate	Meprobamate
Sucralfate	Nifedipine
Theophylline, sustained-release	Theophylline in all its forms
Vitamin C	**No reports**
	Bromide
	Cholestyramine
	Sodium polystyrene sulfonate

From Silbergleit R, Lee DC. Bowel obstruction and radiopaque vitamin B_{12} pseudobezoars. Am J Emerg Med 1995;13:112–113.

The presence of a dose–response relationship between administered dose and hair drug level and the time course of drug appearance in hair have not yet been demonstrated.[39] The American College of Occupational Medicine Committee on Occupational Medical Practice is not aware of any

Table 2–15
Diagnosis of Unknown Poisoning in Knowledgeable Personnel

Poison	Diagnostic Clues
Barbiturates	Characteristic clinical presentation in knowledgeable personnel
	Pill fragments on gastric lavage (refutes other metabolics/central nervous system diagnoses).
	Exclusion of other potential diagnoses through metabolic workup and CT scanning
	Barbiturate level or tox screen
	Hypothermia
	Pinpoint pupils, nystagmus
Carbon monoxide	History of potential exposure (found unconscious in car, garage, at fire)
	New onset of arrhythmias/myocardial ischemia
	New-onset lactic acidosis, altered mental status, seizure
	Equal "cherry-red" coloration of retinal arteries and veins
	Oxygen saturation gap > 5%
Cyanide	Availability to victim in workplace or home
	Aroma of "bitter almonds" to gastric aspirate
	Unexplained "cherry-red" coloration of retinal arteries and veins
	Oxygen saturation gap > 5%
	Anion gap metabolic acidosis (unexplained)
	Fire victims
	New-onset seizures
	Pulmonary edema
Azides	Availability to victim in workplace or home
	Pungent aroma to gastric aspirate
	Unexplained and severe lactic acidosis
	Alternating central nervous system restlessness and atony
	Positive ferric chloride testing of gastric aspirate (red precipitate)
	Headache and nausea in resuscitation team members
Methemoglobin-inducing chemicals	Availability to victim in workplace or home
	Bitter "petrochemical" smell of certain chemicals
	Cyanosis refractory to oxygen
	"Chocolate brown" appearance of blood

From Binder L, Fredrickson L. Poisoning in laboratory personnel and health care professionals. Am J Emerg Med 1991;9:11–15.

published peer-reviewed studies that validate unequivocally the clinical usefulness of hair screening techniques in the face of all the potential confounders (see Problems) encountered in a clinical situation. There is not yet a body to certify laboratories that perform the work.[40]

Analytical Methods

Hair analyses have been performed by radioimmunoassay with confirmation by standard gas chromatography–mass spectrometry (GC–MS) techniques.[41,42] Sampling of hair is subject to contamination by passive means, cross-reaction, or leaching by a component of toiletries. Once incorporated into hair, drugs remain there indefinitely and can be detected as long as the hair is available. A 1½-in. sample of hair may permit the detection of drugs used anytime in the previous 3 months.[43] It may be possible, depending on hair length, to trace the drug intake of an

Table 2–16
Tests Commonly Used in Clinical Assessment of Possible Encephalopathy Secondary to Exposure to Toxic Chemicals (Boston Extended Neurotoxicologic Battery—Clinical)

Domain	Description	Implications
General Intellect		
Wechsler IQ tests (WAIS-R, WISC, WPPSI)	Omnibus IQ measures	Overall level of cognitive function compared with population norms
Peabody Picture Vocabulary Test	Single word comprehension	Robust measure of verbal intelligence in adults, can be sensitive to exposure in children
Stanford–Binet	Omnibus IQ measure	Similar to Wechsler tests
Wide Range Achievement Test—Revised	Academic skills in arithmetic, spelling, reading	Robust estimate of premorbid ability patterns in adults, can be sensitive to exposure in children
Attention, Executive Functioning		(Attention and executive functioning tasks are sensitive to many types of exposure)
Digit Span (WAIS-R)	Digits forward and backward	Measures simple attention and cognitive tracking
Arithmetic (Wechsler tests)	Oral calculations	Assesses attention, tracking, and calculation
Trail Making Test	Connect-a-dot task requiring sequencing and alternating sequences	Measures attention, sequencing, visual scanning, speed of processing
Continuous Performance Test	Acknowledgment of occurrence of critical stimuli in a series of orally or visually presented stimuli	Assesses attention
Paced Auditory Serial Addition	Serial calculation test	Sensitive measure of attention and tracking speed
Wisconsin Card Sorting Test	Requires subject to infer decision-making rules	Tests ability to think flexibly
Verbal, Language		(Language tests are sometimes sensitive to exposure in children but are usually robust in adult exposure, except as noted)
Information (Wechsler tests)	Information usually learned in school	Robust estimate of native abilities in adults
Vocabulary (Wechsler tests)	Verbal vocabulary definitions	Fairly robust estimate of verbal intelligence although sensitive to concreteness associated with brain damage (including toxic encephalopathy)
Comprehension (Wechsler tests)	Proverb definitions, social judgment, problem solving	Sensitive to reasoning skills; can be impaired after exposure to neurotoxicants
Similarities (Wechsler tests)	Inference of similarities between nominative words	Sensitive to reasoning skills; can be impaired after exposure to neurotoxicants
Controlled Oral Word Association	Word list generation within alphabetical or semantic categories	Assesses flexibility, planning, arousal, processing speed, ability to generate strategies, somewhat sensitive to exposure
Boston Naming Test	Naming of objects depicted in line drawings	Sensitive to aphasia, also sensitive to native verbal processing deficits or those acquired through childhood exposure
Reading Comprehension (Boston Diagnostic Aphasia Exam)	A direct screening test of simple reading comprehension	Sensitive to moderate-to-severe dyslexia, usually insensitive to toxic exposure in adults
Writing Sample	Patient writes to dictation or describes a picture	Assesses graphomotor skills, spelling
Visuospatial, Visuomotor		(Visuospatial and visuomotor tasks are frequently sensitive to exposure in adults and children)
Picture Completion (Wechsler tests)	Identification of missing details in line drawing	Measures perceptual analysis
Digit Symbol (Wechsler tests)	Coding task requiring matching symbols to digits	Complex task assessing motor speed, visual scanning, working memory
Picture Arrangement (Wechsler tests)	Sequencing of cartoon frames to represent meaningful stories	Measures visual sequencing, ability to infer relationships from visuospatial/social stimuli
Block Design (Wechsler tests)	Assembly of 3D blocks to replicate 2D representations of designs	Assesses abstract visual construction ability and planning
Object Assembly (Wechsler tests)	Assembly of puzzles	Measure of concrete visual constructional skills, Gestalt recognition
Boston Visuospatial Quantitative Battery	Drawings of common objects spontaneously and to copy	Measures constructional abilities, motor functioning

(continued)

Table 2–16 *(Continued)*

Domain	Description	Implications
Boston Visuospatial Quantitative Battery	Drawing of common objects spontaneously and to copy	Measures constructional abilities, motor functioning
Hooper Visual Organization Test	Identification of correct outline of drawings of cut up objects	Sensitive to Gestalt integration processing
Rey–Osterreith Complex Figure (copy condition)	Drawing of a complicated abstract visual design	Sensitive to deficits in visuospatial planning and construction
Santa Ana Formboard Test	Knobs in a formboard are turned 180° with each hand individually and both hands together	Measures motor speed and coordination
Finger tapping	Speed of tapping with each index finger	Sensitive to lateralized manual motor speed
Memory		(New learning and retention are often sensitive to toxicants; retrograde memory of prior events is more complexly related to exposure)
Logical Memories—Immediate and Delayed Recall (IR, DR) (Wechsler Memory Scales)	Recall of paragraph information read orally on an immediate and 20-minute delayed recall	Sensitive to new learning and retention of newly learned information
Verbal Paired Associate Learning, IR, DR (Wechsler Memory Scales)	Two paired words are presented in a list of pairs; subject must recall second word; test is presented on immediate and delayed recall	Measures abstract verbal list learning, retention
Figural Memory (Wechsler Memory Scales)	Multiple choice recognition of visual designs immediately after initial presentation	Assesses visual recognition memory
Visual Paired Associate Learning, IR, DR (Wechsler Memory Scales)	Six visual designs are paired with six colors; recognition memory is tested immediately after the six are presented on learning trials and at delayed recall	Test of abstract visual learning using recognition (not recall) performance measures
Visual Reproductions, IR, DR (Wechsler Memory Scales)	Visual designs are drawn immediately after presentation and on delayed recall	Measures visual learning and retention
Delayed Recognition Span Test	Based on delayed nonmatching to sample paradigm, disks are moved about on a board to assess recognition memory for words, color, spatial locations	Assesses new learning

From White PF, Proctor SP. Research and clinical criteria for development of neurobehavioral test batteries. J Occup Med 1992(Feb.):140–48.

Table 2–17
Concentrations of Drug in Human Hair (ng/mg)

Drug	Level
Diazepam (1)*	1.37
Nordiazepam (3)	1.04–2.41
Flunitrazepam (1)	0.41
Nitrazepam (1)	0.37
Secobarbital (3)	21.6–58.9
Amobarbital (2)	31.4–41.6
Phenobarbital (4)	21.7–137.3
Amitriptyline (14)	0.04–1.89
Clomipramine (2)	0.37–0.79
Morphine (29)	0.9–27.10
Codeine (3)	0.01–4.21
Benzoylecgonine (3)	1.21–3.41
Amphetamine (3)	0.96–12.71
Fenfluramine (1)	14.1
11-nor-δ8-tetrahydro-cannibinol-9-COOH (32)	0.27–2.91
Betaxolol (5)	0.6–2.8
Nicotine (22 nonsmokers)	0.06–1.82
Nicotine (42 smokers)	0.91–33.89

*Number of cases given in parentheses
(From Kintz P, Tracqui A, Mangin P. Detection of drugs in human for clinical and forensic applications. Int J Leg Med 1992;105:1–4.)

addict over periods longer than 6 months.[44] This is largely due to the absence of drug metabolism in hair and the fairly uniform growth rate of about 1 cm per month.

Sites of Sampling

Drug concentrations differ in head hair, axillary hair, and pubic hair. In one study the highest morphine concentration was found in pubic hair, followed by head hair and axillary hair. Secretion of drugs in perspiration affects this mechanism of deposition and remains a confounding factor.[43]

Potential Uses

If strands of hair are cut into sections (1-month intervals, about 1 cm) it is possible to obtain some information on the pattern of drug use. Hair analysis may ultimately be useful in the screening of personnel in highly sensitive military aviation.[44]

Problems

Analysis of neonatal hair does not detect exposure occurring shortly before birth owing to insufficient time for the drug to enter the hair. In these instances, screening of neonatal urine may reveal the presence of the drug. Because of the relatively low concentrations of most drugs in hair (nanogram per gram quantities) and the modest amount of hair that can be removed, especially from most infants (several milligrams), extraordinarily sensitive assays such as radioimmunoassays and gas chromatography–mass spectrometry must be used. These methods are not routinely available in most clinical laboratories. They are usually not available with a turnaround time sufficient to use the information for clinical purposes. Laboratory analysis of hair is both laborious and tedious. Diffusion of drugs within hair may cause difficulties in interpretation of positive and negative results. No protocols have addressed the stability of drugs in hair, particularly in hair that has been bleached, dyed, or treated with sprays, rinses, or other preparations available to beauticians and to the public. Exposure to automobile exhaust fumes may lead to deterioration of drugs in hair.[45]

SWEAT

Drugs detected after use of a "sweat patch" include cocaine, heroin, methamphetamine, phencyclidine, and tetrahydrocannabinol.

ELECTROCARDIOGRAM

The electrocardiogram can be monitored for drug-induced arrhythmias and potassium, magnesium, and calcium disorders.[44]

BEDSIDE TESTS

Bedside tests for poisoning include odor presentation (see Chapter 1); ferric chloride screening for salicylates (if positive, do stat salicylate serum concentration); nitroprusside (Acetest) test for ketones; visual inspection of blood for red blood cell abnormalities; microscopic evaluation of urine for crystals; dipstick for rhabdomyolysis/hemolysis; use of naloxone diagnostically; chemical dipstick test for ethanol; use of a breathalyzer for ethanol, methanol, and isopropanol; and other tests not fully evaluated (acetaminophen [Chapter 10], cyanide [Chapter 66], lead salicylate [Chapter 67], theophylline [Chapter 45]).

MECONIUM DRUG ANALYSIS

Meconium drug analysis is useful for drug testing in the newborn period. The test is highly specific and sensitive. Meconium analysis can be performed with common laboratory techniques for purposes of mass screening and with capabilities for gas chromatography–mass spectrometry for confirmation. Collection of meconium is easy and noninvasive, and analysis of serial meconium samples can reflect the type, chronology, and amount of in utero drug exposure of the infant. Drugs in meconium are present up to 3 days after birth.[46]

Meconium represents the entire intestinal contents of the fetus before birth and is composed of desquamated epithelial cells from the intestines and skin, bile, pancreatic and intestinal secretions, and the residue of swallowed amniotic fluid. As swallowing can be elicited in the human fetus at about the twelfth week of gestation the deposition of drugs in meconium through fetal swallowing of amniotic fluid and fetal urine can theoretically begin at that point or soon thereafter according to postmortem drug analysis. Serial analysis of meconium may be a useful tool to determine the pattern of drug use by the mother throughout gestation.[47] Meconium is available during the first day of life.[48] Its passage may occur in the first hour of life but usually occurs by the tenth hour of life.[49–51] Preliminary studies suggest that concentrations of cocaine, benzoylecgonine,[50] and morphine in meconium correlate with the amounts of drugs used by the mother during pregnancy.[51] Nicotine metabolites (cotinine and *trans*-3′-hydroxycotinine) may provide a quantifiable measure in meconium of fetal exposure to nicotine[51] by active and passive maternal smoking. Cocaethylene, a metabolite of cocaine and ethanol (see Chapter 21), appears in the meconium. Its presence may clarify the respective roles of cocaine and ethanol in the development of the neurobehavioral abnormalities seen in the cocaine baby syndrome.[50]

DRUG TESTING IN THE WORKPLACE

Components of most drug testing programs include urine collection, shipment to a certified laboratory under chain of custody, initial screening of the urine by immunoassay, confirmation and quantitation of screened-positive specimens by gas chromatography–mass spectrometry, and reporting of positive results to a medical review officer, who then reports true positive results to the federal agency or private company (also see Chapters 19 and 25). Table 2–18 indicates initial cutoff levels for screening immunoassay. Confirmation gas chromatography–mass spectrometry cutoff levels (threshold for positive reporting) are listed in Table 2–19.[52]

Eating food that contains poppy seeds within about 24 hours of the urine collection may result in a urine test that is positive for opioids. Passive exposure to marijuana smoke may result in the appearance of marijuana metabolites in the urine.

The ingestion of several times the recommended therapeutic dose of sympathomimetic amines, such as ephedrine, pseudoephedrine, and phenylpropanolamine, may result in a positive urine test for only methamphetamine. In the case of methamphetamine ingestion, however, methamphetamine and amphetamine are detected in the urine. Some nasal

Table 2–18
Initial Cutoff Levels for a Screening Immunoassay

Drug	Initial Test Cutoff Level (ng/mL)
Marijuana metabolites	100
Cocaine metabolites	300
Opiate metabolites	300*
Phencyclidine	25
Amphetamines	1000

*25 ng/mL if the immunoassay is specific for free morphine
Source: Reference 49.

Table 2-19
Confirmatory Gas Chromatography/Mass Spectrometry Cutoff Levels

Drug	Confirmatory Test Cutoff Level (ng/mL)
Marijuana metabolite*	15
Cocaine metabolite†	150
Opiates	
Morphine	300
Codeine	300
Phencyclidine	25
Amphetamines	
Amphetamine	500
Methamphetamine	500

*δ-9-Tetrahydrocannibinol-9-carboxylic acid.
†Benzoylecgonine
Source: Reference 49.

inhalers contain *l*-methamphetamine, which results in a positive urine test for methamphetamine. A request for chiral separation of the *d* and *l* enantiomers of methamphetamine with subsequent detection of *d*-methamphetamine can rule out the nasal inhaler as a source.[53]

SALIVA

Marijuana, cocaine, phencyclidine, opiates, barbiturates, amphetamines, and benzodiazepines (or their metabolites) have all been detected in saliva by various analytic methods including immunoassay, gas chromatography–mass spectrometry, and thin-layer chromatography. Initial studies with cocaine and phencyclidine suggest a correlation between saliva and plasma concentrations of these drugs, indicating a dynamic equilibrium between saliva and blood. Tetrahydrocannabinol, the active component in marijuana, does not appear to be transferred from plasma to saliva; however, tetrahydrocannabinol is sequestered in the buccal cavity during smoking and can be detected in saliva.

Concentrations of drug are usually lower in saliva than in urine; however, assay methods now available can detect the quantities present. Saliva eliminates the issue of protection of privacy and, to a larger degree, of adulteration during sample collection. Drug concentrations in saliva provide an estimate of the actual circulating amount, and the results can be used for the determination of current intoxication. The pace of data accumulation strongly indicates a place for saliva as a useful future biological medium.[54]

REFERENCES

1. Snyder JW, Vlasses PH. The role of the laboratory in treatment of the poisoned patient. Arch Intern Med 1988;148: 279–280.
2. Brett AS. Implications of discordance between clinical impression and toxicology analysis in drug overdose. Arch Intern Med 1988;148:437–441.
3. Cridland JS. How effective are pharmacologic laboratories in big hospitals? Clin Pharmacol Ther 1994;56:117–121.
4. Di Nubile MJ. The increment in the anion gap: Overextension of a concept? Lancet 1988;2:951–953.
5. Toto RD. Metabolic acid–base disorders. In: Kokko VP, Tanner RL, eds. *Fluids and Electrolytes.* 2nd ed. Philadelphia: WB Saunders 1990:326.
6. Emmett M, Narins RG. Clinical use of the anion gap. Medicine 1977;56:38–54.
7. Oh MS, Carroll HJ. The anion gap. N Engl J Med 1977;297: 814–817.
8. Iberti TJ, Leibowitz AB, Papadokos PJ, Fisher ET. Low sensitivity of the anion gap as a screen to detect hyperlactatemia in critically ill patients. Crit Care Med 1990;18:275–277.
9. Gabow PA, Kachney WD, Fennessey PV, et al. Diagnostic importance of an increased serum anion gap. N Engl J Med 1980;303:854–858.
10. Adrogue HJ, Wilson H, Boyd AE III, et al. Plasma acid–base patterns in diabetic ketoacidosis. N Engl J Med 1982;307: 1603–1610.
11. Oh MS, Carroll HJ, Goldstein DA, Fein IA. Hyperchloremic acidosis during the recovery phase of diabetic ketosis. Ann Intern Med 1978;89:925–927.
12. Kosnett M, Larson S, McCarthy T, Osterloh J. Investigation of an anion gap of minus 88 in a patient taking bromazepam. Clin Chem 1990;36:1040.
13. Winter SD, Pearson JR, Gabow PA, et al. The fall of the serum anion gap. Arch Intern Med 1990;150:311–313.
14. Wrenn K. The delta (δ) gap. An approach to mixed acid–base disorders. Ann Emerg Med 1990;19:1310–1319.
15. Braden GL, Strayhorn CH, Germain MJ, et al. Increased osmolal gap in alcoholic acidosis. Arch Intern Med 1993;153: 2377–2380.
16. Price EA, D'Alessandro A, Kearney T, Olson KR, Blanc PD. Osmolar gap with minimal acidosis in combined methanol and methyl ethyl ketone ingestion. Clin Toxicol 1994;32(1):79–84.
17. Aabakken L, Johansen KS, Rydningen E-B, et al. Osmolal and anion gaps in patients admitted to an emergency medical department. Hum Exp Toxicol 1994;13:131–134.
18. Osterloh JD. Alcoholics and the osmolal gap: Not such a simple diagnostic puzzle. AACT Clin Toxicol Update 1994; 7(3):2.
19. American Academy of Clinical Toxicology Facility Assessment Guidelines for Regional Toxicology Treatment Centers. Clin Toxicol 1993;31:209–210.
20. Wasserberger J, Ordog GJ. Personal communication.
21. Hoffman RS. Comment. Measured serum osmolality—caution: Know your hospital lab. AACT Clin Toxicol Update. Abstract of Eisen TF, et al. Serum osmolality in alcohol ingestions: Differences in availability among laboratories of teaching hospitals, non-teaching hospitals and commercial facilities. Am J Emerg Med 1989;7:256–259.
22. Hoffman RS, Smilkstein MJ, Howland MA, Goldfrank LR. Osmolal gaps revisited: Normal values and limitations. Clin Toxicol 1993;31:81–93.
23. Aabakken L, Johansen KS, Rydningen E-R, et al. Osmolal and anion gaps in patients admitted to an emergency medical department. Hum Exp Toxicol 1994;13:131–134.
24. Flanagan RJ, Widdop B, Ramsey JD, Loveland M. Analytical toxicology. Hum Toxicol 1988;7:489–502.
25. Mahoney JD, Gross PL, Stern TA, et al. Quantitative serum toxic screening in the management of suspected drug overdose. Am J Emerg Med 1990;8:16–22.
26. Gaudreault P, Timberlake S. Toxic compounds quantification: Type of samples and proper timing. Toxic screens, Part I. Clin Toxicol Rev 1989;12(2):32.
27. Hepler BR, Sutheimer CA, Sunshine I. The role of the toxicology laboratory in emergency medicine. J Toxicol Clin Toxicol 1982;19:353–365.
28. Woolf AD, Shannon MW. Clinical toxicology for the pediatrician. Pediatr Clin North Am 1995;42:317–337.
29. Analysis of trace metals for occupationally exposed. MMWR 1984;33:664–665.
30. Savitt DL, Hawkins HH, Roberts DR. The radiopacity of ingested medications. Ann Emerg Med 1987; 16:331–339.

31. Tillman DJ, Ruggles DL, Leikin JB. Radiopacity study of extended-release formulations using digitalized radiography. Am J Emerg Med 1994;12:310–314.
32. Nelson JC, Liu D, Olson KR. Radiopacity of modified release medications. Vet Hum Toxicol 1993;35:317.
33. Woo OF, Jackson GM. Radiopacity of chewable Pepto-Bismol tablets: Report of two patients. Vet Hum Toxicol 1993;35:317.
34. Amitai Y, Silver B, Leikin JB, Frischer H. Visualization of ingested medications in the stomach by ultrasound. Am J Emerg Med 1992;10:18–23.
35. Anderson A, Share J, Woolf A. The use of ultrasound in the diagnosis of toxic ingestions. Pediatr Emerg Care 1989; 5:281.
36. Binder L, Fredrickson L. Poisoning in laboratory personnel and health care professionals. Am J Emerg Med 1991;9:11–15.
37. White PF, Proctor SP. Research and clinical criteria for development of neurobehavioral test batteries. J Occup Med 1992(Feb.):140–148.
38. McBay AJ. Hair drug testing review and update. In: Proceedings, 29th International Meeting of the International Association of Forensic Toxicologists, Copenhagen, June 1991:19–91.
39. Cone EJ. Testing human hair for drugs of abuse. I. Individual dose and time profiles of morphine and codeine in plasma, saliva, urine and beard compared to drug-induced effects on pupils and behavior. J Anal Toxicol 1990;14:1–7.
40. Anstadt GW. Occupational medicine forum: Hair analysis in drug screening. J Occup Med 1990;32:668–669.
41. Baumgartner AM, Jones PF, Baumgartner WA, Black CT. Radioimmunoassay of hair for determining opiate-abuse histories. J Nucl Med 1979;20:749–752.
42. Baumgartner WA, Hill VA, Blahd WH. Hair analysis for drugs of abuse. J Forens Sci 1989;34:1433–1453.
43. Kintz P, Tracqui A, Mangin P. Detection of drugs in human hair for clinical and forensic applications. Int J Leg Med 1992;105:1–4.
44. Shoemaker WC. What should be monitored? The past, present and future of physiological monitoring. Clin Chem 1990;36:1543–1563.
45. Bailey DN. Drug screening in an unconventional matrix: Hair analysis. JAMA 1989;262:3331.
46. Ostrea EM Jr, Knapp K, Romero A, et al. Meconium analysis to assess fetal exposure to nicotine by active and passive maternal smoking. J Pediatr 1994;124:471–476.
47. Ostrea EM Jr, Romero A, Knapp K, et al. Postmortem drug analysis of meconium in early gestation human fetuses exposed to cocaine: Clinical complications. J Pediatr 1994; 124:477–479.
48. Koren G, Klein J, Forman R, et al. Biological markers of intrauterine exposure to cocaine and cigarette smoking. Dev Pharmacol Ther 1992;18:228–233.
49. Wasserman E, Slobody LB. *Survey of Clinical Pediatrics.* 6th ed. International Students Edition. Tokyo: McGraw Hill Kogakusha, 1974.
50. Lewis D, Muldoon K, Leikin JB. Cocaethylene in meconium specimens. Vet Hum Toxicol 1993;35:350.
51. Ostrea EM Jr, Brady M, Gause S, et al. Drug screening of newborns by meconium analysis: A large-scale prospective epidemiologic study. Pediatrics 1992;89:107–113.
52. Code of Federal Regulations: Title 49, Part 40. Procedures for transportation workplace drug testing programs, 1993:528–553. Part 40.29. Laboratory analysis procedures.
53. Lee EJ, Williams KM. Chiralty. Clinical pharmacokinetic and pharmacodynamic considerations. Clin Pharmacokinet 1990; 18:339–345.
54. Schramm W, Smith RH, Craig PA, Kidwell DA. Drugs of abuse in saliva: A review. J Anal Toxicol 1992;16:1–9.

Chapter 3 Gut Decontamination

INTRODUCTION

No gastrointestinal decontamination modalities have been determined to reduce morbidity and mortality by controlled clinical studies.

HISTORICAL RECOMMENDATIONS

Recommendations for the use of methods to decontaminate the gut traditionally have relied on pharmacologic studies in animals and humans rather than on clinical studies on the efficacy and complications of these procedures. Experimental studies in the 1950s and 1960s suggested that syrup of ipecac removed more of an ingested marker (eg, 30–40% between 30 and 60 minutes postingestion) than gastric lavage.[1] For example, when administered immediately, 30 minutes, and 60 minutes after ingestion, syrup of ipecac removed 60, 40, and 20% of an ingested dose of salicylates, respectively.[2] By comparison, gastric lavage removed 45, 26, and 8%, respectively, of the salicylate marker. Based on these and similar studies, syrup of ipecac became the method of choice for treatment of childhood poisoning in the home and the alert patient in the emergency department; however, large variations in the volumes of markers recovered from patients[3] and the use of small-bore orogastric tubes in the animal studies raised questions about the superiority of syrup of ipecac. In human volunteers, gastric lavage recovered 45% of a nontoxic marker when lavage commenced 10 minutes postingestion compared with only 28% recovery after ipecac-induced emesis.[4] Although design factors favored the use of gastric lavage over syrup of ipecac in one study,[5] later studies suggested that the recovery of ingested product from lavage is superior to the recovery from syrup of ipecac.[6]

In the 1980s emergency medical personnel increasingly chose activated charcoal as the initial means of gut decontamination based on the relative lack of adverse effects and on human volunteer studies that demonstrated that activated charcoal reduced the absorption of ingested markers by approximately 50% when administered within 1 hour of ingestion. For example, in a study in human volunteers, the reduction in the absorption of an overdose of ampicillin was as follows: activated charcoal, 57%; ipecac-induced emesis, 38%; gastric lavage, 32%.[7] Several recent studies suggest that the complication rate following the use of emesis and of lavage is greater than the complication rate following the administration of activated charcoal.[8,9] These studies suggest that activated charcoal may be the only decontamination measure needed to treat an overdose,[10] but more studies of serious overdoses are necessary to provide numerical data on toxicokinetics and clinical assessment, to define the optimal measures required to reduce the absorption of ingested drugs.

CURRENT RECOMMENDATIONS

The seminal studies of Saetta et al.[11,12] and Merigian and co-workers[13] have questioned prior approaches to gut decontamination such as syrup of ipecac and gastric lavage.[1–3,14] In adults, many of whom present to the emergency department only 3 to 4 hours after ingestion, a "do nothing approach" may appear to have merit. Dangers inherent in this approach center on the often unreliable history from the suicidal patient, the need for some additional controlled studies to substantiate these approaches, and the possibly distasteful medicolegal consequences of the minimalist approach.

Boston Group

A number of groups have attempted to systematize the approach to gastric and intestinal decontamination. The Boston group (Lovejoy, Shannon, Woolf) has proposed suggestions for general treatment of overdose in children in busy emergency departments[1]:

1. In the symptomatic but alert child with a minor ingestion presenting to the emergency department, activated charcoal alone (for drugs absorbed by activated charcoal) by mouth appears to be sufficient for gastrointestinal decontamination.
2. For the obtunded or comatose child with a potentially serious overdose, lavage followed by activated charcoal via an orogastric or nasogastric tube should be instituted within 1 to 2 hours of ingestion (or longer in the case of sustained-release drugs, gastric concretions, or delayed gastric emptying). Repetitive dosing of activated charcoal should be used when indicated by the substance ingested.
3. For the asymptomatic child who has ingested a minimal amount in the emergency department setting, there is now *initial* information to suggest that relatively little is gained by any removal procedure. Clearly, careful assessment for a sufficiently long period, however, is absolutely necessary. The asymptomatic patient presenting early may in fact have ingested a very large overdose of a toxic substance or may not be forthcoming with a reliable history. In these instances, charcoal should be used. The use of activated charcoal probably is sufficient if the ingested substance is adsorbed by activated charcoal (Table 3–1).[15] Children can be observed for about 2 hours in the emergency department without an

Table 3–1
Adsorption of Drugs and Other Substances to Activated Charcoal in Vitro

Well Adsorbed	Moderately Adsorbed	Poorly or Clinically Inadequately Adsorbed
Aflatoxins	Aspirin and other salicylates	Cyanide
Amphetamine	DDT	Ethanol
Antidepressants	Disopyramide	Ethylene glycol
Antiepileptics	Kerosene, benzene, dichlorethane	Iron
Antihistamines	Malathion	Lithium
Atropine	Many "high-dose" nonsteroidal antiinflammatory drugs, tolfenamic acid	Methanol
Barbiturates	Mexiletine	Strong acids and alkalis
Benzodiazepines	Paracetamol (acetaminophen)	
Beta blocking agents	Polychlorinated biphenyl compounds	
Chloroquine and primaquine	Phenol	
Cimetidine	Syrup of ipecacuanha	
Dapsone	Tolbutamide, chlorpropamide, carbutamide, tolazamide	
Dextropropoxyphene and other opioids		
Digitalis glycosides		
Ergot alkaloids		
Furosemide		
Glibenclamide and glipizide		
Glutethimide		
Indomethacin		
Meprobamate		
Nefopam		
Phenothiazines		
Phenylbutazone		
Phenylpropanolamine		
Piroxicam		
Quinidine and quinine		
Strychnine		
Tetracyclines		
Theophylline		

From Neuvonen PJ, Olkolla KT. Oral activated charcoal in the treatment of intoxications: Role of single and repeated dose. Med Toxicol 1988;3:33–58.

intervention (syrup of ipecac, gastric lavage, cathartics, activated charcoal) and sent home if they are asymptomatic unless there is evidence of ingestion of substantial quantities of a toxic drug. Activated charcoal (50–100 g in adults; 15–30 g in children) should be administered to a patient who has ingested a substantial overdose of a toxic substance less than 1 hour before examination.

4. For the overdose patient in the home setting, compliance with the use of charcoal remains problematic. No study has compared ipecac-induced emesis to observation alone in the home setting, and until that study is carried out, ipecac, as recommended by poison centers or pediatricians, is the logical approach.[16,17]
5. The use of repetitive doses of activated charcoal depends on specific and proved efficacy of this method in removing the drug ingested.
6. Syrup of ipecac should now be abandoned in the hospital as there is little evidence of efficacy even in volunteer studies. Furthermore, the complications that follow the use of syrup of ipecac even in conscious patients, particularly aspiration pneumonia, combined with the diagnostic difficulties that ensue as its effects mimic those of many overdoses, are further compelling reasons to reconsider its role.[18]

SYRUP OF IPECAC

The lack of prospective studies on the clinical outcome of decontamination measures and the lack of efficacy of syrup of ipecac in pharmacologic studies beyond 60 to 90 minutes postingestion have resulted in the increased use of activated charcoal as an alternative to syrup of ipecac.[19] An endoscopic study of overdose patients indicated that neither syrup of ipecac nor lavage removes all intragastric solids, including tablets.[12] The use of syrup of ipecac often delays the administration of activated charcoal in the emergency department,[20] but the administration of activated charcoal via nasogastric tube 10 minutes after a dose of syrup of ipecac does not alter the efficacy of ipecac in volunteers.[21]

INDICATIONS

Administration of syrup of ipecac is recommended for alert patients who would benefit from emesis and who have no contraindication to the use of syrup of ipecac. The use of emesis to reduce absorption usually is not effective more than 4–6 hours after ingestion, unless the toxin itself delays absorption. Additional factors that may delay absorption include food in the stomach, other drugs (anticholinergics, narcotics, ganglionic blockers, aluminum hydroxide), and associated alterations in clinical status (e.g., pain, ulcer, ileus, acute abdomen, trauma, myocardial infarction).

DOSE

For infants 6 to 12 months of age, the dose is 5 to 10 mL plus 15 mL of clear fluids per kilogram body weight.

For children 12 months to 12 years of age, the dose is 15 mL plus 240 mL (8 oz) of clear fluids. In children 1 to 5 years of age, 30 mL of syrup of ipecac reduced the mean time to emesis by 10 minutes (15 versus 25 minutes) compared with 15 mL of syrup of ipecac. Although six episodes of repeated vomiting occurred in the group of children who received 30 mL (none in the group given 15 mL), all patients were asymptomatic by 60 minutes postadministration.[22]

For those over 12 years of age, the dose is 30 mL plus 240 to 480 mL (8–16 oz) of clear fluids. The same dosage may be repeated in 20 to 30 minutes if vomiting has not occurred. The decision to lavage when syrup of ipecac fails to induce vomiting should be based on the need to remove the toxin, as therapeutic doses of syrup of ipecac are not cardiotoxic. Excessive administration of fluids may increase absorption because of the increased tablet dissolution and propulsion of the toxin into the duodenum. Dilution is effective only for corrosive ingestions. Motion does not decrease the time to vomiting, and milk increases the time to emesis (incidence remains the same, probably by delaying gastric emptying).[23] Although the official shelf-life of syrup of ipecac is 5 years, a substantial decrease in potency after 5 years has not been documented.[24]

CONTRAINDICATIONS

Relative

Seizure-inducing drugs, rapid coma-inducing agents, sustained-release theophylline, pregnancy, bleeding diathesis, excessive emesis, serious heart disease, poorly absorbed hydrocarbons, and anticipated use of whole-bowel irrigation are relative contraindications to use of ipecac.

Additional relative contraindications include situations in which too much time has elapsed since the ingestion or the patient has already vomited; the substance ingested has a tendency to cause bradycardia (digitalis, beta blocker, calcium channel blockers); and the patient is very young or very old. The vomiting caused by ipecac may produce or potentiate bradycardia through vagal effects.[25]

Absolute

Absolute contraindications include children under 6 months of age (although there are few clinical data to support this), comatose or seizing patients, corrosive substances, absent or impaired gag reflex, and coingestion of sharp solid objects. Absolute contraindications can also include nontoxic ingestions (eg, single berry or leaf ingestions, vitamins without iron, acetaminophen ingestions under 100 m/kg, some antibiotics, and Ex-Lax ingestion), and ingestions causing altered mental status (antihistamines, opioids, benzodiazepines, ethanol, cyclic antidepressants, phenothiazines), and/or seizures.[25]

There are no good studies in humans either to support or to refute the use of ipecac later than 60 minutes after an ingestion.[25] There are few controlled studies to support the efficacy of ipecac even when administered within minutes of drug ingestion.[26]

INAPPROPRIATE USE OF IPECAC

Wrenn and colleagues found that the most common inappropriate use of ipecac in children was for ingestion of a nontoxic substance, whereas in adults the most common inappropriate use was after ingestion of a substance known to cause altered mental status.[25] The most frequent situation in which ipecac was given inappropriately occurred when too much time had elapsed from the time of ingestion (>60 minutes).[25]

GASTRIC LAVAGE

A prospective controlled study of acutely self-poisoned patients by Merigian and colleagues indicates that little clinical deterioration occurs in asymptomatic patients treated without gastric emptying.[13] Gastric emptying procedures in symptomatic patients did not significantly alter the length of stay in the emergency department, mean length of time intubated, or mean length of stay in the intensive care unit. In fact, gastric lavage was associated with a higher prevalence of medical intensive care unit admissions and aspiration pneumonia. Studies in volunteers indicate that gastric lavage is more effective than syrup of ipecac when performed immediately after exposure,[4,27] but no statistical difference between lavage and emesis exists in the reduction of drug absorption when the markers are administered 1 hour postingestion.[7,28]

EFFICACY

The efficacy of gastric lavage depends on the time elapsed between ingestion and lavage, on the amount ingested, on the inherent toxicity of the substance, and on the rate of absorption. Large amounts of unabsorbed drug will be removed from only a minority of patients who present to an emergency department following an overdose. Unfortunately, identifying the patients who will benefit the most from lavage is difficult.

INDICATIONS

Gastric lavage may be most effective for patients who ingest a life-threatening dose or who exhibit significant morbidity and who present soon (within 1 to 2 hours) after ingestion. Involvement of drugs that delay absorption, ingestion of large quantities of toxic drugs, and absence of bowel sounds on physical examination may lead to increased drug recovery at later times postingestion. Whether these patients benefit from lavage as long as 4 to 6 hours postingestion remains to be determined. Studies suggest that the recovery of drug at this delayed time is small.[17,29] For minor to moderate ingestions of toxic substances that are adsorbed to activated charcoal (Table 3–1), activated charcoal probably is preferred to gastric lavage.[30]

POSITION STATEMENT

The American Academy of Clinical Toxicology and the European Association of Poison Centres and Clinical Toxicology have prepared a draft (to be completed in 1996) of a position paper directed to the use of gastric lavage and authored by Vale,[31] which suggests that gastric lavage should not be employed routinely in the management of poisoned patients. There is no certain evidence that its use will improve outcome and it may cause significant morbidity. Lavage should be considered only if a patient has ingested a life-threatening amount of a toxic substance within 1 hour of presentation. Even then, clinical benefit has not been confirmed in controlled studies. This will, no doubt, be modified in a subsequent publication but it serves to indicate the present direction of thinking in the area. It does not, for the present, address the use of syrup of ipecac, activated charcoal (single or multiple dose), cathartics, or whole-bowel irrigation.

Gastric lavage (see also Position Statement[31]) followed by the instillation of activated charcoal with appropriate tracheal precautions may be useful in patients with altered mental status who present within 1 to 2 hours postingestion. Lavage after this period may be appropriate in the presence of gastric concretions, delayed gastric emptying, or sustained-release preparations.

CAUTIONS

1. Overall, the mortality from acute poisoning is less than 1% and the challenge for clinicians managing poisoned patients is to identify at an early stage those who are most at risk of developing serous complications and who might potentially benefit, therefore, from gut decontamination.
2. Gastric lavage is the passage of a large bore orogastric tube and the sequential administration and aspiration of small volumes of liquid for removal of gastric contents.
3. Gastric lavage should not be considered a routine management procedure in poisoned patients.
4. Gastric emptying studies in experimental animals have shown no impressive drug recovery, particularly if lavage was delayed 60 minutes. Volunteer studies also proved no support for the use of gastric lavage. In the single clinical study in which overall benefit from lavage was demonstrated,[32] patients also received activated charcoal, which may have contributed to the apparent efficacy of lavage when this procedure was undertaken less than 1 hour after overdose.
5. As it is known that the efficacy with which gastric lavage removes gastric contents decreases with time, lavage should be considered only if a patient has ingested a life-threatening amount of a toxic agent up to 1 hour previously.
6. Clinical and experimental studies have not confirmed the benefit of gastric lavage alone even when performed less than 1 hour after toxic ingestion. Drug absorption may be enhanced by its use.
7. In addition, there is no strong clinical evidence to support the view that, overall, lavage later than 1 hour after a toxic ingestion will benefit patients, including those who have ingested a tricyclic antidepressant or aspirin, though anecdotal reports indicate that occasionally impressive returns are achieved.
8. Lavage does not benefit the patient who has ingested a nontoxic agent or a nontoxic amount of a toxic agent.
9. Lavage is not useful as a deterrent to subsequent ingestions.

In conclusion, gastric emptying procedures in the emergency department are usually ineffective, may result in increased morbidity, and appear to offer no clinical advantage over charcoal alone.

CONTRAINDICATIONS

Absolute

Lavage is absolutely contraindicated in patients with an unprotected airway, such as patients with a depressed state of consciousness, and in patients at risk of hemorrhage or perforation due to pathology or recent surgery.[31]

Relative

Relative contraindications to gastric lavage are ingestion of a hydrocarbon, ingestion of an alkaline corrosive, ingestion of acid, and, risk of hemorrhage or perforation due to pathology or recent surgery.

COMPLICATIONS

Complications of gastric lavage include laryngospasm, a fall in the partial pressure of oxygen, aspiration pneumonia, sinus bradycardia, ST elevation on the electrocardiogram, and mechanical injury to the gut (rare).

TECHNIQUE

1. If lavage is considered appropriate, it is essential that the staff (whether they be medical or nursing) undertaking the procedure should be experienced in its execution both to reassure the conscious patient and to reduce the risk of complications. Gastric lavage is not advisable outside of the hospital.[28]
2. The procedure should be explained to the patient if conscious and consent obtained. A patient without previous experience of the procedure should be told, first, that a tube will be passed into her or his stomach so that the poison can be washed out and, second, that although the procedure is uncomfortable it may lead to a faster recovery. If consent is refused for whatever reason the procedure should not be attempted, not only because a technical assault will then be committed, but also because complications are likely to be greater.
3. Before undertaking the procedure it is essential to ensure that suctioning of the airway is available and functioning.
4. Endotracheal or nasotracheal intubation should precede gastric lavage in the comatose patient without a gag reflex. An oral airway should be placed between the teeth to prevent biting of the endotracheal tube if the patient recovers consciousness or convulses during the procedure.
5. The patient should be placed in the left lateral head down position (20° tilt on the table), which has been shown to produce better lavage returns.[33]
6. The length of tube to be inserted is measured and marked before insertion.
7. A wide-bore 36 to 40 French or 30 English gauge tube (external diameter approximately 12–13.3 mm) should be used in adults, and a 16 to 28 French gauge (diameter 5.3–9.3 mm) tube in children. The orogastric tube should be for single use only to avoid the risk of HIV and hepatitis virus transmission. The lavage tube should have a rounded end and be sufficiently firm to be passed into the passage. A nasogastric tube is of insufficient bore to produce a satisfactory lavage as particulate matter including medicines will not pass; moreover, damage to the nasal mucosa may cause severe epistaxis.
8. Force should not be used to pass the tube, particularly if the patient is struggling. Once the tube is passed, its position should be checked either by air insufflation, while listening over the stomach, or by aspiration with pH testing of the aspirate. Traditionally, an aliquot of this sample has been retained for toxicologic analysis though, except in the case of forensic examinations, the majority of laboratories now prefer blood and/or urine.
9. Lavage is carried out using small aliquots of liquid. In an adult, 200 to 300 mL of preferably warm (38°C) fluid such as saline or water should be used. In a child, 10 to 20 mL/kg body weight of warm fluid should be given. Water should preferably be avoided in young children because of the risk of inducing hyponatremia and water intoxication. Small volumes are used to minimize the risk of gastric contents entering the duodenum during lavage, as the amount of fluid affects the rate of gastric emptying. Warm fluids avoid the risk of hypothermia in the very young and very old and those receiving large volumes of lavage fluid.
10. Lavage should be continued until no further particulate matter is seen and the efferent lavage solution is clear.[31]

ACTIVATED CHARCOAL

Product formulations are summarized in Table 3–2. Activated charcoal is emerging as a sole decontamination measure in view of the relative lack of efficacy of both syrup of ipecac and gastric lavage demonstrated in recent controlled clinical trials.[8,20,34,35] The effectiveness of several combined decontamination measures (eg, charcoal–lavage–charcoal, charcoal 5 minutes after 60 mL syrup of ipecac) has not been clinically evaluated in controlled studies. Serial activated charcoal can significantly reduce certain drug half-lives (see Chapter 4).

PRECAUTIONS

The use of multiple doses of activated charcoal has been associated with several cases of intestinal obstruction, particularly in the cecum, both with[36,37] and without[38] the concomitant use of cathartics.

Cathartics should not be administered with each dose of activated charcoal, particularly in infants who are prone to develop electrolyte imbalance. Serious dehydration may result from such repetitive use.[39]

Multiple-dose activated charcoal should not be administered in the presence of diminished bowel sounds, proven ileus, or small bowel obstruction.

The first dose of activated charcoal can be administered through a small-bore nasogastric tube while airway control, intravenous access, blood sampling, cardiac monitoring, and other high-priority procedures are in progress. Once the

Table 3–2
Comparison of Activated Charcoal Products in Ready-to-Use Dosage Units

Product Name	Unit Size	Average Whole Price ($/unit)	Surface Area (m^2/g)	Sorbitol Content (mg/mL)	Charcoal Type
Aqueous Liqui-Char*	12.5 g/60 mL	3.86	950		Norit USP XXII
	25 g/120 mL	5.38			
	30 g/120 mL	5.56			
	50 g/240 mL	8.44			
Sorbitol Liqui-Char*	25 g/120 mL	5.56	950	225	Norit USP XXII
	50 g/240 mL	8.50			
Insta-Char†	15 g/120 mL	3.45	‡		‡
	50 g/240 mL	3.85			
Charcolex§	15 g	1.50	950		Norit USP XXII
	30 g	2.33			
Actidose-Aqua‖	15 g/72 mL	3.25	1500		Norit‡
	25 g/120 mL	4.35			
	50 g/240 mL	5.35			
Actidose with Sorbitol‖	25 g/120 mL	5.35	1500	400	Norit‡
	50 g/240 mL	6.50			
Charcoaid#	30 g/150 mL	5.15	1500	700	Norit B Supra
Activated Charcoal, USP¶	25 g/120 mL	7.30	950		Norit USP XXII
Activated Charcoal, USP¶ in sorbitol base	25 g/120 mL	7.65	950	225	Norit USP XXII

*Jones Medical, Canton, OH.
†Kerr Chemical, Novi, MI.
‡Specific data considered to be proprietary information by manufacturer.
§Lex Pharmaceutical, Medley, FL (product not diluted).
‖Paddock Laboratories, Minneapolis.
#Requa, Greenwich, CT.
¶UDL Laboratories, Rockford, IL.
From McFarland AK III, Chyka PA. Selection of activated charcoal products for the treatment of poisonings. Ann Pharmacother 1993;27:358–361.

patient has been stabilized, lavage with a large-bore orogastric tube can be accomplished.[40]

MULTIPLE-DOSE ACTIVATED CHARCOAL

The use of repeated doses of activated charcoal, as compared with other modalities of gut decontamination, has not been subjected to controlled clinical trials and has generally not been shown to reduce morbidity and mortality. Vale and Proudfoot suggest that in the meantime severely poisoned adults should be given 150 to 200 g of activated charcoal through a nasogastric tube over 4 to 8 hours and have proposed the following guideline: The total dose given may be more critical than the frequency of dosing.[41] At present multiple-dose activated charcoal is probably of value in the treatment of theophylline overdose, but is not likely to be very important in the presence of most other intoxications.[42] It can be considered if a life-threatening amount of phenobarbital, carbamazepine, quinine, dapsone, or aspirin is ingested. Its value in the treatment of digoxin, digitoxin, phenytoin, sodium valproate, meprobamate, dapsone, carbamazepine, and cyclosporine intoxications has yet to be established by controlled studies. It does not hasten the elimination of cyclic antidepressants.

Disadvantages of its use include its unpleasant taste, induction of vomiting, constipation and diarrhea, pulmonary aspiration, and gastrointestinal obstruction in patients with volume depletion. It is contraindicated in the presence of ileus or bowel obstruction and prior to endoscopy after corrosive ingestion unless there is a compelling need to adsorb another ingested toxin.

DOSE

In children the activated charcoal dose of 1 to 2 g/kg is not supported by clinical studies. This dose may lead to error in children because it is difficult to accurately measure 10 g of activated charcoal. Generally, 50 to 100 g is employed to fill the gut in adults. Because of mass action, large doses of activated charcoal (about 1 g/kg) are necessary to promote adsorption and to prevent desorption of the drug. The continuous infusion of activated charcoal or the instillation of activated charcoal in a small nasogastric tube placed in the duodenum may improve the retention of activated charcoal in the overdose situation (eg, theophylline) associated with protracted vomiting.

CATHARTICS

MECHANISM OF ACTION

The two groups of cathartics commonly used to treat patients with overdoses are (1) saline (magnesium citrate, magnesium sulfate, sodium sulfate, disodium phosphate) and (2) saccharides (eg, sorbitol). Saline cathartics act by altering the physicochemical forces within the intestinal lumen. The osmotic retention of fluid within the gastrointestinal tract probably activates motility reflexes and enhances expulsion.[43,44] Sorbitol catharsis can lead to liquid stools and abdominal discomfort.

The time to the first charcoal stool is substantially longer in overdose cases than in healthy volunteers who have been given a charcoal–sorbitol slurry, particularly when drugs with constipating effects are ingested. For example, in a retrospective study of patients presenting to an emergency department, the time to the first charcoal stool was 19.6 hours for ingestion of constipating drugs compared with 4.7 hours for ingestion of nonconstipating drugs.[45]

INDICATIONS

The use of cathartics may reduce the transit time of drugs in the gut and decrease the constipating effects of multiple doses of charcoal, but they have never been shown to improve morbidity and mortality or to decrease hospital stay.[46]

CONTRAINDICATIONS

Contraindications to the use of cathartics include the ingestion of corrosives, severe diarrhea, adynamic or dynamic ileus, serious electrolyte imbalance, and recent bowel surgery. Cathartics should be used with caution when bowel sounds are absent.

SORBITOL

Sorbitol is now the cathartic of choice because it may be more effective than saline cathartics.[47,48] In addition, sorbitol improves the palatability of activated charcoal. Whether it provides a bacteriostatic environment for the activated charcoal remains to be shown.

Each milliliter of 70% sorbitol solution contains 0.9 g sorbitol.[49] The usual dose is 1 to 2 mL of a 70% solution of sorbitol per kilogram body weight. This dose may be diluted 1:1 (ie, 35% solution) for ambulatory adults. Sorbitol dosage in adults is 1 g/kg. Pediatric dosing is controversial, ranging up to 0.5 g/kg. Cathartics are used if indicated with only the first dose of charcoal. Patients, especially children, should be carefully monitored for evidence of impaired fluid and electrolyte balance (eg, hypernatremia) during administration of multiple doses of activated charcoal and sorbitol. Severe dehydration and hypernatremia both developed in a 3-month-old infant following 220 mL of 70% sorbitol/activated charcoal over 3 to 4 hours[37] and in a 23-year-old woman following the administration of 210 mL of 70% sorbitol and 600 mL magnesium citrate over 27 hours.[50] Sorbitol is a sweetener in some medications (eg, valproic acid syrup); consequently, this drug may contribute to fluid and electrolyte imbalance following an overdose of these types of preparations.[51]

SALINE CATHARTICS (MAGNESIUM CITRATE, MAGNESIUM SULFATE, SODIUM SULFATE)

Magnesium citrate (10% solution, 4 mL/kg in a child or 250 mL in an adult) or magnesium sulfate (250 mg/kg in a child or 15–20 g in an adult) can be used in children or debilitated adults. If volume depletion is a problem, cathartics should be withheld. For more aggressive catharsis, whole-bowel irrigation should be used (see below).[52] (See also Chapter 67.)

Hypermagnesemia may follow excessive intake, impaired excretion, or parenteral administration of magnesium.[53,54] Excessive oral intake of magnesium in the absence of either intestinal or renal disease occurs infrequently.[55,56] It has been observed in neonates receiving Mylanta (containing 56 mg of elemental Mg in 4 mL) or Philips Milk of Magnesia (8 teaspoonsful per day, 381.6 mg/kg/d)[55] (Table 3–3). Patients treated for overdose of drugs with frequent oral dosage of magnesium-containing cathartics may develop signs and symptoms of hypermagnesemia[57–59] (Table 3–4). Excessive oral intake of magnesium may induce diarrhea with increased levels of fecal magnesium.[60] Fatal hypermagnesemia has followed rectal administration of magnesium preparations in cases of megacolon and bowel obstruction.[53]

Impaired Excretion

Hypermagnesemia is seen in patients with chronic renal failure who have been receiving magnesium-containing antacids, enemas, or infusions. Excessive dialysate magnesium may also cause symptomatic hypermagnesemia. In acute renal failure, the serum magnesium level ranges from 2.6 to 3.8 mEq/L (1.3–1.9 mmol/L; normal level, 1.4–2.0 mEq/L).[54] Azotemia, acidosis, rhabdomyolysis, and continued magnesium intake are contributing factors.

Parenteral Administration

Symptoms of excess magnesium may be induced by parenteral magnesium therapy. A 250-mL bolus containing 20 g of magnesium sulfate administered to an adult over 15 minutes induced respiratory arrest, hypotension, bradycardia, and QRS and QT prolongation.[61] Errors in administration of intravenous magnesium (50-mL vial of 50% magnesium sulfate instead of 2 mL of 50% solution) may rapidly induce signs and symptoms associated with hypermagnesemia.[62]

Clinical Presentation

Biochemical Effects

The plasma magnesium concentration usually exceeds 4 mEq/L (2 mmol/L) before any signs or symptoms of

Table 3–3
Magnesium Content of Various Drugs

Product	mg	mEq
Oral		
Gelusil Suspension, 5 mL	82	6.8
Gelusil M Suspension, 5 mL	82	6.8
Gelusil II, 5 mL	164	13.7
Maalox Suspension, 5 mL	82	6.8
Maalox Plus, 5 mL	82	6.8
Maalox TC, 5 mL	124	10.3
Milk of magnesia, 10 mL	332	27.0
Mylanta, 5 mL	82	6.8
Mylanta II, 5 mL, parenteral	164	13.7
Magnesium sulfate injection		
10%, 10 mL (1 g)	97.56	8.1
50%, 2 mL (1 g)	97.56	8.1

From Mofenson HC, Caraccio TR. Magnesium intoxication in a neonate from oral magnesium hydroxide laxative. Clin Toxicol 1991;29:215–222.

Table 3–4
Clinical Manifestations of Hypermagnesemia

Level	Serum Mg^{2+} (mEq/L)
Normal serum level	1.4–2.0
Nausea, vomiting, cutaneous flushing	3.0
Decrease in deep tendon reflexes, drowsiness, unsteadiness, diaphoresis	4.0
Electrocardiographic changes (QRS widening, PR prolongation)	5.0
Somnolence, bradycardia, hypotension	6.0–7.0
Absent deep tendon reflexes, voluntary muscle paralysis	10.0
Complete heart block, respiratory paralysis	15.0
Asystole	17.0–20.0

From Jones J, Heiselman D, Dougherty J, Eddy A. Cathartic induced magnesium toxicity during overdose management. Ann Emerg Med 1986;15: 1214–1218.

magnesium excess appear (Table 3–4).[57] Parenteral administration of magnesium lowers plasma calcium concentrations in both normal and hypoparathyroid patients. The anion gap may be unchanged.[63] The osmolal gap can be increased.[64]

Neuromuscular Effects

Excess magnesium decreases impulse transmission across the neuromuscular junction. At blood levels of 4 mEq/L (2 mmol/L), deep tendon reflexes decrease or disappear. Somnolence is observed at 4 to 7 mEq/L (2–3.5 mmol/L) and flaccid paralysis of voluntary muscles at 10 mEq/L (5 mmol/L) or greater levels. This may lead to impairment of respiratory function and apnea, an effect that is antagonized by calcium. When deep tendon reflexes are absent, respiration must be closely monitored.

Cardiovascular Effects

Bradycardia and hypotension due to the direct vasodilating and ganglionic blocking effects of magnesium on peripheral arteries and arterioles may be observed at 4 to 5 mEq/L (2–2.5 mmol/L) (Table 3–4). At plasma magnesium concentrations of 5 to 10 mEq/L (2.5–5 mmol/L), the PR, QRS and QT intervals may increase. Complete heart block and cardiac arrest in asystole may occur at 15 mEq/L (7.5 mmol/L) or greater levels.[54] Cardiopulmonary arrest with coma, nonreactive pupils, flaccid extremities, loss of deep tendon reflexes, and no response to painful stimulus may be observed early after magnesium overdose.[65] In normal humans, 4 g of magnesium sulfate diluted in 20 mL of 5% glucose given intravenously appears to increase cardiac output and heart rate and produce a decrease in systolic arterial pressure and systemic vascular resistance. This is accompanied by vasodilation of the coronary arteriolar bed. The serum magnesium levels increase.[66] Parenteral magnesium sulfate appears to prolong conduction through the sinoatrial and atrioventricular nodal tissues; it also increases atrioventricular nodal refractoriness in healthy humans.[67]

In patients exhibiting Torsade de pointes, single or multiple doses of magnesium sulfate (2 g intravenously over 1–2 minutes followed by a continuous intravenous infusion of 3 to 20 mg Mg/min) have been useful in terminating the arrhythmia.[68,69] For preeclampsia (as an anticonvulsant), a 4.0 g intravenous loading dose followed by 1.0 to 2.0 g IV of a 20% solution has been used.

Gastrointestinal Effects

Hypermagnesemia may be associated with paralytic ileus. A recent report suggested that the ileus was associated with a magnesium level of 8.1 mg/dL on admission. The paralytic ileus resolved when the magnesium level fell below 3.1 mg/dL.[70]

Treatment of Magnesium Excess

1. Discontinue administration of magnesium.
2. Stop other calcium channel blockers which may act synergistically with magnesium.
3. Eliminate magnesium by enema if it is in the bowel. (Activated charcoal does not adsorb magnesium salts.)
4. Monitor serum electrolytes, calcium, phosphorus, renal function, fluid intake, urinary output, and electrocardiogram.
5. Have available intravenous lines, oxygen, and a cardiac monitor.
6. If the patient is symptomatic (hypotonic, central nervous system depression) and has electrocardiographic changes and an elevated serum magnesium level, begin therapy.[71] Therapy with calcium gluconate 10% is administered intravenously (10–20 mL in adults, 100 mg/kg in infants and children up to a maximum of 1 g slowly over 5–10 minutes with electrocardiographic monitoring). This may reverse the hypotension and paralysis. Give calcium in the presence of severe hypermagnesemia even if total serum calcium levels are normal.
7. If renal function is normal, intravenous furosemide (40 mg, adults, 1 mg/kg infants and children) may be administered as alternate therapy with replacement of urine volume by 0.90% saline. Forced diuresis with mannitol (25 g by rapid intravenous infusion) has also been useful.[61]
8. Dialysis and exchange transfusion may be useful in the patient with renal insufficiency and continued high levels of magnesium.
9. Do not administer aminoglycosides as they may potentiate the neuromuscular blockade of magnesium.[72]
10. Pacemaker therapy may be useful.
11. Check magnesium levels in patients who present with paralytic ileus.

PRECAUTIONS

Common undesirable effects of cathartic use include abdominal cramps, excessive diarrhea, and abdominal distension.

WHOLE-BOWEL IRRIGATION

Whole-bowel irrigation (WBI) is probably a useful and rapid method to empty the gut in 4 to 6 hours. It is messy and labor intensive for patients who present to a hospital many hours after an overdose. WBI with high-molecular-weight polyethylene glycol (PEG-3350) and isosmolar electrolyte solution (PEG-ELS) is a safe and efficacious method for gut decontamination introduced in 1980.[73] WBI produces a more thorough cleansing of the entire intestinal tract when compared with cathartics, which are agents that promote defecation rather than eliminate the whole contents of the intestines.

The previously used instillation of large volumes of isotonic saline as a means of preparing the bowel for diagnostic procedures or for gastrointestinal tract surgery was associated with electrolyte and fluid imbalance, and concern about these complications has limited the use of WBI in treatment of overdoses; however, the recent development of isotonic solutions that use polyethylene glycol and sodium sulfate instead of sodium chloride has resulted in a procedure more suitable for clinical trials.[73] This new lavage solution is available as GoLytely and Colyte. The use of PEG-ELS solution in WBI produces no significant changes in serum electrolytes, serum osmolality, body weight, or hematocrit.[74]

MECHANISM OF ACTION

High-molecular-weight polyethylene glycol (PEG-3350) does not produce distension of the abdomen like mannitol, which releases hydrogen in the presence of gut bacteria. The divalent sulfate ion impairs the active transport of sodium, and PEG-3350 prevents the shift of fluid across the intestinal wall by restoring the isotonicity of the solution. Both PEG-3350 and sulfate ions are poorly absorbed from the gastrointestinal tract, even in the presence of inflammatory bowel disease.[75]

INDICATIONS

The efficacy of WBI in reducing the absorption of toxins depends on the type of preparation and on the drug ingested.[6] Activated charcoal does adsorb powdered PEG. The concurrent administration of multiple doses of charcoal does not improve the effectiveness of WBI[76]; however, in vitro data do not exclude the effectiveness of an initial dose of activated charcoal prior to the initiation of WBI.[77] WBI does not increase the clearance of a drug already absorbed into the blood, at least in the aspirin overdose model.[78] Potential uses for WBI as a decontamination measure include ingestion of massive amounts of highly toxic drugs; ingestion of large amounts of drugs in patients presenting late (>4 hours postexposure)[79]; large overdoses of sustained-release preparations,[80] many of which are associated with fatality or significant morbidity (Table 3–5)[81]; ingestion of drug packets by body packers or body stuffers[82]; and ingestion of substances not adsorbed by activated charcoal. An additional possible use may be in ingestion of toxic substances that can be detected by radiography (arsenic, carbon tetrachloride,

Table 3–5
Drugs With Controlled-Release Preparations Associated With Fatality or Significant Morbidity

Drug	Toxic Dose	Comments
Amphetamine	>1 mg/kg	
Dexamphetamine	Variable	
Carbamazepine	>20 mg/kg	Pharmacobezoars; repeat-dose charcoal enhances clearance; charcoal hemoperfusion enhances clearance
Chlorpromazine	>10 mg/kg	Radiopaque*
Clonidine	>0.1 mg/kg	
Dextromethorphan	>10 mg/kg	
Dextropropoxyphene	>10 mg/kg	
Diltiazem	Variable	Pharmacodynamic variation†
Disopyramide	>10 mg/kg	
Felodipine	Variable	Pharmacodynamic variation†
Iron	>20 mg/kg	Radiopaque*; pharmacobezoars: does not bind to charcoal‡
Lithium	>10 mg/kg	Radiopaque*; does not bind to charcoal‡; hemodialysis enhances clearance
Meprobamate	Variable	Pharmacobezoars
Metoprolol	Variable	Pharmacodynamic variation†
Paracetamol (acetaminophen)	>150 mg/kg	
Potassium chloride	>2 mEq/kg if renal function is normal	Radiopaque*; does not bind to charcoal‡
Procainamide	>100 mg/kg	Hemoperfusion enhances clearance
Propranolol	Variable	Pharmacodynamic variation†
Quinidine	>50 mg/kg	
Salicylates	>100 mg/kg	Pharmacobezoars; radiopaque*; hemodialysis enhances clearance
Theophylline	>20 mg/kg	Pharmacobezoars; repeat-dose charcoal§ and charcoal hemoperfusion enhance clearance
Verapamil	Extremely variable	Pharmacodynamic variation†; pharmacobezoars; repeat-dose charcoal enhances clearance§

*Radiopaque medications may lose this property with tablet dissolution. The absence of tablets on plain abdominal x-ray film does not exclude ingestion.
†Pharmacodynamic variation: toxicity from these drugs is significantly determined by patient factors, such as preexisting conditions and concomitant medications. It is therefore difficult to define a safe lower limit for ingestion. All such patients should receive gastrointestinal decontamination.
‡Patients poisoned by controlled-release drugs that do not bind to charcoal should be treated with whole-bowel lavage with polyethylene glycol electrolyte lavage solution (PEG-ELS).
§Increased clearance by using repeat-dose charcoal is clinically significant. The charcoal dose may need to be increased in the presence of PEG ELS.
From Buckley NA, Dawson AH, Reitz DA. Controlled release drugs in overdose: Clinical considerations. Drug Saf 1995;12:73–86.

mercury, thallium). Lead has been removed by WBI from the gastrointestinal tract of a patient suffering from lead toxicity.[83,84]

METALS

Whole-bowel irrigation is a safe and effective decontamination procedure for potentially lethal iron ingestions, especially if the iron tablets have passed the pylorus.[85] Activated charcoal does not adsorb iron or other metal compounds (e.g., lithium, potassium).

FOREIGN BODIES

Whole-bowel irrigation effectively removes miniature disk batteries from the gut and cocaine-filled packets in body packers and body stuffers.[86] Iron, lead, lithium, sustained-release verapamil and theophylline may be cleared from the gastrointestinal tract, but there is little evidence to indicate a lessening of morbidity or mortality from this procedure.

DOSE

The technique for WBI involves the insertion of a nasogastric tube into the stomach and the instillation of PEG-ELS solution while the patient sits on a commode. Alternatively, the solution can be ingested orally. Activated charcoal may be administered prior to WBI. The use of intravenous metoclopramide (10 mg adults, 0.1–0.3 mg/kg body weight) may reduce the incidence of nausea and vomiting. The usual rate of fluid administration is 2 L/hour in adults and 0.5 L/hour (25–40 mL/kg body weight) in children under 12 years of age. PEG-ELS solution should be given at room temperature to prevent hypothermia. The endpoint occurs when the rectal effluent is similar in appearance to the infusate. The usual infusion lasts 2 to 6 hours. This does not ensure that the toxin or foreign body is eliminated.

PRECAUTIONS

Few complications occur following the use of WBI for preparation of the bowel for radiographic examination or for surgery in either adults or children,[87] even in the presence of cardiac, renal, or pulmonary disease.[88] Complaints usually are minor and include nausea, vomiting, abdominal distension and cramps, sleep loss, and anal irritation.[89] Propylene glycol electrolyte lavage solution may occupy activated charcoal binding sites. It may also displace toxin from activated charcoal, leading to a substantial increase in toxin bioavailability.[90]

CONTRAINDICATIONS

Contraindications to the use of WBI include gastrointestinal pathology or dysfunction (obstruction, ileus, hemorrhage, perforation) and inadequate airway protection.

CONTROLLED-RELEASE DRUGS

Serious effects and death may follow as late as 60 hours after overdose of sustained-release forms of drugs including verapamil, aspirin, theophylline, and lithium. Release of drug from the formulation may be further prolonged as a result of formation of a concretion of tablets in the stomach or intestine (eg, theophylline, verapamil, carbamazepine, aspirin). Pharmacobezoars may be diagnosed by a plain abdominal x-ray (for radiopaque medications) or gastroendoscopy.

MONITORING

Treatment nomograms based on plasma concentrations calculated for standard-release formulations of some drugs (eg, aspirin, iron and paracetamol [acetaminophen]) are not appropriate for controlled-release formulations and their application may lead to inappropriate management. Treatment decisions need to be based on clinical toxicity and calculations of the total ingested dose. For drugs, the absolute concentration of which may indicate the need for further treatment (eg, lithium, theophylline, procainamide), the concentration should be measured until there is a sustained decline to nontoxic levels. Poisonings with these preparations have demonstrated multiple peak concentrations indicating continuing and variable absorption for more than 24 hours.[81]

Where there is a significant risk of serious toxicity, gastric lavage should be performed on admission with an orogastric tube large enough to remove whole tablets. Patients presenting with overdose of calcium antagonists or propranolol may require pretreatment with atropine to avoid vagal stimulation, which may precipitate complete heart block or asystole.

ACTIVATED CHARCOAL

The role of activated charcoal in the treatment of controlled-release preparations is still being defined. Repeated doses of activated charcoal can increase the clearance of a number of drugs either by interruption enterohepatic circulation or by direct "dialysis" from capillaries in the gastrointestinal mucosa.[81]

WHOLE-BOWEL IRRIGATION

Use whole-bowel irrigation alone for overdose with those medications not adsorbed to charcoal (Fig. 3–1). Patients with other poisonings receive a single dose of activated charcoal (to adsorb drug that is not held within the controlled-release vehicle), followed by whole-bowel irrigation. Repeated doses of activated charcoal are added only for those drugs where it has clearly been shown to enhance clearance (see Table 3–1).

PHARMACOBEZOARS

Pharmacobezoars may occur with any controlled-release formulation. The presence of pharmacobezoars necessitates prolonged gastrointestinal decontamination to deal with dissociating toxins, or definitive treatment.

Gastric pharmacobezoars have been successfully fragmented or removed via gastroendoscopy. This should be followed by continued gastrointestinal decontamination with activated charcoal and whole-bowel irrigation. Gastric phar-

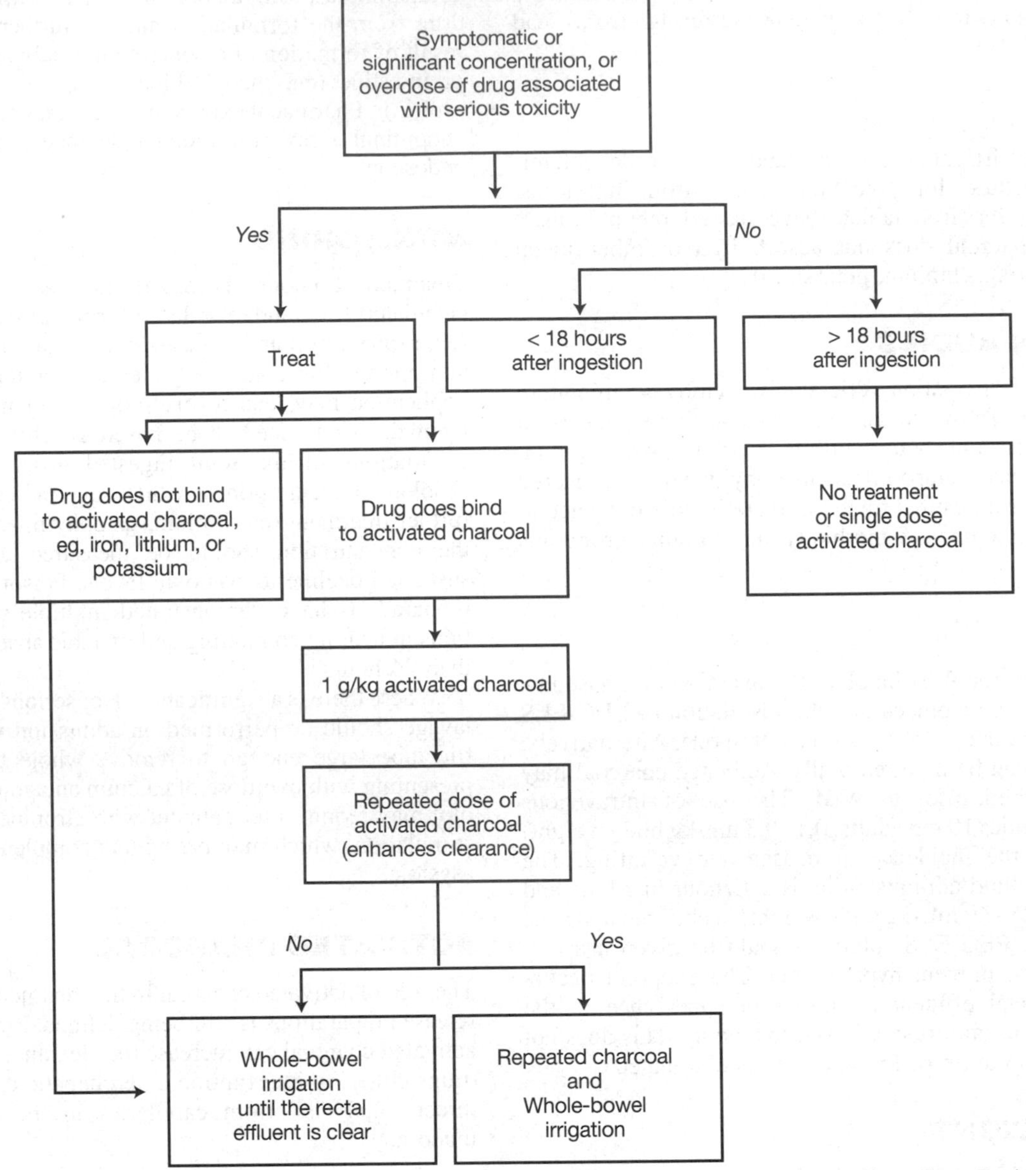

Figure 3–1 Guide to gastrointestinal decontamination for patients with controlled-release formulation overdose. From Buckley NA, Dawson AH, Reitz DA. Controlled release drugs in overdose: Clinical considerations. Drug Saf 1995;12:73–86.

macobezoars can be surgically removed. Surgical removal has most commonly been reported for iron bezoars. It should be considered in patients with bowel obstruction and in those with other contraindications to gastrointestinal decontamination.[81]

SPECIAL REVIEW ARTICLES

Albertson TE, Derlet RW, Foulke GE, et al. Superiority of activated charcoal alone compared with ipecac and activated charcoal in the treatment of acute toxic ingestions. Ann Emerg Med 1989;18:101–104.

Donovan JW. Selective gastric decontamination in the poisoned patient. Top Emerg Med 1993;15:1–12.

Jawary D, Cameron PA, Dziukas L, McNeil JJ. Drug overdose: Reducing the load. Med J Aust 1992;156:343–436.

Neuvonen PJ, Olkolla KT. Oral activated charcoal in the treatment of intoxications: Role of single and repeated dose. Med Toxicol 1988;3:33–58.

Olson KR. Is gut emptying all washed up? Am J Emerg Med 1990; 8:560–561. Editorial.

Perrone J, Hoffman RS, Goldfrank LR. Special considerations in gastrointestinal decontamination. Emerg Med Clin North Am 1994;12:285.

Saetta JP. Gastric decontaminating procedures: Is it time to call a stop? J R Soc Med 1993;86:396–399.

Tenenbein M. Multiple doses of activated charcoal: Time for reappraisal? Ann Emerg Med 1991;20:529–531.

Tenenbein M. Whole bowel irrigation as a gastrointestinal decontamination procedure after acute poisoning. Med Toxicol 1988;3:77–84.

Tenenbein M, Silar DS, Banner W, et al. Symposium: Advances in the management of drug intoxication. Ann RCPSC 1990;23: 453–457.

Vale JA. Clinical toxicology. Postgrad Med J 1993;69:19–32.

Vale JA, Proudfoot AT. How useful is activated charcoal? Studies have left many unanswered questions. Br Med J 1993;308: 78–79.

REFERENCES

1. Lovejoy FH Jr, Shannon M, Woolf AD. Recent advances in clinical toxicology. Curr Problems Pediatr 1992(Mar.):119–129.

2. Abdallah AH, Tye A. A comparison of the efficacy of emetic drugs and stomach lavage. Am J Dis Child 1967;113: 571–574.
3. Corby DG, Lisciandro RC, Lehman RG, et al. The efficacy of methods used to evacuate the stomach after acute ingestions. Pediatrics 1967;40:871–874.
4. Tandberg D, Diven BG, McLeod JW. Ipecac-induced emesis versus gastric lavage: A controlled study in normal adults. Am J Emerg Med 1986;4:205–209.
5. Litovitz TL. Emesis versus lavage for poisoning victims. Am J Emerg Med 1986;4:294–295.
6. Jawary D, Cameron PA, Dziukas L, McNeil JJ. Drug overdose: Reducing the load. Med J Aust 1992;156:343–436.
7. Tenenbein M, Cohen S, Sitar DS. Efficacy of ipecac-induced emesis, orogastric lavage, and activated charcoal for acute drug overdose. Ann Emerg Med 1987;16:838–841.
8. Albertson TE, Derlet RW, Foulke GE, et al. Superiority of activated charcoal alone compared with ipecac and activated charcoal in the treatment of acute toxic ingestions. Ann Emerg Med 1989;18:101–104.
9. Merigian KS, Woodard M, Hedges JR, et al. Prospective evaluation of gastric emptying in the self-poisoned patient. Am J Emerg Med 1990;8:479–483.
10. Olson KR. Is gut emptying all washed up? Am J Emerg Med 1990;8:560–561. Editorial.
11. Saetta JP, Marsh S, Gaunt ME, Quinton DN. Gastric emptying procedures in the self-poisoning patients: Are we forcing gastric content beyond the pylorus? J R Soc Med 1991; 84:274–276.
12. Saetta JP, Quinton DN. Residual gastric content after gastric lavage and ipecacuanha-induced emesis in self-poisoned patients: An endoscopic study. J R Soc Med 1991;84:35–38.
13. Merigian KS, Woodard M, Hedges JR, et al. Prospective evaluation of gastric emptying in the self-poisoned patient. Am J Emerg Med 1990;8:479–483.
14. Robertson WO: Syrup of ipecac: A slow or fast emetic? Am J Dis Child 1962;103:136–139.
15. Neuvonen PJ, Olkolla KT. Oral activated charcoal in the treatment of intoxications: Role of single and repeated dose. Med Toxicol 1988;3:33–58.
16. Litovitz T. In defense of retaining ipecac syrup as an over-the-counter drug. Pediatrics 1988;82(3, pt 2):514–516.
17. Watson WA, Leighton J, Guy J, et al. Recovery of cyclic antidepressants with gastric lavage. J Emerg Med 1989;7:373–377.
18. Vale JA. The relevance of gastrointestinal decontamination in acute poisoning: What should we be advising? Personal presentation, 1994.
19. Litovitz TL, Bailey KM, Schmitz BF, et al. 1990 Annual report of the American Association of Poison Control Centers National Data Collection System. Am J Emerg Med 1991;9:461–509.
20. Kornberg AE, Dolgin J. Pediatric ingestions: Charcoal alone versus ipecac and charcoal. Ann Emerg Med 1991;20:648–651.
21. Freedman GE, Pasternak S, Krenzelok EP. A clinical trial using syrup of ipecac and activated charcoal concurrently. Ann Emerg Med 1987;16:164–166.
22. Dean BS, Krenzelok EP. Syrup of ipecac: 15 mL versus 30 mL in pediatric patients. Clin Toxicol 1985;23:165–170.
23. Varipapu RJ, Oderda GM. Effect of milk on ipecac induced emesis. J Am Pharm Assoc 1977;17:510.
24. Rodgers GC, Matyunas NJ. Gastrointestinal decontamination for acute poisoning. Pediatr Clin North Am 1986;33:261–285.
25. Wrenn K, Rodewald L, Dockstader L. Potential misuse of ipecac. Ann Emerg Med 1993;22:1408–1412.
26. Saincher A, Sitar D, Tenenbein M. Efficacy of ipecac during the feral hour??? After drug ingestion. Vet Hum Toxicol 1993; 36:375.
27. Auerbach PS, Osterloh J, Braun O, et al. Efficacy of gastric emptying: Gastric lavage versus emesis induced with ipecac. Ann Emerg Med 1986;55:692–698.
28. Danel V, Henry JA, Glucksman E. Activated charcoal, emesis, and gastric lavage in aspirin overdose. Br Med J 1988;296: 1507.
29. Comstock EG, Boisaubin EV, Comstock BS, et al. Assessment of the efficacy of activated charcoal following gastric lavage in acute drug emergencies. J Toxicol Clin Toxicol 1982–1983;19:149–165.
30. Hodgkinson DW, Jellett LB, Ashby RH. A review of the management of oral drug overdose in the accident and emergency department of the Royal Brisbane Hospital. Arch Emerg Med 1991;8:8–16.
31. Vale A. Gastric lavage. In: Proceedings, Meeting of American Academy of Clinical Toxicology; European Association of Poison Centres and Clinical Toxicologists; and American Academy of Poison Control Centers, Vienna, April 1994. Draft of position paper.
32. Kulig K, Bar-Or D, Cantrill JV, et al. Management of acutely poisoned patients without gastric emptying. Ann Emerg Med 1984;14:562–567.
33. Burke M. Gastric lavage and emesis in the treatment of ingested poisons: A review and a clinical study of lavage in ten adults. Resuscitation 1972;1:91–105.
34. Palatnick W, Tenenbein M. Activated charcoal in the treatment of drug overdose: An update. Drug Saf 1992;7:3–7.
35. Kulig K. Initial management of ingestions of toxic substances. N Engl J Med 1992;326:1677–1681.
36. Atkinson SW, Young Y, Trotter GA. Treatment with activated charcoal complicated by gastrointestinal obstruction requiring surgery. Br Med J 1992;305:563.
37. Flores F, Battle WS. Intestinal obstruction secondary to activated charcoal. Con Surg 1987;30:57–59.
38. Watson WA, Cremer KF, Chapman JA. Gastrointestinal obstruction associated with multiple-dose activated charcoal. J Emerg Med 1986;4:401–407.
39. Farley TA. Severe hypernatremic dehydration after use of an activated charcoal–sorbitol suspension. J Pediatr 1986;109: 719–722.
40. Linden C. Activated charcoal. Clin Toxicol Rev 1987;9:1–2.
41. Vale JA, Proudfoot AT. How useful is activated charcoal? Studies have left many unanswered questions. Br Med J 1993;308:78–79.
42. Tenenbein M. Multiple doses of activated charcoal: Time for reappraisal? Ann Emerg Med 1991;20:529–531.
43. Harvey RF, Read AE. Mode of action of the saline purgatives. Am Heart J 1975;89:810–813.
44. Cooke AR. Control of gastric emptying and motility. Gastroenterology 1975;68:804–816.
45. Harchelroad F, Cottington E, Krenzelok EP. Gastrointestinal transit times of a charcoal/sorbitol slurry in overdose patients. Clin Toxicol 1989;27:91–99.
46. Riegal JM, Becker CE. Use of cathartics in toxic ingestions. Ann Emerg Med 1981;10:254–258.
47. Minocha A, Herold DA, Barth JT, et al. Activated charcoal in oral ethanol absorption: Lack of effect in humans. Clin Toxicol 1986;24:225–234.
48. Krenzelok EP, Keller R, Stewart RD. Gastrointestinal transit times of cathartics combined with charcoal. Ann Emerg Med 1985;14:1152–1155.
49. Minocha A, Krenzelok EP, Spyker DA. Dosage recommendations for sorbitol–charcoal treatment. Clin Toxicol 1985;23: 579–587.
50. Allerton JP, Strom JA. Hypernatremia due to repeated doses of charcoal–sorbitol. Am J Kidney Dis 1991;17:581–584.
51. Veerman MW. Excipients in valproic acid syrup may cause diarrhea: A case report. DCIP Ann Pharmacother 1990;24: 832–833.
52. Perrone J, Hoffman RS, Goldfrank LR. Special considerations in gastrointestinal decontamination. Emerg Med Clin North Am 1994;12:285–289.
53. Mordes JP, Wacker WEC. Excess magnesium. Pharmacol Rev 1978;29:273–300.
54. Rude RK, Singer FR. Magnesium deficiency and excess. Annu Rev Med 1981;32:245–259.
55. Humphrey M, Kennon S, Pramanik AK. Hypermagnesemia from antacid administration in a newborn infant. J Pediatr 1981;98:313–314.
56. Mofenson HC, Caraccio TR. Magnesium intoxication in a neonate from oral magnesium hydroxide laxative. Clin Toxicol 1991;29:215–222.

57. Jones J, Heiselman D, Dougherty J, Eddy A. Cathartic induced magnesium toxicity during overdose management. Ann Emerg Med 1986;15:1214–1218.
58. Smilkstein MJ, Smolinske SC, Kulig KW, Rumack BH. Severe hypermagnesemia due to multiple dose cathartic therapy. West J Med 1988;148:208–211.
59. Woodard JA, Shannon M, LaCouture PG, Woolf A. Serum magnesium concentrations after repetitive magnesium cathartic administration. Am J Emerg Med 1990;8:297–300.
60. Fine KD, Santa Ana CA, Fordtran JS. Diagnosis of magnesium induced diarrhea. N Engl J Med 1991;324:1012–1017.
61. Bohman VR, Cotton DB. Supralethal magnesemia with patient survival. Obstet Gynecol 1990;76:984–986.
62. Hoffman RS, Smilkstein MJ, Rubenstein F. An 'amp' by any other name: The hazards of intravenous magnesium dosing. JAMA 1989;261:557.
63. Ortiz-Interian CJ, Schlessinger FB, Oster JR. Severe hypermagnesemia without reduction in the anion gap. Magnesium Trace Elem 19910;9:110–114.
64. Gerard SK, Hernandez C, Khayam-Bashi H. Extreme hypermagnesemia caused by an overdose of magnesium-containing cathartics. Ann Emerg Med 1988;17:728–731.
65. McCubbin JH, Sibai BM, Abdulla TN, Anderson GD. Cardiopulmonary arrest due to acute maternal hypermagnesemia. Lancet 1981;1:1058.
66. Vigorito C, Giordano A, Ferraro P, et al. Hemodynamic effects of magnesium sulfate on the normal human heart. Am J Cardiol 1991;67:1435–1437.
67. Kulik DL, Hong R, Ryzen E, et al. Electrophysiologic effects of intravenous magnesium in patients with normal conduction system and no clinical evidence of significant cardiac disease. Am Heart J 1988;115:367–373.
68. Tsivoni D, Banai S, Schuger C, et al. Treatment of Torsade de pointes with magnesium sulfate. Circulation 1988;77:392–397.
69. Tsivoni D, Keren A, Cohen AM, et al. Magnesium therapy for Torsade de pointes. Am J Cardiol 1984;53:528–530.
70. Golzarian J, Scott HW, Richards WO. Hypermagnesemia-induced paralytic ileus. Dig Dis Sci 1994;39:1138–1142.
71. Tsang RC. Neonatal magnesium disturbances. Am J Dis Child 1972;124:282.
72. L'Hommedieu CS, Nicholas N, Armes DA. Potentiation of magnesium sulfate-induced neuromuscular weakness by gentamicin, tobramycin and amikacin. J Pediatr 1983;102: 629–631.
73. Davis GR, Santa Ana CA, Morawski SG, Fordtran JS. Development of a lavage solution associated with minimal water and electrolyte absorption or secretion. Gastroenterology 1980;78:991–995.
74. Tenenbein M, Cohen S, Sitar D. Whole bowel irrigation as a decontamination procedure after acute drug overdose. Arch Intern Med 1987;147:905–907.
75. Brady CE III, DiPalma JA, Morawski SG, et al. Urinary excretion of polyethylene glycol 3350 and sulfate after gut lavage with a polyethylene glycol electrolyte lavage solution. Gastroenterology 1986;90:1914–1918.
76. Hoffman RS, Chiang WK, Howland MA, et al. Theophylline desorption from activated charcoal caused by whole bowel irrigation solution. J Toxicol Clin Toxicol 1991;29:191–201.
77. Kirshenbaum LA, Sitar DS, Tenenbein M. Interaction between whole-bowel irrigation solution and activated charcoal: Implications for the treatment of toxic ingestions. Ann Emerg Med 1990;19:1129–1132.
78. Mayer AL, Sitar DS, Tenenbein M. Multiple-dose charcoal and whole-bowel irrigation do not increase clearance of absorbed salicylate. Arch Intern Med 1992;152:393–396.
79. Tenenbein M. Whole bowel irrigation as a gastrointestinal decontamination procedure after acute poisoning. Med Toxicol 1988;3:77–84.
80. Kirshenbaum LA, Mathews SC, Sitar DS, Tenenbein M. Whole-bowel irrigation versus activated charcoal in sorbitol for the ingestion of modified-release pharmaceuticals. Clin Pharmacol Ther 1989;46:264–271.
81. Buckley NA, Dawson AH, Reitz DA. Controlled release drugs in overdose: Clinical considerations. Drug Saf 1995;12: 73–86.
82. Hoffman RS, Smilkstein MR, Goldfrank LR. Whole bowel irrigation and the cocaine body-packer: A new approach to a common problem. Am J Emerg Med 1990;8:523–527.
83. Boba A. Whole bowel irrigation. Am J Emerg Med 1994;12: 257.
84. Roberge RJ, Martin TG. Whole bowel irrigation in an acute oral lead intoxication. Am J Emerg Med 1992;10:577–583.
85. Tenenbein M. Whole bowel irrigation in iron poisoning. J Pediatr 1987;111:142–145.
86. Tenenbein M. Whole bowel irrigation for toxic ingestions. Clin Toxicol 1985;23:177–184.
87. Sondheimer JM, Sokol RJ, Taylor SF, et al. Safety, efficacy, and tolerance of intestinal lavage in pediatric patients undergoing diagnostic colonoscopy. J Pediatr 1991; 110:148–152.
88. Goldman J, Reichelderfer M. Evaluation of a rapid colonoscopy preparation using a new gut lavage solution. Gastrointest Endosc 1982;28:9–11.
89. DiPalma JA, Brady CE. Colon cleansing for diagnostic and surgical procedures: Polyethylene glycol–electrolyte lavage solution. Am J Gastroenterol 1989;84:1008–1016.
90. Hoffman RS, Chiang WK, Howland MA, et al. Theophylline desorption from activated charcoal caused by whole bowel irrigation. J Toxicol Clin Toxicol 1991;29:191–202.

Chapter 4
Elimination Enhancement

ALKALINE AND ACID DIURESIS

Alkaline diuresis may aid in increasing renal clearance and reducing the elimination half-life of salicylates, phenobarbital, and phenoxyacetate herbicides. Complications include fluid overload, noncardiogenic pulmonary edema (salicylates), cerebral edema, and electrolyte and acid–base disturbances. Patients should be monitored frequently (plasma drug concentrations, urine pH, fluid balance, central venous pressure, electrolytes, serum sodium, potassium, calcium, magnesium). A practical role for diuresis (acid or alkaline) in the treatment of most overdoses has not been determined by controlled studies. The utility of both acid and alkaline diuresis has recently been called into question by the ability of less care-intensive methods such as repeated-dose charcoal to increase the elimination of many toxins.[1]

EXTRACORPOREAL TECHNIQUES

Pond[2] (Table 4–1) and Koppel[3] have summarized the current status of the use of extracorporeal techniques in the treatment of poisoning. Bismuth and Muczinski emphasize that the efficacy of dialysis methods and hemoperfusion in acute poisoning cannot be clinically estimated easily because concomitant intestinal absorption, hepatic metabolism, and urinary excretion must be considered.[4] With supportive treatment alone, spontaneous recovery usually occurs in 98% of the intoxications in intensive care units. Extracorporeal techniques may be limited to use in salicylate, methanol, ethylene glycol, lithium, and theophylline overdose, and are of limited use in sedative–hypnotic, industrial, and household poisonings. When required, such treatment should be available to be able to perform emergency hemodialysis and hemoperfusion within a short time.[5–7]

An American Association of Poison Control Centers (AAPCC) survey found that hemodialysis in 1986 was used predominantly for ethylene glycol, lithium, methanol, and aspirin poisoning. Hemoperfusion was used mostly in theophylline, cyclic antidepressant, and barbiturate overdose. Patient outcome was not determined.[8] By 1992, hemodialysis was used mainly for lithium, aminophylline/theophylline, ethylene glycol, aspirin (formulated alone),

Table 4–1
Compounds for Which Extracorporeal Elimination as a Treatment for Overdose Is Considered Relatively Frequently and the Extracorporeal Procedure Preferred

Toxic Compound	Relative Molecular Mass	Water Soluble	Volume of Distribution (L/kg)	Endogenous Clearance (mL min^{-1} kg^{-1})	Protein Binding	Preferred Method	Comments
Aminoglycosides	>500	Yes	~0.3	~1.5	<10%	Hemofiltration	Useful if clearance decreased due to renal failure
Carbamazepine	236	No	~1.4	~1.3	~74%	Hemoperfusion	Clearance increased in patients on long-term treatment
Ethylene glycol	62	Yes	~0.6	~2	0	Hemodialysis	Clearance decreased as dose increased
Lithium	7	Yes	0.6–1.0	~0.35	0	Hemodialysis	Useful if clearance decreased due to renal failure
Methanol	32	Yes	~0.7	~0.7	0	Hemodialysis	
Paracetamol	151	Yes	~1.0	~5.0	0	Hemodialysis	Useful if clearance decreased due to liver failure
Phenobarbital	232	No	~0.54	~0.06	24%	Hemoperfusion	—
Procainamide	272	Yes	~1.9	~8	~16%	Hemodialysis or hemoperfusion	Clearance decreased in renal failure; active metabolite also removed
Salicylate	138	Yes	~0.17	~0.88	~90%	Hemodialysis	Clearance and binding decrease with increasing dose
Theophylline	180	Yes	~0.5	~0.65	~56%	Hemoperfusion	—

From Pond SM. Extracorporeal techniques in the management of poisoned patients. Med J Aust 1991;154:617–622.

methanol, and ethanol poisoning in that order of frequency. (Table 4–1) Hemoperfusion was used mainly for poisoning by aminophylline/theophylline, long-acting barbiturates, benzodiazepines, and carbamazepine in order of frequency.[9] The toxicokinetics of some drugs removed by extracorporeal techniques are summarized in Tables 4–2[10] and 4–3.[2]

Active drug removal by extracorporeal procedures studied by the AAPCC in the 5-year period from 1987 to 1992 is summarized in Table 4–4.[11,12] Many reports have involved multiple ingestions. Poisons for which hemoperfusion and hemodialysis have been used are listed in Tables 4–5 and 4–6.[13] There appears to be a modest increase in the frequency with which extracorporeal methods have been used for drug removal during the past decade, although many of the older drug indications for their use have now disappeared. Much of the data on usefulness of these procedures continue to be anecdotal.

HEMODIALYSIS

In 1978, Gwilt and Perrier suggested that if the percentage of free drug in the plasma divided by the apparent volume of distribution, V_d (per kilogram of body weight), is greater than 80, 6 hours of hemodialysis should remove a significant amount (20–50%) of a drug.[11] If the percentage of free drug divided by the apparent volume of distribution (per kilogram of body weight) is less than 20, then a small and probably insignificant amount (<10%) of the drug will be removed during 6 hours of hemodialysis. Follow-up controlled clinical studies designed to validate these observations have not been performed.

$$\frac{\%\text{ Free drug}}{V_D\ (\text{L/kg})} > 80 \qquad \text{20–50\% removed by hemodialysis}$$

$$\frac{\%\text{ Free drug}}{V_D\ (\text{L/kg})} < 20 \qquad \text{<10\% removed by hemodialysis}$$

HEMOPERFUSION

Indications

Indications for hemoperfusion in the management of the poisoned patient are as follows:

- An established intoxication causing a severe disturbance of one or more vital functions with a drug having a small distribution volume and displaying a clear relationship between blood levels and toxic effects
- Deterioration of the clinical state of an intoxicated patient with initially less severe symptoms, despite optimal conservative treatment
- Intoxication with a drug known to be metabolized to a more toxic one
- Intoxication with a drug known to produce delayed toxicity[12]
- Severe intoxication with midbrain dysfunction
- Development of complications of coma
- Impairment of normal drug excretory function
- Intoxication with an extractable drug that can be removed at a rate greater than that of endogenous elimination[13]

Table 4–2
Pharmacokinetic Properties of Selected Drugs and Poisons

						Fractional Removal in 4 h (%)		
Drug Name	Apparent Volume of Distribution, V_d (L/kg)	Plasma Clearance (mL/min)	Plasma Protein Binding (%)	Hemodialyzer Clearance (mL/min)	Hemoperfusion Clearance (mL/min)	Normal Patient	With Hemo-dialysis	With Hemo-perfusion
Central Nervous System Agents								
Alcohols								
Ethanol	0.6	170–320	0	120–160	—	76	87	—
Isopropanol	0.6		0	—	—	—	79	—
Methanol	0.6	44	0	98–176	—	22	56	—
Ethylene glycol	0.8	64	—	—	—			—
Sedative hypnotics								
Chloral hydrate	6	600	35–41	120	157–238	29	34	37
Ethchlorvynol	2.8	90	30–50	64	125–300	10	17	23
Glutethimide	2.7	180	45	50	60–250	20	25	32
Meprobamate	0.75	60	0–20	60	85–150	24	42	56
Methyprylon	—	—	20–80	5–171	25–171	50	—	—
Methaqualone	6	140	80	23	216	8	9	18
Pentobarbital	1	36	66	22	50–300	12	18	27
Phenobarbital	0.75	9	25–60	80	80–290	4	33	39
Secobarbital	1.42	5	70	NS	20–119	1	1	16
Analgesics								
Acetaminophen	1	400	10–21*	120	125	75	83	83
Aspirin	0.21	45	73–94	20	90	52	65	89
Anticonvulsant drugs								
Carbamazepine	1	59	70–80	NS	80–129	17	17	36
Ethosuximide	0.7	10	0	140	—	5	52	
Phenytoin	0.57†	25	87–93	NS	76–189	14	14	61
Primidone	0.6	40	0	98	98	20	55	55
Sodium valproate	0.15–0.4	10	90–95	23	—	12	33	—
Psychotherapeutic drugs								
Amitriptyline	20	—	96	NS	14–210	—	—	—
Chloridazepoxide	0.3	25	86–93	NS	—	—	—	—
Chlorpromazine	—	—	90	NS	—	—	—	—
Desipramine	—	—	69–76	NS	—	—	—	—
Diazepam	0.74†	35	90	NS	—	15	15	—
Haloperidol	23	1330	90	NS	—	—	—	—
Imipramine	11	1000	86–96	18	—	27	27	—
Lithium carbonate	0.79	20	0	150	—	8	52	—
Nortriptyline	21	740	94	NS	14–210	11	11	12
Cardiovascular Agents								
Antiarrhythmic drugs								
Bretylium	7	725	1–6	NS	—	—	—	—
Disopyramide	0.83	93	5–65§	123	—	32	40	—
Flecainide	8.7	567	40	NS	—	—	—	—
Lidocaine	1.2	606	66	NS	75–90	82	82	86
Mexiletine	7–10	846	70	NS	—	29	29	—
Procainamide	2	810	15	65	—	75	78	—
N-Acetylprocainamide (NAPA)‖	1.5	200	10	41–97	125	37	49	—
Quinidine	2	270	80–85	11–18	24	37	39	40
Tocainide	3.2	182	10–15	25	—	18	20	—
Antihypertensive drugs								
Acebutolol	1.4	665	11–19	43	—	80	82	—
Atenolol	1.2	176	<5	29–39	—	40	45	—
Diazoxide	0.12	7	94	25	—	18	60	—
Nadolol	2	135	20–30	46–102	—	21	30	—

NS, not significant.
*Data are for the metabolite trichloroethanol.
†Concentration dependent.
‡V_d in uremia is 1.4 L/kg body weight.
§V_d in uremia is 2.2 L/kg body weight.
‖Binding is concentration dependent.
#V_d reduced to 0.42 L/kg in end-stage renal disease.
¶With concurrent L-cysteine infusion.
From Cutler RE, Forland SC, Hammond St JPG, Evans JR. Extracorporeal removal of drugs and poisons by hemodialysis and hemoperfusion. Annu Rev Pharmacol Toxicol 1987;27:169–191.

(continued)

Table 4–2 *(Continued)*

Drug Name	Apparent Volume of Distribution, V_d (L/kg)	Plasma Clearance (mL/min)	Plasma Protein Binding (%)	Hemodialyzer Clearance (mL/min)	Hemoperfusion Clearance (mL/min)	Fractional Removal in 4 h (%) Normal Patient	With Hemo-dialysis	With Hemo-perfusion
Cardiovascular agents—cont'd								
Cardiotonic agents								
Digitoxin	0.5	3	90	NS	19	2	2	14
Digoxin	7.1	160	20–30	20	80	7	8	11
Spasmolytic Agent								
Theophylline	0.45	46	60	70	100–225	30	59	74
Antineoplastic Agent								
Methotrexate	0.64#	52	50–70	—	54–137	24	—	64
Metals and Minerals								
Fluoride	0.5	100	—	100–188	—	—	—	—
Mercury	—	—	99	NS	—	—	—	—
Methylmercury	—	—	99	50–150¶	—	—	—	—
Herbicides and Insecticides								
Paraquat	2.8	28	—	NS	57–156	—	—	—
Demeton-*S*-Methyl-sulfoxide	—	—	—	53	84	—	—	—

#V_d reduced to 0.42 L/kg in end-stage renal disease.
¶With concurrent L-cysteine infusion.

Table 4–3
Kinetic Characteristics of Drugs That Make Them Amenable to Removal by Extracorporeal Procedures

Hemodialysis	Hemoperfusion	Hemofiltration
Relative molecular mass <500	Adsorbed by activated charcoal	Relative molecular mass less than the cutoff of the filter fibers, usually <40,000
Water soluble	Small volume of distribution (<1 L/kg)	Small volume of distribution (<1 L/kg)
Small volume of distribution (<1 L/kg)	Poorly bound to plasma proteins	Single-compartment kinetics
Poorly bound to plasma proteins	Single-compartment kinetics	Low endogenous clearance (<4 mL min^{-1} kg^{-1})
Single-compartment kinetics	Low endogenous clearance (<4 mL min^{-1} kg^{-1})	
Low endogenous clearance (<4 mL min^{-1} kg^{-1})		

Adapted from Pond SM. Extracorporeal techniques in the management of poisoned patients. Med J Aust 1991;154:617–622.

Table 4–4
Active Drug Removal by Extracorporeal Procedures

	Number of patients 1987	1993
Hemodialysis	297	646
Charcoal hemoperfusion	98	>121
Resin hemoperfusion	23	64*

*Charcoal or resin hemoperfusion.

Zilker suggests that the problems that limit the usefulness of hemoperfusion include late initiation of treatment, presence of compounds with a large volume of distribution or with a rapid distribution, poisonings that are more easily treated with hemodialysis, presence of a trained group, and usefulness of symptomatic therapy during the critical phase.[14]

Comparison of Hemoperfusion and Hemodialysis

There is little benefit to hemoperfusion over hemodialysis. Clearance of some drugs may be higher with hemoperfusion than with hemodialysis, but this is probably not clinically significant. Complications of hemodialysis, hemoperfusion, and hemofiltration are summarized in Table 4–7.[2]

PERITONEAL DIALYSIS

Indications

Acute peritoneal dialysis is used principally to treat patients with acute renal failure, especially in patients with bleeding disorders or venous access problems or in centers without access to hemodialysis. Peritoneal dialysis is almost never used in the management of drug overdoses or poisoning and is not an acceptable substitute for hemodialysis. The slow rate of drug removal by this technique is offset by the ability of peritoneal dialysis to be carried out for 24 hours versus the typical 2- to 4-hour cycles of hemodialysis or hemoperfu-

Table 4–5
Drugs and Chemicals Removed With Dialysis

Barbiturates
amobarbital
aprobarbital
barbital
butabarbital
cyclobarbital
pentobarbital
pentobarbital
phenobarbital
quinalbital
(secobarbital)

Nonbarbiturate Hypnotics, Sedatives, Tranquilizers, Anticonvulsants
carbamazepine
carbromal
chloral hydrate
(chlordiazepoxide)
(diazepam)
(diphenylhydantoin)
(diphenylhydramine)
ethiamate
ethchlorvynol
ethosuximide
galamine
glutethimide
(heroin)
meprobamate
(methaqualone)
methsuximide
methyprylon
paraldehyde
primidone
valproic acid

Antidepressants
(amitryptiline)
amphetamines
(imipramine)
isocarboxazid
Monoamine oxidase inhibitors
(pargyline)
(phenelzine)
tranylcypromine
(tricyclics)

Alcohols
ethanol
ethylene glycol
isopropanol
methanol

Analgesics, Antirheumatic Agents
acetaminophen
acetophenetidin
acetylsalicylic acid
colchicine
methylsalicylate
(D-propoxyphene)
salicylic acid

Antimicrobial Agents/ Anticancer Agents
amikacin
dibekacin
fosfomycin
gentamicin
kanamycin
neomycin
netilmicin
sisomicin
streptomycin
tobramycin
(vancomycin)

bacitracin
colistin

ampicillin
amoxicillin
azlocillin
carbenicillin
clavulinic acid
(cloxacillin)
(floxacillin)
mecillinam
mezlocillin
(nafcillin)
penicillin
piperacillin
temocillin
ticarcillin

(cefaclor)
cefadroxil
cefamandole
cefazolin
cefixime
cefmenoxime
(cefonicid)
(cefoperazone)
ceforanide
(cefotaxime)
(cefotetan)
cefotiam
cefoxitin
cefroxadine
cefsulodin
ceftazidime
(ceftriaxone)
cefuroxime
cephacetrile
cephalexin
cephaloridine
cephalothin
(cephapirin)
cephradine

aztreonam
cilastin
imipinem
moxalactam

Antimicrobial Agents/ Anticancer Agents (cont'd)
(chloramphenicol)
ciprofloxacin
(clindamycin)
(erythromycin)
metronidazole
nitrofurantoin
ornidazole
sulfonamides
tetracycline
tinidazole

acyclovir
amantadine
cycloserine
ethambutol
5-fluorocytosine
isoniazid
(chloroquine)
quinine

(azathioprine)
bredinin
cyclophosphamide
5-fluorouracil
(methotrexate)

Cardiovascular Agents
acebutolol
N-acetylprocainamide
atenolol
bretylium
captopril
(diazoxide)
(digoxin)
(lidocaine)
metoprolol
methyldopa
(ouabain)
nadolol
practolol
procainamide
propranolol
(quinidine)
sotalol
tocainide

Metals, Inorganics
(aluminum)*
arsenic
(copper)*
(iron)*
lead
lithium
(magnesium)
(mercury)*
potassium

Metals, Inorganics (cont'd)
phosphate
sodium
strontium
(tin)
(zinc)

bromide
chloride
iodide
fluoride

Miscellaneous Drugs
acipimox
aminophylline
aniline
borates
boric acid
(chlorpropamide)
chromic acid
cimetidine
dinitro-*o*-cresol
folic acid
mannitol
methylprednisolone
potassium dichromate
sodium citrate
theophylline
thiocyanate
ranitidine

Solvents, Gases
acetone
camphor
carbon monoxide
(carbon tetrachloride)
(eucalyptus oil)
thiols
toluene
trichloroethylene

Plants, Animals, Herbicides, Insecticides
alkyl phosphate
amanitin
demeton sulfoxide
dimethoate
diquat
methylmercury complex
(organophosphates)
paraquat
snake bite
sodium chlorate
potassium chlorate

( ), Not well removed; ( )*, removed with chelating agent.
From Winchester JF. Poisoning: Is the role of nephrologist diminishing? Am J Kid Dis 1989;13:171–183.

Table 4–6
Drugs and Chemicals Removed With Hemoperfusion

Barbiturates
amobarbital
butabarbital
hexabarbital
pentobarbital
phenobarbital
quinalbital
secobarbital
thiopental
vinalbital

Nonbarbiturate Hypnotics, Sedatives, Tranquilizers
carbromal
chloral hydrate
chlorpromazine
(diazepam)
diphenhydramine
ethchlorvynol
glutethimide
meprobamate
methaqualone
methsuximide
methyprylon
promazine
promethazine

Analgesics, Antirheumatic Agents
acetaminophen
acetylsalicylic acid
colchicine
methylsalicylate
phenylbutazone
D-propoxyphene
salicylic acid

Antimicrobial Agents/Anticancer Agents
(adriamycin)
ampicillin
carmustine
chloramphenicol
chloroquine
clindamycin
dapsone
doxorubicin
gentamicin
isoniazid
(methotrexate)
thiabendazole

Antidepressants
(amitryptiline)
(imipramine)
(tricyclics)

Plants, Animals, Herbicides, Insecticides
amanitin
chlordane
demeton sulfoxide
dimethoate
diquat
methylparathion
nitrostigmine
organophosphates
paraquat
parathion
phalloidin
polychlorinated biphenyls

Cardiovascular Agents
N-acetylprocainamide
digoxin
(disopyramide)
procainamide
quinidine

Metals, Inorganics
(aluminum)*
(iron)*

Miscellaneous Drugs
aminophylline
cimetidine
(fluoroacetamide)
(phencyclidine)
phenols
(podophyllin)
theophylline

Solvents, Gases
carbon tetrachloride
ethylene oxide
trichloroethanol

( ), Not well removed; ( )*, removed with chelating agent.
From Winchester JF. Poisoning: Is the role of nephrologist diminishing? Am J Kid Dis 1989;13:171–183.

Table 4–7
Complications of Hemodialysis, Hemoperfusion, and Hemofiltration

Complications Common to All Three Procedures
Hypotension
Blood loss
Hematomas
Air embolism
Metabolic disequilibria

Complications Specific to Hemoperfusion:
Thrombocytopenia
Leukopenia
Hypocalcaemia

From Pond SM. Extracorporeal techniques in the management of poisoned patients. Med J Aust 1991;154:617–622.

sion. It does not require anticoagulation and uses minimal equipment.[15]

Physiology

Peritoneal dialysis operates on principles similar to those of hemodialysis, with diffusion of toxins from mesenteric capillaries across the peritoneal membrane into dialysate dwelling in the peritoneal cavity. The blood flow rate depends on intrinsic mesenteric circulation and cannot be adjusted as in hemodialysis. As the clearance of small, dialyzable substances depends on blood and dialysate of low rates, clearance of toxins is consistently higher with hemodialysis than with peritoneal dialysis. Addition of albumin, lipids, or furosemide to the peritoneal dialysate enhances clearance but not to the levels achieved with hemodialysis. Therefore, the role of peritoneal dialysis is limited to the rare patient who is a candidate for hemodi-

Table 4–8
Complications of Acute Peritoneal Dialysis

Pain
Hemorrhage from vascular laceration
Leakage
Inadequate drainage
Perforation of viscus
Superficial subcutaneous infection at catheter insertion site
Bacterial peritonitis
Arrhythmias
Volume depletion
Volume overload
Pneumonia
Pleural effusion
Hyperglycemia and electrolyte disorders

From Health and Policy Committee, American College of Physicians. Clinical competence in acute hemodialysis. Ann Intern Med 1988;108:632–634.

alysis but for whom the treatment is unavailable or contraindicated.[16]

Method

Acute peritoneal dialysis involves either placing a stylet catheter at the bedside under local anesthesia or surgically inserting a Tenckhoff catheter in the abdomen. Dialysate fluid is instilled, and 1 to 2 L is exchanged each hour.

Complications

Multiple complications have been reported with peritoneal dialysis (Table 4–8).[7]

HEMOFILTRATION

During hemofiltration, an arteriovenous pressure difference induces a convective transport of solutes through hollow fiber or flat sheet membrane (Fig. 4–1). This permits a substantial flow of plasma water and a high permeability to compounds with a relative molecular weight less than or equal to 40,000. Hemofiltration is performed similar to hemodialysis except that the blood is pumped through a hemofilter. It can be performed intermittently at high ultrafiltrate rates of up to 6 L/h or continuously at ultrafiltrate flow rates of about 100 mL/h. In the treatment of poisoning, the latter procedure, continuous arteriovenous hemofiltration, has the advantage that it can be performed for a long period.

Efficacy

The advantage of hemofiltration over hemodialysis and hemoperfusion is its ability to remove compounds with a large (<4500–40,000) relative molecular weight. Such compounds include the aminoglycoside antibiotics and metal chelate complexes such as aluminum or iron deferoxamine. The extent of bonding of the toxic compound to plasma protein is a determinant of clearance by hemofiltration. Highly protein-bound compounds include arsenic, calcium channel blockers, diazepam, phenytoin, salicylates and other nonsteroidal antiinflammatory drugs, thyroxine, and the tricyclic antidepressants. Compounds that are poorly protein bound include the alcohols, aminoglycosides, atenolol, and lithium. For highly protein-bound poisons, hemoperfusion offers the best opportunity for rapid removal.[17,18]

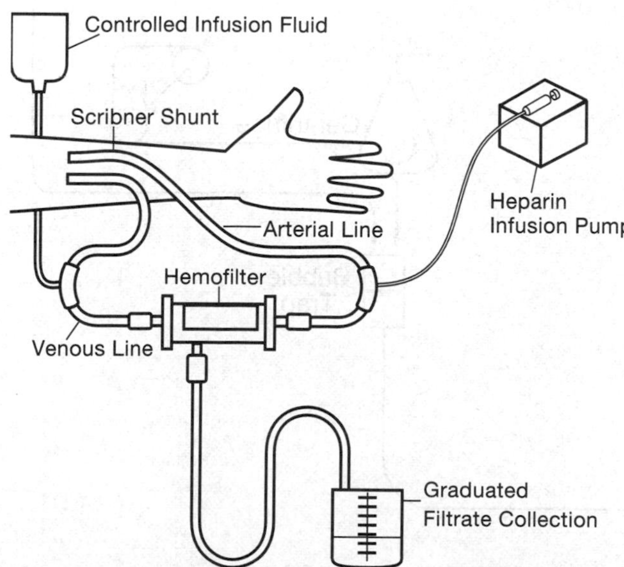

Figure 4–1 Schematic representation of the continuous arteriovenous hemofiltration system. (From Horton MW, Godley PJ. Continuous arteriovenous hemofiltration: An alternative to hemodialysis. Am J Hosp Pharm 1988; 45:1361–1368. Reproduced with permission of the Amicon Division, W.R. Grace & Co., Danvers, MA.)

For dialyzable poisons with a small volume of distribution (eg, aspirin, theophylline), acute hemodialysis appears to be the most reasonable approach. Both hemoperfusion and acute hemodialysis are short-lived procedures. The possibility of post-therapy rebound in blood concentration exists. If a toxin has a large volume of distribution V_D and is filterable or dialyzable, continuous arteriovenous hemofiltration or continuous hemodialysis may be useful.[17] Further controlled studies in this area are indicated.[16]

Complications

Complications of hemofiltration include clotting of the filter and mild bleeding. Horton and Godley have summarized the relative advantages and disadvantages of continuous arteriovenous hemofiltration (CAVH) compared with hemodialysis (Table 4–9).[19] CAVH may be useful for eliminating agents like lithium, methanol, ethanol, ethylene glycol, vancomycin, aminoglycosides, and *N*-acetylprocainamide. Animal studies suggest that CAVH may be a useful technique to remove iron in severe iron intoxication, particularly where renal failure occurs.[20]

Table 4–9
Relative Advantages and Disadvantages of Continuous Arteriovenous Hemofiltration (CAVH) Compared with Hemodialysis

Advantages
CAVH maintains consistent homeostasis through slow, gradual shifts in volume status and serum osmolality.
CAVH avoids hypotensive or dysequilibrium episodes.
CAVH permits continuous control of fluid balance and reduces the need to restrict fluid administration.
CAVH requires a lower volume of blood to be circulating outside the body.
CAVH has no effect on complement or leukocytes.
CAVH does not require expensive equipment or extensive training of personnel.
CAVH has greater clearances of mid-molecular-weight solutes.
Disadvantages
Both CAVH and hemodialysis require some degree of anticoagulation.
Both CAVH and hemodialysis have vascular access complications.
Staff may be unfamiliar with CAVH.
CAVH has lower clearance of low-molecular-weight solutes.
CAVH is not able to maintain nitrogen balance in catabolic patients.

From Horton MW, Godley PJ. Continuous arteriovenous hemofiltration: An alternative to hemodialysis. Am J Hosp Pharm 1988;45:1361–1368.

Status

All the extracorporeal techniques (hemodialysis, hemoperfusion, hemofiltration) have not been subject to controlled clinical trials in poisoned patients. Their clinical benefit remains to be established. The indications to remove toxic compounds by hemofiltration are limited. Clinical studies suggest that CAVH does not appear to substitute for hemodialysis or hemoperfusion. If a compound is amenable to removal by hemodialysis, its clearance will be greater than that achieved by hemofiltration.[17,19] Hemofiltration and plasmapheresis remain potentially hazardous forms of treatment.

PLASMAPHERESIS

Plasmapheresis separates cellular blood components from plasma (Fig. 4–2). The cells are resuspended in either colloids, albumin, or fresh-frozen plasma and then reinfused. The efficacy of plasmapheresis depends on the number of plasma exchanges. It eliminates toxic substances but sacrifices part of the patient's own plasma proteins. Complications (Table 4–10) limit its usefulness.

Individual case reports on the use of plasmapheresis in overdoses of vincristine, inorganic mercury, thyroxine, orellanus, amanita, theophylline, paxillum, iatrogenic antithymocyte globulin, digoxin antibody complexes, phenytoin, dapsone, propoxyphene, hemlock, and carbamazepine do not suggest a practical role for plasmapheresis in clinical toxicology.[3]

HEMODIAFILTRATION

Hemodiafiltration combines continuous hemofiltration with hemodialysis. It is rarely used for detoxification.[21]

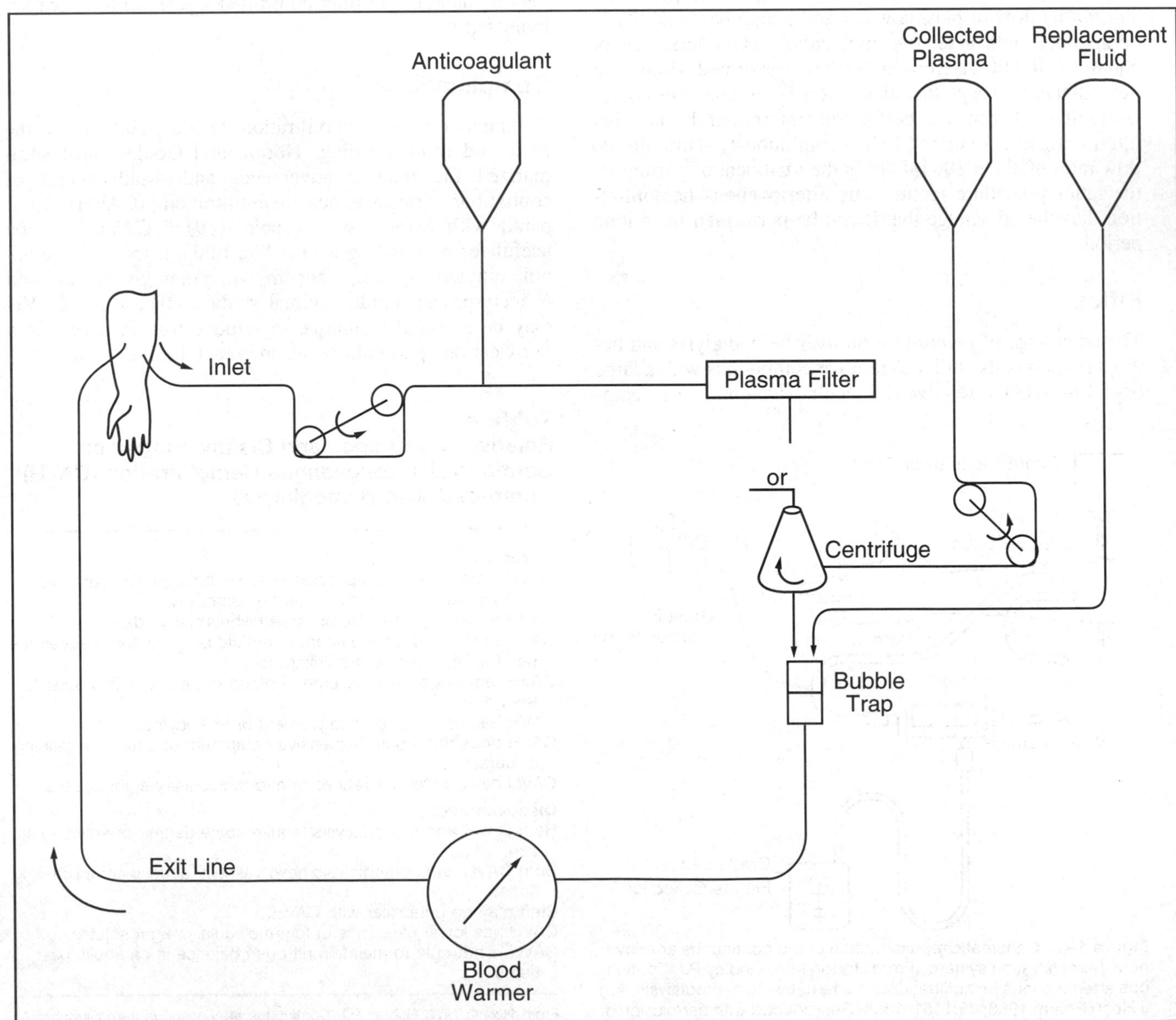

Figure 4–2 Schematic of plasmapheresis circuit for membrane-based (filter) and centrifugal methods. (From Jones JS, Dougherty J. Current status of plasmapheresis in toxicology. Ann Emerg Med 1986; 15:474–482.)

Table 4–10
Complications of Plasmapheresis

Bleeding Disorders
Disseminated intravascular coagulation
Elevated bleeding times
Thrombocytopenia
Citrate Toxicity
Paresthesias
Muscle tetany
Nausea
Chills
Syncope
Cardiac arrhythmias
Dysequilibrium Syndrome
Nausea
Vomiting
Hypovolemia
Fluid Overload
Hypertension
Congestive heart failure
Hypercoagulation
Cerebral thrombosis
Pulmonary embolus
Myocardial infarction
Infection
Pathogenic
Opportunistic
Anaphylaxis
Shock
Urticaria
Angioedema
Vascular Access
Vessel perforation
Pneumothorax
Air embolism
Bacteremia
Miscellaneous
Seizures
Metabolic alkalosis
Cerebral spasm
Adult respiratory distress syndrome
Cardiac arrhythmias (not associated with calcium)

From Jones JS, Dougherty J. Current status of plasmapheresis in toxicology. Ann Emerg Med 1986;15:479–482.

PLASMA PERFUSION

Plasma perfusion is a combination of plasmapheresis and hemoperfusion that has been used in methylparathion poisoning.[22,23]

CARDIOPULMONARY BYPASS

Cardiopulmonary bypass can affect elimination of a drug from the body when the substances are cleared by the lungs, kidneys, or liver. A fall in the total serum concentrations of benzodiazepines, cephalosporins, digoxin, barbiturates, etomidate, isoflurane, nitroglycerin, lidocaine, fentanyl, and propranolol has been demonstrated during or after the bypass procedure (Table 4–11).[24]

Cardiopulmonary bypass continues to be a little used experimental procedure in the treatment of poisoning.[25] Anecdotal reports indicate the potential usefulness of this procedure in the treatment of verapamil intoxication and in other poisonings (eg, lidocaine) that lead to cardiac depression.[26,27] A patient with severe diltiazem poisoning was refractory to cardiopulmonary bypass.[28]

Table 4–11
Possible Alterations to the Disposition of Drugs due to the Physiologic Changes Induced by Cardiopulmonary Bypass

Pharmacokinetic Parameter	Physiologic Change	Expected Alterations
Absorption	Hypotension and blood flow changes	Reduced or delayed absorption
Distribution	Lung sequestration	Decreased volume of distribution; redistribution on restoration of spontaneous circulation
	Hypotension and blood flow changes	Decreased volume of distribution
	Hemodilution and decreased concentration of binding proteins	Increased volume of distribution
	Postbypass α_1-acid glycoprotein increase	Decreased volume of distribution
Elimination		
Hepatic	Decreased hepatic blood flow	Decreased clearance of drugs with flow-dependent elimination
	Decreased concentration of binding proteins	Increased clearance of drugs with restrictive elimination
	Hypothermia, severely decreased hepatic blood flow	Decreased intrinsic clearance (metabolism)
Renal	Hypotension and reduced blood flow	Decreased active tubular secretion
	Decreased concentration of binding proteins	Increased glomerular filtration
	pH and filtration volume changes	Tubular reabsorption changes

From Buylaert WA, Herregots LL, Montier EP, Bogaert MG. Cardiopulmonary bypass and the pharmacokinetics of drugs: An update. Clin Pharmacokinet 1989;17:10–26.

REFERENCES

1. Garrettson LK, Geller RJ. Acid and alkaline diuresis: When are they of value in the treatment of poisoning? Drug Saf 1990;5:220–232.
2. Pond SM. Extracorporeal techniques in the management of poisoned patients. Med J Aust 1991;154:617–622.
3. Koppel C. Position paper: Hemofiltration, plasmapheresis and other techniques. Personal communication at Congress of European Association of Poison Centres and Clinical Toxicologists, Vienna, April 1994.

4. Bismuth C, Muczinski J. Are extracorporeal techniques of elimination validated in acute poisoning? In: *Proceedings, European Association of Poison Centres and Clinical Toxicologists, Istanbul, May 1992*:69.
5. Health and Public Policy Committee, American College of Physicians. Clinical competence in continuous arteriovenous hemofiltration. Ann Intern Med 1988;108:902–907.
6. Health and Public Policy Committee, American College of Physicians. Clinical competence in acute hemodialysis. Ann Intern Med 1988;108:632–634.
7. Health and Public Policy Committee, American College of Physicians. Clinical competence in acute peritoneal dialysis. Ann Intern Med 1988;108:763–765.
8. Litovitz T, Veltri JC. The role of hemoperfusion and hemodialysis in toxicology. Am J Emerg Med 1988;6:80.
9. Litowitz TL, Holm KC, Clancy C, et al. 1992 Annual report of the American Association of Poison Control Centers Toxic Exposure Surveillance system. Am J Emerg Med 1993; 11:494–555.
10. Cutler RE, Forland SC, Hammond St JPG, Evans JR. Extracorporeal removal of drugs and poisons by hemodialysis and hemoperfusion. Annu Rev Pharmacol Toxicol 1987;27:169–191.
11. Gwilt PR, Perrier D. Plasma protein binding and distribution characteristics of drugs as indices of their hemodialyzability. Clin Pharmacol Ther 1978;24:154–161.
12. Rommes JH. Haemoperfusion, indications and side effects. Arch Toxicol 1992;suppl. 15:40–49.
13. Winchester JF. Poisoning: Is the role of nephrologist diminishing? Am J Kid Dis 1989;13:171–183.
14. Zilker T. Personal communication. In: *Proceedings, XVIth International Congress of the European Association of Poison Centres and Clinical Toxicologists, Vienna, April 1994.*
15. Shannon M. Extracorporeal drug removal. II. Other methods. Clin Toxicol Rev 1990;12(9):1–2.
16. Blye E, Lorch J, Cortrell S. Extracorporeal therapy in the treatment of intoxication. Am J Kid Dis 1984;3:321–338.
17. Golper TA, Bennett WM. Drug removal by continuous arteriovenous haemofiltration: A review of the evidence in poisoned patients. Med Toxicol Adverse Drug Experience 1988; 3:341–349.
18. Bressolle F, Kinowski J-M, de la Coussaye JE, et al. Clinical pharmacokinetics during continuous haemofiltration. Clin Pharmacokinet 1994;26:457–471.
19. Horton MW, Godley PJ. Continuous arteriovenous hemofiltration: An alternative to hemodialysis. Am J Hosp Pharm 1988;45:1361–1368.
20. Banner W, Vernon DD, Ward R, et al. Continuous arteriovenous hemofiltration (CAVH) in experimental iron intoxication. Vet Hum Toxicol 1988;30:355.
21. Bellomo R, Kearly Y, Parkin G, et al. Treatment of life-threatening lithium toxicity with continuous arteriovenous hemodiafiltration. Crit Care Med 1991;19:836–837.
22. Cnzhnikov EA, Yasoslavsky AA, Molondenkov MV, et al. Plasma perfusion through charcoal in methylparathion poisoning. Lancet 1977;1:38–39.
23. Berning T, Krummner T, Glaser T, et al. Plasma perfusion in life-threatening exogenous poisoning. Schweiz Med Wochenschr 1987;117:1368–1370.
24. Buylaert WA, Herregots LL, Montier EP, Bogaert MG. Cardiopulmonary bypass and the pharmacokinetics of drugs: An update. Clin Pharmacokinet 1989;17:10–26.
25. Hendren WG, Schieber RS, Garrettson LP. Extracorporeal bypass for the treatment of verapamil poisoning. Ann Emerg Med 1989;18:984–987.
26. Freedman MD, Gal J, Freed CR. Extracorporeal pump assistance: Novel treatment of acute lidocaine poisoning. Eur J Clin Pharmacol 1982;22:129–135.
27. Kennedy JH, Barnette J, Flasterstein A, Higgs W. Experimental barbiturate intoxication: Treatment by partial cardiopulmonary bypass and hemodialysis. Cardiovasc Res Center Bull 1976;14:61–69.
28. Martin TG, Tisherman SA, Stein K. Massive diltiazem OD unresponsive to cardiopulmonary bypass: Personal Communication. In: *Proceedings, XVIth International Congress of European Association of Poison Centres and Clinical Toxicologists, Vienna, April 1994.*

Chapter 5
Antidotes

INTRODUCTION

Antidotes may be lifesaving. They can aid in reducing morbidity and health care costs by shortening the course of treatment. Some antidotes (eg, naloxone, flumazenil) exhibit rapid and dramatic clinical effects. Some do not affect all the toxic effects of a particular poisoning (eg, chelating agents), and a few are useful adjuncts to treatment without specific antidotal effects (eg, diazepam in the treatment of organophosphate poisoning). Controlled clinical studies are limited for ethical reasons. Antidotes are drugs and often precipitate undesirable reactions (eg, naloxone, flumazenil). Meredith and colleagues have prepared a list of antidotes and other agents useful in the treatment of poisoning[1] (Table 5–1). Antidotes appear to reflect national practices (eg, 4-dimethylaminophenol for cyanide intoxication in Germany; hydroxocobalamin for cyanide poisoning in France; silibinin for amanitin poisoning in Austria and Germany), but most antidotes, thanks to widely publicized information (medical toxicology literature, national and international meetings) have been widely used. Governmental regulations, a lack of economic incentives for manufacturers, and a paucity of controlled studies have restricted availability of a number of antidotes (eg, hydroxocobalamin in the United States).

Some antidotes commonly used within the first hour of treatment of a patient with an overdose are summarized in Table 5–2.[2] Antidotes for cardiotoxic drugs and poisons are listed in Table 5–3.

The American Academy of Clinical Toxicology Acute and Intensive Care Committee has proposed facility assessment guidelines for Regional Poison Treatment Centers, which include recommendations for a pharmacy stock of common antidotes in amounts adequate to meet regional needs (Table 5–4).[3]

The World Health Organization through the International Program on Chemical Safety (IPCS) and the Commission of European Communities (CEC) has begun publication of a comprehensive Evaluation of Antidotes series.[1] The National Capitol Center has suggested a list of quantities of recommended stock drugs suggested for an emergency department or pharmacy for use in the treatment of poisoning (Table 5–5).[1]

Table 5–1A
Antidotes and Other Agents Useful in Treatment of Poisoning
Group 1

Antidote	Main Indication of Pathologic Condition	Other Possible Applications
Acetylcysteine	Paracetamol (acetaminophen)	Organochlorine solvents, amanitin
Amyl nitrite	Cyanide	Hydrogen sulfide
Ascorbic acid	Organic peroxides (osmium)	
Atropine	Cholinergic syndrome	
Aurintricarboxylic acid (ATA)	Beryllium	
Benzylpenicillin	Amanitins	
β-Aminopropionitrile	Caustics	
Calcium chloride or other calcium salts	HF, fluorides, oxalates	Calcium antagonists
Dantrolene	Malignant hyperthermia	Malignant neuroleptic syndrome
Deferoxamine	Iron, aluminium	Paraquat
Diazepam	Chloroquine	
Dicobalt edetate	Cyanide	
Digoxin-specific antibody fragments	Digoxin/digitoxin, digitalis glycosides	
Dimercaprol	Arsenic	Copper, gold, mercury (inorganic), lead encephalopathy
4-Dimethylaminophenol (4-DMAP)	Cyanide	Hydrogen sulfide
Ethanol	Methanol, ethylene glycol, glycol ethers	Alkoxysilanes
Flumazenil	Benzodiazepines	
Folinic acid	Folinic acid antagonists	
Glucagon	Beta blockers	
Glucose	Insulin	
Guanidine	Botulism	
Hydroxocobalamin	Cyanide	
Isoprenaline	Beta blockers	
Methionine	Paracetamol (acetaminophen)	
4-Methylpyrazole	Ethylene glycol, methanol	Coprin and disulfiram
Methylthioninium chloride (methylene blue)	Methemoglobinemia	
N-Acetylpenicillamine	Mercury	
Naloxone	Opiates	
Neostigmine	Neuromuscular block (curare type) peripheral anticholinergic poisoning	
Oximes	Organophosphates	
Oxygen	Cyanide, carbon monoxide, hydrogen sulfide	
Oxygen, hyperbaric	Carbon monoxide	Cyanide, hydrogen sulfide, carbon tetrachloride
Penicillamine	Copper	Gold, lead, mercury
Pentetic acid (DTPA)	Radioactive metals	
Phentolamine	Alpha-adrenergic poisoning	
Physostigmine	Central anticholinergic syndrome from atropine and derivatives	Central anticholinergic syndrome from other drugs
Phytomenadione (vitamin K)	Coumarin derivatives	
Potassium hexacyanoferrate (Prussian blue C177520)	Thallium	
Prenalterol	Beta blockers	
Propranolol	Beta-adrenergic poisoning	
Protamine sulfate	Heparin	
Pyridoxine	Isoniazid	Ethylene glycol, gyrometrine, hydrazines
Silibinin	Amanitins	
Sodium nitrite	Cyanide	Hydrogen sulfide
Sodium nitroprusside	Ergotism	
Sodium salicylate	Beryllium	
Sodium thiosulfate	Cyanide	Bromate, chlorate, iodine
Succimer (DMSA)	Lead, mercury	
Tocopherol	Carbon monoxide	Oxygen toxicity
Tolonium chloride (toluidine blue)	Methemoglobinemia	
Trientine (triethylene tetramine)	Copper	
Unithiol (DMPS)	Arsenic	Copper, nickel, lead, cadmium, mercury (methyl and inorganic)

From Meredith TJ, Jacobsen D, Haines JA, Berger J-C, eds. *International Program on Chemical Safety/Commission of the European Communities Evaluation of Antidotes Series.* Vol. 1: *Naloxene, Flumazenil, and Dantrolene as Antidotes.* EUR 14797 EN. Vol. 2. *Antidotes for Poisoning by Cyanide* (van Heijst APVP, guest ed.). EUR 12280 EN. Cambridge: Cambridge University Press, 1993.

Table 5-1B
Group 2: *Agents Used to Prevent the Absorption of Poisons, to Enhance Their Elimination, or to Treat Symptomatically Their Effects on Body Functions*

A. *Emetics*	
Apomorphine	
Ipecacuanha	
B. *Cathartics and solutions used for whole-gut lavage*	
Magnesium citrate	
Magnesium sulfate	
Mannitol	
Sodium sulfate	
Sorbitol	
Whole-gut lavage fluids	
C. *Agents to modify urinary pH*	
Ammonium chloride	
Arginine hydrochloride	
Hydrochloric acid	
Sodium bicarbonate	
D. *Agents to prevent absorption of toxic substances in the gastrointestinal tract*	
Activated charcoal	(For most poisonings) digitalis, coumarin, kepone
Fuller's earth	Paraquat, diquat, potassium, copper, ferrocyanide
Simethicone	Foaming detergents
Sodium bicarbonate	Iron, mercury, organophosphates
Sodium sulfate	Lead, bismuth, barium
Starch	Iodine
E. *Agents to prevent absorption and/or damage in the skin*	
Calcium gluconate gel	Hydrofluoric acid
Macrogol 400	Phenol

Table 5-1C
Group 3: *Other Useful Therapeutic Agents for the Treatment of Poisoning**

Agent	Indication (Symptoms Arising from Poisoning)
Benztropine	Dystonia
Chlorpromazine	Hallucinatory and psychotic states
Corticosteroids	Acute allergic reactions, laryngeal edema, (systemic/topical/bronchoconstriction)
Diazepam	Convulsions, excitation, anxiety, muscular hypertonia
Diphenhydramine	Dystonia
Dobutamine	Myocardial depression
Dopamine	Myocardial depression, vascular relaxation
Epinephrine	Anaphylactic shock, cardiac arrest
Furosemide	Fluid retention, left ventricular failure
Glucose	Hypoglycemia
Haloperidol	Hallucinatory and psychotic states
Heparin	Hypercoagulability states
Lidocaine	Ventricular arrhythmias
Mannitol	Cerebral edema, fluid retention
Oxygen	Hypoxia
Pancuronium	Muscular rigidity, convulsions
Promethazine	Allergic reactions
Salbutamol	Bronchoconstriction (systemic/inhaled)
Sodium bicarbonate	Acidosis, some cardiac disturbances (eg, tricyclic antidepressant poisonings)

*Listed are certain therapeutic agents that are not antidotes according to the accepted definition but that, through their importance and sometimes specific role in the treatment of poisons, border on the concept of "antidotes." In practice, these agents are used very often in cases of poisoning and in other medical circumstances. The usefulness of these agents is in general well established, most of them are considered essential drugs, and they should be available for immediate use.

ACTIVATED CHARCOAL

See section on GI Decontamination.

AMINOPHYLLINE

Mechanism of Action

Aminophylline antagonizes diazepam-induced somnolence[4] and reverses sedation associated with lorazepam[5] by enhancing the level of extracellular adenosine level in the central nervous system,[6] apparently by blocking adenosine reuptake into neuronal and glial cells[7] and antagonizing the depressant action of adenosine.[8] It competitively binds the adenosine receptors. Benzodiazepines increase the activity of adenosine. This depresses neuronal activity by reducing the release of neurotransmitters.[9] Xanthine derivatives without adenosine blocking properties are unable to reverse benzodiazepine-induced sedation.[10] Aminophylline is rarely used for benzodiazepine-induced sedation since the advent of flumazenil (see Flumazenil in this chapter; also see Chapter 41).

Use

Many uses have not been subject to controlled clinical trials. Reports are often anecdotal:

1. May be useful in antagonizing the effects of flurazepam,[9] midazolam,[11] and lorazepam[4,5]
2. Aminophylline improves ventilation in lorazepam-induced neonatal apnea[12]
3. Reversal of coma in cerebral vascular accidents[13]
4. Abolishes Cheyne–Stokes respirations[14]

Table 5-1D
Group 4: *Antidotes and Related Agents Considered Obsolete*

Antidote	Indication
Ascorbic acid	Methemoglobinemia
Cyclophosphamide	Gold–paraquat
Cysteamine	Paracetamol
Diethyldithiocarbamate	Thallium
Fructose	Ethanol
Levallorphan	Opiates
Nalorphine	Opiates
Potassium permanganate	Fluorides
Silibinin	Amanitin
Tannins	Alkaloids
Thioctic acid	Amanitine
Tocopherol (vitamin E)	Paraquat
Universal antidote	Ingested poisons
Copper sulfate	As an emetic
Sodium chloride	As an emetic
Castor oil	As a cathartic
Acetazolamide	As a urinary pH modifier

Table 5-2
Antidotes Commonly Used Within the First Hour of Treatment of a Patient With an Overdose

Toxin	Antidote	Dose and Comments*
Opiates	Naloxone	Starting dose 2 mg. More may be needed for overdoses of some synthetic narcotics; less may be used in addicts to avoid precipitating withdrawal symptoms.
Methanol, ethylene glycol	Ethanol	Loading dose 10 mL of 10% solution per kilogram of body weight. Maintenance dose 0.15 mL per kilogram per hour. Double maintenance dose should be used during dialysis. Titrate to a blood ethanol level of 22 mmol/L (100 mg/dL).
Anticholinergic agents	Physostigmine	1–2 mg intravenously over 5 min. Use only for severe delirium. May be useful to treat seizures or tachydysrhythmias, but strong clinical evidence is lacking.
Organophosphate or carbamate insecticides	Atropine	Test dose 2 mg IV. Repeat in larger increments until drying of pulmonary secretions occurs.
Isoniazid, hydrazine, monomethylhydrazine (in *Gyromitra* species mushrooms)	Pyridoxine	Give in gram-per-gram equivalent doses to what was ingested. If amount ingested is unknown, start with 5 g IV. An overdose of pyridoxine may cause neuropathy.
Beta blockers	Glucagon	Starting dose 5–10 mg IV. Titrate to response (normalization of vital signs). Maintenance dose of 2–10 mg/h may be used.
Tricyclic antidepressants	Bicarbonate	1–2 mmol/kg IV for substantial cardiac conduction delay or ventricular dysrhythmias. Titrate to response and arterial pH.
Digitalis, glycosides	Digoxin-specific antibody fragments	Equimolar to ingestion: the number of miligrams of digoxin ingested divided by 0.6 is the number of vials required. If amount ingested is unknown and the patient has life-threatening dysrhythmias, give 10–20 vials IV. If serum digoxin concentration is known, the number of vials to administer = $\frac{\text{concentration (in ng/mL)} \times 5.6 \times \text{weight in kg}}{600}$
Benzodiazepines	Flumazenil	0.2 mg over 30 s. If there is no response after 30 s, give 0.3 mg over 30 s. If there is no response after 30 s, give 0.5 mg over 30 s at 1-min intervals up to a total dose of 3 mg. Should not be given if the patient shows signs of serious overdose from coingestion of tricyclic antidepressants or was taking benzodiazepines for control of seizures.
Calcium channel blockers, hydrofluoric acid, fluorides	Calcium	1 g calcium chloride given over 5 min by IV infusion with continuous cardiac monitoring. May be repeated often in life-threatening situations, but the serum calcium level should be monitored after the third dose.

*Doses given are for adults.
From Kulig K. Initial management of ingestions of toxic substances. N Engl J Med 1992;326:1677–1681.

5. Causes resistance to neuromuscular blockade by pancuronium[15]
6. May antagonize morphine-[16] and fentanyl-[17]induced respiratory depression
7. Can reduce depth and duration of sedation by thiopental[18]

Cautions

Aminophylline may induce nausea, vomiting, tachycardia, cardiac dysrhythmias, and seizures (see Chapter 45).

Dose

Aminophylline has been administered in doses of 1 to 2 mg/kg intravenously[4,5,7,9] to reverse sedation induced by diazepam,[4,7,8,19] flunitrazepam,[9] lorazepam,[5] and midazolam.

Nonspecific Antagonists

Intravenous aminophylline is a phosphodiesterase inhibitor that acts as a calcium channel facilitator. Aminophylline may reverse adverse effects of nifedipine, a calcium channel blocker, including cor pulmonale.[20]

4-AMINOPYRIDINE (4-AP)

See also Chapter 51.

Mechanism of Action

4-Aminopyridine (4AP) is used as an antagonist of nondepolarizing neuromuscular blocking agents. This agent enhances transmembrane calcium influx, which results in facilitation of synaptic transmission. Aminopyridine also increases the release of acetylcholine at the neuromuscular junction by selective blocking of potassium channels. The rate of efflux of potassium determines the duration of the action potential. Block of the potassium channels prolongs the action potential and allows more calcium to move into the cell. The intracellular uptake of calcium is essential for the release of acetylcholine. Thus, the increased influx following treatment with aminopyridine may result in an increased release of acetylcholine.

4-Aminopyridine is not commercially available in the United States.

Use

1. Pancuronium overdose; potentiates neostigmine and pyridostigmine reversal
2. Verapamil intoxication[21]
3. Possible use in human botulism (improves peripheral but not respiratory paralysis)[22]
4. Of possible use, orally, in disorders of neuromuscular transmission (Eaton–Lambert syndrome, congenital myasthenia, myasthenia gravis[23] and multiple sclerosis)[23,24] Further work is required to validate these uses.

Cautions

1. Overdose with 4-aminopyridine should respond to supportive therapy, prevention of absorption, treatment of seizures with diazepam, and possible use of pancuronium.[25]
2. 4-Aminopyridine may induce central nervous system stimulant effects, including seizures.

Dose

Administer 10 mg by intravenous route slowly infused, or 0.35 to 0.5 mg/kg used with neostigmine or pyridostigmine.[26]

ANTIVENINS

See section on envenomations bites.

ATROPINE

See section on argonophosphate poisoning.

CALCIUM

See Chapter 54.

Table 5–3
Antidotes for Cardiotoxic Drugs and Poisons

Intoxication	Antidote and Dose	Comments
Amphetamines, cocaine, and other stimulants	For tachyarrhythmias: esmolol 25–50 μg/kg/min IV infusion (may give loading bolus 500 μg/kg)	Simple sinus tachycardia may respond to sedation.
	For hypertension: labetalol 10–20 mg IV; phentolamine 2–5 mg IV	Do not use beta-selective beta blocker (eg, propranolol) alone; paradoxical worsening of hypertension may result.
Anticholinergic agents	Physostigmine 0.5–2 mg IV slowly	Caution: may induce atrioventricular block or asystole, especially in patients with tricyclic antidepressant overdose.
Beta blockers	Glucagon 5–10 mg IV bolus, 2–5 mg/h IV infusion	Atropine, isoproterenol, cardiac pacing are usually ineffective.
Calcium antagonists	Calcium chloride 0.5–1 g IV; repeat as needed to raise serum CA^{2+} 2–3 mg/dL	Calcium is more effective for negative inotropic effects, less effective for arteriolar dilation or atrioventricular block.
Cyclic antidepressants	Sodium bicarbonate 50–100 mEq IV boluses	Effective for hypotension, QRS prolongation, and atrioventricular block associated with membrane-depressant effects; not effective for sinus tachycardia, coma, or seizures
Digoxin and other cardiac glycosides	Digoxin-specific antibodies; see package insert or contact poison control center for dosage.	Rapidly effective for all manifestations of cardiotoxicity; dose is based on estimate of body burden of digoxin, not necessarily serum digoxin level.
Iron	Deferoxamine 15 mg/kg/h IV infusion	Higher doses may be needed in patients with serious manifestations.
Metaproterenol and other β_2-adrenergic drugs	Esmolol 25–50 μg/kg/min IV	Lowers heart rate and also reverses hypotension caused by excessive β_2-adrenergic stimulation.
Opioids	Naloxone 0.4–8 mg IV	Larger doses (up to 10–15 mg) may be needed for some resistant opioids.
Organophosphate and carbamate insecticides	Atropine 0.5–2 mg IV initially, repeated doses as needed	Atropine reverses bradycardia and other muscarinic toxicity but does not affect nicotinic toxicity, such as muscle weakness (requires pralidoxime).
Quinidine and other type Ia and Ic antiarrhythmics	Sodium bicarbonate 50–100 mEq IV boluses	Effective for hypotension, QRS prolongation, and atrioventricular block associated with membrane-depressant toxicity
Theophylline, caffeine	Esmolol 25–50 μg/kg/min IV infusion	Lowers heart rate and also reverses hypotension caused by excessive β_2-adrenergic stimulation.

From Callaham ML, ed. *Current Practice of Emergency Medicine.* Philadelphia: Decker, 1991.

Table 5–4
Antidotes for Poison Treatment Centers

N-Acetylcystine 20% (Mucomyst)	Dimercaptosuccinic acid (DMSA)
Activated charcoal	Diphenhydramine hydrochloride
Amantadine (Symmetrel)	Droperidol
Crotalidae polyvalent	Ethyl alcohol 100%
Lactrodectus mactans	Esmolol
Ascorbic acid	Folic acid/leucovorin
Atropine sulfate	Glucagon
Benztropine mesylate	Guanidine
Bromocriptine mesylate	Ipecac syrup
Calcium chloride 10%	Lorazepam
Calcium disodium edetate	Leucovorin
Calcium gluconate 10%	Mannitol 20%
Calcium gluconate gel	Methylene blue 1%
Cathartics	Naloxone hydrochloride (Narcan)
Magnesium citrate	Nicotinamide (niacinamide)
Magnesium sulfate or sodium sulfate	Nitroprusside, sodium
Sorbitol	D-Penicillamine
Cyanide antidote kits	Phentolamine
Amyl nitrite	Physostigmine salicylate
Sodium nitrite 3%	Polyethylene glycol (Golytely, PEG)
Sodium thiosulfate	Pralidoxime chloride (2-PAM, Protopam)
Dantrolene sodium	Propranolol
Dapsone	Protamine sulfate
Deferoxamine mesylate (Desferal)	Prussian blue
Dextrose 50% in water	Pyridoxine hydrochloride
Diazepam (Valium)	Starch
Diazoxide	Thiamine hydrochloride
Digoxin Immune FAB (Digibind)	Vitamin K_1 (AquaMEPHYTON)
Dimercaprol (BAL)	Vitamin K_3

CHELATORS

See Chapter 67.

CYANIDE ANTIDOTES

See section on cyanide.

DANTROLENE

Mechanism of Action

Dantrolene sodium acts in the treatment of hypercatabolic syndromes such as malignant hyperthermia and neuroleptic malignant syndrome by affecting calcium flux across the sarcoplasmic reticulum of skeletal muscle cells, resulting in rapid resolution of hyperthermia, dysrhythmias, muscle rigidity, tachycardia, hypercapnia, and metabolic acidosis.[34]

Use

Dantrolene appears to diminish hyperthermic states and muscle rigidity associated with amphetamine overdose,[27] carbon monoxide poisoning,[28] monoamine oxidase overdose,[29] and organophosphate poisoning and in neuroleptic malignant syndrome.[30] Confirmation of its usefulness for these indications requires further controlled study. Dantrolene was not effective in a controlled study of heat stroke.[31,32] Dantrolene appears to be useful in controlling the hypermetabolic state associated with the rhabdomyolysis secondary to theophylline poisoning.[33]

See Malignant Hyperthermia in Chapter 56.

Cautions

Use of oral dantrolene as a prophylactic drug in patients suspected to be susceptible to malignant hyperthermia may induce nausea, vomiting, dizziness, and diarrhea.

An adult patient given daily doses of dantrolene gradually increasing to 250 mg developed acute pulmonary edema and severe cardiac insufficiency after 11 days of therapy. Myocardial function returned to normal when drug treatment was stopped.[35]

Overdosages of dantrolene in three patients (20-month-old child, 25-year-old adult, and 23-year-old second-trimester pregnant woman) were reported following doses of 10 to 12 mg/kg, comparable to maximal intravenous recommendations. The child and pregnant woman exhibited no symptoms; only lethargy was noted in the 25-year-old. All routine chemistry, hematology, and urinary laboratory tests were normal. The patients were treated supportively and recovered uneventfully. The pregnant patient delivered a healthy child at term.[36]

Animal studies demonstrate an increase in lethality with a concomitant decrease in seizures when dantrolene is added to theophylline.[37] Complete heart block developed in animals pretreated with verapamil who were then given dantrolene.[38]

Dose

Oral

Oral dantrolene is not recommended for prophylaxis or treatment (variability in plasma levels attained, especially in children, delay in achieving therapeutic levels,[39] hepatotoxicity after oral use).

Intravenous

Incremental intravenous administration of dantrolene in a dose of 2.4 mg/kg of body weight in a 2-hour period results in maximal blood levels of 4.2 μg/mL, an elimination half-life of 12.1 hours, and a near steady-state blood level at 5.5 hours.

Watch for dizziness, lightheadedness, drowsiness, phlebitis, muscle weakness, and respiratory failure. A potentially severe hyperkalemia and cardiovascular collapse have been observed in animals after administration of verapamil and dantrolene.[38]

Clinical Presentation

After at least 2 months of therapy with oral dantrolene, patients may develop hepatotoxicity, which can be fatal.[40–43]

Table 5-5
National Capitol Poison Center List of Recommended Stock Drugs for Treatment of Poisonings*

Activated charcoal	At least 500 g *activated* charcoal should be available at all times. Any product labeled "universal antidote" is ineffective and should be discarded. If a premixed charcoal/sorbitol suspension is stocked, it is essential *also* to stock activated charcoal *without* sorbitol (dry powder or aqueous suspension).
Antivenin, *Crotalidae* polyvalent	Snakebite Antivenin (Wyeth) 10 kits, 10 mL/vial
Antivenin, *Lactrodectus mactans*	Black Widow Spider Antivenin (Wyeth) 1 vial
Atropine sulfate	3 20-mL 0.4 mg/mL vials **or** 60 1-mL 0.4 mg/mL ampules **or** 20 10-mL syringes (0.1 mg/mL)
Botulism antitoxin trivalent	Contact local health department office **or** Centers for Disease Control and Prevention in Atlanta, 404–633–3311
Calcium disodium edetate	Calcium EDTA Two ampules 200 mg/mL
Calcium gluconate	1 10-mL vial for injection
Chlorpromazine	1 10-mL 25 mg/mL vial for injection **or** 10 1-mL 25 mg/mL ampules
Cyanide antidote kit	3 Lilly Co. kits or equivalent Kit contains amyl nitrite, sodium nitrite, and sodium thiosulfate
Deferoxamine mesylate	Desferal 10 500-mg 5-mL ampules
Diazepam	Valium 2 10-ml 5 mg/mL vials **or** equivalent in 2-mL ampules or 2-mL syringes
Digoxin immune FAB (ovine)	Digibind 12 vials, each providing 50 mg Digibind
Dimercaprol	BAL 5 3-mL 100 mg/mL ampules
Diphenhydramine hydrochloride	Benadryl 10 1-mL 50 ng/mL ampules
DMSA	Chemet, Succimer 100 100-mg capsules Dose is 10 mg/kg tid × 5 d, then 10 mg/kg bid × 14 d
Ethyl alcohol	One pint 95% Loading dose 1 mL/kg Maintenance dose 0.1 mL/kg/h with close monitoring of blood ethanol levels Target is blood ethanol level of 100 mg/dL
Flumazenil (Mazicon)	10 vials, 10 mL/vial, or 20 vials, 5 mL/vial
Glucagon	Total hospital supply should be at least 50 mg, although up to 130 mg could be required to treat one severely toxic patient for 24 h. Check radiology department for another source, but stock as much as possible in 10-mg vials as it would be difficult to prepare dose from large number of 1-mg vials.
Ipecac syrup	24 30-mL (1-oz) bottles
Magnesium sulfate (crystals)	1 pound of magnesium sulfate or sodium sulfate (250 mg/kg per dose)
Magnesium citrate or sodium sulfate (crystals)	**or** 5 bottles magnesium citrate
Methylene blue	10 10-mL 10 mg/mL ampules
N-Acetylcysteine (Mucomyst)	600 cc (in 10- or 30-mL vials) of 20% Mucomyst Loading dose: 140 mg/kg Maintenance dose: 70 mg/kg × 17 doses
Naloxone hydrochloride (Narcan)	50 1-mL 0.4 mg/mL ampules Pediatric ampules contain 2 mL 0.02 mg/mL Recommendations: 2 mg (5 amps) IV test dose for adults Use 4 mg (10 amps) if propoxyphene is suspected
Physostigmine salicylate	Antilirium 10 2-mL 1 mg/mL ampules Adult test dose is 1–2 mg over 5 min
Pralidoxime chloride	Protopam 3 20-mL vials wth 1 g pralidoxime for reconstitution with sterile water 1 g is the usual adult dose 25–50 mg/kg for pediatric patients
Pyridoxine hydrochloride	Vitamin B_6 25 g (25 vials), in 10-mL 100 mg/mL vials
Sodium bicarbonate	20 50-mL 50 mEq/50 mL ampules or vials
Vitamin K_1	AquaMEPHYTON 2 0.5-mL ampules 2 mg/mL 2 5-mL ampules 10 mg/mL

From Martin TG, Donovan JW. Facility assessment guidelines for regional poison treatment centers. Vet Hum Toxicol 1991;33:394–397.

DICOBALT EDETATE

Mechanism of Action

Cobalt salts may form a relatively nontoxic stable ion complex with cyanide. Used in the United Kingdom; not approved for use in the United States.

Dicobalt edetate is used in the treatment of cyanide poisoning.

Cautions

1. If cyanide toxicity has not been diagnosed, free cobalt ions, which are usually present in solutions of dicobalt edetate, may lead to serious cobalt toxicity.
2. Glucose may protect against cobalt toxicity and should be given at the same time as dicobalt edetate.
3. Vomiting, urticaria, facial laryngeal and neck edema, anaphylactic shock, chest pain, hypotension, and ventricular arrhythmias have been reported with the use of dicobalt edetate.[44,45]
4. Fully conscious patients are unlikely to require dicobalt edetate.
5. There is little experience in pregnancy. Safe use has not been established.

Dose

A suggested dose is 300 mg of dicobalt edetate administered by intravenous injection over 1 minute. If there is no response, a further dose of 300 mg may be given 5 minutes later. Each injection of dicobalt edetate should be followed immediately by 50 mL of 50% glucose intravenously.[46]

DIETHYLENETRIAMINEPENTA-ACETIC ACID (DTPA)

Mechanism of Action

Chelating agents enhance the elimination of radionuclides and metals from the body by a process during which organic compounds exchange less firmly bonded ions for other inorganic ions to form a relatively stable nonionized ring complex which is readily excreted by the kidney.

Use

The U.S. Food and Drug Administration (FDA) has approved an Investigational New Drug (IND) application for the clinical use of zinc trisodium diethylenetriaminepentaacetate (Zn-DTPA) as an experimental drug for the decorporation of plutonium and other actinides. The Medical and Health Science Division of Oak Ridge Associated Universities (ORAU) will manage the IND (telephone 615–576–3131; The U.S. Department of Energy, Office of Health and Environmental Research, Human Health and Assessment Division, Washington, DC, or REAC/TS Center, Oak Ridge, TN 37831–0117).

Diethylenetriaminepentaacetic acid is used for chelation of transuranium metals, plutonium, berkelium, californium, americium, and curium. It may also be useful for chelation of some rare earths (cerium, yttrium, lanthanum, promethium, and scandium) and some transitional metals (zirconium and niobium). The FDA approval of DTPA covers only its use for the transuranium metals.

Cautions

A urinalysis should be performed before each treatment. Potential contraindications to the drug are leukopenia, thrombocytopenia, and serious kidney dysfunction.

Dose

Intravenous

Adults are given 1 g in 250 mL normal saline or 5% glucose in water, infused over 1 hour. Infusions may be repeated on 5 successive days per week.

Aerosol Inhalant

Adults are given 1 g in a 4-mL vial placed in a nebulizer. The entire volume is usually inhaled in 15 to 30 minutes. Inhalation administration can be repeated daily or, if indicated, two to three times per week.

DIGOXIN SPECIFIC ANTIBODY FRAGMENTS

See Chapter on digitalis digoxin.

DIMETHYL-*PARA*-AMINOPHENOL HYDROCHLORIDE (4-DMAP)

Mechanism of Action

Dimethyl-*para*-aminophenol hydrochloride (4-DMAP) rapidly forms methemoglobin.[47] After an intravenous dose of 3.25 mg/kg, 15% of hemoglobin is oxidized to methemoglobin in 5 minutes, and 30% after 10 minutes.[48] After 900 mg of 4-DMAP was administered orally, a 15% methemoglobin concentration was reached in 30 minutes.[49]

Use

1. Restrict use to cyanide-poisoned patients in deep coma, with dilated nonreactive pupils and deteriorating cardiorespiratory function.
2. 4-DMAP has been the drug of choice in Germany for cyanide poisoning. It is no longer used for cyanide poisoning in Sweden.
3. It may possibly be of use in severe hydrogen sulfide poisoning.
4. It may be useful in cyanide poisoning following prolonged use of sodium nitroprusside.[50]

Cautions

1. Even at recommended doses, 4-DMAP may produce an excessive methemoglobinemia ranging up to 70%.[51,52]

2. Hemolysis may occur on the second day after administration of a therapeutic dose.
3. Treatment with 4-DMAP is contraindicated in patients with glucose-6-phosphatase dehydrogenase deficiency.
4. Excess methemoglobinemia may be corrected with methylene blue or toluidine blue. This may release cyanide.[48,53] Exchange transfusion may be useful.
5. In contact with air, 4-DMAP is readily oxidized and the solution changes color to black-brown. Therefore, it must be stored in opaque containers. An open ampule cannot be kept.
6. Headache, dizziness, hyperventilation, cyanosis, and green/brown discoloration of the urine may be seen.
7. Serum bilirubin and serum iron may rise after intravenous use of 4-DMAP.[48]

Dose

A dose of 3.25 mg/kg body weight is given intravenously immediately. This is followed by sodium thiosulfate 150 to 200 mg/kg intravenously. Artificial respiration is implemented as required.

DIMERCAPTOSUCCINIC ACID (DMSA, SUCCIMER)

See also Chapter 67.

Mechanism of Action

Dimercaptosuccinic acid (DMSA) provides two –SH (sulfhydryl groups) which can chelate heavy metals (Fig. 5–1).

Use

An oral medication, DMSA, was approved in 1991 by the FDA for the treatment of severe lead poisoning in children whose blood level is greater than 45 μg/dL (2.17 μmol/L).[54–57] DMSA is specific for arsenic, lead, mercury, methylmercury, and silver but does not bind iron, calcium, or magnesium. DMSA may be of benefit in severe thallium intoxication.[58] It may increase mercury excretion and decrease blood mercury concentrations in mercury vapor poisoning.[59] DMSA may be useful in arsenic poisoning.[60,61]

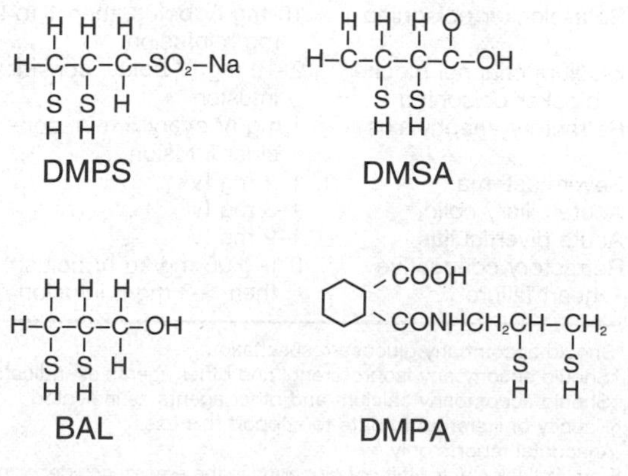

```
 H H H                     H H H O
 | | |                     | | | ‖
H-C-C-C-SO2-Na          H-C-C-C-C-OH
 | | |                     | |
 S S H                     S S
 H H                       H H
 DMPS                      DMSA

 H H H                      COOH
 | | |                  (benzene ring)
H-C-C-C-OH                  CONHCH2CH-CH2
 | | |                          |   |
 S S H                          S   S
 H H                            H   H
 BAL                        DMPA
```

Figure 5–1. Chemical formulas.

Cautions

1. Rashes, nausea, vomiting, and an elevation in the alanine aminotransferase concentration may be seen following DMSA.[48]
2. All patients should be adequately hydrated before treatment.
3. Use of DMSA in the presence of diminished renal function must proceed with great caution.
4. Measure blood lead level before therapy and on day 3, day 7, and weekly for evidence of rebound.
5. Monitor complete blood count and platelets, ferritin, bilirubin, alkaline phosphatase, γ-glutamyltransaminase, aminotransferases, blood urea nitrogen, creatinine, uric acid, calcium, phosphorus, glucose, total protein, albumin, urinalysis, and urine lead. The efficacy of DMSA compared with $CaNa_2EDTA$ for lead poisoning has been questioned (see Chapter 67).
6. A minimum of 2 weeks between courses of therapy is recommended.
7. Therapy should be accompanied by identification and removal of the source of lead exposure, because the drug cannot prevent lead poisoning in a lead-containing environment.

Dose

The dose is 10 mg/kg or 350 mg/m^2 every 8 hours for 5 days. Reduce to 10 mg/kg or 350 mg/m^2 every 12 hours (two-thirds initial dose) for an additional 2 weeks of therapy. A course of therapy lasts 19 days. A minimum of 2 weeks is recommended between courses. In young children who cannot swallow the capsule, open the capsule, and sprinkle the medicated beads on a small amount of soft food or place the beads in a spoon and follow with a soft drink.

In children 1 to 5 years, oral DMSA has been given in doses of 30 mg/kg/d for 5 days, then 20 mg/kg/d for 14 days.[57]

2,3-DIMERCAPTOPROPANE-1-SULFONATE (DMPS)

See also Mercury Poisoning in Chapter 67. Initial clinical studies suggest a decrease in the half-life and blood concentrations, and an increase in the urine concentrations, of metals in patients clinically poisoned with inorganic mercury, copper, chromium, arsenic, lead, cobalt, bismuth, and antimony. Further confirmatory studies are required to delineate the toxicity of DMPS, such as skin rashes, nausea, weakness, and vertigo. It is not available in the United States.

ETHANOL

See chapter on alcohols and glycols.

FLUMAZENIL

Mechanism of Action

Flumazenil antagonizes the actions of benzodiazepines by competitively inhibiting benzodiazepine activity at the GABA/benzodiazepine receptor complex. Flumazenil has little or no agonist activity in man.

Use

Flumazenil is indicated primarily in the treatment of symptoms of benzodiazepine overdose (see also Chapter 41). Flumazenil is possibly effective in improving consciousness in ethanol intoxication, where it may aid in improving blood gas analyses and permitting extubation.[62] Patients anesthetized with diazepam 0.3 mg/kg, or flunitrazepam 0.03 mg/kg, or midazolam 0.3 mg/kg with pentazocine 1 mg/kg, nitrous oxide, and a muscle relaxant regained consciousness within 1 to 6 minutes after administration of flumazenil[63] (see Dosage). Flumazenil may be useful in chronic obstructive pulmonary disease, even in patients with a therapeutic diazepam level.[64]

Cautions

1. Ventricular tachycardia,[65–68] bradycardia,[60] complete heart block, and death may follow flumazenil use.
2. Seizures and acute anxiety states may be provoked in patients dependent on benzodiazepines.
3. Seizures are more common if the patient has taken a tricyclic antidepressant, isoniazid, cocaine, or propoxyphene in addition to the benzodiazepine. Flumazenil antagonizes the anticonvulsant properties of the benzodiazepines, leaving a medication that may be epileptogenic.
4. Acute withdrawal symptoms may be seen in the benzodiazepine-dependent patient given flumazenil in an emergency facility. As return to consciousness after a benzodiazepine overdose may be due to the development of tolerance rather than drug elimination, late use of flumazenil may lead to withdrawal symptoms.
5. Repeated doses may be required because of the short duration of action of flumazenil (<1 hour).

Dose

As a diagnostic tool in the evaluation of comatose drug overdose, flumazenil should be given as a 0.2-mg bolus intravenously, with an additional 0.1 mg/min until the patient is awake. Most patients respond to 3 mg or less. A continuous infusion of flumazenil has not been shown to be superior to a repeat bolus technique, often preferred for routine clinical use.[69–72] An intravenous dose of 5 mg may improve consciousness in alcohol intoxication but does not improve psychomotor function.[73]

FOLIC ACID AND LEUCOVORIN

See Chapter 61.

GLUCAGON

Mechanism of Action

Glucagon stimulates the production of cyclic AMP (cAMP). By increasing myocardial cAMP, glucagon increases the chronotropic and inotropic activity of the heart, and reverses the overdose effects of beta-blockers and calcium-channel blockers.

Use

Potential uses of glucagon in the acute care setting are summarized in Table 5–6.[74] Anecdotal reports suggest a use for glucagon 0.5 mg intravenously over 30 seconds to facilitate passage of a coin from the distal esophagus into the stomach.[75] Preliminary reports indicate a potential usefulness for glucagon in the management of hemodynamic instability associated with calcium channel blocker poisonings.[76–78]

Cautions

Hypokalemia may result from glucagon-induced insulin secretion with intracellular transfer of glucose and potassium. Glucagon should be given cautiously to hypertensive patients, because of catecholamine induction in all patients and particularly in those with pheochromocytoma. Monitor serum glucose levels carefully if glucagon is administered to patients suspected of having an insulinoma or nesidioblastosis. Significant hypoglycemia may occur. Glucagon is relatively safe in pregnancy (FDA Category B). Other adverse reactions may include erythema multiforme,

Table 5–6
Potential Utility of Glucagon for the Emergency Physician

Indication	Dose	Notes
Hypoglycemia	Adults: 1 mg SC, IM, IV	*
	Children: 0.5 mg SC, IM, IV	*
	Neonates: 50 μg/kg SC, IV	*
Hypoglycemia due to sulfonylurea overdose	1 mg SC, IM, IV, consider infusion	*
Esophageal food or coin impaction	1 mg SC, IM, IV; may be repeated	
Beta-blocker poisoning	10-mg IV bolus, then 1 to 5 mg/h infusion	†
Calcium channel blocker blocker poisoning	2–10 mg IV bolus; consider infusion	‡
Refractory anaphylaxis	1 mg IV every 5 min; consider infusion	†
Severe asthma	1–2 mg IV	§
Acute biliary colic	1–3 mg IV	‖
Acute diverticulitis	1–2 mg IV	‖
Refractory congestive heart failure	0.1–0.05 mg/kg IV bolus, then 1–3 mg/h infusion	§

*Should accompany glucose resuscitation.
†Should accompany isoproterenol and other agents as indicated.
‡Should accompany calcium and other agents as indicated.
§Paucity of literature to date to support this use.
‖Anecdotal reports only.
From Pollack CV Jr. Utilty of glucagon in the emergency department. J Emerg Med 1993;11:195–205.

Stevens–Johnson syndrome, hypersensitivity reactions, and thrombophlebitis possibly due to the phenol component of the vehicle. This may be lessened by diluting the drug prior to use in large doses or by continuous infusion.[74,79]

Failure of glucagon therapy in calcium channel blocker overdose may be associated with both hypo- and hypercalcemic states. Careful monitoring of the total serum calcium and, preferably, total serum ionized calcium, as well as supplemental infusion of calcium chloride, may be required.[76]

Dose

Doyon and Roberts suggest that calcium channel blocker overdoses may require glucagon doses higher than those used to reverse the myocardial depression associated with beta blocker overdoses.[76] If an initial bolus of 2–10 mg IV is unsuccessful at increasing blood pressure, it is probably reasonable to double that dose. If glucagon improves the hemodynamic status of the patient, a glucagon infusion should be started at a rate of 2 to 5 mg/h.

HYPERBARIC OXYGEN

See chapter on carbon monoxide poisoning and hydrogen sulfide.

HYDROXOCOBALAMIN

Mechanism of Action

Hydroxocobalamin binds cyanide to form cyanocobalamin (vitamin B_{12}). It does not interfere with tissue oxygenation. Cyanocobalamin is excreted unchanged in urine.[80,81]

Uses

1. Treatment of cyanide poisoning, especially that resulting from excessive sodium nitroprusside infusions
2. Possibly in cyanide-intoxicated smoke inhalation victims
3. As therapeutic treatment after exposure to acetonitrile, propionitrile, potassium, and sodium cyanide by oral, inhalational, or dermal route
4. For improperly prepared cassava [82]
5. For treatment of diseases caused by chronic, low-level cyanide exposure (tobacco amblyopia, Leber's hereditary optic atrophy)[83]

Hydroxocobalamin is an investigational orphan drug in the United States. It is not available commercially in the United States.

Cautions

Anaphylactoid reactions and acne have been observed. Hepatotoxicity, myocardial, and renal changes have been observed in animals. Hydroxocobalamin causes muscle twitching and spasm and hypertension with reflex bradycardia.[84]

A transient reddish discoloration of skin, mucous membranes, and urine is observed. The drug is brownish in color. This discoloration may last 12 hours.[84]

In prolonged infusions, the solution must be protected from light. The presence of hydroxocobalamin in serum interferes with a number of serum chemistry methodologies (bilirubin rises, creatinine falls, serum iron cannot be measured).[85]

Dose

In France a formulation is available that contains 4 g of hydroxocobalamin powder. This is diluted in more than 220 mL of 5% dextrose solution.

An additional formulation in France and Germany now contains 5 g of hydroxocobalamin in 100 mL water for injection.

Give 50 times the estimated cyanide dose. For an approximate fatal dose of 200 mg of cyanide, this would represent a hydroxocobalamin dose of 10 g. If the amount of cyanide ingested is not known, give 50 mg/kg.

A 5-g dose may bind 100 mg of cyanide. Hydroxocobalamin 5 g in combination with sodium thiosulfate 12.5 g appears to be a safe and effective treatment for cyanide poisoning patients.[84] The suggested dose of hydroxocobalamin for preventing nitroprusside-induced cyanide toxicity is 25 mg/h for 10 hours at the end of a nitroprusside infusion. The half-life of cyanide in red cells is about 10 hours.[86] Prolonged nitroprusside infusions of more than 2 μg/kg/min should be avoided. Serum thiocyanate levels should be measured in patients who receive nitroprusside infusions at rates higher than 10 μg/kg/min for longer than 48 hours or who have renal insufficiency.[86]

4-METHYLPYRAZOLE (4 MP)

Use

4-Methylpyrazole (4MP) is used in ethylene glycol poisoning[87] and possibly in methanol poisoning. 4 MP is not currently approved by the FDA.

Mechanism of Action

4-Methylpyrazole is an inhibitor of alcohol dehydrogenase,[88] responsible for metabolizing methanol and ethylene glycol to their toxic metabolites. 4-Methylpyrazole administered by the oral or intravenous route at a dosage of 10 mg/kg/d as long as plasma ethylene glycol is detectable appears to lead to (1) rapid excretion of free ethylene glycol in the urine; (2) an increase in the plasma ethylene glycol half-life; (3) return to normal levels of plasma and urinary oxalate in 2 days; (4) correction of the initial metabolic acidosis within hours; (5) absence of the development of renal failure; and (6) uneventful recovery. Few serious side effects have been observed at doses of 10 to 20 mg/kg/d. 4MP is useful for patients with normal renal function admitted less than 3 hours after ingestion. If renal function is impaired, dialysis may be necessary to remove the toxin.[83,89,90]

A single study in animals suggests that 4MP given 4 hours after a toxic dose of acetaminophen appears to inhibit hepatotoxicity. Further studies will be of interest.[91]

Clinical Presentation

At 4MP doses of 50 and 100 mg/kg, patients may experience nausea, dizziness, and vertigo.[87,89,90,92–94] Multiple doses of 3 mg/kg every 6 hours for 96 hours, after an initial dose of 10 mg/kg,induce a slight rise in blood pressure and hepatic aminotransferase levels. Diarrhea and headache may also be observed.[93]

Cautions

1. Treatment with 4MP is more effective for patients with normal renal function.
2. Patients must be treated soon after ingestion (<3 hours).
3. If renal function is impaired, dialysis may be required.
4. Transient elevations in serum aminotransferase levels have been reported in some subjects treated with multiple dose of 4MP.[83,89]
5. Intravenous bolus dosing may induce a phlebosclerosis with local pain during injection.
6. Nausea, slight dizziness, rashes, and headache may occur in some patients.
7. At doses of 50 to 100 mg/kg, speech and visual disturbances have been observed.[93,94]

Dose

4-Methylpyrazole is administered by the oral or intravenous route at a dose of 10 mg to 20 mg/kg/d, perhaps for 3 to 5 days. Baud and colleagues have administered cumulative doses of 600 to 8650 mg of 4MP intravenously and intramuscularly.[89]

Toxicokinetics

Blood levels have varied from 0 to 55.6 mmol/L and urine levels from 0 to 161 mmol/L.[93] The volume of distribution is 2.4 L/kg. Total clearance is 632 mmol/min. The zero-order kinetics are dose dependent.[95] 4MP is metabolized by cytochrome P450 enzymes to 4-hydroxymethylpyrazole and to glucuronide conjugates, which are excreted in the urine.[93] 4-Carboxypyrazole is a major urinary metabolite.[88]

METHYLENE BLUE

Mechanism of Action

Methylene blue acts as an electron carrier for the hexose monophosphate pathway, which reduces methemoglobin to hemoglobin. In patients with methemoglobinemia, the erythrocyte methemoglobin reductases reduce methylene blue to leukomethylene blue (colorless form), which in turn reduces methemoglobin to hemoglobin.

Use

Methylene blue is administered to symptomatic patients who have been exposed to methemoglobin-forming compounds (e.g. aniline, nitrites, local anesthetics) and whose methemoglobin levels exceed 20 to 30%.

Cautions

1. Large intravenous doses (>7 mg/kg) produce nausea, vomiting, abdominal/chest pain, dizziness, diaphoresis, confusion, and cyanosis as a result of methemoglobin formation. Oxygen saturation and methemoglobin levels should be followed by arterial blood gases.
2. Methylene blue causes hemolysis in glucose-6-phosphate dehydrogenase-deficient patients, and exchange transfusion should be seriously considered as an alternative to methylene blue therapy.
3. As methylene blue is eliminated mostly by renal excretion, the drug should be used cautiously in the presence of renal dysfunction.
4. This drug is contraindicated as an agent to reverse methemoglobinemia after the use of sodium nitrate as an antidote for cyanide poisoning.

Dose

A dose of 0.2 mL/kg of a 1% (10 mg/mL) solution, or 1–2 mg/kg, should be administered over several minutes. The dose may be repeated in 60 minutes.

N-ACETYLCYSTEINE (NAC)

See also Chapter 10.

Mechanism of Action

N-Acetylcysteine may increase oxygen consumption and improve microcirculatory blood flow by stimulating the activity of endothelium-derived relating factor.[96] NAC acts as a glutathione substitute that prevents the formation of an intermediate toxic substance in acetaminophen overdose.

Use

N-Acetylcysteine (NAC) is used for the treatment of acetaminophen overdoses. Survival improves in patients with acetaminophen-induced fulminant hepatic failure given acetylcysteine soon after acetaminophen ingestion; improvement may also be observed after encephalopathy and other signs of severe liver damage, including coagulopathy, have developed.[97] Only the oral form of NAC is approved by the FDA. The intravenous form is available in the United States only through an investigational new drug (IND) protocol. Approval must be obtained through the FDA (301–443–1479). Intravenous NAC is available in the United Kingdom and Canada.

Anecdotal Reports

Potential uses of acetylcysteine in addition to acetaminophen (paracetamol) poisoning include toxicity secondary to halogenated hydrocarbons, which may deplete glutathione (chloroform–phosgene metabolite, carbon tetrachloride, bromobenzene),[98,99] paraquat (in animals, conflicting data suggest diminished glutathione in liver not lung),[101,101] acrylonitrile[98] (formation of cyanoethyacetylcysteine), naphthalene (epoxide metabolite conjugates with glutathione),[98] sulfur mustard, and cytotoxic agents (ifosfamide—intravesical protection,[102] bleomycin—to prevent excess lung fibrosis[103,104]), and prevention of delayed neuropsychiatric complications of carbon monoxide poisoning.[105] Other proposed uses include improvement of alveolar macrophage function in the broncheoalveolar lavage fluid from cigarette smoke,[106] treatment of inflammatory joint disease,[107] prevention of HIV expression (AIDS),[108–111] use in the adult respiratory distress syndrome (free radical scavenger),[112,113] potentiation of the cardiovascular effects of nitroglycerin[114] and organic nitrites,[115] treatment of dichromate intoxication,[116] amanitin poisoning,[117,118] and reduction of lipoprotein.[119–122] No clear conclusions have emerged from these studies to provide definitive guidelines for clinical usefulness. Controlled clinical studies are required to place most of these observations in perspective.

Cautions

After repeated high doses of oral NAC, nausea, vomiting, and diarrhea may occur. Headache, hypotension, and rash rarely occur. Urticaria and hepatotoxicity are seen rarely. High-dose intravenous administration may be accompanied by anaphylactoid reactions beginning about 15 to 60 minutes after starting an infusion in 10% of patients. Asthmatics are especially at risk. A serum sickness-like illness has been described.[123] Treatment is supportive and symptomatic.[124] Activated charcoal administration before oral NAC may not diminish the hepatoprotective effect of NAC.[125]

NALOXONE

See Chapter 25.

OBIDOXIME

See Chapters 59 and 68.

PHENTOLAMINE

Mechanism of Action

Phentolamine mesylate is an alpha-adrenergic blocking vasodilatory agent. It causes peripheral vasodilation by direct relaxation of the smooth muscle and by competitive blocking of alpha receptor sites, both α_1 and α_2. Phentolamine also acts as a weak antagonist of 5-hydroxytryptamine and releases histamine from mast cells.

Use

1. Diagnosis and control of hypertension secondary to a pheochromocytoma
2. Vasopressor (eg, norepinephrine, dopamine) extravasation[128–130]
3. Cocaine-induced myocardial ischemia
4. Naloxone-induced pulmonary edema (anecdotal report)[131]
5. Management of hypertensive crises secondary to overdose with sympathomimetic agents, including the "cheese reaction" to monoamine oxidase inhibitor

Cautions

1. Do not use in hypotension or any condition where sudden hypotension would be undesirable.
2. Do not use with other hypotensive agents.
3. Epinephrine should not be used in a phentolamine overdose, as it may result in hypotension and increase the tachycardia due to its unopposed β_2 action.

Dose

For vasoconstriction, remove the venous access device and inject in a circle around the area where extravasation has occurred, using a new 24-gauge needle for each injection. The recommended dose with this method is a total of 5 to 10 mg (in normal saline) depending on the size of the extravasated area. Phentolamine, 7.5 mL of a solution containing 5 mg of phentolamine in 10 mL of normal saline, slowly infiltrated into the ischemic subcutaneous tissue has been used for dopamine infiltration.[128] Phentolamine may be used as an intravenous infusion in 5% dextrose or saline at a rate of 0.2 to 2 mg/min, titrating the dose to the desired blood pressure response. Blood pressure and pulse should be monitored. A cardiac monitor must be available for continuous use. An intraarterial dose of 1.5 to 5.0 mg given in the radial artery at the level of the wrist may be required.

PHYSIOSTIGMINE

See chapters on anticholinergic poisoning specifically antihistamines diphenhydramine.

PRALIDOXIME

See Chapters 59 and 68.

PROTAMINE

See chapter on anticoagulants.

PRUSSIAN BLUE SALTS

Mechanism of Action

Thallium is exchanged for potassium in the molecular lattice and subsequently the complex is excreted in the feces.

Use

Prussian blue salts have been used as an antidote after radiocesium and thallium contamination in humans. A decomposition product in Prussian blue salts may be cyanide. Ferric(III) hexacyanoferrate(II), $(Fe_4[Fe(CN_6)]_3$, releases cyanide least of the Prussian blue salts.[133]

PYRIDOSTIGMINE

See also Chapter 59.

Mechanism of Action

Pyridostigmine is an anticholinesterase agent that inhibits the hydrolysis of acetylcholine by competing with acetylcholine for attachment to acetylcholinesterase.[134]

Use

1. Used by anesthesiologists to antagonize nondepolarizing neuromuscular blockade[135]
2. As a nerve agent pretreatment under wartime conditions[136]
3. Myasthenia gravis[134]

Cautions

1. Patients may occasionally experience flatus, diarrhea, abdominal cramps, urinary urgency, nausea, headache, vivid daydreams, rhinorrhea, tingling of the extremities, muscle weakness, cramps, and twitching.[136]
2. Patients with a history of asthma may experience bronchospasm.[136]
3. Acute hypertension is rare.[136]

Dose

During anesthesia, 10 to 15 mg/70 kg is administered intravenously with atropine 15 to 20 μg/kg.[135]

For prevention of the effects of anticholinesterase chemical warfare agents, 30 mg is given orally every 8 hours.[136]

For myasthenia gravis initially, depending on physician evaluation, adults are given 60 mg orally three times daily with a maintenance daily dose of 60 mg to 1.5 g. Children may be started on 7 mg/kg or 200 mg/m² daily, divided into five or six doses.[134]

Table 5–7
Dithiocarb Treatment Protocol for Acute Nickel Carbonyl Poisoning

Mild or doubtful exposure (urine nickel level < 10 μg/dL)	Give 2 g dithiocarb orally in divided doses (4-h period)		
Moderately severe to severe exposure (urine nickel level > 10 μg/dL)	Give dithiocarb as follows:		
	First day	2.0 g (10–0.2-g capsules)	0 h
		1.0 g (5–0.2-g capsules)	4 h
		0.6 g (3–0.2-g capsules)	8 h
		0.4 g (2–0.2-g capsules)	16 h
	Subsequent days	0.4 g every 8 h	

From Kurte DL, Dean BS, Krenzelok EP. Acute nickel carbonyl poisoning. Am J Emerg Med 1993;11:64–66.

PYRIDOXINE

Refer to section on antiinfectives, specifically Isoniazid (INH) and chapter on mushrooms, specifically gyromitrin.

SODIUM DIETHYLDITHIOCARBAMATE (DITHIOCARB)

Mechanism of Action

Dithiocarb (DTC) is a chelating agent that increases the excretion of nickel in the urine and feces.[137]

Use

Dithiocarb has been used to treat nickel dermatitis and nickel carbonyl poisoning.[138,139] It is an investigational drug in the United States and is classified as an orphan drug. No manufacturer has taken sponsorship. Where dithiocarb has not been available, disulfiram (Antabuse) has been administered because it is metabolized to two molecules of dithiocarb and is hypothetically of value.[140] The absence of clinical supportive studies and the potential toxicity of disulfiram do not make it an alternative to dithiocarb.[141] Reduction of the incidence of opportunistic infections in patients with symptomatic HIV infection has been attempted.[141]

Cautions

Patients are advised not to drink alcohol from 12 hours before to 48 hours after treatment because of its disulfiram effect.

Patients have reported a metallic taste and abdominal discomfort (gastric complaints, flatulence, diarrhea) following use of dithiocarb.[142]

Dose

Table 5–7 provides a suggested protocol for the use of dithiocarb in acute nickel carbonyl poisoning.[141] For treatment of AIDS opportunistic infections, 400 mg/m² body surface area is administered orally once weekly.[141]

VITAMIN K (PHYTONADIONE)

See section on anticoagulants.

REFERENCES

1. Meredith TJ, Jacobsen D, Haines JA, Berger J-C, eds. *International Program on Chemical Safety/Commission of the European Communities Evaluation of Antidotes Series.* Vol. 1: *Naloxone, Flumazenil and Dantrolene as Antidotes.* EUR 14797 EN. Vol. 2: *Antidotes for Poisoning by Cyanide* (van

Heijst APVR, guest ed.). EUR 14200EN. Cambridge: Cambridge University Press, 1993.
2. Kulig K. Initial management of ingestions of toxic substances. N Engl J Med 1992;326:1677–1681.
3. Martin TG, Donovan JW. Facility assessment guidelines for regional poison treatment centers. Vet Hum Toxicol 1991;33: 394–397.
4. Stirt JA. Aminophylline as a diazepam antagonist. Anesth Analg 1981;60:767–768.
5. Wangler MA, Kirkpatrick DS. Aminophylline is an antagonist of lorazepam. Anesth Analg 1985;64:834–836.
6. Phyllis JW, Edstrom JP, Ellis SW, Kirkpatrick JR. Theophylline antagonizes flurazepam-induced depression of cerebral cortical neurons. Can J Physiol Pharmacol 1979;57:917–920.
7. Meyer BH, Weis OF, Muller FO. Antagonism of diazepam by aminophylline in healthy volunteers. Anesth Analg 1984; 63:900–902.
8. Katz Y, Gavish M. Aminophylline reversal of diazepam intoxication. Lancet 1989;1:900–901.
9. Gurel A, Eleuli IM, Hamulu A. Aminophylline reversal of flumitrazepam sedation. Anesth Analg 1987;66:333–336.
10. Niemand D, Martinell S, Arvidsson S, et al. Aminophylline inhibition of diazepam sedation: Is adenosine blockade of GABA-receptors the mechanism? Lancet 1984;1:463–464.
11. Sibai AN, Sibai AM, Baraka A. Comparison of flumazenil with aminophylline to antagonize midazolam in elderly patients. Br J Anaesth 1991;66:591–595.
12. Kuzemko JA, Paala J. Apnoeic attacks in the newborn treated with aminophylline. Arch Dis Child 1973;48:404–406.
13. Mainzer F. Treatment of incipient apoplexy with intravenous aminophylline. Acon Med Scand 1953;146:362–377.
14. Dowell AR, Heyman A, Sieker HA, Tripathy K. Effect of aminophylline on respiratory center sensitivity in Cheyne–Stokes respiration and in pulmonary emphysema. N Engl J Med 1963;273:1447–1453.
15. Daller JA, Erstad B, Rosado L, et al. Aminophylline antagonizes the neuromuscular blockade of pancuronium but not vecuronium. Crit Care Med 1991;19:983–985.
16. Stirt JA. Aminophylline may act as a morphine antagonist. Anaesthesia 1983;38:275–278.
17. Renzhen-Lia WMD. Aminophylline antagonism of the residual effects of fentanyl anesthesia. Anesth Analg 1985;64:1029.
18. Krintell JJ, Wegmann F. Aminophylline reduces the depth and duration of sedation with barbiturates. Acta Anaesth Scand 1987;31:352–354.
19. Arridsson SB, Ekstrom-Jodal B, Martinell SAGG. Aminophylline antagonizes diazepam sedation. Lancet 1982;2:1467.
20. Bone MF, Kalra L, Phillips A, Ariaraj S. Reversal of the adverse effects of nifedipine by aminophylline, a calcium channel facilitator in cor pulmonale. Thorax 1990;45:328P.
21. TerWee PM, Kremer Horinga TK, Uges DRA, van der Geest S. 4-Aminopyridine and hemodialysis in the treatment of verapamil intoxication. Hum Toxicol 1985;4:327–329.
22. Bull AP, Hopkinson RB, Farrell ID, et al. Human botulism caused by *Clostridium botulinum* Type E: The Birmingham outbreak. Q J Med 1979;48:473–491.
23. Murray NMF, Newson-Davis J. Treatment with oral 4-aminopyridine in disorders of neuromuscular transmission. Neurology 1981;31:265–271.
24. Stefoski D, Davis FA, Fitsimmons WE, et al. 4-Aminopyridine in multiple sclerosis: Prolonged administration. Neurology 1991;4:1344–1348.
25. Spyker DA, Lynch C, Shabanowitz J, Sinn JA. Poisoning with 4-aminopyridine: Report of three cases. Clin Toxicol 1980; 16:487–497.
26. Miller RD, Booij LHDJ, Agoston S, Crul JF. 4-Aminopyridine potentiates neostigmine and pyridostigmine in man. Anesthesiology 1979;50:416–420.
27. Barone JA, Peppers MP. Use of dantrolene in the management of amphetamine-induced hyperthermia. Clin Pharm 1989;8:324–325.
28. Ten Holter JBM, Schellens RLLAM. Dantrolene sodium for treatment of carbon monoxide poisoning. Br Med J 1988;296:1772–1773.
29. Kaplan RF, Feinglass NG, Webster W, Mudra S. Phenelzine overdose treated with dantrolene sodium. JAMA 1986;255:642–644.
30. Shemesh I, Bourvin A, Gold D, Kutscherowsky M. Chlorpyrifos poisoning treated with ipratropium and dantrole: A case report. Clin Toxicol 1988;26:495–498.
31. Bouchama A, Cafege A, Devol EB, et al. Ineffectiveness of dantrolene sodium in the treatment of heat stroke. Crit Care Med 1991;19:176–180.
32. Channa AB, Seraj MA, Saddique AA, et al. Is dantrolene effective in heat stroke patients? Crit Care Med 1990;18: 290–293.
33. Parr MJA, Willatts SM. Fatal theophylline poisoning with rhabdomyolysis: A potential role for dantrolene treatment. Anaesthesia 1991;46:557–559.
34. Van de Kelft E, de Hert M, Heytens L, et al. Management of lethal catatonia with dantrolene sodium. Crit Care Med 1991; 19:1449–1451.
35. Robillart A, Bopp P, Vailly B, Dupeyron JP. Cardiac failure due to dantrolene overdose. Ann Fr Anesth Reanim 1986;5: 617–619.
36. Paloucek FP, Erickson TE, Lundquist S, Ferraro C. Oral dantrolene ingestion: A case series. Vet Hum Toxicol 1991;33: 362.
37. Tayeb OS. A serious interaction of dantrolene and theophylline. Vet Hum Toxicol 1990;32:442–443.
38. Saltzman LS, Kates RA, Corke GC, et al. Hyperkalemia and cardiovascular collapse after verapamil and dantrolene administration in swine. Anesth Analg 1984;63:473–478.
39. Wedel DJ, Quinlan JG, Iaizzzo PA. Clinical effects of intravenously administered dantrolene. Mayo Clin Proc 1995;70: 241–246.
40. Chan CH. Dantrolene sodium and hepatic injury. Neurology 1990;40:1427–1432.
41. Utili R, Boitnott JK, Zimmerman HJ. Dantrolene-associated hepatic injury. Gastroenterology 1977;72:610–616.
42. Wilkinson SP, Portmann B, Williams R. Hepatitis from dantrolene sodium. Gut 1979;20:33–36.
43. Cornett M, Gillard C, Borlee-Hermans G. Hepatite toxique mortelle associee at l'usage du dantrolene. Acta Neurol Belg 1980;80:336–347.
44. Hillman B, Bardham KD, Bain JTB. The use of dicobalt edetate (Kelocyanor) in cyanide poisoning. Postgrad Med J 1974;50:171–174.
45. Naughton M. Acute cyanide poisoning. Anaesth Intensive Care 1974;4:351–356.
46. Reynolds JEF. *Martindale. The Extra Pharmacopoeia.* 30th ed. London: Pharmaceutical Press, 1991:680.
47. Weger NP. Treatment of cyanide poisoning with 4-dimethylaminophenol (DMAP): Experimental and clinical overview. Fundam Appl Toxicol 1983;3:387–396.
48. Weger NP. Aminophenole als Blausaure: Antidote. Arch Toxicol 1968;24:49–50.
49. Klinimek R, Krettek C, Szinicz L, et al. Effects of biotransformation of 4-dimethylaminophenol in man and dog. Arch Toxicol 1983;53:275–288.
50. Ram Z, Spiegelman R, Findler G, Hadani M. Delayed postoperative neurological deterioration from prolonged sodium nitroprusside administration. J Neurosurg 1989;71:605–607. Case report.
51. Van Dijk A, Glerum JH, Van Heijst ANP, Douze JMC. Clinical evaluation of the cyanide antagonist 4-DMAP in a lethal cyanide poisoning case. Vet Hum Toxicol 1987;29(suppl. 2): 38–39.
52. Van Heijst ANP, Douze JMC, Van Kesteren RG, et al. Therapeutic problems in cyanide poisoning. Clin Toxicol 1987; 25:383–398.
53. Kiese M, Lorcher W, Weger N, Zierer A. Comparative studies on the effects of toluidine blue and methylene blue on the reduction of ferrihemoglobin in man and dog. Eur J Clin Pharmacol 1972;4:115–118.
54. Succimer approved to treat severe lead poisoning in children. FDA Med Bull 1991;21(1):5.
55. Graziano JH, Lolacono NJ, Meyer P. Dose–response study of oral 2,3-dimercaptosuccinic acid in children with elevated blood lead concentrations. J Pediatr 1988;113:751–757.
56. Bentur Y, Brook JG, Behar R, Taitelman U. Meso-2,3-dimercaptosuccinic acid in the diagnosis and treatment of lead poisoning. Clin Toxicol 1987;25:39–51.

57. Mortensen ME, Valenzuela PM. Dimercaptosuccinic acid (DMSA) chelation for childhood lead poisoning. Clin Pharmacol Ther 1991;49:162.
58. Hurlbut KM, Dart RC, Sullivan JB, Campbell DC. Use of DMSA in severe thallium toxicity. Vet Hum Toxicol 1990;32:363.
59. Mortensen ME, Valenzuela PM. 2,3-Dimercaptosuccinic acid (DMSA) chelation in mercury (Hg) vapor poisoning. Vet Hum Toxicol 1990;32:382.
60. Kosnett MJ, Becker CE. Dimercaptosuccinic acid: Acute and chronic arsenic poisoning. Vet Hum Toxicol 1988;30:369.
61. Aposhian HV, Maiorino RM, Rivera M, et al. Human studies with the chelating agents, DMPS and DMSA. Clin Toxicol 1992;30:505–528.
62. Lheureux P, Askenasi R. Efficacy of flumazenil in acute alcohol intoxication: Double blind placebo-controlled evaluation. Hum Exp Toxicol 1991;10:235–239.
63. Momose T. A study on the effects of regaining consciousness with flumazenil from anesthesia supplemented with a benzodiazepine and pentazocine. Clin Pharmacol Ther 1991;49:185.
64. Apple M, Bron HNLM, Hooymans DM, Janknegt R. Efficacy of flumazenil in COPD patient with therapeutic diazepam levels. Lancet 1989;1:392.
65. Short TG, Maling T, Galletly DC. Ventricular arrhythmias precipitated by flumazenil. Br Med J 1988;296:1070–1071.
66. Burr W, Sandham P. Death after flumazenil. Br Med J 1989; 298:1713.
67. Marchant B, Wray R, Leach A, Nama M. Flumazenil causing convulsions and ventricular tachycardia. Br Med J 1989; 299:860.
68. Herd B, Clarke F. Complete heart block after flumazenil. Hum Exp Toxicol 1991;10:289.
69. Geller E, Crome P, Schaller MD, et al. Risks and benefits of therapy with flumazenil (Anexate) in mixed drug intoxications. Eur Neurol 1991;31:241–250.
70. Hojer JH, Baehrendtz S, Matell G, Gustafsson LL. Diagnostic utility of flumazenil in coma with suspected poisoning: A double blind, controlled, randomized controlled study. Br Med J 1990;301:1308–1311.
71. Kulka PJ, Lauren PM. Benzodiazepine antagonists. Drug Saf 1992;7:381–386.
72. Weinbroum A, Halpern P, Geller E. The use of flumazenil in the management of acute drug poisoning: a review. Intensive Care Med 1991;17:32–38.
73. Clausen TG, Wolff J, Carl P, Theilgaard A. The effect of benzodiazepine antagonist, flumazenil, on psychometric performance in acute ethanol intoxication in man. Eur J Clin Pharmacol 1990;38:233–236.
74. Pollack CV Jr. Utility of glucagon in the emergency department. J Emerg Med 1993;11:195–205.
75. Blume CM, Thompson MW, Scalzo AJ. Use of IV glucagon to facilitate the passage of a penny from the distal esophagus into the stomach. Vet Hum Toxicol 1993;35:335.
76. Doyon S, Roberts JP. The use of glucagon in a case of calcium channel blocker overdose. Ann Emerg Med 1993;22: 1229–1233.
77. Walter FG, Frye G, Mullen JT, et al. Amelioration of nifedipine poisoning associated with glucagon therapy. Ann Emerg Med 1993;22:1234–1237.
78. Wolf LR, Spadafora MP, Otten EJ. Use of amrinone and glucagon in a case of calcium channel blocker overdose. Ann Emerg Med 1993;22:1225–1228.
79. Linden CH, Aghababian RW. Further uses of glucagon. Crit Care Med 1985;13:248.
80. Baud F, Toffis V, Barriot P, et al. Kinetics of cobalamins in cyanide intoxications treated with hydroxocobalamin. In: *Proceedings, Vth International Congress of Toxicology, Brighton, England, July 16, 1989*. London: Taylor & Francis, 1989.
81. Mueller PD, Hall AH, Osterloh JD, et al. Hydroxocobalamin kinetics and cyanide elimination in heavy smokers. Vet Hum Toxicol 1990;32:361.
82. Espinoza OB, Perez M, Ramirez MS. Bitter cassava poisoning in eight children: A case report. Hum Toxicol 1992;34:65.
83. Bismuth C, Baud FJ, Pontal PG. Hydroxocobalamin in chronic cyanide poisoning. J Toxicol Clin Exp 1988;8:35–38.
84. Forsyth JC, Mueler PD, Becker CE, et al. Hydroxocobalamin as a cyanide antidote: Safety, efficacy and pharmacokinetics in heavily smoking normal volunteers. Clin Toxicol 1993; 31:277–294.
85. Curry SC, Connor DA, Raschke RA. Effect of the cyanide antidote hydroxocobalamin on commonly ordered serum chemistry studies. Ann Emerg Med 1994;24:65–67.
86. Zerbe NF, Wagner BKJ. Use of vitamin B_{12} in the treatment and prevention of nitroprusside-induced cyanide toxicity. Crit Care Med 1993;21:465–467.
87. Bismuth C. 4-Methylpyrazole simplified the treatment of ethylene glycol poisoning. In: *Proceedings, Seventh World Congress on Emergency and Disaster Medicine in Prehospital and Disaster Medicine, Montreal, May 12, 1991* (April–June):203. Abstract.
88. Woodyear WE, Campbell PT, Corey GR. Not so good to the last drop: Ethylene glycol poisoning in a coffee-consuming camper. NC Med J 1992;53:134–136.
89. Baud FJ, Galliot M, Astier A, et al. Treatment of ethylene glycol poisoning with intravenous 4-methylpyrazole. N Engl J Med 1988;319:97–100.
90. Jacobsen D, Sebastian CS, Blomstrand R, McMartin KE. 4-Methylpyrazole: A controlled study of safety in healthy human subjects after single ascending doses. Alcohol Clin Exp Res 1988;12:516–522.
91. Brennan RJ, Mankes RJ, Lefevre R, et al. 4-Methylpyrazole blocks acetaminophen hepatotoxicity in the rat. Ann Emerg Med 1994;23:487–493.
92. McMartin KE, Heath A. Treatment of ethylene glycol poisoning with intravenous 4-methylpyrazole. N Engl J Med 1989;320:125.
93. McMartin KE, Jacobsen D, Sebastian S, Barron SK. Safety and metabolism of multiple doses of 4-methylpyrazole in humans. Vet Hum Toxicol 1988;30:363.
94. Jacobsen D, Sebastian CS, Barron SK, et al. Effects of 4-methylpyrazole, methanol/ethylene glycol antidote in healthy humans. J Emerg Med 1990;8:455–461.
95. Tournoud C, Kopferschmitt J, Sander P, et al. Ethylene glycol poisoning treated with 4-methylpyrazole. In: *Proceedings, European Association of Poison Toxicologists, Istanbul, Turkey, May 24–27, 1992*:30.
96. Harrison PM, Keays R, Bray GP, et al. Improved outcome in paracetamol-induced fulminant hepatic failure following late administration of acetylcysteine. Lancet 1990;335:1572–1573.
97. Keays RT, Gove C, Forbes A, et al. Use of late *N*-acetylcysteine in severe paracetamol overdose. Gut 1989;30: A1512. Abstract.
98. Flanagan RJ. The role of acetylcysteine in clinical toxicology. Med Toxicol 1987;2:93–104.
99. Meredith TJ, Ruprak M, Liddle A, Flanagan RJ. Diagnosis and treatment of acute poisoning with volatile substances. Hum Toxicol 1989;8:277–286.
100. Wegener T, Sandhagen B, Chan KW, Saldien T. *N*-Acetylcysteine in paraquat toxicity: Toxicological and histological evaluation in rats. Ups J Med Sci 1988;93:81–89.
101. Cramp TP. Failure of *N*-acetylcysteine to reduce renal damage due to paraquat in rats. Hum Toxicol 1985;4:107.
102. Holoye PV, Duelge J, Hansen RM, et al. Prophylaxis of ifosfamide toxicity with oral acetylcysteine. Semin Oncol 1983;10(suppl. 1):66–71.
103. Shahzeidi S, Saistrandt B, Jeffery PK, et al. *N*-Acetyl-cysteine partially protects lung fibrosis caused by bleomycin. Thorax 1990;45: 323P.
104. Giri SN, Hyde DM, Schiedt MJ. Effects of repeated administration of *N*-acetyl-L-cysteine on sulfhydryl levels of different tissues and bleomycin-induced lung fibrosis in hamsters. J Lab Clin Med 1988;111:714–724.
105. Howard RJM, Blake DR, Paell H, et al. Allopurinol/*N*-acetylcysteine for carbon monoxide poisoning. Lancet 1987; 2:628–629.
106. Linden W, Wieslander E, Eklund A, et al. Effects of oral *N*-acetylcysteine in cell content and macrophage function in bronchoalveolar lavage from healthy smokers. Eur Respir J 1988;1:645–650.
107. Acetylcysteine. Lancet 1991;337:1069–1070. Editorial.
108. Kalebic T, Kinter A, Poli G, et al. Suppression of human immunodeficiency virus expression in chronically infected monocytic cells by glutathione, glutathione ester, and *N*-acetylcysteine. Proc Natl Acad Sci USA 1991;88:986–990.

109. Roederer M, Staal FJT, Ela SW, et al. *N*-Acetylcysteine: Potential for AIDS therapy. Pharmacology 1993;46:121–129.
110. Droge W. Cysteine and glutathione deficiency in AIDS patients: A rationale for the treatment with *N*-acetylcysteine. Pharmacology 1993;46:61–65.
111. Roederer M, Ela SW, Staal FJT, et al. *N*-Acetylcysteine: A new approach to anti-HIV therapy. AIDS Res Hum Retrovir 1992;8:209–219.
112. Jepsen S, Herlevsen P, Knudsen P, et al. Antioxidant treatment with *N*-acetylcysteine during adult respiratory distress syndrome: A prospective randomized placebo-controlled study. Crit Care Med 1992;20:918–923.
113. Bernard GR. Potential of *N*-acetylcysteine as treatment for the adult respiratory distress syndrome. Eur Respir J 1990; 3(suppl. 11):496–498.
114. Horowitz JD, Antman EM, Lorell BH, et al. Potentiation of the cardiovascular effects of nitroglycerin by *N*-acetylcysteine. Circulation 1983;68:1247–1253.
115. Svendsen JH, Klarlund K, Aldershvile J, Waldorff S. *N*-Acetylcysteine modifies the acute effects of isosorbide-5-mononitrate in angina pectoris patients evaluated by exercise testing. J Cardiovasc Pharmacol 1991;13:320–323.
116. Vassallo S, Howland MA. Severe dichromate poisoning: Survival after therapy with *N*-acetylcysteine and hemodialysis. Vet Hum Toxicol 1988;30:347.
117. Locatelli C, Travaglia CA, Maccarini D, et al. Amanita poisoning: Forced diuresis and intravenous *N*-acetylcysteine combined therapy. In: *Proceedings, 14th International Congress of European Association of Poison Centres, Milan, Italy, September 25–29, 1990*:32.
118. Schneider SM, Vanscoy GJ, Michelson EA. Failure of *N*-acetylcysteine to reduce alpha amanitin toxicity. Vet Hum Toxicol 1989;31:359.
119. Gavish D, Breslow JL. Lipoprotein a reduction by *N*-acetylcysteine. Lancet 1991;337:203–204.
120. Hanson PR. Lipoprotein a reduction by *N*-acetylcysteine. Lancet 1991;337:672–677.
121. Breslow JL, Azrolan N, Boston A. *N*-Acetylcysteine and lipoprotein 1. Lancet 1992;239:126–127.
122. Kroon AA, Demacher PMN, Stalenhoef AFH. *N*-Acetylcysteine and serum concentrations of lipoprotein a. J Intern Med 1991;230:519–526.
123. Mohammed S, Jamal AZ, Robisun LR. Serum sickness-like illness associated with *N*-acetylcysteine therapy. Ann Pharmacother 1994;28:285.
124. Flanagan RJ, Meredith TJ. Use of *N*-acetylcysteine in clinical toxicology. Am J Med 1991;91(suppl. 36):131S–139S.
125. Spiller HA, Krenzelok EP, Grande GA, et al. A prospective evaluation of the effect of activated charcoal before oral *N*-acetylcysteine in acetaminophen overdose. Ann Emerg Med 1994;23:519–523.
126. Simon GA, Tirosk MS, Edery H. Administration of obidoxime tablets to man: Plasma levels and side reactions. Arch Toxicol 1976;36:83–88.
127. Bentur Y, Nutenko I, Tsipiniuk A, et al. Pharmacokinetics of obidoxime in organophosphate poisoning associated with renal failure. Clin Toxicol 1993;31:315–322.
128. Siwy BK, Sadove AM. Acute management of dopamine infiltration injury with regitine. Plast Reconstr Surg 1987;80: 610–612.
129. McCauley WA, Gerace RV, Scilley C. Treatment of accidental digital injection of epinephrine. Ann Emerg Med 1991;20: 665–668.
130. Markovchik V, Burkhart KK. The reversal of the ischemic effects of epinephrine on a finger with local injections of phentolamine. J Emerg Med 1991;9:323–324.
131. Brimacombe J, Archdeacon J, Newell S, Martin J. Two cases of naloxone-induced pulmonary oedema: The possible use of phentolamine in management. Anesth Intensive Care 1991;19:578–580.
132. Rasthaus EM, Landy PJ. Methyl bromide poisoning. Br J Ind Med 1961;18:53–57.
133. Verzijl JM, Joore HCA, van Dijk A, et al. In vitro cyanide release of four Prussian blue salts used for the treatment of cesium contaminated persons. Clin Toxicol 1993;31: 553–562.
134. McEvoy GK, ed. *AHFS Drug Information 94.* Bethesda, MD: American Society of Hospital Pharmacists, 1994:726–728.
135. Wood M. Cholinergic and parasympathomimetic drugs: Cholinesterases and anticholinesterases. In: Wood M, Wood AJJ, eds. *Drugs and anesthesia: Pharmacology for Anesthesiologists.* 2nd ed. Baltimore: Williams & Wilkins, 1990.
136. Keeler JR, Hurst CG, Dunn MA. Pyridostigmine used as a nerve agent pretreatment under wartime conditions. JAMA 1991;266:693–695.
137. Menne T, Kaaber K. Treatment of pompholyx due to allergy with chelating agents. Contact Dermatitis 1978;4:289–290.
138. Sunderman F. The treatment of acute nickel carbonyl poisoning with sodium diethyldithiocarbamate. Ann Clin Res 1971; 3:182–185.
139. Hersh EM, Brewton G, Abrams D, et al. Dithiocarb sodium (diethyldithiocarbamate) therapy in patients with symptomatic HIV infection and AIDS: A randomized, double-blind, placebo-controlled multicenter study. JAMA 1991;265:1538–1544.
140. Kurte DL, Dean BS, Krenzelok EP. Acute nickel carbonyl poisoning. Am J Emerg Med 1993;11:64–66.
141. Hersh EM. Dithiocarb sodium and HIV infection. JAMA 1991; 266:796.
142. Rusinger EC, Kern P, Ernst M, et al. Inhibition of HIV progression by dithiocarb. Lancet 1990;335:679–682.

Chapter 6

Supportive Care

INTRODUCTION

Morbidity and mortality following an overdose are reduced by intensive appropriate symptomatic supportive therapy. A well-trained emergency medical team is required for administration of intensive clinical care, which includes monitoring vital signs, cardiac status, airway, and mental status.

BASIC APPROACH TO THE POISONED PATIENT

1. *Stabilization:* The initial brief patient survey is directed toward correcting immediate life-threatening problems of **a**irway, **b**reathing, **c**irculation, and **d**rug-induced central nervous system depression (ABCD). If the patient is alert with normal speech and pulse, proceed to the definitive patient survey unless immediate eye or skin decontamination is needed. Detection of inadequate oxygenation or circulation with a pulse oximeter demands immediate attention (see Pulse Oximetry in Chapter 66). Other etiologies of pulmonary dysfunction, including those associated with drug abuse, are aspiration pneumonia, noncardiogenic and cardiogenic pulmonary emboli, atelectasis, pneumothorax, pulmonary fibrosis, and, rarely, tetanus-induced respiratory failure. An assessment of neurologic status follows correction of these abnormalities. Give 50 mL 50% dextrose after Dextrostix testing to an adult or 1 mL/kg diluted 1:1 to a child, naloxone 2 mg (see Chapter 25 for precautions), and thiamine 100 mg intravenously to all patients with depressed mental status.
2. *Complete patient evaluation (history, physical examination, laboratory tests):* A complete patient survey directed toward identifying the toxin or possible toxidrome, evaluating the severity of its clinical effects, and searching for associated complications and trauma. The laboratory work complements the history and physical examination.
3. *Appropriate treatment to reduce absorption:* Current methods include skin decontamination, gastric lavage, and administration of oral activated charcoal and possibly cathartics.

4. *Appropriate measures to improve elimination of the toxin:* These may include urine pH alteration, diuresis, hemodialysis, hemoperfusion, peritoneal dialysis, serial (pulsed) activated charcoal.
5. *Consideration of specific antidotes:* Specific antidotes are effective for less than 5% of poisonings.
6. *Continuing care and disposition:* After diagnosis and initial treatment, an adequate observation period should be established. Poison prevention education or psychiatric counseling may be appropriate, and a referral source should be identified for follow-up treatment.

THE AIRWAY

Symptoms of airway obstruction include dyspnea, dysphonia, air hunger, and hoarseness. Signs of airway obstruction include stridor, intercostal and substernal or intercostal retractions, cyanosis, diaphoresis, drooling, and tachypnea. Arterial oxygen tension (Pao_2) and arterial oxygen saturation (Sao_2) are the two dependent parameters that measure the degree of arterial oxygenation. Arterial oxygen tension depends on the fraction of inspired oxygen (Fio_2), alveolar ventilation, and the distribution of ventilation and perfusion in the lungs.

CLINICAL MANIFESTATIONS

Normal oxygen delivery requires adequate hemoglobin oxygen saturation (eg, carbon monoxide reduces arterial oxygen saturation but not Pao_2), adequate hemoglobin levels (anemia reduces oxygen-carrying capacity), normal oxygen-unloading mechanisms (hypothermia, alkalosis, and decreased 2,3-diphosphoglycerate levels reduce oxygen release, as revealed by a leftward shift of the oxyhemoglobin dissociation curve), and an adequate cardiac output. Increasing metabolic acidosis in the presence of a normal Pao_2 suggests a toxin or condition that either decreases oxygen-carrying capacity (eg, carbon monoxide, methemoglobinemia) or reduces tissue oxygen utilization (eg, cyanide, hydrogen sulfide).

OXYGEN TOXICITY

Complications of oxygen therapy result from physical hazards (eg, drying of mucous membranes, fire or explosions, or trauma associated with tubes, catheters, or masks), physiologic effects (ie, atelectasis, hypercarbia), and direct cytotoxicity. There is increased formation of free radicals (eg, superoxide anion, hydrogen peroxide, hydroxyl radicals), which probably interact with cellular enzymes and membranes to produce toxic effects. A number of drugs and toxins, including paraquat, bleomycin, adriamycin, high-dose disulfiram (> 10 mg/kg) or diethyldithiocarbamate (> 250 mg/kg), daunorubicin, and antibiotics, depend on quinoid groups or bound metals, generate free radicals, and potentially enhance oxygen toxicity. Ozone and nitrogen dioxide also are capable of damaging the lungs through free radical formation. The only effective treatment for oxygen poisoning is prevention. Breathing Fio_2 levels of 50% or less for short periods (2–7 days) does not cause pulmonary dysfunction. Pure oxygen can be safely administered for brief periods involved in cardiopulmonary resuscitation or the transport of critically ill patients.

HYPOTENSION

1. Insert a large-bore peripheral intravenous line (16-gauge or larger). A second line is useful in severe cases for the administration of drugs and additional administration of fluid. Give a fluid challenge of 200 mL of saline solution to adults or 10 mL/kg to children and observe for improvement in blood pressure over 10 minutes. Markedly hypotensive children may receive a fluid bolus up to 20 mL/kg. Repeat the fluid bolus if blood pressure fails to normalize, and assess for signs of fluid overload (ie, rales, S_3 heart gallop, neck vein distention). Hemodynamic monitoring should be considered in those adult patients who do not respond to 2-L infusion and short-term, low-dose vasopressors such as dopamine and norepinephrine.
2. Monitor cardiac function in all overdoses and especially in those patients with hypotension or exposure to arrhythmogenic toxins (eg, cardiac glycosides, beta-blocking agents, quinidine, quinine, verapamil, theophylline, cholinesterase inhibitors such as organophosphates and carbamates, tricyclic antidepressants, hydrocarbons, chloral hydrate, lithium, phenothiazines, arsenic, phosphorus).
3. Obtain an electrocardiogram in hypotensive patients and note rate, rhythm, dysrhythmias, and possible conduction delays (PR > 0.2 second, QRS > 0.1 second, or QT interval > 50% of RR interval).
4. An adjunctive measure in treating hypotension includes the Trendelenburg position.
5. In patients who do not respond to initial fluid challenges, monitor central venous pressures and hourly urinary output. Patients with cardiac disease or severe hypotension often need more sophisticated hemodynamic monitoring (pulmonary artery catheter and intraarterial pressure monitoring).

DOPAMINE

Dopamine is the usual vasopressor of choice because it preserves renal perfusion at low doses.

Mechanism of Action

Dopamine acts as an indirect α (vasoconstriction), β_1 (tachycardia, increased myocardial contractility), and β_2 (vasodilation, bronchodilation) adrenoreceptor agonist as well as direct dopamine receptor stimulator depending on dose. At low doses, dopaminergic stimulation dominates, resulting in renal and mesenteric dilation. Medium-range doses cause β_1 stimulation (increased contractility, mildly increased pulse rate). High doses cause primarily α stimulation, producing systemic vasoconstriction including that of renal vessels.

Adverse Effects

Nausea, vomiting, tachydysrhythmias, and, in susceptible patients, angina and gangrene are adverse effects.

Precautions

In drug overdoses with α blocking agents (eg, phenothiazines), unopposed β stimulation would be expected to worsen hypotension. In addition, drugs that inhibit dopamine β-hydroxylase (eg, disulfiram, carbon disulfide) reduce the conversion of dopamine to norepinephrine. Monoamine oxidase inhibitors potentiate dopamine effects, requiring dosages to be decreased by a factor of 10. Alkaline solutions (eg, sodium bicarbonate) inactivate dopamine and should not be administered together in the same intravenous line.

Dose

Use 1 ampule (200 mg) in 250 mL of 5% dextrose in water (D_5W) to make a solution of 800 μg/mL. Start at a low dose range (1–5 μg/kg/min). The medium dose range is 5 to 15 μg/kg/min, and the high dose range is 15 to 30 μg/kg/min. Titrate the dose to maintain systolic blood pressure between 90 and 100 mm Hg using the lowest dose possible. Monitor blood pressure every 15 minutes. To use dopamine in a microdrip infusion pump, multiply the weight of the patient (in kilograms) by 15 and add that number of milligrams of dopamine to 250 mL of D_5W solution. The reading on the microdrip infusion pump (eg, 5) will correspond to the rate of infusion (e.g., 5 μg/kg/min).[1]

NOREPINEPHRINE

Mechanism of Action

A naturally occurring catecholamine with potent α and $β_1$ properties causing both peripheral vascular constriction and increased cardiac contractility.

Dose

Add 2 ampules (8 mg) to 500 mL of 5% dextrose solution (D_5W) to make a concentration of 16 μg/mL. Start at 0.5 to 1 mL/min and titrate to a clinical response. High doses cause intense vasoconstriction, which can result in "normal" blood pressure but decreased tissue perfusion. Low doses (0.25–0.5 mL/min) may be added to medium-range dopamine doses for refractory hypotension, but close hemodynamic monitoring (pulmonary artery catheter and intraarterial pressure monitoring) is advised to assess efficacy. Norepinephrine is the vasopressor of choice for drugs that cause α blockade (eg, phenothiazines, tricyclic antidepressants) and inhibit dopamine β-hydroxylase (eg, disulfiram).

Precautions

Constant cardiac monitoring should be initiated and the blood pressure monitored every 5 minutes until a clear trend is established. An intraarterial monitor may be necessary to monitor blood pressure accurately because of intense vasoconstriction. Excessive blood pressure elevation may result from therapeutic overshoot.

CENTRAL NERVOUS SYSTEM DEPRESSION: COMA

Depressed mental status should be treated promptly with the following antidotes.

The Coma Cocktail (Dextrose, Thiamine, Naloxone)

Hoffman and Goldfrank reviewed extensive data from 1966 to 1994 on the management of the potentially poisoned patient with altered consciousness.[2] Analysis of these data suggests the following tentative and clinically rational conclusions.

Dextrose

When rapid reagent tests are available, all patients with numerical hypoglycemia should receive hypertonic dextrose. Routine administration of hypertonic dextrose is recommended for all patients with nonfocal neurologic examinations and borderline glucose concentrations on rapid reagent testing. When rapid reagent tests are unavailable, all patients without focality should receive hypertonic dextrose.

Other therapeutic modalities such as oral glucose solutions and glucagon should be avoided (except when intravenous access is unavailable) because they are unreliable, may have a delay to onset of action (caused by food), or require the presence of glycogen stores (such as glucagon).

Thiamine (Vitamin B_1)

An empiric dose of 100 mg of thiamine should be given at the time of hypertonic dextrose administration. The routine use of thiamine supplementation is warranted, safe, inexpensive, and cost-effective, and it will prevent the possibility of delayed deterioration secondary to nutritional deficiency.

Naloxone

Naloxone can be administered without demonstrable risk in patients who present with central nervous system and/or respiratory depression and have a low likelihood of opioid addiction and polydrug intoxication (small children). When naloxone is to be used in potentially dependent patients, small doses (0.1–0.2 mg) rather than the doses commonly recommended (0.4–2.0 mg) are advised. This increases arousal and respiratory effort without producing withdrawal.

If ventilation can be adequately supported, then graded dosing of naloxone is usually successful. Administer 0.1 to 0.2 mg as a first dose, and then progress in a doubling fashion until 10 mg has been given. If no response occurs at a total dose of 10 mg, isolated opioid intoxication is unlikely.

Patients whose symptoms recur should be observed in an intensive care setting and given a continuous infusion of naloxone as follows. The hourly infusion rate should deliver a dose of naloxone that is equal to the initial dose required to produce arousal. A repeat bolus of 50% of the initial dose may be needed 20 to 30 minutes after the infusion is started. The repeat dose should be based on clinical findings. Additional naloxone doses often are required in diphenoxylate–atropine (Lomotil), propoxyphene (Darvon), pentazocine (Talwin), or codeine overdoses. If the patient is intubated but an intravenous line cannot be established, 0.8 mg naloxone may be given via the endotracheal tube, followed by several deep ventilations. Naloxone is also absorbed via the subcutaneous and intramuscular routes, with an onset of action of 2 to 5 minutes in normotensive patients.

OXYGEN

All patients with depressed mental status should receive supplemental 100% oxygen (O_2 via mask unless the patient has chronically elevated Pco_2 levels). Always consider agents or conditions that alter hemoglobin-carrying capacity (e.g. carbon monoxide, methemoglobinemia) or alter tissue utilization (cyanide, hydrogen sulfide), and give an appropriate antidote immediately (see Pulse Oximetry in Chapter 66).

CLINICAL PROBLEMS

The medical team familiar with medical toxicology must be aware of the evaluation and treatment of lethargy, agitation, the violent patient, coma, respiratory distress (respiratory depression, aspiration pneumonia, adult respiratory distress syndrome), cerebral edema, seizures, infections, acid–base or electrolyte disorders, osmolar balance problems, agitation, refractory hypertension, hypotension, hyperthermia, hypothermia, maintenance of fluid balance, psychiatric problems, and parental education. Treatment of the poisoned patient may require consultation with specialized services within the hospital or medical community. Reading literature references and liberal use of regional poison control centers are necessary to provide treatment and optimum care. Equipment should be readily at hand to treat the acute anaphylactic reaction, respiratory distress (positive end-expiratory pressure, bronchoscopy, oxygen source), seizures and agitation (diazepam, phenytoin, neuromuscular blockade), and fluid imbalance. Psychiatric support must be available before the patient is discharged. The team will be required to be proficient at endoscopy, central vein cannulization, right heart catheterization, and chest physiotherapy.

QUICK APPROACHES TO CRITICAL SCENARIOS

Angioedema

Swelling of the oropharynx or upper airway may present with hoarseness, dysphagia, wheezing, or inability to handle oral secretions. These symptoms are suggestive of laryngeal edema. Treat with 0.3 and 0.5 mL of 1:1000 epinephrine subcutaneously in the adult. In addition, use vaporized racemic epinephrine 8 to 15 drops aerosolized. The aerosolized solution causes local vasoconstriction and will reduce laryngeal edema. This mode of administration is recommended if there is any suspicion of epiglottitis in children. If the cause is not infectious in origin, diphenhydramine may be useful. The adult dose is 50 mg intravenously or intramuscularly. The pediatric dose is 5 mg/kg/24 h intravenously or intramuscularly or a single dose of 1 mg/kg (0.5–1.5 mg/kg).

SUPPORTIVE CARE: SUMMARY

Acidosis

pH is acutely below 7.35 (see Acid–Base Disorders later in this chapter). Monitor arterial blood gases, serum sodium and potassium levels, and the electrocardiogram. Place a central venous line or Swan–Ganz pulmonary artery catheter to determine the pulmonary capillary wedge pressure if dehydration and hypovolemia are present.

Acute Alcohol Withdrawal

Use restraints if needed. Administer diazepam 5 to 10 mg or another benzodiazepine every 5 to 10 minutes until the patient becomes calm. Establish an intravenous line of normal saline. Thiamine 100 mg should be administered orally, intravenously, or intramuscularly. If the serum potassium level is low, replace potassium at a rate no greater than 20 mEq/h; use a higher rate if there is a central line. Magnesium sulfate can be given as a 2-g dose initially and then 1 g every 12 hours intravenously, provided the patient is not in renal failure or anticoagulated. Search for infection (meningitis) and bleeding (gastrointestinal and intraabdominal) in any patient with an altered level of consciousness. (See Chapter 55).

Acute Dystonic Reaction

Administer intravenous diphenhydramine (2 mg/kg up to 50 mg) over several minutes or intramuscular benztropine mesylate (2 mg in adults). Follow up with diphenhydramine 50 mg orally three times daily or trihexyphenidyl 2 mg orally twice daily. Discontinue etiology (e.g., phenothiazines).

Anaphylaxis

Systemic anaphylaxis in the United States occurs in about 1 in every 3000 patients and may account for more than 500 deaths annually. Table 6–1 lists some mechanisms and agents responsible for systemic anaphylactic reactions.[3] In all patients, an initial assessment of the ABCDs is imperative. Airway, cardiovascular reactions and cutaneous reactions require urgent therapy (Table 6–2). In addition to epinephrine, all patients with an acute allergic reaction should be treated with diphenhydramine 25 to 50 mg intravenously or intramuscularly (5 mg/kg in children) (see Table 6–2). A corticosteroid such as methylprednisolone 125 mg should be administered intravenously simultaneously. The dose in children is 1 to 2 mg/kg. If the patient is not in shock, give epinephrine 0.1 m/kg up to 0.3 to 0.5 mL of 1:1000 epinephrine subcutaneously. Repeat every 15 minutes as required. For patients in shock, give 1 mL of the more dilute 1:10,000 epinephrine (0.1 or 1 mg/10 mL ampules) and administer 1 mg/kg; repeat every 3 minutes as needed to improve the diastolic blood pressure to 90 mm Hg. For adults of normal size, use 10 mL intravenously over 5 to 10 minutes. Start a continuous epinephrine drip at a concentration of 4 μg/mL (1 mg[1 mL]) of a 1:1000 solution in 250 mL 5% dextrose starting at 1 μg/min, increased to a maximum of 4 μg/mL. For children, start at 0.1 μg/kg/min and titrate in increments up to a maximum of 1.5 μg/kg/min. If there is no response, give glucagon 3 to 5 mg intravenously and repeat to a total of 15 mg. Maintain the airway and use fluids as required. Be certain to have access to a basic airway, oxygen, a cardiac monitor, and venous access.

Mild Respiratory Distress Secondary to an Allergen

1. Administer epinephrine (1:1000) 0.3 mg subcutaneously. This may be repeated every 20 minutes × 2.
2. If the patient is wheezing, administer albuterol 2.5 mg/3 mL NS via handheld nebulizer, to be repeated as needed.

3. Administer diphenhydramine 50 to 100 mg by intravenous push; for children, administer 5 mg/kg or 150 mg/m^2/d orally, intramuscularly, or intravenously in divided doses every 6 to 8 hours not to exceed 30 mg/d.
4. Reassess for potential deterioration.

Severe Respiratory Distress/Poor Perfusion

1. Place patient in shock position as needed.
2. Administer epinephrine (1:10,000) 0.2 to 0.3 mg by intravenous push or endotracheally; this may be repeated in 5 minutes.
3. If hypotension is present, administer a fluid challenge.
4. If the fluid challenge is unsuccessful, administer dopamine 200 mg/250 mL NS by intravenous piggyback. Start at 30 µg/min.
5. Consider a second intravenous access site.
6. If the patient is wheezing, consider albuterol 2.5 mg/3 mL NS via handheld nebulizer, to be repeated as needed.

Bradycardia

Bradycardia without hypotension requires close observation. Severe bradycardia with hypotension usually responds to intravenous atropine sulfate. The adult dose is 0.5 to 1 mg. The pediatric dose is 0.01 to 0.03 mg/kg, with a maximum dose of 1 mg and a minimum dose of 0.1 mg. The dose may be repeated up to four times if necessary.

Bronchospasm

The patient with bronchospasm must be treated aggressively. The inciting agent should be eliminated if possible. Albuterol or salbutamol nebulized is recommended as first-line therapy for bronchospasm. The dose is 2.5 mg/3 mL NS nebulized with pressurized air or oxygen. Repeat the dose as necessary. For children, administer 2.5 mg three to four times daily by nebulization.[4] There is a small risk of hypokalemia with large doses which does not appear to be clinically significant (see Chapter 66).

Altered Mental Status (Central Nervous System Depression)

If patients are unable to protect their airway, they require endotracheal intubation and assisted ventilation. The patient with depressed or altered level of consciousness must be evaluated aggressively. The vital signs, serum glucose, electrolytes, and fluid status must be rapidly ascertained. In addition, naloxone 2.0 mg should be administered intramuscularly or intravenously. A thorough physical examination should be done with a focus on a detailed neurological examination and any signs of trauma. The neurologic examination should be repeated numerous times to evaluate and assess for changing status. Intravenous thiamine 100 mg should be given before 1 ampule of D50 (dextrose). Computed axial tomography or magnetic resonance imaging may be required. If no source is found after this extensive workup, lumbar puncture may be required, especially if an infectious cause is suspected. In the initial

Table 6–1
Mechanisms and Agents Responsible for Systemic Anaphylactic Reactions

Mechanism	Agent	Examples
IgE-mediated reaction against native proteins	Venoms	Hymenoptera, fire ant, snake
	Airborne allergens	Pollens, molds, danders
	Foods	Peanuts, milk, egg, seafood, grains
	Enzymes	Trypsin, streptokinase, chymopapain
	Heterologous serum	Tetanus antitoxin, antilymphocyte globulin
	Human proteins	Insulin corticotropin, vasopressin, serum and seminal proteins
	Others	Protamine, latex
IgE-mediated reaction against protein–hapten conjugates	Antibiotics	Penicillins, cephalosporins, sulfonamides
	Disinfectants	Ethylene oxide
Complement activation and generation of anaphylatoxins	Human proteins	Gamma globulins, other blood products
	Dialysis	Contact of blood with some dialysis membranes
Direct activation of mediator release from mast cells, basophils, or both	Hypertonic solutions	Radiocontrast medium, mannitol
	Drugs	Opiates, curare, *d*-tubocurarine, vancomycin
	Others	Dextran, fluorescein for angiography
Unknown	Nonsteroidal antiinflammatory drugs	Aspirin, indomethacin
	Anesthetics	Lidocaine, thiopental
	Preservatives	Metabisulfites, benzoates
	Steroids	Progesterone, hydrocortisone
	Exercise	—
	Exercise and food	—
	Idiopathic anaphylaxis	—

From Bochner BS, Lichtenstein LM. Anaphylaxis. N Engl J Med 1991;324:1785–1790.

Table 6–2
Pharmacologic Treatment of Systemic Anaphylaxis in Adults*

Agent	Indications	Dosage	Goals	Complications
Airway or Cutaneous Reactions				
Initial therapy				
Epinephrine	Bronchospasm, laryngeal edema, urticaria, angioedema	0.3–0.5 mL of 1:1000 dilution (0.3–0.5 mg) SC every 10–20 min	Maintain airway patency, reduce fluid extravasation and pruritus	Arrhythmias, hypertension, nervousness, tremor
Oxygen	Hypoxemia	40–100%	Maintain P_{O_2} ≥60 mm Hg	None
Metaproterenol†	Bronchospasm	0.3 mL (5% solution) in 2.5 mL of saline, inhaled through nebulizer	Maintain airway patency	Same as for epinephrine
Secondary therapy‡				
Aminophylline	Bronchospasm	Loading dose if necessary (6 mg/kg IV over a 30-min period); 0.3–0.9 mg/kg/h IV as maintenance dose§	Maintain airway patency	Arrhythmias, nausea, vomiting, seizures
Corticosteroids	Bronchospasm	250 mg of hydrocortisone or 50 mg of methylprednisolone IV every 6 h for 2–4 doses	Block or reduce prolonged or late-phase reactions	Hyperglycemia, fluid retention
Antihistamines	Urticaria	25–50 mg of hydroxyzine or diphenhydramine IV or PO every 6–8 h as needed	Reduce pruritus, antagonize H_1 effects of histamine	Drowsiness, dry mouth, urinary retention
		300 mg of cimetidine IV or PO every 6 h	Antagonize H_2 effects of histamine	
Cardiovascular Reactions				
Initial therapy				
Intravenous fluids	Hypotension	1 L every 20–30 min as needed	Maintain systolic blood pressure ≥80–100 mm Hg	Congestive heart failure, pulmonary edema
Epinephrine	Hypotension	1 mL of 1:1000 dilution in 500 mL of D_5W IV at a rate of 0.5–5 μg (0.25–2.5 mL)/min	Same as for intravenous fluids	Arrhythmias, hypertension, nervousness, tremor
Secondary therapy				
Norepinephrine	Hypotension	4 mg in 1 L of D_5W IV at a rate of 2–12 μg (0.5–3 mL)/min	Same as for intravenous fluids	Same as for epinephrine
Antihistamines	Hypotension	25–50 mg of hydroxyzine or diphenhydramine IM or PO every 6–8 h as needed	Antagonize H_1 and H_2 effects of histamine on myocardium and peripheral vasculature	Drowsiness, dry mouth, urinary retention
		300 mg of cimetidine IV or PO every 6 h		
Glucagon¶	Refractory hypotension	1 mg in 1 L of D_5W IV at a rate of 5–15 μg (5–15 mL)/min	Increase heart rate and cardiac output	Nausea

*Dosages, choice of specific agents, efficacy, and safety must be individualized. P_{O_2} denotes partial pressure of oxygen, and D_5W 5% aqueous dextrose solution.
†Albuterol (0.5 mL of the 0.5% solution in 2.5 mL of saline) or isoetharine (0.5 mL of the 1% solution in 2 mL of saline) can also be used.
‡These agents have little or no efficacy during the acute anaphylactic reaction; they may reduce or prevent recurrent or prolonged reactions.
§Lower rates are suggested for older patients, those taking medications that reduce metabolism, those with hepatic dysfunction, and those with congestive heart failure; higher rates should be used in younger persons or cigarette smokers.
¶May be particularly useful in patients taking beta-adrenergic blockers, as its ability to stimulate both inotropic and chronotropic cardiac function may be unaltered by beta-adrenergic blockade.
From Bochner BS, Lichtenstein LM. Anaphylaxis. N Engl J Med 1991;324:1785–1790.

physical examination, the gag reflex should be evaluated. (Also, see p 108).

Cerebral Edema

The patient with known or suspected cerebral edema requires aggressive treatment. The patient should be intubated in a manner that does not elevate intracranial pressure and hyperventilated to a P_{CO_2} of 28 to 32 Torr within 2 to 3 minutes. This should be confirmed by arterial blood gas. Furosemide 1 mg/kg may be administered if the patient is in fluid overload.

Circulatory Assistance

Assistance devices available for circulatory support include the intraaortic balloon pump, cardiopulmonary bypass (see Elimination Enhancement), and direct mechanism ventricular assistance (experimental).[5]

Hypovolemic Shock

The patient with gastroenteritis usually presents with problems related to dehydration or hypovolemic shock. The patient with this condition should be given aggressive fluid hydration of either normal saline or Ringer's lactate solution. Potassium chloride supplementation may be required after a baseline serum potassium has been determined. The patient should also have maintenance fluids running at the same time. Reevaluate after the first bolus; administer more fluid as necessary. Follow postural vital signs. Once the patient is no longer in shock, one half of the total fluid deficit should be administered in the first 8 hours. The other half is given over the next 16 hours.

Heart Block

This condition includes not only third-degree heart block, or atrioventricular dissociation, but also second-degree heart block. The asymptomatic patient with this condition should have an external pacer placed and left on standby. The patient with bradycardia with hypotension or worsening heart block may be temporarily treated with atropine. The definitive treatment for this condition also requires elimination of the inciting agent. In refractory cases an intravenous pacing wire should be placed. Any patient with complete heart block or increasing heart block should be admitted to a monitored bed.

Hemorrhagic Gastritis

The patient with hemorrhagic gastritis is at risk for exsanguination and requires aggressive management. Saline lavage may be helpful in reducing bleeding but carries the risk of iatrogenic hypothermia. Antacids may also play a beneficial role. Platelet count and prothrombin and thromboplastin times should be evaluated. The patient should also be typed and crossmatched for packed red cells, platelets, and fresh-frozen plasma. Administer blood products and vitamin K for uncontrolled bleeding.

Hepatic Injury

Hepatic injury may manifest as coagulation abnormalities, late development of electrolyte imbalance, late development of hepatic encephalopathy, early hyperbilirubinemia, and chronic anemia. These conditions are assessed by following the coagulation profiles, complete blood count, serum electrolytes, glucose, creatinine, bilirubin, and liver enzymes. Administer fresh-frozen plasma, vitamin K, careful fluid and electrolyte control, a low-protein diet, neomycin, and lactulose as needed. Hepatic and renal function should be followed for at least 3 days.

Hyperkalemia

The patient with life-threatening hyperkalemia is treated in various ways:

1. Fifty percent dextrose 50 mL with 5 to 10 U of regular intravenous insulin may be given initially. This is followed by 1 L of 20% dextrose with 40 to 80 U of insulin given over the next 2 to 4 hours. Glucose must be monitored every 30 minutes while insulin is being administered.
2. Polystyrene resin or sodium sulfonate resin may be given orally.
3. Ten percent calcium gluconate 10 to 20 mL may be given slowly over 10 to 20 minutes; 0.5 to 1.0 mg/kg may be given intravenously over 2 to 5 minutes in children; this may be repeated in 5 to 10 minutes.
4. Sodium bicarbonate may be given (adults: 50–100 mEq intravenously over 10–20 minutes, children: 1–2 mEq/kg intravenously over 5–10 minutes) and repeated in 15 minutes.

The intravenous medications cause a temporary flow of potassium ions to the intracellular space. The oral medications absorb potassium causing elimination. If the patient does not have adequate renal function, hemodialysis may be required for definitive treatment.

Hypercalcemia

Mild hypercalcemia (< 12 mg/dl) can be managed conservatively by restriction of calcium intake, observation, and treatment of the underlying disorder. Volume depletion should be corrected if present, and vitamin D, calcium supplements, and thiazide diuretics discontinued. These measures will control calcium concentration until the cause can be discovered and treated more specifically. Patients with relatively well-preserved cardiac and renal function may tolerate up to 1 L/h parenteral saline solution, especially if coupled with high-dose (100–200 mg every 2 hours) furosemide. Older patients with impaired cardiac, renal, or pulmonary function, however, require more cautious volume replenishment, often with the aid of a central venous pressure monitor. Simple volume replenishment may decrease the calcium concentration to a far safer level without the need to resort to more dangerous agents. Frequent monitoring of electrolytes—especially potassium, magnesium, and phosphate—is a necessary adjunctive measure.[6]

Hypocalcemia

Administer intravenous calcium gluconate (10% solution) slowly in a dose of 10 mL.

Hypoglycemia

Monitor blood glucose, serum electrolytes, liver and kidney function, glucose balance, and plasma insulin levels. In suspected overdoses, monitor glucose carefully and obtain plasma insulin level. Also, in suspected overdoses, analyze the blood for salicylates and alcohol and the urine for sedative–hypnotic drugs. If insulin overdose is suspected, test for C-reactive protein. Monitor blood glucose, arterial blood gases, serum electrolytes, and liver and kidney function if diabetic or alcoholic ketoacidosis is suspected. Administration of 50% dextrose (D_{50}) should be reserved for those patients in whom hypoglycemia is demonstrated. Preliminary animal and human evidence suggests that glucose-containing intravenous solutions should be avoided in patients at risk for cerebral ischemia, impending cardiac arrest, or severe hypotension or those receiving cardiopulmonary resuscitation.[7]

Hypokalemia

Correct cautiously. In the presence of bradydysrhythmias or tachydysrhythmias, elevation of plasma potassium may enhance conduction defects. Prepare potassium solution in either saline or a glucose-containing solution. The concentration of potassium should not exceed 40 to 60 mEq/L. Give potassium salts at 10 mEq/h or 200 mEq/24 hours. Do not permit serum potassium levels to rise above 4.5 mmol/L (normal, 3.5–5.0 mmol/L). If the patient is severely hypokalemic, saline is the intravenous solution of choice. Glucose enhances the movement of potassium intracellularly. Relative contraindications to potassium use include digitalis toxicity in the presence of renal failure, hyperkalemia, depressed atrioventricular conduction, and second-degree heart block or greater.

Hypoprothrombinemia

Administer vitamin K 2.5 to 5 mg intravenously, intramuscularly, orally, or subcutaneously daily as required.

Neuromuscular Blockade

Polymyxin antibiotics and anesthetic agents may cause this life-threatening condition. Treatment involves ventilatory assistance and intravenous calcium chloride (1 g) or 20 mL 10% calcium gluconate with constant electrocardiographic monitoring.

Psychiatric Review

Suicidal intent can be precipitated by interpersonal crises, depression, a loss of hope, psychosis, drugs, alcohol, and personality disorders. There may be a history of previous suicide attempts or a family history of suicide. Prior to discharge, psychiatric consultation should be obtained in such cases.[50,51,62]

Seizures and Status Epilepticus

Major drugs used to treat status epilepticus are summarized in Table 6–3. A suggested and useful timetable for the treatment of status epilepticus is presented in Table 6–4.[8] If seizures recur, use phenytoin. The loading dose is 17 mg/kg. Administer undiluted by slow intravenous push or dilute 50 mg/mL solution in 50 to 100 mL of 0.9% saline. Watch for hypotension or arrhythmias while administering at a maximum rate of 50 mg/min. Phenobarbital may be used as a second-line agent instead of phenytoin or as a third agent if seizures persist despite above regimen. Monitor urine myoglobin and serum creatine and creatine kinase levels to detect evidence of rhabdomyolysis. The loading dose of phenobarbital is 10 to 20 mg/kg, administered in 50 to 60 mL of 0.9% normal saline over 15 to 20 minutes. Repeat as required. If seizures are refractory to treatment, use a general anesthetic with thiopental or halothane. Monitor the electroencephalogram for seizure activity cessation. Use the above agents cautiously with diazepam because of the development of synergistic respiratory depression. Watch for development of hypoglycemia. Monitor hydration and electrolyte balance. Cerebral edema may be treated with

Table 6–3
A Suggested Timetable for the Treatment of Status Epilepticus

Time* (min)	Action
0–5	Diagnose status epilepticus by observing continued seizure activity or one additional seizure. Give oxygen by nasal cannula or mask; position patient's head for optimal airway patency; consider intubation if respiratory assistance is needed. Obtain and record vital signs at onset and periodically thereafter; control any abnormalities as necessary; initiate ECG monitoring. Establish an IV; draw venous blood samples for glucose level, serum chemistries, hematology studies, toxicology screens, and determinations of antiepileptic drug levels. Assess oxygenation with oximetry or periodic arterial bood gas determinations.
6–9	If hypoglycemia is established or a blood glucose determination is unavailable, administer glucose; in adults, give 100 mg of thiamine first, followed by 50 mL of 50% glucose by direct push into the IV; in children, the dose of glucose is 2 mL/kg of 25% glucose.
10–20	Administer either 0.1 mg/kg lorazepam at 2 mg/min or 0.2 mg/kg diazepam at 5 mg/min by IV; if diazepam is given, it can be repeated if seizures do not stop after 5 min; if diazepam is used to stop the status, phenytoin should be administered next to prevent recurrent status.
21–60	If status persists, administer 15–20 mg/kg phenytoin no faster than 50 mg/min in adults and 1 mg/kg/min in children by IV; monitor ECG and blood pressure during the infusion; phenytoin is incompatible with glucose-containing solutions—the IV should be purged with normal saline before the phenytoin infusion.
>60	If status does not stop after 20 mg/kg phenytoin, give additional doses of 5 mg/kg to a maximal dose of 30 mg/kg. If status persists, give 20 mg/kg phenobarbital by IV at 100 mg/min; when phenobarbital is given after a benzodiazepine, the risk of apnea or hypopnea is great and assisted ventilation is usually required. If status persists, give anesthetic doses of drugs such as phenobarbital and pentobarbital; ventilatory assistance and vasopressors are virtually always necessary.

ECG, electrocardiogram; IV, intravenous line.
*Time starts at seizure onset. Note that a neurological consultation is indicated if the patient does not wake up, convulsions continue after the administration of a benzodiazepine and phenytoin, or confusion exists at any time during evaluation and treatment.
From Recommendations of the Epilepsy Foundation of America's Working Group on Status Epilepticus. Treatment of convulsive status epilepticus. JAMA 1993;270:854–859.

Table 6–4
Major Drugs Used to Treat Status Epilepticus: Intravenous Doses, Pharmacokinetics, and Major Toxic Effects

	Diazepam	Lorazepam	Phenytoin	Phenobarbital
Adult IV dose, mg/kg (range [total dose])	0.15–0.25	0.1 [4–8 mg]	15–20	20
Pediatric IV dose, mg/kg (range [total dose])	0.1–1.0	0.05–0.5 [1–4 mg]	20	20
Pediatric per rectum dose, mg/kg	0.5 mg/kg (max 20 mg)	—	—	—
Maximal administration rate, mg/min	5.0	2.0	50	100
Time to stop status, min	1–3	6–10	10–30	20–30
Effective duration of action, h	0.25–0.5	>12–24	24	>48
Elimination half-life, h	30	14	24	100
Volume of distribution, L/kg	1–2	0.7–1.0	0.5–0.8	0.7
Potential side effects				
Depression of consciousness	10–30 min	Several hours	None	Several days
Respiratory depression	Occasional	Occasional	Infrequent	Occasional
Hypotension	Infrequent	Infrequent	Occasional	Infrequent
Cardiac arrhythmias	—	—	In patients with heart disease	—

From Recommendations of the Epilepsy Foundation of America's Working Group on Status Epilepticus. Treatment of convulsive status epilepticus. JAMA 1993;270:854–859.

mannitol and fluid restriction. (For a discussion of alcohol withdrawal seizures, see Chapter 55). Monitor urine myoglobin.

Torsade de Pointes

Administer magnesium sulfate (20% solution) as a 2-g intravenous bolus. Give 2 to 4 g, 5 to 15 minutes later. If there is no response repeat, then follow with a continuous infusion of 5 to 10 mg/min twice daily for several days. In children, use 25 to 50 mg/kg initially. Monitor serum magnesium. Give slowly with electrocardiographic monitoring. Continue until the QT interval is less than 500 milliseconds. A short-lasting flushing sensation and a mild hypotension may follow the intravenous bolus.[9,10] Note the QT prolongation, short bursts of ventricular tachycardia, and undulating QRS complex that reverses every 4 to 5 beats. Isoproterenol shortens the QT interval. Overdrive pacing is often necessary (see Chapter 32).

SUPPORTIVE CARE: SELECTED TOPICS

THE VIOLENT PATIENT

Talk to the patient. Attempt to address the patient's immediate needs. An offer of food or water may calm the patient and avoid physical confrontation. If these methods fail, medication may be required. Tell the patient that the medication will make her or him calm. A combination of an antipsychotic medication with lorazepam is more effective than an antipsychotic medication alone. Many patients respond to haloperidol 5 mg intramuscularly or thiothixene 10 mg and lorazepam 5 mg intramuscularly in the same syringe (Table 6–5).[11]

Side effects of rapid tranquilization with haloperidol include extrapyramidal symptoms in about 10% of patients. These usually develop within 24 hours and may include combinations of dystonia, torticollis, opisthotonus, oculogyric crises, laryngospasm, and akathisia (inability to sit still). Dystonia may be treated with diphenhydramine 25 to 50 mg intravenously or benztropine 2 mg IM or IV repeated every 5 minutes up to three doses or until resolution of symptoms. Relief usually occurs within 1 to 3 minutes after an intravenous injection. Continue the medication four times daily for 48 hours. In refractory cases, administer diazepam 10 mg intravenously or lorazepam 2 mg intravenously or intramuscularly. Remember that haloperidol has anticholinergic properties and may precipitate malignant hyperthermia in a severely agitated stimulant-using patient.[12]

Wasserberger and colleagues at the Martin Luther King Jr. General Hospital in Los Angeles have proposed a program for handling the violent patient.[13] Staff should maintain a buffer of at least two armlengths between themselves and the violent patient. Hard restraints should be used quickly under a protocol such as presented in Table 6–6.[4]

As soon as possible, the blood sugar level is evaluated (an intravenous line should be established). If the patient is hypoglycemic, 50% dextrose in water is administered. If large doses of diazepam are used the patient may become hypotensive, develop shallow respirations, and become apneic. Once the agitation is diminished, the sedative effects of phencyclidine could lead to cardiovascular collapse and respiratory arrest. In the elderly, only 1 to 2 mg of haloperidol is used. Diazepam is avoided in patients older than 60 because its half-life in this age group may be greatly prolonged. It should be determined if the patient has a metabolic disorder, infectious disease, cardiovascular disorder, intracranial disorder, acute intoxication, acute withdrawal, trauma, environmental injury, or psychiatric disorder.[4]

The intravenous use of haloperidol has not been approved by the U.S. Food and Drug Administration. When used, the intravenous dose is initially 5 to 10 mg with repeated doses of 5 mg as needed. Both the butyrophenones and phenothiazines have alpha-blocking (inhibits vasoconstriction, produces orthostatic hypotension) and anticholinergic (e.g., patient becomes hot) effects. Haloperidol and droperidol should be avoided in patients suffering from an anticholinergic toxic psychosis or who are hot to the touch, especially those who are combative and phencyclidine or cocaine intoxicated. These agents can induce a neuroleptic malignant syndrome, but these medications can be administered to phencyclidine-intoxicated patients who do not have a fever. If high doses of haloperidol or droperidol are employed, extrapyramidal reactions such as spasmodic torticollis, tardive dyskinesias, and oculogyric crises may occur. These reactions can be controlled with diphenhydramine 50 to 100 mg intramuscularly or intravenously or benztropine mesylate 1 to 2 mg intramuscularly.

CIRCULATORY ASSISTANCE

Assistance for patients with circulatory failure not responsive to conservative measures has focused on extracorporeal membrane oxygenation, the intraaortic balloon pump.

Intraaortic Balloon Pump

Intraaortic balloon counterpulsation (IABC) has been used in the management of refractory cardiogenic shock and pulmonary edema resulting from acute myocardial infarction and for refractory ventricular dysrhythmias. IABC may be lifesaving in the treatment of patients whose hemodynamic instability from overdose of myocardial depressant drugs cannot be reversed by pharmacologic means.[14] It has been useful in maintaining adequate cardiac output where conventional therapy has failed for calcium channel blocker-induced cardiogenic shock.[15]

Complications while on the intraaortic balloon pump include delirium, atelectasis, death after IABP placement, ventricular ectopia, lower limb ischemia, bleeding/transfusion, acute renal failure, pneumonia, sepsis, new myocardia infarction, and stroke. The mortality rate is 25%, residual organic brain syndrome 10%, and requirement of a psychiatric consultation is needed in 18% of patients. Defined uses of the IABC have yet to be subjected to controlled clinical trials.[16]

Table 6–5
Rapid Tranquilization of the Violent Patient

Type of Violent Behavior	Tranquilization
Schizophrenia, mania, or other psychosis	Lorazepam 2–4 mg IM combined with haloperidol 5 mg IM or thiothixene 10 mg IM or 20 mg concentrate of haloperidol 5 mg IM or 10 mg concentrate loxapine 10 mg IM or 25 mg concentrate PO
Personality disorder	Lorazepam 1–2 mg PO every 1–2 h or 2–4 mg (0.5 mg/kg) IM every 1–2 h
Alcohol withdrawal	
Agitation, tremors, abnormal vital signs	Chlordiazepoxide 25–50 mg PO q4–6 h >65 years, liver disease: lorazepam 2 mg PO q2h
Extreme agitation	Lorazepam 2–4 mg IM every hour (rapid tranquilization) if not controlled
Cocaine/amphetamine	Mild to moderate agitation: diazepam 10 mg PO q8h Severe agitation: thiothixene 19 mg IM or 20 concentrate of haloperidol 5 mg IM or 10 mg concentrate
Phencyclidine*	
Mild hyperactivity, tension, anxiety, excitement: diazepam 10–30 mg PO or lorazepam 20–4 mg IM (0.5 mg/kg)	
Severe agitation, excitement, hallucinations, bizarre behavior: haloperidol 5–10 mg IM q30–60min	

*All doses given every 30 to 60 minutes, half dose for those >65 years.
Modified from Dubin WR, Weiss KJ. *Handbook of Psychiatric Emergencies.* Springhouse, PA: Springhouse, 1991. Reproduced with permission.

Table 6–6
Patient Management With Use of Restraints

A. Rehearse strategies before employing these techniques.
B. Use restraints sooner rather than later and thoroughly document all actions.
C. Remember universal precautions.
D. Use restraints appropriately. The use of overwhelming force will often be all that is necessary to preclude a fight.
   1. When it is time to subdue the patient, approach him or her with at least five persons, each with a preassigned task.
   2. Grasp the clothing and the large joints to attempt to "sandwich" the patient between two mattresses.
   3. Place the patient on the stretcher face down to reduce leverage and to make it difficult for the patient to lash out.
   4. Remove the patient's shoes or boots.
   5. In exceptional circumstances, as when the patient is biting, grasp the hair firmly.
   6. Avoid pressure to the chest, throat, or neck.
E. The specific type of restraint used (hands, cloth, leather, etc) is determined by the amount of force needed to subdue (ie, use hard restraints for PCP-induced psychosis).
F. Keep in mind, when using physical restraints, that the minimum amount of force necessary is the maximum that ethical practice allows. The goal is to restrain, not to injure. Restraining ties should be adequate but not painfully constricting when applied (being able to slip your finger underneath is a good standard). The restrained patient should be observed in a safe, quiet room away from the other patients; however, the patient must be reevaluated frequently, as restrained patients have been known to deteriorate.

From Wasserberger J, Ordog GJ, Hardin E, et al. Violence in the emergency department. Top Emerg Med 1992;14:71–78.

Extracorporeal Membrane Oxygenation

Sosnowski and colleagues describe extracorporeal membrane oxygenation as a technique for providing prolonged extracorporeal circulation and gas exchange by using extrathoracic cannulation in patients with acute, potentially reversible cardiac, pulmonary, or cardiopulmonary failure. The Extracorporeal Life Support Organization (University of Michigan, Ann Arbor) maintains a worldwide register that indicates the survival rate is 92.5% in those with meconium aspiration syndrome and 83.2% in those with the respiratory distress syndrome.[17] Extracorporeal membrane oxygenation (ECMO) produces temporary support of the heart or lungs and may be ultimately useful in life-threatening poisonings (eg, paraquat, and hydrocarbon aspiration), although it probably is more effective in reversible lung problems.[18,19]

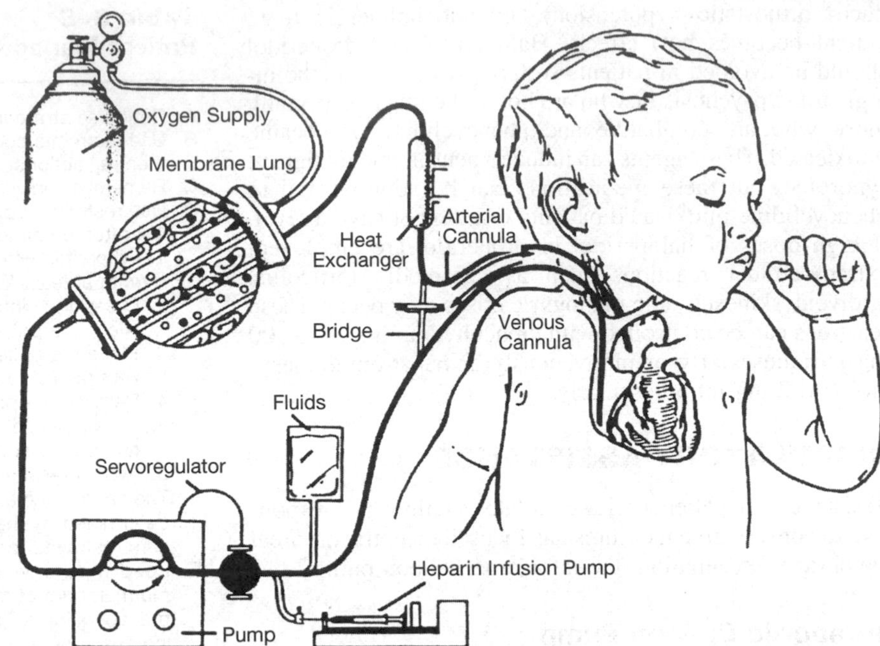

Figure 6–1 Extracorporeal membrane oxygenation. (From Scalzo AJ, Weber TR, Jaeger RW, Connors RH. Extracorporeal membrane oxygenation for hydrocarbon aspiration. Am J Dis Child 1990;144:867–871.)

Indications

1. Infants with a rapidly progressive downward course despite maximal medical treatment, as a last resort
2. Infants who are stable but still hypoxic with maximal medical treatment

Method

Extracorporeal membrane oxygenation may require ligation of the right common carotid artery and right jugular vein and circuit flow rates of 100 to 150 mL/kg/min (Fig. 6–1). Carotid artery and jugular vein reconstruction may lessen the risk after ECMO.[20] Cerebral hemodynamics may be altered. More recently, venovenous bypass has been found to be effective in the presence of normal cardiac function.[17]

Complications

Complications include thromboembolism, hemolysis, liberation of possible toxin from polyvinyl chloride tubing, leukopenia, vocal cord paralysis, hemorrhage associated with systemic heparinization,[21] and heparin bonding of cannulas, tubing, oxygenators, and head exchanges.[19] Chronic lung disease may follow use of ECMO.[22]

Contraindications

1. Immaturity of less than 35 weeks' gestation or weight less than 2000 g
2. Prolonged high-pressure ventilation (> 7 days)
3. Intracranial hemorrhage
4. Congenital heart disease

HYPOTHERMIA (< 35°C [95°F])

Physiologic changes associated with hypothermia are summarized in Table 6–7.[3] The patient should be continuously monitored by measurements of the core temperature, ideally at more than one site. Electronic thermometers with flexible probes are convenient and can record rectal, esophageal, and bladder temperatures. Changes in rectal and bladder temperatures often lag behind fluctuations in the core temperature, and esophageal readings may be elevated during the inhalation of heated air. Drugs associated with hyperthermia are discussed in Chapter 1.

Monitoring

The rectal temperature reflects visceral core temperature, provided the probe is not insulated by stool. Pulmonary artery blood temperature (by pulmonary artery catheter) and esophageal temperature are good measures of core temperature. Tympanic membrane temperature is also a good measure of the visceral core temperature.

The hematocrit typically increases 2% per 1°C decline in temperature. The potassium level should be checked frequently. Hypothermia masks potassium-induced changes in the electrocardiogram. Empiric potassium supplementation can therefore produce a toxic reaction once the patient is rewarmed. Hyperkalemia can be particularly dangerous in a patient with metabolic acidosis, rhabdomyolysis, or renal failure. Persistent hyperglycemia may suggest pancreatitis or diabetic ketoacidosis.

Depending on the degree of hypothermia an arterial line is mandatory for serial blood gas and laboratory assays and to provide a measure of central blood pressure. Pulse oximetry on the digits or earlobes is ineffective due to hypothermia-induced vasoconstriction. Endotracheal intubation should be performed for airway protection if the patient is obtunded. Avoid nasal intubation if possible because of the risk of epistaxis from hypothermia-induced coagulopathy. An orogastric tube should be inserted to aspirate gastric contents. A Foley catheter should be inserted and continuous cardiac monitoring instituted.

Table 6–7
Physiologic Changes Associated with Hypothermia

Severity of Hypothermia	Body Temperature	Central Nervous System	Cardiovascular System	Respiratory System	Renal and Endocrine Systems	Neuromuscular System
Mild	35°C (95°F) to 32.2°C (90°F)	Linear depression of cerebral metabolism; amnesia; apathy; dysarthria; impaired judgment; maladaptive behavior	Tachycardia, then progressive bradycardia; cardiac cycle prolongation; vasoconstriction; increase in cardiac output and blood pressure	Tachypnea, then progressive decrease in respiratory minute volume; declining oxygen consumption; bronchorrhea; bronchospasm	Cold diuresis; increase in catecholamine, adrenal steroids, triiodothyronine, and thyroxine; increase in metabolism with shivering	Increased preshivering muscle tone, then fatiguing shivering-induced thermogenesis; ataxia
Moderate	<32.2°C (90°F) to 28°C (82.4°F)	Electroencephalographic abnormalities; progressive depression of level of consciousness; pupillary dilation; paradoxical undressing; hallucinations	Progressive decrease in pulse and cardiac output; increased atrial and ventricular arrhythmias; nonspecific and suggestive (J-wave) electrocardiographic changes; prolonged systole	Hypoventilation; 50% decrease in carbon dioxide production per 8°C drop in temperature; absence of protective airway reflexes; 50% decrease in oxygen consumption	50% increase in renal blood flow; renal autoregulation intact; no insulin activity	Hyporeflexia; diminishing shivering-induced thermogenesis; rigidity
Severe	<28°C (82.4°F)	Loss of cerebrovascular autoregulation; decline in cerebral blood flow; coma; loss of ocular reflexes; progressive decrease in electroencephalographic activity	Progressive decreases in blood pressure, heart rate, and cardiac output; reentrant dysrhythmias; decreased ventricular arrhythmia threshold; asystole	Pulmonic congestion and edema; 75% decrease in oxygen consumption; apnea	Decrease in renal blood flow parallels decrease in cardiac output; extreme oliguria; poikilothermia; 80% decrease in basal metabolism	No motion; decreased nerve conduction velocity; peripheral areflexia

From Danzl DK, Pozos RS. Accidental hypothermia. N Engl J Med 1994;331:1756–1760.

Rewarming

Blood gas analyzers warm the blood to 37°C (98.6°F) and report the values directly so that arterial blood gas values do not need to be corrected for the patient's lower body temperature. When blood cools, the arterial pH increases and the partial pressure of carbon dioxide (Pco_2) falls. Gradual correction of acid–base imbalances is prudent, as the respiratory and renal components of the bicarbonate buffering system become progressively more efficient as body temperature returns to normal. When the Pco_2 increases by 10 mm Hg at a body temperature of 28°C (87°F), it doubles the decline in pH of 0.08 normally induced at 37°C (98.6°F). The ideal candidate for passive external rewarming is a previously healthy patient with hypothermia.[3]

1. Replete circulatory volume with isotonic solution. The solution's temperature should be less than 41°C (105.8°F).
2. Resuscitate a hypothermic patient until a core temperature of 30°C (86°F) or better before ending a code. Spontaneous cardioversion is more likely if the patient is rewarmed.
3. Severe hypokalemia is a marker of hypothermia. Hypothermia masks potassium-induced changes in the electrocardiogram.
4. Intubation is mandatory if the patient is obtunded.
5. There is no evidence to suggest that intrapleural warm irrigation is more effective than peritoneal lavage. Peritoneal lavage is safer and more easily instituted.
6. Pacemaker insertion cannot be relied on to control the cold myocardium and may precipitate ventricular fibrillation.
7. Electrical defibrillation may be effective at core temperatures of 30°C (86°F) or above.
8. Monitor glucose metabolism and thyroid status.

Cardiac Manifestations

Blood pressure and systemic vascular resistance are preserved until temperatures fall below 25°C (77°F). Arrhythmias are preceded by a characteristic J or Osborn wave (Fig. 6–2) on the electrocardiogram that occurs below 33°C (91.4°F) and becomes more pronounced as temperature decreases. Atrial fibrillation is common below 33°C (91.4°F). The heart becomes asystolic below 20°C (68°F). At 28°C (82.4°F) ventricular fibrillation may occur. Ventricular arrhythmias may occur as the patient is warmed from 28° to 32°C (82.4°–89.6°F).

Hematologic Manifestations

Profound hypothermia (< 28 °C [82.4°F]) leads to granulocytopenia and an increase in hematocrit (hemoconcentration). A diminished platelet count is also noted. Bleeding time is prolonged as temperatures decrease. Tests such as the activated clotting time, prothrombin time, and partial thromboplastin time may be normal even with a clinical coagulopathy, because these tests are performed in heated chambers which warm the blood to normal physiologic temperatures. Disseminated intravascular coagulation has been observed in patients with profound hypothermia.

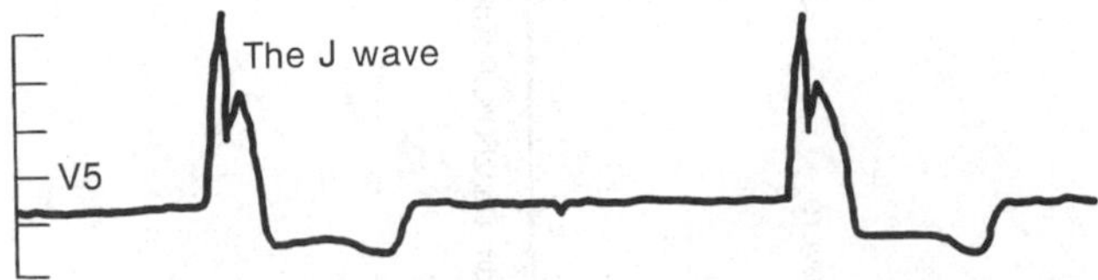

Figure 6–2 Electrocardiogram showing bradycardia with J waves in a patient with hypothermia.

Gastrointestinal Function

Ileus may accompany hypothermia. It resolves rapidly following rewarming. Pancreatitis, characterized by a marked elevation in serum amylase, can be a complication of hypothermia.[23]

Supportive Measures in Hypothermia

1. Always check for sepsis and hypothyroidism.
2. Use drugs cautiously, because metabolism and renal elimination are impaired by hypothermia.
3. Handle severely hypothermic patients carefully, because excessive trauma may induce ventricular fibrillation.
4. Arterial lines simplify blood pressure and arterial blood gas monitoring.
5. Watch for development of cerebral edema.
6. Make notations of the extent of frostbite by noting areas of color, temperature, and skin texture changes. If frostbitten extremities have not been rewarmed, immerse the affected extremity in 42°C water until color and warmth return.

HYPERTHERMIA

See also Drug-Induced Fever in Chapter 1.

Complications

Hyperthermia may be defined as temperatures between 39° and 41°C (102.2° and 105.8°F). Oral temperatures above 41.1°C (106°F) are relatively rare.[24] Besides ethanol, substances involved in hyperthermia include narcotics, sedative–hypnotics (especially barbiturates, chloral hydrate, glutethimide), phenothiazines, tricyclic antidepressants, general anesthetics, carbon monoxide, and insulin. Complications of hyperthermia may include acidosis, hyperkalemia, hypercalcemia, coagulopathy, rhabdomyolysis, myoglobinuria, renal failure, hypotension, tachyarrhythmias, neurologic sequelae, and death.[25]

Cooling Measures

Clothes should be removed and the body, particularly those areas of high blood flow (ie, neck and groin), should be packed in ice. Immersion in an ice water bath is also a highly effective measure to reduce core temperatures, but should be done very carefully in the elderly and in those with heart disease. When possible, evaporative cooling should be used. Warming 500 mL of water from 4 to 40°C removes 18 kcal of heat, and heating the same amount of ice water removes 60 kcal. Evaporation, on the other hand, of 500 mL of water consumes 290 kcal. Cooling measures should be stopped when the core temperature (as measured by rectal probe) falls below 39°C (102°F). Drugs that are associated with hyperthermia are listed in Chapter 1.

EMERGENCY INTRAVENOUS MEDICATIONS

Guidelines for the use of intravenous medications in the Milwaukee County Medical Complex are listed in Table 6–8.[25]

ACID–BASE DISORDERS

Evaluation of Acid–Base Disturbance

1. Assess the patient's clinical status.
2. Obtain arterial blood gas, pH, Pco_2, bicarbonate, and serum electrolyte concentrations.
3. Determine which abnormalities are primary and which are compensatory based on the pH (Tables 6–9 through 6–14). If the pH is less than 7.40, respiratory or metabolic acidosis is primary. If the pH is over 7.40, respiratory or metabolic alkalosis is primary.

Table 6–8
Guidelines for Use of Intravenous Medications: Milwaukee County Medical Complex

Medication	Administration Guidelines	Dosage	Pharmacokinetics
Amrinone lactate (Inocor)	Bolus doses can be administered undiluted; 100 mg in 100 mL 0.9% NaCL Concentration: 1000 µg/mL	Initial: 0.75 mg/kg over 2–3 min; repeat once in 30 min Maintenance: 5–10 µg/kg/min Usual dosage range: 2–20 µg/kg/min Total daily dose: <10 mg/kg/d; wean when discontinuing medication	Onset of action: <5 min Duration of activity: 30 min–2 h
Bretylium tosylate (Bretylol)	Bolus doses can be administered undiluted for life-threatening ventricular arrhythmias; 2 g in 250 mL D_5W or 0.9% NaCl Concentration: 8 mg/mL Keep patient in supine position during drug administration to minimize hypotension	Initial: 5 mg/kg over 1 min for treatment of life-threatening ventricular fibrillation and tachycardia; administer over 5 min for non-life-threatening arrhythmias; repeat 10 mg/kg every 15–30 min PM up to 30 mg/kg Maintenance: 1–2 mg/min infusion	Onset of action: ventricular fibrillation, 1–2 min; ventricular tachycardia, ≥20 min Duration of activity: 6–12 h, longer with multiple doses
Dobutamine HCl (Dobutrex)	500 mg in 250 mL D_5W or 0.9% NaCl Concentration: 2000 µg/ml; do not mix with sodium bicarbonate; administer through a central line	Initial: 2.5 µg/kg/min Maintenance: Increase in 2.5 µg/kg/min increments every 10 min until desired effect obtained Usual dosage range: 2.5–20 µg/kg/min; up to 40 µg/kg/min is rarely necessary; wean when discontinuing medication	Onset of action: <2 min Duration of activity: <10 min
Dopamine HCl (Intropin)	400 mg in 250 mL D_5W or 0.9% NaCl Concentration: 1600 µg/mL; do not mix with bicarbonate; administer through a central line	Initial: for renal perfusion, 0.5–2 µg/kg/min, for shock, 2–5 µg/kg/min Maintenance: Increase in 1–5 µg/kg/min increments every 10 min until desired effect obtained Usual dosage range: 0.5–20 µg/kg/min; doses > 50 µg/kg/min have been used in advanced shock; wean when discontinuing medication	Onset of action: <5 min Duration of activity: <10 min
Epinephrine HCl (Adrenalin)	2 mg in 250 mL D_5W or 0.9% NaCl Concentration: 8 µg/ml Do not use if solution is brown in color or if a precipitate is present; do not mix with sodium bicarbonate; administer through a central line	Initial: 1 µg/min Maintenance: Increase dose until desired effect obtained. Usual dosage range: 1–4 µg/min	Onset of action: Immediate Duration of activity: <10 min

PT, prothrombin time; PTT, partial thromboplastin time; APTT, activated partial thromboplastin time; BP, blood pressure.
From Whipple JK, Medicris-Bringa MA, Schimel RA, et al. Selected vasoactive drugs: A readily available chart reference. Crit Care Nurs 1992;12:23–29.

Table 6-8 *(Continued)*

Medication	Administration Guidelines	Dosage	Pharmacokinetics
Esmolol HCl (Brevibloc)	2.5 g in 250 mL D_5W or 0.9% NaCl Preferably use central line to minimize vein irritation Concentration: 10,000 μg/mL	Initial: 500 μg/kg/min for 1 min, then 50 μg/kg/min Maintenance: Infusion, increase in 50 μg/kg/min increments every 5–10 min; repeat loading dose with each dose increase Usual dosage range: 50–200 μg/kg/min; range use up to 300 μg/kg/min; infusion usually administered ≤24 h; wean when discontinuing medication	Onset of action: immediate Duration of activity: <30 min
Heparin	Bolus doses are administered by direct IV injection Maintenance: 25,000 U in 500 mL D_5W Concentration: 50 U/mL	Initial: 50–75 U/kg over 1 min as bolus Maintenance: for pulmonary emboli use 15–25 U/kg/h; for deep vein thrombus use 110–15 U/kg/h, monitor PTT, and titrate to effect (obtain baseline PT and PTT)	Onset of action: Immediate Duration of activity: Half-life is 0.3–2.0 hours in normal patients & 0.5–3.0 in end-stage renal disease available Goal: Keep APTT in the range of 1.5 to 2.5 times the control value
Isoproterenol HCl (Isuprel)	2 mg in 250 mL D_5W or 0.9% NaCl Concentration: 8 μg/mL Do not use if solution is brownish-pink or pink, or if a precipitate is present; do not mix with sodium bicarbonate	Initial: 2–5 μg/min Maintenance: Increase dose until desired heart rate and BP are obtained Usual dosage range: 0.5–5 μg/min; rates >30 μg/min are used in advanced shock; wean when discontinuing medication	Onset of action: Immediate Duration of activity: <10 min with low dose; ≤50 min with higher doses
Labetolol HCl (Normodyne, Trandate)	May be administered by direct IV injection Infusion: 300 mg in 250 mL D_5W or 0.9% NaCl (total volume approximately 300 mL) Concentration: 1 mg/mL Keep patient in supine position during drug administration and for 3 h after discontinuing medication to prevent orthostatic hypotension	Initial: 20 mg over 2 min Maintenance: 20–30 mg every 10 min until desired effect is obtained or maximum dose is administered; or increase infusion until desired effect is obtained or maximum dose is administered Usual cumulative dose: 50–200 mg for infusion Maximum cumulative dose: 300 mg for direct injection and continuous infusion	Onet of action: 5–10 min Duration of activity: 1–8 h
Lidocaine HCl (Xylocaine)	Administer initial dose as bolus over 2–3 min Maintenance: 2 g in 250 mL D_5W Concentration: 4 mg/mL or 2 g in 500 mL D_5W Concentration: 4 mg/mL	Initial: 1 mg/kg for 1 dose, then 0.5 mg/kg every 10–15 min to a total dose of 3 mg/kg Maintenance: 1–4 mg/min; reduce dose if >70 years old, congestive heart failure, or liver disease is present; monitor serum concentrations When increasing infusion, administer bolus dose of 0.25–0.5 mg/kg	Onset of action: <2 min Duration of activity: 1–20 min Therapeutic serum concentrations: 1.5–5 mg/L Toxic serum concentration: >6 mg/L
Metaraminol (Aramine)	100 mg in 250 mL D_5W or 0.9% NaCl Concentration: 0.4 mg/mL Administer through a large peripheral vein or through central line	Initial: 0.5 mg as bolus Maintenance: Titrate infusion to response; wean when discontinuing medication	Onset of action: 1–2 min Duration of activity: 20 min–1 h
Nitroglycerin (Nitrol, Tridil)	100 mg in 250 mL D_5W or 0.9% NaCl Concentration: 200 μg/ml: use only glass containers	Initial: 5 μg/min Maintenance: Increase in 5 μg/min increments every 3–5 min; if no response at 20 μg/min, increase in 10 μg/min increments and later 20 μg/min increments	Usual dosage range: 50–200 mcg/min Onset of action: Immediate Duration of activity: 10–30 min

Table 6-8 *(Continued)*

Medication	Administration Guidelines	Dosage	Pharmacokinetics
Nitroprusside, sodium (Nipride)	100 mg in 250 mL D_5W Concentration: 400 μg/mL; protect from light; do not use if solution is discolored	Initial: 0.5 μg/min Maintenance: Increase in 0.25–0.5 μg/kg/min increments every 5 min until desired effect obtained Usual dosage range: 0.5–10 μg/kg/min; wean when discontinuing medication to prevent hypertension	Onset of action: 1 min Duration of activity: 3–5 min Toxic thiocyanate concentration: >60 μg/mL; increased incidence of toxicity when therapy >72 h and renal impairment
Norepinephrine bitartrate (Levophed)	4 mg bitartrate in 250 mL D_5W or 0.9% NaCl Concentration: 16 μg/mL (2 mg bitartrate = 1 mg base); do not mix with sodium bicarbonate; do not use if solution is brown in color or precipitate is present; administer through a central line	Initial: 2 μg/min Maintenance: Titrate to response Usual dosage range: 2–12 μg/min; wean when discontinuing medication	Onset of action: Immediate Duration of activity: <5 min
Phenylephrine HCl (Neo-Synephrine)	25 mg in 250 mL D_5W or 0.9% NaCl Concentration: 100 μg/mL	Initial: 100–180 μg/min Maintenance: 40–80 μg/min; wean when discontinuing medication	Onset of action: <2 min Duration of activity: 15–20 min
Procainamide HCl (Pronestyl)	For bolus doses maximum rate of infusion: 25–50 mg/min; 1 g in 250 mL D_5W Concentration: 4 mg/mL; keep patient in supine position during administration	Initial: 50–100 mg every 5 min until arrhythmia responds, adverse effects occur, or 1 g is administered; adverse effects include QRS complex widens >50%, BP decreases >15 mm Hg, and PR interval is prolonged Maintenance: 1–6 mg/min infusion Reduce dose in presence of renal failure or left ventricular dysfunction; monitor serum concentrations	Onset of action: Immediate Duration of activity: 3–4 hours Therapeutic serum concentration 4–10 mg/L Toxic serum concentration: 16 mg/l for procainamide: >30 mg/L for procainamide plus NAPA
Verapamil HCl (Calan, Isoptin)	100 mg in 250 mL D_5W Concentration: 0.4 mg/mL Bolus doses are administered by direct IV injection over a minimum of 2 min	Initial: 0.075–0.15 mg/kg (5–10 mg) over 3 min; if needed, administer second dose of 0.15 mg/kg in 15–30 min Maintenance: 1–10 mg/h infusion	Onset of action: Immediate Duration of activity: 10–20 min

Table 6-9
Primary Acid-Base Disorders

Variable	Primary Disorder	Normal Range, Arterial Gas	Primary Disorder
pH	Acidemia	← 7.35–7.45 →	Alkalemia
P_{CO_2} mm Hg	Respiratory alkalosis	← 35–45 →	Respiratory acidosis
Bicarbonate, mmol/L	Metabolic acidosis	← 22–26 →	Metabolic alkalosis

Rules of Thumb for Recognizing Primary Acid-Base Disorders Without Using a Nomogram

Rule 1

Look at the pH. Whichever side of 7.40 the pH is on, the process that caused it to shift to that side is the primary abnormality

Principle: The body does not fully compensate for primary acid–base disorders.

Rule 2

Calculate the anion gap. If the anion gap is ≥20 mmol/L, there is a primary metabolic acidosis regardless of pH or serum bicarbonate concentration

Principle: The body does not generate a large anion gap to compensate for a primary disorder.

Rule 3

Calculate the excess anion gap (the total anion gap minus the normal anion gap[12 mmol/L]) and add this value to the measured bicarbonate concentration; if the sum is greater than a normal serum bicarbonate (>30 mmol/L), there is an underlying metabolic alkalosis; if the sum is less than a normal bicarbonate (<23 mmol/L), there is an underlying nonanion gap metabolic acidosis

Principle: 1 mmol of unmeasured acid titrates 1 mmol of bicarbonate (+ Δ anion gap = –Δ $[HCO_3^-]$)

From Haber RJ. A practical approach to acid–base disorders. West J Med 1991;155:146-151.

Table 6–10
Acute Respiratory Alkalosis

Variable	Typical Value	Interpretation
pH	7.50	Alkalemia
Pco_2*	29 mm Hg	Respiratory alkalosis
HCO_3^-	22 mmol/L	Normal HCO_3^-

Causes
- Anxiety
- Hypoxia
- Lung disease with or without hypoxia
- Central nervous system disease
- Drug use—salicylates, catecholamines, progesterone
- Pregnancy
- Sepsis
- Hepatic encephalopathy
- Mechanical ventilation

*This is the primary abnormality.
From Haber RJ. A practical approach to acid–base disorders. West J Med 1991;155:146–151.

Table 6–11
Acute Respiratory Acidosis

Variable	Typical Value	Interpretation
pH	7.25	Acidemia
Pco_2*	60 mm Hg	Respiratory acidosis
HCO_3^-	26 mmol/L	Normal HCO_3^-

Causes
- Central nervous system (CNS) depression—drugs, CNS event
- Neuromuscular disorders—myopathies, neuropathies
- Acute airway obstruction—upper airway, laryngospasm, bronchospasm
- Severe pneumonia or pulmonary edema
- Impaired lung motion—hemothorax, pneumothorax
- Thoracic cage injury—flail chest
- Ventilator dysfunction

*This is the primary abnormality.
From Haber RJ. A practical approach to acid–base disorders. West J Med 1991;155:146–151.

Table 6–12
Chronic Respiratory Acidosis With Metabolic Compensation

Variable	Typical Value	Intrepretation
pH	7.34	
Pco_2*	60 mm Hg	Respiratory acidosis
HCO_3^-	31 mmol/L	Metabolic compensation

Causes
- Chronic lung disease—obstructive or restrictive
- Chronic neuromuscular disorders
- Chronic respiratory center depression—central hypoventilation

*This is the primary abnormality.
From Haber RJ. A practical approach to acid–base disorders. West J Med 1991;155:146–151.

Table 6–13
Metabolic Alkalosis With Respiratory Compensation

Variable	Typical Value	Intrepretation
pH	7.50	Alkalemia
Pco_2	48 mm Hg	Respiratory compensation
HCO_3^-	36 mmol/L	Metabolic alkalosis

Causes

Urinary Chloride Level Low	*Urinary Chloride Level Normal or High*
Vomiting, nasogastric suction	Excess mineralocorticoid activity— Cushing's syndrome, Conn's syndrome, exogenous steroids, licorice ingestion, increased renin states, Bartter's syndrome
Diuretic use in past	Current or recent diuretic use
Posthypercapnia	Excess alkali administration
	Refeeding alkalosis

From Haber RJ. A practical approach to acid–base disorders. West J Med 1991;155:146–151.

Table 6–14
Metabolic Acidosis With Respiratory Compensation

Variable	Typical Value	Intrepretation
pH	7.20	Acidemia
Pco_2	21 mm of mercury	Respiratory compensation
HCO_3^-*	8 mmol/L	Metabolic acidosis
		Anion gap = sodium − chloride + bicarbonate
		Normal = 12 ± 2 (SD) mmol/L

Causes

Nonanion Gap	*Anion Gap*
Gastrointestinal bicarbonate loss	Ketoacidosis
Diarrhea	Diabetic
Ureteral diversion	Alcoholic
Renal bicarbonate loss	Renal failure
Renal tubular acidosis	Lactic acidosis
Early renal failure	Rhabdomyolysis
Carbonic anhydrase inhibitors	Toxins
Aldosterone inhibitors	Methanol
Hydrochloric acid administration	Ethylene glycol
Posthypocapnia	Paraldehyde
	Salicylates

*This is the primary abnormality.
From Haber RJ. A practical approach to acid–base disorders. West J Med 1991;155:146–151.

4. Calculate the anion gap: sodium − (bicarbonate + chloride) = anion gap. For example, 140 − (24 + 104) = 12, a normal anion gap. If the anion gap is greater than 20 mmol/L, a metabolic acidosis is present regard-less of the pH or serum bicarbonate concentration.
5. Determine the cause of each primary and secondary disorder (see Chapter 2).
6. Begin cause-specific therapy.[26]

BICARBONATE ADMINISTRATION

Formulation

1. An 8.4% solution (intramuscular) contains 1 mEq each of sodium and bicarbonate ions per milliliter (calculated osmolarity, 2000 mOsm/L).
2. A 7.5% solution contains 0.892 mEq each of sodium and bicarbonate ions per milliliter (calculated osmolarity, 1786 mOsm/L).
3. Ampules (50 mL) of the 8.4 and 7.5% solutions contain 50 and 44.6 mEq of sodium bicarbonate, respectively.

Use

1. Salicylate overdose to alkalinize the urine
2. Tricyclic antidepressant overdose to alkalinize the blood
3. Adjuvant in poisoning with phenobarbital (useful, but not often indicated), chlorpropamide (increases renal clearance), and chlorphenoxy herbicides (enhances renal elimination, increased ionized fractions trapped in both blood and urine)
4. Correction of metabolic acidosis, especially in methanol and ethylene glycol poisoning
5. Potentially useful in a gastric lavage fluid for iron ingestions (Note the danger of hypernatremia with repeat doses of oral sodium bicarbonate)
6. Possible treatment of cocaine-induced wide-complex tachyarrhythmias
7. Drug or toxin-associated myoglobinuria—controversial indication (If the urine pH is not above 6.0, treat with fluid resuscitation and mannitol alone.)
8. Debatable use in lactic acidosis, cardiac resuscitation, and diabetic ketoacidosis
9. Possible use in amantadine, phenothiazine, propoxyphene, cocaine, and carbamazepine overdose

Bicarbonate does not appear to alter the vasopressor effect of epinephrine in cardiopulmonary resuscitation.[27]

In the setting of cardiac arrest its use is limited to severe metabolic acidosis that persists beyond the first 5 to 10 minutes of the resuscitation process or if the patient is known to have severe metabolic acidosis prior to arrest. In this limited setting, the initial dose is 1 mEq/kg (about 1–1.5 ampules). No more than half this amount should be given every 10 minutes. In the postresuscitation phase, sodium bicarbonate administration should be guided by arterial blood gas measurements. Significant metabolic lactic acidosis does not develop in cardiopulmonary arrest for about 5 to 15 minutes after patient collapse.[28]

In the pediatric patient, bicarbonate is administered at half the adult concentration. To achieve this end with a 50-mL ampule of 8.4% $NaHCO_3$, empty half of the ampule (25 mL) and then refill to a total volume of 50 mL with sterile water. This solution now has a concentration of 0.5 mEq/mL. It is not too hypertonic to administer to the pediatric patient. For resuscitation of a newborn, the dose is 6 mL (3 mEq of 4.2% solution [0.5 mEq/mL]); at 6 months (7.5 kg), 7 mL (7 mEq) of 8.4% solution; at 1 year (10 kg), 10 mL (10 mEq); at 6 years (20 kg), 20 mL (20 mEq); and at 10 years (30 kg), 30 mL (30 mEq).[29]

Catecholamines (epinephrine, dopamine, isoproterenol) and calcium salts are inactivated when mixed with sodium bicarbonate. Thoroughly flush the intravenous line after giving sodium bicarbonate before infusing additional drugs.

Bicarbonate Use in the Toxic Patient

Alkaline diuresis in adults can usually be induced by adding 2 to 3 ampules of 8.4% $NaHCO_3$ (50 mEq/50 mL ampule) to 1 L of 5% dextrose in water infused intravenously over 3 to 4.5 hours. Limit the bolus dose to 1 to 2 mEq/kg over 5 minutes in tricyclic antidepressant overdose with a wide QRS complex. In pediatric patients, add 1 to 2 mEq $NaHCO_3$/kg in 15 mL/kg 5% dextrose on 0.45% normal saline over 3 to 4 hours. Limit the bolus dose to 0.5 to 1 mEq/kg over 5 minutes. Monitor arterial blood gases and electrolytes, especially potassium.

Check urine pH in 1 hour. It should be at least 7.5, preferably 8.

Monitor arterial pH.

Correct the potassium deficit. If acidosis is corrected without correcting a potassium deficit, more potassium will move intracellularly and predispose to fatal arrhythmias. In alkalosis, the potassium level should be greater than 3.0 mEq/L; in acidosis, a potassium level of 3 mEq/L is indicative of severe hypokalemia.

Watch for sodium and fluid overload.

Keep the systemic pH below 7.55 to prevent complications of alkalemia.

Maintain alkalinization with continuous infusion of 100 to 150 mEq in 1 L of 5% dextrose in water at 150 to 200 mL/h. This is about twice the maintenance requirements in a child.

Early use of sodium bicarbonate may produce a paradoxical intracellular acidosis that may lead to further depression of myocardial function.

Mechanism of Action

Sodium bicarbonate alters drug ionization of weak acids (eg, salicylate, phenobarbital, chlorpromazine). Alkalinization of the blood prevents movement of ionized drug within the tissues. Cellular membranes are impermeable to ionized compounds. Alkalinization of urine traps the ionized fraction in the urine when the pH is greater than the pK_a.

Sodium bicarbonate changes sodium gradients. The direct sodium effect partially reverses the fast sodium channel blockade manifested by widened QRS complexes, arrhythmias, and hypotension (eg, tricyclic antidepressants, quinidine, procainamide, encainide, flecainide).

Sodium bicarbonate titrates acid and reverses life-threatening acidemia generated during methanol or ethylene glycol intoxication.

INTRATRACHEAL DRUGS

In an emergency, it is sometimes impossible to obtain venous access. The intratracheal administration of drugs provides an alternative that is usually readily available.[30–33] The Resuscitation Council (UK) and the American Heart Association both recommend intratracheal administration of epinephrine and atropine, but, because of the absence of definitive data in humans, fail to agree on the appropriate dose. The American

Heart Association recommends that the same dose of any drug should be given intratracheally as would be used intravenously. The Resuscitation Council recommends that the intratracheal dose should be twice the intravenous dose.

Several drugs are effective when given by the intratracheal route: naloxone, diazepam, lidocaine, adrenaline, isoproterenol, atropine, and terbutaline. If drugs are to be given through an endotracheal tube they should be administered in a suitably large volume of fluid—for an adult, 10 to 20 mL of saline.

In pediatric resuscitation, endotracheal drugs should be diluted in normal saline to a final volume of at least 2 mL, and should be administered through a catheter threaded into the endotracheal tube. Alternatively, the drug may be administered into the endotracheal tube directly and followed with 2 to 5 mL of normal saline to flush the drug into the lower airways. There are conflicting data on the optimal volume of endotracheal fluid to use. The recommended volume should provide adequate delivery to the distal airways while minimizing the risk of significant transient hypoxemia from the instilled saline. In children, when the endotracheal route is the only route available, epinephrine should be given in an initial dose of 0.1 mg/kg (100 μg/kg). The fastest method to administer a drug (intravenous, peripheral, venous, endotracheal) should be employed.

Intratracheal instillation should be followed by five forcible hyperinflations of the lung to ensure distribution throughout the respiratory tract and, thereby, to enhance absorption.[34]

TOTAL PARENTERAL NUTRITION

Within the first 24 hours of coma the body's reserve of carbohydrates is exhausted. This is followed by an intensive catabolism of essential immune, enzymatic, and structural proteins. The daily loss in muscle mass from comatose patients depends on the presence of trauma, but it ranges from 300 to 600 g/d. This loss is often marked by fluid retention. An initial controlled study suggests that some patients with coma due to poisoning appear to have lower serum amino acid levels, more pneumonias, longer hospitalizations, and an increase in disseminated intravascular coagulation. In prolonged coma (more than a few days) with endogenous protein catabolism, consideration should be given to total parenteral nutrition.

Risks

1. Elevation of liver enzymes
2. Hyperbilirubinemia
3. Disturbances of clotting functions
4. Iatrogenic complications of central venous cannulization[35]
5. Excessive alkalemia
6. Hypernatremia
7. Hypokalemia
8. Hypocalcemia, tetany
9. Fluid overload
10. Delay in achieving alkalinization, compared with hyperventilation
11. Pulmonary edema
12. Cerebral edema
13. Hyperosmolality
14. Shifting of oxyhemoglobin dissociation curve leftward (with impaired oxygen release to the tissues)
15. Precipitation of convulsions, ischemia, and/or arrhythmias[36]

Carbon dioxide will accumulate, diffuse across cellular and organ membranes, and enter the brain, where it may produce intracellular acidosis[37] ($H^+ + HCO_3^- \leftrightarrow H_2O + CO_2$). In cells, CO_2 and H_2O combine to form H_2O_3, which then breaks down to HCO_3^- and H^+.[38] Arterial blood gas studies are inaccurate in the presence of cardiac arrest and not a good predictor of intracellular acid–base status.[39] The pH in mixed venous blood most closely reflects the true pH within the cells. Mixed venous acidosis and, hence, intracellular acidosis are usually corrected by hyperventilation.

Contraindications

1. Renal failure
2. Pulmonary edema

TRANSPLANTATION AND THE POISONED PATIENT

Recipients

Transplantation of the liver appears to be a useful therapeutic procedure in toxin-induced hepatic failure. Recipients may include patients with chronic alcoholism who have been sober longer than 6 months and those poisoned with valproic acid, acetaminophen and mushroom[40–53] (Table 6–15).

Donors

Leikin and associates report the success rate for transplantation of kidneys from poisoning victims (alcohol, cocaine, carbon monoxide, barbiturates, lead) to be 93%.[54] For liver transplantation, the success rate was about 71%. A 60% 1-year liver survival rate and 78% kidney 1-year survival rate were observed. Deaths from poisoning, therefore, did

Table 6–15
Transplantation and the Poisoned Patient

Donor	Recipient
Cyanide[41–43,45]	Valproic acid[46]
Ethanol[40]*	Acetaminophen (see also Acetaminophen[47])
Cocaine[40]	Iron[48]
Carbon monoxide[40,44,45]	Mushroom poisoning[49]
Lead[40]	Aminitin[45,50]
Amanita	Cortinarius[51]
Methaqualone[45]	Cyclosporine[52]
Benzodiazepines[45]	Ethanol (most common cause of fulminant hepatic failure leading to transplantation)[53]
Barbiturates[45]	Disulfiram
Insulin[45]	
Methanol[45]	
Sodium cyanide[44]	

*There is little risk of intoxication of the transplanted liver after the fourth day at which time no circulatory amatoxins are detected.

Table 6–16
Drugs With Significant Organ Concentrations in Which Reservoir Effect May Occur

Liver			
Acetaminophen	Chlorpheniramine	Ibuprofen	Morphine
Acetylmethadol	Chlorpyrifos	Imipramine	Nortriptyline
Alphaprodine	Chromium	Iron	Orphenadrine
Alphenolol	Cobalt	Lead	Oxalic acid
Amitriptyline	Cocaine	Lindane	Oxprenolol
Amobarbital	Copper	Lysergic acid diethylamide (LSD)	Oxycodone
Amoxapine	Cyanide	Malathion	Paraldehyde
Anileridine	Cyclobenzaprine	Manganese	Pentobarbital
Antimony	Desipramine	Maprothiline	Pencyclidine
Arsenic	Diazepam	Mepivacaine	Phenmetrazine
Benzphetamine	Diazinon	Meprobamate	Phenobarbital
Borate	2,4-Dichlorophenoxyacetic acid-diphenhydramine	Mercury	Phenylpropanolamine
Buspirane	*N,N*-Diethyl-*m*-toluamide (DEET) dibenzepine	Metadone	Phenytoin
Cadmium	Doxepin	Methamphetamine	Procyclidine
Caffeine	Emetine	Methapyrilene	Propoxyphene
Camphor	Ethanol	Methaqualone	Pyrilamine
Carbaryl	Ethchlorvynol	Methoxyflurane	Quinidine
Carbon tetrachloride	Ethylene glycol	Methylene chloride	Quinine
Carisoprodol	Fenfluramine	Methylenedioxyganphetamine (MDA)	Secobarbital
Chloral hydrate	Fentanyl	Methylfentanyl (China White)	Strychrine
Chlordane	Gasoline	Methylprylone	Thallium
Chlordecone	Glutethimide	Metoprolol	Toluene
Chlordiazepoxide	Halothane	Mianserin	Trazodone
Chlormethiazole	Hydromorphone	Molindone	Tri-*o*-cresyl phosphate
Chlormezanone	Hydroxyzine		Turpentine
Chloroform			Warfarin—and super-warfarin rodenticides
Chloroquine			
Kidney			
Alprenolol	Codeine	Lysergic acid diethylamide (LSD)	Nickel carbonyl
Amikcin	*N,N*-Diethyl-*m*-toluamide (DEET)	Malathion	Notriptyline
Amiodarone	Digoxin	Meprobamate	Pentachlorophenol
Amitriptyline	Diphenhydramine	Mercury	Phenytoin
Amoxaine	Diquat	Methadone	Quinine
Amphetamine	Ethchlorvynol	Methapyrilene	Secobarbital
Arsenic	Ethylene glycol	Methaqualone	Strychnine
Barium	Fluoride	Methoxyflurane	Thallium
Buformin	Gold	Methylene dioxyamphetamine (MDA)	Tolbutamide
Cadmium	Heroin	Methylfentanyl (China White)	Toluene
Chlordane	Ibuprofen	Naloxone	Tri-*o*-cresyl phosphate
Chloroquine	Imipramine		Turpentine
Chlorpromazine	Lithium		
Cocaine			

From Leikin JB, Heyn-Lamb R, Aks S, et al. The toxic patient as a potential organ donor. Am J Emerg Med 1994;12:151–154.

not appear to be a contraindication to donation of the liver or kidney for transplantation.[54–59]

Multiple organs were successfully transplanted from a victim of cyanide poisoning.[40] Corneas have been successfully transplanted from cyanide victims.[41] Renal transplants have been successful following donor death from silver cyanide.[42] Patients who succumb to carbon monoxide poisoning may be kidney donors, provided their renal function is adequate at the time of donation.[43] Deaths have occurred in some patients from chronic hepatitis or renal graft rejection.[44] Transplantation from poisoned donors is still in its preliminary stage of development. Further work is required to define more accurately the criteria for the successful use of organs from such patients[60,61] (Table 6–16).

The Suicidal Patient

Patients who have attempted suicide account for an estimated 0.3 to 1.0% of all emergency department visits, but this figure may be as high as 12% in the adolescent age group. Up to 80% of patients who successfully complete suicide were seen by a physician within the 6 months immediately before their death, and 50% of them within 1 month. Suicide is the ninth leading cause of death in the United States and accounts for 30,000 fatalities annually. It is the second most common cause of death in young adults (15–24 years old) and the third most common cause of death among adolescents.[53]

Stabilization of all life-threatening conditions must be accomplished. The overdose patient is treated with gastrointestinal decontamination procedures according to the specific ingestant (see Chapter 3). Metabolic, renal, and cardiopulmonary status of the patient must be documented. Useful studies include a complete blood count, ethanol, electrolytes, blood urea nitrogen, creatinine, glucose, urinalysis, blood gas, and electrocardiogram. A toxicology screen is indicated for any suicidal patient with an altered level of consciousness or suspected drug ingestion. A drug- or alcohol-intoxicated patient must be monitored and observed until normal mental status returns. Keep the suicidal patient in the emergency department or elsewhere in the hospital until medical and psychological evaluation is complete. All potential weapons, sharp objects, and medications must be removed, and the patient must not have access to anything in the room that might prove to be harmful. Direct observation of the patient is necessary and may require one-on-one nursing or the posting of security personnel at the bedside.

After medical stabilization, the most important aspects of emergency department management of a suicidal patient are determination of the suicide risk and arrangement for appropriate disposition. Potential dispositions can include sending the patient home, general medical admission, voluntary psychiatric unit admission, or involuntary psychiatric hospitalization. Family members should agree to remove all potential weapons, medications, alcohol, and any other obvious means of suicide from the home. A suicide contract (controversial, problematical) should state explicitly that the patient promises to phone the emergency department, his or her physician, or the therapist immediately if suicidal ideation recurs.

Psychiatric admission is necessary for any patient with an unresolved suicidal crisis.

PEDIATRIC DOSES

Pediatric drug doses, where available from the medical literature, have been cited in each chapter in this text. Additional sources of information include the following:

1. Benitz WE, Tatro DC. *The Pediatric Drug Handbook.* 2nd ed. Chicago: Year Book Medical, 1988.
2. McEvoy GK. *AHFS 94: Drug Information.* Bethesda, MD: American Society of Hospital Pharmacists, 1994.
3. *Physicians' Desk Reference.* 49th ed. Montvale, NJ: Medical Economics, 1995.
4. Reynolds JEF. *Martindale: The Extra Pharmacopoeia.* 30th ed. London: The Pharmaceutical Press, 1993.
5. Reisdorff EJ, Roberts MC, Wiegenstein JG. *Pediatric Emergency Medicine.* Philadelphia: WB Saunders, 1993.

REFERENCES

1. McIntyre KM, Lewis AJ, eds. *Textbook of Advanced Cardiac Life Support.* Dallas: American Heart Association, 1983:119.
2. Hoffman RS, Goldfrank LR. The poisoned patient with altered consciousness: Controversies in the use of a "coma cocktail". JAMA 1995;274:562–569.
3. Danzl DK, Pozos RS. Accidental hypothermia. N Engl J Med 1994;331:1756–1760.
4. *Physicians' Desk Reference.* 49th ed. Montvale, N: Medical Economics, 1995:280–286.
5. Martin TG. Personal communication.
6. Brennan S, Lederer ED. Severe electrolyte disturbances. In: Hall JB, Schmidt GA, Wood LDH, eds. *Principles of Critical Care.* New York: McGraw-Hill, 1992:1939–1940.
7. Browning RG, Olson DW, Stueven HA, Mateer JR. 50% dextrose: Antidote or toxin? Ann Emerg Med 1990;19:683–687.
8. Recommendations of the Epilepsy Foundation of America's Working Group on Status Epilepticus. Treatment of convulsive status epileptics. JAMA 1993;270:854–859.
9. Tzivoni D, Banai S, Schuzer C, et al. Treatment of Torsade de pointes with magnesium sulfate. Circulation 1988;77:392–397.
10. Tzivoni D, Keren A. Suppression of ventricular arrhythmias by magnesium. Am J Cardiol 1990;65:1297–1299.
11. Dubin WR, Weiss KJ. *Handbook of Psychiatric Emergencies.* Springhouse, PA: Springhouse, 1991.
12. Wasserberger JL. Drew/UCLA Medical Center, personal communication.
13. Wasserberger J, Ordog GJ, Hardin E, et al. Violence in the emergency department. Top Emerg Med 1992;14:71–78.
14. Freedberg RS, Friedman GR, Palm RN, Feit F. Cardiogenic shock due to antihistamine overdose: Reversal with intraaortic balloon counterpulsation. JAMA 1987;257:660–661.
15. Melanson P, Shih DD, De Roos S, et al. Intraaortic balloon counterpulsation in calcium channel blockers overdose. Vet Hum Toxicol 1993;35:345.
16. Sanders KM, Stern TA, O'Gara PT, et al. Medical and neuropsychiatric complications associated with use of the intraaortic balloon pump. Intensive Care Med 1992;7:154–164.
17. Sosnowski AW, Bonser SJ, Field DJ, et al. Extracorporeal membrane oxygenation: Britain needs units equipped to perform the procedure and a controlled trial. Br Med J 1990; 201:303–304.
18. Kallis P, Al-Sandy NM, Bennett D, Treasure T. Clinical use of intravascular oxygenation. Lancet 1991;337:549.
19. Banner W Jr, Timmons OD, Vernon DD. Advances in the critical care of poisoned paediatric patients. Drug Saf 1994; 10:83–92.
20. Frader J, Lantos S. Extracorporeal membrane oxygenation in neonates. N Engl J Med 1991;324:849–850.
21. Elliott SJ. Neonatal extracorporeal membrane oxygenation: How not to assess novel technologies. Lancet 1991;337: 476–478.
22. Lantos JD, Frader J. Extracorporeal membrane oxygenation and the ethics of clinical research in pediatrics. N Engl J Med 1990;323:409–413.
23. Keamy MF III, Hall J. Hypothermia. In: Hall JB, Schmidt GA, Wood LDH, eds. *Principles of Critical Care.* New York: McGraw-Hill, 1992:848–857.
24. Petersdorf RG. Hypothermia and hyperthermia. In: Wilson JD, Braunwald E, Isselbacker KJ, et al., eds. *Harrison's Principles of Internal Medicine.* 12th ed. New York: McGraw-Hill, 1991:2194–2198.
25. Whipple JK, Medicris-Bringa MA, Schimel RA, et al. Selected vasoactive drugs: A readily available chart reference. Crit Care Nurs 1992;12:23–29.
26. Haber RJ. A practical approach to acid–base disorders. West J Med 1991;155:146–151.
27. Bleske BE, Rice TL, Warren EW, et al. The effect of sodium bicarbonate administration on the vasopressor effect of high-dose epinephrine during cardiopulmonary resuscitation in swine. Am J Emerg Med 1993;11:439–443.
28. Callaham ML. High-dose epinephrine therapy and other advances in treating cardiac arrest. Aust J Med 1990;152: 697–703.
29. Reisdorff EJ, Robert MR, Wiegstein JG. *Pediatric Emergency Medicine.* Philadelphia: WB Saunders, 1993.
30. Intratracheal drugs. Lancet 1988;1:743–747. Editorial.
31. Brown DH, Kasuya A, Leikin JB. Endotracheal drug administration in the critical care setting. J Emerg Med 1987;5: 407–414.
32. Factor P, Sznajder JI. Vascular cannulation. In: Hall JB, Schmidt GA, Wood LDH, eds. *Principles of Critical Care.* New York: McGraw-Hill, 1992:308–321.
33. Zaritsky A. Members of the Medications in Pediatric Resuscitation Panel: Pediatric resuscitation pharmacology. Ann Emerg Med 1993;22 (2, pt 2):445–455.
34. Mueller PS, Vester JW, Fermaglich J. Neuroleptic malignant syndrome: Successful treatment with bromocriptine. JAMA 1983;249:386–388.
35. Kolacinski Z. Early parenteral nutrition in patients unconscious because of acute drug poisoning. J Parenter Enteral Nutr 1993;17:25–29.
36. Mizock BA. Controversies in lactic acidosis: Implications in critically ill patients. JAMA 1987;258:497–501.
37. Bersin RM, Chatterjee K, Arieff AI. Metabolic and hemodynamic consequences of sodium bicarbonate administration in patients with heart disease. Am J Med 1989;87:7–14.
38. Gazmuri RJ, Van Planta M, Weil MH, Rachow EC. Cardiac effects of carbon dioxide-consuming and carbon dioxide-generation buffers during cardiopulmonary resuscitation. J Am Coll Cardiol 1990;15:482–490.

39. Ayers JC, Krothapalli RK. Effect of bicarbonate administration on cardiac function. Am J Med 1989;85:5–6.
40. Bates BA, Burke PA, Jenkins RL, Woolf AD. Toxin associated liver failure: The New England Liver Transplant Service. Vet Hum Toxicol 1992;34:344.
41. Holmdahl J, Blohme I. Renal transplantation after *Cortinarius speciosissimus* poisoning. In: *Proceedings, XVth Congress of European Association of Poison Centres and Clinical Toxicologists, Istanbul, Turkey, May 1992*:102.
42. Bell EA, Shaefer MS, Marin RS, et al. Treatment of valproic acid-associated hepatic failure with orthotropic liver transplantation. Ann Pharmacother 1992;26:18–21.
43. Jaeger A, Kopferschmitt J, Flesch F, et al. Liver transplantation for amanita poisoning. In: *Proceedings, XVth Congress of European Association of Poison Centres and Clinical Toxicologists, Istanbul, Turkey, May 1992*:103.
44. Kern C, Zilker T, v Clarmann M. Successful liver transplantation in a child after amanita poisoning. In: *Proceedings, XVth Congress of European Association of Poison Centres and Clinical Toxicologists, Istanbul, Turkey, May 1992*: 126.
45. Galler GW, Weisenberg E, Brasitus TA. Mushroom poisoning: The role of orthoptic liver transplantation. Clin Gastroenterol 1992;15:229–231.
46. Murphy GE. The physician's responsibility for suicide. I. An error of commission. Ann Intern Med 1975;82:301–305.
47. Mrvos R, Schneide SM, Dean BS, Krenzelok EF. Orthotopic liver transplants necessitated by acetaminophen-induced hepatotoxicity. Vet Hum Toxicol 1992;34:425–427.
48. Comes J, Walter FG, Kozak K, et al. Liver transplantation for fulminant hepatic failure due to iron poisoning. Vet Hum Toxicol 1993;35:337.
49. Polakoff JM, Lacouture PG, Lovejoy FH Jr. The environment away from home as a source of potential poisoning. Am J Dis Child 1984;138:1014–1017.
50. Gardner R, Hanka R, Roberts SJ, et al. Psychological and social evaluation in cases of deliberate self poisoning seen in an accident department. Br Med J 1982;284:491–493.
51. Delong W, Robin E. The communication of suicide intent prior to psychiatric hospitalization: A study of 87 patients. Am J Psychiatry 1961;117:695–705.
52. Butkus DE, Herrera GA, Praju SS. Successful renal transplantation after cyclosporine-associated hemolytic–uremic syndrome following bilateral lung transplantation. Transplantation 1992;54:159–161.
53. Ernst DC. The suicidal patient. Top Emerg Med 1992;14: 45–55.
54. Leikin JB, Heyn-Lamb R, Aks S, Erickson T. Transplantation of organs donated by poisoning victims. Vet Hum Toxicol 1992;34:359.
55. Swanson-Biearman B, Krenzelok EP, Snyder JW, et al. Successful donation and transplantation of multiple organs from a victim of cyanide poisoning. Clin Toxicol 1993;31:95–99.
56. Lindquist T, Oiland D, Weber K. Cyanide poisoning victims as corneal transplant donors. Am J Ophthalmol 1988;106:354–355.
57. Brown P, Buchels J, Jain A, McMaster P. Successful cadaveric renal transplantation from a donor who died of cyanide poisoning. Br Med J 1987;294:1325.
58. Hebert M-J, Boucher A, Beaucage G, et al. Transplantation of kidneys from a donor with carbon monoxide poisoning. N Engl J Med 1992;326:1571.
59. Vekemans M-C, Hantson P, Squifflet JP, et al. Organ procurement from poisoned donors: An 11 case experience. In: *Proceedings, XVth Congress of European Association of Poison Centres and Clinical Toxicologists, Istanbul, Turkey, May 1992:106.*
60. Leikin JB, Heyn-Lamb R, Aks S, Erickson T. The toxic patient as a potential organ donor: One year follow-up. Vet Hum Toxicol 1993;35:318.
61. Alsina AE, Hull D, Bartus SA, Schweizer RT. Liver transplantation for acute fulminant hepatic failure. Conn Med 1992; 56:235–236.
62. Shragg TA. Compelling treatment after suicide attempts. West J Med 1983;138–86.

Chapter 7

Toxicokinetics

INTRODUCTION

DEFINITION

Pharmacokinetics is the mathematical description of the changes in body drug *concentrations* with respect to absorption, distribution, metabolism, and excretion. The duration and intensity of drug effects depend on factors that influence drug movement within the body. Conceptually, these factors are described by following the drug through the body. Remember that drug effect depends on the *active* drug concentration at the receptor site, which is often different anatomically from the central compartment sampling site (i.e., blood, urine). Consequently, drug effect does not always correlate with plasma concentration.

Mathematically, the two-compartment model predicts the changes in plasma concentration for most drugs with predominant renal elimination. The central compartment represents the plasma and organs of high perfusion (heart, brain, kidney), whereas tissue stores and poorly perfused organs account for the peripheral compartment. For calculation purposes, drugs are eliminated from and absorbed into only the central compartment. The resulting plasma concentration (*Cp*), when plotted against time, shows three phases: absorption, distribution, and elimination. $\alpha T_{1/2}$ (distribution half-life) describes the rate of distribution into the peripheral compartment, and $\beta T_{1/2}$ (elimination half-life) describes the rate of drug elimination from the central compartment.

A glossary of terminology used in clinical toxicokinetics (pharmacokinetics) is provided in Appendix 7–1.

DRUG MONITORING

Plasma drug concentrations may be useful in monitoring compliance, individualizing therapy during dosage changes, diagnosing wider treatment, avoiding toxicity, diagnosing toxicity, monitoring and detecting drug interactions, and guiding withdrawal of therapy. Remember to treat the patient, not the plasma drug concentration. Some drugs for which monitoring may be useful are listed in Table 7–1.[1]

FREE DRUG LEVELS

Antiepileptic drugs such as valproic acid, phenytoin, and carbamazepine and a few antiarrhythmic drugs may justify free drug level monitoring; however, there is a considerable lack of data establishing correlations between therapeutic or toxic response and free drug concentrations. Free drug level methods may not easily be available to the local community hospital laboratory.[1] Free drug plus protein bound drug equals total drug concentration. If the percentage of binding fluctuates, it is the free drug that is active. Thus, the total drug concentration may not be helpful.

VOLUME OF DISTRIBUTION

Not a "real" volume, but a hypothetical volume of body fluid that would be required to dissolve the total amount of drug at the same concentration as that found in the blood or plasma. It is a proportionality constant relating the amount of drug in the body to the measured concentration in biological fluid (blood, plasma, plasma water).

A large (V_D) exceeds 1 L/kg, and plasma levels (Cp) usually are measured in nanograms per milliliter. Artificial elimination procedures (e.g., hemodialysis, hemoperfusion) do not effectively enhance the excretion of drugs into a large (V_D). For drugs with a small (V_D), the plasma concentration of drug (Cp) is measured in micrograms per milliliter. Dialysis effectively enhances the elimination of these drugs if they possess good water solubility and poor protein binding.

The volume of distribution (V_d) of drugs during acute overdosage is often different from that during chronic drug overdose. Overdoses with theophylline, salicylate, and lithium may be associated with seizures, arrhythmias and other life-threatening events at serum drug concentrations that are usually therapeutic or mildly toxic.[2]

A decrease in the volume of distribution after a severe overdose may follow limited distribution of the drug due to a decrease in tissue perfusion (procainamide).[3] Salicylate poisoning may lead to an acidosis, which increases the nonionized fraction of salicylates. This enhances tissue penetration by the drug. The volume of distribution increases with increasing salicylate dosage.[4]

Table 7–1
Drugs Worth Monitoring

Cardiac Agents	chloramphenicol
digoxin	gentamicin
disopyramide	tobramycin
lidocaine	vancomycin
procainamide and *N*-acetylprocainamide	**Bronchodilators**
quinidine	caffeine
Antiepileptic Agents	theophylline
carbamazepine	**Psychoactive Agents**
ethosuximide	lithium
phenobarbital	tricyclic antidepressants
phenytoin	**Other Agents**
primidone	acetaminophen
valproic acid	cyclosporine
Antibiotics	methotrexate
amikacin	salicylates

From Longa RJ, Cross RE. Therapeutic drug monitoring. Part 1. Clinical usefulness and total drug concentration. Emerg Med 1987;16:103.

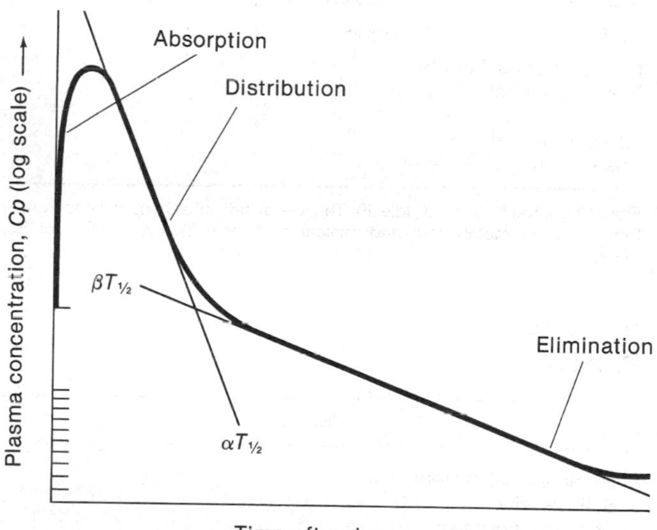

Figure 7–1 Phases of drug movement in a two-compartment model. (From Ellenhorn MJ, Barceloux DG. Medical toxicology: Diagnosis and Treatment of Human Poisoning. New York: Elsevier, 1988:105.)

Table 7–2
Characteristics of Some Human Liver P450s

Gene	Enzyme	Substrates	Probable Inducers
CYP1A2	P450IA2	Acetaminophen, caffeine, theophylline	Cigarette smoke, charcoal-broiled foods, omeprazole
CYP2C	P450IIC*	Mephenytoin, hexobarbital, diazepam, tobultamide, sulfinpyrazone, phenylbutazone	None identified
CYP2D6	P450IID6	Debrisoquine, dextromethorphan, metoprolol, other beta blockers, perhexiline, amitriptyline, other neuroleptics, encainide, flecainide, codeine	None identified
CYP2F1	P450IIE1	Acetaminophen, ethanol	Ethanol, isoniazid
CYP3A4	P450IIIA4	Erythromycin, cyclosporine, steroids, estrogens, midazolam/triazolam, nifedipine, diltiazem, lidocaine, triacetyloleandomycin (TAO), ketoconazole, miconazole, quinidine, lovastatin, FK506	Glucocorticoids, rifampicin, phenytoin, carbamazepine, sulfinpyrazone, phenylbutazone

*Multiple subfamily members whose catalytic properties are incompletely characterized exist.
Adapted from Watkins, PB. Drug metabolism by cytochromes P450 in the liver and small bowel. Gastroenterol Clin North Am 1992;21:511–526.

Table 7–3
CYP2D6 Substrates

Cardiovascular Agents		
Antiarrhythmics	*Beta Blockers*	*Antihypertensive Agents*
Encainide	Bufuralol	Debrisoquine
Flecainide	Metoprolol	Guanoxan
Mexiletine	Propranolol	Indoramin
Propafenone	Timolol	
N-Propylalmaline		
Sparteine		
Psychoactive Agents		
Neuroleptic Agents	*Tricyclic Antidepressants and Related Agents*	*Monoamine Oxidase Inhibitors*
Clozapine	Amitriptyline	Amiflamine
Fluphenazine	Clomipramine	Methoxyphenamine
Perphenazine	Desipramine	
Thioridazine	Imipramine	
Trifluperidol	Nortriptyline	
	Tomoxetine	
Morphine Derivatives		
Analgesics	*Antitussive Agents*	
Codeine	Dextromethorphan	
Miscellaneous Agents		
Methoxyamphet-amine		
Perhexilene		
Phenformin		

From Cholerton S, Daly AK, Idle JR. The role of individual human cytochromes P450 in drug metabolism and clinical response. Trends Pharmacol Sci 1992;13:435.

DRUG-METABOLIZING ENZYMES

CYTOCHROMES P450

The vast majority of phase 1 metabolism is catalyzed by enzymes termed the cytochrome P-450 mixed-function oxidase system, *cytochromes P450,* or simply *P450s* (Table 7–2). This term derives from the fact that these enzymes were initially believed to be similar to mitochondrial cytochromes; they are red in color (pigment) and they maximally absorb light at 450 nm wavelength under certain conditions. More than 20 different P450s have been identified in humans. The majority of P450s involved in drug metabolism appear to belong to three distinct gene families: *CYP1, CYP2,* and *CYP3. CYP2D6* substrates are listed in Table 7–3.[5] Note that acetaminophen is metabolized by cytochromes P4501A2 and P450IIE1.[5,6] Each P450 family is further divided into subfamilies designated by capital letters. Individual P450s are designated by Arabic numbers. P450IA1 and P450IA2 are individual enzymes within the same P450 family and subfamily and, therefore, are closely related.[5]

P450s in the Liver

Many drugs may be largely dependent on single forms of P450 for their metabolism in the liver because each P450 has a unique substrate binding site that determines the affinity with which it binds to and therefore metabolizes a drug. The *CYP1* gene family appears to contain just two genes in humans: *CYP1A1* and *CYP1A2.* Only one of these genes *(CYP1A2)* is consistently expressed in the human liver. The

Table 7–4
Prodrugs

Prodrug	Active Moiety
Gastrointestinal system	
Sulfasalazine	5-Aminosalicylic acid
Stimulant laxatives	
Bisacodyl (diphenol diacetate)	Diphenol
Senna	Sennosides A and B
Cardiovascular system	
Enalapril	Enalaprilat
α-Methyldopa	α-Methylnoradrenaline
Dopamine analogs	
L-γ-Glutamyldopamine	Dopamine
L-γ-Glutamyl-L-dopa	Dopamine
Ibopamine	Epinine
Sulfinpyrazole	Sulfone metabolite
Thrombolytic agents	
Streptokinase	Streptokinase–plasminogen complex
Anistreplase	
(anisoylated plasminogen–streptokinase activator complex)	Deacylated complex
Tetranicotinoyl fructose	Nicotinic acid
Respiratory system	
Theophylline salts (eg, ethylenediamine [aminophylline])	Theophylline
Central nervous system	
Antipsychotic drugs (as enanthates or decanoates)	Active antipsychotic drugs
Fluphenazine	
Zuclopenthixol	
L-Dopa	Dopamine
Diacetylmorphine (heroin)	Morphine
Infectious	
Pivampicillin	Ampicillin
Pivaloyloxymethyl ester	(Formaldehyde; pivalic acid, released)

Table 7–4 *(Continued)*

Prodrug	Active Moiety
Infectious *(Continued)*	
Talampicillin	Ampicillin (carboxybenzaldehyde released)
Pivmecillinam ester	Mecillinam
Chloramphenicol palmitate	Chloramphenicol
Clindamycin palmitate	Clindamycin
Erythrocin stearate or estolate	Erythromycin
Benzoyl metronidazole	Metronidazole
Acyclovir	Triphosphate derivative
Endocrine system	
Glucocorticoids (sodium succinate)	Methylprednisolone, hydrocortisone
Testosterone (propionate, undecanoate, and enanthalate esters)	Testosterone
Malignant disease	
Alkylating agents	
Cyclophosphamide	Phosphoramide mustard
Antimetabolites	
6-Mercaptopurine acid	6-Mercaptopurine ribose phosphate
6-Thioguanine	6-Thioguanine ribose phosphate
5-Fluorouracil	5-Fluorouracil ribose phosphate
Cytarabine	Cytarabine triphosphate
Musculoskeletal and joint disease	
Acetylsalicylic acid (aspirin)	Salicylic acid
Benorylate (aspirin and acetaminophen ester)	Aspirin, acetaminophen
Fenbufen	Biphenylacetic acid and Guanohydroxybiphenylbutanoic acid derivatives
Sulindac	Sulindac sulfide
Nabumetone	6-Methoxy-2-naphthylacetic acid
Dipivoloyl-adrenaline (Dipivefrin)	Adrenaline

From Waller DG, George CF. Prodrugs. Br J Clin Pharmacol 1989;28:497–507.

Table 7–5
Medications and Habits That Increase Cytochrome P450 Drug Metabolism

Barbiturates
Carbamazepine
Chronic alcohol use
Cigarette smoking
Glutethimide
Griseofulvin
Omeprazole
Phenytoin
Polycyclic aromatic hydrocarbons
Primidone
Rifampin

From Mills KC. Essential emergency medicine pharmacokinetics: Prevention of iatrogenic patient poisoning. Top Emerg Med 1993;15:18–29.

catalytic activity of liver P450IA1 is increased (or "induced") in patients who smoke cigarettes or consume charcoal-broiled foods. P450IA2 is an arylhydrocarbon hydroxylase and is the liver P450 that best corresponds to what has previously been termed P448. P450II is the largest family of human cytochrome P450s identified to date. Human P450IIE is inducible by ethanol and corresponds to the microsomal ethanol-oxidizing system (MEOS). P450IIE1 is also induced by isoniazid but not by phenobarbital. P450IIC and P450IID are expressed in the liver, but no induction of these enzymes has been identified. P450III genes are inducible by glucocorticoids, antiseizure medications, and macrolide antibiotics. P450IIIA4 is the major P450III enzyme present in adult liver. In fetal liver P450IIIA7 accounts for the majority of P450 present.

Table 7–6
Medications That Inhibit Cytochrome P450 Drug Metabolism

Acute ethanol ingestion	Metoprolol
Allopurinol	Metronidazole
Amiodarone	Micronazole
Chloramphenicol	Nortriptyline
Chlorpromazine	Omeprazole
Cimetidine	Oral contraceptives
Ciprofloxacin	Phenylbutazone
Danazol (androgens)	Primaquine
Diltiazem	Propoxyphene
Disulfiram	Propranolol
Enoxacin	Quinidine
Erythromycin (macrolides)	Ranitidine
Fluconazole	Trimethoprim–sulfamethoxazole
Fluoxetine	Valproic acid
Imipramine	Verapamil
Ketoconazole	

From Mills KC. Essential emergency medicine pharmacokinetics: Prevention of iatrogenic patient poisoning. Top Emerg Med 1993;15:18–29.

Women have more hepatic P450III activity than men. Drugs shown to be a substrate for P450IIIA should be metabolized at a reduced rate when a patient is also taking a P450IIIA inhibitor. The drug should be metabolized at an increased rate when the patient takes a P450IIIA inducer.[7]

CYPIID6

A substantial number of drugs with a high potential for inhibition are metabolized by the cytochrome P450IID6

Table 7–7
Enzymes Involved in the Metabolic Activation of Various Pulmonary Toxins

Compound	Source	Toxic Effect	Enzymes Involved
Benzo[a]pyrene	Cigarette smoke	Lung cancer	P-448, epoxide hydrolase, PES
4-Ipomeanol	Moldy sweet potatoes	Clara cell necrosis	P-450
3-Methylfuran	Environmental pollutant	Clara cell necrosis	P-450
Parathion	Insecticide	Respiratory edema and failure	P-450, amine oxidase
α-Naphthylthiourea	Rodenticide	Edema	P-450, amine oxidase
Carbon tetrachloride	Organic solvent	Clara and Type II cell damage	P-450
Nitrofurantoin	Antibacterial agent	Fibrosis	P-450 reductase, xanthine oxidase
Paraquat	Herbicide	Type I and II cell damage	P-450 reductase
Naphthalene	Moth balls	Clara cell necrosis	P-450, glutathione *S*-transferase
Butylated hydroxytoluene	Food additive	Type I cell damage (mice)	P-450
3-Methylindole	Bacterial metabolite of tryptophan	Edema, Clara cell necrosis	P-450
p-Xylene	Solvent	Decrease in pulmonary mixed-function oxidases	P-450, deficiency of alcohol and aldehyde dehydrogenase
4-(*N*-Methyl-*N*-nitrosoamino)-1-(3-pyridyl)-1-butanone	Tobacco	Carcinogen	P-450

From Cohen GM. Pulmonary metabolism of foreign compounds: Its role in metabolic activation. Environ Health Perspect 1990;85:31–41.

Table 7–8
Toxic Metabolites: Predictable Formation and Effects

Drug	Metabolite	Effect
Acetaminophen	*N*-Hydroxy-*N*-acetyl *p*-hydroxyaniline	Hepatotoxicity
Carmustine (BCNU, BiCNU)	Active metabolites	Cytotoxicity
Clofibrate (Atromid-S)	Chlorphenoxyisobutyric acid	Myositis
Cyclophosphamide (Cytoxan, Neosar)	4-Hydroxycyclophosphamide → acrolein (in bladder)	Chemical cystitis
Dapsone	*N*-hydroxydapsone	Methemoglobinemia
Furosemide (Lasix)	Reactive intermediate	Nephrotoxicity
Glutethimide	4-Hydroxy-2-ethyl-2-phenylglutarimide	Prolonged coma
Lidocaine (Xylocaine)	Monoethyl-glycine xylidide Glycine xylidide	Seizures
Meperdine (Demerol, Mepergan)	Normeperidine	Central nervous system stimulant with seizures
Methotrexate (Rheumatrex)	7-Hydroxymethotrexate	Nephrotoxicity
Methoxyflurane (Penthrane)	Fluoride ion	Nephrotoxicity
Methsuximide (Celontin)	D-Desmethyl metabolite	Delayed coma in overdose
Nitroprusside (Nipride, Nitropress)	Cyanide Thiocyanate	Cellular hypoxia Altered thyroid function
Propoxyphene (Darvon)	Norpropoxyphene	Cardiotoxicity
Spironolactone (Aldactazide, Aldactone)	Aldadiene	Decreased testosterone synthesis
Sulbenicillin	α-Sulfobenzylpenicilloic acid	Impaired platelet function
Sulfisoxazole (Gantrisin)	*N*-Acetyl sulfisoxazole	Crystalluria

From Macleod CM. Clinical implications of drug metabolism: Toxic metabolites. Res Staff Phys 1992;38:78.

Table 7–9
Toxic Metabolites: Predictable Formation With Unpredictable Effects

Drug	Metabolite	Effect
Acetaminophen	Sulfate conjugate	Thrombocytopenia
Dapsone	Monohydroxyl amines	Hemolysis
Diazepam (Valium, Valrelease)	*N*-Desmethyl diazepam	Adverse autonomic nervous system effects
Halothane (Fluothane)	Trifluoroacetyl halide	Hepatotoxicity
Isoniazid (Laniazid)	*N*-acetylhydrazine	Hepatotoxicity
Lovastatin (Mevacor)	β-Hydroxy acid	Myopathy metabolite
Penicillin	Penicilloic acid	Anaphylaxis
Testosterone	Etiocholanolone	Fever, inflammatory reaction
Thalidomide	Phthalimidophthalmide	Teratogenicity

From Macleod CM. Clinical implications of drug metabolism: Toxic metabolites. Res Staff Phys 1992;38:78.

Table 7-10
Some Examples of Receptors, Their Agonists, and Their Antagonists

Receptor Type	Subtype	Site in Body	Agonists*	Antagonists*
Cholinoceptors	Muscarinic	Tissues innervated by parasympathetic nerves	**Acetylcholine** and analogs (eg, carbachol, bethanechol)	Atropine and analogs Benzhexol Orphenadrine Quinidine Disopyramide Tricyclic antidepressants Pirenzepine (M_1 selective)
	Nicotinic	Neuromuscular junction Postganglionic cells in ganglia	**Acetylcholine** and some analogs (eg, carbachol)	Neuromuscular blocking drugs Ganglion blocking drugs Quinidine Aminoglycoside antibiotics
Adrenoceptors	α/β		**Adrenaline** **Noradrenaline**	Labetalol
	α_1	Vascular smooth muscle Pupillary dilator muscle	Phenylephrine Dopamine (high doses)	Prazosin
	α_2	Presynaptic nerve terminals, CNS	Clonidine	*Yohimbine*
	α_1/α_2			Phentolamine
	β_1	Heart CNS	Dopamine (moderate doses) Dobutamine	Practolol Atenolol Metoprolol
	β_2	Smooth muscle (bronchiolar, vascular, uterine) Pancreatic islets	Salbutamol Terbutaline Rimiterol Fenoterol	
	β_1/β_2		Isoprenaline	Propranolol Oxprenolol
Dopamine receptors	Various (clinical significance uncertain)	CNS Renal vasculature	**Dopamine** (low doses) Bromocriptine Apomorphine	Phenothiazines (eg, chlorpromazine) Thioxanthenes (eg, flupenthixol) Butyrophenones (eg, haloperidol) Metoclopramide
Histamine receptors	H_1	Smooth muscle (bronchiolar, vascular, gastrointestinal)	**Histamine**	Antihistamines (eg, mepyramine, promethazine)
	H_2	Stomach	**Histamine**	Cimetidine Ranitidine
Opioid receptors	Various (clinical significance unclear)	CNS Vascular smooth muscle Gastrointestinal tract Biliary tract Genitourinary tract Pupillary muscle	Morphine and analogs (eg, heroin, buprenorphine) Beta-endorphin Enkephalins Nonopioid narcotics (eg, pentazocine)	Naloxone Naltrexone
5-Hydroxytryptamine receptors	Various (clinical significance unclear)	CNS Vascular smooth muscle	**5-hydroxytryptamine**	Methysergide Cryproheptadine Ketanserin
GABA receptors	$GABA_A$/BDZ complex	CNS	**GABA** Benzodiazepines	*Bicuculine*
	$GABA_B$	CNS (presynaptic)	**GABA** Baclofen	

CNS, central nervous system; GABA, γ-aminobutyric acid; BDZ, benzodiazepines.
*Although the agonists and antagonists are listed according to their relative selectivity for particular subtypes of receptor, it should not be assumed that their selectivity is absolute.
†Agonists printed in bold type are the endogenous agonists which define the receptor type. Nonendogenous compounds printed in italics are not used in routine therapy.
From Aronson JR. Receptors and their relevance to drug therapy. Med Int (Israel Edition) 1989;59:2429–2435.

isoenzyme.[8,9] Fluoxetine and its major metabolite norfluoxetine are strong inhibitors of cytochrome P450IID6 *(CYPIID6)*, impairing hepatic metabolism of P4502D6-dependent drugs, leading to marked elevations in their plasma levels and associated toxicity.[10]

P450s in the Intestine

P450s are present in the crypt cells of the intestine and in highest concentration in enterocytes at the top of the villus. They are located predominantly at the apex of the mature enterocyte, lying in a band just below the microvillous border. The major enterocyte P450 in humans is a member of the P450IIIA family, specifically P450IIIA4. P450IIIA present in enterocytes significantly catalyzes first-pass metabolism of some orally administered drugs. Most lipophilic drugs must traverse a high-density zone of P450s prior to entering the body.[5]

PRODRUGS

Prodrugs are compounds that are inactive in their parent forms but which, after administration, are chemically transformed to the active derivative. The most common prodrug linkage is an ester bond; phosphate salts form most of the rest. Activation of most prodrugs is by an enzymatic process that cleaves off the active moiety.[11] Examples of prodrugs are listed in Table 7–4.[12]

Table 7–11
Drugs That Are Contraindicated During Breastfeeding

Drug	Reported Sign or Symptom in Infant or Effect on Lactation
Bromocriptine	Suppresses lactation
Cocaine	Cocaine intoxication
Cyclophosphamide	Possible immune suppression; unknown effect on growth or association with carcinogenesis; neutropenia
Cyclosporine	Possible immune suppression; unknown effect on growth or association with carcinogenesis
Doxorubicin*	Possible immune suppression; unknown effect on growth or association with carcinogenesis
Ergotamine	Vomiting, diarrhea, convulsions (doses used in migraine medications)
Lithium	One-third to one-half therapeutic blood concentration in infants
Methotrexate	Possible immune suppression; unknown effect on growth or association with carcinogenesis; neutropenia
Phencyclidine (PCP)	Potent hallucinogen
Phenindione	Anticoagulant; increased prothrombin and partial thromboplastin time in one infant (not used in United States)

*Drug is concentrated in human milk.
From Committee on Drugs, American Academy of Pediatrics, Roberts RJ, Chairman. Transfer of drugs and other chemicals into breast milk. Pediatrics 1989;84:924–936.

ENZYME INDUCERS

Enzyme inducers are listed in Table 7–5. Enzyme inducers may induce metabolism of other drugs rapidly (hours, days), but occasionally may require weeks.

ENZYME INHIBITORS

Enzyme inhibitors are listed in Table 7–6.

CARCINOGENS

Carcinogens, unlike drug cytochrome P450 enzyme inducers, undergo oxidative metabolism to yield reactive intermediates that are not readily conjugated and thus react with

Table 7–12
Drugs of Abuse That Are Contraindicated During Breastfeeding*

Drug	Effect
Amphetamine	Irritability, poor sleep pattern
Cocaine	Cocaine intoxication
Heroin	
Marijuana	Only one report in literature; no effect mentioned
Nicotine (smoking)	Shock, vomiting, diarrhea, rapid heart rate, restlessness; decreased milk production
Phencyclidine (PCP)	Potent hallucinogen

*The Committee on Drugs believes strongly that nursing mothers should not ingest any of these compounds. Not only are they hazardous to the nursing infant, but they are detrimental to the physical and emotional health of the mother.
†Drug is concentrated in human milk.
From Committee on Drugs, American Academy of Pediatrics, Roberts RJ, Chairman. Transfer of drugs and other chemicals into breast milk. Pediatrics 1989;84:924–936.

Table 7–13
Radiopharmaceuticals That Require Temporary Cessation of Breastfeeding*

Drug	Recommended Alteration in Breastfeeding Pattern
Gallium-67 (^{67}Ga)	Radioactivity in milk present for 2 wk
Indium-111 (^{111}In)	Small amount present at 20 h
Iodine-125 (^{125}I)	Risk of thyroid cancer; radioactivity in milk present for 12 d
Iodine-131 (^{131}I)	Radioactivity in milk present 2–14 d depending on study
Radioactive sodium	Radioactivity in milk present 96 h
Technetium-99m (^{99m}Tc), ^{99m}Tc macroaggregates, $^{99m}TcO_4$	Radioactivity in milk present 15 h to 3 d

*Consult nuclear medicine physician before performing diagnostic study so that a radionuclide with the shortest excretion time in breast milk can be used. Before study, the mother should pump her breast and store enough milk in freezer for feeding the infant; after study, the mother should pump her breast to maintain milk production but discard all milk pumped for the required time that radioactivity is present in milk.
From Committee on Drugs, American Academy of Pediatrics, Roberts RJ, Chairman. Transfer of drugs and other chemicals into breast milk. Pediatrics 1989;84:924–936.

Table 7–14
Drugs Whose Effect on Nursing Infants Is Unknown but May Be of Concern

Drug	Effect
Psychotropic drugs	Special concern when given to nursing mothers for long periods
Antianxiety	
Diazepam	None known
Lorazepam	None known
Prazepam*	None known
Quazepam	None known
Antidepressant	
Amitriptyline	None known
Amoxapine	None known
Desipramine	None known
Dothiepin	None known
Doxepin	None known
Imipramine	None known
Trazodone	None known
Antipsychotic	
Chlorpromazine	Galactorrhea in adult; drowsiness and lethargy in infant
Chlorprothixene	None known
Haloperidol	None known
Mesoridazine	None known
Chloramphenicol	Possible idiosyncratic bone marrow sup- pression
Metoclopramide* K	None described; potent central nervous system drug
Metronidazole	In vitro mutagen; may discontinue breast-feeding 12–24 h to allow excretion of dose when single-dose therapy given to mother
Tinidazole	See Metronidazole

*Drug is concentrated in human milk.
From Committee on Drugs, American Academy of Pediatrics, Roberts RJ, Chairman. Transfer of drugs and other chemicals into breast milk. Pediatrics 1989;84:924–936.

vital intracellular macromolecules, resulting in necrosis, redox cycling and oxygen radical formation, neoantigen production, and mutations.

PULMONARY TOXINS

Examples of enzymes involved in the metabolic activation of various pulmonary toxins are listed in Table 7–7.[13]

TOXIC METABOLITES

Toxic metabolites may be formed with both predictable and unpredictable effects (Tables 7–8 and 7–9).[14]

RECEPTORS

INTRODUCTION

A receptor is a specific tissue protein (membrane-bound or intracellular) capable of binding the members of a specific group of drugs or endogenous substances.[15] The interaction of a drug with its receptor leads to the pharmacologic effect

Table 7–15
Drugs That Have Caused Significant Effects on Some Nursing Infants and Should Be Given to Nursing Mothers With Caution*

Drug	Effect
Aspirin (salicylates)	Metabolic acidosis (dose related); may affect platelet function; rash
Clemastine	Drowsiness, irritability, refusal to feed, high-pitched cry, neck stiffness (1 case)
Phenobarbital	Sedation; infantile spasms after weaning from milk containing phenobarbital, methemoglo-binemia (one case)
Primidone	Sedation, feeding problems
Salicylazosulfapyridine (sul-fasalazine)	Bloody diarrhea in one infant

*Measure blood concentration in the infant when possible.
From Committee on Drugs, American Academy of Pediatrics, Roberts RJ, Chairman. Transfer of drugs and other chemicals into breast milk. Pediatrics 1989;84:924–936.

through a series of incompletely understood mechanisms. Different types of receptors may be defined according to their most potent endogenous agonist (eg, histamine receptors).

LIGAND

A ligand is a drug or endogenous substance that binds to a receptor (eg, histamine is a ligand at histamine receptors).

AGONIST

An agonist is a ligand that produces an appropriate response when it binds to its receptor (eg, histamine is an agonist at histamine receptors).

ANTAGONIST

An antagonist is a ligand that prevents the effects of an agonist. Pure antagonists do not by themselves cause any effects by binding to receptors (eg, cimetidine is an antagonist of the actions of histamine at one subtype of histamine receptor, H_2).

PARTIAL AGONIST

A partial agonist is a ligand that has both agonist and antagonist properties.

RECEPTOR SUBTYPES

Receptors may be divided into subtypes on the basis of the selectivity of a range of agonists or antagonists (eg, histamine receptors can be divided into two subtypes:

Table 7–16
Maternal Medications Usually Compatible With Breastfeeding*

Drug	Reported Sign or Symptom in Infant or Effect on Lactation
Anesthetics, Sedatives	
Alcohol	Drowsiness, diaphoresis, deep sleep, weakness, decrease in linear growth, abnormal weight gain; maternal ingestion of 1 g/kg daily decreases milk ejection reflex
Barbiturate	See Table 7–15
Bromide	Rash, weakness, absence of cry with maternal intake of 5.4 g/d
Chloral hydrate	Sleepiness
Chloroform	None
Halothane	None
Lidocaine	None
Magnesium sulfate	None
Methyprylon	Drowsiness
Secobarbital	None
Thiopental	None
Anticoagulants	
Bishydroxycoumarin	None
Warfarin	None
Antiepileptic Agents	
Carbamazepine	None
Ethosuximide	None; drug appears in infant serum
Phenobarbital	See Table 7–15
Phenytoin	Methemoglobinemia (one case)
Primidone	See Table 7–15
Thiopental	None
Valproic acid	None
Anthistamines, Decongestants, and Bronchodilators	
Dexbrompheniramine maleate with *d*-isoephedrine	Crying, poor sleep patterns, irritability
Dyphylline†	None
Iodides	May affect thyroid activity; see Miscellaneous Agents, Iodine
Pseudoephedrine†	None
Terbutaline	None
Theophylline	Irritability
Tyriprolidine	None
Antihypertensive and Cardiovascular Drugs	
Acebutolol	None
Atenolol	None
Captopril	None
Digoxin	None
Diltiazem	None
Disopyramide	None
Hydralazine	None
Labetalol	None
Lidocaine	None
Methyldopa	None
Metoprolol†	None
Mexiletine	None
Minoxidil	None
Nadolol†	None
Oxprenolol	None
Procainamide	None
Propranolol	None
Quinidine	None
Timolol	None
Verapamil	None
Antiinfective Drugs (all antibiotics transfer into breast milk in limited amounts)	
Acyclovir†	None
Amoxicillin	None
Aztreonam	None
Cefadroxil	None
Cefazolin	None
Cefotaxime	None
Cefoxitin	None
Ceftazidine	None
Ceftriazone	None
Chloroquine	None
Clindamycin	None
Cycloserine	None
Dapsone	None; sulfonamide detected in infant's urine
Erythromycin†	None
Ethambutol	None
Hydroxychloroquine†	None
Isoniazid	None, acetyl metabolite also secreted; ? hepatoxicity
Kanamycin	None
Moxalactam	None
Nalidixic acid	Hemolysis in infants with glucose-6-phosphate dehydrogenase (G6PD) deficiency)
Nitrofurantoin	Hemolysis in infant with G6PD deficiency
Pyrimethamine	None
Quinine	None
Rifampin	None
Salicylazosulfapyridine (sulfasalazine)	See Table 7–15
Streptomycin	None
Sulbactam	None
Sulfapyridine	Caution in infant with jaundice or G6PD deficiency and in ill, stressed, or premature infant; appears in infant's urine
Sulfisoxazole	Caution in infant with jaundice or G6PD deficiency and in ill, stressed, or premature infant; appears in infant's urine
Tetracycline	None; negligible absorption by infant
Ticarcillin	None
Trimethoprim–sulfamethoxazole	None
Antithyroid Drugs	
Carbimazole	Goiter
Methimazole (active metabolite of carbimazole)	None
Propylthiouracil	None
Thiouracil	None mentioned; drug not used in United States
Cathartics	
Cascara	None
Danthron	Increased bowel activity
Senna	None

(continued)

Table 7–16 *(Continued)*

Drug	Reported Sign or Symptom in Infant or Effect on Lactation	Drug	Reported Sign or Symptom in Infant or Effect on Lactation
Diagnostic Agents		**Muscle Relaxants** ***(Continued)***	
Iodine	Goiter; see Miscellaneous Agents, Iodine	Methadone	None if mother receiving ≤20 mg/24 h
Iopranoic acid	None	Morphine	None
Metrizamide	None	Nefopam	None
Diuretic Agents		Phenylbutazone	None
Bendroflumethiazide	Suppresses lactation	Piroxicam	None
Chlorothiazide, hydrochlorothiazide	None	Prednisolone, prednisone	None
Chlorhalidone	Excreted slowly	Propoxyphene	None
Spironolactine	None	Salicylates	See Table 7n15
Hormones		Suprofen	None
[^{3}H]Norethynodrel	None	Tolmetin	None
19-Norsteroids	None	**Stimulants**	
Clogestone	None	Caffeine	Irritability, poor sleep pattern, excreted slowly; no effect with usual amount of caffeine beverages
Contraceptive pill with estrogen/progesterone	Rare breast enlargement; decrease in milk production and protein content (not confirmed in several studies)	**Vitamins**	
		B_1 (thiamine)	None
		B_6 (pyridoxine)	None
Estradiol	Withdrawal, vaginal bleeding	B_{12}	None
		D	None; follow infant's serum calcium if mother receives pharmacologic doses
Medroxyprogesterone	None	Folic acid	None
Prednisolone	None	K_1	None
Prednisone	None	Riboflavin	None
Progesterone	None	**Miscellaneous Agents**	
Muscle Relaxants		Acetazolamide	None
Baclofen	None	Atropine	None
Methocarbomal	None	Cimetidine†	None
Narcotics, nonnarcotic analgesics, antiinflammatory agents	None	Cisapride	None
Acetaminophen	None	Cisplatin	Not found in milk
Butorphanol	None	Domperidone	None
Codeine	None	Iodine (povidone–iodine/vaginal douche)	Elevated iodine levels in breast milk, odor of iodine on infant's skin
Dipyrone	None		
Flufenamic acid	None		
Gold salts	None	Metoclopramide	See Table 7–15
Hydroxychloroquine	None	Noscapine	None
Ibuprofen	None	Pyridostigmine	None
Indomethacin	Seizure (one case)	Tolbutamide	? Jaundice
Mefenamic acid	None		

*Drugs listed have been reported in the literature as having the effects listed or no effect. The word "none" means that no observable change was seen in the nursing infant while the mother was ingesting the compound. It is emphasized that most of the literature citations concern single case reports or small series of infants.
†Drug is concentrated in human milk.
From Committee on Drugs, American Academy of Pediatrics, Roberts RJ, Chairman. Transfer of drugs and other chemicals into breast milk. Pediatrics 1989;84:924–936.

that for which conventional antihistamines have a high antagonist selectivity, H_1, and that for which drugs such as cimetidine and ranitidine have high antagonist selectivity, H_2).

DOWNREGULATION AND UPREGULATION

Downregulation and upregulation are loose terms used to indicate a decrease or increase, respectively, in the number of receptor sites in a tissue. Changes of this kind often occur in response to long-term administration of a drug or in disease.

Some examples of receptors and their agonists and antagonists are listed in Table 7–10.[15]

BREAST MILK

TOXICOKINETICS

Most substances found in breast milk are accounted for by passive transfer. The efficiency of passive transfer is usually represented by the ratio of the concentration of a substance in milk to the concentration of the substance in plasma: the milk/plasma (M/P) ratio. Agent-specific factors and a maternal factor affect passive transfer.[16]

IONIZATION CONSTANT

Only the un-ionized, lipid-soluble portion of an organic compound diffuses readily into milk. Weak acids tend to give

MP ratios less than 1, whereas weak bases tend to give ratios greater than 1.

PROTEIN BINDING

Highly protein-bound substances tend to partition to a lesser extent into milk than non-protein-bound substances.

MOLECULAR WEIGHT

Agents with molecular weights less than 200 tend to partition more effectively into milk.

CHEMICAL PROPERTIES

Agents chemically similar to milk constituents or transported like milk constituents may be actively excreted in milk.

ELIMINATION/METABOLISM

Metabolism usually produces a less lipid-soluble, less toxic compound. Chemicals that are rapidly metabolized and eliminated from blood have less time to partition into milk and do not reach significant levels. Agents eliminated or metabolized slowly are available for transmission into milk.

LIPID SOLUBILITY

Lipid-soluble compounds are found at higher levels in milk than blood. Those substances that are highly lipid soluble are stored in fat and slowly eliminated from the body.

BLOOD FLOW

The rate of milk formation is 0.8 L/day. With a blood flow of 300 to 400 L/day, even relatively low maternal blood levels of a substance have the potential to produce high levels in milk.

DRUGS AND BREASTFEEDING

The Committee on Drugs of the American Academy of Pediatrics has studied the relationship of drugs, chemicals, foods, and environmental agents to breastfeeding[17] (Tables 7–11 through 7–17). Atkinson and colleagues have summarized drugs that should be avoided during breastfeeding based on likely infant concentration (Table 7–18).[18]

Industrial chemicals detected or excreted in breast milk have been summarized by Giroux and colleagues (Table 7–19).[19] The ratio of some chemical concentrations found in breast milk to that in maternal blood are found in Table 7–20.[20]

Table 7–17
Food and Environmental Agents and Their Effect on Breastfeeding

Agent	Reported Sign or Symptom in Infant or Effect on Lactation
Aflatoxin	None
Aspartame	Caution if mother or infant has phenylketonuria
Bromide	Potential absorption and bromide transfer into milk; see Table 7–16, Anesthetics, Sedatives
Cadmium	None reported
Chlordane	None reported
Chocolate	Irritability or increased bowel activity if excess amounts (16 oz/d) consumed by mother
DDT, benzenehexachlorides, dieldrin, aldrin, hepatachlorepoxide	None
Fava beans	Hemolysis in patient with glucose-6-phosphate dehydrogenase deficiency
Fluorides	None
Hexaclorobenzene	Skin rash, diarrhea, vomiting, dark urine, neurotoxicity, death
Hexachlorophene	None; possible contamination of milk from nipple washing
Lead	Possible neurotoxicity
Methyl mercury, mercury	May affect neurodevelopment
Monosodium glutamate (MSG)	None
Polychlorinated biphenyls and polybrominated biphenyls	Lack of endurance, hypotonia, sullen expressionless facies
Tetrachlorethylene cleaning fluid (perchloroethylene)	Obstructive jaundice, dark urine
Vegetarian diet	Signs of B_{12} deficiency

From Committee on Drugs, American Academy of Pediatrics, Roberts RJ, Chairman. Transfer of drugs and other chemicals into breast milk. Pediatrics 1989;84:924–936.

Table 7–18
Drugs That Should Be Avoided by Breastfeeding Mothers, Based on Likely Infant Concentrations

Avoid Totally at All Ages			
Infant Dose > 100% Maternal Dose (/kg)			
Phenobarbitone	(23–156%)	Thiouracil	(113%)
Avoid at < 52 wk Postconceptional Age			
Infant Dose = 25–100% Maternal Dose (/kg)			
Amiodarone	(37%)	Isoniazid	(50%)
Carbimazole	(27%)	Metronidazole	(0.4–36%)
Ethosuximide	(13–30%)	Theophylline	(8–63%)
Avoid at < 44 wk Postconceptual Age			
Infant Dose = 10–25% Maternal Dose (/kg)			
Atenolol	(16–19%)	Methimazole	(17%)
Ethanol	(19.5%)	Theobromine	(20%)
Metoclopramide	(11.3%)	Tolbutamide	(18%)
Avoid at < 34 wk Postconceptual Age or When Unusually Large Doses Used			
Infant Dose = 5–10% Maternal Dose (/kg)			
Acyclovir	(5–10%)	Disopyramide	(7%)
Amphetamine	(6%)	Gold	(6–8%)
Bacioten	(5%)	Hexamine	(10%)
Caffeine	(10%)	Iodine	(8%)
Chloramphenicol	(7%)	Paracetamol	(8%)
Cimetidine	(5%)	Phenytoin	(4–7%)
Clemastine	(9%)	Piroxicam	(5–10%)
Clonidine	(8%)	Nadolol	(5%)
Codeine	(7%)	Sulfapyridine	(5–7%)
Dapsone	(10%)		

From Atkinson HC, Begg EJ, Darlow BA. Drugs in human milk: Clinical pharmacokinetic considerations. Clin Pharmacokinet 1988;14:217–240.

Table 7–19
Chemicals Detected or Excreted in Milk

Products	Excretion		Detection	
	Human	Animal	Human	Animal
Acetaminophen	+			
Acetone			+	
Acetophenone			+	
Acetylsalicylic acid		+		
Adamantine hydrochloride	+			
Aldrin	+			
Allylcatechol methylene ether		+		
Amidopyrin		+		
4-Amino-10-methyl folic acid	+			
Amitriptyline hydrochloride	+			
Antimony	+			
Antypirin	+			
Barium peroxide	+			
Bentazon				+
Benzene			+	
Benzene hexahydride			+	
Benzo[a]heptalen-9 (5H)-one	+			
Benzo[a]pyrene		+		
2,3-Benzofluoranthene		+		
Bromochlorotrifluoroethane	+			
Butyl alcohol			+	
Cadmium oxide		+		
Caffeine	+			
Calcifero	+			
Carbon tetrachloride			+	
Chloral hydrate	+			
Chlordane			+	
Chloromethane			+	
Choline theophylline salt	+			
Cobalt dibromide	+			
Copper		+		
Copper fumes		+		
Dopper, dusts, and mists (as Cu)		+		
Crufomate		+		
Cyclophosphamide	+			
Cyclosporine	+			
4,4′-DDE	+			
Dehydroacetic acid		+		
1,2-Dehydrocortisone	+			
Di-*sec*-octyl phthalate		+		
Diazepam	+			
Diazinon		+		
1,1-Dichloro-2,2-di(4-chlorophenyl) ethane	+			
Dichlorodifluoromethane			+	
Dichlorodiphenyltrichloroethane			+	
1,2-Dichloroethane	+			
2,4-Dichlorophenoxyacetic acid		+		
Dieldrin	+			
1,8-Dihydroxyanthraquinone	+			
7-(2,3-Dihydroxypropyl)theophylline	+			
1,3-Dimethyl-2,6-dihydroxypurine	+			
meta-Dimethylbenzene			+	
ortho-Dimethylbenzene			+	
para-Dimethylbenzene			+	
Dimethylmercury	+			
Dimezathine		+		
Diphenylbutazone	+			
Erythromycin	+			
Ethyl alcohol	+			
Ethyl butyl ketone			+	
Ethylbenzene			+	
Ethylene trichloride			+	
Ferrous sulfate heptahydrate		+		
Fluorotrichloromethane			+	
Folic acid			+	

(continued)

Table 7–19 *(Continued)*

Products	Excretion		Detection	
	Human	Animal	Human	Animal
Gamma-hexachlorocyclohexane			+	
Glycerylguaiacolate carbamate	+			
Heptachlor	+			
2-Heptanone			+	
β-Hexachlorocyclohexane			+	
1,2,3,4,5,6-Hexachlorocyclohexane			+	
Hexachlorophene		+		
Hexamethylphosphoramide		+		
Iodine	+			
Isonicotinic acid hydrazide	+			
Isopropyl alcohol			+	
Lead acetate		+		
Lead dichloride		+		
Lead nitrate		+		
α-Lindane			+	
Lithium carbonate	+			
Magnesium sulfate	+			
Malathion		+		
Manganese(II) chloride tetrahydrate		+		
Manganous sulfate, monohydrate		+		
Meprobamate	+			
Mercuric chloride		+		
Mercuric nitrate		+		
Methyl chloroform			+	
Methyl cyclopentane			+	
Methyl ethyl ketone			+	
Methyl mercury chloride	+			
Methyl propyl ketone			+	
Methylene chloride	+			
Methylmercury	+			
N-Nitrosodipropylamine		+		
1-Naphthenol methylcarbonate		+		
Niacinamide	+			
Nicotine	+			
Oxychlordan			+	
Oxytetracycline	+			
Perchlorobenzene	+			
Phenacetine	+			
Phenobarbituric acid	+			
3-α-Phenyl β-acetylethyl 4-hydroxycoumarin	+			
Phenyl mercury acetate		+		
2-Phenylphenol				+
Polychlorinated biphenyl	+			
Polychlorinated biphenyl (42 CL)	+			
Polychlorinated biphenyl (54 CL)	+			
Potassium iodide			+	
Potassium penicillin G	+			
Quinidine gluconate	+			
Quinidine sulfate	+			
β-Quinine	+			
Ribavirin	+			
Salicylic acid	+			
Seleninyl chloride	+			
Selenium	+			
Selenium dichloride	+			
Selenium powder	+			
Selenium tetrachloride	+			
Sodium bifluoride	+			
Sodium bromide	+			
Strontium chloride		+		
Strontium chloride hexahydrate		+		
Strontium peroxide	+			
Sulfadimethylisoxazole	+			
3-Sulfanilamido-5-methylisoxazole		+		
2-Sulfanilamidothiazole	+			
Sulfapyridine	+			
Sulfapyrmidine	+			
Sulfisoxazol acetyl	+			
Sulfonamide	+			

Table 7–19 *(Continued)*

Products	Excretion: Human	Excretion: Animal	Detection: Human	Detection: Animal
2,3,7,8-Tetrachlorodibenzo-1, 4-dioxin		+		
Tetrachloroethylene	+			
Thiamine monochloride	+			
DL-.ga-Tocopherol	+			
Toluene			+	
1,1,2-Trichloro-1,2,2-trifluoroethane			+	
Trichloromethane			+	
2,4,5-Trichlorophenoxyacetic acid		+		
Trimethylene	+			
Uranyl nitrate	+			
Urethane		+		
Valproic acid	+			
Vinyl benzene			+	
Vinyl propionate			+	
Xylene			+	
Zinc chloride		+		
Zinc oxide		+		
Zinc oxide fumes		+		
Zirconium		+		

From Giroux D, LaPointe G, Baril M. Toxicological index and the presence in the workplace of chemical hazards for workers who breast-feed infants. Am Ind Hyg Assoc J 1992;53:471–474.

Table 7–20
Ratio of Chemical Concentration in Breast Milk to That in Maternal Blood

Chemical	Milk/Plasma Ratio
Mercury, (inorganic and organic)	0.9
Lead	≤1
Perchloroethylene	3
Polybrominated biphenyls (PBBs)	3
Polychlorinated biphenyls (PCBs)	4–10
Dieldrin	6
o,p-Dichlorodiphenyl trichloroethane (DDT) residues	6–7

From Paul M, Himmelstein J. Reproductive hazards in the workplace: What the practitioner needs to know about chemical resources. Obstet Gynecol 1988;7:921–938.

DRUG INTERACTIONS

Patients particularly susceptible to drug interactions[21] include elderly patients and other patients receiving many drugs, patients who have acute illness (eg, severe anemia, left ventricular failure, status asthmaticus, pneumonia), patients who have unstable disease (eg, epilepsy, diabetes mellitus, cardiac arrhythmia, dementia), patients dependent on drug treatment (eg, transplant recipients, patients with connective tissue disorder, patients with Addison's disease), patients who have considerable renal or hepatic impairment (eg, cirrhosis, congestive cardiac failure, uremia), and patients who have more than one prescribing doctor.

THE ELDERLY

Many of the rapidly increasing population over age 65 receive medical therapy for several chronic conditions simultaneously, often involving treatment with up to eight different drugs per day in addition to use of over-the-counter drugs. Symptoms caused by drug-induced poisonings are often interpreted as normal signs of aging: disorientation, tremors, lethargy, depression, forgetfulness, loss of appetite, and constipation. Failure to take drugs as prescribed is often due to failure to understand the importance of therapy, failure to understand the directions for use, high dosing frequency, cost of medication, and failure to get prescriptions filled. Poor eyesight, failure to read instructions for proper use of a product, eating or swallowing an improperly stored product, taking medicines in the dark, stopping a drug suddenly without physician direction, transferring a drug from its original container to another, and failure to use proper protection when using a dangerous product add to the increasing probability of undesirable drug effects in the elderly. Such factors may increase the number of deaths from drug use in the elderly. Routes of exposure in order of frequency are ingestion, inhalation, ocular contamination, and dermal exposure.[22–32] The majority of poisonings that occur in persons 60 years and older are unintentional and may be amenable to poison prevention education[33] (Tables 7–21, 7–22).

Drugs

Age-related problems most often follow misuse of the benzodiazepines, barbiturates, tricyclic antidepressants, salicylates, acetaminophen, and nonbarbiturate hypnotics.[34]

Drug Interactions

Increasing drug interactions in the elderly may follow an increase in the number of drugs ingested daily, alterations in pharmacokinetics, long-term drug use, alteration in gut surface area, decrease in gastric motility, decreased gastric acid secretion, use of antacids, drugs competing for binding sites on serum albumin (Table 7–23), increase in the proportion of fat to body mass, decreased body water, reduced liver size with diminished ability to metabolize drugs,[27] less efficient renal clearance of drugs, and heightened drug receptor sensitivity, especially to cardiovascular and psychotropic drugs.[35]

Table 7–21
Physiologic Changes and Reported Pharmacokinetic Changes in Elderly Patients

Drug Factor	Physiologic Change	Clinical Effect	Example
Absorption	↓Gastric acidity	↓Absorption of various drugs	Ketoconazole Itraconazole Ferrous sulfate
	↓Small bowel surface area	Clinical relevance unknown	
	↓Blood flow to small bowel	Clinical relevance unknown	
Distribution	↑Adipose tissue and V_d of lipid-soluble drugs	↑$t_{1/2}$ of lipid-soluble drugs	Diazepam Flurazepam
	↓Total body water and V_d of water-soluble drugs	↑Serum or plasma concentration of water-soluble drugs	Ethanol
	↓Lean body mass and V_d of drugs bound to muscle	↓Loading dose required	Digoxin
	↓Plasma albumin	↓Protein-bound (inactive) drug (acidic drugs) ↑Free (active) drug	Phenytoin Warfarin
	↑Plasma α_1-acid glycoprotein	↑Protein-bound (inactive) drug (basic drugs) ↓Free (active) drug	Propranolol
Metabolism	↓Phase I hepatic metabolism	↑$t_{1/2}$ of drugs that undergo phase I metabolism	Diazepam Flurazepam
	Phase II hepatic metabolism unchanged	No change in $t_{1/2}$ of drugs that undergo phase II metabolism	Oxazepam Triazolam
Elimination	↓RPF and ↓GFR	↑$t_{1/2}$ of drugs that undergo renal elimination	Digoxin Gentamicin

GFR, glomerular filtration rate; RPF, renal plasma flow; V_d, volume of distribution.
From Chutka DS, Evans JM, Fleming KC, Mikkelson KE. Drug prescribing for elderly patients. Mayo Clin Proc 1995;70:685–693.

Table 7–22
Important Considerations in Prescribing for the Elderly

Drugs	Pharmacokinetic Considerations	Other Considerations
Analgesics		
Nonnarcotic	Aspirin may have longer duration of action and half-life may be greatly prolonged at higher doses.	Aspirin, nonsteroidal antiinflammatory agents, and acetominophen generally have equal efficacy; the last may be less toxic. Monitoring salicylate blood levels may be helpful.
Narcotic	Morphine blood levels are generally higher, and pain relief lasts longer.	Lower doses of most narcotics may give adequate analgesia and less central nervous system and respiratory depression.
Antimicrobial Agents	Penicillins (except nafcillin), aminoglycosides, cephalosporins, and tetracyclines (except doxycycline) that are eliminated predominantly by kidney may have prolonged half-lives and higher steady-state blood levels.	Monitoring aminoglycoside blood levels may be helpful. Isoniazid toxicity increases with age.
Cardiovascular Agents		
Antiarrhythmics	Lidocaine has prolonged half-life. Quinidine and procainamide have prolonged half-lives and higher steady-state blood levels.	Monitoring lidocaine, quinidine, and procainamide blood levels may be helpful. Disopyramide may have prominent anticholinergic effects, especially blurry vision and urinary retention. Lidocaine may cause confusion at high doses.
Anticoagulants		Lower doses of warfarin are needed for anticoagulation. Bleeding complications may be more frequent.
Antihypertensives		Sodium restriction and weight reduction may be effective when practical.

(continued)

Table 7-22 *(Continued)*

Drugs	Pharmacokinetic Considerations	Other Considerations
Cardiovascular Agents *(Continued)*		
Diuretics		Elderly persons are predisposed to dehydration and electrolyte imbalance. Potassium-sparing agents (or supplementation) are necessary in some persons (especially with digoxin) and may cause hyperkalemia in other persons. Thiazides and furosemide may exacerbate glucose intolerance.
Other agents	Propranolol has prolonged half-life and higher blood levels (immediate and steady-state). Metoprolol may have higher blood levels. Clonidine and methyldopa are eliminated predominantly by kidney and may have prolonged half-life.	Propranolol is often effective despite possible diminished sensitivity to cardiac effects. Incidence of adverse reactions is higher, especially in patients with heart failure, bronchospasm, bradycardia, heart block, and those on hypoglycemic agents. Hydralazine may not cause reflex tachycardia, but may exacerbate angina in some. Postural hypotension occurs in many elderly persons, even before therapy. Clonidine and prazosin usually do not cause postural hypotension with chronic therapy.
Digoxin	Digoxin may have prolonged half-life and higher steady-state blood levels	Monitoring blood levels of digoxin is helpful. Digoxin may not be effective in chronic stable heart failure with sinus rhythm.
Psychoactive Agents		
Antidepressants	Amitriptyline, imipramine, and lithium may have higher blood levels.	Desipramine has the least anticholinergic and sedative effects. Doxepin may have less cardiotoxicity. Monitoring tricyclic blood levels may be helpful. Monitoring lithium blood levels important to avoid toxicity.
Antipsychotic agents	Chlorpromazine blood levels may be higher.	Lower doses of phenothiazines and haloperidol are generally effective and safer
Sedative and hypnotic agents	Diazepam has prolonged half-life, especially in men. Oxazepam and lorazepam kinetics are unchanged, and they have shorter half-lives than other benzodiazepines.	Complaints of sleep disturbance may represent age-related changes in sleep patterns. Nonpharmacologic measures are often effective for sleep disturbances. Increased sensitivity to effects of diazepam. Flurazepam is more toxic in doses >15 mg. Chloral hydrate is generally safe and effective in doses up to 1 g. Diphenhydramine may increase confusion in some persons.
Other Drugs		
Aminophylline	Less needed by intravenous infusion for therapeutic blood levels; half-life may be prolonged.	Monitoring blood levels of aminophylline is helpful.
Cimetidine	Half-life may be prolonged and steady-state blood levels higher.	Cimetidine may cause confusion at higher doses.
Hypoglycemic agents	Eliminated predominately by kidney (except chlorpropamide); tolbutamide has shortest half-life and may be cleared more rapidiy.	Chlorpropramide may cause hyponatremia and prolonged hypoglycemia and is not generally indicated.
Levodopa		Routine doses may cause confusion and postural hypotension.
Phenytoin	Steady-state blood levels may be higher.	Monitoring blood levels of phenytoin is helpful.
Thyroxine	Metabolic clearance may be prolonged.	Maintenance dose may be lower. Thyroid-stimulating hormone level helpful in following response.

From Ouslander JG. Drug therapy in the elderly. Ann Intern Med 1981;95:711–722.

Risk Factors

1. Poor compliance resulting from both accidental (eg, chronic confusional state) and deliberate (eg, depression, altered understanding of risk–benefit) intent and cost of medication.
2. Greater use of more potent drugs (eg, cardiac glycosides) compared with other segments of the population.
3. Respiration: Physiological involution of the alveoli, smoking, asthma, malnutrition, or alcoholism may lead to life-threatening hypoxia and hypercapnia following the use of sedative drugs.
4. Cardiac conduction: A reduction in pacemaker cells, an increase in fat and connective tissue around the conduction system, and atherosclerosis of the coronary vessels can lead to arrhythmias. Tricyclic antidepressants, hydrocarbons, and other arrhythmogenic substances may be less tolerated in the elderly.
5. Circulation: Left ventricular function and vascular homeostasis may be reduced. Antihypertensive drugs and central depressants may have an increased and longer-lasting action on blood pressure and tissue perfusion.

Table 7–23
Clinical Correlations of Diminished Albumin Binding in Old Age

Acetazolamide	Hemolysis due to erythrocyte accumulation
Carbenoxolone	Sodium and water retention
Diazepam	Increased sedation (possibly also a pharmacodynamic effect)
Phenytoin	Osteomalacia, cerebellar toxicity
Warfarin	Bleeding tendency
Tolbutamide	Hypoglycemia
Salicylic acid	Gastrointestinal bleeding
Phenylbutazone	Gastrointestinal toxicity, marrow toxicity
Chlormethiazole	Sedation
Penicillin	Little effect

From Tregaskis BF, Stevenson LH. Pharmacokinetics in old age. Br Med Bull 1990;46:9–21.

Absorption

Decreased absorptive surface, prolonged gastric emptying time, decreased splanchnic blood flow, increased gastric pH, and altered gastrointestinal motility alter the oral absorption of drugs in the elderly.[36]

INFANTS AND CHILDREN

Pharmacokinetic differences observed in infants and children compared with adults are summarized in Table 7–24.[37]

TRANSCUTANEOUS DELIVERY

Currently available medications for transcutaneous delivery include clonidine hydrochloride, scopolamine, estradiol, fentanyl citrate, nitroglycerin, and nicotine. Transcutaneous delivery is being considered for use in the development of antihistamines, antiarthritics, antiaddictives, beta blockers, antiemetics, calcium channel antagonists, tranquilizers, antiasthmatics, antiretroviral agents, hormones, nonsteroidal antiinflammatory agents,[38] and centrally acting cholinergic agents.[39]

Table 7–24
Pharmacokinetics of Drugs in Children Compared With Normal Adults

	Age of Child					
	Newborn Preterm	Term (0–4 wk)	Infancy	1–4 y	5–12 y	Comments
Absorption	↓	↔	↔	↔	↔	No clinical relevance
Distribution						
Body water	↑↑↑	↑↑	↑	↑	↑	Weight-related doses produce lower blood concentrations of water-soluble drugs in the newborn
Body fat	↓↓	↓	↓ Slight	? ↔	? ↔	Minimal clinical effect
Plasma albumin	↓	↓	↓ Slight	↔	↔	Minimal clinical effect
Biotransformation						
Oxidation/ hydrolysis	↓↓↓	↓↓	↑↑ (After some weeks)	↑	↑ Slight	Reduce dosage for newborn and early infancy; increased dosage subsequently
N-Demethylation	↓↓↓	↓	↑↑	↑	↔	Applies to theophylline, caffeine
Acetylation	↓	↓	↑	↑	↔	Reduce dose in newborn, eg, sulfonamides
Conjugation–glucuronidation	↓↓	↓	↑	↑	↔	Reduce dose in newborn, eg, chloramphenicol
Renal excretion						
Glomerular filtration	↓↓	↓	↓ Slight to 6 mo	↔	↔	Reduce dose in first few months
Tubular secretion	↓↓	↓	↓	↔	↔	Reduce dose in first few months

↑, Increased; ↓, decreased; ↔, unaltered.
From Rylance GW. Prescribing for infants and children. Br Med J 1988;296:984–986.

Appendix 7–1. Glossary of Terminology Used in Clinical Toxicokinetics (Pharmacokinetics)*

A

absolute bioavailability For a drug in a dosage form administered by an extravascular route, the fraction of the administered dose that reaches the systemic circulation when the reference is the same dose of drug administered intravenously.

accumulation Increase in drug concentration in whole blood (plasma or serum) or tissue, or the amount of drug in the body, until steady state is reached.

apparent partition coefficient In vitro parameter that is the ratio of the concentrations at equilibrium between a lipoid phase (usually *n*-octanol) and an aqueous phase (usually buffer, pH 7.4). The apparent partition coefficient is uncorrected for dissociation or association in either phase.

area under the curve Concentration of drug in blood (plasma or serum) integrated over time (from zero to time *t* or to infinity) after a single dose or during a dosage interval at steady state.

B

biliary recycling See *enterohepatic recirculation.*

Bioavailability Defined in terms of the relative amount of drug that enters the systemic circulation from an administered dosage form and the rate at which the drug appears in systemic circulation.

bioequivalence Bioequivalence of a drug product is achieved if its extent and rate of absorption (bioavailability) are not substantially different from those of the standard when administered at the same molar dose.

bioequivalence requirement Guide for in vitro and/or in vivo testing of specific drug products that must be satisfied as a condition of marketing.

biological half-life See *elimination half-life.*

biopharmaceutics Physical and chemical properties of a drug, its additives, and its dosage form, and the biological effectiveness of a drug and/or drug product on administration.

biophase Immediate environment surrounding the site of action of a drug in the body.

blood flow Rate of blood perfusion of an organ.

*Adapted from Allen L, Kimura K, Mackichan J, Ritschel WA. Ad Hoc Committee for Pharmacokinetic Nomenclature, American College of Clinical Pharmacology. J Clin Pharmacol 1982;22(suppl.):S3–S6.

C

central compartment Sum of all body regions (organs, tissues, fluids) in which the drug concentration approaches immediate equilibrium with that in blood, plasma, or serum.

chronopharmacokinetics Study of pharmacokinetic drug parameters as affected by circadian rhythm or diurnal variation. Circadian rhythm is affected by endogenous factors, whereas diurnal variation is affected by external synchronizers (Zeitgeber).

clearance Ratio of the overall elimination rate of a drug to its concentration in the reference fluid (ie, plasma). Under steady-state conditions, clearance relates systematically available dose rate (ie, maintenance dose per dosage interval) to the average steady-state concentration of drug in a specified biological fluid. It must be defined according to site of measurement (ie, blood, plasma, plasma water). See *hepatic clearance, renal clearance* or *total clearance.*

clinical pharmacokinetics Application of pharmacokinetic principles to the safe and effective drug therapy of individual patients.

compartment Mathematical entity that can be described by a volume (not necessarily physiologic) and its drug concentration.

concentration Measured amount of drug or metabolite per unit volume of any biological fluid.

creatinine clearance Ratio of the excretion rate of creatinine in urine to the concentration of creatinine in plasma or serum. It is used as a measure of renal function (glomerular filtration rate).

cumulative urinary excretion curves Plots of the cumulative amounts of drug and/or its metabolites excreted into urine versus time after administration of a drug by various routes of administration.

D

disposition All the processes and factors that are involved from the time the drug reaches the circulation to the time when it, or one or more of its metabolites, leaves the body in the urine, feces, bile, expired air, or sweat.

dosage regimen or **dose rate** Dose and dosage interval required to produce clinical effectiveness or to maintain a therapeutic concentration in the body.

dose Amount of drug administered.

dose or **concentration dependency** Change in one or more of the pharmacokinetic processes of absorption, distribution, metabolism, and excretion with changing dose or concentration.

dose–response curve Graphic presentation of the pharmacologic or clinical effectiveness or toxicity (ie, response) versus dose.

dosing interval Time between doses.

drug Substance of synthetic, semisynthetic, natural, or biological origin that prevents, cures, or reduces disease or distress in humans or animals. The effects may be quantified.

drug product or **dosage form** Final pharmaceutical form containing the active ingredient(s) (drug[s]) and vehicle substances necessary in formulating a medicament of desired dosage, desired volume, and desired application form, ready for administration.

drug release or **liberation** Delivery of the active ingredient from a dosage form into solution. The dissolution medium is either a biological fluid (ie, gastric contents) or an artificial test fluid. Drug release is characterized by the speed (dissolution rate constant) and amount of drug in solution.

E

elimination half-life Time necessary to decrease the drug concentration in the blood (plasma or serum) to one half during the elimination phase. It is determined by volume of distribution and total body clearance. It may or may not agree with therapeutic or response half-life.

enterohepatic recirculation Phenomenon in which drugs emptied via bile into the small intestine can be reabsorbed from the intestinal lumen into systemic circulation.

enzyme induction Increase in enzyme content (activity or amount) that may result in faster metabolism of a compound.

enzyme inhibition Decrease in rate of metabolism of a compound (usually by competition) by an enzyme system.

excretion Final elimination of drug from the body's systemic circulation into urine, feces, sweat, air, milk, and so on.

extraction ratio Ratio of organ clearance (ie, hepatic, renal) to blood or plasma flow through the organ.

extravascular administration In pharmacokinetics, all routes of administration except those where the drug is directly introduced into the bloodstream.

Examples of extravascular routes are intramuscular (IM), subcutaneous (SC), peroral (PO), oral, rectal intraperitoneal (IP), and topical, where absolute availability must be considered.

F

feathering Graphic method for obtaining individual exponential slopes (gl) from a polyexponential curve. The term *residual method for curve stripping* is synonymous with feathering.

first-pass effect Phenomenon whereby drugs may be metabolized (not chemically degraded) following absorption but before reaching systemic circulation. Hepatic first-pass effect may occur following peroral and deep rectal administration. It may be avoided by using sublingual and buccal routes of drug administration. Pulmonary first-pass effect cannot be avoided by intravenous buccal or sublingual routes.

flip–flop model Phenomenon whereby the rate constant of input is much smaller than the rate constant of output. This is usually observed when the rate constant of absorption is smaller than the rate constant of elimination.

G

generic product Drug product marketed under the nonproprietary or common name of the drug(s).

H

hepatic clearance Rate of total body clearance accounted for by the liver. The magnitude depends on intrinsic hepatic clearance, fraction of unbound drug in blood, and liver blood flow.

hybrid rate constants Composite rate constants consisting of two or more microconstants. gl (alpha, beta) is a hybrid rate constant, sometimes referred to as an eigenvalue.

I

intravascular administration In pharmacokinetics, all routes of administration where the drug is directly introduced into the bloodstream: intravenous (IV), intraarterial, intracardiac. Bioavailability = 100%, $f = 1$.

intrinsic clearance Theoretical unrestricted maximum clearance of unbound drug by an eliminating organ.

intravenous bolus In common usage, rapid intravenous administration (ie, intravenous injection). Technically, it is a misnomer, a bolus (Greek *bolos* meaning "bite") being something that is swallowed.

L

lag time Interval between drug administration and drug concentration measurable in blood, or the time (other than zero) when the polyexponential function describing the concentration–time relationship commences. Lag times are often found on peroral administration and result from slow disintegration and dissolution of tablets or capsules or delayed gastric emptying.

lean body weight Body weight minus fat mass.

levels (blood, serum, plasma) See *concentration.*

loading dose or **priming dose** Dose used in initiating therapy; usually larger than the maintenance dose and used to provide rapid therapeutic concentrations. The need for a loading dose depends on elimination half-life, dosage interval, and therapeutic concentration to be achieved.

M

maintenance dose Dose required to maintain clinical effectiveness or a therapeutic concentration. It is determined by drug clearance, distribution volume, elimination rate, desired steady-state concentration, and desired therapeutic effectiveness of the drug.

Michaelis–Menten kinetics Certain nonlinear or saturable processes usually involving enzymatic reactions.

microconstants Rate constants of a hypothetical pharmacokinetic model. Hybrid constants are composed of individual microconstants.

multiple-dose administration Use of repeated single doses. It may result in accumulation when a drug is given repeatedly at intervals shorter than those required to eliminate the previously given dose.

N

nonlinear kinetics or **saturation kinetics** The rate of the process is not directly proportional to the concentration, as it is in first-order kinetics. These processes may be described by Michaelis–Menten kinetics, Langmuir equation, and so on.

O

oral administration Strictly speaking, includes buccal, sublingual, and perlingual administration routes where the drug is adsorbed from the mouth cavity (no first-pass effect). Not to be confused with *peroral (PO).*

P

peripheral compartment Sum of all body regions (ie, organs, tissues, or parts of them) to which a drug eventually distributes, but is not in immediate equilibrium with central compartment. The peripheral compartment is sometimes further subdivided into shallow and deep compartments.

peroral administration (PO, per os) Indicates that the dosage form is swallowed and the drug is absorbed from the gastrointestinal tract (first-pass effect possible). Not all drugs are absorbed such as charcoal, kaolin, and some antacids. See *oral administration.*

protein binding Phenomenon that occurs when a drug combines with plasma or tissue protein. It is the unbound drug that is in equilibrium with the biophase.

R

rate-limiting step Process with the slowest rate constant in a system of sequential kinetic processes. If rate constants are nearly identical, then identification of the rate-limiting step may be difficult.

relative bioavailability Term used to indicate both the relative amounts of a drug that reach the general circulation unchanged and the relative rates of appearance of a drug administered to the same subjects or patients in two or more different dosage forms by the same or two different extravascular routes.

relative dosage interval For a specified dosage regimen, the variable period between closely spaced multiple doses given at irregular intervals.

renal clearance Rate of total body clearance accounted for by the kidney. Its magnitude is determined by the net effects of glomerular filtration, tubular secretion and reabsorption, blood flow, and protein binding.

S

single or repeated single-dose administration Does not result kinetically in accumulation. See *maintenance dose.*

steady state Strictly speaking, this is achieved only during constant rate infusion when input and output are equal. The steady-state drug concentrations during multiple-dose administration fluctuate (oscillate) between a maximum (peak) and a minimum (trough) steady-state concentration within each dosage interval.

T

total clearance Usually, the sum of individual clearances of eliminating organs. See *hepatic clearance* and *renal clearance.*

toxicokinetics Deals mathematically with the changes in drug and/or metabolite concentration in the human or animal body after administration.

V

volume of distribution Not a "real" volume, but a hypothetical volume of body fluid that would be required to dissolve the total amount of drug at the same concentration as that found in the blood or plasma. It is a proportionality constant relating the amount of drug in the body to the measured concentration in biological fluid (blood, plasma, plasma water).

REFERENCES

1. Barre J, Didey F, Delion F, Tillement JP. Problems in therapeutic drug monitoring: Free drug level monitoring. Ther Drug Monit 1988;10:133–143.
2. Sue Y-J, Shannon M. Pharmacokinetics of drugs in overdose. Clin Pharmacokinet 1992;23:93–105.
3. Atkinson AJ, Krumlovsky FA, Huang CM, del Greco F. Hemodialysis for severe procainamide toxicity: Clinical and pharmacokinetic observations. Clin Pharmacol Ther 1976;20:585–592.
4. Levy G, Yaffe SJ. Relationship between dose and apparent volume of distribution in children. Pediatrics 1974;54:713–717.
5. Watkins PB. Drug metabolism by cytochromes P450 in the liver and small bowel. Gastroenterol Clin North Am 1992;21:511–526.
6. Murray M. P450 enzymes: Inhibition mechanisms, genetic regulation and effects of liver disease. Clin Pharmacokinet 1992;23:132–141.
7. Kyriakopoulus AA, Greenblatt DJ, Schader RI. Clinical pharmacokinetics of lorazepam: A review. J Clin Psychiatry 1978;39:16–23.
8. Cholerton S, Daly AK, Idle JR. The role of individual human cytochromes P450 in drug metabolism and clinical response. Trends Pharmacol Sci 1992;13:435.
9. Caporaso NE, Shaw GL. Clinical implications of the competitive inhibition of the debrisoquine-metabolizing isozyme by quinidine. Arch Intern Med 1991;151:1985–1992.
10. Otton SV, Wu D, Joffe RT, et al. Inhibition by fluoxetine of cytochrome P450 2D6 activity. Clin Pharmacol Ther 1993;53:401–409.
11. Waller DG, George CF. Prodrugs. Br J Clin Pharmacol 1989;28:497–507.
12. Mazze RI. Metabolism of the inhaled anaesthetics: Implications of enzyme induction. Br J Anaesth 1984;56:365.
13. Cohen GM. Pulmonary metabolism of foreign compounds: Its role in metabolic activation. Environ Health Perspect 1990;85:31–41.
14. Macleod CM. Clinical implications of drug metabolism: Toxic metabolites. Res Staff Phys 1992;38:78.
15. Aronson JK. Receptors and their relevance to drug therapy. Med Int (Israel Edition) 1989;59:2429–2435.
16. Poitrast BJ, Keller WC, Elves RG. Estimation of chemical hazards in breast milk: Aviat Space Environ Med 1988;59(11, suppl.):A87–A92.
17. Committee on Drugs, American Academy of Pediatrics, Roberts RJ, Chairman. Transfer of drugs and other chemicals into breast milk. Pediatrics 1989;84:924–936.
18. Atkinson HC, Begg EJ, Darlow BA. Drugs in human milk: Clinical pharmacokinetic considerations. Clin Pharmacokinet 1988;14:217–240.
19. Giroux D, LaPointe G, Baril M. Toxicological index and the presence in the workplace of chemical hazards for workers who breast-feed infants. Am Ind Hyg Assoc J 1992;53:471–474.
20. Paul M, Himmelstein J. Reproductive hazards in the workplace: What the practitioner needs to know about chemical resources. Obstet Gynecol 1988;7:921–938.
21. Brodie MJ, Feely J. Adverse drug interactions. Br Med J 1988;29:845–849.
22. Dean BS, Krenzelok EP. Poisoning in the elderly: An increasing problem for health care providers. Clin Toxicol 1987;25:411–418.
23. Woolf A, Fish S, Azzara C, Dean D. Serious poisonings among older adults: A study of hospitalization and mortality rates in Massachusetts 1983–1985. Am J Pub Health 1990;8:867–869.
24. Dawling S, Crome P. Clinical pharmacokinetic considerations in the elderly: An update. Clin Pharmacokinet 1989;17:236–263.
25. Owens NJ, Silliman RA, Fretwell MD. The relationship between comprehensive functional assessment and optimal pharmacotherapy in the older patient. DICP Ann Pharmacother 1989;23:847–854.
26. Durnas C, Loi C-M, Cusack BJ. Hepatic drug metabolism and aging. Clin Pharmacokinet 1990;19:359–389.
27. Baldwin JG. Hematopoietic function in the elderly. Arch Intern Med 1988;148:2544–2546.
28. Need we poison the elderly so often. Lancet 1988;2:20–22. Editorial.
29. Vestal RE. Geriatric clinical pharmacology: An overview. In: Vestal RE, ed. *Drug Treatment in the Elderly.* Sydney: ADIS Health Science Press, 1984:12–29.
30. Everitt DE, Avorn J. Drug prescribing for the elderly. Arch Intern Med 1986;146:2393–2396.
31. Ramsay LE, Tucker GT. Clinical pharmacology: Drugs and the elderly. Br Med J 1981;282:125–127.
32. Loi C-M, Vestal ER. Drug metabolism in the elderly. Pharmacol Ther 1988;36:131–149.
33. Kroner BA, Scott RB, Waring ER, Zanga JR. Poisoning in the elderly: Characterization of exposures reported to a poison control center. J Am Geriatr Soc 1993;41:482–486.
34. Flanagan RJ, Caldwell R, Lewis RR, Corless D. Toxicological investigations in the detection of drug-induced decrease in elderly patients. Hum Toxicol 1983;2:371–380.
35. Cadieux RJ. Drug interactions in the elderly: How multiple drug use increases risk exponentially. Postgrad Med 1989;86:179–184.
36. Stevenson IH. Susceptibility of different age groups to toxic damage. In: Volans GN, Sims J, Sullivan FM, Turner P, eds. *Basic Science in Toxicology.* London: Taylor & Francis, 1990:406.
37. Rylance GW. Prescribing for infants and children. Br Med J 1988;296:984–986.
38. Graham R. Transdermal non-steroidal antiinflammatory agents. Br J Clin Pract 1995;49:33–35.
39. Berti JJ, Lipsky JJ. Transcutaneous drug delivery: A practical review. Mayo Clin Proc 1995;70:581–586.

GENERAL REVIEW ARTICLES

Toxicokinetics

Allen L, Kimura K, MacKickin J, Ritschel WA. Manual of symbols, equations and definitions in pharmacokinetics. J Clin Pharmacol 1982;22(suppl.):3S–23S.

Done AK. Helpful half-life. Emerg Med 1977;9(1):211–220. Everything you've always wanted to know about pharmacokinetics but were afraid to ask. Emerg Med 1978;10(6):67–69, 75–76,81. Acid-base disturbances: Aids to evaluation. Emerg Med 1981;13(15):159–171. Acid-base disturbances: Aids to differential diagnosis. Emerg Med 1981;13(17):68–86. Ion trapping in the pathogenesis and treatment of poisoning. Vet Hum Toxicol 1980;22(suppl.):2–9.

George CF. Disease of the alimentary system: Absorption, distribution and metabolism of drugs; effects of disease of the gut. Br Med J 1976;2:742–744.

Gibaldi M, Perrier D. *Pharmacokinetics.* New York: Marcel Dekker, 1982.

Gibaldi M, Levy G. Pharmacokinetics in clinical practice: I. Concepts. JAMA 1976;235:1864–1867; II. JAMA 1976;235:1987–1992.

Greenblatt DJ, Koch-Weser J. Clinical pharmacokinetics. Part I. N Engl J Med 1975;293:702–705; Part II. N Engl J Med 1975;293:963–969.

Mills KC. Essential emergency medicine pharmacokinetics: Prevention of iatrogenic patient poisoning. Top Emerg Med 1993;15:18–29.

Nelson E. Kinetics of drug absorption, distribution, metabolism and excretion. J Pharm Sci 1961;50:181–192.

O'Reilly WJ. Pharmacokinetics in drug metabolism and toxicology. Can J Pharm Sci 1972;7:66–77.

Paxton JW. Pharmacokinetics. NZ Med J 1982;95:150–153.

Sue Y-J, Shannon M. Pharmacokinetics of drugs in overdose. Clin Pharmacokinet 1992;23:93–105.

Wagner JG. Pharmacokinetics. Annu Rev Pharmacol 1968;8:67–94.

Wilkinson GR. Pharmacokinetics of drug disposition: Hemodynamic considerations. Annu Rev Pharmacol 1975;15:11–27.

Apparent Volume of Distribution

Benet LZ, Ronfeld RA. Volume terms in pharmacokinetics. J Pharm Sci 1969;58:639–641.

Gibaldi M, Nagashima R, Levy G. Relationship between drug concentration in plasma or serum and amount of drug in the body. J Pharm Sci 1969;58:193–197.

Niazi S. Volume of distribution as a function of time. J Pharm Sci 1976;65:452–454.

Riegelman S, Loo J, Rowland M. Concept of a volume of distribution and possible errors in evaluation of this parameter. J Pharm Sci 1968;57:128–133.

Clearance Concepts

George CF. Drug kinetics and hepatic blood flow. Clin Pharmacokinet 1979;4:433–448.

Lalka D, Griffith RK, Cronemberger CL. The hepatic first-pass metabolism of problematic drugs. J Clin Pharmacol 1993;33:657–669.

Nies AS, Shand DG, Wilkinson GR. Altered hepatic blood flow and drug disposition. Clin Pharmacokinet 1976;1:135–155.

Rowland M, Benet LZ, Graham GG. Clearance concepts in pharmacokinetics. J Pharmacokinet Biopharm 1973;1:123–136.

Weigand UW, Levy G. Hepatic extraction of endogenous inhibitors of plasma protein binding. J Pharm Sci 1980;69:480–481.

Wilkinson GR, Shand DG. Presystemic hepatic elimination. Acta Pharm Suec 1974;11:648–649.

Half-life

Gibaldi M, Weintraub H. Some considerations as to the determination and significance of biologic half-life. J Pharm Sci 1971;60:624–626.

Wagner JG. Intrasubject variation in elimination half-lives of drugs which are appreciably metabolized. J Pharmacokinet Biopharm 1973;1:165–173.

Urinary Excretion Data

Garrett ER. Pharmacokinetics and clearances related to renal processes. Int J Clin Pharmacol 1978;16:155–172.

Levy G. Effect of plasma protein binding on renal clearance of drugs. J Pharm Sci 1980;69:482–483.

Martin BK. Treatment of data from drug urinary excretion. Nature 1967;56:489–494.

Niebergall PJ, et al. Rapid methods for bioavailability determination utilizing urinary excretion data. J Pharm Sci 1975;64:1721–1722.

Wagner JG. Method for estimating rate constants for absorption, metabolism and elimination from urinary excretion data. J Pharm Sci 1967;56:489–494.

Intravenous Infusion Pharmacokinetics

Kruger-Thiemer E. Continuous intravenous infusion and multicompartment accumulation. Eur J Pharmacol 1968;4:317–324.

Loo JCK, Riegelman S. Assessment of pharmacokinetic constants from post infusion blood curves obtained after IV infusion. J Pharm Sci 1970;59:53–55.

Bioavailability

Azarnoff DL, Huffman DH. Therapeutic implications of bioavailability. Annu Rev Pharmacol Toxicol 1976;16:53–66.

Food and Drug Administration. Drug product bioequivalence requirements and in vivo bioavailability procedures. Fed Regist 1977;42:1624–1653.

Guidelines for biopharmaceutical studies in man. Washington, DC: APHA Academy of Pharmaceutical Sciences, 1972.

Koch-Weser J. Bioavailability of drugs. N Engl J Med (first of two parts) 1974;291:233–236; (second of two parts) 1974;291:503–508.

Ritschel WA. Bioavailability in the clinical evaluation of drugs. Drug Intell Clin Pharm 1972;6:246–256.

Wagner JG. Method of estimating relative absorption of a drug in a series of clinical studies in which blood levels are measured after single and/or multiple doses. J Pharm Sci 1967;56:652–653.

Wagner JG. Design of clinical studies to assess physiological availability. Drug Info Bull 1969;3:45–52.

The Elderly

Feinberg M. The problems of anticholinergic side effects in older patients. Drugs Aging 1993;3:335–348.

Kroner BA, Scott RB, Waring ER, Zanga JR. Poisoning in the elderly: Characterization of exposures reported to a poison center. J Am Geriatr Soc 1993;41:842–846.

Metabolite Pharmacokinetics

Adverse Drug Interaction Program. New Rochelle, NY: The Medical Letter, 1993.

Alvares AP, Kappas A, Eiseman JL, et al. Intraindividual variation in drug disposition. Clin Pharmacol Ther 1979;26:407–419.

Gillette JR. Factors affecting drug metabolism. Ann NY Acad Sci 1971;179:43–66.

Gonzalez FJ, Gelboin HV. Role of human cytochromes P450 in the metabolic activation of chemical carcinogens and toxins. Drug Metab Rev 1994;26:165–183.

Halpert JR, Guengerich FP, Bend JR, Correia MA. Selective inhibitors of cytochrome P450. Toxicol Appl Pharmacol 1994;125:163–175.

Koymans L, D-O de Kelder GM, Koppele TE, JM Vermeulen NPE. Cytochrome P450: Their active-silt structure and mechanisms of oxidation. Drug Metab Rev 1993;25:325–385.

Pang KS, Gillette JR. Metabolite pharmacokinetics: Methods for simultaneous estimates of elimination rate constants of a drug and its metabolites. Drug Metab Dispos 1980;8:39–43.

Watkins PB. Drug metabolism by cytochromes P450 in the liver and small bowel. Gastroenterol Clin North Am 1992;21:511–526.

Wrighton SA, Stevens JC. The human hepatic cytochromes P450 involved in drug metabolism. Crit Rev Toxicol 1992;22:1–21.

Drug Interactions

Adverse interactions of drugs. Med Lett Drugs Ther 1981;23(5):17–28.

Drug interactions update. Med Lett Drugs Ther 1984;26(654):11–14.

Gillette JR, Pang KS. Theoretic aspects of pharmacokinetic drug interactions. Clin Pharmacol Ther 1977;22:623–639.

Levy G. Pharmacokinetic approaches to the study of drug interactions. Ann NY Acad Sci 1976;281:24–39.

Luecke RH, Wosilait WE. Drug elimination interactions: Analysis using a mathematical model. J Pharmacokinet Biopharm 1979;7:629–641.

Chapter 8
The Pregnant Patient

INTRODUCTION

Probabilities of relationships between chemical teratogens and fetal abnormalities are summarized in Table 8–1.[1] There have been, to date, no systematic studies of the toxicokinetics of the overdosed pregnant woman.[2]

TRANSPLACENTAL PASSAGE OF DRUGS

The placental exchange surface can be thought of as a "lipoid barrier."[3] Substances that are highly lipid soluble tend to diffuse easily in a transcellular manner across the exchange membrane. In contrast, hydrophilic (water-soluble) substances are transferred poorly. Drugs having the properties of high lipid solubility, low ionization under physiologic conditions, and relatively low molecular mass (<1000 daltons) will demonstrate rapid and extensive transfer. Examples of such drugs include most barbiturates, digoxin, phenytoins, ritodrine, and magnesium sulfate. Compounds that are hydrophilic, highly ionized, or of more substantial molecular weight (>1000 daltons) will have a much more limited rate and extent of placental transfer. Examples of such drugs are heparin (essentially "excluded" from exchange by its high molecular weight of approximately 1200 daltons), quaternary ammonium compounds such as tubocurare and succinylcholine (whose exchanges are profoundly limited by their high levels of ionization and water solubility), and erythromycin (exchange limited by high molecular weight and water solubility).

DRUG TOXICITY

A cytogenetic investigation of self-poisoning in pregnant women and self-poisoned nonpregnant women suggests that chromatid-type and unstable chromosome-type aberrations appear to increase in the blood cells of pregnant women who attempted suicide by self-poisoning.[4] The frequency of chromatid aberrations in pregnant women relative to nonpregnant women is lower, suggesting a possible protective effect of pregnancy.[4]

Table 8–1
Relationship of Chemical Teratogens to Fetal Abnormalities

Effect	Compound
Definite relationship	Alcohol
	Diphenylhydantoin
	Folic acid antagonists
	Inorganic iodides
	Lithium
	Organic mercury
	Retinoids: vitamin A, isotretinoin (Accutane)
	Sex steroids (including diethylstilbestrol)
	Streptomycin
	Tetracyclines
	Thalidomide
	Thiourea compounds
	Trimethadione
	Warfarin
Probable relationship	Alkylating agents
	Chlorobiphenyls
	Diazepam
	Kanamycin
Questionable relationship	Amphetamines
	Chlordiazepoxide
	Climiphene
	Diphenhydramine
	Ethionamide
	General anesthesia (chronic exposure)
	Gonadotropins
	Haloperidol
	Lysergic acid diethylamide (LSD)
	Meprobamate
	Metronidazole
	Oral hypoglycemic agents
	Penicillamine
	Phenothiazines
	Quinine
	Cigarette smoking
No relationship	Bendectin
	Corticosteroids
	General anesthesia (short-term exposure)
	Heparin
	Isoniazid
	Meclizine
	Penicillin
	Spermicides
	Sulfonamides

From Longo LD. Physiologic assessment of fetal compromise: Biomarkers of toxic exposure. Environ Health Perspect 1987;74:93–101.

ACETAMINOPHEN

Management of the pregnant patient with an acetaminophen overdose should not be different from that of the nonpregnant individual (stabilization, supportive care, gastrointestinal decontamination, *N*-acetylcysteine). If the mother is at risk, *N*-acetylcysteine should not be withheld. The dosage and indications for *N*-acetylcysteine use in newborns have not been established. If the acetaminophen overdose is uncomplicated and the pregnant mother has a viable fetus, immediate delivery should be done only for maternal indications or documented fetal distress.[5–7] Acetaminophen overdose in itself is not an indication for termination of pregnancy.

ANGIOTENSIN-CONVERTING ENZYME INHIBITORS

Fatal anuria, renal tubular dysgenesis, fetal renal malfunction, and acute renal failure has been reported in babies whose mothers have been treated with angiotensin-converting enzyme inhibitors during pregnancy.[8]

ANTIMICROBIAL AGENTS

Wise has summarized data on the relationship between antimicrobial agents (Table 8–2)[7] and pregnancy. Other reviews do not substantially differ.[9,10]

Ofloxacin

Ofloxacin was administered to a 36-year-old woman for 6 days during the 19th week of gestation. The neonate's physical examination and radiographs of the chest and long bones were normal.[11]

Penicillin

Methicillin and ampicillin are effectively transferred across the placenta, but dicloxacillin is not.[7] An anaphylactic response to ampicillin by a pregnant woman at term led to an infant born by caesarean section with metabolic acidosis and Apgar scores of 3, 6, and 7 at 1, 5, and 10 minutes, respectively. Multiform clonic seizures developed. Pronounced neurologic abnormalities were evident at age 6 months. Drugs with the potential to produce anaphylactic reactions should be given with caution to women at term. Intensive fetal monitoring in an anaphylactic reaction is necessary to allow rapid delivery of the newborn if possible.[12] Excretion of penicillins in human milk is usually very limited. Following therapeutic doses, the mean milk concentrations in one study were of 0.4 to 0.6 μg/mL for amoxicillin about 0.5 μg/mL for sulbactam, 2 to 25 μg/mL for ticarcillin, and 0.14 to 0.4 μg/mL for aztreonam.[13]

ANTITHROMBOTIC AGENTS

A recent review of current evidence regarding the safety of antithrombotic agents in pregnancy concludes that[14] heparin is probably safe for the fetus, but oral anticoagulants may not be, especially in the first trimester. Warfarin may be associated with congenital abnormalities. Heparin may cause a persistent anticoagulant effect at the time of delivery, increasing the risk of maternal bleeding. Thus, heparin should be stopped 24 hours before elective induction of labor. The risk of symptomatic fractures is low with heparin, but a subclinical reduction in bone density may occur with long-term therapy. Heparin can be safely given to mothers who are breastfeeding. It is not secreted in breast milk. Heparin is the anticoagulant of choice during pregnancy for indications in which its efficacy is established.

Warfarin also does not appear to induce an anticoagulant effect in the breastfed infant. Low-dose aspirin (<150 mg/dL) during the second and third trimesters appears to be

Table 8–2
Antimicrobial Agents and Their Possible Adverse Effects During Pregnancy

Agent	Use	Adverse Effects on the Fetus: First Trimester	Adverse Effects on the Fetus: Second and Third Trimesters	Comments
Penicillin (benzylpenicillin and phenoxymethylpenicillin)	Probably safe		Allergy; possibility of sensitizing the fetus	All the more common beta-lactams may be described as safe
Long-acting penicillins	Probably safe		Allergy; possibility of sensitizing the fetus	Little information available but no suggestion of increased toxicity
Ampicillin	Probably safe		Allergy; possibility of sensitizing the fetus	
Ampicillin prodrugs: talampicillin, pivampicillin, bacampicillin				Little information available, reasonable to avoid prodrug formulation and use the parent ampicillin
Amoxicillin	Probably safe		Allergy; possibility of sensitizing the fetus	
Amoxicillin and clavulanic acid (Augmentin)	Probably safe		Allergy; possibility of sensitizing the fetus	Little information available; best avoid until more experience reported.
Antipseudomonal penicillins: carbenicillin, mezlocillin, azlocillin, ticarcillin, piperacillin	Probably safe		Allergy; possibility of sensitizing the fetus	Little information available; reserve for treatment of infections caused by susceptible bacteria
Mecillinam	Probably safe		Allergy; possibility of sensitizing the fetus	Little information available; reserve for treatment of serious infections caused by susceptible bacteria
Antistaphylococcal penicillins: flucloxacillin and cloxacillin	Probably safe		Allergy; possibility of sensitizing the fetus	
Cephalosporins				
Oral: cephalexin, cefaclor, cephradine	Probably safe		Allergy; possibility of sensitizing the fetus	Little information available
Injectable	Probably safe		Allergy; possibility of sensitizing the fetus	Little information available. These agents are probably safe and might well be reasonable choices in treatment of severe infection. Agents containing *N*-methyltetrazole sidechains should be avoided on theoretical grounds, that is, they may interfere with vitamin K metabolism (latomoxef and cefamandole in the United Kingdom).
Sulfonamides				
All agents	Probably safe in first trimester; avoid within 2d of delivery		Avoid (within two days of delivery), kernicterus	Risk is greater for more highly protein bound agents, such as sulfafurazole, rather than sulfamethoxazole
Trimethoprim	Probably safe			Theoretical tetratogenic risk of folic acid antagonist; risk of megaloblastic anemia preventable by folinic acid

From Wise R. Prescribing in pregnancy: Antibiotics. Br Med J 1987;294:42–46.

(continued)

Table 8–2 *(Continued)*

Agent	Use	Adverse Effects on the Fetus: First Trimester	Adverse Effects on the Fetus: Second and Third Trimesters	Comments
Co-trimoxazole (trimethoprim and sulfamethoxazole)	Probably safe (but see sulfonamide above)		Kernicterus	Considerable experience of safety in first trimester
Tetracyclines: all agents	Avoid		Discoloration and dysplasia of teeth and bones, cataracts	Possible hepatotoxicity in mother
Aminoglycosides				
Streptomycin	Avoid		Ototoxicity	Little reason to be used; a better choice can be made in tuberculosis and serious sepsis
Gentamicin, tobramycin, netilmicin, amikacin	Caution		Theoretical risk of ototoxicity suggested	Effective in serious sepsis; regular assay required
Spectinomycin	Probably safe			Reserve for treatment of gonorrhea when penicilin resistance or allergy is a problem
Fusidic acid	Probably safe			
Quinolone; nalidixic acid	Caution			Deposition in growing bones of animals; interferes with bacterial DNA; theoretical risk to humans
Recently developed drugs: ciprofloxacin, norfloxacin, enoxacin, ofloxacin, pefloxacin	Avoid			No experience in pregnancy—see quinolones
Nitrofurantoin	Probably safe			Theoretical risk of hemolysis in glucose-6-phosphate dehydrogenase deficiency
Vancomycin	Caution			Safety data not available in humans; reserve for treatment of serious staphylococcal sepsis
Macrolides and lincosamides				
Erythromycin base/stearate	Probably safe			
Erythromycin estolate	Avoid			Maternal hepatoxicity in late pregnancy
Lincomycin and clindamycin	Avoid			Maternal pseudomembranous colitis; avoid unless no other suitable agent available
Metronidazole	Caution	Theoretical risk of teratogenesis		No evidence of teratogenicity in humans; benefit will probably outweigh risk in serious anaerobic sepsis
Chloramphenicol	Avoid		Gray baby syndrome	Little evidence of ill effect to fetus in early pregnancy; remember possible maternal blood dyscrasias; usually a safer choice can be made
Antituberculous agents				
Rifampicin	Caution		Postnatal bleeding	Avoid in mothers with liver disease; high-dosage teratogenicity in animals; benefits probably outweigh risks; vitamin K should be given to mother and neonate

Table 8–2 *(Continued)*

Agent	Use	Adverse Effects on the Fetus: First Trimester	Adverse Effects on the Fetus: Second and Third Trimesters	Comments
Antituberculous agents *(Continued)*				
Isoniazid	Probably safe			
Ethambutol	Probably safe			Observe mother for jaundice
para-Aminosalicylic acid	Probably safe			Now little used
Pyrazinamide	Caution			Little information available
Antifungal agents				
Amphotericin	Caution			
Flucytosine	Avoid	Teratogenic in animals		
Miconazole	Caution			Absorbed from vaginal topical use
Griseofulvin	Avoid	Teratogenic in animals		
Nystatin (topical)	Probably safe			
Antimalarial drugs				
Chloroquine	Probably safe			Safety established in low dose, except for rare reports of hearing loss in children
Quinine	Avoid	Possible abortifacient		
Proguanil	Probably safe			
Pyrimethamine and dapsone (Maloprim)	Avoid			Teratogenicity reported in rats, but no convincing evidence in humans; Maloprim and Fansidar have been associated with fatalities
Pyrimethamine and sulfadoxine (Fansidar)	Avoid			
Primaquine	Avoid			
Antiparasitic agents				
Piperazine	Probably safe			
Mebendazole	Avoid	Possibly teratogenic		
Thiabendazole	Caution			Safety not established
Praziquantel	Caution			Safety not established
Antiviral agents				
Amantadine	Avoid	Embryotoxic in animals		Unless there is a life-threatening infection in the mother it is probably best to avoid antiviral agents in pregnancy
Acyclovir	Caution	Theoretical risk		
Vidarabine	Avoid	Teratogenic in animals		

safe, but the safety of aspirin in higher doses or when taken in the first trimester is still questionable.

BENZODIAZEPINES

An anecdotal report indicates that pregnant women in their second trimester (weeks 20, 22, 22, and 23) and one in the third trimester (week 35) inadvertently received about 10 g of a benzodiazepine (not specifically defined) orally in one dose. The four women in the second trimester vomited part of the dose after ingestion. There was no loss of consciousness. They were discharged in 24 hours. Urine benzodiazepine levels were negative in 4 to 6 weeks. The fetus remained normal. The patient in the third trimester did not vomit, developed respiratory depression with bronchospasm, was provided assisted ventilation in the intensive care unit, and recovered after 5 days of severe drowsiness. The fetus was later assessed as normal. The mother's urine remained positive for benzodiazepine until delivery. All infants were delivered at term, had normal Apgar scores, were morphologically normal, had no apparent deficiency in psychomotor development, and were normal at age 6 months.[15]

BETA BLOCKERS

Beta blockers, frequently cardioselective, have been widely used for the treatment of pregnancy-induced hypertension.

Adverse reactions are believed to be rare and the effects on the fetus or infant have been thought to be minimal.[16,17] Labetalol, given to a mother because of pregnancy-induced hypertension, appeared to induce bradycardia, diminished femoral pulses, a bluish color, and inadequate breathing in a premature infant of 33 weeks' gestational age who was delivered by cesarean section.[16]

CAFFEINE

Pregnancy/Lactation

One retrospective study and one prospective study suggest that women who consume more than one cup of coffee per day are less likely to become pregnant.[19,20] These observations require further validation. Caffeine readily crosses the placenta. The enzyme or enzymes necessary to metabolize caffeine are absent until several days after birth.[21] Fetal arrhythmia may follow excessive intake of caffeine by the mother during pregnancy (200–1800 mg/d).[22]

The Infant

Chronic maternal ingestion of caffeine during pregnancy may lead to neonates who display symptoms of tremulousness (jitteriness), nonbilious vomiting, irritability, intermittent bradycardia, tachypnea, and periodic breathing which can last 38 to 168 hours. The infant's serum caffeine levels may range from 0 to 2.0 ng/L at 13 to 124 hours.[23] There is no definitive evidence of an increase in risk of the more common congenital malformations with moderate caffeine ingestion during pregnancy[24] (see Caffeine in Chapter 52).

CARBON MONOXIDE

During acute carbon monoxide intoxication, maternal carboxyhemoglobin ($HbCO_M$) concentration increases rapidly, then reaches a plateau in 7 to 8 hours. Fetal carboxyhemoglobin ($HbCO_F$) levels show little change during the first hours of maternal intoxication, then increase slowly over 24 hours and may exceed the maternal carboxyhemoglobin levels.[25] During the washout phase at room air, $HbCO_M$ half-life is 466 hours, and $HbCO_F$ half-life is 7 to 9 hours. If the maternal exposure pattern is unknown, the $HbCO_M$ is not helpful in deducing the $HbCO_F$. With normobaric oxygen, $HbCO_M$ and $HbCO_F$ half-lives are respectively 90 minutes and 3 to 4 hours. $HbCO_F$ half-life with pure hyperbaric oxygen is not accurately known. In a prospective randomized study, 2 atmospheres of hyperbaric oxygen for 2 hours did not lead to any evidence of fetal or obstetric morbidity. Because fetal accumulation of carbon monoxide is higher and its elimination is slower than in the maternal circulation, hyperbaric oxygen may decrease fetal hypoxia and improve outcome.[26] Consideration should be given to the use of hyperbaric oxygen in pregnant women with acute carbon monoxide intoxication, irrespective of their $HbCO_M$ or presenting clinical features, although controlled clinical trials to support this treatment are not available.[27]

CARDIOVASCULAR DRUGS

Table 8–3 summarizes some information on cardiovascular drugs and pregnancy.[28]

CIGUATERA

A 20-year-old mother developed ciguatera poisoning in the second trimester. Fetal movements were increased for a few hours. She endured multisystemic symptoms typical of ciguatera for 8 weeks. The newborn at term was normal with adequate respiratory and neurologic reflexes and developed normally during the first 10 months. It is unknown whether ciguatoxin (molecular weight 1112 daltons) can cross the placenta. It may appear in breast milk.[29]

DIGITALIS

Few data are available on intrauterine digitalis toxicity. Digitalis compounds (digoxin, digitoxin) pass through the placenta. Data on the transplacental passage of Fab antibody fragments are not available. The pregnant patient with an acute digitalis overdose should be treated similarly to a nonpregnant patient when indicated. The antidigoxin antibody fragment should be given to the mother when required, although its safety and efficacy for the fetus are unknown. Fetal cardiac rhythm should be monitored. A viable fetus can be delivered as an emergency and the antidote administered to the neonate as indicated by blood levels if necessary.

DRUG ABUSE

A large number of neonates who have been exposed to drugs in utero, particularly those whose mothers denied the use of drugs, appear normal at birth. Detection of the newborn at risk can be enhanced by noting the maternal profile (single, multigravida, no previous maternal care, preoccupation with daily procurement of drugs, prostitution) and drug screening of the newborn by meconium

Table 8–3
Cardiac Drugs and Pregnancy

	Malformation	Placental Passage	Breast Milk
Antiarrhythmic Drugs			
Digoxin	ND	+	+
Quinidine	ND	?	
Procainamide	ND	+	
Lidocaine	ND	+	
Disopyramide	ND*	+	+
Verapamil	ND	+	ND
Antihypertensive Drugs			
Methyldopa	ND	+	ND
Beta blockers	ND	+	+
Hydralazine	ND	+	ND
Prazosin	ND		
Diazoxide	ND	+	ND

*ND, not detectable.
Adapted from Lees KR, Rubin PC. Prescribing in pregnancy: Treatment of cardiovascular disease. Br Med J 1987;294:358–360.

Table 8–4
Indicators Suggesting Drug or Alcohol Dependence in a Pregnant Woman

Behavioral	Medical	Historical
Vague history regarding personal or medical problems	Liver disease, hepatomegaly	Alcohol- or drug-abusing partner
Conflicts with significant others or domestic violence	Pancreatitis	Many emergency department contacts
History of child abuse or neglect	Hypertension	Many physician contacts
Decreased job performance or chronic unemployment	Gastritis, esophagitis	Child with neonatal narcotic abstinence syndrome
Suicidal gestures, thoughts, or attempts	Neurologic disorders	Child with alcohol-related birth defects
Car accidents	Poor nutritional status	Placement of other children outside the home
Cited for driving while intoxicated	Hematologic disorders	Complex perinatal histories and outcomes
Depression	Seropositivity for HIV	Psychiatric treatment or hospital admissions
Irritability or agitation	Bacteremia	Affective disorders
Difficulty concentrating—Mood swings, outbursts of anger	Alcoholic myopathy	Infants with low birth weights
Inappropriate behavior	Sensory impairment	Frequent physician prescriptions for mood-altering drugs
Memory lapses and losses or blackouts	Problems of sepsis, cellulitis	Family history of alcoholism or other drug dependency
Intoxicated behavior	Hepatitis	Sudden infant death syndrome
Smell of alcohol on breath	Abscesses	Family dissolution
Unreliability or unpredictable behavior	Mitral valve disease	
Missed appointments	Septicemia	
Intense daily drama, family chaos	Swelling and erythema of hands	
Slurred speech	Overdose	
Staggering gait	Withdrawal effects	
	Pulmonary infections	
	Hair loss	
	Erratic menses	
	Loss of appetite	
	Poor dental hygiene	
	Anemia	
	Tuberculosis	
	Sexually transmitted disease	
	Obstetric complications, including spontaneous abortion, abruptio placentae, breech presentations, previous cesarean section, eclampsia, intrauterine growth retardation, premature labor and delivery and premature rupture of membranes, intrauterine fetal death, postpartum hemorrhage	

From Jessup M. The treatment of perinatal addiction: Identification, intervention and advocacy. West J Med 1990;152:553–55?.

analysis (radioimmunoassay of metabolites of cocaine, morphine, and cannabinoids).[30]

The pregnant patient may be subject to drug or alcohol dependence (Table 8–4).[31] Maternal complications from narcotic abuse are summarized in Table 8–5.

Table 8–5
Maternal Complications From Narcotic Abuse

Anemia
Subacute bacterial endocarditis
Cellulitis
Hypertension
Phlebitis
Pneumonia
Pyelonephritis
Tuberculosis
Trauma
Psychosocial (prostitution, incarceration, polysubstance abuse)
Sexually transmitted diseases (vaginitis, gonorrhea, syphilis, herpes simplex virus, chlamydia, condylomata)
HIV
Hepatitis A and B

From Dattel BJ. Substance abuse in pregnancy. Semin Perinatol 1990;14:179–198.

Neonatal Withdrawal Syndrome

The onset of neonatal withdrawal syndrome is usually apparent within 1 to 4 days of birth for most drugs except phenobarbital, for which symptoms appear 10 to 14 days after birth, and chlordiazepoxide, for which symptoms may appear 24 days after birth. Drugs with longer elimination half-lives tend to result in withdrawal manifestations later than those with short elimination half-lives. Neonatal withdrawal syndrome does not usually develop in the neonates of mothers who have been drug free for a week or more prior to delivery[32] (Table 8–6). Drugs suggested for use in the treatment of neonatal withdrawal syndrome are listed in Table 8–7.[29]

LINDANE

An anecdotal case report suggests that lindane crosses the placenta, is excreted in human breast milk, and may be fetotoxic.[88]

LITHIUM

A prospective study of 148 women who had consulted teratogen information centers and who had used lithiumduring the first trimester suggests that lithium is not an important human teratogen. Based on this study, the authors suggest that women with major affective disorders who wish

Table 8–6
Nonnarcotic Drugs That Caused Symptoms of Withdrawal In Neonates

Drug	Clinical Symptoms		Clinical Symptoms		Comments		
	General	Central Nervous System	Gastrointestinal	Respiratory	Onset	Duration	Other
Barbiturates: phenobarbital, amobarbital, butalbital, secobarbital	Irritability, poor sleep pattern, diaphoresis, skin abrasions	Excessive crying, hyperreflexia, hyperacusia, hypertonicity, convulsions, severe tremors	Hyperphagia, vomiting, diarrhea	Stuffy nose	First 48 h or at 10–14 d	2–6 mo	
Alcohol	Irritability, poor sleep pattern, diaphoresis	Crying, hyperactivity, hyperacusia, hypertonicity, tremor, seizures	Poor suck, hyperphagia, vomiting, abdominal dyskinesia	Hyperventilation	At birth, first day–18 mo	Brief	High seizure risk
Diazepam	Hypothermia	Hyperactivity, hypotonia, hypertonia, apnea/tremor, hyperreflexia	Poor suck, vomiting, loose stools, poor weight gain	Respiratory depression, tachypnea	2–6 h	8 mo (treatment 10–66 d)	Mother abused several drugs
Chlordiazepoxide	Irritability	Tremors			21 d	9–10 d	Monozygotic twins
Diphenhydramine	Tremulousness		Diarrhea		Age 5 d; 9 d of treatment	3 d	No feeding problem
Hydroxyzine	Irritability	Hyperactivity, jitteriness, tremor, shrill cry, hypotonia, myoclonic jerks	Feeding problems	Increased respiratory rate			Mother had multiple-drug therapy for 5 wks
Ethchlorvynol	Irritability	Hypotonia, jitteriness	Poor suck, hyperphagia		10 d treatment		Mother with multiple-drug treatment
Glutethimide	Irritability, fever, diaphoresis	Hyperactivity, hypertonia, high-pitched cry, opisthotonus	"Colic"	Tachypnea	8 h, but improved after 1 d; renewal of symptoms at 10 d		
Phencyclidine (PCP)	Irritability	Jitteriness, hypertonia, nystagmus	Vomiting, diarrhea		Soon after birth	18 d	Mother also used marijuana
Propoxyphene	Irritability, fever	Hyperactivity, tremor, high-pitched cry	Diarrhea, weight loss, ravenous appetite		20 h of age	Stopped at 56 h of age	
Cocaine	Tremulousness, abnormal sleep pattern	Hypotonia, hyperreflexia	Poor feeding		Mild symptoms from birth		Cocaine intoxication has been associated with tremors, tachycardia, seizures

From Levy M, Spiro M. Neonatal withdrawal syndrome: Associated drugs and pharmacologic management. Pharmacotherapy 1993;13:202–211.

Table 8–7
Drugs and Dosages Used in Treatment of Neonatal Withdrawal Syndrome

Drug	Dosage*
Phenobarbital†	Loading dose 5–10 mg/kg/d PO, IM, or slow IV infusion Maintenance dose 2–6 mg/kg/d q6–8h PO, IM
Diazepam	0.2–1.5 mg/kg PO or slow IV infusion q6–8h, IM q8h
Chlorpromazine	0.5–0.7 mg/kg PO, IM, or slow IV infusion q6h as required
Paregoric USP‡	0.2–0.5 mL/dose (0.08–0.20 mg anydrous morphine) PO q3–4h until control of symptoms
Diluted opium tincture§	Initial dose, 0.2 mL PO q3h, increased by 0.05–1 mL as required
Clonidine	1 μg/kg PO q6h

*Dosage should be tapered after 3–5 days of stabilization of symptoms. A gradual lowering of dose should be followed by prolongation as dosing interval.
†Dosage should be adjusted according to clinical response and drug level.
‡Paregoric USP contains not less than 35 mg of anhydrous morphine and not more than 45 mg in 100 mL. It also contains 43–47% alcohol and other alkaloids.
§Diluted opium tincture contains 1% anhydrous morphine.
From Levy M, Spiro M. Neonatal withdrawal syndrome: Associated drugs and pharmacologic management. Pharmacotherapy 1993;13:202–211.

to have children may, after consultation with their health provider, continue lithium therapy, provided that adequate screening tests, including level II ultrasound and fetal echocardiography, are done.[33]

METALS

Arsenic

Treatment of the pregnant patient poisoned with arsenic is similar to that for the nonpregnant patient.

Iron

Acute iron intoxication in pregnancy poses a dilemma to the clinician. Toxic levels of iron are often associated with severe complications and can be fatal. The effective iron chelator, deferoxamine, has possible teratogenic potential.[34] If delivery occurs, the infant should be evaluated for iron overload or iron deficiency secondary to maternal deferoxamine therapy.[35] The fetus seems to fare better than the mother after maternal iron overdose. Even though the maternal serum iron level is high, little iron appears to pass to the fetus. The risk to the fetus is not from the iron itself, but is secondary to the induced pathophysiologic derangements in the mother. Emergency delivery of a viable fetus should be reserved only for documented maternal or fetal distress.[36]

Lead

Lead crosses the placenta. It is unlikely that edetate calcium disodium ($CaNa_2EDTA$) passes through the placenta. Few studies have been performed during pregnancy following the use of dimercaprol (BAL in Oil) or dimercaptosuccinic acid. During pregnancy, maternal indicators provide the dominant reason to administer lead chelators.

METHYL ISOCYANATE: BHOPAL DISASTER

The Bhopal gas disaster, in which a large amount of methyl isocyanate was liberated, was one of the most damaging industrial accidents in history. It occurred on December 2, 1984, and is considered further in Chapter 58. A study of pregnant women exposed to this toxic gas indicated a high incidence of spontaneous abortion compared with those not exposed. Rates of stillbirths and congenital malformations were not found to be different. Perinatal and neonatal mortality was increased in the affected area.[18]

METHYLENE BLUE

Methylene blue has been used during diagnostic laparoscopy to examine the patency of the fallopian tubes, and during pregnancy to provide a marker in amniocentesis for multiple pregnancies[37] as well as to verify premature rupture of the membranes.[38] The dye is subsequently identified in the vagina. Complications have included a deep blue baby in whom assessment of hypoxia was difficult.[39] Although an inadvertent intrauterine injection of methylene blue during the fifth week of pregnancy did not produce adverse effects,[41] neonatal complications often occur after intervals from intraamniotic injection to delivery of less than 5 weeks.[42] These undesirable effects have included hyperbilirubinemia and secondary hemolysis in the newborn,[43–47] Heinz body formation,[43,45] methemoglobinemia,[44] and a strikingly deep blue baby in whom assessment of hypoxia is difficult.[38,39] When 10 to 30 mg (1–3 mL 1% solution of methylene blue) was injected via an amniocentesis needle into one of two amniotic sacs of twins at 15 to 17 weeks gestation, multiple ileal occlusions were diagnosed in 7 infants born to 21 women with twin pregnancies.[48,49] It appears that methylene blue may be especially hazardous during the second trimester.[47]

Intestinal atresias have been reported,[39,50] but a study of 11 European centers by the EUROCAT Working Group concluded that the use of methylene blue during amniocentesis was not associated with an excess of cases of atresia or stenosis of the ileum or jejunum in neonates. A collaborative follow-up of twin pregnancies in centers where methylene blue has been used, is needed.

MUSHROOM POISONING: AMANITA PHALLOIDES

A 21-year-old pregnant woman ingested *Amanita phalloides*. She developed nausea, vomiting, abdominal pain, and diarrhea within 10 hours of ingestion. Diagnosis was confirmed by measurement of alpha-α-amanitin levels. The mother had an α-amanitin blood level of 18.5 ng/mL by high-performance liquid chromatography. No amatoxins were detected in the amniotic fluid by high-performance liquid chromatography or immunoassay methods. She later gave birth to a healthy baby with no biochemical evidence of hepatocellular danger, suggesting that α-amanitin does not cross the placental barrier during the acute phase of intoxication.[51]

NUTMEG: ANTICHOLINERGIC HYPERSTIMULATION

Ingestion of nutmeg by a 29-year-old primigravida at the 30th week of gestation led to palpitations, agitation, blurred vision, apprehension, chest tightening, and dry mouth. Anticholinergic hyperstimulation caused by nutmeg ingestion should be treated with supportive and symptomatic care early because of its potentially lethal outcome.[52]

OPIATES

Pregnant women addicted to opiates studied at a hospital in the United States revealed an increased incidence of antepartum hemorrhage, premature labor, and intrauterine death, which often occurs during withdrawal. From the infant's point of view, heroin may be preferable to methadone because the abstinence syndrome is less prolonged and severe.[53]

ORGANOPHOSPHATE PESTICIDES

There are few data on the human transplacental passage of many organophosphate pesticides.[60] In addition, little is known regarding cholinesterase development during fetal development. Relative transplacental passage and possibly differing fetal and material sensitivities may be important. Atropine, a principal antidote, has agonist properties and therefore a potential atropine dose may be either subtherapeutic or toxic for the fetus (see Atropine in Chapter 46).

The pregnant patient should be treated like the nonpregnant patient, using life support, gastrointestinal decontamination, thorough respiratory care, atropine, and pralidoxime.[59] The fetus should be monitored closely. If the mother is doing well, but the potentially viable fetus exhibits distress, consideration should be given to immediate delivery and appropriate therapy of the newborn.

PARAQUAT

Nonintervention of a potentially viable pregnancy may be indicated, as the value of hemoperfusion has not been confirmed and, in any case, could be damaging to the fetus.

PROSTAGLANDINS

Prostaglandins are natural products that act as initiators and regulators of labor. When administered at any stage of gestation they cause uterine contractions and expulsion of the conceptus.[34] Three prostaglandins are of interest in pregnancy: prostaglandin $F_{2\alpha}$ (Dinoprost), Prostaglandin E_2 (Dinoprostone), and prostacyclin sodium salt (epoprostenol sodium, prostacyclin, PGI_2).

Prostaglandin $F_{2\alpha}$ and its 15-methyl analog are effective in inducing abortion and labor. Intramyometrial injection of these compounds has been advocated to control postpartum hemorrhage secondary to placenta accreta and uterine hypotonia.

Prostaglandin E_2 is used for similar indications as prostaglandin $F_{2\alpha}$.

A 42-year-old accidentally received a bolus intravenous dose of prostacyclin (250 μg in 50 mL of sterile diluent at 25 mL/h) and became erythematous and profoundly hypotensive. She survived after receiving hydroxyethyl starch, calcium gluconate, and ephedrine intravenously.[61] A 31-year-old woman received 40 mg (normal dose 1–5 mg) of prostaglandin $F_{2\alpha}$ into the lower uterine segment. She developed cardiovascular collapse, acute pulmonary edema, and ventricular premature beats. Treatment included pressor amines, corticosteroids, intravenous fluids, and assisted ventilation.[62] She survived.

Clinical Presentation

Prostaglandins have resulted in life-threatening profound hypotension,[63] myocardial infarction,[64] bronchospasm,[65] seizures in epileptic patients,[66] uterine rupture in midtrimester abortion,[67] amniotic fluid embolism,[68] third-trimester intrauterine deaths,[69] ventricular tachycardia,[70] gastric outlet obstruction in neonates,[71] respiratory distress in a neonate,[72] and uterine hyperstimulation (reversed by B_2 adrenergic therapy),[73] and hypokalemia.[74] Cardiac arrest has followed intramyometrial injection of prostaglandin E_2.[75]

Mechanism of Action

Prostaglandins exert their effect on the smooth muscle of blood vessels, the bronchi, and the uterus. The prostaglandins may have vasodilator effects leading to a decrease in blood pressure with increase in heart rate and cardiac output. Prostaglandins have both inotropic and chronotropic effects on the myocardium.[76] In the bronchi they may cause bronchoconstriction ($F_{2\alpha}$) or dilation of the smooth muscle of the bronchioles (E_2).[77] In the nonpregnant uterus, prostaglandins cause dilation of smooth muscle, but in the pregnant uterus contraction of smooth muscle occurs.[63,78]

Laboratory

An enzyme-linked immunosorbent assay (ELISA) has been developed for the detection of prostaglandin. It can detect as little as 2 pg of 19-hydroxyprostaglandin per 100 mL.

Treatment

Treatment of prostaglandin overdose is largely symptomatic and supportive. Temporary cessation of an intravenous infusion may be adequate. Analgesics may be used for pain.[79]

RADIATION

All x-ray medical exposure should be kept as low as reasonably achievable. Each radiology department should agree on a protocol for examining women in their reproductive years. To minimize unintentional exposure of the fetus, any woman requiring diagnostic irradiation close to the uterus should be asked "Are you or might you be pregnant?" and regarded as pregnant if the answer is other than No. Areas remote from the fetus may be considered to be subject to examination radiologically at any time during pregnancy with the consent of a fully informed radiologist. X-rays directed close to the uterus in women of childbearing ability carry risks to a pregnancy that may occur immediately or up to several weeks after that x-ray examination.[80] Suggested guidelines have been proposed by Popat and colleagues.[75]

RETINOIDS

Three oral retinoids have been associated with possible teratogenic hazards: retinol (vitamin A, found in food and dietary supplements), isotretinoin (Accutane, Roaccutan), and etretinate (Tegison). Accumulated evidence suggests that isotretinoin exposure during pregnancy is highly teratogenic. Retinol may be teratogenic, but the evidence is not conclusive. Data on etretinate do not provide firm evidence that such exposure is highly teratogenic.[54]

RIBAVIRIN

The California Department of Health Services has issued a warning to health care workers who are pregnant and to male and female workers who are attempting to conceive about the dangers of exposure to the antiviral agent ribavirin.[55,56] Animal studies have shown that ribavirin is teratogenic, causing severe malformations in offspring of exposed females. In a recent study, the California Department of Health Services found that exposure of health care workers who tend patients receiving ribavirin aerosol via oxygen tent or mist mask may exceed the recommended safety levels to protect against reproductive harm. Surgical masks and similar respiratory protection are not likely to reduce exposure to the aerosol sufficiently. Hospitals are advised to considered alternative job assignments for health care workers who are at risk and to develop policies to minimize occupational exposure to the drug.

SALICYLATES

Unlike acetaminophen, the parent compound and not the metabolites produces the toxicity of salicylate overdose. This places the fetus at risk. Salicylate traverses the placenta and is found in higher concentrations in the fetus.

Treatment of the mother with salicylate poisoning requires intensive supportive care. Fetal factors such as higher serum concentrations, larger proportion of salicylate in the brain, lower buffering capacity, and decreased salicylate metabolism mitigate against the positive effects of maternal stabilization; gastrointestinal decontamination; fluid, electrolyte, and glucose administration; and extracorporeal removal, all measures that tend to reduce the transplacental migration of salicylates. When the fetus is potentially viable outside of the uterus, consideration should be given to prompt delivery.

TOBACCO: FETAL TOBACCO SYNDROME

Nieburg and colleagues at the Centers for Disease Control and Prevention have suggested the use of the term *fetal tobacco syndrome* for fetal growth retardation when the following conditions are met:[57]

1. The mother smoked five or more cigarettes a day throughout the pregnancy.
2. The mother had no evidence of hypertension during pregnancy, specifically no preeclampsia and documentation of normal blood pressure at least once after the first trimester.
3. The newborn has symmetric growth retardation at term (more than 37 weeks), defined as a birth weight less than 2500 g and a ponderal index (weight in g/length in cm) greater than 2.32.
4. There is no other obvious cause of intrauterine growth retardation (eg, congenital infection or anomaly).

Other relationships between maternal cigarette smoking and adverse pregnancy outcomes have included abruptio placentae, bleeding during pregnancy, premature rupture of membranes, fetal death, neonatal mortality, sudden infant death syndrome and deficits in growth, and intellectual and emotional development and behavior.[57] For congenital malformations overall, the majority of epidemiologic studies have found no association with cigarette smoking;[58] however, a prospective study of 16,583 mothers of 17,152 infants suggests that mothers aged 35 years and older who smoke may have a higher risk of delivering infants with minor malformations.[59]

VITAMIN A

Excessive intake of vitamin A immediately before or during pregnancy substantially increases the risk of birth defects.[154,155] The Teratology Society has recommended that vitamin A supplementation (as retinol or retinal esters) be limited to 8000 IU (2400 μg) per day.[156] A suggestion has been made in the United Kingdom that women who are pregnant or who may become pregnant should not consume more than 50 g of liver a week. Consumption of liver sausage or pate should be limited to about 100 g per week.[157,158]

PREGNANT PATIENTS: ASSOCIATED TOPICS

INDUSTRIAL EXPOSURES

Some adverse reproductive effects in women and men (Tables 8–8 and 8–9) may be associated with industrial exposures.[81]

Increases in late abortions have been noted in operating room nurses, radiology technicians and employees in the agricultural and horticulture industries,[82] female veterinarians,[83] and women employed in plastics manufacture.[84]

The three most common occupational exposures reported by pregnant women are exposures to video display terminals, organic solvents, and lead products. Video display terminals do not appear to represent a reproductive risk. Organic solvents may damage the fetal brain at high exposure levels, such as those encountered in substance abuse. There is no clear evidence to suggest that maternal exposure to legally allowable levels causes fetal damage. In the case of lead, a dose–response fetal risk appears to have been established, and lead levels should be monitored to avoid fetal risk.[85]

Evaluation of the occupationally exposed woman should include the following investigations:[86]

Table 8–8
Exposures Associated with Male Reproductive Dysfunction

Agent	Human Outcomes	Strength of Association in Humans*	Animal Outcomes	Strength of Association in Animals*
Boron	Decreased sperm count	1	Testicular damage	2
Benzene	None	NA†	Decreased sperm motility, testicular damage	1
Benzo[a]pyrene	None	NA	Testicular damage	1
Cadmium	Reduced fertility	1	Testicular damage	2
Carbon disulfide	Decreased sperm count, decreased sperm motility	2,3	Testicular damage	1
Carbon monoxide	None	NA	Testicular damage	1
Carbon tetrachloride	None	NA	Testicular damage	1
Carbaryl	Abnormal sperm morphology	1	Testicular damage	1
Chlordecone	Decreased sperm count, decreased sperm motility	2	Testicular damage	2
Chloroprene	Decreased sperm motility, abnormal morphology, decreased libido	2	Testicular damage	1
Dibromochloropropane (DBCP)	Decreased sperm count, azoospermia, hormonal changes	2	Testicular damage	2
Dimethyl dichlorovinyl phosphate (DDVP)	None	NA	Decreased sperm count	2
Epichlorohydrin	None	NA	Testicular damage	2,3
Estrogens	Decreased sperm count	2	Decreased sperm count	2
Ethylene oxide	None	NA	Testicular damage	1
Ethylene dibromide (EDB)	Abnormal sperm motility	1	Testicular damage	2,3
Ethylene glycol ethers	Decreased sperm count	1	Testicular damage	2
Heat	Decreased sperm count	2	Decreased sperm count	2
Lead	Decreased sperm count	2	Testicular damage, decreased sperm count, decreased sperm motility, abnormal morphology	2
Manganese	Decreased libido, impotence	1	Testicular damage	1,3
Polybrominated biphenyls (PBBs)	None	NA	Testicular damage	1
Polychlorinated biphenyls (PCBs)	None	NA	Testicular damage	1
Radiation, ionizing	Decreased sperm count	2	Testicular damage	2

*1 = limited positive data, 2 = strong positive data, 3 = limited negative data.
†Not applicable because no adverse outcomes were observed.
From Welch LS, Paul ME. Reproductive and developmental hazards.

1. Identify the chemicals in question, by their Material Safety Data Sheets if possible.
2. Identify symptoms and signs reported to be associated with the chemicals.
3. Rule out underlying conditions that may cause a similar clinical picture (eg, morning sickness).
4. Obtain a detailed description of the work performed by the woman, length of exposure, and means of protection (e.g., ventilation system, respirator, mask, gown, gloves, hood, etc).
5. Are there symptoms and signs in fellow workers?
6. What is the pregnancy outcome in other workers?
7. Obtain the most recent levels of the chemicals in question measured in that particular area.
8. Try to understand the attitude of the woman and her supervisors toward her particular work and toward possible change of job. Will it affect her income or promotion?
9. Before reporting to the woman on available information, evaluate the data critically to provide the patient with accurate information.
10. Advise the woman on possible safety measures to reduce exposure (e.g., mask, gloves, ventilation, etc).

The Office of Technology Assessment of the U.S. Congress has published *Reproduction Health Hazards in the Workplace,* Washington, DC: U.S. Government Printing Office, OTA-BA-266, December 1985.

SEIZURES DURING PREGNANCY

Management of the pregnant woman who has had or is having a seizure is similar to that of other seizure patients.[87] Antiepileptic drugs have some teratogenic potential, but there appears to be less risk to the fetus from anticonvulsant exposure than from uncontrolled seizures. The evaluation of a pregnant woman with new-onset seizures should include computed tomography of the head with appropriate abdominal shielding after consultation with a radiologist. Status epilepticus management is based on intravenous benzodiazepine, phenytoin, or phenobarbital. Good fetal outcome is dependent on rapid seizure control.

Table 8–9
Toxic Agents Associated With or Suspected of Reproductive Toxicologic Effects in Women

Chemical	Code*	Suspected Reproductive Effects	Example of Industry of Exposure	Suggested Biological Testing
Organic solvents				
Aromatic hydrocarbons (eg, toluene)	+	Low birth weight Birth defects "Fetal solvent syndrome"	Laboratory reagents Paint thinners Food and hospital sterilization Shoemakers	Compound in blood or expired air metabolites in urine (eg, *o*-cresol in urine)
Ethylene glycol	+	Spontaneous abortions, birth defects	Antifreeze manufacture	
Gases: carbon monoxide	+	Fetal neurologic damage Central nervous system malformation	Firefighters Factories poorly ventilated	Carboxyhemoglobin in blood CO in end-exhaled air
Solvents: carbon disulfide	±	Decrease fertility in women Spontaneous abortion	Viscose rayon Laundries Dry cleaning	Urine sodium azide test 2-Thiothiazolidine-4-carboxylic acid
Sterilizing agents: ethylene oxide	±	Spontaneous abortions Birth defects in animals	Health care Food sterilization Chemical	Hydroxyethyl adducts in hemoglobin
Anesthetic gases				
Halogenated gases	±	Spontaneous abortion	Medical	Compound in urine or blood
Nitrous oxide	±	Low birth weight	Dental Veterinary	
Heavy metals				
Lead	+	Spontaneous abortions	Battery, smelter, foundry workers	Blood lead, blood zinc, protoprophyrin
Mercury	+	Stillbirths	Dentists	Blood mercury
Cadmium	±	Neurodevelopment delay in offspring	Welders	Urine mercury
Manganese	?			Urine cadmium
Cytostatic drugs	±	Spontaneous abortion Congenital malformations	Health care personnel Pharmaceutical industry	Urine thioethers Urinary mutagenicity
Halogenated hydrocarbons				
Dibromochloropropane	+	Neurodevelopmental damage	Chemical oil workers Industrial accidents	
Polybrominated biphenyls	+	Increased infant mortality		Blood analysis
Polychlorinated biphenyls	+	Dark brown pigmentation in offspring, low birth weight, altered menstrual cycles	Electrical equipment fires or explosions	Adipose tissue analysis
Plastics				
Polyurethane	±	Increased spontaneous abortion	Plastics industry	
Styrene				
Polystyrene		Menstrual disorders		
Physical agents				
Electromagnetic fields	±	Spontaneous abortion Malformations	Workers in electricity generation plants and transmission equipment	Measurements of electric and magnetic fields
Low-exposure radiation	0 ±	Carcinogenesis Malformations	Nuclear plants Radiology technicians	Film badges Urine bioassay Plutonium
Heat	±	Fetal distress	Firefighters	Wet bulb Globe temperature index
Ionizing radiation	0	Spontaneous abortion Birth defects not confirmed	Video display terminals (secretaries, clerks)	Measurements of very low and extremely low frequency emissions
Noise	±	Hearing loss	Mothers exposed >100 dB during pregnancy	Noise level measurements
Air travel	±	Increased fetal loss	Flight attendants	
Ozone	?			
Altered biorhythms	±	Menstrual disorders		
Natural radiation	0			
Galactic cosmic radiation	0			

*+, Possible or definite association; ±, questionable.
From Giacoia GR. Reproductive hazards in the workplace. Obstet Gynecol Surv 1992;47:679–687.

PATERNAL EXPOSURES

Exposure of men to a variety of chemicals and drugs can impair their fertility and adversely affect their children.[89–100] Adverse outcomes can include pregnancy loss, malformations evident at birth, and problems detected later in life, such as behavioral abnormalities and cancer. Effects on fetal development can include spontaneous abortion, preterm delivery, or delivery of an infant who is small for gestational age.[96]

Certain paternal occupational exposures, including exposure to fuel combustion products, organic solvents, and metals such as lead and mercury, appear to be more often associated with abnormal outcomes.[96] For example, paternal occupations such as motor vehicle mechanic, firefighting, janitorial services, forestry and logging, printing, plywood milling, and textile industries and exposure to fuel combustion products, organic solvents, and metals such as lead and mercury may result in abnormal pregnancy outcomes. Confounding factors may include exposure of the father to cigarette smoke, alcohol, and cocaine[97] (Table 8–10).

Paternal smoking has been associated with low birth weight and increased perinatal mortality.[94,95] Animal studies of exposure to environmental chemicals (eg, lead, dibromochloropropane) and drugs (e.g., cyclophosphamide) have revealed a higher incidence of adversely affected progeny, behavioral alteration, and a higher incidence of cancer.

Drugs or environmental chemicals to which the father is exposed may be present in his seminal fluid (Table 8–11) and can directly affect the ovulated egg, fertilization, or embryonic development. Further epidemiologic studies are required to identify the site of action of potentially harmful agents. Men occupationally exposed to certain chemicals should be made aware of their increased risks and should be counseled to avoid certain chemical exposures before their partners conceive.[96]

SPERMICIDES

The active ingredient in spermicides is nonoxynol-9. Such contraceptive agents are marketed over the counter as creams, jellies, suppositories, and foam in aerosol containers as well as sponges. These preparations work by providing a physical barrier to sperm penetration as well as a chemical spermicidal action. A meta-analysis of nine studies that investigated teratogenicity suggests that maternal use of

Table 8–10
Some Paternal Pregnancy Associations

Paternal Occupation	Outcome
Motor vehicle mechanic[97]	Spontaneous abortions
Painting (exposure to solvents)[97]	Anencephaly
Firemen, janitorial services, forestry and logging, printing, plywood milling[84,90]	Birth defects
Artists, textile industries[91]	Stillbirth, preterm delivery, small-for-gestational age infant
Exposure to lead, mercury; motor vehicle exhaust fumes; vehicle mechanics, autobody repairmen	Spontaneous abortion Childhood leukemia[96] Wilms' tumor in children[96,97]

Table 8–11
Human Sperm Studies of Occupational Exposures

	Sperm Indicator*			
	Count	Motility	Morphology	F Bodies
Detrimental effects				
Carbon disulfide	+	+	+	
Dibromochloropropane (DBCP)	+	+?	+?	+
Lead	+	+	+	
Inconclusive				
Boron	+?			
Cadmium	+?			
Carbaryl	–			
Ethylene dibromide	+?			
Kepone	+?	+?	+?	
Methylmercury	+?			
Toluene diamine and dinitrotoluene	+?			
No effects				
Anesthetic gases	–		–	
Epichlorohydrin	–		–	
Ethylene glycol monomethyl ether	–			
Formaldehyde	–	–	–	–
Glycerine production	–	+?	–	
Para-tert-Butylbenzoic acid	–			
Polybrominated biphenyls	–	–	–	
Wastewater treatment	–		–	

*+ = detrimental effect observed, +? = detrimental effect with unknown or marginal statistical significance or not clearly related to the exposure, – = no detrimental effect observed.
From Mattison DR, Plowchalk DR, Meadows MJ, et al. Reproductive toxicity: Male and female reproductive systems as targets for chemical injury. Med Clin North Am 1990;74:391–411.

spermicides is not associated with adverse fetal outcome.[101] Warburton and associates reported no increased risk of trisomies with spermicide use.[102]

TOCOLYTIC AGENTS

Pharmacologic inhibition of uterine contractions is the mainstay of treatment for preterm labor. Betamimetics and magnesium sulfate are the common therapeutic agents of choice in the United States today. Prostaglandin synthetase inhibitors, calcium channel blockers, and phosphodiesterase inhibitors are currently undergoing clinical evaluation. In 1980, the U.S. Food and Drug Administration approved ritodrine hydrochloride (Yutopar) for inhibition of premature labor. This is the only drug approved in the United States for this indication.[103–107]

Aminophylline

Aminophylline represents a new class of tocolytic agent whose efficacy remains to be determined.

Alcohol

Ethanol inhibits the secretion of the neurohypophyseal hormones, antidiuretic hormone, and oxytocin. Ethanol appears to suppress uterine activity through inhibition of oxytocin release, reduction of myometrial oxytocin receptors, and noncompetitive antagonism at the uterine level. Nevertheless, in controlled studies, ethanol has been less effective than isoxsuprine, ritodrine, terbutaline, or magnesium sulfate. Children exposed in utero to alcohol as a tocolytic have shown no abnormalities.[108,109]

Betamimetic Agents

Isoxsuprine

Isoxsuprine (Vasodilan) has both β_1- and β_2-adrenergic activity. Maternal hypotension and tachycardia are common side effects. Hypocalcemia, hypoglycemia, hypotension, ileus, and neonatal death are increased after isoxsuprine.[110]

Beta-adrenergic Agonists

Maternal effects of hypotension with reflex compensation tachycardia, increase in stroke volume, increased cardiac output, and increased systolic blood pressure are a result of activation of vascular β_2-adrenergic receptors. There are some inotropic and chronotropic effects. Therefore, betamimetic tocolytic therapy is inadvisable for patients with inherent cardiac disease.[105,106]

Arrhythmias

The most common arrhythmia reported is supraventricular tachycardia, although atrial fibrillation, atrial premature contractions, and ventricular ectopy have also been observed. Continuous electrocardiogram monitoring of a patient receiving intravenous betamimetic therapy should be performed.

Myocardial Ischemia

Chest pain is relatively uncommon. Transient ST-segment depression is the most common observation and appears to be dose related. This usually resolves with discontinuation of therapy. β_2 agonists lower diastolic pressure. Coronary artery perfusion is thereby decreased.

Pulmonary Edema

About 5% of maternal patients receiving intravenous betamimetic therapy develop pulmonary edema. Anemia, hypertension, and the need for blood transfusion are risk factors.

Metabolic Complications

Use of betamimetics may lead to an acute rise in plasma glucose concentration and an increase in insulin release. The oral form of terbutaline, but not ritodrine, may result in an abnormal glucose tolerance test. Significant drops in serum potassium may occur. This is uncommon after oral administration of betamimetic agents. Total body potassium is not decreased. Intravenous potassium replacement can be considered when serum levels drop below 2.0 mmol/100 mL, a cardiac arrhythmia is present, or furosemide is administered. Glycogenolysis and lipolysis lead to increased lactate production. Use of lactated Ringer's solution during betamimetic therapy should be avoided. Maternal pH changes are not usually seen. Neonatal hypoglycemia following cord clamping has been reported with isoxsuprine, salbutamol, and terbutaline, but less after ritodrine. Neonates delivered after recent exposure to maternal betamimetic therapy should be monitored for hypoglycemia.

Calcium Channel Blockers

Nifedipine (Procardia), nicardipine, and verapamil (Colan/Isoftin) are capable of inhibiting uterine contractions. There may be a profound reduction in uteroplacental blood flow. Nifedipine can be used orally or parenterally. After oral use, maximum plasma concentrations are achieved in 15 to 90 minutes with a plasma half-life of 2 to 3 hours. Elimination occurs primarily in the kidneys (70%) and bowel (30%)

Diazoxide

Although diazoxide is a potent inhibitor of myometrial activity, its profound hypotensive effect limits its usefulness as a tocolytic agonist.

Glyceryl Trinitrate

An initial uncontrolled study suggests that glyceryl trinitrate (patches) has tocolytic action. Adverse effects have included headache and minor hypotension.[134,135]

Magnesium Sulfate

Serum magnesium concentrations of 4 to 8 mEq/L appear to be necessary for inhibition of uterine activity.[137–139] After an infusion rate of 3 g/h, a serum magnesium level of about 6 mg/dL is achieved. Magnesium is eliminated almost entirely by renal excretion.[140] Serum magnesium level should be monitored, especially in the presence of depressed renal function. Loss of deep tendon reflexes occurs at serum levels of 4 to 8 mEq/L. Respiratory depression may be seen at 12 to 15 mEq/L. Above this level, cardiac conduction defects and cardiac arrest may occur. Side effects include transient hypotension[141] and a feeling of heat and flushing. Although maternal tachycardia is not observed and cardiac output is unchanged, maternal paralytic ileus, pulmonary edema,[142] and decreased serum concentrations of ionized and nonionized calcium may occur. Transplacental transfer of magnesium to the fetus occurs. Neonatal hypotonia and drowsiness have been observed. Neonatal bone changes have been described.[143,144] Supralethal magnesium concentrations (38.7 mg/dL) have led to weakness, respiratory arrest, and an increase in the QRS and QT duration on the electrocardiogram. Treatment included cessation of administration, mannitol, and calcium.[145]

Cardiac arrest due to acute maternal hypermagnesemia was accompanied by a serum magnesium level of 35.1 mg/dL after a magnesium sulfate infusion. Twelve hours after the arrest, a cesarean section was performed. The infant had Apgar scores of 8 and 9 at 1 and 5 minutes. The maternal and cord magnesium concentration at the time of delivery was 5.8 mg/dL. The electrocardiogram was normal 15 minutes after the serum magnesium had been 35.1 mg/dL. Spontaneous uterine contractions resumed at 11.6 mg/dL. The patient recovered.[146]

Table 8–12
Comparison of Clinical Features Produced by Toluene Versus Alcohol

Clinical Features	Toluene	Alcohol
Growth and development		
Prematurity	+++	+
Small for gestational age	+++	+++
Postnatal growth deficiency	+++	+++
Prenatal microcephaly	±	++
Postnatal microcephaly	+++	+++
Developmental delay	+++	+++
Craniofacial features		
Micrognathia	+++	±
Small palpebral fissures	+++	+++
Abnormal ears	+++	±
Narrow bifrontal diameter	++	+
Abnormal scalp hair patterning	++	±
Thin upper lip	++	+++
Smooth philtrum	+	+++
Small nose	+	+++
Downturned mouth corners	+	–
Large anterior fontanel	+	–
Other features		
Nail hypoplasia	++	+
Abnormal muscle tone	++	+
Hemangiomata	+	+
Renal anomalies	+	±
Altered palmar creases	+	++

From Pearson MA, Hoyme HE, Seaver LH, Rimsza ME. Toluene embryopathy. Delineation of the phenotype and comparison with fetal alcohol syndrome. Pediatrics 1994;93:211–215.

Prostaglandin Synthetase Inhibitors

Indomethacin inhibits preterm labor. Following oral use, peak plasma concentrations are reached in 1 to 2 hours. The half-life of excretion is about 2 hours. Indomethacin is readily transferred across the placental unit to the fetus within 15 minutes. The half-life of excretion of indomethacin in the term neonate is 11 to 15 hours. Maternal side effects are minimal: nausea and heartburn. The main potential fetal and neonatal complications associated with prostaglandin synthetase inhibitors remain premature closure of the ductus arteriosus and neonatal primary pulmonary hypertension.[147,148]

A cohort study suggests that use of indomethacin for preterm labor appears to increase the risk of serious neonatal complications (eg, necrotizing enterocolitis, intracranial hemorrhage, and patent ductus arteriosus) in infants born at or before 30 weeks' gestation.[149]

Ritodrine

Ritodrine is a beta-adrenergic agonist with predominant effects on β_2 receptors.[111,112] Oral administration of 10 mg

Table 8–13
Treatment of Poisoning During Pregnancy

Drug	Fetal Distress Early Delivery	Treatment Same for Pregnant as Nonpregnant Patients	Fetal Monitoring
Acetaminophen	+ (only for maternal indications or fetal distress)	–	+
Carbon monoxide	?	+	+
Digitalis	+ (after Fab fragments?)	+	+
Fluoride	+	+	+
Iron	+	+	+
Organophosphate insecticide	+ (if fetus potentially viable)	+	+
Petroleum distillate	+	+	+
Salicylates	+ (if fetus viable ex utero)	+	+

See References 159 and 160.

Table 8–14
Interim Centers for Disease Control and Prevention Recommendations for Folic Acid Supplementation for Women Who Have Had an Infant or Fetus With Spina Bifida, Anencephaly, or Encephalocele—August 1991

1. Women who have had a pregnancy resulting in an infant or fetus with a neural tube defect should be counseled about the increased risk in subsequent pregnancies and should be advised that folic acid supplementation may substantially reduce the risk for neural tube defects in subsequent pregnancies.
2. Women who have had a pregnancy resulting in an infant or fetus with a neural tube defect should be advised to consult their physician as soon as they plan a pregnancy. Unless contraindicated, they should be advised to take 4 mg per day of folic acid starting at the time they plan to become pregnant. Women should take the supplement from at least 4 weeks before conception through the first 3 months of pregnancy.
3. The 4-mg daily dose should be taken only under a physician's supervision. Tablets containing 1 mg folic acid are available as a prescription item. The folic acid dose should be obtained from pills containing only folic acid. Multivitamin (over-the-counter and prescription) preparations containing folic acid should *not* be used to attain the 4-mg dose because harmful levels of vitamins A and D could also be taken. Prescribing physicians should be aware of the potential for high doses of folic acid to complicate the diagnosis of vitamin B_{12} deficiency. Anemia resulting from vitamin B_{12} deficiency may be prevented with high doses of folic acid; however, the neurologic damage that can result from vitamin B_{12} deficiency could continue.
4. These recommendations are provided only for women who previously have given birth to an infant or had a fetus with a neural tube defect; they are *not* intended for (1) women who have never given birth to an infant or had a fetus with a neural tube defect, (2) relatives of women who have had an infant or fetus with a neural tube defect, (3) women who themselves have spina bifida, or (4) women who take the anticonvulsant valproic acid, a known cause of spina bifida.

From Centers for Disease Control and Prevention. Use of folic acid for prevention of spina bifida and other neural tube defects, 1983–1991. MMWR 1991;40:513–516.

Table 8–15
Centers for Disease Control and Recommendation for Folic Acid Supplementation for Women of Childbearing Age

All women of childbearing age in the United States who are capable of becoming pregnant should consume 0.4 mg of folic acid per day for the purpose of reducing their risk of having a pregnancy affected with spina bifida or other neural tube defects. Because the effects of high intakes are not well known but include complicating the diagnosis of vitamin B_{12} deficiency, care should be taken to keep total folate consumption at <1 mg per day, except under the supervision of a physician. Women who have had a prior neural tube defect-affected pregnancy are at high risk of having a subsequent affected pregnancy. When these women are planning to become pregnant, they should consult their physicians for advice.

From Centers for Disease Control and Prevention. Recommendations for the use of folic acid to reduce the number of cases of spina bifida and other neural tube defects. MMWR 1992;41:1–7.

ritodrine produces peak serum concentrations of 31 ng/mL in about 30 minutes; bioavailability is about 20 to 30%.[113–116] Intravenous ritrodrine is usually given at an initial rate of 50 to 100 μg/min and increased every 15 to 20 minutes until uterine contractions have ceased, unacceptable side effects have developed, or a maximum dosage of 350 μg/min has been achieved. An initial-phase half-life of 6 to 9 minutes is followed by biphasic elimination with a half-life of about 21.3 hours. There is rapid transplacental transfer of intravenous ritodrine. Intramuscular ritodrine (5–10 mg every 2–4 hours) has also been used and leads to a peak ritodrine serum concentration of 97 ng/mL in 10 minutes. Oral sustained-release doses of 120, 240, and 360 mg/d, respectively, led to peak plasma levels of 11, 24, and 32 ng/mL.[117] Maternal pulmonary edema,[118] myocardial ischemia,[119] with ST–T wave changes,[120–122] agranulocytosis,[123,124] salivary gland enlargement,[125] increases in plasma glucose, increases in plasma insulin, and maternal deaths have been observed.[126]

Overdose with ritodrine leads to flushing, tremulousness, tachycardia, hypotension, and hypokalemia. Treatment is symptomatic and supportive.[127]

Salbutamol

Salbutamol is extensively used outside of the United States for inhibition of preterm labor. Its administration, types of side effects, and effectiveness are similar to those of other betamimetic agents. Transplacental transfer occurs.

Terbutaline

Terbutaline (Brethine/Bricanyl) can inhibit uterine contractions and is effective in treating premature labor. A maternal infusion of terbutaline has a half-life of about 4 hours. There is a rapid transplacental transfer within 1 hour. After subcutaneous administration, the absorptive half-life is 7 minutes. Doses of 0.25 mg subcutaneously are used every 20 to 60 minutes until contractions have subsided. Following oral administration, peak serum concentrations of about 1 to 8 ng/mL are reached after 1 hour, lower than after intravenous use (12–30 ng/mL). Maternal side effects such as tachycardia, hypotension, chest pain, atrial arrhythmias,[128] hypokalemia, and jitteriness have occurred with both terbutaline and ritodrine. Sudden maternal death has followed terbutaline use (subcutaneous 0.064 mg/L with 0.2-mg boluses).[129] Myocardial necrosis has been observed in a newborn after maternal subcutaneous terbutaline.[130]

Other β_2-Agonist Agents

Fenoterol, hexaprenaline, and orciprenaline (all β_2-selective agents) produce significant tocolytic effects, but controlled trials are lacking.[131–133] Hexoprenaline appears to produce the least effect on the maternal cardiovascular system, but

Table 8–16
Occupational Reproductive Hazards Resources

Computer Databases
MEDLINE: National Library of Medicine (Bethesda, MD)—contains references from 3000 biomedical journals
TOXLINE: National Library of Medicine (Bethesda, MD)—contains more than 400,000 references to published human and animal toxicologic studies
TOXNET: National Library of Medicine (Bethesda, MD)—toxicology-oriented data bank
REPROTOX: Reproduced Toxicology Center (Washington, DC)—contains referenced summaries of reproductive data for more than 800 physical and chemical agents
ON-LINE CATALOG OF TERATOGENIC AGENTS: Central Laboratory for Human Embryology (Seattle, WA)—free database on teratogenic effects of nearly 2000 substances

Hotlines
Pregnancy/Environmental Hotline (serves primarily Massachusetts, but will accept calls from practitioners nationally)—(800) 322–5014 (MA only); (617) 787–4957. National Birth Defects Center, Kennedy Memorial Hospital (Boston, MA)
Pregnancy Exposure Information Service (serves Connecticut)—(800) 325–5391 (CT only). University of Connecticut Health Center (Farmington, CT)
Washington State Poison Control Network—(800) 732–6985 (Washington only); (206) 526–2121. University of Washington (Seattle, WA)

Regulatory and Related Agencies
Occupational Safety and Health Administration (OSHA) (Washington, DC, regional and local state offices)—responsible for promulgation and enforcement of standards for workplace hazards; will perform workplace inspections at request of employee, union, or health care provider
National Institute for Occupational Safety and Health (NIOSH) (Atlanta, GA, and local state offices)—develops scientific documents for use in standard settings; investigates health and safety hazards in workplaces on request

Written Reference Materials
American College of Obstetricians and Gynecologists/National Institute for Occupational Safety and Health. *Guidelines on Pregnancy and Work.* Washington, DC: U.S. Government Printing Office, 1977
Barlow SM, Sullivan E. *Reproductive Hazards of Industrial Chemicals.* New York: Academic Press, 1982
Brown NA, Scialli AR, eds. *Reproductive Toxicology: A Medical Letter on Environmental Hazards to Reproduction.* Published bimonthly by the Reproductive Toxicology Center, 2425 L Street NW, Washington, DC
Clarkson TW, Nordberg G, Sager PR, eds. *Reproductive and Developmental Toxicity of Metals.* New York: Plenum Press, 1983
National Institute for Occupational Safety and Health. *Registry of Toxic Effects of Chemical Substances, September 1980, With Supplement 1983–84.* Washington, DC: U.S. Government Printing Office, DHHS-86-103, November 1985
Shepard TH. *Catalog of Teratogenic Agents.* Baltimore: Johns Hopkins University Press, 1986
U.S. Congress, Office of Technology Assessment. *Reproductive Hazards in the Workplace.* Washington, DC: U.S. Government Printing Office, OTA-BA-266, December 1985

From Paul M, Himmelstein J. Reproductive hazards in the workplace: What the practitioner needs to know about chemical resources. Obstet Gynecol 1988;7:921–938.

has been associated with fetal tachycardia and pulmonary edema.[131-133]

TOLUENE

Women workers exposed to high air concentrations of toluene (50–150 ppm) appeared to have a higher incidence of spontaneous abortion than a similar group of women with no occupational exposure to toluene.[150] Further studies are required to validate this finding. Animal studies indicate that toluene readily crosses the placenta. Maternal spray paint or glue sniffing leads to maternal complications including renal tubular acidosis, hypokalemia, hypocalcemia, cardiac arrhythmias, rhabdomyolysis, and premature labor.[151] Premature toluene exposure leads to a characteristic pattern of anomalies similar to findings in infants exposed to alcohol in utero (Table 8–12), consisting of an increased incidence of malformations, poor growth, and developmental delays.[152,153]

TREATMENT

Table 8–13 summarizes some suggested approaches to the treatment of poisoning during pregnancy.[159,160]

Table 8–17
The Motherisk Team

Full-time staff
- Director–pediatrician/clinical pharmacologist/toxicologist
- Clinical fellows subspecializing in clinical pharmacology/toxicology
- Coordinator–information specialist
- Medical secretary
- Information specialists

Part-time staff
- Research nurse
- Medical information specialist–pharmacist
- Statistician, PhD
- Sonographer–physician
- Addiction specialist–physician
- Obstetricians and perinatologists
- Clinical pharmacologists–physicians
- Medical toxicologist–physician
- Geneticist–physician
- Prenatal genetics counselor

Students
- Graduate students (pharmacology and toxicology and pharmacy)
- Undergraduate students (pharmacology and toxicology)

From Koren G, Graham K, Feigenbaum A, Einarson T. Evaluation and counseling of teratogenic risk: The Motherisk approach. J Clin Pharmacol 1993;33:405–411.

Table 8–18
Teratogen Information Programs

United States

Arizona
Arizona Teratogen Information Service
Tucson, Arizona
1–800–626–6016 (AZ only); (602) 626–6016

California
California Teratogen Registry
San Diego, California
1–800–532–3749 (CA only); (619) 294–3584

Colorado
Genetics Unit/Teratology Service
Rocky Mountain Drug Information
Denver, Colorado
(303) 394–8741; (303) 893–DRUG: (303) 629–1123

Connecticut
Connecticut Pregnancy Exposure Information Service
Farmington, Connecticut
1–800–325–5391 (CT only); (203) 679–2676

District of Columbia
Reproductive Toxicology Center
Washington, DC
(202) 293–5137

Florida
Genetics Division/The Teratology Service,
Miami, Florida
(305) 547–6006

Teratogen Information Service
Gainesville, Florida
(904) 392–4104

Illinois
Teratogen Helpline
Chicago, Illinois
(312) 791–4451

Iowa
University of Iowa Genetics Division
Iowa City, Iowa
(319) 356–2674

Maryland
FDA Adverse Drug Effects Branch
Rockville, Maryland
(301) 443–6410

Massachusetts
Teratogen Information Service
Boston, Massachusetts
1–800–322–5014 (MA only); (617) 787–4957

Missouri
Washington University School of Medicine Genetics Department
St. Louis, Missouri
(314) 454–7700

Nebraska
Nebraska Teratogen Project
Omaha, Nebraska
1–800–642–6274 (NE only); (402) 559–5070

New York
Prenatal Information Hotline
Hauppauge, New York
(516) 348–2708

Pennsylvania
Pregnancy Healthline
Philadelphia, Pennsylvania
(215) 829–KIDS

Pregnancy Safety Hotline
Pittsburgh, Pennsylvania
(412) 687–SAFE

Magee Womens Hospital Department of Reproductive Genetics
Pittsburgh, Pennsylvania
(412) 647–4168

Texas
Genetics Screening and Counseling Service
Denton, Texas
(817) 383–3561

Utah
Pregnancy Riskline
Salt Lake City, Utah
1–800–822–BABY (UT only); (801) 583–2229

Vermont
Vermont Pregnancy Risk Network
Burlington, Vermont
1–800–531–9800 (VT only); (802) 658–4310

Washington
Washington State Poison Control Network
Seattle, Washington
1–800–732–6985 (WA only); (206) 526–2121 (Alaska, continental U.S.); (206) 543–3373

Wisconsin
Wisconsin Teratogen Project
Madison, Wisconsin
1–800–362–3020 (WI only); (608) 263–1991

Teratogen Information Project
Milwaukee, Wisconsin
(414) 931–4172

Canada

Ontario
Motherisk
Toronto, Ontario
(416) 598–6780

Motherisk
Ottawa, Ontario
(613) 737–1100

Safe Start
Hamilton, Ontario
(416) 525–9140 (x 2278); (416) 521–2100 (x 2780)

FRAME program
London, Ontario
(519) 439–3271 (x 4378)

Quebec
Pregnancy Healthline
Montreal, Quebec
(514) 934–4427

From Vogt BL. Teratogen information programs. In: Koren G, ed. *Maternal–Fetal Toxicology: A Clinician's Guide.* New York: Marcel Dekker, 1990: 332–333.

NEURAL TUBE DEFECTS: PREVENTION

Several studies have indicated that folic acid-containing multivitamins taken during the first 6 weeks of pregnancy prevent, perhaps by more than 50%, the occurrence of neural tube defects in the fetus or infant.[161–163] The Centers for Disease Control and Prevention has issued interim[164] (Table 8–14) and subsequent[165] (Table 8–15) recommendations. Supplemental doses of 0.4 mg of folic acid may be achieved through ingestion of most over-the-counter multivitamin products.[166] A case–control study suggests that use of multivitamins containing folic acid by a mother from 1 month before through 2 months after conception reduces the risk in offspring of orofacial clefts.[167]

Hydantoin Syndrome

Hydantoin and phenobarbital, a metabolite of primidone, are well-established anticonvulsive drugs. When taken in pregnancy, both agents increase teratogenic risk and can produce "hydantoin syndrome" in the fetus. Hydantoin syndrome is a well-known risk of maternal anticonvulsant intake during pregnancy. Typical manifestations are minor craniofacial and digital anomalies such as hypertelorism, epicanthal folds, midface hypoplasia, and hypoplastic distal phalanges and nails.

The sensitive period in embryonic development related to the effect of the hydantoin syndrome is from the 18th to the 56 day after fertilization. About 10% of fetuses exposed to phenytoin show some signs of the hydantoin syndrome. Holoprosencephaly is a rare teratogenic defect of hydantoin intake during pregnancy.[136]

INFORMATION

Occupational and general reproductive hazards resources are listed in Table 8–16.[168] A Reproductive Toxicology Center is located at the Columbia Hospital for Women Medical Center, 2440 M Street NW, Suite 217, Washington, DC 20037–1404. Women may be counseled on reproductive risks of drugs, chemicals, and radiation at the Motherisk Program, Hospital for Sick Children and the University of Toronto, Toronto, Canada (Table 8–17).

TERATOGEN INFORMATION SERVICES

The main function of the a teratogen information service is to provide information and consultation to health care professionals and/or the general public who have concerns with respect to exposure to drugs, chemicals, and radiation during pregnancy to determine any potential risk to the pregnant patient and/or the unborn child.[169] A teratology information service is part of the National Poisons Information Service at Avonley Road, London SE145ER, United Kingdom. Additional teratology information programs in the United States are listed in Table 8–18.[170] Further information is available at local and national poison information centers throughout the world.

Table 8–19
Use-in-Pregnancy Ratings (U.S. Food and Drug Administration, 1979)

Category	Interpretaton
A	Controlled studies show no risk. Adequate, well-controlled studies in pregnant women have failed to demonstrate risk to the fetus.
B	No evidence of risk in humans. Either animal find- ings show risk, but human findings do not; or, if no adequate human studies have been done, animal findings are negative.
C	Risk cannot be ruled out. Human studies are lack- ing, and animal studies are either positive for fetal risk or lacking as well. However, potential benefits may justify the potential risk.
D	Positive evidence of risk. Investigational or post-marketing data show risk to the fetus. Nevertheless, potential benefits may outweigh the potential risk.
X	Contraindicated in pregnancy. Studies in animals or human, or investigational or postmarketing reports, have shown fetal risk which clearly out- weighs any possible benefit to the patient.

From Teratology Society Public Affairs Committee. FDA classification of drugs for teratogenic risk. Teratology 1994;49:446–447.

TERATOGENIC RISK CLASSIFICATION

The Teratology Society has proposed that the current U.S. Food and Drug Administration use-in-pregnancy ratings (Table 8–19)[171] be abandoned and replaced by drug labeling that includes narrative statements that summarize and interpret available data regarding the hazards of development toxicity and provide estimates of potential teratogenic risk.[172]

REFERENCES

1. Longo LD. Physiologic assessment of fetal compromise: Biomarkers of toxic exposure. Environ Health Perspect 1987; 74:93–101.
2. Rubin PC, Craig GF, Gavin K, Sumner D. Prospective survey of use of therapeutic drugs, alcohol and cigarettes during pregnancy. Br Med J 1986;292:81–83.
3. Evans MI, Pryde PG, Reichler A, et al. Fetal drug therapy. West J Med 1993;159:328–332.
4. Huong TTT, Szentesi I, Czeizell A. Lower prevalence of chromosome aberrations and SCE's in self-poisoned pregnant women. Mutat Res 1988;198:255–259.
5. McElhatton PR, Sullivan FM, Volans GM, Fitzpatrick R. Paracetamol poisoning in pregnancy: An analysis of the outcome of cases referred to the teratology information service of the National Poisons Information Service. Hum Exp Toxicol 1990;9:147–153.
6. Riggs BS, Bronstein AC, Kulig K, et al. Acute acetaminophen overdose during pregnancy. Obstet Gynecol 1989;74:247–253.
7. Wise R. Prescribing in pregnancy: Antibiotics. Br Med J 1987;294:42–46.
8. Thorpe-Beeston JG, Armar NA, Dancy M, et al. Pregnancy and ACE inhibitors. Br J Obstet Gynaecol 1993;100:692–693.
9. Safety of antimicrobial drugs in pregnancy. Med Lett Drugs Ther 1987;29:61–63.

10. Chow AW, Jewesson PJ. Use and safety of antimicrobial agents during pregnancy. West J Med 1987;146: 761–767.
11. Peled Y, Friedman S, Hod M, Merlob P. Ofloxacin during the second trimester of pregnancy. DICP Ann Pharmacother 1991;25:1181–1182.
12. Heim K, Alge A, Marth C. Anaphylactic reaction to ampicillin and severe complication in the fetus. Lancet 1991;337: 859–860.
13. Nau H. Clinical pharmacokinetics in pregnancy and perinatology. II. Penicillins. Dev Pharmacol Ther 1987;10:174–198.
14. Ginsberg JS, Hirsh J. Use of antithrombotic agents during pregnancy. Chest 1992;102(suppl. 4):385–390.
15. Cerqueira MJ, Olle C, Bellart J, et al. Intoxication by benzodiazepines during pregnancy. Lancet 1988;1:1341.
16. Haraldsson A, Geven W. Severe adverse effects of maternal labetalol in a premature infant. Acta Paediatr Scand 1989;78: 956–958.
17. Rubin PC. Current concepts: Beta blockers in pregnancy. N Engl J Med 1981;305:1323–1326.
18. Bhandari NR, Syal AK, Kambo I, et al. Pregnancy outcome in women exposed to toxic gas at Bhopal. Indian J Med Res [B] 1990;91:28–31.
19. Wilcox A, Weinberg C, Baird D. Caffeinated beverages and decreased fertility. Lancet 1988;2:1453–1456.
20. Christianson RE, Oechsli FW, Van den Berg BJ. Caffeinated beverages and decreased fertility. Lancet 1989;2:378.
21. Weathersby PS, Lodge JR. Caffeine, its direct and indirect influence on reproduction. J Reprod Med 1977;19:55–63.
22. Oei SG, Vosters RPL, van der Hagen NLJ, et al. Arrhythmia caused by excessive intake of caffeine by pregnant women. Br Med J 1989;298:568.
23. McGowan JD, Altman RE, Kanto WP Jr. Neonatal withdrawal symptoms after chronic maternal ingestion of caffeine. South Med J 1988;81:1092–1094.
24. Myers VAS, Miwa LJ. Caffeine consumption during pregnancy. Drug Intell Clin Pharm 1988;22:614–616.
25. Hill EP, Hill JR, Power GG, Longon LD. Carbon monoxide exchanges between the human fetus and mother: A mathematical model. Am J Physiol 1977;232:311–323.
26. Koren G, Sharav T, Pastuszak A, et al. A multicenter, prospective study of fetal outcome following accidental carbon monoxide poisoning in pregnancy. Reprod Toxicol 1991;5: 397–403.
27. Elkharrat D, Raphael JC, Korack JM, et al. Acute carbon monoxide intoxication and hyperbaric oxygen in pregnancy. Intensive Care Med 1991;17:289–298.
28. Lees KR, Rubin PC. Prescribing in pregnancy: Treatment of cardiovascular disease. Br Med J 1987;294:358–360.
29. Senecal P-E, Osterloh JD. Normal fetal outcome after maternal ciguatera toxin exposure in the second trimester. Clin Toxicol 1991;29:473–478.
30. Ostrea EM Jr, Brady M, Gause S, et al. Drug screening of newborns by meconium analysis: A large-scale prospective epidemiologic study. Pediatrics 1992;89:107–113.
31. Jessup M. The treatment of perinatal addiction: Identification, intervention and advocacy. West J Med 1990;152:553–558.
32. Levy M, Spiro M. Neonatal withdrawal syndrome: Associated drugs and pharmacologic management. Pharmacotherapy 1993;13:202–211.
33. Jacobson SJ, Jones K, Johnson K, et al. Prospective multicenter study of pregnancy outcome after lithium exposure during first trimester. Lancet 1992;339:530–533.
34. Rayburn W, Aronow R, DeLancey B, Hogan MJ. Drug overdose during pregnancy: An overview from a metropolitan poison control center. Obstet Gynecol 1984;64:611–614.
35. Blanc P, Hryhorczuk D, Davel I. Deferoxamine treatment of acute iron intoxication in pregnancy. Obstet Gynecol 1984;65:125–145.
36. Curry S, Bond R, Rashke R, et al. Fetal iron kinetics is a mode of maternal iron poisoning with and without maternal deferoxamine therapy. Vet Hum Toxicol 1988;30:372.
37. Elias S, Gerbie AB, Simpson JL, et al. Genetic amniocentesis in twin gestations. Am J Obstet Gynecol 1980;138:169–173.
38. Alay RD, Southerst JR. Premature rupture of the fetal membranes confirmed by intra-amniotic injection of dye. Am J Obstet Gynecol 1970;108:993.
39. Troche BI. The methylene blue baby. N Engl J Med 1989; 320:1756–1757.
40. Katz Z, Lancet MN. Inadvertent intrauterine injection of methylene blue in early pregnancy. N Engl J Med 1981;30:1427.
41. Nicolini U, Monni G. Intestinal obstruction babies exposed in utero to methylene blue. Lancet 1990;336:1758–1759.
42. Wood SM, Hytten FE. The fate of drugs of pregnancy. Clin Obstet Gynecol 1981;8:255–259.
43. Cowell RM, Hakanson DO, Kocon RW, Oh W. Untoward neonatal effect of intraamniotic administration of methylene blue. Obstet Gynecol 1976;48(suppl.):74S–75S.
44. Serota FT, Bernbaum JC, Schwartz E. The methylene-blue baby. Lancet 1979;2:1142–1143.
45. Crooks J. Hemolytic jaundice in a neonate after intraamniotic injection of methylene blue. Arch Dis Child 1982;57:872–886.
46. McEnerney JK, McEnerney LN. Unfavorable neonatal outcome after intra-amniotic injection of methylene blue. Obstet Gynecol 1983;61:355–375.
47. Vincer MJ, Allen AC, Evans JR, et al. Methylene-blue induced hemolytic anemia in a neonate. Can Med Assoc J 1987;136:503–504.
48. Dolk H. Methylene blue and atresia or stenosis of ileum and jejunum. Lancet 1991;338:1021–1022.
49. McFadyen I. The dangers of intra-amniotic methylene blue. Br J Obstet Gynecol 1992;99:89–90.
50. Van der Pol JG, Wolf H, Boer K, et al. Jejunal atresia related to the use of methylene blue in genetic amniocentesis in man. Br J Obstet Gynecol 1992;99:141–143.
51. Belliardo P, Massano G, Accono S. Amatoxins do not cross the placental barrier. Lancet 1983;1:1381.
52. Levy G. Nutmeg intoxication in pregnancy: a case report. J Reprod Med 1987;32:63–64.
53. Tylden E, Duokens D, Colley N. Pregnancy and opiate addiction. Br Med J 1987;295:551–552.
54. Michell AA. Oral retinoids: What should the prescriber know about their teratogenic hazards among women of childbearing potential? Drug Saf 1992;7:79–85.
55. Koren G. Study of the safety of ribavirin in human pregnancy. Pediatr Infect Dis J 1990;9:S106–S107.
56. Kizer K. Study raises concerns about exposure of health workers to antiviral ribavirin. Action Report 36, California Department of Health Services, March 1989.
57. Nieburg P, Marks JS, McLaren NM, Remington PL. The fetal tobacco syndrome. JAMA 1985;253:2998–2999.
58. Werler MM, Lammer EJ, Rosenberg L, Mitchell AA. Maternal cigarette smoking during pregnancy in relation to oral clefts. Am J Epidemiol 1990;132:926–932.
59. Seidman DS, Ever-Hadani P, Gale R. Effect of maternal smoking and age on congenital anomalies. Obstet Gynecol 1990;76:1046–1050.
60. Tafuri J, Roberts J. Organophosphate poisoning. Ann Emerg Med 1987;16:193–202.
61. Dunne J, Wise C. The pump that gave too much: Accidental overfusion of prostacyclin. Anaesthesia 1991;46:75.
62. Douglas M, Farquharson DF, Ross PLE, Renwich JE. Cardiovascular collapse following an overdose of prostaglandin F_2 alpha: A case report. Can J Anaesth 1989;36: 466–468.
63. Kilpatrick AWA, Thorburn J. Severe hypotension due to intramyometrial injection of prostaglandin E_2. Anaesthesia 1990;45:848–849.
64. Meyer WJ, Benton SL, Moon TJ, et al. Acute myocardial infarction associated with prostaglandin E_2. Obstet Gynecol 1991;165:359–360.
65. Cooley DM, Glosten B, Roberts JR, et al. Bronchospasm after intramuscular 15-methyl prostaglandin F_2 alpha and endotracheal intubation in a nonasthmatic patient. Anesth Analg 1991;73:87–89.
66. Brandenburg H, Jahoda MGJ, Welodminiroff JW, et al. Convulsions in epileptic woman after administration of prostaglandin E_2 derivatives. Lancet 1990;336:1138.
67. Wiener JJ, Evans AS. Uterine rupture in midtrimester abortion: A complication of Gemeprost vaginal pessaries in

oxytocin. Case report. Br J Obstet Gynecol 1990;97:1061–1062.

68. Less A, Goldberger SB, Bernheim J, et al. Vaginal prostaglandin E_2 and fatal amniotic fluid emblem. JAMA 1990;263: 3259–3260.
69. Moran DJ. Gemeprost vaginal pessaries for inducing third trimester intrauterine deaths. Br J Obstet Gynecol 1989;96: 1245–1251.
70. Shoham Z, Ezri T. Ventricular tachycardia associated with injection of prostaglandin F_2 alpha into the uterine cervix during anesthesia. Anesthesiology 1990;72:775–771.
71. Peled N, Dagan O, Babyn P, et al. Gastric outlet obstruction induced by prostaglandin therapy in neonates. N Engl J Med 1992;327:505–512.
72. Andersson S, Paetau P, Hallman M, et al. Neonatal respiratory distress caused by aspiration of a vaginal tablet containing prostaglandin. Br Med J 1987;295:25–26.
73. Egarter CH, Husslein PW, Rayburn WF. Uterine hyperstimulation after low dose prostaglandin E_2 therapy: Tricyclic treatment in 181 cases. Am J Obstet Gynecol 1990;163: 794–796.
74. Burt RL, Connor ED, Davidson IWF. Hypokalemia and cardiac arrhythmia associated with prostaglandin-induced abortion. Obstet Gynecol 1977;50(suppl.):455–465.
75. Popat MT, Suppiah N, White JB. Cardiac arrest following intramyometrial injection of prostaglandin E_2. Anaesthesia 1991;46:236.
76. Zilberstein ME, Gleicher M. Endocrinology. In: Gleicher N, ed. *Principles and Practice of Medical Therapy in Pregnancy.* 2nd ed. Norwalk, CT: Appleton–Lange, 1992:292–293.
77. Burt RL, Connor ED, Davidson IWF. Hypokalemia and cardiac arrhythmia associated with prostaglandin-induced abortion. Obstet Gynecol 1977;50(suppl.):455–465.
78. Douglas M, Farquharson DF, Ross PLE, Renwich JE. Cardiovascular collapse following an overdose of prostaglandin F_2 alpha: A case report. Can J Anaesth 1989;36:466–468.
79. King SJ, Kelly RW, Sutton JG. The development of an enzyme-linked immunosorbent assay for 19-OH-PG F_1 alpha/F_2 alpha. Forens Sci Int 1989;40:211–216.
80. Pearson R. Radiography in women of childbearing ability. Br Med J 1989;299:1175–1176.
81. Hooper K. The hazard evaluation system and information service: A physician's resource in toxicology and occupational medicine. West J Med 1982;137:560–571.
82. McDonald AD, McDonald JC, Armstrong B, et al. Fetal death and work in pregnancy. Br J Ind Med 1988;45:148–157.
83. Schenker MB, Samuels SJ, Green RS, Wiggins P. Adverse reproductive outcome among female veterinarians. Am J Epidemiol 1990;132:96–106.
84. McDonald AD, La Voie J, Cote R, McDonald JC. Spontaneous abortion in women employed in plastics manufacture. Am J Ind Med 1988;14:9–14.
85. Bentur Y, Koren G. The three most common occupational exposures reported by pregnant women: An update. Am J Obstet Gynecol 1991;165:429–437.
86. Mattison DR, Plowchalk DR, Meadows MJ, et al. Reproductive toxicity: Male and female reproductive systems as targets for chemical injury. Med Clin North Am 1990;74:391–411.
87. Jagoda A, Riggio S. Emergency department approach to managing seizures in pregnancy. Ann Emerg Med 1991;20: 80–85.
88. Konje JC, Otolorin EO, Sotunmbi PT, Ladipo OA. Insecticide poisoning in pregnancy: A case report. J Reprod Med 1992;37:992–994.
89. McDonald AD, McDonald JC, Armstrong B, et al. Father's occupation and pregnancy outcome. Br J Ind Med 1989;46: 329–333.
90. Brender JD, Suarez L. Paternal occupation and anencephaly. Am J Epidemiol 1990;131:512–521.
91. Olshan AF, Teschke K, Baird PA. Birth defects among offspring of firemen. Am J Epidemiol 1990;131:312–321.
92. Olshan AF, Teschke K, Baird PA. Paternal occupation and congenital anomalies. Am J Ind Med 1991;20:447–475.
93. Lindbohm ML, Sallmen M, Antilla A, et al. Paternal occupational lead exposure and spontaneous abortion. Scand J Environ Health 1991;17:95–103.
94. Cordier S, Deplan F, Mandereau L, Hemon D. Paternal exposure to mercury and spontaneous abortions. Br J Ind Med 1991;48:375–381.
95. Savitz DA, Schwingl PJ, Kells MA. Influence of paternal age, smoking and alcohol consumption on congenital anomalies. Teratology 1991;44:429–440.
96. Davis DL. Paternal smoking and fetal health. Lancet 1991;1: 123.
97. Robaire B, Hales BF. Paternal exposure to chemicals before conception: Some children may be at risk. Br Med J 1993; 307:341–342.
98. Tomatis L, Narod S, Yamasaki L. Transgeneration transmission of carcinogenic risk. Cardiogenesis 1992;43: 145–151.
99. Dodds L, Marrett LD, Tomkins DJ, et al. Case–control study of congenital anomalies of children of cancer patients. Br Med J 1993;307:164–168.
100. Savitz DA, Whelan EA, Kleckner RC. Effect of parents' occupational exposures on risk of stillbirth, pre-term delivery and small-for gestational-age infants. Am J Epidemiol 1989; 129:1201–1218.
101. Einarson TR, Koren G, Mattice D, Schechter-Isafriri O. Maternal spermicide use and adverse reproductive outcome: A meta-analysis. Am J Obstet Gynecol 1990;162: 655–660.
102. Warburton D, Neugut RH, Lustenberger A, et al. Lack of association between spermicide use and trisomies. N Engl J Med 1987;317:478–482.
103. Besinger RE, Niebyl JR. The safety and efficacy of toxolytic agents for the treatment of pre-term labor. Obstet Gynecol Surg 1990;45:415.
104. Chamberlain G. Pre-term labor. Br Med J 1991;303:44–48.
105. Pisani RJ, Rosenoid EC III. Pulmonary edema associated with toxolytic therapy. Ann Intern Med 1989;110:714–718.
106. Creasy RK. Preventing pre-term birth. N Engl J Med 1991; 325:727–729.
107. Wischnik A. Risk–benefit assessment of tocolytic drugs. Drug Saf 1991;6:371–380.
108. Halmesmaki E, Yiikorkala O. A retrospective study on the safety of prenatal ethanol treatment. Obstet Gynecol 1988; 27:545.
109. Abel EL. Critical evaluation of the obstetric use of alcohol in pre-term labor. Drug Alcohol Depend 1981;7:367.
110. Brazy JE, Pupkin MJ. Effects of maternal isoxsuprine administration on pre-term infants. J Pediatr 1979;94:444.
111. Benedetti TJ. Treatment of pre-term labor with the beta-adrenergic agonist ritodrine. N Engl J Med 1992;327:1758.
112. Ferguson JE II, Dyson DC, Schutz T, Stevenson DC. A comparison of tocolysis with nifedipine or ritodrine: Analysis of efficacy and maternal, fetal and neonatal outcome. Am J Obstet Gynecol 1990;163:105–111.
113. Van Lierde M, Desager JP, Harvengt C, Thomas K. Ritodrine serum levels: Influence of dose and route of administration. Int J Clin Pharmacol Ther Toxicol 1984;22: 382–385.
114. Kuhnert BR, Gross TL, Kuhnert PM, et al. Ritodrine pharmacokinetics. Clin Pharmacol Ther 1986;40:656–664.
115. Caritis SN, Venkataramanan R, Darby MJ, et al. Pharmacokinetics of ritodrine administered intravenously: Recommendations for changes in the current regimen. Am J Obstet Gynecol 1990;162:429–437.
116. Caritis SM, Lin LS, Venkataramanan R, Wong LK. Effect of pregnancy on ritodrine pharmacokinetics. Am J Obstet Gynecol 1988;159:328–332.
117. Witter FR, Benedetti TJ, Petty BG, et al. Pharmacodynamics and tolerance of oral sustained release ritodrine. Am J Obstet Gynecol 1988;159:690–695.
118. Gupta RC, Foster S, Romano PM, Thomas HM. Acute pulmonary edema associated with the use of oral ritodrine for premature labor. Chest 1989;95:479–481.
119. Ben-Shtona I, Zohar S, Marmor A, et al. Myocardial ischemia during intravenous ritodrine treatment: Is it so rare? Lancet 1986;2:917–918.
120. Faidley CK, Dix PM, Morgan MA, Schechter Z. Electrocardiographic abnormalities during ritodrine administration. South Med J 1990;83:503–506.

121. Hendricks SK, Kerves J, Katz M. Electrocardiographic changes associated with ritodrine-induced maternal tachycardia and hypokalemia. Am J Obstet Gynecol 1986;154: 921–923.
122. Hadi HA, Albazzaz SJ. Cardiac isoenzymes and electrocardiographic changes during ritodrine tocolysis. Am J Obstet Gynecol 1989;161:318–321.
123. Ikushima Y, Kobayashi H, Imaishi K, et al. Ritodrine-induced agranulocytosis. Arch Gynecol Obstet 1990;248:53–54.
124. Muro M, Shono H, Oga M, et al. Ritodrine-induced agranulocytosis. Int J Gynecol Obstet 1991;36:329–331.
125. Minakani W, Takahashi T, Izuni A, et al. Enlargement of the salivary gland after ritodrine treatment in pregnant women. Br Med J 1992;304:1668.
126. Spellacy WN, Cruz AC, Buhi WC, Birk SA. The acute effects of ritodrine infusion on maternal metabolism: Measurements of levels of glucose, insulin, glucagon, triglycerides, cholesterol, placental lactogen, and chorionic gonadotropin. Am J Obstet Gynecol 1978;131:637–642.
127. Bricker RSW. Overdose of ritodrine. Anaesthesia 1989;44:864.
128. Levy DL. Morbidity caused by terbutaline infusion during therapy. Am J Obstet Gynecol 1994;170:1835–1836.
129. Hudgens DR, Conradi SE. Sudden death associated with terbutaline sulfate administration. J Obstet Gynecol 1993;169:120–121.
130. Fletcher SE, Fyfer DA, Case CL, et al. Myocardial necrosis in a newborn after long-term maternal subcutaneous terbutaline infusion for suppression of pre-term labor. Am J Obstet Gynecol 991;165:1401–1404.
131. D'Hooghe TM, Odendaal HJ. Severe fatal tachycardia after administration of hexoprenaline to the mother: A case report. S Afr Med J 1991;80:594–596.
132. Rivier G, Nicole A, Stuchi D, Regumy C. Lesional pulmonary edema associated with tocolysis by hexoprenaline sulfate. Schweiz Med Wochenschr 1992;122:237–241.
133. Van Iddekinge B, Gobertz L, Seaward PGR, Hofmeyr GJ. Pulmonary oedema after hexaprenaline administration in preterm labor. S Afr Med J 1991;79:620–622.
134. Lees C, Campbell S, Jauniaux E, et al. Arrest of preterm labour and prolongation of gestation with glyceryl trinitrate, a nitric oxide donor. Lancet 1994;343:1325–1326.
135. Duley L, Elbourne D. Glyceryl trinitrate in management of preterm labour. Lancet 1994;344:553.
136. Kotzot D, Weigl J, Huk W, Rott H-D. Hydantoin syndrome with holoprosencephaly: A possible rare teratogenic effect. Teratology 1993;48:15–19.
137. Cox SM, Sherman L, Levens KJ. Randomized investigation of magnesium sulfate for prevention of pre-term birth. Am J Obstet Gynecol 1990;163:767–772.
138. Carban SJ, O'Brien WF. The effect of magnesium sulfate on the biophysical profile of normal term fetuses. Obstet Gynecol 1991;77:681–684.
139. Kaplan PW, Lesser RP, Fisher RS, et al. A continuing controversy: Magnesium sulfate in the treatment of eclamptic seizures. Arch Neurol 1990;47:1031–1039.
140. Wright JW, Ridgway LE III, Patterson RM. Adjusting the loading dose of magnesium sulfate for tocolysis. Am J Obstet Gynecol 1990;163:889–892.
141. Sherer DM, Cialone PR, Abramowicz JC, Woods JR Jr. Transient symptomatic subendocardial ischemia during intravenous sulfate toxolytic therapy. Am J Obstet Gynecol 1992; 166:33–35.
142. Worrell JA, Brunner JP, O'Donnell DM, Carroll FE. Chest case of the day. Case I. Pulmonary edema associated with toxolytic therapy. Am J Radiol 1992;158:1356–1362.
143. Holcomb WA Jr, Shackeford GD, Petrie RH. Magnesium tocolysis and neonatal bone abnormalities: A controlled study. Obstet Gynecol 1991;78:611–614.
144. Cann CI, Norton KI, Murphy RJC, et al. Congenital rickets associated with magnesium sulfate infusion for tocolysis. J Pediatr 1988;113:1078–1082.
145. Bohman VR, Cotton DB. Supralethal magnesemia with patient survival. Obstet Gynecol 1990;76:984–986.
146. McCubbin JH, Sibai MM, Abdella TN, Anderson GD. Cardiopulmonary arrest due to acute maternal hypermagnesemia. Lancet 1981;1:1058.
147. Moise KJ Jr, Huhta JC, Sharif DS, et al. Indomethacin in the treatment of premature labor: Effects on the fetal ductus arteriosus. N Engl J Med 1988;319:327–331.
148. Demanat E, Legius E, Devlieger H, et al. Prenatal indomethacin toxicity in one member of monozygous twins: A case report. Eur J Obstet Gynecol Reprod Biol 1990;35:267–269.
149. Norton ME, Merrill J, Cooper BAB, et al. Neonatal complications after the administration of indomethacin for preterm labor. N Engl J Med 1993;329:1602–1607.
150. Ng TP, Foo SC, Yoong T. Risk of spontaneous abortion in workers exposed to toluene. Br J Ind Med 1992;49:804–808.
151. Wilkins-Haug L, Gabow PA. Toluene abuse during pregnancy: Obstetric complications and perinatal outcomes. Obstet Gynecol 1991;77:505–509.
152. Pearson MA, Hoyme HE, Seaver LH, Rimsza ME. Toluene embryopathy: Delineation of the phenotype and comparison with fetal alcohol syndrome. Pediatrics 1994;93:211–215.
153. Arnold GL, Kirby RS, Landendoerfer S, Wilkins-Houg L. Toluene embryopathy: Clinical delineation and developmental follow-up. Pediatrics 1994;93:216–220.
154. Hall JG. Vitamin A: A newly recognized human teratogen. Harbinger of things to come? J Pediatr 1984;105:583–584.
155. Rosa FW, Wilk AL, Kiliey FO. Teratogen update: Vitamin A congeners. Teratology 1986;33:355–366.
156. Teratology Society. Recommendations for Vitamin A use during pregnancy. Teratology 1987;35:269–275.
157. Nelson M. Vitamin A, liver consumption and risk of birth defects. Br Med J 1990;301:1176.
158. Klzer KW, Fan AM, Bankowska J, et al. Vitamin A: A pregnancy hazard alert. West J Med 1990; 152:72–87.
159. Tenenbein M. Poisoning in pregnancy. In: Koren G, ed. *Maternal–Fetal Toxicology: A Clinician's Guide.* New York: Marcel Dekker, 1990:89–114.
160. Balaskas TN. Common poisons. In: Gleicher N, ed. *Principles and Practice of Medical Therapy in Pregnancy.* 2nd ed. Norwalk, CT: Appleton–Lange, 1992:236–245.
161. Milunsky A, Jick H, Hick SS, et al. Multivitamin/folic acid supplementation in early pregnancy reduces the prevalence of neural tube defects. JAMA 1989;262:2847–2852
162. MRC Vitamin Study Research Group. Prevention of neural tube defects: Results of the Medical Research Council Vitamin Study. Lancet 1991;338:131–137.
163. Czelzel AE. Prevention of congenital abnormalities by preconsectional multivitamin supplementation. Br Med J 1993; 306:1645–1648.
164. Centers for Disease Control and Prevention. Use of folic acid for prevention of spina bifida and other neural tube defects, 1983–1991. MMWR 1991;40:513–516.
165. Centers for Disease Control and Prevention. Recommendations for the use of folic acid to reduce the number of cases of spina bifida and other neural tube defects. MMWR 1992;41:1–7.
166. Werler MM, Shapiro S, Mitchell AA. Periconceptional folic acid exposure and risk of concurrence of neural tube defects. JAMA 1993;269:1257–1261
167. Shaw GM, Lammer LJ, Wasserman CR, et al. Risks of orofacial clefts in children born to women using multivitamins containing folic acid periconceptionally. Lancet 1995;345: 393–396.
168. Paul M, Himmelstein J. Reproductive hazards in the workplace: What the practitioner needs to know about chemical resources. Obstet Gynecol 1988;7:921–938.
169. Koren G, Graham K, Feigenbaum A, Einarson T. Evaluation and counseling of teratogenic risk: The Motherisk approach. J Clin Pharmacol 1993;33:405–411.
170. Vogt BL. Teratogen information programs. In: Koren G, ed. *Maternal–Fetal Toxicology: A Clinician's Guide.* New York: Marcel Dekker, 1990:332–333.
171. U.S. Food and Drug Administration. Labeling and prescription drug advertising: Content and format for labeling for human prescription drugs. Fed Regist 1979;44(124):3743–3747.
172. Teratology Society Public Affairs Committee: FDA classification of drugs for teratogenic risk. Teratology 1994;49:446–447.

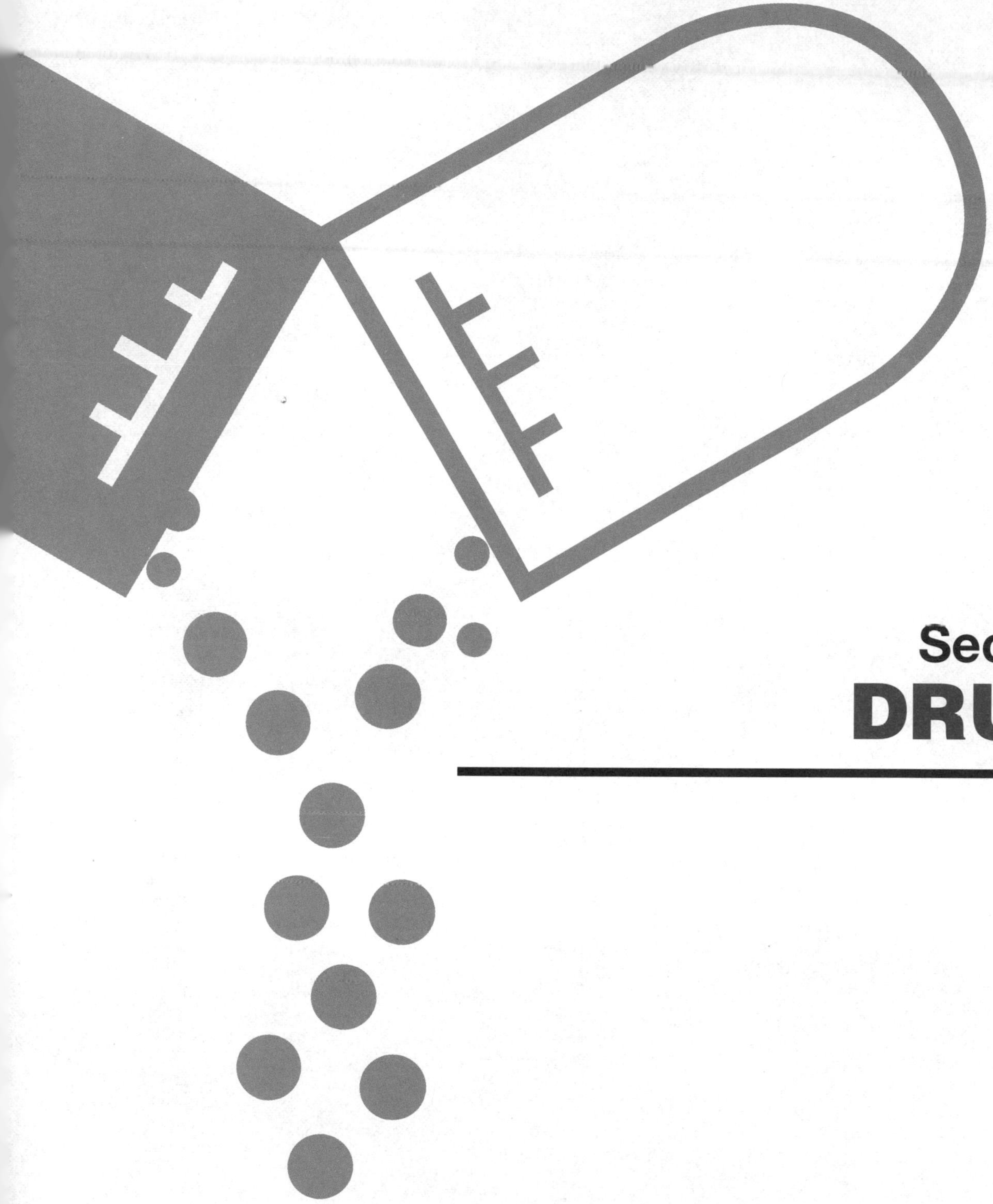

Section II
DRUGS

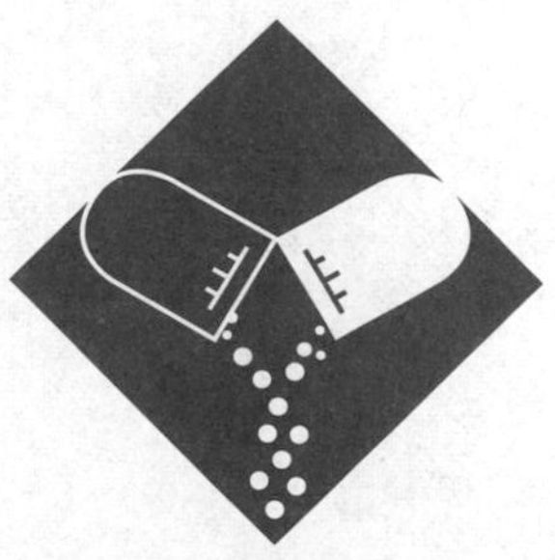

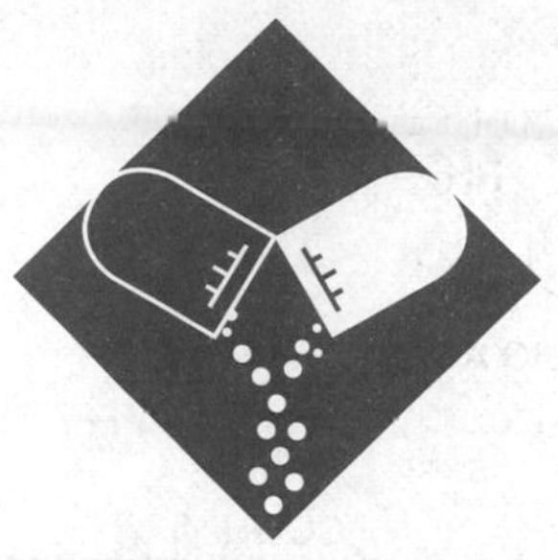

Part A
Analgesics

Chapter 9
Newer Analgesics

GLAFENINE

Glafenine (Fig. 9–1) was marketed in Europe and other countries in 1965 as an analgesic.[1] Acute renal insufficiency following overdose was noted in 1972.[1,2] A number of reports followed.[3–10] In 1978 hepatotoxicity was reported following therapeutic doses of the drug.[11] Additional reports of liver damage followed.[12–17] By 1983 glafenine was withdrawn in Germany because of concern over adverse effects including anaphylaxis and crystallization in the renal tubules.[18] Glafenine was not marketed in Denmark, Ireland, or the United Kingdom. A high relative risk of anaphylactic shock following glafenine use became apparent by 1984[13] and in the following years.[19,20] In December 1989, the European Community Committee on Proprietary Medicinal Products (EC CPMP) recommended stricter controls on glafenine sales, distribution, and warnings. The Belgian and Luxembourg governments requested its withdrawal from sales in 1990.[18,21] By 1991 it was withdrawn from sales in Belgium and its use was restricted in France, Italy, and Switzerland.[22] By early 1992 the EC CPMP recommended withdrawal of the product license from all member states. France, Portugal, and Italy are reviewing the drug; however, it continues to be sold elsewhere throughout the world.[23] It has never been approved for sale in the United States. Worldwide, 14 deaths have been attributed to the drug; perhaps half were caused by it.[21]

Structure and Classification

Glafenine is an anthranilic acid derivative with the chemical name 2,3-dihydroxypropyl-*N*-(7-chloro-4-quinolyl) anthranilate. Its formula is $C_{19}H_{17}C1N_2O_4$ and its molecular weight is 372.8[24] (CAS No. 3820-67-5). Glafenine has been described as glyceryl aminophenaquine,[1] the 4-amino-7-chloro derivative of quinoline.[10]

Use

Glafenine has been used as an analgesic in doses of 200 to 400 mg up to a total of 1 to 1.2 g daily.

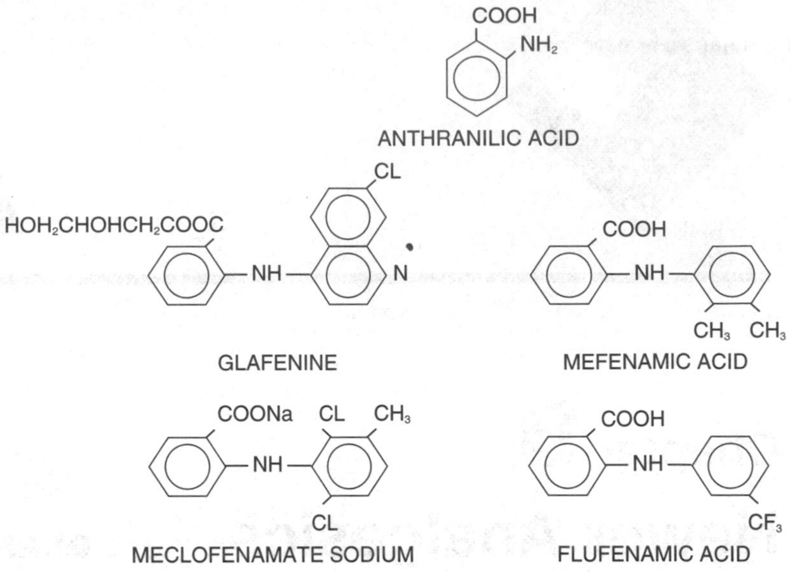

Figure 9–1 Structural formulas of anthranilic acid derivatives. (From Fernandez-Rivas M, de la Hoz B, Cuevas M, et al. Hypersensitivity reactions to anthranilic acid derivatives. Ann Allergy 1993; 71:515–518.)

Toxicokinetics

Glafenine is absorbed rapidly from the gastrointestinal tract, with maximum blood levels appearing within the first hour of ingestion. About 67% is excreted in a 24-hour urine.[1] The half-life is about 75 minutes. It is metabolized to glafenic acid, and yellow crystals of hydroxyglafenic acid may obstruct the collecting tubules.[10]

Clinical Presentation

Ingestions of overdoses of glafenine have been followed, within a few days, by acute renal failure characterized by oliguria or anuria and a rise in the blood urea nitrogen and serum creatinine. Little proteinuria or hematuria has been observed.[8] There is usually no fever, metabolic acidosis, eosinophilia, or hyperkalemia.[6] Biopsy of the kidney often discloses an acute tubulointerstitial nephritis. The glomeruli are usually not affected. Initial vomiting and bilateral lumber pain may precede the renal involvement. Glafenine induces a hemolytic response in patients with glucose-6-phosphate dehydrogenase deficiency.[7] Therapeutic doses may lead to allergic reactions characterized by lymph node swelling, fever, eosinophilia, and rash.[8] The urine in overdosed patients may become bright yellow due to obstruction of the collecting ducts by the yellow-colored crystals of hydroxyglafenic acid.[10] The acute renal failure syndrome generally resolves spontaneously within 1 week, and renal function returns to normal within 3 to 4 weeks.[3–5]

Treatment

Overdose with glafenine has usually responded to symptomatic and supportive treatment with emphasis on fluid supplements and diuretics such as furosemide, although the acute renal failure has generally reverted to normal spontaneously. Hepatotoxicity, allergic reactions, and anaphylactic shock have usually followed therapeutic doses of the drug. These reactions are treated symptomatically.

NEFOPAM

Nefopam (Fig. 9–2) is a unique synthetic analgesic with anticholinergic and sympathomimetic properties. In overdose most reported patients have survived but there have been a number of fatalities. Symptoms include seizures, tachycardia, increase in blood pressure, and hyperreflexia. Treatment is symptomatic and supportive.

Structure and Classification

Nefopam hydrochloride is 3,4,5,6-tetrahydro-5-methyl-1-phenyl-1*H*-2,5-benzoxazocine hydrochloride (Fig. 9–2).[25] It has a molecular formula of $C_{17}H_{19}NO$, HC1 and a molecular weight of 289.8 (CAS No. 1266-9-70-0 for nefopam and 23327-57-3 for the hydrochloride).

Use

Nefopam hydrochloride is an analgesic used for the relief of acute and chronic pain. It also has some anticholinergic and sympathomimetic actions. Nefopam is chemically and pharmacologically distinct from other analgesics.

Product Formulation

It is available as 30-mg tablets of nefopam hydrochloride and, for injection, 1-mL ampoules containing 20 mg/mL.[24]

Therapeutic Dose

The usual dose by mouth is 30 to 90 mg three times daily.

Toxic Dose

A 19-year-old woman who ingested 1.8 g of nefopam survived.[2] A 17-year-old woman ingested 720 mg of nefopam with no overt reaction.[26] A 30-year-old woman who ingested 40 tablets (1200 mg) presented with vomiting, sinus tachycardia, and subsequent seizure but was released after 2 days. A 40-year-old woman ingested 25 tablets (750 mg), and was treated with intravenous fluids and benzodiazepines to control seizures. She was discharged in 2 days.[26] One patient died after an overdose.[27] Several patients who ingested an unknown number of tablets died.[26,27]

Toxicokinetics

Absorption

The absolute bioavailability of the oral form is about 25%.[24] Following a 60-mg oral dose in healthy subjects, peak blood concentrations of 29 to 67 ng/mL are reached in about 2 hours.[25] Similar peak concentrations are achieved about 1.5 hours after an intramuscular dose of 20 mg. Nefopam is about 75% protein bound. The normal therapeutic range of plasma levels is 50 to 100 ng/mL.[24] In one patient, a 60-mg oral dose led to a peak plasma level of 99 ng/mL in 2 hours.[28]

Distribution

The apparent volume of distribution is about 10 L/kg.[24]

Elimination

The three principal metabolic pathways are N-desmethylation, glucuronidation of the N-desmethyl metabolite, and N-oxidation. The metabolites have no analgesic activity.[26] Biotransformation of nefopam is extensive. The metabolites are almost solely excreted via the kidneys. Less than 5% is excreted in the urine in unchanged form. The elimination half-life is 3 to 8 hours (mean, 4 hours) after an oral or intravenous dose. The half-life for the initial portion is about 4 to 5 hours and, for the terminal phase, 10 to 11 hours.[26]

Mechanism of Action

Though chemically and pharmacologically distinct from both narcotic and antiinflammatory agents, nefopam is one fifth to one half as potent as morphine. Its mode of action is unknown.[25,27]

Clinical Presentation

Patients who overdose with nefopam may present with grand mal seizures, sinus tachycardia, metabolic acidosis, and apnea and may remain comatose.[26] A review of several cases of overdose suggests that seizures, hallucinations, and agitation appear to be the neurologic features of overdose;

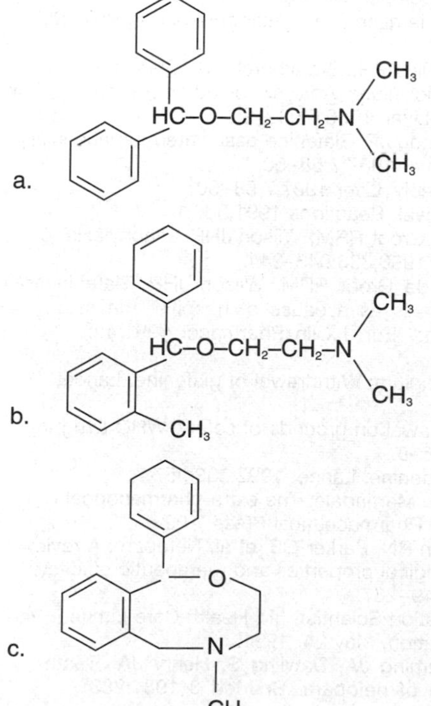

Figure 9–2 Structural formulas of diphenhydramine (a), orphenadrine (b), and nefopam (c). (From Heel RC, Brogden RN, Pakes GE, et al. Nefopam: A review of its pharmacological properties and therapeutic efficacy. Drugs 1980;19:249–267.)

tachycardia with a hyperdynamic circulation is the principal cardiovascular complication.[26]

Nausea, sweating, and sedation are experienced by about 10 to 30% of patients during chronic use of nefopam.[25]

Nine of ten patients studied after an overdose of nefopam recovered with routine supportive treatment.[27]

Laboratory

Analytical Methods

Gas–liquid chromatography with a flame ionization detector has a lower limit of sensitivity of 20 ng/mL with a 2-mL plasma sample.[28]

Blood Levels

A 30-year-old woman developed seizures and renal failure, and suffered a cardiac arrest. She died in 19 hours. The blood nefopam concentration was 1.2 μg/mL.[29] An 18-year-old known drug abuser was found dead; the blood nefopam concentration was 3.8 μg/mL.[30] A 21-year-old woman who died after ingesting an unknown number of tablets had a plasma nefopam level of 31.7 μg/mL and a liver level of 360 μg/g at postmortem examination 15 to 18 hours after death.[26] A 46-year-old woman ingested an unknown number of tablets and died; her postmortem blood level was 15.5 μg/mL. A 44-year-old woman ingested 1.8 g of nefopam and became sweaty, drowsy, and hyperreflexic. She developed a tachycardia and grand mal seizures. Her plasma nefopam concentrations were 3.8 μg/mL at 3 hours and 0.9 μg/mL at 19 hours.[27]

Treatment

Patients generally recover with symptomatic and supportive care. As there is no specific antidote for nefopam poisoning, treatment should be directed primarily to the prompt removal of ingested drug by gastric lavage (with tracheal protection) together with control of seizures and hallucinations (diazepam appears effective). Beta-adrenergic blockade may be useful in controlling cardiovascular complications. Activated charcoal 50 to 100 g in a water suspension should be administered immediately and should bind up to 95% of the dose (up to 10 g) at gastric pH. Induction of vomiting or gastric lavage is unlikely to be more effective.[31,32] Hemodialysis and hemoperfusion are unlikely to be effective in the presence of such high protein binding and volume of distribution.

REFERENCES

1. Gaultier M, Bismuth C, Efthymiou ML, et al. Nephropathie tubulo-interstitielle aigue. Au cours d'une intoxication par la glafenine. Presse Med 1972;1:3125–3128. (Acute tubulointerstitial nephropathy due to glafenine poisoning).
2. Mirouze J, Barjon P, Mion CH, et al. Insuffisance renal aigue consecutive a l'absorption de glafenine. [Acute renal insufficiency following glafenine ingestion.] Therapie 1974; 29:587–592.
3. Gaultier M, Bismuth C, Morel-Maroger M, Dauchy F. Nephropathie tubulo-interstitielle aigue au cours d'intoxications par la glafenine: A propos de 5 cas. [Acute tubulointerstitial nephropathy due to glafenine poisoning.] Therapie 1974;29: 579–585.
4. Duplay H, Mattei M, Barillon D, et al. Nephrite tubulo-interstitielle aigue par intoxication a la glafenine. [Acute tubulointerstitial nephritis due to glafenine poisoning.] Therapie 1974;29:593–597.
5. Chevet D, Rainee M-P, Garre M, et al. Nephropathie aigue tubulo-interstitielle anurique due a une intoxication par la glafenine. [Acute anuric tubulointerstitial nephropathy due to glafenine poisoning.] Therapie 1974;29: 575–578.
6. Renier J-C, Boasson M, Pitois M, Alquier Ph. Insuffisance renale aigue recidivante apres ingestion de glafenine a dose therapeutique. [Recurrent acute renal insufficiency after ingestion of a therapeutic dose of glafenine.] Presse Med 1975;4:670.
7. Bouletreau P, Ducluzeau R, Bui-Xvan B, et al. Acute renal complications of acute intoxications. Acta Pharmacol Toxicol (Copeatu) 1977;41(2):49–63 (suppl.).
8. Geboes K, Stevens E, Bossaert H, Dooms T. Renal injury associated with 'glafenine' overdose. Acta Clin Belg 1978; 33: 401–402.
9. D'Enfert J, Monteil AL, Beraud JJ, Mirouze J. Anurie apres glafenine. Role d'un traitment diuretique associe. [Enhanced renal toxicity of glafenine by diuretics?] Presse Med 1980; 9:716.
10. Proesmans W, Sina JKA, Begucquoy P, et al. Recurrent acute renal failure due to nonaccidental poisoning with glafenine in a child. Clin Nephrol 1981;16:207–210.
11. Ypma RThJM, Festen JJM, De Bruin CD. Hepatotoxicity of glafenine. Lancet 1978;2:480–481.
12. Duche M, Durand H, Boi Ph, et al. Hepatite provoquee par la glafenine. [Hepatitis provoked by glafenine.] Therapie 1982; 37:327–330.
13. Verhamme M, De Wolfe-Peeters C, Van Steenbergen W. Hepatic injury due to glafenine: Report of two cases and review of the literature. Neth J Med 1984;27:35–39.
14. Brissot P, Gie S, Colobert A, et al. Un nouveau cas de'hepatite due a la glafenine. Gastroenterol Clin Bull 1982; 6:948.
15. Stricker BHC, Blok APR, Bronkhorst FB. Glafenine-associated hepatic injury: Analysis of 38 cases and review of the literature. Liver 1986;6:63–72.
16. Danan G, Benhamou JP. Glafenine-associated hepatic injury: 38 or 5 cases? Liver 1987;7:58–60.
17. Stricker BHCh. Reply. Liver 1987;7:58–60.
18. Glafenine withdrawal. Reactions 1991;386:1.
19. Stricker BHC, De Groot RRM, Wilson JHP. Anaphylaxis to glafenine. Lancet 1990;336:943–944.
20. Stricker BH Ch, de Groot RRM, Wilson JHP. Glafenineassociated anaphylaxis as a cause of hospital admission in the Netherlands. Eur J Clin Pharmacol 1991;40: 367–371.
21. Herxheimer A. Belgium: Withdrawal of glafenine. Lancet 1991;337:102.
22. Glafenine: Withdrawal on grounds of safety. WHO Drug Inform 1991;No. 1;5–8.
23. Withdrawal of glafenine. Lancet 1992;339:357.
24. Reynolds JEF, ed. Martindale: The extra pharmacopoeia. 30th ed. London: Pharmaceutical Press, 1993.
25. Heel RC, Brogden RN, Parker GE, et al. Nefopam: A review of its pharmacological properties and therapeutic efficacy. Drugs 1980;19:249–267.
26. Burnett I, Information Scientist, 3M Health Care Limited. Personal communication, May 24, 1991.
27. Piercy DM, Cumming JA, Dawling S, Henry JA. Death due to overdose of nefopam. Br Med J 1981;283: 1508–1509.

28. Schuffan D, Hansen CS, Ober BE. GLC determination of nanogram quantities of a new analgesic nefopam in human plasma. J Pharm Sci 1978;67:1720–1723.
29. Widdop P, Dawling S. Suicidal poisoning by nefopam: A new analgesic drug. Bull Int Assoc Forens Toxicol 1981;16(2): 33–34.
30. Bal TS, Oxley I, Johnson B, Hiscuitt AA. A fatal case involving nefopam and paracetamol. Bull Int Assoc Forens Toxicol 1986;19(1):32–34.
31. Neuvonen PJ. Activated charcoal in nefopam. Br Med J 1984;289:1626.
32. Neuvonen PJ, Jannisto H. Capacity of two forms of activated charcoal to adsorb nefopam in vitro and to reduce its toxicity in vivo. Clin Toxicol 1983/1984;21:333–342.

Chapter 10

Acetaminophen (Paracetamol)

INTRODUCTION

In the United Kingdom, acetaminophen is taken in overdose most frequently by young adults who are not being prescribed psychotropic drugs by their general practitioners.[1] Overall, acetaminophen is involved in some 15 to 30% of deliberate self-poisonings in the United Kingdom.[2] In 1993 about 60,000 inquiries involving acetaminophen were reported by the Toxic Exposure Surveillance System of the American Association of Poison Control Centers.[3] Only a small minority of patients are at risk of severe liver damage and the liver has remarkable powers of regeneration. Recovery from even severe damage is usually rapid and complete, and the overall mortality rate is low.[4]

HEPATOTOXICITY

Although the exact mechanism is unclear, most hepatotoxicity probably results from a toxic intermediary that binds covalently to hepatocytes and causes a centrilobular hepatic necrosis. Alternate explanations of necrosis involve lipid peroxidation and oxidation of thiol groups on key hepatic enzymes such as Ca^{2+} translocases. The liver metabolizes most therapeutic doses of acetaminophen by glucuronide and sulfate conjugation. Only small amounts of acetaminophen are converted to the highly reactive intermediate *N*-acetyl-*p*-benzoquinoneimine (NAPQI) by the cytochrome P_{450} mixed-function oxidase system. Glutathione rapidly detoxifies this intermediate to cysteine and mercapturate conjugates.[5] One explanation of acetaminophen hepatotoxicity is the saturation of the sulfate pathway by the ingestion of an excessive acetaminophen dose, which would then increase the amount of the toxic intermediate formed.[6] When glutathione stores are depleted below a critical value (about 30% of normal stores), NAPQI binds covalently with hepatic cell macromolecules, producing tissue necrosis.[7]

There is significant individual susceptibility to the toxic effects of acetaminophen, as 20% or more of patients with toxic acetaminophen plasma levels do not develop hepatotoxicity. In unselected acetaminophen overdose patients, severe liver damage develops only in about 8% without antidotal therapy, despite the fact that approximately 15%

display plasma acetaminophen levels in the toxic range.[8] Fatal hepatic failure occurs in about 1 to 2% of these patients who have received no specific therapy. Depletion of hepatocellular reduced glutathione alone does not account for acetaminophen-induced hepatotoxicity, as similar experimental reduction of glutathione by other drugs (eg, iodomethane) does not cause hepatic necrosis.[9] Age, diet, nutritional status, metabolic state, and concomitant drug ingestion apparently affect individual changes in cytochrome P_{450} mixed-function oxidase activity and susceptibility to hepatotoxicity.

Drugs that induce hepatic P_{450} enzymes (e.g. phenobarbital, 3-methylcholanthrene) may enhance acetaminophen-induced hepatotoxicity.[9] Survivors of acute overdose rarely develop chronic hepatitis or cirrhosis.

RISK FACTORS

Risk factors that enhance the development of liver toxicity after an overdose of acetaminophen include alcoholism and chronic ingestion of agents that induce hepatic microsomal enzymes (eg, isoniazid,[10] anticonvulsants[11]). Starvation depletes glutathione stores. Patients who consume excessive quantities of acetaminophen in multiple doses usually present with acetaminophen levels in the toxic range.[12] The clinical history is often inaccurate. About 1 in 500 acetaminophen overdoses has a treatable overdose that is not identified by history or in patients with hepatic dysfunction.[13]

TOXIC DOSE

In adults, the single acute threshold dose for severe liver damage is 150 to 250 mg/kg.[8,14] Children under the age of about 10 appear to be much more resistant than adults.[15] Vale and Proudfoot observe that the risk of severe and possibly fatal liver damage after overdose cannot be accurately assessed from the amount of acetaminophen ingested or the symptoms that occur during the period when an antidote provides maximum protection.[16]

Adults	5–15 g (15–45 tablets of 325 mg each)
Adults	<125 mg/kg (no hepatotoxicity)
	250 mg/kg (severe liver damage [50%])
	350 mg/kg (severe liver damage [100%])
Adolescents	125–150 mg/kg (hepatotoxic dose)
Lethal dose	13–25 g (46–75 tablets of 325 mg each)

HEPATIC GLUTATHIONE

Drugs may affect acetaminophen toxicity by reducing glutathione stores or decreasing conjugation. Pharmacokinetic data suggest that the hepatic supply of reduced glutathione begins to be depleted in humans after ingestion of from 0.5 g to 3.0 g acetaminophen and that this depletion is overcome by the administration of *N*-acetylcysteine.[17] Some ethnic difference occurs in the metabolism of acetaminophen. For example, one study indicated that East Indians excrete slightly more glucuronide metabolites and slightly less sulfate metabolites than Chinese. Both ethnic groups excrete less (6% vs 9%) glutathione-derived conjugates than Caucasians of Scottish descent.[18]

Formation of oxidative metabolites and renal excretion appear to follow first-order kinetics (ie, elimination rate is concentration dependent); the conjugation of sulfate and glucuronide metabolites follows Michaelis Menten kinetics (combined zero- and first-order kinetics).[19]

DRUG-INDUCED ALTERATIONS IN METABOLISM

The rate of the formation of the toxic metabolite following ingestion of acetaminophen depends on the rate of absorption of acetaminophen, on the capacity for glucuronide and sulfate conjugation, and on the amount of microsomal enzyme activity (Fig. 10–1). Neither cigarette smoking nor cimetidine pretreatment alters acetaminophen metabolic pathways. The liver biotransforms acetaminophen almost entirely by conjugation rather than cytochrome P_{450}-dependent oxidation. Cimetidine would therefore not affect metabolism of therapeutic acetaminophen doses, as cimetidine primarily inhibits hepatic microsomal oxidative drug metabolism. Therapeutic doses of codeine do not alter the clearance or metabolism of acetaminophen.[20,21] High-dose ranitidine does not affect the metabolic elimination of therapeutic acetaminophen in humans.[22] Cytochromes P4501A2 and P4502E1 are the two principal P450 enzymes that catalyze acetaminophen oxidation to reactive metabolites. P4501A2 activity is reduced by competitive inhibition with theophylline, a factor that may decrease acetaminophen intoxication when both drugs have been ingested.[23]

ACETAMINOPHEN AND AIDS: DRUG INTERACTIONS

Patients with AIDS may have a nutritionally related depletion of glutathione. Multiple doses of acetaminophen should probably be avoided in zidovudine-treated patients who are suspected of having diminished stores of glutathione due to poor nutrition, AIDS, or alcohol consumption or in zidovudine-treated patients who are also receiving therapeutic agents such as anticonvulsants that stimulate cytochrome P450 enzymes.[24] Animal studies suggest that adrenergic agonists deplete hepatic glutathione levels and may potentiate the hepatotoxicity of acetaminophen.[25]

PREGNANCY

Both the mother and the fetus are at risk for hepatotoxicity following an overdose of acetaminophen because acetaminophen, but not the conjugated metabolites, freely diffuses across the placenta in both animals and humans[26]; however, there is no clear evidence that either acetaminophen or *N*-acetylcysteine is teratogenic.[27,28] Treatment of pregnant patients should follow standard protocols. Overdose with acetaminophen in pregnant women is not in itself an indication to terminate a pregnancy[29–31] (see Chapter 8).

FETAL AND NEONATAL METABOLISM

Early in fetal life, fetal hepatocytes possess the ability to oxidize acetaminophen to its toxic metabolite. The ability to conjugate acetaminophen with glutathione ultimately approaches adult levels at maturity.[32] Sulfate conjugation increases with fetal maturity, but glucuronidation is almost

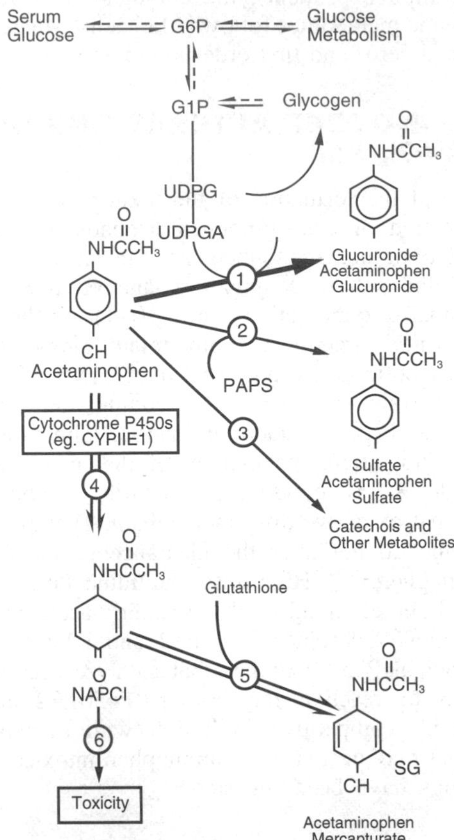

Figure 10–1 Model of acetaminophen metabolism in the liver and effect of fasting and alcohol use. Acetaminophen is metabolized by several major and minor pathways (indicated by circled numbers). Pathway 1 represents metabolism to acetaminophen glucuronide by glucuronusyl transferase. Acetaminophen is conjugated with glucuronide that is provided by uridine(diphospho)acetylglucosamine (UDPGA). The glucuronide is derived from glucose 1-phosphate (G1P), which in turn is derived from either glycogen or glucose 6-phosphate (G6P). In catabolic metabolism (ie, fasting), hepatic metabolic pathways are directed toward gluconeogenesis (dashed lines), thus reducing the amount of glucose precursors available for glucuronidation. Pathway 2 represents metabolism by sulfation, which is dependent on phosphoadenylyl sulfate (PAPS) and hepatic sulfur stores. Pathway 3 represents other minor metabolic pathways that produce only a fraction of acetaminophen metabolites. Pathway 4 represents the mixed-function oxidase system (cytochrome P450, especially 2E1 [CYPIIE1]), and leads to formation of the highly reactive intermediate *N*-acetyl-*p*-benzoquinoneimine (NAPQI). The amount of acetaminophen that passes through this pathway may be increased (gray arrows) by induction of CYPIIE1 by recent alcohol or fasting or because of diminished glucuronidation. Pathway 5 represents the major detoxification pathway. NAPQI is conjugated with glutathione and eliminated until glutathione and available liver sulfur stores become critically low. Pathway 6 represents the fate of NAPQI that is not removed; it binds to critical intracellular molecules and eventually leads to toxicity and cell death. Recent alcohol consumption primarily increases the enzymes in pathway 4, whereas fasting decreases metabolism in pathway 1 and, possibly, pathway 4; increases the amount of enzymes for pathway 4; and decreases available precursors for detoxification of NAPQI through pathway 5, thereby routing more acetaminophen through pathway 6 (see text for details). UDP, uridine diphosphate; UDPG, UDPglucose. (From Whitcomb DC, Block GD. Association of acetaminophen hepatotoxicity with fasting and ethanol use. JAMA 1994;272: 1845–1850.)

undetectable. The decreased ratios of cysteine and mercapturic acid to sulfate and glucuronide conjugates suggest a lower activity of this variant of cytochrome P450 in the neonate.[26] The reduced rate of formation of the toxic metabolite from the cysteine and mercapturic pathways suggests that neonates may be less susceptible to acetaminophen-induced hepatotoxicity than adults.[29] Neonates whose mothers have taken an overdose of acetaminophen experience a relatively lower degree of hepatic damage than adults and older children[31]; however, the fetus remains at risk if a large dose of acetaminophen crosses the placental barrier, because the fetal liver forms the toxic metabolite through oxidation.[31] Although sulfation predominates in the fetus and early life, glucuronidation predominates after age 10. Roberts has diagrammed acetaminophen metabolism in early life[33] (Fig. 10–2).

FULMINANT HEPATIC FAILURE

Fulminant hepatic failure may develop in severely poisoned patients from the third to the sixth day. It is characterized by deepening jaundice, encephalopathy, increased intracranial pressure, grossly disordered hemostasis with disseminated intravascular coagulation and hemorrhage, hyperventilation, acidosis, hypoglycemia, and renal failure. The prognosis is very poor.[34,35]

Acute liver failure in infants, young children, and adults may also be associated with infectious hepatitis (e.g. hepatitis A, hepatitis B, hepatitis C and D, varicella, herpesvirus, Coxsackie virus, echovirus, Epstein–Barr virus, adenovirus); Reye's syndrome[36,37] (characterized by intractable vomiting, associated with abnormal liver histology); acute manifestations of chronic liver disease (Wilson's disease, chronic active hepatitis); and toxic hepatitis (*Amanita phalloides,* pyrrolizidine alkaloids, carbon tetrachloride, chlordane); and drug-induced hepatic injury (isoniazid, *para*-aminosalicylic acid, tetracycline, valproic acid, salicylates, halothane).[38]

Laboratory findings of elevated serum levels of alanine and aspartate transaminase (1500–10,000 U/L), lactic dehydrogenase, and total bilirubin levels; long prothrombin and partial thromboplastin times; hypoalbuminemia; hypoglycemia; and serum ammonia levels more than twice normal in a child should alert the clinician to possible acetaminophen toxicity, as acetaminophen is often given to children with or without a physician's prescription. The severity of the liver function abnormality is not a reliable predictor of outcome.

Patients with concentrations above a line joining plots on a semilogarithmic graph of 1.32 mmol/L (200 mg/L) at 4 hours and 0.20 mmol/L (30 mg/L) at 15 hours after ingestion (called the *treatment line*) have about a 60% chance of developing severe and often fatal liver damage as defined by elevation of the plasma (alanine and aspartate) transaminase activities above 1000 IU/L. In patients with concentrations above a parallel line joining 2 mmol/L (300 mg/L) at 4 hours and 0.33 mmol/L (50 mg/L) at 15 hours, the probability rises to 90%[4,39](Fig. 10–3).

Patients with values above the line often do not develop liver damage, whereas severe liver damage may rarely occur in patients with acetaminophen concentrations as low as 0.83

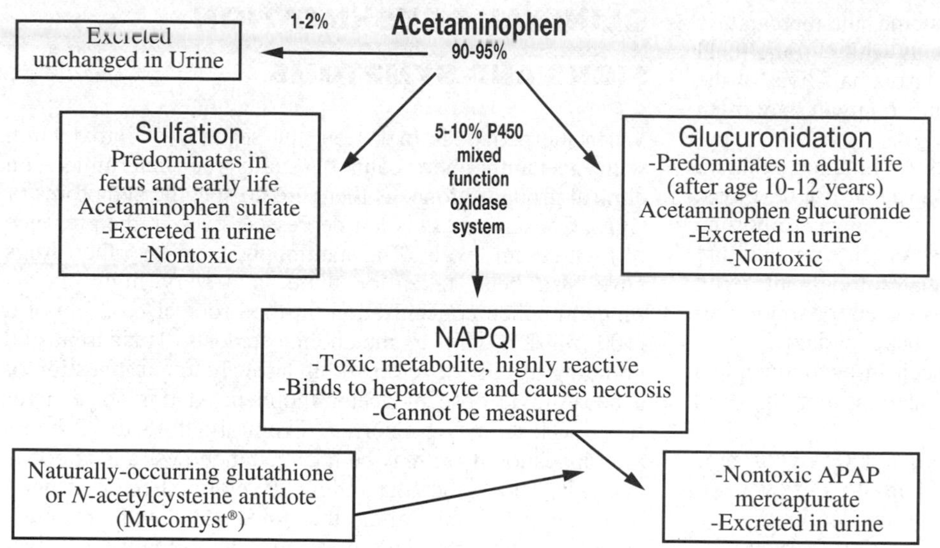

Figure 10–2 Metabolism of acetaminophen. (From Roberts JR. Acetaminophen toxicity: Issues for children and pregnant women. Emerg Med News 1994;16:4–8.

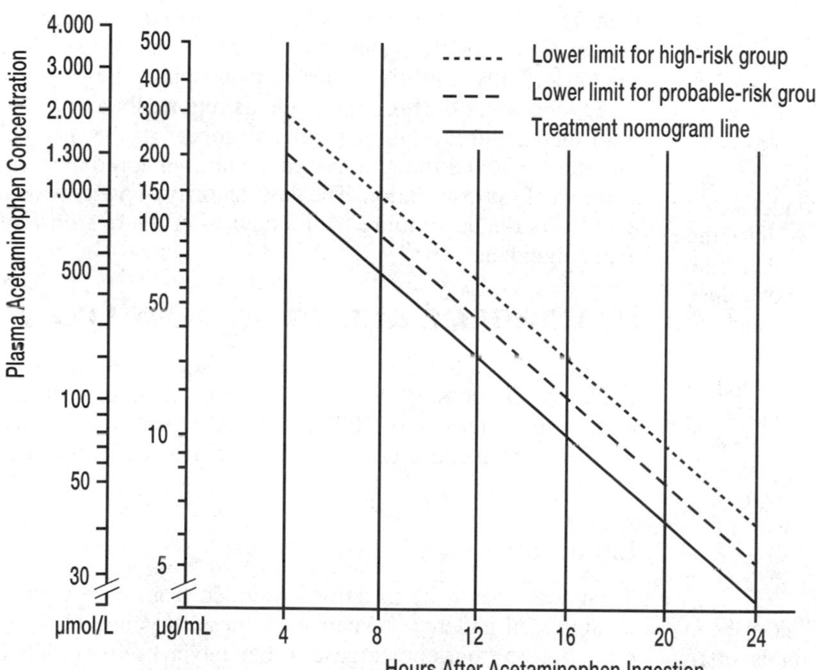

Figure 10–3 Nomogram lines used to define risk groups, according to initial plasma acetaminophen concentration. (From Smilkstein MJ, Bronstein AC, Linden C, et al. Acetaminophen overdose: A 48-hour intravenous *N*-acetylcysteine treatment protocol. Ann Emerg Med 1991;20:1058–1063.)

mmol/L (125 mg/L) at 4 hours. In the United States, patients are given *N*-acetylcysteine when concentrations are above a lower treatment line corresponding to 1 mmol/L (150 mg/L) at 4 hours.[40,41]

NONHEPATIC TOXICITY

RENAL FAILURE

Plasma concentrations of glucuronide and sulfate conjugates increase substantially in patients with moderate renal failure.[42] Renal impairment has been reported in about 1% of patients who have ingested an acetaminophen overdose.[43] The kidney also metabolizes acetaminophen to a toxic intermediate, which binds to renal macromolecules, leading to cell death.[44]

Oliguric renal failure may become apparent within 24 to 48 hours of acetaminophen overdose, and it is almost always associated with back pain, microscopic hematuria, and proteinuria.

Acetaminophen appears to have a role in the causation of analgesic nephropathy and end-stage renal disease.[42,45,46] Renal papillary necrosis may follow consumption of acetaminophen.[47] End-stage renal disease has been reported following the use of more than 1000 acetaminophen pills in a lifetime.[48,49] The fractional urinary recovery of acetaminophen and its glucuronide, sulfate, cysteine, and mercapturic acid conjugates is not altered in patients with chronic renal failure.[42] In such patients the mean plasma half-lives of the acetaminophen glucuronide and sulfate conjugates are often considerably increased.[50]

Although the peak disturbance in liver function occurs 2 to 4 days after an overdose, renal impairment, if it develops, becomes more evident after 1 week and returns to normal about 2 to 3 weeks after ingestion.[51–53] As acute renal failure has been reported despite adequate treatment with *N*-acetylcysteine,[54] a role has been postulated for endotoxin-induced renal toxicity secondary to hepatic damage.[55] A renal concentrating deficit may be seen in acetaminophen poisoning and this appears to be mediated through the renal prostaglandins.[56]

Nonsteroidal antiinflammatory drugs (NSAIDs), now available over the counter, are potent inhibitors of cyclooxygenase and hydroperoxidase, which are necessary for acetaminophen metabolism.[57,58] Combination therapy with both acetaminophen and the NSAIDs appears potentially to subject the kidneys to serious damage.[56] Epidemiologic data are required to validate these observations.

CARDIOTOXICITY

Myocardial changes may include microvesicular fatty degeneration of the myocytes,[59] focal myocardial muscle necrosis and left ventricular dilation,[60] subendocardial necrosis,[61] and focal infiltration of neutrophils into the myocardium.[62] Further studies are required to determine whether these changes are direct toxic effects of an overdose of acetaminophen or secondary changes due to shock or hepatic failure. Acetaminophen-induced cardiotoxicity is rarely clinically significant, but Aronow and Slater suggest that if ST/T-wave abnormalities or a dysrhythmia is present, treatment with *N*-acetylcysteine should be considered, probably irrespective of the plasma acetaminophen level or time lapse since ingestion.[63]

PANCREATOTOXICITY

Doses of acetaminophen as low as 9.75 g have been associated with pancreatitis.[64] Hyperamylasemia is often observed.[65]

HYPERSENSITIVITY REACTIONS

Allergic reactions to acetaminophen are rare, often occuring during the first hour of treatment, and usually involve the skin (bullous, eczematous, or urticarial lesions of the skin or mucous surfaces,[66] exfoliative dermatitis,[67] and urticaria).[68] Bronchospasm and urticaria have been reported in adults[69,70] and children.[71] Dose-dependent anaphylactoid reactions (characterized by vomiting, diarrhea, pruritus, urticaria, angioedema, dyspnea, hypotension) have been reported.[72] Based on clinical experience, only a small percentage of aspirin-sensitive patients cross-react to acetaminophen. The reaction is usually mild because of the weak acetaminophen-induced inhibition of cyclooxygenase compared with aspirin.

CLINICAL PRESENTATION

SIGNS AND SYMPTOMS

When the patient is first seen, the severity of intoxication with acetaminophen cannot usually be determined on clinical grounds alone, as there are no specific symptoms or signs. Consciousness is not depressed, even in the presence of high serum levels of acetaminophen, unless other drugs have also been taken or there is a very high plasma acetaminophen concentration on the order of 6.62 mmol/L (100 mg/L) with a metabolic acidosis.[73] Nausea and vomiting usually develop within a few hours of ingestion of a hepatotoxic dose of acetaminophen. At this stage, liver function tests may be normal. From about 18 to 72 hours after ingestion there may be hepatic tenderness and abdominal pain. Unless hepatic failure develops, there is usually rapid improvement after the third day with eventual complete recovery. The maximum abnormality of liver function tests is usually delayed until the third day.[4] Complications of acetaminophen poisoning may include disturbances of coagulation with disseminated intravascular coagulation,[74] acute pancreatitis,[75] impaired carbohydrate tolerance,[76] myocarditis,[60] and hypophosphatemia.[77]

Several cases of thrombocytopenia reportedly associated with therapeutic acetaminophen use appear in the medical literature.[78] Renal function returns to normal approximately 2 to 3 weeks postingestion. The vast majority of patients who eventually die do so more than 3 days after the overdose of acetaminophen.[35,79,80]

NOMOGRAMS AND TREATMENT LINES

Treatment lines (eg, Fig. 3) have been suggested to offer a guide to the possibility of severe liver damage (plasma transaminase activity of 1000 IU/mL or more) when plasma acetaminophen concentrations are correlated with time after exposure.

Limitations

Treatment lines were initially developed from observations of untreated patients.[16] Their usefulness in young children and after 15 hours postingestion has never been validated. They do not in themselves predict life or death.

Lines

200 line: Joins concentration of 200 mg/L at 4 hours and 30 mg/L at 15 hours on a semilogarithmic graph. The 200 line extended to 24 hours joins 150 mg/L at 4 hours and 30 mg/L at 12 hours.[81]

150 line: Joins 150 mg/L at 4 hours and 30 mg/L at 12 hours.[40]

300 line: Joins a semilogarithmic plot at 3 hours of 300 mg/L at 4 hours and 75 mg/L at 12 hours (fatal hepatic failure case, acute renal failure).[4,39]

100 line: Joins 100 mg/L at 4 hours at 15 mg/L at 15 hours (consider for use in patients with a history of chronic alcohol abuse,[82,83] ingestion of enzyme-inducing drugs such as anticonvulsants,[10,11] isoniazid, and eating disorders [glutathione depletion]).[84,85]

CHRONIC ACETAMINOPHEN OVERDOSE

CHILDREN

Inadvertent overdosage, dose miscalculation, or intentional poisoning may lead to chronic acetaminophen overdosage in either children or adults.[86,87] Doubling the recommended therapeutic dosage of acetaminophen for several days may place children at risk for severe hepatotoxicity. Acetaminophen suppositories (120, 325, and 650 mg) are available over the counter, but should be used with great caution in a child who is vomiting. Persistent vomiting should prompt reexamination of the child.[36]

Chronic overdosage may continue for 24 hours.[36,78,88–91] The amount of acetaminophen administered is in excess of the recommended dosage for children (40–60 mg/kg/d given in divided doses every 4 to 6 hours).[92] The recommended dose in neonates is 5 to 10 mg/kg every 4 to 6 hours.[93] Henretig et al. suggest that the toxic threshold in children is about 150 mg/kg/d for 2 to 4 days.[86]

Symptoms of chronic acetaminophen overdosage in children are nonspecific. They may present with vomiting, lethargy, anorexia, and/or irritability. The temperature is often diminished (35.6–36.8°C). There may be evidence of hepatomegaly and oliguria.

CHRONIC INGESTION

The acetaminophen nomogram (Fig. 3) has not been validated for chronic prolonged ingestions. Hepatic damage may occur despite acetaminophen concentrations in the "nontoxic" range on the nomogram if the time when ingestion was completed rather than the time ingestion commenced is used to plot the results.[94] Chronic, excessive, continuous, or prolonged ingestions do not provide easy predictors, unlike overdose at a single point.[95] An initial nontoxic acetaminophen blood level at 4 hours after ingestion may be followed by a delayed toxic concentration.[95]

ADULTS

Chronic acetaminophen poisoning in adults is uncommon but often results in an encephalopathy together with other clinical and laboratory manifestation of hepatic failure. Chronic excessive use by adults who seek pain relief and fever control may lead to a toxic hepatitis. Simultaneous alcohol abuse, poor nutrition, and AIDS (depletion of glutathione) or ingestion of other medications (cytochrome P450 inducers such as isoniazid, rifampin, phenytoin, carbamazepine, and barbiturates),[96,97] increases individual susceptibility to hepatic damage.[98,99]

Chronic acetaminophen overdosage in adults and children often responds to supportive measures alone (fluids and glucose intravenously, an arterial line for monitoring, fresh-frozen plasma for serious coagulopathies). Gastric emptying procedures and activated charcoal administration are of limited value, if any. *N*-Acetylcysteine is of questionable value as there is little evidence of its efficacy in such cases, especially when administered more than 24 to 48 hours following initial ingestions of acetaminophen in overdosage. Survival has followed supportive care alone without use of *N*-acetylcysteine. There are few definitive studies to support the use of oral or intravenous acetylcysteine after prolonged overdosing.

THE ALCOHOLIC PATIENT

Both animal experimentation[100] and case reports[101] suggest that the alcoholic patient is more susceptible to the hepatic effects of an overdose of acetaminophen.[102,103] In chronic alcoholics glutathione depletion is probably a more important risk factor for hepatotoxicity than increased metabolic activation of acetaminophen.[84,85] Liver toxicity and acute renal tubular necrosis in alcoholics have been associated with daily doses of 4 to 6 g acetaminophen for 3 to 4 days, assuming that the history of ingestion was reliable.[104,105] Most reports of acetaminophen-induced hepatotoxicity in alcoholics involve the use of clearly excessive doses of acetaminophen (5–8 g for several weeks).[85,98] Such exposure may be fatal and may necessitate liver transplantation.[85]

Table 10–1 lists clinical features that help distinguish acetaminophen-induced hepatotoxicity from alcoholic hepatitis. High serum aspartate aminotransferase levels (>1000 IU/L or >10,000 U/L) in an alcoholic suggest acetaminophen toxicity in the presence of negative antibody titers for viral hepatitis. Prothrombin times exceeding 20 to 25 seconds are unusual in most cases of alcoholic hepatitis.[106] Such patients may ingest larger than normal doses over a 24- to 48-hour period simply because they are careless and confused.[107] They also have an increased susceptibility to develop toxic hepatic effects from therapeutic doses of acetaminophen.[85,101,106,108] The alcoholic's lifestyle is disposed to malnutrition, which further depletes hepatic glutathione.

Alcoholics should be cautioned about the use of acetaminophen while they persist in heavy consumption of alcohol. This potentiation appears to be most pronounced in alcoholics or binge drinkers taking acetaminophen in therapeutic doses without suicidal intent. The amount of long-term alcohol consumption required to impair acetaminophen metabolism is not known. The physician should obtain a careful history of alcohol use in any patient with an acetaminophen overdose.[109] The case fatality rate for this syndrome is about 20%. Its incidence appears to be on the rise. In 1993 it was possibly the most frequent single cause of acute liver failure in the United States.[110]

LABORATORY

ASSAY

Acetaminophen may interfere with blood glucose assays, leading to falsely elevated blood glucose concentrations.[111] *N*-Acetylcysteine therapy along with captopril, mesna, and other drugs containing free sulfhydryl groups may produce false-positive ketone readings on urinary dipsticks.[112]

Table 10–1
Laboratory Features Distinguishing Acetaminophen Hepatotoxicity in Chronic Alcoholics from That in Suicide Ingestions and in Alcoholic Hepatitis on Presentation to the Emergency Department

	Alcoholic With Acetaminophen Hepatotoxicity	Suicide Ingestion, Acetaminophen	Alcoholic Hepatitis
AST	Markedly increased	Normal initially, later may be markedly increased	Usually <300
ALT	Increased but less than AST	Normal initially, later may be markedly increased	Slight increase or normal
AST/ALT	>2	<2	>2
Prothrombin time	Increased to markedly increased	Normal initially, later may be markedly increased	Incresed (but usually <20 s)
Acetaminophen level	Normal or slight increase	Increased	Normal

AST, aspartate aminotransferase; ALT, alanine aminotransferase
From Kumar S, Rex DK. Failure of physicians to recognize acetaminophen hepatotoxicity in chronic alcoholics. Arch Intern Med 1991;151:1189–1191.

False-positive cases of suspected acetaminophen overdose may occur when the diagnosis of acetaminophen overdose is based on history alone. The number of potential serious false-negative cases based on history alone is small.[13]

BLOOD

A serum acetaminophen level in all cases of drug overdose can be cost effective. Acetaminophen is widely available, it is usually an initially silent overdose, it is a drug that has the potential for significant morbidity or mortality, and effective treatment is available if the diagnosis is confirmed.[33] The ferric acid procedure is the most reliable, but many factors (eg, acetaminophen metabolites, phenacetin, salicylates, uremia, jaundice) interfere with the colorimetric methods.[113,114] The analytical performance of the TDx immunoassay is comparable to that of high-performance liquid chromatography in the range 15 to 333 mg acetaminophen per liter, and this method is simple and relatively free from interference.[115]

The value of dropping the usual treatment line on the nomogram by 50% (ie, to the 100 line) in patients who are also ingesting enzyme-inducing drugs or who abuse alcohol has not been validated in controlled clinical trials. An acetaminophen blood level should be considered in all alcoholics seen in the emergency department, but the cost may be prohibitive. The physician should consider the use of *N*-acetylcysteine in a patient with active liver disease such as alcoholic hepatitis when blood levels are within the normal range on the acetaminophen nomogram.

ABNORMALITIES

Laboratory Glutathione *S*-S-Transferase β_1 Levels

Centrilobular hepatocytes, which sustain the greatest damage following ingestion of toxic doses of acetaminophen, contain relatively small concentrations of aminotransferases compared with periportal hepatocytes, which sustain much less damage. The glutathione *S*-transferase (GST) β_1 subunit, which has a plasma half-life shorter than 1 hour, is a more sensitive indicator of hepatocellular injury than aminotransferases.[116] Patients with a GST β_1 subunit concentration greater than 10 μg/L develop moderate or severe liver damage despite treatment with *N*-acetylcysteine.[117] The role of GST in the treatment of acetaminophen overdose requires further validation and the development of rapid, inexpensive analytical tests.

Prothrombin Time

The prothrombin time is the best laboratory guide to the severity of hepatic encephalopathy. The development of an encephalopathy is likely when the prothrombin time exceeds 25 seconds at 48 hours postingestion or 40 seconds at 72 hours.[35,78] A peak prothrombin time exceeding 100 seconds or a prothrombin time that continues to increase 4 days after an overdose indicates a poor prognosis (<8% chance of survival) and suggests the need for a liver transplant.[80]

ANCILLARY TESTS

Patients hospitalized for serious ingestions of acetaminophen should be monitored for renal function, hypoglycemia, and electrolyte imbalance. Early signs of hepatotoxicity include hypoglycemia and metabolic acidosis. Impaired hepatic gluconeogenesis and reduced hepatic uptake of lactate produce the hypoglycemic state. A compensated metabolic acidosis may be present even in patients with acetaminophen levels below the toxic range. Hyperlactatemia is common following an overdose of acetaminophen, particularly in severely poisoned patients.[73] A moderate reduction in the platelet count may occur during acute liver failure, but severe thrombocytopenia with a nadir in the platelet count 2 days postingestion may occur in the absence of hepatic encephalopathy.[118] Dysrhythmias and other electrocardiographic abnormalities occur frequently in patients with acetaminophen-induced hepatic coma, but ST-T wave changes develop rarely in nonencephalopathic patients.[119] An assay for 3-(cystein-5-yl) acetaminophen may become a specific marker for acetaminophen hepatotoxicity.[120]

PHOSPHATE LEVELS

Hypophosphatemia correlates with the degree of hepatic damage and is a recognized feature of acute liver failure; however, hypophosphatemia may be present in the absence of hepatic failure.[121] Phosphaturia is a more sensitive marker of renal toxicity than proteinuria.

Renal loss of phosphate after acetaminophen overdose may lead to hypophosphatemia,[115] and this may be a factor in the development of some of the clinical sequelae observed in acetaminophen-induced liver failure such as mental confusion, irritability, and coma.[77] Serum phosphate levels should be obtained in such patients and phosphate replacement therapy considered.

RAPID TESTS

A rapid acetaminophen assay on whole blood may be useful for bedside use. The test uses a disposable reagent strip (one drop of blood containing acetaminophen is applied to the strip, and the acetaminophen is enzymatically hydrolyzed to *p*-aminophenol), and a meter (the *p*-aminophenol is then oxidized by an electrical potential between electrodes, the current being directly proportional to the concentration of acetaminophen). The result is displayed digitally or printed and takes 1 minute. The process appears to be accurate (comparison with high-performance liquid chromatography) over the concentration range 10 to 300 μg/mL. Further studies are in progress.[122] A similar and apparently identical[123,124] preliminary test has indicated rapidity (30 seconds), precision over the serum acetaminophen concentration range 2 to 217 μg/mL, and a high degree of sensitivity (100%). The clinical usefulness of such rapid screening techniques remains to be determined.[125]

TREATMENT

Table 10–2 suggests a management protocol for acetaminophen (paracetamol) poisoning at various times after an overdose.

Bond and colleagues suggest that children less than 6 years of age who ingest pediatric acetaminophen products other than those from packages containing greater than 30 tablets or who ingest less than 200 mg/kg of an adult preparation may be managed at home without referral to a hospital.[126]

GUT DECONTAMINATION: ACTIVATED CHARCOAL

Reduction of Acetaminophen Absorption

Activated charcoal should be given within the first several hours of ingestion of acetaminophen. Activated charcoal may reduce the serum level of acetaminophen even after absorption is complete.[125]

Use of Activated Charcoal and *N*-Acetylcysteine

Activated charcoal adsorbs some of the antidote *N*-acetylcysteine (NAC) in vitro.[127] There is no clinical evidence that the administration of activated charcoal inhibits the efficacy of oral NAC. There is also little evidence to support the practice of increasing the dose of oral NAC therapy after the administration of activated charcoal.[128] There is no contraindication to the administration of activated charcoal and intravenous NAC. NAC dosing is not based on acetaminophen blood levels. The optimal dose of activated charcoal has not been determined.

In summary, Brent suggests that if a patient presents within 1 to 2 hours of an acetaminophen overdose, emesis or

Table 10–2
Management of Paracetamol Poisoning

<8 h After Overdose

- Take blood for plasma paracetamol concentration.
- Give 50 g activated charcoal to adult patients if <1 h has elapsed since substantial overdose.
- Start intravenous NAC if the plasma paracetamol concentration is above the treatment line.
- If the plasma paracetamol concentration is not available by 8 h, begin NAC if >150 mg/kg paracetamol has been ingested.
- Discontinue NAC if the plasma paracetamol concentration is below the treatment line.
- On completion of NAC treatment, check PT (INR), ALT/AST activities, and plasma creatinine concentration.
- If the patient is asymptomatic and the investigations are normal, there is no risk of serious complications and the patient may be discharged.

8–15 h After Overdose

- Take blood for plasma paracetamol concentration, PT (INR), ALT/AST activities, plasma creatinine and bilirubin concentrations, acid–base status (this can be performed on a venous sample), and blood count.
- Start NAC immediately if >150 mg/kg paracetamol has been ingested.
- Discontinue if the plasma paracetamol concentration is below the treatment line.
- On completion of NAC treatment repeat investigations (except paracetamol concentration).
- If the patient is asymptomatic and the investigations are normal, there is little risk of serious complications and the patient may be discharged.

15–24 h After Overdose

- Give standard NAC course of >150 mg/kg paracetamol has been ingested.
- Take blood on admission for plasma paracetamol concentration, PT (INR), ALT/AST activities, plasma creatinine, bilirubin and phosphate concentrations, acid–base status, and blood count.
- Repeat above investigations at end of NAC course.
- If the investigations are abnormal, or if the patient is symptomatic, consider continuing NAC treatment (100 mg/kg in 1 L 5% dextrose over 16 h, repeated until recovery). Repeat investigations as appropriate.

>24 h After Overdose

- Take blood on admission for plasma paracetamol concentration, PT (INR), ALT/AST activities, plasma creatinine, bilirubin and phosphate concentrations, acid–base status, and blood count.
- If the patient has ingested >150 mg/kg paracetamol, is symptomatic or has abnormal investigations, give course of NAC.
- Repeat above investigations at end of NAC standard treatment course and consider continuing NAC (10 mg/kg in 1 L 5% dextrose over 16 h, repeated until recovery) if the patient has or is at risk of developing fulminant hepatic failure.

NAC, *N*-acetylcysteine; ALT, alanine aminotransferase; AST, aspartate aminotransferase; PT, prothrombin time; INR, International Normalized Ratio. From Vale JA, Proudfoot AT. Paracetamol (acetaminophen) poisoning. Lancet 1995;346:547–552.

Table 10–3
Antidote Regimens

Antidote	Route	Regimen	Total Dose (mg/kg)	Length of Treatment (h)
Methionine	Oral	2.5 g (36 mg/kg) 4-hourly for doses	144	12.0
NAC	Oral	140 mg/kg, followed 4 h later by 70 mg/kg 4-hourly for 17 doses	1300	72.0
NAC (20-hour protocol)	IV	150 mg/kg in 200 mL 5% dextrose over 15 min; 50 mg/kg in 500 mL 5% dextrose over 4 h and 100 mg/kg in 1 L 5% dextrose over 16 h	300	20.25
NAC (40-hour protocol)	IV	140 mg/kg in 5% dextrose over 1 h, followed 4 h after initiation of treatment by 12 maintenance doses (70 mg/kg) given over 1 h in 5% dextrose each commencing 4 h after initiation of preceding dose	980	48.0

NAC, *N*-acetylcysetine.
From Vale JA, Proudfoot AT. Paracetamol (acetaminophen) poisoning. Lancet 1995;346:547–552.

activated charcoal therapy will probably reduce the availability of acetaminophen and result in lower blood levels.[129] It seems reasonable to give activated charcoal and to wait for a 4-hour acetaminophen level, as NAC is effective provided it is started within 8 hours of ingestion. If the level is in the potentially toxic range, according to the nomogram, NAC therapy should be initiated. For the patient who presents more than 1 to 2 hours after a pure acetaminophen overdose, it is unlikely that gastrointestinal decontamination will be useful. NAC therapy should be all that is needed provided that toxic levels have been identified. In the patient with known or potential polydrug poisoning, activated charcoal therapy may be sufficient depending on the drugs ingested. Use of a much larger than usual dose of NAC may promote emesis (unpleasant taste, odor), defeating the purpose for which it is administered.[124]

ELIMINATION

Exchange Transfusion

Exchange transfusion has been used in neonates following acetaminophen ingestion by the mother shortly before birth.[130,131]

Arteriovenous Hemofiltration

Arteriovenous hemofiltration has been employed for treatment of the associated hepatic encephalopathy,[132] but there is little evidence that this procedure removes significant amounts of acetaminophen.

Hemodialysis

The primary use of hemodialysis in overdoses of acetaminophen is for the treatment of renal failure. There is little clinical evidence at present that supports the effectiveness of early hemodialysis for overdose therapy. This procedure should not replace antidotal therapy.

Hemoperfusion

Hemoperfusion does not have a well-defined role in the treatment of acetaminophen overdose. This measure has been used in cases of extremely elevated acetaminophen levels to prevent continuing formation of toxic intermediates when the patient presents too late for antidotal therapy.[133] The use of charcoal hemoperfusion in acetaminophen-induced fulminant hepatic failure has not improved survival more than intensive care.[134] Peritoneal dialysis is ineffective.

ANTIDOTE

Methionine

Methionine is an oral antidote used in Great Britain. Experience in the United States has not been sufficient for adequate evaluation of its safety or efficacy (Table 10–3). Methionine is much less expensive than NAC but may exacerbate hepatic encephalopathy when administered more than 1 hour postingestion.[79]

Methionine acts as a glutathione precursor[135–137] and protects against acetaminophen-induced hepatic and renal toxicity, provided that it is administered within 8 to 10 hours of the overdose.[138–140] No significant benefits have been documented in cases where more than 10 hours has elapsed after an acetaminophen overdose.[39,141] Methionine is usually administered orally and it is therefore unsuitable for use in patients who are vomiting and for those in coma.

A preparation is now available commercially that contains 500 mg acetaminophen and 250 mg DL-methionine (Pameton, Sterling Winthrop). The formulation costs more than any other brand of acetaminophen. Its efficacy in preventing liver damage in humans following intentional acetaminophen poisoning has not yet been established.[142]

Oral methionine has been effective in protecting against severe liver damage, renal failure, and death after acetaminophen overdose when given within 10 hours of ingestion.

Indications

Oral methionine is indicated for the treatment of acute acetaminophen poisoning. When 4 hours or more has elapsed after ingestion of an overdose, the plasma concentration of acetaminophen should be measured. Specific treatment with methionine is required if the plasma acetaminophen concentration falls above a line that on a semilog graph joins plots of 200 mg/L (1.32 mmol/L) at 4 hours and 30 mg/L (0.33 mmol/L) 15 hours after the overdose (see Figure 10–3). In cases where plasma concentrations of acetaminophen are not available, methionine should be given if more than 100 mg/kg acetaminophen is taken in a single dose.

If the patient is either vomiting or unconscious, then it is more appropriate to give NAC by the intravenous route.

Dose

Methionine should be given orally in a dose of 2.5 g, followed by three further doses of 2.5 g at 4-hour intervals. If a patient is vomiting and is unable to tolerate oral methionine, intravenous NAC should be given.

Pregnancy

There is no evidence as yet, from the use of methionine in humans, as to whether protection against acetaminophen-induced toxicity results in retardation of fetal growth or even teratogenicity.

Adverse Effects

Oral methionine therapy in the dosage used for acetaminophen poisoning has not been associated in practice with any adverse effects in patients with or without acetaminophen-induced liver failure.

If patients are vomiting or unconscious, intravenous *N*-acetylcysteine should be given in preference to methionine. *N*-acetylcysteine is also the preferred agent in patients with chronic hepatic failure who have taken acetaminophen in overdose.

N-Acetylcysteine

Mechanism of Action

N-Acetylcysteine is the *N*-acetyl derivative of L-cysteine, a naturally occurring amino acid.

Toxicokinetics

The oral bioavailability of NAC is low, probably as a result of extensive first-pass metabolism. At steady state, the volume of distribution of NAC is 0.6 L/kg. The terminal half-life of intravenous NAC is about 6 hours. Elimination occurs primarily by the urinary excretion of inorganic sulfate, with smaller amounts of taurine and unchanged NAC appearing in the urine. Pharmacokinetic studies indicate that the mean maximum plasma concentration of NAC is 554 mg/L during the initial intravenous loading dose (150 mg/kg) when adverse reactions are most likely to occur.[143]

Indications

N-Acetylcysteine is indicated in the treatment of acetaminophen poisoning if:

1. Plasma acetaminophen levels taken between 4 and 12 hours postingestion fall above the "treatment line" indicated in Fig. 3.
2. More than 100 mg/kg acetaminophen has been ingested in a single dose and plasma acetaminophen concentrations are not available.
3. Acute acetaminophen-induced liver failure has developed or is likely to develop (Table 10–2).

Oral NAC is the only antidote currently approved for general use in acetaminophen poisoning in the United States, but intravenous NAC is available under a restricted investigational drug protocol. NAC provides maximum protection against hepatotoxicity when administered within 8 to 10 hours of an acetaminophen overdose.[41] The efficacy of NAC decreases after this period, but no deaths in treated cases occurred when NAC was administered by 16 hours postingestion. The effectiveness of NAC beyond 14 to 36 hours is controversial. Studies from the Liver Unit at King's College Hospital in London have shown that intravenous NAC given up to 72 hours postoverdose decreases progress to grade III/IV hepatic encephalopathy and mortality in fulminant hepatic failure.[144]

Late therapy with NAC is not associated with an increased incidence of adverse effects.[145] NAC therapy probably protects both the liver and the kidney when administered early after an overdose. NAC administration would appear justified in the presence of hepatotoxicity caused by acetaminophen, no matter what the time course or interval since the last dose.

Initiation and Duration of Treatment

Once NAC therapy begins, based on the acetaminophen nomogram, the entire course of NAC should be administered regardless of the location of subsequent levels of acetaminophen on this nomogram. Subsequent plasma levels of acetaminophen that fall below the treatment line are not an indication to stop NAC therapy. Those patients in whom minor ingestions are suspected may await confirmatory plasma levels of acetaminophen, as long as more than 10 to 12 hours does not elapse before NAC administration begins.

A 5% solution of NAC should be given as an oral loading dose of 140 mg/kg. The available commercial preparations of NAC are 10 and 20% solutions and need to be diluted. This can be done using water or a commercial carbonated or still flavored drink. Seventeen further doses of 70 mg/kg NAC should be given as a 5% solution in diluent every 4 hours. The total dose given by this route is 1330 mg/kg over 72 hours.

Intravenous N-Acetylcysteine

Both oral and intravenous NAC are available in the United Kingdom and Canada (Table 10–2). Advantages of intravenous NAC therapy include ease of administration to patients with nausea and vomiting as well as the concurrent administration of activated charcoal without reducing the plasma levels of NAC.[140] Although no prospective clinical trials have compared the intravenous use of NAC with the oral regimen of NAC, one study, which used historical controls, suggested that in patients who present late (>16 hours), oral NAC may be more efficacious than intravenous NAC.[144] The indications for the administration of intravenous NAC are the same as those for oral NAC.

20-Hour Regimen. The regimen consists of intravenous administration of 150 mg/kg made up in 200 mL of 5%

dextrose over 15 minutes, followed by 50 mg/kg in 500 mL of 5% dextrose over 4 hours and 100 mg/kg in 1 L of 5% dextrose over 16 hours. The total dose is 300 mg/kg given over 20 hours. This regimen effectively prevents liver damage, renal failure, and death if started within 8 hours of acetaminophen ingestion, but efficacy falls off rapidly after this time.

In the United Kingdom, intravenous NAC is given in a 5% glucose solution. If patients develop wheezing, flushing, or hypotension during the infusion, the NAC is stopped and the apparent allergic reaction is treated symptomatically.[146]

48-Hour Regimen. In patients admitted 10 to 24 hours after ingestion of acetaminophen, and especially if large amounts are ingested, use of the 48-hour intravenous dosage regimen should be considered. Clinical trials in the United States use a total dose of 980 mg/kg NAC over 48 hours.[40,41] The loading dose is 140 mg IV NAC (3% solution derived by diluting the 20% stock solution with 5% dextrose in water) infused over 1 hour, followed 4 hours later by the first of 12 maintenance doses of 70 mg/kg IV NAC. The maintenance dose also is infused over 1 hour. A nonrandomized trial in the United States indicated that the 48-hour regimen was similar in efficacy to both the 20-hour intravenous and the 72-hour oral regimens when the antidote was administered early.[40] In this study, the 48-hour intravenous protocol appeared more effective than the 20-hour intravenous protocol when the antidote was administered 16 to 24 hours postingestion.

Administration of a 20-hour intravenous NAC protocol (Table 10–2) reduces mortality up to 24 to 36 hours postingestion.[113,147] The late administration (as long as 36 hours after ingestion) of intravenous NAC is safe and may reduce mortality.[148]

Dose

The currently available NAC preparation (Mucomyst) was developed for inhalation use and may contain contaminants. The ability of Millipore filters to remove these contaminants has not been studied. The minimal effective dose has not been determined, although less NAC is administered intravenously than orally. The mean steady-state concentration of NAC after 12 hours of the 20-hour regimen is 35 mg/L. The efficacy of NAC appears similar with both oral and intravenous doses.[140] The optimization of treatment in terms of dosage and duration for high-risk patients receiving treatment more than 16 hours postingestion requires further clinical trials.

In summary, when the results obtained from use of the 20-hour intravenous dosing regimens are compared with those from the 48-hour intravenous and 72-hour oral dosing regimens, no significant differences are observed when endpoints such as mortality and permanent sequelae are considered.[4]

Adverse Effects

Oral Form. *N*-Acetylcysteine has no hepatotoxic effects.[149] Drinking NAC through a straw minimizes its unpleasant odor. Alternatives in patients unable to retain oral NAC include placement of a nasogastric or duodenal (Miller-Abbott, Cantor) tube and intravenous administration of 1 mg metoclopramide per kilogram body weight. Ondansetron improves tolerance to oral NAC in intravenous doses of 0.15 mg/kg repeated every 8 hours for a total of three doses.[150] There are no reports of systemic anaphylactoid reactions following the oral administration of NAC.[151]

Sulfhemoglobinemia (cyanosis without cardiorespiratory distress, elevated sulfhemoglobin level, normal O_2 saturation) rarely occurs.[152]

Intravenous Form. Anaphylactoid reactions (thrombocytopenia, rash, flushing, chest pain, tachycardia, fever, hypotension, angioedema, hypotension, bronchospasm) occur about 15 to 60 minutes after the initiation of intravenous NAC in about 3 to 9% of cases.[153,154] These reactions are serum concentration dependent (usually when the level of NAC exceeds 500 μg/mL) and probably result from histamine release by a nonimmunologic mechanism.[155] Most of these reactions are mild and they usually respond to antihistamines, epinephrine, or a reduction in the rate of infusion of NAC.

"Extended Relief" Acetaminophen

This tablet formulation appears similar to Tylenol Extra Strength caplets (500 mg). The dosage is 2 caplets (total dose, 1300 mg) every 8 hours for adults and children 12 or older. Recommended dose is not to exceed 6 caplets (3900 mg) in 24 hours. The time to peak blood levels following a 1300-mg dose is about 1 to 2 hours. No controlled clinical or toxicokinetic studies of overdose are available. Treatment of acute ingestions over a period less than 8 hours includes standard decontamination procedures, an initial acetaminophen blood level, and blood levels 4 hours or later. If blood levels are above the nomogram levels, NAC should be administered. Levels below 10 μg/mL are probably nontoxic. If levels are below the possible toxicity line but greater than 10 μg/mL, NAC should be started and blood levels repeated in 4 to 6 hours. If patients present late or have a history of a large ingestion, NAC should be started while waiting for the initial levels. The physician should consider extending NAC therapy after the standard 17 doses of acetaminophen if levels are still detectable.[156]

Douglas and colleagues suggest that after a single overdose, the pharmacokinetics of both Extended Relief and Immediate Release acetaminophen are similar, suggesting that overdoses of Extended Relief acetaminophen do not require an alternative diagnostic approach.[157] Graudins and colleagues suggest that measurement of acetaminophen levels after a massive overdose of Extended Relief acetaminophen may lead to underestimation of the need for antidotal therapy if the current nomogram based on an overdose of Immediate Release acetaminophen is used. Delayed absorption may further limit the usefulness of the nomogram. Nontoxic levels of acetaminophen do not exclude the possibility of subsequent hepatotoxicity.[158] Temple and Mrazik suggest that after an overdose with an extended-release acetaminophen product, plasma acetaminophen levels should be measured at least 4 hours after ingestion and again 4 to 6 hours later. If either of these values is above the line on the Rumack-Matthew nomogram indicating potential toxicity, the entire course of antidotal therapy with acetylcysteine should be completed. If neither value is above the nomogram line, toxicity is unlikely. However, if the second value is higher than the first or lies close to the potential toxic range, it would be prudent to consider obtaining additional acetaminophen measurements as well as initiating or continuing acetylcysteine therapy. If the specific type of acetaminophen product ingested is not known, managing the case as if it involved an extended-release product would be prudent.[1]

The nomogram is of value in situations involving an overdose of extended-release acetaminophen in which the initial plasma acetaminophen levels are not in the potentially toxic range.[1]

N-*Acetylcysteine Overdose*

Most severe reactions following the intravenous use of NAC result from the administration of excessive doses. The features of NAC overdose are similar to those of anaphylactoid reactions, but the symptoms are more severe.[159] Cardiovascular collapse and death were temporally associated with the administration of intravenous NAC in a 4-year-old with plasma acetaminophen levels below the toxic line.[160] Several fatalities have occurred following intravenous NAC administration, but the contribution of fulminant hepatic failure to mortality limits conclusions about the causal role of NAC in the death of these patients.

Cimetidine

Cimetidine reduces acetaminophen-induced liver toxicity in animal models, but the amount of cimetidine required to inhibit the formation of toxic metabolites substantially following an overdose of acetaminophen probably is beyond a clinically acceptable dose.[161] A prospective controlled study indicated that the addition of cimetidine therapy to standard NAC therapy does not provide additional hepatoprotection in acutely acetaminophen-poisoned patients when treatment is started later than 8 hours after overdose.[162] Other H_2-receptor antagonists, such as ranitidine, are not effective inhibitors of acetaminophen-induced hepatotoxicity in animal models.[163] The role of cimetidine as adjunctive therapy to NAC is unproven.

4-Methylpyrazole

Animal studies suggest inhibition of acetaminophen-induced hepatotoxicity when 4-methylpyrazole is administered within 4 hours of a toxic acetaminophen dose.[164] 4-Methylpyrazole is an inhibitor of cytochrome P45OIIE1, the main cytochrome P450 enzyme involved in acetaminophen activation in humans. Clinical studies are required to validate this observation.

SUPPORTIVE MEASURES IN ACUTE OVERDOSE

1. Baseline blood tests for hospitalized patients include a complete blood count, liver function tests (hepatic aminotransferase levels, prothrombin time, bilirubin level), glucose, electrolytes, and creatinine. Repeat liver function tests daily for 3 days, then as indicated by the appearance of hepatic encephalopathy. No further tests are necessary for those patients whose acetaminophen levels fall below the toxic line. Repeat acetaminophen levels are unnecessary once serial levels indicate that peak levels have occurred and the last level is below the toxic line. If hepatic or renal dysfunction develops, monitor laboratory values daily until a clear pattern of improvement is seen. Elevations in prothrombin time and unconjugated bilirubin level are the earliest biochemical markers of hepatotoxicity occurring prior to hepatic enzyme elevation.
2. Watch for development of hypoglycemia.
3. Maintain normal hydration and electrolyte balance and avoid forced diuresis.
4. Administer vitamin K_1 for an elevated prothrombin time (1.5× normal). Fresh-frozen plasma should be used for severe prolongation (3× normal). Follow serial hemoglobin and stool guaiac tests for evidence of gastrointestinal bleeding. Prophylactic cimetidine may decrease the incidence of gastrointestinal ulcers.
5. Regular lactulose and enemas assist the elimination of nitrogenous substances and endotoxins from the bowel in encephalopathic patients.
6. Cerebral edema is a major cause of death following the development of hepatic encephalopathy and may be treated with mannitol and fluid restriction.

LIVER TRANSPLANTATION

Fulminant hepatic failure occurs in a small percentage of severely poisoned patients 3 to 6 days after a large acetaminophen overdose. The survival rate for fulminant hepatic failure following acetaminophen overdose depends on age, use of NAC, and degree of encephalopathy on presentation.[165] The increased availability of and improved survival from liver transplantation means that patients with a high risk of fulminant liver failure are candidates for liver transplantation. Delay in performing liver transplantation adversely affects the chances of survival by increasing the risk of cerebral edema, hemorrhage, hypotension, and renal failure.[80] Therefore, candidates for liver transplantation should be identified early, ideally no later than the third to fourth day postingestion. O'Grady and colleagues have suggested indications for transplantation in acute acetaminophen-induced liver failure[134,165](Table 10–4).

FULMINANT HEPATIC FAILURE

Early indicators of fulminant hepatic failure include an uncompensated metabolic acidosis, peak prothrombin time exceeding 100 seconds, continued increase in the prothrombin time on the fourth day,[80] and serum creatinine level greater than 3.4 mg/d. Fulminant hepatic failure after acetaminophen overdose has a mortality of 50%.[134] A plasma factor level less than 10% and a plasma factor VIII/V ratio greater than 30 are not valuable parameters in selecting patients for transplantation.[166,167] Contraindications to liver transplantation in acetaminophen-induced fulminant hepatic failure include active sepsis, refractory systemic hypotension (<90 mm Hg), impaired brainstem function secondary to cerebral

Table 10-4
Criteria for Predicting Death and the Need for Liver Transplantation at King's College Hospital, London*

Cause of Acute Liver Failure	Criteria
Acetaminophen poisoning	pH <7.3 (irrespective of grade or encephalopathy)
	or
	Prothrombin time >100 s and serum creatinine >3.4 mg/dL (300 μmol/L) in patients with grade III or IV encephalopathy
All other causes	Prothrombin time >100 (irrespective of grade of encephalopathy)
	or
	Any of the following variables (irrespective of grade of encephalopathy):
	Age <10 y or >40 y
	Liver failure caused by non-A, non-B hepatitis, halothane-induced hepatitis, or idiosyncratic drug reactions
	Duration of jaundice before onset of encephalopathy >7 d
	Prothrombin time >50 s
	Serum bilirubin >17.5 mg/dL (300 μmol/L)

*Transplantation was considered if the likelihood of survival without it was less than 20%.
From Lee WM. Acute liver failure. N Engl J Med 1993;329:1862–1872. Erratum. N Engl J Med 1994;330:584E.

edema, history of repeated suicide attempt, and repeated requests to die before the onset of encephalopathy.[168]

SUPPORTIVE MEASURES IN FULMINANT HEPATIC FAILURE

1. Monitor the prothrombin time; creatinine, glucose, electrolyte, and hepatic aminotransferase levels; and urine output. Check blood glucose every 4 hours. Check arterial blood gases periodically if the patient's condition does not improve. Any sudden changes in the level of consciousness may be due to hypoglycemia. If this occurs, begin 10 to 20% dextrose.
2. Use Vitamin K_1 if the prothrombin time is elevated. Consider fresh-frozen plasma (see Chapter 27) if there is overt bleeding.
3. Treat cerebral edema with mannitol (0.5 g/kg given over 10 minutes) and repeat if the serum osmolality does not exceed 370 mOsm/kg.
4. Acetaminophen is not teratogenic. Therapeutic abortion is not indicated if the pregnancy is viable. There are no specific indications available for pregnancy termination or early delivery. Measure the INR (International Normalized Ratio, a measure of prothrombin activity) daily and every 12 hours if the initial value is greater than 2 or if it progressively rises.
5. Maintain the central venous pressure with human serum albumin.
6. Continue NAC at doses of 150 mg/kg infused over 24 hours until the INR has fallen below 2.
7. Use intravenous broad-spectrum antibiotics (eg, ceftazidime 1 g three times daily and fluoxacillin 500 mg four times daily).
8. Use sucralfate or an H_2 antagonist to prevent upper gastrointestinal hemorrhage.
9. Avoid sedating agents, benzodiazepines (may precipitate encephalopathy), and nonsteroidal antiinflammatory drugs (provoke gastrointestinal bleeding).

ORGAN DONATIONS

Hearts and corneas are salvagable from patients who die after acetaminophen overdose.[169] Patients dying of acetaminophen overdose should be regarded as potential kidney donors.[38]

BENORYLATE

Benorylate (4-acetamidophenyl-*O*-acetylsalicylate) is the acetylsalicylic ester of acetaminophen. Hydrolysis and deacetylation of this compound produce acetaminophen and salicylic acid.[170] Daily therapeutic doses range from 150 to 234 mg benorylate per kilogram body weight in children to 4 g benorylate in adults. A child survived after developing centrilobular necrosis following the daily ingestion of 6 g benorylate.[171] A 3-year-old child with cystic fibrosis died of massive centrilobular hepatic necrosis following the daily ingestion of 8 g benorylate.[172] Both salicylate and acetaminophen levels should be obtained following the ingestion of excessive doses of benorylate, and treatment should follow the guidelines for both salicylate and acetaminophen toxicity.

REFERENCES

1. Prescott LF, Highley MS. Drugs prescribed for self-poisoners. Br Med J 1985;290:1633–1636.
2. Platt S, Hawton K, Kreitman N, et al. Recent clinical and epidemiological trends in parasuicide in Edinburgh and Oxford: A tale of two cities. Psychol Med 1988; 18:405–418.
3. Litovitz TL, Clark LR, Soloway RA. 1993 Annual Report of the American Association of Poison Control Centers Toxic Exposure Surveillance System. Am J Emerg Med 1994; 12: 546–584.
4. Meredith TJ, Jacobsen D, Haines JA, Berger J-C, eds. *Antidotes for poisoning by paracetamol.* Cambridge: Cambridge University Press, 1995.
5. Corcoran GB, Mitchell Jr, Vaishnaw YN, et al. Evidence that acetaminophen and *N*-hydroxyacetaminophen form a common arylating intermediate, *N*-acetyl-*p*-benzoquinoneimine. Mol Pharmacol 1980;18:536–542.
6. Prescott LF. Drug conjugation in clinical toxicology. Biochem Soc Trans 1984;12:96–99.
7. Mitchell JR, Thorgeirsson SS, Potter WZ, et al. Acetaminophen-induced hepatic injury: Protective role of glutathione in man and rationale for therapy. Clin Pharmacol Ther 1974;16:676–684.
8. Prescott LF. Paracetamol overdosage: Pharmacological considerations and clinical management. Drugs 1983;25:290–314.
9. Mitchell JR, Jollow DJ, Potter WZ, et al. Acetaminophen-induced hepatic necrosis. IV. Protective role of glutathione. J Pharmacol Exp Ther 1973;187:211–217.
10. Crippin JC. Acetaminophen hepatotoxicity: Potentiation by isoniazid. Am J Gastroenterol 1993;88:590–592.
11. Minton NA, Henry JA, Frankel RJ. Fatal paracetamol poisoning in an epileptic. Hum Toxicol 1988;7:33–34.

12. Mathis RD, Walker JS, Kuhns DW. Subacute acetaminophen overdose after incremental dosing. J Emerg Med 1988;6:37–40.
13. Ashbourne JF, Olson KR, Khayam-Bashi H. Value of rapid screening for acetaminophen in all patients with intentional drug overdose. Ann Emerg Med 1989;18:1035–1038.
14. Mitchell JR. Host susceptibility and acetaminophen liver injury. Ann Intern Med 1977;87:377–388.
15. Rumack BH. Acetaminophen overdose in young children. Am J Dis Child 1984;138:428–433.
16. Vale JA, Proudfoot A. Paracetamol (acetaminophen) poisoning. Lancet 1995;346:547–552.
17. Slattery JT, Wilson JM, Kalhorn TF, Nelson SD. Dose-dependent pharmacokinetics of acetaminophen: Evidence of glutathione depletion in humans. Clin Pharmacol Ther 1987;41:413–418.
18. Lee HS, Ti TY, Koh YK, Prescott LF. Paracetamol elimination in Chinese and Indians in Singapore. Eur J Clin Pharmacol 1992;43:81–84.
19. Slattery JT, Koup JR, Levy G, et al. Acetaminophen pharmacokinetics after overdose. Clin Toxicol 1981;18:111–117.
20. Sonne J, Poulsen HE, Loft S, et al. Therapeutic doses of codeine have no effect on acetaminophen clearance or metabolism. Eur J Clin Pharmacol 1988;35:109–111.
21. H_2 receptor antagonists, cytochrome 450 and paracetamol induced hepatotoxicity. Lancet 1985;2:868–870. Editorial.
22. Jack D, Thomas M, Skidmore IF. Ranitidine and paracetamol metabolism. Lancet 1985;2:1067.
23. Tredger JM, Thuluvah P, William R, Murray-Lyon IM. Metabolic basis for high paracetamol dosage without hepatic injury: A case study. Hum Exp Toxicol 1995;14:8–12.
24. Ameer B. Acetaminophen hepatotoxicity augmented by zidovudine. Am J Med 1993;95:342.
25. James RC, Harbison RD, Roberts SM. Phenylpropanolamine potentiation of acetaminophen-induced hepatotoxicity: Evidence for a glutathione-dependent mechanisms. Toxicol Appl Pharmacol 1993;118:159–168.
26. Roberts I, Robinson MJ, Mughal MZ, et al. Paracetamol metabolites in the neonate following maternal overdose. Br J Clin Pharmacol 1984;18:201–206.
27. Settipane RA, Stevenson DD. Cross sensitivity with acetaminophen in aspirin-sensitive subjects with asthma. J Allergy Clin Immunol 1989;84:26–33.
28. Bronstein AC, Rumack BH. Abstract A-12, AAPCC/ABMT/CAPCC Annual Scientific Meeting, October 7, 1984, San Diego, California. Vet Hum Toxicol 1984;26(suppl. 2):44.
29. Ruthrum P, Goel KM. ABC of poisoning: Paracetamol. Br Med J 1984;289:1538–1539.
30. Byer AJ, Traylor TR, Semmer JR. Acetaminophen overdose in the third trimester of pregnancy. JAMA 1982;247:3114–3115.
31. McElhatton PK, Sullivan FM, Volans GN, Fitzpatrick R. Paracetamol poisoning in pregnancy: An analysis of the outcome of cases referred to the Teratology Information Service of the National Poisons Information Service. Hum Exp Toxicol 1990;9:147–153.
32. Rollins DE, von Bahr C, Glaumann H, et al. Acetaminophen: Potentially toxic metabolite formed by human fetal and adult liver microsomes and isolated fetal liver cells. Science 1979;205:1414–1416.
33. Roberts JR. Acetaminophen toxicity: Issues for children and pregnant women. Emerg Med News 1994;16:4–8.
34. Clark R, Thompson RPH, Borirakchanyavat V, et al. Hepatic damage and death from overdose of paracetamol. Lancet 1973;1:66–70.
35. Canalese J, Gimson AES, Davis M, et al. Factors contributing to mortality in paracetamol induced hepatic failure. Br Med J 1981;282:199–201.
36. Gall GD, Cutz E, McLung HJ, et al. Acute liver disease and encephalopathy mimicking Reye syndrome. J Pediatr 1975;87:869–874.
37. Kaul A, Cohen ME, Brottman G, et al. Reye-like syndrome associated with Coxsackie B_2 virus infection. J Pediatr 1979;94:67–69.
38. Andrews PA, Koffman CG. Kidney donation after paracetamol overdose. Br Med J 1993;306:1129.
39. Prescott LF, Illingworth RN, Critchley JAJH, et al. Intravenous *N*-acetylcysteine: The treatment of choice for paracetamol poisoning. Br Med J 1979;2:1097–1100.
40. Smilkstein MJ, Bronstein AC, Linden C, et al. Acetaminophen overdose: A 48-hour intravenous *N*-acetylcysteine treatment protocol. Ann Emerg Med 1991;20:1058–1063.
41. Smilkstein MJ, Knapp GL, Kulig KW, Rumack BH. Efficacy of oral *N*-acetylcysteine in the treatment of acetaminophen overdose: Analysis of the National Multicenter study (1976 to 1985). N Engl J Med 1988;319:1557–1562.
42. Prescott LF, Speirs GC, Critchley JAJH, et al. Paracetamol disposition and metabolite kinetics in patients with chronic renal failure. Eur J Clin Pharmacol 1989;36:291–297.
43. Campbell NRC, Baylis B. Renal impairment associated with an acute paracetamol overdose in the absence of hepatotoxicity. Postgrad Med J 1992;68:116–118.
44. McMurtry RJ, Snodgrass WR, Mitchell JR. Renal necrosis, glutathione depletion and covalent binding after acetaminophen. Toxicol Appl Pharmacol 1978;46:87–100.
45. Bjorck S, Svalander CT, Aurell M. Acute renal failure after analgesic drugs including paracetamol (acetaminophen). Nephron 1988;49:45–53.
46. Sandler DP, Smith JC, Weinberg CR, et al. Analgesic use and chronic renal disease. N Engl J Med 1989;320:1238–1243.
47. Segasothy M, Suleiman AB, Puvaneswary M, Rohana A. Paracetamol: A cause for analgesic nephropathy and end-stage renal disease. Nephron 1988;50:50–54.
48. Ronco PM, Flahault A. Drug-induced end-stage renal disease. N Engl J Med 1994;331:1711–1712.
49. Perneger TV, Whelton PK, Klag MJ. Risk of kidney failure with the use of acetaminophen, aspirin and nonsteroidal anti-inflammatory drugs. N Engl J Med 1994;331:1675–1679.
50. Mofenson HC, Caraccio TR, Nawaz H, Steckler G. Acetaminophen induced pancreatitis. Clin Toxicol 1991;29:223–230.
51. Curry RW, Robinson JD, Sughrue MJ. Acute renal failure after acetaminophen ingestion. JAMA 1982;247:1012–1014.
52. Gabriel R. Paracetamol-induced acute renal failure in the absence of fulminant liver damage. Br Med J 1982;284:505–506.
53. Cobden I, Record CO, Ward MK, Kerr DNS. Paracetamol-induced acute renal failure in the absence of fulminant liver damage. Br Med J 1982; 284:21–22.
54. Davenport A, Finn R. Paracetamol (acetaminophen) poisoning resulting in acute renal failure without hepatic coma. Nephron 1988;50:55–56.
55. Wilkinson SP, Moodie H, Arroya VA, Williams R. Frequency of renal impairment in paracetamol overdose compared with other causes of liver failure. J Clin Pathol 1977;30:141–143.
56. Jones AF, Jolley A, Buckley BM, Vale JA. Effect of indomethacin on polyuria following a paracetamol overdose. Presented at the Meeting of the European Association of Poison Centres, Edinburgh, 1988.
57. Bennett WM, Debroe ME. Analgesic nephropathy: A preventable disease. N Engl J Med 1989;320:1269–1271.
58. Mitchell SR. Tell your kidneys to take a powder. Arch Intern Med 1991;151:617.
59. Mann JM, Pieer-Louis M, Kragel PJ, et al. Cardiac consequences of massive acetaminophen overdose. Am J Cardiol 1989;63:1018–1021.
60. Wakeel RA, Davies HT, Williams JD. Toxic myocarditis in paracetamol poisoning. Br Med J 1987;295:1097.
61. Price LM, Poklis A, Johnson DE. Fatal acetaminophen poisoning with evidence of subendocardial necrosis of the heart. J Forens Sci 1991;36:930–935.
62. Pimstone BL, Uys CJ. Liver necrosis and myocardiopathy following paracetamol overdosage. S Afr Med J 1968;42:259–262.
63. Armour A, Slater SD. Paracetamol cardiotoxicity. Postgrad Med J 1993;69:52–54.
64. Mofenson HC, Caraccio TR, Nawaz H, Steckler G. Acetaminophen-induced pancreatitis. Clin Toxicol 1991;29:223–230.
65. Hord K, Phillips S, McKinney P, Gomez H. The incidence of hyperamylasemia following acetaminophen overdose. Vet Hum Toxicol 1992;34:343.
66. Guin JD, Baker GF. Chronic fixed drug eruption caused by acetaminophen. Cutis 1988;41:106–108.

67. Girdhar A, Bagga AK, Girdhar BK. Exfoliative dermatitis due to paracetamol. Indian J Dermatol Venereal Lepr 1984;50:162–163.
68. Cole FO. Urticaria from paracetamol. Clin Exp Dermatol 1985;10:404.
69. Stricker BHCH, Meyboom RHB. Acute hypersensitivity reactions to paracetamol. Br Med J 1985;291:938–939.
70. Leung R, Plomley R, Czarny D. Paracetamol anaphylaxis. Clin Exp Allergy 1992;22: 831–833.
71. Ellis M, Haydik I, Gilman S, et al. Immediate adverse reactions to acetaminophen in children: Evaluation of histamine release and spirometry. J Pediatr 1989;114:654–656.
72. Diem LV, Grilliat JP. Anaphylactic shock induced by paracetamol. Eur J Clin Pharmacol 1990;38:389–390.
73. Gray TA, Buckley BM, Vale JA. Hyperlactataemia and metabolic acidosis following paracetamol overdose. Q J Med 1987;65:811–821.
74. Clark R, Borirakchanyavat V, Gazzard BG, et al. Disordered haemostatis in liver damage from paracetamol overdose. Gastroenterology 1973;65:788–795.
75. Gilmore IT, Tourvas E. Paracetamol-induced acute pancreatitis. Br Med J 1977;1:753–754.
76. Record CO, Chase RA, Alberti KGMM, Williams R. Disturbances in glucose metabolism in patients with liver damage due to paracetamol overdose. Clin Sci Mol Med 1975;49:473–479.
77. Knockel JP. The pathophysiology and clinical characteristics of severe hypophosphatemia. Arch Intern Med 1977;137:203–220.
78. Skokan JD, Hewlett JS, Hoffman GD. Thrombocytopenic purpura associated with ingestion of acetaminophen (Tylenol). Cleve Clin Q 1973;40:89–91.
79. Saunders JB, Wright N, Lewis KO. Predicting outcome of paracetamol poisoning by using ^{14}C-aminopyrine breath test. Br Med J 1980;280:279–280.
80. Harrison PM, O'Grady JG, Keays RT, et al. Serial prothrombin time as prognostic indicator in paracetamol induced fulminant hepatic failure. Br Med J 1990;301:964–966.
81. Rumack BH, Matthew H. Acetaminophen poisoning and toxicity. Pediatrics 1975;55:871–876.
82. Whitcomb DC, Block GD. Association of acetaminophen hepatotoxicity with fasting and ethanol use. JAMA 1994;272:1845–1850.
83. Bray GP, Mowat DF, Muir DF, et al. The effect of chronic alcohol intake on prognosis and outcome in paracetamol overdose. Hum Exp Toxicol 1992;11:265–270.
84. Lauterburg BH, Velez ME. Glutathione deficiency in alcoholics: Risk factor for paracetamol hepatotoxicity. Gut 1988;29:1153–1157.
85. Lauterburg BH, Davis S, Mitchell JR. Ethanol suppresses hepatic glutathione synthesis in rats in vivo. J Pharmacol Exp Ther 1984;230:7–11.
86. Henretig FM, Selbst SM, Forrest C, et al. Repeated acetaminophen overdosing causing hepatotoxicity in children: Clinical reports and literature review. Clin Pediatr 1989;28:525–528.
87. Greene JW, Craft L, Ghishan F. Acetaminophen poisoning in infancy. Am J Dis Child 1983;137:387.
88. Nogen AG, Bremmer JE. Fatal acetaminophen overdosage in a young child. J Pediatr 1984;92:832–833.
89. Hickson GB, Greene JW, Ghishan FK, Craft LT. Apparent intentional poisoning of an infant with acetaminophen. Am J Dis Child 1983;137:917.
90. Agran PF, Zenk KE, Romansky SG. Acute liver failure and encephalopathy in a 15-month-old infant. Am J Dis Child 1983;137:1107–1114.
91. Swetnam SM, Florman AL. Probably acetaminophen toxicity in an 18-month-old infant due to repeated overdosing. Clin Pediatr 1984;23:104–105.
92. Baeg N-J, Bodenheimer HC Jr, Burchard K. Long-term sequelae of acetaminophen-associated fulminant hepatic failure: Relevance of early histology. Am J Gastroenterol 1988;83:569–571.
93. Temple AR. Pediatric dosing of acetaminophen. Pediatr Pharmacol 1983;3:321–329.
94. Walson PD, Groth JF Jr. Acetaminophen hepatotoxicity after a prolonged ingestion. Pediatrics 1993;91:1021–1022.
95. Tighe TV, Walter FG. Delayed toxic acetaminophen level after initial four hour nontoxic levels. Clin Toxicol 1994;32:431–434.
96. Johnson GK, Tolman KG. Chronic liver disease and acetaminophen. Ann Intern Med 1977;87:302–304.
97. Bidault I, Lagier G, Garnier G, et al. Les hepatites par toxicite subaique du paracetamol existent elles? A propos de 3 cas eventuels. Therapie 1987;42:387–388.
98. Barker JD Jr, de Carle DJ, Anuras S. Chronic excessive acetaminophen use and liver damage. Ann Intern Med 1977;87:299–301.
99. James O, Lesna M, Roberts SH, et al. Liver damage after paracetamol overdose. Lancet 1975;2:579–581.
100. Walker RM, McElligott TF, Power EM, et al. Increased acetaminophen-induced hepatotoxicity after chronic ethanol consumption in mice. Toxicology 1983;128:193–200.
101. Pezzano M, Richard CL, Lampl E, et al. Toxicite hepatique et renale due paracetamol chez l'alcoholique chronique. Presse Med 1988;17:21–24.
102. Seeff LB, Cuccherini BA, Zimmerman HJ, et al. Acetaminophen hepatotoxicity in alcoholics: A therapeutic misadventure. Ann Intern Med 1986;104:399–404.
103. Floren C-H, Thesieff P, Nilsson A. Severe liver damage caused by therapeutic doses of acetaminophen. Acta Med Scand 1987; 222:285–288.
104. Wootton FT, Lee WM. Acetaminophen hepatotoxicity in the alcoholic. South Med J 1990;83:1047–1049.
105. McClain CJ, Holtzman J, Allen J, et al. Clinical features of acetaminophen toxicity. J Clin Gastroenterol 1988;10:76–80.
106. Kunar S, Rex DFK. Failure of physicians to recognize acetaminophen hepatotoxicity in chronic alcoholics. Arch Intern Med 1991;151:1189–1191.
107. Zimmerman HJ. Acetaminophen toxicity in alcoholics. West J Med 1989;150:722.
108. Eriksson LS, Broome U, Kaline M, Lindholm M. Hepatotoxicity due to repeated intake of low doses of paracetamol. J Intern Med 1992;231:567–570.
109. Cheung L, Potts RG, Mayer KC. Acetaminophen treatment nomogram. N Engl J Med 1994;330:1907–1908.
110. Lee WM. Acute liver failure. N Engl J Med 1993;329:1862–1872.
111. Farah DA, Boag D, Moran F, McIntosh S. Paracetamol interference with blood glucose analysis: A potentially fatal phenomenon. Br Med J 1982;285:172.
112. Poon B, Hinberg I, Peterson PG. *N*-Acetylcysteine causes false-positive ketone results with urinary dipsticks. Clin Chem 1990;36:818–820.
113. Bridges RR, Kinniburgh DW, Keehn BJ, et al. An evaluation of common methods for acetaminophen quantitation for small hospitals. Clin Toxicol 1983;20:1–17.
114. Osterloh J. Limitations of acetaminophen assays. Clin Toxicol 1983;20:1–17.
115. Edinboro LE, Jackson GF, Jortani SA, Poklis A. Determination of serum acetaminophen in emergency toxicology: Evaluation of newer methods: Abbott TDx and second derivative ultraviolet spectrophotometry. Clin Toxicol 1991;29:241–255.
116. Beckett GJ, Hayes JD. Plasma glutathione *S*-transferase measurements and liver disease in man. J Clin Biochem Nutr 1987;2:1–24.
117. Beckett GJ, Foster GR, Hussey AJ, et al. Plasma glutathione *S*-transferase and F protein are more sensitive than alanine aminotransferase as markers of paracetamol (acetaminophen)-induced liver damage. Clin Chem 1989;35:2186–2189.
118. Thornton JR, Losowsky MS. Severe thrombocytopenia after paracetamol overdose. Gut 1990;31:1159–1160.
119. Armour A, Slater SD. Paracetamol cardiotoxicity. Postgrad Med J 1993;69:52–54.
120. Hinson JA, Roberts DW, Benson RW, et al. Mechanism of paracetamol toxicity. Lancet 1990;1:732.
121. Jones AF, Harvey JM, Vale JA. Hypophosphatemia and phosphaturia in paracetamol poisoning. Lancet 1989;2:608–609.

122. Jones AF, McAleer JF, Braithwaite RA, et al. Rapid side 100m test for paracetamol. Lancet 1990;335:793–794.
123. Medi Sense (U.K.), Abingdon, Oxfordshire, U.K.
124. Shannon M, Saladino R, McCarty D, et al. Clinical evaluation of an acetaminophen meter for the rapid diagnosis of acetaminophen intoxication. Ann Emerg Med 1990;19:1133–1136.
125. Rose SR, Gorman RL, Oderda GM, et al. Simulated acetaminophen overdose: Pharmacokinetics and effectiveness of activated charcoal. Ann Emerg Med 1991;20:1064–1068.
126. Bond GR, Krenzelok EP, Normann SA, et al. Acetaminophen ingestion in childhood: Cost and relative risk of alternative referral strategies. Clin Toxicol 1994;32:513–525.
127. Klein-Schwartz W, Oderda GM. Adsorption of oral antidotes for acetaminophen poisoning (methionine and *N*-acetylcysteine) by activated charcoal. Clin Toxicol 1981;18: 283–290.
128. Spiller HA, Krenzelok EP, Grande GA, et al. A prospective evaluation of the effect of activated charcoal before oral *N*-acetylcysteine in acetaminophen overdose. Ann Emerg Med 1994;23:519–523.
129. Brent J. Are activated charcoal *N*-acetylcysteine interactions of clinical significance? Ann Emerg Med 1993;22:1860–1861.
130. Lederman S, Fyech WJ, Tredger M, Gamsu AR. Neonatal paracetamol poisoning: Treatment by exchange transfusion. Arch Dis Child 1983;58:631–633.
131. Claas A, Gaude M, Schroeder H. Paracetamol poisoning in an infant. Dtsch Med Wochnschr 1993;118:898–902.
132. Kritharides L, Fassett R, Singh B. Paracetamol associated coma, metabolic acidosis, renal and hepatic failure. Intensive Care Med 1988;14:439–440.
133. Pond SM, Tong TG, Kaysen GA, et al. Massive intoxication with acetaminophen and propoxyphene: Unexpected survival and unusual pharmacokinetics of acetaminophen. J Toxicol Clin Toxicol 1982;19:1–16.
134. O'Grady JG, Gimson AES, O'Brien CJ, et al. Controlled trials of charcoal hemoperfusion and prognostic factors in fulminant hepatic failure. Gastroenterology 1988;94:1186–1192.
135. McLean AEM, Day PA: The effect of diet on the toxicity of paracetamol and the safety of paracetamol–methionine mixtures. Biochem Pharmacol 1975;24:37–42.
136. Vina J, Hems R, Krebs HA. Maintenance of glutathione content in isolated hepatocytes. Biochem J 1978;170:627–630.
137. Vina J, Romero FJ, Estrela JM, Vina JR. Effect of acetaminophen (paracetamol) and its antagonists on glutathione (GSH) content in rat liver. Biochem Pharmacol 1980;29: 1968–1970.
138. Meredith TJ, Crome P, Volans GN, Goulding R. Treatment of paracetamol poisoning. Br Med J 1978;1:1215–1216.
139. Meredith TJ. Paracetamol poisoning in England and Wales. MD thesis, University of Cambridge, 1987:93–112.
140. Vale JA, Meredith TJ, Goulding R. Treatment of acetaminophen poisoning: The use of oral methionine. Arch Intern Med 1981;141:394–396.
141. Meredith TJ, Prescott LF, Vale JA. Why do patients still die from paracetamol poisoning? Br Med J 1986;293:345–346.
142. Paracetamol and methionine: Pameton. Drug Ther Bull 1987; 25:99–100.
143. Prescott LF, Donovan JW, Jarvie DR, Proudfoot AT. The disposition and kinetics of intravenous *N*-acetylcysteine in patients with paracetamol overdosage. Eur J Clin Pharmacol 1989;37:501–506.
144. Makin A, Williams R. The current management of paracetamol overdosage. Br J Clin Pract 1994;48:144–148.
145. Janes J, Routledge PA. Recent developments in the management of paracetamol (acetaminophen) poisoning. Drug Saf 1992;7:170–177.
146. Ferner R. Paracetamol poisoning: An update. Prescribers J 1993;33:45–49.
147. Keays R, Harrison PM, Wendon JA, et al. Intravenous acetylcysteine in paracetamol induced fulminant hepatic failure: A prospective controlled trial. Br Med J 1991;303:1026–1029.
148. Parker D, White JP, Paton D, Routledge PA. Safety of late acetylcysteine treatment in paracetamol poisoning. Hum Exp Toxicol 1990;9:25–27.
149. Beckett GJ, Donovan JW, Hussey AJ, et al. Intravenous *N*-acetylcysteine, hepatotoxicity and plasma glutathione *S*-transferase in patients with paracetamol overdosage. Hum Exp Toxicol 1990;9:183–186.
150. Tobias JD, Gregory DF, Deshpande JK. Ondansetron to prevent emesis following *N*-acetylcysteine for acetaminophen intoxication. Pediatr Emerg Care 1992;8:345–346.
151. Bonfiglio MF, Traeger SM, Hulisz DT, Martin BR. Anaphylactoid reaction to intravenous acetylcysteine associated with electrocardiographic abnormalities. Ann Pharmacother 1992; 26:22–25.
152. Rodgers G, Matyanes N, Ross M, et al. Sulfhemoglobinemia associated with *N*-acetylcysteine (NAC) therapy of acetaminophen (APAP) overdose: A case report. Clin Toxicol 1995;33:475–486.
153. Dawson AH, Henry DA, McEwen J. Adverse reactions to *N*-acetylcysteine during treatment for paracetamol poisoning. Med J Aust 1989;150:329–331.
154. Ho SW, Beilin JJ. Asthma associated with *N*-acetylcysteine infusion and paracetamol poisoning: Report of two cases. Br Med J 1983;287:876–877.
155. Bateman DN, Woodhouse KW, Rawlins MD. Adverse reactions to *N*-acetylcysteine. Hum Toxicol 1984;3:393–398.
156. Temple AR. McNeil Consumer Products Company. Dear Doctor Letter, January 23, 1995.
157. Douglas DR, Smilkstein MJ, Sholar JB. Overdose with 'Extended Relief' acetaminophen: Is a new approach necessary? Ann Emerg Med 1995;2:397–398.
158. Graudins A, Aaron CK, Linden CH. Overdose of extended-release acetaminophen. N Engl J Med 1995;333:196.
159. Mant TGK, Tempowski JH, Volans GN, et al. Adverse reactions to acetylcysteine and effects of overdose. Br Med J 1984;289:217–220.
160. Death after *N*-acetylcysteine, news and notes. Lancet 1984; 1:1421.
161. Slattery JT, McRorie TI, Reynolds R, et al. Lack of effect of cimetidine on acetaminophen disposition in humans. Clin Pharmacol Ther 1989;46:591–597.
162. Burkhart KK, Janco N, Kulig KW, Rumack BH. Cimetidine as adjunctive treatment for acetaminophen overdose. Hum Exp Toxicol 1995;14:229–304.
163. Speeg KV. Potential use of cimetidine for treatment of acetaminophen overdose. Pharmacotherapy 1987;7(6, pt 2): 125S–133S.
164. Brennan RJ, Mankes RF, Lefevere R, et al. 4-Methylpyrazole blocks acetaminophen hepatotoxicity in the rat. Ann Emerg Med 1993;22:894.
165. O'Grady JG, Wendon JA, Tan KC, et al. Liver transplantation after paracetamol overdose. Br Med J 1991;303:221–223.
166. Pereira LMMB, Langley PG, Hayllar KM, et al. Coagulation factor V and VIII/V ratio as predictors of outcome in paracetamol induced fulminant hepatic failure: Relation to other prognostic indicators. Gut 1992;33:98–102.
167. Bradberry SM. Factor V and factor VIII:V ratio as prognostic indicators in paracetamol poisoning. Personal Communication 0-58. In: *Proceedings, XVIth International Congress of European Association of Poison Centres and Clinical Toxicologists, Vienna, April 12, 1994.*
168. O'Grady JG, Alexander GJM, Hayllar KM, Williams R. Early indicators of prognosis in fulminant hepatic failure. Gastroenterology. 1989;97:439–445.
169. Jackson S, Nightingale P, Shelly MP. Organ donation of paracetamol overdose. Br Med J 1993;306:718.
170. Williams FM, Moore U, Seymour RA, et al. Benorylate hydrolysis by human plasma and human liver. Br J Clin Pharmacol 1989;28:703–708.
171. Sacher M, Thaler H. Toxic hepatitis after therapeutic doses of benorylate and D-penicillamine. Lancet 1977;1:481–482.
172. Symon DNK, Gray ES, Hanmer OJ, Russell G. Fatal paracetamol poisoning from benorylate therapy in a child with cystic fibrosis. Lancet 1982;2:1152–1154.

Chapter 11
Nonsteroidal Antiinflammatory Drugs

INTRODUCTION

Although chronic exposure to the nonsteroidal antiinflammatory drugs (NSAIDs) (Fig. 11–1)[1] may lead to acute and chronic renal failure, gastroduodenal damage,[2,3] colitis, infrequent liver injury,[4] occasional neutropenia,[5] elevation of the blood pressure and antagonism to the blood pressure-lowering effect of antihypertensive medication,[6] acute overdoses are relatively benign.

The U.S. Food and Drug Administration (FDA) (1989) has required all manufacturers of NSAIDs to add special warnings regarding the risk of gastrointestinal ulceration, bleeding, and perforation following any NSAID therapy.[7]

Severe poisonings may be complicated by acute renal failure, hepatic dysfunction, seizures, hypotension, apnea, respiratory depression, metabolic acidosis, cardiovascular collapse, cardiac arrest, and coma. Some NSAID overdoses may induce multisystem (gastrointestinal, central nervous system, renal, hepatic, hematopoietic) abnormalities.[8] They are usually reversible.

Ketorolac (Toradol) has been withdrawn from the market in Germany because of concerns relating to adverse reactions affecting the gastrointestinal tract and renal function. In the United States, the FDA requires that doctors be warned about gastrointestinal ulcerations, bleeding, and perforation and impaired renal function.[9] Ketorolac remains on the market in Denmark, France, Italy, Spain, and the United Kingdom.[10] Zomepirac was withdrawn in the United States in 1985 after a number of anaphylactic reactions and deaths.[11]

Table 11–1 summarizes tablet sizes and recommended adult daily doses of NSAIDs.[12]

Toxicokinetics

Metabolism

Four prodrugs of NSAIDs are sulindac, fenbufen, suxibuzone, and acemetacin. Gastrointestinal side effects of sulindac, fenbufen, and acemetacin appear to be weaker than those of aspirin and indomethacin (Table 11–2).[13,14]

Drug Interactions

Elderly people are more likely to have multiple-organ dysfunction.[15] NSAIDs are commonly used in this age

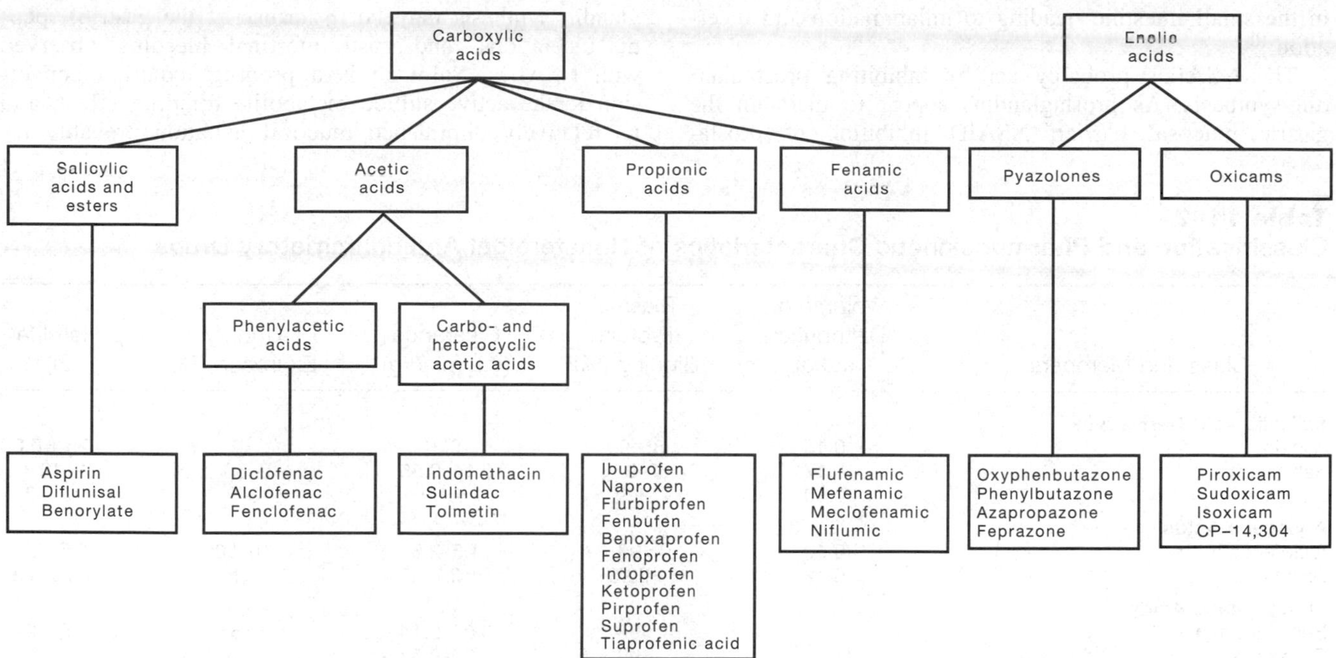

Figure 11–1 Families of nonsteroidal antiinflammatory drugs. (Adapted from Wiseman EH. Pharmacologic studies with a new class of nonsteroidal anti-inflammatory agents—the oxicams—with special reference to piroxicam (Feldene). Am J Med 1982;72(24):3.)

Table 11–1
Tablet Sizes and Maximum Recommended Adult Daily Doses of Nonsteroidal Antiinflammatory Drugs

Drug	Formulation Sizes (mg)				Maximum Recommended Adult Daily Dose (mg)
Diflunisal	250	500			100
Diclofenac	25	50	75	100	150
Fenclofenac	300				1200
Indomethacin	25	50	75	100	200
Sulindac	100	200			400
Tolmetin	200	400			1800
Zomepirac	100				600
Ibuprofen	200	300	400		2400
Naproxen	250	500			1000
Flurbiprofen	50	100			300
Fenbufen	300				900
Benoxaprofen	300				600
Fenoprofen	200	300	600		3000
Ketoprofen	50	100			200
Flufenamic acid	100				600
Mefenamic acid	250	500			1500
Oxyphenbutazole	50	100	250		800
Phenylbutazone	100	200	250	600	800
Azapropazone	300	600			2400
Feproazone	200				600
Piroxicam	10				40

From Court H, Volans GN. Poisoning after overdose with non-steroidal antiinflammatory drugs. Adverse Drug React Acute Poisoning Rev 1984;3:1–21.

group. There is a considerable potential for interactions between NSAIDs and other drugs. These interactions have been recently reviewed.[15–17] Interactions occur with any of the NSAIDs (Table 11–3).[15]

Mechanism of Action

The central event in the initiation of toxicologic damage involves the action of NSAIDs in uncoupling mitochondrial oxidative phosphorylation. During drug absorption, the enterocyte becomes ATP deficient, setting off a cascade of events detrimental to the cell. A combined effect of the uncoupling of oxidative phosphorylation and the inhibition of cyclooxygenase 1 (causing decreased prostaglandin production leading to focal ischemia) is especially damaging. Intestinal permeability increases, allowing back diffusion of acid into the stomach and duodenum and mucosal exposure to luminal aggressive factors in the small intestine, leading to inflammation and ulceration.[18]

The NSAIDs probably act by inhibiting prostaglandin synthesis. As prostaglandins appear to maintain the gastric mucosal barrier, NSAID inhibition of prostaglandin synthesis may be the cause of the gastritis, peptic ulcerations, and gastrointestinal bleeding observed with NSAIDs. Sulindac is a prodrug requiring conversion to the active sulfide metabolite for drug effect, and its relatively diminished mucosal irritation probably re-

Table 11–2
Classification and Pharmacokinetic Characteristics of Nonsteroidal Antiinflammatory Drugs

Class and Members	Volume of Distribution (L/kg)	Plasma Protein Binding (%)	Clearance (mL/min/kg)	Urinary Excretion (%)	Half-life* (h)[a]
Salicylic Acid Derivatives					
Aspirin†	0.15	85–90	9.3	<2	0.25 ± 0.03
Salicylate‡	0.17	80–95§	0.14–0.86	2–30‖	2–19#
Diflunisal	0.10	99.9	0.11	3–9	13 ± 2
Arylacetic Acids					
Alclofenac¶	0.10	>99	1.5–2.5	10–50	1.5–2.5
Diclofenac	0.12	>99.5	3.7	<1	1.1 ± 0.2
Arylpropionic Acids					
Benoxaprofen		>98	0.03–0.14	<5	25–32
Carprofen		>99	0.29–0.57	3–5	9–16
Fenbufen	2–4	>98	2.1–3.6	<2	8–17
Active metabolites:					
γ-Hydroxy-4-biphenylbutanoic acid				<3	7–17
Biphenyl-4-acetic acid				1–15	7–12
Fenoprofen	0.10	>99	0.6–1.3	30	2.5 ± 0.5
Flurbiprofen	0.10	>99	0.3	<1	3.8 ± 1.2
Ibuprofen	0.1–0.15	>99	0.6–1.4	<1	2.0 ± 0.5
Ketoprofen	0.11	>99	1.2	<1	1.8 ± 0.3
Naproxen	0.10–0.12	>99	0.07–0.14	<1	14 ± 2
Oxaprozin¶	0.16	>99	0.04	1–4	58 ± 10
Pirprofen		>99		<5	7.1 ± 1.2
Suprofen	0.17	>99	1.4–1.8	<1	1–3
Tiaprofenic acid	0.1–0.25	98	0.6–1.4	<5	3 ± 0.2
Heterocyclic Acetic Acids					
Etodolac	0.4	>99	0.68	<1	6.5 ± 0.3
Indomethacin¶	0.3–1.6	>99	1–2	16	4.6 ± 0.7
Ketorolac¶	0.1–0.25	>99	0.36–0.57	58	4–10
Sulindac		>99		7	8
Active metabolite:					
Sulindac sulfide	2	93.1	1.5	<1	15.8 ± 11.6
Tolmetin	0.04	>99	1.8	7	1.0 ± 0.3
Zomepirac	1.8	98.5	2.6	0–5	4–8
Pyrazolones					
Azapropazone¶	0.14	>99		62	15 ± 4
Oxyphenbutazone	0.17	>98	0.02	<2	27–64
Phenylbutazone	0.17	>99		1–3	68 ± 25
Oxicams					
Isoxicam	0.17	96	0.001	1–2	29–34
Piroxicam	0.12–0.15	>99	0.04	4–10	57 ± 22
Tenoxicam	0.12–0.15	>98	0.0014	<1	60–75
Fenamic acids					
Flufenamic acid		>90		<1	9
Mefenamic acid	1.3	>99		<6	3–4
Meclofenamic acid		99	2.6–2.9	2–4	3
Nonacidic Drugs					
Nabumetone					
Acitve metabolite:					
6-Methoxy-2-naphtylacetic acid	7.5	99		1	26 ± 5

*Mean ± SD or upper and lower bounds of the range.
†Acetylated; hydrolyzes rapidly forming salicylate.
‡Includes: benorylate, salsalate, and the choline, magnesium, and sodium salts.
§Decreases as plasma concentration increases.
‖Increases as urinary pH increases.
#Increases as plasma concentration increases.
¶Drugs with clinically important renal elimination.
From Murray MD, Brater DC. Renal toxicity of the nonsteroidal anti-inflammatory drugs. Annu Rev Pharmacol Toxicol 1993;33:435–465.

Table 11–3
Interactions of Nonsteroidal Antiinflammatory Drugs (NSAIDs) With Other Drugs

Drug Affected	NSAID Implicated	Effect	Approach to Management
Pharmacokinetic Interactions			
NSAID Affecting Other Drug			
Oral anticoagulants	Phenylbutazone Oxyphenbutazone Apazone	Inhibition of metabolism of *S*-warfarin, increasing anticoagulant effect	Avoid NSAID if possible, or use careful monitoring.
Lithium	Probably all (except possibly sulindac and aspirin)	Inhibition of renal excretion of lithium, increasing plasma lithium concentrations and risk of toxicity	Use sulindac or aspirin if NSAID must be used. Monitor lithium concentration carefully and make appropriate dose reduction.
Oral hypoglycemic agents	Phenylbutazone Oxyphenbutazone Apazone	Inhibition of metabolism of sulfonylurea drugs, prolonging their half-life and increasing the risk of hypoglycemia	Avoid these NSAIDs if possible; if not, monitor blood glucose level closely.
Phenytoin	Phenylbutazone Oxyphenbutazone	Inhibition of metabolism of phenytoin, increasing plasma phenytoin concentration and risk of toxicity	Avoid these NSAIDs if possible; if not, intensify therapeutic-drug monitoring.
	Others	Displacement of phenytoin from plasma protein, reducing total concentration for the same unbound (active) concentration	Interpret total plasma concentration of phenytoin carefully; measuring the unbound concentration may be helpful.
Methotrexate (high, nonrheumatologic dose)	Probably all	Reduced clearance of methotrexate (by unknown mechanism), increasing plasma methotrexate concentration and risk of toxicity	Simultaneous dosing is contraindicated. Use of NSAIDs between cycles of chemotherapy is probably safe. Interaction is not seen with rheumatologic doses of methotrexate.
Sodium valproate	Aspirin	Inhibition of valproate metabolism, increasing plasma valproate concentration	Avoid aspirin; monitor plasma valproate concentration closely if another NSAID is used.
Digoxin	All	Potential reduction in renal function (particularly in very young and very old patients), reducing digoxin clearance and increasing plasma digoxin concentration and risk of toxicity (no interaction if renal function normal)	Avoid NSAIDs if possible; if not, measure plasma digoxin and creatinine concentrations frequently.
Aminoglycosides	All	Reduction in renal function in susceptible persons, lowering aminoglycoside clearance and increasing plasma aminoglycoside concentration	Monitor plasma aminoglycoside concentration closely and adjust the dose accordingly.
Other Drug Affecting NSAID			
Antacids	Indomethacin Others	Variable effects of different preparations: rate and extent of absorption of indomethacin reduced by aluminum-containing antacids, but increased by sodium bicarbonate	No action is required unless markedly reduced absorption results in a poor response to the NSAID; dose may need to be increased. Rate of absorption of other NSAIDs can be slowed by antacids.
Probenecid	Probably all	Reduction in metabolism and renal clearance of NSAIDs and acyl glucoronide metabolites, which are hydrolyzed back to parent drug	
Barbiturates	Phenylbutazone, possibly others	Increased metabolic clearance of NSAID	Higher doses of phenylbutazone may be required.
Caffeine	Aspirin	Increased rate of absorption of aspirin	No action is required.

(continued)

Table 11–3 *(Continued)*

Drug Affected	NSAID Implicated	Effect	Approach to Management
Cholestyramine	Naproxen and probably others	Anion-exchange resin binding of NSAIDs in gut, reducing rate (and possibly extent) of absorption	Separate dosing times by 4 h; larger-than-expected doses of NSAID may be needed.
Metoclopramide	Aspirin and others	Increased rate and extent of absorption of aspirin in patients with migraine	
Pharmacodymamic Interactions			
NSAID Affecting Other Drug			
Antihypertensive agents			
Beta blockers Diuretics Angiotensin-converting enzyme inhibitors	Indomethacin Others (possibly except sulindac)	Reduction in hypotensive effect, probably related to inhibition of prostaglandin synthesis in kidneys (producing retention of salt and water) and blood vessels (producing increased vasoconstriction)	Avoid all NSAID use in patients receiving treatment for hypertension if possible; if not, use sulindac preferentially. Check blood pressure measurements repeatedly after starting NSAID. Additional antihypertensive therapy may be needed.
Diuretics	Indomethacin Others (possibly except sulindac)	Reduction in natriuretic and diuretic effects; may exacerbate congestive cardiac failure	Avoid NSAID use in patients with cardiac failure, if possible; use sulindac and monitor clinical signs of fluid retention.
Anticoagulants	All	Damage to mucosa of gastrointestinal tract and inhibition of platelet aggregation, both increasing risk of gastrointestinal bleeding in patients taking anticoagulants	Avoid all NSAIDs, if possible.
Hypoglycemic agents	Salicylate (high dose)	Potentiation of hypoglycemic effects (by unknown mechanism)	Monitor blood glucose level.
Combination With Increased Risk of Toxicity			
Diuretics			
General	All	Combination associated with increased risk of hemodynamic renal failure	Avoid combination if possible.
Triamterene	Indomethacin	Potentiation of nephrotoxicity, even in subjects with normal renal function	Combination is contraindicated.
Potassium-sparing	All	Potassium retention and hyperkalemia	Avoid combination; monitor plasma potassium level.

From Brooks PM, Day RO. Nonsteroidal antiinflammatory drugs: Differences and similarities. N Engl J Med 1991;324:1716–1725.

sults from reduced drug concentrations in gastromucosal cells.[19]

Clinical Presentation

Ibuprofen Overdose

Ibuprofen overdose is usually benign with a low risk of life-threatening complications, but large ingestions can present with coma, metabolic acidosis,[20] bradycardia, hypotension, seizures, or apnea. Fatalities have been reported mostly in children.[21] Acute reversible renal failure can occur in healthy pediatric patients after a severe toxic ingestion of ibuprofen.[22] There is a poor correlation between ibuprofen serum concentrations and clinical findings.[23] The lack of a specific antidote or definitive treatment and the poor predictive value of an ibuprofen nomogram[23] suggest that routine serum concentration determinations are not considered useful in management of an overdose.[24] Gastric emptying and administration of activated charcoal should be performed in a hospital if 200 to 400 mg/kg has been ingested. Ingestion of more than 400 mg/kg carries a higher risk of serious toxicity.[21]

Gastrointestinal Effects

Nonsteroidal antiinflammatory drug toxicity may involve the stomach and duodenal bulb as well as the small and large intestine.[25] Risk factors for serious gastrointestinal bleeding in NSAID therapy include age (>60 years), history of peptic ulcer disease, dyspepsia with NSAID use, cigarette and alcohol use, high-dose and prolonged NSAID use, concomitant use of steroids, and serious concomitant disease.[26] NSAID gastropathy is likely due to inhibition of prostaglandin production. Ulcers tend to be gastric rather than duodenal. Injury is diffuse: hemorrhages, petechiae, erosions, ulcers. Symptoms do not reflect extent of mucosal damage and occur without demonstrating mucosal injury. Ulcers tend to be "silent" until bleeding/perforation and lesions occur within weeks of therapy. The injury is not prevented with H_2 blockers/sucralfate/antacids, but is possibly prevented with misoprostol and omeprazole. Such lesions heal quickly when drugs are withdrawn, and healing can take place while therapy continues. All NSAIDs have been implicated; the safest are not yet determined (possibly increased risk with NSAIDs of long half-life or those with greatest antiinflammatory effect).[27]

The use of NSAIDs has been associated with small intestinal stricture, ulcerations, perforations, diarrhea, and villous atrophy. Diagnosis can be made by endoscopy or abdominal exploration. Virtually all classes of NSAIDs have been implicated in the development of enteropathy with erosions, ulcerations, blood loss, villous atrophy, and strictures. The pathogenesis is unclear but likely multifactorial.[28]

Neurologic Effects

Following an ingestion of five diclofenac tablets (375 mg total), two ibuprofen tablets (400 mg total), and one indomethacin capsule (75 mg), a 61-year-old woman became disoriented, hallucinated, lost consciousness, and suffered a respiratory arrest. She was treated supportively and discharged the next day.[29]

Respiratory Effects

Most NSAIDs have induced an eosinophilic pneumonia characterized by cough, low-grade fever, dyspnea, malaise, and, less commonly, lymphadenopathy, pleuritic chest pain, pleural effusion, noncardiogenic edema, and diffuse myalgias. Peripheral eosinophilia and an elevated erythrocyte sedimentation rate have also been seen. Bilateral infiltrates are visible on a chest roentgenogram. Patients recover on withdrawal of the offending drug.[30]

Cardiovascular Effects

Atrial fibrillation has been reported following an ibuprofen overdose.[31] A hypertensive effect has occasionally followed the use of NSAIDs in both normotensive and hypertensive patients. NSAID overdose patients, however, infrequently exhibit a significant increase in blood pressure.[32] Such increases in blood pressure are more often seen with indomethacin and naproxen use.[33]

Renal Effects

Acute renal failure has developed after a fenoprofen overdose[34] and a large ibuprofen overdose.[35] Risk factors for acute renal insufficiency include age (>60 years), vascular disease, renal or functional volume depletion, preexisting renal insufficiency, high renin–angiotensin states, and systemic lupus erythematosus.[36] Irreversible renal failure requiring continuous ambulatory peritoneal dialysis has followed therapeutic use of mefenamic acid.[37]

Acute renal failure has followed a simple 60-mg intramuscular dose of ketoralac.[38] Cystitis (characterized by urgency, frequency, dysuria, and hematuria) has frequently followed tiaprofenic acid use, and in some patients symptoms have not resolved despite discontinuation of the agent.[39] Acute renal failure has been described after acute overdose of NSAIDs such as benoxaprofen, fenoprofen, ibuprofen, mefanamic acid, piroxicam, zomepirac, diclofenac, naproxen, and sulindac. The renal impairment is often transient.[40]

Acute renal failure with NSAIDs may follow inhibition of renal prostaglandin synthesis in the face of renal hemodynamics secondary to the volume depletion following binge alcohol drinking.[45] Renal function tests are not routinely required for patients ingesting less than 6 g of ibuprofen.[23] Patients ingesting 3 g or less who remain asymptomatic during 4 hours of observation have little risk of developing any significant delayed toxicity.[23]

Flank Pain Syndrome. Suprofen was marketed in the United States in 1986. Within a few months an unusual syndrome began to be reported consisting of acute flank pain, frequently arising within hours of the first or second dose, often radiating to the abdomen or groin, sometimes accompanied by nausea and vomiting, and usually accompanied by rapidly appearing but reversible renal abnormalities such as azotemia and hematuria.[41] The postulated pathogenic mechanism suggested that the syndrome was due to acute diffuse crystallization of uric acid in the renal tubules.[42] In May 1987, the drug was withdrawn from sales in the United States. A few days earlier, a committee of the European Common Market nations recommended suspension of authorization for suprofen use among member nations.[43]

Sulindac metabolites may be incorporated into renal calculi. This problem is distinct from the flank pain syndrome reported with suprofen. Sulindac crystals have a characteristic "wheat sheaf" appearance. They may form in the urine after increased metabolite excretion, a decrease in urine flow (<240 mL/h), and a urinary pH less than 5.8.[44]

Hepatic Effects

Risk factors for hepatotoxicity following an overdose with a NSAID include advanced age, renal insufficiency, multiple drug use, alcohol use, and higher NSAID drug dose.[46]

Hematologic Effects

A single 0.65-g dose of aspirin may increase the bleeding time of a normal person for 4 to 7 days, probably because of the decreased formation of the platelet aggregation stimulator thromboxane A_2. NSAIDs have a similar mechanism of action but differ in duration of effect from less than 1 day for flurbuprofen, ibuprofen, indomethacin, and sulindac to 2 weeks for piroxicam.[47]

Case reports indicate a low risk of neutropenia following use of NSAIDs.[48]

Dermatologic Effects

Piroxicam and other NSAIDs with photosensitizing potential may exacerbate the severity of collagen diseases, especially those with Sjögren's or sicca syndrome.[49,50]

Laboratory

Blood Levels

A single dose of 50 to 500 mg of diflunisal produces peak plasma concentrations of 9 to 100 μg/mL. A 38-year-old man ingested 4.5 g of diflunisal, lost consciousness, and died. The blood diflunisal concentration was 260 μg/mL.[51]

Toxicity with phenylbutazone is often associated with serum concentrations exceeding 100 μg/mL.[52] A 33-year-old woman ingested 12 g phenylbutazone; her plasma phenylbutazone level was almost 300 μg/mL.[53] A 24-year-old man ingested 17 g of an equine phenylbutazone over a 24-hour period and developed grand mal seizures, coma, hypotension, respiratory and renal failure, and hepatic injury; his serum phenylbutazone concentration 8 hours after admission was 900 μg/mL.[54]

Convulsions, coma, and brainstem signs associated with mefenamic acid overdose were observed in patients with high serum levels of mefenamic acid (462 μg/mL,[55] 72 and 110 μg/mL,[56] 103 μg/mL[57]; therapeutic level = 10 μg/mL).

A 54-year-old woman who ingested a piroxicam overdose of 1800 mg developed multiple superficial ulcerations in the pyloric antrum and first part of the duodenum. Her piroxicam serum concentration reached 241.6 μg/mL (therapeutic level = 5–10 μg/mL).[58]

About 7 hours after a young adult ingested 1500 mg (30 tablets of diclofenac sodium [Voltaren]), the plasma diclofenac concentration was 60.1 μg/mL (189 μmol/L). Fifteen hours after ingestion, only 190 ng/mL (0.6 μmol/L) was detected. The patient was confused and hypotonic but recovered within 2 days of gastric lavage.[59] A peak plasma diclofenac level of about 735 ng/mL is reached 1.5 hours after a 50-mg oral dose.[2] Seven hours after an oral diclofenac dose of 50 mg, the plasma level was 0.015 μg/mL (15 ng/mL).[60] A gas chromatography/mass spectrometry method provides a limit of detection of 2 ng/mL for plasma diclofenac.[61]

Although ibuprofen overdose does not usually result in serious morbidity, acute renal failure, hypotension, metabolic acidosis, seizures, respiratory depression, and coma have been reported.[23] A patient with a plasma ibuprofen concentration of 809 mg/L developed severe hyperkalemia, metabolic acidosis, renal failure, hyperthermia, ventricular tachycardia, and liver and skeletal muscle damage.[62] Death following an ibuprofen overdose was associated with a blood ibuprofen (heart blood, postmortem) level of 518 μg/mL.[63]

An ibuprofen nomogram has been suggested by Hall and colleagues as a possible measure to aid in predicting which initially asymptomatic patients are likely to remain asymptomatic. Its clinical utility is minimal as treatment of ibuprofen overdose, in any case, is supportive and symptomatic. Ibuprofen plasma levels are not necessary for the evaluation and management of most cases of ibuprofen overdose.[23]

Analytical Methods

High-performance liquid chromatography (HPLC) assays have been described for most NSAID drugs in human plasma.[64] An HPLC method for ibuprofen quantitation has been suggested. Its calibration curve in blood is linear from 200 to 20,000 ng/mL.[65]

An HPLC method for determination of plasma indomethacin levels appears accurate to a limit of 50 ng/mL.[66] A liquid chromatography procedure using ultraviolet detection has been suggested for quantitation of sulindac and metabolites in plasma, urine, bile, and gastric fluid. The plasma curves are linear from 0.25 to 10 μg/mL.[67] The ingestion of NSAID drugs may yield positive results on benzodiazepine (from fenoprofen and ibuprofen) and barbiturate (from fenprofen) assays.[68]

A modified reversed-phase HPLC method has been described for analysis of phenylbutazone and its metabolites oxyphenbutazone, γ-hydroxyphenbutazone, and *p*-γ-hydroxyphenbutazone.[69] An HPLC method is available for piroxicam quantitation in plasma, urine, and tissue.[70]

Ancillary Tests

Screening tests in severe overdoses include complete blood counts, electrolytes, creatinine, liver function tests, arterial blood gases (metabolic acidosis), and coagulation studies. Metabolic acidosis occurs rarely and is most frequent in mefenamic acid and phenylbutazone overdoses. Hyperkalemia has been described after indomethacin, ibuprofen, and piroxicam therapy.[71] Hyponatremia and hypoglycemia developed in a neonate (68-hour naproxen level, 78 μg/mL) whose mother ingested 5 grains of naproxen 8 hours prior to delivery.[72] Hypoprothrombinemia without hepatocellular toxicity has been reported with overdoses of aspirin, etodolac, mefenamic acid, indomethacin, naproxen, and ibuprofen.[73]

A fluorescent polarization immunoassay for serum salicylates indicates that a chemical substitution on the 5-position of the salicylate formula enhances cross-reactivity.[74] 5-Methylsalicylic acid, diflunisal, salazosulfapyridine, and 5-aminosalicylic acid show significant cross-reactivity. Diflunisal and salazosulfapyridine, at a similar therapeutic serum level as salicylic acid, can produce false-positive salicylate results.[1] An HPLC assay has a detection limit of 0.5 μg/mL in urine.[75] Renal function tests after an adult ibuprofen overdose do not seem to be indicated unless the patient has ingested 6 to 20 g or more.[23]

Treatment

There is always a possibility of seizures, metabolic acidosis, and other complications. Patients who have any significant symptomatology should be admitted to a hospital for 24 hours, placed on seizure precautions, and evaluated for impaired hepatic function and acid–base balance status. Patients with a history of NSAID ingestion who present with no symptomatology should be given a dose of activated charcoal and observed in the emergency department for 6 hours. If no evidence of symptoms appears, the patient can be discharged from the emergency department with arrangements for follow-up care.

Gut Decontamination

Emesis may be effective within the first several hours postingestion unless contraindicated. (Watch for depressed sensorium, convulsions, and coma.) Mefenamic acid and phenylbutazone overdoses may produce serious symptoms with only several times the therapeutic dose, whereas doses 5 to 10 times the therapeutic dose of other NSAIDs are required to cause significant symptoms. In general, ipecac should not be administered to patients who have ingested an overdose of mefenamic acid, as seizures may occur from 2 hours up to 12 hours after ingestion. Similarly, ipecac should not be administered to children ingesting 400 mg ibuprofen or more: seizures, central nervous system depression, and apnea may follow such ingestions, leading to aspiration and possible pneumonitis.[76]

Ipecac may produce symptoms similar to those of NSAID toxicity; the emesis following ipecac may induce a gastric mucosal tear, and could delay the use of activated charcoal. Gastric lavage with tracheal protection followed by immediate instillation of activated charcoal would appear to be a reasonable approach.[77]

Decontamination measures should be instituted in most cases involving mefenamic acid or phenylbutazone that present within 2 to 4 hours postingestion. Clinical judgment dictates that the necessity of decontamination in other NSAID cases should be based on dosage, weight, time since ingestion, and concomitant drugs. A reasonable guideline for induction of emesis is the ingestion of 10 times the therapeutic dose in adults and 5 times the therapeutic dose in children when the overdose has occurred within the last 4 hours.[78] Patients ingesting less than 100 mg/kg of ibuprofen usually require no emesis.[23]

Activated charcoal (adults, 60–100 g; children, 30–60 g) should be administered to most NSAID overdose victims who present soon after ingestion. Repetitive pulsed charcoal probably is not useful in indomethacin overdose, as enterohepatic recirculation may involve only a small percentage of unchanged drug and metabolites may be devoid of activity. A cathartic (eg, magnesium sulfate: adults, 30 g; children, 250 mg/kg) can be administered concomitantly with activated charcoal. The efficacy of cathartics in NSAID treatment has not been validated.

Elimination Enhancement

The effectiveness of hemodialysis, hemoperfusion, or peritoneal dialysis appears to be limited because of high protein binding. Hemoperfusion, however, was found to reduce the serum half-life and to increase the clearance of phenylbutazone after an overdose.[79] As the kidney excretes only a small proportion of the absorbed NSAIDs in the urine, forced diuresis or alkalinization of the urine would not be expected to increase clearance of NSAIDs.

Cholestyramine (4 g in 200 mL water three times daily) reduced the half-lives of piroxicam and tenoxicam.[80,81] There have been no controlled studies on the use of cholestyramine in NSAID overdoses and few observations in NSAID poisonings. Although its role has not been established, cholestyramine use in some severely symptomatic patients may be of benefit.

Antidote

There is no antidote.

Supportive Measures

Supportive care and symptomatic treatment are the mainstay of therapy. Prognosis is excellent.

- For hypotension, institute a central line, employ positioning, and administer fluids and dopamine.[81]
- For seizures, administer diazepam (5–10 mg IV, 0.1–0.3 mg/kg) in children; use oxygen and suction.
- For respiratory depression, employ assisted ventilation.
- Monitor renal and hepatic function.
- Monitor vital signs.
- Watch for gastrointestinal bleeding by monitoring for a positive stool guaiac. Consider use of an H_2-receptor antagonist or misoprostol.
- In renal failure, consider hemodialysis or hemofiltration.

NEWER NONSTEROIDAL ANTIINFLAMMATORY DRUGS

ACEMETACIN

Acemetacin (Emflex) is a glycolic acid ester of indomethacin; 50 to 90% of a dose of acemetacin is converted to indomethacin. Both compounds are active. Metabolism occurs in the liver. The plasma half-life of acemetacin is 1 to 5 hours; for indomethacin, it is often 3 to 8 hours. The drug has been used for the past 10 years in Germany, 6 years in Japan, and 4 years in Switzerland. There are few reports of overdose.[83]

NABUMETONE

Bioavailability	About 80%
Presystemic metabolism	Almost 100%
Peak plasma level	23 μg/mL (after 1000 mg)
Time to peak plasma level	8.4 hours
Volume of distribution	0.1 L/kg (6-methoxy-2-naphthylacetic acid)
Plasma protein binding	99% (6-methoxy-2-naphthylacetic acid)
Elimination half-life	24 hours (metabolite)
Excreted unchanged	Almost none
Active metabolite	6-methoxy-2-naphthylacetic acid

Gastrointestinal hemorrhage and hypersensitivity reactions have been reported. Nabumetone appears to have a level of safety similar to that of other drugs of this type. Treatment of an overdose with nabumetone should be symptomatic and supportive. No antidote is available.[84–86]

ETODOLAC

Etodolac is a relatively recent addition to the NSAID group. One overdose patient had a noneventful course accompanied by some temporary asymptomatic changes in coagulation parameters and a leukopenia. Treatment of overdose is symptomatic and supportive.

Bioavailability	About 75%[87]
Presystemic metabolism	Almost none
Peak plasma level	12–15 μg/mL (after oral doses of 200 mg)
Volume of distribution	0.4 L/kg[76]
Plasma protein binding	99%[87]
Elimination half-life	6.5 hours (total, 6.3 hours) (free)[87]
Excreted unchanged	<5%

Toxic Dose

A 53-year-old woman ingested from 15 to 46, 200-mg etodolac capsules (3–8.6 g) and remained asymptomatic.[88] No fatal dose has been established.

Treatment

Syrup of ipecac may be used if administered at home immediately after etodolac ingestion. Gastric lavage may be useful if the patient is seen within 1 hour of ingestion or within 4 hours of ingestion with symptoms or following a large overdose (5–10 times the usual dose).[89] Activated charcoal may be of use but neither it nor cathartics or whole-bowel irrigation has been studied systematically. A definitive regimen for treatment awaits further clinical experience with this drug. No specific antidotes are available. Careful monitoring of coagulation parameters (prothrombin time, partial thromboplastin time) and the blood count may prepare the clinician for bleeding episodes.

Forced diuresis, alkalinization of the urine, hemodialysis, and hemoperfusion will probably not be useful due to the high protein binding of etodolac. Etodolac is not dialyzable.

NEDOCROMIL SODIUM

Nedocromil sodium has been available in the United Kingdom since 1986. It is an antiinflammatory agent absorbed from the lung. Few reports are available on overdosage. Its main use appears to be in the prophylactic treatment of bronchial asthma and bronchial hyperresponsiveness.[90–93]

Bioavailability	About 10%
Presystemic metabolism	Almost none
Peak plasma level	3 μg/L
Time to peak plasma level	15 minutes
Volume of distribution	0.7 L/kg
Plasma protein binding	None
Elimination half-life	21 hours (oral)
Excreted unchanged	5%

Clinical Presentation

The most commonly reported adverse effect of nedocromil sodium is an unpleasant taste. Other adverse effects include rhinitis, nausea, upper respiratory tract infection, and occasionally headache. Treatment of an overdose is symptomatic and supportive.

NIMESULIDE

Nimesulide is a NSAID of the sulfonanilide class. Its antiinflammatory, analgesic, and antipyretic activities have been demonstrated in several widely used animal experimental models and in numerous clinical trials.

Nimesulide only weakly inhibits prostaglandin synthesis and appears to exert its effects through various mechanisms. It inhibits the release of oxidants from activated neutrophils and has a scavenging effect on hypochlorous acid without affecting neutrophil function. Nimesulide also decreases histamine release from tissue mast cells and inhibits the production of platelet-activating factor by human basophils. Furthermore, when added in vitro to cultures of human articular chondrocytes, nimesulide inhibits the release of stromelysin and blocks metalloproteinase activity.[94]

After oral administration of 100 mg nimesulide in tablet, granule, or suspension form to healthy volunteers, the drug was rapidly and extensively absorbed. Mean peak plasma concentrations of 2.86 to 4.58 mg/L were achieved within 1.22 to 3.83 hours of administration. The presence of food did not reduce either the rate or the extent of nimesulide absorption. When it was administered in suppository form, peak plasma concentrations were lower and occurred later than those achieved after oral administration; the bioavailability of nimesulide given by suppository ranged from 54 to 96%, relative to that of orally administered formulations.

Nimesulide is rapidly distributed, principally throughout the extracellular fluid compartment; values for volume of distribution ranged from 0.19 to 0.39 L/kg. Nimesulide is extensively bound to plasma proteins; at concentrations ranging from 0.5 to 10 mg/L, the unbound fraction varied between 0.7 to 4.0%.

With oral administration, nimesulide concentrations decline monoexponentially following peak levels. The estimated mean terminal half-life for nimesulide varied from 1.96 to 4.73 hours.

Excretion of unchanged drug in urine and feces is negligible. Nimesulide is eliminated mainly by metabolic transformation and the principal metabolite is the 4′-hydroxy derivative. The presence of other metabolites is being evaluated. Excretion of nimesulide metabolites in the urine and feces accounts for about 80 and 20% of the administered dose, respectively.

Total plasma clearance of nimesulide 100-mg tablets or 200-mg suppositories (steady-state) is achieved within 24 to 36 hours (two to three administrations). With oral nimesulide 100 mg twice daily, only modest accumulation of nimesulide and its 4′-hydroxy derivative occurs.[95]

Overdoses have not been reported.

REFERENCES

1. Dubose TD Jr, Molony DA, Verani I, McDonald GA. Nephrotoxicity of non-steroidal antiinflammatory drugs. Lancet 1994;344:515–518.
2. Loeb DS, Ahlquist DA, Talley NJ. Management of gastroduodenopathy associated with use of non-steroidal antiinflammatory drugs. Mayo Clin Proc 1992;67:354–364.
3. Jick H, Rodriguez LAG. Risk upper gastrointestinal bleeding and perforation associated with individual non-steroidal antiinflammatory drugs. Lancet 1994;343:769–772.
4. Rodriguez LAG, Williams R, Derby LE, et al. Acute liver injury associated with nonsteroidal antiinflammatory drugs and the role of risk factors. Arch Intern Med 1994;154:311–316.
5. Stron BL, Carson JL, Schinnar R, et al. Nonsteroidal antiinflammatory drugs and neutropenia. Arch Intern Med 1993;153:2119–2124.
6. Johnson AG, Nguyen TV, Day RO. Do nonsteroidal antiinflammatory drugs affect blood pressure? A meta-analysis. Ann Intern Med 1994;121:289–300.
7. Important prescribing information. Washington, DC: U.S. Food and Drug Administration, Feb. 3, 1989.
8. Macdougall LG, Taylor-Smith A, Rothberg AD, Thomson PD. Piroxicam poisoning in a 2 year old child: A case report. S Afr Med J 1984;66:31–33.

9. Important drug warning: Toradol[R] (ketoralac tromethamine). Palo Alto, CA: Syntex Laboratories, 1995.
10. Choo V, Lewis S. Ketorolac doses reduced. Lancet 1993; 342:109.
11. Ross-Degman D, Soumerai SB, Fortess EE, Gurwitz JH. Examining product risk in content: Market withdrawal of zomepirac as a case study. JAMA 1993;270:1937–1942.
12. Court H, Volans GN. Poisoning after overdose with nonsteroidal anti-inflammatory drugs. Adverse Drug React Acute Poisoning Rev 1984;3:1–21.
13. Murray MD, Brater DC. Renal toxicity of the nonsteroidal antiinflammatory drugs. Annu Rev Pharmacol Toxicol 1993; 33:435–465.
14. Mizushima Y. Pro-drugs of non-steroidal antiinflammatory agents. Eur J Rheumatol Inflamm 1983;6:141–142.
15. Brooks PM, Day RO. Nonsteroidal antiinflammatory drugs: Differences and similarities. N Engl J Med 1991;324: 1716–1725.
16. Stewart CF, Evans WE. Drug–drug interactions with antirheumatic agents: Review of selected clinically important interactions. J Rheumatol 1990;17(suppl. 22):16–23.
17. Verbeeck RK. Pharmacokinetic drug interactions with nonsteroidal antiinflammatory drugs. Clin Pharmacokinet 1990;19:44–68.
18. Hayllar J, Bjarnason I. NSAIDs, Cox-2 inhibitors and the gut. Lancet 1995;346:521–522.
19. Graham DY, Smith JL, Holmes GI, et al. Non-steroidal antiinflammatory effect of sulindac sulfoxide and sulfide on gastric mucosa. Clin Pharmacol Ther 1985;38:65–70.
20. Downie A, Ali A, Bell D. Severe metabolic acidosis complicating massive ibuprofen overdose. Postgrad Med J 1993;69:575–577.
21. Halperin SM, Fitzpatrick R, Volans GN. Ibuprofen toxicity. A review of adverse reactions and overdose. Adverse Drug React Toxicol Rev 1993;12:107–128.
22. Kim J, Gazarian M, Johnson D. Acute renal failure and ibuprofen overdose: A pediatric case report. Vet Hum Toxicol 1993;35:340.
23. Hall AH, Smolinske SC, Stover B, et al. Ibuprofen overdose in adults. Clin Toxicol 1992;30:23–37.
24. McElwee NE, Veltri JC, Bradford DC, Rollins DE. A prospective population-based study of acute ibuprofen overdose: Complications are rare and routine serum levels are not warranted. Ann Emerg Med 1990;19:657–662.
25. Aabakken L. Review articles: Non-steroidal, anti-inflammatory drugs: Extending the scope of gastrointestinal side effects. Aliment Pharmacol Ther 1992;6:143–162.
26. Bush TM, Shotzhauer TL, Imai K. Nonsteroidal antiinflammatory drugs: Proposed guidelines for monitoring toxicity. West J Med 1991;155:39–42.
27. Sievero W, Stern AI, Lambert JR, Peacock T. Low dose antacids and non-steroidal antiinflammatory drug-induced gastropathy in humans. J Clin Gastroenterol 1991;13(suppl. 1):S145–S148.
28. Kwo PY, Tremaine WJ. Non-steroidal antiinflammatory drug-induced enteropathy: Case discussions and review of the literature. Mayo Clin Proc 1995;70:50–51.
29. Bright TP, McNulty CJ. Suspected central nervous system toxicity from inadvertent nonsteroidal antiinflammatory drug overdose. DICP Ann Pharmacother 1991;25:1066–1067.
30. Khalil H, Molinary E, Stoller JK. Diclofenac (Voltaren)-induced eosinophilic pneumonitis: Case report and review of the literature. Arch Intern Med 1993;153:1649–1652.
31. McCune KH, O'Brien CJ. Atrial fibrillation induced by ibuprofen overdose. Postgrad Med J 1993;69:325–328.
32. Sahloul MZ, d-Kiek R, Ivanovich P, Mujais SK. Non-steroidal antiinflammatory drugs and antihypertensives: Cooperative malfeasance. Nephron 1990;56:345–352.
33. Pope JE, Anderson JJ, Felson DT. A meta-analysis of the effects of non-steroidal antiinflammatory drugs on blood pressure. Arch Intern Med 1993;152:477–484.
34. Appleby DH. Fenoprofen (Nalfon) overdose. Drug Intell Clin Pharm 1981;15:129–130.
35. Lee CY, Finkler A. Acute intoxication due to ibuprofen overdose. Arch Pathol Lab Med 1986;110:747–749.
36. Bush TM, Shotzhauer TL, Imai K. Nonsteroidal antiinflammatory drugs: Proposed guidelines for monitoring toxicity. West J Med 1991;155:39–42.
37. Boletis J, Williams AJ, Shortland JR, Brown CB. Irreversible renal failure following mefenamic acid. Nephron 1989;51: 575–576.
38. Quan DJ, Kaysen SR. Ketoralac-induced acute renal failure following a single dose. Clin Toxicol 1994;32:305–309.
39. Baterman DM. Tiaprofenic acid and cystitis: Grounds for withdrawal? Br Med J 1994;309:552–553.
40. Kulling PEJ, Beckman EA, Skagius ASM. Renal impairment after acute diclofenac, naproxen and sulindac overdoses. Clin Toxicol 1995;33:173–177.
41. Hart D, Ward M, Lifshitz MD. Suprofen-related nephrotoxicity: A distinct clinical syndrome. Ann Intern Med 1987;106: 235–238.
42. Strom BL, West SL, Sim E, Carson JL. The epidemiology of the acute flank pain syndrome from suprofen. Clin Pharmacol Ther 1989;46:693–699.
43. Rossi AC, Bosco L, Faich GA, Tanner A, Temple R: The importance of adverse reaction reporting by physicians: Suprofen and the flank pain syndrome. JAMA 1988;259:1203–1204.
44. Rare complication with sulindac. FDA Drug Bull 1989;19(1):4.
45. Wen S-F, Parthasarathy R, Iliopoalos O, Oberley FD. Acute renal failure following binge drinking and nonsteroidal antiinflammatory drugs. Am J Kidney Dis 1992;30:281–285.
46. Bush TM, Shotzhauer TL, Imai K. Nonsteroidal antiinflammatory drugs: Proposed guidelines for monitoring toxicity. West J Med 1991;155:39–42.
47. Bartley GB, Warndahl RA. Surgical bleeding associated with aspirin and nonsteroidal antiinflammatory agents. Mayo Clin Proc 1992;67:402.
48. Strom BL, Carson JL, Schinnar R, et al. Non-steroidal antiinflammatory drugs and neutropenia. Arch Intern Med 1993; 153:2119–2124.
49. Roura M, Lopez-Gill F, Umbert P. Systemic lupus erythematosus exacerbated by piroxicam. Dermatologica 1990;182: 56–58.
50. Halasz CLG. Photosensitivity to the nonsteroidal antiinflammatory drug piroxicam. Cutis 1987;39:37–39.
51. Levine B, Smyth DF, Caplan YH. A diflunisal related fatality: A case report. Forens Sci Int 1987;35:45–50.
52. Vale JA, Meredith TJ. Acute poisoning due to non-steroidal anti-inflammatory drugs: Clinical features and management. Med Toxicol 1986;1:12–31.
53. De Flines EW, Bolwerk CJ, Komen BJ, Veenhoven WA. Abnormal metabolism of phenylbutazone after overdosage. DICP Ann Pharmacother 1990;24:783.
54. Newton TA, Rose SR. Poisoning with equine phenylbutazone in a racetrack worker. Ann Emerg Med 1991;20:204–207.
55. Hendrickse MT. Mefenamic acid overdose mimicking brainstem stroke. Lancet 1988;2:1019.
56. Robson RH, Balali M, Critchley J, et al. Mefenamic acid poisoning and epilepsy. Br Med J 1979;2:1438.
57. Shipton EA, Muller FO. Severe mefenamic acid poisoning: A case report. S Afr Med J 1985;67:823–824.
58. Mosvold J, Mellem H, Stave R, et al. Overdosage of piroxicam. Acta Med Scand 1984;216:335–336.
59. Netter P, Lambert H, Larcan A, et al. Diclofenac sodium–chlormezanone poisoning. Eur J Clin Pharmacol 1984; 26:535–536.
60. Del Puppo M, Cigghetti G, Kienle MG, et al. Determination of diclofenac in human plasma by selected ion monitoring. Biol Mass Spectrom 1991;20:426–430.
61. Willis JV, Kendall MJ, Flinn RM, et al. The pharmacokinetics of diclofenac sodium following intravenous and oral administration. Eur J Clin Pharmacol 1979;16:405–410.
62. Menzies DG, Conn AG, Williamson IJ, Prescott LF. Fulminant hyperkalaemia and multiple complications following ibuprofen overdose. Med Toxicol Adverse Drug Experience 1989;4: 468–471.
63. Kunsman GW, Rohrig TP. Tissue distribution of ibuprofen in a fatal overdose. Am J Forens Med Pathol 1993;14:48–50.
64. Schultz M, Schmoldt A. HPLC-determination of nonsteroidal anti-inflammatory drugs in human plasma. In: *Proceedings,*

25th International Meeting, International Association of Forensic Toxicologists, Groningen, January 27–30, 1988: 471–479.

65. Rustum AM. Measurement of ibuprofen in human whole blood by reversed-phase ion-paired high-performance liquid chromatography using a pH-stable polymeric column. J Chromatogr Biomed Appl 1990;526:246–253.
66. Johnson AG, Ray JE. Improved high-performance liquid chromatographic method for the determination indomethacin in plasma. Ther Drug Monit 1992;14:61–65.
67. Musson DG, Vincek WC, Constanzer ML, Detty TE. Analytical methods for the determination of sulindac and metabolites in plasma, urine, bile and gastric fluid by liquid chromatography using ultraviolet detection. J Pharm Sci 1984;73:1270–1273.
68. Larsen J, Fogerson R. Nonsteroidal anti-inflammatory drug interference in TDx[R] assays for abused drugs. Clin Chem 1988;34:987–988.
69. De Flines EW, Bolwerk CJ, Komen BJ, Veenhoven WA. Abnormal metabolism of phenylbutazone after overdosage. DICP Ann Pharmacother 1990;24:783.
70. Riedel K-D, Laufen H. High-performance thin-layer chromatographic assay for the routine determination of piroxacam in plasma, urine and tissue. J Chromatogr 1983; 276:243–248.
71. Miller KP, Lazar EJ, Fotino S. Severe hyperkalemia during piroxicam therapy. Arch Intern Med 1984;144:2414–2415.
72. Alun-Jones E, Williams J. Hyponatremia and fluid retention in a neonate associated with maternal naproxen overdosage. Clin Toxicol 1986;24:257–260.
73. Kelker KH. Hypoprothrombinemia without hepatocellular injury in ibuprofen overdose. Clin Toxicol 1995; 33:492. Abstract 17.
74. Koel M, Nebinger P. Specificity data of the salicylate assay by fluorescent polarization immunoassay. J Anal Toxicol 1989;13:358–360.
75. Musson DG, Lin JH, Lyon KA, et al. Assay methodology for quantification of the ester and ether glucuronide conjugates of diflunisal in human urine. J Chromatogr Biomed Appl 1985;337:363–378.
76. Smolinske SC, Hall AH, Vandenberg SA, et al. Toxic effects of nonsteroidal antiinflammatory drugs in overdose: An overview of recent evidence on clinical effects and dose–response relationships. Drug Saf 1990;5:252–274.
77. Roberts JR. NSAIDs: GI protection and overdose. Emerg Med News, May 1990:4–5.
78. Vale JA, Meredith TJ. Acute poisoning due to non-steroidal anti-inflammatory drugs: Clinical features and management. Med Toxicol 1986;1:12–31.
79. Product Information. Upjohn. In: *Physicians' Desk Reference,* 1984. Oradell, NJ: Medical Economics, 1984:2039.
80. Guentert TW, Defoin R, Mosberg H. Accelerated elimination of temoxicam and piroxicam by cholestyramine. Clin Pharmacol Ther 1988;43:179.
81. Narjes H, Heinzel G, Busch U. Cholestyramine affects pharmacokinetics of meloxicam, a new non-steroidal antiinflammatory drug (NSAID), in man. Clin Pharmacol Ther 1991; 49:169.
82. Henry J, Volans G. Analgesic poisoning. I. Salicylates. Br Med J 1984; 289:820–822.
83. Jones RW, Collins AJ, Jotarianni LJ, Sedman E. The comparative pharmacokinetics of acemetacin in young subjects and elderly patients. Br J Clin Pharmacol 1991;31:543–545.
84. Inman WHW, Wilton LV, Pearce GL, Waller PC. Prescription event monitory of nabumetone. Pharm Med 1990;4: 309–317.
85. Bernhard GC. Worldwide safety experience with nabumetone. J Rheumatol 1992;19(suppl. 36):48–57.
86. Friedel HA, Langtry HD, Buckley MM. Nabumetone: A reappraisal of its pharmacology and therapeutic use in rheumatic disease. Drug 1993;45:131–156.
87. Kraml M, Hicks DR, McKean M, et al. The pharmacokinetics of etodolac in serum and synovial fluid of patients with arthritis. Clin Pharmacol Ther 1988;43:571–576.
88. Boldy DAR, Hale KA, Vale JA. Etodolac overdose. Hum Toxicol 1988;7:203–204.
89. Lodine (Etodolac). Product Literature C1 4000-4. Philadelphia: Ayerst Laboratories, Oct. 14, 1991.
90. Foulds RA. An overview of human safety data with nedocromil sodium. J Allergy Clin Immunol 1993;92:202–204.
91. Clark B. General pharmacology, pharmacokinetics and toxicology of nedocromil sodium. J Allergy Clin Immunol 1993;92:200–202.
92. Gonzalez JP, Brogden RN. Nedocromil sodium: A preliminary review of its pharmacodynamic and pharmacokinetic properties and the therapeutic efficacy in the treatment of reversible obstructive airways disease. Drugs 1987;34:560–577.
93. Neal MG, Brown K, Foulds RA, Lal S, et al. The pharmacokinetics of nedocromil sodium, a new drug for the treatment of reversible obstructive airways disease, in human volunteers and patients with reversible obstructive airways disease. Br J Clin Pharmacol 1987;24:493–501.
94. Bevlicqua M, Magni E. Recent contributions to knowledge of the mechanism of action of nimesulide. Drugs 1993; 46(suppl. 1):40–47.
95. Bernareggi A. The pharmacokinetic profile of nimesulide in healthy volunteers. Drugs 1993;46(suppl. 1):64–72.

Chapter 12
Phenazopyridine

INTRODUCTION

Phenazopyridine hydrochloride, used as an analgesic for problems related to the urinary tract mucosa, has, in overdose, produced methemoglobinemia, hemolytic anemia, and acute renal failure. Patients have usually survived with symptomatic supportive and antidotal (methylene blue) therapy.

Phenazopyridine hydrochloride is a synthetic azo dye.[1] It occurs as a light or dark red to dark violet, crystalline powder.[1]

Phenazopyridine is phenylazopyridine-2, 6-diyldiamine hydrochloride. The hydrochloride has a molecular weight of 249.7.[2] The conversion factor between metric and SI units is 4.06.

Use

Phenazopyridine exerts an analgesic effect on the mucosa of the urinary tract and is used to provide symptomatic relief of pain, burning, urgency, frequency, and other discomforts resulting from irritation of the lower urinary tract mucosa caused by infection, trauma, surgery, endoscopic procedures, or the passage of sounds or catheters.[1,2]

Product Formulation

Phenazopyridine hydrochloride is available as 100- and 200-mg tablets. Phenazopyridine hydrochloride combinations include capsules of 50 mg with oxytetracycline hydrochloride 250 mg and sulfamethizole 250 mg (Urobiotic-250); tablets of 150 mg with butabarbital 15 mg and hyoscyamine hydrobromide 0.3 mg (Pyridium Plus); film-coated tablets of 50 mg with sulfisoxazole 500 mg (Azo-Gantrisin, Azo-sulfisoxazole); and film-coated tablets of 100 mg with sulfamethoxazole 500 mg (Azo-Gantanol, Azo-sulfamethoxazole).[1]

Therapeutic Dose

The usual adult dosage of phenazopyridine hydrochloride is 200 mg three times daily. Children may receive 12 mg/kg daily, given in three divided doses.

Toxic Dose

A 15-month-old child ingested 8000 mg and survived.[3] A 19-year-old ingested 6000 mg, was treated conservatively, and survived.[4] As little as 50 mg/kg of oral phenazopyridine has produced human toxicity,[3] and as much as 750 mg/kg has not been lethal in previously healthy patients.[3] As little as 600 mg/d in adults with renal impairment has caused cyanosis.[5]

Fatal Dose

One patient with prior renal dysfunction ingested 2000 mg of phenazopyridine, developed further renal failure, and died of a pulmonary embolism.[6]

Toxicokinetics

Absorption

The toxicokinetics of phenazopyridine have not been thoroughly studied. Phenazopyridine is absorbed from the gastrointestinal tract.

Elimination

Renal clearance appears to be the major route of elimination of phenazopyridine. In one human study, following ingestion of 200 mg three times daily, 90% of an administered dose of phenazopyridine was cleared by the urine in 24 hours; 41% was unchanged phenazopyridine, 6.9% was aniline (known to be linked with methemoglobin in humans),[7] 18% was *N*-acetyl-*p*-aminophenol, and 24% was *p*-aminophenol.[8,9]

Pregnancy/Lactation

Trace amounts of phenazopyridine are believed to cross the placenta and enter the cerebrospinal fluid. It is not known if phenazopyridine is distributed into milk.[1]

Mechanism of Action

The most serious finding in phenazopyridine overdose is progressive oliguric renal failure. This may be due to a direct toxic effect of the drug on the renal tubules, as renal failure may occur as the only adverse effect without hemolysis.[4,6,10–12] The yellow pigmentation in the absence of marked hyperbilirubinemia is probably due to deposition of azo dye in the skin and sclerae and occurs primarily in patients with impaired renal function.[12,13] Hemolysis may follow ingestion of either phenazopyridine or aniline alone (one of the phenazopyridine metabolites).[9,14–16] Methemoglobinemia probably follows phenazopyridine oxidation of hemoglobin iron (Fe^{2+} to Fe^{3+}). A predisposition to hemolysis and methemoglobinemia may be present in patients with a glucose-6-phosphate dehydrogenase deficiency.[14,17] Muscle damage may express itself as rhabdomyolysis and myoglobinuria.[4]

Clinical Presentation

Phenazopyridine, when administered therapeutically or in overdose, may induce the following types of clinical responses.

1. Methemoglobinemia may occur usually with a concomitant hemolytic anemia. Methemoglobinemia may follow a therapeutic dose of phenazopyridine in glucose-6-phosphate dehydrogenase (G6PD)-deficient patients, those with functional renal impairment, and otherwise normal patients. Methemoglobinemia has been reported without hemolytic anemia.[18] Sulfhemoglobinemia has been reported.[19]
2. Hemolytic anemia may occur with and without G6PD deficiency.
3. Nonoliguric acute renal failure usually is associated with evidence of hemolysis and methemoglobinemia.[5]
4. Hypersensitivity hepatitis has been reported (nausea, vomiting, epigastric or right upper quadrant pain, myalgias, fever, jaundice, hepatomegaly, eosinophilia, and elevated liver enzymes). Phenazopyridine has been associated with a centrilobular hepatic neurosis in animals.[3]
5. Muscle damage (rhabdomyolysis)[4] and aseptic meningitis have been reported.[20]

Laboratory

Abnormalities

Because of its properties as an azo dye, phenazopyridine may interfere with urinalysis based on spectrometry or color reactions. It may interfere with the phenolsulfonphthalein excretion test of renal function and with urinary glucose, steroid, and urobilinogen tests.[1]

Ancillary Tests

Diminishing renal function may be evidenced by increases in serum creatinine and blood urea nitrogen, and/or with an abnormal urinalysis (proteins, sediment). Methemoglobinemia may be present early in the course of toxicity. Hemolysis may not occur for 24 to 48 hours (characterized by diminished hemoglobin and hematocrit, increase in reticulocyte count, increase in total bilirubin, anisocytosis, poikilocytosis, "bite" cells or degmacytes, Heinz bodies). The urine may become deep orange-red in color. Rhabdomyolysis (characterized by myoglobinuria, serum myoglobin creatine kinase, and aldolase increased) may be present.[4]

Treatment

Stabilization

Patients should be admitted to an intensive care facility if there is evidence of cyanosis, tachycardia, and rapid shallow respirations. An intravenous line, oxygen, and cardiac monitoring should be immediately available.

Gut Decontamination

Use of induced emesis, gastric lavage, activated charcoal, or whole-bowel irrigation has not been systematically studied in phenazopyridine overdose. Supportive conservative therapy alone has been useful.[4]

Elimination Enhancement

The role of hemodialysis or hemoperfusion has not been evaluated. Peritoneal dialysis has been used for the acute renal failure,[11] but not specifically for phenazopyridine elimination. There are no published reports correlating the urine excretion of phenazopyridine and its metabolites and modalities used for enhancement of drug elimination.

Antidote

Methylene blue IV may be used for treatment of the methemoglobinemia if high levels (>30–45%) of methemoglobin are observed.

Supportive Measures

Supportive and symptomatic measures are usually the mainstay of treatment. Almost all patients have survived with varying treatments ranging from minimal and conservative[4] to use of methylene blue where indicated, gastric lavage, induction of emesis, intravenous fluids, whole blood and packed cell transfusion,[15] exchange transfusion,[21] peritoneal dialysis,[11] diuretics, steroids,[13] and oxygen.[15]

REFERENCES

1. McElroy GK, ed. *AHFS Drug Information 94.* Bethesda, MD: American Hospital Formulary Service, 1994:2333–2334.
2. Reynolds JEF. *Martindale: The Extra Pharmacopoeia.* 30th ed. London: Pharmaceutical Press, 1993:29.
3. Wander HJ, Pascoe DJ. Phenazopyridine hydrochloride poisoning. Am J Dis Child 1965;110:105–107.
4. Gavish D, Knobler H, Gottebrer N, et al. Methemoglobinemia, muscle damage and renal failure complicating phenazopyridine overdose. Isr J Med Sci 1986;22:45–47.
5. Green ED, Zimmerman RC, Ghurabi WH, Colohar DR. Phenazopyridine hydrochloride toxicity: A cause of drug-induced methemoglobinemia. JACEP 1979;8:426–431.
6. Alano FA, Webster GD. Acute renal failure and pigmentation due to phenazopyridine (Pyridium). Ann Intern Med 1970; 72:89–91.
7. Kearney TE, Manoguerra AS, Dunford JV. Chemically induced methemoglobinemia from aniline poisoning. West J Med 1984;140:282–286.
8. Johnson WJ, Chartrand A. The metabolism and excretion of phenazopyridine hydrochloride in animals and man. Toxicol Appl Pharmacol 1976;37:371–376.
9. Fincher ME, Campbell HT. Methemoglobinemia and hemolytic anemia after phenazopyridine hydrochloride (Pyridium) administration in end-stage renal disease. South Med J 1989;82:372–374.
10. Nathan DM, Siegel AJ, Bunn HF. Acute methemoglobinemia and hemolytic anemia with phenazopyridine. Arch Intern Med 1977;137:1636–1638.
11. Feinfeld DA, Ranieri R, Lipnes HI, Avram MM. Renal failure in phenazopyridine overdose. JAMA 1978;240:2661.
12. Eybel CE, Armbruster KFW, Ing TS. Skin pigmentation and acute renal failure in a patient receiving phenazopyridine therapy. JAMA 1974;228:1027–1028.
13. Sharon M, Puente G, Cohen LB. Phenazopyridine (Pyridium) poisoning: Possible toxicity of methylene blue administration in renal failure. Mt Sinai J Med 1986; 53:280–282.
14. Ponte CD, Lewis MJ, Rogers JS II. Heinz-body hemolytic anemia associated with phenazopyridine and sulfonamide. DICP Ann Pharmacother 1989;23:140–142.
15. Cohen BL, Bovasso GJ Jr. Acquired methemoglobinemia and neurologic anemia following excessive Pyridium (phenazopyridine hydrochloride) ingestion. Clin Pediatr 1971; 10:537–540.
16. Zimmerman RC, Green ED, Ghurabi WH, Colohan Dr. Methemoglobinemia from overdose of phenazopyridine hydrochloride. Ann Emerg Med 1980;9:147–149.
17. Galun E, Oren R, Glikson M, et al. Phenazopyridine-induced hemolytic anemia in G-6-PD deficiency. Drug Intell Clin Pharm 1987;21:921–922.
18. Terell JR, Spruill WJ, Parish RC, Jenkins FH. Phenazopyridine-induced methemoglobinemia. Drug Intell Clin Pharm 1988;22:915.
19. Halvorsen SM, Dull WL. Phenazopyridine-induced sulfhemoglobinemia: Inadvertent rechallenge. Am J Med 1991;91:317–319.
20. Herlihy TE. Phenazopyridine and aseptic meningitis. Ann Intern Med 1987;106:172–173.
21. Bruton OC. Exchange transfusion for acute poisoning in children. U.S. Armed Forces Med J 1958;9:1128–1131.
22. Chakraborty TK, Rilshie RJA, Lee Mr. methaemoglobinemia produced by phenozopyridine (Pyridium) in a man with chronic obstructive airways disease. Scot Med J 1987;32:185–186.

Chapter 13

Salicylate

INTRODUCTION

The general accessibility of aspirin has increased with its potential uses as a preventive medication for cerebrovascular ischemic events,[1] colon cancer,[2] angina pectoris,[3] migraine,[4] and recurrent myocardial infarction.[5] Some common sources of salicylates are listed in Table 13–1.

Aspirin Equivalencies

Ingestion of nonaspirin salicylates may be difficult for the poison information specialist to evaluate if the amount of available salicylate is not readily available[6,7] (Table 13–2). Nonaspirin salicylates can be converted to an equivalent weight of aspirin (aspirin equivalent dose [AED]) for comparative purposes. An aspirin conversion factor (ACF) can be calculated for all compounds based on the following equations. For solids,

$$\frac{\text{molecular weight of aspirin}}{\text{molecular weight of compound}} = \text{ACF}$$

For liquids,

$$\text{density of compound} = \text{specific gravity of compound} \times \text{density of water}$$

$$\frac{\text{molecular weight of aspirin}}{\text{molecular weight of compound}} \times \text{density of compound} = \text{ACF}$$

The ACF is used to calculate the AED. The AED is the equivalent amount of aspirin based on weight. For solids,

$$\text{AED (mg)} = \text{mg of nonaspirin salicylate} \times \text{ACF}$$

For liquids,

$$\text{AED (mg)} = \text{mL of nonaspirin salicylate} \times \text{ACF}$$

The calculated AED can be considered as a reasonable estimate of the potential for toxicity if the following assumptions are true: The nonaspirin salicylate is completely

Table 13–1
Common Sources of Salicylates

Proprietary Name (Manufacturer)	Generic and Chemical Names
Prescription	
Darvon Compound (Eli Lilly and Co)	Propoxyphene HCl, aspirin, and caffeine
Empirin with Codeine (Burroughs Wellcome)	Aspirin and codeine phosphate
Fiorinal (Sandoz)	Butalbital, aspirin, and caffeine
Percodan (DuPont)	Oxycodone HCl, oxycodone terephthalate, and aspirin
Over-the-Counter	
Aspirin tablets and suppositories (numerous preparations)	
Alka-Seltzer (Miles Inc)	Aspirin, sodium bicarbonate, citric acid, sodium citrate, and sodium salicylate
Ascriptin (Rhone-Poulenc Rorer)	Aspirin, magnesium hydroxide, dried aluminum hydroxide gel, and calcium carbonate
Aspercreme (Thompson Medical)	Topical cream containing trofamine salicylate
Ben-Gay External Analgesic (Pfizer)	Topical cream containing methyl salicylate and menthol
Bufferin (Bristol-Myers)	Aspirin, calcium carbonate, magnesium oxide, and magnesium carbonate
Cope (Glenbrook)	Aspirin and caffeine
Dristan (Whitehall)	Phenylephrine HCl, chlorpheniramine maleate, and acetaminophen
Ecotrin (SmithKline Beecham)	Enteric-coated aspirin
Excedrin (Bristol-Myers)	Acetaminophen, aspirin, and caffeine
Midol (Glenbrook)	Acetaminophen, pamabrom, and pyrilamine maleate
Oil of Wintergreen	Methyl salicylate
Pepto-Bismol (Procter & Gamble)	Bismuth subsalicylate
Sine-Aid (McNeil)	Acetaminophen and pseudoephedrine HCl
Triaminicin (Sandoz)	Phenylpropanolamine HCl and chlorpheniramine maleate
Vanquish (Glenbrook)	Aspirin, acetaminophen, caffeine, dried aluminum hydroxide gel, and magnesium hydroxide

From Sainsbury SJ. Fatal salicylate toxicity from bismuth subsalicylate. West J Med 1991;155:637–639.

(100%) and instantaneously absorbed; the nonaspirin salicylate is 100% converted in vivo to salicylate; the potency of the nonaspirin salicylate is the same as for aspirin on a mole/mole basis. The more the nonaspirin salicylate deviates from these assumptions, the less reliable is the AED.

Aspirin conversion factors for nonsalicylate compounds listed in Table 13–2 were included where the molecular weight, physical state, and specific gravity or density were available.[7]

EXAMPLE 1 For a 100% pure nonaspirin salicylate, calculate the AED for ingestion of 5 tablets of sodium salicylate (325 mg/tablet):

mg of sodium salicylate × ACF (from Table 13–2) = AED

$$5 \times 325 \text{ mg} \times 1.1252 = 1828.45 \text{ mg}$$

An ingestion of 1625 mg (5 × 325 mg) of sodium salicylate is equivalent to an ingestion of 1828.45 mg of aspirin.

EXAMPLE 2 For a nonaspirin salicylate that is not 100% pure, calculate the AED for ingestion of 10 mL of 35% (w/v) oil of wintergreen (methyl salicylate):

$$35\% \text{ (w/v)} = 35 \text{ g}/100 \text{ mL}$$

Then calculate the amount of pure methyl salicylate:

$$\frac{35 \text{ q}}{100 \text{ mL}} \times \frac{\text{g}}{100 \text{ mL}} = 3.5\text{g}$$

Convert to milliliters using density:

$$\frac{35 \text{ g}}{1.184 \text{ g/mL}} = 2.96 \text{ mL}$$

Calculate the AED:

AED = mL of pure methyl salicylate × ACF (from Table 13–2)

$$\text{AED} = 2.96 \text{ mL} \times 1.3978 = 4.13 \text{ g}$$

Therefore, ingestion of 10 mL of 35% (w/v) oil of wintergreen is equivalent to ingestion of 4.13 g aspirin.

EXAMPLE 3 A 10-kg child was found ingesting a 5-mL (1-tsp) dose of choline salicylate that was set out for grandmother. Calculate the AED of choline salicylate. Assume choline salicylate is 100% bioavailable and completely hydrolyzed and the ACF is 0.7466 (from Table 13–2).

$$\text{AED} = 870 \text{ mg} \times 0.7466 = 649.54 \text{ mg}$$

Glycine

Availability of glycine may be an important factor in the formation of salicyluric acid when salicylates are ingested in toxic amounts. In aspirin overdose, plasma glycine is depleted. Oral glycine (8 g initially followed by 4 g every 2 hours for 16 hours) appears to increase the rate of formation of salicyluric acid after a salicylate overdose.[8,9] The main problems associated with glycine use are the nausea and vomiting it provokes.[9] Oral glycine has not been evaluated as a supplementary treatment for salicylate poisoning.[9]

After a toxic dose of aspirin, salicylate is excreted as salicyluric acid. It appears to be produced together with an increase in elimination as gentisic acid and salicylic acid phenolic glucuronide. This indicates progressive saturation of salicyluric acid formation and raises issues about the in vivo glycine pool when acetylsalicylic acid is taken in overdose.[10]

Table 13–2
Aspirin Conversion Factor for Nonaspirin Salicylate Compounds

Salicylate-Containing Product	MW	Specific Gravity	ACF	Available Form	AED
Acetaminosalol	217.30	—	0.8290	—	—
Aloxiprin	Varies	—	0.8333	Tab 600 mg	500 mg
Aluminum aspirin*	402.30	—	0.8956	Tab 670 mg	600 mg
Aminosalicylic acid	153.14	—	†	Tab 500 mg	—
Ammonium salicylate	155.15	—	1.1611	—	—
Antipyrine salicylate	326.34	—	0.5520	—	—
Aspirin	180.15	—	1.0000	Tab 325 mg	325 mg
Benorylate	313.32	—	0.5750	Tab 750 mg	430 mg
Benzyl salicylate	228.24	1.175	0.9246	—	—
Bismuth subsalicylate	362.11	—	0.4975	Liquid 262.7 mg 15 ml	345.1 mg/15 ml
Bromosalicylic acid acetate	259.06	—	0.6954	—	—
Calcium aminosalicylate	344.34	—	*	Tab 500 mg	—
Calcium carbaspirin	458.40	—	0.3930	—	—
Carbamoylphenoxyacetic acid	195.20	—	0.9229	—	—
Choline salicylate	241.28	—	0.7466	Liquid 870 mg/5 ml	650 mg/5 ml
Diethylamine salicylate	211.30	—	0.8526	Cream 10%	426 mg/5 g
Diflunisal	250.20	—	*	Tab 500 mg	—
Ethyl salicylate	166.06	1.131	1.2244	—	—
Fendosal	381.40	—	0.4723	200 mg	94.47 mg
Glycol salicylate	182.17	—	0.9889	Topical	—
Homosalate	262.36	1.045	0.7154	Sunscreen oil 10%	2.12 g/fl oz
Lithium salicylate	143.98	—	1.2512	—	—
Magnesium salicylate†	298.54	—	1.2068	Tab 325 mg	390 mg
Menthyl salicylate	276.36	—	0.6792	—	—
Methyl salicylate	152.14	1.184	1.3978	Topical 2–35%	28–489 mg/ml
Octyl salicylate	250.37	1.018	0.7303	Sunscreen 3–5%	0.648–1.08 g/fl oz
Phenazone salicylate	326.40	—	0.5519	300 mg	165.6 mg
Phenyl aminosalicylate	229.23	—	*	—	—
Phenyl salicylate	241.21	—	0.7469	Tab 300 mg	224 mg
Physostigmine salicylate	413.17	—	0.4360	Ointment 0.25%	5.45 mg/5 g
Potassium aminosalicylate	191.23	—	*	Tab 500 mg	—
Potassium salicylate	176.21	—	1.0224	—	—
Salicylamide	137.14	—	*	Tab 325 mg	—
Salicylic acid	138.12	—	1.3043	Topical 3–60%	0.196–3.912 g/5 g
Salsalate†	258.22	—	1.3953	Cap 500 mg	697.45 mg
Silver salicylate	244.98	—	0.7354	—	—
Sodium aminosalicylate	175.12	—	*	Tab 500 mg	—
Sodium salicylate	160.11	—	1.1252	Tab 325 mg	358 mg
Sodium thiosalicylate	176.17	—	1.0226	Solution 50 mg/5 ml	51.31 mg/ml for IM use
Sulfasalazine	398.39	—	*	Tab 500 mg	—
Thurfyl salicylate	222.20	—	0.8108	Cream 10–14%	405–568 mg/5 g
Triethanolamine salicylate	286.31	—	0.6292	Cream 10%	314.6 mg/5 g of 10% cream

MW, molecular weight; ACF, aspirin conversion factor; AED, aspirin equivalent dose.
*Hydrolyzed to 2 molecules of salicylate.
†Not converted to salicylate.
From Vandenberg SA, Smolinske SC, Spoerke DG, Rumack BH. Non-aspirin salicylates: conversion factors for estimating aspirin equivalence.

Toxicokinetics

Pregnancy/Lactation/Neonate

The clinical symptoms of a toxic reaction to salicylate in neonates differ from those in adults[11] (Table 13–3). Stimulation of the respiratory center may cause tachypnea in infants, as well as adults. Respiratory alkalosis may not be present or may be transient in infants. Hypoglycemia after salicylate exposure is observed more frequently in infants than in children and adults.[11]

A full-term neonate born to a mother who had ingested analgesics experienced tachypnea, respiratory distress, hypotonia, and metabolic acidosis/respiratory alkalosis with acidemia. Cord and maternal blood concentrations at the time of delivery were 61 and 51 mg/dL, respectively. The urine drug screen was positive for salicylates, and the serum salicylate level was 33 mg/dL on day 4. The fetus concentrates salicylate with fetal/maternal salicylate ratios greater than 1. The neonate has a lower protein binding than an adult, resulting in a larger volume of distribution and higher fraction of free drugs.[12]

Repeated ingestion of aspirin-containing products late in gestation results in the birth of infants with abnormalities in hemostasis, acid–base imbalance, tachypnea, and hemoglycemia.[11]

Preeclampsia (Pregnancy-Induced Hypertension)

Administration of low doses (60 mg/d) of aspirin to women at risk for pregnancy-induced hypertension from the 12th

Table 13–3
Salicylates in Neonates and Adults

	Neonates	Adults
Early respiratory alkalosis	–	+
Hypoglycemia	++	+
Hemorrhage	++	+
Protein binding	Low	High
Rate of salicylate and metabolite excretion	Slow	More rapid
Glomerular filtration rate	Reduced	Reduced
Elimination half-life (h)	4½–11½	3–4

From Buck ML, Grebe TA, Bond GR. Toxic reaction to salicylates in a newborn infant: Similarities to neonatal sepsis. J Pediatr 1993;122:955–958.

week of gestation to delivery appears to be associated with a longer duration of pregnancy and an increase in weight of the newborn. This dose does not appear to expose fetuses or newborns to major hemorrhagic risks.[13–15] Further confirmatory large-scale controlled studies are required. Doses of 100 mg of aspirin daily administered to women during the third trimester of pregnancy have reduced the incidence of pregnancy-induced hypertension and preeclamptic toxemia in women at high risk for these disorders.[16] There were few maternal side effects and no fetal bleeding or circulatory disorders. These authors accept the suggestion that aspirin be stopped at least 5 days before the estimated date of delivery to minimize the risk of induced bleeding disorders.

Aspirin is not curative for mild pregnancy-induced hypertension but may be preventive treatment, which, to be effective, should be started weeks before clinical signs of preeclampsia are present.[17] Low-dose aspirin does not influence the clinical course of women with mild pregnancy-induced hypertension. The use of aspirin in low dose does not avert or alleviate preeclampsia once clinical signs are present. There is as yet insufficient evidence to justify the administration of low-dose aspirin to all primagravid women. The evidence appears sufficiently strong to justify its use in pregnant women judged to be at increased risk of developing toxemia of pregnancy. These would include women with:[18]

- Preexisting chronic hypertension
- Autoimmune disorders (especially systemic lupus erythematosus and the lupus anticoagulant)
- A positive anticardiolipin antibody test
- A history of recurrent toxemia in successive pregnancies
- Hypertension of undetermined nature that developed before 20 weeks' gestation
- An isolated elevated blood pressure reading in the first trimester
- Increased arterial reactivity identified by the angiotensin II infusion test

Neonatal Hemorrhage

A prospective study of infants born at 34 weeks' gestation or earlier or weighing 1500 g or less indicated that aspirin was associated with an increase in intracranial hemorrhage in this group. The authors concluded that use of aspirin during the last 3 months of pregnancy is probably inappropriate.[19]

Congenital Defects

Although two studies have suggested that aspirin use in the first trimester of pregnancy may increase the risk of cardiac malformation,[20,21] a subsequent case-control study indicates that the use of aspirin during the early months of pregnancy, when the fetal heart is developing, is not associated with an increased risk of cardiac defects overall or with an increased risk of aortic stenosis, coarctation, hypoplastic left ventricle, transposition of the great arteries, or constructional defects.[22]

Drug Interactions

Overdose of the tricyclic antidepressant amoxapine together with an overdose of aspirin may lead to formation of a metabolite identified as *N*-acetylamoxapine (Table 13–4). This is an unusual example of a compound formed in vivo by nonenzymatic transacetylation. A 46-year-old woman who died after a combined overdose exhibited *N*-acetylamoxapine in the body fluids postmortem.[23] Topical methylsalicylate ointment can potentiate the anticoagulant effect of warfarin. These actions may be unrelated to the blood salicylate level.[24]

Mechanism of Action

Hyperlactic acidemia or hyperketonemia in adults may be infrequently observed in salicylate poisoning. A disproportionately decreased plasma bicarbonate concentration or fraction lactate or ketoacidosis during salicylate poisoning should arouse suspicion that the patient has a concomitant salicylate-independent disorder.[25]

Clinical Presentation

Metabolic Abnormalities

Most patients poisoned with aspirin (children and adults) have either a simple respiratory alkalosis secondary to direct stimulation of the respiratory center and subsequent hyperventilation or a mixed respiratory alkalosis and metabolic acidosis. Acidemia is frequently associated with neurologic features, pulmonary edema, and a fatal outcome.[26]

A single 0.65-g dose of aspirin may increase the mean bleeding time of a normal person for 4 to 7 days, probably due to the decreased formation of the platelet aggregation stimulator thromboxane A_2. Nonsteroidal antiinflammatory drugs have a similar mechanism of action, although the duration of effect varies widely from less than 1 day for flurbiprofen, ibuprofen, indomethacin, and sulindac to 2 weeks for piroxicam. Impaired coagulation may compromise a surgical result, particularly with grafts, flaps, or microsurgical procedures. Orally administered medications that increase bleeding time are listed in Table 13–5.[27]

Muscle Function

Rhabdomyolysis may be associated with a salicylate-induced hyperthermia. The creatine kinase serum levels are elevated. Diffuse myalgias are observed.[28]

Table 13–4
Salicylate-Drug Interactions

Drug Interactions Related to Absorption
Ulcerogenic and irritating potential
Aspirin in combination enhancing ulcerogenic effects
Caffeine
Phenylbutazone
Indomethacin
Alcohol
Factors reducing ASA absorption
Food
Chelation with iron
Complexation with caffeine
Indomethacin
Drug Interactions Related to Distribution
ASA is protein bound—interactions resulting from displacement
Displacement of bishydroxycoumarin
Displacement of antimicrobial agents
Potentiates penicillins
Potentiates sulfonamides
Displacement of oral hypoglycemia agents
Tolbutamide
Sulfonyureas—chlorpropamide
Displacement of methotrexate
Potentiates PAS toxicity
PABA potentiates ASA
Displacement of bilirubin in neonates
Drug Interactions Related to Salicylate Metabolism
Interactions resulting from glucuronide formation
Excretion of corticosteroids
Potential of interaction by competition for glucoronide metabolism route
Phenothiazines—chlorpromazine
Methocarbamol
Enzyme induction—phenobarbital
Drug Interactions Related to the Excretion of ASA
Effects on excretion of uric acid—ASA antagonizes uricosuric effect of
Probenecid
Sulfinpyrazone
Phenylbutzone
Electrolyte imbalances
Diminishes effects of spironolactone diuretics
Resultant electrolyte retention effects
Supervise salt diets
Supervise diuretic therapy
Supervise digitalis therapy
Acidity potentiated by acetazolamide

ASA, acetylsalicylic acid; PAS, *p*-aminosalicylic acid; PABA, *p*-aminobenzoic acid.
Adapted from Suffness M, Rose BS. Potential drug interactions and adverse effects related to aspirin. Drug Intell Clin Pharm 1974;8:695. Copyright 1974 Drug Intelligence & Clinical Pharmacy, Cincinnati Ohio. Used with permission.

Cardiac Status

Acute salicylate intoxication may induce cardiac depression and asystole. The exact mechanism has not been defined.[29]

Fatalities

Death following salicylate overdose appears to be increased in patients over 70 years of age. Salicylates were the most common agent responsible for single-drug deaths in Ontario during 1984 and 1986.[30] Delayed presentation, coma, hyperpyrexia, pulmonary edema, and acidemia are more common in fatal cases. The mean plasma salicylate concentration in fatal cases is often between 70 and 90 mg/dL. The increased toxicity of higher plasma salicylate concentrations is to be expected, as the rise in the unbound fraction of the drug in the plasma and the volume of distribution both increase as concentrations rise. Failure to hyperventilate may contribute to the development of acidemia. The prognosis of acute salicylate poisoning cannot be determined from the plasma concentration of the blood alone. Clinical features, especially impaired consciousness, and the arterial pH must be evaluated. Hemodialysis and use of activated charcoal should be considered.[31–33]

Acute and Chronic Intoxication

Table 13–6 contrasts acute and chronic salicylate intoxication. A multicenter case-control study suggests that long-term regular use of phenacetin may increase the risk of chronic renal disease; that long-term daily use of acetaminophen, the major metabolite of phenacetin, is associated independently with an increased risk of chronic renal disease; and that there does not appear to be an increased risk of renal disease in daily users of aspirin.[34] These findings require confirmation.[35]

Reye's Syndrome

The Centers for Disease Control and Prevention has provided a definition of Reye's syndrome (Table 13–7).[36] A presumptive case of Reye's syndrome can be excluded by the criteria in Table 13–8.[37]

Trends. The incidence of Reye's syndrome reported through national surveillance has fallen dramatically in the United States from a peak of 0.88 per 100,000 children less than 18 years of age in 1980 to 0.09 per 100,000 in 1989.[38] A similar decline has been observed in the United Kingdom and Australia.[39] Second, an increasing number of inborn errors of fatty acid oxidation have been described. The most common is a medium-chain acyl coenzyme A deficiency. These disorders share the clinical and laboratory features of Reye's syndrome: vomiting, progressive lethargy, hypoglycemia, and fatty infiltration of the liver (Table 13–9).[40,41]

The National Institutes of Health recommends a uniform clinical staging from I (lethargy) to V (flaccid, unresponsive coma). Stage II is a transition from stupor to coma with decortication (stage III) and decerebration (stage IV) (Table 13–10).[42]

Adults. The clinical picture of Reye's syndrome in adults is similar to that seen in children.[43,44] Vomiting and, shortly afterward, encephalopathy develop a few days after influenza, gastroenteritis, or an upper respiratory infection. The association with salicylates seems less strong in adults than in children. About a third of adults die, a mortality similar to that seen in children. In adults, the diagnosis is best confirmed by percutaneous liver biopsy (microvesicular fatty change within the hepatocytes with little or no inflammatory infiltrate or narcosis). The differential diagnosis [45] includes causes of fulminant hepatic failure in adults (e.g., viral hepatitis, isopropanol, amanitin, or carbon tetrachloride poisoning) acetaminophen overdose, halothane anesthesia, and other rare causes including valproate toxicity, urea cycle

Table 13–5
Orally Administered Medications Containing Aspirin or Salicylic Acid Derivatives That Increase Bleeding Time

Adult Analgesic Pain Reliever
Alka-Seltzer
Anacin
Analval
Anodynos
APAC Improved
Arthra-G
Arthritis Pain Formula
Arthropan
ASA
Ascriptin
Aspercin
Aspergum
Aspermin
Aspirin with codeine
AspirTab
Asproject
Axotal
Azdone tablets
B-A-C tablets
Bayer aspirin
Bayer children's cold tablets
BC powder
BC tablets
Buffaprin
Buffasal
Bufferin
Buffets II
Buffex
Buffinol
Cama arthritis pain reliever
Carisoprodol compound tablets
Children's aspirin
Cope
Damason-P
Darvon compound
Darvon compound-65
Darvon with ASA
Darvon-N with ASA
Dasin
Disalcid
Diurex
Doan's
Dolcin
Dolprn #3 tablets
Drinophen
Duradyne
Easprin
Ecotrin
Emagrin
Empirin
Empirin with codeine
Equagesic
Equazine-M
Excedrin
Fiogesic tablets
Fiorgen PF
Fiorinal
Fiorinal with codeine
4-Way Cold tablets
Gelpirin tablets
Gemnisyn
Genprin
Gensan
Goody's Extra Strength
Goody's Headache Powder
Infantol Pink
Isollyl Improved
Lanorinal
Lortab ASA
Magan
Magnaprin
Magsal
Marnal
Measurin
Meprobamate and aspirin
Meprogesic Q
Micrainin
Midol for cramps, maximum strength
Midol Original
Mobidin
Mobigesic
Momentum muscular backache formula
Mono-Gesic
Neogesic
Norgesic
Norgesic Forte
Norwich extra-strength aspirin
Orphenagesic
Orphenagesic Forte
Oxycodone and aspirin
Pabalate-SF
P-A-C
Pain reliever tablets
Panodynes
Pepto-Bismol
Percodan
Percodan-Demi
Persistin
Phenetron compound
Presalin
Propoxyphene compound
Propoxyphene napsylate with ASA
Quiet World tablets
Rexolate
Robaxisal tablets
Roxiprin tablets
St. Joseph
Salabuff
Salatin
Salteo
Salflex
Salicylamide
Salocol
Salsalate
Salsitab
Sine-Off sinus medicine tablets
Soma compound tablets
Soma compound with codeine
Stanback Powder
Supac
Synalgos-DC capsules
Talwin compound
Tenol-Plus
Trigesic
Trilisate
Tri-Pain
Tusal
Ursinus-Inlay-Tabs
Valesin
Vanquish
Verin
Wesprin Buffered
Zorprin

ASA, acetylsalicylic acid
From Bartley GB, Warndahl RA. Surgical bleeding associated with aspirin and non-steroidal antiinflammatory agents. Mayo Clin Proc 1992;67:402–403.

disease such as ornithine transcarbamoylase deficiency, and systemic carnitine deficiency. Pranzatelli and De Vivo have listed drugs and exogenous toxins that induce the Reye's syndrome phenotype (Table 13–11).[41]

Gastric Erosion

Endoscopic studies have shown that all human control subjects who ingest acetylsalicylic acid (ASA) have benign gastric erosions; 60% have duodenal erosions after use of ASA for only 1 day.[46] More prolonged use of ASA can lead to more severe lesions. Surreptitious use of ASA should be considered in the differential diagnosis in patients with recurrent peptic ulcers.[47]

Pepto-Bismol

Bismuth subsalicylate (Pepto-Bismol, etc) has been suggested to minimize salicylate-induced gastric irritation. The salicylate in bismuth subsalicylates is almost entirely available. One tablespoon of Pepto-Bismol contains 130 mg of salicylate. The recommended dose for a 9-year-old is 15 mL up to eight times per 24 hours. If this is added to an antiinflammatory dose regimen of aspirin, serous salicylatc intoxication may follow.[48,49]

Elderly patients who ingest large amounts of Pepto-Bismol daily can develop agitation, confusion, lethargy, disorientation and slurred speech, and acute pulmonary edema. One patient died after ingesting 66 tablets in 24 hours.[50] Such patients may develop a mixed respiratory alkalosis and metabolic acidosis. Barium-like contrast densities may be seen on an abdominal plain film[51,52] (see also Bismuth in Chapter 67).

Sixty milliliters of Pepto-Bismol leads to peak salicylate concentrations of 40.1 μg/mL in 1.8 hours. Aspirin doses of 650 and 1000 mg lead to peak salicylate levels of 4 mg/dL in 1.9 hours and about 60 mg/dL in 2.3 hours, respectively.[53] After 30 mL of Pepto-Bismol (525 mg bismuth subsalicylate) every 30 minutes for eight doses (total daily dose, 4.2 g bismuth subsalicylate), a peak plasma salicylate level of 137 μg/mL is reached in 5 hours.[54] One adult dose of Pepto-Bismol liquid (30 mL of original strength) provides 25 mg of salicylate; one adult dose of Pepto-Bismol tablets (2 tablets) provides 204 mg of salicylate, similar to the salicylate dose delivered by one regular-strength aspirin (249 mg of salicylate). Maximum-strength Pepto-Bismol liquid

Table 13–6
Acute and Chronic Salicylate Toxicity*

Acute	Chronic
Usually young adult Usually suicidal Mortality <2% Use Done nomogram	Most old, very young Therapeutic mistakes Mortality to 25% Cannot use Done Nomogram Mistaken for other illness Myocardial infarction Mesenteric ischemia Upper respiratory infection Encephalopathy/acidosis if unknown etiology
Hemodialysis for 6-h serum salicylate level >120 mg/dL Rx: Multiple dose activated charcoal Seizures—diazepam Pulmonary edema—fluid restriction; mannitol diuresis Hemodialysis, hemoperfusion for serum level >100 mg/dL	Pulmonary edema, cerebral edema More dehydration More central nervous system effects More systemic acidosis: pH > 7.32 More morbidity Rx: Hemodialysis for levels >60 mg/dL in the elderly, in severe acidosis, and with altered mental stability

*At the same blood levels, chronic poisoning is more severe than acute poisoning, with increased hyperventilation, increased dehydration, deeper and non-frequent coma, and seizures. Acute: <35 mg/dL—no signs and symptoms. Chronic: 35–50 mg/dL with systemic acidosis may lead to severe clinical crisis.

contains 460 mg salicylate per dose. Ingestion of 66 tablets by a 36-kg patient resulted in a salicylate dose of 187 mg/kg; the patient died.[50] This may be compared with the recommended dosing schedule of 2 tablets four times a day, which would deliver 11.6 mg of salicylate/kg/d to a 70-kg adult.[52] Bismuth levels may remain elevated for several months[55] (see Chapter 67).

Salicylate overdose has been linked with shock, coagulopathy, and the adult respiratory distress syndrome.[56]

Ototoxicity

Hearing loss and tinnitus are usually reversible and increase progressively with increasing aspirin dosage and increasing concentrations of total and unbound plasma salicylate.[57] Further studies are required to test the concept that unbound plasma salicylate concentration is a better predictor of salicylate-induced ototoxicity than is total plasma salicylate concentration.[58]

Pseudosepsis Syndrome

Patients with chronic salicylate intoxication may present with a syndrome including fever, leukocytosis, a leftward shift in the differential cell count, hypotension, reduced systemic vascular resistance, and multiple-organ system failure (adult respiratory distress syndrome, acute renal failure, coagulopathy [disseminated intravascular coagulation], and encephalopathy). A source of infection is usually not documented in such patients by bacteriologic or

Table 13–7
Centers for Disease Control and Prevention Definition of Reye's Syndrome

- Acute noninflammatory encephalopathy documented clinically by an alteration in consciousness and, if available, a record of cerebrospinal fluid containing <8 leukocytes per millimeter, or by histologic specimen demonstrating cerebral edema without perivascular or meningeal inflammation
- Hepatopathy documented by results of either a liver biopsy or autopsy considered to be diagnostic of Reye's syndrome, or a threefold or greater rise in the levels of either AST, ALT, or serum ammonia
- No more reasonable explanation for the cerebral or hepatic abnormalities

*AST, aspartate aminotransferase; ALT, alanine aminotransferase.
From Rowe PC, Valle D, Brusilow SW. Inborn errors of metabolism in children referred with Reye's syndrome. JAMA 1988; 260:3167–3170.

Table 13–8
Diagnostic Criteria Used to Classify a Presumptive Case of Reye's Syndrome as Unlikely or Excluded

Reye's syndrome was considered unlikely if the case was not already classified as certain, probable, or excluded, or if two or more of the following characteristics were present.
1. Total bilirubin level ≥51 μmol/L
2. Normal ammonia level (if stage 2 or beyond)
3. A threefold or greater rise in creatinine level
4. Focal neurologic signs
5. Myocardial damage
6. No prodromal illness (if ≥12 mo of age)
7. Shock on admission
8. CSF protein level >0.5 g/L

Reye's syndrome was considered excluded if one of the following characteristics was present:
1. Normal AST/ALT
2. No necrosis and inflammation on liver biopsy
3. No steatosis
4. No significant mitochondrial alterations on electron microscopy
5. Other identified cause for the acute illness

CSF, cerebrospinal fluid; AST, aspartate aminotransferase; ALT, alanine aminotransferase.
From Gauthier M, Guay J, Lacroix J, Lortie A. Reye's syndrome: A reappraisal of diagnosis in 49 presumptive cases. Am J Dis Child 1989;143:1181–1185.

pathologic studies. Occult salicylate intoxication should be considered in the differential diagnosis of sepsis syndrome of uncertain origin.[59]

The Elderly

Salicylism should be considered in any elderly patient with unexpected delirium or dementia. Use of the ferric chloride test or the Phenistix Reagent Strip on a urine sample detects the presence of salicylates. When this test is positive, a serum salicylate level should be obtained. Symptoms of chronic salicylism are difficult to diagnose in this age group. These symptoms may include fever, dehydration, confusion, disorientation, hearing loss, falling, agitation, hallucinations, an acute mental status change, lethargy, memory impairment, an inability to care for self, and poor

Table 13–9
Metabolic and Pathologic Comparisons in Reye's-Like Syndromes

Signs and Symptoms	Reye's Syndrome	Carnitine Deficiency	Acyl Coenzyme A Dehydrogenase Deficiencies	Disorders of Urea Synthesis	Branched-Chain Amino Acid Inborn Errors	Hypoglycin Toxicity	Pentanoate Toxicity*	Valproate Toxicity	Salicylate Toxicity
Viral-like early symptoms	+	±	±	±	+	0	0	±	0
Hepatic failure	+	+	+	+	+	+	+	+	+
Myopathy	0	+	+	0	0	0	0	0	0
Coma	+	+	+	±	±	+	+	+	+
Hyperbilirubinemia	L	0	0	0	0	0	0	L	0
Hypertransaminasemia	+	±	+	+	±	+	?	+	±
Ketosis	0	0	0	0	+	±	±	?	±
Hypoglycemia	+	+	+	0	0	+	+	±	±
Amino acidemia	+	+	+	+	+	+	+	+	±
↑ Acyl-carnitine or ↓ plasma carnitine	+	+	+	?	+	?	?	+	?
Hyperammonemia	+	+	+	+	+	+	+	+	±
Fatty acidemia	+	+	+	+	+	+	+	+	+
Mitochondrial swelling	+	+	+	0	0	+	+	+	±
Microsteatosis	+	+	±†	0	0	+	+	+	0
↓ Beta oxidation	+	+	+	±	±	+	?	+	+
Dicarboxylic aciduria	+	+	+	±	+	+	?	+	?
Dehydrogenases affected	+	?	+	0	0	+	±	+	+
↓ Gluconeogenesis	+	+	+	+	+	+	+	+	+
Inhibition of urea cycle	+	+	L	+	L	?	?	+	±
Coenzyme A sequestration	+	+	+	0	0	+	+	+	+
↑ Peroxisome oxidation	+	?	+	0	0	+	?	+	?

L, occasional late effect; +, commonly occurs; ±, may occur; 0, uncommon; ?, unstudied.
*Experimental intoxication
†Macrovesicular
From Osterloh J, Cunningham W, Dixon A, Combest D. Biochemical relationships between Reye's and Reye's-like metabolic and toxicologic syndromes. Med Toxicol Adverse Drug Experience 1989;4:272–294.

Table 13–10
Staging of Reye's Syndrome

Findings	I	II	III	IV	V
Level of consciousness	Lethargic but follows verbal commands	Combative to stuporous, verbalizes inappropriately	Comatose	Comatose	Comatose
Posture	Normal	Normal	Decorticate	Decerebrate	Flaccid
Response to painful stimuli	Purposeful	Purposeful or nonpurposeful	Decorticate	Decerebrate	No response
Pupillary reaction to light	Brisk	Sluggish	Sluggish	Sluggish	No response
Oculocephalic reflex (doll's eyes)	Normal response	Conjugate deviation of eyes	Conjugate deviation of eyes	Inconsistent or no response	No response

From the National Institutes of Health. Diagnosis and treatment of Reye's syndrome. JAMA 1981;246:2441–2444.

Table 13–11
Drugs and Exogenous Toxins* Inducing Reye's Syndrome Phenotype

Acetaminophen	Margosa oil
Aflatoxins	Methylbromides
Atlox	4-Pentenoic acid
Bonkrekate/atractyloside	Phenoformin
Butylated hydroxytoluene	Pyrrolizidine
Chlordane	Salicylates
Diallylacetic acid	Sodium octanoate
Disulfiram	Tetracyclines
Hypoglycin (*Senecia* alkaloid)	Toximul
Isopropyl alcohol	Valproic acid
Lead	

*Insecticides, pesticides, solvents, emulsifiers.
From Pranzatelli MR, DeVivo DC. Pharmacology of Reye's syndrome. Clin Neuropharmacol 1987;10:96–125.

hygiene. Although acid–base disturbances are a common feature of chronic salicylism, many elderly patients have a normal total serum carbon dioxide level and normal serum anion gap on admission. Arterial blood gases are often normal. The elimination half-life of aspirin in healthy elderly patients is often increased. In elderly patients, a low glomerular filtration rate is not reflected by an elevated serum creatinine because of relatively low muscle mass. Because of preexisting hearing loss, elderly patients do not appreciate tinnitus. The effects of chronic salicylism contribute to an impairment in the ability for self-care. This leads to a loss of independent living and the apparent need for nursing home placement. Serum salicylate levels should be monitored in elderly patients in whom salicylate therapy is necessary, as well as those on therapy who have decompensated in a variety of ways (eg, recent impairment of mental function, hearing loss, worsening renal function, or unexplained acid–base disorders).[60]

Most fatal cases of chronic salicylate poisoning occur in infants or the elderly when recommended doses are exceeded in the course of therapy.[61]

Dermal Exposure

Most cases of salicylism from dermal exposure occur in children and in patients with severe skin disorders.[62]

Laboratory

Trinder Method

The Trinder method is a colorimetric test in which the salicylic acid concentration is determined by measuring the absorbance of the ferric iron–salicylate complex formed after total serum protein is precipitated by mercuric chloride and allowed to react with ferric ion supplied by ferric nitrate.[63] With spectrophotometry, the lower limit of detection is about 10 mg/dL. With the Trinder method, salicylic acid, not acetylsalicylic acid, is measured. Other salicylates that produce a positive result with the Trinder reaction are salicylamide and methylsalicylic acid (oil of wintergreen, present in many topical creams, and also in Listerine antiseptic). Both compounds form a similar complex with ferric ion and absorb light at 540 nm.[64]

A rapid bedside salicylate screen test uses urine. A negative result 2 to 4 hours after ingestion indicates the absence of a significant salicylate ingestion. The Trinder reagent is premixed by the laboratory staff. It is a solution of 40 g mercuric chloride and 40 g ferric nitrate in 850 mL of type II deionized water. Concentrated hydrochloric and (10 mL) is added to the solution. Finally, the solution is diluted to a volume of 1 L with type II deionized water. The reagent is stable for 1 year at room temperature. In the Trinder spot test, 1 mL of urine and 1 mL of Trinder reagent are mixed in a test tube. A color change occurs immediately if salicylate is present. All specimens are observed for color change immediately after addition of the Trinder reagent to the urine. If the color change has a discernible violet or purple color, the result is considered positive. If the specimen merely darkens or no color change occurs, the result is considered negative.[65]

Thyroid Function

Salicylates alter thyroid hormone metabolism and can lower protein-bound iodine levels, total serum concentrations of thyroxine and triiodothyronine, and serum thyrotropin concentrations. Patients generally remain euthyroid and values return to normal after cessation of salicylate use.[66]

Done Nomogram

The Done nomogram (Fig. 13–1) applies only to a single ingestion of non-enteric-coated salicylate at a known time.

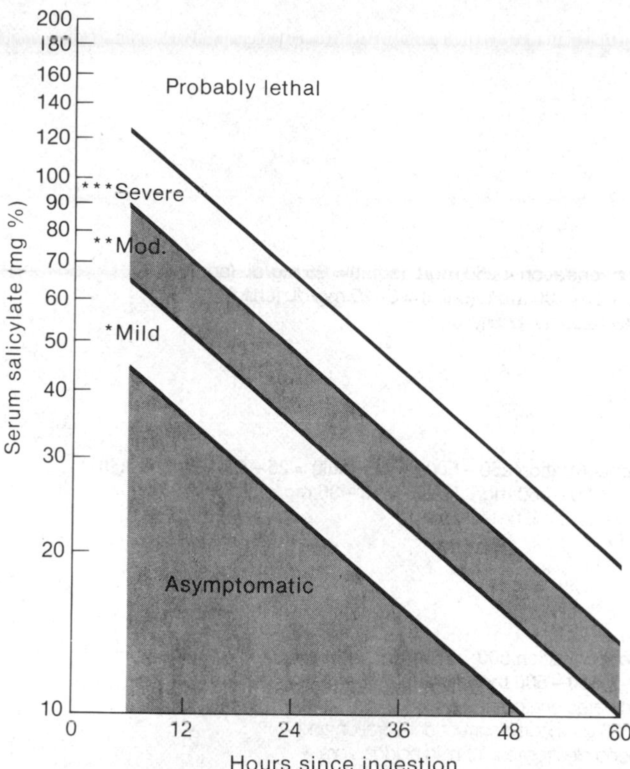

Figure 13–1 Nomogram relating serum salicylate level to severity of intoxication at varying intervals after acute ingestion of single doses of aspirin. Nomogram starts at 6 hours to ensure that levels will not be interpreted before they have reached their peak; it can be used earlier if more than one level is obtained to establish that the salicylate level is declining. *Mild toxicity: mild to moderate hyperpnea without acidosis, lethargy, and vomiting; slight fever may be present. **Moderate toxicity: severe hyperpnea with acidosis, marked lethargy or excitability but no coma or convulsions, and marked gastrointestinal distress. ***Severe toxicity: severe hyperpnea, severe neurologic impairment that may include coma or convulsions, and marked metabolic acidosis. (Adapted from Done AK. Aspirin overdose: Incidence, diagnosis and management. Pediatrics 1978;62(suppl.):895. Reproduced by permission of Pediatrics.)

Dehydration, acidosis, fever, and renal failure complicate its use. Concretions, delayed gastric emptying, and enteric coatings can prolong absorption. A second level several hours later should be drawn to determine if a drop in the salicylate concentration is taking place. In the face of acidemia (do concurrent pH determinations), a falling level indicates redistribution to the central nervous system rather than clearance.[67]

A study of 55 acute salicylate intoxications concludes that (1) the nomogram tends to overpredict the severity of intoxication in the moderate and severe categories and (2) the nomogram has a higher predictive index when used for concentrations drawn 6 to 12 hours after ingestion compared with concentrations drawn more than 12 hours after ingestion.[68]

Treatment

Stabilization

Hydration. Patients with clinically significant symptoms usually are dehydrated. These patients should receive generous fluid replacement with hypotonic glucose solutions (0.25 to 0.5 N saline) using urinary output (3 mL/kg/h or 100–200 mL/h in adults) as a measure of adequate hydration. Renal function (serum creatinine, blood urea nitrogen) should be measured on admission (Fig. 13–2).

Electrolytes. Electrolyte status must be followed closely. Patients usually are hypokalemic and should be given potassium supplements based on serum potassium and creatinine levels. Remember that acidosis may mask hypokalemia. The rate of potassium replacement should be limited to 10 mEq/h in an adult unless severely hypokalemic (<2.5 mEq/L). Urine flow must be established before potassium therapy is given.

Metabolic Acidosis. Acidosis is treated aggressively because decreased serum pH increases tissue penetration of salicylates, especially into the central nervous system. The blood pH should be corrected toward normal levels using the arterial pH as a guide. A bolus of 1 to 1.5 mEq/kg sodium bicarbonate is used if the pH is below 7.2, and then the blood pH is checked. Above pH 7.25, the bicarbonate may be added to the first bottle of fluids. Hypokalemia is corrected concurrently. In deciding whether to institute urine alkalinization and/or dialysis, clinical clues (eg, mental status, tinnitus, tachypnea, acidosis, fluid overload, pulmonary edema, seizures) are much more important than where the patient falls on the nomogram.[67]

Tetany. As ionized calcium may be decreased, intravenous calcium gluconate, 5 to 10 mL in an adult, may be used. Forced alkaline diuresis may worsen hypocalcemia-induced symptoms.

Hypoglycemia. All patients who present with central nervous system depression should receive intravenous glucose (50 mL 50% dextrose or 1 mL/kg) because central nervous system hypoglycemia may occur even with normal serum glucose levels. Blood glucose levels must be measured on admission and whenever central nervous system symptoms develop. Hypoglycemia is corrected immediately with intravenous glucose and dextrose is provided in all intravenous solutions.

Seizures. Convulsions indicate a serious prognosis and suggest the need to enhance elimination by hemodialysis. Seizures are treated with diazepam intravenously, 0.1 to 0.2 mg/kg per dose in children or 5 mg in adults. The physician should look carefully for evidence of metabolic abnormalities (eg hypernatremia, hypoglycemia, hypocalcemia) and cerebral edema (papilledema). The use of glucose and calcium should be considered if seizures do not resolve immediately.

Reye's Syndrome. Management of adults with Reye's syndrome is directed toward the encephalopathy and, in particular, to lowering the raised intracranial pressure. Patients should be admitted to an intensive care unit. The bed is raised to a head-up position of 40° to minimize the effect of raised jugular venous pressure on intracranial pressure. Hypercapnia and painful stimuli must be avoided. Mannitol is infused rapidly in a dose of 0.2 to 1.0 g/kg. Acute

Management of Poisoning Due to Salicylate

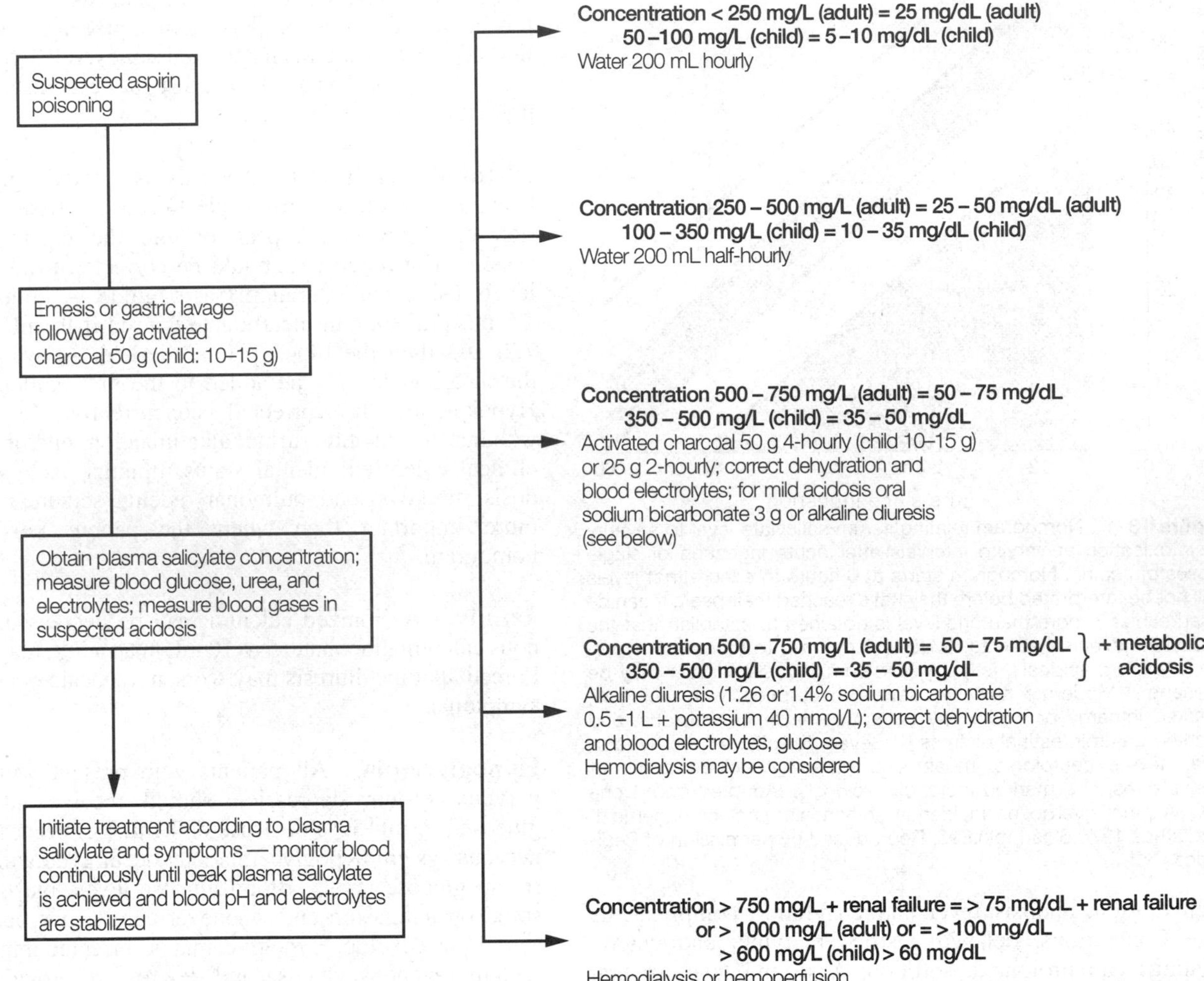

Figure 13–2 Management of salicylate poisoning. (From Notarianni L. A reassessment of the treatment of salicylate poisoning. Drug Saf 1992;7:292–303.)

hyperventilation is helpful. In resistant cases, short-acting barbiturates may be lifesaving. Continuous monitoring of intracranial pressure by surgically placed extradural sensors is useful.[43,44]

Gastric Lesions. Preliminary endoscopic studies in human volunteers challenged with aspirin suggest that proton pump inhibitors prevent morphologic lesions induced by aspirin.[69] Drugs that protect the gastric mucosa, especially antacids, analgesics (eg, misoprostol), prostaglandins, and sucralfate, reduce the hydrogen ion retrodiffusion induced by aspirin. H_2 blockers (eg, omeprazole) may effectively protect the gastric mucosa from lesions induced by aspirin and visualized by gastroscopy.[70–72]

Gut Decontamination

Toxic doses of salicylates cause pylorospasm and decrease the rate of gastric emptying; if enteric-coated or sustained-release preparations are ingested, peak plasma levels do not occur until 24 hours or more. Gastric lavage may remove pill fragments up to 12 hours after ingestion.[9]

Most studies involving the use of activated charcoal after salicylate ingestion have been performed in healthy volunteers.[73–81] In one study, clinically important enhanced salicylate excretion following multiple-dose activated charcoal was not demonstrated.[78] One report summarizes the use of multiple-dose activated charcoal in two patients with salicylate overdose. In each patient serum salicylate concentrations continued to rise after the multiple doses of charcoal had been administered. One patient developed a serum level of 78 mg/dL at 26 hours after ingestion and died in 29.5 hours. The other patient survived.[82] Desorption of aspirin from activated charcoal was suggested in one study,[77] but methodologic flaws challenge its conclusion.[78] Confirmation of the usefulness of activated charcoal in actual salicylate poisoning cases is still required.

A prospective controlled, randomized study performed by Tenenbein and colleagues does not support the use of either multiple-dose charcoal or whole-bowel irrigation to enhance the excretion of previously absorbed salicylate in poisoned patients.[83,84]

Cathartics. Hypermagnesemia has been reported during treatment with multiple doses of activated charcoal–magnesium citrate for acute salicylate intoxication. These results suggest that patients receiving magnesium citrate as part of their management should have serial magnesium measurements monitored during the course of treatment.[85] Four human aspirin studies have not shown any benefit from the addition of cathartics to charcoal.[86–89] Death has followed multiple doses of cathartics.[90]

Urinary Alkalinization. Urinary alkalinization (monitoring urine pH between 7.5 and 8.5) may be as effective and safer than forced alkaline diuresis.

For mild toxicity, 1 mEq/kg sodium bicarbonate is added to the first bottle of 5% dextrose. If alkalinization is not achieved within several hours, the dose may be repeated. Moderate to severe intoxications require additional bolus therapy (50–100 mEq sodium bicarbonate) over 1 to 2 hours plus close monitoring of blood urinary pH. Hypokalemia must be corrected by an intravenous line separate from alkaline therapy, as bicarbonate salts may otherwise form. In addition, hypokalemia must be corrected to alkalinize the urine. Renal sparing of potassium may decrease bicarbonate in the urine. Urinary salicylate excretion increases when the urinary pH is greater than 7.5 and is optimal between 8.0 and 8.5. Some patients with severe intoxications and chronic overdoses may be difficult to alkalinize. The physician should look carefully at the fluid/electrolyte status, especially the potassium level. In moderate to severe poisonings, a chest x-ray and arterial blood gases are ordered. If a significant arterial–alveolar oxygen gradient is present, fluids must be administered cautiously and alternate methods of enhancing elimination should be considered (e.g. hemodialysis). The patient must be watched for signs of hypocalcemia and the development of pulmonary edema. Alkalinization may be stopped when repeat salicylate levels decline below 35 to 40 mg/dL. Remember that rapid electrolyte changes may be more dangerous than the salicylate itself.

Extracorporeal Methods. Hemodialysis effectively increases clearance and improves fluid/electrolyte balance. Patient-specific indications include the presence of cardiac or renal failure, intractable acidosis, and severe fluid imbalance. Serum salicylate levels greater than 100 to 120 mg/dL in single acute ingestions indicate the need for hemodialysis. Seizures indicate a poor prognosis and may indicate the necessity to dialyze at lower levels. Chronic salicylate intoxications may be dialyzed at lower levels (eg, 60–80 mg/dL).[91] Jacobsen and colleagues suggest that hemodialysis offers the theoretical advantage of correcting acid–base and electrolyte disturbances, does not trap platelets, and has a lower heparin requirement than hemoperfusion.[33] A proposed guide to the management of poisoning due to salicylates is presented in Figure 13–2.

Charcoal hemoperfusion produces better salicylate clearance than hemodialysis but does not correct fluid and electrolyte balance like hemodialysis. Peritoneal dialysis is clearly inferior to hemodialysis and hemoperfusion, but does improve salicylate clearance.

Antidote

There are no antidotes for salicylate ingestions, but these patients may have coingested acetaminophen, for which *N*-acetylcysteine is the antidote. If the history does not exclude acetaminophen coingestion, an acetaminophen blood level should be drawn at least 4 hours postingestion.

Supportive Measures

Hypoprothrombinemia. Low prothrombin times usually do not cause serious complications unless there is an underlying bleeding disorder. The relative vitamin K deficiency may be treated with 2.5 to 5 mg vitamin K intravenously every day.

Hyperpyrexia. If rectal temperature is higher than 40°C, a cooling blanket or ice in the axilla and groin must be used. The temperature should be followed closely with a rectal probe and the cooling measures discontinued when rectal temperature falls below 38.5°C. Otherwise, the patient can be left undressed in a cool environment.

REFERENCES

1. SALT Collaborative Group. Swedish aspirin low-dose trial (SALT) of 75 mg aspirin as secondary prophylaxis after cerebrovascular ischaemic events. Lancet 1991;338:1345–1349.
2. Thun MJ, Namboodiri MM, Heath CW Jr. Aspirin use and reduced risk of fatal colon cancer. N Engl J Med 1991;325: 1593–1596.
3. Manson JE, Grobbee DE, Stampfer MJ, et al. Aspirin in the primary prevention of angina pectoris in a randomized trial of United States physicians. Am J Med 1990;89:772–776.
4. Buring JE, Peto R, Hennekens CH. Low-dose aspirin for migraine prophylaxis. JAMA 1990;264:1711–1713.
5. Rummore MM, Goldstein GS. Prevention of recurrent myocardial infarction and sudden death with aspirin therapy. Drug Intell Clin Pharm 1987;21:961–962.
6. Vandenberg SA, Smolinske SC, Spoerke DG. Non-aspirin salicylates: Conversion factors for estimating aspirin equivalence. Vet Hum Toxicol 1989;31:49–50.
7. Vandenberg SA, Smolinske SC, Spoerke DG, Rumack BH. Non-aspirin salicylates: Conversion factors for estimating aspirin equivalence. Vet Hum Toxicol 1987;29:469.
8. Patel DK, Ogunbona A, Notarianni LJ, Bennet PN. Depletion of plasma glycine and effect of glycine by mouth on salicylate metabolism during aspirin overdose. Hum Exp Toxicol 1990;9:389–396.
9. Notarianni L. A reassessment of the treatment of salicylate poisoning. Drug Saf 1992;7:292–303.
10. Patel DK, Hesse A, Ogunbona A, et al. Metabolism of aspirin after therapeutic and toxic doses. Hum Exp Toxicol 1990;8: 131–136.

11. Buck ML, Grebe TA, Bond GR. Toxic reaction to salicylates in a newborn infant: Similarities to neonatal sepsis. J Pediatr 1993;122:955–958.
12. Bond GR, Grebe TA, Arnold-Capell PA. Transplacental salicylate poisoning masquerading as neonatal sepsis. Vet Hum Toxicol 1989;31:346.
13. Wallenburg HC, Dekker GA, Makovitz JW, Rotmans P. Low-dose aspirin prevents pregnancy-induced hypertension and preeclampsia in angiotensin-sensitive primigravidae. Lancet 1986;1:1–3.
14. Wallenburg HC, Rotmans N. Prevention of recurrent idiopathic fetal growth retardation by low-dose aspirin and dipyridamole. Am J Obstet Gynecol 1987;157:1230–1235.
15. Benigni A, Gregorini G, Frascca T, et al. Effects of low-dose aspirin on fetal and maternal generation of thromboxane by platelets in women at risk for pregnancy-induced hypertension. N Engl J Med 1989;321:357–362.
16. Schiff E, Pelel E, Goldenberg M, et al. The use of aspirin to prevent pregnancy-induced hypertension and lower the ratio of thromboxane A_2 to prostacyclin in relatively high risk pregnancies. N Engl J Med 1989;32:351–356.
17. Imperiale TF, Petrulis AS. A meta-analysis of low-dose aspirin for the prevention of pregnancy-induced hypertension disease. JAMA 1991;266:260–264.
18. Lubbe WF. Low dose aspirin in prevention of toxaemia of pregnancy. Does it have a place? Drugs 1987;34:515–518.
19. Rumack CM, Guggenheim MA, Rumack BH, et al. Neonatal intracranial hemorrhage and maternal use of aspirin. Obstet Gynecol 1981;58:525–565.
20. Zierler S, Rothman KJ. Congenital heart disease in relation to maternal use of Bendectin and other drugs in early pregnancy. N Engl J Med 1985;313:347–352.
21. Heinonen DP, Slone D, Shapiro S. *Birth Defects and Drugs in Pregnancy.* Littleton, MA: Publishing Science Corp., 1977.
22. Wexler MM, Michell AA, Shapiro S. The relation of aspirin use during the first trimester of pregnancy to congenital cardiac defects. N Engl J Med 1989;321:1639–1642.
23. Osiewicz RJ, Middleberg R. Detection of a novel compound after overdoses of aspirin and amoxapine. J Anal Toxicol 1989;13:97–99.
24. Yip ASB, Chow WH, Tai YT, Cheung KL. Adverse effects of topical methylsalicylate ointment on warfarin anticoagulation: An unrecognized potential hazard. Postgrad Med J 1990; 66:367–369.
25. Bartels PD, Lund-Jacobsen H. Blood lactate and ketone body concentrations in salicylate intoxication. Hum Toxicol 1986;5:363–366.
26. Proudfoot AT. Metabolic abnormalities: Aspirin poisoning. Personal presentation. Presented at the Scientific Meeting of the European Association of Poison Control Centers and Clinical Toxicologists, Birmingham, UK, May 26–28, 1993.
27. Bartley GB, Warndahl RA. Surgical bleeding associated with aspirin and nonsteroidal antiinflammatory agents. Mayo Clin Proc 1992;67:402–403.
28. Leventhal LJ, Kuritsky L, Ginsburg R, Bomalaski JS. Salicylate-induced rhabdomyolysis. Am J Emerg Med 1989; 7:409–410.
29. Berk WA, Andersen JC. Salicylate-associated asystole: Report of two cases. Am J Med 1989;86:505–506.
30. McGuigan MA. A two-year review of salicylate deaths in Ontario. Arch Intern Med 1987;147:510–512.
31. McGuigan MA. Death due to salicylate poisoning in Ontario. Can Med Assoc J 1986;135:891–894.
32. Chapman BJ, Proudfoot AT. Adult salicylate poisoning: Deaths and outcome in patients with high plasma salicylate concentrations. Q J Med 1989;72:699–707.
33. Jacobsen D, Wiik-Larsen E, Bredeson JE. Hemodialysis or haemoperfusion in severe salicylate poisoning? Hum Toxicol 1988;7:161–163.
34. Sandler DP, Smith JC, Weinberg CR, et al. Analgesic use and chronic renal disease. N Engl J Med 1989;320:1238–1243.
35. Bennett WM, De Broe ME. Analgesic nephropathy: a preventable renal disease. N Engl J Med 1989;320:1269–1271.
36. Rowe PC, Valle D, Brusilow SW. Inborn errors of metabolism in children referred with Reye's syndrome. JAMA 1988;260: 3167–3170.
37. Gauthier M, Guary J, Lacroix J, Lortie A. Reye's syndrome: A reappraisal of diagnosis in 49 presumptive cases. Am J Dis Child 1989;143:1181–1185.
38. Reye's syndrome surveillance— United States, 1989. MMWR 1991;40:88–89.
39. Porter JDH, Robinson PH, Glasgow JFT, et al. Trends in the incidence of Reye's syndrome and the use of aspirin. Arch Dis Child 1990;65:826–829.
40. Orlowski JP, Gillis J, Killam HA. A catch in the Reye. Pediatrics 1987;80:638–642.
41. Pranzatelli MR, De Vivo DC. Pharmacology of Reye's syndrome. Clin Neuropharmacol 1987;10:96–125.
42. National Institutes of Health. Diagnosis and treatment of Reye's syndrome. JAMA 1981;246:2441–2444.
43. Meythalen JM, Varma RR. Reye's syndrome in adults: Diagnostic considerations. Arch Intern Med 1987;147:61–64.
44. Ede RJ, Williams R. Reye's syndrome in adults. Br Med J 1988;296:517–518.
45. Osterloh J, Cunningham W, Dixon A, Combest D. Biochemical relationships between Reye's and Reye's-like metabolic and toxicological syndromes. Med Toxicol Adverse Drug Experience 1989;4:272–294.
46. Ivey KJ. Drugs, gastritis and peptic ulcer. J Clin Gastroenterol 1981;3(suppl. 2):29–34.
47. Perrault J, Fleming CR, Dozois RR. Surreptitious use of salicylates: A cause of chronic recurrent gastroduodenal ulcers. Mayo Clin Proc 1988;63:337–342.
48. Lindsley CR. Use of non-steroidal antiinflammatory drugs in pediatrics. Am J Dis Child 1993;147:229–236.
49. Levy G. Aspirin and bismuth subsalicylate. Am J Dis Child 1993;147:1281.
50. Sainsbury SJ. Fatal salicylate toxicity from bismuth subsalicylate. West J Med 1991;155:637–639.
51. Steffers M, Esnard J, Meyer R, Bellucci A. Salicylate toxicity from bismuth subsalicylate overuse. Clin Res 1989; 32:336A.
52. Ching CK, Long RG, O'Hara R, Richardson J. Iatrogenic bismuth toxicity associated with inadvertent long term De-Nortab ingestion. Int J Pharm Pract 1993;2:111–113.
53. Feldman S, Chew S-L, Pickering LK, et al. Salicylate absorption from a bismuth subsalicylate preparation. Clin Pharmacol Ther 1981;29:788–792.
54. Pickering LK, Feldman S, Ericsson CD, Cleary TG. Absorption of salicylate and bismuth from a bismuth subsalicylate containing compound (Pepto-Bismol). J Pediatr 1981;99: 654–656.
55. Gordon MF, Abrams R, Rubin D, Barr B, Correa D. Bismuth subsalicylate toxicity as a cause for prolonged encephalopathy associated with myoclonus. Neurology 1994;44(suppl. 22):A305.
56. Montgomery H, Porter JC, Bradey RD. Salicylate intoxication causing a severe inflammatory response and rhabdomyolysis. Am J Emerg Med 1994;12:531–532.
57. Brien J-A: Ototoxicity associated with salicylates: a brief review. Drug Saf 1993;9:143–148.
58. Day RO, Graham GG, Bieri D, et al. Concentration–response relationships for salicylate-induced ototoxicity in normal volunteers. Br J Clin Pharmacol 1989;28:695–702.
59. Leatherman JW, Schmitz RG. Fever, hyperdynamic shock and multiple system organ failure: A pseudo-sepsis syndrome associated with chronic salicylate intoxication. Chest 1991;100:1391–1397.
60. Bailey RB, Jones SR. Chronic salicylate intoxication: A common cause of morbidity in the elderly. J Am Geriat Soc 1989;37:556–561.
61. Krause DS, Wolf BA, Shaw LM. Acute aspirin overdose: Mechanisms of toxicity. Ther Drug Monit 1992;14: 441–451.
62. Brubacher JR, Hoffman RS. Salicylism from topical salicylates. Clin Toxicol 1995;33:475–486.
63. Trinder P. Rapid determination of salicylate in biological fluids. Biochem J 1954;57:301–303.
64. Krause DS, Wolf BA, Shaw LM. Acute aspirin overdose: Mechanisms of toxicity. Ther Drug Monit 1992;14:441–451.
65. King JA, Storrow AB, Finkelstein JA. Urine Trinder spot test: A rapid salicylate screen for the emergency department. Ann Emerg Med 1995;26:330–333.

66. McConnell RJ. Abnormal thyroid function test results in patients taking salicylates. JAMA 1992;267:1242–1243.
67. Done AK. Salicylate intoxication: Significance of measurements of salicylates in blood in cases of acute ingestion. Pediatrics 1960;26:800–807.
68. Dugandzic RM, Tierney MG, Dickinson GE, et al. Evaluation of the validity of the Done nomogram in the management of acute salicylate intoxication. Ann Emerg Med 1989; 18:1186–1190.
69. Bergman J-F, Chassany O, Simoneau G, et al. Protection against aspirin-induced gastric lesions by lansoprazole: Simultaneous evaluation by functional and morphologic responses. Clin Pharmacol Ther 1992;52:413–416.
70. Bigard MA, Isal JP. Complete prevention by omeprazole of aspirin-induced gastric lesions in healthy subjects. Gut 1988; 29:A712.
71. Daneshmend TK, Stein AG, Bheskar NK, Haroly CJ. Abolition by omeprazole of aspirin-induced gastric mucosal injury in man. Gut 1990;31:514–517.
72. Loeb DS, Ahlquist DA, Talley NJ. Management of gastroduodenopathy associated with use of non-steroidal anti-inflammatory drugs. Mayo Clin Proc 1992;67:354–364.
73. Danel V, Henry JA, Glucksman E. Activated charcoal, emesis and gastric lavage in aspirin overdose. Br Med J 1988;296: 1507.
74. Danel V, Glucksman E, Henry JA. A comparative study of gastric lavage, emesis and activated charcoal in the management of a simulated aspirin overdose. Vet Hum Toxicol 1987;29(suppl. 2):107.
75. Tenenbein M, Kirschenbaum LA, Sitar DS. Multiple-dose charcoal therapy for salicylate poisoning. Ann Emerg Med 1989;18:444.
76. Yeakel D, Stemple C, Dougherty J. A prospective human crossover study on single versus multiple dose charcoal in salicylate ingestion. Ann Emerg Med 1988;17:439.
77. Filippone GA, Fish SS, Lacouture PG, et al. Reversible adsorption (desorption) of aspirin from activated charcoal. Arch Intern Med 1987;147:1390–1392.
78. Tenenbein M. Desorption of aspirin from activated charcoal. Arch Intern Med 1989;149:717.
79. Tenenbein M, Sitar DS, Kirschenbaum L. Does multiple dose charcoal hemoperfusion enhance salicylate excretion? Vet Hum Toxicol 1989;31:335.
80. Barone JA, Raia JJ, Huang YC. Evaluation of the effects of multiple-dose activated charcoal on the absorption of orally administered salicylate in a simulated toxic ingestion model. Ann Emerg Med 1988;17:34–37.
81. Dillon E, Wilton JH, Barlow J, Watson WA. The effect of two activated charcoal preparations on aspirin absorption in man. Vet Hum Toxicol 1987;39:491–492.
82. Augenstein WL, Kuling KW, Rumack BH. Delayed rise in serum levels in overdose patients despite multiple dose charcoal and after charcoal stool. Vet Hum Toxicol 1987;29: 491.
83. Tenenbein M, Sitar DS, Meyer L. Does oral multiple dose charcoal therapy or whole bowel irrigation increase the clearance of previously absorbed salicylate. Vet Hum Toxicol 1991;33:368.
84. Kirshenbaum LA, Mathews SC, Sitar DS, Tenenbein M. Does multiple-dose charcoal therapy enhance salicylate excretion? Arch Intern Med 1990;150:1281–1283.
85. Gren J, Woolf A. Hypermagnesemia associated with catharsis in a salicylate-intoxicated patient with anorexia nervosa. Ann Emerg Med 1989;18:200–203.
86. Mayersohn M, Perrier D, Pichioni AL. Evaluation of charcoal-sorbitol mixture as an antidote for oral aspirin overdose. Clin Toxicol 1977;11:561–567.
87. Easom JM, Carraccio TR, Lovejoy FH Jr. Evaluation of activated charcoal and magnesium citrate in the prevention of aspirin absorption in humans. Clin Pharm 1982; 1:154–156.
88. Sketris IS, Mowry JB, Czajka PA, et al. Saline catharsis: Effect on aspirin bioavailability in combination with activated charcoal. J Clin Pharmacol 1982;22:59–64.
89. Neuvonen PJ, Oikkola KT. Effect of purgatives on antidote efficacy of oral activated charcoal. Hum Toxicol 1986;5:255–263.
90. Brent J, Kulig K, Rumack BH. Iatrogenic deaths from sorbitol and magnesium sulfate during treatment for salicylism. Vet Hum Toxicol 1989;31:334.
91. Proudfoot AT. *Acute Poisoning: Diagnosis and Management.* 2nd ed. Oxford: Butterworth-Heinemann, 1993:205–209

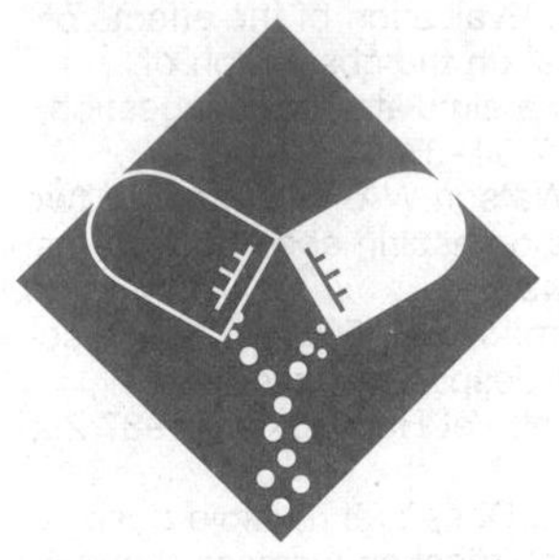

Part B Anti-Infective Drugs

Chapter 14 Introduction

CLOSTRIDIUM DIFFICILE COLITIS

A patient who receives antibiotic therapy that is not active against *Clostridium difficile* is at increased risk of developing pseudomembranous colitis caused by the production of a cytotoxic toxin by this organism during intestinal overgrowth.[1,2] Antibiotic-associated pseudomembranous colitis can arise with almost any antimicrobial agent The relative risk of developing *C. difficile* pseudomembranous colitis after exposure to clindamycin is substantially higher than for third-generation cephalosporins, broad-spectrum penicillins, or any other antibiotic.[3]

Clostridium difficile has been acquired by patients in the hospital setting, and the risk of nosocomial acquisition is probably greater than that in the community, where the carriage rate in healthy adults has been estimated to be about 5%. The incubation period for *C. difficile* colitis ranges from several days up to 6 weeks following antibiotic treatment, so the disease may develop in some patients after discharge from the hospital. *Clostridium difficile* colitis can be distinguished from a benign or nonspecific diarrhea that occurs in some patients given antibiotics in that the latter is not accompanied by fever or leukocytosis and usually disappears promptly on stopping therapy with the offending agent. Stool smears are positive for fecal leukocytes in about 50% of patients with *C. difficile* colitis; however, this is not a specific finding. Pseudomembranes may be observed on sigmoidoscopy or colonoscopy; however, this finding does not establish the etiology. Stools should be cultured for enteric pathogens because they are occasionally acquired nosocomially. The finding of *C. difficile* on culture is insufficient to make a definitive diagnosis of *C. difficile* colitis. The definitive etiologic diagnosis is made by establishing the presence of *C. difficile* toxin in the stool using an in vitro enzyme-linked immunosorbent assay or a cytotoxic assay. Besides stopping the responsible antibiotic, management is directed toward eradicating toxin-producing *C. difficile* with oral vancomycin or metronidazole.[1,2] A treatment algorithm is available (Fig. 14–1).[1]

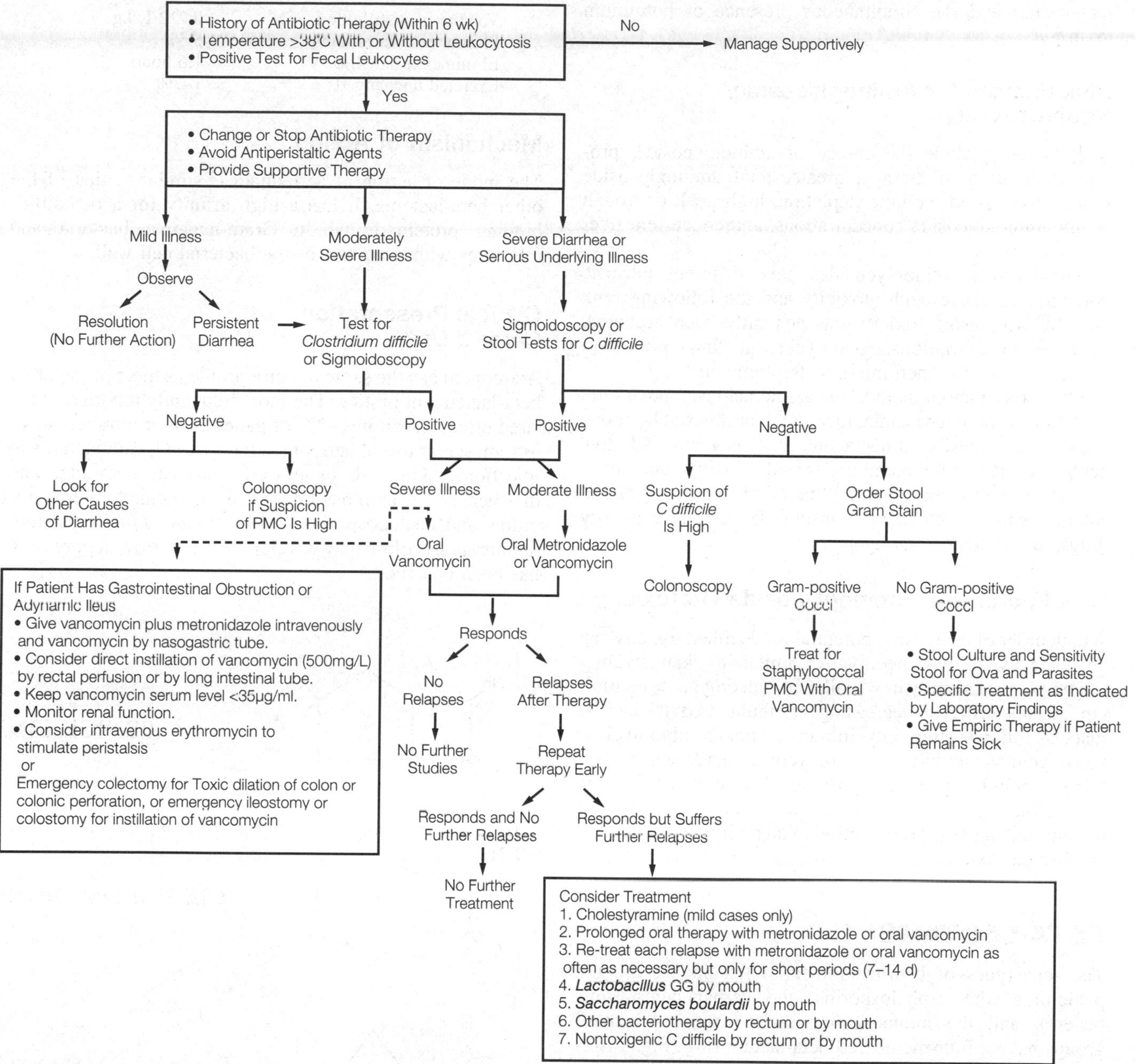

Figure 14–1 Algorithm for management of antibiotic-associated diarrhea and colitis. PMC, pseudomembranous colitis. (From Fekety R, Shah AB. Diagnosis and treatment of *Clostridium difficile* colitis. JAMA 1993;269:71–75.)

AMINOGLYCOSIDES

Ototoxicity

The initial symptom of cochlear damage is often tinnitus, which is usually high-pitched and continuous. By the time hearing loss is reported, significant high-frequency loss has probably already occurred, along with a 25- to 30-dB loss in the lower speech frequencies.[4]

Patients typically develop dysequilibrium if they are ambulatory, with an ataxic gait, stumbling, and loss of balance on turning.

Most clinically observed ototoxicity is, however, of the chronic type, which is generally accepted to be largely irreversible, although estimates of the incidence of reversibility range from 10 to 55%. Streptomycin is predominantly vestibulotoxic, and amikacin appears to be exclusively cochleotoxic.

Neuromuscular Blockade

All the aminoglycosides are capable, in rare circumstances, of causing neuromuscular blockade and resulting paralysis. The mechanism appears to involve blockade of calcium uptake, which results in both inhibition of presynaptic acetylcholine release and blockade of postsynaptic acetylcholine receptors.

Factors known to enhance neuromuscular blockade in association with the use of aminoglycosides include the concurrent use of curare-like drugs, succinylcholine, and magnesium and the simultaneous presence of botulinum toxin.[4]

Risk Factors for Aminoglycoside Nephrotoxicity

Risk factors include the choice of aminoglycoside, prolonged duration of therapy, greater total aminoglycoside dose, hypotension, volume depletion, high peak or trough serum aminoglycoside concentrations, and concurrent liver disease.[4]

The various aminoglycosides have different intrinsic potentials to cause nephrotoxicity and the following rank order of decreasing toxicity has generally been accepted, with minor variations: neomycin > gentamicin > tobramycin > amikacin > netilmicin > streptomycin.[4]

Other risk factors include metabolic acidosis, potassium depletion, hypomagnesemia, increased parathyroid hormone activity, and obesity. Other agents that may have additive nephrotoxicity with the aminoglycosides include amphotericin B, vancomycin, piperacillin, clindamycin, cisplatin, calcium channel blockers, nonsteroidal antiinflammatory drugs, and radiocontrast agents.

Risk Factors for Aminoglycoside Ototoxicity

A rank order of decreasing potential for cochlear toxicity can be made as follows: neomycin > amikacin = kanamycin > tobramycin = kanamycin = amikacin = neomycin > netilmicin. A rank order of decreasing vestibular toxicity can be made as follows: streptomycin > gentamicin > tobramycin = kanamycin = amikacin = neomycin > netilmicin.[4] Risk factors include older age, prolonged duration of therapy, bacteremia, poor physical condition, fever, liver and renal impairment, and the combination of an aminoglycoside with another ototoxic agent.

BETA-LACTAMS

The four types of beta-lactam antibiotics in use are the penicillins, the cephalosporins, the carbapenems (imipenem), and the monobactams (aztreonam).[5] All these groups have a four-membered beta-lactam ring (Fig. 14–2) (Table 14–1).[6]

• AZTREONAM (MONOBACTAMS)

Aztreonam (Azactam) is the first synthetic monobactam to be marked in the United States.[7,8]

Structure

Aztreonam differs from the penicillins and cephalosporins in having a monocyclic rather than bicyclic nucleus.

Toxicokinetics[6–9]

Bioavailability	About 100% (IM) 1% (oral)
Peak plasma level	35–99 μg/mL
Time to peak plasma level	1 hour
Volume of distribution	0.212 L/kg
Plasma protein binding	5.6%
Elimination half-life	1.6 hours
Excreted unchanged	1–7%

Mechanism of Action

The mode of action of aztreonam is similar to that of the other beta-lactams. It has a high affinity for a penicillin-binding protein found in Gram-negative bacteria and interferes with synthesis of the bacterial cell wall.

Clinical Presentation

Chronic Use

Aztreonam has the same toxicity profile as most of the other beta-lactam antibiotics. The most frequently reported undesired effects (seen in 1–2% of patients) after intravenous or intramuscular use of aztreonam have been local reactions to injections, skin rash or pruritus, nausea, vomiting, and diarrhea. Aztreonam has little cross-allergenicity with penicillins and cephalosporins.[10] *Clostridium difficile* pseudomembranous colitis may develop. Bone marrow suppression has been observed.[11]

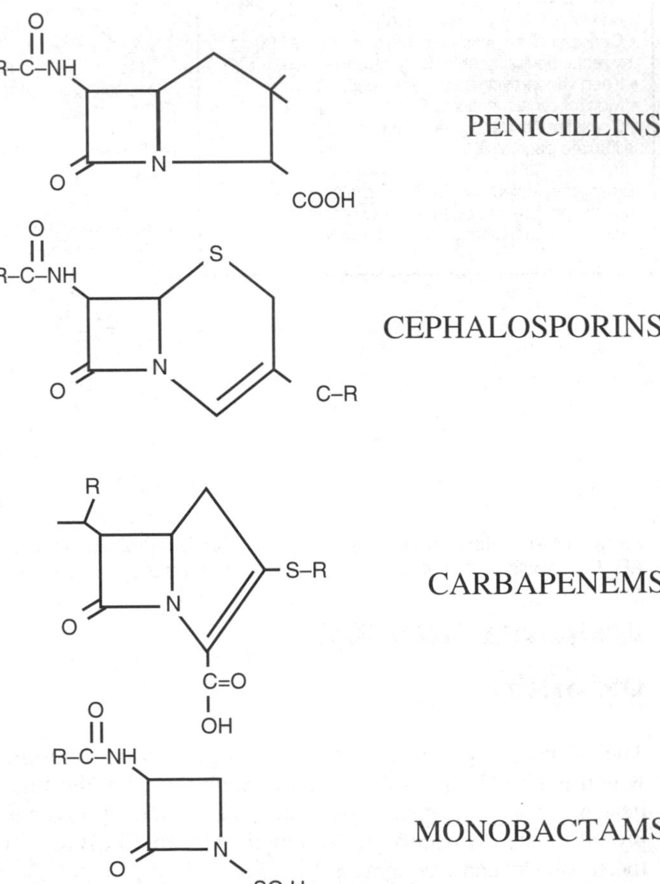

Figure 14–2 General structure of the four classes of beta-lactam antibiotics in use today. Note the four-membered beta-lactam ring common to all of them. (From Saxon A, Beall GN, Rohr AS, Adelman DC. Immediate hypersensitivity reactions to beta-lactam antibiotics. Ann Intern Med 1987;107:204–215.)

Table 14–1
Common Adverse Effects of Beta-lactams

Type of Reaction	Drug	Remarks
Allergic		
Anaphylaxis/rash	Penicillins Cephalosporins Imipenem	Rare anaphylaxis; no rash or anaphylaxis to aztreonam
Contact dermatitis	Ampicillin most common	In patients with Epstein-Barr syndromes, but occurs with all agents
Gastrointestinal (diarrhea) and *Clostridium difficile* colitis	Ampicillin Oral cephalosporins Cefoperazone Cefixime Ceftriaxone	Disturbs normal flora Low incidence of diarrhea Excreted in gut, occasional diarrhea Begin within 4 days Diarrhea in pediatric population
Bacterial or fungal overgrowths	Ceftazidime	Occasional overgrowth with Clostridium, staphylococci, enterococci
Hematologic		
Hemolytic anemia	Penicillin G	At high doses
Neutropenia	Oxacillin Nafcillin Cephalexin	Infrequent with cephalosporins
Platelet dysfunction	Carbenicillin Ticarcillin Moxalactam	Occurs with all β-lactam agents, albeit infrequently
	Cephalosporins	Infrequent
Thrombocytopenia	Penicillin	At high doses
Hypoprothrombinemia	Moxalactam Cefoperazone Cefamandole	Low incidence related to thiomethyl tetrazole moiety
Hepatic		
Rise in transaminase levels	Nafcillin Oxacillin Ticarcillin Aztreonam Imipenem	Rarely to >2–3× normal
Biliary sludging	Ceftriaxone	High biliary excretion, clears spontaneously on withdrawal
Cardiopulmonary	Penicillin G	Excessively rapid administration of K^+ salt causes arrhythmia
Renal		
Hypokalemia	Carbenicillin Ticarcillin	Due to accumulation of nonreabsorbable anion product in distal tubule
Interstitial nephritis	Methicillin	Can occur with all beta-lactams
Neurologic (seizures)	Penicillin G Ceftazidime Imipenem	Can occur with other penicillins also if decreased renal function occurs
Encephalopathy	Cefazolin Cephacetril	At high doses with renal failure
Drug–drug interactions		
Disulfiram-like reactions with alcohol	Moxalactam Cefoperazone Ceftriaxone	Due to thiomethyl tetrazole group (use vitamin K to prevent)
Coagulopathies with anticoagulants	Moxalactam Cefamandole Cefotetan Cefoperazone	

From Neu HC. Third generation cephalosporins: Safety profiles after 10 years of clinical use. Clin Pharmacol 1990;30:396–403.

Overdose

Overdoses with aztreonam have not been reported.

Treatment

In view of the moderate degree of protein binding (56%) and the low volume of distribution (0.2 L/kg) it would appear useful to initiate hemodialysis or hemoperfusion to accelerate elimination of aztreonam from the serum if clinically indicated. There are no antidotes. If there is a clinical concern about possible seizure development (prior history of seizures, very high dose of aztreonam, diminished renal function), then syrup of ipecac would not be advisable. Gastric lavage, activated charcoal, and cathartics have not yet been evaluated in aztreonam overdose.

• IMIPENEM (CARBAPENEMS)

Imipenem is the first of the carbapenems, a new class of beta-lactam antibiotics.[12,13] Imipenem is *N*-formimidyl-thienamycin, an antibiotic produced by *Streptomyces cat-*

teya.[14,15] It is marketed combined with cilastatin, a nonantibiotic enzyme inhibitor that prevents the breakdown of imipenem to nephrotoxic metabolites.[13] The combination is available only for intravenous use.

Therapeutic Dose

The usual adult dosage is 250 mg every 6 hours, with a maximum of 50 mg/kg daily, whichever is lower.

Toxicokinetics[14,16]

	Imipenem	Cilastatin
Bioavailability	<5%	<5%
Peak plasma level	14–80 µg/mL after 250 mg to 1 g IV	
Volume of distribution	0.22 L/kg (0.33 L/kg in children)	0.15 L/kg
Elimination half-life	0.8–1.2 hours	0.8–1.2 hours
Excreted unchanged	5–40% (alone) 70% (with cilastatin)	

Clinical Presentation

Chronic Use

Imipenem should be administered with caution to patients known to be hypersensitive to other beta-lactam antibiotics because of the possibility of cross-reactivity. The most common effects are phlebitis or pain at the site of infusion, nausea, and vomiting, all occurring in less than 3% of patients.[17]

Seizures

Seizures have been reported in up to 5% of patients.[17] Seizures generally begin about 7 days after the onset of therapy. As with other beta-lactam antibiotics, central nervous system lesions and disorders including seizures and renal insufficiency are strong risk factors for seizures. In addition, doses in excess of recommended doses (such as overdoses), particularly in patients with renal insufficiency, are associated with an increased risk of seizures.[18]

Treatment

See Aztreonam. Treatment is symptomatic and supportive. Reduction of potentially elevated serum levels may be afforded by prompt gastric emptying. Cautions must be taken for the potential of seizures in overdose.

• CEPHALOSPORINS

Cephalosporins may have several adverse hematologic effects, including hemolytic anemia, neutropenia, thrombocytopenia, and coagulation defects. Compounds with an *N*-methylthiotetrazole (NMTT) side chain (such as moxalactam, cefotetan, or cefamandole) have been associated with a higher incidence of bleeding. Free NMTT inhibits vitamin K epoxide reductase, thus interfering with the carboxylation of several factors in the coagulation cascade. Cefonicid is a second-generation cephalosporin that does not contain an NMTT chain and is usually considered free of hemorrhagic adverse effects.[19]

MACROLIDES

• AZITHROMYCIN AND CLARITHROMYCIN

Azithromycin and clarithromycin are antimicrobial macrolides similar to erythromycin.

Structure and Classification

Azithromycin is a 15-membered macrolide compound referred to as an azalide; clarithromycin is a 14-membered macrolide similar to erythromycin.

Use

Both azithromycin and clarithromycin have been approved by the U.S. Food and Drug Administration as pantimicrobial agents useful against atypical mycobacterial and toxoplasmal species and, possibly, *Hemophilus influenzae.*

Toxicokinetics

Table 14–2 outlines the toxicokinetics of three macrolides. Drug interactions with the macrolides are summarized in Table 14–3.[20]

Table 14–2
Comparative Pharmacokinetic Variables of Erythromycin, Azithromycin, and Clarithromycin*

	Drug and Dose		
Variable	Erythromycin, 500 mg	Azithromycin, 500 mg	Clarithromycin, 500 mg
Oral bioavailability (%)*	35 ± 25†	37	55 to 68
Taken with food	No	No	Yes
Serum half-life (hr)‡	1.5 to 3	11 to 14	4.9
Frequency of dosing, (×/day)	4	1	2
Alter dose in moderate renal failure	Yes	No	Yes

*Oral bioavailability to the fraction of the parent compound that reaches the systemic circulation.
†Enteric-coated erythromycin base; absorption is dependent on the salt form and temporal relation to meals.
‡The half-life is the time required for the plasma concentration in the body to decline by half.
From Kanatani MS, Guglielmo BJ. The new macrolides: Azithromycin and clarithromycin. West J Med 1994;160:31–37.

Table 14–3
Drug Interactions With Erythromycin, Azithromycin, and Clarithromycin

Interacting Drug	Erythromycin	Azithromycin	Clarithromycin
Digoxin	Increased digoxin levels	Not reported but the potential exists	Not reported but the potential exists
Anticoagulants (warfarin sodium)	Increased therapeutic effects (prothrombin time and international normalized ratio)	Not reported but the potential exists	Not reported but the potential exists
Ergotamines	Possible severe peripheral vasospasm; dysesthesia	Possible severe peripheral vasospasm; dysesthesia	Not reported but the potential exists
Triazolam	Increased pharmacologic effect of triazolam	Not reported but the potential exists	Not reported but the potential exists
Magnesium or aluminum antacids	Possible increase in half-life of erythromycin	Decreased peak serum levels without affecting the extent of absorption	Not reported but the potential exists
Carbamazepine, phenytoin, cyclosporine, hexobarbital, theophylline	Possible increase in serum levels	Not reported but the potential exists	Phase I studies, demonstrated increased plasma levels of theophylline and carbamazepine

From Kanatani MS, Guglielmo BJ. The new macrolides: Azithromycin and clarithromycin. West J Med 1994;160:31–37.

Clinical Presentation
Overdose

Few reports of overdose with these compounds appear in the medical literature. Macrolide antibiotics can be associated with hearing loss and severe nausea, vomiting, and diarrhea.[21,22]

Chronic Use

Gastrointestinal side effects (diarrhea, nausea, abdominal pain, dyspepsia, vomiting or gastritis) have been reported in 10 to 20% of clarithromycin-treated patients and 10% of azithromycin-treated patients compared with 20 to 35% of patients treated with erythromycin.[21]

Treatment

Treatment of an overdose is largely supportive and symptomatic.

• ERYTHROMYCIN
Product Formulation

Six preparations for oral use are available: enteric-coated tablets, enteric-coated pellets and "film"-coated tablets of the base; stearate salts; ethylsuccinate ester and lauryl sulfate salts of the propionyl ester (the estolate). There are two preparations for intravenous use: erythromycin gluceptate and erythromycin lactobionate. Intramuscular administration is avoided because of severe pain on injection. Erythromycin is also available as an ophthalmic ointment and in topical preparations.[23]

Therapeutic Dose

For adults, 1 to 2 g/d in divided doses (max 8 g/d) is given. The recommended pediatric dose is 30 to 50 mg/kg/d in divided doses (max 2 g/d). Intravenously, 15 to 20 mg/kg/d is given in four divided doses (max 4 g/d).

Toxicokinetics

Peak blood levels of 0.1 to 1.9 μg/mL are obtained 3 to 4 hours after a single oral therapeutic dose; levels of 3 to 10 μg follow 1 hour after a single intravenous dose. Erythromycin is about 60% plasma protein bound. Up to 4.5% of an oral dose and 15% of an intravenous dose are recoverable in the urine, but elimination is mainly by biliary excretion of the intact drug. The half-life of the drug is 1.5 hours. The drug is not significantly removed by hemodialysis or peritoneal dialysis. It is excreted in breast milk and transferred across the placenta.[23]

Drug Interactions

Erythromycin can interact with many other drugs through the cytochrome P450 enzyme system. It can increase blood levels of fentanyl, carbamazepine, clozapine, colchicine, cyclosporine, digoxin, ergotamine, midazolam, nadolol, theophylline, triazolam, valproic acid, vinblastine, and warfarin. Concomitant use of erythromycin with astemizole or terfenadine is associated with serious ventricular arrhythmias, Torsade de pointes, and rash.[23]

Gastrointestinal Effects

Abdominal pain, cramps, nausea, vomiting, diarrhea, and flatulence are most frequently associated with both oral and intravenous erythromycin use and are dose related, especially with doses in excess of 4 g/d.

Following an ingestion of 5 g of Erythrocin (20 tablets of Erythrocin 250 mg), a 12-year-old developed acute pancreatitis. She became asymptomatic within 24 hours.[24] A 19-year-old girl ingested 20 erythromycin tablets and developed acute pancreatitis. She recovered.[25]

Cardiovascular Effects

QT prolongation and Torsade de pointes may occur with intravenous administration of erythromycin (Table 14–4). In patients with an underlying cardiac disease the arrhythmia is successfully treated by discontinuing the infusion and giving intravenous lidocaine; fatalities have occurred in seriously ill elderly patients and in premature newborns. QT prolongation can last as long as 4 days after stopping the drug. Susceptibility seems to be related to electrolyte alterations (hypokalemia, hypocalcemia, hypomagnesemia), myocardial ischemia, left ventricular dysfunction, hepatic dysfunction or immaturity, concomitant use of antiarrhythmic agents or other drugs with cardioactive properties (class IA and III antiarrhythmic agents such as amiodarone, disopyramide, flecainide, quinidine, and sotalol; antimicrobial agents such as pentamidine and co-trimoxazole; psychotropic medications like haloperidol, trazadone, and tricyclic antidepressants; antihistaminic agents such as astemizole and terfenadine), and idiopathic prolonged QT interval syndrome. Erythromycin may itself cause action potential prolongation by altering sodium channel function, similar to class IA and III antiarrhythmic agents.[26–29] Hypotension may be observed after both intravenous and oral administration.

Hepatic Effects

Cholestatic hepatitis is described in adults taking the drug for more than 2 weeks. A reversible hepatotoxicity has also been described with erythromycin stearate and erythromycin ethylsuccinate. Fever, rash, and eosinophilia may be observed. The hepatitis generally improves within days of stopping the drug.

Transient Hearing Loss

Ototoxicity is rarely associated with large oral or intravenous doses of erythromycin, more commonly in elderly patients with renal failure, and is apparently related to high serum concentrations of the drug.

Allergic Reactions

Skin rash, Stevens–Johnson syndrome, fixed drug eruptions, and eosinophilia have occasionally been described.

Table 14–4
Adverse Cardiac Effects of Erythromycin Lactobionate Reported to the U.S. Food and Drug Administration

Domestic Reports	Foreign Reports
Prolonged QT interval	Ventricular arrhythmia
Ventricular tachycardia	Electrocardiographic abnormality
Arrhythmia	Prolonged QR interval
Premature ventricular contractions	Ventricular tachycardia
Nodal bradycardia	
Heart arrest	

From Farrar HC, Walsh-Sukys MC, Kyllonen K, Blumer JL, eds. Cardiac toxicity associated with intravenous erythromycin lactobionate: Two case reports and a review of the literature. Pediatr Infect Dis J 1993;12:688–691.

Treatment

Activated charcoal probably is useful in reducing the amount of drug absorbed after an oral overdose, but its role in altering outcome is unknown.

Intravenous erythromycin should be infused over at least 60 minutes, with cardiovascular monitoring in premature newborns and patients with cardiovascular disease. If QT prolongation or any form of ventricular arrhythmias is detected, the infusion should be promptly discontinued. Patients with erythromycin-associated QT prolongation and ventricular arrhythmias or hypotension could possibly benefit by the administration (intravenous push) of 1 mEq/kg sodium bicarbonate to raise the blood pH to 7.45 to 7.50, to be followed by infusion of 0.5 to 1 mEq/kg/h to maintain blood pH at the desired level until the patient stabilizes and arrhythmias cease. Lidocaine (1 mg/kg intravenous bolus) would be the drug of choice for erythromycin-induced ventricular tachycardia or fibrillation. In the group of patients with Torsade de pointes, magnesium sulfate is the drug of choice. The adult dose is 2 g as an intravenous bolus in unstable patients (max 5–10 g) or over 1 to 5 minutes in stable patients.[23]

QUINOLONES AND FLUOROQUINOLONES

Quinolones are antimicrobial agents. Nalidixic acid is a quinolone approved for use in the United States.

Fluoroquinolones are broad-spectrum antiinfective agents active against a wide range of aerobic Gram-positive and Gram-negative organisms. Norfloxacin, ciprofloxacin, and ofloxacin are the fluoroquinolones that have been approved for use in the United States.

The quinolones and fluoroquinolones may induce undesirable effects relating to the gastrointestinal tract and central nervous system. Infrequent allergic reactions and cartilage erosions in weight-bearing joints have been reported.[30]

Structure and Classification

Quinolones exhibiting antibacterial activity contain a 4-quinolone nucleus with a —N at position 1, a —COOH at position 3, and a =O (ketone) at position 4.[31–34]

Subgroups

- Quinolines with carbons at position 2 and 8 (ciprofloxacin, norfloxacin, ofloxacin, pefloxacin)
- Quinolines with a nitrogen at position 2 and carbon at position 8 (cinoxacin)
- Naphthyridine derivatives containing a carbon at position 2 and a nitrogen at position 8 of the 4-quinolone nucleus (enoxacin, nalidixic acid)
- Fluoroquinolones containing a fluorine atom at position 6 of the 4-quinolone nucleus, providing expanded antibacterial activity (ciprofloxacin, enoxacin, norfloxacin, ofloxacin, pefloxacin)

Table 14–5
Pharmacokinetic Properties of Some Fluoroquinolones

Property	Norfloxacin	Ciprofloxacin	Ofloxacin	Pefloxacin	Enoxacin	Temafloxacin
Oral dose (mg)	400	500	400	400	600	600
Peak levels (μg/mL)	1.5	2.5	5.5	4.0	4.0	6.0
Absorption (%)	35–70	75–85	70–80	80–95	80–90	90
Protein binding (%)	15	20–40	10–20	20–30	30–40	26
Urinary recovery (%)	25	30	90	5	60	65
Half-life						
Hours	4	4	7	8–12	6	7–8
C_{cr} <10 mL/min/1.73 m^2	8	10	30	12–15	9.4	>10

C_{cr}, creatinine clearance.
From Walker RC, Wright AJ. The fluoroquinolones. Mayo Clin Proc 1991;66:1249–1259.

Therapeutic Dose

The following dosages are for adults:

Ciprofloxacin	500 mg q12h as required
Nalidixic acid	1 g qid for 1–2 wk
Norfloxacin	400 mg q12h
Ofloxacin	400 mg q12h

Toxicokinetics

The pharmacokinetic properties of some fluoroquinolones are listed in Table 14–5.

Drug Interactions

Drug interactions of fluoroquinolones are summarized in Table 14–6. Quinolones interact with antacids, H_2 antagonists, nonsteroidal antiinflammatory drugs, theophylline, and warfarin.[32,33]

Ofloxacin, nalidixic acid, ciprofloxacin, and norfloxacin potentiate effects by displacing warfarin from albumin binding sites, inhibiting the hepatic metabolism of warfarin and possibly suppressing vitamin K-producing gut bacteria. Bleeding may be precipitated by concomitant use of warfarin with the quinolones.[35]

Table 14–6
Fluoroquinolone Drug Interactions

Drug	Fluoroquinolone*	Comment
Antacids	Norfloxacin, ciprofloxacin, enoxacin, ofloxacin	Decreased absorption with Mg–Al antacids by chelation
H_2 antagonists	Enoxacin, pefloxacin, ciprofloxacin	Decreased metabolism by hepatic cytochrome P450 system
Nonsteroidal antiinflammatory drugs	Enoxacin	Central nervous system excitation, convulsions; synergistic inhibition of γ-aminobutyric acid binding
Theophylline	Enoxacin, ciprofloxacin, pefloxacin, norfloxacin, ofloxacin†	Effect on cytochrome P450, causing raised plasma theophylline concentration
Warfarin	Norfloxacin, ofloxacin, ciprofloxacin	Increase in prothrombin time

*In rank order of reported magnitude of effect.
†At higher than normal dosage only.
From Paton JH, Reeves DS. Clinical features and management of adverse effects of quinolone antibacterials. Drug Saf 1991;6:8–27; erratum: Drug Saf 1991;6:338E.

Pregnancy/Lactation

Ciprofloxacin, ofloxacin, and pefloxacin have not yet been proved safe for the fetus. The fluoroquinolones have been placed in FDA Pregnancy Category C. All three cross the placenta and produce high concentrations in breast milk.[36] Ofloxacin administered in a dose of 200 mg twice daily for 6 days during the 19th week of gestation led to the normal birth of a full-term infant with no teratogenic abnormalities.[37]

Clinical Presentation
Chronic Use (Quinolones)

Immunologic Reactions. Hypersensitivity vasculitis, rashes, hypersensitivity pneumonitis, anaphylaxis, and anaphylactoid reactions have been observed with the quinolones. Some preliminary data indicate that pefloxacin and ciprofloxacin may decrease interleukin-1 production.

Photosensitivity. Photosensitivity may be a phototoxic, nonimmunologic reaction or a photoallergic, immunodependent reaction.

Hematologic Effects. Thrombocytopenia, hemolytic anemia, and leukopenia have been associated with quinolone administration.

Gastrointestinal Effects. Gastrointestinal effects are the most common adverse effect of the quinolones and include, in descending order, nausea, abdominal discomfort, vomiting, and diarrhea. Colitis associated with *Clostridium difficile* toxin has been reported.

Nephrotoxicity. Renal failure, hematuria with red blood cell casts, and crystalluria have been observed. Quinolone-induced crystals have little toxicologic consequences for the kidneys with doses up to 1000 mg for ciprofloxacin, nalidixic acid, norfloxacin, and ofloxacin. Other causes of crystalluria are listed in Table 14–7.

Metabolic Abnormalities. Lactic acidosis and pseudoglycosuria (see Ciprofloxacin) have been observed with the quinolones.

Arthropathy. Arthralgic effects have been reported in children, but the data do not support evidence of permanent damage to the joints.

Central Nervous System Effects. Benign intracranial hypertension, seizures, and organic psychosis have been described and may be a result of blockade of synaptic inhibition mediated by γ-aminobutyric acid.

Neuromuscular Effects. Acute painful proximal myopathy has been associated with nalidixic acid. Increased muscle weakness in myasthenia gravis has followed use of ciprofloxacin.[37–42]

Other Effects

The quinolones have been associated with a variety of nonspecific neurotoxic reactions, for example, seizures, depression, dizziness, euphoria, insomnia, and altered color vision. Such reactions are possibly mediated by inhibition of γ-aminobutyric acid postsynaptic binding sites.

Cross-reactivity between quinolones is manifested by type I hypersensitivity reactions, including generalized urticaria and angioedema.[43]

• NALIDIXIC ACID

Nalidixic acid (NegGram), the first quinolone antibacterial agent, was introduced in 1963. As a result of its narrow antibacterial spectrum, frequent development of resistance, poor absorption from the gastrointestinal tract, and relatively high incidence of side effects, use of nalidixic acid has been limited to lower urinary tract infection caused by a few susceptible bacteria.[44] Acute toxicity resulting from overdose of nalidixic acid continues to be reported and is characterized by vomiting, seizures, hyperglycemia, benign intracranial hypertension, behavior disturbance, and metabolic acidosis.[44–48]

Toxicokinetics

Nalidixic acid is absorbed almost entirely from the gastrointestinal tract, with peak plasma concentrations of 20 to 50 µg/mL reported 2 hours after 1 g has been ingested. It is 90% protein bound, has an elimination half-life of 1 to 2 hours, and is excreted as both the parent compound (5%) and the active metabolite hydroxynalidixic acid (95%). Therapeutic serum levels normally total 15 to 50 µg/mL (nalidixic acid plus hydroxynalidixic acid concentrations).[49] Carboxynalidixic acid may be found in the plasma.[50] Serum levels associated with diminished consciousness and metabolic acidosis in an adult on admission were 297 µg/mL for nalidixic acid and 100 µg/mL for hydroxynalidixic acid.[49] Nalidixic acid has a molecular weight of 232.

Drug Interactions

Simultaneous use of probenecid may increase the serum level of nalidixic acid.[49]

Toxic Dose

An adult ingested 32 g and survived.[50] Nalidixic acid and hydroxynalidixic acid are rapidly excreted after rapid metabolism to inactive glucuronide and dicarboxylic acid derivatives; nearly all of a dose is excreted within 24 hours. Trace amounts appear in the breast milk and trace amounts cross the placenta.[51]

Laboratory

Nalidixic acid may cause false-positive reactions in urine tests for glucose when a copper reduction glucose test is used.

Treatment

Treatment is symptomatic and supportive. If overdosage has occurred less than 2 hours before admission to a health care facility, gastric lavage may reduce possible additional absorption. Seizures can be treated with diazepam. Patients usually recover well enough to be discharged within 24 to 48 hours. There are no available or necessary antidotes, and enhancement of elimination with activated charcoal, cathartics, or extracorporeal methods has not been studied or required.

• TEMOFLOXACIN

Temofloxacin was withdrawn from distribution by the manufacturer after reports of deaths, hemolytic anemia, other hematologic abnormalities, renal failure, hepatic dysfunction, and anaphylaxis.[52]

• CIPROFLOXACIN

Ciprofloxacin, a fluorinated quinolone derivative, is an antibiotic that, in overdose, causes acute renal failure. Treatment is symptomatic and supportive.

Table 14–7
Drugs That Induce Crystalluria

Massive Ingestions	Therapeutic Doses
Primidone	Aspirin
Sulfonamides	Phenacetin
Methotrexate	Sulfonamide
Amoxicillin	Antihistamines
Cephalexin	Ethylene glycol
Ampicillin	Ciprofloxacin

Structure and Classification

Ciprofloxacin is 1-cyclopropyl-6-fluoro-1,4-dihydro-4-oxo-7-(1-piperazinyl)-3-quinolone carboxylic acid. It is a quinolone carboxylic acid derivative, a fluorinated quinolone antibiotic structurally similar to other quinolones including nalidixic acid, cinoxacin, enoxacin, norfloxacin, ofloxacin, and pefloxacin.[53]

On the basis of their spectra of antibacterial activity and pharmacokinetic properties, the 4-quinolone group, derivatives of the original 1,8-naphthyridine agent nalidixic acid, can be subdivided into four classes of compounds:[54]

1. Nalidixic acid
2. Cinoxacin, oxolinic acid, and flumequine
3. Pipemidic acid, norfloxacin
4. Ciprofloxacin, ofloxacin, pefloxacin, enoxacin (These have in common 6-fluoryl, 7-piperazinyl nuclear side chain substitutions, can be taken orally, and have broad-spectrum antibacterial activity.)

Use

Ciprofloxacin is a synthetic antibacterial agent available for oral use in tablets of 250, 500, and 750 mg (Cipro). Ciprofloxacin is effective in treating infections of the upper and lower respiratory tract, urinary tract, gastrointestinal tract, skin, and soft tissues and in osteomyelitis.[55]

Therapeutic Dose

The usual adult dose of ciprofloxacin, depending on the severity of urinary tract infection, is 250 to 500 mg every 12 hours. Doses of 500 to 750 mg orally every 12 hours have been used for other infections. Use of more than 1500 mg/d is not advised.

Toxic Dose

A 33-year-old adult ingested 18.75 g of ciprofloxacin and 25 g of pristinamycin. Fibroscopy showed gastric ulceration. A renal biopsy disclosed a tubular necrosis. The serum creatinine rose on day 4; the serum ciprofloxacin concentration was 3 mg/L. The patient was hemodialyzed and recovered. Acute renal failure has been reported after an overdose with 14 g of ciprofloxacin.[56,57]

Fatal Dose

No lethal dose of ciprofloxacin in humans has been reported.

Toxicokinetics[49,58–61]

Bioavailability	70%
Peak plasma level	1.6–2.8 µg/mL (after 500 mg orally)
Time to peak plasma level	1.0–1.5 hours
Volume of distribution	2.1–3.5 L/kg
Plasma protein binding	16–43%
Elimination half-life	3.5–5.0 hours
Excreted unchanged	15–50%
Active metabolites	Four active metabolites

Drug Interactions

Ciprofloxacin, like enoxacin, inhibits theophylline metabolism at the cytochrome P450 site, resulting in a decrease in theophylline clearance.[61,62] Aluminum- and magnesium-containing antacids and calcium-, iron-, and zinc-containing compounds may decrease ciprofloxacin absorption.[50,63] Crystalluria may follow use of ciprofloxacin with alkalinizing agents[61] (Table 14–7). Probenecid interferes with renal tubular secretion of ciprofloxacin, resulting in a 50% decrease in renal ciprofloxacin clearance, a 50% increase in systemic ciprofloxacin concentration, and a prolonged serum half-life of the drug. Ciprofloxacin may increase caffeine[64] and warfarin[65] serum levels and may increase central nervous system side effects of nonsteroidal antiinflammatory agents. Ciprofloxacin infusions are physically incompatible with heparin and furosemide.[66]

Pregnancy/Lactation

It is not known whether ciprofloxacin crosses the placenta. It is distributed into human milk.[61] Quinolones may damage growing cartilage and epiphyses of long bones, and therefore, are not used in patients less than 18 years of age or in pregnant or nursing women.

Clinical Presentation

Overdose

Overdose with ciprofloxacin may induce acute renal failure, crystalluria, nausea, arthralgias, and possibly gastric ulcer.[67,68] Hepatic failure has been reported.[69]

Chronic Use

Neurologic Effects. All fluoroquinolones are γ-aminobutyric acid inhibitors and may cause seizures.[67,68,70] Myasthenia gravis may be exacerbated following ciprofloxacin use.[71] Benign intracranial hypertension has been described.[72] Reversible visual loss has followed large doses.[73]

Anaphylactic Reactions. Fatal anaphylactic reactions have been reported in AIDS-related complex when oral ciprofloxacin was used.[64,74]

Renal Effects. Interstitial nephritis and acute renal failure have followed ciprofloxacin use.[75–78]

Laboratory

Analytical Methods

A high-performance liquid chromatographic method using fluorescence detection is available for quantitation of ciprofloxacin in human plasma, whole blood, and erythrocytes. The limit of detection for ciprofloxacin is 25 ng/mL. The method appears suitable for therapeutic drug monitoring.[79]

Blood Levels

One day after ingestion of 21,000 mg of ciprofloxacin (28 750-mg ciprofloxacin tablets), the serum ciprofloxacin level was 3 µg/mL.[79]

Abnormalities

Eosinophilia, neutropenia, and elevated levels of serum transaminase activity and creatinine have been reported.[80]

Ancillary Tests

Ciprofloxacin may induce a pseudoglycosuria when tested with the BM-Test-7 (Boehringer-Mannheim), which is based on a specific glucose oxidase/peroxidase reaction. This may be due to a metabolite as direct testing with ciprofloxacin is negative.[81]

Treatment

Stabilization and Gut Decontamination

Syrup of ipecac is not advised for treatment of an overdose, as peak blood levels are reached within 1 hour and there is also the danger of intervening seizures. Gastric lavage may be useful within the first 2 hours of ingestion, but should be accompanied by tracheal protection to avoid early seizure-induced aspiration pneumonitis. There is no evidence that activated charcoal or cathartics are effective.

Elimination Enhancement

The high volume of distribution tends to diminish the effectiveness of hemodialysis or hemoperfusion.

Antidote

There are no antidotes.

Supportive Measures

Seizures. Seizures can be treated with diazepam, phenytoin, and other anticonvulsant drugs.

Renal Dysfunction. Careful periodic evaluation of renal function (urinalysis for crystalluria, serum creatinine, blood urea nitrogen) is indicated. Adequate hydration (intravenous fluids) with careful measurement of fluid intake and output should be instituted. Steroid therapy may ameliorate an interstitial nephritis as well as the arthralgias.

• OFLOXACIN

Ofloxacin is a fluoroquinolone antimicrobial agent that has a propensity to induce symptoms and signs of central nervous system irritability in both therapeutic and toxic doses. The blood level correlates with the clinical course. Treatment is symptomatic and supportive. The prognosis is good for complete recovery after an overdose. No fatalities have been reported after an overdose.

Therapeutic Dose

The usual dosage for ofloxacin is 200 to 400 mg orally every 12 hours for 7 to 14 days.[82,83]

Toxic Dose

A 26-year-old woman inadvertently was administered 4000 mg of ofloxacin intravenously instead of 400 mg. She survived.[84] A 14-year-old ingested an unknown amount of ofloxacin and survived.[85]

Fatal Dose

A fatal dose has not been reported.

Toxicokinetics

The toxicokinetics of ofloxacin are similar to those of the other fluoroquinolones[86] (Table 14–5).

Drug Interactions

Ofloxacin does not interact with ranitidine, cyclosporine, clindamycin, metronidazole, theophylline, or caffeine. Other fluoroquinolones, notably enoxacin, can undergo a marked interaction with these drugs. Quinolones chelate with alkaline earth and transition metal cations, and should not be administered with antacids containing calcium, magnesium, or aluminum, with sucralfate, with divalent or trivalent cations such as iron, or with multivitamins containing zinc. These substances may reduce absorption and plasma concentrations of ofloxacin.[82,83]

Pregnancy/Lactation

Although ofloxacin may be found in breast milk and can pass through the placenta, few reports are available of its use in pregnancy.[56]

Clinical Presentation

Therapeutic Use

Psychotoxic effects including hallucinations, agitation, confusion, headaches, vertigo, depression, visual and olfactory disturbances, ataxia, tremor, paresthesias, anxiety, and insomnia have been reported in about 2 to 4% of patients treated with ofloxacin.[84,85] Seizures occur rarely. Involvement of γ-aminobutyric acidergic and dopaminergic mechanisms has been suggested. Patients with a history of psychiatric disease seem to be at a higher risk of developing psychotoxic effects after ofloxacin. Hepatitis has been observed.[87] Tendon ruptures have followed ofloxacin use.[88]

Overdose

Ofloxacin overdose may be followed by nausea, vomiting, grand mal seizures, anosmia, vertigo, dysgeusia due to cranial nerve involvement, and multiple manifestations of drug-induced psychosis.[89,90] Such symptoms and signs have been associated with an ofloxacin plasma level of 15 μg/mL 12 hours after ingestion. Simultaneous ingestion of anticholinergic agents and production of anticholinergic symptoms together with some psychotic symptoms may be relieved after use of physostigmine.[85,91,92]

Laboratory

Analytical Methods

Ofloxacin is identified in the urine by gas chromatography/ mass spectrometry and in the plasma by high-performance liquid chromatography.[85]

Blood Levels

A serum sample obtained 15 minutes after completion of an infusion of 3 g of ofloxacin revealed an ofloxacin level of 39.3 μg/mL. In 7 hours the level fell to 16.2 μg/mL, and in 24 hours, to 2.7 μg/mL.[85] Following ingestion of an unknown amount of ofloxacin, the plasma levels were 15 μg/mL at 12 hours and 0.2 μg/mL at 24 hours.[85]

Abnormalities

Urinalysis, blood count and differential, electrolytes, hepatic enzymes, uric acid, and creatinine remain within normal limits after an ofloxacin overdose.[84] Transient increases in transaminase levels, eosinophilia, leukopenia, and hematuria have been observed.[47]

Treatment

Stabilization

Patients who have ingested an ofloxacin overdose should be observed for 12 to 24 hours. Treatment is largely symptomatic and supportive.

Gut Decontamination

Agitation may make gastric lavage difficult. Activated charcoal has been employed with a favorable recovery.[85]

Elimination Enhancement

Ofloxacin is eliminated, usually 15 to 25%, by hemodialysis during the first 2 hours of dialysis,[55] but this procedure is rarely required after an ofloxacin overdose.

Antidote

There is no antidote.

TRIMETHOPRIM AND TRIMETHOPRIM–SULFAMETHOXAZOLE

Trimethoprim is an antiinfective that has been used alone and in combination with sulfamethoxazole (TMP–SMX) for synergistic action as an antibacterial agent.[93] Both trimethoprim and TMP–SMX are rarely involved in an overdose. There have been no fatalities from overdose with either product.

Structure and Classification

Trimethoprim is 5-(3,4,5-trimethoxybenzyl) pyrimidine-2,4-diamine. It has a molecular weight of 290.3. Trimethoprim is a dihydrofolate reductase inhibitor.

Trimethoprim may be combined with sulfamethoxazole (Co-Trimoxazole). Sulfamethoxazole is an antibacterial sulfonamide. The commercial product contains a 5 : 1 ratio of sulfamethoxazole to trimethoprim.[94,95]

Use

Trimethoprim and TMP–SMX are used for the treatment of urinary tract infections, *Pneumocystis carinii* pneumonia, enteritis due to susceptible strains of *Shigella flexneri* or *Shigella sonnei,* otitis media, bronchitis, infection in granulocytopenic patients, and, occasionally, *Nocardia* infections.[94,95]

Therapeutic Dose

Trimethoprim is administered in doses of 100 mg every 12 hours. TMP–SMX is administered in doses of 2 tablets every 12 hours (equivalent to trimethoprim 160 mg every 12 hours).[93,95]

Toxic Dose

Trimethoprim has been ingested in an overdose of 8000 mg. The patient survived.[96] TMP–SMX 20 tablets was accidentally administered at one time.[5] The patient was hospitalized and discharged in 2 days.

Fatal Dose

There is no known lethal dose of trimethoprim or TMP–SMX.

Toxicokinetics

Absorption

Trimethoprim is readily and almost completely absorbed from the gastrointestinal tract.[93] A peak serum concentration of about 1 μg/mL is reached 1 to 4 hours after an oral dose. Trimethoprim is 40 to 70% bound to plasma proteins. Steady-state serum concentrations of 1.2 to 3.2 μg/mL follow trimethoprim 160 mg every 12 hours. TMP–SMX is rapidly and well absorbed from the gastrointestinal tract. A single dose of trimethoprim 160 mg and sulfamethoxazole 800 mg produces peak serum concentrations of 1 to 2 μg/mL trimethoprim and 36 to 40 μg/mL sulfamethoxazole in 1 to 4 hours. Sulfamethoxazole is 66% bound to plasma proteins. Sulfamethoxazole crosses the placenta and is distributed into breast milk.[97–100]

Distribution

The apparent volume of distribution for trimethoprim is about 1.4 L/kg, and that of sulfamethoxazole is 0.14 L/kg.[94]

Elimination

From 10 to 30% of trimethoprim is metabolized in the liver to oxide and hydroxylated metabolites. Sulfamethoxazole is also metabolized in the liver, where it is acetylated and conjugated with glucuronic acid. About 40 to 60% of trimethoprim and 20% of sulfamethoxazole is excreted as unchanged drug. The elimination half-life of trimethoprim is 8 to 11 hours, and that of sulfamethoxazole, 10 to 13 hours. The total clearance of trimethoprim is 0.12 L/h/kg.[100,101]

Drug Interactions

Trimethoprim appears to inhibit the hepatic metabolism of phenytoin. It also decreases the renal clearance of procainamide.[102] TMP–SMX should be used with caution with methotrexate, as sulfonamides can displace methotrexate from plasma protein binding sites.

Pregnancy/Lactation

Trimethoprim readily crosses the placenta and is found in breast milk.[95] Sulfamethoxazole also crosses the placenta and appears in breast milk.

Clinical Presentation

Overdose

Trimethoprim poisoning has been characterized by nausea, vomiting, headache, swollen face, epigastric pain, and weakness.[96] TMP–SMX may produce nausea, vomiting, diarrhea, mental confusion, facial swelling, headache, bone marrow depression, and a slight rise in levels of serum transaminases.[97]

Chronic Use

Deaths following TMP–SMX ingestion have been due to drug-induced hemolytic anemia and toxic epidermal necrolysis.[103,104] Trimethoprim alone or with sulfamethoxazole can induce an increased creatinine concentration and renal failure.[105]

Laboratory

Analytical Methods

Trimethoprim may be quantitated in the serum by a high-performance liquid chromatographic (HPLC) method; the limit of detection is 0.2 μg/mL.[106] Simultaneous measurement of trimethoprim and sulfamethoxazole is available with the use of HPLC with sensitivity limits of 0.02 and 0.2 μg/mL, respectively.[107]

Blood Levels

The serum trimethoprim concentration after ingestion of 8000 mg was 19.6 μg/mL. This is about 20 times higher than that observed after a single dose of 200 mg.[96] A suicide following trimethoprim overdose had a blood level of 133 μg/mL postmortem.[108] It is unclear what dose of trimethoprim was ingested.

Abnormalities

Serum transaminase levels may be elevated after overdose with trimethoprim.

Treatment

Stabilization

For most patients with trimethoprim or TMP–SMX overdose, symptomatic and supportive treatment is indicated. Patients require hematologic monitoring.

Gut Decontamination

Gastric emptying, if performed within a few hours of ingestion, may aid in removing some of the drug and prevent rapid induction of toxic serum levels. Activated charcoal has been used,[96] but its efficacy, as well as that of cathartics, has not been studied.

Elimination Enhancement

Acidification of the urine may enhance the elimination of trimethoprim but is generally not recommended.[94] Hemodialysis may remove only moderate amounts of trimethoprim in view of its protein binding and large volume of distribution.[101]

Antidote

There are no antidotes. Leucovorin has not been studied.

Supportive Measures

Patients should be hospitalized where cardiac monitoring, intravenous fluids, and oxygen, if required, are available. Hematologic evaluation should be performed including a bone marrow study according to clinical judgment. Seizures can be treated with diazepam. Electrolytes should be determined and replaced together with adequate fluid replacement. Patients should be followed for any evidence of hematologic depression both in hospital and as outpatients in the following weeks. If patients are asymptomatic and able to eat without difficulty, they can be discharged to be followed as outpatients.

VANCOMYCIN

Vancomycin is a bactericidal glycopeptide antibiotic which may induce acute renal failure when administered in an overdose. It is known to be associated with sensorineural hearing loss.

Use

Intravenous vancomycin hydrochloride is used in the treatment of potentially life-threatening infections and antibiotic-associated pseudomembranous colitis produced by *Clostridium difficile*.[109]

Therapeutic Dose

Intravenous Dose

For adults (with normal renal function), 500 mg every 6 hours or 1 g every 12 hours is administered; for neonates and young children, an initial intravenous dose of 15 mg/kg is followed by 10 mg/kg every 12 hours in neonates younger than 8 days of age and 10 mg/kg every 8 hours in infants 8 days to 1 month of age. Older children receive 40 mg/kg daily in divided dosage.

Oral Dose

For adults, the oral dose is 0.5 to 2 g daily in three or four divided doses, and for children, 40 mg/kg daily in divided doses not to exceed 2 g/d.[109]

Toxic Dose

An adult who received 1 g every 4 hours, a total of 56 g intravenously over 10 days, developed acute renal failure and survived.[110] A 47-day-old premature infant inadvertently received three 12-mg doses of intravenous vancomycin and six 240-mg doses, and survived.[111]

Fatal Dose

A lethal dose has not been established.

Toxicokinetics

Absorption

Minimal absorption of vancomycin follows oral administration. The serum concentration following an intravenous dose reaches a peak of 15 μg/mL in 2 hours.[109]

Distribution

The apparent volume of distribution at steady state is 0.39 to 0.92 L/kg. Protein binding has been reported to be 10 to 82%.[112]

Elimination

Intravenous vancomycin is excreted 80 to 100% unchanged in the urine in the first 24 hours.[112] The elimination half-life is 3 to 10 hours. Total body clearance averages 1 to 3 mL/min/kg. In infants of gestational age less than 36 weeks, total body clearance was 1.07 mL/min/kg and the volume of distribution at steady state was 0.48 L/kg.[113]

Drug Interactions

Patients receiving concurrent vancomycin and aminoglycoside antibiotics are at substantial risk of having a nephrotoxic reaction.[114] Other antibiotics such as amphotericin B, bacitracin, cisplatin, colistin, and polymyxin B, given systemically or topically, may add to the toxicity.[115] Intravenous vancomycin IV enhances the neuromuscular blockade of vecuronium.[116]

Pregnancy/Lactation

Vancomycin has not been systematically studied in pregnant women or lactating mothers. One study in 10 pregnant women suggests that vancomycin use during the second and third trimesters of pregnancy does not produce sensorineural hearing loss or nephrotoxicity in the infant.[116] Methodologic problems require clarification, however, in further studies on the nephrotoxicity of vancomycin in newborns.[117]

Clinical Presentation

Overdose

Vancomycin in overdose may cause oliguria and acute renal failure.[110,111] Rapid intravenous administration may induce cardiopulmonary arrest.[118]

Chronic Use

Vancomycin use may commonly (up to 90%)[119] result in the *red man syndrome* or *red neck syndrome* characterized by hypotension or by pruritus and an erythematous rash or flushing over the face, neck, upper chest, and arms. Red man syndrome may involve histamine release. Basophil histamine release tests will confirm an IgE-mediated reaction to vancomycin.[120] Its severity can be related to the dose of vancomycin, rate of injection, or amount of endogenous histamine released.[121] It can be prevented by giving each intravenous infusion over a period of at least 60 minutes.[122] Red man syndrome has also followed intravenous infusions of teicoplanin,[123] erythromycin,[124] and rifampin (Table 14–8).

Nephrotoxicity, a sensorineural hearing loss, toxic epidermal necrolysis, *Clostridium difficile* colitis, and hematologic depression (leukopenia, neutropenia, thrombocytopenia)[125] have followed vancomycin use.[126–128]

Table 14–8
Differential Diagnosis of Red Man Syndrome

Cutaneous Reddish-Orange Pigmentation
Histamine release
- Rapid infusion of vancomycin
- Drug-induced hypersensitivity reactions

Drugs and chemical agents
- Quinacrine hydrochloride, dinitrophenol
- Saffron, picric acid
- Clofazimine

Lycopenemia (excessive ingestion of vegetables with red-colored carotenoid pigment)
- Tomatoes
- Beets
- Chili beans

Suntanning aids
- Canthaxanthin

Erythroderma
- Atopic dermatitis
- Psoriasis
- Seborrheic dermatitis
- Numular dermatitis
- Mycosis fungoides

Select Causes of Yellow to Yellow-Orange Cutaneous Pigmentation
Carotenemia (excessive ingestion of yellow vegetables) oranges, squash, spinach, yellow corn, beans, carrots, eggs, butter, pumpkins, rutabagas (Swede turnips), papaya, sweet potatoes, yellow turnips)
Jaundice (eg, viral hepatitis)
Hypothyroidism
Uremia
Diabetes mellitus

From Holdiness MR. Neurological manifestations and toxicities of the antituberculosis drugs: A review. Med Toxicol 1987;2:33–51.

Laboratory

Analytical Methods

A high-performance liquid chromatography method is available that is sensitive to 1 μg/mL.[129]

Blood Levels

A patient with acute renal failure following vancomycin ingestion was found to have a serum vancomycin level of 284 μg/mL. Following treatment with continuous arteriovenous hemofiltration, the blood level fell to 140 μg/mL and, later, to below 50 μg/mL.[100] Overdose in an infant led to a peak vancomycin level of 427 μg/mL (peak therapeutic level, 30–50 μg/mL). Levels before and after a 1.5-volume exchange transfusion were 230 μg/mL.[111]

Abnormalities

Serum levels of 25 to 100 μg/mL have been associated with ototoxicity. Contributing factors leading to ototoxicity are renal insufficiency, simultaneous use of other antibiotics, and a history of previous hearing loss.[130]

Ancillary Tests

Serial tests for hearing accuracy may indicate a sensorineural loss.

Treatment

Stabilization

Patients should be hospitalized where they can be monitored for fluid, balance, electrolytes, renal function, hearing function, and hematologic status, especially white blood cells and platelets.

Gut Decontamination

If vancomycin has been used orally, gastric emptying within the first 2 hours may lessen the absorption of vancomycin and reduce the rise in serum concentration of the antibiotic. Multidose activated charcoal may reduce the absorption of an overdose of vancomycin when ingested or administered intravenously.[111] There are no data on the use of cathartics or whole-bowel irrigation after an overdose of vancomycin.

Elimination Enhancement

Continuous arteriovenous hemofiltration may aid in reducing elevated serum levels of vancomycin.[110] Continuous arteriovenous hemofiltration may be effective. The drug is not appreciably removed by hemodialysis.

Antidote

There is no antidote.

Supportive Measures

Acute Renal Failure. Intake and output should be documented, serial serum creatinine levels determined, and urinalysis performed. Furosemide and dopamine may be used to increase urine flow.

Hearing Loss. The patient is followed with serial audiograms. An attempt is made to remove vancomycin with arteriovenous hemofiltration.

Red Man Syndrome. Hydroxyzine 50 mg administered 2 hours before a vancomycin infusion may be of value in mitigating the severity of symptoms.[122] If a second dose is required for a patient with first-dose red man syndrome, the second dose should be given over a period longer than 2 hours after pretreatment with an H_1 blocker. Close observation is mandatory. The infusion must be stopped if there is a clinically significant drop in blood pressure or the onset of chest or muscle pain.

Hematology. Total white blood cell count, neutrophils, and platelets should be followed both in hospital and for several weeks after discharge.

NEUROTOXICITY OF ANTIBACTERIAL THERAPY

Thomas has provided an extensive survey of the neurotoxicity of antibacterial therapy[131] (Tables 14–9 and 14–10). Penicillins, cephalosporins, quinolones, and carbopenems such as imipenem antagonize the inhibitory neurotransmitter γ-aminobutyric-acid. Isoniazid antagonizes and depletes pyridoxine. The optic nerve toxicity associated with ethambutol may be related to chelation of zinc. The neuromuscular syndromes associated with aminoglycosides, polymyxins, and tetracyclines have both presynaptic (eg, tobramycin) and postsynaptic (eg, netilmicin) components; decreasing calcium availability at the synapse or inhibiting transmembrane calcium currents may be important. The aminoglycosides and vancomycin are directly toxic to the cochleovestibular hair cells (toxicity is correlated with high concentrations in the perilymph surrounding the sensory end organs). Aminoglycosides interact with polyphosphoinositides in the hair cell membranes, resulting in the loss of magne-

Table 14–9
Peripheral Neurotoxicity of Antibacterial Therapy

Drug	Type	Comments
Chloramphenicol	S > M	Optic neuropathy more common Occurs only with prolonged use
Colistin	S	Not described with topical use
Dapsone	M	Slow acetylation predisposes Doses <200 mg/d generally safe.
Ethionamide	S	Resolution may take months
Isoniazid	S > M	Slow acetylation predisposes Pyridoxine prevents neurotoxicity
Metronidazole	S	Neurotoxic only with prolonged treatment
Nitrofurantoin	S, M	Avoid in renal failure

S, sensory; M, motor.
From Thomas RJ. Neurotoxicity of antibacterial therapy. South Med J 1994;87:869–874.

Table 14–10
Central Neurotoxicity of Antibacterial Therapy

Syndrome	Drugs
Seizures/encephalopathy/ organic brain syndrome	Bismuth
	Cephalosporins
	Cycloserine
	Erythromycin
	Imipenem–cilastatin
	Isoniazid
	Metronidazole
	Penicillins
	Quinolones
	Rifampin
Cerebellar ataxia	Metronidazole
Benign intracranial hypertension	Nalidixic acid
	Nitrofurantoin
	Tetracyclines
	Trimethoprim–sulfamethoxazole
Optic neuritis	Chloramphenicol
	Ethambutol
	Isoniazid
Cochleovestibular end-organ damage	Aminoglycosides
	Erythromycin
	Minocycline
	Vancomycin
Neuromuscular paralysis	Aminoglycosides
	Ampicillin (?)
	Clindamycin
	Erythromycin
	Polymyxins
	Tetracyclines
Aseptic meningitis	Trimethoprim–sulfamethoxazole

From Thomas RJ. Neurotoxicity of antibacterial therapy. South Med J 1994;87:869–874.

sium, which is necessary for a variety of enzymatic reactions.

Beta-lactam antibiotics may cause neurotoxicity early during clinical use, as shown by studies both in animal models and in vitro using the hippocampal slice mode. Intrathecal administration (eg, >10,000 U of benzyl penicillin daily) and topical application in experimental models are maximally epileptogenic. Risk factors for neurotoxicity are high-dose intravenous use (eg, >30 to 40 million U of benzyl penicillin per day), decreased renal function, abnormal blood–brain barrier, cardiopulmonary bypass, age greater than 50, preexisting disease of the central nervous system, concurrent use of drugs that may lower the seizure threshold (such as theophylline and ciprofloxacin), and concomitant use of nephrotoxic drugs.

Clinical manifestations have included myoclonus, seizures, confusion, hallucinations, encephalopathy, nystagmus, and agitation. Most of the clinically used agents, including benzyl penicillins, ampicillin, amoxicillin, oxacillin, nafcillin, carbenicillin, ticarcillin, piperacillin, cephaloridine, cephalothin, cefazolin, cefonicid, cephalexin, cefmetazole, cephacetrile, cefotaxime, cefuroxime, moxalactam, and imipenem–cilastatin, have been associated with neurotoxicity. Ceftazidime has been reported to cause hallucinations, confusion, encephalopathy, and absence status epilepticus. Ampicillin has been reported to aggravate weakness in myasthenia gravis. Spinal intrathecal beta-lactams have the potential to cause adhesive arachnoiditis. Such use today would be truly exceptional.

Figure 14–3 Clofazimine, 3-(*p*-chloroanilino)-10-(*p*-chlorophenyl)-2, 10-dihydro-2-(isopropylimino)-phenazine. (From Yawalkar SJ, Vischer W. Lamprene (clofazimine) in leprosy. Lepr Rev 1979; 50:135–144.)

LEPROSTATIC DRUGS

CLOFAZIMINE

Clofazimine (Lamprene, B663) is a substituted iminophenazine dye that has been used since 1962 as an antileprosy drug.[132] After prolonged use (months or years) it may lead to abdominal pain, anorexia, vomiting, diarrhea, and weight loss. Clofazimine crystals have been demonstrated in the gut wall tissue and mesenteric lymph nodes.[133] Prolonged use leads to a reddish pigmentation of the skin and viscera, with reddish coloration of the urine, stools, sputum, and sweat.[134] Death has followed development of serious gastrointestinal symptoms. Few overdoses have been reported. Treatment is symptomatic and supportive.

Structure and Classification

Clofazimine (Fig. 14–3) is 2-*p*-chloroanilino-5-*p*-chlorophenyl-3:5-dihydro-3-isopropyl-iminophenazine. It forms dark red crystalline prisms, which are insoluble in water, slightly soluble in ethanol, and soluble in dimethylsulfoxide.[135]

Use

Clofazimine is effective in the prevention and treatment of lepra—erythema nodosum leprosum—reactions and is also useful in the treatment of dapsone-resistant leprosy cases.[136]

Therapeutic Dose

Clofazimine is administered in a dose of 200 mg daily 6 days a week.[132]

Toxicokinetics[132,136,137]

Bioavailability	20%
Peak plasma level	0.5–1.0 μg/mL
Time to peak plasma level	8–12 hours
Elimination half-life	70 days
Excreted unchanged	0.1%

Drug Interactions

Urinary estrogen excretion decreases in pregnancy when clofazimine is administered. Clofazimine reduces rifampin absorption. Plasma levels of vitamin A appear to decrease with increased duration of treatment with clofazimine.[138]

Pregnancy/Lactation

Clofazimine crosses the placenta and is present in breast milk. Infants may be pigmented at birth or from ingesting the drug in maternal milk. Three neonatal deaths have been reported in three pregnancies in which clofazimine was used. The cause of death was not determined.[139]

Clinical Presentation

In general, clofazimine is well tolerated and virtually nontoxic.

Skin Effects

A reversible dose-related pink to brownish skin discoloration, especially on exposed parts, is the most commonly observed side effect of clofazimine. Discoloration of the sweat, hair, sputum, urine, and feces may occur.[140] A late syndrome, commencing some months or years on high dosage (>300 mg daily) with persistent diarrhea, loss of weight, and abdominal pain may lead to death. This syndrome is often associated with the deposition of clofazimine crystals in the submucosa of the small intestine and in the mesenteric lymph nodes. An eosinophilic enteritis has been described in a patient who received up to 600 mg/d for 3 years.[133]

Ocular Effects

A bull's-eye retinopathy has been described.[135] Conjunctival pigmentation was described in a patient who received more than 40 g of clofazimine in 5 months.[141] Generalized retinal degeneration has been observed in a patient with AIDS.[142,143]

Respiratory

Clofazimine crystals may be found within the cytoplasm of alveolar macrophages.[144]

Laboratory

Analytical Methods

A thin-layer chromatography method has a limit of detection of 5 ng/g.[145]

Blood Levels

Blood levels of clofazimine are most likely not available to the community hospital laboratory. This usually serves to confirm presence of the drug (if there is no history related to its use), but is probably not useful in treatment of an overdosage.

Ancillary Tests

Radiologic abnormalities of the small bowel, particularly the ileum, consist of alternating segments of constriction and dilation, cogency of the mucosa folds, and circumscribed "polypoid" areas.[146]

Treatment

Stabilization

Treatment of an overdose is more likely to be symptomatic and supportive. There are no antidotes. Gastric lavage may be useful within the first 6 to 8 hours of ingestion. There are no studies relating to enhancement of elimination of clofazimine.

Supportive Measures

In prolonged clofazimine administration, liver and kidney function tests and serum albumin and globulin and fasting blood sugar levels should be carried out at 3-month intervals. Periodic fundoscopic examination is advised (every 4 months) while the patient receives clofazimine.

ANTITUBERCULOSIS DRUGS

• ETHAMBUTOL

Ethambutol is a tuberculostatic agent, probably acting as an antimetabolite affecting RNA synthesis (Table 14–11). It is 75 to 80% absorbed, with a peak plasma level of 5 μg/mL after a dose of 25 mg/kg. About 80% of the drug and its inactive metabolites is excreted in the urine.[147] Therapeutic toxic effects are restricted largely to the nervous system. Retrobulbar neuritis, manifested by impaired visual acuity and color vision, is reported with dosages of 50 mg/kg/d. There may be constriction of visual fields. Blindness in the elderly has occurred with 15 mg/kg/d. Rarely, allergic reactions, gastrointestinal disturbance, and cholestatic jaundice may occur.[148] It is not used alone, either in the initial treatment or in re-treatment of tuberculosis. When used, it is given as a single oral dose of 15 mg/kg (7 mg/lb) body weight once every 24 hours.[149]

Acute overdosage symptoms include nausea, abdominal pain, fever, mental confusion, visual hallucinations, and optic neuropathy (retrobulbar neuritis) with doses greater than 10 g.[150] Four cases have been reported with no deaths.[151]

• ISONIAZID

Isoniazid (INH) is the cornerstone of the treatment of active tuberculosis as well as the drug of choice for prophylactic therapy of positive tuberculosis skin test reactions.[152–156]

When ingested in overdosage, it produces serious morbidity and mortality. Catastrophe may result from repetitive convulsions or from the massive amounts of sedation often employed to control seizures.[157] The clinical triad of INH overdose consists of repetitive seizures refractory to the usual anticonvulsants, metabolic acidosis often refractory to sodium bicarbonate, and coma.[158] The diagnosis of INH overdosage should be considered in any patient exhibiting otherwise unexplained metabolic acidosis and convulsions.[159] The drug of choice in the treatment of INH

Table 14–11
Some Antituberculosis Drugs

Drug	Adult Dosage (daily)	Pediatric Dosage (daily)	Main Adverse Effects
Isoniazid (INH)*,†	300 mg PO, IM	10–20 mg/kg (max 300 mg)	Hepatic toxicity, peripheral neuropathy
Rifampin*,‡ (Rifadin, Rimactane)	600 mg PO, IV	10–20 mg/kg (max 600 mg)	Hepatic toxicity, flulike syndrome
Pyrazinamide§	1.5–2.5 g PO	15–30 mg/kg (max 2 g)	Arthralgias, hepatic toxicity, hyperuricemia
Ethambutol‖ (Myambutol)	15–25 mg/kg PO	15–25 mg/kg PO	Optic neuritis
Streptomycin¶	15 mg/kg IM	20–30 mg/kg	Vestibular toxicity, renal damage
Combinations			
Rifamate (isoniazid 150 mg, rifampin 300 mg)	2 tablets	Not recommended	
Rifater (isoniazid 50 mg, rifampin 120 mg, pyrazinamide 300 mg)	≤44 kg: 4 tablets 45–54 kg: 5 tablets ≥55 kg: 6 tablets	Not recommended	
Second-Line Drugs			
Capreomycin (Capastat)	15 mg/kg IM	15–30 mg/kg	Auditory and vestibular toxicity, renal damage
Kanamycin (Kantrex and others)	15 mg/kg IM, IV	15–30 mg/kg	Auditory toxicity, renal damage
Amikacin (Amikin)	15 mg/kg IM, IV	15–30 mg/kg	Auditory toxicity, renal damage
Cycloserine# (Seromycin, and others)	250–500 mg bid PO	10–20 mg/kg	Psychiatric symptoms, seizures
Ethionamide (Trecator-SC)	250–500 mg bid PO	15–20 mg/kg	Gastrointestinal and hepatic toxicity, hypothyroidism
Ciprofloxacin (Cipro)	500–750 mg bid PO	Not recommended	Nausea, abdominal pain, restlessness, confusion
Ofloxacin (Floxin)	300–400 mg bid or 600–800 mg/d PO	Not recommended	Nausea, abdominal pain, restlessness, confusion
Aminosalicylic acid (PAS; Teebacin)	4–6 g bid PO	75 mg/kg bid	Gastrointestinal disturbance

*Intravenous preparations of isoniazid and rifampin are available.
†For intermittent use after a few weeks to months of daily therapy, dosage is 15 mg/kg (max 900 mg) twice/week for adults. Pyridoxine 10 to 25 mg should be given to prevent neuropathy in malnourished or pregnant patients and in those with HIV infection, alcoholism, or diabetes.
‡For intermittent use after a few weeks to months of daily therapy, dosage is 600 mg twice/week.
§For intermittent use after a few weeks to months of daily therapy, dosage is 2.5 to 3.5 g twice/week.
‖Usually not recommended for children less than 6 years old because visual acuity cannot be monitored. Some clinicians use 25 mg/kg/d during first 1 or 2 months or longer if organism is isoniazid-resistant. Decrease dosage if renal function diminished. For intermittent use after a few weeks to months of daily therapy, dosage is 50 mg/kg twice/week.
¶Available from Pfizer (800–254–4445) free of charge to physicians, clinics, or hospitals. When oral drugs are given daily, streptomycin is generally given 5 times per week (15 mg/kg or a maximum of 1 g per dose) for an initial 2- to 12-week period, and then (if needed) 2 to 3 times per week (20 to 30 mg/kg, or a maximum of 1.5 g, per dose). For patients >40 years old, dosage is reduced to 500 to 750 mg 5 times per week and 20 mg/kg when given twice per week. Some clinicians change to lower dosage at 60 rather than 40 years old. Dosage should be decreased if renal function is diminished.
#Some authorities recommend pyridoxine 50 mg for every 250 mg of cycloserine to decrease the incidence of adverse neurological effects.
From Drugs for tuberculosis. Med Lett 1995;37:70.

overdosage (seizure, acidosis, coma) is pyridoxine administered in a dose of 1 g for each gram of INH apparently ingested.[160–166] Though rarely used, hemodialysis,[167–170] peritoneal dialysis,[170–173] hemoperfusion,[174] and exchange transfusion[175] have been effective in INH removal. INH overdosages have been reported in the American Indian population, where tuberculosis is common and suicide is prevalent.[165,166,176]

Toxic Dose

Isoniazid 1.5 g (five 300-mg tablets) acutely ingested can induce toxicity in an adult.[165,166,171] Two to three grams acutely ingested at one time is usually toxic.[177] A dosage of 3 mg/kg produced fatal status epilepticus in one patient with prior epilepsy.[178] Six to ten grams acutely ingested (20–30 300-mg tablets) can cause severe toxicity and death. Ten to fifteen grams or more ingested acutely by an adult is often fatal if not treated,[171,179,180] 35 to 40 mg/kg produced seizures in some patients, and 80 to 150 mg/kg induced seizures and a high mortality.[165,176,181] Reported doses taken prior to status epilepticus ranged from 900 mg to 40 g.[171]

Toxicokinetics

Absorption

Isoniazid is absorbed from the gastrointestinal tract and from intramuscular sites. Peak plasma levels of 1 to 7 μg/mL are reached in 1 to 2 hours.[175] Plasma concentrations of rapid INH inactivators are 20 to 50% those of slow inactivators.[182] Protein binding is 10%.[183]

Distribution

Isoniazid is distributed into all body fluids and tissues. Its apparent volume of distribution is 0.6 L/kg.[160]

Peak cerebrospinal fluid levels are 10% of the serum level.[184]

Elimination

Ninety percent of a dose of INH and its metabolites may be excreted unchanged. Excretion is completed in 24 hours.[172] Less than 10% is excreted in the bile. The plasma half-life is 1 to 4 hours in normal subjects,[169,183] 1 to 7 hours in the anephric patient, 2 to 4 hours in the slow acetylator, and 0.7 hour in the rapid acetylator.[182] INH is inactivated in the liver. Its renal clearance is 41 mL/min.[185]

Pregnancy/Lactation

Isoniazid appears in fetal blood if administered during pregnancy. It is found in the breast milk of nursing mothers in a concentration of 0.6 to 1.2 mg/100 mL, 1 to 10 hours after a maternal dose of 5 to 10 mg/kg. Milk concentration is equal to maternal plasma concentration.[186]

Clinical Presentation

Chronic Use

Patients who ingest higher than therapeutic doses of INH over a prolonged period may develop signs and symptoms of chronic INH poisoning. Nausea and vomiting may be an early warning sign, but seizures may occur without previous warning signs of acute INH toxicity, such as coma, severe metabolic acidosis, and hyperglycemia.[187]

Isoniazid-Associated Hepatitis

Incidence. Hepatitis occurs in 0.46% of patients receiving INH as preventive therapy.[188,189] Its incidence is greater with increasing age, it is more frequent in those who regularly use ethanol, and it occurs more often in those patients also receiving phenobarbital or rifampin treatment, but this has not been established.

Clinical Signs and Symptoms. Clinically a prodrome of vague gastrointestinal complaints with anorexia, nausea, vomiting, and abdominal distress may be the early manifestation. Patients, however, may be asymptomatic in the presence of seriously elevated aminotransferase levels. Later, fever, chills, rash, urticaria, dark urine, clay-colored stools, diarrhea, malaise, fatigue, and joint and muscle pains may develop.

Monitoring. Periodic serum transaminase levels should be obtained in all INH patients, especially in those who are ethanol users, those with a history of liver disease, and those receiving other potentially hepatotoxic agents. INH should be discontinued if the transaminase level is two to three times its normal concentration.

Treatment[160–162,164,165,171,177]

Stabilization

Seizures. Seizures may spontaneously occur early in the course of treatment, so that early induction of emesis prior to specific treatment (pyridoxine, diazepam) in a symptomatic patient is not advised. Diazepam (increases brain γ-aminobutyric acid, acts synergistically with pyridoxine to attenuate seizures)[190] 5-10 mg is administered at a rate of 5 mg/min into a large vein; then the vein is flushed with 5% dextrose in water (D_5W) or 5% dextrose in normal saline (D_5NS). If convulsions persist, the same dose of diazepam may be repeated in 10 to 20 minutes. Diazepam should not be injected into the intravenous tubing or mixed or diluted in other solutions or drugs in view of its low solubility, which may cause it to precipitate rapidly.

An airway that is dependable and easily managed must be established. If a severe seizure disorder is present, endotracheal intubation is indicated. In obtunded or unconscious patients, a cuffed endotracheal tube should be inserted. In the unresponsive patient in whom an airway has been established, dependent positioning of the head (Trendelenburg), left lateral position of the body, and gastric suction together with assisted respiration should be instituted. After adequate respirations and normal circulatory status have been established, the tidal volume should be 10 to 15 mL/kg. Mechanically assisted ventilation may be required for respiratory depression.

Intravenous fluids, D_5W or D_5NS, should be started.

Acidosis. If acidosis is not responsive to specific therapy (pyridoxine, diazepam, fluids), sodium bicarbonate 44 to 88 mEq/L is given by intravenous bolus. It should not be mixed with pyridoxine solution. The electrocardiogram is monitored, and the patient observed for signs of hypokalemia or hyperkalemia.

Gut Decontamination

Asymptomatic patients who have ingested a potentially toxic amount of INH should be observed for at least 4 hours after emesis is induced with syrup of ipecac and activated charcoal and cathartics have been administered, as there is often a latent period before toxicity develops. If it can be established unequivocally that toxicity has not occurred when more than 4 hours have elapsed since the ingestion of INH in amounts smaller than 20 mg/kg (1.5 g in an adult), only careful observation may be indicated.

If the patient has had seizures and is postictal, the airway has been protected (endotracheal intubation), and pyridoxine has been administered, the stomach may be emptied by gastric lavage and the lavage returns sent for toxicology evaluation. After the stomach has been emptied, activated charcoal and cathartics should be administered.

Elimination Enhancement

With very little protein binding and a low volume of distribution, INH is a good candidate for dialysis, but in view of its short half-life and efficient antagonist (pyridoxine), such procedures are often unnecessary. If peritoneal dialysis is used, pyridoxine may be added to each liter of fluid used in the dialysis.[173] Hemoperfusion may be useful in reducing the half-life and serum concentration of INH.[174] Exchange transfusion has been successfully used in children.[175]

Elimination procedures are considered in severe intoxications, usually after other procedures (pyridoxine, gut decontamination, fluids, bicarbonate) have been found not to be effective or if the patient has severe renal insufficiency.

Forced diuresis with fluids or furosemide sufficient to produce a urine output of 3 to 6 mL/kg/h has been used, but its efficacy has not been established. Great care must be taken to avoid fluid overload or electrolyte imbalance.

Antidote

If there is doubt whether INH overdosage is the cause of convulsions or coma, an early therapeutic trial of intravenous pyridoxine should be considered, because of its relative safety and potential benefits. Pyridoxine should be given in alleged or definite cases of INH overdosage, even if seizures have not occurred. The optimal pyridoxine dose should be at least equal to the maximum amount of INH allegedly ingested. Pyridoxine is mixed as a 5 or 10% solution with water and administered intravenously over a 5-minute period (5 g/min in a 50-mL volume) and repeated at 5- to 20-minute intervals as needed in a comatose or convulsing patient. Pyridoxine is available commercially in vials of 1 g/10 mL.[158,160,166,173,181,191,192]

If the ingested dose of INH is unknown, 5.0 g of pyridoxine should be administered initially, followed in 30 minutes with an additional 5.0 g until seizures cease or consciousness is regained. Pyridoxine should not be mixed with sodium bicarbonate in an intravenous bottle. When convulsions are controlled, seizure-induced lactic acidosis will resolve and sodium bicarbonate may not be required.

Tachypnea, postural reflex abnormalities, paralysis, and convulsions may follow excessive pyridoxine dosage. Up to 52 g intravenously has been tolerated by INH overdose patients without adverse effects.[165] No adverse effects were observed with pyridoxine in one study at doses from 70 to 357 mg/kg.[191] A pyridoxine solution can be prepared in a 5 or 10% concentration (w/v) in D_5W, filtered through a 0.45-μm filter, and infused over 30 to 60 minutes.[191]

Supportive Measures

Aspiration Pneumonitis. Intermittent positive-pressure breathing is instituted to ensure adequate deep breaths. An endotracheal tube should be in place.

Hypotension. Intravascular volume is restored with fluids.

Hyperglycemia. Diabetic acidosis should be considered.

Urinary retention. The patient is catheterized, and intake and output monitored.

Other Measures. Blood is drawn for arterial blood gases, serum electrolytes, blood urea nitrogen, creatinine, blood glucose, liver function tests, and a complete blood count. Blood is prepared for type and crossmatch so that, if required, there will be no delay in hemodialysis. This is rarely required if pyridoxine is used.

The electroencephalogram (seizures), blood pressure, pulse, respirations, urine (sugar, acetone, albumin), serum electrolytes, blood glucose, visual status, neurologic status, hepatic and renal function tests (aminotransferases, blood urea nitrogen, creatinine), arterial blood gases, and consciousness are monitored.

The patient is hospitalized until findings of liver function tests are normal, neurologic status has returned to its pretoxic state, electrolytes and electroencephalogram are within normal limits, and there is no further evidence of metabolic acidosis.

• THIOACETAZONE

Thioacetazone is one of the mainstays of antituberculosis treatment in the developing world.[193] It is not available in the United States, but is widely used in China, Ethiopia, and India, mainly in combination with isoniazid. Thioacetazone was introduced and continues to be used because of its low cost. This drug is especially toxic to patients with HIV. The tuberculosis unit of the World Health Organization has recommended that thioacetazone not be given to patients at increased risk of HIV infection.[194] Cutaneous, gastrointestinal, and central nervous system toxicity are the predominant toxic responses to thioacetazone. Death has followed its use. Nunn and colleagues have presented a comprehensive review of the present status of thioacetazone.[193]

Structure and Classification

Thioacetazone is a member of the family of thiosemicarbazones. Its molecular formula is $C_{10}H_{12}N_4OS$. It is described chemically as 4-acetylamidobenzaldehyde thiosemicarbazone. The molecular weight is 236.3. Thioacetazone has structural similarities to the toxic histamine antagonist metiamide (both have a thiourea moiety in the side chain) and is related to thiadiazole-containing sulfonamides.[193] Thioacetazone is marketed as TBI, thioacetazone, *p*-acetylamidobenzaldehyde thiosemicarbazone, and amithiozone.

Use

Thioacetazone is a synthetic chemical compound that is available in oral form but is not formulated in any standard dose form.

Thioacetazone is a third-line drug (as is ethionamide, cycloserine, kanamycin, capreomycin, and viomycin) for the treatment of tuberculosis.[195] Its main role is in the prevention of emergence of resistance to other drugs, especially isoniazid. Because of the rate of decline of thioacetazone plasma concentrations, it has been calculated that thioacetazone concentrations capable of inhibiting the multiplication of *Mycobacterium leprae* would be maintained for only about 3 days after the patient has discontinued the drug.[196]

Therapeutic Dose

Thioacetazone is administered orally at a daily dose of 150 mg.

Toxic Dose

Toxicity and death may follow use of therapeutic doses.

Toxicokinetics

Absorption

Peak plasma concentrations during daily treatment are reached in 4 to 5 hours and average 1.8 μg/mL. A concentration of 0.4 μg/mL completely inhibits 75 to 100% of some strains of *Mycobacterium tuberculosis.*[197]

Elimination

The major route of metabolism is probably ring hydroxylation followed by conjugation with glucuronic acid. About 20 to 35% of thioacetazone is excreted unchanged in the urine.[198] The elimination half-life is about 12 to 14 hours. Decline in blood concentrations is biphasic, with a half-life of 21.5 hours after the first 24 hours.

Drug Interactions

Thioacetazone potentiates streptomycin ototoxicity[197] in some patients. Giddiness develops after about 6 weeks of treatment in patients receiving concomitant streptomycin therapy.[197]

Mechanism of Action

Acetylation appears to be defective in patients infected with HIV, and this impairment probably worsens with advancing immunosuppression. Thioacetazone is metabolized to thioacetazone hydroxylamine. The detoxification of this derivative is impaired, especially under conditions of glutathione deficiency such as occur in HIV infection.[193] Either thioacetazone or a reactive metabolite appears to be responsible for cutaneous hypersensitivity reactions in patients treated with tuberculosis, regardless of HIV status.

Clinical Presentation

Gastrointestinal Effects

Nausea, vomiting, and anorexia occur in about 10% of patients taking 200 mg daily and are more common at higher doses.

Ocular Effects

Conjunctivitis is common but not severe.

Skin Reactions

Skin eruption have been classified as mild (uncomplicated pruritus, acneiform eruptions, morbilliform erythema), moderate (extensive maculoerythematous eruptions, urticaria, purpura), and severe (erythroderma, Stevens–Johnson syndrome, Lyell's disease).[195]

Central Nervous System Effects

Giddiness, seizures, choreiform movements, and cerebral edema have been observed.[197]

HIV-Positive Patients

The risk of severe cutaneous hypersensitivity reactions and death is increased in HIV-positive patients.[193]

Laboratory

Analytical Methods

Ultraviolet, colorimetric, and fluorometric methods detect serum and urine thioacetazone concentrations down to 0.3 to 0.6 μg/mL.[199] The preferred analytical method is high-performance liquid chromatography using a reversed-phase column packing with ultraviolet detection. The limit of detection is 3 ng/mL in serum and urine.[196,200]

Blood Levels

Toxic effects have not been correlated with blood levels.

Abnormalities

If hepatotoxicity is involved, serum transaminase concentrations may be increased.

Treatment

Treatment of the toxic effects associated with thioacetazone is symptomatic and supportive. There are no antidotes.

HEPATOTOXICITY OF ANTITUBERCULOSIS DRUGS

Isoniazid, rifampin, pyrazinamide, and ethionamide are known hepatotoxic drugs. In overdose, isoniazid induces seizures which are treated gram for gram with pyridoxine and which may be fatal if pyridoxine is not available.[201] Rifampin overdose may be associated with the red man syndrome and orange-red skin, mucous membranes, urine, feces, sweat, and tears. Death occurs in the presence of underlying liver disease and frequent use or abuse of alcohol. Treatment is symptomatic and supportive. Additive nervous system adverse effects including dizziness and drowsiness occur when cycloserine and ethionamide are added to isoniazid treatment. Pyrazinamide also induces a hypersensitivity-type hepatitis.[202]

BACTERIOSTATIC AGENTS

DAPSONE

Dapsone (4,4′-diaminodiphenylsulfone) has been associated with a number of reports of overdose in children and adults both in the United States and overseas. These are usually observed wherever patients or parents have been under treatment with dapsone for leprosy or dermatitis herpetiformis. Dapsone poisoning is associated with a striking clinical syndrome related to its ability to produce alterations in normal hemoglobin (methemoglobinemia, sulfhemoglobinemia), a deep cyanosis, impairment of oxygen transport and oxygen delivery by the red blood cells, and central nervous system dysfunction. Treatment is only partially successful and depends largely, but not consistently, on the use of repeated doses of activated charcoal and good supportive care. Methylene blue, possibly ascorbic acid, and extracorporeal methods to rid the body of excess dapsone and its metabolites are measures that have yet to prove themselves unequivocally useful. Fatalities have been reported despite of aggressive management.

Treatment

Antidote: Methylene Blue

Methylene blue is a specific treatment for cyanosis resulting from excessive methemoglobinemia such as that induced by dapsone. An effective dose initially is 1 to 2 mg/kg given intravenously over a 5- to 10-minute period. Cyanosis may be lessened temporarily and methemoglobin blood levels decreased, but rebound methemoglobinemia may require multiple injections of methylene blue over several days, as dapsone is continually absorbed and slowly eliminated.

Use of methylene blue must be dictated by clinical evaluation of the patient to determine whether the deep, often dramatic, cyanosis is accompanied by other adverse effects of methemoglobinemia sufficient to warrant the use of this product. If methylene blue is used, methemoglobin levels must be monitored frequently. The cyanosis itself is not a good guide to therapy, as methylene blue may induce a grayish discoloration of the skin. Further, severe anemia may disguise cyanosis even in the presence of elevated methemoglobin levels. Patients, both children[203] and adults,[204] suffering from dapsone overdose, including cyanosis, and treated with the use of methylene blue have recovered.

Supportive Measures

Intramuscular phenobarbital and intramuscular paraldehyde have had no ameliorative effect on decreasing the restlessness observed after dapsone overdose.[205] Intravenous hydrocortisone has not been useful in treatment of the hemolysis.[206] Packed red blood cells in multiple transfusions may be required for symptomatic treatment of the hemolytic anemia. Blurred vision may occur after an initial period of normal vision. This must be immediately evaluated by an assessment of macular function, using fluorescein angiography. Use of prednisolone may be indicated (eg, 75 mg/d for 1 week, then tapered doses).[207]

Hemolysis may develop 3 to 9 days after dapsone ingestion and may continue long after both methemoglobin and sulfhemoglobin levels have returned to normal.[207,208] Patients must therefore be kept under close observation for a more prolonged period.

Oxygen inhalation therapy is not useful in dapsone overdosage.[205,206] Ascorbic acid has not been determined to be clinically useful in dapsone overdose.

Seizures should be treated with diazepam (adult, 5–10 mg intravenously slowly, repeat if required; children, 0.1–0.3 mg/kg slowly). If the patient is unresponsive, phenytoin 15 mg/kg is administered intravenously at 0.5 mg/kg/min with electrocardiographic monitoring.

Patients must be monitored in a hospital unit sufficiently equipped to do the laboratory studies (methemoglobin, lactic acid dehydrogenase, plasma hemoglobin, reticulocyte count, red cell fragility, Heinz bodies) required to evaluate a late-developing (3–days) picture of methemoglobinemia and hemolytic anemia. Tests to determine blood levels of dapsone and monoacetyl dapsone are now available.

NITROFURANTOIN

Nitrofurantoin was introduced 35 years ago for the treatment of urinary tract infections. It is rapidly absorbed from the gastrointestinal tract, well concentrated in the urine, and active against a variety of common urinary tract pathogens.[209] Few reports of nitrofurantoin overdose are available despite its extensive use.

Therapeutic Dose

Recommended doses in adults are 50 to 100 mg four times daily. In children, nitrofurantoin may be administered in doses of 5 to 7 mg/kg body weight per 24 hours in four divided doses. In the elderly, the dose is often reduced to 50 mg four times daily.[209]

Clinical Presentation

Therapeutic Use

Acute pulmonary reactions are more common in the elderly and rare in children.[210] Hepatotoxicity is infrequently observed.[211] Hematologic reactions may be seen in patients of Mediterranean origin who have glucose-6-phosphate dehydrogenase deficiency. Peripheral neuropathy can begin within 6 weeks of starting treatment. Total or partial recovery is common. Hypersensitivity reactions occur in 1 to 5% of patients and may rapidly subside after cessation of therapy. The most frequent adverse reactions to nitrofurantoin are anorexia, nausea, and vomiting, occurring more often in relation to doses greater than 7 mg/kg daily.[209]

Overdose

Excessive doses of nitrofurantoin may be expected to induce nausea and vomiting.

Toxicokinetics[209,212,213]

Bioavailability	90%
Peak plasma level	0.72 μg/mL (after oral 100 mg)
Time to peak plasma level	2 hours
Volume of distribution	0.6 L/kg
Plasma protein binding	90%
Excreted unchanged	30 minutes
Active metabolites	33%

Treatment

Treatment is largely symptomatic and supportive. Vomiting following an overdose should act in expelling most of the ingested dose of nitrofurantoin. There are no antidotes. A high fluid intake should be provided to promote urinary excretion of the drug.

REFERENCES

1. Fekety R, Shah AB. Diagnosis and treatment of *Clostridium* colitis. JAMA 1993;269:71–75.
2. McFarlane LV, Mulligan ME, Kwok RY, Stanm WE. Nosocomial acquisition of *Clostridium difficile* infection. N Engl J Med 1989;320:204–210.
3. Riley TV, Golledge CL. Clindamycin and pseudomembranous colitis. Lancet 1995;346:639.
4. Barclay ML, Begg EJ. Aminoglycoside toxicity and relation to dose regimen. Adverse Drug React Toxicol Rev 1994;13: 207–234.
5. Saxon A, Beall GN, Rohr AS, Adelman DC. Immediate hypersensitivity reactions to beta-lactam antibiotics. Ann Intern Med 1987;107:204–215.
6. Donowitz GR, Mandell GL. Beta-lactam antibiotics (second of two parts). N Engl J Med 1988;318:490–500.
7. Westley-Horton E, Koestner JA. Aztreonam: A review of first monobactam. Am J Med Sci 1991;302:46–49.
8. Aztreonam (Azactam). Med Lett Drugs Ther 1987;29:45–47.
9. McEvoy GK, ed. *AHFS 94.* Bethesda, MD: American Hospital Formulary Service, 1994:164–172.
10. Cadarson AI, Jimenez SAS, Pan CV, Mosquera MR. Aztreonam-induced anaphylaxis. Lancet 1990;336:746–747.
11. Dallal MM, Dzachor JS. Aztreonam-induced myelosuppression during treatment of *Pseudomonas aeruginosa* pneumonia. DICP Ann Pharmacother 1991;25:294–297.
12. Neu HC: Carbapenems: Special properties contributing to their activity. Am J Med 1985:78(suppl. 6A):33–40.
13. Imipenem + cilastatin: A new type of antibiotic. Drug Ther Bull 1991;29(11):43.
14. McEvoy GK, ed. *AHFS Drug Information 94.* Bethesda, MD: American Hospital Formulary Service, 1994:182–190.
15. Reynolds JEF, ed. *Martindale: The Extra Pharmacopoeia.* 30th ed. London: Pharmaceutical Press, 1993:247–250.
16. Boucher BA, Hickerson WL, Kuhl DA, et al. Imipenem pharmacokinetics in patients with burns. Clin Pharmacol Ther 1990;48:130–137.
17. Job ML, Dretler RH. Seizure activity with imipenem therapy: Incidence and risk factors. DICP Ann Pharmacother 1990;24: 467–469.
18. Calandra G, Lydick E, Carrigan J, et al. Factors predisposing to seizures in seriously ill infected patients receiving antibiotics: Experience with imipenem/cilastatin. Am J Med 1988;84:911–918.
19. Riancho JA, Olmos JM, Sedano C. Life-threatening bleeding in a patient treated with cefonicid. Ann Intern Med 1995; 123:472.
20. Kanatani MS, Guglielmo BJ. The new macrolides. Azithromycin and clarithromycin. West J Med 1994;160:31–37.
21. Azithromycin. In: Dollery CT, ed. *Therapeutic Drugs.* Edinburgh: Churchill Livingstone, 1992:18–22.
22. Wallace MR, Miller LK, Nguyer M-T, Shields AP. Ototoxicity with azithromycin. Lancet 1994;343:41.
23. Mondolfi AA. Erythromycin. Clin Toxicol Rev 1995;17(9):1–2.
24. Berger TM, Cook WJ, O'Marcaigh AS, Zimmerman D. Acute pancreatitis in a 12 year old girl after an Erythrocin overdose. Pediatrics 1992;90:624–626.
25. Gumaste UV. Erythromycin-induced pancreatitis. Am J Med 1989;76(part 1):725.
26. Haefeli WE, Schoenenberger RA, Weiss P, Ritz R. Possible risk for cardiac arrhythmias related to intravenous erythromycin. Intensive Care Med 1992;18:469–473.
27. Farrar HC, Walsh-Sukys MC, Kyllonen K, Blumer JL. Cardiac toxicity associated with intravenous erythromycin lactobionate: Two case reports and a review of the literature. Pediatr Infect Dis J 1993;12:688–691.
28. Gitler B, Berger LS, Buffa SD. Torsade de pointes induced by erythromycin. Chest 1994; 105:368–370.
29. Brandress MW, Richardson WS, Barold SS. Erythromycin induced QT prolongation and polymorphic ventricular tachycardia (Torsade de pointes): Case report and review. Clin Infect Dis 1994;18:995–999.
30. Hooper DC, Wolfson JS. Fluoroquinolone antimicrobial agents. N Engl J Med 1991;324:384–394.
31. Percival A, ed. Quinolones: Their future in clinical practice. London: Royal Society of Medicine Services, 1986.
32. Walker RC, Wright AJ. The quinolones. Mayo Clin Proc 1987; 62:1007–1012.
33. Andersen RD, Goldstein EJC. The introduction of the quinolones: A new class of antiinfectives. Hosp Formul 1987; 22:36–47.
34. Paton JH, Reeves DS. Clinical features and management of adverse effects of quinolone antibacterials. Drug Saf 1991;6: 8–27.
35. Baciewicz AM, Ashar BH, Locke TW. Interaction of oflaxacin and warfarin. Ann Intern Med 1993;119:1223.
36. Giamarellou H, Kolokythas E, Petrikkos G, et al. Pharmacokinetics of three new quinolones in pregnant and lactating women. Am J Med 1989;87(suppl. 5A):49.
37. Peled Y, Friedman S, Hod M, Merlob P. Ofloxacin during the second trimester of pregnancy. DICP Ann Pharmacother 1991;25:1181–1182.
38. Christ W. Central nervous system toxicity of quinolones: Human and animal findings. J Antimicrob Chemother 1990; 26(suppl. B):219–225.
39. Bergan T, Rohwedder R, Thorsteinsson SB. Significance of crystalluria caused by quinolones. Rev Infect Dis 1989; 2(suppl. 5):S1395–S1396.
40. Stahlmann R. Safety profile of the quinolones. J Antimicrob Chemother 1990; 26(suppl. D):31–44.
41. Stricker BHC, Slagboom G, Demaeseneer R, et al. Anaphylactic reactions to cinoxacin. Br Med J 1988;297:1434–1435.
42. Henwood JM, Monk JP. Enoxacin: A review of its antibacterial activity, pharmacokinetic properties and therapeutic use. Drugs 1988;36:32–66.
43. Davila I, Diez ML, Quirce S, et al. Cross-reactivity between quinolones: Report of three cases. Allergy 1993;48: 388–390.
44. Islem MA, Sreedharan T. Convulsions, hyperglycaemia and glycosuria from overdose of nalidixic acid. JAMA 1965; 192:1100–1111.
45. Fraser AG, Harrower ADB. Convulsions and hyperglycaemia associated with nalidixic acid. Br Med J 1977;2:1518.
46. Dash H, Mills J. Severe metabolic acidosis associated with nalidixic acid overdose. Ann Intern Med 1976;84:570–571.
47. Mukherjee A, Dutta P, Lahiri M, et al. Benign intracranial hypertension after nalidixic acid overdose in infants. Lancet 1990;1:1602.
48. Leslie PJA, Cregeen RJ, Proudfoot AT. Lactic acidosis, hyperglycaemia and convulsions following nalidixic acid overdosage. Hum Toxicol 1984;3:239–243.
49. Singlas E, Taburet AM, Landru I, et al. Pharmacokinetics of ciprofloxacin tablets in renal failure: Influence of hemodialysis. Eur J Clin Pharmacol 1987;31:589–593.
50. Nix DE, Watson WA, Lener ME, et al. Effects of aluminum and magnesium antacids and ranitidine on the absorption of ciprofloxacin. Clin Pharmacol Ther 1989;46:700–705.
51. Reynolds JEF, ed. *Martindale: The Extra Pharmacopoeia.* 30th ed. London: Pharmaceutical Press, 1993:145–147.
52. Temofloxacin withdrawn. FDA Med Bull 1992;22(2):4.
53. Terp DK, Rybak MJ. Ciprofloxacin. Drug Intell Clin Pharm 1987;21:568–570.
54. Ball AP. Overview of clinical experience with ciprofloxacin. Eur J Clin Microbial 1986;5:214–219.
55. Ciprofloxacin. Med Lett Drugs Ther 1988;30:11–13.
56. Bouchayer D, Vial T, Mercatello A, et al. Acute renal failure secondary to ciprofloxacin overdose. In: *Proceedings, European Association of Poison Centres, Lyon, France, May 22, 1991.*
57. George MJ, Dew RB III, Daly JS. Acute renal failure after an overdose of ciprofloxacin. Arch Intern Med 1991;151:620.
58. Drusano GL, Standiford HC, Plaisance K, et al. Absolute oral bioavailability of ciprofloxacin. Antimicrob Agents Chemother 1986; 30:444–446.
59. Wise R, Lockley RM, Webberly M, Dent J. Pharmacokinetics of intravenous administered ciprofloxacin. Antimicrob Agents Chemother 1984;26:208–210.
60. Wolff M, Boutron L, Decazes J, et al. Diffusion of ciprofloxacin into CSF of patients with purulent meningitis. In: *Program and Abstracts of the 26th Interscience Conference on*

Antimicrobial Agents and Chemotherapy, New Orleans, 1986: 1984. Abstract.

61. Cover DL, Mueller BA. Ciprofloxacin. Penetration into human breast milk: A case report. DICP Ann Pharmacother 1990; 24:703–704.
62. Richardson JP. Theophylline toxicity associated with the administration of ciprofloxacin in a nursing home patient. J Am Geriatr Soc 1990;38:236–238.
63. Polk RE. Drug–drug interactions with ciprofloxacin and other fluoroquinolones. Am J Med 1989; 87(suppl. 5A):76S–81S.
64. Davis H, McGoodwin E, Reed TG. Anaphylactoid reactions reported after treatment with ciprofloxacin. Ann Intern Med 1989;111:1041–1043.
65. Kamada AK. Possible interaction between ciprofloxacin and warfarin. DICP Ann Pharmacother 1990;24:27–28.
66. Jim LK. Physical and clinical compatibility of intravenous ciprofloxacin with other drugs. Ann Pharmacother 1993;27: 704–707.
67. Semel JD, Allen N. Seizures in patients simultaneously receiving theophylline and imipenem or ciprofloxacin or metronidazole. South Med J 1991;84:465–468.
68. Slavich IL, Gleffee RF, Haas EJ. Grand mal epileptic seizures during ciprofloxacin therapy. JAMA 1989;261:558–559.
69. Knapp R, Judmaier W, Frauscher F, Birbamer G. Fatal hepatic failure associated with ciprofloxacin. Lancet 1994;343: 738–739.
70. Karki SD, Bentley DW, Ragharan M. Seizure with ciprofloxacin and theophylline combined therapy. DICP Ann Pharmacother 1990;24:595–596.
71. Mumford CJ, Ginsberg L. Ciprofloxacin and myasthenia gravis. Br Med J 1990;301–318.
72. Winrow AP, Supramaniam G. Benign intracranial hypertension after ciprofloxacin administration. Arch Dis Child 1990;65:1165–1166.
73. Vriabec TR, Sergott RC, Jaeger EA, et al. Reversible visual loss in a patient receiving high-dose ciprofloxacin hydrochloride (Cipro). Ophthalmology 1990;97:707–710.
74. Peters B, Pinching AJ. Fatal anaphylaxis associated with ciprofloxacin in a patient with AIDS related complex. Br Med J 1989;298:605.
75. Rastogi S, Atkinson JLD, McCarthy JT. Allergic nephropathy associated with ciprofloxacin. Mayo Clin Proc 1990;65: 987–989.
76. Murray KM, Wilson MG. Suspected ciprofloxacin-induced interstitial nephritis. DICP Ann Pharmacother 1990;24:379–380.
77. Ying LS, Johnson CA. Ciprofloxacin-induced interstitial nephritis. Clin Pharm 1989;8:518–521.
78. Hootkins R, Fenves AZ, Stephens MK. Acute renal failure secondary to oral ciprofloxacin therapy: A presentation of three cases and a review of the literature. Clin Nephrol 1989;32:75–78.
79. Teja-Isavadham P, Keeratithakul D, Watt G, et al. Measurement of ciprofloxacin in human plasma, whole blood and erythrocytes by high-performance liquid chromatography. Ther Drug Monit 1991;13:263–267.
80. Ball P. Ciprofloxacin, an overview of adverse experiences. J Antimicrob Chemother 1986;18(suppl. D):187–193.
81. Drysdale L, Gilbert L, Thomson A, et al. Pseudoglycosuria and ciprofloxacin. Lancet 1988;2:961.
82. Todd PA, Faulds D. Ofloxacin: A reappraisal of its antimicrobial activity, pharmacology and therapeutic use. Drugs 1991;42:825–876.
83. Lamp KC, Bailey EM, Ryback MJ. Ofloxacin clinical pharmacokinetics. Clin Pharmacokinet 1992;22:32–46.
84. Kohler PB, Arkins N, Tack NJ. Accidental overdose of intravenous ofloxacin with benign outcome. Antimicrob Agents Chemother 1991;35:1239–1240.
85. Koppel C, Hopke T, Menzel J. Central anticholinergic syndrome after ofloxacin overdose and therapeutic doses of diphenhydramine and chlormezanone. Clin Toxicol 1990; 28:249–253.
86. Walker RC, Wright AJ. The fluoroquinolones. Mayo Clin Proc 1991;66:1249–1259.
87. Glum A. Ofloxacin-induced acute severe hepatitis. South Med J 1991;84:1158.
88. Szarfman A, Chen M, Blum MD. More on fluoroquinolone antibiotics and tendon rupture. N Engl J Med 1995;323:193–194.
89. Ofloxacin. Med Lett Drugs Ther 1991;33:71–73.
90. Monk JP, Campoli-Richards DM. Ofloxacin: A review of its antibacterial activity, pharmacokinetic properties and therapeutic use. Drugs 1987;33:346–391.
91. Zaudig M, von Bose M, Weber MM, et al. Psychotic effects of ofloxacin. Pharmacopsychiatry 1989;22:11–15.
92. Zaudig M, von Bose M. Ofloxacin-induced psychosis. Br J Psychiatry 1987; 151:563–564.
93. Cockerill FR III, Edson RS. Trimethoprim–sulfamethoxazole. Mayo Clin Proc 1987;62:921–929.
94. McEvoy GK, ed. *AHFS Drug Information 91.* Bethesda, MD: American Hospital Formulary Service, 1991:461–464, 468–474.
95. Reynolds JEF, ed. *Martindale: The Extra Pharmacopoeia.* 30th ed. London: Pharmaceutical Press, 1993:153–156, 221–223.
96. Hoppu K, Partanen S, Koskela E. Trimethoprim poisoning. Lancet 1980;1:778.
97. Goff O. Renal failure induced by co-trimoxazole. Hosp Ther 1989;14:61–67.
98. Hoppu K, Koskimies O, Turmisto J. Trimethoprim pharmacokinetics in children with renal insufficiency. Clin Pharmacol Ther 1987;42:181–186.
99. Stevens RC, Laizare SC, Stein DS, Holden CL. Pharmacokinetics and toxicity of co-trimexazole following pneumocystis-dosing in healthy subjects. Clin Pharmacol Ther 1991;49: 199.
100. Hutabarat RM, Unadkat JP, Sahajwalla C, et al. Disposition of drugs in cystic fibrosis. 1. Sulfamethoxazole and trimethoprim. Clin Pharmacol Ther 1991;49:402–409.
101. Wathen GG, Winney RJ. High dose co-trimoxazole for patients receiving hemodialysis. Br Med J 1987;295:333.
102. Kosoglou T, Rocci ML, Vlasses PH. Trimethoprim alters the disposition of procainamide and *N*-acetylprocainamide. Clin Pharmacol Ther 1988;44:467–477.
103. Taraszewski R, Harvey R, Rosman P: Death from drug-induced hemolytic anemia. Postgrad Med 1989;85:79–81.
104. Carmichael AJ, Tan CY. Fatal toxic epidermal necrolysis associated with co-trimexazole. Lancet 1989;2:808–809.
105. Smith GW, Cohen SB. Hyperkalemia and non-oliguric renal failure associated with trimethoprim. Br Med J 1994;308:454.
106. Metherall R. High performance liquid chromatographic determination of trimethoprim in serum. Ther Drug Monit 1989; 11:79–83.
107. De Angelis DV, Woolley JL, Sigel CW. High performance liquid chromatographic assay for the simultaneous measurement of trimethoprim and sulfamethoxazole in plasma or urine. Ther Drug Monit 1990;12:382–392.
108. Dawling S, Widdop B. A fatal case involving trimethoprim. Bull Int Assoc Forens Toxicol 1986;19(1):34-35.
109. McEvoy GK, ed. *AHFS Drug Information 94.* Bethesda, MD: American Society of Hospital Pharmacists, 1994:355–359.
110. Walczyk MH, Hill D, Arai A, Wolfson M. Acute renal failure owing to inadvertent vancomycin overdose: Vancomycin removal by continuous arteriovenous hemofiltration. Ann Clin Lab Sci 1988;18:440–443.
111. Burkhart K, Metcalf S, Shurnas E, et al. Exchange transfusion and multidose activated charcoal following vancomycin overdose. Vet Hum Toxicol 1990;32:253.
112. Matzke GR, Zhanel GG, Guay DRP. Clinical pharmacokinetics of vancomycin. Clin Pharmacokinet 1986;11:257–282.
113. Kildoo CW, Lin L-M, Gabriel MH, et al. Vancomycin pharmacokinetics in infants: Relationship to postconceptional age and serum creatinine. Dev Pharmacol Ther 1990;14:77–83.
114. Pauly DJ, Musa DM, Lestico MR, et al. Risk of nephrotoxicity and combination vancomycin–aminoglycoside antibiotic therapy. Pharmacotherapy 1990;10:378–382.
115. Huang KC, Huse A, Shrader AK, Tureda K. Vancomycin enhances the neuromuscular blockade of vecuronium. Anesth Analg 1990;71:194–196.
116. Reyes MP, Ostrea EM Jr, Cabinan AE, et al. Vancomycin during pregnancy: Does it cause hearing loss of nephrotoxicity in the infant? Am J Obstet Gynecol 1989;161:977–981.

117. Gouyon JB, Petion AM. Toxicity of vancomycin given during pregnancy. Am J Obstet Gynecol 1990;163:1375–1376.
118. Glicklich D, Figura I. Vancomycin and cardiac arrest. Ann Intern Med 1984;101:880–881.
119. Wallace MR, Mascola JR, Oldfield EC III. Red man syndrome: Incidence, etiology, prophylaxis. J Infect Dis 1991; 164:1180–1185.
120. Knudsen JD, Pedersen M. IgE-mediated reaction to vancomycin and teicoplanin after treatment with vancomycin. Scand J Infect Dis 1992;24:395–396.
121. Red men should go: Vancomycin and histamine release. Lancet 1990;335:1006–1007. Editorial.
122. Sahai J, Healey DP, Garris R, et al. Influence of antihistamine pretreatment in vancomycin-induced red man syndrome. J Infect Dis 1989;160:876–881.
123. Dubettier S, Boibieux A, Lagable M, et al. Red man syndrome with teicoplanin. Rev Infect Dis 1991;13:770.
124. Estrada V, Algarra J, Vargas E, Jimenez de Diego L. Red neck syndrome induced by erythromycin. Rev Clin Espan 1992;190:100–101.
125. Zenon GJ, Cadle RM, Hamill RJ. Vancomycin-induced thrombocytopenia. Arch Intern Med 1991;151:995–996.
126. Bingley PJ, Harding GM. *Clostridium difficile* colitis following treatment with metronidazole and vancomycin. Postgrad Med J 1987;63:993–994.
127. Hannah BA, Kimmel PL, Dosa S, Turner ML. Vancomycin-induced toxic epidermal necrolysis. South Med J 1990; 83:720–722.
128. Morris A, Ward C. High incidence of vancomycin-associated leucopenia and neutropenia in a cardiothoracic surgical unit. J Infect 1991;22:217–233.
129. Hu MW, Anne L, Forni T, Gottwald K. Measurement of vancomycin in renally impaired patient samples using a new high performance liquid chromatography method with vitamin B_{12} internal standard: Comparison of high performance liquid chromatography, EMIT and fluorescence polarization immunoassay methods. Ther Drug Monit 1990;12: 562–569.
130. Bailie GR, Neal D. Vancomycin in ototoxicity and nephrotoxicity: A review. Med Toxicol 1988;3:376–386.
131. Thomas RJ. Neurotoxicity of antibacterial therapy. South Med J 1994;87:869–874.
132. Yawalker SJ, Vischer W. Lamprene (clofazimine) in leprosy. Lepr Rev 1979;50: 135–144.
133. Mason GH, Ellis-Pegler RB, Arthur JF. Clofazimine and eosinophilic enteritis. Lepr Rev 1977;48:175–180.
134. Jopling WH. Complications of treatment with clofazimine (Lamprene;B663). Lepr Rev 1976;14:1–2.
135. McDougall AC, Horsfall WR, Hede JE, Chaplin AJ. Splenic infarction and tissue accumulation of crystals associated with the use of clofazimine (Lampere; B663) in the treatment of pyoderma gangrenosum. Br J Dermatol 1980;102:227–230.
136. Schaad-Lanyi Z, Dieterle W, Debois JP, et al. Pharmacokinetics of clofazimine in healthy volunteers. Int J Lepr 1987;55: 9–15.
137. Feng PCC, Fenselau CC, Jacobson RR. Metabolism of clofazimine in leprosy patients. Drug Metab Dispos 1981;9:521–524.
138. Holdiness MR. Clinical pharmacokinetics of clofazimine: A review. Clin Pharmacokinet 1989;16:74–85.
139. Farb H, West DR, Pedvis-Leftick A. Clofazimine in pregnancy complicated by leprosy. Obstet Gynecol 1982;59:122–123.
140. Girdhar A, Venkatesan K, Chauhan SL, et al. Red discoloration of the sputum by clofazimine simulating haemoptysis: A case report. Lepr Rev 1992;63:47–50.
141. Craythorn JM, Swartz M, Creel DJ. Clofazimine-induced bull's-eye retinopathy. Retina 1986;6:50–52.
142. Cunningham CA, Friedberg DN, Carr RE. Clofazimine-induced generalized retinal degeneration. Retina 1990;10: 131–134.
143. Forster DJ, Causey DM, Ro NA. Bull's eye retinopathy and clofazimine. Ann Intern Med 1992;116:876–877.
144. Sandler ED, Ng LV, Hadley WK. Clofazimine crystals in alveolar macrophages from a patient with the acquired immunodeficiency syndrome. Arch Pathol Lab Med 1992;116: 541–543.
145. Lanyi Z, Dubois JP. Determination of clofazimine in human plasma by thin-layer chromatography. J Chromatogr Biomed Appl 1982;232:219–223.
146. De Bergeyck E, Janssens PG, de Muynck A. Radiological abnormalities of the ileus associated with the use of clofazimine (Lamprene; B663) in the treatment of skin ulceration due to *Mycobacterium ulcerans.* Lepr Rev 1980;51:221–228.
147. Alford RH. Antimicrobacterial agents. In: Mandell GI, Douglas RG Jr, Bennett JE, eds. *Anti-infective Therapy.* New York: Wiley, 1985:285–286.
148. Gulliford M, Mackay AD, Prowse K. Cholestatic jaundice caused by ethambutol. Br Med J 1986;292:866.
149. Ethambutol hydrochloride. In: *Physicians' Desk Reference.* Montvale, NJ: Medical Economics, 1995:1271.
150. Ducobu J, DuPont P, Laurent M, et al. Acute isoniazid/ ethambutol, rifampicin overdosage. Lancet 1982;1:632.
151. Myambutol. In: *Guide to Recognition and Treatment of Acute Overdosage with Lederle Products.* Lederle Laboratories, Feb. 1976.
152. Coyer JR, Nicholson DP. Isoniazid induced convulsions. Part 1. Clinical. South Med J 1976;69:294–296.
153. Mack RB. Mimi Viletta and the "captain of all the men of death": INH (isoniazid) poisoning. NC Med J 1984;45:321–322.
154. Alford RH. Antimycobacterial agents. In: Mandell GL, Douglas RG Jr, Bennett JE, eds. *Anti-infective Therapy.* New York: Wiley, 1985:281–284.
155. *Handbook of Antimicrobial Therapy.* rev ed. New Rochelle, NY: The Medical Letter, Inc, 1984.
156. McEvoy GK, ed. *AHFS Drug Information* Bethesda, MD: American Society of Hospital Pharmacists, 1994:372–376.
157. Starke H, Williams S. Acute poisoning from overdose of isoniazid: A case report. Lancet 1963;83:406–408.
158. Kingston RL, Saxena K. Management of acute isoniazid overdosages. Clin Toxicol Consult 1980;2:37–44.
159. McBay AJ. Fatal isoniazid poisoning. Bull Int Assoc Forens Toxicol 1968;5(3):2.
160. Sievers ML, Herrier RN, Chin L, et al. Treatment of isoniazid overdose. JAMA 1982;247:583–584.
161. Manoguerra AS. Acute isoniazid toxicity. San Francisco Bay Area Regional Poison Center Newlett 1980;2(3):1–2.
162. Wason S. Isoniazid. Clin Toxicol Rev 1981;3(5):1–2.
163. Yarbrough BE, Wood JP. Isoniazid overdose treated with high dose pyridoxine. Ann Emerg Med 1983;12:303–305.
164. Manoguerra AS. Acute isoniazid toxicity. Clin Toxicol 1980; 16:407–408.
165. Sievers ML, Herrier RN. Treatment of acute isonizid toxicity. Am J Hosp Pharm 1975;32:202–206.
166. Brown CV. Acute isoniazid poisoning. Am Rev Respir Dis 1972;105:206–216.
167. Gold CH, Buchanan N, Tringham V, et al. Isoniazid pharmacokinetics in patients in chronic renal failure. Clin Nephrol 1976;6:365–369.
168. Ducobu J, Dupont P, Laurent M, et al. Acute isoniazid/ ethambutol/rifamicin overdosage. Lancet 1982;1:632.
169. La Greca G, Biasioli S, Boren D, et al. Drugs and dialysis. Int J Artif Organs 1983;6:139–156.
170. Winchester JF, Gelfand MC, Knepshield JH, et al. Dialysis and hemoperfusion of poisons and drugs: Update. Trans Am Soc Artif Intern Organs 1977;23:762–827.
171. Terman DS, Teitelbaum DT. Isoniazid self poisoning. Neurology 1970;20:299–304.
172. Cocco AE, Pazourek LJ. Acute isoniazid intoxication: Management by peritoneal dialysis. N Engl J Med 1963;269:852–853.
173. Katz GA, Jobin GC. Large doses of pyridoxine in the treatment of massive ingestion of isoniazid. Am Rev Respir Dis 1970;101:991–992.
174. Konigshausen TH, Altrogge G, Hein D, et al. Hemodialysis and hemoperfusion in the treatment of most severe INH poisoning. Vet Hum Toxicol 1979;21(suppl.):12–15.
175. Katz BE, Carver MW. Acute poisoning with isoniazid treated by exchange transfusion. Pediatrics 1956;18:72–76.
176. Nelson LG. Grand mal seizures following overdose of isoniazid: A report of four cases. Am Rev Respir Dis 1965;91: 600–604.

177. Sievers ML, Herrier RN. Sensory neuropathy from pyridoxine abuse. N Engl J Med 1984;310:197–198. Letter.
178. Biehl JP, Nimitz HJ. Studies on the use of a high dose of isoniazid: I. Toxicity studies. Am Rev Tuberc 1954;69:759–765.
179. Whitefield CL, Klein RG. Isoniazid overdose: Report of 40 patients with a critical analysis of treatment and suggestions for prevention. Am Rev Respir Dis 1971;103:887.
180. Blanchard PD, Yao JDC, McAlpine DE, et al. Isoniazid overdose in the Cambodian population of Olmsted Country, Minnesota. JAMA 1986;256:3131–3133.
181. Friedman SA. Death following massive ingestion of isoniazid. Am Rev Respir Dis 1969;100:859–862.
182. Jeanes CWL, Schaefer O, Eidus L. Inactivation of isoniazid by Canadian Eskimos and Indians. Can Med Assoc J 1972;106:331–335.
183. Bennett WM, Singer I, Golper T, et al. Guidelines for drug therapy in renal failure. Ann Intern Med 1977;86:754–783.
184. Tuchman AJ, Berger S, Daras M. Cerebrospinal fluid penetration of anti-infective agents. South Med J 1984;77:1443–1445.
185. Kunin CM. A guide to use of antibiotics in patients with renal disease: A table of recommended doses and factors governing serum levels. Ann Intern Med 1967;67:151–158.
186. Chaplan S, Sanders GL, Smith JM. Drug excretion in human breast milk. Adverse Drug React Acute Poison Rev 1982;1:255–287.
187. Rubin DH, Carbone J, Fong B, et al. Chronic isoniazid poisoning. Clin Pediatr 1983;22:518–519.
188. Alexander MR, Louie SG, Guernsey BG. Isoniazid associated hepatitis. Clin Pharmacol 1982;1:148–153.
189. Comstock GW. New data on preventive treatment with isoniazid. Ann Intern Med 1983;98:22:518–519.
190. Chin L, Sievers ML, Laird HE, et al. Evaluation of diazepam and pyridoxine as antidotes to isoniazid intoxication in rats and dogs. Toxicol Appl Pharmacol 1978;45:713–722.
191. Wason S, LaCouture PG, Lovejoy FH Jr. Single high dose pyridoxine treatment for isoniazid overdose. JAMA 1981;246:1102–1104.
192. Sievers ML, Herrier RD. Megavitamin therapy for overdose. Arch Intern Med 1980;140:1676.
193. Nunn P, Porter J, Winstanley P. Thioacetazone: Avoid like poison or use with care? Trans R Soc Trop Med Hyg 1993;87:578–582.
194. World Health Organization. Severe hypersensitivity reactions among HIV-seropositive patients with tuberculosis treatment with thioacetazone. Wkly Epidemiol Rec 1992;67:1–3.
195. Holdiness MR. Adverse cutaneous reactions to antituberculosis drugs. Int J Dermatol 1985;24:280–285.
196. Jenner PJ, Ellard GA, Swai OB. A study of thioacetazone blood levels and urinary excretion in man using high performance liquid chromatography. Lepr Rev 1984;55:121–128.
197. Holdiness MR. Neurological manifestations and toxicities of the antituberculosis drugs: A review. Med Toxicol 1987;2:33–51.
198. Holdiness MR. Clinical pharamcokinetics of the antituberculosis drugs. Clin Pharmacokinet 1984;9:511–544.
199. Ellard GA, Dickinson JM, Gammon PT, Mitchison DA. Serum concentrations and antituberculosis activity of thioacetazone. Tubercle 1974;55:41–54.
200. Jenner PJ. High performance liquid chromatography determination of thioacetazone in body fluids. J Chromatogr Biomed Appl 1983;276:463–470.
201. Scharman EJ, Rosencrance JE. Isoniazid toxicity: A survey of pyridoxine availability. Am J Emerg Med 1994;12:386–388.
202. Corbella X, Vadillo M, Cabellos C, et al. Hypersensitivity hepatitis due to pyrazinamide. Scand J Infect Dis 1995;27:93–94.
203. Nair PM, Philip E. Accidental dapsone poisoning in children. Ann Trop Paediatr 1984;4:241–242.
204. Woodhouse KW, Henderson DB, Charlton B, et al. Acute dapsone poisoning: Clinical features and pharmacokinetic studies. Hum Toxicol 1983;3:507–510.
205. Davis R. Fatal poisoning with Udolac (diaminodiphenyl sulphone). Lancet 1950;1:905–906.
206. Neuvonen PJ, Elonen E, Haapanen EJ. Acute dapsone intoxication: Clinical findings and effect of oral charcoal and haemodialysis on dapsone elimination. Acta Med Scand 1983;214:215–220.
207. Kenner DJ, Holt K, Agnello R, et al. Permanent retinal damage following massive dapsone overdose. Br J Ophthalmol 1980;64:741–744.
208. Lambert M, Sonnett J, Mahieu P, et al. Delayed sulfhemoglobinemia after acute dapsone intoxication. J Toxicol Clin Toxicol 1982;19:45–50.
209. Shah RR, Wade G. Reappraisal of the risk/benefit of nitrofurantoin: Review of toxicity and efficacy. Adverse Drug React Acute Poison Rev 1989;8:183–201.
210. Chudnofsky DR, Otten EJ. Acute pulmonary toxicity to nitrofurantoin. J Emerg Med 1989;7:15–19.
211. Mollison LC, Angus P, Richards M, et al. Hepatitis due to nitrofurantoin. Med J Aust 1992;156:347–349.
212. Mannisto PT, Lamminsiu V. Nitrofurantoin is highly bound to plasma protein. J Antimicrob Chemother 1982;9:327–328.
213. Cunha BA. Nitrofurantoin: Current concepts. Urology 1988;32:67–71.

Chapter 15
AIDS Drugs

INTRODUCTION

Overdoses have been reported following the use of zidovudine, foscarnet, and ganciclovir. Neurologic, renal, and gastrointestinal symptoms predominate (Table 15–1). Few fatalities have been recorded. Antifungal (fluconazole, ketoconazole, amphotericin B, flucytosine), antimycobacterial (isoniazid, rifampin, ethambutol, pyrazinamide, ciprofloxacin), and antiviral (zidovudine, dideoxyinosine, acyclovir, ganciclovir, foscarnet) drugs are used in the treatment of patients with AIDS.[1,2]

INFORMATION SOURCES

Data on information sources regarding AIDS and AIDS drugs are available from the U.S. Food and Drug Administration[3] (Table 15–2).

SUICIDE DRUGS

The HIV-positive patient is subject to polypharmacy, iatrogenic toxicity, unusual drug reactions and interactions, and, possibly, increased drug allergies. The rate of suicide has been reported to be high in persons with chronic and life-threatening illnesses (eg, cancer, Huntington's disease, renal failure). AIDS represents a significant risk factor for suicide.[4–7] Self-poisoning with drugs represents the most common method of committing suicide among AIDS victims.[5] AIDS patients have used barbiturates, cyanide, cocaine,[6] heroin,[7] heroin in combination with methadone,[7] and massive overconsumption of alcohol and medicinal drugs to commit suicide.[7] In addition, several drugs used to treat AIDS-related infections (including pentamidine, isethionate, trimethoprim–sulfamethoxazole, and amphotericin B) have been associated with psychosis and delirium, conditions that increase suicide risk.[6]

INTRAVENOUS DRUG ABUSE

Drug variables associated with HIV infection in intravenous drug abusers include the number of days using nonsterile needles, days in "shooting galleries," sharing of drug

Table 15-1
Major Dose-Limiting Toxic Effects of AIDS Drugs

Zidovudine	Anemia, leukopenia, neutropenia
Didanosine	Pancreatitis, peripheral neuropathy
Zalcitabine	Painful sensorimotor peripheral neuropathy of the lower extremities
Stavudine	Painful sensory peripheral neuropathy

Table 15-2
AIDS Information Sources

General Information	
CDC National AIDS Hotline	
• English service (7 days a week, 24 hours a day)	1-800-342-AIDS (2347)
• Spanish service (7 days a week, 8 AM to 2 AM Eastern time)	1-800-344-7432
• TDD service for the deaf (10 AM to 10 PM Eastern time, Monday through Friday)	1-800-243-7889
CDC National AIDS Clearinghouse P.O. Box 6003 Rockville, MD 20849-6003	1-800-458-5231
• TTY/TDD (Monday through Friday, 9 AM to 7 PM Eastern time)	1-800-243-7012
National Institute on Drug Abuse Hotline	
• English service	1-800-662-HELP (4357)
• Spanish service	1-800-66-AYUDA (662-9832)
Status of U.S. HIV Clinical Trials	
AIDS Clinical Trials Information Service (ACTIS)	1-800-874-2572
• TTY/TDD	1-800-243-7012
• International	1-301-217-0023
• Fax	1-301-738-6616
(Monday through Friday, 9 AM to 7 PM Eastern time)	

For a copy of the 1993 *Surgeon General's Report to the American Public on HIV Infection and AIDS,* call 1-800-342-AIDS.

paraphernalia ("cookers"), and total number of injections of "speed balls" (heroin and cocaine). Nondrug variables include nonwhite race, poverty, prostitution, and a number of intravenous drug abuser sexual partners.[8] The incidence of AIDS may range from 72% in male heterosexual intravenous drug abusers to 0.8% in children whose mothers were sexual partners of intravenous drug abusers.[8]

FRONTLOADING (HALFING)

Frontloading is used by two or more injectors to share out drugs. The injector draws up the drug solution from the preparatory vessel ("cooker") into his or her own syringe and then injects ("spouts") a proportion of the solution directly into the barrel of his or her colleague's syringe. If the first syringe has previously been used, the potential exists for the second "clean" syringe to become inoculated with HIV without sharing even having occurred.[9]

BLEACH DISINFECTION

A 5.25% solution of sodium hypochlorite (household bleach) effectively inactivates HIV. Intravenous drug abusers who share needles are at high risk of acquiring and transmitting HIV. Cleaning needles and syringes with household bleach is used by this group as a strategy to control HIV transmission. The standard procedure includes flushing the syringe twice with undiluted household bleach and then twice with water. The small amounts of sodium hypochlorite remaining in a needle or syringe that may be inadvertently injected after disinfection are relatively nontoxic.[10,11]

Sterile, never-used needles and syringes are safer than bleach-disinfected, previously used needles and syringes. Cleaning injection equipment with disinfectants such as bleach does not guarantee that HIV is inactivated. Disinfectants do not sterilize equipment; however, consistent and thorough cleaning of injection equipment with disinfectants such as bleach should reduce transmission of HIV if equipment is shared.[10–16]

Bleach disinfection of needles and syringes continues to have an important role in *reducing* the risk of HIV transmission for intravenous drug abusers who have no other option but to reuse or share a needle and syringe. The use of full-strength bleach as described should improve the effectiveness of the bleach disinfection.[11–15]

NITRITE INHALANT ABUSE AND KAPOSI'S SARCOMA

Kaposi's sarcoma appears to be concentrated in gay men (especially white gay men) with AIDS and is rare in others. HIV alone does not appear to cause Kaposi's sarcoma in AIDS. Nitrite use by gay men has been on the decline since AIDS was first described. AIDS-related Kaposi's sarcoma found on the face and chest, especially the nose, is consistent with the areas of skin most heavily exposed to inhaled nitrite vapors. Conversion of nitrites to nitrosamines and/or cholesteryl nitrites (known carcinogens) in the skin and blood vessels has been proposed.[17–27] Nitrite inhalants may be a Kaposi's sarcoma cofactor.[28,29]

NITRITE PREPARATIONS

Nitrite can be obtained as a prescription drug (amyl nitrite) used to treat the symptoms of angina (ampules), as liquids (in labeled bottles sold as room deodorizers), and in unlabeled bottles, which usually contain a combination of amyl, butyl, and isobutyl nitrite.[20] The alkyl nitrites have been nicknamed "poppers" because of the sound made when the glass capsules containing amyl nitrite are crushed.[22]

The U.S. Congress enacted a ban on the manufacture and retail sale of butyl nitrites in the Anti-Drug Abuse Act of 1988.[23] To circumvent the clear intent of the law, nitrite manufacturers began to sell other nitrite alkyl congeners, such as isopropyl nitrite, as "new and improved" room deodorizers. In 1990, Congress outlawed manufacture and sale of alkyl nitrites in the Omnibus Crime Bill. Cyclohexyl nitrites are not in the same class asalkyl nitrites and, therefore, may not be banned under current federal law. Underground manufacturers and importers continue to market butyl and isopropyl nitrite illegally.

Table 15–3
Toxicokinetic Features of Selected Nucleoside Analogs with Antiretroviral Activity

Drug	Dose* (mg)	Peak Plasma Level After Dose (μM)	Oral Bioavailability (%)	Volume of Distribution (L/kg)	Terminal Plasma Half-Life (h)	Total Body Clearance (L/kg/h)	Approximate Intracellular Half-Life of Triphosphate (h)	CSF: Plasma Ratio†	Chief Clearance Route
Zidovudine	200	4	63	1.4	1.1	1.3	3	0.60	Liver, kidney
ddC	2	0.1–0.2	87	0.55	1.2	0.34	2.6	0.20	Kidney
ddI	250	8–10	40	NA	0.5	NA	12–24	0.20	NA
Acyclovir	800	7	20	0.68‡	2.9	0.22	1.2	0.50	Kidney
Ribavirin	600	5.1	45	9.2	35§	0.24	NA	0.67‖	Kidney

ddC, 2′,3′-dideoxycytidine; ddI, 2′,3′-dideoxyinosine; CSF, cerebrospinal fluid.
*Dose is typical adult single dose administered orally. For ddI, it is one representative dose that was tested in a phase I trial. Oral doses of ddI were administered with antacids. For acyclovir, the dose has been studied in combination with zidovudine (100 mg) for possible synergistic anti-HIV effect.
†The ratio shown was measured 2 to 4 hours after the dose was administered.
‡Steady-state volume of distribution is shown.
§Ribavirin also accumulates in red cells, where it can reside for several weeks.
‖The CSF: plasma ratio for ribavirin was assessed after several weeks of therapy. The number of hours between the administration of the dose and the collection of these samples is not known.
From Yarchoan R, Mitsuya H, Myers CE, Broder S. Clinical pharmacology of 3′-azido-2′,3′-dideoxythymidine (zidovudine) and related dideoxynucleosides. N Engl J Med 1989;321:726–738. Erratum: 1990;322:280E.

Table 15–4
Interactions of Drugs to Treat Opportunistic Infections in AIDS and Their Use in Pregnancy and Breastfeeding

Drug	Interactions	Pregnancy	Breastfeeding
Acyclovir	Possibility of extreme lethargy with concurrent administration of intravenous acyclovir and zidovudine ↓Acyclovir excretion by probenecid	Fetal abnormalities (animal studies); avoid if possible as risks unknown	Found in breast milk, therefore avoid if possible
Amphotericin B	↑Risk of nephrotoxicity with aminoglycosides, cefalothin, and cyclosporine; avoid concomitant use ↓Effect of miconazole (suggested but not proven)		
Clindamycin	↓Effect of neostigmine and pyridostigmine ↑Effect of tubocurarine ↑Nephrotoxicity of gentamicin	Safety not established	Safety not established
Dapsone	↓Dapsone excretion by probenecid ↓Effect by rifampicin (rifampin) ↓Dapsone absorption by didanosine buffers	Can be used; need folate supplements; caution, especially late pregnancy	Not recommended
Fluconazole	↑Fluconazole concentrations by hydrochlorothiazide ↓Fluconazole concentrations by rifampicin ↑Effect of nicoumalone, warfarin, sulfonylureas, and phenytoin ↑Concentrations of cyclosporine and theophylline	Contraindicated (teratogenic in animal studies)	
Foscarnet	Beware concomitant nephrotoxic drugs Beware cumulative toxicity with zidovudine ↑Hypocalcemia by pentamidine	Contraindicated	Contraindicated
Ganciclovir	↑Myelosuppression with zidovudine Beware concomitant myelosuppressive drugs	Contraindicated (reversible hypospermatogenesis); barrier contraception in men for 90 d after last dose	Contraindicated; no feeding until >72 h after last dose
Isoniazid	↓Isoniazid concentrations by antacids and corticosteroids; reduced efficacy ↑Effect of some anticonvulsants (carbamazepine, ethosuximide and phenytoin) ↑Concentrations of diazepam and theophylline		Caution: monitor infant for possible toxicity; prophylactic pyridoxine advised for infant as well as mother
Itraconazole	↓Itraconazole concentrations by rifampicin, antacids, adsorbents, and H_2 antagonists ↑Effect of warfarin ↑Concentrations of cyclosporine	Safety not established; appears safe in animal studies, but best avoided	Found in breast milk
Ketoconazole	↓Ketoconazole concentrations by antacids, absorbents, H_2 antagonists, rifampicin, phenytoin, and didanosine ↑Effect of nicoumbalne, warfarin, and phenytoin ↑Concentrations of cyclosporine and terfenadine ↓Concentrations of antimuscarinic agents Disulfiram-type reaction with alcohol	Teratogenic in animal studies, therefore contraindicated	Avoid (insufficient data)
Pyrazinamide	↓Effect of uricosurics		
Rifampicin	↓Rifampicin concentrations by antacids ↓Effect of methadone, some antiarrhythmics (disopyramide, mexiletine, propafenone, quinidine), chloramphenicol, warfarin, antidiabetics (chlorpropamide and tolbutamide especially), phenytoin, some antifungals (fluconazole, itraconazole, ketoconazole), haloperidol, propranolol, verapamil, digoxin, corticosteroids, cyclosporine, sex hormones (particularly oral contraceptives), theophylline, thyroxine, and cimetidine		

(continued)

Table 15–4 *(Continued)*

Drug	Interactions	Pregnancy	Breastfeeding
Sulfadiazine	↑Effect of thiopental, nicoumalone, warfarin, sulfonylureas, phenytoin, and methoxtrexate ↑Concentrations of cyclosporine Antifolate effect: beware cumulative effect with other antifolates	Embryotoxic in animal studies; kenicterus (late pregnancy); avoid if possible	
Trimethoprim	↑Effect of nicoumalone, warfarin, sulfonylureas, and phenytoin Antifolate effect: beware cumulative effect with other antifolates Beware concomitant myelosuppressive drugs	Teratogenic risk, therefore contraindicated	Caution
Trimethoprim–sulfamethoxazole (Co-trimoxazole) and sulfonamides	↑Effect of thiopentone (thiopental), warfarin, sulfonylureas and phenytoin ↑Risk of nephrotoxicity with cyclosporine ↑Antifolate effect with phenytoin, pyrimethamine, and methotrexate Folic acid ↓ effects of sulfur drugs and must not be used	Avoid: possible teratogenesis	Caution: small risk of kernicterus in jaundiced infants and of hemolysis in glucose-6-phosphate dehydrogenase (G6PD)-deficient infants

From Peters BS, Carlin E, Weston RJ, et al. Adverse effects of drugs used in the management of opportunistic infections associated with HIV infection. Drug Saf 1994;10:439–454.

Table 15–5
Drugs That Cause Severe Cutaneous Reactions in HIV-Positive Individuals

Trimethoprim–sulfamethoxazole	Amoxillin and clavulanic acid
Trimethoprim and dapsone	Isoniazid
Pyrimethamine	Rifampicin
Sulfadiazine	Streptomycin
Dideoxycytidine	Thioacetazone

Toxicity of Nitrite Abuse

The acute toxic effects of inhaled and ingested nitrites in humans include skin irritations (especially around the nose and lips), tracheobronchial irritation, headache, hypotension, cyanosis, methemoglobinemia, intoxication, and, rarely, death. Other effects include development of habitual use patterns, tolerance, and burns resulting from inadvertent ignition of the vapor.

Epidemiology of Nitrite Abuse

Nitrites have been proposed to enhance HIV transmission by their association with risky sexual behaviors and HIV infection among gay men. Nitrite use has been associated with immunosuppression. Finally, nitrite inhalant use has been associated with the development of AIDS-related Kaposi's sarcoma.[29]

GENERAL PROPERTIES OF AIDS DRUGS

Toxicokinetics

Yarchoan and colleagues (Table 15–3) have summarized the toxicokinetic properties of nucleoside analogs and their metabolites.[30]

Drug interactions (see individual drug descriptions) leading to adverse reactions are frequently seen in patients with AIDS, as multiple drugs are commonly prescribed to these individuals. A summary of drug interactions involving AIDS drugs and their use in pregnancy and breastfeeding is presented in Table 15–4.[31] Lee and Safrin provide a comprehensive summary of drug interactions as well.[2,32]

Clinical Presentation[33]

Drug Reactions

The incidence of drug reactions (eg, rash, hypersensitivity,[34] pancreatitis)[35] in HIV-infected patients is high. Increased incidences of reactions have followed the use of trimethoprim–sulfamethoxazole, amoxicillin–clavulanate,[36] and thalidomide. Altered drug metabolism may account for the increased incidence of adverse reactions to drugs in AIDS patients with acute illnesses,[37] but specific mechanisms have not been evaluated.

Cutaneous Reactions

Patients with AIDS infection who have received multiple medications appear to be at increased risk of developing Stevens–Johnson syndrome, toxic epidermal necrolysis, and scalded skin syndrome, particularly if they have had previous cutaneous drug reactions (Table 15–5).[38–40] A generalized morbilliform exanthem is the most commonly observed drug reaction, occurring 7 to 10 days after therapy initiation; it resolves rapidly after drug withdrawal. Long-term prospective trials are required to more accurately determine the incidence of risk factors for acute morbidity from these adverse cutaneous reactions.

Table 15-6
Psychiatric and Neurologic Side Effects of Medications Used in HIV Spectrum Disease

Drug	Side Effect
Trimethoprim–sulfamethoxazole	Psychosis, mutism, bizarre mannerisms, depression, loss of appetite, insomnia, apathy, headache, neuritis
Ketoconazole	Headache, dizziness, photosensitivity
Amphotericin B	Delirium, peripheral neuropathy, blurred vision, diplopia, weight loss, loss of appetite, headache
Azidothymidine	Mania, agitation, headache, insomnia, myostitis
Dideoxyinosine, dideoxycytidine	Sensory neuropathies, pancreatitis (with neurologic complications)
Acyclovir	Depression, agitation, auditory and visual hallucinations, depersonalization, tearfulness, confusion, hyperesthesia, hyperacusis, insomnia, intrusive thoughts, headache
Interferons	Depression, confusion, delirium, memory and psychomotor impairment, fatigue suggestive of frontal lobe changes, reversible impairment of higher cognitive functions, acute encephalitis, chills, myalgias, arthralgias, headache, extrapyramidal symptoms, mania, neurasthenia with catatonia
Interleukin-2	Disorientation, cognitive deterioration
Isoniazid	Depression, agitation, auditory and visual hallucinations, paranoia, peripheral neuropathy, memory impairment
Ethambutol	Headache, dizziness, confusion, visual disturbances
Rifampin	Headache, fatigue, loss of appetite, visual disturbances
Cycloserine	Anxiety, depression, confusion, disorientation, hallucinations, paranoia, loss of appetite, fatigue
Sulfonamides	Headache, neuritis, insomnia, loss of appetite, photosensitivity
Baclofen	Interacts with haloperidol to induce delusional depression and pseudoparkinsonism
Disulfiram/diethyldithiocarbamate	Peripheral neuropathy
Methotrexate	Headaches, blurred vision, fatigue, photosensitivity, aseptic meningitis, encephalopathy
Procarbazine	Mania, loss of appetite, headaches, insomnia, nightmares, confusion, malaise
Flucytosine	Confusion, headache, sedation
Vincristine	Hallucinations, headache, neuritis, ataxia, sensory loss, peripheral neuropathy, autonomic and cranial neuropathy
Vinblastine	Depression, loss of appetite, headache, neuritis
Etoposide	Neuropathy, loss of appetite
5-Fluorouracil	Cerebellar ataxia
Cytosine arabinoside	Peripheral neuropathy, cerebellar ataxia
L-asparaginase	Reversible encephalopathy

From Whitaker RED, Ostrow DG. Psychiatric and psychopharmacologic problems in HIV-1 infection. Hosp Formul 1991;26:948–959.

AIDS Clinical Trials

A database search has been prepared by the AIDS Clinical Trials Information Service, a service of the U.S. Public Health Service, P.O. Box 6421, Rockville, MD 10850. Telephone: 1-800–TRIALS-A; fax: 1-301-738-6616.[41]

Reactions to Trimethoprim–Sulfamethoxazole

The frequency of severe adverse reactions (skin rashes, cytopenias, hepatotoxicity, vomiting, diarrhea) to trimethoprim–sulfamethoxazole in patients with AIDS (40–80%) is much higher than in patients without AIDS.[37] Some evidence points to the hydroxylamine derivatives of sulfamethoxazole as the reactive metabolites that predispose to such adverse reactions. HIV-positive individuals have a systemic glutathione deficiency and may have a reduced capacity to scavenge such metabolites, leading to an increased exposure to these metabolites.[42–45]

Pancreatitis

Didanosine, pentamidine, trimethoprim–sulfamethoxazole, anticonvulsants, and HIV-related diseases such as cytomegalovirus, mycobacteriosis, cryptosporidosis, and tumors are reported causes of pancreatitis in AIDS patients.[35]

Neurologic Effects

Psychiatric and neurologic side effects of drugs used in HIV-spectrum disease are listed in Table 15–6.[46] Delirium in AIDS may follow intoxication with drugs (e.g., hypnotics, opiates, phencyclidine or alcohol) and alcohol or drug withdrawal.[47]

Extrapyramidal Symptoms. Patients with AIDS who have taken dopamine blocking agents appear to be more susceptible to extrapyramidal symptoms than psychotic patients without AIDS. Neuroleptic agents should be used cautiously and in lower doses in patients with AIDS.[48,49]

Pathophysiology

Activity of cytochrome P450, intimately involved in the biotransformation of drugs, is depressed during the course of some viral infections in animals and humans. This depression results from the production of interferon and subsequent inhibition of cytochrome P450 synthesis at a pretranslational step.[50]

Antidotes and Glutathione in HIV

Diethyldithiocarbamate (Dithiocarb)

A controlled prospective study suggests that dithiocarb reduces the incidence of opportunistic infections in patients with symptomatic HIV infections, in addition to reducing lymphadenopathy and splenomegaly. Dithiocarb is a strong antioxidant.[51–53]

N-Acetylcysteine and Glutathione

Herzenberg and colleagues at Stanford University[54–61] and Buhl and colleagues[62,63] have demonstrated a diminished glutathione level in the immune system of the AIDS patient. Glutathione appears to be critical to the function of natural killer cells and important for lymphocyte-mediated cytotoxicity. This appears to protect cells against reactive oxygen intermediates.[52] Lack of glutathione and oxidative injury have been identified during acetaminophen poisoning, adult respiratory distress syndrome, idiopathic pulmonary fibrosis, and AIDS.[64] Glutathione is the major source of plasma cysteine. AIDS patients have low plasma cysteine concentrations and low acid-soluble thiol concentrations. Glutathione, glutathione ester, and *N*-acetylcysteine suppress HIV expression, decrease HIV protein synthesis, and decrease HIV RNA synthesis.[65] The excessive use of acetaminophen in HIV-infected patients will doubtless require serious consideration.

In addition to thiol products, consideration has also been given to the use of penicillamine[55,65] as an anti-HIV therapy. Controlled clinical studies have not been performed.

Drug hypersensitivity may result from the glutathione deficiency and slow acetylation of some drugs. Acutely ill patients with HIV infections are slow acetylators of trimethoprim–sulfamethoxazole and dapsone.[66] Exaggerated insect bite reactions have also been reported in HIV-positive patients.[67]

Sudden Death

Remember that sudden death in a drug user who is HIV positive may not be the result of a drug overdose. Other causes (pneumonitis, encephalitis) must be considered.[68]

REFERENCES—AIDS DRUGS

1. Drugs for AIDS and associated infections. Med Lett Drugs Ther 1993;35:79–81.
2. Lee BL, Safrin S. Drug interactions and toxicities in patients with AIDS. Curr Opin Infect Dis 1992;5:231–240.
3. FDA Consumer 1993;27:14.
4. McKegney FP, O'Dowd MA. Suicidality and HIV status. Am J Psychiatry 1992;149:396–398.
5. Cote TC, Biggar RJ, Dannenberg AL. Risk of suicide among persons with AIDS: A national assessment. JAMA 1992; 268:2066–2068.
6. Marzuk PM, Tierney H, Tardiff K, et al. Increased risk of suicide in persons with AIDS. JAMA 1988;259:1333–1337.
7. Rajs J, Fugelstad A. Suicide related to human immunodeficiency virus infection in Stockholm. Acta Psychiatr Scand 1992;85:234–239.
8. Sobel JD. Acquired immunodeficiency syndrome in intravenous drug abusers. In: Levine DP, Sobel JD, eds: *Infections in Intravenous Drug Abusers.* New York: Oxford University Press, 1990:342–379.
9. Green ST, Taylor A, Frischer M, Goldberg DJ. "Frontloading" ("halfing") among Glasgow drug injectors as a continuing risk behavior for HIV transmission. Addiction 1993;88:1581–1582.
10. Froner GA, Rutherford GW, Rokeach M. Injection of sodium hypochlorite by intravenous drug users. JAMA 1987; 258:325.
11. Morgan DL: Intravenous injection of household bleach. Ann Emerg Med 1992;21:1394–1395.
12. Use of bleach for disinfection of drug injection equipment. MMWR 1993;42:418–419.
13. Centers for Disease Control and Prevention, Center for Substance Abuse Treatment, National Institute of Drug Abuse. HIV/AIDS Prevention Bulletin, April 19, 1993.
14. Curran JW. CDC, Public Health services letter, May 24, 1993.
15. Watters JK, Jones TS, Shapshak P, et al. Household bleach as disinfectant for use by injecting drug users. Lancet 1993;342:742–743.
16. Krepcho MA, Fernandez-Esquer ME, Fleeman AC, et al. Predictors of bleach use among current African-American injecting drug users: A community study. J Psychoactive Drugs 1993;25:135–141.
17. Haverkos HW. Nitrite inhalant abuse in AIDS-related Kaposi's sarcoma (KS). AIDS Res Hum Retroviruses 1992;8:878.
18. Haverkos HW, Dougherty JA, eds. *Health Hazards of Nitrite Inhalants.* NIDA Research Monograph 83. DHHS Publication No. (ADM) 89-1573. Washington, DC: Alcohol, Drug Abuse and Mental Health Administration, 1988.
19. Haverkos HW. Nitrite inhalant abuse and AIDS-related Kaposi's sarcoma. J Acquir Immune Defic Syndr 1990;3(suppl. 1): S47–S50.
20. Seage GR III, Mayer KH, Horsburgh CR, et al. The relation between nitrite inhalants, unprotected receptive anal intercourse, and the risk of human immunodeficiency virus infection. Am J Epidemiol 1992;135:1–11.
21. Haverkos HW, Dougherty J. Health hazards nitrite inhalants. Am J Med 1988;84:479–482.
22. Haverkos HW. The search for cofactors in AIDS including an analysis of the association of nitrite inhalant abuse and Kaposi's sarcoma. In: Geminara D, Watson RR, eds. *Alcohol, Immunomodulation and AIDS.* New York: Alan R. Liss, 1990:93–102.
23. Drotman DP, Haverkos HW. What causes Kaposi's sarcoma? Inquiring epidemiologists want to know. Epidemiology 1992;3:191–193.
24. Haverkos HW, Drotman DP, Morgan WM. Kaposi's sarcoma in patients with AIDS: Sex, transmission node, and race. Biomed Pharmacother 1990;44:461–466.
25. Berel V, Peterman TA, Berkelman RL, Jaffe HW. Kaposi's sarcoma among persons with AIDS: A sexually transmitted infection? Lancet 1990;335:123–128.
26. Archibald CP, Schechter MT, Craib KJP, et al. Risk factors for Kaposi's sarcoma in the Vancouver Lymphadenopathy–AIDS study. J Acquir Immune Defic Syndr 1990; 3(suppl. 1): S18–S28.
27. Cockerill FR III, Edson RS. Trimethoprim–sulfamethoxazole. Mayo Clin Proc 1991;66:1260–1269.
28. Mirvish SS, Williamson J, Babcock D, Chen S-C. Mutagenicity of iso-butyl nitrite vapor in the Ames test and some relevant chemical properties including the reaction of isobutyl nitrite with phosphate. Environ Mol Mutagen 1993; 21:247–252.
29. Haverkos HW, Kopstein AN, Wilson H, Drotman P. Nitrite inhalants: History, epidemiology and possible links to AIDS. Environ Health Perspect 1994;102:858–861.
30. Yarchoan R, Mitsuya F, Myers CE, Broden S. Clinical pharmacology of 3′-azido-2′-3′-dideoxythymidine (zidovidine) and related dideoxynucleosides. N Engl J Med 1989;34:726–738.
31. Peters BS, Carlin E, Weston RJ, et al. Adverse effects of drugs used in the management of opportunistic infections associated with HIV infection. Drug Saf 1994;10439–454.
32. Lee BL, Safrin S. AIDS commentary: Interactions and toxicities of drugs used in patients with AIDS. Clin Infect Dis 1992; 14:773–779.
33. Pluda JM, Mitsuya H, Yarchoan R. Hematologic effects of AIDS therapies. Hematol/Oncol Clin North Am 1991;5: 229–248.
34. Williams I, Weller IVD, Malin A, et al. Lancet 1991;337:436–437.

35. Jost R, Stey C, Salomon F. Fatal drug-induced pancreatitis in HIV. Lancet 1993;341:1412.
36. Battogay M, Opravil M, Wulfrich B, Luthy R. Rash with amoxicillin–clavulanate therapy in HIV-infected patients. Lancet 1989;2:110.
37. Lee BL, Wong D, Benowitz NL, Sullain PM. Altered patterns of drug metabolism in patients with acquired immunodeficiency syndrome. Clin Pharmacol Ther 1993;53:529–535.
38. Porteous DM, Berger TG. Severe cutaneous drug reactions (Stevens–Johnson syndrome and toxic epidermal necrolysis) in human immunodeficiency virus infection. Arch Dermatol 1991;127:740–741.
39. Coopman SA, Stern RS. Cutaneous drug reactions in human immunodeficiency virus infection. Arch Dermatol 1991;127: 714–717.
40. Saiag P, Caumes E, Chosidow O, et al. Drug-induced toxic epidermal necrolysis (Lyell syndrome) in patients infected with the human immunodeficiency virus. J Am Acad Dermatol 1992;26:567–574.
41. AIDS drugs being studied. FDA Consumer 1992;26(3):8–9.
42. Van der Ven AJAM, Koopmans PP, Vree TB, Van der Meer JWM. Adverse reactions to Co-trimoxazole in HIV infection. Lancet 1991;338:431–433.
43. Toma E, Fournier S. Adverse reactions to Co-trimoxazole in HIV infection. Lancet 1991;338:954.
44. Pozniak A, Weinberg J, MacLeod G. HIV and Co-trimoxazole toxicity. Lancet 1991;338:760–761.
45. Slattery JT, Unadkat JD. Adverse reactions to Co-trimoxazole in HIV infection. Lancet 1991;338:1216.
46. Whitaker RED, Ostrow DG. Psychiatric and psychopharmacologic problems in HIV-1 infection. Hosp Formul 1991; 26:948–959.
47. Cohen MAA. Biopsychosocial approach to the human immunodeficiency virus epidemic: A clinician's primer. Gen Hosp Psychiatry 1990;12:98–123.
48. Pozniak AL, McLeod GA, Mahari M, et al. The influence of HIV status on single and multiple drug reactions to antituberculosis therapy in Africa. AIDS 1992;6:809–814.
49. Hriso E, Kuhn T, Masdeu JC, Grundman M. Extrapyramidal symptoms due to dopamine-blocking agents in patients with AIDS encephalopathy. Am J Psychiatry 1991;148:1558–1101.
50. Renton KW, Cribb AE, Armstrong S. Role of altered drug metabolism in viral drug interactions. Rev Infect Dis 1991;13: 1256–1257.
51. Hersh EM, Brewton G, Abrams D, et al. Dithiocarb sodium (diethyldithiocarbmate) therapy in patients with symptomatic HIV infection and AIDS: A randomized double-blind, placebo-controlled, multicenter study. JAMA 1991;265:1538–1544.
52. Gougerot-Pocidalo M-A, Levacher M. Glutathione and HIV infection. Lancet 1990;335:234.
53. Dupuy J-M, Revillard J-P, Hersh EM, et al. Glutathione and HIV infection. Lancet 1990;335:234–235.
54. Staal FJT, Roederer M, Israelski DM, et al. Intracellular glutathione levels in T-cell subsets decrease in HIV-infected individuals. AIDS Res Hum Retroviruses 1992;8:305–311.
55. Roederer M, Ela SW, Staal FJT, et al. *N*-Acetylcysteine: A new approach to anti-HIV therapy. AIDS Res Hum Retroviruses 1992;8:209–219.
56. Staal FJT, Roederer M, Herzenberg LA, Herzenberg LA. Intracellular thiols regulate activation of nuclear factor KB and transcription of human immunodeficiency virus. Proc Natl Acad Sci USA 1990;87:9943–9947.
57. Roederer M, Staal FJT, Raju PA, et al. Cytokine-stimulated human immunodeficiency virus replication is inhibited by *N*-acetyl-L-cysteine. Proc Natl Acad Sci USA 1990;87:4884–4888.
58. Roederer M, Raju PA, Staal FJT, et al. *N*-Acetylcysteine inhibits latent HIV expression in chronically infected cells. AIDS Res Hum Retroviruses 1991;7:491–495.
59. Roederer M, Staal FJT, Osado H, et al. CD4 and CD8 T-cells with high intracellular glutathione levels are selectively lost as the HIV infection progresses. Int Immunol 1991;3: 933–937.
60. Staal FJT, Ela SW, Roederer M, et al. Glutathione deficiency and human immunodeficiency virus infection. Lancet 1992;339:909–912.
61. Roederer M, Staal FJT, Ela SW, et al. *N*-Acetylcysteine: Potential for AIDS therapy. Pharmacology 1993;46:121–129.
62. Buhl R, Jaffe HA, Holvoyd KJ, et al. Systemic glutathione deficiency in symptom-free HIV-seropositive individuals. Lancet 1989;2:1294–1298.
63. Buhl Jaffe HA, Holroyd KJ, Wells FB, et al. Glutathione deficiency and HIV. Lancet 1990;335:546.
64. Ruffman R, Wendel A. GSH rescue by *N*-acetylcysteine. Klin Wochenschr 1991;69:857–862.
65. Kalebic T, Kinter A, Poli G, et al. Suppression of human immunodeficiency virus expression in chronically infected monocytic cells by glutathione, glutathione ester, and *N*-acetylcysteine. Proc Natl Acad Sci USA 1991;88:986–990.
66. Harb GE, Jacobson MA. Human immunodeficiency virus (HIV) infection: Does it increase susceptibility to adverse drug reactions? Drug Saf 1993;9:1–8.
67. Smith KJ, Skelton HG III, Vogel P, et al. Exaggerated insect bite reactions in patients positive for HIV. J Am Acad Dermatol 1993;29:269–272.
68. Jones ME, Brettle PP, Busuttil A, et al. Sudden death in HIV infected drug users: Presumptive overdose in an HIV-positive narcotic addict. J Infect 1993;27:79–81.

ZIDOVUDINE (AZT)

Zidovudine was the first drug approved in the United States for use in the management of HIV infections.[1–7] Zidovudine therapy delays progression to AIDS and late stages of HIV disease, increases CD4 cell counts, and suppresses viral replication in patients with asymptomatic or mildly symptomatic HIV infection who have 200 to 500 CD4 cells/μL. Overdoses of zidovudine alone have been relatively asymptomatic; when the drug is combined with sedative–hypnotics or other drugs of abuse, central nervous system depression and mild hepatotoxicity may be observed. There have been no fatalities following zidovudine overdoses. Overdoses have often occurred within a month of the first positive HIV test.[8]

Structure and Classification

Zidovudine is 3′-azido-3′-deoxythymidine (ZDV, AZT, Retrovir). Its metabolite is zidovudine glucuronide, 3′-azido-3′-deoxy-5′-*O*-β-D-glucopyranuronosylthymidine (ZDVG, GAZT). The molecular weight of zidovudine is 267.24; the conversion factor (SF) is 3.74.

Product Formulation

Zidovudine is available for oral use in capsules, 100 mg (Retrovir); in solution, 50 mg/5 mL (Retrovir Syrup); and in parenteral injection for intravenous infusion, 10 mg/mL (Retrovir Infusion).[9] It is a synthetic chemical product.

Therapeutic Dose

The current recommended therapeutic dose is 100 mg five or six times daily (500–600 mg/d).[9] For patients with asymptomatic HIV infection, 100 mg every 4 hours while awake (500 mg/d) may be effective.[10] The currently recommended pediatric dose is 180 mg/m^2 (up to 200 mg) every 6 hours for children 3 months to 12 years old.[2] A syrup (50 mg/5 mL) is available for patients unable to swallow capsules.[11] Zidovudine appears to be safe and possibly effective in asymptomatic patients with more than 200 and less than 500 CD4-positive T lymphocytes per microliter.[1,3,4]

Clinical Presentation

Doses up to 25,000 mg (450 mg/kg) have been ingested with few, if any, abnormal symptoms or signs.[12–15] After ingesting 36,000 mg, one patient experienced a grand mal seizure.[16] Patients may develop symptoms of ocular nystagmus, lethargy, and ataxia at lower doses (5000—7500 mg) when sedative–hypnotic agents, benzodiazepines, and marijuana are also ingested.[17–20] A 27-month-old child ingested 130 mg of zidovudine and survived.[21] A 24-year-old ingested 6 g of zidovudine with 2 g of acyclovir; temporary bone marrow failure developed over the next 10 days.[22] No lethal dose for zidovudine has been reported.

Occupational Exposure

Accidental needlesticks are a potentially serious threat to the health of medical and nursing personnel.[23–26] There is no convincing clinical data that offer proof of prophylactic success in the prevention of HIV virus infection. A number of failures of zidovudine prophylaxis have been reported when zidovudine was administered within 1 hour of an accidental exposure.[27–30] As there are possibly serious side effects following zidovudine therapy, initiating such use as an emergency procedure should be preceded by careful counseling.

Chronic Use

Long-term administration of zidovudine is associated with myopathy, manifested by myalgia, proximal muscle wasting, and an increase in serum creatine kinase concentration. Long-term therapy is also associated with progressive HIV disease, declines in CD4 cell counts, and emergence of viral strains with decreased susceptibility to zidovudine.

Toxicokinetics[31–37]

Absorption

Rapid and nearly complete absorption from the gastrointestinal tract follows oral administration (Table 15–3). The systemic bioavailability of zidovudine capsules and solution is about 63% and reflects a substantive first-pass metabolism.[33]

Drug Interactions

Acetaminophen concurrently administered with zidovudine increases the rate of bone marrow suppression,[7] but has no effect on peak times, half-lives, or area under the curve of zidovudine or its metabolite.[38] Acetaminophen glucuronidation is competitively inhibited by zidovudine, but zidovudine glucuronidation is only slightly inhibited by acetaminophen. Acetaminophen hepatotoxicity is probably augmented by zidovudine through its competition for glucuronidation metabolic pathways.[39] Patients are able to tolerate concurrent therapy with zidovudine and antimycobacterial agents without unacceptable toxicity.[40]

Cefoperazone, piperacillin, amoxicillin, chloramphenicol, probenecid, vancomycin, miconazole, rifampicin, phenobarbital, carbamazepine, phenytoin, valproic acid, quinidine, phenylbutazone, ketoprofen, probenicid, and propofol,[41] which are subject to glucuronidation, may alter the glucuronidation of zidovudine.[40]

Pregnancy/Lactation

Zidovudine and its glucuronide metabolite cross the placenta,[42–44] and are found in therapeutic levels in all body fluids of the infant.[45] Use of zidovudine throughout pregnancy in a known HIV-infected mother did not prevent transmission of the virus to the fetus.[46]

A retrospective study in 43 women who had ingested zidovudine during pregnancy (12 in the first trimester) indicated that all newborns (45) were born alive with a birth weight of 3000 g. No pattern of intrauterine growth retardation, asphyxia, or serious hematologic toxicity was observed in the infants.[47] A Zidovudine in Pregnancy Registry is available: telephone (800) 722–9292, extension 8465, in the United States, and (919) 315–8465 from countries outside the United States.

Laboratory

Analytical Methods

A radioimmunoassay procedure is available to allow simultaneous determination of both zidovudine and its metabolite zidovudine glucuronide. The lower detection limit of the radioimmunoassay is 0.27 μg/L.[48] A high-performance liquid chromatography method analyzes both the drug and its metabolite simultaneously. It has a linearity of 20 to 5000 ng/mL.[49]

Blood Levels

A 27-month-old who ingested 130 mg (10.2 ng/kg) had a blood level of 1.9 μg/mL 75 minutes later. Two hours later after induced emesis, the level was 0.6 μg/mL, dropping further to 0.1 μg/mL in 24 hours.[21] Following a 7200-ng ingestion, the blood levels of zidovudine and zidovudine glucuronide were 1.4 and 3.4 μg/mL, respectively.[15] The serum level after an oral dose of 250 mg zidovudine is usually less than 5 mmol/L.

Ancillary Tests

Cerebrospinal fluid examination after overdose is usually within normal limits.[17] Electroencephalograms taken 3 days postoverdose were normal in a patient who suffered a grand mal seizure.[16] The electrocardiogram may exhibit a mild sinus tachycardia.[17] Serum transaminase levels were elevated but normal after severe overdoses of 20,000 mg[18] and 36,000 mg.[16]

Treatment

Stabilization

Patients who have ingested an overdose of solely zidovudine are usually alert and have normal vital signs. They should be treated symptomatically and supportively in hospital, where they should be observed for at least 24 hours.

Patients who have ingested an overdose of zidovudine together with a sedative–hypnotic agent may have varying presentations relating to central nervous system depression. Patients should receive an intravenous line and have access to oxygen and cardiac monitoring as necessary.

For both of the preceding groups it is of paramount importance that there be proper maintenance of a normal airway and respiratory and circulatory status.

Gut Decontamination

Seizures have occurred within 3 hours of ingestion of high doses of zidovudine,[16] and therefore use of syrup of ipecac is not advisable. If gastric lavage is contemplated, adequate tracheal protection should be provided. If a toxicology screen or history indicates that a sedative–hypnotic drug has been ingested together with zidovudine, then activated charcoal may be beneficial. There is no clinical evidence that activated charcoal or cathartics are useful in zidovudine overdose treatment.

Elimination Enhancement

With the high volume of distribution and relatively benign course following supportive therapy, hemodialysis and hemoperfusion are not likely to be used very often. There are no data reported thus far to support the usefulness of these procedures. Whole-bowel irrigation has not been used, but may possibly be beneficial in high-volume ingestions. This procedure requires study before it can be recommended.

Antidote

There is no antidote for zidovudine overdose.

Supportive Measures

Patients should be treated symptomatically and supportively. On admission to an emergency facility, blood should be drawn for complete blood counts including neutrophil and platelet counts, liver function tests, and renal function studies.

Many patients who overdose have AIDS and are also intravenous drug abusers. Therefore, a urine screen should be obtained for barbiturates, benzodiazepines, cannabinols, and other drugs known to the local drug culture.

Seizures may be treated with diazepam. Electroencephalography and computed brain scans may be indicated.

Blood may be drawn to confirm the presence of zidovudine; subsequent samples may be drawn to follow the clinical course. Blood levels often return to normal therapeutic levels within 24 hours. Follow-up blood counts, including neutrophil and platelet counts, should be performed during the first few weeks.

Multiple doses of acetaminophen should be avoided in zidovudine-treated patients who are suspected of having diminished stores of glutathione due to poor nutrition, HIV infection, or alcohol consumption, and in zidovudine-treated patients who are also receiving therapeutic agents that stimulate P450 enzymes, such as anticonvulsants.[39]

REFERENCES—ZIDOVUDINE

1. Moore RD, Creagh-Kirk T, Keruly J, et al. Long-term safety and efficacy of zidovudine in patients with advanced human immunodeficiency virus disease. Arch Intern Med 1991; 151:981–986.
2. McKinney RE Jr, Maha MA, Connor FM, et al. A multicenter trial of oral zidovudine in children with advanced human immunodeficiency virus disease. N Engl J Med 1991;324: 1018–1025.
3. Fischl MA, Parker CB, Pettinelli C, et al. A randomized controlled trial of a reduced daily dose of zidovudine in patients with the acquired immunodeficiency syndrome. N Engl J Med 1990;323:1009–1014.
4. Volberding PA, Lagakos SW, Koch MA, et al. Zidovudine in asymptomatic human immunodeficiency virus infection: A controlled trial in persons with fewer than 500 CD-4 positive cells per cubic millimeter. N Engl J Med 1990;322:941–949.
5. Fischl MA, Richman DD, Hansen N, et al. The safety and efficacy of zidovudine (AZT) in the treatment of subjects with mildly symptomatic human immunodeficiency virus type 1 (HIV) infection: A double-blind, placebo-controlled trial. Ann Intern Med 1990;112:727–731.
6. Coller AC, Bozzette S, Coombs RW, et al. A pilot study of low dose zidovudine in human immunodeficiency virus infection. N Engl J Med 1990;323:1015–1021.
7. Richman DD, Fischl MA, Grieco MH, et al. The toxicity of azidothymidine (AZT) in the treatment of patients with AIDS and AIDS-related complex. N Engl J Med 1987;317:192–197.
8. Valentine C, Williams O, Davis A, et al. Case study of zidovudine overdose. AIDS 1993;7:436–437.
9. Zidovudine. In: McEvoy GK, ed. *AHFS Drug Information 94.* Bethesda, MD: American Society of Hospital Pharmacists, 1994:438–451.
10. Swart AM, Weller I, Darbyshire JH. Early HIV infection: to treat or not to treat? Cautiously until trials produce answers on long term efficacy and safety. Br Med J 1990;301:825–826.
11. Zidovudine. Med Letter Drugs Ther 1990;32:78.
12. Terragna A, Mazzarello G, Anselmo M, et al. Suicidal attempts with zidovudine. AIDS 1990;4:88.
13. Selwyn PA, Iezza A. Zidovudine overdose in an intravenous drug user. AIDS 1990;4:822–824.
14. Staszewski S, Rehmet S, Odewald J, et al. Overdosage of zidovudine. Lancet 1989;1:385.
15. Heard JM, Slovis CM. Zidovudine (AZT) (Retrovir®) overdose. Vet Hum Toxicol 1988;30:365–366.
16. Routy JP, Prajs E, Blanc AP, et al. Seizure after zidovudine overdose. Lancet 1989;1:384–385.
17. Spear JB, Kessler HA, Lehrman SN, de Miranda P. Zidovudine overdosage. Ann Intern Med 1988;109:76–77.
18. Hargreaves M, Fuller G, Costello C, Gazzard B. Zidovudine overdose. Lancet 1988;2:509.
19. Casals A, Ribelles N, Clotet B, Fox M. Zidovudine overdose. Med Clin 1989;5:199.
20. Pickus OB. Overdose of zidovudine. N Engl J Med 1988;318: 1206.
21. Moore EC, Cohen F, Kauffman RE, Aravind MK. Zidovudine overdose in a child. N Engl J Med 1990;322:408–409.
22. Lefeuillade A, Poizot-Martin I, Dhiver C, et al. Zidovudine overdose: A case with bone marrow toxicity. AIDS 1991;5: 116–117.
23. Sacho H, Schoub BD. Guidelines for the use of zidovudine for post-exposure prophylaxis after needlestick injuries in health care settings. S Afr Med J 1990;77:619–622.
24. Henderson DK, Gerberding JL. Prophylactic zidovudine after occupational exposure to the human immunodeficiency virus: An interim analysis. J Infect Dis 1989;160:321–327.
25. Jeffries DJ. Zidovudine after occupational exposure to HIV: Hospitals should be able to give it within an hour. Br Med J 1991;302:1349–1351.

26. Elkharrat D, Wautier JI, Caulin C, Bonnet N. Zidovudine after occupational exposure to HIV. Br Med J 1991;303:309.
27. Lange JMA, Boucher CAB, Hollak CEM, et al. Failure of zidovudine prophylaxis after accidental exposure to HIV-1. N Engl J Med 1990;322:1375–1377.
28. Lucey D, Milum S, Lindquist C, et al. Pseudofailure of zidovudine prophylaxis after a human immunodeficiency virus: Positive needlestick. J Infect Dis 1990;162:1211–1212.
29. Durand E, Le Jeunne C, Hughes F-C. Failure of prophylactic zidovudine after suicidal self-inoculation of HIV-infected blood. N Engl J Med 1991;324:1062.
30. Zidovudine and needlestick exposure. Lancet 1990;335: 1271. Editorial.
31. Singlas E, Pioger JC, Taburet AM, et al. Comparative pharmacokinetics of zidovudine (AZT) and its metabolite (GAZT) in healthy subjects and HIV seropositive patients. Eur J Clin Pharmacol 1989;36:639–640.
32. Klecker RW, Collins JM, Yarchoan R, et al. Plasma and cerebrospinal fluid pharmacokinetics of 3′-azido-3′-deoxythymidine: A novel pyrimidine analog with potential application for the treatment of patients with AIDS and related diseases. Clin Pharmacol Ther 1987;41:407–412.
33. Collins JM, Unadkat JD. Clinical pharmacokinetics of zidovudine: An overview of current data. Clin Pharmacokinet 1989;17:1–9.
34. Blum MR, Liao SHT, Good SS, de Miranda P: Pharmacokinetics and bioavailability of zidovudine in humans. Am J Med 1988;85(suppl. 1A):189–194.
35. Yarchoan R, Mitsuya H, Myers CE, Broder S. Clinical pharmacology of 3′-azido-2′,3′-dideoxythymidine (zidovudine) and related dideoxynucleosides. N Engl J Med 1989;321:726–738.
36. Balis FM, Pizzo PA, Murphy RF, et al. The pharmacokinetics of zidovudine administered by continuous infusion in children. Ann Intern Med 1989;110:279–285.
37. Watts DH, Brown ZA, Tartaglione T, et al. Pharmacokinetic disposition of zidovudine during pregnancy. J Infect Dis 1991;163:226–232.
38. Steffe EM, King H, Inciardi JF, et al. The effect of acetaminophen on zidovudine metabolism in HIV-infected patients. J Acquir Immune Defic Syndr 1990;3:691–694.
39. Ameer B. Acetaminophen hepatoxicity augmented by zidovudine. Am J Med 1993;95:342.
40. Kavesh NG, Holzman RS, Seidlin M. The combined activity of azidothymidine and antimycobacterial agents: A retrospective study. Annu Rev Respir Dis 1989;139:1094–1097.
41. Rajaonarison JF, Lacarelle B, Catalin J, Rahmani R. 3′-Azido-3′-deoxythymidine drug interactions: Screening for inhibitors in human liver microsomes. Drug Metab Disp 1992;20: 578–584.
42. Liebes L, Mendoza S, Wilson D, Dancis J. Transfer of zidovudine (AZT) by human placenta. J Infect Dis 1990;161: 203–207.
43. Schenker S, Johnson RF, King TS, et al. Azidothymidine (zidovudine) transport by the human placenta. Am J Med Sci 1990;299:16–20.
44. Gillet JY, Garraffo R, Barar D, et al. Fetoplacental passage of zidovudine. Lancet 1989;2:269–270.
45. Chavanet P, Diquet B, Waldner A, Bortier H. Perinatal pharmacokinetics of zidovudine. N Engl J Med 1989;321: 1548–1549.
46. Bernard N, Boulley A-M, Perol R, et al. Failure of zidovudine prophylaxis after exposure to HIV-1. N Engl J Med 1990; 323:916.
47. Sperling RS, Stratton P, O'Sullivan MJ, et al. A survey of zidovudine use in pregnant women with human immunodeficiency virus infection. N Engl J Med 1992;326: 857–861.
48. Tadapalli SM, Puchett L, Jeal S, et al. Differential assay of zidovudine and its glucuronide metabolite in serum and urine with a radioimmunoassay kit. Clin Chem 1990;36:897–900.
49. Lacroix C, Hoang TP, Wojciechowski F, et al. Simultaneous quantification of zidovudine and its metabolites in serum and urine by high performance liquid chromatography using a column-switching technique. J Chromatogr 1990;525:240–245.
50. Tadapalli SM, Puchett L, Jeal S, et al. Differential assay of zidovudine and its glucuronide metabolite in serum and urine with a radioimmunoassay kit. Clin Chem 1990;36: 897–900.
51. Lacroix C, Hoang TP, Wojciechowski F, et al. Simultaneous quantification of zidovudine and its metabolites in serum and urine by high performance liquid chromatography using a column-switching technique. J Chromatogr 1990;525: 240–245.

2′,3′-DIDEOXYCYTIDINE (ddC, ZALCITABINE)

2′,3′-Dideoxycytidine is a reverse transcriptase inhibitor of HIV type 1, similar to zidovudine (AZT).[1–6] Zalcitabine may induce adverse effects such as rash, fever, and aphthous stomatitis during the first month of treatment. The major clinical toxic effects are a painful sensorimotor peripheral neuropathy involving predominantly the lower extremities and, less frequently, pancreatitis.[7] The recommended dose is two 0.375-mg tablets every 8 hours. Overdose with zalcitabine has not been reported. Toxicokinetics are summarized in Table 15–3. Symptoms of peripheral neuropathy typically resolve over several weeks.

REFERENCES—2′,3′-DIDEOXYCYTIDINE (ddC, ZALCITABINE)

1. Broder S. Dideoxycytidine (ddC): A potent antiretroviral agent for human immunodeficiency virus infection: An introduction. Am J Med 1990;88(suppl. 5B):5B–1S.
2. Broder S. Pharmacodynamics of 2′,3′-dideoxycytidine: An inhibitor of human immunodeficiency virus. Am J Med 1990; 88(suppl. 5B):5B-2S–5B-7S.
3. Merigian TC, Skowron G. ddC Study Group of the AIDS Clinical Trials Group of the National Institute of Allergy and Infectious Diseases. Safety and tolerance of dideoxycytidine as a single agent: Results of early-phase studies in patients with acquired immunodeficiency syndrome (AIDS) or advanced AIDS-related complex. Am J Med 1990;88(suppl. 5B):5B-11S–5B-15S.
4. Broder S, Yarchoan R. Dideoxycytidine: Current clinical experience and future prospects. Am J Med 1990;88(suppl. 5B):5B-31S–5B-33S.
5. Yarchoan R, Perno CF, Thomas RV, et al. Phase I studies of 2′,3′-dideoxycytidine in severe human immunodeficiency virus infection as a single agent and alternating with zidovudine (AZT). Lancet 1988;1:76–81.
6. Yarchoan R, Mitsuya H, Myers CE, Broder S. Clinical pharmacology of 3′-azido-2′,3′-dideoxycytidine (zidovudine) and related dideoxynucleosides. N Engl J Med 1989;321: 726–738.
7. Nightingale SL. Zalcitabine approved for use in combination with zidovudine for HIV infection. JAMA 1992;268:705.

2′,3′-DIDEOXYINOSINE (ddI, DIDANOSINE)

2′,3′-Dideoxyinosine, a purine nucleoside analog, is a potent inhibitor of the replication of HIV in culture systems, and appears to have promise as a therapeutic agent against HIV in humans.[1,2] There seems to be a correlation between the clinical response (p24 antigen, CD4 cell counts) in children with symptomatic HIV infection and the plasma concentration of didanosine.[3] Didanosine is a treatment option for adults and children with severe HIV infection who are unable to tolerate, or whose condition has deteriorated on, zidovudine. Overdoses have not been reported.

Therapeutic Dose

Dideoxyinosine may be administered to adults in doses of 250 mg twice daily or 10 mg/kg/d, with decreasing doses based on weight.[4] The recommended dose in children is dependent on body surface area (m^2): < 0.4 m^2, 25 mg twice daily; 0.5–0.7 m^2, 50 mg twice daily; 0.8–1.0 m^2, 75 mg twice daily; 1.1–1.4 m^2, 100 mg twice daily.[5]

Doses investigated have ranged from 0.4 mg/kg every 12 hours to 33.0 mg/kg every 12 hours.[1]

Toxicokinetics

The absorption of ciprofloxacin is dramatically reduced when it is coadministered with didanosine (Table 15–3). This interaction is caused by complexation between the magnesium and aluminum cations and the ciprofloxacin molecule, which results in the formation of a nonabsorbable complex.[6]

Clinical Presentation

Intravenous Administration

Mild phlebitis, a maculopapular rash, palpitations, and a mild headache have been observed.[2]

Oral Administration

Major toxic effects are pancreatitis[7–9] (usually nonfatal) and peripheral neuropathy in patients receiving more than 20 mg/kg/d.

Neurologic Effects

Peripheral neuropathy (pain, burning, aching in the soles of the feet) has been the primary dose-limiting toxicity seen in patients receiving more than 20 mg/kg/day.[10] Seizures with electrolyte abnormalities have been observed.[2,11]

Fulminant hepatic failure ending fatally was observed in an adult receiving 12 mg/kg body weight once daily.[12]

Ocular Effects

Amblyopia, diplopia, optic atrophy, and blindness have been reported.[13]

Cardiac Effects

Conduction abnormalities[14] and cardiac arrest[15] have been noted. Heart failure has been reported after 2 to 3 months of treatment. Improvement follows cessation of use.[16]

Laboratory

Analytical Methods

A paired-ion high-performance liquid chromatography method is available to quantitate 2′,3′-dideoxyinosine concentrations in human plasma, urine, and cerebrospinal fluid. The lower limit of detection is 0.1 μM.[17]

Blood Levels

Elevation in serum transaminase levels, hypertriglyceride levels, hyperuricemia, hypokalemia, and increases in serum amylase and glucose have been reported.[2,18] A few patients have a rise in neutrophil and lymphocyte counts and hemoglobin values. Hypokalemia, hypocalcemia, and hypomagnesemia have been observed.[15] Severe electrolyte abnormalities have been associated with seizures and cardiac arrest.[15]

Treatment

Treatment of an overdose (either oral or intravenous) is symptomatic and supportive and similar to that following overdose with other synthetic nucleoside antiviral agents (acyclovir, ganciclovir, zidovudine). Early (within 1 hour) gastric decontamination may lessen the probability of high and, perhaps, toxic blood levels. Extracorporeal procedures (hemodialysis, hemoperfusion) may be useful (low volume of distribution). There are no antidotes. The use of drugs that produce pancreatic toxicity such as pentamidine, sulfonamides, alcohol, and cimetidine should be avoided.[19] Careful cardiac monitoring should be instituted in patients with known cardiac dysfunction.

REFERENCES—2′,3′-DIDEOXYINOSINE (ddI, DIDANOSINE)

1. Lambert JS, Seidlin M, Reichman RC, et al. 2′,3′-Dideoxyinosine (ddI) in patients with the acquired immunodeficiency syndrome or AIDS-related complex: A phase 1 trial. N Engl J Med 1990;322:1333–1340.
2. Dolin R, Lambert JS, Morse GD, et al. 2′,3′-Dideoxyinosine in patients with AIDS or AIDS-related complex. Rev Infect Dis 1990;12(suppl. 5):S540–S551.
3. Butler KM, Husson RN, Balis FM, et al. Dideoxyinosine in children with symptomatic human immunodeficiency virus infection. N Engl J Med 1991;324:137–144.
4. Bouvet E, Casalino E, Prevost MH, Vachon F. Fatal case of 2′,3′-dideoxyinosine-associated hypokaelemia. Lancet 1990; 336:1515.
5. *Videx (Didanosine) Dosing Guide.* Princeton, NJ: Bristol Laboratories, 1991:B-B 384-10-91.
6. Sahai J. Avoiding the ciprofloxacin–didanosine interaction. Ann Intern Med 1995;123;394–395.
7. Manson SJ, Greenfield SM, Turner JL. Acute dideoxyinosine pancreatitis as a common complication of 2′,3′-dideoxyinosine therapy in the acquired immunodeficiency syndrome. Am J Gastroenterol 1992;87:708–713.
8. Pancreatitis with ddI. FDA Consumer 1990;24:5.
9. Schindzielorz A, Pike I, Daniels M, et al. Rates and risk factors for adverse events associated with didanosine in the expanded access program. Clin Infect Dis 1994;19:1076–1083.
10. Rozencweig M, McLaren C, Beltangady M, et al. Overview of phase I trials of 2′,3′-dideoxyinosine (ddI) conducted in adult patients. Rev Infect Dis 1990;12(suppl. 5):S570–S575.
11. Bach MC. Clinical response to dideoxyinosine in patients with HIV infection resistant to zidovudine. N Engl J Med 1990;323:275.
12. Lai KK, Gang DL, Zawacki JK, Cooley TP. Fulminant hepatic failure associated with 2′,3′-dideoxyinosine (ddI). Ann Intern Med 1991;115:283–284.

13. Whitcup SM, Butler KM, Pizzo PA, Nussenblat RB. Retinal lesions in children treated with dideoxyinosine. N Engl J Med 1992;326:1226–1227.
14. Cooley TP, Kunches LM, Saunders CA, et al. Treatment of AIDS and AIDS-related complex with 2′,3′-dideoxyinosine given once daily. Rev Infect Dis 1990;12(suppl. 5):S552–S560.
15. Dunkle LM. Bristol Myers Squibb. Letter to Videx (ddl) Investigators. March 28, 1990.
16. De Jong MD, Borleffs JCC. Didanosine and heart failure. Lancet 1992;339:806–807.
17. Carpen ME, Poplock DG, Pizzo PA, Balis FM. High-performance liquid chromatographic method for analysis of 2′,3′-dideoxyinosine in human body fluids. J Chromatogr 1990;526:69–75.
18. Katlama C, Tubiana R, Rosenheim M, et al. Dideoxyinosine-associated hypokalaemia. Lancet 1991;337:183.
19. Sachs MK. Antiretroviral chemotherapy of human immunodeficiency virus infections other than with azidothymidine. Arch Intern Med 1992;152:485–501.

FOSCARNET

Foscarnet sodium is active against both cytomegalovirus and HIV type 1 (HIV).[1–6] It has also been effective in herpes simplex virus and varicella–zoster.[7,8] Its most serious adverse effect is impairment of renal function. Foscarnet is an investigational drug in the United States. There have been no published reports of overdose. Foscarnet is available (as Foscavir) from Astra Pharmaceuticals (1–800–225–6333) on a compassionate use basis for treating refractory cytomegalovirus or herpes simplex virus infections.

Structure and Classification

Foscarnet has a molecular weight of about 192. It is used as the hexahydrate with a molecular weight of 300. Conversion factor is 3.33.

Therapeutic Dose

Dosages of 40 to 60 mg/kg every 8 hours intravenously for 14 to 21 days (lower in patients with decreased renal function) have been useful, but an optimal dosage and duration of therapy have not been established.[6] A lethal dose for foscarnet has not been reported.

Administration

Caution: Foscarnet should not be administered by rapid or bolus intravenous injection. Toxicity may be increased as a result of excessive plasma levels. Care should be taken to avoid unintentional overdose by carefully controlling the rate of infusion. Therefore, an infusion pump must be used. Despite the use of an infusion pump, overdoses have occurred.

Clinical Presentation

In controlled clinical trials performed in the United States, 1 of 10 patients died after receiving a total daily dose of 12.5 g, instead of the intended 10.9 g, for 3 days. Overdose may result in seizures, renal function impairment, paresthesias either in the limbs or periorally, and electrolyte disturbances involving primarily calcium and phosphate.[9]

Laboratory

Analytical Methods

Plasma and urine may be analyzed employing steps to eliminate infectious virus. Ultrafiltration removes proteins from plasma. Phosphonoformic acid is determined in the ultrafiltrate by reversed-phase liquid chromatography on a Spherisorb ODS-2 column with electrochemical detection. The limit of detection is 33 μmol/L (10 μg/mL).[10]

Blood Levels

The degree of malaise, nausea, vomiting, fatigue, and headache may be associated plasma concentrations above 350 μmol/L (about 100 μg/mL).[11]

Treatment

Patients who have overdosed should be ensured an adequate airway and efficient respiratory and circulatory status. Preparation should be made for possible seizure onset. Blood should be drawn for renal function tests and electrolyte levels (calcium and phosphorus). Fluid balance should be determined for at least 24 hours. Renal function (serum creatinine, creatine clearance) should also be determined. Gastric lavage and activated charcoal may lessen the probability of development of high serum levels of foscarnet. For serious overdose, hemodialysis may be useful, as it appears to clear foscarnet in acute renal failure.[12] Follow-up of renal function for several weeks may be indicated.

There is no specific antidote for foscarnet overdose. Hemodialysis and hydration may be of benefit in reducing drug plasma levels in patients who receive an overdosage of foscarnet, but these have not been evaluated in a clinical trial setting. The patient should be observed for signs and symptoms of renal impairment and electrolyte imbalance. Medical treatment should be instituted if clinically warranted.

REFERENCES—FOSCARNET

1. Chrisp P, Clissold SP. Foscarnet: A review of its antiviral activity, pharmacokinetic properties and therapeutic use in immunocompromised patients with cytomegalovirus retinitis. Drugs 1991;41:104–129.
2. Minor JR, Baltz JK. Foscarnet sodium. DICP Ann Pharmacother 1991;25:41–47.
3. Balfour HH Jr. Management of cytomegalovirus disease with antiviral drugs. Rev Infect Dis 1990;12(suppl. 7):S849–S860.
4. Ringden O, Lonnqvist B, Paulin T, et al. Pharmacokinetics, safety and preliminary clinical experiences using foscarnet in the treatment of cytomegalovirus infections in bone marrow and renal transplant recipients. J Antimicrob Chemother 1986;17:373–387.
5. Bergdal S, Sonnerborg A, Larsson A, Strannegard O. Declining levels of HIV P24 antigen in serum during treatment with foscarnet. Lancet 1988;1:1052.
6. Foscarnet: Drugs for viral infections. Med Lett Drugs Ther 1990;32:75–76.
7. Safrin S, Crumpacker C, Chatis P, et al. A controlled trial comparing foscarnet with vidarabine for acyclovir-resistant mucocutaneous herpes simplex in the acquired immunodeficiency syndrome. N Engl J Med 1991;325:551–555.
8. Safrin S, Berger TG, Gilson I, et al. Foscarnet therapy in five patients with AIDS and acyclovir-resistant Varicella–zoster virus infection. Ann Intern Med 1991;115:19–21.

9. Foscarnet Product Literature (Foscarnet Sodium Injection), Westborough, MA. Astra Pharmaceutical Products.
10. Sjovall J, Karlsson A, Ogenstad S, et al. Pharmacokinetics and absorption of foscarnet after intravenous and oral administration to patients with human immunodeficiency virus. Clin Pharmacol Ther 1988;44:65–73.
11. Sjovall J, Bergdahl S, Movin G, et al. Pharmacokinetics of foscarnet and distribution to cerebrospinal fluid after intravenous infusion in patients with human immunodeficiency virus infection. Antimicrob Agents Chemother 1989;1023–1031.
12. Dercey G, Cacoub P, LeHoang P, et al. Foscarnet-induced acute renal failure and effectiveness of haemodialysis. Lancet 1987;2:216.

GANCICLOVIR

Ganciclovir, also known as 9-[[2-hydroxy-1-(hydroxymethyl)ethoxy]methyl]guanine, BWB795U, 2′-NDG, DHPG, and Biolf-62, is an acyclic deoxyguanosine analog. It was approved in the United States in 1989 for intravenous treatment, and in 1995 for prevention, of cytomegalovirus retinitis in immunocompromised patients.[1]

Structure and Classification

Ganciclovir resembles acyclovir except for the addition of a 3′-hydroxymethyl group, a change that may enable the compound to be incorporated into both viral and host DNA.[2]

Product Formulation

Ganciclovir sodium is available for parenteral use, as a sterile solution for intravenous infusion preparation (500 mg of ganciclovir, Cytovene, Syntex). It is administered by intermittent slow intravenous infusion. Ganciclovir sodium is reconstituted by adding 10 mL of sterile water for injection to a vial labeled as containing 500 mg of ganciclovir to provide a solution containing 50 mg/mL. Bacteriostatic water for injection containing parabens should not be used. The reconstituted solution is then withdrawn from the vial and diluted in 50 to 250 (usually 100) mL of a compatible intravenous infusion solution. The product has a high pH (approximately 9–11).[3,4]

Therapeutic Dose

The usual initial induction dosage of intravenous ganciclovir for treatment of cytomegalovirus retinitis in adults and children older than 3 months with normal renal function (creatinine clearance of 80 mL/min per 1.73 m^2 or more) is 5 mg/kg as a 1-hour infusion every 12 hours.[3] Induction therapy is usually continued for 14 to 21 days. Patients have received up to 15 mg/kg/d for 6 to 35 days.[5] Following induction treatment, ganciclovir is administered in maintenance doses of 5 mg/kg once daily for 7 days each week or 6 mg/kg once daily for 5 days each week.

Toxicokinetics

Patients who have received up to 5 to 7 g subsequently developed acute renal failure and have survived. A single dose of 60 mg/kg in an 18-month-old was not associated with adverse symptoms. No fatalities have been reported from ganciclovir overdose.[6]

Occupational Exposure

In animal studies ganciclovir has been shown to be mutagenic, carcinogenic, and teratogenic.[3] The manufacturer states that the drug should be handled and disposed of in accordance with guidelines issued for cytotoxic drugs,[4] including the use of latex gloves and protective eyewear. Some hospitals are now preparing solutions of ganciclovir in a biological safety cabinet, issuing warning labels on vials of ganciclovir that are dispensed to ambulatory-care patients, and requesting that used vials be returned to the pharmacy department for disposal.[7]

Drug Interactions

Ganciclovir with zidovudine may be additive or synergistic in producing myelosuppression.[8,9] With probenecid or other drugs that inhibit renal tubular secretion or absorption, ganciclovir renal clearance may be reduced. With antimitotic drugs there may be additive effects with ganciclovir on inhibition of replication of rapidly dividing cell populations (hematopoietic precursors, spermatogonia, germinal layers of skin, and gastrointestinal mucosa).

Pregnancy/Lactation

Ganciclovir is teratogenic and carcinogenic and causes aspermatogenesis in animals. Therefore, it carries a high risk of damage to fetuses. Ganciclovir should not be given to pregnant women. It inhibits spermatogenesis in men and suppresses fertility in women. It is not known whether ganciclovir is excreted in breast milk. A mother receiving ganciclovir should not breastfeed until at least 72 hours after the last dose of ganciclovir.[3]

Clinical Presentation

Therapeutic/Chronic Use

Neutropenia appears to be the most important dose-limiting adverse effect[2]; the occurrence of significant neutropenia (absolute count $< 1 \times 10^9$/L) averages 30%. The neutropenia is both dose related and idiosyncratic and appears to be reversible, starting approximately 14 days after therapy is begun and resolving 23 days after its discontinuation.[10]

Overdose

A number of overdoses have been reported to the manufacturer.[6] Such overdoses reflect toxic effects of ganciclovir on the bone marrow, kidney, and gastrointestinal tract (Table 15–7).

Laboratory

Analytical Methods

Reverse-phase high-performance liquid chromatography is the most commonly used method of quantifying ganciclovir

Table 15–7
Overdoses With Ganciclovir

Dose	Age	Adverse Effect
7 × 22 mg/kg in 3-d period	—	None
2 × 9 mg/kg/d		None
2 × 500 mg	21 mo	None
2 × 5 mg/kg × 14 d + 8 mg/kg/d		Neutropenia, reversible: 17 d
One dose: 1675 mg (~24 mg/kg)		Neutropenia, reversible: 1 d
One dose: 60 mg/kg	18 mo	Exchange transfusion; no adverse effects
500 mg (inadvertent dose)	19 y	History of renal dysfunction; hematuria possibly drug related
20 mg/kg (inadvertent dose)	60 y	Increase in preexisting neutropenia
5–7 g (suicide attempt)	33 y (AIDS)	Serum creatinine 5.2 mg/dL; hyperkalemia (possible acute renal failure)
3000 mg/d × 2 d	38 y (AIDS)	Abdominal pain, retching, vomiting, diarrhea without melena, substernal pain, lethargy, oliguria, serum creatinine 5.9 mg/dL, pancytopenia; *therapy:* hemodialysis × 2, packed red blood cells, platelets, granulocyte colony-stimulating factor, erythropoietin, immunoglobulin G

From Erice A, Jordan MC, Chace BA, et al. Ganciclovir treatment of cytomegalovirus disease in transplant recipients and other immunocompromised hosts. JAMA 1987;257:3082–3087.

concentrations in body fluids. Radioimmunoassay and enzyme-linked immunosorbent assay systems are also available.[11]

Blood Levels

Treatment of adults with AIDS for cytomegalovirus infections with 1-hour infusions of 1.0 and 2.5 mg/kg/dose every 8 hours yields mean peak serum concentrations of 1.8 and 5.0 μg/mL, respectively, with corresponding mean and rough serum concentrations of 0.15 to 0.48 μg/mL.[12] Blood levels appear dose related.[13]

Abnormalities

Neutropenia, thrombocytopenia, and anemia are frequently observed in ganciclovir-treated patients. Hematopoietic parameters should be followed periodically for at least 1 month following an overdose.

Ancillary Tests

Hepatocellular enzyme studies, blood glucose determinations, and renal function tests (serum creatinine, blood urea nitrogen) should be periodically obtained in the overdose patient.

Treatment

Stabilization

Patients who have overdosed with ganciclovir should be considered for intensive care treatment. Attention should be directed to the airway, especially in patients with preexisting cytomegalovirus respiratory disease. Respiratory rates and circulatory stability should be monitored. Reverse isolation procedures may be indicated (profound myelosuppression).

Gut Decontamination

Syrup of ipecac may be of assistance in the home if administered within the first few hours to a patient who has overdosed with ganciclovir, is not obtunded, not pregnant, and has no obvious gastrointestinal signs or symptoms. Gastric lavage with adequate airway protection may be useful within the first 4 hours of ingestion. Caution should be exercised in the patient who is already vomiting or has evidence of gastrointestinal dysfunction.

Use of syrup of ipecac, gastric lavage, activated charcoal, cathartics, and whole-bowel irrigation has not been systematically studied in patients with ganciclovir overdose.

Elimination Enhancement

Hemodialysis appears to effectively reduce ganciclovir plasma concentrations.[14] Continuous arteriovenous hemodialysis, useful in the treatment of renal failure in critically ill patients, has shown a low morbidity compared with other techniques[15] and is also useful in eliminating ganciclovir from plasma.[16] This is not surprising in view of the characteristics of the drug: molecular weight of 225 daltons, solubility in water approximately 3 mg/mL,[17] and low volume of distribution.[14]

An exchange transfusion was administered to an 18-month-old child who received a single dose of approximately 60 mg/kg of ganciclovir during a clinical trial. No adverse events were noted.[6] No data are available on the usefulness of hemoperfusion or other extracorporeal methods.

Antidote

There is no antidote.

Supportive Measures

Patients with a history of ganciclovir overdose should be hospitalized and monitored for evidence of bone marrow suppression and renal, hepatic and gastrointestinal function. Daily complete blood counts include platelet counts and daily studies of renal function (blood urea nitrogen, serum creatinine) and electrolytes. Stool samples are tested for gross or occult blood. Periodic bone marrow studies are performed in accordance with clinical judgment. Neutrophil counts should be followed frequently during the first month after ingestion.

Where necessary, antibiotics and antifungal agents are administered. Packed red blood cells, platelet packs, granulocyte colony-stimulating factor, erythropoietin, and immunoglobulin infusions may be required. Severe neutropenia may be ameliorated with recombinant human granulocyte–macrophage colony-stimulating factor (rhGM-CSF)[18,19] 5μg/kg/d once or twice daily.

REFERENCES—GANCICLOVIR

1. Nightingale SC. Ganciclovir approved. Lancet 1989;2:281.
2. Balfour HH Jr. Management of cytomegalovirus disease with antiviral drugs. Rev Infect Dis 1990;12(suppl. 7):S849–S860.
3. Ganciclovir. In: McEvoy GK, ed. *AHFS Drug Information 94.* Bethesda, MD: American Society of Hospital Pharmacists, 1994:407–418.
4. Saks BJ, Siegel J, eds. *Product Monograph: Cytovene® (Ganciclovir Sodium).* Palo Alto, CA: Syntex Laboratories, 1989.
5. Masur H, Lane HC, Palestine A, et al. Effect of 9-(1,3-dihydroxy-2-propoxymethyl)-guanine on serious cytomegalovirus disease in eight immunosuppressed homosexual men. Ann Intern Med 1986;104:41–44.
6. Dorfman JS, Syntex Laboratories, Medical Services Department. Personal communication, April 19, 1991.
7. Haas DP, Hale KN. Policies and procedures for handling ganciclovir. Am J Hosp Pharm 1990;47:511–512.
8. Jacobson MA, de Miranda P, Gordon SM, et al. Prolonged pancytopenia due to combined ganciclovir and zidovudine therapy. J Infect Dis 1988;158:489–490.
9. Hochster H, Dieterich D, Bozzette S, et al. Toxicity of combined ganciclovir and zidovudine for cytomegalovirus disease associated with AIDS. Ann Intern Med 1990;113:111–117.
10. Erice A, Jordan MC, Chace BA, et al. Ganciclovir treatment of cytomegalovirus disease in transplant recipients and other immunocompromised hosts. JAMA 1987;257:3082–3087.
11. Faulds D, Heel RC. Ganciclovir: A review of its antiviral activity, pharmacokinetic properties and therapeutic efficacy in cytomegalovirus infections. Drugs 1990;39:597–638.
12. Laskin OL, Stahl-Bayliss CM, Kalman CM, Rosecan LR. Use of ganciclovir to treat serious cytomegalovirus infections in patients with AIDS. J Infect Dis 1987;155:323–327.
13. Shepp DH, Dandliker PS, Miranda P, et al. Activity of 9-[2-hydroxy-1-(hydroxymethyl)-ethoxymethyl] guanine in the treatment of cytomegalovirus pneumonia. Ann Intern Med 1985;103:368–373.
14. Sommadossi JP, Bevan R, Ling T, et al. Clinical pharmacokinetics of ganciclovir in patients with normal and impaired renal function. Rev Infect Dis 1988;10(suppl. 3):507–514.
15. Stevens PE, Davies SP, Brown EA, et al. Continuous arteriovenous hemodialysis in critically ill patients. Lancet 1988;2:150–152.
16. Rello J, Roglan A, Garcia-Cases C, et al. Effect of continuous hemodialysis on ganciclovir pharmacokinetics. DICP Ann Pharmacother 1990;24:544–545.
17. Jisor GC, Lin LH, Jackson SE, et al. Stability of ganciclovir sodium (DHPG sodium) in 5% dextrose or 0.9% sodium chloride injections. Am J Hosp Pharm 1986;43:2810–2812.
18. Grossberg HS, Bonnem EM, Buhles WC. GM-CSF with ganciclovir for the treatment of CMV retinitis in AIDS. N Engl J Med 1989;320:1560.
19. Sulicki M, Rosenfeld CS, Przepiorka D, et al. Treatment of ganciclovir-induced neutropenia with recombinant human GM-CSF. Am J Med 1991;90:401–402.

PENTAMIDINE ISETHIONATE

Pentamidine isethionate is an aromatic diamidine derivative structurally similar to stilbamidine and procainamide and to "potassium-sparing" diuretics such as amiloride, tricumtrenes, and trimethoprim.[1] Pentamidine has been used for many years in the treatment of African trypanosomiasis and leishmaniasis.[2] For the past 30 years it has also been effective therapy for *Pneumocystis carinii* pneumonia. Infection with HIV is commonly complicated by *P. carinii* pneumonia. At present, therapy for this protozoal pneumonia is limited to trimethoprim–sulfmethoxazole and pentamidine isethionate. With parenteral administration of pentamidine there is a high risk of toxicity.[3] Inhaled pentamidine produces higher concentrations of the drug on the bronchoalveolar surface with minimal systemic absorption. Routine prophylaxis with inhaled pentamidine may become the accepted treatment of this potentially lethal disorder.[3–7] There have been no reports of overdose with the intravenous, intramuscular, or inhaled forms of pentamidine. Overdoses, when they occur, may reflect an intensification of many aspects of pentamidine toxicity (cardiovascular, renal, pancreatic) already experienced.

Structure and Classification

The molecular weight is 592.7 and the conversion factor is 1.68.[8]

Use

Pentamidine isethionate is designated an orphan drug by the U.S. Food and Drug Administration and is used for the treatment of pneumonia caused by *P. carinii.* It is also administered by inhalation for the prevention of *P. carinii* pneumonia in high risk, HIV-infected patients.

Therapeutic Dose

Intravenous pentamidine 3 and 4 mg/kg/d has been used for 14 to 21 days in both the adult and pediatric populations,[2,9,10] in the treatment of *P. carinii* pneumonia.[4,5]

Fatal Dose

No lethal dose has been established.

Toxicokinetics[2,9,11,12]

Peak plasma level	0.2–1 μg/mL (IV)
Volume of distribution	3 L/kg
Elimination half-life	9 hours (IM)
	6 hours (IV)
Excreted unchanged	30–60%
Active metabolites excreted	>2.5–5%

Concentrations in the bronchoalveolar sediment 18 to 24 hours after administration are greater following treatment with 300 mg aerosolized pentamidine than with intravenous doses of 4 mg/kg.[12]

The mean pentamidine concentration in bronchoalveolar lavage fluid for patients receiving aerosolized pentamidine (600 mg) is 96.6 ng/mL, compared with 14.4 ng/mL for patients receiving 3 mg/kg/d intravenously. Trough concentrations of pentamidine in plasma increased from 0–25.4 ng/mL at the end of 1 week of intravenous therapy to 61.1 ng/mL at the end of 3 weeks.[5]

Occupational Exposure

Health care workers are exposed to an estimated annual pentamidine aerosol dose of 4.9×10^{-3} mg. In contrast, up to 36 mg is deposited into the lungs of a patient receiving a single dose of 300 mg of nebulized pentamidine.[13] Health care workers who administer aerosolized pentamidine should wear masks and gloves and ensure that they have proper ventilation.[14] Risk to other patients is decreased by using separate treatment rooms with closed doors, preparing the drug in a vertical-flow hood using latex gloves, and instructing patients to exhale through the mouth and to turn off the nebulizer if the mouthpiece is removed.

Pregnancy/Lactation

Pentamidine isethionate appears to be embryocidal in rats.[15] Few pregnancy studies have been done in large human populations. Pentamidine has been placed in Pregnancy Category C by the U.S. Food and Drug Administration. Pentamidine should not be given to a pregnant woman or nursing mother unless the potential benefits are judged to outweigh the unknown risks.[16] Pregnant health care workers should avoid pentamidine exposure.[14]

Mechanism of Action

The mechanism of action of pentamidine is still unknown.[17] It may be a folic acid antagonist and may bind to DNA, inhibiting DNA polymerase and ribosomal function, as well as synthesis of nucleic acids, proteins, phospholipids, and polyamines, but the exact mechanism has not yet been determined.[17]

Clinical Presentation

Chronic Parenteral Use

Intramuscular pentamidine 4 mg/kg/d administered to children with cancer and *P. carinii* pneumonia induced mild azotemia (47%), hypoglycemia (40%), injection site reactions (67%), leukopenia (13%), and rash (20%). Studies comparing inhaled pentamidine with trimethoprim–sulfamethoxazole have not been completed.[17]

Reactions immediately following its use have included hypotension, tachycardia, nausea and vomiting, metallic taste, hallucinations, and syncope.[17,18] Hypoglycemia (27%), which may be fatal,[19,20] nephrotoxicity (up to 25%), leukopenia, thrombocytopenia, hallucinations, hypotension, ventricular tachycardia, and Torsade de pointes[10,21–23] have been observed.

Torsade de pointes, QT_c interval prolongation, and ventricular fibrillation developed in one patient receiving intravenous pentamidine 4 mg/kg/d. The electrocardiographic abnormalities completely normalized when the intravenous preparation was discontinued and replaced by aerosol pentamidine.[13]

Pancreatitis, which may be fatal,[1,24–26] may follow parenteral pentamidine therapy.[17] Hypomagnesemia[27] and hypocalcemia may occur.[28,29] Insulin-dependent diabetes mellitus has followed intravenous use.[20,30] Hypokalemia and hyperkalemia have been reported.[31]

Chronic Inhalation Use

Significant systemic effects have followed inhalation of pentamidine. There have been isolated reports of pancreatitis, maculopapular rash, hypoglycemia, pneumothorax, atypical pulmonary *P. carinii* infection, and extrapulmonary pneumocystosis. Cough and bronchospasm are frequently observed. Acute renal failure has been observed.[32] Bronchial bleeding has followed use of the aerosol.[33] *Pneumocystis carinii* choroiditis may develop during treatment.[34] Torsade de pointes has been reported following inhalation.[35]

As of 1985, only five reported pentamidine-associated deaths have been reported. In one case, an 8-year-old child experienced convulsions, bradyarrhythmia, and respiratory arrest during a pentamidine infusion.[18] Since 1985, additional reports of death have followed acute pancreatitis[24,25] or hypoglycemia.[19]

Laboratory

Analytical Methods

A high-performance liquid chromatography method is available for quantitation of pentamidine in whole blood, plasma, and urine. A reversed-phase chromatographic system with fluorescence detection is used. This method has been validated for concentrations down to 16 nmol/L in plasma and hemolyzed blood and to 27.7 nmol/L in urine. The standard curves are linear from 7 to 700 nmol/L.[36,37] A bioassay is also available that appears sensitive and specific.[38]

Inhalation Therapy. Available clinical pharmacology data suggest that a dose up to 40 times the recommended inhaled dose (300 mg every 4 weeks) would be required to produce systemic levels similar to a single 4 mg/kg intravenous dose.[16]

Intravenous Therapy. There has been no evidence correlating the clinical picture with blood levels.

Ancillary Tests

Electrocardiographic findings of bradyrhythmias, marked QT_c interval prolongation, precordial T-wave abnormalities, and ST-segment changes, often with a mild hypomagnesemia, have been observed with both intravenous and inhaled pentamidine.[21]

Treatment

Stabilization

Patients with an overdose of intravenous or inhaled pentamidine are usually in a health care facility. An intravenous line, oxygen, and cardiac monitoring should be available. Ventricular arrhythmias may be life threatening. The patient will probably be conscious and breathing, although the presence of *P. carinii* pneumonia may chronically compromise respiration. The patient should be admitted to an intensive care facility where adequate precautions are taken by health care workers to protect themselves and other patients.

Elimination Enhancement

In view of the high apparent volume of distribution of pentamidine, it is less likely that hemodialysis, hemoperfusion, or other extracorporeal methods appreciably aid in the rapid elimination of pentamidine.

Antidote

There is no antidote for pentamidine overdosage.

Supportive Measures

Torsade de Pointes. Patients who develop polymorphic or monomorphic ventricular tachycardia during pentamidine therapy may benefit from bolus magnesium sulfate injection.[39] If the arrhythmia persists, rapid overdrive pacing or isoproterenol infusion may be useful.[23] Lidocaine may be useful in treatment.[23] Hypomagnesemia and hypokalemia may predispose to the development of Torsade de pointes. Potassium and magnesium levels should be closely followed and aggressively replaced. Frequent electrocardiograms should be monitored, and electrolyte imbalance, bradycardia, and other medications that may potentiate the development of arrhythmias (eg, procainamide) should be avoided.[10]

Hypoglycemia. Severe hypoglycemia may occur during pentamidine therapy or even days after the last dose. Patients must be closely monitored for hypoglycemia during treatment and for several weeks thereafter.[19]

Diabetes Mellitus. The diabetogenic effects of pentamidine are likely to be dose dependent, time dependent, and irreversible.[30] A rise in serum creatinine or a fall in blood sugar frequently precedes the onset of frank diabetes.

Daily monitoring of blood for blood urea nitrogen, creatinine, glucose, potassium, magnesium, calcium, and serum amylase levels, electrocardiography, and urine collection for glucose should be instituted.

REFERENCES—PENTAMIDINE ISETHIONATE

1. Kleyman TR, Roberts C, Ling BN. A mechanism for pentamidine-induced hyperkalemia: Inhibition of distal nephron sodium transport. Ann Intern Med 1995;122:103–106.
2. Wood G, Hogan P, Wetzig N, Whitby M. Survival from pentamidine induced pancreatitis and diabetes mellitus. Aust NZ J Med 1991;21:341–342.
3. Monk JP, Benfield P. Inhaled pentamidine: An overview of its pharmacological properties and a review of its therapeutic use in *Pneumocystis carinii* pneumonia. Drugs 1990;39:741–756.
4. Hoo GWS, Mohsenifar Z, Meyer RD. Inhaled or intravenous pentamidine therapy for *Pneumocystis carinii* pneumonia in AIDS. Ann Intern Med 1990;113:195–202.
5. Conte JE Jr, Chernoff D, Feigal DW Jr, et al. Intravenous or inhaled pentamidine for treating *Pneumocystis carinii* pneumonia in AIDS. Ann Intern Med 1990;113:203–209.
6. Leoung GS, Feigal DW Jr, Montgomery AB, et al. Aerosolized pentamidine for prophylaxis against *Pneumocystis carinii* pneumonia: The San Francisco Community Prophylaxis Trial. N Engl J Med 1990;323:769–775.
7. Hirschel B, Lazzarin A, Chopard P, et al. A controlled study of inhaled pentamidine for primary prevention of *Pneumocystis carinii* pneumonia. N Engl J Med 1991;324:1079–1083.
8. Reynolds JEF, ed. *Martindale. The Extra Pharmacopoeia.* 30th ed. London: Pharmaceutical Press, 1993:524–525.
9. Pentamidine isethionate. In: McEvoy GK, ed. *AHFS Drug Information 91.* Bethesda, MD: American Society of Hospital Pharmacists, 1991:480–488.
10. Taylor AJ, Hull RW, Coyne PE, et al. Pentamidine-induced Torsade de pointes: Safe completion of therapy with inhaled pentamidine. Clin Pharmacol Ther 1991;49:698–700.
11. Otterness IG, Torchia AJ, Doshan HD. Complement inhibition by amidines and guanidines: In vivo and in vitro results. Biochem Pharmacol 1978;27:1873–1878.
12. Conte JE Jr. Pharmacokinetics of intravenous pentamidine in patients with normal renal function or receiving hemodialysis. J Infect Dis 1991;163:169–175.
13. Montgomery AB, Corkery KJ, Brunette ER, et al. Occupational exposure to aerosolized pentamidine. Chest 1990;98:386–388.
14. Conover B, Goldsmith JC, Buehler BA, et al. Aerosolized pentamidine and pregnancy. Ann Intern Med 1988;109:927.
15. Harshad TW, Little BB, Bawdon RE, et al. Embryofetal effects of pentamidine isethionate administered to pregnant Sprague-Dawley rats. Am J Obstet Gynecol 1990;163:912–916.
16. *Pentamidine Isethionate Product Monograph.* Rosemont, IL: Lyphomed, June 1989.
17. Wispelwey B, Pearson R. Pentamidine: A risk-benefit analysis. Drug Saf 1990;5:212–219.
18. Sands M, Kron MA, Brown RB. Pentamidine: A review. Rev Infect Dis 1985;7:625–634.
19. Sattler FR, Waskin H. Pentamidine and fatal hypoglycemia. Ann Intern Med 1987;107:789–790.
20. Yurdakok M. Diabetogenic effect of pentamidine. JAMA 1987;257:1177.
21. Wharton JM, Demopulos PA, Goldschlager N. Torsade de pointes during administration of pentamidine isethionate. Am J Med 1987;83:571–576.
22. Mitchell P, Dodek P, Lawson L, et al. Torsade de pointes during intravenous pentamidine isethionate therapy. Can Med Assoc J 1989;140:173–174.
23. Stein KM, Haronian H, Mensah GA, et al. Ventricular tachycardia and Torsade de pointes complicating pentamidine therapy of *Pneumocystis carinii* pneumonia in the acquired immunodeficiency syndrome. Am J Cardiol 1990;66:888–889.
24. Kumar S, Schnadig VJ, MacGregor MG. Fatal acute pancreatitis associated with pentamidine therapy. Am J Gastroenterol 1989;451–453.
25. Zuger A, Wolf BZ, El-Sadr W, et al. Pentamidine associated fatal acute pancreatitis. JAMA 1986;256:2383–2385.
26. Herer B, Chinet T, LaBrune S, et al. Pancreatitis associated with pentamidine by aerosol. Br Med J 1989;298:605.
27. Gradon JD, Fricchione L, Sepkowitz D. Severe hypomagnesemia associated with pentamidine therapy. Rev Infect Dis 1991;13:511–512.
28. Youle MS, Clarbour J, Gazzard B, Chanas A. Severe hypocalcemia in AIDS patients treated with foscarnet and pentamidine. Lancet 1988;1:1455–1456.
29. Shah GM, Alvarado P, Kirschenbaum MA. Symptomatic hypocalcemia and hypomagnesemia with renal magnesium wasting associated with pentamidine therapy in a patient with AIDS. Am J Med 1990;89:380–382.

30. Collins RJ, Pien FD, Houk JH. Case report: Insulin dependent diabetes mellitus associated with pentamidine. Am J Med Sci 1989;297:174–175.
31. Peltz S, Hashimi S. Pentamidine induced severe hyperkalemia. Am J Med 1989;87:698–699.
32. Miller RF, Delany S, Semple SJG. Acute renal failure after nebulized pentamidine. Lancet 1989;1:1271–1272.
33. Miller RF, Semple SJG. Bronchial bleeding with nebulized pentamidine. Lancet 1988;2:1488.
34. Sneed SR, Blodi CF, Berger BB, et al. *Pneumocystis carinii* choroiditis in patients receiving inhaled pentamidine. N Engl J Med 1990;322:936–937.
35. Engrav MB, Coodley G, Magnusson AR. Torsade de pointes after inhaled pentamidine. Ann Emerg Med 1992;21:1403–1405.
36. Ericsson O, Rais M. Determination of pentamidine in whole blood, plasma and urine by high performance liquid chromatography. Ther Drug Monit 1990;12:362–365.
37. Conte JE Jr, Upton RA, Phelps RT, et al. Use of a specific and sensitive assay to determine pentamidine pharmacokinetics in patients with AIDS. J Infect Dis 1986;154:923–929.
38. Bernard EM, Donnelly HJ, Maher MP, Armstrong D. Use of a new bioassay to study pentamidine pharmacokinetics. J Infect Dis 1985;152:750–754.
39. Tzivoni D, Banai S, Schuger C, et al. Treatment of Torsade de pointes with magnesium sulfate. Circulation 1988;77:392–397.

TRIMETHOPRIM–SULFAMETHOXAZOLE

See Chapter 14.

ATOVAQUONE

Atovaquone was approved by the U.S. Food and Drug Administration Antiviral Drugs Advisory Committee in September 1992.[1,2] No reports of overdose or poisoning are available in the medical literature.

Atovaquone appears to have activity against *Pneumocystis carinii* that is not fully understood. It has also been shown to have good in vitro activity against *Toxoplasma gondii.*

Product Formulation

Atovaquone (Mepron) is available in tablets of 150 mg (United States) and 250 mg (Canada).

Therapeutic Dose

The usual adult and adolescent dose is 750 mg taken with food three times a day for 21 days. The usual pediatric dose has not been established.

Toxicokinetics

Bioavailability	Increased with meals
Time to peak blood level	1–8 hours, second peak in 24–96 hours
Protein binding	>99.9%
Fatal blood level	>5.0 μg/mL
Half-life	2.2–2.9 days
Elimination	Fecal >94%

Pregnancy/Lactation

Studies have not been done in pregnant women. It is not known whether atovaquone is distributed in human breast milk.

Drug Interactions

Atovaquone is very highly plasma protein bound, and could potentially displace other medications that are also very highly plasma protein bound.

Laboratory

Because atovaquone may cause anemia and neutropenia, hemoglobin concentrations and neutrophil counts should be monitored periodically. Liver function tests, including serum levels of alanine and aspartate transaminases, and serum amylase concentration should be monitored periodically. A reversible increase in serum transaminase levels may be observed.[3]

Clinical Presentation

Fever, skin rash, cough, diarrhea, headache, insomnia, nausea, vomiting have been reported.[3]

Treatment

Treatment is symptomatic and supportive. Liver function tests should be followed for about 1 week after ingestion.[4]

REFERENCES—ATOVAQUONE

1. FDA Consumer 1993;27:8.
2. Atovaquone, systemic. USD DI Update 1993:413–414.
3. Epstein LJ, Mohsenifar Z, Daar ES, et al. Clinical experience with atovaquone: A new drug for treating *Pneumocystis carinii.* Am J Med Sci 1994;308:5–8.
4. Spencer CM, Goa GL. Atovaquone: A review of its pharmacological properties and therapeutic efficacy in opportunistic infections. Drug Saf 1995;50: 176–196.

STAVUDINE

Stavudine (Zerit), formerly known as d4T, a nucleoside analog of thymidine, was approved by the U.S. Food and Drug Administration in 1994 for treatment of adults with advanced HIV infection who are intolerant of approved therapies with proven clinical benefit or who have experienced significant clinical or immunologic deterioration while receiving these therapies or for whom such therapies are contraindicated.[1]

Therapeutic Dose

The recommended doses are 40 mg twice daily for patients more or less than 60 kg, and 30 mg twice daily for patients less than 60 kg. The maximum tolerated dose is about 4.0 mg/kg/d due to peripheral neuropathy.[2]

Toxicokinetics

Bioavailability is about 90%. Peak plasma levels reach about 1.5 μg/mL in less than 1 hour. The volume of distribution is about 0.9 L/kg. Plasma half-life is 1.5 hours. About 40% of a dose is excreted in the urine as unchanged drug.

Clinical Presentation

Peripheral neuropathy-related symptoms are the most serious adverse events, occurring more often at doses of 2.0 mg/kg/d. Symptoms are reversible. Chills and fever, nausea and vomiting, insomnia, depression, anorexia, and dyspepsia have been reported. Chronic features of overdose will likely include peripheral neuropathy and hepatotoxicity.[1–3]

Laboratory

Analysis of plasma by reversed-phase high-performance liquid chromatography with ultraviolet detection is sensitive to stavudine levels of 3 to 10 ng/mL.[4] Elevated hepatic transaminase concentrations may be observed after a few weeks of therapy. Neutropenia is observed after 40 mg twice daily.[3]

Treatment

Treatment is mainly symptomatic and supportive. Gastric evacuation may be useful if the patient is seen within 1 to 2 hours of ingestion. There is no antidote. No data are available on the use of extracorporeal methods to hasten elimination (eg, hemodialysis, hemoperfusion). Patients may be discharged in 6 hours if liver function tests have stabilized.

REFERENCES—STAVUDINE

1. U.S. Food and Drug Administration. Stavudine approved for certain patients with advanced HIV. JAMA 1994; 272:382.
2. Fischl MA. Treatment of HIV disease in 1993/1994. AIDS Clin Rev 1993:167–187.
3. *Safety Profile of Stavudine (Zerit®) in Clinical Trials.* Monograph P9-W003. Bristol-Meyers Squibb, August 1994.
4. Burgen DM, Rosing H, van Gijn R, et al. Determination of stavudine, a new antiretroviral agent, in human plasma by reversed-phase high-performance liquid chromatography with ultraviolet detection. J Chromatogr Biomed Appl 1992;584:239–247.

Chapter 16
Antifungal Drugs

INTRODUCTION

There are three major groups of antifungal drugs (Fig. 16–1). The polyene antifungal drug group includes amphotericin B, natamycin, and nystatin. Though all are used topically for treating superficial candidiasis, only amphotericin B is used intravenously; it is an important agent for therapy of systemic fungal infections.[1] Overdoses with amphotericin B may be fatal.[2–6] Flucytosine is a synthetic nucleotide analog, and is the only member of the second group of antifungal drugs. There have been no reports of overdosage with flucytosine. The imidazoles are the third major group of antifungal drugs. Most are used topically (clotrimazole, miconazole, econazole, isoconazole, tioconazole); ketoconazole and itraconazole[7] are active systemically after oral administration. Miconazole must be administered parenterally. Reports of overdose with miconazole reflect the clinical toxicology of the imidazole group.[8,9] Griseofulvin has also been used in the treatment of dermatophyte infections as well as a number of nonfungal disease states (Raynaud's phenomenon, progressive systemic sclerosis, lichen planus, mycosis fungoides, herpes zoster, eosinophilic fasciitis, and molluscum contagiosum).[7–10] Systemic fungal infections are largely treated by amphotericin B, flucytosine, miconazole, and ketoconazole.

Systemic fungal infections are increasing because of AIDS, immunocompromised patients who are living longer, addiction to intravenous drugs, and greater use of invasive procedures and broad-spectrum antibiotics (Table 16–1). Use of systemic antifungal agents may increase over the next decade. Newer antifungal agents have little tendency to be abused. These include bifonazole,[11] naftifine,[12,13] nystatin,[14] sulconazole,[15] terbinafine,[16] terconazole,[17,18] and tioconazole.[7]

Como and Dismukes have summarized the toxicokinetics and adverse effects of systemic antifungal agents[19] (Tables 16–2 and 16–3).

AMPHOTERICIN B

Amphotericin B, a polyene antibiotic, is considered the "gold standard" of antifungal therapy, especially for the systemic mycoses.[20–22] Its drawbacks, however, include the

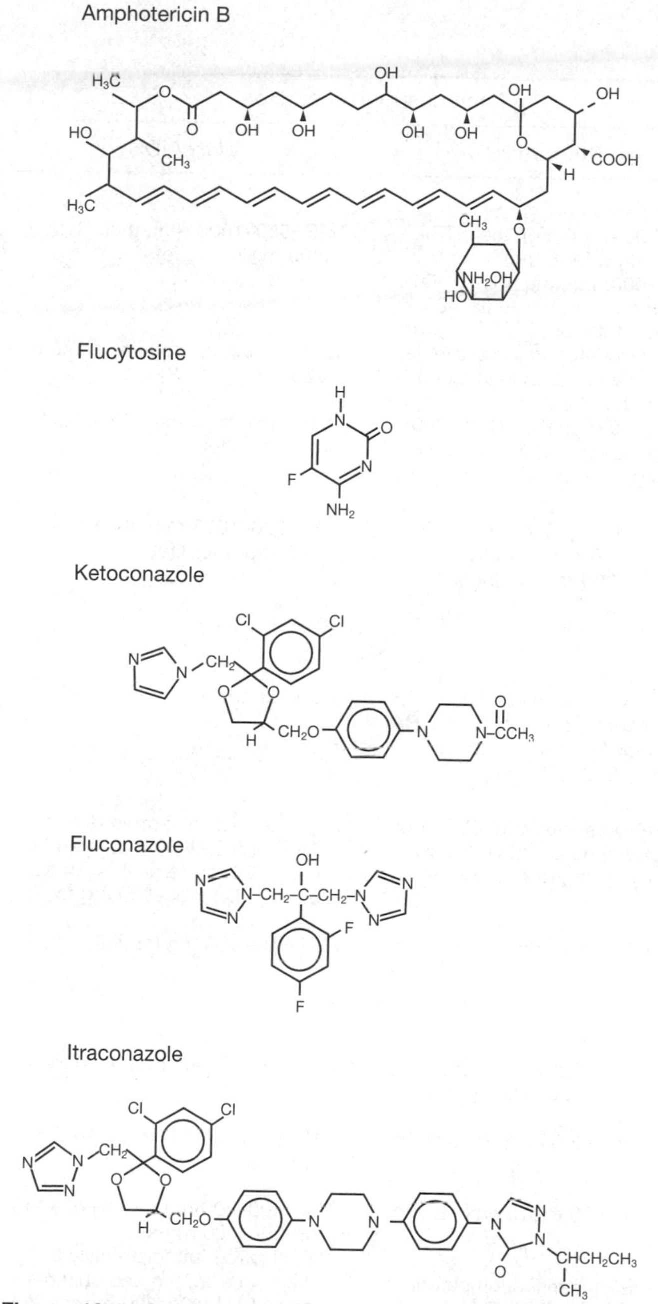

Amphotericin B

Flucytosine

Ketoconazole

Fluconazole

Itraconazole

Figure 16-1 Structures of drugs used to treat patients with systemic fungal infections. (From Como JA, Dismukes WE. Oral azole drugs as systemic antifungal therapy. N Engl J Med 1994;330: 263–272.)

need for intravenous administration, and intolerance by many patients because of side effects such as fever, chills, headache, myalgias, and poor penetration into the cerebrospinal fluid.[20,23] Although renal dysfunction and bone marrow suppression frequently follow chronic use, overdosed infants and children have developed life-threatening arrhythmias and death.[2–6]

Source

Amphotericin A and B are produced together during fermentation of *Streptomyces nodosus,* but only amphotericin B is used clinically.

Product Formulation

Amphotericin B is available in the United States as a powder for intravenous use and as a topical cream 3% and lotion 3% (Fungizone, with parabens, propylene glycol, and thimerosol) and as an ointment 3% (Fungizone). It is available as Fungilin in the United Kingdom, where it is also formulated in pessaries and lozenges.[24]

Therapeutic Dose

Intravenous therapy with amphotericin B is usually 0.5 mg/kg/d and may range up to 1.0 mg/kg/d on alternate days[20] (Table 16–1). It is usually given as a slow intravenous infusion over 4 to 6 hours.

Toxic Dose

Up to 14 mg in infants[2] and 200 mg in adults[5] have been ingested with moderate sequelae (Table 16–5). Cardiac arrest and death have followed 5 mg intravenously. Serious overdose effects of systemic antifungal drugs are listed in Table 16–2.

Toxicokinetics

The toxicokinetics of antifungal agents[1,25–32] are summarized in Table 16–3.

Drug Interactions

Antagonism between amphotericin B and the imidazoles miconazole and ketoconazole has been observed.[1] Amphotericin B with gentamicin may induce a synergic nephrotoxicity.[33,34] Similarly, other drugs with a nephrotoxic potential may be additive to the nephrotoxic effects of amphotericin. These drugs include other aminoglycosides, capreomycin, colistin, cisplatin, methoxyflurane, polymyxin B, and vancomycin.[35] As amphotericin B may cause hypokalemia, this effect may be potentiated by corticosteroids. The hypokalemia may potentiate digoxin toxicity,[1] may be associated with rhabdomyolysis,[36] and may enhance the effect of nondepolarizing (curariform) drugs.[1] The manufacturer cautions against concomitant use with antineoplastic drugs.[37]

Pregnancy/Lactation

The U.S. Food and Drug Administration has placed amphotericin in Pregnancy Category B. Controlled clinical studies have not been conducted with amphotericin in pregnant women. There are few data on levels of amphotericin B in human milk.

Mechanism of Action

Amphotericin B exerts its antifungal activity by binding to sterols in the fungal cell membrane. The membrane ceases to function as a selective barrier, and potassium and other cell constituents are lost.[20,38]

Table 16–1
Summary of Usual Therapy for Systemic Mycoses

Type of Infection	Immunocompetent Host	Immunosuppressed Host: Without AIDS	Immunosuppressed Host: With AIDS
Histoplasmosis			
Acute	Observe	AMB (500–1000 mg), then ITRA (400 mg/d for 6 mo)	AMB (500–1000 mg), then ITRA (400 mg/d for life)
Acute, with ventilatory failure	AMB (500–1000 mg until improvement noted)	AMB (1000 mg), then ITRA (400 mg/d for 6 mo) or AMB (40 mg/kg, total dose)	Same as above
Cavitary	ITRA (400 mg/d for 6 mo), or KETO (400–800 mg/d for 6 mo), or AMB (35 mg/kg, total dose)	No specific information available; probably same as in immunocompetent host	No information; probably same as above
Progressive disseminated	AMB (500–1000 mg until stable), then ITRA (400 mg/d for 6 mo) or AMB (40 mg/kg, total dose)	AMB (1000 mg), then ITRA (400 mg/kg/d for 6 mo) or AMB (40 mg/kg, total dose)	AMB (1000 mg), then ITRA (400 mg/d for life)
Blastomycosis			
Acute	Observe only if clinically improving at diagnosis, otherwise ITRA (400 mg/d for 6 mo) or KETO (400–800 mg/d)	AMB (1000 mg), then ITRA (400 mg/d for 6 mo) or AMB (2000–3000 mg, total dose)	AMB (500–1000 mg), then ITRA (400 mg/d for life)
Acute, with ventilatory failure	AMB (500–1000 mg until stable), then ITRA (400 mg/d) or KETO (400–800 mg/d)	Same as above	Same as above
Chronic pulmonary or extrapulmonary nonmeningeal	ITRA (400 mg/d for 6 mo), or KETO (400–800 mg/d for 6 mo), or AMB (2000 mg, total dose)	AMB (500–1000 mg until improvement noted), then ITRA (400 mg/d for 6–12 mo) or AMB (2000–3000 mg)	Same as above
Coccidioidomycosis			
Acute	Observe, except "high-risk" patients*: rapid disease—AMB (1500–2000 mg, total dose); slow disease—FLU (400–800 mg for 12 mo)	Rapid disease—AMB (1500–2000 mg, total dose); slow disease—FLU (400 mg/d for 6–12 mo)	High-risk patients: rapid disease—AMB (1500–2000 mg), then FLU (400–800 mg for life); slow disease—FLU (400–800 mg for life)
Thin-walled cavity	Observe if stable; symptomatic, enlarging—FLU (400 mg/d for 6 mo) or resect; high risk, even without symptoms—same as above	FLU (400–800 mg/d for 6–12 mo)	FLU (400–800 mg for life)
Ruptured cavity with empyema and pneumothorax	AMB (1500–2500 mg, total dose)	AMB 1500–2500 mg, total dose), then FLU (400–800 mg/d for 12 mo)	AMB (2000–3000 mg), then FLU (for life)
Rapidly progressive miliary	AMB (2000–3000 mg, total dose)	AMB (2000–3000 mg, total dose)	AMB (2000–3000 mg), then FLU (for life)
Meningeal			
Patient awake	FLU (400–800 mg/d for 12 mo or longer, depending on symptoms)	FLU (400–800 mg/d, probably for life)	FLU (400–800 mg for life) or AMB (2000–3000 mg systemically + intracisternally 3×/wk); once awake and cultures neg—FLU (400–800 mg for life)
Patient confused	AMB (2000–3000 mg systemically + intracisternally 3×/wk until cultures neg, then decrease frequency); with improvement, FLU (400–800 mg/d for at least 12 mo)	Same as in immunocompetent host, but continue FLU (400–800 mg/d) for life (?)	
Cryptococcosis			
Pulmonary	Observe if LP neg; alternatively, FLU† (200–400 mg/d)	AMB (0.7 mg/kg/d) wth or without 5-FC (150 mg/kg/d) for 6 wk or until stable, then FLU (200–400 mg/d for 12 mo)	AMB (0.7 mg/kg/d) + 5-FC (100 mg/kg/d) until stable, then FLU (200–400 mg for life)
Extrapulmonary nonmeningeal	If stable—FLU (400 mg/d for 6 mo); if sick—AMB (0.4 mg/kg/d) + 5-FC (150 mg/kg/d) for 4 wk	Same as above	Same as above
Meningeal	AMB (0.4 mg/kg/d) + 5-FC (150 mg/kg/d) for 4 wk; if awake and stable—FLU† (400 mg/d for 6–12 mo)	AMB (0.7 mg/kg/d) + 5-FC (150 mg/kg/d) for 6 wk; if awake and stable—FLU† (400 mg/d for 6–12 mo)	Same as above

AMB, amphotericin B; 5-FC, 5-fluorocystosine (flucytosine); FLU, fluconazole; ITRA, intraconazole; KETO, ketoconazole; LP, lumbar puncture; neg, negative.
*Blacks and those with immunosuppression but without AIDS.
†Role of this drug untested.
From Sarosi Ga, Davies SF. Therapy for fungal infections. Mayo Clin Proc 1994;69:1111.

Table 16–2
Common or Serious Adverse Effects of Systemic Antifungal Drugs

Organ or System	Amphotericin B	Flucytosine	Miconazole	Ketoconazole	Fluconazole	Itraconazole
Gastrointestinal tract	Nausea, vomiting, anorexia	Nausea and vomiting (5% of patients), diarrhea, abdominal pain	Nausea and vomiting (<15% of patients)	Nausea and vomiting (<10% of patients), abdominal pain, anorexia	Nausa and vomiting (<5% of patients)	Nausea and vomiting (<10% of patients)
Skin	—	Rash	Pruritus, rash	Pruritus, rash	Rash, possibly exfoliative (Stevens–Johnson syndrome)	Pruritus, rash
Liver	—	Asymptomatic elevations of plasma transaminases (7% of patients), hepatitis (rare)	—	Asymptomatic elevations of plasma transminases (2–10% of patients), hepatitis	Asymptomatic elevations of plasma transaminases (<1–7% of patients), hepatitis (rare)	Asymptomatic elevations of plasma transaminases (<1–5% of patients), hepatitis (rare)
Bone marrow	Anemia	Anemia (less common), leukopenia, thrombocytopenia	Anemia, leukopenia, thrombocytosis or thombocytopenia	—	—	—
Kidney	Azotemia (80% of patients), renal tubular acidosis, hypokalemia, hypomagnesemia	—	—	—	—	—
Endocrine system	—	—	Hyperlipidemia, hyponatremia	Adrenal insufficiency (rare), decreased libido, impotence, gynecomastia, menstrual irregularities	—	Hypokalemia, hypertension, edema, impotence (rare)
Other	Thrombophlebitis, headache, fever and chills	Confusion, headache	Phlebitis, fever, psychosis	Headache, fever and chills, photophobia	Headache, seizure	Headache, dizziness

From Como JA, Dismukes WE. Oral azole drugs as systemic antifungal therapy. N Engl J Med 1994;330:263–272.

Table 16–3
Selected Pharmacologic Properties of Systemic Antifungal Agents

Property	Amphotericin B	Flucytosine	Miconazole	Ketoconazole	Itraconazole	Fluconazole
Oral bioavailability (%)	<5	≥80	25	75*	>70*	>80
Protein binding (%)	91–95	4	91–93	99	>99	11
Apparent volume of distribution (L/kg)	4.0	0.6–0.7	—†	—‡	—‡	0.7–0.8
Peak plasma concentration (μg/mL)	1.2–2.0	30–45	1.2–2.5	1.5–3.1	0.2–0.4	10.2
Dose (mg)	50 IV	2000 PO	400 IV	200 PO	200 PO	200 PO
Time to peak plasma concentration (h)	—	2	—	1–4	4–5	2–4
Terminal elimination half-life	15 d	3–6 h	20–24 h	7–10 h§	24–42 h§	22–31 h
Unchanged drug in urine (%)	3	>75	1	2–4	<1	80
Cerebrospinal fluid or plasma concentration (%)	2–4	>75	5–10	<10	<1	>70

*The absolute bioavailability of ketoconazole and itraconazole has not been determined because of the absence of a form suitable for intravenous use. The values reported represent the bioavailability of these agents relative to that of an oral solution in normal subjects.
†The mean apparent volume of distribution of miconazole in one study of normal subjects was 1474 L/kg of body weight.
‡The apparent volume of distribution was not assessed in humans because of the absence of a form suitable for intravenous use. In dogs, the apparent volumes of distribution of ketoconazole and itraconazole were 0.87 and 17 L/kg, respectively.
§Itraconazole and ketoconazole exhibit dose-dependent elimination. Longer terminal elimination half-lives are possible with large daily doses.
From Como JA, Dismukes WE. Oral azole drugs as systemic antifungal therapy. N Engl J Med 1994;330:263–272.

Clinical Presentation
Chronic Use

The most commonly reported cardiovascular effects of amphotericin B are tachycardia and changes in blood pressure, including hypertension.[39] Sinus bradycardia is uncommon. Ventricular fibrillation has been reported after rapid infusions of the drug, especially in patients with renal insufficiency (Table 16–4).

Amphotericin B almost invariably causes a decrease in renal function, including a decline in glomerular filtration rate, renal tubular acidosis, decreased serum potassium, and diminished renal concentrating ability.[40] This does not alter its pharmacokinetics.[40] Similarly, a normochromic normocytic anemia accompanied by a depression of erythropoietin production almost always occurs in patients on prolonged amphotericin treatment.[41,42] In many patients amphotericin B causes fever, chills, hypotension, and tachypnea, often beginning 1 to 3 hours after starting an infusion and lasting 1 or more hours.

Overdose

In infants and very young children doses of 2.5 to 8 mg/kg produced no obvious adverse effects.[43,44] In an 8-week-old baby who received 14 mg of amphotericin B, abdominal distention, bloody diarrhea, and thrombocytopenia were observed within 12 hours of overdose; the patient recovered.[45] A neonate (1 month/24.5 weeks' gestation) inadvertently received a 50-fold overdose of amphotericin over a 3-day period. Hypokalemia and elevated levels of γ-glutamyl transferase and aspartate transaminase were observed, but there was no evidence of bone marrow depression or depressed renal function. The terminal half-life was calculated to be 148 days. Blood levels were normal.[45] No permanent renal or bone marrow function abnormalities have been reported following amphotericin overdose. Four infants and children developed cardiac arrest and died after up to 10 to 50 times the recommended dose (Table 16–5).

Table 16–4
Complications of Amphotericin B Therapy

Gastrointestinal	Rare diarrhea, nausea, vomiting
Neurologic	Leukoencephalopathy,[40] hypokalemic paralysis[36]
Renal	Impairment of renal function in up to 80% of treated patients,[42] increased serum urea nitrogen and creatinine concentrations, decreased glomerular filtration rate and urinary concentrating ability, distal renal tubular acidosis, hypermagnesuria, hyponatriuria, hyperkaluria, decreased serum potassium and magnesium levels; rare hematuria, pyuria, proteinuria[43]; recurrent reversible acute renal failure[44]
Intrathecal	Headache, nausea and vomiting, urinary retention, pain along lumbar nerves, paresthesia, vision changes, arachnoiditis
Skin	Red man syndrome rash[45]
Heart	Ventricular fibrillation with hyperkalemia after rapid infusion in anuric patient,[46] transient asystole,[47] premature ventricular contraction in a neonate,[48] malignant hypertensive episodes[49]
Hepatic	Acute fetal hepatic necrosis[40]
Lungs	Pulmonary hypertension with liposomal amphotericin B,[51] bronchiolitis obliterans[52]
Hematologic	Normochromic normocytic anemia, thrombophlebitis, pain at injection site; rare thrombocytopenia, leukopenia, agranulocytosis, eosinophilia, coagulation defects

Laboratory
Analytical Methods

Concentrations of amphotericin B in biological fluids have usually been measured by bioassay[25,46–54] or high-pressure liquid chromatography.[55]

Table 16–5
Overdoses with Amphotericin B

Age	Weight	Dose of Amphotericin B	Adverse Effects
21 d*	0.6 kg	2.5 mg/kg	None
2 y*	13.5 kg	3.7 mg/kg	None
Neonate*	3 kg	8 mg/kg	None
8 wk*	Unknown	14 mg	Abdominal distention, bloody diarrhea, thrombocytopenia
5 mo	7 kg	4.4 mg/kg	None (blood level 4 µg/mL)
32 d (24.5-wk gestation)	690 g at birth	15 mg/kg (total dose)	Hypokalemia Elevated γ-glutamyl transpeptidase and aspartate transaminase levels enzymes Half-life 148.1 d
21 y*		200 mg	No sequelae
5 y*		3 mg/kg	Nausea, vomiting
—*		25 mg in 250 mL infusion (instead of 5 mg in 500 mL)	No sequelae
2 y		5 mg IV	Vomiting, seizure, cardiac arrest, survived
7 y		10-fold overdose	Cardiac arrest, death
4.5 wk		25 times higher than intended	Cardiac arrest, death
7 wk		50 times higher than intended	Cardiac arrest, death

*Manufacturer's case reports (Squibb, 1988).
Source: References 42–44.

Ancillary Tests

Renal function tests (blood urea nitrogen, serum creatinine or endogenous creatinine clearance) and liver function tests may become elevated during therapy. A normochromic normocytic anemia, hypokalemia, hypomagnesemia and elevated liver function tests may be observed during therapy.

Treatment

Stabilization

Patients with amphotericin B overdose should be hospitalized for symptomatic and supportive treatment. In most cases the patient has been inadvertently administered an intravenous overdose and is already in a health care facility. Rare acute hepatotoxicity, cardiac arrhythmia, and central nervous system lesions represent the greatest immediate threats to life. Immediate intravenous access should be established along with cardiac monitoring for all patients with serious vital sign abnormalities. Chest x-ray and arterial blood gases should be obtained where there is evidence of respiratory depression or distress.

Gut Decontamination

There is no indication for gastrointestinal contamination, as amphotericin B is generally administered by the intravenous route. No studies are presently available relative to secretion into the intestinal tract. Emesis, lavage, and activated charcoal or cathartics may be useful if large amounts of ointment, creams, or lozenges are orally ingested; however less than 10% of amphotericin is absorbed orally and there are no clinically controlled data to support use of gastric or intestinal emptying procedures.

Elimination Enhancement

Amphotericin B behaves as a colloid in aqueous solution and is poorly dialyzable. Its poor dialyzability and high protein binding result in clearance of only negligible amounts by hemodialysis.[56] There are no clinical data to support the use of forced diuresis or of other extracorporeal methods.

Antidote

There is no antidote.

Supportive Measures

Chills/Fever. Chills and fever are frequent.[57] Agents that appear to aid in preventing amphotericin B-induced chills include ibuprofen 10 mg/kg given orally 30 minutes before amphotericin B infusion, hydrocortisone 25 mg given intravenously before infusion, and meperidine hydrochloride 0.5 mg/kg administered intravenously about 20 minutes before the reaction would be expected to begin,[58] (patients on chronic amphotericin treatment could theoretically become addicted).[59] Dantrolene does not appear to ameliorate the fever or chills of these patients.[60]

Hypokalemia. Amiloride 5 mg twice daily can reduce the amount of potassium wasting and thus enable retention of higher potassium levels.[50,61]

Nephrotoxicity

Sodium Supplementation. One liter of 0.9% sodium chloride is administered daily to patients receiving 40 mg of amphotericin B per day or more to help reduce the incidence of nephrotoxicity.[62,63] There is no clinical evidence for the efficacy of this procedure in treatment of the overdose patient.

Mannitol. Mannitol has not been evaluated in the overdose patient as a treatment for amphotericin B nephrotoxicity.

The patient must be monitored daily for renal function (serum creatinine, blood urea nitrogen); electrocardiographic and other cardiac monitoring and repeat serum electrolyte (sodium, potassium) determinations are also necessary. Hepatic function tests should be obtained periodically as should complete blood counts including platelet counts. Periodic neurologic evaluation should be performed to rule out impending neurologic deficits. Depending on clinical judgment, respiratory function studies and an x-rays of the lungs may be obtained to rule out parenchymal or bronchial pathology.

FLUCYTOSINE

Flucytosine, a synthetic fluorinated pyrimidine analog (Fig. 16–1), is associated with bone marrow suppression, hepatic dysfunction, and diarrhea. Rapid development of fungal resistance has limited its use. Acute or chronic toxicity due to overdose may be manifested by severe bone marrow suppression or gastrointestinal disorders.

Therapeutic Dose

Flucytosine is usually administered in doses of 150 mg/kg/d in four divided doses. Patients with a creatinine level of 1.7 mg/dL or greater usually require dose reductions.[22] A fatal colitis-like condition with multiple intestinal perforations and peritonitis was observed in one patient given flucytosine.[64]

Toxicokinetics

Tables 16–3 and 16–6 summarize flucytosine pharmacokinetics.[65] Flucytosine is teratogenic to rats.

Mechanism of Action

Flucytosine is deaminated to 5-fluorouracil and then converted to 5-fluorodeoxyuridylic acid monophosphate, an inhibitor of thymidylate synthetase that interferes with DNA synthesis.[22]

Table 16–6
Toxicokinetics of Flucytosine and Griseofulvin

	Flucytosine	Griseofulvin
Therapeutic dose	150 mg/kg/d PO	500 mg–1 g/d (microsize) 330–750 mg/d (ultramicrosize)
Peak serum level (μg/mL)	30–40	0.4–2.0 (in 4–8 h)
Volume of distribution (L/kg)	0.68	—
Protein binding (%)	2–4	—
Half-life	2.5–6	9–24
Excreted unchanged in urine (%)	75–90	<1
Cerebrospinal fluid/ serum	$\frac{0.6\text{–}1.0}{1}$	—
Oral bioavailability (%)	75–90	25–70
Cleared by hemodialysis	+	–?

Clinical Presentation

Flucytosine toxicity is especially manifest in rapidly proliferating tissues, particularly the bone marrow and the lining of the gastrointestinal tract.[66] The risk of bone marrow toxicity appears to be increased with prolonged high serum flucytosine concentrations (≥100 μg/mL). Adverse gastrointestinal effects may include nausea, vomiting, anorexia, abdominal bloating, diarrhea, and, rarely, bowel perforation. Elevations of serum hepatic enzyme levels appear to be dose related and reversible.

In the presence of azotemia or concomitant amphotericin B, leukopenia, thrombocytopenia, and enterocolitis may occur and may be fatal.[22] Such complications appear to be more frequent among patients whose flucytosine blood level is greater than 100 to 125 μg/mL.[67] Anaphylactic reactions have been reported in a patient with AIDS.[68]

Laboratory
Analytical Methods

Bioassay[69] and gas chromatographic[70] methods are available.

Blood Levels

Peak serum levels of 30 to 45 μg/mL are reached within 6 hours following a single 2-g oral dose.

Abnormalities

Crystalluria has been observed with doses of 200 mg/kg body weight.[71]

Treatment
Stabilization

Airway, breathing, and circulation should be evaluated on examination. Blood studies should include a complete blood count (red blood cells, leukocytes, differential count, platelet count), hepatic function tests, enzyme tests, and an evaluation of renal function. If facilities are available, a flucytosine serum level can be determined and periodically monitored. All patients should be hospitalized until evidence of bone marrow suppression, serious gastrointestinal disturbance, and hepatic or renal dysfunction has been fully evaluated. Follow-up hematology studies should be scheduled.

Gut Decontamination

As absorption is slow (2–6 hours) but relatively complete from the gastrointestinal tract and toxic effects following flucytosine ingestion may be dose related, gastric emptying should be considered if the patient is conscious, has a gag reflex, and has no obvious internal abdominal pathology after physical examination. The usefulness of activated charcoal, cathartics, syrup of ipecac, and gastric lavage has not been clinically confirmed.

Elimination Enhancement

Flucytosine may be removed more quickly with the use of extracorporeal methods such as hemodialysis and peritoneal dialysis, but clinical confirmation is required.

Antidote

No antidote is available.

Supportive Measures

As flucytosine is metabolized to the antimetabolite 5-fluorouracil, overdoses should be treated with all necessary precautions and a detailed follow-up, as required in a cytotoxic drug overdose (see Chapter 61).

GRISEOFULVIN

Griseofulvin is an oral fungistatic antibiotic produced by *Penicillium griseofulvin* that is effective in the treatment of dermatophytoses.[10] It has been available for several decades but has recently been joined by the imidazoles (ketoconazole, itraconazole, fluconazole). The incidence of adverse reactions to therapeutic doses is very low; there are no overdose reports in the medical literature. Interest in griseofulvin, which may have waned with the appearance of the newer imidazoles, has increasingly focused on its use in a number of nonfungal diseases such as Raynaud's phenomenon, progressive systemic sclerosis, lichen planus, mycosis fungoides, herpes zoster, eosinophilic fasciitis, and molluscum contagiosium.[10] Use of griseofulvin for these diseases has not been approved by the U.S. Food and Drug Administration. In view of these developments, the scope for use of griseofulvin may increase.

Therapeutic Dose

The usual adult dose of microsize griseofulvin is 500 mg to 1 g daily, and that of ultramicrosize, 330 to 750 mg daily. Pediatric doses for the microsize formulation are usually 10 to 11 mg/kg/d, and for the ultramicrosize, 73 mg/kg/d.[72] A toxic or lethal dose in humans has not been established.

Toxicokinetics[72–75]

Drug Interactions

Alcohol. Conconcomitant use of griseofulvin with alcohol may cause tachycardia and flushing.[76]

Phenobarbital. Blood griseofulvin concentrations decrease.

Coumarin Anticoagulants. There is a decrease in warfarin effectiveness.

Oral Contraceptives. Concomitant use with oral contraceptives may enhance metabolism of the estrogenic component of the oral contraceptive and lead to amenorrhea, increased breakthrough bleeding, and decreased contraceptive efficacy.

Pregnancy/Lactation

Griseofulvin may be fetotoxic in the pregnant patient.[72,77]

Mechanism of Action

Although the precise mechanism of action of griseofulvin is still unknown, it is presumed to disrupt the fungal mitotic spindle structure and arrest fungal growth in the M phase of the life cycle (Table 16–6).

Clinical Presentation

Therapeutic use can lead to headaches, nausea, vomiting, anorexia, abdominal cramps, flatulence, and diarrhea.[72,73] Hypersensitivity reactions to griseofulvin that may be life threatening include urticaria, erythema multiforme, angioedema, and a reaction resembling serum sickness.[72] Erythroid hypoplasia, allergic interstitial nephritis,[78] and a fatal toxic epidermal necrolysis[79] occur rarely. Persistent-cold urticaria, an acute allergic reaction that often follows a reaction to penicillin, has also been reported following griseofulvin.[80] Disabling neurologic phenomena such as vertigo, blurry vision, mental depression, lethargy, and insomnia have been observed.[78] Rarely, life-threatening hepatotoxicity has been reported.[78] Griseofulvin may exacerbate attacks of acute porphyria. Renal[81] and hematopoietic toxicity following griseofulvin use is extremely rare.[78] As griseofulvin is produced by a species of *Penicillium,* the possibility of cross-sensitivity with penicillins should be considered.

Laboratory

Serums levels have not been correlated with toxic effects.

Treatment

There are no specific data suggesting specific therapeutic measures for treatment of a griseofulvin overdose. Supportive and symptomatic therapy are indicated. After prompt evaluation of the airway, breathing, and circulatory status, attention must focus on any life-threatening complication such as a hypersensitivity reaction (angioedema, serum sickness) or a serious hepatotoxic reaction.

Treatment of a hypersensitivity response may require intravenous fluids, monitoring of central venous pressure and/or pulmonary wedge pressure in patients with underlying cardiovascular disease, electrocardiographic monitoring, epinephrine, diphenhydramine, or either aminophylline or beta-adrenergic agonists for bronchospasm. If anaphylaxis, with hypotension and bradycardia, is unresponsive to epinephrine and fluid challenge, then consideration should be given to use of dopamine, dobutamine, or atropine.

There is no antidote. Gastric emptying with airway protection may be useful. There is no evidence to support the use of activated charcoal, cathartics, or extracorporeal aids to elimination.

Supportive Measures

Patients with serious renal, hepatotoxic, hemapoietic, or hypersensitivity reactions should be admitted to the hospital and, if required, followed in an intensive care facility with careful respiratory and cardiovascular monitoring. Depending on the clinician's judgment, patients may be discharged after renal, hepatic, and hematopoietic functions have been stabilized, the patient has no neurologic deficit, vital signs are normal, and there is no imminent threat of a recurrent hypersensitivity response. Follow-up is suggested for evaluation of all the above parameters.

FLUCONAZOLE

Fluconazole (Diflucan), a synthetic bistriazole derivative (Fig. 16–1),[82] differs from other azoles with respect to its toxicokinetic (Table 16–7) and toxicity profiles. Fluconazole is one of the more recent members of the azole family to be licensed for the treatment of systemic fungal infections. It may be administered orally or parenterally, is water soluble, has a long serum half-life and low protein binding, and penetrates well into the cerebrospinal fluid. There are no published reports of overdose in humans. Fatal hepatic necrosis, however, has followed its use.[82–86]

Therapeutic Dose

Dosage reduction is advised for patients with impaired renal function. A minimum lethal dose has not been determined.

Toxicokinetics

Elimination

Fluconazole is virtually completely eliminated by the kidney. As the glomerular filtration rate diminishes, even without significant change in the apparent volume of distribution, the half-life (normally approximately 30 hours) becomes prolonged. Dosage should be reduced accordingly. Hemodialysis reduces the plasma concentrations of fluconazole in severely impaired patients by a mean of 48% during the dialysis period.[94] See Table 16–7.[95]

Drug Interactions

The absorption of fluconazole, area under the concentration curve, and mean maximum concentration values are unchanged when fluconazole is administered with cimetidine.[90] Other drug interactions involving oral azole antifungal drugs are summarized in Tables 16–8 and 16–9.[89,94–98]

Pregnancy/Lactation

There are no adequate and controlled studies in pregnant women.[83] Fluconazole attains concentrations in breast milk that may be harmful to the nursing infant.[99]

Mechanism of Action

The azole antifungal agents interrupt the conversion of lanosterol to ergosterol, the main sterol of yeast and fungal cell membranes.[100] Fluconazole acts by binding to fungal cytochrome P450, thus inhibiting the demethylase enzyme involved in the synthesis of ergosterol.

Clinical Presentation

Fluconazole has been associated with abdominal discomfort and nausea and, less commonly, with signs of liver damage. In rare instances, it has been linked to severe skin rashes and two cases of fatal hepatic necrosis.[84,97] Dizziness, headache, somnolence, delirium/coma, psychiatric disturbances, malaise, fatigue, and seizures have been reported. There are rare reports of fever, edema, pleural effusion, oliguria, arthralgia/myalgia, and finger stiffness.[83] Alopecia is commonly associated with higher doses (400 mg/d) of fluconazole given for 2 months or longer. This effect may be severe but is reversed by discontinuing fluconazole therapy or substantially reducing the daily dose.[101]

Laboratory

Analytical Methods

Fluconazole is analyzed by a high-performance liquid chromatography assay.

Table 16–7
Toxicokinetics of Antifungal Imidazoles

	Fluconazole	Itraconazole	Ketoconazole	Miconazole
Therapeutic dose	50–400 mg/d	100–200 mg	200–400 mg/d	1.8–3 g/d × 1–2 wk IV (adults); 20–40 mg/kg/d (children); individual doses not over 15 mg/kg
Peak serum level (μg/mL)	0.8–1	0.13	2–35	2 mg/L (after 1 g IV)
Volume of distribution (L/kg)	0.65–0.8		0.36	21
Protein binding (%)	12	99.8	99	90–93
Half-life (h)	25–30[a]		6.5–8	1.68 (oral) 24 (IV)
Excreted unchanged in urine (%)	65–80[b,c]	<1	<1	1
Cerebrospinal fluid/serum	$\frac{0.5\text{–}0.9^{d,e}}{1}$	$\frac{<0.1}{1}$	$\frac{<0.1}{1}$	$\frac{0.05}{1}$
Relative bioavailability (%)	85 in 2 h	99.8	75	27

[a]Ormerod AD, White MI. Cold urticaria triggered by griseofulvin. Br Med J 1987;295:612.
[b]Brammer KW, Farrow PR, Faulkner JK. Pharmacokinetics and tissue penetration of fluconazole in humans. Rev Infect Dis 1990;12(suppl.3):S318–S326.
[c]Toon S, Ross CE, Gokal R, Rowland M. An assessment of the effects of impaired renal function and haemodialysis on the pharmacokinetics of fluconazole. Br J Clin Pharm 1990;29:221–226.
[d]Kowalsky SF, Dixon DM. Fluconazole: A new antifungal agent. Clin Pharm 1991;10:179–194.
[e]Galgiani JN. Fluconazole, a new antifungal agent. Ann Intern Med 1990;113:177–179.

Table 16–8
Fluconazole Drug Interactions

Drug/Class	Results
Cimetidine	Slightly reduced fluconazole absorption
Oral contraceptives	No significant pharmacokinetic change in estrogen or progesterone components
Rifampin	Significant decrease in fluconazole's AUC and half-life
Warfarin	Slight but significant increase in AUC and prothrombin time
Tolbutamide	Significant increase in AUC of tolbutamide and prolongation of half-life
Testosterone	No significant changes in testosterone levels
Adrenocorticotropic hormone	No change in adrenal response
Cyclosporin A	Minimal change in levels
Phenytoin	Phenytoin metabolism inhibited

AUC, Area Under the Concentration Curve.
From Lazar JD, Hilligoss DM. The clinical pharmacology of fluconazole. Semin Oncol 1990;17(suppl.6):14–18.

Blood Levels

Mean maximum serum concentrations after fluconazole 200 mg orally are 3.43 ± 0.67 μg/mL, with a corresponding mean time to maximum serum concentration of 4.0 hours.[87,89]

Abnormalities

Eosinophilia, anemia, leukopenia, neutropenia, thrombocytopenia,[84] hypokalemia requiring replacement potassium therapy and/or discontinuance of fluconazole,[102,103] increased serum creatinine and blood urea nitrogen concentrations, and elevated levels of serum bilirubin and transaminases have been observed.[85]

Treatment

Stabilization

Limited information is available on the acute toxicity of fluconazole in humans. If acute overdosage occurs, supportive and symptomatic treatment should be initiated. There is no evidence to support the use of gastric lavage.

If clinical judgment indicates the presence of symptoms of overdose, the patient should be carefully observed in a hospital facility for at least 24 hours. If there is no evidence of overdose or other unexplained clinical signs or symptoms in the first 8 hours after ingestion, consideration may be given to discharge from intensive observation. Airway, breathing, and circulatory status should be monitored until it becomes evident that the patient is awake, breathing normally, and otherwise stable.

Gut Decontamination

Activated charcoal and cathartics may be of value, but no confirmatory studies are available.

Elimination Enhancement

As most of fluconazole is excreted unchanged by the kidney, consideration should be given to hemodialysis for serious overdoses.[88] There are no data to substantiate the use of forced diuresis, peritoneal dialysis, exchange transfusion, charcoal or resin hemoperfusion, plasmapheresis, or whole-bowel irrigation after a fluconazole overdose.

Table 16–9
Drug Interactions Involving Oral Azole Antifungal Drugs

	Azole Involved	
Effect and Drug Involved	Clinically Important Interaction*	Potentially Clinically Important Interaction†
Decreased Plasma Concentrations of Azole		
Decreased absorption of azole		
Antacids	Ketoconazole, itraconazole	
H_2-receptor antagonist drugs	Ketoconazole, itraconazole	
Sucralfate		Ketoconazole
Increased metabolism of azole		
Isoniazid	Ketoconazole	
Phenytoin	Ketoconazole, itraconazole	
Rifampin	Ketoconazole, itraconazole	Fluconazole
Increased Plasma Concentration of Coadministered Drug		
Cyclosporine	Ketoconazole	Fluconazole, itraconazole
Digoxin		Itraconazole
Phenytoin	Ketoconazole, fluconazole	Itraconazole
Sulfonylurea drugs, especially tolbutamide		Ketoconazole, itraconazole, fluconazole
Terfenadine	Ketoconazole, Itraconazole	
Astemizole	Ketoconazole, itraconazole	
Warfarin		Ketoconazole, itraconazole, fluconazole

*The interaction is likely to be clinically important in most patients on the basis of results of controlled studies or corroborative clinical observations. If the concomitant administration of azole and another drug cannot be avoided, monitoring of plasma drug concentrations and possible adjustment in the dose are indicated.
†The interaction is less likely to be clinically important on the basis of results of controlled studies or limited observations in patients. Monitoring of plasma drug concentrations and an adjustment in the dose may be indicated.
From Como JA, Dismukes WE. Oral azole drugs as systemic antifungal therapy. N Engl J Med 1994;330:263–272.

Antidote

No antidote is available.

Supportive Measures

The patient should be observed for clinical or laboratory signs of hepatic or renal damage. Serum potassium levels must be monitored. If there is evidence of renal or hepatic damage, the patient should be admitted until evaluation indicates that there is no imminent danger to these organ systems. Blood counts should include platelet determination.

KETOCONAZOLE

Ketoconazole, a synthetic substituted imidazole derivative structurally related to clotrimazole, miconazole, tioconazole, and econazole (Fig. 16–1), was the first broad-spectrum oral antifungal drug synthesized and has been used in the United States for more than a decade and in the United Kingdom since 1981.[104] It has not been associated with overdose, although fatalities have been reported in association with hepatotoxic reactions.[104]

Therapeutic Dose

Ketoconazole is taken orally in a dose of 400 mg once daily for deep mycoses and 300 mg for chronic mucocutaneous candidiasis or *Candida* esophagitis. Deep mycoses not responding to 400 mg daily may require 600 to 800 mg daily for 6 to 12 months.[105] Deaths associated with hepatotoxicity have followed treatment with therapeutic doses.[106–108] Doses up to 1600 mg have been ingested without apparently serious toxic effects.

Toxicokinetics[109,110]

See Table 16–3.

Drug Interactions

Ketoconazole is poorly absorbed in the absence of gastric acidity.[105] Cimetidine (Tagamet), ranitidine (Zantac), famotidine (Pepcid), and nizatidine (Axid) decrease its absorption. Concurrent use of rifampin (Rifadin, Rimactane) and ketoconazole markedly decreases the effects of both drugs. Ketoconazole may increase the effect of oral anticoagulants,[23,111] the toxicity of cyclosporine[108] (Sandimmune), and the toxicity of corticosteroids.[112] When ketoconazole is used with phenytoin, the serum concentrations of both drugs may be altered. A disulfiram-like reaction can occur with alcohol.[105] Transient increases in quinidine concentrations have been observed.[108,113] Triazolam concentrations are increased by ketoconazole.[114]

Pregnancy/Lactation

Ketoconazole is embryotoxic in rats when administered in the first trimester of pregnancy. To date there are no adequate and controlled studies on use of ketoconazole by pregnant women. Ketoconazole is probably distributed into human milk, suggesting that lactating women receiving the drug should not breastfeed until definitive studies reflect its safety. In the United States ketoconazole is in Food and Drug Administration Pregnancy Category C.[115]

Mechanism of Action

Ketoconazole probably exerts its antifungal effects by inhibiting the biosynthesis of ergosterol, the main sterol in the membranes of fungi.[108]

In addition, ketoconazole may inhibit the synthesis of cholesterol in mammalian cells.[116] Finally, it appears to interfere with cytochrome P450 enzyme systems in several organs (testes, ovaries, adrenal glands, kidneys, liver).[116]

Clinical Presentation

Chronic use of ketoconazole may lead to anorexia, nausea or vomiting, pruritus, rash, and dizziness. Anaphylaxis rarely occurs after the first dose.[105] As ketoconazole appears to interfere with gonadal function, it may suppress testosterone concentrations and can lead to gynecomastia, decreased libido, loss of potency in men, and menstrual irregularities in women. High doses may lower plasma cortisol concentrations.[110] Adrenal crisis has followed.[117,118] An IgG-mediated hemolytic anemia has followed its use,[119] and hypoglycemia has been observed.[120]

When high dosages (400 mg orally every 6 to 8 hours) of ketoconazole are used in the treatment of prostatic cancer, hypertension may be induced secondary to increases in mineralocorticoid levels.[121] Hallucinations have been infrequently associated with ketoconazole and may reflect its penetration into the central nervous system.[122] Serious hepatic toxicity is estimated to be about 1 in 15,000 exposed patients.[104] Hepatitis associated with ketoconazole is usually reversible when treatment is stopped. Fatalities have followed continued use of the drug after the onset of jaundice and other symptoms of hepatitis. Interestingly, acetaminophen is one of the many metabolites of ketoconazole in the dog.[104]

Laboratory

Analytical Methods

Serum and plasma levels of ketoconazole have been determined by bioassay[123] and by more sensitive high-performance liquid chromatography methods.[124]

Blood Levels

In normal subjects given a single oral 200- or 400-mg dose of ketoconazole, peak serum concentrations occur at 2 hours and reach 8 µg/mL.[108] Higher levels are found in patients taking 800 to 1200 mg/d.[116] The drug is undetectable at 24 hours.

Treatment

Stabilization

For most ketoconazole acute overdosage patients, supportive symptomatic therapy, maintenance of life support measures (airway, respiration, circulation), and administration of sufficient fluids to maintain a urine flow of 3 to 6 mL/kg per hour would appear to be adequate. Caution must be exercised to avoid fluid overload and pulmonary edema.

Gut Decontamination

There is no clinical evidence to support the efficacy of emesis or gastric lavage.

Elimination Enhancement

As most of the parent drug ketoconazole is metabolized and little unchanged drug is found in the urine, extracorporeal methods to enhance elimination would not appear useful.

Antidote

There is no antidote. Although acetaminophen may be a metabolite found in animals, confirmatory studies in humans have not been performed and there is no clinical evidence to support the use of *N*-acetylcysteine at present.

Supportive Measures

If hepatic and renal function tests are normal, and there is no evidence of adrenal or gonadal dysfunction, hypoglycemia, hemolytic anemia, hypertension, or central nervous system abnormalities, the patient can be discharged after being monitored for 24 hours (cardiovascular function, fluids, electrolytes). These suggested guidelines may be altered with further clinical experience.

ITRACONAZOLE

Itraconazole (Table 16–2) has recently been licensed in the United Kingdom (Sporanox). It can be used orally,[125,126] is well absorbed, and undergoes extensive hepatic metabolism.[127] It does not penetrate the brain or cerebrospinal fluid in therapeutic concentrations, is highly specific for fungal cytochrome P450, has no effect on mammalian steroid biosynthesis or hepatic drug metabolism, and does not appear to alter pituitary–testicular or adrenal function. It is not recommended for pregnant or lactating mothers. Serious toxicity has not been experienced with itraconazole except for mild gastrointestinal intolerance.[7,8] Serum concentrations of itraconazole are reduced by concomitant administration of rifampin. In doses of 200 to 400 mg/d it has been useful in invasive aspergillosis.[128] A safe and effective pediatric dose has not been established. Other reactions observed include hypertriglyceridemia, hypokalemia, and hepatic enzyme elevations. No fatal reactions have been noted.[129] Gynecomastia and rashes are infrequent occurrences. At doses of 600 mg/d hypokalemia and hypertension were observed in five of eight patients studied.[129] Further studies are required to evaluate the possible relationship of dose to toxicity.

MICONAZOLE

Miconazole has been used in both intravenous and topical forms. The intravenous form is now used less frequently since ketoconazole has become available. Overdosage with the intravenous form of miconazole may lead to arrhythmias, hyponatremia, lethargy, and seizures (Table 16–10).

Structure and Classification

Miconazole is a synthetic imidazole-derivative antifungal drug available for parenteral use and as miconazole nitrate for topical and vaginal use.[130,131]

Table 16–10
Miconazole Overdoses

Age	31 wk[a]	4 months[b]
Sex	Female	Male
Diagnosis	*Candida* septicemia	? Systemic candidiasis
Dose	50 mg/kg q8h IV (instead of 50 mg/kg/d)	500 mg IV
Serum levels	12 μg/mL (6 h)	—
Signs and symptoms	Bradycardia 72 h Ectopic atrial rhythm Delayed intraventricular conduction Dusky Lethargic Apneic Hyponatremia	Tonic–clonic convulsions
Treatment	Fluid restriction	Diazepam (rectal, IVP)

[a]Davey PG. New antiviral and antifungal drugs. Br Med J 1990;300:793–798.
[b]Kanarek KS, Williams PR. Toxicity of intravenous miconazole overdosage in a pre-term infant. Pediatr Infect Dis 1986;5:486–488.

Therapeutic Dose

See Table 16–7.

Toxic Dose

Two reports of overdose, one in a premature neonate of 31 weeks and one in a 4-month-old infant, have been reported.[8,9] Both survived (Table 16–10). A lethal dose has not been reported.

Toxicokinetics

Data available following overdose in a premature infant[8] indicate that the serum level reached 12 μg/mL 6 hours after the last dose (Table 16–7). The infant had received 150 mg/kg/d. The level receded to 8.5 μg/mL at 16 hours and 1.4 μg/mL at 40 hours after the last dose.

Drug Interactions

There appears to be an antagonism between miconazole and amphotericin B.[131] Miconazole may prolong prothrombin time in patients on warfarin or other coumarin anticoagulants.[131] Severe hypoglycemia has been reported when miconazole has been used with an oral sulfonylurea and diabetic agent. Drug interactions with cyclosporine, phenytoin, and rifampin may occur based on the structural similarity of miconazole to ketoconazole.

Pregnancy/Lactation

Safe use of miconazole in pregnant women or nursing mothers has not been established.[131]

Mechanism of Action

Miconazole, similar to other imidazoles, exerts its antifungal action by altering fungal cell membranes and interfering with intracellular enzymes.

Clinical Presentation

Adverse effects following intravenous miconazole have included nausea, vomiting, thrombophlebitis, anemia, and hyponatremia. Adverse reactions attributed to the vehicle (Cremophor EL) include hyperlipemia, pruritus, thrombocytosis, and, with too rapid infusion, cardiorespiratory arrest.[132] There is one report of three cases of grand mal seizures following miconazole.[133]

Following overdose in infants (Table 16–10), cardiorespiratory depression with bradycardia, delayed intraventricular conduction, seizures, and hyponatremia have been observed. There was a concomitant rise in serum miconazole values. These signs have responded to supportive and symptomatic therapy. Because the commercial miconazole injection contains, in each milliliter, 0.5 mg of methylparaben and 0.05 mg of propylparaben as bactericidal agents, 1 mg of lactic acid as a buffering agent, and 0.115 mL of polyethoxylated castor oil, it is not possible to exclude one or more of these agents as a cause of seizure activity.[9]

Blood Levels

Serum levels of miconazole may reflect evidence of an overdosage. Confirmatory studies are not available.

Abnormalities

Cardiac monitoring in an overdose may disclose bradycardia, prolonged intraventricular conduction, and premature atrial beats.

Ancillary Tests

Laboratory examination in an overdose should include complete blood count including platelet count, serum electrolytes, blood lipid profile, chest x-ray, electrocardiogram, cardiac monitoring, and appropriate diagnostic neurologic examinations.

Treatment

Stabilization

The major life-threatening complications of miconazole when given intravenously either too fast (< 60 minutes) or insufficiently diluted (< 200 mL of fluid) include cardiac arrest, respiratory arrest, and anaphylaxis.[132] Severely intoxicated patients should receive an intravenous line, cardiac monitoring, electrocardiogram, and oxygen. Mechanical ventilation may be required. If acute shortness of breath, choking, hypotension, cyanosis, or laryngeal edema is observed, immediate treatment with epinephrine, oxygen, and an adequate airway may be indicated.

Gut Decontamination

Gastric or intestinal decontamination procedures have not been evaluated in imidazole overdoses.

Elimination Enhancement

In view of its substantial apparent volume of distribution, high protein binding, extensive metabolism, and minimal renal excretion of unchanged drug, hemodialysis is probably ineffective after an overdose. Extracorporeal procedures including hemoperfusion have not been evaluated after an imidazole overdose.

Antidote

No antidote is available.

Supportive Measures

Patients receiving intravenous miconazole usually are in a hospital, where they will have been administered repetitive daily doses of the drug. Adequate facilities should be immediately available for evaluating and treating cardiorespiratory arrest, anaphylaxis, and shock. Seizures appear to respond best to diazepam.[9] Hyponatremia may respond to fluid retention.

REFERENCES

1. Daneshmend TK, Warnock DW. Clinical pharmacokinetics of systemic antifungal drugs. Clin Pharmacokinet 1983;8:17–42.
2. Brent J, Hunt M, Kulig K, Rumack BH. Amphotericin B overdoses in infants: Is there a role for exchange transfusion? Vet Hum Toxicol 1990;32:124–125.
3. Brent J, Hunt M, Kulig K, Rumack BH. Amphotericin B overdoses in infants: Is there a role for exchange transfusion? Vet Hum Toxicol 1989;31:347. Abstract.
4. Koren G, Lau A, Kenyon CF, et al. Clinical course and pharmacokinetics following a massive overdose of amphotericin B in a neonate. Clin Toxicol 1990;28:371–378.
5. Spoerke DG. Amphotericin B. Poisindex[R] Toxicologic Management, July 1990.
6. Cleary JD, Hayman J, Sherwood J, et al. Amphotericin B overdose in pediatric patients with associated cardiac arrest. Ann Pharmacother 1993;27:715–719.
7. Davey PG. New antiviral and antifungal drugs. Br Med J 1990;300:793–798.
8. Kanarek KS, Williams PR. Toxicity of intravenous miconazole overdosage in a pre-term infant. Pediatr Infect Dis 1986;5: 486–488.
9. Coulthard K, Martin J, Matthew N. Convulsions after miconazole overdose. Med J Aust 1987;146:57–58.
10. Araujo DE, Flowers FP, King MM. Griseofulvin: A new look at an old drug. DICP Ann Pharmacother 1990;24:851–854.
11. Lackner TE, Clissold SP. Bifonazole: A review of its antimicrobial activity and therapeutic use in superficial myoses. Drugs 1989;38:204–225.
12. Naftifine for fungal skin infections. Med Lett Drugs Ther 1988;30:(177):98–99.
13. Stoughton RB, Sefton J, Zeleznick L. In vitro and in vivo cutaneous penetration and antifungal activity of naftifine. Cutis 1989;44:333–335.
14. McEvoy GK, ed. *AHFS Drug Information 94.* Bethesda, MD: American Society of Hospital Pharmacists, 1994:94–95, 2288–2289.
15. Benfield P, Clissold SP. Sulconazole: A review of its antimicrobial activity and therapeutic use in superficial dermatomycoses. Drugs 1988;35:143–153.
16. Lever LR, Thomas R, Dykes PJ, et al. Investigation of the pharmacokinetics of oral and topical terbinafine. Clin Res 1989;37(2):726A. Onychomycosis and terbinafine. Lancet 1990;1:636. Editorial.
17. Terconazole for candida vaginitis. Med Lett Drugs Ther 1988; 30(782):118–119.
18. Moebius U. Influenza-like syndrome after terconazole. Lancet 1988;2:966–967.
19. Como JA, Dismukes WE. Oral azole drugs as systemic antifungal therapy. N Engl J Med 1994;330:263–272.

20. McEvoy GK, ed. *AHFS Drug Information 94.* Bethesda, MD: American Society of Hospital Pharmacists 1994:70–71, 2270–2271.
21. Graybill JR, Carven PC. Antifungal agents used in systemic mycoses: Activity and therapeutic use. Drugs 1983;25: 41–62.
22. Douglas KG Jr, Bennett JE. *Anti-infective Therapy.* New York: Wiley, 1985:307–324.
23. Dismukes WE. Azole antifungal drugs: Old and new. Ann Intern Med 1988;109:177–179.
24. Reynolds JEF, ed. *Martindale: The Extra Pharmacopoeia.* 30th ed. London: Pharmaceutical Press, 1993:315–319.
25. Louria DB. Some aspects of the absorption, distribution and excretion of amphotericin B in man. Antibiot Med Chem Ther 1958;5:295–301.
26. Atkinson AJ Jr, Bennett JE. Amphotericin B pharmacokinetics in humans. Antimicrob Agents Chemother 1978;13: 271–276.
27. Atkinson AJ Jr, Bindschadler DD. Pharmacokinetics of intrathecally administered amphotericin B. Am Rev Respir Dis 1969;99:917–924.
28. Starkie JR, Mason EO Jr, Kramer WG, Kaplan SL. Pharmacokinetics of amphotericin B in infants and children. J Infect Dis 1987;155:766–774.
29. Katikaneni LP. Amphotericin B eliminations and serum levels in very low birth weight infants. Clin Res 1989;37:342A.
30. Drugs for treatment of deep fungal infections. Med Lett Drugs Ther 1988;30(761):30–32.
31. Drugs for treatment of fungal infections. Med Letter Drugs Ther 1990;32(820):58–60.
32. Koren G, Lau A, Klein J, et al. Pharmacokinetics and adverse effects of amphotericin B in infants and children. J Pediatr 1988;113:559–563.
33. Baley JE, Meyers C, Kliegman RM, et al. Pharmacokinetics, outcome of treatment and toxic effects of amphotericin B and 5-fluorocytosine in neonates. J Pediatr 1990;116: 791–797.
34. Churchill DN, Seely J. Nephrotoxicity associated with combined amphotericin B–gentamicin therapy. Nephron 1977;19: 176–181.
35. Antoniskis D, Larsen RA. Acute rapidly progressive renal failure with simultaneous use of amphotericin B and pentamidine. Antimicrob Agents Chemother 1990;34:470–472.
36. Drutz DJ, Fan JH, Tai TY, et al. Hypokalemic rhabdomyolysis and myoglobinuria following amphotericin B therapy. JAMA 1970;211:824–826.
37. *Physicians' Desk Reference.* 49th ed. Oradell, NJ: Medical Economics, 1995:523–525.
38. Christiansen KJ, Bernard EM, Gold JWM, Armstrong D. Distribution and activity of amphotericin B in humans. J Infect Dis 1985;152:1037–1043.
39. Katz PZ, Cohn RA. Amphotericin B and hypertension. Pediatr Infect Dis J 1994;13:839–840.
40. Maddux MS, Barrier SL. A review of complications of amphotericin B therapy: Recommendations for prevention and management. Drug Intell Clin Pharm 1980;14:177–181.
41. Walker RW, Rosenblum MK. Amphotericin B (AMB)-related leukoencephalopathy. Neurology 1991;41(suppl. 1):199.
42. MacGregor RR, Bennett JE, Erslev AJ. Erythropoietin concentration in amphotericin B-induced anemia. Antimicrob Agents Chemother 1978;14:270–273.
43. Hoitsma AJ, Wetzels JFM, Koene RAP. Drug induced nephrotoxicity: Aetiology, clinical features and management. Drug Saf 1991;6:131–147.
44. Sabra R, Branch RA. Amphotericin B nephrotoxicity. Drug Saf 1990;5:94–108.
45. Sacks P, Fellner SK. Recurrent reversible acute renal failure from amphotericin. Arch Intern Med 1987;147:593–595.
46. Ellio ME, Tharpe W. Red man syndrome associated with amphotericin B. Br Med J 1990;300:1468.
47. Craven PC, Gemillion DH. Risk factors of ventricular fibrillation during rapid amphotericin B infusion. Antimicrob Agents Chemother 1985;27:868–871.
48. DeMonaco HJ, McGovern B. Transient asystole associated with amphotericin B infusion. Drug Intell Clin Pharm 1983;17: 547–548.
49. Googe JH, Walterspiel JN. Arrhythmia caused by amphotericin B in a neonate. Pediatr Infect Dis 1988;7:73.
50. Dukes CS, Perfect JR. Amphotericin B-induced malignant hypertensive episodes. J Infect Dis 1990;161:588.
51. Carnecchia BM, Kurtzke JF. Fatal toxic reaction to amphotericin B in cryptococcal meningo-encephalitis. Ann Intern Med 1960;53:1027–1036.
52. Levine SJ, Walsh TJ, Martinez A, et al. Cardiopulmonary toxicity after liposomal amphotericin B infusion. Ann Intern Med 1991;114:664–666.
53. Roncoroni AJ, Corrado C, Besuschio S, et al. Bronchiolitis obliterans possibly associated with amphotericin B. J Infect Dis 1990;161:589.
54. Bindschadler DD, Bennett JE. A pharmacologic guide to the clinical use of amphotericin B. J Infect Dis 1969;120:427.
55. Mayhew JW, Fiore C, Murray T, et al. An internally standardized assay for amphotericin B in tissues and plasma. J Chromatogr 1983;274:271.
56. Block ER, Bennett JE, Livoti LG, et al. Flucytosine and amphotericin B: Hemodialysis effects on the plasma concentration and clearance. Ann Intern Med 1974;80:613–617.
57. Burnett RJ, Reents SB. Premedication for amphotericin B-induced chills. Clin Pharm 1989;8:836–837.
58. Oldfield EC III, Burnett RJ, Reents SB. Meperidine for prevention of amphotericin B-induced chills. Clin Pharm 1990;9: 251–252.
59. Fincannon J. Meperidine addiction associated with amphotericin treatment in leukemia: Case study and staff reaction. Arch Psychiatr Nurs 1988;2:302–306.
60. DaCamara CC, Lane TW. Dantrolene for amphotericin B-induced rigors. Arch Intern Med 1987;147:2220.
61. Smith SR, Galloway MJ, Reilly JT, et al. Amiloride prevents amphotericin B related hypokalemia in neutropenic patients. J Clin Pathol 1988;41:494–497.
62. Branch RA. Prevention of amphotericin B-induced renal impairment: A review on the use of sodium supplementation. Arch Intern Med 1988;148:2389–2394.
63. Stein RS, Alexander JA. Sodium protects against nephrotoxicity in patients receiving amphotericin B. Am J Med Sci 1989;298:299–304.
64. Harder EJ, Hermans PE. Treatment of fungal infections with flucytosine. Arch Intern Med 1975;135:231–237.
65. Harper KJ, Sawyer WT. Malabsorption of flucytosine in a pediatric patient with Shwachman syndrome. DICP Ann Pharmacother 1989;23:782–783.
66. McEvoy GK, ed. *AHFS Drug Information 94.* Bethesda, MD: American Society of Hospital Pharmacists, 1994:74–81, 2104–2106.
67. Kauffman C, Frame PT. Bone marrow toxicity associated with 5-fluorocytosine therapy. Antimicrob Agents Chemother 1977;11:244–247.
68. Kotani S, Hirose S, Niiya K, et al. Anaphylaxis to flucytosine in a patient with AIDS. JAMA 1988;260:3275–3276.
69. Kaspar RL, Drutz DJ. Rapid simple bioassay for 5-fluorocytosine in the presence of amphotericin B. Antimicrob Agents Chemother 1975;7:462–465.
70. Harding SA, Johnson GF, Solomon HM. Gas chromatographic determination of 5-fluorocytosine in human serum. Clin Chem 1976;22:772–776.
71. Williams KM, Chinwah M, Cobcroft R. Crystalluria during flucytosine therapy. Med J Aust 1979;2:617.
72. McEvoy GK, ed. *AHFS Drug Information 91.* Bethesda, MD: American Society of Hospital Pharmacists, 1991:80–82.
73. Becker LE. Griseofulvin. Dermatol Clin 1984;2:115–120.
74. Anderson DW. Griseofulvin: Biology and clinical usefulness. Ann Allergy 1965;23:103–110.
75. Liu C-C, Magat J, Chang R, et al. Absorption, metabolism and excretion of ^{14}C-griseofulvin in man. J Pharmacol Exp Ther 1973;187:415–422.
76. Vasiliou V, Malamas M, Marselos M. The mechanism of alcohol intolerance produced by various therapeutic agents. Acta Pharmacol Toxicol 1986;58:305–310.
77. Metneki J, Czeizel A. Griseofulvin teratology. Lancet 1987;1: 1042.
78. Haskell LP, Mennemyer RP, Greenman R, Pelezar C. Isolated erythroid hypoplasia and renal insufficiency induced by

long-term griseofulvin therapy. South Med J 1990;83:1327–1330.
79. Mion G, Verdon R, Le Gulluche Y, et al. Fatal toxic epidermal necrolysis after griseofulvin. Lancet 1989;2:1331.
80. Ormerod AD, White MI. Cold urticaria triggered by griseofulvin. Br Med J 1987;295:612.
81. Yang DJ, Rankin GO. Nephrotoxicity of antifungal agents. Adv Drug React Ac Pois Rev 1985;1:37–49.
82. Kowalsky SF, Dixon DM. Fluconazole: A new antifungal agent. Clin Pharm 1991;10:179–194.
83. Antifungal: Fluconazole. In: McEvoy GK, ed. *AHFS Drug Information 94* Bethesda, MD: American Society of Hospital Pharmacists, 1994:74–81.
84. Fluconazole. Med Lett Drugs Ther 1990;32 (818):50–52.
85. Franklin IM, Elias E, Hirsch C. Fluconazole-induced jaundice. Lancet 1990;336:565.
86. Fluconazole (systemic). USP DI Update 1990, August 8:466–469.
87. Brammer KW, Farrow PR, Faulkner JK. Pharmacokinetics and tissue penetration of fluconazole in humans. Rev Infect Dis 1990;12(suppl. 3):S318–S326.
88. Toon S, Ross CE, Gokal R, Rowland M. An assessment of the effects of impaired renal function and haemodialysis on the pharmacokinetics of fluconazole. Br J Clin Pharmacol 1990;29:221–226.
89. Debruyne D, Ryckelynck J-P, Moulin M, et al. Pharmacokinetics of fluconazole in patients undergoing continuous ambulatory peritoneal dialysis. Clin Pharmacokinet 1990;18:491–498.
90. Blum RA, D'Andrea DT, Florentino BM, et al. Increased gastric pH and the bioavailability of fluconazole and ketoconazole. Ann Intern Med 1991;114:755.
91. Ebden P, Neill P, Farrow PR. Sputum levels of fluconazole in humans. Antimicrob Agents Chemother 1989;33:963–964.
92. Arndt CA, Walsh TJ, McCully CL, et al. Fluconazole penetration into cerebrospinal fluid: Implications for treating fungal infections of the central nervous system. J Infect Dis 1988;157:178–180.
93. Foulds G, Brennan DR, Wajszczuk C, et al. Fluconazole penetration into cerebrospinal fluid in humans. J Clin Pharmacol 1988;28:363–366.
94. Lazar JD, Hilligoss DM. The clinical pharmacology of fluconazole. Semin Oncol 1990;17 (suppl. 6):14–18.
95. Richardson K, Cooper K, Marriott MS, et al. Discovery of fluconazole, a novel antifungal agent. Rev Infect Dis 1990;12(suppl. 3):S267–S271.
96. Saxen H, Hoppu K, Pohjavuori M. Pharmacokinetics of fluconazole in very low birth weight infants during the first two weeks of life. Clin Pharmacol Ther 1993;54:269–277.
97. Lazar JD, Wilner KD. Drug interactions with fluconazole. Rev Infect Dis 1990;12(suppl. 3):S327–S333.
98. Blum RA, Wilton JH, Hilligoss DM, et al. Effect of fluconazole on the disposition of phenytoin. Clin Pharmacol Ther 1991;49:420–450.
99. Force RW. Fluconazole concentrations in breast milk. Pediatr Infect Dis 1995;14:235–236.
100. Pasko MT, Piscitelli SC, Van Slooton AD. Fluconazole: A new triazole antifungal agent. DICP Ann Pharmacother 1990;24:860–867.
101. Pappas PG, Kauffman CA, Perfect J, et al. Alopecia associated with fluconazole therapy. Ann Intern Med 1995;123:354–357.
102. German GE. FDA approves the drug fluconazole (alternate treatment for AIDS). FDA Information Bulletin, January 29, 1990.
103. Kidd D, Ranaghan EA, Morris TCM. Hypokalaemia in patients with acute myeloid leukaemia after treatment with fluconazole. Lancet 1989;1:1017.
104. Lake-Bahaar G, Scheuer PJ, Sherlock S. Hepatic reactions associated with ketoconazole in the United Kingdom. Br Med J 1987;294:419–422.
105. Drugs for treatment of fungal infections. Med Lett Drugs Ther 1990;32(82a):58–60.
106. Tabor E. Hepatotoxicity of ketoconazole in men and in patients under 50. N Engl J Med 1987;316:1606–1607.
107. Gradnor JD, Sepkowitz DV. Massive hepatic enlargement with fatty change associated with ketoconazole. DICP Ann Pharmacother 1990;24:1175–1176.
108. Van Tyle JH. Ketoconazole. Mechanism of action, spectrum of activity, pharmacokinetics, drug interactions, adverse reactions and therapeutic use. Pharmacotherapy 1984;4:343–373.
109. Jacobs PH, Nael N. The action and safety of ketoconazole: A brief literature review. Cutis 1988;42:276–282.
110. Daneshmend TK. Diseases and drugs but not food decrease ketoconazole 'bioavailability'. Br J Clin Pharmacol 1990;29:783–784.
111. Wali JP, Aggarwal P, Gupta V, et al. Ketoconazole in treatment of visceral leishmaniasis. Lancet 1990;2:810–811.
112. Glynn AM, Slaughter RL, Brass C, et al. Effects of ketoconazole on methylprednisolone pharmacokinetics and cortisol secretions. Clin Pharmacol Ther 1986;39:654–659.
113. McNulty RM, Lazor JA, Sketch M. Transient increase in plasma quinidine concentrations during ketoconazole–quinidine therapy. Clin Pharm 1989;8:222–225.
114. Varhe A, Olkkola T, Neuvonen PJ. Oral triazolam is potentially hazardous to patients receiving systemic antimycotics: Ketoconazole as itraconazole. Clin Pharmacol Ther 1994;56:601–607.
115. McEvoy GK, ed. *AHFS Drug Information 94.* Bethesda, MD: American Society of Hospital Pharmacists, 1994:87–91, 2282–2284.
116. Sonino N. The use of ketoconazole as an inhibitor of steroid production. N Engl J Med 1987;317:812–818.
117. McCance DR, Ritchie CM, Sheridan B, Atkinson AB. Acute hypoadrenalism and hepatotoxicity after treatment with ketoconazole. Lancet 1987;1:573.
118. Khosla S, Wolfson JS, Demerjian Z, Godine JE. Adrenal crises in the setting of high-dose ketoconazole therapy. Arch Intern Med 1989;149:802–804.
119. Umstead GS, Babiak LM, Tejwani S. Immune hemolytic anemia associated with ketoconazole therapy. Clin Pharm 1987;6:499–500.
120. Lobo BL, Miwa LJ, Jungnickel PW. Possible ketoconazole-induced hypoglycemia. Drug Intell Clin Pharm 1988;22:632.
121. Aabo K, De Coster R. Hypertension during high-dose ketoconazole treatment: A probably mineralocorticosteroid effect. Lancet 1987;2:637–638.
122. Fisch RZ, Lahad A. Adverse psychiatric reaction to ketoconazole. Am J Psychiatry 1989;146:939–940.
123. Jorgensen JH, Alexander GA, Graybill JR, Drutz DJ. Sensitive bioassay for ketoconazole in serum and cerebrospinal fluid. Antimicrob Agents Chemother 1981;20:59–63.
124. Turner CA, Turner A, Warnock DW. High performance liquid chromatographic determination of ketoconazole in human serum. J Antimicrob Chemother 1986;18:757–763.
125. Blomley M, Teare EL, de Belder A, et al. Itraconazole and anti-tuberculosis drugs. Lancet 1990;336:1255.
126. Sachs MK, Paluzzi RG, Morre JH Jr, et al. Amphotericin-resistant *Aspergillus* osteomyelitis controlled by itraconazole. Lancet 1990;335:1475.
127. Frontling RA. Overview of medically important antifungal azole derivatives. Clin Microbiol Rev 1988;1:187–217.
128. Denning DW, Tucker RM, Hanson LH. Treatment of invasive aspergillosis with itraconazole. Am J Med 1989;86(suppl. 2):791–800.
129. Tucker RM, Hag Y, Denning DQ, Stevens DA. Adverse events associated with itraconazole in 189 patients on chronic therapy. J Antimicrob Chemother 1990;26:561–566.
130. Smith AG. Potentiation of anticoagulants by ketoconazole. Br Med J 1984;288:188–189.
131. McEvoy GK, ed. *AHFS Drug Information 94.* Bethesda, MD: American Society of Hospital Pharmacists, 1994:91–94, 2284–2286.
132. Fainstein V, Bodey GP. Cardiorespiratory toxicity due to miconazole. Ann Intern Med 1980;93:432–433.
133. Jordan WM, Bodey GP, Rodriguez V, et al. Miconazole therapy for treatment of fungal infections in cancer patients. Antimicrob Agents Chemother 1979;16:792–797.

Chapter 17

Antiparasitic Drugs and Antimalarial Drugs

INTRODUCTION

Common antiparasitic and antimalarial drugs can be classified as follows[1]:

- 4-Aminoquinolines, eg, chloroquine, hydroxychloroquine, and amodiaquine
- 8-Aminoquinolines, eg, primaquine
- Cinchona alkaloids, eg, quinine
- Dihydrofolate reductase inhibitors, eg, proguanil and pyrimethamine
- Dihydrofolate reductase inhibitor plus a sulfonamide or sulfone, eg, pyrimethamine plus sulfadoxine (Fansidar) and pyrimethamine plus dapsone (Malparim)
- Antibiotics, eg, tetracycline and erythromycin
- Quinoline methanol, eg, mefloquine

The toxic effects of some antiparasitic drugs are listed in Table 17–1.[2] Few reports of overdose with anthelmintic drugs are available.

Overview of Common Antiparasitic and Antimalarial Drugs

Amodiaquine is a 4-aminoquinoline antimalarial agent.[3] Reports of agranulocytosis[4] and hepatitis[5] have dampened enthusiasm for use of amodiaquine and it is no longer recommended for malaria prophylaxis.[3]

Chloroquine, a synthetic 4-aminoquinoline derivative, is a primary drug for the treatment of malaria[6–9] and is available in tablet form as chloroquine hydrochloride. It causes severe poisoning in overdosage that may be rapidly fatal without therapeutic intervention. Chloroquine has some antiinflammatory activity. In vitro, it has antihistaminic, antiserotonin, and prostaglandin inhibitory activity.

Halofantrine, an amino alcohol, together with mefloquine and artemisinine derivatives, is used in the treatment of chloroquine-resistant malaria.[10–12]

Hydroxychloroquine, a synthetic 4-aminoquinoline derivative, is used for the suppression or chemoprophylaxis of malaria and for treatment of rheumatoid arthritis and lupus erythematosus.[13] It is commercially available as the

Table 17–1
Summary of Antimicrobial Agents Used for Treating Parasitic Infections and Their Main Side Effects

Agent	Indications	Contraindications	Primary Side Effects
Albendazole	Hydatid cyst, intestinal nematodes	Not approved by FDA	Minimal
Allopurinol	Leishmaniasis	Not approved by FDA	Hypersensitivity reactions
Amodiaquine	Malaria	Not available in the United States	Similar to chloroquine
Amphotericin B	Amebic meningoencephalitis, leishmaniasis	Not approved by FDA	Immediate febrile reactions, nephrotoxicity
Azithromycin	Cryptosporidiosis, toxoplasmosis	Not approved by FDA	Unknown
Benznidazole	American trypanosomiasis	Not approved by FDA	GI upset, dermatitis, neuritis, myelosuppression
Bithionol	*Fasciola hepatica*	Not approved by FDA	Minimal
Chloroquine	Malaria	—	GI upset, pruritus, dermatitis, myelosuppression, hemolysis
Clindamycin	Malaria, babesiosis, toxoplasmosis	Not approved by FDA	Antibiotic-associated diarrhea
Dapsone	*Pneumocystis carinii* pneumonia	Not approved by FDA	GI upset, rash, hemolysis in G6PD deficiency methomoglobinemia
Diethylcarbamazine	Filariasis (not onchocerciasis)	—	Mazzotti reaction (hypersensitivity to dying microfilariae)
Diloxanide furoate	Amebiasis (asymptomatic)	Pregnancy; available from CDC	GI upset, flatulence
Doxycycline	Malaria (prophylaxis)	Pregnancy, children <8 y old	GI upset, rash from photosensitivity
Eflornithine (DFMO)	West African CNS trypanosomiasis	—	Anemia, leukopenia
Emetine	Amebic liver abscess	Pregnancy, children <5 y old	GI upset, cardiac toxicity (ECG monitoring needed)
Iodoquinol	Amebiasis (asymptomatic), balantidiasis, *Dientamoeba*	Sensitivity to iodine	GI upset, acne, rash
Ivermectin	Onchocerciasis	Pregnancy, children <5 y old	Mazzotti reaction (less than diethylcarbamazine)
Ketoconazole	Leishmaniasis	—	Hepatitis
Mebendazole	Ascariasis, trichuriasis, hookworms, pinworms	Pregnancy	Minimal at usual dose; primarily GI upset
Mefloquine	Malaria	Pregnancy, children <5 y old, beta-blocker drugs	GI upset, seizures, acute brain syndrome
Meglumine antimonate	Leishmaniasis	Not approved by FDA	GI upset, rash, pruritus, nephrotoxicity
Melarsoprol (arsenical)	African trypanosomiasis (CNS stage)	—	Encephalopathy, local skin irritation
Metronidazole	Amebiasis, giardiasis	Not approved by FDA for giardiasis	GI upset, disulfiram-like effect
Niclosamide	Tapeworms, especially *Diphyllobothrium latum* and *Taenia splium*	—	GI upset, pruritus
Nifurtimox	American trypanosomiasis	Not approved by FDA; available from CDC	GI upset, polyneuritis, seizures, psychologic disturbances
Pentamidine	*P. carinii* pneumonia, leishmaniasis	—	Abscesses at site of IM injection; with IV therapy, fever, hypotension, hypoglycemia, hypocalcemia, nephrotoxicity
Piperazine	Ascariasis	Seizure disorder	Hypersensitivity, neurotoxicity
Praziquantel	Most flukes, tapeworms, and cases of cysticercosis	Ocular cysticercosis	GI upset, dizziness, hypersensitivity to dying cysticerci
Primaquine	Malaria	Pregnancy	Hemolysis in G6PD deficiency, GI upset
Propamidine	*Acanthamoeba* keratitis (topical application)	—	—
Pyrantel pamoate	Alternative for ascariasis, hookworms, pinworms	Pregnancy	GI upset
Pyrimethamine	Malaria, toxoplasmosis (use with clindamycin or sulfadiazine)	—	Mild; sulfa toxicity when combined with sulfadoxine (as Fansidar)
Quinacrine	Giardiasis	Pregnancy, psoriasis	GI upset, yellow staining of skin, psychologic disturbances

CDC, Centers for Disease Control and Prevention; CNS, central nervous system; DFMO, α-difluoromethylornithine; ECG, electrocardiographic; FDA, Food and Drug Administration; GI, gastrointestinal; G6PD, glucose-6-phosphate dehydrogenase.
From Rosenblatt JE. Antiparasitic agents. Mayo Clin Proc 1992;67:276–287.

Table 17–1 *(Continued)*

Agent	Indications	Contraindications	Primary Side Effects
Quinidine, quinine	Malaria, babesiosis	—	Cinchonism, urticaria, GI upset; with IV therapy, hypotension, heart block
Spiramycin	Cryptosporldiosis, toxoplasmosis	Avaiable from FDA	
Stiboglucanate sodium (antimonial)	Leishmaniasis	Not approved by FDA; available from CDC	GI upset, nephrotoxicity, ECG changes
Sulfonamides Sulfadiazine Sulfadoxine Sulfamethoxazole	Malaria, toxoplasmosis, *P. carinii* pneumonia (treatment and prophylaxis when combined with pyrimethamine or trimethoprim)	Pregnancy, newborns	Allergic reactions including fever and severe dermatitis, serum sickness, crystalluria, neurotoxicity, and hepatotoxicity
Suramin	African trypanosomiasis (early hemolymphatic stage)	—	GI upset, pruritus, nephrotoxicity (albuminuria), photophobia, paresthesias
Tetracycline	Malaria, balantidiasis	Pregnancy, children <8 y old	GI upset, rash from photosensitivity
Thiabendazole	Strongyloidiasis, trichinosis, toxocariasis, trichostrongyliasis, cutaneous larva migrans	Pregnancy	GI upset, rash, pruritus, headache, hypoglycemia, hypotension
Trimethoprim	*P. carinii* pneumonia (treatment and prophylaxis when combined with sulfamethoxazole)	—	See side effects of sulfonamides
Trimetrexate	*P. carinii* pneumonia	Not approved by FDA	Antifolate; must be given with leucovorin to prevent hematotoxicity
Tryparsamide (arsenical)	West African CNS trypanosomiasis (when combined with suramin)	—	Encephalopathy, local skin irritation

sulfate salt.[13,14] Overdoses and suicide attempts with *hydroxychloroquine* are rare. Few published data are available on the toxicokinetics of this compound after an overdose.[15]

Ivermectin (Mectizan) is a semisynthetic macrocyclic lactone (fermentation antibiotic, a derivative of one of the avermectins, a group of macrocyclic lactones produced by *Streptomyces avermitilis).*[16–18] It is widely used in Africa and Latin America, where it is a major agent in the treatment of onchocerciasis, one of the leading causes of blindness in humans. It is not marketed in the United States or the United Kingdom. Ivermectin overdose is infrequent. A number of patients have experienced inadvertent injections and have recovered. There have been no fatalities.

Mefloquine hydrochloride (Lariam), a 4-quinoline methanol derivative, is an antimalarial drug chemically related to quinine. It is available in the United States in white tablets, each containing 250 mg of mefloquine hydrochloride, for the prevention and treatment of *Plasmodium falciparum* and *Plasmodium vivax* malaria.

Proguanil hydrochloride is a synthetic antimalarial agent that may, after long-term use, lead to renal failure and megaloblastic anemia. Overdoses are generally followed by complete recovery, although deaths have been reported. Treatment is symptomatic and supportive.

Pyrimethamine–sulfadoxine is currently the drug of choice for the prophylaxis of malaria caused by chloroquine-resistant *P. falciparum.* Pyrimethamine can be used with dapsone as an alternative. In conjunction with a sulfonamide (sulfadiazine, sulfisoxazole, sulfamethoxazole, trisulfapyrimidines), pyrimethamine is used for the treatment of toxoplasmosis.[9,19,20]

Pyrimethamine is a folic acid antagonist. It binds to and reversibly inhibits dihydrofolate reductase in the parasite, preventing the reduction of dihydrofolic acid to tetrahydrofolic acid (folinic acid).[21] Poisonings with pyrimethamine have been observed in areas indigenous to its use. In France, most pyrimethamine intoxications are due to prolonged overdosages in infants treated for congenital toxoplasmosis. A nonfatal inadvertent administration of 10 times the usual dosage of pyrimethamine for 10 days in a 7-week-old infant treated for congenital toxoplasmosis resulted in a pyrimethamine plasma concentration of 6.22 μg/mL, by high-pressure liquid chromatography with a sensitivity limit of 65 ng/mL.[22]

Quinine poisoning has been increasingly reported during the past 10 years.[23–26] Quinine overdoses continue to occur because of abortion attempts, suicidal attempts, and accidental ingestions. It continues to be a major cause of death in women using it as an abortifacient. Death generally follows renal failure, acute hemolytic anemia,[27,28] and respiratory arrest. The major causes of morbidity in nonfatal cases of quinine overdose[9,29–32] include reversible renal failure, cinchonism, prolonged hearing deficits, and blindness.

Heroin addicts who inject heroin diluted with quinine intravenously may develop convulsions, coma, or death.[33] Drug screening for employment has frequently included testing urine for quinine as an indirect indication of heroin or other drug abuse. An 8-oz bottle of tonic mixer contains approximately 2.2 mg of quinine per fluid ounce mixed with 2.5 oz of gin and a twist of lime. An individual who has recently had a gin and tonic may be suspected of heroin usage.[34]

Even though quinine is not used as often for adulteration of heroin as previously (expense, availability), narcotic addicts presenting with "idiopathic" atrioventricular conduction defects should have the urine examined for quinine. Alcohol intake may exacerbate quinine toxicity.[35]

Toxic and Fatal Doses

Toxic and fatal doses of antiparasitic drugs are summarized in Table 17–2.

Toxicokinetics

The toxicokinetics of the major antiparasitic drugs are summarized in Table 17–3.

Clinical Presentation

See Table 17–4 for signs and symptoms of overdoses with some anthelmintic drugs.

Amodiaquine. Syncope, spasticity, speech problems, seizures, involuntary movements,[36] agranulocytosis,[4] and hepatitis [5] have been reported.

Chloroquine. The clinical effects of an acute chloroquine poisoning episode may develop within 30 minutes of ingestion and lead to death if the stomach is not quickly emptied.[37,38] Recent experience suggests several possible predictors for death from chloroquine poisoning: systolic blood pressure less than 85 mm Hg, dose ingested greater than 5 g, QRS prolongation of at least 0.12 second, and blood chloroquine concentration greater than 25 μmol/L (8 μg/mL).[39]

Acute chloroquine intoxication is associated with a hypokalemia that is correlated with the severity of the intoxication. Plasma potassium levels should be followed closely, particularly in patients receiving catecholamine infusions. The physician should avoid repleting with too much potassium and thereby inducing a hyperkalemia.[40]

Halofantrine. Acute effects include abdominal pain, diarrhea, intravascular hemolysis,[41] increases in liver enzymes levels,[42] and pruritis. Prolongation of the QT interval has also been reported.[43–45] Halofantrine is not available in the United States.

Hydroxychloroquine. Cardiotoxicity is rarely observed, but increased abuse of hydroxychloroquine may impair conductivity and decrease excitability. This may be associated with elevated serum hydroxychloroquine concentrations.[46]

Seizures, vomiting, arrhythmias, cardiac arrest, death,[15, 47–49] acute necrotizing eosinophilic myocarditis,[50] myopathy,[51] ventricular arrhythmias,[52] and hepatic failure have been reported. Patients receiving daily doses of hydroxychloroquine of less than 6.5 mg/kg of body weight may tolerate massive total doses (1054–3923 g) without the development of functionally significant retinal toxicity.[53]

Ivermectin. Ocular irritation, injection site irritation, nausea, vomiting, tachycardia, hypotension, hypothermia,[54–59] prolonged prothrombin time,[60] leukocytosis, elevated liver enzymes, and ST–T wave changes[61,62] have been reported.

Table 17–2
Antiparasitic Drugs: Doses

	Therapeutic	Toxic	Fatal	Survival
Amodiaquine	200–400 mg[a]			
Chloroquine	mg base/kg/24 h (in children)		0.75–1 g (children 2–3 g (adults)[c,d] (death in 2–3 h)	4 g[b]
Halofantrine	8 mg/kg (children)			
Hydroxychloroquine	500–800 mg/wk		10–12 g[e,f]	
Ivermectin	0.05–0.20 mg/kg[g]			
Mefloquine	1250 ng[h]	900–1000 ng[i]		
Proguanil	100–200 ng/d	up to 1,400 mg[j] (survived)	900 mg, and 5 g[k] 900 mg (children) 1.8–8 g (adults)	

[a]Reynolds JEF, ed. *Martindale: The Extra Pharmacopoeia.* 30th ed. London: Pharmaceutical Press, 1993:395–396.
[b]Havena PL, Splaingard ML, Borisonis D, Hofman GM. Survival after chloroquine ingestion in a child. Clin Toxicol 1988;26:381–388.
[c]Torrey EF. Chloroquine seizures: Report of four cases. JAMA 1968;204:867–870.
[d]Riou B, Barriot P, Rimailho A, Baud FJ. Treatment of severe chloroquine poisoning. N Engl J Med 1988;318:1–6.
[e]Kemmenoe AJ. An infant fatality due to hydroxychloroquine poisoning. J Anal Toxicol 1990;14:186–188.
[f]Overdose of hydroxychloroquine. Pharm J, June 1, 1963, p. 504.
[g]Ette EI, Thomas WOA, Achumba JJ. Ivermectin: A long acting microfilaricidal agent. DICP Ann Pharmacother 1990;24:426–433.
[h]Product Literature: Lariam. Roche Laboratories, February 1990.
[i]Patchen LC, Campbell CC, Williams SB. Neurologic reactions after a therapeutic dose of mefloquine. N Engl J Med 1989;321:1415–1416.
[j]Webster LT Jr. Drugs used in the chemotherapy of protozoal infections. In: Gilman AG, Rall TW, Nies AS, Taylor P, eds. *Goodman and Gilman's The Pharmacologic Basis of Therapeutics.* 8th ed. New York: Pergamon Press, 1991:684–795.
[k]Maegrath BG, Tottey MM, Adams ARD, et al. The absorption and excretion of paludrine in the human subject. Ann Trop Med Parasitol 1946;40:493–501.

Table 17–3
Antiparasitic Drugs: Toxicokinetics[a–gg]

	Amiodaquine	Chloroquine	Halofantrine	Hydroxychloroquine	Ivermectin	Mefloquine	Proguanil hydrochloride	Pyrimethamine	Quinine
Bioavailability (%)	High	90		>90	90	70–80	>90	High	90
Time to peak plasma level (h)	0.6–1.3 3–5 (metabolite)	1.5–3	18	17	4	7–24	3	2	1–3
Volume of distribution (L/kg)		92	100		0.5	13–41		2.8	1.2–1.7
Protein binding (%)	90			50	2	98	75	80	70
Elimination Half-life (h)	5–8 h 3–6 h (metabolite)	3–300 h	1–2 d	3 h (30 h after overdose)		13–40 d	16–20 h	4–6 d	20 h
Excreted unchanged (%)		10–20			23		60	20	<25

[a]Ette EI, Thomas WOA, Achumba JJ. Ivermerctin: A long acting microfilaricidal agent. DICP Ann Pharmacother 1990;24:426–433.
[b]Winstanley PA, Edwards G, Orme ML'E, Breckenridge AM. Effect of dose size on amodiaquine pharmacokinetics after oral administration. Eur J Clin Pharmacol 1987;33:331–333.
[c]Karbwang J, Ward SA, Milton KA, et al. Pharmacokinetics of halofantrine in healthy Thai volunteers. Br J Clin Pharmacol 1991;32:639–640.
[d]Broom C. The human pharmacokinetics of halofantrine hydrochloride. In: Warhurst DC, Schofield CJ, eds. *Halofantrine in the Treatment of Multidrug Resistant Malaria.* Cambridge: Elsevier, 1989:15–20.
[e]Bryson HM, Goa KL. Halofantrine: A review of its antimalarial activity, pharmacokinetic properties and therapeutic potential. Drugs 1992;43:236–258.
[f]Miller DR, Fiechtner JJ, Carpenter JR, et al. Plasma hydroxychloroquine concentrations and efficacy in rheumatoid arthritis. Arthritis Rheum 1987;30:567–571.
[g]Villalobos D. Plaquenil (hydroxychloroquine) plasmapheresis (PPR) in an overdose. Vet Hum Toxicol 1991;33:364.
[h]Hall AH, Spoerke DG. Bronsten AC, Kulig KW, Rumack BH: Human ivermectin exposure. J Emerg Med 1985;3:217–219.
[i]*Mectizan (Ivermectin MSD).* Rahway, NJ: Merck, 1988:35–85.
[j]*Ivermectin Poison Control Monograph.* West Point, PA: Merck Sharp & Dohme, Division of Merck, 1985:1–18.
[k]Azia MA, Diallo S, Diop IM, et al. Efficacy and tolerance of ivermectin in human onchocerciasis. Lancet 1982;2:171–173.
[l]Azia MA, Diallo S, Lariviere M, et al. Ivermectin in onchocerciasis. Lancet 1982;2:1456–1457.
[m]Campbell WC, ed. *Ivermectin and Abamectins.* New York: Springer-Verlag, 1989.
[n]Edwards G. Pharmacokinetics of antifilarial drugs. Trop Med Parasitol 1987;38:64–65.
[o]Edwards G, Breckinridge AM. Clinical pharmacokinetics of anthelmintic drugs. Clin Pharmacokinet 1988;15:67–93.
[p]Edwards G, Dingsdale A, Helsley N, et al. The relative systemic availability of ivermectin after administration as capsule, tablets and oral solution. Eur J Clin Pharmacol 1988;35:681–684.
[q]Karbwang J, White NJ. Clinical pharmacokinetics of mefloquine. Clin Pharmacokinet 1990;19:264–279.
[r]Nosten F, Karbwang J, White NJ, et al. Mefloquine antimalarial prophylaxis in pregnancy: Dose finding and pharmacokinetic study. Br J Clin Pharmacol 1990;30:79–85.
[s]Helsby NA, Ward SA, Edwards G, et al. The pharmacokinetics and activations of proguanil in man: Consequences of variability in drug metabolism. Br J Clin Pharmacol 1990;30:593–598.
[t]Maegrath BG, Tottey MM, Adams ARD, et al. The absorption and excretion of paludrine in the human subject. Ann Trop Med Parasitol 1946;40;493–501.
[u]Wattanagoon Y, Taylor RB, Moody RR, et al. Single dose pharmacokinetics of proguanil and its metabolites in healthy subjects. Br J Clin Pharmacol 1987;24:775–780.
[v]Taylor RB, Moody RR, Ochekpe NA. Determination of proguanil and its metabolites cycloguanil and 4-chlorphenyl-biguanide in plasma, whole blood and urine by HPLC. J Chromatog 1987;416:394–399.
[w]Smith CC, Hirig J. Persistent excretion of pyrimethamine following oral administration. Am J Trop Med Hyg 1959;8:60–62.
[x]Bennett WM, Singer I, Golper T, et al. Guidelines for drug therapy in renal failure. Ann Intern Med 1977;86:754–783.
[y]Maher JF. Pharmacological aspects of renal failure and dialysis. In: Drukker W, Parsons FM, Maher JF, eds. *Replacement of Renal Function by Dialysis.* Boston: Martinus Nijhoff, 1983:770.
[z]La Greca G, Biasioli S, Borin D, et al. Drugs and dialysis. Int J Artif Organs 1983;6:135–156.
[aa]White NJ. Clinical pharmacokinetics of antimalarial drugs. Clin Pharmacokinet 1985;10:187–215.
[bb]Bateman DN, Blain PG, Woodhouse KW, et al. Pharmacokinetics and clinical toxicity of quinine overdosage: Lack of efficacy of techniques intended to enhance elimination. Q J Med N Ser 1985;54:125–131.
[cc]Rollo IM. Drugs used in the chemotherapy of malaria. In: Goodman LS, Gilman A, eds. *The Pharmacological Basis of Therapeutics.* 5th ed. New York: MacMillan, 1975:1062–1065.
[dd]McEvoy GK, ed. *AHFS Drug Information 86.* Bethesda, MD: American Society of Hospital Pharmacists, 1986:346–349.
[ee]White NJ, Looareesuwan S, Warrell DA, et al. Quinine pharmacokinetics and toxicity in cerebral and uncomplicated falciparum malaria. Am J Med 1982;73:564–572.
[ff]Brodie BB, Baer JE, Craig LC. Metabolic products of the cinchona alkaloids in human urine. J Biol Chem 1951;188:567–581.
[gg]Bennett WM, Singer I, Golper T, et al. Guidelines for drug therapy in renal failure. Ann Intern Med 1977;86:754–783.

Table 17–4
Overdoses With Some Anthelmintic Drugs

	Age	Toxic Dose	Overdose: Clinical Signs and Symptoms
Mebendazole	8-wk	50 mg bid × 3 d	Staring, opisthotonos, respiratory arrest, tachyrhythmias, seizures[a]
Oxamniquine	Adult	6.25 g	Dizziness, convulsions, semicoma, vomiting, diffuse electroencephalograph abnormalities
Pyrantel pamoate		>2500 mg	Doses of up to 15,000 mg/d for 10 d taken with no untoward systemic toxicity; diarrhea and nausea may occur with doses >2500 mg
Thiabendazole	Adult	>3 g	May have transient disturbances of vision and psychic alterations; seizures

[a]Jaeger A, Sauder P, Kopferschmitt J, Flesch F. Clinical features and management of poisoning due to antimalarial drugs. Med Toxicol 1987;2:242–273.

Mefloquine. Effects include seizures, vertigo, nausea, dizziness, fatigue, and acute psychosis.[63] Two major clinical features have been described.[63] The first is an "acute brain syndrome," which consists of an encephalopathy with disorientation and mental dysfunction, sometimes complicated by status epilepticus and coma. The second consists of a group of psychiatric symptoms, including acute psychosis, memory loss, confusion, hallucinations, and behavioral abnormalities, such as aggression, agitation, and hyperactivity or hypoactivity. Depression can be severe, with suicide attempts, and may persist as long as 9 months. The other psychiatric symptoms generally do not last more than 10 days.

Proguanil Hydrochloride. Mouth ulcers, diarrhea,[64] vomiting, abdominal pain, chronic renal failure, megaloblastic anemia, and pancytopenia[65,66] have been observed.

Pyrimethamine. Folic acid deficiency, reversible bone marrow depression, nausea, vomiting, and hemolytic anemia have been reported.[67]

Quinine. Effects include reversible visual damage,[26,68] seizures, muscle weakness, coma, cardiac arrhythmias, cinchonism, tinnitus, dizziness, headache, fever, hypersensitivity reaction, hearing loss, immune thrombocytopenia, coma, hemolytic uremic syndrome,[69] disseminated intravascular coagulation,[70] hypoglycemia, peripheral neuropathy,[71] and a prolonged QT interval.[72]

Laboratory

Analytical Methods

Amodiaquine	High-performance liquid chromatography[73]
Chloroquine	High-performance liquid chromatography[74]
Halofantrine	High-performance liquid chromatography[75]
Hydroxychloroquine	High-performance liquid chromatography
Ivermectin	High-performance liquid chromatography or fluorescence detection[76]
Mefloquine	High-performance liquid chromatography[77]
Proguanil hydrochloride	High-performance liquid chromatography (2 ng/mL limit of detection)[66,78]
Pyrimethamine	High-performance liquid chromatography (65 ng/mL limit of detection)
Quinine	High-performance liquid chromatography (18 ng/mL sensitivity)[79]

Toxic Blood Levels

Mefloquine	> 1000 ng/mL[80] (Levels > 1000 ng/mL penetrate the central nervous system.[82])
Proguanil hydrochloride	> 100 ng/mL[72]
Quinine	9–60 μg/mL (fatal)[82] > 15 μg/mL (toxic)[23,24]

Treatment Aspects of Specific Drugs

Treatment is symptomatic and supportive.

Amodiaquine and Halofantrine

Watch QT interval.

Hydroxychloroquine

Avoid class I antiarrhythmic agents.

Ivermectin

Observe for seizures.

Chloroquine

Patients have survived following severe chloroquine poisoning when treatment is begun early and includes the following:

1. Epinephrine administered through a syringe-type pump, in an initial dose of 0.25 μg/kg of body weight per minute followed by increments of 0.25 μg/kg per minute until an adequate systolic arterial pressure (about 100 mm Hg) is obtained. (The epinephrine is administered with intravenous 5% glucose to ensure adequate epinephrine dilution in the vein, ie, > 1:10,000.)[83]

2. Rapid intubation after intravenous thiopental 5 mg/kg.
3. Mechanical ventilation with a fractional inspired oxygen concentration of 40%, a tidal volume of 10 mL/kg, and a ventilatory rate of 14/min.
4. Diazepam 2 mg/kg administered over 30 minutes through a motor-driven syringe type pump.[83]

Diazepam is difficult to dissolve. A separate intravenous line and a motor-driven syringe-type pump are used for its administration. The administration of diazepam by intravenous infusion is not recommended in the United States but has been used in some protocols to treat status epilepticus.[84] Following these general treatment guidelines, two patients survived who had potentially fatal findings after chloroquine overdose (QRS > 0.12 second, chloroquine blood level > 25 mmol/L [8 μg/mL], and ingested dose > 6 g).[85,86] Further work is awaited to determine a rational basis for using these drugs (eg, epinephrine and diazepam) together in a patient whose cardiac muscle may already be compromised.

Stabilization. Patients should be admitted to a hospital where an oxygen supply, cardiac monitoring, and an intravenous line may be established. Patients should remain in hospital for at least 48 hours after signs and symptoms of chloroquine overdose appear to have returned to normal.

Treatment is largely supportive. Cardiac and respiratory arrest may quickly supervene. Therefore, preparations should be made for tracheal airway protection (endotracheal intubation) and mechanical ventilation. Defibrillators and cardiac pacemakers may be required. The adequacy of the tidal volume should be checked (normal, 10–15 mL/kg). Seizures, if present, should be controlled before the stomach is emptied. The seizures may result from the following:

- Anoxia: Administer 100% oxygen. Begin assisted ventilation.
- Cerebral stimulation: Administer diazepam (up to 10 mg intravenously slowly in adults; 0.1–0.3 mg/kg intravenously slowly in child). If the patient is unresponsive, administer phenytoin 15 mg/kg intravenously at up to 0.5 mg/kg/min, with electrocardiographic monitoring. Studies in rats and one clinical report show that diazepam may have a protective effect in chloroquine intoxication.[87]
- Hypotension: Administer intravenous fluids. Place the patient in Trendelenburg position. If the patient is not responsive, administer dopamine or norepinephrine. For dopamine (Intropin), 1 ampule (200 mg) is added to 500 mL normal saline or 5% dextrose in water (concentration is 400 μg/mL); start with 2 to 5 μg/kg/min, progressing as required to 50 μg/kg/min; watch for ventricular arrhythmias. For norepinephrine (Levophed), a 4-mL vial is added to 1000 mL 5% dextrose in water to make a solution of 4 μg/mL; start an intravenous drip at the rate of 0.1 to 0.2 μg/kg/min; titrate as required.

Gut Decontamination. Emesis should be avoided because of rapid onset of symptoms. If gastric emptying is preferred it should be performed with prior endotracheal intubation. The drug is rapidly absorbed, however, and if symptoms are already present, gastric aspiration may not be effective. Gastric lavage may precipitate cardiac manifestations.

Kivisto and Neuvonen suggest that gastric lavage and syrup of ipecac are not as effective in an acute chloroquine overdose as the early use of activated charcoal. Activated charcoal can prevent absorption of more than 95% of the fraction of an ingested chloroquine dose still in the stomach[88] and should be administered as soon as possible after oral ingestion of chloroquine.[89]

Activated charcoal (adults, 60–100 g; children, 30–60 g) may be placed into the gastric lavage tube after lavage followed by cathartic.

Elimination Enhancement. Forced diuresis and/or urinary acidification cannot be recommended. Exchange transfusion may prove to be useful: chloroquine concentrations are high in red blood cells, whole blood cells, and platelet. No studies are available to validate this concept.[90]

Antidote. Patients who have ingested more than 5 g of chloroquine, have a systolic blood pressure less than 80 mm Hg, and have a QRS interval longer than 120 milliseconds should receive high-dose intravenous epinephrine and diazepam immediately.[91]

Supportive Measures. Levels of electrolytes (especially potassium)[92] and liver and renal function must be monitored. A chest x-ray is required to detect diffuse changes of pulmonary edema, and cardiac monitoring (ECG) is needed to check for arrhythmias.[93,94] Hypotension is possible. Endomyocardial biopsy findings may reveal histologic features diagnostic of chloroquine cardiomyopathy including large secondary lysosomes, mycloid bodies, and curvilinear bodies.[95] These findings may appear after long-term chronic treatment with chloroquine.

Hypokalemia. If serum levels fall or there is electrocardiographic evidence of hypokalemia, potassium is administered. The dosage is 0.25 mEq/kg/h for a patient weighing less than 40 kg. If the patient weighs more than 40 kg and the potassium level is less than 3.7 mEq/L, a maximum of 10 mEq/h potassium chloride should be administered in 2 hours. In all cases, the potassium level must be checked after each 2-hour dose.

Intraventricular Block. Treatment consists of isoproterenol 4 mg (4 mL 1:5000) in 250 mL 5% dextrose in water or 0.9% saline (concentration of 16 μg/mL) at 0.3 μg/kg/min, increasing by 0.2 μg/kg to a maximum of 1.3 ug/kg/min, to decrease the afterload, and alkalinization with sodium bicarbonate to a pH of 7.5. A pacemaker may be necessary.

Ventricular Tachycardia or Fibrillation. Direct-current cardioversion is instituted. Rapid pacemaker stimulation (120/min) is needed if ventricular tachycardia recurs.

Cardiac Arrest. Cardiac massage, assisted ventilation, 100% oxygen, and epinephrine intravenously or via endotracheal tube are instituted.

Refractory Shock. An anecdotal report suggests that amrinone (bolus dose of 75 mg over 5 min and then 16.6 μg/kg/min infusions) may be useful for refractory cardiogenic shock following chloroquine poisoning.[96]

Other Measures. Diazepam is used for seizures. For methemoglobinemia greater than 30%, methylene blue is administered. For hemolysis, transfusion, alkalinization, and diuresis are employed.[97]

Cardiac and renal function must be monitored. Chloroquine blood or urine levels confirm its presence. Arrhythmias may require lidocaine. Class IA antiarrhythmic agents (e.g. quinidine, disopyramide, procainamide) should be avoided. Hospitalization and observation should be continued until cardiovascular and neurologic status is stable. Aggressive supportive measures are sufficient to obtain a complete recovery in many cases.[98]

Mefloquine

Watch for seizures.

Pyrimethamine

Calcium leucovorin 3–9 mg intramuscularly for 3 days is administered,[20] as is folic acid 10 mg/d. Hematologic monitoring is instituted.

Quinine

Treatment comprises eye examinations (visual fields, electroretinography, electrooculogram, visual evoked potentials, dark adaptions, color testing) and periodic electrocardiograms. Stellate ganglion block is controversial.[99–102] Class I, II, and III antiarrhythmic agents should be avoided.[103]

REFERENCES—ANTIPARASITIC AND ANTIMALARIAL DRUGS

1. Salako LA. Pharmacokinetics of antimalarial drugs: Their therapeutic and toxicological implications. Ann Ist Super Sanita 1985;21:315–326.
2. Rosenblatt JE. Antiparasitic agents. Mayo Clin Proc 1992;67:276–287.
3. Winstanley PA, Edwards G, Orme ML'E, Breckenridge AM. Effect of dose size on amodiaquine pharmacokinetics after oral administration. Eur J Clin Pharmacol 1987;33:331–333.
4. Hatton C, Peto T, Bunch C, et al. Frequency of severe neutropaenia associated with amodiaquine prophylaxis against malaria. Lancet 1986;1:411–414.
5. Neftel KA, Woodtly W, Schmid M, et al. Amodiaquine-induced agranulocytosis and liver damage. Br Med J 1986; 292:721–723.
6. Mack RB. 4-Aminoquinolines can be dangerous to your health: Chloroquine (Aralen) intoxication. NC Med J 1984;45: 245–246.
7. Chloroquine and other antimalarials. In: Reynolds JEF, ed. *Martindale: The Extra Pharmacopoeia.* 30th ed. London: Pharmaceutical Press, 1993:393–411.
8. Chloroquine hydrochloride. Chloroquine phosphate. In: McEvoy GK, ed. *AHFS Drug Information 94.* Bethesda, MD: American Society of Hospital Pharmacists, 1994:452–456.
9. Marr JJ. Antiparasitic agents. In: Mandell GL, Douglas RG Jr, Bennett JE, eds. *Anti-Infective Therapy.* New York: Wiley, 1985:381–383.
10. Halofantrine in the treatment of malaria. Lancet 1989;2:537–538. Editorial.
11. Watkins WM, Oloo JA, Lury JD, et al. Efficacy of multiple dose halofantrine in treatment of chloroquine-resistant falciparum malaria in children in Kenya. Lancet 1988;2:247–250.
12. Bandon D, Bernard J, Moulia-Pelat JP, et al. Halofantrine to prevent falciparum malaria on return from malarious areas. Lancet 1990;336:377–378.
13. Hydroxychloroquine. In: McEvoy GK, ed. *AHFS Drug Information 94.* Bethesda, MD: American Society of Hospital Pharmacists, 1994:456–458.
14. Hydroxychloroquine. In: Reynolds JEF, ed. *Martindale: The Extra Pharmacopoeia.* 30th ed. London: Pharmaceutical Press, 1993:401–402.
15. Miller D, Fiechtner J. Hydroxychloroquine overdosage. J Rheumatol 1989;16:142–143.
16. Ivermectin. In: Reynolds JEF, ed. *Martindale: The Extra Pharmacopoeia.* 30th ed. London: Pharmaceutical Press, 1993: 43–44.
17. Ette EI, Thomas WOA, Achumba JJ. Ivermectin: A long acting microfilaricidal agent. DICP Ann Pharmacother 1990; 24:426–433.
18. Ivermectin. In: Dollery CF, ed. *Therapeutic Drugs.* Edinburgh: Churchill Livingstone, 1991;1:1128–1131.
19. Pyrimethamine. In: McEvoy GK, ed. *AHFS Drug Information 94.* Bethesda, MD: American Society of Hospital Pharmacists, 1994:460–464.
20. Calcium leucovorin. In: McEvoy GK, ed. *AHFS Drug Information 94.* Bethesda, MD: American Society of Hospital Pharmacists, 1994:2465–2467.
21. Hitchings GH. The utilisation of biochemical differences between host and parasites as a basis for chemotherapy. In: Goodwin LG, Nimmo-Smith RH, eds. *Drugs, Parasites and Hosts.* London: J & A Churchill, 1962:200.
22. Tracqui A, Mikail I, Kintz P, Mangin P. Non-fatal prolonged overdose of pyrimethamine in an infant: Measurement of plasma and urine levels using HPLC with diode-array detection. J Anal Toxicol 1993;17:248–250.
23. Boland ME, Roper SMG, Henry JA. Complications of quinine poisoning. Lancet 1985;1:384–385.
24. Dyson EH, Proudfoot AT, Prescott LF, et al. Death and blindness due to overdose of quinine. Br Med J 1985;291: 31–33.
25. Murray SF, Jay JL. Loss of sight after self poisoning with quinine. Br Med J 1983;287:1700.
26. Bateman DN, Blain PG, Woodhouse KW, et al. Pharmacokinetics and clinical toxicity of quinine overdosage: Lack of efficacy of techniques intended to enhance elimination. Q J Med N Ser 1985;54:125–131.
27. Dannenberg AL, Dorfman SF, Johnson J. Use of quinine for self induced abortion. South Med J 1983;76:846–849.
28. Licciardello AT, Stanbury JB. Acute hemolytic anemia from quinine used as an abortifacient. N Engl J Med 1948; 238:120–121.
29. Rollo IM. Drugs used in the chemotherapy of malaria. In: Goodman LS, Gilman A, eds. *The Pharmacological Basis of Therapeutics.* 5th ed. New York: MacMillan, 1975:1062–1065.
30. Quinine. In: McEvoy GK, ed. *AHFS Drug Information 94.* Bethesda, MD: American Society of Hospital Pharmacists, 1994:464–467.
31. *Handbook of Antimicrobial Therapy.* rev ed. New Rochelle, NY: Medical Letter, 1984:101.
32. Quinine. In: Reynolds JEF, ed. *Martindale: The Extra Pharmacopoeia.* 30th ed. London: Pharmaceutical Press, 1993:408–411.
33. Winek CL, Davis ER, Collom WD, et al. Quinine fatality: Case report. Clin Toxicol 1974;7(2):129–132.
34. Winek CL, Schweighardt FK, Fochtman FW, et al. Quinine in urinalysis for heroin. JAMA 1971;217:1243–1244.
35. Lupovich P, Pilewski R, Sapira JD, et al. Cardiotoxicity of quinine as adulterant in drugs. JAMA 1970;212:1216.
36. Akindele O, Odejide AO. Amodiaquine-induced involuntary movements. Br Med J 1976;2:214–215.

37. Kjaer K. Effects of an overdose of chloroquine in a pregnant woman. Am J Trop Med Hyg 1955;4:259–262.
38. Frisk-Holmberg M, Bergqvist Y, Englund U. Chloroquine intoxication. Br J Clin Pharmacol 1983;15:502–503.
39. Wilkinson R, Mahatane J, Wade P, Parvol G. Chloroquine poisoning. Br Med J 1993;307:504.
40. Chemmessy JL, Favier C, Borrow SW, et al. Hypokalemia related to acute chloroquine ingestion. Clin Toxicol 1995;33: 475–486. Abstract 73.
41. Vachon F, Fajac I, Gachot B, et al. Halofantrine and acute intravascular haemolysis. Lancet 1992;340:909–910.
42. Hallwood PM, Horton RJ, O'Sullivan KM, Parr SN. Halofantrine and pruritus. Lancet 1989;2:397–398.
43. Halofantrine in the treatment of malaria. Lancet 1989;2:537–538. Editorial.
44. Wisekegle FY. *A Survey of Antimalarial Drugs 1941–1945.* Ann Arbor MI: JW Edwards, 1946:309–324.
45. Nosten F, Ter Kuik FA, Luxemburger C, et al. Cardiac effects of antimalarial treatment with halofantrine. Lancet 1993; 341:1054–1056.
46. Wang R. Hydroxychloroquine cardiotoxicity. Clin Toxicol 1995;33:475–486. Abstract 164.
47. Kemmenoe AJ. An infant fatality due to hydroxychloroquine poisoning. J Anal Toxicol 1990;14:186–188.
48. Overdose of hydroxychloroquine. Pharm J, 1 June 1 1963, p. 504.
49. Dalley RA, Hainsworth D. Fatal plaquenil poisoning. J Forens Sci Soc 1965;5:99–101.
50. Getz MA, Subramanian R, Logemann T, Bellantyne F. Acute necrotizing eosinophilic myocarditis as a manifestation of severe hypersensitivity myocarditis. Ann Intern Med 1991;115: 201–202.
51. Kunze K, Kauerz V, Scholdt A. Drug induced myopathy by hydroxychloroquine. Vet Hum Toxicol 1987;29(suppl. 2): 59–60.
52. Makin AJ, Wendon J, Fitt S, et al. Fulminant hepatic failure secondary to hydroxychloroquine. Gut 1994;35:569–571.
53. Johnson MW, Vine AK. Hydroxychloroquine therapy in massive total doses without retinal toxicity. Am J Ophthalmol 1987;104:139–144.
54. Hall AH, Spoerke DG, Bronsten AC, et al. Human ivermectin exposure. J Emerg Med 1985;3:217–219.
55. *Mectizan (Ivermectin MSD).* Rahway, NJ: Merck, 1988:35–85.
56. *Ivermectin Poison Control Monograph.* West Point, PA: Merck, Sharp and Dohme, Division of Merck, 1985:1–18.
57. Awadzi K, Dadzie KY, Shulz-Key H, et al. The chemotherapy of onchocerciasis. X. An assessment of four simple dose treatment regimens of MK-933 (ivermectin) in human onchocerciasis. Am Trop Med Parasitol 1985;79:63–78.
58. Dadzie KY, Bird AC, Awadzi K, et al. Ocular findings in a double-blind study of ivermectin versus diethylcarbamazine versus placebo in the treatment of onchocerciasis. Br J Ophthalmol 1987;7:78–85.
59. Bryan RF, Stoles SL, Spencer HC. Expatriates treated with ivermectin. Lancet 1991:337:304.
60. Homeida MMA, Bagi IA, Ghalib HW, et al. Prolongation of prothrombin time with ivermectin. Lancet 1988;1:1346–1347.
61. White AT, Newland HS, Taylor HR, et al. Controlled trial and dose finding study of ivermectin for treatment of onchocerciasis. J Infect Dis 1987;156:463–470.
62. Iliff-Sizemore SA, Partlow MR, Kelley ST. Ivermectin toxicology in a rhesus macaque. Vet Hum Toxicol 1990;32:530–532.
63. Hennequin C, Bouree P, Bazin N, et al. Severe psychiatric side effects observed during prophylaxis and treatment with mefloquine. Arch Intern Med 1994;154:2360–2362.
64. Drysdale SF, Phillips-Howard PA, Behrens RH. Proguanil, chloroquine and mouth ulcers. Lancet 1990;335:164.
65. Boots M, Phillips M, Curtis JR. Megaloblastic anemia and pancytopenia due to proguanil in patients with chronic renal failure. Clin Nephrol 1982;18:106–108.
66. Maegrath BG, Tottey MM, Adams ARD, et al. The absorption and excretion of paludrine in the human subject. Ann Trop Med Parasitol 1946;40:493–501.
67. Luzzi GA, Peto TEA. Adverse effects of antimalarials: An update. Drug Saf 1992;8:295–311.
68. Hla KK, Leahy N, Henry J. Accidental quinine poisoning in children under five. Vet Hum Toxicol 1987,29(suppl. 2): 121–123.
69. Gottschall JL, Elliott W, Lianos E, et al. Quinine-induced immune thrombocytopenia associated with hemolytic uremic syndrome: A new clinical entity. Blood 1991;77:306–310.
70. Spearing RL, Hickton CM, Sizeland P, et al. Quinine-induced disseminated intravascular coagulation. Lancet 1990;336: 1535–1537.
71. Banerji NK, Martin VAF. Myelo-optico-neuropathy following quinine poisoning. J Irish Med Assoc 1974;67:46–47.
72. White NJ, Looareesuwan S, Warrell DA, et al. Quinine pharmacokinetics and toxicity in cerebral and uncomplicated falciparum malaria. Am J Med 1982;73:564–572.
73. Winstanley PA, Edwards G, Orme ML'E, Breckenridge AM. The disposition of amodiaquine in man after oral administration. Br J Clin Pharmacol 1987;33:1–7.
74. Bergqvist Y, Frisk-Holmberg M. Sensitive method for the determination of chloroquine and its metabolite desethylchloroquine in human plasma and urine by high performance liquid chromatography. J Chromatogr 1980;221:119–127.
75. Broom C. The human pharmacokinetics of halofantrine hydrochloride. In: Warhurst DC, Schofield CJ, eds. *Halofantrine in the Treatment of Multidrug Resistant Malaria.* Cambridge: Elsevier, 1989:15–20.
76. Chiou R, Stubbs RJ, Bayre WF. Determination of ivermectin in human plasma and milk by fluorescence detection. J Chromatogr 1987;416:196–202.
77. Arnold PJ, Stetten OV. High performance liquid chromatographic analysis of mefloquine and its main metabolite by direct plasma injection with pre-column enrichment and column switching techniques. J Chromatogr 1986;353:193–200.
78. Helsby NA, Ward SA, Edwards G, et al. The pharmacokinetics and activations of proguanil in man: Consequences of variability in drug metabolism. Br J Clin Pharmacol 1990;30: 593–598.
79. Zoest AR, Wanwinolruk S, Hung CT. Simple high performance liquid chromatographic method for the analysis of quinine in human plasma without extraction. J Liq Chromatogr 1990;13:3481–3491.
80. Patchen LC, Campbell CC, Williams SB. Neurologic reactions after a therapeutic dose of mefloquine. N Engl J Med 1989;321:1415–1416.
81. Rouveix B, Bricaire F, Michon C, et al. Mefloquine and an acute brain syndrome. Ann Intern Med 1989;110:577–578.
82. Hall A. Dangers of high dose quinine and overhydration in severe malaria. Lancet 1985;1:1453.
83. Riou B, Barriot P, Rimailho A, Baud FJ. Treatment of severe chloroquine poisoning. N Engl J Med 1988;319:50.
84. Mofenson H, Caraccio TR. Treatment of severe chloroquine poisoning. N Engl J Med 1988;319:50.
85. Stiff G, Robinson D, Cugnosi HL, et al. Massive chloroquine overdose: A survivor. Postgrad Med J 1991;67:678–679.
86. Bauer P, Maine B, Weber M, et al. Full recovery after a chloroquine suicide attempt. Clin Toxicol 1991;29:12–30.
87. Crouzette J, Vicaut E, Palombo S, et al. Experimental assessment of the protective activity of diazepam on the acute toxicity of chloroquine. J Toxicol Clin Toxicol 1983;20:271–279.
88. Kivisto KT, Neuvonen PJ. Activated charcoal for chloroquine poisoning. Br Med J 1993;307:1068.
89. Neuvonen PJ, Kivisto K, Laine K, Pyykko K. Prevention of chloroquine absorption by activated charcoal. Clin Pharmacol Ther 1991;49:132.
90. Laurenson IF, Lalloo DG, Naragi S, et al. Chloroquine overdose in Papua New Guinea. Br Med J 1993;307:564.
91. Meearan K, Jacob MG. Discussion group: Chloroquine poisoning rapidly fatal without treatment. Br Med J 1993; 307:49–50.
92. Kelly JC, Wasserman GS, Bernard WD, et al. Chloroquine poisoning in a child. Ann Emerg Med 1990;19:47–50.
93. Sanghri LM, Mathur BB. Electrocardiogram after chloroquine and emetine. Circulation 1965;32:281–289.
94. Michael TAD, Aiwazzadeh S. The effects of acute chloroquine poisoning with special reference to the heart. Am Heart J 1976;79:831–842.

95. Ratliff NB, Estes ML, Myles JL, et al. Diagnosis of chloroquine cardiomyopathy by endomyocardial biopsy. N Engl J Med 1987;316:191–193.
96. Hantson P, Ronveau JL, Coninck B, et al. Amrinone for refractory cardiogenic shock following chloroquine poisoning. Intens Care Med 1991;17:430–431.
97. Mofenson HC, Caraccio TR, Brody G, et al. Chloroquines and aminoquinolones. PP/T News. NCMC Regional Poison Control Center 1990 (Sept/Oct);9:(9–10):230–232.
98. Garnier R, Elmalem J. Haemoperfusion in chloroquine poisoning. Br Med J 1985;291:141.
99. Robertson DH, Raman KRK. Quinine poisoning: An unusual indication for stellate ganglion blockade. Anesthesia 1979;34: 1041–1042.
100. Boscoe MJ, Calver DM, Keyte C, et al. Quinine overdose: Prevention of visual damage by stellate ganglion block. Anesthesia 1983;38:1669–1671.
101. Scott DL, Ghia JN, Teeple E. Aphasia and hemiparesis following stellate ganglion block. Anesth Analg 1983;62:1038–1040.
102. Bacon P, Spalton DJ, Smith SE. Blindness from quinine toxicity. Br J Ophthalmol 1988;72:219–224.
103. Jones RG, Sue-Ling HM, Kear C, et al. Severe symptomatic hypoglycaemia due to quinine therapy. J R Soc Med 1986;79;426–428.

QUININE

Toxicokinetics

Placental Transfer

Quinine passes through the placenta. Use of quinine as an abortifacient can produce poisoning in the fetus with frequent infant deafness.[1] Other suspected teratogenic effects of quinine are blindness and physical malformation.[2] Quinine passes into breast milk.

Drug Interactions[3]

Digoxin	Increased serum digoxin, decreased renal clearance of digoxin
Antacids with aluminum	Delayed or decreased absorption of oral quinine
Neuromuscular blocking agents Pancuronium Succinylcholine Tubocurarine	Potentiate effects, respiratory difficulties
Hepatic synthesis of vitamin K-dependent coagulation factors	Hypoprothrombinemia
Oral anticoagulants	Effect is enhanced
Sodium bicarbonate, acetazolamide	Increased urinary pH, increased plasma concentration of quinine, increased toxicity Hyperthermia
Alcohol[4]	Potentiates quinine toxicity[5]

Mechanism of Action

Quinine appears to interfere with the function of plasmodial DNA.[3] It has a local anesthetic action. Quinine acts on all body muscle groups. On cardiac muscle it acts similar to quinidine when given intravenously and may cause severe hypotension. On uterine muscle it may be oxytocic to the pregnant uterus.[6] On skeletal muscle, it decreases tetanic response, excitability of the motor end plate, and calcium distribution. Quinine is a local irritant. When ingested orally, it produces gastric pain, nausea, and vomiting. Subcutaneously or intramuscularly it is very painful. When administered intravenously it may induce thrombosis of a vein. In the kidney it may induce tubular damage. Quinine may cause inappropriate insulin release, leading to symptomatic hypoglycemia.[7]

Clinical Presentation

Eye Changes

Eye changes may appear the next day or after the patient awakens from a heavy sleep or from a comatose state following ingestion.[4,8–11] Patients complain of seeing badly in a bright light and of "misty" vision. The mean time of onset of blindness was 6 hours later than that of other features of cinchonism. The initial plasma quinine concentration may be a useful predictor of subsequent visual toxicity. Eye changes may also begin ¼ to ½ hour after a quinine overdose. Partial or complete blindness is often sudden. It may pass after 14 to 24 hours; however, such changes may last up to 10 weeks or longer. Generally, there is full recovery in 1 to 3 weeks. Central vision tends to recover without treatment.[12] Patients may remain permanently blind.

Ophthalmoscopic changes include the following:

- Pallor of the optic disks (Their appearance suggests optic atrophy. This begins to appear several days after ingestion. Optic nerve, retina, and retinal vessels may be normal when the patient is first seen.[3])
- Extreme contraction of the arteries and veins of the retina, often after the first day
- Cherry spot at the macula
- Retinal edema

In the acute stages of the initial marked loss of vision, the electroretinogram may remain almost normal; it becomes abnormal during the phase of visual improvement and parallels the changes in visual acuity on the second or third day. Visual evoked potential, dark adaptation, and color testing measurements are often abnormal.

Ear Changes

Deafness is an early sign. It usually passes quickly and completely. Deafness may also be accompanied by tinnitus, a feeling of fullness in the head, headache, giddiness, and dizziness. Quinine may reduce high-tone auditory acuity, resulting in flattening of the audiograms. This effect is rapid in onset, is usually unnoticed, and usually resolves.[13] The patient may present with acute deafness and mutism.[14]

Electrocardiographic Changes

The cardiotoxicity of quinine is similar to that of class IA antiarrhythmic drugs. Cardiotoxicity is usually the cause of death from overdose. Quinine has a negative inotropic action; it slows the rate of depolarization and conduction;

finally, it increases the action potential duration and the effective refractory period in the myocardium.[15]

Sinus tachycardia, high-degree atrioventricular heart block, prolongation of the PR interval, sinoatrial block and arrest, complete dissociation, ventricular fibrillation, Torsade de pointes, and prominent U waves may be seen. Quinine also has alpha-adrenergic blocking effects. Hypotension may follow the vasodilation, myocardial depression, or dysrhythmia.[15]

Laboratory

On admission, blood is drawn for a complete blood count, blood sugar, prothrombin time, renal function tests, urinalysis, and electrolytes. Periodic eye examinations should include visual fields, electroretinography, electrooculogram, visual evoked potentials, dark adaptation, and color testing. Periodic electrocardiograms are done as indicated.

Treatment

Stabilization

The patient is admitted to an intensive care facility, where attention to vital signs (blood pressure, pulse, respirations) with careful monitoring of the electrocardiogram and ventilation should be instituted. Assisted ventilation should be prepared for. Blood is drawn to determine the plasma quinine level if visual symptoms are absent. In general, supportive care remains the mainstay of treatment for quinine toxicity.

Gut Decontamination

Early emesis induction is indicated after a single ingestion of 1.5 to 2 g or more in an adult or approximately 25 mg/kg in a child, and should be instituted within 4 hours of ingestion, if possible, in view of the rapidity of absorption. Gastric lavage and/or repeated administration of activated charcoal may be preferable for patients in whom rapid clinical deterioration is suspected. Repeated activated charcoal reduces the plasma half-life of quinine and should be administered early in quinine overdosage. It may be the only effective way to lessen the potentially disastrous consequences of permanent blindness and fatal cardiotoxicity.[16]

Elimination Enhancement

Measures to enhance the elimination of quinine have been generally ineffective.[17] Hemodialysis combined with resin hemoperfusion may be effective in the treatment of quinine blindness refractory to the usual therapy.[18] Exchange transfusion has not been successful.[17]

Antidote

There is no effective antidote.

There is no evidence that any treatment affects the visual prognosis.[19] For angioedema, epinephrine and diphenhydramine may be useful. Fluid and electrolyte levels should be monitored and evaluations of renal function repeated. Hyperbaric oxygen has been suggested but not thoroughly evaluated.[20]

Class I, II, and III antidysrhythmics should be avoided in treating cardiotoxicity. Direct-current cardioversion is used to treat ventricular tachycardia or ventricular fibrillation. Overdrive pacing or isoproterenol may be useful for Torsade de pointes. Transvenous pacing can be useful for complete heart block or marked prolongation of the QRS complex. Serum alkalinization with sodium bicarbonate may be useful for QRS prolongation. Acidosis, electrolyte imbalance, and hypoxia must be treated aggressively to halt the progression of the cardiotoxicity.[15]

REFERENCES—QUININE

1. Dannenberg AL, Dorfman SF, Johnson J. Use of quinine for self induced abortion. South Med J 1983;76:846–849.
2. Nishimura H, Tanimura T. *Clinical Aspects of the Teratogenicity of Drugs.* Amsterdam: Excerpta Medica, 1976:140–143.
3. Quinine. In: McEvoy GK, ed. *AHFS Drug Information 94.* Bethesda, MD: American Society of Hospital Pharmacists, 1994:464-467.
4. Elliott RH. Quinine poisoning: Its ocular lesions and visual disturbances. Am J Ophthalmol 1918;1:547–560, 650–658.
5. Quinine. In: Reynolds JEF, ed. *Martindale: The Extra Pharmacopeia.* 30th ed. London: Pharmaceutical Press, 1993:408–411.
6. Rollo IM. Drugs used in the chemotherapy of malaria. In: Goodman LS, Gilman A, eds. *The Pharmacological Basis of Therapeutics.* 5th ed. New York: MacMillan, 1975:1062–1065.
7. Browne GF, Coppel DL. Management of quinine overdose. Hum Toxicol 1984;3:399–402.
8. Banerji NK, Martin VAF. Myelo-optico-neuropathy following quinine poisoning. J Irish Med Assoc 1974;67:46–47.
9. Diamondstone AH, Braveman BL, Baker LA. Ventricular tachycardia and bilateral amaurosis produced by quinine poisoning. Arch Intern Med 1947;80:763–770.
10. La Greca G, Biasioli S, Borin D, et al. Drugs and dialysis. Int J Artif Organs 1983;6:139–156.
11. Grant WM. *Toxicology of the Eye.* 3rd ed. Springfield, IL: Charles C Thomas, 1986:778–784.
12. Brinton GS, Norton EWD, Zahn JR, et al. Ocular quinine toxicity. Am J Ophthalmol 1980;90:403–410.
13. Roche RJ, Silamut K, Pukrittayakamee S, et al. Quinine induces reversible high tone hearing loss. Br J Clin Pharmacol 1990;29:780–782.
14. Schonwald S, Shannon M. Unsuspected quinine intoxication presenting as acute deafness and mutism. Am J Emerg Med 1991;9:318–320.
15. Wolf LR, Otten EJ, Spadafora MP. Cinchonism: Two case reports and review of acute quinine toxicity and treatment. J Emerg Med 1992;10:295–301.
16. Prescott LF, Hamilton AR, Heyworth R. Treatment of quinine overdosage with repeated oral charcoal. Br J Clin Pharmacol 1989;27:95–97.
17. Bateman DN, Blain PG, Woodhouse KW, et al. Pharmacokinetics and clinical toxicity of quinine overdosage: Lack of efficacy of techniques intended to enhance elimination. Q J Med N Ser 1985;54:125–131.
18. Gibbs JL, Trafford A, Sharpstone P. Quinine amblyopia treated by combined haemodialysis and activated resin haemoperfusion. Lancet 1985;1:752–753.
19. Canning CR, Hague S. Ocular quinine toxicity. Br J Ophthalmol 1988;72:23–26.
20. Lupovich P, Pilewski R, Sapira JD, et al. Cardiotoxicity of quinine as adulterant in drugs. JAMA 1970;212:1216.

Chapter 18

Antiviral Drugs

INTRODUCTION

Drugs used in the treatment of viral infections in the United States are listed in Table 18–1.[1] Overdose with fatalities has been reported following acyclovir and amantadine. Treatment is largely symptomatic and supportive (see also Chapter 15).

ACYCLOVIR

Acyclovir (Zovirax) (Fig. 18–1) is a synthetic purine nucleoside derived from guanine, a prodrug, and its active form is acyclovir triphosphate, which accumulates in infected cells as a result of activation trapping by the virus-specified thymidine kinase.

It is currently the only antiviral agent approved by the U.S. Food and Drug Administration for the treatment of genital herpes simplex virus infection.[2,3]

Therapeutic Dose

Oral

For treatment of initial genital herpes infections, the recommended adult dosage is 200 mg every 4 hours (while awake) for 7 to 10 days. For treatment of acute herpes zoster in nonimmunocompromised adults, 800-mg doses are used orally every 4 hours, five times daily (4 g/d), for 7 to 10 days.

Parenteral

The usual intravenous dosage is 5 mg/kg every 8 hours (15 mg/kg/d) for adults and children over 12 years of age. For treatment of herpes simplex encephalitis, the usual intravenous dosage for adults and children is 10 mg/kg every 8 hours (30 mg/kg/d) for at least 10 days. For adults and children undergoing hemodialysis, the manufacturer recommends 5 mg/kg acyclovir be administered intravenously once daily after each dialysis period. For end-stage renal disease, an initial dose of 250 mg/m^2, a maintenance dose of 250 to 500 mg/m^2 every 48 hours, and a dose of 150 to 500 mg/m^2 immediately after dialysis have been suggested.

Table 18-1
Drugs for Treatment of Viral Infections

Viral Infection	Drug of Choice	Dosage
Cytomegalovirus		
Retinitis, colitis, esophagitis	Ganciclovir (Cytovene)	5 mg/kg IV bid for 14–21 d[a]
	or Foscarnet (Foscavir)	60 mg/kg IV q8h or 90 mg/kg IV q12h for 14–21 days[b]
Chronic suppression of retinitis[c]	Ganciclovir	5 mg/kg IV daily or 6 mg/kg 5×/wk[a]
	or Foscarnet	90–120 mg/kg IV daily[b,d]
Hepatitis B virus		
Chronic hepatitis	Interferon alfa-2b (Intron A)	5×10^6 U/d or 10×10^6 U 3×/wk SC or IM for 4 mo
Hepatitis C virus		
Chronic hepatitis	Interferon alfa-2b	3×10^6 U SC or IM 3×/wk for 24 wk[e]
Herpes simplex virus		
Genital herpes		
First episode	Acyclovir (Zovirax)	400 mg PO tid for 7–10 d[f]
Recurrence	Acyclovir	400 mg PO tid for 5 d[g]
Frequent recurrences	Acyclovir	400 mg PO bid
Encephalitis	Acyclovir[h]	10 mg/kg IV q8h for 14–21 d
Mucocutaneous disease in immunocompromised	Acyclovir	5 mg/kg IV q8h[i] for 7–14 d or 400 mg PO 5×/d
Neonatal	Acyclovir[j]	10 mg/kg IV q8h for 10–21 d
Acyclovir-resistant	Foscarnet	40 mg/kg IV q8h
Keratoconjunctivitis	Trifluridine[k] (Viroptic)	1 drop of 1% solution topically every 2 h, up to 9 drops/d for 10 d
Influenza A virus	Amantadine—generic (Symmetrel)	100 mg PO bid for 4 d[l]
	or Rimantadine (Flumadine)	200 mg PO qd or 100 mg PO bid for 5 d[m]
Respiratory syncytial virus	Ribavirin (Virazole)	Aerosol treatment 12–18 h/d for 3–7 d[n]
Varicella–zoster virus		
Varicella	Acyclovir	20 mg/kg (800 mg max) PO qid for 5 d
Herpes zoster	Acyclovir[o]	800 mg PO 5×/d for 7–10 d
Varicella or zoster in immunocompromised	Acyclovir	10 mg/kg IV q8h for 7 d[p]
Acyclovir-resistant	Foscarnet	40 mg/kg IV q8h

[a]Dosage reduction is recommended for creatinine clearance <80 mL/min.
[b]Dosage reduction is recommended for creatinine clearance <1.6 mL/min/kg.
[c]In AIDS and in other highly immunocompromised patients with retinitis, chronic suppression is recommended after acute treatment.
[d]Over 2 hours. Higher doses (120 mg/kg/d) appear to be more effective (Jacobson MA, et al. J Infect Dis 168:444, 1993).
[e]Some experts recommend stopping the drug if no response in transaminase activity by 16 weeks. The optimal dosage and duration of therapy are still under study.
[f]FDA-approved dosage is 200 mg five times a day. For severe initial genital herpes, intravenous acyclovir (5 mg/kg q8h for 5–7 days) can be used. Dosage reduction is recommended for creatinine clearance <50 mL/min.
[g]Only modest benefit. FDA-approved dosage is 200 mg five times a day.
[h]Pediatric dosage is 500 mg/m² q8h. Vidarabine 15 mg/kg/d as an intravenous infusion over 12–24 hours for 10 days is a generally less effective alternative.
[i]Pediatric dosage is 250 mg/m² IV q8h for 7–14 days.
[j]Not approved by the FDA for this indication. For premature infants, 20 mg/kg/d in two divided doses has been used (Englund JA, et al. J Pediatr 119:129, 1991). Vidarabine (Vira-A) 15 mg/kg/d as an IV infusion over 12–24 hours for 10 days is an FDA-approved alternative.
[k]Vidarabine 3% ointment, ½-inch ribbon 5 times/d, is an equally effective alternative treatment. An ophthalmic preparation of acyclovir is available in some countries. Treatment of herpes simplex virus ocular infections should be supervised by an ophthalmologist; duration of therapy and dosage depend on response.
[l]The recommended pediatric dosage is 4.4 mg/kg/d up to a maxium of 150 mg/d. Dosage should be decereased in patients with diminished renal function (creatinine clearance <80 mL/min), and those older than 65 years should receive 100 mg/d.
[m]Pediatric dosage is 5 mg/kg/d up to a maximum of 150 mg. Dosage of 100 mg/d is recommended for older nursing home residents and for patients with severe hepatic dysfunction or creatinine clearance ≤10 mL/min.
[n]Reservoir concentration of 20 mg/mL. Requires special aerosol-generating device (SPAG-2, Viratek, Inc.) available from manufacturer and expert respiratory therapy monitoring for administration.
[o]Effectiveness established in ophthalmic zoster and in localized zoster of less than 3 days' duration.
[p]Pediatric dosage is 500 mg/m² q8h for 7–10 days. Vidarabine 10 mg/kg/day IV over 12–24 hours for 5 days is a less effective alternative.
From Drugs for non-HIV viral infections. Med Lett Drug Ther 1994;36:27–31.

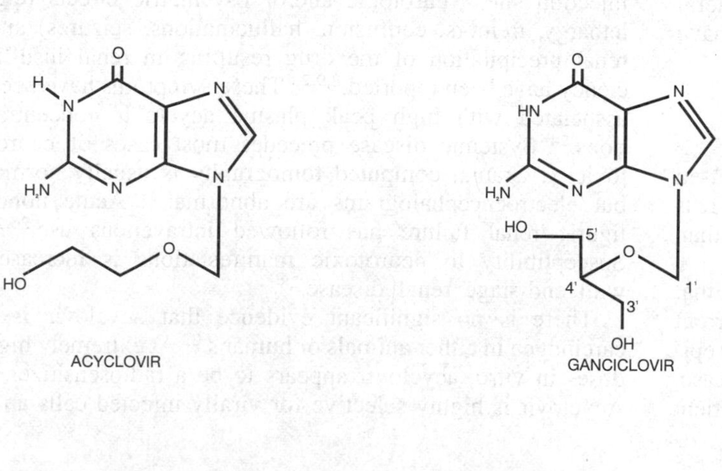

Figure 18-1 Chemical structures of acyclovir and ganciclovir. (From Fan-Howard P, Nahata MC, Brady MT. J Clin Pharm Ther 1989;14:329–340.)

Toxic Dose

High oral doses[4] of 800 to 4800 mg/d[5] appear to be generally well tolerated. Neurotoxicity may be seen with high doses in the patient with compromised renal function. This is accompanied by high plasma acyclovir levels (eg, approximately 90 μmol/L). Diarrhea, nausea and vomiting, and elevated serum creatinine levels may be observed and will recede with diminished doses.

Parenteral doses up to 3.6 g/m^2 (84 mg/kg) have been tolerated by some patients for up to 2 weeks.[5] Peak serum acyclovir concentrations up to 10 μg/mL following oral administration and up to 80 μg/mL following intravenous administration have been reported. Acyclovir crystals may precipitate in the renal tubules, resulting in renal dysfunction, renal failure, or anuria[6]. A 70-year-old woman received 4000 mg of acyclovir daily together with dextropropoxyphene napsylate 100 mg every 6 hours. She developed acute renal failure, became unresponsive and later improved without specific therapy.[7]

Toxicokinetics[5,8–14]

Bioavailability	25–30%
Peak plasma level	2–5 μM (0.6–1.3 μg/mL)
Time to peak plasma level	2 hours
Volume of distribution	0.8 L/kg
Plasma protein binding	15–20%
Elimination half-life	3 hours
Excreted unchanged	90–92%

Drug Interactions

Zidovudine. Profound drowsiness and lethargy have been reported when both drugs were used together.[15]

Probenecid. Competitive inhibition of renal secretion of acyclovir results in an increased half-life (up to 40%) and decreased urinary excretion and renal clearance of acyclovir.[9]

Antifungal Agents. Amphotericin B and ketoconazole potentiate the antiviral effects of acyclovir.

Interferon. Interferon has an additive or synergic antiviral effect to acyclovir in vitro. Parenteral acyclovir must be used with caution in patients who have had a prior neurologic reaction to interferon.

Methotrexate. The manufacturer states that parenteral acyclovir should be used with caution in patients who have exhibited prior neurologic reactions to methotrexate.

Pregnancy/Lactation

Acyclovir crosses the placenta. At doses 30 times that used clinically, acyclovir is a teratogen in animal studies.[16] It is distributed into breast milk at concentrations higher than maternal plasma concentrations.

The Centers for Disease Control and Prevention state that systemic acyclovir treatment should *not* be used for recurrent genital herpes episodes or for prophylaxis of recurrent episodes in pregnant women without life-threatening disease. Acyclovir has been successfully used in a pregnant patient with herpes simplex virus encephalitis; she delivered a healthy newborn.[17] Trials in pregnancy are proceeding.[18] Newborns less than 1 month of age with herpes simplex virus infection who received acyclovir 30 mg/kg intravenously developed rash, tremulousness, and vomiting.[19] All formulations of acyclovir are assigned to Food and Drug Administration Pregnancy Category C, which indicates that safety in human pregnancy has not been determined. No formal testing has been performed in pregnant women.[21]

Pregnancy Registry. An Acyclovir in Pregnancy Registry is managed by the Burroughs Wellcome Company at 3030 Cornwallis Road, Research Triangle Park, NC 27709. Telephone: (800) 722–9292, extension 58465 (from the United States) or (919) 315–8465 from other countries.[20] The registry has indicated that there is no increased risk of birth defects and no pattern of birth defects among infants born to women exposed to acyclovir during pregnancy.

Mechanism Of Action

Acyclovir is an antiviral agent only after it is phosphorylated to the diphosphate and triphosphate forms in infected cells by a virus-induced thymidine kinase.[14] After phosphorylation, it becomes an inhibitor of the viral DNA polymerase. Acyclovir incorporated into the growing viral deoxyribonucleic acid chain causes its termination. It is, in fact, the first antiviral drug to require a viral enzyme for activation.[22]

Clinical Presentation

Topical Use

There may be occasional burning or stinging on application with mild erythema on drying.

Oral Use

Short-term use has most commonly been associated with occasional nausea and vomiting.[4,8] Long-term (1-year) use is equally well tolerated, with nausea, vomiting, diarrhea, abdominal pain, rash, and headache occurring in less than 5% of patients.[8]

Intravenous Use

The adverse reactions most frequently reported with intravenous acyclovir are inflammation and phlebitis at the injection site. Neurologic and/or psychiatric effects (e.g. lethargy, tremors, confusion, hallucinations, seizures) and renal precipitation of the drug resulting in renal insufficiency have been reported.[8,9,23] These symptoms have been associated with high peak plasma acyclovir concentrations.[24] Systemic disease precedes most cases of neurotoxicity. Cranial computed tomography is usually normal but electroencephalograms are abnormal.[25] Acute nonoliguric renal failure has followed intravenous use.[26,27] Susceptibility to neurotoxic manifestations is increased with end-stage renal disease.[28]

There is no significant evidence that acyclovir is a carcinogen in either animals or humans.[22] At extremely high doses in vitro, acyclovir appears to be a radiosensitizer.[29] Acyclovir is highly selective for virally infected cells and, unlike ganciclovir, zidovudine, and interferon, has no dose-related effect on human bone marrow in the recommended dosage range.[30]

Overdose[24,31–33]

Several patients have ingested up to 100 capsules of oral acyclovir with no apparent adverse effects.[34] Overdose has followed the administration of bolus injections or of high doses in patients whose fluid and electrolyte balance was not properly monitored.[24] This has been followed by elevation of the levels of blood urea nitrogen and serum creatinine and development of renal failure. One adult ingested 4800 mg with no apparent adverse effects.[5]

An 8-day-old 3235-g newborn accidentally received an overdose of approximately 220 mg (65 mg/kg) of acyclovir (recommended dose, 32 mg [10 mg/kg]). Treatment with oral activated charcoal and increase in intravenous fluid rate was begun 6.5 hours after the overdose. Although the serum acyclovir level was 26 μg/mL 5.5 hours after the overdose, there were no overt neurologic abnormalities or evidence of renal toxicity. Both overdoses are examples of 10-fold formulation errors in the pharmacy.[31]

Laboratory

Analytical Methods

Serum levels of acyclovir can be measured with accuracy using radioimmunoassay,[35,36] high-performance liquid chromatography,[34] or bioassay.[35]

Blood Levels

In neonates, intravenous infusions of 5,10, and 15 mg/kg have resulted in mean peak acyclovir concentrations of 6.8, 13.8, and 19.4 μg/mL.[31] Plasma concentrations greater than 2 μg/mL in infants follow oral doses of 1340 mg/m^2 given at 12-hour intervals.[37] A peak serum acyclovir level of 51.8 μg/mL (22.99 μmol/L) was attained in a 77-year-old patient with coma and nonoliguric renal failure following intravenous acyclovir 51 g three times daily. Neurotoxicity developed with a delay of 24 to 48 hours after the acyclovir peak serum concentration.[19] The manufacturer considers 4.5 μg/mL as a threshold for neurotoxicity (normal peak range is 0.4-2 μg/mL).[38]

Abnormalities

Elevated levels of serum creatinine are observed following intravenous doses greater than 5 mg/kg every 8 hours.[22] Dehydration, preexisting renal insufficiency, and high-dose bolus infusion can result in crystallization of acyclovir within leukocytes in renal tubules or collecting ducts, causing a reversible crystalline nephropathy.[7,22,36] Oral acyclovir has not been associated with renal dysfunction. Symptoms of lethargy, tremor, disorientation, and transient hemiparesis appear at plasma levels between 10 and 60 μg/mL.[24]

Ancillary Tests

Depressed white cell counts and elevated levels of serum creatinine, bilirubin, aspartate transaminase, alanine transaminase, and serum alkaline phosphatase have been observed in less than 20% of patients receiving the drug for several years.[30]

Treatment

Stabilization

After an intravenous overdose, an intravenous line should be maintained with normal saline, renal function (watch intake, output, serum creatinine, blood urea nitrogen) should be evaluated, and supportive care should be instituted. Extravasation phlebitis (see Chapter 61) should be treated by discontinuing the infusion and by the application of warm compresses. Adverse hemodynamic effects generally have not been observed.

Gut Decontamination

Following an oral overdose, gut decontamination procedures may decrease the possibility of the development of neurotoxic and renal changes, especially in the patient with prior evidence of neurotoxicity and diminished renal function. Early (within 2 hours of ingestion) emesis or gastric lavage may lessen, but not entirely eliminate, the toxic effects. There is no evidence to support the usefulness of activated charcoal. Following intravenous overdose, there is no evidence that gut decontamination procedures would be of value.

Elimination Enhancement

Removal of acyclovir is accelerated during hemodialysis.[22,39,40] A 6-hour hemodialysis results in a 60% decrease in plasma acyclovir concentration.[34] Therefore, if severe overdose has occurred and/or renal impairment exists, hemodialysis should be considered.[41] There have been no controlled clinical studies of its usefulness in acyclovir overdose. Laskin and colleagues reported on an adult with acyclovir-induced central nervous system toxicity and a blood level of 3.4 μg/mL who clinically improved after hemodialysis with a simultaneous decrease in blood level.[42] With normal renal function and no evidence of cardiovascular instability, simply increasing fluid flow (intravenous saline) may be sufficient to preclude crystal deposit formation. There is no evidence to support the need for hemoperfusion procedures. Exchange transfusions and peritoneal dialysis do not remove the drug.[24]

Antidote

No antidote is available.

Supportive Measures

Patients may require long-term monitoring and symptomatic treatment for neurotoxic sequelae (abnormal behavior) and for follow-up of renal function stability. Such patients should be hospitalized for initial observation and clinical evaluation (neurologic, renal) and released, depending on clinical judgment, after ruling out such conditions as meningitis, encephalitis (lumbar puncture), and renal dysfunction (urinalysis for crystals, serum blood urea nitrogen and creatinine). There is no clinical evidence to support increases in steroid doses after an acyclovir overdose. Symptomatic treatment (e.g. with neuroleptic agents) may assist in controlling unusual behavioral symptomatology. Careful correlation of overdose management with control of the underlying viral infection is indicated.[41,42]

REFERENCES—ACYCLOVIR

1. Drugs for non-HIV viral infections. Med Lett Drugs Ther 1994;36(919):27–31.
2. Nilsen AE, Aasen T, Halsos AM, et al. Efficacy of oral acyclovir in the treatment of initial and recurrent genital herpes. Lancet 1982;2:571–572.
3. Johnson RE, Mullooly JP, Valanus BG, et al. Acyclovir use and its surveillance in a general population. DICP Ann Pharmacother 1990;24:624–628.
4. Fletcher CV, Chnnock BJ, Chace B, Balfour HH Jr. Pharmacokinetics and safety of high-dose oral acyclovir for suppression of cytomegalovirus disease after renal transplantation. Clin Pharmacol Ther 1988;44:158–163.
5. Acyclovir. In: McEvoy G, ed. *AHFS Drug Information 94.* Bethesda, MD: American Society of Hospital Pharmacists, 1994:383–391, 2268–2670.
6. Fischer A, Fellay G, Regamey C. Toxicite renale et neurologique de l'acyclovir. Schweiz Med Wochenschr 1990;120: 1200–1203.
7. Centers for Disease Control and Prevention. Pregnancy outcome following systemic prenatal acyclovir exposure: June 1, 1984–June 1, 1993. MMWR 1993;42:806–809.
8. O'Brien JJ, Campoli-Richards DM. Acyclovir: An updated review of its antiviral activity, pharmacokinetic properties and therapeutic efficacy. Drugs 1989;27:233–309.
9. Blum MR, Liao SHT, De Miranda P. Overview of acyclovir pharmacokinetic disposition in adults and children. Am J Med 1982;73(1A):186–192.
10. Hopefl AW. The diurnal use of intravenous acyclovir. Drug Intell Clin Pharm 1983;17:623–628.
11. De Miranda P, Good SS, Krsney HC, et al. Metabolic fate of radioactive acyclovir in humans. Am J Med 1982;73(1A):215–220.
12. Laskin OL, Longstreth JA, Whelton A, et al. Acyclovir kinetics in end-state renal disease. Clin Pharmacol Ther 1982;31: 594–601.
13. Laskin OL. Acyclovir pharmacology and clinical experience. Arch Intern Med 1984;144:1241–1246.
14. King DH. History, pharmacokinetics and pharmacology of acyclovir. J Am Acad Dermatol 1988;18:176–179.
15. Bach MC. Possible drug interaction during therapy with azidothymidine and acyclovir in AIDS. N Engl J Med 1987;316:547.
16. Klug S, Lewandowski C, Blankenburg G, et al. Effect of acyclovir on mammalian embryonic development in culture. Arch Toxicol 1985;58:29–96.
17. Frieden FJ, Ordorica SA, Goodgold AL, et al. Successful pregnancy with isolated herpes simplex virus encephalitis: Case report and review of the literature. Obstet Gynecol 1990;175:511–513.
18. Brocklehurst P, Carney O, Helson K, et al. Acyclovir, herpes and pregnancy. Lancet 1990;226:1594–1595.
19. Haefeli WE, Schoenenberger PAZ, Weiss P. Acyclovir-induced neurotoxicity: Concentration–side effect relationship in acyclovir overdose. Am J Med 1993;94:212–215.
20. Centers for Disease Control and Prevention. Pregnancy outcomes following systemic prenatal acyclovir exposure: June 1, 1984–June 30, 1993. Arch Dermatol 1994; 130:153–154.
21. Centers for Disease Control and Prevention. From the MMWR: Pregnancy outcomes following systemic prenatal acyclovir exposure: June 1, 1984–June 30, 1993. Arch Dermatol 1994;130:153–154.
22. Dorsky DI, Crumpacker CS. Drugs five years later: Acyclovir. Ann Intern Med 1987;107:859–871.
23. Wade JC, Meyers JD. Neurologic symptoms associated with parenteral acyclovir treatment after marrow transplantation. Ann Intern Med 1983;98:921–925.
24. Rubin J. Overdose with acyclovir in a CAPD patient. Perit Dial Bull 1987;7:42–53.
25. Adair JC, Gold M, Bond RE. Acyclovir neurotoxicity: Clinical experience and review of the literature. South Med J 1994; 87:1227–1231.
26. Giustina A, Romanelli G, Cimino A, Brunori G. Low dose acyclovir and acute renal failure. Ann Intern Med 1988;108: 312.
27. Rashed A, Azedeh B, Abu Romeh SH. Acyclovir-induced acute tubulo-interstitial nephritis. Nephron 1990;56:436–438.
28. Gill MJ, Burgess E. Neurotoxicity of acyclovir in end state renal disease. J Antimicrob Chemother 1990;25:300–301.
29. Sougawa M, Akagik K, Murata T, et al. Enhancement of radiation effects of acyclovir. Int J Radiat Oncol Biol Phys 1986;12:1537–1540.
30. Davey PG. New antiviral and antifungal drugs. Br Med J 1990;300:793–798.
31. Englund JA, Fletcher CV, Johnson D, et al. Effect of blood exchange on acyclovir clearance in an infant with neonatal herpes. J Pediatr 1987;110:151–153.
32. Eck P, Silver SM, Clark EC. Acute renal failure and coma after a high dose of oral acyclovir. N Engl J Med 1991;325: 1178.
33. McDonald L, Tartaglione TA, Mendelman PM, et al. Lack of toxicity in two cases of neonatal acyclovir overdose. Pediatr Infect Dis J 1989;8:529–532.
34. Collins GE. Personal correspondence from Drug Information Department, Burroughs Wellcome Co., March 7, 1991.
35. Quinn RP, De Miranda GL, Good SS. A sensitive radioimmunoassay for the antiviral agent BW248U(9-(2-hydroxyethoxymethyl)guanine). Anal Biochem 1979;98:319–328.
36. Skubitz KM, Quinn RP, Lietman PS. A rapid acyclovir radioimmunoassay using charcoal adsorption. Antimicrob Agents Chemother 1982;21:352–354.
37. Rudd C, Rivadeneira ED, Gutman LI. Dosing considerations for oral acyclovir following neonatal herpes disease. Acta Pediatr 1994;83:1237–1243.
38. Leikin JB, Schicker L, Orlowski J, et al. Hemodialysis removal of acyclovir. Vet Hum Toxicol 1995;37:233–234.
39. Moore DF, Taylor SC, Bryson YJ. Virus inhibition assay for measurement of acyclovir levels in human plasma and urine. Antimicrob Agents Chemother 1981;20:787–792.
40. Keeney RE, Kirk LE, Bridgen D. Acyclovir tolerance in humans. Am J Med 1982;73(1A):176–181.
41. Laskin OL, Longstreth JA, Whelton A, et al. Effect of renal failure on the pharmacokinetics of acyclovir. Am J Med 1982; (1A):197–201.
42. Krasney HC, Liao SHT, De Miranda P, et al. Influence of hemodialysis on acyclovir pharmacokinetics in patients with chronic renal failure. Am J Med 1982;73(1A):202–204.

AMANTADINE

Amantadine poisoning has been reported infrequently over the past 20 years. When it occurs, it can lead to fatalities. There is no specific treatment. Management is largely supportive.

Structure and Classification

Amantadine (1-adamantanamine hydrochloride) is a synthetic water-soluble primary amine with a uniquely structured tricyclic 10-carbon ring (Fig. 18–2).[1,2]

Use

Amantadine is used for the prophylaxis and symptomatic treatment of respiratory infections caused by influenza A virus strains.[2,3] It does not inhibit strains of influenza B.[4] Amantadine is also used in the symptomatic treatment of all

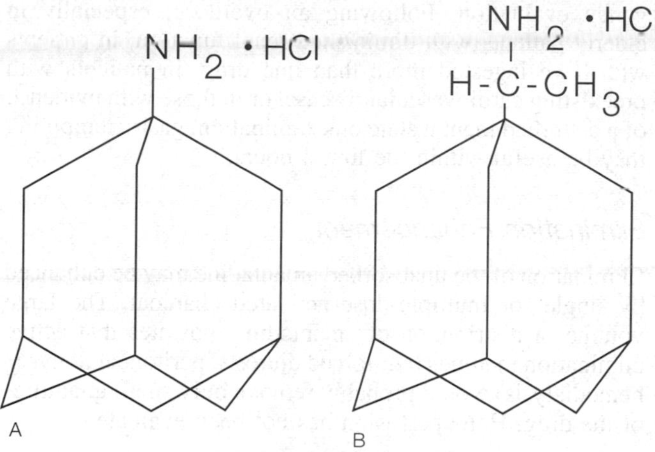

Figure 18–2 Chemical structures of amantadine hydrochloride **(A)** and rimantadine hydrochloride **(B)**. (From Tominack RL, Hayden FG. Rimantadine hydrochloride and amantadine hydrochloride use in influenza A virus infections. Infect Dis Clin North Am 1987;1: 459–478.)

forms of the parkinsonian syndrome, including the postencephalitic, idiopathic, and arteriosclerotic types, and for the relief of parkinsonian signs and symptoms in carbon monoxide poisoning and antipsychotic agent-induced (eg, phenothiazines) extrapyramidal effects.[5,6] It has been studied as an aid in the ambulatory treatment of cocaine withdrawal symptoms.[7,8]

Therapeutic Dose

Amantadine is administered for influenza A and parkinsonism in doses of 200 mg daily, though some clinicians use doses of 100 mg daily as prophylaxis.

Toxic Dose

Amantadine administered in doses of more than 2 g is potentially lethal.[9–12] Death may not occur for several days,[9–21] and it may not be preceded by clear abnormalities in respiration or cardiac function.[11,19] Survival has followed ingestions of 1.2 g[17] and 2.8 g.[14]

Toxicokinetics[13,14,22–26]

Bioavailability	>80%
Peak plasma level	0.08 μg/mL (after 50 mg)
Time to peak plasma level	1–4 hours
Volume of distribution	4–10 L/kg
Plasma protein binding	65%
Elimination half-life	12 hours
Excreted unchanged	56%

Absorption

Whole blood concentrations of amantadine are 32% or more greater than plasma concentrations because of its binding to red blood cells.[22]

Elimination

Acidification of urine may increase the rate of excretion of amantadine. However, this method is generally *not* advised.[15]

Drug Interactions

Renal clearance of amantadine was reduced and plasma concentrations were elevated in a patient who was simultaneously taking hydrochlorothiazide–triamterene.[27] Toxic delirium was reported in a patient who was concurrently taking amantadine and trimethoprim–sulfamethoxazole.[16,27] Serious central nervous system side effects such as confusion and hallucinations frequently result from the addition of anticholinergic drugs to an amantadine management program.[17]

Pregnancy/Lactation

Embryotoxic and teratogenic effects have been described in rats receiving 15 times the usual human dose. Treatment with amantadine in women of childbearing age is not justified except perhaps in life-threatening influenza pneumonia.[4] Nevertheless, a 34-year-old woman who used amantadine to prevent relapse of her multiple sclerosis throughout two of her pregnancies delivered two normal infants.[18]

Mechanism of Action

Amantadine produces a virostatic effect by preventing penetration of absorbed virus into the host cell. It blocks reuptake of dopamine into the presynaptic neurons, as well as altering the accumulation, release, and further uptake of catecholamines in the central and peripheral nervous systems. These dopamine-enhancing properties probably account for its beneficial effect in patients with parkinsonian symptoms.

Clinical Presentation

Chronic Use

Chronic use of therapeutic doses (200 mg daily) in the patient with diminished renal function leads to symptoms of and signs of neurotoxicity (hallucinations, central and peripheral nervous system deficits).[20] Delirium and disorientation, weakness, fatigue, and falling in elderly patients with diminished renal function usually follow therapeutic doses of amantadine administered for influenza prophylaxis in nursing homes.[2] Rarely, ocular toxicity with blurred vision, sudden loss of vision, visual hallucinations, oculogyric crises, and mydriasis have been reported following therapeutic amantadine use. Amantadine may be secreted in the tear film, causing corneal deposits and corneal irritation.[28] Long-term use of amantadine has been associated with livedo reticularis, peripheral edema, congestive heart failure,[29,30] and urinary retention. Amantadine may increase seizure activity in patients with a preexisting seizure disorder.[31]

Overdose

In acute overdose, dry mouth, pupillary dilation, toxic psychosis,[12,14,17] and urinary retention have been observed, all of which indicate anticholinergic activity.[32] The toxic effects of amantadine overdose appear to center around the cardiovascular, central nervous, and respiratory systems.[33] Cardiopulmonary arrest, ventricular fibrillation, prolonged QT intervals, Torsade de pointes, ventricular tachyarrythmias, and death can follow ingestion of 2.5 g of amantadine. Such cardiac abnormalities may begin up to 36 hours after an overdose.[9] Central nervous system manifestations include agitation, acute toxic psychosis,[14] increased motor activity, tremors, disorientation, hallucinations, and seizures.[34] Finally, although respiratory toxicity is the least common concomitant of overdose, two deaths have been reported secondary to adult respiratory distress syndrome,[12] and a third death was believed to be secondary to pulmonary hemorrhage and pulmonary edema.[33]

Laboratory

Analytical Methods

Amantadine is analyzed in biological samples by gas chromatography,[19] and a pentafluoropropionic anhydride derivative has been analyzed by gas chromatography–mass spectrometry.[20]

Blood Levels

Patients who received 300 mg daily for 3 weeks had plasma concentrations of 0.68 to 1.01 μg/mL.[35] Following overdoses, blood levels appear generally to correlate with the dose ingested: 2.37 μg/mL after 1.2-g ingestion,[17] 4.8 μg/mL after 3.0-g ingestion,[10] and 23.4 μg/mL after 12-g overdose.[12] Levels of 21 μg/mL[19] and 30 μg/mL[20] have been recorded, but there is no indication of the amount ingested; both cases were fatalities.

Abnormalities

Neurotoxic effects have been associated with amantadine plasma concentrations of 1 to 5 μg/mL.[24,27] Aggressive behavior was observed in patients receiving 300 mg daily with steady-state plasma levels of 0.68 to 1.01 μg/mL.[35]

Ancillary Tests

The cerebrospinal fluid concentration of amantadine following an oral overdose of 1.2 g was 1.2 μg/mL, approximately half the blood concentration (2.37 μg/mL).[14]

Treatment

Stabilization

Treatment of most patients with amantadine toxicity is expectant and supportive.[17] Usually simple observation and occasional sedation may be all that is required, but each patient should be admitted to an intensive care facility where cardiac monitoring and immediate attention to airway, breathing, and circulation are available.

Gut Decontamination

Although there have been no controlled studies on the efficacy of syrup of ipecac or gastric lavage in amantadine-poisoned patients, the clinician must exercise judgment in deciding which procedure is indicated for a specific patient, recognizing that fatalities do occur, that the history is often inaccurate, that seizures may occur, that blood levels rise quickly after amantadine ingestion, and that renal insufficiency may not be immediately apparent on a first emergency evaluation. Following an overdose, especially in elderly patients with diminished renal function, in patients who have ingested more than one drug, in patients with preexisting cardiovascular disease, or in those with evidence of a disturbed mental state on examination, gastric emptying may be useful within the first 4 hours.

Elimination Enhancement

Elimination of the unabsorbed amantadine may be enhanced by single- or multiple-dose activated charcoal. The large volume of distribution of amantadine indicates that active elimination methods (eg, forced diuresis, peritoneal dialysis, hemodialysis) would probably remove only small quantities of the drug. Hemoperfusion has not been evaluated.

Antidote

There is no antidote. Physostigmine (0.5 mg intravenously given twice) ameliorated the agitation, tremors, hallucinations, and increased motor activity seen in a 2½-year-old who ingested 600 mg of amantadine.[36] Physostigmine in 1-mg doses rapidly reversed the delirium and myoclonus in a 67-year-old treated for amantadine intoxication.[36] Caution, however, must be exercised with the use of physostigmine (seizures, bronchospasm, bradycardia, asystole)[37] (see Chapter 38).

Supportive Measures

As serious ventricular tachyarrhythmias may appear up to 36 hours following an overdose of amantadine, continuous electrocardiographic cardiac monitoring is indicated for at least 36 to 48 hours.[8,9]

In the overdose patient with agitated behavior, sedation should be considered after the patient has been admitted, is on a cardiac monitor, and is under close continual care with special consideration for sudden shifts in blood pressure (hypotension, shock), pulse, and temperature (hyperthermia). Symptoms of toxicity in the elderly, particularly hallucinations and disorientation, can appear with therapeutic doses.

Blood pressure should be maintained by placing the patient in the Trendelenburg position and beginning an infusion of normal saline intravenously. Care must be taken to avoid exacerbating any impending fluid overload.

Bicarbonate prevents the excretion of amantadine into an acid urine, its only route of elimination.[12]

Care must be taken when using adrenergic agents to maintain a normal heart rate, as these agents, in combination with amantadine, further dispose the patient to serious ventricular tachyarrhythmias. Lidocaine may be the drug of choice to terminate ventricular arrhythmias in the overdose patient.[34] Class I antiarrhythmics may exacerbate an arrhythmia with abnormalities of cardiac repolarization and attendant prolonged QT intervals. Isoproterenol was ineffective in a case of amantadine-induced Torsade de pointes.[9]

REFERENCES—AMANTADINE

1. Baselt RC, Cravey RH. *Disposition of Toxic Drugs and Chemicals in Man.* Chicago: Year Book Medical, 1989:32.

2. Tominack RL, Hayden FG. Rimantadine hydrochloride and amantadine hydrochloride use in influenza A virus infections. Infect Dis Clin North Am 1987;1:459–478.
3. Zuckerman MA, Oxford JS. Amantadine for influenza A. Br Med J 1991;302:1022.
4. Nicholson KG, Wiselka MJ. Amantadine for influenza A. Br Med J 1991;302:425–426.
5. Schwab RS, England AC, Poskanzer DC, et al. Amantadine in the treatment of Parkinson's disease. JAMA 1969;208: 1168–1170.
6. Di Mascio A, Bernardo DL, Greenblatt DJ, et al. A controlled trial of amantadine in drug-induced extrapyramidal disorders. Arch Gen Psychiatry 1976;33:599–602.
7. Tennant FS Jr, Sagherian AA. Double blind comparison of amantadine and bromocriptine for ambulatory withdrawal from cocaine dependence. Arch Intern Med 1987;147: 109–112.
8. Handelsman L, Chordia PL, Escovar IM, et al. Amantadine for treatment of cocaine dependence in methadone-maintained patients. Am J Psychiatry 1988;145:533.
9. Sartori M, Pratt CM, Young JB. Torsade de pointes: Malignant cardiac arrhythmia induced by amantadine poisoning. Am J Med 1984;77:388–391.
10. Cook PE, Dermer SW, McCurg T. Fatal overdose with amantadine. Can J Psychiatry 1986;31:757–758.
11. Simpson DM, Ramos F, Ramirez LF. Death of a psychiatric patient from amantadine poisoning. Am J Psychiatry 1988;145:267–268.
12. Brown CR, Hernandez S, Kelly MT. Hyperthermia and death from amantadine overdose. Vet Hum Toxicol 1987;29:463.
13. Bleidner WE, Harmon JB, Hewes WE, et al. Absorption, distribution and excretion of amantadine hydrochloride. J Pharmacol Exp Ther 1965;150:484–490.
14. Fahn S, Craddock G, Kuman G. Acute toxic psychosis from suicidal overdosage of amantadine. Arch Neurol 1971;25: 45–48.
15. Amantadine. In: McEvoy GK, ed. *AHFS Drug Information 94.* Bethesda, MD: American Society of Hospital Pharmacists, 1994:392–395, 2426–2428.
16. Speeg KV, Leighton JA, Maldonado AL. Case report: Toxic delirium in a patient taking amantadine and trimethoprim sulfmethoxazole. Am J Med Sci 1989;298:410–412.
17. Snoey ER, Bessen HA. Acute psychosis after amantadine overdose. Ann Emerg Med 1990;19:668–670.
18. Levy M, Pastuszak A, Koren G. Fetal outcome following intrauterine amantadine exposure. Reprod Toxicol 1991;5:79–81.
19. Reynolds PC, Van Meter S. A death involving amantadine. J Anal Toxicol 1984;8:100.
20. Priddis C. A fatal case involving amantadine. Bull Int Assoc Forens Toxicol 1986;19(1):35-36.
21. Ing TS, Daugirdas JT, Soung LS, et al. Toxic effects of amantadine in patients with renal failure. Can Med Assoc J 1979; 120:695–698.
22. Haradam VW, Sharp JG, Smilack JD, et al. Pharmacokinetics of amantadine hydrochloride in subjects with normal and impaired renal function. Ann Intern Med 1981;94(pt 1):454–458.
23. Aoki FY, Sitar DS, Ogilvie RI. Amantadine kinetics in healthy young subjects after long-term dosing. Clin Pharmacol Ther 1979;16:729–736.
24. Sande MA, Mandell GL. Antimicrobial agents. In: Gilman AG, Goodman LS, Rall TW, Murad F, eds. *The Pharmacological Basis of Therapeutics.* New York: Macmillan, 1985:1232.
25. Pacific GM, Nardini M, Ferrari P, et al. Effects of amantadine on drug-induced parkinsonism: Relationship between plasma levels and effect. Br J Clin Pharmacol 1976;3:883–889.
26. Liu P, Cheng PJ, Ing TS, et al. In vitro binding of amantadine to plasma proteins. Neuropharmacology 1962;2:149.
27. Wilson TW, Rajput AH. Amantadine–dyazide interaction. Can Med Assoc J 1983;129:974–975.
28. Degelau S, Somani S, Cooper SL, Irvine PW. Occurrence of adverse effects and high amantadine concentrations with influenza prophylaxis in the nursing home. J Am Geriatr Soc 1990;33:428–432.
29. Frauenfelder FT, Meyer SM. Amantadine and corneal deposits. Am J Ophthalmol 1990;110:96–97.
30. Vale JA, Maclean KS. Amantadine induced heart failure. Lancet 1976;1:548.
31. Parkes JD, Marsden CD, Price P. Amantadine induced heart failure. Lancet 1977;1:904.
32. Atkinson WL, Arden NH, Patriarca PA, et al. Amantadine prophylaxis during an institutional outbreak of type A (HINI) influenza. Arch Intern Med 1986;146:1751–1756.
33. Douglas RG. Prophylaxis and treatment of influenza. N Engl J Med 1990;322:443–450.
34. Pimental L, Hughes B. Amantadine toxicity presenting with complex ventricular ectopy and hallucinations. Pediatr Emerg Care 1991;7:89–92.
35. Rizzo M, Biandrate P, Tognoni G, Morselli PL. Amantadine in depression: Relationship between behavioral effects and plasma levels. Eur J Clin Pharmacol 1973;5:226–228.
36. Berkowitz CD. Treatment of acute amantadine toxicity with physostigmine. J Pediatr 1979;95:144–145.
37. Casey DE. Amantadine intoxication reversed by physostigmine. N Engl J Med 1978;278:516.

FIALURIDINE (FIAU)

In patients with chronic hepatitis B, treatment with fialuridine, an investigational nucleoside analogue, induces a severe toxic reaction characterized by hepatic failure, lactic acidosis, pancreatitis, neuropathy, and myopathy. This toxic reaction is probably caused by widespread mitochondrial damage and may occur infrequently with other nucleoside analogs.[1]

The clinical picture of hepatic failure resembles that of Reye's syndrome in its progression of symptoms and in the early appearance of hepatic synthetic dysfunction, hyperammonemia, and lactic acidosis, despite minimal increases in transaminase levels and mild jaundice. The toxicity affects predominantly organs and tissues that have a slow turnover of cells and a major dependence on mitochondrial function. Light microscopy of liver specimens shows marked accumulation of microvascular fat, with scant hepatocellular necrosis.[1,2]

REFERENCES—FIALURIDINE

1. McKenzie R, Fried MW, Sallie R, et al. Hepatic failure and lactic acidosis due to fialuridine (FIAU), an investigational nucleoside analogue for chronic hepatitis B. N Engl J Med 1995;333:1099–1105.
2. Swartz MN. Mitochondrial toxicity: New adverse drug effects. N Engl J Med 1995;333:1146–1148.

GANCICLOVIR

Neutropenia, usually reversible, is the principal adverse effect of ganciclovir (Fig. 18–1). Other undesirable effects include thrombocytopenia, confusion, and seizures. Probenecid increases ganciclovir half-life secondary to decreased renal excretion.[1] High-dose intravitreal administration may lead to rapidly deteriorating vision.[2] Ganciclovir crosses the placenta.[3] (See Chapter 15.)

REFERENCES—GANCICLOVIR

1. Morris DJ. Adverse effects and drug interactions of clinical importance with antiviral drugs. Drug Saf 1994;10: 281–291.
2. Saran BR, Maguire AM. Retinal toxicity of high dose intravitreal ganciclovir. Retina 1994;14:248–252.

3. Gilstrap LC, Lawdon RE, Robert SW, Sohh S. The transfer of the nucleoside analog ganciclovir across the perfused human placenta. Am J Obstet Gynecol 1994;170:967–973.

RIBAVIRIN

Animal studies have shown that ribavirin is teratogenic, causing severe malformations in offspring of exposed females.

The Infectious Diseases and Immunization Committee of the Canadian Paediatric Society made the following recommendations regarding occupational exposure to aerosolized ribavirin:

- Switch off the aerosol generator before entering the hood or tent in which the child is being treated.
- Special precautions are unnecessary for anyone in the room.
- Pregnant women should not enter the tent while ribavirin is flowing.
- Gloves should be worn when preparing ribavirin for aerosolization or when cleaning contaminated equipment.[1]

REFERENCES—RIBAVIRIN

1. Infectious Diseases and Immunization Committee, Canadian Paediatric Society. Ribavirin: Is there a risk to hospital personnel? Can Med Assoc J 1991;144:285–286.

RIMANTADINE HYDROCHLORIDE

Rimantadine (α-methyl-1-adamantanemethylamine hydrochloride) is a closely related derivative of amantadine that shares the compact hydrocarbon structure but differs in the substitution on the ring (Fig. 18–2). Oral rimantadine is currently marketed as Flumadine in some European countries and is an investigational drug in the United States.[1] It has been used extensively in the Soviet Union,[2] where investigators believe it to be more effective and less toxic than amantadine in prophylaxis against influenza.[2] Rimantadine, like amantadine, also only inhibits strains of influenza type A but not influenza type B.[3] Unlike amantadine, rimantadine is extensively metabolized and undergoes both hydroxylation of the ring and glucuronidation.[4]

The mean elimination half-life of rimantadine is 29 hours. It is weakly bound to plasma proteins (40%), its volume of distribution is 15-25 L/kg, and its nonrenal clearance is 703 mL/min. It has a renal clearance of 55 mL/min, and approximately 8% is excreted in the urine as unchanged drug. The mean peak concentration in plasma following a single dose to healthy adults is approximately 80 ng/mL, and that following multiple doses is about 420 ng/mL.[5] These levels are reached in 2 to 6 hours after a single oral dose. Plasma concentrations are 15 to 20% higher in patients taking cimetidine (1200 mg/d).[6] Therapeutic doses are 200 to 300 mg/d.[7] The infrequent occurrence of central nervous system side effects, such as seizures,[8] may be correlated with plasma levels. Rimantadine in doses of 200 to 300 mg/d causes the same frequency of gastrointestinal effects as amantadine.[7]

Theoretically, inhibitors of glucuronidation such as acetaminophen and probenecid could increase the plasma levels and potential toxicity of rimantadine.[9]

There have been no reports of overdosage with rimantadine; however, the extensive volume of distribution would tend to render hemodialysis or other extracorporeal procedures of elimination relatively ineffective.[10]

REFERENCES—RIMANTADINE HYDROCHLORIDE

1. Dolin R. Antiviral chemotherapy and chemoprophylaxis. Science 1985;227:1296–1303.
2. Zlydnikov DM, Kubar OI, Ovaleva TP. Kamforin: Study of rimantadine in the USSR: A review of the literature. Rev Infect Dis 1981;3:408–421.
3. Nicholson KG, Wiselka MJ. Amantadine for influenza A. Br Med J 1991;302:425–426.
4. Wills RJ, Belshe R, Tomlinson D, et al. Pharmacokinetics of rimantadine hydrochloride in patients with chronic liver disease. Clin Pharmacol Ther 1987;42:449–454.
5. Tominack RL, Wills RJ, Gustavson LE, Hayden FG. Multiple dose pharmacokinetics of rimantadine in elderly adults. Antimicrob Agents Chemother 1988;32:1813–1819.
6. Holazo AA, Choma N, Brown SY, et al. Effect of cimetidine on the disposition of rimantadine in healthy subjects. Antimicrob Agents Chemother 1989;33:820–823.
7. Douglas RG. Prophylaxis and treatment of influenza. N Engl J Med 1990;322:443–450.
8. Bentley DW, Karki ISD, Betts RF. Rimantadine and seizures. Ann Intern Med 1989;110:323–324.
9. Tominack RL, Hayden FG. Rimantadine hydrochloride and amantadine hydrochloride use in influenza A virus infections. Infect Dis Clin North Am 1987;1:459–478.
10. Fillastre J-P, Singlas E. Pharmacokinetics of newer drugs in patients with renal impairment, Part 1. Clin Pharmacokinet 1991;20:294–310.

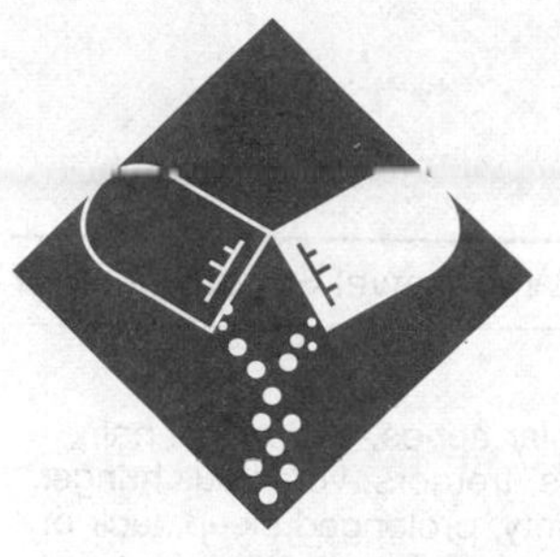

Part C
Drugs of Abuse

Chapter 19
Introduction

OVERVIEW

Symptoms and signs of drug abuse and withdrawal symptoms after both acute intoxication and overdose are summarized in Table 19–1.[1] Criteria for drug dependence are listed in Tables 19–2.[2] Drugs of abuse are compared in Table 19–3.[3] A major set of problems appears to be related to primary pattern intoxicants such as alcohol, nicotine, cocaine, opioids, and cannabis involving both sexes and producing public health and social problems of great magnitude. Risk factors for substance abuse in teenagers are listed in Table 19–4.[14]

STREET DRUGS: CURRENT USE

It is estimated that almost 21 million Americans have used cocaine.[4] About 3.5 million are annual cocaine users and are 18 to 25 years old. There are perhaps 65 million lifetime and 21 million recent marijuana users including 50% of high school seniors (7% use marijuana daily) and eighth grade students.[5] Up to 40% of high school seniors use other drugs. In 1988 in New York City, there were 690,000 weekly substance abusers, an increase of 79% from 1979 estimates. Medical students reported that 27, 11, and 10% have used marijuana, cocaine, and tranquilizers, respectively. In 1980, U.S. citizens spent $79 billion on the purchase of illicit substances.[6,7] Approximately 12% of resident physicians reported increased use of alcohol, marijuana, or cocaine, and 7% reported increased use of sedatives, stimulants, or opiates when compared with the period prior to residency training.[8–10] For most substances, the majority of residents state that they began their use in college, high school, or earlier. In a large number of patients, death was the initial relapse symptom of parenteral opioid abuse.[8–10]

An estimated 3% of the U.S. population deliberately has misused or abused psychoactive medication often with severe consequences.[7] The increase in emergency room risks for drug abuse is illustrated in Figure 19–1.[5]

Table 19–5 lists the street names for drugs of abuse.[11]

"ROOFIES"

According to a recent national news report, "Roofies" are being abused by Florida teens. *Roofies* is the slang term for

Table 19–1
Symptoms and Signs of Drug Abuse*

Drug	Acute Intoxication and Overdose	Withdrawal Syndrome
CNS Stimulants Cocaine, amphetamine, dextroamphetamine, methylphenidate, phen- metrazine, phenylopropanolamine, 2,5-dimethoxy-4-methylamphetamine (STP), 3,4-methyledioxymethamphetamine (MDMA), 4-bromo-2,5-dimethoxyamphetamine (bromo-DMA), diethylpropion, most amphetamine-like antiobesity drugs	**Vital Signs:** temperature elevated, heart rate increased, respiration shallow, BP elevated. **Mental Status:** sensorium hyperacute or confused, paranoid ideation, hallucinations, delirium, impulsivity, agitation, hyperactivity, sterotypy. **Physical Exam:** pupils dilated and reactive, tendon reflexes hyperactive, cardiac arrhythmias, dry mouth, sweating, tremors, convulsions, coma, stroke.	Muscular aches, abdominal pain, chills, tremors, voracious hunger, anxiety, prolonged sleep, lack of energy, profound depression, sometimes suicidal, exhaustion
Opioids Heroin, morphine, codeine, meperidine, methadone, hydromorphone, opium, pentazocine, propoxyphene, fentanyl, sufentanyl	**Vital Signs:** temperature decreased, respiration depressed, BP decreased, sometimes shock. **Mental Status:** euphoria, stupor. **Physical Exam:** pupils constricted (may be dilated with meperidine or extreme hypoxia), reflexes diminished to absent, pulmonary edema, constipation, convulsions with propoxyphene or meperidine, cardiac arrhythmias with propoxyphene, coma.	Pupils dilated, pulse rapid, gooseflesh, lacrimation, abdominal cramps, muscle jerks, "flu" syndrome, vomiting, diarrhea, tremulousness, yawning, anxiety
CNS Depressants Barbiturates; benzodiazepines, glutethimide; meprobamate; methaqualone; ethchlorvynol; chloral hydrate; methyprylon; paraldehyde	**Vital Signs:** respiration depressed, BP decreased, sometimes shock. **Mental Status:** drowsiness or coma, confusion, delirium. **Physical Exam:** pupils dilated with gluthethimide or in severe poisoning, tendon reflexes depressed, ataxia, slurred speech, nystagmus, convulsions or hyperirritability with methaqualone, signs of anticholinergic poisoning with glutethimide, cardiac arrhythmias with chloral hydrate.	Tremulousness, insomnia, sweating, fever, clonic blink reflex, anxiety, cardiovascular collapse, agitation, delirium, hallucinations, disorientation, convulsions, shock
Hallucinogens LSD (*d*-lysergic acid diethylamide), psilocybin, mescaline, PCP	**Vital Signs:** temperature elevated, heart rate increased, BP elevated. **Mental Status:** euphoria, anxiety or panic, paranoia, sensorium often clear, affect inappropriate, illusions, time and visual distortions, visual hallucinations, depersonalization, with PCP hypertensive encephalopathy. **Physical Exam:** pupils dilated (normal or small with PCP); tendon reflexes hyperactive; with PCP, cyclic coma or extreme hyperactivity, drooling, blank stare, mutism, amnesia, analgesia, nystagmus (sometimes vertical), gait ataxia, muscle rigidity, impulsive or violent behavior, violent, scatologic, pressured speech.	None
Cannabis Group Marijuana, hashish, THC (Δ^9-tetrahydrocannibinol), hash oil, sinsemilla	**Vital Signs:** heart rate increased, BP decreased on standing. **Mental Status:** anorexia, then increased appetite; euphoria, anxiety, sensorium often clear; dreamy, fantasy state; time–space distortions; hallucinations may be rare. **Physical Exam:** pupils unchanged; conjunctiva injected; tachycardia, ataxia, and pallor in children.	Nonspecific symptoms including anorexia, nausea, insomnia, restlessness, irritability, anxiety, depression
Anticholinergic Agents Atropine; belladonna; henbane; scopolamine; trihexyphenidyl; benztropine mesylate; procyclidine; propantheline bromide; jimson weed seed	**Vital Signs:** temperature elevated; heart rate increased; possibly decreased BP. **Mental Status:** drowsiness or coma, sensorium clouded, amnesia, disorientation, visual hallucinations, body image alterations, confusion; with propantheline, restlessness, excitement. **Physical Exam:** pupils dilated and fixed; decreased bowel sounds; flushed, dry skin and mucous membranes; violent behavior; convulsions; with propantheline, circulatory failure, respiratory failure, paralysis, coma	Gastrointestinal and musculoskeletal symptoms

LSD, *D*-lysergic acid diethylamide; PCP, phencyclidine. BP, blood pressure.
*Mixed intoxications produce complex combinations of signs and symptoms.
From Symptoms and signs of drug abuse. Med Lett Drugs Ther 1987;29(748):86.

Table 19–2
Criteria for Substance Dependence Established by the American Psychiatric Association

Maladaptive pattern of substance use with impairment or distress, as manifested by three or more of the following factors during a 12-month period:

1. Tolerance: need for greater amounts or experiencing less effect with same amount
2. Withdrawal: symptoms of withdrawal or substance taken to relieve or avoid symptoms
3. Substance taken in greater amounts or for a longer period than intended
4. Persistent desire or unsuccessful efforts to decrease or control use
5. Considerable time spent to obtain substance (eg, visiting multiple physicians or driving long distances), using the substance (such as chain-smoking), or recovering from its effects
6. Important social, occupational, or recreational activities given up or decreased because of use of substance
7. Use of substance despite knowledge of persistent or recurrent physical or psychologic harm that is likely to be caused or exacerbated by it

Specify whether with or without physiologic dependence, that is, whether 1 or 2 is present or not

From Juergens SM. Prescription drug dependence among elderly persons. Mayo Clin Proc 1994;69:1215–1217. Editorial

Table 19–3
Attributes of Drug Addiction: Comparison

	Nicotine	Heroin	Cocaine	Alcohol	Caffeine
Psychoactive effects	+	+	+	+	+
Drug-reinforced behavior	+	+	+	+	+
Compulsive use	+	+	+	+	–/+
Use despite harmful effects	+	+	+	+	–/+
Relapse after abstinence	+	+	+	+	–
Recurrent drug cravings	+	+	+	+	+
Tolerance	+	+	+	+	+
Physical dependence	+	+	+	+	+
Agonist useful in treating dependence	+	+	–	+	–

From Benowitz NL, Cigarette smoking and nicotine addiction. Med Clin North Am 1992;76:415–437.

Table 19–4
Potential Risk Factors for Substance Abuse

Maternal or twin alcoholism
Parental alcohol or other drug use
Family history of alcoholism
Family history of antisocial behavior
Child abuse and neglect (intrafamilial or extrafamilial)
Parents with poor parenting skills
Poor relationship with parents
Drug use by sibling
Drug use by best friend
Perceived peer drug use
School failure
Low interest in school and achievement
Rebelliousness and alienation
Low self-esteem
Early antisocial behavior
Psychopathology, particularly depression
Negative character traits (eg, frequent lying, lack of empathy toward feelings of others, favoring immediate over delayed gratification, need to seek sensation, insensitivity to punishment)
Previous dependence on alcohol or other drugs
Disorganization in community
Delinquent behavior
Low religiosity
Early alcohol use
Early experimentation with alcohol and other drugs
Early sexual activity

From Schydlower M, Chairman, Committee on Substance Abuse, 1992–1993, American Academy of Pediatrics. Role of the pediatrician in prevention and management of substance abuse. Pediatrics 1993;91:1010–1013.

a diazepam (Valium)-type sedative, flunitrazepam, not legally available in the United States. The drug is commonly abused in Europe, Asia, and South America. Flunitrazepam is legally available as Rohipnol in other countries. Although Roofies and diazepam are both benzodiazepines, there are slight differences in their chemical structures. Roofies have more hypnotic and amnesic effects than diazepam. Roofies are commonly sniffed or snorted in Chile, where they may be legally bought without a prescription.

A glossary of more than 1500 street terms that refer to specific drug types or drug activity has been compiled by the Drugs and Crime Data Center and Clearinghouse of the U.S. Department of Justice (telephone 1–800–666–3332).

COSTS

Los Angeles County

Cocaine

One ounce price of cocaine (rock form) is $425 (50–70% pure). A bulk bag of 100 kg or more costs $14,000 per kilogram; a single kilogram costs $17,000 and is about 87% pure.

Heroin

Black tar has sold for $2500 an ounce, with the purity level around 7%. A gram of heroin powder (Mexican Brown) may sell for $160, and a "Mexican Oz" (25 g) for

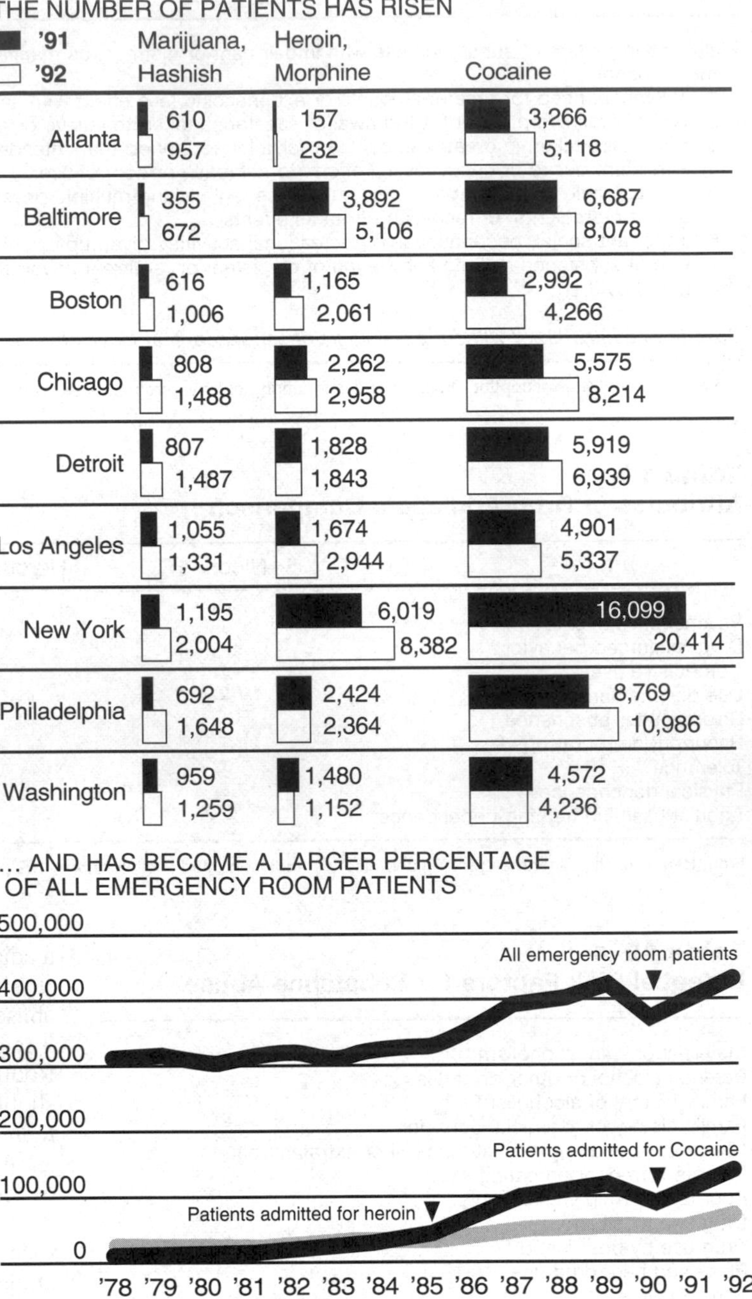

Figure 19–1 Drugs and emergency room visits. (From Treaster JB. U.S. reports rise in drug emergencies. NY Times, October 5, 1993.)

$3000 to $3500. The purity level of the Mexican Brown is 40% or less. White heroin is not used much; however, Southeast Asian heroin (86–92% pure) may cost up to $150,000 to $200,000 per kilogram and $1000 to $2000 per ounce. Southwest Asian heroin has run $92,000 to $100,000 per kilogram.

Marijuana

Commercial-type marijuana costs $700 to $1900 per pound, $100 to $300 per ounce, and $10 to $20 per gram or baggie. Sinsemilla brands cost $1500 to $5000 per pound or $250 to $350 per ounce.

Amphetamine

An ounce of powder or crystal amphetamine sells for $800 to $1000. One gram sells for $80 to $100; a quarter-gram sells for $20 to $25.

Phencyclidine

An ounce of liquid phencyclidine sells for $100 to $200.

London

In London, an addict spends an average £100 a day on drugs, £36,500 a year. Most of this money is raised by theft. The

Table 19–5
Street Names for Drugs of Abuse

San Diego	Crank	Heroin, IV amphetamines
Los Angeles	Stuff, Smack, Junk	Heroin
	Coke, Snow, Cola	Cocaine
	Sherms, Dust, Juice, Wack, Angel Dust	PCP
	Loads	Codeine with glutethimide
San Francisco	Crank, Crystal, Speed	Methamphetamines
	Speed	Amphetamines
	T's and Blues	Talwin and tripelennamine
Oregon	Toot, Snow	Cocaine
Seattle	Black beauties	Caffeine and phenylpropanolamine or ephedrine
Phoenix	Coke	Cocaine
	Tootsie Roll	Heroin (Mexican brown)
	Hitting rags	Solvent sniffing
	Sherm	PCP mixed with marijuana, soaked in formaldehyde or embalming fluid, then smoked
	Shrooms	*Psilocybe* mushrooms
Denver	Yo-yo	Yohimbine
	Crank	Decongestant inhalers (Vicks = levomethamphetamine, Benzedrex = propylhexedrine)
	Crystal, Rock	Other amphetamines or methamphetamines
	Chiva	Mexican brown heroin
	Mud	Heroin in molasses
	Apples	Marijuana
Dallas	WACs	Marijuana cigarettes sprayed with Black Flag roach killer (delayed, prolonged schizophrenic-like reaction)
	Speed, Crank	Phenmetrazine, synthetic amphetamines, methamphetamines
	Eve	Derivative of Ecstasy
	T's and Purples	Pentazocine (Talwin) containing naloxone plus 100 mg tripelennamine tablets (increase over the usual 50 mg)
Louisiana	Pinkhearts, Speckled Birds, Black Molly	Look-alikes simulating amphetamines
	Clickers	Marijuana soaked in embalming fluid or PCP
Kansas City	1 & 1	Pentazocine (Talwin) and tripelennamine, or methylphenidate (Ritalin) and pentazocine, or methylphenidate and diazepam (Valium)
	Tic and Tac, Angel Dust, Dusted Parsley, Hawaiian Wood Rose, Super Grass	PCP
	Shermans, Shermans	PCP or PCP with marijuana
	Green, Purple, Mauve, Jet, Super K, Super C, Special LA	Ketamine
	Ketamine Green, Purple	LSD
	Mickey Mouse, The Wizard, Window Pane	LSD
	Pink Hearts, Robin's Egg	Look-alikes
	Christmas Trees	Depressants or stimulants
	Whippet	Used in restaurants to make whipped cream, contains nitrous oxide
	Jamestown Weed	Jimson weed
Chicago	Coast, West Coast	Methylphenidate (Ritalin) IV
	Syrup and Beans	Codeine-containing cough syrup plus a depressant (glutethimide or diazepam [Valium])
	Happy Sticks, Joy Sticks	Marijuana dipped in liquid PCP
	Tolley	Toluene
Detroit	Crack	Rock cocaine, a form of free-base cocaine
Miami	Crack	Rock cocaine, free-base cocaine
	Vitamin C, Lady, Lady Snow, White, Peruvian White, Rock, Snow Candy, Nose Candy	Cocaine
	Sinsemilla	Marijuana cultivated without seeds
Atlanta	Crank	Cocaine
	Speed	Amphetamines or methamphetamines
	Crystal	MDA (the hallucinogenic amphetamine)
Washington, DC	Loveboat	PCP put on marijuana
	Love, Lovely, Boat, Butt Naked, John Hinckley	PCP
	Mexican Maid	Heroin
	Maze	Designer heroin (fentanyl derivatives)

(continued)

Table 19–5 *(Continued)*

Washington, DC (continued)	Newboy, Breakin', USDA, President, Watergate, NASA, Silent Partner, Thriller, Risking High, Dishrag	Heroin
	Bam	Heroin plus phenmetrazine (Preludin)
	Speedballing	Heroin plus cocaine IV
	Coke, Girl, Snow	Cocaine
	Disco Hits, Mr. Natural, Unicorn Acid, Window Pane	LSD
Philadelphia	Monster	Methamphetamines
New York	Crack	Rock cocaine, free-base cocaine
	Bazooka, Pasta	Coca paste (raw cocaine washed in an acid base)
	Snort, Snuff	Cocaine powder
	Speedballing	Cocaine and heroin injected IV together
	Fours and Doors	Glutethimide plus analgesics with codeine
Long Island, NY	Cocaine plus PAM cooking oil spray IV, Happy Dust, Star Dust, White Dust	Cocaine
	Coca Paste	Raw cocaine washed in an acid base
	Bazooka Paste	Marijuana mixed with procaine
Boston	Packs, Loads	Glutethimide plus analgesics with codeine

PCP, phencyclidine; LSD, D-lysergic acid diethylamide, MDA, methylene dioxyamphetamine.
Source: See Reference 11.

actual value of the goods stolen is probably substantially greater than the cash the addict gets for it.[12,13]

DRUG ABUSE TERMINOLOGY

A pool of 99 experts from 23 organizations representing disciplines and professions relevant to substance abuse has proposed a glossary of 50 substance abuse terms.[15]

DRUG ABUSE GROUPS

THE DRUG-SEEKING PATIENT

Patients who wish to obtain prescriptions from a doctor for the sole purpose of continuing a pattern of drug abuse attempt to do this by feigning physical problems (bleeding, self-inflicted skin lesions, renal colic [pain on left side of body, burning sensation on urination, pricking finger to drop blood into the urine], toothache, tic douloureux), feigning psychological problems (anxiety, insomnia, fatigue, depression), practicing deception (prescription theft, forgery, requesting refills prematurely, claiming medication is lost or stolen), pressuring the physician (coercive tactics eliciting sympathy or guilt, threats of physical or financial harm, offer of bribes, using the names of family members or friends), forging prescriptions (altering a prescription written by a physician, forging a prescription on a piece of paper or stolen prescription blank), pretending that they are from out of town and have lost their prescription or have had it stolen, and using extraordinary persuasive and dramatic abilities to convince the physician of their need for drugs.[7]

DRUG ABUSE EVOLUTION: STEPS

Drug taking usually occurs in steps leading from use to abuse, then to dependency.[16,17] Initially, the seeking of drugs and their low-level use are highly volitional. Progression is not inevitable. A minority of users progress to abuse, fewer still to dependency. Dependence is a chronic, relapsing disorder. Abuse can also assume this character. About 5.5 million people in the United States were dependent on or abusing drugs according to a 1990 report.[2] Almost half the clear-cut cases are in the criminal justice system.

PREDICTION OF DRUG ABUSE

Increase in later substance abuse appears to be related to certain risk factors in children and adolescents (Table 19–4).

DRUG-EXPOSED INFANTS

There are indications that approximately 1 in 10 infants may be exposed to illicit drugs during pregnancy. The Committee on Substance Abuse of the American Academy of Pediatrics has made the following recommendation:[18]

1. Pediatricians can be involved in organizing community-based social service or child protective service systems, designed to provide essential services for drug-abusing women and their children.
2. A comprehensive medical and psychosocial history including specific inquiry regarding maternal drug use should be a part of every newborn evaluation.
3. Newborn urine toxicology should be regarded only as a potential adjunct to a thorough maternal drug history. Universal toxicologic screening is not recommended.
4. The pediatrician should include maternal drug use in the differential diagnosis of any neonate with suggestive symptomatology.
5. The pediatrician should be knowledgeable about state and local child protection reporting requirements.
6. In most circumstances, when a drug-exposed infant or drug-abusing mother is identified, the pediatrician should consider recruiting the assistance of local child protective services to provide multidisciplinary treatment and support for the affected mother, child, and family.
7. The pediatrician should evaluate the drug-exposed infant for other medical conditions associated with

maternal drug use, including the possibility of concurrent sexually transmitted diseases in the mother and infant.

8. As adverse effects of drug exposure may not be evident at birth, the pediatrician should be alert to potential long-term consequences that may become apparent during ongoing care.
9. The American Academy of Pediatrics supports the development and evaluation of models of coordinated multidisciplinary prevention, intervention, and treatment services that improve access to early comprehensive care for all substance-abusing pregnant women and their children. Evaluation of current and new treatment modalities is imperative to determine their effectiveness.
10. Funds for research, prevention, and treatment should be made available to address issues of drug-exposed infants.
11. The public must be assured of nonpunitive access to comprehensive care that will meet the needs of the substance-abusing pregnant woman and her infant.
12. Pediatricians are encouraged to become actively involved in policy issues related to drug-exposed infants and children at the federal, state, and local levels.

Sudden Infant Death Syndrome

Sudden infant death syndrome (SIDS) has been observed more frequently in infants of substance-abusing mothers (ISAM). The rates per thousand live births are 8.36 for cocaine, 18.38 for opiates and 3.73 for phencyclidine, versus that for non-ISAM births, 1.22.[7] A population-based study also suggests that a greater incidence of symptomatic apnea was reported before SIDS for the ISAM (1 in 5) than for the non-ISAM population (1 in 20).[19]

CHILDREN AND ADOLESCENTS

Screening for Drug Abuse

The American Academy of Pediatrics Committee on Adolescence, Committee on Bioethics and Provisional Committee on Substance Abuse have reviewed the subject of drug abuse in children and adolescents and concluded the following:[20]

1. The Academy condemns the nontherapeutic use of psychoactive drugs by children and adolescents.
2. Voluntary screening for purposes of treatment is within the ethical tradition of health maintenance, but the psychosocial risks of such screening in the area of drug abuse warrant particularly careful attention to the requirements for informed consent and the maintenance of confidentiality.
3. "Voluntary" screening may be a deceptive term in that there are often consequences for those who decline to volunteer.
4. Parental consent may be sufficient for the involuntary screening of the younger child who lacks the capacity to make informed judgments. Parental permission is not sufficient for involuntary screening of the older, competent adolescent, and the Academy opposes such involuntary screening. Consent from the older adolescent may be waived when there is reason to doubt competency or in those circumstances in which information gained by history or physical examination is strongly suggestive of a young person at high risk from substance abuse.
5. Referral of a child or adolescent to a health care professional for evaluation, counseling, and treatment would be the appropriate response to suspicion of drug use within an educational or vocational environment.
6. The pediatrician's major role in this area should be counseling and treatment, not police work. He or she should, therefore, not perform drug screening for the primary purpose of detecting illegal use.
7. Student athletes should not be singled out for involuntary screening for drugs of abuse. Except for health-related purposes, such testing should not be a condition for participation in sports or any school function.

High School Students

A recent survey of 9th to 12th grade students noted that the median value for smoking during the preceding 30 days was 31%; for using smokeless tobacco, 11%; for having at least one alcoholic drink 54%; for having five or more drinks on one occasion, 35%; for using marijuana at least once, 12%; and for using any form of cocaine including powder, crack, or free-base, 2%.[21] A survey of nearly 50,000 students from 420 public and private high schools nationwide found that one in four high school sophomores and one in three seniors said they had smoked marijuana at least once within the last year.[22]

Needlestick Injuries

Children have begun to present themselves to hospitals with needlestick injuries from discarded used needles found in public places.[23]

Eighth Grade Students and Self-Care

Self-care is an important risk factor in eighth grade students for alcohol, tobacco, and marijuana use. In one study, 9.1% smoked one or more packs of cigarettes, 16.7% had drunk 11 or more alcoholic drinks, and 18.4% had tried marijuana.[21]

The survey also found that eighth graders were using marijuana at a higher rate than in prior years. Students reported using cocaine, crack, hallucinogenic drugs, heroin, and stimulants at least once in the last year at marginally higher rates for a second consecutive year. Still, the levels of illegal drug use were below those found in the late 1970s and early 1980s.[22]

Drug-using adolescents do not often admit that they have a dependency problem. The physician is likely to encounter toxin-related problems in teenagers as an acute drug or alcohol overdose; as chronic outward effects of chemical dependency and/or detoxification; by detection by history, physical examination, or laboratory analysis during health maintenance visits; or from other injuries (eg, motor vehicle accidents, falls, near drowning) or diseases (eg, AIDS, hepatitis, endocarditis) in which drug or alcohol use had played a significant secondary role. The period of highest risk for initiation of drug use peaks at 18 years of age and declines thereafter. Exceptions include cocaine and prescribed psychoactive drugs for which the period of new experimentation extends through the midtwenties.[24] Drugs most commonly abused by adolescents with trauma are alcohol, benzodiazepines, cocaine, and cannabinoids.[25]

WOMEN

Perhaps more than 70% of mothers in many inner cities have been subject to drug abuse by the age of 16 years, have a lack of self-esteem, live in inadequate and unsafe housing, are single parents, are in some sort of legal difficulty, have dysfunctional family relationships, and poor educational and vocational skills, are in economic distress, do not enjoy good health, have a partner or spouse who is also a drug abuser, and may have psychiatric disturbances, depression, or be suffering from a posttraumatic rape syndrome.

Rh-Negative Women

Women with Rh-negative blood (16% of population) who share needles when they inject illicit drugs carry a high risk of being exposed to and forming a strong immune response against Rh-positive blood. Subsequent pregnancies may be threatened because of Rh disease.[26] Of 9 perinatal deaths in 67 cases of blood sampling and intravascular fetal transfusion for severe alloimmune hemolytic disease between May 1986 and November 1989, 3 occurred in the fetuses of two intravenous drug abusers who become alloimmunized by sharing needles with their Rh-positive boyfriends. The female drug abuser should be made aware of this risk of sharing needles with her boyfriend. Provision of clean needles and syringes may aid in reducing the risk of alloimmunization as well as preventing the spread of viral infection.[27]

The Pregnant Patient

Indicators that suggest drug or alcohol dependence in a pregnant woman have been summarized[28] (see Chapter 8). About 1 of every 10 children in the state of New York is estimated to be a child of drug abusers.[29] An estimated 50% or more of female intravenous drug abusers in New York City have been exposed to HIV and could therefore transmit the virus to their children in utero or at birth.[29]

Toxicokinetics in the Pregnant Woman

The toxicokinetics of all drugs are altered during pregnancy. Illicit drugs tend to be of low molecular weight and pass freely from the maternal through the placental and into the fetal compartment.[30] There is a reduction in the maternal concentration of a drug late in gestation due to an increase in maternal blood volume (and, therefore, the volume of distribution) and an increase in total clearance from increased renal (but not hepatic) perfusion. The fetoplacental unit is a part of this increase in total volume. Therefore, a reduction in maternal drug concentration reflects, in part, fetal exposure. This, in turn, leads to a reduced elimination half-life for maternally ingested substances. Most drugs (antibiotics, barbiturates, ethanol, meperidine, local anesthetics) cross the placenta within minutes. Drug concentrations in the fetus are usually 50 to 100% of maternal levels. Transfer from the fetal to the maternal compartment also exists. Chronic maternal addiction does not appear to induce metabolic pathways in the placenta for the biotransformation of drugs of abuse.[31]

Laboratory

Study of meconium from the infants of drug-dependent mothers suggests that meconium specimens (first 3 days of stool) show metabolites of cocaine, morphine, and cannabinoids more often (within days 1 and 2) than a urine screen.[32] The Abbott TDx is an effective assay method for meconium.[33] Infants of substance-abusing mothers appear to have an increase in blood norepinephrine levels at 2 months of age. This may account for an increase in sympathetic nervous system tone in these babies.[34]

HEALTH PROBLEMS

An overall perspective of the problems consequent to drug abuse that are experienced by the individual drug abuser and by the society in which that person lives is given in Table 19–6.[35]

DRUGS AND CHEMICALS ABUSED INDUCING CHILDHOOD ADDICTION

Europe

Self-adhesive stickers impregnated with D-lysergic acid diethylamide (LSD), strychnine, ± a phenothiazine are offered to children to cause dependency and create new customers for Europe's illegal drug trade.[36] This tactic was first seen in The Netherlands and Switzerland, then in the United Kingdom. The stickers are a blue star on a white background; a small token named "window pane" with motifs to cut out; and a small card with the name "rote pyramide" (red pyramid) printed on it.

Signs and symptoms from exposure to these stickers include headaches, vomiting, hallucinations, and/or fluctuating temperature.

United States

Cocaine has been given to schoolchildren to induce addiction.

PHENACETIN

Effects of phenacetin abuse include increased mortality with death from urologic or renal disease, cancer, and cardiovascular disease[37] and hypertension.[38]

Analgesic abuse (Germany), five or more tablets a week for 2 or more years, has caused papillary necrosis.

INHALERS

Adrenaline

Excessive chronic self-medication with an adrenaline-containing inhaler used for asthma may lead to a catecholamine-induced cardiomyopathy.[39] Cessation of use leads to clinical improvement.

Table 19–6
Types of Health Problems Consequent to Drug Abuse That Occur With a Frequency That Is Significant from the Standpoint of Public Health

Event	Comment
Biological	
Trauma	
Accidents	Includes accidents in cars, planes, boats, and trains; industrial accidents; electrocution, head injury, loss of limbs; injury from falling, etc.
Fires	Evidence exists that intoxicants contribute substantially to the risk of fire
Drownings	Intoxicants frequently involved
Cardiovascular disease	
Hypertension	
Stroke	
Coronary heart disease	
Gastrointestinal and biliary disease	
Ulcer	
Pancreatitis	
Carcinomas of the oropharynx, esophagus, and other parts of gastrointestinal tract	
Cirrhosis of the liver	
Pulmonary	
Carcinoma	
Chronic obstructive pulmonary disease	
Central nervous system/neurologic	
Dementia	
Neuropathy	
Hematopoietic	
Anemias	
Immune system	Alcohol, cannabis, and nicotine are known to impair the function of macrophages, so infections are more frequent in populations of users than in nonusers Opioids may also have similar effects on immune function, as infections are more frequent in opioid users than in the general population
Death from overdose	
Psychological/psychiatric	
Abuse	
Dependence	
Psychiatric disorders	Drug effects may mimic many common psychiatric disorders, most notably depression
Suicide	There is a strong relationship between use of intoxicants and suicide
Homicide	Many are committed under the influence of intoxicants
Social and economic	
Loss of productivity	
Crime	At least half of all criminals have substance abuse problems, and many crimes are committed under the influence of intoxicants
Family disruption	Family treatment centers accept that intoxicants are a serious problem in disturbed families
Child abuse	
Rape	

From Senay EC: Drug abuse and public health: A global perspective. Drug Saf 1991;6(suppl. 1):1–65.

Salbutamol

Abuse of salbutamol inhalers has been reported in asthmatics dependent on the propellant (a fluorinated hydrocarbon).[40,41]

NONTRADITIONAL SOURCES OF ALCOHOL

Nontraditional sources of alcohol include Listerine mouthwash, hairsprays, Lysol Disinfectant spray (*O*-phenylphenol 0.1%, ethyl alcohol 79%). Lysol has been mixed with orange juice and drunk by children (Senate Hearings on Indian Affairs) on Indian reservations.[42]

ILLICIT ANESTHETIC USE

Illicit use of anesthetics (e.g. halothane, enflurane, isoflurane[43]) by ingestion, intravenous injection, sniffing, and topical application has been reported, with frequent deaths especially after sniffing (Japan).[44] Mostly hospital-related personnel are involved.

DRUGS ABUSED BY PERSONS WITH ANOREXIA NERVOSA AND BULIMIA NERVOSA

Emetine is eliminated slowly from the body, with up to 35% of the drug still retained after 35 days.[45,46] Its presence can be detected in stool and urine long after ipecac use is stopped. Both high-pressure liquid chromatography and thin-layer chromatography can be used to identify the drug.[47] Surreptitious ipecac consumption may also be diagnosed by physical symptoms (e.g. proximal muscle weakness and a waddling gait) and a characteristic abnormal muscle biopsy in addition to the medical history of drug abuse, chemical signs and symptoms, laboratory studies, and diagnostic workup.[48]

Clinical Presentation

Up to one third of patients with bulimia have a history of anorexia nervosa. A minority have coexistent anorexia nervosa and present with a low body weight and other features of anorexia nervosa such as fear of fatness, vigorous exercising, and amenorrhea. Calluses may form on the back of the hand (Russel's sign) due to repeated abrasion of the skin. Painless enlargement of the parotid and submandibular glands may be correlated with self-induced vomiting. Hematemesis, gastric dilation, and, rarely, perforation can occur. Other complications include impaired renal function, tetany, and seizures.[49–51]

Rare complications include myopathies from misuse of ipecac, ruptured esophagus, and pneumomediastinum associated with vomiting and subtle abnormalities in neuroendocrine regulatory systems.[52,53]

Diuretics

The bulimic patient may ingest potassium in the belief that it may act as a diuretic as well as conventional diuretics in an attempt to lose weight.[54]

Poisonings

Anorexia and bulimia nervosa are often associated with depression and suicide attempts.[55] Poisonings in anorexia nervosa are often complicated by frequent delays to presentation, misrepresentation or omission of the toxins involved, frequent presence of such life-threatening toxins as the tricyclic antidepressants or aspirin, frequent electrolyte disturbances, problem of decontamination, and frequent need of hospitalization for medical and psychiatric monitoring and treatment.[56]

Treatment

For anorexia nervosa there appears to be little if any role for pharmacotherapy. Drugs used to promote food intake and weight gain, such as cyproheptadine, amitriptyline, clonidine, and opiate antagonists, have provided disappointing results. For bulimia, tricyclic antidepressants (eg, imipramine, desipramine), monoamine oxidase inhibitors, bupropion, nerve antidepressants such as trazodone,[57] amfebutamone, and fluoxetine[58,59] may be useful. Anticonvulsants, benzodiazepines, lithium, fenfluramine, and opiate antagonists[60] require further study.[61]

Bulimia

All bulimic patients should have a thorough medical history and physical examination. Screening laboratory tests should include a complete blood count, serum electrolytes, blood urea nitrogen, creatinine, serum glucose, and uric acid and calcium determinations. An electrocardiogram with rhythm strip is desirable. If the history of physical examinations suggests misuse of ipecac, a thorough cardiac assessment is indicated. Muscle enzyme value, lipid levels, magnesium and zinc concentrations, electromyography, chest roentgenogram, abnormal flat plate, and endoscopic evaluation may be indicated. If marked alkalosis or hypokalemia is present, hospitalization should be considered to interrupt the bulimic behavior, correct electrolyte abnormalities, and monitor for cardiac complications. Dental consultation may be indicated to help avoid the progression of enamel erosion. Physicians must assume that laxative abuse, diuretic abuse, or misuse of ipecac may be present.[52]

TOPICAL OCULAR ANESTHETICS

Keratitis and persistent epithelial defects are the effects of abuse. These agents are obtained by theft or prescription. The individual usually has a history of psychoactive substance abuse. All topical ocular anesthetics are used.[62]

CYCLOPENTOLATE HYDROCHLORIDE (CYCLOGYL)

This mydriatic and cycloplegic drug has been approved for topical use. In chronically excessive dosages producing ataxia, visual hallucinations, keratitis, photophobia, tearing, and redness. The presence of a dimethylated side chain (-N-$[CH_3]_2$) in cyclopentolate that is also found in the hallucinogens hordenine and bufatenine may in part explain the abuse.[63]

ANTACIDS

Abuse of an aluminum hydroxide/magnesium hydroxide antacid preparation (21 g each) for 18 to 24 months led to bilateral renal calculi and hypophosphatemia.[64] To treat severe osteomalacia, antacid ingestion is discontinued, and vitamin D_2, calcium phosphate, and possibly sodium fluoride are administered.

CYCLIZINE

In opiate-dependent individuals receiving methadone, cyclizine causes intensive stimulation, often with hallucinations, occasionally aggressive behavior, and seizures. Tolerance is reported. There is no clear-cut withdrawal syndrome.[65]

γ-HYDROXYBUTYRIC ACID

γ-Hydroxybutyric acid is marketed illicitly nationwide to body builders. It allegedly produces a "high" and also produces gastrointestinal symptoms, central nervous system and respiratory depression, and uncontrolled movements.[66–69] GHB is sold through mail-order outlets, health food stores, body building gyms, and fitness centers.[69] On November 8, 1990, the U.S. Food and Drug Administration warned consumers to discontinue use of the illegally marketed substance. As of November 28, 1990, 25 cases of GHB toxicity have been reported to poison control centers in California. No reliable estimate of GHB consumption in the general population is available. Marketing or promotion of the drug is now illegal in California.[70] There are no documented or anecdotal reports of long-term adverse effects or fatalities, nor any evidence of physiologic addiction.[71]

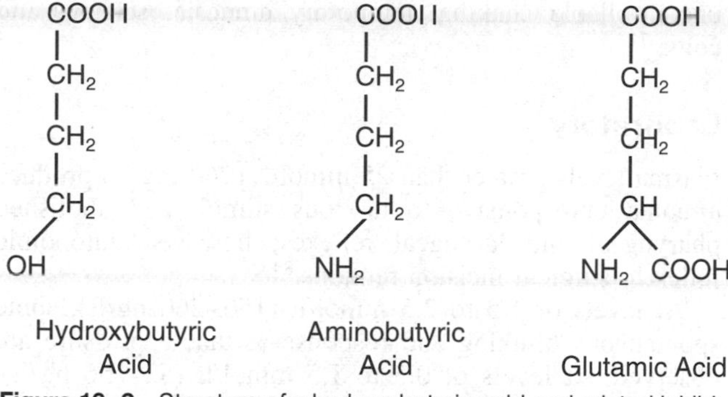

Figure 19–2 Structure of γ-hydroxybutyric acid and related inhibitory neurotransmitter γ-hydroxybutyric acid and excitatory neurotransmitter glutamic acid. (From Dyer JE. Gamma-hydroxybutyrate: A health-food product producing coma and seizurelike activity. Am J Emerg Med 1991; 9:321–324.)

Structure and Classification

γ-Hydroxybutyric acid is a four-carbon compound derived from and similar to γ-aminobutyric acid[72,73] (Fig. 19–2).

γ-Hydroxybutyric acid is gaining popularity as an illicit street drug in the eastern United States. There is no accurate method for assessing the amount or quality of the GHB consumed. Despite Food and Drug Administration interdiction, this substance is still available to, marketed for, and used by body builders, dieters, and persons suffering from insomnia. There are no documented or anecdotal reports of long-term adverse effects or fatalities, nor any evidence of physiologic addiction.

Uses

γ-Hydroxybutyric acid is promoted as a "steroid alternative" and for weight control, because it is alleged to increase muscle mass and reduce body fat by stimulating the production of human growth hormone. Its role in the increase in muscle mass has not been subject to clinical trials. Sales promotions indicate that 30 to 50 mg/kg GHB taken at bedtime provides 2 to 3 hours of sleep while growth hormone is being released.[74] GHB allegedly produces a "high," making it attractive as a drug of abuse; in this context it may be taken with alcohol or other drugs. It has also been used as an anesthetic agent in Africa,[75] as treatment for ethanol and opiate withdrawal,[76] and as treatment for ischemic conditions.[77]

Product Formulation

γ-Hydroxybutyric acid is sold as a sodium salt, in either powder or granular form, and is commonly dissolved in water before use.[68]

Common product names and distribution of GHB in the United States are outlined in Table 19–7.[71] The amount of GHB contained in marketed products is not known.

Source

γ-Hydroxybutyric acid is available legally under investigational new drug applications, almost all of which involve the use of GHB in narcoleptic patients,[67,68] produced by metabolism of the neurotransmitter γ-aminobutyric acid[71] (Fig. 19–2).[74]

Table 19–7
γ-Hydroxybutyrate: Product Names and Distributors

Common Product Name	Currently Known Distributors
γ-Hydroxylbutyric acid	Biosky
Sodium oxybate	Biotonic Formulary
Sodium oxybutyrate	Hi-Tech Bodybuilding
γ-Hydroxybutyrate sodium	
γ-OH	
4-Hydroxy butyrate	
γ-Hydrate	
Somatomax PM	

From Chin MY, Kreutzer RA, Dyer JE. Acute poisoning from gamma-hydroxybutyrate in California. West J Med 1992;156:380–384.

Toxic Dose

At doses of 10 mg/kg, amnesia and hypotonia may be observed. Doses of 20 to 30 mg/kg are associated with a normal sequence of rapid eye movement (REM) and non-REM sleep. A dose of 50 mg/kg induces abrupt unconsciousness and coma. More than 50 mg/kg of GHB decreases cardiac output, often leading to severe respiratory depression, seizurelike activity, and/or coma.[68,73,78]

An intravenous dose of 65 mg/kg induced sleepiness within 5 minutes, descending into a comatose state that lasted 1 or 2 hours or longer, after which there was a rapid awakening.[79]

Toxicokinetics

γ-Hydroxybutyric acid is well absorbed orally, readily crosses the blood–brain barrier, and is later metabolized to carbon dioxide and water without active metabolites.[73,80]

Absorption

The absorption from the gastrointestinal tract is rapid and the onset of systemic effects occurs within 15 minutes. Oral doses in humans of 75 to 100 mg/kg produce peak blood levels of 0.87 and 1.15 mmol/L (90 and 120 ng/L) in 1.5 to 2 hours.[74,81]

Distribution

The apparent volume of distribution is 0.4 to 0.58 L/kg.[74]

Elimination

γ-Hydroxybutyric acid is metabolized to carbon dioxide, which is eliminated in the expired air. Initial oxidation produces carbon fragments that enter the tricarboxylic acid cycle. Less than 1 to 5% of GHB is eliminated in the urine.

Drug Interactions

γ-Hydroxybutyric acid acts synergistically with ethanol to produce central nervous system and respiratory depression.

Ethanol also increases endogenous levels of GHB.[74] GHB may potentiate the effects of narcotic analgesics and skeletal muscle relaxants and may be potentiated by the action of benzodiazepines and neuroleptics.[73] Antagonism may occur with D-amphetamine, naloxone, haloperidol, and drugs used for absence seizures.[74] These drugs have not been assessed as possible treatments for GHB overdose. Naloxone has not been effective.

Mechanism of Action

γ-Hydroxybutyric acid is produced by the body as a normal metabolite and is not a nutritional requirement.[68] It is found naturally in the central nervous system and, in higher concentrations, in the peripheral tissues. γ-Aminobutyric acid (GABA) is catabolized via transamination to succinate semialdehyde, which is then oxidized to succinate. Brain tissue is capable of reducing succinate semialdehyde to GHB.[71] It exhibits the properties of a neurotransmitter in humans, but its effects have not been associated with specific neuronal tracts. GHB crosses the blood–brain barrier. In the brain, GHB increases dopamine levels, exerts effects through the endogenous opioid system, and probably acts by other independent receptor-dependent mechanisms.[73] GHB is a precursor of the neurotransmitter GABA.[67]

High concentrations of GHB are detected in cerebrospinal fluid, plasma, and urine of patients with succinic semialdehyde dehydrogenase deficiency.[81,82] Vigabatrin appeared to induce biochemical (decreased cerebrospinal fluid GHB) and clinical improvement in one patient.[85]

Clinical Presentation

Numerous side effects have been reported in connection with the use of GHB at doses ranging from 2 g to more than 30 g. These include vomiting, drowsiness, hypnagogic state, amnesia, hypotonia, and vertigo. Loss of consciousness, irregular and depressed respirations, or involuntary movements may follow. Seizurelike activity, bradycardia, and/or respiratory arrest have also been reported.[67]

Severity and duration of symptoms appear to depend on the use of GHB and/or other drugs such as alcohol, benzodiazepines, cannabis, and amphetamines. One death has been reported when GHB was administered with heroin.[83] Some patients have required respiratory support or other intensive care.[67]

An acute comatose state may follow GHB intoxication within 15 to 20 minutes of ingestion, followed by spontaneous resolution in 2 to 96 hours.

Coma has occurred in patients after the ingestion of 1 to 6 teaspoons of GHB. Tonic–clonic seizurelike activity occurred in two patients after 1 teaspoon and 4 tablespoons of GHB, respectively. All patients recovered from the acute symptoms (nausea, vomiting, dizziness, bradycardia, confusion, agitation, and hallucinations) within 7 hours. Dizziness has been reported to continue for up to 14 days.[71] Patients report a pleasurable sensation of "high" and that it made them "feel good".

Symptoms reported to poison centers have included drowsiness, dizziness, a "high," headache, convulsion, nausea, vomiting, diarrhea, incontinence, trouble breathing, uncontrollable shaking, temporary amnesia, seizure, and coma.[71]

Laboratory

Plasma levels greater than 25 mmol/L (260 mg/L) produce a coma unresponsive to noxious stimuli and abolished pharyngeal and laryngeal reflexes; however, autonomic reflex to surgical incision remains.[84]

At levels of 1.5 to 2.5 mmol/L (156–260 ng/L), some spontaneous blinking and response to tactile pressure are observed. At levels of 0.5 to 1.5 mmol/L (52–156 ng/L), occasional eye opening and spontaneous movement are observed. At levels less than 0.5 mmol/L (50 ng/L), patients remained awake.

Treatment

Initial removal of GHB from the patient must be ensured. Treatment is largely symptomatic and supportive. Vigabatrin[85] may have a role in treatment of an overdose, but insufficient data have been accumulated to recommend its use.

ELEMENTAL MERCURY

Self-injection of elemental mercury to "get high" led to painful arm, anorexia, myalgia, and weakness. The blood mercury level was 79 ng/mL (normal, <1.0), and the urine mercury level 380 ng/nL (normal, <20).[86]

INTRAVENOUS SLOW-RELEASE OPIATES

Intravenous use of oral slow-release morphine tablets has been reported.[87]

BUPRENORPHINE

Buprenorphine is the preferred drug of more than half of intravenous drug users in contact with drug services in eastern Glasgow. This figure rises to 69% when temazepam is added.[88]

MUNCHAUSEN'S SYNDROME

Chemical abuse has been reported in a case of Munchausen's syndrome by proxy.[89] A preschooler was abused by parents with phenytoin and carbamazepine (see also Laxatives).

DEXTROMETHORPHAN

Robitussin DM abuse has been reported among teenagers. The acute health risks appear to be minimal.[90] The abuse potential is real, as a "high" was experienced after one 4-oz bottle.[91] Abuse of Benylin DM led to recurrent mania.[92]

DIMENHYDRINATE

Dimenhydrinate (Dramamine) is associated with dependency and tolerance.[93,94] Abuse of antihistamines (e.g. tripelennamine IV alone or with paregoric or pentazocine, diphenhydramine hydrochloride IV with butorphanol, cyclizine with buprenorphine) may be common among young women with anorexia or bulimia and among people with a history of drug dependence.[93] Abusers may develop symptoms of withdrawal (acute dystonia),[94] poor appetite, "sick stomach," and emotional lability.[95]

POPPY SEEDS

Excessive poppy seed consumption is associated with elated feelings. This is prevalent in Eastern Europe. Withdrawal symptoms are observed.[96,97] (See also Chapter 25.)

PROPOXYPHENE

Dextropropoxyphene and acetaminophen suppositories induce rectal lesions when abused for long periods.[98] Effects of withdrawal from the chronic abuse of dextropropoxyphene include nausea, tremor, agitation, insomnia, diaphoresis, fever, headache, confusion, psychotic reactions, and seizures.[99]

ERYTHROPOIETIN

Erythropoietin is abused to enhance athletic performance. The increase in hematocrit increases the risk of encephalopathy, seizures, vascular distention, impairment of blood flow with tissue hypoxia, and more rapid clotting (possible phlebothrombosis, pulmonary embolism, myocardial infarction, stroke, and exacerbation of chronic lung disease).[100] (See also Chapter 29.)

STEROIDS

Euphoria and apparent dependence may follow use of androgenic anabolic steroids. Some may have withdrawal symptoms (depression, fatigue, craving for steroids).[101] Some experience wide mood swings with periods of aggression. Betamethasone nosedrop abuse has resulted in Cushing's syndrome[102] (see Anabolic Steroids, Page 319).

COUGH SYRUPS

Cough syrups containing codeine phosphate, ephedrine hydrochloride, and promethazine hydrochloride are readily available in India without prescription (Phensedyl). Several cases of dependence are described.[103]

L-THYROXINE

Factitious hyperthyroidism with sudden death may be due to deliberate intake of excessive amounts of L-thyroxine.[104]

BENZODIAZEPINES

Lorazepam and alprazolam are more diazepam-like in having relatively high abuse liability, whereas oxazepam, halazepam, and possibly chlordiazepoxide are relatively low in this regard.[105]

BUSPIRONE

Buspirone may have a lesser abuse potential than lorazepam.[106]

ANTIMUSCARINIC AGENTS

Centrally active antimuscarinic agents (trihexyphenidyl, benztropine, procyclidine, biperiden) may have antidepressant and mood-elevating properties and may be liable to abuse. Although much of the evidence is anecdotal, it suggests that psychological or physiologic dependence may be induced, that tolerance occurs, and that withdrawal may result in myalgias, diaphoresis, malaise, coryza, paresthesias, gastrointestinal distress, headaches, anxiety, insomnia, terrifying dreams, fatigue, dysphoria, and a rebound exacerbation of the motor dysfunction for which the agent was originally used.[107]

TRANYLCYPROMINE

Tranylcypromine may be subject to abuse in patients with psychiatric disorders because of its capacity to exert amphetamine-like effects.[108] A withdrawal syndrome has been described for tranylcypromine and other monoamine oxidase inhibitors similar to that seen with amphetamine withdrawal.[109] Symptoms include psychosis, delirium, and severe sleep disturbances.[110]

NITROUS OXIDE

Dentists use nitrous oxide and the food industry uses nitrous oxide as a propellant for whipped cream.[111] Chronic exposure to nitrous oxide induces a myeloneuropathy whose early symptoms include mild numbness of the hands and feet, impaired equilibrium, loss of coordination, and mild muscular weakness. Late symptoms and signs include ataxia, sphincter impairment, decreased vibratory sense, headaches, poor memory, decreased tendon reflexes, altered mood, impotence, peripheral anesthesia, and a positive Lhermitte sign (electric shock-like sensation provoked by neck flexion). Other clinical states reported with chronic abuse of nitrous oxide include pneumodiastinum, oral frostbite, prolonged delirium with inappropriate behavior, and hallucinations and paranoid delusions. Megaloblastic bone marrow due to vitamin B_{12} deficiency is induced by nitrous oxide's blocking of vitamin B_{12}, a cofactor in the conversion of homocystine to methionine, catalyzed by methionine synthetase.[110]

LOPERAMIDE, FENTANYL, AND NALTREXONE

Loperamide,[112] oral fentanyl,[113] and naltrexone[114] have been implicated in anecdotal reports indicating drug dependence.

MUSCLE RELAXANTS

Centrally acting muscle relaxants, despite their unrelated chemical structures, possess sedative properties and are abused mainly for this effect. They are frequently used in combination with other central nervous system depressants.[115]

Skeletal Muscle Relaxants

Baclofen (Lioresal) is a γ-aminobutyric acid derivative. Carisoprodol (Soma) is chemically related to meprobamate. Cyclobenzaprine hydrochloride (Flexeril) is closely related to the tricyclic antidepressants. All of these agents possess sedative properties and are abused mainly for this effect. Abusers demonstrate signs of tolerance and also suffer withdrawal symptoms of anxiety, tremors, insomnia, and occasionally hallucinations or seizures.[114,116,117]

Carisoprodol abuse can cause signs and symptoms of depressant intoxication such as ataxia, slurred speech, stupor, and drowsiness. Mydriasis and nystagmus may also be noted. As carisoprodol is neither a controlled substance nor (at present) a commonly known abused pharmaceutical, the laboratory may not look for this drug. If the laboratory *does* detect meprobamate, the physician should look for the concurrent presence of the parent drug carisoprodol. Carisoprodol also may be combined with codeine; these tablets are manufactured by numerous pharmaceutical companies. Tablets marked with the number "3" contain 30 mg of codeine; the number "4" products contain 60 mg of codeine. If carisoprodol with codeine is consumed in increased doses, the effects of the opiate, that is, pupillary constriction and lowered body temperature, may not be present. Codeine, however, causes additive depressant effects such as drowsiness, ataxia, and decreased pulse and blood pressure. Laboratory findings may reveal only the presence of the opiate codeine.[118]

ANTIPARKINSONISM DRUGS

The antiparkinsonism drug most frequently abused appears to be trihexyphenidyl (Artane), followed by biperiden (Akineton), benztropine (Cogentin), procyclidine (Renaadrin), and orphenadrine.[119]

LEVODOPA

Levodopa therapy may induce euphoria and relaxation in the patient with Parkinson's disease. Dosage may be gradually increased. On discontinuation, mood disturbances, dysphoria, and anxiety may be experienced. This mild abuse potential should be considered in patients with prior addictive behavior.[124]

ERGOTAMINE

Ergotamine may be abused by patients with migraine headaches. If it is used for a long period, the development of a rebound headache constitutes a major clinical use, alleviated only by continued use of the drug.

ESTROGEN

Estrogens are psychoactive; they lift mood, can be given by injection, and have powerful psychological effects.[1] Such dependence is disputed.[120]

TEMAZEPAM

Temazepam is marketed in the United Kingdom as opaque yellow oval soft capsules with liquid centers (Normison) or as green soft gelatin capsules with liquid centers (Eunhypnos). In the Scottish drug abuse community they are known as "eggs" or "goosies."[121] The drug abuser draws off the contents of a temazepam capsule using a syringe and injects it intravenously, where it may cause vascular problems.

NIFEDIPINE

Nifedipine is an unlikely candidate as a drug of abuse.[122] It is not hallucinogenic, stimulant, or sedative in effect and should hold no attraction for addicts. In the United Kingdom, nifedipine capsules resemble temazepam capsules. Several deaths due to nifedipine have occurred in intravenous drug abusers who mistook nifedipine for temazepam.[123]

INHALATION ABUSE

Fluorinated hydrocarbons, collectively referred to as Freons, have been shown to result in widespread systemic toxicity after accidental or intentional inhalation. Freon inhalation may lead to the production of cardiac arrhythmias, in particular ventricular ectopy and ventricular fibrillation. (See also Chapter 65.)

Similar agents available to the consumer are being intentionally abused by teenagers and adults. Solvent sniffing, or volatile substances abuse (VSA), refers to the intentional inhalation of volatile hydrocarbons. Compounds may include ethers, ketones, and aromatic and aliphatic hydrocarbons found in adhesives, aerosols, cleaning fluids, and fuels. The American Academy of Poison Control Centers (AAPCC) reported 5236 cases of Freon exposure in 1991. Of these, 146 were reported as intentional, resulting in 6 deaths. AAPCC 1992 figures indicate 5962 cases of Freon exposure. Of these, 214 were reported as intentional, resulting in 4 deaths.[125] About 30% of all adolescent poisoning fatalities are secondary to inhalant abuse (AAPCC Toxic Exposure Surveillance System).

ANALGESIC NEPHROPATHY

The role of phenacetin (phenacetin nephritis) in the production of analgesic-associated nephropathy (AAN) has largely diminished since its removal from many products worldwide. There has been little decline in AAN since the phenacetin removal. The nephrotoxicity of analgesic mixtures may depend on the practice of adding potentially addictive components (caffeine, codeine, barbiturates). Most patients now who admit an overconsumption of analgesics use mixtures. Restriction of over-the-counter sales of all analgesic mixtures may have led to a decrease in the incidence of AAN.[126] Few studies have suggested the development of AAN from abuse of aspirin, acetaminophen, and nonsteroidal antiinflammatory drugs.[127]

SUBSTANCE ABUSE BY ATHLETES

Drugs

Most of the substances commonly abused used by athletes in the hope of enhancing athletic performance appear to have a potential for the rapid development of tolerance, short duration of action, rapid onset of action, abrupt release at the termination of action, some anticholinergic action, production of a pleasurable euphoria, and ritualistic administration.[128,129] Three categories of drugs are generally used by athletes:

1. Street drugs: alcohol, tobacco, marijuana, cocaine.
2. Ergogenic drugs: central nervous system stimulants, anabolic steroids, "designer substances," nutritional supplements.
3. Performance continuance drugs: analgesics, antiinflammatory agents (see Chapter 11). Woolley and Barnett[128,129] and Mofenson[130] have provided a comprehensive background of their experience.

Agents Taken to Increase Lean Muscle Mass and Strength

Anabolic Steroids. Anabolic steroids are human or veterinary products of androgenic anabolic steroidal hormones and synthetic testosterone-like drugs. *Oral preparations* include ethylestrenol (Maxibolin), methandrostenolone (Dianabol), nandrolone (Durabolin, among others), oxymetholone (Androyd, Anadrol-50), and stanazolol (such as Winstrol). *Parenteral preparations* include nandrolone phenpropionate, nandrolone decanoate, testosterone enanthate, and testosterone cypromate.

Epidemiology. There are reported to be more than 1 million current or former illicit anabolic androgenic steroid users in the United States. Their use is often associated with use of other illicit drugs, cigarettes, and alcohol.[128]

Androgen Use. It appears that athletes may be taking doses of androgen in 100- to 1000-fold excess over physiologic doses. Often, several preparations are taken. Oral and parenteral forms may be used together. Athletes often "stack the pyramid" with increases and decreases of dosages over days and weeks, with drug holidays sometimes interspersed. Veterinary preparations of unknown toxicity are often used by humans. Drugs from foreign countries that may be too toxic for approval by the U.S. Food and Drug Administration or about which little is known are used. Needles may be shared; AIDS may follow. Physicians are often the source of the drugs, sometimes by prescription. Users may abstain for months before competition and use a diuretic before the actual drug test to dilute the urine and disguise the steroid.

Risk Behavior Syndrome. Anabolic steroid use in high school students is part of a 'risk' behavior syndrome which includes sexual behaviors, suicidal behaviors, frequency of not wearing a passenger seat belt, riding a motorcycle, not wearing a helmet while riding a motorcycle, driving after drinking alcohol, riding with a driver who has been drinking alcohol, fighting, and carrying a weapon.[131]

Detection of Androgens. Detection is difficult due to the availability of numerous preparations with numerous degradative products. Samples are presently separated by chromatography. Peaks detected are analyzed by mass

Table 19–8
Olympic Committee-Banned Drugs Classified According to Detection Procedure

Procedure I	
Stimulants	
Amfepramone (diethylpropion)	Furfenorex
Amiphenazole	Mefenorex
Amphetamine	Methoxyphenamine
Amphetaminil	Methamphetamine
Benzphetamine	Methylephedrine
Caffeine	Methylphenidate
Cathine (norpseudoephedrine)	Morazone
Chlorphentermine	Nikethamide
Chlorprenaline	Pentetrazol (cardiazole)
Clobenzorex	Phendimetrazine
Cropropamide	Phenmetrazine
Dimethamphetamine	Phentermine
Ephedrine	Phenylpropanolamine (norephedrine)
Etafedrine	Pipradol
Etilamfetamine	Prolintane
Fencamfamine	Propylhexedrine
Fenetylline	Strychnine
Fenproporex	
Narcotic Analgesics	
Alpha-prodine	Ethoheptazine
Dextromoramide	Methadone
Dextropropoxyphene	Pethidine (meperidine)
Dipipanone	
Beta Blockers	
Acebutolol	Atenolol
Procedure II	
Stimulants	
Cocaine	Ethamivan
Narcotic Analgesics	
Anileridine	Levorphanol
Buprenorphine	Methadone
Codeine	Morphine
Dihydrocodeine	Nalbuphine
Ethylmorphine	Pentazocine
Heroin	Phenazocine
Beta Blockers	
Acebutolol	Nadolol
Alprenolol	Oxprenolol
Labetalol	Propranolol
Metoprolol	Sotalol
Procedure III	
Diuretics	
Acetazolamide	Dichlorphenamide
Amiloride	Ethacrynic acid
Benzthiazide	Furosemide
Bendrofluazide	Hydrochlorothiazide
Bumetanide	Spironolactone
Canrenone	Triamterene
Chlorthalidone	
Procedure IV	
Free Fraction	
Bolasterone	Metandienone
Dehydrochloro-methyltestosterone	Oxandrolone
Fluoxymesterone	Stanozolol
Conjugated Fraction	
Bolasterone	Nandrolone
Boldenone	Norethandrolone
Clostebol	Oxymesterone
Mesterolone	Oxymetholone
Methyltestosterone	Testosterone

From Park J, Park S, Lho D, et al. Drug testing at the 10th Asian Games and 24th Seoul Olympic Games. J Anal Toxicol 1990;14(2):66–72.

spectrometry.[4] Olympic Committee-banned drugs and analytical procedures are listed in Table 19–8.[132]

Adverse Effects

1. Hepatic effects: with oral or 17 α-alkylating agents; common—abnormal values on tests for liver injury and liver function, cholestatic jaundice; rare—hepatomas, peliosis hepatis, benign and malignant tumors
2. Endocrine effects: decreased production of luteinizing hormone, follicle-stimulating hormone, and testosterone; males—testicular atrophy, decreased sperm production, sterility, gynecomastia, hypertension, acne, baldness; women—hoarseness, hirsutism, menstrual irregularities, enlarged clitoris, decreased breast size, alopecia, usually nonreversible; both sexes—acne, gynecomastia, altered glucose tolerance, hyperinsulinism
3. Cardiovascular effects: elevated blood pressure, increased low-density lipoprotein cholesterol levels, changes in triglyceride concentrations, decreased high-density lipoprotein cholesterol levels, fluid and water retention; thrombotic complications (stroke, acute myocardial infarction) temporally linked with androgen abuse in athletes[133,134]; platelet aggregation[135]
4. Musculoskeletal effects: premature epiphyseal closure and short stature
5. Behavioral effects: excessive aggressiveness, changes in libido, psychotic symptoms, bipolar affective disorder, anxiety, irritability, anger, dependence, dependence in conjunction with psychosis
6. Immunologic system: decreased immunoglobulins and T-cell changes
7. Neurologic changes: cerebrovascular hemorrhage, intracranial hypertension, transient ischemic attacks[133,136]

Human Growth Hormone. This lyophilized polypeptide hormone formerly was extracted from the pituitary glands of cadavers. The formulation includes follicle-stimulating hormone, luteinizing hormone, adrenocorticotropic hormone, thyrotropin, prolactin, and mannitol. Seven cases of Creutzfeldt–Jakob disease and some deaths prompted the U.S. Food and Drug Administration (FDA) to recall the product in 1985 because of the enzymatic viruslike contamination. Later, a recombinant DNA-produced hormone extract was approved by the FDA.[137] No cases of Creutzfeldt–Jakob disease have since been reported. Antibodies to human growth hormones are produced in 30 to 40% of individuals who take this drug.

Adverse effects include acromegaly, joint pain, osteoarthritis, limitation of joint range and/or function, soft organ growth, and premature prostatic hypertrophy.

Cyproheptadine. Cyproheptadine hydrochloride (Periactin) is a serotonin and histamine antagonist that is supposed to increase the appetite and produce weight gain (average 1 lb/wk). It may stimulate the release of luteinizing hormone and, thus, testosterone production. These observations are uncontrolled and lack scientific validity.

Ginseng. This herb is sold with the message that it helps the athlete adapt to environmental and social stresses. Both species of ginseng contain two 17β-hydroxylated steroids.

Adverse effects include central nervous system stimulation, hypertension, paradoxical hypotension, fluid and electrolyte imbalance, gynecomastia, and possibly toxic effects on the heart and kidneys.

Amino Acids. These highly nitrogenous compounds are believed by athletes to cause nitrogen retention and to enhance cellular protein formation and, thus, muscle growth. Free-form amino acids (single levoisomer crystalline compounds manufactured individually and then combined) and hydrolysate amino acids (from natural protein, eg, casein, lysed by enzymatic action to provide amino acids in the same ratio as those found in protein) vie for the athlete's attention. No clinical data support the usefulness of either or one over the other.

Adverse effects include possible renal damage.

Methods Used to Increase Oxygen Depth and Capacity[138,139]

Blood Doping (Induced Erythrocythemia). Blood doping is used to elevate the number of red blood cells in the circulatory system and by so doing increase the oxygen-carrying capacity of blood. It is believed by athletes to enhance endurance.

Methods. Fresh red blood cells are infused from a matched donor; or whole blood is drawn from the athlete and frozen until the blood volume has returned to normal, when it is then reinfused; or most commonly, 2 units of the athletes blood are drawn and stored, and after a period of at least 5 weeks the packed cells are reinfused 1 to 7 days before competition. Blood doping is banned by both the International Olympic Committee and the National College Athletic Association.

Adverse Effects. With incorrectly typed blood, the effects include rash, fever, acute hemolytic reaction with renal damage, delayed transfusion reaction with fever, jaundice, transmission of infectious disease (viral hepatitis, AIDS), circulatory overload, and metabolic shock.

Methylating Agents. Trimethylglycine and dimethylglycine are believed by athletes to be the biochemical catalysts that may infuse oxygen delivery to the muscles. Pangamic acid, which contains dimethylglycine, is sometimes known as vitamin B_{15} but is not a vitamin. All these chemicals are supposed to release methyl groups. There are no restrictions on the use of methylating agents, but there are no controlled clinical studies relating to their efficacy in athletic performance or muscle function.

100% Oxygen. No advantage was shown in a prospective study.[140]

Erythropoietin. Erythropoietin may be used by athletes to enhance red cell production and oxygen-carrying capacity. It may be difficult to detect before competition.

Agents that Increase Energy

Athletes believe stimulants may allow them to perform at higher levels of performance for longer periods and may make them more aggressive. The International Olympic Committee (IOC) divides stimulants into the following groups:

- Psychomotor agents: local anesthetics, certain sympathomimetic drugs, xanthines (eg, coffee)
- Sympathomimetic amines
- Direct central nervous system stimulants

Local Anesthetics. Cocaine, procaine hydrochloride, lidocaine hydrochloride, and other synthetic anesthetics fall into this group. Only cocaine is currently banned by the IOC. There are some restrictions on the use of the others.

Certain Sympathomimetic Drugs. These include phenylethylamines (eg, amphetamine and related products).

Xanthines. Caffeine is the only substance in this group banned by the IOC (above a urinary concentration of 12 μg/mL) and the NCAA (above a urinary concentration of 15 μg/mL). See Table 19–8 for a list of drugs banned by the International Olympic Committee.

Adverse effects of xanthines include jitters, powerful diuresis, dehydration, irritability, insomnia, and dry mouth. Heart disease, pancreatic cancer, and birth defects, although suspected, have not been shown to be caused by caffeine ingestion.

Sympathomimetic Amines. These agents are restricted by most international sports governing bodies. The NCAA has dropped them from their list of banned drugs.

Direct Central Nervous System Stimulants. These are usually banned. Stimulants such as cocaine may be associated with fatal cardiac dysrhythmias, myocardial infarction, pneumothorax, and intracranial hemorrhage (see Chapter 21). Adverse effects include the following

- Behavioral changes: hyperactivity, tremulousness, agitation, restlessness, insomnia, anxiety, paranoid toxic psychosis (large doses)
- Cardiovascular system: tachycardia, hypertension, life-threatening dysrhythmias, myocardial infarction
- Central nervous system: dilated pupils, intracranial hemorrhages, convulsions
- Gastrointestinal system: anorexia, diarrhea, constipation, weight loss.
- Hyperthermia (large doses)

Agents that Purportedly Decrease Recovery Time After Exertion

The following agents have not been subject to carefully controlled prospective clinical trials. Data are lacking to establish the safety or efficacy of these compounds in pregnant or lactating women.

Octacosanol. Octacosanol is a 28 straight-carbon chain alcohol expressed from wheat germ oil. Presumed to improve stamina, strength, and reaction time.

Guarana. Guarana is prepared from the seeds of the *Parellinia cupana* tree from Brazil. It contains 2.5 to 5% caffeine. An octacosanol–guarana combination is called Boost.

γ-Oryzanol. One of four isomers of oryzanol, γ-oryzanol is extracted from rice bran oil. It is supposed to neutralize free radicals released during heavy exercise. γ-Oryzanol is often taken with vitamin E.

Proteolytic Enzymes. These include chymotrypsin, trypsin–chymotrypsin, and papain (obtained from *Carica papaya*). Proteolytic enzymes are supposed to reverse the decrease in tissue permeability and edema of athletic performance.

Adverse effects include rash, pruritus, buccal tingling, menorrhagia, and metrorrhagia.

Dimethyl Sulfoxide. Adverse effects include garlic taste, garliclike odor on skin, burning sensation and heat on application, urticaria, angioedema, transient disturbance of color vision, lens opacities, photophobia, headache, nausea, diarrhea, dizziness, sedation, and burning on urination. Its safety has not been established, and preparations that have not been purified for human use may be dangerous. (See Chapter 65.)

Bee Pollen. Bee pollen is purported to improve athletic and sexual performance; prevent allergy, infection, and cancer; prolong life; improve digestion; and improve weight gain. There are no substantive prospective well-controlled clinical studies to support these claims.

Nutritional Supplements. Although not drugs of abuse, athletes ingest excessive amounts of vitamins B, C, and E to improve their athletic performance. There have been no published reports of controlled clinical studies to support their safe and effective use in improving endurance, muscle efficiency, or motor performance.

Alkalizers

Drugs such as sodium bicarbonate may be taken a few days before and after an athletic event to reduce the lactic acid that results from intensive exercise and that the body clears spontaneously through anabolic metabolism. Alkalinization of the urine increases tubular reabsorption of weak bases, such as stimulants, and induces their urinary excretion. The belief is that the weak base that is reabsorbed may act longer and may be more difficult to detect in the urine.

Danazol

Danazol, 17α-pregna-2, 4-dien-20-yno [2, 3D]isoxazol-17β-ol,[1] is a weak androgen structurally related to the anabolic steroid stanazolol used in the treatment of endometriosis and benign breast disorders.[141]

Danazol has been associated with pseudotumor cerebri and hepatocellular adenomas.[142] Side effects include weight gain, menometrorrhagia, amenorrhea, mild alopecia, altered libido, hot flashes, deepened voice, hirsutism, and acne. Additionally, myalgias or cramps, headaches, anxiety, tremulousness, elevated transaminase levels, microscopic hematuria, dizziness, and nausea have been reported.[137,143] A gas chromatography–mass spectrometry method for determination of danazol metabolites in now available. Ethisterone, 2-hydroxymethylethisterone, and 2 hydroxymethyl-1,2-dehydroethisterone are the main urinary metabolites of the 30 metabolites reported. It is problematic whether danazol either enhances or perhaps even detracts from athletic performance.

Vanadium

Vanadyl sulfate tablets (7.5 mg) are used by athletes as a "natural" over-the-counter preparation to enhance muscle strength. Athletes are often not aware of its anabolic effects and its possible long-term effects including mental illness and effects on glucose metabolism.[144]

Table 19–9
Drugs Associated With Stroke

Heroin
Cocaine (crack, free-base cocaine)
Amphetamines
Lysergic acid diethylamide (LSD)
Phencyclidine (PCP)
T's and Blues
Over-the-counter sympathomimetic decongestants, cold remedies, and diet aids
- Phenylpropanolamine
- Ephedrine
- Pseudephedrine

Adapted from Sloan MA, Kittner SJ, Rigamonti D, Price ER. Occurrence of stroke associated with use/abuse of drugs. Neurology 1991;41: 1358–1364.

DRUG IMPURITIES AND ADDITIVES

Diluents and *adulterants* are terms that refer to exogenous substances (either active or inactive) added to a specimen after its chemical synthesis or refinement, but before its retail sale. Information on drug contaminants derives largely from a number of databases.[145] Additives that may be added to cocaine, heroin, and phencyclidine are discussed in those chapters.

ADVERSE EFFECTS IN DRUG ABUSERS

Drugs that when abused cause stroke are listed in Table 19–9. Recreational drugs associated with seizures are summarized in Table 19–10.[146] Thrombocytopenia in drug abusers can be associated with hypersplenism, chronic hepatitis, bacterial or fungal sepsis, AIDS, disseminated intravascular coagulation, cocaine, and an automimune thrombocytopenia in heroin addicts.

HALLUCINOGENS

Chemical classes of hallucinogens are listed in Table 19–11. Therapeutic drugs associated with hallucinations are listed in Table 19–12.[147] Plants of abuse (hallucinogens, stimulants) are listed in Table 19–13.[148]

ANTICHOLINERGIC AGENTS

Fentanyl Smokes

Abusers may try to obtain a high by applying multiple fentanyl patches, licking them, swallowing them, or injecting the solution. The patches contain fentanyl base and are available as 2.5-, 5.0-, 7.5-, and 10-mg patches delivering 25, 50, 75, and 100 μg/h, respectively. Analgesia can be obtained at doses of 64 to 318 μg of fentanyl base. About 10% of a nebulized dose probably reaches the lungs.[149]

Trihexyphenidyl

In the United Kingdom, trihexyphenidyl was available without prescription prior to 1964 and was used by young people for its hallucinogenic properties.[150] Similar use in the

Table 19–10
Recreational Drugs Associated With Seizures

Drug	Single-Drug Use	Polydrug Use	Route*	Time Interval†
Cocaine	+	+‡	Intranasal	10 min–2 h
			Intravenous	10 min–12 h
			Smoked	<24 h
			Oral	<8 h
Amphetamine	+	+	Intravenous	0–24 h
			Intranasal	2–24 h
			Oral	<12 h
Heroin	+	+	Intravenous	1–24 h
			Intraarterial	<2 h
Phencyclidine	+	+	Smoked	1–3 h
Marijuana	–	+	Smoked	—
LSD (D-lysergic acid diethylamide)	–	+	Oral	—

*In some cases, recreational drugs were used by more than one route.
†Time interval between recreational drug use and onset of seizures.
‡May occur with concomitant methylphenidate or oral diazepam use.

Table 19–11
Chemical Classification of Hallucinogens

Common Name	Chemical Name
Indole Alkaloid Derivatives	
Psilocin	Dimethyl-4-hydroxytryptamine
Psilocybin	Dimethyl-4-phosphoryltryptamine
Harmine	7-Methoxy-1-methyl-9*H*-pyridol[3,4b]indole
Ibogaine	
LSD	D-Lysergic acid diethylamide
	Lysergic acid amide
	Isolysergic acid amide
DMT	Dimethyltryptamine
DPT	Dipropyltryptamine
AMT	α-Methyltryptamine
DET	Diethyltryptamine
	6-Hydroxymethyltryptamine
Butotenine	Dimethyl-5-hydroxytryptamine
Piperidine Derivatives	
Atropine	*N*-Ethyl-2-pyrrolidylmethylphenylcyclopentyl-glycolate
Hyoscine (scopolamine)	
Hyoscyamine	
Cocaine	
Ditran	
Phencyclidine (PCP)	1-(1-Phencyclohexyl)piperidine
Ketamine	2-(*O*-Chlorophenyl)-2-(methylamino)cyclohexanone
Phenylethylamine Derivatives	
Mescaline	3,4,5-Trimethoxyphenylethylamine
STP/DOM	2,5-Dimethoxy-4-methylamphetamine
DOE	2,5-Dimethoxy-4-ethylamphetamine
DOB	2.5-Dimethoxy-4-bromoamphetamine
MDA	Methylenedioxyamphetamine
DOET	Dimethoxyethylamphetamine
MMDA	3 Methoxy-4,5-methylenedioxyamphetamine
PMA	*p*-Methoxyamphetamine
TMA	3,4,5-Trimethoxyamphetamine
Cannabinols	
Marijuana	Δ^9-Tetrahydrocannabinol

From Leikin JB, Krantz AJ, Zell-Kanter M, et al. Clinical features and management of intoxication due to hallucinogenic drugs. Med Toxicol Adverse Drug Experience 1989;4:324–350.

United States has been sporadic. It is generally available only by prescription; other hallucinogens may be cheaper and more pleasant.[151]

Trihexyphenidyl has been widely enjoyed by prison inmates as a drug of abuse: "If I take five Artanes I can see my mother. If I take 10 Artanes, I can see my girlfriend."[152] Some inmates crush the trihexyphenidyl tablets, mix the powder with tobacco, and smoke the mixture in an attempt to obtain a high. Trihexyphenidyl tablets serve as a type of prison currency for which the inmates gamble.[153,154]

With respect to its use as an antiparkinsonian drug, trihexyphenidyl has been replaced by L-dopa, and some of the toxic reactions associated with its abuse may be missed in psychiatric populations where such symptoms are common.[151]

Benztropine Mesylate

Other similar drugs that may be abused include biperiden hydrochloride, 2-mg tablets (Akineton oral); biperiden lactate, parenteral 5 mg/mL (Akineton); orphenadrine citrate (see Muscle Relaxants); and procyclidine hydrochloride (Kemadrine).[155,156]

Table 19–12
Therapeutic Drugs Associated With Hallucinations

Drug	Type of Hallucination
Acyclovir	V,T
Amantidine	A,V
Baclofen	A,V
Benztropine	V
Biperiden	V
Bromocriptine	A,V
Carbamazepine	V
Chlordiazepoxide	V
Chlorpheniramine	A,V
Chlorpromazine	A,V
Cimetidine	A,V
Clonazepam	A,V,T
Clonidine	A,V
Cyclosporine	V
Dantrolene	A,V
Dextromethorphan	A,V
Diethylpropion	A
Digoxin	A,V
Dimenhydrinate	A,V
Diphenhydramine	V
Disopyramide	A,V
Ephedrine	A,V
Gentamicin	NS
Griseofulvin	A
Hyoscine (scopolamine)	NS
Imipramine	V
Indomethacin	V,O
Isosorbide	V
Levodopa	A,V
Lorazepam	V
Metaproterenol	V,G
Methyldopa	V
Methylphenidate	V
Methylprednisolone	V
Minocycline	V
Pemoline	A,V,T
Phenylzine	A,V
Phenylephrine	A,V
Pindolol	A
Procainamide	V
Propranolol	V
Quinidine	NS
Ranitidine	A,V
Streptokinase	NS
Sulfasalazine	V
Timolol	NS
Triazolam	A,V,T
Trihexyphenidyl	A,V
Vidarabine	NS

A, auditory; V, visual; T, tactile; G, gustatory; O, olfactory; NS not specified. From Leikin JB, Krantz AJ, Zell-Kanter M, et al. Clinical features and management of intoxication due to hallucinogenic drugs. Med Toxicol Adverse Drug Experience 1989;4:324–350.

Clinical Diagnosis

Antiparkinsonian drug ingestion may result in central and peripheral nervous system side effects similar to those seen with other anticholinergic agents. Mild side effects

Table 19–13
Miscellaneous Plants of Abuse

Plant	Part Used	Toxic Agent
Argyreia nervosa	Seed	Ergoline hallucinogens
Atropa belladonna	Seed	Tropane alkaloids
Banistereopsis species	Various	Harmaline (hallucinogen)
Cola nitida	Seed	Caffeine
Datura species	Seed	Tropane alkaloids
Hyoscyamus niger	Whole plant	Tropine alkaloids
Ilex paraguarensis	Leaf	Caffeine
Mandragora officinarum	Whole plant	Tropane alkaloids
Methysticodendron amesianum	Stems/leaf	Tropane alkaloids
Mimosa hostilis	Root	Phenylamine hallucinogens
Olmedioperebea sclerophylla	Fruit	Unknown hallucinogen
Passiflora incarnata	Stem/leaf	Harmaline (hallucinogen)
Pelganum harmala	Seed	Harmaline (hallucinogen)
Piper methysticum	Root	Methysticin/kawain
Piptadenia colubrina	Seed	Phenylamine hallucinogens
Piptadenia excelsa	Seed	Phenylamine hallucinogens
Piptadenia macrocarpa	Seed	Phenylamine hallucinogens
Piptadenia peregrina	Seed/bark	Phenylamine hallucinogens
Salvia divinorum	Leaf	Unknown hallucinogen
Sophora secundiflora	Seed	Cytisine (stimulant)
Tabernanthe iboga	Root	Ibogaine (hallucinogen)
Trichocereus pachanoi	Cactus	Mescaline
Virola calophylla	Bark	Phenylamine hallucinogens

From Spoerke DG, Hall AH. Plants and mushrooms of abuse. Emerg Med Clin North Am 1990;8:579–593.

include dilated pupils, hyperpyrexia, dry skin, flushed facies, constipation, tachycardia, nervousness, dizziness, dryness of the mouth, ataxia, and urinary retention. There is one anecdotal report on memory and cognitive impairment.[157] The toxic psychosis consists of confusion, excitement, restlessness, hallucinations, paranoid ideation, disorientation in time, and, occasionally, euphoria.[158,159]

An overdosage may be used specifically to induce this type of toxic state. At dose ranges below the toxic level, these drugs are usually used to achieve euphoriant, antidepressant, and socially stimulating effects.[157]

Tolerance may develop following the misuse of trihexyphenidyl and benztropine. Patients may stop taking their required neuroleptic medication and increase their dose of trihexyphenidyl for its euphoriant effects. A type of physiologic addiction may be evident if such withdrawal results in myalgias, diaphoresis, gastrointestinal distress, anxiety, hallucinations, and rebound exacerbation of motor dysfunction in patients with parkinsonism or neuroleptic-induced extrapyramidal effects.[160]

Treatment

Clinicians need to be aware of the potential for such drug abuse.[161] Drug-seeking behavior, feigning of extrapyramidal adverse effects, hallucinations, or unusual excitability should alert the health care provider to a possible drug abuse state. The prophylactic use of anticholinergic agents in patients using antipsychotic drugs is to be avoided unless such patients develop extrapyramidal signs.[161] In young polydrug abusers with poor social relationships, considerable thought should be given before prescribing anticholinergic drugs.[162] It is, however, important not to withhold these drugs from patients who need them.[151]

There are specific dangers inherent in physostigmine use (see Chapter 38).[159]

JIMSON WEED

Jimson weed is a ubiquitous plant that grows in fields and along roadsides. In the fall, seed pods produce multiple small, black seeds that teenagers sometimes abuse for a hallucinogenic high. As jimson weed parties are not uncommon, often multiple teenagers are involved when exposures occur. Although the seeds can cause hallucinations, numerous adverse effects are also involved. Frightened teenagers usually seek treatment at the local emergency department within several hours of ingestion when the unpleasant adverse effects do not resolve.

CLENBUTEROL

Clenbuterol, chemical name[163] 4-amino-α-[(*tert*-butylamine)methyl]-3,5-dichlorobenzyl alcohol hydrochloride, is a sympathomimetic bronchodilator[164–166] that can affect muscle mass and function. Clenbuterol stimulates protein deposition in striated muscle (20% increase) and simultaneously increases energy expenditure and hence reduces muscle glycogen and body fat deposition (20% decrease).[164] These properties are often seen with other classic beta-adrenoceptor agonists. The effects on cardiac muscle are propranolol sensitive, and probably β_1-adrenoceptor-mediated skeletal muscle may respond to β_2-adrenoceptors, atypical adrenoceptors, and even non-receptor-mediated pathways. Clenbuterol induces a true hypertrophy of muscle (type II fibers) and an increase in the 1-glycolytic capacity of the muscle as a whole, giving rise to an increase in force and a reduction in relaxation time.[167,168] Clenbuterol and similar beta agonists taken in large doses can induce a protein anabolic response that may enhance performance.[164] Athletes feel that they can derive 10 to 25% of the effect of anabolic steroids by taking between 60 and 100 μg of clenbuterol per day. Some take as much as 600 μg per day.

Clenbuterol has also been used as a uterine relaxant without noticeable side effects on the fetus.[169] Its half-life is 29 hours.[169] The Sports Council has considered β_2-agonists to be related to androgenic anabolic steroids.[170]

Therapeutic Dose

Clenbuterol is used as a β_2-receptor agonist in obstructive lung disease[171,172] where it is administered in doses of 20 to 40 μg twice daily.[173] It may improve pulmonary function equal to the action of terbutaline.

Toxicokinetics

About 34 to 43% of an administered dose is excreted in the urine as unchanged drug.[172]

Laboratory

Analytical Methods

Clenbuterol can be quantitated in the urine using high-performance thin-layer chromatography and capillary gas chromatography with electron-capture detection. The detection limit is 0.2 ppb.

Adverse Effects

Clenbuterol is a self-limiting compound because headaches can be disturbing to the user. Clenbuterol may lead to a dose-dependent tremor and palpitations.[163,171,172] Tardive dyskinesia has been described after long-term treatment.[165] At high doses it is associated with headaches, nervousness, lightheadedness,[165] an increase in heart rate, and a slight rise in systolic blood pressure.[163] A decrease in T-wave amplitude may be seen on the electrocardiogram.[163]

CODEINE–ACETYLSALICYLIC ACID

Drug abusers have found that codeine is easily separated from some drugs containing acetylsalicylic acid and codeine. The codeine can be used orally or intravenously.[173]

LAXATIVES

Use of castor oil orally to induce labor was noted by the ancient Egyptians and has also been recommended as a home remedy.[174] A 33-year-old gravida 4, para 2, 40-week gestation ingested about 30 mL of castor oil in an attempt to induce labor. In approximately 60 minutes, the patient experienced spontaneous rupture of her membranes and suffered a cardiorespiratory arrest, secondary to an amniotic fluid embolism with disseminated intravascular coagulation (see also Chapter 52).

Clinical Presentation

The major findings in a laxative abuse patient include chronic diarrhea, vomiting, abdominal pain, lassitude, thirst, weakness (15%), edema, bone pain resulting from osteomalacia, and weight loss.[175,176]

Findings may disclose a protein-losing enteropathy, steatorrhea, pathologic colon changes associated with featureless radiologic findings (10–30%), acid–base abnormalities (20–25%), and hypokalemia (20–25%).[177]

Such patients do not readily comply with treatment recommendations. Metabolic problems may be secondary to chronic potassium depletion, a toxic effect on the nerve supply to the colon, or an injury to the liver.[177]

Magnesium-Containing Cathartics

Laxative abuse with magnesium-containing cathartics may induce hypermagnesemia, quadriparesis, and neuromuscular junction defects.[178,179] A 25-day-old infant was "limp" and "would not wake up" following administration of magnesium hydroxide (Philip's Milk of Magnesia, 8 teaspoonfuls per day, equivalent to 1297.4 mg of elemental magnesium or 381.6 mg/kg/d). (The recommended doses of magnesium hydroxide are 40 mg/kg/dose or 0.5 mL/kg/dose as needed for children older than 5 years; 0.4 to 1.2 g in 2- (to 5-year-olds; and 1 to 2 teaspoonfuls in infants older than 6 months.) The infant's serum magnesium level was 7.7 mEq/L (normal, 1.6–2.4 mEq/L). After treatment with 5% glucose in 0.33% saline with 30 mEq potassium chloride intravenously and calcium gluconate 100 mg/kg intravenously IV with electrocardiographic monitoring, the sensorium improved within 5 hours. At 18 hours, the serum magnesium was 3.2 mEq/L and the infant was easily arousable.

Management consists of discontinuing administration of magnesium and elimination of magnesium as a source of enema if it is in the bowel. Activated charcoal does not absorb magnesium salts. Monitoring of blood electrolyte, calcium, and phosphorus levels, renal function, fluid intake, urine output, and an electrocardiogram is indicated.[180] If the patient is symptomatic (hypotonic, central nervous system depression) or has electrocardiographic changes and the serum magnesium is above 2.9 mg/dL (2.3 mEq/L or 1.1 μmol/L), therapy should be considered.[181] Therapy consists of the intravenous administration of 10 to 20 mL of 10% calcium gluconate solution in adults or 100 mg/kg in infants and children up to a maximum of 1 g slowly over 5 to 10 minutes with electrocardiographic monitoring. If renal function is normal, alternate therapy includes intravenous furosemide 40 mg in adults or 1 mg/kg in infants and children with replacement of the urine volume with 0.89% saline intravenously. Dialysis may be useful in the management of severe symptomatic hypermagnesemia or in cases of renal failure. Exchange transfusion may be useful in newborns suffering from severe magnesium intoxication. Blood pressure support and assisted ventilation may be required. A decrease in the deep tendon reflexes may predict impending respiratory failure. Absence of the deep tendon reflexes indicates a serum magnesium level of 12 mg/dL or greater (10 mEq/L or 5 μmol/L). Aminoglycosides should be avoided as they potentiate the neuromuscular blockade of magnesium.[182]

Laboratory

Once the diagnosis of laxative abuse is considered, several approaches may be taken to confirm the etiology (Table 19–14).

Liver function tests may be abnormal in patients with senna abuse.[183]

A high-performance thin-layer chromatography method has been proposed for urine screening of all phenolic and

Table 19–14
Laboratory Evaluation for Laxative Abuse

- Barium enema to test for cathartic colon (ahaustral right colon)
- Sigmoidoscopy for gross presence of melanosis coli (microscopic form is often a normal variant)
- Alkalinization assay of stool: phenolphthalein, some anthraquinones, and rhubarb turn red; bisacodyl turns purple-blue
- Spectrophotometry* or thin-layer chromatography* of urine or stool water: detects anthraquinones, bisacodyl, phenolphthalein; can detect anthraquinones >32 h after one dose
- Measurement of stool osmolality: only useful if <250 mOsm/kg (implying dilution of stool with water or urine)
- Measurement of stool sodium and potassium; calculation of fecal osmotic gap: 290 – 2 × (stool sodium concentration + stool potassium concentration)
- Stool osmotic gap: if >50 mOsm/kg, measure stool magnesium (normally <45 mmol/L or <30 mEq/L)
- Measurement of stool sulfate and phosphate

*These tests are usually done in a commercial or referral laboratory. The stool specimen should be liquid and frozen. A "laxative survey" request will usually result in chromotographic, spectrophotometric, and other methods of detecting anthraquinones, bisacodyl, phenolphthalein, castor oil, mineral oil, magnesium, and phosphate. Docusate sodium, the active ingredient in Colace, can be detected by thin-layer chromatography but is not measured in the currently available laxative screens.
From Donowitz M, Kokke FT, Saidi R. Evaluation of patients with chronic diarrhea. N Engl J Med 1995;332:725–729.

anthraquinone laxatives.[184] A gas chromatography method with multiple ion detection has been useful in obtaining a positive urine identification of dioxyanthraquinone phenolphthalein, oxyphenacetin, and bisacodyl.[185]

A qualitative test for urinary detection of anthraquinone excretion products has been described.[186]

The Fecal Osmotic Gap

In some patients the sum of stool electrolytes is equal to or less than the stool osmolality and the total stool electrolytes can be estimated by the equation 2 × (stool sodium concentration plus stool potassium concentration), 2([Na] + [K]). In the patient with so-called osmotic diarrhea, the stool osmolality is greater than 2 ([Na] + [K]), and in the patient with so-called secretory diarrhea, the stool osmolality is equal to total stool electrolytes. A gap of less than 10 mOsm/kg indicates secretory diarrhea and a gap less than 50 indicates osmotic diarrhea. An osmotic gap of 50 provides a discrimination between osmotic diarrhea and experimental secretory diarrhea with one exception: the osmotic gap in all subjects who receive phenolphthalein is less than 50, and in those who receive magnesium hydroxide, polyethylene glycol, lactulose, or sorbitol, the osmotic gap is >50. Thus, an osmotic gap of 50 discriminates between pure osmotic diarrhea and pure secretory diarrhea.[180,187–189]

Treatment

Physician empathy, psychiatric intervention, and continuous psychosocial support while investigation proceeds constitute treatment.

MUNCHAUSEN'S SYNDROME

Some of the following features may help to identify a Munchausen's patient:

1. Pseudologica fantastica is habitual and uncontrollable pathologic lying with content intriguing to the listener, characterized by fantastic details, such as being a military commander captured by the enemy, an undersea diver working with Jacques Cousteau, a fighter pilot, a former member of underground resistance forces, a submarine commander tortured by the Gestapo, a wrestling champion, a criminal lawyer, a private investigator, or even a physician. The usually dramatic medical histories, however, are vague in their details, inconsistent, and embellished with ready excuses for discrepancies.
2. Evidence, often visible, of previous medical or surgical care, such as scarring of all superficial veins, venous cutdown scars, gridiron abdomen, and cranial burrholes may be observed. The patient often has actually wandered from hospital to hospital, to different cities, different parts of the country, or even to foreign countries.
3. These patients are medically sophisticated and can often recount textbook descriptions of the onset and causes of their alleged illnesses.
4. These patients flaunt hospital rules, shift complaints from one organ system to another, and require additional consultations.
5. They demand medication, most frequently narcotic and nonnarcotic analgesics.
6. Despite long hospital stays, these patients rarely have visitors. If they do, more often than not the visitor turns out to be an accomplice supplying necessary paraphernalia to continue the simulation.
7. These patients are truculent and evasive.
8. The immediate medical history portrays acute and harrowing events, but yet is not entirely convincing. No real evidence of a pathologic lesion or dysfunction is discernable, despite an apparent acute presentation of illness. Examples include overwhelmingly severe abdominal pain of an uncertain type, cataclysmal blood loss unsupported by corresponding pallor, and or dramatic loss of consciousness.
9. The family or medical history proves to be unreliable.[190,191]

Munchausen's syndrome by proxy[192] describes those parents who, by falsification, cause their children innumerable painful hospital procedures. The disorder is a form of child abuse.[193] Criteria for the diagnosis include (1) illness in a child is fabricated by a parent or someone who is in loco parentis; (2) presentation of a child for medical assessment and care, usually persistently, often resulting in multiple medical procedures; (3) denial of the etiology of the child's illness by the perpetrator; and (4) cessation of acute symptoms and signs of illness when the child is separated from the perpetrator (almost always the mother).[177,194]

Malignant Munchausen's syndrome describes patients who present with fabricated stories and signs, often with heavily scarred abdomens, and are diagnosed as having malignant disease. Such patients may be seen at multiple institutions.[177]

Cases of fictitious AIDS have been reported with increasing frequency since the onset of the AIDS epidemic. Patients typically give a complete history of opportunistic infections and present with acute neurologic or psychiatric complaints. Most are members of groups at high risk for HIV infection.[195]

Diagnosis

Poisoning as a part of Munchausen's syndrome has been reported with vitamin D (hypercalcemia),[196] carbamazepine (Munchausen's syndrome by proxy),[197] ipecac-induced starvation in a child (of an anorexic mother with a prior history of Munchausen's syndrome by proxy), phenolphthalein-induced diarrhea in three siblings,[198] self-injection of corn starch (sudden death) by a 31-year-old man with a history of Munchausen's,[199] and phenolphthalein-induced diarrhea in a 34-month-old child.[200] An 18-year-old woman with subcutaneous emphysema of the face injected air, and recovered.[201] Munchausen's syndrome by proxy is also known as Polle syndrome, named after the sole son of Baron von Munchausen who died at 1 year of age.[185]

INTRAVENOUS DRUG ABUSERS

How Do Intravenous Drug Abusers Die?

Autopsy reviews of the cause of death of 274 patients with evidence of intravenous drug abuse admitted to a large public hospital indicate that 127 died from diseases unrelated to intravenous drug abuse. In 41% of these deaths, chronic alcoholism was implicated. Deaths from overdose syndromes and drug-related organ pathology constituted only 11% of all cases. The mean age at death was 39 years. Half of all patients died from infection, 72 from AIDS.[202] AIDS has, in fact, replaced hepatitis as the major nonbacterial infection associated with intravenous drug abuse. HIV-infected drug abusers may die from bacterial infections before clinical AIDS develops. Transmission of HIV by blood is highly efficient, often requiring only one exposure.[203] Mortality reports on alcoholics and drug addicts suggest that there is no evidence that narcotic misuse has life-threatening chronic effects comparable to those of alcohol abuse. Joint misuse of drugs and alcohol affects mortality adversely.

Non-HIV Infections

Non-HIV infections of intravenous drug abusers (IVDAs) are presented in Table 19–15.[204] Respiratory complications suffered by IVDAs are summarized in Table 19–16.[205]

"Cotton Fever"

"Cotton fever" is a febrile reaction seen in drug abusers who have injected dry suspensions that have been filtered through cotton balls. It appears to be a benign self-limited condition that begins 10 to 20 minutes after injection. Symptoms may include headache, malaise, chills, dyspnea, palpitations, nausea, vomiting, abdominal pain, low back pain, myalgias, and arthralgias. The patient appears acutely ill, and develops a temperatures of 38.5 to 40.3°C within the first hours after injection. Tachycardia and tachypnea are present despite normal cardiorespiratory examination and chest radiographs. Abdominal, muscle, and joint tenderness may be present. The serum leukocyte counts range from 5700 to 35,000/mm^3. Liver enzyme levels may be moderately elevated. Arterial blood gases are normal and blood cultures show no growth. The syndrome usually resolves spontaneously in 12 to 24 hours. It has perhaps declined with the use of crack cocaine; as heroin makes its comeback, it may once again be seen in the emergency department. It is difficult to diagnose a drug abuser with a high fever prospectively. A vigorous

Table 19–15
Non-HIV Infections of Intravenous Drug Abusers

Viral hepatitis	Endocarditis
Hepatitis A	Central nervous system infection
Hepatitis B	Tetanus
Hepatitis C	Wound botulism
Delta hepatitis	Fungal meningitis
Sexually transmitted disease	Fungal cerebritis
Gonorrhea	Endophthalmitis
Syphilis	Spinal abscess
Bone and joint infection	Epidural abscess
Septic arthritis	Brain abscess
Osteitis pubis	Cerebral mucormycosis
Osteoarticular candidiasis	Tubercular meningitis
Osteomyelitis	Systemic candidiasis
Skin and soft tissue infection	Candidal meningitis
Cellulitis	Human T-lymphotropic virus type I and II infections
Phlebitis	Tuberculosis
Jugular venous thrombosis	Tickborne relapsing fever†
Penile gangrene	
Pyomyositis	
Gas gangrene	

Adapted from Haverkos HW, Langer WR. Serious infections other than human immunodeficiency virus among intravenous drug abusers. J Infect Dis 1990;161:894–902.

*Ostrea EM, Jr, Porter T, Balun J, et al. Effects of chronic maternal drug addiction on placental drug metabolism. Dev Pharmacol Ther 1989;12:42–48.

†Lopez-Cortes L, Lozano de Leon F, Gomez-Mateos JM, et al. Tick-borne relapsing fever in intravenous drug abusers. J Infect Dis 1989;159:804.

Table 19–16
Effects of Intravenous Drug Abuse on the Respiratory System

Lung abscess
  Single: due to narcotic or sedative–hypnotic stupor with aspiration
  Multiple: IV drug abuse, right-sided endocarditis, or septic thrombophlebitis; *Staphylococcus aureus* most common
Tuberculosis, in heroin addicts
  Pulmonary
  Extrapulmonary
Allergic bronchopulmonary aspergillosis: marijuana contamination
Bronchiolitis obliterans: smoking free-base cocaine
Respiratory failure
Injury to upper airway: sniffing
Pulmonary edema
Pulmonary talcosis
Pulmonary embolization of needle fragments
Pulmonary fibrosis: talc
Bullous parenchymal changes
Atelectasis
Pulmonary vascular changes
Empyema
Pneumothorax
Bronchopleural fistula
Pneumomediastinum (free-base cocaine smoking, marijuana smoking, heroin intravenous injection)

Adapted from Glassroth J, Adams GD, Schnoll S. The impact of substance abuse on the respiratory system. Chest 1987;91:596–602.

investigation must be made for a source of infection in all such patients. Perhaps "cotton fever" is a retrospective diagnosis.[206]

Fever

Fever in the IVDA may be associated with both infectious and noninfectious causes (Table 19–17).[207]

Stroke

Stroke associated with drug abuse has become a serious neurologic problem (Table 19–9). Symptoms usually occur within 48 hours of exposure.[208]

Donation and Sale of Blood

Intravenous drug abusers continue to donate and sell their blood. About 20% of those IVDAs who had donated or sold blood since 1985 tested positive for antibodies to HIV type I, and about 6% tested positive for antibodies to human T-lymphotropic virus types I and II. Increased effort is required to screen prospective donors and sellers, particularly at commercial blood banks.[209]

Table 19–17
Potential Causes of Fever in the Intravenous Drug Abuser

- I. Infectious
  - A. Intravenous Drug Abuse-related
    - 1. Common
      - Cardiovascular: endocarditis/endovascular infection
      - Pulmonary: pneumonia, septic pulmonary emboli, abscess, empyema, aspiration
      - Skin and soft tissue: cellulitis, subcutaneous abscess
      - Hepatitis
      - Sexually transmitted disease
      - Osteomyelitis
      - Septic arthritis
      - Transient bacteremia
      - Septic thrombophlebitis
      - HIV-related opportunistic infection
      - Mycotic aneurysm
    - 2. Uncommon
      - Meningitis, brain abscess
      - Tetanus
      - Botulism
      - Malaria
  - B. Non–drug-related
    - Viral, bacterial, mycobacterial, parasitic
- II. Presumed noninfectious: particular to the intravenous drug abuser
  - Acute drug withdrawal syndrome
  - Acute drug intoxication (eg, cocaine)
  - "Cotton fever"
  - "Musculoskeletal syndrome"
  - Brown (Mexican) heroin
  - Drug hypersensitivity reactions
- III. Miscellaneous
  - Neoplasms
  - Connective tissue disease
  - Granulomatous disease
  - Endocrine disorders
  - Metabolic/inherited disease
  - Drug fevers

From Levine DP, Sobel JD. *Infections in Intravenous Drug Abusers.* New York: Oxford University Press, 1991.

Fingerstick Blood Screening

Surveillance of HIV type I disease in IVDAs may be facilitated by the fingerstick paper absorption method of blood collection and analysis. The method is simple, rapid, safe, easy to perform, and may be useful for street outreach, outpatient screening programs for IVDAs and their contacts, and large-scale epidemiologic surveys.[210]

Other Diseases

Tuberculosis (from reactivation of latent tuberculosis infection),[211] Hodgkin's disease,[212] and Reye's syndrome,[213] have been described in IVDAs with HIV infection.

Purified protein derivative (PPD) tuberculin positivity (induration ≥5 mm) is less likely to be positive in HIV-I seropositive patients than in HIV-I seronegative patients. Skin test anergy (to mumps and *Candida*) is higher in the HIV-I seropositive group and increases as the CD4+ lymphocyte count falls. Delayed-type hypersensitivity is seriously depressed in HIV-I seropositive IVDAs. Anergy testing appears mandatory to assess a negative PPD test result.[214] IVDAs continue to be at higher risk for tuberculosis both because of drug use[215] and because of HIV-related immunosuppression.[216,217]

Sodium Hypochlorite Injections

A 5.25% solution of sodium hypochlorite (household bleach) effectively inactivates HIV. IVDAs who share needles are at high risk of acquiring and transmitting HIV. Cleaning needles and syringes with household bleach is used as a strategy to control HIV transmission in this group. Usually, the syringe is flushed twice with undiluted household bleach and then twice with water. An IVDA who attempted suicide with an intravenous injection of a 0.3 mL of a 5.25% sodium hypochlorite solution suffered few toxic effects from the bleach.[218] Others have injected 0.5 mL[27] and 1.8 mL[28] of this solution into tissue and experienced pain and edema that subsided in 1 week. One patient who was inadvertently administered 30 mL of sodium hypochlorite by intravenous infusion experienced a cardiorespiratory arrest but recovered.[219] Perhaps these experiences may be used to reassure the IVDA who may inadvertently inject some residual bleach that remains in the syringe or a needle after the disinfecting procedure outlined above.[218]

KETAMINE

Ketamine hydrochloride is available in vials containing 10 to 50 mg and 100 mg of ketamine per milliliter. It is available as Ketalar in the United States and other countries and also as Ketaject in the United States and Ketanest in Germany. (See also Chapter 56.)

Sources

Ketamine hydrochloride is a synthetic drug. Street names for ketamine solutions include K, Jet, Super Acid, and 1980. Powders are called Green, Purple, Mauve, Special LA Coke, Super C, and Super K.[220] Ketamine has a green crystalline appearance; a color results from its mixture with vitamin B_{12} which is thought to minimize adverse reactions.[220]

Clinical Presentation

Ketamine use may be followed by hallucinations, delirium, irrational behavior, blurred vision, nausea, vomiting, respiratory stimulation or depression, tachycardia or bradycardia, hypertension or hypotension, seizures, and cardiac arrhythmias.[221]

Ketamine induces a clinical state of "dissociative anesthesia" during which the patient is dissociated from his environment but not necessarily asleep.

Spontaneous involuntary movement, nystagmus, and hypertonus may occur.[222] Disadvantages of ketamine use include its slow onset of action, increased muscle tone, jerky spontaneous muscular movements that occur during induction and anesthesia, cardiovascular stimulation, slow recovery, and postoperative nausea and vomiting. Emergency sequelae may include auditory and visual hallucinations, restlessness, disorientation, confused and irrational behavior, and vivid dreams and may last up to 24 hours after ketamine anesthesia.[222]

Acute toxic effects include the following:

- Cardiovascular: increase in mean aortic pressure, pulmonary artery pressure, central venous pressure, heart rate, cardiac index, myocardial depressant effect; reduction in ejection fraction; arrhythmias including supraventricular tachycardias[223]
- Respiratory: laryngospasm, coughing (pharyngeal and laryngeal reflexes remain active during ketamine anesthesia), increase in pharyngeal secretions, bronchodilation, transient apnea, reduction in respiratory rate and tidal volume
- Psychic: hallucinations, alterations in perception of body image, unpleasant dreams
- Muscular: increased muscle tone, sudden jerky movements that may interfere with surgery
- Neurologic: seizures, polyneuropathies, ataxia, visual distortions and illusions, and slurring of speech (reported in recreational users)
- Eyes: increased intraocular pressure, blurred vision
- Mouth: hypersalivation
- Gastrointestinal: nausea and vomiting (may follow low doses of 0.25 and 0.5 g/kg of intramuscular ketamine)

There does not appear to be strong evidence to support any permanent changes in personality or intellectual function (decrease in memory) following the one-time use of ketamine as an anesthetic[226,227]; however, no controlled clinical studies are available. Hallucinatory recurrence without additional use of the drug may occur in drug abusers[228–230]; similarly, the possibility of psychosis exists from recurrent use of ketamine.

Treatment

Stabilization

1. Admit to an intensive care unit.
2. Available equipment and expertise for advanced airway management (e.g., intubation) are mandatory.[231]
3. Any form of unconsciousness or deep sedation should be followed by periodic vital sign measurement and continuous cardiac and respiratory monitoring or oximetry.
4. A physician or nurse must be in constant attendance from the time of injection until recovery is well established.
5. Alpha and beta blocking agents, verapamil, and benzodiazepines have been shown to block cardiovascular stimulation.[224]
6. Use of ketamine in young potentially drug-abusing patients is not advisable. Death has apparently occurred in patients who had misrepresented their drug habits.[232] Special close observation in the recovery room and in the period thereafter for at least 48 hours will alert the staff to any secondary respiratory depression.
7. Ketamine anesthesia and unconsciousness should be managed with naloxone, glucose, oxygen, and mechanical ventilation according to clinical discretion.
8. Naloxone may counteract ketamine anesthesia.[233] Further confirmation of these data is required.[234]

Elimination Enhancement

Only a minor fraction of the ketamine dose is eliminated during hemodialysis (10%) or hemofiltration (4%).[223]

Antidote

There is no antidote.

Supportive Measures

Hypersalivation following ketamine use can be minimized with concurrent atropine (0.01 mg/kg, maximum total dose 0.5 mg) or glycopyrrolate (0.005 mg/kg, maximum total dose 0.25 mg).[225,231]

Mild disequilibrium may persist for 1 to 4 hours after ketamine administration. Close professional or parental observation should be maintained during this period.

Seizures respond to diazepam, phenytoin, phenobarbital, or paralysis. Emergency delirium usually responds to benzodiazepines, or droperidol.[235] Dystonic reactions may be managed with diphenhydramine.[220] Hypertension may respond to beta blockers, especially if patients are also receiving thyroid replacement therapy.[236]

Patients should be placed in a quiet, darkened room until they recover. Diazepam may be given for unresponsive panic attacks.[237]

LABORATORY

Screening for and diagnosis of substance abuse are outlined in Table 19–18.

Table 19–18
Screening for and Diagnosis of Substance Abuse

History of Substance Abuse	
Substances used	Opioids (eg, heroin, prescription analgesics)
	Stimulants (eg, cocaine, prescription stimulants)
	Alcohol (eg, beer, wine, spirits, nonbeverage sources)
	Sedative–hypnotics (eg, benzodiazepines, barbiturates)
	Tobacco (eg, cigarettes, chewing tobacco)
	Other (eg, marijuana, hallucinogens, solvents)
Route of administration	Injection (eg, intravenous, subcutaneous, intramuscular)
	Intranasal
	Inhaled
	Oral
Pattern of use	Amount
	Frequency
	Duration
	Most recent use
	Needle sharing or shooting gallery use
Treatment history	Setting (outpatient, inpatient, residential)
	Drug treatment program
	Pharmacologic treatment
	Treatment outcome
Complications of Substance Abuse	
Medical	Needle-induced: viral, bacterial, and fungal infections, peripheral vascular disease
	Drug-induced: overdose, withdrawal, organ-specific complications (eg, nephropathy due to heroin, cardiac ischemia due to cocaine, gastrointestinal, cardiac, and neurologic disease due to alcohol)
	Other: tuberculosis, sexually transmitted disease
Social	Unemployment
	Family disruption
	Legal problems
	Homelessness
Physical Examinations	
Signs of injection drug use	Recent: "tracks," cellulitis, abscess
	Past: "track" or abscess scars
Signs of intoxication	Opioids (lethargy, pinpoint pupils)
	Cocaine (hypertension, tachycardia, agitation)
	Alcohol, benzodiazepines, other drugs
Signs of withdrawal	Opioids (tachycardia, hypertension, lacrimation, piloerection)
	Cocaine (depressed mood)
	Alcohol, benzodiazepines, other drugs
Evidence of medical complications	
Laboratory Tests	
Toxicologic screening of urine	
Screening for medical complications	

From O'Connor PG, Selwyn PA, Schottenfeld RS. Medical care for injection-drug users with human immunodeficiency virus infection. N Engl J Med 1994;331:450–459.

Table 19–19
Cutoff Levels Established by the Department of Health and Human Services Testing of Drugs and Their Metabolites

	Cutoff Level (ng/mL)	
Drug or Metabolite	Initial Test	Confirmatory Test
Marijuana metabolites	100	15
Cocaine metabolites	300	150
Opiates	300	
Morphine		300
Codeine		300
Phencyclidine	25	25
Amphetamines	1000	
Amphetamine		500
Methamphetamine		500

Source: U.S. Department of Transportation, October 1990, Code of Federal Regulations, Title 40, Subtitle A, Part 40, p. 540, October 1, 1993.

URINE TESTS

Urine tests for drugs of abuse comprise two types of analytical procedures: screening tests and confirmatory tests (Table 19–19). Screening tests are usually rapid and inexpensive. Confirmatory tests may be able to reduce the number of false-positive results.[238]

Workplace

The Mandatory Guidelines for Federal Workplace Drug Testing Programs require the use of immunoassay techniques for initial drug tests and gas chromatography–mass spectrometry for a confirmatory test[239] (Table 19–19).

Screening Tests

Indications

Marked deterioration or aberration in a young person's behavior, mood, rationality, and thought (hallucinations, paranoia, schizophrenia); deterioration in academic performance or school or work attendance; conduct or antisocial disorders such as repetitive lying, stealing, and disrespect of the rights of others; recurrent violence toward other individuals or toward property; serious depressive or biphasic mood disorders; some suicide attempts; unexplained fatigue in a person whose life is deteriorating; chronic vasomotor rhinitis; seizure disorder or coma of unexplained etiology; and graduation from treatment facilities for cannabis, cocaine, or opiate dependence are all good indications for a screening test for drugs of abuse.[238]

Specimen Collection

Chain of Custody. A urine specimen for drugs of abuse must be documented from the time it has been passed from the body, through its transport in a labeled, sealed container, and during its laboratory analysis. An unsupervised urine sample should have a urine pH, temperature, and specific gravity recorded immediately after voiding. If the specimen is freshly voided, the urine temperature should range between 33 and 36°C and the urinary pH between 4.6 and 8.0.

Storage. A urine specimen can be stored at room temperature for up to 3 days or in the refrigerator for 1 week, but is best frozen at –6.6°C or lower for a prolonged period (weeks to months). Samples to be analyzed for LSD should be protected from strong light.

Follow-up

If a single urine specimen is positive, additional tests at periodic and irregular intervals may be more meaningful than the single test.

Cutoff Point

A cutoff point is the threshold value set by the manufacturer of the drug analyzing equipment that indicates at what point there is a demonstrably high statistical probability that the drug will be detected if present (Table 19–19). Results that fall below the cutoff point are recorded as negative even though a more sensitive method or lower cutoff (detection) point would give a positive result.[238] Cutoff points are based on limits of detection by the particular analytical method used, cross-reactivity considerations, experience, and the confirmation technology (usually the gas chromatography–mass spectrometry procedure).

Table 19–20
Potential Cross-reacting Drugs for the Five Major Drug Types

Enzyme Immunoassay/ Radioimmunoassay	Potential Cross-Reacting Substance
Marijuana (cannabinoids)	Ibuprofen (Advil, Nuprin, Motrin)
	Fenoprofen (Nalfon)
	Naproxen (Naprosyn)
Cocaine	Coca leaf tea*
Opiates	Dextromethorphan
	Chlorpromazine (Thorazine)
	Poppy seeds (large amounts)
Phencyclidine	Chlorpromazine
	Thioridazine (Mellaril)
	Meperidine (Demerol)
	Detromethorphan
	Diphenhydramine (Benadryl)
	Doxylamine (Unisom)
Amphetamines	Ephedrine
	Methylphenidate (Ritalin)
	Phenylpropanolamine (PPA)
	Other weight-reducing and decongestant drugs

*Note: This is not actually a cross-reactivity but the presence of cocaine in the tea.
Source: U.S. Department of Transportation, October 1990. Code of Federal Regulations, Title 40, Subtitle A, Part 40, p. 540, October 1, 1993.

Confirmatory Tests

Gas chromatography–mass spectrometry (GC/MS) is the standard reference method for confirmation of toxicologic analysis. It can detect most drugs in low nanogram-per-milliliter concentrations and can detect a single metabolite of a drug. A positive test by an immunoassay or the most precise use of GC/MS involves electron impact ionization, three-ion monitoring, and ion rationing.

Thin-layer chromatography (TLC) can be verified for nonforensic purposes by high-performance liquid chromatography (HPLC) or gas–liquid chromatography (GLC). GLC is useful for the detection of alcohol and volatile inhalants in blood or urine specimens. In HPLC, with the aid of ultraviolet, fluorescent, or electrochemical changes, a detector can be employed at the terminal end of the column that can measure drugs with greater sensitivity and specificity than TLC. GLC also employs several types of detectors such as nitrogen phosphorus detector.

Cross-Reactive Drugs

Common cross-reacting drugs in screening immunoassays are summarized in Table 19–20.[240]

Turnaround Time

Turnaround times for detecting drugs in urine after use at cutoff concentrations are listed in Tables 19–21 and 19–22.[238,241] Detection limits of commonly abused drugs are listed in Table 19–23.[149] Problems and challenges in performing drug analysis or urine samples in the industrial setting are summarized in Table 19–23.[149] Problems and challenges in performing drug analysis or urine samples in

Table 19–21
Urine Screening Tests for Drugs of Abuse

Test Procedure	Name of Test	Manufacturer (Location)	Turnaround Time	Average Per Test Cost to Patient
Enzyme immunoassay	EMIT	Syva Co. (Palo Alto, CA)	1 h (stat) 1 d normally	$25*
Radioimmunoassay	Abuscreen	Roche Diagnostics (Nutley, NJ)	1–2 d	$25*
Thin-layer chromatography	Toxi-Lab	Analytical Systems (Laguna Beach, CA)	3–4 h (stat) 1 d normally	$25–$40
Fluorescence polarization immunoassay	TDx	Abbott Laboratories, Diagnostics Division (Irving, TX)	1–2 h (stat) 1 d normally	$25

*Screening panels can be obtained in some major commercial laboratories at a cost of $30 to $40 for five classes of drugs.
From Schwartz RH. Urine testing in the detection of drugs of abuse. Arch Intern Med 1988;148:2407–2412.

Table 19–22
Time Intervals for Detecting Drugs in Urine After Use at Cutoff Concentrations

	Days Detectable After Use
NIDA-Recommended Drug Tests	
Marijuana metabolite	
Single use	< 7
Ongoing abuse	<30
Cocaine metabolite	< 3
Opiate metabolite	< 2
Phencyclidine	< 7
Amphetamines	< 2
Others	
Alcohol	< 1
Barbiturates	< 2
Phenobarbital	< 7
Benzodiazepines	< 3
Methaqualone	< 7
Methadone	< 4

NIDA, National Institute on Drug Abuse.
From Osterloh JD, Becker CE. Chemical dependency and drug testing in the workplace. West J Med 1990;152:506–513.

Table 19–23
Detection Limits of Commonly Abused Drugs*

Drug	Limit of Sensitivity (µg/mL)	Approximate Duration of Detectability (d)
Amphetamine	0.5	2
Methamphetamine	0.5	2
Barbiturates		
Short-acting		1
Hexobarbital	1.0	
Pentobarbital	0.5	
Secobarbital	0.5	
Thiamylal	1.0	
Intermediate-acting		2–3
Amobarbital	1.0	
Aprobarbital	1.5	
Butabarbital	0.5	
Butalbital	1.5	
Long-acting		<7
Barbital	5.0	
Phenobarbital	1.0	
Benzodiazepines	1.0	3
Cocaine metabolites		2–3
Benzoylecgonine	0.5	
Ecgonine methyl ester	1.0	
Methadone	0.5	3
Codeine	0.5	2
Propoxyphene	0.5	1–2
Cannabinoids	20 ng/mL	3–5†
Methaqualone	1.0	<7
Phencyclidine	0.5	8

*Factors of dose, frequency, route of administration, and the person's health have dramatic effects on these values.
†In rare circumstances, these substances may be present for up to 2 weeks in heavy users.
From McCunney RJ. Drug testing: Technical complications of a complex social issue. Am J Ind Med 1989;15:589–600.

Table 19–24
Caveats for Urinary Drug Screening

1. Determine the *need* for urinary drug testing. Are these positions involving public safety or is there evidence of a drug abuse problem in the workplace?
2. Determine the *purpose* of the testing. Will urinary drug testing be part of an overall program that attempts to control the effects of other mind-altering substances such as alcohol and over-the-counter and prescription medications?
3. Determine the *type of testing* that is necessary. Which drugs will be included?
4. Determine the *frequency of testing.* Will testing be done at preplacement evaluation, at periodic intervals, or at the time of work-related accidents? At present, there appears to be little legal challenge to the issue of conducting preplacement urinary drug screens; however, the major area that is open to legal challenge is *random* drug screening.
5. *Select an appropriate laboratory* that can ensure chain-of-custody and conduct the *confirmatory tests* following a positive initial screen.
6. *Establish a protocol* for dealing with positive results *before* the program is instituted. (It is unwise to evaluate results of urine testing done during preplacement evaluations "after-the-fact.")
7. Consider the *costs* of the program, including the need for confirmatory tests.
9. Consider *other substances* that can also affect work performance such as *alcohol,* over-the-counter medications, and prescription drugs.
10. Be aware of the *limitations of testing.* False-positive reactions can occur. Ideally, drug testing should be combined with a substance abuse program that includes employee education and supervisory education.
11. *Be realistic.* Drug screening will not eliminate drug problems.

From McCunney RJ. Drug Testing: Technical complications of a complex social issue. Am J Ind Med 1989;15:589–600.

Table 19–25
Sources of Error in Testing Urine Specimens for Drugs of Abuse

- Substitution of urine from a non–drug-using individual or of apple juice for the urine of the person being tested
- Adulteration of the specimen by the addition of water, sodium chloride, vinegar, ammonia water, sodium hydrochlorite, or soap solution
- Interference from nonprescription medications or foods, especially when testing for amphetamine (sympathomimetics) or opiate drugs
- Collection or storage error caused by an unclean container, failure to filter cloudy urine, storage at room temperature for 4 or more days, or, in the case of LSD analysis, exposure to strong light
- Technical error resulting from questionable reliability of equipment, insufficiently frequent calibrations, insufficient positive or negative controls, lack of warm-up time, overused solvents (thin-layer chromatography), temperature variation (enzyme multiplied immunoassay technique), or reuse of material from previous positive samples
- Administration error due to testing the wrong sample, improper labeling of specimen, inaccurate recording of results, or faulty transcription

From Schwartz RH. Urine testing in the detection of drugs of abuse. Arch Intern Med 1988;148:2402–2412.

Table 19–26
Attempted or Accidentally Adulterated Urine Drug Abuse Samples

1. Adding water may reduce the concentration below the detection point (but most samples have so much drug it does not matter).
2. Adding commercial cleaner, ammonia, bleach, lye, or Drano will change urine pH radically and, thus, is easily detectable. So check the pH, it will be very high.
3. Measure the temperature of the sample at the time of collection. It is almost impossible to dilute the sample and still have the correct body temperature.
4. Diluted urine looks pale—a clue.
5. If the specific gravity of the urine is 1.000 to 1.001, it is probably diluted. Couple specific gravity check with a temperature check.
6. Ammonia in a urine sample produces an easily detectable odor.
7. Odor of furniture polish or Pine Sol is detectable.
8. Drano does not produce a distinctive odor and does not produce a color change. The sodium hydroxide dissolves to a colorless solution.
9. If a little acid or base is added to urine, neutralize it.
10. For dilute urine, extract a greater volume of urine. It improves the sensitivity of test.
11. If substitution of another fluid for urine is suspected, check if creatinine is present.
12. Witness urine sample procedures.
13. Confirm with gas chromatography–mass spectrometry.
14. Drug concentrations in urine may be decreased by adding hydrogen peroxide, Joy detergent, sodium bicarbonate, or $NaHClO_4$. False-positive results were caused by hydrogen peroxide and Joy. Sodium bicarbonate causes a suspiciously high urine pH; $NaHClO_4$, an apparently low pH.
15. A prospective study with nonsteroidal antiinflammatory drugs disclosed two false-positive urine tests for cannabinoids by enzyme-mediated immunoassay. Of 510 urine samples collected from 102 individuals, one from a patient who took 1200 mg of ibuprofen in three divided doses for 1 day and one from a patient who took naproxen on a chronic basis, none were falsely positive for benzodiazepines. Two urine tests were false positive for barbiturates by fluorescence polarization Immunoassay in a patient taking ibuprofen and one in a patient taking Naprosyn.
16. Individuals may place various chemical substances under their fingernails and release them into the urine sample to affect subsequent analysis.
17. Placing a pinhole in the bottom of the urine container would result in a leak that would not be detected at the collection site. During shipping, however, most or all of the urine could leak out.
18. Use of a fluid-filled bulb placed under the arm with a tube leading to the genital area enables the subject to squeeze the bulb and release water or other substances that would dilute or contaminate the urine.
19. The subject can obtain urine from friends not using drugs or save his or her own urine from drug-free periods to be placed in a container during the collection period.
20. The subject can scoop water from the commode into the collection container and dilute the urine. The water in the toilet can, however, be dyed, or the toilet can be a chemical one, eliminating in both cases the availability of water for dilution.
21. Creatinine is normally present in a urine sample.
22. Drinking large volumes of water or other liquid several hours prior to the urine collection can result in a tenfold dilution of urine, lowering the concentration of drug sufficiently so that it might not be detectable by a laboratory analysis.
23. UrinAID (glutaraldehyde) is a commercial product sold for the purpose of defeating urine drug tests. The major component has been identified as glutaraldehyde. UrinAid can be effective in preventing the detection of drugs in the urine by the EMIT test, but does not defeat other immunoassays such as the Abuscreen, radioimmunoassay, and Online.

Sources: References 242–249.

the industrial setting are summarized in Table 19–24.[241] Sources of error are listed in Table 19–25.[238] Methods of adulterating urine samples are listed in Table 19–26.

Urine samples used in drug abuse testing should be tested for creatinine. If the creatinine level is less than 4.0 mmol/L, negative results for drugs may not be valid.[250]

HAIR ANALYSIS

Analysis of hair for drugs of abuse by radioimmunoassay and GC/MS may be an effective means of identifying drug abusers.[251] Comparison with a urine assay shows it to be useful after some days have passed following exposure. Morphine and codeine may appear in the beard approximately 7 to 8 days after drug administration at a time when drug is not detectable in urine, plasma, and saliva and drug-induced effects have disappeared. Data suggest that hair analysis may provide evidence of time and degree of drug exposure.[252] The absence of drug metabolism in hair and the fairly uniform hair growth rate of about 1 cm per month may provide a historic account of drug use from analysis of hair samples.[253]

Conclusions related to the use of hair for analysis must be validated by further controlled studies. Analytical refinements yet to be performed must include standardization of the assay procedures for screening and confirmation, establishment of appropriate cutoffs, development of reliable quality control programs, and proficiency testing. This step must be taken before this method of analysis will be able to be used to determine the status of employment or liberty.[253]

ELECTROENCEPHALOGRAM

Alpha activity on an electroencephalogram is usually associated with wakefulness. It is seen in patients in coma usually with pontomesencephalic infarction or diffuse posthypoxic cerebral cortical necrosis. The prognosis in such cases is dismal. It has, however, also been observed in comatose states resulting from overdoses of sedative–hypnotic drugs. With aggressive therapy, these patients have recovered.[254,255]

SALIVA

Marijuana, cocaine, phencyclidine, opiates, barbiturates, amphetamines, and benzodiazepines (or their metabolites) have all been detected in saliva by various analytical methods including immunoassay, GC/MS, and TLC. Initial studies with cocaine and phencyclidine suggest a correlation between saliva and plasma concentrations of these drugs, indicating a dynamic equilibrium between saliva and blood. Tetrahydrocannabinol, the active component in marijuana, does not appear to be transferred from plasma to saliva; however, tetrahydrocannabinol is sequestered in the buccal cavity during smoking and can be detected in saliva.

Concentrations of drug are usually lower in saliva than in urine; however, assay methods now available can detect the quantities present. Saliva eliminates the issues of protection of privacy and, to a large degree, of adulteration during sample collection. Drug concentrations in saliva provide an estimate of the actual circulating amount and the results can be used for the determination of current intoxication. Many drugs are retained for a shorter time in saliva than in urine. The pace of data accumulation strongly indicates a place for saliva as a useful future biological medium.[256]

SWEAT TESTS

The first sweat patch test for amphetamines, cocaine, and opiates has received Food and Drug Administration marketing clearance for use by trained drug abuse testing professionals in clinical and rehabilitation centers.

The test system consists of application of a patch to the skin to collect sweat and an assay to detect drugs.

The patch is a waterproof, adhesive pad about the size of a playing card. It can be worn up to 7 days on the back, upper arm, or lower chest and will collect drugs of abuse used during that period.[257]

The Sudormed Sweat Specimen Containter is manufactured by Sudormed of Santa Ana, California. The SolarCare Technologies Corporation EIA Micro-Place Assay is made by SolarCare Technologies Corporation, Bethlehem, Pennsylvania.

TREATMENT OF DRUG ABUSE

OBJECTIVES

Complete abstinence from illicit drugs is a desirable goal. The ability to function in society is a more realistic and perhaps appropriate definition of recovery. The day-to-day substantial reduction of a patient's consumption of illicit drugs compared with what would be experienced without treatment is a modest but attainable goal. Other goals include reduction of street crime, developing educational or vocational capabilities, restoring employment, averting fetal exposure to drugs, and improving general health, psychological functioning, and family life.

EFFECTIVENESS

There are four major methods of drug treatment: methadone maintenance, residential therapeutic communities, outpatient nonmethadone treatment, and chemical dependency programs. No details are available regarding the efficacy of mutual self-help groups such as Narcotics Anonymous.

METHADONE MAINTENANCE

Methadone maintenance is an ambulatory treatment for opiate dependence. A daily oral dose of 30 to 100 mg of methadone hydrochloride yields a stable level of active metabolite. Eventually, the dose produces neither subjective intoxication nor clinically detectable behavioral impairment. Toxic side effects are rare; general health improves. Patients become more amenable to counseling, environmental changes, and support services. It is a controversial treatment because many clients continue to use heroin and other drugs intermittently and to commit crimes, including the sale of take-home methadone. Half to two thirds of those admitted to methadone maintenance programs remain in treatment 1 year or longer. Programs very in reaching their goals.

THERAPEUTIC COMMITTEES

Therapeutic committees are usually residential programs with 9- to 18-month courses of treatment followed by continuing contact during a variable period of reentry. These programs are designed for people with major behavioral and social impairments, including a history of serious criminal behavior. The communities involve psychotherapy, behavioral modification, an internal hierarchy of jobs and progressive responsibilities, and a variety of medical, educational, and vocational services. In the past most individuals have been heroin dependent, but cocaine is now becoming dominant. Features of the program include strict prohibitions against drugs and violent behavior during treatment, close supervision, testing, and expulsion on detection. Attrition and early discharge are high: only about 15 to 25% of those admitted complete the full course. Behavior improves (avoiding drugs and crime, holding employment). The minimal retention necessary to sustain improvement after leaving treatment is at least 3 months.

OUTPATIENT NONMETHADONE PROGRAMS

These programs involve a 6-month course of one or two visits per week for individual or group psychotherapy or counseling. Those admitted to such programs are usually not dependent on opiates, but otherwise cover all categories of drug abuse and patterns of dependency. Attrition is rapid. Outcomes are better during and after treatment than before admission, and are positively related to the duration of treatment.

CHEMICAL DEPENDENCY PROGRAMS

Chemical dependency programs are general residential or in-hospital programs, with a 3- to 5-week course, followed by up to 2 years of prescribed attendance at self-help or weekly therapy groups. These programs are based on the 12-step model of personal change of Alcoholics Anonymous. Treatment is devoted largely to primary alcoholism. Those with primary drug problems appear to have poorer outcomes than those with primary alcohol problems. There is no evidence that hospital programs are more or less effective in treatment drug problems than residential chemical dependency programs.

DETOXIFICATION

Detoxification begins with emergency admission for an overdose. Much drug detoxification now takes place in hospital beds. It can usually be undertaken safely on a

Table 19-27
Treatment of Drug Abuse Reactions

Obtain blood alcohol level. See chapter pertaining to the specific drug.

	Treatment
Cocaine/Central Nervous System Stimulants	
Acute	
Cocaine	
Paranoia	Haloperidol
Seizures	Diazepam
Amphetamines	Benzodiazepine Haloperidol
Hypertension	Nitroprusside Phentolamine Labetalol
Hyperthermia	Rapid cooling
Withdrawal	Amantadine, bromocriptine
Opioids	
Acute	
Apnea, coma	Naloxone (for heroin, morphine, codeine, meperidine, propoxyphene, methadone, ?pentazocine)
Pulmonary edema	Naloxone ineffective
Withdrawal	Methadone, clonidine
Hallucinogens	
Acute	Hypersuggestibility
Seizures	Diazepam
Agitation	Haloperidol
Withdrawal	Not after hallucinogen
Cannabis	
Acute	Adults, no treatment

residential, partial daycare, or ambulatory basis. Hospitalization is needed for addicted newborns or persons with heavy dependence on sedatives, concurrent medical or serious psychiatric problems, or a documented history of complications or flight (Table 19–27).

CURRENT STATUS

Problems relate to private insurance (often inadequate), hospital inpatient treatment (excess acute care costs), detoxification (often unnecessary hospitalization), and data on drug treatment programs (inadequate, and often not current).

REFERENCES

1. Symptoms and signs of drug abuse. Med Lett Drugs Ther 1987;29(748):86.
2. U.S. Department of Health and Human Services, Public Health Service. The health consequences of smoking nicotine addiction: A report of the Surgeon General. Washington, DC: U.S. Government Printing Office, 1988.
3. American Psychiatric Association. *Diagnostic and Statistical Manual of Mental Disorders.* 3rd ed., rev. Washington, DC: American Psychiatric Association, 1987.
4. Hoffman RS. Street drugs. Prehosp Dis Med 1991;6(2):252.
5. Treaster JB. U.S. reports rise in drug emergencies. NY Times, October 5, 1993.
6. Current tobacco, alcohol, marijuana, cocaine use. MMWR 1991;40:659–663.
7. Wilford BB. Abuse of prescription drugs. West J Med 1990; 152:609–612.
8. Koran L, Litt I. House staff well-being. West J Med 1988;148: 97–101.
9. Hughes PH, Conard SE, Baldwin DC Jr, et al. Resident physician substance use in the United States. JAMA 1991; 265:2069–2073.
10. Menk EJ, Baumgarten RK, Kingsley CP, et al. Success of reentry into anesthesiology training programs by residents with a history of substance abuse. JAMA 1990;263:3060–3062.
11. The drugs on the street where you live. Emerg Med 1986; 18(3):129–177.
12. Ammon TK, Anglin MD. Update on illicit drug use in Los Angeles County. In: *Proceedings, Community Epidemiology Work Group, Epidemiologic Trends in Drug Abuse.* National Institute on Drug Abuse, U.S. Department of Health and Human Services, June 1992 and December 15–18, 1992 meeting.
13. Golding AMP. Two hundred years of drug abuse. J R Soc Med 1993;86:282–286.
14. Schydlower M, Chairman, Committee on Substance Abuse, 1992–1993, American Academy of Pediatrics. Role of the pediatrician in prevention and management of substance abuse. Pediatrics 1993;91:1010–1013.
15. Rinaldi RC, Steindler EM, Wilford BB, Goodwin D. Clarification and standardization of substance abuse terminology. JAMA 1988;259:555–557.
16. Gerstein DR, Harwood HJ, eds. *Treating Drug Problems.* Washington, DC: National Academy Press, 1990.
17. Gerstein DR, Lewin LS. Special report: Treating drug problems. N Engl J Med 1990;323:847–848.
18. Pruitt AW, Chairman and Committee on Substance Abuse. Drug-exposed infants. Pediatrics 1990;86:639–642.
19. Ward SLD, Bautista D, Chan L, et al. Sudden infant death syndrome in infants of substance-abusing mothers. J Pediatr 1990;117:876–881.
20. Committee on Adolescence, Committee on Bioethics, also Provisional Committee on Substance Abuse. Screening for drugs of abuse in children and adolescents. Pediatrics 1989;84:396–398.
21. Richardson JL, Dwyer K, McGuigan K, et al. Substance abuse among eighth grade students who take care of themselves after school. Pediatrics 1989;84:556–566.
22. Janofsky M. Drug use rising among teenagers, study says. NY Times, December 13, 1994.
23. Walsh SS, Pierce AM, Hart CA. Drug abuse: A new problem. Br Med J 1987;295:526–527.
24. Woolf A. The epidemiology of poisonings and drug abuse in adolescents and adults. Clin Toxicol Rev 1988;10(4):1–2.
25. Loiselle JM, Baker MD, Templeton MJ Jr, et al. Substance abuse in adolescent trauma. Ann Emerg Med 1993;22:1530–1534.
26. Harman C. Rh-negative women who share needles run risk of being childless, MD says. Can Med Assoc J 1990;142: 975.
27. Bowman JM, Manning FA, Harman CR. Alloimmunization and intravenous drug abuse. Can Med Assoc J 1990; 142:439.
28. Jessup M. The treatment of perinatal addiction, identification, intervention and advocacy. West J Med 1990;152:553–558.
29. Deren S, Frank B, Schneidler J. Children of substance abusers in New York State. NY State J Med 1990;90:179–184.
30. Dattel BJ. Substance abuse in pregnancy. Semin Perinatol 1990;14:179–187.
31. Ostrea EM Jr, Brady MJ, Parks PM, et al. Drug screening of meconium in infants of drug-dependent mothers: An alternative to urine testing. J Pediatr 1989;115:474–477.
32. Ostrea EM Jr, Porter T, Balun J, et al. Effects of chronic maternal drug addiction on placental drug metabolism. Dev Pharmacol Ther 1989;12:42–48.
33. Rosenzweig IV, Clark GD, Thiersch NJ, Raisys VA. Neonatal drugs of abuse screening in meconium: A comparison between Abbot TDx and Syva ETS. Clin Chem 1990;36:1023.
34. Ward SLD, Schuetz S, Wachsman L, et al. Elevated plasma norepinephrine levels in infants of substance-abusing mothers. Am J Dis Child 1991;145:44–48.
35. Senay EC. Drug abuse and public health: A global perspective. Drug Saf 1991;6(suppl. 1):1–65.

36. Drugs on stickers. Lancet 1991;336:1501.
37. Duback DC, Rosner B, Sturmer T. An epidemiologic study of abuse of analgesic drugs: Effects of phenacetin and salicylate on mortality and cardiovascular morbidity (1968–1987). N Engl J Med 1991;324:155–160.
38. Kuster G, Ritz E. Analgesic abuse and hypertension. Lancet 1989;2:1105.
39. Stewart MJ, Fraser DM, Boon N. Dilated cardiomyopathy associated with chronic overuse of an adrenaline inhaler. Br Heart J 1992;68:221–222.
40. Whitehouse AM, Novosel S. Salbutamol psychosis. Biol Psychiatry 1989;26:631–633.
41. Brennan PO. Inhaled salbutamol: A new form of drug abuse? Lancet 1983;2:1030–1031.
42. Add Lysol[R] to list of abused drugs. Forens Drug Abuse Advisor 1991;3(3):19–20.
43. Kuhlman JJ Jr, Magluilo J Jr, Levine B, Smith ML. Two deaths involving isoflurane abuse. J Forens Sci 1993;38: 968–971.
44. Yamashita M, Matsuki A, Oyama T. Illicit use of modern volatile anesthetics. Can Anaesth Soc J 1984;31:76–79.
45. Kunkel DB. The toxic toll of keeping thin. Emerg Med 1985; 17(1):176–180.
46. Pellini EJ, Wallace GB. The pharmacology of emetine. Am J Med Sci 1916;152:325–336.
47. Santangelo WC, Richey JE, Rivera L, Fordtran JS. Surreptitious ipecac administration simulating intestinal pseudo obstruction. Ann Intern Med 1989;110:1031–1032.
48. Tolstoi LG. Ipecac-induced toxicity in eating disorders. Int J Eating Disorders 1990;9:371–375.
49. Bulimia nervosa: common in women. Drug Ther Bull 1992; 30:13–15.
50. Garner DM. Pathogenesis of anorexia nervosa. Lancet 1933; 341:1631–1635.
51. Beumont PJV, Russell JD, Touyz SW. Treatment of anorexia nervosa. Lancet 1993;341:1635–1640.
52. Mitchell JE, Seim HC, Colon E, Pomeroy C. Medical complications and medical management of bulimia. Ann Intern Med 1987;107:71–77.
53. Devlin MJ, Walshin DT, Kral JG, et al. Metabolic abnormalities in bulimia nervosa. Arch Gen Psychiatry 1990;47:144–148.
54. Franko DL, Banitt PF. Abusing potassium by a patient with bulimia nervosa. Am J Psychiatry 1991;48:682.
55. Jebbink RJA, Zwaveling JH. Self-poisoning in eating disorders. Lancet 1988;1:1276.
56. Woolf AD, Gren JM. Acute poisonings among adolescents and young adults with anorexia nervosa. Am J Dis Child 1990;144:785–788.
57. Hudson JI, Poper HG Jr, Keck PE Jr, McElroy SL. Treatment of bulimia nervosa with trazodone: Short-term response and long-term follow-up. Clin Neuropharmacol 1989; 12(suppl. 1):538–546.
58. Solyom L, Solyom C, Ledwidge B. The fluoxetine treatment for low weight chronic bulimia nervosa. J Clin Psychopharmacol 1990;110:421–425.
59. Fava M, Herzog DB, Hamburg P, et al. Long-term use of fluoxetine in bulimia nervosa: A retrospective study. Ann Clin Psychiatry 1990;2:53–56.
60. Mitchell JE, Christenson G, Jennings J, et al. A placebo controlled double-blind crossover study of naltrexone hydrochloride in outpatients with normal-weight bulimia. J Clin Psychopharmacol 1989;9:94–97.
61. Kennedy SH, Goldblood DS. Current perspectives on drug therapies for anorexia nervosa and bulimia nervosa. Drugs 1991;4:367–377.
62. Rosenwasse GOD, Holland S, Pfugfelder SC, et al. Topical anesthetic abuse. Ophthalmology 1990;97:967–972.
63. Sato EH, de Freitas D, Foster CS. Abuse of cyclopentolate hydrochloride (Cyclogyl) drops. N Engl J Med 1992;326: 1363–1364.
64. Harmelin DL, Martin FIR, Wark JD. Antacid induced phosphate depletion syndrome presenting as nephrolithiasis. Aust NZ J Med 1990;20:803–805.
65. Ruben SM, McLean PC, Melville J. Cyclizine abuse among a group of opiate dependents receiving methadone. Br J Addict 1989;84:929–934.
66. Multistate outbreak of poisonings associated with illicit use of gamma hydroxybutyrate. MMWR 1990;39:861–863.
67. Warning about GHB: Food and Drug Administration. JAMA 1991;265:1802.
68. Centers for Disease Control and Prevention. Multistate outbreak of poisonings associated with illicit use of gamma hydroxy butyrate. MMWR 1990;39:861–863.
69. Illness with GHB use. FDA Consumer 1991;25(2):5.
70. Adornato BT, Tse V. Another health food hazard: gamma hydroxy butyrate induced seizures. West J Med 1992;157: 471.
71. Chin M-Y, Kreutzer RA, Dyer JE. Acute poisoning from gamma-hydroxybutyrate in California. West J Med 1992;56: 380–384.
72. Dyer JE. Gamma-hydroxybutyrate a health food product producing coma and seizure-like activity. Am J Emerg Med 1991;9:321–326.
73. Mamelak M. Gamma hydroxy butyrate: An endogenous regulator of energy metabolism. Neurosci Biobehav Rev 1989; 13:187–190.
74. Gilmore DA, Freed CR, Bronstein AC. Central nervous system depression and weakness following ingestion of gamma hydroxybutyrate. Vet Hum Toxicol 1991;33:366.
75. Lane RB. Gamma hydroxy butyrate (GHB). JAMA 1991;265: 2959.
76. Gallimberti L, Canton G, Gentile N, et al. Gamma hydroxy butyric acid for treatment of alcohol withdrawal syndrome. Lancet 1989;2:787–789.
77. Auerbach SB, Noj EK, Falk H. Gamma hydroxy butyrate (GHB). JAMA 1991;265:2959.
78. U.S. Pharmaceutical Convention Inc. *USP Dispensing Information:* vol. 1B: *Drug Information for the Health Care Professional.* Easton, PA: Mack, 1990:2914.
79. Vickers MD. Gamma hydroxybutyric acid. Proc R Soc Med 1968;61:821–824.
80. Vayer P, Mandel P, Maitre M. Mini review: Gamma hydroxybutyrate, a possible neurotransmitter. Life Sci 1987;41:1547–1557.
81. Hoes MJ, Vree TB, Guelen RJ. Gamma-hydroxybutyric acid as hypnotic. Encephale 1980;6:93–99.
82. Jaeken J, Casaer P, de Cock P, Francois B. Vigabatrin in GABA metabolism disorders. Lancet 1989;1:1074.
83. Ferrara SD, Tedeschi L, Frison G, Rossi A. Fatality due to gamma hydroxybutyric acid (GHB) and heroin intoxication. J Forens Sci 1995;40:501–504.
84. Helrich M, McAslan Tc, Skolnik S, et al. Correlation of blood levels of 4-hydroxybutyrate with state of consciousness. Anesthesiology 1964;25:771–775.
85. Gibson KM, DeViro DC, Jakobs C. Vigabatrin therapy in patient with succinic semialdehyde dehydrogenase deficiency. Lancet 1989;2:1105–1106.
86. Jensen D, Burton BT, Magnusson AB. Recreational intravenous injection of elemental mercury. Vet Hum Toxicol 1988;30:372.
87. Bloor RN, Smalldridge NJF. Intravenous use of slow release morphine sulfate tablets. Br Med J 1990;300:640–641.
88. Gray RF, Ferez A, Janhar P. Emergence of buprenophine dependence. Br J Addict 1989;84:1373–1374.
89. Mahesh VK, Stern HP, Kearns GL, Stroh SE. Application of pharmacokinetics in the diagnosis of chemical abuse in Munchausen's syndrome by proxy. Clin Pediatr 1988; 27:243–246.
90. McElwee NE, Veltri JC. Intentional abuse of dextromethorphan (DM) products: 1985 to 1988 statewide data. Vet Hum Toxicol 1990;32:355.
91. Helfer J, Kim OM. Psychoactive abuse potential of Robitussin-DM[R]. Am J Psychiatry 1990;147:672.
92. Walker J, Yatham LN. Beylin (dextromethorphan) abuse and mania. Br Med J 1993;306:896.
93. Young GB, Body D, Kreeft J. Dimenhydrinate: Evidence for dependence and tolerance. Can Med Assoc J 1988;138:437–438.
94. Bartlik B, Galanter M, Angrist B. Dimenhydrinate addiction in a schizophrenic woman. J Clin Psychiatry 1989;50:476.
95. Craig DL, Mellor CS. Dimenhydrinate dependence and withdrawal. Can Med Assoc J 1990;142:970–973.

96. Kaplan R. Poppy sead dependence. Med J Aust 1994;161: 176.
97. Unnithan S, Strang J. Poppy tea dependency. Br J Psychiatry 1993;163:813–814.
98. Rotenberg A, Chaveinc L, Rault P, et al. Lesions rectales secondaire a l'abus de suppositoires de dextropropoxyphene et paracetamol: Deux nouvelles observations. Presse Med 1988;17(30):1545.
99. Hedenmalm K. A case of severe withdrawal syndrome due to dextropropoxyphene. Ann Intern Med 1995;123:473.
100. Scott WC. Abuse of erythropoietin to enhance athletic performance. JAMA 1990;264:1660.
101. Tennant F, Black DL, Voy RO. Anabolic steroid dependence with opioid type features. N Engl J Med 1988;319:578.
102. Stevens DJ. Cushing's syndrome due to the abuse of betamethasone nasal drops. J Laryngol Otol 1988;102: 219–221.
103. Borde M, Nizamie SH. Dependence on a common cough syrup. Lancet 1988;1:760.
104. Bhasin S, Wallace W, Lawrence JB, Lesch M. Sudden death associated with thyroid hormone abuse. Am J Med 1981; 71:887–890.
105. Griffiths RR, Wolf B. Relative abuse liability of different benzodiazepines in drug abusers. J Clin Psychopharmacol 1990; 10:237–243.
106. Schneiderman JF, Romach MK, Kaplan HL, Sellers EM. Comparative abuse liability of lorazepam (L), buspirone (B) and secobarbital (S). Clin Pharmacol Ther 1989;45:187.
107. Dilsaver SC. Antimuscarinic agents as substances of abuse: A review. J Clin Psychopharmacol 1988;8:14–22.
108. Brady KT, Lydiard RB, Kellner C. Tranylcypromine abuse. Am J Psychiatry 1991;148:1268–1269.
109. Dilsaver SC. Heterocyclic antidepressant monoamine oxidase inhibitor and neuroleptic withdrawal phenomena. Prog Neuropsychopharmacol Biol Psychiatry 1990;14:137–161.
110. Briggs NC, Jeffereson JW, Koeneck FH. Tranylcypromine addiction: A case report and review. J Clin Psychiatry 1990; 51:426–429.
111. Jastak JT. Nitrous oxide and its abuse. J Am Dent Assoc 1991;122:48–52.
112. Hill MA, Greason FC. Loperamide dependence. J Clin Psychiatry 1992;53:450.
113. Hays LR, Stillner V, Littrel R. Fentanyl dependence associated with oral ingestion. Anesthesiology 1992;77:819–821.
114. Lerner AG, Sigal M, Baculu A, Gelkopf M. Naltrexone abuse potential. J Nerv Ment Dis 1992;180:734–754.
115. Elder NC. Abuse of skeletal muscle relaxants. Am Fam Phys 1991;44:1223–1226.
116. Goldstein ET, Murray KB, Preskorn SH. Baclofen induced delirium. Ann Clin Psychiatry 1990;2:223–224.
117. Luehr JG, Meyerle KA, Larson EW. Mail-order (veterinary) drug dependence. JAMA 1990;236:657.
118. Good PJ. Soma (carisoprodol): A challenge to a DRE evaluation. Phoenix: The DRE (Drug Recognition Expert), 1995;7: 14–15.
119. Schifance F, Marra R, Magni G. Orphenadrine abuse. South Med J 1988;81:546–547.
120. Semley S, Bewly TH. Drug dependency with oestrogen replacement therapy. Lancet 1992;339:290–291.
121. Hammersley R, Lavelle T, Forsyth A. Buprenophine and temazepam: Abuse. Br J Addict 1990;85:301–303.
122. Purdue NN, Fernando GCA, Busuttil A. Two deaths from intravenous nifedipine abuse. Int J Legal Med 1991;104: 289–291.
123. Purdes BN, Fernando GCA, Buscettil A. Two deaths from intravenous nifedipine abuse. Int J Legal Med 1991;104: 289–291.
124. Soyka M, Huppert D. L-Dopa abuse in a patient with former alcoholism. Br J Addict 1992;87:117–118.
125. Brady WJ, Stremski E, Eljaiek L, Aufderheide TP. Freon inhalational abuse presenting with ventricular fibrillation. Am J Emerg Med 1994;12:533–536.
126. De Broe ME, Elseviers MM: Analgesic nephropathy: Still a problem? Nephron 1993;64:505–513.
127. Nanra RS. Analgesic nephropathy in the 1990's: An Australian perspective. Kidney Int 1993;44(suppl. 42):S-86–S-92.
128. Woolley BH. The latest fads to increase muscle mass and energy. Postgrad Med 1991;89:199–205.
129. Woolley BH, Barnett DW. The use and misuse of drugs by athletes. Houston Med J 1986;2:29–35.
130. Mofenson HC: Substance abuse in sports. Pediatr Ther Toxicol (Suppl.) 1988 2(6):S5–S8.
131. Middleman AB, Faulkner AH, Woods ER, et al. High-risk behaviors among high school students in Massachusetts who use anabolic steroids. Pediatrics 1995;96:268–272.
132. Park J, Park S, Lho D, et al. Drug testing at the 10th Asian games and 24th Seoul Olympic games. J Anal Toxicol 1990; 14:66–72. Park J, Chung B. Drug abuse in sports (doping): Analytical Procedures: 41st Meeting of the American Academy of Forensic Scientists, Feb. 14, 1989: 1–244. DCC-KAIST, PO Box 131, Cheongryang, South Korea.
133. Rockhold BRW. Cardiovascular toxicity of anabolic steroids. Annu Rev Pharmacol Toxicol 1993:497–520.
134. Kennedy MC, Lawrence C. Anabolic steroid use and cardiac death. Med J Aust 1993;158:346–348.
135. Bray GP, Tredger JM, Williams R. Resolution of danazol-induced cholestasis with *S*-adenosylmethionine. Postgrad Med J 1993;69:237–239.
136. Moss-Newport J. Anabolic steroid use and cerebellar hemorrhage. Med J Aust 1993;158:794.
137. Fradkin JE, Schonberger LB, Mills JL, et al. Creutzfeldt-Jakob disease in pituitary growth hormone recipients in the United States. JAMA 1991;265:880–884.
138. Winter FD Jr, Snell PG, Stray-Gunderson J. Effects of 100% oxygen on performance of professional soccer players. JAMA 1989;262:227–229.
139. Murray TM. Erythropoietin: Another violation of ethics. Phys Sports Med 1989;17:39–40.
140. Donaldson VH. Danazol. Am J Med 1989;87:3-49N–3-55N.
141. Lee YJ, Horstman LL, Ahn YS. Danazol for Henoch-Schönlein pupura. Ann Intern Med 1993;118:827.
142. Kahn H, Manzarbeitia C, Theise N, et al. Danazol-induced hepatocellular adenomas. Arch Pathol Lab Med 1991; 115:1054–1057.
143. Ferenchik G, Schwartz D, Ball M, Schwartz K. Androgenic-anabolic steroid abuse and platelet aggregation: A pilot study in weight lifters. Am J Med Sci 1992;303:78–82.
144. Gerrard DF, Fawcett JP, Farquhar SJ. Venadium use by athletes. NZ Med J 1993;106:259.
145. Shesser R, Jotte R, Olshaker J. The contribution of impurities to the acute morbidity of illegal drug use. Am J Emerg Med 1991;9:336–342.
146. Orser B. Thrombocytopenia and cocaine abuse. Anesthesiology 1991;74(1):195–196.
147. Leikin JB, Krantz AJ, Zell-Kanter M, et al. Clinical features and management of intoxication due to hallucinogenic drugs. Med Toxicol Adverse Drug Experience 1989;4:324–350.
148. Spoerke DG, Hall AH. Plants and mushrooms of abuse. Emerg Med Clin North Am 1990;8:589.
149. Marquardt KA, Tharratt RS. Fentanyl smokes. Vet Hum Toxicol 1993;35:362.
150. Stephens DA. Psychotoxic effects of benzhexol hydrochloride (Artane). Br J Psychiatry 1967;113:213–218.
151. Macvicar K. Abuse of antiparkinsonian drugs by psychiatric patients. Am J Psychiatry 1977;134:809–811.
152. Lowry TP. Trihexyphenidyl abuse. Am J Psychiatry 1977;134: 1315.
153. Goggin DA, Solomon GF. Trihexyphenidyl abuse for euphorigenic effect. Am J Psychiatry 1979;136:459–460.
154. Rouchell AM, Dixon SP. Trihexyphenidyl abuse. Am J Psychiatry 1977;134:1315.
155. McEvoy GK. *AHFS Drug Information 90.* Bethesda, MD: American Hospital Formulary Service, 1990.
156. Smith JM. Abuse of the antiparkinson drugs: A review of the literature. J Clin Psychiatry 1980;41:351–354.
157. Kajimura N, Nizuki Y, Kai S, et al. Memory and cognitive impairments in a case of long-term trihexyphenidyl abuse. Pharmacopsychology 1993;26:59–62.
158. Rubinstein JS. Abuse of antiparkinsonian drugs. JAMA 1978; 239:2365–2366.
159. Craig DH, Rosen P. Abuse of antiparkinsonian drugs. Ann Emerg Med 1981;10:98–100.

160. Hidalgo HA, Mowers RM: Anticholinergic drug abuse. DICP Ann Pharmacother 1990;24:40–41.
161. Kaminer Y, Munitz H, Wijsenbee K. Trihexyphenidyl (Artane) abuse: Euphoriant and anxiolytic. Br J Psychiatry 1982; 140:473–474.
162. Crawshaw JA, Mullen PE. A study of benzhexol abuse. Br J Psychiatry 1984;145:300–303.
163. Whitsett TL, Manion CV, Wilson MF. Cardiac, pulmonary and neuromuscular effects of clenbuterol and terbutaline compared with placebo. Br J Clin Pharmacol 1981;12: 195–200.
164. Muscling in on clenbuterol. Lancet 1992;340:403. Editorial.
165. Reynolds JEF, ed. *Martindale: The Extra Pharmacopoeia.* 29th ed. London: Pharmaceutical Press, 1989:1458.
166. Whitsett TL, Manion CV, Wilson MF. Cardiac, pulmonary and neuromuscular effects of clenbuterol and terbutaline compared with placebo. Clin Pharmacol Ther 1980;27:294–295.
167. MacLennan PA, Edward RHT. Effect of clenbuterol and propranolol on muscle mass: Evidence that clenbuterol stimulates muscle beta-adrenoceptors to induce hypertrophy. Biochem J 1989;264:573–579.
168. Delday MI, Williams PE, Maltin CA. Effect of clenbuterol on immobilized muscle. J Neurol Sci 1990;98:376.
169. Zahn V, Krumbacher G. Clenbuterol: A long term uterine relaxant. J Perinat Med 1981;9:96–100.
170. Beckett AH. Clenbuterol and sports. Lancet 1992;340:1165.
171. Blom-Bulow P, Boe J, Bulow K, Hagelqvist I. A comparison of oral beta$_2$-agonists clenbuterol and salbutamol in obstructive lung disease: A double blind cross-over study. Curr Ther Res 1985;37:51–57.
172. Micheli F, Gatto E, Gene R, Pardal MF. Clenbuterol-induced tardive dyskinesia. Clin Neuropharmacol 1991;14:427–431.
173. Jensen S, Hansen AC. Abuse of codeine separated from over-the-counter drugs containing acetylsalicylic acid and codeine. Int J Legal Med 1993;105:279–281.
174. Davis L. The use of castor oil to stimulate labor in patients with premature rupture of membranes. J Nurse-Midwifery 1984;29:366.
175. Cummings M. Types of laxatives. FDA Consumer 1991 (April):34.
176. Asher R. Munchausen's syndrome. Lancet 1951:1:339–341.
177. Chapman JS. Peregrinating problem patients: Munchausen's syndrome. JAMA 1957;165:927–933.
178. Castelbaum AB, Donofrio PD, Walker FA, Troost BT. Laxative abuse causing hypermagnesemia, quadriparesis and neuromuscular junction defect. Neurology 1989;39:746–747.
179. Mofenson HC, Caraccio TR. Magnesium intoxication in a neonate from oral magnesium hydroxide laxative. Clin Toxicol 1991;29:215–222.
180. Eherer AJ, Fordtran JS. Fecal osmotic gap and pH in experimental diarrhea of various causes. Gastroenterology 1992; 103:545–551.
181. Tsaing RC. Neonatal magnesium disturbances. Am J Dis Child 1972;124:202.
182. L'Hommedieu CS, Nicholas D, Armes DA. Potentiation of magnesium sulfate-induced neuromuscular weakness by gentamicin, tobramycin and amikacin. J Pediatr 1983;102: 629–631.
183. Beuers B, Spengler U, Pape GR. Hepatitis after chronic abuse of senna. Lancet 1991;337:372–373.
184. De Wolff TA, de Haas EJM, Verweij M. A screening method for establishing laxative abuse. Clin Chem 1981;27:914–917.
185. Faber DB, Kok RM. The comparison of TLC with GLC and GC/MS as well as TLC/GLC as screening methods for synthetic chemical stimulating laxatives in case of abuse. In: *Proceedings, Annual European Meeting of International Association of Forensic Toxicologists, Glasgow, August 1979.* Bull Int Assoc Forens Toxicol 1979;15(1):15–16.
186. Silk DBA, Gibson JA, Murray CRH. Reversible finger clubbing in a case of purgative abuse. Gastroenterology 1975;6: 790–794.
187. Binder HJ. The gastroenterologist's osmotic gap: Fact or fiction? Gastroenterology 1992;103:702–704.
188. Duncan A, Robertson C, Russell RI. The fecal osmotic gap: Technical aspects regarding its calculation. J Lab Clin Med 1992;119:359–363.
189. Donowitz M, Kokke FT, Said R. Evaluation of patients with chronic diarrhea. N Engl J Med 1995;332:725–729.
190. Giorgi DF. Munchausen syndrome. NY State J Med 1992;92: 301–303.
191. Hunter SE, Sussman N. Chronic factitious disorder with physical symptoms (Munchausen syndrome). Psychiatr Clin North Am 1981;4:365–377.
192. Rosenberg DA. Web of deceit: A literature review of Munchausen's syndrome by proxy. Child Abuse Negl 1987; 11:547–563.
193. Parker G, Barrett E. Factitious patients with fictitious disorders: A note on Munchausen's syndrome. Med J Aust 1991;155:772–773.
194. Meadow R. Munchausen's syndrome by proxy. Arch Dis Child 1982;57:92–98.
195. Zuger A, O'Dowd MA. The Baron has AIDS: A case of factitious human immunodeficiency virus infection and review. Clin Infect Dis 1992;14:211–216.
196. Belchetz PE, Cohen RD, O'Riordan JLH, Tomlinson S. Factitious hypercalcemia. Br Med J 1976;1:690–691.
197. Makesh VK, Stern HP, Kearns GL, Stroh SE. Application of pharmacokinetics in the diagnosis of chemical abuse in Munchausen's syndrome by proxy. Clin Pediatr 1988; 27:243–246.
198. Feldman KW, Christopher DM, Oppenheim KE. Anorexia nervosa/Munchausen's syndrome by proxy and ipecac. Vet Hum Toxicol 1987;29:482.
199. Nichols GR, Davis GJ, Coney TG. In the shadow of the Baron: Sudden death due to Munchausen's syndrome. Am J Emerg Med 1990;8:216–219.
200. Ackerman NB Jr, Strobel CT. Polle syndrome: Chronic diarrhea in Munchausen's child. Gastroenterology 1981;81: 1140–1142.
201. Karnik AM, Farah S, Khadadalh M, et al. A unique case of Munchausen's syndrome. Br J Clin Pract 1990;44:699–700.
202. Klatt EC, Mills NA, Noguchi TT. Causes of death in hospitalized intravenous drug abusers. J Forens Sci 1990;25: 1143–1148.
203. Perkins HA, Samson S, Garner J, et al. Risk of acquired immunodeficiency syndrome (AIDS) for recipients of blood components from donors who subsequently developed AIDS. Blood 1987;70:1604–1610.
204. Nelson KE, Vlahov D, Margolick J, et al. Blood and plasma donations among a cohort of intravenous drug users. JAMA 1990;263:2194–2197.
205. Glassroth J, Adams GD, Schnoll S. The impact of substance abuse on the respiratory system. Chest 1987;91:596–602.
206. Harrison DW, Walls RM. 'Cotton fever': A benign febrile syndrome in intravenous drug abusers. J Emerg Med 1990;8: 135–139.
207. Levine DP, Sobel JD. *Infections in Intravenous Drug Abusers.* New York: Oxford University Press, 1991.
208. Sloan MA, Kittner SJ, Rigamonti D, Price TR. Occurrence of stroke associated with use/abuse of drugs. Neurology 1991;41:1358–1364.
209. Chitwood DD, Page JB, Comerford M, et al. The donation and sale of blood by intravenous drug users. Am J Pub Health 1991;81:631–633.
210. Steger KA, Craven DE, Shea BF, et al. Use of paper-absorbed fingerstick blood samples for studies of antibody to human immunodeficiency virus type I in intravenous drug users. J Infect Dis 1990;162:964–967.
211. Goodwin FK. Tuberculosis in drug users. JAMA 1989;262: 1439.
212. Rothmann S, Tourani J-M, Andrieu J-M. Hodgkin's disease in HIV-infected intravenous drug abusers. N Engl J Med 1990;323:275–276.
213. Joliet P, Widmann J-J. Reye's syndrome in adult with AIDS. Lancet 1990;335:1457.
214. Graham NMH, Nelson KE, Solomon L, et al. Prevalence of tuberculin test positivity and skin test anergy in HIV-I-seropositive and -seronegative intravenous drug users. JAMA 1992;267:369–373.
215. Reichman L, Felton C, Edsall J. Drug dependence a possible new risk factor for tuberculosis disease. Arch Intern Med 1979;139:337–339.

216. Handwerger S, Mildvan D, Senie R, McKinley F. Tuberculosis and the acquired immunodeficiency syndrome at a New York City Hospital: 1978–1985. Chest 1987;91:176–180.
217. O'Donnell A, Pappas LS. Pulmonary complications of intravenous drug abuse: Experience at an inner-city hospital. Chest 1988;94:251–253.
218. Froner GA, Rutherford GW, Rokeach M. Injection of sodium hypochlorite by intravenous drug users. JAMA 1987;258: 325.
219. Becker GL, Cohen S, Borer R. The sequelae of accidentally injecting sodium hypochlorite beyond the root apex. Oral Surg Oral Med Oral Pathol 1974;38:633–638.
220. Felser JM, Orban DJ. Dystonic reaction after ketamine abuse. Ann Emerg Med 1982;11:673–673.
221. Baselt RC, Cravey RH. *Disposition of Toxic Drugs and Chemicals in Man.* 3rd ed. Chicago: Year Book, 1989:444–446.
222. Wood M. Intravenous anesthetics. In: Wood M, Wood AJJ, eds. *Drugs and Anesthesia: Pharmacology for Anesthesiologists.* 2nd ed. Baltimore: Williams & Wilkins, 1990:179–223.
223. Koppel C, Arndt I, Ibe K. Effects of enzyme induction, renal and cardiac function on ketamine plasma kinetics in patients with ketamine long-term analgosedation. Eur J Drug Metab Pharmacokinet 1990;15:259–263.
224. Reich DL, Silvay G. Ketamine: An update on the first twenty-five years of clinical experience. Can J Anaesth 1989;36: 186–197.
225. Green SM, Johnson NE. Ketamine sedation for pediatric procedures: Part 2: Review and implications. Ann Emerg Med 1990;19:1033–1046.
226. Schorn TOF, Whitwann JG. Are there long-term effects of ketamine on the central nervous system? Br J Anaesth 1980; 52:967–968.
227. Johnstone RE. A ketamine trip. Anesthesiology 1973;39:460–461.
228. Ketamine abuse. FDA Drug Bull 1979;9:24.
229. Ahmed SN, Petchkovsky L. Abuse of ketamine. Br J Psychiatry 1980;137:303.
230. Fine J, Firestone SC. Sensory disturbances following ketamine anesthesia: Recurrent hallucinations. Anesth Analg 1973;52:428–430.
231. Green SM, Nakamura R, Johnson NE. Ketamine sedation for pediatric procedures: Part 1: Prospective series. Ann Emerg Med 1990;19:1024–1032.
232. Bloomquist E. Drug dangers. JAMA 1971;218:1301.
233. Stella L, Crescenti A, Torn G. Effect of naloxone on the loss of consciousness induced by IV anaesthetic agents in man. Br J Anaesth 1984;56:369–373.
234. Amiot JF, Bouju P, Palacci JH. Effect of naloxone on loss of consciousness induced by IV ketamine. Br J Anaesth 1985;57:930.
235. Bescey L, Malamed S, Radnay P, et al. Reduction of the psychotomimetic and circulatory effects of ketamine by droperidol. Anesthesiology 1972;37:536–542.
236. Kaplan JA, Cooperman LJ. Alarming reactions to ketamine in patients taking thyroid medication: Treatment with propranolol. Anesthesiology 1971;35:229–230.
237. Jansen KLR. Non-medical use of ketamine: Dissociative states in unprotected settings may be harmful. Br Med J 1993;306:601–602.
238. Schwartz RH. Urine testing in the detection of drugs of abuse. Arch Intern Med 1988;148:2402–2412.
239. Goldberger BA, Cone EJ. Confirmatory tests for drugs in the workplace by gas chromatography–mass spectrometry J Chromatogr A 1994:674:73–86.
240. Osterloh JD, Becker CE. Chemical dependency and drug testing in the workplace. West J Med 1990;152:506–513.
241. McCunney RJ. Drug testing: Technical complications of a complex social issue. Am J Ind Med 19089;15:589–600.
242. Adulterated urine samples: An interview with Bob Fogerson. Syva Monitor 1987;5(2):1–3.
243. Person NB, Ehrenkranz JRL. Fake urine sample for drug analysis: Hot, but not hot enough. JAMA 1988;259:841.
244. Johnson CA, Cary PL. Intentional adulteration of urine specimen for drugs of abuse testing to produce false positive results. J Anal Toxicol 1990;14:195–196.
245. Warner A. Interference of common household chemicals in immunoassay methods for drugs of abuse. Clin Chem 1989; 35:648–651.
246. Rollins DE, Jennison TA, Jones G. Investigation of interference by non-steroidal anti-inflammatory drugs in urine tests for abused drugs. Clin Chem 1990;36:602–606.
247. Hawks RL, Chiang CN. *Urine Testing for Drugs of Abuse.* NIDA Research Monograph No. 73, DHHS Publication No. (ADM) 87-1481,1981.
248. Goldberger BA, Caplan YH. Effect of glutaraldehyde (UrinAID) on detection of abused drugs in urine by immunoassay. Clin Chem 1994;40:1605–1606.
249. Sanson HL, Fraser MD, Botelho C, et al. Detection of urine specimens adulterated with UrinAID. In: Proceedings, California Association of Toxicologists, October 1993.
250. La Fole P, Beck O, Blennow G, et al. Importance of creatinine analysis of urine when screening for abused drugs. Clin Chem 1991;37:1927–1931.
251. Baumgarten WA, Hill VA, Blahd WH. Hair analysis for drugs of abuse. J Forens Sci 1989;34:1433–1453.
252. Cone EJ. Testing human hair for drugs of abuse: 1. Individual dose and time profiles of morphine and codeine in plasma, saliva, urine and beard compared to drug-induced effects on pupils and behavior. J Anal Toxicol 1990;14:1–7.
253. Strang J, Marsh A, Desonza N. Hair analysis for drugs of abuse. Lancet 1990;1:740.
254. Carroll WM, Mastiglia FL. Alpha and beta coma in drug intoxication. Br Med J 1977;2:1518–1519.
255. Kuroiwa Y, Furukawa T. EEG prognostication in drug-related alpha cone. Arch Neurol 1981;38:200.
256. Schramm W, Smith RH, Craig PA, Kidwell DA. Drugs of abuse in saliva: A review. J Anal Toxicol 1992;16:1–9.
257. FDA Consumer 1995;29:5.

Chapter 20
Amphetamines and Designer Drugs

INTRODUCTION

Amphetamine (phenylisopropylamine) is the prototype of a class of noncatecholamine compounds (Table 20–1) that produce strong central nervous system stimulation (Fig. 20–1).

MEDICAL USES

Methylphenidate and amphetamines are accepted for chronic therapeutic use in properly documented narcolepsy in adults and attention deficit disorder in children. Occasionally, both these drugs may be indicated when the attention disorder extends into adulthood. In addition, they may be useful as 2- to 3-day trials to gauge the effectiveness of certain tricyclic antidepressants in mild depression or senile withdrawn behavior in the elderly. The medical and nonmedical use of methylphenidate is prohibited in Japan and Sweden. The use of amphetamines for short-term (8–12 weeks) suppression of appetite remains a legal indication, although this use is highly controversial. Long-term benefit of amphetamines for appetite suppression is clinically insignificant because of tolerance and is potentially harmful because of the common complication of abuse. These drugs cannot be legally prescribed for the treatment of drug dependence, fatigue, anxiety reactions, or chronic anxiety or to generate a sense of well-being. The illicit hallucinogens *p*-methoxyamphetamine and the methylenedioxyamphetamine compounds (3,4-methylenedioxyamphetamine [MDA], 3,4-methylenedioxymethamphetamine [MDMA], 3,4-methylenedioxy-*N*-ethylamphetamine [MDEA], 3-methoxy-4,5-methylenedioxyamphetamine [MMDA]) have no legal indications. The structurally similar, amphetamine-like, anorectic drugs are approved for short-term (a few weeks) use in obesity and are less tightly controlled by the U.S. government because of the lower abuse potential.

Schedule III anorectic drugs include chlorphentermine, clortermine, mazindol, and phenmetrazine; Schedule IV anorectic agents include diethylpropion, fenfluramine, and phentermine. An estimated 80% of the legal use of amphetamines is for weight reduction. Conversely, about

Table 20–1
Common Legal Amphetamine Products

DEA Schedule	Generic Name	Trade Name	Usual Therapeutic Dose	Formulation
Amphetamines and Their Isomers				
II	Amphetamine	Benzedrine	2.5–10 mg one to three times daily	5-10-mg tablets
		Biphetamine		15-mg slow-release tablets
		Others		20-, 50-mg tablets
II	Dextroamphetamine	Dexamyl	2.5–5 mg one to three times daily	5-, 10-mg tablets
		Dexedrine		15-mg slow-release tablets
				1 mg/mL elixir
II	Methamphetamine HCl	Desoxyn	2.5–5 mg one to three times daily or 5–15 mg of extended-release once daily	2.5-, 5-mg tablets
		Fefamine		5-, 10-, 15-mg slow-release capsule
		Others		
Amphetamine Analogs				
III	Benzphetamine HCl	Didrex	25–50 mg once daily to a maximum of 50 mg tid	25-, 50-mg tablets
III	Chlorphentermine HCl	Pre-Sate	65 mg once daily	No longer available
III	Clortermine	Voranil	50 mg once daily	No longer available
IV	Diethylpropion HCl	Tenuate	25 mg tid or 75 mg extended-release once daily	25-mg tablets
				75-mg slow-release tablets
		Tepanil		
		Dospan		
		Ten-Tab		
IV	Fenfluramine HCl	Pondimin	20 mg tid to a maximum of 40 mg tid	20-mg tablets
III	Phendimetrazine tartrate	Plegine	35 mg bid or tid: maximum = 70 mg tid	35-mg tablets
				105-mg slow-release capsule
II	Phenmetrazine HCl	Preludin	25 mg bid or tid: maximum = 25 mg tid or 75 mg of extended-release once daily	25-mg tablets
				75-, 105-mg slow-release capsules
IV	Phentermine	Ionamin	15–30 mg of resin complex once daily	8-, 15-, 30-mg tablets
II	Methylphenidate	Ritalin	Adults: 20–30 mg daily Children: 5 mg bid to start	5-, 10-, 20-mg tablets
				25-mg sustained-release tablets
IV	Pemoline	Cylert	37.5–112.5 mg daily	18.75-, 37.5-, 75-mg tablets

Adapted from Oderda GM, Schwartz WK: Management of poisonings with central nervous system stimulants. Clin Toxicol Consult 1979;1:74.

25% of the reported cases of amphetamine abuse in 1978 resulted from the excessive consumption of legitimate prescriptions.

Mephentermine (Wyamine) is an intravenous solution previously used as a pressor agent for hypotension, but now is superseded by more effective and less dangerous drugs.

MISUSE AND ABUSE

Amphetamines are especially appealing to individuals who interact poorly in social settings and have difficulty internalizing new experiences. These drugs reduce the need for external stimuli by increasing internal arousal mechanisms. In contrast to asocial, schizoid personalities who tend to *abuse* amphetamines (ie, the drug interferes with their social, economic, or medical welfare), *misuse* of amphetamines (ie, using these drugs for nonmedically indicated purposes) occurs frequently in individuals trying to enhance performance.

Intermittent Low-Dose Misuse

Many individuals occasionally take 5 to 20 mg of oral amphetamines to allay fatigue, elevate mood, or prolong wakefulness. Students studying for exams, military personnel on extended exercises, athletes wanting to excel, and truck drivers on prolonged trips commonly use amphetamines. Professional football players have consumed these drugs to induce analgesia and rage, improve speed, and reduce weight. These drugs do seem to improve the performance of tired individuals on repetitive tasks, unless jitteriness or impaired judgment adversely affects the outcome. Most sporadic users do not develop a habitual craving for amphetamines. Rarely, hallucinations and sudden death occur during strenuous exercise in warm envi-

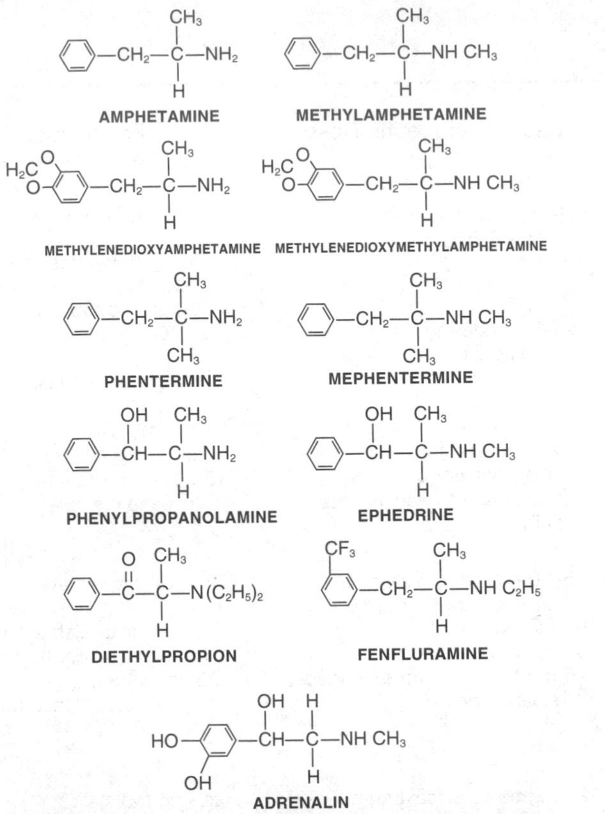

AMPHETAMINE METHYLAMPHETAMINE

METHYLENEDIOXYAMPHETAMINE METHYLENEDIOXYMETHYLAMPHETAMINE

PHENTERMINE MEPHENTERMINE

PHENYLPROPANOLAMINE EPHEDRINE

DIETHYLPROPION FENFLURAMINE

ADRENALIN

Figure 20-1 Structures of amphetamine and its analogs. (From Colbert DL. Drug abuse screening with immunoassays: Unexpected cross-reactivities and other pitfalls. Br. J Biomed Sci 1994;51:136–146.)

ronments. In addition, these drugs may push the user to greater expenditures of energy, resulting in excessive fatigue. The hazardous consequences of fatigue and the subsequent reduced physical performance may not be recognized by the patient, because of drug-induced impaired judgment. Such situations may lead to unfortunate accidents.

Sustained Oral Misuse

Some people who have been using amphetamines either illicitly or through legitimate prescriptions continue to ingest them in regular daily doses of 20 to 40 mg. Attempts to reduce the dose result in depression and lethargy. Unfortunately, such patients may become incapable of accurately evaluating the physical or psychological effects of amphetamine use. Individuals who enjoy the euphoric effects are particularly vulnerable to excessive doses, as tolerance develops, leading to the consumption of daily doses ranging from 50 to 150 mg.[1] An additional risk is polydrug abuse, as alcohol and sedative–hypnotic agents commonly are used to combat the insomnia associated with habitual amphetamine misuse.[2]

High-Dose Intravenous Abuse

Individuals who relish the euphoria discover that intravenous injections produce a more intense feeling of pleasure. The "rush" or "flash" has been compared with sexual orgasm. Other attractive feelings apparent between injections include a sense of power, hyperactivity, hyperexcitability, euphoria, and heightened sexual awareness. Although the abuse pattern involves fewer individuals as compared with oral use, violent and bizarre behavior, slovenly dress, emaciated appearance, and major medical complications have focused public and professional attention on this abuse pattern. Tolerance and cravings for the "flash" lead to repeated injections during a "speed run" of 1000 mg at a time and up to 5 g within 24 hours. *Speed* is the term given to methamphetamine. A *speed freak* is a compulsive speed user. Stereotyped behavior, which includes skin picking, bead stringing, pacing, and interminable chattering, often is apparent. During the action phase, the speed freak often does not sleep, ignores body care, and rarely eats. Orgasm and ejaculation are difficult or impossible to achieve, leading to marathon sexual activity in some but not all users. High methamphetamine doses result in extreme suspiciousness or even an overt paranoid psychosis, which, along with hyperactivity and poor impulse control, may produce unpredictable violent behavior. The person continues to perpetuate the "high" by repeated intravenous injection (1–10 per day) until fatigue, paranoia, confusion, or lack of drug terminates use (usually several days to 1 week).

During the reaction phase, exhaustion develops; the user sleeps for 24 to 48 hours and subsequently eats ravenously. Unfortunately, once the hunger is satisfied, severe depression starts. To relieve the depression, the amphetamine addict starts intravenous use again, thus beginning another cycle or "speed binge."[3] Certain individuals feel too anxious on amphetamines and turn to the compulsive, polydrug intravenous use of barbiturate–amphetamine or heroin–amphetamine ("poor man's speedball") combinations. Particularly in the Pacific Northwest, methylphenidate (Ritalin) may be substituted for methamphetamine.

When the intravenous dosage is increased too rapidly, the individual develops a peculiar condition and is called "overamped"; that is, he or she is conscious but unable to speak or move. Elevated blood pressure, temperature, and pulse, as well as chest distress, occur in this setting. Death from overdose is infrequent in tolerant individuals. In fact, habitual large-dose users commonly exhibit no obvious physical signs of dependence other than the obvious signs of economic, social, and emotional deterioration. The person becomes unreliable, irritable, paranoid, and unstable, leading to social (family problems), physical (unkempt appearance), and economic (job loss, bankruptcy) deficits. Suicide may occur from either loss of impulse control or severe depression during the exhaustion phase. Adverse psychological reactions include anxiety reactions, amphetamine psychosis, exhaustion syndrome, prolonged depression, and persistent hallucinosis (perhaps as a result of the unmasking of underlying psychiatric disorders).[4]

Inhalant Abuse

One Benzedrine inhaler contains the equivalent of 250 mg of racemic amphetamine. The usual method was to chew and swallow the paper strip, preferably with chewing gum to reduce the irritant properties of the base. Occasionally, the strips were soaked in beverages (ie, coffee, alcohol) or swallowed whole. One study of an incarcerated population in the 1940s revealed that 25% used the inhalant material for intoxication.[5] The 1959 Food and Drug Administration ban on over-the-counter amphetamine inhalants led to introduction of the Benedrex inhaler, which contains 250 mg of propylhexedrine, 12.5 g methanol, and various aromatic compounds. By the mid-1970s, both oral and intravenous abuse of these inhalers had been reported in the medical literature. Several patients who habitually used methamphetamines chewed or swallowed 2 to 11 inhalers to support their abuse pattern. Patients with previous amphetamine experience compared the euphoria induced by the intravenous injection of Benedrex extracts with that induced by 15 mg of methamphetamine or 75 mg of phenmetrazine.[6] Benedrex abuse usually is associated with documented polydrug abuse and homosexual activities. Euphoria apparently does not result from inhalation.[7] Sudden death during strenuous exercise and homicides and suicides during drug-induced psychosis have been reported.[6] Most methamphetamine and amphetamine analogs have been voluntarily removed from inhalants; however, Vicks Nasal Inhaler, a nasal decongestant, contains 50 mg of *l*-desoxyephedrine together with menthol, camphor, methyl salicylate, and bornyl acetate. (*l*-Desoxyephedrine is *l*-methamphetamine.) This product may have high abuse potential, as the racemic mixture has been extensively abused.[8]

Acute Toxic Dose

The minimal lethal amphetamine dose varies with age and animal species. Children appear more susceptible than adults. In humans, death has been reported with as little as 1.5 mg/kg methamphetamine,[9] whereas survival occurred after an ingestion of 28 mg/kg amphetamine.[10] An adult fenfluramine death resulted after an oral dose of 1.6 g. Because of tolerance, amphetamine addicts can inject 1 to 5 g of amphetamine intravenously.

On the basis of animal data, 3,4-methylenedioxymethamphetamine (MDMA) is one to six times more potent than mescaline and 1.5 to 3 times less toxic than MDA.

3,4-Methylenedioxymethamphetamine is a psychoactive amphetamine derivative. Although hallucinogenic and sympathomimetic effects are limited at therapeutic doses, those who overdose on MDMA (ie, 500–1000 mg) demonstrate an amphetamine-like reaction, which includes anxiety, dysphoria, tachycardia, hypertension, hypertonicity, and seizures. The U.S. Drug Enforcement Administration currently is considering reclassifying this drug to allow medical investigation of its properties.

Drug Interactions

Interactions of stimulants with commonly used psychotropic agents are listed in Table 20–2.

STRUCTURE

Substitution of a methoxyl group on the 4-position of amphetamine enhances the hallucinogenic properties of methylenedioxymethamphetamine and its structural relative, *p*-methoxyamphetamine. Both products are capable of producing hyperthermia, seizures, rhabdomyolysis, coma and death.[11] 2,5-Dimethoxy-4-bromoamphetamine (DOB) is the brominated derivative of 2,5-dimethoxy-4-methylamphetamine (STP, DOM), which itself has hallucinogenic properties similar to those of lysergic acid diethylamide (LSD) in doses of 1 to 4 mg. Recently, MDMA, which has been nicknamed the "yuppie psychedelic" because of its popularity among students and young professionals, was added to the list of Schedule I drugs (ie, no medical use). The closely related synthetic amphetamine compound 3-methoxy-4,5-methylenedioxyamphetamine (MMDA) causes hallucinations in high doses, but MDMA produces primarily sympathomimetic effects in overdose without hallucinations. A new synthetic amphetamine derivative is 3,4-methylenedioxy-*N*-ethylamphetamine, (MDEA), which is called "Eve" on the street.

CLANDESTINE PRODUCTION

In recent years the most popular primary precursor for the production of illegal amphetamine and methamphetamine has been phenyl-2-propanone, a nonpsychoactive substance now placed in Schedule II of the Controlled Substance Act.[12–14] Many clandestine laboratory operators who in the past had been producing only methamphetamine now synthesize phenyl-2-propanone either alone or in combination with methamphetamine.[15] In California, illicit production of methamphetamine has become an immense export industry.[16]

The second most frequently encountered clandestine synthesis of methamphetamine uses ephedrine converted to chlorpseudoephedrine followed by reduction.[17] An unusual clandestine reduction of ephedrine to methamphetamine employs lithium metal and ammonium gas.[18] This reaction also converts phenylpropanolamine to amphetamine and methylephedrine to dimethyamphetamine.

Impurities found in the ephedrine reduction method provide intelligence concerning illicit production methods, identification of samples of common origin (ie, conspiracy links), and the origin of possible harmful effects on the methamphetamine user. For example, possible methamphetamine impurities so discovered may appear to be responsible for cases exhibiting choreiform movements.[15] Many modifications of each method exist.[19]

Table 20–2
Interactions of Stimulants With Commonly Used Psychotropic Agents

Medication	Comments
Sympathomimetics (ie, ephedrine, pseudoephedrine)	Potentiate effects of both medications
Antihistamines	May diminish effectiveness of stimulants
Monoamine oxidase inhibitors	Decrease stimulant metabolism; potentiate effects of both medications; may cause hypertensive crisis
Tricyclic antidepressants (TCAs)	May alter TCA levels; potentiate effects of both medications; with imipramine may cause confusion, lability, aggressiveness
Anticonvulsants	May increase anticonvulsant level; may decrease absorption

From Wilens TE, Biederman J. The stimulants. Psychiatr Clin North Am 1992;15:191–222.

Use of essential oils as precursor products, such as 3-methoxy-4,5-methylenedioxyamphetamine (nutmeg oil, mace oil, or parsley seed oil), 2,5-dimethoxy-3,4-methylenedioxyamphetamine (parsley seed oil), and 2,3-demethoxy-4,5-methylenedioxyamphetamine (dill seed oil), may be contemplated.[20] 2,5-Dimethoxy-4-ethoxyamphetamine has now been detected as a street drug in Canada.[21] 4-Ethoxyamphetamine has been known in Canada since 1986. It is structurally similar to 4-methoxyamphetamine, considered by some as the most dangerous of all amphetamines.[22]

Ephedrone, 2-methylamino-l-phenylpropane-l-one, also known by its street name "Jeff," is an oxidation product of ephedrine and has become a substantial drug of abuse in the former Soviet Union, where it is responsible for numerous drug overdose deaths.[23]

ICE: METHAMPHETAMINE

"Ice," also known as "Glass," originated in the Far East (Korea, the Philippines, and given the name *shabu* in Japan) for the synthesis of large crystals of methamphetamine with the ephedrine reduction method. It is a major drug problem in Japan. Ice is in the form of a translucent crystal similar in appearance to rock candy or rock salt. Ice is a very pure form of methamphetamine hydrochloride (98–100% pure) and is a controlled substance (Schedule II). It first appeared in Hawaii in 1985, where it was called *batu* and has since come to the U.S. mainland.[24–27]

Methamphetamine powder can be injected, inhaled, smoked, or ingested.[28] In the Honolulu area, Ice is smoked using a glass pipe (Fig. 20–2). The translucent form (Ice) appears to be water based, burns quickly, and leaves a milky white residue inside the bowl. A yellowish crystal methamphetamine, said to be oil based, burns slower and leaves a brownish or black residue in the pipe.

In Hawaii, Ice has surpassed cocaine as the drug of choice. It eliminates use of a needle; is longer lasting; is often odorless, colorless, and tasteless; is easy to transport; and is more expensive than cocaine, but cheaper to produce.

Dose

The amounts of smokable methamphetamine used by high-dose abusers ranges between 2.5 and 15 g/d. This is approximately 150 to 1000 times the recommended daily dose for therapeutic use and at least three times the average quantity used by high-dose intravenous amphetamine abusers.[28]

Clinical Presentation

Effects of the drug last 2 to 24 hours depending on the dose. Highs may last 2 to 3 days. Chronic abusers of Ice resemble chronic abusers of other amphetamines and amphetamine-like drugs (delusions, paranoia, aggressive behavior); suicide and homicide are not uncommon. Tics, bruxism, and compulsive behavior are often observed. Gastrointestinal problems may include anorexia, weight loss, and malnutrition. Myocardial infarction,[29] caudal thalamic infarcts,[30] transient cortical blindness,[31] systemic vasospasm, irreversible cardiomyopathy,[32] acute pulmonary edema[33] and death have followed its use.[34] Withdrawal results in abdominal cramps, gastroenteritis, headache, lethargy, dyspnea, increase in appetite, and profound depression, occasionally terminating in suicide.[20]

Ethanol–Methamphetamine Combination

Ethanol is the drug most commonly associated with complications of methamphetamine.[35] The combination of methamphetamine with ethanol results in increased cardiac work. This may increase cardiac toxicity. Nicotine, cocaine, and amphetamine produce similar cardiovascular responses when combined with ethanol. The combination of methamphetamine and ethanol may produce more adverse cardiovascular or cerebrovascular events than either drug taken alone at the same dose.

Tobacco–Methamphetamine Combination

In the last decade, abuse of methamphetamine has been perhaps the most serious drug problem in Japan.[36–38] Recently, abusers have begun to inhale methamphetamine by smoking a cigarette containing tobacco mixed with methamphetamine. Pyrolysis products produced included a number of amphetamine analogs.

Pregnancy

Intrauterine growth abnormalities, complications of pregnancy and delivery including maternal death,[39] and neurophysiologic and neurobehavioral abnormalities in neonates have been described with antenatal methamphetamine drug exposure.[40] Such findings are similar to those seen after cocaine abuse. This is not surprising in view of their similar pharmacologic propensities in producing vasoconstriction and hypertension. Amphetamine ingestion may present as eclampsia.[41] Intrauterine death has followed an intravenous injection of amphetamine.[42]

Methamphetamine studies in pregnancy describe an increased incidence of intrauterine growth retardation, prematurity, and perinatal complications.[43,44] Body weight, length, and head circumference changes in the infant are described.[45] At birth, withdrawal symptoms may include abnormal sleep patterns, tremors, hypertonicity, a high-pitched cry, poor feeding patterns, sneezing, frantic sucking, and tachypnea.[44] During the first year, the infant may exhibit lethargy, poor feeding, poor alertness, and severe lassitude. Development, however, is usually within normal limits during the first year. There is no evidence of an increased incidence of congenital anomalies.[45]

A relatively benign neonatal course is not a good predictor of later findings, which may include oculomotor apraxia, a parkinsonian dystonia, a severe tactile-elicited dystonia, pronounced intention tremor, severe active hypotonia, and hemiparesis.[44]

"CRYSTAL"

Crystal, also known as "Crank" or "Meth" or "Crystal Meth" on the street, is a white to yellow product easily created in amateur laboratories. Crude, the powder has the odor of rotten eggs; pure, it may be odorless. Laboratories set

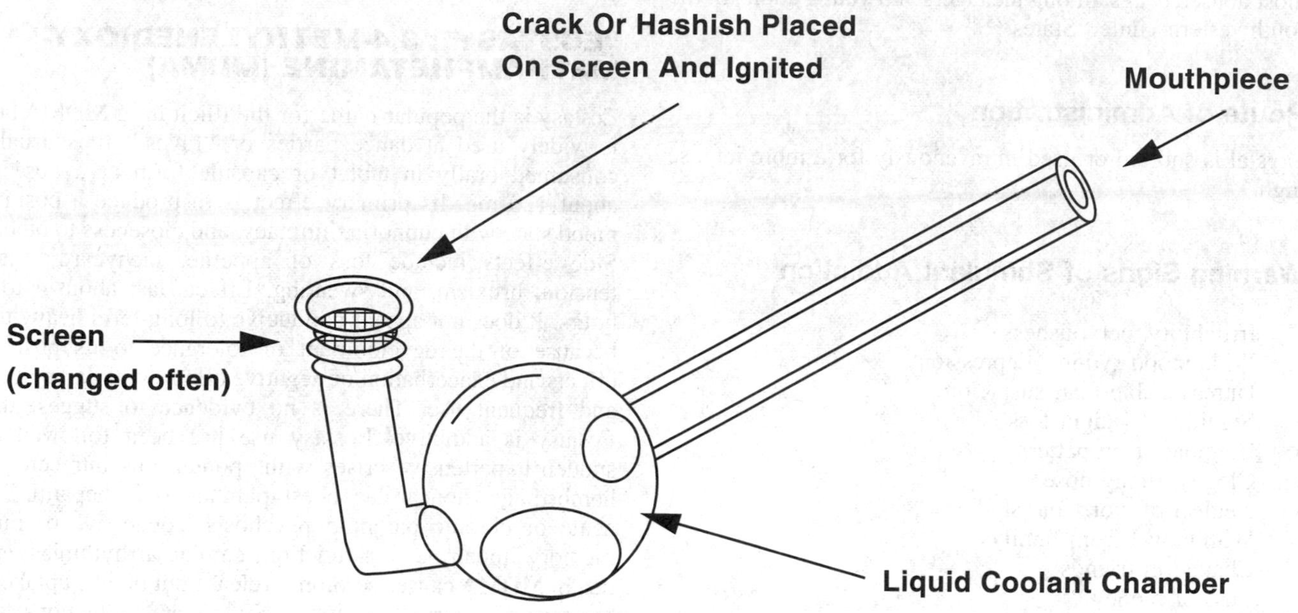

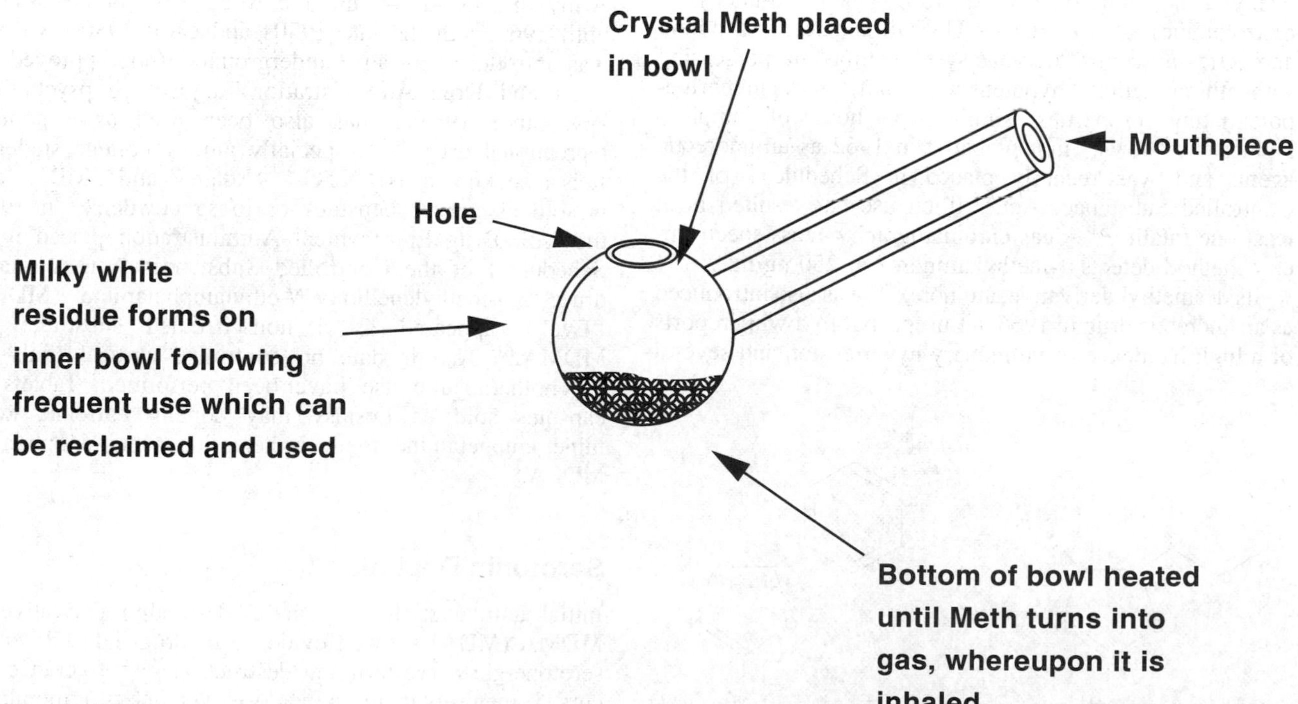

Figure 20-2 Crack and methamphetamine pipes. (From the Division of Law Enforcement, Office of the Attorney General, Sacramento, CA.)

up in garages and houses can be easily dismantled. Pounds are made for a few dollars. Crystal has become one of the most abused drugs among teenagers and young adults in the southwestern United States.[25,46]

Route of Administration

Crystal is snorted or used intravenously for a more intense high.

Warning Signs of Stimulant Addiction

- Irritability, nervousness
- Wide mood swings, depression
- Unreasonable fear, suspicion
- Significant weight loss
- Irregular sleep pattern
- Cloggy, runny nose
- Neglect of work and studies
- Withdrawal from family
- Change in friends
- Loss of money

In addition to classic symptoms of amphetamine abuse, ischemic stroke and thalamic infarction, as well as myocardial infarction, have been reported following inhalation use of pulverized Crystal Meth.

ICE: 4-METHYLAMINOREX

4-Methylaminorex (Fig. 20–3), *cis*-2-amino-4-methyl-5-phenyl-2-oxazoline (*cis*-4,5-dihydro-4-methyl-5-phenyl-2-oxazolamine), also known as U4EUh and Ice, is a potent anorectic and central nervous system stimulant, possessing sympathomimetic, hypotensive, and norepinephrine-potentiating properties similar to those of amphetamines.[47–49] It was first prepared in 1962 as an anorectic agent, and was recently placed in Schedule I of the Controlled Substances Act.[50] Illicit use has resulted in at least one fatality.[51] A gas chromatography–mass spectrometry method detects 4-methylaminorex at 250 ng/mL.[52]

Its desmethyl derivative, aminorex,[53] was also introduced as an anorectic drug in 1966 in Europe, but following reports of a high incidence of pulmonary hypertension and several deaths,[54,55] it was withdrawn from sale in 1968. It has reappeared recently as a designer drug.[53]

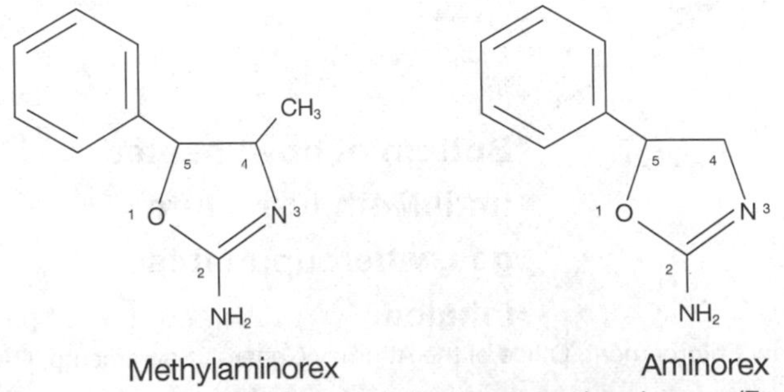

Methylaminorex   Aminorex

Figure 20-3 Structures of methylaminorex and aminorex. (From Brewster ME, Davis FT. Case report: Appearance of aminorex as a designer analog of methylaminorex. J Forens Sci 1991;36:587–592.)

"ECSTASY": 3,4-METHYLENEDIOXY-METHAMPHETAMINE (MDMA)

Ecstasy is the popular name for the illicit drug MDMA and is widely used at dance parties or "raves." It is usually consumed orally in tablet or capsule form at a dose of about 120 mg. Its primary effect is to produce a positive mood state with euphoria, intimacy, and closeness to others. Side effects include loss of appetite, tachycardia, jaw tension, bruxism, and sweating. Effects last about 4 to 6 hours. It does not appear conducive to long-term heavy use because of the development of tolerance to its positive effects and exacerbation of negative effects with large doses and frequent use. There is no evidence to suggest that Ecstasy is addictive. Ecstasy use has been followed by sudden hypertensive crises with spontaneous intracerebral hemorrhage, noncardiac chest pain, a toxic hepatitis, an acute or chronic paranoid psychosis, congestive or mild memory impairment in function, cardiac arrhythmias, and death. MDMA causes serotonin release but blocks uptake at serotonergic nerve terminals. Significant reductions are observed in cerebrospinal fluid levels of 5-hydroxindole-acetic acid, a presynaptic marker of serotonin.[56]

3,4-Methylenedimethoxyamphetamine is a ring-substituted amphetamine derivative that is chemically related to both hallucinogens and stimulants.[57,58] It was first developed as an appetite suppressant in 1914 after it was synthesized in Germany by E. Merck and Company, but it was never marketed.[59] The first biological data appeared in 1973 based on work in animals conducted by the U.S. Army in 1953–1954, but the work was not declassified until 1969.[60] In the late 1970s and early 1980s, MDMA was introduced as an "underground" (not approved by Food and Drug Administration) adjunct to psychotherapy. Since 1983 it has also been used as a popular recreational drug,[58,59] especially among college students. It is also known as "XTC," "Adam," and "MDA" and is sold as gelatin capsules or loose powder.[61] In 1985, the U.S. Drug Enforcement Administration placed it on Schedule I of the Controlled Substances Act. A related drug, 3,4-methylenedioxy-*N*-ethylamphetamine (MDEA, "Eve"), appeared as a nonscheduled substitute for MDMA.[61] To this date no controlled clinical trials for psychotherapeutic use have been performed. Tablets or capsules sold as Ecstasy may contain caffeine, ketamine, amphetamine, methamphetamine, acetaminophen, or MDEA.[62]

Serotonin Depletion

Initial animal studies on the *N*-desmethyl derivative of MDMA (MDA) showed evidence of drug-induced central serotonergic nerve terminal destruction.[63,64] Tolerance occurs. Some users increase the dose over weeks or months of use to as many as 10 or more tablets during the course of an evening. Subsequent data indicate that MDMA, like MDA, is toxic to serotonergic nerve terminals in the rodent brain.[65,66] (See also Chapter 49.)

Clinical Presentation

Anecdotal reports indicate that MDMA induces euphoria, verbosity, and a feeling of closeness with others. By the second day, drowsiness, muscle aches, facial muscle pain, depression, and difficulty in concentrating may be experienced. Such effects may follow a single dose of 60 to 250 mg (approximately 1–4 mg/kg).[58]

There are similar manifestations to both fatal Ecstasy ingestion and severe hyperthermia: muscle rigidity, trismus, hyperthermia, sinus tachycardia, sweating, cardiac arrhythmia, cardiac arrest, tachypnea, cyanosis, metabolic acidosis, rhabdomyolysis, myoglobinuria, and disseminated intravascular coagulation. Signs can develop several hours after Ecstasy ingestion. These complications appear to occur unpredictably and require prompt action, with a treatment plan possibly similar to that used by anesthetists to treat severe hyperthermia, including use of dantrolene.[67] No pharmaceutical company has ever made MDMA, nor has the Food and Drug Administration given its approval. In 1985, the Drug Enforcement administration classified MDMA as a Schedule I compound, believed to have a high potential for abuse and without any currently accepted medical use.[68]

Although there are no data to indicate that such recreational doses of MDMA permanently damage the human brain, observations on recreational users suggest that MDMA may differ from other recreational drugs: (1) Users usually wait at least 2 to 3 weeks between doses of the drug; more frequent use diminishes the desirable effects while enhancing undesirable side effects. (2) Desirable effects begin to change with each successive dose: freshmen love it, sophomores like it, juniors are ambivalent, and seniors are afraid of it. (3) There appear to be no reports of individuals who take frequent and large amounts of MDMA for an extended period. These reports would tend to indicate that there is a long-term, potentially irreversible effect of MDMA on the human brain.[58]

Doses/Blood Levels/Fatalities

A 32-year-old woman ingested between 100 and 150 mg of MDMA, developed a serum level of 6500 ng/mL, and lived.[69] A 40-year-old man ingested a single 50-mg dose, and 2 hours later, his MDMA plasma level peaked at 105.6 ng/mL.[69]

Five deaths have been associated with finding MDMA or MDEA in the blood.[59] One death was due to trauma; MDMA was found in the blood, but the quantity was not measured. Another death was also due to trauma; butalbital 0.8 mg/L (3.6 μmol/L) as well as MDEA 950 ng/mL (4.6 μmol/L) was detected in the blood. One death was associated with a history of recent alcohol use; the blood MDMA level was 1.1 mg/L (5.7 μmol/L). A fourth fatality was a healthy 18-year-old woman who ingested approximately 150 mg of MDMA and an unknown amount of alcohol; she developed ventricular fibrillation and died; her blood showed an MDMA concentration of 1.0 mg/L (5.1 μmol/L) and an ethanol level of 40 mg/dL (8.7 μmol/L). The fifth death followed ingestion of three Ecstasy capsules (approximately 300 mg), alcohol, and propoxyphene; the postmortem blood level of MDEA was 2.0 mg/L (9.7 μmol/L). Thus, one patient appears to have died directly from MDMA (ventricular fibrillation), and the other four deaths may have resulted from trauma or an underlying disease exacerbated by the use of MDMA or MDEA.[61] Similarly, a 34-year-old man with a history of Wolff–Parkinson–White syndrome died; postmortem toxicology revealed MDMA in the blood (2000 ng/mL) and urine (50,000 ng/mL).[70] Ingestion of MDMA may result in life-threatening events or exacerbation of coronary artery disease, asthma, or underlying cardiomyopathy.

Drug Interactions

After ingesting MDMA and the monoamine oxidase inhibitor phenelzine, a 50-year-old man developed marked hypertension, diaphoresis, altered mental status, and hypertonicity lasting 5 to 6 hours; he recovered with supportive treatment.[71] Exaggerated sympathomimetic effects are seen when ingestion of monoamine oxidase inhibitors precedes that of other sympathomimetic agents such as amphetamine, methamphetamine, phenylpropanolamine, metaraminol, mephentermine, methylphenidate, ephedrine, phenylephrine, and dopamine.[17] Similar effects might be expected with MDMA.

Chronic Paranoid Psychosis

Two patients developed a chronic paranoid psychosis after chronic abuse of repeated (usually high) doses (eg, 80–85 mg) of MDMA.[72,73] Misuse of MDMA has also been associated with flashbacks, anxiety, panic confusion, suicidal depression, and insomnia.[74,75]

These reports suggest that individuals with prior psychiatric histories may have an increased susceptibility to the adverse effects of MDMA. In such individuals a single dose of MDMA may be sufficient to produce an enduring psychiatric illness.[76–79] A toxic psychosis has followed ingestion of 140 mg of MDEA (Eve).[80]

Complications

Acute severe complications may follow use of MDMA and include convulsions, collapse, hyperthermia,[81,82] disseminated intravascular coagulation, rhabdomyolysis, acute renal failure,[83] cerebral infarcts,[84] hemorrhage,[85] and death.[86–90] Some who take the drug for the first time may experience paranoia, hallucinations, insomnia, tachycardia, or muscle stiffness including trismus and bruxism. These acute effects usually resolve within 48 hours.[86] Regular users often chew gum to overcome the effects on their jaw muscles; they may present with weight loss, exhaustion, jaundice, flashbacks, irritability, paranoia, depression, or psychosis. Repeated use may endanger hepatic function.[86] Chest pain,[91] tachycardia, hyperkalemia,[92] and spontaneous intracranial hemorrhage have been observed.[93] The hyperthermia may be mediated by serotonin receptors.[94–96] Rarely, fulminant hepatic failure may require liver transplantation.[97]

AMPHETAMINES: GENERAL INFORMATION

Mechanism of Action

Serotonergic Toxicity

Amphetamine derivatives, including *p*-chloramphetamine, fenfluramine, 3,4-methylenedioxyamphetamine, and MDMA, in addition to causing an acute release of serotonin, also lead to long-term depletion of serotonin that correlates with morphologic damage to serotonergic nerve endings.[98]

Dopaminergic Toxicity

Amphetamine-related ingestions block reuptake of dopamine in therapeutic doses, but in overdose may act as dopamine receptor blockers, resulting in typical movement disorders. These usually resolve in the acute setting without any specific intervention.[99]

Lead Poisoning

Illicit methamphetamine may be synthesized by a method that involves the reaction of lead acetate and phenylacetic acid to form phenyl-2-propanone, a precursor methamphetamine in the amalgam process.[100] Subsequent use of methamphetamine adulterated with lead can result in lead poisoning.[100–102]

A suspected case of intravenous methamphetamine-associated lead poisoning may be defined by three or more of the following symptoms in an intravenous methamphetamine user[102]: abdominal pain, nausea, vomiting, lower back and leg pains, weakness, weight loss, and anorexia. A confirmed case is defined as one with seronegativity for both acute hepatitis A and acute hepatitis B and a blood lead level greater than 40 μg/dL (1.93 μmol/L) and/or an erythrocyte protoporphyrin level greater than 60 μg/dL (1.06 μmol/L) in an intravenous methamphetamine user.

Laboratory

Blood and Urine Levels

A person arrested for erratic driving demonstrated a blood level of 0.5 mg/mL, 12 hours postingestion.[103] The administration of 5-15 mg of dextroamphetamine to nonfatigued adults does not result in generalized improvement of psychomotor skills. Some improvement does occur in selected tasks that require rapid responses or increased alertness.[104]

Therapeutic plasma concentrations of fenfluramine are usually in the range 0.05 to 0.15 μg/mL. Toxic effects appear at concentrations greater than 0.5 μg/mL and death has occurred at concentrations greater than 6.0 μg/mL.[105]

Vapor inhalation of methamphetamine results in mean peak methamphetamine plasma concentrations of about 40 ng/mL within 2.5 hours of initiation of drug inhalation. This level declines to about 3 ng/mL over 40 hours. Subjective effects ("high") and cardiovascular effects are most prominent during the first 30 minutes, suggesting rapid development of tachyphylaxis.[106]

Death following illicit phendimetrazine use has been associated with a blood concentration of 300 ng/mL. Therapeutic phendimetrazine levels following ingestion of one 35-mg tablet or one 105-mg sustained-release formulation rarely exceed 100 to 240 ng/mL.[107]

Analytical Methods

Immunoassay-positive results for amphetamine are not absolutely specific for the drug and could be caused by a number of other phenethylamines. Such positive results may also have been caused by an amphetamine analog. In suspect cases, samples with depressed counts (by radioimmunoassay) should be tested for illicit amphetamine analogs.[108]

Confirmation of all presumed positive results in urine samples by various high-performance liquid chromatography (HPLC) or gas chromatography is labor intensive, prone to interference from artifacts, and usually insensitive to secondary amines.[109] A rapid sensitive test for confirmation of both amphetamine and methylamphetamine in urine also detects related sympathomimetic agents such as MDMA and methoxyphenamine. The method uses HPLC with a precolumn derivatization using the fluorophore FMOC chloride (9-fluorenylmethyl chloroformate) and fluorescence detection.[110]

Urine samples may be analyzed for amphetamine, methamphetamine, and MDMA by solid-phase extraction, derivatization, and gas chromatography–mass spectrometry. The detection limit for amphetamine, methamphetamine, and MDMA with this procedure is 50 ng/mL.[49,111,112]

False-Positive Urine Test for Amphetamine. Simultaneous use of amantadine, desipramine, and cocaine prolongs the high and decreases the adverse effects of cocaine. High concentrations of desipramine and amantadine are sufficiently cross-reactive to cause a false-positive amphetamine test.[113]

Methamphetamine radioimmunoassay methods continue to evolve[114–118] in an attempt both to quantitate methamphetamine and its metabolite amphetamine and to separate the psychoactive *d* isomer of methamphetamine from its nonscheduled *l* isomer.[117] False-positive test results require confirmation by gas chromatography–mass spectrometry. Methamphetamine has also been detected and quantified in hair, nails, sweat, and saliva by electron-impact mass fragmentography.[118]

Methamphetamine Isomers. Methamphetamine may occur as a racemic mixture of *d* and *l* optical isomers. *d*-Methamphetamine, a Schedule II controlled substance, is a potent central nervous system stimulant subject to illicit drug abuse, whereas *l*-methamphetamine (*l*-desoxyephedrine) is an alpha-adrenergic stimulant available in over-the-counter Vicks Nasal Inhaler as a nasal decongestant. Therefore, use of Vicks inhalers may pose potential problems for laboratories conducting urine drug testing for methamphetamine abuse. For laboratories relying solely on immunoassay testing, cross-reactivity of *l*-desoxyephedrine may lead to erroneous results.[119] The TDx assay is stereoselective for the *d* isomers of amphetamine and methamphetamine. Persons using Vicks inhalers as per the stated directions on the package would not be expected to yield false-positive results when their urine is tested by the TDx assay. Persons using Vicks inhalers at *double the recommended dose* on the package may yield false-positive amphetamine results. Urine specimens collected following excessive inhaler use (12–20 times the indicated dose) contained *l*-desoxyephedrine concentrations sufficient to produce a false-positive amphetamine results with the TDx assay.[119]

Treatment

Stabilization

The major life-threatening complications of acute amphetamine overdose include hyperthermia, hypertension, convulsions, cardiovascular collapse, and self-inflicted trauma.[120] Severely intoxicated patients should receive an intravenous line, cardiac monitoring (electrocardiogram), and oxygen. Respiratory depression is uncommon in pure amphetamine intoxication, but either cardiogenic pulmonary edema or the adult respiratory distress syndrome may develop. Most patients tolerate sinus tachycardia well, but propranolol may be used to slow tachydysrhythmias in symptomatic patients. Hypotension may respond to fluid challenges, but often a vasopressor is needed. Shock is a poor prognostic sign and indicates the need for right-sided heart catheterization to measure right-sided filling pressures and cardiac output.

Supportive Measures

For the patient who is acutely ill, management is urgent and includes control of seizures, (airway management, ventilatory support, and intravenous diazepam), measurement of core temperature, rapid rehydration, and the possible use of active cooling measures and dantrolene.[83,93] Mannitol diuresis may enhance myoglobin clearance and prevent acute renal failure.[92] Panic disorders and depression may respond to serotonin-active drugs such as fluvoxamine (100 mg daily), amitriptyline, and tranylcypromine; however, the use of monoamine oxidase inhibitors in amphetamine overdose is not advised.[111] Dantrolene (3 mg/kg over 1 hour) may reduce the hyperthermia while having little effect on the clinical outcome.[121,122]

In patients who present within 4 hours of ingestion, hemodynamic parameters, renal and clotting function, rectal temperature, and psychological and neurologic status should be monitored and gastric lavage should be considered with appropriate tracheal precautions.

Agitation. Anxiety, agitation, and hyperactivity should generally be controlled by the use of repeated small doses of intravenous diazepam. Haloperidol was proposed as safer and more effective than chlorpromazine and has been used successfully in MDMA overdose. Because of their potential for enhanced toxicity, however, neither of these agents is recommended.

Seizures. Seizures should be treated with airway management, ventilatory support, and intravenous diazepam. Convulsions refractory to diazepam may be controlled with phenytoin. Curarization may be necessary when hyperthermia and rhabdomyolysis complicate the clinical course.

Hypertension. Tachycardia and hypertension should be treated with beta blockers (eg, atenolol) and alpha blockers (eg, phentolamine) respectively. Labetalol, a combined alpha and beta blocker, may be even more suitable.

Volume Depletion. Vigorous fluid replacement is necessary to correct volume depletion and to facilitate thermoregulation by sweating.

Fever. Mild fever should be treated with cool compresses and sponging. Rectal temperatures exceeding 39°C should be treated more aggressively with hypothermic blankets and ice baths as well as administration of dantrolene. Dantrolene infusions were shown to rapidly correct hyperpyrexia and the hypermetabolic state seen in MDMA overdose. If dantrolene is ineffective in controlling the fever, the patient should be paralyzed and mechanically ventilated.[123] Neuromuscular paralysis is rapidly effective for severe hyperthermia associated with muscle rigidity or hyperactivity. If the patient remains rigid despite neuromuscular blockade, a defect at the muscle cell should be considered (ie, malignant hyperthermia), and dantrolene should be given.[124]

Complications

Severe amphetamine intoxication may be complicated by a variety of problems, including acute renal failure, rhabdomyolysis, acute compartment syndrome, subarachnoid hemorrhage, intracerebral hematoma, cerebral edema with transtentorial herniation, disseminated intravascular coagulation, and adult respiratory distress syndrome. Laboratory examinations and repeat physical examinations are necessary to diagnose these conditions early. Management is primarily supportive, but surgery may be required for intracranial lesions or compartment syndromes.

Body Packing. Body packing of amphetamines with type 1 packages (fingercots, cellophane, condoms) may result in symptoms of toxicity and could require surgical intervention.[125] (See also Chapter 21.)

"Speed" Addiction

Methamphetamine "speed" addicts may respond to treatment with oral dextroamphetamine (20–80 mg daily) mixed with orange juice prescribed to assist the subject over the "craving" or "withdrawal" phase.[126] The program is of interest but further experience is required to substantiate its usefulness.[127]

Illicit Methamphetamine Manufacture

Any responder to an illicit laboratory should use personal protective equipment such as impervious rubber boots or synthetic boots, chemical-resistant impervious gloves, positive-pressure self-contained breathing apparatus or cartridge respirators with appropriate filters, goggles, and chemical resistant overalls, all of which should be disposable.[128]

REFERENCES—AMPHETAMINES

1. Cohen S. Amphetamine abuse. JAMA 1975;231:414–415.
2. Council on Scientific Affairs. Clinical aspects of amphetamine abuse. JAMA 1978;240:2317–2319.
3. Smith DE. Physical vs psychological dependence and tolerance in high dose methamphetamine abuse. Clin Toxicol 1969;2:99–103.

4. Smith DE, Fisher CM. An analysis of 310 cases of acute high dose methamphetamine toxicity in Haight Ashbury. Clin Toxicol 1970;3:117–124.
5. Monroe RR, Drell HJ. Oral use of stimulants obtained from inhalers. JAMA 1947;135:909–915.
6. Anderson RJ, Reed WG, Hillis LD, et al. History, epidemiology, and medical complications of nasal inhaler abuse. J Toxicol Clin Toxicol 1982;19:95–107.
7. Di Maio VJM, Garriott JC. Intravenous abuse of propylhexedrine. J Forens Sci 1977;22:152–158.
8. Gal J. Amphetamines in nasal inhalers. J Toxicol Clin Toxicol 1982;19:577–578.
9. Zalis EG, Parmley LF. Fatal amphetamine poisoning. Arch Intern Med 1963;101:822–826.
10. Kendrick WC, Hull AR, Knochel JP. Rhabdomyolysis and shock after intravenous amphetamine administration. Ann Intern Med 1977;86:381–387.
11. Shulgin AT. 3-Methoxy-4,5-methylenedioxyamphetamine: A new psychotomimetic agent. Nature 1964;201:1120–1121.
12. Sottolano SM. The quantitation of phenyl-2-propanone using high-performance liquid chromatography. J Forens Sci 1988;33:1415–1420.
13. Dal Cason TA, Angelos SA, Rancy JK. A clandestine approach to the synthesis of phenyl-2-propanone from phenylpropenes. J Forens Sci 1984;29:1187–1208.
14. Frank RS. The clandestine drug laboratory situation in the United States. J Forens Sci 1983;28:18–31.
15. Cantrell TS, John B, Johnson L, Allen AC. A study of impurities found in methamphetamine synthesized from ephedrine. Forens Sci Int 1988;39:39–53.
16. Arax M, Gorman T. California's illicit farm belt export. Los Angeles Times, March 13, 1995, pp. A1, A15.
17. Allen AC, Kiser WO. Methamphetamines from ephedrine: 1. Chloroephedrines and aziridines. J Forens Sci 1987;32:953–962.
18. Ely RA, McGrath DC. Lithium–ammonia reduction of ephedrine to methamphetamine: An unusual clandestine synthesis. J Forens Sci 1990;35:720–723.
19. Allen A, Cantrell TS. Synthetic reductions in clandestine amphetamine and methamphetamine laboratories: A review. Forens Sci Int 1989;42:183–199.
20. Dal Cason TA. An evaluation of the potential for clandestine manufacture of 3,4-methylenedioxyamphetamine (MDA) analogs and homologs. J Forens Sci 1990;35:675–697.
21. By AW, Dawson BA, Lodge BA, et al. Synthesis and spectral properties of 2,5-dimethoxy-4-ethoxyamphetamine and its precursors. J Forens Sci 1990;35:316–335.
22. By AW, Duhaime R, Lodge BA. The synthesis and spectra of 4-ethoxyamphetamine and its isomers. Forens Sci Int 1991;49:159–170.
23. Zhingel KY, Dovensky W, Crossman A, Allen A. Ephedrone: 2-Methylamino-l-phenylpropan-l-one (Jeff). J Forens Sci 1991;36:915–920.
24. Smith DE. Physical vs psychological dependence and tolerance in high dose methamphetamine abuse. Clin Toxicol 1979;2:99–103.
25. Mineo RM. *Facts About . . . CRYSTAL.* La Jolla, CA: Scripps Memorial Hospital, the McDonald Center for Alcoholism and Drug Addiction Treatment, 1992.
26. Jackson JG. Hazards of smokable methamphetamine. N Engl J Med 1989;321:907.
27. Largent DR, Desha A, Stevenson P, et al. *"Ice": Crystal methamphetamine.* California Department of Justice, Bureau of Narcotic Enforcement, September, 1989.
28. Monroe RR, Drell HJ. Oral use of stimulants obtained from inhalers. JAMA 1947;135:909–915.
29. Hong R, Matsuyama E, Nur K. Cardiomyopathy associated with the smoking of crystal methamphetamine. JAMA 1991;265:1151–1154.
30. Sachdeva K, Woodward KG. Caudal thalamic infarction following intranasal methamphetamine use. Neurology 1989;39:305–306.
31. Gospe SM Jr. Transient cortical blindness in an infant exposed to methamphetamine. Ann Emerg Med 1995;26:380–382.
32. Furst SR, Fullon SP, Reznik GN, Shah PK. Myocardial infarction after inhalation of methamphetamine. N Engl J Med 1990;323:1147–1148.
33. Nestor TA, Tamamotoa WI, Kam TH, Schultz T. Acute pulmonary edema caused by crystalline methamphetamine. Lancet 1989;2:1277–1278.
34. Bailey DN, Manoguerra AS. Survey of drug abuse patterns and toxicology analysis in an emergency room population. J Anal Toxicol 1980;4:199–203.
35. Mendelson J, Jones RT, Upton R, Jacob P III. Methamphetamine and ethanol interactions in humans. Clin Pharmacol Ther 1995;57:559–568.
36. Mack RB. The iceman cometh and killeth: Smokable methamphetamine. NC Med J 1990;51:276–278.
37. Sekine H, Nakahara Y. Abuse of smoking methamphetamine mixed with tobacco: 1. Inhalation efficiency and pyrolysis products of methamphetamine. J Forens Sci 1987;32:1271–1280.
38. Sekine H, Nakahara Y. Abuse of smoking methamphetamine mixed with tobacco, II: The formation mechanism of pyrolysis products. J Forens Sci 1990;35:580–590.
39. Catanzarite VA, Stein DA. 'Crystal' and pregnancy: Methamphetamine-associated maternal deaths. West J Med 1995;162:454–457.
40. Dixon SD, Bejar R. Echoencephalographic findings in neonates associated with maternal cocaine and methamphetamine use: Incidence and clinical correlates. J Pediatr 1989;115:770–778.
41. Elliott RH, Rees GB. Amphetamine ingestion presenting as eclampsia. Can J Anaesth 1990;37:130–133.
42. Dearlove JC, Betteridge TJ, Henry JA. Stillbirth due to intravenous amphetamine. Br Med J 1992;304:548.
43. Oro AS, Dixon SD. Perinatal cocaine and methamphetamine exposure: Maternal and neonatal correlates. J Pediatr 1987;111:571–578.
44. Dixon SD. Effects of transplacental exposure to cocaine and methamphetamine in the neonate. West J Med 1989;150:436–442.
45. Bost RO, Kemp P, Hnilica V. Tissue distribution of methamphetamine and amphetamine in premature infants. J Anal Toxicol 1989;13:300–302.
46. Rothrock, JF, Rubenstein R, Lyden PD. Ischemic stroke associated with methamphetamine inhalation. Neurology 1988;38:589–592.
47. Klein RFX, Sperling AR, Cooper DA, Kram TC. The stereoisomers of 4-methylaminorex. J Forens Sci 1989;34:962–979.
48. Yelnosky J, Katz R. Sympathomimetic actions of *cis*-2-amino-4-methyl-5-phenyl-2-oxazoline. J Pharmacol Exp Ther 1963;141:180–184.
49. Patil PN, Yamauchi D. Influence of optical isomers of some centrally acting drugs on norepinephrine responses. Eur J Pharmacol 1970;12:132–135.
50. Lawn JC. Schedules of controlled substances: Temporary placement of 2-amino-4-methyl-5-phenyl-2-oxazoline (4-methylaminorex) into Schedule I. Fed Regist 1987;52:30174–30175.
51. Davis FT, Brewster ME. A fatality involving U4Euh, a cyclic derivative of phenylpropanolamine. J Forens Sci 1988;33:549–553.
52. Sudmeier SJ, Smith FP, Reuschel SA, Kidwell DA. Four isomers of methylaminorex in urine examined by immunoassay and GC/MS. In: *Proceedings American Academy of Forensic Sciences, 44th Annual Meeting, New Orleans, February 17–22, 1992:*Abstract K-47, p. 198.
53. Brewster ME, Davis FT. Appearance of aminorex as a designer analog of methylaminorex. J Forens Sci 1991;36:587–592.
54. Gurtner H. Aminorex and pulmonary hypertension. Cor Vasa 1985;27:160–171.
55. Seiler K. Aminorex and pulmonary circulation. Arzneitmittelforschung 1975;25:837.
56. Solowij N. Ecstasy (3,4-methylenedioxymethamphetamine). Curr Opin Psychiatry 1993;6:411–415.
57. Peroutka SJ. Incidence of recreational use of 3,4-methylenedimethoxymethamphetamine (MDMA, 'Ecstasy') on an undergraduate campus. N Engl J Med 1987;317:1542–1543.

58. Peroutka SJ. 'Ecstasy': A human neurotoxin? Arch Gen Psychiatry 1989;416:191.
59. Dowling GP, McDonough ET, Bost RO. 'Eve' and 'Ecstasy': A report of five deaths associated with the use of MDEA and MDMA. JAMA 1987;257:1615–1617.
60. Davis WM, Hatoum HT, Waters W. Toxicity of MDA (3,4-methylenedioxyamphetamine) considered for relevance to hazards of MDMA (ecstasy) abuse. Alcohol Drug Res 1987;7: 127–134.
61. Brown C, Osterloh J. Multiple severe complications from recreational ingestion of MDMA ("Ecstasy"). JAMA 1987;258: 780–781.
62. Wolff K, Hay AWM, Sherlock K, Conner M. Contents of 'Ecstasy.' Lancet 1995;346:1100–1105.
63. Ricaurte GA, Gorno LS, Wilson MA, et al. (+/–)-3,4-Methylenedioxymethamphetamine selectively damages central serotonergic neurons in nonhuman primates. JAMA 1988; 260:51–55.
64. Ricaurte C, Bryan G, Strauss L, et al. Hallucinogenic amphetamine selectively destroys serotonin nerve terminals. Science 1985;229:986–988.
65. Battaglia G, Yeh SY, O'Hearn E, et al. 3,4-Methylenedioxymethamphetamine and 3,4-methylenedioxymethamphetamine destroy serotonin terminals in rat brain: Quantification of neurodegeneration by measurement of [^{3}H]paroxetine-labeled serotonin uptake sites. J Pharmacol Exp Ther 1987;242:911–916.
66. Stikker W Jr, Ali SF, Scallet AC, et al.: Neurochemical and neurohistological alterations in the rat and monkey produced by orally administered methylenedioxymethamphetamine (MDMA). Toxicol Appl Pharmacol 1988;94:448–457.
67. Rittoo DB, Rittoo D. Complications of "Ecstasy" misuse. Lancet 1992;340:725–727.
68. Randall T. Ecstasy-fueled 'rave' parties become dances of death for English youths. JAMA 1992;268:1505–1506.
69. Verebey K, Alrazi J, Jaffe JH. The complications of 'Ecstasy' (MDMA). JAMA 1988;259:1649–1650.
70. Suarez RV, Riecmersma R. "Ecstasy" and sudden cardiac death. Am J Forens Med Pathol 1988;9:339–341.
71. Smilkstein MJ, Smolinske SC, Rumack BH. A case of MAO inhibitor/MDMA interaction: Agony after Ecstasy. Clin Toxicol 1987;25:149–159.
72. McGuire P, Fahy T. Chronic paranoid psychosis after misuse of 'MDMA' ("Ecstasy"). Br Med J 1991;302:697.
73. Greer G, Strassman RJ. Information on "Ecstasy." Am J Psychiatry 1985;142:1391-1411.
74. Creighton FJ, Black DL, Heyde CE. 'Ecstasy' psychosis and flashbacks. Br J Psychiatry 1991;159:713–715.
75. Benazzi F, Mazzoli M. Psychiatric illness associated with 'Ecstasy'. Lancet 1991;338:1520.
76. McCann UD, Ricaurte GA. MDMA ("Ecstasy") and panic disorder: Induction by a single dose. Biol Psychiatry 1992;32: 950–953.
77. Pallanti S, Mazzi D. MDMA (Ecstasy): Precipitation of panic disorder. Biol Psychiatry 1992;32:91–95.
78. McCann UD, Ricaurte GA. Lasting neuropsychiatric sequelae of (+–)-methylenedioxymethamphetamine ("Ecstasy") in recreational users. J Clin Psychopharmacol 1991;11:302–305.
79. Schifano F. Chronic atypical psychosis associated with MDMA ("Ecstasy") abuse. Lancet 1991;338:1335.
80. Gouzoulis E, Borchardt D, Hermle L. A case of psychosis induced by 'Eve' (3,4-methylene-dioxyethylamphetamine). Arch Gen Psychiatry 1993;50:75.
81. Screaton GR, Singer M, Cairns HG, et al. Hyperpyrexia and rhabdomyolysis after MDMA ("Ecstasy") abuse. Lancet 1992; 339:677–678.
82. Woods JD, Henry JA. Hyperpyrexia induced by 3,4-methylenedioxyamphetamine ("Eve"). Lancet 1992;340:305.
83. Better OS, Stein JH. Early management of shock and prophylaxis of acute renal failure in traumatic rhabdomyolysis. N Engl J Med 1990;322:825–829.
84. Manchanda S, Connolly MJ. Cerebral infarction in association with ecstasy abuse. Postgrad Med J 1993;69:874–889.
85. Harries DP, De Silva R. Ecstasy and intracerebral hemorrhage. Scot Med J 1992;37:150–152.
86. Whitaker-Azmitia PM, Aronson TA. "Ecstasy" (MDMA)-induced panic. Am J Psychiatry 1989;146:119.
87. Henry JA. Ecstasy and the dance of death: Severe reactions are unpredictable. Br Med J 1992;305:566.
88. Chadwick IS, Curry PD, Linsley A, et al. Ecstasy, 3-4 methylenedioxymethamphetamine (MDMA), a fatality associated with coagulopathy and amphetamine. J R Soc Med 1991;8: 371.
89. Campkin NTA, Davies VM. Another death from Ecstasy. J R Soc Med 1992;85:861.
90. Gorard DA, Davier SE, Clark ML. Misuse of Ecstasy. Br Med J 1992;305:309.
91. Henry JA, Jeffreys KJ, Dawling S. Toxicity and deaths from 3,4-methylenedioxymethamphetamine ("Ecstasy"). Lancet 1992;340:384–387.
92. Fahal I, Sallomi DF, Yaqoob M, Bell GM. Acute renal failure after Ecstasy. Br Med J 1992;35:29.
93. Rittoo D, Rittoo DR, Rittoo D. Misuse of Ecstasy. Br Med J 1992;305:309–310.
94. Sawyer J, Stephens WP. Misuse of Ecstasy. Br Med J 1992; 305:310.
95. De Silva RN, Harries DP. Misuse of Ecstasy. Br Med J 1992; 305:310.
96. Schmidt CJ, Black CK, Abbate GM, Taylor VL. Methylenedioxyamphetamine-induced hyperthermia and neurotoxicity are independently mediated by 5-HT_2 receptors. Brain Res 1990;529:85-90.
97. Garbino J, Jollet P, Metha G. Liver transplantation after fulminant hepatic failure due to 'Ecstasy' hepatitis. In: *Proceedings, 5th World Congress of the World Federation of Association of Clinical Toxicology Centers and Poison Control Centers, Taipei, November 8, 1994:* Abstract H28.
98. Rudnick G, Wall SC. The molecular mechanism of Ecstasy [3,4-methylenedioxymethamphetamine (MDMA)]: Serotonin transporters are targets for MDMA-induced serotonin release. Proc Natl Acad Sci USA 1992;89:1817–1821.
99. Warder C, Winger J. Choreoathetoid reaction associated with a methylphenidate reaction in a toddler. Clin Toxicol 1995; 33:475–486 (Abstract 94).
100. Allcott JV III, Barnhart RA, Mooney LA. Acute lead poisoning in two users of illicit methamphetamine. JAMA 1987;258: 510–511.
101. Norton RL, Kauffman KW, Chandler DB, et al. Intravenous lead poisoning associated with methamphetamine use. Vet Hum Toxicol 1989;31:379.
102. Lead poisoning associated with intravenous methamphetamine use: Oregon, 1988. MMWR 1989;38:830–831.
103. Kintz P, Mangin P. Toxicological findings after fatal fenfluramine self-poisoning. Hum Exp Toxicol 1992;11:51–52.
104. Evans MA, Martz R, Lemberger L, et al. Effects of dextroamphetamine on psychomotor skills. Clin Pharmacol Ther 1976;19:777–781.
105. Perez-Reyes M, White WL, McDonald SA, et al. Clinical effects of methamphetamine vapor inhalation. Life Sci 1991;49:953–959.
106. Hood I, Monforte J, Gault R, Mirchandani H. Fatality from illicit phendimetrazine use. Clin Toxicol 1988;26:249–255.
107. Bost RO, Sutheimer CA, Sunshine I. Relative merits of some methods for amphetamine assay in biological fluids. Clin Chem 1976;22:789–801.
108. Christophersen AS, Bugge A, Dahlin E, et al. Interference with analysis of amphetamine in blood by *N*-ethylbenzenamine from rubber septums. J Anal Toxicol 1988;12:147–149.
109. Lewis JH. The use of HPLC fluorescence detection and FMOC in the detection of amphetamine and methylamphetamine in the urine of drug abusers. In: Uges DRA, de Zeeuw RA, eds. *TIAFT, Proceedings of the 25th International Meeting, International Association of Forensic Toxicologists, Groningen, 1988:*272–276.
110. Rasmussen S, Cole R, Spiehler V. Methamphetamine antemortem blood and urine by radioimmunoassay and GC/MS. J Anal Toxicol 1989;13:263–267.
111. Gan BK, Baugh D, Liu RH, Walia AS. Simultaneous analysis of amphetamine, methamphetamine and 3,4-dioxymethamphetamine (MDMA) in urine samples by solid-phase ex-

traction, derivatization and gas chromatography/mass spectrometry. J Forens Sci 1991;36:1331–1341.
112. Paton DM, Bell JI, Yee R, et al. Pharmacology and toxicity of 3,4-methylenedioxyamphetamine, paramethoxamphetamine and related dimethoxyamphetamines. Proc West Pharmacol Soc 1975;18:229–231.
113. Merigian KS, Browning RG. Desipramine and amantadine causing false-positive urine test for amphetamine. Ann Emerg Med 1993;22:1927–1928.
114. Shaw RF. The forensic toxicoloty of methamphetamine in San Diego County, 1989. Calif Assoc Toxicol Newslett 1991 (Spring):23.
115. Hornbeck CL, Czarny RJ. Evaluation of a fluorescence polarization immunoassay for methamphetamine/amphetamine. In: *Proceedings of Meeting of American Academy of Forensic Sciences, Anaheim, California, 1990:* 133 (Abstract K6).
116. Carrico J, Freeman J, Graham B, Jones C. A new Emit[R] assay for amphetamine/methamphetamine. In: *Proceedings of Meeting of American Academy of Forensic Sciences, 1990:*141–142 (Abstract K37).
117. Gaff SL, Ward CD, Vitone S, Wu R, et al. Abuscreen radioimmunoassay for methamphetamine (high specificity): A selective RIA for detection of *d*-methamphetamine abuse. In: *Proceedings of Meeting of American Academy of Forensic Sciences, Anaheim, California, 1990:* 164 (Abstract K23).
118. Suzuki S-I, Inoue T, Hori H, Inayama S. Analysis of methamphetamine in hair, nail, sweat and saliva by mass fragmentography. J Anal Toxicol 1989;13:176–178.
119. Poklis A, Moore KA. Stereoselectivity of the TDxADx/Flx amphetamine/methamphetamine II amphetamine/methamphetamine immunoassay: Response of urine specimens following nasal inhaler use. Clin Toxicol 1995;33:35–41.
120. Gary NE, Saidi P. Methamphetamine intoxication: A speedy new treatment. Am J Med 1978;64:537–540.
121. Singarajah C, Lavies NG. An overdose of Ecstasy: A role for dantrolene. Anaesthesia 1992;47:686–687.
122. Barrett PJ. 'Ecstasy' misuse: Overdose or normal dose? Anaesthesia 1993;48:83.
123. Cregg MT, Tracey JA. Ecstasy abuse in Ireland. Irish Med J 1993;86:118–120.
124. Callaway CW, Clark RF. Hyperthermia in psychostimulant overdose. Ann Emerg Med 1994;24:68–76.
125. Watson CJE, Thomson HJ, Johnston PS. Body-packing with amphetamines: An indication for surgery. J R Soc Med 1991;84:311–312.
126. Nichol AM. The nontherapeutic use of psychoactive drugs: A modern epidemic. N Engl J Med 1983;308:925–933.
127. Sherman JP. Dexamphetamine for "speed" addiction. Med J Austral 1990;153:306.
128. Skeers VM. Illegal methamphetamine drug laboratories: A new challenge for environmental health personnel. J Environ Health 1992;55:6–10.

METHCATHINONE ("CAT")

Methcathinone (see also Chapter 74: Khat) is an illicit drug commonly known by its street name "Cat."[1–3] It is similar in structure and effect to methamphetamine, looks like cocaine, and produces the same euphoria as crack. A designer drug, it has been abused in the former Soviet Union[1] since 1982, when home synthesis began in Leningrad, under the name ephedrone ("Jeff") (Fig. 20–4)[4] and has been used in the rural U.S. Midwest since 1991.[3,5,6] Cases have appeared in other states, allegedly spread by motorcycle gangs who have expertise in making and distributing methamphetamine. The recipe uses readily available, legal ingredients (e.g., ephedrine), and it is easier to make than methamphetamines. According to addicts, methcathinone is more potent and addictive than other psychostimulants. Intoxicating effects may last up to 6 days.[6] In the United States, the Drug Enforcement Administration has placed this drug in Schedule I of the Controlled Substances Act.[7,8] Deaths following its use have been reported in the former Soviet Union.[6,9]

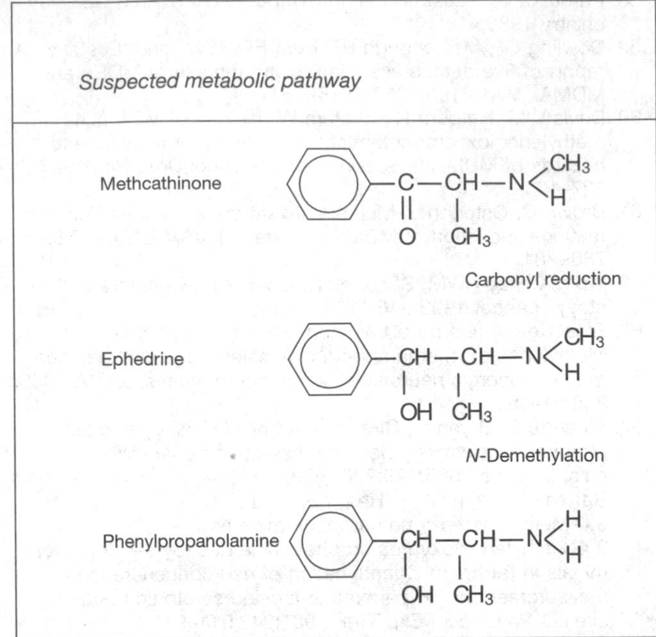

Figure 20-4 Metabolic pathway of methcathinone. (From Emerson TS, Cisek JE. Methcathinone: A Russian designer amphetamine infiltrates the rural Midwest. Ann Emerg Med 1993;22:1897–1903. Erratum. 1994;23:790E.)

Structure and Classification

Methcathinone is a phenylisopropylamine that can produce a variety of pharmacologic effects depending on the presence and location of substituent groups. The parent compound of this family of agents, phenylisopropylamine itself (ie, amphetamine), is a psychostimulant. A metabolic pathway is suggested in Figure 20–4.[9] Four of these agents encountered in the clandestine market are not truly designer drugs: one (cathinone) is the active constituent of a shrub (Khat, *Catha edalis*) that has been abused for centuries. The others (aminorex, 4-methylaminorex[U4EUh, 4-MAX], and the *N*-methyl derivative of cathinone) were originally developed as potential anorectic agents by the pharmaceutical industry.[1] They are related to one another and are distinct from amphetamine in possessing a benzylic oxygen function. Certain methoxy-substituted derivatives, for example, 1-(2,5-dimethoxy-4-methylphenyl-2-aminopropane) (Dom), are hallucinogenic in humans.[2] Animal studies suggest that the descending rank order of stimulation compared with cocaine is aminorex, methcathinone, cathinone, 4-methylaminorex, and cocaine.[1]

Use

Methcathinone is used for its potent central nervous system-stimulant properties.

Product Formulation

A white powdery substance, methcathinone may contain other active ingredients such as toluene (alone toluene may cause an encephalopathy, ventricular arrhythmia, dermatitis, hypokalemia and renal tubular acidosis); potassium permanganate or sodium dichromate (may cause chromium toxicity and have a caustic potential); sulfuric acid; and ephedrine (either as an unreactive original agent or as a diluent, it may cause overdose reactions similar to those of over-the-counter products containing ephedrine). Ingredient-related problems may be experienced by users of incompletely processed "green" Cat. The usual off-white powder takes on a green tinge when it has been crudely processed with sodium dichromate.

Source

Methcathinone is produced by clandestine laboratories.

Dose

The typical dose of Cat is 0.5 to 1 g/d by the intranasal or intravenous route. The cost is $100 per gram.[6,10]

Toxicokinetics

Elimination

Active metabolites include ephedrine and phenylpropanolamine.[3]

Drug Interactions

Beta blockers administered to Cat users with cardiac problems may leave the users susceptible to malignant hypertension and subsequent stroke.[5]

Mechanism of Action

Methcathinone appears to act primarily in the central nervous system through dopaminergic pathways and may have active metabolites (ephedrine and phenylpropanolamine) with strong peripheral action.[3]

Clinical Presentation

Overdose

Prominent findings include visual and auditory hallucinations, fever, and tachycardia, followed by periods of bradycardia and hypotension (6–12 hours) as acute symptoms resolve.[3] Cat produces a euphoric high with reports of increased sexuality, creativity, and garrulousness. As dosage or time of usage increase, anxiety, disorientation, and paranoia develop.[5] Psychomotor activity, impulsivity, and aggression have been observed.

Chronic Use

Chronic use may result in the development of a paranoid psychosis, decline in personal hygiene, muscle-wasting anorexia, hypertrophied lingual papillae, acrocyanosis, acne, hepatomegaly, antisocial behavior, and parkinsonism.[1] Death has been reported in Russia from cardiac arrhythmia and violent suicides. Life-threatening high fevers; seizures; mydriasis with diminished light reaction, loss of accommodation, and fine horizontal and vertical nystagmus; flushing; sweating palms; upgoing Babinski reflex; and brisk deep tendon reflexes have been observed. Some users have open lesions in their arms and hands from exposure to the caustic chemicals during manufacturing. Users may develop nose lesions or epistaxis following intranasal insufflation (snorting) of the drug.

Users snort, ingest, smoke, or inject Cat. They marginally use the drug over 15 to 60 minutes during binges lasting 5 days and then rest for several days.[5]

Withdrawal

Withdrawal may involve cardiovascular collapse with hypotension and bradycardia, lethargy, irritability, miosis, craving for sweets, coryza, myalgias, muscle spasms, and arthralgias especially involving the knees.[5]

Laboratory

Few commercial tests can detect methcathinone. Testing chronic users for suspected metabolites such as phenylpropanolamine and ephedrine may provide a clue. Such tests are not conclusive of methcathinone use because these drugs are available without prescription.

Treatment

Treatment requires supportive measures similar to those used for the methamphetamines or cocaine. Most adverse effects are self-limited on withdrawal of the drug. Differential diagnosis should include central nervous system infection; sepsis; thyrotoxicosis; withdrawal from sedatives, hypnotics, or alcohol; and toxic reactions to other drugs including theophylline, salicylates, monoamine oxidase inhibitors (reactions with other drugs), nitrophenols, halogenated hydrocarbons, MDMA (Ecstasy), LSD, mescaline, phencyclidine (PCP), and cocaine.

Benzodiazepines are indicated for patients with hallucinations, hyperactivity, seizures, or extreme agitation. Fever responds to lorazepam and cooling measures. Lorazepam's effects last 5 to 8 hours, about as long as methcathinone. Acetaminophen is useful (orally or rectally). Hypotension and bradycardia respond to conservative traditional supportive therapy. Psychosis during the detoxification process is managed by antipsychotic agents. Following detoxification, the patient dependent on methcathinone should be enrolled in a comprehensive drug abuse treatment program.

REFERENCES—METHCATHINONE ("CAT")

1. Young R, Glennon RA. Cocaine-stimulus generalization to two new designer drugs; Methcathinone and 4-methylaminorex. Pharmacol Biochem Behav 1993;45:229–231.
2. Glennon FA, Yousif M, Naiman N, Kalix P. Methcathinone: A new and potent amphetamine-like agent. Pharmacol Biochem Behav 1987;26:547–551.

3. Emerson TS, Cisek JE. Methcathinone ("Cat"): A Russian designer amphetamine infiltrates the rural Midwest. Vet Hum Toxicol 1993;34:362.
4. Zhingel KY, Dovensky W, Crossman A, Allen A. Ephedrone: 2-Methylamino-1-phenylpropan-1-one (Jeff). J Forens Sci 1991;36:915–920.
5. Carrell S. Methcathinone: The next drug epidemic? Emerg Med News 1993;15:1–24.
6. Goldstone MS. "Cat: Methcathinone—a new drug of abuse. JAMA 1993;269:2508.
7. Bonner RC. Schedule of controlled substances: Temporary placement of methcathinone into Schedule I. Fed Regist 1992;57:9080–9081.
8. Bonner RD. Schedules of controlled substances: Temporary placement of methcathinone into Schedule I. Fed Regist 1992; 18824–18825.
9. Emerson TC, Cisek JE. Methcathione: A Russian designer amphetamine infiltrates the rural midwest. Ann Emerg Med 1993;22:1897–1903.
10. Bowles S. Designer drugs' potency dwarfs crack cocaine: 'Cat' produces high that can last up to six days. Seattle Times, September 28, 1992, p. A1.

PEMOLINE

Pemoline (2-imino-5-phenyl-4-oxazolidinone) is a central nervous stimulant used principally in children with attention deficit disorder and in adults with memory deficit or narcolepsy (Table 20–1). It induces an increase in the availability of dopamine and norepinephrine at the synaptic cleft, similar to the amphetamines.

Toxicokinetics

A single 2 mg/kg oral dose of pemoline leads to a maximum plasma concentration of 4.3 μg/mL in 2.8 hours. The elimination half-life is 8.6 hours, and total body clearance is 0.65 mL/min/kg.[1]

Clinical Presentation

Chronic use has induced adverse effects such as addiction, paranoid psychosis, and precipitation of Gilles de la Tourette's syndrome. Hepatotoxicity, which may be fatal, has followed use.[2] Pemoline may be associated with abnormal involuntary movements[3–5] after exposure to 1.5 to 2 mg/kg/d for 3 weeks to 3 months.[6] It may precipitate a psychosis and has a potential for drug abuse and dependency.[7]

REFERENCES—PEMOLINE

1. Sallee F, Stiller R, Perel J, Bates F. Oral pemoline kinetics in hyperactive children. Clin Pharmacol Ther 1985;37:606–609.
2. Nehra A, Mullich F, Ishak KG, Zimmerman HJ. Pemoline-associated hepatic injury. Gastroenterology 1990;99:1517–1519.
3. Briscoe JG, Curry SC, Gerkin RD, Ruiz PR. Pemoline-induced choreoathetosis and rhabdomyolysis. Med Toxicol 1988;3:72–76.
4. Merrian AE. Pemoline-induced abnormal involuntary movement. J Clin Psychopharmacol 1990;10:302–303.
5. Singh BK, Singh A, Chusid E. Chorea in long-term use of pemoline. Ann Neurol 1983;13:218.
6. Sallee FR, Stiller RL, Perel JM, Everett G. Pemoline-induced abnormal involuntary movements. J Clin Psychopharmacol 1989;9:125–129.
7. Polchert SE, Morse RM. Pemoline abuse. JAMA 1985;254:946–947.

CLOBENZOREX HYDROCHLORATE

Clobenzorex hydrochlorate, supplied under the trade name Aselin, is an anorectic drug manufactured in Mexico (Fig. 20–5). This product is metabolized to amphetamine. Laboratories doing drug screens for clients near the border with Mexico should be aware that clobenzorex hydrochlorate will cause a positive drug screen for amphetamine.[1]

REFERENCE—CLOBENZOREX HYDROCHLORATE

1. Tarver JA. Amphetamine-positive drug screens from use of clobenzorex hydrochlorate. J Anal Toxicol 1994;18:183.

PROPYLHEXEDRINE

Propylhexedrine is a potent alpha-adrenergic sympathomimetic agent with one-twelfth the central nervous system stimulatory effect and less than one-eighth the pressor effect of amphetamine.[1] Propylhexedrine is found in Benzedrex Nasal Inhaler, an over-the-counter nasal decongestant. Propylhexedrine was substituted for amphetamine in the over-the-counter Benzedrine inhaler in 1970.

Propylhexedrine Recovery

The Benzedrex inhaler contains 250 mg propylhexedrine, 4.5 mg menthol, and various aromatic compounds soaking a cotton wick. The extraction process usually involves separating the wick and soaking it in hydrochloric acid. The wick is then squeezed out and the liquid is heated to yield propylhexedrine contaminated with various impurities. If the correct process is followed, up to 98% propylhexedrine can be recovered. The extraction process likely boils off ingredients such as menthol and other aromatic compounds. The remaining liquid is highly acidic and corrosive if not properly neutralized. This "stove-top speed" may also be contaminated with a significant amount of fibrous residue from the wick.

Street Names

Common street names include "Bathtub Crystal," "Peanut Butter Meth," "Bathtub Crank," and "Bathtub Speed." Intravenous injection is the preferred route of administration for this substance.

Clinical Presentation

Corrosive effects include local erythema, induration, edema, ulceration, and necrosis at the injection site. Other toxic effects include tachycardia, palpitations, myocardial infarction, diplopia, brainstem dysfunction, psychosis, severe headache, nausea, and sudden death.

Common pulmonary autopsy findings among intravenous propylhexedrine abusers include fibrosis, edema, foreign body granulomas, hypertension, and cor pulmonale. Ventricular hypertrophy is a common cardiac finding [1]

Treatment

Propylhexedrine abusers presenting to the emergency department should be examined closely for evidence of neck injection and potential extravasation. Any patient with extravasation of propylhexedrine in the neck should be admitted to the hospital and monitored closely for airway compromise and local tissue necrosis, in addition to systemic drug toxicity.[1]

REFERENCE—PROPYLHEXEDRINE

1. Perez J, Burton BT, McGirr JG. Airway compromise and delayed death following attempted central vein injection of propylhexedrine. J Emerg Med 1994;6:795–797.

Chapter 21
Cocaine

INTRODUCTION

HISTORY

Cocaine has been used for many centuries (Table 21–1) but its toxic effects have only been elucidated in the past 10 years.

EPIDEMIOLOGY

The smoking of coca paste (coca leaves mashed with alkali, kerosene, and sulfuric acid) in Latin America and South America led to the coca paste syndrome and its accompanying stepwise development of euphoria, dysphoria, hallucinations, and paranoid psychosis. The widespread use of "crack" in the United States today is probably a direct result of the coca paste experience. When a Colombia coca paste sample is smoked it behaves more like free cocaine than a cocaine sulfate salt.[1]

Infants

Cocaine intoxication may occur in infants who are breastfed by mothers recently exposed to cocaine or by mothers who have rubbed cocaine on their nipples to relieve soreness.[2] The infant may experience irritability, vomiting, diarrhea, dilated pupils, hyperactivity, marked hyperventilation, and continuous movements of the extremities. Cocaine intoxication should be suspected in any infant presenting acutely with ventricular arrhythmias, hyper- or hypotension, seizures, or respiratory distress.[3]

Inner-City Crack Use

A recent national household survey of drug use found that approximately 1 million Americans, including 1.0% of those between 18 and 25 years of age, had used crack during the previous year. Unlike injection drug use, which is practiced predominantly by men, the use of crack cocaine is widespread among both men and women. Increasing evidence suggests that the widespread use of crack cocaine has increased the spread of sexually transmitted disease, including infection with HIV, because of high-risk sexual practices among crack users.[4]

Table 21–1
Cocaine History

Historical	Pre-Inca inhabitants discover mind-altering properties of *Erythroxylon coca*
1507	Indians chew coca with alkaline ash
16th century	Coca leaves brought to Spanish court
1859	Alkaloid cocaine characterized; anesthetic properties recognized
Late 19th century	Sigmund Freud uses cocaine to relieve depression; cocaine recognized as corneal anesthetic; peripheral nerve-blocking properties observed; Coca Cola marketed (cocaine–caffeine mixture)
1891	Reports of cocaine intoxication, deaths
1906	United States controls cocaine use (Pure Food and Drug Act)
1914	Harrison Narcotic Act labels cocaine as narcotic
1960s	Intravenous drug users use "speedball" (heroin and cocaine); sniff, smoke cocaine
1970	Cocaine becomes Schedule II drug
1980	Cocaine use and fatalities widen in United States; fatalities increase
1993	Price reduced

Table 21–2
Causes of Cocaine Infant Deaths

- Acute maternal cocaine abuse (intrauterine death)
- Anoxic encephalopathy at birth (short survival)
- Traumatic compression asphyxia
- Infectious cardiomyopathy in early years (maternal cocaine abuse at birth)
- Malnutrition, dehydration (during parental cocaine abuse)
- Sibling lacing of milk bottle with cocaine

Mortality

Death of infants related to cocaine use may occur at various periods of child development (Table 21–2). Syndromes following cocaine intoxication in the newborn period include necrotizing enterocolitis and bowel perforation, infantile colic (an abstinence syndrome), and possible respiratory abnormalities.[5] Fetal or newborn deaths associated with maternal cocaine use appear to occur at about the 30th week of pregnancy.[6] Fetal blood cocaine and benzoylecgonine levels in one series were 0.26 and 1.73 μg/mL, respectively. The average maternal levels were 0.14 and 1.80 μg/mL, respectively.[7]

Sudden Infant Death Syndrome (SIDS)

The risk of SIDS among cocaine-exposed infants may be elevated[8,9] and may be associated with respiratory pattern abnormalities,[10] but further studies are necessary to clarify the methodologic problems encountered in earlier observations.[11,12] The efficacy of home monitoring is unclear.[11]

Children

Children may be exposed to cocaine by breastfeeding, accidental ingestion, intentional administration, and passive inhalation of crack vapors. They may be asymptomatic with positive assays for cocaine or exhibit evidence of an abnormal respiratory pattern, sudden infant death syndrome, visual impairment, abnormal motor development, poor reading and mathematical skills, and impaired social and emotional development. Many live in an environment where adults regularly use cocaine. The central nervous system of such children may become sensitized ("kindling") following repeated exposure to cocaine. Eventually central nervous system stimulation occurs in response to relatively low levels of the drug.[3,13–18]

Adolescents

Cocaine abuse occurs in both healthy and chronically ill adolescents. Acts of self-destruction may be observed in both groups including attempted suicide, a manifestation of cocaine withdrawal, and acts of aggression and violence, signs of cocaine intoxication.[19] Syndromes of cocaine intoxication now seen in older children and adolescents include the malignant hyperthermia or hypermetabolic syndrome and cocaine colitis. Cocaine abstinence syndrome may include hyperprolactinemia. Cocaine should be considered in the differential diagnosis of chest pain in an adolescent. This may be due to spontaneous pneumomediastinum, pneumothorax, myocardial ischemia or infarction, myocarditis, and severe arrhythmias. Generalized and partial seizures, cerebrovascular infarction, and hemorrhage have also been observed.[5]

EMERGENCY DEPARTMENT

The cocaine/crack epidemic has brought a number of concomitant problems into the emergency department including effects on the newborn, chest pain and myocardial infarction and ischemia in young adults, the increasing incidence of HIV infection associated with crack and prostitution, severe child abuse and neglect, an increase in penetrating trauma, an increase in deaths in utero and in infants, and direct effects on infants and children relating to passive cocaine inhalation.[20]

SOURCE

The coca plant, *Erythroxylon coca,* should not be confused with the cocoa plant, which contains caffeine rather than cocaine (Fig. 21–1).[21]

STRUCTURE

Cocaine is an ester type of local anesthetic and belongs to the tropane family of natural alkaloids. Other members of the family include scopolamine and atropine (Fig. 21–2).

PURITY

The street drug contains a variety of adulterants (Table 21–3). A number of compounds may appear in illicit cocaine and may form the basis for identifying the source of clandestine cocaine processing.[22–27] Acidic, basic, and neutral impurities introduced from the coca plant and from the processing of cocaine in clandestine laboratories may be

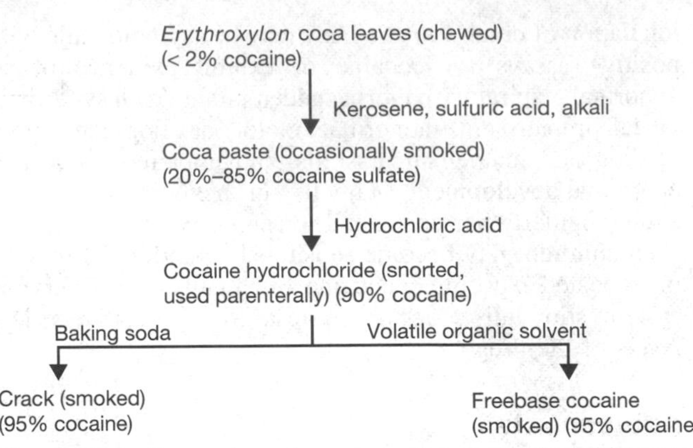

Figure 21-1 Processing of cocaine starts with chewable coca leaves and ends with nearly pure smokable cocaine. (From Bouknight LG, Bouknight RR. Cocaine: A particularly addictive drug. Postgrad Med 1988;83(4):115–118, 121–124, 131.)

SCOPOLAMINE

HC—CH—CH_2 CH_2OH; O; N • CH_3; CH—OCO—C(H); HC—CH—CH_2

COCAINE

CH_3—CO_2; HC—CH—CH; N • CH_3; CH—OCO; HC—CH—CH_2

Ecgonine | Benzoic acid

Figure 21-2 Structures of scopolamine and cocaine

analyzed and may form the basis for a chromatographic impurity signature profile analysis (CISPA).[28]

USE

Medical uses include local vasoconstriction, ophthalmologic anesthesia and severe pain, and topical anesthesia.

ECONOMICS OF CRACK[29]

- *Harvesting:* In Bolivia, one cargo of leaves or about 100 pounds fetches between \$38 and \$51.
- *Refining:* Before it leaves South America, a kilogram of powder, or 2.2 pounds, is worth between \$950 and \$1200.
- *Shipping:* Shippers charge their Los Angeles connections between \$12,000 and \$14,000 per kilogram.
- *Wholesaling:* When resold in 1-ounce packets, each kilogram can bring between \$25,000 and \$35,000.
- *Retailing:* The standard curbside price is \$20 per rock, a small nugget that averages about 0.2 g. A kilogram broken into these individual rocks generates at least \$100,000, and as much as \$200,000 if cut with adulterants such as lidocaine and procaine.
- *Using:* The average crack user smokes about seven or eight rocks a day, a habit that runs about \$1050 per week.

Table 21-3
Cocaine Additives

Pharmacologically Active	Inert
Lidocaine	Inositol
Cyproheptidine	Mannitol
Methephedrine	Lactose
Diphenhydramine	Dextrose
Benzocaine	Starch
Mepivacaine	Sucrose
Aminopyrine	Sodium bicarbonate
Methapyrilene	Barium carbonate
Tetracaine	Mannose
Nicotinamide	**Volatile Compounds**
Ephedrine	Benzene
Phenylpropanolamine	Methyl ethyl ketone
Acetaminophen	Ether
Procaine base	Acetone
Caffeine	
Acetophenetidin	
1-(1-Phenylcyclohexyl)pyrrolidine	
Methaqualone	
Dyclonine	
Pyridoxine	
Codeine	
Stearic acid	
Piracetum	
Rosin (colophonum)	
Fencanfamine	
Benzoic acid	
Phenothiazines	
L-Threonine	
Heroin	
Boric acid	
Aspirin	
Dibucaine	
Propoxyphene	
Heroin*	
Amphetamine*	
Methamphetamine*	

*Considered frequent additives/coinjectants; absolute frequency unknown. From Shesser R, Jotte R, Olshaker J. The contribution of impurities to the acute morbidity of illegal drug use. Am J Emerg Med 1991;9:336–342.

ABUSE PATTERNS

About half of patients who have a diagnosis of cocaine dependence may be marijuana (cannabis) dependent. Cocaine addicts also may be alcohol and heroin dependent. Multiple-drug dependency requires consideration at the time of admission and before discharge.[30]

Differential effects dependent on routes of cocaine administration are summarized in Table 21–4.

Cardiopulmonary symptoms including chest pain may be seen more often in patients who have snorted cocaine.[31]

CRACK COCAINE

Cocaine freebase is prepared from cocaine hydrochloride (the usual cocaine preparation available on the street) by

Table 21–4
Differential Effects Dependent on Routes of Cocaine Administration

Administration		Initial Onset of Action (s)	Duration of "High" (min)	Average Acute Dose (mg)	Peak Plasma Level (ng/mL)	Purity (%)	Bioavailability (% absorbed)
Route	Mode						
Oral	Coca leaf chewing	300–600	45–90	20–50	150	0.5–1	—
Oral	Cocaine HCl	600–1800		100–200	150–200	20–80	20–30
Intranasal	"Snorting" cocaine HCl	120–180	30–45	5 × 30	150	20–80	20–30
Intravenous	Cocaine HCl	30–45	10–20	25–50 >200	300–400 1000–1500	7–100	100
Smoking, intrapulmonary	Coca paste	8–10	5–10	60–250	300–800	40–85	6–32
	Freebase			250–1000	800–900	90–100	
	Crack				?	50–95	

From Taylor WA, Gold MS. Pharmacologic approaches to the treatment of cocaine dependence. West J Med 1990;152:573–577.

Table 21–5
Pulmonary Pathology Associated With Cocaine Use

Pulmonary hemorrhage
Pulmonary edema
Vascular lesions
  Microemboli
  Arterial medial hypertrophy
  Spasm with thrombosis and pulmonary infarction
Interstitial diseases
  Granulomatosis
    Cellulose
    Talc
  Pneumoconiosis-like interstitial fibrosis
    Silica
Immunologically mediated diseases
  Hypersensitivity pulmonary disease
  Asthma
Bronchiolitis obliterans organizing pneumonia (BOOP)
Barotrauma
  Pneumothorax
  Pneumomediastinum
Inhalation injuries
  Carbonaceous deposits
  Aspiration of foreign bodies
  Thermal injury

From Laposata EA, Mayo GL. A review of pulmonary pathology and mechanisms associated with inhalation of freebase cocaine ("crack"). Am J Forens Med Pathol 1993;14:1–9.

extracting the cocaine with an alkaline solution (buffered ammonia) and adding a solvent such as ether or acetone. The mixture separates into two layers, the top solvent layer containing the dissolved cocaine. The solvent is then evaporated, leaving almost pure cocaine crystals. All contaminants are not removed. Freebase cocaine is sometimes further adulterated by the producer. The cocaine alkaloid (freebase) is a colorless, odorless, transparent, crystalline substance that makes a popping or cracking sound when heated (hence the term *crack*). It can be mixed into a cigarette and smoked or heated in a water pipe and inhaled. A solution of cocaine hydrochloride can also be heated in a pan with baking soda added until a solid "rock" is formed, pieces of which can be smoked directly through paraphernalia. Freebase cocaine smoke is composed of 6.5% cocaine vapor and 93.5% particulate cocaine with an average particle size of 2.3 μm; this small size allows all components of the respiratory system to be exposed to freebase cocaine during inhalation. Pulmonary pathology associated with cocaine use is summarized in Table 21–5.[32]

PYROLYSIS PRODUCTS

Cocaine probably undergoes significant decomposition during the process of smoking. A number of pyrolysis products are formed including benzoic acid, methyl benzoate, *N*-methylbenzimide, methylcycloheptatriene carboxylate isomers, and methyl-4-(3-pyridyl) benzoate isomers of anhydroecgonine methyl ester (AEME) (methylecgonidine). AEME is the major pyrolysis product, and the major thermal decomposition product of cocaine. AEME may contribute to the adverse effects of cocaine smoking but this has not been evaluated.[33] Little if any AEME is excreted in the urine after cocaine is administered by the intravenous or intranasal routes.[34] AEME is structurally similar to arecoline and anabasine and may be a cholinergic agent.[33]

COCAINE ABUSE

Toxicokinetics

Absorption

Oral Ingestion. Cocaine is rapidly and well absorbed from the nasal, oral, and pulmonary routes (Fig. 21–3). Oral ingestion of crack cocaine leads to an adrenergic crisis with hypertension, tachycardia, hyperthermia, agitation, and generalized seizure activity. Patients may exhibit electrocardiographic evidence of cardiac ischemia, without elevations in serum creatine phosphokinase MB fraction. Treatment includes lorazepam and esmolol. Patients recover in 48 to 72 hours.[35]

Intravenous Injection. Peak plasma levels after intravenous use or smoking of the usual doses appear to be in the range of 500 to 1000 μg/mL (Fig. 21–3).[36]

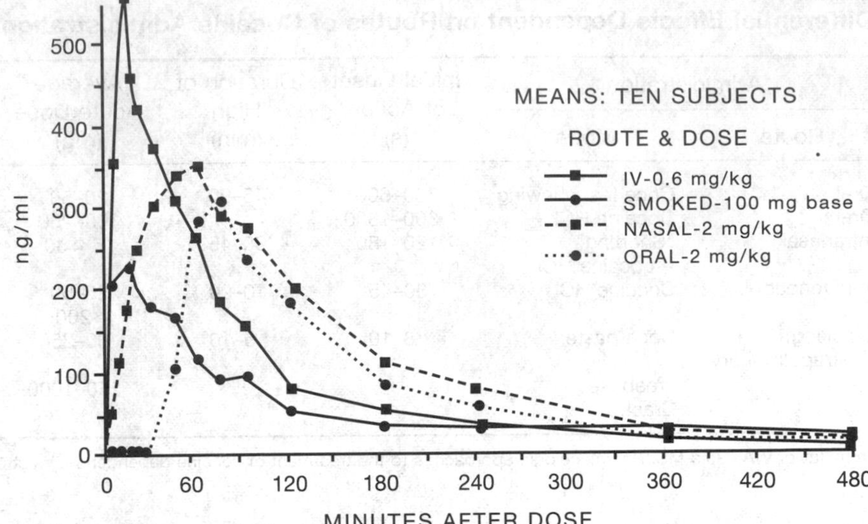

Figure 21-3 Plasma levels of cocaine. (From Jones RT. The pharmacology of cocaine smoking in humans. In: *Research Findings on Smoking of Abused Substances.* NIDA Research Monograph 99. Washington, DC: National Institute on Drug Abuse, 1990:30–41.)

Topical Application. Topical application of a 3-mL solution of tetracaine 0.5%, adrenaline 0.05%, and cocaine 11.8% (TAC) in children led to peak plasma cocaine levels of 0 to 274 ng/mL, with most less than 50 ng/mL.[37] No change in heart rate or blood pressure was detected.[37]

Elimination

Metabolic Pathways. See Figure 21–4. In total, 11 metabolites of cocaine have been identified. Four—ecgonidine, norecgonidine methyl ester, norecgonine methyl ester, and *m*-hydroxybenzoylecgonine—have recently been identified

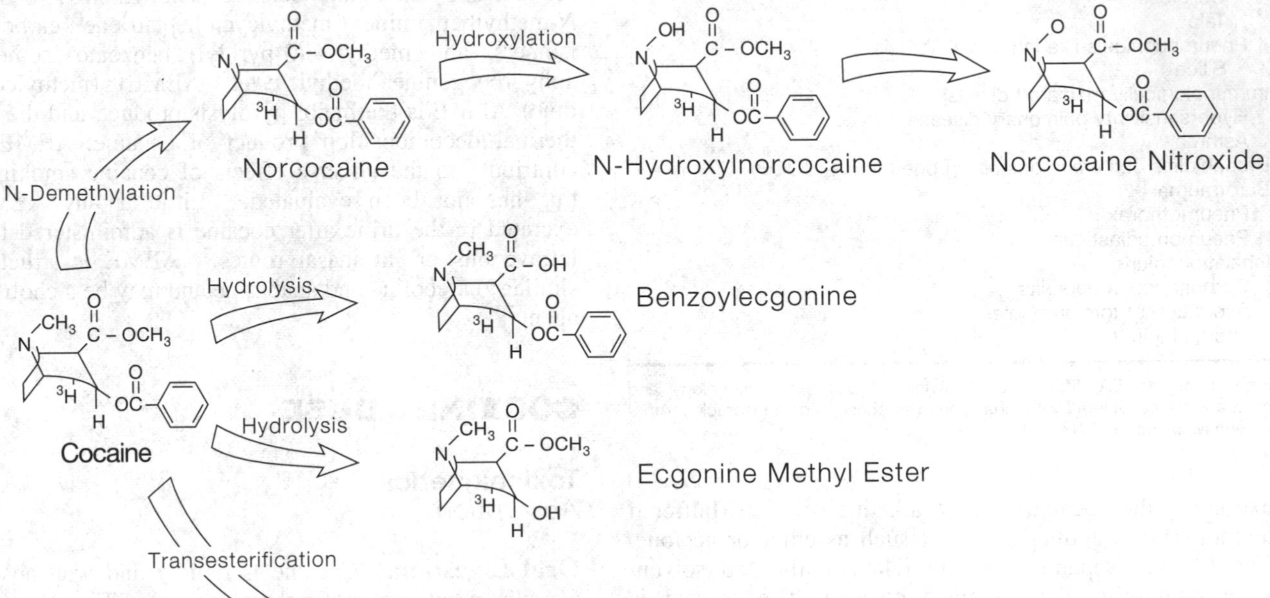

Hydroxylation

Norcocaine

N-Hydroxylnorcocaine

Norcocaine Nitroxide

N-Demethylation

Hydrolysis

Benzoylecgonine

Cocaine

Hydrolysis

Ecgonine Methyl Ester

Transesterification

C_2H_5OH
Ethanol

Cocaethylene

Figure 21-4 Metabolism of cocaine. Cocaine is either deesterified to produce benzoylecgonine or ecgonine methyl ester or demethylated to form norcocaine, which is further metabolized to produce *N*-hydroxynorcocaine and norcocaine nitroxide. In the presence of ethanol, cocaine is metabolized to cocaethylene. Norcocaine and cocaethylene possess pharmacologic activities similar to those of cocaine. [^{3}H] Cocaine used in our studies was labeled at the 4-position on the tropane ring; the label would thus be retained on major cocaine metabolites. (From Schenker S, Yang Y, Johnson RF, et al. The transfer of cocaine and its metabolites across the term human placenta. Clin Pharmacol Ther 1993;53:329–339.)

in the urine by gas chromatography and mass spectrometry.[38] Mixing cocaine with ethanol produces cocaethylene.

Urinary Excretion. Benzoylecgonine can be detected in the urine at levels of 300 ng/mL or above for up to 22 days after the last cocaine use.[39] A prospective study on the urine of cocaine smokers indicates that substantial quantities of AEME, a major pyrolysis product of cocaine, are excreted in the urine. Its toxicologic importance is not known.[33,40]

A positive finding of benzoylecgonine in the urine is generally considered evidence of illicit cocaine use. A coca tea leaf imported into the United States and sold over the counter in health food stores as Health Inca Tea or Mate de Coca has an average cocaine content of 1.8 mg in 180 mL of tea and may induce excretion of up to 2400 ng/mL of benzoylecgonine in the urine.[41] On the morning after use of TAC (tetracaine, adrenaline, and cocaine) as a topical anesthetic, 83% of urines analyzed by gas chromatography–mass spectrometry were positive for benzoylecgonine. Some were still positive 36 hours later. Physicians who use TAC solution as a local anesthetic should caution their patients that they may fail a urine drug screen for cocaine if they are tested within 36 to 48 hours of use of TAC.[42] This may be true for patients treated for epistaxis with topical cocaine.

Pregnancy. Cocaine abuse may injure the fetus and newborn infant exposed to cocaine by the mother during pregnancy, at the time of birth, during lactation, and by passive exposure to cocaine smoke during infancy and childhood.[43–56] Risk factors associated with fetal and neonatal cocaine exposure are listed in Table 21–6. The effects on the new life can be devastating (Table 21–7). Teratogenic effects may follow cocaine use by the mother during pregnancy (Table 21–8); a specific teratogenic syndrome has not been identified. The pathogenesis of fetal injury is summarized in Figure 21–5. Disturbances in human brain development may occur (Table 21–9). Cardiac abnormalities are often associated with in utero cocaine exposure (Table 21–10).[57] The drug has also caused intoxication in breastfeeding infants.[58]

Prenatal Cocaine Exposure. Prenatal cocaine exposure increases the risk of smaller infants, whether from shortened gestation, intrauterine growth retardation, or both.[59]

"Crack baby" data are inconclusive: children with a history of prenatal cocaine exposure are not inevitably and permanently damaged and may not develop developmental and behavioral deficits.[60]

A positive result on a cocaine urine toxicology test at the time of delivery is associated with prematurity and possibly low birth weight.[61]

During the first year of life, very low birth weight cocaine-exposed infants are at an increased risk of intraventricular hemorrhage, are more likely to be placed outside maternal care, and exhibit cognitive and motor delays.[62] Follow-up studies to confirm these observations are not yet available. Healthy, cocaine-exposed infants born at term may be at risk for only subtle deficits in later life.[63]

A significant amount of the maternal dose of cocaine and benzoylecgonine is retained by the placenta, which later leaches out into both fetal and maternal circulation.[64]

Table 21–6
Risk Factors: Fetal and Neonatal Cocaine Exposure

Fetal Exposure
Cocaine passes placental barrier
Plasma and hepatic cholinesterases: diminished capacity
Uterine and fetal vasoconstriction

Neonatal Exposure
Premature labor: intense uterine contractions
Fetal oxygenation diminished: uterine vasoconstriction
Poor maternal nutrition
HIV or other infectious exposures
Maternal use of other drugs of abuse

Table 21–7
Conditions With Increased Incidence in Pregnant Women Exposed to Cocaine

Spontaneous abortion
Placenta previa
Abruptio placentae
Fetal death
Prematurity (preterm labor, delivery)
Congenital malformations
Placental infarcts
Intrauterine growth retardation
Birth of small-for-gestation age infant (smaller head circumference, decreased birth length)
Low birth weight
Ischemic infarct of bowel (necrotizing enterocolitis)
Multiple intestinal atresias

Table 21–8
Teratogenic Effects Reported in the Offspring of Women Who Used Cocaine During Pregnancy

Body Area	Anomalies
Cranial–spinal	Exencephaly, hydrocephaly, porencephaly, cephalomalacia, encephalocele, myelomeningocele, hypoplastic corpus callosum, parietal lobe cleft, heterotopias
Facial	Unilateral oro-orbital cleft, cleft lip, cleft palate, facial diplegia, blepharophimosis, ptosis, skin tags, cutis aplasia, Pierre Robin syndrome
Cardiovascular	Atrial septal defect, ventricular septal defect, transposition of the great arteries, pulmonary artery stenosis, hypoplastic right heart syndrome, biventricular hypertrophy, cardiomegaly
Gastrointestinal and genitourinary tracts	Ileal atresia, inguinal hernia, prune belly syndrome, renal agenesis, multicystic kidneys, hydronephrosis, hydroureter, hypospadias, undescended testis, hydrocele
Extremities	Limb reduction defects, phocomelia, polydactyly, syndactyly

From Young SL, Vosper HJ, Phillips SA. Cocaine: Its effects on maternal and child health. Pharmacotherapy 1992;12:2–17.

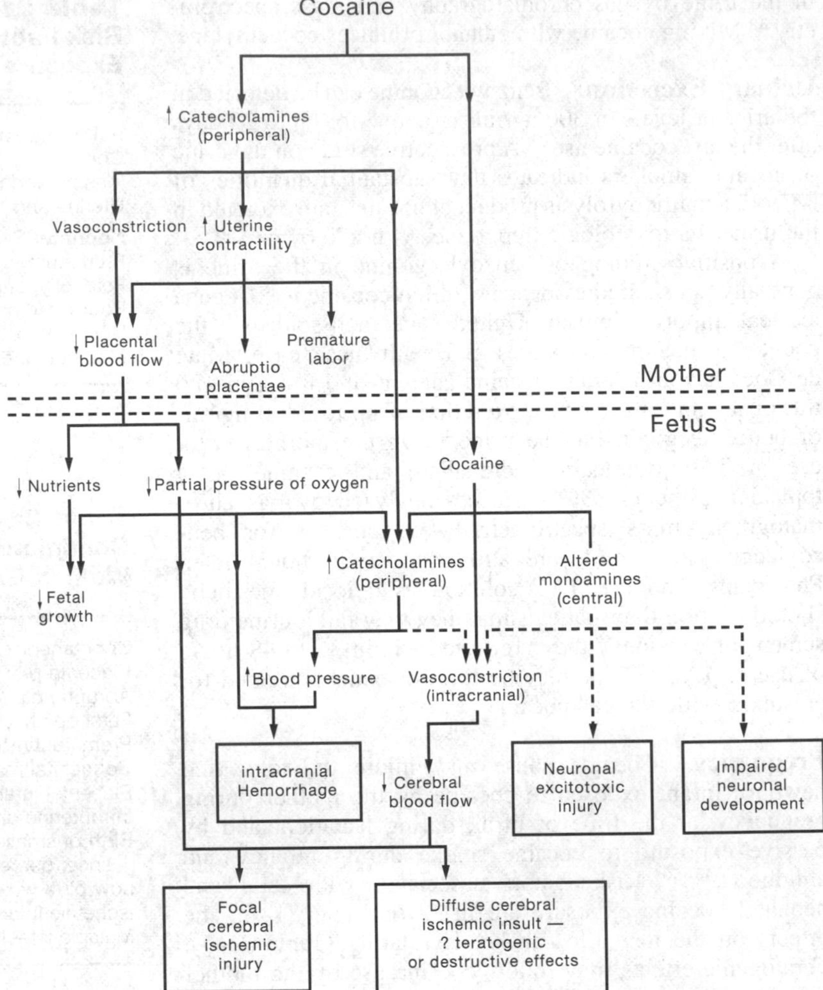

Figure 21-5 Deleterious effects of maternal cocaine use on fetuses. Effects that appear plausible on the basis of current information but whose confirmation requires more supporting evidence are indicated by dotted lines. ↑ denotes increased, and ↓ decreased. (From Volpe JJ. Effect of cocaine use on the fetus. N Engl J Med 1992;327:399–407. Erratum. 1992;327:1039E.)

Table 21-9
Disturbances in Human Brain Development Reported after Intrauterine Exposure to Cocaine

Event	Peak Gestational Period	Abnormality Reported After Cocaine Exposure
Neural tube formation	3–4 wk	Myelomeningocele, encephalocele
Prosencephalic development	2–3 mo	Agenesis of corpus callosum; agenesis of septum pellucidum; septo-optic dysplasia
Neuronal proliferation	3–4 mo	Microcephaly
Neuronal migration	3–15 mo	Schizencephaly, neuronal heterotopias
Neuronal differentiation	5 mo postnatal	Abnormal cortical neuronal cytodifferentiation (preliminary)
Myelination	After birth	None

From Volpe JJ. Effect of cocaine use on the fetus. N Engl J Med 1992;327:399–407. Erratum. 1992;327:1039E.

Table 21-10
Cardiac Abnormalities Associated With In Utero Cocaine Exposure in Humans

Pulmonary atresia	Hypoplastic heart syndrome
Pulmonary stenosis	Biventricular hypertrophy
Atrial septal defect	Right-sided valve changes
Ventricular septal defect	Patent ductus arteriosus
Aortic valve leaflet prolapse	Conduction defects

From Kain ZN, Kain TS, Scarpelli EM. Cocaine exposure in utero: Perinatal development and neonatal manifestations: Review. J Toxicol Clin Toxicol 1992;30:607–636.

Fetal Growth. Cocaine, norcocaine, and cocaethylene are rapidly transferred across the placenta.[65] Characteristics of drug-dependent and social cocaine users in pregnancy have been proposed by Koren (Table 21–11).[66]

It is difficult to evaluate the effect of maternal cocaine use on fetal growth due to the compounding factors of tobacco and marijuana smoking, the use of alcohol and other illicit substances, and differences in nutritional status and prenatal care. Despite these limitations, fetal growth appears to be decreased in women who use cocaine throughout pregnancy.

Table 21-11
Characteristics of Pregnant Cocaine Users

Drug-Dependent Users	Social Users
Use cocaine throughout pregnancy	Stop cocaine use with onset of pregnancy
Use other hard drugs	Rarely use other hard drugs
Use intravenous route	Rarely use intravenous route
Are of low socioeconomic status	Are of higher socioeconomic status
Receive generally poor medical and prenatal care	Receive generally good medical and prenatal care
Have adverse pregnancy outcomes	Have a normal pregnancy and newborn

Adapted from Graham K, Koren G. Characteristics of pregnant women exposed to cocaine in Toronto between 1985 and 1990. Can Med Assoc J 1991;144:563–568.

These effects are not manifest in the infants of women who use cocaine only in the first trimester of pregnancy.[58]

A study conducted by the Centers for Disease Control and Prevention suggests that cocaine use during pregnancy is an independent contributor to the risk of placental abruptio, decreased fetal growth, and prematurity, and perhaps to urinary congenital anomalies and neonatal neurobehavioral deficits.[67,68] Evidence linking prenatal cocaine use and an increase in incidence of perinatal cerebral infarction or sudden death syndrome is lacking.[68]

Fetal Cocaine Syndrome? A well-defined "fetal cocaine syndrome" does not exist. A prospective study at the Motherisk Program in Toronto suggests that first-trimester exposure to cocaine in nonaddicts is not associated with a substantially increased teratogenic risk,[69,70] but other studies suggest that first-trimester fetal cocaine exposure appears to be associated with facial alterations (increased intercanthal distance and increased midface retrusion in boys).[71] Prospective studies are required to substantiate these findings. Even a single exposure during pregnancy may produce infarction, edema, and tissue necrosis. The loss of vascular supply may produce fetal damage that cannot be repaired.[72]

Lactation. Cocaine is excreted in breast milk and can induce cocaine intoxication in the breastfed infant.[73,74] Apnea and seizures have been induced in an infant from the direct ingestion of cocaine used as a topical anesthetic for nipple soreness.[75] Cessation of cocaine exposure early in pregnancy by social cocaine users does not appear to be associated with any subsequent adverse pregnancy outcomes[76] (Table 21–7).

Meconium. Meconium from premature infants of cocaine-dependent mothers contains cocaine but not benzoylecgonine, ecgonine, and ecgonine methyl esters. This suggests that metabolism of cocaine in the premature neonate is limited.[77] Radioimmunoassay of infants' hair and gas chromatography–mass spectrometry of meconium appear to be more sensitive than immunoassay of urine, which failed to identify 60% of cocaine-exposed infants in one series.[78] A fluorescence polarization immunoassay (FPIA) is available to screen for benzoylecgonine in an extract of meconium. The FPIA is sensitive to 0.6 μg benzoylecgonine per gram of meconium. A gas chromatography–mass spectrometry confirmation is sensitive to less than 0.25 mg cocaine or 0.15 mg benzoylecgonine per gram meconium.[79] Meconium analysis provides no advantage over urine analysis for prenatal cocaine exposure when equivalent assays are used, and neither method reliably detects exposure when the last reported use is before 3 weeks prior to delivery.[80]

Urine Screen Test. A rapid latex agglutination inhibitor screening method (the Abuscreen On Trak) has been useful in detecting cocaine in the first infant urine specimen with results in 3 to 5 minutes. Its sensitivity and specificity are 96 and 100%, respectively, but unlike the enzyme-mediated immunoassay technique (EMIT), it does not detect metabolites (eg, benzoylecgonine). Gas chromatography–mass spectrometry can be used to confirm a positive result.[81] Further tests of clinical usefulness are indicated.

Amniotic Fluid. Amniotic fluid levels of androstenedione and testosterone are decreased in males born to cocaine users. Females may not be affected. Follicle-stimulating hormone is increased in both males and females. Luteinizing hormone is increased only in males. Therefore, cocaine passes through the placenta and affects the fetal testis–hypophyseal endocrine system.[82]

Child Development. Evidence from the newborn period has been too inadequate and inconsistent to allow any clear predictions about the effects of prenatal exposure to cocaine on the development and behavior of the child.[83] Many of the initial observations of high rates of sudden infant death syndrome, congenital abnormalities, and neonatal neurobehavioral dysfunction have not been confirmed consistently in subsequent studies.[84] Chasnoff and colleagues, using an appropriate control group and a consistent well-standardized assessment tool administered by blind examiners, showed no difference on the Bayley Scales of Infant Development at 2 years of age when cocaine-exposed children are compared with social class-matched controls.[85] The long-term neurologic and cognitive outcomes remain unknown (Table 21–12).[86] Neurologic functions most likely to be affected by intrauterine cocaine exposure are difficult to quantify with conventional tests.[86]

Seizures. Children of cocaine-using mothers who ultimately develop seizures exhibit postdelivery tremulousness, irritability, and excessive startle responses. Shortly after birth some of these children may develop seizures. Many continue to have seizures after the first year of life. Further studies are indicated to determine the long-term potential for the induction of epilepsy by cocaine. Infants discharged from a hospital may continue to be at risk for cocaine-related seizures if the mother still uses the drug. Continued exposure to crack smoke or to breast milk from a cocaine-using mother may place the infant in additional jeopardy for seizures.[87]

Drug and Disease Interactions

Marijuana. Combinations of cocaine and marijuana increase (up to 50 beats/min) the heart rate above levels seen with either drug alone. Increases in mean arterial pressure following the drug combination are equivalent to those produced by cocaine alone.[88]

Plasma Pseudocholinesterase Deficiency. Preliminary observations suggest that patients with low plasma cholinesterase levels may be more likely to have seizures, to develop cardiovascular complications, and to die.[89,90] Some cocaine-related deaths may be due to genetic inheritance of an atypical pseudocholinesterase. Testing of parental plasma may indicate such a predisposition in the children. Patients with a documented succinylcholine sensitivity (prolonged apnea) due to an atypical serum cholinesterase may be vulnerable to cocaine toxicity.[91] In vitro studies also suggest that cocaine may be a competitive inhibitor of plasma cholinesterase.[92]

Lower mean pseudocholinesterase values were observed in patients with complications such as ischemic chest pain, convulsions, and cardiac arrest associated with cocaine. Further studies are required before this enzyme can be considered a significant predictor and as a causative factor for populations at risk for severe complications or sudden death.[93,94]

Drugs and chemicals that inhibit plasma cholinesterase include organophosphate and carbamate insecticides, organophosphorus eyedrops (eg, echothiophate), and antimyasthenia gravis agents (neostigmine, pyridostigmine).

Patients may ingest an organophosphate insecticide while smoking crack (crystalline) in an effort to prevent the rapid breakdown of cocaine by inhibition of plasma cholinesterase, thereby leading to a prolonged or intensified high. One pregnant woman who did this developed nausea and weakness in 1 hour, then vomited, developed fasciculations, and had a generalized tonic–clonic seizure. She delivered a normal baby, and was treated with tracheal intubation, atropine 4 mg, diazepam 10 mg, phenobarbital 900 mg, and pralidoxime chloride 2 g followed by 1 g every 8 hours for 24 hours.[95] There is no substantial clinical evidence that administration of pseudocholinesterase decreases the toxic effects of cocaine. Hepatic disease may also compromise synthesis of pseudocholinesterase.

Table 21–12
Neurologic Findings in Cocaine-Exposed Infants (Including Withdrawal Findings)*,†,‡

Tremulousness	Abnormal electroencephalograms
Startle responses increased	Cerebral infarction
Deficient interactive behavior	Echoencephalographic abnormalities
Irritability	Visual disturbances
Abnormal sleep patterns	Neurobehavioral disturbances
Poor feeding	Hyperactivity
Athetoid movements	Brief attention span
Microcephaly	Sleep disturbances
Growth retardation	High-pitched crying
Seizures	Increased muscle tone
Hypotonia	
Abnormally dilated or tortuous vessels in iris‡	

*Oro AS, Dixon SD. Perinatal cocaine and methamphetamine exposure: Maternal and neonatal correlates. J Pediatr 1987;111:571–578.
†Livesay S, Ehrlich S, Finnegan LP. Cocaine and pregnancy: Maternal and infant outcome. Pediatr Res 1987;21:238A.
‡Isenberg SJ, Spierer A, Inkelis SH. Ocular signs of cocaine intoxication in neonates. Am J Ophthalmol 1987;103:211–214.

Calcium Channel Antagonists

Nifedipine pretreatment potentiates the incidence of seizures and death after cocaine administration. A calcium channel antagonist (diltiazem) given to healthy humans prior to cocaine did not alter the increase in blood pressure, heart rate, pupil size, or subjective "high" ratings produced by the cocaine.[96,97]

Cardiovascular Disease

Overdoses of cocaine are associated with inotropic and chronotropic changes with a propensity to induce cardiovascular depression and dysrhythmias (Table 21–13) (see Pathophysiology and Clinical Presentation).

Cocaethylene

Cocaethylene, the ethyl homolog of cocaine (ethylbenzoylecgonine), chemically synthesized more than 100 years ago but recently clinically evaluated, is a pharmacologically active metabolite of cocaine (Fig. 21–6), and is found in

Table 21–13
Cardiovascular Toxicity of Cocaine

Hypertension
Tachycardia
Ventricular arrhythmias
Supraventricular arrhythmias
Congestive heart failure
Myocarditis
Myocardial ischemia
Myocardial infarction
Coronary artery dissection*

*Jaffe BD, Broderick TM, Leier CV. Cocaine-induced coronary artery dissection. N Engl J Med 1994;330:510–511.

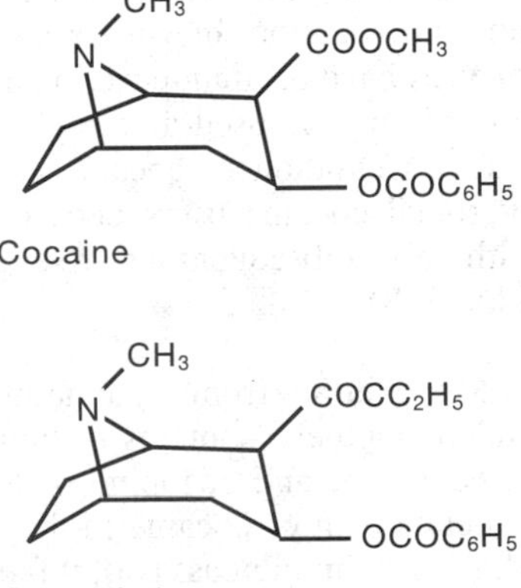

Figure 21-6 In the presence of cocaine and ethanol, the liver metabolizes cocaine to its ethyl homolog, cocaethylene. Cocaethylene provides the same pleasurable effects as cocaine, and is more lethal than the parent drug. (From Randall T. Cocaine, alcohol mix in body to form even longer lasting, more lethal drug. JAMA 1992;267:1043–1044.)

cocaine users who have simultaneously consumed cocaine and ethanol.[98–101] It has been found in the blood and urine[102] of healthy patients. Cocaethylene is formed in the liver from cocaine and ethanol by transesterification (Fig. 21–6).[101,103] Its concentration in blood may approach or surpass that of cocaine (highest found in one study, 1600 μg/mL). The longer half-life (2 hours) compared with cocaine (38 minutes) may explain why some individuals whose cocaine blood levels are low experience cocaine-related strokes or heart attack.

Cocaethylene may be more cardiotoxic than cocaine or ethanol alone,[104,105] but Pirwitz and colleagues have found that intravenous ethanol, given immediately after intranasal cocaine, prevents early and recurrent coronary vasoconstriction. The increased morbidity and mortality associated with concomitant cocaine and ethanol consumption does not appear to be due to ethanol-induced potentiation of cocaine-related coronary vasoconstriction.[106] Cocaethylene penetrates the blood–brain barrier.[107] Cocaethylene may explain why so many cocaine users use alcohol. They apparently get a higher and longer high.

Cocaethylene is found in the blood and brain when cocaine and ethanol are present. Cocaethylene may be active at cocaine binding sites in the central nervous system (dopamine, norepinephrine, serotonin, opioid sigma and muscarinic cholinergic receptors) and may be active at the sodium channel.[100,103,108,109]

Cocaethylene probably hydrolyzes to ecgonine ethyl ester (EEE) in a manner similar to the hydrolysis of cocaine to ecgonine methyl ester.[98] Detection of EEE in the blood may indicate the presence of cocaethylene. When urine is analyzed, cocaethylene and EEE are detected in all patients positive for cocaine and ethanol.[110] Quantification of cocaethylene and cocaine in blood and urine may be performed by gas chromatography–ion trap mass spectrometry and gas chromatography with electron-capture detection.[100] An alternate method uses high-performance liquid chromatography with ultraviolet detection (235 nm). Cocaethylene is also present in meconium.[111] The presence and concentration of cocaethylene cannot be accurately deduced from simultaneous serum levels of cocaine or ethanol. Cocaethylene appears in greater concentrations in meconium than in urine and may be a useful analytical indicator of fetal alcohol exposure.[112]

Speedballs

Speedball is the street name for heroin laced with cocaine. It combines the initial high "kick" of cocaine with the subsequent euphoric sleep "rush" of heroin. The mixture may be "cut" with sugars, local anesthetics, caffeine, amphetamines, phencyclidine, and quinine. The mixture (speedball) is frequently injected. Naloxone is contraindicated because it may precipitate acute narcotic withdrawal and induce pulmonary edema and ventricular dysrhythmias in the presence of residual cocaine.[113–115] The patient should be allowed to awaken slowly, employing mechanical ventilation as long as necessary. Anesthesiologists should be aware of preoperative self-administration of illicit substances by anxious and drug-dependent patients and must consider this in their evaluation of an otherwise unexplained intraoperative tachycardia and hypertension.[114,116]

Phenytoin Adulteration

Crack cocaine is often adulterated with phenytoin. Determination of phenytoin levels in cocaine-intoxicated patients with lethargy, nystagmus, or ataxia may aid in management.[117]

Mechanism of Action

β_1-Adrenergic stimulation results in tachycardia, hypertension, and arrhythmia. β_2-Adrenergic stimulation can lead to hypotension after vasodilation. Alpha-adrenergic stimulation induces hypertension with a reflex bradycardia. Central nervous system stimulation leads to anxiety psychoses and seizures. An increased metabolic rate and hyperactivity can induce hyperthermia and rhabdomyolysis.

Central Nervous System

Cocaine initially causes euphoria, hyperactivity, restlessness, and garrulity. Later tremor, hyperreflexia, and convulsions are observed. Finally, coma, hyporeflexia, and respiratory and/or cardiovascular depression may occur. Death results from either respiratory depression or cardiac arrest.

Figure 21–7 summarizes a suggested pathophysiologic mechanism for the production of new-onset multifocal tics in chronic cocaine abusers.[118]

Cardiovascular System

Intravenous cocaine drug users are at increased risk for developing endocarditis. Whether this is due to an effect of cocaine on immunity or is related to the technique of injection by cocaine users is not clear.[119,120]

Intranasal administration of cocaine may induce vasoconstriction of the coronary arteries, with a decrease in coronary blood flow despite an increase in myocardial oxygen demand. Extreme elevations in heart rate and blood pressure are likely to cause subendocardial ischemia even in the absence of underlying coronary obstruction, purely on the basis of excessive myocardial oxygen demand[121] (Table 21–13). These effects are probably mediated by alpha-adrenergic stimulation. Phentolamine has been used experimentally to reverse these effects.[122] Cocaine-induced activation of platelets may induce myocardial ischemia by occlusion and spasm of diseased small coronary vessels.[123]

Hemodynamic Effects

Most "social" or "recreational" cocaine users ingest less than 250 mg (2–4 mg/kg) at a sitting.[124] This dose may cause coronary artery vasoonstriction and a modest decrease in coronary blood flow.[122] Hemodynamic studies in a series of patients given intranasal cocaine (2–3 mg/kg) show that this dose causes a modest increase in heart rate (17%), mean arterial pressure (8%), cardiac index (18%), and the first derivative of left ventricular pressure (*DP/dt*) (18% positive and 15% negative). No change in pulmonary capillary wedge, pulmonary artery, and left ventricular end-diastolic

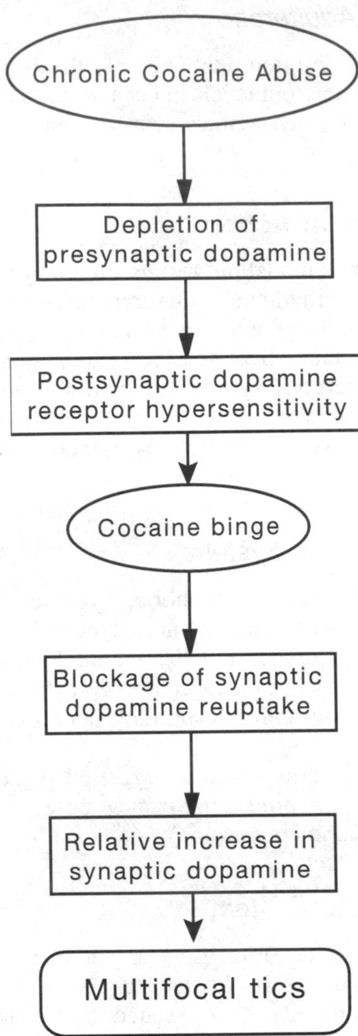

Figure 21-7 Flow diagram summarizing a possible pathophysiologic mechanism for new-onset multifocal tics in chronic cocaine abusers. Note that Gilles de la Tourette's syndrome is thought to be associated with a postsynaptic dopamine receptor hypersensitivity. (From Pascual-Leone A, Dhuna A, Anderson DC. Longterm neurological complications of chronic, habitual cocaine abuse. Neurotoxicology 1991;12:393–400.)

pressures or in systemic and pulmonary vascular resistance has been observed.[125] Benzoylecgonine, but not ecgonine methyl ester, is a potent long-lasting vasconstrictor.[126]

Respiratory System

Cocaine smoking appears to induce acute respiratory symptoms, exacerbation of asthma, thermal airway injury, deterioration in lung function, pneumothorax, pneumomediastinum, bronchiolitis obliterans, noncardiogenic pulmonary edema, pulmonary infiltrates (interstitial pneumonitis), pulmonary vascular disease, and pulmonary hemorrhage[127] (Table 21–14). Nearly one third of patients dying suddenly after cocaine inhalation may have autopsy evidence of hemosiderin-laden macrophages in lung tissue,[128] and 26% of freebase cocaine users report episodes of blood-streaked sputum after smoking the drug.[129] Intense cocaine-induced vasconstriction may be the mechanism for pulmonary hemorrhage as well as rhabdomyolysis.[127]

Table 21–14
Respiratory Complications of Smoking Cocaine

Crack lung (lung infiltrates, fever, bronchospasm, eosinophilia, elevated IgE level; hemoptysis often in a cigarette smoker)
Pneumothorax
Pneumopericardium secondary to barotrauma
Reactive airway disease (tracheobronchial constriction, mucous plugging of small airways)
Pulmonary function test abnormalities, reversible
Bronchitis
Fatal bronchospasm in asthmatics
Bronchiolitis obliterans
Pneumomediastinum
Pulmonary edema
Hypodermic needle aspiration (into an anesthetized airway)
Necrotizing thermal injury to base of tongue, epiglottis, and piriform sinus
Retropharyngeal emphysema
Inhalational injury (intratracheal ignition of either vehicle used in freebasing cocaine)
Increased frequency of respiratory pauses
Decrease in minute ventilation

Tashkin and colleagues have observed that frequent crack use is associated with a high prevalence of at least occasional occurrences of acute cardiorespiratory symptoms within 1 to 12 hours of smoking cocaine (cough productive of black sputum, hemoptysis, chest pain usually worse with deep breathing, cardiac palpitations, and a mild but significant impairment in the diffusing capacity of the lung).[130] Blackened bronchoalveolar lavage fluid indicates the possibility of crack cocaine smoking and its associated sequelae.[131]

Liver

Abnormal liver function tests in humans taking cocaine have been reported.[132] Patients have been observed with clinical evidence of hepatic necrosis after cocaine use. The severe zone 3 necrosis is indistinguishable from the toxic necrosis commonly seen with acetaminophen.[133] A rapid increase in serum transaminase levels develops within a few hours of intravenous cocaine usage and is followed by a rapid decrease within a few days. Prolongation of prothrombin time, elevation of serum bilirubin level, and an increase in serum creatine phosphokinase concentration with myoglobinuria are also seen. Crack users, probably via sexual exposure, may be at increased risk of developing hepatitis B and D infection.[134]

Clinical Presentation

Cocaine use is associated with multiple systemic acute and chronic complications (Table 21–15) including sympathetic storm (Table 21–16).[135] Numerous nonrespiratory complications are associated with crack cocaine (Table 21–17).

Cocaine is probably the most commonly mentioned illicit drug associated with admissions to emergency departments. Cocaine intoxication or withdrawal may complicate the treatment of injured patients through its ability to cause acute cardiac events, vascular ruptures, excited delirium, agitation, hyperthermia, seizures, blood glucose abnormalities, and other symptoms and signs.[136]

Table 21-15
Common Complications of Cocaine

Central Nervous System
Central nervous system sympathomimetic storm
Tremors
Seizures
Migraine headaches
Cerebral vasculitis
Cerebral infarction
Intracranial hemorrhage
Subarachnoid hemorrhage

Cardiovascular
Hypertension
Cardiac arrhythmias from sympathetic storm
Cardiac arrhythmias from sodium channel blockade
Global myocardial ischemia
Regional myocardial ischemia
Myocardial infarction
Regional transmural myocardial infarction
Cardiomyopathies
Myocarditis
Endocarditis
Aortic rupture
Diffuse microaneurysms (throughout the body)

Pulmonary
Alveolar hemorrhage
Adult respiratory distress syndrome
Pneumomediastinum
Pneumothorax
Pulmonary thrombosis
Hypersensitivity lung reaction

Obstetric
Abruptio placentae
Spontaneous abortion

Pediatric
Prematurity
Long-term fetal hypoxia
Intrauterine growth retardation
Neonatal behavioral dysfunction
Congenital malformations
Seizures from fetal hypoxia
Seizures from passive inhalation
Seizures from accidental ingestation of rock cocaine
Child neglect

Gastrointestinal
Mesenteric ischemia
Ingestion of crystalline cocaine for smuggling (body packer)
Ingestion of rock cocaine to avoid arrest (body stuffer)
Malnutrition

Renal
Rhabdomyolysis-induced renal failure

Ear, Nose, and Throat
Nasal septal necrosis
Rhinitis
Sinusitis
Laryngitis

Psychiatric
Severe depression
Severe paranoia
Violent behavior

Trauma
Impaired judgment
Accidents
Violent behavior

Metabolic
Hypoxia
Hyperthermia
Hypoglycemia
Lactic acidosis
Hypokalemia
Hyperkalemia

Infections from Intravenous Drug Use
Hepatitis B
HIV
Endocarditis

From Wassberger J, Ellenhorn MJ, Landers S, et al. The emergency management of acute cocaine toxicity. Top Emerg Med 1993;15(3):27–40.

Table 21-16
Differential Diagnosis of Sympathomimetic Storm

Trauma
Head trauma

Drugs
Cocaine
Phencyclidine (PCP)
Amphetamine
Phenylpropanolamine
Ethanol withdrawal
Ethanol intoxication
Theophylline

Medical Illness
Thyrotoxicosis
Thyroid storm
Pheochromocytoma
Hypoglycemia
Sepsis
Malignant hypertension
Heat stroke
Malignant neuroleptic syndrome
Malignant hyperthermia
Acute psychiatric disease
Paranoid schizophrenia
Acute mania

From Wassberger J, Ellenhorn MJ, Landers S, et al. The emergency management of acute cocaine toxicity. Top Emerg Med 1993;15(3):27–40.

Table 21-17
Nonrespiratory Complications of Free-Basing Cocaine (Crack Cocaine)

- Hemolytic–uremic syndrome
- Acute gastroduodenal perforation (no prior ulcer history)
- Esophagitis, epiglottis: burns from chemicals used for freebasing; child abuse
- Central nervous system complications
  - Transient neurologic symptoms in infants and children passively exposed (drowsiness, unsteadiness of gait, seizures)
  - Seizures
  - Intracerebral and subarachnoid hemorrhage
  - Psychosis (schizophrenic paranoid)
  - Ischemic cerebral infarction
  - Violence (homicides)
  - Acute dystonic reaction
  - "Crack" smiles (facial lacerations inflicted by drug pusher—facial nerve injury)
  - Pontine hemorrhage
  - Bilateral amblyopia
  - Crack dependence in psychiatric patients
  - Anorexia
  - Unilateral unreactive, dilated pupils (rubbing eye after smoking crack cocaine)
- Hyperactivity
- Weight loss
- Manic euphoria
- Depressive dysphoria
- Skin infarction
- Muscle infarctions
- Rhabdomyolysis
  - Myoglobinuria
  - Renal failure
- Hyperthermia
- Increases in crime
- Increases in admissions to drug treatment programs
- Increases in sexually transmitted diseases (failure to use condom, sex for drugs, sexual activity with drug use)
  - HIV
  - Hepatitis B
- Increased child abuse, child neglect
- Cardiac complications
  - Ventricular fibrillation
  - Tachycardia
  - Myocardial infarction
  - Death
  - Cardiomyopathy (embolic stroke)
  - Decreased cardiac output at birth
- "Crack vial" ingestions (symptomatic, poorly radiopaque)
- Lactic acidosis
- Obsessive–compulsive disorders
- "Crack packing" (sudden ingestion of "crack" cocaine)
- Child development problems
  - Trouble interpreting nonverbal signals
  - Easily frustrated
  - Hard to concentrate
  - Seizures
  - Cerebral paresis
  - Mental retardation
  - Slow language acquisition
  - Hyperactivity
  - Sudden mood swings
  - Extreme passivity
  - Apparent lack of emotion
  - Overwhelmed by stimuli such as noise and piles of toys

Mortality

Dopamine Depletion. Rapid death may resemble the neuroleptic malignant syndrome, though the cocaine-associated syndrome is atypical in having minimal rigidity. As there may be a relative dopamine depletion, dopamine antagonists are contraindicated. Chlorpromazine can worsen the neuroleptic malignant syndrome following levodopa withdrawal and might be expected to have a similar worsening effect on this syndrome in cocaine abusers. Dopamine agonists may reverse this rapidly fatal syndrome. Further corroborative studies are required to clarify this approach before it is translated to general clinical use.[137]

Sudden Death (Catecholamine Release). Death may follow cardiac arrhythmias due to massive catecholamine release with or without myocardial ischemia. Seizures can cause catecholamine release leading to life-threatening arrhythmias. Respiratory arrest may occur with high concentrations of cocaine. In some cases of sudden death there is an intracerebral hemorrhage or a ruptured aorta, both following cocaine-induced hypertension. Cases of excited delirium exhibit intense paranoia followed by bizarre and violent behavior, accompanied by hyperthermia, leading to sudden death.[138,139]

Cardiovascular Complications

Table 21–13 summarizes the cardiovascular toxicity of cocaine.

Sex–Cocaine Syndrome. Acute cardiac events may be precipitated by the sex–cocaine syndrome. Sex-induced cardiodynamic surges, the higher demands of a hyperdynamic circulation in pregnancy, and vasoactive stresses with high levels of cocaine may be the substrates for the induction of malignant arrhythmias, cardiac failure, and death.[140] In areas where the level of HIV-I infection in heterosexual intravenous drug users is high and the use of crack cocaine is common, increased sexual activity (including the exchange of drugs or money for sex) may result in increased heterosexual transmission of HIV-I.[141]

Myocardial Infarction. Although 5 million Americans are thought to use cocaine regularly, about 155 cases of cocaine-related acute myocardial infarction have been reported in the North American literature. Because of this, many patients with cocaine-related chest pain are admitted to the hospital with a diagnosis of possible myocardial infarction.[142]

Cocaine-related myocardial infarction is associated with a high prevalence of coronary thrombi and anterior wall involvement in otherwise normal coronary arteries.[122,143–145] Cocaine-induced myocardial infarction may follow cocaine abuse by the intranasal, intravenous, and inhalation routes.[146] About half of these patients who experience a myocardial infarction have had previous chest pain; 9 of 10 have been cigarette smokers and two thirds have had their myocardial infarcts within 3 hours of use of cocaine (range, 1 minute to 4 days).[147] Most patients presenting to an emergency department with cocaine-induced chest pain do not have a myocardial infarction.

Proposed mechanisms for cocaine-induced myocardial infarction include coronary artery spasm, in situ thrombus formation and platelet aggregation, direct myocardial injury, accelerated atherosclerosis, nonatherosclerotic intimal proliferation, and increased myocardial oxygen demand.[145,146] Cocaine-induced myocardial infarction in patients with normal coronary arteries probably involves adrenergically mediated increases in myocardial oxygen consumption, vasoconstriction of large epicardial arteries or small coronary resistance vessels, and coronary thrombosis. Accelerated atherosclerosis and impairment of endothelium vasodilator function may occur after chronic cocaine use.[148]

Coronary Vasoconstriction. Intranasal cocaine induces recurrent coronary vasoconstriction. The initial vasoconstriction is noted 30 minutes after drug administration, and is temporally related to the peak blood concentration of cocaine. As the blood concentration of cocaine declines, this vasoconstriction is alleviated. At 90 minutes after drug administration, coronary vasoconstriction recurs and is temporally related to increased concentrations of the principal metabolites of cocaine, benzoylecgonine and ethyl methyl ecgonine. Angina pectoris and myocardial infarction occurring hours after cocaine inhalation may be due to the coronary vasoconstrictive influence of such metabolites.[149]

Platelets. Biogenic amines such as serotonin and epinephrine are known to stimulate platelet aggregation. Cocaine increases thromboxane production and platelet aggregation, which may exacerbate ischemia by increasing vasoconstriction activity. Abnormal coronary resistance vessels (small epicardial vessels on endomyocardial biopsy) indicate that when a chronic change in coronary blood vessels reaches a critical stage, presumably chest pain can be induced by plugging of the small vessels by platelet thrombi activated by further cocaine abuse. Release of thromboxane A_2 from stimulated platelets could also exacerbate ischemia by increasing vasoconstrictor activity.[150]

Risk Factors. Risk factors associated with cocaine-induced myocardial infarction include known cardiac ischemic risk factors such as tobacco use, a family history of cardiac disease, hypertension, hypercholesterolemia, and diabetes mellitus.

Dysrhythmias. Most dysrhythmias following cocaine use are supraventricular. No specific treatment is required unless the patient is hemodynamically unstable.

Laboratory Tests. Serial serum creatine kinase MB band (CK-MB) values may aid clinical decision making in the management of chest pain patients without electrocardiographic ST-segment elevation. Newer serum markers that are not yet universally available include cardiac troponin-T, cardiac troponin-I, CK-MB isoforms, and cardiac myosin light chains.[151] It is not known how these markers react in cocaine-induced ischemia/infarction. Single or serial normal or nondiagnostic electrocardiograms do not rule out ischemia or injury in this group of patients.[152]

Postmyocardial Infarct Evaluation. Recurrent ischemic chest pain has been reported in patients who continue to abuse cocaine as well as in those who do not.[145] Exercise treadmill test, ST elevations on Holter monitoring, cardiac catheterization, and provocative testing with ergonovine have not been consistently useful in predicting patients at risk (see also Treatment section later in this chapter).

Chest Pain. Chest pain of presumed cardiac origin in a cocaine-abusing individual should be considered an ischemic event. Patients may require admission to the coronary care unit.[142] Chest pain is the most frequent cocaine-associated complaint, occurring in as many as 40% of such patients presenting to the emergency department.[153] Chest pain may often be seen in emergency departments following insufflation, inhalation, or intravenous use of cocaine. Such pain in the cocaine user may be due to pneumomediastinum and pneumothorax (inhalation use), foreign particle or septic emboli (intravenous use), associated trauma, and myocardial ischemia and infarction (any route). All patients presenting to the emergency department with acute chest pain should be questioned about cocaine use.

Hollander and colleagues found that cocaine-associated chest pain begins about 60 minutes after cocaine use and persists for about 120 minutes.[154] The chest pain is mostly substernal and pressurelike. Shortness of breath and diaphoresis are common. There are no clinical differences between patients who subsequently have myocardial infarctions and those who do not. Patients are usually young male cigarette smokers with histories of repetitive cocaine abuse. Few traditional cardiac risk factors are found in this patient population. The electrocardiogram is less sensitive in identifying myocardial infarction in patients with cocaine-induced than in other patients presenting with chest pain. Recurrent myocardial infarction may occur in patients with normal coronary angiograms who use cocaine.[145] An elevated CK-MB level within 3 hours of emergency department presentation is often associated with a subsequent ischemic event in the clinically stable chest pain patient without ST-segment elevation.[155]

Recurrent chest pain following cocaine use in one multicenter prospective study occurred in about half of patients. Myocardial infarction is infrequent in these patients.[156] Mortality in such patients is often ultimately related to HIV disease. As cocaine has been shown to accelerate atherosclerosis, patients with chest pain secondary to cocaine may be at risk for delayed complications of ischemic heart disease.

The ST-segment and T-wave changes can mimic acute myocardial injury. The quality of acute chest pain related to cocaine use is indistinguishable from that experienced in acute myocardial ischemia (see Treatment, Chest Pain, later in this chapter).

Contraction Bands. Contraction band necrosis in the heart is probably a characteristic histologic feature of catecholamine toxicity and may be seen in the acute period after myocardial infarction, during severe stress reactions, and after the administration of catecholamines or sympathomimetic agents, including cocaine.[157]

Cardiomyopathy. Long-term use of cocaine may induce a cardiomyopathy.[158] Contraction band necrosis heals with scarring and fibrosis, which may result in a biventricular dilated cardiomyopathy similar to that seen in pheochromocytoma patients.[159] When an acutely dilated cardiomyopathy appears that is temporally related to smoking crack cocaine, cessation of exposure over the next few weeks may be followed by reversal of the cardiomyopathy and improvement in left ventricular systolic function.[160]

Neurologic Complications

About 10 to 30% of strokes in young adults are associated with drug use, rising to 90% of patients in the third and fourth decades[161–163] (Table 21–17). For this reason drug screens should be part of the evaluation of young people presenting with stroke. Drugs most often implicated in stroke are sympathomimetic agents such as the amphetamines, phenylpropanolamine, phencyclidine, methylphenidate, cocaine, and opiates such as heroin.[162,163] In the past decade cocaine has become the most common agent implicated in drug-related stroke. Neurologic symptoms develop immediately or within 3 to 6 hours of use of cocaine in most cases of cocaine-related strokes.[163,164] Cocaine-associated strokes occur in both first-time users and long-time users and are independent of the route of administration (Table 21–18).

The alkaloid form of cocaine has been associated with both occlusive and hemorrhagic strokes. The hydrochloride form has been related mainly to hemorrhagic strokes.[161] Both subarachnoid and intracerebral hemorrhages have been associated with cocaine use. In about 80% an aneurysm or arteriovenous malformation has been detected. Cerebral angiographic examination is recommended in cases of cocaine-related intracerebral hemorrhage, especially if the hemorrhage is lobar or intraventricular.

Cocaine is now implicated as the most common illicit drug associated with cerebrovascular disease in adults.[165] Crack cocaine sniffers seem to be associated with both ischemic and hemorrhagic cerebrovascular disease, divided approximately evenly. Cocaine hydrochloride (intranasal, intravenous) is more commonly associated with hemorrhagic stroke.[164,166]

Subarachnoid Hemorrhage. Patients with sudden onset of a severe headache several minutes to hours after

Table 21–18
Mechanisms of Cocaine-Related Stroke

Ischemic Strokes	Hemorrhagic Strokes
Vasoconstriction of pial vessels	Acute hypertension with or without associated cerebral vascular anomaly
Cardioembolic	Reperfusion of ischemic, softened brain
Vasospasm following subarachnoid hemorrhage	Hemorrhage into cerebral neoplasm
Vasculopathy with endothelial cell sloughing	Thrombocytopenia
Nonhypertensive vasculopathy	Venular vasospasm with rupture of postcapillary venules
Hypercoagulability	Pial arteriole vasodilation
?Vasculitis	
Reduction of cerebral blood flow of uncertain mechanism	
Hemorrhagic infarction	

From Levine SR, Brust JC, Futrell N, et al. A comparative study of the cerebrovascular complications of cocaine: Alkaloidal versus hydrochloride: A review. Neurology 1991;41:1173–1177.

cocaine use, especially if it is associated with nausea, vomiting, neck stiffness, or loss of consciousness, should be admitted for evaluation of a possible subarachnoid hemorrhage. Preexisting lesions (cerebral aneurysm or arteriovenous malformation) form the substrate for this complication. Patients may arrive either hypertensive or normotensive.

Intracerebral Bleed. Intracerebral bleeds secondary to cocaine may present with headache, transient or persistent loss of consciousness, altered mental status, or abnormal neurologic examination with lateralizing signs. Some patients may have an underlying lesion (aneurysm, arteriovenous malformation, tumor). Computed tomography usually shows the hemorrhage.

Ischemic Cerebrovascular Accident. Cocaine can induce an ischemic cerebrovascular accident in some abusers, probably arising from cocaine-induced hypertension, subsequent vasospasm, and finally ischemia. Cocaine blocks serotonin reuptake and acutely increases serotonin levels. Serotonin is a strong vasoconstrictor and may contribute to decreasing blood flow to the brain. Cerebral vasculitis may also induce a cerebrovascular accident.[167] This can be diagnosed by an arteriogram or by a biopsy. The vasculitis may follow crack use.[168] Patients may present with hemiplegia, aphasia, paresthesia, and dysarthria. Computed tomography usually shows the infarct area, but it may be initially negative. Anterior spinal artery syndrome and lateral medullary syndrome may also follow cocaine use.[168,169] Embolic stroke has followed crack use.[170]

Transient Ischemic Attack. Following cocaine abuse, transient ischemic attacks may occur in the distribution of the middle cerebral and vertebrobasilar arteries.[169] By the time the patient presents to the hospital for examination, the neurologic examination may be normal. Computed tomography and cerebrospinal fluid examination are probably normal. This condition is probably secondary to vasospasm.

Cerebral Infarction. A newborn developed a cerebral infarction shortly after delivery. The mother had used 5 g of cocaine over a 3-day period prior to delivery and 1 g in the 15 hours preceding birth. At about 16 hours of age the child became apneic and cyanotic and experienced multiple focal seizures and a right-sided hemiparesis. The stroke was confirmed with computed tomography. Benzoylecgonine was present in the infant's urine for 4 days.[171,172]

Seizures. Between approximately 2 and 10% of patients presenting to an emergency department with cocaine toxicity have seizures. Cocaine-related seizures have been defined as seizures occurring within 90 minutes of cocaine use as per a witness report. Cocaine-related grand mal seizures have been reported as long as 12 hours after cocaine use.[173] Those with no history of prior seizures usually experience single generalized convulsions occurring after intravenous or crack cocaine use. Cranial computed tomography (CT) scans and electroencephalograms are usually normal. These patients usually recover without neurologic deficits. If the patient experiences focal seizures there will usually be a cerebral infarction, subarachnoid hemorrhage, or intraparenchymal hemorrhage. Status epilepticus is usually observed in cocaine users with no prior seizure history who have used large amounts of cocaine (2–8 g). Patients with a history of non-cocaine-related seizures, will, after using cocaine, usually experience focal motor seizures, which are usually multiple.[174] These frequently occur after intranasal use. If they have a single generalized seizure they usually have a normal cranial CT scan, electroencephalogram, and neurologic outcome (Table 21–19).

Table 21–19
Causes of Cocaine Seizures*

Adrenergic "surge"
Acute hypertensive episodes
Cerebral vasospasm
Hyperthermia
Intracranial hemorrhage, aneurysm, arteriovenous malformation
Vasculitis?
"Cutting agents" (epileptogenic agents: lidocaine, procaine, phencyclidine, amphetamines, quinidine)
Metabolic acidosis from intense muscular activity, hypoxemia, rhabdomyolysis, or lactate acidosis, which sensitize and potentiate the effects of catecholamines (This may result in dysrhythmias, hypotension, cerebral hypoperfusion, anoxia, and seizures.)
Hyperthermia from peripheral vasoconstriction, increased skeletal muscle activity, increased cardic output, and central thermoregulatory dysfunction
Pharmacologic "kindling effect" when repeat doses of cocaine are administered

*Seizures may occur after use of intravenous, intranasal, free-base, oral, topical, rectal, or intravaginal cocaine.

A patient with cocaine-induced seizures may present with a history of seizure and a normal examination or be postictal or actively seizing. Seizures are usually generalized tonic–clonic.

Children presenting to an urban emergency department with an unexplained seizure may represent a group at risk for cocaine intoxication. This may be an indication for toxicology screening.[175,176] In many cases it is the first seizure the patient has had. Seizures may also be associated with a hyperadrenergic state (hypertension, hyperthermia, and acidosis) and lead to respiratory arrest.[177] This hyperadrenergic state may lead to hypertension, an intracerebral bleed, cardiac arrhythmias, myocardial ischemia, and/or severe hyperthermia.

Risk Factors. Those at risk for cocaine-related seizures include (1) individuals who experience direct convulsant effects, usually after exposure to massive doses (2–8 g); (2) females, who are at greater risk for cocaine-related seizures than males (but cocaine-related chest pain appears to occur predominantly in males); (3) individuals with a history of epilepsy who may have their typical seizure precipitated by cocaine (even intranasally through a lowering of the seizure threshold;) and (4) those with chronic habitual cocaine abuse, which may result in "chemical" kindling of epilepsy.

Headache. Cocaine may trigger migraine headaches. Withdrawal from cocaine may likewise trigger headaches that are relieved by further cocaine administration.[178] In addition, headache may be related to head trauma during a cocaine-induced seizure or trauma to the head from problems related to a drug deal. Subdural or epidural hematoma or skull fracture must be considered. If the drug is used intravenously or the patient has AIDS, headache can also be caused by central nervous system infections.[179]

Cerebrospinal Fluid Rhinorrhea. Chronic intranasal use of cocaine may lead to vasospasm, chronic inflammatory changes, and damage to the cribriform plate. Surgical repair may be necessary.

Fungal Cerebritis. Intravenous cocaine users have experienced fungal cerebritis, and such cases have usually terminated fatally.[180]

Movement Disorders. Cocaine abuse has been associated with stereotyped movements, such as picking and stroking, tics,[181] Tourette's syndrome, chorea, and dystonic reactions[182]; the latter may follow the use of crack cocaine.[183]

Brain Abscess. Cocaine snorting leading to frontal sinusitis may subsequently be followed by a lethal brain abscess. The initial CT scan may be negative. Sinus pathology and intracranial symptoms in a cocaine abuser should alert the clinician to the possibility of brain abscess.[184]

Cerebral Atrophy. Chronic cocaine abusers with no discrete evidence of cerebral infarction or history of significant head trauma, HIV infection, or other neurologic disease may have CT evidence of diffuse frontotemporal cerebral atrophy.[185]

Cocaine Washed-Out Syndrome. Patients often present after a several-day cocaine binge with a diagnosis of decreased level of consciousness. They are arousable only after vigorous stimuli are applied and even then they may be unable to speak, say their name, or follow simple commands. They seem too exhausted to even talk or move. Deep tendon reflexes, Babinski's sign, cranial nerve examination, pupillary size and reactivity, doll's eyes, and cold calorics are usually normal. A metabolic and structural workup is usually normal. Most have no sedative drug on their toxicologic screen. Routine electrolytes, blood count, lumbar puncture, and CT scan of the head are all normal. In 12 to 18 hours, they become less lethargic and are discharged.[186]

Massive Overdose (Cocaine Packers)

Life-threatening toxic effects are associated with cocaine use (Table 21–20).

Body stuffers are compared with body packers in Table 21–21.[187] The sudden ingestion of crack cocaine when confronted by law enforcement personnel is often observed in teenagers who develop otherwise unexplained alterations of mental status, cardiovascular symptomatology, or acute abdominal complaints. Digital rectal examination may disclose a firm mass if crack packets have been ingested many hours before hospitalization, and plain radiography may disclose discrete packets if the crack has been wrapped in condoms, balloons, latex rubber, or aluminum foil or surrounding air or liquid is trapped in the packaging material. The drug itself is radiolucent.[188,189] The typical cocaine package may contain 5 to 7 g of cocaine. The lethal oral dose of cocaine in humans is about 1 to 1.2 g. Rupture of a single package carries the risk of death. Often, these patients are initially asymptomatic. This history is unreliable. Whole-bowel irrigation may be useful.[190] "Minipackers" are drug dealers who swallow drug-filled containers to avoid arrest. The drug is typically enclosed in small plastic bags. Death may occur if the package, rather than entering the esophagus, obstructs the upper airway or if the bag ruptures in the stomach, releasing a lethal amount of the drug.[191]

Table 21–20
Criteria for Life-Threatening Toxicity

Vital Signs
Systolic blood pressure >200 mm Hg (return to normal after acute event)
Systolic blood pressure <90 mm Hg (after fluid resuscitation)
Diastolic blood pressure >150 mm Hg (return to normal after acute event)
Pulse <40 or >180 (with systolic blood pressure >90 mm Hg)
Temperature >40.5°C (without other signs of acute infection)
Central Nervous System Events
Subarachnoid, intraparenchymal, or intraventricular hemorrhage
Cerebral infarction
Seizure(s)
Agitated delirium with hyperthermia (38.9°C or higher) requiring sedation with 10 mg diazepam IV or more or its equivalent
Ischemia or infarction of the spinal cord
Cardiovascular Events
Cardiac arrest
Myocardial ischemia or infarction
Aortic dissection
Ventricular tachycardia
Unstable supraventricular arrhythmias
Pulmonary Events
Pulmonary thrombosis
Pneumothorax or pneumomediastinum
Gastrointestinal Events
Bowel ischemia or infarction
Muscle Events
Rhabdomyolysis (defined as creatine phosphokinase level of 10,000 IU/L or higher)
Other Organ System Events
Splenic infarction
Renal infarction
Hepatic infarction
Obstetric Events
Abruptio placentae
Spontaneous abortion

From Hoffman RS, Henry GC, Howland MA, et al. Association between life-threatening cocaine toxicity and plasma cholinesterase activity. Ann Emerg Med 1992;21:247–253.

Medical Complications of Abuse

Insufflation. Reactive hyperemia of nasal mucosa causes a persistent rhinitis. Erosions and, less often, nasal perfora-

Table 21–21
Body Packers Versus Body Stuffers

	Body Packers	Body Stuffers
Background	Hired specifically to smuggle drugs, eg, heroin or cocaine	User or seller, on verge of arrest, swallows the evidence
Wrapping	Carefully wrapped (latex, sometimes condoms, with or without covering of aluminum foil)	May not be carefully wrapped or in aluminum foil; may be in an open porous container such as a sandwich bag, glass, or plastic "crack vials"; sometimes swallowed
Detection	Most escape detection	
Toxicity	Few toxic effects	Initially asymptomatic; later may be seizing, comatose, or dead in a jail cell
Radiograph	Carefully wrapped package with air or liquid trapped in packaging material (useful in 75–80% of cases)	Not always useful; number of ingested containers small; little liquid or air in packaging material
History	Inaccurate	Inaccurate
Coingestants	Usually not; most are not drug abusers, transport one drug	Present (users, street sellers)
Treatment	Gastric emptying, activated charcoal, whole-bowel irrigation	Gastric emptying, hazardous; careful induction of emesis; activated charcoal with whole-bowel irrigation
Surgery	If severely symptomatic	If severely symptomatic risk of obstruction is less
Endoscope	Encourage gastrointestinal transit	Empty bags will pass through on normal gastrointestinal transit

Adapted from Pollack CV, Biggers DW, Carlton FB Jr, et al. Two crack cocaine body stuffers. Ann Emerg Med 1992;21:1370–1380.

tion complicate chronic use.[192] Attempts at rhinoplasty in such users may lead to surgical complications including septal collapse, delayed mucosal healing, and inadequate correction of septal defect.[193] Sniffing high doses of cocaine (up to about 1500 mg) may unmask or aggravate myasthenia gravis.[194] Pain, photophobia, and decreased visual acuity associated with an iritis may develop a few hours after using intranasal cocaine.[195] Deep inhalation may deposit adulterants near the ethmoid sinuses, leading to sinusitis.[196] Bilateral optic neuropathy with decreased visual acuity and optic nerve head swelling may occur secondary to osteolytic sinusitis.[197] Optic disk swelling, optic atrophy, an apparent Foster Kennedy syndrome, and visual field defects may be related to intranasal cocaine use. Long-term cocaine snorters develop rebound nasal stuffiness after intranasal use that is often self-treated with nasal inhalers, sprays, and drops containing phenylephrine, oxymetazoline, beclomethasone, and flunisolide, all vasoconstrictors that can contribute to nasal mucoperichondrial necrosis and septal perforations.[198] Botulism has followed *Clostridium botulinum* maxillary sinusitis after intranasal cocaine abuse.[199] In addition, pulmonary granulomas,[200] abdominal colic, dyspnea on exertion, cough, pulmonary opacities, and cerebrospinal fluid rhinorrhea[201] have been reported after administration via the nasal route. Following nasal insufflation of cocaine, material may be drawn into the nasopharynx and from there into the mouth, resulting in a mixture of cocaine with saliva. The end product is an acid capable of dissolving the predominant dental mineral, calcium phosphate hydroxyapatite, from both enamel and dentin.[202] Inhalation of cocaine may precipitate an attack of acute porphyria.[203]

IV Injection. Although life-threatening bleeding is a rare occurrence, severe thrombocytopenia with a purpura-like syndrome may be observed beginning 21 days following the last use of intravenous cocaine (Table 21–22). Normalization of the platelet count follows corticosteroid therapy or splenectomy.[204] Intravenous injection of 4 to 5 g/d cocaine was followed by a central retinal artery occlusion.[205]

Table 21–22
Differential Diagnosis of Thrombocytopenia in Drug Abusers

Hypersplenism
Chronic hepatitis
Bacterial or fungal sepsis
AIDS
Disseminated intravascular coagulation
Cocaine
Autoimmune thrombocytopenia in heroin addicts

Adapted from Orser B. Thrombocytopenia and cocaine abuse. Anesthesiology 1991;74:195–196.

Cocaine and HIV Infection. An increasing number of people who inject cocaine intravenously are at risk of HIV infection through needle sharing, perhaps because of the frequency of injection during binges of cocaine use—up to 15 to 25 times in a single day. Some who inject every 10 to 15 minutes may leave the needle sitting in the vein to top it up every few minutes.[206] Though estimates indicate that there are 60,000 HIV-positive drug users in New York, distribution of clean needles and syringes is still illegal in some states. In South America, HIV infection is now seen in 36 to 57% of cocaine injectors.[207] Those who smoke cocaine in the form of crack are at higher risk of HIV infection (and sexually transmitted diseases) from sex-for-drug transactions.[207] In the sex-for-drugs group, increases in rates of syphilis and congenital syphilis have been observed.[208,209]

Other links between cocaine use and HIV infection, (in addition to the sharing of paraphernalia, and of injections, the sharing of "cookers,"[206–210] and the use of shooting galleries,) are the association between "speedballing" (simultaneous injection of heroin and cocaine among intravenous drug abusers in the New York area) and HIV infection,[211] a possibly increased incidence of Kaposi's sarcoma in those who have ever used cocaine, and an association between cocaine and depression of helper/suppressor T-lymphocyte ratios.[212,213]

Rhabdomyolysis

Some degree of rhabdomyolysis and an elevated creatine phosphokinase level are almost always found in serious cocaine toxicity. Rhabdomyolysis should be suspected in any cocaine-abusing patient with coma, seizures, hyperpyrexia hypotension, or severe agitation. Patients with rhabdomyolysis, acute renal failure, liver dysfunction, and disseminated intravascular coagulation have a high mortality rate.

Clinical signs or symptoms of rhabdomyolysis may be absent, making laboratory evaluation an essential diagnostic step.[214] Rhabdomyolysis and acute myoglobinuric renal failure have been associated with intoxication with amphetamines, tricyclic antidepressants, barbiturates, phenylpropanolamine, heroin, methadone, phencyclidine, mercuric chloride, lindane, sea snake venom, peanut oil, carbenoxolone, marijuana, carbon monoxide, alcohol, loxapine, and vasopressin.[215]

Drug overdose may cause rhabdomyolysis after (1) an extended period (sometimes only 20–30 minutes on a hard surface) of immobilization causing pressure-induced muscle necrosis; (2) a reaction resembling malignant hyperthermia; and (3) a chronic drug abuse state (alcohol, heroin, cocaine).

There appears to be no correlation between the amount of muscle mass damaged and the amount of renal dysfunction. Factors such as hyperuricemia, hypocalcemia, hypokalemia, hypophosphatemia, disseminated intravascular coagulation, hypotension, hepatic damage, and acidosis may be related. Creatine kinase serum levels are often elevated. Urine myoglobin may be present. A urine dipstick is a simple test for myoglobinuria, although a negative test does not rule out rhabdomyolysis.[214]

Smoking

Chronic cough and bronchitis productive of black or blood-tinged sputum frequently result from habitual freebase smoking. Pneumomediastinum and pneumothoraces have been reported after the prolonged Valsalva maneuvers associated with freebasing.[216] Pulmonary complications related to freebase cocaine smoking are summarized in Tables 21–5 and 21–14.[217]

A controlled study of heavy, habitual smokers of cocaine (mean 6.5 g/wk for an average of 53 months) indicated a high prevalence of at least occasional occurrences of acute cardiorespiratory symptoms within 1 to 12 hours of smoking cocaine (cough productive of black sputum, hemoptysis, chest pain, usually worse on deep breathing, cardiac palpitations) and a mild but significant impairment in the diffusing capacity of the lung that persisted after cessation of cocaine use.[218] There is a disparity between the high prevalence of acute respiration symptoms in temporal association with freebase use and the absence of a high prevalence of chronic respiratory symptoms. Further studies are required to clarify the possible damage incurred at the gas-exchanging surface of the lung. Table 21–17 lists nonrespiratory complications of smoking cocaine.

Cocaine Callus. A callus on the ulnar side of the right thumb can follow repeated contact of the thumb with the serrated wheel that ignites the lighter used to ignite crack cocaine in a paper.[219]

General Medical Conditions

Thyrotoxicosis has been observed in chronic cocaine users.[220] Hypocalcemia (to calcium levels as low as 3.6 mg/dL), hyperuricemia, and elevated serum creatine phosphokinase levels (as high as 763,000 IU/L), with evidence of severe rhabdomyolysis, may be seen in intravenous cocaine recreational users.[221]

Arsenic Poisoning

Cocaine may be "cut" with compounds containing arsenic. The occurrence of nausea, vomiting, and diarrhea and the presence of a sensorimotor neuropathy in a crack cocaine abuser may indicate arsenic intoxication.[222]

Intraurethral Use

Intraurethral use of cocaine, to enhance sexual performance, has been associated with severe disseminated intravascular coagulation, necessitating amputation of extremities and a necrotic penis.[223]

Psychiatric Complications

Distorted thought processes can cause aggressive suicidal and homicidal behavior; impaired judgment and attentional deficits increase the chance of accidental trauma.

Withdrawal

Myocardial infarction in the presence of disease-free coronary arteries may follow withdrawal from cocaine.[224,225] In one report the patient had been drinking large amounts of alcohol.[164] Vasospasm during cocaine withdrawal may be the result of dopamine depletion or receptor downregulation with an increased sensitivity to alpha-adrenergic receptor stimulation.[226] Dystonia may also follow cocaine withdrawal.[227] Further studies of biogenic amines are required to clarify these observations.

Cocaine users frequently develop silent myocardial ischemia with ST-segment elevation on the electrocardiogram during the first weeks of withdrawal. Coronary vasospasm may be a factor.[226]

Craving appears greatest in the 24 hours before admission and is associated with intense psychological depression. No definite crash may be observed. Mood states, craving, and sleep disturbances gradually improve during the initial 4 weeks.[228] This cocaine abstinence syndrome is usually medically benign and requires little medication for detoxification in an inpatient setting.

Cocaine abuse is a major problem among methadone-maintained opiate addicts. A prospective study demonstrates that increasing the patient's methadone dose by 5 mg in response to each cocaine-positive urine screen (to a maximum of 120 mg/d) resulted in abstinence from cocaine for up to 10 weeks (81% positive urine screens to 10.8% positive) at methadone doses of 115 mg/d.[229]

Laboratory

Analytical Methods

Analytical methods for cocaine determination are summarized in Table 21–23.[230–236]

Saliva. Cocaine and benzoylecgonine concentrations are 5 and 2.5 times higher, respectively, in saliva than in serum in individuals who have used cocaine in the previous 24 hours. Simultaneous measurement of cocaine and benzoylecgonine in saliva is useful in screening for recent cocaine use.[237]

Hair. Cocaine, benzoylecgonine, and ecgonine methyl ester may be analyzed in human hair by gas chromatography–mass spectrometry[238–240] and radioimmunoassay. This has been used as an adjunct to the usual analyses performed or to document exposure to drugs in situations where traditional specimens, such as blood and urine, have not been collected in a timely fashion.[241]

Scalp hair cocaine analysis may be useful in confirming the presence of cocaine either in an adult or in an infant whose mother was a possible cocaine user. Koren and colleagues have observed that pyrolysis of crack results in accumulation in hair of cocaine, but not its benzoylecgonine metabolite. After admitted cocaine use, both species are detectable in hair. External contamination with crack smoke is washable, whereas systemic exposure is not.[242] Contamination of hair by environmental cocaine may be difficult to distinguish from active drug use. Though hair cocaine may sometimes be positive when a urine test is negative, cocaine use occurring only in recent days would not yet be detectable by hair analysis. Further confirmatory studies will be of interest, especially in frequent users.[243]

Urine. Detection of cocaine and its metabolites in abuse screening is about 95% efficient at a cutoff point of 300 mg/L when any of the following tests are used: a latex agglutination inhibition assay (Abuscreen On Trak); mass spectrometry; an automated homogeneous immunoassay technique (ETC system); a manual enzyme-mediated immunoassay technique (EMIT-st); and a fluorescent polarization immunoassay (TDx).[244]

Street Samples. About 5% of young children (1 month to 5 years) in an urban pediatric emergency department without signs or symptoms suggestive of cocaine exposure have measurable benzoylecgonine in the urine by both enzyme-mediated immunoassay technique and radioimmunoassay.[245]

Body Stuffers. High plasma cocaine concentrations (> 1 μg/mL) are usually associated with toxicity, although such levels in fatal overdoses may range from 0.1 to 20.9 μg/mL.[246] The time since the last dose can be roughly estimated by examination of urinary ratios of benzoylecgonine to cocaine. A ratio less than 100 in urine suggests that cocaine was ingested less than 10 hours before the sample was collected.[247]

Pregnancy. A method of analysis involving solid-phase extraction and high-performance liquid chromatography is sensitive for the detection of cocaine and benzoylecgonine in amniotic fluid. The minimum detection level is 30 ng/mL.[248] The concentration of benzoylecgonine, a potent vasoconstrictor,[249] in amniotic fluid is several times higher than in neonatal urine. The amniotic fluid may act as a reservoir for

Table 21–23
Analysis of Cocaine and Its Metabolites

Method	Sample	Analyte	Approximate Detection Limit (ng/mL)	Usual Use
Immunoassay	Urine	Benzoylecgonine	300*	Qualitative or semi-quantitative Drug abuse screening Presumptive identification only
Thin-layer chromatography	Urine	Benzoylecgonine Ecgonine methyl ester Cocaine	500	Qualitative Drug abuse screening Presumptive identification only
Gas chromatography	Urine	Benzoylecgonine Ecgonine methyl ester Cocaine	Variable, approximately 50	Quantitative Drug abuse screening Presumptive or confirmation
Gas chromatography	Blood	Benzoylecgonine Ecgonine methyl ester Cocaine	Variable, 5–50	Quantitative Clinical correlation Kinetics
High-pressure liquid chromatography	Urine	Benzoylecgonine Cocaine	50	Quantitative Limited use for drug abuse screening
High-pressure liquid chromatography	Blood	Cocaine Benzoylecgonine	50	Quantitative Clinical correlation Kinetics
Gas chromatography–mass spectrometry	Urine	Benzoylecgonine Ecgonine methyl ester Cocaine	≤5	Quantitative Definitive identification and confirmation
Gas chromatography–mass spectrometry	Blood	Benzoylecgonine Ecgonine methyl ester Cocaine	≤5	Quantitative Clinical correlation Kinetics

*Can be lower; cutoff set to minimize false-positive results.
From Jatlow P. Cocaine: Analysis, pharmacokinetics, and metabolic disposition. Yale J Biol Med 1988;61:(2):105–113.

benzoylecgonine. Radioimmunoassay of newborn hair and gas chromatography–mass spectrometry of meconium are more sensitive than immunoassay of newborn urine in identifying the cocaine-exposed infant. These methods only identify infants exposed within the last 12 weeks of pregnancy.

Cocaine can be detected in neonatal urine for 12 to 24 hours after delivery if the drug was consumed within 2 days of delivery. Benzoylecgonine can be detected up to 5 days. Urine testing is negative if cocaine use was terminated several days before delivery. Meconium may be positive for up to 3 days after delivery.[78] Analysis of hair from the neonate provides information regarding long-term rather than recent cocaine use. The results remain positive for 5 to 6 months until the infant fetal hair is shed.[250]

Abnormalities

Cardiovascular Effects. Non-Q-wave myocardial infarction, with the presence of a T-wave infarct electrocardiographic pattern, is often seen in cocaine abusers.[251] During acute cocaine abuse, abnormalities are more prevalent and the QT interval is prolonged.[252]

Acid–Base Effects. Acid–base abnormalities would be expected to accompany hypoxemia and the reduced peripheral perfusion caused by cardiac depression or dysrhythmias. Arterial blood gases in most patients using cocaine by crack smoking, intravenous injection, and nasal insufflation show a pH from 7.35 to 7.5. Alkalosis (ph >7.45) is seen in about 15% of patients and is usually caused by hyperventilation, as evidenced by tachypnea and a low $Paco_2$. Acidosis is observed in about 33% of patients. The acidosis is primarily respiratory, with hypoventilation secondary to chest trauma or decreased mental status rather than pulmonary disease. A metabolic acidosis can also occur and may be associated with seizures, trauma, or agitation. Respiratory alkalosis is uncommon and is usually associated with tachypnea. Patients with a history of potential cocaine toxicity should be evaluated for both metabolic and respiratory acid–base abnormalities.[253,254]

Blood Levels

In evaluation of blood cocaine levels, a number of variables must be considered, including tolerance, previous history of cocaine use, individual susceptibility (eg, cardiovascular disease, pseudocholinesterase deficiencies), concomitant drug use (illicit or licit), role of adulterants, storage techniques, and time between administration and death.

Nonfatal Blood Levels. Smoked cocaine and intravenous cocaine appear to produce similar increases in heart rate, blood pressure, and subjective effects at similar venous plasma cocaine levels. The potency of smoked cocaine is about 60% that of intravenous cocaine; that is, a 50-mg dose of smoked cocaine has effects similar to those of a 32-mg dose of intravenous cocaine. Plasma cocaine levels may reach 425 ng/mL about 20 minutes after a 32-mg intravenous dose and 380 ng/mL after a 50-mg dose of smoked cocaine.[255]

Fatal Blood Levels. High plasma concentrations are rarely seen because of the short half-life of cocaine. Concentrations greater than 1 μg/mL are usually associated with toxicity.

Urine Levels

Cocaine may be detected in the urine of newborns up to 3 to 5 days following delivery if exposure occurs in utero.[256] Rosenberg and colleagues have observed the cocaine metabolite benzoylecgonine in the urine of 5% of toddlers and children treated for routine pediatric complaints.[13] The most likely route of exposure is second-hand smoke inhaled when adult caretakers use freebase or crack cocaine. None of the children had any signs or symptoms that would have indicated exposure. A urine test becomes positive at a threshold concentration of 50 ng/mL. The National Institute on Drug Abuse (NIDA) considers a urine test for cocaine positive when it scores in excess of 300 ng/mL for cocaine metabolites.[13]

In the collection of a random untimed urine specimen, the dose, serum concentration, and effects or impairment cannot be predicted exactly from the measurement of urine drug concentrations. This is largely due to the lack of a scientifically established relationship between these parameters. Sources of variability include timing (with respect to prior events or to urine flow), usage patterns (long or short term, intravenous, pulmonary, etc), physiologic variability, pathologic interactions, and other drug information. Route of absorption, cholinesterase activity, metabolic pathways, contaminants and hydrolysis products, and cocaethylene formation are additional considerations. Peak benzoylecgonine concentrations appear in the urine over a 3- to 24-hour period. The half-life of benzoylecgonine formation averages 1.9 hours, and its elimination half-life is 7.5 hours.[257]

Topical Application

A 5-mg dose of cocaine freebase applied to the volar forearm skin surface resulted in a maximal urinary benzoylecgonine concentration of 55 ng/mL at 48 hours. When 5 mg of cocaine hydrochloride was similarly applied, a maximal urinary benzoylecgonine concentration of 15 ng/mL was observed at 24 hours.[258]

Electroencephalography, Echoencephalography, and Computed Tomography

Intrauterine exposure to cocaine subjects the newborn to neurologic and electroencephalographic abnormalities, which may remain abnormal for 3 to 12 months.[259] Electroencephalographic abnormalities in cocaine-exposed infants may include intraventricular hemorrhage, echodensities known to be associated with necrosis, and cavitary lesions found mostly in the basal ganglia, frontal lobes, and posterior fossa.[260] Ventricular dilation, absence of cerebral hemispheres (by CT scan), microcephaly, and microphthalmia have been described in an infant whose mother had used cocaine in the first trimester of pregnancy.[261]

Roentgenography

Plain films of the abdomen with the suspect in the supine and upright positions may be useful in the diagnosis of body packing, but false-negative results may occur.[262] Urine samples tested for benzoylecgonine and a contrast study of the bowel with follow-up abdominal roentgenograms 5 hours after the oral ingestion of a water-soluble contrast compound (eg, 50 mL meglumine amidotrizoate [Gastrografin]) may be useful in detecting drug packages.[263] A daily view is performed thereafter. The patient may be discharged with negative views after the passage of two packet-free stools.[264]

Table 21–24
Treatment to Avoid If Possible in Management of Cocaine Toxicity

Drug	Possible Adverse Reaction
Beta blockers (labetalol)	Coronary artery constriction
Haloperidol	Hyperpyrexia
Lidocaine, procainamide, quinidine	Seizures and arrhythmias
Nifedipine (in body packer and body stuffer)	Increased gastrointestinal absorption
Mineral oil (body packer)	Dissolve rubber balloon
High-dose naloxone, flumazenil	Seizures
Temperature > 108°C	
Dantrolene	Cardiac insufficiency
Bromocriptine	Coronary artery constriction
Tachycardia	
Aspirin	Increased thyroxine, thyroid storm

From Wassberger J, Ellenhorn MJ, Landers S, et al. The emergency management of acute cocaine toxicity. Top Emerg Med 1993;15(3):27–40.

Treatment

For most patients with mild cocaine-induced stimulation, central nervous system sedation with a benzodiazepine (eg, diazepam) should be effective. Where clinically applicable, addition of an adrenergic blocking agent, preferably one with both alpha and beta blocking properties (eg, labetolol), may be useful, although beta blockers (eg, propranolol) have also been effective, but care must be taken when using a beta blocker to avoid the unopposed manifestations of alpha stimulation with its concomitant hypertension.

Treatments to avoid are listed in Table 21–24. Management of complications is summarized in Table 21–25.

Stabilization

Determine the blood glucose. Normalize if low. Get a rectal temperature to rule out a malignant type of hyperthermia. Follow with a CT scan to exclude an intracranial bleed. Treat seizures aggressively with diazepam (0.1–0.3 mg/kg up to an adult dose of 10 mg). Phenytoin may be ineffective. Phenobarbital acts slowly. Endotracheal intubation, assisted ventilation, and neuromuscular blockers (with electroencephalographic monitoring) are required for persistent seizures and subsequent acidosis. Use the neuromuscular blockers until the electroencephalogram is normal for 2 or more hours.

Hyperthermia. The most life-threatening presentation of acute cocaine intoxication is a severe hyperthermia with temperatures of 106° to 114°F. Give 10 mg diazepam IV. Hyperthermia can prevent gluconeogenesis causing hypoglycemia. In these patients, 50 to 100 mL of 50% dextrose, and 100 mg of thiamine intravenously, are indicated.

Table 21–25
Management of Cocaine Complications

Pulmonary edema	Intubate and ventilate. Monitor fluids with pulmonary artery catheter. For inotropes, monitor electrocardiogram.
Hypertension	Administer benzodiazepines (high doses). Institute nitroprusside drip. Administer phentolamine (nitroglycerin drip if chest pain also). If all fails and tachycardia is severe, give small dose of beta blockers.
Ventricular dysrhythmias	In first few hours, use non-sodium channel blocker. If wide QRS arrhythmia, give diazepam, magnesium sulfate, sodium bicarbonate, bretylium, amiodarone. After first 2 hours, administer lidocaine, procainamide (?myocardial ischemia).
Seizures	Administer benzodiazepines, IV barbiturates, phenytoin. For neuromuscular paralysis, intubate. Institute mechanical ventilation. Obtain computed axial tomography scan.
Hyperthermia (most life-threatening complication)	Use cool mist and evaporative fans. Administer benzodiazepines. Apply body ice packs; lower temperature to 102°C or lower. Give acetaminophen 2000 mg rectally. If temperature >108°C, administer dantrolene (questionable), bromocriptine (watch for cardiovascular collapse, coronary artery spasm). Do not give aspirin (binds with protein-bound thyroxine, may aggravate a misdiagnosed thyroid storm).
Chest pain	Avoid beta blockers and lidocaine. Decrease afterload. Administer benzodiazepines. Institute nitroglycerin drip. Administer nifedipine? Administer thrombolytic agents? Oxygen/nitroglycerin tablets, spray or patch? Give morphine as required and one aspirin (unless hyperthermic).
Metabolic acidosis	Use of IV bicarbonate is controversial; it may further depress the myocardium and paradoxically decrease arterial and intracellular pH.
Body packers	Avoid beta blockers. Administer high-dose benzodiazepines. Institute cooling measures. Hydrate. Avoid mineral oil. Administer Golytely? Avoid endoscopy. Surgical removal is necessary if patient is symptomatic after benzodiazepines.
Combative	Administer benzodiazepines (decrease catecholamines?)—lorazepam. Check blood sugar—50% dextrose IV as needed. Give oxygen. Do not administer haloperidol or phenothiazines (risk of malignant hyperthermia, seizures).
Altered level of consciousness	Administer naloxone in small increments. Monitor respiration. Give IV glucose as required. If no response to naloxone and glucose, consider multidrug overdose.
"Speedball"	Rule out intracranial lesion.
Sinus tachycardia	Do not use beta blockers. Administer diltiazem (continuous IV).

Patients who do not respond to diazepam, acetaminophen 2000 mg (in the form of 500-mg rectal suppositories), and vigorous cooling measures (eg, ice packs) or those who maintain temperatures above 108°F have been treated with dantrolene 1 mg/kg every 6 hours or bromocriptine orally via a nasogastric tube. The efficacy of dantrolene in the treatment of cocaine-induced hyperthermia has not been established. It can lead to cardiac insufficiency and pulmonary edema. Dantrolene and bromocriptine are now rarely used. Hyperthermia may induce rhabdomyolysis: administer aggressive fluid therapy to maintain a high urine output. Investigate for sepsis.

Hypertension. Ingestion of 20 g of cocaine by an adult induced a heart rate of 185 beats/min and a blood pressure of 230/110. Intravenous labetolol 20 mg administered over a 10-minute period, followed by a labetolol drip over 8 hours, controlled the heart rate at less than 100 beats/min and the diastolic pressure at less than 100 mm Hg.[265]

Esmolol is a short-acting intravenous cardioselective B_1 blocker with an elimination half-life of about 10 minutes. It must be diluted to 10 mg/mL and administered at the rate of 50 µg/kg/min, increasing up to 100 µg/kg/min for about 4 minutes; 500 µg/kg has been administered as a loading dose. It is not a specific antidote. Watch for paradoxical hypertension, bronchospasm, and hypotension.[266] Esmolol and beta-specific antagonists may either exacerbate hypertension (paradoxical hypertension) or induce hypotension.[267]

Hypertension Without Tachycardia. Use a vasodilator:

- Phentolamine 0.02 to 0.1 mg/kg intravenously (blocks coronary artery vasoconstriction caused by cocaine)
- Nifedipine 0.1 to 0.2 mg/kg intravenously (renal)
- Nitroprusside 2 to 10 µg/kg/min intravenously

Nifedipine, verapamil, and diltiazem may dilate abdominal and cerebral vasculature, permitting more cocaine to be absorbed. They are not recommended for either hypertension or chest pain in patients who have ingested either rock cocaine or packets of cocaine.

Hypertension With Tachycardia. If hypertension with tachycardia is not controlled by the above medications, use beta blockers plus intravenous nitroglycerin to offset coronary artery vasoconstriction. Propranolol is not advised because blockage of B_2 receptors opposes vasodilation. Its unopposed alpha action may result in paradoxical hypertension. It may also worsen cocaine-induced coronary artery vasospasm.

Labetalol 10 to 20 mg intravenously repeated at 10-minute intervals up to a total of 300 mg is under evaluation for control of life-threatening hypertension and tachycardia.

For a hypertensive emergency without tachycardia or ventricular arrhythmia, institute a nitroprusside drip 10 µg/kg/min for 10 minutes only; follow with a maintenance drip of 0.5 to 2 µg/kg/min.

Hypertension with Chest Pain. Institute a nitroglycerin drip. Avoid beta blockers. Use benzodiazepines to reduce excess production of catecholamines by the central nervous system. Avoid lidocane. Administer oxygen by nasal cannula at 5 L/min. Monitor cardiac status and initiate an intravenous line. If systolic blood pressure is greater than 120 mm Hg, administer nitroglycerin sublingually (up to 3 tablets or 3 sprays of 0.4 mg each). Apply a nitroglycerin patch to the chest. If pain is refractory to nitroglycerin, use morphine. Cocaine-induced chest pain with coronary artery spasm not responsive to nitroglycerin may respond to sublingual nifedipine,[268] but its role has yet to be defined. Phentolamine may ameliorate myocardial ischemia by relieving cocaine-induced coronary artery constriction.[145] Obtain an electrocardiogram. Give one aspirin with 10 mL of an antacid. Benzodiazepine (diazepam, lorazepam) can be used to control cocaine-induced sympathetic status. Observe for 24 hours to differentiate global myocardial ischemia from a localized, regional transmural infarction. If signs of a regional transmural myocardial infarction are not present or confirmed by the electrocardiogram, the patient may not require admission to a coronary care unit.

If the chest pain is strongly suggestive of a myocardial infarction, or an electrocardiogram with a current injury showing marked hyperactive ST-segment elevations is not responsive to nitroglycerin and nifedipine, consider thrombolytic therapy. If hyperacute anterolateral myocardial infarction with seizures is present, do a CT scan to rule out an intracerebral bleed before instituting thrombolytic therapy.[269]

Myocardial Ischemia and Infarction

Beta-adrenergic Blockade. Some of the routine pharmaceutical interventions for the treatment of acute myocardial infarction may be harmful in a patient with cocaine-induced ischemia.[270] Beta-adrenergic blockade in cocaine-induced coronary vasoconstriction may induce a further decrease in coronary artery diameter, but the effect of beta blockers on mortality has not been studied in patients with cocaine-associated infarction. As the period of myocardial ischemia may persist up to 2 weeks following cessation of cocaine abuse,[271] it would be prudent to avoid beta blockers in patients with suspected cocaine-induced myocardial ischemia. In addition, such beta blockade should probably be avoided for as long as 2 weeks following withdrawal of the toxin. Beta blockade may be considered in myocardial infarctions associated with tachycardias to relieve myocardial oxygen demand.

Lidocaine. Lidocaine and procaine share pharmacologic characteristics with cocaine and the possibility exists that they may enhance cocaine toxicity. Few data are available on the use of these products in treatment of complications of cocaine-induced myocardial infarction. No adverse effects have yet been reported. Cocaine toxicity may be short-lived. Lidocaine can be considered for the treatment of ventricular ectopy following a cocaine-induced myocardial infarction.

Phenytoin. Phenytoin may be useful for the treatment of ventricular dysrhythmias, but there may be a delay in reaching therapeutic levels rapidly.

Thrombolytic Therapy. In an acute myocardial infarction of less than 6 hours' duration with evolving or changing ST–T wave elevations and without any contraindications such as marked hypertension and bleeding, thrombolytic agents should be considered.[145,272,273]

Dysrhythmias. Cardioversion should be considered for all unstable dysrhythmias. Unstable supraventricular dysrhythmias may be treated by correcting ischemia, administering calcium channel blockers and alpha or beta adrenergic blockers, or cardioversion. Adenosine may be ineffective.

Supportive Therapy. Early therapy of cocaine-induced myocardial infarction should be similar to that of the typical patient with myocardial ischemia. Establish intravenous access and administer oxygen. Give aspirin to inhibit platelet aggregation. If the systolic blood pressure is greater than 100 mm Hg, administer nitroglycerin sublingually for the relief of pain. If pain does not resolve with nitroglycerin, administer nifedipine 10 mg orally or phentolamine 1 to 5 mg intravenously, followed by a drip of 10 mg in 1000 mL of 5% dextrose in water at 10 mL/min while monitoring the blood pressure. Administer thrombolytic agents if required.[145,272,273] For life-threatening dysrhythmias, consider use of type IA antidysrhythmic agents with caution. Stress cessation of cocaine and tobacco use.

Calcium channel blockers may alleviate coronary spasm (experimental data). Beta blockers can potentiate cocaine-induced coronary vasoconstriction. Phentolamine may be useful if propranolol has induced unopposed alpha-adrenergic receptor stimulation. Cocaine users may sustain myocardial infarction with normal coronary arteries.

Acute myocardial infarction after cocaine use should be treated as myocardial infarction in non-cocaine users except for the use of beta blockers.

Thrombolysis. Thrombolysis may be useful if manifestations of myocardial infarction are not relieved by coronary vasodilation therapy with nitrates, calcium channel blockers, or phentolamine.[274] The classic indications for the treatment of acute myocardial infarction with thrombolysis are chest pain characteristic of infarction lasting 30 minutes or longer but less than 6 hours, with 0.1-mV or greater ST-segment elevation in two or more contiguous leads on the electrocardiogram, in a patient younger than 75 years[275] (Table 21–26). Cocaine users are at high risk for subarachnoid hemorrhage and aortic dissection, however. If this is suspected, avoid thrombolysis.

The success of thrombolysis is not universal. Approximately 20% of infarct-related arteries fail to open with thrombolytic regimens, and approximately 15% of reperfused arteries reclose in subsequent hours and days.[275]

The onset of chest pain may not correspond to true total occlusion of the infarct-related artery, and some time may pass before complete occlusion develops. Furthermore, coronary arteries may open and close several times during the early period of infarction, even though chest pain appears to be nearly continuous. For these reasons, it is appropriate to consider thrombolysis for patients with acute Q-wave infarctions who present "late" after the onset of chest pain, beyond 6 to 12 hours or even up to 24 hours, if there is evidence of ongoing ischemia and if there are no contraindications (Table 21–26).[275]

Table 21–26
Criteria for Thrombolysis in Acute Myocardial Infarction

Chest pain consistent with acute myocardial infarction
Electrocardiographic changes
- ST-segment elevation >0.1 mV in at least two contiguous leads
- New or presumably new left bundle-branch block
- ST-segment depression with prominent R wave in leads V_2 and V_3, if this is thought to indicate a posterior infarction (benefit is doubtful if it is thought to indicate unstable angina)

Time from onset of symptoms
- <6 h: most beneficial
- 6–12 h: lesser but still important benefits
- >12 h: diminished benefits but possibly still useful for continuing chest pain or "stuttering" pain course

Age
- Physiologic age more important than chronologic age
- <75 y: clear-cut benefits
- ≥75 y: fewer clear-cut benefits

From Anderson HV, Willerson JT. Thrombolysis in myocardial infarction. N Engl J Med 1993;329:703–709.

Do not use thrombolysis in a hypertensive patient or in a cocaine-using patient with seizures until a head CT scan is proven to be normal.[276]

Aortic Dissection. Aortic dissection can follow an acute severe elevation of systolic blood pressure after cocaine use. Calcium channel blockers and nitroprusside are useful to control the hypertension.

Endocarditis. Left-sided more than right-sided valves are involved in cocaine users. Watch for paravalvular abscess with transesophageal echocardiography.

Cardiomyopathy. Repeat cocaine use leads to depression of left ventricular function. Calcium channel blockers may be useful, but their use has not been studied in a controlled setting.

Cardiac Arrest. The Advanced Cardiac Life Support recommends intravenous epinephrine for asystole. Epinephrine further increases the cocaine adrenergic surge.[277] Labetolol (0.25 mg/kg intravenously over 2 minutes) alleviates the increase in systemic arterial pressure caused by cocaine but does not influence cocaine-induced coronary artery vasoconstriction.[278]

The Combative Patient. It may be impossible to insert an intravenous line into a very combative patient. In such cases, give lorazepam 8 mg/kg intramuscularly. If possible, start an intravenous line thereafter. Give diazepam 10 to 20 mg or lorazepam 2 to 8 mg acutely and repeat if needed with continuous cardiorespiratory monitoring until the effects of both the cocaine and the sedative cease. Much larger doses, of diazepam up to 100 to 150 mg, have been suggested for control of the extremely combative patient.[279] Experience with these doses is limited. Patients may become apneic from large doses of benzodiazepines. Flumazenil may precipitate seizures. Treat respiratory depression with intubation and ventilation. Use hard restraints as required (see Chapter 4). Once the patient is under sufficient control to start an intravenous line, obtain a blood sugar evaluation. If the patient is hypoglycemic, then give 50 to 100 mL of 50% dextrose in water together with thiamine 100 mg. Diazepam, oxygen, and normalization of the blood sugar usually enable the management team to institute routine critical care.[135] Sedatives with butyrophenones (such as haloperidol and droperidol) or phenothiazines (such as chlorpromazine) are not recommended. These agents are anticholinergic atropine-like drugs that can cause a patient to become hot and precipitate malignant hyperthermia. These drugs also lower the seizure threshold by blocking inhibitory central nervous system dopaminergic receptors. Benzodiazepines reduce blood pressure, pulse, and agitation.[135]

Rhabdomyolysis. Monitor the patient with serial serum creatine kinase and urine myoglobin studies. Attempt to differentiate rhabdomyolysis-induced enzyme increases from those due to myocardial infarction. Use alkalinization, diuretics (eg, mannitol, furosemide), and fluids to diminish the precipitation of myoglobin in the urine and lessen the resultant renal failure.

Renal Failure. Perhaps one third of patients with rhabdomyolysis develop renal failure following myoglobin-induced tubular injury. Hemodialysis aids in reversing the renal failure. Dopamine (3μm/kg/day) and furosemide (60 mg three times daily) may reduce renal vascular resistance and assist in reducing the number of hemodialyses required to reverse oliguria.[284] Further studies are required to corroborate these observations.

Dysrhythmias

Sinus Tachycardia. Most dysrhythmias are supraventricular. If chest pain is not present, it is not usually necessary to treat. If mild elevation of blood pressure is not present, treatment is usually not required. If the tachycardia is uncomplicated, do not use beta blockers. Specific management is indicated for the hemodynamically unstable patient.

Ventricular Dysrhythmia. Lidocaine, procainamide, quinidine, and cyclic antidepressants are sodium channel blockers and can enhance arrhythmias and seizures. Sodium bicarbonate may be considered for wide-complex arrhythmias due to cocaine overdoses.[280] Although acidosis may depress myocardial function and potentiate ventricular dysrhythmias, the use of bicarbonate remains controversial. Benzoylecgonine may be critical in producing vasoconstrictive effects after cocaine use. Gastric alkalinization may accelerate benzoylecgonine production and lead to precipitation or worsening of ischemic and behavioral complications.[126] Intravenous bicarbonate may further impair a depressed myocardium and may paradoxically decrease arterial and intracellular pH.[281] Avoid lidocaine and procainamide in the treatment of ventricular ectopy in the first 1 or 2 hours after acute use of cocaine.[282] Ventricular ectopy occurring more than 2 hours after an acute cocaine exposure may be an indication for use of lidocaine and procainamide. The role of magnesium sulfate is not established. Consider cardioversion for unstable dysrhythmias. Administration of nifedipine after cocaine use did not induce an improvement in left ventricular function or coronary blood flow in dogs.[283]

Chest Pain. Criteria for admitting cocaine abusers with chest pain to rule out myocardial infarction should include sustained or persistent chest pain, chest pain with known risk factors for coronary artery disease, or chest pain with electrocardiographic changes suggestive of ischemia. A suggested protocol for patients admitted to rule out myocardial infarction comprises cardiac enzymes every 8 hours for 24 hours, daily electrocardiograms, and repeat electrocardiograms with recurrent or increased chest pain as well as with new findings consistent with a potential change in cardiovascular status.[285]

COCAINE CHEST PAIN SYNOPSIS

1. The incidence of infarction in patients who present to the emergency department with cocaine-associated chest pain is about 5 to 6%.[286–290] The optimal approach to patients with cocaine-associated chest pain has not yet been defined.
2. The low incidence of myocardial infarction indicates that routine coronary care and admission may not be cost effective.[286]
3. Patients with cocaine-associated chest pain who are immediately released from a hospital may continue to use cocaine or tobacco, predisposing them to recurrent coronary artery vasoconstriction,[286,288] but they are unlikely to sustain a myocardial infarction or die within the subsequent year.[286]
4. Most cocaine-associated myocardial infarctions occur within 12 hours of emergency department arrival.[286]
5. Delayed complications are indicated by ST-segment elevation, early rise in CK-MB, or complications in the first 12 hours after presentation. Therefore, a 12-hour observation period with CK-MB and electrocardiograms is probably the most cost-effective approach to optimum patient care.[286]
6. Patients with chest pain should be questioned about cocaine use.
7. Two thirds of patients with cocaine-associated myocardial infarctions have greater than 50% coronary artery stenosis. One of four has two-vessel coronary disease; 1 in 10 has three-vessel disease.[290]

Altered Level of Consciousness: Speedballs

1. Administer naloxone 2 mg intravenously. Titrate naloxone in 0.4-mg increments while monitoring respiration rate, depth, and pattern. Indications for use of naloxone include cocaine and heroin abuse, altered level of consciousness, miotic pupils, and shallow respiration. Use caution in agitation, acute withdrawal, seizures, hypertensive crisis with an acute pulmonary edema, arrhythmias, and cardiac arrest.
2. Determine the blood sugar level. If the patient has hypoglycemia, give 50 mL (25 g) to 100 mL (50 g) of 50% dextrose intravenously for adults and 25% dextrose 2 mL/kg intravenously for children.
3. If there is no response to naloxone and glucose, consider multidrug overdose. Rule out structural intracranial lesion.

Body Stuffers. If rock cocaine has been ingested, gut decontamination with activated charcoal 1 g/kg is preferred. Give sorbitol with the first dose to promote excretion from the gastrointestinal tract. Surgery is not indicated to remove a few small disintegrated rocks ingested by a body stuffer.

Body Packers. If the patient is relatively asymptomatic, use activated charcoal. Mineral oil and endoscopy are contraindicated: latex condoms or rubber balloons containing cocaine may dissolve. Consider surgery in a symptomatic body packer to remove large numbers of cocaine packages.

Craving. No specific drugs have been shown conclusively to block the euphoriant properties of cocaine or to reduce the effects of withdrawal or craving. Bromocriptine, amantadine, levodopa, methylphenidate, and ibocaine should be considered experimental.[291]

Elimination Enhancement

Preliminary data suggest that asymptomatic cocaine body packers with a delayed presentation may be aided by the use of whole-bowel irrigation with polyethylene glycol electrolyte lavage solution, followed by contrast radiography to confirm the adequacy of removal. This technique should be confirmed by further studies; it has not been shown to be safe and effective with early presentations, with poorly wrapped substances, or for symptomatic cocaine body packers.[292] Rapid hydrolysis of cocaine to its inactive metabolite in an alkalinized gastric medium in vitro may indicate a role for gastric alkalinization in the acute management of body packer breakage,[293] but acceleration of benzoylecgonine (a vasoconstrictor) production by alkalinizing fluids containing cocaine can lead to precipitation or worsening of ischemic and behavioral problems. Further controlled studies are required to validate safe use of alkalinization.[126]

Antidote

Butylcholinesterase is present in the blood at low levels and metabolizes cocaine to inactive compounds. A method for isolating butylcholinesterase from human plasma has been developed. Increasing the amount of butylcholinesterase in the blood may be a possible approach to enhancing more rapid inactivation of cocaine.[294]

Supportive Measures

Seizures. Seizures should be controlled with diazepam. If diazepam is not effective then phenytoin loading should be tried. If phenytoin is not effective, phenobarbital loading and pentobarbital general anesthesia may be tried.[295] After seizures are controlled, an investigation of the patient should rule out other causes of seizures, stroke, subarachnoid hemorrhage, and infection. A CT scan, lumbar puncture, and electroencephalogram may be of value if indicated. Cocaine-associated status epilepticus is a relatively rare complication of cocaine abuse. It may follow all methods of cocaine use. Frequently it follows unusually large doses of cocaine and often concurrent use of other drugs (eg, heroin, amphetamines, or marijuana). Cocaine-associated status epilepticus is often resistant to medical treatment.[296]

SEIZURE SUMMARY

1. For seizures of short duration, administer intravenous benzodiazepines.
2. If seizures are repeated, administer intravenous phenytoin and/or barbiturates.
3. Determine blood glucose. Normalize if low.
4. Determine rectal temperature. Rule out malignant hyperthermia.
5. Order a CT scan to exclude intracerebral bleed.
6. For persistent seizures with hyperthermia, institute neuromuscular paralysis with a nondepolarizing agent, intubation, and mechanical ventilation.

Chronic Dependency. Fenfluramine, trazodone, local anesthetics, and neuroleptic agents either have not yet demonstrated clinical effectiveness in ameliorating the signs and symptoms of cocaine withdrawal or have caused unacceptable side effects. Monoamine oxidase inhibitors, when used concurrently with stimulants such as cocaine, may induce a hypertensive crisis.[297] Initial studies with fluoxetine are of interest, but treatment may worsen the craving in some patients.[298] Several studies indicate a possible role for carbamazepine in decreasing craving[299] for cocaine and reducing cocaine use among methadone maintenance patients.[300] Caution should be exercised as carbamazepine may increase heart rate and blood pressure in cocaine smokers.[301] An initial but not yet confirmed controlled study suggests that phenytoin induces sustained abstinence from cocaine.[302] Ibogaine, an investigational drug, requires further study.

Intravenous Drug Users and HIV. Intravenous cocaine users tend to inject more frequently (up to five times within 1 hour) than intravenous heroin users, who take 1 hour or longer between "hits." The high from cocaine is of much shorter duration than the high from heroin. The craving for more cocaine occurs much sooner ("binging"). Because of the frequency of injection, cocaine users may be less consistent in using bleach to decontaminate needles and, therefore, less likely to inactivate HIV. In addition, cocaine users are often less willing to share their needles because they need them more often. Increasing the availability of sterile needles and syringes would lessen the need to share equipment.[303] An obvious form of AIDS risk reduction that intravenous cocaine users might adopt is switching from injecting cocaine hydrochloride to smoking crack or free-base. However, this is obviously not without numerous other risks.[304]

REFERENCES

1. Elsohly MA, Brenneisen R, Jones AB. Coca paste: Chemical analysis and smoking experiments. J Forens Sci 1991;36: 93–103.
2. Cravey RH. Cocaine deaths in infants. J Anal Toxicol 1988; 12:354–355.

3. Garland JS, Smith DS, Rice TB, Siker D. Accidental cocaine intoxication in a nine-month-old infant: Presentation and treatment. Pediatr Emerg Care 1989;5:245–247.
4. Edlin BR, Irwin KL, Faruque S, et al. Intersecting epidemics: Crack cocaine use and HIV infection among inner-city young adults. N Engl J Med 1994;331:1422–1427.
5. Lovejoy FH Jr, Shannon M, Woolf AD. Recent advances in clinical toxicology. Curr Prob Pediatr 1992;22:119–129.
6. Sturner WQ, Sweeney KG, Callery RT, Haley NR. Cocaine babies: The scourge of the 90s. J Forens Sci 1991;36:34–39.
7. Meeker JE, Reynolds PC. Fetal and newborn death associated with maternal cocaine use. J Anal Toxicol 1990;14:379–382.
8. Chasnoff IJ, Burns KA, Burns WJ. Cocaine use in pregnancy: Perinatal morbidity and mortality. Neurotoxicol Teratol 1987; 9:291–293.
9. Durand DJ, Espinoza AM, Nickerson BG. Association between prenatal cocaine exposure and sudden infant death syndrome. J Pediatr 1990;117:909–911.
10. Chasnoff IJ, Hunt CE, Kletter R, Kaplan D. Prenatal cocaine exposure is associated with respiratory pattern abnormalities. Am J Dis Child 1989;143:583–587.
11. Bauchner H, Zuckerman B. Cocaine, sudden infant death syndrome, and home monitoring. J Pediatr 1990;117: 904–906.
12. Bauchner H, Zuckerman B, McClain M, et al. Risk of sudden infant death syndrome among infants with in utero exposure to cocaine. J Pediatr 1988;113:831–834.
13. Rosenberg NM, Meert KL, Knazik SR, et al. Occult cocaine exposure in children. Am J Dis Child 1991;145:1430–1432.
14. Kharasch SJ, Glotzer D, Vinci R, et al. Unexplained cocaine exposure in young children. Am J Dis Child 1991;145: 204–206.
15. Dinnies JD, Darr CD, Saulys AJ. Cocaine toxicity in toddlers. Am J Dis Child 1990;144:743–744.
16. Heagarty MC. Crack cocaine: A new danger for children. Am J Dis Child 1990;144:756–757.
17. Conway EE, Mezey AP, Powers K. Status epilepticus following the oral ingestion of cocaine in an infant. Pediatr Emerg Care 1990;6:189–190.
18. Riggs D, Weibley RE. Acute hemorrhagic diarrhea and cardiovascular collapse in a young child owing to environmentally acquired cocaine. Pediatr Emerg Care 1991;7:154–155.
19. Shannon M, Lacouture PG, Roa J, Woolf A. Cocaine exposure among children seen at a pediatric hospital. Pediatrics 1989;83:337–342.
20. Bateman DA, Heagarty MC. Passive freebase cocaine ("crack"): Inhalation by infants and toddlers. Am J Dis Child 1989;143:25–27.
21. Bouknight LG, Bouknight RR. Cocaine: A particularly addictive drug. Postgrad Med 1988;83:122.
22. Brewer LM, Allen A. *N*-Formylcocaine: A study of cocaine comparison parameters. J Forens Sci 1991;36:697–707.
23. Janzen KE. Ethylbenzoylecgonine: A novel component in illicit cocaine. J Forens Sci 1991;36:1224–1228.
24. Ensing JG, Hummelen JC. Isolation, identification and origin of three previously unknown congeners in illicit cocaine. J Forens Sci 1991;36:1666–1687.
25. Ensing JG, de Zeeuw RA. Detection, isolation and identification of truxilles in illicit cocaine by means of thin layer chromatography and mass spectrometry. J Forens Sci 1991; 36:1299–1311.
26. Casale JF. Detection of pseudoecgonine and differentiation from ecgonine in illicit cocaine. Forens Sci Int 1990;47: 277–287.
27. Le Belle M, Callahan S, Latham D, et al. Comparison of illicit cocaine by determination of minor components. J Forens Sci 1991;36:1102–1120.
28. Casale JF, Waggoner RW Jr. A chromatographic impurity signature profile analysis for cocaine using capillary gas chromatography. J Forens Sci 1991;36:1312–1330.
29. U.S. Drug Enforcement Administration. Los Angeles Times, December 20, 1994, p. A21.
30. Miller NS, Klahr AL, Gold MS, et al. The prevalence of marijuana (cannabis) use and dependence in cocaine dependence. NY State J Med 1990;90:491–492.
31. Rich JA, Singer DE. Cocaine-related symptoms in patients presenting to an urban emergency department. Ann Emerg Med 1991;20:616–621.
32. Laposata EA, Mayo GL. A review of pulmonary pathology and mechanisms associated with inhalation of freebase cocaine ("crack"). Am J Forens Med Pathol 1993;14:1–9.
33. Jacob P, Jones RT, Benowitz NL, et al. Cocaine smokers excrete a pyrolysis product, anhydroecgonine methyl ester. Clin Toxicol 1990;28:121–125.
34. Jacob P, Lewis ER, Elias-Baker BA, Jones RT. A pyrolysis product, anhydroecgonine methyl ester (methylecgonidine), is in the urine of cocaine smokers. J Anal Toxicol 1990; 14:353–357.
35. Merigian KS, Park LJ, Leeper KW, et al. Adrenergic crisis from crack cocaine ingestion: Report of five cases. J Emerg Med 1994;12:485–490.
36. Paly D, Jatlow P, Van Dyke C, et al. Plasma cocaine concentrations during cocaine pack smoking. Life Sci 1982;30: 731–738.
37. Tendrup TE, Walls HC, Mariani PJ, et al. Plasma cocaine and tetracaine levels following application of topical anesthesia in children. Ann Emerg Med 1992;21:162–166.
38. Zhang JY, Foltz RL. Cocaine metabolism in man: Identification of four previously unreported cocaine metabolites in human urine. J Anal Toxicol 1990;14:201–205.
39. Burke WM, Ravi NV. Urinary excretion of cocaine. Ann Intern Med 1990;112:548–549.
40. Martin BR, Lue LP, Boni JP. Pyrolysis and utilization of cocaine. J Anal Toxicol 1989;13:158–162.
41. Jackson GF, Snady JJ, Poklis A. Urinary excretion of benzoylecgonine following ingestion of Health Inca Tea. Forens Sci Int 1991;49:57–64.
42. Altieri M, Bogema S, Schwartz RH. TAC topical anesthetic produces positive urine tests for cocaine. Ann Emerg Med 1990;19:577–579.
43. Handler A, Kiston N, Davis F, Ferri C. Cocaine use during pregnancy: Perinatal outcomes. Am J Epidemiol 1991;133: 818–825.
44. Collins E, Hardwich RJ, Jeffrey H. Perinatal cocaine intoxication. Med J Aust 1989;150:331–334.
45. Chasnoff I, Griffith DR, MacGregor S, et al. Temporal patterns of cocaine use in pregnancy: Perinatal outcome. JAMA 1989;261:1741–1744.
46. Hadeed AJ, Siegel SR. Maternal cocaine use during pregnancy: Effect on the newborn infant. Pediatrics 1989;84: 205–210.
47. Rosenak D, Diamont YZ, Haffe H, Hornstein E. Cocaine: maternal use during pregnancy and its effect on the mother, the fetus, and the infant. Obstet Gynecol Surv 1990;45: 348–359.
48. Telsey AM, Merrit A, Dixon SD. Cocaine experience in a term neonate: Necrotizing enterocolitis as a complication. Clin Pediatr 1988;27:547–550.
49. Spinazzola R, Kenigsberg K, Usmani SS, Harper RG. Neonatal gastrointestinal complications of maternal cocaine abuse. NY State J Med 1992;92:22–23.
50. Van den Anker JN, Cohen-Overbeek TE, Wladimiroff JW, Sauer PJJ. Prenatal diagnosis of limb reduction defects due to maternal cocaine use. Lancet 1991;338:1332.
51. Hoyme HE, Lyons Jones K, Dixon SD, et al. Prenatal cocaine exposure and fetal vascular disruption. Pediatrics 1990;85: 743–747.
52. Lyons Jones K. Developmental pathogenesis of defects associated with prenatal cocaine exposure: Fetal vascular disruption. Clin Perinatol 1991;18:139–146.
53. Hannig VL, Phillips JA III. Maternal cocaine abuse and fetal anomalies: Evidence for teratogenic effects of cocaine. South Med J 1991;84:498–499.
54. Spires MC, Gordon EF, Choudhuri M, et al. Intracranial hemorrhage in a neonate following prenatal cocaine exposure. Pediatr Neurol 1989;5:324–326.
55. Maynard EC, Dreyer SA, Oh W. Prenatal cocaine exposure and hyaline membrane disease (HMD). Pediatr Res 1989;24: 223A.
56. Zuckerman B, Maynard EC, Cabral H. A preliminary report of prenatal cocaine exposure and respiratory distress syn-

drome in premature infants. Am J Dis Child 1991;145: 695–698.
57. Kain ZN, Kain TS, Scarpell EM. Cocaine exposure in utero: Perinatal development and neonatal manifestations—review. Clin Toxicol 1992;30:607–636.
58. Young SL, Vosper HJ, Phillips SA. Cocaine: Its effects on maternal and child health. Pharmacotherapy 1993;12: 2–17.
59. Zuckerman B, Frank DA. Prenatal cocaine exposure: Nine years later. J Pediatr 1994;124:731–733.
60. Griffith DR, Azuma SD, Chasnoff IJ. Three-year outcome of children exposed prenatally to drugs. J Am Acad Child Adolescent Psychiatry 1994;33:20–27.
61. Kliegman RM, Madura D, Kiwi R, et al. Relation of maternal cocaine use to the risks of prematurity and low birth weight. J Pediatr 1994;124:751–756.
62. Singer LT, Yamashita TS, Hawkins S, et al. Increased incidence of intraventricular hemorrhage and developmental delay in cocaine-exposed, very low birthweight infants. J Pediatr 1994;124:756–771.
63. Chasnoff IJ, Griffith DR, Frier C, Murray J. Cocaine/polydrug use in pregnancy: Two year follow-up. Pediatrics 1992;89: 284–289.
64. Simone C, Derewlany LO, Oskamp M, et al. Transfer of cocaine and benzoylecgonine across the perfused human placental cotyledon. Am J Obstet Gynecol 1994;170:1404–1410.
65. Schenker S, Yang Y, Johanson RF, et al. The transfer of cocaine and its metabolites across the term human placenta. Clin Pharmacol Ther 1993;53:329–339.
66. Koren G. Personal communication.
67. Plessinger MA, Woods JR Jr. The cardiovascular effects of cocaine use in pregnancy. Reprod Toxicol 1991;5:99–113.
68. Slutsker L. Risks associated with cocaine use during pregnancy. Obstet Gynecol 1992;79:778–779.
69. Graham KA, Dimitrakoudis D, Pellegrini E, Koren G. Outcome of pregnancy after first trimester exposure to cocaine. Vet Hum Toxicol 1988;30:376.
70. Koren G, Graham K. Cocaine in pregnancy. Vet Hum Toxicol 1992;34:263–265.
71. Astley SJ, Clarren SK, Little RE, et al. Analysis of facial shape in children gestationally exposed to marijuana, alcohol and/or cocaine. Pediatrics 1992;89:67–77.
72. Plessinger MA, Woods JR Jr. Maternal placental and fetal pathophysiology of cocaine exposure during pregnancy. Clin Obstet Gynecol 1993;36:267–278.
73. Chasnoff IJ, Lewis DE, Squires L. Cocaine intoxication in a breast fed infant. Pediatrics 1987;80:836–838.
74. Giacoia GP. Cocaine in the cradle: A hidden epidemic. South Med J 1990;83:947–951.
75. Chaney NE, Franke J, Wadlington WB. Cocaine convulsions in a breast-feeding baby. J Pediatr 1988;112:134–135.
76. Graham K, Dimitrakoudis D, Pellegrini E, Koren G. Pregnancy outcome following first trimester exposure to cocaine in social users in Toronto, Canada. Vet Hum Toxicol 1989;31:143–148.
77. Browne SP, Tebbett JR, Moore SM, et al. Analysis of meconium for cocaine in neonates. J Chromatogr Biomed Appl 1992;575:158–161.
78. Callahan CM, Grant TM, Phipps P, et al. Measurement of gestational cocaine exposure: Sensitivity of infants' hair, meconium and urine. J Pediatr 1992;120:763–768.
79. Clark GD, Rosenzweig IB, Raisys VA, et al. The analysis of cocaine and benzoylecgonine in meconium. J Anal Toxicol 1992;16:261–263.
80. Casanova OQ, Lombardero N, Behnke M, et al. Detection of cocaine exposure in the neonate: Analyses of urine, meconium and amniotic fluid from mothers and infants exposed to cocaine. Arch Pathol Lab Med 1994;118:988–993.
81. Welch E, Fleming LE, Peyser I, et al. Rapid cocaine screening of urine in a newborn nursery. J Pediatr 1993;123: 468–470.
82. Ahluwalia SS, Clark JFJ, Westney SL, et al. Amniotic fluid and umbilical artery levels of hormone and prostaglandins in human users. Reprod Toxicol 1992;6:57–62.
83. Zuckerman B, Bresnahan K. Developmental and behavioral consequences of prenatal drug and alcohol exposure. Pediatr Clin North Am 1991;38:1387–1406.
84. Zuckerman B, Frank DA. "Crack kids" not broken. Pediatrics 1992;89:337–339.
85. Chasnoff IJ, Burns WJ, Schnoll SH, et al. Cocaine use in pregnancy. N Engl J Med 1985;313:666–669.
86. Volpe JJ. Effect of cocaine use on the fetus. N Engl J Med 1992;327:399–407.
87. Kramer LD, Locke GE, Ogunyemi A, Nelson L. Neonatal cocaine-related seizures. J Child Neurol 1990;5:60–64.
88. Foltin RW, Fischman MW, Pedroso JJ, Pearlson GD. Marijuana and cocaine interactions in humans: Cardiovascular consequences. Pharmacol Biochem Behav 1987;28: 459–464.
89. Anton AH. Unexpected cocaine-induced fatalities: A possible cause. Drug Intell Clin Pharm 1988;22:914.
90. Hoffman RS, Henry GC, Howland MA, et al. Association between life-threatening cocaine toxicity and plasma cholinesterase activity. Ann Emerg Med 1992;21:247–253.
91. Jatlow P, Barash PG, Van Dyke C, et al. Cocaine and succinylcholine sensitivity: A new caution. Anesth Analg 1978; 58:235–238.
92. Delaney K, Hoffman RS. Effects of cocaine on the in vitro determination of plasma cholinesterase activity: Analysis of kinetics of inhibition. Vet Hum Toxicol 1991;33:385.
93. Devenyi P: Cocaine complications and pseudocholinesterase. Ann Intern Med 1989;110:167–168.
94. Henry GC, Hoffman RS, Thompson T, et al. Effects of low dose short-term cocaine use on human plasma cholinesterase activity. In: *Proceedings, International Congress* on *Clinical Toxicology, New York, September 8–13, 1993:* Abstract 132.
95. Hershman Z, Aaron C. Prolongation of cocaine effect. Anesthesiology 1991;74:631–632.
96. Rowbotham MC, Hooker WD, Mendelson J, Jones RT. Cocaine–calcium channel antagonist interactions. Psychopharmacology 1987;93:152–154.
97. Derlet RW, Albertson TE. Potentiation of cocaine toxicity with calcium channel blockers. Am J Emerg Med 1989;7:464–468.
98. Dean RA, Harper ET, Dumaual N, et al. Effects of ethanol on cocaine metabolism: Formation of cocaethylene and norcocaethylene. Toxicol Appl Pharmacol 1992;117:1–8.
99. Lewis D, Muldoon K, Leikin JB. Cocaethylene in meconium specimens. Vet Hum Toxicol 1993;35:351.
100. Hime GW, Hearn WL, Rose S, Cofino J. Analysis of cocaine and cocaethylene in blood and tissues of GC-NPD and GC-ion trap mass spectrometry. J Anal Toxicol 1991;15: 241–245.
101. Hearn WL, Hime GW, Cofino J, Rose S. Detection of cocaethylene as a major metabolite. In: *Proceedings, American Academy of Forensic Sciences, February 18–23, 1991:* 174 (Abstract K18).
102. De la Torre R, Farre M, Ortuno J, et al. The relevance of urinary cocaethylene following the simultaneous administration of alcohol and cocaine. J Anal Toxicol 1991;15:223.
103. Rose S, Cofino J, Hearn WL, Hime GW. Investigation of the metabolite formation of cocaethylene. In: *Proceedings, American Academy of Forensic Sciences, February 18–23, 1991:*174 (Abstract K19).
104. Uszenski RT, Grillis RA, Schaer GL, et al. Additive myocardial depressant effects of cocaine and ethanol. Am Heart J 1992;124:1276–1283.
105. Randall T. Cocaine, alcohol mix in body to form even longer lasting, more lethal drug. JAMA 1992;267:1043–1044.
106. Pirwitz MJ, Willard JE, Landau C, et al. Influence of cocaine, ethanol or their combination on epicardial coronary arterial dimensions in humans. Arch Intern Med 1995;155:1186–1191.
107. Hearn WL, Rose S, Wagner J, et al. Cocaethylene is more potent than cocaine in mediating lethality. Pharmacol Biochem Behav 1991;39:531–533.
108. Mash DC, Flynn DD, Wetli CV, Hearn WL. Potency of cocaethylene at monoamine neurotransmitter uptake sites and neuroreceptors in the human brain. In: *Proceedings, Ameri-*

can Academy of Forensic Sciences, February 18–23, 1991: 174 (Abstract K20).

109. Woodward JJ, Mansbach R, Carroll FI, Balster RL. Cocaethylene inhibits dopamine uptake and produces cocaine-like actions in drug discrimination studies. Eur J Pharmacol 1991;197:235–236.
110. Wu AHB, Onigbirde TA, Johnson KG, Winbish GH. Alcohol specific cocaine metabolites in serum and urine of hospitalized patients. J Anal Toxicol 1992;16:132–136.
111. Brookoff D, Shaw L, Campbell E, Fields L. Cocaethylene, cocaine and ethanol levels in trauma patients. Ann Emerg Med 1993;22:989.
112. Lewis DE. Cocaethylene in meconium specimens. J Toxicol Clin Toxicol 1994;32:697–703.
113. Kissner DG, Lawrence WD, Selis JE, Flint A. Crack lung: Pulmonary disease caused by cocaine abuse. Am Rev Respir Dis 1987;136:1250–1252.
114. Samuels J, Schwalbe SS, Marx GF. Speedballs: A new cause for intraoperative tachycardia and hypertension. Anesth Analg 1991;72:397–398.
115. Merigian KS. Cocaine-induced ventricular arrhythmias and rapid atrial fibrillation temporally related to naloxone administration. Am J Emerg Med 1993;11:96–97.
116. Shesser R, Jotte P, Olshaker J. The contribution of impurities in the acute morbidity of illegal drug use. Am J Emerg Med 1991;9:336–342.
117. Katz A, Hoffman RS, Silverman R. Phenytoin toxicity from smoking "crack" cocaine adulterated with dilantin. Vet Hum Toxicol 1992;34:347.
118. Pascual-Leone A, Dhuna A, Anderson DC. Long term neurological complications of chronic habitual cocaine abuse. Neurotoxicology 1991;12:393–402.
119. Chambers HF, Morris L, Tauber MG, Modin G. Cocaine use and the risk for endocarditis in intravenous drug users. Ann Intern Med 1987;106:833–836.
120. Rezkalla SH, Hale S, Kloner RA. Cocaine-induced heart disease. Am Heart J 1990;120:1403–1408.
121. Heuter DC. Cardiovascular effects of cocaine. JAMA 1987; 257:979–980.
122. Lange RA, Cigarroa RG, Yancy CW Jr, et al. Cocaine-induced coronary artery vasoconstriction. N Engl J Med 1989;321:1557–1562.
123. Majid P, Cheirif JB, Rolley R, et al. Does cocaine cause coronary vasospasm in chronic cocaine abuser? A study of coronary and systemic hemodynamics. Clin Cardiol 1992;15: 253–258.
124. Chitwood DD. Patterns and consequences of cocaine use. Natl Inst Drug Abuse Res Monogr Ser 1985;61:111–129.
125. Boehrer JD, Moliterno DJ, Willard JE, et al. Hemodynamic effects of intranasal cocaine in humans. J Am Coll Cardiol 1992;20:90–93.
126. Konkol RJ, Olsen GD, Aks S, et al. Gastric alkalinization in the treatment of cocaine toxicity. Ann Emerg Med 1993; 22:1238–1239.
127. Godwin JE, Harley RA, Miller KS, Hefner JE. Cocaine, pulmonary hemorrhage, and hemoptysis. Ann Intern Med 1989; 110:843.
128. Murray R, Smialek J, Golle M, et al. Pulmonary vascular abnormalities in cocaine users. Am Rev Respir Dis 1988;137: 459.
129. Suhl J, Gorelick A. Pulmonary function in male freebase cocaine users. Am Rev Respir Dis 1988;137:488.
130. Tashkin DP, Khalsa M-E, Gorelick D, et al. Pulmonary status of habitual cocaine smokers. Am Rev Respir Dis 1992; 145:92–100.
131. Greenebaum E, Copeland A, Grewal R. Blackened bronchoalveolar lavage fluid in crack smokers: A preliminary study. Am J Clin Pathol 1993;100:481–487.
132. Marks V, Chapple PAL. Hepatic dysfunction in heroin and cocaine users. Br J Addict 1967;62:189–195.
133. Wanless IR, Dore S, Gopinath N, et al. Histopathology of cocaine hepatotoxicity: Report of four patients. Gastroenterology 1990;98:497–501.
134. Comer GM, Mittal MK, Donelson SS, Lee T-P. Cluster of fulminant hepatitis B in crack users. Am J Gastroenterol 1991;86:331–334.
135. Wasserberger J, Ellenhorn MJ, Landers S, et al. The emergency management of acute cocaine toxicity. Top Emerg Med 1993;15:27–40.
136. Hanzlick R, Gowitt GT. Cocaine metabolite detection in homicide victims. JAMA 1991;265:760–761.
137. Klosten TR, Kleber HD. Rapid death during cocaine abuse: A variant of the neuroleptic malignant syndrome? Am J Drug Alcohol Abuse 1988;14:335–346.
138. Benowitz NL. Clinical pharmacology and toxicology of cocaine. Pharmacol Toxicol 1993;72:3–12.
139. Prahlow JA, Davis GJ. Death due to cocaine intoxication initially thought to be a homicide. South Med J 1994;87:295–298.
140. Burkett G, Bandstra ES, Cohen J, et al.: Cocaine-related maternal death. Am J Obstet Gynecol 1990;163:40–41.
141. Chiasson MS, Stoneburner RL, Hidebrand DS, et al. Heterosexual transmission of HIV-I associated with the use of smokable freebase cocaine (crack). AIDS 1991;5:1121–1121.
142. Goldfrank L. Consultations. Ann Emerg Med 1987;16:240.
143. Lange RE, Flores EP, Cigarroa RG, Hillis LD. Cocaine-induced myocardial ischemia and infarction. Cardiology 1990;8:74–79.
144. Gitter MJ, Goldsmith SR, Dunbar DN, Sharkey SW. Cocaine and chest pain: Clinical features and outcome of patients hospitalized to rub out myocardial infarction. Ann Intern Med 1991;115:277–282.
145. Hollander JE, Hoffman RS. Cocaine-induced myocardial infarction: An analysis and review of the literature. J Emerg Med 1992;10:169–177.
146. Hollander JE, Carter WA, Hoffman RS. Use of phentolamine for cocaine-induced myocardial ischemia. N Engl J Med 1992;327:361.
147. Minor RL Jr, Winniford MD. Cocaine and coronary artery thrombosis. Ann Intern Med 1992;116:776–777.
148. Minor RL Jr, Scott BD, Brown DD, Winniford MD. Cocaine-induced myocardial infarction in patients with normal coronary arteries. Ann Intern Med 1991;115:797–806.
149. Brogan WC III, Lange RA, Glamann B, Hillis LD. Recurrent coronary vasoconstriction caused by intranasal cocaine: Possible role for metabolites. Ann Intern Med 1992;116:556–561.
150. Flores ED, Lange RA, Ciguaroa RG, et al. Effect of cocaine on coronary artery dimensions in atherosclerotic coronary artery disease: Enhanced vasoconstriction at sites of significant stenoses. J Am Coll Cardiol 1990;16:74–79.
151. Hockstra JW. Diagnosis of myocardial ischemia and infarction. Acad Emerg Med 1994;1:143–146.
152. Tokarski GF, Paganussi P, Urbanski R, et al. An evaluation of cocaine-induced chest pain. Ann Emerg Med 1990;19: 1088–1092.
153. Brody SL, Slovis CM, Wrenn KD. Cocaine-related medical problems: Consecutive series of 233 patients. Am J Med 1990;88:325–331.
154. Hollander JE, Hoffman RS, Gennis P, et al. Prospective multicenter evaluation of cocaine-associated chest pain. Acad Emerg Med 1994;1:330–339.
155. Hedges JR, Young GP, Henkel GK, et al. Early CK-MB elevations predict ischemic events in stable chest pain patients. Acad Emerg Med 1994;1:9–16.
156. Hollander JE, Hoffman RS, Fairweather P, et al. Cocaine associated chest pain: Long term follow-up. Vet Hum Toxicol 1993;35:350.
157. Southern JF. Case records of the Massachusetts General Hospital: Case 15-1988. N Engl J Med 1988;318:970–981.
158. Hogya PT, Wolfson AB. Chronic cocaine abuse associated with dilated cardiomyopathy. Am J Emerg Med 1990;8:203–204.
159. Karch SB, Billingham ME. The pathology and etiology of cocaine-induced heart disease. Arch Pathol Lab Med 1988; 112:225–230.
160. Chokshi SK, Moore R, Pandian NG, Isner JM. Reversible cardiomyopathy associated with cocaine intoxication. Ann Intern Med 1989;111:1039–1040.
161. Tapia JF. Weekly clinicopathological exercises: Case 27-1993. N Engl J Med 1993;329:117–124.

162. Sloan MA, Kittner JK, Rigamonti D, Puce TR. Occurrence of stroke associated with use/abuse of drugs. Neurology 1991;41:1358–1364.
163. Kaku DA, Lowenstein DH. Emergence of recreational drug abuse as major risk factor for stroke in young adults. Ann Intern Med 1990;113:821–827.
164. Levine SR, Brust JCM, Futrell N, et al. Cerebrovascular complication of the use of the "crack" form of alkaloidal cocaine. N Engl J Med 1990;323:699–704.
165. Levine SR, Brust JCM, Futrell N, Brass LM, et al. A comparative study of the cerebrovascular complications of cocaine: Alkaloidal versus hydrochloride—a review. Neurology 1991;41:1173–1177.
166. Peterson PL, Roszler M, Jacobs I, Wilner HI. Neurovascular complications of cocaine abuse. J Neuropsychiatry 1991; 3:143–149.
167. Krendel DA, Ditter SM, Frankel MR, Ross WK. Biopsy-proven cerebral vasculitis associated with cocaine abuse. Neurology 1990;40:1092–1094.
168. Mody CK, Miller BL, McIntyre HB, et al. Neurological complications of cocaine abuse. Neurology 1988;38:1189–1193.
169. Spivey WH, Euerle B. Neurologic complications of cocaine abuse. Ann Emerg Med 1990;19:1422–1428.
170. Petty GW, Brust JCM, Tatemichi TK, Barr MC. Embolic stroke after smoking "crack" cocaine. Stroke 1990;21:1632–1635.
171. Chasnoff IJ, Bussey ME, Savich R, Stack CM. Perinatal cerebral infarction and maternal cocaine use. J Pediatr 1986; 108:456–459.
172. Chasnoff IJ, MacGregor S. Maternal cocaine use and neonatal morbidity. Pediatr Res 1987;21:356A.
173. Lowenstein DH, Massa SM, Rowbotham MC, et al. Acute neurologic and psychiatric complications associated with cocaine abuse. Am J Med 1987;83:841–846.
174. Dhuna A, Pascual-Leone A, Langendorf F, Anderson DC. Epileptogenic properties of cocaine in humans. Neurotoxicology 1991;12:621–626.
175. Ernst AA, Sanders WM. Unexpected cocaine intoxication presenting as seizures in children. Ann Emerg Med 1989;18: 774–777.
176. Krug SE, Marble RD, Lubitz DL, Long TJ. Screening for cocaine intoxication in children with unexplained seizures in the emergency department. Ann Emerg Med 1991;20:448.
177. Jonsson S, O'Meara M, Young JB. Acute cocaine poisoning. Am J Med 1983;75:1061–1064.
178. Cooper LJ, Bloom FE, Roth RH. *The Biochemical Basis of Neuropharmacology.* New York: Oxford University Press, 1986.
179. Roberts JR. Discussion. In: *Year Book of Emergency Medicine.* Chicago: Year Book, 1991:182.
180. Pearigen PD. Medical complications of cocaine abuse. N Engl J Med 1986;315:1495–1500.
181. Pascual-Leone A, Dhuna A. Cocaine-associated multifocal tics. Neurology 1990;40:999–1000.
182. Hegarty AM, Lipton RB, Meriam AE, Freeman K. Cocaine as a risk factor for acute dystonic reactions. Neurology 1991; 41:1670–1672.
183. Habal R, Sauter D, Olowe O, Duras M. Cocaine and chorea. Am J Emerg Med 1991;9:618–620.
184. Rao AN. Brain abscess: A complication of cocaine inhalation. NY State J Med 1988;88:548–550.
185. Pascual-Leone A, Dhuma A, Anderson DC. Cerebral atrophy in habitual cocaine abusers: A planimetric CT study. Neurology 1991;41:34–38.
186. Sporer KA, Lesser SH. Cocaine washed-out syndrome. Ann Emerg Med 1992;21:112.
187. Pollack CV, Biggers DW, Carlton FB Jr, et al. Two crack cocaine body stuffers. Ann Emerg Med 1992;21:1370–1380.
188. Roberts JR, Wason S, Merigian KS. Crackpacking: A new radiographic diagnosis. Ann Emerg Med 1989;18:800–801.
189. Riggs D, Weibley RE. Acute toxicity from oral ingestion of crack cocaine: A report of four cases. Pediatr Emerg Care 1990;6:24–26.
190. Makosiej FJ, Hoffman RS, Howland MA, Goldfrank LR. An in vitro evaluation of cocaine hydrochloride absorption by activated charcoal and desorption upon addition of polyethylene glycol electrolyte lavage solution. Clin Toxicol 1993;31: 381–395.
191. Introna F Jr, Smialek JE. The "mini-packer" syndrome: Fatal ingestion of drug containers in Baltimore, Maryland. Am J Forens Med Pathol 1989;10:21–24.
192. Vilensky W. Illicit and licit drugs causing perforation of the nasal septum. J Forens Sci 1982;27:958–962.
193. Slavin SA. The cocaine user: The potential problem patient for rhinoplasty. Plast Reconstr Surg 1990;86:436–442.
194. Berciano J, Oterino A, Rebollo M, Pascual J. Myasthenia gravis unmasked by cocaine abuse. N Engl J Med 1991;326: 892.
195. Wang SJ. Cocaine-induced iritis. Ann Emerg Med 1991;20: 192–193.
196. Cohen S. Cocaine: Acute medical and psychiatric complications. Psychiatr Ann 1984;14:747–749.
197. Newman NM, DiLoreto DA, Ho JT, et al. Bilateral optic neuropathy and osteolytic sinusitis: Complications of cocaine abuse. JAMA 1988;259:72–74.
198. Schweitzer VG. Osteolytic sinusitis and pneumomediastinum: Deceptive otolaryngological complications of cocaine abuse. Laryngoscope 1985;96:206–210.
199. Kudrow DB, Henry DA, Haake DA, et al. Botulism associated with *Clostridium botulinum* sinusitis after intranasal cocaine abuse. Ann Intern Med 1988;109;984–985.
200. Cooper CB, Bai TR, Heyderman E, et al. Cellulose granulomas in the lung of a cocaine sniffer. Br Med J 1983;286: 2021–2022.
201. Sawicka EH, Trosser A. Cerebrospinal fluid rhinorrhea after cocaine sniffing. Br Med J 1983;286:1476–1477.
202. Krutchkoff DJ, Eisenberg E, O'Brien JE, Ponzillo JJ. Cocaine induced dental erosion. N Engl J Med 1990;322:408.
203. Dick AD, Prentice MG. Cocaine and acute porphyria. Lancet 1987;2:1150.
204. Leissinger CA. Severe thrombocytopenia associated with cocaine use. Ann Intern Med 1990;112:708–709.
205. Devenyi P, Schneiderman JF, Devenyi RG, Lawby L. Cocaine induced central retinal artery occlusion. Can Med Assoc J 1988;138:129–130.
206. Joseph SC. A methadone clone for cocaine. New York Times, January 11, 1989.
207. Farrell M. Cocaine and HIV. Br Med J 1991;303:330.
208. Nanda D, Feldman J, Delke I, et al. Syphilis among parturients at an inner city hospital: Association with cocaine use and implications for congenital syphilis rates. NY State J Med 1990;90:448–490.
209. Minkoff HL, McCalla S, Delke I, et al. The relationship of cocaine use to syphilis and human immunodeficiency virus infections among inner city parturient women. Obstet Gynecol 1990;163:521–526.
210. Marmor M, Des Jarlais DC, Cohen H, et al. Risk factors for infection with human immunodeficiency virus among intravenous drug abusers in New York City. AIDS 1987;1:39–44.
211. Weiss SH. Links between cocaine and retroviral infection. JAMA 1989;261:607–608.
212. Marmor M, Friedman-Kiens E, Laubenstein L, et al. Risk factors to Kaposi's sarcoma in homosexual men. Lancet 1982; 1:1083–1086.
213. Biggar RJ, Melbye M, Elbesen P, et al. Low T-lymphocyte ratios in homosexual men. JAMA 1984;251:1441–1446.
214. Welch RD, Todd K, Krause GS. Incidence of cocaine-associated rhabdomyolysis. Ann Emerg Med 1991;20:154–157.
215. Merigian K, Roberts JR. Cocaine intoxication: Hyperpyrexia, rhabdomyolysis and acute renal failure. Clin Toxicol 1987; 25:135–148.
216. Shessor R, Davis C, Edelstein S. Pneumomediastinum and pneumothorax after inhaling alkaloidal cocaine. Ann Emerg Med 1981;10:213–215.
217. Ettinger NA, Albin RJ. A review of the respiratory effects of smoking cocaine. Am J Med 1989;87:655.
218. Tashkin DP, Khalsa M-E, Gorelick D, et al. Pulmonary status of habitual cocaine smokers. Am Rev Respir Dis 1992; 145:92–100.
219. Larkin RF. The callus of crack cocaine. N Engl J Med 1990; 323:685.

220. Burton KR, Marin CA, Murray FT, Muniz CE. Hyperthyroidism in a cocaine-dependent patient. J Clin Psychiatry 1989;50: 305–306.
221. Goetz C, Harchelroud F. Severe hypocalcemia associated with cocaine-induced rhabdomyolysis. Vet Hum Toxicol 1991;33:387.
222. Lombard J, Levin IH, Weiner WJ. Arsenic intoxication in a cocaine abuser. N Engl J Med 1989;320:869.
223. Mahler JC, Perry S, Sutton B. Intraurethral cocaine administration JAMA 1988;259:3126.
224. Del Aguila C, Rosman H. Myocardial infarction during cocaine withdrawal. Ann Intern Med 1990;112:712.
225. Levine MAH, Nishikawa J. Acute myocardial infarction associated with cocaine withdrawal. Can Med Assoc J 1991; 144:1139–1140.
226. Nademanee K, Gorelick DA, Josephson MA, et al. Myocardial ischemia during cocaine withdrawal. Ann Intern Med 1989;111:876–880.
227. Choy-Kwong M, Lipton RB. Dystonia related to cocaine withdrawal: A case report and pathogenic hypothesis. Neurology 1989;39:996–997.
228. Miller NS, Summers GL, Gold MS. Cocaine dependence: Alcohol and other drug dependence and withdrawal characteristics. J Addict Dis 1993;12:25–35.
229. Stine SM, Burns B, Kosten T. Methadone dose for cocaine abuse. Am J Psychiatry 1991;148:1268.
230. Wallace JE, Hamilton HE, Christenson JG, et al. An evaluation of selected methods for determining cocaine and benzoylecgonine in urine. J Anal Toxicol 1977;1:20–25.
231. Budd RD, Mathis DF, Yang FC. TLC analysis of urine for benzoylecgonine and norpropoxyphene. Clin Toxicol 1980;16: 1–5.
232. Rafla FK, Epstein RL. Identification of cocaine and its metabolites in human urine in the presence of ethyl alcohol. J Anal Toxicol 1979;3:59–63.
233. Kogan MJ, Verebey KG, De Pace AC, et al. Quantitative determination of benzoylecgonine and cocaine in human biofluids by gas–liquid chromatography. Anal Chem 1977;49: 1965–1969.
234. Wallace JE, Hamilton HE, King DE, et al. Gas–liquid chromatographic determination of cocaine and benzoylecgonine in urine. Anal Chem 1976;48:34–48.
235. Masoud AN, Knipski DM. High performance liquid chromatographic analysis of cocaine in human plasma. J Anal Toxicol 1980;4:305–310.
236. Jatlow P. Cocaine: Analysis, pharmacokinetics and metabolic disposition. Yale J Biol Med 1988;61:105–113.
237. Schramm W, Craig PA, Smith RH, Berger GE. Cocaine and benzoylecgonine in saliva, serum and urine. Clin Chem 1993; 39:481–487.
238. Harkey MR, Henderson GL, Zhou C. Simultaneous quantitation of cocaine and its major metabolites in human hair by gas chromatography/chemical ionization mass spectrometry. J Anal Toxicol 1991;15:260–265.
239. Cone EJ, Youselnejad D, Darwin WD, Maguire T. Testing human hair for drugs of abuse: II. Identification of unique cocaine metabolites in hair of drug abusers and evaluation of decontamination procedures. J Anal Toxicol 1991;15: 250–255.
240. Reuschel SA, Smith FP. Benzoylecgonine (cocaine metabolite) detection in hair sample of jail detainees using radioimmunoassay (RIA) and gas chromatography/mass spectrometry (GC/MS). J Forens Sci 1991;36:1179–1185.
241. Martz R, Donnelly B, Fetterolf D, et al. The use of hair analysis to document a cocaine overdose following sustained survival period before death. J Anal Toxicol 1991;15:279–281.
242. Koren GB, Klein J, Forman R, Graham K. Hair analysis of cocaine: Differentiation between systemic exposure and external contamination. J Clin Pharmacol 1992;32:671–675.
243. Graham K, Koren G, Klein J, et al. Determination of gestational cocaine exposure by hair analysis. JAMA 1989; 262:3328–3330.
244. Trinler WA, Reuland DJ. Unequivocal determination of cocaine in simulated street drugs by a combination of high performance liquid chromatography and infrared spectrophotometry. J Forens Sci 1978;23:37–43.
245. Rosenberg NM, Meert KL, Knazik S, et al. Occult cocaine exposure. Pediatr Emerg Care 1991;7:393.
246. Isner JM, Estes NAM, Thompson PD, et al. Acute cardiac event temporally related to cocaine abuse. N Engl J Med 1986;315:1438–1443.
247. Malbrain MLMG, De Medts P, Wanters A, et al. Drug smuggler's delirium. Br Med J 1993;306:102.
248. Madder JA, Powers RH. Effect of cocaine and cocaine metabolites on cerebral arteries in vitro. Life Sci 1990;44: 1109–1114.
249. Jain L, Meyer W, Moore C, et al. Detection of fetal cocaine exposure by analysis of amniotic fluid. Obstet Gynecol 1993; 81(p 1):787–790.
250. Szeti HH. Kinetics of drug transfer to the fetus. Clin Obstet Gynecol 1993;36:246–254.
251. Kossowsky WA, Lyon AF, Chou S-Y. Acute non-Q wave cocaine-related myocardial infarction. Chest 1989;96:617–621.
252. Chakko S, Sepulveda S, Kessler KM, et al. Frequency and type of electrocardiographic abnormalities in cocaine abusers (electrocardiogram in cocaine abuse). Am J Cardiol 1994;74:710-713.
253. Watson WA, Stevens DK, Campbell JP, Carter JE. Acid–base effects associated with cocaine use in emergency department (ED) patients. Personal communication at Scientific Meeting of European Association of Poison Centers and Clinical Toxicologists, Birmingham, UK, May 26–28, 1993.
254. Stevens DC, Campbell JP, Carter JE, Watson WA. Acid–base abnormalities associated with cocaine toxicity in emergency department patients. Clin Toxicol 1994;32:31–39.
255. Foltin RW, Fischman MW. Smoked and intravenous cocaine in humans: Acute tolerance, cardiovascular and subjective effects. J Pharmacol Exp Ther 1991;257:247–261.
256. Hamilton HE, Wallace JE, Shimak EL, et al. Cocaine and benzoylecgonine excretion in humans. J Forens Sci 1977;22: 697–707.
257. Osterloh J. Testing for drugs of abuse: Pharmacokinetic considerations for cocaine in urine. Clin Pharmacokinet 1993; 24:355–361.
258. Baselt RC, Chang JY, Yoshikawa DM. On the dermal absorption of cocaine. J Anal Toxicol 1990;14:383–384.
259. Doberczak TM, Shanzer S, Senie RT, Kandall SR. Neonatal neurologic and electroencephalographic effects of intrauterine cocaine exposure. J Pediatr 1988;113:354–358.
260. Dixon SD, Bejar R. Echoencephalographic findings in neonates associated with maternal cocaine and amphetamine use: Incidence and clinical correlates. J Pediatr 1989; 115:770–778.
261. Rais-Bahrami K, Nagvi M. Hydroencephaly and maternal cocaine use: A case report. Clin Pediatr 1990;29:729–730.
262. McCarron MM, Wood JD. The cocaine 'body-packer' syndrome. JAMA 1983;250:1417–1420.
263. Gherardi R, Marc B, Alberti X, et al. A cocaine body packer with normal abdominal plain radiograms: Value of drug detection in urine and contrast study of the bowel. Am J Forens Med Pathol 1990;11:154–157.
264. Marc B, Baud FJ, Aelion MJ, et al. The cocaine body-packer syndrome: Evaluation of a method of contrast study of the bowel. J Forens Sci 1990;35:345–355.
265. Gay GR, Loper KA. The use of labetalol in the management of cocaine crisis. Ann Emerg Med 1988;17:282–283.
266. Polan S, Tadjziechy M. Esmolol in the management of epinephrine- and cocaine-induced cardiovascular toxicity. Anesth Analg 1989;69:663–664.
267. Sand IC, Brody SL, Wrenn KD, Slovis CM. Experience with esmolol for the treatment of cocaine-associated cardiovascular complications. Am J Emerg Med 1991;9:161–163.
268. Abol FI. The effects of nifedipine in cocaine toxicity. Am J Med Sci 1992;303:372–378.
269. Ramoska E, Sacchetti AD. Propranolol-induced hypertension in treatment of cocaine intoxication. Ann Emerg Med 1985; 14:112–113.
270. Patel R, Harder B, Ahmed S, Regan TJ. Cocaine related myocardial infarction: High prevalence of occlusive coronary

thrombi without significant obstructive atherosclerosis. Circulation 1988;78(suppl. II):II-430.
271. Kossowsky WA, Lyon AF. Cocaine and acute myocardial infarction: A probable connection. Chest 1984;86:729–731.
272. Smith HWB III, Liberman HA, Brody SL, et al. Acute myocardial infarction temporally related to cocaine use: Clinical, angiographic and pathophysiologic observations. Ann Intern Med 1987;107:13–18.
273. Hadjimitiades S, Covalesky V, Manno BV, et al. Coronary arteriographic findings in cocaine abuse-induced myocardial infarction. Cathet Cardiovasc Diagn 1988;14:33–36.
274. Hadjimellicides S, Covalesky V, Manno BV. Coronary arteriographic findings in cocaine abuse induced myocardial infarction. Cathet Cardiovasc Diagn 1988;14:33–36.
275. Anderson HV, Willerson JT. Thrombolysis in myocardial infarction. N Engl J Med 1993;329:703–709.
276. Wasserberger J. The ten commandments of treating cocaine chest pain. King/Drew Medical Center, 1995.
277. Om A, Ellahhan S, Di Sciascio G. Management of cocaine-induced cardiovascular complications. Am Heart J 1993;125: 469–475.
278. Boehrer JD, Moliterno DJ, Willard JE, et al. Influence of labetalol on cocaine-induced coronary vasoconstriction in humans. Am J Med 1993;94:608–618.
279. Hoffman B, Derlet R. Cocaine intoxication considerations, complications and strategies: Point and counterpoint. Emerg Med 1992;1:1–6.
280. Bechman KJ, Parker RB, Hariman RJ, et al. Hemodynamic and electrophysiological actions of cocaine: Effects of sodium bicarbonate as an antidote in dogs. Circulation 1991; 83:1799–1807.
281. Kaukonen L, Hoffman RS. Cocaine. NY State J Med 1990; 90:39.
282. Derlet RW, Albertson TE, Tharratt RS. Lidocaine potentiation of cocaine toxicity. Ann Emerg Med 1991;20:135–138.
283. Hale SL, Alker KJ, Rezkalla SH, et al. Nifedipine protects the heart from the acute deleterious effects of cocaine if administered before but not after cocaine. Circulation 1991;83: 1437–1443.
284. Lucatello A, Sturani A, Cocchi R, Fusaroli M. Dopamine plus furosemide in cocaine-associated acute myoglobinuric renal failure. Nephron 1991;60:242–243.
285. Zimmerman JL, Dellinger RP, Majid PA. Cocaine-associated chest pain. Ann Emerg Med 1991;20:611–615.
286. Hollander JE, Hoffman RD. Letter to editor. Acad Emerg Med 1995;2:232.
287. Hollander JE, Hoffman RS, Gennis P, et al. Cocaine associated chest pain: One year follow-up. Acad Emerg Med 1995; 2:179–184.
288. Hollander JE, Thone HC Jr, Hoffman RS. Chest discomfort, cocaine and tobacco. Acad Emerg Med 1995;2:238.
289. Hollander JE, Hoffman RS, Shiti DR. Cocaine-associated MI (CAMI) study group. Acad Emerg Med 1995;2:456.
290. Pitts S. ST-segment elevation as a discrimination in cocaine-associated chest pain. Acad Emerg Med 1995;2:331–332.
291. Michels R, Narzuk PM. Progress in psychiatry. N Engl J Med 1993;329:634.
292. Hoffman RS, Smilkstein MJ, Goldfrank LR. Whole bowel irrigation and the cocaine body-packer: A new approach to a common problem. Am J Emerg Med 1990;8:523–527.
293. Aks S, Vanden Hoek T, Tebbett I, et al. Cocaine liberation from body packets in an in vitro model. Vet Hum Toxicol 1991;33:354.
294. Dretcher K. Butyrylcholinesterase in cocaine overdose. In: *Proceedings, FASEB Meeting, Anaheim, California, April 5–9, 1992.*
295. Bouskey HA, Warnock DG, Smith LH. Neurologic aspects of cocaine abuse. West J Med 1988;149:442–448.
296. Dhuna A, Pascual-Leone A. Cocaine-associated status epilepticus. J Epilepsy 1990;3:165–169.
297. Garvin FH, Ellinwood EH Jr. Cocaine and other stimulants. Actions, abuse and treatment. N Engl J Med 1988;318:1173–1182.
298. Weiss RD. Relapse to cocaine abuse after initiating desipramine treatment. JAMA 1988;260:2545–2546.
299. Halikas JA, Crosby RD, Carlson GA, et al. Cocaine reduction in unmotivated crack users using carbamazepine versus placebo in a short-term, double-blind crossover design. Clin Pharmacol Ther 1991;50:81–95.
300. Halikas JA, Kuhn KL, Maddux TL. Reduction of cocaine use among methadone maintenance patients using concurrent carbamazepine maintenance. Ann Clin Psychiatry 1990; 2:3–6.
301. Hatsukami D, Keenan R, Halikas J, et al. Effects of carbamazepine on acute responses to smoked cocaine-base in human cocaine users. Psychopharmacology 1991;104:120–124.
302. Crosby RD, Pearson MT, Eller C. A double-blind study of phenytoin in the treatment of cocaine abuse. Clin Pharmacol Ther 1995;57:160 (Abstract PI-102).
303. Friedman SR, Stark C, Sulfian M, DesJarlais DC. Will bleach decontaminate needles during cocaine binges in shooting galleries? JAMA 1989;262:1467.
304. DesJarlais DC. Intravenous cocaine, crack and HIV infection. JAMA 1988;259:1945–1956.

Chapter 22

Hallucinogenic Drugs

INTRODUCTION

Chemical classes of hallucinogens are listed in Table 22–1. Therapeutic drugs associated with hallucinations are listed in Table 22–2.[1] Toxicokinetic properties of many hallucinogenic drugs of abuse are summarized in Table 22–3.[1]

Hallucinogens exhibit agonist or partial agonist effects at the 5-HT_2, 5-HT_{1A}, and 5-HT_{1C} receptors (5-HT = serotonin).[2,3] Levels of growth hormone, prolactin, β-endorphin, corticotropin, and cortisol are increased with hallucinogen use presumably related to the serotonergic properties of the drugs.

Leikin and colleagues have studied the clinical features and management of intoxication due to hallucinogenic drugs.[1] Each hallucinogen produces behavioral effects related to its serotonergic, dopaminergic, or adrenergic activity. A flashback is a recurrence of imagery associated with hallucinogen use that occurs after the acute effects of the drug have worn off. They have been described with L-lysergic acid diethylamide (LSD), mescaline, phencyclidine, and marijuana use and may occur months to years after cessation of use.

LYSERGIC ACID DIETHYLAMIDE (LSD)

From 1988 to 1990, while cocaine, marijuana, and alcohol were losing some of their popularity among high school seniors, there was a concomitant rise in the number of people admitted to hospital emergency rooms because of bad experiences with LSD[4] (Table 22–4). In 1993, after some decline in use, LSD (Fig. 22–1) was again sold in large quantities (5–10 million doses per month) by LSD distributors. Some pills contain less than 3 μg of LSD.[5]

Toxic Dose

An 8-month-old ingested 5 blotters of LSD and developed a tachycardia. The neurologic examination was normal. He was discharged in 24 hours after intravenous fluids were administered and a nasogastric tube was inserted to obtain a gastric aspirate, which, together with the urine, was positive for LSD.[6]

Table 22–1
Chemical Classification of Hallucinogens

Common Name	Chemical Name
Indole Alkaloid Derivatives	
Psilocin	Dimethyl-4-hydroxytryptamine
Psilocybin	Dimethyl-4-phosphoryitryptamine
Harmine	7-Methoxy-1-methyl-9*H*-pyridol-[3,4b]-indole
Ibogaine	
LSD	D-Lysergic acid diethylamide
	Lysergic acid amide
	Isolysergic acid amide
DMT	Dimethyltryptamine
DPT	Dipropyltryptamine
AMT	α-Methyltryptamine
DET	Diethyltryptamine
	6-Hydroxymethyltryptamine
Bufotenine	Dimethyl-5-hydroxytryptamine
Piperidine Derivatives	
Atropine	*N*-Ethyl-2-pyrrolidylmethylphenylcyclopentylglycolate
Hyoscine (scopolamine)	
Hyoscyamine	
Cocaine	
Ditran	
Phencyclidine (PCP)	1-(1-Phencyclohexyl) piperidine
Ketamine	2-(*O*-Chlorophenyl-2-methylamino)-cyclohexanone
Phenylethylamine Derivatives	
Mescaline	3,4,5-Trimethoxyphenylethylamine
STP/DOM	2,5-Dimethoxy-4-methylamphetamine
DOE	2,5-Dimethoxy-4-ethylamphetamine
DOB	2,5-Dimethoxy-4-bromoamphetamine
MDA	Methylenedioxyamphetamine
DOET	Dimethoxyethylamphetamine
MMDA	3-Methoxy-4,5-methylenedioxyamphetamine
PMA	*p*-Methoxyamphetamine
TMA	3,4,5-Trimethoxyamphetamine
Cannaboids	
Marijuana	Δ^9-Tetrahydrocannabinol

From Leikin JB, Krantz AJ, Zell-Kanter M, et al. Clinical features and management of intoxication due to hallucinogenic drugs. Med Toxicol Adverse Drug Exp 1989;4:324–350.

Toxicokinetics

Patients taking fluoxetine and lithium in therapeutic doses may develop seizures after adding LSD for recreational use.[7] Patients with a history of LSD use may experience flashbacks or hallucinatory episodes if they use selective serotonin reuptake inhibitor drugs (eg, sertraline, paroxetine).[8]

Mechanism of Action

L-Lysergic acid diethylamide is a potent agonist at 5-HT_{1A} receptors, but mescaline and other phenylethylamines have little affinity for 5-HT_{1A} receptors. Indoleamine (eg, LSD, *N,N*-dimethyltryptamine [DMT]) and phenethylamine hallucinogens (eg, mescaline, 2,5-dimethoxy-4-methylamphetamine [DOM]) (Fig. 22–1) have an affinity for postsynaptic 5-HT_2 receptors in the locus ceruleus and the cerebral cortex. Most 5-HT_2 receptors in the brain are located in the cerebral cortex, where hallucinogens exert an effect on perceptual and cognitive functions.

Table 22–2
Therapeutic Drugs Associated With Hallucinations

Drug	Type of Hallucination
Acyclovir	V,T
Amantadine	A,V
Baclofen	A,V
Benztropine	V
Biperiden	V
Bromocriptine	A,V
Carbamazepine	V
Chlordiazepoxide	V
Chlorpheniramine	A,V
Chlorpromazine	A,V
Cimetidine	A,V
Clonazepam	A,V,T
Clonidine	A,V
Cyclosporine	V
Dantrolene	A,V
Dextromethorphan	A,V
Diethylpropion	A
Digoxin	A,V
Dimenhydrinate	A,V
Diphenhydramine	V
Disopyramide	A,V
Ephedrine	A,V
Gentamicin	NS
Griseofulvin	A
Imipramine	V
Indomethacin	V,O
Isosorbide	V
Levodopa	A,V
Lorazepam	V
Orciprenaline (metaproterenol)	V,G
Methyldopa	V
Methylphenidate	V
Methylprednisolone	V
Minocycline	V
Pemoline	A,V,T
Phenylzine	A,V
Phenylephrine	A,V
Pindolol	A
Procainamide	V
Propranolol	V
Quinidine	NS
Ranitidine	A,V
Scopolamine	NS
Streptokinase	N,S
Sulfasalazine	V
Timolol	NS
Triazolam	A,V,T
Trihexyphenidyl	A,V
Vidarabine	NS

A, auditory; V, visual; T, tactile; G, gustatory; O, olfactory; NS, not specified. From Leikin JB, Krantz AJ, Zell-Kanter M, et al. Clinical features and management of intoxication due to hallucinogenic drugs. Med Toxicol Adverse Drug Experience 1989;4:324–350.

The 5-HT_2 antagonists offer promise as a potential treatment for the acute adverse reactions ("bad trips") experienced by some individuals who use LSD and other psychodelic hallucinogens. There are no Food and Drug Administration-approved selective 5-HT_2 antagonists. Cyproheptadine, clozapine, and risperidone may ultimately become useful in blocking the electrophysiologic and behavioral effects of hallucinogenic drugs.[9]

Table 22–3
Principal Pharmacologic Properties of Hallucinogenic Drugs

Drug, Chemical Structure	Duration of Acute Effect (h)	pK_a	Route of Metabolism/ Excretion	Half-life	Protein Binding (%)	V_d *(L/kg)*	Urine Screen Positive for	Duration of Psychotropic Effects	Dose of Abuse	Fatal Dose
Phencyclidine (PCP), arylcyclohexylamine	4–6	8.5	Hepatic/urine	1 h	65	6.2–0.3	2 wk	≤ 1 mo	1–9 mg	1 mg/kg
Cocaine, tropane alkaloid	0.5	5.6	Plasma hydrolysis*	48–75 min	8.7	1.2–1.9	144 h	≤ 5–7 d	20–200 mg (intranasally)	1–12 g
Cannabis, monoterpenoid	0.5–3	10.6	Hepatic hydroxylation	25–57 h	97–99	10	≤ 6 d	≤ 6 h	5–15 mg THC	
Lysergic acid diethylamide (LSD), indole alkylamine	0.7–8	7.8	Hepatic hydroxylation	2.5 h		0.27	120 h	May last days	100–300 μg	0.2 mg/kg
Psilocybin, tryptamine	0.5–6						Not detected	12 h	20–100 mushrooms	5–15 mg
Mescaline, phenylalkylamine	4.6	Not known	Hepatic/urine†	6 h	None	Not known		12 h	5 mg/kg	20 mg/kg
Morphine, alkaloid/ derivative of opium	4–5	8.05	Glucuronidation/ urine	1.9–3.1 h	35	3.2	48 h	≤ 6 h	2–20 mg	Variable, dependent on tolerance; nontolerant fatal dose is 120 mg orally or 30 mg parenterally
Heroin, diacetylmorphine	3.4	7.6	Hepatic‡	3 min	40	25	40 h	≤ 6 h	2.2 mg	Variable, dependent on tolerance
Amphetamine, β-(phenylisopropyl)-amine	Variable	9.93	Hepatic§	12 h‖	16–20	3–6	2–4 d	Delusions may remain for months	100–1000 mg daily	Variable, dependent of tolerance

*V_d, volume of distribution; THC, Δ^9-tetrahydrocannibinol.
*By serum cholinesterase.
†60% excreted unchanged.
‡Converted to morphine.
§Converted to phenylacetone.
‖Urine pH-dependent.
From Leikin JB, Krantz AJ, Zell-Kanter M, et al. Clinical features and management of intoxication due to hallucinogenic drugs. Med Toxicol Adverse Drug Experience 1989;4:324–350.

Table 22-4
Hallucinogen History

1943	Hoffman accidentally discovers hallucinogenic properties of LSD
1961	LSD observed to interact with brain serotonin
1966	Hallucinogens banned in United States
1970	Psychodelic drugs placed in Schedule I
1970s, 1980s	Young people using lower doses; more ritualized use
1988–1990	Rise in emergency department admissions for bad experience with LSD
1993	LSD sold in large quantities

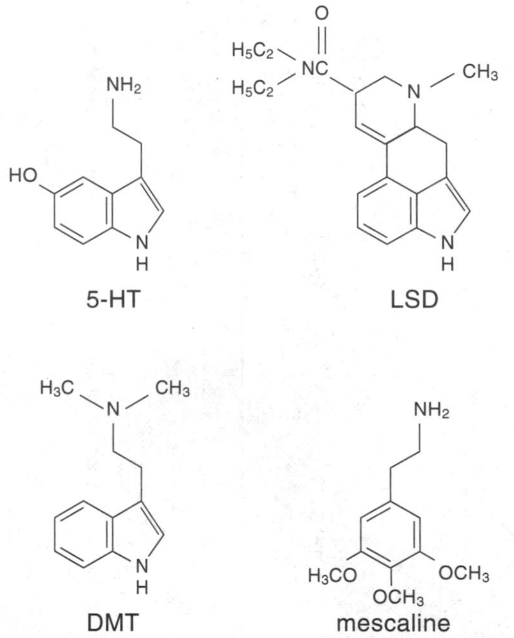

Figure 22-1 Structural formulas for serotonin (5-HT), lysergic acid diethylamide (LSD), mescaline, and the simple indoleamine hallucinogen *N,N*-dimethyltryptamine (DMT). The chemical structures are drawn to emphasize common structural features such as the indolethylamine nucleus of 5-HT, LSD, and DMT and the phenethylamine nucleus shared by LSD and mescaline. From Aghajanian GK. Serotonin and the action of LSD in the brain. Psychiatr Ann 1994;24:137–141.

Clinical Presentation

Chronic Reactions

Smith and Seymour describe four chronic reactions to LSD that were reported in the 1960s: (1) prolonged psychotic reactions, (2) depression sufficiently severe so as to be life-threatening, (3) flashbacks, and (4) exacerbations of preexisting psychiatric illness.[10] Since then, a fifth chronic reaction has been listed in the *Diagnostic and Statistical Manual; Third Edition, Revised* (DSM-III-R): posthallucinogen perceptual disorder.

Prolonged psychotic reactions have similarities to schizophrenic reactions and appear to occur most often in people with preexisting psychological difficulties, primarily prepsychotic or psychotic personalities. Psychedelic drug-induced personality disorganizations can be quite severe and prolonged. Appropriate treatment often requires antipsychotic medication and residental care in a mental health facility followed by outpatient counseling.

Posthallucinogen Perception Disorder

Individuals with posthallucinogen perception disorder (PHPD) experience a persistent perceptual disorder that they describe as like living in a bubble under water. They also describe trails of light and images following movement of their hands, and often describe living in a "purple haze." This perceptual disorder is aggravated by use of any psychoactive drug, including alcohol and marijuana, and is distinguished from flashbacks, which are episodic rather than chronic phenomena. With PHPD, the individual often suffers anxiety, even panic, and becomes phobic and depressed. Individuals with PHPD do not have a disturbed psychiatric history prior to the onset of psychedelic drug use. PHPD can occur even after a single dose.

Tolerance

Tolerance develops rapidly among patients given LSD. An initial dose of 50 μg, with weekly or twice weekly administration, often leads within a few weeks to an eventual dose of 400 or even 800 μg.[11]

Hyperthermia

Neuroleptic malignant syndrome may be observed following LSD use. Muscle biopsy may show a myoedema, focal necrosis, and glycogen and lipid depletion. Dantrolene may reduce the high temperature and rigidity and can lead to an improved level of consciousness.[12]

Laboratory

Gas chromatography–mass spectrometry (GC–MS) is useful in confirming positive LSD urine levels to a lower limit of 5 pg/mL urine.[13] An instrumental high-performance thin-layer chromatographic (HPTLC) technique for determination of LSD can detect less than 1 μg/L urine. Immunocross-reactive metabolites provide a positive response in a radioimmunoassay, but the HPTLC remains negative.[14] LSD can be detected in the urine by radioimmunoassay after 3 days at the 0.1 ng/mL cutoff level.[15]

McCarron and colleagues analyzed the serum and urine specimens of patients with suspected LSD intoxication by both radioimmunoassay (limit of detection, 0.1 ng/mL) and high-pressure liquid chromatography (limit of detection, 0.5 ng/mL). Radioimmunoassay tends to give higher readings than high-pressure liquid chromatography because the radioimmunoassay cross-reacts with LSD metabolites. The average quantitative LSD serum value by high-pressure liquid chromatography was 1.2 ng/mL; urine values averaged 2.9 ng/mL. LSD concentrations in isolated serum or urine specimens are of limited value except to confirm the presence of LSD. Specimens for LSD radioimmunoassay may be collected and stored frozen for batch analysis at a convenient time.[16]

Treatment

Stabilization

1. Monitor vital signs. Ensure airway and circulatory status.

2. Avoid restraints.
3. Sedate the patient with quiet reassurance and diazepam.
4. Avoid phenothiazines (they diminish threshold for seizures).
5. Avoid gastric lavage; it is ineffective and may exacerbate the psychotic reaction.

No reliable data are available on hemoperfusion or hemodialysis.

Acute Panic Attack. Supportive care, reassurance, and the reduction of sensory stimuli are the most important aspects of management. The patient should be placed in a safe, quiet environment, preferably with a familiar person who can provide constant reassurance (ie, "talk the patient down"). Restraints should be avoided if possible but may become necessary to avoid destructive behavior. Diazepam (5–10 mg intravenously in an adult) is the drug of choice for sedation. Haloperidol may be administered as a second-line drug if the above measures fail to calm the patient and continued agitation represents an increased medical risk.

All patients who require the continued use of restraints should have the first-voided urine specimen sent for myoglobin and urinalysis. A positive dipstick test for hematuria in the absence of microscopic evidence of red blood cells suggests myoglobinuria.

Acute Psychotic Reactions. Neuroleptic drugs should be administered cautiously in this setting. Phenothiazine use has been associated with hypotension, sedation, potentiation of anticholinergic effects, decreased seizure threshold, and extrapyramidal reactions. Frequently, the actual psychedelic drug involved is not known, and phenothiazines can potentiate drugs with anticholinergic effects. The use of chlorpromazine in 2,5-dimethoxy-4-methylamphetamine (STP) ingestions reportedly caused several cases of cardiovascular collapse.[17] Most visual hallucinations are actually illusions rather than true hallucinations, and the patients understand that what they are seeing is drug induced. When antipsychotic drugs are necessary, haloperidol probably is the safest neuroleptic agent.

Flashbacks. Psychotherapy, antianxiety agents, and neuroleptic drugs are used.

Gut Decontamination

The usual methods of decontamination almost always are unnecessary, as LSD is rapidly absorbed, and their use intensifies behavior abnormalities.

Elimination Enhancement

Because of the short half-life and few serious medical reactions, hemoperfusion, hemodialysis, and peritoneal dialysis have not been used for LSD intoxication.

Antidote

There are no specific antidotes for LSD intoxication. Phenothiazines are not antidotes and may cause serious adverse effects such as diminishing the threshold for seizure.

REFERENCES—HALLUCINOGENIC DRUGS

1. Leikin J, Krantz AJ, Zell-Kanter M, et al. Clinical features and management of intoxication due to hallucinogenic drugs. Med Toxicol Adverse Drug Experience 1989;40:324–352.
2. Strassman RJ, Qualls CR. Dose–response study of *N,N*-dimethyltryptamine in humans: I. Neuroendocrine, autonomic and cardiovascular effects. Arch Gen Psychiatry 1994;56: 85–97.
3. Strassman RJ, Qualls CR. Dose–response study of *N,N*-dimethyltryptamine in humans: II. Subjective effects and preliminary results of a new rating scale. Arch Gen Psychiatry 1994;56:98–108.
4. Treaster JB. Use of LSD, drug of allure and risk, rises with new generation's interest. NY Times, December 27, 1991, p. A11.
5. Drug dealings: LSD is back. Forens Drug Abuse Advisor 1993;5(8):63.
6. Maslanta AM, Scott SK. LSD overdose in an eight-month-old boy. J Emerg Med 1992;10:481–483.
7. Jackson TW, Hornfeldt CS. Seizure activity following recreational LSD use in patients treated with lithium and fluoxetine. Vet Hum Toxicol 1991;33:387.
8. Markel H, Lee A, Holms RD, Domino EF. LSD flashback syndrome exacerbated by selective serotonin reuptake inhibitor antidepressants in adolescents. J Pediatr 1994;125:817–819.
9. Aghajanian GK. Serotonin and the action of LSD in the brain. Psychiatr Ann 1994;24:137–141.
10. Smith DE, Seymour RD. LSD: History and toxicity: Today, there is group concern over long-term post hallucinogenic disorder. Psychiatr Ann 1994;24:145–147.
11. Madden JS. LSD and post-hallucinogen perceptual disorder. Addiction 1994;89:762–763.
12. Behan WMH, Bakheit AMO, Behan PO, More IAR. The muscle findings in the neuroleptic malignant syndrome associated with lysergic acid diethylamide. J Neurol Neurosurg Psychiatry 1991;54:741–743.
13. Sun JV, Bonelli EJ. Lysergic acid diethylamide (LSD): Specificity: Sensitivity and linearity of HP5971A MSD. In: *Proceedings, American Academy of Forensic Sciences, 1989:* Abstract K4.
14. Blum LM, Carenzo EF, Rieders F. Determination of lysergic acid diethylamide (LSD) in urine by instrumental high-performance thin-layer chromatography. J Anal Toxicol 1990; 14:285–287.
15. Vu-Duc T, Vermay A, Calamca A. Detection de l'acide lysergique diethylamide (LSD) dans l'urine humaine: Elimination, depistage et confirmation analytique. Schweiz-Med Wochenschr 1991;121:1887–1890.
16. McCarron MM, Walberg CB, Baselt RC. Confirmation of LSD intoxication by analysis of serum and urine. J Anal Toxicol 1990;14:165–167.
17. Solursh LP, Clement WR. Hallucinogenic drug abuse: Manifestations and management. Can Med Assoc J 1968;98:407–413.

N,N-DIMETHYLTRYPTAMINE (DMT)

N,N-Dimethyltryptamine (Fig. 22–1) is an endogenous mammalian hallucinogen and drug of abuse. Intravenous dimethyltryptamine fumarate is a hallucinogen at doses of 0.2 and 0.4 mg/kg. Effects are felt almost instantaneously, peak within 2 minutes, and resolve within 20 to 30 minutes and include visual hallucinatory phenomena, bodily dissociation, extreme shifts in mood, and auditory effects in about 50% of subjects. Plasma levels of DMT are correlated with the psychological effects. A 0.4 mg/kg injection leads to peak plasma levels of 32 to 300 ng/mL. A dose of 0.2 mg/kg is a threshold dose for hallucinogenic effects. DMT, like other classic hallucinogens, induces pupillary dilation, which may be 5-HT_2 mediated. Diastolic blood pressure may rise transiently.[1,2]

Structure and Classification

N,N-Dimethyltryptamine is 3-[2-(dimethylamino) ethyl]indole, empirical formula $C_{12}H_{16}N_2$. Its molecular weight is 188.3, and CAS number, 61-50-7.

Source

N,N-Dimethyltryptamine is obtained from the seeds and leaves of *Piptadenia pergyina* (Mimosaceae) and other South American plants. It may be present in the tropical legume *Mucuna pruriens.*

Toxicokinetics

Dimethyltryptamine fumarate 0.2 to 0.4 mg/kg elicits nearly instantaneous onset of visual hallucinatory phenomena, bodily dissociation and extreme shifts in mood, a "rush". Auditory effects are often noted. Effects peak within 2 minutes after injection and resolve quickly within 20 to 30 minutes. Lower doses, 0.05 and 0.1 mg/kg, are not hallucinogenic. Emotional and somesthetic effects predominate. At doses of 0.4 mg/kg, visual imagery predominates. Auditory effects are observed in about half of individuals using DMT. There is an almost complete loss of control. The threshold dose for hallucinogenic effects is 0.2 mg/kg. Visual hallucinations occur; auditory ones are less common. At 0.05 mg/kg, no auditory or visual effects are experienced.

Mechanism of Action

Hallucinogens are agonists or partial agonists at serotonin (5-HT) receptors, specifically at 5-HT_2, 5-HT_{1A}, and 5-HT_{1C} subtypes.[1,2] The hyperthermic effects of DMT are probably mediated by the 5-HT_2 subtype; 5HT_{1C} agonists are hypothermic in humans.[3]

Clinical Presentation

Pupils typically are dilated. Temperature may increase and heart rate and mean arterial blood pressure are elevated.

Laboratory

Analytical Methods

Blood levels of DMT (free base) are assayed by a gas chromatography–mass spectrometry technique whose limit of detectability is 1 ng/mL.[4]

Blood Levels

The time course of blood DMT levels matches the development of subjective effects,[1,2] peaking at 2 minutes after completion of an injection. Peak values range from 32 to 200 ng/mL after a 0.4 mg/kg injection.

Ancillary Tests

Levels of pro-opiomelanocortin peptides (corticotropin and β-endorphin) parallel subjective effects and blood DMT concentrations, lagging 5 to 10 minutes behind these changes. Prolactin levels rise in a dose-dependent manner.

Treatment

1. Place the patient in a quiet dark room. Talk the patient down.
2. Treat symptomatically.
3. Monitor cardiac status.
4. Avoid phenothiazines to diminish potential for seizures.

REFERENCES—*N,N*-DIMETHYLTRYPTAMINE (DMT)

1. Strassman RJ, Qualls CR. Dose–response study of *N,N*-dimethyltryptamine in humans: I. Neuroendocrine, autonomic and cardiovascular effects. Arch Gen Psychiatry 1994;56: 85–97.
2. Strassman RJ, Qualls CR. Dose–response study of *N,N*-dimethyltryptamine in humans: II. Subjective effects and preliminary results of a new rating scale. Arch Gen Psychiatry 1994;56:98–108.
3. Anderson I, Cowan P, Grahame-Smith D. The effects of gepirone on neuroendocrine function and temperature in humans. Psychopharmacology 1990;100:498–503.
4. Walker R, Mandell L, Kleinman J, et al. Improved selective ion monitoring mass-spectrometric assay for the determination of *N,N*-dimethyltryptamine in human blood utilizing capillary column gas chromatography. J Chromatogr 1979;162:539–546.

COLORADO RIVER TOAD

The dried venom of *Bufo alvarius* contains 5-methoxy-*N,N*-dimethyltryptamine (Meo-DMT), a hallucinogen related to *N,N-* dimethyltryptamine.[1] "Smoking toad" induces hallucinations lasting about 5 minutes. A clinical picture of profound drooling, seizure activity, arrhythmias, and cyanosis follows the oral application of a toad (toad kissing).[2]

REFERENCES—COLORADO RIVER TOAD

1. Gallagher L. Smoking toad. NY Times Mag, June 5, 1994, pp. 48–49.
2. Hitt M, Ettinger DD. Toad toxicity. N Engl J Med 1986;314:1517–1518.

PEYOTE

In the United States, the hallucinogenic peyote cactus grows almost exclusively in "peyote gardens," a narrow strip of the South Texas chaparral country east of Laredo. In its natural form the cactus, whose scientific name is *Lophophora williamsii,* is a squat ground-hugging plant about an inch tall and 2 to 3 in. across, with a tapering, turnip-shaped root.

Dealers known as *peyoteros* clip off the above-ground portion of the plant and dry it. The dried plant, or button, is generally chewed, although it is sometimes used to brew a hallucinogenic tea.

Chapter 23

Marijuana and Other Cannabinoids

MARIJUANA

Marijuana is the most commonly used illicit drug in the United States. Of the 19.5 million people in 1991 who used marijuana (at least once) 5.3 million used the drug once a week or more and 3.1 million used it daily or almost daily.[1]

Like tobacco, marijuana consists of dried, chopped plant parts. Its source is *Cannabis sativa,* the hemp plant. The principal psychoactive agent in marijuana is Δ^9-tetrahydrocannabinol (THC), which sometimes constitutes more than 7% of marijuana material (Fig. 23–1).

Product Formulations

Cannabis

Collective term for psychoactive compounds derived from *C. sativa.*

Marijuana

Also spelled *marihuana,* marijuana refers to any part of the plant or its extract that is used to induce psychotomimetic or therapeutic effects. Synonyms include pot, Mary Jane, MJ, weed, grass, puff, hagga, and macohna.

Hashish

This natural product is the dried resin collected from flower tops and contains varying concentrations of THC up to 10%. This form is commonly used in the Middle East and North Africa. Hashish oil is a dark viscous alcohol or gasoline extract that can contain up to 20% THC.

Bhang

Bhang consists of dried mature leaves and flower stems that are less potent than hashish.

Ganja

Ganja is the resinous mass composed of small leaves and bracts of inflorescence from female plants.

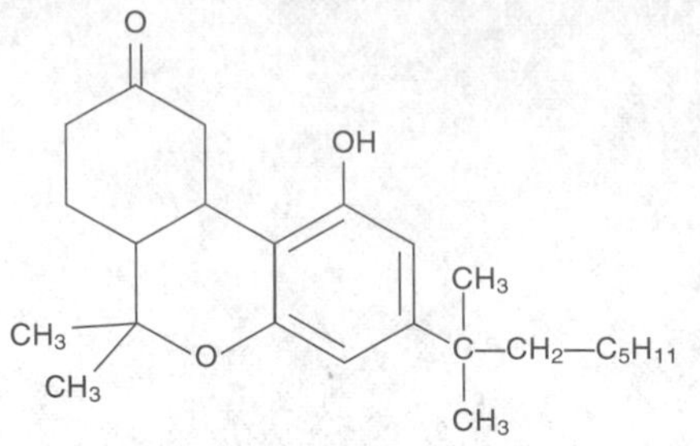

Nabilone

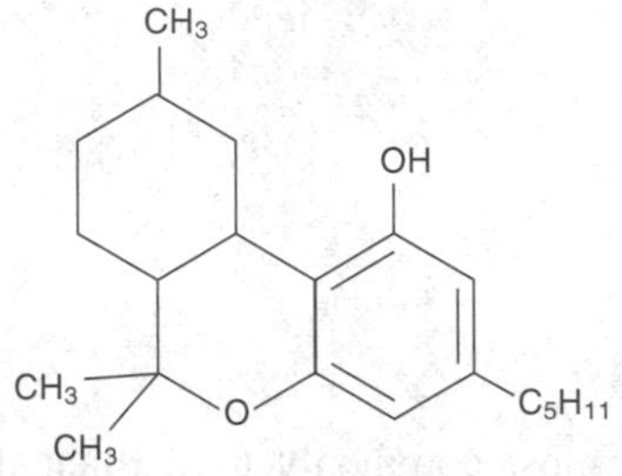

Δ9 Tetrahydrocannabinol

Figure 23-1 Chemical structures of nabilone and Δ^9-tetrahydrocannibinol. (From Ward A, Holmes B. Nabilone: A preliminary review of its pharmacological properties and therapeutic use. Drugs 1985; 30:127–144.)

Sinsemilla

Seedless (unpollinated female) marijuana that grows widely, especially in California, and accounts for about 85% of domestic production. The THC content averages about 5%.

History

In September 1989, the Drug Enforcement Administration rejected a petition to reschedule marijuana in smoked form from Schedule I (prohibited) to Schedule II (available only by prescription) status under the Controlled Substances Act.[2–4] Controversy continues on the acceptability of marijuana, in smoked form, for the control of nausea in patients receiving chemotherapy.[5]

The Drug Enforcement Administration issued a final order in March 1992, stating that the plant marijuana has no currently accepted medical use.[6] It refused to reschedule marijuana from Schedule I to Schedule II of the Controlled Substances Act. The Public Health Service also concluded that smoked marijuana is potentially more harmful than helpful to patients with compromised immune systems.[7] Nevertheless, in early 1994, a sharp increase in use of marijuana among eighth graders and high school students was reported.[8] "Pot" has become America's number one cash crop, with earnings estimated at $32 billion a year. Careful cultivation has made it an indoor industry both in the United States and elsewhere.[9]

Marijuana "Blunts"

Sales of cheap cigars are booming, in the Philadelphia region and across the United States, because young adults, teenagers, and even younger children slice the cigars open and pack them with the drug.[10] Blunts are fat, 5-in. smokes that sell for as little as 25 cents. Because their wrappers are easily resealed, the cigars can be filled with marijuana, crack cocaine, or other drugs. The combination also can stretch the use of small quantities of cheap marijuana. The harsh stench of the cheap cigar is prized for its ability to mask the sweet smell of marijuana. A single blunt cigar can contain $10 to $20 worth of marijuana.

Toxicokinetics

Elimination

Clinical studies have reported that heavy cannabis users show positive urinary cannabinoid levels for many weeks after discontinuation from the drug. This prolonged excretion could be explained by accumulation of THC in deep tissue compartments such as fat, followed by return of THC to plasma with subsequent elimination. The mean terminal elimination half-life of THC in plasma (4.3 days) of frequent marijuana users is longer than previously reported (range, 2.6–12.6 days).[11]

Drug Interactions

Although additive/or superadditive effects on psychomotor performance may follow concomitant use of marijuana and ethanol, a substantial decrease in the duration of subjective effects of ethanol and marijuana is consistent with a reduction of the maximum ethanol levels and a delay in peak plasma ethanol levels. Further studies are required to determine the clinical effects or usefulness of such combinations.[12]

Combinations of cocaine and marijuana appear to increase heart rates above levels seen with either drug alone. Increases plateau at about 50 beats/min above normal. Increases in mean arterial pressure following combinations of cocaine and marijuana are equivalent to those produced by cocaine alone.[13] Multiple-drug abuse (alcohol, amphetamines, benzodiazepines, cocaine, opiates) continues to be a problem with marijuana users. Trauma and inadequate methadone maintenance are by-products of such self-induced polypharmacy.[14] Cocaine-dependent individuals often appear to be dependent on marijuana (cannabis), a fact that must be carefully elicited on admission by a detailed history.[15,16] Phencyclidine may be intentionally combined with marijuana ("superweed") to obtain a more intense hallucinogenic experience.[17]

Pregnancy

A prospective study of marijuana use and pregnancy suggested that infants whose mothers had positive urine assays for marijuana exhibited impaired fetal growth (lower birth weight, decrease in length) when compared with infants of nonusers.[18] The study did not demonstrate a cause-and-effect relationship.

Richardson and colleagues later concluded that there is no increased risk of spontaneous abortion, effects on birth weight or head circumference, or effects on the rate of minor or major physical anomalies as a result of prenatal marijuana use. There do not appear to be significant effects on the neurobehavioral outcome of newborns. There are insignificant effects on long-term development.[19] Long-term development and behavioral effects remain to be determined.[18]

An initial unconfirmed case–control study suggests that there is a 10-fold increased risk of leukemia in the offspring of mothers who had smoked marijuana just before or during pregnancy.[20]

A cannabinoid receptor gene in the brain has been cloned.[21] This development may lead to some specific pharmaceutical agents that may provide analgesia, anticonvulsant effects, or other symptomatic relief while avoiding the undesirable side effects of cannabinoids.[22]

Clinical Presentation

Clinical manifestations due to marijuana smoking have included long-term impairment of memory in adolescents, a sixfold increase in the incidence of schizophrenia, cancer of the mouth, jaw, tongue, and lungs in 19- to 30-year-olds, fetotoxicity, and nonlymphoblastic leukemia in children of marijuana-smoking mothers.[23]

Childhood Ingestions

Cannabis ingestion in children should be suspected if a combination of the following clinical signs is present, and particularly if siblings develop symptoms simultaneously: rapid onset of drowsiness, moderate pupillary dilation, marked hypotonia with other neurologic involvement, presence of small dark particles (eg, granules, leaves, or resin) in the mouth, significant lid lag, and the absence of a history and/or symptoms indicative of trauma, central nervous system infection, or seizures.

Hashish resin ingestion in children in amounts ranging from 0.25 to 1 g has led to a rapid onset of obtundation (30–75 minutes); some children have developed opisthotonic-like movements alternating with hypotonia, and others may have meningismus. About one third of children experience tachycardia (>150 beats/min). Occasional cyanosis, right bundle-branch block, and apnea with bradycardia may be observed. All children usually recover without sequelae from 10 to 36 hours after ingestion. The acute ingestion of cannabinoids is potentially life-threatening. Acute supportive care and decontamination may be required.[24]

Acute Psychosis

Acute toxic psychosis associated with the use of marijuana was reported in U.S. soldiers during the Vietnam War, one of whom shot an individual on guard duty.[25] Suicidal ideation, anxiety, and paranoia accompanied the organic psychosis, which lasted 1 to 11 days. The development of acute psychosis after chronic use remains controversial because of questions about the contribution of premorbid personalities and multiple-drug use (eg, phencyclidine [PCP]).[26] Undifferentiated manic, schizophreniform, and confusional psychoses have been reported in heavy marijuana users admitted to psychiatric hospitals.[27] Comparison between psychotic men with high urinary cannabinoid levels and negative control groups suggests that high THC intake is associated with a rapidly resolving psychosis characterized by hypomania and occasionally schizophrenic symptoms.[28] Flashbacks can occur.

Chronic Effects

Respiratory System. Quantitative studies on products of marijuana smoking suggest that, compared with smoking tobacco, smoking marijuana is associated with a nearly fivefold greater increment in the blood carboxyhemoglobin level, an approximately threefold increase in the amount of tar inhaled and retained in the respiratory tract. These observations may account for previous findings that smoking only a few marijuana cigarettes a day (without tobacco) has the same effect on the prevalence of acute and chronic respiratory toxicity and the extent of tracheobronchial epithelial histopathology as smoking more than 20 tobacco cigarettes a day (without marijuana).[29]

Cancer. Several initial studies suggest an association between chronic marijuana smoking and cancer of the mouth and larynx.[30,31]

Marijuana smoking may also be associated with an increased risk for the development of respiratory tract malignancy.[32] Several cases have been reported of respiratory tract malignancy (tongue, tonsil, piriform sinus, paranasal sinus, larynx, lung) in young long-term marijuana smokers.[32] The smoking of one marijuana cigarette (800–900 mg, 1–3% THC) leads to the deposition in the lower respiratory tract of about a fourfold greater quantity of insoluble smoke particulates (tar) than smoking a filtered tobacco cigarette of comparable weight.[29]

Aspergillosis. Studies have shown that most illegally obtained marijuana is contaminated with *Aspergillus* species, most often *A. flavus* and *A. fumigatus*. *Aspergillus* spores easily pass through contaminated marijuana that is smoked.[33] For immunocompetent individuals, such exposure is unlikely to be associated with disease. In immunocompromised patients, invasive pulmonary aspergillosis may ensue.[34] *Aspergillus* in marijuana may be eliminated by baking marijuana at minimum temperature of 150°C (300°F) 15 minutes before smoking. Similar conditions do not degrade THC.[35]

Digital Clubbing. Studies of patients who chronically use hashish suggest that the hashish may elevate catecholamine levels, causing vasodilation of peripheral arteries, followed by digital clubbing.[36]

Pharmacokinetic parameters after intravenous THC have revealed no difference between frequent and infrequent marijuana users in the area under the curve, volume of distribution, elimination half-life of parent THC and metabolites in plasma and urine, and metabolic and renal clearances.[37]

Laboratory

Urine Levels

Prompt urine screening for the presence of cannabinoids and rapid reporting of results may obviate the need for invasive measures such as lumbar puncture, expensive biochemical studies, and computed tomography. An unexplained coma in a child requires a full workup, which should not be delayed inappropriately; a broad toxic screen is advised to rule out other toxic agents.[38]

A 4½-year-old developed euphoria, nausea, hypotonia, and increasing drowsiness. The Glasgow Coma Scale score was 6/15. The toxicology screen showed cannabinoids in the blood and urine. An 18-month-old who had been eating hashish developed coma. Cannabinoids (11-nor-delta-7-THC-9-carboxylic acid) were present in the blood (41 ng/mL) and urine (332 ng/mL).[39] Both children recovered.

Δ^9-Tetrahydrocannabinol is stored largely in adipose tissue and may accumulate faster than it can be removed in persistent users. Stein states that after using three or more joints per day, an individual who then stops smoking marijuana completely and adopts an excessive fitness program mobilizing body fat will test positive for urinary THC at 50 to 100 ng/mL for more than 2 months. An individual who smokes an occasional joint will test positive at from 500 to 1000 ng/mL or more for 3 to 4 days. Passive inhalation of marijuana smoke by nonusers occasionally results in a urine concentration of 20 ng/mL and rarely as high as 40 ng/mL.[40]

U.S. Government Standards

Title 49 of the Code of Federal Regulations Subtitle A (10–1–93 edition) defines U.S. government standards for the determination of initial and confirmatory cutoff levels (Tables 23–1 and 23–2).

Initial Test

1. The initial test shall use an immunoassay which meets the requirements of the Food and Drug Administration for commercial distribution. The initial cutoff levels shall be used when screening specimens to determine whether they are negative for these five drugs or classes of drugs.
2. These cutoff levels are subject to change by the Department of Health and Human Services as advances in technology or other considerations warrant identification of these substances at other concentrations.

Confirmatory Test

1. All specimens identified as positive on the initial test shall be confirmed using gas chromatography–mass spectrometry (GC–MS) techniques at the cutoff levels listed for each drug. All confirmations shall be by quantitative analysis. Concentrations that exceed the linear region of the standard curve shall be documented in the laboratory record as "greater than highest standard curve value."

2. These cutoff levels are subject to change by the Department of Health and Human Services as advances in technology or other considerations warrant identification of these substances at other concentrations.

Positive urine tests indicate only the likelihood of prior use and do not correlate with psychomotor impairment. The urine cannabinoid concentration is at best a poor guide to the amount actually taken, as a low level may result from either a large dose taken a long time previously or a small dose taken recently. Cannabinoids are detectable for an average of 1 to 2 days and as long as 7 days after a single marijuana cigarette. Smoking an additional marijuana cigarette extends the detection time 1 to 2 days. The enzyme-mediated immunoassay technique (EMIT-dau: sensitivity, 20 ng/mL) detected urine cannabinoids for an average of 27 days (maximum, 46 days) after cessation of chronic marijuana use.[41] Urine cannabinoid levels fluctuate, and as many as 77 days were required before these levels dropped below the detectable level for 10 consecutive days. Passive inhalation of marijuana smoke is unlikely to result in a positive cannabinoid urine screening test, except for heavy prolonged exposure (eg, the equivalent of 16 marijuana cigarettes in a small room for 1 hour on 6 consecutive days.)[42] Nonsmoking subjects who were confined to a room or a car did not develop psychotomimetic symptoms at maximum levels of tolerable smoke.[43] Even when nonsmokers were tested daily for accumulation, only 3 of 80 urine samples were positive at the 20 ng/mL level and none were positive at the 50 ng/mL level.[44]

An EMIT screen may test false negative if a specimen is adulterated by the acidity of bleach, detergent, salt, or vinegar or diluted in water from a tap or a toilet bowl.

A combination of screening by EMIT (specificity, 90%; sensitivity, 95%) and confirmation by GC–MS (specificity >99.9%, sensitivity >99.9%) will yield almost 100% accuracy in testing for marijuana.[40]

Ritodrine may interfere in GC–MS urine confirmation of the THC metabolite 11-nor-Δ^9-THC-α-carboxylic acid.[45]

Blood Levels and Driving

Although marijuana is composed of more than 60 constituents called cannabinoids, the principal psychoactive agent in cannabis is THC. THC is metabolized by microsomal hydroxylation to 11-hydroxy-THC (11-OH-THC), which is also believed to be pharmacologically active. Little 11-OH-THC is excreted in urine. The major urinary metabolite is

Table 23–1
Initial Test Cutoff Levels (ng/mL)

Marijuana metabolites	100
Cocaine metabolites	300
Opiate metabolites	300*
Phencyclidine	25
Amphetamine	1000

*25 ng/mL if immunoassay is specific for free morphine.

Table 23–2
Confirmatory Test Cutoff Levels (ng/mL)

Marijuana metabolites	15
Cocaine metabolites	150
Opiates	
Morphine	300
Codeine	300
Phencyclidine	25
Amphetamines	500
Amphetamine	500
Methamphetamine	500

11-nor-Δ^9-carboxy-THC (THC-COOH) from the subsequent oxidation of 11-OH-THC. THC-COOH has been most often measured to determine the presence and involvement of marijuana in traffic fatalities; however, THC-COOH is not pharmacologically active. Measurement of THC and 11-OH-THC in blood is therefore more likely to be a better indicator of possible impairment of motor coordination than measurement of THC-COOH in blood or urine. The mean concentrations of THC and 11-OH-THC in blood of 13 drivers were 5.4 and 18 ng/mL, respectively. Plasma levels of THC have been shown to fall rapidly within an hour of smoking to about 10% of peak concentration and, after 3 to 4 hours, are typically less than 1 ng/mL. The metabolite THC-COOH reportedly appears in blood in higher concentrations for a number of hours after smoking marijuana but well after the psychoactive effects of marijuana have worn off.[46]

Studies of aircraft pilot performance following the smoking of one cigarette containing 20 mg of THC suggest that impairment of performance can last as long as 24 hours after smoking. The user may be unaware of the drug's influence.[47]

REFERENCES—MARIJUANA

1. *National Household Survey on Drug Abuse.* Washington, DC: National Institute of Drug Abuse, 1991.
2. Young FL. Opinion and recommended ruling, marijuana rescheduling petition. Washington, DC: Department of Justice, Drug Enforcement Administration, September 1988: Docket 86-22.
3. Marijuana scheduling petition: Denial of petition remand. Fed Regist 1992;57:10503.
4. Grinspoon L, Bakalar JB, Doblin R. Marijuana, the AIDS wasting syndrome and US government. N Engl J Med 1995; 333:670–671.
5. Doblin R, Kleiman MAR. Medical use of marijuana. Ann Intern Med 1991;114:809–810.
6. U.S. Department of Justice, Drug Enforcement Administration. Marijuana scheduling petition: Final order. Fed Regist 1992;57:10499–10508.
7. U.S. Public Health Service. Denying new requests for medicinal marijuana. Int Med News Cardiol News 1992;25:31.
8. Treaster JB. Survey finds marijuana use is up in high schools. NY Times, February 1, 1994.
9. Pollan M. How pot has grown. NY Times Mag, February 19, 1995, pp. 31–57.
10. Senkowsky S. Marijuana 'blunts': The adolescent craze. City of Phoenix: The DRE 1995;7:11–13.
11. Johansson E, Halldin MM, Agurell S, et al. Terminal elimination plasma half-life of delta^9-tetrahydrocannabinol (delta^9-THC) in heavy users of marijuana. Eur J Clin Pharmacol 1989;37:273–277.
12. Lukas SE, Benedikt R, Mendelson JH, et al. Marijuana attenuates the rise in plasma ethanol levels in human subjects. Neuropsychopharmacology 1992;7:77–81.
13. Foltin RW, Fischman MW, Pedroso JJ, Pearlson GD. Marijuana and cocaine interactions in humans: Cardiovascular consequences. Pharmacol Biochem Behav 1987;28:459–464.
14. Soderstrom CA, Trifillis AL, Shankar DS, et al. Marijuana and alcohol use among 1,023 trauma patients. Arch Surg 1988; 123:733–737.
15. Du Pont RL, Saylor KE. Marijuana and benzodiazepines in patients receiving methadone treatment. JAMA 1989; 2611:3409.
16. Miller NS, Klahr AL, Gold MS, et al. The prevalence of marijuana (cannabis) use and dependence in cocaine dependence. NY State J Med 1990;90:491–492.
17. Lanska DJ, Lanska MJ. PCP use among adolescent marijuana users. J Pediatr 1988;113:950–951.
18. Zuckerman R, Frank DA, Kingson R, et al. Effects of material marijuana and cocaine use on fetal growth. N Engl J Med 1989,320:767–768.
19. Richardson GA, Day NL, McGaughey PJ. The impact of prenatal marijuana and cocaine use on the infant and child. Clin Obstet Gynecol 1993;36:302–328.
20. Robison LL, Buckley JD, Daigle AE, et al. Maternal drug use and risk of childhood non-lymphoblastic leukemia among offspring: An epidemiologic investigation implicating marijuana (a report from the Children's Cancer Study Group). Cancer 1989;63:1904–1910.
21. Matsuda LA, Lolait J, Brownstein MJ, et al. Structure of a cannabinoid receptor and functional expression of the cloned DNA. Nature 1990;346:561–564.
22. Cannabinoid receptor gene cloned. JAMA 1990;264:1384.
23. Nahas G, Latour C. The human toxicity of marijuana. Med J Aust 1992;15:495–497.
24. Johnson D, Convadi A, McGuigan M. Hashish ingestion in toddlers. Vet Hum Toxicol 1991;33:393.
25. Talbot JA, Teague JW. Marihuana psychosis: Acute toxic psychosis associated with the use of cannabis derivatives. JAMA 1969;210:299–302.
26. Halikas JA, Goodwin DW, Gage SB. Marijuana use and psychiatric illness. Arch Gen Psychiatry 1972;27:162–165.
27. Carney MWP, Bacelle L, Robinson B. Psychosis after cannabis use. Br Med J 1984;288:1047.
28. Rottanburg D, Robins AH, Ben-Arie O, et al. Cannabis-associated psychosis with hypomanic features. Lancet 1982; 2:1364–1366.
29. Wu T-C, Tashkin DP, Djahed B, Rose JE. Pulmonary hazards of smoking marijuana as compared with tobacco. N Engl J Med 1988;318:347–351.
30. Caplan GA. Marijuana and mouth cancer. J R Soc Med 1991;84:386.
31. Taylor FM. Marijuana as a potential respiratory tract carcinogen: A retrospective analysis of a community hospital population. South Med J 1988;81:1213–1216.
32. Tashkin DP. Is frequent marijuana smoking harmful to health? West J Med 1993;158:635–636.
33. Kagen SL, Kurup VP, Sohnle PG, Fink JN. Marijuana smoking and fungal sensitization. J Allergy Clin Immunol 1983;71: 389–393.
34. Chesid MJ, Gelfand JA, Nutter C, Fauci AS. Pulmonary aspergillosis, inhalation of contaminated marijuana smoke, a chronic granulomatosis disease. Ann Intern Med 1975; 82:682–683.
35. Levitz SM, Diamond RD. Aspergillosis and marijuana. Ann Intern Med 1991;115:578–579.
36. Baris YI, Tan E, Kalyoncu F, et al. Chest 1990;98:1545–1546.
37. Kelly P, Jones PT. Metabolism of tetrahydrocannabinol in frequent and infrequent marijuana users. J Anal Toxicol 1992; 16:228–235.
38. MacNab A, Anderson E, Susak L. Ingestion of cannabis: A cause of coma in children. Pediatr Emerg Care 1989;5:238–239.
39. Rubio F, Quintero S, Hernandez A, et al. Flumazenil for coma reversal in children after cannabis. Lancet 1993;341:1028–1029.
40. Stein IN. Marijuana testing. West J Med 1988;148:78.
41. Ellis BM Jr, Mann MA, Judson BA, et al. Excretion patterns of cannabinoid metabolites after last use in a group of chronic users. Clin Pharmacol Ther 1985;38:572–578.
42. Cone EJ, Johnson RE. Contact highs and urinary cannabinoid excretion after passive exposure to marijuana smoke. Clin Pharmacol Ther 1986;40:245–256.
43. Morland J, Bugge A, Shuterud B, et al. Cannabinoids in blood and urine after passive inhalation of cannabis smoke. J Forens Sci 1985;30:997–1002.
44. Perez-Reyes M, Di Guiseppi S, Mason AP, et al. Passive inhalation of marijuana smoke and urinary excretion of cannabinoids. Clin Pharmacol Ther 1983;34:36–41.
45. Podkowik B-I, Repka ML, Smith MC. Interference by ritodrine in GC/MS confirmation of delta-9-tetrahydrocannabinol-9-carboxylic acid in urine. Clin Chem 1991;37: 1305–1306.

46. Gerostamoulos J, Drummer OH. Incidence of psychoactive cannabinoids in drivers killed in motor vehicle accidents. J Forens Sci 1993;38:649–656.
47. Leirer VO, Yesavage JA, Morrow DG. Marijuana carry-over effects on aircraft pilot performance. Aviat Space Environ Med 1991;62:221–227.

DRONABINOL

Dronabinol (Marinol) is Δ^9-tetrahydrocannabinol (Fig. 23–1) and has been available since 1985 to treat nausea and vomiting associated with cancer chemotherapy in patients who fail to respond adequately to conventional antiemetic therapy. It was approved by the U.S. Food and Drug Administration in 1992 for the treatment of anorexia associated with weight loss in patients with AIDS. Dronabinol has an antiemetic efficacy similar to that of prochlorperazine but less than that of metoclopramide. There are anecdotal reports that smoking marijuana is of benefit in patients with multiple sclerosis. The results of small clinical trials of THC suggest that it can reduce tremor and spasticity in some patients with multiple sclerosis.[1] Large amounts may induce seizure activity.[2]

Overdose may be accompanied by disturbing psychotic symptoms such as hallucinations, delusions, and paranoid feelings. Few deaths have been reported from the use of dronabinol, although two deaths have been reported from the use of Indian hemp. One death has followed the smoking of cannabis herb or resin. Another cannabinoid available as an antiemetic agent, nabilone (Cesamet), is administered orally in doses of 1 to 2 mg 1 to 3 hours before and every 8 to 12 hours after chemotherapy.[3,4]

Product Formulation

Dronabinol is supplied as a round soft gelatin capsule containing either 2.5, 5, or 10 mg.

Source

Dronabinol is naturally occurring and has been extracted from *Cannabis sativa* (marijuana).

Therapeutic Dose

The initial oral dose for appetite stimulation in patients with AIDS is 5 mg/m^2 body surface area daily with increments of 2.5 mg/m^2 to a maximum dose of 15 mg/m^2. The average daily dose is 5 to 20 mg daily.[5] Doses of 20 to 30 mg/m^2 daily are used in the management of emesis in chemotherapy.[6]

Fatal Dose

The estimated lethal human dose of intravenous dronabinol is 30 mg/kg (2100 mg/70 kg). Significant central nervous system symptoms have followed oral doses of 0.4 mg/kg (28 mg/70 kg).[7]

Toxicokinetics

Absorption

Dronabinol is slowly absorbed from the gastrointestinal tract. It undergoes first-pass metabolism and its bioavailability after oral administration is 10 to 20%. It is 97 to 99% bound to plasma proteins.

Distribution

Dronabinol has a large volume of distribution (about 10 L/kg).

Elimination

Dronabinol is metabolized to 11-hydroxydronabinol, which is similar in activity to the parent compound; less than 5% of an oral dose is recovered unchanged in the feces. The half-life of nabilone is about 2 hours. Nabilone is eliminated in the feces (65%) and urine (20%).[8]

Pregnancy/Lactation

The Food and Drug Administration has placed dronabinol in Pregnancy Category C. Dronabinol is concentrated in and secreted in human breast milk.

Mechanism of Action

Dronabinol is a centrally acting sympathomimetic drug that acts at cannabinoid receptor sites in the brain.

Clinical Presentation

Signs and symptoms following dronabinol intoxication include drowsiness, euphoria, heightened sensory awareness, altered time perception, reddened conjunctiva, dry mouth, and tachycardia. Following moderate intoxication, memory impairment, depersonalization, mood alteration, urinary retention, and reduced bowel motility may be present; following severe intoxication, symptoms and signs include decreased motor coordination, lethargy, slurred speech, and postural hypotension. Apprehensive patients may experience panic reaction and seizures may occur in patients with existing seizure disorders. Visual difficulties have been reported.[6,7]

Drug Abuse and Dependence

Psychological and physiologic dependence has been noted in healthy individuals. Addiction is uncommon and may follow prolonged high-dose administration.

Abstinence Syndrome

Abrupt discontinuation of 210 mg/d after 12 to 16 days leads to irritability, insomnia, and restlessness. Later "hot flashes," rhinorrhea, loose stools, hiccoughs, and anorexia are observed. Symptoms abate over 48 hours.

The most serious side effects of nabilone are depersonalization and dysphoria. Other common effects observed include vertigo, dizziness, drowsiness, dry mouth, and difficulty in concentration. Nabilone increases the psychomotor impairment produced by diazepam, alcohol, and codeine.[8]

Laboratory

Analysis of body fluids can be performed by either enzyme-mediated immunoassay (EMIT) or radioimmunoassay (RIA) of metabolites in urine. Each is capable of detecting cannabinoids in the range 20 to 100 ng/mL. Metabolites may remain for a few days or longer after a single dose and up to a month after chronic exposure. Laboratory tests do not differentiate acute from chronic intoxication.

Treatment

A potentially serious oral ingestion, if recent, should be managed with gut decontamination. In unconscious patients with a secure airway, instill activated charcoal (30–100 g in adults, 1–2 g/kg in infants) via a nasogastric tube. A saline cathartic or sorbitol may be added to the first dose of activated charcoal. Patients experiencing depressive, hallucinatory, or psychotic reactions should be placed in a quiet room and offered reassurance. Benzodiazepines (5–10 mg diazepam orally) may be used for the treatment of extreme agitation. Hypotension responds to Trendelenburg position and intravenous fluids. Pressors are rarely required.

REFERENCES—DRONABINOL

1. Martyn CN, Illis LS, Thom J. Nabilone in the treatment of multiple sclerosis. Lancet 1995;345:579
2. Bhargava HN. Potential therapeutic application of naturally occurring and synthetic cannabinoids. Gen Pharmacol 1978; 9:195–213.
3. Abromowicz M, ed. Nabilone and other antiemetics for cancer patients. Med Lett Drugs Ther 1988;29:1–3.
4. Brunton LL. Agents affecting gastrointestinal water flux and motility, digestants and bile acids. In: Gilman AG, Rall TW, Nies AS, Taylor P, eds. *Goodman and Gilman's the Pharmacological Basis of Therapeutics.* 8th ed. New York: Pergamon Press, 1990:914-932.
5. Hellinger FJ. The cost of Marinol (dronabinol). JAMA 1993; 270:2810.
6. Jaffe JH. Drug addiction and drug abuse. In: Gilman AG, Rall TW, Nies AS, Taylor P, eds. *Goodman and Gilman's the Pharmacological Basis of Therapeutics.* 8th ed. New York: Pergamon Press, 1990:549–553.
7. Schwartz RH, Hawks RI. Laboratory detection of marijuana use. JAMA 1985;254:788–792.
8. Rubin A, Lemberger L, Warrick P, et al. Physiologic disposition of nabilone, a cannabinol derivative, in man. Clin Pharmacol Ther 1977;22:85–91.

Chapter 24
Phencyclidine

INTRODUCTION

STREET NAMES

Table 24–1 lists some current street names for phencyclidine.[1] The number of phencyclidine (PCP) emergency room visits declined in both Los Angeles and the rest of the United States between 1985 and 1989.[2]

SAMPLE COMPOSITION/PURITY

Active, inert, and volatile additives found in phencyclidine are summarized in Table 24–2.[3] Little is known about the relative toxicity of the drug versus that of the impurities or additives.

PHENCYCLIDINE ABUSE

Toxicokinetics

Distribution

The volume of distribution of phencyclidine is 6.2 L/kg. It is highly lipid soluble and accumulates in adipose tissue and in the brain.[4] Plasma protein binding is about 65%.[5]

Metabolism

Metabolism of adipose tissue may cause the release of PCP. This contributes to the recurrence of symptoms and fluctuations in clinical status.[6]

Elimination

An initial rapid decrease in urine phencyclidine levels during the first 9 days is followed by a more gradual decline. Urine samples are PCP positive an average of 2 weeks, and most samples are PCP negative by 30 days.[7] During this period, differentiating among accidental exposure, new use, and abstinence may be difficult. Pre-op tests for surgical procedures within this 30-day period have resulted in positive urine phencyclidine levels in chronic users despite abstinence.[8]

Table 24–1
Street Names for Phencyclidine

Angel dust	Mint weed
Angel hair	Mist
Angel mist	Monkey dust
Animal tranquilizer	PCP
Cadillac	Peace
C.J.	Peace Pill
Crystal joints	Rocket fuel
Cyclones	Scuffle
Dust	Selma
Elephant tranquilizer	Sherman
Embalming fluid	Snorts
Goon	Soma
Gorilla biscuits	Supercools
Hog	Superweed
Horse tranquilizers	Surfer
Jet fuel	T
Kay Jay	TAC
K.J.	TIC
Killer weed	Tranks
Krystal joint	Whacky weed
K.W.	Zombie dust
Lovely	

From Milhorn HT Jr. Diagnosis and management of phencyclidine intoxication. Am Fam Physician 1991;43:1293–1302.

Pregnancy

Infants exposed to PCP in utero may develop symptoms of neonatal narcotic withdrawal, temperament problems, and sleep problems during the first year of life. They appear to be largely within normal limits for growth and development at 1 year. Further studies are needed to determine later effects of in utero PCP exposure.[9]

Drug Interactions

Animal studies suggest that antipsychotic drugs can block PCP receptor-mediated neurotoxicity. This requires confirmation in human studies.[10]

Clinical Presentation

Patients may present with various combination of central nervous system stimulation and depression, cholinergic and anticholinergic effects, and adrenergic effects. The most common physical findings are nystagmus (horizontal, vertical, or rotatory) and hypertension.[11]

Extremely high blood pressure levels are unusual as are hypertension-induced complications. Tachycardia occurs in approximately one third of patients. Cholinergic signs (diaphoresis, miosis, bronchospasm, salivation) and anticholinergic or adrenergic signs (tachycardia, mydriasis, urinary retention) may be present.[6]

Major Intoxication Patterns

Coma. The level of consciousness ranges from fully alert to comatose. Coma may occur suddenly but often develops after a period of bizarre or violent behavior. It may be of relatively short duration but can last up to a week. Some patients with prolonged coma have been found to have continued drug absorption from ruptured packets of ingested PCP. On emergence from coma, abnormalities such as agitation and psychosis are common.

Table 24–2
Phencyclidine Additives

Active	Inert
Phenylpropanolamine	Magnesium sulfate
Benzocaine	Ammonium chloride
Procaine	Ammonium hydroxide
Ephedrine	Phenyllithium halide
Caffeine	Phenylmagnesium halide
Piperidine	**Volatile**
PCC (1-piperidinocyclohexanecarbonitrile)	Ethyl ether
TCP (1-[1-(2-thienyl)cyclohexyl]-piperidine)	Toluene
PCE (cyclohexamine)	Cyclohexanol
PHP (phenylcyclohexylpyrrolidine)	Isopropanol
Ketamine	

From Shesser R, Jotte R, Olshaker J. The contribution of impurities to the acute morbidity of illegal drug use. Am J Emerg Med 1991;9:336–342.

Mental Status Change. Mental status changes induced by PCP include confusion, disorientation, auditory and visual hallucinations, and delusions. Acute PCP intoxication can produce a psychosis identical to acute schizophrenia. Patients may develop catatonia, with unusual posturing, mutism, and staring. Myoclonic and dystonic movements, including opisthotonos and torticollis, may be seen, as may choreoathetoid movements.

Acute Toxic Psychosis. Phencyclidine-intoxicated patients are alert but display bizarre behavior, agitation, or violence. They may be extremely combative and require physical or chemical restraints. Intoxicated patients are prone to sustaining significant injuries. A patient who appears calm one minute may be agitated or violent the next. Symptoms often resolve within hours, although some patients have symptoms lasting days or even weeks. Recovery from psychosis may be very gradual over weeks to months.

Acute Brain Syndrome. Acute brain syndrome after use of PCP has been reported.[6]

Minor Intoxication Patterns

Generally, patients with minor patterns of toxicity recover more quickly than patients with major patterns and usually do not require hospitalization. Such patterns may be manifested by lethargy or stupor and bizarre behavior.

Violent Reactions. The most frequent causes of chemically induced psychosis are amphetamines, cocaine, and phencyclidine. Other common drugs that cause violent reactions are ethanol (intoxication, intolerance, and withdrawal), anticholinergic agents, aromatic hydrocarbons, corticosteroids, lysergic acid diethylamide (LSD), and sedative–hypnotic agents (intoxication or withdrawal). Conditions that may contribute to violent behavior are anemia, dementia, electrolyte abnormalities, endocrinopathies, head trauma, hypoglycemia, hypoxia, postictal status, and vitamin deficiencies.

Agitation. These patients have clear sensoriums and nonviolent behavior associated with increased motor activity. Generally, the agitation resolves by 6 hours. Rarely, apnea has developed.[11]

Euphoria. Phencyclidine toxicity may mimic mild ethanol intoxication.

Minimal Behavioral Impairment. Some patients display evidence of nystagmus, ataxia, loss of muscle coordination, and vital sign abnormalities without obvious signs of behavioral toxicity. Incidental intoxication has been documented in a chronically depressed elderly lady who lived above a clandestine phencyclidine laboratory.[12] Positive blood phencyclidine levels were reported in law enforcement officers who handled phencyclidine confiscated during drug raids.[13]

Children

Children may become intoxicated by ingesting the butts of used PCP-impregnated cigarettes or from passive inhalation of sidestream smoke. Children aged 5 years and younger often present with lethargy, severe depression of consciousness, ataxia, nystagmus, and staring episodes. Presenting signs may also include apnea, seizures, opisthotonos, and choreoathetosis. Miosis may be present. In children, unexplained stupor or coma, seizures, ataxia, nystagmus, strange behavior, staring spells, or unusual posturing can indicate possible PCP intoxication.[6]

Medical Complications

Complications include seizures, hyperthermia, rhabdomyolysis and acute renal failure, intracranial hemorrhage, apnea, aspiration pneumonia, and cardiac arrest.

Differential Diagnosis

Phencyclidine-intoxicated patients share many features with overdoses of cocaine, amphetamines, anticholinergic agents, and hallucinogens and withdrawal from alcohol or other sedative–hypnotic agents. These include a psychotic or delirious state with agitation, hypertension, hyperthermia, tachycardia, disorientation, and hallucinations.[6] The differential diagnosis should include primary psychiatric disorders, head trauma, hypoxia, hypoglycemia, hyponatremia, sepsis, meningitis and encephalitis, hyperthermia, thyroid storm, and the neuroleptic malignant syndrome.[6]

Fatalities

Most deaths in PCP-intoxicated patients occur not because of direct effects of the drug but because of its behavioral toxicity. The bizarre and violent behavior induced by PCP, along with analgesic effects and lack of muscular coordination, may cause drowning or significant trauma. Nontraumatic causes of death include cardiopulmonary arrest after status epilepticus, primary respiratory arrest, intracranial hemorrhage, and cardiac arrest after hyperpyrexia. Hyperkalemia from rhabdomyolysis is another potential cause of death.[6]

Laboratory

Phencyclidine blood levels do not correlate well with clinical findings and do not guide clinical management.

A "body stuffer" (see Chapter 21) of phencyclidine developed rigidity, diaphoresis, and a temperature of 41.3°C. The serum PCP concentration reached 1879 ng/mL; his cerebrospinal fluid phencyclidine concentration was 245 ng/mL. Thirteen days after ingestion he passed two plastic bags per rectum, one of which was ruptured. He recovered.[14]

As part of the U.S. National Institute on Drug Abuse (NIDA) guidelines for laboratories performing federal workplace drug testing, laboratories are required to detect, identify, and quantitate PCP down to urine concentrations of 25 ng/mL. The initial test cutoff level is 25 ng/mL; the confirmatory test cutoff level is also 25 ng/mL.

Diphenhydramine in urine concentrations of 50 to 1200 µg/L may cause a urine specimen to test positive for PCP by fluorescence polarization immunoassay with apparent PCP concentrations up to 32 to 37 µg/L.[15]

Treatment

Gut Decontamination

Patients who inhale, insufflate, or ingest phencyclidine more than several hours prior to medical attention probably do not benefit from the usual measures of decontamination (syrup of ipecac/lavage, activated charcoal, cathartics). The possibility of significant enterohepatic circulation suggests that serial activated charcoal may interrupt this recirculation. The need for syrup of ipecac or lavage is a matter of clinical judgment, as the procedure itself may cause excessive agitation in the PCP-intoxicated patient.

Elimination Enhancement

Urinary acidification has been recommended to achieve "ion trapping" and enhance urinary PCP excretion. Although the amount of PCP excreted in the urine can be increased by this method, urinary acidification is virtually never indicated. Only a small percentage of PCP is excreted in the urine. Acidification will not affect liver metabolism, the major route of drug elimination, and thus will not significantly increase the overall removal of the drug. Induction of metabolic acidosis may itself cause complications. Rhabdomyolysis is a potential complication of PCP intoxication, and an acidic urine increases the risk of myoglobinuric renal failure.

Seizures caused by PCP should be treated with intravenous benzodiazepines; the use of other anticonvulsants has not been evaluated. Refractory seizures can cause hypoxia, severe metabolic acidosis, hyperthermia, and rhabdomyolysis; therefore, neuromuscular blockade may occasionally be required. Aggressive cooling measures are necessary in hyperthermic patients.

Urine should be screened for myoglobin by dipstick testing for heme. Serum creatine phosphokinase levels should be measured in patients with heme-positive urine. Because the present of urinary myoglobin may be transient, serum creatine phosphokinase levels should be measured when rhabdomyolysis is strongly suspected on clinical grounds, even with heme-negative urine.[6]

Antidote

Neither propranolol nor haloperidol is a specific antidote. Experimental animal data suggest that the administration of PCP-specific antigen binding fragments (Fab) produced substantial changes in the volume of distribution (10-fold decrease) of PCP and in its unbound fraction (from 50% to <1%). Within 10 minutes of administration of anti-PCP Fab fragments to dogs, the serum concentration of PCP increased 17- to 56-fold.[16] These data suggest that high-affinity anti-PCP Fab fragments could reverse the toxicity of PCP. Further confirmatory work is, no doubt, in progress.[17] This product has not been developed for clinical use.

Supportive Measures

Hypertension. Specific antihypertensive therapy is indicated in patients with persistent severe blood pressure elevations and those with hypertension-induced end-organ damage.[6]

Agitated Violent Behavior. Once a patient is controlled, staff must obtain a complete history, perform a thorough physical examination, and obtain laboratory tests and roentgenograms to determine the underlying problem. Emphasis should be placed on determining if a patient has a metabolic disorder, infectious disease, cardiovascular disorder, intracranial disorder, acute intoxication, acute withdrawal, trauma, environmental injury, or psychiatric disorder.[18–22]

Wasserberger and colleagues at the Martin Luther King Jr. General Hospital in Los Angeles have proposed a program for handling the violent patient (see Table 6–6). Staff should allow a buffer of at least two arm lengths between themselves and the patient. Hard restraints should be used quickly under a protocol.[22] As soon as possible, the blood sugar level should be evaluated (an intravenous line will be needed for treatment). If the patient is hypoglycemic, 50% dextrose in water should be administered. If large doses of diazepam are used the patient may become hypotensive, develop shallow respirations, and become apneic, especially if the source of the agitation is PCP. Once the agitation is diminished, PCP's sedative effects can lead to cardiovascular collapse and respiratory arrest. In the elderly, only 1 to 2 mg of haloperidol should be used. Diazepam is not used in patients over age 60 because its half-life in this age group may be greatly prolonged. The use of intravenous haloperidol is not approved by the Food and Drug Administration. It must be determined if the patient has a metabolic disorder, infectious disease, cardiovascular disorder, intracranial disorder, acute intoxication, acute withdrawal, trauma, environmental injury, or psychiatric disorder.[22]

Rhabdomyolysis and Renal Failure. Once volume depletion is corrected, a liter of 5% dextrose in water containing 25 g of mannitol and 100 mEq of sodium bicarbonate should be run at 250 mL/h. This should be continued until myoglobinuria disappears, assuming a flow rate of 40 mL/h. The patient should be monitored for hypokalemia. Hemodialysis should be considered for worsening renal function.[23]

Indications for Hospitalization. Seizures, rhabdomyolysis, hyperthermia, and significant injuries require hospitalization. Pediatric patients who are symptomatic from PCP exposure should be admitted. Patients with altered mental status or behavioral toxicity should be considered for hospitalization.

Discharge. Patients should be observed until their mental status has remained normal for several hours.[6] Patients with mild to moderate symptomatology will improve rapidly and can be discharged from the emergency department.

REFERENCES

1. Milhorn HT. Diagnosis and management of phencyclidine intoxication. Am Fam Physician 1991;43:1293–1302.
2. UCLA Drug Abuse Research Groups funded by the National Institute of Justice. Los Angeles Times, June 17, 1991.
3. Shesser R, Jotte R, Olshaker J. The contribution of impurities to the acute morbidity of illegal drug use. Am J Emerg Med 1991;9:336–342.
4. Cook CE, Brine DR, Jeffecote AR. Phencyclidine deposition after intravenous and oral doses. Clin Pharmacol Ther 1982;31:625–634.
5. Giles HG, Corrigall WA, Khouw V, et al. Plasma protein binding of phencyclidine. Clin Pharmacol Ther 1982;31:77–82.
6. Baldridge EB, Bessen HA. Phencyclidine. Emerg Med Clin North Am 1990;8:541–550.
7. Simpson GM, Khajawall AM, Alatorre E, et al. Urinary phencyclidine excretion in chronic abusers. J Toxicol Clin Toxicol 1982/1983;19:1051–1059.
8. Khajawall AM, Simpson GM. Peculiarities of phencyclidine urinary excretion and monitoring. J Toxicol Clin Toxicol 1982/1983;19:835–842.
9. Wachsman L, Schuetz S, Chan LS, Wingert WA. What happens to babies exposed to phencyclidine (PCP in utero?) Am J Drug Alcohol Abuse 1989;15:31–39.
10. Farber NB, Price MT, Labruyer J, et al. Antipsychotic drugs block phencyclidine receptor-mediated neurotoxicity. Biol Psychiatry 1993;34:119–121.
11. McCarron MM, Schulze BW, Thompson GA, et al. Acute phencyclidine intoxication: Incidence of clinical findings in 1,000 cases. Ann Emerg Med 1981;10:237–242.
12. Aniline O, Pitts FN, Allen RE, et al. Incidental intoxication with phencyclidine. J Clin Psychiatry 1980;41:393–394.
13. Pitts FN Jr, Allen RE, Aniline O, et al. Occupational intoxication and long-term persistence of phencyclidine (PCP) in law enforcement personnel. Clin Toxicol 1981;18:1015–1020.
14. Jackson JE. Phencyclidine pharmacokinetics after a massive overdose. Ann Intern Med 1989;111:613–615.

15. Levine BS, Smith ML. Effects of diphenhydramine or immunoassay of phencyclidine in urine. Clin Chem 1990;36:1258.
16. MacDonald DI. New treatment for PCP? JAMA 1987;257: 3188.
17. Owens SM, Mayersohn M. Phencyclidine-specific Fab fragments alter phencyclidine disposition in dogs. Drug Metab Dispos 1986;14:52–58.
18. Wasserberger J, Ordog GJ, Hardin E, et al. Violence in the emergency department. Top Emerg Med 1992;14:71–78.
19. Mofenson HC, Caraccio TR. The agitated, violent or acutely psychotic patient: PP/T Review. Nassau County Medical Center Regional Poison Control Center. 1992; 11(5):301–306.
20. Thomas H, Schwartz E, Petrilli R. Droperidol versus haloperidol for chemical restraint of agitative and combative patients. Ann Emerg Med 1992;21:407–413.
21. Dubin WR, Weiss KJ. *Handbook of Psychiatric Emergencies.* Springhouse, PA: Springhouse, 1991.
22. Wasserberger JL. Personal communication, Drew/UCLA Medical Center.
23. Jerrard DA. "Designer drugs": A current perspective. J Emerg Med 1990;8:733–741.

Chapter **25**

The Opiates

INTRODUCTION

Opiate overdose produces constricted pupils, respiratory depression, and coma and is treated with naloxone and good supportive care.[1]

CLASSIFICATION

I. Older opiates
   A. Natural opium
      Opium
      Tincture of opium
      Paregoric (camphorated opium tincture)
      Morphine
      Codeine
   B. Synthetic Derivatives
      1. Morphine and congeners
         Heroin
         Hydromorphone (Dilaudid)
         Oxymorphone (Numorphan)
         Hydrocodone
         Oxycodone
      2. Meperidine and Congeners
         Meperidine hydrochloride (Pethidine, Demerol)
         Anileridine (Leritine)
         Diphenoxylate hydrochloride and atropine sulfate (Lomotil)
         Fentanyl (Innovar, Sublimaze), fentanyl derivatives, and "China White"
         Loperamide (Imodium)
         Alphaprodine (Nisentil)
      3. Others
         Pentazocine hydrochloride (Talwin)
         Butorphanol tartrate (Stadol)
         Nalbuphine hydrochloride (Nubain)
         Naloxone (Narcan)
         Naltrexone (Trexan)
         Buprenorphine (Buprenex)

II. New opiates
   Dextromoramide (Palfium)
   Dezocine (Dalgan)
   Ketobemidone (Ketogin)
   Meptazinol hydrochloride (Meptid)

Nalmefene (Revex)
Pentamorphone
Tilidine hydrochloride (Valoron)
Tramadol hydrochloride (Ultram)

Opiates are controlled substances in the United States (Table 25–1).

Figure 25–1 presents the structural formulas of some opioids, describing the common γ-phenyl-*N*-methylpiperidine chemical backbone.[2]

Toxicokinetics

Table 25–2 is a summary of toxicokinetic and clinical data on some opioids in common use.[2]

Therapeutic Dose

Table 25–3 summarizes dosages of opioid analgesic agents for adults and children weighing 50 kg or more who have not previously received opioid agents.[3]

Mechanism of Action

Beta endorphins (endogenous opioids) are elevated in healthy men who run until they collapse without being sensitive to discomfort. Such men can run until they become confused, dehydrated, hyperthermic, and hypophosphatemic without experiencing any intolerable discomfort.[4] Signs of opiate addiction intoxication are listed in Tables 25–4 and 25–5. Opioid receptor interactions are listed in Table 25–6. Physiological effects of opioids are summarized in Table 25–7.

Clinical Presentation

A distinction can be made between the maladaptive behavior associated with the regular use of opiates and the direct effects of opiates on the central nervous system. The former consists of opioid dependency and opioid abuse. The latter includes the medical syndromes of opioid intoxication and opioid withdrawal. Acute overdose is a medical emergency and is a complication of acute intoxication.[5]

Opioid Dependence

The American Psychiatric Association has established diagnostic criteria for opioid dependency, criteria for severity of opioid dependency, and diagnostic criteria for opioid abuse (Table 25–8).

Opioid Abuse

Opioid abuse is now considered a residual category of the maladaptive pattern of opioid use that does not meet the diagnostic criteria of opioid dependence. The central feature is continued use of the drug despite persistent and recurrent social, occupational, psychological, or physical problems caused by the use of the drug. A time element is also included.

Proconvulsant Effects

Anecdotal reports suggest that morphine, meperidine, fentanyl, sufentanil, and alfentanil are proconvulsant in nonepileptics. Morphine has also been proconvulsant in epileptics. Anticonvulsants (eg, phenytoin, phenobarbital, and

Table 25–1
The Controlled Substances Act: Schedules of Controlled Substances

Schedule I Substances
Drugs in this schedule are those that have no accepted medical use in the United States and have a high abuse potential. Some examples are heroin, marijuana, LSD, peyote, mescaline, psilocybin, tetrahydrocannabinoids, ketobemidone, levomoramide, racemoramide, benzylmorphine, dihydromorphine, morphine methylsulfonate, nicocodeine, nicomorphine, acetylmethadol, fenethylline, tilidine, and methaqualone.

Schedule II Substances
The drugs in this schedule have a high abuse potential with severe psychic or physical dependence liability. Schedule II controlled substances consist of certain narcotic drugs and drugs containing amphetamines or methamphetamines as the single active ingredient or in combination with each other. Examples of Schedule II controlled substances are opium, morphine, codeine, hydromorphone, methadone, pantopon, meperdine, cocaine, oxycodone, anileridine, oxymorphone, and straight amphetamines and methamphetamines. Also in Schedule II are phenmetrazine, methylphenidate, amobarbital, pentobarbital, secobarbital, etorphine hydrochloride, phenylacetone, and phencyclidine.

Schedule III Substances
The drugs in this schedule have an abuse potential less than that of those in Schedules I and II and include compounds containing limited quantities of certain narcotic drugs and nonnarcotic drugs, such as derivatives of barbituric acid, except those that are listed in another schedule, glutethimide, methyprylon, chlorhexadol, sulfondiethylmethane, sulfonmethane, nalorphine, benzphetamine, chlorphentermine, clortermine, mazindol, and phendimetrazine. Paregoric is in the schedule as well. Any suppository dosage form containing amobarbital, secobarbital, or pentobarbital is in this schedule.

Schedule IV Substances
The drugs in this schedule have an abuse potential less than that of those listed in Schedule III and include such drugs as barbital, phenobarbital, methylphenobarbital, chloral betaine, chloral hydrate, ethchlorvynol, ethinamate, meprobamate, paraldehyde, methohexital, fenfluramine, diethylpropion, phentermine, dextropropoxyphene, pentazocine, mebutamate, chlordiazepoxide, diazepam, oxazepam, clorazepate, flurazepam, clonazepam, prazepam, alprazolam, halazepam, temazepam, triazolam, and lorazepam.

Schedule V Substances
The drugs in this schedule have an abuse potential less than that of those listed in Schedule IV and consist of preparations containing moderate, limited quantities of certain narcotic drugs, generally for antitussive and antidiarrheal purposes, which may be distributed without a prescription order.

Adapted from Drug Enforcement, July 1985.

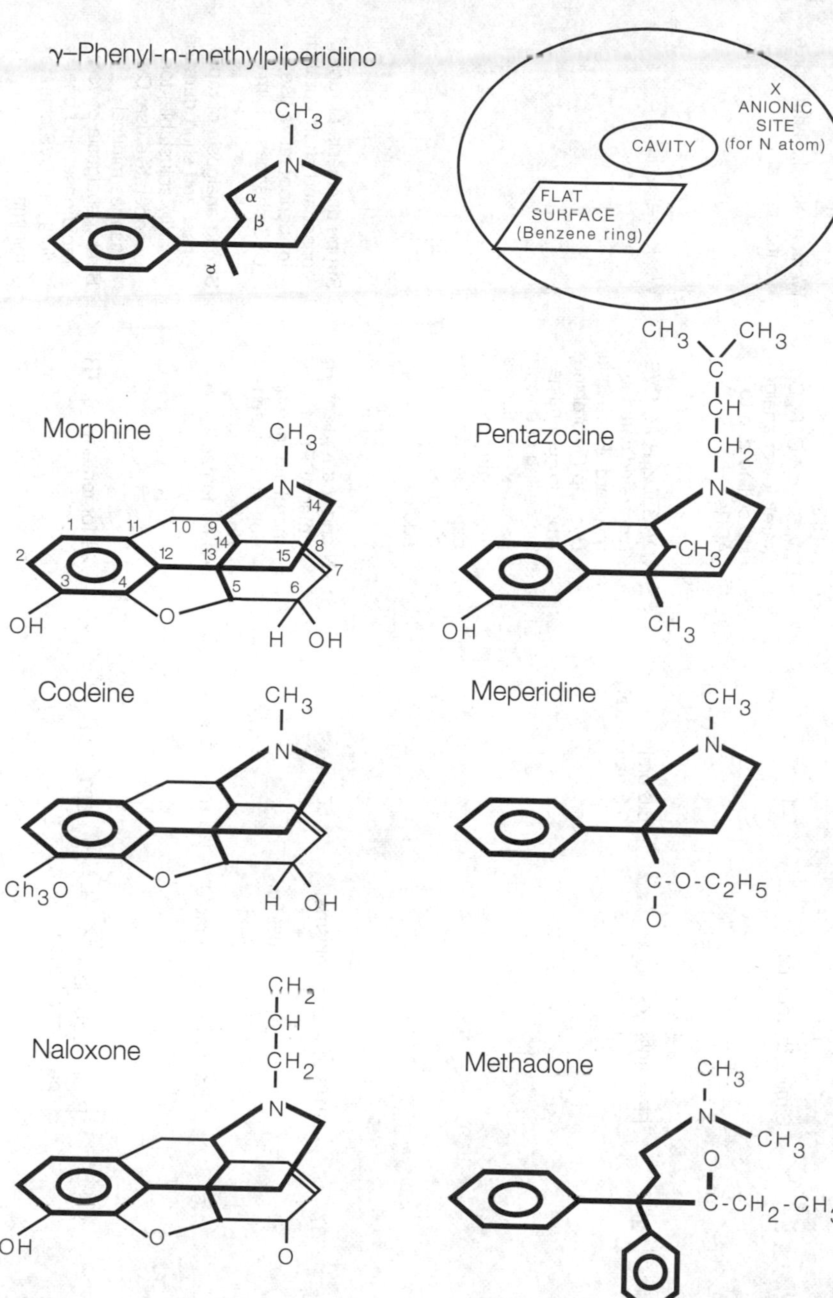

Figure 25–1 Structural formulas of some opioids. **Top left:** Note that γ-phenyl-*N*-methylpiperidine forms the common chemical "backbone" in all the compounds shown, although in some, for example, methadone, the piperidine ring has been opened. **Top right:** shows the main features of the opioid receptor. The main topographic features of the receptor are shown and by mentally transposing the formula of, for example, pentazocine over the diagram, it becomes evident how the main parts of the chemical structure relate to the key areas of the receptor. (From Thompson JW. Clinical pharmacology of opioid agonists and partial agonists. In: Doyle D, ed. *Opioids in the Treatment of Cancer Pain.* International Congress and Symposium Series No. 146. London: (Royal Society of Medicine Services, 1990: 17–38.)

phenothiazines) increase the conversion of meperidine to normeperidine,[6] a proconvulsant.

Withdrawal Syndrome Treatment

Diagnostic criteria for opioid withdrawal of the American Psychiatric Association are listed in Table 25–9.

Clonidine (Catapres)

An initial study with clonidine hydrochloride and naltrexone hydrochloride given in combination appeared to aid 12 of 14 heroin users to withdraw successfully from opioids.[7–10] Clonidine ameliorates symptoms of the opioid withdrawal syndrome mediated via noradrenergic pathways such as watery eyes, runny nose, sweating, diarrhea, chills, and goose flesh. Bone and muscle pain, insomnia, and craving for the euphoriant effect of opioids are not relieved by clonidine or its structural analog lofexidine (licensed in the United Kingdom).[11]

Nitrous Oxide

Withdrawal from alcohol and opioids has been treated with promising results with nitrous oxide inhalation.[12–14] The gas is given on one occasion only as follows: 20 minutes oxygen, 20 minutes carefully titrated nitrous oxide, 20 minutes oxygen washout period. The patient is fully conscious throughout. Further studies and evaluation of its dangers are indicated before this method passes into routine use. Experience has been restricted to adults.

Table 25–2
Comparative Data on Some Opioids in Clinical Use

Drug and Dose (oral or other)	Duration of Action (h)	% Protein Bound	$t_{1/2\beta}$ (h)	Elimination	Analgesic Potency (morphine-1)	Unwanted Effects (ADRs)	Comments
Weak Analgesic							
μ Agonists							
Codeine methylmorphine 10–60 mg	4	7	3	A prodrug; 10% demethylated to morphine	0.08	N, V, S, *Dz*, C, B, R, Dp (rare); lower analgesic ceiling due to ADRs	Weak analgesic; antitussive; antidiarrheal
Dihydrocodeine) 30–60 mg	4		3	Similar to codeine	0.1	N, V, S, *Dz*,* C, R, Dp (rare); lower analgesic ceiling due to ADRs	Weak analgesic; antitussive; antidiarrheal
Mixed κ and σ Agonist and μ Antagonist							
Pentazocine (Fortral) 25–100 mg oral 30–60 mg parenteral	2	60–70	2	FPM 80%; O + G	0.6 oral 0.3 parenteral	N, V, S, *Dz*, P, *M*, CVS (contraindicated in myocardial ischemia), Dys, Dp (nalorphine type); lower analgesic ceiling due to partial κ-agonist; partial μ-antagonism can precipitate morphine withdrawal in addict	Weak analgesic
Strong-Analgesic, Short-Acting							
μ Agonists							
Fentanyl (Sublimaze) 50–200 μg IV spontaneous respirations 0.3–0.5 mg IV assisted respirations	0.5	84	37	91% ionized in plasma; rapid hepatic metabolism; <10% unchanged	50	N and V ambulant; *R*; other ADRs of morphine; cumulation on repeated doses	Strong analgesia of rapid onset and short duration; for perioperative use; CVS changes minimal
Alfentanil (Rapifen) 500 μg IV (over 30s) +250 μg/4–5 min IV	0.3	92	1.6	89% un-ionized in rapid hepatic metabolism	16.5	As for fentanyl	Strong analgesia of rapid onset and short duration; readily adjustable; for perioperative use; CVS changes minimal
Sufentanil	Minutes		2.5	Rapid redistribution; hepatic metabolism	600–700	As for fentanyl; S, TR	Strong analgesia of very rapid onset and brief duration; CVS changes minimal
Strong Analgesic, Long-Acting							
μ Agonists							
Morphine 8–20 mg	4	34	3	Renal hepatic Cg	1	N, V, S, C, R, Mi, Dp	Strong and effective analgesic that remains the standard of reference

Papaveretum (Omnopon) 10–20 mg	As for morphine		As for morphine		0.5	Indistinguishable from morphine	Contains 50% morphine, codeine 2.5–5%, narcotine 16–22%, and papaverine 2.5–7% as hydrochlorides; It has been claimed that this mixture of alkaloids causes less respiratory depression than morphine alone this is unsubstantiated
Diamorphine, (Diacetylmorphine, heroin) 5–10 mg	4		Very short	Rapidly deacetylated to morphine	1.5	As for morphine; but IV acts faster than morphine and causes less V but more S	Strong and effective analgesic (a prodrug) that is orally indistinguishable from morphine; oral solutions unstable
Pethidine (Meperidine, USA) 50–150 mg oral 25–100 mg SC IM	2	65–75	2.5	N-demethylation to norpethidine; then Cg	0.125	N, V, S, ?<C, R, My, Dp; overdose causes tremors and convulsions due to norpethidine	Strong analgesic for acute but not chronic pain; analgesic ceiling lower than that of morphine; atropine-like actions * reduced risk of biliary colic
Methadone (Physeptone) 5–10 mg	6–8	71–87	15† 48–72‡	N-demethylation; cumulation due to long $T_{1/2\beta}$	1† 3‡	N, V, Sr, R, Mi, Dp	Strong analgesic for acute or, more especially, lchronic pain; probably less euphoria but cumulation may produce sedation
Phenazocine (Narphen) 5 mg	6		Presumed long		5	N, V, S < morphine; less C and B; Dp	Strong long-acting analgesic; sublingual use; dependence, but withdrawal less severe than for morphine probably due to cumulation
Levorphanol (Dromoran) 1.5–4.5 mg oral 2–4 mg SC, IM	6		12–16	Cg; cumulation in fat	5	Less N, V; R prolonged with overdose; Dp	Strong long-acting analgesic. Possibly less sedative.
μ Partial Agonist							
Buprenorphine 0.4–0.8 mg sublingual; 0.2–0.6 mg IM	8	96	3.5	N-alkylation and G	25–50	N, V; R ?	Strong long-acting analgesic; sublingual use; naloxone partial reversal; use doxapram for R
κ and σ agonist and μ antagonist							
Nalbuphine (Nubain) 10–20 mg SC, IM, or IV No oral preparation	5		5	N-dealkylation + Cg FPM high	1	N, V, R ceiling effect; S, Dz, Dys, P, headache, dry mouth	Strong analgesic for moderately severe acute pain with limited ceiling; nalorphine-like unwanted effects

ADR, adverse drug reaction; FPM, first-pass metabolism; O, oxidation; G, glucuronidation; Cg, conjugation; N, nausea; V, vomiting; S, sedation; Dz, dizziness; C, constipation; B, biliary colic; R, respiratory depression; Mi, miosis; Dp, dependence; P, psychotomimetic effects; M, mood changes; Dys, dysphoria; TR, truncal rigidity; H, histamine release (urticaria, pruritius, sneezing, hypotension); CVS, cardiovascular changes; My, mydriasis.
*Italics indicate a high incidence.
†Single dose.
‡Repeated dosing.
From Thompson JW. Clinical pharmacology of opioid agonists and partial agonists. In: Doyle D, ed. *Opioids in the Treatment of Cancer Pain.* International Congress and Symposium Series No. 146, London: Royal Society of Medicine Services, 1990:17–38.

Table 25-3
Dosage of Opioid Analgesic Agents for Adults and Children Weighing 50 kg or More Who Have Not Previously Received Opioid Agents*

	Approximate Equianalgesic Dose		Usual Starting Dose for Moderate-to-Severe Pain	
Drug	Oral	Parenteral	Oral	Parenteral
Opioid Agonists†				
Morphine‡	30 mg q3–4h (for around-the-clock dosage) 60 mg q3–4h (for single dose or intermittent dosage)	10 mg q3–4h	30 mg q3–4h	10 mg q3–4h
Controlled-release morphine‡	90–120 mg q12h	Not available	90–120 mg q12h	Not available
Hydromorphone‡	7.5 mg q3–4h	1.5 mg q3–4h	6 mg q3–4h	1.5 mg q3–4h
Levorphanol	4 mg q6–8h	2 mg q6–8h	4 mg q6–8h	2 mg q6–8h
Meperidine	300 mg q2–3h	100 mg q3h	Not recommended	100 mg q3h
Methadone	20 mg q6–8h	10 mg q6–8h	20 mg q6–8h	10 mg q6–8h
Oxymorphone‡	Not available	1 mg q3–4h	Not available	1 mg q3–4h
Combination Opioid–NSAID Preparations§				
Codeine	180–200 mg every 3–4 hr¶	75 mg q3–4h	60 mg q3–4h	60 mg q2h (IM or SC)
Hydrocodone	30 mg q3–4h	Not available	10 mg q3–4h	Not available
Oxycodone	30 mg q3–4h	Not available	10 mg q3–4h	Not available

NSAID, nonsteroidal antiinflammatory drug.
*Published data on the doses that are equivalent in analgesic effect (equianalgesic) to morphine vary. Clinical response is the criterion that must be used for each patient, and adjustment according to clinical response is necessary. Because there is not complete cross-tolerance among these drugs, it is generally necessary to use a lower dose than the equianalgesic dose when changing drugs and to adjust it according to the response once again.
†The recommended doses do not apply to patients with renal or hepatic insufficiency or other conditions affecting drug metabolism and pharmacokinetics.
‡For morphine, hydromorphone, and oxymorphone, rectal administration is an alternative route for patients unable to take oral medications; equianalgesic doses may differ from the oral and parenteral doses, however, because of pharmacokinetic differences. Transdermal fentanyl is also available; dosage conversion has not been calculated with respect to single doses of morphine. See the package insert for conversion calculations.
§When aspirin or acetaminophen is given in combination with an opioid–NSAID preparation, the doses must be adjusted according to the patient's body weight. Aspirin is contraindicated in children in the presence of fever or other viral disease because of its association with Reye's syndrome.
¶Doses of codeine above 65 mg are often not appropriate because analgesia diminishes incrementally with increasing doses, but nausea, constipation, and other side effects increase continually.
From Jacox A, Carr DB, Payne R. New clinical-practice guidelines for the management of pain in patients with cancer. N Engl J Med 1994;330: 651–655.

Table 25-4
Signs of Opiate Addiction*

1. Look for unusual changes in behavior—wide mood swings, periods of depression, anger, and irritability—alternating with periods of euphoria.
2. Addiction is a disease of loneliness and isolation. Addicts quickly withdraw from family, friends, and leisure activities.
3. Denial is the primary symptom of addiction. When directly confronted by a spouse, the addict may become defensive, vehemently rejecting accusations.
4. Domestic strife, fights, and arguments may increase in number and intensity.
5. Addicts need to be near their drug source. For a health care professional addicted to narcotics or other medical drugs, this means long hours at the hospital, even when off duty. For alcoholics, it means frequently calling in sick to work. Alcoholics may disappear without explanation to bars or hiding places to drink secretly.
6. Watch for unexplained overspending, legal problems (such as DWI [driving while intoxicated]), gambling, extramarital affairs, and increased problems at work.
7. Sexual drive may decrease significantly.
8. Pills, syringes, or alcohol bottles found around the house are another sign of addiction.
9. Bloody swabs or tissues found at home may indicate an intravenous drug user.
10. Addicts suddenly may develop the habit of locking themselves in the bathroom or other rooms while they are using drugs.
11. An obvious physical sign of alcoholism is the frequent smell of alcohol on the breath.
12. Narcotic addicts often have pinpoint pupils.
13. They also may display evidence of withdrawal, especially diaphoreses (sweating) and tremors.
14. Weight loss and pale skin are also common.
15. Undetected addicts are found comatose.
16. Untreated addicts are found dead.

*The spouse of an addicted doctor or nurse may detect a number of addiction symptoms, some similar to those found in the workplace and some additional signs. Addiction to potent narcotics progresses very quickly (in a few weeks or months), giving little time for symptoms to develop. For addiction to drugs, signs may appear over a period of years.
From Silverstein JH, Silva DA, Iberti TJ. Opioid addiction in anesthesiology. Anesthesiology 1993;79:354–375. Erratum 1993;79:1160E.

Table 25-5
Medical Syndromes in Opiate Abusers*

Syndrome (Onset and Duration)	Characteristics
Opiate intoxication	Conscious, sedated, "nodding"; mood normal to euphoric; pinpoint pupils; history of recent opiate use
Acute overdose	Unconscious; pinpoint pupils; slow, shallow respirations
Opiate withdrawal	
Anticipatory† (3–4 h after last "fix")	Fear of withdrawal; anxiety; drug craving; drug-seeking behavior
Early (8–10 h after last "fix")	Anxiety, restlessness; yawning; nausea, sweating; nasal stuffiness, rhinorrhea; lacrimation; dilated pupils; stomach cramps; drug-seeking behavior
Fully developed (1–3 d after last "fix")	Severe anxiety; tremor; restlessness; piloerection‡; vomiting, diarrhea; muscle spasm§; muscle pain; increased blood pressure, tachycardia; fever, chills; impulse-driven drug-seeking behavior
Protracted abstinence (may last up to 6 mo)	Hypotension; bradycardia; insomnia; loss of energy, appetite; stimulus-driven opiate cravings

*The times given in the table refer to heroin. Withdrawal will develop more slowly with long-acting opiates such as methadone.
†Anticipatory symptoms begin as the acute effects of heroin begin to subside.
‡The piloerection has given rise to the term *cold turkey.*
§The sudden muscle spasms in the legs have given rise to the term *kicking the habit.*
From Ling W, Wesson DR. Drugs of abuse: Opiates. West J Med 1990;152:565–572.

Table 25-6
Opioid Receptors

Receptor	Location	Actions	Drugs	Comments
Mu	Cerebral cortex (lamina IV), thalamus, periaqueductal gray	Mu-1: analgesia; Mu-2: respiratory depression, physical dependence	Morphine Fentanyl Codeine Naloxone	Classic effects of opioids act at this receptor, Mu-1 present in low concentrations at birth
Delta	Frontal cortex, limbic system, olfactory tubercle	Analgesia, respiratory depression, euphoria, dependence	Enkephalin, endogenous opioid peptides	Functional significance unclear
Kappa	Spinal cord	Spinal analgesia, sedation, low physical dependence	Dynorphin, mixed antagonists (eg, butorphanol, nalbuphine, pentoazocine)	Ceiling effect, may cause withdrawal
Sigma		Psychotomimetic, hallucinations dysphoria Tachycardia, hypertension, respiratory and vasomotor stimulation	Phencyclidine Ketamine Pentazocine	

Adapted from Yaster M, Deshpande JK. Management of pediatric pain with opioid analgesics. J Pediatr 1988;113:421–429.

Table 25-7
Physiologic Effects of Opioids by Organ System

Central nervous system Analgesia Sedation Nausea and vomiting Miosis Antitussive Seizures Dysphoria Respiratory system depression CO_2 response Minute ventilation, rate, tidal volume	Cardiovascular system Bradycardia (fentanyl, morphine) Tachycardia (meperidine) Histamine release (morphine) Gastrointestinal system Decreased motility and peristalsis Increased sphincter tone: Oddi, ileocolic

From Yaster M, Deshpande JK. Management of pediatric pain with opioid analgesics. J Pediatr 1988;113:421–429.

Table 25-8
Diagnostic Criteria for Opioid Dependence and Severity of Opioid Dependence

Opioid Dependence (At least three must be present):
1. Opioids are taken in larger amounts or over a longer period than the person intended.
2. A desire for the drug persists, or the patient has made one or more unsuccessful efforts to cut down or to control opioid use.
3. A great deal of time is spent in activities necessary to obtain opioids (such as theft), taking the drug, or recovering from its effects.
4. The patient is frequently intoxicated or has withdrawal symptoms when expected to fulfill major role obligations at work, school, or home (eg, does not go to work, goes to school or work "high," is intoxicated while taking care of his or her children) or when opioid use is physically hazardous (such as driving under the influence).
5. Important social, occupational, or recreational activities are given up or reduced.
6. Marked tolerance; needs greatly increased amounts of the drug—at least a 50% increase—to achieve the desired effect, or a notably diminished effect occurs with continued use of the same amount.
7. Has characteristic withdrawal symptoms (see opioid withdrawal syndrome in Table 25-9).
8. Opioids are often taken to relieve or avoid withdrawal symptoms.

In addition, some symptoms of the disturbance have persisted for at least a month or have occurred repeatedly over a longer period.

Severity of Opioid Dependence

Mild	Few, if any symptoms are present in excess of those required to make the diagnosis, and the symptoms result in no more than mild impairment in occupational functioning or in usual social activities or relationships with others.
Moderate	Functional impairment of symptoms is between "mild" and "severe."
Severe	Many symptoms are present in excess of those required to make the diagnosis, and the symptoms greatly interfere with occupational functioning or usual social activities or relationships with others.
Partial remission	During the past 6 months, there has been some use of the substance and some symptoms of dependence.
Full remission	During the past 6 months, either there has been no use of opioids, or opioids have been used and there were no symptoms of dependence.

Source: Ling W, Wesson DR. Drugs of abuse: opiates. In: *Addiction Medicine* (Special Issue). West J Med 1990;152:565-572.

Table 25-9
DSM-III-R Diagnostic Criteria for Opioid Withdrawal

A. Cessation of prolonged (several weeks or more) moderate or heavy use of an opioid or reduction in the amount of opioid used (or administration of an opioid antagonist after a brief period of use), followed by at least three of the following:
   1. Craving for an opioid
   2. Nausea or vomiting
   3. Muscle aches
   4. Lacrimation or rhinorrhea
   5. Pupillary dilation, piloerection, or sweating
   6. Diarrhea
   7. Yawning
   8. Fever
   9. Insomnia

B. Not due to any physical or other mental disorder

From the *Diagnostic and Statistical Manual of Mental Disorders.* 3rd ed., rev. Washington, DC: American Psychiatric Association, 1987.

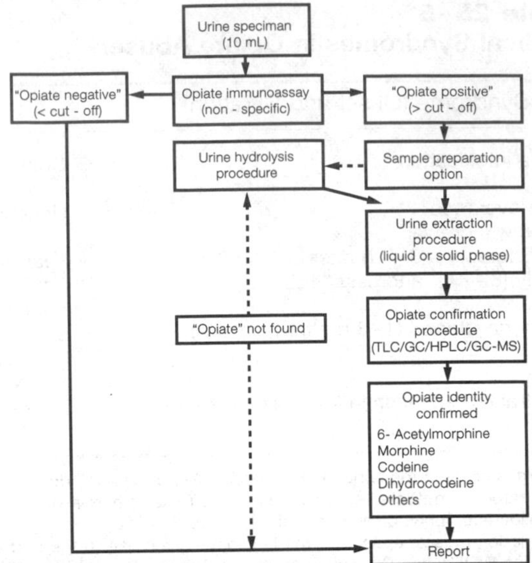

Figure 25-2 Flow diagram of opiate screening procedure. (From Braithwaite RA, Jarvie DR, Minty PSB, et al. Screening for drugs of abuse: I. Opiates, amphetamines and cocaine. Ann Clin Biochem 1995;32:123-153.)

Opiate Screening

Braithwaite and colleagues summarized the opiate screening procedure in a flow diagram (Figure 25-2).[15]

REFERENCES—INTRODUCTION

1. Opiates or opioids. Lancet 1983;1:687. Editorial.
2. Thompson JW. Clinical pharmacology of opioid agonists and partial agonists. In: Doyle D, ed. *Opioids in the Treatment of Cancer Pain.* International Congress and Symposium Series No. 146. London: Royal Society of Medicine Services. 1990:17-38.
3. Jacox A, Carr DB, Payne R. New clinical practice guidelines for the management of pain in patients with cancer. N Engl J Med 1994;330:651-655.
4. Dale G, Fleetwood JA, Weddell A, et al. Beta-endorphin: A factor in "fun run" collapse? Br Med J 1987;294:1004.
5. Ling W, Wesson DR. Drugs of abuse: opiates. In: *Addiction Medicine* (Special Issue). West J Med 1990;152:565-572.
6. Tempelhoft R, White PF. Pro and anticonvulsant effects of anesthetics: Part I. Anesth Analg 1990;70:303-315.
7. Traub SL. Clonidine for opiate withdrawal. Hosp Formul 1985;20:77-80.
8. Washton AM, Resnick RB. Outpatient opiate detoxification with clonidine. J Clin Psychiatry 1982;43:39-41.
9. Bakris GL, Cross PD, Hammarsten JE. The use of clonidine for management of opiate abstinence in a chronic pain patient. Mayo Clin Proc 1982;57:657-660.
10. Kleber HD, Topazan M, Gaspari J, et al. Clonidine and naltrexone in the outpatient treatment of heroin withdrawal. Am J Drug Alcohol Abuse 1987;13:1-17.
11. Cox S, Alcorn R. Lofexidine and opioid withdrawal. Lancet 1995;345:1385-1386.
12. Gillman MA, Lichtigfeld FJ. Analgesic nitrous oxide for alcohol withdrawal: A critical review after 10 year's use. Postgrad Med J 1990;66:543-546.
13. Gillman MA, Lichtigfeld FJ. The drug management of severe alcohol withdrawal syndrome. Postgrad Med 1990;66: 1005-1010.
14. Ojutkangas R. Analgesic nitrous oxide: Rapid, safe therapy for addictive withdrawal. Postgrad Med J 1991;67:1027-1030.
15. Braithwaite RA, Jarvie DR, Minty PSB, et al. Screening for drugs of abuse: I. Opiates, amphetamines and cocaine. Ann Clin Biochem 1995;32:123-153.

ANILERIDINE

Use/Structure/Classification

Anileridine (Leritene) is a synthetic narcotic analgesic similar in structure to but several times more potent than meperidine. Its chemical formula is ethyl 1-(4-aminophenethyl)-4-phenylpiperidine-4-carboxylate. Its empirical formula is $C_{22}H_{28}N_2O_2$ and its molecular weight is 352.5. The CAS number is 144-14-9.[1]

Therapeutic Dose

Anileridine is supplied as the dihydrochloride in 25-mg tablets for oral administration (25–50 mg every 4–6 hours) and as the phosphate in a 25 mg/mL injectable solution (5–10 mg intravenously or 25–50 mg subcutaneously).[2]

Toxicokinetics

Anileridine is metabolized in humans by deesterification and *N*-acetylation. About 5% of a single dose is excreted unchanged in a 24-hour urine.[2] Anileridine is partially metabolized to noranileridine (normeperidine).[3]

Laboratory

Anileridine may be analyzed in body fluids using procedures similar to those used for meperidine or codeine.[2]

Blood levels in two deaths following intentional ingestion were 0.9 μg/mL[4] and 2 μg/mL.[5] (Therapeutic anileridine concentrations in the blood or plasma probably do not exceed 2 μg/mL.)

Treatment

Therapy for overdose is similar to that for meperidine overdose.

REFERENCES—ANILERIDINE

1. Reynolds JEF, ed. *Martindale: The Extra Pharmacopoeia.* 30th ed. London: Pharmaceutical Press, 1993:1067.
2. Baselt RC, Cravey RH. *Disposition of Toxic Drugs and Chemicals in Man.* 3rd ed. Chicago: Year Book, 1989:56–57.
3. Lin SC, Way EL. N-dealkylation of anileridine to normeperidine. J Pharmacol Exp Ther 1965;150:209–215.
4. Peclet C, Rousseau JJ, Rousseau M. Anileridine intoxication. Bull Int Assoc Forens Toxicol 1981;16(1):27–28.
5. Peat MA, Kopjak L. An anileridine death. Bull Int Assoc Forens Toxicol 1979;14(3):19.

BUPRENORPHINE

Use

Buprenorphine (Buprenex, Temgesic), a derivative of thebaine, is an opioid with mixed agonist–antagonist properties that is being investigated as a potential detoxification and maintenance agent for the treatment of opiate dependence.[1] At times of short heroin supply, buprenorphine is the drug of choice.[2] Buprenorphine is a partial mu agonist and a potent antagonist at kappa receptor sites. In humans, buprenorphine produces typical mu-opioid agonist effects of long duration, including analgesia, euphoria, sedation, and pupillary constriction.

Buprenorphine may be an acceptable alternative to methadone for heroin dependence treatment.[3–5]

Clinical Presentation

One patient ingested 35 to 40, 0.4-mg tablets of buprenorphine (14–16 mg) and survived.[6] Respiratory depression did not occur; the patient was conscious on admission, and became somewhat drowsy.[6] Psychotomimetic symptoms are experienced after total doses of 900 to 1200 μg of buprenorphine administered epidurally.[7] Prolonged nausea and vomiting develop after intravenous buprenorphine.[8] A dose of 0.8 mg of sublingual buprenorphine for postoperative analgesia was associated in one case with late-onset, prolonged respiratory depression,[9] whereas 0.4 mg of sublingual buprenorphine was not followed by any changes in respiratory function in one randomized double-blind, placebo study.[10]

Drug Abuse

Reports of buprenorphine abuse from India,[11] New Zealand, Australia, Germany, and Britain[12,13] suggest an increasing trend. In the United Kingdom, buprenorphine sublingual tablets are crushed and snorted like snuff.[14]

Laboratory

Analytical Methods

A radioimmunoassay method is available for quantitation of buprenorphine in urine. It has sensitivity to concentrations of 1 ng/mL.[15] Buprenorphine and its major metabolite *N*-desalkylbuprenorphine can be simultaneously determined in urine by reverse-phase high-performance liquid chromatography with urine level electrochemical detection. The sensitivity of the assay is 0.2 ng/mL for unconjugated buprenorphine and 0.15 ng/mL for the metabolite.

Urine Levels

Buprenorphine and its dealkylated metabolite norbuprenorphine can be detected in urine only within 1 to 3 days of intake. After sublingual administration, doses of 400 μg led to mean total urine buprenorphine concentrations of 12.7 ng/mL; 800 μg led to 14.0 ng/mL; 1600 μg led to 27.2 ng/mL; and 2000 μg led to 11.3 ng/mL.[16]

Blood Levels

Adults were given 0.4-mg sublingual doses of buprenorphine 3 hours after a 0.3-mg intravenous dose. Plasma buprenorphine concentration 2 hours after the sublingual dose were 450 to 840 ng/mL, decreasing to 470 μg/mL in 6.5 hours and 310 ng/mL in 10 hours.[17]

Hair Levels

Preliminary results suggest a dose–response relationship between hair concentration and administered dose.[18] Hair analysis may be useful but data confirming this are scarce. Detection limits by coulometry are 0.01 ng/mL for norbuprenorphine and 0.02 ng/mL for buprenorphine.[19]

REFERENCES—BUPRENORPHINE

1. Heel RC, Brogden RN, Speight TM, et al. Buprenorphine: A review. Drugs 1979;17:82–110.
2. Debrabandere L, Van Boven M, Daenens P. Development of a fluoroimmunoassay for the detection of buprenorphine in urine. J Forens Sci 1995;40:250–253.
3. Resnick RB, Galanter M, Pycha C, et al. Buprenorphine: An alternative to methadone for heroin dependency treatment. Psychopharmacol Bull 1993;28:109–113.
4. Johnson RE, Cone EJ, Hemingfield JE, Fudala PJ. Use of buprenorphine in the treatment of opiate addiction: I. Psychologic and behavioral effects during a rapid dose induction. Clin Pharmacol Ther 1989;46:335–347.
5. Johnson RE, Jaffe JH, Fudala PJ. A controlled trial of buprenorphine treatment for opioid dependence. JAMA 1992; 287:2750–2755.
6. Banks CD. Overdosage of buprenorphine: Case Report. NZ Med J 1979;89:255–256.
7. MacEvilly M, O'Caurall C. Hallucinations after epidural buprenorphine. Br Med J 1989;298:928–929.
8. Fullerton T, Tinu EG, Kolski GB, Bertius JS. Prolonged nausea and vomiting associated with buprenorphine. Pharmacotherapy 1991;11:90–93.
9. Thorn SE, Rowal N, Wennhager M. Prolonged respiratory depression caused by sublingual buprenorphine. Lancet 1988; 1:179–180.
10. Tantucci C, Paoletti F, Bruni B, et al. Acute respiratory effects of sublingual buprenorphine: Comparison with intramuscular morphine. Int J Clin Pharmacol Ther Toxicol 1992;30:202–207.
11. Chowdhury AN, Chowdhury S. Buprenorphine abuse: Report from India. Br J Addict 1990;85:1349–1350.
12. Strang J. Abuse of buprenorphine (Temgesic) by snorting. Br Med J 1991;302:969.
13. Sakol MS, Stark C, Sykes R. Buprenorphine and temazepam abuse by drug takers in Glasgow: An increase. Br J Addict 1989;84:439–441.
14. O'Connor JJ, Moloney E, Travers R, Campbell A. Buprenorphine abuse among opiate addicts. Br J Addict 1988;83: 1085–1087.
15. Debrabandere L, Van Boven M, Daenens P. Analysis of buprenorphine in urine specimens. J Forens Sci 1991;37: 82–89.
16. Hand CW, Ryan KE, Dutt SK, et al. Radioimmunoassay of buprenorphine in urine: Studies in patients and in a drug clinic. J Anal Toxicol 1989;33:100–104.
17. Bullingham RES, McQuay HJ, Porter EJB, et al. Sublingual buprenorphine used postoperatively: Ten hour plasma drug concentration analysis. Br J Clin Pharm 1982;13:665–673.
18. Kintz P, Cirimele V, Edel Y, et al. Hair analysis for buprenorphine and its dealkylated metabolite by RIA and confirmation by LC/ECD. J Forens Sci 1994;39:1497–1503.
19. Kintz P, Tracqin A, Pfitzinger H, Mangin P. Hair analysis for buprenorphine and its dealkylated metabolites. In: *Proceedings, American Academy of Forensic Sciences, February 1994:*192 (Abstract K25).

BUTORPHANOL TARTRATE

Use/Product Formulation

Studies with butorphanol (Stadol) (Figure 25–3) administered in doses of 0.5 to 3 mg appear to indicate effectiveness in the acute treatment of migraine, severe headaches, cancer pain, musculoskeletal pain, and postcesarean section pain.

Butorphanol tartrate is available as a nasal spray (Stadol-NS) and has been approved by the U.S. Food and Drug Administration to be used in any type of pain for which an opioid analgesic is appropriate. It is being marketed for migraine headache and postoperative pain.[1]

Clinical Presentation

Use of butorphanol nasal spray for migraine treatment has been associated with hallucinations, feelings of being "extremely stoned" or "stuporous," and feelings of inability to move for hours.[2] Sedation, dizziness, nausea, vomiting, insomnia, and nasal congestion have been observed.[3] Hypotension, syncope, and severe hypertension have been reported.[1]

Overdose may induce respiratory depression and cardiovascular changes including increased pulmonary artery pressure, pulmonary wedge pressure, left ventricular end-diastolic pressure, systemic arterial pressure, and pulmonary vascular resistance.[4]

Laboratory

Analytical Methods

Butorphanol has been analyzed in biological fluids by radioimmunoassay,[5] electron-capture gas chromatography

Figure 25–3 Structural formulas of dezocine, pentazocine, butorphanol, and morphine. (From O'Brien JJ, Benfield P. Dezocine: A preliminary review of its pharmacodynamic and pharmacokinetic properties, and therapeutic efficacy. Drugs 1989;38:226–248.)

with heptafluorobutynic anhydride derivatization,[6,7] and gas chromatography–mass spectrometry and trimethylsilyl derivatization.[5]

Blood Levels

A 1-mg intravenous injection of butorphanol is followed within 15 minutes by plasma butorphanol concentrations up to 1.3 μg/L, declining to 0.6 μg/L by 1 hour.[6] One hour after a 2-mg intravenous injection, the serum concentration averages 1.5 μg/L.[5] A 2-mg intramuscular dose produces a peak plasma level of 2 μg/L in 45 minutes, declining to 1.3 μg/L by 4 hours.[6] Death from cardiopulmonary arrest has followed use of butorphanol in surgery.[8] the butorphanol blood level was 6 μg/L.[5]

Treatment

Naloxone, oxygen, intravenous fluids, vasopressors, controlled respiration, gastric lavage, and activated charcoal are indicated.

REFERENCES—BUTORPHANOL TARTRATE

1. Butorphanol nasal spray for pain. Med Lett Drugs Ther 1993; 35(909):105–106.
2. Robbins L. Stadol[R] nasal spray: Treatment for migraine? Headache 1993;33:220.
3. *Physicians' Desk Reference.* 49th ed. Montvale, NJ: Medical Economics, 1994:739–742.
4. Heel RC, Brogden RN, Speight TM, et al. Butorphanol: A review of its pharmacological properties and therapeutic efficacy. Drugs 1978;16:473–505.
5. Pittman KA, Smyth RD, Mayol RF. Serum levels of butorphanol by radioimmunoassay. J Pharm Sci 1980;69:160–163.
6. Gaver RC, Vasiljer M, Wong H, et al. Disposition of parenteral butorphanol in man. Drug Metab Disp 1980;8:230–235.
7. Pfeffer M, Smyth RD, Pittman KA, Nardella PA. Pharmacokinetics of subcutaneous and intramuscular butorphanol in dogs. J Pharm Sci 1980;69:801–803.
8. Hearn WL, Rose S, Andollo W, Hime G. Fatality associated with enflurane and butorphanol. In: *Proceedings, American Academy of Forensic Sciences, 43rd Annual Meeting, February 18–23, 1991:* Abstract K35.

CODEINE (METHYLMORPHINE), HYDROCODONE, AND DIHYDROCODEINE

Source

Illicit laboratories in New Zealand have produced morphine and heroin from commercially available codeine-based pharmaceutical preparations. The codeine demethylation procedure is based on the use of pyridine hydrochloride. Simple laboratory equipment and reagents are required. These can be used by individuals with little or no chemical background following a recipe-like procedure. The process yields a characteristic product known as "homebake."[1]

Toxicokinetics

After a single 30-mg dose of codeine, maximum plasma concentrations are observed at about 1 hour (codeine) and 1.28 hours (codeine 6-glucuronide).[2] Activity of the glucuronide has not yet been determined.

Elimination

Codeine is metabolized to codeine-6-glucuronide (80%), norcodeine (2%), morphine (0.5%), morphine-3-glucuronide (2%), morphine-6-glucuronide (0.8%), and normorphine (2.5%). Some individuals cannot O-dealkylate codeine into morphine; they lack the required cytochrome P450 II DC isoenzyme.[3]

Morphine-6-glucuronide has a stronger analgesic effect than morphine itself. Its plasma concentration is higher than that of morphine. Codeine-6-glucuronide probably possesses an activity similar to codeine. The plasma concentration of codeine-6-glucuronide is probably higher than that of codeine.

The half-life of codeine is 1.5 hours, that of codeine-7-glucuronide is 2.75 hours, that of morphine-3-glucuronide is 2.75 hours, and that of morphine-3-glucuronide is 1.7 hours. The systemic clearance of codeine is 2300 mL/min; the renal clearance is 94 mL/min, and that of codeine-6-glucuronide is about 120 mL/min. Protein binding of codeine is 56% and that of codeine-6-glucuronide, 34%.[3]

Urine Codeine Levels

For the first 10 to 20 hours following an ingestion of codeine, the urinary codeine:morphine ratio is greater than 1. The presence of norcodeine indicates that codeine was taken as the primary drug. Between 20 and 40 hours after codeine ingestion, the ratio of codeine to morphine is less than 1 and norcodeine is not detectable. Three days after codeine use, the urine shows only morphine and is identical to those following heroin or morphine use.[4]

The renal clearance of codeine is about 180 mL/min and is inversely correlated with urine pH. The renal clearance of codeine glucuronide is about 50 mL/min and is not correlated with urine pH. After a single dose, 12% is excreted in the urine as unchanged codeine.[2] Detection times for total codeine and total morphine after 60- and 120-mg doses, respectively, are 27 and 39 hours (total codeine) and 23 and 34 hours (total morphine). Urine codeine:morphine ratios are not reliable indices of the type of opiate exposure.[5]

Clinical Presentation

Codeine–Glutethimide Combinations

In northwest Pennsylvania, oral combinations of glutethimide and codeine are known as "sets." Nine fatalities were reported between 1985 and 1987 due to this combination. All deaths occurred in known "sets" abusers.[6,7]

Dihydrocodeine

Dihydrocodeine use (10–16 mg) has been followed by acute renal failure.[8]

Laboratory

Analytical Methods

Codeine. Codeine, norcodeine, morphine, and normorphine with their corresponding *O*-glucuronide conjugates can be quantitated in human plasma and urine by high-performance liquid chromatography with electrochemical detection. The detection limits for codeine, codeine-6-glucuronide, and norcodeine are 5 ng/mL in plasma and 25 ng/mL in urine. Detection limits for morphine are 5 ng/mL in plasma and 20 ng/mL in urine; for morphine-3-glucuronide, 10 ng/mL in plasma and 70 ng/mL in urine, and for morphine-6-glucuronide, 5 ng/mL in plasma and 50 ng/mL in urine.[9,10]

Dihydrocodeine. One method for isolation and identification of dihydrocodeine uses gas chromatography and mass spectrometry.[11] Blood and urine concentrations may be quantitated by gas chromatography with a nitrogen–phosphorus detector.[12]

Hydrocodone. A procedure for the determination of hydrocodone (dihydrocodeine) in serum uses electron-capture gas chromatography with pentafluorophenylhydrazine derivatives. The method is sensitive to 1 ng/mL of hydrocodone in serum.[13]

Blood Levels

Dihydrocodeine. An adult dihydrocodeine suicide victim exhibited a blood dihydrocodeine level of 40 μg/mL.[12,14]

Hydrocodone. On oral administration of 10 mg to normal humans, hydrocodone concentration reaches a maximum of about 24 ng/mL in 2.3 hours.[15] A 3-year-old received 15 mg of hydrocodone, developed respiratory depression, and died. The blood concentration of hydrocodone was 200 ng/mL.[16,17] Two fatal overdoses in adults were associated with blood hydrocodone concentrations of 300 ng/mL.[18]

Treatment

Overt signs of opioid toxicity respond to naloxone.[19]

REFERENCES—CODEINE (METHYLMORPHINE), HYDROCODONE, AND DIHYDROCODEINE

1. Bedford KR, Nolan SL, Onrust R, Siegers JD. The illicit preparation of morphine and heroin from pharmaceutical products containing codeine: 'Homebake' Laboratories in New Zealand. Forens Sci Int 1987;34:197–204.
2. Chen ZR, Somagy AA, Reynolds G, Bochner F. Disposition and metabolism of codeine after single and chronic doses in one poor and seven extensive metabolisers. Br J Clin Pharmacol 1991;31:381–392.
3. Vree TB, Verwey-Van Wissen CPWGM. Pharmacokinetics and metabolism of codeine in humans. Biopharm Drug Dispos 1991;13:445–460.
4. Posey BL, Kimble SN. High-performance liquid chromatographic study of codeine, norcodeine and morphine is indication of codeine ingestion. J Anal Toxicol 1984;8:68–74.
5. Cone EJ, Welch F, Paul BD, Mitchel JM. Forensic drug testing for opiates: III. Urinary excretion rates of morphine and codeine following codeine administration. J Anal Toxicol 1991;15:161–166.
6. Havier RG, Lin R. Deaths as a result of a combination of codeine and glutethimide. J Forens Sci 1985;30:563–566.
7. Bender FH, Cooper JV, Dreyfus R. Fatalities associated with an acute overdose of glutethimide (Doriden) and codeine. Vet Hum Toxicol 1988;30:332–333.
8. Park GR, Shelly MP, Ammum K, Roberts P. Dihydrocodeine: A reversible cause of renal failure? Eur J Anaesthesiol 1989;6:303–334.
9. Gjerde H, Fongen U, Gundersen H, Christophersen AS. Evaluation of a method for simultaneous quantification of codeine, ethylmorphine and morphine in blood. Forens Sci Int 1991;51:105–110.
10. Verwez-Van Wissen CPWGM, Koopman-Kimenai PM. Direct determination of codeine, norcodeine, morphine and normorphine with their corresponding *O*-glucuronide conjugates by high-performance liquid chromatography with electrochemical detection. J Chromatogr Biomed Appl 1991;570:309–320.
11. Nakamura GR, Stoll WJ, Meeks RD. Analysis of dihydrocodeine for urine using Sep-Pak^R C_{18} cartridges for sample cleanup. J Forens Sci 1987;32:535–538.
12. Dawling S, Widdop B. A fatal case involving dihydrocodeine. Bull Int Assoc Forens Toxicol 1981;16(1):25–26.
13. Barnhart JW, Caldwell WJ. Gas chromatographic determination of hydrocodone in serum. J Chromatogr 1977;130:234–249.
14. Rogers JF, Findlay JWA, Hill JH, et al. Codeine disposition in smokers and non-smokers. Clin Pharmacol Ther 1982;32:218–227.
15. Baselt R, Cravey RH. A compendium of therapeutic and toxic concentrations of toxicologically significant drugs in human biofluids. J Anal Toxicol 1977;1:81–103.
16. Vivian D. Three deaths due to hydrocodone in a resin complex cough medicine. Drug Intell Clin Pharmacol 1979;13:445–446.
17. Morrow PL, Faris EC. Death associated with inadvertent hydrocodone overdose in a child with a respiratory tract infection. Am J Forens Med Pathol 1987;8:60–63.
18. Park JL, Nakamura GR, Griesimer EG, et al. Hydromorphine detected in bile following hydrocodone ingestion. J Forens Sci 1982;27:223–224.
19. Hart LM, Dean BS, Krenzelok EP. Massive pediatric codeine overdose with survival. Vet Hum Toxicol 1993;35:341.

DESIGNER DRUGS: SYNTHETIC DRUGS OF ABUSE

I. FENTANYL, FENTANYL DERIVATIVES, AND "CHINA WHITE"

Designer drugs" (Table 25–10) are chemical substances intended for recreational use that have been modified from legitimate pharmaceutical agents.[1] Such forms of these chemicals are popular with illicit drug users because they can circumvent legal restrictions.[2] They are usually stronger and cheaper than the parent compound and can be easily produced by clandestine laboratories.[3] Initially these drugs were sufficiently different from parent compounds to render them temporarily immune from the control of the Drug Enforcement Agency.[4,5] Until a drug was isolated, studied, and scheduled, no laws could apply to it. Although this is no longer possible under the Controlled Substances Analogue (CSA) Enforcement Act of 1986, these substances continue to appear on the street, posing a serious health risk.[6] Emergency and intensive care physicians became aware of overdoses with these products, the characteristics of which

Table 25–10
Designer Drugs

Phenylethylamines (Mescaline IV)
Amphetamines
Methamphetamine: speed, crank meth, crystal, ice
3,4-Methylenedioxymethamphetamine (MDMA): ecstasy, Adam, XTC, MDM, M&M
3,4-Methylenedioxyamphetamine (MDA): love drug
Tetramethoxyamphetamine (TMA-2)
2,5-Dimethoxy-4-methylamphetamine (DOM)
p-Methoxyamphetamine (PMA)
Brom-DOM (DOB)
4-Bromo-2, 5-methoxyloxyphenylethylamine (2-CB/MFT)
3,4-Methylenedioxyethamphetamine (MDEA); Eve
4-Methylaminorex
Synthetic opioid derivatives
  Fentanyl derivatives
    α-Methylfentanyl: China White
    3-Methylfentanyl
  Meperidine derivatives
    1-Methyl-4-phenyl-4-propionoxypiperidine (MPPP)
    1-Methyl-4-phenyl-1,2,3,6-tetrahydropyridine (MPTP)
Arylhexylamines
  Phencyclidine (PCP)
Methaqualone derivatives
  Mecloqualone
  Nitromethaqualone

they had not seen before. For example, in the late fall of 1988, 18 people died as a result of a China-White (fentanyl derivative) outbreak in the city of Pittsburgh.[7] (See also Chapter 56.)

The concept of designer drugs does not include new forms or new dosing routes of old drugs, such as cocaine used in the crystalline freebase form (crack). It also does not include legal, although abused, alternatives to controlled substances, for example, phenylpropanolamine, ephedrine, caffeine, and butylnitrite. It does not include drug combinations such as T's and Blues (pentazocine and tripelennamine), speedballs (cocaine or amphetamine and heroin), and Star Search (cocaine and phencyclidine).[8] Few of these compounds are currently in use. Those in use in the San Francisco area include U4EUh (ie, euphoria).[8]

Some criteria for diagnosing designer drug intoxication are included in the revised third edition of the *Diagnostic and Statistical Manual of Mental Disorders* (DSM-III-R).[9]

Clandestine Drug Laboratories

What Is a Clandestine Drug Laboratory

The clandestine drug laboratory or clan lab is a mini-chemical laboratory designed for one purpose: to make deadly, illegal drugs quickly and cheaply[10] (Table 25–11). Clan lab chemists can produce lysergic acid diethylamide (LSD), synthetic heroin, and other drugs, but their drug of choice is methamphetamine, commonly called speed or crank.

What Do You Do If You Spot a Clan Lab

1. Leave the area at once. Stay at least 500 feet away from any suspected clandestine laboratory.
2. Immediately contact the police or sheriff.
3. Do not investigate. Most law enforcement agencies have special narcotics teams.

Table 25–11
Detection of a Clandestine (Clan) Lab

Signs of a Possible Lab
1. Strong or unusual chemical odors; laboratory equipment (glass tubes, beakers, Bunsen burners, funnels)
2. Fortifications on houses or outbuildings, such as heavily barred windows or doors
3. Chemical cans or drums in the front or back yard (these containers often have the labels marked or painted over)
4. Automobile or foot traffic at all hours of the day or night
5. People going outside the building only long enough to smoke, especially at motels or during bad weather
6. New high fences with no visible livestock or animals

Locations of Clan Labs
1. Rural rentals with absentee landlords (homes, barns, mobile homes, or outbuildings)
2. Lower-income urban homes or apartment rentals with absentee landlords
3. Trailers and motor homes
4. Motel rooms
5. Houseboats and mini-storage units (these are used to store chemicals, drugs, lab equipment and weapons)

Booby Traps
1. Exterior/interior trip wires designed to set off alarms
2. Exterior/interior trip wires designed to set off explosive or toxic chemical devices
3. Hidden pungee sticks (these are buried wooden plants with large nails or spikes protruding upward)
4. Light switches, refrigerators, VCRs, or other electrical appliances wired to explosive devices

Dangers

Explosion and fire are probably the most common hazards. Actions such as knocking over the wrong container, having a lit cigarette, and switching on electrical equipment that makes a simple spark are enough to cause an explosion.

Fentanyl

Fentanyl (Fig. 25–4) has been sniffed and smoked, rubbed on the buccal mucosa, and gargled. Overdosage with inhaled fentanyl as with all opioids, by any route, can be treated with naloxone.[11] Patients are often found unconscious with needles and attached syringes in their antecubital vein. (See also Chapter 56 for commercial fentanyl anesthetics.)

Fentanyl Analogs

Individuals having access to fentanyl in the operating room and intensive care areas of the hospital may be potential users. Think of this when health care providers present to the emergency department with signs and symptoms of drug overdose. Fentanyl and its designer derivatives (*para*-fluorofentanyl, α-methylfentanyl, and 3-methylfentanyl) are often more potent than street heroin or morphine.[12]

A dramatic rise in unintentional drug overdose deaths (16) in Allegheny County, Pennsylvania, in 1988 was traced to an illicit manufacturer of 3-methylfentanyl (China White).[13] Other drugs detected in individuals dying of 3-methylfentanyl included cocaine, alcohol, morphine, qui-

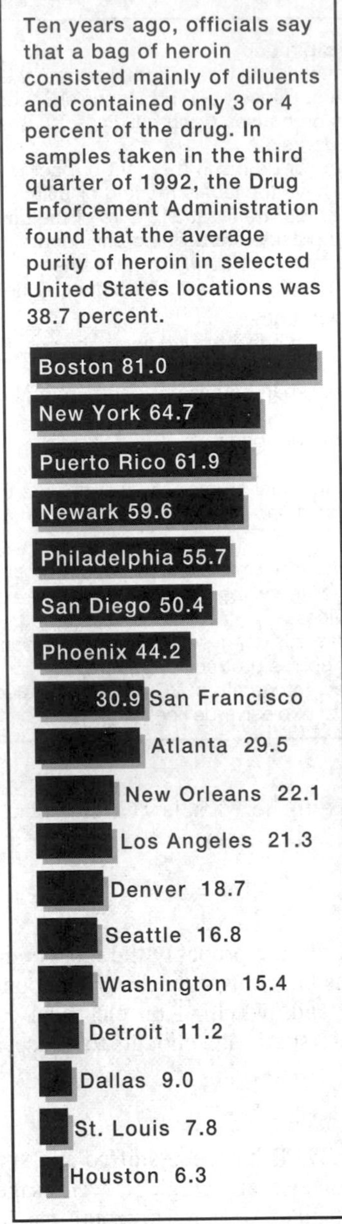

Figure 25–4 Purity of heroin available on the street as of 1992. (Source: Drug Enforcement Administration. Reprinted from Treaster JB. With supply and purity up heroin use expands. NY Times, August 1, 1993.)

nine, benzodiazepine, propoxyphene, acetaminophen, codeine, and an antidepressant[14] (see Laboratory). The minimal lethal dose of α-methylfentanyl is 125 μg; that of *p*-fluorofentanyl, 250 μg; and that of 3-methylfentanyl, a few micrograms (6000 × potency of morphine).[12]

Toxicokinetics

Elimination

Secondary peaks in the plasma concentration of fentanyl and sufentanil have been observed.[15]

Drug Interactions

Erythromycin may reduce alfentanil clearance.[16] Alfentanil potentiates midazolam-induced unconsciousness.[17] Regular alcohol consumption may lead to pharmacodynamic tolerance to alfentanil.[18] Alcohol and drugs that produce respiratory or central nervous system depression may potentiate the effect of fentanyl or its analogs.

Table 25–12 summarizes toxicokinetic data for fentanyl, alfentanil, and sufentanil.[19]

Mechanism of Action

The fentanyl derivatives quickly cross the blood–brain barrier. In the central nervous system, they act as mu receptor agonists, leading to respiratory insufficiency or arrest, profound central nervous system depression, and extreme euphoria.

Clinical Presentation

Many patients who are given fentanyl (50–75 μg), sufentanil (15 μg), or alfentanil (500 μg) begin to cough before any other drug is given.[20] Seizurelike activity may be associated not only with fentanyl but also with alfentanil and sufentanil during induction of anesthesia as well as postoperatively.[21,22] Dose-related muscular rigidity of the chest wall, trunk, and extremities may be observed.

Respiratory arrest occurred after a single caudal epidural dose of sufentanil 50 μg and bupivacaine 0.25% with epinephrine 1 : 200,000, 20 mL for repair of a perineal fistula; the patient responded to oxygen and naloxone.[23] Respiratory arrest can follow intravenous administration of a transdermal fentanyl patch (total dose/patch-5 mg) after aspiration of its contents.[24] "Tango and Cash" is the name given to a batch

Table 25–12
Toxicokinetic Data for the Fentanyl Derivatives

Analog	$t_{1/2}$ *(min)* α	$t_{1/2}$ *(min)* β	Clearance (mL/min)	Volume of Distribution (L/kg)
Fentanyl	13–28	90–360	150–575	60–300
Alfentanil	16	100	178–560	40–70
Sufentanil	17	150	730	150

Adapted from Poklis A. Fentanyl: A review for clinical and analytical toxicologists. Clin Toxicol 1995;33:439–447.

of methylfentanyl-containing drugs that resulted in a number of deaths on the East Coast in early 1991.[25]

Dependence

Oral fentanyl citrate results in a rapid increase in plasma fentanyl concentration, with accompanying dose-related sedation, analgesia, respiratory depression, opioid side effects (pruritus, nausea, vomiting), and difficulty in micturition. Hays and colleagues suggest that oral fentanyl may also be abused by anesthesia and operating room personnel.[26]

Fentanyl-Related Deaths

Henderson has reviewed 112 overdose deaths related to fentanyl and its analogs. Nearly all the deaths occurred in California. The incidence has decreased markedly since 1984, but clandestine laboratories have been discovered outside of California. Pulmonary edema and congestion and needle puncture sites were consistent postmortem findings. Morphine and codeine were seldom found in the blood, suggesting that the victims had not used heroin recently. Factors that heighten the risk of death for the fentanyl user are diminished tolerance and concurrent use of ethanol. Mean fentanyl concentrations in the blood (3.0 ng/mL) and urine (3.9 ng/mL) were quite low.[27]

Laboratory

A urine screen for opioids may be negative.

Analytical Methods

Alfentanil. An alfentanil radioimmunoassay has been described.[28]

Sufentanil. Sufentanil blood and cerebrospinal fluid concentrations are quantitated by a radioimmunoassay method sensitive to 0.05 ng/mL.[28,29] A gas chromatography–mass spectrometry method is also available.[30]

Fentanyl. A radioimmunoassay assay method with solvent extraction is able to detect 0.2 ng/10 mL urine.[31] A solid-phase[125] radioimmunoassay (Coat-a-Count) can detect fentanyl in blood and urine with a sensitivity to less than 0.2 ng/mL.[32] A gas chromatography/nitrogen-sensitive detection method is sensitive in whole blood assays to 0.25 ng/mL.[33,34]

α-Methylfentanyl and China White Fentanyl Analogs. A radioimmunoassay method modified by Henderson is able to detect α-methylfentanyl at 1 μg/g in powder samples and between 1 and 10 ng/mL in the body fluids of China White in overdose victims.[12,35] The Coat-a-Count solid-phase fentanyl radioimmunoassay can be successfully used as a rapid screening method for China White powder samples. Analogs found by this procedure include, in addition to fentanyl, α-methylfentanyl, fluorofentanyl, 3-methylfentanyl, thienylfentanyl, and 3-methylthienylfentanyl.[36]

Table 25-13
Therapeutic Plasma Levels of Alfentanil, Fentanyl, and Sufentanil

Alfentanil*	Fentanyl	Sufentanil
100–200 ng/mL (superficial surgery) 200–400 ng/mL (intraabdominal surgery)	1–3 ng/mL (analgesia) 4–10 ng/mL (analgesia for surgery combined with nitrous oxide) >20 ng/mL (unconsciousness, satisfactory for anesthesia if used as sole agent†)	0.05–1 ng/mL

*Larijani GE, Goldberg ME. Alfentanil hydrochloride: A new short acting narcotic analgesic for surgical procedures. Clin Pharm 1987;6:275–282.
†Woods M. Opioid agonists and antagonists. In: Woods M, Wood AJJ, eds. *Drugs and Anesthesia: Pharmacology for Anesthesiologists.* Baltimore: Williams & Wilkins 1990:151.

Blood Levels

At about 34 ng/mL fentanyl in plasma, loss of consciousness has been observed.[37] Serum or plasma levels greater than 100 ng/mL fentanyl have been measured after intravenous infusion of high doses to patients.[38] Death was associated with a fentanyl concentration of 17.7 ng/mL[34] (Table 25–13).

Treatment

The duration of respiratory depression following overdosage with fentanyl or its derivatives may be longer than the duration of action of an opioid antagonist.[15] Repeated doses of naloxone may be required. It may be necessary to give up to 10 mg of naloxone by intravenous push before the need to start with a naloxone infusion becomes apparent. Administration of naloxone should not preclude immediate establishment of a patient airway, administration of oxygen, and assisted or controlled ventilation as indicated for hypoventilation or apnea. If respiratory depression is associated with muscular rigidity, a neuromuscular blocking agent may be required to facilitate assisted or controlled ventilation.[39] Intravenous fluids and vasoactive agents may be required to manage hemodynamic instability. Fentanyl and its analogs should be used cautiously in intoxicated patients and in those given other drugs that have central nervous system respiratory depressant effects. Slow intravenous administration of fentanyl may help prevent muscular rigidity.[40]

REFERENCES—FENTANYL, FENTANYL DERIVATIVES, AND "CHINA WHITE"

1. Henderson GL. Pharmacology and toxicology of fentanyl and related compounds. Calif Assoc Toxicol Newslett, July 1983.
2. Sternbach GL, Varon J. 'Designer drugs': Recognizing and managing their toxic effects. Postgrad Med 1992;92:169–176.
3. Ford M, Hoffman RS, Goldfrank LR. Opioids and designer drugs. Emerg Med Clin North Am 1990;8:495–511.

4. Jerrard DA. 'Designer drugs': A current perspective. J Emerg Med 1990;8:733–741.
5. Sidford C. Designer drugs. Clin Toxicol Rev 1989;11(11):1–2.
6. U.S. Congress CSA (Controlled Substance Analogue) Enforcement Act (21 Provision USC813: Treatment of CSA) Defor 21 USC 802 32A. Public Law 990570. 99th Congress, Oct. 27, 1986.
7. Martros M, Hecker J, Clark R, et al. "China White" epidemic: An eastern United States emergency department experience. Ann Emerg Med 1989;18:441.
8. Buchanan JF, Brown CR. 'Designer drugs': A problem in clinical toxicology. Med Toxicol 1988;3:1–17.
9. Beebe DK, Walley E. Substance abuse: The designer drugs. AFP 1991;43:1689–1698.
10. Bureau of Narcotic Enforcement, California Department of Justice, Statement, November 1989.
11. Marquardt KA, Tharratt RS. Inhalation abuse of fentanyl patch. Clin Toxicol 1994;32:75–78.
12. Henderson GL. Designer drugs: Past history and future prospects. J Forens Sci 1988;33:569–575.
13. Martin M, Hecker J, Clark R, et al. China White epidemic: An eastern United States emergency department experience. Ann Emerg Med 1991;20:158–164.
14. Hibbs J, Perper J, Winek CL. An outbreak of designer drug-related deaths in Pennsylvania. JAMA 1991;265:1011–1013.
15. Hudson RJ. Apnoea and unconsciousness after apparent recovery from alfentanil-supplemental anaesthesia. Can J Anaesth 1990;37:255–257.
16. Bartkowski R, Mcdonnell E. Prolonged alfentanil effect following erythromycin administration. Anesthesiology 1990;73: 566–568.
17. Kissin I, Vinik HR, Castillo R, Bradley EL Jr. Alfentanil potentiates midazolam-induced unconsciousness in subanalgesic doses. Anesth Analg 1990;71:65–69.
18. Lammens HJM, Bovill JG, Hennis PJ, et al. Alcohol consumption alters the pharmacodynamics of alfentanil. Anesthesiology 1989;71:669–679.
19. Poklis A. Fentanyl: A review for clinical and analytical toxicologists. Clin Toxicol 1995;33:439–447.
20. Ananthanrayan C. Tissue effect of fentanyl. Anaesthesia 1990;45:595.
21. Strong WE, Matson M. Probable seizure after alfentanyl. Anesth Analg 1989;68:692–693.
22. Rosenberg M, Lisman SR. Major seizure after fentanyl administration: Two case reports. J Oral Maxillofac Surg 1986;44:577–579.
23. Steinstra R, van Poorten F. Immediate respiratory arrest after caudal epidural sufentanil. Anesthesiology 1989;71:993–994.
24. De Sio JM, Bacon Dr, Peer G, Lema MJ. Intravenous abuse of transdermal fentanyl therapy in a chronic pain patient. Anesthesiology 1993;79:1139–1141.
25. Nieves E. 6 addicts die and police warn of toxic drug. NY Times, Feb. 3, 1991.
26. Hays LR, Stillner V, Littrell R. Fentanyl dependency associated with oral ingestion. Anesthesiology 1992;77:819–820.
27. Henderson GL. Fentanyl related deaths: Demographics, circumstances and toxicology of 112 cases. J Forens Sci 1991; 36:422–433.
28. Michiels M, Hendriks R, Heykants JJ. Radioimmunoassay of the new opioid analgesics alfentanil and sufentanil. J Pharm Pharmacol 1983;35:86–93.
29. Hansdottir V, Hedner T, Woestenborghs R, Nordberg G. The CSF and plasma pharmacokinetics of sufentanil after intrathecal administration. Anesthesiology 1991;74:264–269.
30. Ferslew KE, Hagordorn AN, McCormick WF. Postmorten determination of the biological distribution of sufentanil and midazolam after an acute intoxication. J Forens Sci 1989;34: 249–257.
31. Stiller RL, Scierka AM, Davis PJ, et al. A method to increase recovery of fentanyl from urine. Clin Toxicol 1989;27:101–108.
32. Henderson GL, El Shanni AS, Wilson HA, et al. Fentanyl in urine and serum by solid phase 125-1 radioimmunoassay. In: Uges DRA, de Zeeuw RA, eds. *Proceedings, 25th International Meeting, International Association of Forensic Toxicologists, Groningen, 1988.*
33. Watts V, Caplan Y. Determination of fentanyl in whole blood at subnanogram concentrations by dual capillary column gas chromatography with nitrogen sensitive detectors and gas chromatography/mass spectrometry. J Anal Toxicol 1988;12: 246–254.
34. Chaturvedi AK, Rao NGS, Baird JR. A death due to self-administered fentanyl. J Anal Toxicol 1990;14:385–387.
35. Henderson GL. Blood concentrations of fentanyl and its analogs in overdose victims. Proc West Pharmacol Soc 1983; 26:287–290.
36. Henderson GL, Harkey MR, Jones AD. Rapid screening of fentanyl (China White) powder samples by solid-phase radioimmunoassay. J Anal Toxicol 1990;14:172–175.
37. Lunn JK, Stanley SH, Eisele J. High dose fentanyl anesthesia for coronary artery surgery: Plasma fentanyl concentrations and influence of nitrous oxide on cardiovascular responses. Anesth Analg 1979;58:390–395.
38. Bovill JG, Sebel PS. Pharmacokinetics of high-dose fentanyl. Br J Anaesth 1980;52:795–801.
39. Owen H, Brose WG. Delayed respiratory depression following alfentanyl. Anesthesiology 1989;70:1037–1038.
40. Chudnofsky CR, Wright SW, Dronen SC, et al. The safety of fentanyl use in the emergency department. Ann Emerg Med 1989;18:635–639.

II. MEPERIDINE ANALOGS

Clinical Presentation

1-methyl-γ-phenyl-1,2,3,6 tetrahydropyridine (MPTP) is a synthetic designer drug designed to act like meperidine. Metabolic activation by monoamine oxidase of MPTP to MPP has produced a Parkinsonian-like syndrome in a number of individuals using MPTP intravenously.

MPTP-Induced and Clinical Parkinsonism: Similarities and Differences

Similarities

1. MPTP induces all the major clinical signs of Parkinson's disease with the possible exception of tremor.
2. The motor deficits induced by MPTP in primates are reversed by dopamine agonist drugs in a manner identical to that observed in humans.
3. Repeated administration of L-dopa to MPTP-treated primates produces all the long-term complications (dyskinesias, dystonia, "on–off" phenomena) associated with its use in the treatment of Parkinson's disease.[1,2]

Differences

1. The motor deficits induced by MPTP in primates slowly disappear over a period of months. This contrasts with the slowly progressive nature of Parkinson's disease.
2. The pathologic changes induced by MPTP are largely restricted to the substantia nigra. Other areas such as the locus ceruleus, which die in Parkinson's disease, are spared.
3. Lowy bodies, the pathologic marker of Parkinson's disease, are not observed in MPTP-treated primate brains.[1]

III. PHENYLETHYLAMINES: MESCALINE-AMPHETAMINE HYBRIDS (NONOPIATES)

Blood concentrations of 3,4-methylenedioxymethamphetamine (MDMA) in acute fatal overdoses have ranged from 1.0 to 2.0 μg/mL.[3–6] A simple oral dose of 50 mg of MDMA produced a peak plasma concentration of 106 ng/mL.[2] Two persons who died following MDMA use were found to have blood concentrations of 10.9 and 0.58 μg/mL.[7]

Some 3,4-methylenedioxyamphetamine (MDA) analogs have been chemically characterized.[8] Methods for the detection of amphetamine-like designer drugs has been compared.[9] (See also Chapter 20.)

REFERENCES—MEPERIDINE ANALOGS AND PHENYLETHYLAMINES

1. Jenner P. MPTP-induced Parkinsonism: Chemical basis of an age related disease. In: Volans GN, Sims J, Sullivan FM, Turner P, eds. *Basic Science in Toxicology.* London: Taylor & Francis, 1990:615–625.
2. Maret G, Testa B, Jenner P, et al. The MPTP story: MDA activates tetrahydropyridine derivatives to toxins causing parkinsonism. Drug Metab Rev 9990;22:291–332.
3. Shulgin AT. What is MDMA. Pharm Chem Newslett 1985;14: 3–5, 10–11.
4. FDA Consumer 1985;19(7):36–37.
5. Buchanan J. Ecstasy in the emergency department. San Francisco Bay Area Region Poison Center Clin Toxicol Update 1985;7(4):1–3.
6. Rohrig TP, Prouty RW. Tissue distribution of methylenedioxymethamphetamine. J Anal Toxicol 1992;16:52–53.
7. Verebey K, Alrazi J, Jaffe JH. The complications of "ecstasy" (MDMA). JAMA 1988;259:1649–1650.
8. Dalcason TA. The characterization of some 3,4-methylenephenylisopropylamine (MDA) analogs. J Forens Sci 1989;34: 928–961.
9. Ruagyuttiharn W, Samathanun G, Moody DW. Comparison of RIA, ENRI[R], and TDX[P] detection for amphetamine-like designer drugs. In: *Proceedings, 2nd International Meeting, International Association of Forensic Toxicologists, Banff, July 28–31, 1987:*213–217.

IV. ICE: 4-METHYLAMINOREX

4-Methylaminorex[1] (*cis*-2-amino-4-methyl-5-phenyl-2-oxazoline, 4,5-dihydro-4-methyl-5-phenyl-2-oxazolamine), also known as U4EUh and Ice, is a potent anorectic and central nervous system stimulant, possessing sympathomimetic,[2] hypotensive, and norepinephrine-potentiating properties similar to those of amphetamines.[3] It was first prepared in 1962 as an anorectic agent, and was recently placed in Schedule I under the Controlled Substances Act.[4] Illicit use has resulted in at least one fatality.[5] A gas chromatography–mass spectrometry method detects 4-methylaminorex at 250 ng/mL.[6]

Its desmethyl derivative, aminorex,[7] was also introduced as an anorectic drug in 1966 in Europe, but following reports of a high incidence of pulmonary hypertension and several deaths,[8,9] it was withdrawn from sale in 1968. It has reappeared as a designer drug.[7] (See also Chapter 20.)

REFERENCES—ICE: 4-METHYLAMINOREX

1. Klein RFX, Sperling AR, Cooper DA, Kram TC. The stereoisomers of 4-methylaminorex. J Forens Sci 1989;34:962–979.
2. Yelnosky J, Katz R. Sympathomimetic actions of *cis*-2-amino-4-methyl-5-phenyl-2-oxazoline. J Pharmacol Exp Ther 1963;141:180–184.
3. Patil PN, Yamauchi D. Influence of optical isomers of some centrally acting drugs on norepinephrine responses. Eur J Pharmacol 1970;12:132–135.
4. Lawn JC. Schedules of controlled substances: Temporary placement of 2-amino-4-methyl-5-phenyl-2-oxazoline (4-methylaminorex) into Schedule I. Fed Regist 1987;52: 30174–30175.
5. Davis FT, Brewster ME. A fatality involving U4EUh, a cyclic derivative of phenylpropanolamine. J Forens Sci 1988;33: 549–553.
6. Sudmeier SJ, Smith FP, Reuschel SA, Kidwell DA. Four isomers of methylaminore in urine examined by immunoassay and GC/MS. In: *Proceedings, American Academy of Forensic Scientists, New Orleans, 44th Annual Meeting, February 17–22, 1992:*198 (Abstract K-47).
7. Brewster ME, Davis FT. Appearance of aminorex as a designer analogue of methylaminorex. J Forens Sci 1991; 36:587–592.
8. Gurtner H. Aminorex and pulmonary hypertension. Cor Vasa 1985;27:160–171.
9. Seiler K. Aminorex and pulmonary circulation. Arzneitmittelforschung 1975;25:837.

DEXTROMORAMIDE

Dextromoramide, a strong opioid narcotic analgesic, has become a popular substitute or alternative drug of abuse for drug-dependent individuals in some countries. Dextromoramide was removed from sale in the United States in the 1960s.[1] Those who inject or ingest this drug may quickly succumb without knowing their own lack of tolerance to it. Subcutaneously, it is approximately 10 times more potent than methadone, 10 to 25 times more potent than morphine, and about 50 times more potent than meperidine.[1]

Use

Dextromoramide tartrate is an analgesic related to methadone and is used in the treatment of severe pain. It is not recommended for use in obstetric analgesia. The compound is about five times as potent as morphine and is used in surgery, intensive care, or at home.[2,3]

Product Formulation

Dextromoramide tartrate is available in the United Kingdom as Palfium for injection of 5 and 10 mg/mL in ampules of 1.1 mL and as tablets containing 5 mg (white) or 10 mg (peach-colored tablet containing the artificial coloring agent sunset yellow).[4,5] A suppository form is available containing 10 mg of dextromoramide in a uritepsol H15 base.[5] Dextromoramide is also known under the proprietary names Jetrium and Narcolo.[4]

Source

Dextromoramide and dextromoramide tartrate are synthetic compounds.

Therapeutic Dose

The usual therapeutic dose is the equivalent of dextromoramide 5 mg by mouth or by injection, increased as required up to 20 mg by mouth or 15 mg by injection.[4] A dose equivalent to not more than 80 μg/kg body weight has been suggested for use in children.[4] Therapy should commence with reduced dosage in the elderly and in those with impaired hepatic, renal, or thyroid function. The dose should be reduced gradually if dependence is suspected.

Fatal Dose

Dependence on dextromoramide has been described.[6,7] Oral doses of 100 mg (20 tablets) and injections of 15 to 25 mg have led to fatalities with high blood levels indicating chronic or repetitive dosing.[8]

Toxicokinetics[9–11]

Presystemic metabolism	>50%
Peak plasma level	68–177 ng/mL (after 7.5-mg oral dose) 10–80 mg/L (after 5 mg IV)
Time to peak plasma level	0.5–4.0 hours
Volume of distribution (L/kg)	0.6–2.4 L/kg
Elimination half-life	0.5–1.6 hours (first phase) 6–29 hours (second phase)
Excreted unchanged	<0.06%

Drug Interactions

Dextromoramide is a narcotic analgesic and may potentiate the central nervous system depressant effect of other drugs such as the opiates, other narcotics, benzodiazepines, phenothiazines, butyrophenones, and other psychoactive drugs.

Pregnancy/Lactation

Malformations (exencephaly, craniorrhachischisis, kinking of the spinal cord, dilation of the fourth brain ventricle, and ectopia of the neural tube) have been demonstrated in a mouse embryo experimental model.[12] There are no adequate controlled studies of dextromoramide in human pregnancy. Regular use of the compound during pregnancy may induce a state of dependence in the neonate. Dextromoramide should not be administered to the lactating mother: use by the lactating mother of this drug may be associated with significant clinical effects (eg, central nervous system depression) in the nursing baby.

Mechanism of Action

Dextromoramide is an opioid agonist with strong analgesic activity; it is apparently an agonist mainly at the mu receptor.[13,14]

Clinical Presentation

Almost all reports of overdose involve individuals who have been found unconscious or dead following oral ingestion or injections of dextromoramide.[6,7,15,16] The drug is a powerful central nervous system depressant. Many who succumb are dependent on the drug or have also ingested or injected other central nervous system depressant drugs simultaneously.

Laboratory

Analytical Methods

A direct gas chromatographic assay is available for analyses of dextromoramide in human plasma,[2] with a lower limit of detectability in plasma of 2 ng/mL.

Ancillary Tests

A single dose of 10 mg of dextromoramide led to a urine concentration of 70 ng/mL 8 hours postingestion.[17]

Treatment

Stabilization

Treatment of dextromoramide overdose is similar to treatment of methadone overdose. Close monitoring in a hospital for at least 72 hours is essential.

There is no evidence that cathartics, activated charcoal, and whole-bowel irrigation are an effective decontaminating procedure.

Elimination Enhancement

Dextromoramide has a high apparent volume of distribution. It is unlikely to be responsive to dialysis or hemoperfusion procedures; however, these procedures have not been attempted in any overdose case to date.

Antidote

Naloxone may be useful as the antidote to dextromoramide central nervous system depression; however, trials of naloxone have not yet been attempted in a dextromoramide overdose. In view of the long elimination half-life of dextromoramide, it is conceivable that repeat doses or intravenous infusion of an antagonist may be required.

Supportive Measures

Treatment should include establishment of an airway, maintenance of adequate respiratory ventilation, precise supportive care to maintain fluid and electrolyte balance, administration of an opioid antagonist (eg, naloxone), and prevention of aspiration of gastric contents. Babies born to dextromoramide-dependent mothers exhibit withdrawal signs many hours after birth and should be carefully observed for at least 7 days.

Patients who are admitted following a dextromoramide overdose should be continuously monitored, provided adequate sources of oxygen, and observed in an intensive care unit until they regain consciousness, have stable vital signs, and have had a psychiatric consultation.

REFERENCES—DEXTROMORAMIDE

1. Brower C. A dextromoramide related fatality. J Forens Sci 1990;35:483–489.
2. Kintz P, Tracqui A, Mangin P, et al. Toxicological findings after fatal dextromoramide injection. Clin Toxicol 1989;27:385–388.
3. Kintz P, Tracqui A, Mangin P, et al. Fatal intoxication by dextromoramide: A report on two cases. J Anal Toxicol 1989; 13:238–239.
4. Reynolds JEF, ed. *Martindale: The Extra Pharmacopoeia.* 30th ed. London: Pharmaceutical Press, 1993:1071.
5. Dollery C, ed. *Therapeutic Drugs.* Edinburgh: Churchill Livingstone, 1991:D66–D69.
6. Carmack J. Dependence on dextromoramide. Br Med J 1967;1:362.
7. Juby BA. Dependence on dextromoramide. Br Med J 1967; 1:362–363.
8. Hansson RC. Fifteen deaths associated with dextromoramide. Bull Int Assoc Forens Toxicol 1986;19(1):39–41.
9. Kintz P, Mangin, Lugnier AA, Chaumont AJ. Gas chromatographic assay for dextromoramide in human plasma. J Chromatogr 1988;432:329–333.
10. Pagani I, Barzaghi N, Crema F, et al. Pharmacokinetics of dextromoramide in surgical patients. Fundam Clin Pharmacol 1989;3:27–35.
11. Kintz P, Tracqui A, Mangin P, et al. Tissue distribution of dextromoramide in the rat. Fundam Clin Pharmacol 1990;4: 163–167.
12. Jurand A, Martin LVH. Teratogenic potential of two neurotropic drugs, haloperidol and dextromoramide, tested on mouse embryos. Teratology 1990;42:45–54.
13. Wuster M, Schulz R, Herz A. Specificity of opioids towards the mu, delta and epsilon opiate receptors. Neurosci Lett 1978;15:193–198.
14. Janssen PAJ, Jageneau AH. A new series of potent analgesics: Dextro-2.2-diphenyl-3-methyl-4-morpholino-butyrylpyrrolidine and related amides, Part I. J Pharm Pharmacol 1957;9:381–400.
15. Chaumant AJ, Mangin P, Lugnier AA. Intoxications mortelles par le dextromoramide et toxicomanie. J Med Leg Droit Med 1981,24:687–692.
16. Ashton, Franc, Haynes: Home Office Forensic Science Laboratory, Aldermaston, Berks, UK. Two fatalities involving dextromoramide. Bull Int Assoc Forens Toxicol 1978;14 (2): 22–23.
17. Sheehan TMT. Dextromoramide: A challenge to the analyst. In: *Proceedings, 25th International Meeting, International Association of Forensic Toxicologists, Banff, July 28–31, 1987:* 436–440.

DEZOCINE

Dezocine (Dalgan) (Fig. 25-3) is a synthetic opioid agonist–antagonist analgesic of the aminotetralin series.[1] After parenteral administration of therapeutic doses it is approximately equipotent with morphine and is similar in effectiveness to morphine, meperidine, and butorphanol as an analgesic for moderate to severe postoperative pain. In single analgesic doses, dezocine is a more potent respiratory depressant than morphine. Dependence-producing properties have not yet been observed. Dezocine shows structural similarities to some other mixed opioid agonist–antagonist drugs such as pentazocine and butorphanol.[1] In morphine-addicted animals dezocine caused withdrawal symptoms, and it should not be given to patients physically dependent on narcotics. Treatment of an overdose is similar to that for morphine overdose. Dezocine is available in the United States and is not a controlled substance.

Use

Dezocine is indicated for the short-term relief of pain and chronic moderate to severe pain as a result of advanced cancer.[2] A patient who has developed a significant degree of tolerance to other opioids during long-term treatment is probably not a suitable candidate for dezocine treatment.

Product Formulation

- 5 mg/mL Dalgan (sodium metabisulfite)[3]
- 10 mg/mL Dalgan (sodium metabisulfite)
- 15 mg/mL Dalgan (sodium metabisulfite)

Therapeutic Dose

A single intramuscular dose of 5 to 20 mg (adjusted according to the patient's weight, severity of pain, physical status, and other medication being received) may be repeated every 2 to 4 hours.[4] The initial dose in most studies has been 10 mg intramuscularly or 5 mg intravenously.

The safety and efficacy of dezocine in children and adolescents up to 18 years of age have not been established.

Toxicokinetics[1,5,6]

Peak plasma level	10–38 ng/mL (after 10 mg IM)
Time to peak plasma level	10–90 minutes
Volume of distribution	9-11 L/kg
Elimination half-life	2.5 hours
Excreted unchanged	1–4%

Drug Interactions

Potential problems (e.g., central nervous system depression, respiratory depression, hypotension) may occur when dezocine is used with antidiarrheal agents and antiperistaltic agents such as difenoxin–atropine, diphenoxylate–atropine, kaolin, pectin, belladonna alkaloids and opium, loperamide, opium tincture, and paregoric; central nervous system depression-producing medications; monoamine oxidase inhibitors; and hydroxyzine. Naloxone may antagonize the analgesic and central nervous system and respiratory depressant effect of dezocine. Naloxone may precipitate withdrawal symptoms in physically dependent patients: the dosage should be carefully titrated when used to treat opioid overdosage in dependent patients.[4] Dezocine may be ineffective if administered to a patient receiving naltrexone therapy. If dezocine is administered prior to another mu-receptor agonist, dezocine may reduce the therapeutic effect of the other opioid.

Pregnancy/Lactation

It is not known whether dezocine is excreted in breast milk. Adequate and well-controlled studies have not been done in pregnant women. Dezocine has been placed in Pregnancy Category C. Regular use during pregnancy may cause physical dependence in the fetus, leading to withdrawal symptoms (seizures, irritability, excessive crying, tremors, hyperactive reflexes, fever, vomiting, diarrhea, sneezing, and yawning) in the neonate.[4]

Mechanism of Action

Dezocine has its primary effect at the mu receptor, which mediates supraspinal analgesia, euphoria, and respiratory depression. Secondary activity may take place at the delta receptor, which may modify the mu receptor. Dezocine does not appear to have the same affinity for the kappa and sigma receptors as other agonist–antagonist opioids. It does not exhibit any antagonistic effects at therapeutic doses.[5]

Clinical Presentation

Nausea, vomiting, and sedation occur with dezocine about as often as with other opioid analgesics.[6,7] Dizziness, anxiety, disorientation, hallucinations, sweating, tachycardia, and skin reactions at the injection site have also been reported. Acute respiratory depression, which can be reversed with naloxone, can occur after intravenous dezocine. Respiratory effects are dose related up to 30 mg/70 kg body weight, where they reach a ceiling.[8] Fatal respiratory depression has not been reported, but in patients with limited respiratory reserve, dezocine may be dangerous.

Dezocine may increase the cardiac index, pulmonary artery pressure, and left ventricular stroke wave. It may be dangerous in patients with coronary artery disease.[9]

Abuse Potential

Dezocine appears to cause subjective effects in nondependent drug users similar to those of morphine and different from those of nalbuphine (Nubain) or pentazocine.[9]

Overdose

Symptoms of overdose of opioid analgesics include cold clammy skin, confusion, nervousness or restlessness, severe convulsions, severe dizziness and drowsiness, low blood pressure, pinpoint pupils, bradycardia, dyspnea or hypopnea, loss of consciousness (coma), and severe weakness.

Laboratory

Analytical Methods

Dezocine may be quantitated in plasma by high-performance liquid chromatography with electrochemical detection.[10] The lower limit of detection of dezocine is 1 to 2 ng/mL.[11]

Blood Levels

Side effects are more frequent when the dezocine plasma concentration is 45 ng/mL or higher.[2]

Treatment

There has been little experience with dezocine overdose. Treatment of overdose of all opioid analgesics should include the following measures:

1. Establish an adequate respiratory exchange by providing a patent airway and instituting assisted or controlled respirations.
2. Administer the opioid antagonist naloxone (400 μg [0.4 mg] to 2 mg as a single dose), preferably intravenously. Naloxone injection may be repeated at 2- to 3-minute intervals as needed. Naloxone may also antagonize the analgesic action of opioid analgesics and may precipitate withdrawal symptoms in physically dependent patients.
3. Administer intravenous fluids and/or vasopressors and use other supportive measures as required.
4. Monitor the patient. Administer additional naloxone as required. Alternatively, initial treatment may be followed by continuous intravenous infusion of naloxone, with the rate of infusion adjusted according to patient response.[4]

REFERENCES—DEZOCINE

1. O'Brien JJ, Benfield P. Dezocine. A preliminary review of its pharmacodynamic and pharmacokinetic properties and therapeutic efficacy. Drugs 1989;38:226–248.
2. Stambaugh JE Jr, McAdams J. Comparison of intramuscular dezocine with butorphanol and placebo in chronic cancer pain: A method to evaluate analgesia after both single and repeated doses. Clin Pharmacol Ther 1987;42:211–219.
3. Dezocine (systemic). USP DI Update 1991;1:106–109.
4. Dezocine (Dalgan®), Astra. Calif Assoc Toxicol Newslett Spring 1991:12–13.
5. Locniskar A, Greenblatt DJ, Zinny MA. Pharmacokinetics of dezocine, a new analgesic: Effect of dose and route of administration. Eur J Clin Pharmacol 1986;30:121–123.
6. Locniskar A, Greenblatt DJ, Zinny MA. Pharmacokinetics of dezocine, a new analgesic: Effect of dose and route of administration. Eur J Clin Pharmacol 1986;30:121–123.
7. Dezocine. Med Lett Drugs Ther 1990;32(829):95–96.
8. Romagnoli A, Keats AS. Ceiling respiratory depression by dezocine. Clin Pharmacol Ther 1984;35:367–373.
9. Rothbard RL, Schreiner BF, Yu PN. Hemodynamic and respiratory effects of dezocine, ciramadol and morphine. Clin Pharmacol Ther 1985;38:84–88.
10. Jasinski DR, Preston KC. Assessment of dezocine for morphine-like subjective effects and miosis. Clin Pharmacol Ther 1985;38:544–548.
11. Locniskar A, Greenblatt DJ. Determination of ciramadol and dezocine, two new analgesics, by high performance liquid chromatography using electrochemical detection. J Chromatogr Biomed Appl 1986;374:215–220.

DIPHENOXYLATE HYDROCHLORIDE AND ATROPINE SULFATE (LOMOTIL)

Lomotil poisoning is representative of a unique opiate-anticholinergic overdose combination that appears to be more serious and often more fatal in children than in adults, has delayed deleterious effects, and, at least in children, appears to present no correlation between dose ingested and severity of toxicity.[1–3]

The 1990 Annual Report of the American Association of Poison Control Centers National Data Collection System lists 1654 cases of diphenoxylate–atropine poisonings, including 1004 cases involving children less than 6 years old, and 2 deaths.[4]

In the 1991 Annual Report of the American Association of Poison Control Centers National Data Collection System, 1644 cases of diphenoxylate–atropine ingestion are listed, including 51 moderate cases and 10 major cases. No fatalities were reported that year.[5]

Structure and Classification

Diphenoxylate is a synthetic phenylpiperidine derivative closely related to meperidine (Demerol), alphaprodine (Nisentil), anileridine (Leritine), fentanyl (Sublimaze), and fentanyl derivatives (China White).

Source

Lomotil is a synthetic product. Commercial names in the United States include Lomotil (Searle), Diphenatol (Rugby), Elmotil (Elder), Enoxa (Reid-Provident), Lofene (Lannett), Lonox (Geneva Generics), LoTrol (Vanguard), Low-Quel (Halsey), and SK Dipenoxylate (Smith, Kline & French). Names outside the United States include Diarsed (France), Reasec (Italy, Switzerland), and Retardin (Denmark, Norway, Sweden).

Use

Diphenoxylate–atropine is an antidiarrheal agent often used to treat traveler's diarrhea. It prolongs the transit time of intestinal contents by its action on the smooth muscle of the gut.

Product Formulation

Each tablet, or 5 mL of liquid, contains 2.5 mg diphenoxylate hydrochloride and 0.025 mg (25 μg) atropine sulfate (a subtherapeutic amount of the latter is added to discourage its abuse).[6]

Therapeutic Dose

The initial adult dosage is 5 mg four times daily. Children aged 1 to 12 years should take an oral solution, 0.3 to 0.4 mg/kg, daily in divided doses. The maintenance dose is one-fourth the daily dose.[6]

Toxic Dose

The lowest dose reported associated with signs and symptoms of poisoning was 2 tablets.[7] Six tablets produced poisoning in another series.[8] The lowest fatal dose reported was 1.2 mg/kg.[9] Ingestion of 20 tablets by a 2-year-old resulted in respiratory and cardiac arrest and death, whereas the same dose in another 2-year-old did not produce any symptoms.[10] Possibly, the reported size of the alleged dose was inaccurate. In adults, 15 to 30 tablets did not produce respiratory depression or coma.[7]

Toxicokinetics

Absorption

After oral ingestion, diphenoxylate–atropine is easily absorbed through the gastrointestinal tract. Absorption is slowed in overdose because of a delay in gastrointestinal motility. Such delays may be as long as 30 hours. Diphenoxylate and its salts are largely insoluble, thus making parenteral abuse less likely.[11]

Distribution

The apparent volume of distribution of diphenoxylate is 4.6 L/kg, and that of atropine, approximately 2 to 4 L/kg. Peak plasma levels of both diphenoxylate and diphenoxylic acid, an active metabolite, are reached in 2 hours.[12] Enterohepatic recycling may be important in the metabolism of diphenoxylate.[13]

Elimination

The major metabolite, diphenoxylic acid, formed in the liver, is five times more active than diphenoxylate as an antidiarrheal agent.[12] The half-life of diphenoxylate is 2.5 hours, and that of diphenoxylic acid, 4.4 hours, after therapeutic dosage. The half-life in overdose may be prolonged to more than 12 hours. Diphenoxylate is excreted in the feces (49.2%) and urine (13.7%) as conjugated products, over a 96-hour period. Less than 0.1% of diphenoxylate and less than 0.8% of diphenoxylic acid are excreted in the urine unchanged.

Drug Interactions

Diphenoxylate inhibits the microsomal hepatic enzyme system and has the potential to prolong the half-lives of drugs whose rate of elimination is dependent on this system.[6]

Lactation

The compounds are excreted in breast milk.

Clinical Presentation

Atropine may exert its effects in children before, during, or after opioid effects.[3,14]

Moderate to severe diphenoxylate (opiate) symptoms appear 2 to 3 hours after ingestion and include slow pulse, slow depressed respirations, drowsiness, convulsions, and coma. There may be abdominal pain or pancreatitis.[15] The pupils are constricted and cortical blindness secondary to cerebral hypoxia may occur.[2] Cyanotic skin, hypothermia, and muscle fasciculation may be present. Respiratory depression and coma are the most prevalent components of diphenoxylate–atropine poisoning.[2] Adults do not appear to have the same susceptibility to opiate toxicity as do children.[3] Symptoms, especially coma and respiratory depression, may be delayed up to 30 hours because of delayed gastrointestinal motility. Opiate overdose (central nervous system and respiratory depression with miosis) may predominate or occur without signs of atropine toxicity. All patients appear to exhibit opioid effects sometime during the course of the overdose. Diphenoxylate–atropine intoxication can be considered to be an overdose of a long-acting opioid that may include manifestations of atropine toxicity.

There appears to be little correlation between dose ingested and severity of signs or symptoms in diphenoxylate–atropine overdose.[3] Children may develop signs of atropinism even with a normal dose.[2] It is not possible to predict which dose is toxic to children.[3] Symptoms may respond to treatment only to recur many hours later (24–36 hours). Because of the long elimination half-life (12–24 hours) of difenoxine (diphenoxylic acid) in overdose, it seems likely that the recurrence of respiratory depression and opioid symptoms after apparent recovery from diphenoxylate–atropine overdose is due to the accumulation of diphenoxylic acid.[16]

Diphenoxylate abuse has been reported in two cases.[17] In one case, it was substituted for methadone. Receiving doses of 100 to 125 tablets plus 2 oz of tincture of opium daily, the patient, an adult, developed dry mouth, blurred vision, and tachycardia—all attributable to the atropine component in the Lomotil. When the product was not available, he experienced an opiate abstinence syndrome.

A report on eight children with diphenoxylate–atropine (Lomotil) overdose and a review of 28 additional overdoses in young children described in the literature indicated the following:

- Small children intoxicated with diphenoxylate–atropine do not always have signs of atropinism followed in a few hours by signs of opioid overdose. Only 4 of 36 patients (11%) followed this pattern. Twenty-one (58%) had atropine symptoms before, during, or after opioid symptoms, and 15 patients (42%) had only opioid symptoms.
- All have opioid effects sometime during the course of the overdose. Diphenoxylate–atropine intoxication should be considered an overdose of a long-acting opioid that may include manifestations of atropine toxicity.
- In most cases, atropine effects last from 2 to 12 hours. In one patient atropinism developed 18 hours after the ingestion.
- Delayed gastric emptying and gastrointestinal atony may be a factor in the occurrence of central nervous system and respiratory depression 15 to 18 hours after an ingestion. The recurrence of respiratory depression after apparent recovery from diphenoxylate–atropine overdose may be due to accumulation of the active metabolite of diphenoxylate (diphenoxylic acid or difenoxamine), a compound whose serum half-life is twice as long as that of diphenoxylate.[16]

Laboratory

Plasma diphenoxylate levels are not easily obtained at most clinical laboratories. Plasma or urinary diphenoxylate levels have little clinical usefulness in the management of overdose (see Clinical Presentation), because the rapid conversion of diphenoxylate to diphenoxylic acid generally renders diphenoxylate undetectable. Arterial blood gases (pH, $Paco_2$, Pao_2) must be serially monitored as a guide to respiratory adequacy. No effect on serum electrolytes, blood urea nitrogen, hemoglobin, hematocrit, white cell count, blood glucose, or spinal fluid glucose was observed in one series of poisonings.[6]

Analytical Methods

The determination of plasma diphenoxylic acid, the major metabolite of diphenoxylate, has been performed by gas chromatography–mass spectrometry and radioimmunoassay.[18,19]

Treatment

Treatment depends on the recognition that a diphenoxylate–atropine combination has been ingested. Airway, breathing, and circulation must be intact. Tidal volume should be maintained between 10 and 15 mL/kg. An artificial airway should be created by endotracheal intubation as required. If there is respiratory embarrassment, adequate oxygenation must be instituted.

Gut Decontamination

Administration of an emetic is undesirable because of the rapidity with which the patient may become apneic and drowsy, increasing the possibility of aspiration.[3] Activated charcoal may be useful.[20] Caution must be exercised in using induced emesis if there is respiratory depression, depression of consciousness, obtundation, or loss of the gag reflex. In such cases, gastric lavage with endotracheal intubation would appear safer. Intravenous infusion of naloxone may be an alternative to oral activated charcoal when the patient has intestinal ileus or gastric atony.[16]

Antidote (Naloxone)

Respiratory depression and coma are indications for initiating naloxone. The dosage in the adult is 0.4 to 2.0 mg intravenously (1–5 ampules) repeated every few minutes up to a total of 10 mg; in the child, the initial dose is 0.01–0.1 mg/kg intravenously followed by an additional dose of 0.1 mg/kg as required. If there is no response, consideration must be given to exclusion of diphenoxylate–atropine, propoxyphene, or methadone as the causative agent. If there is a response, multiple doses of naloxone every 20 to 45 minutes may be required, as the half-life of naloxone is short and an opioid antagonist may be effective for only 45 to 70 minutes.[21] If frequent intravenous boluses are required to maintain adequate respiration and consciousness, a continuous intravenous naloxone infusion should be instituted. Naloxone 4 to 8 mg (from a 10-mL multiple-dose vial containing 0.4 mg/mL) is added to each liter of 5% dextrose in water or similar fluid, and the solution is infused at a rate of 100 mL/h (0.4–0.8 mg naloxone per hour). Forced diuresis, hemodialysis, hemoperfusion, and peritoneal dialysis are not useful in removing diphenoxylate or its metabolites, in view of the high volume of distribution.

Supportive Measures

Patients with signs of atropinism or central nervous system depression should be admitted. For urinary retention, catheterization may be required. Intensive care monitoring of vital signs (pulse rate, respiratory rate and depth, blood pressure), fluid balance (intake and output), level of consciousness, pupil size, and arterial blood gases must be continually recorded to guide patient status with regard to naloxone administration and fluid infusions (cerebral and pulmonary edema). This should be maintained for at least 24 hours.

Parents should be instructed to keep such tablets out of the reach of any children in the house. Patients should not be discharged until respiratory rate and depth and state of consciousness have returned to normal and other opioid symptoms are absent. Symptomatic patients should be kept under intensive observation for at least 24 hours irrespective of whether they have already responded to the above modalities and appear asymptomatic. They may still be in danger. Cardiovascular and pulmonary examination should indicate normal function.

REFERENCES—DIPHENOXYLATE AND ATROPINE SULFATE (LOMOTIL)

1. Wasserman G. Antidiarrheal agent can be toxic to children. JAMA 1974;230:14. Editorial.
2. Wasserman GS, Green VA, Wise GW. Lomotil ingestions in children. Am Fam Physician 1975;1:93–97.
3. Curtis JA, Goel KM. Lomotil poisoning in children. Arch Dis Child 1979;54:222–225.
4. Ahmad SR. Lomotil overdose. Pediatrics 1992;89:980–981.
5. Litovitz T, Holm KC, Bailey KM, Schuster BB. 1991 Annual Report of the American Association of Poison Control Centers National Data Collection System. Am J Emerg Med 1992;10:452–505.
6. McEvoy GK, ed. *AHFS Drug Information 94.* Bethesda, MD: American Society of Hospital Pharmacists, 1994:1877–1879.
7. Rumack BH, Temple AR. Lomotil poisoning. Pediatrics 1974; 53:495–500.
8. Henderson W, Psaila A. Lomotil poisoning. Lancet 1969;1: 306–307.
9. Ginsberg CM, Angle CR. Diphenoxylate–atropine (Lomotil) poisoning. Clin Toxicol 1969;2:377–382.
10. Penfold D, Volans GN. Overdose from Lomotil. Br Med J 1977;2:1401–1402.
11. Berkowitz BA. The relationship of pharmacokinetics to pharmacological activity: Morphine, methadone and naloxone. Clin Pharmacokinet 1976;1:219–230.
12. Baselt R. *Disposition of Toxic Drugs and Chemicals in Man.* 3rd ed. Chicago: Year Book, 1989:295–296.
13. Karim A, Ranney RE, Evensen KL, et al. Pharmacokinetics and metabolism of diphenoxylate in man. Clin Pharmacol Ther 1972;13:407–419.
14. Snyder R, Mofenson HC, Greensher J. Toxicity from Lomotil: Accidental ingestion by a 22 month old child. Clin Pediatr 1973;12:47–49.
15. McCormick RA, O'Donoghue D, Brennan N. Diphenoxylate and pancreatitis. Lancet 1985;1:752.
16. McCarron MM, Challoner KR, Thompson GA. Diphenoxylate–atropine (Lomotil) overdose in children: An update (Report of 8 cases and review of the literature). Pediatrics 1991;87P; 694:697–700.
17. Ives TJ. Illicit use of diphenoxylate hydrochloride to prevent narcotic withdrawal symptoms. Drug Intell Clin Pharmacol 1980;14:715–716.
18. Ford GC, Haskins NJ, Palmer RF, et al. The measurement of diphenoxylic acid in plasma following administration of diphenoxylate. Biomed Mass Spect 1976;3:45–47.
19. Jackson LS, Stafford JE. The evaluation and applications of a radioimmunoassay for the measurement of diphenoxylic acid, the major metabolite of diphenoxylate hydrochloride (Lomotil) in human plasma. J Pharmacol Methodol 1987;18: 189–197.
20. Mack RB. Toxic encounters of the dangerous kind. Diphenoxylate (Lomotil). NC Med J 1981;42:858.
21. McGuigan M, Lovejoy FH Jr. Overdose of Lomotil. Br Med J 1978;1:990.

HEROIN

In early 1994 there was a resurgence in the use of heroin in the United States. The product became more easily available and of sufficient purity (Fig. 25–4) to be used by snorting, similar to cocaine.[1] Heroin additives may be inadvertently used by heroin users (Table 25–14). Nonfatal overdoses are common. Overdoses are frequent in subjects who have used heroin with alcohol, benzodiazepines, cannabis, or amphetamines. Heroin laced with phencyclidine (Angel Dust) has led to deaths in New York.[2] In New York, symptoms of agitation, hallucinations, paranoia, sinus tachycardia, mild hypertension, dilated pupils, dry skin and mucous membranes, and diminished bowel sounds have followed insufflation of heroin sold as "point on point" and "sting" containing scopolamine.[3]

Table 25–14
Heroin Additives

Alkaloids	Inert
Thebaine	Starch
Acetylcodeine	Sugar
Papaverine	Calcium tartrate
Noscapine	Calcium carbonate
Narceine	Sodium carbonate
Active Nonalkaloids	Sucrose
Tolmectin	Dextrin
Quinine	Magnesium sulfate
Phenobarbital	Dextrose
Methaqualone	Lactose
Lidocaine	Barium sulfate
Phenolphthalein	Silicon dioxide
Caffeine	Vitamin C
Dextromoramide	**Volatile**
Chloroquine	Rosin
Diazepam	Toluene
Nicotinamide	Methanol
N-Phenyl-2-naphthylamine	Acetaldehyde
Phenacetin	Ethanol
Acetaminophen	Acetone
Fentanyl	Diethyl ether
Doxepin	Chlorofrm
Naproxen	Acetic acid
Promazine	
Piracetom	
Procaine	
Diphenhydramine	
Aminopyrine	
Allobarbital	
Indomethacin	
Glutethimide	
Scopolamine	
Sulfonamide	
Arsenic	
Strychnine	
Cocaine*	
Amphetamine*	
Methamphetamine*	

*Considered frequent additives/coinjectants; absolute frequency unknown.
From Shesser R, Jotte R, Olshaker J. The contribution of impurities to the acute morbidity of illegal drug use. Am J Emerg Med 1991;9:336–342.

Aflatoxins

Heroin is produced in subtropical countries from plants and may be susceptible to contamination by aflatoxins. Urine from intravenous heroin users may contain aflatoxins. Users risk direct systemic exposure to aflatoxin B, a consequence of which may be suppression of cell-mediated immunity.[4]

Body Packers

Heroin body packers are drug smugglers or "mules" who transport large amounts of concentrated heroin from foreign centers by swallowing wrapped packages or inserting packages into the rectum or vagina. After they reach their destination, the "mules" use strong cathartics, rectal suppositories, or disposable enemas to retrieve the packages rectally. The danger of death from heroin intoxication is the major concern in heroin body packing. McCarron and colleagues studied 14 body packers carrying 2 to 112 heroin packages.[5] Nine swallowed the packets, and five inserted them rectally. Three of 20 body packers reported in the medical literature died, probably from absorption of heroin from ruptured packages.

Heroin Packages

Heroin packages may be as large as 3 × 1.5 cm or 5 × 2.5 cm. The larger packages may lead to obstruction, initially at the pylorus or later at the ileocecal valve.

Clinical Diagnosis

Patients may have no symptoms, or they may exhibit diffuse abdominal tenderness and a distended abdomen with palpable packages.

Simple manual examination, anoscopy, and rectal lavage usually disclose rectally inserted packs of drugs and often indicate smuggling for personal use. Professional smugglers are more liable to swallow narcotics, in which case the method of choice is abdominal x-ray. In uncertain cases, fecal examination over a period of a few days may be necessary.[6]

Laboratory Tests

Heroin urine tests are usually negative. A negative urine toxicologic screen does not exclude the possibility of body packing. A heroin body packer with heroin detectable in the urine probably either has used heroin recently or is absorbing heroin from the packages. A normal abdominal roentgenogram does not preclude further investigation if there is a high possibility of body packing.

Care

Obtain an abdominal roentgenogram to confirm the diagnosis, determine the location of the packages in the gastrointestinal tract, and follow the movements of the package. Establish an intravenous line and place the patient on a cardiac monitor. Monitor oxygen saturation by pulse oximetry. If required, perform an endotracheal intubation, transfer to the intensive care unit, and proceed with assisted ventilation.

Ingested Packages

Stomach. Syrup of ipecac or gastric lavage should not be used for patients who have ingested heroin packages because of the large size of the packages. Vomiting may cause package obstruction of the proximal esophagus. Endoscopic removal of packages in the stomach may induce heroin intoxication if the snare used for removal causes a package to break. Any signs of heroin absorption (heroin toxicity) should be treated with intravenous naloxone (see Naloxone, Continuous Infusion later in this chapter).[7,8] If the desired respiratory rate is not obtained, a bolus dose of naloxone may be given, or the concentration of naloxone can be increased by 0.4 mg or more for each hourly aliquot of intravenous fluid. For example, a naloxone drip can contain 0.8 mg (later 1.2 ng) per 100 mL 5% dextrose in water given at the rate of 100 mL/h.

Activated charcoal, 60 g in 250 or 500 mL of 3% sodium sulfate solution, is administered orally. Activated charcoal 60 g can be given orally every 6 hours.

Colon. If foreign bodies are located in the colon, low-volume phosphosoda enemas or high-volume saline enemas are indicated. Food ingestion is not permitted until all packages are determined to be in the large intestine. The first bundle obtained is opened to examine the wrappings and test the core material for heroin and cocaine. Metoclopramide 10 mg every 8 hours is used to encourage gastric emptying, but is contraindicated in bowel obstruction.

Initially a bisacodyl (Dulcolax) suppository is inserted to empty the rectum. No attempt is made to remove rectal packages manually. Patients who have ingested drug packages are given 60 g of activated charcoal in 200 to 500 mL of 3% sodium sulfate solution orally. Whole-bowel irrigation is not performed. The polyethylene glycol in Go-Lytely can dissolve the heroin from a package, rupturing it and increasing absorption of heroin.

Heroin toxicity is treated with intravenous naloxone. The patient is monitored for heroin-induced pulmonary edema. Arterial blood gases and a chest x-ray are obtained if the patient develops dyspnea or tachypnea or if the pulse oximeter shows a decrease in oxygen saturation. Indications for surgical consultation are repeated bouts of heroin toxicity, radiologic evidence of retention of packages in the stomach, and bowel obstruction. A surgical consult should be obtained early. Urine toxicology screens are performed on all patients. Patients are not discharged until all packages are accounted for and negative abdominal radiographs are obtained.[5]

Polyethylene Glycol. Polyethylene glycol (as Go-Lytely) may solubilize heroin from some packages while they are retained in the stomach. In addition, it may interfere with heroin adsorption by activated charcoal, resulting in heroin toxicity.

Heroin Lung. Heroin lung is an occasional complication of heroin intoxication. It causes a rapidly reversible form of pulmonary edema.[9] Treatment is supportive and symptomatic.

Delayed Encephalopathy. A delayed encephalopathy may become evident after an overdose. Magnetic resonance imaging a few weeks later may disclose bilateral infarcts in the putamen and caudate. Initial physical and radiographic findings may not predict the outcome.[10]

Toxicokinetics

A recent shift from intravenous injection to intranasal use ("snorting") has been observed among heroin addicts. Peak levels of heroin, similar to those observed after intramuscular administration, are attained with intranasal administration of 6 mg of heroin (Fig. 25–5). Physiologic, behavioral, and performance effects following the intranasal route are similar to those after intramuscular use. Intranasal heroin is about one-half as potent as intramuscular heroin.[11]

Clinical Presentation

Heroin Withdrawal

A 5-day protocol using clonidine (0.1–0.3 mg) and naltrexone (1–4 mg) three times daily may have potential for the outpatient treatment of heroin withdrawal.[12]

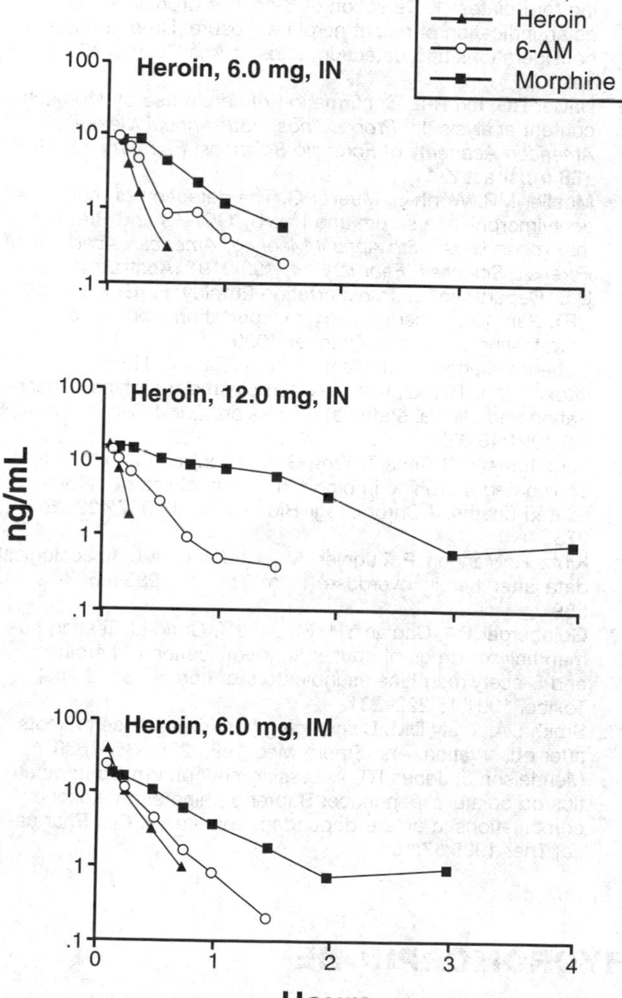

Figure 25–5 Mean blood concentrations of heroin, 6-acetylmorphine (6-AM), and morphine following administration of heroin hydrochloride by the intranasal (IN) and intramuscular (IM) routes. (From Cone EJ, Holicky BA, Grant TM, et al. Pharmacokinetics and pharmacodynamics of intranasal "snorted" heroin. J Anal Toxicol 1993;17:327–337.)

Immune Dysfunction (AIDS)

Natural Killer cell activity is reduced in parenteral heroin abusers who are HIV negative compared with methadone maintenance patients. This suggests that abnormalities of cellular immunity in parenteral heroin abusers may be normalized by long-term methadone treatment.[13]

Immune Dysfunction and the Addict

Acquired immunodeficiency syndrome and intravenous drug abuse[14] are discussed in Chapter 19.

Laboratory

Analytical Methods

A gas chromatography–mass spectrometry (GC–MS) assay method for quantitation of urinary 6-acetylmorphine (6-AM), free morphine, and total morphine is available. The limit of sensitivity for 6-AM is 0.81 ng/mL. Following heroin administration, 6-AM is excreted rapidly with a half-life of 0.6 hour. The half-life of free morphine is 3.6 hours, and that of total morphine, 7.9 hours. After administration of morphine and codeine, no 6-AM is detected by GC–MS above the 0.81 ng/mL detection limit of the assay. Presence of 6-AM in the urine indicates that heroin or 6-AM was administered within 24 hours of specimen collection and that the 6-AM in the urine is not due to morphine or codeine administration.[15]

Blood Levels

The blood level of 6-monoacetylmorphine (6-MAM) is usually very low or not detectable; stomach content can be used as a substitute in heroin detection.[16] The detection of 6-MAM in blood or urine shows recent, but single drug use. After more frequent or chronic heroin use, 6-MAM can be detected in hair. GC–MS and radioimmunoassay are the preferred analytical methods.[17] GC—MS detection of 6-MAM in the urine supports the conclusion that heroin was ingested. Because it is so rapidly metabolized, the absence of detectable levels of 6-MAM does not exclude the possibility of heroin ingestion[18] (Fig. 25–6).

In heroin intoxication the total plasma morphine concentration appears to provide a better correlation with the clinical condition of the patient than the plasma level of free morphine.[19]

In a series of deaths suspected to be heroin related, conjugated morphine was found in the blood in all cases.[20] The presence of free morphine in blood indicates a recent heroin injection. Detection of conjugated morphine in blood indicates that life was sustained over a longer period. In most cases of fatal heroin overdoses, 6-MAM has been identified.[21]

Ancillary Tests

Analysis of hair for 6-AM can be used to differentiate heroin users from users of other opiates (eg, poppy seed, licit morphine, and codeine).[22]

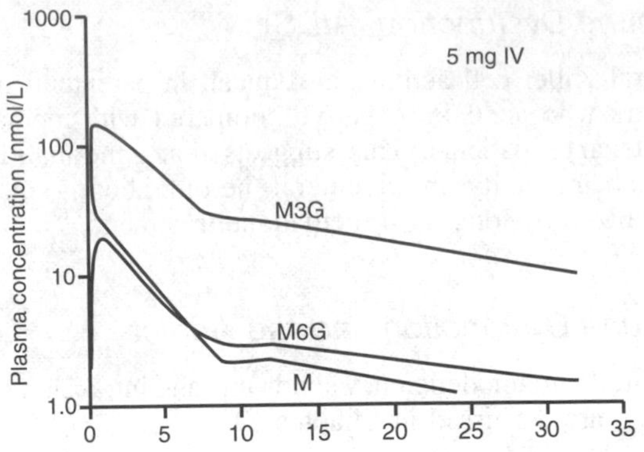

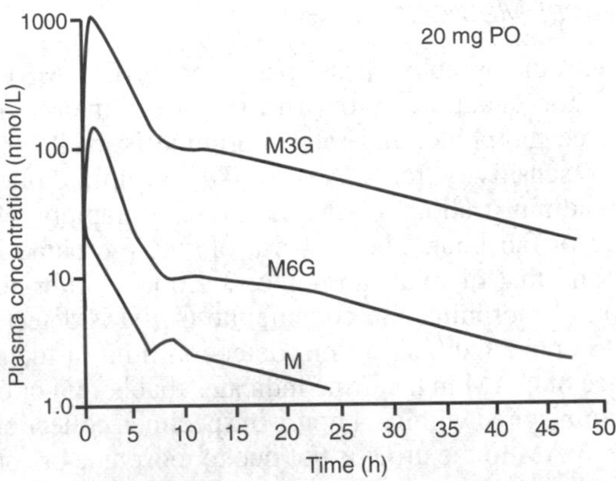

Figure 25-6 Mean plasma concentrations of morphine (M), morphine-6-glucuronide (M6G), and morphine-3-glucuronide (M3G) in seven healthy volunteers receiving single 5-mg intravenous (IV) and 20-mg oral (PO) doses of morphine. (From Hasselstrom J, Sawe J. Morphine pharmacokinetics and metabolism in humans: Enterohepatic cycling and relative contribution of metabolites to active opioid concentrations. Clin Pharmacokinet 1993;24: 344-354.)

Treatment

Following an intravenous heroin overdose and treatment with naloxone, prolonged observation may not be required for patients who are awake and alert and have no evidence of pulmonary involvement after the first several hours. Prospective studies are still required to ascertain whether or not mandatory 24-hour observation is necessary.[23] Buprenorphine and naloxone combinations of 2 and 0.4 mg intravenously were useful in one controlled study of heroin-dependent individuals.[24]

REFERENCES—HEROIN

1. Treaster JB. With supply and purity up heroin use expands. NY Times, August 1, 1993.
2. Treaster B. 7 hospitalized in Bronx after using heroin mix: Police warn users of potent new blend. NY Times, March 18, 1995, p. 9.
3. Hamilton R, Perrone J, Meggs WJ, et al. Epidemic anticholinergic poisoning from scopolamine tainted heroin. Clin Toxicol 1993;33:475–486 (Abstract 42).
4. Hendrickse RG, Maxwell SM, Young R. Aflatoxins and heroin. Br Med J 1989;299:492–493.
5. Utrecht MJ, Stone AF, McCarron MM. Heroin body packers. J Emerg Med 1993;11:33–40.
6. Karhunen PJ, Pennttila A, Panula A. Detection of heroin "body-packers" at Helsinki airport. Lancet 1987;1: 1265.
7. Mofenson HC, Caraccio TR. Continuous infusion of intravenous naloxone. Ann Emerg Med 1987;16:600.
8. Goldfrank L, Weisman RS, Errick JK, Lo M-W. A dosing nomogram for continuous infusion intravenous naloxone. Ann Emerg Med 1986;15:566–570.
9. Wang M-L, Lin JL, Liau S-J, Bullard RJ. Heroin in lung: Report of two cases. J Formosa Med Assoc 1994;93: 170–172.
10. McDonald FW, Cienki JJ, Horowitz RS, et al. Delayed encephalopathy after heroin use. Clin Toxicol 1995;33:478–485 (Abstract 20).
11. Cone EJ, Holicky BA, Grant TM, et al. Pharmacokinetics and pharmacodynamics of intranasal "snorted" heroin. J Anal Toxicol 1993;17:327–337.
12. Kleber HD, Topazian M, Gaspari J, et al. Clonidine and naltrexone in the outpatient treatment of heroin withdrawal. Am J Drug Alcohol Abuse 1987;13:1–17.
13. Novick DM, Ochshorn M, Ghali V, et al. Natural killer cell activity and lymphocyte subsets in parenteral heroin abusers and long-term methadone maintenance patients. J Pharmacol Exp Ther 1989;250:606–610.
14. Update: Acquired immunodeficiency syndrome—United States. MMWR 1985;34:245–248.
15. Cone EJ, Welch P, Mitchell JM, Paul BD. Forensic drug testing for opiates: 1. Detection of 6-acetylmorphine in urine as an indication of recent heroin exposure: Drug and assay considerations and detection times. J Anal Toxicol 1991; 15:1–7.
16. Havier RG, Lin R-L. Confirmation of heroin use by stomach content analysis. In: *Proceedings, 46th Annual Meeting, American Academy of Forensic Sciences, February 14, 1994:* 188 (Abstract K-11).
17. Moeller MR, Worth S, Mueller C. The detection of monoacetylmorphine in serum and hair by GC/MS and RIA. In: *Proceedings, 46th Annual Meeting, American Academy of Forensic Sciences, February 14, 1994:*191 (Abstract K31).
18. U.S. Department of Transportation Employers' Guide to 49 CFT. Part 40: Procedures for transportation workplace drug testing programs. October 1989.
19. Gutierrez-Cebollada J, Cami J, de la Torre R. Heroin intoxication: The relation between plasma morphine concentration and clinical status at admission. Eur J Clin Pharmacol 1991;40:635.
20. Lora-Tomayo C, Tena T, Tena G. Concentrations of free and conjugated morphine in blood in twenty cases of heroin-related deaths. J Chromatogr Biomed Appl 1987;422:267–273.
21. Kintz P, Mangen P, Lugnier AA, Chument AJ. Toxicological data after heroin overdose. Hum Toxicol 1989;8:587–589.
22. Goldberger BA, Caplan YH, Maguire T, Cone IJ. Testing human hair for drugs of abuse: III. Identification of heroin and 6-acetylmorphine as indicators of heroin use. J Anal Toxicol 1991;15:222–231.
23. Smith DA, Yealy DM. Discharging heroin overdose patients after observation. Ann Emerg Med 1993;22:1638–1639.
24. Mendelson J, Jones RT. Assessing new pharmacotherapeutics on opiate dependence: Buprenorphine and naloxone combinations in opiate-dependent volunteers. Clin Pharmacol Ther 1995;57:160.

HYDROMORPHONE

Hydromorphone (Dihydromorphinone, Dilaudid) has a high analgesic potency—five to six times that of morphine and three times that of heroin. Hydromorphone concentrations with subcutaneous infusions are 70% those with intravenous infusion and may be preferable to intravenous opioid infusions for management of severe cancer pain.[1]

Toxicokinetics

The minimally effective plasma concentration of hydromorphone in patients with chronic severe pain is about 4 ng/mL.[2,3] Oral hydromorphone is metabolized to hydromorphone-3-glucuronide, which accumulates in renal failure.[4]

Laboratory

Two fatalities exhibited postmortem blood hydromorphone concentrations of 0.5 and 1.2 mg/L, respectively. Plasma concentrations (in normal human volunteers) reached an average peak of 0.022 ng/L 0.8 hour after a single 4-mg dose.[5] Lethal blood concentrations of hydromorphone (> 0.01 mg/dL) were present in all 12 individuals who died from the intravenous use of Dilaudid.[6] A high-performance liquid chromatography method using an ESA coulometric detection set can be used for plasma hydromorphone determination; the detection limit is 0.1 ng/mL.[7]

Treatment

Clonazepam is useful in the treatment of myoclonus after high doses of hydromorphone and other opioids.[8] Naloxone is an effective antidote.

REFERENCES—HYDROMORPHONE

1. Moulin DE, Kreeft JH, Murray-Poisons N, Bouqillon AJ. Comparison of continuous subcutaneous and intravenous hydromorphone infusions for management of cancer pain. Lancet 1991;337:465–468.
2. Baselt RC. *Disposition of Toxic Drugs and Chemicals in Man.* 3rd ed. Chicago: Year Book, 1989:415–416.
3. Reidenberg MM, Goodman H, Erle H, et al. Hydromorphone levels and pain control in patients with severe chronic pain. Clin Pharmacol Ther 1988;44:376–382.
4. Babal N, Hager N, Thirdwell M, et al. Steady-state disposition of hydromorphone and hydromorphone-3-glucuronide in cancer patients. Clin Pharmacol Ther 1995;57:165.
5. Baselt RC. Two hydromorphone fatalities. Bull Int Assoc Forens Toxicol 1978;14(2):20.
6. CDS: Dilaudid[R]-related deaths—District of Columbia 1987. MMWR 1988;37:425–427.
7. Hill HF, Coda BA, Tanaka A, Schaffer R. Multiple-dose evaluation of intravenous hydromorphone pharmacokinetics in normal human subjects. Anesth Analg 1991;72:330–336.
8. Eisele JH Jr, Grigsby EJ, Dea G. Clonazepam treatment of myoclonic contractions associated with high dose opioids: Case report. Pain 1992;49:231–232.

KETOBEMIDONE

Ketobemidone, 1-[4-(3-hydroxyphenyl)-1-methyl-4-piperidyl]-propan-1-one, is an opioid analgesic with actions similar to those of morphine. In Scandinavia, ketobemidone is available only in combination with an antispasmodic substance, 3-dimethylamino-l-diphenylbutane, as Ketogin. In Denmark, Ketogin is abused by drug addicts. Deaths have been reported following its use.

REFERENCES—KETOBEMIDONE

1. Simmsen KW. Four cases involving ketobemidone. Bull Int Assoc Forens Toxicol 1992;22(4):28–31.

l-α-ACETYLMETHADOL HYDROCHLORIDE (LAAM)

A narcotic maintenance drug, *l*-α-acetylmethadol hydrochloride (LAAM) was approved by the U.S. Food and Drug Administration in July 1993. Experience in maintenance clinics suggests that LAAM is comparable to methadone in reducing the use of narcotics. Initial studies suggest that patients can be treated every other day instead of every day as is required with methadone. Adverse reactions include arrhythmias, flulike symptoms, abdominal cramps, diarrhea, and muscle aches. LAAM can be dispensed only by a narcotic treatment program approved by the Food and Drug Administration, Drug Enforcement Administration, and state methadone authorities.

It is distributed under the name ORLAAM Oral Concentrate.[1]

REFERENCE—LAAM

1. LAAM approved to treat drug dependence. FDA Consumer 1993;27:5–6.

MEPERIDINE HYDROCHLORIDE

Toxicokinetics

α-acid glycoprotein (AAG) is the main plasma protein that binds meperidine (Demerol, Pethidine). Plasma AAG concentration may be increased in patients with myocardial infarction, trauma, necrotizing enterocolitis, surgery, arthritis, Crohn's disease, and obesity. It is considered as an "acute phase reactant." Meperidine is frequently administered to patients in stress. Increased meperidine protein binding in these patients may partially explain the various degrees of response among individuals to any specific meperidine concentration.[1]

Lactation

Postcesarean patient-controlled analgesia with meperidine leads to accumulation of normeperidine in breast milk, which is often associated with neonatal neurobehavioral depression on the third day of life.[2]

Metabolism

Meperidine undergoes metabolism in the liver to normeperidine, a convulsant. In patients with alcoholic hepatitis and cirrhosis, multiple doses of meperidine lead to central nervous system excitation.[3]

Clinical Presentation

High doses of meperidine produce convulsions because of its conversion to normeperidine. Myoclonus usually precedes convulsions.[4,5] Plasma normeperidine levels and central nervous system irritability are significantly correlated.[5,6] Predisposing factors for meperidine-induced seizures include doses greater than 100 mg every 2 hours for longer than 24 hours, renal failure, an alkaline urine (decreased excretion), coadministration of enzyme-inducing drugs, coadministration of phenothiazines that lower seizure threshold, and a history of seizures.[7]

Daily doses of meperidine greater than 25 mg/kg may be associated with seizures due to normeperidine toxicity especially in the presence of renal impairment or if meperidine has been taken orally, when high first-pass clearance results in rapid conversion to normeperidine. As the plasma half-life of normeperidine with normal renal function is 15 to 30 hours, normeperidine concentrations may take about 3 days to reach 90% of the final plateau values.[8] Other neuropsychiatric manifestations of meperidine toxicity are summarized in Table 25–15.[19]

Laboratory

Table 25–16 correlates levels of central nervous system toxicity after meperidine use with plasma normeperidine concentrations.[9]

Treatment

Discontinue the drug. Establish an adequate airway; monitor breathing and circulation. Intravenous barbiturates, particularly pentobarbital, have been effective in quieting the agitated state and multifocal myoclonus with meperidine toxicity. Treat seizures with diazepam. Rule out epilepsy. Carbamazepine may also be useful in managing hypomanic symptoms.[9] Naloxone does not antagonize the tremors, twitching, or seizures caused by normeperidine, but it does antagonize the opiate effects (sedation, respiratory depression, hypotension, coma).

Table 25–15
Neuropsychiatric Manifestations of Meperidine Toxicity

Psychiatric symptoms
Shaky feelings
Irritability
Auditory and visual hallucinations
Psychiatric signs
Agitation
Hypomania
Paranoia
Delirium
Complex partial seizure
Neurologic signs
Tremor
Muscle twitches
Myoclonus
Generalized seizure

From Shochet RB, Murray GB. Neuropsychiatric toxicity of meperidine. J Intensive Care Med 1988;3:246–252.

REFERENCES—MEPERIDINE

1. Julius HC, Levine HL, Williams WD. Meperidine binding to isolated alpha$_1$ acid glycoprotein and albumin. DICP Ann Pharmacother 1989;23:568–572.
2. Wittels B, Scott DT, Sinatra RS. Exogenous opioids in human breast milk and acute neonatal neurobehavior: A preliminary study. Anesthesiology 1990;73:864–869.
3. Danziger LH, Martin SJ, Blum RA. Central nervous system toxicity associated with meperidine use in hepatic disease. Pharmacotherapy 1994;14:235–238.
4. Goetting MG. Neurotoxicity of meperidine. Ann Emerg Med 1985;14:1007–1009.
5. Kaiko R, Foley K, Heidrich G, et al. Normeperidine plasma levels and central nervous system (CNS) irritability in cancer patients. Fed Proc 1978;37:568.
6. Hershey LA. Meperidine and central neurotoxicity. Ann Intern Med 1983;98:548–549.
7. Tang R, Shimomura S, Rotblatt M. Meperidine induced seizures in sickle cell patients. Hosp Formul 1980;15:764–772.
8. Pryre BJ, Grech H, Stoddart PA, et al. Toxicity of norpethidone in sickle cell crisis. Br Med J 1992;304:1478–1479.
9. Shochet RB, Murray GB. Neuropsychiatric toxicity of meperidine. J Intens Care Med 1988;3:246–252.

MEPTAZINOL HYDROCHLORIDE

Meptazinol is an analgesic capable of relieving severe pain after intravenous dosage or moderate pain after oral dosage.[1] Given parenterally, meptazinol is one fifth to one twentieth as potent as morphine.[2,3] It is claimed to cause less respiratory depression, constipation, and miosis than other opioids. Reports of opioid antagonist activity, receptor selectivity, multiple modes of action, lesser respiratory depression, constipation, miosis, and lack of psychotropic activity suggest that meptazinol may have limited abuse potential compared with other opioids.[2] Dysphoric effects clearly distinguish meptazinol from other morphinelike drugs. An overdose of meptazinol may cause significant respiratory depression, which may not be reversed by naloxone.[4]

Table 25–16
Central Nervous System Toxicity of Meperidine: Correlation With Normeperidine Levels in 67 Patients

Level of Toxicity	Clinical Symptoms	Plasma Normeperidine Level (ng/mL)	Normeperidine/Meperidine Ratio
I	Asymptomatic	56 (6–190)	0.2 (0.02–0.58)
II	Shaky feelings	422 (128–1290)	1.3 (0.32–3.05)
III	Tremors	463 (146–1141)	2.2 (0.43–9.77)
IV	Twitches Myoclonus Grand mal seizures	814 (424–1856)	3.0 (0.79–5.4)

From Shochet RB, Murray GB. Neuropsychiatric toxicity of meperidine. J Intensive Care Med 1988;3:246–252.

Structure and Classification

Meptazinol is a synthetic hexahydroazepine derivative.[5] It is available in Europe as Meptid. Meptazinol is structurally related to meperidine.[6]

Product Formulation

Meptazinol is available in the United Kingdom as tablets of 200 mg and as an injection of 100 ng/mL (as the hydrochloride).[7]

Therapeutic Dose

At 70 mg, meptazinol produces a profile of response similar to that of 15 mg of morphine.[2] At 140 mg, the profile of morphinelike effect is greater that with the 70-mg dose. This may be reflected by hypothermia, nervousness, and feelings of turning of the stomach.[2] Similar findings followed doses of 280 mg, including decreased feeling of relaxation, increase in an LSD scale score, and nervousness.

Toxic Dose

A 61-year-old woman ingested 1000 mg (5, 200-mg tablets) of meptazinol together with a quarter bottle of whisky. She experienced respiratory arrest and survived after supportive care.[4]

Fatal Dose

No fatal dose in humans has been established.

Toxicokinetics

Absorption

Gastric emptying is a major determinant of the rate of absorption and magnitude of plasma concentration.[8] Following a single 200-mg oral dose, peak plasma levels of 43 ng/mL (range, 9.1–110 ng/mL) are reached in about 0.5 to 2 hours.[1,8,9] Following intravenous administration of 25 mg, peak plasma concentrations of about 80 to 90 ng/mL are reached in 0.5 hour. The bioavailability after oral dosage is low, 8.69%. In this respect, meptazinol is similar to other phenolic analgesics such as morphine, pentazocine, and butorphanol, all of which have low bioavailability due to extensive first-pass conjugation. Meptazinol is 27.1% bound to plasma membranes. This contrasts with the plasma protein binding of other analgesics such as butorphanol (80%) and buprenorphine (98%) and may minimize the probability of interaction with other more highly protein-bound drugs.[1]

Distribution

The apparent volume of distribution is about 5 L/kg,[1] which is similar to the volume of distribution of the structurally related narcotic analgesic meperidine.

Elimination

The elimination half-life after an intravenous dose of 25 mg averages about 2 hours. After an oral dose of 200 mg, the plasma clearance is 2.2 L/min. Elimination of meptazinol appears to occur primarily by metabolism to the glucuronide conjugate.[8,10]

Drug Interactions

In combination with anesthetics, meptazinol produces the same pattern of respiratory depression as other potent analgesics such as meperidine and pentazocine.[11,12] Ethanol appeared to have no effect on the ventilatory response to hypercapnia alone or in combination with one oral dose of 200 mg of meptazinol.[2,13]

Pregnancy/Lactation

Meptazinol may pass into breast milk, but the safety of its use during pregnancy or lactation has not been established.

Mechanism of Action

Meptazinol has both opioid agonist and antagonist activity and selectively binds at a subpopulation of mu receptors, designated mu_1. The reported central cholinergic activity appears to reside primarily in the l-isomer.[2,7,13] Meptazinol effects are opioid-like at lower doses and different at higher doses, in contrast to morphine.[2]

Clinical Presentation

At doses that approach 280 mg, the profile of effects after meptazinol use is not like that of morphine. Patients report less relaxation and an increase in nervousness. The dysphoria with meptazinol is usually not seen with other morphine-like drugs.[2] Pupillary diameters decrease after the 70- and 140-mg doses but do not decrease further at the 280-mg dose. Its abuse potential appears to be less than that of morphine, codeine, or propoxyphene.[2]

The majority of discomfort after a 200-mg oral dose concerns the gastrointestinal tract (nausea, vomiting, stomachache, indigestion/heartburn, diarrhea, and constipation).[1] There have been no reports of any major central nervous system effects (eg, euphoria, dysphoria) although giddy/dizzy feelings were experienced.[7]

Respiratory depression appears dose related and in one study was reversed by naloxone.[12] Following ingestion of 1000 mg with whisky, a 61-year-old woman experienced respiratory arrest. Naloxone in doses up to 10 mg was not effective in restoring spontaneous respiration. She began to breathe spontaneously 5 hours after admission and made a full recovery.[4]

Laboratory

Analytical Methods

Plasma concentrations of meptazinol are determined by high-performance liquid chromatography using fluorescence detection. The lower limit of sensitivity is 3 ng/mL.[10]

Blood Levels

Two and one-half hours following ingestion of 100 mg of meptazinol, the serum meptazinol concentration was 20.1

μg/mL (20,000 ng/mL). This level fell to 69 ng/mL, 15.5 hours after the overdose.[4]

Treatment

Stabilization

Treatment is largely symptomatic and supportive. Patients should be placed in an intensive care unit where monitoring facilities, a central line, and oxygen are available. Prolonged (4–8 hours) assisted ventilation may be required after intubation. Continuous monitoring of respiratory rate, pulse, blood pressure, and level of consciousness should be ongoing until the patient begins to breathe spontaneously.

Gut Decontamination

The degree of respiratory depression may be related to the dose of meptazinol ingested. Therefore, gastric emptying should begin preferably within 4 hours of an ingestion. The airway must be protected. There is no clinical evidence that activated charcoal or cathartics are useful after a meptazinol overdose.

Elimination Enhancement

Although meptazinol has a relatively low degree of protein binding it is widely distributed. Hemodialysis and hemoperfusion are not likely to be useful in treating the overdose patient.

Antidote

Naloxone was not effective in reversing respiratory depression following one meptazinol overdose[4]; however, it should be tried in increasing doses because it appears to reverse dose-related respiratory depression.[12]

Supportive Measures

Patients who begin spontaneous respiration should be observed for 24 hours. By that time they should be alert, awake, and responsive and have relatively normal physical findings. They may then be discharged after a psychiatric consultation.

REFERENCES—MEPTAZINOL HYDROCHLORIDE

1. Norbury HM, Franklin RA, Graham DF. Pharmacokinetics of the new analgesic meptazinol after oral and intravenous administration to volunteers. Eur J Clin Pharmacol 1983;25: 77–80.
2. Johnson RE, Jasinski DR. Human pharmacology and abuse potential of meptazinol. Clin Pharmacol Ther 1987;41: 426–433.
3. Holmes B, Ward A. Meptazinol: A preview of its pharmacodynamic and pharmacokinetic properties and therapeutic efficacy. Drugs 1985;30:285–212.
4. Davison AG, Collinson PO, Asseti AR, Clarke SW. Meptazinol overdose producing near fatal respiratory depression. Hum Toxicol 1987;6:331.
5. Price PKJ, Lathan AN. Meptazinol: A side effect profile compared to placebo in general practice. J Int Med Res 1982; 10:219–224.
6. Spiegel K, Pasternak GW. Meptazinol: A novel Mu-1 selective opioid analgesic. J Pharmacol Exp Ther 1984;228: 414–419.
7. Reynolds JEF, ed. *Martindale: The Extra Pharmacopoeia.* 30th ed. London: Pharmaceutical Press, 1993:1080–1081.
8. Franklin RA. The influence of gastric emptying on plasma concentrations of the analgesic meptazinol. Br J Pharmacol 1977;59:565–569.
9. Franklin RA, Aldridge A, White C de B. Studies on the metabolism of meptazinol, a new analgesic drug. Br J Clin Pharmacol 1976;3:497–502.
10. Frost T. Determination of meptazinol in plasma by high performance liquid chromatography with fluorescence detection. Analyst 1981;106:999–1001.
11. Hardy DAJ. Meptazinol and respiratory depression. Lancet 1983;2:576.
12. Slattery RJ, Harmer M, Rosen M, Vickers MD. Naloxone reversal of meptazinol-induced respiratory depression. Anaesthesia 1982;37:1163–1166.
13. Ali NA, Marshall RW, Allen EM, et al. Comparison of the effects of therapeutic doses of meptazinol and a dextropropoxyphene/paracetamol mixture alone and in combination with ethanol on ventilatory function and saccadic eye movements. Br J Clin Pharmacol 1978;20:631–637.

METHADONE

Fatalities

In 1992, Drummer et al. in Melbourne reported 10 deaths occurring 2 to 6 days after initiation of methadone maintenance.[1] The mean starting dose was 53 mg. The mean blood methadone level at death was 2.1 μmol/L. When initial doses higher than 15 to 30 mg are used in an unsupervised setting, respiratory depression may ensue. Death may occur during induction of methadone maintenance when tolerance is incorrectly assessed, and during maintenance when several days' doses are combined. Death can also follow accidental ingestion.[2]

Methadone Maintenance

Guidelines on the use of methadone in maintenance and detoxification treatment of narcotic addicts were issued by the National Institute on Drug Abuse in March 1989,[3] and can be obtained from the U.S. Food and Drug Administration (telephone: 301–295–8029).

Laboratory

A good correlation exists between plasma methadone concentrations (ng/mL) and dose (mg/kg/d) at steady state over a wide dosage range (3–100 mg of methadone per day).[4]

A high-performance liquid chromatography method for quantitation of plasma methadone levels has a detection limit of 5 ng.[5] Plasma methadone concentration appears to increase by 263 ng/mL for every milligram of methadone consumed per kilogram of body weight.[6] A gas chromatography–mass spectrometry assay is available to determine both methadone and its metabolite 2-ethyl-1-5-dimethyl-3,3-diphenylpyrrolidine (EDDP) in the urine.[7]

Errors

Several reports of errors have appeared in the literature in which antibiotics have been reconstituted with methadone instead of distilled water. Naloxone should be given to any patient with decreased level of consciousness and miosis, whether or not there is a history of opiate ingestion.[8,9]

Treatment

Admit to hospital and provide respiratory support. Institute gastric emptying while airway is protected. Administer naloxone.[10]

As adverse effects from methadone can be delayed as long as 5 hours after ingestion, observe the patient in the hospital at least 6 hours.[11]

REFERENCES—METHADONE

1. Drummer OH, Opeskin K, Syrjanen M, Cordner SM. Methadone toxicity causing death in the subjects starting on a methadone maintenance program. Am J Forens Med Pathol 1992;13:346–350.
2. Harding-Pink D. Methadone: One person's maintenance dose is another poison. Lancet 1993;341:665–666.
3. Section 291.501: Methadone in the maintenance treatment of narcotic addicts. Part 310: New Drugs. Recodification of Methadone Regulations. Title 21: Food and Drugs. Fed Regist 1977;42:46698–46710.
4. Wolff K, Hay A. Methadone concentrations in plasma and their relationship to drug dosage. Clin Chem 1992;38:438–439.
5. Baselt R. *Disposition of Toxic Drugs and Chemicals in Man.* 3rd ed. Chicago: Year Book, 1989:512–516.
6. Wolff K, Sanderson M, Hay AWM, Raistrick D. Methadone concentrations in plasma and their relationship to drug dosage. Clin Chem 1991;37:205–209.
7. Baugh LD, Liu RH, Walia AS. Simultaneous gas chromatography/mass spectrometry assay of methadone and EDP in urine. J Forens Sci 1991;36:548–555.
8. Roland EK, Lickitch G, Dunn HG, et al. Methadone poisoning due to accidental contamination of prescribed medication. Can Med Assoc J 1984;131:1357–1358.
9. Rayle MO, Ryan CA, Nazarli S. Unusual cause of methadone poisoning. Acta -Paediatr Scand 1991;80:486–487.
10. Binchy JM, Molyneux EM, Manning J. Accidental ingestion of methadone by children in Merseyside. Br Med J 1994;308:1335–1336.
11. Garrettson LK. Delayed onset of toxicity after methadone ingestion due to therapeutic error. Vet Hum Toxicol 1994;36:367.

MORPHINE

Structure

Morphine is an alkaloid and a phenanthrene derivative of opium. Plasma levels after 5 and 20 mg of morphine are shown in Figure 25–6.

Toxicokinetics

Elimination

Half-lives of morphine, morphine-3-glucuronide (M3G), and morphine-6-glucuronide (M6G) are 15, 11, and 13 hours, respectively. The terminal half-life of normorphine is 24 hours after oral administration.[1] The elimination half-life of morphine is inversely correlated with gestational age (9.3 hours in the preterm newborn baby and 6 to 7 hours in the term newborn).[2]

Plasma concentration–time curves following oral and intravenous administration of morphine disclose the M6G: morphine ratio to be about 2.6, and the M3G:morphine ratio, above 30.[1]

Metabolism

Metabolism of morphine to morphine glucuronides proceeds extremely rapidly, and, in the majority of subjects, detectable quantities of M6G and M3G are found in the plasma 5 minutes after dosing. Mean plasma levels of M3G and M6G exceed those of morphine at 0.1 and 0.5 hour after dosing, respectively, and remain higher than morphine levels at all times thereafter. In conjunction with the recent demonstration of the pharmacologic activity of M6G in human subjects, the findings strongly suggest that the majority of the clinical effects of morphine treatment after oral treatment (and other enteral routes of treatment) are mediated by the active metabolite. A considerable proportion of the effects of a parenteral dose of morphine are probably also attributable to this substance.[3]

Morphine-6-glucuronide appears to be 10- to 20-fold more potent than the parent drug in the central nervous system. After a single oral dose of morphine, the ratio of M6G to morphine is 3:1. Chronic oral dosing suggests that the ratio is considerably higher (about 6:1).[4]

Mechanism of Action

Morphine is metabolized in the liver to its 2- and 6-glucuronides, both of which bind to opiate receptors. The 6-glucuronide is a more potent analgesic than morphine itself; the 3-glucuronide antagonizes the analgesic activity of 6-glucuronide in experimental animals. Patient analgesic response to morphine appears to depend on the 3-glucuronide:6-glucuronide ratio, the 6-glucuronide being responsible for the analgesic effect. In some cases of paradoxical pain, patients with chronic nociceptive pain that does not respond to morphine, the ratio (usually 45:1) is much higher. Lesser quantities of active 6-glucuronide are produced in proportion to the active or even antagonistic 3-glucuronide.[5] These preliminary observations require further clinical validation.[6]

Laboratory

Ingestion of Poppy Seeds

Ingestion of a number of baked goods that contain poppy seeds can lead to positive screening tests for opiates. This is due to the presence of morphine and codeine as well as other natural products (eg, phenanthrene or benzylisoquiloline) especially on the surface of inadequately washed poppy seeds. *O*-6-Monoacetylmorphine (6-MAM) is rapidly produced by hepatic catabolism of heroin (diacetylmorphine) and small amounts are excreted in the urine. 6-MAM has not been detected in the urine after the ingestion of codeine, morphine, or poppy seeds.[7,8] Therefore, its presence in urine may be considered as a legally defensible evidence of heroin use or of 6-MAM itself.[7] Detection of 6-MAM in urine is important for ruling out poppy seed ingestion as a cause of a "false"-positive result in immunoassay screens for opiates. 6-MAM is not present in poppy seeds or in urine after the ingestion of poppy seeds.[9] Codeine is metabolized to morphine. The use of prescription and nonprescription medicine containing codeine can lead to positive immunoassay screening results. Simultaneous determination of 6-MAM, morphine, codeine, and other opiates by gas chromatography–mass spectrometry is sensitive for all components to about 10 ng/mL.[8]

Two to six hours after ingestion of cakes containing 25 g of poppy seeds, urine morphine values ranged from 0.0 to 300.0 ng/mL. No significant change in pupil size, body temperature, blood pressure, pulse rate, nystagmus, or typical field sobriety tests is observed.[10] Analysis of the urine can be performed on the Syva ETS analyzed with a low cutoff value of 300 ng/mL for the opiate assays. Therefore, consumption of large amounts of poppy seeds does not lead to symptoms of opiate impairment in such individuals even though they may have positive urine results.[8] The amount of morphine in poppy seeds may vary from 450 μg/g (white seeds) to 30 μg/g (black seeds). Ingestion of 1 g of the white poppy seeds led to positive tests for opiates in a urine screening assay.[11] Ingestion of poppy seed rolls containing 2 g of Australian seeds (108 μg morphine/g seed) led to excretion of less than 150 ng/mL total opiates, 24 hours after ingestion. Ingestion of 15 g of seeds (159 μg/morphine/g seed) led to total morphine levels greater than 300 ng/mL for about 24 hours, with the highest levels of 2010 ng/mL morphine and 78 ng/mL codeine obtained 9 hours after ingestion.[12] Ingestion of three poppy seed bagels led to a urine codeine concentration of 214 ng/mL and urine morphine concentration of 2797 ng/mL at 3 hours, with 16 ng/mL codeine and 676 ng/mL morphine at 22 hours.[13]

Ruling Out Poppy Seed Ingestion

Conditions that can rule out poppy seed ingestion as the sole source for morphine and codeine in urine include the following:

1. Codeine levels exceeding 300 ng/mL
2. Morphine:codeine ratio less than 2 (A lower morphine: codeine ratio would indicate the use of codeine).
3. High levels of morphine (>1000 ng/mL/L) with no codeine detected (Following poppy seed ingestions leading to levels of morphine of 100 ng/mL or more, all urine samples contain detectable amounts of codeine [>25 ng/mL]. Most laboratories do not report codeine concentrations below 300 ng/mL.)
4. Morphine levels in excess of 5000 ng/mL (but Meneely[10] showed higher levels) (The presence of 6-MAM would also rule out poppy seeds as the source.)[14]

Treatment

Treatment is similar to that for other narcotic drugs.

REFERENCES—MORPHINE

1. Hasselstrom J, Sawe J. Morphine pharmacokinetics and metabolism in humans: Enterohepatic cycling and relative contributions of metabolites to active opioid concentrations. Clin Pharmacokinet 1993;24:344–354.
2. Mikkelsen S, Feilberg VL, Christensen CB, Lundstrom KE. Morphine pharmacokinetics in premature and mature newborn infants. Acta Paediatr 1994;83:1025–1028.
3. Osborne R, Joel S, Trew D, Slevin M. Morphine and metabolite behavior after different routes of morphine administration: Demonstration of the importance of the active metabolite morphine-6-glucuronide. Clin Pharmacol Ther 1990;47:12–19.
4. McQuay JH, Carrol D, Faura CC, et al. Oral morphine in cancer pain: Influences on morphine and metabolite concentration. Clin Pharmacol Ther 1990;48:236–244.
5. Bowsher D. Parodoxical pain: When the metabolites of morphine are in the wrong ratio. Br Med J 1993;306:473–474.
6. Morley JS, Miles JB, Walls JC, Bowsher D. Paradoxical pain. Lancet 1992;540:1045.
7. Fehn J, Megges G. Detection of O^6-monoacetylmorphine in urine samples by GC/MS as evidence for heroin use. J Anal Toxicol 1985;9:134–138.
8. Mule SJ, Casella GA. Rendering the poppy seed defence defenceless: Identification of 6-monoacetylmorphine in urine by gas chromatography/mass spectroscopy. Clin Chem 1988;34:1427–1430.
9. Bowie LJ, Kirkpatrick PB. Simultaneous determination of monoacetylmorphine, morphine, codeine and other opiates by GC/MS. J Anal Toxicol 1989;13:326–329.
10. Meneely KD. Poppy seed ingestion: The Oregon perspective. J Forens Sci 1992;37:1158–1162.
11. Beck O, Vitols S, Stensio M. Positive urine screening for opiates after consumption of sandwich bread with poppy seed flavoring. Ther Drug Monit 1990;1:585–586.
12. El Sohly NH, El Sohly MA, Stanford DF. Poppy seed ingestion and opiates urinalysis: A closer look. J Anal Toxicol 1990;14:308–310.
13. Struempler PE. Excretion of codeine and morphine following ingestion of poppy seeds. J Anal Toxicol 1987;11:92–99.
14. Salerno S, Wisniewski HM, Rudelli RD. Effect of poppy seed ingestion on the TDx opiates assay. Ther Drug Monit 1990; 12:210–213.

NALBUPHINE HYDROCHLORIDE

Use

Nalbuphine (Nubaine) appears to be a useful and safe analgesic drug when administered by paramedics in the prehospital setting: 15 mg (0.75 mL) intravenously over 15 seconds if judged to be less than 60 kg body weight; 20 mg (1.0 mL) intravenously if judged to be equal to or greater than 60 kg.[1]

Toxicokinetics

The elimination half-life after intravenous administration of nalbuphine was 0.9 hour in children (after 0.2 mg/kg) and 2.3 hours in the elderly (10 mg) in one study. Clearance after intravenous administration was greater in children (2.7 L/h/kg) than in adults (1.78 L/h/kg) or the elderly (1.4 L/h/kg). Following oral administration (30 mg) mean peak nalbuphine concentrations were higher in the elderly (49 μg/L) than in adult volunteers (7 μg/L).[2]

Administration of nalbuphine to the mother during parturition may induce a reversible respiratory depression in the newborn baby. The placental transfer of nalbuphine is highly variable and rapid, with a fetal-to-arterial ratio ranging from 0.5 to 6. Fetal plasma concentrations are about the same or higher than maternal concentrations and may be associated with respiratory and cardiac depression.[3]

REFERENCES—NALBUPHINE HYDROCHLORIDE

1. Steve JK, Stofberg L, MacDonald G, et al. Nalbuphine analgesia in the prehospital setting. Am J Emerg Med 1988;6: 634–639.
2. Jaillon P, Gardin ME, Lecocq B, et al. Pharmacokinetics of nalbuphine in infants, young healthy volunteers and elderly patients. Clin Pharmacol Ther 1989;46:226–233.
3. Guillonneau M, Jacqz-Aigrain E, de Crey A, Zeggout H. Perinatal adverse effects of nalbuphine given during parturition. Lancet 1990;1:1588.

NALMEFENE

Nalmefene is a naltrexone derivative (Revex) that is a pure opiate antagonist without agonist effects. It appears to have a longer duration of effect than naloxone and is a more potent antagonist than naloxone at all three main types of opioid receptors.[1] Overdoses with nalmefene have not been reported, but consideration should be given to the possibility of naloxone-like catecholamine stimulation, which may induce arrhythmias and hypertension. Treatment of an overdose will probably be symptomatic and supportive.

Use

Because of its prolonged duration of action, nalmefene (nalmetrene) has potential advantages over naloxone. Fewer complications are expected to occur as a result of fluctuations in levels of consciousness (eg, sedation, aspiration, occult respiratory insufficiency). Less risk of renarcotization is expected in the patient who leaves the emergency department against medical advice soon after regaining consciousness. Maintenance infusion is indicated far less often, making calculation of infusion rates and monitoring of intravenous lines unnecessary in busy emergency departments. A prolonged opiate effect may follow overdose with propoxyphene and methadone, both of which have longer half-lives than naloxone. Peak plasma levels with pentazocine, diphenoxylate, and some other drugs occur later than with heroin and much later than with naloxone. Hepatic insufficiency, renal failure, and unusually large doses of opiates can prolong opiate toxicity. Intravenous nalmefene at both 0.5- and 1.0-mg doses reverses opiate toxicity, rapidly, completely, and for at least 4 hours.[2]

Therapeutic Dose

A single oral dose of nalmefene (50 mg) completely blocked fentanyl-induced (2 μg/kg intravenously) respiratory depression, analgesia and subjective effects for up to 48 hours.[3–5] Intravenous nalmefene 0.4 mg appeared effective in antagonizing respiratory depression induced by morphine.[6] One milligram intravenously appeared more effective than naloxone in reversing meperidine-induced sedation up to 240 minutes after administration of nalmefene.[7,8] Nalmefene is well tolerated in intravenous doses up to 24 mg without changes in vital signs.[9] A simple 50-mg oral dose totally prevents the effects of intravenous opiates for 48 hours.[10] A single 1-mg dose prevents the respiratory depressant effect of intravenous fentanyl for up to 4 hours. A 2-mg dose prevents respiratory depression for 8 hours.[10,11]

Toxicokinetics

Absorption

Unlike naloxone with a plasma half-life of 1 to 2 hours, nalmefene is active after both oral and parenteral administration and has a plasma half-life of 8 to 9 hours, similar to that of naltrexone. Its serum half-life is 10 to 12 hours, compared with 63 minutes for naloxone. Although the serum half-life of nalmefene is longer than 10 hours, a 1.0-mg dose prevents respiratory depression from fentanyl challenge for only 4 hours; one 2.0-mg dose prevents respiratory depression for up to 8 hours. If a narcotic with a duration of action of 4 hours is used, a 1.0-mg dose of nalmefene should provide reversal of sedation and respiratory depressant effects for the period.[7,8]

Distribution

The volume of distribution after 0.5 to 2.0 mg intravenously was 9.1 to 11.2 L/kg.[9]

Elimination

Following an intravenous dose of 0.5 mg of nalmefene, the elimination half-life was 9.5 hours; after 10 mg, 7.8 hours; and after 2.0 mg, 2.9 hours in one study.[9]

Mechanism of Action

Nalmefene does not produce mu-opiate agonist (morphine-like) effects in an opiate-abusing population. Nalmefene has opiate antagonist, not agonist, properties.[3,4] Nalmefene is four times as potent acutely as naloxone in antagonizing effects at the mu receptor, and more potent than naloxone in antagonizing effects at the kappa receptor.[7,8] The mu receptor is "morphinelike" and mediates supraspinal analgesia, respiratory depression, miosis, physical dependency, and euphoria. Kappa receptors mediate spinal analgesia, miosis, sedation, and limited respiratory depression.

Clinical Presentation

Nalmefene is occasionally associated with dizziness, lightheadedness, fatigue and lassitude, agitation, irritability, muscle tension, and a "hangover feeling," which is not dose related.[3,4] Drowsiness or sleepiness is the most common drug effect observed after administration of nalmefene. Other adverse effects include myalgia, arthralgia, nausea, paranoia, and paresthesias.[10] Oral nalmefene does not produce typical morphinelike effects and has no apparent abuse potential.[3] Further experience may indicate that nalmefene will precipitate opiate withdrawal in dependent patients, much like naloxone.

Where doses of 5 to 40 mg of nalmefene were administered to patients with primary biliary cirrhosis, all experienced a severe opioid withdrawal reaction. Pruritus was improved, fatigue was less, and plasma bilirubin showed a small fall.[12] All experienced anorexia, nausea, colicky abdominal pain, and constipation.

REFERENCES—NALMEFENE

1. Thornton JR, Losowsy MS. Opioid peptides and primary biliary cirrhosis. Br Med J 1988;297:1501–1503.
2. Kaplan JL, Marx JA. Effectiveness and safety of intravenous nalmefene for emergency department patients with suspected narcotic overdose: A pilot study. Ann Emerg Med 1993;22:187–190.
3. Fudala PJ, Johnson RE, Heishman SJ, Henningfield JE. Evaluation of the abuse liability of nalmefene. Clin Pharmacol Ther 1991;49:167.
4. Fudala PJ, Heishman SJ, Henningfield JE, Johnson RE. Human pharmacology and abuse potential of nalmefene. Clin Pharmacol Ther 1991;49:300–306.
5. Gal TJ, di Fazio CA, Dixon R. Prolonged blockade of opioid effects with oral nalmefene. Clin Pharmacol Ther 1986;40:537–542.
6. Konieczko KM, Jones JG, Barrowcliffe MP, et al. Antagonism of morphine-induced respiratory depression with nalmefene. Br J Anesth 1988;61:318–323.
7. Barsan WG, Seger D, Danzl DF, et al. Duration of antagonistic effects of nalmefene and naloxone in opiate-induced sedation for emergency department procedures. Ann Emerg Med 1987;16:477.
8. Barsan WG, Seger D, Danzl DF, et al. Duration of antagonistic effects of nalmefene and naloxone in opiate-induced sedation for emergency department procedures. Am J Emerg Med 1989;7:155–161.
9. Levinson B, Reynolds R, Kisiski J, Lee JW. The pharmacokinetics of nalmefene, an opioid antagonist. Anesthesiology 1990;73:A355.
10. Dixon R, Howes J, Gentile J, et al. Nalmefene: Intravenous safety and kinetics of a new opioid antagonist. Clin Pharmacol Ther 1986;39:49–53.
11. Reynolds JEF, ed. *Martindale: The Extra Pharmacopoeia.* 30th ed. London: Pharmaceutical Press, 1993:685.
12. Gal TJ, di Fazio CA. Prolonged antagonism of opioid action with intravenous nalmefene in man. Anesthesiology 1986;64:175–180.

NALOXONE

Figure 25–1 shows the structure of naloxone (*N*-allynoroxymorphone; Narcan). Also see Chapter 5.

Use

A prospective, randomized, double-blind, placebo-controlled study showed that 0.4 to 1.2 mg naloxone intravenously was no better than placebo in amelioration of hypotension in septic shock.[1] Continuous naloxone administration may aid in suppressing opiate withdrawal symptoms in human opiate addicts during detoxification treatment.[2] An anecdotal report suggests that intravenous naloxone 1.6 mg reversed the hypotension associated with a captopril overdose.[3] Anecdotal evidence suggests that naloxone with activated charcoal may be useful in improving degree of consciousness following a valproic acid overdose.[4]

Preliminary Studies

Naloxone induces an increase in cortisol secretion. Acute alcoholism may induce an increase in endogenous opioids in the plasma and cerebrospinal fluid. Preliminary studies tend to suggest that naloxone may reverse the effect of alcohol by its ability to increase cortisol secretion. The ultimate answer to this relationship remains to be determined.[5]

A World Health Organization study suggests that there is inadequate evidence that repeated naloxone administration without added neuroleptic medication is more effective than placebo in treatment of patients with the symptoms of schizophrenia.[6]

Naloxone may be an additional modality of use in the treatment of captopril-induced hypotension. The mechanism of its effectiveness in one anecdotal report is not clear. Further clinical studies are indicated.[3]

Intramuscular naloxone 0.4 ng/kg had no readily apparent benefit in the resuscitation of asphyxiated newborn infants in a clinical trial of 85 infants.[7]

Naloxone Therapy[8]

Dose

Preliminary studies with oral naloxone administered in doses from 0.5 to 16 mg once daily indicate possible efficacy in the treatment of opioid-induced constipation. All patients should be monitored for the signs and symptoms of systemic withdrawal. Adverse reactions can be managed with single dose reduction or lengthening of the interval.[9] When given orally, naloxone is extensively metabolized and may have greater bioavailability at the enteric wall than systemically. Naloxone can be titrated up to 12 mg at dose intervals of 6 hours or longer, and this procedure should be used if multiple daily doses are required.

If attempts at intravenous access for naloxone injection are unsuccessful, an injection of 0.4 mg naloxone with a 22-gauge needle into the midventral surface of the tongue after aspiration with no blood return and intubation can be considered in the treatment of narcotic-induced respiratory depression.[10] If, however, the patient has a normal blood pressure, this route may be unnecessary, as naloxone is absorbed efficiently and is rapid acting when the patient is not in shock and an adequate dose is administered by the intramuscular route. In addition, a sublingual injection may have the potential to cause intraoral bleeding and possible airway compromise. There is also the possibility that a paramedic or other health care professional planning to use the sublingual route may be bitten by a patient who may be at high risk of having AIDS.[11]

Continuous Infusion

Mofenson and Caraccio have offered a method for infusion therapy with naloxone after the bolus dosing has been determined.[12]

- Step 1: Determine maintenance fluid requirements for 24 hours.
- Step 2: To determine amount of naloxone (in mg) to add to the maintenance fluid for a 24-hour period, take the amount required for the initial response in mg × ⅔ × 24 hours.
- Step 3: To determine the desired rate of naloxone infusion (in mL/h) take the maintenance fluid (Step 1)/24 hours.

This method may reduce the risk of possible fluid overload in young children and the potential for pulmonary edema from opioids. Naloxone should not be mixed with preparations containing bisulfite, metabisulfite, long-chain or high-molecular-weight anions, or any solution having an alkaline pH. A naloxone mixture should not be used after 24 hours from the time prepared.

Infusions of naloxone may be indicated When (1) repeated bolus therapy is required; (2) a large initial bolus is required; (3) a large amount of opiate or a long-acting opiate (eg, propoxyphene, methadone) has been ingested; or (4) opioid metabolism is decreased, as in liver disease.[12]

Neonates and Children

Caution should be exercised before administering naloxone to infants of mothers who received meperidine during labor. Naloxone is not recommended in the treatment of meperidine-induced seizures and may be detrimental.[13] Continuous naloxone infusions have been used in infants aged 12 months and 3 days who were intoxicated with 100 ng normethadone[14] and 5 mg morphine, respectively. Administration of naloxone to the infant of an opioid-dependent patient may induce seizures and features of opioid withdrawal (eg, hyperactivity, irritability, restlessness).[15]

The currently recommended dose of naloxone is 0.1 mg/kg for infants and children from birth to 5 years of age or 20 kg of body weight. Children older than 5 years of age or weighing more than 20 kg may be given 2.0 mg. These doses may be repeated as needed to maintain opiate reversal. The higher dose recommendation is based, in part, on a concern that 0.01 mg/kg, currently recommended in approved labeling, may not provide optimal opiate reversal in some infants. In addition, it is intended to simplify naloxone dosing and provide greater probability of optimal opiate reversal in most patients.

Because doses as high as 0.4 mg/kg have been administered to newborns without ill effect, it is felt that the higher dose poses no increased risk. Naloxone doses ranging from 0.005 to 0.4 mg/kg have been reported in the pediatric literature. Individual doses up to 0.4 mg/kg and constant intravenous infusion of 0.16 mg/kg/h for 5 days have not been associated with naloxone-related adverse effects. The average half-life of naloxone in premature newborns is 70 minutes.

Although there are no well-controlled studies in infants and children directly comparing the intravenous and intratracheal versus intramuscular or subcutaneous routes of administration, the Committee on Drugs of the American Academy of Pediatrics' recommendation is based on a concern that absorption of intramuscularly and subcutaneously injected medication may be erratic or delayed in the patient who is hypotensive, hypoperfused, and/or peripherally vasoconstricted.[16]

Pathophysiology

Naloxone appears to modulate the release of catecholamines presumably from chromaffin cells. Plasma epinephrine, norepinephrine, and dopamine concentrations were increased in a patient with pheochromocytoma after intravenous naloxone 10 mg was administered.[17]

Naloxone and Morphine Metabolism

Animal studies with naloxone and morphine suggest that morphine acts mainly on the dopaminergic system in the brain, interacting with naloxone preferential receptors. Its action is also induced through the noradrenergic system in some areas of the brain. No biochemical action of morphine is apparent in the central serotonergic system.[18]

Kappa Receptor Activators

Kappa receptor activators (pentazocine, butorphanol) may result in sedative and psychotomimetic effects, which are antagonized by high doses of naloxone.[19]

Toxicokinetics/Clinical Presentation

Pregnancy

Intravenous naloxone 0.4 mg may induce severe hypertension during labor in a patient with a history of previous mild hypertension. Patients with mild to moderate hypertension who receive narcotic antagonists during labor should be carefully monitored.[20]

Drug Interactions

Buprenorphine. The antagonism of buprenorphine requires large doses of naloxone and is characterized by gradual onset of the reversal effects and decreased duration of action of the normally prolonged respiratory depression.[21]

Methohexital. The acute onset of withdrawal symptoms induced by naloxone in opiate addicts appears to be blocked by the acute action of the barbiturate methohexital.[22] This observation requires clinical confirmation in opiate withdrawal states.

Clonidine and Yohimbine. These α_2-receptor ligands (agonist and antagonist) appear to alter the effect of naloxone by reducing noradrenergic release (clonidine) or enhancing noradrenergic release (yohimbine). The effects of naloxone–clonidine and naloxone–yohimbine combinations remain to be clinically validated.[23]

Naloxone may induce an acute rise in blood pressure in a patient receiving clonidine chronically. This may be critical in an unconscious elderly hypertensive person who would not be in a position to give a history of clonidine use.[24]

Effects of Naloxone

Table 25–17 summarizes some results of naloxone-precipitated violence.

Table 25–17
Naloxone-Precipitated Violence

Physical discomfort of withdrawal
Confusion on regaining consciousness in a hospital setting
Anger at interruption of the "high"
Unmasking of other toxins
Unmasking of underlying personality disorder

Naloxone has been associated with hypertension, cardiac arrhythmias, cardiac arrest, and sudden death, all of which may be provoked by sympathetic stimulation. Seizures, by an as yet undetermined mechanism, may also follow naloxone use.[25] Even low doses of 40 to 80 mg of naloxone may precipitate pulmonary edema in otherwise healthy young people.[26] Large doses may induce an acute pulmonary edema in the older age groups.[27]

Phentolamine. Phentolamine is a competitive alpha-blocking drug with a similar affinity for α_1 and α_2 receptors. It also blocks serotonin receptors and causes mast cells to release histamine. Many features of acute pulmonary edema may be explained by massive catecholamine release. Anecdotal reports of naloxone-induced pulmonary edema suggest a possible use of phentolamine in its management. Further data are required to validate this observation.[28]

Laboratory

Analytical Methods

A 20-mg bolus of naloxone followed by a 0.24 mg/min infusion led to plasma naloxone levels of about 60 to 80 ng/mL 5 hours after the start of infusion. A high-performance liquid chromatography method with electrochemical detection has a detection limit of 1 ng/mL.[29]

Ancillary Tests

Conjunctival Test for Opiate Dependence. Pupillary diameter transparencies by the eye are obtained pretreatment with a Polaroid CV5 camera under constant conditions of reduced ambient lighting. Two drops of naloxone hydrochloride (1 mg/mL in normal saline) are applied 1 minute apart to one conjunctival sac and two drops of normal saline are instilled contralaterally as a control measure. At 20 and 45 minutes after naloxone instillation, further photographs of both eyes are taken. Significant pupillary dilation is observed in opiate addicts on maintenance methadone treatment. No pupillary response is seen in nonaddict subjects given an opiate premedication before elective surgery. This test may be useful to identify the physically dependent opiate user.[30]

Nasal Test for Opiate Dependency. A significant increase in withdrawal distress and pupillary dilation was observed after nasal administration of 1 mg (1 mg/400 mL) naloxone in all subjects who showed opiate-positive urine samples. In control subjects, no reaction to naloxone was observed.[31]

Treatment

Treatment is symptomatic and supportive.

REFERENCES—NALOXONE

1. DeMaria A, Hefferman JJ, Grindlinger GA, et al. Naloxone versus placebo in treatment of spetic shock. Lancet 1985;1:1363–1365.
2. Loimer N, Schmid RW, Presslich O, Leuz K. Continuous naloxone administration suppresses opiate withdrawal symptoms in human opiate addicts during detoxification treatment. J Psychiatr Res 1989;23:81–86.
3. Varon J, Dumas SR. Naloxone reversal of hypotension due to captopril overdose. Ann Emerg Med 1991;20:1125–1127.
4. Elberto G, Erickson T, Popiel R, et al. Central nervous system manifestations of a valproic acid overdose responsive to naloxone. Ann Emerg Med 1989;18:889–891.
5. Cami J, de la Torre R, Garcia-Sevilla L, et al. Alcohol antagonism of hypercortisolism induced by naloxone. Clin Pharmacol Ther 1988;43:559–604.
6. Pickar D, Bunney WE, Douillet P, et al. Repeated naloxone administration in schizophrenia: A Phase II World Health Organization study. Biol Psychiatry 1989;25:440–448.
7. Chernick V, Manfreda J, de Booy V, et al. Clinical trial of naloxone in birth asphyxia. J Pediatr 1988;113:519–525.
8. Kunkel DB. Narcotic antagonist update. Emerg Med 1987;19:97–108.
9. Culpepper-Morgan JA, Inturris CE, et al. Treatment of opioid-induced constipation with oral naloxone: A pilot study. Clin Pharmacol Ther 1992;52:90–95.
10. Maio RF, Gaukel B, Freeman B. Intralingual naloxone injection for narcotic-induced respiratory depression. Ann Emerg Med 1987;16:572–577.
11. Wasserberger J, Ordog GJ, Kolodny M. Intralingual naloxone injections. Ann Emerg Med 1988;17:874.
12. Mofenson HC, Caraccio TC. Continuous infusion of intravenous naloxone. Ann Emerg Med 1987;16:600.
13. Bonfiglio MF, Mauro VC. Naloxone in the treatment of meperidine-induced seizures. Drug Intell Clin Pharm 1987;21:174–175.
14. Tenenbein M. Continuous naloxone infusion for opiate poisoning in infancy. J Pediatr 1984;105:645–648.
15. Gibbs J, Newson T, Williams J, Davidson DC. Naloxone hazard in infant of opioid abuser. Lancet 1989;2:159–160.
16. Committee on Drugs: Kaufman RE, Banner W Jr, Blumer JL, et al. Naloxone dosage and route of administration for infants and children: Addendum to energy drug doses for infants and children. Pediatrics 1990;86:484–485.
17. Manmell M, Maggi M, de Feo ML, et al. Naloxone administration releases catecholamines. N Engl J Med 1983;308:654–655.
18. Shibanoki S, Kubo T, Kogura M, Ishikawa K. Naloxone affects both pharmacokinetics and pharmacodynamics of morphine: Application of direct correlation analysis. Biochem Pharmacol 1991;42:1107–1114.
19. Peters G, Gaylor S. Human central nervous system effects of a selective kappa opioid agonist. Personal communication. American Society of Clinical Pharmacology and Therapeutics, Nashville, TN, 19th Annual Meeting, March 1990.
20. Schoenfeld A, Friedman S, Stein LB, et al. Severe hypertensive reaction after naloxone injection during labor. Arch Gynecol 1987;240:45–47.
21. Gal TJ. Naloxone reversal of buprenorphine-induced respiratory depression. Clin Pharmacol Ther 1989;45:66–71.
22. Loimer N, Schmid R, Lenz K, et al. Acute blocking of naloxone-precipitated opiate withdrawal symptoms by methohexitone. Br J Psychiatry 1990;157:748–752.
23. Rockford J, Daves P. Clonidine and yohimbine modulate the effects of naloxone on novelty-induced hypoalgesia. Psychopharmacology 1992;107:575–580.
24. Brimacomber J, Archdeacne J, Newell S, Martin J. Two cases of naloxone-induced pulmonary oedema: The possible use of phentolamine in management. Anaesth Intensive Care 1991;19:578–582.
25. Wasserberger J, Ordog GJ. Naloxone-induced hypertension in patients on clonidine. Ann Emerg Med 1988;17:557.
26. Mariani RJ. Seizure associated with low-dose naloxone. Am J Emerg Med 1989;7:127–128.
27. Partridge BL, Ward CP. Pulmonary edema following low-dose naloxone administration. Anesthesiology 1986;65:709–710.
28. Schwartz JA, Koenigsberg MD. Naloxone-induced pulmonary edema. Ann Emerg Med 1987;16:1294–1296.
29. Reid RW, Deakin A, Lechey DJ. Measurement of naloxone in plasma using high performance liquid chromatography with electrochemical detection. J Chromatogr Biomed Appl 1993;614:117–122.
30. Crighton FJ, Ghodse AH. Naloxone applied to conjunctiva as a test for physical opiate dependency. Lancet 1989;1:748–750.

31. Loimer N, Hofmann P, Chaudhry HR. Nasal administration of naloxone for detection of opiate dependence. J Psychiatr Res 1992;26:39–43.

NALTREXONE

Use

Receptors for the opiate system, mainly of the mu type, are reported to be closely involved in the regulation of hypothalamic gonadotropin-releasing hormone neurons. Naltrexone (Trexan), an opioidergic antagonist with a high affinity for the mu receptor, has been used in functional hypothalamic amenorrheic patients to reestablish ovulation and menses.[1]

Naltrexone at dose levels of 1.5 to 2 mg/kg daily appears to be useful in regulating self-injurious behavior in autistic children.[2,3] At these dose levels, naltrexone (in autistic children 4–12 years of age) had no significant effects on heart rate, systolic blood pressure, transaminase levels, and electrocardiogram.[4]

Naltrexone appears to curtail abnormal sexual behavior in Tourette's syndrome,[5] diminishes seizures associated with Rett syndrome,[6] and has been useful in a patient with neurotic excoriations (50 mg orally at bedtime).[7]

Naltrexone 50 mg daily, in a controlled study of bulemic women, was not associated with a significant reduction in binge eating or vomiting episodes.[8]

Opioid receptor antagonists decrease alcohol craving, alcohol consumption, and loss of control over drinking.[9] Reduction in ethanol consumption by alcoholics following naltrexone administration (50 mg/d) may occur because of greater subjective intoxication, greater aversive effects, or less positive reinforcement from ethanol.[10–12]

Therapeutic Dose

Oral naltrexone may be useful prophylactically to prevent pruritus associated with epidural morphine. The 50 mg tablet is crushed and dissolved in 50 mL of water. Five to six milliliters of the solution (5–6 mg) plus 4 mL of any flavored syrup is given orally within 5 minutes of administration of morphine. The solution is stable for 24 hours.[13] Naltrexone (6 mg) is effective orally as a prophylactic against the pruritus and vomiting associated with intrathecal morphine for analgesia after cesarean section.[14] The recommended dose of naltrexone for treatment of alcohol dependence is 50 mg once a day for 12 weeks.[15]

Clinical Presentation

Patients ingesting up to 300 mg of naltrexone daily develop feelings of well-being, increased alertness, euphoria, and mild hypomania.[16]

Laboratory

A procedure for the analysis of naltrexone and 6-β-naltrexol in plasma and urine uses negative ion chemical ionization mass spectrometry and capillary column chromatography to achieve a limit of quantitation of 0.1 ng/mL.[17]

REFERENCES—NALTREXONE

1. Remorgida V, Venturini RL, Anserini P, et al. Naltrexone in functional hypothalamic amenorrhea and in the normal luteal phase. Obstet Gynecol 1990;76:1115–1120.
2. Leboyer M, Bouvard MP, Dugas M. Effects of naltrexone on infantile autism. Lancet 1988;1:715.
3. Campbell M, Anderson LT, Small AM, et al. Naltrexone in autistic children: A double blind and placebo-controlled study. Psychopharmacol Bull 1990;26:130–135.
4. Herman BH, Hannock MK, Smith AA, et al. Effects of acute administration of naltrexone on cardiovascular function, body temperature, body weight and serum concentrations of liver enzymes in autistic children. Dev Pharmacol Ther 1989;12: 118–127.
5. Sandyk R. Naltrexone suppresses abnormal sexual behavior in Tourette's syndrome. Neurology 1988;38(suppl 1):291.
6. Thompson DF, Thompson GD. Naltrexone in the management of seizures associated with Rett syndrome. Drug Intell Clin Pharm 1987;21:874.
7. Smith KC, Pittelbow RR. Naltrexone for neurotic excoriations. J Am Acad Dermatol 1985;20:861–866.
8. Mitchell JE, Christenson G, Jennings J, et al. A placebo-controlled, double-blind crossover study of naltrexone hydrochloride in outpatients with normal weight bulimia. J Clin Psychopharmacol 1989;9:94–97.
9. Froehlich JC, Li TK. Recent developments in alcoholism: Opioid peptides. Recent Dev Alcohol 1993;11:187–205.
10. Swift RM, Whelihan W, Kuznetsov O, et al. Naltrexone-induced alterations in human ethanol intoxication. Am J Psychiatry 1994;151:1463–1467.
11. O'Brien CP. Treatment of alcoholism as a chronic disorder. EXS 1994;71:349–359.
12. Volpicelli JR, Alterman AI, Hayashida M, O'Brien CP. Naltrexone in the treatment of alcohol dependence. Arch Gen Psychiatry 1992;49:876–880.
13. Abboud TK. Preparation of oral naltrexone solution. Anesthesiology 1990;73:190–191.
14. Abboud TK, Lee K, Zhu J, et al. Prophylactic oral naltrexone with intrathecal morphine for cesarean section: Effects on adverse reactions and analgesia. Anesth Analg 1990;71:367–370.
15. Naltrexone for alcohol dependence. Med Lett Drugs Ther 1995;37(953):64–66.
16. Lerner AG, Sigal M, Bacolu A, Gelkopf M. Naltrexone abuse potential. J Nerv Ment Dis 1992;180:734–735.
17. Monti KM, Foltz RL, Chinn DM. Analysis of naltrexone and 6-beta-naltrexol in plasma and urine by gas chromatography–negative ion chemical ionization mass spectrometry. J Anal Toxicol 1991;15:136–140.

OXYCODONE

Toxicokinetics

Oxycodone (Percocet) by intravenous bolus exhibits a half-life of about 4 hours, clearance of 0.78 L/min, and volume of distribution at steady state of 2.6 L/kg. Clearance and volume of distribution at steady state are 0.78/min and 2.60 L/kg, respectively. The elimination half-life is about 4 hours.[1]

Clinical Presentation

Noncardiogenic pulmonary edema has been described after overdose with heroin; with use of intravenous nalbuphine and morphine; and with oral propoxyphene, methadone, codeine, and oxycodone overdose. Treatment is symptomatic with added oxygen and naloxone. Mechanical ventilation and positive end-expiratory pressure may not be required. An adult ingested 6 Percocet tablets (each containing 5 mg oxycodone with 325 mg acetaminophen) and developed noncardiogenic pulmonary edema; the patient received naloxone and recovered.[2]

Laboratory

Therapeutic concentrations of oxycodone range up to 0.1 mg/L. Death has usually been associated with blood levels greater than 4 mg/L. Two patients were found dead with blood levels of 0.6 and 0.7 mg/L, respectively.[3]

REFERENCES—OXYCODONE

1. Poyhia R, Olkkola KT, Sepalla T, Kalso E. The pharmacokinetics of oxycodone after intravenous injection in adults. Br J Clin Pharmacol 1991;32:516–518.
2. Turturro MA, O'Toole KS. Oxycodone-induced pulmonary edema. Am J Emerg Med 1991;9:201–207.
3. Drummer OH. Deaths involving oxycodone. Bull Int Assoc Forens Toxicol 1993;23(2):20–22.

PENTAMORPHONE

Pentamorphone (14β-pentylaminomorphinone) is a morphinan derivative.[1] It is a potent analgesic with a duration of action similar to that of fentanyl.[2] It has a limited ventilatory depressant effect in humans in doses that have been associated with clinically effective analgesia.[3] Pentamorphone, similar to fentanyl, produces postoperative analgesia, sedation, and respiratory depression when administered at a dose of 0.15 μg/L (0.12–0.24 μg/kg). It has two to eight times the analgesic activity of fentanyl.[4,5] In one double-blind study, intravenous pentamorphone 0.08 to 0.24 μg/kg was ineffective in treating and postoperative pain after major surgery.[1] Nausea and vomiting may follow doses of 0.08 to 0.16 μg/kg.[1]

REFERENCES—PENTAMORPHONE

1. Wong HY, Parker RK, Fragen R, White PF. Pentamorphone for management of postoperative pain. Anesth Analg 1991;72:656–666.
2. Ruds FG, Wynn RL, Ossipov M, et al. Antinociceptive activity of pentamorphone, a 14 beta-amino morphone derivative, compared to fentanyl and morphine. Anesth Analg 1989;69: 450–456.
3. Afifi MS, Glass PSA, Cohen WA, et al. Depression of ventilatory responses to hypoxia and hypercapnia after pentamorphone. Anesth Analg 1990;71:377–383.
4. Goldberg JS, Martz MD, Berend JS. A comparison of pain sedation and respiratory depression following pentamorphone or fentanyl general anesthesia. Clin Pharmacol Ther 1991;49:182.
5. Glass PSA, Camporesi EM, Shafron D, et al. Evaluation of pentamorphone in humans: A new potent opiate. Anesth Analg 1989;68:302–307.

PENTAZOCINE HYDROCHLORIDE

Use

Pentazocine (Talwin) acts as both an agonist and an antagonist at mu receptors (mediates supraspinal [brain] analgesia, central nervous system depression, miosis) and, unlike other opioids, as an agonist at sigma receptors (mediates psychotomimetic effects: dysphoria, hallucinations, delusions, hypertension, tachycardia and tachypnea). Naloxone has more affinity for mu opioid receptors than for kappa and sigma receptors.[1] Smaller doses of naloxone should antagonize mu effects, and larger doses may be needed to counteract kappa and sigma effects.[2]

Clinical Presentation

Pentazocine Alone

Many patients who ingest pentazocine alone do not have the classic opioid syndrome of central nervous system and respiratory depression with miosis. Most are awake. Other findings include grand mal seizures.[3] Few patients who receive intravenous naloxone show improvement. The major treatment is supportive care.[2]

Pentazocine With Other Substances

With alcohol, a sedative–hypnotic drug, or an antihistamine, there is increased toxicity (apnea, deep coma, recurrent seizures). One patient developed opioid pulmonary edema. One died.

Laboratory

A high-performance liquid chromatography method using fluorometric detection rapidly quantified pentazocine in plasma. The limit of detection is 1 ng/mL of plasma.[4]

Treatment

Patients who have overdosed on pentazocine should be closely monitored for late development of opioid pulmonary edema. Three of five patients with coma and inadequate respiration responded to intravenous naloxone in doses of 0.4 to 1.2 mg.[2]

REFERENCES—PENTAZOCINE HYDROCHLORIDE

1. Martin W. Naloxone. Ann Intern Med 1976;85:765–768.
2. Challoner KR, McCarron MM, Newton EJ. Pentazocine (Talwin®) intoxication: Report of 57 cases. J Emerg Med 1990;8:67–74.
3. Roytblat L, Bear R, Gesztes T. Seizures after pentazocine overdose. Isr J Med Sci 1986;27:385–386.
4. Moeller N, Dietzel K, Nuernberg B, et al. High performance liquid chromatographic determination of pentazocine in plasma. J Chromatogr Biomed Appl 1990;530:200–205.

PENTAZOCINE AND METHYLPHENIDATE

The combination of crushed pentazocine (Talwin) tablets and methlyphenidate (Ritalin) is called T's and Blues in Kansas City, Missouri. The clinical picture is similar to that following intravenous abuse with pentazocine–tripelennamine combinations.[1]

REFERENCE—PENTAZOCINE AND METHYLPHENIDATE

1. Carter HS, Watson WA. IV pentazocine/methylphenidate abuse: The clinical toxicity of another T's and Blues combination. Clin Toxicol 1994;32:541–554.

PENTAZOCINE AND TRIPELENNAMINE (T'S AND BLUES)

Infection complications, central nervous system toxicity, and a characteristic drug reaction (chest pain, anxiety, muscle spasms, dizziness, and nausea) have been observed after use of this combination of drugs.[1]

Chest pain began in one patient after injection of about 2 to 3 mL of a mixture of 150 mg of pentazocine and 50 mg of tripelennamine dissolved in water and filtered through cotton. The patient developed an acute Q-wave anteroseptal myocardial infarction. Both pentazocine and tripelennamine may increase serum catecholamine levels. Administration of beta-adrenergic blocking agents may theoretically be contraindicated due to resultant unopposed alpha-adrenergic stimulation. Alpha-adrenergic blocking drugs (eg, phentolamine) calcium channel blocking agents, and possibly intravenous nitroglycerin or nitroprusside may be more rational therapeutic choices.[2]

REFERENCES—PENTAZOCINE AND TRIPELENNAMINE (T'S AND BLUES)

1. Showalter CV. T's and Blues: Abuse of pentazocine and tripelennamine. JAMA 1980;244:1224–1225.
2. McGwier BW, Altert MA, Panayiotou H, Lauber CR. Acute myocardial infarction associated with intravenous injection of pentazocine and tripelennamine. Chest 1992;101:1730–1732.

PROPOXYPHENE

Structure

Propoxyphene, a synthetic chemical, is structurally and pharmacologically related to methadone.[1]

Clinical Presentation

Dextropropoxyphene–Acetaminophen Combination

Vomiting usually settles within a few hours. If it should persist or remain 24 to 36 hours after ingestion of these combined preparations, there may be associated pain and tenderness in the right hypochondrium. This may indicate the onset of hepatocellular necrosis. Less frequently, renal tubular necrosis and acute renal failure may develop. Death is usually due to hepatic failure with encephalopathy, cerebral edema, intercurrent infection, or hemorrhage secondary to hypoprothrombinemia.[2]

Intramuscular Abuse

Prolonged intramuscular abuse of dextropropoxyphene leads to fibrous myopathy, atrophy of muscles used for the intramuscular injection, radial neuropathy, ulceronecrotic lesions at injection sites, and a lobular panniculitis.[3]

Laboratory

Some data suggest that the plasma concentration propoxyphene : norpropoxyphene ratios are greater than one in suicides. In accidents the metabolite concentration may be greatest (propoxyphene : norpropoxyphene <1).

Treatment

A treatment guide for dextropropoxyphene and dextropropoxyphene–acetaminophen overdoses has been proposed by Lawson and Northridge[5] (Fig. 25–7). An anecdotal report suggests that wide QRS complex dysrhythmia responds to sodium bicarbonate.[6]

REFERENCES—PROPOXYPHENE

1. Jaffe JH, Martin WR. Opioid analgesics and antagonists. In: Gilman AG, Goodman LS, Rall TW, et al., eds. *Goodman and Gilman's the Pharmacological Basis of Therapeutics.* 7th ed. New York: MacMillan, 1985:519–520.
2. Proudfoot AT. Clinical features and management of distalgenic overdose. Hum Toxicol 1984;3(suppl.):85S–94S.
3. Restrepo JF, Guzman R, Pena MA, et al. Fibrous myopathy induced by propoxyphene injections. J Rheumatol 1993; 20:596–597.
4. Strom J. Acute propoxyphene self-poisoning with special reference to propoxyphene cardiotoxicity and treatment. Dan Med Bull 1989;36:316–336.
5. Lawson AAH, Northridge DB. Dextropropoxyphene overdose, epidemiology, clinical presentation and management. Med Toxicol 1987;2:430–444.
6. Stork GM, Redd JT, Fine K, Hoffman RS. Propoxyphene-induced wide QRS complex dysrhythmia responsive to sodium bicarbonate: A case report. Clin Toxicol 1995;33: 179–183.

TILIDINE HYDROCHLORIDE

Tilidine hydrochloride is an analgesic agent with properties closely related to those of dextropropoxyphene.[1] Respiratory depression is dose related. Fifty milligrams intravenously does not appear to depress respiration; 100 mg intravenously causes a respiratory depression that can be compared with that induced by 10 mg of intravenous morphine.[2] Toxic doses may involve decreased consciousness, coma, respiratory paralysis, and convulsions.[1] Tilidine is approximately half as potent as meperidine.[2] Overdoses should be treated symptomatically and supportively. Naloxone appears to effectively antagonize respiratory depression induced by tilidine.[2]

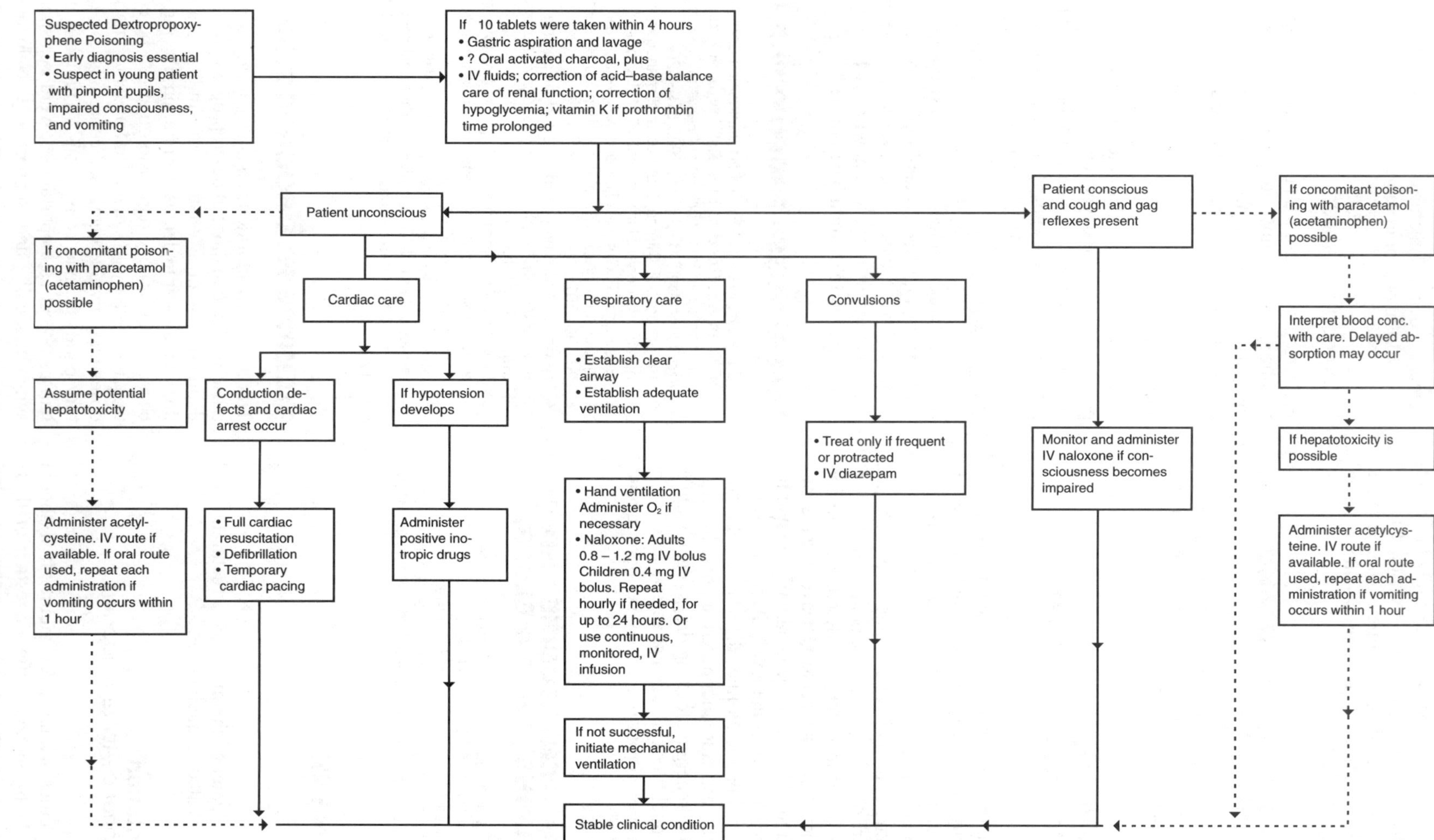

Figure 25–7 Management of acute dextropropoxyphene poisoning. (From Lawson AA, Northridge DB. Dextropropoxyphene overdose: Epidemiology, clinical presentation and management. Med Toxicol Adverse Drug Experience 1987;2:430–444.)

Structure and Classification

Tilidine is ethyl DL-*trans*-2-dimethylamino-1-phenyl-cyclohex-3-*trans*-1-carboxylate hydrochloride. Its empirical formula is $C_{17}H_{23}NO_2 \cdot HCl$, and its molecular weight is 318.8. The CAS number for the base is 20380-58-9 and that for the hydrochloride 27107-79.5.[3]

Product Formulation

Valoron is a combination of tilidine and naloxone (50 mg tilidine hydrochloride and 4 mg naloxone) given to prevent abuse by drug-dependent individuals.

Therapeutic Dose

Oral doses are usually 100 to 200 mg daily.[1] Tilidine may also be administered in doses of 50 mg intravenously.

Toxic Dose

Ingestion of 1.0 g by a 20-year-old man has been reported; the patient survived.[4]

Fatal Dose

A 44-year-old woman was found in a semicomatose state after she ingested 750 mg of tilidine. She also ingested barbiturates. The patient died in 1 hour.[1]

Toxicokinetics

Absorption

Tilidine is rapidly absorbed from the gastrointestinal tract. A peak blood concentration of 90 ng/mL is observed 90 minutes after oral administration of 50 mg. Tilidine is a prodrug from which the active metabolite nortilidine is formed by demethylation.[5] Systemic availability of the parent drug is 6%, and of the active metabolite nortilidine, 99%.[6]

Distribution

The apparent volume of distribution of tilidine is 4.0 L/kg.[5]

Elimination

Nortilidine and bisnortilidine are the major metabolites. The terminal half-life of nortilidine is 3.3 hours following a single oral administration, 4.9 hours after intravenous administration, and 3.6 hours following multiple dosing.[5] Renal elimination of unchanged drug is 1.6% of the dose following intravenous administration and less than 0.1% of the dose after oral administration. Total clearance is 1139 mL/min.[5]

Mechanism of Action

Radioreceptor assays reveal that nortilidine, rather than tilidine and bisnortilidine, exhibits affinity for opiate receptors.[5] Affinity for the mu opiate receptor is more than 10 times higher for the (+) enantiomer than for the (–) enantiomer.

Clinical Presentation

Toxic doses may induce a lowering of consciousness, coma, respiratory paralysis, and seizures.[1,4,7]

Laboratory

Analytical Methods

A method for quantitation of tilidine uses gas chromatography with nitrogen–phosphorus detection. The lower limits of sensitivity of the assay method are about 1 to 2 ng/mL for tilidine and nortilidine and 5 ng/mL for bisnortilidine.[5]

Blood Levels

Blood levels of tilidine in a fatal overdose were 4.3 μg/mL, with 0.30 μg/mL nortilidine and 0.6 μg/mL bisnortilidine. Tolerance is rapidly built up in cases of abuse, and blood levels of 30 to 40 μg/mL may be measured.[1]

Treatment

Stabilization

Treatment is largely symptomatic and supportive. Naloxone may counteract respiratory depression.

Gut Decontamination

Activated charcoal given 3 to 25 minutes after tilidine ingestion appears to adsorb tilidine.[8] Syrup of ipecac alone has not been effective in preventing tilidine absorption.[8,9]

REFERENCES—TILIDINE HYDROCHLORIDE

1. Van Boven M, Daenens P, Bruneel N. A death case involving tilidine. Arch Toxicol 1976;36:121–125.
2. Romagnoli A, Keats AS. Comparative respiratory depression of tilidine and morphine. Clin Pharmacol Ther 1975;17: 523–528.
3. Reynolds JEF, ed. *Martindale: The Extra Pharmacopoeia.* 30th ed. London: Pharmaceutical Press, 1993:1097.
4. Klapetek J. Valoron intoxikation by selbsmod vers. Munch Med Wochenschr 1973;115:113–115.
5. Vollmer K-A, Thomann P, Hengy H. Pharmacokinetics of tilidine and metabolites in man. Aznneimittelforschung 1989;39: 1283–1288.
6. Vollmer K-A, Poisson A. On the metabolism of ethyl-DL-*trans*-2-dimethylamino-1-phenyl-cyclohex-3-ene-*trans*-l-carboxylate hydrochloride (tilidine HCl). Second communication: studies with ^{14}C-labelled substances in rats and dogs. Arzneimittelforschung 1976;26:1827–1836.
7. Klapatek J. Critical comments on a case history 'A death case involving tilidine'. Arch Toxicol 1978;40:1–4.
8. Condonnier JA, van den Heede MA, Heyndrickx AM. In vitro adsorption of tilidine HCl by activated charcoal. Clin Toxicol 1986/1987;24:503–517.
9. Condonnier JA, van den Heede M, Heyndrickx AM. Activated charcoal and ipecac syrup in prevention of tilidine absorption in man. Vet Hum Toxicol 1987;29(suppl. 2):105–106.

TRAMADOL HYDROCHLORIDE

Tramadol is an orally active synthetic opioid agonist analgesic marketed in Europe and in the United States

(Ultram).[1] It produces clinical analgesia as effectively as codeine, pentazocine, meperidine, and propoxyphene.

Structure and Classification

Tramadol hydrochloride is *trans*-2-dimethylaminomethyl-1-(3-methoxyphenol) cyclohexanol hydrochloride. Its empiric formula is $C_{16}H_{25}NO_2 \cdot HCl$. It has a molecular weight of 299.8. The CAS number is 27203-92-5.[2] Tramadol, an opioid analgesic, is marketed as Crispin in Japan and Tramal in Germany and Switzerland.

Product Formulation

Tramadol is given by mouth; by intramuscular, subcutaneous, or intravenous injection; and by suppository.

Therapeutic Dose

Usual doses are 50 mg orally, 50 to 100 mg by injection, and 100 mg rectally. Total daily dose does not exceed 400 mg. Tramadol hydrochloride 150 mg appears to be significantly more effective than the combination of 650 mg of acetaminophen and 100 mg of propoxyphene.[1]

Toxic Dose

An accidental rectal administration of 27 mg/kg to a few-week-old infant resulted in severe cerebral depression. Naloxone was required for 48 hours. The child recovered.[3] At effective analgesic doses of 200 mg, nausea, vomiting, somnolence, and dizziness have been observed.[4] A 6-month-old child was erroneously given 100 mg tramadol by suppository. Seizures, acidosis, and respiratory depression followed. The child survived with supportive therapy and naloxone.[5]

Toxicokinetics

Absorption

Peak plasma levels occur at about 1.5 hours.[1] Therapeutic blood levels in adults are about 100 to 300 ng/mL (0.1–0.2 μg/mL).[3]

Distribution

Tramadol completely penetrates the blood–brain barrier. Cerebrospinal fluid concentrations of tramadol appear to follow closely the serum elimination curve.[5]

Elimination

Tramadol has a plasma elimination half-life of 5 to 6 hours.[1] It is metabolized to an active desmethyl derivative and several inactive compounds.[1] Most excretion takes place through the kidneys.[6]

Mechanism of Action

Tramadol attaches to the mu receptor and blocks norepinephrine and serotonin reuptake.[1]

Clinical Presentation

Acute overdose may induce miosis, respiratory depression, hypotonicity, and acidosis.[3,5] Chronic side effects include fatigue, dizziness, vertigo, headache, visual disorders, nausea, vomiting, sweating, dry mouth, constipation, premature beats, euphoria, dysphoria, hallucinations, and changed body perception.[5] A relative absence of dependence on tramadol was evident in early clinical trials.[7] Minimal withdrawal signs are observed in naloxone precipitation studies.[1]

Laboratory

Analytical Methods

Tramadol concentrations in the cerebrospinal fluid, serum, and urine can be measured by gas chromatography–mass spectrometry.[5]

Blood Levels

Administration of a 100-mg suppository to a 6-month-old child led to serum and cerebrospinal fluid concentrations of 2.0 μg/mL, which decreased to less than 1.0 μg/mL in 17 hours. Urine tramadol levels reached 20 ug/mL, descending to below 10 μg/mL in 13 hours.[15]

Abnormalities

The electroencephalogram may show a flattened trace, which resolves within 1 week.[5]

Treatment

Treatment is largely symptomatic and supportive. Repeated doses of naloxone may be required. Early gastric lavage has been useful after a substantial overdose with tramadol.[5]

Gut Decontamination

Gastric lavage with airway protection may be useful early after an overdose (within 3–4 hours). Activated charcoal and cathartics have not been used in tramadol overdoses.

Antidote

Administration of intravenous naloxone 10 μg/kg to a child with a tramadol overdose resulted in pupil widening and rapid restoration of alert behavior.[5] Naloxone may need to be administered repeatedly over a 48-hour period.[3]

Supportive Measures

Assisted ventilation, a source of oxygen, a central line, and fluids constitute the basic initial treatment of an overdose with tramadol.

REFERENCES—TRAMADOL HYDROCHLORIDE

1. Sunshine A, Olson NZ, Zighelboim I, et al. Analgesic oral efficacy of tramadol hydrochloride in postoperative pain. Clin Pharmacol Ther 1992;51:740–746.
2. Reynolds JEF, ed. *Martindale: The Extra Pharmacopoeia.* 30th ed. London: Pharmaceutical Press, 1993:1097–1098.
3. Bianchetti MG, Beutler A, Ferrier PE. Intoxication severe avec uoprace (tramadol) chez un nourisson de cinque semaines. Helv Paediatr Acta 1988;43:241–244.
4. Fricke JR, Minn F, Cunningham PD, et al. Tramadol HCl: Dose response to pain from oral surgery. Clin Pharmacol Ther 1991;59:182.
5. Riedel F, v Stockhausen H-B. Severe cerebral depression after intoxication with tramadol in a 6 month old infant. Eur J Clin Pharmacol 1984;26:631–632.
6. Lee SR, McTavish D, Sorkin EM. Tramadol: A preliminary review of its pharmacodynamic and pharmacokinetic properties and therapeutic potential in acute and chronic pain status. Drugs 1993;46:313–347.
7. Richter W, Barth H, Flohe L, Giertz H. Clinical investigation in the development of dependence during oral therapy with tramadol. Arzneimittelforschung 1985;35:1742–1744.

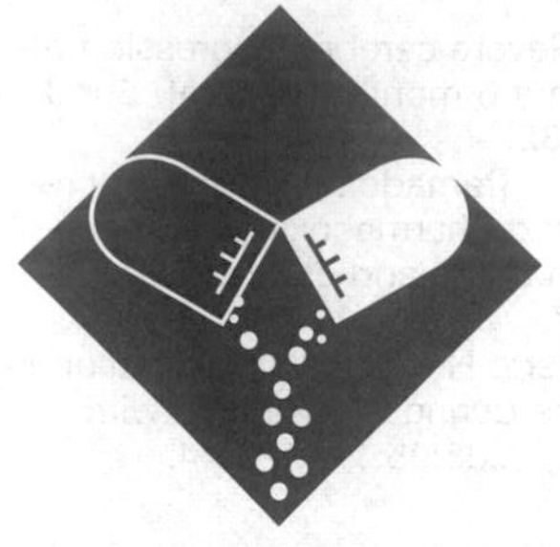

Part D Systems Toxicology

Chapter 26 Bone Disorders and the Bisphosphonates

BONE

Long term effects of medications on bone formation are summarized in Table 26–1.[1] Management of disorders of bone metabolism is described in Table 26–2.[1]

BISPHOSPHONATES

Bisphosphonates are synthetic analogs of pyrophosphate (Fig. 26–1), a naturally occurring substance that inhibits the mineralization of bone. These compounds are used mainly to inhibit bone resorption, both endogenous and resorption stimulated by parathyroid hormone, calcitriol, cytokines, and prostaglandins.[1–4]

In order of increasing potency of antiresorption activity, the main bisphosphonates are etidronate, tiludronate, clodronate, pamidronate, alendronate, and risendronate.[5] Newer bisphosphonates include alendrolate, meridronate, and tiludronate.[4] Cancer-associated hypercalcemia can be divided into three clinical groups on the basis of different pathogenetic mechanisms: patients with hematologic cancer (eg, myeloma), patients with solid tumor and bone metastases (eg, breast cancer), and patients with solid tumors without metastases (i.e., simulates primary hyperparathyroidism).

Structure and Classification

See Figure 26–1.[5]

Product Formulation

Etidronate Disodium

- EHDP
- Didronel (United Kingdom, United States): oral tablets, 200 mg, 400 mg; intravenous, mg/mL (300 mg)
- Na_2EHDP

Pamidronate Disodium

- APD
- Aredia (United Kingdom, United States): 30-mg intravenous infusion

Sodium Clodronate

- Bonefos, Loron (United Kingdom)

Therapeutic Dose

Etidronate 5 to 10 mg/kg/d is continued, if a symptomatic or biochemical response is seen, for about 6 months. Doses of 20 mg/kg/d have been given for 1 month only. More prolonged treatment leads to bone pain and spontaneous fractures.

Pamidronate 30 mg given intravenously as a single infusion in 250 mL saline over 4 hours leads to a fall in serum calcium concentration after about 24 hours.

Clodronate is administered as daily infusions of 300 mg in 500 mL saline over 2 hours and is continued until the serum calcium is normal, usually between 3 and 5 days. Oral doses of 800 to 1600 mg daily for 1 to 6 months produce effective suppression of Paget's disease.

Use

Bisphosphonates have been used to treat Paget's disease of bone, hypercalcemia of malignant disease, and osteoporosis (vertebral crush fractures).[4]

Table 26–1
Mechanisms of Action of Drugs Toxic to the Bone

Agent	Mechanism
Aluminum	Inhibition of osteoblasts Impaired skeletal mineralization
Anticonvulsants	Interference with vitamin D metabolism through decreased formation and increased breakdown of 25-hydroxyvitamin D_3 Decreased gut absorption of calcium (independent of the above)
Bisphosphonates	Impaired skeletal mineralization [etidronic acid (etidronate)]
Corticosteroids	Multifactorial: decreased calcium absorption, increased urinary calcium loss, and direct inhibition of osteoblasts
Cyclosporine	High-turnover osteoporosis
Fluoride	Impaired skeletal mineralization
Heparin	? Direct inhibition of 1α-hydroxylase, leading to decreased active vitamin D
Methotrexate	Inhibition of osteoblasts ? Effect on vitamin C metabolism

From Jones G, Sambrook PN, Drug-induced disorders of bone metabolism: Incidence, management and avoidance. Drug Saf 1994;10:480–489.

Table 26–2
Overview of the Management of Drug-Induced Disorders of Bone Metabolism

Agent	Management
Aluminum	Awareness of problem Dialysate aluminum <10 μg/L Consider deferoxamine
Anticonvulsants	Vitamin D and calcium supplementation
Bisphosphonates	Lower dose or cyclical therapy Consider newer bisphosphonates
Corticosteroids	Minimize dose Consider calcitriol, bisphosphonates Consider bone-sparing alternatives
Cyclosporine	Minimize dose and duration of therapy Consider cyclosporin G
Fluoride	Cease use
Heparin	Aim for <3 months treatment Consider low-molecular-weight heparin Effect is reversible on cessation
Methotrexate	Cease use Effect is reversible on cessation

From Jones G, Sambrook PN. Drug-induced disorders of bone metabolism: Incidence, management and avoidance. Drug Saf 1994;10:480–489.

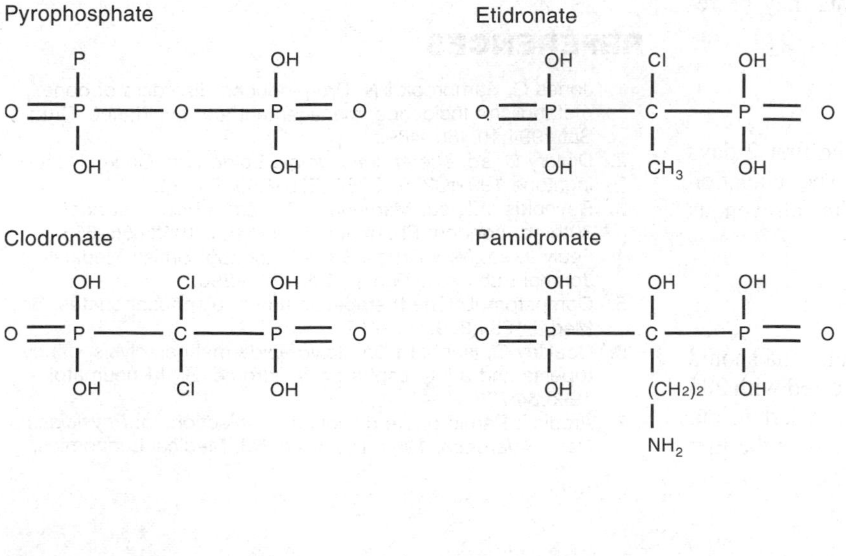

Figure 26–1 Chemical structure of pyrophosphate and three bisphosphonates. (From Compston JE. The therapeutic use of bisphosphonates. Br Med J 1994;309:711–715.)

Toxicokinetics

Bisphosphonates are not metabolized. They are absorbed, excreted, and stored unchanged. Intestinal absorption is poor (1–10%) and is further reduced by concurrent ingestion of food, especially products containing calcium (Table 26–3). Plasma clearance is rapid (half-life of about 2 hours) because of the rapid uptake of 20 to 60% of the absorbed fraction into the skeleton. The remainder is excreted in the urine. Some bisphosphonates may remain in the skeleton for life.[2]

Table 26–3
Toxicokinetics of the Biphosphonates

	Clodronate	Etidronate	Pamidronate
Oral absorption	1–4%	0–8.7%	Poor
Presystemic metabolism	Nil	Nil	Nil
Plasma half-life	1.8–2.3 h	2–6 h	30 min
Volume of distribution	0.2–0.5 L/kg	0.3–1.3 L/kg	
Plasma protein binding	2.1–7.1%	—	<14%

Source: Dollery[2] and Reynolds.[3]

Mechanism of Action

Bisphosphonates have a strong affinity for hydroxyapatite crystals. In high doses they inhibit calcification of bone.[5] They inhibit growth and dissolution of hydroxyapatite crystals in bone, and may impair osteoclast activity. They diminish bone resorption and bone formation.[4]

Clinical Presentation

Reduced intestinal absorption of calcium, iron, and antacids occurs with concurrent administration of bisphosphonates. Severe hypocalcemia has been reported in patients taking aminoglycosides and bisphosphonates. The oral forms may lead to nausea, vomiting, a transient fever, leukopenia, and an increase in C-reactive protein. Pancytopenia and aplastic anemia are rare but serious complications.[6] Rapid intravenous administration may lead to renal failure. Asymptomatic hypercalcemia may be observed. Etidronate can inhibit bone mineralization when given continuously for periods greater than 6 to 12 months, resulting in bone pain and fractures. This effect is dose dependent and reversible. This has not been described after use of alendronate, tiladronate, and pamidronate, which may even stimulate bone mineralization.[5]

Acute overdoses may lead to nausea and vomiting. Treatment is symptomatic and supportive. Prolonged chronic overdosage may result in the nephrotic syndrome and fractures.

Clodronate

For 2 to 3 days after an overdose, there may be a tendency toward hypercalcemia. Serum calcium should be monitored. Oral or parenteral calcium supplements may be required.

Etidronate

An overdose may induce hypocalcemia in the first 2 days with paresthesias and carpopedal spasm. The chelation effects of etidronate should be reversible with intravenous calcium gluconate.

Pamidronate

No overdoses have been reported. The hypocalcemia should be treated with calcium gluconate. An adult treated with 285 mg/d for 3 days experienced fever (39.5°C), hypertension, and transient taste difficulties lasting 6 hours after the first infusion.[7] Bone mineralization defects,[8] rickets,[9] asthma[10] in aspirin-sensitive asthma patients, and lymphopenia[11] have been described. Reports of serious ocular morbidity and loss of vision secondary to inflammatory eye disease following intravenous pamidronate use have been submitted to the Committee on Safety of Medicines of the United Kingdom.[12]

Laboratory

Hypocalcemia, hypokalemia, hypomagnesemia, hypophosphatemia, and evidence of hepatic dysfunction have been reported with etidronate and pamidronate.[3] There is little evidence of any correlation between the plasma concentration of bisphosphonates and their therapeutic effects.

Treatment

Following an acute overdose with clodronate, gastric lavage may remove unabsorbed drug. Conventional methods are used for the treatment of hypocalcemia. Treatment of acute hypercalcemia centers on adequate hydration, maintenance of high urinary sodium and calcium excretion, correction of hypophosphatemia, a low-calcium diet, furosemide, glucocorticoids, calcitonin, and bisphosphonates. Rarely, acute renal failure follows intravenous etidronate. Reduction in dose should be considered for patients with serum creatinine levels of 2.5 to 4.9 mg/dL; doses should be withheld when the serum creatinine is above 5.0 mg/dL.[7]

REFERENCES

1. Jones G, Sambrook PN. Drug-induced disorders of bone metabolism: Incidence, management and avoidance. Drug Saf 1994;10:480–489.
2. Dollery C, ed. *Therapeutic Drugs.* Edinburgh: Churchill Livingstone 1991;C276–C282, E88–E93, P1–P4.
3. Reynolds JEF, ed. *Martindale: The Extra Pharmacopoeia.* 30th ed. London: Pharmaceutical Press, 1993:655–666.
4. Feely J, ed. *New Drugs.* 3rd ed. London: British Medical Journal Publishing Group, 1994:288–290.
5. Compston JE. The therapeutic use of bisphosphonates. Br Med J 1994;309:711–715.
6. Coakley G, Isenberg DA. Toxic epidermal necrolysis, pancytopenia and adult respiratory syndrome. Br J Rheumatol 1995;34:739.
7. Aredia[R]: Pamidronate disodium for injection. In: *Physicians' Desk Reference, 1994.* Montvale, NJ: Medical Economics,

1994:813–815. Didronel[R] I.V. Infusion: Etidronate disodium, p. 1272. Didronel[R]; Etidronate disodium, pp. 1808 1810.

8. Adamson BB, Gallacher SJ, Byars J, et al. Mineralisation defects with pamidronate therapy for Paget's disease. Lancet 1993;342:1459–1461.
9. Silverman SL, Hurvitz EA, Nelson VS, et al. Rachites syndrome after disodium etidronate therapy in an adolescent. Arch Phys Med Rehab 1994;75:118–120.
10. Rolla G, Bucca C, Brussino L. Bisphosphonate induced bronchoconstriction in aspirin-sensitive asthma. Lancet 1994; 343:426–427.
11. Liotz F, Boval-Boizard B, Fritz P, Kuntz D. Lymphocyte subgroups in lymphopenia induced by pamidronate. Therapie 1994;46:63.
12. O'Donnell NP, Rao GP, Aguis-Fernandez A. Paget's disease ocular complications of disodium pamidronate treatment. Br J Clin Pract 1995;49:272–273.

Chapter 27

Anticoagulants, Antifibrinolytic Agents, and Thrombolytic Agents

ANTICOAGULANTS

Drugs affecting blood coagulation factors include oral anticoagulants, heparin, defibrinating enzymes from snake venoms, plasma volume expanders, drugs that cause hepatic injury, and drugs that stimulate increased plasma coagulation factors.[1,2] Overdosage and poisoning arising from the use or misuse of these chemicals have been largely confined to the ingestion of anticoagulants for human use[3–11] and rodenticides[12–17] and the parenteral use of heparin[18,19] (Table 27–1).

General Pathophysiology

Factor V is usually normal during an oral anticoagulant overdose. If the prothrombin time (PT) and activated partial thromboplastin time (APTT) are both prolonged, diagnostic possibilities include a circulating anticoagulant, liver disease, vitamin K deficiency, and oral anticoagulant overdose. Oral anticoagulants affect vitamin K_1-dependent clotting factors at different rates.[20] Factor VII (proconvertin) is the first to decrease in concentration in the plasma, followed by factors IX (Christmas factor), X (Stuart factor), and II (prothrombin). For oral anticoagulant overdosage, the one-stage PT is most useful.[21] The APTT is the most specific indicator of heparin action and overdose[22,23] (Table 27–2).

Anticoagulant Rebound

Coumadin

Cerebral infarction and stroke may occur after sudden cessation of coumadin therapy.[24]

Heparin

"Heparin rebound" is a common cause of bleeding in the postcardiac bypass period.[25,26] The amount of protamine sulfate required to neutralize the heparin is about two and a half times the amount of heparin given. Clotting of blood returns to normal after adequate neutralization of heparin with protamine sulfate.

Table 27-1
Antithrombotic Therapy Guidelines: Quick Reference

I. Warfarin
Oral anticoagulant
Rapidly absorbed from gastrointestinal tract
Half-life, 36–42 h
Inhibits vitamin K–dependent coagulation factors (II, VII, IX, X)

II. Unfractionated Heparin
Anticoagulant
Accelerates inhibitory interaction between antithrombin III and coagulation proteins (especially thrombin and factor Xa)
Intravenous or subcutaneous administration

III. Fractionated Heparin
Anticoagulant
Low molecular weight
Predictable bioavailability (half-life)
Inhibits factor Xa > IIa
Intravenous or subcutaneous administration

IV. Aspirin
Inhibits platelet aggregation (cyclooxygenase)
Inhibits vascular prostacyclin
Rapid onset of action (30–40 min)
Long-lasting effect

V. Ticlopidine
Inhibits adenosine diphosphate–mediated platelet aggregation
Delayed onset of action (24–48 h)
Most severe adverse reaction is neutropenia

VI. Antiplatelet Agents
Aspirin has been shown to be beneficial in
- Preventing cardiac events in men and women >50 y of age
- Stable angina
- Unstable angina
- Myocardial infarction
- TIA and noncompleted stroke
- Coronary angioplasty
- Coronary artery bypass
- Mechanical heart valves (in combination with warfarin)
- Prosthetic tissue valves in high-risk patients (in combination with warfarin)
- Atrial fibrillation (less beneficial than warfarin)

Ticlopidine has been shown to be beneficial in
- Unstable angina
- Coronary artery bypass
- TIA and noncompleted stroke
- Completed stroke

VII. Prevention of Venous Thrombosis
High-risk patients
- Adjusted dose heparin
  or
- Low-molecular-weight heparin
  or
- Low-dose warfarin (INR, 2.0–3.0; starting day of surgery)

Medium-risk patients
- Standard low-dose heparin (5000 U SC beginning 2 h after surgery)
- External pneumatic compression (if contraindications for anticoagulants)

VIII. Treatment of Venous Thromboembolism
Intravenous heparin (5000-U bolus) followed by a continuous infusion or twice-daily subcutaneous injections (17,500 U) to APTT 1.5 to 2.5 times control
In most cases, heparin and warfarin can be started simultaneously, overlapping for 3 to 5 d
Warfarin should be continued for at least 3 mo
Caval interruption is indicated if anticoagulant therapy is contraindicated

IX. Atrial Fibrillation
The following associated conditions increase the risk of stroke:
- Increasing age
- Left ventricular dysfunction
- Female sex
- Hypertension
- Valvular heart disease
- Previous thromboembolism

Warfarin is indicated, particularly in high-risk patients, unless contraindications to its use exist
Aspirin should be used in low-risk patients

X. Valvular Heart Disease
Rheumatic mitral valve disease
- Systemic embolism or atrial fibrillation: warfarin (INR, 2.0–3.0)

Aortic valve disease
- Systemic embolism or atrial fibrillation: warfarin (INR, 2.0–3.0)

Mitral valve prolapse
- TIA (aspirin, 325 mg/d)
- TIA while receiving aspirin, systemic embolism, or atrial fibrillation; warfarin (INR, 2.0–3.0)
- TIA while receiving aspirin (contraindication for warfarin): ticlopidine (250 mg bid)

Mitral annular calcification
- Systemic embolism or atrial fibrillation: warfarin (INR, 2.0–3.0)

XI. Prosthetic Heart Valves
Mechanical prosthetic valves: warfarin (INR, 2.5–3.5). (The combined use of warfarin and aspirin should be considered strongly in high-risk patients.)
Mechanical prosthetic valve with systemic embolism: warfarin plus aspirin (100–160 mg/d)
or
Warfarin plus dipyridamole (400 mg/d)
Mechanical prosthetic valve with high risk of bleeding: warfarin (INR, 2.0–3.0) with or without aspirin (100–160 mg/d)
Mechanical prosthetic valve with endocarditis: continue warfarin (INR, 2.5–3.5)
Bioprosthetic heart valves
- Bioprosthetic in mitral position: warfarin for 3 mo (INR, 2.0–3.0)
- Bioprosthetic in aortic position: aspirin (325 mg/d)
- Bioprosthetic and atrial fibrillation, systemic embolism, or atrial thrombus (high-risk patients): warfarin (INR, 2.0–3.0) plus aspirin (100 mg/d)

XII. Acute Myocardial Infarction
Antiplatelet Therapy
- Non-enteric-coated aspirin (160–325 mg/d) should be given to all patients with suspected myocardial infarction
- Aspirin (160–325 mg/d) should be given to all patients for an indefinite period (unless warfarin is used)

Heparin
- Patients with myocardial infarction, whether or not thrombolytic therapy is given, should receive heparin
- Patients at high risk for mural thrombosis/systemic embolism should receive heparin

Warfarin
- Patients at high risk for mural thrombosis/systemic embolism should receive warfarin for 1–3 mo (INR, 2.0–3.0)

Combination therapy
- The safety and efficacy of combination therapy are being investigated

(continued)

Table 27–1 *(Continued)*

XIII. Coronary Bypass Grafts
Dipyridamole before surgery is optional
Aspirin (325 mg/d) alone, started 6 h after surgery is recommended
Ticlopidine (250 mg bid) is indicated for patients allergic to or intolerant of aspirin
Coronary angioplasty
Aspirin (325 mg/d) should be initiated at least 24 h before the procedure and continued indefinitely
Ticlopidine (250 mg bid) is indicated for patients with aspirin allergy
Dipyridamole is optional
Heparin to maintain the ACT >300 s should be provided during the procedure
Heparin should be continued for 12–24 h after a complicated procedure (the benefits of warfarin are unknown)

XIV. Peripheral Vascular Disease/Surgery
Aspirin (325 mg/d) should be given (starting preoperatively) to patients undergoing prosthetic femoropopliteal surgery
Aspirin (160–325 mg/d) should be given to all patients with peripheral vascular disease because of their high risk for myocardial infarction and stroke
Aspirin (325–650 mg bid) should be given to patients undergoing carotid endarterectomy (preoperatively and postoperatively for 30 d); after 30 days, the dose may be decreased to 160 to 325 mg/d

XV. Cerebrovascular Disease
Asymptomatic carotid bruit: aspirin (325 mg/d)
Symptomatic carotid stenosis: aspirin (325 mg/d) (endarterectomy should be considered strongly if >70% stenosis)
TIA: aspirin (325–975 mg/d); if aspirin allergy, ticlopidine (250 mg twice daily)
Completed stroke: (aspirin 325–975 mg/d); if aspirin allergy, ticlopidine (250 mg bid) (some evidence suggests that ticlopidine may be the preferred agent in patients with completed stroke)
Acute cardioembolic stroke: (1) small to moderate sized, no evidence of hemorrhage on computed tomography or magnetic resonance imaging performed ≥48 h later: intravenous heparin followed by warfarin (INR, 2.0–3.0); (2) large or in the presence of poorly controlled hypertension: delay anticoagulation for 5–14 d

TIA, transient ischemic attack; INR, international normalized ratio; APTT, activated partial thromboplastin time; ACT, activated clotting time.
From Becker RC, Ansell J. Antithrombotic therapy. An abbreviated reference for clinicians. Arch Intern Med 1995;155:149–161.

Table 27–2
Causes of Abnormal Prothrombin Time and Partial Thromboplastin Time

Disseminated intravascular coagulation*
Liver disease (factors II, VII, IX, and X deficiencies)*
Coumadin anticoagulation (II, VII, IX, and X)*
Heparin anticoagulation (II, XII, IX, X, XI, and XII)*
Factor X (Stuart–Prower) deficiency
Factor V deficiency (Owren's disease, parahemophilia)
Hereditary afibrinogenemia
Congenital dysfibrinogenemia
Primary fibrinolysis
Malabsorptive states
Antibiotic use (II, VII, IX, X)
Vitamin K deficiency

*Common disorder.
From Abell TL, Merigian KS, Lee JM, et al. Cutaneous exposure to warfarin-like anticoagulant causing an intracerebral hemorrhage: A case report. J Toxicol Clin Toxicol 1994;32(1):69–73.

Warfarin Rodenticide Poisoning

Most childhood exposures to warfarin rodenticides are asymptomatic.[27] Reports of poisoning with superwarfarin rodenticide coumarin anticoagulants indicate a prolonged morbidity and the necessity for aggressive therapy.[28,29]

Structure and Classification

Oral anticoagulants are either synthetic 3-substituted coumarin derivatives of 4-hydroxycoumarin, rodenticides (eg, brodifacoum or difenacoum), or synthetic derivatives of indan-1,3-dione.[23,30] In a coumarin-overdosed patient, the warfarin *S*(–) enantiomorph would appear to have a predominant role in the production of hypoprothrombinemia with its associated clinical toxicity.

Rodenticides: Commercial Products

Coumarins include warfarin, coumafene, zoocoumarin, coumafuryl, bromadiolone, coumachlor, difenacoum, brodifacoum, indandiones, diphacinone, chlorophacinone, and pindone or pivaldione.[23]

Factor IX Complex

Factor IX complex is a concentrate of blood coagulation factors II, VII, IX, and X. It may produce transient fever, chills, headache, flushing, tingling, and changes in pulse rate or blood pressure; however, because it is prepared from pooled plasma it may also contain the causative agents of viral hepatitis and AIDS.

Therapeutic Dose

Therapeutic maintenance dosages for anticoagulant drugs are listed in Table 27–3.

Toxicokinetics[10,31–37]

Bioavailability	About 100%
Time to peak plasma level	1 hour
Volume of distribution	0.126 L/kg
Plasma protein binding	98–99%
Elimination half-life	40 hours (warfarin); 120–160 hours (phenprocoumon)

There is no correlation between prothrombin time and concentration of free warfarin in serum.[38]

Drug Interactions

Drugs with significant interactions with oral anticoagulants are listed in Table 27–4.[32,39–41]

Pregnancy

Warfarin is a small molecule (molecular weight, 1000) and crosses the placenta. The heparin molecule is comparatively large (molecular weight, 20,000) and probably does not cross the placenta.[42]

Coumarin derivative exposure in the first trimester of pregnancy results in a specific malformation syndrome[43] known as warfarin embryopathy. Deformations of the central nervous system have been observed following warfarin therapy during any trimester of pregnancy.[44] In the late third trimester, exposure to coumarin anticoagulants may result in late prenatal, perinatal, or postnatal hemorrhage.[45,46]

Vitamin K Cycle

Vitamin K is a cofactor in the postribosomal synthesis of clotting factors II, VII, IX, and X as well as proteins C and

Table 27–3
Therapeutic Maintenance Dosage*

	Daily Initial Dose (mg)			Daily Maintenance Dose (mg)
	Day 1	Day 2	Day 3	
Anisindione	300	200	100	25–250
Dicoumarol	200–300		25–200	
Phenprocoumon	24			0.75–6
Warfarin	10–15	10–15	10–15	2–10
Other anticoagulants†				
Acenocoumarol	8–12	4–8		1–8
Diphenadione	20–30	10–15		2.5–5
Ethylbiscoumacetate	1.2	1.2	1.2	300–600
Phenindione	200	100		25–150

*Dependent on prothrombin level.
†Griffith MJ. Heparin catalyzed inhibitor/protease reactions: Kinetic evidence for a common mechanism of action of heparin. Proc Natl Acad Sci USA 1983;80:5460–5464.

Table 27–4
Drugs With Significant Interactions With Oral Anticoagulants Where There is a Decrease (D), Increase (I), or No Change (NC) in Reported Prothrombin Time

Antibacterials	
Carbenicillin	I
Chloramphenicol	I
Ciprofloxacin	I
Dicloxacillin	D
Enoxacin	I
Erythromycin	I
Metronidazole	I
Nafcillin	D
Nalidixic acid	I
Norfloxacin	I
Ofloxacin	I
Sulfamethazole	I
Sulfafurazole (sulfisoxazole)	I
Tetracycline	I
Trimethoprim–sulfamethoxazole (Cotrimoxazole)	I
Antituberculars	
Isoniazid	I, NC
Rifampicin (rifampin)	I
Antifungals	
Fluconazole	I
Griseofulvin	D
Itraconazole	I
Miconazole	I
Antimalarials	
Proguanil	I
Antiarrhythmics	
Amiodarone	I
Disopyramide	D
Propafenone	I

Anticonvulsants	
Carbamazepine	D
Phenobarbital (phenobarbitone)	I, D
Phenytoin	I, D
Antihyperlipidemics	
Cholestyramine	D
Clofibrate	I
Lovastatin	I
Analgesics/Antipyretics	
Paracetamol (acetaminophen)	I
Paracetamol–dextropropoxyphene	I
Antineoplastics	
Aminoglutethimide	D
Broxuridine (bromodeoxyuridine)	I
Ifosfamide	I
Mitotane	I
Mercaptopurine	D
Sulofenur	I
Nonsteroidal Antiinflammatories	
Aspirin (acetylsalicylic acid)	I, NC
Halofenate	I, NC
Indomethacin	I, NC
Ketoprofen	I, NC
Methylsalicylate (topical)	I, NC
Oxyphenbutazone	I, N
Phenylbutazone	I, NC
Tolmetin	I, NC

H_2-Receptor Antagonists	
Cimetidine	I
Ranitidine	I
Immunosuppressives	
Azathioprine	D
Cyclosporine	I, D, NC
Sedative/Hypnotics	
Chloral hydrate	I
Secobarbital (Quinalbarbitone)	D
Miscellaneous	
Allopurinol	I
Danazol	I
Diazoxide	I
Digibind	I
Dipyridamole	I
Disulfiram	I
Omeprazole	I
Oral contraceptives	D
Ponalrestat	I
Stanozalol	I
Sucralfate	D
Thyroxine	I
Ticlopidine	I, NC
Triclofos	I
Vitamin A (retinol)	I
Vitamin C (ascorbic acid)	D

From Freedman MD, Olatidoye AG. Clinically significant drug interactions with the oral anticoagulants. Drug Saf 1994;10:381–394.

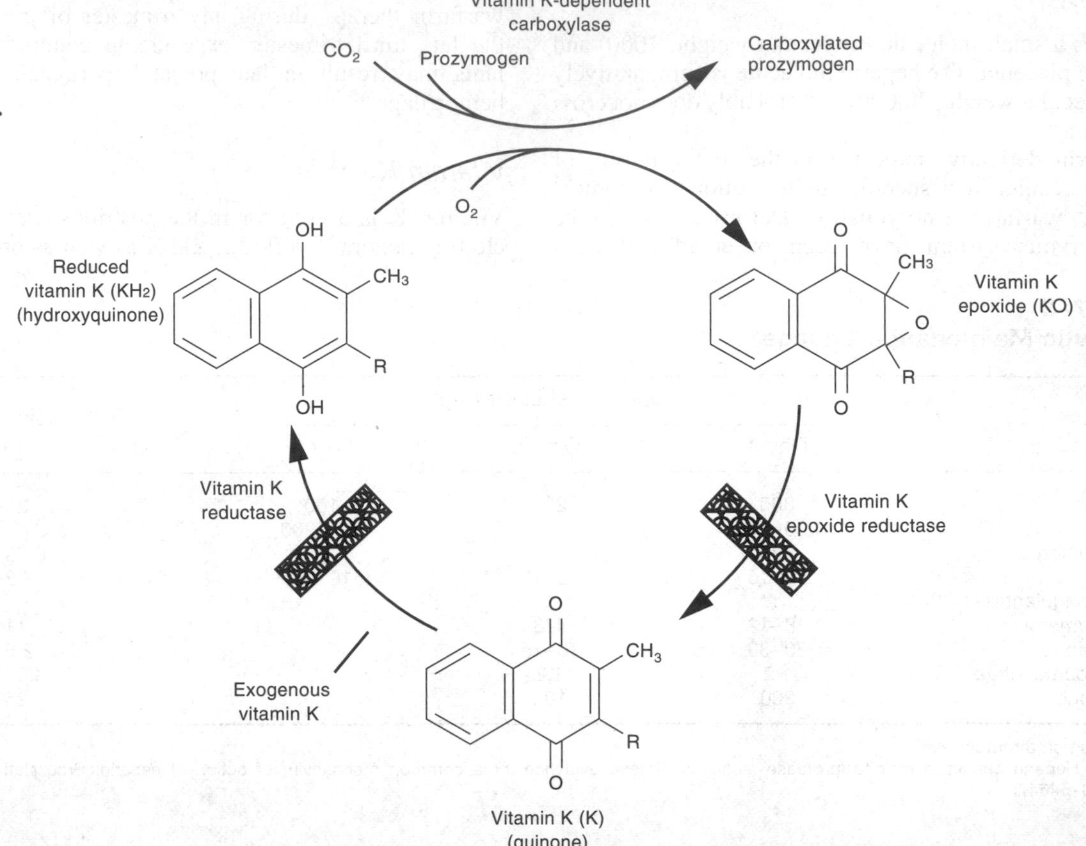

Figure 27–1 The vitamin K cycle and the effect of warfarin and exogenous vitamin K (phytomenadione). Vitamin K (quinone) is converted to reduced vitamin K (KH_2, hydroxyquinone) by vitamin K reductase. Vitamin KH_2 is the substrate for the carboxylation of prozymogens (eg, factors II, VII, IX, X) to active enzymes. Carbon dioxide and oxygen are required for this reaction and vitamin KH_2 is converted to vitamin K epoxide (KO). Vitamin K is regenerated from vitamin KO by vitamin K epoxide reductase. Warfarin inhibits vitamin K epoxide reductase and, to some extent, vitamin K reductase (hatched areas). Exogenous vitamin K in large doses overcomes the blockage by warfarin presumably because vitamin K reductase is less sensitive to warfarin than is vitamin K epoxide reductase (arrow). (From Pineo GF, Hull RD. Adverse effects of coumarin anticoagulants. Drug Saf 1993;9:263–271.)

S. Coumarins depress protein C. This may be associated with coumarin skin necrosis[47] (Fig. 27–1).

Toxicokinetics of Vitamin K[48]

Bioavailability	10–62%
Peak plasma level	K_1-2,3-epoxide in normal people (<20 ng/mL); after brodifacoum poisoning (to 600 ng/mL)
Volume of distribution	0.07 L/kg
Elimination half-life	1–4 hours

Clinical Presentation

Oral Anticoagulant Medication

Overdose with anticoagulants classically leads to bleeding in multiple organ sites (Table 27–5).

Protein C and Protein S Deficiency

Skin necrosis associated with warfarin may be associated with an inherited heterozygous form of protein C deficiency. Cutaneous reactions associated with coumarin derivatives manifest in one of four ways: ecchymosis and purpura from hypocoagulation; macular, papular, vesicular, urticarial, and purpuric skin eruptions; the "purple toe" syndrome; and frank tissue necrosis. Lesions appear within 3 to 6 days of initiation of warfarin sodium therapy. Obese women around 50 years of age who are under therapy for thrombophlebitis or pulmonary thromboembolism are at the highest risk. Skin necrosis tends to occur in adipose tissue, mainly in the thighs, breasts, and buttocks. Therapy is primarily supportive. Discontinuation of warfarin sodium has not been shown

Table 27–5
Overdose of Warfarins

Abnormal	Normal
White blood cells elevated[1]	Bleeding time[12]
Prothrombin time elevated[12,13]	Blood calcium
Coagulation time elevated	Capillary fragility[13]
Hemoglobin decreased[13]	Fibrinogen
Red blood cells decreased	Platelets
Bleeding time may be prolonged[13]	Liver function tests
Activated partial thromboplastin time prolonged	Factor V level[17]
Cystoscopy: "meat juice" at ureteral ostia[13]	Electrolytes
Stool for occult blood positive	Kidney function tests
Decrease in factors II, VII, IX, X	

to alter the course or recurrence of disease. The benefits of administering vitamin K or steroids remain unproved. Surgical intervention may be required. The cause of skin necrosis resulting from warfarin sodium and other warfarin congeners remains a mystery.[49]

Protein C has anticoagulant and profibrinolytic activity. Protein S, a cofactor for protein C, potentiates protein C activity at the endothelial cell surface. Reductions in either protein C or S may be a contributing factor to thromboembolic complications.[50–52] A protein C concentrate available from Immuno in Vienna accelerated healing in a person with warfarin-induced skin necrosis with a protein C deficiency.[53]

Covert Oral Anticoagulant Ingestion (Surreptitious, Factitious, and Munchhausen Syndrome Types)

Patients exhibit an unexplained acquired hemorrhagic diathesis associated with low prothrombin complex activity (II, VII, IX, X). They are often individuals who have access to coumarin or indandione compounds, either as a medication (nurses, doctors, pharmacists, or other medical personnel) or as a rodenticide.[54,55] Clinical recognition of this disorder may not occur for months or years. Diagnosis is supported by finding decreased vitamin K-dependent blood clotting factors (II, VII, IX, X) and by a good therapeutic response to vitamin K_1. Confirmation of the diagnosis is provided by chemical detection of the drug in the patient's plasma. Factors V and VIII are usually normal. The one-stage prothrombin activity is reduced in most patients to less than 10% of normal activity.

Superwarfarins

The long-acting anticoagulant rodenticides are 4-hydroxycoumarin derivatives with a 4-bromo (1,1-biphenyl) side chain. Children produce abnormal prothrombin times which may not be observed until 48 hours postingestion.[56] The occurrence of an abnormal prothrombin time may not be predicted based on a history of the amount ingested or on the presence of the characteristic green-blue product dye in or around a child's mouth. Acute toxicity may be evidenced by transient abdominal pain, vomiting, or heme-positive stools. Some rodenticides (superwarfarins) may have far longer action on vitamin K-dependent clotting factors than does warfarin. Vitamin K therapy may be required for 2 to 3 months.

Animal studies suggest that one-time ingestions of brodifacoum rat bait can cause severe coagulation abnormalities that require large doses of vitamin K_1 and can last months, as well as clinical bleeding; in contrast, a single ingestion of warfarin-containing bait does not usually induce abnormalities in coagulation. Fatalities have followed brodifacoum ingestion.[57] Vitamin K_1 must be administered in high doses and at frequent intervals until clotting factor tests are normal (days or weeks), and the tests must be monitored for several months after they have initially returned to normal.

Difenacoum, Brodifacoum, Chlorphacinone

Difenacoum, brodifacoum, and chlorphacinone produce a diminution in vitamin K-dependent gamma-carboxylation of glutamic acid residues in prothrombin factor precursors that is 100 times greater on a molar basis than that of warfarin. This follows reduction of vitamin K_1-2,3-epoxide reductase. In addition, they may have a half-life up to 120 days[16] (warfarin, 42 hours).[32]

Laboratory

Abnormal and normal results follow an overdose of warfarins (see Table 27–5). A simple high-performance liquid chromatographic method has been developed for detection and quantification of brodifacoum. The limit of detection for plasma is 2 μg/mL. A liquid chromatographic method can simultaneously measure the serum levels of five anticoagulant rodenticides: brodifacoum, bromadiolone, coumatetralyl, difenacoum, and warfarin.[58] Plasma or urine brodifacoum levels can be provided free by phoning Zeneca Emergency Information Network at 1–800–327–8633.

International Normalized Ratio

In an effort to standardize the results of the prothrombin time test, the World Health Organization introduced the International Normalized Ratio (INR).

Values of INR are independent of the reagents and methods and, therefore, are comparable between laboratories across the country and abroad. The INR is defined as the patient/normal prothrombin time (PT) ratio that would result if the World Health Organization's primary international thromboplastin was used to test the patient sample:

$$\text{INR} = \left(\frac{\text{patient PT}}{\text{normal PT}}\right)^{\text{ISI}}$$

where ISI = the International Sensitivity Index of the thromboplastin used in the local laboratory.[59]

Treatment

Stabilization

Morgan indicates that the average child eating a few mouthfuls (or 25-g packet) of 0.005% rat bait at a single sitting is generally not at risk[22] and no treatment is necessary.[27,28,60] If more than 25 g of a 0.005% concentration has been consumed (either acutely or over a few days in small amounts), then treatment should begin (Fig. 27–2).

Patients who have overdosed on an oral anticoagulant or who have ingested an undetermined amount of drug or rodenticide should be admitted to an intensive care facility where careful follow-up with adequate laboratory testing capabilities for clotting parameters is available. Close observation is necessary to detect the development of airway obstruction secondary to hemorrhage. All oral anticoagulant ingestion should cease immediately. Clandestine sources should be removed.

Following an extensive study of anticoagulant rodenticides over 5 years, a Washington State group recommends that for one-time ingestions of plain warfarin-related or superwarfarin-related rodenticides, no decontamination, no dilution, no emergency department visits, no in-hospital

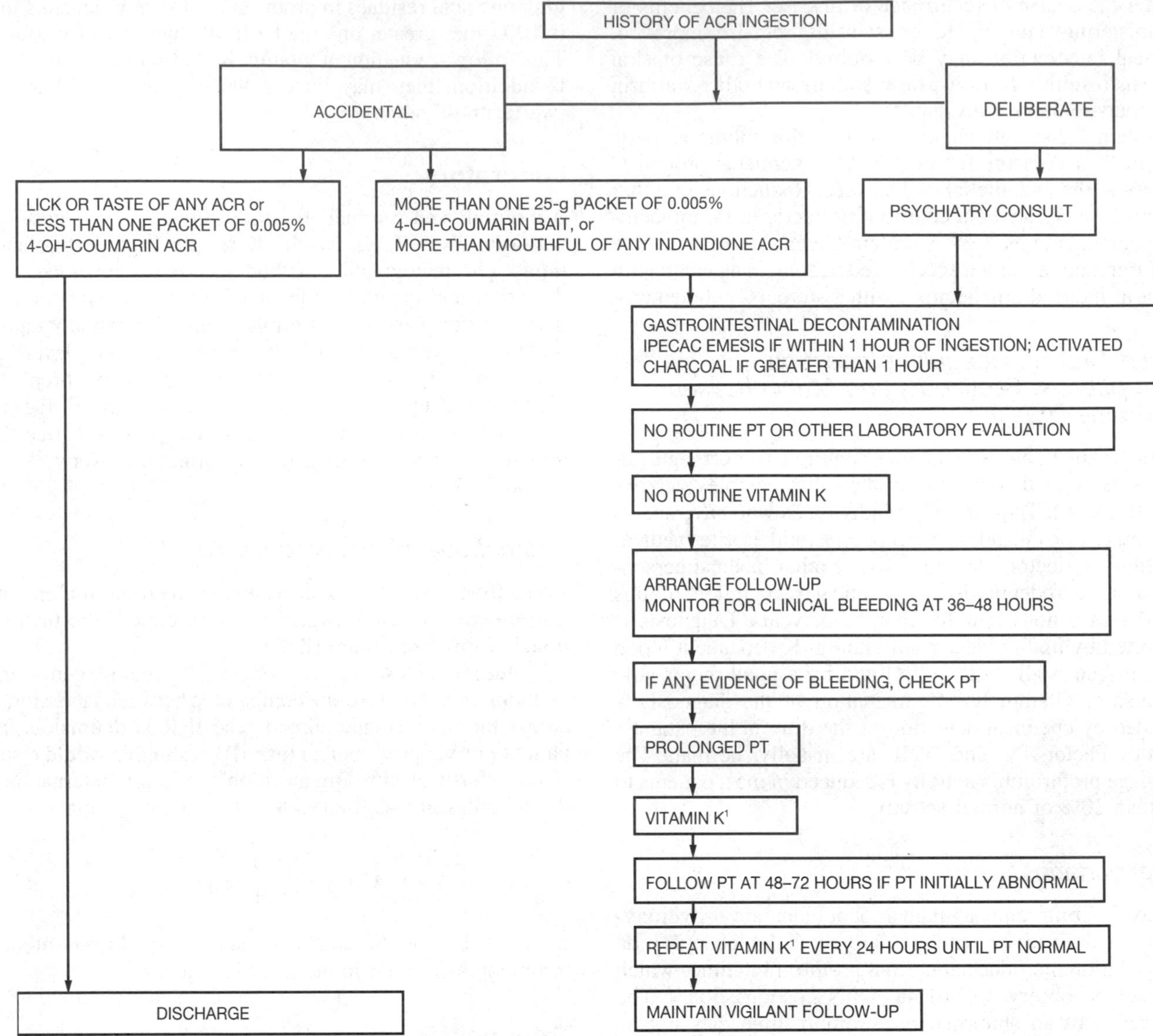

Figure 27–2 Recommended treatment for anticoagulant rodenticide (ACR) ingestion. PT, prothrombin time. (From Katona B, Wason S. Superwarfarin poisoning. J Emerg Med 1989;7:627–631.)

treatment, and no prothrombin time determinations are necessary in the absence of clinical symptoms. They focus on urging parents and parent–surrogates to observe the child for signs of bleeding or bruising.

For suicide attempts by teenagers or adults or for repetitive ingestions, especially those including other animals (eg, dogs), traditional emergency management can be critical.[61] Draw blood for an immediate prothrombin time, complete blood count, and activated partial thromboplastin time. Prothrombin times should be obtained every 12 hours for several days even if a severe prolongation is not observed in a baseline study. If hemorrhage is severe, replace deficiencies in factors II, VII, IX, and X with whole blood or plasma (including fresh-frozen plasma). None of the clotting factors II, VII, IX, and X are labile on storage, so the use of whole blood or plasma, fresh or frozen, is not absolutely necessary. Recognize the potential risks of acquiring viral hepatitis and AIDS. Vitamin K can usually reverse deficiencies in vitamin K-dependent coagulation factors II, VII, IX, and X as well as proteins C and S.[62]

Warfarin overdose in patients with prosthetic heart valves requires prolonged, controlled partial reversal of anticoagulation until warfarin and metabolites decline to the therapeutic plasma level of 3.0 μg/mL.[7] Use of fresh-frozen plasma infusions every 12 hours by Toolis and co-workers in two patients resulted in half-lives of 80 and 45 hours.[7] No bleeding was observed at any time. The prothrombin ratio must be monitored several times daily (every 12–24 hours after baseline) to assist in determining quantity and times of plasma dosage. Plasma warfarin concentrations are useful for determining the approximate duration of therapy.

Gut Decontamination

Ipecac may precipitate intracranial hemorrhage by raising intracranial blood pressure. Ipecac-induced emesis may provoke gastrointestinal bleeding.

Gastric lavage should be used with suction available or by prior-cuffed endotracheal intubation in an obtunded or unconscious patient. Gastric lavage may also provoke bleeding. The efficacy of gastric emptying has not yet been established.

Activated charcoal in an aqueous slurry may be administered through the lavage tube. Suggested doses are 50 to 100 g for adults and 15 to 50 g for children.

Cathartics have not been evaluated.

Elimination Enhancement

Forced diuresis, hemodialysis, and peritoneal dialysis are not useful. Hemoperfusion has not been used.

Cholestyramine 12 to 16 g daily in divided doses is effective in reducing the half-life and in increasing the total clearance of oral anticoagulants.[36,63] There is evidence that it may be effective in warfarin overdose, possibly by interrupting the enterohepatic recirculation of warfarin.[9]

Exchange transfusions may possibly be effective in a serious life-threatening overdose in a child but inadequate data exist to substantiate this.

Antidote

Vitamin K_1 (phytonadione) is useful in restoring the prothrombin time to normal levels and in decreasing or stopping the bleeding episodes.

If an overdose of an oral anticoagulant drug or an unknown dose of an oral anticoagulant pesticide (eg, brodifacoum, difenacoum) has been ingested, vitamin K_1 (phytonadione [Mephyton]) is administered orally in doses of 10 to 25 mg/d for adults and 5 to 10 mg for children. Vitamin K_1 has a short duration of action and so must be given repeatedly. The turnover rate of K_1 is 30 to 50% per hour; that is, all the body vitamin K_1 is replaced every 2 to 3 hours[64] (Fig. 27–1). Intramuscular phytonadione (Aquamephyton) can be given to adults in doses of 5 to 10 mg and to children under 12 in doses of 1 to 5 mg. Doses up to 100 to 125 mg/d for many weeks or months may be required in a severe rodenticide overdose.

Intravenous vitamin K_1 can be administered in a 0.9% sodium chloride or glucose infusion slowly. Too rapid infusion may result in flushing, cyanosis, dizziness, hypotension, and bronchoconstriction.[64] Prothrombin times will guide subsequent doses but will often not begin to return to normal for at least 3 to 4 days. Intramuscular or oral vitamin K_1, 10 mg three to five times daily, can then be instituted.[13,64] Anaphylactic reactions may occur during or a few minutes after direct intravenous infusion of undiluted vitamin K_1.[65]

Phytonadione is absorbed rapidly by the subcutaneous route. The subcutaneous route is preferable to the intravenous route unless problems are anticipated with subcutaneous absorption.[66]

If the hematologic risk is low, intramuscular K_1 (5–10 mg) alone can be given in divided doses.[13]

Vitamin K_3 (menadione) is ineffective for the treatment of warfarin and superwarfarin toxicity.[15] It elicits a poor response and should not be used.[20,67]

Factor II/IX/X concentrate and intravenous vitamin K_1 2.5 mg are used to reverse overdoses of oral anticoagulants. Both products improve the prothrombin time and partial thromboplastin time and raise the depressed levels of factors II, VII, and X. The concentrate acts maximally at 30 minutes, except for factor VII activity. Vitamin K_1 begins to correct these values, including factor VII, in 2 hours and overcorrects by 24 hours. The concentrate is more easily controlled but carries with it the risk of transmission of non-A, non-B hepatitis[68] and AIDS.[69,70] Therefore, its use in oral anticoagulant reversal should be limited to correcting life-threatening hemorrhage.[71]

Prothrombin times should be monitored frequently. In severe poisonings vitamin K_1 should be continued until the plasma warfarin level is in the therapeutic range (<1 μg/mL) to avoid a rebound to dangerous prothrombin times.

The decision to reverse excessive warfarin anticoagulation with vitamin K assumes that short-term elevations in INR are associated with a significant risk of bleeding.

Characteristics associated with an increased risk of bleeding during long-term warfarin anticoagulation are age above 65; a history of cerebrovascular disease, stroke, or gastrointestinal bleeding; heart disease; concurrent aspirin therapy; and hypertension. High-intensity warfarin therapy has also been associated with an increased risk of bleeding.

Administration of vitamin K parenterally to correct the INR in overanticoagulated patients is not without risks. Rapid intravenous administration may be associated with facial flushing, diaphoresis, chest pain, hypotension, or dyspnea associated with or without anaphylaxis. Cerebral thrombosis and death have been associated with intravenous and intramuscular administration of vitamin K.

Administration of vitamin K may interfere with subsequent attempts to achieve oral anticoagulation

Conservative treatment of nonbleeding patients without the use of vitamin K is safe and may eliminate problems associated with vitamin K administration. A randomized prospective study is required to determine in overanticoagulated patients the utility of parenteral or oral vitamin K compared with conservative management.[72]

Supportive Measures

1. Monitor the coagulation time, bleeding time, and one-stage prothrombin time. Keep patients in the hospital under continuous observation until laboratory and clinical evidence of control of bleeding is obtained.[16,17,73]
2. Phenobarbital 100 to 120 mg/d is useful in inducing hepatic microsomal metabolism of coumarins[57]; it has not been carefully evaluated and cannot be recommended at present.
3. For patients requiring emergency surgery after an oral anticoagulant overdose, exchange transfusions, whole blood, or plasma may need to be employed together with frequent determinations of hematocrit; frequent analyses for blood in urine, vomit, and stool; frequent evaluation of pulse, respirations, and blood pressure; and frequent inspection of skin and muscles for any evidence of recurrent bleeding.
4. Ferrous sulfate therapy may be useful in replenishing red blood cell mass.
5. Prior to discharge, obtain a psychiatric consultation.

Table 27-6
International Normalized Ratio (INR) and Reversal of Anticoagulant Effects of Warfarin

INR	Bleeding	Treatment
>2.0 <6.0	No	Rapid reversal not indicated
6.0–10.0	No	Vitamin K 0.5–1 mg slow IV injection
10.0–20.0	No	Vitamin K 3–5 mg slow IV injection Check INR every 6–12 h
>20.0		Vitamin K 10 mg slow IV Check INR every 6 h
Life-threatening bleeding		Vitamin K 10 mg IV
Serious warfarin overdose		Fresh-frozen plasma or factor concentrates

From Becker RC, Ansell J. Antithrombotic therapy: An abbreviated reference for clinicians. Arch Intern Med 1995;155:149–161.

6. The patient should not be discharged until a follow-up program (hematologic and psychiatric care) is established.

Table 27–6 summarizes the relationship of the INR to the reversal of the anticoagulant effects of warfarin.[74]

HEPARIN

Heparin overdosage in the clinical setting occurs frequently but few poisoning cases have been reported. Overdosage can usually be controlled with good supportive therapy. If bleeding is severe, protamine sulfate administered alone or together with fresh whole blood or plasma may be effective. Heparin administered surreptitiously,[75] heparin rebound,[26] and heparin-induced thrombosis–thrombocytopenia syndrome (HITTS)[76–84] are all problems requiring immediate evaluation and care.

Therapeutic Dose

The initial intravenous injection can contain up to 12,500 U of heparin; this is followed by 5000 to 10,000 U every 4 hours sufficient to keep the clotting time at two to three times the pretreatment figure, or to keep the activated partial thromboplastin time at 1.5 to 2.5 times the control value.

Continuous infusion of an initial loading of 4000 Units intravenously is followed by 20,000 to 40,000 U of heparin given in 1 L of dextrose or 0.9% sodium chloride injection over 24 hours, and continued as required.

Subcutaneous dosage therapy is initiated with 4000 U intravenously, followed by 10,000 U every 8 hours or 15,000 U every 12 hours.

In children, an initial dosage is 50 U/kg body weight intravenously, followed by 100 U/kg every 4 hours as required.

Heparin is not administered intramuscularly because of pain, irritation, and hematoma formation at the injection site.[2,30,85]

Toxicokinetics[2,10,82,85–87]

Bioavailability	Complete after intravenous use
Peak plasma level	0.2–0.6 U/m4L
Volume of distribution	0.06 L/kg
Elimination half-life	0.3–2 hours

Drug Interactions

Drugs that affect platelet function (aspirin, nonsteroidal antiinflammatory drugs, dipyridamole, dextran)[85] and thrombolytic agents (streptokinase, urokinase) used with heparin may increase the risk of hemorrhage. More than 0.1 mL of heparin left in a syringe for each 3 to 4 mL of arterial blood drawn may result in a decrease in P_{CO_2}, P_{O_2}, and HCO_3 and base excess in the sample.[88]

Pregnancy/Lactation

Cases in which heparin was used during pregnancy indicate that less than two thirds of such pregnancies resulted in normal children. Heparin use, however, has not been associated with fetal anomalies.[89] Excessive maternal deaths, fetal loss, premature deliveries (22%), and neonatal deaths (13%) appear to be substantially more frequent with heparin than with the coumarin derivatives.[90,91] Long-term use of heparin during pregnancy is associated with reversible bone loss.[92] Heparin does not appear to cross the placenta[85] and is not distributed into breast milk.[93]

Mechanism of Action

Anticoagulant Effects

Heparin interacts with antithrombin III heparin cofactor to produce a substance that immediately neutralizes thrombin by forming a complex with it at its active serine center.

Non-anticoagulant Effects

Heparin also inhibits platelet function, increases the permeability of vessel walls, inhibits the proliferation of vascular smooth muscle cells, inhibits delayed hypersensitivity reactions, and is involved in the regulation of angiogenesis.[94]

Risk Factors in Heparin-Induced Bleeding

- Age greater than 60 years of age (9.7%)
- Females (10.6%) affected more than males (7.3%)
- Median dose greater than 50 U/kg (25.3%)
- Blood urea nitrogen greater than 50 mg/dL (13.8%).
- Heavy drinking (15%)
- Concomitant intake of aspirin (14.2%)[95]

Clinical Presentation

Overdoses of heparin result in rapid prolongation of the coagulation time and active bleeding. Overdosage with heparin should be considered in a neonate with a bleeding diathesis whose partial thromboplastin time is greater than 2 minutes, prothrombin time is longer than 60 seconds, clotting time is markedly prolonged, and platelet count is normal.

Surreptitious Use

When confronted with unexpected laboratory findings and response to treatment, patients may admit to their surreptitious use of heparin.

Aldosterone Suppression: Hyperkalemia

Heparin and its congeners are predictable, potent inhibitors of aldosterone production (Fig. 27–3). Aldosterone suppression occurs within a few days of initiation of therapy, is reversible, and is independent of either anticoagulant effect or route of administration. Decreases in aldosterone levels may occur with heparin dosages as low as 5000 U twice daily. Aldosterone suppression results in natriuresis and, less predictably, in decreased excretion of potassium. Greater than normal serum potassium levels occur in about 7% of patients, but marked hyperkalemia generally requires the presence of additional factors perturbing potassium balance (in particular, renal insufficiency, diabetes mellitus, and use of certain medications). Serum potassium levels should be monitored periodically in patients being given heparin for 3 or more days, and in patients at relatively high risk for hyperkalemia, the monitoring interval should probably be no greater than 4 days.

The most straightforward way to reverse heparin-induced hyperkalemia is to discontinue heparin administration. Clinically important hyperkalemia can be avoided by instituting other potassium-lowering measures, for example, discontinuing other potassium-elevating drugs (such as angiotensin-converting enzyme inhibitors), decreasing potassium intake, and enhancing urinary potassium excretion (eg, by administering furosemide or fludrocortisone). If heparin is continued, the resultant hyperkalemia may be prolonged.[96]

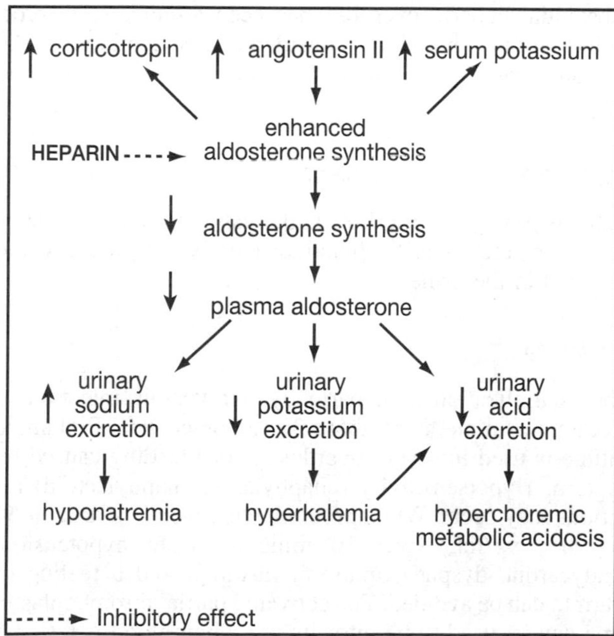

Figure 27–3 A schema for the pathogenesis of heparin-induced aldosterone suppression and resulting electrolyte abnormalities. Although heparin inhibits aldosterone synthesis stimulation by corticotropin, angiotensin II, and potassium, the precise mechanisms accounting for the suppression of aldosterone are unknown. The most important mechanism appears to involve a reduction in both the number and affinity of the angiotensin II receptors in the zona glomerulosa. (From Oster JR, Singer I, Fishman LM. Heparin-induced aldosterone suppression and hyperkalemia. Am J Med 1995;98:575–586.)

Heparin-Induced Thrombosis–Thrombocytopenia Syndrome

Heparin may fail to control pathologic thrombosis. This may be due to a hypercoagulable state associated with malignancy, antithrombin III deficiency, inadequate heparin dosage, or heparin-induced thrombosis.[84]

Complications. Complications of heparin-induced thrombosis–thrombocytopenia syndrome (HITTS) may be thrombotic (deep venous thrombosis, pulmonary emboli, myocardial infarction, cerebral thrombosis, digital vasculitis, adrenal infarct/hemorrhage, renal artery embolism, spinal artery thrombosis, priapism, skin necrosis, aortic and limb arterial thrombosis) or hemorrhagic (cerebral hemorrhage, gastrointestinal bleeding, adrenal hemorrhage, skin bruising, epistaxis, hematuria, intramuscular hematoma, or wound hematoma). HITTS has a 30% death rate.[97]

Diagnosis. Typically, a patient on therapeutic or prophylactic heparin suddenly deteriorates 5 to 10 days after commencing heparin therapy and begins to require increasing doses of heparin to maintain anticoagulation as disclosed by the activated partial thromboplastin time. Antithrombin III levels fall. A low platelet count (as low as 5000–29,000) is frequently detected in HITTS. Vague low back, thigh, or abdominal pain and distention 1 or 2 days prior to clinically evident vascular obstruction may be warnings of a large-vessel thrombosis.

Treatment. Promptly withdraw heparin therapy. There is an added risk of further thrombosis and embolism when heparin therapy is discontinued. Warfarin has a long latent period so is not immediately useful. Consider dextran therapy, antiplatelet drugs such as aspirin and dipyridamole, and substitution of low-molecular-weight heparin. Intravenous streptokinase therapy (loading dose of 250,000 U intravenously, followed by continuous infusion of 100,000 U/h for 72 hours) has led to the reversal of near-gangrenous changes in both the upper and lower extremities resulting from venous thrombosis secondary to heparin therapy.[98] Tissue plasminogen activator may also be useful[99] (see Ancrod later in this chapter).

Intravenous immunoglobulin 0.4 g/kg body weight followed by a platelet transfusion appeared to restore normal platelet counts in a patient with severe heparin-associated thrombocytopenia.[100] Patients with heparin-associated antiplatelet antibodies should not receive heparin or heparin-coated pulmonary artery catheters.[101] If thromboemboli have already formed, additional anticoagulation is immediately required. For this purpose, warfarin is too slow; corticosteroids are of no benefit[84]; antiplatelet agents, though untested, may be useful; and platelet transfusions have been recommended if the patient is actively bleeding but may be otherwise detrimental. Protamine sulfate has no value because the problem is not due to the anticoagulating

Table 27–7
Low-Molecular-Weight Heparins

Heparin	Mean Molecular Weight
Enoxaprin	3500–5550
Kabi-265 (Tedelprin)	4000–6000
OP 2123	3500–5000
CY216 (Nadroprine)	4500
Sandoz CH-8140	4500–8000
Novo LHN-1	4900

properties of heparin, but rather to its antigenic properties.[78] Hirulog, a direct thrombin inhibitor and hirudin analog, may be useful for the prevention of progressive thrombi.[102]Low-

Low-Molecular-Weight Heparins. Low-molecular-weight heparins. (LMWHs) have been separated with an average molecular weight of 4000 to 6500 (Table 27–7). They have an attenuated effect on coagulation and prolongation of the activated partial thromboplastin time compared with unfractionated heparin. Whether they produce less bleeding for an equivalent antithrombotic effect than unfractionated heparin remains to be established.[103]

The only LMWH product approved at present in the United States is enoxaprin injection (Lovenox). LMWH inhibits aldosterone production and produces hyperkalemia, as does standard heparin.[104] All LMWH are neutralized by protamine. Hematomas, urticaria, angioedema, and skin necrosis have been reported at the injection site. Enoxaprins are associated with a lower rate of major bleeding episodes than standard heparins, and with moderate thrombocytopenia, fever, local irritation, pain, hematuria, erythema, and thrombolytic episodes.[105]

The recommended dose is 30 mg twice daily by subcutaneous injection only.

Heparin Flush Syndrome

The heparin flush syndrome indicates that an iatrogenic hemorrhage can be induced by routine and unmonitored use of heparin in "flush" solutions given to "flush" arterial and venous catheters to maintain patency and thus vascular access.[106,107] Ampules with different strengths of heparin may appear identical.[107] A normal reptilase time is a quick test used to implicate heparin as the active inhibitor of coagulation and will clot fibrinogen even in the presence of heparin. Protamine sulfate rapidly halts bleeding and normalizes coagulation tests.[106]

Heparin Withdrawal

Within the first 24 hours of heparin discontinuation, patients not already taking aspirin or warfarin may be at increased risk for transient ischemic attack, stroke, or clinical deterioration.[108]

Laboratory

Periodic platelet counts should be obtained. If the counts begin to drop or unexplained recurrent thromboembolic phenomena begin to occur, the presence of a heparin-dependent antiplatelet antibody should be suspected and heparin should be promptly discontinued.[76,80] An activated partial thromboplastin time and an antithrombin III level should be obtained. Thrombocytopenia is observed after continuous or intermittent intravenous or subcutaneous heparin use.[60] It occurs 2 to 4 days after heparin treatment is begun, is mild and transient, and may resolve even if heparin is continued.

Heparin assays may underestimate drug levels in neonatal plasma unless the neonatal antithrombin III deficiency is fully corrected in the test system. Use of standard assays may lead to overheparinization of newborn infants, thereby placing them at a higher risk of bleeding.[109]

Treatment

Stabilization

The patient should be admitted to an intensive care facility where careful monitoring of blood clotting parameters is available. Parenteral heparin should be discontinued. (Oral heparin is not dangerous because it is inactivated by gastric acid.) The patient must be observed closely for the development of airway obstruction secondary to hemorrhage.

Airway, breathing, and circulatory status must be immediately evaluated and assisted where required. Tidal volume should be at least 10 to 15 mL/kg.

Blood should be drawn for baseline complete blood count, platelet count, coagulation profile (bleeding time, clotting time), and activated partial thromboplastin time.

If bleeding is minimal, administration of heparin should be stopped (short half-life). If bleeding is severe or a substantial heparin overdose has been administered, protamine sulfate should be considered (see Antidote). The activated partial thromboplastin time should be monitored frequently.

Elimination Enhancement

Dialysis procedures (peritoneal dialysis, hemodialysis) have not been effective.[110] Inactive metabolic products are excreted in the urine.

Antidote

The neutralization of heparin by intravenous injection of protamine sulfate takes about 30 to 60 seconds. Protamine sulfate is used in severe overdosage or bleeding caused by heparin. Hypersensitivity (anaphylaxis, anaphylactoid) reactions may occur. When protamine is given in a dose of 50 mg (10 mg/mL) over 10 minutes, acute hypotension, bradycardia, dyspnea, transient flushing, and a feeling of warmth can be avoided. The activated partial thromboplastin time can be used to monitor its use when blood is tested 5 to 15 minutes after administration. About 1 mg of protamine sulfate neutralizes 90 to 115 U of heparin. If given within a few minutes of intravenous heparin injection, 1 to 1.5 mg of protamine sulfate can be used for each 100 U of heparin administered. If 1 hour has elapsed since the heparin injection, 0.5 to 0.75 mg of protamine sulfate can be given for every 100 U of heparin; if more than 2 hours have elapsed, 0.25 to 0.375 mg of protamine sulfate can be given for each 100 U of heparin. For commercial heparin, 1 mg is approximately equivalent to 120 U.[85]

Heparin rebound is defined as the resurgence of anticoagulant activity in a patient whose blood heparin has been adequately neutralized with protamine. It is a potential bleeding disorder associated with cardiopulmonary bypass and either protamine sulfate or protamine chloride use.[111]

Supportive Measures

1. Monitor clotting parameters, especially the activated partial thromboplastin time and the platelet count, daily.
2. If thrombocytopenia begins to develop, consider HITTS. Platelet transfusions may be useful.
3. If bleeding is severe, whole blood or plasma may be required. Follow-up care with supplemental ferrous sulfate may be required to replenish the red blood cell mass.
4. If bleeding has not been severe, the patient should be hospitalized until clotting parameters are normal, he or she is asymptomatic, and there is no obvious source of bleeding.
5. Posthospital care should include careful follow-up for development of heparin rebound or heparin-induced thrombosis.

ANTIFIBRINOLYTIC AGENTS

Figure 27–4 is a schematic representation of the fibrinolytic system.

APROTININ

The basic proteinase inhibitor from bovine organs, aprotinin (Trasylol), can only be administered intravenously, and has a half-life of about 2 hours.[112] When it is administered at the start of cardiopulmonary bypass surgery it appears to reduce blood loss[113] and to protect against global myocardial ischemia. The recommended loading dose is 15,000 to 20,000 KIU (Kallikrein Inactivator Units)/kg body weight intravenously followed by 50,000 KIU/h by continuous infusion. Doses as high as 2,000,000 KIU have been administered.[107,114] At a constant intravenous infusion rate of 250,000 KIU/h, a steady-state plasma concentration of 40 to 50 KIU/mL is obtained,[103] equivalent to a concentration of about 1 μmol/L. At the high dose,[113,114] plasma concentrations of 150 KIU/mL are obtained and are associated with fibrinolysis inhibition and reduction of blood loss and blood use[115] after cardiopulmonary bypass and orthoptic liver transplantation.[116] A combination of high-dose aprotinin and profound hypothermia with low blood blow or circulatory arrest may lead to a disseminated intravascular coagulopathy.[117]

A dose of 625,000 KIU of aprotinin administered intravenously can lead to a decrease in arterial pressure, and metabolic acidosis. Noradrenaline, steroids, and sodium bicarbonate may be useful.[118] Hypersensitivity reactions after repeated doses occur in approximately 10% of patients. A radioallergosorbent test (RAST) with aprotinin before repeated administration may be useful.[119]

ε-AMINOCAPROIC ACID

ε-amino-*N*-caproic acid (EACA) is an inhibitor of fibrinolysis that has been used for more than 20 years to control bleeding in a variety of situations including hematuria and postpartum hemorrhage.[120] Acute renal failure, myopathy,[121,122] rash, nausea, diarrhea, and prolongation of bleeding time with high doses have been reported.[123] There have been no published reports of overdosage with EACA but the manufacturer has received reports of infusion rate errors leading to 10- to 20-fold overdoses, almost all of which were asymptomatic and resolved without sequelae.[124,125]

Structure and Classification

ε-Aminocaproic acid is a synthetic monoamine carboxylic acid. At injection it has a pH of 6 to 7.6. EACA is also known

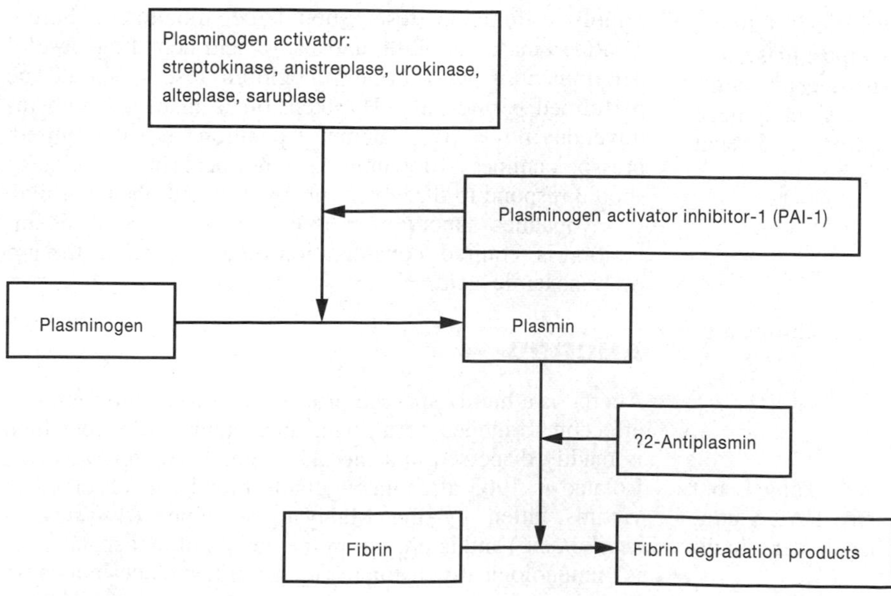

Figure 27–4 Schematic representation of the fibrinolytic system. (From Verstraete M. Use of thrombolytic drugs in non-coronary disorders. Drugs 1989;38:801–821.)

as 6-aminohexanoic acid and is marketed as Amicar, and Capracid in Italy; Capralense in France; Capramol in Belgium and France; Epsikapron; and Hemocaptrol.

Toxic Dose

The minimum lethal dose is unknown. Toxicity has been associated with intravenous doses as small as 2 g.[126] Prolongation of bleeding times was observed in all patients receiving 48 g/d.[123]

Toxicokinetics[127–128]

Time to Peak plasma level	2 hours
Volume of distribution	0.39 L/kg
Excreted unchanged	About 70–80%

Pregnancy/Lactation

Safe use of the drug with respect to adverse effects on fetal development has not been established. Clinical studies have not been performed on breast milk excretion.

Mechanism of Action

ϵ-Aminocaproic acid is an antifibrinolytic agent whose action has been attributed to the inhibition of plasmin synthesis from plasminogen.[130] Its primary action may be inhibition of activation of profibrinolysis.

Clinical Presentation

Toxic effects following therapeutic doses include nausea, vomiting, diarrhea, conjunctival hyperemia, delirium, impotence,[131] seizures,[132] dizziness, hypotension, and arrhythmias.[133] Use of EACA has been associated with thrombosis of the pulmonary artery,[134] renal artery,[135] and cerebral vasculature.[136] Bleeding has followed use of 36 to 48 g/d.[123] Renal[122] and hepatic[125] failure may follow high doses of EACA taken for long periods.

Myopathy[121,122,130] associated with weakness, fatigue, and elevated serum concentrations of creatine kinase and creatine phosphokinase, aldolase, and aspartate transaminase have followed EACA use. EACA has occasionally been associated with rhabdomyolysis, myoglobinuria, and renal failure.[122]

Laboratory
Analytical Methods

Blood EACA levels may be assayed by gas chromatography.[137,138]

Blood Levels

Plasma EACA concentrations greater than 130 mg/L but less than 300 mg/L are desirable.[138] Plasma EACA concentrations are not easily measured in health care facilities.

Abnormalities

Tests should include coagulation time, fibrinogen levels, and platelet counts.

Treatment
Stabilization

Patients receiving EACA should be hospitalized where monitoring of fibrinolytic activity and renal, hepatic and muscle function assays are available, and where a rapid response to thrombosis (renal, pulmonary, cerebral, cardiac) will be able to mitigate adverse clinical effects. Attention is immediately given to adequacy of the airway, breathing, and circulation with awareness of tidal volume, blood pressure, pulse, and respiratory rate. Intravenous lines, oxygen, and cardiac monitoring should be available.

Gut Decontamination

Gastric emptying may be useful within the first several hours of ingestion of an overdose of oral EACA. There have been no clinical studies on the use of syrup of ipecac, gastric lavage, cathartics, or whole-bowel irrigation in EACA overdose.

Elimination Enhancement

ϵ-Aminocaproic acid is not metabolized and is excreted largely unchanged in the urine. There are no systematic controlled studies on the use of hemodialysis or hemoperfusion in EACA overdosage.

Antidote

There is no antidote.

Supportive Measures

In symptomatic patients with significant EACA exposure, arterial blood gases, complete blood counts, urinalysis, liver and kidney function tests, bleeding times, and fibrinolytic function tests should be monitored. Serum creatine kinase, aldolase, and lactic acid dehydrogenase[124] determinations with urine myoglobin testing should be performed periodically. Hypotension is managed with intravenous fluids, Trendelenburg position and, if required, pressor amines (dopamine, norepinephrine). Seizures should respond to diazepam, phenytoin, and phenobarbital. If myopathies supervene and continuous fibrinolysis inhibition is required, consideration may be given to the use of tranexamic acid.[120]

ANCROD

Ancrod is a highly specific protease that has a thrombinlike effect on fibrinogen, resulting in an unstable fibrin clot which is readily dispersed and rapidly lysed.[139] Ancrod was first isolated in 1963 after incoagulable blood was observed in victims bitten by the Malayan pit viper (*Agkistrodon rhodostoma*) and is present in the venom of that snake.[140] It is immunologically distinct from heparin and does not cause immune thrombocytopenia. Ancrod is rarely associated with significant bleeding.[141]

Product Formulation

One ampule of the first International Reference Preparation (1976) contains 55 U in 16.90 mg with lactose and albumin.[142] It is available in Canada, Spain, and the United Kingdom as Arvin with 70 U/mL in ampules of 1 mL. Ancrod is derived from the Malayan pit viper.

Mechanism of Action

Ancrod induces rapid depletion of plasma fibrinogen by clearing the fibrinogen in a thrombinlike fashion. This leads to circulation of soluble non-crosslinked ancrod–fibrin, which appears to stimulate endogenous tissue plasminogen activator (t-PA) release from vessel walls.[143]

Laboratory

Ancrod in doses of 0.5 U/kg body weight administered in 250 mL normal saline over 6 to 24 hours or subcutaneously reduces the fibrinogen level, increases levels of fibrin degradation products, and decreases plasminogen. This occurs without evidence of bleeding. Ancrod is an investigational drug in the United States.

Therapeutic Dose

Ancrod is given in amounts sufficient to maintain plasma fibrinogen in the range 200 to 400 μg/mL. This is followed by a maintenance dose of 1 to 2 U/kg every 24 hours with the dose adjusted to maintain a fibrinogen level between 0.5 and 1.0 g/L. It is discontinued when concomitant warfarin has produced prolongation of the INR (see Laboratory) to 2 to 3 for 24 hours[144,145] (Table 27–8).

Clinical Presentation

There have been no reports to date of ancrod overdose. Treatment of bleeding usually requires symptomatic and supportive measures. Hematologic parameters should be obtained in all bleeding patients to rule out other causes of bleeding (see Hirudin).[146]

HIRUDIN

Leeches (*Hirudo medicinalis*) contain a substance with anticoagulant properties (hirudin).[147,148] Hirudin is a polypeptide comprising 65 amino acids and has a molecular weight of above 8000.

Mechanism of Action

Both the natural and recombinant hirudins are highly selective thrombin inhibitors. Venous thromboses and thromboses in the arterial and extracorporeal circulation (with 5–50 times higher doses) are completely inhibited in animal and some human studies.[147,149,150]

Toxicokinetics[151]

Time to peak plasma level	1 hour
Volume of distribution	0.20 L/kg
Elimination half-life	1 hour
Excreted unchanged	50%

Clinical Presentation

Hirudin given as a bolus of 0.6 mg/kg followed by 0.2 mg/kg/h is associated with a significant risk of major hemorrhage.[152]

Treatment

Overdose with hirudin can be expected to induce bleeding. In a bleeding patient a thrombin time, prothrombin time, activated partial thromboplastin time, complete blood count including platelet count, peripheral smear for review, and bleeding time should be obtained. Hirudin bleeding responds to prothrombin complex concentrate.[153]

Table 27–8
Characteristics of Thrombolytic Agents

	Streptokinase	Urokinase	Alteplase	Anistreplase	Saruplase	BM-06022
Source	Group C streptococci	Recombinant, human fetal kidney	Recombinant, human	Group C streptococci plasminogen, anisoylated	Recombinant, human	Recombinant, human mutant
Molecular weight	47,000	35,000–55,000	63,000–70,000	131,000	47,000	39,000
Fibrin specificity	No	No	Yes	No	Yes	Yes
Metabolism	Hepatic	Hepatic	Hepatic	Hepatic		Renal
Half-life (min)	18–23	14–20	3–4	70–120	6–8	14
Mode of action	Activator complex	Direct	Direct	Direct	Direct	Direct
Antigenicity	Yes	No	No	Yes	No	No
Blood viscosity	Decreased	Unknown	No change	Decreased	Unknown	Unknown
Estimated hospital cost per dose ($US)	$300/1.5 mU	$2000/3 mU	$2200/100 mg	$1800/30 U	Not determined	Not determined

From Granger CB, Califf RM, Topol EJ. Thrombolytic therapy for acute myocardial infarction: A review. Drugs 1992;44:293–325. Erratum. 1993;45:894.

TRANEXAMIC ACID

Tranexamic acid (*trans*-4-(aminomethyl)-cyclohexane carboxylic acid, AMCA),[154] a synthetic lysine analog,[155] is an antifibrinolytic agent[156] that inhibits fibrinolysis similar to EACA by saturating the lysine binding sites at which plasminogen and plasmin bind to fibrinogen and fibrin. It is available in the United States and in many parts of the world as Cyklokapron.[157] Tranexamic acid may decrease the need for transfusions and factor replacement in hemophiliacs having dental extractions.[155] Tranexamic acid has been used intravenously and orally in doses of 3 to 6 g/d[158] to reduce problems with upper gastrointestinal hemorrhage, although doses of 4 to 16 g daily have been used.[159] It may also serve to reduce blood product usage due to blood loss following fibrinolysis during orthoptic liver transplantation.[160]

Toxicokinetics

Bioavailability	30–40%
Peak plasma level	7 μg/mL
Time to peak plasma level	2 hours
Elimination half-life	2 hours
Excreted unchanged	100%

Tranexamic acid passes through the placenta.[161]

Clinical Presentation

Nausea, vomiting, diarrhea, reversible acute renal failure, disturbances of color vision, central venous stasis retinopathy, subarachnoid hemorrhage, and massive pulmonary thromboembolism have been observed.[162]

Laboratory

Analysis of tranexamic acid is made by electron-capture gas chromatography.[163]

Treatment

Treatment of overdose is supportive and symptomatic (see ϵ-Aminocaproic Acid).

REFERENCES—ANTICOAGULANTS AND ANTIFIBRINOLYTIC AGENTS

1. O'Reilly RA. Anticoagulant, antithrombotic and thrombolytic drugs. In: Gilman AG, Goodman LS, Rall TW, Murad F, eds. *The Pharmacological Basis of Therapeutics.* 7th ed. New York: Macmillan, 1985:1338–1357.
2. Giddings JC, Evans BK. Drugs affecting blood coagulation and hemostasis. Int Anesthesiol Clin 1985;23(2):103–123.
3. Katz J, Metz J. Hemorrhages in a young boy due to unsuspected diphenadione (Didandin) intoxication. Clin Pediatr 1969;8:291–293.
4. Seiler K, Duckert F. Intoxication with phenprocoumon (Marcoumar): Pharmacokinetics and side effects. Thromb Diath Haemorrh 1969;21:320–324.
5. De Wolff FA, van Kempen GMJ. Three cases of phenprocoumon (Marcoumar®) intoxication. Proc Eur Soc Toxicol 1977;18:189–191.
6. Hvidzala EV, Gellady AM. Intentional poisoning of two siblings by prescription drugs. Clin Pediatr 1978;17:480–482.
7. Toolis F, Robson RH, Critchley JAJH. Warfarin poisoning in patients with prosthetic heart valves. Br Med J 1981;283:581–582.
8. Saunderson H, Fernandez L. Confusion between warfarin and propranolol leading to warfarin overdosage. Can Med Assoc 1981;124:366.
9. Renowden S, Westmoreland D, White JP, et al. Oral cholestyramine increases elimination of warfarin after overdose. Br Med J 1985;291:513–514.
10. Hackett LP, Ilett KF, Chester A. Plasma warfarin concentrations after a massive overdose. Med J Aust 1985;142:642–643.
11. Olchovsky D, Pines A, Zwas ST, et al. Apathetic thyrotoxicosis due to hemorrhage into a hyperfunctioning thyroid nodule after excessive anticoagulation. South Med J 1985;78:609–611.
12. Holmes RW, Love J. Suicide attempt with warfarin, a bishydroxycoumarin like rodenticide. JAMA 1952;148:935–937.
13. Fristedt B, Sterner N. Warfarin intoxication from percutaneous absorption. Arch Environ Health 1965;11:205–208.
14. Barlow AM, Gay AL, Park BK. Difenacoum (Neosorexa) poisoning. Br Med J 1982;285:541.
15. Murdoch DA. Prolonged anticoagulation in chlorphacinone poisoning. Lancet 1983;1:355–356.
16. Lipton RA, Klass EM. Human ingestion of a 'superwarfarin' rodenticide resulting in a prolonged anticoagulant effect. JAMA 1984;252:3004–3005.
17. Jones EC, Growe GH, Naiman SC. Prolonged anticoagulation in rat poisoning. JAMA 1984;252:3005.
18. Pachman DJ. Accidental heparin poisoning in an infant. Am J Dis Child 1965;110:210–212.
19. Schreiner RL, Wynn RJ, McNulty C. Accidental heparin toxicity in the newborn intensive care unit. J Pediatr 1978;92:115.
20. Kwaan HC, Simon NM, del Greco F. Hemorrhagic diathesis induced by surreptitious ingestion of coumarin drugs. Med Clin North Am 1972;56:263–273.
21. Moster KM, Hajjar GL. Effect of heparin on the one-stage prothrombin time. Ann Intern Med 1967;66:1207–1213.
22. Morgan DP. *Recognition and Management of Pesticide Poisonings.* 3rd ed. EPA-540/9-80-005. Washington, DC: USEPA, 1982.
23. Mandel HG, Cohn VH. Fat soluble vitamins: Vitamin A, K_1 and E. In: Gilman AG, Goodman LS, Rall TW, Murad F, eds. *The Pharmacological Basis of Therapeutics.* 7th ed. New York: Macmillan, 1985:1582–1586.
24. Hart RG, Coull BM. Hypercoagulability following coumadin withdrawal. Am Heart J 1983;106:169–170.
25. McLean J. The thromboplastin action of heparin. Am J Physiol 1916;41:250–257.
26. Purandare SV, Parulkar GB, Panday SR, et al. Heparin rebound: A cause of bleeding following open heart surgery. J Postgrad Med 1979;25(2):70–74.
27. Katona B, Sigell LT, Wason S. Anticoagulant rodenticide poisoning. Vet Hum Toxicol 1986;28:478. Abstract.
28. Katona B, Wason S. Anticoagulant rodenticide. Clin Toxicol Rev 1986;8(12):1–2.
29. Chen TW, Deng JF. A brodifacoum intoxication case of mouthful amount. Vet Hum Toxicol 1986;28:488. Abstract.
30. Heparin and other anticoagulants. In: Reynolds JEF, ed. *Martindale: The Extra Pharmacopoeia.* 30th ed. London: Pharmaceutical Press, 1993:225–242.
31. Serlin MJ, Breckenridge AM. Drug interactions with warfarin. Drugs 1983;25:610–620.
32. Koch-Wesser J, Sellers EM. Drug interactions with coumarin anticoagulants. N Engl J Med 1971;285:487–498, 547–558.
33. Abell TL, Merigian KS, Lee JM, et al. Cutaneous exposure to warfarin-like anticoagulant causing an intracerebral hemorrhage: A case report. Clin Toxicol 1994;34:69–73.
34. Yacobi A, Udall JA, Levy G. Serum protein binding as a determinant of warfarin body clearance and anticoagulant effect. Clin Pharmacol Ther 1976;19:552–558.
35. Meinertz T, Gilfrich H-J, Groth U, et al. Interruption of the enterohepatic circulation of phenprocoumon by cholestyramine. Clin Pharmacol Ther 1977;21:731–735.

36. Jahnchen E, Meinertz T, Gilfrich H-J, et al. Enhanced elimination of warfarin during treatment with cholestyramine. Br J Clin Pharmacol 1978;5:437–440.
37. Lewis RJ, Trager WF. Warfarin metabolism in man: Identification of metabolites in urine. J Clin Invest 1970;49:907–913.
38. Yacobi A, Levy G. Pharmacokinetics of the warfarin enantiomers in rats. J Pharmacokinet Biopharm 1974;2:239–255.
39. Solomon HM, Schrogie JJ, Williams D. The displacement of phenylbutazone-^{14}C and warfarin-^{14}C from human albumin by various drugs and fatty acids. Biochem Pharmacol 1968;17:143–151.
40. Standing Advisory Committee for Haematology of the Royal College of Pathologists. Drug interaction with coumarin derivative anticoagulants. Br Med J 1982;285:274–275.
41. Robinson DS, Benjamin DM, McCormack JJ: Interaction of warfarin and non-systemic gastrointestinal drugs. Clin Pharmacol Ther 1971;12:491–495.
42. Bailie M, Allen ED, Elkington AR. The congenital warfarin syndrome: A case report. Br J Ophthalmol 1980;64:633–635.
43. Disaia PJ. Pregnancy and delivery of a patient with a Starr-Edwards mitral valve prosthesis. Obstet Gynecol 1966;28:469–472.
44. Ginsberg JS, Hirsh J, Turner DC, et al. Risks to the fetus of anticoagulant therapy during pregnancy. Thromb Haemost 1989;61:197–203.
45. Quenneville G, Barton B, McDevitt E, et al. The use of anticoagulants for thrombo-phlebitis during pregnancy. Am J Obstet Gynecol 1959;77:1135–1149.
46. Villasanta U. Thromboembolic disease in pregnancy. Am J Obstet Gynecol 1965;93:142–160.
47. Kazmier FJ. Thromboembolism, coumarin necrosis and protein C. Mayo Clin Proc 1985;60:673–674.
48. Menon IS. Side effects of phenindione. Br Med J 1968;2:622.
49. Sternberg ML, Pettyjohn FS. Warfarin sodium-induced skin necrosis. Ann Emerg Med 1995;26:94–97.
50. Sheth SB, Carvalho AC. Protein S and C alterations in acutely ill patients. Am J Hematol 1991;36:14–19.
51. Rick ME. Protein C and protein S. Vitamin K-dependent inhibitors of blood coagulation. JAMA 1990;263:701–703.
52. Israels SJ, Seshia SS. Childhood stroke associated with protein C or S deficiency. J Pediatr 1987;111:562–563.
53. Lewandowski K, Zawilsky K. Protein C concentrate in the treatment of warfarin-induced necrosis in the protein C deficiency. Thromb Haemost 1994;71:395–399.
54. O'Reilly RA, Aggeler PM. Surreptitious ingestion of coumarin anticoagulant drugs. Ann Intern Med 1966;64:1034–1041.
55. O'Reilly RA, Aggeler PM. Covert anticoagulant ingestion: Study of 25 patients and review of world literature. Medicine 1976;55:389–399.
56. Smolinske SC, Scherger DL, Kearns PS, et al. Superwarfarin poisoning in children: A prospective study. Pediatrics 1989;84:490–494.
57. Kruse JA, Carlson RW. Fatal rodenticide poisoning with brodifacoum. Ann Emerg Med 1992;21:331–336.
58. Felice LJ, Chalermchaikit T, Murphy MJ. Multicomponent determination of 4-hydroxycoumarin anticoagulant rodenticides in blood serum by liquid chromatography with fluorescence detection. J Anal Toxicol 1991;15:126–129.
59. Poller L. The effect of low-dose warfarin on the risk of stroke in patients with nonrheumatic atrial fibrillation. N Engl J Med 1991;325:129–130.
60. Warfarin. Poisindex. Englewood, Colo, Micromedex, Inc. Reviewed by Rumack BH (02/82, 12/84), Troutman WG (01/85). Revised by Flomenbaum N (10/84), Smolinske SC (01/85).
61. Morrissey B, Burgess JL, Robertson WO. Washington's experience and recommendations. Re: Anticoagulant rodenticides. Vet Hum Toxicol 1995;37:362–363.
62. Consensus Conference: Fresh-frozen plasma indications and risks. JAMA 1985;253:551–553.
63. Meinertz T, Kaspar W, Kahl C, Ahnrchen E. Anticoagulant activity of the enantiomers of acenocoumarol. Br J Clin Pharmacol 1978;5:187–188.
64. Bjornsson TD, Blaschke TF. Vitamin K_1 disposition and therapy of warfarin overdose. Lancet 1978;2:846–847.
65. De la Rubia J, Grau E, Montserrat I, et al. Anaphylactic shock and vitamin K_1. Ann Intern Med 1989;110:943.
66. Hirsh J, Poller L. Subcutaneous or intravenous phytonadione? Arch Intern Med 1995;135:1337.
67. Finkel MJ: Vitamin K_1 and vitamin K analogues. Clin Pharmacol Ther 1961;2:794–814.
68. Centers for Disease Control. Non-A, non-B hepatitis associated with a factor IX complex infused during cardiovascular surgery—Arizona. MMWR 1986;35(24):391–399.
69. Jason J, Holman RC, Dixon G, et al. Effects of exposure to factor concentrates containing donations from identified AIDS patients. JAMA 1986;256:1758–1762.
70. Safer factor VII and IX. Lancet 1986;2:255–256. Editorial.
71. Taberner DA, Thomson JM, Poller L. Comparison of prothrombin complex concentrate and vitamin K_1 in oral anticoagulant reversal. Br Med J 1976;2:83–85.
72. Glover JJ, Morrill GB. Conservative treatment of overanticoagulated patients. Chest 1995;108:987–990.
73. Ikeda M, Conney AH, Burns JJ. Stimulatory effect of phenobarbital and insecticides on warfarin metabolism in the rat. J Pharmacol Exp Ther 1968;162:338–343.
74. Becker RC, Ansell J. Antithrombotic therapy: An abbreviated reference for clinicians. Arch Intern Med 1995;155:149–161.
75. Martin CM, Engstrom PF, Barrett O Jr. Surreptitious self-administration of heparin. JAMA 1970;212:475–476.
76. Olin JW, de Wolfe VG. Paradoxical thromboembolism associated with heparin therapy. Cleve Clin Q 1981;48:378–384.
77. Weisman RE, Tobin RW. Arterial embolism occurring during systemic heparin therapy. Arch Surg 1958;76:219–227.
78. Rice L, Jackson D. Can heparin cause clotting? Heart Lung 1981;10:331–335.
79. Cipolle RJ, Rodvold KA, Seifert R, et al. Heparin associated thrombocytopenia: A prospective evaluation of 211 patients. Ther Drug Monit 1983;5:205–211.
80. Herring WB, Shelburne PF. Heparin induced thrombosis. NC Med J 1984;45:159–162.
81. Smith JP, Walls JT, Muscato MS, et al. Extracorporeal circulation in a patient with heparin induced thrombocytopenia. Anesthesiology 1985;62:363–365.
82. Ansell J, Deykin D. Heparin induced thrombocytopenia and recurrent thromboembolism. Am J Hematol 1980;8:325–332.
83. Kakkaseril JS, Cranley JJ, Panke T, et al. Heparin induced thrombocytopenia: A prospective study of 142 patients. J Vasc Surg 1985;2:382–384.
84. Arthur CK, Isbister JP, Aspery EM. The heparin induced thrombosis–thrombocytopenia syndrome (H.I.T.T.S.): A review. Pathology 1985;17:82–86.
85. Coagulants and anticoagulants. In: McEvoy GK, ed. *AHFS Drug Information 94*. Bethesda, MD: American Society of Hospital Pharmacists, 1994:874–888.
86. Jaques LB. Heparin: A unique misunderstood drug. Trends Pharmacol Sci 1982;56:263–273.
87. Bennett WM, Mutner RS, Parker RA, et al. Drug therapy in renal failure: Dosing guidelines for adults. Ann Intern Med 1980;93:286–325.
88. Ordog GJ, Wasserberger J, Balasubramaniam S. Effect of heparin on arterial blood gases. Ann Emerg Med 1985;14:233–238.
89. Stevenson RE, Burton AM, Ferlauto GJ, et al. Hazards of oral anticoagulants during pregnancy. JAMA 1980;243:1549–1551.
90. Pauli RM, Hall JG, Wilson KM. Risks of anticoagulation during pregnancy. Am Heart J 1980;100:761–762.
91. Merrill LK, VerBurg DJ. The choice of long-term anticoagulants for the pregnant patient. Obstet Gynecol 1976;47:711–717.
92. Dahlman TC, Sjoberg KE, Ringertz H. Bone mineral density during long-term prophylaxis with heparin in pregnancy. Am J Obstet Gynecol 1994;170:1315–1320.
93. Chaplin S, Sanders GL, Smith JM. Drug excretion in human breast milk. Adverse Drug React Acute Poison Rev 1982;1:255–287.
94. Hirsh J. Heparin. N Engl J Med 1991;324:1565–1574.
95. Walker AM, Jick H. Predictors of bleeding during heparin therapy. JAMA 1980;244:1209–1212.

96. Oster JR, Singer I, Fishman LM. Heparin-induced aldosterone suppression and hyperkalemia. Am J Med 1995;98: 575–586.
97. Hougardy N, Machiels J-P, Ravo ETC. Heparin-induced thrombocytopenia. N Engl J Med 1995;333:1007.
98. Mehta DP, Yoder EL, Appel J, Bergsman KL. Heparin-induced thrombocytopenia and thrombosis: Reversal with streptokinase: A case report and review of literature. Am J Hematol 1991;36:275–279.
99. Dieck JA, Rizo-Patron C, Unisa A, et al. A new manifestation and treatment alternative for heparin-induced thromboses. Chest 1990;98:1524–1526.
100. Frame JM, Mulvey KP, Phares JC, Anderson MJ. Correction of severe heparin-associated thrombocytopenia with intravenous immunoglobulin. Ann Intern Med 1989;111:946–947.
101. Laster JL, Nichols WK, Silver D. Thrombocytopenia associated with heparin-coated catheters in patients with heparin-associated antiplatelet antibodies. Arch Intern Med 1989;149:2285–2287.
102. Chamberlin JR, Lewis B, Leya F, et al. Successful treatment of heparin-associated thrombocytopenia and thrombosis using Hirulog. Can J Cardiol 1995;11:515–517.
103. Verstraete M. Pharmacotherapeutic aspects of unfractionated and low molecular weight heparins. Drugs 1990;40: 498–530.
104. Levesque H, Verdier S, Cailleux N, et al. Low molecular weight heparins and hypoaldosteronism. Br Med J 1990;300: 1437–1438.
105. Eichinger S, Kyrle PA, Brenner B, et al. Thrombocytopenia associated with low-molecular-weight heparin. Lancet 1991; 337:1425–1426.
106. Passannante A, Macik BG. The heparin flush syndrome: A cause of iatrogenic hemorrhage. Am J Med Sci 1988;296:71–73. Case report.
107. Williams PE, Dawes J, Dearden NM, et al. Coagulation disorder due to apparent inadvertent heparin administration. Clin Lab Haematol 1989;11:101–104.
108. Slivka A, Levy DE, Lapinski RH. Risk associated with heparin withdrawal in ischaemic cerebrovascular disease. J Neurol Neurosurg Psychiatry 1989;52:1332–1336.
109. Schmidt B, Mitchell L, Ofosu F, Andrew M. Standard assays underestimate the concentration of heparin in neonatal plasma. J Lab Clin Med 1988;112:641–643.
110. Maner JR. Pharmacological aspects of renal failure and dialysis. In: Drukker W, Parsons FM, Maher JF, eds. *Replacement of Renal Function by Dialysis.* 2nd ed. Boston: Martinus Nijhoff, 1983:781.
111. Kuitunen AH, Salmenpera MT, Heinonen J, et al. Heparin rebound: A comparative study of protamine chloride and protamine sulfate in patients undergoing coronary artery bypass surgery. J Cardiothorac Vasc Anesth 1991;5:221–226.
112. Verstraete M. Clinical application of inhibitors of fibrinolysis. Drugs 1985;29:236–261.
113. Bidstrup BP, Royston P, Sapsford RN, et al. Reduction in blood loss and blood use after cardiopulmonary bypass with high dose aprotinin (Trasylol). J Thorac Cardiovasc Surg 1989;97:364–372.
114. Van Coveren W, Jansen NJG, Bidstrup BP, et al. Effects of aprotinin on hemostatic mechanisms during cardiopulmonary bypass. Ann Thorac Surg 1987;44:640–645.
115. Bidstrup B. Aprotinin for bleeding after cardiopulmonary bypass. Lancet 1990;335:1535–1536.
116. Mallet SV, Cos E, Burroughs AK, Rolles K. Aprotinin and reduction of blood loss and transfusion requirements in orthotopic liver transplantation. Lancet 1990;336:886–887.
117. Saffitz JE, Strohl DJ, Sundt TM, et al. Disseminated intravascular coagulation after administration of aprotinin in combination with deep hypothermic circulatory arrest. Am J Cardiol 1993;22:1080–1082.
118. Bohrer H, Bach A, Fleischer F, Lang J. Adverse haemodynamic effects of high dose aprotinin in a pediatric cardiac surgical patient. Anaesthesia 1990;45:853–854.
119. Withrich B, Schmid P, Schmid ER, et al. IgE-mediated anaphylactic reaction to aprotinin during anaesthesia. Lancet 1992;340:173–174.
120. Kane MJ, Silverman LR, Rand JH, et al. Myonecrosis as a complication of the use of epsilon aminocaproic acid: A case report and review of the literature. Am J Med 1988;85:861–863.
121. Randall J, Taylor K. Epsilon-aminocaproic acid myopathy. Aust NZ J Med 1990;20:851.
122. Biswas CK, Milligan DAR, Agte SD, et al. Acute renal failure and myopathy after treatment with aminocaproic acid. Br Med J 1980;2:115–116.
123. Glick R, Green D, Ts'ao C-h, et al. High dose ϵ-aminocaproic acid prolongs the bleeding time and increases rebleeding and intraoperative hemorrhage in patients with subarachnoid hemorrhage. Neurosurgery 1981;9:398–401.
124. Steffen RO. Lederle Laboratories. Personal communication. March 21, 1991.
125. McEvoy GK, ed. *AHFS Drug Information 94.* Bethesda, MD: American Society of Hospital Pharmacists, 1994:890–892.
126. Wysenbeak AJ, Sella A, Vardi M, Yeshurun D. Acute delirious state after ϵ-aminocaproic acid. Lancet 1978;1:221.
127. Burchiel KJ, Schmer G. A method for monitoring antifibrinolytic therapy in patients with ruptured intracranial aneurysms. J Neurosurg 1981;54:12–15.
128. Frederiksen MC, Bowsher DJ, Ruo TI, et al. Kinetics of epsilon-aminocaproic acid distribution, elimination, and antifibrinolytic effects in normal subjects. Clin Pharmacol Ther 1984;35:387–393.
129. Pagliano LA, Benet LZ. Critical compilation of terminal half-lives, percent excreted unchanged and changes of half-life in renal and hepatic dysfunction for studies in humans with references. J Pharmacokinet Biopharm 1975;3:333–383.
130. Vanneste JAL, van Wijngaarden GK. Epsilon-aminocaproic acid myopathy. Eur Neurol 1982;21:242–248.
131. Evans BE, Aledort LM. Inhibition of ejaculation due to epsilon-aminocaproic acid. N Engl J Med 1978;298:166–167.
132. Rabinovici R, Heyman A, Kluger Y, Shinar E. Convulsions induced by aminocaproic acid infusion. DICP Ann Pharmacother 1989;23:780–781.
133. Quandt CM, De Los Reyes RA, Diaz FG, Ausman JI. Pharmacologic management of subarachnoid hemorrhage. Drug Intell Clin Pharm 1982;16:909–915.
134. Johansson S-A. Acute right heart failure during treatment with epsilon-aminocaproic acid (E-ACA). Acta Med Scand 1967;182:331–334.
135. Tubbs RR, Benjamin SP, Dohn DE. Recurrent subarachnoid hemorrhage associated with aminocaproic acid therapy and acute renal artery thrombosis. J Neurosurg 1979;51:94–97. Case report.
136. Hoffman ER, Koo AH. Cerebral thrombosis associated with Amicar[R] therapy. Radiology 1979;131:687–689.
137. Keucher TR, Solow EB, Metaxas J, Campbell RL. Gas chromatographic determination of an antifibrinolytic drug, ϵ-aminocaproic acid. Clin Chem 1976;22:806–809.
138. Haug MT, Mauro VF, Davis HH. Effect of renal failure and hemodialysis on aminocaproic acid plasma concentrations. DICP Ann Pharmacother 1989;23:922–923.
139. Becker GJ. Ancrod in glomerulonephritis. Q J Med 1988;69: 849–850.
140. Reid HA, Thean PC, Chan KE, Baharam AR. Clinical effects of bites by Malayan viper (*Agkistrodon rhodostoma*). Lancet 1963;1:617–621.
141. Kim S, Wadhwa NK, Kant KS, et al. Fibrinolysis in glomerulonephritis treated with ancrod: Renal, functional, immunologic and histopathologic effects. Q J Med 1988;69:879–895, 896–905.
142. Reynolds JEF, ed. *Martindale: The Extra Pharmacopoeia.* 30th ed. London: Pharmaceutical Press, 1993:225.
143. Pollak VE, Glas-Greenwalt P, Olinger CP, et al: Ancrod causes rapid thrombolysis in patients with acute stroke. Am J Med Sci 1990;299:319–325.
144. Derners C, Ginsberg JS, Brill-Edwards P, et al. Rapid anticoagulation using ancrod for heparin-induced thrombocytopenia. Blood 1991;28:2194–2197.

145. Hirsh J, Dalen JE, Deykin D, Poller L. Heparin: Mechanism of action, pharmacokinetics, dosing considerations, monitoring, efficacy and safety. Chest 1992;102 (suppl.):337S–351S.
146. Wallerstein RO Jr. Laboratory evaluation of a bleeding patient. West J Med 1989;150:51–58.
147. Meyer BH, Luus HG, Muller FO, et al. The pharmacology of recombinant hirudin, a new anticoagulant. South Afr Med J 1990;78:268–270.
148. Markwardt F. Pharmacology of hirudin: One hundred years after the first report of the anticoagulant agent in medicinal leeches. Biomed Biochim Acta 1985;44:1007–1013.
149. Wallis RB. Hirudins and the role of thrombin: Lessons from leeches. Trends Pharm Sci 1988;9:425–427.
150. Bittl JA, Strony J, Brinker JA, et al. Treatment with bivalirudin (Hirulog) as compared with heparin during coronary angioplasty for unstable or postinfarction angina. N Engl J Med 1995;333:764–769.
151. Meyer BH, Muller FO, Luus HG. The clinical pharmacology of anticoagulant DNA-hirudin. Clin Pharmacol Ther 1991;49:189.
152. Conrad KA. Clinical pharmacology and drug safety: Lessons from hirudin. Clin Pharmacol Ther 1995;58:123–126.
153. Irani MS, White HJ Jr, Sexon RG. Reversal of hirudin-induced bleeding diathesis by prothrombin complex concentrate. Am J Cardiol 1995;75:422–423.
154. Reynolds JEF, ed. *Martindale: The Extra Pharmacopoeia.* 30th ed. London: Pharmaceutical Press, 1993:924–925.
155. Tranexamic acid. Med Lett Drugs Ther 1987;29(749):89–90.
156. Arrisati G, TenCate JW, Buller HR, Mandelli F. Tranexamic acid for control of hemorrhage in acute promyelocytic leukemia. Lancet 1989;2:122–124.
157. Reynolds JEF. *Martindale: The Extra Pharmacopoeia.* 30th ed. London: Pharmaceutical Press, 1993:338.
158. Henry DA, O'Connell DL. Effects of fibrinolytic inhibitors on mortality from upper gastrointestinal hemorrhage. Br Med J 1989;298:1142–1146.
159. Ramirez-Lassepas M. Antifibrinolytic therapy in subarachnoid hemorrhage caused by ruptured intracranial aneurysm. Neurology 1984;31:316–322.
160. Boylan JF, Sandler AN, Sheiner P, et al. Reduced blood product usage with tranexamic acid prophylaxis in primary liver transplantation. Anesthesiology 1992;7:A1092.
161. Kullander S, Nilsson IM. Human placental transfer of an antifibrinolytic agent (AMCA). Acta Obstet Gynecol Scand 1970;49:241–242.
162. Woo KS, Tse LKK, Woo JLF, Vallance-Owen J. Massive pulmonary thromboembolism after tranexamic acid antifibrinolytic therapy. Br J Clin Pract 1989;43:465–466. (Also, Ann Emerg Med 1989;18:116–117.)
163. Vessman J, Stromberg S. Determination of tranexamic acid in biological material by electron capture gas chromatography after direct derivatization in an aqueous medium. Anal Chem 1977;49:369–373.

THROMBOLYTIC AGENTS

Overdose with thrombolytic agents can be associated with severe hemorrhage, which may be fatal. Bleeding may especially occur at puncture sites. Treatment involves the use of antifibrinolytics, cryoprecipitates, fresh-frozen plasma, whole blood, or platelets.

Four thrombolytic agents are in clinical use in the United States[1]: streptokinase (SK), urokinase (UK), alteplase or recombinant tissue plasminogen activator (r-TPA), and anistreplase (APSAC) (Table 27–8).

Structure and Classification

Table 27–8 summarizes the characteristics of thrombolytic agents.

Therapeutic Dose

The therapeutic dose of alteplase is 100 mg as a 10-mg intravenous bolus followed by continuous infusion over 3 hours.[2]

Toxicokinetics (Alteplase)[2,3]

Peak plasma level	1000–4000 ng/mL
Volume of distribution	0.07 L/kg
Elimination half-life	5–10 minutes

Pregnancy/Lactation

Few controlled studies on use in pregnancy and lactation have been performed with thrombolytic agents.

Mechanism of Action

Thrombolytic agents activate the proteolytic enzyme plasminogen. Once plasminogen is activated, fibrin dissolution follows[4] (Fig. 27–4).

Clinical Presentation

Bleeding is the most common adverse event of thrombolytic therapy[4–7] (Table 27–9). The risk of bleeding is high in patients in whom invasive procedures are performed or who are given heparin concurrently or subsequently. Strokes and intracerebral bleeding have occurred.[8] Major bleeds require transfusion. Minor bleeds include gross hematuria, hematemesis, hematomas, and oozing from intravenous access.[9] Fatal hemorrhages range from 0 to 4%. A fall in fibrinogen levels to less than 100 mg/mL during or after thrombolytic therapy has been associated with an increased risk of bleeding.[10] Hypersensitivity responses follow streptokinase use and anistreplase infusion in 1 to 8 patients.[4,11] Hypotension follows use of all thrombolytic agents in 10 to 20% of patients following either rapid infusion or high-dose infusion. Other symptoms include serum sickness, headaches, backaches, renal dysfunction,[12] reversible hepatic dysfunction, nausea, vomiting, and fever. Streptokinase has been associated with the Guillain–Barré syndrome[8] and, rarely, with hemolysis.[13]

Laboratory

Alteplase has been assayed in human plasma using spectrophotometry, enzyme-linked immunosorbent assay, antibody radioimmunoassay, and an enzyme immunoassay.[2]

Treatment

Bleeding

1. Discontinue the lytic agent and other anticoagulants. If bleeding occurs within 4 hours of heparin administration, consider the use of protamine sulfate.[4]
2. Replace volume as required.
3. Apply normal pressure for 15 to 30 minutes to compressible bleeding sites.
4. If bleeding continues, administer transfusion products. Cryoprecipitate 10 U may be given. Fibrinogen levels guide further doses.

Table 27–9
Risk Factors for Bleeding With Thrombolytic Regimens

Risk Category	Peripheral or Systemic Bleeding	Intracranial Bleeding
Major (thrombolytic therapy contraindicated)	Major surgery or organ biopsy within 6 wk Major trauma within 6 wk Gastrointestinal or genitourinary bleeding within 6 mo History of a bleeding diathesis Known or suspected aortic dissection Known or suspected pericarditis	Known intracranial tumor Previous neurosurgery Stroke within 6 mo Head trauma within 1 mo
Important (a relative contraindication to thrombolysis)	Puncture of a noncompressible vessel Cardiopulmonary resuscitation for >10 min	Acute severe hypertension Remote thrombotic stroke Recent transient ischemic attacks
Minor (increased risk of bleeding, but no definite contraindication to thrombolysis)	Diabetic retinopathy Cardiopulmonary resuscitation for <10 min Older age Female sex Small body size	Older age History of hypertension Small body size Female sex

From Anderson HV, Willerson JT. Thrombolysis in acute myocardial infarction. N Engl J Med 1993;329:703–709.

5. Transfusion is usually not required if the level of fibrinogen is 100 mg/dL or more.
6. If the patient continues to bleed or has fibrinogen levels greater than 100 mg/dL, 2 to 6 U of fresh-frozen plasma may be necessary.
7. If bleeding continues after cryoprecipitate and fresh-frozen plasma are administered obtain a bleeding time to assess platelet function. If the bleeding time is longer than 7 minutes, 10 U of platelets and antifibrinolytic drugs are recommended. If the bleeding time is under 9 minutes, only antifibrinolytic agents are required. ϵ-Aminocaproic acid and tranexamic acid are available antifibrinolytic agents.[14]

Hypotension

Discontinue the infusion. Reinstitute at a slower rate.

REFERENCES—THROMBOLYTIC AGENTS

1. Fears R. Biochemical pharmacology and therapeutic aspects of thrombolytic agents. Pharmacol Rev 1990;42: 201–222.
2. Ziller FP, Spinler SA. Alteplase: A tissue plasminogen activator for acute myocardial infarction. Drug Intell Clin Pharm 1988;22:6–14.
3. Verstraete M. The pharmacokinetics of anisoylated plasminogen streptokinase activation complex, tissue-type plasminogen activator, and simple-chain urokinase-type plasminogen activator. In: Julian DG, Kubler W, Norris RM, et al., eds. *Thrombolysis in Cardiovascular Disease.* New York: Marcel Dekker, 1989:69–86.
4. Nazar J, Davison R, Kaplan K, Fintel D. Adverse reactions to thrombolytic agents: Implications for coronary reperfusion following myocardial infarction. Med Toxicol 1987;2:274–286.
5. Guidry JR, Raschke RA, Mortunas AE. Anticoagulants and thrombolytics. Crit Care Clin 1991;7:533–554.
6. Sane DC, Califf RM, Topol EJ, et al. Bleeding during thrombolytic therapy for acute myocardial infarction: Mechanisms and management. Ann Intern Med 1989;111:1010–1022.
7. Verstraete M, Vaughan DE. Latest update in thrombolysis. In: Julian DG, Kubler W, Norris RM, et al., ed. *Thrombolysis in Cardiovascular Disease.* New York: Marcel Dekker, 1989: 409–431.
8. Califf RM, Topol EJ, George BS, et al. Hemorrhagic complications associated with use of intravenous tissue plasminogen activator in treatment of acute myocardial infarction. Am J Med 1988;85:353–359.
9. Cairns JA, Collins R, Fuster V. Coronary thrombolysis. Chest 1989;95:235.
10. Fletcher AP, Alkjaersig NR. The hematologic consequences of thrombolytic therapy. Proc Hematol 1986;14:183–200.
11. Tisdale JE, Stringer KA, Antalek M, Matthews GE. Streptokinase-induced anaphylaxis. DICP Ann Pharmacother 1989;23:984–987.
12. Kalra PA, Coady AM, Iqbal A, et al. Acute tubular neurosis induced by coronary thrombolytic therapy. Postgrad Med 1991;67:212.
13. Mathiesen O, Grunner N. Haemolysis after intravenous streptokinase. Lancet 1989;1:1016–1017.
14. Tissue-type plasminogen activator for acute coronary thrombosis. Med Lett Drugs Ther 1987;29(754):107–109.

Chapter 28
Blood and Blood-forming Drugs

CITRATE

Whole Blood Storage

Whole blood is treated with a citrate solution to prevent coagulation and to preserve the blood. Citrate–phosphate–dextrose (CPD) has been approved by the U.S. Food and Drug Administration for blood storage up to 21 days when the blood is maintained between 1° and 6°C. Citrate–phosphate–dextrose–adenine (CPD-1) permits storage up to 35 days at that temperature. Citrate retards glycolysis and prevents coagulation by binding ionized calcium.[1]

Use

Sodium citrate and citric acid are used when collecting blood to chelate calcium which prevents blood clotting.[2] Rapid infusion of blood or plasma can lead to a fall in ionized calcium.

Therapeutic Dose

Citric acid is a normal constituent of blood plasma (normal concentration, 0.8 mg/dL). A 1 mg/kg/min citric acid infusion produces an elevation of plasma citric acid of 8 mg/100 dL.[3]

Massive Transfusion

The term *massive transfusion* is usually described as the use of 10 U or more of whole blood or packed red cells in a 24-hour period.[4] The definition can also be expanded to include the transfusion of more than one blood volume in 24 hours.[5,6]

Citrate intoxication can occur in patients receiving blood at a rate greater than 1 U in 5 to 10 minutes.[7,8] This amount may be greater than that required to bind ionized calcium, resulting in hypocalcemia.[1] This effect is of special concern in hypothermic patients who may have serum citrate concentrations 40 to 140 times normal after large-volume transfusion.[1] In general, when blood is being transfused at a rate less than 30 mL/kg/h, that is, less than 8 U/h, compensating mechanisms ensure that ionized calcium concentration remains within normal limits.[5]

An inadvertent injection of 400 mL of citrate–phosphate–dextrose administered in a 50-minute interval led to cardiac arrest with electromechanical dissociation that responded to calcium chloride therapy. The estimated peak serum citrate level was greater than 120 mg/dL.[9]

In children, calcium replacement has led to hypercalcemia and death.[7] The use of calcium should be reserved for the massively transfused patient with profound liver disease or acute heart failure, two situations in which metabolism of citrate may be impaired. Citrate also binds magnesium, and hypomagnesemia, another cause of cardiac arrhythmia (long QT syndrome, Torsade de pointes),[8,10] has been reported in massively transfused patients.[11,12] Magnesium toxicity has also been described in patients with massive transfusions.[4]

Laboratory

When citrate is rapidly administered intravenously (or bank blood is given at a rate greater than 120 mL/min)[6] there may be a decrease in total blood calcium.[3] The majority of patients, however, may become hypokalemic during massive transfusion often after initial hypercalemia.[4] Serum potassium should be monitored in all patients who receive a massive transfusion. Monitoring is mandatory in patients with renal compromise.

Plasma Ionized Calcium

A toxic plasma citrate level of 50 mg/dL can result in a calculated plasma ionized calcium level of about 0.5 mM, which could lead to marked depression of myocardial function.[8] Normal serum calcium and citrate concentrations are listed in Table 28–1.[13]

The normal range of ionized calcium is 0.9 to 1.6 mM (1.8–3.2 mEq/L). The total calcium level in the blood following the injection of citrate usually remains normal or may even increase. A deficiency of ionized calcium may increase the irritability of muscle and may induce fasciculations, tetany, seizures, or cardiac failure if the level is reduced for more than a few seconds. Ventricular fibrillation and cardiac asystole (after QT prolongation) have been the most serious cardiac complications of citrate-induced depression of ionized calcium. Arterial hypotension may be resistant to further blood transfusion or pressor agents.[8] It may also cause some impairment of the coagulation mechanism.[14] Acute disturbances in ionized calcium homeostasis may not be apparent from total calcium measurement. This emphasizes the need for repeated ionized calcium measurements.[15]

Table 28–1
Normal Serum Calcium and Citrate Concentrations*

Total	2.12–2.50 mmol/L
Protein-bound, nondiffusible	0.8–1.1 mmol/L (35–45% of total)
Ionized	1–1.25 mmol/L
Complex-bound	0.25 mmol/L
Citrate	0.09–0.14 mmol/L

*Ultrafiltrable = ionized + complex-bound.

From Abbott TR. Changes in serum calcium fractions and citrate concentrations during massive blood transfusions and cardiopulmonary bypass. Br J Anaesth 1983;55:753–760.

Transfusion of not more than 50 mL every 30 minutes has shown no evidence of citrate intoxication. If the rate at which citrate is infused remains below 0.5 mg/kg body weight per minute, the serum concentration of citrate ion remains below 9 mg/dL (0.5 mM/L) and the calculated ionized calcium level remains above 0.85 mM/L, which is within the normal range.[16]

Toxicokinetics

Metabolism

Citric acid is generally metabolized very rapidly, primarily by the liver, adrenal cortex, and muscle. About 18 to 20% of infused citrate is excreted in the urine. Peak plasma citrate levels are generally related to the rate of infusion and not to the total amount of citric acid infused.[17] A citrate infusion rate of 1 mL/kg/min produces plasma citrate levels of between 8 and 25 mg/dL.[3] One patient received 8.6 mg/kg/min citric acid over 20 minutes, resulting in a peak plasma citrate level of 79.6 mg/dL, which returned to normal 40 minutes after the infusion.[3] An infusion of 9.5 mg/kg can result in an estimated plasma citrate level in the range 76 to 120 mg/dL.[9]

Acid–citrate–dextrose (ACD) solution given at the rate of 6.25 to 8.6 mg/kg/min has caused prolongation of the QT_c interval on the electrocardiogram.[3]

Pregnancy

The plasma citric acid level is lower in the third than in the second trimester of pregnancy.[7]

Clinical Presentation

Early signs of citrate intoxication commonly seen during hemopheresis procedures may include perioral and acral numbness and tingling, feelings of tenseness or lightness of muscles, and a sense of "twitchiness." The adverse effects of severe citrate intoxication are not inadequate coagulation but bradycardia, decreased cardiac output, and possible arrhythmia. These problems may be enhanced if cold blood is infused. Patients with severe osteoporosis (decreased calcium stores) or severe liver disease (inability to mobilize

Table 28–2
Hazards of Blood Transfusion

- Hemolytic reactions
- Chill/fever reactions
- Contaminated blood
- Noncardiac pulmonary edema
- Circulation overload
- Allergic reactions (urticarial, anaphylactoid)
- Infectious diseases
- Air embolism
- Massive transfusion problems
  - Fluid overload
  - Adult respiratory distress
  - Electrolyte abnormalities
  - Hypothermia
  - Platelet and factor dilution

From Nolan TE, Gallup DG. Massive transfusion: A current review. Obstet Gynecol Surv 1991;46(5):289–295.

citrate to bicarbonate) may be at increased risk.[7] Some hazards of blood transfusion are listed in Table 28–2.[4]

A 5-year-old boy received an inadvertent infusion of 400 mL of citrate–phosphate–dextrose solution (10.52 g sodium citrate, 10.2 g dextrose, 1308 mg citric acid, 888 mg sodium bisphosphate). The infusion of anticoagulant was immediately discontinued. Postoperatively, an infusion of calcium gluconate at 60 mg/h was continued for 2 hours until a serum calcium level greater than 9 mg/dL was maintained for five determinations.[18]

Calcium Infusion

Skeletal stores of calcium are immense and, as a rule, calcium salts are not needed for treatment. Intravenous infusion of calcium may cause disturbances in the cardiac rhythm and should be avoided. An exception is exchange transfusion in newborns, where the electrocardiogram and

Table 28–3
Intervals Between Last Dose of Drug and Safe Blood Donation

Drug	Safe Interval	Drug	Safe Interval
Ampicillin	24 h	Etretinate	24 mo
Cloxacillin	48 h	Piroxicam	28 d
Aspirin	7 d*	Quinine	7 d*
Cimetidine	0	Salbutamol inhaler	0
Clomiphene	3 mo	Tiaprofenic acid (sustained release)	4 d*
Dothiepin	0		
Diazepam	7 d		

*Do not use donation for platelet transfusion within 10 days of last dose.
These guidelines are in addition to usual clinical exclusions, eg, active infection, pregnancy, rheumatoid arthritis, and active ulcer.
From Ferner RE, Chaplin S, Dunstan JA, Baird GM. Drugs in donated blood. Lancet 1989;2:93–94.

Table 28–4
Mechanisms and Effects of Antiplatelet Agents

Mechanism of Antiplatelet Action	Effects	Effective Agents
Increased concentration of cAMP	Inhibits platelet aggregation Inhibits release reaction (of platelet granules) Change in platelet shape Inhibits platelet adhesion	Activators of membrane adenylate cyclase Adenosine PGI_2, PGE_2, PGD_2 Phosphodiesterase inhibitors Dipyridamole Caffeine Theophylline Increased endothelial PGI_2 production Glyceryl trinitrate
Inhibition of arachidonic acid metabolism	Decreases TXA_2*: platelet aggregation, secretion of granules, and vasoconstricton PGI_2: inhibits platelet function and causes vasodilation	Phospholipase inhibitors Steroids Mepacrine Cyclooxygenase inhibitors Aspirin NSAIDs Sulfinpyrazone Thromboxane synthetase inhibitors Imidazole derivatives Dazoxiben
Inhibition of thrombin	Inhibits platelet aggregation Inhibits thrombus formation in extracorporeal circulation Inhibits thrombus formation in arteries	Coumarin Heparin
Inhibition of calcium channels†		Calmodulin-independent Verapamil Nifedipine Diltiazem Calmodulin-dependent Chlorpromazine Trifluperazine
Inhibition of adrenaline binding	Potentiation of other stimuli‡ Possible role in thrombus formation	Dihydroergocryptine Yohimbine Nicergoline Phentolamine
Inhibition of ADP-induced aggregation	Inhibits platelet activation Reduces availability of fibrinogen receptor on platelet membrane	Ticlopidine Pyridoxal derivatives Penicillins§

PG, prostaglandin; TX, thromboxane; NSAID, nonsteroidal antiinflammatory drug.
*Arachidonic acid, derived from platelet membrane phospholipids, undergoes enzymatic transformations to produce the prostaglandin endoperoxides (PGG_2, PGH_2), TXA_2, and vascular prostacyclin. These labile products are converted into the stable prostaglandins (PGE_2, PGD_2, and PGF_{2a} and TXB_2.)
†Calcium transport across the platelet membrane activates platelets secondary to a number of stimuli.
‡Adrenaline potentiates the effects of other stimuli by facilitating calcium transport.
§Penicillins compete for adrenaline, ADP, and factor VIII: von Willebrand factor receptors.
From Saltiel E, Ward A. Ticlopidine: A review of its pharmacodynamic and pharmacokinetic properties, and therapeutic efficacy in platelet-dependent disease states. Drugs 1987;34:222–262.

serum calcium levels can be carefully monitored. Excess citrate is usually metabolized quickly. As long as adequate circulatory volume is maintained, as guided by the central venous pressure or pulmonary artery wedge pressure, depression of calcium ion during transfusion may be devoid of clinical significance.[19]

During the management of massive hemorrhage, (1) coagulation tests and platelet counts should be monitored frequently; (2) aggressive correction of hypovolemia should be instituted to avoid the coagulation defect associated with prolonged shock; and (3) where a large wound will necessitate major surgery shortly, or where there is a head injury, administration of fresh-frozen plasma colloid solutions on a one-to-one ratio with red cell concentrates is indicated, to avoid a dilutional coagulopathy.[20]

Overdosage

There is a real danger of calcium overdosage with aggressive treatment of citrate-induced hypocalcemia.[16,21] Harmful effects of citrate infusion may occur if the dosage exceeds 250 mg/kg/h.[9]

Prevention

All pharmacologically active solutions should be labeled boldly in color with nontoxic dye and positioned so as not to be confused with other preparations. There should be clear instructions on the bottle regarding the proper dose of citrate–phosphate–dextrose and the danger of citrate toxicity.[9]

Donated Blood

Ferner and colleagues have listed intervals between the last dose of some drugs and safe blood donation. These data do not provide for variations in drug dose, distribution, or disposition in individuals, nor do they consider metabolites. Further work is required to validate these calculations[22] (Table 28–3).

Anti–Platelet Drugs

Mechanisms effects of antiplatelet agents are listed in Table 28–4. See also chapters on salicylates, NSAID's, and anticoagulants for additional information.

REFERENCES—CITRATE

1. Rudolph R, Boyd CR. Massive transfusion: Complications and their management. South Med J 1990;83:1065–1070.
2. Westphal RG. *Handbook of Transfusion Medicine.* Washington, DC: The American Red Cross Blood Series. Fayetteville, NY: Roberts Press, 1990:76.
3. Hwland WS, Belleville JW, Zucker MB, et al. Massive blood replacement: V. Failure to observe citrate intoxication. Surg Gynecol Obstet 1957;105:529–540.
4. Nolan TE, Gallup DG. Massive transfusion: A current review. Obstet Gynecol Surv 1991;46:289–295.
5. Rutledge R, Sheldon GF, Collins ML. Massive transfusion. Crit Care Clin 1986;2:791–805.
6. Michelsen T, Salmela L, Tigerstedt I, et al. Massive blood transfusion: Is there a limit? Crit Care Med 1989;17:699–700.
7. Wolf PL, McCarty LJ, Hafleigh B. Extreme hypercalcemia following blood transfusion combined with intravenous calcium. Vox Sang 1970;19:544–545.
8. Ludbrook J, Wynn W. Citrate intoxication: A clinical and experimental study. Br Med J 1985;2:523–528.
9. Lee-Chow BL, Auerbach PS, Olson KR, et al. Cardiac arrest following direct intravenous administration of a citrate anticoagulant solution. Vet Hum Toxicol 1985;28:296.
10. Kulkaris P, Bhattacharya S, Petros AJ. Torsade de Pointes and long QT syndrome following major blood transfusion. Anaesthesia 1992;47:125–127.
11. McLellan BA, Reid SP, Lane PC. Massive blood transfusion causing hypomagnesemia. Crit Care Med 1984;12:146–147.
12. Kruskall MS, Mintz PD, Bergin JJ, et al. Transfusion therapy in emergency medicine. Ann Emerg Med 1988;17:327–335.
13. Abbott TR. Changes seen in calcium fractions and citrate concentrations during massive blood transfusions and cardiopulmonary bypass. Br J Anaesth 1983;55:753–760.
14. Hubbard TF, Neis DD, Barmore JL. Severe citrate intoxication during cardiovascular surgery. JAMA 1956;162:1534–1535.
15. Stulz PM, Scheidegger D, Drop LJ, et al. Ventricular pump performance during hypocalcemia: Clinical and experimental studies. J Thorac Cardiovasc Surg 1979;78:185–194.
16. Bunker JP, Dendixen HH, Murphy AJ. Hemodyamic effects of intravenously administered sodium citrate. N Engl J Med 1962;266:372–377.
17. Jennings ER, Beland AJ, Cope JA, et al. Citrate toxicity and the use of anticoagulant and citrate dextrose blood for extracorporeal circulation. Surg Gynecol Obstet 1965;120:997–1008.
18. Lee BL, Auerbach PS, Olson KR, et al. Cardiac arrest following intravenous administration of a citrate anticoagulant solution. Ann Emerg Med 1986;15:1352–1356.
19. Kahn RC, Jascott D, Carlon GC, et al. Massive blood replacement: Correlation of ionized calcium, citrate and hydrogen in concentration. Anesth Analg 1979;58:274–278.
20. Hewson JR, Neame PB, Kumar N, et al. Coagulopathy related to dilution and hypotension during massive transfusion. Crit Care Med 1985;13:387–391.
21. Bunker JP, Stetson JB, Coe RC, et al. Citric acid intoxication. JAMA 1955;157:136–137.
22. Ferner RE, Chaplin S, Dunstan JA, Baird GM. Drugs in donated blood. Lancet 1989;2:93–94.

IRON–DEXTRAN

Iron–dextran preparations may be used intramuscularly or intravenously for treatment of iron deficiency anemia. Hypersensitivity reactions (immediate or delayed) follow high intravenous doses. Overdoses of iron–dextran may produce meningitis symptoms. There have been no deaths. Poisoning with iron–dextran presents an altered clinical course compared with inorganic iron poisoning.

Structure and Classification

Iron–dextran is a complex of ferric hydroxide with dextran of average molecular weight between 5000 and 7500.[1] About 98% of the iron in iron–dextran is present as a stable iron–dextran complex.[2]

Use

Iron–dextran is used in the treatment of microcytic hypochromic anemia resulting from iron deficiency, especially in those patients in whom oral administration of iron is not feasible or ineffective because of intolerance, poor absorption, gastrointestinal disease, or refusal or inability to take the oral medication.

Product Formulation

A parenteral injection for intramuscular use only is equivalent to 50 mg elemental iron per milliliter (Imferon) and contains phenol 0.5%.[2] The injections have a pH of 5.2 to 6.5.[1]

The average molecular weight of the dextran used in the manufacture of Imferon is 5000, but the molecular weight of the iron complex may be many times this figure.[3] Imferon contains 50 mg of elemental iron and 20 mg of dextran per milliliter.[4]

Source

Fisons Corporation USA has temporarily ceased production and supply of Imferon in the United States as a result of manufacturing difficulties. More supplies are available elsewhere. Emergency requests can be made to the U.S. Food and Drug Administration at 1-301-443-0487.[2]

Therapeutic Dose

For iron replacement secondary to blood loss, the dosage of iron–dextran (50 mg iron/mL) is calculated as follows:

0.02 × blood loss (in mL) × hematocrit (decimal fraction) = total dosage of iron–dextran in mL

For iron deficiency anemia the following formula is employed:

0.0476 × (normal hemoglobin − observed hemoglobin in g/dL) (±) 1 mL/5 kg body weight (up to maximum of 14 mL), which accounts for storage iron = total dosage of iron–dextran in mL

Iron–dextran may be injected intravenously undiluted at a rate not exceeding 50 mg iron/min (1 mL/min). If no reaction to the test dose occurs, subsequent intravenous doses may be increased up to 100 mg of iron daily until the total calculated dose has been administered. Large intravenous doses may be followed by arthralgia, myalgia, and fever. Iron–dextran may be given intramuscularly.[2]

Toxic Dose

A 32-mL dose administered intravenously induced meningitis symptoms. The patient survived.[5] A child received 1300 mg of elemental iron intravenously as iron dextrose. In 8 hours the serum iron level was 1830 μg/L. The serum iron levels returned to normal over 3 days with a serum half-life of 18.7 hours. The patient remained asymptomatic and survived.[6]

Fatal Dose

A 4-year-old child was inadvertently given 2.0 g instead of 0.3 g and died of sepsis.[7]

Toxicokinetics

Absorption

Following rapid infusion of up to 2.5 g iron as iron–dextran, iron accumulates in the liver,[8] bone marrow, and spleen, and appears rapidly in circulating red cells. The complex is cleared from the plasma with a half-life of 2 to 3 days.[3] The iron–dextran is rapidly broken down in the reticuloendothelial system, and then released into a pool that exchanges freely with plasma transferrin.[9] This is carried in the bone marrow and is imported into hemoglobin. During the first days of treatment with iron–dextran, serum iron concentrations may reach 50,000 μg/100 mL. When the total serum iron level is greater than 1000 μg/100 mL the serum turns brown.[3]

Elimination

Trace quantities of iron–dextran appear in the urine.[3] The half-life of the complex in plasma is 2 to 3 days.[3] During pregnancy the mean half-life is 42 hours.[10] Only traces of unmetabolized iron–dextran are excreted in the urine, bile, or feces.

Clinical Presentation

Overdose

Following an overdose muscle cramps, bilateral frontal headache, neck stiffness, opisthotonus, and photophobia may be observed. After delayed onset of 12 to 24 hours, arthralgias, vomiting, metabolic acidosis, bradycardia, and depressed central nervous system sensorium can be seen with death due to sepsis.[7] The serum hemoglobin does not rise during the infusion. This results in abnormally high concentrations of free iron, which crosses into the cerebrospinal fluid and is responsible for meningitis symptoms.[5]

Hypersensitivity Reactions

Hypersensitivity reactions range from 1% to nearly 50% in different studies.[11] These reactions appear to occur more frequently after large intravenous doses of iron–dextran. The most dangerous complication is an anaphylactoid (anaphylactic-like) reaction. Similar to contrast medium reactions, the anaphylactoid reaction manifests during the first few minutes of an infusion and resembles a type I (IgE-mediated) allergic reaction. IgE-mediated reactions to dextran are rare.[12] The most common hypersensitivity reaction, occurring in more than 30% of patients given dextran, is the development of arthralgias and fever within 24 to 48 hours of initiation of intravenous therapy. Other rare systemic hypersensitivity reactions occur 1 to 2 weeks after initiation of iron–dextran therapy and include generalized lymphadenopathy, malaise, fever, elevated erythrocyte sedimentation rate, leukocytes with neutrophilia, splenomegaly and arthralgia/arthritis.[10] Infrequent reactions following iron–dextran use include rhabdomyolysis[13] and systemic lupus erythematosus.[14,15] Local reactions may occur at the intramuscular site of injection. In patients with renal failure and marked hyperparathyroidism, iron–dextran injections have been followed by severe intramuscular calcification.[16] Sarcomas have been reported following use of iron–dextran, but such observations have not been confirmed.[17]

Laboratory

Analytical Methods

The iron–dextran complex is present in the circulation for 2 to 3 weeks after administration and interferes with all colorimetric iron assays.[18] In patients receiving iron–dextran therapy, transferrin-based iron, total iron binding capacity (TIBC), total iron (except hemoglobin–iron), and dextran-bound iron levels can be measured by a colorimetric technique using dithionite.[19,20]

Abnormalities

Iron–dextran may, even if administered within the previous 3 weeks, produce false-positive and abnormally elevated readings of serum iron.[4] The total iron binding capacity may be markedly increased in response to iron–dextran therapy.[14] A fatal dose of iron–dextran resulted in a total serum iron level (including iron–dextran) of 54,500 μg/dL (normal, 50–160 μg/d). At an iron level of 14,500 μg/d, the total iron binding capacity was 322 μg/dL.

Treatment

Stabilization

Treatment of an iron–dextran overdose is symptomatic and supportive. Monitoring of serum iron and TIBC is indicated.

Elimination Enhancement

The drug is negligibly removed by hemodialysis. Whole blood exchange transfusion may be useful if administered early.[7]

Antidote

Deferoxamine may decrease the side effects of iron–dextran treatment, but because the iron probably remains substantively bound to the dextran, chelation with deferoxamine may be ineffective.[6]

REFERENCES—IRON-DEXTRAN

1. Reynolds JEF, ed. *Martindale: The Extra Pharmacopoeia.* 30th ed. London: Pharmaceutical Press, 1993:851–853.
2. McEvoy GK, ed. *AHFS Drug Information 94.* Bethesda, MD: American Society of Hospital Pharmacists, 1994:1642–1644.
3. Wood JK, Milner PFA, Pathak UN. The metabolism of iron–dextran given as a total-dose infusion to iron-deficient Jamaican subjects. Br J Haematol 1968;14:119–129.
4. McIntosh ME, Lynn JK, Meyerriecks N, Contant I. Serum iron determination in patients receiving therapy with iron–dextran ("Imferon"). Clin Chem 1976;22:524–527.
5. Shuttleworth D, Spence C, Slade R. Meningism due to intravenous iron–dextran. Lancet 1983;2:453.
6. Rodgers G, Matyunas N, Ross M. Lack of toxicity following a large inadvertent overdose of iron–dextran: A case report. Clin Toxicol 1995;33:475–486 (Abstract 76).
7. Davidar SM, Snodgrass WR. Fatal iron–dextran poisoning: A combined iron toxicity and dextran induced immune block. Vet Hum Toxicol 1989;31:34L.
8. Fleming LW, Hopwood D, Shepherd AN, Stewart WK. Hepatic iron in dialysed patients given intravenous iron–dextran. J Clin Pathol 1990;43:119–124.
9. Kanakakorn K, Cavill I, Jacobs A. The metabolism of intravenously administered iron–dextran. Br J Trace Haematol 1973;25:637–643.
10. Duke AB, Kelleher J, Walters G. Serum iron and iron binding capacity after total dose infusion of iron–dextran for iron deficiency anaemia in pregnancy. J Obstet Gynaecol Br Commonw 1974;81:895–900.
11. Bielory L. Serum sickness from iron–dextran administration. Acta Haematol 1990;83:166–168.
12. Altman LC, Petersen PE. Successful prevention of an anaphylactoid reaction to iron–dextran. Ann Intern Med 1988; 109:346–347.
13. Foulkes WD, Sewry C, Calam J, Hodgson HJC. Rhabdomyolysis after intramuscular iron–dextran in malabsorption. Ann Rheum Dis 1991;50:184–186.
14. OH VMS. Iron–dextran and systemic lupus erythematosus. Br Med J 1992;305:1000.
15. Harchelroad F, Rice S. Iron–dextran: Treatment or overdose. Vet Hum Toxicol 1992;34:329.
16. Rees JKH, Coles GA. Calciphylaxis in man. Br Med J 1969; 2:670–672.
17. Weinbren K, Salm R, Greenberg G. Intramuscular injections of iron compounds and oncogenesis in man. Br Med J 1978; 1:683–685.
18. Hvisman W. Interference of Imferon in colorimetric tests for iron. Clin Chem 1980;26:635–637.
19. Jacobs JC, Alexander NM. Colorimetric and constant-potential colorimetry determinations of transferrin-bound iron, total iron binding capacity, and total iron in serum containing iron–dextran with use of sodium dithionite and alumina columns. Clin Chem 1990;36:1803–1807.
20. Vercammen M, Goedhuys W, Boeyckens A, et al. Iron and total iron-binding capacity in serum of patients receiving iron–dextran: Kodak Ektachen methodologies, spectrophotometry and atomic absorption spectrometry compared. Clin Chem 1990;36:1812–1815.

Chapter 29
The Cytokines

INTRODUCTION

Cytokines are soluble factors that can act as supportive, cytotoxic, or immune modulators[1,2] (Table 29–1).[2,3] More than 30 peptides have been purified and sequenced and the coding genes cloned. The cytokines are divided into five main groups[2]:

- *Interferons* (alpha, beta, and gamma): originally recognized by their ability to protect cells from viral infection
- *Interleukins* (1–9): diverse immunoregulatory factors named in historical sequence
- *Hematopoietic colony-stimulating factors* (erythropoietin, granulocyte–macrophage colony-stimulating factor [GM-CSF], granulocyte colony-stimulating factor [G-CSF], and macrophage colony-stimulating factor [M-CSF]): structurally dissimilar, but functionally related in controlling hematopoiesis
- *Tumor necrosis factors* (alpha and beta): structurally related proteins with cytotoxic activity in vitro
- *Assorted growth factors* (eg, platelet-derived growth factor): named according to the cell system in which their activity was discovered

INTERFERONS

Use

Interferons have been used in the treatment of hairy cell leukemia, chronic myelogenous leukemia, Kaposi's sarcoma, malignant melanoma, renal cell carcinoma, cutaneous T-cell lymphoma, and bladder cancer. They are not active alone against breast, colon, lung, and prostate cancers[4–6] (Table 29–2).[6]

Toxicokinetics[2,7]

Time to peak plasma level	1–8 hours
Volume of distribution	12–40 L/kg
Elimination half-life	4–6 hours (alpha)
	1–2 hours (beta)
	25–35 minutes (gamma)

Table 29–1
New Immunomodulators and Peptide Regulatory Factors

Immunomodulator	Therapeutic Potential	Preparation	Route and Dose
Cyclosporine	Transplant surgery Bone marrow transplant Autoimmune diseases	Oral suspension Capsules IV infusion	PO/IV Enema 5–100 mg/kg
Levamisole	Aphthous stomatitis Leprosy Sarcoidosis T-cell anergy	50-mg tablet	PO 150 mg once weekly
HuGM-CSF rHG-CSF	Leukopenia Cyclic neutropenia Agranulocytosis AIDS With cancer chemotherapy With ganciclovir for cytomegalovirus Retinitis myelodysplasia	Recombinant protein in aqueous buffer	IV SC 3 μg/kg/d
Erythropoietin rhEPO	Dialysis anemia Aplastic anemia	Powder	IV SC 100 U/kg weekly
Interferons	Melanoma Leukemia Cancer Kaposi's sarcoma Autoimmune diseases Pulmonary hemangiomatosis Hyper IgE syndrome Hepatitis B with HB vaccine for nonresponders	Powder in vials (mega-units)	Intranasal SC IV Intralesional 100 μg/m² body surface thrice weekly
Immunoglobulin	Passive immunoprophylaxis Hypogammaglobulinemia	Freeze-dried powder	IV IM 0.02–0.12 mL/kg
Interleukin-2	Metastatic melanoma Advanced cancer of lung and bowel	Powder	IV

HuGM-CSF, human granulocyte–macrophage colony-stimulating factor; rHG-CSF, recombinant human granulocyte colony-stimulating factor; rhEPO, recombinant human erythropoietin.
From James DG. Immunotherapy, Br J Clin Pract 1989;43(12):433–437.

Drug Interactions

Interferons may reduce hepatic microsomal cytochrome P450 activity. A reduction in clearance and a prolongation of the half-life of theophylline have been observed.

Clinical Presentation

Toxic effects appear to be similar for all interferons (alpha, beta, gamma).[3,8] These include a flulike syndrome of fever, chills, arthralgias, myalgias, and headache (Table 29–3).[9] Chronic side effects include fatigue, anorexia, nausea, vomiting, diarrhea, suppression of blood counts, elevation of hepatic enzymes, and central nervous system and cardiovascular toxicity. Severity of toxicity is usually dose related and is often enhanced when interferon is given by the intravenous route or administered to older patients. Potentially life-threatening toxic effects induced by high doses of interferon include central nervous system and cardiovascular toxicity. Central nervous system toxic effects such as anxiety, agitation, somnolence, altered cognitive function, seizures, coma, and electroencephalographic abnormalities have been observed.

Cardiovascular toxic effects include cardiac arrhythmias, cardiomyopathy, myocardial ischemia, acute myocardial infarction, and hypo- or hypertension. High intravenous doses may lead to some prolongation of the prothrombin time and partial thromboplastin time. Interferon alfa induces a reversible acute renal failure.[10] The toxic effects induced by interferon are usually reversible on discontinuation of the drug.[11]

Thrombocytopenia and some prolongation of the prothrombin time and partial thromboplastin time are common.

Treatment

Treatment requires discontinuation of cytokine use. Management is largely symptomatic and supportive. Late toxicity may appear 2 to 6 weeks after therapy.

INTERLEUKINS

Toxicokinetics

After intravenous administration, recombinant interleukin-2 disappears from the plasma with a distribution half-life of 6 to 13 minutes. The mean peak plasma concentration is reached 90 to 240 minutes after an intramuscular injection. Bioavailability after an intramuscular administration is 37%.

Distribution

The volume of distribution is 0.1 L/kg.[12]

Excretion

Total body clearance is 120 mL/min. The plasma beta-phase elimination is 30 to 120 minutes.

Clinical Presentation (Interleukin-2)

Cardiovascular Effects

Non-life-threatening and life-threatening toxic effects are common. Hypotension (transiently responsive to fluid administration), increase in heart rate and cardiac output, and decrease in systemic peripheral resistance have been observed. A capillary leak syndrome contributes to the hypotension by efflux of fluid from the intravascular space into the interstices. Other cardiovascular toxic effects include a decrease in left ventricular stroke work and ejection fraction, ventricular and supraventricular arrhythmias, myocardial ischemia, infarction, and death (if underlying coronary artery disease is present). Anuria, pulmonary edema, and adult respiratory distress syndrome have been observed. Treatment of hypotension and capillary leak syndrome may be instituted with combinations of dopamine and other pressor agents (eg, phenylephrine), judicious fluid administration, and diuretics. Such toxicity regresses after discontinuation of interleukin-2. Corticosteroids may be useful in reversing the capillary-leak syndrome.[13,14]

Central Nervous System Effects

Acute neuropsychiatric toxicity is often observed and includes severe behavioral changes, cognitive changes,

Table 29–2
Different Types of Cytokines

Cytokine	Alternative Name	Associated Cell	Function and Therapeutic Potential
Interleukin (IL)		Macrophage T lymphocyte	Mediates inflammation causing fever, acute phase protein release
IL-1	Hemopoietin 1	Fibroblast	Activates neutrophils and macrophages Stimulates T cells
IL-2	T-cell growth factor	T	Supports T-cell growth and expansion Enhances lymphokine-activated killer (LAK) activity
IL-3	Hemopoietin 2	T	Promotes hemopoietic progenitors
IL-4	B-cell-stimulating factor 1	T	Activates B cells to proliferate and to differentiate into plasma cells
IL-5	Eosinophil factor	T	Promotes proliferation of eosinophils and eosinophil degranulation
IL-6	B-cell-stimulating factor 2	T Fibroblast	Stimulates B cell to plasma cell and to antibody production
Interferon (IFN) α-IFN β-IFN γ-IFN	 Leukocyte IFN Fibroblast IFN Immune IFN	 Monocyte/macrophage Fibroblast T lymphocyte	 Activates intracellular oligoadenylate synthetase to break down RNA, hence antiviral activity
Tumor Necrosis Factor TNF-α TFN-β	 Cachectin Lymphotoxin	 Monocyte/macrophage T lymphocyte	 A polypeptide responsible for septicemia-induced endotoxin shock A specific monoclonal antibody neutralizes shock
Colony-Stimulating Factor (CSF) Granulocyte CSF Macrophage CSF Granulocyte–macrophage CSF	 GC-CSF M-CSF rHu-GM-CSF	 Fibroblast/endothelium Fibroblast/endothelium T lymphocyte	 Growth factor responsible for proliferation and maturation of bone marrow stem cells. rHu-GM-CSF successful in treating leukopenic states
Erythropoietin	EPO	Kidney	Corrects dialysis anemia

rHU, recombinant human.
From James DG. Immunotherapy. Br J Clin Pract 1989;43:433–437.

Table 29-3
Management of Interleukin-2-Induced Toxicity

General toxicity	
Fever and chills	Prevention and treatment with paracetamol (acetaminophen) and nonsteroidal antiinflammatory agents
	Intravenous pethidine (meperidine) for severe chills
Gastrointestinal effects	Prevention with H_2-receptor antagonists and antinausea agents (eg, metoclopramide)
	Atropine diphenoxylate or diarrhea
	Fluid replacement and bicarbonate administration if diarrhea is severe
Cardiac toxicity	
Myocardial toxicity	Exclude patients with coronary artery disease
	Cardiac monitoring during treatment
Arrhythmias	Discontinuation of IL-2 if sustained ventricular tachycardia or electrical evidence of cardiac ischemia
	Unsustained ventricular ectopy and supraventricular tachyarrhythmias require conventional antiarrhythmics (eg, digoxin, verapamil)
Hypotension	Initial management with feet elevation and prudent fluid replacement with crystalloid or colloid solutions or low-dose dopamine to maintain systolic blood pressure between 85 and 100 mm Hg
	Avoid arrhythmogenic vasopressors and prefer phenylephrine use if patient remains hypotensive or develops tachycardia (heart rate >150/min)
	Reduce or discontinue IL-2 if hypotension persists or blood pressure is below 70 mm Hg
Capillary leak syndrome	Weigh patients twice daily
	Fluid restriction (1–1.5 L/d) and furosemide in cases of excessive weight gain and oliguria
Dermatologic toxicity	H_1-receptor antagonists (eg, diphenhydramine), emollients, and topical treatment
Hematologic toxicity	Red cell transfusions to maintain hemoglobin level above 110 g/L
Hepatic toxicity	Consider discontinuation of IL-2 for bilirubin level more than 100 µmol/L
Infectious complications	Early treatment for any clinical suspicion of infection using broad-spectrum or antistaphylococcal antibiotics
	Prophylactic antibiotics may prevent infection for patients with surgically tunnelled intravenous catheters
Neuropsychiatric toxicity	Exclude patients with central nervous system metastases
	Benzodiazepines for anxiety
	Low-dose haloperidol for mild agitation and hallucinations
	Discontinuation of IL-2 for patients with marked perturbation (disorientation, confusion) or altered mental state
	Prudent readministration of IL-2 following complete resolution of symptoms
Pulmonary toxicity	Discontinuation of IL-2 for partial oxygen pressure less than 60 mm Hg
	Intermittent exogenous oxygen or intubation with mechanical ventilatory support if necessary
Renal toxicity	Maintain renal perfusion with low-dose dopamine infusions
	Avoid nephrotoxic drugs
	Consider discontinuation of IL-2 for creatinine level more than 500 µmol/L

From Vial T, Descotes J. Clinical toxicity of interleukin-2. Drug Saf 1992;7:417–433.

disorientation, and confusion. These resolve within 48 to 72 hours of discontinuation of interleukin-2. Coma and seizures have been observed. Rarely, an acute fatal leukoencephalopathy has been reported.[15,16]

Anecdotal reports have associated interleukin-2 with the nephrotic syndrome, acute pancreatitis, thrombocytopenia, elevated plasma concentration of adrenocorticotropic hormone, cortisol, epinephrine and norepinephrine, hypothyroidism, and an increase in the incidence of hypersensitivity to iodine-containing radiographic contrast media. Interleukin-4 may induce acute gastric mucosal injury; this may occur even with concomitant ranitidine administration.[17]

Treatment

Management of toxicity with interleukin-2 indicates a use for ibuprofen (600 mg orally every 6 hours) in the reduction of fever, chills, myalgias, nausea, and vomiting.[18,19] Vial and Descotes have suggested a management program for interleukin-2-induced toxicity (Table 29-3).[18] Patients receiving high doses of interleukin-2 should be monitored in an intensive care unit. Treatment is symptomatic and supportive.[20]

TUMOR NECROSIS FACTORS

Toxic effects are similar to those of interferon, with fatigue, fever, chills, headache, anorexia, nausea, vomiting, diarrhea, and pain at the injection site. Suppression of blood counts and liver function abnormalities occur frequently. Modest hypotension is correctable with intravenous fluids. Lethargy, confusion, and disorientation may be observed.

COLONY-STIMULATING FACTORS

Granulocyte–macrophage colony-stimulating factor may lead to fever, arthralgias, myalgia, a capillary leak syndrome with generalized edema, pleural and pericardial effusions, erythroderma, and, at high doses, thromboses at the site of venous catheters. G-CSF toxic effects include bone pain, hypotension, and renal dysfunction at the highest doses.

Doses of up to 100 µg/kg/d (4000 µg/m^2/d) have led to increases in the white blood cell count to 200,000 cells/m^3. Adverse reactions include dyspnea, malaise, nausea, fever, rash, sinus tachycardia, headache, and chills, reversible after discontinuation. Treatment comprises discontinuation and monitoring for an increase in white blood cells and respiratory syncope.

ERYTHROPOIETIN

Erythropoietin (EPO) is a glycosylated protein that is normally produced by the human body in response to renal hypoxia. It stimulates erythroid precursors in the marrow to increase red cell production and this provides a simple control mechanism.[21] Erythropoietin deficiency is associated with end-stage renal failure; such patients are anemic because of an impaired marrow response. Use of erythropoietin appears to improve the quality of life (less fatigue and improvement in exercise tolerance)[21–23] of hemodialysis patients.[24] Serious life-threatening side effects may follow the use of commercial erythropoietin (recombinant human erythropoietin)[25–27] (Table 29–4). In an attempt to increase the oxygen-carrying capacity of their blood, healthy endurance athletes (eg. runners, cyclists, and cross-country skiers) have reportedly begun to use erythropoietin. This may have contributed to the death of cyclists in the Netherlands.[28] The Medical Commission of the International Olympic Committee (IOC) has recently classified erythropoietin as a doping substance.[29–31]

Structure and Classification

Erythropoietin is a glycoprotein made up of 165 amino acids and four complex carbohydrate chains that are rich in sialic acid and account for 40% of the total molecular weight of 34,000. The amino acid sequence is identical to that of human erythropoietin.[32,33]

Use

Recombinant human erythropoietin is used in the treatment of anemia associated with chronic renal failure, including patients on dialysis (end-stage renal disease) and patients not on dialysis. It is also indicated for the treatment of anemia related to therapy with zidovudine (AZT) in HIV-infected patients.[34]

Product Formulation

Erythropoietin is available in the United States as epoetin alfa (Epogen). It is commercially available in Europe as Eprex, which is identical to Epogen. A similar product, epoetin beta, is marketed in Japan as Marogen. The molecular formula appears to be the same as that of epoetin alfa.[35]

Table 29–4
Adverse Effects Associated With Recombinant Human Erythropoietin Therapy

Increased extracorporeal blood clotting (vascular access thrombosis)
Development or exacerbation of hypertension
Hypertensive encephalopathy
Grand mal seizures
Iron deficiency
Headache, visual disturbances
Flulike syndrome (may include aches and pains of limbs and pelvis, diaphoresis, shivering, abdominal pain)
Exacerbation of acne
Conjunctival inflammation
Possible increased predialysis serum potassium, creatinine, and urea nitrogen concentrations

From Schwenk MH, Halstenson CE. Recombinant human erythropoietin. DICP Ann Pharmacother 1989;23:528–536.

Source

Erythropoietin is manufactured commercially as a recombinant human erythropoietin. It is synthesized by Chinese hamster ovary cells into which the human erythropoietin gene has been introduced.[36]

Therapeutic Dose

Epoetin alfa is administered intravenously or subcutaneously to adults in doses of 50 to 100 U/kg body weight three times a week. The maximum recommended maintenance dose is 300 U/kg body weight three times a week.[37]

Toxic Dose

The maximum amount of epoetin alfa that can safely be administered in single or multiple doses has not been determined. Doses of up to 1500 U three times weekly for 3 to 4 weeks have been administered without any direct toxic effects from the epoetin alfa itself.[36]

Fatal Dose

A fatal dose has not been established. No specific data are available on the cyclist deaths referred to earlier.

Toxicokinetics

Absorption

Serum concentrations of erythropoietin peak about 13 to 18 hours after a subcutaneous dose, and bioavailability over 72 hours is 20 to 36%.[38] Serum concentrations are still detectable after 4 days.[39] Serum concentrations after subcutaneous administration are about 5 to 10% of those found after the same intravenous dose. Peak serum levels of 1000 to 3000 U/L are measured after intravenous administration, and 32 to 484 U/L, after subcutaneous injection.[39]

Distribution

The apparent volume of distribution of epoetin alfa is about 40 to 90 mL/kg.[39,40]

Elimination

The half-life of recombinant human erythropoietin is 4 to 11 hours after intravenous use and 25 hours after subcutaneous administration.[40,41] Clearance values range from 4 to 15 mL/kg/h. Only a few nanograms are excreted unchanged in the urine.[39] The role of the liver in the metabolism of recombinant human erythropoietin is unclear.

Drug Interactions

Aluminum intoxication during hemodialysis may cause resistance to erythropoietin by interference with heme

Table 29–5
Registered Hematopoietic Colony-Stimulating Factors

Native Molecule	Generic Name	Brand Name	Manufacturer	Form
GM-CSF	Molgramostim	Leucornax	Schering Plough/Sandoz	Nonglycosylated
GM-CSF	Sargramostim	Leukine	Immunex	Glycosylated
GM-CSF	Sargramostim	Prokine	Immunex*	Glycosylated
G-CSF	Filgrastim	Neupogen	Amgen†	Nonglycosylated
G-CSF	Lenograstim	Neutrogin‡	Chugai	Glycosylated

GM-CSF, granulocyte–macrophage colony-stimulating factor; G-CSF, granulocyte colony-stimulating factor.
*Distributed by Hoechst-Roussel in the United States and to be distributed by Behringwerke in Europe.
†Distributed in conjunction with Roche outside the United States.
‡Brand name in Japan. Brand name to be Granocyte when distributed in Europe.
From Steward WP. Granulocyte and granulocyte–macrophage colony-stimulating factors. Lancet 1993;342:153–157.

synthesis, with accumulation of protoporphyrin.[41] Desmopressin may contribute to the improvement in bleeding time during treatment with recombinant human erythropoietin.[42] Theophylline appears to suppress production of erythropoietin by the kidneys.[43] Amphotericin B may blunt the erythropoietin response to anemia.[44]

Pregnancy/Lactation

Adequate and well-controlled studies during pregnancy in humans have not been done. Epoetin alpha has been placed in Pregnancy Category C. It is not known whether epoetin alpha is excreted in human breast milk.[38]

Mechanism of Action

Erythropoietin, which under normal conditions is present in small amounts in the plasma (12–21 mU/mL),[45] binds to specific receptor sites of erythroid progenitor cells (CFU-E), causing the cells to proliferate and differentiate into the morphologically recognized normoblasts. By this process, approximately 20 mL of new red blood cells is produced each day. The mechanism of action of recombinant human erythropoietin is identical to that of natural erythropoietin. The anemia of chronic renal failure is due primarily to a deficiency of renal-derived erythropoietin.[46]

Clinical Presentation

Hematocrits greater than 0.55 may be associated with encephalopathy, hypertensive seizures, vascular distension, impairment of blood flow resulting in hypoxia, and more rapid clotting possibly leading to phlebothrombosis, pulmonary embolism, myocardial infarction, or stroke. The hematocrit may continue to rise for 5 to 10 days after the last dose of recombinant human erythropoietin is administered, thus overshooting recommended maximum levels.

In an Olympic marathon, a male runner might begin the race with a hematocrit of 42 or 43%. With an outdoor temperature of 50° to 55°C he might finish with a hematocrit of 55% because of fluid loss. If the runner uses recombinant human erythropoietin he might begin the race with a hematocrit of 52 to 58%, and end the race with a hematocrit in the high sixties.[32] Unlike blood doping, recombinant human erythropoietin can be administered in private without medical personnel involved.[46]

Laboratory

Analytical Methods

At present there is no way to identify someone who uses the recombinant human erythropoietin. The recombinant hormone is virtually indistinguishable biochemically and immunologically from the native molecule.[47] A radioimmunoassay is available to measure serum or plasma erythropoietin levels. Its lower detection limit is 3 U/L.[48]

Blood Levels

Normal serum erythropoietin levels are about 10 to 20 U/L.[48] No correlation appears to exist between erythropoietin concentration and hematocrit excess or blood volume in polycythemia vera patients.[48]

Treatment

If excess hematocrits are observed, during routine serial hematocrit observations that accompany recombinant human erythropoietin administration, withhold the drug and perform a phlebotomy to decrease the hematocrit. Monitoring of blood pressure, cardiac and renal function, and neurologic status is paramount in the use of recombinant human erythropoietin. There are no antidotes. Elimination enhancement procedures (hemodialysis, hemoperfusion) may not be effective; however, clinical trials have not evaluated excess responses to recombinant human erythropoietin.

RECOMBINANT GRANULOCYTE AND GRANULOCYTE–MACROPHAGE COLONY-STIMULATING FACTORS

Registered hematopoietic colony-stimulating factors are listed in Table 29–5.[49]

Use

Neutrophil counts rise in a dose-proportional fashion in response to recombinant G-CSF in patients who are neutropenic after cancer chemotherapy.[50]

Clinical Presentation

At doses of 5 μg/kg/d or 25 μg/m^2/d, the most common unwanted effect is mild to moderate bone pain. About

20 to 30% of patients may have myalgia, malaise, rash, or injection site reactions.[51] Intravenous boluses and short infusions of GM-CSF are more likely to produce adverse effects. Effects are dose related. A syndrome of flushing, hypotension, tachycardia, dyspnea, nausea, and vomiting with arterial oxygen desaturation may occur after the first injection and is reversed by oxygen and intravenous fluids. At doses greater than 20 μg/kg/d, GM-CSF has been associated with pleural and pericardial effusions, venous thrombosis, and pulmonary embolism.[52] G-CSF has led to stimulation of multiple myeloma growth.[52]

A life-threatening hyperleukocytosis was introduced by GM-CST in an acute myelomonocytic leukemia patient.[53]

REFERENCES

1. Galvani DN. Cytokines, biological function and clinical use. J R Coll Physicians Lond 1988;22:226–231.
2. Windebaal KP. The cytokines are coming. Arch Dis Childh 1990;65:1285–1286.
3. Henderson B, Blake S. Therapeutic potential of cytokine manipulation. Trends Pharm Sci 1993;14:145–146.
4. Balmer LM. Clinical use of biological response modifies a cancer treatment: An overview. Part I. The interferons. DICP Ann Pharmacother 1990;24:761–769.
5. Goldstein D, Laszlo J. The role of interferons in cancer therapy: A current perspective. CA J Clinipharm 1988;38:258–265.
6. Stuart-Harris RC, Lauchlan P, Day P. NSW therapeutic assessment group. Med J Aust 1992;156:869–872.
7. Wills RJ. Clinical pharmacokinetics of interferons. Clin Pharmacokinet 1990;19:390–399.
8. Renault PF, Hoofnagle JH. Side effects of alpha interferon. Semin Liver Dis 1989;9:273–277.
9. Fent K, Zbinden G. Toxicity of interferon and interleukin. Trends Pharm Sci 1987;8:100–105.
10. Miranda-Guardiola F, Fdez-Liama P, Badia JR, et al. Acute renal failure associated with alpha-interferon therapy for chronic hepatitis B. Nephrol Dial Transplant 1995;10:1441–1443.
11. Crum E. Biological response: Modified-induced emergencies. Semin Oncol 1989;16:579–587.
12. Hamblin TJ. Interleukin 2: Side effects are acceptable. Br Med J 1990;300:275–276.
13. Kintzel PE, Colis KJ. Recombinant interleukin-2: A biological response modifier. Clin Pharm 1991;10:110–128.
14. Kragel AH, Travis WD, Stein RG, et al. Myocarditis or acute myocardial infarction associated with interleukin-2 therapy for cancer. Cancer 1990;66:1513–1516.
15. Denicoff KD, Rubinow DR, Papa MZ, et al. The neuropsychiatric effects of treatment with interleukin-2 and lymphokine-activated killer cells. Ann Intern Med 1987;107:293–300.
16. Vecht CJ, Keohane C, Manon RS, et al. Acute fatal leukoencephalopathy after interleukin-2 therapy. N Engl J Med 1990;323:1146–1147.
17. Rubin JT, Lotze MT. Acute gastric mucosal injury associated with systemic administration of interleukin-4. Surgery 1992;111:274–280.
18. Vial T, Descotes J. Clinical toxicity of interleukin-2. Drug Saf 1992;7:417–433.
19. Eberlein TJ, Schoof DD, Michie HR, et al. Ibuprofen causes reduced toxic effects of interleukin-2 administration in patients with metastatic cancer. Arch Surg 1989;124:542–547.
20. Lee RE, Lotze MT, Skibbher JM, et al. Cardiorespiratory effects of immunotherapy with interleukin-2. J Clin Oncol 1989;7:7–20.
21. Adamson JW, Vapnek D. Recombinant erythropoietin to improve athletic performance. N Engl J Med 1991;324:698–699.
22. Brien AJ, Simon TL. The effect of red blood cell infusion on 10 km race time. JAMA 1987;257:2761–2765.
23. Evans RW, Rader B, Manninen DL and Cooperative Multicenter EPO Clinical Trial Group. JAMA 1990;263:825–830.
24. Canadian Erythropoietin Study Group. Association between recombinant human erythropoietin and quality of life and exercise capacity of patients receiving haemodialysis. Br Med J 1990;300:573–578.
25. Wong KC, Li PKT, Lui SF, et al. The adverse effects of recombinant human erythropoietin therapy. Adverse Drug React Acute Poison Rev 1990;9:183–206.
26. Watson AJ. Adverse effects of therapy for the correction of anemia in hemodialysis patients. Semin Nephrol 1989;9(suppl. 1):30–34.
27. Schwenk MH, Halstenson CE. Recombinant human erythropoietin. DICP Ann Pharmacother 1989;23:528–536.
28. Undetectable dialysis drug is tied to athletes' deaths. Los Angeles Times, May 22, 1990, p. 1.
29. Berglund B, Ekblom B. Effect of recombinant human erythropoietin treatment on blood pressure and some haematological parameters in healthy men. J Intern Med 1991;229:125–130.
30. International Olympic Committee. Preliminary minutes from the Meeting of the IOC Medical Commission, Lausanne, April 7, 1990.
31. Cowart V. Erythropoietin: A dangerous new form of blood doping? Physician Sports Med 1989;17:115–118.
32. Lai P-H, Everett R, Wang F-F, et al. Structural characterisation of human erythropoietin. J Biol Chem 1986;261:3116–3121.
33. Hambley H, Mufti GJ. Erythropoietin: An old friend revisited. Br Med J 1990;300:621–622.
34. Product Literature. Epogen[R]: Epoetin Alfa. Thousand Oaks, CA: Amgen, 1989.
35. Epoetin Beta, Epoetin Alfa. USAN Council List No. 316. New names. Clin Pharmacol Ther 1990;47:667.
36. New biotechnology product treats anemia associated with renal disease; also under study for AIDS patients. FDA Drug Bull 1990;20(1):8.
37. Epoetin alpha, recombinant (systemic). USPDI Update 1990;1(3):113–116.
38. Macdougall IC, Roberts DE, Coles GA, Williams JD. Clinical pharmacokinetics of epoetin (recombinant human erythropoietin). Clin Pharmacokinet 1991;20:99–113.
39. Salmonson T, Danielson BG, Wikstrom B. The pharmacokinetics of recombinant human erythropoietin after intravenous and subcutaneous administration of healthy subjects. Br J Clin Pharmacol 1990;29:709–713.
40. Flaherty KK, Caro J, Erslev A, et al. Pharmacokinetics and erythropoietin response to human recombinant erythropoietin in healthy men. Clin Pharmacol Ther 1990;47:557–564.
41. Rosenlof K, Fyhrquist F, Tenhunen R. Erythropoietin, aluminum and anemia in patients on hemodialysis. Lancet 1990;335:247–249.
42. Jacquot C, Masselot JP, Berthelot JM, et al. Addition of desmopressin to recombinant human erythropoietin in treatment of haemostatic defect of uremia. Lancet 1988;1:420.
43. Bakris GL, Sauter ER, Hussey JL, et al. Effects of theophylline on erythropoietin production in normal subjects and in patients with erythrocytosis after renal transplantation. N Engl J Med 1990;323:86–90.
44. Lin AC, Goldwasser E, Burnard EM, Chapman SW. Amphotericin B blunts erythropoietin response to anemia. J Infect Dis 1990;161:348–351.
45. Eschbach JW, Adamson JW. Guidelines for recombinant human erythropoietin therapy. Am J Kid Dis 1989;14(suppl. 1):2–8.
46. Scott WC. The abuse of erythropoietin to enhance athletic performance. JAMA 1990;264:1660.
47. Egrie JC, Strickland TW, Lane J, et al. Characterization and biological effects of recombinant human erythropoietin. Immunobiology 1986;172:213–224.
48. Schlageter M-H, Toubert M-E, Podgorniak M-P, Najean Y. Radioimmunoassay of erythropoietin: Analytical performance and clinical use in hematology. Clin Chem 1990;36:1731–1735.

49. Steward WP. Granulocyte and granulocyte–macrophage colony stimulating factors. Lancet 1993;342:153–157.
50. Hollingshead LM, Goa KL. Recombinant granulocyte colony-stimulating factor (rG-CSF): A review of its pharmacological properties and prospective role in neutropenic conditions. Drugs 1991;42:300–330.
51. Stern AC, Jones TC. The side effect profile of GM-CSF. Infection 1992;20(suppl. 2):S124–S127.
52. Sal Rubia J, Bonanad S, Palau J, et al. Rapid progression of multiple myeloma following G-CSF mobilization. Bone Marrow Transplant 1994;14:475–476.
53. Einzig AI, Dutcher JP, Wiernik PH. Life-threatening hyperleucocytosis and pulmonary compromise after priming with recombinant human granulocyte–macrophage colony-stimulating factor in patient with acute myelomonocytic leukemia. J Clin Oncol 1995;13:304–305.

Chapter 30
Plasma Volume Expanders

INTRODUCTION

The choice of primary agents for volume replacement is limited. Blood and blood products have limited availability. There is increasing concern over infectious and immunologic risks, and the costs involved in obtaining, storing, crossmatching, processing, and dispersing blood and blood products continue to rise.[1] Blood and plasma substitutes provide a cost-effective alternative to blood products.

Suggested guidelines for the use of albumin and nonprotein colloid and crystalloid solutions are listed in Table 30–1.[2]

CRYSTALLOIDS

Electrolyte solutions containing sodium (crystalloids such as isotonic saline and Ringer's lactate solution) have no inherent oncotic pressure and, therefore, are relatively inefficient volume expanders (Table 30–2). The lowered osmotic pressure favors fluid movement to the interstitial compartment, setting the stage for interstitial pulmonary edema.[3] After intravascular infusion, these products are distributed over the entire extracellular fluid space. Only about 25% of the infused volume remains intravascular. If used alone to maintain blood volume, they will cause significant hypoalbuminemia.[4] Large volumes are required to result in effective plasma volume expansion. Studies by Shoemaker et al. indicate that colloid therapy may improve cardiac performance and oxygen transport.[5,6]

Shoemaker and colleagues believe the endpoint rather than the type of fluid used has become the principal question. The basic problem is how to increase oxygen transport at a cellular level in the critically ill. The aim is to increase cardiac index 50% above normal (>4.5 L/min/m^2), oxygen consumption 30% greater than normal (>170 mL/min/m^2), oxygen delivery greater than normal (>600 mL O_2/min/m^2), and blood volume 500 mL in excess of the norm (3.2 L/m^2 for males and 2.8 L/m^2 for females).[5,6] Wagner and D'Amelio have extensively reviewed these topics.[7]

Table 30–1
University Hospital Consortium Guidelines for the Use of Albumin, Nonprotein Colloid, and Crystalloid Solutions

Indication	Guideline
Hemorrhagic shock	Crystalloids should be considered the initial resuscitation fluid of choice. Colloids are appropriate for resuscitation in conjunction with crystalloids when blood products are not immediately available. On the basis of cost-effectiveness considerations,* nonprotein colloids are favored over albumin, except in the following cases: • If sodium restriction is required, the use of 25% albumin, diluted to 5% with 5% dextrose solution is recommended. • If nonprotein colloids are contraindicated, use of 5% albumin solution is recommended.† Crystalloid and colloid solutions should not be considered substitutes for blood or blood components when oxygen-carrying capacity is reduced and/or when replenishment of clotting factors or platelets is required. Patients who experience symptoms of shock while undergoing hemodialysis are included in this guideline and should receive crystalloid solutions as the resuscitation fluid of choice.
Nonhemorrhagic (maldistributive) shock	Crystalloids should be considered first-line therapy for nonhemorrhagic shock. The effectiveness of colloid solutions in the treatment of sepsis has not been demonstrated in clinical trials; however, in the presence of capillary leak with pulmonary and/or peripheral edema, or following the administration of at least 2 L of crystalloid solution without effect, nonprotein colloid may be used. If nonprotein colloids are contraindicated, albumin may be used.
Hepatic resection	Crystalloid use to maintain effective circulating volume following major hepatic resection (>40% resected) is recommended. The use of nonprotein colloid solutions and albumin is also appropriate, depending on the function of the residual liver and hemodynamic status. If crystalloids are not used, nonprotein colloids are recommended as the most cost-effective alternative.
Thermal injury	Crystalloid solutions should be used for initial fluid resuscitation (within the first 24 hours). Colloids should be administered in conjunction with crystalloids if all of the following are true: • Burns cover more than 50% of the patient's body surface. • At least 24 hours have passed since the burn occurred. • Crystalloid therapy has failed to correct hypovolemia. Based on cost-effectiveness considerations, nonprotein colloids are recommended. If nonprotein colloids are contraindicated, albumin may be used.
Cerebral ischemia	Colloid solutions are of no demonstrated value and should not be used in the treatment of ischemic stroke or subarachnoid hemorrhage. Their use for these indications should be discouraged, except in patients with hematocrit levels lower than 40% on admission. Patients with elevated hematocrit levels on admission should receive crystalloid solutions to increase intravascular volume, creating a state of hypervolemia and hemodilution (hematocrit levels of approximately 30% to maximize cerebral perfusion). Additional interventions (eg, blood removal) may be needed in such cases. Colloid solutions (both nonprotein and albumin) should be discouraged on the basis of cost-effectiveness considerations.
Nutritional intervention	Albumin should not be used as a supplemental source of protein calories in patients requiring nutritional intervention; however, patients with diarrhea associated with enteral feeding intolerance may benefit from the administration of albumin if all of the following conditions are met: • Significant diarrhea (>2 L/d) occurs. • Serum albumin is less than 20 g/L (2.0 g/dL). • Continued diarrhea occurs despite trial of short-chain peptide and elemental formulas; other causes of diarrhea have been considered and ruled out.
Cardiac surgery	Crystalloids should be the fluid of choice as the priming solution for cardiopulmonary bypass pumps. The use of nonprotein colloids in addition to crystalloids may be preferable in cases in which it is extremely important to avoid pulmonary interstitial fluid accumulation. For postoperative volume expansion, crystalloids should be considered the first-line solution, followed by nonprotein colloids, and finally albumin. Nonprotein colloids may be beneficial if reduction in systemic edema is required.
Hyperbilirubinemia of the newborn	Albumin should not be administered in conjunction with phototherapy. Albumin should not be used prior to exchange transfusion. Albumin has been used with mixed results as an adjuvant to exchange transfusions and should be administered only with concurrent transfusion of blood. Crystalloids and nonprotein colloids do not have bilirubin-binding properties and should not be considered as alternatives to albumin.
Cirrhosis and paracentesis	Albumin, administered alone or in conjunction with diet modification and diuretics, should be avoided for the treatment of cirrhosis with ascites removal of less than 4 L. Crystalloids should be considered the solution of choice to prevent complications associated with large-volume paracentesis, such as reduced effective plasma volume and renal dysfunction. Nonprotein colloids and albumin should be considered second-line agents for the prevention of complications following the removal of 4L or more of ascitic fluid.

*Therapeutic equivalence between products has been identified in several guidelines. In those instances, products are recommended based on economic considerations. Thus, nonprotein colloids (which are currently less expensive than albumin) are preferred over albumin. Changes in the relative cost of these products (eg, albumin becoming less costly than nonprotein colloids) should be reflected through modifications to the guidelines.

†Relative contraindications to the use of nonprotein colloids include, but may not be limited to, the following: (1) previous hypersensitivity to the components of the solution, (2) underlying bleeding disorders, (3) risk of serious intracranial hemorrhage, and (4) renal failure with either oliguria or anuria.

Table 30-1 *(Continued)*

Indication	Guideline
Nephrotic syndrome	Short-term albumin use, in conjunction with diuretic therapy, is appropriate for patients with acute, severe, peripheral, or pulmonary edema.
Organ transplantation	Albumin and/or nonprotein colloid administration has not been demonstrated conclusively to be effective during and/or after renal transplantation surgery. Albumin may be useful for postoperative liver transplant patients in the control of ascites and peripheral edema if all of the following conditions are met: • Serum albumin is less than 25 g/L (2.5 g/dL). • Pulmonary capillary wedge pressure is less than 12 mm Hg. • Hematocrit is more than 30%. In these cases, albumin may also be used to replace ascitic fluid lost through drainage catheters following liver transplantation. The use of albumin in liver transplantation is not well documented in the biomedical literature.
Plasmapheresis	Albumin, in conjunction with large-volume plasma exchange, is appropriate. Large-volume plasma exchange is defined as more than 20 mL/kg in one session, or more than 20 mL/kg per week in repeated sessions. Crystalloid solutions and albumin/crystalloid combinations should be considered as cost-effective alternatives for small-volume exchanges.
Indications with limited or inconclusive published supportive evidence, considered appropriate based on the results of the consensus exercise	Granulocytapheresis: Nonprotein colloid solution is appropriate as a sedimenting agent for donation of granulocytes and for acute cytareduction in chronic myelogenous leukemia (chronic granulocytic leukemia). Stem cell cryopreservation: Nonprotein colloid solution is appropriate as part of a cryopreservation solution for frozen storage of hematopoietic stem cells: • Pretreatment of Dacron aortic grafts: Albumin is appropriate to make grafts impervious to blood before insertion. • Red blood separation for major blood type incompatible bone marrow transplantation: Nonprotein colloids are appropriate. • Severe necrotizing pancreatitis: Albumin is appropriate.
Indications with limited or inconclusive published supportive evidence, considered inappropriate based on the results of the consensus exercise	Severe hypoalbuminemia; impending hepatorenal syndrome; increasing drug efficacy; uncomplicated pancreatitis

From Vermeulen LC Jr, Ratko TA, Erstad BL, et al. A paradigm for consensus: The University Hospital Consortium guidelines for the use of albumin, nonprotein colloid, and crystalloid solutions. Arch Intern Med 1995;155(4):373–379.

Table 30-2
Some Crystalloid and Colloid Preparations

	Normal Saline	Lactated Ringer's	5% Albumin	Dextran 70 6% Normal Saline	Hetastarch 6% Normal Saline
Na (mOsm L^{-1})	154	147	130–160	154	154
Cl (mOsm L^{-1})	154	109		154	154
Osmolality (mOsm L^{-1})	308	278	300	308	310
Plasma expansion per 500 mL (mL)	100	100	500	500–700	500–700
Large molecule size (means)	—	—	62,000–69,000	20,000–200,000 (70,000)	10–1,000,000 (70,000)
Elimination	—	—	Hepatic	Plasma hydrolysis Renal	Reticuloendothelial system Renal
Duration of expansion, approximate (h)	(Very transient)		24	24	36
Effect on coagulation	—	—	—	Impaired	?
Allergic reactions	—	—	0.011	0.03–4.7	0.85
Anaphylaxis	—	—	—	0.08–0.6*	0.006
Recommended maximum dose (mL kg^{-1} 24 h^{-1}	—	—	—	20	20
Cost to Emory University Hospital Pharmacy ($US)†	0.60/L	0.74/L	36.00/500 mL	7.22/500 mL	38.45/500 mL

*Preventable by prior administration of dextran.
†In Canada the cost of albumin is absorbed through the funding of the Red Cross, thus, only dextran and hetastarch use is reflected in the hospital or departmental budget.
From Ramsay JG. Methods of reducing blood loss and non-blood substitutes. Can J Anaesth 1991;38:595–612.

Table 30–3
Properties of Plasma Volume Expanders

Solution	Half-life	Distribution (%) EV	Distribution (%) IV	Osmotic Activity	Sodium Content (mOsm/L)
Albumin	5–10 d	20	80*	Depends on dilution	Depends on diluent
Dextran 40 (Rheomacrodex)	6–9 h		100	Hyperosmotic	154
Dextran 70 (Macrodex)	12 h		100	Hyperosmotic	154
Fluosol-DA 20%†	Short (h)		100	Isosmotic	
Fresh-frozen plasma	As for plasma components		100	Isosmotic	170–190
Hydroxyethyl starch	24 h		100	Isosmotic	154
Modified gelatins					
Urea-linked gelatin (Haemaccel)	4 h	50	50	Isosmotic	145
Succinylated gelatin (Gelofusin)	5 h	50	50	Isosmotic	154
Stable plasma protein solution	5–10 d	20	80*	Isosmotic	130–150

EV, extravascular; IV, intravascular
*Depends on permeability of the capillary endothelium.
†Fluorinated hydrocarbon whole blood substitute.
From Fisher MM, Brady PW. Adverse reactions to plasma volume expanders. Drug Saf 1990;5:86–93.

COLLOIDS

Synthetic colloids are confined mainly to the intravascular space because they contain colloid osmotic particles, which, because of their size, are largely retained by the normal capillary endothelial cells in the basement membrane. The osmotic pressure exerted by the molecules across the capillary endothelium ensures that the solution is confined to the intravascular space. These colloidal macromolecules are suspended in an electrolyte solution with a sodium concentration similar to that of plasma. The three main groups of synthetic colloids are the dextrans, the gelatins, and hydroxyethyl starch. For the medical toxicologist the major problems resulting from the use of plasma expanders fall into four major categories: anaphylactoid reactions, pulmonary edema, renal failure, and problems in blood clotting.

The physiochemical properties of several colloids are summarized in Table 30–3.

Types of Colloids

Dextrans

Two dextran solutions are now most widely used: a 6% solution with an average molecular weight of 70,000 (dextran 70) and a 10% solution with an average weight of 40,000 (dextran 40, low-molecular-weight dextran). The molecular weights are averages. Dextran solutions contain a range of various-sized dextran molecules. The colloid osmotic pressure is 268 mm Hg. Brand names include Rheomacrodex (dextran 40) and Macrodex (dextran 70). Dextran has a molecular weight lower than those of other plasma substitutes and a prolonged effect.

Hydroxyethyl Starch

Commercially available hydroxyethyl starch (HES, Hetastarch) solutions contain a heterogeneous solution of HES molecules, with an average molecular weight of 69,000, similar to albumin. Molecular size ranges from 1000 to 100,000. Hetastarch is available in the United States as a 6% solution in 0.9% sodium chloride. Pentostarch (average molecular weight, 250,000) is available in the United Kingdom as a 10% solution.[1]

Albumin

Albumin is available for intravenous infusion in 5% (50 mg/mL) and 25% (250 mg/mL) solutions.[8]

Gelatin

Gelatin is available as a 4% solution with electrolytes in the United Kingdom.[9] The two most commonly used modified gelatin solutions are Haemaccel, in which the gelatin is crosslinked by urea, and Gelofusin, in which it is crosslinked by succinylation.[10] Haemaccel has a 10-fold higher content of calcium and potassium than Gelofusin. This higher calcium content can lead to clotting in warming coils when Haemaccel is infused with blood.[10]

Use

Plasma volume expanders are used for plasma volume expansion, for antithrombotic effects,[11] and to improve microcirculatory blood flow.[1] Dextrans have also been studied as possibly effective modalities in the treatment of patients with myocardial ischemia, cerebral ischemia, and peripheral vascular disease and in maintaining vascular graft potency.[1] Oral dextran sulfate (UADD1), a low-molecular-weight (7000–8000) dextran, may have antiretroviral activity against human immunodeficiency virus type I.[12,13]

Source

Dextrans

Dextrans are produced by a specially developed strain of bacterium, *Leuconostoc mesenteroides*. The molecules produced by the bacteria are very large, with molecular weights of several millions.[1]

Hydroxyethyl Starch

Starch is the energy storage polysaccharide of plants and is analogous functionally and structurally to glycogen, the energy storage polysaccharide molecule of animals. Starch is composed of two types of glucose polymers: amylase, a linear molecule, and amylopectin, a highly branched molecule that structurally resembles glycogen. Amylopectin is rapidly hydrolyzed enzymatically by amylase hydrolysis with a half-life of only about 20 minutes. In the 1960s, the amylopectin molecule was modified to make it more stable within the plasma. This was done by substituting hydroxyethyl groups to create hydroxyethyl starch,[1] but its use in severe anemia has been disappointing.[14]

Gelatin

The gelatins are prepared by hydrolysis of bovine collagen with subsequent chemical modification.

Perfluorocarbons

Perfluorocarbons are 8- to 10-carbon fluorinated hydrocarbons. Oxygen is highly soluble in liquid perfluorocarbons. The perfluorocarbons have been considered to be useful as an "artificial blood."[1]

Stroma-Free Hemoglobin

Human hemoglobin solutions as oxygen-carrying blood substrates have been under research for about 70 years. Problems have included renal toxicity due to the erythrocytic stromal components of the early hemoglobin preparation and not to the hemoglobin itself. This has led to stroma-free hemoglobin solutions with erythrocytic membrane fragments removed.[1]

Albumin

Human albumin solutions are used as plasma volume expanders. They are prepared from pooled blood, plasma, serum, or placentas obtained from healthy human donors.

Therapeutic Dose

- Dextran 40 (10% Solution): Initial intravenous doses are often 500 to 1000 mL (50–100 g) rapidly over 30 to 60 minutes or occasionally over 4 to 6 hours. Subsequent doses of 500 mL are given on alternate days. Infants may be given 5 mL/kg body weight, and children, 10 mL/kg.[9]
- Dextran 70 (6% Solution): Initial doses are 500 to 1000 mL (30–60 g). A 32% solution of dextran 70 has been instilled in the uterus, at a dose of 50 to 100 mL, as a rinsing and dilation fluid for air hysteroscopy.
- Hetastarch (6% solution): 500 to 1000 mL[1] (30–60 g).[15]
- Gelatin (4% solution): Doses up to 2000 mL (80 g) for adults or 30 mL/kg body weight for children.[15]

Toxicokinetics

Absorption

Toxicokinetic properties of plasma volume expanders are listed in Table 30–3.[10]

Elimination

Hydroxyethyl Starch. Smaller molecules are excreted unchanged in the urine. Larger molecules diffuse into the interstitium, where slow enzymatic degradation occurs.[1] The plasma elimination half-life is about 17 hours, but has been as long as 48 days.[1,16–19] HES is metabolized by α-amylase in the blood.

Gelatin. Half-lives of 1.1 and 6.2 hours have been recorded. About 49% of a dose is recovered in the urine within 24 hours.[16]

Pregnancy/Lactation

A dextran 70 infusion in a pregnant woman induced an anaphylactic reaction.[20] After 100 mL of a dextran 40 solution was administered to a mother before an epidural block, an anaphylactoid reaction was observed with apparent death of the fetus. The fetus was delivered and recovered after vigorous cardiopulmonary resuscitation.[21] Similar cases due to modified fluid gelatin have been less frequent. There appears to be a substantial difference between clinical signs in the mother and those in the fetus.[21] In France there have been 32 reports of dextrans administered to pregnant women, including 18 neonatal deaths.[21]

Mechanism of Action

Dextran

Dextran inhibits platelet aggregation and renders fibrin more susceptible to fibrinolytic enzymes, features that make it useful in preventing venous thrombosis. Infusion of more than 20 mL/kg (1500 mL/70 kg) can reduce factor VIII levels, mimicking the changes of von Willebrand's disease. Dextran 70 is thus not the best choice for a plasma substitute where large volumes are needed. It also interferes with blood crossmatching, so that a blood sample must be taken before a transfusion is started.

Gelatin

The colloid osmotic pressure of Haemaccel (350–390 mOsm/L H_2O) is similar to that of plasma. That of Gelofusin (succinylated gelatin) is 405 H_2O mOsm/L. These products are marketed in the United Kingdom. Their more rapid glomerular filtration leads to osmotic diuresis and a shorter half-life: about 5 hours for Haemaccel and 5 hours for Gelofusin. Neither preparation appears to affect bleeding time or coagulation factors except through dilution.

Hydroxyethyl Starch

The particle size (molecular weight 70,000) and colloid osmotic pressure of HES are similar to those of 5% serum albumin. Forty percent of the starch is excreted within 24 hours. The plasma half-life, about 12 days, is longer than those of other plasma substitutes. Partial thromboplastin times and factor VIII activities may be decreased.

Clinical Presentation

Overdose

Excess intravenous doses of dextran 40 have resulted in acute anuric renal failure,[22–24] tachycardia, hypotension and hypoxia, pulmonary edema, adult respiratory distress syndrome,[25] coagulopathy,[26–28] congestive heart failure,[29] and fluid overload.

Anaphylactoid Reactions

Anaphylaxis has followed use of many of the colloids.[30,31] The reaction is mediated by IgG (type III Gell and Coombs response).[27] Ring and Messner determined that the incidence of anaphylactoid reaction was 0.85% with hydroxyethyl starch, 0.14% with gelatin, 0.007% with dextran 40, 0.069% with dextran 60/75, and 0.011% with human serum albumin.[32,33] The reactions can be severe and even fatal. With dextran infusions, the anaphylactoid reactions occur during infusion of the first 100 mL. Severe anaphylactoid reactions occur with no previous reactions to dextran given intravenously.[1] Haemaccel, a gelatin colloid, has been associated with severe anaphylactoid reactions, some of which have resulted in death. Reactions are more likely if Haemaccel is infused rapidly and if the patient is normovolemic.[34]

Coagulopathy

Fatal disseminated intravascular coagulation has followed infusion of HES[35] (see Laboratory). Low doses of dextran (less than 15 g/kg body weight) are not associated with clinical bleeding, but platelet adhesiveness and plasma levels of clotting factors are decreased. Larger doses are associated with bleeding complications.

Low doses of HES have no effect on coagulation. Moderate doses (20 mL/kg) transiently decrease platelet counts, prolong prothrombin and partial thromboplastin times, and decrease fibrinogen levels. Bleeding times remain normal, and platelet adhesiveness remains intact.[1] When very large doses (>20 mL/kg) of HES are administered there can be increased incisional bleeding, increased intraoperative blood loss, and spontaneous serosal bleeding.[1] HES has been associated with acquired von Willebrand's disease when administered in doses greater than 1 L.[36]

Perfluorocarbons

Perfluorocarbons induce a transient leukopenia, elevated liver function test values, increased pulmonary artery pressure, transient hypotension, hyperthermia, and pulmonary failure. An emulsifying agent in Fluosol is probably responsible for some of these adverse effects.[1,37]

Human Serum Albumin

Reported adverse events following albumin administration are summarized in Table 30–4.[38] The incidence of severe hypersensitivity reactions relating to human serum albumin appears to be small.[38]

Table 30–4
Reported Adverse Events Following Albumin Administration

System/Disorder	Adverse Events
Immune	Anaphylactoid reactions
Coagulation	Platelet aggregation inhibition
	Heparin-like activity
	Increased PT and PTT
	Decreased concentrations of fibrinogen, factor VIII, prothrombin, and antithrombin
Renal	Decreased sodium elimination, clearance, and filtered load
	Decreased osmolar clearance
	Decreased GFR
Metal loading	Increased aluminum, nickel, and chromium concentrations
Hepatic disease	Gastrointestinal bleeding
	Increased ascites
Cardiovascular	Increased CVP and PCWP
	Decreased LVSWI, CWUs, CWU:CVP, and LVSWI:PCWP
	Decreased ionized and total calcium
	Negative inotropic effect
	Postresuscitation hypertension
Respiratory	Increased F_{IO_2}:P_{O_2} ratio
	Increased pulmonary shunting
Serum amino acids	Decreased ILe:Leu ratio

CVP, central venous pressure; CWU, cardiac work unit; F_{IO_2}:P_{O_2}, inspired: arterial oxygen tension ratio; GFR, glomerular filtration rate; Ile:Leu, isoleucine: leucine; LVSWI, left ventricular stroke work index; PCWP, pulmonary capillary wedge pressure; PT, prothrombin time; PTT, partial thromboplastin time. From Gales BJ, Erstad BL. Adverse reactions to human serum albumin. Ann Pharmacother 1993;27(1):87–94.

Renal Failure

Renal failure has been observed after dextran 40 but has not been reported after dextran 70.[27] A similar result has followed infusion of gelatin,[39] but this observation has been subject to controversy.[40] The terms *osmotic nephrosis* and *hyperoncotic acute renal failure*[41] have been used to describe the renal failure following dextran administration. Dextran may induce vacuolization of the proximal tubular cells.[41] Birefringent particles have been observed in a number of tissues after dextran administration.[42]

Laboratory

Analytical Methods

Analytic techniques often do not distinguish between the different fractions of dextran. Residual plasma levels of dextran have been estimated by hydrolyzing the dextran to glucose, which is then determined by the anthrone method.[43,44] More accurate methods specific for molecular size include gel permeation chromatography, high-performance liquid chromatography, and nephelometric methods.[17] Grootendorst and colleagues suggest that measurement of the colloid osmotic pressure in the intensive care setting is preferable to measurement of the albumin concentration.[45]

Blood Levels

Following an intravenous infusion of 575 g of dextran 40, plasmapheresis blood levels of dextran fell from 18.75 to

7.75 mg/mL.[22] Infusion of 90 g of dextran 40 led to a serum dextran level of 13.7 mg/mL, which fell to 7 mg/mL after 12 hours of continuous arteriovenous hemofiltration and to 2.8 mg/mL following plasmapheresis.[23] Plasma oncotic pressure (normal, 22 mm Hg) rose to 31 mm Hg after an overdose of dextran 40. A pressure of 34 mm Hg was reached after an overdose of dextran 40.[24] In both patients, plasmapheresis led to reduction of the plasma oncotic pressure to normal levels.

Abnormalities

Bilateral pulmonary infiltrates were observed after a large dose of 32% dextran 70 in 10% dextrose was introduced into the uterus. This was accompanied by prolongation of the prothrombin time.[26] Prolonged prothrombin time and activated partial thromboplastin times, shortened thrombin and reptilase times, accelerated fibrinolysis, decreased levels of factor VIII, and functional platelet defects rarely follow HES infusion.[35,46,47] Macroamylasemia has followed infusion of 500 mL of 6% HES.[48]

Ancillary Tests

Dextran produces a turbidity that interferes with *ortho*-toluidine glucose measurements, resulting in a "factitious" elevation in blood glucose.[49] Hyperkalemia may follow HES infusions.

Treatment

Stabilization

Anaphylactoid Reaction. Treatment of anaphylactoid reaction is the same as that for true anaphylaxis and may require oxygen, sympathomimetic drugs, asthmatic drugs, and volume replacement, preferably with an alternative plasma volume expander.[10,34]

Pulmonary Edema. Pulmonary edema is treated symptomatically and supportively with oxygen, furosemide, and other medications as required.

Renal Failure. Renal failure is treated conservatively.

Coagulopathy. Coagulopathies are treated with multiple blood transfusions, including fresh-frozen plasma, platelet concentrates, cryoprecipitates, and packed red cells.[35]

Elimination Enhancement

Plasmapheresis has appeared to rapidly lower increased dextran levels, reduce plasma oncotic pressure, and improve glomerular filtration of urine after dextran overdoses and renal failure.[4,23] More specifically, renal function appears to return to normal not when the plasma colloidal osmotic pressure is normalized but when the concentration of dextran 40 is lowered to allow the tubular epithelium to recover. The increased oncotic pressure is the consequence, not the cause, of impaired renal function and decreased elimination of colloid.[24]

HUMAN SERUM ALBUMIN

Overzealous use of human albumin may lead to acute pulmonary edema or circulatory failure.

Structure and Classification

Albumin is a 580- to 585-amino-acid protein with a molecular weight of about 65,000. It is the major protein produced by the liver and its major functions include transport of a variety of substances in the blood and maintenance of osmotic pressure. The serum albumin level reflects its synthesis, degradation, and distribution.[50]

Use

Unlike synthetic colloids, human albumin binds reversibly with anions, cations, and some substances that are active or toxic only in the free form. It has anticoagulant properties, inhibiting platelet aggregation and enhancing the inhibition of factor Xa by antithrombin III. It may also have a role in preserving microvascular integrity.[51] There is no convincing evidence that albumin is better than synthetic alternatives for volume replacement; nor is there clear evidence for maintaining the serum albumin concentration above a certain level.[51] Some criteria for albumin use are listed in Table 30–5.[52]

Product Formulation

Commercial preparations of albumin usually contain no preservatives or antimicrostabilizers. Both 5 and 25% solutions of human albumin contain 130 to 160 mEq of sodium per liter. Five percent human albumin solutions are isoncotic with human plasma; 25% solutions are oncotically equivalent to five times their volume of human plasma. Five percent human albumin contains 50 mg/mL; 25% contains 250 mg/mL.

Source

The normal adult liver produces 200 mg/kg/d albumin or about 15 g/d in a 70-kg man. Infusion of colloids such as dextran and excess production of gamma globulin result in a rapid decrease in the rate of albumin synthesis. Infusion of excess albumin does not alter albumin synthesis but can increase the rate of degradation. Stress, trauma, malnutrition, infection, and irradiation decrease albumin synthesis, whereas cortisone and thyroid hormones stimulate albumin synthesis.[50]

Therapeutic Dose

The usual initial dose of human albumin is 25 g. This can be repeated in 15 to 30 minutes if the response is not adequate (pulse, blood pressure, presence and degree of shock, plasma protein content on oncotic pressure, hemoglobin or hematocrit values, degree of venous and pulmonary congestion). No more than 250 g of albumin (5 L of a 5% solution or 1 L of a 25% solution) should be administered within 24 hours.[8] In emergencies, the usual dose of human albumin for children is 25 g. In nonemergency situations, 25 to 50% of

Table 30–5
Criteria for Appropriate Albumin Use

Criterion	Conditions*	
	Clinical	Administration-Related
Shock		
Hemorrhagic	SBP <80 mm Hg, CVP <6 mm Hg, or PCWP <10 mm Hg	At least 1 L of crystalloid solution administered before second vial of albumin; blood or blood products are not available at or before albumin administration time; administered within first 2 h of blood loss
Nonhemorrhagic	SBP <80 mm Hg, CVP <6 mm Hg, or PCWP <10 mm Hg; hemoglobin and hematocrit concentrations stable (<10% decrease over preceding 24 h)	Concomitant administration of crystalloid solution; at least 1 L of crystalloid solution administered before second vial of albumin
Paracentesis	Removal of >3 L fluid; absence of peripheral edema	
Open-heart surgery		As cardiopulmonary pump prime; no greater than 37.5 g of albumin used per procedure
Post-liver transplantation		In intensive care unit immediately posttransplantation
Nephrotic syndrome	>3 g urine protein in 24 h; presence of peripheral edema	No greater than 25 g of albumin used; diuretic administered within 1 h following albumin
Hemodialysis-associated hypotension	SBP <80 mm Hg, CVP <6 mm Hg, or PCWP <10 mm Hg	Albumin used during or immediately following hemodialysis session; no greater than 25 g of albumin used per hemodialysis session
Burn injury	Involves >40% of body surface area, or full-thickness burn involving 20% of body surface area, or other cases to be reviewed by burn unit medical codirector	

CVP, central venous pressure; PCWP, pulmonary capillary wedge pressure; SBP, systolic blood pressure.
*All conditions must be met.
From Stumpf JL, Lechner JL, Ryan ML. Use of albumin in a university hospital: The value of targeted physician intervention. DICP Ann Pharmacother 1991;25:239–243.

the usual adult dose has been used. Premature infants have received 1 g/kg.

Toxicokinetics

Distribution

About 31 to 42% of the exchangeable albumin pool is located in the plasma compartment.[50] There is complete distribution of intravenous albumin within the intravascular space in 7 to 10 days.

Drug Interactions

Table 30–6 summarizes drugs bound to albumin and to α_1-acid glycoprotein. Conditions associated with a decrease or increase in levels of albumin and α_1-acid glycoprotein are listed in Table 30–7. Free drug level monitoring may be useful for valproic acid, phenytoin, carbamazepine, lidocaine, and disopyramide overdoses.

Table 30–6
Drugs That Bind to Albumin and α_1-Acid Glycoprotein

Albumin	α_1-Acid Glycoprotein
Midazolam	Dipyridamole
Warfarin (binds to site I)	Quinidine
Diazepam (binds to site II)	Alprenolol
Phenylbutazone	Imipramine
Dicumarol	Propranolol
Tolbutamide	Lignocaine (Lidocaine)
Indomethacin	Etidocaine
Salicylate	Bupivacaine
Phenobarbital	Methadone
Theophylline	Disopyramide
	Ketosteroid hormones
	Nortriptyline
	Chlorpromazine
	Meperidine

Clinical Presentation

Rapid infusion of human albumin solutions may cause vascular overload (Table 30–3).[38]

Laboratory

False elevations of serum alkaline phosphatase have been reported following the infusion of human serum albumin from placental sources due to the presence of heat-stable alkaline phosphatase in the products.[8] Human albumin solutions have contained aluminum and ammonium as contaminants.[53] These contaminants may accumulate in patients with impaired renal function. Plasma aluminum concentration may be considerably increased in infants receiving aluminum-containing antacids even in the presence of normal renal function. Careful monitoring of aluminum dosage and plasma aluminum concentration is indicated.[54]

Table 30-7
Some Conditions Associated With Altered Protein Concentration in Plasma

	Decrease	Increase
Albumin	Age (neonate, elderly) Burns Cancer Cirrhosis Enteropathy Liver abscess Malnutrition Nephrotic syndrome Pregnancy Renal failure Surgery Trauma	Benign tumor Neurosis Paranoia Psychosis Schizophrenia
α_1-Acid glycoprotein	Age (neonate) Severe cirrhosis Nephrotic syndrome Oral contraceptive Pregnancy	Age (elderly) Cancer Celiac disease Crohn's disease Infections Inflammatory states Myocardial infarction Obesity Renal failure Rheumatoid arthritis Stress Surgery Trauma
Lipoprotein	Hyperthyroidism Malnutrition	Alcoholism Hypothyroidism Obstructive liver diseases

From Barre J, Didey F, Delion F, Tillement JP. Problems in therapeutic drug monitoring: Free drug level monitoring. Ther Drug Monitor 1988;10:133–143.

Treatment

Observe patients (especially those with normal or increased circulatory volume) for signs of hypervolemia such as pulmonary edema or circulatory failure.

SPECIAL REFERENCES

- Mishler JM. Synthetic plasma volume expanders: Their pharmacology, safety and clinical efficacy. Clin Haematol 1984;13:75–92.
- Moss GS, Gould SA. Plasma expanders: An update. Am J Surg 1988;155:425–434.
- Estal BL, Gales BJ, Rappaport WD. The use of albumin in clinical practice. Arch Intern Med 1991;151: 901–911.

REFERENCES

1. Waxman K, Tremper KK, Mason GR. Blood and plasma substitutes: Plasma expansion and oxygen transport properties. West J Med 1985;143:202–206.
2. Vermuelen LC Jr, Ratko TA, Erstad BL, Brecker ME, Matuszewski KA, and members of the University Hospital Consortium Consensus Exercise on the use of albumin, nonprotein colloid and crystalloid solutions. Arch Intern Med 1995;155:373–379.
3. Moss GS, Gould SA. Plasma expanders: An update. Am J Surg 1988;155:425–434.
4. Machin S. Developments in plasma volume expanders. In: *Proceedings of a Symposium: Recent Advances in Plasma Volume Expanders, Royal College of Surgeons, Dublin,* May 1989.
5. Shoemaker WC, Appel PL, Karin HB, et al. Prospective trial of supernormal values of survivors as therapeutic goals in high-risk surgical patients. Chest 1988;94:1176–1186.
6. Shoemaker WC. Monitoring and management of acute circulatory problems: The expanded role of the physiologically oriented critical care nurse. Am J Crit Care 1992;1:38–53.
7. Wagner BKJ, D'Amelio LF. Pharmacologic and clinical considerations in selecting crystalloid, colloidal and oxygen-causing resuscitation fluids, part I. Clin Pharmacol 1993;12: 335–346.
8. McEvoy GK, ed. *AHFS Drug Information 94.* Bethesda, MD: American Society of Hospital Pharmacists, 1994:864–865.
9. Reynolds JEF, ed. *Martindale: The Extra Pharmacopoeia.* 30th ed. London: Pharmaceutical Press, 1993:652–653.
10. Fisher MM, Brady BW. Adverse reactions to plasma volume expanders. Drug Saf 1990;5:86–93.
11. Bergqvist D. Dextran in the prophylaxis of deep vein thrombosis. JAMA 1987;258:324–325.
12. Abrams DI, Kuno S, Wong R, et al. Oral dextran sulfate (UADDI) in the treatment of the acquired immunodeficiency syndrome (AIDS) and AIDS-related complex. Ann Intern Med 1989;110:183–188.
13. Lorentsen KJ, Hendrix CW, Collins JM, et al. Dextran sulfate is poorly absorbed after oral administration. Ann Intern Med 1989;111:561–566.
14. Kale PB, Sklar GE, Wesloocicz LA, Di Lisio E. Flusol: Therapeutic failure in severe anemia. Ann Pharmacother 1993; 27:1452–1453.
15. Reynolds JEF, ed. *Martindale: The Extra Pharmacopeia.* 30th ed. London: Pharmaceutical Press, 1993:653.
16. Klotz V, Kroemer H. Clinical pharmacokinetic considerations in the use of plasma expanders. Clin Pharmacokinet 1987; 12:123–135.
17. Boon JC, Jench F, Ring J, Messmer K. Intravascular persistence of hydroxyethyl starch in man. Eur Surg Res 1976;8: 497–503.
18. Yacobi A, Staill RG, Sum CY, et al. Pharmacokinetics of hydroxyethyl starch in normal subjects. J Clin Pharmacol 1982; 22:206–212.
19. Maguire LS, Strauss RG, Koepke JA, et al. The elimination of hydroxyethyl starch from the blood of donors experiencing single or multiple intermittent-flow centrifugation leukapheresis. Transfusion 1981;24:347–353.
20. Berg EM, Fasting S, Sellerold OFM. Serious complications with dextran 40 despite prophylaxis. Anaesthesia 1991; 46:1033–1035.
21. Barbier P, Jonville A-P, Autret E, Coureau C. Fetal risks with dextrans during delivery. Drug Saf 1992;7:71–73.
22. Zwaveling JH, Meulenbelt J, Van Xanten NHW. Effectiveness of plasma exchange in reversing elevated plasma osmotic pressure associated with dextran 40 overdose. In: *Proceedings, European Association of Poison Centres and Clinical Toxicologists, 1988:*71; Zwaveling JH, Meulenbelt J, Van Xanten NWW, Heine RJ. Renal failure associated with the use of dextran 40. Neth J Med 1989;35:321–326.
23. Kurnik BRC, Singer F, Groh WC. Dextran-induced acute anuric renal failure. Am J Med Sci 1991;302:28–30. Case report.
24. Druml W, Polzleitner D, Laggner AN, et al. Dextran 40, acute renal failure and elevated plasma oncotic pressure. N Engl J Med 1988;318:252–253.
25. Taylor MA, Diblasi SL, Bender RM, et al. Adult respiratory distress syndrome complicating intravenous infusion of low molecular weight dextran. Cathet Cardiovasc Diagn 1994;32: 249–253.
26. Choban MJ, Kalhan SB, Anderson RJ, Collins R. Pulmonary edema and coagulopathy following intrauterine instillation of 32% dextran 70 (Hyskar). J Clin Anesth 1991;3:317–319.

27. Ljungstrom K-G, Revenas B, Smedegard G, et al. Histopathological lung changes in immune complex mediated anaphylactic shock in humans elicited by dextran. Forens Sci Int 1988;38:251–258.
28. Mangar D. Documentation of high molecular weight dextran (Hyskan) solution entering the serum during hysteroscopy. Am J Obstet Gynecol 1992;166:771.
29. Golan A, Siedner M, Bahar M, et al: High output left ventricular failure after dextran use in an operative hysteroscopy. Fert Steril 1990;54:939–941.
30. Cron TA, Gerber H. Anaphylactoid reaction to Physiogel (Rm) SRK 5%: A contribution to the plasma substitutes controversy. Schweiz Med Wochenschr 1991;21:1773–1776.
31. Cullen MJ, Singer M. Severe anaphylactoid reaction to hydroxyethyl starch. Anaesthesia 1990;45:1041–1042.
32. Ring J, Messmer K. Incidence and severity of anaphylactoid reactions to colloid volume substrates. Lancet 1977;1: 466–469.
33. Ring J, Seifert J, Messmer K, Brendel W. Anaphylactoid reactions due to hydroxyethyl starch infusion. Eur Surg Res 1976;8:389–399.
34. Prevedoros HP, Bradburn NT, Harrison GA. Three cases of anaphylactoid reaction to Haemacce. Anaesth Intensive Care 1990;18:409–412.
35. Chang JC, Gross HM, Jang NS. Disseminated intravascular coagulation due to intravenous administration of Hetastarch. Am J Med Sci 1990;300:301–303.
36. Dalrymple-Hay M, Aitchison R, Collins P, et al. Hydroxyethyl starch induced acquired von Willebrand's disease. Clin Lab Haematol 1992;14:209–211.
37. Spence RK, McCoy S, Costabile J, et al. Fluosol DA-20 in the treatment of severe anemia: Randomized, controlled study of 46 patients. Crit Care Med 1990;18:1227–1230.
38. Gales BJ, Ersted BL. Adverse reactions to human serum albumin. Ann Pharmacother 1992;27:87–94.
39. Hussain SF, Drew PJT. Acute renal failure after infusion of gelatin. Br Med J 1989;299:1137–1138.
40. Frazer RS, MacMillan RR. Acute renal failure after infusion of gelatin. Br Med J 1989;299:1399.
41. Moran M, Kapsner C. Acute renal failure associated with elevated plasma oncotic pressure. N Engl J Med 1987;317: 150–153.
42. Bergonzi G, Paties C, Vassolo G, et al. Dextran deposits in tissues of patients undergoing hemodialysis. Nephrol Dial Transplant 1990;5:54–58.
43. Weet JF, Cobb CA, Lebrie SJ. A sensoautomated micromethod for dextran in the presence of glucose. J Lab Clin Med 1976;87:898–902.
44. Gabel LF, Kerkkamp HEM, Nederstigt JN. Dextran determination in human serum with the aid of an enzymatic glucose method. J Clin Chem Clin Biochem 1988;26: 655–658.
45. Grootendorst AF, Van Wilgenburg MGM, de Laat PHJM, van der Howen B. Albumin use in intensive care medicine. Intensive Care Med 1988;14:554–557.
46. Plasma substitute: The choice during surgery and intensive care. Drug Ther Bull 1987;25(10):37–39.
47. Stump DC, Strauss RG, Henriksen RA, et al. Effects of hydroxyethyl starch or blood coagulation particularly factor VIII. Transfusion 1985;29:349–350.
48. Kohler H, Kirch W, Horstman HJ. Hydroxyethyl starch-induced macroamylasemia. Int J Clin Pharmacol 1977;15: 428–431.
49. Mangar D. Letter. Anesth Analg 1992;75:644–645.
50. Guthrie RD Jr, Hines C Jr. Use of intravenous albumin in the critically ill patient. Am J Gastroenterol 1991;86: 255–263.
51. Soni N. Wonderful albumin? Not all it is cracked up to be. Br Med J 1995;310:887–888.
52. Stumpf JL, Lechner JL, Ryan ML. Use of albumin in a university hospital: The value of targeted physician intervention. DICP Ann Pharmacother 1991;25:239–243.
53. Chamubeau RAFM, Jorning GGA, Korse FG, Roos PJ. Ammonium in intravenous albumin preparations. Lancet 1993;342:1110–1111.
54. Tsou VM, Young RM, Hart MH, Vanderhoof JA. Elevated plasma aluminum levels in normal infants receiving antacids containing aluminum. Pediatrics 1991;87:148–151.

Chapter 31 Ticlopidine Hydrochloride

INTRODUCTION

Ticlopidine hydrochloride (Fig. 31–1) is a synthetic chemical inhibitor of platelet function that can cause both hematologic and gastrointestinal side effects.[1,2] In overdose, it has increased the bleeding time and induced life-threatening hemodynamic effects and coagulopathy. Treatment is symptomatic and supportive. The increase in bleeding time as well as the possible development of aplastic anemia may respond to corticosteroids. Ticlopidine is marketed as Triclid, Tiklind, and Ticlodone.[1]

Use

Well-controlled studies show that ticlopidine is of benefit in the reduction of nonfatal and fatal events in the heart, brain, and peripheral arteries.[3,4] It is indicated in the prevention of subsequent vascular events and in patients with transient ischemic attacks, completed atherothrombotic strokes, unstable angina, and, probably, intermittent claudication.[1,5,6] It is also used to prevent platelet loss during extracorporeal circulatory procedures.

Product Formulation

Ticlopidine hydrochloride is available as a white 250-mg film-coated tablet for oral administration.

Therapeutic Dose

The recommended therapeutic dosage is 500 mg/d in two divided doses taken with food.[2]

Toxic Dose

A 38-year-old ingested about 24 standard 250-mg tablets (total dose, 6000 mg). He survived without special therapy.[7] Ingestion of 10 g resulted in life-threatening hemodynamic instability and coagulopathy.[8]

Fatal Dose

A fatal dose has not been established.

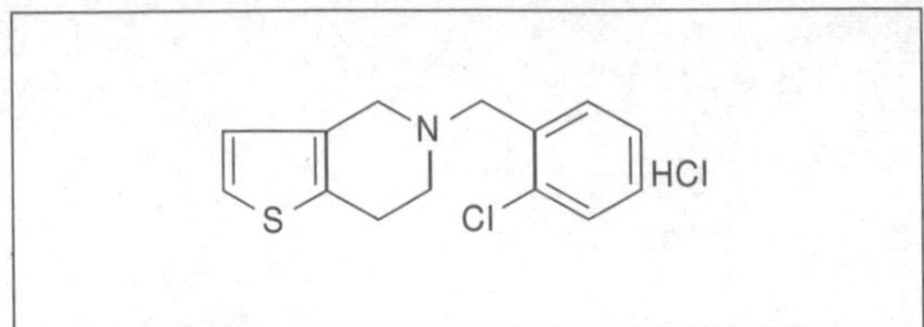

Figure 31–1 Structure of ticlopidine.

Toxicokinetics[2]

Bioavailability	90%
Peak plasma level	0.3–2.0 μg/mL
Time to peak plasma level	1–3 hours
Plasma protein binding	90%
Elimination half-life	24–36 hours
Excreted unchanged	<1%
Active metabolites	2-Keto derivative

Maximum effects on ADP aggregation and bleeding occur in 4 to 8 hours.[9]

Drug Interactions

Ticlopidine appears to reversibly inhibit the metabolic clearance of theophylline. Ticlopidine may induce a fall in mean cyclosporine concentration.[2] Prolongation of bleeding time caused by ticlopidine therapy is antagonized by orally and intravenously administered corticosteroids.[10] Ticlopidine appears to decrease digoxin serum levels .[11]

Pregnancy/Lactation

Ticlopidine is classified in Pregnancy Category B on the basis of animal studies. No controlled studies have been conducted in pregnant women or in women who are breastfeeding.

Mechanism of Action

Ticlopidine inhibits platelet aggregation induced by adenosine diphosphate (ADP), collagen, arachidonic acid, thrombi, and platelet aggregation factor.[3] It also reduces plasma fibrinogen (and, therefore, blood viscosity) and increases red cell deformation. These effects are associated with a dose-dependent prolongation of bleeding time, which peaks in 3 days and persists for up to 10 days after treatment. Unlike aspirin, ticlopidine does not interfere with the prostacyclin–thromboxane pathway.[5,12] Mechanisms and effects of antiplatelet agents are summarized in Table 28–4.[13]

Clinical Presentation

Overdose

Abnormalities may include an increased bleeding time and increased alanine transaminase concentration. Patients have been reported to recover without sequelae.[7]

Chronic Use

Chronic use has been associated with diarrhea,[14,15] rashes, neutropenia, prolongation of bleeding time,[16] decreased platelet function,[16] and hepatic dysfunction. All blood counts usually return to normal within 3 weeks of stopping the drug.[3] Gastrointestinal symptoms usually subside spontaneously. Cholestasis is infrequent.[17]

Ticlopidine is a known inducer of myelotoxicity and of aplastic anemia.[18,19] After 3 to 8 weeks of ticlopidine therapy, typical features of thrombotic thrombocytopenic purpura have developed.[20–22] A functional thrombasthenia state in normal platelets may follow administration of ticlopidine.[22]

Laboratory

Analytical Methods

A gas chromatography method with nitrogen–phosphorus detection is available for analysis of ticlopidine in plasma.[23] The lower limit of reliable measurement is 10 mg/mL.

Abnormalities

The major adverse effect of ticlopidine is a severe, reversible neutropenia, generally during the first 3 months of therapy.

Ancillary Tests

Although bleeding time is prolonged, serious hemorrhage is uncommon.

Blood Levels

There is no correlation between the plasma level of ticlopidine and its effect on platelet function.[9]

Treatment

Patients are treated largely with symptomatic and supportive measures. High doses of corticosteroids may be useful in aplastic anemia.[19] An intravenous injection of methylprednisolone or oral treatment with prednisolone counteracts the prolongation of bleeding time, but does not interfere with the inhibition of platelet aggregation brought about by ticlopidine. This may be due to the vasoconstrictive effect of corticosteroids, possibly through reduction of vascular prostacyclin release.[10] Granulocyte colony-stimulating factor improves the neutropenia.[24]

Frequent observation is required during the first 3 months of treatment to check for blood, skin, and liver toxicity.[7]

REFERENCES

1. Reynolds JEF, ed. *Martindale: The Extra Pharmacopoeia.* 30th ed. London: Pharmaceutical Press, 1993:234–235.
2. Ito MK, Smith AR, Lee ML. Ticlopidine: A new platelet aggregation inhibitor. Clin Pharm 1992;11:603–617.
3. Ticlopidine. Lancet 1991;337:459–460. Editorial.
4. Gent M, Blakely JA, Easton JD, et al. The CATS Group, The Canadian American Ticlopidine Study (CATS) in thromboembolic stroke. Lancet 1989;1:1215–1220.
5. Haynes RB, Sandler RS, Larson EB, et al. A critical appraisal of ticlopidine: a new antiplatelet agent: Effectiveness and clinical indications for prophylaxis of atherosclerotic events. Arch Intern Med 1992;152:1376–1378.
6. Macko R. Ticlopidine hydrochloride and prevention of stroke. West J Med 1993;159:182.
7. Lewis RH. Personal communication, Syntex Laboratories, Palo Alto, CA, June 3, 1992.

8. Horowitz RS, Bogart T, McCubbin T, et al. Cardiopulmonary instability, mental status changes and hemorrhage associated with overdose of ticlopidine (Ticlod[R]). Vet Hum Toxicol 1993;35:344.
9. Picard-Fraire C. Pharmacokinetic and metabolic characteristics of ticlopidine in relation to its inhibitory properties on platelet function. Agents Actions Suppl 1984;15:68–75.
10. Ticlopidine for prevention of stroke. Med Lett Drugs Ther 1992;34(874):65.
11. Vargas R, Reitran M, Teitelbaum P, et al. Study of the effect of ticlopidine on digoxin blood levels. Clin Pharmacol Ther 1988;43:176.
12. Coller BS. Platelets and thrombolytic therapy. N Engl J Med 1990;322:33–42.
13. Saltiel E, Ward A. Ticlopidine: A review of its pharmacodynamic and pharmacokinetic properties and therapeutic efficacy in platelet-dependent disease states. Drugs 1987;34: 222–262.
14. Guedon C, Bruna T, Ducrotte P, et al. Altered small bowel motility in severe chronic diarrhea with ticlopidine. Gastroenterol Clin Biol 1989;13:934–937.
15. Chasany O, Bacq Y, Metman EH, et al. Chronic severe diarrhea in the course of ticlopidine treatment. Gastroenterol Clin Biol 1989;11:950.
16. Balsano F, Cocchei S, Libretti A, et al. Ticlopidine in the treatment of intermittent claudication: A 21 month double-blind trial. J Lab Clin Med 1989;114:84–91.
17. Grimm IS, Litynski JJ. Cholestasis associated with ticlopidine. Am J Gastroenterol 1994;8:279–280.
18. Garnier G, Taillan B, Pesce A, et al. Ticlopidine and severe aplastic anemia. Br J Haematol 1992;81:1459–1460.
19. Mataix R, Ojeda E, Perez MDC, Jimenez S. Ticlopidine and severe aplastic anemia. Br J Haematol 1992;80:125–132.
20. Ellie E, Durrieu C, Besse P, et al. Thrombotic thrombocytopenia purpura associated with ticlopidine. Stroke 1992;23: 922–923.
21. Tardy B, Page Y, Tardy-Poncet B, et al. Thrombotic thrombocytopenia purpura related to ticlopidine. Thromb Haemostas 1991;65(suppl.):1082.
22. Di Minno G, Cerbone AM, Mattioli PL, et al. Functionally thrombasthenia state in normal platelets following the administration of ticlopidine. J Clin Invest 1985;75:328–338.
23. Shah J, Teitelbaum P, Molony B, et al. Single and multiple dose pharmacokinetics of ticlopidine in young and elderly subjects. Br J Clin Pharmacol 1991;32:761–764.
24. Ruiz-Irastorza G, Alonso JJ, Iglesias JJ, Aguirre C. Granulocyte colony-stimulating factor for neutropenia secondary to ticlopidine. Acta Haematol 1994;91:106–107.

Chapter 32
Antiarrhythmic Drugs

INTRODUCTION

Classes of Antiarrhythmic Drugs

The classification of antiarrhythmic drugs in outline in Table 32–1. The relationship between phases of the cardiac action potential and the surface electrocardiographic (ECG) recording are noted in Figure 32–1. Major ion currents underlying the cardiac action potential are outlined in Table 32–2.

Potassium and Class I Drugs

Hyperkalemia decreases automaticity, conduction, and contractility in myocardial cells. Hypokalemia increases the duration of the action potential and the refractory period leading to the occurrence of ventricular arrhythmias. In the initial phase of acute poisonings, either hyperkalemia (ajmaline, nadoxolol) or hypokalemia (disopyramide, ajmaline, cibenzoline, flecainamide) may be observed. In chronic overdoses, the toxicity of class I antiarrhythmic drugs may be enhanced by hyperkalemia (Table 32–2, Fig. 32–1).

Atypical Ventricular Tachycardia
Torsade de Pointes

Etiology. Antiarrhythmic agents in classes I and III of the modified Vaughan Williams classification are by far the most commonly reported drugs in association with this arrhythmia. Other nonarrhythmic medications and conditions that may be associated with Torsade de pointes are listed in Tables 32–3 and 32–4.

Definition. Torsade de pointes is a ventricular tachycardia characterized by QRS complexes of progressively changing amplitude and contour that seem to revolve around the isoelectric line (Fig. 32–1). The peaks of these complexes are successively located on one side of the baseline and then on the other, and this positive, then negative polarity in the frontal plane of the electrocardiogram creates the typical twisting-about-a-point appearance. Rates are 180 to 250/min. Long–short RR interval cycle sequences commonly precede the onset of Torsade de pointes. The diagnosis of Torsade de pointes is based on the characteristic ventricular

Table 32–1
Vaughan Williams' Classification of Antiarrhythmic Drugs

Class and Mechanism of Action	Examples
I. Sodium channel blockers	
A. Moderate-to-marked sodium channel blockade; prolongs refractoriness by blocking several types of potassium channel	Quinidine, procainamide, disopyramide
B. Mild-to-moderate sodium channel blockade; has little effect on refractoriness, as there is essentially no blockade of potassium channels	Lidocaine, phenytoin, mexiletine, tocainide
C. Marked sodium channel blockade; prolongs refractoriness by blocking outward-rectifying potassium channels	Encainide, flecainide, propafenone, moricizine
II. β-Adrenergic blockers Indirect blockade of calcium channel opening by attenuating adrenergic activation	Propanolol, metoprolol, atenolol, esmolol, timolol
III. Potassium channel blockers Prolongs refractoriness and delays repolarization by blocking potassium channels; has little direct effect on sodium channels	Amiodarone, bretylium, sotalol
IV. Calcium channel blockers Slows sinoatrial node pacemaker cells and atrioventricular conduction by direct blockade of calcium channels	Verapamil, diltiazem, nifedipine, nicardipine

From Katz AM. Cardiac ion channels. N Engl J Med 1993;328:1244–1251.

tachycardia and prolonged ventricular repolarization time, with QT intervals usually exceeding 500 milliseconds. Additional features that are sometimes present include a prominent U wave, abnormal contour of T or TU waves, T wave alternans, a subnormal spontaneous sinus rate (especially in children), and sinus pauses.[1]

Proarrhythmia

Aggravation or provocation of arrhythmias is known as *proarrhythmia*.[2] All types of bradyarrhythmia and tachyarrhythmia, whether supraventricular or ventricular, can be worsened or provoked by antiarrhythmic drugs (Table 32–5). Torsade de pointes is the prototype of ventricular tachyarrhythmias provoked by antiarrhythmic drugs. Incessant monomorphic ventricular tachycardia is another common form of proarrhythmia; this arrhythmia is often caused by class IC antiarrhythmic agents and usually has a QRS complex with a very long duration so that it appears "sinusoidal" in contour. During therapy with class IA drugs, the risk of developing proarrhythmia is increased by the presence of bradycardia, hypokalemia, or hypomagnesemia. Atrial fibrillation also seems to increase the risk of proarrhythmia.

Patients with quinidine-induced Torsade de pointes usually have QT intervals exceeding 550 ms. Patients at risk are probably those with preexisting QT prolongation, bradycardia not corrected by a pacemaker, hypokalemia or hypomagnesemia, a history of Torsade de pointes with similar drugs (because of cross-sensitivity), and genetic abnormalities in drug metabolism.

Other risk factors for proarrhythmia include toxic blood levels due to old age, renal disease, hepatic disease, heart disease, severe ventricular dysfunction (usually defined as an

Table 32–2
Major Ion Currents Underlying the Cardiac Action Potential

Action Potential Phase	Current	Direction	Effect of Current on Action Potential
Phase 0 (upstroke; inward >> outward currents)	I_{Na}	Inward	Rapid upstroke of action potential in atrial, ventricular, and Purkinje fibers
	$I_{Ca\text{-}L}$	Inward	Slow upstroke in many sinus and atrioventricular nodal cells
	$I_{Ca\text{-}T}$	Inward	Small component of rapid upstroke of action potential in atrial, ventricular, and Purkinje fibers
Phase 1 (initial repolarization; outward > inward currents)		Outward	Rapid early repolarization after overshoot of action potential
Phase 2 (plateau; inward ≈ outward currents)	$I_{Ca\text{-}L}$	Inward	Slow inactivation maintains early plateau phase
	I_{Na}	Inward	Slow inactivation maintains early plateau phase
	I_{NaCa}	Inward	May assist in maintenance of plateau phase
		Outward	Residual slowly inactivating outward current during plateau phase
Phase 3 (rapid repolarizaton; outward > inward currents)	I_K	Outward	Delayed rectifier repolarizes membrane to near resting potential
Phase 4 (diastole; inward ≈ or > outward currents)	I_{K1}	Outward	Maintains high negative resting potential near –90 mV
	I_f	Inward	Partially responsible for diastolic depolarization
	$I_{Na\text{-}B}$	Inward	Partially responsible for diastolic depolarization

I_{Na} = fast inward sodium current; $I_{Ca\text{-}L}$ = slow inward calcium current through L-type channels; $I_{Ca\text{-}T}$ = slow inward calcium current through T-type channels; I_{TO} = transient outward potassium current; I_{NaCa} = electrogenic sodium–calcium exchange current; I_K = outward delayed rectifer potassium current; I_{K1} = outward potassium current that exhibits anomalous (inward-going) rectification; I_f = inward pacemaker current; $I_{Na\text{-}B}$ = inward background sodium content.
From Tan HL, Hou CJ, Lauer MR, Sung RJ. Electrophysiologic mechanisms of the long QT interval syndromes and Torsade de pointes. Ann Intern Med 1995;122:701–714.

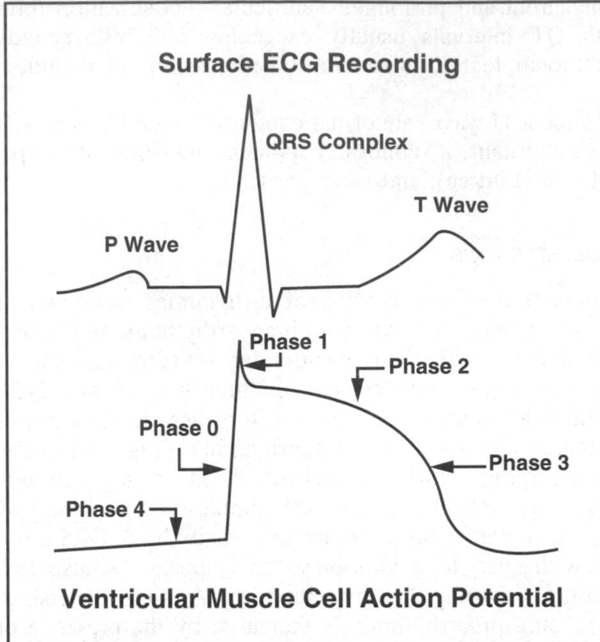

Figure 32-1 Relationship between phases of the cardiac action potential and the surface electrocardiographic (ECG) recording. The QT interval roughly corresponds to the plateau phase of the action potential. The broad T wave is inscribed as a result of the rapid repolarization occurring nonsimultaneously throughout the ventricles. The QT interval is prolonged by agents or conditions that delay repolarization in the ventricular cells. (From Tan HL, Hou CJ, Laver MR, Sung RJ. Electrophysiological mechanisms of the long QT interval and Torsade de pointes. Ann Intern Med 1995;122:701–714.)

ejection fraction <35%), serious presenting arrhythmia (ie, sustained ventricular tachycardia or fibrillation), concomitant digitalis therapy, hypokalemia or hypomagnesemia, bradycardia or intermittent long RR intervals on background electrocardiogram, and certain drug combinations (eg, class IA plus class IA, class IA plus class III, and class IA plus a tricyclic antidepressant drug).[2]

In general, drug-induced ventricular tachyarrythmias develop soon after drug therapy begins. Onset of proarrhythmia after a period of stable, long-term drug treatment is probably due to an intervening event such as ischemia, hypokalemia, addition of another drug, or change in drug dose.

Treatment

Avoidance of the precipitating drug is mandatory.

Intravenous magnesium and temporary atrial or ventricular pacing are the initial choices in therapy. Temporary pacing suppresses the ventricular tachycardia, which often does not recur even after cessation of pacing. Administration of isoproterenol to increase heart rate can be tried cautiously until pacing is instituted.

Class IB drugs can also be tried, as they decrease action potential duration. The vasodilators pinacidil and cromakalim decrease cardiac action potential duration by activating the ATP-dependent potassium current.

Prostaglandins are other therapeutic possibilities.

If drug discontinuance does not result in clinical improvement, then intravenous magnesium therapy may be of value.[3] Intravenous magnesium sulfate (single bolus of 1 g) suppresses the acquired form of Torsade de pointes in 2 to 5 minutes. A second bolus of 1 to 4 g may be given 5 to 15 minutes later. Continuous infusion of 2 to 20 mg/min is administered for up to 48 hours until the QT regresses below 0.50 seconds.[1,4,5] Hypokalemia is treated with oral or

Table 32–3
Etiology of Torsade de Pointes

I. Congenital QT prolongation syndromes
   Jervell and Lang–Nielson
   Romano–Ward
II. Cardiac
   Myocardial ischemia
   Myocardial infarction
   Myocarditis
   Bradycardia
   Atrioventricular block
III. Electrolyte abnormalities
   Hypokalemia
   Hypomagnesemia
   Hypocalcemia
   Liquid protein diet
IV. Neurologic
   Subarachnoid hemorrhage
   Cerebrovascular accident
   Pneumoencephalography
V. Environmental/toxin
   Hypothermia
   Arsenic
   Organophosphate insecticides
VI. Pharmacologic agents
   A. Psychotropic agents
      Phenothiazines
      Thioridazine
      Trifluperazine
      Chlorpromazine
   B. Antidepressants
      Amitriptyline
      Imipramine
      Maprotiline
   C. Antiarrhythmic agents
      1. Sodium (fast channel) antagonists
         a. Quinidine
            Procainamide
            Disopyramide
            Ajmaline
         b. Lidocaine
            Mexilitene
            Tocainide
            Aprinide
         c. Encainide
      2. Sympathetic antagonists
         a. Propranolol
      3. Antifibrillatory agents
         a. Amiodarone
         b. *N*-Acetylprocainamide
         c. Sotalol
      4. Calcium (slow channel) antagonists
         a. Lidoflazine
         b. Bepridil
         c. Nifedipine
      5. Anion antagonists
         a. None
   D. Vasodilators
      Prenylamine
      Fenoxidil
   E. Miscellaneous
      Diuretics
      Corticosteroids
      Atropine
      Isoproterenol

From Vukmir RB. Torsade de pointes: A review. Am J Emerg Med 1991;19: 250–255.

intravenous potassium supplements.[3] Hypomagnesemia is usually not present.[3] The only common side effect of magnesium sulfate is a short-lasting flushing sensation during the intravenous bolus.[5] Mild hypotension may also be observed. Common cardiovascular effects of excess magnesium include hypotension, transient tachycardia followed by bradycardia, electrocardiographic change (increased PR, QRS, and QT intervals, variable decrease in P-wave voltage, variable degree of T-wave peaking), heart block at high concentrations, and arrest in asystole at high concentrations. If magnesium sulfate therapy is unsuccessful, ventricular or atrial pacing may be appropriate where an existing arrhythmia is aggravated by an antiarrhythmic agent. Direct-current cardioversion may be necessary.[2]

Patients may require no treatment, especially if the rate is slow and the ventricular complex is an escape beat. Multifocal or multiple (5–10/min) ventricular premature beats usually respond to lidocaine. Alternative antiarrhythmic drugs include procainamide, bretylium, and propranolol. When the rhythm is slow and the ventricular complexes are escape beats, antiarrhythmic drugs should not be administered because they may suppress the escape pacemakers.

Table 32-4
Nonarrhythmic Medications With Reported Proarrhythmic Effects

Antimicrobial Agents
Pentamidine
Amantadine
Erythromycin
Trimethoprim–sulfamethoxazole
Chloroquine
Central Nervous System Agents
Antidepressants (tricyclics, amoxapine, maprotiline, trazodone)
Monoamine oxidase inhibitors
Steroids
Miscellaneous Agents
Organophosphates
Anesthetics
Probucol
Coronary vasodilators (prenylamine, lidoflazine, bepridil)
Inotropic agents (amrinone, milrinone, dobutamine)
Sotalol

From Martyn R, Sumberg JC, Kerin NZ. Proarrhythmia of nonantiarrhythmic drugs. Am Heart J 1993;126:201–205.

Laboratory Identification

Blood levels of antiarrhythmic drugs are discussed under their appropriate drug headings. A urine screen has been elaborated for identification of the antiarrhythmic drugs ajmaline, aprindine, diltiazem, disopyramide, flecainide, ballopamil, lidocaine, lorcainide, mexiletine, phenytoin, prajmaline, propafenone, quinidine, sparteine, tocainide, and verapamil and their metabolites. After acid hydrolysis of the conjugates, extraction, and acetylation, the urine samples are

Table 32-5
Proarrhythmic Effects of Agents Used for Treating Atrial Fibrillation or Flutter

Adverse Effect	Agents Most Commonly Causing Adverse Effect	Comments
Torsade de pointes	Quinidine, disopyramide, procainamide, sotalol	Almost all antiarrhythmic agents can cause Torsade but it is most common with IA agents and sotalol. Hypokalemia and bradycardia are precipitating factors. Risk of 1–2% in patients prescribed quinidine (fatal in 0.5–1%).
Monomorphic ventricular tachycardia or ventricular fibrillation	All antiarrhythmic agents implicated	Rare unless significant ventricular dysfunction present. Risk factors same as those for ventricular tachycardia in patients treated for ventricular arrhythmias.
Increased frequency or duration of paroxysmal atrial fibrillation or flutter	Digoxin, verapamil, diltiazem	Prevalence unknown. Clinical significance depends on severity of symptoms during atrial arrhythmia.
Acceleration of ventricular rate by enhanced AV nodal conduction, decreased atrial rate or conversion of fibrillation to flutter	Quinidine, disopyramide, flecainide, propafenone, lidocaine	Increase in rate may be associated with aberrant conduction, hemodynamic compromise, or both. Flutter with 1:1 conduction may occur in 1–2% of patients treated for atrial fibrillation or flutter with IC agents, many of whom will develop significant symptoms.
Acceleration of ventricular rate in the WPW syndrome with atrial fibrillation	Verapamil, digoxin, lidocaine, propranolol	Intravenous drug most commonly involved. Verapamil and digoxin may cause life-threatening arrhythmias. Lidocaine and propranolol have been associated with increased ventricular rate, but this is very rare.
Aggravation of sinus node disease in the tachycardia–bradycardia syndrome	Virtually all antiarrhythmic agents including digoxin, calcium blockers, and beta blockers in susceptible patients	Tends to occur at the onset of a paroxysm of atrial arrhythmia. Suspect in a patient with paroxysmal atrial fibrillation and worsening or new dizziness with drug therapy. Prevalence varies with drug and severity of sinus node disease.
High-degree AV block	Digoxin Type IA or IC agents	Uncommon complication. Generally occurs in patients with severe AV nodal or infra-His conduction system disease. May be life-threatening if complete block occurs.
Aberrant ventricular conduction	Flecainide, propafenone	Main significance is difficulty differentiating atrial flutter from ventricular tachycardia. Aberration is most frequently tachycardia related.

AV, atrioventricular; WPW, Wolff–Parkinson–White.
From Falk RH. Proarrhythmia in patients treated for atrial fibrillation or flutter. Ann Intern Med 1992;117:141–150. Erratum. 1992;117:446E.

analyzed by computed gas chromatography–mass spectrometry.[6]

Cardiovascular Function*

Preload/Intravascular Volume

Physiologic determinants and examples of toxic effects include (1) fluid intake, which is influenced by many toxic causes of impaired mental status or ability to drink and hormonal (eg, antidiuretic hormone) effects such as the syndrome of inappropriate antidiuretic hormone secretion (eg, chlorpropamide, phenformin, vasopressin), and (2) fluid losses, which can be due to gastrointestinal bleeding (metals, corrosives, alcohols, salicylates), anticoagulation (long-acting rodenticides, coumadin), hepatic failure (acetaminophen, amatoxins), and disseminated intravascular coagulation, which may be induced by crotalid envenomation or hyperthermia.

Gastrointestinal fluid losses may be secondary to the following:

- Vomiting, local effects: chemical burns, metals, salicylates, fluoride, soaps and detergents, colchicine, mushrooms, staphylococcal food poisoning
- Vomiting, central effects: opioids, nicotine, cardiac glycosides
- Vomiting, local and central effects: theophylline, caffeine, ipecac
- Stool losses, local effects: chemical burns, metals, mushrooms, colchicine, podophyllin, solanine plants
- Stool losses, cholinergic stimulation: organophosphates, carbamates, physostigmine
- Iatrogenic stool losses due to cathartics or laxatives

Insensible losses may be secondary to sweat (eg, cholinergic excess, sympathomimetic excess, black widow envenomation, salicylates, dinitrophenol) and respiratory loss (observed in salicylate and dinitrophenol poisoning). Urinary loss may be secondary to diuretics or diabetes insipidus (eg, lithium, demeclocycline) and edema or effusions secondary to chemical burns, arsenic, mercury, or iron. Intraluminal fluid loss is observed with sorbitol. Losses due to dermal chemical burns and anaphylaxis secondary to antibiotics, aspirin, *Hymenoptera* stings, or antivenins have also been observed. Venous smooth muscle tone is affected by sympathetic α_1 constriction or β_2 dilation. The main effect of most vasodilators is usually arterial, but venodilators include nitrites and nitrates (amyl, isobutyl, ethyl, and butyl nitrites and antiangina agents) and iron.

Afterload/Vascular Resistance

Arterial/arteriolar smooth muscle tone is influenced by sympathetic (α_1, peripheral α_2 constriction, β_2 antagonists, and central α_2 dilation) and cholinergic effects resulting in slight dilation and coronary constriction.

- α_1 **agonists** (hypertension): epinephrine, norepinephrine, dopamine (high dose), phenylephrine, methoxamine (*direct*); amphetamines, cocaine, dopamine (medium dose), monoamine oxidase inhibitors (*indirect*); ephedrine, phenylpropanolamine, pseudoephedrine (*direct/indirect*).
- α_1 **antagonists** (hypotension): phentolamine, prazosin, cyclic antidepressants, phenothiazines (*receptor blockers*); guanethidine (*postganglionic reuptake blockade*); reserpine (*norepinephrine depletion*).
- α_2 **agonists** (transient hypertension from peripheral stimulation, persistent hypotension from central stimulation): clonidine, guanabenz, methyldopa, oxymetazoline/tetrahydrozoline.
- α_2 **antagonists** (transient hypotension, then hypertension): yohimbine.
- β_2 **agonists:** Hypotension is rare because nonspecificity usually balances β_2 vasodilation with β_1 increased cardiac output. Theophylline-induced hypotension is probably due to β_2 vasodilation.
- β_2 **antagonists:** Hypertension is rare because of concomitant decrease in cardiac output. Beta blockade in setting of cocaine may result in hypertension.
- Vasoconstrictors: (hypertension) ergot agents, vasodilators; (hypotension) ethanol, nitrates, nitrites, angiotensin-converting enzyme inhibitors, hydralazine, diazoxide, minoxidil, magnesium.

Inotropy/Cardiac Pump Function

Toxicity is affected by synchronization and rapidity of cardiac conduction, force of cardiac contraction, for example, actin–myosin contraction associated with increased available calcium (increased contractility/hypertension: catecholamines, glucagon, theophylline/caffeine, digitalis glycosides (therapeutic), or calcium antagonists; decreased contractility/hypotension: calcium channel blockers, magnesium, profound hypocalcemia, relaxation, sarcoplasmic reticulum uptake of calcium [efflux of calcium reduces sarcoplasmic reticulum calcium], decrease in calcium–troponin C binding). The increased troponin–tropomyosin inhibition of actin–myosin leads to actin–myosin relaxation, which may be rapid (increases contractility) secondary to catecholamine production or delayed (decreases contractility) as observed with profound hypercalcemia and massive digitalis glycosides (overdose).

Viability of cardiac tissue is dependent on its nutrient supply (eg, oxygen), which is in turn affected by coronary vasoconstrictors such as cocaine, ergot agents, sympathomimetic agents, nicotine, and metabolic function (eg, enzymatic, mitochondrial, microtubular) affected by cyanide, carbon monoxide, arsenic, iron, selenious acid, sodium monofluoroacetate, colchicine/podophylline, and miscellaneous injury (eg, secondary to doxorubicin and ipecac).

Heart Rate and Rhythm

Sinus rate is influenced by autonomic input due to sympathetic tone (β_1 increases rate) and cholinergic tone (decreases rate). Toxic effects may be secondary to β_1 agonists (increase rate) including epinephrine, amphetamines, cocaine, theophylline/caffeine, albuterol (hypoxia, hypotension); β_1 antagonists (decrease rate) following beta blocker exposure; α_2 agonists (decrease central sympathetic output, decrease rate) including clonidine, guanabenz, methyldopa, and

*This section is adapted from Smilkstein[7] and Ellenhorn and Barreloux.[8]

oxymetazoline/tetrahydrozoline; and cholinergic stimulation (decreases rate) due to cholinesterase inhibitors, digitalis glycosides, centrally increased vagal tone (many causes), and cholinergic inhibition (increases rate) caused by anticholinergic agents or cyclic antidepressants. Decreased automaticity, which decreases the rate, may be due to digitalis glycosides (high dose), calcium channel blockers, hyperkalemia, high-dose cyclic antidepressants, cocaine, and type IA, IB, and IC antidysrhythmic agents. Decreased atrioventricular conduction (atrioventricular block) may be induced by digitalis glycosides, calcium channel blockers, adenosine, class IC/III (bretylium) antidysrhythmic agents, and dysrhythmias due to changes in normal automaticity. Triggered rhythms are due to early afterdepolarizations (Torsade caused by class Ia and III antidysrhythmic agents) and delayed afterdepolarizations (ventricular dysrhythmias caused by digitalis glycosides). Examples of reentry effects include atrioventricular nodal reentry (digitalis), ventricular dysrhythmias (ventricular tachycardia caused by cyclic antidepressants and other antidysrhythmic agents), and marked conduction block/bradyasystole, often the end result of many exposures (cyclic antidepressants, cocaine, antidysrhythmic agents, antihistamines, digitalis, etc).

Pregnancy

With few exceptions, antiarrhythmic medications appear to be relatively safe. Most are U.S. Food and Drug Administration (FDA) Category C, meaning that either there are animal studies suggesting risk but no confirmatory human studies or there are no controlled studies in both human beings and animals. Of the class IA agents, quinidine has the longest record of safe use during pregnancy. Procainamide appears to be equally safe, is well tolerated over short-term therapy (months), and has the advantage of intravenous dosing. Class IB drugs include lidocaine, which appears to be relatively safe as an intravenous antiarrhythmic agent. Phenytoin is contraindicated because of the risk of birth defects (FDA category X). Class IC agents, which include flecainide and propafenone, appear to be relatively safe, although experience is limited.[9]

Table 32–6
Antiarrhythmic Drugs in Pregnancy

Drug	Class: Vaughan-Williams	Class: FDA*	Placental Transfer	Adverse Effects	Teratogenic	Transfer to Breast Milk	Risk†
Quinidine	IA	C	Yes	Thrombocytopenia, rarely oxytocic	No	Yes‡	Minor
Procainamide	IA	C	Yes	None	No	Yes‡	Minor
Disopyramide	IA	C	Yes	Uterine contraction	No	Yes‡	Minor (L)
Lidocaine	IB	C	Yes	Bradycardia, central nervous system side effects	No	Yes‡	Minor
Mexiletine	IB	C	Yes	Bradycardia; low weight	No	Yes‡	Minor (L)
Tocainide	IB	C	Unknown	Unknown	Unknown	Unknown	Minor (L)
Phenytoin	IB	X	Yes	Mental and growth retardation, fetal hydantoin syndrome	Yes	Yes‡	Significant
Flecainide	IC	C	Yes	None	No	Yes‡	Minor (L)
Propafenone	IC	C	Yes	None (L)	No	Unknown	Minor (L)
Moricizine	I	B	Unknown	Unknown	No	Yes	Minor (L)
Propranolol	II	C	Yes	Growth retardation, bradycardia, apnea, hypoglycemia	No	Yes‡	Minor
Sotalol	III	B	Yes	Beta-blocker effects	No	Yes‡	Minor (L)
Amiodarone	III	D	Yes	Hypothyroidism, growth retardation, premature birth, large fontanelle	Yes?	Yes	Significant
Bretylium	III	C	Unknown	Unknown	Unknown	Unknown	Moderate (L)
Verapamil	IV	C	Yes	Bradycardia, heart block, hypotension	No	Yes‡	Moderate
Diltiazem	IV	C	No	Unknown	Unknown	Yes‡	Moderate (L)
Digoxin	NA	C	Yes	Low birth weight	No	Yes‡	Minor
Adenosine	NA	C	No (L)	None	No	Unknown	Minor (L)

(L), Very limited experience; NA, not applicable.
*FDA class (use-in-pregnancy ratings): (A) Controlled studies show no risk. Adequate, well-controlled studies in pregnant women have failed to demonstrate risk to the fetus. (B) No evidence of risk in human beings. Either animal findings show risk, but human findings do not or, if no adequate human studies have been done, animal findings are negative. (C) Risk cannot be ruled out. Human studies are lacking, and animal studies are either positive for fetal risk, or lacking as well; however, potential benefits may justify the potential risk. (D) Positive evidence of risk. Investigational postmarketing data show risk to the fetus. Nevertheless, potential benefits may outweigh the potential risk. (X) Contraindicated in pregnancy. Studies in animals or humans or investigational or postmarketing reports have shown fetal risk that clearly outweighs any possible benefit to the patient.
†Risk of causing injury to fetus.
‡American Academy of Pediatrics considers drug to be "usually compatible with breast feeding."
From Page RL. Treatment of arrhythmias during pregnancy. Am Heart J 1995;130:871–876.

Class II (beta-adrenergic blocking) agents generally have been well tolerated. Cardioselective agents such as metoprolol and atenolol might interfere less with β_2-mediated peripheral vasodilation or uterine relaxation and are the preferred agents. Class III agents are characterized by delay of repolarization. Sotalol appears to be relatively safe, although there is a risk of Torsade de pointes (polymorphic ventricular tachycardia in the setting of a prolonged QT interval).[9]

Amiodarone is associated with serious adverse effects on the fetus, including hypothyroidism, growth retardation, and premature delivery. The effects of bretylium during pregnancy are unknown.[9]

With respect to the calcium channel blocking agents (Vaughan Williams Class IV), especially verapamil, there are reports of maternal and/or fetal bradycardia, heart block, depression of contractility, and hypotension during treatment of fetal arrhythmias.[9]

Although classified in FDA Category C, digoxin is perhaps the safest agent for use in pregnancy. The serum concentration in the third trimester may be difficult to assess as a result of a circulating digoxin-like substance that interferes with the radioimmunoassay. Near term, a stable dose may give the false impression of toxicity and prompt inappropriate dose reduction.[9]

Table 32–6 summarizes effects of antiarrhythmic drugs in pregnancy.

REFERENCES–INTRODUCTION

1. Ben-David J, Zipes DP. Torsade de pointes and proarrhythmia. Lancet 1993;341:1578–1582.
2. Campbell TJ. Proarrhythmic actions of antiarrhythmic drugs: A review. Aust NZ J Med 1990;20:275–282.
3. Tzivoni D, Banai S, Schuger C, et al. Treatment of Torsade de pointes with magnesium sulfate. Circulation 1988;77:392–399.
4. Tzivoni D, Keren A. Suppression of ventricular arrhythmias by magnesium. Am J Cardiol 1990;65:1397–1399.
5. Perticone F, Adinolfi L, Bonaduce D. Efficacy of magnesium sulfate in the treatment of Torsade de pointes. Am Heart J 1986;112:847–849.
6. Maurer HH. Identification of antiarrhythmic drugs and their metabolites in urine. Arch Toxicol 1990;64:218–230.
7. Smilkstein MJ. Presentation on Cardiovascular Pharmacology, North American Congress of Clinical Toxicology—94, Salt Lake City, Utah, September 1994.
8. Ellenhorn MJ, Barceloux DG. *Medical Toxicology.* New York: Elsevier Science, 1988.
9. Page RL. Treatment of arrhythmias during pregnancy. Am Heart J 1995;130:871–876.

ADENOSINE

Adenosine (Adenocard) has been approved by the FDA for use in the acute termination of supraventricular tachycardia.[1] It has also been used in the differential diagnosis of tachyrhythmias.[2] It produces transient slowing of the sinus rate and delay in atrioventricular nodal conduction, with lengthening of the PR segment on the electrocardiogram and of the AH interval in a His bundle recording.[3–5] It has no direct effects on ventricular tissue (Fig. 32–2).

Therapeutic Dose

Adenosine must be given intravenously, as it has an ultrashort half-life of seconds. For adults 6 mg (one vial) is given as a rapid intravenous bolus. The recommended dose in infants and children is 37.5 μg/kg, with increments of 37.5 μg/kg until a maximum of 350 μg/kg is reached.[6] Although the maximal recommended dose of 12 mg may be ineffective when administered through a small peripheral vein, a dose of 6 mg administered through a central vein in the same patient may have a very potent effect.[6] Cairns and Niemann administered one 12-mg dose of adenosine to patients with suspected paroxysmal supraventricular tachycardia (PSVT).[7] This single dose is most likely to convert all patients with PSVT in which the atrioventricular node is a critical component of the reentrant circuit. If PSVT recurs, additional doses of adenosine are not likely to maintain a sinus rhythm. In patients taking dipyridamole or carbamazepine, an initial bolus dose of 3 mg may be sufficient. Adenosine should be used cautiously in patients with right-to-left shunting and should not be administered into the distal port of a Swan–Ganz catheter.[8]

Toxicokinetics

Pregnancy

Adenosine has not been systematically studied in pregnant patients, although it has been safely used in some pregnant patients.

Tachyrhythmias during pregnancy are rare. Management of supraventricular tachycardias in pregnancy include vagal maneuvers (often unsuccessful); beta blockade (eg, esmolol), which may produce hypotension and transient neonatal hypoglycemia and hypotonia; and electrical cardioversion. Administration of adenosine, in one anecdotal case report, was successful in terminating a supraventricular tachycardia in a 39-week pregnant patient.[9]

Drug Interactions

Dipyridamole potentiates the dromotropic effects of adenosine, causing prolonged atrioventricular nodal blockade.[10] Verapamil may be potentially dangerous in elderly patients with atrial flutter. If therapy is required, overdrive atrial pacing is the treatment of choice.[11] Theophylline acts as an antagonist.[12] Carbamazepine increases the strength of adenosine-induced heart block and asystole.[13]

Mechanism of Action

Adenosine decreases spontaneous depolarization (ie, pacemaker activity) in the sinus node and conduction velocity in the atrioventricular node. Its direct negative chronotropic and dromotropic properties are the basis for its wide diagnostic and therapeutic application in patients with supraventricular tachycardia. In atrial tissue, adenosine produces a negative inotropic effect by activating the adenosine-sensitive potassium channel under basal conditions, as well as by attenuating catecholamine-stimulated contractility and cyclic AMP accumulation under enhanced autonomic conditions. In ventricular tissue, adenosine minimally affects the ventricular inotropic state under basal

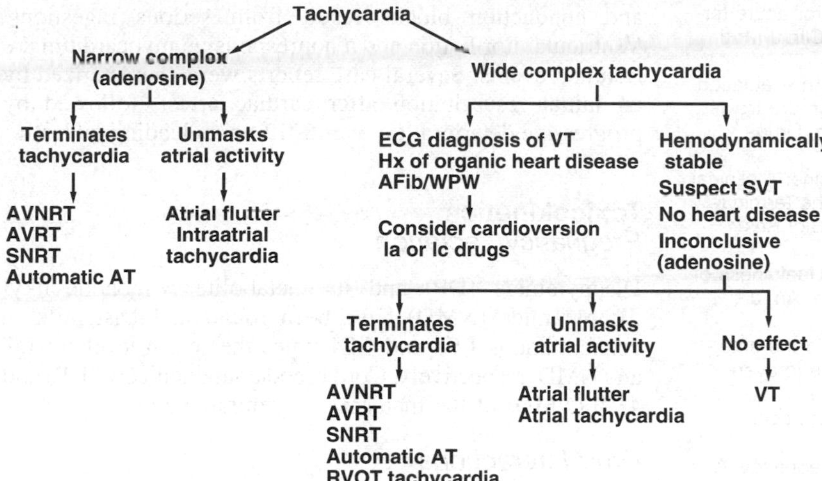

Figure 32-2 Use of adenosine in diagnosis of and therapy for tachyarrhythmias (see text for discussion). *AFib/WPW,* atrial fibrillation/Wolff–Parkinson–White syndrome; *AT,* atrial tachycardia; *AVNRT,* atrioventricular nodal reentrant tachycardia; *AVRT,* atrioventricular reentrant tachycardia; *ECG,* electrocardiographic; *Hx,* history; *Ia drugs,* disopyramide, procainamide, and quinidine; *Ic drugs,* propafenone and flecainide; *RVOT,* right ventricular outflow tract; *SNRT,* sinus node reentrant tachycardia; *SVT,* supraventricular tachycardia; *VT,* ventricular tachycardia. Transient suppression. (From Shen WK, Kurachi Y. Mechanisms of adenosine-mediated actions on cellular and clinical cardiac electrophysiology. Mayo Clin Proc 1995;70:274–291.)

conditions; however, it negates the catecholamine-induced activity by inhibiting adenylate cyclase activity and cyclic AMP production.[14]

Clinical Presentation

Undesirable effects include cutaneous flushing, dyspnea and chest pain, nausea, lightheadedness, headache, and dizziness in about 20% of patients. The frequency and severity of the symptoms are usually dose related.[14]

Proarrhythmias

Bradycardia, transient atrial flutter or fibrillation, sinus arrest, varying degrees of atrioventricular block, and ventricular premature beats have been recorded. Adenosine has rarely been associated with a transient hypotension. Prolonged bradysystole and seizures have followed its use.[10] Inhaled adenosine causes bronchospasm.[15] Proarrhythmic responses are also common after a bolus injection of adenosine. Premature atrial and ventricular beats are most common. Nonsustained polymorphic ventricular tachycardia and atrial fibrillation have been reported. Episodes of transient asystole and heart block are frequently observed, but these are usually short-lived and resolve spontaneously without intervention.[14] Pauses with ventricular standstill of several seconds may occur. Sustained bradycardia requiring temporary pacing followed a bolus of 150 μg/kg given to a 10-year-old with Down's syndrome.[6] Adenosine should not be administered in the presence of congenital or acquired prolonged QT syndrome; its negative chromotropic and dromotropic actions may induce a Torsade de pointes polymorphic ventricular tachycardia.[16,17] Every patient with tachycardia should have a full 12-lead electrocardiogram before adenosine treatment. Rarely, adenosine may transiently increase the ventricular response rate when used to terminate an episode of paroxysmal atrial fibrillation.[18] Transient atrioventricular block can precipitate ventricular fibrillation in patients with the Wolff–Parkinson–White syndrome and atrial fibrillation administered adenosine.[19]

Nonarrhythmic medication may also induce proarrhythmic effects (Table 32–3).

Overdose

Overdoses have not been reported in the published literature.

Contraindications

- Sick sinus syndrome, which may induce loss of consciousness[20]
- Second- or third-degree atrioventricular block, unless a functioning pacemaker is in place[21]

Cautions

- History of asthma or wheezing (Inhaled adenosine causes bronchospasm in patients with asthma.)[22]
- Presence of bronchoconstriction.[23]
- Administration of adenosine via central venous catheter (Further study is required. It may be advisable to reduce the recommended dose to half of the initial 6 mg (to 3 mg) to avoid the potential for a more profound effect on atrioventricular conduction.)[8,16]

Treatment

Treatment is symptomatic and supportive. External pacing should be immediately available.[11] Patients and nurses should be mentally prepared for briefly symptomatic high-grade heart blocks of several seconds' duration.[12] In situations of prolonged adenosine-induced chest pain in patients with ischemic heart disease, theophylline may alleviate the chest pain.[14]

REFERENCES—ADENOSINE

1. Adenosine approved for treatment of paroxysmal supraventricular tachycardia. Clin Pharm 1990;9:79.
2. Cabrera R, Lucas FJ, Pevalver C, et al. Adenosine triphosphate as a diagnostic to identify tachycardias at the emergency room. Chest 1993;104(suppl.):167S.

3. Pinski SL, Maloney JD. Adenosine: A new drug for acute termination of supraventricular tachycardia. Cleve Clin J Med 1190;57:383–388.
4. Faulds D, Chrisp P, Buckley MM-T. Adenosine: An evaluation of its use in cardiac diagnostic procedures and in the treatment of paroxysmal supraventricular tachycardia. Drugs 1991;41:596–624.
5. Sellers TD, Kirchhoffer JG, Modesto TA. Adenosine: A clinical experience and comparison with verapamil for the termination of supraventricular tachycardias. Prog Clin Biol Res 1987;230:283–299.
6. Overhold ED, Rheuban KS, Gutgesell HP, et al. Usefulness of adenosine for arrhythmias in infants and children. Am J Cardiol 1988;61:336–340.
7. Cairns CB, Niemann JT. Intravenous adenosine in the emergency department: Management of paroxysmal supraventricular tachycardia. Ann Emerg Med 1991;20:717–721.
8. Roelke M, Yurchak PM. Adenosine and supraventricular tachycardia. N Engl J Med 1992;326: 1221.
9. Podolsky SM, Varon J. Adenosine use during pregnancy. Ann Emerg Med 1991;20:1027–1028.
10. Webster DR, Daar AA. Prolonged bradysystole and seizures following intravenous adenosine for supraventricular tachycardia. Am J Emerg Med 1993;11:192–194.
11. White RD. Acceleration of the ventricular response in paroxysmal bone atrial fibrillation following the injection of adenosine. Am J Emerg Med 1993;11:245–246.
12. Camm AJ, Garratt CJ. Adenosine and supraventricular tachycardia. N Engl J Med 1992;226:1221–1222.
13. Reed R, Falk JL, O'Brien J. Untoward reactions to adenosine therapy for supraventricular tachycardia. Am J Emerg Med 1991;9:566–570.
14. Shen W-K, Kurachi Y. Mechanisms of adenosine-mediated actions on cellular and clinical cardiac electrophysiology. Mayo Clin Proc 1995;70:274–291.
15. Cushley MJ, Tattersfield AE, Holgate ST. Adenosine-induced bronchoconstriction in asthma: Antagonism by inhaled theophylline. Am Rev Respir Dis 1984;129:380–384.
16. Harrington GR, Froelich EG. Adenosine-induced Torsade de pointes. Chest 1993;103:1299–1301.
17. Wesley RC, Turaquest P. Torsade de pointes after intravenous adenosine in the presence of prolonged QT syndrome. Am Heart J 1992;123:794–796.
18. Adenosine and the diagnosis of tachycardias. Lancet 1992; 339:464–465.
19. Exner DV, Muzylla T, Gillis AM. Proarrhythmia in patients with the Wolff–Parkinson–White syndrome after standard doses of intravenous adenosine. Ann Intern Med 1995; 122:351–352.
20. Rankin AC, McGovern BA. Adenosine or verapamil for the acute treatment of supraventricular tachycardia. Ann Intern Med 1991;114:513–515.
21. Sobel RM. Untoward reaction to adenosine therapy for supraventricular tachycardia. Am J Emerg Med 1992;10:393.
22. Nathan J. Terminating paroxysmal supraventricular tachycardias with adenosine. West J Med 1991;156:290–291.
23. Burkhart KK. Respiratory failure following adenosine administration. Am J Emerg Med 1993;11:249–250.

CLASS IA DRUGS

DISOPYRAMIDE

Clinical Presentation

Ingestion by healthy adults of less than 2.5 g usually causes hemodynamically minor changes in conduction (e.g., QT, PR prolongation). Minor anticholinergic side effects occur, including urinary retention, blurred vision, and dry mouth. Cardiovascular collapse and apnea usually appear within several hours afer a serious overdose, but the anticholinergic properties of disopyramide may theoretically delay symptoms. A variety of ventricular supraventricular dysrhythmias and conduction blocks result from serious ingestions. Ventricular fibrillation and a nonresponsive myocardium are terminal events. Several case reports were characterized by an initial resuscitation after cardiac arrest, followed by progressive deterioration over 6–12 hours leading to death.[7]

Toxicokinetics

Pregnancy/Lactation

Disopyramide (DP) and its metabolite *N*-monodesalkyl disopyramide (NMD) have been found in breast milk in concentrations 1.06 and 6.24 times the serum levels of DP and NMD, respectively. Cord blood contained 26% (DP) and 43% (NMD) of the maternal concentrations.[1]

Drug Interactions

Erythromycin added to a regimen of disopyramide may induce QT_c prolongation, polymorphic ventricular tachycardias, and elevation of disopyramide serum levels. Erythromycin interferes with the hepatic *N*-dealkylation of disopyramide to its mono-*N*-dealkylisopyramide metabolite, thus increasing disopyramide and decreasing metabolite serum levels.[2] Rifampin decreases serum levels of disopyramide when administered concurrently.[3]

Laboratory

Analytical Methods

Quantitation of disopyramide is accomplished by gas chromatography using a flame ionization detector (GC/FID). Identification of the compound is performed by thin-layer chromatography and ultraviolet spectrophotometry.[4]

Blood Levels

A 41-year-old who ingested disopyramide developed fatal cardiac arrest and died. Concentrations of postmortem blood disclosed a disopyramide concentration of 49 μg/mL and a mono-*N*-dealkylated metabolite concentration of 9 μg/mL.[5]

Treatment

Hemodialysis

Hemodialysis is effective in reducing the serum half-life in chronic hemodialysis patients and may be useful in cases where supportive care is not effective.[6] Clinical experience is not adequate to guide therapy.

Hemoperfusion

Gosselin et al. suggest that clearance is greater with hemoperfusion than with hemodialysis, but their data were limited to dogs and one patient.[7] Jaeger et al. reported that hemoperfusion increased clearance by only 5% in two patients.[8]

Supportive Measures

1. Consider dialysis early if the clinical condition deteriorates with supportive care.
2. High doses of calcium chloride (0.5 g every 5 minutes up to a total dose of 3.0 g), in combination with conventional therapy and cardiopulmonary resuscitation, appeared to reverse the electromechanical dissociation following a 2000-mg disopyramide overdose.[9]

3. A fatal Torsade de pointes type of ventricular arrhythmia may follow disopyramide use in patients with acute hepatocellular dysfunction. Discontinue disopyramide administration when jaundice or acute hepatocellular dysfunction occurs.[10]

REFERENCES—DISOPYRAMIDE

1. Ellsworth AJ, Horn JR, Raisys VA, et al. Disopyramide and *N*-monodesalkyl disopyramide in serum and breast milk. DICP Ann Pharmacother 1989;23:56–57.
2. Ragosta M, Weihl AC, Rosenfeld LE. Potentially fatal interaction between erythromycin and disopyramide. Am J Med 1989;86:465–466.
3. Staum JM. Enzyme induction: Rifampin–disopyramide interaction. DICP Ann Pharmacother 1990;24:701–703.
4. Michaelek RW, Rejent TA, Spencer RA. Disopyramide fatality: Case report and GC/FID analysis. J Anal Toxicol 1982;6: 255–257.
5. Orloff KG, Thompson BC, Caplan YH. Fatal dose with disopyramide. Bull Int Assoc Forens Toxicol 1980;15:4–5.
6. Karim A. Disopyramide dialyzability. Lancet 1978;2:214.
7. Gosselin B, Matthieu D, Chopin C, et al. Acute intoxication with disopyramide: Clinical and experimental study by hemoperfusion on amberlite XAD 4 resin. Clin Toxicol 1980;17: 439–449.
8. Jaeger A, Sauder PH, Kopferschmitt J, et al. Acute disopyramide poisoning: A multicenter study of 106 cases. Vet Hum Toxicol 1982;24:285. Abstract.
9. Accomero F, Pellanda A, Ruffini C, et al. Prolonged cardiac resuscitation during acute disopyramide poisoning. Vet Hum Toxicol 1993;35:231–237.
10. Schattner A, Gindin J, Geltner D. Fatal Torsade de pointes following jaundice in a patient treated with disopyramide. Postgrad Med J 1989;65:333–334.

MORICIZINE

Moricizine hydrochloride is a phenothiazine derivative first synthesized in the Soviet Union in 1964, where it was released for general use in 1971.[1] It was approved as a new antiarrhythmic agent by the FDA in June 1990 (Ethmozine, DuPont) for the treatment of documented life-threatening ventricular arrhythmias. Moricizine is a Vaughan Williams class I agent with potent local anesthetic and membrane-stabilizing properties.[2] It does not quite fit any of the usual subclasses of antiarrhythmic drugs. The drug suppresses abnormal automaticity and prolongs the PR and QRS intervals; thus, it has some properties of subclasses IA and IC.[3]

Structure and Classification

Moricizine is ethyl [10-(3-morpholinopropionyl) phenothiazin-2-yl] carbamate, a phenothiazine derivative.[4] On the basis of clinical and cellular electrophysiologic studies, Vaughan Williams has concluded that it is a class IC agent.[5]

Use

Moricizine is indicated for the treatment of documented life-threatening ventricular arrhythmias, such as sustained ventricular tachycardia. Because of its proarrhythmic effects, it is recommended only for those patients for whom clinical judgment indicates that the benefits outweigh the risks.[6]

Product Formulation

Moricizine hydrochloride (Ethmazine) is available in film-coated tablets of 200 mg (light green), 250 mg (light orange), and 300 mg (light blue).[6]

Source

Moricizine is a synthetic product.

Therapeutic Dose

The usual adult dose is between 600 and 900 mg per day given every 8 hours in three equally divided doses. Patients with significant renal or hepatic dysfunction are started at doses of 600 mg or below.

Fatal Dose

Deaths have occurred after accidental or intentional overdoses of 2250 and 10,000 mg of moricizine hydrochloride, respectively.[6]

Toxicokinetics

Absorption

Moricizine is well absorbed from the gastrointestinal tract after oral administration, with peak plasma levels following a 300-mg oral dose reaching a maximum concentration of approximately 0.5 μg/mL (0.2–1.2 μg/mL) at between 1 and 2.5 hours after ingestion.[7] There is a high first-pass metabolism, and bioavailability is only 34 to 38%.

Distribution

The apparent volume of distribution after an oral dose is approximately 300 L (4.3 L/kg).[7] It is highly protein bound (approximately 95%) to α_1-acid glycoprotein, albumin, and peripheral tissue.[8]

Elimination

Moricizine is extensively metabolized before elimination, mainly by sulfur oxidation, hydroxylation, *N*-dealkylation, and glucuronide or sulfate conjugation.[9] Two metabolites are pharmacologically active: moricizine sulfoxide and phenothiazine-2-carbamic acid ethyl ester sulfoxide. These two metabolites represent less than 1% of the administered dose and have plasma half-lives of approximately 3 hours. The elimination half-life of moricizine after a single oral dose is about 2 hours. Approximately 56% of the drug and its metabolites is excreted in the feces and 39% in the urine, with only 0.14% excreted unchanged in the urine. Some moricizine is also recycled through the enterohepatic circulation.[6]

Drug Interactions

Cimetidine reduces moricizine clearance to approximately one half, and increases its plasma concentration to 1.4 times its normal value.[6] Plasma theophylline half-life is decreased 19 to 33% and its clearance is increased 44 to 66% when given together with moricizine.

Pregnancy/Lactation

There are no adequate well-controlled studies in pregnant women. The FDA has placed moricizine hydrochloride in Pregnancy Category B. It should be used in pregnancy only if clearly needed. It is excreted in human milk and has potentially adverse effects on the nursing infant.

Mechanism of Action

In controlled clinical trials moricizine has been shown to have antiarrhythmic effects similar to those of disopyramide, quinidine, and propranolol. Moricizine prolongs the PR interval by 20% and the QRS duration by 19%, but has little effect on the duration of the QT interval.[9] The arrhythmias sometimes associated with QT prolongation (long QT syndrome, Torsade de pointes) and frequently seen with quinidine are relatively rare with moricizine.[10] Moricizine produces a dose-dependent prolongation of conduction in the atrium, atrioventricular node, His-Purkinje system, and ventricular myocardium.[11] Its major electrophysiologic effects are a decreased maximum rate of phase 0 depolarization, increased rates of phase 2 and 3 repolarization and decreased effective refractory period. (See Figure 32–1)

Clinical Presentation

Chronic Use

The most frequent noncardiac adverse effects have been nausea and dizziness, seen in about 10 to 15% of patients.[12] Drug fever, thrombocytopenia, and elevated liver function tests, all reversible, have been infrequently observed.

Moricizine exhibits proarrhythmic effects in approximately 3% of patients.[13] Pairs and runs of ventricular premature contractions seen in a patient on moricizine therapy are a strong indication for alternative therapy.[1]

Overdose

Deaths have occurred after accidental and intentional overdoses of 2250 and 10,000 mg of moricizine hydrochloride, respectively. Overdose may produce emesis, lethargy, coma, syncope, hypotension, conduction disturbances, exacerbation of congestive heart failure, myocardial infarction, sinus arrest, arrhythmias (including junctional bradycardia, ventricular tachycardia, ventricular fibrillation, and asystole), and respiratory failure.[6]

Laboratory

Blood Levels

Antiarrhythmic and electrophysiologic effects of moricizine are not correlated with its plasma concentration or with those of its metabolites.

Abnormalities

A few patients exhibit an increase in bilirubin or transaminase levels. Less than 1% have had evidence of renal failure.

Treatment

Stabilization

Serious poisoning with moricizine may present with cardiovascular collapse. Treatment is supportive. The patient is hospitalized, with first priority given to intravenous lines, oxygen, and cardiac monitoring. Continuous monitoring is conducted for cardiac, respiratory, and central nervous system changes. Advanced cardiac life support systems, including an intracardiac pacing catheter, should be available.

Gut Decontamination

If the patient can be reached within the first few hours, an attempt should be made to lavage the stomach with adequate tracheal protection. Activated charcoal may be able to absorb some of the enterohepatic recycled drug and its metabolites, but controlled studies have not yet been performed.

Elimination Enhancement

In view of its high protein binding, extensive volume of distribution, and formation of multiple metabolites, it appears that hemodialysis or hemoperfusion would not be effective after an overdose.

Antidote

There is no antidote for moricizine overdose.

Supportive Measures

1. Hypotension should be treated with fluids, and, if required, vasopressors. Persistent hypotension should be managed with a pulmonary catheter and arterial lines in a coronary care unit. An intraaortic balloon pump may be effective, but supportive data are lacking at present.
2. Bradycardia and hypotension may respond to sodium lactate or sodium bicarbonate, but confirmatory clinical studies have not been performed.

REFERENCES—MORICIZINE

1. Grubb BP. Moricizine: A new agent for the treatment of ventricular arrhythmias. Am J Med Sci 1991;301:298–401.
2. Vaughan Williams EM. A classification of antiarrhythmic actions reassessed after a decade of new drugs. J Clin Pharmacol 1984;24:129–147.
3. Moricizine for cardiac arrhythmias. Med Lett Drugs Ther 1990;32(830):99–100.
4. Reynolds JEF, ed. *Martindale: The Extra Pharmacopoeia.* 30th ed. London: Pharmaceutical Press, 1993:69.
5. Vaughan Williams EM. Classification of antiarrhythmic action of moricizine. J Clin Pharmacol 1991;31:216–221.
6. *Physicians' Desk Reference.* 45th ed. Oradel, NJ: Medical Economics, 1991:923–926.
7. Mann HJ. Moricizine: A new class 1 antiarrhythmic. Clin Pharm 1990;9:842–852.
8. Siddoway LA, Schwartz SL, Barbey JT, et al. Clinical pharmacokinetics of moricizine. Am J Cardiol 1990;65:21D–25D.
9. Rosenshtraukh L, Anyukhovsky E, Nesterenko V. Electrophysiologic aspects of moricizine HCl. Am J Cardiol 1987;60:27–34.
10. Bigger T. Cardiac electrophysiologic effects of moricizine hydrochloride. Am J Cardiol 1990;65:15–20.
11. Ruffy R, Rosenshtraukh L, Elharrar V, Zipes D. Electrophysiologic effects of ethmozine on the canine myocardium. Cardiovasc Res 1979;13:354–363.
12. Kennedy H. Noncardiac adverse effects and organ toxicity of moricizine during short term and long term studies. Am J Cardiol 1990;65:47–50.
13. Morganroth J, Pratt C. Prevalence and characteristics of proarrhythmia from moricizine. Am J Cardiol 1989;63:172–176.

PRAJMALINE

Prajmaline (prajmalium bitartrate, *N*-propyl ajmalinium hydrogen tartrate) is a class IC antiarrhythmic drug with class IA properties similar to those of ajmaline and quinidine. It is the *N*-propyl derivative of ajmaline and is given in doses of 40 to 80 mg daily. Prajmaline has been available since the 1970s, and a number of overdose reports[1–3] have indicated a high fatality rate. Clinical symptoms following overdose are similar to those of ajmaline. It has an oral bioavailability of 80%, a distribution half-life of 10 minutes, and an elimination half-life of 6 hours. It is 60% bound to plasma proteins, and has a volume of distribution of 4 to 5 L/kg. There are two main metabolites, 21-carboxyprajmaline and hydroxyprajmaline, and about 20% is eliminated renally as the unchanged drug.[1] Overdoses with less than 20 of the 20-mg tablets have been fatal.[2] Blood levels do not correlate well with clinical outcome. Treatment is largely supportive. Resin hemoperfusion in one case appeared to assist in survival,[2] but in two others did not prevent a fatality.[1] There are no antidotes.

REFERENCES—PRAJMALINE

1. Koppel C, Oberdisse V, Heinemeyer G. Clinical course and outcome in classic antiarrhythmic overdose. Clin Toxicol 1990;28: 433–444.
2. Lederle RM, Harbig K, Wermuth G, Klaus D. Hamoperfusion mit Kunsharz-Adsorben bei schwerer Intoxikation mit *N*-Propyl-Ajmalinium-Bitartrat. Intensivmed 1981;18:77–82.
3. Gelbke HP, Schlicht HJ. Suicide by an overdose of *N*-propylajmalinium bitartrate. Arch Toxikol 1977;37:135–141.

PROCAINAMIDE

Drug Interactions

Respiratory failure due to extreme neuromuscular weakness was produced by procainamide intoxication in a patient with preexisting neuropathy caused by aminodarone.[1] Cimetidine treatment appeared to increase the average steady-state blood concentrations of procainamide and *N*-acetylprocainamide (NAPA). Such interaction may lead to toxic procainamide levels.[2] Amiodarone added to a *N*-procainamide regimen led to an increase in serum procainamide levels with development of occasional clinical signs of toxicity.[3] Trimethoprim decreased the renal clearance of procainamide and NAPA, resulting in increased plasma concentrations of both drugs and increase in the QT_c interval after procainamide.[4] Trimethoprim increases the plasma concentrations of procainamide and NAPA by decreasing their renal clearances and allowing more conversion of procainamide to NAPA.[4] This may be secondary to competition for renal tubular cationic secretion[5]; however, a 76-year-old man receiving oral procainamide 750 mg every 6 hours developed Torsade de pointes. The drug was discontinued and subsequently the patient responded to ventricular pacing.[6]

Clinical Presentation

Minor side effects include gastrointestinal disturbances, headache, mild hypotension, rash, insomnia, dizziness, ataxia, hallucinations, weakness, and slight prolongation of the QT interval and QRS complex.

Respiratory arrest and myasthenic crisis developed following administration of procainamide to a myasthenia gra vis patient.[7] Procainamide therapy administered to control recurrent ventricular arrhythmias may retard removal of ventilatory support following chest surgery because of its tendency to produce muscle weakness and associated respiratory insufficiency.[8] Pure red cell aplasia has followed prolonged use of sustained-release procainamide.[9]

Laboratory

Analytical Methods

A sensitive modified enzyme-mediated immunoassay technique (EMIT) is available for detection of procainamide and NAPA in plasma, serum, and urine. A sample volume of 100 μL is adequate for the required sensitivity of 0.1 μg/mL with minimal sample interference.[10]

Blood Levels

Occasionally, procainamide levels up to 16 μg/mL are required to suppress ventricular dysrhythmias. Mild toxicity may occur in the range 12 to 16 μg/mL, and serious toxicity occurs when procainamide levels exceed 16 μg/mL.[11] The presence of active metabolite (NAPA) complicates interpretation of a true therapeutic procainamide level; therefore, both levels (procainamide and NAPA) are necessary to predict accurate therapeutic concentrations. Plasma levels are only guidelines for therapy, as the interpretation of toxic levels is complicated by active metabolites. NAPA production depends on the rate of acetylation, which is genetically determined and variable between races. Total procainamide and NAPA therapeutic levels range from 5 to 25–30 μg/mL. True in vivo plasma procainamide levels may differ from measured levels when freshly drawn and separated blood samples are not used for analysis. In storage, procainamide continues to diffuse into red blood cells and undergoes metabolism to both active (NAPA) and inactive metabolites.[12] IgG antibodies to histone complex H2A–H2B appear to be sensitive and specific markers of procainamide-induced lupus.[13]

Electrocardiogram

Torsade de pointes, although usually infrequent following procainamide use, may be observed more often when there is a change in renal status and when NAPA values rise. QT_c prolongation may be associated in such cases with elevated NAPA values.[14] In an overdose case, junctional tachycardia and conduction defects appeared at total procainamide and NAPA levels exceeding 42 μg/mL, and severe hypotension and lethargy, at levels above 60 μg/mL.[15] Measures of QT interval and QRS prolongation together with hypotension are sensitive measures of serious poisoning.

Treatment

Treatment is supportive:

1. Apply the usual supportive measures.
2. Avoid quinidine and disopyramide.
3. Consider pacemaker insertion early with signs of increasing atrioventricular block.

REFERENCES—PROCAINAMIDE

1. Miller B, Skupin A, Rubenfire M, Bigman O. Respiratory failure produced by severe procainamide intoxication in a patient with preexisting peripheral neuropathy caused by amiodarone. Chest 1988;94: 663–665.
2. Bauer LA, Black D, Gensler A. Procainamide–cimetidine during interaction in elderly male patients. J Am Geriatr Soc 1990;38:467–469.
3. Saal AK, Werner JA, Greene HL, et al. Effect of amiodarone on serum quinidine and procainamide levels. Am J Cardiol 1984;53:1264–1267.
4. Kosoglou T, Rocci ML Jr, Vlasses PH. Trimethoprim alters the disposition of procainamide and *N*-acetyl procainamide. Clin Pharmacol Ther 1988;44:467–477.
5. Vlasses PH, Kosoglou T, Chase SL, et al. Trimethoprim inhibition of the renal clearance of procainamide and *N*-acetylprocainamide. Arch Intern Med 1989;149:1350–1353.
6. Habbab MA, El-Sherif N. Drug-induced Torsade de pointes: Role of early afterdepolarizations and dispersion of repolarization. Am J Med 1990;89:241–246.
7. Godley PJ, Morton TA, Karbhoski JA, Tami JA. Procainamide-induced myasthenia crisis. Ther Drug Monit 1990;12:411–414.
8. Putnam JB, Bolling SF, Kirsch MM. Procainamide-induced respiratory insufficiency after cardiopulmonary bypass. Ann Thorac Surg 1991;51:482–483.
9. Giannone L, Kugler JW, Krantz SB. Pure red cell aplasia associated with administration of sustained-release procainamide. Arch Intern Med 1987;147:1179–1180.
10. Henry PA, Dhruv RA. More sensitive enzyme mediated immunoassay technique for procainamide and *N*-acetylprocainamide in plasma, serum and urine. Clin Chem 1988;34:957–960.
11. Koch-Weser J, Klein SW. Procainamide dosage schedules, plasma concentrations and clinical effects. JAMA 1971;215: 1454–1460.
12. Chen ML, Loo MG, Chiou WL. Pharmacokinetics of drugs in blood: III. Metabolism of procainamide and storage effects of blood samples. J Pharm Sci 1985;72:572–574.
13. Totoritis MC, Tan EM, McNally EM, Rubin RL. Association of antibody to histone complex H2A–H2B with symptomatic procainamide induced lupus. N Engl J Med 1988;318:1431–1436.
14. Heiselman DE, Litman GI. Risk factors for procainamide-induced Torsade de pointes. Clin Res 1986;34:7A.
15. Atkinson AJ, Krumlovsky FA, Huang CM, et al. Hemodialysis for severe procainamide toxicity: Clinical and pharmacokinetic observations. Clin Pharmacol Ther 1976;20:585–592.

QUINIDINE

Quinidine is one of the cinchona alkaloids derived from cinchona bark. These compounds include the structural isomer of quinidine, quinine, clonidine, and cinchonine. Although it has been used medicinally since the 17th century for a variety of illnesses, the current clinical indications for quinidine are limited to the suppression of atrial and ventricular dysrhythmias. The medical use of quinine involves primarily malaria prophylaxis and suppression of nocturnal cramps. Quinine toxicity now occurs predominantly as a complication of its lay use as an abortifacient.

Structure/Classification/Use

Quinidine is a weak base and is the dextrorotatory isomer of quinine, a member of the quinoline group of natural alkaloids. Quinidine is one of the class IA antiarrhythmic drugs, which include procainamide and disopyramide.

Product Formulation

Oral products include the sulfate (200-mg tablet), gluconate, and polygalacturonate salts. Intravenous quinidine is available as the gluconate, but hypotension severely limits its clinical usefulness.

Toxic Dose

The usual adult dose of quinidine sulfate is 200 to 300 mg three or four times per day. An adult who ingests 2.5 to 4 g would be expected to exhibit serious toxic effects. The ingestion of 8 g of quinidine by an adult led to severe hypotension and dysrhythmias, which required overdrive pacing and an intraaortic balloon pump for control.[1] A 4-g ingestion by a 57-year-old woman who had no previous history of cardiovascular disease produced conduction delays, hypotension, coma, and convulsions.[2] A patient who reportedly ingested 20 g survived with supportive care, despite hypotension and anuria.[3] Quinine sulfate displays similar toxicity, with an average toxic dose of 4 g.

Absorption

The bioavailability of quinidine is 70 to 80% after oral use but varies between individuals and preparations. The sulfate salt is rapidly absorbed in 60 to 90 minutes. Polygalacturonate salts produce peak quinidine concentrations in 5 to 6 hours; gastrointestinal absorption of gluconate salts is intermediate (peak of 3–4 hours).

Distribution

The apparent volume of distribution is 2.7 to 3.0 L/kg with a brief initial distribution phase (6–12 minutes). Congestive heart failure reduces the volume of distribution by one third, and chronic liver disease increases it by 30%. Quinidine is a basic drug highly bound (90%) to α_1-acid glycoprotein. Chronic liver disease increases the portion of unbound drug due to decreased protein binding, and this results in lower therapeutic levels.

Elimination

The usual plasma half-life of approximately 7 hours after intravenous administration increases in the presence of chronic liver disease.[4] The elimination kinetics of hydroquinidine appear to be similar to those of quinidine.[5] Hepatic biotransformation by hydroxylation accounts for 60 to 80% of the elimination of an absorbed quinidine dose, whereas the kidneys excrete 20 to 40% unchanged. Congestive heart failure reduces clearance by one half compared with clearance at a urine pH of 6 to 7. Quinidine metabolites include 3-hydroxyquinidine *N*-oxide, 2′-oxoquinidinone, desmethylquinidine, and quinidine *N*-oxide. Although metabolism is highly variable between individuals, at least in cases of quinidine-induced Torsade de pointes, the metabolites do not appear to contribute to the formation of dysrhythmias.[6]

Drug Interactions

Cimetidine induces elevations in quinidine serum concentrations. This may follow decreased hepatic quinidine clearance as a consequence of enzyme inhibition.[7] A similar quinidine serum elevation is observed when ketoconazole is concurrently administered.[8] Verapamil impairs the metabolism of quinidine to 3-hydroxyquinidine and reduces the oral clearance and half-life of quinidine.[9]

Pregnancy

A patient at 33 weeks of gestation was administered quinidine for treatment of a fetal supraventricular tachycardia. The patient had evidence of quinidine toxicity at low to midtherapeutic serum levels of quinidine, but markedly elevated levels of 3 (*S*)-3-hydroxyquinidine (3-hydroxyquinidine). The elevated levels of 3-hydroxyquinidine may be associated with quinidine toxicity even in the presence of a nontoxic serum quinidine level. Quinidine and metabolite levels were measure by high-pressure liquid chromatography.[10]

Mechanism of Action

Cardiac Conduction

Quinidine produces clinical and toxic effects similar to those of procainamide.[11] The conduction velocity decreases progressively as drug concentration rises, as reflected by increases in the PR interval, QRS duration, and QT interval.[12] High plasma quinidine levels cause high-grade atrioventricular block, bundle-branch block, and asystole resembling that of hyperkalemia. In contrast to procainamide, QT prolongation with quinidine occurs at therapeutic levels. The intensity of the electrical effect is enhanced by increasing potassium concentration. In therapeutic doses quinidine decreases phase 4 depolarization and, therefore, spontaneous cell firing; however, in high doses, quinidine *increases* the slope of phase 4 depolarization, and this is reflected clinically by increased ventricular dysrhythmias after overdose. Procainamide displays similar but weaker effects.

Hypotension

Intravenous quinidine depresses contractility and decreases systemic vascular resistance primarily by alpha-adrenergic receptor blockade. Procainamide has a similar but weaker effect. High blood levels of quinidine increase left ventricular end-diastolic pressure through its negative inotropic effect. Cardiovascular collapse has resulted from depression of contractility.

Respiratory Failure

Pulmonary edema developed after a suicidal 8-g quinidine ingestion with normal pulmonary capillary wedge pressures.[1]

Clinical Presentation

Allergic or Idiosyncratic Reaction

These adverse reactions are not related to plasma concentration and include drug fever, cholestatic hepatitis, systemic lupus erythematosus,[13] asthma, anaphylaxis, thrombocytopenia, hemolytic anemia (especially in glucose-6-phosphate dehydrogenase deficiency), and hypoprothrombinemia. Skin changes range from maculopapular eruption to thrombocytopenic purpura, cutaneous vasculitis,[14] photosensitivity, and bullous lesions.

Chronic Use

Gastrointestinal symptoms, especially diarrhea, are the most frequent adverse reactions. Cinchonism is a toxic syndrome following prolonged, excessive use of *Cinchona* alkaloids (quinidine, quinine); symptoms appear similar to those following salicylate or atropine overdose. This syndrome may develop at relatively low quinidine levels. Clinical manifestations include headache, fever, mydriasis, visual field and visual acuity changes, tinnitus, hearing loss, organic brain syndrome that varies from memory impairment to delirium, nausea, vomiting, rash, and hot flushed skin. Chronic organic brain syndrome may be the only symptom of cinchonism.[15] Coma, convulsions, and cardiorespiratory arrest occur in patients with severe cinchonism. Quinine amblyopia is a visual loss that may be complete and sudden. *Cinchona* alkaloid toxicity should be suspected in patients with sudden visual loss and widely dilated nonreactive pupils. Although some recovery occurs, loss may be permanent.[16] Stellate ganglion block, vasodilators, and adrenocorticotropic hormone have been suggested, but treatment is unlikely to be successful more than 24 hours after ingestion.[1]

Overdose

Massive acute poisoning results in both cardiovascular and neurologic signs and symptoms.[2] Cardiovascular effects result from delayed conduction and myocardial depression. Toxic effects are often superimposed on underlying cardiovascular disease. Increased conduction defects lead to atrioventricular block and widening of the QT, PR, and QRS complexes, idioventricular rhythm, and asystole.[17] Demand pacemakers may not capture the heart following severe overdose. Conduction defects are always present in overdose, although QT prolongation may be present at therapeutic levels.

Myocardial depression and decreased peripheral vascular resistance lead to hypotension and shock. Ventricular tachycardia and fibrillation complicate serious overdose. Quinidine syncope results from bursts of polymorphous or atypical ventricular tachycardia—*Torsade de pointes*—which may occur at therapeutic levels. Central nervous system symptoms (eg, lethargy, delirium, convulsions, and coma) may appear without cardiovascular depression,[15] although QT prolongation always occurs in poisoning.

Laboratory

Plasma Levels

The use of plasma levels to manage overdose is not often successful, because of different sensitivities between laboratory methods and individual patient variation in protein binding. Therapeutic quinidine levels range from 2 to 6 μg/mL. Levels greater than 8 μg/mL may be associated with toxic symptoms, and levels above 14 μg/mL have been associated with cardiac toxicity in a majority of patients.

Analytical Methods

Quinidine assay methods include fluorometry, high-pressure liquid chromatography (HPLC), gas chromatography–mass spectrometry, and enzyme immunoassay techniques. Quinine does not interfere with the EMIT immunoassay method for quinidine, but does interfere with HPLC when quinine is the internal standard. Compared with HPLC, EMIT is less sensitive because it does not discriminate between the parent compound and metabolites (eg, 3-hydroxyquinidine, *O*-desmethylquinidine).[18]

Electrocardiogram

QT and QRS prolongation is an excellent marker of significant ingestion if recorded after peak plasma levels. Widening of QT and QRS intervals usually begins to occur when plasma levels exceed 2 μg/mL and is definitely evidenced at plasma levels above 8 μg/mL.[19] A 50% increase in the QT interval or QRS complex indicates the presence of toxic quinidine levels. Serum levels of electrolytes (potassium, calcium, phosphorus, magnesium) should be checked in all cases of serious poisoning.

Treatment

Stabilization

Serious poisoning may present early with cardiovascular collapse. Therefore intravenous lines, oxygen, and cardiac monitoring are first priority. Convulsions are often responsive to diazepam. Failure to respond to the usual anticonvulsant drugs is an indication to check serum levels of electrolytes (particularly calcium) and glucose levels. Respiratory distress may result from either respiratory depression, aspiration pneumonia, or the adult respiratory distress syndrome. In patients with underlying cardiovascular disease, pulmonary edema may result from depressed myocardial contractility.

Gut Decontamination

The usual measures of emesis/lavage, activated charcoal, and cathartics within the first several hours (longer if sustained-release preparations are ingested) are indicated. Repeated doses of activated charcoal (every 3–4 hours) may enhance the elimination of quinidine trapped in the acid medium of the stomach.

Elimination Enhancement

Although renal excretion of unmetabolized quinidine increases in acid urine, the usefulness of acid diuresis has not been clinically evaluated.[20] Dialysis does not remove a clinically significant amount of quinidine because of the high degree of protein binding, and should be used only in the presence of renal failure. Hemoperfusion may be useful if hepatic failure reduces metabolism.

Antidote

Glucagon has a positive inotropic effect in dogs, but its clinical efficacy has not been evaluated. Bretylium antagonizes quinidine-induced toxic effects on ventricular fibers, but it may enhance quinidine-induced reduction in atrioventricular conduction.[21]

Supportive Measures

1. Treat hypotension initially with fluids, if required, vasopressors. Both isoproterenol and norepinephrine have been used successfully, and a resistant case has responded to the placement of an intraaortic balloon pump.[1] Persistent hypotension should be managed with a pulmonary catheter and arterial lines in a coronary care unit.
2. Treat ventricular dysrhythmias with class IB drugs (lidocaine, phenytoin), and avoid class IA drugs (procainamide, disopyramide). Bretylium should be used with caution because of synergistic atrioventricular nodal suppression.
3. When atypical ventricular tachycardia presents, the goal is to reduce the QT interval. Infusion of isoproterenol at 2 to 8 μg/min may be effective, but usually overdrive pacing (120–140/min) is necessary. Lidocaine and procainamide are not effective and may be deleterious. Be sure to correct electrolyte imbalances (especially hypokalemia).

REFERENCES—QUINIDINE

1. Shub C. Gau GT, Sidell PM, et al. The management of acute quinidine intoxication. Chest 1978;73:173–178.
2. Kerr F, Kenoyer G, Bilitch M. Quinidine overdose: Neurological and cardiovascular toxicity in normal person. Br Heart J 1971;33:629–631.
3. Woic L, Oyri A. Quinidine intoxication treated with hemodialysis. Acta Med Scand 1974;195:237–239.
4. Conrad KA, Molk BL, Chidsey CA. Pharmacokinetic studies of quinidine in patients with arrhythmias. Circulation 1977;55:1–7.
5. Lesne M, Devas DM, Reynaert M. Enterogastric cycle and intoxication with hydroquinidine: A case report. Clin Toxicol 1981;18:659–662.
6. Thompson KA, Murray JJ, Blair IA, et al. Plasma concentrations of quinidine, its major active metabolites and dihydroquinidine in patients with Torsade de pointes. Clin Res 1986;34:408A. Abstract.
7. Mackichan JJ, Badoulas H, Schaal SF. Effect of cimetidine on quinidine bioavailability. Biopharm Drug Dispos 1989; 10:121–125.
8. McNulty RM, Lazor JA, Sketch M. Transient increase in plasma quinidine concentrations during ketoconazole–quinidine therapy. Clin Pharm 1989;8:222–225.
9. Edwards D, Lavoie R, Beckman H, et al. The effect of coadministration of verapamil on the pharmacokinetics and metabolism of quinidine. Clin Pharmacother 1987;41:68–73.
10. Killeen AA, Bowers LD. Fetal supraventricular tachycardia treated with high dose quinidine: Toxicity associated with marked elevation of the metabolite, 3 (S) -3-hydroxyquinidine. Obstet Gynecol 1987;70:445–449.
11. Hoffman BF, Rosen MR, Wit AL. Electrophysiology and pharmacology of cardiac arrhythmias: VII. Cardiac effects of quinidine and procainamide. Am Heart J 1975;90:117–122.
12. Finnegan TRL, Traince JR. Depression of the heart by quinidine and its treatment. Br Heart J 1954;16:341–350.

13. Lavie CJ, Biundo J, Quinet RJ, et al. Systemic lupus erythematosus (SLE) induced by quinidine. Arch Intern Med 1985;145:446–448.
14. Shalit M, Flugelman MY, Harats N, et al. Quinidine induced vasculitis. Arch Intern Med 1985;145:2051–2052.
15. Summers WK, Allen RE, Pitts FN. Does physostigmine reverse quinidine delirium. West J Med 1981;135:411–412.
16. Murray SB, Jay JL. Loss of sight after self poisoning with quinine. Br Med J 1983;281:1700.
17. Bailey DJ. Cardiotoxic effects of quinidine and their treatment. Arch Intern Med 1960;105:13–22.
18. Dextraze PG, Foreman J, Griffiths WC, et al. Comparison of an enzyme immunoassay and a high performance liquid chromatographic method for quantitation of quinidine in serum. Clin Toxicol 1981;18:291–297.
19. Phillips RE, Warrell DA, White NJ, et al. Intravenous quinidine for the treatment of severe falciparum malaria: Clinical and pharmacokinetic studies. N Engl J Med 1985;312:1273–1278.
20. Gaudreault P. Quinidine. Clin Toxicol Rev 1982;4(12):1–2.
21. De Azevedo RM, Watanabe Y, Dreifus LS. Electrophysiologic antagonism of quinidine and bretylium tosylate. Am J Cardiol 1974;33:633–638.

CLASS IB DRUGS

LIDOCAINE

Clinical Presentation

Lidocaine causes toxic cardiovascular and central nervous system effects, with symptoms of the latter appearing in some patients near the upper limit of therapeutic plasma lidocaine levels. Early central nervous system symptoms include lightheadedness, dizziness, drowsiness, confusion, dysarthria, ataxia, hearing loss, and euphoria. Visual disturbances, agitation, and muscle fasciculations indicate more toxic plasma lidocaine levels and portend the development of convulsions and coma. Seizures may present with plasma levels above 8 μg/mL.[1] Apnea and hypotonia occur in massive overdose. Large intravenous doses in adults (1–2 g) result in immediate asystole, apnea, and multiple convulsions.[2,3] Cardiovascular toxicity occurs primarily in massive overdose when large lidocaine doses depress myocardial contractility and delay bundle-branch conduction. Case reports associate the therapeutic use of lidocaine with the onset of adult respiratory distress syndrome[4] and the development of acute methemoglobinemia in a patient with a normal hemoglobin electrophoresis and methemoglobin reductase level.[5] Symptoms of toxicity after an acute overdose with lidocaine may persist hours or days after the levels of lidocaine have become subtherapeutic, possibly because of persistent metabolites.[1]

Laboratory

Following an inadvertent overdose of 2 g of intravenous lidocaine hydrochloride, hypotension, decreased heart rate, tremors and nonresponsiveness to stimuli were observed at plasma and unbound concentration of 17.7 and 12.0 μg/mL, respectively. The elimination half-lives of plasma and unbound lidocaine were 3.8 and 2.7 hours, respectively. The patient moved his extremities when suctioned at a total plasma level of 8.9 μg/mL and an unbound concentration of 4.98 μg/mL. The patient became alert and recovered spontaneous respirations when the total and unbound concentrations were 6.8 and 3.7 μg/mL, respectively. The central nervous system effects induced by lidocaine required support when the total plasma lidocaine concentration was above 7 μg/mL. Complete recovery was observed at a total plasma level less than 5 μg/mL.[6]

Postmortem lidocaine levels after overdose range from 6 to 33 μg/mL, but in most cases the blood lidocaine level exceeds 15 μg/mL.[7] Blood concentrations of 40 and 53 μg/mL were consistent with a fatal outcome in two adults.[8] An estimated 1.2-g intravenous dose over 1 hour in a 20-kg man produced hypotension and asystole; the serum lidocaine level was 19.2 μg/mL 1¾ hours postarrest.[9] An intravenous bolus of 50 mg of lidocaine (12 mg/kg) administered to a 6-month-old child produced cardiovascular collapse, respiratory arrest, seizures for 48 hours, and coma with recovery; the plasma levels of lidocaine 1.2 and 3.5 hours after administration were 3.8 and 1.5 μg/mL, respectively. The patient recovered with supportive care.[1] A 13-month-old child died after an oral lidocaine overdose. The serum lidocaine concentration was 19.5 μg/mL, and that of the metabolite (monoethylglycylxylidide), 6.5 μg/mL.[10]

Treatment

1. Diazepam is the drug of choice to treat seizures. Adequate ventilation and acid–base balance must be ensured, because hypoxia and hypercapnia may increase cerebral penetration of the basic drug lidocaine.[11]
2. Avoid the use of phenytoin, because of its synergistic cardiac effects.
3. Supportive care should suffice for most overdoses in view of the short half-life of lidocaine. Fluids, dopamine, intubation, epinephrine, atropine, and cardiac pacing may be necessary for massive doses resulting in asystole.
4. A cardiac pacing wire may be necessary for heart block.
5. An extracorporeal pump to support circulation may be useful in reducing patient mortality from acute massive lidocaine overdose.[12]

REFERENCES—LIDOCAINE

1. Jonville AP, Barbier P, Blond MH, et al. Accidental lidocaine overdosage in an infant. Clin Toxicol 1990;28:101–106.
2. Poklis A, Mackell MA, Tucker EF. Tissue distribution of lidocaine after fatal accidental injection. J Forens Sci 1984;29:1229–1236.
3. Finkelstein F, Kreeft J. Massive lidocaine poisoning. N Engl N Med 1979;301:50.
4. Howard JJ, Mohsenufar Z, Simons SM. Adult respiratory distress syndrome following administration of lidocaine. Chest 1982;81:644–645.
5. O'Donohue WJ, Moss LM, Angelillo VA. Acute methemoglobinemia induced by topical benzocaine and lidocaine. Arch Intern Med 1980;140:1508–1509.
6. Armstrong DK, Bremseth DL, Lima JJ. Clinical response and total and unbound plasma concentrations after lidocaine overdose. Ther Drug Monit 1988;10:499–500.
7. Peat MA, Deyman ME, Crouch DJ, et al. Concentrations of lidocaine and monoethylglycylxylidide (MEGX) in lidocaine associated deaths. J Forens Sci 1985;30:1048–1057.

8. Dawling S, Flanagan RJ, Widdop B. Fatal lignocaine poisoning: Report of two cases and review of the literature. Hum Toxicol 1989;8:389–392.
9. Edgren B, Tilelli J, Gehrz, R. Intravenous lidocaine overdosage in a child. Clin Toxicol 1986;24:51–58.
10. Amitai Y, Whitesell L, Lovejoy FH Jr. Death following accidental lidocaine overdose in a child. N Engl J Med 1986;314: 182–183.
11. Moore DC, Crawford RD, Scurlock JE. Severe hypoxia and acidosis following local anesthetic induced convulsions. Anesthesiology 1980;53:259–260.
12. Freedman MD, Gal J, Freed CR. Extracorporeal pump assistance: Novel treatment for acute lidocaine poisoning. Eur J Clin Pharmacol 1982;22:129–135.

LIDOCAINE ANALOGS

Mexiletine Overdose

A suicidal ingestion of 4400 mg of mexiletine resulted in paresthesias of the tongue, nausea, seizures, asystole, and death in 2½ hours.[1] Following ingestion of 2400 mg of mexiletine by two adults and 1000 mg by another, dizziness, drowsiness, and mild disorientation persisted for about 6 hours; two experienced bradycardia.[2] Sudden cardiac arrest and hypokalemia following ingestion of 8000 mg of mexiletine responded to treatment with gastric lavage, atropine, and cardiopulmonary resuscitation.[3,4] Survival followed an attempted suicide with ingestion of 12,400 mg of mexiletine, 620 mg of nifedipine, and 50 to 100 tablets of sublingual nitroglycerin. Initial presentation included mental obtundation, vomiting, tonic-clonic seizure, high-degree atrioventricular block, profound vasodilation, and cardiovascular collapse. The patient responded to intravenous calcium gluconate, continuous phenylephrine, dopamine, and epinephrine and aggressive fluid management.[5] Status epilepticus has been observed without cardiovascular disorders.[6]

Toxicokinetics

Tocainide

Tocainide appears to be concentrated in breast milk and, in one case, was administered at approximately 6 months gestation. The patient delivered a normal baby 1 month prematurely.[7] Therapeutic plasma concentrations are in the range 4 to 10 µg/mL.[8]

Mexiletine

Postmortem blood taken immediately after death showed a mexiletine level of 34 to 37 µg/mL.[2] Blood levels of 16, and 17 mmol/L (therapeutic, 4.7–9.3 mmol/L) measured 4 hours after ingestion of a mexiletine overdose by three adults were associated with sinus bradycardia and no other cardiac signs.[3] The postmortem blood level of mexiletine in an adult found dead was 37 µg/mL.[3–5]

Drug Interactions

Mexiletine has no significant effect on plasma digoxin concentrations. Cimetidine has no significant effect on the pharmacokinetics of mexiletine. Proarrhythmic effects may be enhanced in patients receiving mexiletine and theophylline concurrently.[9]

Mechanism of Action

Class IB agents are noted for their ability to produce blockade of the fast inward sodium channel, thus slowing impulse conduction through myocardial tissue. They reduce the duration of the action potential, shorten the effective refractory period, and reduce both the frequency and duration of ventricular dysrhythmias.[6]

Clinical Presentation

Adverse reactions to mexiletine include nausea, vomiting, heartburn, esophageal spasm, tremor, seizures, ataxia, and dyskinesia.[10]

Laboratory

Tocainide

A rapid HPLC assay can determine free and total plasma tocainide levels.[11] A tocainide serum level of 68 µg/mL was measured in a comatose patient with ventricular tachyrhythmias who died.[12] A rapid assay can determine free and total plasma tocainide levels.[11]

Mexiletine

Thrombocytopenia has been associated with the therapeutic use of mexiletine.[13]

Treatment

One patient ingested 400 mg of tocainide and developed a blood level of 34 µg/mL. Hemodialysis for 4 hours appeared to be useful in enhancing clinical recovery and reducing the blood level.[8] There are no antidotes to poisoning by these compounds.

REFERENCES—LIDOCAINE ANALOGS

1. Jequier P, Jones R, Mackintosh A. Fatal mexiletine overdose. Lancet 1976;1:429.
2. Chambers SC, Milsom SM, Ikram H. Mexiletine overdose. NZ Med J 1982;95:898–899.
3. Blackmore RC, Oselton MD. Fatal mexiletine poisoning. Bull Int Assoc Forens Toxicol 1982;16(3):7–8.
4. Hruby K, Missliwetz J. Poisoning with oral antiarrhythmic drugs. Int J Clin Pharmacol Ther Toxicol 1985;23:253–257.
5. Frank SE, Snyder JT. Survival following severe overdose with mexiletine, nifedipine and nitroglycerin. Am J Emerg Med 1991;9:43–46.
6. Nelson LS, Hoffman RS. Mexiletine overdose producing status epilepticus without cardiovascular abnormalities. Clin Toxicol 1994;32:731–736.
7. Wilson JH. Breast milk tocainide levels. J Cardiovasc Pharmacol 1988;12:497.
8. Cohen A. Accidental overdose of tocainide successfully treated. Angiology 1987;38:614.
9. Monk JP, Brogden RN. Mexiletine: A review of its pharmacodynamic and pharmacokinetic properties and therapeutic use in the treatment of arrhythmias. Drugs 1990;40:374–411.
10. Kerin NZ, Aragon A, Marinescu G, et al. Mexiletine: Long term efficacy and side effects in patients with chronic drug-resistant potentially lethal ventricular arrhythmias. Arch Intern Med 1990;150:381–384.

11. Harris SC, Guerra C, Wallace JE. Assay of free and total tocainide by high performance liquid chromatography (HPLC) with ultraviolet (UV) detection. J Forens Sci 1989;34:912–917.
12. Sperry K, Wohlenberg N, Standefer JC. Fatal intoxications by tocainide. J Forens Sci 1987;32:1440–1446.
13. Fasola GP, D'Osvaldo F, De Pangher V, et al. Thrombocytopenia and mexiletine. Ann Intern Med 1984;100:162.

CLASS IC DRUGS

AJMALINE

Ajmaline monoethanolate is a class IC antiarrhythmic drug with class IA properties whose adverse cardiovascular effects are similar to those of quinidine.[1–5] It is a synthetic drug consisting of a white or slightly yellowish powder with an odor similar to that of alcohol. Ajmaline was first discovered among the rauwolfia alkaloids in 1931 and has been marketed for about three decades.[6] Considerable experience has, therefore, been accumulated.[5,7–11] In Paris, ajmaline was responsible for 38 cases of poisoning resulting in 9 deaths.[7] In Germany, the most frequently used class IC drugs are ajmaline, prajmaline, propafenone, and flecainide.[8] In the German series (Berlin), overdoses with ajmaline led to 4 deaths.[8] Acute intoxication tends to be suicidal in adults and accidental in children.[3,7,9] Similar to other drugs that have adverse effects on the cardiac conduction system and/or cardiac contractility (eg, quinine, quinidine, digitalis, glycosides, chloroquine, ajmaline overdose is associated with a high mortality.[8]

Source

Ajmaline is a pure alkaloid isolated from rauwolfia. It does not appear to have the sedative qualities of other rauwolfia alkaloids.[2]

Use

Ajmaline is used in ventricular arrhythmia of acute onset refractory to lidocaine and in preexcitation syndromes.[3,12,13]

Product Formulation

Ajmaline injection is prepared as a sterile solution in water for injection with a pH of 4 to 6. Ajmaline is available orally as Cardiorythmine (France), and each dose contains 200 or 500 mg. There is also a combination product with butabarbital.

Toxic Dose

The therapeutic maintenance dose is 150 to 400 mg daily. A 56-year-old woman died 1½ hours after ingesting 2500 mg of ajmaline[4] and a 4-year-old succumbed after ingesting 850 mg.[14] Three patients, however, survived doses of 1050 mg,[15] 2240 mg, and 750 mg.[16] There is no correlation between ingested overdose and fatal outcome.[8] Fatal intoxications have been observed with as little as 10 times the single therapeutic dose of 50 mg.[8]

Toxicokinetics

Absorption

Ajmaline is administered by the oral route and by intravenous infusion. Approximately 5% of an oral dose is bioavailable.

Distribution

The distribution half-life of ajmaline is 6 minutes. The apparent volume of distribution is 2 to 3 L/kg.[8] Approximately 75% of ajmaline in plasma is bound to plasma protein with a strong affinity to β_1-acid glycoprotein.[17]

Metabolism

Twenty different acetylated metabolites have been extracted from the urine.[17,18] The main metabolite is hydroxyajmaline. There is also an *N*-oxide.[8] The toxicity of oral ajmaline may be due to saturation of a metabolic enzyme with resultant rise in plasma concentrations.[8]

Elimination

After infusion of 50 mg over 5 minutes ajmaline displays an elimination half-life of 95 minutes.[8] About 5% of an ajmaline dose is excreted unchanged in the urine.[8] Impairment of liver function or cardiogenic shock leads to a reduced total plasma clearance of ajmaline. After enzyme induction with phenobarbital, the total plasma clearance of ajmaline is increased by a factor of 5.[17]

Drug Interactions

Hepatic microsomal enzyme inducers such as phenobarbital accelerate metabolism of ajmaline and increase its excretion.[17] Patients under halothane or fluothane anesthesia appear to be more sensitive to ajmaline.

Pregnancy/Lactation

There have been no controlled studies demonstrating clinical evidence of safety of either the mother or the fetus when ajmaline is administered during pregnancy.

Mechanism of Action

Ajmaline is a class IC antiarrhythmic drug similar to flecainide, encainide, and cibenzoline, but it has properties of a class IA antiarrhythmic agent (eg, quinidine, procainamide, disopyramide). It diminishes cardiac excitability, slows the heart rate, and increases atrioventricular conduction time. In high doses, ajmaline appears to have a negative inotropic effect; both atrioventricular and intraventricular blocks are not uncommon. Similar to quinidine, it has led to asystole ventricular fibrillation and circulatory collapse after rapid intravenous injection. The drug may affect the central nervous system, resulting in respiratory depression, convulsions, and death.[9]

Clinical Presentation

Accidental intoxication has been reported, particularly in children.[19] A 4½-year-old child developed grade 1 atrioventricular block with QT prolongation. He was treated with supportive measures and recovered. A 24-year-old ingested 2240 mg of ajmaline, became unconscious, went into shock, and, after clonic–like generalized convulsions, recovered with the aid of metaraminol and intravenous fluids. His QRS measured 0.28 second and QT interval 0.92 second on admission. A left bundle-branch block pattern developed and, after 30 hours, the electrocardiogram returned to normal and he recovered. A similar course was observed in another 24-year-old who ingested 750 mg of ajmaline and recovered.[16,20] Cardiac arrest has been observed after intravenous use in elderly patients.[20] A 4-year-old infant died 3 hours after ingesting about 850 mg of ajmaline.[14] Cardiac arrest was observed in 9 of 38 overdoses.[7] The patient may present with cardiac conduction disturbances, including bradycardia and tachycardia. Cardiac signs are most pronounced 1 to 2 hours after an overdose.

Ajmaline overdose may also be characterized by gastrointestinal symptoms (nausea, vomiting). Ataxia, clonic–tonic seizures, loss of consciousness, and apnea were observed in a 17-month-old after ingestion of 250 mg.[9]

Laboratory

Analytical Methods

Radioactive labeling of the ajmaline molecule is very difficult. Urine extracted with dichloromethanol/isopropanol is associated with glucuronide cleavage. The extracts are acetylated and analyzed by gas chromatography–mass spectrometry.[2,19]

Blood Levels

Blood levels of ajmaline measured after intravenous administration indicate that the desirable therapeutic level ranges from 1 to 3 μg/dL and that 15 μg/dL is a toxic dose.[13,21] After oral administration, levels are undetectable. A blood ajmaline concentration of 5.5 μg/mL was measured in a 4-year-old girl who died 3 hours after ingesting 850 mg of the drug.[14] A blood level of 10 μg/mL was measured in a woman aged 56 years who died 2½ hours after ingesting 2500 mg of ajmaline.[22] Within 150 minutes of ingestion of 1000 mg of ajmaline by a 57-year-old man, a blood level of 3 μg/mL and a urine level of 12.6 μg/mL were observed; by day 2, no further ajmaline was detected in the blood, whereas the urine level was 6.09 μg/mL.[11]

Treatment

Stabilization

As cardiac arrest and other serious life-threatening arrhythmias may occur early after an overdose, intravenous lines, cardiac monitoring, and evaluation of the tidal volume and oxygenation are first priority on admission.

Gut Decontamination

Placement of a transvenous pacemaker may be advisable before gastric lavage with its attendant vagal stimulation and induction of bradycardia, especially in patients with bradycardia on admission or with signs of an antiarrhythmic-induced conduction disturbance.

Gastric lavage with prior endotracheal intubation should be initiated, if it is to be used, within the first few hours of overdose, in view of the sudden rapid appearance of cardiac arrhythmias. Activated charcoal may be of value.[23] Neither gastric lavage nor activated charcoal in ajmaline overdose has been subjected to controlled clinical trials. No further therapy is necessary if the patient has no clinical symptoms with a normal electrocardiogram. Intraventricular block (QRS > 0.12 second) can be treated with intravenous sodium bicarbonate. In ventricular arrhythmias, resistance to sodium bicarbonate should be followed by an attempt at cardioversion. Cardiac arrest requires the usual cardiopulmonary resuscitation procedures.

Elimination Enhancement

The large volume of distribution and high plasma protein binding tend to preclude effective extracorporeal detoxification (eg, hemodialysis, hemoperfusion, peritoneal dialysis).[24]

Antidote

There are no known antidotes.

Supportive Measures

All persons who overdose with ajmaline should be admitted to an intensive care unit. Continuous electrocardiographic monitoring should be instituted on admission. Installation of a cardiopulmonary bypass may be required in certain cases.[8] Ventricular arrest and fibrillation may occur and may follow widening of the QRS complex.

REFERENCES—AJMALINE

1. Reynolds JEF, ed. *Martindale: The Extra Pharmacopoeia.* 30th ed. London: Pharmaceutical Press, 1993:58.
2. Koppel C, Tenczer J, Arndt I. Metabolic disposition of ajmaline. Eur J Drug Metab Pharmacokinet 1989;14:309–316.
3. Grenadier E, Alpan G, Keidar S, et al. The efficacy of ajmaline in ventricular arrhythmias after failure of lidocaine therapy in the acute phase of myocardial infarction. Angiology 1983;34:204–214.
4. Lengfelder W, Senges J, Rizos I. Intraindividual comparison of intravenous ajmaline and quinidine in patients with sustained ventricular tachycardia: Effects on normal myocardium and on arrhythmia characteristics. Eur Heart J 1985;6:312–322.
5. Chiale PA, Przybylski J, Halpern MS, et al. Comparative effects of ajmaline on intermittent bundle branch block and the Wolff–Parkinson–White syndrome. Am J Cardiol 1977;39: 651–657.
6. Kleinsorge H. Klinische untersuchungen uber die wirkungsweise des rauwolfia-alkaloids ajmaline by herzhythmusstorungen insbesondere der extrasystole. Med Klin 1959;54: 409.
7. Riboulet G, Efthymiou ML, Conso F, et al. Acute intoxication by ajmaline. Vet Hum Toxicol 1979;2:(suppl.):91–92.
8. Koppel C, Oberdisse V, Heinemeyer G. Clinical course and outcome in class IC antiarrhythmic overdose. Clin Toxicol 1990;28:433–444.
9. Ben Schachar C, Kishon Y. Intoxication with ajmaline in an infant. Chest 1979;76:97–98.

10. Binder C, Wimmer M. Einfall von ajmalin intoxication in klein kindes alter. Wien Klin Wochenschr 1972;84:67–69.
11. Almog C, Maidan A, Pik A, Schlesinger Z. Acute intoxication with ajmaline. Isr J Med Sci 1979;15:570–572.
12. Jonrod JC, Barrelet JA. Suicidal attempt by overdosage of ajmaline. Am Heart J 1965;70:719–720.
13. Kleinsorge H, Gaida P. Das verhalten des serumspiegels nach intravenoeser injektion von ajmaline. Klin Wochenschr 1962;40:149.
14. Ikeda N, Umetsu K, Suzuki T, et al. An infant fatality involving ajmaline. J Forens Sci 1988;33:558–561.
15. Hager W, Friedreich KH, Wink K, Wegehaupt L. Suizidversuch mit ajmalin. Dtsch Med Wochenschr 1968;93: 1809–1812.
16. Hruby K, Missliwetz J. Poisoning with oral antiarrhythmic drugs. Int J Clin Pharm Ther Toxicol 1985;23:253–257.
17. Koppel C, Wagemann A, Martens F. Pharmacokinetics and antiarrhythmic efficacy of intravenous ajmaline in ventricular arrhythmias of recent onset. Eur J Drug Metab Pharmacokinet 1989;14:161–167.
18. Koppel C, Tenczer J. Mass spectral characterization of urinary metabolites of ajmaline. Pharamcol Toxicol 1988;65:25.
19. Kallfelz HC, Rotthauwe HW. Ajmalin-intoxikation in kindesalter. Med Klin 1964;59:336–342.
20. Rautenburg HW, Menner K, Knothe W. Herzstillstand nach ajmaline injection bei Herz Katheterisierung unter Halothane. Narkose Med Welt 1962;27:2329.
21. Batalow Z, Apostolov L. Sur certaines actions toxiques de l'ajmaline avec contribution de deux cas. Folia Med 1968;10: 403.
22. Clarke EGC, ed. *Isolation and Identification of Drugs.* London: Pharmaceutical Press, 1969:177.
23. Nitsch J, Kohler U, Luderlitz B. Hemmung der flecainid-resorption durch Aktivkohle. Z Kardiol 1987;76:289–291.
24. Riegger AJG, Dilger J, Roth W, et al. Elimination von ajmalin durch verschiedene entgiftungsverfahren. Intensivmed 1980;17:57–60.

CIBENZOLINE

Cibenzoline, (±)-2-(2,2-diphenylcyclopropyl)-2-imidazoline, is a new antiarrhythmic agent, chemically unrelated to other antiarrhythmic drugs. It is an investigational drug in the United States, but is available in France as Cipralan.[1] Its electrophysiologic properties are similar to those of quinidine.[2–5] It possesses class IC, III, and IV activity.[3]

Cibenzoline lengthens AH and HV intervals and ventricular myocardial effective refractory periods.[6] Electrocardiographic findings reflect a dose-related prolongation of the PR and QRS intervals with slight prolongation of the QT_c interval; this principally reflects QRS prolongation.[6–8]

Therapeutic Dose

Cibenzoline succinate is given by mouth in a dose equivalent to cibenzoline base 130 mg initially, then 4 to 6 mg/kg body weight or 260 to 390 mg daily. It is given parenterally in initial doses of 1 mg/kg cibenzoline base over 2 minutes followed either by 8 mg/kg after 24 hours by infusion or by oral therapy.[1]

A minimum lethal dose has not been established.

Toxicokinetics

Cibenzoline is well absorbed after oral administration and has a systemic bioavailability of approximately 85%.[2,9] It reaches peak plasma levels in 1 hour,[2] and becomes approximately 50% bound to plasma protein.[10] Plasma cibenzoline concentrations correlate well with its antiarrhythmic effect; levels of 215 to 405 ng/mL result in a 90% reduction of premature ventricular complex frequency.[5] Its apparent volume of distribution at steady state is approximately 4 to 6 L/kg.[2,9] Cibenzoline is eliminated primarily by renal excretion. The elimination half-life is 6 to 15 hours and is independent of dose.[9] In renal failure, its half-life increases to 22 hours.[2] Approximately 40 to 60% of an oral or intravenous dose is recovered in the urine.[2,9] Total clearance is approximately 9 mL/min/kg.[9]

Doses of cibenzoline in toxicokinetic studies have ranged from 130 to 190 mg every 12 hours.

Drug Interactions

Cimetidine, but not ranitidine, increased the area under the curve and decreased the total body clearance and apparent volume of distribution of cibenzoline.[11]

Clinical Presentation

Adverse effects with cibenzoline are infrequent and include gastrointestinal disturbances (vomiting, diarrhea), central nervous system side effects (headache, visual disturbances, tremor), anticholinergic effects (dry mouth, urinary retention), asymptomatic liver enzyme elevation, and a negative inotropic effect.[12]

Overdose with cibenzoline led to hypotension, loss of consciousness, nausea, vomiting, and intraventricular block in one 60-year-old man who was refractive to potassium loading, intravenous sodium lactate 500 mL, and intravenous calcium chloride 2 g. The cardiogenic shock was refractory to dobutamine 10 mg/kg/min, glucagon 3 mg, and additional sodium lactate. The patient died in 12 hours with a serum level of 2550 ng/mL. Sodium lactate, reported elsewhere as being effective with other class I agents,[13] was ineffective in this patient.[14]

Hypoglycemia, also seen with class IA antiarrhythmic agents, has been reported following cibenzoline use.[12,15,16] It is reversible after discontinuation of the drug.

Laboratory

Cibenzoline is analyzed by high-performance liquid chromatography with ultraviolet detection at 214 nm (plasma) and 254 nm (urine).[17] A gas chromatography–negative ion chemical ionization mass spectrometry method is also available.[18]

Treatment

Stabilization

Patients who have overdosed with cibenzoline should be hospitalized and provided with an intravenous line, oxygen, and cardiac monitoring and with an evaluation of tidal volume as first priority.

Gut Decontamination

It is unlikely that gastric lavage will be effective 1 to 2 hours following an overdose. Anticholinergic properties, however, suggest that gut decontamination may be beneficial more than several hours after a large overdose.

Elimination Enhancement

Pharmacokinetic properties suggest that hemodialysis is not likely to be an effective therapy for cibenzoline overdose.[2] Hemoperfusion has not been reported following cibenzoline overdose.

Antidote

There is no antidote.

Supportive Measures

Sodium lactate 500 mL may be of assistance[13] in treating arrhythmias following an overdose, although one report indicated it was of no value.[14] Calcium chloride was also ineffective; however, the patient was also receiving nicardipine. Cardiogenic shock may be treated with pressor amines or glucagon, but there is no clinical evidence of their efficacy in this overdose.

REFERENCES—CIBENZOLINE

1. Reynolds JEF, ed. *Martindale: The Extra Pharmacopoeia.* 30th ed. London: Pharmaceutical Press, 1993:62.
2. Aronoff G, Brier M, Mayer ML, et al. Bioavailability and kinetics of cibenzoline in patients with normal and impaired renal function. J Clin Pharmacol 1991;31:38–44.
3. Miller JS, Vaughan Williams EM. Effects on rabbit nodal, atrial, ventricular and Purkinje cell potentials of a new antiarrhythmic drug, cibenzoline, which protects against action potential shortening in hypoxia. Br J Pharmacol 1982; 75:469–478.
4. Kostis JB, Krieger S, Moreynra A, Cosgrove N. Cibenzoline for treatment of ventricular arrhythmias: A double blind placebo controlled study. J Am Coll Cardiol 1984;4:372–377.
5. Brazzell RK, Aogaiche K, Heber JJ, et al. Cibenzoline plasma concentrations and antiarrhythmic effect. Clin Pharmacol Ther 1984;35:307–316.
6. Browne KF, Prystowsky EN, Zipes DP, et al. Clinical efficacy and electrophysiologic effects of cibenzoline therapy in patients with ventricular arrhythimas. J Am Coll Cardiol 1984; 3:857–864.
7. Nolan PE Jr. The new antiarrhythmics: Cibenzoline, moricizine, and pirmenol. Hosp Ther 1990;15:323–331.
8. Manz M, Pfitzner P, Luderitz b. Cibenzoline: Electrophysiologic effects in patients with supraventricular tachycardia. Eur Heart J 1989;10(suppl):302.
9. Massarella JW, Khoo K-C, Aogaichi K, et al. Effect of renal impairment on the pharamcokinetics of cibenzoline. Clin Pharmacol Ther 1988;43:317–323.
10. Reidenberg MM, Lorenzo BJ, Drayer DE, et al. A nonradioactive iothalamate method for measuring glomerular filtration rate and its use to study the renal handling of cibenzoline. Ther Drug Monit 1988;10:434–437.
11. Massarella JW, Defeo TM, Liguori J, et al. The effects of cimetidine and ranitidine on the pharmacokinetics of cifenline. Br J Clin Pharmacol 1991;31:481–483.
12. Hilleman DE, Mohbiuddin SM, Ahmed IS, Dahl JM. Cibenzoline-induced hypoglycemia. Drug Intell Clin Pharm 1987;21:38–40.
13. Chouty F, Funck-Brentano CF, Leenhardt A, et al. Treatment of new class I anti-arrhythmic agent poisoning with intravenous sodium molar lactate or bicarbonate. Eur Heart J 1989;10(suppl.):302 (Abstract 1521).
14. Wyss E, Karp P, Mons P, et al. Cardiogenic shock resistant to sodium lactate during cibenzoline overdosage. Therapie 1990;45:455.
15. Lefort G, Haissaguerre M, Floro J, et al. Hypoglycemies au cours de surdosages par un novel antiarrhythmique: La cibenzoline. Presse Med 1988;17:687–691.
16. Jeandel C, Preiss MA, Pierson H, et al. Hypoglycemia induced by cibenzoline. Lancet 1988;1:1232–1233.
17. Hachman MR, Lee TL, Brooks MA. Determination of cibenzoline in plasnma and urine by high pressure liquid chromatography. J Chromatogr 1983;273:347–356.
18. Min BH, Garland WA. Quantitation of cibenzoline in human plasma by gas chromatography/negative ion chemical ionization mass spectrometry. J Chromatogr 1984;336:403–409.

DETAJMIUM

Ajmaline and some of its derivatives such as prajmaline and detajmium are class IA/IC antiarrhythmic drugs according to the classification of Vaughan Williams. Detajmium has been used in the former German Democratic Republic.[1] Recommended therapeutic doses of detajmium bitartrate (3 × 25 mg/d) are similar to those of prajmaline bitartrate (3–6 × 20 mg/d). Detajmium overdose may lead to asystole and cardiac arrest associated with high detajmium concentrations.

REFERENCE—DETAJMIUM

1. Tenczer J, Lappenberg-Pelzer M, Schneider V, et al. Fatal poisoning with detajmium: Identification of detajmium and its metabolites and artifacts by gas chromatography–mass spectrometry and quantification by high-performance liquid chromatography. J Chromatogr 1994:661:47–55.

ENCAINIDE

Toxicokinetics

Encainide has two major active metabolites, *O*-demethylencainide (ODE) and 3-methoxy-*O*-demethylencainide (MODE), which have longer half-lives and equal or greater potency than the parent compound.[1–3] Encainide has two distinct phenotypes for metabolism, extensive (approximately 92%) and nonextensive (8%).[1,2]

Extensive metabolizers have an encainide half-life of 1.7 hours, producing the two active metabolites ODE and MODE. Nonextensive metabolizers have an encainide half-life of 9.8 hours, producing the inactive metabolite *N*-demethylencainide (NDE). Effective plasma levels of ODE for suppression of arrhythmia are 100 to 300 ng/mL, whereas plasma levels of MODE are 60 to 280 ng/mL during long-term therapy in extensive metabolizers. Nonextensive metabolizers require concentrations of encainide greater than 265 ng/mL for therapeutic effects. Plasma levels of encainide are 250 to 1000 ng/mL in nonextensive metabolizers, 20 times higher than those in extensive metabolizers due to the greater oral bioavailability and longer half-life of elimination. Toxicity with ODE is seen at concentrations above 300 ng/mL. Protein binding is 70.5 and 78% for extensive and nonextensive metabolizers, respectively.[3]

Toxic Dose

A 3- to 4-g overdose of encainide in an adult produced central nervous system (obtundation, seizures) and cardiovascular (QT prolongation, bradycardia, hypotension) toxic effects similar to those of class IA antiarrhythmic drugs (quinidine) and tricyclic antidepressants.[4] Encainide differs from the latter drugs in its lack of anticholinergic, alpha-adrenergic antagonist, and vasodilator properties. The bradycardia and hypotension in this case appeared to respond to intravenous sodium bicarbonate, as in tricyclic antidepressant overdose.[5] A 6-month-old infant ingested a single 25-mg encainide tablet. Within 30 minutes the infant developed a wide-complex sinus tachycardia (QRS, 0.16 second) and acutely decompensated with development of ventricular tachycardia.

Treatment

Hypertonic sodium bicarbonate or sodium chloride may be beneficial in reversing encountered cardiotoxic overdose. Because encainide is readily absorbed and has a rapid onset of action, induced emesis is probably contraindicated. Gastric lavage may induce vagal stimulation and asystole. Activated charcoal is of limited use when an ingestant is absorbed rapidly. Transport personnel should not delay transport until toxic signs appear, especially in infants or children in whom a single tablet could be lethal. Similarly, an adult who reports intentionally ingesting "just a minimal" dose of a rapidly and high toxic substance deserves prompt transport for evaluation and treatment.[5] Withdrawal of encainide led to a fatal episode of ventricular tachycardia leading to fibrillation.[6] Hospital admission should be considered for selected patients in whom encainide or flecainide is to be discontinued.[6]

Encainide exacerbates hyperglycemia in some patients. It is not known whether this is due to the parent compound or its metabolites.[7] Serum glucose levels should be monitored when encainide therapy is begun in patients with type II diabetes mellitus and when encainide is discontinued in patients receiving insulin therapy.[7]

FLECAINIDE

Toxicokinetics

The liver metabolizes about 50% of an absorbed therapeutic dose; the kidney excretes about 30% unchanged. Like other antiarrhythmic agents, flecainide may cause proarrhythmic effects.[8] Flecainide prolongs the AH, HV, PR, and QRS intervals, as well as (to a lesser extent) the effective refractory period in the ventricular myocardium.

Drug Interactions

Patients receiving concomitant flecainide and amiodarone have a significantly increased flecainide plasma concentration.[9] The clearance and volume of distribution of flecainide are significantly greater in smokers than nonsmokers, though there is no difference between the two groups with respect to terminal plasma half-life or renal clearance.[10]

Pregnancy/Lactation

A patient who received 200 mg of flecainide and 160 mg of sotalol daily delivered a normal baby by cesarean section 3 weeks before term. There were no teratogenic effects, although an umbilical cord: maternal plasma ratio of 0.86 : 1 showed placental transfer of flecainide. The maternal milk : maternal plasma ratio was 1.57 : 1 to 2.18 : 1, indicating excretion of flecainide in breast milk.[11] This experience appeared to be corroborated by others.[12] Intravenous flecainide (110 mg) was administered to a woman at 30 weeks' gestation and successfully suppressed a fetal tachycardia.[13] Sudden withdrawal of flecainide and encainide may be associated with serious life-threatening ventricular arrhythmias.[14]

Based on the pharmacokinetics of flecainide in infants, the expected average steady-state plasma concentration in a newborn consuming all the milk products of its mother (approximately 700 mL/d) would not be expected to exceed about 62 ng/mL. Few toxic effects have been observed at plasma levels ranging from 100 to 900 ng/mL. The risk to the suckling infant is very low.[15]

Clinical Presentation

In one series of patients with a history of serious ventricular dysrhythmias, the flecainide dose of 200 mg twice daily was associated with the development of ventricular tachycardia demonstrating an unusual sinusoidal QRS complex.[16] Flecainide overdose has led to cardiorespiratory failure, ventricular fibrillation, asystole atrioventricular block, marked prolongation of the QRS, QT, and T wave, coma, and bradycardia.

Generalized tonic–clonic seizures followed ingestion of 1500 mg of flecainide.[17] This was followed by a period of unconsciousness, with hypotonic limbs and extensor plantar responses.[17] The patient recovered. The initial flecainide level was greater than 4 μg/mL.

Laboratory

Analytical Methods

A simple, sensitive (10 ng/mL) HPLC method is available to measure plasma flecainide levels.[10] A HPLC method for the quantification of encainide and its metabolites in plasma and urine indicates limits of detection of 5 ng/mL in plasma and 25 ng/mL in urine.[19] A reverse-phase HPLC technique can also analyze the parent compound and its metabolites with a minimum detection limit of 10 ng/mL.[3] Methods to enhance elimination probably do not remove significant amounts of this drug from the blood.[20]

Ancillary Tests

The PR, QRS, and QT intervals may be markedly prolonged on the electrocardiogram following a flecainide overdose.[17]

Blood Levels

Cardiac arrest developed in a patient with a postmortem blood level of 16 μg/mL.[21] The patient died about 1 hour after he appeared intoxicated. Cardiac arrest terminated the course of an adult patient who exhibited a postmortem flecainide level of 13 μg/mL.[22] A blood concentration of 1.8 μg/mL was measured in a patient who died in acute respiratory distress and cardiogenic shock unresponsive to dopamine, dobutamine, and sodium nitroprusside.[23]

On the basis of current data, plasma levels exceeding 1 μg/mL are probably toxic.[24] Atrioventricular nodal block with escape rhythm and QRS interval prolongation developed in a patient who had a flecainide plasma level of 3.0 μg/mL.[25] The therapeutic serum range of flecainide is 200 to 1000 ng/mL (0.42–2.1 μmol/L).[26] A fluorescence polarization immunoassay (Abbott TDx)[2] is calculated with flecainide acetate (therapeutic range, 200–1000 ng/mL).[27]

Electrocardiogram

Ingestion of 900 mg of flecainide daily by an adult led to symptoms of blurred vision, headache, photophobia, paresthesias, and generalized weakness. The electrocardiogram showed broadening of P waves, prolongation of the PR interval, and widening of the QRS with a plasma level of 2.5 μg/mL. The QT interval lengthened at levels of 1.86 to 1.1 μg/mL. At 0.49 μg/mL, the QT interval normalized and giant T waves appeared. The patient survived with supportive therapy.[28] Blurred vision, dry mouth, dizziness, nausea, and fatigue occurred in another patient 10 minutes after ingestion of 1800 mg of flecainide. The electrocardiogram disclosed no P wave, but a wide QRS complex and an increased QT interval. The patient was treated supportively and survived.[29]

A patient ingested 3800 mg of flecainide with 50 mg of diazepam, 20 mg of loperamide, and 100 g of ethanol. In 2 hours the flecainide serum level was 3.7 μg/mL. The electrocardiogram showed a prolonged QT interval, prolonged QRS interval, and prolonged PR interval with a ventricular tachycardia, which deteriorated to polymorphous ventricular tachycardia. Sinus rhythm was restored without pacing, cardioversion, or dopamine, sodium bicarbonate, and physostigmine. Normalization of the electrocardiogram was correlated with diminishing serum levels of flecainide.[30]

Treatment

Stabilization

Stabilization (airway, respiration, circulatory status) with oxygen, cardiac monitoring, and intravenous lines is first priority in an intensive care facility. Rapid gastric emptying (within 1 hour of ingestion) may assist in removing flecainide sufficient to avoid its wide tissue distribution and cardiotoxic effects; however, this must be tempered by knowledge of the occasional occurrence of seizures within 2 hours of a flecainide overdose.[16] Care must be taken to protect the airway before gastric lavage.

Hypertonic sodium bicarbonate (100 mL of 1 mEq/mL) is well tolerated by patients taking therapeutic doses of flecainide or encainide for ventricular arrhythmias, but in one study it appeared to have no significant effect on the duration of the QRS, PR, or QT interval when compared with normal saline.[31]

Intravenous administration of molar sodium lactate (500 mL over 30 minutes) with intravenous potassium chloride to three flecainide overdose patients resulted in an improvement in clinical status with narrowing of the QRS. Similar effects were observed in two patients who had overdosed with propafenone and four with cibenzoline.[32]

Cardioversion has not been evaluated in patients with elevated flecainide plasma levels. Pacing may be time consuming if hemodynamic collapse is impending.[30] Cardiogenic shock and Torsade de pointes may respond to intubation, mechanical ventilation, dopamine, and a sodium load (see Torsade de Pointes in the Introduction to this chapter). Proarrhythmic effects of flecainide acetate (sympathomimetic ventricular tachycardia) may be suppressed by high-dose intravenous amiodarone.[33]

Elimination Enhancement

Hemodialysis did not prevent death in an individual who had a flecainide plasma concentration of 6500 ng/mL (therapeutic range, 200–980 ng/mL).[34,35] Hemodialysis and hemoperfusion are not effective in the treatment of flecainide overdose.[36,37]

Gotz and colleagues proposed prophylactic use of a pacemaker (extrathoracic or intravenous), gastric lavage, activated charcoal, forced diuresis with acidification of the urine, and, in the case of electromechanical dissociation, immediate hemoperfusion, even though its efficacy has not yet been demonstrated.[38]

The Cast Study

The Cardiac Arrhythmic Suppression Trial (CAST) was the first long-term, multicenter, multidrug, placebo-controlled trial of the safety and efficacy of antiarrhythmic drug therapy in reducing the risk of sudden death. Results indicate that the use of encainide and flecainide, both class IC antiarrhythmic agents, to treat asymptomatic or minimally symptomatic ventricular arrhythmias in patients after myocardial infarction is associated with a substantial increase in the rate of sudden death and total mortality. These data suggest that encainide and flecainide, by exerting a proarrhythmic effect, may induce lethal ventricular arrhythmias,[39,40] a theory that is at present controversial.[41] The FDA has urged physicians to use these drugs only for life-threatening arrhythmias.[42] A subsequent study indicated that there was no excess mortality when both of the drugs were used in patients with supraventricular arrhythmias.[43] Finally, atrial life-threatening proarrhythmic effects appeared to follow use of class IC antiarrhythmic drugs in a recent study.[44]

REFERENCES—ENCAINIDE AND FLECAINIDE

1. Harrison DC, Kates RE, Quart BD. Relation of blood level and metabolites to the antiarrhythmic effectiveness of encainide. Am J Cardiol 1986;58:66C–73C.
2. Woosley RL, Wood AJJ, Roder DM. Encainide. N Engl J Med 1988;318:1107–1115.
3. Dasgupta A, Rosenzweig IB, Turgeon J, Raisys V. Encainide and metabolites analysis in serum or plasma using a reversed phase high performance liquid chromatographic technique. J Chromatogr 1990;526:260–265.
4. Pentel PR, Goldsmith SR, Salerno DM, et al. Effect of hypertonic sodium bicarbonate on encainide overdose. Am J Cardiol 1986;57:878–879.
5. Mortensen ME, Bolon CE, Kelley MT, et al. Encainide overdose in an infant. Ann Emerg Med 1992;21:998–1001.
6. Thomas GS. Death following withdrawal of encainide. N Engl J Med 1989;321:393.
7. Salerno DM, Fifield J, Krejci J, Hodges M. Encainide-induced hyperglycemia. Am J Med 1988;84:39–44.
8. Nappi JM, Anderson JL. Flecainide: A new prototype antiarrhythmic agent. Pharmacotherapy 1985;5:209–218.
9. Leclercq JF, Denjoy L, Mentere F, Coumel P. Flecainide acetate dose concentration relationship in cardiac arrhythmias: Influence of heart failure and amiodarone. Cardiovasc Drug Ther 1990;4:1161–1165.

10. Holtzman JL, Weeks CE, Kvam DC, et al. Identification of drug interactions by meta-analysis of premarketing trials: The effect of smoking on the pharmacokinetics and dosage requirements of flecainide acetate. Clin Pharmacol Ther 1989; 46:1–8.
11. Wagner X, Jouglard J, Moulin M, et al. Coadministration of flecainide acetate and sotolol during pregnancy: Lack of teratogenic effects, passage across the placenta and excretion in human breast milk. Am Heart J 1990;119: 700–702.
12. Palmer CM, Norris MC. Placental transfer of flecainide. Am J Dis Child 1990;144:144.
13. Wren C, Hunter S. Maternal administration of flecainide to terminate and suppress fetal tachycardia. Br Med J 1988;296:249.
14. Woodburn JD Jr. Cardiac arrest from a daily newspaper article. Ann Emerg Med 1989;18:1375–1376.
15. McQuinn RL, Pisani A, Wafa S, et al. Flecainide excretion in human breast milk. Clin Pharmacol Ther 1990;48:262–267.
16. Sellers TD, Di Marco JP. Sinusoidal ventricular tachycardia association with flecainide acetate. Chest 1984;85:647–649.
17. Kennerdy A, Thomas P, Sheridan DJ. Generalized seizures as the presentation of flecainide toxicity. Eur Heart J 1989;10: 950–954.
18. Plomp TA, Boom HT, Maes RAA. Measurement of flecainide plasma concentrations by high performance liquid chromatography with fluorescence detection. J Anal Toxicol 1986;10:102–106.
19. Bartek MJ, Mayol RF, Boarman MP, et al. Analysis of encainide and metabolites in plasma and urine by high-performance liquid chromatography. Ther Drug Monit 1988; 10:446–452.
20. Conrad GJ, Ober RE: Metabolism of flecainide. Am J Cardiol 1984;53:41B–51B.
21. Forrest ARW, Marsh I, Galloway JH, Gray PB. A rapidly fatal dose with flecainide. J Anal Toxicol 1991;15:41–43.
22. Levine B, Chute D, Caplan YH. Flecainide intoxication. J Anal Toxicol 1990;14:335–336.
23. Forbes WP, Hee TT, Mohiuddin SM, Hillman DE. Flecainide-induced cardiogenic shock. Chest 1988;94:1121.
24. Rosen DM, Woosely RL. Drug therapy: Flecainide. N Engl J Med 1986;315:36–41.
25. Holmes B, Heel RC. Flecainide: A preliminary review of its pharmacodynamic properties and therapeutic efficacy. Drugs 1985;29:1–33.
26. Malikin G, Murphy M, Lam S. Assay of flecainide in serum by high performance liquid chromatography after microscale protein precipitation. Ther Drug Monit 1989;11:210–213.
27. Ray J. Flecainide. What are we measuring? Ther Drug Monit 1990;12:416.
28. Crijns HJGM, Kingma JH, Viersma JW, Lie KI. Transient giant inverted T waves during flecainide ingestion. Am Heart J 1987;113:214–215.
29. Xing-Sheng Y, Jing-Ping S, Guang Z. Acute flecainide toxicity. Chin Med J 1990;103:606–607.
30. Winkelmann BR, Leinberger H. Life-threatening flecainide toxicity: A pharmacodynamic approach. Ann Intern Med 1987;106:807–814.
31. Pentel PR, Fifield J, Salerno DM. Lack of effect of hypertonic sodium bicarbonate on QRS duration in patients taking therapeutic doses of class IC antiarrhythmic drugs. J Clin Pharmacol 1990;301:789–794.
32. Chouty F, Funck-Brentano C, Leehardt A, et al. Intravenous sodium lactate as a treatment for class 1 anti-arrhythmic agents overdose. Circulation 1989;80(suppl. II):II-430.
33. Sagie A, Strasberg B, Kusniec J, et al. Rapid suppression of flecainide induced incessant ventricular tachycardia with high dose intravenous amiodarone. Chest 1988;93:879–880.
34. Palitzcsch KD, Bode H, Huck K, Vsadel KH. Multiple successful resuscitations after flecainide intoxication with suicidal threat. Dtsch Med Wochenschr 1992;117:56–60.
35. Schaller M-D, Fischer AP, Wasserfallen JB, et al. Cardiac arrest after volunteer intoxication with flecainide: Resuscitation by prolonged partial extracorporeal circulation. Schweiz Med Wochenschr 1992;122:786.
36. Braun J, Kollert JR, Gessler V, Becker JV. Failure of haemoperfusion to reduce flecainide intoxication: A case study. Med Toxicol 1987;2:463–467.
37. Wurzberger R, Witter E, Avenhaus H, et al. Hamoperfusion bei flecainidintoxikation. Klin Wochenschr 1986;64:442–444.
38. Gotz D, Pohle S, Barchow D. Primary and secondary detoxification in severe flecainide intoxication. Intensive Care Med 1991;17:181–187.
39. Ruskin JN. The Cardiac Arrhythmia Suppression Trial (CAST). N Engl J Med 1989;321:386–388.
40. The Cardiac Arrhythmia Suppression Trial (CAST) investigators. Preliminary report: Effect of encainide and flecainide on mortality in a randomized trial of arrhythmic suppression after myocardial infarction. N Engl J Med 1989;321:406–412.
41. Echt DS, Liebson PR, Mitchell LB, et al. Mortality and morbidity in patients receiving encainide, flecainide or placebo. The cardiac arrhythmic suppression trial. N Engl J Med 1991;324:781–788.
42. Change urged in use of two drugs. FDA Consumer 1989; 23(6):2.
43. Pritchett ELC, Wilkinson WE. Mortality in patients treated with flecainide and encainide for supraventricular arrhythmias. Am J Cardiol 1991;67:976–980.
44. Feld GK, Chen P-S, Nicod P, et al. Possible atrial proarrhythmic effects of class IC antiarrhythmic drugs. Am J Cardiol 1990;66:378–383.

LORCAINIDE

Lorcainide is a class IC antiarrhythmic agent available in Belgium. Toxicokinetic studies indicate up to 100% bioavailability, protein binding of 85%, volume of distribution of 5 to 10 L/kg, elimination half-life of 7 to 13 hours, largely hepatic, and production of norlorcainide, an active metabolite with a longer half-life, preceded by bradycardia, shock, coma, and seizures. Death has followed ingestion of 2500 mg.[1] Treatment is similar to that for other class 1C antiarrhythmic agents.

REFERENCES—LORCAINIDE

1. Evers J, Buttner-Belz. Fatal lorcainide poisoning. Clin Toxicol 1995;33:157–159.

PROPAFENONE

Propafenone has been available in West Germany and Europe since 1977 and in the United States since 1990. Overdoses have been reported following its use and fatalities have occurred. Symptomatic and supportive care is paramount in treatment of serious toxicity following propafenone poisoning.

Structure and Classification

Propafenone (2′-[2-hydroxy-3-(propylamino)propoxy]-3-phenylpropiophenone is a class IC antiarrhythmic agent.[1] The structure of propafenone is similar to that of many beta blockers. Propafenone appears as a racemic of D and L isomers and has a bitter taste.[2] Its molecular weight is 377.91.

Use

Propafenone has been marketed in the United States for oral treatment of life-threatening ventricular arrhythmias such as sustained ventricular tachycardia (see The CAST Study under Flecainide). It is not recommended in the United States for treatment of less severe arrhythmias such as nonsustained ventricular tachycardias and frequent premature ventricular contractions, even if patients are symptomatic.[3] It may have a role in treating supraventricular arrhythmias but has not been approved by the FDA for this indication.[4,5]

Product Formulation

Propafenone (Rhythmol) is supplied as 150-and 300-mg tablets.[3]

Therapeutic Dose

Most patients respond to oral doses of propafenone of 150 to 300 mg every 8 hours.[4] Because of nonlinear kinetics, a threefold increase in dosage may lead to a tenfold elevation in plasma concentration (as in changing from 150 mg twice a day to 300 mg three times a day).[6]

Toxic Dose

A 57-year-old patient ingested 1350 mg of propafenone and survived.[7] A 20-year-old ingested 4500 mg and survived.[8] A 2-year-old child ingested 180 mg, went into cardiopulmonary collapse, and recovered.[9] A 26-year-old ingested 6000 mg and survived.[10] A dose of 2700 mg led to hypotension, seizures, and conduction disturbances; the patient survived.[11] Doses of 4800 mg[12] and 9000 mg[13] were associated with fatal outcomes. A 27-year-old ingested 8.1 g of propafenone and survived.[14]

Toxicokinetics

Absorption

Propafenone is well absorbed (95%) with a bioavailability of 11 to 39%, indicating an extensive presystemic clearance.[15,16] The peak plasma concentration of propafenone after a single dose of 300 mg is approximately 400 ng/mL; for 5-hydroxypropafenone (5-HP), it is almost 180 ng/mL.[17] After 150 mg three times a day the steady-state plasma propafenone level is about 400 ng/mL, the 5-HP level is about 240 ng/mL, and *N*-depropylpropafenone level is approximately 90 ng/mL.[4] Peak plasma concentrations of the drug and its metabolite are reached in 1 to 4 hours.[17] Following 1 month of treatment, blood levels of the drug and its 5-HP metabolite rise. 5-HP is rapidly absorbed. After 300 mg of oral 5-HP, a peak level of 150 ng/mL is reached after 36 minutes.[18,19] No good correlation exists between plasma propafenone concentration and suppression of arrhythmias[4] although some authors consider serum propafenone levels of 500 to 2000 ng/mL to be within the therapeutic range.[20]

Distribution

Propafenone has a large apparent volume of distribution of 1.1 to 3.6 L/kg and is 97% protein bound,[21] mainly to α_1-acid glycoprotein.[22] The therapeutic plasma level of propafenone has been suggested to be 0.5 to 2.0 μg/mL.[6]

Elimination

Propafenone exhibits extensive first-pass metabolism by a hepatic oxidative pathway and is extensively metabolized into two active metabolites—5-HP and *N*-depropylpropafenone—both of which have activity comparable to that of propafenone.[23] Formation of the 5-HP metabolite is mediated by the cytochrome P450 II (D6[CYP2D6]) isozyme. Propafenone half-life ranges from 2 to 32 hours.[24,25] Extensive metabolizers have half-lives of 2 to 10 hours; poor metabolizers, 10–32 hours. In the 10% of patients who are poor metabolizers, 5-HP is absent or largely diminished.

The renal clearance of propafenone is approximately 12 mL/min/kg.[26] The terminal half-life of 5-HP is 8 to 16 hours.[18] Less than 1% of the dose is eliminated unchanged in the urine.[27]

Drug Interactions

- *With local anesthetics*[3]: Concurrent use with propafenone may increase the risk of nervous system side effects.
- *With other antiarrhythmic drugs:* Concurrent use with propafenone may result in increased cardiac effects.
- *With quinidine:* Quinidine decreases propafenone clearance and its metabolic clearance to 5-HP.[28]
- *With rifampicin:* Rifampin lowers the plasma concentration of propafenone and reduces its antiarrhythmic effect.[29]
- *With metoprolol:* Propafenone increases metoprolol blood levels and metoprolol beta blocking activity.[30]
- *With warfarin:* Propafenone increases warfarin plasma concentration and enhances anticoagulant effect.[31]
- *With digoxin:* Propafenone increases the total and renal clearance of digoxin and increases digoxin serum concentrations, requiring a reduction in digoxin maintenance dosage with careful monitoring of serum concentrations of the cardiac glycoside.[32,33] There is a decrease in heart rate and shortening of the QT_c interval.[33] The volume of distribution and nonrenal clearance of digoxin appear to be decreased.[34] In clinical practice, if propafenone concentrations are not readily available, digoxin serum levels should be monitored.[35]

Pregnancy/Lactation

Propafenone has been placed in FDA Pregnancy Category C. Both propafenone and 5-HP are detectable in newborn plasma and in maternal milk, though at concentrations lower than those in maternal plasma.[36]

Mechanism of Action

Propafenone is a fast sodium channel blocker with weak beta-adrenoceptor blocking activity.[25] Its kinetics of interaction with cardiac sodium channels are similar to those of flecainide and encainide.[4] It suppresses nonsustained ventricular arrhythmias. Its major metabolites, 5-HP and *N*-depropylpropafenone, share its sodium channel blocking properties. Propafenone slows intraatrial and atrioventricular nodal conduction by prolonging atrial refractoriness.[37] It also prolongs, to a lesser extent, the ventricular effective refractory period.

Arrhythmia suppression occurs at the same dose level in both extensive and poor metabolizers.[24] Increases (15–25%) in PR, QRS, QT_c, AH, and HV intervals follow its use.[4] After a 300-ng dose of 5-HP, there is significant prolongation of the PQ and QRS intervals.[18]

The degree of beta blockade after propafenone use is increased in those 7 to 10% of the population with a genetic deficiency in the ability to metabolize the parent drug to its metabolite, 5-HP.[38]

Both (*R*)- and (*S*)-propafenone have comparable effects on sodium current-dependent conduction in the atrial and ventricular myocardium, whereas the calcium current-dependent excitations in the atrioventricular node are affected more by (*S*)-propafenone than (*R*)-propafenone. The currently used (*R,S*)*-propafenone is a racemic mixture. The two isomers have equal effects on the sodium channel. Pure* (*S*)-propafenone has much more beta-adrenergic blocking activity than the (*R*) form.[39,40]

Clinical Presentation

Adverse Effects

Gastrointestinal Effects. About 20% of patients experience some mild side effects, which may include constipation, nausea, vomiting, and, rarely, diarrhea. A bitter taste is noted by 5 to 10% of patients.[6]

Neurologic Effects. At a plasma propafenone concentration of 900 ng/mL or higher, visual blurring, dizziness, and paresthesias may be observed.[24] At a level of 450 ng/mL, such effects are minimal. Poor metabolizers have increased side effects.[24] Propafenone may induce generalized myasthenic symptoms in patients with ocular myasthenia.[41]

Asthma. Because of its beta-blocker activity, propafenone may induce severe reactive airway disease.[42,43] Rare cases of cholestatic hepatitis have been reported.[44]

Conduction Defects. Propafenone can cause cardiac conduction abnormalities such as new left or right bundle-branch block, atrioventricular block, and sinus node dysfunction.

Myocardial Depressant Effects. Propafenone may cause worsening of congestive heart failure.[4] These effects (conduction and myocardial depression) are dose dependent and occur most often in patients with advanced underlying heart disease. Propafenone may cause lethal arrhythmias.[45]

Proarrhythmias. Clinically significant proarrhythmias (increase in ventricular premature contractions, conversion of nonsustained to sustained ventricular tachycardia, or new appearances of ventricular tachycardia or ventricular fibrillation) may occur in 5% of patients.[46]

Overdose

Signs of overdose, usually most severe within 3 hours of ingestion, include hypotension, somnolence, bradycardia, atrioventricular dissociation, and intraatrial and intraventricular conduction disturbances; asystole may occur. Convulsions and high-grade ventricular arrhythmias have been reported.[7–13,14,47–50]

Laboratory

Analytical Methods

Plasma concentrations of propafenone and its two major metabolites, 5-HP and *N*-depropylpropafenone, are analyzed by high-performance liquid chromatography.[51]

Blood Levels

Patients who had overdosed with propafenone and survived had propafenone blood levels of 1888 ng/mL,[10] 3000 ng/mL,[8] 3185 ng/mL,[11] 3449 ng/mL,[7] 3737 ng/mL,[43] and 4702 ng/mL.[13] Blood levels in nonsurvivors were 7700 ng/mL[12] and 21,000 ng/mL.[48] One patient died with a blood level of 800 ng/mL; this patient had also overdosed with propranolol.[49]

Abnormalities

A positive antinuclear antibody titer may be observed.[6]

Treatment

Stabilization

Early recognition of poisoning, preferably within the first 1 to 2 hours, is important. Hypotension, seizures, and shock may occur within 1 to 2 hours of ingestion. An intravenous line, oxygen, and cardiac monitoring and careful evaluation of tidal volume are available in an intensive care facility.

Gut Decontamination

Gastric emptying should be performed early after an overdose to lessen the amount of propafenone absorbed and thereby aid in keeping blood levels from rising to dangerously high levels. As seizures may occur within 1 hour of an overdose, caution must be exercised to maintain an adequate airway (endotracheal intubation). Activated charcoal may be useful but there is no controlled clinical evidence to support this. Plasma levels of propafenone and its active metabolites may not peak for up to 4 hours[17]; decontamination procedures may be useful for up to 4 to 6 hours after ingestion.

Elimination Enhancement

Hemodialysis[7,26] and hemoperfusion[13,48] have not been useful in removing propafenone. The strong protein binding and extensive volume of distribution mitigate against such measures. Plasma exchange appeared useful in one case.[7]

Antidote

There is no antidote.

Supportive Measures

1. Advanced cardiac life support, including atropine and pressor amines (dopamine, dobutamine), should be available. Isoproterenol (isoprenaline) has been useful.[49]
2. With the wide QRS, prolonged QT interval, and possible interference with cardiac sodium channels, sodium loading has been proposed. Molar sodium lactate has been used in an overdose; the patient survived.[49] In other cases, sodium loading with sodium bicarbonate[8] or hypertonic saline[13] was followed by survival.[8,13] Care must be taken to prevent acute pulmonary edema secondary to sodium overload.
3. Diazepam is useful in treating seizures. Phenytoin was useful in one overdose patient[9]; however, phenytoin has class IB antiarrhythmic properties and must be used with great caution in the presence of preexisting conduction defects.
4. Cardiac pacing may be necessary for heart block.
5. Use of other class IC drugs for treatment (flecainide, tocainide) may exacerbate conduction problems and should be avoided.
6. A combination of bolus and continuously infused epinephrine with temporary internal pacing appeared effective in one patient.[14]

REFERENCES—PROPAFENONE

1. Dukes ID, Vaughn Williams EM. The multiple models of action of propafenone. Eur Heart J 1984;5:115–125.
2. Chow MSS, Lebsack C, Dillerman D. Propafenone: A new antiarrhythmic agent. Clin Pharm 1988;7:869–877.
3. Propafenone (systemic). USP DI update 1990;10:660–662.
4. Funch-Brentano C, Kroemer HK, Lee JT, Roden DM. N Engl J Med 1990;322:518–525.
5. Pritchett ELC, McCarthy EA, Wilkinson WE. Propafenone treatment of symptomatic paroxysmal supraventricular arrhythmias: A randomized, placebo-controlled crossover trial in patients tolerating oral therapy. Ann Intern Med 1991; 114:539–544.
6. Shen EN. Propafenone: A promising new antiarrhythmic agent. Chest 1990;98:434–441.
7. Conte F, Latini R, Meroni M, Castel JM. Propafenone acute intoxication removed by plasma exchange. In: *Proceedings of the Fourteenth International Congress of the European Association of Poison Centers, September 25, 1990:*117.
8. Ohayon J, Colle J-P, Besse P. Intoxication volontaire a la propafenone sur coeur sain (A propos d'une observation). Coeur 1985;16:629–634.
9. McHugh TP, Perina DG. Propafenone ingestion. Ann Emerg Med 1987;16:437–440.
10. Hettinger M, Siebner H. Intoxikation mit propafenone. Mediz Welt 1989;40:1495–1497.
11. Friocourt P, Martin C, Lozach L. Intoxication volontaire par la propafenone: A propos d'un cas. Ann Cardiol Angeiol 1988;37(3):133–136.
12. Brzezinka H, Holtz J, Goenechea S. Propafenone fatality. Bull Int Assoc Forens Toxicol 1988;20(1):30–32.
13. Budde T, Meyer M, Breithardt G, et al. Therapie der schweren propafenoneintoxikation: Eliminations versuch mittels hamoperfusion. Z Kardiol 1986; 75:764–769.
14. Kerns W, English B, Ford M. Severe adult propafenone toxicity. Vet Hum Toxicol 1992;34:329.
15. Hii JTY, Duff HJ, Burgess ED. Clinical pharmacokinetics of propafenone. Clin Pharmacokinet 1991;21:1–10.
16. Somberg JC, Tepper D, Landau S. Propafenone: A new antiarrhythmic agent. Am Heart J 1988;115:1274–1279.
17. Giani P, Landolina M, Giudici V, et al. Pharmacokinetics and pharmacodynamics of propafenone during acute and chronic administration. Eur J Clin Pharmacol 1988;34:187–194.
18. Haefeli WE, Vozeh S, Ha H-R, et al. Concentration effect relations of 5-hydroxypropafenone in normal subjects. Am J Cardiol 1991;67:1022–1026.
19. Haefeli W, Vozeh S, Ha H-R, et al. Pharmacodynamics of 5-hydroxypropafenone. Clin Pharmacol Ther 1990;47:139.
20. Tyberg J, Macnab J, Giesbrecht E, McGuigan M. Toxicokinetics of propafenone and its metabolites in a near fatal overdose. Vet Hum Toxicol 1993;35:344.
21. Parker RB, McCollam PL, Bauman JL. Propafenone: A novel type IC antiarrhythmic agent. DICP Ann Pharmacother 1989;23:196–203.
22. Gilles AM, Yee YG, Kates RE. Binding of antiarrhythmic drugs to purified human alpha 1-acid glycoprotein. Biochem Pharmacol 1985;34:4279–4282.
23. Zoble RG, Kirsten EB, Brewington J, Propafenone Research Group. Pharmacokinetics and pharmacodynamic evaluation of propafenone in patients with ventricular arrhythmia. Clin Pharmacol Ther 1989;45:535–541.
24. Siddoway LA, Roden DM, Woosley RL. Clinical pharmacology of propafenone: Pharmacokinetics, metabolism and concentration response relations. Am J Cardiol 1984;54:9D–12D.
25. Siddoway LA, Thompson KA, McAllister CB, et al. Polymorphism of propafenone metabolism and disposition in man: Clinical and pharmacokinetic consequences. Circulation 1987;75:785–791.
26. Burgess E, Duff H, Wilkes P. Propafenone disposition in renal insufficiency and renal failure. J Clin Pharmacol 1989; 29: 112–113.
27. Seipel L, Breithardt G. Propafenone: A new antiarrhythmic drug. Eur Heart J 1980;1:309–313.
28. Funck-Brentano C, Kroemer H, Pavlou H, et al. Inhibition of propafenone metabolism by low doses of quinidine in man. Clin Res 1988;36:363A.
29. Castel JM, Cappiello E, Leopaldi D, Latini R. Rifampicin lowers plasma concentrations of propafenone and its antiarrhythmic effect. Br J Clin Pharmacol 1990;30:155–156.
30. Wagner F, Kalusche D, Trenk E, et al. Drug interaction between propafenone and metoprolol. Br J Clin Pharmacol 1987;24:213–220.
31. Kates RE, Yee T-G, Kirsten ER. Interaction between warfarin and propafenone in healthy volunteer subjects. Clin Pharmacol Ther 1987;42:305–311.
32. Zalzstein E, Koren G, Bryson SM, Freedom RM. Interaction between digoxin and propafenone in children. J Pediat 1990; 116:310–312.
33. Calvo MV, Martin-Suarez A, Luengo CM, et al. Interaction between digoxin and propafenone. Ther Drug Monit 1989;11: 10–15.
34. Nolan PE Jr, Marcus FI, Erstad BL, et al. Effects of coadministration of propafenone on the pharmacokinetics of digoxin in healthy volunteer subjects. J Clin Pharmacol 1989; 29:46–52.
35. Birgot M-C, Debruyne D, Bonnefoy L, et al. Serum digoxin levels related to plasma propafenone levels during concomitant treatment. J Clin Pharmacol 1991;31: 521–526.
36. Libardoni M, Piovan D, Busato E, Padrini R. Transfer of propafenone and 5-hydroxypropafenone to foetal plasma and maternal milk. Br J Clin Pharmacol 1991;32:527–528.
37. Connolly SJ, Kates RE, Lebsack CS, et al. Clinical efficacy and electrophysiology of oral propafenone for ventricular tachycardia. Am J Cardiol 1983;52:1208–1213.
38. Lee JT, Kroemer HK, Silberstein DJ, et al. The role of genetically determined polymorphic drug metabolism in the beta blockade produced by propafenone. N Engl J Med 1990; 322:1764–1768.
39. Stoschitzky K, Klein W, Stark G, et al. Different stereoselective effects of (*R*)- and (*S*)-propafenone: Clinical pharmacologic, electrophysiologic and radioligand binding studies. Clin Pharmacol Ther 1990;47:740–746.
40. Burnett DM, Gal J, Zahniser NR, Nies AS. Propafenone interacts stereoselectively with beta-1 and beta-2 adrenergic receptors. J Cardiovasc Pharmacol 1988;12:615–619.

41. Looky BRF, Weir D, Chong E. Exacerbation of myasthenia by propafenone. J Neurol Neurosurg Psychiatry 1991;54:377.
42. Veale D, McComb JM, Gibson GJ. Propafenone. Lancet 1990;335:979.
43. Olm M, Jimenez MJ, Munne P. Efficacite de la methosamine par voie veineuse los des intoxications a la propafenone. [Efficacy of intravenous methoxamine in propafenone poisoning.] Presse Med 1989;18:1124.
44. Schlepper M. Propafenone: A review of its profile. Eur Heart J 1987; 8(suppl.A):27–32.
45. Nathan AW, Bexton RS, Hellstrand KJ, Camm AJ. Fatal ventricular tachycardia in association with propafenone, a new class IC antiarrhythmic agent. Postgrad Med J 1984;60:155–156.
46. Ravid S, Podrid PJ, Novrit B. Safety of long term propafenone therapy for cardiac arrhythmia: Experience with 774 patients. J Electrophysiol 1987;1:580–590.
47. Siebenlist D, Nurnberger M, Hermann G, Gattenlohner. Intoxikation mid propafenone. Intensivmed 1982;19:151–156.
48. Bosche J, Mattern R. Todlichen vergiftungstall mid dem antiarrhythmikum propafenone. Beitr Geriche Med 1980;38: 231–234.
49. Dimopoulos G. A case of fatal propafenone poisoning. Bull Int Assoc Forens Toxicol 1987;19(3):31–32.
50. Camous JP, Ichai C, Meyer P, et al. Traitement des intoxications aux nouveaux antiarrhythmiques (cibenzoline, flecainide, propafenone). Presse Med 1987;16:2076.
51. Kates RE, Yee YG, Winkle RA. Metabolite cumulation during chronic propafenone dosing in arrhythmia. Clin Pharmacol Ther 1984;37:610–614.

CLASS II DRUGS: BETA BLOCKERS

Table 32–7 outlines the pharmacokinetic characteristics and usual therapeutic dosages of selected beta blockers. See also Chapter 33.

Clinical Presentation

Acute beta blocker poisoning is characterized by depression of cardiac conduction and contractility, respiratory depression, coma, seizures, and, in some patients, hypoglycemia. Symptoms occur within 1 to 2 hours of ingestion. Management includes ventilatory support; treatment of hypoglycemia; use of competitive beta-adrenoceptor agonists, vasopressors, and glucagon; and cardiac pacing.[1] Remember that beta blockers have been associated with a high risk of anaphylactic reactions.[2] Radiocontrast medium infusion is the most common cause of anaphylactoid reactions (non-IgE-mediated anaphylaxis). Intravenous infusion of conventional contrast agents can promote systemic histamine release, subclinical bronchospasm, and oxygen desaturation. In this host environment, beta-blocker exposure is associated with greater risk of moderate to severe anaphylactoid reactions.[2]

Alprenolol

A 12.8-g suicidal ingestion resulted in death.

Atenolol

Ingestions of 1- and 1.2-g doses by adults produced little clinical effect[3] except for mild bradycardia and hypotension.[4] Ingestion of 4 to 6.5 g by an adult led to ventricular asystole; the patient responded to cardiac massage and a temporary pacemaker.[5] A 61-year-old patient ingested 3 g of atenolol and collapsed with no obtainable blood pressure. The electrocardiogram exhibited a nodal rhythm of 20 beats/min. After glucagon, atropine, and dopamine, activated charcoal after gastric lavage, isoproterenol, and intravenous crystalloids, the patient responded to hemodialysis.[6]

Bisoprolol

An adult who ingested 140 mg of bisoprolol (normal dose, 20 mg/d) developed sinus bradycardia and survived.[7] Bisoprolol has greater cardioselectivity than atenolol.[5,8] It has a high oral bioavailability (90%) and a long elimination half-life (about 11 hours). Peak concentrations of about 50 ng/mL are reached about 3 hours after a therapeutic dose.[5,9] It is bound to plasma proteins to the extent of 30%, and has an apparent volume of distribution of 3.3 L/kg. Approximately 50% of the dose is excreted unchanged.

Labetolol

A 43-year-old ingested 5.6 to 7 g of labetolol and developed profound hypotension. The patient responded after multiple 5-mg boluses of adrenaline and a 20-mg adrenaline bolus. In

Table 32–7
Pharmacokinetic Characteristics and Usual Therapeutic Dosages of Selected Beta Blockers

Beta Blocker	Oral Availability (%)	Volume of Distribution (L/kg)	Urinary Excretion (%)	Elimination Half-life (h)	Protein Binding (%)	Lipid solubility	Usual Daily Dose (mg)
Acebutolol	50	1.2	40	3.0	30–40	Low	200–800
Atenolol	40	1.1	90	6.5	<5	Low	25–100
Labetalol	25	9.4	<5	6.2	50	Low	200–800
Metoprolol	50	5.5	7.5	5.0	12	Moderate	25–200
Nadolol	30	2.4	18	18.0	30	Low	20–80
Oxprenolol	40	1.5	5	2.5	80	Moderate	60–320
Pindolol	90	2.3	54	3.5	57	Moderate	5–30
Propranolol	30	4.0	<1	4.5	93	High	40–320
Sotalol	60	0.7	60	9.0	0	Low	80–480
Timolol	50	2.1	15	4.5	10	Low	5–40

From Browning RG, Merigian KS. Acute beta-blocker poisonings. Top Emerg Med 1993;15(3):1–14.

her 24-hour intensive care stay, she received a total of 174 mg of adrenaline. She recovered.[10]

An adult ingested a 6-g overdose, developed severe renal failure, was hemodialyzed, treated with isoprenaline and glucagon, and survived.[11]

Esmolol

Administration of 5000 μg/kg/min instead of the recommended loading dose of 500 μg/kg/min over 1 minute to a patient with atrial flutter led to immediate bradycardia, hypotension, and drowsiness. The infusion rate was decreased to 5 μg/kg/min, and the bradycardia, hypotension, and drowsiness disappeared within 15 minutes.[12] An intravenous dose of 1.3 g led to asystole followed by rapid recovery with standard Advanced Cardiac Life Support therapy and supportive care.[13]

Timolol

Two to nine drops of timolol 0.25% in each eye may lead to weakness, dizziness, balance problems, stumbling, nausea, and near syncope in patients above 70 years of age.[14]

Pregnancy/Lactation

Beta blockers, frequently cardioselective, have been widely used for the treatment of pregnancy-induced hypertension. Adverse reactions are believed to be rare, and the effects on the fetus or infant have been thought to be minimal.[15,16] Labetalol, given to a mother because of pregnancy-induced hypertension, appeared to induce bradycardia, diminished femoral pulses, a bluish color, and inadequate breathing in a premature infant of 33 weeks' gestational age who was delivered by cesarean section.[15]

Sotalol is excreted in breast milk; an infant received up to 23% of the maternal dose.[17] Other beta blockers that have been found in breast milk include acebutolol, atenolol, labetalol, pindolol, metoprolol, nadolol, oxprenolol, propranolol, and timolol.[18]

Withdrawal Symptoms

Abrupt withdrawal of beta blockers without intrinsic sympathomimetic activity (eg, nadolol, propranolol) may result in acute precipitation of angina and myocardial infarction in hypertensive patients with no prior history of coronary heart disease.[19] It appears that beta blockers with intrinsic sympathomimetic activity (such as oxprenolol and pindolol, and calcium channel blockers are less likely to cause withdrawal syndromes than those without intrinsic sympathomimetic activity)[20–22] although healthy volunteers in a controlled study showed no evidence of central nervous withdrawal syndrome following abrupt withdrawal of propranolol.[23] Abrupt cessation of propranolol therapy, which had controlled symptoms in a psychotic patient, led to a resumption of psychotic symptoms.[24] There appears to be a period of hypersensitivity to isoproterenol following abrupt withdrawal of atenolol and a small overshoot of heart rate with exercise and position change. Bopindolol produced a prolonged state of decreasing sensitivity to isoproterenol.[25]

Laboratory

Acebutolol

Fatalities following acebutolol do not exhibit a correlation between the amount ingested and the blood level.[26] Similarly, there is no close correlation between ingested dose and toxic effects.

Atenolol

Following ingestion of 4 to 6.5 g of atenolol, serum atenolol concentrations were 849 pg/L (36 hours) and 564 pg/L (96 hours).[5] The concentrations at these times after ingestion of 50 mg of atenolol would be about 20 and 10 pg/L.

Metoprolol

The postmortem metoprolol level of a patient who was found hypotensive and unresponsive in bed was approximately 50 times the therapeutic level (4.7 μg/mL) after 10 hours of resuscitation.[27] Hyperkalemia[28] and hypoglycemia[29] occur rarely.

Propranolol

Blood propranolol levels confirm toxicity but do not aid immediate management. Therapeutic plasma levels range from 30 to 200 ng/mL. In fatal propranolol overdose, the plasma level ranges from 4000 to 28,000 ng/mL; survival has been reported at 2300 and 2800 ng/mL.

Sotalol

Ingestion of 14.4 g of sotalol led to a plasma concentration of 6500 ng/mL (65 μg/mL) in a 58-year-old woman who died.[30] This drug is a nonselective beta-adrenergic agonist in beta-blocker overdose.

Treatment

Browning and Merigian have suggested a useful plan for management[31] (Table 32–8).

Stabilization

If symptomatic treatment fails, then antidotes should be administered as follows: high doses of glucagon followed by isoproterenol, epinephrine and the new phosphodiesterase inhibitors. Mechanical ventilation should be started at the same time as pharmacologic treatment in cases of severe collapse or prolonged QRS.

Elimination

Minimal protein binding (5–15%) appears to enhance the effectiveness of hemodialysis in a life-threatening atenolol overdose, especially if renal function is diminished.[6] Sotalol-induced Torsade de pointes was successfully treated with hemodialysis after failure of conventional therapy (magnesium sulfate,[32] isoproterenol, and overdrive pacing).[33] Extracorporeal circulatory support using a femoral vein–femoral artery bypass is useful in supplementing pharma-

Table 32–8
Treatment of Cardiotoxicity Induced by Beta Blocking Agents

Hypotension*	Fluids Correct bradyarrhythmia if severe Glucagon Sympathomimetic drugs such as isoproterenol, dopamine, adrenaline, prenalterol
Bradycardia†	Atropine Isoproterenol Pacemaker
Ventricular tachyarrhythmias	Increase heart rate for escape rhythms Lignocaine‡ Direct-current cardioversion

*Selection of therapy should, when possible, be guided by the placement of a pulmonary artery catheter and measurement of ventricular filling pressure, cardiac output and peripheral vascular resistance.
†Only if symptomatic.
‡Could precipitate seizures if administered rapidly.
From Pentel PR, Salerno DM. Cardiac drug toxicity: Digitalis glycosides and calcium-channel and beta-blocking agents. Med J Aust 1990;152(2):88–94.

cologic treatment (isoprenaline and glucagon). A patient who ingested 2 g of propranolol recovered.[34]

Antidote

Isoproterenol. Start at 4 μg/min in adults; some patients may require a higher dosage (eg, 200 μg/min, or 10 times the usual therapeutic dose, was necessary in a severe propranolol overdose case).[35] Over 65 hours, 260 mg of isoproterenol was administered to the survivor of a massive overdose.[36] Follow the blood pressure closely, as isoproterenol may aggravate peripheral vasodilation as a result of its β_2 effects at high doses. Consider glucagon and norepinephrine, as isoproterenol is often ineffective in correcting hypotension.

Glucagon. Glucagon is probably the drug of choice to treat massive beta-blocker overdose. A loading dose of up to 10 mg followed by infusion of up to 5 mg/h may be required.[37]

Supportive Measures

1. Most overdoses are mild and respond to supportive care. Observe mild overdose cases at least 4 hours for the development of signs of poisoning.
2. Hypotension: Multiple intravenous boluses of adrenaline may lead to a rise in blood pressure after dopamine, glucagon, sodium bicarbonate, and calcium have not been successful.[10] Amrinone 5 to 15 μg/kg/min is a positive inotropic agent with intrinsic vasodilator activity that may be as effective as glucagon in reversing depressed myocardial function.[38]
3. Electromechanical dissociation: Calcium chloride 1 g, repeatedly administered, may restore blood pressure and narrowing of the QRS complexes after a propranolol overdose that has not responded to conventional treatment.[39]
4. Beta blockers should be discontinued in patients who are at risk for anaphylaxis, in conditions such as idiopathic anaphylaxis and *Hymenoptera* venom sensitivity, and in individuals who are to undergo allergy skin tests (inhalant, food, or drug) or receive allergen immunotherapy or contrast medium infusion.[2]
5. Patients receiving beta blockers who experience anaphylaxis are at increased risk for potentiated, "epinephrine-resistant" anaphylaxis. Beta blockers exert their effects by competitive inhibition of catecholamine binding at beta-adrenoceptor sites, such that the dose–response curve for the agonist is shifted to the right. The use of higher than customary doses of a beta agonist may be required for managing bronchospasm in an asthmatic patient undergoing anaphylaxis to achieve therapeutic effects. A lower dose of epinephrine may be appropriate for the management of beta-blocker-associated anaphylaxis, to avoid unopposed alpha-adrenergic effects leading to a paradoxical hypertension and coronary vasoconstriction.[2]
6. Glucagon increases cAMP levels via noncatecholamine mechanisms and can exert potent chronotropic and inotropic effects.[2] This likely explains its use as an antidote in beta–blocker and calcium channel blocker overdoses.

REFERENCES—CLASS II DRUGS: BETA BLOCKERS

1. Browning RG, Merigian KS. Acute beta blocker poisoning. Top Emerg Med 1993;15:1–14.
2. Lang DM. Anaphylactoid and anaphylactic reactions: Hazards of beta blockers. Drug Saf 1995;12:299–304.
3. Shanahan FLJ, Counihan TB. Atenolol self-poisoning. Br Med J 1978;2:773.
4. Weinstein RS, Cole S, Knaster HB, et al. Beta blocker overdose with propranolol and with atenolol. Ann Emerg Med 1985;14:161–163.
5. Stinson J, Walsh M, Feely J. Ventricular asystole and overdose with atenolol. Br Med J 1992;305:693.
6. Saitz R, Williams BW, Farber HW. Atenolol-induced cardiovascular collapse treated with hemodialysis. Crit Care Med 1991;19:116–118.
7. Trancqui A, Kintz P, Mangin P, Lenoir B. Self-poisoning with a beta-blocker bisoprolol. Hum Exp Toxicol 1990;9:255–256.
8. Bisoprolol: Another cardioselective beta-blocker. Drug Ther Bull 1989;27:55.
9. Lancaster SG, Sorkin EM. Bisoprolol: A preliminary review of its pharmacodynamic and pharmacokinetic properties and therapeutic efficacy in hypertension and angina pectoris. Drugs 1988;36:256–285.
10. Hicks PR, Rankin APN. Massive adrenaline doses in labetolol overdose. Anaesth Intensive Care 1991;19:447–449.
11. Kovzets A, Danby P, Edmunds ME, et al. Acute renal failure associated with a labetolol overdose. Postgrad Med J 1990;66:66–67.
12. Product literature: Brevibloc (esmolol HCl). DuPont Critical Care.
13. Miller A, White S. Survival following massive intravenous esmolol overdose. Clin Toxicol 1995;533:475–486.
14. Hayes LP, Stewart CJ, Kim J, Mohr JA. Timolol side effects and inadvertent overdose. J Am Geriatr Soc 1989;37:261–262.
15. Haraldsson A, Geven W. Severe adverse effects of maternal labetalol in a premature infant. Acta Paediatr Scand 1989;78:956–958.
16. Rubin PC. Current concepts: Beta blockers in pregnancy. N Engl J Med 1981;305:1323–1326.
17. Hackett LP, Wojnar-Hutton RE, Dusci LJ, et al. Excretion of sotalol in breast milk. Br J Clin Pharmacol 1990;29:277–278.
18. Atkinson HC, Begg EJ, Darlow BA. Drugs in human milk: Clinical pharmacokinetic considerations. Clin Pharmacokinet 1988;14:217–240.

19. Psaty BM, Koepsell TD, Wagner EH, et al. The relative risk of incident coronary heart disease associated with recently stopping the use of beta blockers. JAMA 1990;263:1653–1657.
20. Bolli P, Buhler FR, Raeder EA. Lack of beta adrenoreceptor hypersensitivity after abrupt withdrawal of long-term therapy with oxprenolol. Circulation 1981;64:1130–1134.
21. Walden RJ, Hernandez J, Yu Y, et al. Withdrawal of beta-blocking drugs. Am Heart J 1982;104:515–520.
22. Egstrup K. Transient myocardial ischemia after abrupt withdrawal of antianginal therapy in chronic stable angina. Am J Cardiol 1988;61:1219–1222.
23. Al-Qassat H, Cleeves LA, Francis PL, et al. Is there a central nervous system withdrawal syndrome associated with discontinuing long-term treatment with propranolol? Hum Toxicol 1988;7:249–254.
24. Rosenthal S, Ellison J. Propranolol withdrawal in psychosis. Am J Psychiatry 1990;147:534.
25. Walden RJ, Tomlinson B, Graham B, et al. Withdrawal phenomena after atenolol and bopindolol: Haemodynamic responses in healthy volunteers. Br J Clin Pharmacol 1990;30:557–565.
26. Trancqui A, Kintz P, Wendling P, et al. Toxicological findings in a fatal case of acebutolol self-poisoning. J Anal Toxicol 1992;16:398–400.
27. Stajic M, Granger RH, Beyer JC. Fatal metoprolol overdose. J Anal Toxicol 1984;8:228–230.
28. Ashouri OS. Metoprolol-induced hyperkalemia in a diabetic with advanced renal failure. Arch Intern Med 1985;145:578.
29. Hesse B, Pederson JG. Hypoglycaemia after propranolol in children. Acta Med Scand 1973;193:551–552.
30. Perrot D, Bui-Xuan B, Lang J, et al. A case of sotalol poisoning with fatal outcome. Clin Toxicol 1988;26:384–396.
31. Browning RG, Merigian KS. Acute beta-blocker poisoning. Top Emerg Med 1993;15:1–14.
32. Cristall MA, Hii JRY, Lehman RG, Horowitz JD. Sotalol-induced Torsade de pointes: Management with magnesium infusion. Postgrad Med J 1992;68:289–290.
33. Singh SN, Lazin A, Cohen A, et al. Sotalol-induced Torsade de pointes successfully treated with hemodialysis after failure of conventional therapy. Am Heart J 1991;121:601–602.
34. McVey FK, Corke CF. Extracorporeal circulation in the management of massive propranolol overdose. Anaesthesia 1991;46:744–746.
35. Agura ED, Wexler LF, Witzburg RA. Massive propranolol overdose: Successful treatment with high dose isoproterenol and glucagon. Am J Med 1986;180:755–757.
36. Lewis M, Kallenbach J, Germond C, et al. Survival following massive overdose of adrenergic blocking agents (acebutolol and labetalol). Eur Heart J 1983;4:328–332.
37. DeLima LGR, Kharasch ED, Butler S. Successful pharmacologic treatment of massive atenolol overdose: Sequential hemodynamics and plasma atenolol concentrations. Anesthesiology 1995;83:204–207.
38. Kollef MP. Labetalol overdose successfully treated with amrinone and alpha-adrenergic receptor agonists. Chest 1994;105:626–627.
39. Brimacomber JR, Scully M, Swanston R. Propranolol overdose: A dramatic response to calcium chloride. Med J Aust 1991;155:267–268.

CLASS III DRUGS

AMIODARONE

Amiodarone is an iodinated benzofuran derivative with a chemical structure similar to that of thyroxine. Recent clinical interest centers around its ability to suppress resistant supraventricular and ventricular dysrhythmias and to improve intractable congestive heart failure. The most serious adverse reaction to therapeutic use is the development of a rapidly progressive adult respiratory distress syndrome.[1]

Therapeutic Dose

Therapeutic loading and maintenance doses display wide variability (400–2000 and 200–800 mg/d, respectively). Acute overdose has rarely been reported. The ingestion of 8 g of amiodarone by a healthy adult produced a slight bradycardia (second to third day), QT prolongation, and diaphoresis without changes in the blood pressure.[2] Side effects of therapeutic doses (eg, photosensitivity, hypothyroidism, gynecomastia, hepatotoxicity, hyperthyroidism, pulmonary fibrosis, skin pigmentation, corneal deposits) did not occur after the acute overdose. In this case, symptoms and signs were delayed up to several days, probably as a result of the slow absorption and prolonged half-life of amiodarone. In one patient who ingested 15 g of amiodarone, sinus bradycardia was followed by first-degree heart block requiring pacing.[3] An attempted suicide with 2600 mg did not cause any clinical symptoms, or changes in heart rate or blood pressure. No ventricular arrhythmias were observed, but the QT interval was lengthened with T-wave inversion in the precordial leads and transient disappearance of the R wave in leads V_1 to V_4, simulating an anteroseptal infarction.[4] Following ingestion of 3.4 g of amiodarone by an adult, the electrocardiogram was normal. After gastric lavage and a short run of ventricular tachycardia, the patient recovered.[5]

Toxicokinetics

Oral absorption of therapeutic doses is slow, with a wide range of bioavailability (22–86%).[6] Plasma amiodarone is highly protein bound (98%).[7] In human volunteers given therapeutic doses the volume of distribution is large (9–17 L/kg), and the elimination half-life is long (3–21 hours after a single dose and 52 days after long-term administration).[8] One overdose case displayed an elimination half-life of 31 hours.[9] In patients treated long term, serum levels of amiodarone and *N*-desethylamiodarone are approximately equal.[10]

The therapeutic plasma concentration is about 1 to 2.5 mg/L. Renal excretion is responsible for less than 1% the administered dose.[11]

Drug Interactions

Amiodarone can increase the serum concentrations, pharmacologic effects, and toxicity of digoxin, diltiazem, quinidine, procainamide, oral anticoagulants, and phenytoin.[12,13]

Pregnancy

Amiodarone undergoes transplacental passage. The fetal amiodarone blood level is about 10 to 25% of the maternal blood level, suggesting a transplacental barrier. Serious adverse effects of amiodarone on the fetus produced by maternal ingestion include neonatal hypothyroidism, small size for gestational age, and prematurity. Hormonal substitute therapy may be required soon after birth in infants with biochemical and clinical evidence of hypothyroidism at birth.[14]

In six instances where a mother was administered amiodarone during pregnancy, all infants at birth appeared healthy, without a goiter, corneal microdeposits, hepatic dysfunction, or pulmonary fibrosis.[15] During pregnancy, goiter and hypothyroidism many be diagnosed in utero in the fetus by ultrasonography and measurement of the thyroid-stimulating hormone level in the amniotic fluid.[16] If thyroid enlargement is identified, consideration should be given to cesarean section.

Mechanism of Action

Amiodarone prolongs the action potential duration of myocardial cells without altering the resting membrane potential. Consequently, the drug alters repolarization (QT prolongation) without affecting spontaneous (phase 4) depolarization. As neither class I nor class II antiarrhythmic drugs possess both these properties, amiodarone is classified as a class III antiarrhythmic agent. The effect of amiodarone on thyroid metabolism remains unclear but probably involves an intracellular rather than a central or peripheral action.[2] Amiodarone also possesses noncompetitive alpha and beta sympathetic receptor blocking properties, which result in systemic and coronary vasodilation.[17]

Clinical Presentation

Serious adverse reactions to therapeutic doses of amiodarone include a rapidly fatal adult respiratory distress syndrome,[18] polymorphous ventricular tachycardia[19] (*Torsade de pointes*), hypothyroidism, and hyperthyroidism.[2] Adverse clinical effects are usually experienced after long-term administration of amiodarone; are mostly extracardiac, linked to dosage and tissue concentrations; and are usually reversible. Generally, they occur when the plasma concentration of amiodarone (or desethylamiodarone, its main metabolite) is greater than 1.5 μg/mL.

Skin

Photosensitivity of the skin and blue coloration of the nails occur infrequently.

Eyes

Amiodarone microdeposits accumulate in the cornea in almost all amiodarone patients; they are visible on slit-lamp examination and rarely lead to impaired vision.

Thyroid

From 2 to 7% of patients develop hypothyroidism and 5 to 16% develop hyperthyroidism with potential worsening of any arrhythmia. Hyperthyroidism appears to occur more often in patients with a goiter. Amiodarone, when given chronically at 200 mg/d, releases 5 to 10 mg iodide into the circulation. Amiodarone thyrotoxicosis is characterized by weight loss, weakness, restlessness, hyperkinesia, and recurrence of the arrhythmia for which the patient uses the drug. Eye signs and thyroid enlargement are frequently absent. The thyrotoxicosis may occur weeks or months after the drug has been withdrawn. Hypothyroidism may be transient or persistent and develops in patients with or without underlying thyroid disorders.[20]

Lungs

Most cases of amiodarone pulmonary toxicity occur when doses greater than 400 mg/d are used for periods of at least 2 months.[21–25] Risk factors include advanced age (>60 years), lower pretreatment DLco (<80%), and higher plasma desethylamiodarone concentrations (>2.3 μg/mL).[26] A preexisting abnormality in pulmonary function, the chest x-ray, or the drug–dose relationship has been shown to be useful in predicting drug toxicity in individual patients. The pulmonary syndrome may be a hypersensitivity response.[24] Pulmonary toxicity often presents as an interstitial or alveolar infiltration, which is usually bilateral. Pulmonary toxicity complicates clinical use in about 5 to 7% of patients. Symptoms develop either acutely, resembling an infectious pneumonitis,[23] or slowly, with cough, dyspnea on exertion, and weight loss. Fever may supervene. Because of the long half-life of amiodarone (up to 54 days), toxic effects may persist despite drug withdrawal. Treatment consists of discontinuing the drug or lowering the dose to less than 400 mg/d. Corticosteroids have led to resolution of the pulmonary infiltrates.

Liver

Hepatic abnormalities associated with amiodarone therapy vary from transient increases in routine liver function test results to severe hepatic failure. Hepatic failure, occasionally fatal, has been reported.[27] When it occurs, onset of liver enzyme abnormalities was reported after an average of 10.4 months of therapy following a mean cumulative dose of 104 g.[27]

Laboratory

Ancillary Methods

Frequently, bronchoscopy with bronchoalveolar lavage and transbronchoscopic lung biopsy is performed to support the diagnosis of amiodarone pulmonary toxicity and to exclude other diagnostic possibilities, such as infection and malignancy. The clinician must also consider whether additional studies, such as pulmonary artery catheterization, pulmonary angiography, and even open lung biopsy, are necessary.

Thyroid Function Tests

Elevation of thyroid-stimulating hormone levels is transient, and levels gradually return to pretreatment values. In contrast, thyroxine and free thyroxine levels remain elevated. This condition can be confused with hyperthyroidism, which also occurs in a few patients receiving amiodarone. It can be difficult to distinguish between a euthyroid patient receiving amiodarone and an amiodarone-treated patient who has become hyperthyroid. Ultrasensitive thyroid-stimulating hormone assays and measurement of triiodothyronine and free triiodothyronine levels can be useful in this setting.[28–31]

Liver Function Tests

With doses of 200 to 400 mg/d and blood amiodarone or desethylamiodarone levels less than 1 to 5 μg/mL, approximately 10 to 20% of patients show asymptomatic increases in bilirubin, transaminase, and alkaline phosphatase levels. Though severe hepatic toxicity is rare, six deaths have followed prolonged use of between 200 and 600 mg/d.[32,33]

Proarrhythmic Effect

A proarrhythmic effect (eg, Torsade de pointes) is infrequent except in older patients, in those with hypokalemia, and in those receiving treatment disposing to bradycardia or interfering with ventricular repolarization.[34]

Amiodarone may provoke malignant arrhythmias or conduction abnormalities in patients with hypertrophic cardiomyopathy.[35]

Treatment

Patients should respond to general therapeutic measures. Decontamination measures may be useful beyond several hours postingestion because of the toxicokinetics of amiodarone. Treatment of amiodarone pulmonary toxicity consists of simply discontinuing the drug, although corticosteroids may speed recovery.[23] Very rapid withdrawal of corticosteroids has led to a recurrence in some patients.

Severe cardiovascular collapse may be accompanied by a wide-complex bradycardia in patients with Wolff–Parkinson–White syndrome following intravenous amiodarone. Treatment includes isoprenaline and direct-current cardioversion.[32]

If bradycardia ensues, a beta-adrenergic agonist or a pacemaker may be indicated. Hypotension with inadequate tissue perfusion may respond to vasopressors. Neither amiodarone nor its metabolite is dialyzable.[36] With its high degree of protein binding and its extensive volume of distribution, amiodarone does not appear to be a good candidate for hemoperfusion; however, there are insufficient data on which to draw a final conclusion regarding this management. Cholestyramine has been suggested as a means to reduce the enterohepatic circulation of amiodarone.[37] Plasma levels of amiodraone and its metabolite desmethylamiodarone, as well as levels of free thyroxine and thyroxine, appear to decrease in response to plasmapheresis.[38]

Activated charcoal reduces amiodarone absorption.[1] Gastric lavage should be performed while the patient is connected to a cardiac monitor.[43] Profound bradycardia may occur during the procedure. The patient should be observed 1 to 2 days in a coronary care unit for signs of arrhythmia, bradycardia, and heart block.[5] Further antiarrhythmic drugs should be avoided if possible. If bradycardia compromises the patient's hemodynamic state, cardiac pacing should be considered.[44]

It is not clear whether prophylactic pacing should be done if significant lengthening of the PR interval develops. Oral cholestyramine (4 g each hour for 4 hours) may reduce the half-life of amiodarone.[5] Further dosing may be considered for up to 12 hours due to the potential for delayed absorption of amiodarone. Cholestyramine appears to reduce the enterohepatic circulation of amiodarone.[37]

BRETYLIUM

Bretylium tosylate is a quaternary benzylammonium compound (class III antiarrhythmic) used to treat ventricular arrhythmias refractory to lidocaine. It is used in complex, life-threatening clinical settings in which many drugs are often given and its individual clinical effects may be difficult to interpret.

Clinical Presentation

A 3-day-old child with ventricular fibrillation received 12 mg/kg/h for 43 hours instead of 1 mg/kg/h. The blood level of bretylium was 17 μg/mL about 12 hours after the drug was discontinued (therapeutic level, 1.3 μg/mL). During infusion, the child exhibited dilated, nonreactive pupils, no response to sound or light, no spontaneous motor activity, and absent oculocephalic, oculovestibular, corneal, and gag reflexes. An electroencephalogram, however, showed only mildly attenuated activity. Within 26 hours of discontinuation of bretylium, neurologic findings were normal. At 12 months, his development was normal. Treatment was supportive and symptomatic.[39] A prolonged neurologic depression with eventual neurologic recovery was observed in a 74-year-old who received an 81.5 mg/kg overdose of bretylium tosylate.[40]

A 58-year-old man with ventricular fibrillation received one 30 mg/kg bolus of bretylium tosylate instead of 10 mg/kg. The blood pressure rose to 310/90 mm Hg, and fell in 90 minutes to 90/40 mm Hg. He developed anuria and asystole, and died. The blood level of bretylium was 8.8 μg/mL 3 hours after the bolus and 6.18 μg/mL 15 hours after the bolus. This high level was probably associated with the anuria.[41] Hypotension due to adrenergic blockade after bretylium appears to be its most common side effect.

Treatment

Treatment of bretylium overdose is symptomatic and supportive. Although bretylium is dialyzable,[42] there is no published evidence that hemoperfusion or hemodialysis is useful in an acute overdose.

REFERENCES—AMIODARONE AND BRETYLIUM

1. Martin WJ, Miller FA Jr. Amiodarone toxicity. Mayo Clin Proc 1985;60:638–639.
2. Alves LE, Rose EP, Cahill TB. Amiodarone and the thyroid. Ann Intern Med 1985;102:412.
3. Garson A, Gillette PC, McVey P, et al. Amiodarone treatment of critical arrhythmia in children and young adults. J Am Coll Cardiol 1984;4:749–755.
4. Oreto G, Lapresa V, Melluso C, et al. Amiodarone overdose: A case report. Arch Mal Coeur Vasseaux 1980;73:857–862.
5. Goddard DJR, Whorwell PJ. Amiodarone overdose and its management. Br J Clin Pract 1989;34:184–186.
6. Riva E, Gerna M, Latini R, et al. Pharmacokinetics of amiodarone in man. J Cardiovasc Pharmacol 1982;4:264–269.
7. Harris L, McKenna WJ, Krikler SJ, et al. Renal elimination of amiodarone and its desethyl metabolite. Postgrad Med J 1983;59:440–442.

8. Middlekauff NR, Wiener I, Saxon LA, Stevenson WG. Low dose amiodarone for ventricular fibrillation: Time for a prospective study? Ann Intern Med 1992;116(12, pt 1):1017–1020.
9. Bonati M, D'Aronno V, Galletti F, et al. Acute overdosage of amiodarone in a suicide attempt. J Toxicol Clin Toxicol 1983; 20:181–186.
10. Flannagan RJ, Storey GCA, Holt DW, et al. Identification and measurement of desethylamiodarone in blood plasma specimens from amiodarone treated patients. J Pharm Pharmacol 1982;34:638–643.
11. Gill J, Heel RC, Fitton A. Amiodarone: An overview of its pharmacological properties and review of its therapeutic use in cardiac arhythmias. Drugs 1992;43:69–110.
12. Estes MAM III. Evolving strategies for the management of atrial fibrillation: The role of amiodarone. JAMA 1992; 267:3332–3333.
13. Lesko JL. Pharmacokinetic drug interactions with amiodarone. Clin Pharmacokinet 1989;17:130–140.
14. Widerhorn J, Bhandai A, Bughi S, et al. Fetal and neonatal adverse effects profile of amiodarone treatment during pregnancy. Am Heart J 1991;122:1162–1166.
15. Rey E, Bachrach LK, Burrow GN. Effects of amiodarone during pregnancy. Can Med Assoc J 1987;136:959–960.
16. Kourides IAS, Berkowitz RL, Pang S, et al. Antepartum diagnosis of goitrous hypothyroidism by fetal ultrasonography and amniotic fluid thyrotropin concentration. J Clin Endocrinol Metab 1984;59:1016–1018.
17. Marcus FI, Fontaine GH, Frank F, et al. Clinical pharmacology and therapeutic applications of the antiarrhythmic agent amiodarone. Am Heart J 1981;101:480–493.
18. Wood DL, Osborn MJ, Rooke J, et al. Amiodarone pulmonary toxicity: Report of two cases associated with rapidly progressive fatal adult respiratory distress syndrome after pulmonary angiography. Mayo Clin Proc 1985;60:601–603.
19. Sclarovsky S, Lewin RF, Kracoff O, et al. Amiodarone induced polymorphous ventricular tachycardia. Am Heart J 1985;105:6–12.
20. Unger J, Lambert M, Jonckheer MH, Dehayer P. Amiodarone and the thyroid: Pharmacological, toxic and therapeutic effects. J Intern Med 1993;233:435–443.
21. McNeil KD, Firouz-Abadi A. Amiodarone pulmonary toxicity: Three unusual manifestations. Aust NZ J Med 1992;22: 14–18.
22. Pitche WD. Southwestern Internal Medicine Conference: Amiodarone pulmonary toxicity. Am J Med Sci 1992; 303:206–212.
23. Retz JL, Martin WJ II. Amiodarone pulmonary toxicity. Intensive Care Med 1992;18:388–390.
24. Rubin DA, McAllister A, Sorbera C, Kay RH. Subacute pulmonary toxicity from amiodarone. NY State J Med 1991; 9:403–405.
25. Fraire AE, Guntupalli KK, Greenberg SD, et al. Amiodarone pulmonary toxicity: A multidisciplinary review of current status. South Med J 1993:86:67–77.
26. Dusman RE, Stanton MS, Miles WM, et al. Clinical features of amiodarone-induced pulmonary toxicity. Circulation 1990; 82:51–59.
27. Richer M, Robert S. Fatal hepatotoxicity following oral administration of amiodarone. Ann Pharmacother 1995;29:582–586.
28. Ahmed Z, Goldman JM. Reevaluation of amiodarone. Ann Intern Med 1995;123:809.
29. Nadamanee K, Piwonka RW, Singh BN, Hershman JM. Amiodarone and thyroid function. Prog Cardiovasc Dis 1989; 31:427–437.
30. Wiersinga WM, Trip MD. Amiodarone and thyroid hormone metabolism. Postgrad Med J 1986;62:909–914.
31. Lombardi A, Martino E, Braverman LE. Amiodarone and the thyroid. Thyroid Today 1990;13:1–7.
32. Till JA, Baxenda IIM, Benetar A. Acceleration of the ventricular response to actual flutter by amiodarone in an infant with Wolff–Parkinson–White syndrome. Br Heart J 1993;70: 84–87.
33. Flaherty KK, Chase SL, Yaghezian HM, Rubin R. Hepatotoxicity associated with amiodarone therapy. Pharmacotherapy 1989;9:30 44.
34. Lwakatare JML, Morris-Jones S, Knight EJ. Fatal fulminating liver failure possibly related to amiodarone treatment. Br J Hosp Med 1990;44:60–61.
35. Fananapazir L, Leon MB, Bonow RO, et al. Sudden death during empiric amiodarone therapy in symptomatic hypertrophic cardiomyopathy. Am J Cardiol 1991;67:169–174.
36. Wilson FS. Wyeth-Ayerst Laboratories. Personal communication. Feb. 19, 1991.
37. Nitsch J, Luderlt Z. Enhanced elimination of amiodarone by cholestyramine. Dtsch Med Wochenschr 1986;111:1241–1244.
38. Uzzan B, Pussard E, Leon A, et al. The effects of plasmapheresis on thyroid hormone and plasma drug concentrations in amiodarone-induced thyrotoxicosis. Br J Clin Pharmacol 1991;31:371–372.
39. Thompson AE, Sussman JB. Bretylium intoxication resembling clinical brain death. Crit Care Med 1989;17:194–195.
40. Gibson JS, Munter DW. Intravenous bretylium overdoses. Am J Emerg Med 1995;13:177–179.
41. Bodnar T, Nowak R, Tomlanovich C. Massive intravenous bolus: Bretylium tosylate. Ann Emerg Med 1980;9:630–633.
42. Reynolds JFK, ed. *Martindale: The Extra Pharmacopoeia.* 30th ed. London: Pharmaceutical Press, 1993:61–62.
43. Kivisto KT, Neuvonen PJ. Effect of activated charcoal in the absorption of amiodarone. Hum Exp Toxicol 1991;10:327–329.
44. Henry J, Volans G. ABC of poisoning: Cardiac drugs. Br Med J 1984;289:1062–1064.

N-ACETYLPROCAINAMIDE

N-Acetylprocainamide (Acecainide), the *N*-acetylated metabolite of procainamide, is a class III antiarrhythmic agent that can be given intravenously or orally and is eliminated primarily by renal excretion.[1] It appears to reduce premature ventricular beats and prevent induction of ventricular tachycardia. *N*-Acetylprocainamide does not appear to induce systemic lupus erythematosus and antinuclear antibodies.

Toxicokinetics

The mean peak plasma concentration 2.5 hours after the administration of 1000 mg of *N*-acetylprocainamide was 5.4 μg/mL. Bioavailability in healthy subjects is 85%. The apparent steady-state volume of distribution ranges from 1.25 to 1.7 L/kg[2]; *N*-acetylprocainamide is 10% bound to plasma proteins. The elimination half-life is approximately 8 hours.[3] Following oral administration, 59 to 87% of a dose is excreted unchanged in the urine. Renal clearance is 0.15 to 0.176/h/kg in healthy subjects. *N*-Acetylprocainamide does not form the reactive metabolite nitrosoprocainamide, thought to play a role in the lupus reaction.[1,2,4]

Clinical Presentation

Reported adverse effects have involved mainly the gastrointestinal tract (nausea, vomiting, diarrhea, anorexia) and central nervous system (paresthesias, somnolence, fatigue, vivid dreams, lightheadedness). Adverse effects usually resolve within 24 hours of stopping therapy. Sudden death possibly associated with *N*-acetylprocainamide occurred in 24% of patients in one study.[1] Proarrhythmic events including Torsade de pointes, polymorphic ventricular tachycardia, and ventricular fibrillation have been reported.[1] Other unwanted effects include blurry vision, rash, and decreased sexual function. These adverse effects tend to be within the therapeutic range, 10 to 37 μg/mL.

Laboratory

Torsade de pointes was associated with a plasma level of 32.4 μg/mL.[5]

Treatment

Therapy for *N*-acetylprocainamide overdose is largely similar to that for procainamide and requires an intravenous line, oxygen, and cardiac monitoring in an intensive care setting. The usual measures of gastric emptying and activated charcoal may be useful within the first 3 to 4 hours of oral ingestion, but controlled clinical studies supporting this recommendation have not yet been performed. Life-threatening intoxication may respond to hemoperfusion,[6] continuous arteriovenous hemofiltration, or continuous arteriovenous hemodiafiltration.[7] A hemodialyzer and hemoperfusion cartridge placed in series appear to achieve a more rapid reduction of serum *N*-acetylprocainamide levels than the above methods.[8]

REFERENCES—N-ACETYLPROCAINAMIDE

1. Harron DWG, Brogden RN. Acecainide (*N*-acetylprocainamide): A review of its pharmacodynamic and pharmacokinetic properties, and therapeutic potential in cardiac arrhythmias. Drugs 1990;39:720–740.
2. Atkinson AJ Jr, Ruo TI, Piergies AA, et al. Pharmacokinetics of *N*-acetylprocainamide in patients profiled with a stable isotope method. Clin Pharmacol Ther 1989;46:182–189.
3. Piergies AA, Ruo TI, Jansyn EM, et al. Effect kinetics of *N*-acetylprocainamide-induced QT interval prolongation. Clin Pharmacol Ther 1987;42:107–112.
4. Utrecht JP. Reactivity and possible significance of hydroxylamine and nitroso metabolites of procainamide. J Pharmacol Exp Ther 1985;232:420–425.
5. Stratmann HG, Walter KE, Kennedy HL. Torsade de pointes associated with elevated *N*-acetylprocainamide levels. Am Heart J 1985;109:375–376.
6. Braden GL, Fitzgibbons JP, Germain MJ, Ledewitz HM. Hemoperfusion for *N*-acetylprocainamide intoxication. Ann Intern Med 1986;105:965–966.
7. Domoto DT, Brown WW, Bruggensmith KP. Removal of toxic levels of *N*-acetylprocainamide with continuous arteriovenous hemofiltration or continuous arteriovenous hemodiafiltration. Ann Intern Med 1987;106:550–552.
8. Karr RM, Kellner K, Ing TS, Leehey DJ. Combined high efficiency hemodialysis and charcoal hemoperfusion in severe *N*-acetylprocainamide intoxication. Am J Kidney Dis 1992;20:403–406.

CLASS IV DRUGS: CALCIUM CHANNEL BLOCKERS

Hypotension and bradycardia (sinus node depression, atrioventricular nodal depression, dysrhythmias) are often seen with calcium channel blocker overdose. Serious overdoses with diltiazem and nifedipine are infrequent. (See Chapter 33.)

Structure and Classification

Calcium channel blockers available in the United States include the phenylalkylamines (verapamil), the dihydropyridines (nifedipine, nicardipine, nimodipine, amlodipine, bepridil, felodipine, isradipine), and the benzothiazepines (diltiazem).[1]

Flunarizine, a difluorinated piperazine derivative with calcium entry blocking properties, has therapeutic potential in a number of neurologic and cerebrovascular disorders including migraine, seizures, and vertigo,[2–4] but can induce parkinsonism.[5] Cinnarizine is an H_1-receptor antagonist with calcium channel blocking properties.[6]

Toxic Dose

An overdose of diltiazem 4.8 g led to a reduction in serum calcium.[3] A single 10-mg nifedipine capsule proved fatal in a 14-month-old child.[7] Toxicity has not depended on plasma levels.[2]

Diltiazem

An 18-year-old man ingested 720 mg of diltiazem and developed sinus tachycardia; one 300-mg ingestion of diltiazem by a 50-year-old was nontoxic. Similarly, a 120-mg diltiazem ingestion by an 18-month-old was nontoxic.[9] A 50-year-old ingested 5880 mg of diltiazem with beer, became hypotensive, and had a short period of ventricular asystole; he survived.[8]

Nifedipine

An 800-mg (70 mg/kg) nifedipine ingestion by a 14-month-old child caused coma, hypotension, hyperglycemia, third-degree atrioventricular block, cardiac arrest, seizures, and visual field defects[9]; the child slowly recovered. A dose of 200 mg of nifedipine in a 1-year-old resulted in sinus tachycardia, and in a 72-year-old man, it led to hypotension. A 9-year-old ingested 100 mg of nifedipine without toxic symptoms. A 25-year-old ingested 50 mg without symptoms. In an adult with chronic renal failure, a 280-mg nifedipine ingestion produced profound hypotension but tissue perfusion remained adequate.[10]

Verapamil

A 960-mg dose of a slow-release preparation of verapamil in a 66-year-old led to bradycardia, dizziness, and respiratory depression. A 1.9-g dose in a 33-year-old woman was nontoxic. A 2-year-old ingested 240 mg of verapamil without any evidence of toxicity.[11]

A review of 18 cases of calcium channel blocker ingestion in children suggests that ingestion of up to one tablet of nifedipine (10 mg) or verapamil (80 mg or 120 mg) is generally not significant in children,[12] but fatalities have followed verapamil ingestion in by toddler less than 2 years of age. A 73-year-old woman ingested sustained-release verapamil 2.88 g and presented 24 hours later. Intravenous glucagon 5 mg, then 3 mg/h appeared to be beneficial in treating hemodynamic irritability.[13]

Fatal Dose

Doses of diltiazem up to 12 g have been followed by bradycardia; hypotension; first-, second-, and third-degree atrioventricular block; sinus bradycardia; sinus arrest with junctional escape; accelerated junctional rhythm; and asystole. Most patients have had an improvement in signs and symptoms within 3 days. Six of thirty-nine overdoses have died.[14–16]

A 33-year-old man ingested verapamil 4.16 g, developed asystole, and died after treatment with gastric lavage, syrup of ipecac, activated charcoal, calcium chloride, atropine, naloxone, intravenous fluids, dopamine, transcutaneous pacing, intravenous potassium, and epinephrine.[17] A 22-year-old ingested 7.2 to 9.6 g of sustained-release verapamil, developed respiratory depression, and died.[18] A single 10-mg nifedipine capsule proved fatal in a 14-month-old child.[19]

Toxicokinetics

Calcium channel blockers are well absorbed orally but undergo extensive hepatic metabolism and first-pass clearance. They are all highly protein bound, but the volume of distribution varies with each agent. The protein binding of diltiazem is 80 to 90%, and the volume of distribution is approximately 5.3 L/kg. Clearance of diltiazem after oral ingestion follows first-order kinetics, with a half-life of 5 to 10 hours, independent of the amount ingested. In sustained-release preparations, however, the peak absorption time is delayed and the half-life may be very prolonged because of continued gastrointestinal absorption. The toxic effects of sustained-release calcium channel blockers may be delayed more than 12 hours after ingestion. All patients with sustained-release calcium channel blocker overdose should be admitted to the hospital for observation, even if they are asymptomatic.[20]

Pregnancy/Lactation

A patient received diltiazem throughout pregnancy with twins. The infants were delivered at 37 weeks' gestation. There were no apparent maternal or fetal adverse effects throughout pregnancy, through the neonatal period, and up to 6 months later.[21] Nifedipine is excreted into human milk in an amount less than 5% of a therapeutic dose.[22] Its pyridine metabolite is also excreted in human milk. Both nifedipine and its metabolite may reach peak levels similar to that of maternal blood.[23]

Drug Interactions

See Table 32–9 for a summary of drug–drug interactions involving calcium channel blockers.

Mechanism of Action

Cardiovascular and renal, metabolic, and adverse effects of calcium channel blockers are reviewed in Tables 32–10 and 32–11.[24] Calcium ions (Ca^{2+}) are critical in the regulation of cellular movement and transport, electrical activation of excitable cells, and different enzymatic reactions. Calcium channels regulate Ca^{2+} movement from the extracellular space to the intracellular space. There are three basic types of calcium channels: receptor-operated calcium channels, stretch-operated calcium channels, and voltage-sensitive (potential-operated) calcium channels. Receptor-operated calcium channels are stimulated by certain ligands, such as neurohormones. Stretch-operated calcium channels can be stimulated when certain vascular walls are stretched. Voltage-sensitive calcium channels respond to voltage changes across cellular membranes, such as depolarization of the membrane by the opening of the sodium channels. Voltage-sensitive calcium channels are composed of homologous protein subunits also found in sodium and potassium channels.[21]

There are at least three subtypes of voltage-sensitive calcium channels classified by their conductance and sensitivity to voltages: L, N, and T subtypes. Only the L channels are affected by calcium channel blockers.[21]

Extracellular Ca^{2+} concentration is approximately 5000 to 10,000 times greater than inside the cell, and this gradient is maintained by $Ca^{2+}/2H^+$ -ATPase and $3Na^{2+}/Ca^{2+}$ exchange pumps. Calcium channel opening allows an influx of Ca^{2+} and increases the cytosolic Ca^{2+} concentration.[21]

The calcium channel antagonists form a heterogeneous class of drugs that block the inward movement of calcium into cells through so-called "slow channels" from extracellular sites. Structurally, these agents vary significantly. They inhibit phase 0 depolarization in cardiac pacemaker cells and the phase 2 plateau in myocytes, Purkinje cells, and vascular smooth muscle cells. In doing so, they cause vasodilation and serve to depress myocardial contractility and sinus and atrioventricular nodal conduction.[21]

The various agents within the calcium channel blocker class vary in their pharmacologic effects. Nifedipine has a more profound peripheral smooth muscle vasodilatory effect than the other agents. Verapamil tends to have a more potent central cardiac effect, decreasing atrioventricular node conduction and myocardial contractility. Diltiazem has both central and peripheral circulatory effects, although the central effects appear to predominate, placing it closer to the verapamil end of the spectrum. Diltiazem and verapamil have negative inotropic effects.[21]

Clinical Presentation

Factors predisposing to calcium channel blocker toxicity are listed in Table 32–12.[25]

Withdrawal Effects

Withdrawal of calcium channel blocking drugs from severely hypertensive patients, even in the absence of previous angina or myocardial infarction, may precipitate myocardial infarction.[26] Worsening angina and myocardial infarction have been described after the withdrawal of calcium channel blocking agents in patients with normal coronary angiography who are being treated for ischemic chest pain.[27] A specific mechanism of toxicity has not been evaluated.

Sustained-release preparations of verapamil may induce concretions because of the gelatinous nature of the pills.[28] Hypotension and bradyrhythmias may develop up to 18 hours after ingestion despite gastric lavage and use of

Table 32–9
Drug–Drug Interactions Involving Calcium Entry Blockers

Drug	Interacting Drug	Effect	Probable Mechanism	Comments
Verapamil (other calcium entry blockers possible but less likely)	Beta blockers	Heart block, cardiac failure, asystole (after IV verapamil)	Additive depression of AV conduction, myocardial contractility	Primarily seen with verapamil; should be used with caution in patients on beta-blockers
	Digitalis (toxicity)	Aggravates heart block; asystole	Additive depression of cardiac conduction	Avoid use of calcium blockers in patients with digitalis toxicity
Verapamil, diltiazem	Propranolol	Reduced oral clearance with increased concentrations of propranolol	Inhibition of first-pass metabolism	Propranolol dose may need to be reduced
Verapamil, diltiazem	Digoxin	Reduced digoxin clearance, increased digoxin concentrations	Inhibition of metabolism and renal excretion of digoxin	Reduce digoxin dose after starting verapamil or diltiazem; monitor SDC
Verapamil, diltiazem	Cyclosporine	Increased cyclosporine concentrations	Uncertain	Reduce cyclosporine dose after starting verapamil or diltiazem; monitor cyclosporine concentrations
Verapamil	Quinidine	Hypotension (after IV verapamil)	Additive alpha-adrenergic blockade	Use IV verapamil cautiously in patients taking quinidine or other drugs with alpha blocking activity
Verapamil	Prazosin	Increased prazosin concentrations; greater hypotensive effect	Reduced clearance; additive alpha blocking effect	Use combination cautiously; may need to decrease prazosin dose
Verapamil	Halothane	Bradycardia, hypotension	Additive depression of sinus node function and myocardial contractility	Avoid coadministration
Verapamil, diltiazem	Disopyramide, flecainide	Cardiac failure	Additive depression of myocardial contractility	Avoid use if possible, particularly in patients with impaired myocardial function
Verapamil, diltiazem	Amiodarone, flecainide	Sinus arrest, heart block	Additive depression of sinus node function and AV nodal conduction	Use combination with extreme caution
All calcium blockers	Cimetidine	Increased oral bioavailability of calcium blockers	Inhibition of metabolism, reduce presystemic metabolism	Reduce calcium entry blocker dose 30–40%
Verapamil	Rifampicin, sulfinpyrazone	Reduced oral bioavailability of verapamil	Accelerated metabolism, increased presystemic metabolism	Increase verapamil dose, use alternative calcium blocker with less presystemic metabolism

AV, atrioventricular; SDC, serum digoxin concentration.
From Pearigen PD, Benowitz NL. Poisoning due to calcium antagonists: Experience with verapamil, diltiazem and nifedipine. Drug Saf 1991;6(6):408–430.

activated charcoal.[29] Sustained-release verapamil intoxication may lead to atrioventricular block,[30] bradycardia leading to asystole[31] or hypotension,[32] asystolic arrest,[33] or functional rhythms with atrioventricular dissociation,[34] up to 26 hours after initial decontamination and supportive procedures appear to have stabilized the patient. Severe hypotension may lead to cerebral infarction after verapamil overdose.[35]

Slow-Release Verapamil

Manifestations of immediate and sustained-release verapamil overdoses are similar. Sustained-release verapamil overdose is frequently associated with a delayed and prolonged course of toxic signs and symptoms.[36]

Clinical effects usually develop within 30 to 60 minutes of ingestion of an overdose of 5 to 10 times the therapeutic dose. Central nervous system features include drowsiness, confusion, and, rarely, seizures. If coma occurs, it is usually secondary to cardiovascular collapse. Gastrointestinal features may include nausea and vomiting. Metabolic effects include hyperglycemia secondary to the reduced release of insulin and metabolic acidosis secondary to lactic acidosis resulting from poor tissue perfusion. Hypotension is the most common cardiovascular finding and is caused principally by vasodilation and, to a lesser extent, by reduced myocardial contractility.[37]

Laboratory

Routine drug testing does not detect calcium channel blockers.

Analytical Methods

A useful reversed-phase HPLC assay is available for determination of verapamil, norverapamil, and its dealkylated metabolites in plasma. The limit of detection is less than 5 ng/mL for all compounds.[38]

Diltiazem and its metabolites may be quantified by gas chromatography or HPLC. An HPLC method indicates that diltiazem is stable for at least 6 weeks at temperatures below 25°F.[39]

Table 32–10
Cardiovascular Effects of Calcium Channel Blockers

	Amlodipine	Diltiazem	Felodipine	Isradipine	Nicardipine	Nifedipine	Nitrendipine	Verapamil
Heart rate	↔	↓	↑↔	↔	↔	↑	↔	↓
Sinus node activity	↔	↓	↔	↓	↔	↔	↔	↓
Atrioventricular node conduction	↔	↓	↔	↔	↔	↔	↔	↓
Myocardial contractility	↔	↓↓	↔	↔	↔	↔	↔	↓↓
Cardiac output	↑	Variable	↑	↑	↑	↑	↑	Variable
Coronary blood flow	↑	↑↔	↑	↑	↑	↑↑	↑	↑
(H) In Humans, (A) in Animals	(A)	(H)	(H)	(A)	(H)	(A), (H)	(A)	(A)
Peripheral vasodilation	↑↑	↑	↑↑	↑↑	↑	↑↑	↑	↑
Myocardial O_2 demand	↓	↓	↓	↓	↓	↓	↓	↓
Platelet aggregation (in vitro)	↓	↓	↔	↓	↔	↓	↓	↓

↑, Increased; ↓, decreased; ↔, remains the same.
From Purcell H, Waller DG, Fox K. Calcium antagonists in cardiovascular disease. Br J Clin Pract 1989;43(1):369–379.

Table 32–11
Renal, Metabolic, and Other Adverse Effects of Calcium Channel Blockers

	Amlodipine	Diltiazem	Felodipine	Isradipine	Nicardipine	Nifedipine	Nitrendipine	Verapamil
Renal effects								
Plasma flow	↑	↑	↑	↑	↑	↔	↑↔	↔
Glomerular filtration	↑	↑	↑	↑	↑	↔	↑↔	↑↔
Vascular resistance	↓	↓	↓	↓	↓	↓	↓	↓
Diuretic/natriuretic (acute)	↑	↔	↑	↑	↑	↑	↑	↔
Renin activity (chronic)	↔	↑	↑	↑	↔	↑	↑	↔
Glucose/insulin effects	↔	Variable	↔	↔	Variable	Variable	↔	Variable
Serum lipid effects	↔	↔	↔	↔	↔	↔	↔	↔
Potential adverse reactions in addition to those attributed to vasodilation (eg, headache, flushing, edema, hypotension)	Fatigue, nausea	AV block, bradycardia, congestive heart failure, nausea, gingival hyperplasia	Fatigue, nausea, tachycardia	Dizziness, palpitations, fatigue	Fatigue, nausea, insomnia	Nausea, weakness, muscle cramps, dyspnea	Fatigue, insomnia	AV block, constipation, bradycardia, nausea, dizziness, congestive heart failure

AV, atrioventricular.
↑, Increased; ↓, decreased; ↔, remains the same.
From Purcell H, Waller DG, Fox K. Calcium antagonists in cardiovascular disease. Br J Clin Pract 1989;43(10):369–379.

Table 32–12
Factors Predisposing to Calcium Channel Blocking Agent Toxicity

Underlying Cardiac Disease
Sinus node dysfunction
Atrioventricular block
Congestive heart failure

Impaired Drug Elimination
Hepatic failure

Drug Interactions
Additive effects on myocardial contractility or heart rate
  Diuretic agents (dehydration), beta-blocking agents, class I antiarrhythmic drugs
Impaired drug elimination
  Drugs that impair cardiac output, for example, beta-blocking agents
  Drugs that impair hepatic blood flow

From Pentel PR, Salerno DM. Cardiac drug toxicity: Digitalis glycosides and calcium-channel and beta-blocking agents. Med J Aust 1990;152:88–94.

Blood Levels

Verapamil. Verapamil levels confirm toxicity but usually do not aid acute management.

Diltiazem. The therapeutic range of blood diltiazem concentrations is about 100 to 200 μg/L.[11] A review of the literature indicates that with blood levels up to 500 μg/L, first-degree heart block and sinus bradycardia may be observed in an asymptomatic patient. From 500 to 1000 μg/L, hypotension is observed. From 1000 to 1500 μg/L, conduction abnormalities and hypotension have been observed. At levels above 1500 μg/L, cases require temporary pacemakers. At levels above 6100 μg/L, most patients die.[40]

Nifedipine. Approximately 2 hours following a 250-mg nifedipine overdose accompanied by ethanol, a 34-year-old patient's nifedipine level was 181 ng/mL (therapeutic level, 25–100 ng/mL). In 2 hours it was reduced to 70 ng/mL. The patient recovered.[41] The blood concentration of nifedipine 10 hours after an overdose with 600 mg of nifedipine delayed-release tablets rose to 604 ng/mL, with its principal metabolite at a level of 100 ng/mL.[42]

Hyperglycemia

Hyperglycemia and metabolic acidosis can develop in severe verapamil overdoses.[43] Hyperglycemia has also followed overdoses of nifedipine.[44] Ca^{2+}, Mg^{2+}, K^{+}, and Na^{+} levels should be checked in severe overdose.

Serum Calcium

Overdose is typically associated with an abnormal serum calcium level. Following ingestion of 4 g of verapamil, a 24-year-old man had a serum Ca^{2+} level of 1.5 mmol/L (6.1 mg/dL). The electrocardiogram showed a third-degree atrioventricular block. Ten milliliters of 10% intravenous calcium gluconate converted the cardiac rhythm to a second-degree atrioventricular block. Calcium may improve conduction but usually has little effect on hypotension. If severe hypocalcemia is present high doses of calcium can be beneficial[45]; however, although calcium salts are often useful as part of the first-line treatment of verapamil overdose, early use of inotropic drugs or cardiac pacing should be considered in resistant cases.[46]

Electrocardiogram

Electrocardiographic abnormalities after verapamil overdose involve prolonged conduction (QRS, PR, QT intervals), various degrees of atrioventricular block, and asystole.

Treatment

Pearigen and Benowitz have suggested a management protocol for poisoning due to calcium antagonists (Fig. 32–3).[47] Patients with symptoms, especially those who have taken sustained-release preparations, should be admitted to an intensive care unit for continuous electrocardiographic monitoring.[38]

The optimum emergent treatment of calcium channel blocker overdose has yet to be defined. Good reversal and clinical improvement have not been consistently demonstrated.[21]

Stabilization

Animal studies indicate that hypotension and bradycardia following overdose with calcium channel blockers may be due to peripheral vasodilation (nifedipine) or a direct effect of diltiazem and verapamil on cardiac output. This indicates that different therapeutic interventions may be necessary for the management of an overdose of each subclass of calcium channel blockers.[48]

Gut Decontamination

The use of ipecac in a patient with hypotension may be dangerous. The yield is often poor; a vagally induced decrease in heart rate in a hemodynamically unstable patient should discourage its use. Gastric lavage is as effective and safer in these patients.[49] Activated charcoal should be administered via the oral or nasogastric route.[50] Calcium administration for diltiazem overdose has not usually been beneficial in improving hypotension.[11,51,52] Multiple-dose activated charcoal may be useful after a sustained-release overdose, but did not appear useful in one patient following a diltiazem overdose.[52] Delayed toxicity with sustained-release preparations may be observed despite apparently good initial decontamination (with gastric lavage and charcoal administration).[53] Polyethylene glycol whole-gut lavage is effective in sustained-release overdose.[30]

Elimination Enhancement

Calcium channel blockers are highly protein bound, extensively distributed in the tissues, and rapidly metabolized by the liver to inactive metabolites. Consequently, techniques such as hemofiltration and dialysis are of no value in managing overdose.[38]

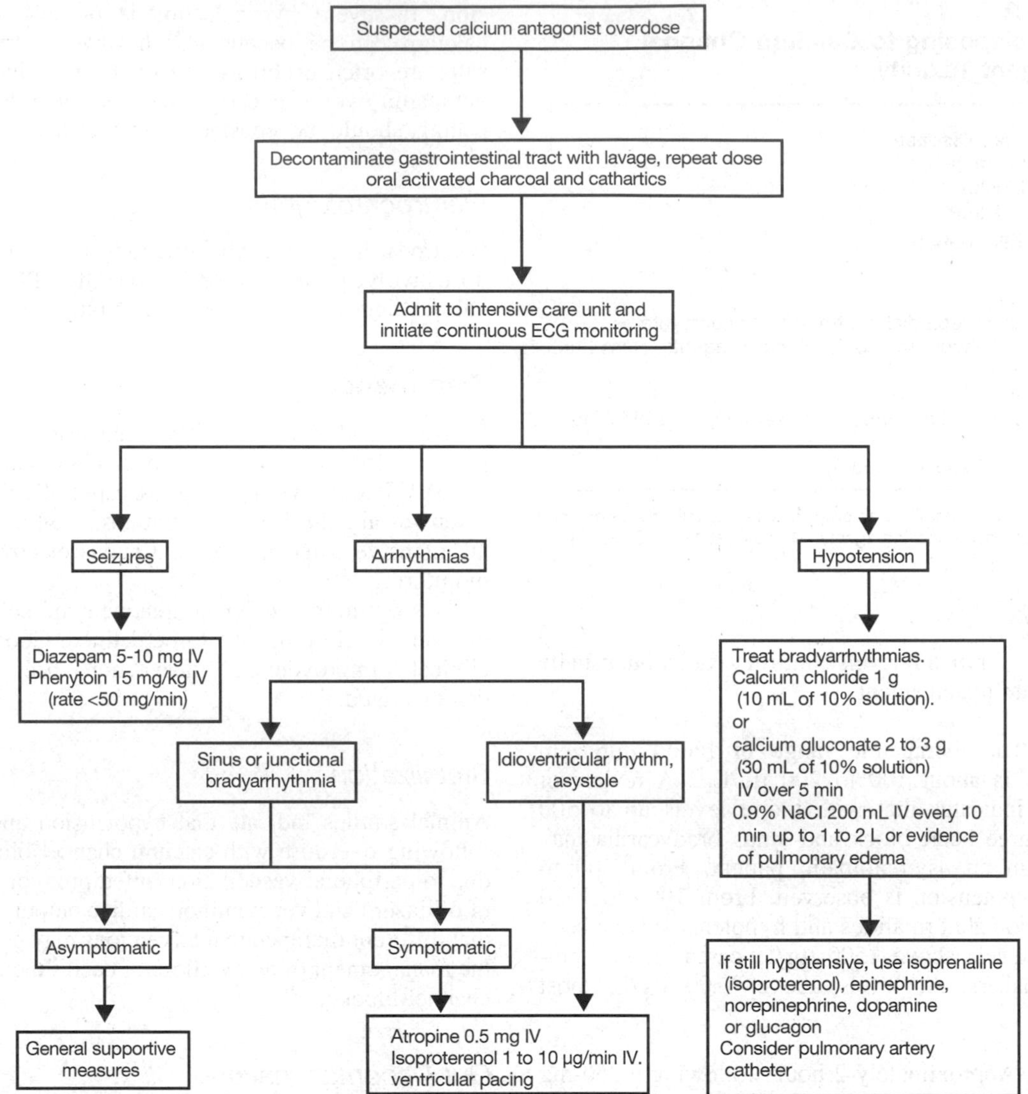

Figure 32-3 Protocol for management of poisoning due to calcium antagonists. (From Pearigen PD, Benowitz NL. Management of poisoning due to calcium antagonists. Drug Saf 1991;6:424.)

Antidote

Calcium Gluconate. An adult dose of 10 mL of 10% calcium gluconate over 5 minutes may be used to reverse hypotension with careful monitoring of rhythm. A repeat bolus (after 10–15 minutes) or intravenous drip (10–20 mL/h of the 10% calcium gluconate solution) may be needed. Calcium levels must be monitored. The optimal calcium dosage required for the treatment of calcium channel blocker toxicity has not been determined. Hypercalcemia may be significant if more than 45 mEq of calcium is administered acutely.[21]

Atropine. There may be a lack of response to atropine until calcium is administered. Calcium given intravenously with or without normal saline can assist in reversing the cardiac and vasodilatory response of calcium antagonist overdose,[30] but atropine is a commonly used vagolytic agent for the treatment of bradycardia and atrioventricular nodal blockade. There are occasional reports of therapeutic effects in calcium channel blocker toxicity.[21]

Glucagon. Glucagon exhibits chronotropic and inotropic effects in calcium channel blocker overdose. The binding of glucagon to its specific catecholamine-independent receptors activates adenyl cyclase and converts intracellular ATP to cyclic AMP. The intracellular cylic AMP stimulates the uptake of calcium by the sarcoplasmic reticulum and plasma membrane-enriched fraction. Calcium is important for the coupling of the action potential of the contraction press. Increased intracellular calcium leads to increased myocardial contractility. This effect on myocardial cells appears to be influenced by the amount of circulating ionized calcium, the presence of phosphodiesterase inhibitors, and the degree of heart failure. Normal serum ionized calcium may be a prerequisite for full responsivity of myocardial cells to glucose.

Intravenous glucagon 0.5 to 5 mg is often followed by a rise in blood pressure.[14,54] If an initial bolus of 3 to 5 mg is unsuccessful at increasing blood pressure, it appears reasonable to double that dose. If the hemodynamic status improves, a glucagon infusion can be started at a rate of 2 to 5 mg/h. Glucagon can be administered safely for as long as 48 hours with few ill effects.[14] The most common adverse drug reactions associated with its use are nausea, emesis, and hyperglycemia.[55] Careful monitoring of total serum calcium and preferably of total serum ionized calcium, as well as supplemental infusions of calcium chloride, appear to constitute an optimal management program. If these modalities do not restore the hemodynamic status, a bolus infusion of amrinone may be useful.[14] Some recent literature reports anecdotal success with glucagon, although other reports describe the use of up to 10 mg of glucagon intravenously without clinical improvement.[21]

4-Aminopyridine. 4-aminopyridine is not available for general clinical use in the United States. The drug is a competitive antagonist of nondepolarizing neuromuscular blocking agents and also is a competitive antagonist of verapamil. In one anecdotal report, 4-aminopyridine restored blood pressure and cardiac rhythm in 90 minutes in a patient unresponsive to atropine, calcium, and isoproterenol.[56]

Catecholamines and Sympathomimetic Agents. Various catecholamines and sympathomimetic agents, including isoproterenol, dopamine, dobutamine, epinephrine, and norepinephrine, have been used to counter the hypotensive effects of calcium channel blocker overdose, all with mixed results. It remains unclear which catecholamine or combination of catecholamines is better for the treatment of calcium channel blocker toxicity based on current data in the literature. On the basis of their pharmacologic profiles, beta-adrenergic receptor agonists such as dobutamine and isoproterenol would be logical choices when primarily cardiac chronotropy and inotropy are affected. Direct alpha-adrenergic receptor agonists may be a better choice if the toxicity is related primarily to decreased systemic vascular resistances. Combining alpha- and beta-adrenergic receptor agonists (such as dobutamine and norepinephrine) or using agents with both alpha- and beta-adrenergic effects (such as epinephrine) may ameliorate both cardiac dysfunction and decreased systemic vascular resistance.[21]

Supportive Measures/Notes

1. With adequate cardiovascular function and in the presence of blood levels many times higher than therapeutic concentrations, patients with diltiazem overdose appear to have a good prognosis.[11,57]
2. Sustained-release verapamil overdoses may be followed by a matted lump of tablets (bezoar) in the stomach. Gastroscopy followed by gastric lavage should be performed to break down these bezoars.[34]
3. Bradycardia, second- and third-degree atrioventricular block, idioventricular rhythm, and hypokalemia have been treated with potassium supplementation and intravenous calcium gluconate, and atropine in addition to mannitol.
4. Amrinone and glucagon (10 mL intravenously) were safe and effective in the management of hemodynamic instability following ingestion of sustained-release verapamil 3.6 g.[57] Further studies are necessary to validate the role of amrinone.
5. There is insufficient clinical evidence at present to recommend the use of 4-aminopyridine or aminophylline in the routine treatment of a calcium channel blocker overdose.
6. For hypotension, institute fluid replacement with 0.9% saline. Administer calcium chloride (10 mL 10% calcium chloride intravenously every 5 minutes at 0.2 mg/kg to a total dose of 10 mL) or calcium gluconate 20 to 30 mL. Repeat every 15 to 20 minutes. Monitor serum calcium.
7. Administer glucagon 10 mL intravenously if an initial 3–5 mg bolus is unsuccessful at increasing blood pressure.
8. If hypotension is severe, insert a Swan–Ganz catheter.
9. Administer isoprenaline, dopamine, dobutamine, or noradrenaline.
10. Watch pulmonary capillary wedge pressure to prevent pulmonary edema.
11. For pulmonary edema, administer diuretics and institute mechanical ventilation.
12. An intraaortic balloon pump may be able to maintain adequate cardiac output when conventional therapy has failed for calcium output when conventional therapy has shock.[58]
13. If therapeutic measures for diltiazem overdoses are successful the patient usually recovers within 36 hours, allowing the discontinuation of pacing or inotropic infusions.[41]
14. Dopamine is an initial pressor of choice (75% response) for diltiazem overdose. Isoproterenol produces a therapeutic response in 50% of patients. Pacing leads to a response in most cases of diltiazem overdose.
15. Monitor blood pressure and the electrocardiogram for at least 3 days after a verapamil overdose and for a longer period when sustained-release verapamil has been ingested.[59]

Ingestion of a few tablets of sustained-release calcium channel blocker by children was not associated with symptoms in one series. Recommendations regarding a duration of observation vary from less than 6 hours to 24 hours in pediatric cases.[60]

Hemodynamic Monitoring

Patients with hemodynamic compromise from calcium channel blocker overdose that does not respond to initial therapy should receive invasive hemodynamic monitoring. Specific cardiac output and systemic vascular resistance measurement may determine the optimal pharmacologic therapy and fluid supplement.[21]

Pulmonary Artery Catheterization

There is minimal information in the literature with regard to pulmonary artery catheterization measurements and calcium channel blocker toxicity in humans. Pulmonary artery catheterization measurements demonstrate hyperkinetic cardiac output and decreased systemic vascular resistances on pressor agents. The accumulation of data or pulmonary artery catheterization in calcium channel blocker toxicity will help physicians gain better insight into calcium channel blocker toxicity and the choice of pharmacologic therapy.[21]

Electromechanical Supports

Cardiac pacing is indicated for significant bradycardia and high-grade conduction blocks. The increase in heart rate alone induced by cardiac pacing can improve cardiac output. Cardiac pacing (both external and internal) does not always capture or improve the hemodynamics in calcium channel blocker toxic patients. Intraaortic balloon counterpulsation directly augments cardiac output in the failing heart. By temporarily providing adequate cardiac output, it provides a window of opportunity for the metabolism and elimination of the offending calcium channel blocker. Cardiac pacing may be used in concert with intraaortic balloon counterpulsation for significant bradycardia and high-grade blocks.[21]

REFERENCES—CALCIUM CHANNEL BLOCKERS

1. Clark CF, Hanna TC. Calcium channel blocker toxicity. Top Emerg Med 1993;15:15–26.
2. Todd PA, Benfield P. Flunarizine: A reappraisal of its pharmacological properties and therapeutic use in neurological disorders. Drugs 1989;38:481–499.
3. Diamond S, Freitag DO, Diamond MD. Flunarizine in migraine therapy. Clin Pharmacol Ther 1990;47:165.
4. Shimell CJ, Fritz VU, Levien SL. A comparative trial of flunarizine and propranolol in the prevention of migraine. South Afr Med J 1990:77–78.
5. Benvenuti F, Baroni A, Bandinelli S, et al. Flunarizine-induced parkinsonism in the elderly. J Clin Pharmacol 1988;28:600–608.
6. Reynolds JFK, ed. *Martindale: The Extra Pharmacopoeia.* 30th ed. London: Pharmaceutical Press, 1993:734.
7. Pearigen PD. Death from accidental nifedipine ingestion in a toddler. Vet Hum Toxicol 1993;35:345.
8. Ferner RE, Odemuyiwa O, Field AB, et al. Pharmacokinetics and toxic effects of diltiazem in massive overdose. Hum Toxicol 1989;8:497–499.
9. Wells TG, Graham CJ, Moss M, Kearns GC. Nifedipine poisoning in a child. Pediatrics 1990;86:91–94.
10. Schiffl H, Ziupa J, Schollmeyer P. Clinical features and management of nifedipine overdosage in a patient with renal insufficiency. Clin Toxicol 1984;22:387–395.
11. Ramoska EA, Spiller HA, Myers A. Calcium channel blocker toxicity. Ann Emerg Med 1990;19:649–653.
12. Riggs BS, Hall AH, Kulig KW, et al. Calcium channel blockers in children: A review of 18 cases. Vet Hum Toxicol 1987;29:484–485 (Abstract 127).
13. Doyon S, Roberts JR. The use of glucagon in a case of calcium channel blocker overdose. Ann Emerg Med 1993;22:1229–1233.
14. Erickson FC, Ling LJ, Grande GA, Anderson DL. Diltiazem overdose: Case report and review. J Emerg Med 1991;9:357–366.
15. Harchelroad F. ARDS associated with calcium channel blocker overdose. Vet Hum Toxicol 1992;34:328.
16. Beno JM, Nemeth DR. Diltiazem and metoclopramide overdose. J Anal Toxicol 1991;15:285–286.
17. Minella RA, Schulman DS. Fatal verapamil toxicity and hypokalemia. Am Heart J 1991;121:1810–1812.
18. MacDonald D, Alguire PC. Case report: Fatal overdose with sustained release verapamil. Am J Med Sci 1992;303:115–117.
19. Pearigen PD. Death from accidental nifedipine ingestion in a toddler. Vet Hum Toxicol 1993;35:345.
20. Proano L, Chiang WK, Wang RY. Calcium channel blocker overdose. Am J Emerg Med 1995;13:444–450.
21. Lubbe WF. Use of diltiazem during pregnancy. NZ Med J 1987;100:121.
22. Ehrenkranz RA, Ackerman BA, Hulse JD. Nifedipine transfer into human milk. J Pediatr 1989;114:478–479.
23. Penny WJ, Leurs MJ. Nifedipine is excreted in human milk. Eur J Clin Pharmacol 1989;36:427–428.
24. Purcell H, Waller DG, Fox K. Therapeutic focus: Calcium antagonists in cardiovascular disease. Br J Clin Pract 1989;34:369.
25. Pentel PR, Salerno DM. Cardiac drug toxicity: Digitalis, glycosides and calcium channel and beta blocking agents. Med J Aust 1990;152:88–94.
26. Dimmitt SB, Beilin LJ, Hockings BEF. Verapamil withdrawal as a possible cause of myocardial infarction in a hypertensive woman with a normal coronary angiogram. Med J Aust 1988;149:218.
27. Heupler FA, Proudfoot WL. Nifedipine therapy for refractory coronary arterial spasm. Am J Cardiol 1979;44:798–803.
28. Sporer KA, Manning JJ. Massive ingestion of sustained release verapamil with a concretion and bowel infarction. Ann Intern Med 1993;22:603–605.
29. Buckley N, Dawson AH, Howarth D, Whyte IM. Slow-release verapamil poisoning: Use of polyethylene glycol whole-bowel lavage and high-dose calcium. Med J Aust 1993;158:202–204.
30. Spiller HA, Meyers A, Ziemba T, Riley M. Delayed onset of cardiac arrhythmias from sustained release verapamil. Ann Emerg Med 1991;20:201–203.
31. Quezado Z, Lippmann M, Wertheimer J. Severe cardiac, respiratory and metabolic complications of massive verapamil overdose. Crit Care Med 1991;19:436–438.
32. Krick SE, Gums JG, Grauer K, Cooper GR. Severe verapamil (sustained release) overdose. DICP Ann Pharmacother 1990;24:705–706.
33. Rankin RJ, Edwards IR. Overdose of sustained release verapamil. NZ Med J 1990;103:165.
34. Kozlowski JH, Kozlowski JA, Shuller D. Poisoning with sustained release verapamil. Am J Med 1988;85:127.
35. Samniah N, Schlaeffer F. Cerebral infarction associated with oral verapamil overdose. Clin Toxicol 1988;26:365–369.
36. Shah AR, Passalacqua VR. Sustained-release verapamil overdose causing stroke: An unusual complication. Am J Med Sci 1992;304:357–359. Case report.
37. Kenny J. Treating overdose with calcium channel blockers. Br Med J 1994;308:992–993.
38. Koppel C, Wagemann A. Plasma level monitoring of D,L-verapamil and three of its metabolites by reversed-phase high-performance liquid chromatography. J Chromatogr Biomed Appl 1991;570:229–234.
39. Caille G, Duke LM, Theoret Y, et al. Stability study of diltiazem and two of its metabolites using a high performance liquid chromatographic method. Biopharm Drug Dispos 1989;10:107–114.
40. Roper TA, Sykes R, Gray C. Fatal diltiazem overdose: Report of four cases and review of the literature. Postgrad Med J 1993;69:474–476.
41. Welch RD, Todd K. Nifedipine overdose accompanied by ethanol intoxication in a patient with congenital heart disease. J Emerg Med 1990;8:169–172.
42. Ferner RE, Monkman S, Riley J, et al. Pharmacokinetics and toxic effects of nifedipine in massive overdose. Hum Exp Toxicol 1990;9:309–311.
43. Silva OA, DeMelo RA, Filko JPJ. Verapamil acute self-poisoning. Clin Toxicol 1979;14:361–369.
44. Herrington DM, Insley BM, Weinmann GG. Nifedipine overdose. Am J Med 1986;81:344–346.
45. Kvo MJ, Tseng YZ, Chen TF, Fong DE. Verapamil overdose and severe hypocalcemia. Clin Toxicol 1992;30:309–311.
46. Watson NA. Management of massive verapamil overdose. Med J Aust 1991;55:728.
47. Pearigen PD, Benowitz NL. Poisoning due to calcium antagonists: Experience with verapamil, diltiazem and nifedipine. Drug Saf 1991;6:408–430.
48. Spivey WH, Schoffstall JM, Gambone LM, et al. Effects of calcium channel blocker overdose-induced toxicity on systemic hemodynamics and cardiac output distribution in the conscious dog. Ann Emerg Med 1988;17:402.
49. Spurlock BW, Virani NA, Henry CA. Verapamil overdose. West J Med 1991;154:208–211.

50. Watson NA, Fitzgerald CP. Management of massive verapamil overdose. Med J Aust 1991;155:124–125.
51. Roberts D, Honcharik N, Sitar DS, Tenenbein M. Diltiazem overdose: Pharmacokinetics of diltiazem and its metabolites and effect of multiple dose charcoal therapy. Clin Toxicol 1991;29:45–52.
52. Jakubowski AT, Mizgala HF. Effect of diltiazem overdose. Am J Cardiol 1987;60:932–933.
53. Kirshenbaum LA, Mathews SC, Sitar DS, Tenenbein M. Whole bowel irrigation versus activated charcoal in sorbitol for the ingestion of modified-release pharmaceuticals. Clin Pharmacol Ther 1989;46:264–271.
54. Walter FG, Frye G, Mullen JT, et al. Amelioration of nifedipine poisoning associated with glucagon therapy. Ann Emerg Med 1993;22:1234–1237.
55. Wolf LR, Spadaforo MP, Otten EJ. Use of amrinone and glucagon in a case of calcium channel blocker overdose. Ann Emerg Med 1993;22:1225–1228.
56. TerWee PM, Kremer-Hovinga TK, Uges DRA, van der Geest S. 4-Aminopyridine and hemodialysis in the treatment of verapamil intoxication. Hum Toxicol 1985;4:227–229.
57. Jaeger A, Sauder P, Bianchetti G, et al. Intoxications aigues par le diltiazem etude cinetique et hemodynamique. J Toxicol Clin Exp 1990;10:243–248.
58. Melanson P, Shih RD, De Roos F, et al. Intraaortic balloon counterpulsation in calcium channel blocker overdose. Vet Hum Toxicol 1993;35:345.
59. Tom PA, Morrow CT, Kelen GD. Delayed hypotension after overdose of sustained release verapamil. J Emerg Med 1994; 12:621.
60. Brayer A, Wax P. Accidental ingestions of sustained release calcium channel blockers in children. Clin Toxicol 1995; 33:475–486 (Abstract 75).

DIGITALIS

Product Formulation

Digoxin is by far the most commonly prescribed digitalis preparation in the United States. Digitoxin is more popular in Latin countries, Europe, and Canada. Its toxicity is significantly different because of its nonpolar structure and resulting toxicokinetic properties. Rarely used digitalis preparations include digitalis leaf, ouabain, lanatoside C, deslanoside, and gitalin. Cardiac glycoside-containing plants include common oleander *(Nerium oleander)*, foxglove *(Digitalis purpurea)*, lily of the valley *(Convallaria majalis)*, yellow oleander *(Thevetia peruviana)*, and red squill *(Urginea maritima)*. Digoxin is available in 0.125-, 0.25-, and 0.5-mg tablets and as a 0.05 mg/mL elixir.

Toxic Dose

Ingestion of 0.05 mg/kg (eg, one 0.5-mg tablet) by a 10-kg child would be expected to produce a digoxin blood level above the upper therapeutic limit of 2 ng/mL. Although children tolerate acute digoxin ingestions better than adults, the serious sequelae of digoxin mean that any potential or suspected ingestion above this range should be treated with gut decontamination and observation in an emergency department.

Any suicidal ingestion in a patient chronically taking digoxin should be considered a serious ingestion. Toxic effects in such patients are difficult to predict because of a variety of factors that predispose to digitalis poisoning.

Toxicokinetics

Significant differences exist between digoxin and digitoxin kinetics.

Absorption

Digoxin. Bioavailability depends on tablet dissolution; this factor is now more standardized and ranges from 50 to 80%. Patient factors that reduce absorption include coadministration of food, malabsorption syndromes, antacids, and decreased gastrointestinal motility.

Digitoxin. Excellent absorption occurs after oral doses. Following an oral dose, the latency period is 1 to 2 hours and effects peak in 4 to 12 hours.

Distribution

Digoxin. Digoxin has a large apparent volume of distribution (adults, 7–8 L/kg; neonates, 10 L/kg; infants, 16 L/kg). The volume of distribution is reduced in renal disease, hypothyroidism, and quinidine therapy and in the elderly (loss of muscle mass). The initial volume of distribution is small, and this may result in excessively high levels immediately after administration. Most digoxin is distributed to the skeletal muscle (approximately 65% of the absorbed dose). The myocardium : plasma ratio is about 30 : 1.

Digitoxin. Digitoxin is highly protein bound and has a relatively small apparent volume of distribution.

Elimination

Digoxin. The kidney excretes 60 to 80% of digoxin unchanged. The terminal elimination half-life averages about 36 hours.[1] Biliary excretion and enterohepatic circulation may not be significant in therapeutic doses. Studies show variability in biliary excretion due to liver disease and collection methods. Depending on the collection method, biliary excretion accounts for 8 to 30% of a therapeutic oral dose in 24 hours.[2]

Digitoxin. The liver metabolizes digitoxin by removing sugar (digitoxose) to form epidigitoxigenin, which is conjugated to an inactive metabolite. Digoxin is a by-product of digitoxin metabolism (about 8%). Enterohepatic circulation probably is responsible for the long elimination half-life (about 100 hours). Verapamil and diltiazem, but not nifedipine, reduce the nonrenal clearance by an average of 29 and 21%, respectively.[3]

Pregnancy

Ingestion of 8.9 mg of digitoxin by a woman in the eighth month of pregnancy resulted in clinical evidence of maternal and fetal digitalis intoxication. The newborn infant died 3 days postpartum.[4]

Drug Interactions

Table 32–13 summarizes interactions affecting the toxicokinetics of digitalis cardiac glycosides.

Table 32-13
Agents Affecting the Pharmacokinetics of Digitalis

Alteration	Agents
Decreased absorption	Activated charcoal, antacids, cholestyramine, colestipol, cytotoxic agents (cyclophosphamide, doxorubicin [adriamycin]), dietary fiber, kaolin–pectin, metoclopramide, neomycin, sulfasalazine
Increased absorption	Antibiotics (by inhibiting gut flora), anticholinergics (propantheline)
Inhibition of serum protein binding	Clofibrate, phenobarbital, phenylbutazone, prazosin, sulfonamides, tolbutamide, warfarin
Enhanced hepatic metabolism	Phenobarbital, phenylbutazone, phenytoin, rifampicin (rifampin)
Enhanced renal excretion	Hydralazine, levodopa, nitroprusside
Inhibition of renal tubular secretion	Quinidine, spironolactone, triamterene, trimethoprim, verapamil
Inhibition of extrarenal clearance	Diltiazem, quinidine, verapamil
Decreased volume of distribution	Quinidine
Increased serum digoxin concentrations (mechanism unknown)	Amiodarone, aspirin, bepridil, diltiazem, flecainide, ibuprofen, indomethacin, nifedipine, nicardipine, nisoldipine, nitrendipine, propafenone

From Mooradian AD. Digitalis: An update of clinical pharmacokinetics, therapeutic monitoring techniques and treatment recommendations. Clin Pharmacokinet 1988;15(3):165–179.

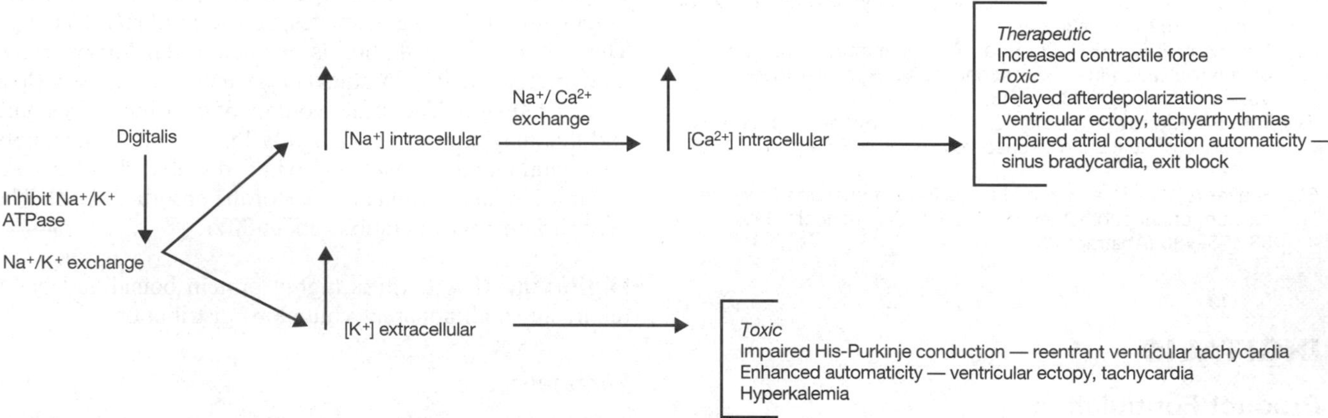

Figure 32-4 Postulated direct cardiac effects of digitalis. (From Pentel PR, Salerno DM. Cardiac drug toxicity: Digitalis glycosides and calcium-channel and beta-blocking agents. Med J Aust 1990;152:88–94.)

Erythromycin. Erythromycin causes inhibition of *Eubacterium lentum,* which converts digoxin into digoxin reduction products in the gut. This may lead to an increase in serum digoxin concentrations.[5,6]

Erythromycin–Tetracycline. Erythromycin and tetracycline can double the digoxin concentration in some patients, probably by eliminating gut flora that normally reduce digoxin and decrease its absorption.[6,7]

Mechanism of Action

Figure 32–4 depicts a postulated direct cardiac effect of digitalis. Hypomagnesemia may be a more frequent contributor to digoxin toxicity than hypokalemia.[8,9]

Clinical Presentation

Factors predisposing to digitalis toxicity are summarized in Table 32–14. Mortality increases in patients exhibiting five prognostic features: advanced age, heart disease, male sex, high-degree atrioventricular block, and hyperkalemia.[10] Differences between acute and chronic digoxin poisoning are outlined in Table 32–15.

Table 32-14
Factors Predisposing to Digitalis Toxicity

Increased cardiac sensitivity
Acute hypoxia
Electrolyte abnormalities
  Hypokalemia, hyperkalemia,* hypercalcemia, hypomagnesemia
Respiratory alkalosis
Myocardial ischemia
  Acute
  Recent myocardial infarction
Increased sympathetic tone
Advanced age
Direct-current cardioversion
Increased serum digitalis concentration
Overdose—accidental or intentional
Impaired renal or hepatic clearance
Drug interactions
  Quinidine, verapamil, amiodarone, quinine, spironolactone, propafenone, erythromycin, tetracycline

*Both hypokalemia and hyperkalemia may aggravate digoxin toxicity.
From Pentel PR, Salerno DM. Cardiac drug toxicity: Digitalis glycosides and calcium-channel and beta-blocking agents. Med J Aust 1990; 152:88–94.

Table 32–15
Differences in Acute and Chronic Digoxin Poisoning

	Acute Intoxication	Chronic Toxicity
Types of patients most commonly involved	In many cases the patients are normal with no history of cardiac disease.	Patients are ill with cardiac abnormalities underlying the toxic state. The symptoms may mimic the condition for which the drug is being used.
Symptoms on admission	Nausea and vomiting are the most consistent findings. Diarrhea is occasionally observed.	Anorexia, nausea, vomiting, headache, malaise, fatigue, weakness, and drowsiness are common. Diarrhea is less commonly seen. Paresthesias and neuritic pain along with confusion, disorientation, aphasia, delirium, hallucinations, and rarely convulsions are all reported. Visual changes and skin rashes are also noted.
Findings on admission	Electrocardiogram findings indicate supraventricular arrhythmias, in general, with heart block and bradycardia most commonly noted. There is a general lack of ventricular arrhythmias.	All types of arrhythmias have been attributed to digitalis glycosides. The most common arrhythmias are nonparoxysmal nodal tachycardia, atrial tachycardia with atrioventricular dissociation, and bidirectional ventricular tachycardia.
Serum potassium	Levels are normal or increased depending on the magnitude of the overdose and the relative time course.	Normal to decreased depending on the use of potent loop diuretics, nutrition status of the patient, and presence of other factors known to affect the potassium level.
Serum digoxin determinations	High levels are always expected and seem to roughly correlate with the magnitude of the rise in serum potassium and the presence of serum cardiac arrhythmias.	The levels may not clearly identify therapeutic ranges but are generally elevated in any prominent toxic state. Borderline normal values may represent toxicity.
Serum half-life of digoxin	It has been reported to be shortened in both adults and children, although conflicting reports have been published.	The half-life determinations for both adults and children are similar.

From Elkins BR. Management of acute digoxin overdosage. Clin Toxicol Consult 1979;4:96.

Chronic Use

Chronic digitalis toxicity often is minor and may be difficult to diagnose because side effects mimic underlying disease states.

Cardiovascular Effects. Any dysrhythmia may result from digitalis toxicity.[11] The classic digoxin toxic rhythm is a combination of suppressant and excitatory effects (eg, nonparoxysmal atrial tachycardia with 2:1 block). Premature ventricular extrasystoles are the most common digitalis toxic rhythm disturbance, with premature atrial and junctional extrasystoles occurring less frequently. These extrasystoles may be miltifocal or bigeminal. The most common sustained rhythms are junctional escape rhythms, followed in incidence by ectopic atrial tachycardia with some degree of atrioventricular block. Regularization of rate in the setting of atrial fibrillation and digoxin administration suggests the development of a digitalis toxic junctional rhythm. Further intoxication causes an increased irregular rate (enhanced automaticity), junctional tachycardia, and Wenckebach exit block. All grades of atrioventricular block can occur in digitalis toxicity and may require temporary pacing. Hypokalemia often accompanies rhythm disturbances. Ventricular tachycardia and ventricular fibrillation are the most serious digitalis-induced dysrhythmias.

Nonspecific and Gastrointestinal Effects. Common nonspecific and gastrointestinal symptoms of digitalis toxicity include malaise, fatigue, weakness, anorexia, nausea, vomiting, and headache.

Visual Effects. Visual symptoms include scotoma, blurred vision, color aberrational photophobia, and transient blindness.

Psychosensorial Effects. Mental confusion, hallucinations, and delirium occur regularly, but convulsions are rare.

Overdose

Serious Prognostic Factors

Age. Older patients, especially with underlying disease, are at higher risk. Children often have a more benign course and tolerate much higher peak digoxin levels. An 18-month-old infant with a peak digoxin level of 48 μg/mL exhibited only mild effects of digoxin poisoning (serum potassium of 5.2 mEq/L, mild bradycardia, and brief periods of junctional rhythm, sinus arrest, and second-degree Wenckebach atrioventricular block).[12]

Hyperkalemia. Many adult patients with a digoxin level of 10 ng/mL have potassium levels about 6 mEq/L.

High-Grade Atrioventricular Block. This is a serious prognostic factor.

Plasma Digoxin Level. Concentrations exceeding 15 ng/mL indicate a serious prognosis.

Ventricular Tachycardia. The presence of this rhythm carries a 60 to 65% mortality rate.

Clinical Effects. Nausea and vomiting are the most consistent gastrointestinal findings in digitalis poisoning. Mental status changes may be present. Cardiovascular symptoms are the most frequent effects and may be delayed up to 6 hours. In children, bradycardia and conduction delays occur commonly but endogenous pacemakers usually capture adequately and prevent hemodynamic compromise. The common rhythm disturbances include bradycardia (21–75%), heart block (23–56%), and tachydysrhythmias (30–42%). Ventricular arrhythmias occur less frequently in children.

Fatalities. Death from massive overdose in adults results from the exacerbation of therapeutic effects:

- Pump failure secondary to negative inotropic effects (10% of deaths)
- Conduction impairment with severe atrioventricular block (20% of deaths)
- Ventricular arrhythmias from increased automaticity (70% of deaths)

Laboratory

Analytical Methods

Free digoxin concentrations appear to be quantitated most accurately in the presence of Fab at multiple doses with use of ultrafiltration with fluorescene polarization immunoassay. Radioimmunoassay should not be used to measure free or total serum digoxin concentrations as it reports spurious results when Fab has unoccupied binding sites.[13]

Serum Digoxin Levels

Red blood cell K^+ depletion by cardiac glycoside may be a useful marker of the effect of digitalis on Na^+, K^+-ATPase.[14,15] In acute digitoxin poisoning red blood cell K^+ depletion may allow prediction of the severity of digitalis poisoning; it appears to reflect the myocardial cell K^+ depletion, which can occur in parallel with tachyarrhythmia and conduction disturbances.[16] The clinical usefulness of this marker requires confirmatory studies.

Serum Digitoxin Levels

An adult who ingested 35 mg of digitoxin was treated with digitalis antibody Fab fragments (Digitalis Antidote BM, 80 mg). A total of 11, 80-mg doses of Fab fragment were administered. The free fraction of serum digitoxin was assayed with the Baxter–Status fluorescence enhanced enzyme partition immunoassay and the total digitoxin was analyzed with the Abbott TDx fluorescence polarization immunoassay.[17] The patient recovered.

Ingestion of digitoxin 250 mg by a young adult resulted in elevation of the serum digitoxin level to 360 mmol/L 8 hours after ingestion. Digoxin-specific Fab fragments (Digitalis Antidote BM, 480 mg) were administered at three separate times (total, 1440 mg). Sinus rhythm was stabilized and the patient remained asymptomatic.[18]

Digitoxin-specific monoclonal antibody Fab fragments have been shown to be useful in induced digitoxin poisoning in animals.[19]

Treatment

Stabilization

A suggested plan for management of low-, intermediate-, and high-risk digitalis intoxications is outlined in Table 32–16.[20]

Gut Decontamination

Cholestyramine 12 to 16 g orally per day appears to be useful in enhancing digoxin elimination, probably by interrupting the enterohepatic recycling of digoxin.[21]

Activated charcoal (may require repeated doses) appeared to be more effective than cholestyramine and colestipol in a randomized study on preventing absorption of digoxin.[22,23] Cholestyramine and colestipol in a 94-year-old patient presumably interrupted the enterohepatic recycling of digoxin.[21]

Antidote

Once the sheep-derived digoxin-specific antibodies are administered, (1) check repeatedly for hypokalemia in the first few hours; (2) observe for evidence of congestive heart failure from loss of digitalis-mediated inotropy; and (3)

Table 32–16
Treatment of Digitalis Intoxication

Low-Risk Patients
There is no evidence of electrocardiographic rhythm disturbances.
Serum digoxin levels are mildly elevated.
There is no history of severe cardiac disease.
Left ventricular function is good.
Digoxin is used for uncomplicated atrial fibrillation.

Treatment
Manage as outpatient.
Withhold digitalis temporarily.
Repeat ECGs: look for effects of digitalis withdrawal.

Intermediate-Risk Patients
Cardiac toxicity is confirmed by ECG in patients without life-threatening complications

Treatment
Observe in monitored setting.
Obtain potassium and magnesium levels.
Institute replacement therapy if there is marked depression in blood potassium or magnesium level.
Potassium replacement may exacerbate atrioventricular block.
Hypercalcemia (like hypokalemia and hypomagnesemia) increases ventricular automaticity.
Avoid antiarrhythmic drug therapy unless hemodynamically significant dysrhythmias or high-grade ectopy exists.

High-Risk Patients
Serum digitalis levels are very high.
Life-threatening arrhythmias occur.

Treatment
Admit to coronary care unit.
Empty stomach of oral ingestion within 6 to 8 hours.
Use charcoal slowly.
Anion-exchange resins may shorten half-life of digitoxin from the gastrointestinal tract.
Use atropine for marked sinus bradycardia, sinoatrial arrest, and second- or third-degree heart block.
Insert temporary pacemaker if patient is hemodynamically unstable and does not respond to atropine.
Use of Digoxin–Specific Fab Fragments

Dick M, Carwin J, Tepper D. Digitalis intoxication recognition and management. J Clin Pharmacol 1991;31:444–447.

monitor for allergic reactions, particularly in patients with known allergy to sheep proteins and in patients who have previously been given digitalis immune Fab.[20]

Indications. Fab fragments also neutralize lanatoside C_4 and proscillaridin and scilliroside poisoning, as well as that of other glycosides found in *Nerium oleander* leaves.[10] Fab should be used in the treatment of digitalis poisoning of infants and young children without heart disease who ingest more than 0.3 mg/kg, who have underlying heart disease, or who have a serum digoxin concentration greater than 0.5 ng/mL, threatening dysrhythmias, hemodynamic instability, or rapid progressive toxicity. Earlier use of Fab therapy, before cardiac pacing or treatment with antidysrhythmic agents, has been advocated. Patients require close monitoring after Fab therapy because a second dose may be necessary if the toxicity recurs or fails to resolve. Adolescents are more sensitive to digitalis and may require Fab therapy at lower plasma digoxin concentrations.

General indications for Fab therapy include the following:

- Imminent cardiac arrest, cardiac arrest, or shock, or rapid progression of clinical findings (progressive obtundation, worsening conduction defects, rapidly rising serum potassium in the context of digitalis poisoning history alone)
- Hyperkalemia with digitalis poisoning (Fab therapy rapidly reverses hyperkalemia)
- Serum digoxin level greater than 10 ng/mL at steady state 6 to 8 hours postingestion in adults, or serum digoxin level greater than 0.5 ng/mL in children (Administration should be based on the symptoms and not solely on the serum digoxin level.)
- Hemodynamically unstable life-threatening dysrhythmias (eg, ventricular fibrillation, ventricular tachycardia, atrial tachycardia, variable atrioventricular block, accelerated junctional, conduction defects)
- Ingestion of more than 10 mg (40, 0.25-mg tablets) in adults or 4 mg (16, 0.25-mg tablets [or >0.3 mg/kg]) in a child or lower doses (0.2 mg/kg) in adolescents
- Bradycardia or second- or third-degree heart block unresponsive to atropine[24]

Fab therapy is indicated in the treatment of digitalis poisoning in infants and young children who have ingested 0.3 mg/kg body weight of digoxin, who have underlying heart disease, or who have a serum digoxin concentration greater than 6.4 nmol/L (>5.0 ng/mL) in the elimination phase and who also have a life-threatening arrhythmia, hemodynamic instability, hyperkalemia over 6 mEq/L, or rapidly progressive toxicity.[24,25] Fab therapy may be useful for noncardiac manifestations of digitalis toxicity, such as an acute psychosis "digitalis delirium," which is characterized by severe agitation, delusional thinking, assaultive behavior, and even death.[26]

Adolescents who are more sensitive to the toxic effects of digoxin than younger children may require treatment with Fab therapy after ingesting lower doses.

Administration of Fab fragments should be based on symptoms and signs and not only on the serum digoxin level.[27]

Those who have preexisting acute or chronic renal failure are at higher risk for severe digitalis intoxication.[29]

Fab therapy has been useful in digitoxin intoxication and oleander poisoning.[30]

Ineffective Use. Digoxin Fab fragments, although effective against cardiac glycosides derived from plants such as oleander, foxglove, and lily-of-the-valley, were not immediately effective in treating a child who was poisoned after ingesting yew berries. Yew contains taxine, a cardiac glycoside unlike those found in oleander, foxglove, and lily-of-the-valley, which does not cause hyperkalemia and is not associated with measurable serum digoxin levels. A very small dose of Fab (20 mg) was enough to bind only 0.03 mg of digoxin. The child was also paced and recovered.

Dosage. Taboulet and colleagues have observed that if initial administration of 800 mg of Fab fails to reduce digitoxin-induced arrhythmias, another dose of 500 mg should be tried.[10] For chronic overdosage, a mean dose of 80 to 160 mg Fab is generally adequate. Extrapolation of this experience with digitoxin to digoxin must be done with caution.

Calculation of Body Load of Glycoside. From the ingested amount:

$$\text{Ingested amount (mg)} \times \text{digoxin bioavailability (60\%) or digitoxin bioavailability (100\%)}$$

From the serum glycoside concentration:

$$\text{Serum glycoside concentration (ng/mL)} \times \text{volume of distribution } (V_d) \times \text{weight (kg), with } V_d = 5.6 \text{ L/kg for digoxin and } 0.56 \text{ L/kg for digitoxin}$$

A small test dose usually is administered, although hypersensitivity reactions have not been reported. Digoxin-specific Fab fragments are expensive ($1000 per average suicidal ingestion). Contact your local poison control center for availability. The Burroughs Wellcome Digibind Hot Line is 1–800–334–4828.

Fab fragments are also available in Europe (Digidot, Boehringer–Ingelheim). In France, one vial of Fab fragments contains 80 mg of Fab and neutralizes 1 mg of digoxin or digitoxin. When no data on amount ingested or urine glycoside levels are available, 10 vials are administered, with another 10 vials as required.[31] In Germany, Fab fragments have been given as a bolus of 80 to 160 mg and then 320 mg infused over 7 to 24 hours.[32] Massive digitoxin intoxications may require treatment with prolonged and repeated intravenous infusions of Fab.[30]

Digoxin Overdose: Calculation of Dosage of Fab Fragments. If the amount and type of digoxin are known,[33]

$$\text{Total body load} = \text{amount ingested (mg)} \times 0.8^{a}$$
$$\text{Total body load}/0.6\ \text{mg}^{b} = \text{number of vials of Fab needed}$$

If the steady-state serum digoxin (or digitoxin) concentration is known,

Total body load = serum digoxin/digitoxin concentration (ng/mL) × V_d^c × weight (kg)/1000

Total body load/0.6 mg = number of vials of Fab needed[d]

a. This reflects 80% bioavailability for the tablets. A factor of 1.0 can be used for digoxin elixir or capsules or digitoxin.
b. 0.6 mg is neutralized by each 40-mg vial of Fab fragments.
c. V_d = 5.6 L/kg for digoxin, 0.56 L/kg for digitoxin.
d. Calculation of an equimolar dose of Fab:

$$\frac{\text{Molecular Weight Fab} = 50{,}000}{\text{Molecular Weight Digoxin} = 781} = 64 \times \text{body load (mg)} = \text{Fab Fragment Dose (mg)}$$

Calculation Error: The Acute Overdose. If the serum digoxin concentration is used to calculate the number of vials required in an acute digoxin overdose, the calculations may lead to an inaccurate number of vials of Fab needed. The serum digoxin concentration assumed in calculations based on total body load of digitalis is a steady-state value. An acutely intoxicated patient is not in a steady state for at least 6 hours. In severe digoxin poisoning, losses of digoxin through vomiting, gastric lavage, activated charcoal, or metabolism may result in less than 60% of an acute, ingested dose entering the systemic circulation. Heath maintains that 10 vials (400 mg) is adequate for 75% of patients. Even less may be needed as full stoichiometric equivalence may not be necessary to produce a satisfactory clinical response in the early (distribution) phase of an acute poisoning. In the first hours the volume of distribution may be smaller. An initial dose of 6 to 8 mg/kg of Fab fragments, repeated as required in 30 to 60 minutes, may be sufficient. Further work is required to confirm these observations.[34]

Supportive Measures

Chronic Toxicity. Magnesium should be considered as a temporizing antiarrhythmic agent until digoxin Fab fragments become available. Magnesium possesses significant antiarrhythmic properties in the setting of digoxin toxicity. Intravenous magnesium may be a lifesaving adjunct in the treatment of digoxin-induced ventricular fibrillation.[35,36]

Treatment of patients with signs or symptoms of digitoxin toxicity should be guided by the specific toxic effect. It may include insertion of a pacemaker or administration of potassium, antiarrhythmic agents, Fab fragments, or possibly multiple oral doses of charcoal. Clinically stable patients receiving digoxin who have elevated serum digoxin concentrations but are without signs or symptoms of digoxin toxicity appear to be at low risk of developing serious digoxin toxicity and may not require treatment beyond the discontinuation of digoxin therapy.[37]

Adults With Digoxin Toxicity

1. Give 2 g magnesium sulfate (10%) intravenously over 2 minutes.
2. Follow with 1 to 2 g/h.
3. Check serum magnesium level every 2 hours. Maintain magnesium level of 4 to 5 mEq/L.
4. Monitor for neuromuscular dysfunction, respiratory compromise, or both.
5. Depression of deep tendon reflexes or respiration is an indication for immediately stopping a magnesium sulfate infusion and for repeating the serum magnesium.[38]
6. Administer Fab Fragments as outlined above.

Ventricular Arrhythmias. Taboulet and colleagues suggest that ventricular pacing (difficult to handle, may increase risk of fatal outcome) should be reserved for those patients not responding to Fab therapy.[10,39,40] Ventricular arrhythmias induced by digitalis toxicity are very sensitive to magnesium therapy. Magnesium can suppress ventricular arrhythmia in patients with both normal magnesium levels and hypomagnesemia[36] and can be used where there is likely to be a delay in the availability of digoxin antibodies.[41]

Hyperkalemia. Hyperkalemia (> 6 mEq/L) inhibits the Na^+, K^+-ATPase pump in acute digoxin intoxication. The presence of hyperkalemia indicates up to 50% mortality without Fab therapy. Potassium blood levels greater than 7 mEq/L are associated with electrocardiographic changes of peaked T waves, depressed ST segment, wide QRS, and prolonged PR interval.

Treatment of hyperkalemia in digitalis overdose (> 6 mEq/L) should include the following:

1. Give intravenous 5 to 10% glucose 0.5 g/kg, sodium bicarbonate 1 mEq/kg, and intravenous insulin 0.1 g/kg for each 200 to 400 mg/kg glucose.
2. Avoid calcium.
3. Administer a sodium polystyrene sulfonate retention enema 0.5 g/kg orally (25% on sorbitol or Kayexalate) in severe cases. Kayexalate enema acts in 30 minutes and may be repeated every 4 hours if the previous doses have not been evacuated.
4. Hemodialysis is the treatment of choice for severe or refractory hyperkalemia or in the presence of renal failure.

If Fab fragments and glucose/insulin/bicarbonate are administered simultaneously, severe hypokalemia may result.[40,42,43]

Admission

1. Admit acute ingestions if the digoxin serum level is expected to exceed 2 ng/mL or if conduction disturbances or arrhythmias occur within 6 hours of observation.
2. Chronic toxicity usually requires hospitalization to monitor arrhythmias and correct predisposing factors.
3. Digoxin-specific Fab fragments interfere with clinical immunoassays for digitalis, and therefore such serum tests are unreliable for at least 5 to 7 days postadministration.
4. Stable patients receiving digoxin who have elevated serum digoxin concentrations appear to be at a lower risk of developing serum digoxin toxicity and do not generally require treatment beyond discontinuation of digoxin therapy.[44]

SCILLIROSIDE AND PROSCILLARIDIN

Scilliroside and proscillaridin are glycosides derived from red squill. Scilliroside is a convulsant and cardiotoxic rodenticide. Proscillaridin (Talusin, Scillacriot) is used in the treatment of cardiac failure in subjects with impaired renal function. In vitro data suggest a potential usefulness for specific antidigoxin Fab fragments in the treatment of scilliroside and proscillaridin poisoning.[45]

DIGOXIN-LIKE IMMUNOREACTIVE SUBSTANCE (DLIS)

Investigators[46–48] have elucidated a substance present in body fluids (blood,[49] saliva,[50] urine,[51] cerebrospinal fluid,[52] bile acids,[53] amniotic fluid,[54] follicular fluid[55]) that produces false-positive interferences with digoxin immunoassays, and may be present when there is no history of ingestion of digoxin—digoxin-like immunoreactive substance (DLIS).[49] DLIS has also been found in the hypothalamus, hypophysis, placenta, and adrenal glands.[48]

Digoxin-like immunoreactive substance has also been referred to as endoxin, digoxin-like substance, cardiodigin, endocardin, endalin, ouabain-like substance,[56] digoxin-like immunoreactive factor, endogenous digoxin-like immunoreactivity, and endogenous digitalis-like substance. The name digoxin-like immunoreactive substance has also been proposed.[57]

Mechanism of Action

Cardiac glycosides act as specific inhibitors of Na^+, K^+-ATPase (the sodium pump) to induce their therapeutic and toxic effects. This concept suggests a receptor site for which an endogenous ligand could exist.[48] Inhibition of Na^+ transport may lead to an increase in intracellular Ca^{2+} and to vascular contraction and a rise in blood pressure. DLIS has been associated with increased blood volume states, increases in cardiac output, congestive heart failure, exercise, and stress.

Identity of DLIS

A number of candidates for endogenous digitalis-like substances have been proposed.[48,52,58–60] None has yet been isolated and chemically characterized in clinical states associated with obvious DLIS presence.

Laboratory

Blood Levels

No standard yet exists to ease comparative measurements between laboratories, each of which has its own reference values. Values in normotensive pregnancies for total DLIS average approximately 900 pg/mL, and levels up to 1143 pg/mL have been measured in patients pregnant with twins.[61–63] Therapeutic values of digoxin may overlap with levels of DLIS. The importance of DLIS and its role in digoxin therapy and therapeutic monitoring is, therefore, of interest to clinicians. Nonpregnant patients have had levels of 100 pg/mL and below.[50] Neonates exhibit levels up to 1500 pg/mL,[52] decreasing to 0 on day 45.[64]

Free and Total DLIS Levels

Total DLIS levels remain stable throughout pregnancy at 700 to 800 pg/mL. Free DLIS rises from 30 to 240 pg/mL in the third trimester and falls to zero within 24 hours of delivery.[65,66]

Assay Methods: Cross-Reactivity

Digoxin assays are extensively used for therapeutic drug monitoring. Radioimmunoassay (RIA) and non-RIA methods are employed. A study of five RIA and five non-RIA methods indicated that the Coat-a-Count RIA (Diagnostic Products Corporation) and the EMIT column method (Syva) run on the Cobas MIRA (Roche) showed the least interference, and the DELFIA Method (LKB/Wallace) appeared to show the greatest cross-reactivity with DLIS.[49] A recently developed RIA method for digoxin uses a monoclonal antibody that recognizes digoxin and exhibits no reactivity with DLIS. It appears to be a rapid, sensitive, specific, and reproducible assay method for digoxin and its metabolites.[60]

Drug Interference

Drug ingestions may also interfere with the digoxin assay. Digitoxin, and possibly steroids such as prednisone, progesterone, testosterone, spironolactone, and its metabolites, and digoxin immune Fab (ovine) may cause false-positive results.[67,68]

Clinical Presentation

Digoxin-like immunoreactive substance has been observed in patients with renal insufficiency,[69] liver dysfunction,[70,71] congestive heart failure,[72,73] hypertension, aneurysmal subarachnoid hemorrhage, acromegaly,[74] and in pregnant women, neonates, and children.[75] Serum levels of DLIS rise during pregnancy, then quickly fall off in the mother after delivery. Neonates have high levels but these fall to zero by the end of the second month of life.

Therapeutic Use

A 31-year-old patient with severe toxemia at 25½ weeks gestation, unresponsive to nifedipine and hydralazine and not receiving digoxin had a serum digoxin (DLIS) level of 300 pg/mL. Digoxin immune Fab (ovine) (Digibind) 10 mg was administered intravenously. Within 30 minutes there was a significant decline in blood pressure.[76,77] Further work is needed to clarify the possible role of digoxin and immune Fab in this and similar conditions.

Toad Poisoning and DLIS

A ouabain-like compound (resibufogenin) found in the skin of the toad, *Bufo viridis,* inhibits Na^+, K^+-ATPase activity and has the characteristics of a cardiac glycoside.[78] High concentrations of digitalis-like activity are present and circulate normally in the plasma of the toad, *Bufo marinus.*[79] A 31-year-old man consumed a bowl of toad soup (*Bufo melanosticus* Schneider) and within 30 minutes experienced nausea, vomiting, dizziness, blurred vision, perioral numbness, unconsciousness, and pulmonary arrest. He was resuscitated. An electrocardiogram indicated a high-grade atrioventricular block; the QRS was normal. The serum digoxin level (no history of digoxin ingestion) was 2.1 ng/mL (probably a DLIS). The patient's symptoms were similar to those of severe digitalis intoxication.[80]

A Chinese medicine known as Kyushin cross-reacts with digoxin in immunoassays. A constituent of Kyushin is chansu, the dried venom of the Chinese toad, *Bufo bufo gargarizans* Cantor. Bufalin and cinobufaginal, the main components of chansu, have chemical structures similar to that of digoxin.[69] Herbal teas may contain digoxin-like factors.[81]

DIGOTOXIN-LIKE IMMUNOREACTIVE SUBSTANCE (DTLIS)

Digotoxin-like immunoreactive substance does not increase in value in patients with renal insufficiency. The normal therapeutic serum range for digitoxin is approximately 10 to 35 ng/mL. The highest level of DTLIS found by a sensitive assay was 3.05 ng/mL. There is therefore little clinical overlap and probably little chemical or laboratory significance for this substance.[57]

REFERENCES—DIGITALIS

1. Lalonde RL, Deshpande R, Hamilton PP, et al. Acceleration of digoxin clearance by activated charcoal. Clin Pharmacol Ther 1985;37:367–371.
2. Caldwell JH, Clin CT. Biliary excretion of digoxin in man. Clin Pharmacol Ther 1976;19:410–415.
3. Kuhlmann J. Effects of verapamil, diltiazem and nifedipine on plasma levels and renal excretion of digitoxin. Clin Pharmacol Ther 1985;38:667–673.
4. Sherman JL, Locke RV. Transplacental neonatal digitalis intoxication. Am J Cardiol 1960;6:834–837.
5. Morton MR, Cooper JW. Erythromycin-induced digoxin toxicity. DICP Ann Pharmacother 1989;23:668–670.
6. Maxwell DL, Gilmour-White SK, Hall MR. Digoxin toxicity due to interaction of digoxin with erythromycin. Br Med J 1989; 298:572.
7. Linday L, Dobkin JF, Wang TC, et al. Digoxin inactivation by the gut flora in infancy and childhood. Pediatrics 1987;79: 544–548.
8. Whang R, Oei TO, Watanabe A. Frequency of hypomagnesemia in hospitalized patients receiving digitalis. Arch Intern Med 1985;145:655–656.
9. Sonnenblick M. Correlation between manifestations of digoxin toxicity and serum calcium, magnesium and potassium concentrations and arterial pH. Br Med J 1983;286: 1089–1091.
10. Taboulet P, Baud FJ, Bismuth C. Clinical features and management of digitalis poison: Rationale for immunotherapy. Clin Toxicol 1993;31:247–260.
11. Moorman JR, Pritchett ELC. The arrhythmias of digitalis intoxication. Arch Intern Med 1985;145:1289–1291.
12. Springer M, Olson KR, Feaster W. Acute massive digoxin overdose: Survival without use of digitalis-specific antibodies. Am J Emerg Med 1986;4:364–368.
13. Ukhelyi MR, Cummings DM, Green P, et al. Effect of digoxin Fab antibodies on five digoxin immunoassays. Ther Drug Monit 1990;12:288–292.
14. Ingelfinger JA, Goldman P. The serum digitalis concentration: Does it diagnose digitalis toxicity? N Engl J Med 1976;294: 867-870.
15. Lasagna L. How useful are serum digitalis measurements? N Engl J Med 1976;294:898–899.
16. Urtizberea M, Rochdi M, Sabourand A, et al. Relationship between red blood cell potassium and plasma digitoxin concentrations in intoxicated patients. Pharmacol Toxicol 1991; 68:237–242.
17. Wood WG, Farber P, Kurowski V. A case of divergent digitoxin values under treatment of a patient with acute digitoxin overdose with digitalis antibody fragments. Klin Wochenschr 1990;68:324–327.
18. Hess T, Zeugin T, Wess M. Swizidale digitalis intoxikation: Uberlegnungen zur behandlungs strategie mit antikorpern. Schweiz Med Wochenschr 1989;199:1466–1469.
19. Urtizberea M, Sabourand A, Terrien N, Schermann M. Reversal of advanced digitoxin poisoning in rabbits by monoclonal anti-digitoxin Fab fragment. In: *Abstracts of Vth International Congress of Toxicology, Brighton, England, July 16, 1989.* London: Taylor & Francis, 1989.
20. Dick M, Curwin J, Tepper D. Digitalis intoxication recognition and management. J Clin Pharmacol 1991;31:444–447.
21. Henderson RP, Solomon CP. Use of cholestyramine in the treatment of digoxin intoxication. Arch Intern Med 1988;148: 745–746.
22. Neuvonen PJ, Kivisti KT. Activated charcoal should replace the resins in the treatment of digoxin intoxication. Arch Intern Med 1989;149:2603–2604.
23. Neuvonen PJ, Kivisto K, Hirvisalo EL. Effects of resins and activated charcoal on the absorption of digoxin, carbamazepine and furosemide. Br J Clin Pharmacol 1988;25:229–233.
24. Woolf AD, Wenger T, Smith TW, Lovejoy FH Jr. The use of digoxin-specific Fab fragments for severe digitalis intoxication in children. N Engl J Med 1992;326:1734–1744.
25. Woolf AD, Wenger T, Smith TW, Lovejoy FH Jr. Results of multicenter studies of digoxin specific antibody fragments in managing digitalis intoxication in the pediatric population. Am J Emerg Med 1991;9(suppl. 1):16–20.
26. Varriole P, Mossari A. Rapid reversal of digitalis delirium using digoxin immune Fab therapy. Clin Cardiol 1995;18: 351–352.
27. Scumaik GM. Oleander poisoning: Treatment with digoxin-specific Fab antibody fragment. Ann Emerg Med 1988; 17:732–735.
28. Clark RF, Selden BS, Curry SC. Digoxin-specific Fab fragments in treatment of oleander toxicity in the canine model. Ann Emerg Med 1991;20:1073–1077.
29. Woolf AD. Digoxin specific Fab antibody fragments. Clin Toxicol Rev 1991;13(10):1–2.
30. Kurowski V, Iven H, Djonlagic H. Treatment of a patient with severe digitoxin intoxication by Fab fragments of antidigitalis antibodies. Intensive Care Med 1992;18:439–442.
31. Taboulet P, Baud FJ, Bismuth C. Clinical features and management of digitalis poisoning: Rationale for immunotherapy. In: *Proceedings, European Association of Poison Control Centers Meeting, Lyon, France, May 22, 1991.*
32. Zilker T, Bihlmayr J, Felgenhauer N, v. Clarmann M. Comparison of cases of digitalis intoxications before and after introduction of anti digoxin FAB fragments (ADFABF) into therapy. *In: Proceedings, European Association of Poison Centres Meeting, Lyon, France, May 22, 1991.*
33. Martiny SS, Phelps SJ, Massey KC. Treatment of severe digitalis intoxication with digoxin-specific antibody fragments: A clinical review. Crit Care Med 1988;16:629–635.
34. Heath AJ. How do we dose Fab antibody fragments in digitalis intoxication? In: *Proceedings, European Association of Poison Centres Meeting, Lyon, France, May 22, 1991.*
35. Green SM, Nefbl J. Antiarrhythmic efficacy of magnesium in the setting of life-threatening digoxin toxicity. Am Emerg Med 1989;7:374–378.
36. Tzivoni D, Keren D. Suppression of ventricular arrhythmia by magnesium. Am J Cardiol 1990;65:1397–1399.
37. Park GD, Spector R, Goldberg MJ, Feldman RD. Digoxin toxicity in patients with high serum digoxin concentrations. Am J Med Sci 1987;294:423–428.
38. Reisdorff EJ, Clark MR, Walters BL. Acute digitalis poisoning: The role of intravenous magnesium sulfate. Ann Emerg Med 1986;4:463.
39. Taboulet P, Baud FJ, Bismuth C, Vicaut E. Acute digitalis intoxication: Is pacing still appropriate? Clin Toxicol 1993;31: 261–273.
40. Woolf A. Revising the management of digitalis poisoning. Clin Toxicol 1993;31:275–276. Editorial.

41. Kinlay S, Buckley NA. Magnesium sulfate in the treatment of ventricular arrhythmias due to digoxin toxicity. Clin Toxicol 1995;33:55–59.
42. Johnston LN. Digoxin toxicity presenting with visual disturbance and trigeminal neuralgia. Neurology 1990;40: 1469–1470.
43. Sharff JA, Bayer MJ. Acute and chronic digitalis toxicity: Presentation and treatment. Ann Emerg Med 1982;11:327–330.
44. Park GD, Spector R, Goldberg MJ, Feldman RD. Digoxin toxicity in patients with high serum digoxin concentrations. Am J Med Sci 1987;294:423–428.
45. Sabourand A, Urtizberrea M, Cano N, et al. Specific anti-digoxin Fab fragments: An available antidote for proscillaridin and scilliroside poisoning. Hum Exp Toxicol 1990;9:191–193.
46. Gruber KA, Whitaker JM, Buckalew VM Jr. Endogenous digitalis-like substance in plasma of volume-expanded dogs. Nature 1980;28:743–745.
47. Graves SW, Brown B, Valdes R Jr. An endogenous digoxin-like substance in patients with renal impairment. Ann Intern Med 1983;99:604–608.
48. Schoner W. Endogenous digitalis-like factors. Trends Pharmacol Sci 1991;12:209–211.
49. Morris RG, Frewin DB, Saccoia NC, et al. Interference from digoxin-like immunoreactive substances in commercial digoxin kit assay methods. Eur J Clin Pharmacol 1990;39: 359–363.
50. Jakobi P, Krivoy N, Schwartz K, et al. Digoxin-like immunoreactivity in saliva and plasma of pregnant women. Clin Chem 1991;37:135–136.
51. Siegfried BA, Valdes R Jr. Excretion of endogenous digoxin-like immunoreactive factors in human urine is a function of urine flow rate. Clin Chem 1988;34:960–964.
52. Krivoy N, Lalkin A, Jakobi P. Digoxin-like immunoreactivity detected in cerebrospinal fluid of humans with fever. Clin Chem 1990;36:703–704.
53. Toseland PA, Oldfield PR, Murphy GM, Lawson AM. Tentative identification of a digoxin-like immunoreactive substance. Ther Drug Monit 1988;10:168–171.
54. Graves SW, Valdes R, Brown BA, et al. Endogenous-like immunoreactive substance in human pregnancies. J Clin Endocrinol Metab 1984;58:748–751.
55. Jakobi P, Krivoy N, Eibschitz I, et al. Digoxin-like immunoreactive factors(s) in human gonadotropin stimulated follicular fluid. J Clin Endocrinol Metab 1989;69:209–211.
56. Valdes R. Endogenous digoxin-like immunoreactive factors impact on digoxin measurements and potential physiological implications. Clin Chem 1985;31:1525–1532.
57. Mueller BA, Bussey HI, Casto DT, et al. Lack of endogenous crossreactivity with three radioimmunoassays in adults with renal insufficiency. Clin Pharm 1988;7:825–828.
58. Virge E, Ekman R. Partial characterization of endogenous digoxin-like substance in human urine. Ther Drug Monit 1988;10:8–15.
59. Goto A, Yamada K, Ishi M, Sugimoto T. Release of endogenous digitalis-like factor with sodium loading. N Engl J Med 1989;320:124–125.
60. Wahyono D, Piechaczyk M, Scherrmann JM, et al. Highly specific radioimmunoassay for digoxin using a monoclonal antibody selected for lack of interference by digoxin-like immunoreactive substances in cord blood sera. Ther Drug Monit 1991;13:113–119.
61. Krivoy N, Jakobi P, Paldi E, Alroy G. Total digoxin-like immunoreactive factor(s) in healthy population, uncomplicated term pregnancies and neonates. J Endocrinol Invest 1990; 13:9–12.
62. Jakobi P, Krivoy N, Weissman A, Paldi E. Digoxin-like immunoreactive factor in twin and pregnancy-associated hypertensive pregnancies. Obstet Gynecol 1989;74:29–33.
63. Morris RG, Frewin DB, Sarcoia NC, et al. Digoxin-like immunoreactive substance levels in cord blood obtained from twins. Eur J Clin Pharmacol 1991;40:199–200.
64. Wolach B, Carmi D, Shilo L, et al. Endogenous digoxin-like factor in neonates: Effect of age and relation to serum bilirubin levels. Acta Paediatr Scand 1989;78:364–368.
65. Jakobi P, Lewit N, Kol S, Krivoy N. Protein bound and free digoxin-like immunoreactive factor in normal pregnancy: A longitudinal study. *In: Proceedings, Society of Perinatal Obstetricians, Tenth Annual Meeting, Houston, Texas, Jan. 23, 1990.*
66. Jakobi P, Kol S, Weissman A, Krivoy N. Peripartum changes in free and protein bound digoxin-like immunoreactive factor. In: *Proceedings, Society of Perinatal Obstetricians, Tenth Annual Meeting, Houston, Texas, Jan. 23, 1990.*
67. Yosselson-Superstine S. Drug interferences with plasma assays in therapeutic monitoring. Clin Pharmacokinet 1984; 9:67–87.
68. Pleasants RA, Williams DM, Porter RS, Gadsden RH Sr. Reassessment of cross-reactivity of spironolactone metabolites with four digoxin immunoassays. Ther Drug Monit 1989; 11:200–204.
69. Fushimi R, Tachi J, Amino N, Miyai K. Chinese medicine interfering with digoxin immunoassays. Lancet 1989;1:339.
70. Kim JQ, Lee DH, Kim SI. The effect of digoxin-like immunoreactive substance on therapeutic drug monitoring of digoxin in patients with liver diseases. Clin Chem 1990;36:1032.
71. Gervais A, Nanji AA, Greenway DC, McLean W. Digoxin-like immunoreactive substance (DLIS) in liver disease: Comparison of clinical and laboratory parameters in patients with and without DLIS. Drug Intell Clin Pharm 1987;21:450–452.
72. Shilo L, Adawi A, Solomon G, Shenkman L. Endogenous digoxin-like immunoreactivity in congestive heart failure. Br Med J 1987;295:415–416.
73. Dasgupta A, Saldana S, Heimann P. Monitoring free digoxin instead of total digoxin in patients with congestive heart failure and high concentrations of digoxin-like immunoreactive substances. Clin Chem 1990;36:2121–2123.
74. Ng LL, Hockaday TDR. Endogenous digitalis-like factors in acromegaly. N Engl J Med 1987;317:572–573.
75. Stone J, Bentur Y, Zalstein E, et al. Effect of endogenous digoxin-like substances on the interpretation of high concentrations of digoxin in children. J Pediatr 1990;117:321–325.
76. Goodlin RC. Antidigoxin antibodies in eclampsia. N Engl J Med 1988;318:518–519.
77. Goodlin RC, Makowski EL. Fetal endotoxins and complications of pregnancy. West J Med 1988;148:590–592.
78. Lichtstein D, Kachalsky S, Deutsch J. Identification of a ouabain-like compound in toad skin and plasma as a bufodienolide derivative. Life Sci 1986;38:1261–1270.
79. Flier JS, Maratos-Flier E, Pallotta JA, McIsaac D. Endogenous digitalis-like activity in the plasma of the toad *Bufo marinus*. Nature 1979;279:341–343.
80. Chern M-S, Ray C-Y, Wu D. Biologic intoxication due to digitalis-like substance after ingestion of cooked toad soup. Am J Cardiol 1991;67:443–444.
81. Longerich L, Johnson E, Gault MH. Digoxin-like factors in herbal teas. Clin Invest Med 1993;16:210–218.

PAPAVERINE

Papaverine (6,2-dimethoxy-1-veratrylisoquineoline hydrochloride), found in crude opium, is a peripheral vasodilator and a direct smooth muscle relaxant. Although it has been used for angina pectoris and cerebral ischemia, its use for treatment of these conditions is considered obsolete. Presently it appears useful when injected intracavernously (in doses of 10–30 mg) into the penis for patients with problems of sexual impotency.[1–4]

Toxicokinetics

Papaverine has an elimination half-life of 0.5 to 2 hours. After intramuscular injection, the peak serum level occurs after 1 to 2 hours. After intravenous administration a dose of 1 mg/kg produces a plasma concentration of 1 mg/L in 5 minutes. The drug is metabolized by the liver and is excreted mainly in the urine, primarily as metabolites. Less than 1% of the dose is excreted unchanged. After intravenous use the volume of distribution is 0.9 to 1.5 L/kg. The drug is highly protein bound at 87%.

Laboratory

A high-performance liquid chromatography method is specific and has good reproducibility with a sensitivity of 1 μg/L.[9–11]

Clinical Presentation

Complications of intracavernous therapy include prolonged erection, thickening at injection site, bleeding at injection site, pain at injection site, diaphoresis, and urethral bleeding.[5] Oral administration of relatively large doses of papaverine has been shown to be associated with minimal side effects, although headache, nausea, and vomiting can occur. Hepatotoxicity and cardiac arrhythmias have been reported after intravenous use.[6] A 61-year-old woman developed severe lactic acidosis after ingesting about 15 g of papaverine.[6] This was associated with intense respiratory alkalosis, elevated plasma pyruvate, mild hyperglycemia, and hypokalemia. A 21-year-old man received 80 mg papaverine intramuscularly. Within 2 hours he became dizzy and weak and lost consciousness (Glasgow coma scale 8–10). He awoke 3 hours later.[7]

Large doses of papaverine can depress the atrioventricular node and intraventricular conduction, produce serious arrhythmias, and increase the rate and depth of respiration. Fatalities have followed intravenous use.[7] Polymorphous ventricular tachycardia with prolongation of the QT_c interval has followed infusion of 6 to 10 mg into the coronary arteries.[8]

Treatment

Treatment of papaverine overdose is supportive and symptomatic.

REFERENCES—PAPAVERINE

1. Mooradian AD, Morly JE, Kaiser FE, et al. Biweekly intracavernous administration of papaverine for erectile dysfunction. West J Med 1989;151:515–517.
2. Al-Juburi AZ, O'Donnell DD. Follow-up outcome of intracavernous papaverine. J Ark Med Soc 1990;86:383–385.
3. Vasoactive intracavernous pharmacotherapy for impotence: Papaverine and phentolamine: Diagnostic and therapeutic technology assessment. JAMA 1990;264:752–754.
4. Fried FA. The use of vasoactive agents in the treatment of erectile impotence. NC Med J 1990;51:295–296.
5. Corriere JN Jr, Fishman IJ, Benson GS, Carlton CE Jr: Development of fibrotic penile lesions secondary to the intracorporeal injection of vasoactive agents. J Urol 1988;140: 615–617.
6. Vaziri ND, Stokes J, Treadwell TR. Lactic acidosis, a complication of papaverine overdose. Clin Toxicol 1981;18:417–423.
7. Ilan Y, Gemer O. Papaverine-induced coma. Eur J Clin Pharmacol 1988;33:651.
8. Talman CL, Winniford MD, Rasser JD, et al. Polymorphous ventricular tachycardia: a side effect of intracoronary papaverine. J Am Coll Cardiol 1990;15:275–278.
9. Belpaire FM, Rossul MT, Gogaert MG. Pharmacokinetics of papaverine IV: Urinary elimination of papaverine metabolites in man. Xenobiotica 1978;8:297–300.
10. Kramer WG, Romagnoli A. Papaverine disposition in cardiac surgery patients. Eur J Clin Pharmacol 1984;27:127–130.
11. Garrett ER, Roseboom H, Green JR, Schuermann W. Pharmacokinetics of papaverine hydrochloride and the biopharmaceutics of its oral dosage forms. Int J Clin Pharmacol Biopharm 1978;16:192–208.

Chapter 33

Antihypertensive Drugs

INTRODUCTION

Dosages and mechanisms of action of antihypertensive drugs are outlined in Table 33–1. Drug interactions and adverse effects of antihypertensive drugs are summarized in Table 33–2 and 33–3, respectively.[1]

ANGIOTENSIN-CONVERTING ENZYME INHIBITORS

New Angiotensin-Converting Enzyme Inhibitors

In the past few years a number of new angiotensin-converting enzyme (ACE) inhibitors have been investigated (Table 33–4).[2–14]

Toxicokinetics

The Toxicokinetics of the new ACE inhibitors are presented in Table 33–5.[2–14]

Clinical Presentation

The principal adverse effect of ACE inhibitor overdose is hypotension, although hyperkalemia and renal failure may occur. Therefore, following gut decontamination, treatment is primarily supportive to maintain an adequate blood pressure.

Defects in skull ossification, pulmonary hypoplasia, oligohydramnios, neonatal hypertension, renal failure, anuria, and fetal death have been reported after fetal exposure during pregnancy to ACE inhibitors.[15,16] Fatal acute enterocolitis in a neonate followed in utero exposure to captopril throughout pregnancy.[17] Congenital renal dysgenesis may have resulted from the ingestion of captopril throughout pregnancy.[18]

Treatment

Reported treatments have included gut decontamination, intravenous fluids, vasopressors, and naloxone. Naloxone

Table 33–1
Antihypertensive Drugs*

Drug	Usual Dosage Range (Total mg/d)†	Frequency (times/d)	Mechanisms	Comments
Initial Antihypertensive Agents				
Diuretics				For thiazide and loop diuretics, lower doses and dietary counseling should be used to avoid metabolic changes
Thiazides and related agents			Decreased plasma volume and decreased extracellular fluid volume; decreased cardiac output initially, followed by decreased total peripheral resistance with normalization of cardiac output; long-term effects include slight decrease in extracellular fluid volume	More effective antihypertensive than loop diuretics except in patients with serum creatinine ≥221 μmol/L (2.5 mg/dL) Hydrochlorothiazide or chlorthalidone is generally preferred; used in most clinical trials
Bendroflumethiazide	2.5–5	1		
Benzthiazide	12.5–50	1		
Chlorothiazide	125–500	2		
Chlorthalidone	12.5–50	1		
Cyclothiazide	1.0–2	1		
Hydrochlorothiazide	12.5–50	1		
Hydroflumethiazide	12.5–50	1		
Indapamide	2.5–5	1		
Methyclothiazide	2.5–5	1		
Metolazone	0.5–5	1		
Polythiazide	1.0–4	1		
Quinethazone	25.0–100	1		
Trichlormethiazide	1.0–4	1		
Loop diuretics			See Thiazides	Higher doses of loop diuretics may be needed for patients with renal impairment or congestive heart failure.
Bumetanide	0.5–5	2		
Ethacrynic acid	25.0–100	2		Ethacrynic acid is only alternative for patients with allergy to thiazide and sulfur-containing diuretics
Furosemide	20.0–320	2		
Potassium-sparing			Increased potassium resorption	Weak diuretics
Amiloride	5–10	1 or 2		Used mainly in combination with other diuretics to avoid or reverse hypokalemia from other diuretics
Spironolactone	25–100	2 or 3	Aldosterone antagonist	Avoid when serum creatinine ≥221 μmol/L (2.5 mg/dL)
Triamterene	50–150	1 or 2		May cause hyperkalemia, and this may be exaggerated when combined with ACE inhibitors or potassium supplements
Adrenergic inhibitors				
Beta-blockers			Decreased cardiac output and increased total peripheral resistance; decreased plasma renin activity; atenolol, betaxolol, bisoprolol, and metoprolol are cardioselective	Selective agents will also inhibit β_2 receptors in higher doses, eg, all may aggravate asthma
Atenolol	25–100‡	1		
Betaxolol	5–40	1		
Bisoprolol	5–20	1		
Metoprolol	50–200	1 or 2		
Metoprolol (extended release)	50–200	1		
Nadolol	20–240‡	1		
Propranolol	40–240	2		
Propranolol (long acting)	60–240	1		
Timolol	20–40	2		
Beta blockers with ISA				
Acebutolol	200–1200‡	2	Acebutolol is cardioselective	No clear advantage for agents with ISA except in those with bradycardia who must receive a beta blocker; they produce fewer or no metabolic side effects
Carteolol	2.5–10‡	1		
Penbutolol	20–80‡	1		
Pindolol	10–60‡	2		
Alpha/beta blocker				
Labetalol	200–1200	2	Same as beta blockers, plus α_1 blockade	Possibly more effective in blacks than other beta blockers May cause postural effects; titration should be based on standing blood pressure
Alpha blockers			Block postsynaptic α_1 receptors and cause vasodilation	All may cause postural effects; titration should be based on standing blood pressure
Doxazosin	1.0–16	1		
Prazosin	1.0–20	2 or 3		
Terazosin	1.0–20	1		

Table 33–1 *(Continued)*

Drug	Usual Dosage Range (Total mg/d)†	Frequency (times/d)	Mechanisms	Comments
ACE inhibitors				
Benazepril	10.0–40‡	1 or 2	Block formation of angiotensin II, promoting vasodilation and decreased aldosterone; also increased bradykinin and vasodilatory prostaglandins	Diuretic doses should be reduced or discontinued before starting ACE inhibitors whenever possible to prevent excessive hypotension Reduce dose of those drugs marked with double dagger in patients with serum creatinine ≥221 μmol/L (2.5 mg/dL) May cause hyperkalemia in patients with renal impairment or in those receiving potassium-sparing agents Can cause acute renal failure in patients with severe bilateral renal artery stenosis or severe stenosis in artery to solitary kidney
Captopril	12.5–150‡	2		
Cilazapril	2.5–5.0	1 or 2		
Enalapril	2.5–40‡	1 or 2		
Fosinopril	10.0–40	1 or 2		
Lisinopril	5.0–40‡	1 or 2		
Perinodopril	1.0–16‡	1 or 2		
Quinapril	5.0–80‡	1 or 2		
Ramipril	1.25–20‡	1 or 2		
Spirapril	12.5–50	1 or 2		
Calcium antagonists			Block inward movement of calcium ion across cell membranes and cause smooth muscle relaxation	
Diltiazem	90–360	3		These agents also block slow channels in heart and may reduce sinus rate and produce heart block
Diltiazem (sustained release)	120–360	2		
Diltiazem (extended release)	180–360	1		
Verapamil	80–480	2		
Verapamil (long acting)	120–480	1 or 2		
Dihydropyridines				Dihydropyridines are more potent peripheral vasodilators than diltiazem and verapamil and may cause more dizziness, headache, flushing, peripheral edema, and tachycardia
Amlodipine	2.5–10	1		
Felodipine	5–20	1		
Isradipine	2.5–10	2		
Nicardipine	60–120	3		
Nifedipine	30–120	2		
Nifedipine (GITS)	30–90	1		
Supplemental Antihypertensive Agents				
Centrally acting α_2 agonists				
Clonidine	0.1–1.2	2	Stimulate central α_2 receptors that inhibit efferent sympathetic activity	Clonidine patch is replaced once/wk None of these agents should be withdrawn abruptly; avoid in patients who do not adhere to treatment
Clonidine (patch)§	0.1–0.3	1 weekly		
Guanabenz	4–64	2		
Guanfacine	1–3	1		
Methyldopa	250–2000	2		
Peripheral acting adrenergic antagonists				
Guanadrel	10–75	2	Inhibits catecholamine release from neuronal storage sites	May cause serious orthostatic and exercise-induced hypotension
Guanethidine	10–100	1		
Rauwolfia alkaloids				
Rauwolfia serpentina	50–200	1	Depletion of tissue stores of catecholamines	
Reserpine	0.05‖–0.25	1		
Direct vasodilators				
Hydralazine	50–300	2–4	Direct smooth muscle vasodilation (primarily arteriolar)	Hydralazine is subject to phenotypically determined metabolism (acetylation)
Minoxidil	2.5–80	1 or 2		For both agents, should treat concomitantly with diuretic and beta blocker due to fluid retention and reflex tachycardia

ACE, angiotensin-converting enzyme; ISA, intrinsic sympathomimetic activity; GITS, gastrointestinal therapeutic system.
*In all patients, lifestyle modifications should also be advised.
†The lower dose indicated is the preferred initial dose, and the higher dose is the maximum daily dose. Most agents require 2 to 4 weeks for complete efficacy, and more frequent dosage adjustments are not advised except for severe hypertension. The dosage range may differ slightly from the recommended dosage in the *Physician's Desk Reference* or package insert.
‡Indicates drugs that are excreted by the kidney and require dosage reduction in the presence of renal impairment (serum creatinine ≥221 μmol/L [≥2.5 mg/dL]).
§Weekly patch is 1, 2, 3, equivalent to 0.1 to 0.3 mg/d.
‖A 0.1-mg dose may be given every other day to achieve this dosage.
From the Fifth Report of the Joint National Committee on Detection, Evaluation and Treatment of High Blood Pressure (JNICV). Arch Intern Med 1993;153:154–163.

Table 33–2
Selected Drug Interactions With Antihypertensive Therapy*

Diuretics
Possible situations for decreased antihypertensive effects
  Cholestyramine and colestipol decrease absorption.
  NSAIDs (including aspirin and over-the-counter ibuprofen) may antagonize diuretic effectiveness.
Possible situations for increased antihypertensive effects
  Combinations of thiazides (especially metolazone) with furosemide can produce profound diuresis, natriuresis, and kaliuresis in renal impairment.
Effects of diuretics on other drugs
  Diuretics can raise serum lithium levels and increase toxic effects by enhancing proximal tubular resorption of lithium.
  Diuretics may make it more difficult to control dyslipidemia and diabetes.

Beta Blockers
Possible situations for decreased antihypertensive effects
  NSAIDs may decrease effects of beta blockers.
  Rifampin, smoking, and phenobarbital decrease serum levels of agents metabolized primarily by liver due to enzyme induction.
Possible situations for increased antihypertensive effects
  Cimetidine may increase serum levels of beta blockers that are metabolized primarily by liver due to enzyme inhibition.
  Quinidine may increase risk of hypotension.
Effects of beta blockers on other drugs
  Combinations of diltiazem or verapamil with beta blockers may have additive sinoatrial and atrioventricular node depressant effects and may also promote negative inotropic effects on failing myocardium.
  Combinations of beta blockers and reserpine may cause marked bradycardia and syncope.
  Beta blockers may increase serum levels of theophylline, lidocaine, and chlorpromazine due to reduced hepatic clearance.
  Nonselective beta blockers prolong insulin-induced hypoglycemia and promote rebound hypertension due to unopposed alpha stimulaton; all beta blockers mask adrenergically mediated symptoms of hypoglycemia and have potential to aggravate diabetes.
  Beta blockers may make it more difficult to control dyslipidemia.
  Phenylpropanolamine (which can be obtained over the counter in cold and diet preparations), pseudoephedrine, ephedrine, and epinephrine can cause elevations in blood pressure due to unopposed alpha receptor–induced vasoconstriction.

ACE Inhibitors
Possible situations for decreased antihypertensive effects
  NSAIDs (including aspirin and over-the-counter ibuprofen) may decrease blood pressure control.
  Antacids may decrease the bioavailability of ACE inhibitors.
Possible situations for increased antihypertensive effects
  Diuretics may lead to excessive hypotensive effects (hypovolemia)
Effect of ACE inhibitors on other drugs
  Hyperkalemia may occur with potassium supplements, potassium-sparing agents, and NSAIDs.
  ACE inhibitors may increase serum lithium levels.

Calcium Antagonists
Possible situations for decreased antihypertensive effects
  Serum levels and antihypertensive effects of calcium antagonists may be diminished by these interactions: rifampin–verapamil; carbamazepine–diltiazem and verapamil; phenobarbital and phenytoin–verapamil.
Possible situations for increased antihypertensive effects
  Cimetidine may increase pharmacologic effects of all calcium antagonists due to inhibition of hepatic metabolizing enzymes resulting in increased serum levels.
Effects of calcium antagonists on other drugs
  Digoxin and carbamazepine serum levels and toxic effects may be increased by verapamil and possibly by diltiazem.
  Serum levels of prazosin, quinidine, and theophylline may be increased by verapamil.
  Serum levels of cyclosporine may be increased by diltiazem, nicardipine, and verapamil; cyclosporine dose may need to be decreased.

Alpha Blockers
Possible situations for increased antihypertensive effects
  Concomitant antihypertensive drug therapy (especially diuretics) may increase chance of postural hypotension.

Sympatholytic Agents
Possible situations for decreased antihypertensive effects
  Tricyclic antidepressants may decrease effects of centrally acting and peripheral norepinephrine depleters.
  Sympathomimetics, including over-the-counter cold and diet preparations, amphetamines, phenothiazines, and cocaine, may interfere with antihypertensive effects of guanethidine and guanadrel.
  Severity of clonidine withdrawal reaction can be increased by beta blockers.
  Monoamine oxidase inhibitors may prevent degradation and metabolism of norepinephrine released by tyramine-containing foods and may cause hypertension; they may also cause hypertensive reactions when combined with reserpine or guanethidine.
Effects of sympatholytics on other drugs
  Methyldopa may increase serum lithium levels.

NSAID, nonsteroidal antinflammatory drug; ACE, angiotensin-converting enzyme.
This table does not include all potential drug interactions with antihypertensive drugs.
From the Fifth Report of the Joint National Committee on Detection, Evaluation and Treatment of High Blood Pressure (JNICV). Arch Intern Med 1993;153:154–163.

Table 33–3
Adverse Drug Effects*

Drugs	Selected Side Effects†	Precautions and Special Considerations
Diuretics‡		
Thiazides and related diuretics	Hypokalemia, hypomagnesemia, hyponatremia, hyperuricemia, hypercalcemia, hyperglycemia, hypercholesterolemia, hypertriglyceridemia, sexual dysfunction, weakness	Except for metolazone and indapamide, ineffective in remal failure (serum creatinine ≥221 μmol/L [≥2.5 mg/dL]); hypokalemia increases digitalis toxic effect; may precipitate acute gout
Loop diuretics	Same as for thiazides except loop diuretics do not cause hypercalcemia	Effective in chronic renal failure
Potassium-sparing agents	Hyperkalemia	Danger of hyperkalemia in patients with renal failure and in patients treated with ACE inhibitors or NSAIDs
Amiloride		
Spironolactone	Gynecomastia, mastodynia, menstrual irregularities, diminished libido in males	
Triamterene		Danger of renal calculi
Adrenergic Inhibitors		
Beta blockers‡	Bronchospasm, possible aggravation of peripheral arterial insufficiency, fatigue, insomnia, exacerbation of CHF, masking of symptoms of hypoglycemia, hypertriglyceridemia, decreased high-density lipoprotein cholesterol (except for drugs with ISA), reduced exercise tolerance	Should not be used in patients with asthma, COPD, CHF with systolic dysfunction, heart block (greater than first degree), and sick sinus syndrome; use with caution in insulin-treated diabetics and patients with peripheral vascular disease; should not be discontinued abruptly in patients with ischemic heart disease
Alpha/beta blocker		
Labetalol	Bronchospasm, possible aggravation of peripheral vascular insufficiency, orthostatic hypotension	Should not be used in patients with asthma, COPD, CHF, heart block (greater than first degree), and sick sinus syndrome; use with caution in insulin-treated diabetics and patients with peripheral vascular disease
Alpha blockers	Orthostatic hypotension, syncope, weakness, palpitations, headache	Use cautiously in older patients because of orthostatic hypotension
ACE Inhibitors	Cough, rash, angioneurotic edema, hyperkalemia, dysgeusia	Hyperkalemia can develop, particularly in patients with renal insufficiency; hypotension has been observed with initiation of ACE inhibitors, especially in patients with high plasma renin activity or receiving diuretic therapy; can cause reversible, acute renal failure in patients with bilateral renal arterial stenosis or unilateral stenosis in solitary kidney and in patients with cardiac failure and with volume depletion; rarely can induce neutropenia or proteinuria; absolutely contraindicated in second and third trimesters of pregnancy
Calcium Antagonists		
Dihydropyridines Amlodipine Felodipine Isradipine Nicardipine Nifedipine	Headache, dizziness, peripheral edema, tachycardia, gingival hyperplasia	Use with caution in patients with CHF; may aggravate angina and myocardial ischemia
Diltiazem Verapamil	Headache, dizziness, peripheral edema (less common than with dihydropyridines), gingival hyperplasia, constipation (especially verapamil), atrioventricular block, bradycardia	Use with caution in patients with cardiac failure; contraindicated in patients with second- or third-degree heart block, or sick sinus syndrome
Centrally Acting α_2 Agonists		
Clonidine Guanabenz Guanfacine hydrochloride	Drowsiness, sedation, dry mouth, fatigue, orthostatic dizziness	Rebound hypertension may occur with abrupt discontinuance, particularly with previous administration of high doses or with continuation of concomitant beta-blocker therapy
Clonidine patch	Same as for clonidine, localized skin reactions to patch	
Methyldopa		May cause liver damage, fever, and Coombs-positive hemolytic anemia

(continued)

Table 33–3 *(Continued)*

Drugs	Selected Side Effects†	Precautions and Special Considerations
Peripheral-Acting Adrenergic Antagonists		
Guanadrel sulfate Guanethidine monosulfate	Diarrhea, orthostatic and exercise hypotension	Use cautiously because of orthostatic hypotension
Rauwolfia alkaloids Reserpine	Lethargy, nasal congestion, depression	Contraindicated in patients with history of mental depression or with active peptic ulcer
Direct Vasodilators	Headache, tachycardia, fluid retention	May precipitate angina pectoris in patients with coronary artery disease; generally, use with diuretic and beta blocker
Hydralazine	Positive antinuclear antibody test	Lupus syndrome may occur (rare at recommended doses)
Minoxidil	Hypertrichosis	May cause or aggravate pleural and pericardial effusions

ACE, angiotensin-converting enzyme; NSAID, nonsteroidal antiinflammatory drug; COPD, chronic obstructive pulmonary disease; ISA, intrinsic sympathomimetic activity; CHF, congestive heart failure.
*See Table 33–1 for a list of drugs.
†The listing of side effects is not all-inclusive, and clinicians are urged to refer to the package insert for a more detailed listing. Sexual dysfunction, particularly impotence in men, has been reported with the use of all antihypertensive agents. Few data are available on the effect of antihypertensive agents on sexual function in women.
‡Some of the metabolic side effects of diuretics and beta-blockers can be minimized by appropriate dietary counseling.
From the Firth Report of the Joint National Committee on Detection, Evaluation and Treatment of High Blood Pressure (JNICV). Arch Intern Med 1993;153:154–163.

Table 33–4
New Angiotensin-Converting Enzyme Inhibitors

Benazepril*
Cilazepril*
Delapril*
Enalapril*
Fosinopril*
Lisinopril†
Pentopril*
Perindopril*
Quinapril*
Ramipril†,*
Spirapril

*Prodrugs.
†Approved in United States.

has not been shown to be an effective antidote. Close monitoring of vital signs, as well as serum potassium and creatinine concentrations, must be included in the management of an ACE inhibitor overdose. A prospective study of captopril, enalapril, and lisinopril overdose in children less than 6 years of age at one regional poison center suggests home management of patients under 6 years of age who ingest less than 4 mg/kg captopril, less than 1 mg/kg enalapril, or less than 1 mg/kg lisinopril.[19]

Hypotension

Administration of intravenous colloids and/or crystalloids to expand intravascular fluid volume has been successful alone in restoring and maintaining blood pressure in several ACE inhibitor overdoses and is usually the initial choice for blood pressure support.

If volume resuscitation is unsuccessful or not tolerated, vasopressors, for example, dopamine and norepinephrine or epinephrine, may be used.

Angiotensin II Infusion

An angiotensin II infusion seems ideally suited for treating ACE inhibitor-induced hypotension. Angiotensin amide is pharmacologically and physiologically identical to naturally occurring angiotensin II, and was first approved by the Food and Drug Administration in June 1962. It is currently available by contacting CIBA–Geigy, who will ship the drug to the prescribing physician. Most patients require an infusion of angiotensin II at 3 to 10 μg/min or higher rates. Blood pressure, heart rate, and the electrocardiogram should be monitored continuously during an angiotensin II infusion. The administration of naloxone has been evaluated in the treatment of ACE inhibitor overdose, with equivocal results.[20]

Cough

A controlled study suggests that sodium cromoglycate is effective in the treatment of ACE inhibitor-induced cough.[21]

Angioedema

Treatment of patients with angioedema depends on the severity of the edema.[22] The airway must be maintained and is the initial concern. A nasopharyngeal airway might be all that is needed, depending on the site of obstruction. If the situation dictates, oral or nasal intubation with direct visualization may be necessary. The emergency physician must be prepared for surgical intervention if the edema worsens and respiratory embarrassment ensues. If the soft tissues of the neck are too edematous for safe intubation or cricothyroidotomy, fiberoptic bronchoscopic nasal intubation or retrograde intubation over a guidewire passed through the cricothyroid membrane may be attempted. Fortunately, most cases are effectively controlled by standard antiallergic drug therapy. ACE inhibitor-induced angioedema is not associated with an increase in IgE. Standard pharmacologic treat

Table 33–5
Toxicokinetics of New Angiotensin-Converting Enzyme Inhibitors

	Benazepril	Cilazepril	Delapril	Eosinopril	Lisinopril	Pentopril	Perindopril	Quinapril	Ramopril	Spirapril
Absorption (bioavailability)	ND	57–77%	ND	30%	29%	ND	19%	60%	60%	ND
Time to peak serum concentration	0.5 h 1.5 h (M)	1 h 3 h (M)	1 h 2 h (M)	2.8 h (M)	6–8 h	1.28 h 7.50 h (M)	2–6 h (M)	2 h	3 h (M)	0.65 h 1.8 h (M)
Volume of distribution	0.4 L/kg (M)	0.36 L/kg	ND	0.15 L/kg	1.6 L	0.8 L/kg 0.5 L/kg (M)	4.3 L/kg	ND	ND	ND
Half-life (elimination)	0.6 h 2.2 h (M)	24–168 h (M)	0.3 h 1.2 h (M) 1.4 h (M)	2.1 h	>30 h	ND	1.9 h (M)	2 h 2 h (M)	13–17 h (M)	ND
Protein binding	97% 95% (M)	ND	ND	97.4% (M)	ND	ND	42% 7% (M)	97%	73% 56% (M)	ND
Renal clearance	1.79 L/h (M)	14–15 L/h	ND	25.8 mL/min	6.3 L/h	12.78 L/h 15.30 L/h (M)	6.6 L/h	ND	10 mL/min 100 mL/min (M)	ND
Metabolism	L	L/R	L	L	—	L	L	L	L	ND
Urine excreted unchanged	20% (M)	ND	2.4% 21.2% (M) 23.7% (M)	ND	29%	ND	2.6%	ND	<2%	ND
Placental transfer	ND	ND	ND	ND	ND	ND	ND	ND	<1%	ND
Breast milk	Negligible (M)	ND	ND	ND	ND	ND	ND	ND	<0.25% (animal)	ND
Removed by hemodialysis	ND	ND	ND	ND	ND	ND	ND	ND	ND	ND

M, metabolite; R, renal; L, liver. ND, No data.

ment (epinephrine, antihistamines, and steroids) may not be effective. The physician should be alert to a possible rebound phenomenon and closely observe the patient.

REFERENCES—INTRODUCTION AND ANGIOTENSIN-CONVERTING ENZYME INHIBITORS

1. Fifth Report of the Joint National Committee on Detection, Evaluation and Treatment of High Blood Pressure (JNICV). Arch Intern Med 1993;153:154–163.
2. Raia JJ Jr, Barone JA, Byerly WG, Lacy CR. Angiotensin-converting enzyme inhibitors: A comparative review. DICP Ann Pharmacother 1990;24:506–525.
3. Kelly JG, O'Malley K. Clinical pharmacokinetics of the newer ACE inhibitors: A review. Clin Pharmacokinet 1990;19:177–196.
4. Kelly JG, Doyle GD, Carmody M, et al. Pharmacokinetics of lisinopril, enalapril and enalprilat in renal failure: Effects of hemodialysis. Br J Clin Pharmacol 1988;26:781–786.
5. Harrigan JR, Lees KR, Meredith PA. Age and the physiologically realistic characterization of benazeprilate pharmacokinetics. Br J Clin Pharmacol 1990;29:589P.
6. Deget F, Grogden RN. Cilazapril: A review of its pharmacodynamic and pharmacokinetic properties and therapeutic potential in cardiovascular disease. Drugs 1991;41:799–820.
7. Hvik K, Duchin KL, Kripalani KJ, et al. Pharmacokinetics of forsinopril in patients with various degrees of renal function. Clin Pharmacol Ther 1991;49:457–467.
8. Shionioiri H, Yasuda G, Ikeda A, et al. Pharmacokinetics and depressor effect of delapril in patients with essential hypertension. Clin Pharmacol Ther 1987;41:74–79.
9. Van Schaik BAM, Geyskes GG, Van der Wauw PA, et al. Pharmacokinetics of lisinopril in hypertensive patients with normal and impaired renal function. Eur J Clin Pharmacol 1988;34:61–65.
10. Lecocq B, Funck-Brentano C, Lecocq V, et al. Influence of food on the pharmacokinetics of perindopril and the time course of angiotensin-converting enzyme inhibitor in serum. Clin Pharmacol Ther 1990;47:397–402.
11. Macfadyen RJ, Lees KR, Reid JL. Perindopril: A review of its pharmacokinetics and clinical pharmacology. Drugs 1990; 39(suppl. 1):49–63.
12. Lees KR, Green ST, Reid JL. Influence of age on the pharmacokinetics and pharmacodynamics of perindopril. Clin Pharmacol Ther 1988;44:418–425.
13. Cetnarowski-Cropp AB. Quinapril: A new second-generation ACE inhibitor. DICP Ann Pharmacother 1991;25:499–504.
14. Todd PA, Benfield P. Ramipril: A review of its pharmacological properties and therapeutic efficacy in cardiovascular disorders. Drugs 1990;39:110–135.
15. Use of ACE inhibitors in pregnancy and neonate. Int Pharm J 1990;4:95.
16. Brent RL, Beckman DA. Angiotensin-converting enzyme inhibitors: An embryopathic class of drugs with unique properties: Information for clinical teratology counselors. Teratology 1991;43:543–546.
17. De Carolis MP, Muzii U, Romagnoli C, et al. Neonatal necrotizing enterocolitis (NEC) and maternal treatment with captopril. Clin Exp Hypertension 1991;Pt B10:264.
18. Knott PD, Thorpe SS, Lamont CAR. Congenital renal dysgenesis possibly due to captopril. Lancet 1989;1:451.
19. Hogue-Murray K, Horowitz R, Dart RC. Outcome of ACE inhibitor ingestion in children under the age of six years. Clin Toxicol 1995;33:475–486 (Abstract 61).
20. Trilli LE, Johnson KA. Lisinopril overdose and management with intravenous angiotensin II. Ann Pharmacother 1994;28: 1165–1168.
21. Hargreaves HR, Berson MK. Inhaled sodium cromoglycate in angiotensin-converting enzyme inhibitor cough. Lancet 1995;345:13–16.
22. Finley CJ, Silverman MA, Nunez AE. Angiotensin-converting enzyme inhibitor-induced angioedema if unrecognized. Am J Emerg Med 1992;10:550–552.

ANGIOTENSIN II TYPE 1 RECEPTOR ANTAGONISTS (LOSARTAN)

Angiotensin II has been demonstrated to be important in the pathogenesis and/or pathophysiology of several common hypertensive diseases, including essential hypertension, renal hypertension, and renovascular hypertension. Angiotensin II has also been demonstrated to be important in the pathophysiology of several common clinical syndromes, including congestive heart failure and coronary insufficiency, and in a variety of renal diseases associated with albuminuria.[1]

Losartan (Cozaar), the potassium salt of 2-*n*-butyl-4-chloro-5-hydroxymethyl-1-[(s′-(1H-tetrazol-5-yl) biphenyl-4-yl)methyl]imidazole, was the first described orally active, nonpeptide specific angiotensin II antagonist with specificity and high affinity for type 1 receptors. A maximal blood pressure response is obtained with 50 mg, given once daily, with the peak response occurring within 6 hours of dosing. Losartan is rapidly absorbed; peak plasma concentrations are achieved within 1 hour. It has a relatively short terminal half-life (1.5–2.5 hours). Oral bioavailability is approximately 33%. Losartan undergoes extensive first-pass hepatic metabolism to the predominant circulating form of the drug, a 5-carboxylic acid metabolite (EXP-3174); peak plasma concentrations of EXP-3174 are achieved within 2 to 4 hours. The metabolite EXP-3174 is more potent (15–30 times) and has a longer terminal half-life than does losartan. Losartan is a competitive antagonist. It is marketed in doses of 25, 50, and 100 mg, with a recommended starting dose of 50 mg given once daily.[1]

The most likely manifestations of overdose are hypotension and tachycardia. Bradycardia may occur from parasympathetic (vagal) stimulation. If hypotension is symptomatic, it should be treated supportively. Neither losartan nor its active metabolite is removed by hemodialysis.[2,3]

REFERENCES–ANGIOTENSIN II TYPE 1 RECEPTOR ANTAGONISTS (LOSARTAN)

1. Bauer JH, Reams GP. The angiotensin II type 1 receptor antagonists: A new class of antihypertensive drugs. Arch Intern Med 1995;155:1361–1368.
2. Product information: Losartan. Merck and Company, April 1995; J5C001 (908).
3. Hartenbaum D. Losartan potassium (COZAAR[R]). Merck and Company, personal communication, November 20, 1995.

BETA BLOCKERS IN HYPERTENSION

Beta-adrenergic receptor blocking drugs have an established position in the treatment of hypertension and coronary heart disease[1,2] (Table 33–6). More than 30 different beta antagonists (beta blockers) are now commercially available. First-generation nonselective beta blockers such as propranolol, sotalol, and labetalol are antagonists at human cardiac β_1 and β_2 adrenoceptors. These drugs block β_2 adrenoceptors in bronchial smooth muscle, predisposing to bronchoconstriction, and they also block β_2 adrenoceptors in the liver and muscle, inhibiting carbohydrate and lipid metabolism; most beta blockers increase total peripheral resistance

Table 33–6
Beta Blockers for Hypertension

Drug	Activity	Maintenance Dose
Acebutolol (Sectral)	β_1 selective, intrinsic sympathomimetic	400 mg once/d
Atenolol (Tenormin)	β_1 selective	50 mg once/d
Betaxolol (Kerlone)	β_1 selective	10 mg once/d
Bopindolol	Nonselective, intrinsic sympathomimetic	1–2 mg/d
Carteolol (Cartol)	Nonselective, intrinsic sympathomimetic	2.5 mg once/d
Celiprolol	β_1 selective, intrinsic sympathomimetic	200–300 mg once/d
Dilevalol	Nonselective, intrinsic sympathomimetic	200–800 mg/d
Labetalol (Normodyne, Trandate)	Nonselective β and selective α_1 blocking activity	200 mg bid
Metoprolol (Lopressor)	β_1 selective	100 mg once/d
Nadolol (Corgard)	Nonselective	40 mg once/d
Penbutolol (Levatol)	Nonselective, intrinsic sympathomimetic	20 mg once/d
Pindolol (Visken)	Nonselective, intrinsic sympathomimetic	10 mg bid
Propranolol (Inderal, generic)	Nonselective	60 mg bid
Timolol (Blocadren, generic)	Nonselective	10 mg bid

Modified from Betaxolol for hypertension. Med Lett Drugs Ther 1990;32(821):61.

by inhibiting β_2-mediated arteriolar vasodilation. First-generation beta-blockers are contraindicated in patients with asthma, obstructive airway disease, diabetes mellitus, and/or peripheral artery disease.[3]

Second-generation beta blockers such as atenolol, acebutolol, and metoprolol are relatively selective for β_1 adrenoceptors, do not attenuate catecholamine-induced vasodilatation, and are less likely to induce bronchoconstriction. Recently, a third generation of β_1-selective beta blockers have been produced that have an increased ability to induce arterial vasodilation without bronchoconstriction.

All beta blockers are capable of being ingested in overdose and all produce severe hypotension as a response. Betaxolol is well-described in a case study example of an antihypertensive beta-blocker overdose.[4]

Toxicokinetics

Beta blockers are also discussed in Chapter 32. Table 33–7 summarizes the toxicokinetics of some antihypertensive beta blockers.

Clinical Presentation

Signs of beta-blocker toxicity are usually present within 2 hours of ingestion.[5]

Overdose

Two reports have been made available of overdose associated with betaxolol use. A 16-year-old girl took 460 mg (23 tablets) of betaxolol in a suicide attempt. She developed hypotension but had no abnormal electrocardiographic signs and was discharged the following day. A 22-year-old woman ingested an overdose of both betaxolol and disopyramide. She developed cardiogenic shock, an intraventricular block, and diffuse intravascular coagulation and was treated supportively with isoprenaline, glucagon, and pressor amines. A temporary pacemaker was inserted.[4]

Chronic Use

Betaxolol. Bradycardia, vasomotor disorders of extremities, heart failure, faintness, minor gastrointestinal complaints, dyspnea, and impotence are occasionally observed.[4,6,7]

Bopindolol. Fatigue, sleeplessness, vivid dreams, depression, dizziness, gastrointestinal upset, palpitations, and headache are observed with long-term treatment.[8–10]

Celiprolol. Dizziness, fatigue, and tiredness are seen occasionally.[3]

Dilevalol. Dizziness, headache, and diarrhea occur in less than 10% of patients on chronic therapy. Cold extremities, dyspnea, bradycardia, and heart block occur infrequently. Elevated transaminase levels and a positive antinuclear antibody titer are occasionally observed, similar to other beta blockers.[10]

Labetalol. Hypotension following a labetalol overdose may require massive doses of epinephrine (>5 mg). One patient received 175 mg of adrenaline in 24 hours.[11]

Laboratory

Blood levels do not seem to correlate well with the therapeutic or toxic activity of most beta blockers.[5]

Treatment
Stabilization

Respiration must be established and ventilation assisted with endotracheal intubation as required. The patient may develop sudden bradycardia, severe hypotension, or cardiac failure. Patients should be followed in an intensive care facility where oxygen, intravenous fluids, and cardiac monitoring are available.

Table 33–7
Toxicokinetics of Some Antihypertensive Beta Blockers

	Betaxolol[5,6]	Bopindolol[7–9]	Dilevalol[9,10]	Penbutolol[1,11]	Celiprolol[3]
Absorption (bioavailability)	80–90%	66–70%	30%	95%	30% (at 100 mg), 70% (300–400 mg)
Time to peak serum concentration	3–4 h	ND	50 min	1 h	ND
Volume of distribution	5–8 L/kg	2–3 L/kg	25 L/kg	0.5–0.6 L	ND
Half-life (elimination)	14–20 h	10 h	8–12 h	17–26 h	4–5 h
Protein binding	45–60%	ND	75%	88–95%	ND
Total clearance	18.5 L/h	16–99 L/h	23–30 mL/min/kg	ND	ND
Metabolism	Liver	Liver	Liver	Liver	Liver
Excreted in urine unchanged	16%	ND	1.25%	<4–6%	10–15%
Placental transfer	+	ND	ND	ND	ND
Breast milk	+	ND	+	ND	ND

Gut Decontamination

There is no controlled clinical evidence that syrup of ipecac, gastric lavage, activated charcoal, or cathartics are of value in the treatment of overdose with this group of drugs. Peak serum concentrations may be reached (in ≤ 1 hour) before any attempt can be made to mitigate absorption. This group of drugs is well absorbed orally.

Elimination Enhancement

There is no evidence that extracorporeal assistance (eg, hemodialysis, hemoperfusion) is useful. Furthermore, the extensive volumes of distribution and high protein binding tend to preclude the efficacy of such treatment.

Antidote

As has been noted previously (see chapter on antiarrhythmics) glucagon is an effective antidote in beta-blocker overdoses. Glucagon enhances cardiac contractility and reverses negative inotropic and chronotropic effects.

Supportive Measures

Supportive care provides the mainstay of treatment for overdose with the antihypertensive beta blockers. For hypotension, position change, intravenous fluids, and pressor amines may assist in maintaining blood pressure. The electrocardiogram, pulse, blood pressure, neurobehavioral status, and intake and output for fluid balance must be monitored. Care must be taken not to fluid overload the patient.[12,13] (See also Chapter 32.)

REFERENCES—BETA BLOCKERS IN HYPERTENSION

1. Schlanz KQ, Thomas RL. Penbutolol: A new beta-adrenergic blocking agent. DICP Ann Pharmacother 1990;24:403–408.
2. Van den Meiracker AH, Man in't Veld AJ, Van Eck HJR, et al. The clinical pharmacology of bopindolol, a new long-acting beta-adrenoceptor antagonist in hypertension. Clin Pharmacol Ther 1987;42:411–419.
3. Milne RJ, Buckley MMT. Celiprolol: An updated review of its pharmacodynamic and pharmacokinetic properties and therapeutic efficacy in cardiovascular disease. Drugs 1991; 4:941–969.
4. Steck JD. Betaxolol. Lorex Pharmaceuticals, personal communication, March 12, 1991.
5. Love JN. Beta blocker toxicity: A clinical diagnosis. Am J Emerg Med 1994;12:356–357.
6. Boutroy MJ, Morselli PL, Bianchetti G, et al. Betaxolol: A pilot study of its pharmacological and therapeutic properties in pregnancy. Eur J Clin Pharmacol 1990;38:535–539.
7. Morselli PL, Boutroy MJ, Bianchetti G, et al. Placental transfer and perinatal pharmacokinetics of betaxolol. Eur J Clin Pharmacol 1990;38:477–483.
8. Harron DWC, Goa KL, Langtry HD. Bopindolol: A review of its pharmacodynamic and pharmacokinetic properties and therapeutic efficacy. Drugs 1991;41:130–149.
9. Perkins SL, Tattrie B, Johnson PM, Rabin EZ. Analytical problems encountered during high-performance liquid chromatographic separation and coulometric detection of bopindolol metabolites in human plasma. Ther Drug Monit 1988;10:480–485.
10. Chrisp P, Goa KL. Dilevalol: A review of its pharmacodynamic and pharmacokinetic properties and therapeutic potential in hypertension. Drugs 1990;39:234–263.
11. Hicks PR, Rankin APN. Massive adrenaline doses and labetalol overdose. Anesth Intensive Care 1991;19:447–449.
12. Donnelly R, MacPhee GJA. Clinical pharmacokinetics and kinetic–dynamic relationships of dilevalol and labetalol. Clin Pharmacokinet 1991;21:95–106.
13. Aguirre C, Calvo R, Saiain JMR. Serum protein binding of penbutolol in patients with hepatic cirrhosis. Int J Clin Pharmacol Ther Toxicol 1988;26:566–569.

CALCIUM CHANNEL BLOCKERS AS ANTIHYPERTENSIVE DRUGS

In the past 10 years calcium antagonists (Fig. 33–1) have attained an important place in the therapy of supraventricular arrhythmias, angina, essential hypertension, and other cardiovascular disorders.[1,2] All calcium antagonists decrease the concentration of intracellular calcium, but each calcium antagonist has unique characteristics[3] (Table 33–8). Like the beta blockers, a second generation of calcium antagonists (Table 33–9) have been developed with more specific selectivity for vascular smooth muscle in preference to cardiac muscle.[1] The older calcium antagonists have actions on both vascular and nonvascular smooth muscle. The newer calcium antagonists are potent vasodilators selective for peripheral vasculature, but they have variable effects on cerebral (see nimodipine in Table 33–8) and coronary vasculature. Reports of overdose have been restricted largely to nicardipine. All patients survived after symptomatic and supportive therapy for varying degrees of hypotension, somnolence, bradycardia, drowsiness, and confusion. (See also Chapter 32.)

Toxicokinetics

The toxicokinetics of antihypertensive calcium channel blockers are summarized in Table 33–10. A number of similar pharmacokinetic characteristics are apparent: (1) an incomplete bioavailability due to hepatic first-pass metabolism; (2) hepatic biotransformation as the main route of elimination; (3) unchanged urinary excretion usually less than 5%; (4) high protein binding; and (5) a high apparent volume of distribution. Peak serum concentrations are usually reached within 1 to 1.5 hours of ingestion.

Drug Interactions

Potentiation of drugs listed in Table 33–9 may follow concurrent use of other calcium channel blockers and other hypotensive agents including anesthetic agents. Felodipine plasma concentrations are reduced in patients taking anticonvulsants.[4] Nicardipine plasma concentration may rise with concurrent cimetidine use.[5] Nimodipine may induce phenytoin toxicity.[6] Nisoldipine metabolism is moderately inhibited by cimetidine.[7] Nisoldipine and nitrendipine cause an increase in serum digoxin values.[8]

Pregnancy/Lactation

Only nimodipine has been studied in pregnant and lactating animals. No drug of this group has been subject to controlled clinical studies in pregnant or lactating women. The U.S.

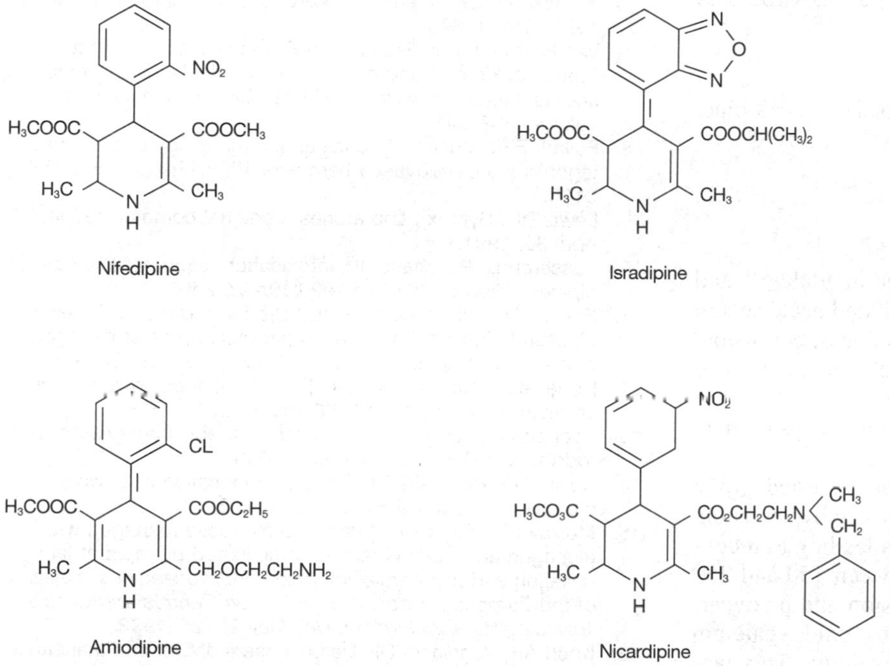

Nifedipine

Isradipine

Amiodipine

Nicardipine

Figure 33–1 Chemical structures of dihydropyridine calcium antagonist drugs. (From Meredith PA, Elliot HL. Clinical pharmacokinetics of amlodipine. Clin Pharmacokinet 1992;22:22–31.)

Table 33–8
Pharmacologic Effects of Calcium Antagonists*

	Vasoselectivity	Systemic Vasodilation	Negative Inotropic Effects	Negative Dromotropic Effects	Nonvascular Smooth Muscle Side Effects	Vasodilatory Side Effects
Diltiazem	+	+	+	+	+	+
Nifedipine	+++	++	+	0	0	+++
Verapamil	0	+	+++	++	+++	+
Felodipine	++	++	+	+	+	++
Nicardipine	++++	++	0	0	0	++
Nimodipine	+++	+	0	†	—	+
Nisoldipine	+++	++	0	0	—	++
Nitrendipine	+++	++	0	0	0	++
Isradipine	+++	++	0	0	0	++

*Values are based on a scale from 0 to 4 (++++), where 0 = least and 4 = most.
†Data not available.
Adapted from Pepine C. Nicardipine, a new calcium channel blocker: Role for vascular selectivity. Clin Cardiol 1989;12:240–246.

Table 33–9
Second-Generation Calcium Antagonists*

	Molecular Weight	Usual Starting Dose
Amlodipine	408.9	5–10 mg once/d
Felodipine (Plendil)	384.3	5 mg bid
Isradipine* (Dynacirc)†	371.4	2.5–5 mg bid
Nicardipine hydrochloride† (Cardene, Loxen)‡	516.0	20 mg tid (maximum 40 mg tid)
Nimodipine† (Nimotop)§	418.4	60 mg q4h
Nisoldipine	388.4	2.5–2.0 mg/d
Nitrendipine	360.4	10 mg bid

*All are dihydropyridine derivatives.
†Available in United States.
‡Available in France.
§Nimodipine is indicated for the improvement of neurologic deficits due to spasm following subarachnoid hemorrhage from ruptured congenital intracranial aneurysms in patients who are in good neurologic condition postictus (eg, Hunt and Hess grades I–III).

Food and Drug Administration has placed isradipine, nicardipine, and nimodipine in Pregnancy Category C.

Clinical Presentation

Overdose

Nicardipine overdoses have been observed in adults[9,10] and children.[11] Symptoms and signs have included acute severe hypotension, profound bradycardia, drowsiness, confusion, sinus tachycardia, and cardiovascular shock. Doses ingested vary from 180 to 2500 mg. The patient who took 2500 mg was found dead.[12] A simple 10-mg nifedipine capsule may be fatal to a toddler.[13]

A 2.5-mg capsule of isradipine was ingested by a 2-year-old child. This led, within 30 minutes, to hypotension, which was treated with intravenous fluids leading to recovery.[14] A 66-year-old woman ingested between 150 and 250 mg of isradipine and developed hypotension and bradycardia, which were treated with intravenous fluids, calcium gluconate, intravenous glucagon, and dopamine. This was followed by atrial fibrillation and evidence of left ventricular failure, which resolved on cessation of the glucagon and dopamine infusions.[15] She developed an acute non-Q-wave myocardial infarction. Hyperglycemia and metabolic acidosis are also seen.[16]

Chronic Use

Chronic exposure to the calcium channel blockers may induce dizziness, flushing, headache, edema, gingival hyperplasia,[17] and palpitations, most of which appear to be dose dependent.[1]

Treatment

All overdose patients who have survived have responded to supportive and symptomatic care with pressor amines, intravenous fluids, and intensive care. Use of calcium salts requires evaluation by further controlled studies. Intravenous glucagon (5- to 10-mg bolus) resolved hypotension in one anecdotal trial of nifedipine poisoning,[18] but has been erratic in relieving bradycardia and hypotension with other calcium channel blockers. Its role remains to be determined. (See also Chapter 32.)

REFERENCES—CALCIUM CHANNEL BLOCKERS AS ANTIHYPERTENSIVE DRUGS

1. Parmley WW. New calcium antagonists: Relevance of vasoselectivity. Am Heart J 1990;120:1408–1413.
2. Weiner DA. Calcium channel blockers. Med Clin North Am 1988;72:83–115.
3. Pepine C. Nicardipine, a new calcium channel blocker: Role for vascular selectivity. Clin Cardiol 1989;12: 240–246.
4. Capewell S, Freestone S, Critchley JAJH, et al. Reduced felodipine bioavailability in patients taking anticonvulsants. Lancet 1988;2:480–482.
5. Nicardipine: A new calcium entry blocker. Med Lett Drugs Ther 1989:31 (791):41–43.
6. Nimodipine. In: McEvoy GK, ed. *AHFS Drug Information 94.* Bethesda, MD: American Society of Hospital Pharmacists, 1994:1182–1187.
7. Van Harten J, Ban Brummelen P, Lodewijks MTM, et al. Pharmacokinetics and hemodynamic effects of isoldipine and its interaction with cimetidine. Clin Pharmacol Ther 1988;43:332–341.
8. Follath F, Taeschner W. Clinical pharmacology of calcium antagonists. J Cardiovasc Pharmacol 1988;12(suppl. 6):S98–S100.
9. Lewis RH. Syntex Laboratories, personal communication, April 30, 1991.
10. Passeron D, Peschaud JL. Intoxication aigue par le nicardipine. J Toxicol Clin Exp 1990;10:257–259.
11. French Antipoison Centers and Droy JM, Daridon E, Leroy J, Massari P. Intoxications aigues par nicardipine et nifedipine etude multicentrique. J Toxicol Clin Exp 1990;10:249–256.
12. Nagasaki Y, Kotani J, Funao T, et al. Fatal poisoning by nicardipine. Kitasata Med 1988;18:287–291.
13. Pearigen PD. Death from accidental nifedipine ingestion in a toddler. Vet Hum Toxicol 1993;35:345.
14. Spiller HA, Ramoska EA. Isradipine ingestion in a two year old child. Vet Hum Toxicol 1993;35:233.
15. Murray LM, Seger DL. Isradipine overdose managed with glucagon and dopamine and complicated by rapid atrial fibrillation and myocardial infarction. In: *Proceedings, Meeting of the European Association of Poison Centrés and Clinical Toxicologists, Birmingham, UK, May 26–28, 1993.*
16. Koch AR, Vogelaers DP, Decruyenaere JM, et al. Fatal intoxication with amlodipine. Clin Toxicol 1995;33:253–256.
17. Clavijo GA, De Clavijo IV, Weart CW. Amlodipine: A new calcium antagonist. Am J Hosp Pharm 1994;51:59–68.
18. Walter FG, Frye G, Mullen JT, et al. Amelioration of nifedipine in poisoning associated with glucagon therapy. Ann Emerg Med 1993;22:1234–1237.

AMLODIPINE

Amlodipine (Table 33–9) is an unusual dihydropyridine calcium channel blocker useful in the treatment of hypertension. It exhibits toxicokinetic differences from the other dihydropyridines (eg, slow absorption, high volume of distribution, slow rise to peak plasma level, long half-life). Overdoses may be followed by hypotension, bradyrhythmias, and conduction delays.

Structure and Classification

Amlodipine (amlodipine besylate) is a 1,4-dihydropyridine calcium channel blocking agent. Unlike other 1,4-dihydropyridine agents it has a structural difference that renders the molecule more than 90% ionized at physiologic pH. This may account for the differences in physiochemical, pharmacologic, and toxicokinetic properties from other agents (eg, nifedipine, nitrendipine, nimodepine, isradepine).[1,2]

Amlodipine is marketed as Norvasc in the United States and Istin in the United Kingdom. All calcium channel blockers available in the United States except diltiazem and verapamil are dihydropyridines.[3]

Use

Amlodipine is used in the treatment of hypertension, chronic stable angina pectoris, and vasospastic angina.

Product Formulation

Amlodipine is available in 5- and 10-mg tablets.[4]

Source

Amlodipine is a synthetic chemical.

Therapeutic Dose

The usual initial dose is 5 mg once daily.

Toxic Dose

Patients have ingested up to 250 mg of amlodipine and survived.[4] A patient who ingested 120 mg was hospitalized, underwent gastric lavage, and remained normotensive. A patient ingested 105 mg, was hospitalized, and developed hypotension that normalized following plasma expansion. A 29-month-old child ingested 30 mg of amlodipine (about 2 mg/kg). There was no hypotension, but the heart rate reached 180. Ipecac was administered 3.5 hours after ingestion. No sequelae were noted.[5]

Fatal Dose

About 70 mg of amlodipine was ingested together with benzodiazepine by a patient who died with high benzodiazepine plasma levels.[4,6] The highest measured levels were reached 10.5 h after intake. Serum levels of amlodipine remained high throughout the clinical course up to the time of irreversible shock 24 hours after ingestion.[7]

Toxicokinetics

Absorption

Following oral administration the bioavailability is about 50 to 88%. Food has no effect on toxicokinetic parameters. Peak plasma concentrations of 6 to 7 ng/mL occur in 6 to 7

Table 33–10
Toxicokinetics of Antihypertensive Calcium Channel Blockers

	Amlodipine	Felodipine	Isradipine	Nicardipine	Nimodipine	Nisoldipine	Nitrendipine
Absorption (bioavailability)	60–65%	15%	15–24%	6.5–30%	3–30%	3.7–8.4%	8–11%
Time to peak serum concentrations	6–12 h	0.6–1.1 h	1.5 h	1 h	1–9 h	1.5 h	1.5 h
Volume of distribution	21 L/kg	10 L/kg	4 L/kg	11.6 L/kg	0.9–2.3 L/kg	1.6–5.9 L/kg	4–8 L/kg
Half-life (elimination)	35–45 h	10–15 h	7 h	1.5–2 h (one dose); 8.6 h (long term)	1–2 h	2–15 h	2.5 h (PO) 11.7 h (IV)
Protein binding	95%	99%	95%	95%	95%	99%	~90%
Total clearance	20 L/h	45–60 L/h	317 L/h	7.8 L/h/kg	0.5–1.8 L/h/kg	0.5–0.95 L/h/kg	1.3 L/h/kg
Metabolism	Liver	Liver	Liver	Liver	Liver	Liver	Liver
Excreted in urine unchanged	<10%	<0.5%	0	<1%	<1%	0	3–4%
Placental transfer	ND	ND	ND	ND	+ (in animals)	ND	ND
Breast milk	ND	ND	ND	ND	+ (in animals)	ND	1.7 μg/d
Peak plasma level	1.2–1.4 ng/mL	1.0 ng/mL	1 ng/mL/mg dose (multiple dose)	10–12 ng/mL	30 ng/mL	2.0–4.0 ng/mL	11.4 ng/mL

Aronoff GR, Sloan RS. Nitrendipine kinetics in normal and impaired renal function. Clin Pharmacol Ther 1985;38:212–218.
Blychert E, Edgar B, Elmfeldt D, Hedner T. A population study of the pharmacokinetics of felodipine. Br J Clin Pharmacol 1991;31:15–24.
Clifton DG, Blouin RA, Dilea C, et al. The pharmacokinetics of oral isradipine in normal volunteers. J Clin Pharmacol 1988;28:36–42.
Cook E, Clifton GG, Vargas R, et al. Pharmacokinetics, pharmacodynamics and minimum effective clinical dose of intravenous nicardipine. Clin Pharmacol Ther 1990;47:706–718.
Edgar B, Lundborg P, Regardh CG. Clinical pharmacokinetics of felodopine: A summary. Drugs 1987;34(suppl. 3):16–27.
Friedel H, Sorkin EM. Nisoldipine: A preliminary review of its pharmacodynamic and pharmacokinetic properties and therapeutic efficacy in the treatment of angina pectoris, hypertension and related cardiovascular disorders. Drugs 1988;36:682–731.
Murdock D, Heel RD. Amlodipine: A review of its pharmacodynamic and pharmacokinetic properties, and therapeutic use in cardiovascular disease. Drugs 1991;41:378–505.
Nimodipine for cerebral vasospasm after subarchnoid hemorrhage. Med Lett Drugs Ther 1989;31(792):47–48.
Singh BN, Josephson MA. Clinical pharmacology, pharmacokinetics and hemodynamic effects of nicardpine. Am Heart J 1990;119:427–434.
Soons PA, de Boer AG, van Brummelen P, Breimer DD. Oral absorption file of nitrendipine in healthy subjects: A kinetic and dynamic study. Br J Clin Pharmacol 1989;27:179–189.
Vinger E, Andersson K-E, Brandt L, et al. Pharmacokinetics of nimodipine in patients with aneurysmal subarachnoid hemorrhage. Eur J Clin Pharmacol 1986;30:421–425.
White WB, Yeh SC, Krol GJ. Nitrendipine in human plasma and breast milk. Eur J Clin Pharmacol 1989;36:531–534.
Wells TG, Sinaiko AR. Anithypertensive effect and pharmacokinetics of nitrendipine in children. J Pediatr 1991;118:638–643.

hours.[8] Amlodipine is 97 to 99% protein bound. It is subjected to extensive hepatic metabolism.

Distribution

Amlodipine is rapidly distributed into tissue, then slowly released. Unlike other dihydropyridines amlodipine has a high volume of distribution, about 20 L/kg.[3]

Elimination

The elimination half-life of amlodipine is 40 to 50 hours.[3] There are no active metabolites. Less than 5% of an oral dose is excreted unchanged in the urine.[8] The remainder is metabolized to a number of inactive metabolites excreted in the urine and feces. The rate of oxidative metabolism is relatively slow and so amlodipine does not exhibit extensive "first-pass" or presystemic metabolism after oral administration.[8] Total body clearance is 7 mL/min/kg.[3]

Drug Interactions

Amlodipine, like other dihydropyridine agents, is less likely than diltiazem or verapamil to adversely interact with beta blockers, antiarrhythmic agents, or digoxin. Digoxin and cimetidine do not affect amlodipine toxicokinetics.

Mechanism of Action

All calcium channel blockers impede the movement of calcium ions into vascular smooth muscle and cardiac muscle. Amlodipine is a potent vasodilator, like other dihydropyrines. Except for verapamil and diltiazem, all calcium channel blockers are dihydropyridines. As it is more than 90% ionized at physiologic pH, amlodipine, unlike other unchanged dihydropyridines, slowly associates with the dihydropyridine receptor site. This may be the basis for its long plasma half-life and duration of action.[9]

Clinical Presentation

Therapeutic Use

The dihydropyridines (Table 33–9) can cause significant edema. This also occurs with amlodipine but, unlike the other calcium channel blockers, amlodipine does not cause reflex tachycardia.[8,10] Flushing, dizziness, and palpitations have been reported.

Overdose

An overdose may be expected to cause excessive peripheral vasodilation with marked hypotension and, possibly, a reflex tachycardia. Bradyrhythmias, conduction system delay (primarily atrioventricular nodal), and congestive heart failure may occur following an overdose.

Laboratory

Analytical Methods

A gas chromatography assay with electron capture has a limit of detection of 0.2 μg/L.[11] A gas chromatography–mass spectrometry method has also been described to assay amlodipine and its major metabolites.[12]

Abnormalities

A small decrease in serum potassium (0.1–0.2 mEq/L) and infrequent increases in serum creatinine, glucose, uric acid, hepatic transaminases, and creatine phosphokinase have been observed.[13]

Treatment

Stabilization

With large overdoses, patients should be hospitalized where cardiac and respiratory monitoring can be instituted, and a central line placed. Intravenous calcium gluconate may be useful.

Gut Decontamination

In view of the slow absorption of amlodipine, gastric lavage may be instituted up to 6 to 8 hours after an overdose. There are no data to support the use of activated charcoal or cathartics.

Elimination Enhancement

In view of the high volume of distribution and high degree of protein binding, hemodialysis is unlikely to be useful.

Antidote

Although calcium gluconate may be considered, there are few data to support its use after an amlodipine overdose. An anecdotal report suggests that hypotension following a nifedipine poisoning was resolved after addition of intravenous glucagon therapy.[14]

Supportive Measures

Hypotension can be treated by elevation of the extremities and fluid administration. If required, vasopressors (such as phenylephrine) should be considered. Vital signs and urine output should be monitored.

Atropine may be administered if there is a conduction system delay. If an acceptable heart rate and/or cardiac output cannot be otherwise maintained, temporary cardiac pacing may be useful.

REFERENCES—AMLODIPINE

1. Selevan J, Cada D. Review of amlodipine (Norvasc[R]). Hosp Pharm 1992;27:440–449.
2. Stopher DA, Beresford AP, Macrae PV, Humphrey MJ. The metabolism and pharmacokinetics of amlodipine in humans and animals. J Cardiovasc Pharmacol 1888;12(suppl. 7): S55–S59.
3. Meredith PA, Elliott HL. Clinical pharmacokinetics of amlodipine. Clin Pharmacokinet 1992;22:22–31.
4. Product Literature. Norvasc[R]. Pfizer Laboratories, August 1992.
5. Amlodipine: A new calcium channel blocker. Med Lett Drugs Ther 1992;34(882):99–102.
6. Campbell MG. Pfizer Laboratories, personal communication, January 21, 1993.
7. Koch AR, Vogelaers DP, Decruyenaere JM, et al. Fatal intoxication with amlodipine. Clin Toxicol 1995;33:253–256.

8. Elliott HL, Meredith PA. The clinical consequences of the absorption, distribution, metabolism and excretion of amlodipine. Postgrad Med J 1991;67(suppl. 3):S20–S23.
9. Burges RA. The pharmacological profile of amlodipine in relation to ischaemic heart disease. Postgrad Med J 1991; 67(suppl. 3):S9–S15.
10. Amlodipine besylate. In: McEvoy GK, ed. *AHFS Drug Information 94.* Bethesda, MD: American Society of Hospital Pharmacists, 1994:974–978.
11. Beresford AP, Macrae PV, Stopher DA, Wood SA. Analysis of amlodipine in human plasma by gas chromatography. J Chromatogr 1987;20:178–183.
12. Beresford AP, McGibney D, Humphrey MJ, et al. Metabolism and kinetics of amlodipine in man. Xenobiotica 1988;18: 245–254.
13. Osterloh I. The safety of amlodipine. Am Heart J 1989;118: 1114–1120.
14. Walter FG, Frye G, Mullen JT, et al. Amelioration of nifedipine poisoning associated with glucagon therapy. Ann Emerg Med 1993;22:1234–1237.

CLONIDINE TRANSDERMAL PATCH

Transdermal application of clonidine requires a long period (usually 48–72 hours) to achieve therapeutic drug plasma concentrations, and transdermal application must usually be supplemented with oral clonidine therapy early in the treatment of hypertension and chemical withdrawal states. The oral form of clonidine is generally associated with a higher incidence of adverse effects than the transdermal form. The most common adverse effects are drowsiness and dry mouth. Acute toxicity associated with clonidine overdose includes profound hypotension, weakness, emesis, emotional lability, hypo- and areflexia, lethargy, somnolence, hypothermia, symptomatic bradycardia, miosis, hypoventilation, apnea, and seizures. Symptoms may last up to 72 hours. Following removal of excess amounts of the drug by emesis, gastric lavage, and activated charcoal slurry, symptomatic and supportive therapy involves fluids, administration of atropine, and, occasionally, external cardiac pacing for hemodynamically compromising bradycardia.[1] Whole-bowel irrigation in one patient resulted in passage of the clonidine patch in the rectal effluent.[2]

REFERENCES—CLONIDINE TRANSDERMAL PATCH

1. Raber JH, Shinar, C, Finkelstein S. Clonidine patch ingestion in an adult. Ann Pharmacother 1993;27:719–722.
2. Henretig F, Wiley J, Brown L. Clonidine patch toxicity: The proof's in the poop! Clin Toxicol 1995;33:475–485.

GUANFACINE

Guanfacine, an α_2-adrenoceptor agonist similar to clonidine, guanabenz, and methyldopa and a phenylacetyl-guanidine derivative,[1] is marketed as Tenex 1 mg (guanfacine hydrochloride) for the treatment of hypertension. Ingestion of 4 mg (0.35 mg/kg) by a 2-year-old child (approximately 30 times the normal adult dosage) resulted in lethargy, diaphoresis, and hypotension. Adult therapeutic blood levels range from 1.5 to 2 ng/mL. The child had blood levels on admission and 2 hours later of 39.5 and 16.9 ng/mL, respectively.[2] Treatment included gastric lavage, activated charcoal, and intravenous infusion of fluids with cardiac monitoring. Except for a short period of sinus arrhythmia, the course was uneventful and the child was discharged 24 hours after admission. Guanfacine has a half-life of approximately 12 hours.

A 25-year-old ingested 60 mg of guanfacine and experienced severe drowsiness and bradycardia (45 beats/min). The patient recovered after gastric lavage and isoproterenol over a 12-hour period.[3] A 28-year-old ingested 30 to 40 mg of guanfacine, became lethargic, was treated with activated charcoal and a cathartic, and was discharged in 24 hours. Blood chemistries (blood urea nitrogen, glucose, serum electrolytes) and a complete blood count were within normal limits.[4] A 2-year-old ingested 5 mg (5 tablets) of guanfacine, was lethargic for 24 hours, and recovered.[4]

Patients should be treated with symptomatic and supportive measures and should be admitted for 24 hours. No antidotes are available.[1]

REFERENCES—GUANFACINE

1. Mosqueda-Garcia R. Guanfacine: A second generation alpha$_2$ adrenergic blocker. Am J Med Sci 1990;299:73–76.
2. Van Dyke MW, Bonace AL, Ellenhorn MJ. Guanfacine overdose in a pediatric patient. Vet Hum Toxicol 1990;32:46–47.
3. Granier P, Arsac P, Debru JL. Intoxication par la guanfacine. Nouv Presse Med 1982;11:1636–1637.
4. Coyne ME. Wyeth–Ayerst Laboratories, personal communication, May 29, 1991.

MAGNESIUM

Magnesium (see also Chapters 52 and 67) is commonly used to control hypertension and prevent seizures in preeclampsia, to stop premature labor, to treat cardiac arrhythmias after surgery and myocardial infarction,[1] and to maintain normal circulating concentrations of calcium and magnesium.[2]

Use

Investigations are underway on the use of magnesium to control hypertension following acute cocaine ingestion,[3] to provide brain protection during periods of ischemia,[4] and to prevent changes in spinal cord sensory processing leading to chronic pain.[5] Magnesium may exert an inhibiting effect on spinal cord glucose utilization.[6] Magnesium has been observed to have a bronchodilating effect in some cases of bronchial asthma.[7,8] It has been an effective adjunct in ameliorating arrhythmias that develop after digoxin poisoning[9] and in the treatment of quinidine toxicity and Torsade de pointes.[10,11] Supraventricular tachycardia has responded to magnesium sulfate (2 g) as a rapid intravenous bolus.[12] Termination was mediated by blocking the atrioventricular node and in accessory pathways.

Product Formulation

Oral and parenteral preparations of magnesium are listed in Table 33–11.[13]

Table 33–11
Oral and Parenteral Preparations of Magnesium

Oral
Magnesium gluconate (Almora, Magnate, Magonate), 500-mg tablets (27 mg magnesium)
Magnesium amino acid chelate (chelated magnesium), 500-mg tablets (100 mg magnesium)
Magnesium carbonate (Nephro-Mag), 250-mg tablets
Magnesium chloride (Slow-Mag), delayed-release tablets (64 mg magnesium)

Parenteral
Magnesium sulfate, available in 2-, 10-, or 20-mL ampules or vials as 10% (0.8 mEq/mL), 12.5% (1 mEq/mL), or 50% (4 mEq/mL) solution
Magnesium chloride, available in 30- and 50-mL vials as 20% (1.97 mEq/mL) solution

From DiPalma JR. Magnesium replacement therapy. Am Fam Physician 1990;42:173–176.

Mechanism of Action

Cardiovascular Effects

High concentrations of circulating magnesium (5- to 20-fold above normal) depress myocardial contractility.[14] Magnesium has a direct vascular action. Hypomagnesemia increases vascular tone; hypermagnesemia decreases vascular tone by reducing calcium entry into vascular smooth muscle and thereby diminishing contractility.[15,16] Magnesium also interferes with the vasoconstrictive but not the inotropic actions of epinephrine.[17] In addition, it diminishes the contractile response of vascular tissue to vasoconstrictors such as norepinephrine and angiotensin II.[18] Hypotension associated with epidural anesthesia in women receiving magnesium may be resistant to vasopressor therapy.[2]

Neuromuscular Effects

Magnesium decreases acetylcholine release from the prejunctional motor neuron, decreases motor endplate sensitivity of acetylcholine, and decreases muscle membrane excitability. It does not cross the blood–brain barrier, but it can create a flaccid weakened state.[19] Hypomagnesemia without hypocalcemia may be associated with seizures, which respond to magnesium sulfate (3 g intravenously over 4 hours, 2 g after 30 hours, in one patient).[20]

Pregnancy

Animal studies suggest that magnesium has a greater vasodilatory action on uterine blood vessels than on systemic blood vessels.[21]

Toxic Dose

As a tocolytic agent, magnesium sulfate has been administered as 4.0 g intravenously as a loading dose, followed by 1.0 to 2.0 g/h. By error, 1.5 g/h (maximum, 3 g) was infused into the epidural space of a 40-week pregnant patient in early labor. A normal infant was delivered by cesarean section. The patient exhibited no paresthesia or motor weakness.[19]

Laboratory

Serum Magnesium Levels

Total serum magnesium concentrations reflect free or ionized (55%), chelated (12%), and protein-bound (33%) fractions.[22] The free form is the active form of magnesium. A decrease in albumin lowers total serum levels without affecting the ionized level. Alkalosis increases and acidosis decreases protein binding. Low serum magnesium levels may not indicate cellular magnesium deficiency. Tissue magnesium deficiency may exist with normal serum magnesium levels.[23]

Correlation With Illness

Although a high prevalence of hypomagnesemia (10–65%) has been reported in critically ill patients, most patients remain asymptomatic and no correlation has been found between the serum magnesium level and the severity of illness or clinical outcome (eg, intensive care unit stay, mortal arrhythmias, neuromuscular abnormalities).[24] Such patients often have normal ionized calcium levels and normal potassium levels, which may partly account for the lack of symptoms. Severe hypomagnesemia (about 1 mg/dL) is often associated with hypokalemia and an increase in mortality.

Intracellular Magnesium

Magnesium is primarily an intracellular (46%) and skeletal (53%) ion; less than 1% of total body magnesium is found in the extracellular compartments. Serum levels may not reflect tissue levels.

Cardiopulmonary arrest has been associated with a serum magnesium level of 35.1 mg/dL.[24] At a serum level of 14.1 mg/dL no deep tendon reflexes were reported; these were again active at 8.1 mg/dL. Torsade de pointes may be associated with hypomagnesemia.[25]

Serum Calcium

Total body magnesium is partitioned in bone (60%), skeletal muscle (20%), and other tissues (20%). As serum phosphate levels decrease, serum magnesium concentrations fall; conversely, low serum calcium concentrations can be associated with an elevated serum magnesium level. Magnesium is known to act as a calcium antagonist.[26] Magnesium causes clinical changes similar to those seen with administration of a calcium blocking agent: peripheral vasodilation, flushing, decrease in blood pressure, and decrease in strength of cardiac conduction.

Serum Potassium

Magnesium depletion can, by itself, induce hypokalemia that is responsive to magnesium therapy alone.[25]

Summary

A low serum magnesium level nearly always indicates a severe deficiency and a high level nearly always indicates toxicity, but a normal level does not rule out inadequate body stores.[27]

REFERENCES—MAGNESIUM

1. Abraham AS, Rosenmann D, Kramer M, et al. Magnesium in the prevention of lethal arrhythmias in acute myocardial infarction. Arch Intern Med 1987;147:753–755.
2. Zaloga G, Eisenbach JC. Magnesium, anesthesia and hemodynamic control. J Anesthesiol 1991;74:1–2.
3. Weaver K, Merrell CL, Griffin G. Effect of magnesium on cocaine induced, catecholamine-mediated platelet and vascular response in term pregnant ewes. Am J Obstet Gynecol 1989;161:1331–1337.
4. Goldman RS, Finkbeiner SM. Therapeutic use of magnesium sulfate in selected cases of cerebral ischemia and seizure. N Engl J Med 1988;319:1224–1225.
5. Kafiluddi R, Kennedy RH, Seifen E. Effects of buffer magnesium on positive inotropic agents in guinea pig cardiac muscle. Eur J Pharmacol 1989;165:181–189.
6. Szabo MD, Crosby G. Central nervous system effects of magnesium. Anesth Analg 1989;69:691–692.
7. Okayama H, Aikawa T, Okayama M, et al. Bronchodilating effect of intravenous magnesium sulfate in bronchial asthma. JAMA 1987;257:1076–1078.
8. Noppen M, Vanmuele L, Impens N, Schandevyl W. Bronchodilating effect of intravenous magnesium sulfate in acute severe bronchial asthma. Chest 1990;97:272–276.
9. Reisdorff EJ, Clark MR, Walters BL. Acute digitalis poisoning: The role of intravenous magnesium sulfate. J Emerg Med 1986;4:463–469.
10. Tsivoni D, Banai S, Schuger C, et al. Treatment of Torsade de pointes with magnesium sulfate. Circulation 1988;77:392–397.
11. Tsivoni D, Keren A, Cohen AM, et al. Magnesium therapy for Torsade de pointes. Am J Cardiol 1984;53:528–530.
12. Wesley RC Jr, Haines DE, Lerman BR, et al. Effect of intravenous magnesium sulfate on supraventricular tachycardia. Am J Cardiol 1989;63:1129–1131.
13. DiPalma JR. Magnesium replacement therapy. Am Fam Physician 1990;42:173–176.
14. Paddle BM, Haugaard N. Role of magnesium in effects of epinephrine on heart contraction and metabolism. Am J Physiol 1971;221:1178–1184.
15. Altura BM, Altura BT. Ouabain, membrane Na^+K^+-ATPase and the extracellular action of magnesium ions in arterial smooth muscle. Artery 1977;3:72–83.
16. Altura BM, Altura BT. Magnesium, electrolyte transport and coronary vascular tone. Drugs 1984;28:120–142.
17. Prielipp RC, Zaloga GP, Butterworth JF, et al. Magnesium inhibits the alpha-1 but not the beta-1 adrenergic actions of epinephrine in postoperative coronary artery bypass graft patients. Anesthesiology 1990;73:A282.
18. Cohen L, Kitzes R. Magnesium sulfate in the treatment of variant angina. Magnesium 1984;3:46–49.
19. Dror A, Henriksen E. Accidental magnesium sulfate injection. Anesth Analg 1987;66:1020–1021.
20. Matthey F, Gelder CM, Schon FEG. Isolated hypomagnesemia presenting as focal seizures in diabetes mellitus. Br Med J 1986;293:1409.

Table 33–12
Management of Hypertensive Crisis: Emergencies and Urgencies*

Drug	Dose	Onset	Cautions
Parenteral Vasodilators			
Sodium nitroprusside	0.25–10 μg/kg/min as IV infusion; maximal dose for 10 min only	Instantaneous	Nausea, vomiting, muscle twitching; with prolonged use may cause thiocyanate intoxication, methemoglobinemia acidosis, cyanide poisoning; bags, bottles, and delivery sets must be light resistant
Nitroglycerin	5–100 μg as IV infusion	2–5 min	Headache, tachycardia, vomiting, flushing, methemoglobinemia; requires special delivery system due to drug binding to polyvinyl chloride tubing
Diazoxide	50–150 mg as IV bolus, repeated, or 15–30 mg/min by IV infusion	1–2 min	Hypotension, tachycardia, aggravation of angina pectoris, nausea and vomiting, hyperglycemia with repeated injections
Hydralazine	10–20 mg as IV bolus 10–40 mg IM	10 min 20–30 min	Tachycardia, headache, vomiting, aggravation of angina pectoris
Enalaprilat	0.625–1.25 mg every 6 h IV	15–60 min	Renal failure in patients with bilateral renal artery stenosis, hypotension
Parenteral Adrenergic Inhibitors			
Phentolamine	5–15 mg as IV bolus	1–2 min	Tachycardia, orthostatic hypotension
Trimethaphan camsylate	1–4 mg/min as IV infusion	1–5 min	Paresis of bowel and bladder, orthostatic hypotension, blurred vision, dry mouth
Labetalol	20–80 mg as IV bolus over 10 min; 2 mg/min as IV infusion	5–10 min	Bronchoconstriction, heart block, orthostatic hypotension
Methyldopa	250–500 mg as IV infusion every 6 h	30–60 min	Drowsiness
Oral Agents			
Nifedipine (not extended release)	10–20 mg PO, repeat after 30 min	15–30 min	Rapid uncontrolled reduction in blood pressure may precipitate circulatory collapse in patients with aortic stenosis
Captopril	25 mg PO, repeat as required	15–30 min	Hypotension, renal failure in bilateral renal artery stenosis
Clonidine	0.1–0.2 mg PO, repeated every hour as required to a total dose of 0.6 mg	30–60 min	Hypotension, drowsiness, dry mouth
Labetalol	200–400 mg PO, repeat every 2–3 h	30 min–2 h	Bronchoconstriction, heart block, orthostatic hypotension

*It is sometimes appropriate to administer a diuretic agent with any of these drugs.
From the Fifth Report of the Joint National Committee on Detection, Evaluation and Treatment of High Blood Pressure (JNICV). Arch Intern Med 1993;153:154–163.

Table 33-13
Treatment of Hypertensive Emergencies in Pediatric Patients

Drug	Onset of Action	Dosage and Route	Comments
Nifedipine	Minutes	0.25–0.5 mg/kg per dose; sublingual	Excellent first-line drug; avoids abrupt declines in BP
Captopril	Minutes	Infants: 0.01–0.25 mg/kg per dose, PO Children: 0.1–0.2 mg/kg per dose, PO	May abruptly decrease BP, may cause acute renal failure in patients with renovascular disease
Hydralazine hydrochloride	Minutes	0.1–0.2 mg/kg, IV	Tachycardia, headache
Diazoxide	Minutes	1–3 mg/kg, IV bolus	Usually, furosemide also given because of salt and water retention. Do not repeat within 1 h
Labetalol hydrochloride	Minutes	0.25–1.5 mg/kg/h, IV	May abruptly decrease BP
Nitroprusside	Seconds	1–8 μg/kg/min, IV	Remains a drug of choice but necessitates admission to intensive care unit
Phentolamine mesylate	Seconds	0.1–0.2 mg/kg, IV	Alpha-adrenergic blocking agent, for treatment of pheochromocytoma

From Lieberman E. Pediatric hypertension: Clinical perspective. Mayo Clin Proc 1994;69:1098–1107. Comment: Mayo Clin Proc 1995;70:406–407.

21. Vincent RD Jr, Chestnut DH, Sipes SL, et al. Magnesium sulfate decreases maternal blood pressure but not uterine blood flow during epidural anesthesia in gravid ewes. Anesthesiology 1990;74: 77–82.
22. Elin RJ. Assessment of magnesium status. Clin Chem 1987;33: 1965–1970.
23. Zaloga GP. Interpretation of the serum magnesium level. Chest 1989;95:257–258.
24. McCubbin JH, Sibai BM, Abdella TN, Anderson GD. Cardiopulmonary arrest due to acute maternal hypermagnesemia. Lancet 1981;1:1058.
25. Grant HI, Yeston NS. Cardiac arrest secondary to emotional stress and Torsade de pointes in a patient with associated magnesium and potassium deficiency. Crit Care Med 1991; 19:292–294.
26. Levine BS, Coburn JW. Magnesium, the mimic/antagonist of calcium. N Engl J Med 1984;310:1253–1255. Editorial.
27. Higgins GL III. Magnesium medicine comes of age. Emerg Med 1991;23(4):83–95.

YOHIMBINE

Experience to date suggests a benign course even after massive overdose. Observation would seem to be the management of choice.[1]

REFERENCE—YOHIMBINE

1. Friesen K, Palatnick W, Tenenbein M. Benign course after massive ingestion of yohimbine. J Emerg Med 1993; 11:287–288.

THE HYPERTENSIVE CRISIS

Hypertensive crisis is defined as a blood pressure greater than 120 to 140 mm Hg diastolic without evidence of acute central nervous system, cardiac, or renal damage. The patient may have minimal or no complaints and is often noncompliant with treatment. Therapeutic goals include gradual reduction of blood pressure (diastolic) within 24 hours. Oral agents are sufficient. Frequently used agents include clonidine and nifedipine.

A hypertensive emergency is defined as increased blood pressure with evidence of end-organ damage (brain, heart, kidneys) or dysfunction. Evidence of altered organ function, not the blood pressure, is the basis for diagnosis. Immediate reduction of blood pressure, usually by parenteral agents, is necessary.

Treatment of hypertensive emergencies in adults and pediatric patients is outlined in Tables 33–12 and 33–13, respectively.

Chapter 34 Vasodilators

INTRODUCTION

Vasodilators are commonly used in Europe. Many have not been approved for use in the United States. Table 34–1 lists drugs with vasodilator properties.

PHOSPHODIESTERASE III INHIBITORS: INOTROPES

The rate and force of myocardial contraction is related to the myocardial concentration of cyclic AMP. Enoximone, milrinone, and amrinone inhibit the phosphodiesterase (Table 34–2),[1] which inactivates cyclic AMP. The increase in cyclic AMP tends to lead to an enhanced slow Ca^{2+} inward current with an increase in force of myocardial contractility. These drugs are noncatecholamine inotropic agents. They exhibit both arteriodilator and venodilator activities.[2]

Unwanted Effects

Intravenous[3] and oral[4] milrinone were noted in large-scale multicenter studies to cause supraventricular and ventricular arrhythmias or excess mortality.[5] There is little evidence that the phosphodiesterase inhibitors improve survival.[6,7] Thrombocytopenia, agranulocytosis,[8] insomnia, seizures, agitation, anxiety, and headache have followed the use of enoximone.[9] Amrinone is no longer available because of its adverse effects.[10] The application for enoximone is not being pursued in the United States.[11] Overdose probably leads to enhancement of undesirable arrhythmias.

Toxicokinetics

The toxicokinetics of the phosphodiesterase III inhibitors are summarized in Table 34–3.

Clinical Presentation

Amrinone

A patient with severe congestive heart failure was given a total of 840 mg of amrinone by bolus and infusion over 3 hours and died in 2 weeks.[12]

Table 34-1
Vasodilators

Adenosine
Amrinone, enoximone, milrinone (phosphodiesterase III inhibitors)*
Bepridil*
Buflomedil*
Cinnarizine*
Cyclandelate
Diltiazem
Dipyridamole*
Flosequinan*
Flunarizine*
Glyceryl trinitrate
Isosorbide nitrate
Isoxuprine
Naftidofuryl*
Nifedipine
Nimodipine
Nitrendepine
Pentoxifylline*
Pentaerythritol tetranitrate
Prajmaline
Tolazoline

*Discussed in this chapter.

Table 34-2
Drug Inhibiting Phosphodiesterase

Group	Selectivity
Imidazalone derivatives	
Enoximone	PDE III
Piroximone	
Bipyridine derivatives	
Amrinone	PDE III
Milrinone	
Pyridazinones	
Pimobendan	PDE III
Imadazodan	
Opium alkaloids	
Papaverine	PDE I–V
Alkylxanthines	
Theophylline	PDE I–V
Isobutyl methyl xanthine	
Caffeine	

PDE, phosphodiesterase.
From Skoyles JR, Sherry KM. Pharmacology, mechanisms of action and uses of selective phosphodiesterase inhibitors. Br J Anaesth 1992;68:293–302.

Enoximone

In infants, enoximone infusion of 20 μg/kg/min induced a rise in serum osmolality due to the propylene glycol (41.3% w/v) in the preparation.[13] Toxicity due to propylene glycol may manifest as hyperosmolarity, lactic acidosis, hemolysis, hemoglobinuria, skin irritation, deafness, and other neurologic disturbances. A 2-year-old child ingested an unknown number of enoximone capsules. The child was hospitalized for 18 hours. There were no sequelae.[10]

Treatment

Treatment is symptomatic and supportive. Seizures may respond to diazepam. Infusion of the phosphodiesterase III drug should be discontinued. Blood pressure, electrocardiogram, and capillary wedge pressure must be monitored.[3] There are no antidotes. The efficacy of hemodialysis or hemoperfusion in assisting elimination has not been evaluated.

REFERENCES—PHOSPHODIESTERASE III INHIBITORS: INOTROPES

1. Skoyles JR, Sherry KM. Pharmacology: Mechanisms of action and uses of selective phosphodiesterase inhibitors. Br J Anaesth 1992;68:293–302.
2. Estafanous FG. Con: Amrinone is not a first-choice inotrope following cardiopulmonary bypass. J Cardiothorac Vasc Anesth 1991;5:184–186.
3. Enoximone and milrinone: Inotropic vasodilators for severe heart failure. Drug Ther Bull 1991;9(20):39–40.
4. Picker M, Carver JR, Rodeheffer RJ, et al. The effect of oral milrinone on mortality in severe chronic heart failure. N Engl J Med 1991;23:325:1468–1475.
5. Anderson JL, Baim DS, Fein SA, et al. Efficacy and safety of sustained (48 hours) intravenous infusions of milrinone in patients with severe congestive heart failure: A multicenter study. J Am Coll Cardiol 1987;9:711–722.
6. Poole-Wilson PA, Lindsay D. Advances in the treatment of chronic heart failure: Two steps forward, one step back. Br Med J 1992;304:1069–1070.
7. Feldman AM. Can we alter survival in patients with congestive heart failure? JAMA 1992;267:1956–1961.
8. Vernon MW, Heel RC, Brogden RN. Enoximone: A review of its pharmacological properties and therapeutic potentials. Drugs 1991;42:997–1017.

Table 34-3
Toxicokinetics of Phosphodiesterase III Inhibitors

	Amrinone	Enoximone	Milrinone
Bioavailability (%)		53–60	85–92
Time to peak plasma concentration (h)		2.5	2–3
Volume of distribution (L/kg)	1.3–1.5	1.8	0.3
Half-life (h)	2.6	1–2	0.8
Clearance (L/h/kg)	0.28–0.4	10 mL/min/kg	0.15
Protein binding (%)		65%	70%
Excreted in urine unchanged (%)	<1		
Dosage	0.75 mg/kg IV loading dose, then 5–10 μg/kg/min	10 μg/kg/min	25 μg/kg bolus; or IV 0.7 μg/kg/min (or 2.5–5 mg q6h)

9. Appardurai I, Edmunds M, Wyatt R, Spyt TJ. Convulsions induced by enoximone administered as a continuous intravenous infusion. Br Med J 1990;300:613–614.
10. Gershick AH: Commentary. Adverse effects of milrinone for heart failure. ACP J Child 1992;March/April:46.
11. Schleman MM. Marian Merrell Dow, personal communication, March 12, 1992.
12. Reich L. Winthrop Pharmaceuticals, personal communication, May 29, 1991.
13. Huggon I, James I, Macrae D. Hyperosmolarity related to propylene glycol in an infant treated with enoximone infusion. Br Med J 1990;301:19–30.

AMRINONE

Amrinone, a bipyridine derivative, is a noncardiac glycoside and noncatecholamine cardiotonic agent with positive inotropic effects and vasodilatory properties[1,2] and was approved for intravenous use by the U.S. Food and Drug Administration in 1984.[3] There have been few reports of overdose with amrinone.[4] Because of the vasodilatory effects of amrinone, overdose may result in severe hypotension.[5]

Structure and Classification

Amrinone, 5-amino-3, 4′-bipyridin-6-(^{1}H)-one, is the prototype of a new class of cardiotoxic agents, the bipyridines; one other analog, milrinone, is now under investigation.[6,7] Amrinone is chemically distinct from the digitalis glycosides or catecholamines.[4]

Use

Amrinone is mainly used commercially as the 2-hydroxypropanate to treat pulmonary hypertension,[8,9] congestive heart failure, and postoperative heart failure.[10,11] It may be used to support the circulation after cardiopulmonary bypass in adults and children.[8] Treatment with amrinone is reserved largely for those patients with congestive heart failure refractory to conventional treatment with digitalis glycosides, diuretics, and often also vasodilators.[1] Long-term use of amrinone over 72 hours may become less effective because of tachyphylaxis.[2]

Product Formulation

Amrinone lactate is available for parenteral use containing 5 mg of amrinone per milliliter with sodium metabisulfite 0.25 mg/mL (Inocor lactate).[5]

Source

Amrinone, its *N*-acetyl metabolite (*N*-[1, 6-dihydro-5-oxo)(3,4′-bipyridin)-5-yl]acetamide, and the internal standard for the assay (1,6-dihydro-6-oxo[3,4^{1}-bipyridin]-5-carboxamide) are synthetic products.[12]

Therapeutic Dose

For the short-term management of congestive heart failure or to improve cardiac output in advanced cardiac life support treatment for adults (this indication is not in the currently approved labeling as reviewed by the U.S. Food and Drug Administration), an initial amrinone dose of 0.75 mg/kg is injected intravenously over a 2- to 3-minute period.[5] A continuous infusion of amrinone is then maintained at 5 to 10 µg/kg/min. An additional loading dose of 0.75 mg/kg may be given 30 minutes after initiation of therapy. Total dose of amrinone, including initial, supplemental, and cumulatively infused doses, usually should not exceed 10 mg/kg/d. Higher doses (up to 18 mg/kg/d) have been used for short periods.

Studies in infants indicate that to obtain a plasma amrinone concentration of 2 to 7 µg/mL, infants should receive initial boluses of 3.0 to 4.5 mg/kg in divided doses followed by an infusion of 10 µg/kg/min, whereas neonates should receive a 0.75 mg/kg initial bolus followed by a lower infusion rate of 3 to 5 µg/kg/min.[13]

High Dose

A 2.25 mg/kg loading dose and 20 µg/kg/min infusion were administered to extubated patients 24 hours after coronary artery bypass graft surgery. At this dose, amrinone significantly decreased systemic vascular resistance and significantly increased the cardiac index.[8] Although amrinone significantly increased heart rate, both the recommended dose and the high dose resulted in decreased mean arterial, mean pulmonary artery, central venous, and pulmonary artery occlusion pressures.[8]

Fatal Dose

A fatal dose may have been infused when 840 mg was administered over 3 hours by initial bolus and subsequent infusion, with death ensuing 2 hours later.[14] The patient had a history of renal and heart failure.

Toxicokinetics

Absorption

There is a dose-related increase in peák plasma levels up to a concentration of approximately 4 µg/mL after oral doses of up to 3.5 mg/kg. No further increases in plasma concentration were seen in one study at doses greater than 200 mg/d.[12] A 1.5 mg/kg intravenous bolus followed by a 5 µg/kg/min infusion for 6 hours resulted in a level of 1.7 µg/mL.[15] In the serum, amrinone is 30% protein bound.[16]

Distribution

The volume of distribution has ranged from 0.64 to 1.65 L/kg after oral administration, and was 0.04 L/kg after administration of a 5 mg/kg intravenous bolus dose to patients in congestive heart failure.[15] Following an intravenous bolus injection of 0.68 to 1.2 mg/kg in normal volunteers, amrinone lactate had an apparent volume of distribution of 1.2 L/kg.[4]

Elimination

Amrinone is eliminated by conjugative pathways (eg, glucuronidation, glutathione addition, acetylation) and not by oxidative pathways.[1] Terminal elimination of amrinone from the bloodstream appears to follow first-order kinetics with a mean half-life of 2.6 hours[12] to 3.6 hours.[4] During the first 24 hours, 10 to 40% of the dose of the drug is excreted as unchanged amrinone.[12] In patients with congestive heart failure receiving infusions of amrinone lactate, the mean apparent first-order terminal elimination half-life is about 5.8 hours.[4] In infants the elimination half-life decreases with patient age, from 12.7 to 14.6 hours in 1-week-old infants to 3.8 to 6.4 hours in 28- to 38-week-old infants. Amrinone clearance averaged 2.93 mL/min/kg and the volume of distribution was 1.7 L/kg.[13]

Drug Interactions

With cardiac glycosides (eg, digoxin), amrinone produces additive inotropic effects. With disopyramide, amrinone may induce excessive hypotension. With lidocaine, quinidine, metoprolol, propranolol, hydralazine, prazosin, isosorbide dinitrate, nitroglycerin, chlorthalidone, ethacrynic acid, furosemide, hydrochlorthiazide, spironolactone, captopril, heparin, warfarin, potassium supplements, insulin, and diazepam, amrinone has been reported to be used in a limited number of patients without unusual adverse effects.[5]

Pregnancy/Lactation

Amrinone is known to have induced fetal abnormalities in rabbits and other pregnancy-related problems in rats. There are no adequate and well-controlled studies in pregnant women. The Food and Drug Administration has placed amrinone in Pregnancy Category C. Amrinone should be used during pregnancy only if the potential benefit justifies the potential risk to the fetus. Because it is not known whether amrinone is excreted in human milk, the drug should be used with caution in nursing women.[5]

Mechanism of Action

Amrinone is a potent cardiac inotropic agent and also has direct vasodilatory properties in systemic and pulmonary vessels. Its inotropic action results from the selective inhibition of phosphodiesterase III, with a subsequent increase in cardiac cyclic AMP concentration.[6] Amrinone does not, unlike cardiac glycosides such as digoxin, appear to inhibit the cardiac sodium- and potassium-dependent ATP. Further studies are required to elucidate the exact mechanism of action of amrinone.

Clinical Presentation

Chronic Use

Thrombocytopenia. Although the manufacturer noted thrombocytopenia in 2.4% of the patient population, oral amrinone resulted in platelet counts below 200,000/mm^3 in 34% of patients.[3] One patient experienced a platelet level of 23,000/mm^3 and was given platelet transfusions. Bleeding did not occur. Similar experience has been reported elsewhere.[17] The thrombocytopenia may be dose dependent.[5] Pancytopenia has been reported following short-term, high-dose intravenous amrinone.[18] Thrombocytopenia has been associated in one study of 18 children with an increased concentration of the metabolite *N*-acetylamrinone.[19]

Hypotension. Hypotension has been observed after intravenous use. This may become significant and require appropriate therapy.[17,20]

Ventricular Arrhythmias. Following intravenous infusion, ventricular arrhythmias may occur. Such arrhythmias may, however, reflect the serious underlying pathology for which amrinone may be used.[20,21] Further studies are indicated to evaluate this.

Gastrointestinal Effects. Nausea, vomiting, diarrhea,[22] abdominal pain, and anorexia may occur infrequently during intravenous therapy.

Hepatotoxicity. Dose-related hepatotoxicity has been reported in dogs. [5] Approximately 0.2% of patients receiving amrinone intravenously develop evidence of hepatotoxicity.[3,5]

Hypersensitivity Reactions. Hypersensitivity occurs rarely and has followed 2 weeks of therapy. Pericarditis, pleuritis, ascites, myositis, hypoxemia, nodular pulmonary densities, and jaundice have been reported.[4]

Sensitivity Sodium Metabisulfite. Patients known to be sensitive to sulfites, especially asthmatics, should not receive the commercial amrinone preparation, which contains sodium metabisulfite. Fatal allergic reactions may result.

Overdose

Acute overdoses may lead to severe hypotension, ventricular arrhythmias, thrombocytopenia, and, possibly hepatotoxicity. In addition, metabolic acidosis, cardiac arrest, oliguria, and death have been reported following an overdose 10 times the prescribed dose in an infant.[23,24]

Laboratory

Analytical Methods

An isocratic high-performance liquid chromatography method for the assay of plasma amrinone has been described.[16]

Blood Levels

In adult studies, a relationship exists between the plasma amrinone concentration and the cardiac index: a 30% increase in cardiac output from baseline occurs at a concentration of 1.5 μg/mL, and a 50% increase at 3.7 μg/mL.[15,16] The recommended dosing regimen can be expected to result in a plasma amrinone concentration of approximately 3 μg/mL.

Ancillary Tests

Potassium loss due to excessive diuresis may predispose patients on digitalis to arrhythmias. Hypokalemia should be corrected by potassium supplementation in advance of or during amrinone use. Fluid electrolyte changes, renal and hepatic function, and hematology, including platelets, should be monitored carefully during amrinone therapy.

Treatment

Stabilization

Patients should be in a cardiac intensive care facility where continuous cardiac parameters may be recorded including the cardiac index, pulmonary capillary wedge pressure, central venous pressure, and electrocardiogram. Airways should be patent and, dependent on clinical judgment, endotracheal intubation should be performed as required for mechanical ventilation.

Hypotension may occur any time following an overdose. Preparations should be made for an intravenous line with use of fluids (careful monitoring of fluid balance) and pressor agents as required. Continuous recording of blood pressure, pulse, and respiration is required. Circulatory support without fluid overloading is desirable.

Elimination Enhancement

No clinical studies are available to support the use of extracorporeal elimination procedures (eg, hemodialysis, hemoperfusion, or plasmapheresis). One case report suggests use of continuous arteriovenous hemofiltration in patients with renal and hepatic dysfunction who are receiving amrinone infusions.[25]

Antidote

No antidote is available for the treatment of amrinone overdose.

Supportive Measures

Supportive therapy is the mainstay of treatment for an overdose of amrinone. As patients usually have serious underlying cardiac pathology when treated with amrinone, all such patients should be in an intensive cardiac care unit with appropriate cardiology staff available and in attendance. Oxygen, ventilatory support, careful fluid balance, electrolyte studies (especially for potassium levels), monitoring of electrocardiogram, central venous pressure, cardiac indices (see Stabilization), complete blood count (including platelets), and hepatic and renal function tests are required after appropriate consultations with a nephrologist and cardiologist.

REFERENCES—AMRINONE

1. Ward A, Brogden RN, Heel RC, et al. Amrinone: A preliminary review of its pharmacological properties and therapeutic use. Drugs 1983;26:468–502.
2. Maisel AS, Wright CM, Carter SM, et al. Tachyphylaxis with amrinone therapy: Association with sequestration and down-regulation of lymphocyte beta-adrenergic receptors. Ann Intern Med 1989;110:195-201.
3. Treadway G. Clinical safety of intravenous amrinone: A review. Am J Cardiol 1985;56:39B–40B.
4. Product Literature: Inocor[R] lactate injection. Brand of amrinone lactate: Sterile intravenous solution. Winthrop Pharmaceuticals, September 1989:1W161-X.
5. Amrinone. In: McEvoy GK, ed. *AHFS Drug Information 94.* Bethesda, MD: American Society of Hospital Pharmacists, 1994:974–978.
6. Fita G, Gomar C, Jimenez MJ, et al. Amrinone in perioperative low cardiac output syndrome. Acta Anaesthesiol Scand 1990;34:482–485.
7. Braunwald E, Julian D, eds. *The Acute Therapy of Heart Failure. Intravenous Milrinone: A New Therapeutic Option.* London: Royal Society of Medicine, 1991.
8. Prielipp RC, Butterworth JF IV, Zaloga GP, et al. Effects of amrinone on cardiac index, venous oxygen saturation and venous admixture in patients recovering from cardiac surgery. Chest 1991;99:820–825.
9. Berner M, Jaccard C, Oberhansli I, et al. Hemodynamic effects of amrinone in children after cardiac surgery. Intensive Care Med 1990;16:85–88.
10. Hess W, Arnold B, Veit S. The haemodynamic effects of amrinone in patients with mitral stenosis and pulmonary hypertension. Eur Heart J 1986;7:800–807.
11. Hess W. Effects of amrinone on the right side of the heart. J Cardiothorac Anesth 1989;3:38–44.
12. Kullberg MP, Freeman GB, Biddlecome C, et al. Amrinone metabolism. Clin Pharmacol Ther 1981;29:394–401.
13. Lawless S, Burckart G, Diven W, et al. Amrinone pharmacokinetics in neonates and infants. J Clin Pharmacol 1988; 28:283–284.
14. Reich L. Winthrop Pharmaceuticals, personal communication, May 29, 1991. Submitted to the U.S. Food and Drug Administration as a Drug Experience Report, December 4, 1984.
15. Edelson J, LeJemtel TH, Alousi AA, et al. Relationship between amrinone plasma concentration and cardiac index. Clin Pharmacol Ther 1981;29:723–728.
16. Lawless S, Burckart G, Piccola G, et al. Simplified assay of amrinone in plasma by high-performance liquid chromatography. Ther Drug Monit 1990;12:570–573.
17. Wilmshurst PT, Webb-Peploe MM. Side effects of amrinone therapy. Br Heart J 1983;49:447–451.
18. Mattingly PM, Burnette PK, Weston MW, Manhy RP. Pancytopenia secondary to short-term, high-dose intravenous infusion of amrinone. DICP Ann Pharmacother 1990;24:1172–1174.
19. Ross MP, Allen-Webb EM, Pappas JB, McGough EC. Amrinone-associated thrombocytopenia: Pharmacokinetic analysis. Clin Pharmacol Ther 1993;53:661–667.
20. Franciosa JA. Intravenous amrinone: An advance or a wrong step? Ann Intern Med 1985;102:399–400.
21. Mancini D, LeJemtel T, Sonnenblick E. Intravenous use of amrinone for the treatment of the failing heart. Am J Cardiol 1985;56:8B–15B.
22. Silverman BD, Merrill AJ Jr, Gerber L. Clinical effects and side effects of amrinone: A study of 24 patients with chronic congestive heart failure. Arch Intern Med 1985;145:825–829.
23. Case 460: American Association of Poison Control Centers Annual Report 1990. Am J Emerg Med 1991;9:507.
24. Lebovitz DJ, Lawless ST, Weise KL. Fatal amrinone overdose in a pediatric patient. Crit Care Med 1995;23:977–986.
25. Lawless S, Restaino I, Azin S, Corddry D. Effects of continuous arteriovenous haemofiltration on pharmacokinetics of amrinone. Clin Pharmacokinet 1993;25:80–82.

BEPRIDIL

Bepridil hydrochloride (Vascor, United States; Cordium, France) is a calcium channel blocking agent that is not chemically related to verapamil, nifedipine, or diltiazem.[1,2] It has been used in Europe since 1980.[3] It is used for the oral treatment of chronic stable angina pectoris[4–7] only in patients who fail to respond optimally or are intolerant of other antianginal agents.[1]

Therapeutic Dose

Dosage for therapeutic use is 200 to 400 mg/d.

Toxicokinetics

Approximately 90% of an oral dose of bepridil is absorbed, but because of a substantial first-pass effect, its bioavailability is 60%. Following absorption, bepridil reaches peak serum levels in 2 to 3 hours that are dose related: 200 mg, 764 ng/mL; 300 mg, 1268 ng/mL; 400 mg, 1631 ng/mL. It is 99% protein bound, mostly to α_1-acid glycoprotein. Bepridil is extensively metabolized in the liver to 17 metabolites, of which one, 4-hydroxy-*N*-phenylbepridil, has some pharmacologic activity. It has an extensive apparent volume of distribution, 8 L/kg, and has an elimination half-life of 33 hours after a single oral dose and 42 hours after multiple doses.[8] Its pharmacokinetics is compared with those of other calcium channel blockers in Table 34–4.

Mechanism of Action

Bepridil blocks both the slow inward calcium channel and the fast inward sodium channel in the myocardium.[2] It has the action of both class IV (calcium channel blockers) and class I (membrane-stabilizing agents) antiarrhythmic drugs.[4] Bepridil prolongs effective refractory periods of the atrioventricular node, atria, and ventricles and prolongs retrograde refractory periods in accessory conduction pathways.[2] It slows the heart rate and lowers the blood pressure 3 to 6%; it decreases myocardial oxygen consumption and increases myocardial perfusion.[2]

Clinical Presentation

Bepridil may cause dizziness, nausea, dyspepsia, headache, tremor, asthenia, diarrhea, nervousness, interstitial pulmonary fibrosis,[9] and, rarely, agranulocytosis.[1,2] Unlike other calcium channel blockers, bepridil induces some degree of prolongation of the QT and QT_c intervals on the electrocardiogram. A number of patients have developed Torsade de pointes arrhythmias, which are more often found in association with advanced age, hypokalemia (< 4 mmol/L), and high plasma bepridil concentrations.[2,10,11] Pulmonary fibrosis is a known side effect of four cardiovascular agents: amiodarone, flecainide, tocainide, and bepridil.[9]

Laboratory

A high-performance liquid chromatography method is available for quantitation of bepridil. It is precise and accurate over the range 10 to 2000 ng/mL.[12] A gas chromatography assay with nitrogen-sensitive detection has a sensitivity threshold as low as 10 ng/mL plasma.[13]

Treatment

Stabilization

Following an overdose close observation in a cardiac care facility for a minimum of 48 hours is indicated. An intravenous line, oxygen, and cardiac monitoring should be available.

Symptomatic and supportive treatment is the mainstay of management of an overdose. If patients can be treated prior to 2 hours after an overdose, gastric emptying may be of value. There is no evidence that activated charcoal is of value. It would appear prudent to avoid the use of antiarrhythmic drugs that prolong the QT_c interval, such as class IA drugs (eg, quinidine, procainamide), class IC drugs (eg, flecainide), and class III drugs (eg, amiodarone).[2] Accumulated data suggest that the risk for development of ventricular arrhythmias and torsade de pointes with bepridil use is increased in the elderly and in those with high blood bepridil concentrations, decreased liver function, hypokalemia, prolonged baseline QT intervals, serious ventricular arrhythmias, acute myocardial infarction, hypotension, overt congestive heart failure, and second- or third-degree atrioventricular block.[14]

Beta-adrenergic stimulation or parenteral administration of calcium solutions may increase transmembrane calcium influx. Hypotensive reactions and high-degree atrioventricular block should be treated with vasopressors and cardiac pacing, respectively. Ventricular tachycardia should be managed by cardioversion and, if persistent, by overdrive pacing.[15]

Antidote

There are no antidotes.

Table 34–4
Toxicokinetics of Bepridil: Comparison With Other Calcium Channel Blockers

	Bepridil	Diltiazem	Nifedipine	Verapamil
Oral bioavailability (%)	60	44	45	19
Clearance, IV dose (mL/min/kg)	5	11	10	12
Half-life, single oral dose (h)	33	3	3	5
Excreted in urine unchanged (%)	<0.1	<4	0	<3
Active metabolites	4-OH-*N*-phenyl bepridil	Desacetyl-diltiazem	None reported	Norverapamil
Protein bound (%)	>99	80	98	90
Volume of distribution (L/kg)	8	5	1.5	5

Adapted and modified from Benet LZ. Pharmacokinetics and metabolism of bepridil. Am J Cardiol 1985;55:8C–13C.

Elimination Enhancement

In view of the extensive volume of distribution and high protein binding of bepridil, measures such as hemodialysis and hemoperfusion would probably not be effective in removing significant quantities of the drug. Pharmacokinetic observations of half-life, total body clearance, and protein binding following ingestion of bepridil by hemodialysis patients suggest that bepridil is not removed by hemodialysis.[16] A comprehensive review of bepridil has been prepared by Hollingshead and colleagues.[17]

REFERENCES—BEPRIDIL

1. Bepridil for angina pectoris. Med Lett Drugs Ther 1991; 33(84S):53–54.
2. Bepridil. Lancet 1988;1:278–279. Editorial.
3. Lanneyde Courien JF, Martin J, Richalet A. Etude clinique d'un nouvel anti-angineux le bepridil (a propos de 92 cas). Vie Med 1979;60:1675–1676.
4. Funck-Brentano C, Coudray P, Planellas J, et al. Effects of bepridil and diltiazem on ventricular repolarization in angina pectoris. Am J Cardiol 1990;66:812–817.
5. Deedwania P, Carbajal E, Bobba V, Linn L. Calcium channel block by bepridil compared to propranolol in the treatment of patients with chronic stable angina. Clin Pharmacol Ther 1987;41:241.
6. Shapiro W, Di Bianco R, Thadani U, Bepridil Collaborative Study Group. Comparative efficacy of 200, 300 and 400 mg of bepridil for chronic stable angina pectoris. Am J Cardiol 1985;55:36C–42C.
7. Hill JA, O'Brien JT, Alpert JS, et al. Effect of bepridil in patients with chronic stable angina: Results of a multicenter trial. Circulation 1985;71:98–103.
8. Benet LZ. Pharmacokinetics and metabolism of bepridil. Am J Cardiol 1985;55:8C–13C.
9. Vasilomanolakis EC, Goldberg NM. Bepridil-induced pulmonary fibrosis. Am Heart J 1993;126:1016–1017.
10. Malicier D, Malicier F, Gallet M, et al. Troubles du rythme ventriculaire graves lors d'un surdosage en bepridil (Cordium): A propos de deux observations. J Med Leg Droit Med 1986,29:157–164.
11. Coumel P. Safety of bepridil: From review of the European data. Am J Cardiol 1992;69:75D–78D.
12. Ng K-T, Plutte JA, Galante LJ. Determination of bepridil in biological fluids by high performance liquid chromatography. J Chromatogr Biomed Appl 1984;309:125–131.
13. Vink J, Van Hal HJM, Pognat J-F, Bouquet des Chaux J-L. Determination of the anti-ischemic drug bepridil in human plasma using gas chromatography with nitrogen-sensitive detection. J Chromatogr Biomed Appl 1983;272: 87–94.
14. Singh BN. Bepridil therapy: Guidelines for patient selection and monitoring of therapy. Am J Cardiol 1992;69:79D–85D.
15. Product Literature: Vascor (bepridil hydrochloride). McNeil Pharmaceuticals, December 27, 1990.
16. Nayak RK, Halstenson CE, Opsahl JA, et al. Pharmacokinetics of bepridil in hemodialysis patients. Clin Pharmacol Ther 1987;41:238.
17. Hollingshead LM, Faulds D, Fitton A. Bepridil: A review of its pharmacological properties and therapeutic use for stable angina pectoris. Drugs 1992;44:835–857.

BUFLOMEDIL

Buflomedil hydrochloride, a synthetic chemical, is an adjunct to conservative treatment used in the treatment of peripheral and central vascular insufficiency.[1] It has been used in France since 1976. Overdose has been associated with convulsions, central nervous system depression, arrhythmias, and death. Treatment is largely symptomatic and supportive (Fig. 34–1).

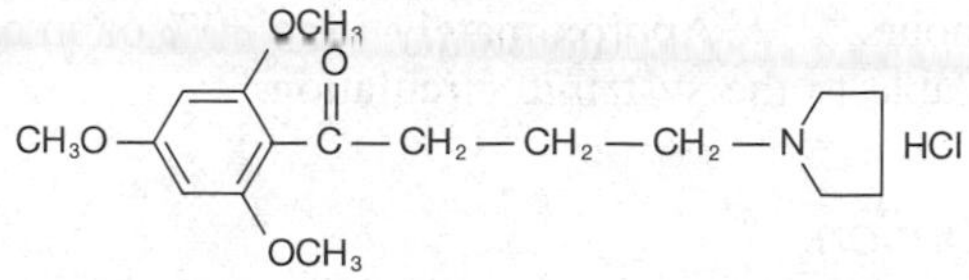

OCH$_3$ / CH$_3$O–C$_6$H$_2$–C(=O)–CH$_2$–CH$_2$–CH$_2$–N(pyrrolidine) HCl / OCH$_3$

Figure 34-1 Structure of buflomedil. (From Ghysel MH, Haguenoer JM. Three cases of fatal intoxication by buflomedil associated with alcohol or paracetamol. In: *Proceedings, 29th International Meeting, International Association of Forensic Toxicology, Copenhagen, Denmark, June 24–27, 1991*:435–439.)

Use

Buflomedil hydrochloride has been used to treat peripheral vascular insufficiency including intermittent claudication, Raynaud's phenomenon, and frostbite. It has been tried in diabetic retinopathy, cerebrovascular insufficiency, and cochleovestibular disturbances.[1]

Product Formulation

Buflomedil hydrochloride is administered orally in the form of 150-mg tablets. Ampules of 50 mg in 5 mL of saline are also available.[2] Proprietary names include Befedil, Bufene, Buflon, Defluina, Flomed, Fonzylane, Hemoflux, Irroden, Lofton, Loftyl, and Sinoxis.[2]

Therapeutic Dose

For the treatment of peripheral vascular or cerebrovascular disease, the usual dosage is 450 to 600 mg/d, usually in two or three divided doses. From 50 to 200 mg/d may be used intravenously either in divided doses or as a slow intravenous infusion in 500 mL of isotonic glucose or saline solution. Buflomedil 50 mg can also be given intramuscularly.[1]

Toxic Dose

Fourteen children, average age 34 months, were given from 150 to 900 mg of buflomedil. All survived.[3] One adult ingested 900 mg/d for 4 days, developed myoclonic seizures, and recovered.[4] A similar outcome followed use of buflomedil (450 mg/d) with haloperidol and clomipramine.[5] A 21-year-old woman ingested 3750 mg, experienced generalized seizures 4 hours later, and responded to supportive treatment.[5] An 80-year-old woman ingested 1800 mg/d, developed myoclonic seizures, and survived.[6] Twelve adults ingested an average of 4650 mg and survived.[3]

Fatal Dose

Fatalities have followed ingestion of 9000 mg,[3] 6750 mg,[7] 2250 mg,[8] and 3000 mg.[9,10]

Toxicokinetics

Absorption

Buflomedil is quickly absorbed from the gastrointestinal tract, reaching maximum plasma levels of 2 to 4 μg/mL in

3 to 4 hours.[1,11,12] Approximately 50 to 80% of an oral dose is available to the systemic circulation.[1]

Distribution

The apparent volume of distribution of buflomedil is 1.3 to 1.4 L/kg.[12] At therapeutic plasma concentrations in humans, buflomedil is 60 to 80% bound to plasma proteins.

Elimination

Following oral administration, almost 90% of the dose is excreted in the urine after 4 days, with approximately 20% as unchanged buflomedil.[1,12] The elimination half-life of buflomedil is about 2 to 3 hours.[12,13] Approximately 20% of an absorbed dose of buflomedil undergoes first-pass metabolism by demethylation on the trimethoxybenzene ring to a metabolite, *para*-desmethyl buflomedil.[12] Total body clearance is 15 to 40 L/h.[1] The mean recovery of unchanged drug and metabolite in the urine after oral dosage is 18 and 15%, respectively.[12]

Pregnancy/Lactation

There have been no controlled studies on the use of buflomedil during pregnancy and lactation.

Mechanism of Action

The major pharmacologic actions of buflomedil suggest that it acts on vascular smooth muscle by nonselective competitive inhibition of alpha adrenoceptors. It appears to increase mostly peripheral arterial flow. It may also increase erythrocyte deformability, inhibit platelet aggregation, and increase oxygen levels in the muscles in peripheral arterial occlusive disease.[1,14]

Clinical Presentation

Chronic Use

The most frequent side effects reported to the manufacturer during treatment with buflomedil include flushing, headache, vertigo, gastrointestinal discomfort, and dizziness.[6]

Overdose

The most frequent clinical features in reports of overdose include convulsions, coma, drowsiness, agitation, sinus tachycardia and vomiting; ventricular fibrillation, pulmonary edema, and peripheral vasodilation have each been reported.[3–8,10] A 19-year-old ingested 3 grams of buflomedil developed seizures, pulmonary edema, and ventricular fibrillation and died 2.5 hours later.[10]

Laboratory

Analytical Methods

A high-performance liquid chromatography method is available for the quantitation and ultraviolet spectrum identification of buflomedil in whole blood and plasma.[9] The detection limit for plasma and whole blood is 40 ng/mL. Prolongation of the QRS interval may be seen in the electrocardiogram.[15]

Blood Levels

Following a fatal 3000-mg ingestion of buflomedil, a blood level of 80 μg/mL was observed.[9] This value is about 20 times higher than the maximum concentration of 3.80 μg/mL, which followed oral ingestion of 450 mg of the drug,[13] and twice the value (43 μg/mL) measured in the plasma before death of a patient who had ingested 6750 mg.[7] Ingestion of 3000 mg of buflomedil led to a blood level of 63.4 μg/mL in an adult who died.[10] Ingestion of 2250 mg was associated with a blood level of 43 μg/mL in a patient who was found dead.[8] Three patients who died after buflomedil ingestion exhibited plasma levels of 34, 36.3, and 1.26 μg/mL. In the last case, high blood levels of paracetamol were also measured.[16]

Treatment

Stabilization

Patients with buflomedil overdose may present with minimal-appearing symptoms such as agitation, drowsiness, vomiting, and sinus tachycardia. Within 3 to 4 hours of admission the sudden onset of seizures may be accompanied by pulmonary edema, ventricular arrhythmia, and death. All patients who have ingested more than 450 mg should immediately receive an intravenous line and cardiac monitoring. Patients with altered mental status should receive oxygen, naloxone, glucose, and, if indicated, thiamine. Initial evaluation of adequacy of ventilation (ie, tidal volume, arterial blood gases, cyanosis) should be performed. Serious toxicity may result from pulmonary edema or ventricular arrhythmias.

Gut Decontamination

Gastric emptying, if it is to be attempted, should be performed within 2 hours of overdose with tracheal protection. Sudden seizures may lead to aspiration pneumonia in an unprotected patient following any decontamination procedure (eg, gastric lavage, syrup of ipecac, activated charcoal). Removal of medication from the stomach, however, may offer the patient some protection from the later development of seizures, arrhythmias, and death, complications that can be associated with high blood levels of buflomedil. There is no controlled clinical evidence that activated charcoal or cathartics are useful in the treatment of buflomedil overdosage.

Elimination Enhancement

The moderately high apparent volume of distribution and high protein binding of buflomedil may tend to preclude the usefulness of hemodialysis or hemoperfusion after an overdose. There have, however, been no trials with these procedures.

Antidote

There is no antidote.

Supportive Measures

1. All patients with a history of buflomedil overdose should be admitted for continuous observation for at least 24 hours if there is any sign of major toxicity (eg, depressed consciousness or respirations, hypotension, dysrhythmias, seizures). Patients should be observed until they are symptom free for 24 hours.
2. Treatment of buflomedil overdose is largely supportive and symptomatic. Seizures usually respond to intravenous diazepam. Phenytoin may be a second-line drug. Respiratory depression and aspiration pneumonia are particularly hazardous in comatose patients. Management requires intubation and positive-pressure ventilation.
3. Admission laboratory and monitoring procedures should include electrocardiograms, blood electrolytes, arterial blood gases, serial vital signs, and cardiac monitoring.
4. In patients with repeated seizures, the urine should be checked for myoglobin.
5. Serial serum drug levels may confirm an overdose or help to predict duration of symptoms.
6. Comatose patients may require a urinary catheter to check urinary output and prevent urinary retention.

REFERENCES—BUFLOMEDIL

1. Clissold SP, Lynch S, Sorkin EM. Buflomedil: A review of its pharmacodynamic and pharmacokinetic properties and therapeutic efficacy in peripheral and cerebral vascular diseases. Drugs 1987;33:430–460.
2. Reynolds JEF, ed. *Martindale: The Extra Pharmacopoeia.* 30th ed. London: Pharmaceutical Press, 1993:1308.
3. Medernach C, Garnier R, Efthymiou M-L. Intoxication aigue par le buflomedil. Presse Med 1981;10:3496.
4. Leys D, Pavy G, Bourgeois P, Petit H. Myoclonies au cours d'un traitement par buflomedil. Therapie 1985;40:481.
5. Otmane-Telba M, Gury B, Paulien R, et al. Toxicite neurologique reversible du surdosage au buflomedil. Presse Med 1985;14:286.
6. Treves R, Desproges-Gotteron R. Encephalopathie myoclonique chez une malade traitee par une dose excessive de buflomedil. Presse Med 1983;12:645.
7. Danel V, Saviuc P, Vincent F, et al. Intoxication aigue mortelle au buflomedil. J Toxicol Clin Exp 1988;8:243–246.
8. Bohn G, Ogbuihi S, Audick W. Buflomedil intoxication. Bull Int Assoc Forens Toxicol 1990;20(3):32–34.
9. Rop PP, Bresson M, Antoine J, et al. Quantitation and ultraviolet spectrum identification of buflomedil in whole blood and plasma by HPLC. J Anal Toxicol 1990;14:18–21.
10. Athanaselis S, Maravetias C, Michalodimitrakis M, Koutselinis A. Buflomedil concentrations in blood and viscera in a case of fatal intoxication. Clin Chem 1984;30:157.
11. Rey E, Barrier G, D'Athis P, et al. Pharmacokinetics of buflomedil after intravenous and oral administration. Int J Clin Pharmacol Ther Toxicol 1980;18:437–441.
12. Gundert-Remy U, Weber E, Lam G, et al. The clinical pharmacokinetics of buflomedil in normal subjects after intravenous and oral administration. Eur J Clin Pharmacol 1981; 20:459–463.
13. Fredj G, Clenet M, Rousselet F. Dosage du buflomedil dans les millieux biologiques: Determination des differents parametres pharmacocinetiques. Therapie 1978;33:321–332.
14. Bachand RT, Dubourg AY. A review of long-term safety data with buflomedil. J Int Med Res 1990;18:245–252.
15. Martinez-Sierra R, Lara B, Torres A. Buflomedil intoxication: The little-known risk. Clin Toxicol 1992;30:305–308.
16. Ghysel MH, Haquenoer JM. Three cases of fatal intoxication by buflomedil associated with alcohol or paracetamol. In: *Proceedings, 29th International Meeting, International Association of Forensic Toxicologists, Copenhagen, Denmark, June 24-27, 1991*:435–439.

DIPYRIDAMOLE

Dipyridamole is a vasodilator and antiplatelet agent widely used in the treatment of cerebral, peripheral, and coronary vascular disease.[1] Although patients with preexisting cardiovascular disease may develop further cardiac symptoms after normal or slightly increased doses of dipyridamole, ingestion of five- to sevenfold overdoses of the drug have not produced serious problems related to coronary blood flow. Hypotension and tachycardia are the only cardiovascular signs that appear to follow excess ingestion of the drug. A fatality has followed use of a therapeutic dose in a patient with cardiovascular disease. No overdose has terminated fatally. No antidotes are available.

Structure and Classification

Dipyridamole is 2, 6-bis(diethanolamino) -4,8-dipiperidino-pyrimido-(5,4-*d*)-pyrimidine (Fig. 34–2).[2–5]

Use

Dipyridamole is approved in the United States for use as an adjunct to coumarin anticoagulants in the prevention of postoperative thromboembolic complications of cardiac valve replacement.[6] Other nonapproved uses of dipyridamole have included trials to decrease platelet aggregation in other thromboembolic disorders. Dipyridamole alone does not prolong the survival of patients with acute myocardial infarction, reduce the incidence of deep-vein thrombosis postoperatively, prevent thromboembolism after hip surgery, or benefit patients with transient cerebral ischemic attacks.[5,7] Dipyridamole has also been studied together with thallium-201 cardiac imaging as a test for detecting coronary artery disease in patients unable to exercise effectively.[7,8] Experimental studies indicate a possible role for dipyridamole in cancer chemotherapy as a potentiating agent for cytotoxic drug therapy. Preliminary data suggest that dipyridamole is associated with a reversibility of thallium-201 myocardial scan deficits in patients with sarcoidosis.[9]

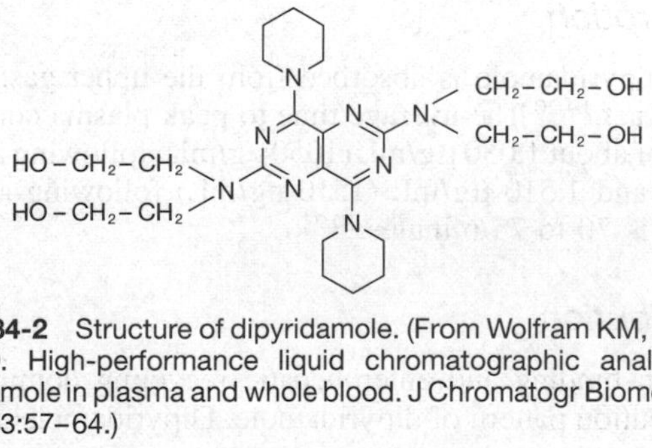

CH_2-CH_2-OH
CH_2-CH_2-OH
$HO-CH_2-CH_2$
$HO-CH_2-CH_2$

Figure 34-2 Structure of dipyridamole. (From Wolfram KM, Bjornsson TD. High-performance liquid chromatographic analysis of dipyridamole in plasma and whole blood. J Chromatogr Biomed Appl 1980;183:57–64.)

Product Formulation

Dipyridamole (Persantine) is available as oral tablets containing 25, 50, or 75 mg.[4] The tablets are orange, round, and stamped "B1" on one side and "17," "18," and "19," respectively, on the other side.[6,8,10] Ampules containing 10 and 50 mg in 2 mL yellow solution for intravenous injection are available in Europe but not in the United States.[3] Dipyridamole is stable if protected from light, heat, and moisture.

Source

Dipyridamole is a synthetic chemical.

Therapeutic Dose

The therapeutic dose is 75 to 100 mg four times daily as an adjunct to the usual warfarin therapy.[6]

Toxic Dose

Patients with unstable angina, multivessel coronary disease, and epicardial coronary collaterals appear to be at risk of dipyridamole-induced myocardial ischemia when doses of 75 to 100 mg are administered prior to planned coronary bypass surgery.[11–14] Chest pain may develop in about 4 to 20% of patients who receive 200 to 400 mg of dipyridamole prior to thallium imaging.[8,12] Intravenous dipyridamole 0.56 mg/kg was followed by chest pain and bradycardia; the patient survived.[15] A 64-year-old patient received dipyridamole 300 mg and developed anginal jaw pain; he survived.[16,17] A 62-year-old patient ingested 5000 mg of dipyridamole, developed a myocardial infarction, and survived.[18]

Eight children ingested overdoses of up to 625 mg (tablets) and survived.[10] One 13-year-old ingested 225 mg (tablets) and survived.[9,10] An elderly woman (age unknown) inadvertently given 75-mg tablets four times daily, instead of the prescribed 25 mg four times daily, survived.[9] A man who ingested 750 mg of dipyridamole survived.[10] A woman aged 17 years attempted suicide by ingesting 1.5 to 2.5 g of dipyridamole and survived.[10]

Fatal Dose

A 77-year-old patient received dipyridamole 400 mg orally prior to a thallium imaging test. She developed a fatal electromechanical dissociation.[9]

Toxicokinetics

Absorption

Oral dipyridamole is absorbed from the upper gastrointestinal tract.[19,20] The average time to peak plasma concentrations of about 1.050 μg/mL (1050 ng/mL) following a 50-mg tablet and 1.510 μg/mL (1510 ng/mL) following a 75-mg tablet is 70 to 75 minutes.[10,21]

Distribution

Protein binding and enterohepatic recycling dominate the distribution pattern of dipyridamole. Dipyridamole is bound primarily to α_1-acid glycoprotein to the extent of almost 99%.[21,22] The coefficient of dipyridamole distribution between human plasma and erythrocytes is 6.53.[23] Very little of the free or conjugated drug crosses the blood–brain barrier.[20–23] The volume of distribution is approximately 2 L/kg.[3,21]

Elimination

Dipyridamole is converted in the liver to the monoglucuronide conjugate and is excreted with the bile into the duodenum. In the intestine, dipyridamole glucuronide is partly reconverted to free dipyridamole. Both dipyridamole and its glucuronide are absorbed by the intestinal mucosa and returned to the liver via enterohepatic recirculation.[24,25]

Dipyridamole exhibits a decline in plasma levels that fits a two-compartment model. The alpha half-life, the initial decline after the peak concentration, is about 40 minutes. The beta half-life, the terminal decline in the plasma concentration, is approximately 10 to 11 hours.[10,21] The terminal half-life constitutes only about 20% of the total area under the curve. No free dipyridamole is found in the urine. About 90% of a dose is recovered in the feces.[21] Total body clearance in intravenous studies has been rapid at approximately 15 L/h (50–250 mL/min.)[21]

Drug Interactions

Dipyridamole may inhibit platelet aggregation. Heparin given concomitantly with dipyridamole may induce bleeding.[5] In vitro studies suggest that dipyridamole potentiates the anti-HIV effects of zidovudine and of dideoxycytidine in human monocyte–macrophages.[26,27] Dipyridamole at therapeutic concentrations may induce significant inhibition of adenosine metabolism,[28] leading to an increase in plasma adenosine levels.[1] Caffeine may inhibit the hemodynamic changes (increase in systolic blood pressure, pulse, pressure, and heart rate) induced by dipyridamole.[29]

Pregnancy/Lactation

Safe use of dipyridamole during pregnancy has not been established. It has been placed in Pregnancy Category B by the U.S. Food and Drug Administration. Few congenital abnormalities have followed administration of dipyridamole and aspirin to pregnant patients.[30–32] One of eight pregnancies yielded a live infant with bilateral incurving fifth fingers.[33] Spontaneous abortions have been observed in some pregnancies in the first and second trimesters.[33,34] One of eleven pregnancies yielded a fetus with multiple chromosomal abnormalities; the newborn died.[34] Dipyridamole may, when added to a warfarin regimen during pregnancy, result in an increase in fetal wastage.[35] Dipyridamole is distributed into breast milk. Caution should be exercised in treating nursing women.[5,6,10]

Mechanism of Action

Platelet adhesion and aggregation appear to be reduced below the lower limit of normal at blood dipyridamole levels above 3.5 μmol/L (about 1.5 μg/mL).[36] Known biochemical properties of dipyridamole include inhibition of adenosine transport and accumulation in the plasma (leading to coronary vasodilation), inhibition of cyclic AMP and phosphodiesterase, and stimulation of prostacyclin (prostaglandin I_2) synthesis.[1]

Clinical Presentation

A total of 11 cases of overdose with dipyridamole tablets have been reported to the manufacturer.[10] Symptoms and signs of overdose included drowsiness, weakness, fainting, nausea, gastrointestinal distress, flushing with hypotension, and tachycardia. There were no fatalities.[10]

Laboratory

Analytical Methods

A sensitive and specific high-performance liquid chromatography method is available for measuring dipyridamole in whole blood and plasma using paired ion chromatography and fluorescence detection. The lower limit of sensitivity for dipyridamole is 1 ng/mL.[2] A fluorometric assay has also been developed by Boehringer–Ingelheim.[36]

Abnormalities

Serum from a patient taking dipyridamole gave very high readings when lipoproteins were measured by nephelometry.[10] Dipyridamole imparts a yellowish-blue fluorescence to solutions and could interfere with other laboratory tests involving fluorescence or nephelometry measurements.[37]

Ancillary Tests

Electrocardiographic changes following dipyridamole use may show ST–T wave elevations.

Treatment

Stabilization

Patients who have overdosed with dipyridamole usually respond to symptomatic and supportive treatment. Attention to the airway, breathing, and circulation together with cardiac monitoring, availability of oxygen, and careful observation for incipient hypotension usually form the basis for treatment. Patients should be observed in the emergency department and should be able to be discharged after 6 hours if all vital signs are within normal limits and an electrocardiogram indicates stability.

Gut Decontamination

Activated charcoal (possibly multiple dose) may accelerate excretion of dipyridamole by interfering with its enterohepatic cycle. There is no evidence that syrup of ipecac, gastric lavage, cathartics, or whole-bowel irrigation accelerates or improves the chance of recovery.

Elimination Enhancement

Dipyridamole is highly protein bound and has a high apparent volume of distribution; hemodialysis or hemoperfusion is not likely to be of benefit.

Antidoto

There is no specific antidote.

Supportive Measures

Bradycardia should respond to intravenous atropine.[16] Anginal symptoms and ischemic electrocardiographic changes usually resolve with sublingual nitroglycerin therapy.[12] If the patient does not respond to nitroglycerin treatment, intravenous theophylline may be effective.[9,12] Complex ventricular arrhythmias, an infrequent complication, are generally transient and readily treated.[9] Severe chest pain following dipyridamole administration, which is relieved by aminophylline and antianginal medications, should be considered an indication of significant ischemia and treated accordingly. Thrombolysis may be required.[17] Patients presenting with suspected coronary artery disease in the setting of aortic stenosis may be at increased risk for life-threatening complications from oral dipyridamole and should be preferentially referred to cardiac catheterization.[9] Accumulated data suggest that preoperative dipyridamole should not be a routine therapy in patients with unstable angina undergoing coronary bypass surgery or coronary angioplasty, especially if coronary collateral vessels are identified.[11,13,15,19] Clinical data suggest that intravenous dipyridamole may induce severe bronchospasm in asthmatic patients. Intravenous aminophylline should be readily available if a dipyridamole–thallium test is planned for a patient known to have asthma.[37–40]

REFERENCES—DIPYRIDAMOLE

1. German DC, Krechich VM, Bjornsson TD. Oral dipyridamole increases plasma adenosine levels in human beings. Clin Pharmacol Ther 1989;45:80–84.
2. Wolfram KM, Bjornsson TD. High-performance liquid chromatographic analysis of dipyridamole in plasma and whole blood. J Chromatogr Biomed Appl 1980;183:57–64.
3. Reynolds JEF, ed. *Martindale: The Extra Pharmacopoeia.* 30th ed. London: Pharmaceutical Press, 1993:225–226.
4. Dollery C, ed. *Therapeutic Drugs.* Edinburgh: Churchill Livingstone, 1991:D175–D177.
5. Dypyridamole. In: McEvoy GK, ed. *AHFS Drug Information 94.* Bethesda, MD: American Society of Hospital Pharmacists, 1994:1180–1181.
6. *Physicians' Desk Reference.* 49th ed. Montvale, NJ: Medical Economics, 1994:43.
7. Beeley L. Dipyridamole in prevention of myocardial infarct and strokes. Br Med J 1987;295:1553.
8. Friedman HZ, Goldberg SF, Hauser AM, O'Neill WW. Death with dipyridamole thallium imaging. Ann Intern Med 1988; 109:990–991.
9. Tellier P, Paycha F, Antony I, et al: Reversibility by dipyridamole of thallium-201 myocardial scan defects in patients with sarcoidosis. Am J Med 1988;85:189–193.
10. Bowers PA. Boehringer–Ingelheim Pharmaceuticals, personal communication, January 23, 1992.
11. Keltz TN, Gitler B, Cooper JA. Dipyridamole-induced myocardial ischemia. JAMA 1987;258:203–204.
12. Castello R, Hidalgo R. Dipyridamole-induced myocardial ischemia. JAMA 1988;259:1179.
13. Keltz TN, Gitler B, Cooper JA. Dipyridamole-induced myocardial ischemia. JAMA 1988;259:1179.
14. Ranhosky A. Dipyridamole-induced myocardial ischemia. JAMA 1987;258:203.
15. Pennell DJ, Underwood SR, Ell PJ. Symptomatic bradycardia complicating the use of intravenous dipyridamole for thallium-201 myocardial perfusion imaging. Int J Cardiol 1990;27:272–274.

16. Keltz TN, Innerfield M, Gitler B, Cooper JA. Dipyridamole-induced myocardial ischemia. JAMA 1987;257:1516–1517.
17. Kwai AH, Jacobson AF, McIntyre KM, et al. Persistent chest pain following oral dipyridamole for thallium-201 myocardial imaging. Eur J Nucl Med 1990;16:745–746.
18. Jahangiri M, Holdright DR. Myocardial infarction secondary to dipyridamole overdose. Arch Emerg Med 1992;9:62–64.
19. Yamamoto S, Matsuura H, Umezawa T, et al: Dipyridamole-induced ischemia in a child with jeopardized collaterals after Kawasaki syndrome. Jpn Heart J 1990;31:867–874.
20. Mellinger TJ, Bohorfusch JG. Pathways and tissue distribution of dipyridamole (Persantin®). Arch Int Pharmacodyn 1965;156:380–388.
21. Bjornsson TD, Mahony C. Clinical pharmacokinetics of dipyridamole. Thromb Res 1983;suppl. IV:93–104.
22. Kopitar Z, Weisenberger H. Spezifische bindung von dipyridamol an ein menschliches serumprotein. Arzneimitte/forschung 1971;21(6):859–862.
23. Kubler W. Die bindung des koronarcilatators dipyridamol and die plasma eiweisskorper des menschen. Arch Kreislaufforsch 1971;64:115–128.
24. Beisenherz G, Koss F, Klatt L, Binder B. The absorption and excretion of 2,6-bis(diethanolamino)-4, 8-dipiperidinopyrimido-(5,4-*d*)pyrimidine after oral administration. Arch Int Pharmacodyn 1965;158:380–388.
25. Beisenherz G, Koss FW, Schule A, et al. Das schicksal des 2,6-bis(diathanlamino)-4,8-dipiperidine-pyrimido (5,4-d) pyrimidin im menschlichen und tierischen organismus. Arzneimittelforschung 1960;10:307–312.
26. Wyngaarden JB. Dipyridamole may enhance effectiveness of AIDS therapy. JAMA 1989;262:17.
27. Szebeni J, Wahl SM, Popovic M, et al. Dipyridamole potentiates the inhibition by 3'-azido-3'-deoxythymidine and other dideoxynucleosides of human immunodeficiency virus replication in monocytes–macrophages. Proc Natl Acad Sci USA 1989;86:3842–3846.
28. Klabunde RE. Dipyridamole inhibition of adenosine metabolism in human blood. Eur J Pharmacol 1983;93:21–26.
29. Smits P, Straatman C, Pijpers E, Thien T. Dose-dependent inhibitions of the hemodynamic response to dipyridamole by caffeine. Clin Pharmacol Ther 1991;50:529–537.
30. Taguchi K. Pregnancy in patients with a prosthetic heart valve. Surg Gynecol Obstet 1977;145:206–208.
31. Biale Y, Cantor A, Lewenthal H, Gueron M. The course of pregnancy in patients with artificial heart valves treated with dipyridamole. Int J Gynaecol Obstet 1980;18:128–132.
32. Ibara-Perez C, Arevalo-Toledo N, Alvarez de la Cadena O, Noriega-Guerra L. The course of pregnancy in patients with artificial heart valves. Am J Med 1976;61:504–512.
33. Chen WWC, Chan CS, Lee PK, et al. Pregnancy in patients with prosthetic heart valves: An experience with 45 pregnancies. Q J Med 1982;51:358–365.
34. Deviri E, Levinsky L, Yechezkel M, Levy MJ. Pregnancy after valve replacement with porcine xenograft prosthesis. Surg Gynecol Obstet 1985;160:437–443.
35. Sareli P, England MJ, Berk MR, et al. Maternal and fetal sequelae of anticoagulation during pregnancy in patients with mechanical heart valve prostheses. Am J Cardiol 1989; 63:1462–1465.
36. Rajah SM, Crow MJ, Penny AF, et al. The effect of dipyridamole on platelet function: Correlation with blood levels in man. Br J Clin Pharmacol 1977;4:129–133.
37. Wiener K. Interference in fluorescene/nephelometry assays by dipyridamole. Lancet 1981;2:634.
38. Eagle KA, Boucher CA. Intravenous dipyridamole infusion causes severe bronchospasm in asthmatic patients. Chest 1989;95:258–259.
39. Keech AC, McCarthy JS, Norcott CJ. Adverse respiratory reactions to intravenous dipyridamole for myocardial stress thallium studies. Br Heart J 1990;64:93.
40. Lette J, Cerino M, Laverdiere M, et al. Severe bronchospasm followed by respiratory arrest during thallium–dipyridamole imaging. Chest 1989;95:1345–1349.

FLOSEQUINAN

Flosequinan, a fluoroquinolone derivative, is used for the treatment of congestive heart failure.[1–3]

Structure and Classification

Flosequinan (Manoplax)[4] is a 7-fluoro-1-methyl-3-methylsulfinyl-4-quinolone. Its empirical formula is $C_{11}H_{10}$-FNO_2S. The molecular weight is 239.3.[1]

Use

Flosequinan has been used for the treatment of congestive heart failure in patients who cannot tolerate or have not responded adequately to an angiotensin-converting enzyme (ACE) inhibitor, digitalis glycosides, and diuretics.[1,2,5]

Product Formulation

Flosequinan is available in 50-, 75-, or 100-mg tablets.

Source

Flosequinan is a synthetic chemical product.

Therapeutic Dose

Patients use between 50 and 100 mg/d flosequinan.

Fatal Dose

The Prospective Randomized Flosequinan Longevity Evaluation (PROFILE) trials indicate that patients with congestive heart failure who received flosequinan 100 mg/d had a greater risk of death than those who received lower doses or a placebo.[5] As of July 1993, the British manufacturer has withdrawn the drug.[6]

Toxicokinetics

Absorption

After oral administration, flosequinan is rapidly and extensively absorbed. Oral bioavailability exceeds 98%. The peak plasma concentration of flosequinan is reached in 0.8 hour, and that of the sulfone metabolite (flosequinoxan), 7.4 hours.[2]

Elimination

Flosequinan undergoes first-pass metabolism in the liver to a sulfone derivative (flosequinoxan). The pharmacokinetics of these compounds differ. Less than 2% is excreted unchanged in the urine.[1]

Drug Interactions

Some patients taking warfarin have required a reduction in dose to maintain control. Cimetidine, by its action on cytochrome P450 enzymes, may decrease the conversion of flosequinan to its sulfone metabolite.[2]

Pregnancy/Lactation

Flosequinan is in Pregnancy Category C. There are no adequate and well-controlled studies of the drug in pregnant or nursing women.[1]

Mechanism of Action

Flosequinan acts directly on vascular smooth muscle, probably by modifying the availability of intramuscular free (ionized) calcium. The drug has a balanced action as a vasodilator on both venous and arterial beds.[2]

Clinical Presentation
Overdose

One person received an 800-mg dose resulting in prolonged hypotension, tachycardia, and nausea, which resolved without sequelae. Symptoms expected to occur following an overdose of flosequinan include those relating to the vasodilatory properties of the drug, such as hypotension, tachycardia, headache, dizziness, generalized flushing, nausea, and vomiting. Prolonged coagulation times have been observed in animals receiving high doses of flosequinan.[2]

Chronic Use

Chronic ingestion of flosequinan may lead to headaches, palpitations, dizziness, and taste disturbances.[2] Flosequinan is associated with arrhythmogenesis including right and left bundle-branch blocks and ventricular tachycardias.[7] Flosequinan can cause renal failure in patients with bilateral renal artery stenosis.[8]

Laboratory

Increased transaminase activity has been reported.

Treatment
Elimination Enhancement

Up to 30% of flosequinan and its major metabolite is removed after 4 hours of hemodialysis.[9]

Antidote

There is no specific antidote.

Supportive Measures

In case of an overdose, standard care should be used to manage the hypotension (cardiac and respiratory monitoring, intravenous fluids, and pressor amines). Coagulation status must be monitored. Coagulation abnormalities may respond to vitamin K. As the sulfone metabolite of flosequinan has a half-life of between 30 and 40 hours, careful observation and monitoring should extend over several days.

REFERENCES—FLOSEQUINAN

1. Med Lett Drugs Ther 1993;35(892):23–24.
2. Barnett DB. Flosequinan. Lancet 1993;341:733–736.
3. Haynes WG, Webb DJ. Flosequinan in heart failure. Lancet 1993;341:1100–1101.
4. Reynolds JEF, ed. *Martindale: The Extra Pharmacopoeia.* 30th ed. London: Pharmaceutical Press, 1993:360.
5. Mayor GH. Boots Pharmaceuticals, Lincolnshire, IL, Dear Doctor Letter, April 23, 1993.
6. Flosequinan withdrawn. Lancet 1993;342:235.
7. Noble J, Farrer M, McComb JM. Flosequinan and arrhythmogenesis. Lancet 1993;341:1100.
8. Wood SM, Dudley CRK, DeVaney AM, Winearles CG. Flosequinan and renovascular disease. Lancet 1993;341:116–117.
9. Mayor GH. Boots Pharmaceuticals, Lincolnshire, IL, personal communication, June 28, 1993.

FLUNARIZINE AND CINNARIZINE

In some European countries cinnarizine and flunarizine are prescribed for "chronic cerebrovascular disease" and are considered to be "cerebral vasodilators." Controlled clinical studies of both flunarizine and cinnarizine have not yet established their efficacy as cerebral vasodilators.[1] Few cases of deliberate overdose with cinnarizine or flunarizine have been reported.

Structure and Classification

Flunarizine is a difluorinated piperazine derivative, a selective calcium antagonist structurally related to cinnarizine[2] (Fig. 34–3).

Use

Flunarizine has been used as a prophylactic treatment for migraine and to reduce seizures in epilepsy, treat vertigo, and treat cerebrovascular insufficiency.[2]

Therapeutic Dose

Therapeutic doses of flunarizine are 10 mg/d in adults and 5 mg/d in children weighing less than 40 kg.[2]

Toxic Dose

Adverse extrapyramidal effects follow the use of flunarizine at doses of 10 to 20 mg/d and cinnarizine at doses of 45 to 180 mg/d.

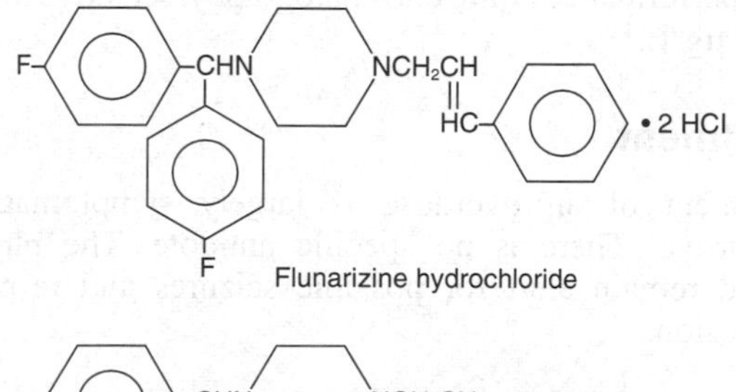

Flunarizine hydrochloride

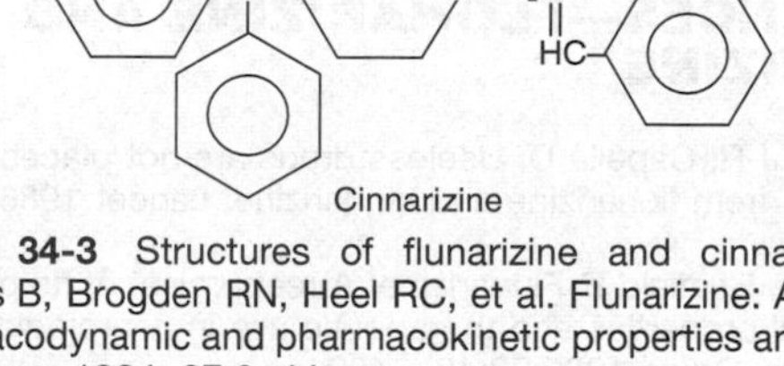

Cinnarizine

Figure 34-3 Structures of flunarizine and cinnarizine. (From Holmes B, Brogden RN, Heel RC, et al. Flunarizine: A review of its pharmacodynamic and pharmacokinetic properties and therapeutic use. Drugs 1984; 27:6–44.

Fatal Dose

A fatal dose has not been established.

Toxicokinetics

Absorption

Peak plasma flunarizine concentrations of 39 to 115 μg/L occur 2 to 4 hours after oral administration of one daily 10-mg dose. About 90% is bound to plasma proteins.

Distribution

The mean volume of distribution is about 43 L/kg.

Elimination

Flunarizine is extensively metabolized. The main route of metabolic excretion appears to be the bile. The terminal half-life is about 18 days. The plasma half-life of cinnarizine is about 3 hours.

Drug Interactions

Hepatic enzyme inducers (eg, phenytoin, carbamazine, valproic acid) increase the metabolism of flunarizine.

Mechanism of Action

Cinnarizine is a selective calcium entry blocker with antihistaminic, antiserotoninergic, and antidopaminergic activity.[3]

Clinical Presentation

Patients receiving flunarizine or cinnarizine develop drowsiness. Weight gain, headache, depression, nausea, dry mouth, and rash are occasionally observed. Extrapyramidal reactions including dyskinesia, akathisia, and depression that frequently mimic parkinsonism have been described.[3]

Laboratory

A preferred analytical method for cinnarizine in plasma is high-performance liquid chromatography, sensitive to a level of 20 μg/L.[4]

Treatment

Treatment of an overdose is largely symptomatic and supportive. There is no specific antidote. The physician should remain alert for possible seizures and respiratory depression.

REFERENCES—FLUNARIZINE AND CINNARIZINE

1. Laporte J-R, Capella D. Useless drugs are not placebos: Lessons from flunarizine and cinnarizine. Lancet 1986;2: 853–854.
2. Todd PA, Benfield P. Flunarizine: A reappraisal of its pharmacological properties and therapeutic use in neurological disorders. Drugs 1989;38:487–499.
3. Micheli F, Pardal MF, Gatto M, et al. Flunarizine and cinnarizine-induced extrapyramidal reactions. Neurology 1987;37:881–884.
4. Nitsche V, Mascher H. Rapid high-performance liquid chromatographic assay of cinnarizine in human plasma. J Chromatogr 1982;227:521–525.

NAFTIDOFURYL OXALATE

Naftidofuryl is a synthetic 5-HT_2 antagonist with vasodilator properties that has been associated with seizures, electrocardiographic abnormalities, and death after overdose (Fig. 34–4).[1]

Naftidofuryl is marked as nafronyl oxalate, Praxilene (United Kingdom), Di-actane (France), and Dusodril (Germany).

Use

Naftidofuryl is used as a vasodilator for peripheral and cerebral vascular disorders, although there is little evidence for its cerebroprotective action.[2,3] It may be of value in intermittent claudication due to peripheral vascular disease and in Raynaud's syndrome,[4] and in leg cramps at rest.[5]

Product Formulation

In the United Kingdom, naftidofuryl is available in oral and parenteral forms (tablets, 200 mg; capsules, 100 mg; parenterally, 40 mg/5 mL and 200 mg/10 mL).

Therapeutic Dose

The usual dose for cerebrovascular disorders is 100 mg three times daily by mouth. The usual dose for peripheral vascular disorders is 100 to 200 mg three times daily.[1] A dose of 200 to 400 mg may be administered by intravenous infusion.[4] The highest therapeutic oral dose known to have been used is 1600 mg in one day.

Toxic Dose

A 35-year-old woman ingested 6 g, experienced auricular and ventricular arrhythmias, and survived. Doses of 360 to 1000 mg have been associated with seizures and death.[6] A patient received 10 g and survived.

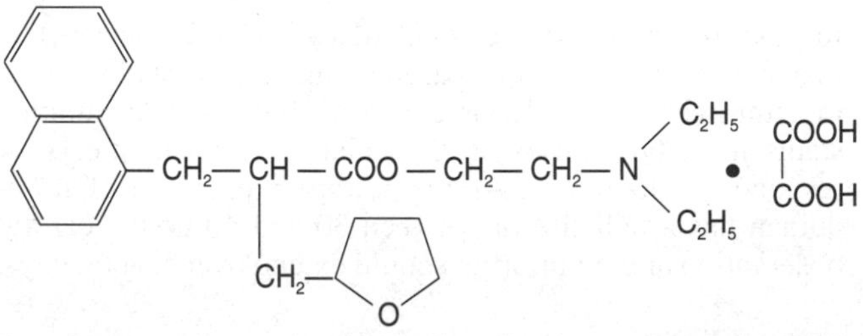

Figure 34-4 Structure of naftidofuryl. (From Walmsley LM, Wilkinson PA, Brodie RR, Chasseaud LF. Determination of naftidofuryl in human plasma by high-performance liquid chromatography with fluorescence detection. Chromatogr 1985;338:433–437.)

Fatal Dose

Death has followed doses of 360 to 1000 mg of naftidofuryl.[6]

Toxicokinetics

Absorption

About 24% of the drug is absorbed from the gastrointestinal tract. The peak plasma level is reached about 0.5 hour after an oral dose. There is some presystemic metabolism. Approximately 80% is protein bound, mostly to albumin. The drug penetrates the brain.[4]

Distribution

Naftidofuryl undergoes enterohepatic recirculation. Following intravenous administration, the apparent volume of distribution is 0.8 to 1 L/kg.

Elimination

Metabolites are not active. The plasma half-life is about 1 hour.

Drug Interactions

Intravenous naftidofuryl should be used with caution in a patient who is receiving antiarrhythmic or beta-adrenoceptor blocking drugs.[4]

Pregnancy/Lactation

No controlled studies have been performed on the pregnant or lactating female.

Mechanism of Action

Naftidofuryl is a 5-HT_2 antagonist. Its vasodilatory action follows its effect on the 5-HT_2 receptors of smooth muscle cells.[4] Naftidofuryl possesses class IA and IC electrophysiologic properties. Naftidofuryl is also a potent local anesthetic and is four times more active than lidocaine.[7] Animal studies suggest a protective effect on ischemic neuronal damage.[3,8]

Clinical Presentation

Overdose after rapid infusion may lead to loss or impairment of consciousness, seizures, and hypotension. Nausea and epigastric pain may occur. A 60-year-old woman was found unconscious after an overdose of naftidofuryl tablets; she died. In a study of 10 cases of naftidofuryl poisoning, seizure, heart block, bradycardia, and cardiac arrest were prominent.[9] Serious cardiovascular complications appear to be associated with intravenous rather than oral administration of the drug and they may occur in patients free of preexisting cardiac conduction irregularities.[10] A 93-year-old man developed a respiratory rate of 48 breaths/min after accidentally chewing (instead of swallowing) a naftidofuryl capsule 30 minutes earlier.[7] A 35-year-old woman with a normal heart swallowed 6 g of naftidofuryl. She developed disorders of atrioventricular conduction and ventricular-like arrhythmia with collapse that resolved after mechanical ventilation. Acute renal failure may follow both oral and intravenous naftidofuryl.[11–13]

Laboratory

Analytical Methods

A high-performance liquid chromatography assay method with fluorescence detection at 286 nm is available with a limit of detection of 4 ng/mL.[1] A gas chromatography–mass spectrometry method is available for analysis of tissue and blood concentration.[9]

Blood Levels

Postmortem blood levels in five of seven fatal cases were 3, 6.5, 8.4, 11, and 75 μg/mL.[9]

Abnormalities

QRS widening has been observed after an overdose. Other electrocardiographic findings include sinus tachycardia, bradycardia, atrioventricular block (first degree),[6] and cardiac arrest.

Ancillary Tests

Moderate hypokalemia has been observed after overdose.[6] Urinalysis may indicate the presence of oxalate crystals, especially in patients who have received intravenous naftidofuryl for several weeks before developing acute renal failure.[11]

Treatment

Stabilization

Overdose with naftidofuryl must be considered serious and requires immediate hospitalization. Patients should be in an intensive care facility where vital signs (blood pressure, pulse, respirations) can be followed, and oxygen and cardiac monitoring are available. Overdoses are largely treated symptomatically and supportively. Class I antiarrhythmic drugs should be avoided.

Gut Decontamination

Early (within 2 hours) gastric lavage with tracheal protection may be useful in reducing peak blood levels.

Antidote

There is no antidote.

Supportive Measures

Type I antiarrhythmic drugs (eg, quinidine, disopyramide, procainamide) may enhance the arrhythmogenic properties of naftidofuryl. Patients should be observed for at least 24 hours after the electrocardiogram has returned to normal.

REFERENCES—NAFTIDOFURYL OXALATE

1. Walmsley LM, Wilkinson PA, Brodie RR, Chasseaud LF. Determination of naftidofuryl in human plasma by high performance liquid chromatography with fluorescence detection. J Chromatogr Biomed Appl 1985;338:433–437.
2. Steiner TJ. Naftidofuryl in the treatment of recent stroke: Results of a controlled clinical trial. Vasa Suppl 1988;24:44–47.
3. Krieglstein J, Sauer D, Nuglisch J, et al. Naftidofuryl protects neurons against ischemic damage. Eur Neurol 1989;29: 224–228.
4. Dollery CF, ed. *Therapeutic Drugs.* Edinburgh: Churchill Livingstone, 1991:n8–n10.
5. Connolly MJ, Young JB, Naylor JR. Treating leg cramps: Naftidofuryl is a safe and effective alternative. Br Med J 1995;310:1138.
6. Rey JL, Marek A, Tribouilloy C, et al. Massive naftidofuryl poisoning with severe disorders of cardiac rhythm and conduction. Arch Mal Coeur 1989;82:1467–1471.
7. Khan SA, Pace JE, Cox ML. Respiratory distress secondary to naftidofuryl. Br Med J 1990;301:1219.
8. Fujikura H, Kato H, Nakano S, Kogure K. A serotonin S_2 antagonist, naftidofuryl, exhibited a protective effect on ischemic neuronal damage in the gerbil. Brain Res 1989;494: 387–390.
9. Sadler DW, Quigley C. A fatal overdose of naftidofuryl (Praxilene®). Bull Int Assoc Forens Toxicol 1991;21(4):29–32.
10. Ducloux G, Marchand X, Lasurent JM, et al. Cardiovascular complications due to naftidofuryl overdose. Ann Cardiol Angeiol 1985;34:167–169. Case report.
11. Moesch C, Rince M, Daudon M, et al. Renal intratubular crystallization of calcium oxalate and naftidofuryl oxalate. Lancet 1991;338:1219–1220.
12. Cuvelier C, Goffin E, Cosyns J-P, et al. Acute renal failure due to naftidofuryl oxalate (Praloxine[R]) overdose in a kidney transplant recipient. Nephrol Dial Transplant 1995;10: 1756–1758.
13. Le Meur Y, Moesch C, Rince M, et al. Potential nephrotoxicity of intravenous infusions of naftidofuryl oxalate. Nephrol Dial Transplant 1995;10:1751–1755.

PENTOXIFYLLINE

Pentoxifylline is used for compromised vascular blood flow states. In overdose it may induce evidence of gastrointestinal, cardiovascular, and central nervous system symptoms and signs. There have been no fatalities. Patients recover within 24 hours.

Structure and Classification

Pentoxifylline, 3,6-dimethyl-1-(5-oxohexyl)xanthine, belongs to the family of trialkylxanthines. Its molecular formula is $C_{13}H_{18}N_4O_3$ and its molecular weight is 278.3. It is a weak acid with a pH of 0.9.

Pentoxifylline is marketed as pentifylline, oxpentifylline, Trental, Torental, Tarontal, and Terental.[1,2]

Use

There is a report that pentoxifylline may improve the symptoms of intermittent claudication[3]; however, a review of 12 randomized trials suggests that the data are inadequate to show a positive or negative effect in this condition.[4] It may be useful in cerebrovascular disease and sickle cell anemia,[5] and may improve survival of experimental skin flaps. Preliminary trials indicate a potential usefulness in counteracting the acute respiratory distress syndrome and diminishing symptoms of septic or hemorrhagic shock.[6] Pentoxifylline appears to be associated with an improvement in the healing of venous ulcers of the leg,[7] livedo vasculitis,[8] and diabetic neuropathy.[9]

Product Formulation

The product is commercially available as 400-mg oral, extended-release, film-coated tablets, containing benzyl alcohol and povidone.[2,10]

Source

Pentoxifylline is a synthetic xanthine derivative.[11]

Therapeutic Dose

The usual therapeutic dose is 1 tablet (400 mg) three times daily.

Toxic Dose

Infants of 12 to 24 months who have ingested 10 to 15 tablets of pentoxifylline have developed nausea, profuse vomiting, arterial hypotension, sinus tachycardia, myoclonia, and seizures.[12] One 18-month-old had nausea after 100 mg; a 13-month-old developed vomiting after only 400 mg. Both recovered. A 22-year-old woman ingested 4000 to 6000 mg of pentoxifylline and survived.[12] A series of children and adults ingested 10 to 80 mg/kg and survived.[13] An 11-year-old ingested 1800 mg and developed vomiting and a rapid pulse; she recovered.[14] In adults, doses from 300 to 12,000 mg ultimately led to recovery.[15] Gastrointestinal symptoms followed a dose of 10 mg/kg in children and adults; hemodynamic changes may follow doses of 60 to 80 mg/kg. Seizures are observed at 75 mg/kg.[13]

Fatal Dose

A lethal dose has not been established.

Toxicokinetics

Absorption

Pentoxifylline is rapidly absorbed. Following a single oral dose of 400 mg, a mean pentoxifylline plasma concentration of 1,102 μg/L is reached at 1.05 hours. Following ingestion of the sustained-release formulation (400 mg), the mean peak plasma concentration was 299 μg/L at about 3 hours.[11,15] Maximum levels may be reached between 2 and 6 hours after ingestion.[13]

Distribution

An apparent volume of distribution in normal subjects is 3.6 L/kg.[15] There is little evidence to suggest a significant degree of plasma protein binding with pentoxifylline.

Elimination

The elimination half-life is about 0.93 hour after a 100-mg intravenous infusion. After oral administration of a sustained-release formulation of pentoxifylline, the terminal half-life is increased to 3.4 hours with an absolute bioavailability of 20%.[15,16] Pentoxifylline is metabolized in the liver to a number of inactive metabolites.[15] Less than 1% of the dose is excreted in the urine as unchanged compound. Metabolite I, a methylxanthine derivative, is assumed to be active.[14]

Drug Interactions

There have been reports of bleeding and/or prolonged prothrombin time when pentoxifylline is used with anticoagulants or drugs that inhibit platelet aggregation.[2] Clinically significant interactions have not occurred in patients receiving pentoxifylline concurrently with beta-adrenergic blocking agents, cardiac glycosides, diuretics, antidiabetic agents, and/or antiarrhythmic drugs.[2] Pentoxifylline and aspirin appear, in initial studies, to slow the progression of dementia due to cerebrovascular disease.[17] Pentoxifylline appeared to prevent cyclosporine-induced nephrotoxicity in animals.[18]

Pregnancy/Lactation

No systematic studies of pentoxifylline use by pregnant women have been performed. Pentoxifylline, similar to other methylxanthines, rapidly crosses into breast milk. The parent compound and metabolite are detectable 2 hours after administration to lactating females.[19] The quantities of pentoxifylline ingested by a nursing infant are unlikely to be of clinical significance.

Mechanism of Action

An exact mechanism of action in humans has not been determined. Studies suggest that pentoxifylline (1) increases red blood cell deformability, leading to increased blood flow and decreased whole blood viscosity; (2) increases prostacyclin release, which may decrease microcirculatory flow disturbance in sepsis[11]; (3) decreases adhesiveness of polymorphonuclear leukocytes in the endothelium, which may lead to an increase in tissue oxygenation[20]; (4) decreases endotoxin-induced synthesis of tumor necrosis factor (TNF), possibly the essential effector molecule in septic shock[21,22]; (5) inhibits platelet aggregation and increases white cord cell deformability[3]; (6) prevents an increase in pulmonary vascular permeability to protein induced by endotoxin[23]; (7) appears to modulate cachectic activity in cancer patients[24]; and (8) inhibits phosphodiesterase, leading to relaxation of the smooth muscle of the vascular wall.[14]

Clinical Presentation

The first signs and symptoms of overdose may be observed in 4 to 5 hours. Initially, overdose of pentoxifylline may induce gastrointestinal symptoms (eg, nausea, vomiting, and abdominal pain). At higher dose levels, hemodynamic instability (eg, hypotension, bradycardia, tachycardia) may be observed. Central nervous system changes (seizures preceded by somnolence and followed by coma and hypothermia) have been described.[14] Agitation, sleeplessness, mydriasis, and hyperthermia may be seen.[14]

Laboratory

Analytical Methods

High-performance liquid chromatography for pentoxifylline and its main metabolite (1-(5-hydroxylexyl-3,7-dimethylxanthine)) has a limit of detection of 5 ng/mL for both compounds.[25,26] A similar method (liquid chromatography) is useful for analyzing pentoxifylline and three of its metabolites in plasma and urine.[27]

Blood Levels

There is no evidence that blood levels are correlated with signs and symptoms after pentoxifylline poisoning.

Abnormalities

Liver function tests, renal function tests, coagulation parameters, blood sugar, uric acid, complete blood count, sedimentation rates, and platelet function are usually within normal limits. There may be an increase in basal insulinemia.[14] Blood calcium and magnesium levels may decrease.[14] The electrocardiogram is usually normal. After an overdose of 4000 to 6000 mg, bradycardia and first- and second-degree atrioventricular block (Mobitz type II) were observed.[13]

Treatment

Treatment is largely symptomatic and supportive and includes gastric evacuation, activated charcoal, correction of hypotension, and correction of dehydration. Care must be taken to protect the airway as seizures may occur. There is no antidote. Seizures may respond to benzodiazepines (diazepam). Vital signs, blood sugar, serum calcium and magnesium, and the electrocardiogram should be carefully monitored. Crystalloids may be administered through a central venous line. Atropine has been used for bradycardia.[13] Hemodialysis may be considered, but there is little experience with this modality in human poisoning. Signs and symptoms usually remit within 12 hours.

REFERENCES—PENTOXIFYLLINE

1. Reynolds JEF, ed. *Martindale: The Extra Pharmacopoeia.* 29th ed. London: Pharamceutical Press, 1989:1514–1515.
2. Pentoxifylline. In: McEvoy GK, ed. *AHFS Drug Information 92.* Bethesda, MD: American Society of Hospital Pharmacists, 1992:796–799.
3. Ambrus JL, Anain JM, Anain SM, et al. Dose–response effects of pentoxifylline on erythrocyte filterability: Clinical and animal model studies. Clin Pharmacol Ther 1990;48:50–56.
4. Radack K, Wyderski AJ. Conservative management of intermittent claudication. Ann Intern Med 1990;113:134–146.
5. Dannenhoffer MA, Rozek S. Pentoxifylline in sickle cell anemia. Drug Intell Clin Pharm 1987;21:620.
6. Cocci AMT, Waxman K, Soliman MH, et al. Pentoxifylline improves survival following hemorrhagic shock. Crit Care Med 1989;17:36–38.

7. Colgan M-P, Dormandy JA, Jones PW, et al. Oxpentifylline treatment of venous ulcers of the leg. Br Med J 1990;30: 972–975.
8. Ely H, Bard JW. Therapy of livedo vasculitis with pentoxifylline. Cutis 1988;42:448–453.
9. Cohen KL, Harris S. Pentoxifylline and diabetic neuropathy. Ann Intern Med 1987;107:600–601.
10. Garnier R, Riboulet-Delmas G, Chatenet T, Efthymiou ML. Acute pentoxifylline poisoning in children. Ann Pediatr (Paris) 1986;33:62–63.
11. Ward A, Clissold SP. Pentoxifylline: A review of its pharmacodynamic and pharmacokinetic properties and its therapeutic efficacy. Drugs 1987;34:50–97.
12. Szinajder IJ, Bentur Y, Taitelman U. First and second degree atrioventricular block in oxpentifylline overdose. Br Med J 1984;288:26.
13. Chatenet T. Bilan de sept annees d'observation de torentel (pentoxifylline) par le Centre Anti-Poisons de Paris These de Medecine. [Balance sheet of seven years of observation of Torental® (pentoxifylline) by the Paris Anti-Poison Center.] Paris: Anti-Poison Center, 1983.
14. Fischer JM. Hoechst-Roussel Pharmaceuticals, Somerville, NJ, personal communication, December 1, 1988.
15. Rames A, Poirier J-M, Le Coz F, et al. Pharmacokinetics of intravenous and oral pentoxifylline in healthy volunteers and in cirrhotic patients. Clin Pharmacol Ther 1990;47: 354–359.
16. Bearman B, Ings R, Mansky J, et al. Kinetics of intravenous and oral pentoxifylline in healthy subjects. Clin Pharmacol Ther 1985;37:25–28.
17. Barclay LL, Blass JP, Bondy DA. Pentoxifylline and aspirin in circulatory dementias. Clin Res 1989;37:527A.
18. Brunner LJ, Vadiei K, Iyer LV, Luke DR. Prevention of cyclosporine-induced nephrotoxicity with pentoxifylline. Renal Failure 1989;11:97–104.
19. Witter FR, Smith RV. The excretion of pentoxifylline and its metabolites into human breast milk. Am J Obstet Gynecol 1985;151:1094–1097.
20. Rao KMK, Somel DL, Crawford J, et al. Leukocyte function and blood viscosity in patients receiving pentoxifylline. Clin Res 1989;37:341A.
21. Sarina PSA. Pentoxifylline in septic shock. Postgrad Med J 1990;66:980–982.
22. Mandell GL. ARDS, neutrophils and pentoxifylline. Am Rev Respir Dis 1988;1103–1105.
23. Welsh CH, Lien D, Worthen S, Weil JV. Pentoxifylline decreases endotoxin-induced pulmonary neutrophil sequestration and extravascular protein accumulation in the dog. Am Rev Respir Dis 1988;138:1106–1114.
24. Deizube BJ, Fridovich-Keil JL, Bouvard I, et al. Pentoxifylline and well-being in patients with cancer. Lancet 1990; 335:662.
25. Grasela DM, Rocci M Jr. High performance liquid chromatographic analysis of pentoxifylline and 1-(5'-hydroxylexyl)-3, 7-dimethylxanthine in whole blood. J Chromatogr 1987;419: 368–379.
26. Garnier-Moiroux A, Poirier J-M, Cheymol G. High performance liquid chromatographic determination of pentoxifylline and its hydroxy metabolite in human plasma. J Chromatogr Biomed Appl 1987;416:183–188.
27. Lambert WE, Yousouf MA, Van Liedekerke BM, et al. Simultaneous determination of pentoxifylline and three metabolites in biological fluids by liquid chromatography. Clin Chem 1989;35:298–311.

Chapter 35
Lipid-Lowering Drugs

The lipid-lowering drugs are effective in lowering serum cholesterol levels,[1,2] but there are no convincing data indicating their ability to reduce cardiovascular morbidity or mortality.[3]

The hyperlipidemic agents that have been commonly employed throughout the world include the fibric acids (eg, clofibrate, gemfibrozil, fenfibrate, and bezafibrate) and the 3-hydroxy-3-methylglutaryl-coenzyme A (HMG-CoA) reductase-inhibiting drugs (eg, lovastatin, simvastatin, pravastatin, fluvastatin).[4] Probucol is also widely used. Other lipid-lowering drugs include nicotinic acid and its analogs and the omega-3 fatty acids.[5]

Chronic usage of these drugs may lead to gastrointestinal complaints, hepatotoxicity, skin rashes, myopathies, eye toxicity, depression, and sleep disturbance. Overdose may result in myalgias, chest pain, blurred vision, nausea, and diarrhca.[6] Treatment is largely symptomatic and supportive.

Source

Bezafibrate and probucol are synthetic chemicals. Lovastatin is a metabolite derived from the fungus *Aspergillus terreus.* Pravastatin is produced by microbial transformation of compactin by *Nocardia autotropica.* Simvastatin is a chemical derivative of lovastatin. Fluvastatin is a synthetic mevalonolactone derivative.

Therapeutic Dose

Bezafibrate	200 mg tid
Gemfibrozil	1000–1200 mg/d
Fluvastin	20–40 mg/d
Lovastatin	20–40 mg/d
Probucol	500 mg bid
Pravastatin	10–20 mg/d
Simvastatin	10–40 mg/d

Fatal Dose

Fatal doses have not been reported.

Toxicokinetics

The toxicokinetics of the lipid-lowering drugs are summarized in Table 35–1.[7–16] There is no correlation between

Table 35–1
Toxicokinetics of Lipid-Lowering Drugs

	Bezafibrate	Gemfibrozil	Lovastatin	Pravastatin	Simvastatin	Probucol	Fluvastatin
Bioavailability (%)	100	100	5	17–34		2–8	
Time to peak plasma concentration (h)	2	1–2	2–4	1–2	1–2.5		
Protein binding (%)	94–96	97	95	50	95		98
Volume of distribution (L/kg)	0.2			0.5			
Half-life (h)	2.1	7–8	2.9	1.3–2.6	2.5		0.5–0.8
Breast milk				Neglible		+ (animals)	
Crosses blood–brain barrier			Yes	No			No
Excreted in urine unchanged (%)		48*	10	80	13		6
Total clearance (mL/min/kg)				13.5†			
Renal clearance				6.3%			
Active metabolite					+		

*Todd PA, Ward A. Gemfibrozil: A review of its pharmacodynamics and pharmacokinetic properties, and therapeutic use in dyslipidaemia. Drugs 1988;36:314–339.
†Singvhi SM, Pan HY, Morrison RA, Willard DA. Disposition of pravastatin sodium, a tissue selective HMG-CoA reductase inhibitor in healthy subjects. Br J Clin Pharmacol 1990;29:239–243.

plasma levels of probucol and the degree of serum cholesterol reduction. Probucol accumulates in the adipose tissue and may persist there and in the circulation for more than 6 months. It is eliminated mainly in the bile and feces.[17]

Absorption

Lovastatin. Plasma concentration peaks within 2 to 4 hours. Only 5% of an oral dose reaches the circulation due to first-pass hepatic extraction.

Pravastatin. Mean peak plasma concentrations are 9.1 ng/mL after a single 10-mg dose, 26.5 ng/mL after 20 mg, and 45.8 ng/mL after up to 40 mg at steady state. Mean peak plasma concentrations are 6.1, 10.6, and 30.6 mg/mL after doses of 10, 70, and 40 mg. Mean time to reach peak plasma concentration after a single dose is 0.9 to 1.6 hours. Bioavailability is 12 to 34% due to a first-pass effect.[18]

Distribution

The apparent volume of distribution of pravastatin is 0.54 to 0.9 L/kg. Fifty percent of the drug is protein bound. Unlike lovastatin, pravastatin is not detected in the cerebrospinal fluid.[18]

Elimination

Metabolites of pravastatin have 2 to 10% of the potency of the parent drug. About 80% is excreted in 24 hours. The terminal elimination half-life is 1.3 to 2.6 hours; the corresponding value for its main metabolites is 0.8 to 1.3 hours. There are few changes in the presence of renal impairment.[19]

Drug Interactions

The fibric acid derivatives (eg, gemfibrozil) appear to potentiate the action of coumadin anticoagulants[5] because they bind extensively to plasma albumin, which displaces other acidic drugs (Table 35–2).[20,21] Simvastatin does not appear to potentiate anticoagulant status.[21] Lovastatin potentiates the effect of warfarin because it is strongly protein bound and may displace warfarin from its binding sites.[22] Myopathy with HMG-CoA reductase inhibition may be enhanced by concomitant use of cyclosporine, gemfibrozil, or niacin. Concurrent use of cimetidine, ranitidine, or omeprazil increases the serum concentration of fluvastatin. Concurrent use of rifampin increases clearance and decreases serum concentrations.

Pravastatin does not induce hepatic metabolizing enzymes.[11] Cholestyramine decreases the bioavailability of pravastatin,[23] but may enhance its lipid-lowering effect.[11]

Pregnancy/Lactation

Lovastatin has been placed in Pregnancy Category X: "Studies in animals or human beings have demonstrated fetal abnormalities" and "the drug is contraindicated in women who are or may become pregnant.[24] An anecdotal report suggests congenital abnormalities in an infant whose mother received lovastatin in the first trimester of pregnancy.[24]

Negligible amounts of pravastatin are found in breast milk.[18]

Mechanism of Action

Lipid-lowering drugs are competitive inhibitors of HMG-CoA reductase, which catalyzes the conversion of HMG-CoA to mevalonate. They act primarily in the liver, where they reduce cholesterol synthesis. This, in turn, increases the number of hepatic low-density lipoprotein receptors, resulting in an overall decrease in total blood cholesterol, low-density lipoproteins, triglycerides, and very low density lipoprotein cholesterol.[8]

Clinical Presentation
Chronic Use

Therapeutic adverse effects seen with the lipid lowering drugs include headache, abdominal pain, diarrhea, nausea, fatigue, rash, myopathy, hepatotoxicity, depression, eye toxicity, paresthesias and neuropathy, and pancreatitis (Table 35–3). Bezafibrate may also induce loss of libido, headache, and rash or pruritus.[5] Bezafibrate is related structurally to clofibrate and has also been associated with cholelithiasis, a disorder frequently observed with hyperlipoproteinemia.[25]

Two large trials suggested an increased incidence of malignant disease, particularly of the liver, gallbladder, and rectum, and an increased incidence of ectopic ventricular activity, angina, and intermittent claudication with clofibrate. Its clinical use has diminished.[3]

Long-term treatment with HMG-CoA reductase inhibitors including lovastatin and simvastatin is a potential cause of drug-induced lupus syndrome. Antinuclear antibodies are positive in a homogenous pattern; anti-DNA antibodies, anti-smooth muscle antibodies, and antiribonucleotide protein antibodies are negative.[22,26]

Transient symptomatic hypotension[27] and nephrotoxicity evidenced by a selective glomerular-type proteinuria have been observed after long-term treatment with simvastatin.[21]

No cataractogenesis has been observed with pravastatin, simvastatin, or lovastatin.[18,28]

Paresthesias and neuropathies have been described after use of simvastatin and gemfibrozil.[29]

Skeletal muscle toxicity (myalgia, creatine phosphokinase levels more than 10 times the upper normal limit) is

Table 35–2
Antihyperlipidemic Drug Interactions

Antihyperlipidemic Agent	Manifestations of Drug Interaction	Interactive Agents
Bile acid sequestrants (cholestyramine, colestipol)	Binding and decreased absorption of interactive agents	Thiazide diuretics, digitalis glycosides, beta-blockers, coumarin anticoagulants (warfarin), thyroid hormones, fibric acid derivatives, oral antihyperglycemic agents (sulfonylureas)
Nicotinic acid	Increased concentration of nicotinic acid in the circulation	Aspirin (high dosage)
	Decreased efficacy of interactive agents	Uricosuric agents (sulfinpyrazone)
	Hepatocellular necrosis	Drugs that adversely affect hepatic structure or function
	Elevations in liver enzymes; possible muscle necrosis	HMG-CoA reductase inhibitors
HMG-CoA reductase inhibitors (fluvastatin, lovastatin, pravastatin, simvastatin)	Rhabdomyolysis	Cyclosporin, prednisone, fibric acid derivatives, erythromycin
	Elevations in liver enzymes; possible muscle necrosis	Nicotinic acid
Fibric acid derivatives (bezafibrate, ciprofibrate, clofibrate, fenofibrate, gemfibrozil)	Binding and decreased absorption of fibrates	Bile acid sequestrants
	Rhabdomyolysis	HMG-CoA reductase inhibitors
	Increased anticoagulant activity	Warfarin
Probucol	Possible amplification of HDL cholesterol reduction	Androgens, progestins, beta blockers, other HDL cholesterol-lowering agents
	Possible amplification of QT_c prolongation	Group IA antiarrhythmic agents (quinidine, procainamide, disopyramide), tricyclic antidepressants, phenothiazines

HMG-CoA, 3-hydroxy-3-methylglutaryl-coenzyme A; HDL, high-density lipoprotein.
From Farmer JA, Gotto AM Jr. Antihyperlipidaemic agents: Drug interactions of clinical significance. Drug Saf 1994;11:301–309.

Table 35–3
Adverse Reactions With Chronic Use of Lipid-Lowering Drugs

	Gastrointestinal Effects	Myopathy	Hepatotoxicity	Rash	Impotence	Depression	Eye Toxicity	Paresthesias and Neuropathy
Gemfibrozil		+[50]			+[42]			+
Bezafibrate	+[51]	+						
Fenofibrate	++							
Lovastatin	+++	+[52,53]	+[46,47]				0 to +[48,49]	
Pravastatin		+	+	++		+[41]	++	
Probucol	+							
Simvastatin	+	+	+		+	+		+

rarely observed when the HMG-CoA reductase inhibitors are administered alone, but is increased in patients also receiving cyclosporine or fibric acid derivatives.[18]

Lovastatin is associated with significant myopathy when ingested in conjunction with cyclosporine, fibric acid derivatives, niacin, or erythromycin.[23] Some patients who have received lovastatin in combination with gemfibrozil, niacin, or cyclosporine have developed a clinical rhabdomyolysis.[9]

Minor transient increases in laboratory indices or hepatic function have been observed with long-term pravastatin treatment.

Acipimox. Acipimox is chemically related to nicotinic acid and has been used in hypertriglyceridemic states at a dose of 250 mg three times daily. It is readily absorbed from the gastrointestional tract. Plasma concentration peaks within 2 hours. It does not bind to plasma proteins. The plasma half-life is about 2 hours. Acipimox is not significantly metabolized and is excreted in the urine unchanged. Most adverse reactions reported have included transient flushing and mild gastrointestional disturbances. Both nicotinic acid and acipimox appear to exert at least some of their actions by inhibiting fat store lipolysis and reducing fasting plasma free fatty acid levels, limiting very low density lipoprotein synthesis. Acipimox is synergistic with cholestyramine as a lipid-lowering agents.[34,35]

Overdose

Probucol. A 15-kg 3-year-old boy ingested 5 g of probucol. This was followed by a brief episode of diarrhea. The child remained well.[30]

Gemfibrozil. A 7-year-old child accidentally ingested 7.5 to 9.0 g of gemfibrozil (Lopid), which resulted in one episode of vomiting. The child was otherwise asymptomatic.

A 47-year-old man intentionally ingested 3.6 g of gemfibrozil in addition to 6 tablets of paracetamol, 6 tablets of isosorbide mononitrate, and an unspecified amount of ethanol. This patient was hospitalized for 2 days and suffered no ill effects. A 21-year-old man intentionally ingested 12 to 15 g of gemfibrozil with an unspecified amount of ethanol. This patient developed generalized myalgias, pleuritic chest pain, blurred vision, nausea, and diarrhea. He was hospitalized and these symptoms resolved within 24 hours.[6]

Lovastatin. A review of the medical literature has failed to identify any reports of an overdose with lovastatin; however, five healthy human volunteers have received up to 200 mg of lovastatin as a single dose without clinical significant adverse experiences. A few cases of accidental overdose have been reported; no patients had any specific symptoms, and all patients recovered without sequelae. The maximum dose taken was 52, 20-mg tablets (1.04 g).[31]

Laboratory

Analytical Methods

Bezafibrate. A gas chromatography method for plasma determination has a lower limit of detection of 0.2 μg/mL.[16]

Gemfibrozil. Plasma and urine concentrations of gemfibrozil and its metabolites have been assayed by both gas and liquid chromatography.[32,33] Limits of detection are 0.5 μg/mL for the gas chromatographic assay in plasma and 5 μg/mL for that in urine. For the high-performance liquid chromatography method, the limit of detection is 50 ng/mL.

Lovastatin. A reverse-phase high-pressure liquid chromatography assay is available for lovastatin and its metabolite in plasma and bile.[36]

Pravastatin. A useful assay procedure depends on extraction and purification of the drug or its metabolites with C_{18} disposable solid-phase columns. After derivatization, pravastatin and its metabolites are quantified by capillary gas chromatography–mass spectrometry with a limit of sensitivity of 0.5 ng/mL.[37] A thin layer radiochromatography assay has detection limits of 4.3 ng/mL and 0.3 μg/mL for plasma and urine, respectively.[10]

Probucol. An automated high-performance liquid chromatography method is available for determination of probucol in plasma and lipoprotein fractions.[38]

Fluvastatin. Blood and plasma concentrations may be determined with high-performance liquid chromatography and fluorescence detection, a method whose limit of quantitation is 1 to 2 ng/mL.[39]

Abnormalities

Elevations in hepatic function tests (eg, alkaline phosphatase, transaminases) and creatine kinase have been observed after therapeutic doses.[4] Prolongation of the QT interval with polymorphic ventricular tachycardia (Torsade de pointes) has followed use of probucol.[40,41]

Treatment

Stabilization

Treatment of overdose with lipid-lowering drugs is largely symptomatic and supportive.

Antidote

There is no antidote for probucol, the fibric acid agents, or the HMG-CoA inhibitors.

Supportive Measures

Torsade de pointes following probucol use has responded to propranolol.[42,43] (See also Chapter 32.) Persons who have overdosed on HMG-CoA inhibitors should be observed for symptoms suggestive of a myopathy (muscle tenderness, weakness or pain), rhabdomyolysis (darkened urine), or hepatotoxicity (anorexia, abdominal pain, jaundice). Serum transaminase levels should be checked periodically. Initial and follow-up ophthalmologic examinations for lens opacities may be indicated in the long-term user. For lovastatin, pravastatin, and simvastatin overdoses,

Table 35–4
Various Drugs Reported to Affect Lipoprotein Levels

Agents	Total Cholesterol	LDL	HDL	VLDL	Triglyceride
Amiodarone	↑	–	–	–	↑
Antacid	↓	↓	↓ –	–	–
Aspirin	–	–	–	–	↓ –
Biguanides	↓	↓	–	–	↓
Cimetidine*/ranitidine	–	–	↑ –	–	–
Interferons	↓	↓	↓	↑	↑
Ketoconazole (high dose)	↓	↓	–	–	–
Neomycin	↓	↓	–	–	–
Nicotinic acid/nicotinamide†	–	↓	↑	–	↓

LDL, low-density lipoprotein; HDL, high-density lipoprotein; VLDL, very-low-density lipoprotein; dashes, no substantial change, inconsistent results, or insufficient data; up arrow, increase; down arrow, decrease.
*Only cimetidine showed increased high-density lipoprotein levels in some studies.
†When used as a vitamin or as the amide derivative (nicotinamide), nicotinic acid has little effect on lipoprotein levels; however, in pharmacologic doses, niacin increases high-density lipoprotein levels and reduces low-density lipoprotein and triglyceride levels.
From Henkin Y, Como JA, Oberman A. Secondary dyslipidemia: Inadvertent effects of drugs in clinical practice. JAMA 1992;267:961–968.

supportive and symptomatic treatment remains the mainstay of management. Other drugs reported to alter lipoprotein values are summarized in Table 35–4.[44]

REFERENCES

1. Walker JF, Shapiro DR. Hydroxymethylglutaryl coenzyme A reductase inhibitors as monotherapy in the treatment of hypercholesterolemia. Am J Cardiol 1990;65:19F–22F.
2. Maker VMG, Thompson GR. HMG CoA reductase inhibitors as lipid-lowering agents: Five years experience with lovastatin and an appraisal of simvastatin and pravastatin. Q J Med 1990;74:165–175.
3. Dunnigan MG. Should clofibrate still be prescribed? Further trials with harder end points are needed for all lipid-lowering drugs. Br Med J 1992;205:379–380.
4. Krukemyer JJ, Talbert RL. Lovastatin: a new cholesterol-lowering agent. Pharmacotherapy 1987;7:198–210.
5. Smellie WAS, Lorimer AR. Adverse effects of the lipid-lowering drugs. Adverse Drug React Toxicol Rev 1992;11:71–92.
6. Boselli BA. Parke-Davis, personal communication, March 1991.
7. Pan HY. Clinical pharmacology of pravastatin, a selective inhibitor of HMG-CoA reductase. Eur J Clin Pharmacol 1991;40(suppl. 1):515–518.
8. Henwood JM, Heel RC. Lovastatin: A preliminary review of its pharmacodynamic properties and therapeutic use in hyperlipidaemia. Drugs 1988;36:429–454.
9. Grundy SM. HMG-CoA reductase inhibitors for treatment of hypercholesterolemia. N Engl J Med 1988;319:24–32.
10. Singhvi SM, Pan HY, Morrison RA, Willard DA. Disposition of pravastatin sodium, a tissue selective HMG-CoA reductase inhibitor in healthy subjects. Br J Clin Pharmacol 1990; 29:239–243.
11. Pan HY, de Vault AR, Swites BJ, et al. Pharmacokinetics and pharmacodynamics of pravastatin alone and with cholestyramine in hypercholesterolemia. Clin Pharmacol Ther 1990;48:201–207.
12. Pravastatin and simvastatin for hypercholesterolemia. Med Lett Drugs Ther 1991;33(830):18–20.
13. Mauro VF, MacDonald JL. Simvastatin: A review of its pharmacology and clinical use. DICP Ann Pharmacother 1991;25: 257–264.
14. Pentikainen PJ, Saraheimo M, Schwartz JI, et al. Comparative pharmacokinetics of lovastatin, simvastatin, pravastatin in humans. J Clin Pharmacol 1992;32:136–140.
15. Endele R. A gas chromatographic method for the determination of bezafibrate in serum and urine. J Chromatogr 1978; 154:261–263.
16. Okerholm RA, Keeley FJ, Peterson FE, Glazko AJ. The metabolism of gemfibrozil. Proc R Soc Med 1976;69(suppl. 2):11–14.
17. Zimetbaum P, Eder H, Frishman W. Probucol: Pharmacology and clinical application. J Clin Pharmacol 1990;30:3–9.
18. McTavish D, Sorkin EM. Pravastatin: A review of its pharmacological properties and therapeutic potential in hypercholesterolemia. Drugs 1991;42:65–89.
19. Halstenson CE, Triscari J, de Vault A, et al: Single dose pharmacokinetics of pravastatin and metabolites in patients with renal impairment. J Clin Pharmacol 1992;32: 124–132.
20. Farmer JA, Gotto AA Jr. Antihyperlipidaemia agents: Drug interactions of clinical significance. Drug Saf 1994;11: 301–309.
21. Gaw A, Wosornu D. Simvastatin during warfarin therapy in hyperlipoproteinemia. Lancet 1992;340:979–980.
22. Ahmad S. Lovastatin-induced lupus erythematosus. Arch Intern Med 1991;151:1667–1668.
23. Broisman L, Englster P, Chow MSS. Focus on pravastatin, an HMG-CoA reductase inhibitor for the treatment of hypercholesterolemia. Hosp Formul 1991;76:552–563.
24. Ghidini A, Sicherer S, Willner J. Congenital abnormalities/ (VATER) in baby born to mother using lovastatin. Lancet 1992;339:1416–1417.
25. Armstrong K, Kelly AJ. Bezafibrate and cholelithiasis. Eur J Gastroenterol Hepatol 1993;5:665.
26. Bannwarth B, Miremont G, Papapietro P-M. Lupus-like syndrome associated with simvastatin. Arch Intern Med 1992; 152:1093.
27. French J, White H. Transient symptomatic hypotension in patients on simvastatin. Lancet 1989;2:807–808.
28. Deslypere JP, Delanghe J, Vermeulen A. Proteinuria as complication of simvastatin treatment. Lancet 1990;336: 1093.
29. Paresthesias and neuropathy with hypolipidemic agents. Aust Adverse Drug React Bull 1993;12(2):6.
30. Probucol (Lorelco[R]): Product literature. Merrell Dow, November 1985.
31. Milander JH. Merck Sharp Dohme, personal communication, January 1989.
32. Randinitis E, Kirkel AW, Nelson C, Parker TD. Gas chromatographic determination of gemfibrozil and its metabolites in plasma and urine. J Chromatogr 1984;307: 210–215.
33. Hengy H, Kolle V. Determination of gemfibrozil in plasma by high performance liquid chromatography. Arzneimittelforschung 1985;35:1637–1639.
34. Lavazzari M, Milanesi G, Oggioni E, Pamparana F. Results of a phase IV study carried out with acipimox in type II dia-

betic patients with concomitant hyperlipoproteinemia. J Int Med Res 1989;17:373–380.
35. Series JJ, Gaw A, Kilday C, et al. Acipimox in combination with low dose cholestyramine for the treatment of type II hyperlipidaemia. Br J Clin Pharmacol 1990;30:49–54.
36. Stubbs RJ, Schwartz M, Bayne WM. Determination of mevinolin and merivolinic acid in plasma and bile by reverse phase HPLC. J Chromatogr 1986;383:438–443.
37. Fimke PT, Ivashkir E, Arnold HE, Cohen AI. Determination of pravastatin sodium and its major metabolites in human serum/plasma by capillary gas chromatography/negative ion chemical ionization mass spectrometry. Biomed Environ Mass Spectrom 1989;18:949–959.
38. Schoneshofer M, Heilmann P, Schwab L, Schwartzkopff W. Automatic column liquid chromatographic determination of probucol in human serum and lipoprotein fraction. J Chromatogr 1989;49:230–235.
39. Smith HT, Jokabaitis LA, Troendle AJ, et al: Pharmacokinetics of fluvastatin and specific drug interaction. Am Hypotension 1993;6:375S–382S.
40. Pirarro S, Bargoy V, D'Agostin P. Gemfibrozil-induced impotence. Lancet 1990;336:155.
41. Ohya Y, Kumamoto K, Trubota Y, Fujishima M. Factors related to QT interval prolongation during probucol treatment. Eur J Clin Pharmacol 1993;345:47–52.
42. Kajinami K, Takekoshi M, Mabuchi H. Propranolol for probucol-induced QT prolongation with polymorphic ventricular tachycardia. Lancet 1993;34:124–125.
43. Gohn DC, Simmons TW. Polymorphic ventricular tachycardia (Torsade de pointes) associated with the use of probucol. N Engl J Med 1992;326:1435–1436.
44. Henkin Y, Como JA, Oberman A. Secondary dyslipidemia: Inadvertent effects of drugs in clinical practice. JAMA 1992;267:961–968.

Chapter 36
Anticonvulsants

INTRODUCTION

Commonly used anticonvulsants in children are summarized in Table 36–1.[1] Dosages of anticonvulsant drugs used in the treatment of seizures are listed in Table 36–2.

Major problems associated with poisoning by the antiepileptic drugs include the anticonvulsant hypersensitivity syndrome and undesirable effects observed during and after pregnancy. Characteristics of conventional and new anticonvulsants are listed in Table 36–3. French has compared the toxicokinetics of common antiepileptic drugs (Table 36–4).[1]

Table 36–5 outlines plasma concentrations that may be associated with severe anticonvulsant poisoning. Patients must be treated on the basis of clinical rather than biochemical findings. Data for some of these concentrations are sparse.[2]

THE ANTICONVULSANT HYPERSENSITIVITY SYNDROME

Phenytoin, carbamazepine, primidone, and phenobarbital can all produce an identical, multisystem hypersensitivity reaction. The onset of the reaction is usually between 4 weeks and 3 months of starting the drug, with a more rapid onset on challenge. A patient who develops the syndrome with one anticonvulsant may develop it with other drugs, even though the drugs may be pharmacologically distinct.[3,4]

The initial features are mucocutaneous eruptions and fever. The cutaneous eruptions include morbilliform rashes, erythema multiforme, exfoliative dermatitis, and toxic epidermal necrolysis. Facial edema has been observed. Mucosal involvement includes a conjunctivitis with scarring and synechiae. Lymphadenopathy, hepatitis, eosinophilia, and lymphocytosis are frequently observed. Nephritis, bone marrow suppression, pneumonitis, and myopathy have been reported.

The initial step in management is discontinuation of the causative agent. The reaction appears to resolve quickly after initiation of prednisolone. Treatment otherwise is symptomatic and supportive.[5]

Table 36–1
Commonly Used Anticonvulsants in Children

Drug	Indications	Starting Dose (mg/kg per 24 h)	Target Dose for Initial Assessment of Effect (mg/kg per 24 h)	Incremental Dose		Usually Effective Dose (mg/kg per 24 h)	Frequency of Dosing (times per 24 h)	Target Range (mg/L; μmol/L)
				Size (mg/kg per 24 h)	Interval (d)			
Carbamazepine	Partial and generalized tonic–clonic seizures	5	12.5	2.5	7	10–25	2 or 3	4–10; 17–42
Clobazam	Adjunctive therapy in refractory epilepsy	0.25	0.25	0.125	15	0.25–0.5	2 or 3	Not helpful
Clonazepam	Myoclonic epilepsy; Lennox–Gastaut syndrome; infantile spasms; status epilepticus	0.025	0.05	0.025	7	0.025–0.1	2 or 3	Not helpful
Diazepam	Status epilepticus		—	—	—	—	—	—
Ethosuximide	Generalized absence	10	15	5	5	15–40	1	40–100; 280–700
Phenobarbital	Generalized tonic–clonic seizures; newborn seizures; febrile seizures; status epilepticus	4	6	2	10	4–9	1	10–35; 40–80
Phenytoin	Generalized tonic–clonic seizures; partial seizures; status epilepticus	5	7	1	10	5–9	1 or 2	10–20; 40–80
Sodium valproate	Generalized tonic–clonic seizures; generalized absence; myoclonic epilepsy; febrile seizures	10	20	10	10	15–40	1 or 2	Not helpful

From Rylance GW. Treatment of epilepsy and febrile convulsions in children. Lancet 1990;336:488–491.

Table 36–2
Treatment of Seizures

Seizure Disorder	Drugs	Usual Daily Dosage Adults (mg)	Usual Daily Dosage Children (mg/kg)	Usual Therapeutic Serum Concentration* (μg/mL)
Primary Generalized Tonic–Clonic (Grand Mal)				
Drugs of choice	Valproate†	1000–3000	15–60	50–120
	or Carbamazepine	800–1600‡	10–30	6–12§
	or Phenytoin	300–400‖	4–8	10–20 μg/ml
Alternatives	Lamotrigine	100–500	Not approved	Not established
	Primidone	750–1250	10–20	6–12
	Phenobarbital	90–150	2–5	15–35
Partial, Including Secondarily Generalized				
Drugs of choice:	Carbamazepine	800–1600‡	10–30	6–12§
	or Phenytoin	300–400‖	4–8	10–20
	or Valproate†	1000–3000	15–60	50–120
Alternatives	Primidone	750–1200#	10–20	6–12
	Phenobarbital	90–150	2–5	15–35
	Lamotrigine (as adjunct)	100–500	Not approved	Not established
	Gabapentin (as adjunct)	900–2400¶	Not approved	Not established
Absence *(Petit Mal)*				
Drugs of choice	Ethosuximide	750–1250	20–40	40–100
	or Valproate	1000–3000	15–60	50–120
Alternatives	Clonazepam	1.5–20	0.05–0.2	20–80 ng/mL
	Lamotrigine	100–500	Not approved	Not established
Atypical Absence, Myoclonic, Atonic				
Drug of choice	Valproate†	1000–3000	15–60	50–120
Alternatives	Clonazepam	1.5–20	0.05–0.2	20–80 ng/mL
	Felbamate (as adjunct)	1200–3600	15–60	Not established

*Some patients obtain complete seizure control at lower concentrations, and occasional patients need higher concentrations. Serum concentrations may be altered by concurrent use of other drugs.
†Not FDA-approved unless absence is involved.
‡Intolerance to carbamazepine can often be avoided by starting with 100 to 200 mg bid and increasing the dosage at weekly intervals in increments of 100 to 200 mg/d, up to the usual maintenance dosage.
§Monitoring serum concentrations of carbamazepine alone may occasionally be misleading because the assay does not account for an active metabolite, carbamazepine-10, 11-epoxide, which contributes to antiepileptic activity and also causes toxic effects. Serum measurements of the active metabolite are available but may be too expensive for routine use.
‖Adjustments in dosage above 300 mg/d for adults should usually be made in 25- or 30-mg increments because of saturation kinetics.
#Start with 50–100 mg daily and increase gradually 2- to 3-day intervals.
¶Start with a dose of 300 mg once or twice daily and increase rapidly up to maintenance dosage.
From Drugs for epilepsy. Med Lett 1995;37(947):37–40.

Table 36–3
Conventional and New Antiepileptic Drugs

Generic Name	Trade Name	Indications (Seizure Types)	Typical Dose (mg/d)	Half-life (h)	% Bound	Most Common Side Effects
Phenytoin	Dilantin	Partial with or without seizure generalization; generalized tonic–clonic*	300–400	24–30	90	Gum hyperplasia, hirsutism
Carbamazepine	Tegretol	Partial with or without seizure generalization; generalized tonic–clonic*	600–1200	8–12	75	Neutropenia, rash, hyponatremia
Phenobarbital	Luminal	Partial with or without seizure generalization; generalized tonic–clonic*	60–120	72	50	Behavioral changes
Divalproex sodium (valproate)	Depakote	Partial with or without seizure generalization; generalized tonic–clonic; absence, myoclonic*	750–3000	6–12	90–95	Weight gain, hair loss, GI complaints
Felbamate	Felbatol	Partial with or without seizure generalization; generalized tonic–clonic; absence; myoclonic*	2400–3600	20–24	25	Insomnia, weight loss, GI complaints
Gabapentin	Neurontin	Partial with or without seizure generalization in patients >12	900–1800	5–6	0	Somnolence, dizziness
Lamotrigine	Lamictal	Pending†	300–700	24‡	55	Rash, dizziness
Vigabatrin	Sabril	Pending†	3000–4000	NA§	0	Drowsiness, irritability

GI, gastrointestinal; NA, not applicable.
*Approved for use as monotherapy.
†Probably will be approved with indications similar to those for gabapentin.
‡Excretion half-life increases to about 72 h with concomitant administration of valproate and decreases to about 13 h when used with hepatic enzyme-inducing medications.
§Excretion half-life is not equal to pharmacodynamic half-life.
From Laxer KD. Treating epilepsy. West J Med 1994;161:309–319.

Table 36–4
Pharmacokinetics of Common Antiepileptic Drugs

Drug	Plasma Half-life (h)	Therapeutic Range (µg/mL)	Special Pharmacokinetic Issues
Phenytoin	Dose dependent	5–20	90% protein bound; only free fraction is active; may be displaced by other drugs; at mid–high therapeutic levels, enters zero-order kinetics, and serum level may rise rapidly
Carbamazepine	18–54 (initial); 10–20 (after chronic administration)*	4–12	Induces its own metabolism; dose needs to be increased after initiation of therapy; half-life variable from one individual to another
Phenobarbital	53–140	15–40	Extremely long half-life permits once-a-day dosing
Primidone	5–15	5–12	Metabolized to phenobarbital: primidone and phenobarbital levels need to be monitored; coadminstration of enzyme-inducing drugs may increase phenobarbital levels
Sodium valproate	5 to 20	50–150	Plasma half-life may not reflect central nervous system half-life; steady serum levels not as important
Ethosuximide	30 (children 7–9 y) 60 (adults)	40–100 40–60 (adults)	Half-life twice as long in adults as children
Clorazepate	18–60	20–80 mg/mL	Rapid withdrawal may precipitate convulsions or status epilepticus

*Undergoes autoinduction.
From French J. The long-term therapeutic management of epilepsy. Ann Intern Med 1994;120:411–422.

Table 36–5
Plasma Level Interpretation

Anticonvulsant	Therapeutic Concentration		Concentration That May Be Associated With Severe Toxicity	
	µmol/L	mg/L	µmol/L	(mg/L)
Carbamazepine	<40	<10	200	50
Ethosuximide	<750	<100	1750	250
Phenobarbital	<180	<40	450	100
Phenytoin	<80	<20	160	40
Primidone*	<50	<12	225	50*
Valproic acid	<700	<100	1000	140

*Phenobarbital should also be measured.
Adapted from Yersky MS, Friel RN, McCormick K. Antiepileptic drug disposition during pregnancy. Neurology 192;42(suppl. 5):12–16.

PREGNANCY

There is an increased incidence of congenital malformations in children born to epileptic women who have taken an anticonvulsant drug during pregnancy. If a mother has epilepsy and is taking anticonvulsant drugs, her chance of having a child with a major congenital abnormality is just over 6%. Several studies suggest that abnormalities are more likely if more than one anticonvulsant is used or if particularly large doses are taken.[6]

PARADOXICAL INTOXICATION

"Paradoxical intoxication" may follow the use of an anticonvulsant agent that, at blood levels generally above the "therapeutic" range, induce seizures without the prior presence of the usually dose-related side effects.

SEIZURE EXACERBATION

Exacerbation of seizures in adults and children may follow treatment with phenytoin, carbamazepine, benzodiazepines, and vigabatrin.[7,8]

TREATMENT

Overdose with both the classic and the newer anticonvulsant drugs generally responds to supportive and symptomatic management. There are no antidotes. Extracorporeal methods of elimination are not usually clinically effective.

REFERENCES—ANTICONVULSANTS

1. French J. The long-term therapeutic management of epilepsy. Ann Intern Mod 1994;120.411-422.
2. Morrow JI, Routledge PA. Poisoning by anticonvulsants. Adverse Drug React Acute Poison Rev 1989;8(2):97-109.
3. Alldredge BK, Knutsen AP, Ferriero D. Antiepileptic drug hypersensitivity syndrome: In vitro and clinical observations. Pediatr Neurol 1994;10:169-171.
4. Scerri L, Shall L, Zaki I. Carbamazepine-induced anticonvulsant hypersensitivity syndrome: Pathogenic and diagnostic considerations. Clin Exp Dermatol 1993;18:540-542.
5. Handfield-Jones SE, Jankins RE, Whittaker SJ, et al. The anticonvulsant hypersensitivity syndrome. Br J Dermatol 1993;129:175-177.
6. Meadow R. Anticonvulsants in pregnancy. Arch Dis Child 1991;66:62-65.
7. De Krom MCTFM, Verduin N, Visser E, et al. Three cases with status epilepticus during vigabatrin treatment. J Neurol Neurosurg Psychiatry 1994;57:1294-1295.
8. Liporace JD, Sperling MP, Dichter MA. Absence seizures and carbamazepine in adults. Epilepsia 1994;35:1026-1028.

CARBAMAZEPINE

Overdoses are not frequent and seldom fatal. Supportive measures and charcoal hemoperfusion have been useful in treatment. Overdoses with carbamazepine may, because of slow absorption, lead to delayed onset of coma with compromise of respiration. There is no antidote. Carbamazepine, like meprobamate, may lead to gastric mass formation.[1] Common toxic effects include neurologic abnormalities (eg, ataxia, seizures, coma), cardiorespiratory problems (eg, dysrhythmias, conduction disorders, respiratory depression), and eye abnormalities such as nystagmus and ophthalmoplegia.[2]

Structure and Classification

Carbamazepine (Tegretol) is chemically and stereospatially related to the tricyclic antidepressants and is also spatially similar to phenytoin. In overdose, many of the effects of carbamazepine are shared by the tricyclic antidepressants and phenytoin.

Toxicokinetics[3–14]

Time to peak plasma level	6–24 hours
Volume of distribution	1–2 L/kg
Plasma protein binding	75–80%
Elimination half-life	8–13 hours
Excreted unchanged	23%

Drug Interactions

Fluoxetine may inhibit the metabolism of carbamazepine and its epoxide metabolite.[15] Erythromycin can inhibit the hepatic metabolism of carbamazepine, resulting in carbamazepine toxicity.[16] Dextropropoxyphene, isoniazid, and calcium channel blockers[2] increase the serum carbamazepine concentration.[17] Carbamazepine may reduce effective blood levels of drugs metabolized by the hepatic microsomal P450 oxidative system such as phenytoin, haloperidol, clonazepam, and alprazolam.[18]

Pregnancy/Lactation

Teratogenic Effects. Malformations have been described in infants born to mothers taking carbamazepine alone. These include spina bifida (in 1% of cases),[19] congenital heart disease, diaphragmatic hernia, and digital hypoplasia and hydronephrosis.[19] Growth retardation, facial abnormalities (eg, prominent forehead, palpebral fissures slanted downward, flat nasal bridge, anteverted nostrils), and developmental delay have been observed.[20,21] The metabolite of carbamazepine, an epoxide, may be mutagenic. A retrospective and prospective study after exposure to carbamazepine in utero disclosed the familiar pattern of minor craniofacial defects, fingernail hypoplasia, and neurodevelopmental delay that has been reported in the past with other anticonvulsant drugs.[21] This study awaits confirmation. There have been methodologic problems with the report.[22]

Neonates. Cholestatic hepatitis may develop in infants of mothers receiving carbamazepine during pregnancy or nursing.[23]

Clinical Presentation

Overdose

Neurologic Effects. Study of a series of carbamazepine overdose patients suggests four clinically distinct stages: (I) coma, seizures (carbamazepine levels > 25 μg/mL [105 μmol/L]); (II) combativeness, hallucinations, choreiform movements (15–25 μg/mL [65–105 μmol/L]); (III) drowsiness, ataxia (11–15 μg/mL [45–65 μmol/L]); (IV) potentially catastrophic relapse (< 11 μg/mL [45 μmol/L]).[24]

Cardiovascular Effects. Carbamazepine exhibits class I antiarrhythmic properties. Kasarskis and colleagues define two forms of carbamazepine-associated cardiac dysfunction. One group developed sinus tachycardias in the setting of a massive carbamazepine overdose. The second group, mostly elderly women, developed life-threatening bradyarrhythmias or atrioventricular conduction delay, associated with either therapeutic or modestly elevated carbamazepine serum levels.[25] Ingestion of 10 g of carbamazepine by an adult led to T-wave flattening after 12 hours and T-wave inversion after 4 days; the patient survived.[26]

Respiratory Effects. Respiratory depression, irregular respirations, or apnea may occur within the first 24 hours. Pulmonary edema may occur.[27,28]

Fatalities. Death may result from severe cardiovascular effects, aspiration pneumonitis, severe hepatitis, or aplastic anemia.[29,30] These complications have also been seen after chronic therapeutic use.

Chronic Use

Adverse effects of carbamazepine use may include neutropenia, thrombocytopenia, skin rashes, water intoxication, inappropriate secretion of antidiuretic hormone, hyponatremia,[31] ataxia, lupus syndrome, hepatitis, and aplastic anemia, which may be fatal.[32] Tourette's syndrome may be exacerbated by carbamazepine at therapeutic levels.[33]

Renal Effects. Acute tubular necrosis has been reported.[34] Carbamazepine may rarely induce antinuclear antibodies and a systemic lupus erythematosus-like syndrome.[35]

Pseudolymphoma Syndrome. A pseudolymphoma syndrome similar to that following phenytoin use may occur with carbamazepine. The clinical features are lymphadenopathy, fever, rash, and, less commonly, hepatosplenomegaly and eosinophilia. The syndrome occurs between 4 and 30 days after first exposure to the drug. No instances of progression to malignant lymphoma have been reported.[36,37]

Laboratory

Analytical Methods

The Acculevel carbamazepine therapeutic drug monitoring test is an in-office noninstrumented whole blood test whose limit of sensitivity is 2 μg/mL.[38] Blood is obtained by fingerstick (12 μL) and mixed with a reagent. A plastic cassette containing a chromatographic paper strip is used to read the plasma carbamazepine level.

Therapeutic plasma levels of carbamazepine range from 6 to 8 mg/L (25–34 μmol/L). Ataxia and nystagmus may occur at levels exceeding 10 mg/L (42 μmol/L).[2]

In overdose, peak serum concentrations have ranged from 18 to 70 μg/mL (78–285 μmol/L). Serum carbamazepine levels equal to or above 40 μg/mL (170 μmol/L) are associated with an increased risk of serious complications such as coma, seizures, respiratory failure, and cardiac conduction defects.[39] Children 1 to 12 years of age are at risk of serious morbidity from carbamazepine overdose at lower serum concentrations than adults.[40]

Ancillary Studies

In chronic overdoses with carbamazepine, such as may be found in epileptics, there may be an increase in paroxysmal abnormalities. During the acute phase of toxicity following an overdose of carbamazepine, the electroencephalogram (EEG) may be dominated by occipital delta activity.[41]

Hyperglycemia, hypokalemia, and hyponatremia are related to high drug concentrations. About half of overdosed patients experience transient evidence of hepatic dysfunction, which is usually of little clinical significance.[42] Prolonged QT intervals, followed by an increased QRS, intraventricular conduction defects, and prolonged PR intervals are seen with carbamazepine toxicity.[43]

Treatment

Stabilization

1. Establish respiration and airway.
2. If the patient is comatose, insert an endotracheal tube and connect to a source of mechanical ventilation. The tidal volume should be 10 to 15 mL/kg.
3. If hypotension exists, exercise care in forcing fluids (water retention). Place the patient in Trendelenburg position. Pressor amines (eg, dopamine or norepinephrine) may be required.
4. Admit patients to an intensive care facility if they are symptomatic, have ingested more than several grams, or have high or rising plasma levels.[44]

Gut Decontamination

Wason and colleagues studied the use of multiple-dose activated charcoal in five children with carbamazepine overdose and recommend no more than two to three appropriate doses (1 g/kg per dose) after a carbamazepine overdose to prevent concretion formation or continued absorption of the drug.[45] Multiple doses of activated charcoal appeared to increase the clearance of carbamazepine but were not associated with clinical benefits.

Elimination Enhancement

Forced diuresis, hemodialysis, and peritoneal dialysis are ineffective and potentially dangerous (antidiuretic hormone action of carbamazepine).

Charcoal hemoperfusion may be useful[46–50] for removal of both carbamazepine and its metabolites; it has been employed after adequate supportive care has been provided without amelioration of the clinical condition. In three patients who underwent hemoperfusion[46,48,51] the total amounts of carbamazepine removed were less than 1 g in one case after 5 hours[46] and 0.44 and 0.87 g after 4 hours in the other two cases.[48]

Antidote

An anecdotal report suggests that administration of intravenous flumazenil 2.0 mg was followed by opening of the eyes and led to total awakening of a patient, which lasted 25 minutes, after which the patient again lost consciousness.[52] This requires validation by further controlled studies.

Supportive Measures

1. Monitor the complete blood count, vital signs, electrolytes, liver enzymes, and electrocardiogram periodically for at least 24 hours after admission of the overdose patient.
2. Monitor status of consciousness (including a coma scale) and deep tendon reflexes.
3. For coma, institute endotracheal intubation and mechanically assisted ventilation.
4. For dystonic and athetoid posturing, observe and protect the airway.
5. For hypotension, institute a fluid challenge intravenously; place the patient in Trendelenburg position; and, if required, administer dopamine (Intropin) and/or norepinephrine (Levophed). Watch for ventricular arrhythmias.
6. Seizures infrequently occur. Initiate therapy with an intravenous diazepam bolus (adults, 0.25 mg/kg up to 20 mg per dose). Repeat every 15 to 20 minutes as required. If seizures recur, use phenytoin or phenobarbital.
7. Treat oliguria symptomatically.
8. Correct electrolyte abnormalities.

REFERENCES—CARBAMAZEPINE

1. Coutselinis A, Poulos L. An unusual case of carbamazepine poisoning with a near-fatal relapse after two days. Clin Toxicol 1980;16:385–387.
2. Bridge TA, Norton RL, Robertson WA. Pediatric carbamazepine overdose. Pediatr Emerg Care 1994;10:200–263.
3. Eadie MJ. Anticonvulsant drugs: An update. Drugs 1984;27: 328–362.
4. Morselli PL, Frigerio A. Metabolism and pharmacokinetics of carbamazepine. Drug Metab Rev 1975;4:97–113.
5. Sullivan JB Jr, Rumack BH, Peterson RG. Acute carbamazepine toxicity resulting from overdose. Neurology (NY) 1981;31:621–624.
6. Rey E, d'Athis P, deLauture D, et al. Pharmacokinetics of carbamazepine in the neonate and in the child. Int J Clin Pharmacol Biopharm 1979;17:90–96.
7. Tomson T, Tybring G, Bertilsson L. Single dose kinetics and metabolism of carbamazepine-10, 11-epoxide. Clin Pharmacol Ther 1983;33:58–65.
8. Yerby MS, Friel PN, Miller DQ. Carbamazepine protein binding and disposition in pregnancy. Ther Drug Monit 1985;7: 269–273.
9. Eichelbaum M, Ekbom K, Bertilsson L, et al. Plasma kinetics of carbamazepine and its epoxide metabolite in man after single and multiple doses. Eur J Clin Pharmacol 1974; 8:337–341.
10. Luke DR, Rocci ML Jr, Schaible DH, et al. Toxicokinetics of carbamazepine and its 10,11-epoxide. Vet Hum Toxicol 1985;28:315.
11. Pynnonen S, Sillanpaa M, Frey H, et al. Carbamazepine and 10,11-epoxy carbamazepine levels in children. Proc Eur Soc Toxicol 1977;18:192–194.
12. Westenberg HGM, Van der Kleijn E, Oei TT, et al. Kinetics of carbamazepine and carbamazepine-epoxide determined by use of plasma and saliva. Clin Pharmacol Ther 1978;23: 320–328.
13. Tegretol[R] (carbamazepine). In: *Physicians' Desk Reference.* 41st ed. Oradell, NJ: Medical Economics, 1987:962–964.
14. Valsalan VC, Cooper GL. Carbamazepine intoxication caused by interaction with isoniazid. Br Med J 1982;285:261–262.
15. Grimsley SR, Jann MW, D'Mello AP, et al. Pharmacodynamics and pharmacokinetics of fluoxetine/carbamazepine interaction. Clin Pharmacol Ther 1991;49:135.
16. Mitsch RA. Carbamazepine toxicity precipitated by intravenous erythrocin. DICP Ann Pharmacother 1989;232:878–879.
17. Allen S. Cerebella dysfunction following dextropropoxyphene-induced carbamazepine toxicity. Postgrad Med J 1994;70:764–769.
18. Arana GW, Epstein S. Molloy M, Greenblatt DJ. Carbamazepine-induced reduction of plasma alprazolam concentrations: A clinical case report. J Clin Psychiatry 1988;49:448–449.
19. Rosa FW. Spina bifida in infants of women treated with carbamazepine during pregnancy. N Engl J Med 1991;324: 674–677.
20. Vestermark V, Vestermark S. Teratogenic effect of carbamazepine. Arch Dis Child 1991;66:641–642.
21. Jones KL, Lacro RV, Johnson KA, Adams J. Pattern of malformations in the children of women treated with carbamazepine during pregnancy. N Engl J Med 1989;320:1661–1666.
22. Donaldson JO. The pregnant epileptic fetal risks from anticonvulsant therapy. JAMA 1990;264:1044.
23. Frey B, Schubiger G, Musy JP. Transient cholestatic hepatitis in a neonate associated with carbamazepine exposure during pregnancy and breast feeding. Eur J Pediat 1990;150: 136–138.
24. Weaver DF, Camfield P, Fraser A. Massive carbamazepine overdose: Clinical and pharmacologic observations in five episodes. Neurology 1988;38:755–759.
25. Kasarskis EJ, Juo C-S, Berzer R, Nelson KR. Carbamazepine-induced cardiac dysfunction: Characterization of two distinct clinical syndromes. Arch Intern Med 1992;152:186–191.
26. Meissner C. Carbamazepine (Finlepsin[R]): Vergiftung mit toxischer Myokardschadigung. Eine Kasuitsik. Z Klin Med 1990;45:261–264.
27. Kitson GE, Wauchob TD. Pulmonary oedema following carbamazepine overdose. Anaesthesia 1988;43:967–969.
28. Begley JP. Pulmonary oedema after carbamazepine overdose. Anaesthesia 1989;44:789–790.
29. O'Neal W Jr, Whitten KM, Baumann RJ, et al. Lack of serious toxicity following carbamazepine overdosage. Clin Pharmacol 1984;3:545–547.
30. Zucker P, Daum F, Cohen MI. Fatal carbamazepine hepatitis. J Pediatr 1977;91:667–668.
31. Appleby L. Rapid development of hyponatremia during low dose carbamazepine therapy. J Neurol Neurosurg Psychiatry 1984;47:1138–1140.
32. Livingston S, Pauli L, Berman W. Carbamazepine (Tegretol) in epilepsy. Dis Nerv Syst 1974;35:103–107.
33. Mack RB. Julius seizure: Carbamazepine (Tegretol) poisoning. NC Med J 1985;46(1):41–42.
34. Jubert P, Almirall J, Casanovas A, Garcia M. Carbamazepine-induced acute renal failure. Nephron 1994;66:121.
35. Di Giorgio CM, Rabinowicz AL, Olivas RD. Carbamazepine-induced antinuclear antibodies and systemic lupus erythematosus-like syndrome. Epilepsia 1991;32:128–129.
36. Carbamazepine and "pseudolymphoma." Aust Adverse Drug React Bull 1991;10(1):3.
37. Sinnige HAM, Boender CA, Kuypers EW, Ruitenberg HM. Carbamazepine-induced pseudolymphoma and immune dysregulation. J Intern Med 1990;227:355–358. Case Report.
38. Cochran EB, Massey KL, Phelps SJ. A rapid noninstrumented whole blood carbamazepine assay for pediatric patients. J Pediatr 1990;116:307–310.
39. Hojer J, Malmlund H-A, Berg A. Clinical features in 28 consecutive cases of laboratory confirmed massive poisoning with carbamazepine abuse. Clin Toxicol 1993;25:449–458.
40. Spiller HA, Krenzelok EP. Carbamazepine overdose: Serum concentration less predictive in children. Clin Toxicol 1993; 31:459–460.
41. Howard RS, Trend PSTJ, Townsend HRA. EEG appearances in acute carbamazepine toxicity. Hum Exp Toxicol 1990;9: 313–315.
42. Seymour JF. Carbamazepine overdose: Features of 33 cases. Drug Saf 1993;8:81–88.
43. Apfelbaum JD, Caravati EM, Kerns WP, et al. Cardiovascular effects of carbamazepine toxicity. Ann Emerg Med 1994; 33:31.
44. Lahr MB. Hyponatremia during carbamazepine therapy. Clin Pharmacol Ther 1985;37:693–696.
45. Wason S, Baher RC, Carolan P, et al. Carbamazepine overdose: The effects of multiple dose activated charcoal. Clin Toxicol 1992;30:39–48.
46. Leslie PJ, Heyworth R, Prescott LF. Cardiac complications of carbamazepine intoxication: Treatment by haemoperfusion. Br Med J 1983;286:1018.
47. Gary NE, Byra WM, Eisinger RP. Carbamazepine poisoning: Treatment by haemoperfusion. Nephron 1981;27:202–203.
48. De Groot, Van Heijst ANP, Maes RAA. Charcoal hemoperfusion in the treatment of two cases of acute carbamazepine poisoning. Clin Toxicol 1984;22:349–369.
49. Chan KM, Aguanno JJ, Jansen R, et al. Charcoal hemoperfusion for treatment of carbamazepine poisoning. Clin Chem 1981;27(7):1300–1302.
50. Vuignier BI, Woo OF, Becker CE. Fatal carbamazepine overdose with seizures: Role of charcoal hemoperfusion. Vet Hum Toxicol 1986;28(5):304 (Abstract 158).
51. Nilsson C, Sterner G, Idvall J. Charcoal hemoperfusion for treatment of serious carbamazepine poisoning. Acta Med Scand 1984;216:137–140.
52. Zuber M, Elsasser S, Ritz R, Scollo-Lavizzari G. Flumazenil (Anexate[R]) in severe intoxication with carbamazepine (Tegretol[R]). Eur Neurol 1988;28:161–163.

CLONAZEPAM

Clonazepam is a synthetic benzodiazepine derivative in use as an anticonvulsant in the United States since 1975.[1]

It is a Schedule IV (C-IV) drug under the Federal Controlled Substances Act of 1970.[2]

Product Formulation

Clonazepam is available orally as Klonopin in tablets of 0.5, 1, and 2 mg.

Therapeutic Dose

The pediatric dose (up to 10 years of age or up to 30 kg body weight) is 0.01 to 0.03 mg/kg/d. Pediatric maintenance doses should not exceed 0.2 mg/kg/d. The adult dose is up to 4 to 8 mg daily.[2] Adult maintenance dose should not exceed 20 mg/d.[2]

Toxic Dose

Overdoses of up to 60 mg of clonazepam have been taken without serious sequelae. Drowsiness and ataxia develop without serious respiratory depression.[3] A 4-year-old boy who may have ingested 14 to 32 mg of clonazepam survived.[4]

Toxicokinetics[1,5–7]

Bioavailability	80%
Peak plasma level	7–24 ng/mL
Time to peak plasma level	1–4 hours
Volume of distribution	1.5–4.4 L/kg
Plasma protein binding	80%
Elimination half-life	20–80 hours
Excreted unchanged	<0.5%

Drug Interactions

Additive central nervous system depression may occur when clonazepam is used with other central nervous system depressants, anticonvulsants, or alcohol. Phenytoin concentrations may be increased when both drugs are used together.[2]

Pregnancy/Lactation

Safe use of clonazepam during pregnancy or lactation has not been established.

Mechanism of Action

Clonazepam has a high affinity for central benzodiazepine receptors. It is a facilitator of the γ-aminobutyric acid system (GABA) and also increases central synthesis of serotonin.[8]

Clinical Presentation

Overdose

Overdose with clonazepam may produce somnolence, confusion, ataxia, diminished reflexes, or coma.

Chronic Use

Physical or psychological dependence may follow long-term use by those who have been dependent on other drugs or by alcoholic patients. Sudden withdrawal after long-term administration may lead to dysphoria, restlessness, irritability, sleepiness and hand tremors, oral dyskinesias, muscle rigidity, and seizures.[9] Such symptoms may not begin for several days after the drug is discontinued, because of its long half-life. Depression, acute excitation, intrusiveness, and belligerence may reflect behavioral disinhibition associated with clonazepam.[10] Anorgasmia, impaired erectile functioning, and inability to ejaculate have been observed with chronic use of clonazepam.[8] An idiosyncratic nonhypersensitivity-type liver damage has been reported.[11] Respiratory, gastrointestinal, genitourinary, and hematologic dysfunction may occur during chronic use of clonazepam.

Laboratory

Chromatographic methods are available for clonazepam quantitation. High-performance liquid chromatography (HPLC) appears most precise. The detection limit of the HPLC method is 4 ng/mL.[12]

Treatment

Treatment of clonazepam overdose is largely symptomatic and supportive. Gastric lavage, activated charcoal, and cathartics may be useful but supportive studies are lacking.[4] The high protein binding and extensive volume of distribution suggest that diuresis, hemodialysis, or hemoperfusion would not be effective in accelerating removal of clonazepam. The long half-life requires observation and monitoring of the patient for a minimum of 48 hours. (See also Diazepam).

REFERENCES—CLONAZEPAM

1. Baselt RC, Cravey RH. *Disposition of Toxic Drugs and Chemicals in Man.* 3rd ed. Chicago: Year Book, 1989: 199–201.
2. McEvoy GK, ed. *AHFS Drug Information 94.* Bethesda: American Society of Hospital Pharmacists, 1994:1353–1355.
3. Browne TR. Clonazepam. Arch Neurol 1976;3:326–332.
4. Welch TR, Rumack BH, Hammond K. Clonazepam overdose resulting in cyclic coma. Clin Toxicol 1977;10:433–436.
5. Greenblatt DJ, Miller LG, Schader RI. Clonazepam pharmacokinetics, brain uptake and receptor interactions. J Clin Psychiatry 1987;48(10, suppl.):4–9.
6. Berlin A, Dahlstron H. Pharmacokinetics of the anticonvulsant drug clonazepam evaluated from single oral and intravenous doses and by repeated oral administration. Eur J Clin Pharm 1975;9:155–159.
7. Andre M, Boutray MJ, Bianchetti G, et al. Clonazepam in neonatal seizures: Dose regimens and therapeutic efficacy. Eur J Clin Pharmacol 1991;40:193–195.
8. Cohen LS, Rosenbaum JF. Clonazepam: New uses and potential problems. J Clin Psychiatry 1987;48(10, suppl): 50–55.
9. Jaffe R, Gibson E. Clonazepam withdrawal psychosis. J Clin Psychopharmacol 1986;6:193.
10. Binder RL. Three case reports of behavioral disinhibitors with clonazepam. Gen Hosp Psychiatry 1987;9:151–153.
11. Olsson R, Zettergron L. Anticonvulsant-induced liver damage. Am J Gastroenterol 1988;83:576–577.
12. De Carvalho D, Lancote VL. Measurement of plasma clonazepam for therapeutic control: A comparison of chromatographic methods. Ther Drug Monitor 1991;13:55–61.

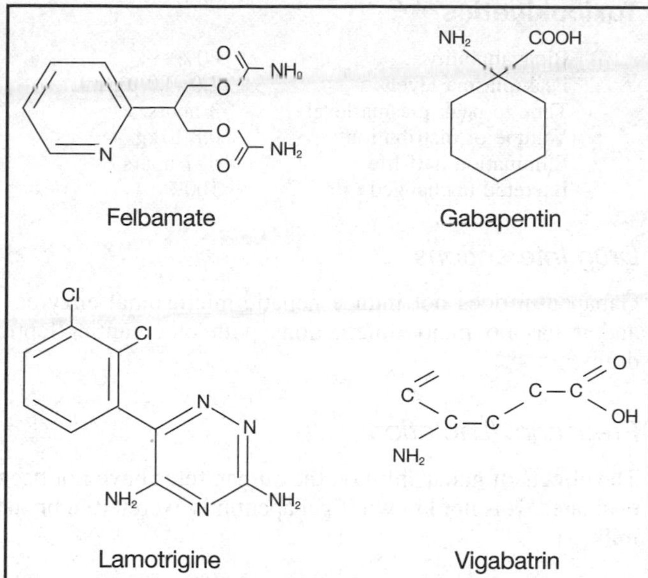

Figure 36-1 Structures of the four major new antiepileptic drugs. (From Fisher RS. Emerging antiepileptic drugs. Neurology 1993; 43(11,suppl. 5):S12–20.)

FELBAMATE

Felbamate (Fig. 36–1) is a synthetic dicarbamate related to meprobamate.[1] Overdose is accompanied by mild gastric distress. No fatalities have been reported following overdoses. Felbamate was approved by the Food and Drug Administration in August 1993. Based on reports of patients who developed life-threatening aplastic anemia following the use of felbamate, the Food and Drug Administration has recommended that patients be withdrawn from treatment with felbamate. They are urged to consult their physicians first and to avoid abrupt withdrawal.[2,3]

Use

Felbamate is indicated as monotherapy and adjunctive therapy in the treatment of partial seizures with and without generalization in adults with epilepsy and as adjunctive therapy in the treatment of partial and generalized seizures associated with the Lennox–Gastaut syndrome in children.

Product Formulation

Felbamate is available as 400- and 600-mg tablets and as a 600 mg/5 mL suspension for oral administration.

Therapeutic Dose

In adults, felbamate is initiated at 1200 mg/d. Adjustment upward is made weekly while other antiepileptic drugs are reduced. In children aged 2 to 14 years with Lennox–Gastaut syndrome, felbamate is added at 15 mg/kg/d in divided doses while reducing present antiepileptic drugs with careful control of plasma levels.

Toxic Dose

Doses up to 3600 mg/d have been associated with fatigue, fever, headache, dizziness, somnolence, rash, and dyspepsia (see Clinical Presentation). A dose of 12,000 mg was followed by mild gastric distress and tachycardia. Movement disorders have been observed.[4]

Toxicokinetics[5,6]

Bioavailability	About 10%
Peak plasma level	2.5–4 μg/mL
Time to peak plasma level	1–4 hours
Volume of distribution	0.75 L/kg
Plasma protein binding	25%
Elimination half-life	20 hours
Excreted unchanged	40–50%

Drug Interactions

Felbamate causes an increase in steady-state phenytoin and valproate concentrations, but also a decrease in steady-state carbamazepine plasma concentrations. Phenytoin and carbamazepine cause a doubling of the clearance of felbamate.

Pregnancy/Lactation

Felbamate is listed in Pregnancy Category C by the Food and Drug Administration.

Mechanism of Action

Felbamate may have inhibitory effects on GABA receptor binding, benzodiazepine receptor binding, and binding at the *N*-methyl-D-aspartate (NMDA) receptor–ionophore complex.

Clinical Presentation

Chronic Use

Treatment with felbamate may lead to weight gain, weakness, malaise, influenza-like symptoms, palpitations, tachycardia, agitation, psychological disturbance, aggressive reaction, pruritus, and Stevens–Johnson syndrome.[7]

Overdose

An acute overdose was followed by mild gastric distress and tachycardia. The patient recovered.

Withdrawal

Abrupt withdrawal of felbamate may be followed by status epilepticus.[8]

Laboratory

Increases in serum transaminase and alkaline phosphatase levels, leukopenia, leukocytosis, thrombocytopenia, granulocytopenia, hypokalemia, and hyponatremia have been infrequently reported.

Treatment

Treatment of signs and symptoms of overdose is symptomatic and supportive. It is not known if felbamate is dialyzable. There are no antidotes.

REFERENCES—FELBAMATE

1. Brodie MJ, Porter RJ. New and potential anticonvulsants. Lancet 1990;336:425–426.
2. Kessler D, FDA Director, Statement, August 1994.
3. Ahmad SR. Felbamate and aplastic anemia. Lancet 1994; 344:465.
4. Luciano D, Devinsky O, Raguthu S, et al. Movement disorders during felbamate therapy. Epilepsia 1994;35(suppl.18):159.
5. Felbamate product literature. Cranbury, NJ: Wallace Laboratories, July 31, 1993.
6. Wilensky AJ, Friel PN, Ojemann LM, et al. Pharmacokinetics of W-554 (ADD 03055) in epileptic patients. Epilepsia 1985; 26:602–606.
7. Jachel RA. Stevens–Johnson syndrome after treatment with felbamate. Epilepsia 1994;35:98.
8. De Giorgio CM, Lopez J, Lekht ZN, Rabinowicz A. Status epilepticus induced by felbamate withdrawal. Neurology 1995;45:1021–1022.

GABAPENTIN

Gabapentin (Neurontin), a synthetic cyclohexane acetic acid derivative, has been approved by the Food and Drug Administration for use in addition to other antiepileptic drugs in patients with partial (focal) seizures with or without secondary generalization.[1,2] Gabapentin (Fig. 36–1) is structurally related to GABA, the major endogenous inhibitory neurotransmitter in the brain, but unlike vigabatrin, another GABA analog, gabapentin is not an agonist at GABA receptors, but rather binds to a unique receptor in the brain.[2] Overdoses are followed by lethargy, sedation, dizziness, double vision, slurred speech, and occasionally diarrhea, all of which resolve within 18 hours with few aftereffects.[3,4]

Product Formulation

Gabapentin is available in 300-mg dosage forms for oral use.

Therapeutic Dose

Gabapentin is started with a single dose of 300 mg on day 1 and the dosage is raised each day by 300 mg to a maximum of 2400 mg.[2]

Toxic Dose

Doses up to 48.9 g have been tolerated with few symptoms including moderate sedation, dizziness, fatigue, and slurred speech.[3,4,5]

Fatal Dose

There have been no reports of death following an overdose. Acute life-threatening toxicity has not been observed with doses equal to or less than 20 times the recommended human dose.[4]

Toxicokinetics[3,5,6]

Bioavailability	60%
Peak plasma level	2.0–3.0 μg/mL
Time to peak plasma level	3 hours
Volume of distribution	0.8 L/kg
Elimination half-life	5–7 hours
Excreted unchanged	100%

Drug Interactions

Gabapentin does not induce hepatic microsomal enzymes, and it has no major interactions with other antiepileptic drugs.[5–8]

Pregnancy/Lactation

The effects of gabapentin on the human fetus have not been evaluated. It is not known if gabapentin is excreted in breast milk.

Clinical Presentation

Somnolence, fatigue, dizziness, ataxia, fatigue, nystagmus, and weight gain have followed long-term use and have been observed when gabapentin was added to other antiepileptic drugs.[1,9] Symptoms generally resolve within 18 hours.[3,4] Pancreatic tumors seen in rodent studies were benign, occurred only with large doses, and were not thought to occur to humans.[10,11]

Laboratory

Analytical Methods

Assays or measurements of gabapentin concentration in biological fluids have included high-performance liquid chromatography,[12] which has a detection level of 0.02 mg/L in plasma, and gas chromatography, which has sensitivity limits of 0.2 mg/L in plasma and 50 mg/L in urine.[13]

Blood Levels

A dose–response pattern is apparent for plasma gabapentin concentrations and related clinical effects within the dosage range 600 to 1800 mg/d. Plasma concentrations range from 2 to 15 μg/mL.[3,14] Monitoring of plasma levels is usually unnecessary.[5] Eight hours following an ingestion of 48.9 g of gabapentin, the plasma concentration was 62 μg/mL. The disappearance of symptoms by 18 hours postingestion corresponded to the decrease in gabapentin plasma concentrations. Minimal clinical effects have been associated with a serum concentration of 44 μg/mL.[15]

Ancillary Tests

Serum electrolytes, liver function indices, creatinine, albumin, complete blood count, and urinalysis are within normal limits after an overdose.[3]

Treatment

Following an overdose, vital signs should be monitored. If the patient is seen with 3 hours, gastric lavage with endotracheal protection and an initial dose of activated charcoal with sorbitol appears useful, together with careful observation for about 24 to 48 hours. There are no antidotes and there are no reports of the use of hemodialysis or hemoperfusion following an overdose. Treatment is largely symptomatic and supportive.

REFERENCES—GABAPENTIN

1. Gabapentin: A new anticonvulsant. Med Lett Drugs Ther 1994;36(921):39–40.
2. Gabapentin: A new antiepileptic drugs. Drug Ther Bull 1994; 32(4):29–30.
3. Fischer JH, Barr AN, Rogers SL, et al. Lack of serious toxicity following gabapentin overdose. Neurology 1994;4:982–983.
4. Garofalo E, Koto E, Feuerstein T. Experience with gabapentin overdose: Five case studies. Epilepsia 1993;34:157.
5. Goa KL, Sorkin EM. Gabapentin. Drugs 1993;46:409–427.
6. Chadwick D. Gabapentin. Lancet 1994;343:89–91.
7. Tyndel F. Interaction of gabapentin with other antiepileptics. Lancet 1994;242:1363–1364.
8. Radulovic LL, Wilder BJ, Leppik IE, et al. Lack of interaction of gabapentin with carbamazepine or valproate. Epilepsia 1994;35:155–161.
9. UK Gabapentin Study Group. Gabapentin in partial epilepsy. Lancet 1990;335:1114–1119.
10. *Martindale: The Extra Pharmacopoeia.* 30th ed. London: Pharmaceutical Press, 1993:300.
11. New drugs for epilepsy on the way. Pharm J 1991;247:534.
12. Hengy WD, Kavanagh MC, Diskinson RB. Determination of gabapentin in plasma and urine by high-performance liquid chromatography and pre-column labelling for ultraviolet detection. J Chromatogr 1985;341:473–478.
13. Harper WD, Kavanagh MC, Diskinson RB. Determination of gabapentin in plasma and urine by capillary column gas chromatography. J Chromatogr 1990;529:167–174.
14. Browne TR. Efficacy and safety of gabapentin. In: Chadwick D, ed. *New Trends in Epilepsy Management.* London: Royal Society of Medicine Series, 1993:47–57.
15. Fernandez M, Walter F, Peterson L, Walkotte S. Gabapentin overdose: Elevated levels with minimal clinical effects. Clin Toxicol 1995;33:475–486 (Abstract 92).

LAMOTRIGINE

Lamotrigine (Lamital) is a newer synthetic anticonvulsant phenyltriazine compound chemically unrelated to other agents currently used in epilepsy (Fig. 36–1). It may produce headache, vomiting, and ataxia related to elevated plasma levels. Few patients with overdose have been reported. Treatment is symptomatic and supportive.

Use

Lamotrigine appears useful in the treatment of refractory epilepsy, partial epilepsy, and primary generalized epilepsy.[1]

Therapeutic Dose

Therapeutic doses without use of other anticonvulsants start at 50 mg daily for 2 weeks, then 50 to 100 mg twice daily (up to as much as 400 mg/d).[2,3] When used with other anticonvulsants, lamotrigine is started at 50 mg twice daily, with maintenance doses of 100 to 200 mg twice daily. Children under 2 years of age are started with 2 mg/kg/d, with maintenance doses of 5 to 15 mg/kg/d. Lower doses are used if sodium valproate is also administered.[4,5]

Toxicokinetics[4,6]

Bioavailability	100%
Peak plasma level	1–4 μg/mL
Time to peak plasma level	2 hours
Volume of distribution	1.2 L/kg
Plasma protein binding	55%
Elimination half-life	1 day
Excreted unchanged	10%

Drug Interactions

Hepatic drug enzyme inducers such as carbamazepine, phenytoin, and phenobarbital reduce the half-life of lamotrigine to 15 hours.[7,8] Sodium valproate reduces the total clearance of lamotrigine about 21% and increases its half-life to 59 hours.[4] Lamotrigine may increase blood levels of carbamazepine.[9] Acetaminophen induced a decrease in the half-life of lamotrigine by a mechanism not yet elucidated.[10]

Pregnancy/Lactation

Lamotrigine has not been studied in the pregnant or lactating woman.

Mechanism of Action

Lamotrigine acts mainly by inhibiting excitatory amino acid release. It stabilizes neuronal membrane via blockade of voltage-sensitive sodium channels.

Clinical Presentation

In overdose, lamotrigine induces nausea, vomiting, headache, and ataxia, symptoms that appear to reflect increases in blood levels.[4,11] Adverse effects include dizziness, diplopia, blurred vision, somnolence, headache, ataxia, asthenia, nausea, vomiting, rash, and depression.[11] Angioedema is rarely observed. A few deaths have been reported after status epilepticus with disseminated intravascular coagulation and multiorgan failure.[3,4,11] Abrupt withdrawal may lead to rebound seizures.

Laboratory

Analytical Methods

A reverse-phase high-performance liquid chromatography method is sensitive to 5 μg/mL.[11] A radioimmunoassay method is sensitive to 20 μg/mL.[12]

Blood Levels

There is no evidence of an increase in frequency of the most frequent side effects with an increase in blood lamotrigine levels. Nausea and vomiting have been observed at 6 to 7 μg/mL. Headache and ataxia may be seen at blood levels above 10 μg/mL.[10] Some patients tolerate plasma levels greater than 10 μg/mL (39 μmol/L) without toxic effects. Leukopenia has been reported.[13]

Abnormalities

First-degree heart block has been described.[14]

Treatment

Treatment of a lamotrigine overdose is largely symptomatic and supportive. There is no antidote. Gastric lavage may be useful in the first several hours after ingestion to reduce the likelihood of high blood concentrations. Activated charcoal may also be useful, but there are no data to support its use. Hemodialysis and hemoperfusion are not likely to be useful (due to high protein binding, high volume of distribution). Close electrocardiographic monitoring for patients with lamotrigine overdose with QRS prolongation is recommended because of the drug's possible arrhythmogenic effect in overdose.[15] Blood counts should be monitored for 2 to 3 weeks for possible development of leukopenia.

REFERENCES—LAMOTRIGINE

1. Timmings PL, Richens A. Lamotrigine in primary generalised epilepsy. Lancet 1992;339:1300–1301.
2. Goa KL, Ross SR, Chrisp P. Lamotrigine: A review of its pharmacological properties and clinical efficiacy in epilepsy. Drugs 1993;46:152–176.
3. Mikati MA, Schachter SC, Schomer DL, et al. Long-term tolerability, pharmacokinetic and preliminary efficacy study of lamotrigine in patients with resistant partial seizures. Clin Neuropharmacol 1989;12:312–321.
4. Brodie MJ, Porter RJ. New and potential anticonvulsants. Lancet 1990;2:425–426.
5. Binnie CD, Ven Ende Boas W, Kasteleijn-Nolste-Tremited GA, et al. Acute effect of lamotrigine (BW 430C) in persons with epilepsy. Epilepsia;1986;27:348–357.
6. Cohen AF, Land GS, Breimer DD, et al. Lamotrigine, a new anticonvulsant: Pharmacokinetics in normal humans. Clin Pharmacol Ther 1987;42:535–541.
7. Yuen AWC, Land GS, Weatherby BC, Peck AW. Sodium valproate acutely inhibits lamotrigine metabolism. Br J Clin Pharmacol 1992;33:511–513.
8. Jawad S, Yuen WC, Peck AW, et al. Lamotrigine: Single-dose pharmacokinetics and initial 1 week experience in refractory epilepsy. Epilepsy Res 1987;1:194–201.
9. Warner T, Patsalos PN, Prevett M, et al. Lamotrigine-induced carbamazepine toxicity: An interaction with carbamazepine-10,11-epoxide. Epilepsy Res 1992;11:147–150.
10. Depot M, Powell JR, Messenheimer JA Jr, et al. Kinetic effects of multiple oral doses of acetaminophen on a single oral dose of lamotrigine. Clin Pharmacol Ther 1990;48: 346–355.
11. Cociglio M, Alric R, Bouvier O. Performance analysis of a reversed-phase liquid chromatographic assay of lamotrigine in plasma using solvent-demixing extraction. J Chromatogr Biomed Appl 1991;572:269–276.
12. Biddlecombe RA, Dean KL, Smith CD, Jeal SC. Validation of a radioimmunoassay for the determination of human plasma concentrations of lamotrigine. J Pharm Biomed Analg 1990;8:691–694.
13. Nicholson RJ, Kelly KP, Grant IS. Leucopenia associated with lamotrigine. Br Med J 1995;310:504.
14. Betts T, Goodwin G, Withers RM, Yuen AWC. Human safety of lamotrigine. Epilepsia 1991;32(suppl. 2):S17–S21.
15. Buckley A, White JM, Dawson AH. Self-poisoning with lamotrigine. Med J Aust 1993;159:488.

PARALDEHYDE

Paraldehyde toxicity may be observed during treatment of status epilepticus.[1]

Therapeutic Dose

For seizures, 5 mL paraldehyde, well diluted, may be administered intravenously; 10 mL may be given by gastric tube as required every 4 hours. Bostrom has advocated the control of seizures with the use of 200 mg/kg paraldehyde initially in an intravenous infusion over a 5-minute period, followed by a drip of 20 mg/h to maintain a steady-state screen level of about 200 μg/mL.[1]

Toxicokinetics[1–5]

Bioavailability	95%
Time to peak plasma level	0.5 hour
Volume of distribution	0.9 L/kg
Elimination half-life	7 hours (3–10 hours)
Excreted unchanged	3%

Clinical Presentation

Abdominal pain, central nervous system depression, a severe high-anion-gap metabolic acidosis, and a leukocytosis of 24,000 to 65,000 may be observed.[6]

Hematologic Effects

Increase in blood coagulability, general arterial thrombosis,[7] and leukocytosis have been observed.

Acid–Base Balance

Increase in anion-gap metabolic acidosis[6,8] and dehydration have been reported.

Intramuscular Effects

Pain, tissue necrosis, and sciatic nerve damage may occur.[9]

Tolerance

Chronic paraldehydism in the alcoholic may manifest as tolerance, tremulousness, restlessness, mental anxiety, agitation, and substitution for alcoholism. Alcoholics may become chronically dependent on paraldehyde.[10] Withdrawal from paraldehyde may result in delirium tremens and hallucination, similar to withdrawal in alcoholism. Treatment of paraldehyde withdrawal is similar to that of alcohol withdrawal (sedatives, anticonvulsants, correction and monitoring of fluid, electrolyte, and carbohydrate balance).[10]

Skin Effects

Sterile abscesses have been observed at injection sites.

Laboratory

Analytical Methods

A quantitative method employing ultrafiltration and gas chromatography with a wide-bore capillary column exhibits sensitivity, specificity, precision, accuracy, and linearity for therapeutic drug monitoring and toxicologic purposes.[11] In general, such levels reflect the severity of overdose, but treatment must be based mainly on clinical evaluation.

Ancillary Tests

Electrocardiographic and other cardiac indices of right ventricular failure may be observed with overdose. The anion gap should be calculated to detect high-anion-gap metabolic acidosis. A chest x-ray is indicated if signs of pulmonary involvement are evident.

Treatment

Treatment is directed toward maintenance of airway, breathing, and circulation. Supportive care is the mainstay of therapy. Patients are often critically ill and must be under constant supervision.

Gut Decontamination

Paraldehyde is locally corrosive to the mouth and upper gastrointestinal tract. Emesis induction would appear only to add local insult to prior injury and, therefore, should probably not be performed.

There is no evidence to support the effectiveness of activated charcoal.

Elimination Enhancement

Extracorporeal detoxification methods would appear to be of limited use. Where improvement has accompanied dialysis, this may have resulted from correction of the metabolic acidosis.[12–14]

Antidote

There is no antidote.

Supportive Measures

Supportive clinical care is the mainstay of treatment. Patients should be treated in an intensive care facility.

Monitoring of arterial blood gases and serum electrolytes with estimation of the anion gap, electrocardiogram, hepatic and renal function tests, respiratory function studies, chest x-rays, physical examination of the chest, cardiac function studies, complete blood counts, and clotting parameters should be ongoing until there is clinical evidence of improvement.

REFERENCES—PARALDEHYDE

1. Bostrom B. Paraldehyde toxicity during treatment of status epilepticus. Am J Dis Child 1982;136:414–415.
2. Anthony RM, Andorn AC, Sunshine I, et al. Paraldehyde pharmacokinetics in ethanol abusers. Fed Proc 1977;36:285.
3. Thurston JH, Liang HS, Smith JS, et al. New enzymatic method for measurement of paraldehyde: Correlation of effects with serum and CSF levels. J Lab Clin Med 1968; 72:699–704.
4. Levine H, Gilbert AJ, Bodansky M. The pulmonary and urinary excretion of paraldehyde in normal dogs and in dogs with liver damage. J Pharm Exp Ther 1940;69:316–323.
5. Hitchcock P, Nelson EE. The metabolism of paraldehyde. 1943;79:286–294.
6. Emmett M, Narins PG. Clinical use of the anion gap. Medicine 1977;56:38–54.
7. Gooch WM III, Kennedy J, Banner W Jr, et al. Generalized arterial and venous thrombosis following intra-arterial paraldehyde. Clin Toxicol 1979;15:39–44.
8. Waterhouse C, Stern EA. Metabolic acidosis occurring during administration of paraldehyde. Am J Med 1957;23: 987–989.
9. Browne TR. Drug therapy reviews: Drug therapy of status epilepticus. Am J Hosp Pharm 1978;35:915–927.
10. Mendelson J, Wexler D, Leiderman PH, et al. A study of addiction to nonethyl alcohols and other poisonous compounds. Q J Stud Alcohol 1957;18:561–580.
11. Hessel DW. The analysis of blood serum for paraldehyde by ultrafiltration and gas chromatography with a wide-bone capillary column. J Anal Toxicol 1988;12:350–353.
12. Beier LS, Pitt WH, Gonick HC. Metabolic acidosis occurring during paraldehyde intoxication. Ann Intern Med 1963;58: 155–158.
13. Gutman RA, Burnell JM, Solak F. Paraldehyde acidosis. Am J Med 1967;42:435–440.
14. Seyffart G. Paraldehyde. In: Haddad LM, Winchester JF, eds. *Clinical Management of Poisoning and Drug Overdose.* Philadelphia: WB Saunders, 1983:410–413.

PHENYTOIN (DIPHENYLHYDANTOIN)

Phenytoin overdose is debilitating and has rather specific features (eg, nystagmus, ataxia, drowsiness) in the initial and mild stage. The overdose is rarely fatal and is treated by immediately discontinuing phenytoin. There is no specifically useful antidote. Laboratory tests to gain a more accurate indication of clinical status (free phenytoin blood levels) are not widely available, but total phenytoin blood levels can be measured. At high doses, phenytoin half-life is increased, but gut decontamination procedures are probably the safest and most effective method of treatment. Methods used to enhance elimination (eg, fluid diuresis, hemodialysis, peritoneal dialysis, charcoal hemoperfusion) are usually ineffective. Patience, often for 3 to 5 days, with good symptomatic supportive care, is its own reward.

Extravasation

Injectable phenytoin is extremely alkaline (pH 12) and irritating to soft tissues when it extravasates from an intravenous infusion. It may also precipitate when it comes into contact with blood or saline solution, causing venous occlusion and secondarily increasing the likelihood of leakage from an intravenous catheter site.[1,2] Propylene glycol, the water-miscible vehicle used to maintain phenytoin solution, is itself reported to be a tissue irritant.[3]

Toxicokinetics[4–8]

Bioavailability	20–90%
Peak plasma level	1.6–2.8 μg/mL
Time to peak plasma level	2 and 10 hours
Volume of distribution	0.5–0.8 L/kg
Plasma protein binding	5–6 L/kg (unbound)
Elimination half-life	8–60 hours
Excreted unchanged	<4%

At toxic doses, metabolism is linear (zero-order kinetics), governed by saturable enzyme systems in the liver.

Free Phenytoin Levels

Gordon and Gerstenblitt have concluded that impairment of protein binding to phenytoin may occur in neonatal or elderly patients; during the late phase of pregnancy; in patients with hyperbilirubinemia, hepatic disease, uremia, nephrotic syndrome, burns, surgery, malnutrition, or other conditions associated with hypoalbuminemia; as well as during combination therapy with valproic acid, aspirin, sulfonamides, and tolbutamide by displacing phenytoin from its albumin binding sites. The unbound fraction of phenytoin also increases with increasing temperature. In these clinical settings of impaired protein binding, the total plasma concentration of phenytoin may result in underestimation of the free fraction and inadvertent phenytoin toxicity. Thus, measurement of the free phenytoin fraction is the preferred index of available anticonvulsant activity. Free phenytoin levels less than 2.1 μg/mL typically do not lead to phenytoin-induced neurotoxicity.[9]

Phenytoin–Drug Interactions

Interactions of phenytoin with other drugs are outlined in Table 36–6.

Pregnancy

Teratogenic effects have been observed[22–25] (Table 36–7).

Clinical Presentation

The earliest signs of overdose with phenytoin (generally a serum level >20–30 μg/mL) include nystagmus on lateral gaze, ataxia, and drowsiness. Onset of symptoms is usually within 1 to 2 hours of ingestion and these may persist for about 4 to 5 days.[26,27] As blood levels increase (>30 μg/mL), nystagmus becomes vertical, speech becomes slurred, drowsiness is more intense, ataxia and lurching gait are observed, coarse tremors of the extremities or involuntary movement become apparent, and many patients cannot walk or even stand. With increasing dose, consciousness is lessened and the patient becomes confused, disoriented, or even hyperactive or manic. The pupils may remain normal or become dilated and reactive; deep tendon reflexes may become briskly reactive. A totally unresponsive state or respiratory depression is unusual with phenytoin intoxication. If the patient is found in coma, a search should be made for an additional drug.[28]

"Paradoxical intoxication" is observed when, as serum levels of phenytoin increase, an increase in seizures is observed without any evidence of the usual toxic effects seen with phenytoin overdose (eg, nystagmus, ataxia). This phenomenon is observed in patients who are already on chronic phenytoin therapy. Treatment for such seizures requires stopping the phenytoin and not increasing it. Diazepam is useful. Serum levels of phenytoin confirm the diagnosis and should be monitored before reinstating phenytoin therapy.

Differential Diagnosis

In a patient who has evidence of nystagmus, ataxia, hyperactivity, and disturbances in consciousness, the following conditions should be considered in addition to drug overdose: posterior fossa tumor, acute viral cerebellitis, Guillain–Barré syndrome, botulism, hysteria. The most common cause of acute ataxia in all age groups is an overdose of toxic drugs.[28] Death is rare after phenytoin overdose, and when it occurs, it is usually due to cardiac arrest or ventricular fibrillation. Respiratory arrest is rare.

Laboratory

Toxic effects are more closely related to the free concentrations.[29] Minor signs appear at free phenytoin levels of 1.5 to 3.5 μg/mL, and are usually serious above 5 μg/mL. Patients who are critically ill and hypoalbuminemic may exhibit phenytoin toxicity with elevated free phenytoin serum concentrations greater than 4 μg/mL but may also have total phenytoin levels within the normal therapeutic range.[30] Renal abnormalities and hypoalbuminemia associated with

Table 36–6
Phenytoin–Drug Interactions

Drugs That Increase Plasma Phenytoin Level
Amiodarone[10,11]
Clobazam[12]
Fluconazole[13]
Ranitidine[14]
Drugs That Decrease Plasma Phenytoin Level
Carboplatin[15]
Rifampicin[16]
Theophylline[17]
Drugs That Decrease Free Plasma Phenytoin Fraction
Influenza vaccine[18]
Tolbutamide[19,20]
Drugs Whose Plasma Level Is Decreased by Phenytoin
Doxorubicinol (metabolite of doxorubicin)[21]

Table 36–7
Fetal Hydantoin Syndrome

Chest Abnormalities	
Congenital breast disease	
Widespread hypoplastic nipples	
Rib/sternal abnormality	
Performance deficits	
Mental retardation	Ocular hypertelorism
Craniofacial abnormalities	Microcephaly
Broad nasal bridge	Cleft lip/palate
Wide fontanelle	Abnormal or low-set ears
Low-set hairline	Epicanthal folds
Broad alveolar ridge	Ptosis of eyelids
Metopic ridging	Coloboma
Short neck	Coarse scalp hair
Limb Abnormalities	
Small or absent nails	Altered palmar crease
Hypoplasia of distal phalanges	Digital thumb
	Dislocated hip
Other	
Pilonidal sinus	Acne vulgaris
Hernia (umbilical or inguinal)	Hemorrhagic disease
Optic nerve hypoplasia	Hirsutism
Abnormal genitalia	Melanotic neuroectodermal tumor
Neuroblastoma	Retinoschisis

AIDS may place patients at risk for elevated free fractions of phenytoin and subsequent toxicity.[31]

Blood Levels

Blood levels greater than 95 μg/mL (total phenytoin) are associated with death, although one child with a level of 108 μg/mL survived an accidental overdose.[32] Deaths have been recorded at levels of 50 to 70 μg/mL.[33]

If a patient presents with any signs or symptoms of overdose and an initial serum level greater than 30 μg/mL, phenytoin should be withdrawn for 72 to 84 hours before restarting.[34] Admission phenytoin serum levels following an overdose are not a useful predictor of length of hospital stay.[35]

Patients under treatment for phenytoin overdose should be monitored with serum or plasma total phenytoin levels, serum free phenytoin levels, if available, blood glucose, urine glucose, serum creatinine, urinalysis, aspartate and alanine transaminases, bilirubin, electrocardiogram, electromyogram as indicated, computer tomogram of the skull if required, blood levels of other drugs used concomitantly, and basal thyroid function tests.[36]

Treatment

Stabilization

1. Correct hypotension by position change (Trendelenburg), fluid infusion to correct volume deficits, or pressor amines (eg, dopamine) if required.
2. Treat complete heart block with intravenous atropine (0.5–1 mg) or a pacemaker.
3. For seizures, discontinue phenytoin immediately. Administer diazepam 0.1–0.3 mg/kg intravenously to a maximum of 20 mg per dose in an adult. This may be repeated in 10 to 20 minutes if required.
4. For hyperglycemic nonketotic coma, administer fluids intravenously, inject small amounts of insulin, and carefully monitor blood glucose.

Gut Decontamination

Activated charcoal in an aqueous slurry should be administered after gastric lavage: 50 to 100 g to an adult, 30 to 50 g to a child. Serial doses of activated charcoal may be effective.[37] Toxicokinetic studies are suggestive of a positive effect of multiple-dose oral activated charcoal in increasing the clearance of phenytoin for the body.[38] Multiple-dose activated charcoal appears to have shortened the time to peak phenytoin concentration, the half-life, and the course of phenytoin intoxication in two children.[39]

Elimination Enhancement

Forced fluid diuresis, peritoneal dialysis, exchange transfusion, hemodialysis, and plasmapheresis are ineffective. There is little renal elimination and a danger of fluid overload.

Antidote

There is no antidote.

Supportive Measures

All patients suspected of phenytoin intoxication should be admitted. With careful supportive treatment, decontamination measures, and observation, most phenytoin intoxications can be successfully managed.

Folic acid supplementation appears to lessen the incidence of teratogenic abnormalities resulting from anticonvulsant drugs. Folic acid is added to the regimen of an epileptic woman who wishes to become pregnant, and vitamin K is administered to the newborn.[40]

Routine electrocardiographic monitoring is probably not required in patients with an uncomplicated phenytoin overdose.[41]

Intravenous Phenytoin

Deaths have been reported in patients aged 44 to 85 who have received intravenous phenytoin. Rapid manual infusion of phenytoin and inclusion of the infusion vehicle, propylene glycol, have been suggested as factors leading to hypotension and cardiac arrhythmias.[42]

REFERENCES—PHENYTOIN

1. Haga HJ III, Hastings H. Extravasation of phenytoin in the hand. J Hand Surg 1988;13A:942–943.
2. Spengler RF, Arrowsmith JB, Kilarski DJ, et al. Severe soft-tissue injury following intravenous infusion of phenytoin: Patient and drug administration risk factors. Arch Intern Med 1988;148:1329–1333.
3. MacCara ME. Extravasation: A hazard of intravenous therapy. Drug Intell Clin Pharm 1983;17:713–717.
4. Wilder BJ, Buchanan RA, Serrano EE. Correlation of acute diphenylhydantoin intoxication with plasma levels and metabolic excretion. Neurology 1973;23:1329–1332.
5. Jung D, Powell JR, Walson P, et al. Effect of dose on phenytoin absorption. Clin Pharmacol Ther 1980;28:479–485.
6. Kutt H. Interactions of antiepileptic drugs. Epilepsia 1975;16: 393–402.
7. Robinson JD, Morris BA, Aherne GW, et al. Pharmacokinetics of a single dose of phenytoin in man measured by radioimmunoassay. Br J Clin Pharmacol 1975;2:345–349.
8. Gugler R, Manion CV, Azarnoff D. Phenytoin: Pharmacokinetics and bioavailability. Clin Pharmacol Ther 1976;19:135–142.
9. Gordon MF, Gerstenblitt D. The use of free phenytoin levels in averting phenytoin toxicity. NY State J Med 1990;90: 469–470.
10. Lesko LJ, Ruangtrakool T. In vitro displacement of phenytoin from protein binding sites by amiodarone. Clin Pharmacol Ter 1987;41:238.
11. Nolan PE, Marcus FI, Hoyer GL, et al. Pharmacokinetic interaction between intravenous phenytoin and amiodarine in healthy volunteers. Clin Pharmacol Ther 1989;46:43–50.
12. Zifkin B, Sherwin A, Andermann F. Phenytoin toxicity due to interaction with clobazan. Neurology 1991;41:313–314.
13. Blum RA, Wilton JH, Hilligoss DM, et al. Effect of fluconazole on the disposition of phenytoin. Clin Pharmacol Ther 1991; 49:420–425.
14. Bramhall D, Levine M. Possible interaction of ranitidine with phenytoin. Drug Intell Clin Pharm 1988;22:979–980.
15. Dofferhoff ASM, Berendsen HH. Decreased phenytoin level after carboplatin treatment. Am J Med 1990;89:247–248.
16. Abajo FJ. Phenytoin interaction with rifampicin. Br Med J 1988;297:1048.
17. Hendeles L, Wyatt R, Weinberger M, et al. Decreased oral phenytoin absorption following concurrent theophylline administration. J Allergy Clin Immunol 1979;63:156.
18. Smith CD, Bledsoe MA, Curran R, et al. Effect of influenza vaccine on serum concentrations of total and free phenytoin. Clin Pharm 1988;7:828–832.

19. Wesseling H, Mols-Thurkow I. Interaction of diphenylhydantoin (DPH) and tolbutamide in man. Eur J Clin Pharmacol 1975;8:75.
20. Beech E, Mathur SVS, Harrold BP. Phenytoin toxicity produced by tolbutamide. Br Med J 1988;297:1613–1614.
21. Cusack BJ, Tesnohlidek DA, Loeske VL, et al. The effect of phenytoin on doxorubicin and doxorubicinol pharmacokinetics. Clin Res 1988;36:117A.
22. Hvidberg EF, Dam M. Clinical pharmacokinetics of anticonvulsants. Clin Pharmacokinet 1976;1:161–188.
23. Lander CM, Smith MT, Chalk JB. Bioavailability and pharmacokinetics of phenytoin during pregnancy. Eur J Clin Pharmacol 1984;27:105–110.
24. Bodendorfer TW. Fetal effects of anticonvulsant drugs and seizure disorders. Drug Intell Clin Pharm 1978;12:14–21.
25. Committee on Drugs, American Academy of Pediatrics. Anticonvulsants and pregnancy. Pediatrics 1977;63:331–333.
26. Wilson JT, Huff JG, Kilroy AW. Prolonged toxicity following acute phenytoin overdose in a child. J Pediatr 1979;95:135–138.
27. Briggs GG, Bodendorfer TW, Freeman RK, et al. *Drugs in Pregnancy and Lactation: A Reference Guide to Fetal and Neonatal Risk.* Baltimore: Williams & Wilkins, 1983:288.
28. Mack RB. Medical exorcism: Acute dilantin intoxication. NC Med J 1984;45(2):99–100.
29. Booker HE, Darcey B. Serum concentrations of free diphenylhydantoin and their relationship to intoxication. Epilepsia 1973;14:177.
30. Discoll DF, McMahon M, Blackburn GL, Bistrian BR. Phenytoin toxicity in a critically ill hypoalbuminemic patient with normal serum drug concentrations. Crit Care Med 1988;16:1248–1249.
31. Toler SM, Wilkerson MA, Porter WH, et al. Severe phenytoin intoxication as a result of altered protein binding in AIDS. DICP Ann Pharmacother 1990;24:698–700.
32. Pruitt AW, Zwiren GT, Patterson JH, et al. A complex pattern of disposition of phenytoin in severe intoxication. Clin Pharmacol Ther 1975;18:112–120.
33. Subik M, Robinson DS. Phenytoin overdose with high plasma levels. West VA Med J 1982;78(11):781–782. Case Report.
34. Baird-Lambert J, Jager-Roman E, Buchanan N. Phenytoin elimination after intoxication during long term treatment. Med J Aust 1982;2:228–229.
35. Curtis DL, Pilbe R, Ellenhorn M, et al. Phenytoin toxicity: Predictions of clinical course. Vet Hum Toxicol 1989;31:162–163.
36. Kushnir M, Weinstein R, Landau B, et al. Hypothyroidism and phenytoin intoxication. Ann Intern Med 1984;102:341–342.
37. Weichbrodt GD, Elliott DR. A treatment of phenytoin toxicity with repeated doses of activated charcoal. Ann Emerg Med 1987;16:1387–1389.
38. Rowden AM, Spoor JE, Bertino JS Jr. The effect of activated charcoal on phenytoin pharmacokinetics. Ann Emerg Med 1990;19:1144–1147.
39. Dolgin JG, Nix DE, Sanchez J, Watson WA. Pharmacokinetic simulation of the effect of multiple-dose activated charcoal in phenytoin poisoning: Report of two pediatric cases. DICP Ann Pharmacother 1991;25:646–649.
40. Biale Y, Lewenthal H. Effect of folic acid supplementation on congenital malformations due to anticonvulsive drugs. Eur J Obstet Gynecol Reprod Biol 1984;18:211–216.
41. Curtis DL, Pirbe R, Ellenhorn MJ, et al. Phenytoin toxicity: A review of 94 cases. Vet Hum Toxicol 1989;31:164–165.
42. Earnest EP, Marx JA, Drury LR. Complications of IV phenytoin for acute treatment of seizures: Recommendations for usage. JAMA 1983;6:762–765.

PRIMIDONE

Primidone (Mysoline) is often used with other anticonvulsants in the treatment of epilepsy. Few cases of primidone overdose have been reported. As phenobarbital is an active metabolite of primidone, treatment is similar to that for phenobarbital overdose. Fatalities have been reported.

Toxicokinetics[1–5]

Bioavailability	60-80%
Peak plasma level	5–15 μg/mL, 10–20 μg/mL (phenobarbital), 7–10 μg/mL (phenylethylmalonamide [PEMA])
Time to peak plasma level	3 hours
Volume of distribution	0.6 L/kg
Plasma protein binding	To 10%
Elimination half-life	10–12 hours
Excreted unchanged	1%

Drug Interactions

Primidone's interactions with other drugs are similar to those of phenobarbital. The ratio of derived phenobarbital to unmetabolized primidone in the serum is higher in epileptic patients treated with primidone and phenytoin than in those treated with primidone alone.[6,7]

Pregnancy/Lactation

No unusual toxic effects have been reported in epileptic pregnant women taking primidone. Most pregnant women on antiepileptic drugs deliver normal infants. The effects of primidone on fetal and neonatal development have not been established. Neonatal hemorrhage with a coagulation defect resembling vitamin K deficiency has been described in newborns whose mothers took primidone and other anticonvulsants.[8] Primidone is found in breast milk in concentrations sufficient to induce somnolence in nursing newborns.[9] During the second trimester of pregnancy, primidone plasma levels rise and phenobarbital levels fall. This ratio is reversed in the last week of pregnancy and in the postpartum period.[10]

Mechanism of Action

Primidone may be an anticonvulsant in its own right, but it also exerts its anticonvulsant properties through the metabolite phenobarbital. Central nervous system depression appears to be due to primidone and not to its metabolites.[11,12]

Clinical Presentation

Symptoms of poisoning may include sedation, vertigo, dizziness, nausea, vomiting, ataxia, diplopia, and nystagmus.

Massive crystalluria (hexagonal crystals) indicates severe poisoning with primidone.[13] The crystals result from precipitation of primidone in the urine, and this is observed at serum levels greater than 80 μg/mL.[13,14]

Treatment

Treatment is supportive and symptomatic. The use of gastric lavage, activated charcoal, and cathartics has not been studied. Stabilization comprises the following measures:

1. Maintenance of airway, breathing, and circulatory integrity
2. Endotracheal intubation as needed
3. Assisted ventilation as required

REFERENCES—PRIMIDONE

1. Hvidberg EF, Dam M. Clinical pharmacokinetics of anticonvulsants. Clin Pharmacokinet 1976;1:161–188.
2. Schottelius DD. Primidone: Absorption, distribution and excretion. In: Woodbury DM, Penry JK, Pippenger CE, eds. *Antiepileptic Drugs.* New York: Raven Press, 1982:405–413.
3. Booker HE, Hosokawa K, Burdette RD, et al. A clinical study of primidone levels. Epilepsia 1970;11:395–402.
4. Lee CC, Marbury TC, Perchalski RT, et al. Pharmacokinetics of primidone elimination by uremic patients. J Clin Pharmacol 1982;22:301–308.
5. Houghton GW, Richens A, Toseland PA, et al. Brain concentrations of phenytoin, phenobarbital and primidone in epileptic patients. Eur J Clin Pharmacol 1975;9:73–78.
6. Reynolds EH, Fenton G, Fenwick P, et al. Interaction of phenytoin and primidone. Br Med J 1975;2:594–595.
7. Finchman RW, Schottelius DD, Salis AL. The influence of diphenylhydantoin on primidone metabolism. Arch Neurol 1974;30:259.
8. *Physicians' Desk Reference.* 49th ed. Oradell, NJ: Medical Economics, 1995:2692–2693.
9. O'Brien TE. Excretion of drugs in human milk. Am J Hosp Pharm 1974;31:844–854.
10. Battino D, Binelli S, Bossi L. Changes in primidone/phenobarbital ratio during pregnancy and the puerperium. Clin Pharmacokinet 1984;9:252–260.
11. Gallagher BB, Baumel IP, Mattson RH, et al. Primidone, diphenylhydantoin and phenobarbital aspects of acute and chronic toxicity. Neurology 1973;23:145–149.
12. Brillman J, Gallagher BB, Mattson RH. Acute primidone intoxication. Arch Neurol 1974;30:255–258.
13. Van Heijst ANP, de Jong W, Seldenrijk R, et al. Coma and crystalluria: A massive primidone intoxication treated with hemoperfusion. J Toxicol Clin Toxicol 1983;20(4):307–318.
14. Bailey DN, Jatlow PI. Chemical analysis of massive crystalluria following primidone overdose. Am J Clin Pathol 1972; 58:583–589.

VALPROIC ACID AND SODIUM VALPROATE

Valproic acid, 2-propylpentanoic acid (Depakene, Depakote), a synthetic chemical, was approved in 1978 in the United States for the treatment of epilepsy. Since then, reports of overdose and poisoning have appeared,[1–5] sufficient to indicate the generally mild nature of its central nervous system depression although drowsiness and coma may occur; its propensity for interaction with other anticonvulsants[6,7]; its response to simple supportive care; and its unpredictable though infrequent tendency to produce hepatic necrosis (Reye-like syndrome)[8–11] and acute pancreatitis.[12–16]

Toxic Dose

Toxic effects are frequently associated with daily doses greater than 1800 mg[1,2] and blood levels greater than 100 μg/mL.[12] Unconsciousness occurs when more than 200 mg/kg has been ingested.[5]

Toxicokinetics[17–19]

Peak plasma level	50–100 μg/mL
Time to peak plasma level	1–4 hours
Volume of distribution	0.15–0.40 L/kg
Plasma protein binding	90%
Elimination half-life	7–15 hours
Excreted unchanged	1–3%

Drug Interactions

Valproic acid does not induce hepatic microsomal drug-metabolizing enzymes. Phenobarbital serum levels increase when valproic acid is also administered, enhancing the sedative effect. The mechanism is not known. Therefore, when phenobarbital is given with sodium valproate, the dose of phenobarbital may need to be reduced.[7,20] Primidone blood levels are increased initially when administered with sodium valproate, but return to normal within 1 to 3 months.[21]

When valproic acid and phenytoin are given together, blood levels (total and free) of phenytoin should be determined and the dosage adjusted as required.

Pregnancy/Lactation

Valproic acid is found in the placental circulation. It is dysmorphogenic in animals.[22] Valproic acid exposure during the first trimester of pregnancy appears to be associated with an increase in neural tube defects (spina bifida).[23] The risk of spina bifida after valproic acid use during pregnancy appears to be 1 to 2%. There is no substantial evidence that valproic acid use increases the risk for other specific major malformations above the increased risk due to maternal epilepsy.[24] Minor facial malformations have been described, including epicanthal folds with an infraorbital crease, flat nasal bridge, small upturned nose, long upper lip with a relatively shallow philtrum, thin upper vermillion border, and downturned angles of the mouth (a fetal valproate syndrome).[25]

Higher valproate doses (1200–2000 mg daily) resulting in higher valproate serum concentrations (73 μg/mL versus 44 μg/mL in other mothers) may be associated with an increased risk of spinal bifida.[26]

Withdrawal symptoms begin 12 to 48 hours after delivery and include irritability, jitteriness, abnormal tone, seizures, and feeding problems.

Clinical Presentation

Acute valproic acid poisoning is observed infrequently but is not rare. Patients usually exhibit drowsiness; unconsciousness appears to occur only if more than 200 mg/kg body weight of valproic acid has been ingested. There is little correlation between central nervous system effects (depth of coma, seizures) and plasma valproate levels. Encephalopathy, stupor, and coma without hepatic toxicity have been reported in adults. Children have developed a reversible dementia and apparent brain atrophy.[27] Such patients exhibit nontoxic valproate plasma levels, lack of fever, hyperammonemia, and normal liver function tests.[28] Seizures occur rarely when 100 to 700 mg/kg valproic acid is administered daily in the treatment of epilepsy.[21] Valproate causes reversible proximal tubular dysfunction and Fanconi syndrome.[29]

Hepatotoxicity Following Chronic Use

Hepatotoxicity associated with valproic acid use manifests as asymptomatic elevations in serum concentrations of liver enzymes (fairly common); hyperammonemia associated with lethargy, vomiting, stupor, or coma but generally not accompanied by hepatocellular damage; and acute hepatotoxicity that may terminate fatally.[12]

Laboratory

Blood Levels

When plasma levels of valproic acid exceed the upper therapeutic blood level of 100 μg/mL, the free drug fraction increases as binding sites become saturated.[21] Multiple-dose activated charcoal appears to be more effective if a toxin is not extensively bound to plasma proteins.[30] Repeated doses of activated charcoal have been used to increase the elimination of valproate despite its high protein binding.[31]

Ancillary Tests

Serum valproate levels, liver function, serum amylase levels, and complete blood counts, including platelets and bleeding time, should be monitored in the overdosed patient. The electroencephalogram is usually normal. Slight thrombocytopenia with inhibition of the second phase of platelet aggregation may be seen. Both the erythrocyte sedimentation rate and the fibrinogen level may be decreased. An abnormal bleeding, partial thromboplastin, and prothrombin times may be observed.

Treatment

Stabilization

An airway and breathing should be established and circulatory status evaluated. If respiratory depression is present on admission, the patient may require assisted mechanical ventilation after endotracheal intubation. Tidal volume adequacy should be checked (normal, 10–15 mL/kg).

Gut Decontamination

Emesis inducers are not ordinarily advisable as the patient will be somnolent or stuporous on admission. The patient should be observed for aspiration.

Gastric lavage may be of limited value in view of the very rapid absorption of the drug.

Activated charcoal (adults, 50–100 g; children, 15–30 g) may adsorb valproate still in the gut, but its efficacy has not been evaluated.

Elimination Enhancement

No systematic studies are available to support the usefulness of forced diuresis, hemodialysis, peritoneal dialysis, exchange transfusion, or hemoperfusion.

Anecdotal reports indicate that a patient with persistent hemodynamic instability was refractory to naloxone, activated charcoal, fluid resuscitation, and a dopamine drip. Seizures responded to lorazepam. Hemodialysis led to a reduction in the valproic acid level and return of responsiveness.[32] Charcoal hemoperfusion in one patient increased valproic acid clearance associated with clinical improvement.[33] The relatively small volume of distribution would tend to favor extracorporeal removal. In view of the good recovery with supportive treatment, extracorporeal removal is of questionable benefit in valproic acid intoxication without renal failure.

Antidote

An adult with depressed consciousness following an overdose of valproic acid became alert and responsive within 1 minute of administration of naloxone 2 mg by intravenous push.[34] Little effect has been observed after administration of naloxone in patients with high serum valproic acid levels.[35]

Supportive Measures

Supportive treatment is the mainstay of valproate overdose.

Adequate urine output should be maintained. All anticonvulsive drugs and all hepatic enzyme inducers should be discontinued. This should be sufficient for rapid recovery within the next 24 to 72 hours.

Seizures should be managed by determination of the serum levels of valproic acid, discontinuation of the drug if serum levels of valproate are elevated, and use of intravenous diazepam (0.1–0.3 mg/kg) to a maximum of 20 mg in an adult. This may be repeated in 10 to 20 minutes if required.

If patients are stuporous, somnolent, or drowsy, but otherwise have normal vital signs and liver function tests, simple observation for 24 to 72 hours in a hospital intensive care unit may be sufficient.

There is one anecdotal report of a patient with valproic acid-associated fulminant failure who responded to orthotopic liver transplantation.[36]

There are few data to support the usefulness of L-carnitine either as treatment of overdose or for prevention of valproate-related hepatotoxicity.

REFERENCES—VALPROIC ACID AND SODIUM VALPROATE

1. Chadwick DW, Cumming WJK, Livingstone I, et al. Acute intoxication with sodium valproate. Ann Neurol 1978;6: 552–553.
2. Steiman GS, Woerpel RW, Sherard ES Jr. Treatment of an accidental sodium valproate overdose with an opiate antagonist. Ann Neurol 1979;6:274.
3. Eeg-Olofsson O, Lindskog U. Acute intoxication with valproate. Lancet 1982;1:1306.
4. Karlsen RL, Kett K, Henriksen O. Intoxication with sodium valproate: A case report. Acta Med Scand 1983;213: 405–406.
5. Garnier R, Boudignat O, Fournier PE. Valproate poisoning. Lancet 1982;2:97.
6. Closson RG. Interaction between valproic acid and phenytoin. West J Med 1983;138:108.
7. Keys PA. Valproic acid: Interactions with phenytoin and phenobarbital. Drug Intell Clin Pharm 1982;16:737–739.
8. Palm R, Silseth C, Alvan G. Phenytoin intoxication as the first symptom of fatal liver damage induced by sodium valproate. Br J Clin Pharmacol 1984;17:597–599.
9. Sugimoto T, Nishida N, Yasuhara A, et al. Reye-like syndrome associated with valproic acid. Brain Dev 1983;5: 334–337.
10. Hojer B, Rane A. Fatal hepatic failure in a child treated with phenytoin and valproic acid. Dev Med Clin Neurol 1980; 24:846–849.
11. Ware S, Milward-Sadler CH. Acute liver disease associated with sodium valproate. Lancet 1980;2:1110–1113.
12. Turnbull DM. Adverse effects of valproate. Adverse Drug React Acute Poison Rev 1983;2:191–216.

13. Schmidt D. Adverse effects of valproate. Epilepsia 1984; 25(suppl.1):S44–S49.
14. Isom JB. On the toxicity of valproic acid. Am J Dis Child 1984;138:901 000.
15. Wyllie E, Wyllie R, Cruse RP, et al. Pancreatitis associated with valproic acid therapy. Am J Dis Child 1984;138: 912–914.
16. Williams IHP, Reynolds RP, Emery JL. Pancreatitis during sodium valproate treatment. Arch Dis Child 1983;58:543–544.
17. Loiseau P, Bracket A, Henry P. Concentration of dipropylacetate in plasma. Epilepsia 1974;16:609–615.
18. Bauer LA, Davis R, Wilensky A, et al. Valproic acid clearance: Unbound fraction and diurnal variation in young and elderly patients. Clin Pharmacol Ther 1985;32:697–700.
19. Bryson SM, Verma N, Scott PJW, et al. Pharmacokinetics of valproic acid in young and elderly subjects. Br J Clin Pharmacol 1983;16:104–105.
20. Hvidberg EF, Dam M. Clinical pharmacokinetics of anticonvulsants. Clin Pharmacokinet 1976;1:161–188.
21. Gugler R, von Unruh GE. Clinical pharmacokinetics of valproic acid. Clin Pharmacokinet 1980;5:67–83.
22. Pinder RM, Borgden RN, Speight TM, et al. Sodium valproate: A review of its pharmacological and therapeutic efficacy in epilepsy. Drugs 1977;13:81–123.
23. Lindhout D, Schmidt D. In utero exposure to valproate and neural tube defects. Lancet 1986;1:1392–1393.
24. Lammer EJ, Sever LE, Oakley GP Jr. Teratogen update: Valproic acid. Teratology 1987;35:465–473.
25. DiLiberti JD, Farndon PA, Dennis NR, Curry CJR. The fetal valproate syndrome. Am J Med Genet 1984;19:473–481.
26. Omtzigt JGC, Nau H, Los FJ, Pijpers L, Lindhout D. The disposition of valproate and its metabolites in the late first trimester and early second trimester of pregnancy in maternal serum, urine and amniotic fluid: Effect of dose, comedication, and the presence of spina bifida. Eur J Clin Pharmacol 1992;43:381–388.
27. Papazian O, Canizales E, Alfonso I, et al. Reversible dementia and apparent brain atrophy during valproate therapy. Ann Neurol 1995;38:687–691.
28. Settle EC. Valproate and associated encephalopathy with coma. Am J Psychiatry 1995;152:1236–1237.
29. Lande MB, Kim MS, Bartlett C, Guay-Woodford LM. Reversible Fanconi syndrome associated with valproate therapy. J Pediatr 1993;123:320–322.
30. Pond SM. Role of repeated oral doses of activated charcoal in clinical toxicology. Med Toxicol 1986;1:3–11.
31. Neuvonen PJ, Olkolla KT. Oral activated charcoal in the treatment of intoxications: Role of single and repeated doses. Med Toxicol 1988;3:33–58.
32. Williams SR, Clark RF. Hemodialysis of a valproic acid poisoning. Clin Toxicol 1995;33:475–486 (Abstract 13).
33. Graudins A, Aaron CK. Delayed peak serum valproic acid level in massive divalproex overdose: Successful treatment with charcoal hemoperfusion. Clin Toxicol 1995;33:475–486.
34. Alberto G, Erickson T, Popiel R, et al. Central nervous system manifestations of a valproic acid overdose responsive to naloxone. Ann Emerg Med 1989;18:889–891.
35. Anderson GO, Ritland S. Life threatening intoxication with sodium valproate. Clin Toxicol 1995;33:279–284.
36. Bell EA, Shaefer MS, Markin RS, et al. Treatment of valproic acid-associated hepatic failure with orthotopic liver transplantation. Ann Pharmacother 1992;26:118–121.

MAGNESIUM VALPROATE

Magnesium valproate appears similar in efficacy to sodium valproate in initial trials. The therapeutic serum level range is 40 to 100 μg/mL. No significant increase in serum concentration is found. The effective dosage appears to be 20 to 30 mg/kg/d. Magnesium valproate is rapidly absorbed with a half-life of 8.25 hours and a volume of distribution of 0.1 L/kg.[1]

VALPROMIDE

Valpromide (VPD, 12-dipropylacetamide, 2-propylvaleramide) has been used as an antiepileptic drug for the past 25 years in several European countries. Valpromide is a prodrug of valproic acid.

Product Formulation

Valproic acid is a liquid; sodium valproate is a hygroscopic solid; valpromide is a nonhygroscopic solid. It is available as an enteric-coated 300-mg tablet (Depamide, France; Vistora, Spain).

Toxicokinetics

The fraction of valpromide biotransferred to valproic acid is approximately 0.8 after both oral and intravenous use. The bioavailability of valpromide relative to valproic acid is 80%.

	Valproic Acid	Valpromide
Clearance (L/h/kg)	0.007	1
Volume of distribution (L/kg)	0.15	0.60
Beta half-life (hours)	7–15	0.8
Excreted unchanged in urine (%)	1–3	<1.0

Drug Interactions

Valpromide increases the plasma concentration of carbamazepine 10,11-epoxide by inhibition of the enzyme epoxide hydrolase. Valpromide may increase amitriptyline and nortriptyline levels in the blood when given together.[2]

REFERENCES–MAGNESIUM VALPROATE, VALPROMIDE

1. Xie KJ, Xiao B, Yan CX, He ZW. Several studies on magnesium valproate. Clin Pharmacol Ther 1991;49:137.
2. Bialer M. Clinical Pharmacology of valpromide. Clin Pharmacokinet 1991;1:20:114–122.

VIGABATRIN

Severe behavioral disturbances, drowsiness, irritability, and weight gain may be dose dependent.

Structure and Classification

Vigabatrin is a synthetic structural analog of GABA, which is an inhibitory neurotransmitter (Fig. 36–1). Vigabatrin exists as a racemic mixture of two enantiomers. Only the *S*(+) enantiomer is pharmacologically active.[1]

Use

Vigabatrin appears to be most effective in partial seizures whether or not they also become generalized.

Product Formulation

Vigabatrin is available in the United Kingdom as Sabril.[2]

Therapeutic and Toxic Doses

Therapeutic starting doses of vigabatrin are 500 mg twice daily. A common daily dose is 3 g, with a maintenance range of 2 to 4 g. One patient developed a psychosis after ingesting 8 to 12 g of vigabatrin.[3] A fatal dose has not been determined. In one series psychosis developed after ingestion of 500 to 5000 mg. The period from initiation of therapy to the onset of psychosis varied from 5 days to 21 weeks. In all cases, the psychosis followed the cessation of vigabatrin.[4] Vertigo and tremor followed ingestion of 14 g/d for 3 days; recovery was uneventful.[5]

Toxicokinetics[6,7]

Bioavailability	60–80%
Peak plasma level	13–20 μg/mL
Time to peak plasma level	2 hours
Volume of distribution	0.6–1 L/kg
Elimination half-life	5–7 hours
Excreted unchanged	100%
Active metabolite	*S* (+) enantiomer

Drug Interactions

Vigabatrin does not induce liver enzymes. When it is given to patients already receiving phenytoin, plasma concentrations of phenytoin fall by about 20% by an unknown mechanism and may lead to an increase in seizure frequency.[8] None of the enzyme-inducing anticonvulsants (eg, carbamazepine, phenytoin, primidone, phenobarbital) influence vigabatrin elimination.

Pregnancy/Lactation

There are no published studies on use of vigabatrin in pregnancy and lactation. Safe use in pregnancy or lactation has not been established.

Mechanism of Action

Studies suggest that vigabatrin inhibits irreversibly the enzyme GABA transaminase, which itself inactivates GABA, an inhibitory neurotransmitter, thus permitting an increase in the concentration of GABA at GABAergic synapses in the brain. Vigabatrin is itself inactive but is converted in vivo to its active form by GABA aminotransferase.[9]

Clinical Presentation

Chronic Use

Long-term use of vigabatrin is associated with drowsiness, headache, fatigue, irritability, depression, dizziness, confusion, and weight gain. These adverse effects appear to be dose dependent.[10–12] Excitation in children and hallucinations and paranoia in adults have been reported.[13] Short temper and behavioral disturbances have been observed with doses of 3 g/d or more.[11,14–18] Visual, auditory, and somatosensory evoked potentials are unchanged in human subjects.[11] A history of psychiatric illness commonly predisposes patients to a psychotic reaction pattern.[18,19] Myoclonus that subsides after dose reduction has been observed.[20]

Microvacuoles are seen within white matter tracts in the brain of rats given vigabatrin for 12 months or longer. The lesions appear to be reversible on cessation of therapy. Such evidence has not been observed in humans.[2,21,22] An acute encephalopathy after vigibatrin use may be related to a preexisting cerebral abnormality.[23]

Withdrawal

As with all antiepileptic drugs, an acute exacerbation of seizures may occur after the sudden withdrawal of vigabatrin.[24] In addition, withdrawal of vigabatrin has been followed by acute psychosis.

Overdose

One patient developed a psychotic episode lasting 36 hours after having taken an overdose of 8 to 12 g of vigabatrin during postictal confusion.[3]

Laboratory

Analytical Methods

An isocratic high-performance liquid chromatography method using fluorescence detection is available for determination of vigabatrin in 50 μL of plasma. The minimum detection limit is 0.08 μg/ml and the minimum quantitation limit is 0.54 μg/mL.[1]

Blood Levels

No clear relationship between blood concentration and clinical effect of the drug has been shown.[25]

Abnormalities

Slight decreases in hemoglobin and hematocrit have been observed with decreases in serum transaminase concentrations.[1] Vigabatrin appears to induce increased excretion in the urine of β-alanine, GABA, and β-aminoisobutyric acid.[26] Pyroglutamic aciduria may follow vigabatrin use.[27] Its significance is still not clear.

Plasma alanine transaminase activity is an unreliable marker of liver function in patients taking this drug. Plasma alanine transaminase activity within the reference range does not discount the possibility of liver disease.[28]

Treatment

Patients who overdose with vigabatrin should be treated with symptomatic and supportive management. There is no antidote. Consideration should be given to use of elimination enhancement procedures, such as hemoperfusion and hemodialysis, in a serious overdose, in view of the minimal protein binding, low volume of distribution, and largely unchanged renal excretion.[29]

Patients should be monitored with visual evoked potential studies in view of the uniformity of visual pathway involvement of intramyelinic edema in lower species.[22] Vigabatrin should not be used by patients with a history of behavioral disturbances or severe mental illness.[16]

REFERENCES—VIGABATRIN

1. Tsanaclis LM, Wichs J, Williams J, Richens A. Determination of vigabatrin in plasma by reversed-phase high-performance liquid chromatography. Ther Drug Monit 1991;13:251–253.
2. Vigabatrin. Lancet 1989;1:532–533. Editorial.
3. Sander JWAS, Hart YM, Sharvon SD. Vigabatrin and epilepsy. J Neurol Neurosurg Psychiatry 1992;55:245.
4. Sander JWAS, Hart YM, Trimble MR, Sharvon SD. Vigabatrin and psychosis. J Neurol Neurosurg Psychiatry 1991;54:435–439.
5. Clinical Investigation Brochure 1988: Vigabatrin (GABA transaminase inhibitor). Cincinnati, OH: Merrell Dow Research Institute. Merrell Dow Pharmaceuticals, 1988.
6. Brodie MJ. Established anticonvulsants and treatment of refractory epilepsy. Lancet 1990;336:350–354.
7. Hoke JF, Ruberg SJ, Antony KK, Okerholm RA. Pharmacokinetics and dose proportionality of gamma-vinyl GABA (vigabatrin) following multiple oral doses. Neurology 1991;41(suppl. 1):139.
8. Tassinan CA, Michelucci R, Ambrosetto G, Salvi F. Double blind study of vigabatrin in the treatment of drug resistant epilepsy. Arch Neurol 1987;44:907–910.
9. Sjoerdsma A. Suicide enzyme inhibitors as potential drugs. Clin Pharmacol Ther 1981;30:3–22.
10. Remy C, Beaumont D. Efficacy and safety of vigabatrin in the long term treatment of refractory epilepsy. Br J Clin Pharmacol 1989;27:125S–129S.
11. Ring HA, Reynolds EHJ. Vigabatrin and behavior disturbance. Lancet 1990;335:970.
12. Ring HA, Heller AJ, Farr IN, Reynolds EH. Vigabatrin: Rational treatment for chronic epilepsy. J Neurol Neurosurg Psychiatry 1990;53:1051–1055.
13. Olive G, Rey E, Pons G, Richard MO, et al. Pharmacokinetics of R(–) and S(+) vigabatrin (GVG) in children. Clin Pharmacol Ther 1989;45:39.
14. Robinson MK, Richens A, Oxley R. Vigabatrin and psychiatric disturbances. Lancet 1990;2:504.
15. Sander JWAS, Hart YM. Vigabatrin and behavior disturbances. Lancet 1990;335:57.
16. Brodie MJ, McKee PJW. Vigabatrin and psychosis. Lancet 1990;1:1279.
17. Dann M. Vigabatrin and behavior disturbances. Lancet 1990;335:605–606.
18. Grant SM, Heel RC. Vigabatrin: A review of its pharmacodynamic and pharmacokinetic properties and therapeutic potential in epilepsy and disorders of motor control. Drugs 1991;41:889–926.
19. Liegeois-Chauvel C, Marquis P, Gisselbrecht D, et al. Effects of long term vigabatrin on somatosensory evoked potentials in epileptic patients. Br J Clin Pharmacol 1989;27:69S–72S.
20. Neufeld MY, Vishnevska S. Vigabatrin and multifocal myoclonus in adults with partial seizures. Clin Neuropharmacol 1995;18:280–283.
21. Paljarvi L, Vapalahti M, Sivenius J, Riekkonen P. Neuropathological findings in 5 patients with vigabatrin treatment. Neurology 1990;40(suppl. 1):151.
22. Graham D. Neuropathology of vigabatrin. Br J Clin Pharmacol 1989;27:43S–45S.
23. Sharief MK, Sander JWA, Shorvon SD. Acute encephalopathy with vigabatrin. Lancet 1993;342.
24. Staples CI, King MA, Boyle RS. Acute psychosis after withdrawal of vigabatrin. Med J Aust 1992;156:291.
25. Gram L, Lyon BB, Dam M. Gamma-vinyl GABA: A single blind trial in patients with epilepsy. Acta Neurol Scand 1983;68:34–39.
26. Shih VE, Tenanbaum A. Aminoaciduria due to vinyl-GABA administration. N Engl J Med 1990;323:1353.
27. Bonham JR, Rattenbury JM, Meeks A, Pollitt RJ. Pyroglutamic aciduria from vigabatrin. Lancet 1989;1:1452–1453.
28. Williams A, Goldsmith R, Coakley J. Profound suppression of plasma alanine aminotransferase activity in children taking vigabatrin. Aust NZ J Med 1993;23:65.
29. Reynolds EH. Vigabatrin: Rational treatment for chronic epilepsy. Br Med J 1990;300:177–178.

ZONISAMIDE

Zonisamide (AD-810, CI-912) is a substituted 1,2-benzisoxazole anticonvulsant that originated in Japan, where it is now marketed.[1] It is effective in myoclonic epilepsy, complex partial seizure, absence seizures, and single partial seizures.[1,2] Trials in the United States have been stopped because the drug has been associated with renal calculi.[1]

Therapeutic Dose

Doses of 6 to 7 mg/kg/d have been used.[2,3]

Toxicokinetics[4–7]

Peak plasma level	20–30 μg/L
Time to peak plasma level	1½–4 hours
Elimination half-life	56 hours

Drug Interactions

In overdose, zonisamide does not appear to alter the half-life of carbamazepine.[7]

Clinical Presentation

Chronic Use

Toxic effects from chronic use include weight loss, anorexia, nausea, drowsiness, tremor, dizziness, numbness, and decrease in mental acuity. Hypochromic anemia and elevated levels of serum pyruvic transaminase[8] and serum glutamic transaminase[3] have been observed.

Overdose

A 26-year-old woman with a history of epileptic seizures was maintained with 400 mg/d zonisamide as well as 12 mg/d clonazepam (CZP) and 1000 mg/d carbamazepine. Blood levels of 37.2 μg/mL, 87.8 ng/mL, and 6.6 μg/mL, respectively, were obtained 1 day before she was found unconscious, with bradycardia, hypotension, and depressed respiration. Spontaneous horizontal nystagmus and myoclonus were evident 13 hours later. The patient became alert 4 days later. She continued to seize with plasma zonisamide, clonazepam, and carbamazepine levels of 40.7 μg/mL, 43.6 ng/mL, and 0.3 μg/mL, respectively. The patient ultimately was discharged.[7]

Laboratory

Plasma concentrations of zonisamide and carbamazepine are measured by high-performance liquid chromatography, and that of clonazepam by gas chromatography.

Treatment

Patients should be treated symptomatically and supportively. Oxygen, intravenous lines, and cardiac monitoring should be available. The patient should be admitted to an intensive care facility where pulse, blood pressure, complete blood counts, liver function tests, and neurologic status can be continuously monitored. Periodic electroencephalogram studies should be performed as indicated. If the patient is seen within

4 hours of ingestion, an attempt should be made to empty the stomach (eg, gastric lavage). There are no controlled studies to support the use of activated charcoal or cathartics.

REFERENCES—ZONISAMIDE

1. Brodie MJ, Porter RJ. New and potential anticonvulsants. Lancet 1990;2:425–426.
2. Shimizu A, Yamamoto J, Yamada Y, et al. The antiepileptic effect of zonisamide in patients with refractory seizures. Curr Ther Res 1987;42:147–155.
3. Wilensky AJ, Friel NP, Ojemanni LM, et al. Zonisamide in epilepsy: A pilot study. Epilepsia 1985;26:212–220.
4. Matsumoto K, Miyazaki H, Fujii T, et al. Absorption, distribution and excretion of 3-(sulfamoyl [^{14}C]methyl)-1,2-benzisoxazole (AD-810) in rats, dogs and monkeys and of AD-810 in men. Arzneimitt-Forschung Drug Res 1983;33:961–968.
5. Taylor CP, McLean JR, Bockbrader HN, et al. Zonisamide (AD-810, C1-912). In: Meldrum BS, Porter RJ, eds. *New Anticonvulsant Drugs.* London: John Wiley, 1986:277–294.
6. Berent S, Sackellares JC, Giordani B, et al. Zonisamide (C1-912) and cognition: Results from preliminary study. Epilepsia 1987;28:61–67.
7. Naito H, Itoh N, Matsui N, Eguchi T. Monitoring plasma concentrations of zonisamide and clonazepam in an epileptic attempting suicide by an overdose of the drugs. Curr Ther Res 1988;43:463–467.
8. Sackellares JC, Donofrio PD, Wagner JG, et al. Pilot study of zonisamide (1,2-benzisoxazole-3-methanesulfonamide) in patients with refractory partial seizures. Epilepsia 1985; 26:206–211.

PSEUDOSTATUS EPILEPTICUS

Many patients who present with apparent status epilepticus in fact have pseudostatus epilepticus, a condition that mimics status epilepticus but in which repeated seizures are psychogenic.[1–3]

Pseudostatus epilepticus is also called hysterical seizures, simulated seizures, pseudoseizures, and nonorganic seizures.[1]

Diagnosis

Physical Examination

1. The patient often does not have the classic features of convulsive seizures.
2. There are often vocalization, bizarre behavior, and preservation of consciousness despite the apparent convulsion.
3. Incontinence, tongue biting, and cyanosis may occur but are less common than in true status epilepticus.[3,4]

History

1. Often there is a long history of personality disorder.
2. The patient may have had hysterical features, such as a nonorganic paralysis and suicidal gestures.
3. The history of epilepsy is usually highly atypical, with an unusual pattern, odd responses to treatment, and normal (or nonspecifically abnormal) electroencephalographic recordings.
4. In the record there is often evidence of earlier pseudoseizure or pseudostatus.
5. The patients are frequently female.[1]

Laboratory

1. Electroencephalography during an episode is of considerable value.
2. In pseudostatus the electroencephalogram may show minor abnormalities or signs of medication, but no ongoing epileptic activity or typical postictal activity.[3]

Treatment

Patients usually receive intravenous anticonvulsants (eg, benzodiazepines), which curtail the seizures only after consciousness is abolished. As the patient recovers consciousness, seizures recur. Then more medication is administered. Some patients are sent to an intensive care facility. Some patients are paralyzed and ventilated before a correct diagnosis is made. Treatment ultimately requires in-depth prolonged psychiatric management.[1]

REFERENCES—PSEUDOSTATUS EPILEPTICUS

1. Pseudostatus epilepticus. Lancet 1989;1:485. Editorial.
2. Toone BK, Roberts J. Status epilepticus: An uncommon hysterical conversion syndrome. J Nerv Ment Dis 1979;167: 548–552.
3. Howell SJ, Owen L, Chadwick DW. Pseudostatus epilepticus. Q J Med 1989;266:507–519.
4. King DW, Gallagher BB, Murvin AJ, et al. Pseudoseizures: Diagnostic evaluation. Neurology 1982;32:18–23.

NEW ANTICONVULSANTS

Vigabatrin, oxcarbamazepine, lamotrigine, gabapentin, zonisamide, flunarizine, felbamate, stiripentol, topiramate, and eterobarb are new drugs in various phases of investigation as anticonvulsants.[1] Several are structural analogs of GABA, an inhibitory neurotransmitter.

REFERENCE—NEW ANTICONVULSANTS

1. Brodie MJ, Porter RJ. New and potential anticonvulsants. Lancet 1990;336:425–426.

Chapter 37 Antidepressant Agents

INTRODUCTION

Antidepressant drugs are among the most commonly encountered causes of self-poisoning. These drugs include tricyclic, tetracyclic, bicyclic, and monocyclic antidepressants, as well as monoamine oxidase (MAO) inhibitors and selective serotonin reuptake inhibitors (SSRIs). Of these, the tricyclic antidepressants (TCAs) are generally more toxic in overdose, with major toxicity usually manifesting within the first 6 hours of overdose.[1] Toxicity following overdose of antidepressant drugs is most likely to be seen with the classic TCAs and classic MAO inhibitors, followed by the newer cyclic antidepressants. Toxicity is rarely seen with the newer MAO-A inhibitors and SSRIs when these drugs are taken in isolation.[1]

Table 37–1 summarizes classes of psychotropic drugs with examples of the "newer" drugs discussed in this chapter. Table 37–2 summarizes some pharmacologic effects of the antidepressant drugs.[2] Tables 37–3 and 37–4 list antidepressant drugs available in the United States and the United Kingdom.

Therapeutic Dose

Typical doses and estimated relative potency of antipsychotic drugs available in the United States are presented in Table 37–5.

Fatality Toxicity Index

On the basis of the Fatality Toxicity Index (FTI), which ranks dothiepin, amitriptyline, and tranylcypromine as drugs with "unacceptable risks" (more than 40 deaths per million prescriptions), maprotiline as "very dangerous" (more than 30 deaths per million), phenelzine and imipramine as "clearly dangerous" (more than 20 deaths per million), and clomipramine, protriptyline, and trazodone as "potentially dangerous" (more than 10 deaths per million), lofepramine, mianserin, fluvoxamine, fluoxetine, and viloxazine are ranked as "relatively safe," being associated with fewer than 10 deaths per million prescriptions. De Jonghe and Swinkels have used similar methodology to identify fluoxetine, fluvoxamine, mianserin, paroxetine, and trazodone as "safe antidepressants," on the basis that overdose with a 14-day

Table 37–1
The Central Nervous System and Psychotropic Drugs

- Cyclic antidepressants
  - Tricyclic antidepressants
  - Amineptine
  - Dothiepin
  - Lofepramine
  - Metapramine
  - Minaprine
- Neuroleptic agents
  - Clozapine
  - Methotrimeprazine
  - Propericiazine
  - Remoxipride
  - Zuclopenthixol
- Dopamine receptor drugs
  - Bupropion
  - Dobutamine
  - Dopexomine
  - Levodopa–carbidopa
  - Lisuride
  - Sulpiride
- Monoamine oxidase inhibitors
  - Moclobemide
  - Pimozide
  - Selegiline
  - Toloxatone
- Serotonin receptor drugs
  - Buspirone
  - Cyproheptadine
  - Fluoxetine
  - Fluvoxamine
  - Oxaflozane
  - Oxetorone fumarate
  - Paroxetine
  - Pizotifen
  - Risperidone
  - Sertraline
  - Sumatriptan
- H_2-receptor antagonists
  - Cimetidine
  - Famotidine
  - Nizatidine
  - Ranitidine
- Hallucinogens
  - Lysergic acid diethylamide (LSD)
  - Phencyclidine (PCP)
  - Marijuana
- Central nervous system stimulants

supply of medication is likely to be tolerated without significant toxicity.[3]

Toxicokinetics

A survey of the toxicokinetics of antidepressant agents is presented in Tables 37–6 and 37–7. Note the large volume of distribution and high protein binding of these drugs, indications that extracorporeal methods of elimination may be relatively ineffective.

Mechanism of Action

Antidepressant agents are active at adrenergic, serotonin, dopamine, histamine H_1, and muscarnic receptors (Table 37–8). This is reflected in their toxic effects (Table 37–9).

Clinical Presentation

Schizophrenia

Evidence suggests that the dopamine D_2 receptor (DRD2) gene is a candidate gene for schizophrenia.[4–8] Dopamine D_2 receptor blockade also is responsible for the extrapyramidal syndromes induced by neuroleptic agents.[2,9]

Neuroleptic-Induced Deficit Syndrome

Antipsychotic drugs (eg, haloperidol) are associated with a deficit syndrome characterized by sedation, extrapyramidal signs, indifference to internal and external stimuli, passivity, and reduced initiative.[10] Such impairment of cognitive, social, and affective function has been termed the

Table 37–2
In Vitro Short-Term Biochemical Activity of Selected Older and Newer Antidepressant Drugs

	Reuptake Inhibition			Receptor Affinity				
Drug	NA	5-HT	D	α_1	α_2	H_1	MUSC	D_2
Older Drugs*								
Amitriptyline	±	++	0	+++	±	++++	++++	0
Clomipramine	±	+++	0	++	0	+	++	++
Desipramine	+++	0	0	+	0	±	+	0
Dothiepin	±	±	0	±	0	+++	+++	0
Doxepin	++	+	0	+++	0	++++	++	0
Imipramine	+	+	0	++	0	+	++	0
Nortriptyline	++	±	0	++	0	+	++	0
Trimipramine	+	0	0	+++	±	++++	++	++
Newer Drugs								
Amfebutamone (bupropion)	±	0	++	0	0	0	0	0
Amoxapine	++	0	0	++	0	+	0	++
Citalopram	0	+++	0	0	0	0	0	0
Fluoxetine†	0	+++	0	0	0	0	0	0
Fluvoxamine	0	+++	0	0	0	0	0	0
Lofepramine	+++	0	0	+	0		+	++
Maprotiline	++	0	0	++	0	+++	+	+
Mianserin	0	0	0	+++	++	++++	0	0
Paroxetine†	0	++++	0	0	0	0	±	0
Sertraline†	0	+++	0	0	0	0	0	0
Trazodone	0	+	0	+++	±	±	0	0

NA, noradrenaline (norepinephrine); 5-HT, 5-hydroxytryptamine (serotonin); D, dopamine; α_1, α_1 adrenergic receptor; α_2, α_2-adrenergic receptor; H_1, H_1 histamine receptor; MUSC, muscarinic (cholinergic) receptor; D_2, D_2 dopamine receptor; 0, no effect; ±, equivocal effect; +, small effect; ++, moderate effect; +++, large effect; ++++, maximal effect.

From Rudorfer MW, Manji HE, Poter WZ. Comparative tolerability profiles of the newer versus older antidepressants. Drug Saf 1994;10:18–42.

Table 37–3
Antidepressants Available in the United States

Monoamine oxidase inhibitors	
Phenelzine sulfate	Nardil
Tranylcypromine sulfate	Parnate
Serotonin reuptake inhibitors	
Fluoxetine hydrochloride	Prozac
Paroxetine hydrochloride	Paxil
Venlafaxine hydrochloride	Effexor
Tricyclic antidepressants	
Amitriptyline hydrochloride	Elavil, Endep, Etrafon, Triavil (with perphenazine), Limbitrol (with chlordiazepoxide)
Clomipramine hydrochloride	Anafranil
Desipramine hydrochloride	Norpramin
Doxepin hydrochloride	Adapin, Sinequan
Imipramine hydrochloride	Tofranil
Nortriptyline hydrochloride	Pamelor
Protriptyline hydrochloride	Vivactil
Trimipramine maleate	Surmontil
Miscellaneous	
Bupropion hydrochloride	Wellbutrin
Trazodone hydrochloride	Desyrel

Source: *Physicians' Desk Reference.* 49th ed. Montvale, NJ: Medical Economics, 1995.

Table 37–4
Antidepressants Available in the United Kingdom

Tricyclic antidepressants	
Amitriptyline hydrochloride	Domical, Elavil, Lentizol, Saroten, Tryptizol
Amoxapine	Asendin
Butriptyline	
Clomipramine hydrochloride	Anafranil
Desipramine hydrochloride	
Dothiepin	Prothiaden
Lofepramine	Gamenil
Viloxazine hydrochloride	Vivalan
Monoamine oxidase inhibitors	
Isocarboxazide	Maplan
Tranylcypromine	Parnate
Other antidepressant drugs	
Flupenthixol	Fluanxol
Tryptophan	
Serotonin reuptake inhibitors	
Fluoxetine hydrochloride	Prozac
Fluvoxamine maleate	Faverin
Paroxetine	Seroxat
Sertraline	Lustrol
Tetracyclic antidepressants	
Maprotiline	Ludiomil
Miscellaneous	
Trazodone	Molipaxin

Source: British National Formulary, September 1988. Feel J, ed. *New Drugs.* 3rd ed. London: BMJ, 1994.

Table 37–5
Typical Doses and Estimated Relative Potency of Antipsychotic Drugs Available in the United States

Drug	Equivalent Dose* (mg)	Usual Total Daily Dose (mg/d): Short-term Therapy	Usual Total Daily Dose (mg/d): Maintenance Therapy
Phenothiazines			
Chlorpromazine	100	200–1000	50–400
Thioridazine	100	200–800	50–400
Mesoridazine	50	100–400	25–200
Acetophenazine	20	60–150	40–80
Prochlorperazine	15	60–200	20–60
Perphenazine	10	12–64	8–24
Trifluoperazine	5	10–60	4–30
Triflupromazine	25	30–150	20–100
Fluphenazine	2	5–50	1–15
Thioxanthenes			
Thiothixene	5	10–60	6–30
Chlorprothixene	100	50–600	50–400
Butyrophenones			
Haloperidol	2	5–50	1–15
Dibenzoxazepines			
Loxapine	10	20–160	10–60
Dihydroindolones			
Molindone	10	40–225	15–100
Dibenzodiazepines			
Clozapine	50	300–900	200–400
Benzisoxazoles			
Risperidone	1	4–8	Unknown
Long-acting injectable preparations			
Fluphenazine decanoate	—	—	6–100 every 2–4 wk
Haloperidol decanoate	—	—	50–200 every 4 wk

*Numbers shown are the numbers of milligrams of the drug required for the dose to be equivalent to the doses of the other drugs in the table (eg, 100 mg of chlorpromazine is equivalent to 2 mg of haloperidol). Relative potency may not be the same at higher dosages as at lower ones.
From Kane JM. Schizophrenia. N Engl J Med 1996;334:34–41.

Table 37–6
Toxicokinetics of Antidepressant Agents

	Bioavailability (%)	Protein Binding (%)	Volume of Distribution (L/Kg)	Half-life (h)	Clearance (L/h/kg)	Excretion (%) Urine	Feces	Unchanged	Main Metabolite(s)
Tricyclic antidepressants									
Imipramine	40–45	96	14–21	10–29	0.5–1	80	20	n.s.	Desmethyl-(A) = desipramine
Clomipramine	40–70	98	16	20–40	0.7	60	30	1–3	Desmethyl-(A)
Opiramol	n.s.	91	n.s.	6–23	n.s.	70	30	n.s.	Dehydroxyethyl-(A?)
Trimipramine	n.s.	95	31	9–23	n.s.	n.s.	n.s.	n.s.	Yes (A)
Lofepramine	7	99	n.s.	5	n.s.	n.s.	n.s.	n.s.	Desipramine- (A)
Amitriptyline	45	94	5–22	3–36	0.8–1.9	n.s.	n.s.	n.s.	*N* Desmethyl (A) = nortriptyline
Nortriptyline	30–80	92	21–57	17–93	0.4	n.s.	n.s.	n.s.	10-Hydroxy (A)
Protriptyline	77–93	92	22	54–92	n.s.	n.s.	n.s.	n.s.	Desmethyl- (A?)
Dothiepin	30	n.s.	11–70	14–25	1.4–3.8	n.s.	n.s.	0.5	Desmethyl-, dothipen *S* oxide
Desipramine	60–70	73–90	20–26	14–62	0.6–1.8	n.s.	n.s.	n.s.	n.s.
Doxepin	13–45	n.s.	9–33	8–24	n.s.	n.s.	n.s.	n.s.	Desmethyl- (A)
Tetracyclic antidepressants									
Maprotiline	66–75	88	15–28	27–58	0.4	60	30	n.s.	Desmethyl- (A)
Mianserin	20	96	18	30	0.7	70	20	4–7	Hydroxy-, desmethyl-, *N*-oxide- (A?)
Selective serotonin reuptake inhibitors									
Paroxetine	50	95	17	10–24	0.5–1	64	36	<2	Numerous (NA)
Citalopram	100	50	14–16	33	0.4	n.s.	n.s.	12	Desmethyl- (A)
Fluvoxamine	60	77	5–20	15–22	0.6–1	94	n.s.	<4	Numerous (NA)
Fluoxetine	72	95	20–42	46	0.2–0.5	80	15	11	Desmethyl- (A) = Norfluoxetine
Sertraline	40	99	>20	26	1.4	44	44	<0.2	Desmethyl- (A)
Reverse inhibitory monoamioxidase A									
Moclobemide	45–80	50	1.2	1–3	0.4–0.6	mainly	n.s.	<0.5	*N*-oxidation (A/NA)

n.s., not stated; (A), active; (NA), not active.
From Knudsen K. Tricyclic antidepressant poisoning: Aspects of pharmacologic treatment of severe overdose. Goteborg, 1994.

Table 37–7
Pharmacokinetic Parameters of Different Classes of Antidepressants

Pharmacokinetic Parameter	Tricyclic Antidepressants (TCAs)	Serotonin Selective Reuptake Inhibitors (SSRIs)	Bupropion	Trazodone	Monoamine Oxidase Inhibitor
T_{max}	Occurs within 1–3 h for tertiary amine TCAs and 4–8 h for secondary amine TCAs. Associated with sedation, orthostatic hypotension, and impairment of intracardiac conduction.	Slow rate of absorption: typically 4–8 h. Nausea can occur within <1 h of SSRI administration, suggesting a direct gastric effect. Given long T_{max}, shifting dose to minimize insomnia is unlikely to be helpful.	Occurs within 1–3 h. Associated with complaints of nausea (gastrointestinal or central) and stimulant effects. Highest incidence of seizures overlaps with T_{max} interval.	Occurs within 1–2 h. Associated with sedation.	Occurs within 1–3 h. Some cardiovascular adverse effects occur maximally during this interval.
Half-life	All TCAs have half-lives of 24 h or more in physically healthy, normal metabolizers when the half-lives of the parent drug and its active metabolites are considered together. Hence, TCAs can be given once per day unless there is concern about C_{max} (eg, cardiac patients). Steady state achieved within 7 days in most young, physically healthy adults.	Substantial differences among SSRIs: fluoxetine (2–4 d), norfluoxetine (7–15 d), paroxetine at initial dose (≈ 1 d but is prolonged at higher doses due to autoinhibition), sertraline over clinically relevant dose range (≈ 1 d). Time to achieve steady state in young, physically healthy adults: fluoxetine (10–20 d), norfluoxetine (35–75 d), sertraline (7 d) paroxetine (7 d at 20 mg/d and longer at higher doses). With the long half-lives of fluoxetine and norfluoxetine, there can be gradual buildup of effects over many weeks and persistence for a sustained interval after drug discontinuation. Dose titration can be difficult.	Half-life (mean ± SD) of bupropion, 9.8 ± 6.8 h; hydroxybupropion, 22.2 ± 5.6 h; erythrothydrobupropion, 26.8 ± 9.4 h; and erythrohydrobupropion, 19.8 ± 8.2 h. Half-life of parent drug plus concerns about seizure incidence and height of C_{max} make mutliple daily dosing necessary for acute and maintenance therapy.	5–9 h. Short half-life necessitates multiple daily dosing to induce a remission. Unknown whether multiple daily dosing is needed to maintain remission. In absence of evidence to contrary, multiple daily dosing is recommended for maintenance therapy. Steady state reached within 2–3 d.	2–4 h. Long biological effects due to irreversible deactivation of enzyme. Full disassociation of plasma concentration–response–time curve.
Active metabolites	TCAs have numerous metabolites whose pharmacologic profiles can differ in a clinically meaningful way from that of the parent drug. The secondary amine TCAs (eg, desipramine, nortriptyline) are demethylated metabolites of the tertiary amine TCAs (eg, imipramine, amitriptyline). They are perhaps more potent as antidepressants than tertiary amine TCAs; however, their adverse effect profile is more favorable: less anticholinergic, antihistaminic, anti-α_1-adrenergic, and direct membrane stabilization effects. There are also hydroxylated metabolites.	The SSRIs differ substantially from each other in this regard. Fluoxetine has a metabolite (norfluoxetine) that is equipotent to the parent drug in terms of both serotonin reuptake inhibition and inhibition of the hepatic isoenzyme IID6. Neither sertraline nor paroxetine has metabolites that contribute in a clinically meaningful way to serotonin reuptake inhibition. Both have metabolites that can inhibit the enzyme IID6; the concentrations of these metabolites and their potential for this effect are such as to be of no apparent clinical consequence.	The three biologically active metabolites may contribute more to the seizure risk than to antidepressant efficacy.	*m*CPP is the principal biologically active metabolite, having a pharmacologic profile substantially different from that of trazodone. It has been implicated an anxiogenic and other effects.	Metabolites are structurally and pharmacologically like amphetamines and may mediate some of the stimulant effects of MAOIs that occur shortly after ingestion (ie, 2–5 h).

(continued)

Table 37–7 *(Continued)*

Pharmacokinetic Parameter	Tricyclic Antidepressants (TCAs)	Serotonin Selective Reuptake Inhibitors (SSRIs)	Bupropion	Trazodone	Monoamine Oxidase Inhibitor
Dose–plasma drug level proportionality	Over the clinically relevant dose range, TCAs follow linear pharmacokinetics in most patients. Approximately 7% of whites are genetically slow metabolizers of TCAs due to functional deficiency in the hepatic isoenzyme IID6. Therefore, dose increases in these patients result in disproportionally greater increases in TCA plasma levels. Age, disease, concomitant drug therapy, and unusually high doses of TCAs can also cause nonlinear pharmacokinetics with TCAs.	Sertraline follows linear pharmacokinetics over its clinically relevant dosing range, whereas fluoxetine and paroxetine do not. Dose increases of the latter result in disproportionally greater increases in plasma drug levels and longer half-lives. Their nonlinear pharmacokinetics reflect their inhibition of hepatic isoenzymes responsible for their biotransformation prior to elimination.	Inadequately studied to make definitive statements. Of potential clinical relevance due to the dose-dependent (and hence plasma drug level-dependent) risk of seizure and the complex metabolism of bupropion.	Inadequately studied to make definitive statement. Could be relevant to effects associated with C_{max}.	Suggestive evidence for nonlinear pharmacokinetics over clinically relevant dose range, but no known clinical significance.
Special populations					
Age	Patients over 60 develop approximately twice the plasma TCA concentration on the same dose as younger individuals on amitriptyline, nortriptyline, and presumably the other TCAs.	Age has a negligible effect on plasma sertraline levels, but a greater effect on paroxetine and fluoxetine plus norfluoxetine levels. Physically healthy, elderly (≥65 y) individuals can develop higher plasma levels of these two drugs than do young individuals.	Not adequately studied.	There is a decrease in *m*CPP clearance with age due to decline of renal function.	Minimal to no information about pharmacokinetic differences in children, adolescents, or elderly. Caution recommended.
Disease states	Impairment of left ventricular cardiac function and liver function decreases clearance of tertiary and secondary amine TCAs. Impairment of renal function decreases clearance of hydroxylated metabolites of TCAs.	This area has not been systematically studied. Significant liver impairment triples and doubles the half-lives of fluoxetine and norfluoxetine, respectively. As hepatic clearance is dependent on hepatic arterial blood flow, clearance is also likely to decrease with impairment in left ventricular cardiac function.	Not adequately studied. Would predict greater accumulation in metabolites in patients with renal disease.	*m*CPP clearance is dependent on renal and left ventricular cardiac function.	Not adequately studied. Doubtful that there would be clinically meaningful pharmacokinetic consequences. There can be pharmacodynamic consequences.

Drug-drug interactions					
As target drug	Metabolism of TCAs can be induced and inhibited by a variety of drugs. Inducers include carbamazepine, phenobarbital, and phenytoin. Steady-state plasma TCA levels may fall by 50% or more with the resultant risk of relapse. Inhibitors include fluoxetine, paroxetine, quinidine, and neuroleptics. Steady-state plasma TCA levels may increase 4–10 times with the resultant risk of serious toxicity (eg, delirium, seizures, cardiac arrhythmias). Discontinuation of concomitantly administered inducers or inhibitors will result in an increase or decrease, respectively, in plasma TCA levels.	Fluoxetine and paroxetine inhibit their own metabolism and hence are likely to inhibit each other. Fluoxetine inhibits the metabolism of sertraline. The effect of paroxetine is unknown.	Little systematic study, some case report data. Likely that parent drug and/or metabolite levels lowered by carbamazepine and related inducers of P450 isoenzymes. Case report of substantial elevation of hydroxybupropion and threohydrobupropion by fluoxetine. Paroxetine has not been studied but would be a potential concern. Levels of bupropion and/or metabolites might also be affected by cimetidine and beta blockers.	Little systematic study. Given wide therapeutic index and short half-life, clinically significant interaction in terms of serious adverse outcome is unlikely.	No known effect by other drugs on the MAOI pharmacokinetics.
As protagonist drug	No evidence.	Fluoxetine and paroxetine at 20 mg/d produce clinically meaningful inhibition of the hepatic isoenzyme IID6 leading to increased plasma levels of drugs metabolized via this enzyme. Sertraline at 50 mg/d does not. These differences will be amplified by dose increases due to the nonlinear pharmacokinetics of fluoxetine and paroxetine versus the linear pharmacokinetics of sertraline, and in the elderly due to the age-related decline in fluoxetine and paroxetine clearance versus the minimal effect of age on sertraline clearance. Fluoxetine also inhibits the biotransformation of alprazolam to 4-hydroxyalprazolam, which is dependent on hepatic isoenzyme IIIA4. Other drugs dependent on IIIA4 should be similarly affected.	No evidence that bupropion induces or inhibits the metabolism of other drugs in a clinically meaningful way.	No evidence that trazodone induces or inhibits the metabolism of other drugs in a clinically meaningful way.	No known effect of MAOIs on the metabolism or elimination of other drugs, but do inhibit one enzyme and so may affect hepatic isoenzymes.

*m*CPP, 1-m-chlorophenylpiperazine; MAOI, monoamine oxidase inhibitor.
From Preskorn SH. Pharmacokinetics of antidepressants: Why and how they are relevant to treatment.

Table 37–8
Pharmacological Properties of Antidepressants and Their Possible Clinical Consequences

Property	Possible Clinical Consequences
Blockade of norepinephrine uptake at nerve endings	Alleviation of depression Tremors Tachycardia Erectile and ejaculatory dysfunction Blockade of the antihypertensive effects of guanethidine (Ismelin and Esimil) and guanadrel (Hylorel) Augmentation of pressor effects of norepinephrine
Blockade of serotonin uptake at nerve endings	Alleviation of depression Anorectic effects
Blockade of dopamine uptake at nerve endings	Psychomotor activation Antiparkinsonian effect Aggravation of psychosis
Blockade of histamine H_1 receptors	Potentiation of central depressant drugs Sedation drowsiness Weight gain Hypotension
Blockade of muscarinic receptors	Blurred vision Dry mouth Sinus tachycardia Constipation Urinary retention Memory dysfunction
Blockade of α_1-adrenergic receptors	Potentiation of the antihypertensive effect of prazosin (Minipress) Postural hypotension, dizziness Reflex tachycardia
Blockade of α_2-adrenergic receptors	Blockade of the antihypertensive effects of clonidine (Catapres), guanabenz (Wytensin), and α-methyldopa (Aldomet)
Blockade of dopamine D_2 receptors	Extrapyramidal movement disorders Endocrine changes (prolactin elevation)
Blockade of serotonin 5-HT_2 receptors	Ejaculatory disturbances Hypotension Alleviation of migraine headaches

From Richelson E. Synaptic pharmacology of antidepressants: An update. McLean Hosp J 1988;13:67–88.

Table 37–9
Side Effects of Antidepressant Drugs*

Drug	Sedation	Insomnia	Anticholinergic Effects	Orthostatic Hypotension	Delay in Cardiac Conduction or Arrhythmia	Nausea
Tricyclic drugs						
Amitriptyline	+++	0	+++	+++	Yes	0
Trimipramine	+++	0	+++	++	Yes	0
Desipramine	+	+	+	+	Yes	0
Doxepin	+++	0	++	+++	Yes	0
Imipramine	++	0	++	++	Yes	0
Nortriptyline	++	0	+	+	Yes	0
Protriptyline	+	++	++	+	Yes	0
Monoamine oxidase inhibitors						
Phenelzine	+	+	0	+++	Very rare	0
Tranylcypromine	0	++	0	+++	Very rare	+
Isocarboxazid	0	++	0	++	Very rare	0
Newer agents						
Amoxapine	++	0	+	++	Low	0
Fluoxetine	0	++	0	0	Low	++
Maprotiline	++	0	+	++	Yes	0
Trazodone	+++	0	0	++	Low	+
Alprazolam	+	0	0	0	None	0
Bupropion	0	++	0	0	Low	+

*Zero denotes no side effect, + a minor side effect, ++ a moderate side effect, and +++ a major side effect.
From Poter WZ, Rudorfer MV, Manji H. The pharmacologic treatment of depression. N Engl J Med 1991;325:633–642.

neuroleptic-induced deficit syndrome (NIDS).[11,12] Some patients switched to the newer antipsychotic agents such as clozapine experience an "awakening" effect. Delineation of NIDS from other treatment effects such as drug-induced parkinsonism and akathisia, sedation, and depressive features of schizophrenia is still a major problem. The cognitive impairment due to the underlying disease may improve with therapy, but may then be replaced by a cognitive impairment caused by neuroleptic therapy.[8]

Type I and II Schizophrenia

Two syndromes of schizophrenia can be distinguished.[13] Each may be associated with a specific pathologic process. The type I syndrome, equivalent to acute schizophrenia, and characterized by the positive symptoms (delusions, hallucinations, and thought disorder) is in some way associated with a change in dopaminergic transmission. The type II syndrome is characterized by negative symptoms (affective flattening and poverty of speech) and is unrelated to dopaminergic transmission but may be associated with intellectual impairment and, perhaps, structural changes in the brain. Type I symptoms are reversible; type II symptoms may be irreversible. Type I syndrome predicts a potential response to neuroleptic agents. Type II syndrome is associated with a poor long-term outcome. Episodes of type I symptoms may be followed by development of the type II syndrome, and both may be present together. Type II symptoms, however, define a group of illnesses of graver prognosis.

Laboratory

Only the TCAs need to be identified and quantified in acute antidepressant overdose situations. Quantification of other cyclic antidepressants, MAO-A inhibitors, or SSRIs is not warranted. Qualitative identification of MAO-A inhibitors and SSRIs may be justified if these drugs are suspected of being present in combination.[1]

REFERENCES—PSYCHOTROPIC DRUGS

1. Power BM, Hackett LP, Dusci LJ, Ilett KF. Antidepressant toxicity and the need for identification and concentration monitoring in overdose. Clin Pharmacokinet 1995;29: 154–171.
2. Rudorfer MW, Manji HE, Potter WZ. Comparative tolerability profiles of the newer versus older antidepressants. Drug Saf 1994;10:18–42.
3. De Jonghe F, Swinkels JA. The safety of antidepressants. Drugs 1992;43(suppl. 2):40–47.
4. Carpenter WT, Buchanan BRN. Schizophrenia. N Engl J Med 1994;330:681–690.
5. Rosenthal RM, Hellerstein DJ, Minter CR. Positive and negative syndrome typology in schizophrenic patients with psychoactive substance use disorder. Compr Psychiatry 1994;35:91–98.
6. Arinami T, Itokawa M, Engushi M, et al. Association of dopamine D2 receptor molecular variant with schizophrenia. Lancet 1994;343:703–704.
7. Kerwin R, Dumon V. Dopamine receptor genes and schizophrenia: The tail wags the dog? Lancet 1994; 343:686.
8. Seeman P, Van Tol HHM. Dopamine receptor pharmacology. Trends Pharm Sci 1994;15:264–270.
9. Lewander T. Neuroleptics and the neuroleptic-induced deficit syndrome. Acta Psychiatr Scand 1994;89(suppl. 380):8–13.
10. Lader MW. Neuroleptic-induced deficit syndrome (NIDS). J Clin Psychiatry 1993;54:496–500.
11. Carpenter WT Jr. The deficit syndrome. Am J Psychiatry 1994;15:327–328.
12. Weller MPI. Neuroleptic-induced deficit syndrome. Postgrad Med J 1993;69:957–958.
13. Crow TJ. Molecular pathology of schizophrenia: More than one disease process. Br Med J 1980;280:66–86.

Chapter **38**

Cyclic Antidepressants

INTRODUCTION

SUICIDES

About half of the patients who commit suicide are depressed. Most depressed patients who commit suicide are not taking antidepressants immediately before death. Therapeutic failure (newer, less toxic antidepressants) appears to be a greater problem with antidepressants than toxicity.[1] European studies suggest that amitriptyline, imipramine, nortriptyline, and desipramine are associated with a greater incidence of suicides than mianserin or trazodone.[2]

CHEMICALLY UNIQUE ANTIDEPRESSANTS

Trazodone is a triazolopyridine derivative that is structurally and pharmacologically different from the previously described antidepressants. The cardiotoxicity, neurotoxicity, and respiratory depression frequently encountered in tricyclic overdoses do not occur in trazodone overdose.[3]

Nomifensine is a chemically unique tetrahydroisoquinoline derivative that exhibits a low incidence of convulsions and cardiotoxicity; however, the occurrence of severe adverse reactions (eg, fatal hemolytic anemia, hepatic necrosis, cardiac dysrhythmias) led to the voluntary recall of this drug by the manufacturer in 1986.

Bupropion was recently approved by the Food and Drug Administration (December 1985); it is a unicyclic phenylaminoketone with antidepressant effects, probably the result of its weak inhibition of presynaptic dopamine reuptake. After reports of seizures in 4 of 50 nondepressed bulimic patients receiving the drug in a clinical trial, marketing was delayed pending a new study.[4]

Zimeldine was withdrawn from sale in Europe and America in 1983 because of its association with impaired liver function, loss of motor control, Guillain–Barré syndrome and other neuropathies, and myalgias.[5–9]

PRODUCT AVAILABILITY

During the past few years, the number of antidepressants under clinical investigation has expanded rapidly. The older tertiary and secondary amine tricyclic compounds have been used extensively and their acute toxicity is well reported. Maprotiline, trimipramine, trazodone, and amoxapine are recently released compounds for which clinical data are more limited. Nonetheless, the latter two drugs appear to have significantly different effects in severe overdose.

ACUTE TOXIC DOSAGE

Following ingestion of 350 mg of trazodone a 72-year-old woman developed hyponatremia, hypertension, and seizures.[10] A 63-year-old woman ingested 3 to 4.5 g of trazodone and developed lethargy, sinus bradycardia, a prolonged corrected QT interval (QT_c), and torsade de pointes leading to a cardiac arrest after which she suffered from coma, renal failure, and cardiac instability, which led to her death.[11] Her serum trazodone level on admission was 5680 ng/mL (therapeutic concentration, 1600 ng/mL).[12]

CLASSIC CYCLIC ANTIDEPRESSANTS

Toxicokinetics

Tricyclic antidepressants (TCAs) taken in large quantities during suicide attempts exhibit altered toxicokinetics.[13–27] Their absorption may be delayed by inhibition of gastric emptying and peristalsis. Significant enterohepatic recirculation delays final elimination of a large fraction of the drug. The enzymes responsible for TCA benzylhydroxylation can become saturated and thus reduce TCA elimination to zero-order kinetics. TCA unbound to plasma proteins may also increase because of acidemia resulting from respiratory depression after overdose. Other compounds are ingested in suicide attempts that greatly change TCA toxicokinetics.[28]

Distribution

Cyclic antidepressants are highly lipophilic and possess large and variable volumes of distribution (ie, 15–40 L/kg). After absorption, these drugs are rapidly distributed to tissue, where high concentrations occur in the liver, kidney, lungs, and myocardium. Generally, the tissue: plasma ratio exceeds 10:1.[29]

Amitriptyline is distributed predominantly in plasma, nortriptyline in the red blood cells. The differential distribution is dose dependent and reflects the higher binding of amitriptyline to α_1-acid glycoprotein when compared with nortriptyline. Interpretation of TCA blood levels is clarified by assaying red blood cells and plasma.[30] Amitai and colleagues suggest that in an acute overdose, TCA antidepressant red blood cell metabolites are the best markers of impaired intraventricular conduction.[31]

Elimination

Plasma concentrations of antidepressant drugs that are more than 95% metabolized are not altered by decreased renal function. Concentrations of drugs that are mostly excreted unchanged in the urine are greatly increased in patients with reduced renal function. Metabolites that account for 10% or more of the dose of the parent in urine are usually increased in the urine.[32]

Hydroxylated Metabolites. Tricyclic antidepressants and some other antidepressants are among the psychotropic drugs that undergo hydroxylation reactions (Table 38–1). Hydroxylated metabolites (OHMs) of antidepressant drugs are pharmacologically active. Hepatic hydroxylation is a major metabolic pathway for TCAs and other antidepressants. The OHMs are less lipophilic than their parent compounds. This may account for their smaller volume of distribution. The cerebrospinal fluid:total plasma concentration ratio is typically greater for OHMs than for their parent compounds. This may indicate a strong contribution of OHMs to central effects after TCA use.[33]

At therapeutic levels, demethylation varies considerably between adults (25–89% in one study). This indicates that the quantities of parent drug and active metabolite may also vary significantly between individuals given the same dose.[16] Amitriptyline elimination half-life in overdose ranges from 25 to 81 hours,[34] whereas half-lives in imipramine overdose vary between 12 and 21 hours.[19]

Viloxazine. Following an oral dose of 100 mg, peak blood levels of 0.8 to 3.56 μg/mL are reached in about 2 hours.[35–40] The elimination half-life is 2 to 5 hours.[41] A gas chromatography procedure sensitive to 0.1 μg/mL is available for the quantitation of viloxazine plasma levels.[42] Viloxazine is metabolized mainly by hydroxylation.[43,44] When viloxazine is used with either theophylline[45] or carbamazepine,[46] competition for the same hepatic microsomal enzymes appears to inhibit elimination of the latter two drugs, resulting in elevated blood levels and an increase in their toxicity.

Drug Interactions

At Therapeutic Levels. Neuroleptic drugs directly inhibit TCAs by hydroxylation (Table 38–2). Fluoxetine significantly prolongs elimination and increases flow levels of TCAs. Toxic hepatic metabolites of acetaminophen may

Table 38–1
Metabolism of Antidepressants to Active Moieties

Demethylation to Active Metabolites	
Imipramine	→ Desipramine
Amitriptyline	→ Nortriptyline
Maprotiline	→ Desmethylmaprotiline
Doxepin	→ Desmethyldoxepin
Demethylated: parent-drug ratio 0.1–3	
Hydroxylation to Active Metabolites	
Imipramine	→ 2-Hydroxyimipramine
Desipramine	→ 2-Hydroxydesipramine
Amitriptyine	→ 10-Hydroxyamitriptyline
Nortriptyline	→ 10-Hydroxynortriptyline
Amoxapine	→ 8-Hydroxyamoxapine
	→ 7-Hydroxyamoxapine

From Ereshefsky L, Tran-Johnson T, Davis DM, LeRoy A. Pharmacokinetic factors affecting antidepressant drug clearance and clinical effect: Evaluation of doxepin and imipramine: New data and review. Clin Chem 1988;34:863–880.

Table 38–2
Common Drug Interactions Involving Tricyclic Antidepressants

Interaction With	Consequence
Antipsychotic agents	↑Level of TCA
Disulfiram	↑Level of TCA
Cimetidine	↑Level of TCA
Estrogen	↑Level of TCA
Methylphenidate	↑Level of TCA
Smoking	↓Level of TCA
Barbiturates	↓Level of TCA
Phenytoin	↑Phenytoin
Guanethidine/clonidine	Antagonize hypotensive effects
Monoamine oxidase inhibitors	5-Hydroxytryptamine enhancement
Sympathomimetics	Hypertension: hyperpyrexia
Alcohol: central nervous system depressants	Additive sedation
Anticholinergic agents	Additive

TCA, tricyclic antidepressant.
From Tollefson GD. Adverse drug reactions/interactions in maintenance therapy. J Clin Psychiatry 1993;54(suppl.):48–58; discussion: 59–60.

delay TCA elimination. The elderly have slower rates of drug elimination.[47] Fluvoxamine added to imipramine or desipramine may result in a dramatic increase in the plasma concentrations of the TCAs with associated adverse effects. Fluvoxamine appears to inhibit the demethylation of imipramine and, possibly, the hydroxylation of desipramine.[48] All antidepressants that are not monoamine oxidase inhibitors and some that are reduce the seizure thresholds. Newer antidepressants, such as selective 5-hydroxytryptamine uptake inhibitors, have not yet been adequately evaluated in epileptics.[49]

Some additional TCA interactions include the following:

Drug	TCA	Effect
Captopril	Desmethyl-imipramine	Shortens QRS duration in rats[50]
Carbamazepine	TCA	Induces hepatic metabolism, lowers plasma TCA level[51]
Fluoxetine	TCA	Decreases TCA hepatic metabolism[52]
Fluvoxamine	TCA	Inhibits demethylation of TCA[53]
Morphine	TCA	Increases plasma morphine level and half-life[54]
Propafenone	Desipramine	Increases serum desipramine level[55]
Propranolol	Maprotiline	Increases serum maprotiline level to toxic levels[56] (inhibition of hepatic hydrolase and reduction of hepatic blood flow by propranolol)

At Overdose Levels. The combination of a TCA and a neuroleptic drug overdose may increase the plasma TCA level, may result in a greater percentage of patients with intraventricular conduction delays and first-degree atrioventricular block, and, to a lesser extent, may increase the incidence of conduction delay and ventricular arrhythmias.[57] Three times as many patients may manifest abnormally prolonged QT_c intervals when a neuroleptic drug is also ingested with a TCA.[57] Monoamine oxidase inhibitors such as phenelzine may induce fever, muscle contractions, hypotension, metabolic acidosis, and cardiovascular collapse unresponsive to pressors and inotropes.[58]

Pregnancy/Lactation

Reports of nursing mothers treated with amitriptyline showed that their infants had nondetectable blood levels of amitriptyline/nortriptyline and no adverse effects.[1] Nortriptyline was not detected in the sera of infants breastfed by nortriptyline-treated mothers.[59] Although two of four infants evaluated developed low concentrations of 10-hydroxynortriptyline, no adverse effects were observed.[59]

In a study of 15,000 births, there was no evidence of gross congenital abnormalities in infants born to women who received TCAs during the first trimester.[60] In a study of 19 women taking imipramine and 28 women receiving amitriptyline hydrochloride during the first trimester of pregnancy, there was no evidence of congenital malformations.[61] In the immediate postpartum period, a newborn can show the effects of antidepressants received in utero. There are reports of infants showing signs of respiratory distress, urinary retention, myoclonus, tachycardia, and heart failure. Some of these infants have later shown signs of withdrawal.[62]

Mechanism of Action

Trazodone inhibits serotonin uptake and inhibits serotonin receptors (5-HT_2) in addition to moderately inhibiting alpha-adrenergic receptors and exhibiting some antihistamine (H_1) activity.[63] Its active metabolite, *m*-chlorophenylpiperazine (mCPP), acts both as a serotonin receptor agonist and antagonist, inhibits serotonin reuptake, and interacts with alpha-adrenergic, dopamine, acetylcholine, and beta-adrenergic receptors.[64]

Elevated catecholamine levels and QRS widening without a commensurate blood pressure response in a study of cyclic antidepressant patients suggests desensitization of adrenergic receptors.[65]

Clinical Presentation

Common drugs and plants that may produce an anticholinergic syndrome are listed in Table 38–3. Remember that all TCAs have the potential to cause seizures and arrhythmias in overdose.

Tricyclic Compounds

Central Nervous System. Patients with impaired drug clearance, including geriatric patients and alcoholics, may show signs of confusion, agitation, and nervousness even without prominent anticholinergic symptoms.[66]

Duration of coma generally is short: one series revealed a mean coma duration of 6.4 hours.[67] Prolongation of coma more than 24 hours is rare and suggests complications or coingestion of central nervous system depressants.[68]

Elderly patients receiving antidepressants may develop a memory deficit.[69] A patient with coma profound enough to

Table 38–3
Common Drugs and Plants That May Produce the Anticholinergic Syndrome

Chemical Classification	Representative Examples
Tricyclic antidepressants	Amitriptyline HCl (Elavil)
	Amitriptyline HCl and perphenazine (Triavil, Etrafon)
	Amitriptyline HCl and chlordiazepoxide (Limbitrol)
	Desipramine HCl (Norpramine, Pertofrane)
	Doxepin HCl (Sinequan, Adapin)
	Impramine HCl (Tofranil)
	Imipramine Pamoate (Tofranil)
	Nortriptyline HCl (Aventyl)
	Protriptyline HCl (Vivactil)
Antipsychotic drugs	Phenothiazines (especially thioridazine)
	Butyrophenones (Haloperidol)
Antihistamines	Chlorpheniramine maleate (Ornade, Teldrin)
	Diphenhydramine HCl (Benadryl)
	Orphenadrine HCl (Disipal)
	Promethazine HCl (Phenergan)
Ophthalmic preparations	Atropine 1% ophthalmic solution
	Cyclopentolate (Cyclogel)
	Tropicamide (Mydriacyl)
Antispasmodic agents	Methantheline Br (Banthine)
	Propantheline Br (Pro-Banthine)
Antiparkinsonian agents	Benztropine mesylate (Cogentin)
	Biperiden HCl (Akineton)
	Ethopropazine HCl (Parsidol)
	Procyclidine HCl (Kemadrin)
	Trihexyphenidyl HCl (Artane Pipanol, Tremin)
Proprietary (hypnotics, analgesics, antiasthmatics)	Asthmador (belladonna or stramonium alkaloids)
	Compōz (scopolamine, methapyrilene, pyrilamine)
	Excedrin-PJ (salicylamide, acetaminophen, methapyrilene)
	Sleep-Eze (scopolamine, methapyrilene)
	Sominex (scopolamine, methapyrilene, salicylamide)
Belladonna alkaloids	Atropine sulfate
	Scopolamine HBr
	Tincture of belladonna
	Belladonna extract
Plants	Bittersweet *(Solanum dulcamara)*
	Black henbane *(Hyoscyamus niger)*
	Deadly nightshade *(Atropa belladonna)*
	Jimson weed *(Datura stramonium)*
	Jerusalem cherry *(Solanum pseudocapsicum)*
	Potato leaves, sprouts, tubers *(Solanum tuberosum)*

eliminate brainstem function rarely recovers; however, patients with drug overdose may make a full recovery despite neurologic findings. This demonstrates the need for continuing aggressive treatment in any patient who has overdosed on TCAs despite their appearance or the initial assessment of having suffered an irreversible brain insult.[69] Acute dystonia and extrapyramidal symptoms have followed the therapeutic use of amitriptyline. Intravenous procyclidine 10 mg may terminate the attack.[70]

Seizures. A report to the Committee on Safety of Medicines in the United Kingdom in November 1979 indicated that few seizures were reported with amitriptyline and imipramine (introduced before 1970) when compared with maprotiline and mianserin (introduced after 1970).[71]

Most seizures associated with cyclic antidepressant toxicity occur soon after admission, are brief, and terminate without specific anticonvulsant therapy. Even when brief, however, seizures may occasionally lead to hypotension,[72] abrupt cardiovascular deterioration, and death. TCA-induced seizures appear to be associated with elevated total plasma TCA concentrations.[73] Risk factors predisposing to seizures are listed in Table 38–4.[74] Reports of antidepressant-related seizures suggest the following[75]:

Table 38–4
Risk Factors Predisposing to Seizures

Primary Factors	Secondary Factors
History of seizures	Electroencephalographic abnormalities
Family history of seizures	Brain injury, CNS neoplasms, head trauma
	Secondary dementia
Mental retardation	Substance abuse or withdrawal
Birth difficulties	CNS vascular disease
Advanced age	Electroconvulsive or insulin shock therapy
Primary dementia	Polypharmacy

CNS, central nervous system.
From Skowron DM, Stimmel GL. Antidepressants and the risk of seizures. Pharmacotherapy 1992;12:18–22.

1. A significant proportion of antidepressant-related seizures occur in individuals with identifiable predisposing

factors such as family history of seizures, neurologic and medical conditions, concurrent medications, and substance abuse.

2. Seizure risk is increased following overdose, suggesting a dose-dependent relationship between antidepressant drugs and seizures.
3. Seizure risk following overdose is higher for amoxapine and maprotiline than for other antidepressant drugs, but similar comparisons for bupropion, fluoxetine, and clomipramine have not been reported.
4. Seizure risk has an observable dose-dependent relationship with some antidepressants at therapeutic doses.
5. Rapid dose escalation may increase the risk of seizures.
6. Cumulative risk, which takes duration into account, has seldom been examined and may be confounded by changes in dose.

Tremor, akathisia, myoclonus, dyskinesia, delirium, sedation, memory disturbances,[76] neuroleptic malignant syndrome,[77] and mania[78,79] have been reported after therapeutic use of TCAs.

Peripheral Nervous System. Peripheral neuropathies and polyradiculoneuropathy have followed amitriptyline overdoses (eg, 1.25 and 2.2 g).[80,81]

Causative agents of both seizures and tachycardias include amphetamines, belladonna alkaloids, cocaine, sympathomimetic drugs, xanthines, and anticholinergic drugs.[82] About three fourths of patients with maprotiline overdose (tetracyclic antidepressants) develop seizures within 2 to 5 hours of ingestion. About 10% of these patients with normal electrocardiograms develop seizures.[83]

Rhabdomyolysis. Seizures and coma are risk factors for the development of rhabdomyolysis. The occurrence of seizures or coma alone is not a good predictor of risk.[84]

Pulmonary Edema. Tricyclic antidepressant-induced pulmonary edema can develop between 5 and 48 hours after ingestion. Similarities exist between the adult respiratory distress syndrome following a TCA overdose, the "heroin lung syndrome," and pulmonary injury secondary to methadone ingestion. These similarities include diffuse bilateral pulmonary infiltrates on chest x-ray, hypoxemia, noncardiogenic pulmonary edema, and postmortem findings consisting of alveolar septal thickening, lymphocytic infiltrates, and edema.[85]

Radiographic evidence of pulmonary edema is observed in about 10% of TCA overdose patients. Patients in one study with elevated mean plasma tricyclic drug levels greater than 2000 ng/mL on admission appeared to have a greater tendency to develop bilateral alveolar infiltrates consistent with acute lung injury. A second chest film may be justified in those patients with significant peak plasma TCA levels even though the admission film may have appeared normal. Some patients with relatively low admission plasma TCA levels may go on to develop radiographic abnormalities. Fatalities involving noncardiogenic pulmonary edema underscore the potential for development of adult respiratory distress syndrome after severe TCA overdose.[86] Such pulmonary edema may not be correlated with hypotension on admission.[87] Shannon and Lovejoy suggest that one of every three patients with severe TCA overdose will develop a pulmonary complication; one of six will develop an aspiration pneumonia; and one of seven will develop pulmonary edema. Clinical and radiographic findings consistent with adult respiratory distress syndrome were noted in one series in 9% of patients with TCA overdose.[88]

Cardiovascular Status. The majority of TCA overdose deaths occur before or soon after arrival at a hospital. Life-threatening arrhythmias and/or cardiac arrest usually occur in a setting of marked electrocardiographic changes, hypotension, respiratory depression, coma, or convulsions and are generally uncommon as sole events.[89]

Hypotension is common after severe TCA overdose. A 22-year-old woman ingested 300 mg of amitriptyline, which led to a myocardial infarction from which she recovered. Hypotension appeared to be a predicting factor.[90] Hypotension often occurs independently of the blood TCA concentration and prolongation of the QRS interval. Hypotension may be strongly associated with the development of arrhythmias and pulmonary edema. Admission hypotension may appear after therapeutic doses of TCAs.[91] Hypotension alone is not of significant prognostic value. Potential electrocardiographic findings after overdose with cyclic antidepressants are outlined in Table 38–5.[92]

Cardiovascular toxicity with intractable myocardial depression, ventricular tachycardia, and ventricular fibrillation are common mechanisms of death. In human overdoses with fatal outcomes, mainly bradycardias are seen prior to death; however, tachyarrhythmias and ventricular fibrillation are the most often reported causes of death. Major arrhythmias may develop suddenly in patients who on arrival are normotensive and who have only minor electrocardiographic changes.[89]

Hepatic Function. Cholestatic and hepatic reactions associated with use of TCAs represent an idiosyncratic hypersensitivity reaction and are generally mild and revers-

Table 38–5
Potential Electrocardiogram Findings With Overdoses of Cyclic Antidepressants

Sinus tachycardia
Prolonged PR, QRS, QT_c intervals
ST-T wave changes
Bundle branch block
Second- or third-degree atrioventricular block
Supraventricular dysrhythmias
Atrial and atrioventricular junctional tachycardias
Atrial fibrillation
Atrial flutter
Bradycardia
Ventricular dysrhythmias
Premature ventricular contractions
Idioventricular rhythm
Ventricular tachycardia
Ventricular fibrillation
Torsade de pointes
Terminal 40-ms frontal QRS vector between 130° and 270°
Asystole

From Groleau G, Jotte R, Barsh R. The electrocardiographic manifestations of cyclic antidepressant therapy and overdose: A review. J Emerg Med 1990;8:597–605.

ible. Severe hepatic injury with fulminant hepatic failure and death has been reported.[93]

Gastrointestinal Status. Bowel ischemia requiring resection may follow a TCA overdose.[94] Acute intestinal pseudo-obstruction, spontaneous cecal perforation, and fecal peritonitis may follow a TCA overdose, especially in the elderly and in those with concomitant neurologic disease.[95] Repeated doses of activated charcoal used as therapy for an amitriptyline overdose led to a charcoal bezoar and small bowel obstruction.[96]

Withdrawal Syndromes. Withdrawal of TCAs may lead to syndromes related to cholinergic rebound. These syndromes include (1) anorexia, nausea, emesis, diarrhea, diaphoresis, myalgias, malaise, headache, chills, fatigue, and anxiety; (2) insomnia accompanied by vivid dreams; (3) akathisia or parkinsonism; and (4) hypomania or mania.[97–100] Anecdotal reports suggest that transient behavioral aberrations have followed the abrupt cessation of therapeutic use of TCAs and have included delirium after doxepin use,[101] mania/hypomania,[102] panic anxiety[103] and symptoms suggestive of cholinergic hyperactivity[104] after amitriptyline, and extreme motor activity clinically indistinguishable from akathisia after imipramine.[105]

Death. A study comparing the number of poisoning deaths in the United Kingdom associated with antidepressants with the estimated prescriptions dispensed for those antidepressants suggests that prescriptions for amitriptyline, dothiepin, doxepine, trimipramine, and maprotiline are more likely to result in death from overdose at all ages than are prescriptions for mianserin and carpipramine. There are methodologic weaknesses with this type of study (different population samples, hospitals versus general practice, use of more than one substance, etc).[106] The fatal toxicity indices of some tricyclic and second-generation antidepressants suggest a somewhat greater toxicity of the older TCAs when compared with second-generation drugs of the same therapeutic class.[107–109] Further studies in other countries will enhance the value of such fatal toxicity index data (Tables 38–6 and Table 38–7).

Newer Cyclic Antidepressants

Amoxapine/Loxapine. Amoxapine overdose may abolish brainstem reflexes and still lead to recovery. Corneal reflexes return 24 hours after ingestion; oculocephalic and oculovestibular responses may not return for 36 to 48 hours. Screening patients in whom oculocephalic and corneal reflexes were absent suffered persistent neurologic deficits.[110] A 37-year-old woman ingested about 875 mg of amoxapine and developed neuroleptic malignant syndrome.[111]

Although amoxapine is alleged to have fewer cardiac effects than other TCAs, amoxapine overdose may be a precipitating cause of both heart failure and arrhythmias.[112–114]

Maprotiline. The combination of a high maprotiline dose together with sinus tachycardia and a pathologic electrocardiogram appears to indicate a high risk for single or multiple seizures.[115] The minimum toxic dose of maprotiline is 425 to 750 mg. The lowest acute lethal dose of maprotiline is estimated to be 3 g but survival has been seen with ingestions as large as 5 g.[116] A 50-year-old

Table 38–6
Antidepressants and Overdose

Relatively Safe Fewer than 10 deaths per million prescriptons: lofepramine, mianserin, fluvoxamine, fluoxetine, viloxazine	**Very Dangerous** More than 30 deaths per million: maprotiline
Potentially Dangerous More than 10 deaths per million: clomipramine, protriptyline, trazodone	**Unacceptable Risk** More than 40 deaths per million: dothiepin, amitriptyline, tranylcypromine
Clearly Dangerous More than 20 deaths per million: phenelzine, imipramine	

From Montgomery SA, Baldwin D, Green M. Why do amitriptyline and dothiepin appear to be so dangerous in overdose? Acta Psychiatr Scand Suppl 1989;354:47–53.

Table 38–7
Fatal Toxicity Indices (1982–1986) for Antidepressant Drugs in England, Scotland, and Wales

Drug	Year	Fatal Toxicity Index (number of deaths per million prescriptions)	
Early Tricyclic Drugs Introduced up to and Including 1970			
Desipramine	1963	148.9	•••
Dothiepin	1969	59.6	•••
Amitriptyline	1961	56.1	•••
Nortriptyline	1963	42.3	NS
Doxepin	1969	40.6	NS
Imipramine	1959	30.0	•
Trimipramine	1966	30.0	NS
Clomipramine	1970	9.9	•••
Protriptyline	1966	6.5	•
Iprindole	1967	0.0	NS
Monoamine Oxidase Inhibitors			
Tranylcypromine	1960	43.8	NS
Phenelzine	1959	20.0	•
Isocarboxazid	1960	11.0	NS
Iproniazid	1958	0.0	NS
Antidepressants Introduced After 1973			
Maprotiline	1974	19.8	•
Trazodone	1980	12.3	••
Viloxazine	1974	0.0	NS
Butriptyline	1975	0.0	NS
Mianserin	1976	7.8	•••
Nomifensine	1977	2.4	•••
Lofepramine	1983	0.0	•••
All antidepressants		37.6	

•Significantly different at 5% level from all antidepressants ($P < .05$).
••Significantly different at 1% level from all antidepressants ($P < .01$).
•••Significantly different at 0.1% level from all antidepressants ($P < .001$).
NS, Not significantly different ($P > .05$).
From Reid F, Henry JA. Lofepramine overdosage. Pharmacopsychiatry 1990;23(suppl. 1):23–27.

woman was found dead with a blood maprotiline level of 1 μg/mL.[117]

Mianserin. Although cardiac arrhythmias with mianserin use are unusual, life-threatening ventricular arrhythmias including polymorphous ventricular tachycardia following an overdose with an unknown amount of mianserin were associated with serum mianserin concentrations 20 to 50 times the therapeutic value. The therapeutic concentration of mianserin (plus desmethylmianserin) is 100 ng/mL and serious toxicity has been associated with concentrations above 500 ng/mL.[118] Pinpoint pupils followed a mianserin overdose of 1200 mg. The small pupils did not respond to naloxone. Within 6 hours the patient was alert with pupils 2 mm in diameter. Twenty-four hours later the pupils were normal. Two hours after the overdose, the blood mianserin concentration was 390 ng/mL, and the desmethylmianserin level, 7 ng/mL.[118] The patient was treated symptomatically and recovered.[119]

Trazodone. Seizures and hyponatremia followed an overdose of trazodone. The patient survived.[10,64] Severe cardiac toxicity (sinus bradycardia, prolonged QT_c interval, torsade de pointes, cardiac arrest), coma, and renal failure led to death after a significant overdose (4.5 g) of trazodone.[11] Respiratory depression is most common in the presence of other central nervous system depressants, but respiratory arrest has been reported following 2.2 and 3.0 g of trazodone.[120]

Viloxazine. Ingestion of viloxazine in doses of 1 to 6.5 g together with a benzodiazepine was followed by hypotension and coma from which patients appeared to recover within 24 hours.[121] Few patients have shown abnormalities on the electrocardiogram after overdose, although there have been anecdotal reports of cardiogenic shock with conduction difficulties[122] and inferior coronary ischemia.[123] There is one report of seizures following therapeutic use of 300 mg/d.[124] No fatalities have been reported following overdose with viloxazine. Sedation, hypotension, anticholinergic unwanted effects, and weight gain have not usually been a problem when viloxazine has been administered in therapeutic doses.[125] Nausea appears to occur in 20 to 50% of patients and is the main reason patients stop using the drug.[127,126]

Carpipramine. Acute carpipramine poisoning has been studied by the Paris group. The clinical features are those of TCA overdose: many anticholinergic signs and prolongation of intraventricular conduction. Such conduction defects appear when the 1 g or more is ingested.[127] A fatality following the ingestion of carpipramine and ethyl alcohol was associated with a blood carpipramine concentration of 2.0 mg/L (2 μg/mL).[128]

Predictors of Toxicity

Some possible predictors of severe TCA toxicity are listed in Table 38–8.

Table 38–8
Some Possible Predictors of Severe Tricyclic Antidepressant (TCA) Toxicity[123]

Age >30
Serum TCA level more or less than 800 ng/mL (2880 mmol/L)
Ingestion of amitriptyline
Heart rate more or less than 120
QRS duration more or less than 100 ms
QRS axis >90°
Terminal 40-ms axis more or less than 135°
QT_c interval >48 ms
Amplitude of terminal R wave in lead aVR (RaVR) and R wave/S wave ratio in lead aVR (R/S ratio) of 1.4 and R wave >5 mm[129]

Laboratory

Analytical Methods

Homogeneous enzyme immunoassays provides a rapid and sensitive qualitative method for the detection of TCAs in plasma, serum, and whole blood.[130] The minimum detectable concentration of most of the TCAs is in the range 15 to 50 ng/mL. A fluorescent polarization immunoassay (FPLA, TDx assay) is useful in rapid evaluation (within 30 minutes in an ADx analyzer) of patient compliance and detection of therapeutic excessive drug concentrations (imipramine/desipramine concentrations >300 ng/mL; amitriptyline/nortriptyline >360 ng/mL). The TDx assay exhibits cross-reactivity for a variety of tricyclic and tetracyclic antidepressants and several metabolites of these compounds.[131] A high-performance liquid chromatography method provides good precision, sensitivity, and selectivity for routine confirmation of TDx results.[132,133]

Maprotiline and *N*-desmethylmaprotiline in plasma may be quantitated by gas chromatography with nitrogen–phosphorus detection.[132,133]

Plasma Cyclic Antidepressant Levels

Therapeutic blood level ranges for antidepressant drugs available in the United States are listed in Table 38–9.[134] Patients with plasma TCA levels greater than 450 ng/mL tend to develop cognitive or behavioral toxicity (agitation, disorientation, confusion, memory impairments, fragmented speech, pacing, decreased concentration). This may be related to the ability of TCAs to antagonize central muscarinic cholinergic receptors.[135]

Amitriptyline. Following ingestion of 9000 mg of amitriptyline, the serum amitriptyline level was 2350 ng/mL (therapeutic range, 75–225 ng/mL).[136] Plasma TCA concentrations in one study of 67 parents with TCA overdose were of no added value in predicting toxic complications or deciding when patients could leave the intensive care unit. The development of serious complications was unlikely in patients whose level of consciousness is grade II or less (Matthews–Lawson scale) and who are admitted to a hospital more than 6 hours after an overdose. An alert and oriented patient with a QRS duration less than 100 milliseconds appears to be the best indicator for safe transfer to a medical or psychiatric ward.[137] Arterial and venous differences in concentrations of amitriptyline and its me-

Table 38–9
Suggested or Expected Therapeutic Ranges for the Antidepressant Drugs Available in the United States

Drug	Therapeutic Range (μg/L)
Tricyclic drugs	
Imipramine + desipramine	150–250
Nortriptyline	50–150
Amitriptyline + nortriptyline	80–250
Desipramine	125–300
Protriptyline	70–260
Doxepin + desmethyldoxepin	150–250
Trimipramine	Similar to other tricyclic drugs
Other antidepressant drugs	
Maprotiline	200–600
Amoxapine + 8-hydroxyamoxapine	200–600
Trazodone	800–1600
Alprazolam	20–55
Fluoxetine	Not available

From Orsulak PJ. Therapeutic monitoring of antidepressant drugs: Guidelines updated. Ther Drug Monit 1989;11:497–507.

tabolites may exist following an overdose.[138] The amitriptyline plus nortriptyline plasma concentration was higher than the venous blood sample in one series of patients.

Trazodone. Three trazodone-related fatalities had blood trazodone concentrations ranging from 0.96 to 4.56 μg/mL.[139] A reverse-phase liquid chromatography method for analysis of trazodone is sensitive to 0.1 μg/mL.[140]

Maprotiline. Maprotiline may be detectable in serum by either gas–liquid chromatography, gas chromatography–mass spectrometry, or high-performance liquid chromatography. It may not be included in a routine toxic screen. A clinical diagnosis of maprotiline overdose (in absence of history) can be considered if a patient presents with signs of TCA overdose (coma, seizures, prolonged QRS intervals) and the toxic screen does not detect a TCA.[116]

Nortriptyline. Lethal blood nortriptyline concentrations have been reported as 10 to 26 μg/mL.[141] A 31-year-old man died with a heart blood concentration of 86.4 μg/mL.[142] Generally, in TCA fatalities the ratio of parent drug to desmethyl metabolite is greater than 2 in blood as well as in tissues.[143]

Imipramine. Cardiac and respiratory toxicity after imipramine overdose leading to death has been associated with combined blood concentrations (imipramine, desipramine, and 2-hydroxyimipramine) greater than 1.0 μg/mL in a 26-year-old woman who died after an imipramine overdose. The sum of the three components was 14 μg/mL.[144]

Cardiotoxic Parameters

A study of amitriptyline poisoning suggests that early in the course of the intoxication (all serious complications—ventricular arrhythmias, seizures, and severe hypotension—developed within 4 hours of admission), the QRS duration correlated with plasma, unbound, and red blood cell nortriptyline concentrations. The QRS duration also correlated with the unbound but not the plasma amitriptyline concentration. The level of consciousness correlated with plasma and unbound amitriptyline concentrations in both alpha and beta phases and with red blood cell amitriptyline concentration in the alpha phase. There was no correlation between nortriptyline concentration and level of consciousness. No correlation between coma grade or QRS duration and cerebral spinal fluid amitriptyline concentration was found. It is not possible to predict outcome based on a simple TCA concentration because of the wide range of concentrations of amitriptyline and amitriptyline metabolites observed between individuals. Generally, patients wake up within 24 hours, even after a severe TCA overdose.[145] Amitai and colleagues, in an initial study, suggested that TCA metabolites in red blood cells reflect the tissue distribution of the drug and are the best markers of cardiotoxicity.[146,147]

Postmortem Blood Levels

In overdose cases in which the sum of blood TCA parent drug and major active metabolite concentrations is in excess of 1.0 μg/mL, toxicity and resulting fatality are probable.[148] Postmortem blood concentrations can be substantially higher than concentrations at the time of death.[149] The liver parent drug : major metabolite ratio may aid in the decision process for cases in which the manner of death was ambiguous. The assumption that postmortem blood concentrations mirror drug concentrations at the time of death cannot be assumed to be valid.[150]

Postmortem blood concentrations ranged from 1.7 to 25.3 μg/mL in one autopsy series, whereas liver tissue levels of TCAs generally exceeded those in the myocardium.[151]

Five of 77 patients with TCA overdose were alert and oriented at 24 hours with plasma concentrations greater than 1000 ng/mL. Coma grade in this series was the best predictor. Plasma concentration adds nothing to the predictive value of the coma grade and QRS interval. A coma grade of II or less 6 hours or later predicted a benign course. Quantitative plasma concentrations are of little help in the immediate management of a TCA overdose.[152]

Abnormalities

Electrocardiogram. Electrocardiogram (ECG) changes are almost always noted early in the hospital course; subsequent unexpected cardiac complications in TCA overdose are rare.[57] A rightward deviation of the vector of the terminal 4 milliseconds of the QRS complex between 130° and 270° (> 137°) (which will produce an ECG negative in lead I and positive in lead aVR) has been demonstrated to have a sensitivity of 83 to 100% and a specificity of 63 to 98% for the presence of clinical TCA toxicity.[153] In one study, patients with a QRS axis greater than 90° were over 3.5 times more likely to demonstrate major toxicity than those with a normal axis.[154] This was the result of the right-axis deviation of the terminal 40-millisecond QRS vector (T40-ms negative deflector in lead I) in the more severely intoxicated patients. Patients with a QRS interval greater than 100 milliseconds were more than 2.5 times likely to demonstrate severe toxicity (seizures, endotracheal intubation, coma, arrhythmias requiring treatment, hypotension, or death) than those with a normal axis.[155] Other ECG parameters with increased likelihood of severe toxicity were a sinus tachycardia greater than 120 beats/min and a prolonged QT_c interval greater than 480 milliseconds.

There is a need to increase the ability to predict toxicity rapidly without relying on TCA levels. Liebelt and colleagues suggest that the amplitude of the terminal R wave in lead aVR (R_{aVR}), and R wave/S wave ratio in lead aVR (R/S) are greater in patients with TCA levels higher than 300 ng/mL and in patients who develop seizures and/or arrhythmias (Table 38–8). The R_{aVR} and R/S reflect aberrant right ventricular conduction. An R/S ratio of 1.4 and an R wave of 3 mm or more appear to be related to subsequent seizures or arrhythmia development[129] (Fig. 38–1).[156]

A retrospective analysis of TCA overdoses revealed that ECG parameters (QRS duration, QT interval, T40-ms QRS vector) cannot be relied on to include or exclude the diagnosis of TCA overdose, and TCA levels do not correlate with ECG parameters. The sensitivity and specificity of the T40 axis were found to be only 29 and 83%, respectively.[157] Initial clinical findings of TCA overdose are not adequately replaced by initial ECG parameters in making this diagnosis. The sensitivity and specificity of the QRS duration are 44 and 83%, respectively. The initial heart rate has a sensitivity and specificity of 68 and 59%, respectively. When compared with imipramine, trazodone does not produce any PR or QRS interval prolongation. Trazodone may be arrhythmogenic in patients with two underlying factors for adverse cardiac reactions.[64]

Pediatric Patients. Admission TCA serum concentrations correlated with electrocardiographic changes (QT_c, ORS) in pediatric patients. High TCA concentrations are more frequently associated with acidosis in acute poisoning, as patients who present with seizures are more likely to have significant atrioventricular conduction delays. In pediatric patients the triad of acidosis, seizures, and electrocardiographic abnormalities identifies a group who are at increased risk of significant morbidity from acute TCA ingestion.[158]

Enzyme and Cholesterol Levels. Modest elevation in creatine kinase or lactic acid dehydrogenase may occur after a TCA overdose. These enzymes do not appear to originate from the myocardium and are of no utility in assessment of antidepressant cardiotoxicity or prediction of clinical course.[159] Imipramine treatment leads to a significant increase in total serum cholesterol, decrease in high-density lipoprotein cholesterol, and increase in the cholesterol: high-density lipoprotein cholesterol ratio.[160] Anecdotal reports indicate that hypoglycemia may occur with imipramine or amitriptyline.[161] Fatigue, dizziness, loss of weight, and increase in appetite have been observed. There is no history of ingestion of alcohol or hypoglycemic agents. Symptoms resolve with intravenous glucose and cessation of medication.[162] TCAs may cause hypoglycemic unawareness in diabetic patients.

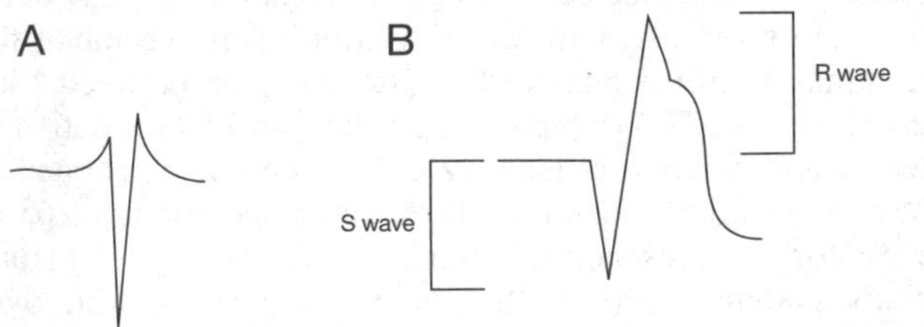

Figure 38-1 **A.** Normal QRS interval in lead aVR. **B.** An abnormal QRS interval as it appears in a patient with severe tricyclic antidepressant poisoning. R_{aVR} was measured as the maximal height in millimeters of the terminal upward deflection in the QRS complex, with the PQ segment used as the baseline. The S wave was measured in millimeters as the depth of the initial downward deflection. (From Liebelt EL, Francis PD, Woolf AD. ECG lead aVR versus QRS interval in predicting seizures and arrhythmias in acute tricyclic antidepressant toxicity. Ann Emerg Med 1995;26:195–201.)

N-Acetylamoxapine. A 46-year-old woman ingested 100 aspirin, 32 Nytol[R] diphenhydramine (Nytol) and 50 amoxapine (Asendin). She died in 24 hours. *N*-Acetylamoxapine is a novel by-product resulting from the transacetylation of amoxapine by aspirin.[163]

Ancillary Tests

Repeat analyses of amitriptyline and amitriptyline metabolites are unlikely to contribute to the clinical management of patients with amitriptyline overdose. That more significant correlations have been observed between cerebrospinal fluid concentrations than between cerebrospinal fluid and total plasma concentrations suggests that cerebrospinal fluid concentrations are determined by the unbound concentration.[164]

Treatment

Admittance to Hospital: Criteria

The decision to admit should be based on evaluation of the presence of central nervous system depression, respiratory depression, hypotension, dysrhythmias, conduction block, and seizures. Most major complications develop within 6 hours of arrival. The patient should be observed for 6 hours and discharged (with transfer to a psychiatric service when appropriate) after a final dose of charcoal only if none of the previously mentioned complications has appeared. Transient sinus tachycardia is a nonspecific finding that probably need not alter the decision to discharge; however, persistent tachycardia demands a thorough evaluation[90,165] (Table 38–10).

Stabilization

Cyclic antidepressants represent a drug group in which a patient with an acute overdose may present to the emergency department with trivial symptoms, yet may subsequently deteriorate rapidly despite maximum medical therapy. All patients who may have ingested more than 10 to 20 mg of TCAs per kilogram should immediately receive an intravenous line and cardiac monitoring. Those patients with altered mental status should receive oxygen, naloxone, glucose, and, if indicated, thiamine. Initial attention should be directed toward evaluation of the adequacy of ventilation (ie, tidal volume, arterial blood gases, cyanosis). Serious toxicity usually results from ventricular dysrhythmias, hypotension, seizures, or respiratory insufficiency. Prolonged cardiac massage may be necessary in cases of asystole, as successful recovery has occurred in both children and adults despite periods of asystole exceeding 90 minutes.[166–168]

Table 38–10
Management of Tricyclic Antidepressant Overdose

1. Immediately evaluate the patient and administer oxygen.
2. Monitor vital signs (include ECG monitoring).
3. Insert an intravenous line.
4. Support vital functions:
   - Respiratory depression
     Maintain airway
     Monitor arterial blood gases
     Intubate and hyperventilate if indicated
   - Hypotension
     Infuse crystalloid
     Alkalinize
     Inotropes (dobutamine or dopamine)
     Vasopressors (noradrenaline)
   - Coma: maintain airway
5. Reduce TCA absorption:
   - Ipecac or gastric lavage within first 6 h
   - Activated charcoal (1 g/kg) in all cases
6. Increase TCA elimination:
   - Multiple doses of activated charcoal (0.5–1.0 g/kg) q4h in major overdose
7. Treat convulsions:
   - Diazepam (0.1 mg/kg IV) as required
   - Phenytoin infusion (15 mg/kg IV) over 30 min to prevent further convulsions
8. Observe ECG changes (prolonged PR, QRS, or QT interval, bundle-branch block). Treat arrhythmias:
   - Sinus tachycardia—supportive measures only
   - Supraventricular arrhythmias
     Alkalinize to a pH of 7.40–7.45
     Synchronized cardioversion if supraventricular tachycardia is prolonged, alkalinization is ineffective, and there is major hemodynamic disturbance
     Supraventricular tachycardia with widened QRS often closely resembles ventricular tachycardia or can be indistinguishable from it (if in doubt, treat as ventricular tachycardia)
   - Ventricular tachycardia
     Alkalinize to a pH of 7.45–7.5
     Lignocaine (1 mg/kg IV bolus, then infusion of 2–4 mg/min)
     Synchronized cardioversion if these measures are ineffective
     Isoprenaline infusion (0.5–5.0 µg/min) and overdrive placing for torsade de pointes
   - Ventricular fibrillation
     Defibrillate
     Early use of sodium bicarbonarte (1–3 mmol/kg) and hyperventilation aiming for a pH of 7.45–7.5
     1:1000 adrenaline (0.5–1.0 mg IV)
     Lignocaine (as for ventricular tachycardia)
     Beta blockers if these measures are ineffective
   - Bradycardia or heart block (Mobitz II second and third degree)
     Alkalinize to a pH of 7.4–7.45
     Isoprenaline
     Pacemaker
9. Refractory cardiac arrest:
   - Give basic and advanced life support for a minimum of 1 h
   - Alkalinize to a pH of 7.50

From Dziukas LJ, Vohra J. Tricyclic antidepressant poisoning. Med J Aust 1991;154:344–350.

Hypotension. As with any case of suspected overdose, the ABCs are the initial consideration, with early attention to gastric decontamination. Respiratory depression is common and may necessitate intubation. Intravenous access should be secured rapidly and blood pressure supported with fluid boluses followed by pressors as needed. For refractory hypotension, direct-acting sympathomimetic agents such as norepinephrine and phenylephrine may effectively counter cyclic antidepressant-induced alpha blockade. Agents such as dopamine are less effective because of norepinephrine depletion at synaptic terminals and failure of the agent to be taken up into cells. Pure beta-adrenergic agonists, such as isoproterenol and dobutamine, and even combination alpha- and beta-adrenergic agonists like dopamine can result in unopposed beta-adrenergic activity in the face of alpha-adrenergic blockade and may worsen hypotension and arrhythmias. Sodium bicarbonate has been demonstrated to increase blood pressure and should be administered concomitantly. There are anecdotal reports of success with extracorporeal bypass and an intraaortic balloon pump.[169]

Animal studies suggest that myocardial depression is a more serious problem than cardiac dysrhythmias in TCA intoxication and that this is a major cause of hypotension and stroke. TCA-induced vasodilation does not appear to be a significant factor. Norepinephrine is effective in reversing myocardial depression during severe TCA intoxication. Glucagon (10-mg bolus followed by an infusion of 10 mg over 6 hours) may lead to an immediate and sustained rise in blood pressure.[170]

Dysrhythmias. Sodium loading may be the most important factor in reducing TCA toxicity and may be required because of the overwhelming TCA-induced sodium channel blockade.[171]

Sodium Chloride. Use of intravenous sodium chloride has resulted in narrowing of the QRS complexes, diminished tendency to ventricular tachycardia and ventricular fibrillation, and an increase in blood pressure.[172]

Sodium Bicarbonate. Sodium bicarbonate therapy has successfully reversed bradyrhythmias, multifocal premature ventricular ectopy, ventricular tachycardia, conduction delays, varying degrees of heart block, and hypotension.[173,174] The exact mechanism of action is controversial. In vitro studies indicate that both blood pH and extracellular sodium concentrations contribute to the beneficial therapeutic effects of sodium bicarbonate on cardiotoxicity.[175] Increasing the pH reduces the percentage of unbound amitriptyline.[18] Sodium bicarbonate has become the treatment of choice. It should be administered as an intravenous bolus of 1 to 2 mEq/kg followed by continuous infusion (titrated to pH) immediately on the discovery of conduction abnormalities or, specifically, a QRS duration exceeding 100 milliseconds.[89]

The two most common methods of alkalinization are mechanical hyperventilation and intravenous sodium bicarbonate. Although hyperventilation is a more rapid and titrable method of alkalinization than bicarbonate, it is probably not as effective as bicarbonate. When the two treatments are combined, profound alkalosis may result, with life-threatening consequences such as neuromuscular irritability, ionized hypocalcemia, and cardiac dysrhythmias.[176] A profound alkalemia can result in a shift in the oxygen dissociation curve to the left, impairing tissue oxygen delivery, cerebral vasoconstriction, an increase in myocardial sensitivity to catecholamines, and an intracellular shift of potassium (hypokalemia).[177] These effects can predispose the patient to arrhythmias. If the pH rises above 7.6 there is a marked increase in the potential for serious effects. Close repetitive monitoring of the plasma pH to maintain the pH below 7.55 but above 7.45 is indicated.[178]

Torsade de Pointes (Ventricular Arrhythmias). Ventricular dysrhythmias may be exacerbated by other drugs with membrane-stabilizing effects, namely, type Ia and Ic antiarrhythmic agents; therefore, these should be avoided. Phenytoin may improve conduction but has not been shown to be more effective than alkalinization, cannot be infused rapidly, and increases the likelihood of ventricular tachycardia; it also should be avoided. Lidocaine is probably the safest, most effective agent,[169] followed by magnesium sulfate (see below).

Respiratory Insufficiency. Management of respiratory insufficiency may resemble sedative/hypnotic-induced adult respiratory distress syndrome and involve intubation and positive-pressure ventilation.

Seizures. Benzodiazepines are considered the agent of choice, providing rapid central nervous system penetration without prolonged sedation. If benzodiazepines fail to control seizure activity, phenobarbital (15–20 mg/kg) is a good second-line agent. Physostigmine, a carbamate anticholinesterase, is a nonspecific central nervous system analeptic that has been used in this setting but is associated with a 10% incidence of seizures, a 10% incidence of cholinergic crisis (hypotension, vomiting, diarrhea, and increased respiratory secretions), and a worsening of preexisting conduction block that can result in bradycardia, asystole, and death. Therefore, it is not recommended.[169] An anecdotal report suggests that when high-dose benzodiazepine therapy fails to control seizure activity in amoxapine-induced refractory status epilepticus, propofol (Diprivan) (see Chapter 56) is effective when given in a dose of 2.5 mg/kg as an intravenous bolus followed by infusion of 0.2 mg/kg/min.[179]

Magnesium. Magnesium has been administered as a 2-g intravenous bolus of magnesium sulfate. If necessary, a 2- to 4-g bolus is then given 5 to 15 minutes later to suppress the torsade de pointes and ventricular premature beat. In some, the magnesium sulfate infusion has been given at a rate of 3 to 20 mg/min and continued until the QT interval is less than 500 milliseconds, a process that takes 7 to 48 hours. Hypomagnesemia is usually not present.[180,181] The only obvious side effect of magnesium sulfate is a short-lasting flushing sensation. Mild hypotension may also be observed.[182]

Dopamine. Dopamine effects are less defined in TCA overdose. There is, with dopamine, a risk of developing ventricular arrhythmias, which appears greater than with isoproterenol, but less than with dobutamine. At low doses (< 5 mg/kg/min), vasodilation of the renal, mesenteric, coronary, and intracerebral vascular beds is observed. At intermediate doses (5–10 μg/kg/min) dopamine beta-adrenergic agonist properties predominate: augmentation of myocardial contractility and heart rate resulting from the release of norepinephrine from myocardial storage sites. When large doses (> 10 mg/kg/min) are infused, alpha-adrenergic-mediated vasoconstriction predominates. Dopamine must not be added to sodium bicarbonate or other alkaline solutions, as it may precipitate. Like norepinephrine, dopamine should be infused through a central vein if possible.

Dobutamine. Dobutamine has not been studied in TCA-induced hypotension. Dobutamine is supplied in 2-mL vials containing 250 mg of drug. The vial must be diluted to at least 50 mL and is incompatible with sodium bicarbonate. The infusion rate should be initiated at 2.5 mg/kg/min and titrated as necessary to 20 mg/kg/min. As long as 10 minutes may be required to obtain the fuel effect of an increase in the infusion rate. Peripheral β_2-receptor stimulation may occur resulting in vasodilation. A combination of dopamine and isoproterenol may be useful, but has not been studied in humans.[183] Sodium bicarbonate has not yet been evaluated in TCA-induced hypotension in the absence of arrhythmias.[183]

Clonidine. Clonidine may be harmful in TCA poisoning.[184]

Catecholamines. Blockage of endogenous norepinephrine reuptake by TCAs may result in a state of catecholamine depletion. This suggests use of a direct-acting catecholamine such as norepinephrine, instead of an indirect-acting agent such as dopamine, which depends on the release of endogenous catecholamines for its clinical effect.[185] Animal studies suggest that myocardial depression, rather than vasodilation, is a more important cause of hypotension after TCA use. Both dopamine and norepinephrine are effective in reversing myocardial dysfunction associated with TCA intoxication. To determine which the clinician should use, variables such as the response to bicarbonate and fluids, the specific TCA taken, and other connected drugs may influence the effectiveness of these agents. Further hemodynamic monitoring studies may offer solutions to these questions.[186]

Gut Decontamination

Gastric decontamination should begin as early as possible, with large-volume (at least 5 L) gastric lavage followed by charcoal administration. Pills have been recovered as late as 18 hours after a cyclic antidepressant ingestion and after lavage with up to 10 L of saline. Charcoal has been shown to decrease plasma levels. One gram per kilogram is given initially with a cathartic (eg, sorbitol) and then, if bowel sounds are present, every 2 to 4 hours, alone. A multidose regimen may reduce elimination half-life to as little as 4 hours. The half-life is directly proportional to the delay before charcoal administration. Finally, because cyclic antidepressants are highly protein and tissue bound, hemodialysis and charcoal hemoperfusion are of little value, although hemoperfusion may have a rare role in acute refractory cardiovascular instability.[169]

Clinical studies suggest that if gastric lavage is performed it is unlikely to be effective after the first 4 to 5 L of lavage fluid has been instilled. Unless drug particulate is seen in lavage return, gastric lavage with 5 L of fluid should be considered adequate.[187]

Repeat doses of activated charcoal may, in a setting of TCA overdose, induce diminished bowel motility and produce an obstructing charcoal bezoar.[96] Multiple-dose activated charcoal administered after an acute TCA overdose may lead to pulmonary aspiration. Obtunded, intubated patients who have ingested TCAs should receive an initial dose of charcoal, but repetitive doses should be withheld if bowel sounds remain absent. Gastric aspiration should be performed prior to extubation of these patients.[188] Charcoal was recovered from the airway of 18 of 72 patients who received activated charcoal slurry by nasogastric tube in the emergency room after endotracheal intubation.[189]

Antidote

Animal studies suggest that anti-imipramine antibodies may be able to redistribute imipramine and reduce target imipramine concentrations.[190] Similar nortriptyline antibodies are in the preparatory stage.[191] The use of equimolar amounts of Fab to neutralize TCA, as in Digibind treatment, would appear to require excessive amounts of Fab. Titration with Fab to reduce the free TCA level may be an approach to control the toxic effects of an overdose of TCA and avoid administration of excessively large amounts of protein.[192] Desmethylimipramine (DMI) cardiotoxicity in rats is reduced by binding of a small fraction of DMI body burden to anti-TCA monoclonal antibody. Anti-TCA may alter the pattern of DMI tissue distribution and reduce the QRS prolongation by increasing efflux of DMI from a cardiotoxic compartment.[193]

The combination of anti-TCA Fab and sodium bicarbonate reduces DMI-induced QRS prolongation in rats to a greater extent than either treatment alone. Both anti-TCA Fab abuse and sodium bicarbonate alone significantly reduce QRS prolongation in rats 10 minutes after treatment. Anti-TCA Fab increases the total DMI concentration in the serum and reduces DMI concentration in the brain and heart. None of the treatments alter the unbound DMI concentration.[194]

Lethality due to amitriptyline was reduced in actively immunized rabbits. For TCAs, neutralizing the ingested dose with an equimolar dose of Fab fragments would require an excessive amount of Fab fragments.[195] High-affinity monoclonal and polyclonal antibodies have been developed in animals and purified by affinity chromatography.[196] Techniques to develop antibodies of high binding constant are underway; however, at present, it is still not possible to treat overdoses of cyclic antidepressants with Fab fragments: the quantities of protein that would have to be injected would be excessive.[197]

Supportive Measures

1. All patients with severe TCA ingestion should receive a chest x-ray within 24 hours of admission.[97]
2. A Glasgow Coma Scale score less than 8 was the most sensitive predictor of serious complications in one series of patients who overdosed on TCAs (sensitivity, 86%; specificity, 89%). This was significantly better than the QRS interval (QRS >100 milliseconds; sensitivity, 59%; specificity, 76%). Patients responsive to verbal stimuli on leaving the emergency department appear to be at very low risk of developing complications.[198]
3. Most patients who develop cardiovascular or central nervous system complications do so within 1 hour of admission. Few develop arrhythmias after they become alert and their electrocardiogram readings have been normal for 1 hour. Therefore, 24 hours of cardiac monitoring is considered sufficient, provided that no underlying cardiac disease exists.[199,200]
4. The elimination half-life of amitriptyline after serious overdose was 15 to 43 hours in one study while peak plasma levels were found between 2 and 4.5 hours after drug intake. In another study, 11 of 77 patients with TCA intoxication presented with plasma concentrations exceeding 1000 ng/mL 24 hours after admission to the hospital.[138] After 24 hours, 2 of these patients were in light coma (Matthews–Lawson Coma Scale, grades 2 and 1). Six patients needed assisted ventilation, most because of bronchopneumonia following aspiration. None had cardiovascular symptoms, and all had normalized ECGs. Within 36 hours of admission to a hospital most patients were transferred. No serious toxic symptoms were reported after the patients left the intensive care unit. Plasma concentrations are of limited value in determining length of stay in the intensive care unit.[199]
5. Other causes of the anticholinergic syndrome should be considered (Table 38–3).
6. In a patient with mild or moderate depression and ischemic heart disease or arrhythmias, consideration should be given to the use of a selective serotonin receptor inhibitor or perhaps bupropion in view of the risk of sudden death from TCAs.[201]
7. An initial anecdotal report suggests that patients with hemodynamic collapse unresponsive to advanced life support measures, fluid and vasopressor therapy, and other measures to decontaminate and enhance elimination of the agent may respond to femoral–femoral extracorporeal circulation (ECC), which can provide hemodynamic support until toxic cardiovascular effects abate.[202] Intravenous glucagon 10 mg followed by an infusion of 10 mg over 6 hours resulted in a sustained rise in blood pressure following imipramine-induced hypotension.[170] This was accompanied by shortening of the QRS interval. A study in animals suggests that treatment of TCA overdoses with inotropic agents improves hemodynamic status and decreases the incidence of arrhythmias. Both epinephrine and norepinephrine can be used to treat TCA poisoning. If serious arrhythmias occur, they can be treated with magnesium sulfate.[203]
8. Amoxapine overdose is associated with a high incidence of seizures. Propofol (Diprivan) 2.5 mg/kg as an intravenous bolus, followed by infusion (0.2 mg/kg/min), has been effective in an anecdotal study of amoxapine-induced refractory status epilepticus.[204]

Discharge Criteria

The patient is observed for 6 hours and discharged after a final dose of charcoal if no central nervous system depression, respiratory depression, hypotension, dysrhythmias, conduction block, or seizures persist. Persistent tachycardia should be evaluated before discharge.[169]

General Review Articles

- Rudorfer MV, Potter WZ. Antidepressants: A comparative review of the clinical pharmacology and therapeutic use of the 'newer' versus the 'older' drugs. Drugs 1989;37:713–738.
- Preskorn SH. Pharmacokinetics of antidepressants: Why and how they are relevant to treatment. J Clin Psychiatry 1993;54(9, suppl.):14–34.
- Dziukas LJ, Vohra J. Tricyclic antidepressant poisoning. Med J Aust 1991;154:344–350.

REFERENCES—CYCLIC ANTIDEPRESSANTS

1. Isacsson G, Holmgren P, Wasserman D, Bergman U. Use of antidepressants among people committing suicide in Sweden. Br Med J 1994;308:506–509.
2. Antidepressant drugs and the risk of suicide. WHO Drug Inform 1995;7:18–20.
3. Lesar T, Kingston R, Dahms R, et al. Trazodone overdose. Ann Emerg Med 1983;12:221–223.
4. Burroughs-Wellcome Company. Personal communication, July 31, 1986.
5. Fagius J, Osterman PO, Siden A, Wiholm B-E. Guillain–Barré syndrome following zimeldine treatment. J Neurol Neurosurg Psychiatry 1985;48:65–69.
6. Pomara N, Coffman KL, Bush DF, Gerhon S. Myalgia and elevation in muscle creatine phosphokinase during zimeldine treatment. J Clin Psychopharmacol 1984;4:220–222.
7. Dexter LL. Zimeldine induced neuropathies. Hum Toxicol 1984;3:141–143.
8. Langlois R, Cournoyer G, de Montigny C, Caille G. High incidence of multisystemic reactions to zimeldine. Eur J Clin Pharmacol 1985;28:67–71.
9. Simpson GK, Davidson MM. Possible hepatotoxicity of zimeldine. Br Med J 1983;287:1181.
10. Balestrieri G, Cerudelli B, Ciaccio S, Rizzoni D. Hyponatremia and seizures due to overdose of trazodone. Br Med J 1992;304:686.
11. Augenstein WL, Smolinske SC, Kulig KW, Rumack BH. Trazodone overdose and severe cardiac toxicity. Vet Hum Toxicol 1987;29:478.
12. Baughan E, Jawod SSM. Effects of overdose of trazodone. Br Med J 1992;303:1114.
13. Goldberg MJ, Park GD, Spector R, et al. Lack of effect of oral activated charcoal on imipramine clearance. Clin Pharmacol Ther 1985;38:350–353.
14. Nagy A, Johansson R. Plasma levels of imipramine and desipramine in man after different routes of administration. Naunyn Schmiedeberg's Arch Pharmacol 1975;290:145–160.
15. Schulz P, Dick P, Blaschke TF, et al. Discrepancies between pharmacokinetic studies of amitriptyline. Clin Pharmacokinet 1985;10:257–268.
16. Rollins DE, Alvan G, Bertilsson L, et al. Interindividual differences in amitriptyline demethylation. Clin Pharmacol Ther 1980;28:121–129.
17. Heel RC, Avery GS. Drug data information, Appendix A. In: Avery GS, ed. *Drug Treatment.* 2nd ed. Sydney: ADIS Press, 1980:1217.
18. Levitt MA, Sullivan JB, Owens SM, et al. Amitriptyline plasma protein binding: Effect of plasma pH and relevance to clinical overdose. Am J Emerg Med 1986;4:121–125.
19. Alexanderson B. Pharmacokinetics of desmethylimipramine and nortriptyline in man after single and multiple oral doses: A cross-over study. Eur J Clin Pharmacol 1972;5:1–10.
20. Ziegler VE, Biggs JT, Wylie LT, et al. Protriptyline kinetics. Clin Pharmacol Ther 1978;23:580–584.
21. Ziegler VE, Biggs JT, Wylie LT, et al. Doxepin kinetics. Clin Pharmacol Ther 1978;23:573–579.
22. Joyce PR, Sharman JR. Doxepin plasma concentrations in clinical practice: Could there be a pharmacokinetic explanation for low concentrations? Clin Pharmacokinet 1985;10: 365–370.
23. Jauch R, Kopitar Z, Prox A, et al. Pharmakokinetik und stoffwechsel von trazodone beim menschen. Arzneimittelforschung 1976;26:2084–2089.
24. Ankier SI, Martin BK, Rogers MS, et al. Trazodone: A new assay procedure and some pharmacokinetic parameters. Br J Clin Pharmacol 1981;11:505–509.
25. Dugas JE, Weber SS. Amoxapine. Drug Intell Clin Pharm 1982;16:199–204.
26. Cooper TB, Kelly RG. GLS analysis of loxapine, amoxapine and their metabolites in serum and urine. J Pharm Sci 1979;68:216–219.
27. Riess W, Dubey L, Funfgelt EW, et al. The pharmacokinetic properties of maprotiline (Ludiomil[R]) in man. J Intern Med Res 1974;3(suppl. 2):16–41.
28. Jarvis MR. Clinical pharmacokinetics of tricyclic antidepressant overdose. Psychopharmacol Bull 1991;27:541–550.
29. Jandhyala BS, Steenberg ML, Pered JM, et al. Effects of several tricyclic antidepressants on the hemodynamics and myocardial contractility of the anesthetized dog. Eur J Pharmacol 1977;42:403–410.
30. Amitai Y, Kennedy EJ, De Sandre P, Frischer H. Distribution of amitriptyline and nortriptyline in blood: Role of alpha-1-glycoprotein. Ther Drug Monit 1993;15:267–273.
31. Amitai Y, Erickson T, Kennedy EJ, et al. Tricyclic antidepressants in red cells and plasma: Correlation with impaired intraventricular conduction in acute overdose. Clin Pharmacother 1993;54:219–227.
32. Lane EA. Renal function and the disposition of antidepressants and their metabolites. Psychopharmacol Bull 1991;27: 533–540.
33. Young RC. Hydroxylated metabolites of antidepressants. Psychopharmacol Bull 1991;27:521–532.
34. Spiker PG, Biggs JT. Tricyclic antidepressants: Prolonged plasma levels after overdose. JAMA 1976;236:1711–1712.
35. Brosman RD, Busby AM, Holland PRC. Cases of overdosage with viloxazine hydrochloride (Vivalen). J Int Med Res 1976; 4:83–85.
36. Faller JP, Feissel M, Ruyes O, et al. Cardiogenic shock with conduction difficulties in the course of a serious intoxication with viloxazine. Presse Med 1988;17:1412.
37. Regouby Y. Inferior coronary ischemia during massive viloxazine and clotrazepam intoxication. Therapie 1991;46: 409–410.
38. Langs T, Thomas F, Jupas JJ, Ravard Y. Seizures with viloxazine. Presse Med 1991;20:477.
39. Update of antidepressants: Lofepramine, amoxapine and viloxazine. Drug Ther Bull 1990;28(2):82–83.
40. Tsegos IK, Ekdani MY. A double blind controlled study of viloxazine and imipramine in depression. Curr Med Res Opin 1974;2:455–460.
41. Bayliss PFC, Case DE. Blood level studies with viloxazine hydrochloride in man. Br J Clin Pharmacol 1975;2:209–214.
42. Groppi A, Papa P. One stage extraction procedures for gas chromatography determination of viloxazine as its acetyl derivative in human plasma. J Chromatogr 1985;337:142–145.
43. Pinder RM, Bragden RN, Speight TM, Avery RS. Viloxazine: A review of its pharmacological and therapeutic efficacy in depressive illness. Drugs 1977;13:401–421.
44. Reynolds JEF, ed. *Martindale: The Extra Pharmacopoeia.* 29th ed. London: Pharmaceutical Press 1989:384–385.
45. Thomson AH, Addus GJ, McGobern EM, McDonald NJ. Theophylline toxicity following coadministration of vitoxazine. Ther Drug Monit 1988;10:359–360.
46. Pisani F, Narbone MC, Fazio A, et al. Effect of viloxazine on serum carbamazepine levels in epileptic patients. Epilepsia 1984;25:482–485.
47. Jarvis RR. Clinical pharmacokinetics of tricyclic antidepressant overdose. Psychopharmacol Bull 1991;27:541–550.

48. Spina E, Campo GM, Avenoso M, et al. Interaction between fluvoxamine and imipramine/desipramine in four patients. Ther Drug Monit 1992;14:194–196.
49. Dolan RJ. Answer. Br Med J 1990;301:171.
50. Li P, Benitez J, Roden D, Branch RA. Angiotensin II facilitates tricyclic antidepressant-induced changes in QRS duration in the rat. Clin Toxicol 1992;30:83–98.
51. Baldessarini RJ, Teicher MH, Cassidy JW, Stein MH. Anticonvulsant co-treatment may increase toxic metabolites of antidepressants and other psychotropic drugs. J Clin Psychopharmacol 1988;8:381–382.
52. Bergstrom RF, Peyton AL, Lemberger L. Quantification and mechanism of the fluoxetine and tricyclic antidepressant interaction. Clin Pharmacol Ther 1991;51:239–248.
53. Bertschy G, Vandel S, Vandel B, et al. Fluvoxamine-tricyclic antidepressant interaction. An accidental finding. Eur J Clin Pharmacol 1991;40:114–120.
54. Ventafridda V, Ripamont C, De Conno F, et al. Antidepressants increase bioavailability of morphine in cancer patients. Lancet 1987;1:1204.
55. Katz MP. Raised serum levels of desipramine with the antiarrhythmic propafenone. J Clin Psychiatry 1991;52:432–433.
56. Saiz-Ruiz J, Moral L. Delirium induced by association of propranolol and maprotiline. J Clin Psychopharmacol 1988;8:77–78.
57. Wilens TE, Stern TA, O'Gara PT. Adverse cardiac effects of combined neuroleptic ingestion and tricyclic antidepressant overdose. J Clin Psychopharmacol 1990;10:51–54.
58. Johnson PN, Lewander WJ, Mello MJ, Savitt DL. A fatal drug interaction: Phenelzine/imipramine. Vet Hum Toxicol 1988;30:351.
59. Wisner KL, Perel JM. Serum nortriptyline levels in nursing mothers and their infants. Am J Psychiatry 1991;148:1234–1236.
60. Kuennsberg EV, Knox JD. Imipramine in pregnancy. Br Med J 1972;2:292.
61. Crombie DL, Pinsent RJ, Fleming DM, et al. Fetal effects of tranquilizers in pregnancy. N Engl J Med 1975;293:198–199.
62. Guze BH, Guze PH. Psychotropic medication use during pregnancy. West J Med 1989;151:296–298.
63. Gold PW, Goodwin FK, Chrousos GP. Clinical and biochemical manifestations of depression: Relation to the neurobiology of stress (first of two parts). N Engl J Med 1988;319:413–420.
64. Mills KC. Trazodone toxicity: Current concepts. Top Emerg Med 1993;15:37–46.
65. Merigian KG, Hedges JR, Kaplan LA, et al. Plasma catecholamines in cyclic antidepressant overdose. Ann Emerg Med 1988;17:403.
66. Giller EJ Jr, Bialos DS, Docherty JP, et al. Chronic amitriptyline toxicity. Am J Psychiatry 1979;136:4518–4519.
67. Noble J, Matthew J. Acute poisonings by tricyclic antidepressants: Clinical features and management of 100 patients. Clin Toxicol 1969;2:403–421.
68. Hulten BA, Heath A. Clinical aspects of tricyclic antidepressant poisoning. Acta Med Scand 1983;213:275–278.
69. Marcoupoulos BA, Graves RE. A depressant effect on memory in depressed older persons. J Clin Exp Neuropsychol 1990;12:655–663.
70. Ornadel D, Barnes EA, Dick DJ. Acute dystonia due to amitriptyline. J Neurol Neurosurg Psychiatry 1992;55:44.
71. Edward JG. Antidepressants and convulsions. Lancet 1979;2:1368–1369.
72. Lipper B, Bell A, Gaynor B. Recurrent hypotension immediately after seizures in nortriptyline overdose. Am J Emerg Med 1994;12:451–457.
73. Preskorn SH, Fast GA. Tricyclic antidepressants induced seizures and plasma drug concentration. J Clin Psychiatry 1992;53:160–162.
74. Skowron DM, Stimmel LL. Antidepressants and the risk of seizures. Pharmacotherapy 1992;12:18–22.
75. Rosenstein DL, Nelson JC, Jacobs SC. Seizures associated with antidepressants: A review. J Clin Psychiatry 1993;54:289–299.
76. Lejoyeux M, Rouillon F, Ades J, Gorwood P. Neural symptoms induced by tricyclic antidepressants: Phenomenology and pathophysiology. Acta Psychiatr Scand 1992;85:249–256.
77. Baoa L, Martinelli L. Neuroleptic malignant syndrome: A unique association with a tricyclic antidepressant. Neurology 1990;40:1797–1798.
78. Lipschitz A. Antidepressants and mania. Am J Psychiatry 1990;147:372.
79. Sugarman P, Hughes T. Assault after ingestion of antidepressants. Br Med J 1991;303:720.
80. Leys D, Pasquirer F, Lamblin MD, et al. Acute polyradiculoneuropathy after amitriptyline overdose. Br Med J 1982;294:608.
81. Marley J. Acute polyradiculoneuropathy after amitriptyline overdose. Br Med J 1987;294:1616.
82. Tribble J, Weinhouse E, Garland J, Wendelberger K. Treatment of a severe imipramine poisoning complicated by a negative history of drug ingestion. Pediatr Emerg Care 1989;5:234–237.
83. Wyss PA, Serena S, Meier PJ. Dose-dependency of seizures in maprotiline (Ludiomil[R]) intoxications. Vet Hum Toxicol 1993;35:321–341.
84. Donovan JW, Britt A. Incidence and risk factors of rhabdomyolysis in anticholinergic toxicity. In: *Proceedings, International Congress of European Association Poison Centres and Clinical Toxicologists, Birmingham, UK, May 1993.*
85. Zuckerman GB, Conway EE Jr. Pulmonary complications follow tricyclic antidepressant overdose in an adolescent. Ann Pharmacother 1993;27:572–574.
86. Roy TM, Ossorio MA, Cipolla LM, et al. Pulmonary complications after tricyclic antidepressant overdose. Chest 1989;96:852–856.
87. Shannon M, Lovejoy FH Jr. Pulmonary consequences of severe tricyclic antidepressant ingestion. Clin Toxicol 1987;24:443–461.
88. Varnell RM, Godwin JD, Richardson ML, Vincent JM. Adult respiratory distress syndrome from overdose of tricyclic antidepressants. Radiology 1989;170:667–670.
89. Power BM, Hackett LP, Dusci LJ, Ilett KF. Antidepressant toxicity and the need for identification and concentration monitoring in overdose. Clin Pharmacokinet 1995;29:154–171.
90. Chamsi-Pasha H, Barner PC. Myocardial infarction: A complication of amitriptyline overdose. Postgrad Med J 1988;64:968–970.
91. Shannon M, Merola J, Lovejoy FH Jr. Hypotension in severe tricyclic antidepressant overdose. Am J Emerg Med 1988;6:439–442.
92. Groleau G, Jotte R, Barish R. The electrocardiographic manifestations of cyclic antidepressant therapy and overdose: A review. J Emerg Med 1990;8:597–605.
93. Keegan AD. Doxapine-induced recurent acute hepatitis. Aust NZ J Med 1993;23:523.
94. Wallace DE. Bowel ischemia in two patients following tricyclic antidepressant overdose. Vet Hum Toxicol 1989;31:377.
95. McMahon AJ. Amitriptyline overdose complicated by intestinal pseudo-obstruction and caecal perforation. Postgrad Med J 1989;65:948–949.
96. Ray MJ, Padin DR, Condie JD, Halls JM. Charcoal bezoar: Small bowel obstruction secondary to amitriptyline overdose therapy. Dig Dis Sci 1988;33:1061–1067.
97. Stokes PE. Fluoxetine: A five-year review. Clin Ther 1993;15:216–246.
98. Dilsaver SC, Greden JF. Antidepressant withdrawal phenomena. Biol Psychiatry 1984;19:237–256.
99. Ceccherini Nelli A, Bardellini L, Cur A, et al. Antidepressant withdrawal: Prospective findings. Am J Psychiatry 1993;150:165.
100. Davison P, Wardrope J. Acute amitriptyline withdrawal and hypotension. Drug Saf 1993;8:78–80.
101. Santos AB, McCurdy L. Delirium after abrupt withdrawal from doxepin. Am J Psychiatry 1980;137:239–240. Case Report.
102. Mirin SM, Schatzberg AF, Creasey DE. Hypomania and mania after withdrawal of tricyclic antidepressants. Am J Psychiatry 1981;138:87–89.

103. Gawain FH, Markoff RA. Panic anxiety after abrupt discontinuation of amitriptyline. Am J Psychiatry 1986;138:117–118.
104. Davison P, Wardrofe J. Acute amitriptyline withdrawal and hyponatremia: A case report. Drug Saf 1993;8:78–80.
105. Sathananthan GL, Gershon S. Imipramine withdrawal: An akathesia-like syndrome. Am J Psychiatry 1973;130:1286–1287.
106. Farmer RDT, Piner RM. Why do fatal overdose rates vary between antidepressants? Acta Psychiatr Scand 1989; 8(suppl. 354):25–35.
107. Leonard BE. Toxicity of antidepressants in overdose. Int J Clin Pharm Res 1989;9:101–110.
108. Cassidy SL, Henry JA. Fatal toxicity of antidepressant drugs in overdose. Br Med J 1987;295:1021–1024.
109. Henry JA. A fatal toxicity index for antidepressant poisoning. Acta Psychiatr Scand 1989;80(suppl. 354):37–45.
110. Nosko MG, McLean DR, Chin WDN. Loss of brainstem and pupillary reflexes in amoxapine overdose: A case report. Clin Toxicol 1988;26:117–122.
111. Taylor NE, Schwartz II. Neuroleptic malignant syndrome following amoxapine overdose. J Nerv Ment Dis 1988;176:244–251.
112. Sorensen MR. Acute myocardial failure following amoxapine intoxication. J Clin Psychopharmacol 1988;8:75.
113. Genser AS, Marcus SM. Progressive cardiac conductive defects due to amoxapine overdose. Vet Hum Toxicol 1987; 29:481.
114. Burckhardt D, Raeder E, Muller U, et al. Cardiovascular effects of tricyclic and tetracyclic antidepressants. JAMA 1978; 239:213–216.
115. Wyss PA, Serena S, Meier PJ. Dose-dependency of seizures in maptrotiline (Ludiomil[R]) intoxications. Vet Hum Toxicol 1993;35:341.
116. Jackson B, Shannon M. Maprotiline. Clin Toxicol Rev 1988; 11(1):1-2.
117. Dimopoulos GD. Maprotiline (Ludiomil) poisoning. Bull Int Assoc Forens Toxicol 19912;21:32–34.
118. Fuller GN, Calibour J. Pinpoint pupils in mianserin overdose. Br Med J 1987;294:1233.
119. Haefeli WE, Schoenenberger RA. Recurrent ventricular fibrillation in mianserin intoxication. Br Med J 1991;302:415–416.
120. Gamble DE, Peterson LG. Trazodone overdose: Four years of experience from voluntary reports. J Clin Psychiatry 1986; 47:544–546.
121. Kuhn R. The treatment of depressive states with G 223JJ (imipramine hydrochloride). Am J Psychiatry 1959;115:459–464.
122. Mann AM, Catterson Ag, McPherson AS. Toxicity of imipramine: Report of serious side effects and massive overdosage. Can Med Assoc J 1959;81:23–28.
123. Noack CH. A death from overdosage of "Tofranil." Med J Aust 1960;2:182.
124. Lee FI. Imipramine overdosage: Report of a fatal case. Br Med J 1961;1:338–339.
125. Steel CM, O'Duffy J, Brown SS. Clinical effects and treatment of imipramine and amitriptyline poisoning in children. Br Med J 1967;3:663–667.
126. Callaham M, Kassel D. Epidemiology of fatal tricyclic antidepressant ingestion: Implications for management. Ann Emerg Med 1985:14:1–9.
127. Carlier P, Garnier R, Benzaken C, et al. Acute carpipramine overdosage: Report of 26 cases. Therapie 1982;37:89–94.
128. Fraser AD, Isner AF. A carpipramine related fatality. J Forens Sci 1987;32:1103–1108.
129. Liebelt FL, Francis PD, Woolf AD. ECG lead RaVR improves prediction of acute tricyclic antidepressant (TCA) toxicity. Vet Hum Toxicol 1993;35:368.
130. Asselin WM, Leslie JM. Direct detection of therapeutic concentrations of tricyclic antidepressants in whole hemolyzed blood rising to EMIT serum tricyclic antidepressant assay. J Anal Toxicol 1991;15:167–173.
131. Nebinger P, Koel M. Specificity data of the tricyclic antidepressant assay by fluorescent polarization immunoassay. J Anal Toxicol 1990;14:219–221.
132. Poklis A, Soghoian D, Crooks CR, Sandy JJ. Evaluation of the Abbot ADx total serum tricyclic immunoassay. Clin Toxicol 1990;28:235–248.
133. Drebit R, Baker GB, Dewhurst GB. Determination of maprotiline and desmethylmaprotiline in plasma and urine by gas chromatography with nitrogen–phosphorus detection. J Chromatogr 1988;432:334–339.
134. Orsulak PJ. Therapeutic monitoring of antidepressant drugs: Guidelines updated. Ther Drug Monit 1989;11:497–507.
135. Meador-Woodruff JH, Akil M, Wisner-Carlson R, Grunhaus L. Behavioral and cognitive toxicity related to elevated plasma tricyclic antidepressant levels. J Clin Psychopharmacol 1988; 8:28–32.
136. Yang KL, Dantzkes DR. Reversible brain death: A manifestation of amitriptyline overdose. Chest 1991;99:1037–1038.
137. Hulten RA, Adams R, Askenasi R, et al. Predicting severity of tricyclic antidepressant overdosage. Clin Toxicol 1992;30: 161–171.
138. Hulten BA, Martensson E, Knudsen K, Heath A. Difference in arterial and venous concentrations of amitriptyline and its metabolites after overdose. Vet Hum Toxicol 1987;29:484.
139. Hadac JP, An TL, Konakai Y, et al. Analysis of blood and tissue in three trazodone related deaths. In: *Proceedings, American Academy of Forensic Sciences, 43rd Annual Meeting, Chicago, February 18–23, 1991:* Abstract K37.
140. Brown P, Tribby P. Analysis of trazodone by normal phase liquid chromatography. Clin Chem 1990;36:1045 (Abstract 0436).
141. Stead AH, Moffat AC. A collection of therapeutic, toxic and fatal blood drug concentrations in man. Hum Toxicol 1983;3: 437–464.
142. Rohrig TP, Prouty RW. A nortriptyline death with unusually high tissue concentrations. J Anal Toxicol 1989;13:303–304.
143. Tracqui A, Kintz P, Ritter-Lohrer S, et al. Toxicological findings after fatal amitriptyline self-poisoning. Hum Exp Toxicol 1990;9:257–261.
144. Fraser AJ, Susnik E, Isner AF. Analysis of 2-hydroxyimipramine in an imipramine-related fatality. J Forens Sci 1987;32:543–545.
145. Hulten BA, Heath A, Knudsen K, et al. Severe amitriptyline overdose: Relationship between toxicokinetics and toxicodynamics. Clin Toxicol 1992;30:171–179.
146. Amitai Y, Erickson T, Leikin JB, et al. Acute tricyclic antidepressant overdose: Cardiac toxicity and levels in red cells and plasma. Vet Hum Toxicol 1993;35:340.
147. Amitai Y, Erickson T, Kennedy EJ, et al. Tricyclic antidepressants in red cells and plasma correlation with impaired intraventricular conduction in acute overdosage. Clin Pharmacol Ther 1993;54:219–227.
148. Frommer DA, Kulig KW, Marx JA, Rumack B. Tricyclic antidepressant overdose: A review. JAMA 1987;257:521–526.
149. Apple FS, Bandt CB. Liver and blood post-mortem tricyclic antidepressant concentrations. Am J Clin Pathol 1988;89: 794–796.
150. Apple FS. Post-mortem tricyclic antidepressant concentrations: Assessing cause of death using parent drug to metabolite rate. J Anal Toxicol 1989;13:197–198.
151. Bailey DN, Shaw RF. Tricyclic antidepressants: Interpretation of blood and tissue levels in fatal overdoses. J Anal Toxicol 1979;3:43–46.
152. Hulten BA, Dawling S, Volans GM, Heath AJW. Predicting severity of tricyclic antidepressant overdose. In: *Proceedings, 14th International Congress of European Association of Poison Centres, Milan, Italy, September 25–29, 1990:* 149.
153. Niemann JT, Bessen HA, Rothstein RJ, Lake MM. Electrocardiographic criteria for tricyclic antidepressant cardiotoxicity. Am J Cardiol 1986;57:1154–1159.
154. Wolfe FR, Caravati EM, Rollins DE. Terminal 40 ms frontal plasma QRS axis as a marker for tricyclic antidepressant overdose. Ann Emerg Med 1989;18:348–351.
155. Caravati EM, Bossart DJ. Demographic and electrocardiographic factors associated with severe tricyclic antidepressant toxicity. Clin Toxicol 1991;29:31–43.
156. Liebelt FL, Francis PD, Woolf AD. ECG lead AVR versus QRS interval in predicting seizures and arrhythmias in acute tricyclic antidepressant toxicity. Ann Emerg Med 1995;26:195–206.
157. Lavoie FW, Gansert GG, Weiss RE. Value in initial ECG findings and plasma drug levels in cyclic antidepressant overdose. Ann Emerg Med 1990;19:696–702.

158. Phillips L, Kearns G. Pediatric tricyclic antidepressant ingestions: Predictors of morbidity. Clin Res 1992;40:838A.
159. Shannon M. Serum enzyme disturbances after tricyclic antidepressant overdose. Vet Hum Toxicol 1989;31:171–172.
160. Yergani WK, Pohl R, Balon R, et al. Increased serum total cholesterol to HDL-cholesterol ratio after imipramine. Psychol Res 1990;21:207–209.
161. Shrivatstava RK, Edwards D. Hypoglycemia associated with imipramine. Biol Psychiatry 1983;18:1509–1510.
162. Sherman KE, Bornemann M. Amitriptyline and asymptomatic hypoglycemia. Ann Intern Med 1988;109:683–684.
163. Osiewicz RJ, Middleberg R. Detection of a novel compound after overdoses of aspirin and amoxapine. J Anal Toxicol 1989;13:97–99.
164. Hulten PA, Heath A, Knudsen K, et al. Amitriptyline and amitriptyline metabolites in blood and cerebrospinal fluid following human overdose. Clin Toxicol 1992;30:181–201.
165. Dziukas LJ, Vohra J. Tricyclic antidepressant poisoning. Med J Aust 1991;154:344–350.
166. Orr DA, Bramble MG. Tricyclic antidepressant poisoning and prolonged external cardiac massage during asystole. Br Med J 1981;283:1107–1108.
167. Tokarski GF, Young J. Criteria for admitting patients with tricyclic antidepressant overdose. J Emerg Med 1988;6:121–124.
168. Ware WR. Tricyclic antidepressant overdose: Pharmacology and treatment. South Med J 1987;80:1410–1415.
169. Newton EH, Shih RD, Hoffman RS. Cyclic antidepressant overdose: A review of current management strategies. Am J Emerg Med 1994;12:376–379.
170. Sener EK, Gabe S, Henry JA. Response to glucagon in imipramine overdose. Clin Toxicol 1995;33:51–53.
171. McCabe JL, Cobaugh DJ, Menegazzi JJ, Fata JM. A comparison of hypertonic saline, sodium bicarbonate and hyperventilation in severe tricyclic antidepressant overdose in swine. Vet Hum Toxicol 1993;35:367.
172. Hoegholm A, Clenetsen P. Hypertonic sodium chloride in severe antidepressant overdosage. Clin Toxicol 1991;29:297–298.
173. Brown TCK. Sodium bicarbonate treatment for tricyclic antidepressant arrhythmias in children. Med J Aust 1976;2:380–382.
174. Hoffman JR, McElroy CR. Bicarbonate therapy for dysrhythmia and hypotension in tricyclic antidepressant overdose. West J Med 1981;134:60–65.
175. Pentel PR, Benowitz NL. Tricyclic antidepressant poisoning management of arrhythmias. Med Toxicol 1986;1:101–121.
176. Wrenn K, Smith BA, Slovis CM. A potential hazard of combined hyperventilation and intravenous bicarbonate. Ann Emerg Med 1992;10:553–555.
177. Martin JG, Roberg RJ. Hypokalemia and electrolyte imbalance associated with antidepressant overdoses. Vet Hum Toxicol 1993;35:340.
178. Wrenn K, Smith BA, Slovis CM. Profound alkalemia during treatment of tricyclic antidepressant overdose: A potential hazard of combined hyperventilation and intravenous bicarbonate. Am J Emerg Med 1992;10:553–559.
179. Merigian KS, Browning RG, Leeper KV. Successful treatment of amoxapine-induced refractory status epilepticus with propofol (Diprivan[R]). Acad Emerg Med 1995;2:128–133.
180. Tzivoni D, Banai S, Schuzer C, et al. Treatment of Torsade de pointes with magnesium sulfate. Circulation 1988;77:392–397.
181. Perticone F, Adinolfi L, Bonaduce D. Efficacy of magnesium sulfate in the treatment of Torsade de pointes. Am Heart J 1986;112:847–849.
182. Tsivoni D, Keren A. Suppression of ventricular arrhythmias by magnesium. Am J Cardiol 1990;65:1297–1399.
183. Buchman AL, Dauer J, Geiderman J. The use of vasoactive agents in the treatment of refractory hypotension seen in tricyclic antidepressant overdose. J Clin Psychopharmacol 1990;10:409–413.
184. Knudsen K, Ricksten S-E, Heath A. Clonidine interaction in amitriptyline poisoning. Clin Toxicol 1988;26:223–232.
185. Teba L, Schiebel F, Dedhic HV, Lazzell VA. Beneficial effect of norepinephrine in the treatment of circulatory shock caused by tricyclic antidepressant overdose. Am J Emerg Med 1988; 6:566–568.
186. Vernon DD, Banner W, et al. Efficacy of dopamine and norepinephrine for treatment of hemodynamic compromise in amitriptyline intoxication. Crit Care Med 1991;19:544–549.
187. Watson WA, Leighton J, Guy J, et al. Recovery of cyclic antidepressants with gastric lavage. J Emerg Med 1989;7:373–377.
188. Givens T, Holloway M, Wason S. Pulmonary aspiration of activated charcoal after tricyclic antidepressant overdose. Vet Hum Toxicol 1990;32:375.
189. Ray TM, Ossorio HA, Cipolla LM, et al. Pulmonary complications after tricyclic antidepressant overdose. Chest 1989; 96:852–856.
190. Keyler DE, Brunn GJ, Pentel PB. Monoclonal antibody effects on imipramine distribution in rats. Vet Hum Toxicol 1989;31:364.
191. Sullivan JB, Egen NB. Methods in production and isolation of antibodies to nortriptyline. Vet Hum Toxicol 1987;29:483.
192. Hursting MJ, Opheim KE, Raisys VA, et al. Tricyclic antidepressant-specific Fab fragments alter the distribution and elimination of desipramine in the rabbit: A model for overdose treatment. Clin Toxicol 1989;27:53–66.
193. Pentel PR, Brunn GJ, Pond SM, Keyler DE. Pretreatment with drug-specific antibody reduces desipramine cardiotoxicity in rats. Ann Emerg Med 1991;20:1083.
194. Brunn GJ, Keyler DE, Pond SM, Pentel PR. Interaction of drug-specific antibody Fab fragment and $NaHCO_3$ for reversal of desipramine cardiotoxicity in rats. Vet Hum Toxicol 1991;33:359.
195. Sabouraud A, Urtizberea M, Chaffey O, et al. Nortriptyline-specific active immunization in the rabbit: A mode to study the effect of antibodies on amitriptyline toxicity and disposition. In: *Proceedings, International Congress of Clin Toxicol, Pois Cont, Anal Toxicol, Lux Tox, 90, Luxembourg, May 2–5, 1990:* 233–237.
196. Denis H, Marulo S, Terrien N, et al. Specific IgG and Fab as main tool in tricyclic antidepressant animal poisoning. Vet Hum Toxicol 1987;29(suppl. 2):157.
197. Liu D, Purssell R, Levy JG. Production and characterization of high affinity monoclonal antibodies to cyclic antidepressants. Mol Clin Toxicol 1987;25:527–538.
198. Emerman CL, Connors AF Jr, Burma GM. Loss of consciousness as a predictor of complications following tricyclic overdoses. Ann Emerg Med 1987;16:326–330.
199. Pentel P, Sioric L. Incidence of late arrhythmias following tricyclic antidepressant overdose. Clin Toxicol 1981;18:543–548.
200. Hulten BA. TCA poisoning treated in the intensive care unit. Pharmacopsychiatry 1990;23:16–18.
201. Glassman AH, Roose SP, Bigger JT Jr. The safety of tricyclic antidepressants in cardiac patients: Risk–benefit reconsidered. JAMA 1993;269:2673–2675.
202. Williams JM, Hollingshead MJ, Vasilakis A, et al. Extracorporeal circulation in the management of severe tricyclic antidepressant overdose. Am J Emerg Med 1994;12:456–488.
203. Knudsen K, Abrahamsson J. Effects of amrinone, norepinephrine, magnesium sulfate and milrinone in survival on the occurrence of arrhythmias in amitriptyline poisoning in the rat. Crit Care Med 1994;22:1851–1855.
204. Merigian KS, Browning RG, Leeper KV. Successful treatment of amoxapine-induced refractory status epilepticus with propofol (Diprivan[R]). Acad Emerg Med 1995;2:128–133.

THE NEWER CYCLIC ANTIDEPRESSANTS

AMINEPTINE HYDROCHLORIDE

Amineptine is a TCA used in France since 1978 (Survector)[1] and in Italy since 1983.[2] It is distinguished from other TCAs by an amino acid side chain containing seven carbon atoms attached to the middle ring.[3] The recommended therapeutic dose is 100 to 200 mg/d. By 1990 about 30 cases of chronic overdose were reported to the Paris Poison Control Center.[4] In chronic overdose metabolites appear (molecules beta oxidized in the side chain and a lactam form).[4]

Toxicokinetics

Amineptine is rapidly absorbed, and approximately 1 hour after an oral dose of 100 mg, it reaches a maximum plasma concentration of 1.066 μg/L.[3,5–7] Its apparent volume of distribution is 2.44 L/kg and it is eliminated with a half-life slightly less than 1 hour after an oral dose of 100 mg. One of the active metabolites has similar pharmacokinetic properties.[5] Plasma levels are determined by high-performance liquid chromatography.[3]

Clinical Presentation

Amineptine may induce a hypersensitivity type of hepatotoxicity which begins within a few weeks of the onset of treatment and is characterized by an intrahepatic cholestasis during which patients develop fever, pruritus, abdominal pain and jaundice.[2] Recovery follows within a few weeks of discontinuing medication. A direct hepatotoxicity may follow overdose.[8] Pancreatitis has also been observed.[9] Skin changes appear in some patients after several months to years of drug use (a rosaceaform acne on the face, back, and chest). This often follows a chronic self-increased overdose with high doses.[4,10,11] Metabolites of amineptine are found in the lesions.[4] Patients often become dependent on the drug and take 1000 to 4000 mg/d.[4,12–14] Such dependence appears more often among patients treated for substance abuse. In such patients, amineptine metabolites may be detected in the urine,[4] and steroid excretion patterns may be altered.[4] One patient developed anaphylaxis following one capsule of amineptine.[14]

Treatment

Lesions on the skin following a chronic overdose often recede over a few months, but may leave residual deformities. Symptoms of hepatitis recede within several weeks of discontinuing the drug. Treatment of acute overdose is similar to that for other TCAs discussed in this chapter.

REFERENCES—AMINEPTINE HYDROCHLORIDE

1. Bismuth C, Baud FJ, Conso F, et al. *Toxicologie Clinique.* 4th ed. Paris: Medicine-Sciences, Flammarion, 1987:176.
2. Rosselini SR, Grilli F, Gaudio M, et al. Hepatic injury associated with amineptine therapy. Ital J Gastroenterol 1990;22: 40–43.
3. Lachatre G, Pira C, Riche C, et al. Single-dose pharmacokinetics of amineptine and of its main metabolite in healthy young adults. Fundam Clin Pharmacol 1989;2:19–26.
4. Vexiau P, Gourmel B, Castot A, et al. Severe acne due to chronic amineptine overdose. Arch Dermatol Res 1990;282: 103–107.
5. Poignant JC. Revue pharmacologique sur l'amineptine. Encephale 1979;5:709–720.
6. Sbarra C, Castelli MG, Noseda A, Fanelli R. Pharmacokinetics of amineptine in man. Eur J Drug Metab Pharmacokinet 1981;6:123–126.
7. Sbarra C, Negrini P, Fanelli R. Quantitative analysis of amineptine (S1694) in biological samples by gas chromatography–mass fragmentography. J Chromatogr 1979;162:31–38.
8. Andrieu J, Doll J, Coffinier C. Hepatites dues a l'aminoptine: Quatre observations. Gastroenterol Clin Biol 1982;6:915–918.
9. Domingo JJS, Marco AS, Echeberria RV. Hepatic and pancreatic injury associated with amineptine therapy. J Clin Gastroenterol 1994;18:168–169.
10. Jeanmougin M, Civatte J, Cavellier-Balloy B. Toxidermie Rosacieforme a l'amineptine (Survector*). Ann Dermatol Venereol 1988;115:1185–1186.
11. Levigne V, Faisant M, Mourier C, et al. Acne monstreuse de l'adulte: Role inducteur du survector? Ann Dermatol Venereol 1988;115:1184–1185.
12. Vandel S, Bertschy G, Bizouard P, et al. Modalite d'installation d'une dependance a l'amineptine. Therapie 1990;45:47–52.
13. Castot A, Benzaken C, Wagniart F, Erthymious ML. Amineptine abuse: Analysis of 155 cases: An official cooperative report of the Regional Centre of Pharmacovigilance. Therapie 1990;45:399–405.
14. Sgro C, Lacroix D, Waldner A, et al. Anaphylactic shock with amineptine: First report. Rev Med Intern 1989;10:461–462.

CLOMIPRAMINE

Clomipramine, a synthetic tricyclic antidepressant analog of imipramine, was approved in the United States in January 1990 for the treatment of obsessive–compulsive disorder (OCD).[1,2] It has been marketed in Switzerland since 1966, in France since 1967, in the United Kingdom since 1970,[3] and in Canada since 1973.[4] This medication may require 2 to 3 months before it begins to have an impact on OCD,[5] during which time the patient with OCD may contemplate suicide. Clomipramine appears to be often associated with death following overdose, although many patients survive after ingesting quite high doses.

Use

Clomipramine is available in the United States for the treatment of OCD. It has been available in Europe and Canada for many years for the treatment of depression.[6]

Therapeutic Dose

The initial dosage of clomipramine hydrochloride, 25 mg once a day, can be increased, if tolerated, in 25-mg increments to 75 mg in the first week, 100 mg in the second, 150 mg in the third, and 200 ng in the third. The usual therapeutic range is 75 to 250 mg daily in divided doses.[6]

Toxic Dose

Doses of up to 5000 mg have been ingested with complete recovery.[7]

Fatal Dose

The lowest dose of clomipramine associated with a fatality was 750 mg.[7] A 57-year-old patient ingested about 1050 mg of clomipramine together with alprazolam and ethyl alcohol and was found dead.[8] An adult aged 27 years ingested between 5000 and 5750 mg of clomipramine, became unconscious in 2 hours, developed apnea and asystole, and died.[9] One patient who may have ingested 7000 mg of clomipramine died.[7]

Toxicokinetics

Absorption

Although it is well absorbed from the gastrointestinal tract, clomipramine is subject to extensive first-pass metabolism; this decreases its oral bioavailability to about 50%.[10,11] First-pass demethylation converts clomipramine to its primary active metabolite, desmethylclomipramine. Peak plasma concentrations of clomipramine occur 3 to 4 hours after a 150-mg dose, whereas levels of desmethylclomipramine peak after 4 to 6 hours. Mean steady-state concentrations (achieved in 7–14 days) after 238 mg of clomipramine are 148 ng/mL; desmethylclomipramine, 313 ng/mL; 8-hydroxyclomipramine, 56 ng/mL; and 8-hydroxydesmethylclomipramine, 153 ng/mL.[12] Plasma drug concentrations are not correlated with efficacy. There is some evidence that concentrations considered "too low" (ie, <150 μg/L) are usually associated with nonresponse. "Too high" concentrations (ie, >450 μg/L) are often associated with a higher frequency of side effects and even with nonresponse.[10] Therefore, clomipramine is an antidepressant with a fairly narrow therapeutic range, lending itself as an ideal candidate for blood concentration monitoring.[10]

Distribution

The mean apparent volume of distribution is 12 L/kg (range, 7–20 L/kg).[13] Clomipramine is 98% bound to plasma proteins, and its major metabolite, desmethylclomipramine, is 97% bound.[14]

Elimination

Clomipramine has an elimination half-life of about 39 hours[15]; the elimination half-life of desmethylclomipramine has been reported to range from 4.4 to 233 days.[16]

Drug Interactions

Lithium may augment the effects of clomipramine when used in patients with obsessive and panic symptoms.[17]

Pregnancy/Lactation

Clomipramine has been placed in Pregnancy Category C by the Food and Drug Administration. Clomipramine has been detected in human milk; therefore, consideration should be given to discontinuing its use during breastfeeding, although the American Academy of Pediatrics and other authors consider clomipramine compatible with breastfeeding.[18,19] Infants exposed in utero to clomipramine should be followed carefully during the neonatal period. Use of clomipramine by the mother during late pregnancy may lead to a full-term infant displaying a withdrawal syndrome consisting of tachypnea, intermittent hypertonia, and marked diaphoresis in the first hours of life. Such symptoms disappear within 10 days.[18,20]

Mechanism of Action

Clomipramine appears to be an inhibitor of serotonin reuptake.[21] This property may distinguish those antidepressant drugs that are active in OCD from those that are not.[6] Clomipramine decreases the concentration of the primary metabolite of serotonin, 5-hydroxyindoleacetic acid (5-HIAA), in the cerebrospinal fluid. It also reduces the concentration of 3-methoxy-4-hydroxyphenylglycol, the major metabolite of norepinephrine, in the cerebrospinal fluid.[22] The ability of clomipramine to reduce OCD symptoms may also be due to a downregulation of serotonin receptors. Clompramine may also cause dopamine antagonism, suppress rapid eye movement sleep,[23] elevate plasma prolactin,[24] and induce an increase in the heart rate and PR interval. It may cause flattening of T waves, a prolonged preejection period, and shortening of the left ventricular ejection time.[25]

Clinical Presentation

Chronic Use

The adverse effect profile of clomipramine closely follows those of other TCAs. Anticholinergic effects are most frequently reported and include dry mouth, constipation, blurred vision, urinary retention, and mydriasis.[26] Hyponatremia, excessive sweating, myoclonus, manic episodes,[27] hyperprolactinemia, amenorrhea, anorgasmia,[28] glactorrhea, disruption of glucose control in patients with diabetes mellitus,[29] pancreatitis (rarely),[30] and seizures[31] have been reported.[26]

Rebound withdrawal symptoms may occur in adults[32] and in neonates.[20] Clomipramine dependence may lead to anxiety attacks, perspiration, abdominal pain, and loss of efficacy following attempts to withdraw or to decrease the dose.[33]

Overdose

Clinical features of overdose are similar to those observed with other TCAs. Mild intoxication generally appears within 4 hours and is characterized by dry mouth, blurred vision, dilated pupils, sinus tachycardia, pyramidal neurologic signs, and either drowsiness or excitation. With more severe overdose, hypotension, convulsions, coma, respiratory depression, and electrocardiographic abnormalities such as prolonged PR interval and widened QRS complex may occur.[34] Clomipramine appeared to have a lower fatality index (deaths per million prescriptions) after overdose when compared in one retrospective study with TCAs.[35] Fatalities have been reported.[8,9,36–40]

Laboratory

Analytical Methods

High-pressure liquid chromatography has been used to identify the plasma and urinary concentrations of clomipramine and its metabolites.[41]

Blood Levels

Deaths following clomipramine overdose have been associated with blood clomipramine levels ranging from 540 to

6560 ng/mL and desmethylclomipramine levels ranging from 580 to 9900 ng/mL.[8,9,33–37]

Electrocardiographic abnormalities similar to those found after overdose with other TCAs may be observed with clomipramine.

Treatment

Immediate medical intervention is mandatory. Airway and circulatory support should be instituted immediately, with monitoring of vital signs, electrocardiogram, and clinical parameters. Ventilaton and other life support measures may be required. As seizures can occur, means for treating them must be available; benzodiazepines or barbiturates usually terminate the seizures. Close monitoring of cardiopulmonary status and hydration is important. Toxicologic screening of blood and urine may be useful to assess the degree of poisoning and to rule out the presence of other toxic substances.[42]

REFERENCES—CLOMIPRAMINE

1. Clomipramine approved for severe obsessive compulsive disorder: From the FDA. JAMA 1990;263:1896.
2. German GE. USFDA: FDA's approval of prescription drug clomipramine for severe obsessive–compulsive disorder, January 10, 1990.
3. Shader RI, Greenblatt DJ. Newly marketed medications: ABCs and mind your Qs. J Clin Psychopharmacol 1990;10: 81–82.
4. Kahne GJ, Wray RW. Clomipramine for bowel obsessions. Am J Psychiatry 1989;146:120–121.
5. Obsessive–compulsive disorder. Harvard Med School Health Lett 1990;15(6):4–8.
6. Clomipramine for obsessive compulsive disorder. Med Lett Drugs Ther 1988;30(778):102–104.
7. Umrath T. CIBA-Geigy Corporation. Personal communication.
8. Fraser AD, Isner AF, Moss MA. A fatality involving clomipramine. J Forens Sci 1986;31:762–767.
9. Swanson-Bierman B, Goetz M, Dean BS, Krenzelok EP. Anafranil overdose: A fatal outcome. Vet Hum Toxicol 1990; 31:378.
10. Balant-Gorgia AE, Gex-Fabry M, Balant LP. Clinical pharmacokinetics of clomipramine. Clin Pharmacokinet 1991;20: 447–462.
11. De Cuyper HJA, van Praag HM, Mulder-Hajonides WREM, et al. Pharmacokinetics of clomipramine in depressive patients. Psychol Res 1981;4:147–156.
12. Linnoila M, Insel T, Kilts C, et al. Plasma steady-state concentrations of hydroxylated metabolites of clomipramine. Clin Pharmacol Ther 1982;32:208–211.
13. Nagy A, Johansson R. The demethylation of imipramine and clomipramine as apparent from their plasma kinetics. Psychopharmacology 1977;54:125–131.
14. Bertilsson L, Braithwaite R, Tybring G, et al. Techniques for plasma protein binding of desmethylclomipramine. Clin Pharmacol Ther 1979;26:265–271.
15. Burch JE, Shaw DM, Michalakeas A, et al. Time course of plasma drug levels during one-daily oral administration of clomipramine. Psychopharmacology 1982;77:344–347.
16. Kuss HJ, Jungkunz G. Nonlinear pharmacokinetics of clomipramine after infusion and oral administration in patients. Prog Neuropsychopharmacol Biol Psychiatry 1986;10:739–748.
17. Feder R. Lithium augmentation of clomipramine. J Clin Psychiatry 1988;49:458.
18. Schimmell MS, Katz EZ, Shaag Y, et al. Toxic neonatal effects following maternal clomipramine therapy. Clin Toxicol 1991;29:479–484.
19. Committee on Drugs, American Academy of Pediatrics. The transfer of drugs and other chemicals into human breast milk. Pediatrics 1983;72:375–383.
20. Singh S, Gulati S, Narang A, Bhakoo ON. Non-narcotic withdrawal syndrome in a neonate due to maternal clomipramine therapy. J Paediatr Child Health 1990;26:110.
21. Peters MD, Davis SK, Austin LS. Clomipramine: An antiobsessional tricyclic antidepressant. Clin Pharmacol 1990;9: 165–178.
22. Asberg M, Ringberger VA, Sjoqvist F, et al. Monoamine metabolites in cerebrospinal fluid and serotonin uptake inhibition during treatment with clomipramine. Clin Pharmacol Ther 1977;21:201–207.
23. Chen CN. Sleep, depression and antidepressants. Br J Psychiatry 1979;135:385–402.
24. Jones RB, Luscomber DK, Groom BV. Plasma prolactin concentrations in normal subjects and depressive patients following oral clomipramine. Postgrad Med J 1977;55(suppl. 4): 166–171.
25. Burckhardt D, Raeder E, Muller V, et al. Cardiovascular effects of tricyclic and tetracyclic antidepressants. JAMA 1978; 239:213–216.
26. McTavish D, Benfield P. Clomipramine: An overview of its pharmacological properties and a review of its therapeutic use in obsessive compulsive disorder and panic disorder. Drugs 1990;39:136–153.
27. Vieta E, Bernardo M, Vallejo J. Clompiramine-induced mania in obsessive–compulsive disorder. Hum Psychopharmacol Clin Exp 1991;6:72–73.
28. Price J, Grunhaus LJ. Treatment of clomipramine-induced anorgasmia with yohimbine: A case report. J Clin Psychiatry 1990;51:32–33.
29. Katz LM, Fochtmann LK, Pato MT. Clomipramine, fluoxetine and glucose control. Ann Clin Psychiatry 1991;3:271–274.
30. Roberge RJ, Martin TG, Hodgman M, Benitez JG. Acute chemical pancreatitis associated with a tricyclic antidepressant (clomipramine) overdose. Clin Toxicol 1994;32:425–429.
31. Tunca Z, Tunca MI, Dilsiz A, et al. Clomipramine-induced pseudocyanotic pigmentation. Am J Psychiatry 1989; 146:552–553.
32. Diamond BI, Borison RL, Katz R, De Veaugh-Geiss J. Rebound withdrawal reactions due to clomipramine. Psychopharmacol Bull 1989;25:209–212.
33. Nores JM, Befort JP, Remy JM. A case of clomipramine addiction. Acta Ther 1991;17:311–312.
34. Matthews HJS: The management of self-poisoning due to clomipramine (Anafranil). J Int Med Res 1973;1:485–488.
35. Cassidy S, Henry J. Fatal toxicity of antidepressant drugs in overdose. Br Med J 1987;295:1021–1024.
36. Meatherall RC, Guay DRP, Chalmers JL, Keenan JR. A fatal overdose with clomipramine. J Anal Toxicol 1983;7:168–171.
37. Hucker RS. Fatal clomipramine and trimipramine poisoning. Bull Assoc Forens Toxicol 1983;17(2):20–22.
38. Ward N, Dawling S. A fatal case involving chlorpromazine and clomipramine. Bull Int Assoc Forens Toxicol 1987;19(2): 16–17.
39. Haqqani MT, Gutteridge DR. Two cases of clomipramine hydrochloride (Anafranil) poisoning. Forens Sci 1974;3:83–87.
40. Edelbroek PM, Koelma IA, de Wolff FA. A fatal multi-dose poisoning: The role of clomipramine. In: *Proceedings, International Congress of Clin Toxicol Poison Control Anal Toxicol, Lux-Tox '90, Luxembourg May 2–5, 1990:* PO 3.15.
41. Gaskell SJ. Gas chromatography/high resolution mass spectrometry as a reference method for clomipramine determination. Postgrad Med J 1980;56(suppl. 1):90–93.
42. James WA, Lippmann SB. Clomipramine for obsessive–compulsive disorder: Prescribing guidelines. South Med J 1991;84:1242–1245.

CLOTHIAPINE

Clothiapine, 2-chloro-11-(4-methyl-1-piperazinyl)dibenzo [*b,f*] [1,4]thiazepine, is a dibenzothiazepine tricyclic antipsychotic agent used in Italy for the treatment of acute and chronic schizophrenia. The toxicity of clothiapine is not well documented. Serum concentrations greater than 0.3 μg/mL are associated with central nervous system depression.[1] Ingestion of 2.5 g of clothiapine was followed by coma and pronounced hypotension. Twenty-four hours after ingestion a serum level of 384 ng/mL was detected and hypotension developed followed by death. Treatment of an overdose is symptomatic and supportive. There is no antidote.[2]

REFERENCES—CLOTHIAPINE

1. Baldi ML, Rocchi L, Papa P, et al. Clothiapine poisonings: Toxic versus therapeutic serum drug levels. In: *Proceedings, XIVth International Congress of European Association of Poison Centres, Milan, Italy, September 25–29, 1990:49.*
2. Romano G, Di Bono G. A fatality involving clothiapine and clomipramine. J Forens Sci 1994;34:877–882.

DOTHIEPIN HYDROCHLORIDE

Dothiepin (Fig. 38–2) is a synthetic TCA which is a thio derivative of amitriptyline.[1,2] Dothiepin is available commercially in the United Kingdom as Prothiaden. Dothiepin is not available in the United States.

Product Formulation

Dothiepin hydrochloride is available in capsules of 25 mg and tablets of 75 mg.

Therapeutic Dose

For depression, dothiepin hydrochloride is given by mouth in doses of 25 mg three times daily, which are gradually increased to 50 mg three times daily as required or 75 or 150 mg as a single nighttime dose.[3] Doses up to 225 mg daily have been given to severely depressed patients.[4]

Toxic Dose

Ingestion of 1 to 4.5 g of dothiepin by a series of eight adults was followed by impaired consciousness (7/8), grand mal seizures (2/8), and tachycardia (7/8). All survived.[5] An adult man ingested 1.5 g of dothiepin and became comatose, developing cardiac arrest within minutes of arrival at a hospital; he survived.[6]

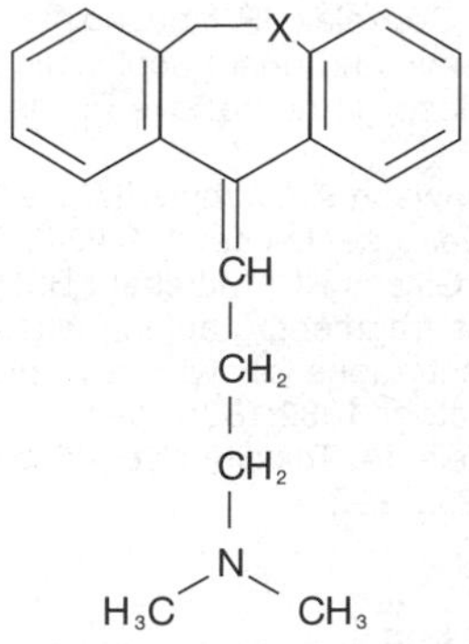

X
CH
CH$_2$
CH$_2$
N
H$_3$C CH$_3$

X = CH$_2$ Amitriptyline
X = S Dothiepin
X = O Doxepin

Figure 38-2 Structure of dothiepin in relation to amitriptyline and doxepin. (From Maguire KP, Burrows GD, Norman TR, Scoggins BA. Metabolism and pharmacokinetics of dothiepin. Br J Clin Pharmacol 1981;12:405–409.)

Fatal Dose

Death has followed ingestion of 50 25-mg capsules of dothiepin (total dose, 1250 mg).[7,8] Analyses of fatalities from TCA overdoses suggest that amitriptyline and dothiepin are the drugs most likely to be associated with death.[9,10]

Toxicokinetics

Absorption

Dothiepin is readily absorbed in the gastrointestinal tract. The mean half-life of absorption is 1.2 hours.[1,11–13] A mean peak plasma concentration of 47 ng/mL is reached in 3 hours. The distribution half-life is 2.6 hours. First-pass metabolism has been demonstrated for nortriptyline, desipramine, and maprotiline, but studies have not been carried out for dothiepin.[1] The mean blood:plasma ratio is 0.7. Following a single 75-mg oral dose, the mean peak concentration of dothiepin is 47 ng/mL at 3 hours, and that of dothiepin-*S*-oxide is 81 ng/mL at 5 hours. Plasma protein binding is about 80 to 90%.

Distribution

The mean volume of distribution is about 45 L/kg.[1]

Elimination

The beta half-life (elimination) is about 20 hours. Dothiepin-*S*-oxide is the major metabolite. Northiaden (desmethyldothiepin) is an *N*-demethylated derivative. Both metabolites have antidepressant activity.[6,7]

Pregnancy/Lactation

Controlled clinical studies in pregnancy have not been performed with dothiepin. Dothiepin and its metabolites have been detected in breast milk.[15] The mean total daily infant exposure amounts to about 4.4% of the maternal dothiepin dosage. This compares with calculated instant doses of 3.3% for amitriptyline alone, 1.9% for amitriptyline plus nortriptyline, 1% for desipramine alone, 2.2% for doxepin plus desmethyldoxepin, 0.3% for imipramine plus desipramine, and 2.3% for nortriptyline alone.[11]

Clinical Presentation

A 36-year-old woman ingested 2 to 3 g of dothiepin, developed ventricular tachycardia, and was treated with gastric lavage and charcoal hemoperfusion, but she began to hallucinate 48 hours after ingestion. At 56 hours postoverdose, she became apneic with ventricular fibrillation. The plasma dothiepin level was 4.5 µg/mL, with the northiaden metabolite at 1.28 µg/mL.[16] Patients with only mild sedation and normal limb–lead QRS width may still have complications[17] (see Toxic Dose).

Laboratory

Analytical Methods

A useful analytical method is high-performance liquid chromatography (HPLC) with ultraviolet detection (sensitivity, 10 ng/mL).[1,8] Gas–liquid chromatography analysis can detect 26 ng/L; mass fragmentography can detect 0.5 ng/mL.[15] An HPLC method quantifies dothiepin and nordothiepin (sensitive to 2 ng/mL). Dothiepin-*S*-oxide and nordothiepin-5-oxide are sensitive to 5 ng/mL by this method.[11] A gas chromatography–mass spectrometry fragmentography method is also available.[18]

Blood Levels

Following ingestion of 1 to 4.5 g, the peak plasma concentration of dothiepin ranges from 819 to 385 ng/mL (steady-state therapeutic level, 68 ng/mL). Plasma dothiepin levels greater than 900 ng/mL (0.9 μg/mL) are associated with typical signs of TCA poisoning such as depressed consciousness, seizures, and tachycardia. In one series of eight overdose patients, only one exhibited slight widening of the QT_c interval; all others had normal sinus rhythm.[19] Death is usually associated with plasma levels greater than 1000 ng/mL.[12] In a series of three fatalities after dothiepin overdose, blood levels ranged from 1.4 to 2.5 μg/mL.[5,7] In a later series of three fatalities, blood levels ranged from 0.3 to 2.2 μg/mL.[9]

Ancillary Tests

After ingestion of 1.5 g of dothiepin, an adult man developed wide QRS complexes, ventricular tachycardia, ventricular fibrillation, and cardiac arrest.[5]

Treatment

Gut Decontamination

Treatment consists largely of gastric lavage and activated charcoal[3,6] (either single or multiple doses). Although use of activated charcoal suggests a role in decreasing the half-life of dothiepin, other studies with TCAs show little or no such significant decrease in half-life.[13–15,18]

Elimination Enhancement

The high degree of protein binding, together with the extensive volume of distribution, tends to preclude the potential usefulness of hemodialysis and hemoperfusion.

Antidote

There is no antidote.

Supportive Measures

Following a dothiepin overdose leading to ventricular fibrillation and cardiac arrest, an adult was treated with intravenous sodium bicarbonate, dopamine, and lidocaine with hyperventilation. His condition remained unstable. One hour later, intravenous sodium chloride (170 mM) was given over 5 minutes. The blood pressure rose immediately; the QRS complexes narrowed and cardiac abnormalities became less frequent. Similar episodes of hypotension and cardiac abnormalities over the following days were reversed by rapid infusions of sodium chloride 100 mM.[5]

REFERENCES—DOTHIEPIN

1. Maguire KP, Burrows GD, Norman TR, Scoggins BA. Metabolism and pharmacokinetics of dothiepin. Br J Clin Pharmacol 1981;12:405–409.
2. Zusky P, Manschreck TC, Blanchard C, et al. Dothiepin hydrochloride: Treatment of efficacy and safety. J Clin Psychiatry 1986;47:504–507.
3. Ilett KF, Hackett LP, Dusci LJ, Paterson JW. Disposition of dothiepin after overdose: Effects of repeated-dose activated charcoal. Ther Drug Monit 1991;13:485–489.
4. Reynolds JEF, ed. *Martindale: The Extra Pharmacopoeia.* 30th ed. London: Pharmaceutical Press, 1993:253.
5. Hoegholm A, Clementsen P. Hypertonic sodium chloride in severe antidepressant overdosage. J Toxicol Clin Toxicol 1991;29:297–298.
6. Robinson AE, Coffee AI, McDowall RD. Toxicology of some autopsy cases involving tricyclic antidepressant drugs. Z Rechtsmedizin 1974;74:261–266.
7. Robinson AE, McDowell RD, Sattar H, et al. Tricyclic and tetracyclic antidepressant drugs: Forensic toxicology of some autopsy cases. J Anal Toxicol 1979;23:3–13.
8. Maguire KP, Norman TR, Burrows GD, Scoggins BA. Simultaneous measurement of dothiepin and its major metabolites in plasma and whole blood by gas chromatography–mass fragmentography. J Chromatogr 1981;222:399–409.
9. Montgomery SA, Baldwin D, Green M. Why do amitriptyline and dothiepin appear to be so dangerous in overdose Acta Psychiatr Scand 1989;80(suppl. 354):47–52.
10. Cassidy S, Henry J. Fatal toxicity of antidepressant drugs in overdose. Br Med J 1987;295:1021–1024.
11. Ilett KF, Lebeders TH, Wojnar-Horton RE, et al. The excretion of dothiepin and its primary metabolites in breast milk. Br J Clin Pharmacol 1992;3:635–639.
12. Tracqui A, Kintz P, Mangin P. A fatal case of dothiepin self-poisoning. Bull Int Assoc Forens Toxicol 1992;22:28–30.
13. Goldberg MJ, Park GD, Spector R, et al. Lack of effect of oral activated charcoal on imipramine clearance. Clin Pharmacol Ther 1985;38:350–352.
14. Schemin M, Virtanen R, Tisalo E. Effect of activated charcoal on the pharmacokinetics of doxepin. Int J Clin Pharmacol Ther Toxicol 1985;23:38–42.
15. Karkkainen S, Neuvonen PJ. Pharmacokinetics of amitriptyline influenced by oral charcoal and urine pH. Int J Clin Pharmacol Ther Toxicol 1985;24:326–332.
16. Lancaster SG, Gonzalez JP. Dothiepin: A review of its pharmacodynamic and pharmacokinetic properties and therapeutic efficacy in depressive illness. Drugs 1989;38: 123–147.
17. Buckley NA, Dawson AH, Whyte IM, Henry DA. Toxicity of dothiepin in overdose. Lancet 1994;343:735.
18. Crampton EL, Glkass RC, Marchant B, Rees JA. Chemical ionisation mass fragmentographic measurement of dothiepin placebo concentrations following a single oral dose in man. J Chromatogr 1980;183:141–148.
19. McGrady H, Reis JA. Toxicity of dothiepin in overdose. Lancet 1944;343:292–293.

LOFEPRAMINE

First-generation TCAs are cheap and effective but often cause unwanted effects. The second-generation antidepressants are not necessarily more effective, but may have fewer or milder unwanted effects. Examples of the latter group include lofepramine (Fig. 38–3), viloxazine, and amoxapine.[1] Lofepramine in overdose is not usually accompanied by hy-

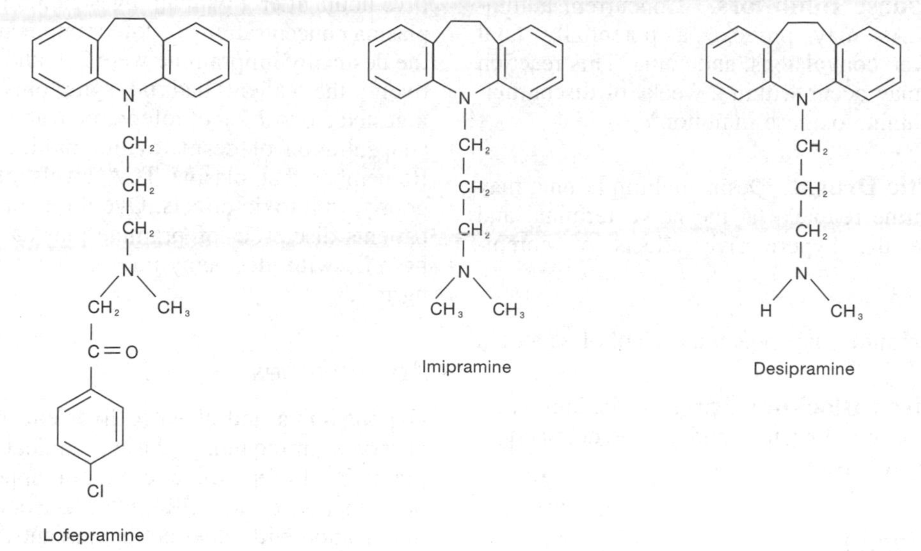

Figure 38-3 Structures of lofepramine, imipramine, and desipramine. (From Lancaster SG, Gonzalez JP. Lofepramine: A review of its pharmacodynamic and pharmacokinetic properties, and therapeutic efficacy in depressive illness. Drugs 1989;37(2):123–140.

potension, arrhythmias, or coma. No deaths have definitely been attributed to lofepramine alone or in combination.

Structure and Classification

Lofepramine is a synthetic TCA structurally similar to imipramine; it is extensively metabolized to desipramine[2,3] (Fig. 38–3).

Product Formulation

Lofepramine hydrochloride is available in the United Kingdom as Gamanil tablets, which are scored and contain lofepramine 70 mg (as the hydrochloride).

Therapeutic Dose

In the treatment of depression, lofepramine is given by mouth in divided doses of 140 to 210 mg daily. Use of a daily dose as high as 490 mg has been reported.[4] At the usual dose (140–210 mg daily) lofepramine appears as effective as imipramine 75 to 150 mg daily, amitriptyline 30 to 150 mg daily, clomipramine 100 mg daily, maprotiline 150 mg daily, and mianserin 30 to 60 mg daily.[1]

Toxic Dose

Twenty-one patients ingested between 0.14 and 4.9 g of lofepramine. Seven were asymptomatic (mean dose 1.85 g) and 14 patients had mild symptoms. One had a deep coma, suffered from respiration depression, and required ventilation for 36 hours. Five had mild hypertension, 5 had tachycardia, and several had anticholinergic symptoms. Hypotension, convulsions, and cardiac arrhythmias were not reported.[5] When lofepramine was ingested with other drugs, hypotension, arrhythmias, and coma were observed.

Fatal Dose

In the United Kingdom few deaths have been reported from lofepramine when taken alone.[5] One death has been attributed to ingestion of both dothiepin and lofepramine.[5]

Toxicokinetics

Absorption

Following oral administration of a single dose of 210 mg to healthy subjects, lofepramine is rapidly absorbed, with peak plasma concentrations of 140 ng/mL (lofepramine) and 5 ng/mL (desipramine) achieved within 1 and 4 hours, respectively.[2,6–8] Desmethylimipramine is itself an antidepressant.

Distribution

Lofepramine is highly bound to plasma proteins (99.3%); the active metabolite desipramine is also highly bound (98.6%). An approximate apparent volume of distribution is 2.3 L/kg.[7]

Elimination

Lofepramine is partially metabolized to desipramine by a cytochrome P450-dependent enzyme system on first pass through the liver. It is metabolized by *N*-dealkylation, hydroxylation, and glucuronidation. The plasma clearance of lofepramine is 686 L/h. Its main urinary metabolites are desipramine, 2-hydroxydesipramine, and its glucuronide (2-hydroxyimodibenzyl), and the glycine conjugate of *p*-chlorobenzoic acid. The mean elimination half-lives are 1.7 hours for a 70-mg dose and 2.5 hours for a 140-mg dose.[2] Lofepramine has a half-life in the beta phase of about 5 hours (compared with 24 hours for other TCAs).[9,10]

Drug Interactions

Monoamine Oxidase Inhibitors. Concurrent administration with TCAs may provoke a potentially fatal syndrome with fever, convulsions, and coma. This reaction with lofepramine may occur within 2 weeks of discontinuation of the monoamine oxidase inhibitor.[4,11]

Sympathomimetic Drugs. Desmethylimipramine may inhibit norepinephrine reuptake at the nerve terminal and thereby potentiate the hypertensive effects of norepinephrine.

Alcohol. Lofepramine may potentiate alcohol sedation.

Adrenergic Neuron Blocking Drugs. The antihypertensive effects of guanethidine, bethanidine, and debrisoquin may be reduced by TCAs.

Pregnancy/Lactation

There have been no controlled studies in pregnancy or during lactation. TCAs are excreted in breast milk. The metabolite desmethylimipramine may be excreted in breast milk.[12]

Mechanism of Action

Lofepramine is highly lipophilic; however, its low bioavailability and delayed absorption may contribute to the low toxicity of lofepramine when taken in overdose.[13] Lofepramine inhibits the reuptake of monoamines in peripheral adrenergic nerves.

Clinical Presentation

Lofepramine overdose in humans may be associated with tachycardia, hypertension, dry mouth, dilated pupils, ileus, blurred vision, dizziness, flushing, hypersalivation, muscle weakness, and vomiting.[5] Only 1 of 55 cases studied had deep coma requiring ventilation. Hypotension, convulsions, and cardiac arrhythmias were not reported.[5]

Dry mouth is the most common side effect.[14] Constipation, dizziness, sweating, nausea/vomiting, tremor palpitation, blurred vision, drowsiness, fatigue, headache, and insomnia were also observed during clinical studies.[2] There does not appear to be a correlation between plasma lofepramine levels and adverse effects.[7] Reversible peripheral neuropathy has been reported after doses of 210 mg/d.[15] Sudden cardiac death occurred in a 39-year-old male jogger who was ingesting 210 mg/d lofepramine.[16] He had been experiencing anticholinergic adverse effects and palpitations prior to this episode.

Laboratory

Analytical Methods

Gas chromatography (lowest detectable plasma level, 1 ng/mL)[17] and high-performance liquid chromatography with electrochemical detection (limit of detection, plasma concentration of 0.5 ng/mL) methods are available.

Blood Levels

Five hours after a woman ingested 3.5 g of lofepramine the plasma concentrations of lofepramine and its main metabolite desmethylimipramine were 259 and 235 ng/mL, respectively; the patient had no symptoms.[18] Another patient ingested 5.6 to 7.2 g of lofepramine and vomited; the plasma concentration of desmethylimipramine was 190 ng/mL.[18] Remember that plasma TCA levels generally correspond poorly with toxic effects. Overdoses of lofepramine in five patients disclosed lofepramine plasma levels of 10 to 394 ng/mL, with desmethylimipramine levels of 34 to 235 ng/mL.[5]

Abnormalities

Hyponatremia and elevated liver enzyme activities[11] were observed infrequently during clinical studies with lofepramine.[2] Lofepramine does not appear to produce the prolongation of the QRS interval characteristic of milder intoxication with other antidepressants.[9] Patients who overdosed with up to 4.9 g of lofepramine remained awake (not in coma). One of 13 patients had a widened QRS interval. No arrhythmias or convulsions were seen.[19] In most patients, any rise in liver enzyme abnormalities is transient.[20]

Treatment

Stabilization

Treatment of lofepramine overdose is largely symptomatic and supportive. Intubation and ventilation should be provided where indicated.

Gut Decontamination

Gastric lavage may be effective even up to 24 hours after an attempt at self-poisoning, as most TCAs have an anticholinergic effect and the bowel is atonic. The lavage should be performed with an orogastric with a line wide enough to remove the tablets. The lavage may be terminated by instilling 20 to 50 g of activated charcoal into the stomach. The charcoal may interrupt the enterohepatic recirculation cycle.

Elimination Enhancement

Measures such as hemodialysis and hemoperfusion are not likely to be of value in view of the high degree of protein binding and the extensive volume of distribution.

Antidote

There is no antidote.

Supportive Measures

Level of consciousness, respiration, and bowel sounds should be monitored and symptomatic treatment provided as indicated. Blood sodium and liver function tests should be performed on admission.

REFERENCES—LOFEPRAMINE

1. Update of antidepressants: Lofepramine, amoxapine and viloxazine. Drug Ther Bull 1990;28(21):82–84.
2. Lancaster SG, Gonzalez JP. Lofepramine: A review of its pharmacodynamic and pharmacokinetic properties and therapeutic efficacy in depressive illness. Drugs 1989;37: 123–140.
3. Virgili P, Henry JA. Determination of lofepramine and desipramine using high performance liquid chromatography and electrochemical detection. J Chromatogr 1989;496: 228–233.
4. Dollery DF, ed. *Therapeutic Drugs.* Edinburgh: Churchill Livingstone, 1991;2:653–655.
5. Reid F, Henry JA. Lofepramine overdose. Pharmacopsychiatry 1990;23(suppl. 1):23–27.
6. Forshell GP, Siweris B, Tucks JR. Pharmacokinetics of lofepramine in man: Relationship to inhibition of noradrenaline uptake. Eur J Clin Pharmacol 1976;9:291–298.
7. Ghose K, Spragg BP. Pharmacokinetics of lofepramine and amitriptyline in elderly healthy subjects. Int Clin Psychopharmacol 1989;4:201–215.
8. Dollery CT, ed. *Therapeutic Drugs.* Edinburgh: Churchill Livingstone, 1991;2:D208–D211.
9. Heath A. Suicidal overdoses of antidepressants with special reference to lofepramine. Int Med 1984;suppl. 10:27–30.
10. Plym Forshell G. The absorption, excretion and plasma protein binding of lofepramine in the rat, dog and man. Zenobiotica 1977;7:153–164.
11. D'Arcy PF. Drug reactions and interactions. Int Pharm J 1989;3:3.
12. Anderson PO. Drug use during breastfeeding. Clin Pharm 1991;10:594–624.
13. Hla KK, Virgili P, Henry JA. Is decreased bioavailability of lofepramine the cause of its safety in overdose? In: *Proceedings, 14th International Congress of European Association of Poison Centres, Milan, Italy, September 25–29, 1990:*45.
14. Dutt JE. On the clinical response/serum level relationship for antidepressants: II. Lofepramine and imipramine. Psychopharmacol Bull 1982;18:17–27.
15. Hewitt JA, Glinn J. Lofepramine and motor neuropathy. Br Med J 1989;299:1223–1224.
16. Lock T, Konyon W, Abou-Saleh MT. Sudden cardiac death and antidepressants. Br J Psychiatry 1991;159:736–737.
17. Lundgren R, Olsson A, Forshell GP. Gas chromatographic determination of lofepramine and desmethylimipramine in plasma. Acta Pharm Suec 1977;14:81–94.
18. Crome P, Ali C. Clinical features and management of self poisoning with newer antidepressants. Med Toxicol 1986;1: 411–420.
19. Heath A, Hutton BA. Lofepramine toxicity in overdose. In: *Proceedings, VI World Congress of Psychiatry, Vienna, 1983.* Abstract.
20. Kelly C, Roche S, Naguib M, et al. A prospective evaluation of the hepatotoxicity of lofepramine in the elderly. Int Clin Psychopharmacol 1983;8:83–86.

METAPRAMINE

Metapramine (Fig. 38–4) is a synthetic TCA marketed in France in 1984 that is rapidly absorbed and distributed and is extensively metabolized. Overdoses are characterized by central nervous system depression and cardiac repolarization changes. There have been no reports of fatalities. Metapramine is marketed in Europe as Timaxel.

Product Formulation

The drug is available for oral administration (50-mg tablets) in the form of metapramine fumarate, and is available in solution as the hydrochloride.[1]

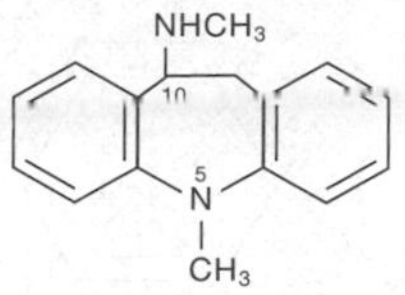

NHCH3
10
5
N
CH3

Metapromine

Figure 38-4 Structure of metapramine. (From Viala A, Cano JP, Durand A, Monjanel S. Qualitative and quantitative determination of metapramine and its metabolites in biological materials. J Chromatogr 1979;168:195–201.)

Therapeutic Dose

The recommended daily dosage ranges from 150 to 300 mg.[2]

Toxic Dose

A 23-year-old woman ingested 1.50 g of metapramine with prochlorperazine and meprobamate. She became comatose and was treated with mechanical ventilation and gastric lavage. Within 48 hours the patient awoke with cardiac repolarization disturbances.[2] A 34-year-old patient found responsive after ingestion of 300 to 500 mg of metapramine together with 150 mg of clobazen remained lethargic after gastric lavage. The next day vital signs were stable, although cardiac repolarization disturbances made electrocardiographic controls necessary for 48 hours. She awoke in 3 days and was discharged.

Fatal Dose

No fatal dose has been reported.

Toxicokinetics

Absorption

Metapramine exhibits very rapid distribution in the body so that only low concentrations are found in blood serum samples. The average steady-state plasma levels after infusions of 1.18, 2.36, and 4.71 mg/h were 15.6, 28.5, and 51.2 mg/mL, respectively.[3]

Distribution

The apparent volume of distribution ranges from 0.6 to 1.3 L/kg.[3] During the first phase of distribution the plasma drug level decreases very rapidly with a half-life of 4.4, followed by a slower distribution phase with an approximate half-life of 1.2 hours.

Elimination

Demethylation leads to *N*-desmethylmetapramine concentration, the main method of histamine formation of metapramine.[4] Metapramine undergoes considerable metabolism in the liver so that it is present in urine samples only in low concentrations and heavily masked by metabolites. In plasma the half-life is 5 to 6 hours. Plasma clearance after intravenous infusions of 1.18, 2.36, and 4.71 mg/h varied from 68 to 107 L/h in one study.[3]

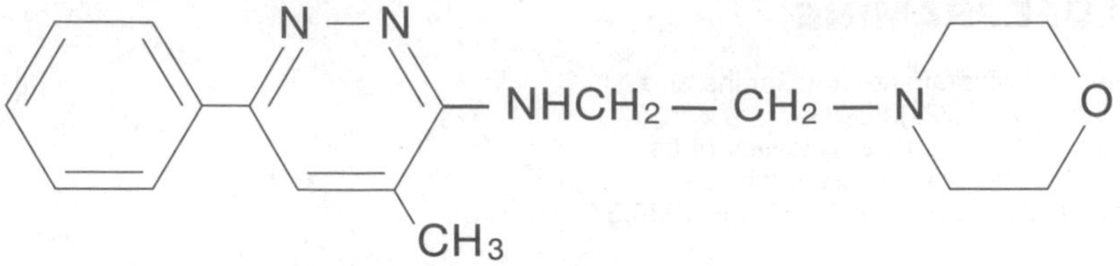

Figure 38-5 Structure of minaprine.

Mechanism of Action

Metapramine differs biochemically from other TCAs in that it markedly enhances the turnover of norepinephrine without notably inhibiting its reuptake.[3]

Clinical Presentation

Patients may be found unresponsive. Coma may intervene within 2 hours of ingestion. Lethargy continues for 48 to 72 hours. Two overdose patients recovered in 48 to 72 hours with slow resolution of cardiac repolarization disturbances.[2] No fatalities have been reported.

Laboratory

Analytical Methods

A HPLC procedure with ultraviolet detection is quick, reproducible, and sensitive: requires a small sample size; and has a detection limit in plasma of about 3 mg/mL.[2] An HPLC method with fluorometric detection is useful.[4] The detection limit for thin-layer chromatography is about 100 mg.[5]

Blood Levels

Plasma concentrations of metapramine were 73 ng/mL following ingestion of 1.50 g and 921 ng/mL following ingestion of 300 to 500 mg. Urine concentrations were 2000 and more than 4000 ng/mL in both patients, respectively. The drug may be detected in gastric contents by thin-layer chromatography.

Treatment

Treatment is symptomatic and supportive. Careful cardiac monitoring is required. Patients should not be discharged until at least 48 hours after they have become alert and have no residual electrocardiographic changes.

REFERENCES—METAPRAMINE

1. Viala AR, Cano J-P, Durand AG, et al. Determination of metapramine in plasma by gas chromatography with nitrogen-selective and electron-capture detection. Anal Chem 1977;49:2354–2357.
2. Rouquette C, Hecquet D, Pommereau X, et al. Metapramine overdose: Report of two cases and analytical determinations. J Anal Toxicol 1985;9:275–277.
3. Sumirtapura YC, Leroux Y, Komar AR, et al. Pharmacokinetics of metapramine (1956ORP) in man after infusion and intravenous ingestion. Eur J Clin Pharmacol 1983;25:673–677.
4. Decouvelaere B, Terlain B, Bieder A. Biotransformation of metapramine in three animal species (dog, rabbit, rat) and in man. Therapie 1982;37:249–257.
5. Sommadossi JP, Lemar M, Necciari J, et al. High performance liquid chromatographic method for determination of plasma and urine metapramine after demethylation. J Chromatogr 1982;228:205–231.

MINAPRINE HYDROCHLORIDE

Minaprine hydrochloride is an antidepressant glycine antagonist available in France and Italy[1] (Fig. 38–5). It has stimulant properties and is administered orally in doses of 100 to 300 mg daily. An 18-year-old woman ingested 7.5 g of minaprine and developed seizures refractory to benzodiazepines but responsive to thiopental sodium. Her condition was complicated by ventricular arrhythmias, bradycardia, torsade de pointes, ventricular tachycardia, and asystole. She died after she developed hypokalemia, disseminated intravascular coagulation, rhabdomyolysis, renal insufficiency, and cerebral edema.[2] A 21-year-old adult ingested 6 g of minaprine and developed seizures, respiratory distress requiring assisted ventilation, and hypokalemia with a prolonged QT interval on the electrocardiogram; the patient survived.[3] Agranulocytosis has been reported following the use of 100 to 200 mg/d for 4 to 6 weeks.[4]

REFERENCES—MINAPRINE HYDROCHLORIDE

1. Reynolds JF, ed. *Martindale: The Extra Pharmacopoeia.* 30th ed. London: Pharmaceutical Press, 1993:265.
2. Roynard JL, Pouirriat JL, Fournier JL, et al. Fatal intoxication with minaprine. Press Med 1989;18:986.
3. Bertrand J, Deny N, Weber B, et al. Emergency therapy in acute minaprine intoxication. Presse Med 1983;12:2057.
4. Bastim Y, Vial T, Espinouse D, et al. Three cases of acute agranulcytosis: Was minaprine the culprit? Presse Med 1993; 22:82–93.

VENLAFAXINE

Venlafaxine (Effexor) is a new synthetic antidepressant useful in the treatment of depression and possibly in obsessive–compulsive disorder[1] and chemically related to bupropion[2] (Fig. 38–6). It was approved by the Food and Drug Administration in December 1993.[3]

Product Formulation

Venlafaxine hydrochloride is available as tablets of 25, 37.5, 50, 75, and 100 mg.

Therapeutic Dose

The initial dosage is 75 mg/d divided into two or three doses. This is raised as required by 75 mg/d at 4-day intervals to a maximum of 375 mg/d.[4]

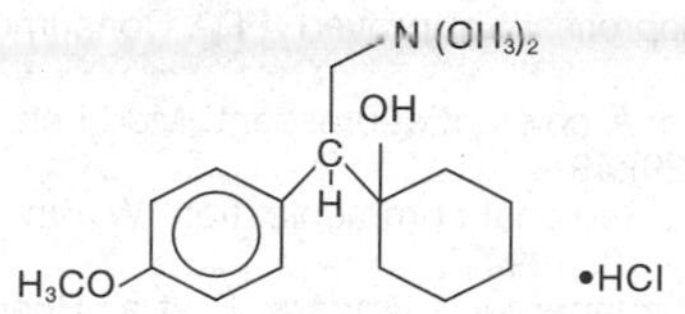

Figure 38-6 Structure of venlafaxine hydrochloride.

Toxic Dose

Doses of 2.75 g have led to seizures and coma. A dose of 6.75 g with lithium 15 g was followed by nausea, vomiting, and diarrhea. After 1.5 g an adult became unresponsive to verbal commands but responsive to painful stimuli. The patient developed sinus tachycardia. Ingestion of 2.5 g led to loss of consciousness, stupor, and sinus tachycardia. All patients have recovered.[5]

Fatal Dose

A fatal dose has not been reported.

Toxicokinetics

Absorption

Venlafaxine is well absorbed from the gastrointestinal tract. Peak serum concentrations are reached from 1 to 2 hours after oral administration.[6,7] Peak levels of *o*-desmethylvenlafaxine, its major active metabolite, are reached 3 to 4 hours after oral administration of venlafaxine.[7] After single oral doses of 25, 75, and 150 mg, mean peak serum concentrations of 37, 102, and 163 ng/mL, respectively, were observed. Simultaneous levels of *o*-desmethylvenlafaxine were 61, 168, and 325 ng/mL.[7] Following oral administration, venlafaxine undergoes first-pass metabolism to its active metabolite *o*-desmethylvenlafaxine.[7]

Distribution

Venlafaxine is about 30% protein bound.[7] The apparent volume of distribution of venlafaxine is about 6 to 7 L/kg. The volume of distribution of its major active metabolite is about 4 to 6 L/kg.

Elimination

The drug is metabolized by cytochrome $P_{450}IID_6$ in the liver, and about 1 to 10% is excreted in the urine as unchanged drug. The elimination half-life of the parent drug is about 5 hours, and that of the metabolite, 11 hours. The mean total body clearance is about 2 L/h/kg, and that of the metabolite, 0.2 L/h/kg.[7]

Drug Interactions

Drugs that inhibit cytochrome $P_{450}IID_6$ such as quinidine may increase serum concentrations and possibly the toxicity of venlafaxine in extensive metabolizers. Venlafaxine should not be started until at least 14 days after a monoamine oxidase inhibitor has been discontinued because of its adrenergic and serotonergic activity. Venlafaxine should be stopped at least 7 days before a monoamine oxidase inhibitor is started.[6] Hyperthermia, rigidity, myoclonus, autonomic instability, mental status changes including extreme agitation progressing to delirium and coma, and features resembling neuroleptic malignant syndrome have been reported with concomitant selective serotonin reuptake inhibitor/monoamine oxidase inhibitor therapy. Severe hyperthermia and seizures, sometimes fatal, have been reported with concomitant TCA/monoamine oxidase inhibitor therapy.[8]

Pregnancy/Lactation

There are no adequate and well-controlled studies in pregnant women.[5]

Mechanism of Action

Venlafaxine inhibits norepinephrine and serotonin reuptake and weakly inhibits dopamine reuptake. Animal studies suggest that it has no affinity for muscarinic, cholinergic, histaminergic, α_1-adrenergic receptors, opioid (mu), or benzodiazepine receptors. It lacks monoamine oxidase inhibitory activity. It has no affinity for beta-adrenoceptor, serotonin-1, serotonin-2, and dopamine-2 receptors.[7,9]

Clinical Presentation

Adverse effects of venlafaxine resemble those of fluoxetine (Prozac) and the other selective serotonin reuptake inhibitors and include nausea, headache, anxiety, anorexia, nervousness, sweating, dizziness, insomnia, and somnolence.[4] Sexual dysfunction and weight loss have occurred. At doses of 300 mg/d some patients develop a sustained increase in diastolic blood pressure. Seizures have been observed. All overdose patients have recovered without sequelae.[5] Ingestion of 2.75 g led to generalized seizures.[5] In overdose, severe central nervous system depression has been observed.[10] Extrapyramidal effects can occur with as little as one or two therapeutic doses of venlafaxine.[11]

Laboratory

Analytical Methods

Venlafaxine and its *o*-desmethyl metabolite are analyzed by high-performance liquid chromatography with ultraviolet detection, a method that is sensitive to as little as 10 ng/mL of both the drug and its metabolite.[8]

Blood Levels

After ingestion of 2.75 and 2.5 g, peak plasma levels were 6.24 and 2.35 μg/mL, respectively. The peak plasma levels of *o*-desmethylvenlafaxine were 3.37 and 1.30 μg/mL, respectively.[8]

Abnormalities

Ingestion of 2.75 g of venlafaxine led to prolongation of the QT_c interval to 500 milliseconds.[8]

Ancillary Tests

Small increases in serum cholesterol have been reported.[12] Electroencephalographic effects are similar to those caused by other antidepressants such as imipramine.[6]

Treatment

Treatment should include maintenance of an adequate airway, oxygenation, and ventilation. Bicarbonate has not been used. Cardiac rhythm and vital signs must be monitored. Treatment is largely supportive and symptomatic. Activated charcoal or gastric lavage should be considered, but the airway must be secured because of possible seizures. Venlafaxine has a large volume of distribution; therefore, forced diuresis, dialysis, hemoperfusion, and exchange transfusion are unlikely to be of benefit. There is no antidote. Multiple-drug involvement is a possibility.

REFERENCES—VENLAFAXINE

1. Zajecka JM, Fawcett J, Guy C. Coexisting major depression and obsessive–impulsive disorder treated with venlafaxine. J Clin Psychopharmacol 1990;10:152–153.
2. Montgomery, SA. Venlafaxine: A new dimension in antidepressant pharmacotherapy. J Clin Psychiatry 1993;54:119–126.
3. New antidepressant approved. FDA Consumer 1994; 28:2.
4. Venlafaxine: A new antidepressant. Med Lett Drugs Ther 1994;36(929):49–51.
5. Albano DL. Personal communication. Wyeth–Ayerst Laboratories, May 12, 1994.
6. Saletu B, Grunberger J, Anderer P, et al. Pharmacodynamics of venlafaxine evaluated by EEG grain mapping, psychometry and psychophysiology. Br J Clin Pharmacol 1992;33: 589–601.
7. Klamerus KJ, Maloney K, Rudolph RL, et al. Introduction of a composite parameter to the pharmacokinetics of venlafaxine and its active *o*-desmethyl metabolite. J Clin Pharmacol 1992;32:714–724.
8. Product Information: Effexon. Wyeth–Ayerst Laboratories, 1994.
9. Product Information: Effexon. Wyeth–Ayerst Laboratories, December 19, 1993.
10. Fantasky A, Burkhart KK. A case report of venlafaxin toxicity. Clin Toxicol 1995;33:359–361.
11. Tzallas PJ, Rynn KO. Extrapyramidal side effects secondary to venlafaxine. Clin Toxicol 1995;33:475–489.
12. Venlafaxine: A new dimension in antidepressant pharmacotherapy. J Clin Psychiatry 1993;54:119–121.

Chapter 39

Monoamine Oxidase Inhibitors

INTRODUCTION

New Medications

Monoamine oxidase (MAO) inhibitors currently in clinical use are listed in Table 39–1.[1,2] Deprenyl (selegiline), a derivative of methamphetamine, is a selective MAO-B inhibitor. Its dopaminergic effect confers efficacy in Parkinson's disease (see Selegiline). Clorgyline is a selective MAO-A inhibitor, which, at high doses, induces orthostatic hypotension. It is also subject to the MAO inhibitor tyramine and sympathomimetic restrictions. The drug is at present not being commercially pursued. The manufacturer discontinued the manufacture of isocarboxazid (Marplan) in December 1993. The drug continues to be available on special request.[3] Foods (Table 39–2) and drugs (Table 39–3) may interact with MAO inhibitors and lead to life-threatening hypertension, subarachnoid hemorrhage, and death.

Second-Generation Monoamine Oxidase Inhibitors

Monoamine oxidase (Table 39–1) exists in two catalytically discrete forms: MAO-A (substrates: 5-hydroxytryptamine and norepinephrine) and MAO-B (substrates: phenylethylamine and benzylamine). Tyramine and dopamine are good substrates for both forms. MAO-A predominates in the intestines and MAO-B in the platelets. The brain has a predominance of MAO-B.[1,2] The differential diagnosis of a MAO inhibitor overdose must include any condition that can produce a hyperadrenergic state (Table 39–4).

Selegiline and Nonselective Monoamine Oxidase Inhibitors

A serious drawback to the use of nonselective irreversible monoamine oxidase inhibitors (MAOIs) such as phenelzine, isoniazid, and tranylcypromine is their potential for interactions that result in increased concentrations of pressor amines and, in some cases, life-threatening hypertension. This response may occur with other prescribed and over-the-counter drugs, including tricyclic antidepressants, sympathomimetic amines (eg, pseudoephedrine and phenylpro-

Table 39–1
Monoamine Oxidase Inhibitors in Clinical Use

Monoamine Oxidase Inhibitor	Amine Oxidase Type Preferentially Inhibited	Preferred Monoamine Substrate	Clinically Effective Dosage Range (mg/d)	Relative Liability to Induce Tyramine "Cheese" Effect
Phenelzine	A and B, irreversible	Tyramine Tryptamine Other monoamines	45–90	Moderate
Tranylcypromine	A and B, irreversible	Tyramine Tryptamine Other monoamines	20–60	High
Isocarboxazid	A and B, irreversible	Tyramine Tryptamine Other monoamines	30–70	Moderate
Deprenyl	B, at low dosage; non-selective at high dosage (>15 mg/d), irreversible	Phenylethylamine Benzylamine Other monoamines	15–30	Low
Moclobemide	A, rapidly reversible	5-Hydroxytryptamine Norepinephrine Other monoamines	300–600	Low

From Cooper AJ, O'Reilly RL. Update on the monoamine oxidase inhibitors (MAOIs). J New Dev Clin Med 1991;9:35–54.

Table 39–2
Foods Interacting With Monoamine Oxidase Inhibitors

Food Containing Tyramine	
Avocados	Particularly if overripe
Bananas	Reactions can occur if eaten in large amounts; tyramine levels high in peel
Bean curd	Fermented bean curd, fermented soya bean, soya bean pastes, soy sauces, and miso soup, prepared from fermented bean curd, all contain tyramine in large amounts; miso soup has caused reactions.
Beer and ale	Major domestic brands do not contain appreciable amounts; some imported brands have had high levels; nonalcoholic beer may contain tyramine and should be avoided
Caviar	Safe if vacuum-packed and eaten fresh or refrigerated only briefly
Cheese	Reactions possible with most, except unfermented varieties such as cottage cheese; in others, tyramine concentration is higher near rind and close to fermentation holes
Figs	Particularly if overripe
Fish	Safe if fresh, dried products should not be eaten; caution required in restaurants; vacuum-packed products are safe if eaten promptly or refrigerated only briefly
Liver	Safe if very fresh, but rapidly accumulates tyramine; caution required in restaurants
Milk products	Milk and yogurt appear to be safe
Protein extracts	See also Soups; avoid liquid and powdered protein dietary supplements
Meat	Safe if known to be fresh; caution required in restaurants
Sausage	Fermented varieties such as bologna, pepperoni, and salami have a high tyramine content
Shrimp paste	Contains large amounts of tyramine
Soups	May contain protein extracts and should be avoided
Soy sauce	Contains large amounts of tyramine; reactions have occurred with teriyaki
Wines	Generally do not contain tyramine, but many reactions have been reported with Chianti, champagne, and other wines
Yeast extracts	Dietary supplements, eg, Marmite, contain large amounts; yeast in baked goods, however, is safe
Food Not Containing Tyramine	
Caffeine	A weak pressor agent; large amounts may cause reactions
Chocolate	Contains phenylethylamine, a pressor agent that can cause reactions in large amounts
Fava beans (broad beans, "Italian" green beans)	Contain dopamine, a pressor amine, particularly when overripe
Ginseng	Some preparations have caused headache, tremulousness, and maniclike symptoms
Liqueurs	Reactions reported with some, eg, Chartreuse and Drambuie; cause unknown
New Zealand prickly spinach	Single case report; patient ate large amounts
Whiskey	Reactions have occurred; cause unknown

From Food interacting with MAO inhibitors. Med Lett Drugs Ther 1989;31(785):11–12.

panolamine, found in decongestant remedies), and meperidine, and with foods rich in tyramine (the cheese reaction). MAO-A preferentially oxidizes noradrenaline and 5-hydroxytryptamine, whereas MAO-B oxidizes phenylethylamine. Tyramine is oxidized by either form of MAO; however, when there are high concentrations of amine substrates, selectivity of metabolism is lost.[4]

The selective MAOI selegiline preferentially inhibits

Table 39–3
Monoamine Oxidase Inhibitor–Drug Interactions

Drug	Interaction
Sympathomimetic agents	MAOIs potentiate the effects of all these agents, but dangerous interactions with CNS stimulation, hypertension, organ damage, or intracranial bleeding are more likely when indirect-acting drugs of this class are used.
CNS depressants	
Meperidine (Demerol)	Dangerous interaction with MAOIs, characterized by hyperpyrexia, seizures, and coma.
Dextromethorphan (in many over-the-counter cough suppressants)	
Other narcotics	MAOIs potentiate the effects of all of these agents, leading to CNS depression and, at times, intoxication.
Other CNS depressants	
Anesthetics	
Alcohol	
Antihistamines,	
Barbiturates	
Nonbarbiturate sedatives	
Benzodiazepines (e.g., diazepam)	
Neuroleptics (e.g., haloperidol)	
Anticonvulsants (e.g., phenytoin)	
Antihypertensive agents	
Reserpine (Serpasil)	Combination of these agents with MAOIs can lead to paradoxical hypertension and CNS excitation.
α-Methyldopa (Aldomet)	
Guanethedine (Esimil and Ismelin)	
Clonidine (Catapres)	MAOIs may potentiate its effects.
Hydralazine (Apresoline)	MAOIs potentiate its effects.
Diuretics (eg, hydrochlorothiazide)	Combination with an MAOI can lead to hypotension.
Sympathetic receptor blocking agents	
Alpha antagonists (eg, phentolamine)	MAOIs may potentiate the effects of these agents.
Beta blockers (eg, propranolol)	MAOI effects on these agents are unpredictable. Frequently, effects are inhibited early and potentiated later.
Antiarrhythmic agents	
Bretylium (Bretylol)	Additive adrenergic effects.
Anticholinergic and antiparkinsonian agents	
Atropine, scopolamine (eg, Donnatal)	MAOIs potentiate these agents and can lead to atropine intoxication syndrome. These agents may also decrease the metabolism of MAOIs.
L-dopa (Dopar, Larodopa)	MAOIs potentiate its effects and can lead to unpredictable changes in blood pressure and may induce CNS excitation or intoxication.
Antibiotics	
Nitrofurans (Macrodantin)	These antimicrobial agents have MAO inhibitory activity and can cause additive toxicity with increased or decreased blood pressure, CNS excitation, and hyperpyrexia when given to MAOI-treated patients.
Sulfisoxazole (Gantrisin)	Combination with phenelzine has led to ataxia, vertigo, tinnitus, muscle pains, and parethesias.
Neuromuscular blocking agents	
Succinylcholine (Anectine)	Phenelzine may reduce cholinesterase leading to prolonged apnea.
Atracurium (Tracrium)	May cause severe hypertension when combined with tranylcypromine.
Anticoagulants	
Coumarins (eg, warfarin)	MAOIs may potentiate their effects.
Antidiabetics	
Insulin, oral hypoglycemics (eg, chlorpropamide)	MAOIs may potentiate effects leading to hypoglycemia.
Chemotherapeutic agents	
Procarbazine (Matulane)	This drug has MAO inhibitory activity and can cause additive toxicity with increased or decreased blood pressure, CNS excitation, and hyperpyrexia when given to MAOI-treated patients.
Other psychopharmacologic agents	
Tricyclic antidepressants* (eg, imipramine)	Combination of MAO inhibitory effects can lead to additive toxicity with hypertension, hypotension, CNS excitation, and hyperpyrexia.
Carbamazepine (Tegretol)	
Fluoxetine (Prozac)	Additive toxicity from serotonergic excess.
Neuroleptics (eg, haloperidol)	Increased anticholinergic side effects and extrapyramidal side effects.

MAOI, monoamine oxidase inhibitor; CNS, central nervous system.
*There are reports of safe use of tricyclic antidepressant (TCA)–MAOI combinations in treating refractory depression. TCA and MAOI must be started simultaneously or the MAOI must be added to the TCA.
From Lipson RE, Stern TA. Management of monoamine oxidase inhibitor-treated patients in the emergency and critical care setting. J Intens Care Med 1991;6:117–125.

MAO-B and is thought to be less likely to provoke hypertensive crises with amine-rich foods or when coprescribed with other catecholamine-enhancing drugs in doses up to 10 mg per day.[4]

Selective Monoamine Oxidase Inhibitors

The newer selective MAOIs may be implicated in the production of life-threatening paroxysmal hypertension induced by noradrenaline; this condition is known as

Table 39–4
Differential Diagnosis of Monoamine Oxidase Inhibitor Overdose

Intoxications	Withdrawal States	Infectious Diseases
Cocaine	Sedative–hypnotic	Meningitis
Phencyclidine	α_2-Agonists	Encephalitis
Amphetamines	Alcohol	Tetanus
Methylphenidate	Beta blockers	Rabies
α_2-Agonists	**Psychiatric Disorder**	Sepsis
Theophylline	Lethal catatonia	**Adverse Drug Reactions**
Phenylpropanolamine	**Medical Conditions**	Neuroleptic malignant syndrome
Strychnine	Hypoglycemia	Malignant hyperthermia
Salicylates	Pheochromocytoma	Dystonic reaction
Nicotine	Hyperthyroidism	
Anticholinergic agents	Heat stroke	

From Mills KC. Monoamine oxidase inhibitor toxicity. Top Emerg Med 1993;15(3):58–71.

pseudopheochromocytoma. Noradrenaline concentrations rose significantly after treatment with selegiline and toloxatone given in conjunction with other medications known to affect the metabolically linked catecholamine and indoleamine systems, for example, terbutaline, phenylephrine, fluoxetine, and tricyclic antidepressants.[4]

Use of Opioids in Patients Taking Monoamine Oxidase Inhibitors

The following are guidelines for using opioids in patients on MAOIs[5]:

1. Avoid meperidine or dextromethorphan in patients.
2. Use morphine or fentanyl if patient requires opioids.
3. A sensitivity test is suggested in morphine recipients.
4. Encourage discontinuation of MAOIs at least 2 weeks before receiving opioid analgesics.
5. Suggest that patients wear medical alert bracelets.

Clinical Presentation

Classical MAOIs may be associated with lethal toxicity in overdose. After a "latent" period of some hours, patients may progressively develop motor uneasiness, agitation, violent motor activity with moaning and grimacing, profuse sweating, and hallucinations. Death may result from hyperthermia, which may peak as late as 24 hours postpresentation. Patients should be closely monitored for 24 hours with strict control over dietary and drug intake. Davis et al. suggest that deaths have most commonly followed interaction of therapeutic MAOIs with dietary agents, tricyclic antidepressants, or sympathomimetic amines.[6,7]

The Serotonin Syndrome

The serotonin syndrome involves use of selective MAOIs with serotonin receptor drugs (see Chapter 49). Patients can develop central nervous system irritability, hyperreflexia, and myoclonus. The blood pressure may be normal. Fatalities have been reported.[8]

Monoamine Oxidase Inhibitor Abuse

Phenelzine and tranylcypromine have been abused by patients who often have a past history of prior substance abuse or a severe character disorder. The medications were used in excessive amounts, exceeding the therapeutic ranges and safety limits, often with disregard for potential or actual harmful results. Evidence of excessive dosage (irritability, anger, teeth grinding) is often present with little evidence of tolerance to these side effects. Withdrawal symptoms may include anxiety, depression, confusion, hallucinations, tremulousness, nausea, vomiting, diarrhea, and chills.[9] Tapering of doses, rather than abrupt discontinuation, appears to reduce the likelihood of withdrawal symptoms.

Laboratory

Blood Levels

Plasma MAOI levels are not well characterized in either therapeutic or excessive doses. Plasma tranylcypromine levels peak at about 25 ng/mL 2 hours after ingestion of a 20-mg oral dose. Postmortem blood tranylcypromine levels in fatal overdose cases were 0.25 mg/L (850-mg overdose) and 3.7 mg/L (300-mg overdose). Plasma MAOI levels can confirm ingestion but neither guide clinical management nor predict clinical outcome. Drug screens typically do not detect MAOIs.

Abnormalities

Adverse laboratory changes reported in the setting of MAOI overdose include a consumptive coagulopathy, thrombocytopenia, decreased fibrinogen, elevated fibrin split products, depressed prothrombin and partial thromboplastin times, hemolysis, leukocytosis, elevated serum muscle enzymes (creatine phosphokinase, aldolase), and acute renal failure. Peaked T waves in the absence of hyperkalemia appeared on the electrocardiogram of a patient who overdosed on tranylcypromine. Sinus bradycardia also developed during the first 4 to 8 hours postingestion and resolved by 24 hours.

Ancillary Tests

Patients who develop moderate to severe toxicity after a MAOI overdose should receive a complete blood count, serum electrolytes, serum creatinine, urinalysis, serum muscle enzymes, an electrocardiogram, and a coagulation profile (prothrombin time, partial thromboplastin time, fibrinogen, fibrin split products).

Treatment

Stabilization

Monoamine oxidase inhibitor overdoses or the concurrent ingestion of certain foods or medications with a MAOI may cause a life-threatening emergency resulting from severe cardiovascular or central nervous system reactions. Patients who exhibit vital sign abnormalities should receive an intravenous line, cardiac monitor, oxygen, and assisted ventilation as needed. Initial attention should be directed toward assessment of the adequacy of ventilation and blood pressure and correction of abnormalities.

Hypertension. Patients may present with seriously elevated blood pressure. The decision to lower blood pressure is a clinical judgment based on underlying cardiovascular disease, the extent of the increase in blood pressure, and evidence of end-organ failure (myocardial ischemia, intracranial hemorrhage, decreased visual acuity, congestive heart failure, renal failure). Sodium nitroprusside and intravenous phentolamine are the drugs of choice for severe hypertension in this setting. Practolol successfully reversed the vital sign abnormalities after a tranylcypromine overdose, but the use of propranolol and its effect on blood pressure (ie, unopposed alpha-adrenergic action as a result of beta-adrenergic blockade) have not been well studied.

Hypotension. A direct-acting alpha-adrenergic agonist (eg, norepinephrine, high-dose dopamine) is preferable to an indirect-acting agent (eg, low-dose dopamine) for the treatment of hypotension unresponsive to fluids. In the presence of shock, hemodynamic monitoring (pulmonary artery catheter, intraarterial line) may be necessary to maximize right ventricular filling, cardiac output, and peripheral vascular resistance.

Ventricular Tachyarrhythmias. Lidocaine, phenytoin, and procainamide are the safest antiarrhythmic agents in this setting. Bretylium may enhance the clinical effects of MAOIs and probably should not be administered in this setting.

Gut Decontamination

Monoamine oxidase inhibitor doses that exceed 1 mg/kg are potentially dangerous. Patients who ingest these amounts should receive gut decontamination (emesis/lavage, activated charcoal, cathartics) if they present within 4 hours postexposure. Either no symptoms or minimal symptoms would be expected in patients within the first 4 hours because of the delayed onset of MAOI actions.

Antidote

There is no specific antidote to MAOI poisoning. Phenothiazine compounds have reversed the agitation and muscle rigidity associated with MAOI overdose; however, the use of intramuscular chlorpromazine in tranylcypromine overdose was temporally associated with cardiac arrest.

Elimination Enhancement

Urinary acidification can enhance the renal elimination of tranylcypromine, but renal excretion probably accounts for only a small amount of the total drug elimination. The use of hemodialysis was temporally associated with clinical improvement in a tranylcypromine overdose case, but toxicokinetic data were not available to judge the effect of dialysis in clearance.

Supportive Measures

Hyperthermia. Moderately elevated body temperatures may be treated with acetaminophen and external cooling. A malignant hyperthermia-type condition (tachycardia, tachypnea, metabolic acidosis, hypercapnia, temperatures exceeding 40°C, and muscle rigidity) may develop in MAOI overdose patients. Intravenous dantrolene successfully reversed the malignant hyperthermia syndrome in a phenelzine overdose case. The intravenous dose administered was 2.5 mg/kg, which was repeated every 6 hours for 24 hours. Bromocriptine is an alternative drug used in cases of malignant hyperthermia.

Muscle Rigidity. Diazepam is the initial drug of choice to control muscle rigidity; phenytoin is an alternative. Neuromuscular paralysis with pancuronium may be necessary when excessive muscle tone contributes to respiratory failure or hyperthermia. The use of succinylcholine should be avoided because of its association with malignant hyperthermia.

Observation. All patients suspected of ingesting toxic doses of MAOIs should be observed in a monitored setting for 24 hours because of the potential for delayed onset of reactions. Vital signs and cardiac rhythm should be monitored regularly.

Drug Interactions. Patients should be placed on special diets low in tyramine-containing foods. Sympathomimetic drugs and sedative–hypnotic drugs should be avoided because of potentiation of MAOI overdose effects and central nervous system depression, respectively. Meperidine may produce paradoxical central nervous system excitation when administered with MAOIs. Precautions for food and drug interactions should remain in effect for 1 to 2 weeks postexposure.

REFERENCES—INTRODUCTION

1. Cooper AJ, O'Reilly RL. Update on the monoamine oxidase inhibitors (MAOI's). J New Dev Clin Med 1991;9:35–54.
2. Rudorfer MV. Monoamine oxidase inhibitors: Reversible and irreversible. Psychopharmacol Bull 1992;28:45–57.
3. Medd BH. Discontinuation of manufacture of isocarboxazid.
4. Livingston MG. Interactions with selective MAOIs. Lancet 1995;345:533–534.
5. Rossiter A, Souney PF. Interaction between MAOIs and opioids: Pharmacologic and clinical considerations. Hosp Formul 1993;28:692–698.
6. Davis JM, Bartlett E, Termini BA. Overdosage of psychotropic drugs: A review. Part II: Antidepressants and other psychotropic agents. Dis Nerv Syst 1968;29:246–256.
7. Power BM, Hackett LP, Dusci LJ, Ilett KF. Antidepressant toxicity and the need for identification and concentration monitoring in overdose. Clin Pharmacokinet 1995;29:154–171.
8. Livingston MG. Interactions and selective MAOIs. Lancet 1995;345:533–534.
9. Baumbacher G, Hansen MS. Abuse of monoamine oxidase inhibitors. Am J Drug Alcohol Abuse 1992;18:399–406.

ETRYPTAMINE

α-Etryptamine (formerly marketed as Monase) is a nonhydrazine reversible MAOI used as an antidepressant.[1-3] It was withdrawn from the market in 1962 because of agranulocytosis. The drug is rapidly absorbed with a half-life of about 8 hours, is widely distributed (1 L/kg), and is excreted by the

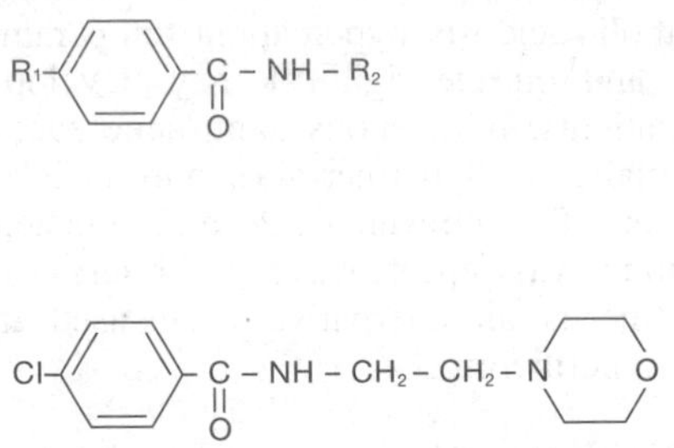

R_1–C₆H₄–C(=O)–NH–R_2

Cl–C₆H₄–C(=O)–NH–CH_2–CH_2–N(morpholine)O

Moclobemide

Figure 39-1 Structures of the benzamide nucleus and the benzamide derivative moclobemide. (From Fitton A, Faulds D, Goa KL. Moclobemide: A review of the pharmacological properties and therapeutic use in depressive illness. Drugs 1992;43:561–596.)

kidneys.[3] Metabolites are not active. A dose of 700 mg was fatal. A fatality was reported in Arizona in 1993.[1] The drug can be detected in the urine by gas–liquid chromatography, gas chromatography–mass spectrometry, high-performance liquid chromatography, and thin-layer chromatography. Malignant hyperthermia has been noted. α-Etryptamine may induce serotonin neurotoxicity similar to 3,4-methylenedioxymethamphetamine (MDMA) and *p*-chloroamphetamine (PSA).[2]

REFERENCES—ETRYPTAMINE

1. Morano RA, Spies C, Walker FB, Plant SM. Fatal intoxication involving etryptamine. J Forens Sci 1993;38:721–725.
2. Huang X, Johnson MP, Nicholes DE. Reduction in brain serotonin markers by alpha-ethyltryptamine (Monase). Eur J Pharmacol 1991;200:187–190.
3. Daldrup T, Heller C, Matthiesen V, et al. Etryptamine: Eine neue Designes-DRoge mit fataler Wirkung. Z Rechtsmed 1986;97:61–68.

MOCLOBEMIDE

Moclobemide is *p*-chloro-*N*-(2-morpholinoethyl)benzamide. The chemical formula is $C_{13}H_{17}ClN_2O_2$, and the molecular weight, 268.7 (CAS 73120-77-9). It is a reversible, selective inhibitor of MAO-A,[1,2] which constitutes about 70% of the MAO activity in the brain.[3] It appears to have about the same efficacy in depression as the tricyclic antidepressants and has found use in endogenous depression,[4] bipolar depression, agitated depression, melancholia (*Diagnostic and Statistical Manual of American Psychiatric Association,* third edition, revised), and psychotic depression. Its relative lack of sedative properties may make it suitable for the treatment of elderly depressed patients.[5] It is used in doses 100 to 400 mg daily and sold in Europe under the name Auroxix[6,7] (Fig. 39–1).

Toxicokinetics

Absorption

Moclobemide is readily absorbed (>95%) through the gastrointestinal tract.[8,9] Within 1 to 2 hours of oral use, a peak plasma level of about 1 μg/mL is reached.[5] It is protein bound to the extent of 50%.

Distribution

The volume of distribution at steady state is 0.8 to 1.25 L/kg.[10]

Elimination

The elimination half-life is 1 to 2 hours. Moclobemide appears to be eliminated (after first-pass hepatic metabolism) by first-order kinetics, resulting in urinary excretion of the monoamine metabolites homovanillic acid (HVA), dihydroxyphenylacetic acid (DOPAC), 3-methoxy-4-hydroxyphenyl glycol (DOPEG), and 5-hydroxyindoleacetic acid (5-HIAA).[9,10] Approximately 1% of a maternal dose appears in breast milk on a milligram/kilogram basis.[9] Less than 0.5% appears in the urine in unchanged form. The drug has a relatively high systemic clearance (700–1200 mL/mg).[10] A high-performance liquid chromatography method with ultraviolet detection has been described.[8] The sensitivity of the method is 0.07 μg/mL.

Drug Interactions

Dingemanse has described the following interactions with moclobemide[11]:

Serotonin Reuptake Inhibitors. When moclobemide is combined with fluvoxamine, more patients report headache, fatigue, nausea, and dizziness than those who receive fluvoxamine and placebo. The combination of moclobemide and fluoxetine is associated with fewer cases of fatigue, headache, nausea, and restlessness compared with fluoxetine monotherapy. Fatal cases of serotonin syndrome have been reported after moclobemide–citalopram and moclobemide–clomipramine overdoses.[12] Many antidepressants obviously carry a risk of a serious interaction if combined with MAOIs such as citalopram, fluoxetine, fluvoxamine, and sertraline and inhibitors of serotonin reuptake such as clomipramine, trazodone, imipramine, meperidine, and dextromethorphan. Death may follow a few hours after ingestion. Ingestion of other MAOIs (eg, isocarboxazid) with sertraline has led to serotonin syndrome.[13]

Antiparkinsonian Agents. When levodopa–bensierazide (1:4) (Madopar) is combined with moclobemide or selegiline, tolerability is poor, necessitating a reduction in the dose of Madopar. The most frequently occurring adverse events are nausea, vomiting, and dizziness, with the intensity of the events being more severe during treatment with the selegiline combination. The adverse events resolve completely over a short time. Concomitant moclobemide and selegiline result in supraadditive tyramine potentiation, necessitating dietary tyramine restrictions in practice.

Ephedrine. When ephedrine is administered alone, there is an overt increase in blood pressure; this is more pronounced when ephedrine is added to moclobemide at steady-state concentrations. The moclobemide/ephedrine combination is associated with an increase in the number of adverse events reported including palpitations, headache, and lightheadedness.

Clinical Presentation

Side Effects

Somnolence, sweating, headache, a moderate rise in systolic blood pressure, and a rise in body temperature to 38°C have been observed within 10 to 12 hours of drug administration. Symptoms vanish within 24 hours.[5]

Overdose

The manufacturer states that as of 1992, more than 3900 patients with various forms of depression had been treated with moclobemide.[7,14–17] Of this group, 18 patients attempted suicide by overdose, with or without other drugs. The highest overdose was more than 20 g. Benzodiazepines, tricyclic antidepressants, alcohol, chloral hydrate, haloperidol, acetaminophen, paracetamol, lithium, and barbiturates were some of the drugs taken concomitantly. Hypotension, fever (38.5°C), disorientation, drowsiness, nausea, and reduced reflexes followed a 950-mg dose in one patient. The patient recovered in 7 days.[15] In another patient the blood pressure returned to normal without treatment in 24 hours.[1] The most common signs of drug intoxication ranged from deep sedation to coma in one patient who also ingested benzodiazepines. At a dose of more than 600 mg, a blood pressure of 150/100 mm Hg was observed with a pulse of 88/min.

Patients ingesting up to 2000 mg of moclobemide have shown only mild gastrointestinal symptoms or no symptoms at all. At 3000 to 4000 mg, depressed consciousness and a slight increase in blood pressure have been observed. At 7000 to 8000 mg, patients show fatigue, agitation, tachycardia, increased blood pressure, and dilated slow-reacting pupils. Both central nervous system depression and excitation (seizures) have been observed. Tremor, mydriasis, hyperthermia, hypertension, and acidosis may be seen. There may be an additive effect with tricyclic antidepressants. In massive overdoses (>2000–6000 mg), seizures, hyperthermia, muscle rigidity, and pain, together with rhabdomyolysis, resemble classical MAOI intoxication as well as the unusual neuroleptic malignant syndrome.[18] There have been no reports of death when moclobemide was taken as the sole drug in overdose.[19] Deaths occur when tricyclic antidepressants and/or alcohol are taken in overdose together with moclobemide.[19]

Laboratory

An increase in white blood cells were observed at a dose of 950 mg.[2] This returned to normal in 3 days. Electrocardiographic findings of broad T waves and a slightly prolonged ST interval were observed after ingestion of 1500 mg, although the electrocardiogram and electroencephalogram were normal in one patient who had ingested 1550 mg. The patient recovered in 7 hours.[14] There may be an increase in serum creatine kinase, a transient myoglobinuria, increased transaminase levels, a slight leukocytosis, and a slight decrease in the platelet count.

Treatment

With symptomatic and supportive treatment in a hospital, moclobemide overdose patients who were treated with gastric lavage, activated charcoal, and intravenous fluids appeared to recover usually within 24 hours and, in two cases, within 5 and 7 days.[1] Seizures may require diazepam, thiopental, and mechanical ventilation. Dantrolene may be useful for hyperthermia. Blood pressure must be monitored in all moclobemide overdose patients.[20]

REFERENCES—MOCLOBEMIDE

1. Hetzel W. Safety of moclobemide taken in overdose for attempted suicide. Psychopharmacology 1992;106:S127–S129.
2. Guelfi JD, Payan C, Fermanian J, et al. Moclobemide versus clomipramine in endogenous depression: A double-blind randomised clinical trial. Br J Psychiatry 1992;160:519–524.
3. Freeman H. Moclobemide. Lancet 1993;342:1528–1532.
4. Angst J, Stabl M. Efficacy of moclobemide in different patient groups: A meta-analysis of studies. Psychopharmacology 1992;106:S109–S113.
5. Wiesel F-A, Raaflaub J, Kettler R. Pharmacokinetics of oral moclobemide in healthy human subjects and effects on MAO-activity in platelets and excretion of urine monoamine metabolites. Am J Clin Pharmacol 1985;28:89–95.
6. Reynolds JEF, ed. *Martindale: The Extra Pharmacopoeia.* 29th ed. London: Pharmaceutical Press, 1989:374.
7. Fitton A, Faulds D, Goa KL. Moclobemide: A review of the pharmacological properties and therapeutic use in depressive illness. Drugs 1992;43:561–596.
8. Raaflaub J, Haefelfinger P, Trautmann KH. Single dose pharmacokinetics of the MAO-inhibitor moclobemide in man. Arzneimittelforschung 1984;34:80–82.
9. Pons G, Schoerlin MP, Tam YK, et al. Moclobemide excretion in human milk. Br J Clin Pharmacol 1990;29:27–31.
10. Schoerlin M-P, Mayersohn M, Korn A, Eggers H. Disposition kinetics of moclobemide, a monoamine oxidase-A enzyme inhibitor: Single and multiple dosing in normal subjects. Clin Pharmacol Ther 1987;42:395–404.
11. Dingemanse J. An update of recent moclobemide interaction data. Clin Psychopharmacol 1993;7:167–180.
12. Neuvonen PJ, Pohjola-Sintonen S, Tacke V, Vuori E. Five fatal cases of serotonin syndrome after moclobemide–citalopram or moclobemide–clomipramine overdoses. Lancet 1993;342:1410.
13. Brannan SK, Talley BJ, Bouden CL. Sertraline and isocarboxazide cause a serotonin syndrome. J Clin Psychopharmacol 1994;14:144–145.
14. Vine R, Norman TR, Burrows GD. A case of moclobemide overdose. Int Clin Psychopharmacol 1988;3:325–326.
15. Heinze G, Sanchez A. Overdose with moclobemide. J Clin Psychiatry 1986;47:438.
16. Beaumond G, Hetzel W. Patients at risk of suicide and overdose. Psychopharmacology 1992;106:S123–S126.
17. Myvenfors PG, Eriksson T, Sandstedt LS, Sjoberg G. Moclobemide overdose. J Intern Med 1993;233:113–115.
18. Hackett LP, Joyce DA, Hall RW, et al. Disposition and clinical effects of moclobemide and three of its metabolites following overdose. Drug Invest 1993;5:281–284.
19. Chen DT, Ruch R. Safety of moclobemide in clinical use. Clin Neuropharmacology 1993;16(suppl. 2):S63–S68.
20. Coulter DM, Pillans PI. Hypertension with moclobemide. Lancet 1995;346:1032.

SELEGILINE

Selegiline is an antiparkinsonian drug that may delay the appearance of the disease.[1–6] It has also shown some antidepressant action and may improve cognitive function in Parkinson's disease.[7]

In the United States, interest in selegiline increased after discovery of its ability to antagonize the effects of 1-methyl-4-phenyl-1,2,3,6-tetrahydropyridine (MPTP), a "designer

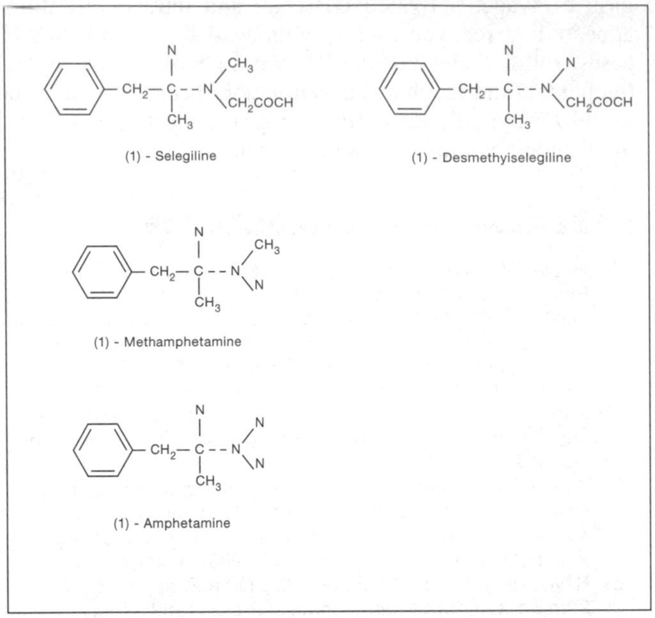

(1) - Selegiline

(1) - Desmethyiselegiline

(1) - Methamphetamine

(1) - Amphetamine

Figure 39-2 Metabolic pathway of selegiline. (From Meeker JE, Reynolds PC. Postmortem tissue methamphetamine concentrations following selegiline administration. J Anal Toxicol 1990;14:330–331.)

drug" that causes the symptoms of Parkinson's disease.[8] MAO-B converts MPTP to MPP^+ (1-methyl-4-phenylpyridium ion), a toxic metabolite. This step can be eliminated with the use of MAOIs, suggesting that dopamine levels in the brain can be increased with selegiline.

Selegiline (Eldepryl) may be mistaken for trifluoperazine (Stelazine), with resultant worsening of parkinsonian symptoms.[9] Selegiline has no pressor effects when administered in doses of 10 mg/d,[2] although 20 mg/d in one patient led to headache and hypertension after a meal high in tyramine.[10] Selegiline is metabolized to methamphetamine and amphetamine and, in overdose, may exhibit clinical effects related to these substances[11] (Fig. 39–2).

Structure and Classification

Selegiline is chemically *R*-(–)-*N*,α-dimethyl-*N*-2--propynylphenethylamine hydrochloride or *N*,α-dimethyl-*N*-2-propynbenzeneethanamine. It is commonly referred to as deprenyl.[11–15] Its empirical formula is $C_{13}H_{12}N_1HCl$ and its molecular weight is 223.7. The CAS numbers are 14611-51-9 (selegiline) and 14611-52-0 (hydrochloride).[14] Selegiline is marketed in the United States and the United Kingdom as Eldepryl.

Use

Selegiline is used as an adjunct in the management of parkinsonian patients being treated with levodopa–carbidopa who exhibit deterioration in the quality of their response to this therapy.[16]

Product Formulation

Selegiline is commercially available as 5-mg tablets.

Source

Selegiline is a synthetic chemical.

Therapeutic Dose

Selegiline is administered to those parkinsoniam patients who are receiving levodopa–carbidopa therapy in a dose of 5 mg twice daily. After 2 or 3 days of selegiline treatment, an attempt may be made to reduce the dose of levodopa–carbidopa.

Toxic Dose

Exposure to doses of 600 mg may result in severe hypotension and psychomotor agitation.

Fatal Dose

A 72-year-old woman was found dead after apparently consuming twelve 5-mg tablets of selegiline together with some antidepressants.[11]

Toxicokinetics

Absorption

Selegiline is readily absorbed following oral administration (half-life of absorption, 0.3 hour). A single oral dose of 10 mg produced mean peak concentrations of 0.04 and 0.03 μg/mL of methamphetamine and amphetamine, respectively.[17] The maximum time to reach the peak methamphetamine concentration is 3.1 hours. Amphetamine peaks at 4.6 hours.[11]

Distribution

Selegiline is highly bound to plasma protein and has a high volume of distribution at steady state, 4.7 L/kg.[15]

Elimination

Selegiline hydrochloride is extensively metabolized to form methamphetamine (half-life, 20.5 hours) and amphetamine and *N*-desmethylselegiline (half-life, 2 hours) (Fig. 39–2). The metabolites are excreted by the kidneys. Little or no selegiline is found in the urine.[8,11] The half-life of the drug and its metabolites is 39 hours. Plasma clearance is 1.7 mL/mg/kg.

Drug Interactions

Ingestion of selegiline with fluoxetine by an adult led to mania, diaphoresis, and hypertension.[18] Combination of selegiline with meperidine resulted in increased restlessness and irritability, progressing to delirium, with muscular rigidity, sweating, and a raised temperature (maximum, 38°C). The patient remained normotensive.[19] Combinations of selegiline with tricyclic antidepressants or serotonin reuptake inhibitors may be associated with fever, tremors, agitation, restlessness, reduced levels of consciousness, and, rarely, fatalities.[20]

Pregnancy/Lactation

Studies of selegiline during pregnancy or lactation have not been performed. It is not known whether selegiline is excreted in breast milk or is subject to placental transfer.

Mechanism of Action

Selegiline is a MAOI with selective action against the B form of the enzyme. Its administration prevents the degradation of dopamine in the human brain, where this is a substrate for MAO-B. It leaves those peripheral mechanisms intact that normally prevent a hypertensive response following tyramine administration.[21] In addition to its antiparkinsonian activity, selegiline has been shown to have antidepressant potential.[22] In humans, MAO in the gastrointestinal tract is predominantly type A (MAO-A), whereas most of the MAO in the brain is type B (MAO-B).[8] The beneficial action of MAO-B inhibitors appears to result from the preservation of endogenous norepinephrine, serotonin, and dopamine in the brain. Selegiline is not associated with the tyramine reaction that has limited other nonselective MAOIs in the treatment of Parkinson's disease.[23]

Clinical Presentation

Overdoses are likely to cause significant inhibition of both MAO-A and MAO-B. Signs and symptoms of overdose may resemble those observed with nonselective MAOIs, for example, tranylcypromine (Parnate), isocarboxazid (Marplan), and phenelzine (Nardil).[16] Death has been reported following overdose.[11]

Therapeutic use may lead to increased tremor, bradykinesia, falling, dystonic symptoms, dyskinesias, hallucinations, confusion, sleep disturbance, headache, dry mouth, blurred vision, orthostatic hypotension, hypertension, poor appetite, urinary retention, and diaphoresis. Hypomanic behavior may be due to the L-amphetamine and L-amphetamine metabolites of selegiline.[24]

Signs and symptoms of overdose may include drowsiness, dizziness, faintness, irritability, hyperactivity, agitation, severe headache, hallucinations, trismus, opisthotonus, seizures and coma, rapid and irregular pulse, hypertension, hypotension and vascular collapse, precordial pain, respiratory depression and failure, hyperpyrexia, diaphoresis, and cold, clammy skin.[6]

Laboratory
Analytical Methods

Methamphetamine may be assayed in the urine by immunoassay and gas–liquid chromatography.[11]

Blood Levels

Following the ingestion of about 60 mg of selegiline, the postmortem blood concentration of methamphetamine was 0.17 to 0.28 μg/mL; the blood amphetamine level was 0.07 μg/mL.[11]

Treatment

Patients who have ingested an overdose of selegiline should be immediately admitted to a hospital, where blood pressure, body temperature, and fluid and electrolyte balance may be closely monitored. Induction of emesis or gastric lavage with instillation of a charcoal slurry under airway protection may be useful in early poisoning. Signs and symptoms of central nervous system stimulation, including seizures, should be treated with intravenous diazepam. Phenothiazine derivatives and central nervous system stimulants should be avoided. Hypotension and vascular collapse should be treated with intravenous fluids and, if necessary, a pressor agent. Adrenergic agents may induce a markedly increased pressor response. Respiration should be supported by airway management, use of supplemental oxygen, and mechanical ventilatory assistance as required. It is unlikely that extracorporeal methods to enhance elimination (hemodialysis, hemoperfusion) will be effective (high protein binding, extensive volume of distribution). Treatment is largely symptomatic and supportive. There is no antidote.

REFERENCES—SELEGILINE

1. Raub W. Selegiline delays progression of early Parkinson's. JAMA 1990;213:21.
2. Parkinson Study Group. Effect of deprenyl on the progression of disability in early Parkinson's disease. N Engl J Med 1989;321:1364–1371.
3. Elizan TS, Yahr MD, Moros DA, et al. Selegiline as an adjunct to conventional levodopa therapy in Parkinson's disease: Experience with this type B monoamine oxidase inhibitor in 200 patients. Arch Neurol 1989;46:1208–1283.
4. Rinne JO, Royta M, Paljarri L, et al. Selegiline (Depryl) treatment and death of nigra neurons in Parkinson's disease. Neurology 1991;41:859–861.
5. Wessel K, Szelenyi I. Selegiline: An overview of its role in the treatment of Parkinson's disease. Clin Invest 1992;70:460–462.
6. Golbe LI, Langston JW, Shoulson I. Selegiline and Parkinson's disease: Protective and symptomatic considerations. Drugs 1990;39:646–651.
7. Hietanen MH. Selegiline and cognitive function in Parkinson's disease. Acta Neurol Scand 1991;84:407–410.
8. Calesnick B. Selegiline for Parkinson's disease. Am Fam Physician 1990;41:589–591.
9. Kurth MC, Langston JW, Tetrud JW. "Stelazine" versus "selegiline": A hazard in prescription writing. Arch Intern Med 1990;150:2379–2384.
10. McGrath BJ, Stewart JW, Quitker FM. A possible L-deprenyl induced hypertension reaction. J Psychopharmed 1989;9: 310–311.
11. Meeker JE, Reynolds PC. Postmortem tissue methamphetamine concentrations following selegiline administration. J Anal Toxicol 1990;14:330–331.
12. British National Formulary Number 24. British Medical Association and Royal Pharmaceutical Society of Great Britain, September 1992:195.
13. *Physicians' Desk Reference.* 49th ed. Montvale, NJ: Medical Economics, 1994:2430–2432.
14. Reynolds JEF, ed. *Martindale: The Extra Pharmacopoeia.* 30th ed. London: Pharmaceutical Press, 1993:849–850.
15. Dollery CT, ed. *Therapeutic Drugs.* Edinburgh: Churchill Livingstone, 1991:S7–S11.
16. Waters CH. Selegiline (Eldepryl) for Parkinson's disease. West J Med 1991;155:68–69.
17. Eldepryl Investigators Product Profile. Denville, NJ: Somerset Pharmaceuticals.
18. Suchowersky O, de Vries JD. Interaction of fluoxetine and selegiline. Canad J Psychiatry 1990;35:571–572.
19. Zornberg GL, Bodkin JA, Cohen BM. Severe adverse interactions between pethidine and selegiline. Lancet 1991;337: 246.
20. Blume CD. Inc. Dear Doctor Letter. Denville, NJ: Somerset Pharmaceuticals, November 14, 1994.

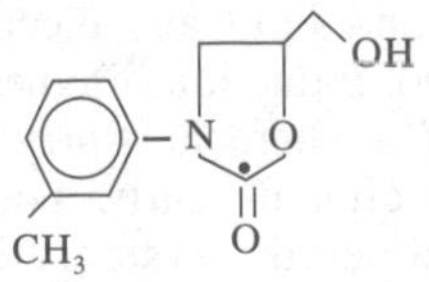

Figure 39-3 Structure of toloxatone. (From Benedetti MS, Rovei V, Dencker SJ, et al. Pharmacokinetics of toloxatone in man following intravenous and oral administrations. Arzneimittelforschung 1982; 32:276–280.)

21. Reynolds GP, Elsworth JD, Blau K, et al. Deprenyl is metabolized to methamphetamine and amphetamine in man. Br J Clin Pharmacol 1978;6:542–544.
22. Mann JJ, Aarons SF, Wilner PJ, et al. A controlled study of the antidepressant efficacy and side effects of (–)-deprenyl: A selective monoamine oxidase inhibitor. Arch Gen Psychiatry 1989;46:45–50.
23. Fuller MA, Tolbert SR. Selegiline: Initial or adjunctive therapy of Parkinson's disease? DICP Ann Pharmacother 1991;25: 36–40.
24. Boyson SJ. Psychiatric effects of selegiline. Arch Neurol 1991;48:902.

TOLOXATONE

Toloxatone is a MAOI antidepressant often ingested in overdose with other antidepressants. Although an overdose may be symptomatically benign, serious cardiac and central nervous system toxicity has been observed. Fatalities may occur. Treatment is supportive and symptomatic.

Structure and Classification

Toloxatone is 5-(hydroxymethyl)-3-(3-methylphenyl)-2-oxazolidinone (Fig. 39–3). The empirical formula is $C_{11}H_{13}NO_3$.[1] It has a molecular weight of 207.2. The CAS number is 29218-27-7. Toloxatone is marketed in Europe as Humoryl and Perenum. Toloxatone is an antidepressant which reversibly inhibits Type A monoamine oxidase.

Use

Toloxatone is used in Europe as an antidepressant. It has not been approved in the United States.

Product Formulation

Toloxatone is available in gelules of 200 mg each for oral use.[2]

Source

Toloxatone is a synthetic chemical product.

Therapeutic Dose

Toloxatone is administered in doses of 200 mg. Effective daily doses have varied from 600 to 1400 mg.[3]

Toxic Dose

The normal toxic dose is 2 g.[2,4]

Fatal Dose

One patient ingested 6 g of toloxatone together with clomipramine and lorazepam. The patient became comatose, developed bilateral mydriasis and hyperthermia, and died in asystole.[2]

Toxicokinetics

Absorption

Toloxatone is rapidly absorbed from the gastrointestinal tract. The absorption half-life is 0.12 to 0.33 hour. The bioavailability of the oral form is about 50 to 60% that of an intravenous infusion. Peak plasma concentrations of 384 to 640 ng/mL are observed 0.5 to 1.0 hours after a single 1 mg/kg dose is ingested. There are few data to confirm a correlation between plasma concentration and clinical efficacy. Protein binding to plasma proteins, almost entirely to albumin, is approximately 50%.

Distribution

Toloxatone has an apparent volume of distribution between about 1 and 1.6 L/kg.

Elimination

Toloxatone is rapidly cleared from the plasma with a beta half-life of 0.96 to 1.81 hours. In acute overdose the toxicokinetic parameters (half-life, 1.5 hours; total body clearance, 653 mL/min) were not significantly different from those reported with the usual therapeutic doses. Toloxatone is extensively metabolized in humans. About 80% of a 200-mg dose is excreted in the urine mainly as metabolic products. The elimination half-life is 0.96 to 1.81 hours.

Pregnancy/Lactation

Few data are available on toloxatone use in pregnant or lactating women.

Drug Interactions

Life-threatening reactions may take place when toloxatone is used with phenylephrine. The "new" MAOIs (eg, toloxatone, selegiline) are not immune to the usual interactions of "old" MAOIs.[5]

Mechanism of Action

Toloxatone is a reversible inhibitor of MAO-A.[3] Significant increases in brain 5-hydroxytryptamine, noradrenaline, and dopamine levels have been observed in animal studies.

Clinical Presentation

Azoyan and colleagues reviewed 122 patients with toloxatone overdose.[2,4] Symptoms following an overdose of toloxatone begin within 1 hour of ingestion. In most cases, drowsiness, sinus tachycardia, and diminished respiration may be observed. In massive overdose, coma, myoclonic jerk, trismus, mydriasis, hyperthermia, and cardiovascular collapse have been seen. Fatalities have followed a toloxatone overdose, especially when other antidepressants have also been ingested.[2,4]

A fatal fulminant hepatitis has followed long-term use of toloxatone in several patients.[6]

Laboratory

Analytical Methods

A modified thin-layer chromatography technique has been described for analysis of toloxatone in plasma. The limit of sensitivity of the technique is 5 ng/mL.[3]

Blood Levels

Plasma concentrations in symptomatic patients after overdose are usually greater than 2 μg/mL.[2] A symptomatic patient following overdose exhibited a peak plasma level of about 1.5 μg/mL. Severe intoxication is associated with plasma levels greater than 20 μg/mL.[2]

Abnormalities

Hypokalemia (2.5–2.5 mEq/L), leukocytosis (11,000–12,000 white blood cells/mm^3), hyperglycemia, and hypoglycemia have been observed in toloxatone overdose. Transaminase levels have been increased in patients developing hepatotoxicity after toloxatone treatment.[6]

Ancillary Tests

In two patients who overdosed on toloxatone, cerebrospinal fluid:blood ratios were 1:2 and 1:3.[2]

Treatment

The usual course of a toloxatone overdose is benign, but cardiovascular collapse and death have occurred. Treatment is largely symptomatic and supportive. Patients should be admitted to an intensive care facility where they will have access to cardiac monitoring, oxygen, and a central line. An airway must be established (endotracheal intubation) and assisted ventilation may be required. Gastric lavage may be useful if performed within 4 hours of ingestion. Activated charcoal may be used but is not supported by clinical studies. The high volume of distribution, high plasma protein binding, and rapid elimination would tend to preclude the usefulness of hemodialysis or hemoperfusion. Hyperthermia may require cooling measures. Transaminase levels should be monitored. Patients should be closely monitored (pulse, respiration, blood pressure, temperature) and not discharged until 24 hours after all symptoms have disappeared and the electrocardiogram has returned to normal. Such precautions are necessary in view of the propensity of these patients to ingest more than one medication, after including other antidepressants. There is no antidote. Blood potassium and blood glucose concentrations should be periodically determined. Discharge should follow normalization of these parameters.

REFERENCES—TOLOXATONE

1. Reynolds JEF, ed. *Martindale: The Extra Pharmacopoeia.* 30th ed. London: Pharmaceutical Press, 1993:271.
2. Azoyan P, Garnier R, Baud FJ, Efthymiou ML. Acute toloxatone intoxication: Report of 122 cases. Therapie 1990; 45:139–144.
3. Benedetti MS, Rovei V, Dencker SJ, et al. Pharmacokinetics of toloxatone in man following intravenous and oral administration. Arzneimittelforschung 1982;32:276–280.
4. Azoyan P, Garnier R, Baud FJ, Efthymiou ML. Toxicokinetics of toloxatone in overdose. In: *Proceedings, XIVth International Congress of the European Association of Poison Centres, Milan, Italy, September 26–29, 1990*:47.
5. Lefebre H, Richard R, Noblet C, Moore N, Wolf L-M. Life-threatening pseudo-phaeochromocytoma after toloxatone, terbutaline and phenylephrine. Lancet 1993;341:555–556.
6. Pateron D, Babany G, Hadengue A, et al. Toloxatone-induced fulminant hepatitis. Gastroenterol Clin Biol 1990;14: 504–506.

Chapter 40
Neuroleptic Drugs

NEUROLEPTIC DRUGS IN GENERAL

Toxicokinetics
Pregnancy/Lactation

Contradictory findings relate both an increase in major congenital anomalies when exposure to phenothiazines occurs during the first trimester[1] and no significant increase in severe congenital anomalies following similar exposure.[2] Toxic effects reported in newborns include restlessness, abnormal movements, hypertonia, and an extrapyramidal syndrome, which may persist for as long as 6 months and which includes tremor, hypertonia, weakness, poor sucking, and sluggish primitive reflexes.[3] It would appear prudent to avoid antipsychotic drugs during the first trimester and to consider their use during subsequent trimesters only in urgent circumstances.[3]

The ratio of concentration of neuroleptic drugs in breast milk to that in serum is about 1.[4,5]

Drug Interactions

Coingestion of an overdose of neuroleptic drugs and tricyclic antidepressants (TCAs) may result in an increase in the plasma TCA level, with intraventricular conduction delays, first-degree atrioventricular block, and ventricular arrhythmias. There is a higher prevalence of prolongation of the QRS duration and a threefold increase in the prevalence of QT_c prolongation.[6]

Known interactions with antipsychotic agents are listed in Table 40–1.[7]

Clinical Presentation
Neurotoxicity

Thioridazine. The manufacturer reported on 223 cases of acute thioridazine overdose.[8] The usual therapeutic dosage ranges from 25 to 800 mg daily for adults. In children, the upper level is between 2 and 4 mg/kg daily. Overdoses have ranged from 10 mg (12-day-old infant) to 50 mg. The most frequent signs and symptoms of acute overdose include, in decreasing order of frequency, impairment of consciousness, arrhythmias and/or electrocardiographic changes, extrapyramidal symptoms, confusional

Table 40–1
Interactions With Antipsychotic Agents

Drug	Interaction
Alcohol	Additive sedation, lack of coordination HAL increases alcohol levels Alcohol may worsen EPS
Antacids	Impair absorption of CPZ
Anticholinergic agents	Additive anticholinergic effects Inconsistent effects on APD levels Inconsistent effects on APD efficacy
Anticonvulsants	
Carbamazepine	Markedly decreases HAL levels May induce delirium
Phenytoin	May decrease HAL and CLZ levels
Phenobarbital	Lowers CPZ levels Additive sedative effects
Valproic acid	Levels increased by CPZ
Antidepressants	
Tricyclics	Increase levels of CPZ, PPZ, and HAL Nortriptyline levels increased by HAL and PPZ Desipramine levels increased by APDs Inconsistent effects on APD efficacy
Fluoxetine	Increases HAL levels (~20%) May cause EPS
Anxiolytic agents	
Alprazolam	Increases levels of HAL and FPZ
Buspirone	Increases HAL levels (~26%)
Antidiarrheal agents	
Attapulgite	Impairs absorption of PMZ
Aluminum salts	May lower CPZ levels
Antihypertensive agents	
α-Methyldopa	CPZ and HPL may increase hypotension Added to APDs may cause confusion, behavioral deterioration
Guanethidine	CPZ reverses antihypertensive effect
Propranolol	Levels increased by CPZ Increases CPZ and THZ levels
Cimetidine	Lowers CPZ levels
Disulfiram	Lowers levels of PPZ
Lithium	Increases molindone levels May cause EPS May cause neurotoxicity
Orphendrine	CPZ may cause hypoglycemia
Tobacco	Decreases levels of HAL, FPZ, and CPZ Decreases parkinsonism

APD, antipsychotic drug; FPZ, fluphenazine; CLZ, clozapine; HAL, haloperidol; PMZ, promazine, EPS, extrapyramidal symptoms; PPZ, perphenazine; THZ, thioridazine.
From Goff DC, Baldessarini RJ. Drug interactions with antipsychotic agents. J Clin Psychopharmacol 1993;13:57–67.

states, hypotension, agitation, and respiratory disorders. Seizures have occurred in adults who have ingested more than 2 g of thioridazine. The lowest lethal dose was 900 mg. Death follows cardiac arrhythmias, cardiac arrest, respiratory arrest, and aspiration pneumonia. Patients have survived ingestion of 10 g and died after as little as 1500 mg/d.[9]

Seizures. Probably all neuroloeptic drugs lower the seizure threshold. This becomes a problem when patients have taken an overdose, have underlying seizure disorders, take other proconvulsant drugs, or withdraw from sedative–hypnotic agents.[10]

Table 40–2
Neuroleptic Malignant Syndrome Etiologic Agents

I. Neuroleptic Drugs
- A. Phenothiazines
- B. Butyrophenone
- C. Thioxanthenes
- D. Other dopamine antagonists
  - Metoclopramide (Reglan)
  - Sulpride
  - Sultopride
  - Zuclopenthixol
  - Tetrabenazine

II. Nonneuroleptic agents
- A. Tricyclic antidepressants
  - Desipramine (Norpramin, Pertofrane)
  - Anoxapine (Asendin)
  - Maprotiline (Ludiomil)
  - Trimipramine
  - Dothiepin
  - Amitriptyline (Elavil)
  - Fluoxetine (Prozac)
- B. Monoamine oxidase inhibitors
  - Phenelzine (Nardil)
- C. Anticonvulsants
  - Carbamazepine (Tegretol)
  - Phenytoin (Dilantin)
- D. Withdrawal parkinsonian medication
  - Ethopropazine (Parsidol)
  - Levadopa/carbidopa (Sinemet)
  - Amantadine
  - B promocriptine (Parlodel)
- E. Lithium
  - With clozapine
  - With carbamazepine
  - With phenelzine
  - With chlorpromazine
  - With antiparkinsonian agents
  - With doxepin
- F. Estrogen
  - Possible trigger in patient on neuroleptics

From Lev R, Clark RF. Neuroleptic malignant syndrome presenting without fever: Case report and review of the literature. J Emerg Med 1994;12:49–55.

Thermal Dysregulation

Use of anticholinergic and antihistaminic agents in hyperthermic syndromes is controversial because of their potential to alter the thermoregulatory mechanism by inhibiting the dissipation of heat. Caution should be exercised when using these agents in the presence of fever greater than 101°F.[11] Recovery from temperatures as high as 108°F after seizures and death from temperatures of 109.5°F (complicated by acute compartment syndromes, rhabdomyolysis, and acute tubular necrosis) have been reported.[12,13]

Neuroleptic Malignant Syndrome

Etiology. Table 40–2 summarizes etiologic agents associated with the neuroleptic malignant syndrome (NMS) (see also Haloperidol). Haloperidol, phenothiazines, butyrophenones, and thioxanthines are the most commonly associated agents.[14] Criteria for the diagnosis are listed in Table 40–3.[15]

Symptoms. Neuroleptic malignant syndrome is a tetrad of fever, rigidity, altered sensorium, and autonomic dysfunction. Temperature typically ranges from 38.5° to 42°C. Fever may not be present.[14] The rigidity is classically described as leadpipe. Other disorders include tremor, sialorrhea, bradykinesia, festinating gait, dystonia, chorea, trismus, opisthotonos, and dysphagias. Mental status ranges from mild confusion and agitation to lethargy, stupor, and coma. Autonomic dysfunction is manifested by tachycardia, labile blood pressure, tachypnea, urinary incontinence, respiratory stridor, diaphoresis, pallor, and cardiac arrest. Patients who present early in their course may not have all the classic features.

Neuroleptic malignant syndrome frequently occurs 3 to 9 days after initiation of neuroleptic treatment or after the addition of a second neuroleptic medication. Symptoms of NMS usually develop over 24 to 72 hours and last 5 to 10 days after the neuroleptic drug is discontinued.[14]

Neuroleptic Withdrawal. Withdrawal syndrome associated with antipsychotic drugs includes autonomic and behavioral symptoms, parkinsonism, withdrawal dyskinesia, and covert dyskinesias.[16,17] The neuroleptic withdrawal syndrome has followed use of haloperidol and pimozide and sudden cessation of amantadine.

Laboratory Tests. There are no diagnostic laboratory findings in NMS.

Complications.[16,18–20] The most common complication is rhabdomyolysis, which results from muscle rigidity and breakdown. Other reported complications include aspiration pneumonia, pulmonary embolism, pulmonary edema, adult respiratory distress syndrome, sepsis, disseminated intravascular coagulation, seizures, myocardial infarction, peripheral neuropathy, and death. Periarticular ossification has been reported following NMS and other central nervous system disturbances, but the exact mechanism is unknown. The anticholinergic properties of neuroleptic drugs and TCAs promote intestinal ileus, which may lead to necrotizing enterocolitis.[14]

Table 40–3
Diagnostic Criteria for Neuroleptic Malignant Syndrome

1. Treatment with neuroleptic agents within 7 d of onset (2–4 wk for depot neuroleptics)
2. Hyperthermia (≥38°C)
3. Muscle rigidity
4. Five of the following:
   - Change in mental status
   - Tachycardia
   - Hypertension or hypotension
   - Tachypnea or hypoxia
   - Diaphoresis or sialorrhea
   - Dysarthria or dysphagia
   - Tremor
   - Incontinence
   - Creatine phosphokinase elevation or myoglobinuria
   - Leukocytosis
   - Metabolic acidosis
5. Not due to other drug-induced, systemic, or neuropsychiatric illness

From Caroff SN, Mann SC, Lazarus A, et al. Neuroleptic malignant syndrome: Diagnostic issues. Psychiatr Ann 1991;21:130–147.

Differential Diagnosis. The differential diagnosis of NMS includes causes of fever, leukocytosis, and rigidity[2] (Table 40–4). In a patient with fever, stiff neck, and altered mentation (all seen in NMS), meningitis must be ruled out. Other etiologies to consider are encephalitis, sepsis, thyrotoxicosis, heat stroke, drug overdose, delirium, malignant hyperthermia, lethal catatonia, and extrapyramidal reactions. Table 40–5 differentiates NMS from malignant hyperthermia and lethal catatonia. Table 40–6 compares the serotonin syndrome, the neuroleptic malignant syndrome, and Ecstasy (3,4-methylenedioxymethamphetamine [MDMA]).

Neuroleptic malignant syndrome is a life-threatening medical emergency. Patients require monitored intensive care management (Table 40–7).[21]

Tardive Dyskinesia

This extrapyramidal reaction is the most serious side effect of phenothiazine and haloperidol treatment. It has rarely been associated with the use of molindone, a dopamine D_2-receptor site binder.[22] Permanent dyskinesias that involve involuntary and repetitive movements characterize this adverse reaction. The face and mouth are often involved but the limbs and trunk also may display these movements. Lip smacking, protrusion of the tongue, chewing and jaw deviations, facial grimacing, eye blinking, and furrowing of the eyebrows are typical kinetic disorders.[23] Sleep abolishes all movements, and voluntary activity of the involved muscle group markedly reduces the frequency of involuntary repetitive movements. This disorder affects 3 to 6% of phenothiazine-treated psychiatric outpatients and up to 40% of institutionalized patients. Chronically treated elderly women appear to be the most susceptible group.[24] Dyskinesias may appear at any time during treatment, but particularly occur when drug treatment is discontinued after 2 years.

Rabbit Syndrome

Rabbit syndrome is a late-onset neuroleptic drug-induced extrapyramidal syndrome characterized by rhythmic 5/s to 5.5/s second involuntary movements of the oral and masticatory musculature that mimic the chewing movements of a rabbit. It is reversible when neuroleptic drug therapy is discontinued and responds to antiparkinsonian drug therapy. The high frequency of the perioral movements and the absence of lingual movements distinguish the rabbit syndrome from tardive dyskinesia. Physostigmine may worsen the symptoms of rabbit syndrome but reduces those of tardive dyskinesia.[25–27]

Table 40–4
Differential Diagnosis of Neuroleptic Malignant Syndrome

Primary Central Nervous System Disorders
Infections (viral encephalitis, AIDS, postinfectious encephalomyelitis)
Tumors
Cerebrovascular accidents
Trauma
Seizures
Major psychoses (lethal catatonia)

Systemic Disorders
Infections
Metabolic conditions
Endocrinopathies (thyroid storm, pheochromocytoma)
Autoimmune disease (systemic lupus erythematosus)
Heat stroke
Toxins (carbon monoxide, tetanus, strychnine)
Drugs (salicylates, dopamine inhibitors and antagonists, stimulants psychedelics, monoamine oxidase inhibitors, anesthetics, anticholinergics, alcohol or sedative withdrawal)

From Caroff SN, Mann SC, Lazarus A, et al. Neuroleptic malignant syndrome: Diagnostic issues. Psychiatr Ann 1991;21:130–147.

Neuroleptic Supersensitivity Psychosis

Chouinard has proposed diagnostic criteria for this disorder: a minimum of 3 months treatment with oral neuroleptic drugs, a progressive decrease in responsiveness to neuroleptic drugs, and development of psychotic symptoms within 6 weeks of the abrupt discontinuation of treatment.

A common neurochemical abnormality differing only in site of action may account for dopamine receptor supersensitivity mediating neuroleptic withdrawal psychosis (mesolimbic region), tardive dyskinesia (neostriatal region), and Tourette's disorder (basal ganglia, frontal and cingulate regions). Treatment may require restoring a neuroleptic drug to manage symptoms.[28,29]

Cardiovascular Effects

Conduction delays, hypotension, and ventricular dysrhythmias are common to TCA overdose but can be seen after phenothiazine ingestion. The severity and incidence of these complications are much less after neuroleptic drug overdose.

QT prolongation and life-threatening ventricular tachycardia (torsade de pointes) have been reported following overdoses of haloperidol. Temporary overdrive pacing may be required. Patients who have ingested an overdose of haloperidol must be considered at risk for life-threatening cardiac arrhythmias and should be carefully monitored.[30]

The electrophysiologic effects of thioridazine and other phenothiazine tranquilizers are similar to those of quinidine and include a decrease in the maximum rate of rise of action potential during phase 0 depolarization, a depression in the amplitude and duration of phase 2, and prolongation of phase 3 repolarization. The resulting electrocardiographic changes are a prolonged QT interval, flattening or depression of the T wave, and an increase in the U-wave amplitude.

Table 40–5
Differentiating Neuroleptic Malignant Syndrome From Malignant Hyperthermia and Lethal Catatonia

	Neuroleptic Malignant Syndrome	Malignant Hyperthermia	Lethal Catatonia
Central mechanism	+	–	+
Peripheral mechanism	–	+	–
Fever	+	+	+
Muscle rigidity	+	+	+
Associated neuroleptic medications	+	–	–
Associated anesthetics	–	+	–
Autonomic dysfunction (hypertension, diaphoresis, incontinence)	+	±	–
Response to dantrolene	±	+	–

From Schneider SM. Neuroleptic malignant syndrome: Controversies in treatment. Am J Emerg Med 1991;9:360–362.

Respiratory Depression

Respiratory depression requiring intubation occurs rarely, but the coingestion of sedative–hypnotic drugs and TCAs significantly increases the necessity for intubation.

Pulmonary Edema

The diagnosis of phenothiazine-induced pulmonary edema should be suspected in any patient with potential access to these drugs who presents with coma and diffuse pulmonary infiltrates.[31] Treatment is supportive.

Eye Signs

Cataracts, retinal damage, and corneal edema may be associated with chronic phenothiazine use. Welders receiving phenothiazines may develop retinal damage after short periods (minutes) of unprotected exposure to a manual metal arc welding unit.[32]

The muscle isoenzyme of creatinine kinase may also be raised by intramuscular injection, hyperactivity, and catatonia and in medically ill patients taking neuroleptic drugs. Thus, it is not a specific indicator of NMS. Its importance in early detection of the syndrome and in other forms of neuromuscular disturbance remains doubtful.[33] Symptoms develop rapidly over 24 to 72 hours and last 5 to 10 days after cessation of oral neuroleptic drug therapy. Depot injections

Table 40–6
Comparison of Serotonin Syndrome, Neuroleptic Malignant Syndrome, and MDMA

	Serotonin Syndrome	Neuroleptic Malignant Syndrome	Ecstasy (MDMA)
Cause	Drugs that enhance brain serotonin activity MAOI–tryptophan MAOI–fluoxetine Fluoxetine–tryptophan MAOI–meperidine hydrochloride Moclobemide–clomipramine Fluoxetine–carbamazepine	Dopamine blocking agents	3,4-Methylenedioxymeth-amphetamine
Clinical	Hyperthermia, tachycardia, autonomic instability, agitation, diaphoresis, myoclonus, shivering, tremor, confusion, or delirium ± hyperthermia, disseminated intravascular coagulation, rhabdomyolysis, acute renal failure	Hyperthermia, rigidity, fluctuating consciousness, autonomic instability	Hyperthermia, tachycardia, disseminated intravascular coagulation, rhabdomyolysis, acute renal failure
Mechanism of action	Hyperstimulation of 5-HT_{1A} receptor in brainstem and spinal cord	Acute depletion of dopamine (rigidity), hyperthermia, tachycardia, elevated creatinine phosphokinase levels, renal failure from rhabdomyolysis	Affects both dopamine- and serotonin-containing neurons. Stimulates neuronal serotonin release
Treatment	Benzodiazepine; beta blocker	Discontinuation of medication; bromocriptine; dantrolene sodium; cooling blankets; hydration; respiratory support	Removal of medication; cooling and dantrolene sodium for hyperthermia; anticonvulsants for seizures; monitoring in intensive care unit; benzodiazepines cyproheptadine?

MAOI, monoamine oxidase inhibitor.
Source: Ames D. Wirshing WC. Ecstasy, the serotonin syndrome and neuroleptic malignant syndrome: A possible link? JAMA 1993;269:869. Friedman R. Ecstasy, the serotonin syndrome and neuroleptic malignant syndrome: a possible link? JAMA 1993;269:869–870.

Table 40–7
Treatment of Neuroleptic Malignant Syndrome

Termination of the dopamine antagonist
Supportive measures
 Reducing body temperature
 Treating secondary infections
 Maintaining pulmonary, cardiovascular, and renal functions
 Sedation
Dantrolene sodium
 1–3 mg/kg/d IV, in four divided doses
 May be increased to 10 mg/kg/d IV in four divided doses
 Oral maintenance doses range from 50 to 200 mg/d
Bromocriptine
 2.5–10 mg PO tid initially
 If no improvement in 24 h, increase up to 20 mg PO qid
Therapy with dantrolene or bromocriptine or both is started immediately and continued until the patient's condition improves clinically or creatinine kinase levels return to normal
Consideration of electroconvulsive therapy

From Epperly TD, McGlaughlin VG, Leo KU. A hazardous side effect of neuroleptics: Diagnosis and treatment. Geriatrics 1990;45(8):58–62.

of fluphenazine can prolong the syndrome as long as 21 days after administration.[34]

Death

Estimates of mortality from NMS range from 20 to 30%. Death usually occurs 3 days after the development of symptoms. Causes of death include respiratory failure, cardiovascular collapse, renal failure, arrhythmias, and thromboembolism.

Extrapyramidal Reactions

Symptoms following a haloperidol overdose begin within 12 to 24 hours of ingestion. Clinical improvement is seen in 6 days. Transient thrombocytosis has been observed. Long-term follow-up (1–9 months) reveals a residual of restlessness, aggressiveness, unprovoked violence, agitation, and irritability.[35] The frequency of extrapyramidal symptoms and anticholinergic effects with neuroleptic drugs is summarized in Table 40–2.[36]

Renal Dysfunction

Acute reversible oliguria with or without acute interstitial nephritis may follow overdoses of chlorprothixene.[37–39]

Laboratory

Analytical Methods

Because of high volume of distribution (11–25 L/kg) of haloperidol and the relatively low serum concentration, preferred methods of analysis include high-performance liquid chromatography (HPLC) with electrochemical detection.[40] A HPLC method for quantitation of haloperidol and reduced haloperidol has detection limits of 0.5 ng/mL in plasma and 5 ng/mL in urine.[41]

Blood Levels

The relationship between serum concentration and therapeutic response is minimal. In patients whose condition responds to haloperidol, a serum concentration of at least 5 ng/L is associated with a positive response. The therapeutic range is about 5 to 16 ng/mL.[40] Most potent antpsychotic agents (such as haloperidol and perphenazine) yield total plasma concentrations of about 1 to 25 ng/mL. Low-potency agents (such as chlorpromazine and thioridazine) yield levels that typically range 5 to 10 times higher with a complex assortment of metabolic byproducts.

Optimum patient response in schizophrenia was associated, in one study, with plasma haloperidol levels of 4.2 to 11.0 ng/mL for the first 2 weeks of treatment[42]; improvement in choreiform movements in Huntington's disease in another study was associated with serum haloperidol concentrations between 2 and 5 ng/mL.[43] Haloperidol (H) is metabolized in humans to reduced haloperidol (RH), which is present in both plasma and red blood cells. Assays for both H and RH may provide a more accurate method for monitoring this drug.[44] H and RH can also be measured in hair.[45]

Thiothixene. A high-performance thin-layer chromatography method is available for quantitation of thiothixene plasma values.[46] Sensitivity is about 0.1 ng/mL.

Thioridazine. Serum concentrations of thioridazine and its metabolites mesoridazine, sulfonidazine, and the ring sulfoxide are quantitated by an HPLC method,[47] as modified.[48]

Loxapine. A plasma level of 0.192 mg/L was reported in a stuporous woman.[49] Postmortem blood concentrations of 7.7 mg/L have been reported.[50] A 2500-mg ingestion, which later proved fatal, resulted in an admission plasma level of 1.9 mg/L.

Clothiapine. Ingestion of 2.4 g of clothiapine induced coma and hypertension, with a blood level of 384 ng/mL 24 hours after ingestion. Analysis is performed by gas chromatography with nitrogen–phosphorus detection and electron capture detection.[51]

Lupus Anticoagulant: Immune Abnormalities

A lupus anticoagulant may appear in long-term (months or years) phenothiazine users. Such patients may develop prolongation of the activated partial thromboplastin time and, less frequently, the prothrombin time. A hypercoagulable state may manifest as thrombotic phenomena.[52,53] Long-term chlorpromazine therapy may be associated with a high incidence of antinuclear antibodies and increased levels of IgM.[54] High serum IgM titers with chlorpromazine may require a change to other antipsychotic medication.[55]

Treatment

Stabilization

Obtunded patients should receive the usual measures of glucose, naloxone, and, if indicated, thiamine. The adequacy of respiration should be evaluated by clinical and laboratory means (ie, tidal volume, arterial blood gases) as dictated by clinical judgment. Stuporous or comatose patients should be intubated and placed on a ventilator to prevent aspiration. Patients with vital sign or cardiac abnormalities should receive cardiac monitoring and an intravenous line with Ringer's lactate.

Low Blood Pressure. Hypotension is the most common sign of cardiotoxicity and usually responds to the Trendelenburg position and Ringer's lactate fluid challenges. Alpha-adrenergic agonists (eg, norepinephrine, methoxamine) are probably the vasopressors of choice. Vasopressors with mixed alpha- and beta-adrenergic function (eg, epinephrine, dopamine) may worsen hypotension because of the unopposed beta-adrenergic stimulation from phenothiazine-induced alpha blockade.

Dysrhythmias. Quinidine, procainamide, and disopyramide are contraindicated. Isoproterenol is contraindicated because of the exacerbation of hypotension by its beta-adrenergic agonist effects.

A 12-lead electrocardiogram should be performed at admission and repeated 12 and 24 hours after ingestion of the drug. If atrioventricular blocks or arrhythmias are detected, cardiac monitoring should be initiated. Thioridazine in high doses exhibits a beta-adrenoceptor and a calcium channel blocking effect. Drugs with these types of properties are contraindicated. Amiodarone may facilitate torsade de pointes and, therefore, should be used with caution. Lidocaine-like agents are often ineffective even if electrolyte imbalance is corrected. In addition, these types of drugs may not prevent recurrence. The most appropriate treatment of thioridazine-induced arrhythmias is probably temporary pacing.[32–35] This cardiac pacing should last approximately 10 days, especially in patients who have presented with ventricular tachycardia associated with atrioventricular blocks I or II.[8]

Gut Decontamination

Up to 4 to 6 hours postingestion, children should receive the usual decontamination measures (lavage or charcoal, with only a single dose of cathartics) if they have consumed more than several tablets. Remember, tracheal protection must be provided. Seizures may suddenly develop during gut decontamination, therefore ipecac is contraindicated.

Elimination Enhancement

The high protein binding and large volume of distribution make it unlikely that hemodialysis and forced diuresis will be useful.

Following ingestion of 10 g of chlorprothixene, hemoperfusion/hemodialysis removed about 160 mg (1.6%) of the estimated dose from the plasma compartment. Despite this, the patient's clinical condition improved.[55]

Antidote

There is no antidote.

Supportive Measures

Admission Criteria. Patients with a history of significant neuroleptic ingestion should receive gut decontamination, an electrocardiogram, and vital sign and cardiac monitoring. Symptomatic patients (eg, hypotension, conduction delay, dysrhythmia) should be admitted until the electrocardiogram is normal for 24 hours. Asymptomatic patients can be released after a 4-hour observation period. Any other somatic illness that may be causing a fever should be ruled out.

Seizures. Diazepam and phenytoin are the anticonvulsant drugs of choice. Loxapine in particular may produce recurrent and prolonged seizures. Urine myoglobin and serum muscle enzyme levels should be checked in all patients with prolonged muscle rigidity or seizures.

Acute Dystonic Reactions. Intravenous diphenhydramine (2 mg/kg up to 50 mg over several minutes) and intramuscular benztropine mesylate (2 mg in adults) are the drugs of choice and should relieve symptoms in 5 and 15 20 minutes, respectively.[56] Mild sedation is the main side effect. An anticholinergic agent (eg, Benadryl 50 mg orally three times daily or trihexylphenidyl 2 mg orally twice daily) should then be given for the next 3 days because of the long half-life of major tranquilizers.

Akathisias and Parkinsonian-like Syndrome. These may be relieved by reduction of the dose or addition of antiparkinsonian drugs (eg, Artane). Propranolol 20 to 50 mg daily has been effective in reducing motor hyperactivity following haloperidol use.[57]

There is no clear evidence that one antiparkinsonian drug is more effective than another. These drugs should be used with caution in patients with prostatic hypertrophy, urinary retention, narrow-angle glaucoma, tachycardia, myasthenia gravis, and respiratory difficulties and in pregnant patients.

Hyperthermia. For malignant hyperthermia, dantrolene may be administered at an initial intravenous dose of 2.5 mg/kg up to a maximum of 10 mg/kg. The maintenance dantrolene dose is 2.5 mg/kg every 6 hours until the crisis resolves. Arterial blood gases, serum electrolytes, glucose, and creatine kinase must be monitored carefully.

Tardive Dyskinesia. No drugs used for the treatment of tardive dyskinesia are uniformly safe and effective over extended periods. The long list of drugs used to treat tardive dyskinesia attests to their general lack of therapeutic benefits. These drugs include the serotonergic agents, such as tryptophan and cyproheptadine hydrochloride (Periactin); noradrenergic agents such as lithium carbonate (Lithane, Eskalith); the beta-adrenergic receptor antagonist propranolol hydrochloride (Inderal); and the alpha-adrenergic agonist clonidine hydrochloride (Catapres). Trials with morphine, naloxone hydrochloride (Narcan), estrogen, pyridoxine, fusaric acid, manganese chloride, phenytoin (Dilantin), ergoloid mesylate (Hydergine), and papaverine hydrochloride have produced no or only sporadic benefits.[58]

Dopamine. Resetting dopaminergic hypersensitivity back to normal sensitivity with dopamine agonists (bromocriptine mesylate [Parlodel]) or dopamine precursors (levodopa) has not been consistently successful.

Acetylcholine. Anticholinergic agents usually aggravate existing tardive dyskinesia or unmask covert tardive dyskinesia. Trials with physostigmine (anticholinesterase inhibitor) and dietary choline and lecithin supplements have been disappointing.

γ-Aminobutyric Acid. Drugs used to enhance γ-aminobutyric acid (GABA) activity by direct agonism or by inhibiting the catalytic enzyme GABA transaminase all have produced inconsistent results. Baclofen (Lioresal) and sodium valproate (Depakene) are not recommended for routine use.

Benzodiazepines. Benzodiazepines often temporarily reduce tardive dyskinesia but rarely may aggravate it. Diazepam is not recommended because of potential problems with dependence during extended use.

Rigidity. Anticholinergic and antihistaminic agents are first-line choices to reverse severe neuroleptic-induced rigidity. Their use is not recommended in the presence of fever.

Agranulocytosis. Granulocyte colony-stimulating factor (G-CSF) has been effective in treatment of chlorpromazine- and clozapine-induced agranulocytosis.[59]

REFERENCES—NEUROLEPTIC DRUGS IN GENERAL

1. Rumeau-Rouquette C, Goujard J, Huel G. Possible teratogenic effects of phenothiazines in human beings. Teratology 1977;15:57–64.
2. Milkovich L, van den Berg BJ. An evaluation of the teratogenicity of certain antinauseant drugs. Am J Obstet Gynecol 1976;125:244–248.
3. Guze BH, Guze PA. Psychotropic medication use during pregnancy. West J Med 1989;151:296–298.
4. Olesen OV, Bartels U, Poulson JH. Perphenazine in breast milk and serum. Am J Psychiatry 1990;147:1378–1379.
5. Whalley LJ, Blain PG, Prime JK. Haloperidol secreted in breast milk. Br Med J 1981;282:1746–1747.

6. Wilens TE, Shirn TA, O'Gara PT. Adverse cardiac effects of combined neuroleptic ingestion and tricyclic antidepressant overdose. J Clin Psychopharmacol 1990; 10:51–54.
7. Goff DC, Baldessarini RJ. Drug interactions with antipsychotic agents. J Clin Psychopharmacol 1993;13:58–66.
8. Le Blaye I, Donatini B, Hall M, Krupp T. Acute overdosage with thioridazine: A review of the available clinical exposure. Vet Hum Toxicol 1993;35:147–150.
9. Hulisz DT, Dasa SL, Black LD, Heiselman DE. Complete heart block and torsade de pointes associated with thioridazine poisoning. Pharmacotherapy 1994;14:239–245.
10. Gelenberg AJ. Major complications of neuroleptic drug use. West J Med 1994;160:55–56.
11. Gratz SS, Levinson DF, Simpson GM. The treatment and management of neuroleptic malignant syndrome. Prog Neuropsychopharmacol Biol Psychiatry 1992;16:425–443.
12. Shapiro MF. Despair, trifluoperazine, exercise and temperature of 108°F. Am J Psychiatry 1967;124:705–707.
13. Platts MM, Maher A, Stentiford NH. Phenelzine and trifluoperazine poisoning. Lancet 1965;2:738.
14. Lev R, Clark RF. Neuroleptic malignant syndrome presenting without fever: Case report and review of the literature. J Emerg Med 1994;12:49–55.
15. Caroff SN, Mannh SC, Lazarus A, et al. Neuroleptic malignant syndrome: Diagnostic issues. Psychiatr Ann 1991; 21:130–147.
16. Lang AE. Withdrawal akathisia: Case reports and proposed classification of chronic akathisia. Move Disord 1994; 9:188.
17. Bower DJ, Chalasani P, Ammons JC. Withdrawal induced neuroleptic malignant syndrome. Am J Psychiatry 1994;151: 451–452.
18. Malprotra AK, Litman RE, Pickar D. Adverse effects of antipsychotic drugs. Drug Saf 1993;9:429–436.
19. Tolten VY, Hirschenstein E, Hew P. Neuroleptic malignant syndrome presenting without initial fever: A case report. J Emerg Med 1994;12:43–47.
20. Schneider SM. Neuroleptic malignant syndrome: Controversies in treatment. Am J Emerg Med 1991;9:360–362.
21. Epperly TD, McGlaughlin VG, Leok VA. Hazardous side effects of neuroleptics: Diagnosis and treatment. Geriatrics 1990;45:58–62.
22. Katz SE. Tardive dyskinesia associated with molindone treatment. Am J Psychiatry 1990;147:124–125.
23. Kobayashi RM. Drug therapy of tardive dyskinesias. N Engl J Med 1977;296:257–260.
24. Crane GE. Persistent dyskinesias. Br J Psychiatry 1973;172: 395–405.
25. Sovner R, Dimascio A. The effect of benztropine mesylate in the rabbit syndrome and tardive dyskinesia. Am J Psychiatry 1977;134:1301–1302.
26. Deshmukh DK, Joshi VS, Agarwal MR. Rabbit syndrome: A rare complication of long-term neuroleptic medication. Br J Psychiatry 1990;157:293.
27. Weiss KJ, Ciranto DA, Shader RI. Physostigmine test in rabbit syndrome and tardive dyskinesia. Am J Psychiatry 1980;137:627–628.
28. Silva RR, Fridhoff AJ, Alpert M. Neuroleptic withdrawal psychosis in Tourette's disorder. Biol Psychiatry 1993;34:341–342.
29. Chouinard G. Severe cases of neuroleptic-induced supersensitivity psychosis, diagnostic criteria for the disorder and its treatment. Schizophrenia Res 1990;5:21–33.
30. Henderson RA, Lane S, Henry JA. Life-threatening ventricular arrhythmia (torsade de pointes) after haloperidol overdose. Hum Exp Toxicol 1991;10:59–62.
31. Li C, Gefter WB. Acute pulmonary edema induced by overdosage of phenothiazines. Chest 1992;101:102–104.
32. Power WJ, Travers SP, Mooney DJ. Welding arc maculopathy and fluphenazine. Br J Ophthalmol 1991;75:433–435.
33. Bristow MF, Kohen D: How "malignant" is the neuromuscular malignant syndrome? In early mild cases it may not be malignant at all. Br Med J 1993;307:1223–1224.
34. Bond WS. Detection and management of the neuroleptic malignant syndrome. Clin Pharm 1984;3:302–307.
35. Yoshida I, Sakaguchi Y, Matsuishi T, et al. Acute accidental overdosage of haloperidol in children. Acta Paediatr 1993;82: 877–880.
36. Bezchlibryk-Butler KZ, Remington GJ. Antiparkinsonian drugs in the treatment of neuroleptic induced extrapyramidal symptoms. Can J Psychiatry 1994;39:74–84.
37. Scheithauer W, Ulrich W, Kovarik J, Stummvol H-K. Acute oliguria associated with chlorprothixene overdosage. Nephron 1988;48:71–73.
38. Morgan JP, Baltch AL. Acute oliguria from overdose of chlorprothixene. NY State J Med 1979;69:1340–1342.
39. Rossen B, Steiness I. The pathophysiology of acute renal failure after chlorprothixene overdosage. Acta Med Scand 1981;209:525–527.
40. Lawson GM. Monitoring of serum haloperidol. Mayo Clin Proc 1994;69:189–190.
41. Park KH, Lee MH, Lee MG. Simultaneous determination of haloperidol and its metabolite, reduced haloperidol, in plasma, blood, urine and tissue homogenates by high-performance liquid chromatography. J Chromatogr Biomed Appl 1991;572:259–267.
42. Mavroidis ML, Kanter DR, Hirschowitz J, Garver DL. Clinical response and plasma haloperidol levels in schizophrenia. Psychopharmacology 1983;81:354–356.
43. Barr AN, Fischer JH, Koller WC, et al. Serum haloperidol concentrations and choreiform movements in Huntington's disease. Neurology 1988;38:84–88.
44. Vatassery GT, Herzan LA, Dyskin MW. Liquid chromatographic determination of reduced haloperidol and haloperidol concentrations in packed red blood cells from humans. J Anal Toxicol 1990;14:25–28.
45. Matsuno H, Uematsu T, Nakashima M. The measurement of haloperidol and reduced haloperidol in hair as an index of dosage history. Br J Clin Pharmacol 1990;29:187–194.
46. Davis CM, Harrington CA. Quantitation of thiothixene in plasma by high-performance thin layer chromatography and fluorometric detection. Ther Drug Monit 1988;10:215–223.
47. McKay G, Cooper JK, Gurnsey T, Midha KK. A simple, sensitive and simultaneous assay of thioridazine, sulphoridazine and mesoridazine in plasma by HPLC. Liq Chromatogr 1985; 3:256–258.
48. Von Bahr C, Movin G, Nordin C, et al. Plasma levels of thioridazine and metabolites are influenced by the debrisoquine hydroxylation phenotype. Clin Pharmacol Ther 1991;49:234–240.
49. Vasilrades J, Sahawneh TM, Owens C. Determination of therapeutic and toxic concentrations of doxepin and loxapine using gas–liquid chromatography with a nitrogen-sensitive detector and gas chromatography–mass spectrometry of loxapine. J Chromatogr 1979;164:457–470.
50. Reynolds PC, Som LW, Hurman PW. Loxapine fatalities. Clin Toxicol 1979;14:181–185.
51. Baldi ML, Rocchi L, Papa P, et al. Clothiapine poisonings: Toxic versus therapeutic serum drug levels. In: *Proceedings, XIVth International Congress of European Association of Poison Centres, Milan, Italy, September 25–29, 1990:*49.
52. El-Mallakh RS, Donaldson JO, Kranzler HR, Racy A. Phenothiazine associated lupus anticoagulant and thrombotic disease. Psychosomatics 1988;29:109–113.
53. Kaslow KA, Rosse RB, Zeller JA, et al. Phenothiazine-induced lupus anticoagulant. J Clin Psychiatry 1992;53:103–104.
54. Zucker S, Zarrabi HM, Schubach WH, et al. Chlorpromazine-induced immunopathy: Progressive increase in serum IgM. Medicine 1990;69:92–100.
55. Koppel C, Schirop T, Ibe K, et al. Hemoperfusion in severe chlorprothixene overdose. Intensive Care Med 1987;13:358–360.
56. Ott DA, Goeden SR. Treatment of acute phenothiazine reaction. J Am Coll Emerg Physicians 1979;8:471–472.
57. Dorevitch A, Durst R, Ginath Y. Propranolol in the treatment of akathisia caused by antipsychotic drugs. South Med J 1991;84:1505–1506.
58. Casey DE. Tardive dyskinesia. West J Med 1990;153:535–541.

59. Kendra JR, Rugman FP, Flaherty TA, et al. First use of G-CSF in chlorpromazine-induced agranulocytosis: A report of two cases. Postgrad Med J 1993;69:885–887.

CLOZAPINE

Clozapine was released in the United States in February 1990 for patients with refractory schizophrenia. Its use has been limited by a 1 to 2% incidence of agranulocytosis and by deaths due to neutropenic sepsis.[1–3] Overdose with clozapine may lead to fatalities. There is no antidote.

Structure and Classification

Clozapine is a member of the dibenzodiazepine class of antipsychotic drugs[4,5] (Fig. 40–1).

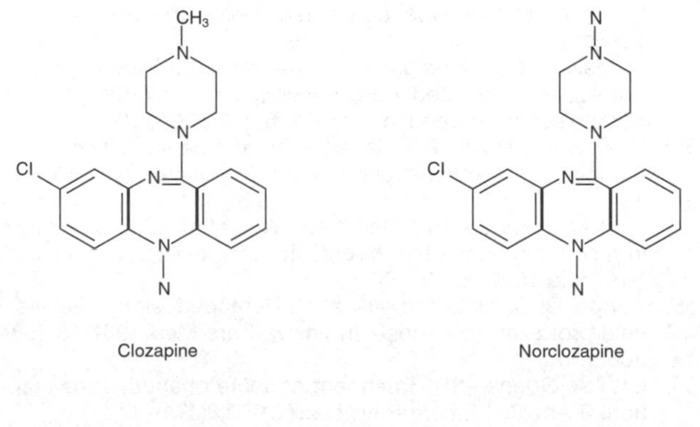

Use

Clozapine is indicated in the management of severely ill schizophrenic patients who have failed to respond to other neuroleptic agents or who cannot tolerate the adverse effects produced by those agents.[6] Because of the significant risk of agranulocytosis and seizures with clozapine, the patient should be given an adequate trial with at least two different standard antipsychotic medications before clozapine therapy is initiated.[6]

Product Formulation

Clozapine is available in 25- and 100-mg oral tablets. It is marketed as Clozaril (United States) and Leponex.

Source

Clozapine is a synthetic chemical product.

Therapeutic Dose

Oral doses begin at 25 mg one to two times daily and are increased in increments of 25 to 50 mg/d, if tolerated, to achieve a dose of 300 to 450 mg/d by the end of 2 weeks. Some patients have required up to 900 mg/d.[6]

Clozapine

Norclozapine

Figure 40–1 Structures of clozapine and norclozapine. (From Meeker JE, Herrmann PW, Som CW, Reynolds PC. Clozapine tissue concentrations following an apparent suicidal overdose of Clozaril. J Anal Toxicol 1992;16:54–56.)

Toxic Dose

Seizures tend to occur at clozapine doses greater than 600 mg/d.[7,8] A linear relationship appears to exist between the dose of clozapine and plasma concentration.[9] Eleven patients have survived ingestion of more than 4000 mg.[10] One patient survived an ingestion of 10,000 mg.[11] A 33-year-old man ingested 2250 mg and survived.[12]

Fatal Dose

A 25-year-old man ingested 200 mg of clozapine and died in several hours.[5] One patient committed suicide with an oral dose of 3000 mg.[10] Overdoses of 300 to 400 mg may be fatal.[13]

Toxicokinetics

Absorption

Following single and multiple doses, plasma concentrations of clozapine peak at 1 to 4 hours.[14] Because of moderate hepatic first-pass metabolism, the bioavailability of orally administered clozapine (50–200 mg) ranges from 27 to 50%. A linear correlation exists between clozapine dosage and plasma clozapine concentration.[14]

At steady-state dose levels of 300 to 400 mg/d, plasma concentrations of clozapine and norclozapine were 374 (range, 4–1667 ng/mL) and 116 (range, 15–400 ng/mL), respectively.[4] Schizophrenic patients appear to respond to plasma concentrations above 350 mg/mL.[15]

A rule of thumb is that plasma concentrations of clozapine average about 40 to 50 ng/mL per milligram of drug given per kilogram, so that a typical daily dose of 300 to 400 mg (about 5 mg/kg) yields levels of about 200 to 400 ng/mL.[16,17]

Distribution

Clozapine is approximately 95% bound to plasma proteins in vitro.[14] Clozapine and its *N*-desmethyl metabolite are preferentially retained in the lungs in animals. The initial distribution half-life of clozapine is 1 to 5 hours.[17] Its apparent volume of distribution is about 5 L/kg body weight.[17]

Elimination

In humans, clozapine is extensively metabolized by *N*-oxidation, *N*-demethylation, and dehalogenation to yield pharmacologically inactive products. Unchanged clozapine accounts for approximately 2 to 5% of the cxcreted drug.[18] The terminal elimination half-life is approximately 12 hours (range, 6–30 hours).[17]

Drug Interaction

Clozapine induces an increase in central nervous system depressant effects when used with alcohol or central nervous system depression-producing medications (sedative–

hypnotic agents, opiates). Clozapine potentiates the anticholinergic effects of atropine-type drugs and may potentiate the hypotensive effects of antihypertensive drugs. Epinephrine should not be used in the treatment of clozapine-induced hypotension because of a possible reverse epinephrine effect.[6] Highly protein bound medications such as digoxin, heparin, phenytoin, and warfarin are displaced from their binding sites by clozapine, resulting in adverse clinical effects. The reverse may also occur. Clozapine may potentiate the myelosuppressive effects of bone marrow depressants. Such drugs may enhance the agranulocytosis following clozapine use. Smoking may decrease the serum concentration of clozapine.[14] Cimetidine, by inhibiting the oxidative system of cytochrome P450, increases serum clozapine levels and leads to adverse clinical effects.[19] Phenytoin has induced a decrease in plasma clozapine concentration.[20] Fluvoxamine elevates serum levels of clozapine.[21] Valproic acid results in a decrease in serum clozapine concentration.[22]

Pregnancy/Lactation

Clozapine crosses the placenta. The Food and Drug Administration has placed clozapine in Pregnancy Category B. Clozapine may be excreted in breast milk.

Mechanism of Action

Clozapine is a "broad-spectrum" receptor antagonist at dopamine D_1 and D_2 receptors, α_1 and α_2 adrenoreceptors, and serotonin (5-HT_2), histamine (H_1), and acetylcholine (muscarinic) receptors. It differs from some of the classic antipsychotic agents in animal studies (eg, haloperidol) by blocking D_1 more than D_2 receptors, by raising plasma prolactin levels only transiently, and by its inability to induce supersensitivity in striatal dopamine systems.[23,24] Clozapine may exert its effects by differentially modulating D_1 and D_2 receptors in the extrapyramidal, limbic, and mesocortical systems.[24] Clozapine causes a greater antagonism of serotonin S_2 receptors relative to D_2 receptors. The lower incidence of acute extrapyramidal effects with clozapine compared with other antipsychotic drugs is likely to result from its relatively weak antagonism of striatal dopamine D_2 receptors. Tardive dyskinesia does not seem to occur, even with long-term use.[25] A candidate for the locus of action of clozapine is the recently cloned dopamine D_4 receptor.[26]

Clinical Presentation

Overdose

Symptoms of acute overdose include drowsiness, restlessness, lethargy, areflexia, hyperreflexia, agitation, confusion, disorientation, delirium, blurred vision, mydriasis, convulsions, and coma; hypotension, hypertension,[27] arrhythmia, tachycardia, and heart block; respiratory depression; hypersalivation; hypothermia[10,12]; hypoactive bowel sounds, dry skin, and inability to urinate[24]; adult respiratory distress syndrome, pancreatitis,[28] and myocarditis.[10,12,29–32] Sudden death has been reported.[29]

A 25-year-old man ingested 20 100-mg tablets (2000 mg) of clozapine. Six hours later in a hospital, he died. On autopsy he exhibited an eosinophilic myocarditis.[5] Acute overdose of 50 to 200 mg (½ to 2 tablets) of clozapine in young children has led to confusion, ataxia, muscle rigidity, nystagmus, torticollis, drooling, slurred speech, agitation, screaming, crying, and stupor. Recovery usually follows symptomatic care.[33–35] Abrupt discontinuation of clozapine in a psychotic patient may lead to rapid and prolonged relapse in psychotic symptoms.[36]

Gossweiler reviewed 199 cases of overdose. Severe symptoms followed ingestion of 600 mg in 3 of 16 cases, in 13 patients who had ingested 600 to 1500 mg, and in 19 patients who had ingested 1500 to 5000 mg.[30]

Chronic Use

Common undesirable effects following chronic use include nausea and vomiting, weight gain, transient hyperthermia, hypotension, hypersalivation, dizziness, constipation, tachycardia, and drowsiness.[6] A paradoxical hypertension has been described.[27] Approximately 3 to 4% of patients receiving 300 to 600 mg/d clozapine develop seizures. The incidence increases sharply for doses of 600 to 900 mg/d.[7,8] Clozapine can cause neutropenia and agranulocytosis. Up to 3% of patients taking the drug for 1 year develop neutropenia.[37,38] Eosinophilia may follow long-term use of clozapine.[39] This may terminate fatally. Neuroleptic malignant syndrome has been reported following doses of 200 to 500 mg/d taken for several weeks to months.[40–42] Clozapine has been associated with the induction of tardive dyskinesia[43] (see Mechanism of Action). Several studies suggest amelioration of tardive dyskinesia in some patients after initiation of clozapine therapy.[44,45] Clozapine may induce obsessive–compulsive symptoms, which subside within 1 to 3 weeks of cessation of drug use.[46] An anecdotal report suggests an association with acute dystonia.[47] Known causes of death are cardiac failure, aspiration pneumonia, and renal failure.[48]

Laboratory

Analytical Methods

A high-performance liquid chromatography method is available for the simultaneous quantitation of clozapine and its *N*-desmethylclozapine metabolite in human plasma.[4] Detection limits of 15 ng/mL for clozapine and 30 ng/mL for desmethylclozapine have been achieved.

Blood Levels

Plasma levels of 1313 and 2194 ng/mL were associated with grand mal seizures in two patients.[49] Approximately 2.5 hours following ingestion of 2250 mg of clozapine by a 33-year-old patient, the plasma clozapine level was 2916 ng/mL (therapeutic range, 200–400 ng/mL). One day later, after supportive therapy, the level was 413 ng/mL. The patient recovered.[12] Sudden death in an adult was associated with a plasma level of 4460 ng/mL.[29,31] Ingestion of 10,000 ng was followed by a peak plasma level of 2190 ng/mL. A 25-year-old man ingested 2000 mg of clozapine and died in several hours.[5] Antemortem and postmortem (death occurred within 6 hours) blood concentrations of clozapine were 1.94 μg/mL (4 hours after ingestion) and 5.81 μg/mL, respectively. Similar values for norclozapine were 10.8 and 12.0%

of the areas of response relative to clozapine.[5] Ingestion of 100 to 200 mg by children leads to serum clozapine levels of about 500 ng/mL.[33,34]

Abnormalities

Patients receiving clozapine should have a white blood cell count each week throughout treatment and for 4 weeks after its discontinuation.[10]

The manufacturer requires that a patient's weekly leukocyte count be above an "agranulocytosis threshold" of 2×10^9/L (2000/μL) before each week's supply of medication is released. Monitoring the granulocyte count to a threshold of 1×10^9/L (1000/μL) may be a more sensitive indicator. Half of reported episodes of agranulocytosis occur within 3 months of starting treatment, but weekly monitoring of leukocyte counts continues indefinitely.[50]

Several anecdotal reports suggest that hyponatremia may have been a possible epileptogenic trigger.[13] Clozapine alters the electroencephalogram in a majority of patients treated, with seizure frequency as high as 5 to 10% at doses above 600 ng/d. This may lead to prolonged postictal encephalopathy.[51] Clozapine differs from other neuroleptic drugs in increasing plasma norepinephrine levels.[52] Severe hypoglycemia has been associated with high doses of clozapine.[53]

Treatment

Stabilization

Treatment is largely symptomatic and supportive. Patients should be admitted to a unit where an adequate oxygen supply, intravenous fluids, and cardiac and respiratory monitoring are available. Staff should be prepared for the sudden onset of seizures, agitation, anticholinergic toxicity, and paradoxical sialorrhea.[12]

Gut Decontamination

Syrup of ipecac is not recommended in view of the possibility of sudden seizures in the clozapine overdose patient. There is no evidence that gastric lavage is effective; however, physical removal of tablets during the first hour may tend to reduce the possibility of high plasma levels. If gastric lavage is contemplated, tracheal protection must be provided as seizures may intervene unpredictably. Activated charcoal with a single dose of cathartics may be of use, but controlled studies are not available to substantiate their efficacy.

Elimination Enhancement

In view of the extensive protein binding of clozapine and its high apparent volume of distribution, it appears that measures such as forced diuresis, peritoneal lavage, dialysis, hemoperfusion, and exchange transfusion are unlikely to be of benefit.

Antidote

There is no specific antidote.[54,55]

Supportive Measures

Admission Criteria. Patients with a history of significant clozapine ingestion should receive gut decontamination, cardiac and respiratory monitoring, and observation for at least 100 hours with periodic evaluation of electrolytes and acid–base balance (special attention for metabolic acidosis).[10]

Seizures. Diazepam and phenytoin are the anticonvulsant drugs of choice. Valproic acid may be used.[7] Carbamazepine, which may cause agranulocytosis or aplastic anemia, is contraindicated in conjunction with clozapine.[7] Temperature, oxygenation, and urine myoglobin must be followed in cases of recurrent and prolonged seizures.

Hypotension. Change in position, intravenous fluids, plasma expanders, albumin, and vasopressors (e.g., dopamine and norepinephrine) may be effective. Epinephrine and its derivatives are contraindicated.[6]

Arrhythmia. Lidocaine and phenytoin are the antiarrhythmic drugs of choice for ventricular dysrhythmias. Intractable ventricular dysrhythmias may require pacing. Quinidine, procainamide, and disopyramide are contraindicated. Digitalis, sodium bicarbonate, or potassium may be required according to clinical judgment. Their use in clozapine overdoses is limited.

Neuroleptic Malignant Syndrome. Hyperthermia is treated with cooling measures and antipyretics (aspirin or acetaminophen) as indicated. Dehydration is managed with fluids and electrolytes. Blood pressure and cardiac rhythm must be closely monitored for evidence of cardiovascular instability. An adequate oxygen supply must be ensured with airway insertion and assisted ventilation as required. Muscle rigidity is treated with dantrolene sodium (100–300 mg/d orally in divided doses, or 1.25–1.5 mg/kg body weight intravenously) or by administering amantadine (100 mg twice daily) or bromocriptine (5 mg three times a day) to restore the central balance of dopamine and acetylcholine at their receptor sites. Serum creatine phosphokinase, renal function, and urine myoglobin should be monitored.

Tardive Dyskinesia. There has been no effective treatment demonstrated in controlled clinical studies (see Neuroleptic Drugs in General for additional comments).

Agranulocytosis. Agranulocytosis following clozapine use has been successfully treated with granulocyte colony-stimulating factor (G-CSF).[56] G-CSF should be started within 48 hours of the onset of agranulocytosis.[57]

REFERENCES—CLOZAPINE

1. Gerson SL, Lieberman JA, Friedenberg WR, et al. Polypharmacy in fatal clozapine-associated agranulocytosis. Lancet 1991;338:262–263.
2. Idanpaan-Heikkila J, Alhava E, Olkinuora M, Palva IP. Agranulocytosis during treatment with clozapine. Eur J Clin Pharmacol 1977;11:193–198.
3. Report on Clozaril[R] (clozapine). East Hanover, NJ: Sandoz Pharmaceuticals, February 1991:CLO-0291-01.

4. Lovdahl MJ, Perry PJ, Miller DD. The assay of clozapine and *N*-desmethylclozapine in human plasma by high performance liquid chromatography. Ther Drug Monit 1991;13:69–72.
5. Meeker JE, Herrmann PW, Som SW, Reynolds PC. Clozapine tissue concentrations following an apparent suicidal overdose of Clozaril[R]. J Anal Toxicol 1992;16:54–56.
6. Clozapine (systemic). USP DI Update 1990;1(4):243–246.
7. Devinsky O, Honigfeld G, Patin J. Clozapine-related seizures. Neurology 1991;41:369–371.
8. Haller E, Binder RL. Clozapine and seizures. Am J Psychiatry 1990;147:1069–1071.
9. Haring C, Fleischacker W, Schett P, et al. Influence of patient related variables on clozapine plasma levels. Am J Psychiatry 1990;147:1471–1475.
10. Krassner MB. Personal communication, East Hanover, NJ: Sandoz Pharmaceuticals, February 26, 1991.
11. Pall H, Kleinberger G, Kotzaurek R, et al. Schwere Leponex[R]: Vergiftung und ihre intensive behandlung. Wien Klin Wochenschr 1976;88:179–182.
12. Wolf LR, Otten EJ. A case report of clozapine overdose. Vet Hum Toxicol 1991;33:370.
13. Ogilvie AD, Croy MF. Clozapine and hyponatremia. Lancet 1992;340:672.
14. Fitton A, Heel RC. Clozapine: A review of its pharmacological properties and therapeutic use in schizophrenia. Drugs 1990;40:722–747.
15. Perry PJ, Miller DD, Arndt SV, Cadoret RJ. Clozapine and norclozapine plasma concentrations and clinical response of treatment-refractory schizophrenic patients. Am J Psychiatry 1991;148:231–235.
16. Baldessarini RJ, Frankenburg FR. Clozapine: A novel antipsychotic agent. N Engl J Med 1991;324:746–754.
17. Choc MG, Lehr RG, Hsuan F, et al: Multiple dose pharmacokinetics of clozapine in patients. Pharm Res 1987;4:402–405.
18. Gauch R, Michaelis W. The metabolism of 8-chloro-11-(4-methyl-4-piperzinyl)-5*H*-dibenzo[*b,c*] [1,4]diazepam (clozapine) in mice, dogs, and human subjects. Farmaco 1971;26:667–681.
19. Szymanski S, Lieberman JA, Picou D, et al. A case report of cimetidine-induced clozapine toxicity. J Clin Psychiatry 1991;52:21–22.
20. Miller DD. Effect of phenytoin on plasma clozapine concentrations in two patients. J Clin Psychiatry 1991;52:23–25.
21. Hiemke C, Weigmann H, Hartter S, et al. Elevated levels of clozapine in serum after addition of fluvoxamine. J Clin Psychopharmacol 1994;14:279–281.
22. Finley P, Warner D. Potential impact of valproic acid therapy on clozapine disposition. Biol Psychiatry 1994;36:487–488.
23. Clozapine and loxapine for schizophrenia. Drug Ther Bull 1991;29(11):41–42.
24. Ereshefsky L, Watanabe MD, Tran-Johnson TK. Clozapine: An atypical antipsychotic agent. Clin Pharm 1989;8:691–709.
25. Hirsch SR, Puri BK. Clozapine: Progress in treating refractory schizophrenia. Side effects, but a cost-benefit analysis supports treatment. Br Med J 1993;306:1427–1428.
26. Shaikh S, Collier D, Kerwin RW, et al. Dopamine D_4 receptor subtypes and response to clozapine. Lancet 1993; 116–341.
27. Gupta S. Paradoxical hypertension associated with clozapine. Am J Psychiatry 1994;131:148.
28. Jubert P. Clozapine-related pancreatitis. Ann Intern Med 1994;121:722–723.
29. Kaempe B, Vesterby A, Thomsen NJ, Rosenthal J. Clozapine–a fatal case. Bull Int Assoc Forens Toxicol 1979;15(1):15–16.
30. Gossweiler B. Vergiftungen mit Leponex[R]. Personal communication. Swiss Toxicological Information Center, January 14, 1992.
31. Vesterby A, Pedersen JH, Kaempe B, Thomsen NJ. Sudden death during clozapine (Leponex[R]) therapy. Ugeskr Laeg 1980;142:170–171.
32. Schuster P, Gabriel E, Keifferle B, et al. Reversal by physostigmine of clozapine-induced delirium. Clin Toxicol 1977;10:437–441.
33. Goetz CM, Love RC, Schuster P. Overdose of clozapine in a child. Vet Hum Toxicol 1993;35:338.
34. Mady SP, Wax P. Clozapine intoxication in a young child. Vet Hum Toxicol 1993;35:338.
35. Hadley CM, Walson PD. Pediatric clozapine (Clozaril[R]) ingestion. Vet Hum Toxicol 1993;35:338.
36. Parsa MA, Al-Lahham YH, Ramirez LF, Meltzen HY. Prolonged psychotic relapse after abrupt clozapine withdrawal. J Clin Psychopharmacol 1993;13:154–155.
37. Kane J, Honigfeld G, Singer J, et al. Clozapine for the treatment-resistant schizophrenic: A double blind comparison with chlorpromazine. Arch Gen Psychiatry 1988;45:789–796.
38. Krupp P, Barnes P. Leponex-associated granulocytopenia: A review of the situation. Psychopharmacology 1989;99: S118–S121.
39. Tiihonen J, Paanila J. Eosinophilia associated with clozapine. Lancet 1992;339:488.
40. DasGupta K, Young A. Clozapine-induced neuroleptic malignant syndrome. J Clin Psychiatry 1991;52:105–107.
41. Anderson ES, Powers PS. Neuroleptic malignant syndrome associated with clozapine use. J Clin Psychiatry 1991;52: 102–104.
42. Miller DD, Sharafuddin MJA, Kathol RG. A case of clozapine-induced neuroleptic malignant syndrome. J Clin Psychiatry 1991;52:99–101.
43. Dave M. Clozapine related tardive dyskinesia. Biol Psychiatry 1994;36:886–887.
44. Lieberman JA, Saltz BL, Johns CA, et al. The effect of clozapine on tardive dyskinesia. Br J Psychiatry 1991;158:503–510.
45. Van Putten T, Wirshing WC, Marder SR. Tardive Meige syndrome responsive to clozapine. J Clin Psychopharmacol 1990;10:381–382.
46. Patil VJ. Development of transient obsessive compulsive symptoms during treatment with clozapine. Am J Psychiatry 1992;149:272.
47. Kastrup O, Gastpar M, Schwarz M. Acute dystonia due to clozapine. J Neurol Neurosurg Psychiatry 1994;57:119.
48. Le Blaye I, Donatini B, Hall M, Krupp P. Acute overdose with clozapine: A review of the available clinical experience. Pharm Med 1992;6:169–178.
49. Simpson GM, Cooper TA. Clozapine plasma levels and convulsions. Eur J Psychiatry 1978;135:99–100.
50. Beal M. Clozapine update. West J Med 1994;160:53–54.
51. Karper PP, Salloway SP, Seibyl JP, Krystal JH. Prolonged postictal encephalopathy in two patients with clozapine-induced seizures. J Neuropsychiatry Clin Neurosci 1992;4:454-457.
52. Breier A, Buchanan RW, Waltrip RW II, et al. The effect of clozapine on plasma norepinephrine: Relationship to clinical efficacy. Neuropsychopharmacology 1994;10:1–7.
53. Kamras A, Doraiswany PM, Jane JL, et al. Severe hyperglycemia associated with high doses of clozapine. Am J Psychiatry 1994;131:1395.
54. Levinson B. Clozapine (Leponex) overdosage. South Afr Med J 1975;49:5.
55. Norris DL, Israelstam K. Clozapine (Leponex) overdosage. South Afr Med J 1975;49:385.
56. Weide R, Koppler H, Heymanns J, et al. Successful treatment of clozapine induced agranulocytosis with granulocyte-colony stimulating factor (G-CSF). Br J Haematol 1992;80: 557–559.
57. Gerson SL, Gullion G, Yeh H-S, Moson C. Granulocyte colony-stimulating factor for clozapine-induced agranulocytosis. Lancet 1992;340:1097.

CYAMEMAZINE

Cyamemazine is an aliphatic phenothiazine derivative marketed in France since 1972 under the name Tercian. It is used in the management of neuropsychiatric disorders with a daily dose of 200 to 300 mg orally or by intramuscular injection in doses of 25 to 200 mg daily.[1]

Clinical Presentation

Death has followed an overdose of 7.5 g.

Laboratory

Therapeutic steady state plasma concentrations of the drug usually range from 0.05 to 0.040 ng/mL where 200 to 300 mg are taken daily. Following the ingestion of 7.5 g a blood level of 9.8 ug/mL by high performance liquid chromatography was observed.

Treatment

Treatment is symptomatic and supportive. Watch for seizures and treat appropriately.

REFERENCE—CYAMEMAZINE

1. Tracqui A, Kintz P, Jamey C, Mangin P. Toxicological data in a fatality involving cyamemazine. J Anal Toxicol 1993;17:386–388.

HALOPERIDOL

Haloperidol is an antipsychotic agent. Long-term (at least 12 months) use leads to extrapyramidal side effects including tardive dyskinesia in about 30% of patients. After discontinuation of the drug, tardive dyskinesia remains as a chronic disease in up to 50% of patients.[1] Overdose is associated with severe extrapyramidal symptoms, hypotension, and sedation. The risk of torsade de pointes should be considered.[2,3]

Use

Haloperidol is used to treat patients with psychotic disorders (e.g., schizophrenia); to control tics and verbal utterances associated with Gilles de la Tourette's syndrome; and to manage hyperexcitable children whose condition is not responsive to other treatment modalities.

Product Formulation

Haloperidol is available as tablets (0.5, 1, 2, 5, 10, and 20 mg) and as the decanoate for intramuscular injections of 50 and 10 mg/mL.

Therapeutic Dose

The recommended daily dose for patients with moderate symptoms is 1 to 6 mg, and for patients with severe symptoms, 6 to 15 mg.[4]

Toxicokinetics

Absorption

Haloperidol is well absorbed from the gastrointestinal tract but first-pass hepatic metabolism decreases oral bioavailability to 40 to 75%. Serum concentration peaks 0.5 to 4 hours after an oral dose.[4]

Distribution

The apparent volume of distribution is about 20 L/kg, consistent with the high lipophilicity of the drug. Haloperidol circulates in blood bound predominantly (90–94%) to plasma proteins.[4]

Elimination

Clearance occurs almost exclusively by hepatic metabolism. Renal excretion is negligible. A metabolite, reduced haloperidol, has minimal pharmacologic activity compared with the parent drug.

Haloperidol is similar in structure to the dopaminergic proneurotoxin 1-methyl-4-phenyl-1,2,3,4-tetrahydropyridine (MPTP), which probably causes parkinsonism in humans. MPTP undergoes monoamine oxidase P450-catalyzed oxidation to the neurotonic 1-methyl-4-phenylpyridinium species (MPP^+), which has selectivity for dopaminergic neurons. HPP^+ and $RHPP^+$, a pyridinium metabolite, are found in the plasma, blood, and urine of every patient receiving haloperidol. Their steady-state concentrations are related to the daily dose of haloperidol and to the corresponding plasma concentration. Urinary excretion data suggest that oxidation to these pyridinium species constitutes a minor pathway for haloperidol elimination compared with conjugation or formation of reduced haloperidol.[1]

The elimination half-life of haloperidol ranges from 13 to 35 hours.

Clinical Presentation

Accidental overdose of haloperidol in 24 children led to disturbance in consciousness, tremors, hyperreflexia, akathisia, opisthotonus, oculogyric crisis, and drooling. Most patients recover, but some may retain extrapyramidal side effects.[5]

Laboratory

Analytical Methods

Gas chromatography is sensitive to 500 μg/L.[3] Because of the high volume of distribution and the relatively low serum concentration of haloperidol, measurements are restricted to high-sensitivity methods of analysis including radioimmunoassay, gas chromatography, and high-performance liquid chromatography with electrochemical detection.[4]

Blood Levels

Establishing a definitive relationship between serum haloperidol concentrations and therapeutic effect has been difficult. For those patients who respond to haloperidol, a serum concentration of at least 5 ng/mL is advisable to ensure a positive response.[4] A maximum serum haloperidol level of 28 ng/mL was associated with haloperidol toxicity in an accidental haloperidol poisoning in 24 children.[2] Side effects increased in incidence with plasma concentrations greater than 6 ng/mL at 12 to 14 hours after the final administration.

Abnormalities

Transient thrombocytosis, elevated serum transaminase levels, and electrocardiographic evidence of a prolonged QT interval have been described.

Ancillary Tests

Hair analysis (distal segment) for haloperidol may provide data helpful in evaluation of haloperidol regimens and compliance.[6]

Treatment

1. Respiratory and circulatory competence should be established.
2. Respiratory depression may require assisted ventilation.
3. Hypotension and circulatory collapse should be treated by the use of intravenous fluids plasma expanders.
4. Sympathomimetic vasoconstriction with beta-adrenergic agonists (e.g., epinephrine) may aggravate hypotension or arrhythmias.
5. Gastric lavage should be performed if the patient is seen within 4 hours of ingesting the drug.
6. Activated charcoal may be useful, but no systematic study has been devoted to its evaluation.
7. There is no antidote.
8. Anticholinergic and antiparkinsonian medications given parenterally may relieve extrapyramidal reactions.
9. Vital signs and the electrocardiogram should be monitored for signs of QT prolongation or dysrhythmias. Monitoring should continue in-hospital until the electrocardiogram is normal for 24 hours.
10. Severe arrhythmia should be treated with appropriate antiarrhythmic agents.
11. Forced diuresis, hemodialysis, and hemoperfusion will most likely be ineffective (high volume of distribution).

REFERENCES—HALOPERIDOL

1. Eyles DW, McLennan HR, Jones A, et al. Quantitative analysis of two pyridinium metabolites of haloperidol in patients with schizophrenia. Clin Pharm Ther 1994;56:512–520.
2. Yoshida I, Sakaguchi Y, Matsuishi T, et al. Acute accidental overdosage of haloperidol in children. Acta Paediatr 1993;82:855–880.
3. Dollery C, ed. *Therapeutic Drugs.* Edinburgh: Churchill Livingstone, 1991:H1–H4.
4. Lawson GM. Monitoring of serum haloperidol. Mayo Clin Proc 1994;69:189–190.
5. Sinaniotis CA, Spyrides P, Vlachos P, Papdatos C. Acute haloperidol poisoning in children. J Pediatr 1978;9:1038–1039.
6. McMullin MM, Selavka CM, Wheeler MT, et al. Forensic hair testing for haloperidol: A tale of two cases. In: *Proceedings, American Academy of Forensic Sciences, 46th Annual Meeting, San Antonio, February 14–19, 1994:* Abstract 3.

METHOTRIMEPRAZINE

In Europe, methotrimeprazine (levomepromazine) is widely used as an antipsychotic drug.[1,2] In the United States it is usually employed as an analgesic. Methotrimeprazine in overdose may lead to death.[3] Treatment of overdose is largely supportive and symptomatic.

Structure and Classification

Levomepromazine is marketed as Nozinon and Veractil in the United Kingdom and Levoprome in the United States. Structures of methotrimeprazine and its metabolites are shown in Fig. 40–2.[4]

Use

Methotrimeprazine has been suggested for the control of symptoms in patients dying of advanced cancer.[5] It may have a use in the treatment of migraine.[6]

Product Formulation

Methotrimeprazine hydrochloride is available for intramuscular use in the United States (20 mg methotrimeprazine/mL with benzyl alcohol 0.9% and sodium metabisulfite 0.3%).[7] Nozinon contains 25 mg of methotrimeprazine maleate.

Source

Methotrimeprazine is a chemical synthetic product.

Therapeutic Dose

The tablets may be given in doses of 25 to 50 mg daily. The initial dose may be increased to 100 to 200 mg, divided into three doses. It may be increased to a total of 1 g daily as required.[8]

II I III

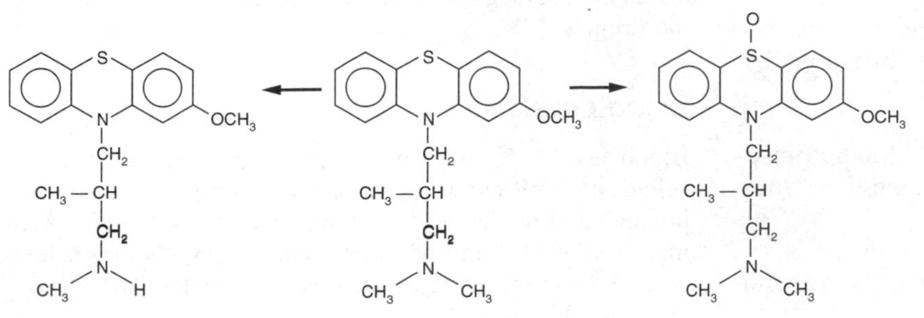

S N OCH$_3$ CH$_2$ CH$_3$—CH CH$_2$ N CH$_3$ H

S N OCH$_3$ CH$_2$ CH$_3$—CH CH$_2$ N CH$_3$ CH$_3$

O S N OCH$_3$ CH$_2$ CH$_3$—CH CH$_2$ N CH$_3$ CH$_3$

Figure 40–2 Structures of methotrimeprazine **(I)**, *N*-monodesmethyl methotrimeprazine **(II)**, and methotrimeprazine sulfoxide **(III)**. (From Dahl SG, Bratlid T, Lingjaerde O. Plasma and erythrocyte levels of methotrimeprazine and two of its nonpolar metabolites in psychiatric patients. Ther Drug Monit 1982;4:81–87.)

Fatal Dose

Ingestion of 1100 and 5000 mg of methotrimeprazine was fatal in a 24-year-old woman and a 54-year-old woman, respectively.[9]

Toxicokinetics

Absorption

The bioavailability of the oral dose is 50% that of the intramuscular dose.[10] The plasma concentration of methotrimeprazine (after a 25-mg intramuscular injection) peaks at 22 to 29 ng/mL after 30 to 90 minutes. Following a single oral dose of 50 mg, peak plasma methotrimeprazine concentrations of 16 to 40 ng/mL are reached after 1 to 4 hours. Methotrimeprazine sulfoxide concentrations of 14 to 63 ng/mL are reached in 1 to 4 hours. The concentration of the sulfoxide in plasma usually exceeds the concentration of the parent drug. Following long-term doses of 200 to 400 mg/d, the plasma levels are 36 to 40 ng/mL.[9]

Distribution

The apparent volume of distribution is 23 to 42 L/kg.[9]

Elimination

The elimination half-life of methotrimeprazine is 15 to 30 hours.[9] The half-life of the active metabolite, methotrimeprazine sulfoxide, ranges from 13 to 31 hours.[11] Less than 1% of a dose of methotrimeprazine is excreted unchanged in a 24-hour urine.[12] About 99% of the drug is eliminated within 4 to 8 days of termination of maintenance therapy.[9] The sulfoxide is pharmacologically active. Sulfoxidation may take place in the gut before the drug reaches the systemic circulation.[10] The drug is metabolized by ring sulfoxidation and *N*-demethylation.[13] The metabolites 3-OH-levomepromazine, 7-OH-levomepromazine, and *N*-desmethyllevomepromazine are pharmacologically active.[10,14]

Drug Interactions

Epinephrine. Phenothiazines can remove the pressor effects of epinephrine due to their alpha-adrenergic blocking action.

Hypotensive Agents. Methotrimeprazine has an alpha-adrenergic blocking action and may enhance the effects of hypotensive drugs.

Anticholinergic Agents. Anticholinergic activity including extrapyramidal symptoms may be increased by methotrimeprazine.

Central Nervous System Depressants. Methotrimeprazine may enhance the effects of other central nervous system depressants and alcohol.

Opiate Analgesics. Methotrimeprazine may be a useful addition to opiate analgesic use.[8]

Monoamine Oxidase Inhibitors. Unexplained fatalities have occurred in patients receiving methotrimeprazine together with pargyline and with tranylcypromine.[15]

Pregnancy/Lactation

Safe use in pregnancy and during lactation has not been established. Phenothiazines may be secreted in breast milk and induce extrapyramidal symptoms and irritability in the neonate.

Mechanism of Action

Methotrimeprazine has antidopaminergic, anadrenergic, serotoninergic, antihistaminic, and anticholinergic actions. It binds to dopamine D_2 receptors with an affinity equal to that of chlorpromazine.[14] The exact mechanism of the analgesic is not known, but the site of action does not seem to be the opiate receptors, as there is no antagonism by naloxone.[16]

Clinical Presentation

Overdose

Methotrimeprazine overdose may be manifested by seizures, severe extrapyramidal symptoms, central nervous system depression, hypotension, coma, and death.[9] Thrombocytopenia may be induced.[17] An acute respiratory distress syndrome has been described.[18]

Chronic Use

Adverse reactions to methotrimeprazine include sedation, dizziness, vomiting, weakness, orthostatic hypotension, hepatotoxicity, agranulocytosis, extrapyramidal symptoms, and weight gain.[6]

Laboratory

Analytical Methods

High-performance liquid chromatography (HPLC) with electrochemical detection is used to analyze levomepromazine in plasma and urine. The limit of detection is 100 pg at a concentration of 500 μg/L.[19] Gas chromatography–mass spectrometry (GC–MS) has been used to detect the drug and several of its non-hydroxylated metabolites in plasma and urine.[20,21] *O*-demethylated and ring-hydroxylated metabolites are identified in the urine with GC–MS.[19] A reverse-phase HPLC method based on ion-pair formation with dodecyl sulfate analyzes levomepromazine (detection limit, 15 nM) and its metabolites in serum and urine.[12] Blood levels are useful mainly for confirmation of the presence of the drug.

Blood Levels

Blood levels of 1800 ng/mL have been observed in fatal suicides.[22] Following ingestion of 500 mg of methotrimeprazine, a blood level of 3000 ng/mL was measured.[9] After ingestion of 1100 mg of methotrimeprazine, the blood level was 7500 ng/mL. A fatal dose was associated with a blood level of 700 ng/mL.[9]

Abnormalities

Electrocardiographic changes in overdose may include sinus tachycardia, atrioventricular block, left bundle-branch block, and intraventricular block.[9]

Ancillary Tests

The sulfuric acid–ferric chloride reagent (Forrest test) displays a blue-purple color in urine samples from patients receiving more than 50 to 100 mg of methotrimeprazine daily.[12]

Treatment

Stabilization

Patients with severe overdose may quickly develop severe hypotension. Treatment requires insertion of a central line, provision of oxygen, and establishment of a patent airway. Mechanical ventilation may be required. Hypotension can be managed by a supine or head-down position, intravenous fluids, or pressor amines. Epinephrine should be avoided as phenothiazines may reverse the effect of epinephrine, enhancing the hypotension. Dopamine may be of use.

Gut Decontamination

An effort should be made to provide gastric emptying. Syrup of ipecac is not advisable as seizures may intervene and emesis may induce an aspiration pneumonia.

Elimination Enhancement

The large volume of distribution largely precludes the usefulness of hemodialysis or hemoperfusion.[23]

Antidote

There is no antidote.

Supportive Measures

Hypothermia may predispose to cardiac arrhythmias. The patient should be observed for evidence of intestinal or urinary bladder distension. Seizures may be treated with diazepam.

REFERENCES—METHOTRIMEPRAZINE

1. Deshaies G, Lanteri-Laura G, Fargeon A. The therapeutic use of levopromazine in psychiatry. Ann Med Psychol 1958;5:965–979.
2. Lambert PA, Beaujard M, Achaintre A, et al. Therapeutic trials using a new phenothiazine derivative: Levomepromazine. Ann Med Psychol 1957;2:291–296.
3. Nasilowski W, Sybirska H, Gajdzinska H. Legal–medical and toxicological evaluation of 18 lethal cases of poisoning by phenothiazine derivatives. Z Rechtsmedizin 1974;74:293–299.
4. Dahl SG, Bartlid T, Lingjaerde O. Plasma and erythrocyte levels of methotrimeprazine and two of its non-polar metabolites in psychiatric patients. Ther Drug Monit 1982;4:81-87.
5. Oliver DJ. The use of methotrimeprazine in terminal care. Br J Clin Pract 1985;39:339–340.
6. Shell IG, Dufour DG, Moher D, et al. Methotrimeprazine versus meperidine and dimenhydrinate in the treatment of severe migraine: A randomized controlled trial. Ann Emerg Med 1991;20:1201–1205.
7. McEvoy GK, ed. *AHFS Drug Information 94.* Bethesda, MD: American Society of Hospital Pharmacists, 1994:1530–1531.
8. Dollery DT, ed. *Therapeutic Drugs.* Edinburgh: Churchill Livingstone 1991;1:M110–M114.
9. Freislederer A, Mallach JH, Moosmayer A. Fatal levomepromazine poisoning. Med Welt 1988;39:1473–1476.
10. Dahl SG. Pharmacokinetics of methotrimeprazine after single and multiple doses. Clin Pharmacol Ther 1976;19:435–442.
11. Dahl SG, Strandjord RE, Siggusson S. Pharmacokinetics and relative bioavailability of levomepromazine after repeated administration of tablets and syrup. Eur J Clin Pharmacol 1977;11:305-310.
12. Allgen LG, Hellstrom L, Sant'orp CJ. On the metabolism and elimination of the psychotropic phenothiazine drug levomepromazine 537 (Nozinan[R]) in man. Acta Psychiatr Scand Suppl 1963;39:366–381.
13. Johnsen H, Dahl SG. Identification of *o*-demethylated and ring-hydroxylated metabolites of methotrimeprazine (levomepromazine) in man. Drug Metab Disp 1982;10:63–67.
14. Loennechen T, Andersen A, Hals PA, Dahl SG. High performance liquid chromatographic determination of levopromazine (methotrimeprazine) and its main metabolites in serum and urine. Ther Drug Monit 1990;12:574–581.
15. Sjoqvist F. Psychotropic drugs: 2. Interaction between MAO inhibitors and other substances. Proc R Soc Med 1965;58:967–978.
16. St John AE, Born CK. Characterization of analgesic activity effects of methotrimeprazine and morphine. Res Commun Chem Pathol Pharmacol 1979;26:25–34.
17. Amore M, Montanari M, Cerisoli M. Severe immune thrombocytopenia induced by neuroleptic. Am J Psychiatry 1991;148:1266.
18. Eshel G, Usher M, Barr J, et al: Phenothiazine treatment and respiratory distress syndrome in a child. J Toxicol Clin Toxicol 1994;32;191–197.
19. Murakami K, Murakami K, Ueno T, et al. Simultaneous determination of chlorpromazine and levomepromazine in human plasma and urine by high performance liquid chromatography using electrochemical detection. J Chromatogr 1982;227:103–112.
20. Dahl SG, Garle M. Identification of nonpolar methotrimeprazine metabolites in plasma and urine by GLC–mass spectrometry. J Pharm Sci 1977;66:190–193.
21. Baselt RC, Cravey RH. *Disposition of Toxic Drugs and Chemicals in Man.* Chicago: Year Book, 1989:535–537.
22. Bonnichsen R, Geertinger P, Maehly AC. Toxicological data on phenothiazine drugs in autopsy cases. Z Rechtsmedizin 1970;67:158–169.
23. Anderson S-B, Forshell GP, Schulman A, et al. Levomepromazine elimination in patients during active and sham hemodialysis. Artif Organs 1982;7:340–343.

PIMOZIDE

Pimozide, a new antipsychotic drug, appears to be somewhat benign in overdose, although it may lower the seizure threshold and predispose to fatal cardiac arrhythmias. Treatment of overdose is largely symptomatic and supportive.

Structure and Classification

Pimozide is the first of a new series of psychotropic drugs, the diphenylbutylpiperidines.[1] Its molecular weight is 461.6. Its conversion factor to SI units is 2.16 ($\mu g/mL \times 2.16 = \mu mol/L$, $\mu mol/L \div 2.16 = \mu g/mL$).[2–4] Pimozide is structurally similar to the butyrophenones.[5]

Use

Pimozide is advocated for once daily use as maintenance therapy in chronic schizophrenia and for the treatment of psychic and functional disorders induced by personality traits.[2] It has been reported to be particularly effective in treating monosymptomatic hypochondriacal psychosis and delusional jealousy[6,7] and has been used in Tourette's syndrome.[1]

Product Formulation

Pimozide is available in tablets of 2, 4, and 10 mg as Orap.[3] It is approved for use in the United States and United Kingdom.

Source

Pimozide is a synthetic chemical product.

Therapeutic Dose

Pimozide is intended for oral administration in an initial dose of 2 to 4 mg, which may be increased until a maintenance level (usually about 6 mg) is reached. The recommended maximum daily dose is 10 mg. The recommended daily dose in patients with psychic and functional disorders is 2 mg.[2]

Toxic Dose

A 17-year-old woman ingested 100 mg and survived.[2] A 2½-year-old child ingested 60 mg and survived.[1] Two sudden deaths, possibly due to cardiac arrhythmias, followed rapid titration of pimozide dose to 70 to 80 mg daily over a 2 week period.[8]

Fatal Dose

A fatal dose has not been established.

Toxiconetics

Absorption

Pimozide is slowly absorbed from the gastrointestinal tract, reaching a peak plasma level of about 5 ng/mL (after 0.86 mg orally) in approximately 8 hours. A 2-mg dose is followed by peak plasma levels of 18 to 20 ng/mL in about 3 to 6 hours.[2]

Elimination

Pimozide is metabolized in the liver by oxidative *N*-dealkylation to two main metabolites, both of which are inactive.[1,2,9] About 1% of a dose is excreted as unchanged pimozide and about two thirds as 4-bis(4-fluorophenyl)butyric acid.[2] The plasma half-life is about 18 hours in healthy volunteers. The half-life reached 53 hours in a study of chronic schizophrenic patients.[10] Pimozide is excreted in breast milk.

Drug Interactions

Pimozide may potentiate the action of drugs that have central nervous system depressant or sedative activities such as barbiturates, narcotic analgesics, antihistamines, alcohol, and other antipsychotic drugs. Pimozide may antagonize the action of anticonvulsant drugs.[2] Anticholinergic agents may be synergistic with pimozide, increasing anticholinergic activity. Antidepressants may increase sedative, hypotensive, and anticholinergic effects. Propranolol and cimetidine may decrease hepatic metabolism of pimozide, increasing clinical and toxic effects. As pimozide may lead to prolongation of the QT_c interval, extra caution is required when prescribing pimozide in combination with drugs such as antidepressants and antiarrhythmic agents.[11] Concurrent therapy with phenothiazines or chloral hydrate may have been a predisposing factor in three fatal cardiac disorders in patients less than 37 years old.[2]

Pregnancy/Lactation

Controlled studies have not been performed in pregnant or lactating women.

Mechanism of Action

Pimozide is a selective blocker of dopaminergic (D_2) receptors at central, probably striatal, sites. It has lesser effects on blocking serotonin and α_1-adrenergic receptors, and weakly antagonizes muscarinic acetylcholine receptors.[1,2]

Clinical Presentation

A 17-year-old woman ingested 100 mg of pimozide. Following gastric lavage, the patient exhibited only slight tremors of the extremities, with all laboratory and electroencephalographic studies remaining normal.[2] A 2½-year-old child who ingested pimozide 60 mg experienced mild extrapyramidal symptoms that later resolved.[3] Two sudden deaths were observed in schizophrenic patients whose doses were titrated up to 70 to 80 mg/d over a 2-week period. Cardiac arrhythmia was suspected as the cause of death in both cases.[8] A 6-year-old boy ingested 100 mg, developed a prolonged QT_c interval, and survived.[12]

About 10 to 15% of patients experience extrapyramidal symptoms (eg, tremor, rigidity, salivation, and masked facies).[1] Tinnitus and anticholinergic effects such as blurred vision and dry mouth are observed. Infrequently reported effects include anorexia, nausea, abdominal pain, diarrhea, constipation, hypotension, sedative, drowsiness, insomnia, anxiety, agitation, excitement, hallucinatory experience, amenorrhea with glactorrhea, focal swelling, edema of the eyelids, and erythematous rashes. Most are dose related and have occurred when the daily dose exceeded 10 mg.[2] Three patients had epileptiform seizures while receiving pimozide.[11] Prolongation of the QT_c interval may lead to life-threatening arrhythmias such as torsade de pointes.[5]

Laboratory

Analytical Methods

Plasma pimozide levels may be estimated by a radioimmunoassay technique with which the major metabolites of pimozide do not interfere.[13] The detection limit is 50 pg/mL.

Blood Levels

Blood levels are not easily available in most hospital laboratories. They can be used to confirm drug presence, but there is no evidence that they would be useful in guiding management. Four people found dead had pimozide blood levels within the therapeutic range.[14] A 6-year-old who ingested 200 mg (100 2-mg tablets) had a serum pimozide concentration of 18 ng/mL.

Abnormalities

Pimozide has been associated with electrocardiographic abnormalities including prolongation of the QT_c interval and torsade de pointes,[15] as well as T-wave and U-wave abnormalities.[11]

Ancillary Tests

Eosinophilia and increased lactate dehydrogenase, aspartate transaminase, and cholesterol levels were observed in a few patients in one study.[1,10]

Treatment

Stabilization

Patients should be provided with immediate access to an intravenous line, cardiac monitor, and oxygen, and observed for sudden seizures and possible development of torsade de pointes. Special attention should be given to airway patency (tidal volume), respiration, and circulation. Treatment is largely symptomatic and supportive. After an overdose, patients should be carefully observed for up to 4 days before consideration is given to discharge.

Gut Decontamination

Gastric lavage may be useful with tracheal protection. Use of syrup of ipecac for emesis induction is not advised because of the possible depression of the seizure threshold with pimozide.

Elimination Enhancement

There is no evidence to support the use of extracorporeal methods of elimination (hemodialysis, hemoperfusion) in pimozide poisoning.

Antidote

There is no antidote.

Supportive Measures

Excessive dosage may lead to prolongation of the QT_c interval with precipitation of torsade de pointes. Torsade de pointes is treated with magnesium sulfate followed by pacing and connecting electrolyte abnormalities. Such patients should be carefully monitored until the electrocardiogram is within normal limits for at least 24 hours.

Seizures may be managed with diazepam. Patients should be carefully followed for deepening of sedation. Dystonias can be treated with intravenous diphenhydramine. Mechanically assisted ventilation may be required. Hypotension and circulatory collapse should be treated with intravenous fluids, plasma, or concentrated albumin and vasopressor agents such as metaraminol, phenylephrine, and norepinephrine. Epinephrine should not be used.[16]

REFERENCES—PIMOZIDE

1. Colvin CL, Tankonow RM. Pimozide: Use in Tourette's syndrome. Drug Intell Clin Pharm 1985;19:421–424.
2. Pinder RM, Brogden RM, Sawyer PR, et al. Pimozide: A review of its pharmacological properties and therapeutic uses in psychiatry. Drugs 1976;12:1–40.
3. Reynolds JEF, ed. *Martindale: The Extra Pharmacopoeia.* 30th ed. London: Pharmaceutical Press, 1993:610–611.
4. Dollery CT, ed. *Therapeutic Drugs.* Edinburgh: Churchill Livingstone, 1991:P-111–P114.
5. Opler LA, Feinberg SS. The role of pimozide in clinical psychiatry: A review. J Clin Psychiatry 1991;52:221–233.
6. Holmes VF. Treatment of nonsymptomatic hypochondriacal psychosis with pimozide in an AIDS patient. Am J Psychiatry 1989;164:554–555.
7. Debray P, Messerschmitt P, Longchamp D, Herbault M. The use of pimozide in pediatric psychiatry. Presse Med 1972; 1:2917–2918.
8. Shapiro AK, Shapiro E, Fulop G. Pimozide treatment of tic and Tourette disorders. Pediatrics 1987;79:1032–1039.
9. McCreadie RG, Heykants JJP, Chalmers A, Anderson AM. Plasma pimozide profiles in chronic schizophrenics. Br J Clin Pharmacol 1979;7:533–534.
10. Kline F, Burgoyne RW, Yamomoto J. Comparison of pimozide, trifluoroperazine as once-daily therapy in chronic schizoprenic outpatients. Curr Ther Res 1974;16:696–705.
11. Fulop G, Phillips RA, Shapiro AK, et al. ECG changes during haloperidol and pimozide treatment of Tourette's disorder. Am J Psychiatry 1987;144:673–678.
12. Salness RA, Goetz CM, Gorman RL, et al. Two cases of pimozide ingestion. Vet Hum Toxicol 1992;34:334.
13. Michiels LJM, Heykants JJP, Knaeps AG, Janssen JAJ: Radioimmunoassay of the neuroleptic drug pimozide. Life Sci 1975;16:937–944.
14. Peclet C, Rousseau JJ, Gaudet M, Picotte P. Four cases involving pimozide. Bull Int Assoc Forens Toxicol 1991;21: 26–28.
15. Krahenbuhl SI, Sauter B, Kupferschmidt H, et al. Reversible QT prolongation with torsade de pointes in a patient with pimozide intoxication. Am J Med Sci 1995;309:315–316. Case Report.
16. *Physicians' Desk Reference.* 49th ed. Montvale, NJ: Medical Economics, 1995:2510–2513.

REMOXIPRIDE

Remoxipride is a substituted benzamide neuroleptic drug with few anticholinergic effects. It is a dopamine receptor (D_2) antagonist. In overdose it may be fatal. Treatment is symptomatic and supportive. Following a number of reports of the association of aplastic anema with remoxipride use, the Committee on Safety of Medicine in the United Kingdom recommended monitoring for blood dyscrasias.[1–4] Subsequently, the manufacturer withdrew the product from the worldwide market, but the drug is available for compassionate use for those patients who are refractory to conventional schizophrenic therapy.[1,2]

REFERENCES—REMOXIPRIDE

1. Kerwin R. Adverse reaction reporting and new antipsychotics. Lancet 1993;342:1440.
2. Laidlaw ST, Snowden JA, Brown MJ. Aplastic anemia and remoxipride. Lancet 1993;342:1244–1245.
3. Philpott NJ, Marsh JCW, Gordon-Smith EC, Bolton JS. Aplastic anemia and remoxipride. Lancet 1993;342:1244–1245.
4. Murphy PT, Sivakumaran M, Ghosh K, et al. Cytopenia and remoxipride. Lancet 1994;343:352–353.

THIORIDAZINE

Thioridazine (Melleril, Mellaril) is a phenothiazine with potent anxiolytic and antipsychotic properties. The side effect profile of thioridazine is well documented. The most frequent side effects are sedation and orthostatic hypotension. As with other phenothiazines, arrhythmia may rarely develop in patients treated with thioridazine.[1]

Toxic Dose

Patients have survived after ingestion of 10 g of thioridazine and have died after as little as 1500 mg/d.[2]

Mechanism of Action

The electrophysiologic effects of thioridazine and other phenothiazine tranquilizers are similar to those of quinidine and include a decrease in the maximum rate of rise of action potential during phase 0 depolarization, a depression in the amplitude and duration of phase 2, and prolongation of phase 3 repolarization. The resulting electrocardiographic changes are a prolonged QT interval, flattening or depression of the T wave, and an increase in U-wave amplitude. Actions of thioridazine are numerous and include antagonism of cholinergic, α_1-adrenergic, dopamine (D_2), histamine (H_1), and serotonin-2 receptors.

Clinical Presentation

The most frequent feature after an acute overdose is impairment of consciousness. Clinical features of toxicity vary but often include progression of somnolence to a comatose state. Syncope may result within hours of ingestion. Hyperthermia may or may not be present. Both hypertensive and hypotensive syndromes have been reported. Hypotension can be explained in part by potent peripheral alpha-adrenergic blockade and may be managed by volume replacement and alpha agonists. Cardiac manifestations include prolonged QT interval, T-wave changes, varying degrees of atrioventricular block, sinus and ventricular tachycardia (including torsade de pointes), and asystole. Thioridazine may exert a quinidine-like effect on ventricular repolarization and may inhibit sinoatrial or atrioventricular nodal cholinergic stimulation. The persistent third-degree atrioventricular block in one patient was somewhat different relative to previously reported cases.[2] Compared with other neuroleptic drugs, thioridazine has been shown to be more likely to cause tachycardia, prolonged QT interval, prolonged QT_c, widened QRS complex (>100 milliseconds), and arrhythmias.[3]

Treatment

Management of thioridazine overdose includes prevention or limitation of intestinal drug absorption, airway maintenance, and supportive and therapeutic treatment of cardiovascular and neurologic complications.[2] Hypotension resistant to physical measures should be controlled by dopamine infusion combined, if needed, with inotropic drugs.[1] Treatment of ventricular tachyrhythmias associated with a prolonged QT interval should include rapid correction of metabolic and electrolyte disturbances (eg, hypokalemia and hypomagnesemia). Isoproterenol can be administered to shorten the QT interval in patients without severe coronary artery disease. Intravenous magnesium may be the drug of choice in managing torsade de pointes.[2]

Thioridazine in high doses exhibits a beta-adrenoceptor and a calcium channel blocking effect; drugs with these types of properties are contraindicated. Amiodarone may facilitate torsade de pointes and, therefore, should be used with caution. Lidocaine-like agents are often ineffective, even if electrolyte imbalance is corrected. In addition, these types of drugs may not prevent recurrence. It would appear that the most appropriate treatment of thioridazine-induced arrhythmias is temporary pacing. This cardiac pacing should last approximately 10 days, especially in patients who present with ventricular tachycardia associated with atrioventricular block I or II.[1]

REFERENCES—THIORIDAZINE

1. Le Blaye I, Donatini B, Hall M, Krupp P. Acute overdosage with thioridazine: A review of the available clinical exposure. Vet Hum Toxicol 1993;35:147–150.
2. Hulisz DT, Dasa SL, Black LD, Heiselman DE. Complete heart block and Torsade de pointes associated with thioridazine poisoning. Pharmacotherapy 1994;14:239–245.
3. Buckley NA, Whyte IA, Dawson AH. Cardiotoxicity more common in thioridazine overdose than with other neuroleptics. Clin Toxicol 1995;33:199–204.

ZUCLOPENTHIXOL

Zuclopenthixol (Fig. 40–3) is a thioxanthene with general properties similar to those of phenothiazine and chlorpromazine.[1,2] Extrapyramidal reactions and sedation may follow

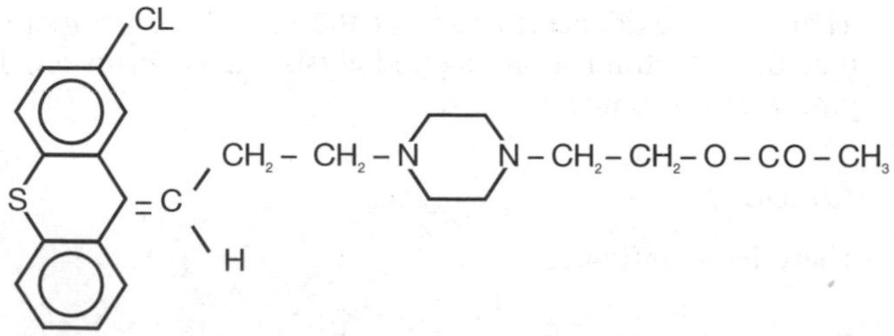

Figure 40–3 Structure of zuclopenthixol acetate (From Matar AM, Abdel-Mawgoud M, Skov S. Zuclopenthixol: A new generation of antipsychotic drugs: An open clinical trial. J Clin Psychopharmacol 1990;10:283–286.)

an overdose. Treatment is symptomatic and supportive (see Treatment under Neuroleptic Drugs in General). No fatalities have been reported.

Structure and Classification

Zuclopenthixol decanoate is structurally related to fluphenazine decanoate.[3] *cis(Z)*-Clopenthixol is the neuroleptically active isomer of clopenthixol, which is a 1:2 mixture of *cis(Z)*- and *trans(E)*-clopenthixol.[4,5] The current product used has only the *cis(Z)* isomer.[6] The *trans(E)* isomer is not active.[7] The factor for conversion to the SI system is 2.11 (ng/mL × 2.11 = nmol/L; nmol/L ÷ 2.11 = ng/mL).

Related drugs are flupenthiol (Depixol, Fluanxol) and zuclopenthixol acetate (Clopixol Acuphase). These drugs are not available in the United States. They are available in the United Kingdom and Europe.

Use

Zuclopenthixol is an antipsychotic neuroleptic drug used especially for psychotic patients with hallucinations and delusions accompanied by hostility, agitation, and increased psychomotor activity.[5–18]

Product Formulation

Zuclopenthixol hydrochloride (Clopixol) is available in 2-mg tablets for oral use. Zuclopenthixol acetate (Clopixol Acuphase) is available for intramuscular use (50 mg/mL). Zuclopenthixol decanoate (Clopinoxol) is available for intramuscular injection containing 200 ng/mL.[2]

Source

Zuclopenthixol is a synthetic chemical.

Therapeutic Dose

The usual dose of the hydrochloride for the treatment of psychosis is the equivalent of 20 to 50 mg of the base daily in divided doses. In severe schizophrenia, up to 150 mg daily has been given. Doses of the hydrochloride are expressed in terms of the base, and those of the decanoate in terms of the ester.[1] Doses of 50 to 150 mg daily of zuclopenthixol acetate appear sufficient for most acute patients.

Toxic Dose

Ingestion of zuclopenthixol hydrochloride 200 to 500 mg by a 35-year-old led to severe coma, respiratory depression, dry mouth, and abnormal vision. The patient recovered in 1½ days. A 17-month-old infant ingested 25 mg of zuclopenthixol hydrochloride and recovered after some decrease in consciousness. A 40-year-old adult ingested zuclopenthixol deconoate 500 mg (equivalent to an oral dose of zuclopenthixol 300 mg) and recovered. A 21-year-old received injections of zuclopenthixol acetate 600 mg for 6 days, in addition to 60 mg of zuclopenthixol hydrochloride orally over 2 days. The patient recovered in 9 days after a coma lasting 4 days.[19]

Toxicokinetics

Absorption

A dose of 100 mg leads to a peak serum level of 41 ng/mL after about 36 hours, decreasing to 15 ng/mL after 72 hours.[20] Steady-state serum levels of 12 to 16 ng/mL have been measured after administration of 100 mg twice daily.[7] Following an oral dose of 20 mg/d zuclopenthixol, steady-state serum concentrations of 2.8 to 12 ng/mL (7–30 nmol/L) were observed.[19]

Elimination

The mean elimination half-life is about 40 to 90 hours.

Pregnancy/Lactation

Following use of oral or intramuscular zuclopenthixol decanoate, zuclopenthixol levels in milk are about 29% of serum levels. The daily dose to a nursing infant is estimated as 0.5 to 5 μg, corresponding to a dose of 0.01 to 0.1 mg in an adult and probably insufficient to cause any side effects.[21] The ratio of milk to serum concentration is 0.12.[21]

Clinical Presentation

Therapeutic Use

The most frequently occurring side effects include dystonia, rigidity, akinesia, tremors, and reduced salivation.[8] Transient or persistent sedation has been observed in addition to weight gain or weight loss.[4]

Overdose

Very high doses of zuclopenthixol result in an exacerbation of side effects, both extrapyramidal and sedative.[22] Seizures, hyperthermia, and hypothermia may be observed. In addition, respiratory depression, anticholinergic symptoms (dry mouth, abnormal vision), hypotension, tachycardia, and hypersalivation have been observed.[19]

Laboratory

Analytical Methods

Serum concentrations of zuclopenthixol can be determined by high-performance liquid chromatography.[23] The lower limit of sensitivity is about 0.5 ng/mL.[7] A liquid chromatography method with mass spectrometry has a resolution limit of 100 pg for clopenthixol.[24]

Blood Levels

Ingestion of 2.5 g of clopenthixol led to a peak blood level of 0.90 μg/mL, about 60 times the maximum clopenthixol (*cis(Z)* + *trans(E)*) level observed after a single oral dose of 30 mg.[24] Over 7 days the level decreased to 0.04 μg/mL. Blood levels appear dose dependent.[22] Ingestion of 200 to 500 mg of zuclopenthixol hydrochloride led to a zuclopenthixol blood level of 290 ng/mL (722 nmol/L).[19] Following an intramuscular dose of zuclopenthixol acetate (600 mg in 6 days), the zuclopenthixol blood level was 1.6 ng/mL (about 4 nmol/L).

Abnormalities

Posttreatment eosinophilia, transient elevated serum triglyceride levels, and altered levels of hepatic enzymes have been seen.[4] Creatine phosphokinase does not rise[7] unless multiple injections are administered by the intramuscular route at the same site.[19] Zuclopenthixol is a potent uricosuric agent.[25] The electrocardiogram may exhibit a sinus arrhythmia or tachycardia.[19]

Treatment

Stabilization

Treatment is symptomatic and supportive and should follow guidelines for the neuroleptic drugs. Patients should be observed for adequacy of respiration (monitor tidal volume and arterial blood gases) for at least 12 to 24 hours as indicated by clinical judgment. Tracheal support (endotracheal tube) should be provided as required.

Patients with a history of significant zuclopenthixol ingestion should receive gut decontamination and an electrocardiogram. Vital signs and cardiac monitoring require admission to a hospital for at least 24 hours. Symptoms (extrapyramidal, sedative) may require observation and treatment for the first 24 to 36 hours, after which patients may be discharged provided there are no seizures, hyperthermia, coma, or respiratory depression.[19]

Gut Decontamination

Gastric lavage should be performed early (within the first 6 to 12 hours) after an overdose. Activated charcoal with a single dose of cathartics may be of use, but there are no controlled clinical studies to support their efficacy.

Elimination Enhancement

Whole-bowel irrigation may be useful in treatment of this delayed-absorption drug, but clinical studies have not yet been pursued to support this concept.

Antidote

There is no antidote.

Supportive Measures

For severe hyperthermia, maintenance of fluid and electrolyte balance and control of seizures require prompt attention (see Thermal Dysregulation under Clinical Presentation of Neuroleptic Drugs in General).

REFERENCES—ZUCLOPENTHIXOL

1. Reynolds JEF, ed. *Martindale: The Extra Pharmacopoeia.* 29th ed. London: Pharmaceutical Press, 1989:775.
2. British National Formulas. Number 24, September 1992. Zuclopenthixol dihydrochloride, p. 153; zuclopenthixol decanoate, p. 155.
3. Viala A, Ba B, Durand A, Gouezo F, et al. Comparative study of pharmacokinetics of zuclopenthixol decanoate and fluphenazine decanoate. Psychopharmacology 1988;94:293–297.
4. Serafetinides EA, Collins S, Clark ML. Haloperidol, clopenthixol and chlorpromazine in chronic schizophrenia: Chemically unrelated antipsychotics as therapeutic alternatives. J Nerv Ment Dis 1972;154:31–42.
5. Chakravarti SK, Muthu A, Muthu PK, et al. Zuclopenthixol acetate (5% in Viscolea): Single dose treatment for acutely disturbed psychotic patients. Curr Med Res Opin 1990;12:58–65.
6. Aaes-Jorgensen T. Serum concentrations of *cis(Z)*- and *trans(E)*-clopenthixol after administration of *cis(Z)*-clopenthixol and clopenthixol to human volunteers. Acta Psychiatr Scand 1986;64:64–77.
7. Aaes-Jorgensen T, Gravem A, Jorgensen A. Serum levels of the isomers of clopenthixol in patients given *cis(Z)*-clopenthixol or *cis(Z)/trans(E)*-clopenthixol. Acta Psychiatr Scand 1981;64(suppl. 294):70–77.
8. Matar AM, Abdel-Mawgoud M, Skov S. Zuclopenthixol: A new generation of antipsychotic drugs: An open clinical trial. J Clin Psychopharmacol 1990;10:283–287.
9. Amdisen A, Nielsen MS, Dencker SJ, et al. Zuclopenthixol acetate in Viscoleo[R]: A new drug formulation: An open Nordic multi-centre study of zuclopenthixol acetate in Viscoleo[R] in patients with acute psychoses including mania and exacerbation of chronic psychoses. Acta Psychiatr Scand 1987;75:99–107.
10. Gravem A, Elgen K. *cis(Z)*-Clopenthixol: The neuroleptically active isomer of clopenthixol: A presentation of five double-blind clinical investigations and other studies with *cis(Z)*-clopenthixol (Cisordinal[R], Clopixol[R]). Acta Psychiatr Scand 1981;64(suppl. 294):5–12.
11. Gravem A, Bugge A. *cis(Z)*-Clopenthixol and clopenthixol in the treatment of acute psychoses and exacerbations of acute psychoses: A double-blind clinical investigation. Acta Psychiatr Scand 1981;64(suppl. 294):13–19.
12. Sechter D, Caillard V, Cuche H, Deniker P. Open clinical study of *cis(Z)*-clopenthixol. Acta Psychiatr Scand 1981;64(suppl. 294):20–24.
13. Heikkila L, Karsten D, Valli K. A double-blind clinical investigation of *cis(Z)*-clopenthixol and clopenthixol in chronic schizophrenia patients. Acta Psychiatr Scand 1986;64(suppl. 29):25–29.
14. Heikkila L, Laitinen J, Vartianen H. *cis(Z)*-Clopenthixol and haloperidol in chronic schizophrenic patients: A double blind clinical multicentre investigation. Acta Psychiatr Scand 1981;64(suppl. 294):30–38.
15. Karsten D, Kivimaki T, Linna S-L, et al. Neuroleptic treatment of oligophrenic patients: A double-blind clinical multicentre trial of *cis(Z)*-clopenthixol and haloperidol. Acta Psychiatr Scand 1981;64(suppl. 294):39–45.
16. Gotestam KG, Ljunghall S, Olsson B. A double-blind comparison of the effects of haloperidol and *cis(Z)*-clopenthixol in senile dementia. Acta Psychiatr Scand 1981;64(suppl. 294): 46–53.
17. Gotestam KG. A geriatric rating scale empirically derived from three rating scales for geriatric behaviour. Acta Psychiatr Scand 1981;64(suppl. 294):54–63.
18. Aaes-Jorgensen T. Serum concentrations of *cis(Z)*- and *trans(E)*-clopenthixol after administration of *cis(Z)*-clopenthixol and clopenthixol to human volunteers. Acta Psychiatr Scand 1981;64(suppl. 294):64–69.
19. Larsen N, Prof Services. Personal communication, Copenhagen, Luncbeck and Co, January 6, 1993.
20. Amdisen A, Aaes-Jorgenson T, Thomsen NJ, et al. Serum concentrations and clinical effects of zuclopenthixol in acute disturbed, psychotic patients treated with zuclopenthixol acetate in Viscoleo[R]. Psychopharmacology 1986;90: 412–416.
21. Aaes-Jorgensen T, Bjorndal F, Bartels U. Zuclopenthixol levels in serum and breast milk. Psychopharmacology 1986; 90:417–418.
22. Jorgensen A, Aaes-Jorgensen T, Gravem A, et al. Zuclopenthixol decanoate in schizophrenia: Serum levels and clinical state. Psychopharmacology 1985;87:364–367.

23. Aes-Jorgensen T. Specific high-performance liquid chromatography method for estimation of *cis(Z)*- and *trans(E)*-isomers of clopenthixol and a *N*-dealkyl-metabolite. J Chromatogr 1980;183:239–245.
24. Tas AC, van der Greef J, ten Noever de Brauw MC, et al. LC/MS determination of bromazepam, clopenthixol and reserpine in serum of a non-fatal case of intoxication. J Anal Toxicol 1986;10:46–48.
25. Bloch M, Gur E, Shaler AJ. Hypouricemic effect of zuclopenthixol: A potential marker of drug compliance? Psychopharmacology 1992;109:377–378.

Chapter 41 Sedative–Hypnotic Drugs

GENERAL TREATMENT OF OVERDOSES

Stabilization

Oxygenation. A clear airway must be established and adequate ventilation maintained as required. A cuffed endotracheal tube should be inserted if gag reflex or central nervous system depression prevents adequate protection of the airway. The patient is then placed on a ventilator and arterial blood gases are monitored.

Cardiovascular System. Intravenous access must be provided and fluids (Ringer's lactate) initiated at a maintenance rate for adults of 150 mL/h. Hypotension is initially corrected with fluid boluses of 200 mL, up to 2-L positive balance or until the systolic blood pressure reaches 100 mm Hg. Vasopressors such as dopamine and levarterenol should be used if fluids do not raise the systolic blood pressure to 90 to 100 mm Hg. Patients who require vasopressors to maintain blood pressure should have hemodynamic monitoring (preferably an arterial line and pulmonary artery catheter) to guide fluid and drug management. Fluid balance is followed by inserting a Foley catheter to measure hourly urine volume, urine specific gravity, and urine electrolytes. Care must be taken not to give excessive fluids because of the propensity of sedative–hypnotic drugs to produce pulmonary edema. Reduced urine output usually results from hypovolemia so that diuretics generally are not appropriate. All obtunded patients should receive glucose and naloxone. (Thiamine also should be given to chronic alcoholics.)

Be aware that respiratory arrest may occur suddenly (eg, during lavage procedure) and that mental status may fluctuate, leading to respiratory arrest after initial lightening of coma (eg, meprobamate). Most deaths after sedative–hypnotic overdose result from progressive respiratory insufficiency secondary to either adult respiratory distress syndrome or bacterial pneumonia.[1] An elevated respiratory rate may indicate aspiration pneumonia, adult respiratory distress syndrome, or, less often, a pulmonary embolus or pneumothorax.

Gut Decontamination

Comatose patients should be lavaged only after a cuffed endotracheal tube has been inserted and the patient has been placed in the left lateral, head-down position. The initial gastric aspirate is saved for drug analysis. Coma reduces gastrointestinal mobility and this may permit effective lavage 6 to 12 hours after ingestion.

Elimination Enhancement

In general, hemoperfusion clearance is superior to hemodialysis clearance, except for long-acting barbiturates. The decision on which measure to use depends on clinical judgment based on both the drug level and the clinical response of the patient. Factors that suggest the use of hemodialysis or hemoperfusion include the failure of supportive care to maintain vital signs; the presence of underlying disease, which contraindicates a prolonged coma; and the documentation of lethal blood levels.

Antidote

Respiratory and central nervous system stimulants should not be used, as the hazards of hyperpyrexia and convulsions outweigh the benefits of such drugs.

Supportive Measures

Differential Diagnosis. Knowledge of the exact sedative drug is usually not necessary because supportive care suffices in the vast majority of cases and no safe, effective antidotes exist. Physical signs help differentiate the involved sedative–hypnotic drug.

Ethchlorvynol	Prolonged, deep coma; hypothermia; sweet odor on breath; hypotension; pulmonary edema; prolonged apnea
Glutethimide	Fluctuating coma lasting several days; anticholinergic signs; pulmonary complications
Meprobamate	Deep, fluctuating coma lasting more than 24 hours; gastric mass; hypotension; pulmonary edema
Methyprylon	Hyperthermia; tachycardia; paradoxical excitement; respiratory depression
Methaqualone	Muscle twitching; myoclonus; coma lasting 2 to 4 days; extravasation of blood (purpura, retinal hemorrhage, gastrointestinal tract bleeding)

Blood Levels. Blood levels confirm drug ingestion but rarely improve patient management, except perhaps in severe poisoning where lethal levels suggest the need for hemoperfusion. Because of tolerance, coingested drugs, large tissue stores, underlying medical disease, and (active) metabolites, clinical evaluation correlates better with outcome than blood levels. Ethanol and other sedative–hypnotic drugs should always be screened for when the clinical picture does not correlate with blood levels, as most central nervous system depressants have synergistic actions (ie, general anesthetics, alcohols, narcotics, sedative–hypnotic drugs). Excessively high blood levels may help decide on the necessity for hemodialysis or hemoperfusion.

Abnormalities. Prolonged coma (ie, >12 hours) is associated with an increased incidence of chest x-ray abnormalities (atelectasis, pneumonia, adult respiratory distress syndrome), leukocytosis with or without infection, hypoxemia, myoglobinuria, elevated serum creatine kinase, abnormal body temperature, and skin lesions.[2] The incidence of pneumonitis, however, is low even in the presence of an abnormal chest x-ray, leukocytosis, positive sputum cultures, or elevated body temperature.

Observation. Coma often lasts for days so patience is necessary as long as the vital signs remain stable. Physicians should watch for the development of complications (pulmonary edema, aspiration pneumonia, skin bullous lesions, withdrawal). The differential diagnosis of clinical deterioration in sedative–hypnotic overdose includes the following; the appropriate treatments are also listed.

Increased respiratory depression	Assisted ventilation
Hypotension	Cautious fluid repletion, dopamine/norepinephrine
Pulmonary edema	Oxygen, positive end-expiratory pressure, assisted ventilation
Hypothermia	Passive rewarming with blankets
Cerebral edema (convulsions, apnea, papilledema)	Hyperventilation, mannitol
Dysrhythmias	Lidocaine, propranolol, phenytoin

Hyperthermia is treated with cooling blankets or sponging rather than antipyretics, because antipyretics have frequently unpredictable and sometimes paradoxical effects.

Withdrawal. Most sedative–hypnotic drugs (including barbiturates, glutethimide, meprobamate, methyprylon, and chloral hydrate) produce physical and psychological dependence when taken in 3 to 10 times the sedative dose for 1 to 2 months. Abstinence syndromes produce major (psychosis, seizures, death) and minor (apprehension, sympathetic hyperactivity, weakness, anorexia, sweating, insomnia, postural hypotension) withdrawal symptoms.[3]

Any sedative–hypnotic drug, with the exception of the opiates, can be withdrawn with the use of phenobarbital or benzodiazepines because of cross-tolerance. Phenobarbital has a wider margin of safety in the setting of barbiturate withdrawal than short-acting barbiturates. The stabilizing dose of phenobarbital can be calculated by knowing its equivalency with 30 mg phenobarbital. Phenobarbital in a stabilizing dose is given for 2 days in three to four divided doses based on the drug history[4] (Wesson method). After stabilization, the phenobarbital dose is reduced 30 mg/d. If minor withdrawal symptoms develop, 200 mg of pentobarbital is administered intramuscularly and the daily phenobarbital dosage is increased by 25%. If signs of phenobarbital toxicity appear, the daily dosage is reduced by 50% and withdrawal is continued. Co-addiction to opiates should be considered in difficult cases as opiate withdrawal may be difficult to differentiate from sedative–hypnotic withdrawal.

REFERENCES—GENERAL TREATMENT OF OVERDOSES

1. Jay SJ, Johanson WG Jr, Pierce AK. Respiratory complications of overdose with sedative drugs. Am Rev Respir Dis 1975;112:591–598.
2. Glauser FL, Smith R. Physiologic and biochemical abnormalities in self induced overdosage. Arch Intern Med 1975;135: 1468–1473.
3. Khantzian EJ, McKenna GJ. Acute toxic and withdrawal reactions associated with drug use and abuse. Ann Intern Med 1979;80:361–372.
4. Smith DE, Wesson DR. Phenobarbital technique for treatment of barbiturate dependence. Arch Gen Psychiatry 1971; 24:56–60.

BARBITURATES

Pulmonary embolism has been reported following a barbiturate overdose. The patient was treated with anticoagulants and recovered.[1]

Electroencephalogram

Generally, the electroencephalogram (EEG) displays a predictable progression of changes depending on the depth of coma. In severe cases, the EEG may be isoelectric without the presence of irreversible brain damage.

Henry Matthew and colleagues identified seven grades of encephalographic activity seen in patients who had overdosed with sedatives or tricyclic antidepressants (Table 41–1).[2] EEG grades I and II appear to be associated with conscious or drowsy patients; EEG grade III and IV patients are unconscious but respond to painful stimulation. Grades V to VII are associated with deep coma. Grade VI (isoelectric record, totally unresponsive to all stimuli) can last up to 28 hours, and, in most cases, the patients make a full clinical recovery. There appears to be a correlation between the EEG guide of coma and the clinical assessment of depth of coma, body temperature, duration of coma, and serum levels of some long-lasting barbiturates and methaqualone.

Alpha activity in the EEG of some patients in coma may be normally associated with wakefulness. This apparently paradoxical combination of behavioral and electroencephalographic features has been termed *alpha coma* and is seen mainly in cases of pontomesencephalic infarction, diffuse posthypoxic cerebral cortical necrosis, toxic insult, and head injury. The prognosis in such cases is dismal. In patients who have become stuporous or comatose after a sedative–hypnotic or other toxic insult and who do not have appreciable cerebral hypoxia an EEG pattern dominated by frequencies in the alpha range is usually associated with recovery without neurologic sequelae.[3–7]

Table 41–1
Grades of Encephalographic Changes

Grade I	Alpha rhythm or predominant alpha rhythm with beta or some rare theta waves
Grade II	Predominant theta rhythm with some alpha, beta, and low-voltage delta activity
Grade III	Predominant low/high-voltage delta activity mixed with some theta waves
Grade IV	Delta activity with or without brief isoelectric intervals
Grade V	Suppression–burst activity, namely, where 3–10 cycle/s activity of several seconds' duration alternates with electrical silence
Grade VI	Near silence but with isolated and low-voltage 3–7 cycle/s waves occurring singly or in bursts of half a second
Grade VII	An isoelectric record, totally unresponsive to all stimuli

Toxicokinetics

Drug interactions affecting sodium phenobarbital concentrations are listed in Table 41–2.

Laboratory

Blood levels of sedative–hypnotic drugs are summarized in Table 41–3.

Treatment

Stabilization

1. Respiratory arrest is the major cause of early death. Assess the patency of the airway and the adequacy of ventilation first. Appropriate corrective measures include supplemental oxygen, head tilt–chin lift, intubation, and assisted ventilation.
2. Establish an intravenous line with Ringer's lactate and give a fluid challenge up to 2 L for patients who are

Table 41–2
Miscellaneous Interactions Affecting Serum Phenobarbital Concentrations

Drug	Serum Phenobarbital Concentration	Mechanism
Activated charcoal	↓	DA
Ammonium chloride	↓	Reduction in tubular reabsorption
Antacids	↓	DA
Acetazolamide	↑	INH
Chloramphenicol	↑	INH
Dextropropoxyphene	↑	INH
Dicoumarol	↓	IND
Folic acid	↓	IND
Furosemide (frusemide)	↑	INH
Methsuximide	↑	INH
Methylphenidate	↑	INH
Pheneturide	↑	INH
Pyridoxine	↓	IND?
Thioridazine	↑↓	INH/IND
Valproic acid (sodium valproate)	↑*	Decreased serum protein binding

*Free non–protein-bound concentration (however, the major effect of valproic acid is to inhibit phenobarbital metabolism).
DA, decreased absorption; IND, hepatic induction; INH, hepatic inhibition; ↑, increased concentration; ↓, decreased concentration.
From Patsalos PN, Duncan JS. Antiepileptic drugs: A review of clinically significant drug interactions. Drug Saf 1993;9:156–184.

Table 41-3
Sedative–Hypnotic Drug Blood Levels

	Blood Level (mg/100 mL)		
	Therapeutic	Toxic	Lethal
Barbiturates			
Short-acting	0.1–0.8	0.7–1.4	3–4
Intermediate-acting	0.1–0.5	1–3	3
Phenobarbital	ca. 1.0	4–6	8–15
Barbital	ca. 1.0	6–8	10–20
Chloral hydrate	1.0	10	25
Chlordiazepoxide	0.1–0.2	0.55	2
Diazepam	0.05–0.25	0.5–2.0	2.0
Ethanol	—	0.15	0.35
Ethchlorvynol	ca. 0.5	2	15
Glutethimide	0.02	1–9	3–10
Meprobamate	1	8–12	20
Methaqualone	0.5	1–3	3
Methyprylon	1.0	3–6	10
Oxazepam	0.1–0.2	—	—
Paraldehyde	ca 5.0	20–40	50

From Ellenhorn MJ, Barceloux DG. *Medical Toxicology.* New York: Elsevier, 1988:579.

hypotensive. Cardiac dysrhythmias are rare but were reported in 3 of 1140 overdose cases.[8]

3. Be sure to give glucose, naloxone, and thiamine to all patients with depressed mental status.
4. Take a careful history, estimating the amount of drugs and alcohol ingested and the time of ingestion.
5. Evaluate for trauma and signs of drug abuse.
6. Order urine, blood, and toxicology screens specifically for central nervous system depressants, stimulants, and psychoactive drugs. Obtain electrolyte and glucose levels, renal and liver function tests, and arterial pH and blood gases.

Gut Decontamination

Gastric lavage should be performed with a large-bore, double-lumen tube, preferably one with multiple distal openings. Multiple-dose activated charcoal (1 g/kg, then three doses of 0.5 g/kg 4 hours apart) was useful in a 28-day-old infant.[9]

Elimination Enhancement

Due to a tenfold error in preparing the medication, a 28-day-old male infant received an overdose of phenobarbital and presented as a floppy lethargic infant. He was treated with 3 g (1 g/kg) aqueous superactivated charcoal followed by three doses of 1.5 g (0.5 g/kg) 4 hours apart and one dose of 3 mL (1 mL/kg) 20% sorbitol, through a nasogastric tube. Twelve hours after admission, the patient was awake, alert, and normothermic.[9] The calculated elimination half-life was 11.2 hours. Data on charcoal use and dosage in infants are limited. In a newborn, multiple doses of activated charcoal reduced the half-life of phenobarbital from about 250 to 22 hours.[10]

Vale and colleagues have used 50 to 100 g oral activated charcoal followed by 50 g every 4 hours. The plasma half-life of phenobarbital is reduced from 110 to 12 hours. The mean total body clearance of 84 mL/min compares favorably with that obtained by using hemodialysis (74 mL/min) and hemoperfusion (79 mL/min). Diarrhea and constipation were the only side effects noted and depended on the type of charcoal use. This treatment should be seriously considered as a treatment of choice for severe phenobarbital poisoning.[11,12]

Supportive Measures

Patients must be monitored for complications of alkalosis and fluid overload. These include pulmonary and cerebral edema, hypokalemia, hypomagnesemia, hypernatremia, and hypocalcemia.[12] The minimum renal clearance of phenobarbital achieved by alkaline diuresis is about 17 mL/min, which compares poorly with that found with repeated dose charcoal therapy.[13]

REFERENCES—BARBITURATES

1. Toscano J, Kussin PS, Samuelson W, Fulkerson WJ. Pulmonary embolism complicating barbiturate overdose. Crit Care Med 1990;18:777–778.
2. Haider I, Matthew H, Oswald I. Electroencephalographic changes in acute drug poisoning. Electroencephalogr Clin Neurophysiol 1971;30:23–31.
3. Guterman B, Sebastian P, Sodha N. Recovery from alpha coma after lorazepam overdose. Clin Electroencephalogr 1986;12:205–208.
4. Carroll WM, Mastiglia FL. Alpha and beta coma in drug intoxication. Br Med J 1977;2:1518–1519.
5. Tomassen W, Kamphuisen HAC. Alpha coma. J Neurol Sci 1986;76:1–11.
6. Austin EJ, Wikus RJ, Longstreet WT Jr. Alpha coma with sedative overdose. Neurology 1989;38:156–157.
7. De Boer WB, Kendall PA, Breheny FX. Alpha coma and barbiturate poisoning. Anaesth Intens Care 1989;17:503–504.
8. McCarron MM, Schulze BW, Walberg CB, et al. Short-acting barbiturate overdosage correlation of intoxication score with serum barbiturate concentration. JAMA 1982; 248:55–61.
9. Amitai Y, Degani Y. Treatment of phenobarbital poisoning with multiple dose activated charcoal in an infant. J Emerg Med 1990;5:450–499.
10. Veerman M, Espejo MG, Christopher MA, Knight M. Use of activated charcoal to reduce elevated serum phenobarbital concentration in a neonate. Clin Toxicol 1991;29:53–58.
11. Vale JA, Ruddock FS, Boldy DAR. Multiple doses of activated charcoal in the management of phenobarbitone and carbamazepine poisoning. Vet Hum Toxicol 1987;29(suppl. 2):152.
12. Lindberg MC, Cunningham A, Lindberg NH. Acute phenobarbital intoxication. South Med J 1992;85:803–807.
13. Boldy DAR, Vale JA, Prescott LF. Treatment of phenobarbitone poisoning with repeated oral administration of activated charcoal. Q J Med 1986;61:997-1002.

BENZODIAZEPINES

Acute overdose toxicity has been observed more often with the short-acting benzodiazepines midazolam and triazolam and the intermediate-acting flunitrazepam than with diazepam, lorazepam, and nitrozepam.[1] Death caused by benzodiazepines alone in the absence of other significant toxicologic agents or pathology is uncommon, although benzodiazepines alone can cause death in the absence of significant natural disease or advanced age.[2] Death has been reported after flunitrazepam, diazepam, nitrazepam, alprazolam, triazolam, temazepam, and flurazepam.

Use

Benzodiazepines are used as anxiolytic agents, sedative–hypnotic agents, anticonvulsants, and muscle relaxants.

Toxicokinetics

See Table 41–4 and Figures 41–1, 41–2, and 41–3.

Pregnancy/Lactation

A causal relationship between teratogenicity and benzodiazepine use has not been established. High concentrations of diazepam and its active metabolites have been demonstrated for up to 12 days after birth in neonates whose mothers had received moderate (10–15 mg) to large (90 mg) doses of diazepam.[3] Significant depression is seen in the neonates, ranging from the floppy baby syndrome characterized by hypotonia, lethargy, respiratory depression, hypothermia, and poor reflexes to simply lethargy and poor feeding.[4] Seizures, prolonged hypotonia, and prolonged respiratory depression are seen in newborns after treatment with lorazepam.[5]

Laegreid and associates in Sweden, in a case–control study, described neurologic abnormalities in infants during the neonatal period after maternal benzodiazepine used during early pregnancy.[6] Dysmorphic features include craniofacial abnormalities including a low nasal bridge, short palpebral fissures, epicanthine folds, a short upturned nose, slightly malformed and/or low-set ears, and a hypoplastic mandible. This observation was not confirmed in another Swedish study.[7] Confounding factors may be the concomitant use of alcohol and substance abuse.[8] Additional controlled studies are required.

Benzodiazepine neonatal exposure from breast milk is about 5% of the maternal dose.[9] Withdrawal symptoms (irritability, crying, sleep disturbance, tremors, seizures) may occur in a neonate following exposure to a benzodiazepine in utero and then in breast milk. A mother ingested alprazolam for 9 months while breastfeeding; she withdrew herself over a period of 3 weeks. The baby suffered apparent withdrawal symptoms.[10] Onset of withdrawal symptoms may be delayed for 1 to 2 weeks.[11]

Children

Benzodiazepine ingestions are rarely life threatening in children. Benzodiazepine toxicity should be considered in

Table 41–4
Mean (Range) Pharmacokinetic Parameters of the Major Benzodiazepines

Drug	V_d (L/kg)	Protein binding (%)	t_{max} (h)	$t_{1/2}$ (h)	CL (L/h/kg)	Metabolism oxi	Metabolism conj	Active Metabolites
Alprazolam	0.7–1	70	1.2–1.7	12 (9–15)	0.073	x		Hydroxyprazolam
Chlordiazepoxide	0.3–0.6	95	1–4 (0.5–6)	10 (6–28)	0.012–0.030	x		Demethylchlordiazepoxide, desmethyldiazepam, oxazepam
Clobazam	0.9–1.8	90	1–4	25 (10–49)	0.024–0.036	x		Demoxepam, demethylclobazam
Diazepam	1–2	98	0.5–2	32 (14–61)	0.024–0.030	x		*N*-Desmethyldiazepam, oxazepam, 3-hydroxydiazepam
Desmethyldiazepam (active metabolites of halazepam, medazepam, pinazepam, prazepam)	0.9–1.3	98		51 (51–120)		x		Oxazepam
Flurazepam (dealkylflurazepam)			1	80 (40–200)		x		Hydroxyflurazepam, flurazepam aldehyde
Lorazepam	0.8–1.6	92	1–2	13 (8–25)	0.048–0.078		x	None
Loprazolam	4	80	1–3 (0.5–12)	11 (5–22)	0.012	x		None
Midazolam	1.1	95	0.5–1	2 (1.5–2.5)	0.240–0.488	x		1-Methylhydroxymidazolam
Nitrazepam	1.5–2.8	86	2	26 (18–48)		x		None
Oxazepam	0.5–2	97	1–4	7 (5–13)	0.036–0.174		x	None
Temazepam	1.4	97	2.4 (0.8–5)	13 (7–17)	0.060–0.084		x	Oxazepam
Triazolam	1.3	90	1.3 (0.3–4)	2.5 (2–5)	0.222–0.528	x		1-Methylhydroxytriazolam

V_d, apparent volume of distribution; t_{max}, time to peak plasma concentration; $t_{1/2}$, elimination half-life; CL, total drug clearance; oxi, oxidation; conj, conjugation.
From Gaudreault P, Guay J, Thivierge RL, Verdy I. Benzodiazepine poisoning: Clinical and pharmacological considerations and treatment. Drug Saf 1991;6:247–265.

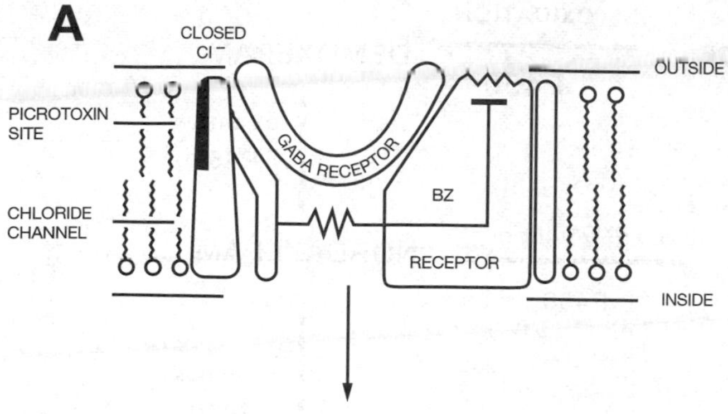

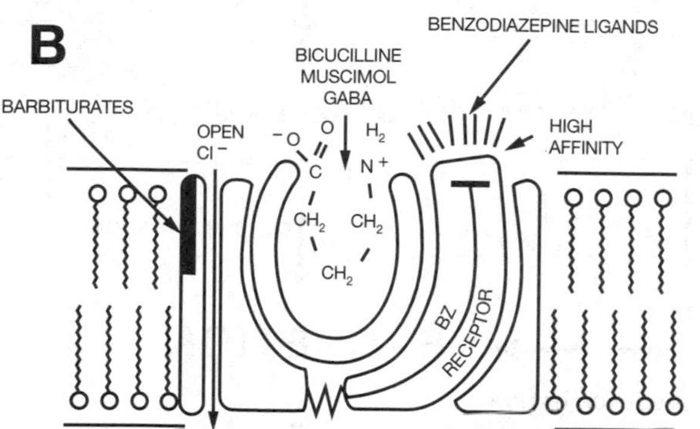

Figure 41-1 GABA$_A$/benzodiazepine receptor–chloride ionophore complex. Receptors are depicted for GABA, barbiturates, and benzodiazepine ligands. GABA receptor agonists (eg, GABA, muscimol) and GABA receptor antagonists (eg, bicuculline) bind to GABA$_A$ receptors; barbiturates are thought to bind to specific recognition sites near the chloride ionophore; benzodiazepine receptor agonists (eg, diazepam), benzodiazepine receptor antagonists (eg, flumazenil), and benzodiazepine receptor inverse agonists (eg, 6,7-dimethoxy-4-ethyl-3-carbomethoxy-β-carboline) bind to benzodiazepine receptors. **A.** Receptor complex in an inactivated state with the Cl^- channel closed. **B.** Receptor complex in an activated state with the Cl^- channel open. Activation is induced by GABA or GABA agonists binding to GABA receptors or by barbiturates. Activation of the receptor complex is associated with conformational changes and the opening of the Cl^- channel. Consequent entry of Cl^- into the neuron results in hyperpolarization. The frequency of chloride channel opening in the presence of GABA is increased by benzodiazepine receptor agonists. GABA, γ-aminobutyric acid; BZ, benzodiazepine. (From Amrein R, Hetzel W. Pharmacology of drugs frequently used in ICU's: Midazolam and flumazenil. Intens Care Med 1991;17:S1–S10.)

the differential diagnosis of isolated ataxia. Deliberate parent administration must be considered in children with benzodiazepine ingestions.[12]

Mechanism of Action

Stimulation of the γ-aminobutyric acid b (GABA$_b$) receptors opens the chloride ion channel in the receptor complex and thereby increases conductance of chloride ion across the nerve cell membrane. This reduces the potential difference between the inside and outside of the cell and blocks the ability of the cell to conduct nerve impulses[13] (Fig. 41–1). (See Flumazenil in this chapter.)

Clinical Presentation

Alprazolam

The therapeutic dose is 0.25 to 1 mg. Following ingestion of 10 mg of alprazolam, a 34-year-old exhibited dangerously aggressive behavior.[14] Five months later he presented with evidence of major depression. Other reactions that have been observed include mania, amnesia, agitation, depersonalization, and perceptual distortion. Two patients who attempted suicide with alprazolam ingested 20 to 30 1-mg tablets and 60 1-mg tablets, respectively.[15] Therapeutic plasma levels of alprazolam are about 20 to 30 ng/mL. The patients described had serum alprazolam levels 10 times greater following therapeutic doses. Neither patient demonstrated any alteration in vital signs or central nervous system depression. Both recovered. In three apparent cases of suicide by alprazolam ingestion, postmortem concentrations averaging 230 ng/mL were observed.[16]

Bromazepam

A 36-year-old man was found dead with blood bromazepam concentration of 51 ng/mL.[17] A 60-year-old woman was found dead with a blood bromazepam level of 5 μg/mL.[18] Serum bromide levels may be increased in patients who ingest bromazepam. This may be associated with a decrease in the anion gap.[19]

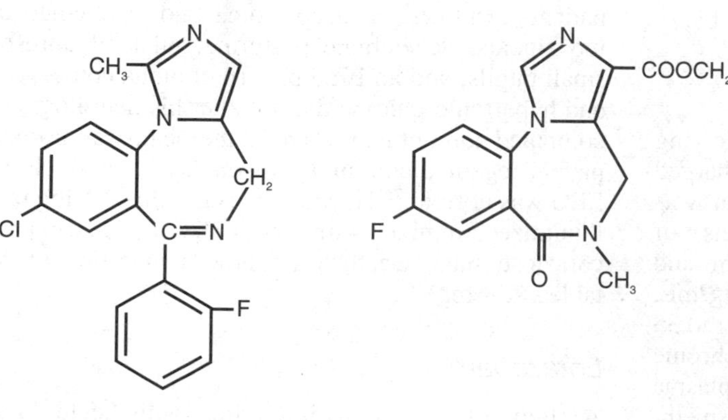

Figure 41-2 Chemical structures of midazolam and flumazenil. Midazolam is a 1,4-benzodiazepine that acts as an agonist at the benzodiazepine receptor. Flumazenil is a 1,4-imidazobenzodiazepine that acts as an antagonist (and weak partial agonist) at the benzodiazepine receptor. The relationship of flumazenil to benzodiazepine agonists is analogous to the relationship between naloxone and opiates such as morphine. (From Jones EA, Gammal SH, Martin P. Hepatic encephalopathy: New light on an old problem. Q J Med 1988;69:851–867.)

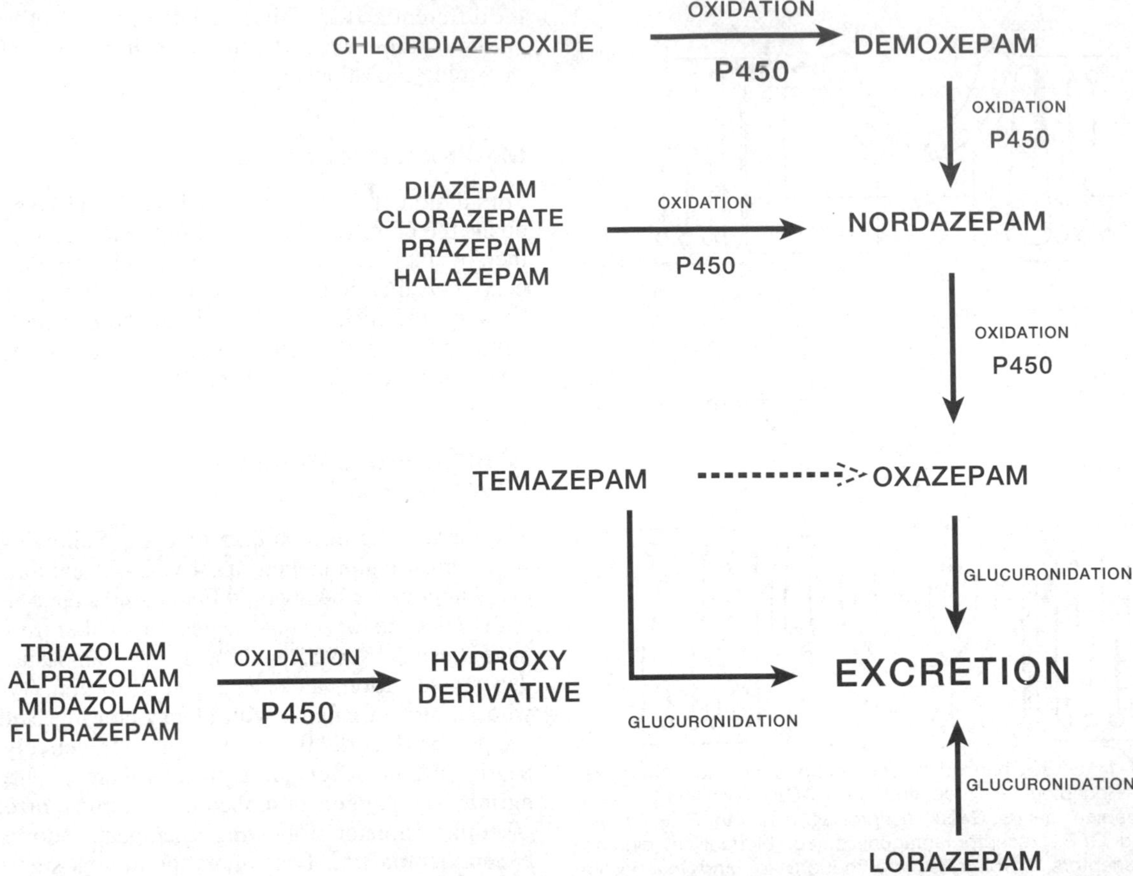

Figure 41-3 Basic metabolic pathways leading to benzodiazepine elimination in humans. Oxidation P450 indicates metabolism by hepatic cytochrome P450 mixed-function oxidase system. Broken arrow indicates possible metabolic pathway. Compared with oxidation, glucuronidation is generally rapid and unaffected by impaired liver function. (From Skinner MH, Thompson DA. Pharmacologic considerations in the treatment of substance abuse. South Med J 1992;85:1207–1219.)

Chlordiazepoxide

A 45-year-old woman was administered 5.2 g of chlordiazepoxide (CDX) and, 4.5 days after cessation of therapy, presented in coma with respiratory depression. She was treated with assisted ventilation and survived. Toxicity appeared to be due to the blood concentration of a metabolite of CDX, demoxepam.[20] The active metabolites of CDX are desmethyl-CDX, demoxepam, nordazepam, and oxazepam. All influence the toxicologic potency of CDX when the concentration of demoxepam falls below 10 µg/mL. The patient was able to extubated. Below 1 µg/mL, transfer from the intensive care unit to an ordinary ward is possible.[20]

Diazepam

A 58-year-old man ingested 1250 mg of diazepam following which preexisting delusions ceased.[21] He was discharged after receiving supportive care. A 25-year-old man was found dead with an empty blister pack (10 tablets) of diazepam nearby. The concentrations of diazepam and metabolites in the blood were (diazepam) 3.7 µg/mL, (desmethyldiazepam) 1.6 µg/mL, (oxazepam, free) 0.35 µg/mL, and (temazepam, free) 0.25 µg/mL.[22] After chronic oral doses of 30 mg three times daily, steady-state plasma diazepam concentrations average 1.03 µg/mL and desmethyldiazepam 0.43 µg/mL.[23]

Estazolam

Ten attempted suicides with estazolam (ProSom, 4 to 10 mg) (therapeutic dose, 1–2 mg) led to coma and respiratory depression in two patients, one of whom required assisted ventilation. All were discharged from the hospital within 4 days.[24]

Flunitrazepam

A 60-year-old man was found unconscious after ingesting 25 2-mg tablets of flunitrazepam (therapeutic dose, 2 mg). The patient exhibited a deep coma, no spontaneous limb movements, decerebrate posturing, bilateral unresponsive small pupils, and an EEG pattern of alpha coma. Naloxone and hypertonic glucose did not alter his neurologic state. A computed tomography scan of the head was normal. The patient regained consciousness on day 2, at which time the EEG was normal.[25] Heyndrickx states that 3 4-mg tablets of flunitrazepam mixed with food, milk, or juice can produce a comatose state. Death has followed ingestion of 7 to 14 tablets (28 mg).[26]

Lorazepam

A study of 277 of 425 children with acute lorazepam (Ativan) intoxication showed that a mean ingested dose of 1 mg/kg (therapeutic dose, 2–6 mg/d in adults) led to central nervous system depression (drowsiness or coma). Nausea and vomiting were observed in 35 children. None experienced respiratory depression. Agitation and hallucinations, observed in children more than adults, were present in 32 of the children.[27] A 70-year-old patient ingested 100 mg of lorazepam, exhibited an alpha coma rhythm on the EEG, and recovered in 2 days.[28] The fatal adult dose may be about 1.85 g.[29] A 6-year-old boy ingested 30 mg of lorazepam, was treated by gastric lavage, and hallucinated 4 hours later. Within 27 hours the child was alert without abnormal neurologic signs and was discharged.[30]

Midazolam

A 20-year-old received 110 mg of midazolam and 1180 mg of lidocaine by intravenous infusion over 16 hours. She died in 25 hours. The blood level of midazolam was 800 μg/L.[31] The plasma midazolam concentration required to obtain a sedative effect is about 400 μg/L.[32] A 25-year-old chronic alcoholic received a dose of 2850 mg (therapeutic dose, 1–2 mg) of midazolam (Versed) over 5 days for the treatment of delirium tremens. Respiratory depression was not observed. On the fifth day he became conscious and oriented. Tachycardia and diaphoresis resolved.[33]

A 71-year-old man inadvertently received midazolam 5 mg intraarterially. Saline 10 mL was administered. No adverse effects resulted.[34] As of March 31, 1990, domestic (U.S.) midazolam-associated cardiorespiratory deaths reported to the manufacturers totaled 81 patients. Routes of midazolam administration were intravenous, 69; intramuscular, 8; intravenous and intramuscular, 1; and intranasal, 1.[35] Prolonged sedation of infants with intravenous midazolam, especially those infants receiving concomitant fentanyl or aminophylline therapy, or in the presence of hypotension, may sometimes lead to a reversible encephalopathy.[36]

Nitrazepam

Nitrazepam (Mogadon) is an epileptic medication that has not been approved for use in the United States. Side effects in young children include drooling, aspiration, hypotonia, and lethargy. Unexplained deaths occurred in six children with a mean age of 27.8 months who received an initial dose of 0.3 to 0.6 mg/kg/d nitrazepam.[37] Six cases of fatal overdose (therapeutic dose, 5–10 mg) have been reported, one of which involved the ingestion of 250 mg of nitrazepam. Blood concentrations of 1.2 to 1.9 mg/L were observed (therapeutic level, 0.035–0.084 mg/L).[38]

Oxazepam

Oxazepam (Serax) is the 3-hydroxy metabolite of nordiazepam. It is administered orally in doses of 30 to 60 mg. A 75-year-old man ingested 200 mg of oxazepam and became comatose; he responded for a few minutes to flumazenil 1 mg. Spontaneous recovery was observed 24 hours later. Skin blisters appeared on the forearm the next day and regressed spontaneously 9 days later.[39] A 2-year-old girl ingested 90 mg of the drug. Eighteen hours after ingestion, the serum oxazepam concentration was 0.5 mg/L at which time the patient was lethargic (therapeutic concentration, 0.31 mg after one 15-mg dose of oxazepam). The patient recovered.

Triazolam

Anecdotal reports of triazolam-associated amnesia,[29,40] anxiety, bizarre behavior, confusion, depression, paranoid reactions, hallucinations, hostility, and delusions with special sensitivity in the elderly[41] appeared during the late 1980s. The manufacturer reduced the recommended dose from 1 to 0.5 to 0.25 mg. The Food and Drug Administration issued new labeling, which was approved in November 1991, emphasizing triazolam use for short-term (7–10 days) treatment of insomnia. They consider a dose of 0.125 mg adequate for geriatric or debilitated patients.[42]

Triazolam (Halcion) has been used as a hypnotic drug in doses as low as 0.125 mg.[43,44] Following an oral dose of 0.25 mg, a mean peak plasma concentration of 30 μg/L is achieved within 0.75 to 15 hours.[45] A 53-year-old man was found dead after ingesting 46 0.125-mg tablets of triazolam; his serum triazolam level was 140 μg/L.[46] A 76-year-old woman found dead after ingesting triazolam had a blood triazolam concentration of 47 mmol/L.[47] A 58-year-old woman ingested 70 0.25-mg triazolam tablets, became unconscious, and died; her blood triazolam concentration was 870 nmol/L (peak therapeutic concentration, 50 nmol/L).[48] A 36-year old woman ingested 5 mg of triazolam, only two times the usual therapeutic dose, and was found unresponsive; she later recovered. Overdose has been reported to the manufacturers with doses from 2 to 20 mg resulting in lethargy and coma.[49]

On October 2, 1991, all products containing triazolam were withdrawn from the market in the United Kingdom because adverse effects reported over the years appeared more marked with triazolam than other benzodiazepines. These include anxiety between doses and rebound insomnia on ending treatment, serious paradoxical reactions such as aggression, excitation and features of psychosis, marked mental impairment, and fatal overdose.[50]

Elderly

Juergens observes that all benzodiazepines can cause memory-related problems.[51] In most studies, the ability of patients to learn new information is impaired (anterograde amnesia) after benzodiazepine therapy. Anterograde amnesia becomes more severe with increased dose, faster absorption, intravenous administration, and higher potency of the benzodiazepines. Elderly patients are more sensitive than young patients to the effects of benzodiazepines on memory. The long-term use of benzodiazepines in elderly patients commonly exacerbates underlying dementia and may cause excessive morbidity. Elderly patients seem to be at increased risk of benzodiazepine-induced psychomotor impairment, and the impairment may gradually worsen with stable therapeutic levels. Use of alcohol and high doses of benzodiazepines and administration of other drugs such as anticholinergic agents are associated with increased sensitivity for cognitive and psychomotor effects.

Table 41–5
Comparison of Syndromes Related to Benzodiazepine Withdrawal

Syndrome	Symptoms	Course
Acute sedative–hypnotic-type withdrawal	Anxiety, insomnia, nightmares, seizures, psychosis, hyperpyrexia, death	Onset: 1–2 d after stopping short-acting benzodiazepines; 2–4 d after stopping long-acting benzodiazepines
Subacute, prolonged benzodiazepine withdrawal	Anxiety (including somatic manifestations) insomnia, nightmares, muscle spasm, psychosis	Symptoms begin 1 d after stopping benzodiazepines; can continue for weeks to months, but will improve with time
Symptom reemergence	Varible but should be the same as symptoms prior to taking benzodiazepines	Symptoms emerge when benzodiazepine is stopped and will continue unabated

From Landry MJ, Smith DE, McDuff DR, Baughman OL III. Benzodiazepine dependence and withdrawal: Identification and medical management. J Am Board Fam Pract 1992;5:167–175.

Withdrawal

Landry and associates have provided some useful definitions.[52] Benzodiazepine abuse is defined as benzodiazepine use that causes impairment and dysfunction in the patient's social, occupational, emotional, psychological, or physical well-being. The impairment and dysfunction range from mild to severe and often are self-limiting. Benzodiazepine addiction is a chronic, progressive, pathologic process with biopsychosocial components that generally include (1) a compulsion to use a benzodiazepine, (2) loss of control over benzodiazepine use (or over drug-induced behavior), and (3) continued use of the drug despite adverse consequences. In contrast, benzodiazepine dependence relates to the development of physical tolerance and withdrawal.[52]

Benzodiazepine withdrawal syndromes are described in Table 41–5.[52] Typically, symptoms develop 1 to 11 days after withdrawal (average, 3–4 days) and usually are minor compared with those of ethanol and barbiturate withdrawal. Symptoms include anxiety, insomnia, headache, muscle spasm, anorexia, vomiting, nausea, tremor, postural hypotension, and weakness. A spectrum of affective disorders (psychosis, agitation, confusion, hallucinations, delirium) and motor dysfunction (tremor, restlessness, myoclonic jerk, seizures) may develop in serious cases after withdrawal from high daily doses (60–300 mg).[53,54] Seizures are rare and most commonly develop 7 to 8 days after withdrawal (range, 2–12 days). The most common symptoms in minor to moderate withdrawal are mood swings and convulsion. Withdrawal symptoms usually peak in 5 to 6 days and resolve by 4 weeks, but minor symptoms may persist for months.[55] The presence of tinnitus, involuntary movements, or perceptual changes helps differentiate benzodiazepine withdrawal from anxiety.[56,57]

Rebound insomnia may occur after sudden withdrawal of short-acting benzodiazepines (eg, lorazepam),[58] perhaps because of a lag in replacement of endogenous benzodiazepine compounds. Recent studies in Britain indicate that benzodiazepines may produce pharmacologic dependence at the therapeutic dosage, but the syndrome is atypical with little drug-seeking behavior, rapid tolerance, or escalation of dosage.[59] Nonspecific withdrawal symptoms can last for months with unusual perceptual distortions as well as quite prominent somatic symptoms.[60]

Table 41–6
Determination of Benzodiazepines in Blood by Gas Chromotography With Electron Capture Detection

Species	Detection Limit (µg/mL)	Recovery (%)	Linearity (µg/mL)
Brotizolam	0.008	40	0–10
Flunitrazepam	0.02	45	0–8
Midazolam	0.03	60	0–12
Triazolam	0.04	43	0–8

Laboratory

Toxicologic screening is inconsistent in identifying children with known benzodiazepine ingestion.[8]

Gas chromatography–mass spectrometry methods are available to analyze diazolo- (chlordiazepoxide, clorazepate, diazepam, temazepam, prazepam, halazepam) and triazolo- (alprazolam, triazolam, midazolam) benzodiazepines in the urine. The limits of detection are 50 ng/mL for all the diazolobenzodiazepines and 5 to 20 ng/mL for the triazolobenzodiazepines.[61]

Benzodiazepines are also analyzed by gas chromatography with electron capture detection (GC-ECD). Most benzodiazepines are strongly protein bound. The analytical method must determine the free fraction rather than the total because drug clearance, distribution, biotransformation, and toxicity refer to the free fraction in the blood. Artifacts may be introduced by heparin or plasticizers on storage for extended periods. The analytical characteristics of the method for fast-acting benzodiazepines have been studied by Wong and Lee in Hong Kong and are summarized in Table 41–6.[62]

Treatment

Antidote

Single intravenous doses of aminophylline 1 to 2 mg/kg may reverse the sedation induced by diazepam, lorazepam, flunitrazepam, flurazepam, and midazolam. The longer

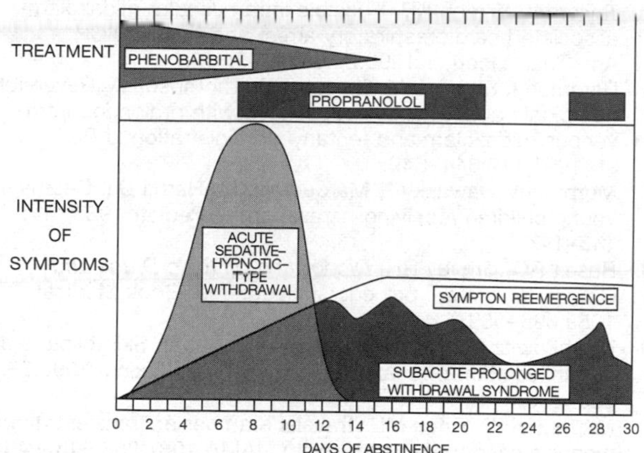

Figure 41-4 Treatment of benzodiazepine withdrawal syndromes. (From Smith DE, Wesson DR. Benzodiazepine dependency syndromes. J Psychoactive Drugs 1983;15:85–95, as adapted by Landry MJ, Smith DE, McDuff DR, Baughman OL III. Benzodiazepine dependency and withdrawal: Identification and medical management. J Am Board Fam Pract 1992;5:167–176.)

Table 41-7
Benzodiazepine Equivalency

Benzodiazepine	Dose (mg)
Chlordiazepoxide	25
Clonazepam	2
Diazepam	5
Oxazepam	30
Flurazepam	15
Lorazepam	1
Triazolam	0.5
Chlorazepate	3.75
Alprazolam	0.25

Landry MJ, Smith DE, McDuff DR, Baughman OL III. Benzodiazepine dependence and withdrawal: Identification and medical management. J Am Board Fam Pract 1992;5:167–175.

half-life of theophylline (4–8 hours) may be advantageous in decreasing the incidence of rebound sedation observed with the benzodiazepine antagonist flumazenil, which has a half-life of 1 hour. Further comparative studies might confirm the clinical usefulness of this concept[63–65] (see also Flumazenil).

Supportive Measures

Most patients require only medical observation. Patients who are ambulating after 6 to 8 hours of observation may be discharged after appropriate psychiatric counseling.

Withdrawal

Treatment of benzodiazepine withdrawal syndromes is depicted in Figure 41–4.[52,57] Smith and Wesson have developed a benzodiazepine equivalency scale for use in benzodiazepine withdrawal (Table 41–7).

The phenobarbital substitution technique for benzodiazepine withdrawal can be used for all benzodiazepines, benzodiazepine–polydrug combinations, polybenzodiazepine combination dependence, high-dose benzodiazepine dependence, and all sedative–hypnotic drugs. The phenobarbital substitution method uses propranolol for acute and subacute somatic complaints and symptoms. Phenobarbital is used during acute benzodiazepine withdrawal and detoxification.[53] There is, however, the possibility of developing dependency on the barbiturates.[57,66] Controlled clinical studies have not compared the relative effectiveness of phenobarbital versus chlordiazepoxide, clonazepam, or diazepam.[67] Phenobarbital withdrawal conversion for benzodiazepines is summarized in Table 41–8.

Table 41-8
Phenobarbital Withdrawal Conversion for Benzodiazepines and Other Sedative–Hypnotic Drugs

Generic Name	Dose (mg)	Phenobarbital Withdrawal Conversion (mg)
Benzodiazepines		
Alprazolam	1	30
Chlordiazepoxide	25	30
Clonazepam	2	15
Clorazepate	15	30
Diazepam	10	30
Flurazepam	15	30
Halazepam	40	30
Lorazepam	1	15
Oxazepam	10	30
Prazepam	10	30
Temazepam	15	30
Barbiturates		
Amobarbital	100	30
Butabarbital	100	30
Butalbital	50	15
Pentobarbital	100	30
Secobarbital	100	30
Glycerol		
Meprobamate	400	30
Piperidinedione		
Glutethimide	250	30
Quinazoline		
Methaqualone	300	30

From Smith DE, Wesson DR. Benzodiazepine dependency syndromes. J Psychoactive Drugs 1983;15:92.

REFERENCES—BENZODIAZEPINES

1. Meier PJ, Wyss PA, Radovanovic DI. Differential acute overdose toxicity of various benzodiazepine derivatives. Vet Hum Toxicol 1993;35:338.
2. Drummer OH, Syrjanen ML, Cordner SM. Deaths involving the benzodiazepine flunitrazepam. Am J Forens Med Pathol 1993;14:238–243.
3. Cree JE, Meeger J, Hailey DM. Diazepam in labor: Its metabolism and effect on clinical condition and thermogenesis in the newborn. Br Med J 1973;4:251–260.
4. Roman TSR, Krishnamurthy L. Diazepam intoxication in neonates. Indian Pediatr 1993;30:377–379.
5. Reiter PD, Stiles AD. Lorazepam toxicity in a premature infant. Ann Pharmacother 1993;27:727–730.
6. Laegried L, Olegard R, Conradi N, et al. Congenital malformations and maternal consumption of benzodiazepines: A case control study. Dev Med Child Neurol 1990;32: 432–444.

7. Bergman V, Boethius G, Swartling PG, et al. Teratogenic effects of benzodiazepine use during pregnancy. J Pediatr 1990;116:490–492.
8. Bergman V, Rosa FW, Baum C, et al. Effects of exposure to benzodiazepines during fetal life. Lancet 1992;340:694–696.
9. Dusci LJ, Good SM, Hall RW, Ilett KF. Excretion of diazepam and its metabolites in human milk during withdrawal from combination high dose diazepam and oxazepam. Br J Clin Pharmacol 1990;29:123–126.
10. Sutton LR, Hinderliter SA. Diazepam abuse in pregnant women on methadone maintenance: Implications for the neonate. Clin Pediatr 1990;29:108–111.
11. Anderson PO, McGuire GG. Neonatal alprazolam withdrawal: Possible effect of breast feeding. DICP Ann Pharmacother 1989;23:614.
12. Wiley J, Wiley C. Benzodiazepine ingestions in children. Clin Toxicol 1995;33:475–486 (Abstract 87).
13. Gaudreault P, Guay J, Thivierge RL, Verdy I. Benzodiazepine poisoning: Clinical and pharmacological concentrations and treatment. Drug Saf 1991;6:247–265.
14. French AP. Dangerously aggressive behavior as a side effect of alprazolam. Am J Psychiatry 1989;146:276.
15. McCormick SR, Nielsen J, Jatlow PI. Alprazolam overdose: Clinical findings and serum concentrations in two cases. J Clin Psychiatry 1985;416:247–248.
16. Munoz M, Johnson R. Suicide by alprazolam (Zanax[R]). Calif Assoc Toxicol Newslett, Summer 1988:28–29.
17. Kintz P, Boukhabza A, Tracqui A, et al. Tissue disposition after bromazepam, secobarbital and amobarbital self poisoning. Bull Int Assoc Forens Toxicol 1991;21:34–38.
18. Brehmer C, Hem PX. A fatal bromazepam poisoning. Bull Int Assoc Forens Toxicol 1992;24(4):21–22.
19. Kosnett M, Larson S, McCarthy T, Osterloh J. Investigation of an anion gap of minus 88 in a patient taking bromazepam. Clin Chem 1990;36:1040.
20. Minder EI. Toxicity in a case of acute and massive overdose of chlordiazepoxide and its correlation to blood concentration. Clin Toxicol 1989;27:117–127.
21. Sandvik H. Clearance of paranoid schizophrenic delusions after diazepam. Lancet 1991;337:237–238.
22. Goenechea S, Brzezinka H, Holtz J. A fatal case involving diazepam. Bull Int Assoc Forens Toxicol 1988;20:19–20.
23. Van der Kleijn E, van Rossum JM, Mustens ETJM, Rijntjes NVM. Pharmacokinetics of diazepam in dogs, mice and humans. Acta Pharmacol Toxicol 1971;29:109–127.
24. Dumont D, Mathe D, Piva C. Poisoning by a new benzodiazepine estazolam (France). Med Leg Toxicol 1980;23:257–259.
25. Deleu D, de Keyser J. Flunitrazepam intoxication simulating a structure brainstem lesion. J Neurol Neurosurg Psychiatry 1987;50:236–237.
26. Heyndrickx B. Fatal intoxication due to flunitrazepam. J Anal Toxicol 1987;11:278.
27. Garnier R, Medernach C, Harbach S, Fournier E. Agitation and hallucination in children with acute lorazepam poisoning: Report of 65 cases. Ann Pediatr 1984;3:286–289. [in French]
28. Guterman B, Sebastian P, Sodha N. Recovery from alpha coma after lorazepam overdose. Clin Electroencephalogr 1981;12:205–208.
29. Bixler EO, Kalis A, Manfredi RC, et al. Next-day memory impairment with triazolam use. Lancet 1991;337:827–831.
30. Jeffrey DI, Whitfield MF. Lorazepam poisoning. Br Med J 1974;2:719.
31. Bogusz M. Fatal lidocaine and midazolam overdose in the course of diphenhydramine poisoning therapy. Bull Int Assoc Forens Toxicol 1992;22:32–33.
32. Crevat-Pisano P, Dragna S, Granthil C, et al. Plasma concentrations and pharmacokinetics of midazolam during anaesthesia. J Pharm Pharmacol 1986;38:578–582.
33. Lineaweaver WC, Anderson K, Hing DN. Massive doses of midazolam infusion for delirium tremens without respiratory depression. Crit Care Med 1988;16:294–295.
34. Marsch SCU, Schafer HG. Accidental intraarterial injection of midazolam through a 3-way stopcock in arterial line. Anesthetist 1990;39:337–338.
35. Taylor JW, Simon KB. Possible intramuscular midazolam-associated cardiorespiratory arrest and death. DICP Ann Pharmacother 1990;24:695–697.
36. Bergman I, Steeves M, Burchart G, Thompson A. Reversible neurologic abnormalities associated with prolonged intravenous midazolam and fentanyl administration. J Pediatr 1991;119:644–649.
37. Murphy JV, Sawasky F, Marquardt KM, Harris DJ. Deaths in young children receiving nitrazepam. J Pediatr 1987;111:145–147.
38. Baselt RC, Cravey RH. *Disposition of Toxic Drugs and Chemicals in Man.* 3rd ed. Chicago: Year Book Medical, 1989:598–599.
39. Moshkowitz M, Pines A, Finkelstein A, et al. Skin blisters as a manifestation of oxazepam toxicity. Clin Toxicol 1990;28:383–386.
40. Marris HH III, Estes ML. Traveler's amnesia: Transient global amnesia secondary to triazolam. JAMA 1987;258:945–946.
41. Greenblatt DJ, Harmatz JS, Shapiro L, et al. Sensitivity to triazolam in the elderly. N Engl J Med 1991;324:1691–1698.
42. New Halcion labeling. FDA Med Bull 1992;22(1):7–8.
43. Wretlind M, Pilbrandt A, Sundwell A, Vessman J. Disposition of three benzodiazepines after single oral administration in man. Acta Pharmacol Toxicol 1977;40:28–39.
44. Zileli MS, Teletor F, Deniz S, et al. Oxazepam intoxication simulating non-ketotic diabetic coma. JAMA 1986;21:1971.
45. Baktir G, Fisch HV, Huguenin P, Bircher J. Triazolam concentration effect relationships on healthy subjects. Clin Pharmacol Ther 1983;24:195–201.
46. Robins AJ. A fatality due to carbon monoxide poisoning associated with triazolam overdose. Bull Int Assoc Forens Toxicol 1990;20(3):18–20.
47. Sunter JP, Bal TS, Cowan WK. Three cases of fatal triazolam poisoning. Br Med J 1988;297:719.
48. O'Dowd JJ. Fatal triazolam poisoning. Br Med J 1988;297:1048.
49. Olson KR, Yin L, Osterloh J, Tani A. Coma caused by trivial triazolam overdoses. Am J Emerg Med 1985;3:210–211.
50. The sudden withdrawal of triazolam: Reasons and consequences. Drug Ther Bull 1991;29:89–90.
51. Juergens SM. Problems with benzodiazepines in elderly patients. Mayo Clin Proc 1993;68:818–820.
52. Landry MJ, Smith DE, McDuff DR, Baughman OL III. Benzodiazepine dependence and withdrawal: Identification and medical management. J Am Board Fam Pract 1992;5:167–176.
53. Leung FW, Guze PA. Diazepam withdrawal. West J Med 1983;138:98–101.
54. Preskorn SH, Denner LJ. Benzodiazepines and withdrawal psychosis. JAMA 1977;237:36–38.
55. Higgitt AC, Lader MH, Fonagy P. Clinical management of benzodiazepine dependence. Br Med J 1985;291:688–690.
56. Busto U, Sellers EM, Naranjo CA, et al. Withdrawal reaction after long-term therapeutic use of benzodiazepines. N Engl J Med 1986;315:854–859.
57. Smith DE, Wesson DR. Benzodiazepine dependency syndromes. J Psychoactive Drugs 1983;15:85–95.
58. Walsh JK, Schweitzer PK, Parwatikar S. Effects of lorazepam and its withdrawal on sleep, performance and subjective states. Clin Pharmacol Ther 1983;34:496–500.
59. Ashton H. Benzodiazepine withdrawal: An unfinished story. Br Med J 1984;288:1135–1140.
60. Tyrer PJ. Benzodiazepines on trial. Br Med J 1984;288:1601–1602.
61. Mule SJ, Casella GA. Quantitation and confirmation of the diazolo- and triazolobenzodiazepines in human urine by gas chromatography/mass spectrometry. J Anal Toxicol 1989;13:179–184.
62. Wong Y-S, Lee C-W. Fatalities involving fast-acting benzodiazepines in Hong Kong. In: Kaemp B, ed. *Proceedings, 29th International Meeting of International Association of Forensic Toxicologists Copenhagen, June 1991:*418–434.
63. Bonfiglio MF, Daste JF. Clinical significance of the benzodiazepine–theophylline interaction. Pharmacotherapy 1991;11:85–87.
64. Gallen JS. Aminophylline reversal of midazolam sedation Anesth Analg 1989;69:260–268.

65. Katz Y, Goviah M. Aminophylline reversal of diazepam intoxication. Lancet 1989;1:1990–1991.
66. Treatment of benzodiazepine dependence. Lancet 1987;1: 78–79. Editorial.
67. Roy-Byrne PP. Benzodiazepine dependence. J Am Board Fam Pract 1992;5:245–247. Editorial.

CHLORAL HYDRATE

Chloral hydrate 30 mg/kg rectally every 2 hours was effective in the treatment of status epilepticus in adults when other conventional anticonvulsants (diazepam, diphenylhydantoin, sodium valproate, and fluobarbital) were ineffective. This observation requires confirmation in a controlled study.[1] Animal studies suggest that chloral hydrate, a reactive metabolite of trichloroethylene, a known carcinogen, may itself be potentially carcinogenic. Clinical studies have not indicated any evidence of carcinogenicity in humans.[2]

Clinical Presentation

Case reports of patients who have taken overdoses of chloral hydrate have three recurring features in common: the high mortality of an overdose when this is accompanied by arrhythmias, repeated failure of antiarrhythmic therapy, and abolition or suppression of arrhythmias with beta blockade.[3]

Dependence

High-dose long-term use results in tolerance and physical dependence. Sudden withdrawal results in a serious abstinence syndrome similar to delirium tremens (seizures and psychosis) and responds to barbiturates or other sedative–hypnotic drugs.

Childhood Sedation

Repetitive dosing of chloral hydrate is of concern because of accumulation of the metabolites, trichloroethanol and trichloracetic acid, which may produce excessive central nervous system depression, predispose newborns to conjugated and unconjugated hyperbilirubinemia, decrease albumin binding of bilirubin, and contribute to metabolic acidosis.[4]

Laboratory

A gas chromatographic method with electron capture detection allows the identification and quantitation of chloral hydrate and both its metabolites, 2,2,2-trichloroethanol and trichloroacetic acid.[5]

Treatment

Gut Decontamination

Controlled studies that support or refute the use of multiple doses of activated charcoal in overdose with chloral hydrate do not exist.[3]

Antidote

An adult who ingested 10 g of chloral hydrate became unconscious with respiratory depression and hypotension. The pupils were constricted. Intravenous naloxone (0.4 mg × 4 doses) produced no improvement. Flumazenil 200 μg followed at 1-minute intervals by three further 100-μg doses produced a dramatic response with an increased level of consciousness, verbalization, and pupillary dilation. The respiratory rate returned to normal. Further controlled studies are required to establish this as a specific treatment for chloral hydrate overdose.[6]

Supportive Measures

Bretylium may be an effective alternative to lidocaine and beta blocker therapy for ventricular arrhythmias.[7]

There have been no controlled trials of antiarrhythmic therapy in chloral hydrate overdose. Most anecdotal case reports indicate that (1) the mortality rate is high after an overdose of chloral hydrate when this is accompanied by arrhythmias, (2) standard antiarrhythmic therapy may often fail, and (3) arrhythmias may be abolished or suppressed with beta blockade, which may be the treatment of choice for life-threatening arrhythmias.[2]

REFERENCES—CHLORAL HYDRATE

1. Lampi Y, Eshol Y, Gilad F, Saroua-Pinchas I. Chloral hydrate in intractable status epilepticus. Ann Emerg Med 1990;19: 674–676.
2. Salmon AG, Kizer WW, Zeise L, et al. Potential carcinogenicity of chloral hydrate: A review. Clin Toxicol 1995;33:115–121.
3. Graham SR, Day RO, Lee R, Fulder GWO. Overdose with chloral hydrate: A pharmacological and therapeutic review. Med J Aust 1988;149:668–688.
4. Committee on Drugs and Committee on Environmental Health, American Academy of Pediatrics. Use of chloral hydrate for sedation in children. Pediatrics 1993;92:471–473.
5. Meyer E, Van Bocxlaer JF, Lambert WE, et al. Determination of chloral hydrate and metabolites in a fatal intoxication. J Anal Toxicol 1995;19:124–126.
6. Donovan KL, Fisher DJ. Reversal of chloral hydrate overdose with flumazenil. Br Med J 1989;298:1253.
7. Kovacs G, Gerau R, Dreyer J, et al. Bretylium in the treatment of chloral hydrate induced ventricular arrhythmias. Vet Hum Toxicol 1993;35:339.

CHLORMETHIAZOLE

Chlormethiazole was developed following studies that demonstrated that the thiazole portion of the thiamine (vitamin B_1) molecule had sedative and anticonvulsant properties.[1,2] It has been a popular drug for alcohol withdrawal in the United Kingdom, but, as with all sedative and hypnotic drugs used in treating alcohol withdrawal, it may induce tolerance, dependency, and potentially lethal interactions with alcohol.[3,4] Overdoses with chlormethiazole are not infrequent in this population group and may be fatal. Intravenous use may cause death from respiratory depression.[5] Treatment is largely symptomatic and supportive.

Structure and Classification

Chlormethiazole is a thiazole derivative, related to the thiazole part of the vitamin B_1 (thiamine) molecule.[6,7]

The conversion factor for the chlormethiazole base is 6.18 (μg/mL) × 6.18 = μmol/L; μmol/L ÷ 6.18 = μg/mL.

The conversion factor for chlormethiazole edisylate is 1.95 (μg/mL) × 1.95 = μmol/L; μmol/L ÷ 1.95 = μg/mL.

Use

Chlormethiazole has been used as a sedative–hypnotic drug, as an anticonvulsant (eg, in status epilepticus), as an aid in withdrawal from alcohol and other drugs,[3] and in the treatment of acute alcoholic toxicity (eg, delirium tremens).[7] Alcoholics may ingest 3 to 12 chlormethiazole tablets daily for many years, although they continue to drink heavily.[8] Chlormethiazole has also been used intravenously in the treatment of preeclampsia as a sedative and anticonvulsive agent.[1]

Product Formulation

Chlormethiazole edisylate is available in the United Kingdom and elsewhere in capsules (192 mg), as a syrup (250 mg/5 mL), for intravenous infusion (8 mg/mL in bottles of 500 mL), and as a tablet (500 mg, Heminevrin). It is also marketed as Distraneurine and Hemineurin.[6]

Source

Chlormethiazole edisylate is a synthetic chemical product.

Therapeutic Dose

The usual hypnotic dose is 1 or 2 capsules (192 or 384 mg of the base). For alcohol withdrawal the patient is hospitalized and may be given 9 to 12 capsules, or the equivalent, divided into four doses on the first day; the dosage is gradually reduced over the following 5 days.[4,6] Administration over 7 days may induce dependence.[7] Alcohol abuse may lead to a continual increase in the dose of chlormethiazole required to produce the desired effect, that is, reducing the excitatory state that characterizes withdrawal from alcohol. Some alcoholics may take more than 25 g daily.[9]

Toxic Dose

One patient ingested 90 capsules (192 mg base), equivalent to 17,280 mg of chlormethiazole base, and survived.[8] An intravenous dose of 4000 mg was administered inadvertently to a preeclamptic patient over 30 minutes; she recovered.[1] An adult ingested 15 tablets (75 g) of chlormethiazole and survived.[2]

Fatal Dose

One patient died within 1 hour of ingesting 10 g of the drug.[10] A 39-year-old man who may have ingested 50 tablets (192 mg base each) of chlormethiazole, a total of 9600 mg of the base, together with alcohol, was found dead.[11]

Toxicokinetics

Absorption

Absorption is rapid from the gastrointestinal tract, with peak plasma concentrations of 0.58 (ages 25–28 years) to 1.90 (age 70 years) μg/mL reached about 40 minutes to 1 hour, respectively, following administration of 600 mg of chlormethiazole ethanedisulfonate.[12] About 70% of chlormethiazole is bound to plasma proteins. The maximum systemic bioavailability of an orally administered dose is about 15% due to significant first-pass hepatic extraction.[13] Intravenous infusion of 1.20 to 2.25 g of chlormethiazole ethanedisulfonate at rates varying from 11.9 to 25.0 mg/min gave rise to plasma concentrations between 0.3 and 40 μg/ml at the cessation of infusion.

Distribution

The average volume of distribution is about 5 L/kg.[13] The elimination half-life of chlormethiazole is about 4 to 6 hours.[12,13] The half-lives of the two metabolites, 5-acetyl-4-methylthiazole (AMT) and 5-(1-hydroxyethyl)-4-methylthiazole, are about 5.5 hours and 18 hours, respectively.[12] The pharmacologic activity of the metabolites is not known. Less than 5% of chlormethiazole appears unchanged in the urine after extensive metabolism by a first-pass effect in the liver. Plasma clearance is about 23 mL/min/kg.[13]

Drug Interactions

Alcohol increases the bioavailability of chlormethiazole probably by altering its extensive first-pass hepatic metabolism.[14,15] Chlormethiazole-induced depression can be additive to the action of other central nervous system depressant drugs (eg, barbiturates, other sedative–hypnotic drugs, anesthetics, opiates, alcohols).

Pregnancy/Lactation

Chlormethiazole crosses the placenta.[1] Respiratory depression has been observed in neonates whose mothers received intravenous chlormethiazole for preeclampsia.[1] It is cleared from the neonatal circulation slowly. Data on chlormethiazole in breast milk are not available.

Mechanism of Action

Chlormethiazole has hypnotic, anxiolytic, and anticonvulsant properties similar to those of the barbiturates and probably has a similar mechanism of action, although this has not been elucidated.

Clinical Presentation

Patients who have been exposed to an oral overdose of chlormethiazole may be admitted in deep coma, with absent muscle tone or deep tendon reflexes, respiratory depression, hypotension, hypothermia, and an increase in salivation. Tachycardia is often present with normal bowel sounds. Aspiration pneumonitis is a frequent concomitant.[8] After intravenous use, transient burning sensations in the face, sneezing, phlebitis proximal to the infusion site, and hypothermia (seen in both preeclamptic mothers and neonates) have been observed.[1] Known alcoholics may be found dead with empty bottles of chlormethiazole nearby.[11,16]

Laboratory

Analytical Methods

A gas chromatography method for the underivatized drug is available using mass spectrometry sensitive to 1 ng.[12] Detection methods using flame ionization and nitrogen–phosphorus detection are also available.[10] Liquid chromatography has also been used.

Blood Levels

Plasma levels from nine adult patients in coma who ingested an overdose of chlormethiazole ranged from 8 to 66 μg/mL.[17] In one series, patients admitted in coma had plasma levels of 7 to 36 μg/mL, whereas those admitted still conscious had levels up 11.5 μg/mL. All survived.[8] Deaths were associated with plasma levels up to 60 μg/mL without evidence of ethanol and of up to 18 μg/mL with ethanol levels present.[16] Blood levels roughly correlate with dose ingested and clinical course, but are useful largely for confirmation of diagnosis.

Ancillary Tests

Electrocardiograms in one series of overdose patients who survived were all normal.[8] Baseline laboratory tests should include a complete blood count, serum electrolytes, serum hepatic transaminases, and serum creatinine.

Treatment

Stabilization

Severe intoxication with chlormethiazole resembles barbiturate coma. Immediate protection of the airway, ventilation, and circulation should be provided together with administration of glucose, naloxone, and thiamine. An intravenous line, oxygen, and cardiac monitor should be provided. Mechanical ventilation may be required.

Gut Decontamination

Although chlormethiazole has a rapid absorption half-life, fatalities reveal residuals of many tablets in the stomach. In view of the long elimination half-life, an attempt should be made to institute gastric emptying in the first 6 to 8 hours postingestion in obtunded patients after endotracheal intubation. There are no data to support the use of whole-bowel irrigation, cathartics, or activated charcoal.

Elimination Enhancement

Chlormethiazole has a high degree of protein binding (70%) and is extensively distributed (5 L/kg). This would tend to preclude forced diuresis, peritoneal dialysis, hemodialysis, or hemoperfusion. In one patient, less than a quarter of the dose in one capsule was removed by charcoal column hemoperfusion in 5 hours.[18]

Antidote

There is no available antidote.

Supportive Measures

Patients who have ingested an overdose of chlormethiazole may remain in coma for up to 4 days.[8] Patients should be observed for development of aspiration pneumonia and respiratory arrest. Respiratory depression may require intubation and assisted ventilation. Hypotension unresponsive to fluid infusions may require pressor amines. Hemodynamic monitoring should be instituted as required, similar to treatment following a barbiturate overdose.

REFERENCES—CHLORMETHIAZOLE

1. Tischler E. Intravenous chlormethiazole in the management of severe pre-eclampsia. Aust NZ J Obstet Gynaecol 1973;13:137–142.
2. Burmeister H, Ibe K, Beyer K-H. Klinik under toxicologie einer akuten chlormethiazole (Distraneurin®)-intoxikation. Arch Toxikol 1966;22:137–149.
3. McInnes GT. Chlormethiazole and alcohol: A lethal cocktail. Br Med J 1987;194:592.
4. Shaw GK. Chlormethiazole and alcohol: A lethal cocktail. Br Med J 1987;294:975.
5. Chich J. Delirium tremens. Br Med J 1989;298:3–4.
6. Reynolds JEF, ed. *Martindale: The Extra Pharmacopoeia.* 30th ed. London: Pharmaceutical Press, 1993:371.
7. Glatt MM. Chlormethiazole ("Heminevrin"). Prescribers J 1966;5:90–91.
8. Illingworth RN, Stewart MJ, Jarvie DR. Severe poisoning with chlormethiazole. Br Med J 1979;2:902–903.
9. Foster A. Sedatives for alcoholics. Br Med J 1977;1:1355.
10. Baselt RC, Cravey RH. *Disposition of Toxic Drugs and Chemicals in Man.* 3rd ed. Chicago: Year Book Medical, 1989:159–161.
11. Baxt R. Fatal chlormethiazole and alcohol poisoning. Bull Int Assoc Forens Toxicol 1974;14(3):31–32.
12. Nation RL, Vine J, Triggs EJ, Learoyd B. Plasma level of chlormethiazole and two metabolites after oral administration to young and aged human subjects. Eur J Clin Pharmacol 1977;12:137–145.
13. Moore RG, Triggs EJ, Shanks CA, Thomas J. Pharmacokinetics of chlormethiazole in humans. Eur J Clin Pharmacol 1975;8:353–357.
14. Neuvonen PJ, Pentikainen PJ, Jostell KG, Syvalahti E. The pharmacokinetics of chlormethiazole in healthy subjects as affected by ethanol. Clin Pharmacol Ther 1981;29:268–269.
15. Linnoila M, Mattila MJ, Kitchell BS. Drug interactions with alcohol. Drugs 1979;18:299–311.
16. Horder JM. Fatal chlormethiazole poisoning in alcoholics. Br Med J 1978;1:693–694.
17. Flanagan RJ, Lee TD, Rutherford DM. Analysis of chlormethiazole, ethchlorvynol and trichloroethanol in biological fluids by gas–liquid chromatography as an aid to the diagnosis of acute poisoning. J Chromatogr 1978;153:473–479.
18. Ferner RE, Pottage A, Ryan DW, Bateman DN. Charcoal-column haemoperfusion does not significantly enhance chlormethiazole removal. Hum Toxicol 1986;5:367–368.

ETHCHLORVYNOL

Gradual stepwise reduction from abuse levels should be carried out on an inpatient basis. A long-acting barbiturate such as phenobarbital may be substituted for ethychlorvynol (Placidyl), with one sedative dose of 30 mg of phenobarbital for each 100 mg of ethychlorvynol.[1]

REFERENCE—ETHCHLORVYNOL

1. Yell RP. Ethychlorvynol overdose. Am J Emerg Med 1990;8:246–250.

FLUMAZENIL

Flumazenil is a specific antagonist at the benzodiazepine receptor site. Its users must be carefully monitored for respiratory and circulatory compromise. It does not obviate the need for intensive symptomatic and supportive care which is required for the treatment of a benzodiazepine overdose. Deaths have followed its use in mixed overdoses. (See Chapter 5.)

Structure and Classification

Flumazenil is an imidazobenzodiazepine similar to, for example, midazolam.[1,2] The conversion factor is 3.30. To convert from SI units: nmol/L ÷ by 3.30 = ng/mL. To convert to SI units: ng/mL × 3.30 = nmol/L.

Flumazenil is marketed as R015-1788 and Anexate in Europe. In the United States, the product is available as Romazicon.[3]

Use

1. In patients being treated for tetanus, flumazenil reverses iatrogenic benzodiazepine overdose.
2. Flumazenil is ineffective when sedation is not induced, in part, by a benzodiazepine agonist.[4] It is ineffective in coma caused by tricyclic antidepressants or barbiturates alone.[5]
3. In a patient in coma because of liver disease and benzodiazepine overdose, flumazenil may facilitate the diagnosis by removal of the drug-induced component.
4. In coma due to multiple-drug overdose, flumazenil reverses the benzodiazepine component of central nervous system depression and may help in the diagnosis; however, because flumazenil is associated with such risks as seizures, arrhythmias, and withdrawal symptoms, it cannot be recommended for the patient with coma of unknown origin and a possibly mixed toxic ingestion.
5. There may be potential for use of flumazenil in the treatment of acute hepatic encephalopathy associated with an increased concentration of benzodiazepine agonist.[6–14]
6. Flumazenil reverses the sedative effects of benzodiazepines, but may not be effective in treatment of benzodiazepine-induced respiratory depression.
7. Flumazenil reverses overdose symptoms of zolpidem.[15]
8. Flumazenil lessens but does not obviate the need for endotracheal intubation in some patients. Respiratory and hemodynamic monitoring should be performed whenever flumazenil is used. It may lessen the need for gastric lavage, mechanical ventilation, arterial and urinary catheterization, frequent passive position changes, computed tomography of brain, blood culture, lumbar puncture, and electroencephalograms in selected patients.[16–18]
9. In coma of unknown cause, slow administration of flumazenil 1 to 2 mg may aid in the diagnosis of drug-induced coma involving a significant benzodiazepine effect. Positive response can obviate the need for a toxicology screen, computed tomography, and so forth. The patient can be questioned about the drugs ingested.
10. Flumazenil antagonizes some cerebral effects of volatile anesthetics in animals[19]: isoflurane,[20] but not halothane.[21]
11. In respiratory depression due to combined intake of benzodiazepine and an opioid, flumazenil will antagonize the benzodiazepine component but respiration will remain depressed due to the opioid.
12. Flumazenil permits interruption of continuous sedation for diagnostic purposes or to terminate benzodiazepine sedation definitely.
13. Cost of care may be lessened. Where indicated these procedures (see No. 9 above) should still be performed.[16–18]
14. Flumazenil has been used in the empiric treatment of nonspecific alterations in mental status, particularly in the presence of possible drug overdose.[22] Although flumazenil is effective in reversing diazepam-induced sedation, it is only partially effective in reversing diazepam-induced depression of hypoxic ventilatory drive.
15. Flumazenil may be useful where benzodiazepine sedation during regional anesthesia has become excessive or suddenly unnecessary, for example, with benzodiazepines paradoxical excitement, where prompt return to full consciousness is required in day-stay surgery.[23]

Strong Clinical Supporting Evidence for Use of Flumazenil

1. Flumazenil reverses sedation and anterograde amnesia with midazolam.[24,25] It does not reverse retrograde amnesia.[26]
2. Flumazenil stopped recurrent apnea in a neonate whose mother had ingested benzodiazepines prenatally.[27]
3. Flumazenil has been used for intraoperative arousal during spine fusion.[28]

*Anecdotal Reports**

1. Chloral hydrate overdose.[29]
2. Zopiclone.[30,31]
3. Zopildem.[15]
4. Paradoxical reaction to benzodiazepines.
5. In transurethral resection, to differentiate disorientation caused by water intoxication versus benzodiazepines.
6. Baclofen is an agonist for GABAergic receptors. Flumazenil may affect a baclofen-induced coma.[32]
7. Cardiovascular depression associated with benzodiazepine may be reversed with flumazenil.
8. A useful test in the differential diagnosis of the encephalopathies may be the response of a patient to the administration of a benzodiazepine receptor antagonist.[11]
9. Flumazenil may reverse the acute dystonia induced by midazolam.
10. Flumazenil (3 mg) induces a reduction in interictal epileptic activity on the electroencephalogram. Flumazenil in high doses may exert an anticonvulsant action in full seizures.[33,34]
11. Carbamazepine overdose.[35]
12. Ketamine anesthesia.[36]

13. Flumazenil use as "diagnostic tool" in paradoxical reaction to benzodiazepines.
14. Flumazenil has been used for failure to return to full consciousness at the termination of an often benign procedure. This may indicate that a cerebral accident has occurred.
15. Flumazenil may help wean patients from ventilators.
16. Flumazenil may be helpful for the young child who ingests only benzodiazepines and presents in coma.
17. Flumazenil may be useful in preventing or reversing tolerance to benzodiazepine agonists.

Unsubstantiated Evidence

1. Ethanol overdose reports have been anecdotal and uncontrolled.[21] Chronic alcohol abuse may increase the number and responsiveness of benzodiazepine receptors. Flumazenil does not improve the central nervous system depression induced by ethanol intoxication and has no effect on performance after ethanol intoxication.[37–40]
2. Flumazenil has anticonvulsant action in high doses. Interruption of seizures has been reported.[34]
3. With respect to hepatic encephalopathy, fulminant hepatic failure, and hepatic coma, anecdotal reports have been conflicting.[3,8] The arousal effect of flumazenil in hepatic encephalopathy may be a prognostic factor predicting short-term survival in severe hepatic encephalopathy.[41]
4. Flumazenil does not alter the effects of substances such as opiates and barbiturates that do not act through benzodiazepine receptor sites.[12]
5. Flumazenil has been used in benzodiazepine withdrawal but may precipitate withdrawal in chronic benzodiazepine abusers.

Product Formulation

Flumazenil is supplied in the United States as a 0.1 mg/mL solution in 5- and 10-mL vials.[3]

Source

Flumazenil is a synthetic chemical product.

Therapeutic Dose

For reversal of conscious sedation or in general anesthesia, the initial dose is 0.2 mg intravenously over 15 seconds, repeated at 1-minute intervals to a maximum dose of 1 mg.

In benzodiazepine overdose, flumazenil 0.2 mg is given over 30 seconds, followed by 0.3 and 0.5 mg at 1-minute intervals to a maximum dose of 3 mg. Some patients have received up to 5 mg.

For recurrent sedation, 0.2 mg flumazenil is administered intravenously as required, to a total of 1 mg/h, or is infused at 0.5 mg/h. Patients sedated mainly with benzodiazepines may remain awake without further treatment. Many treated patients who have regained consciousness have become resedated, are easily reawakened and remain alert with repeated injections of flumazenil. The appropriate dose for children has not been established. A recent report stated that 0.01 mg/kg was used.[42] The duration of action of flumazenil in children (9 hours) may be longer than that in adults.[42]

Failure of a patient with unconsciousness of unknown origin to respond to intravenous doses of flumazenil greater than 5 mg may indicate the involvement of agents other than benzodiazepines or another etiology.

Pure benzodiazepine overdose requires a small dose of flumazenil to reverse overdose symptoms and signs: 0.5 to 0.7 mg. Those with mixed-drug overdoses require higher doses: 0.8 to 2 mg. For a neonate with recurrent apnea, the loading dose is 0.02 mg/kg intravenously, followed by a maintenance dose of 0.05 mg/kg/h for 6 hours,[27] or a continuous infusion 0.5 mg/h. The patient should be in an intensive care facility. About one third of patients with severe benzodiazepine overdose reenter coma shortly after an effective injection of flumazenil. In some patients, especially the elderly, when a continuous infusion is started, signs of severe resedation or impaired ventilation are seen.

Slow drug titration under close observation is used to avoid anxiety and agitation and is preferable to injection of large boluses. Patients should be observed for resedation and anxiety reaction after awakening. Those patients with a history of seizure disorder or clinical evidence suggestive of impending seizures should not be given flumazenil. An electrocardiogram finding typical of tricyclic antidepressant poisoning is a relative contraindication to flumazenil. Before flumazenil is started, any severe hemodynamic or respiratory abnormalities must be corrected.[43]

Once it is administered, the duration of a single dose of flumazenil usually does not exceed 1 hour.[44–46] Repeat doses are often required except with short-acting benzodiazepines, for example, triazolam. Continuous intravenous infusion may be required. Respiratory and hemodynamic monitoring are still necessary.

Flumazenil can make gastric lavage and administration of activated charcoal possible and safer without lessening the need for endotracheal intubation. It improves consciousness, permits return of protective airway reflexes, and lessens the potential for pulmonary aspiration.

Toxicokinetics

Absorption

The bioavailability of flumazenil through the oral route is low (16%) because of extensive first-pass metabolism.[47–51] A mean maximum concentration of 70.1 mg/mL is reached in 0.64 hour.[2] Following 10 mg of intravenous flumazenil, the distribution half-life is 4.5 minutes.[52] The protein-bound fraction of flumazenil is approximately 40 to 50%.[53] Binding at the benzodiazepine receptor is diagrammed in Figures 41–1 and 41–2.[11,54] The time to reach a steady state with flumazenil is about 5 hours. There is no apparent reason to use a continuous infusion. Continuous infusion has not been shown to be superior to repeat bolus doses. Duration of action after a single intravenous injection has varied from 15 to 140 minutes, depending on the dose.[45,46] Peak levels of flumazenil necessary to achieve reversal of benzodiazepine-induced coma are 20 to 25 nmol/L (6 ng/mL). Maintenance levels of flumazenil are about 10 to 20 nmol/L.

Distribution

The initial volume of distribution is 16 L (about 0.2 L/kg) and the volume of distribution at steady state is 64.8 L (about 1 L/kg).[52] Following initial distribution according to cerebral blood flow, flumazenil is taken up by gray matter structures in the brain (cerebral cortex, cerebellum, thalamus, and basal ganglia). Cerebral levels of flumazenil decrease with a half-life of 25 to 38 minutes.[51]

Elimination

The elimination half-life after oral administration is 0.88 hour in normal subjects and 1.3 hours in patients with cirrhosis.[51] Following intravenous use the respective half-lives are 0.79 and 1.4 hours.[2,55] In chronic lung disease there is a two- to four-fold increase in elimination half-life and a two- to four-fold decrease in plasma clearance.[56]

Less than 0.2% of an intravenous dose of flumazenil is recovered as unchanged drug in the urine, indicating extensive metabolism of the drug.[49,57] Metabolites are inactive.[54] Hepatic elimination is rapid (short elimination half-life, 0.9 hour); total plasma and blood clearance rates are high (691 and 617 mL/min, respectively). The toxicokinetics of flumazenil are not significantly altered in benzodiazepine overdose.[58] Flumazenil and its metabolites are completely eliminated in 48 to 72 hours.[58]

Drug Interactions

The disposition of flumazenil is not affected by the coadministration of midazolam, lorazepam, flunitrazepam, and alcohol.[48] In patients suffering from respiratory depression due to the combined effects of a benzodiazepine and an opioid, flumazenil safely antagonizes the benzodiazepine component. This does not necessarily mean that respiration is fully restored. The effect of the opioid may still be present.[54]

Pregnancy/Lactation

Flumazenil easily crosses the placenta. No teratogenicity has been observed. Safe use during pregnancy has not been established.[45]

Mechanism of Action

No clinically important hemodynamic changes or increases in levels of plasma catecholamines, glucose, cortisol, vasopressors, or β-endorphins have followed the use of flumazenil.[59–61]

GABA–Benzodiazepine Receptor Complex

A neuronal cell surface protein complex contains a benzodiazepine receptor, a GABA receptor, and a chloride channel (Fig. 41–1).[54] The three sites are anatomically distinct but closely related functionally.[21] Flumazenil acts at the central nervous system but not at peripheral benzodiazepine receptor binding sites to competitively block the effects of benzodiazepines on GABAergic pathway-mediated inhibitors in the central nervous system.

Flumazenil does not block the pharmacologic effects of GABA, GABA-mimetics, or barbiturates but it does antagonize the action of benzodiazepines, imidazopyridines, and other compounds that bind to benzodiazepine receptors.

Benzodiazepines facilitate the inhibitory effects of both GABA at the presynaptic junction and glycine at the postsynaptic junction. GABA and glycine are the two major inhibitory neurotransmitters. They act as neurotransmitters at 50 to 75% of all synapses in the central nervous system. Their effects at receptor sites are competitively antagonized by flumazenil.[62]

Benzodiazepines increase the affinity of GABA for its receptor sites, as well as increase the coupling of GABA receptors to the Cl^- channel. When the channel is opened, Cl^- diffuses inside, down its concentration gradient, and hyperpolarizes the cell membrane. This hyperpolarized membrane is more resistant to neuronal excitation.[53]

Clinical Presentation

Therapeutic Use

Side effects reported after flumazenil use include nausea, dizziness, headache, blurred vision, increased sweating, anxiety, and panic attacks.[63] Ventricular tachycardia may be induced by seizures, resulting in increased concentrations of circulatory catecholamines and possibly hypercapnia and hypoxia. In the presence of cardiac sensitization by a tricyclic antidepressant, arrhythmias may be precipitated.[64] Agitation, nonspecific discomfort, tearfulness, anxiety, and a sensation of coldness may be seen in patients receiving flumazenil for reversal of benzodiazepine overdose, long-term sedation, multiple intoxications, and coma not due to benzodiazepine overdose.[44,65]

Seizures

Seizures and acute anxiety with flumazenil are seen in patients dependent on benzodiazepines, especially if there has also been a tricyclic antidepressant overdose. Flumazenil antagonizes the anticonvulsant properties of benzodiazepines and may reveal the epileptogenic activity of a tricyclic antidepressant or any other seizure-inducing drug. An individual with an unknown overdose who may have ingested cyclic antidepressant drugs may be at risk from treatment with flumazenil. Flumazenil can provoke seizures in epileptics in the presence of convulsant drugs such as tricyclic antidepressants. It may exhibit a proconvulsant effect when used with isoniazid.[66] Flumazenil may induce an increase in intracranial pressure in patients with severe head injury.[42]

Withdrawal

Benzodiazepine-dependent patients in acute withdrawal may undergo withdrawal following flumazenil use postoperatively in the recovery room. In "late" use, return to consciousness after an accidental benzodiazepine overdose may be due to the development of acute tolerance rather than drug metabolism. Hence, "late" use of flumazenil may be more likely to precipitate a withdrawal reaction rather than its use shortly before onset of benzodiazepine intoxication. Flumazenil precipitates withdrawal signs and symptoms (excitement, combativeness) which may require very large doses of diazepam for control.[67]

Arrhythmias

Flumazenil can precipitate a cardiac arrhythmia in a patient who has overdosed on both a benzodiazepine and a tricyclic antidepressant. There is one report of bradycardia followed by asystole and death in a patient who ingested a benzodiazepine–antidepressant mixture and received flumazenil.[68] Flumazenil 500 μg, administered to reverse the effects of temazepam, led to a complete heart block in 1 minute; the patient was given atropine and reverted to sinus rhythm.[69]

Flumazenil does not protect against chloral hydrate arrhythmogenesis.[40] There is one report of nonfatal ventricular tachycardia following administration of flumazenil to a patient who had ingested a benzodiazepine–chloral hydrate mixture.[40] Cardiac arrest has been reported following flumazenil use.

Death

Deaths have been reported after flumazenil use for a multiple-drug overdose. Wearing off of reversal effects has been followed by recurrence of intoxication. Flumazenil may reverse the sedative effects of benzodiazepines but not their respiratory depressant effects. Flumazenil alone in benzodiazepine intoxication is inadequate treatment. Partial reversal could lead to a fatal delay in instituting rapid tracheal intubation and ventilatory assistance.[70] Resedation following flumazenil use may be characterized by drowsiness, mild confusion, stupor, and coma.

Postoperative use of flumazenil may exacerbate the sensation of pain with a concomitant increase in consciousness.[65] Nausea and vomiting may occur in 1 to 10% of patients.[22,42] Patients may awaken with an endotracheal tube in place. This can be avoided by using small repeated doses of flumazenil.[7] In a patient with tetanus who requires benzodiazepines in high doses, flumazenil may induce a severe tetanospasm.[71]

Flumazenil has led to a moderate increase in blood pressure and elevation of left ventricular end-diastolic pressure in patients with ischemic heart disease who have received a benzodiazepine. Flumazenil may induce an increase or decrease in blood pressure and an increase in heart rate.[72]

Hepatic Encephalopathy

Oral flumazenil in hepatic encephalopathy can induce an acute psychosis (anxiety, restlessness, insomnia, crying fits, panic disorientation, hallucinations, and abusive aggressive behavior). The serum ammonium concentration and electroencephalogram may remain unchanged.[73]

Overdose

Large intravenous doses given to healthy volunteers in the absence of benzodiazepine overdose led to no serious adverse reactions, severe signs or symptoms, or significant laboratory test abnormalities. Reversal of benzodiazepine effects with an excessively high dose may produce anxiety, agitation, increased muscle tone, hyperesthesia, and possibly convulsions.[13]

Laboratory

Analytical Methods

High-performance liquid chromatography and gas–liquid chromatography with nitrogen phosphorus detection have been used to quantify plasma flumazenil concentrations.[74,75] A gas chromatography–mass spectrometry method is sensitive to 1.0 ng/mL in plasma.[76] No interference of flumazenil with detection of benzodiazepines by immunologic assay could be found.[75]

Blood Levels

During the anhepatic stage of a liver transplantation, flumazenil plasma concentrations are higher than those in cirrhotic patients and healthy volunteers.[77] There is an increase in plasma flumazenil concentration in cirrhosis.[2]

Abnormalities

Flumazenil administered intravenously in a dose of 10 mg produces a significant change in the electroencephalogram.[52,78]

Treatment

Flumazenil should be withheld if there is a history or physical findings suggestive of seizure or if there are electrocardiographic signs of tricyclic antidepressant overdose. Flumazenil should not be used to shorten the period of observation even though it may decrease the need for ventilatory support and intensive monitoring. The cardiotoxic effects of flumazenil in those multiple-drug ingestions that may include a cardiogenic toxin are not known. Before using flumazenil the physician must ascertain[43] that oxygenation is intact, the airway is open, and the patient is hemodynamically stable and is monitored with pulse oximetry.[24,79] Reversal of diazepam sedation does not modify ventricular performance in patients with cardiac disease.[59] Flumazenil should be used only if continued observation for recurrence of sedation can be ensured. Incremental doses (0.1–0.2 mg) should be titrated to the individual patient's need. Seizures may be precipitated in multiple-drug ingestions involving proconvulsant drugs as well as in chronic benzodiazepine users as a manifestation of a severe withdrawal reaction. Such seizures may then respond to a small dose of benzodiazepines.[59]

There may be a continued need for endotracheal intubation in cases where gastric lavage is indicated (ie, poisoning with benzodiazepines in combination with other and more toxic drugs).[17] Remember that the sedative action of benzodiazepines may be depressing a more serious side effect of another component of the overdose.[79]

Despite rapid reversal of sedation and memory loss with flumazenil, requirements for narcotic analgesic[80] administration in the postoperative setting are no different than for other postoperative patients. When there is neurologic deterioration in a benzodiazepine patient with chronic obstructive pulmonary disease, flumazenil may be helpful even when serum benzodiazepine levels are not raised.[81] Flumazenil has no influence on regional or total hemispheric cerebral blood flow when injected alone. Following benzodiazepine use, flumazenil antagonizes the depressant effects on cerebral circulation or even increases blood flow.[82]

Flumazenil can reverse the sedation but not the amnesia for gastroscopy induced by benzodiazepines.[83] It can be used to reverse adverse effects of midazolam in ophthalmic surgical procedures, for example, paradoxical reaction and upper airway obstruction.[84]

Remember that reversal of benzodiazepine-induced sedation can be accompanied by adrenergic stimulation.[85]

Patients must be observed for resedation until the agonist effects have worn off. This period of observation should continue for 2 to 4 hours after a midazolam infusion has been stopped. The patient must remain under close observation in an intensive care unit until both agonist and antagonist levels have declined to subtherapeutic levels.[86] "Resedation" after benzodiazepine reversal should be called "residual sedation." When the effect of flumazenil declines, patients only return to the level of sedation that would have been present had they not received flumazenil.[83]

General Review Article

- Sugarman JM, Paul RI. Flumazenil: A review. Pediatr Emerg Care 1994;10:37–43.

REFERENCES—FLUMAZENIL

1. Reynolds JEF, ed. *Martindale: The Extra Pharmacopoeia.* 30th ed. London: Pharmaceutical Press, 1993:682.
2. Janssen U, Walker S, Maier K, et al. Flumazenil disposition and elimination in cirrhosis. Clin Pharmacol Ther 1989;46: 317–323.
3. Benzodiazepine antagonist approved by FDA. Clin Pharm 1992;1:287–288. Editorial.
4. Galletly DC, Ure R, Turley A. Flumazenil: A twelve-month survey on use in a New Zealand public hospital. Anaesth Intens Care 1990;18:229–233.
5. O'Sullivan GF, Wade DN. Flumazenil in the management of acute drug overdosage with benzodiazepines and other agents. Clin Pharmacol Ther 1987;42:254–259.
6. Grimm G, Katzenschlager R, Holzner F, et al. Effect of flumazenil in hepatic encephalopathy. Eur J Anaesth 1988;suppl. 2:147–149.
7. Grimm G, Ferenci P, Katzenschlager R, et al. Improvement of hepatic encephalopathy treated with flumazenil. Lancet 1988;2:1392–1394.
8. Basile AS, Gammal SH. Evidence for the involvement of the benzodiazepine receptor complex in hepatic encephalopathy: Implications for treatment with benzodiazepine receptor antagonists. Clin Neuropharmacol 1988;11:401–422.
9. Jones EA, Basile AS, Mullen KD, Gammal SH. Flumazenil: Potential implications for hepatic encephalopathy. Pharmacol Ther 1990;45:331–343.
10. Jones EA, Skolnick P, Gammal SH, et al. The gamma-aminobutyric acid A ($GABA_A$) receptor complex and hepatic encephalopathy: Some recent advances. Ann Intern Med 1989;110:532–546.
11. Jones EA, Gammal SH, Martin P. Hepatic encephalopathy: New light on an old problem. J Med 1988;69:857–867.
12. Record CO. Neurochemistry of hepatic encephalopathy. Gut 1991;32:1261–1263.
13. Scollo-Lavizzari G, Steinmann E. Reversal of hepatic coma by benzodiazepine antagonist (Ro 15-7788). Lancet 1985;1:324.
14. Bosman DK, Van den Bults ACG, De Haan JG, et al. The effects of benzodiazepines, receptor antagonists and partial agonists in acute hepatic encephalopathy in the rat. Gastroenterology 1991;101:772–781.
15. Naef MM, Forster A, Nahory A, et al. Flumazenil antagonizes the sedative action of zolpidem, a new iminoazopyridine hypnotic. Anesthesiology 1989;4(3A):A297.
16. Hojer J, Baehrendtz S, Magnusson A, Gustafsson LL. A placebo-controlled trial of flumazenil given by continuous infusion in severe benzodiazepine overdosage. Acta Anaesthesiol Scand 1991;35:584–590.
17. Hojer J, Baehrendtz S. The effect of flumazenil (RO15-1788) in the management of self-induced benzodiazepine poisoning: A double-blind controlled study. Acta Med Scand 1988;224:357–365.
18. Hojer J, Baehrendtz S, Matell G, Gustafsson LL. Diagnostic utility of flumazenil in coma with suspected poisoning: A double blind randomised controlled study. Br Med J 1990; 301:1308–1311.
19. Roald OK, Forsman M, Steen PA. Partial reversal of the cerebral effects of isoflurane in the dog by the benzodiazepine antagonist flumazenil. Acta Anaesthesiol Scand 1988;32: 209–212.
20. Murayana T, Shingu K, Ogawa T, et al. Flumazenil does not antagonize halothane thiamylal or propofol anaesthesia in rats. Br J Anaesth 1992;69:61–64.
21. Votey SR. Flumazenil: A new benzodiazepine antagonist. Ann Emerg Med 1991;70:181–188.
22. Mora ST, Torjman A, White PF. Effects of diazepam and flumazenil on sedation and hypoxic ventilatory response. Anesth Analg 1989;68:473–478.
23. Sage DJ. Reversal of sedation with flumazenil in regional anaesthesia: A review. Eur J Anaesthesiol 1988;suppl. 2:201–207.
24. Whitman JG. Flumazenil: A benzodiazepine antagonist: Many uses possibly including withdrawal from benzodiazepines. Br Med J 1988;297:999–1000.
25. Whitman JG. The use of midazolam and flumazenil in diagnostic and short surgical procedures. Acta Anaesthesiol Scand 1990;34(suppl. 92):16–20.
26. McKay AC, McKinney MS, Clarke RSJ. Effect of flumazenil on midazolam-induced amnesia. Br J Anaesth 1990;65:190–196.
27. Richard P, Autret E, Bardol J, et al. The use of flumazenil in a neonate. Clin Toxicol 1991;29:137–141.
28. Eldar I, Lieberman N, Shiber R, et al. Use of flumazenil for intraoperative arousal during spine fusion. Anaesth Analg 1992;75:580–583.
29. Donovan KL, Fisher DJ. Reversal of chloral hydrate overdose with flumazenil. Br Med J 1989;298:1253.
30. Ahmad Z, Herepath M, Ebden P. Diagnostic utility of flumazenil in coma with suspected poisoning. Br Med J 1991;302:292.
31. Lariviere L. Personal communication. Rhone–Poulenc Pharmaceuticals, October 21, 1992.
32. Saissy JM, Vitris M, Demaziere J, et al. Flumazenil counteracts intrathecal baclofen-induced central nervous system depression in tetanus. Anesthesiology 1991;76:1051–1053.
33. Scollo-Lavizzari G. The clinical anticonvulsant effect of flumazenil, a benzodiazepine antagonist. Eur J Anaesthesiol 1988;suppl. 2:129–138.
34. Scollo-Lavizzari G. The anticonvulsant effects of the benzodiazepine antagonist, RO15-1788: An EEG study in 4 cases. Eur Neurol 1984;23:1–6.
35. Zuber M, Elsasser S, Ritz R, Scollo-Lavizzari G. Flumazenil (Anexate[R]) in severe intoxication with carbamazepine (Tegretol[R]). Eur Neurol 1988;28:161–163.
36. Restall J, Johnston IG, Robinson DN. Flumazenil in ketamine and midazolam anaesthesia. Anaesthesia 1990;45:938–940.
37. Flukiger A, Hartmann D, Leishman B, Ziegler WH. Lack of effect of benzodiazepine antagonist flumazenil (RO 15-1788) on the performance of healthy subjects during experimentally induced ethanol intoxication. Eur J Clin Pharmacol 1988;34: 273–276.
38. Clausen TG, Wolff J, Carl P, Theilgaard A. The effect of the benzodiazepine antagonist, flumazenil, on psychometric per-

formance in acute ethanol intoxication in man. Eur J Clin Pharmacol 1990;38:233–236.
39. Lhoureux P, Askenasi R. Flumazenil in acute alcohol intoxication: A randomized double blind study. In: *Proceedings, Int Cong Clin Toxicol Pois Cont Anal Toxicol, Lux Tox'90, Luxembourg, May 25, 1990:* 488.
40. Short TG, Maling T, Galletly DC. Ventricular arrhythmia precipitated by flumazenil. Br Med J 1988;2906:1070–1071.
41. Bansky G, Meier PJ, Riederer E, et al. Effects of a benzodiazepine antagonist in hepatic encephalopathy in man. Hepatology 1987;7:1103.
42. La Fleche RF. Flumazenil. Clin Toxicol Rev 1990;12(5):1–2.
43. Weinbroum A, Halpern P, Geller E. The use of flumazenil in the management of acute drug poisoning: A review. Intens Care Med 1991;17:S32–S38.
44. Amrein R, Leishman B, Bentzinger C, Roncer G. Flumazenil in benzodiazepine antagonism: Actions and clinical use in intoxications and anaesthesiology. Med Toxicol 1987;21:411–429.
45. Amrein R. Discussion. Eur J Anaesthesiol 1988;suppl. 2:123–125.
46. Amrein R, Hetzel W: Pharmacology of Dormicum[R] (midazolam) and Anexate[R] (flumazenil). Acta Anaesthesiol Scand 1990;34(suppl. 92):6–15.
47. Katz JA, Fragen RJ, Dunn KL. Flumazenil reversal of midazolam sedation in the elderly. Region Anesth 1991;16: 247–252.
48. Klotz V, Kanto J. Pharmacokinetics and clinical use of flumazenil (RO15-1788). Clin Pharmacokinet 1988;14:1–12.
49. Klotz V, Ziegler G, Reimann N. Pharmacokinetics of the selective benzodiazepine antagonist RO15-1788 in man. Eur J Clin Pharmacol 1984;27:115–117.
50. Klotz V. Drug interactions and clinical pharmacokinetics of flumazenil. Eur J Anaesthesiol 1988;suppl. 2:103–108.
51. Basile AS, Hughes PD, Harrison PH, et al. Elevated brain concentrations of 1,4-benzodlazepines in fulminant hepatic failure. N Engl J Med 1991;325:475–478.
52. Breimer LTM, Hennis PJ, Burm AGL, et al. Pharmacokinetics and EEG effects of flumazenil in volunteers. Clin Pharmacokinet 1991;30:491–496.
53. Kasson BJ. Flumazenil: A specific benzodiazepine antagonist. J Am Assoc Nurse Anaesth 1992;60:472–476.
54. Amrein R, Hetzel W. Pharmacology of drugs frequently used in ICU's: Midazolam and flumazenil. Intensive Care Med 1991;17:S1–S10.
55. Marshall DE, Haradona AN, Orcutt RH, et al. GC/MS method for the determination of flumazenil in plasma and urine. Res Commun Substance Abuse 1991:12:228–236.
56. Van der Rijk CCD, Drost RH, Schalen SW, Schramel M. Pharmacokinetics of flumazenil in fulminant hepatic failure. Eur J Clin Pharmacol 1991;41:501.
57. Whitwan JG. Flumazenil: A benzodiazepine antagonist: Many uses, possibly including withdrawal from benzodiazepines. Br Med J 1988;297:999–1000.
58. Rodwell PJL, Maclaren HM, Hughes EW, et al. The pharmacokinetics of flumazenil used as a bolus and an infusion regimen in the treatment of major benzodiazepine self-poisonings. Ann Emerg Med 1992;21:471.
59. Geller E. Flumazenil in clinical medicine: Indications and precautions. Eur J Anaesthesiol 1988;suppl. 2:325–329.
60. Geller E, Halpern P, Chernilas J, et al. Cardiorespiratory effects of antagonism of diazepam sedation with flumazenil in patients with cardiac disease. Anesth Analg 1991;72:207–211.
61. Geller E, Niv D, Weinbrun A, et al. The use of flumazenil in the treatment of 34 intoxicated patients. Resuscitation 1988; 16(suppl.):S57–S62.
62. Stolarek IH, Ford MJ. Acute dystonia induced by midazolam and abolished by flumazenil. Br Med J 1990;30:614.
63. Nutt D, Costello M. Flumazenil and benzodiazepine withdrawal. Lancet 1987;2:463.
64. Marchant B, Wray R, Leach A, Nama M. Flumazenil causing convulsions and ventricular tachycardia. Br Med J 1989; 299:860.
65. Karavokivos KAT, Tsipis GB. Flumazenil: A benzodiazepine antagonist. DICP Ann Pharmacother 1990;24:976–981.
66. Weisman RS, Hoffman RS, Howland MA, Goldfrank L. Flumazenil's effect on the isoniazid seizure threshold in mice. Vet Hum Toxicol 1992;34:345.
67. Lopez A, Rebollo J. Benzodiazepine withdrawal syndrome after a benzodiazepine antagonist. Crit Care Med 1990; 18:1480–1481.
68. Burr W, Sandham P. Death after flumazenil. Br Med J 1989; 298:1713.
69. Herd B, Clarke F. Complete heart block after flumazenil. Hum Exp Toxicol 1991;10:289.
70. Lim AG. Death after flumazenil. Br Med J 1989;299:858–859.
71. Mapelli A, Bellinzona G, Lorini FL, et al. Diagnostic and therapeutic use of flumazenil in emergency medicine. Eur J Anaesth 1988;(suppl. 2):295–317.
72. Marty J, Nitenberg A. The use of midazolam and flumazenil in cardiovascular diagnostic and therapeutic procedures. Acta Anaesthesiol Scand 1990;34(suppl. 92):33–34.
73. Seebach J, Jost R. Flumazenil-induced psychotic disorder in hepatic encephalopathy. Lancet 1992;339:488–489.
74. Abernethy DR, Arendt RM, Lauven PM, Greenblatt DJ. Determination of RO15-1788, a benzodiazepine antagonist, in human plasma by gas liquid chromatography with nitrogen-phosphorus detection. Pharmacology 1983;26:285–289.
75. Koppel C, Wagemann A, Tencze RJ. Identification of the benzodiazepine antagonist flumazenil in plasma and urine after treatment of patients with benzodiazepine overdose. In: Uges DRA, de Zeeuw RA, eds. *Proceedings, International Association of Forensic Toxicologists, 25th International Meeting, Groningen, June 27–30, 1988:*326–334.
76. Kintz P, Mangin P. Plasma determination of flumazenil, a benzodiazepine antagonist, by immunotoxicology and by capillary gas chromatography/mass spectrometry. J Anal Toxicol 1991;15:202–203.
77. Park GR, Podkowik Bl. Plasma concentrations of flumazenil during liver transplantation. Anaesthesia 1992;47:887–889.
78. Hart YM, Meinardi H, Sander JWAS, et al. The effect of intravenous flumazenil on electroencephalographic activity: Results of a placebo-controlled study. J Neurol Neurosurg Psychiatry 1991;54:305–309.
79. Pollard BJ, Masters AP, Bunting R. The use of flumazenil (Ancrate, RO15-1788) in the management of drug overdose. Anaesthesia 1989;44:137–138.
80. Olsen KM, Pablo CS, Ackerman BH. Postoperative analgesic requirements following flumazenil administration. DICP Ann Pharmacother 1990;24:1159–1163.
81. Appel M, Bron HNL, Hooymans PM, Janknegt R. Efficacy of flumazenil in COPD patient with therapeutic diazepam levels. Lancet 1989;1:392.
82. Wolff J. Cerebrovascular and metabolic effects of midazolam and flumazenil. Acta Anaesth Scand 1990;34(suppl. 92):75–77.
83. Pearson RC, McCloy RF, Morns P, Bardhas KD. Midazolam and flumazenil in gastroenterology. Acta Anaesthesiol Scand 1990;34(suppl. 92):21–24.
84. Gobeaux D, Sardnal F. Midazolam and flumazenil in ophthalmology. Acta Anesthesiol Scand 1990;34(suppl. 92):35–38.
85. Flache WE, Ritter J. Lack of adrenergic response to flumazenil: Reversal of midazolam sedation. Clin Pharmacol Ther 1988;43:149.
86. Fisher GC, Clapham MCC, Hutton P. Flumazenil in intensive care: The duration of arousal after an assessment dose. Anaesthesia 1991;41:413–416.

GLUTETHIMIDE

Discontinued drugs such as glutethimide (Doriden) may still be found in the community. Cessation of use after ingestion of quantities exceeding the recommended dose may be followed by seizures, confusion, agitation, nausea, anxiety, and sleep disturbance. Diazepam in high doses may be required for amelioration of the seizures.[1]

REFERENCE—GLUTETHIMIDE

1. Lucas RE, Montgomery WS. Glutethimide withdrawal: The ethics of supply and demand. Aust NZ J Med 1992;22:708.

HEXAPROPYMATE

Hexapropymate is a carbamate sedative–hypnotic drug that, in overdose, resembles meprobamate or barbiturate intoxication and may lead to fatalities. Hypothermia, severe respiratory depression, and prolonged coma may require a long period of assisted ventilation. Treatment is largely supportive and symptomatic.[1]

Toxic Dose

A 75-kg man ingested 3.6 g of hexapropymate and survived.[2] A 28-year-old man who ingested 16 g became deeply comatose, was treated supportively, and survived.[3] A 20-year-old man who ingested 9.2 g died in 12 hours,[4] and a 32-year-old man who ingested 40 g lapsed into a deep coma before he died on the third day after overdose.[5] Coma with respiratory depression has been reported following doses as small as 4 g. Doses of 8 g or more appear to involve an increased risk of serious cardiovascular disorders (hypotension, shock).[6]

Toxicokinetics

Absorption

Hexapropymate is absorbed by the gastrointestinal route. Few toxicokinetic studies are available.[7] Toxicokinetic data largely derive from data obtained after overdose of the drug.

Distribution

The apparent volume of distribution has been reported to vary between 1.5 and 3.5 L/kg.[7]

Elimination

The elimination half-life of hexapropymate in normal volunteers ranges from 2.7 to 8.1 hours. After one overdose, the half-life was 21 hours.[7]

Mechanism of Action

Hexapropymate is a carbamate hypnotic substance with properties similar to those of the barbiturates and meprobamate.

Clinical Presentation

Following an overdose with hexapropymate, patients may develop clinical evidence of serious cardiovascular, respiratory, and central and peripheral nervous system impairment. Tachycardia, bradycardia, cardiac arrhythmias, and hypotension may lead to cardiac arrest. Respiratory depression can be followed by apnea, with atelectatic areas in the lung and bronchopneumonia. Cyanosis may be present. Patients may be initially agitated with myosis or mydriasis, absence of corneal, gag, and cough reflexes, seizures, depressed or absent deep tendon reflexes, general muscular hypotonicity, and electroencephalographic abnormalities. Coma is deep and lasts several days or even longer if other central nervous depressants have been abused simultaneously. Hypothermia, metabolic acidosis, and oliguria have been described.[6] Patients are often found dead.[2]

Laboratory

Analytical Methods

A gas chromatographic method for hexapropymate quantitation has a limit of detection of 2.7 mg/L (15 µmol/L).[7]

Blood Levels

Maximum serum concentrations after hexapropymate overdoses have varied from 7.6 to 54.4 mg/L. Serum concentrations less than 20 mg/L have usually been associated with survival. There is no relationship, however, between the serum concentration and the depth or duration of coma.[7]

Abnormalities

Serum lactate concentrations may be elevated and probably account for the metabolic acidosis observed in severe overdose.[3]

Ancillary Tests

The electrocardiogram may exhibit supraventricular tachycardia, intraventricular block, bradycardia, and premature ventricular beats.[3,6] A Wolff–Parkinson–White pattern has been observed. Blood glucose, urea, creatinine, electrolytes, and amylase concentrations are usually normal. Hepatic enzyme (transaminases) levels may be slightly elevated.

Treatment

Stabilization

Treatment of hexapropymate overdose is symptomatic and supportive with special cognizance of the long period during which the patient may remain in coma. The initial evaluation for airway, ventilation, and circulation after a hexapropymate overdose is similar to that after other sedative–hypnotic overdoses. Endotracheal intubation, intravenous lines, oxygen, and cardiac monitor should be provided as necessary. Profound hypothermia may be present.

Gut Decontamination

Obtunded patients should be lavaged after the trachea has been protected with a cuffed endotracheal tube and after the patient has been placed in the left lateral, head-down position. The initial gastric aspirate should be saved for gastric analysis. As coma may be associated with reduced gastrointestinal mobility, gastric lavage may still be useful 6 to 12 hours after ingestion. There is no clinical evidence to support the efficacy of activated charcoal or cathartics in the hexapropymate-overdosed patient.

Elimination Enhancement

The extensive volume of distribution of hexapropymate probably precludes hemoperfusion or hemodialysis, but failure of supportive care to maintain vital signs, an underlying disease that contraindicates a prolonged coma, or the documentation of lethal blood levels may provide the basis for an initial trial of one of these measures based on the clinician's judgment.

Antidote

There is no antidote.

Supportive Measures

Supportive measures are summarized under General Treatment of Overdoses at the beginning of this chapter. Special attention should be given to the use of serial arterial blood gases to monitor hypoxemia, cautious rewarming of the hypothermic patient, careful observation for the development of atelectatic changes or bronchopneumonia, and prolonged assisted ventilation (for several days or more as required). Remember that the patient may also have ingested ethanol and/or other central nervous system depressant drugs. Urine should be obtained for sedative–hypnotic screening. Serum salicylates, acetone, methanol, ethanol, acetaminophen, and isopropanol should be determined. Intravenous sodium bicarbonate may assist in reversing the metabolic acidosis. Hypotension may be ameliorated by position change and Ringer's lactate or normal saline intravenous infusion (150 mL for an adult over a 30-minute to 1-hour period if the systolic blood pressure is less than 80 mm Hg). Fluid boluses of 200 mL may be added up to 2-L positive balance or until the systolic blood pressure reaches 100 mm Hg. Vasopressors such as dopamine should be used if fluids do not raise the systolic blood pressure to 90 of 100 mm Hg. Patients should be monitored with an arterial line, pulmonary artery catheter, and Foley catheter to measure hourly urine volume, urine specific gravity, and urine electrolytes. Careful observation for evidence of pulmonary edema is necessary.

REFERENCES—HEXAPROPYMATE

1. Reynolds JEF, ed. *Martindale: The Extra Pharmacopoeia.* 30th ed. London: Pharmaceutical Press, 1993:600.
2. Noirfalise A. Cinq cas de suspicion d'intoxication par l'hexapropymate. J Eur Toxicol 1971;1:50–52.
3. Robbins G, Brown AK. Hexapropymate self-poisoning. Br Med J 1978;1:1593.
4. Yamarellos P, Dimopoulos G. Three cases of hexapropymate (Merinax) poisoning. Bull Int Assoc Forens Toxicol 1979; 14(3):29–30.
5. Hassoun A, Van Binst R. Fatal hexapropymate intoxication. Bull Int Assoc Forens Toxicol 1979;14(3):28.
6. Addlerfligel C. Personal communication: Report on 31 cases of hexapropymate poisoning. Brussels: Centre Antipoisons, November 2, 1989.
7. Gustaffson LL, Berg A, Magnusson A, et al. Hexapropymate self-poisoning causes severe and long lasting clinical symptoms. Med Toxicol Adverse Drug Experience 1989;4:295–301.

MEPROBAMATE

Toxicokinetics

Bismuth and colleagues have calculated the 24-hour hepatic metabolism of meprobamate as follows[1]:

$$\text{Serum meprobamate (day 1 − 2)} = x \text{ mg/L}$$
$$x \text{ mg/L} \times \text{weight (kg)} \times V_D \text{ (0.75 1/kg)} = Y \text{ g}$$
$$\text{24-hour urine excretion of meprobamate} = Z \text{ g}$$
$$Y - Z = \text{24-hour hepatic metabolism in grams.}$$

Laboratory

A gas chromatographic method for determination of meprobamate in human plasma is sensitive to concentration of 1 mg/L.[2]

Screening for the presence of meprobamate by the classic method (thin-layer chromatography) may be important as this compound cannot be detected by high-performance liquid chromatography using ultraviolet detection.[3]

Treatment

Stabilization

The initial evaluation for airway, ventilation, and circulation after meprobamate overdose is similar to that after all sedative–hypnotic overdoses, with endotracheal intubation, intravenous lines, oxygen, and cardiac monitors provided as needed. Hypotension may be out of proportion to depth of coma and must be treated cautiously with fluids because the use of forced diuresis has been complicated by pulmonary edema.[4] Seriously overdosed patients who do not respond to initial fluid replacement (2 L of Ringer's lactate) should be given vasopressors.

Gut Decontamination

Delayed gastric emptying and formation of drug masses suggest that lavage is useful up to 12 hours after ingestion. Fluctuating vital signs or levels of consciousness may indicate continuous absorption from stomach drug masses and, therefore, the need for endoscopy. Activated charcoal and cathartics should follow gastric lavage and syrup of ipecac.

Elimination Enhancement

Hemoperfusion is indicated only after severe ingestions in patients who do not respond to supportive care, who cannot tolerate prolonged coma, or who ingest massive doses (>40 g). Meprobamate blood levels greater than 100 mg/L suggest the need for hemoperfusion. A limited study on one patient suggests that continuous arteriovenus charcoal hemoperfusion can remove substantial amounts of meprobamate even in a patient with profound hemodynamic instability.[5]

Antidote

There is no antidote.

REFERENCES—MEPROBAMATE

1. Bismuth C, Baud FJ, Muczynski J. Meprobamate hepatic metabolism: Its calculation in clinical toxicology. In: *Proceedings, XVth Congress of European Association of Poison Centres and Clinical Toxicologists, Istanbul, May 24–27, 1992*:67.
2. Trenque T, Lamiable D, Millart H, et al. Gas chromatographic determination of meprobamate in human plasma. J Chromatogr Biomed Appl 1993;615:343–346.
3. Lambert WE, de Leenheer AP, Van Bocxlaer JF, Piette M. Meprobamate intoxication: Rare and difficult to find. Clin Toxicol 1992;30:683–684.
4. Axelson JA, Hagaman JF. Meprobamate poisoning and pulmonary edema. N Engl J Med 1977;296:1481.
5. Lin J-L, Lim P-S, Lai B-C, Lin W-L. Continuous arteriovenous hemoperfusion in meprobamate poisoning. Clin Toxicol 1993;31:645–652.

METHYPRYLON

Laboratory

A reverse-phase high-performance liquid chromatography–ultraviolet assay of plasma methyprylon (Noludar) concentrations is sensitive to less than 1.0 μg/mL.[1]

As for most sedative–hypnotic drugs, clinical status is a better guide to management than plasma methyprylon levels. Generally observed clinical effects do not necessarily correlate with plasma level and blood levels must be interpreted with caution.[2] Approximate blood levels include a therapeutic plasma level of 10 μg/mL and a toxic plasma level of 30 to 60 μg/mL at which patients may be responsive only to a painful stimulus. Levels above this range often result in deeper stages of coma. Lethal plasma levels occur near 100 μg/mL. Baseline tests for serious ingestions include a complete blood count, electrolytes, glucose, creatinine, chest x-ray, and arterial blood gases.

Treatment

Gut Decontamination

Alert adult patients who ingest more than 800 mg of methyprylon and present within 4 hours of ingestion should undergo gastric decontamination. Patients asymptomatic after 4 hours require no decontamination. Obtunded patients who require lavage may benefit from the procedure up to 8 hours after ingestion because of decreased gastrointestinal mobility.

Elimination Enhancement

Hemodialysis reduces the elimination half-life, which is considerably prolonged in overdose,[3] but whether coma is shortened is not clear. The question of whether an active metabolite exists and whether it is dialyzable remains unanswered. Hemodialysis should be considered in cases of large ingestions that fail to respond to supportive care. Peritoneal dialysis in one patient recovered 80% of the unmetabolized drug.[4] Hemoperfusion also increases clearance and reduces elimination half-life, but experience is too limited to draw conclusions. Forced diuresis is contraindicated because of the propensity of methyprylon to cause pulmonary edema.

Antidote

There is no antidote.

REFERENCES—METHYPRYLON

1. Contos DA, Dixon KF, Guthrie RM, et al. Nonlinear elimination of methyprylon (Noludar) in an overdosed patient: Correlation of clinical effects with plasma concentration. J Pharm Sci 1991;80:768–771.
2. Bailey DN, Jatlow PI. Methyprylon overdose: Interpretation of serum drug concentrations. Clin Toxicol 1973;6:563–569.
3. Pancorbo AS, Palagi PA, Piecoro JJ, et al. Hemodialysis in methyprylon overdose: Some pharmacokinetic considerations. JAMA 1977;237:470–471.
4. Polin RA, Henry D, Pippinger CE. Peritoneal dialysis for severe methyprylon intoxication. J Pediatr 1977;90:831–833.

METHAQUALONE

The combination of methaqualone with wine ("luding out") produces diminished proprioception, a sense of well-being, ataxia, and paresthesias that lead to feelings of indestructibility and euphoria. Methaqualone is similar to all sedative–hypnotic drugs in its ability to reduce both inhibitions and sexual performance.

Recently, legal production of methaqualone ceased in the United States and the reduction in toxic exposures paralleled a voluntary decrease in prescribing and, eventually, reduction in availability.

As for all sedative–hypnotic overdoses, initial evaluation is directed toward ensuring the adequacy of the ABCs (airway, breathing, and circulation) and administration of glucose, naloxone, and thiamine.

MONOUREIDES

The monoureide hypnotics such as bromvalerylurea (BVU), bromodiethylacetylurea (BDU), and allylisopropylacetylurea (AIU) are widely used in Japan, where many acute poisonings with these hypnotic drugs have been observed. A high-performance liquid chromatography method with multiwavelength ultraviolet detection is available for analysis of serum and urine.[1] Detection limits for BVU, BDU and AIU are 5, 10, and 10 mg, respectively.[2] Hepatitis and pancreatitis have been described following overdose with BVU.[3]

REFERENCES—MONOUREIDES

1. Hayashida M, Nihira M, Kurose M, et al. Investigation of acute poisoning substances and its medico-legal practice of emergency analysis. Jpn J Leg Med 1985;39:539.
2. Miyauchi H, Ameno K, Fuke C, et al. Simultaneous determination of bromvalerylurea, bromodiethylacetylurea and allylisopropylacetylurea in serum and urine by high performance liquid chromatography with a multiwavelength UV detection and thin-layer chromatography. J Anal Toxicol 1991;123–125.
3. Kageyama Y, Yamauchi H, Nakayama S, et al. A case of bromvalerylurea intoxication associated with acute hepatitis and pancreatitis. Jpn J Med 1990;29:121.

PYRITHYLDIONE

Pyrithyldione (3,3-diethyl-2,4-dioxo-1,2,3,4 tetrahydropyridine) has been sold commercially as Persedon for use as a sedative–hypnotic drug. It has activity similar to that of the barbiturates. Pyrithyldione was used for several years in combination with other drugs such as aspirin, phenacetin, and codeine. It has been administered in doses of 200 and 400 mg at night.[1] Assay methods available include gas chromatography and mass spectroscopy. A therapeutic blood level is 590 ng/mL.[2] In combination with heroin, pyrithyldione led to the death of a heroin addict.[1]

REFERENCES—PYRITHYLDIONE

1. Jorens PG, Coucke V, Selala M, Schepens PJC. Fatal intoxication due to the combined use of heroin and pyrithyldione. Hum Exp Toxicol 1992;11:296–297.
2. Langer-Groetzbach R, Martens V, Hochrein H. Chronische intoxikation mit pyrithyldine. Notfallmedizin 1985;11:1410–1411.

ZOLPIDEM

Zolpidem, an imidazopyridine derivative, is a novel, rapid-onset, short-acting hypnotic drug marketed in several European countries.[1] It is chemically unrelated to the benzodiazepines. In overdose it may result in coma, pinpoint pupils, and respiratory depression, which does not respond to naloxone but does respond to flumazenil. No fatalities have been reported.

Structure and Classification

Zolpidem hemitartrate is an imidazopyridine derivative.[2] It is commercially available in France as Stilnox. In the United States it is manufactured as Ambien. Approval by the Food and Drug Administration has been pending since January 1989, and zolpidem was recently awarded approvable status in April 1992.[3] In February 1992, the FDA's Drug Abuse Advisory Committee classified zolpidem as a Schedule V drug.[4] It has now been approved as a Schedule IV drug.[5]

Use

Zolpidem is a sedative–hypnotic drug with fast onset of action and short half-life.

Product Formulation

Zolpidem is manufactured in doses of 10 mg.[1,6]

Source

Zolpidem is a synthetic chemical product.

Therapeutic Dose

The recommended dose will probably be 10 mg administered before retiring at night, with a dose of 5 mg for patients over age 65 years of age and those with hepatic or renal insufficiency.[4]

Toxic Dose

A 50-year-old man ingested 30 tablets (300 mg) of zolpidem with about 600 mg of prothipendyl and alcohol. He responded (improvement of consciousness, correction of miosis and normalization of respiratory pattern and blood gas analysis) to flumazenil and recovered within 1 day.[7]

Fatal Dose

A fatal dose has not been reported.

Toxicokinetics

Absorption

A peak blood level of 200 ng/mL was reached 30 minutes after oral administration of 20 mg of zolpidem.[8] After oral administration zolpidem is rapidly and completley absorbed from the gastrointestinal tract. Although some first-pass biotransformation of the drug results in a bioavailability of about 70%,[4] after doses of 7 to 20 mg, zolpidem is 92% bound to plasma proteins.

Distribution

The apparent volume of distribution after a 5-mg intravenous dose was 0.5 L/kg. Brain concentrations reach one third to one half of those achieved in the plasma.[9]

Elimination

Zolpidem is completely metabolized. Less than 1% of an administered dose is excreted unchanged in the urine.[4] Three metabolites have been identified but have no pharmacologic activity after an 8-mg intravenous dose. Systemic clearance of zolpidem was 0.26 L/kg/g and the elimination half-life was 1.5 hours.[4]

Drug Interactions

Chlorpromazine, haloperidol, imipramine, and cimetidine have little effect on zolpidem toxicokinetics, although potentiation of the sedative effect of zolpidem was observed when it was given in combination with chlorpromazine and imipramine. No pharmacodynamic interactions have been observed with concomitant administration of cimetidine or ranitidine.[4]

Pregnancy/Lactation

The excretion of zolpidem in breast milk represents 0.004 to 0.019% of an administered dose.[10]

Mechanism of Action

Imidazopyridines are thought to interact with the same GABA receptor/chloride channel complex as the benzodiazepines by high affinity with the "central-type" benzodiazepine receptors.[7,11] Like the benzodiazepine hypnotic drugs, zolpidem appears to potentiate GABAergic transmission, thus increasing the frequency of chloride channel opening, resulting in the inhibition of neuronal excitation.[4] Zolpidem appears to cause only sedation, but is devoid of significant myorelaxant, anxiolytic, and anticonvulsant activity.[4] It also appears to be free of monoaminergic and histaminergic activity.[11] Benzodiazepines exert both their clinical and side effects through nonselective interaction with a family of benzodiazepine recognition sites on neuronal membranes. One of these sites, the so-called benzodiazepine or omega site, appears to mediate sedation, whereas other sites may mediate anticonvulsant, anxiolytic, and other effects. Zolpidem appears to be relatively selective for the omega site.[12]

Clinical Presentation

Therapeutic Use

At higher dosage, zolpidem is associated with adverse effects such as nausea and vomiting, headache, lightheadedness/dizziness, confusion, anterograde amnesia, and queasiness.[4,6,13] Zolpidem increases sleep stages III and IV and is virtually devoid of tolerance, rebound insomnia, and dependence, although there are still insufficient data on long-term abuse potential or tolerance following zolpidem use. Several reports have described chronic abuse, tolerance, withdrawal symptoms, and hallucinatory phenomena[14] with zolpidem.[15,16]

An anecdotal report of psychotic symptoms in two patients beginning within 30 minutes of ingesting 10 mg of zolpidem indicates that the symptoms lasted less than 30 minutes. After wakening they could not recall the events.[17] Similar amnesic events have been described for several benzodiazepines, particularly triazolam.[18] As zolpidem and triazolam share similar toxicokinetic profiles with rapid absorption and very short elimination half-life, the amnesic psychotic reactions may depend more on the toxicokinetic profile of the hypnotic drug than on specific binding to benzodiazepine receptor subtypes.[17]

Overdose

Coma, pinpoint pupils and respiratory depression have been described.[7] Somnolence, vertigo, and vomiting may be observed.[18] In one patient ingestion of 39 tablets was not followed by coma, even though treatment was not begun for 6 hours.[18] Hand, limb, and perioral tremor, muscle twitching, myoclonic jerks, diplopia, gastric and abdominal pain, and swallowing difficulties have been reported.[15] Seizures may follow withdrawal.

Laboratory

Analytical Methods

A high-performance liquid chromatographic method with fluorometric detection is available for the detection of zolpidem in body fluids (urine, serum). It is sensitive to 1 ng/mL in plasma or blood.[8,19]

Blood Levels

Following the ingestion of 300 mg of zolpidem, a plasma level of about 800 ng/mL was observed within 3 hours.[19]

Ancillary Tests

Increased transaminase levels, a leukocytosis, a mild transient hypokalemia, and thrombocytopenia were observed in a large series studied by Garnier and colleagues.[20] The French study suggests that when intoxication occurs with zolpidem alone at doses less than 100 mg, no therapeutic measures are required other than psychiatric referral of suicidal patients. When higher doses of zolpidem are ingested, gastric lavage and medical monitoring over a minimum period of 12 hours are recommended for all patients with signs of intoxication, as well as for asymptomatic patients who have been rapidly hospitalized following intoxication.[20]

Treatment

Stabilization

Treatment should be largely symptomatic and supportive, similar to that following a benzodiazepine overdose.

Gut Decontamination

Gastric lavage may decrease the absorption of zolpidem if it is performed within 1 hour of ingestion. Tracheal protection must be provided. Activated charcoal was used in one patient, but there are no systematic studies supporting its use.

Elimination Enhancement

Extracorporeal methods of treatment (hemodialysis, hemoperfusion) would probably not be useful in the clinical setting (high protein binding, rapid onset of action and elimination, availability of an effective antidote).

Antidote

In a controlled study flumazenil 0.04 mg/kg rapidly reversed the decrease in alertness, psychometricity, and electroencephalographic changes induced by zolpidem.[21] In one overdose patient who had ingested 300 mg of zolpidem followed by coma, pinpoint pupils, and respiratory depression requiring assisted ventilation, intravenous flumazenil 1 mg (0.2 mg/min) was followed by arousal of the patient, correction of the miosis, and normalization of the respiratory pattern and blood gas analysis.[6] Naloxone appears to be ineffective in diminishing coma or respiratory acidosis.[7] Repeated doses of flumazenil may be required.

REFERENCES—ZOLPIDEM

1. Langtry HD, Benfield P. Zolpidem: A review of its pharmacodynamic and pharmacokinetic properties and therapeutic potential. Drugs 1990;40:291–313.
2. Meram D, Descotes J. Intoxication aigue par le zolpidem. Rev Med Intern 1989;10:466.
3. Reynolds JEF, ed. *Martindale: The Extra Pharmacopoeia.* 30th ed. London: Pharmaceutical Press, 1993:622.
4. Fullerton T, Frost M. Focus on zolpidem: A novel agent for the treatment of insomnia. Hosp Formul 1992;27: 773–791.
5. *Physicians' Desk Reference.* 49th ed. Montvale, NJ: Medical Economics, 1995:2304–2307.

6. Wheatley D. Zolpidem: A new imidazopyridine hypnotic. Psychopharm Bull 1989;25:124–127.
7. Lheureux P, Debailleul G, De Witte O, Askenazi R. Zolpidem intoxication mimicking narcotic overdose: Response to flumazenil. Hum Exp Toxicol 1990;9:105–107.
8. Guinebault P, Dubruc C, Hermann P, Thenot JP. High performance liquid chromatographic determination of zolpidem, a new sleep inducer, in biological fluids with fluorometric detection. J Chromatogr Biomed Appl 1986;383: 208–211.
9. Thenot JP, Hermann P, Durand A, et al. Pharmacokinetics and metabolism of ZOLPIDEM in various animal species and in humans. In: Sauvanet JP, Langer SP, Morsell RL, et al., eds. *Imidazopyridines in Sleep Disorders.* New York: Raven Press, 1988:139–153.
10. Pons G, Francoual C, Guillet P, et al. Zolpidem excretion in breast milk. Eur J Clin Pharmacol 1989;37:245–248.
11. Nicolson AN, Pascoe PA. Hypnotic activity of an imidazopyridine (Zolpidem). Br J Clin Pharmacol 1986;21:205–211.
12. Gillin JC. The long and the short of sleeping pills. N Engl J Med 1991;324:1733–1735.
13. Maarek L, Cramer P, Attali P, et al. The safety and efficacy of zolpidem in insomniac patients: A long-term open study in general practice. J Int Med Res 1992;20:162–170.
14. Pirs RW. Dose-related sensory disturbances with zolpidem. J Clin Psychiatry 1995;51:35–36.
15. Cavallaro R, Regazzetti MG, Covelli G, Smeraldi E. Tolerance and withdrawal with zolpidem. Lancet 1993;342:374–375.
16. Gericke CA, Ludolph AC. Chronic abuse of zolpidem. JAMA 1994;272:1721–1722.
17. Ansseau M, Pitchot W, Hansenne M, Moreno AG. Psychotic reactions to zolpidem. Lancet 1992;339:809.
18. Oswald I. Triazolam syndrome 10 years on. Lancet 1989;2: 451.
19. Debailleul G, Khalil FA, Lheureux P. HPLC quantification of zolpidem and prothipendyl in a voluntary intoxication. J Anal Toxicol 1991;15:35–37.
20. Garnier R, Guerault E, Muzard D, et al. Acute zolpidem poisoning: Analysis of 344 cases. Clin Toxicol 1994;32:391–404.
21. Naef MM, Forster A, Mahory A, et al. Flumazenil antagonizes the sedative action of zolpidem as new imidazopyridine hypnotic. Anesthesiology 1989;71:A297.

ZOPICLONE

Following the barbiturates and benzodiazepines is a new group of rapidly eliminated hypnotic drugs ("third generation"),[1] which includes the triazolodiazepines, the imadazodiazepines, and a new chemical group, the cyclopyrrolones, of which zopiclone is an example. Zopiclone differs chemically from barbiturates and benzodiazepines but has the same pharmacologic actions—a sedative–hypnotic profile together with anticonvulsant, muscle relaxant, and antiaggressive properties. Although it is not a benzodiazepine it binds with benzodiazepine receptors in the central nervous system.[2] Zopiclone is similar in its hypnotic effects to nitrazepam 5 to 10 mg and flurazepam 15 and 30 mg.[3] Zopiclone appears to have dependence-producing properties and may lead to undesirable effects after sudden withdrawal. Overdose with zopiclone may lead to a rapid loss of consciousness.

Structure and Classification

Zopiclone is marketed in Europe as Imovane. The conversion factor is 2.57: nmol/L ÷ 2.57 = ng/mL; 1 ng/mL × 2.57 = nmol/L.[4,5]

Use

Zopiclone is effective in the treatment of patients with insomnia,[6,7] producing a sleep pattern similar to those produced by temazepam[7] and triazolam.[2,8]

Source

Zopiclone is a synthetic chemical.

Therapeutic Dose

About 7.5 mg of zopiclone appears to be the optimum dose for most patients, both young and old.

Toxic Dose

An adult ingested 30 mg and survived.[9]

Fatal Dose

A fatal dose has not been reported.

Toxicokinetics

Absorption

Zopiclone is absorbed rapidly after oral administration. Its oral bioavailability in humans is about 80%. A peak plasma zopiclone concentration of 65 ng/mL (167 nmol/L) is reached 1.4 hours after a dose of 7.5 mg. Following a 15-mg dose, peak plasma levels up to 68 mg/mL are reached at 9 hours.[10] The absorption half-life is 0.27 hour.[11] Zopiclone is about 5 to 38% bound to plasma protein, mainly serum albumin.

Distribution

Zopiclone has a volume of distribution of 1.5 L/kg.[12]

Elimination

The only active metabolite of zopiclone, zopiclone-*N*-oxide, is assumed to exert 50% of the activity of the parent drug.[11,13] Blood levels decline to 3 ng/mL (7.71 nmol/L) by 24 hours after dosage.[13] The drug has an initial half-life of 2 hours and a terminal half-life of 6 hours.[13–15] Zopiclone and its metabolites are eliminated within 24 to 48 hours of the final dose.[16] Zopiclone undergoes extensive hepatic metabolism; only 4 to 5% is excreted unchanged in the urine. Plasma clearance is about 14 L/h and is not altered by hemodialysis.[17]

Drug Interactions

When carbamazepine is given together with zopiclone, the absorption of both drugs is retarded.[18] Drugs that alter the rate of gastric emptying may affect the hypnotic activity of zopiclone.[16] Alcohol does not alter the plasma concentration of zopiclone and does not alter its toxicokinetics.[16]

Pregnancy/Lactation

The drug is excreted into breast milk. The milk–plasma area under the curve rate is about 0.6.[11] The kinetic profiles in plasma and breast milk are similar. Assuming a daily milk intake of 0.15 L/kg and 100% absorption, the average infant dose of zopiclone in milk is 1.4% of the weight-adjusted dose ingested by the mother.[12]

Mechanism of Action

Zopiclone, like several other nonbenzodiazepines, is linked to benzodiazepine receptors in the central nervous system. Zopiclone acts at a site close to rather than identical to that occupied by benzodiazepines.[19,20] In animals zopiclone possesses marked anticonvulsant, myorelaxant, antiaggressive, sedative–hypnotic, and "anticonflict" activity.[21]

Clinical Presentation

Chronic Use

Zopiclone can cause a metallic taste.[2] Other adverse effects include dry mouth, gastrointestinal effects, and drowsiness.[22] Jitteriness and difficulty in concentrating have been reported after 7.5 mg of zopiclone.[23]

Overdose

Overdose may lead to drowsiness and a loss of consciousness.[9]

Withdrawal

Withdrawal of zopiclone after regular treatment for 3 weeks may be associated with rebound insomnia.[19] The incidence of withdrawal symptoms appears low,[5,24] but similar to that for other sedative–hypnotic drugs. Physical dependence liability is described.[5,25–27] Reemergence of physical symptoms of craving for narcotics can occur after a single dose of zopiclone.

Laboratory

Analytical Methods

Quantitation of zopiclone in serum and urine is performed by high-performance liquid chromatography. The method is sensitive to a plasma level of 2 ng/mL and urine level of 200 ng/mL.[11] A modification of this method has a limit of detection of 15 ng/mL.[28]

Blood Levels

A 61-year-old woman ingested 187.5 mg of zopiclone, which led to a serum zopiclone concentration of 38 ng/mL. A 34-year-old man who ingested 225 mg of zopiclone developed blood levels of 303, 196, and 163 ng/mL 10, 12, and 14 hours, respectively, after intake.[28] A 25-year-old man ingested 300 mg of zopiclone and developed a maximum plasma concentration of 1600 ng/mL. The plasma elimination half-life was 3.5 hours.[9]

Abnormalities

The electroencephalogram exhibits a decrease in alpha low-frequency waves.[8] After ingestion of about 127.5 mg of zopiclone, a 28-year-old developed first-degree atrioventricular block on the electrocardiogram.[29] Hyperkalemia, hyperglycemia, and hyperbilirubinemia have been reported after an overdose, although in usual doses zopiclone does not appear to alter thyroid, liver, or renal function.[30]

Treatment

Zopiclone is rapidly absorbed. Most ingestions produce mild symptoms but loss of consciousness may follow an overdose. If the coma does not respond to a painful stimulus a search should be made for coingested drugs, trauma, or an underlying medical disease.

Gut Decontamination

Lavage should be considered for all ingestions greater than the therapeutic dose with central nervous depression evident within 3 hours of ingestion. Activated charcoal (10 times the estimated ingested dose or 1 g/kg body weight) and a cathartic should be administered when the patient presents within 3 to 4 hours of ingestion. Care should be taken to protect the trachea.

Elimination Enhancement

Hemoperfusion and hemodialysis have not been studied in zopiclone overdose but are unlikely to be effective in view of the extensive volume of distribution and moderately high protein binding.

Antidote

A rapid return to consciousness followed administration of an intravenous bolus of flumazenil 200 μg to a 55-year-old man who had overdosed with zopiclone. Complete recovery was achieved after an intravenous infusion of flumazenil 100 μg/h was started for a second episode of unconsciousness.[31,32]

Supportive Measures

Most patients require only medical observation. If the patient is ambulatory after 8 to 12 hours of observation, discharge may be considered after appropriate psychiatric counseling. Hypotension should be treated with fluid challenges (see General Treatment of Overdoses at the beginning of this chapter).

General Review Articles

- Goa KL, Heel RC. Zopiclone: A review of its pharmacodynamic and pharmacokinetic properties and therapeutic efficacy as a hypnotic. Drugs 1986;32:48–65.
- Wadworth AN, McTavish D. Zopiclone: A review of its pharmacological properties and therapeutic efficacy as an hypnotic. Drugs Aging 1993;3:441–459.

REFERENCES—ZOPICLONE

1. Nicholson AN. Zopiclone: A third generation of hypnotics. Pharmacology 1983;27(suppl. 2):1–2.

2. Zopiclone: Another carriage in the tranquilizer train. Lancet 1990;335:507–508. Editorial.
3. Autret E, Maillard F, Autret A. Comparison of the clinical hypnotic effects of zopiclone and triazolam. Eur J Clin Pharmacol 1987;31:621–623.
4. Reynolds JEF, ed. *Martindale: The Extra Pharmacopoeia.* 30th ed. London: Pharmaceutical Press, 1993:622.
5. Boissl K, Dreyfus JF, Delmotte M. Studies in the dependence-inducing potential of zopiclone and triazolam. Pharmacology 1983;27(suppl. 2):242–247.
6. Fleming JAE, Bourgouin J, Hamilton P. A sleep laboratory evaluation of the long-term efficacy of zopiclone. Can J Psychiatry 1988;33:103–107.
7. Wheatley P. Zopiclone: A non-benzodiazepine hypnotic: Controlled comparison to temazepam in insomnia. Br J Psychiatry 1985;146:312–314.
8. Aantaa R, Salmen M, Nyrte T. Difference in action between oral triazolam and zopiclone. Eur J Clin Pharmacol 1990; 38:47–51.
9. Royer-Morrat MJ, Rambourg M, Jacob I, et al. Determination of zopiclone in plasma using column liquid chromatography with ultraviolet detection. J Chromatogr Biomed Appl 1992;581:291–299.
10. Boniface PJ, Martin IC, Nolan SL, Tan S. Development of an HPLC method of analysing for zopiclone in biological samples. In: Kaempe B, ed. *Proceedings, 29th International Meeting, International Association of Forensic Toxicologists, Copenhagen, June 1991:*334–339.
11. Gaillot J, Heusse P, Houghton GW, et al. Pharmacokinetics and metabolism of zopiclone. Pharmacology 1983; 2(suppl. 2):76–91.
12. Matheson I, Sunde HA, Garillot J. The excretion of zopiclone into breast milk. Br J Clin Pharmacol 1990;30:267–271.
13. Houghton GW, Dennis MJ, Templeton R, Martin BK. A repeated dose pharmacokinetic study of a new hypnotic agent, zopiclone (Imovane®). Int J Clin Pharmacol Ther Toxicol 1985;23:97–100.
14. Treatment of insomnia. Drug Ther Bull 1990;28:98.
15. Kelly F, Cross NL, Sheffield F. Zopiclone. Lancet 1990;335: 1033–1034.
16. Fairweather DB, Hindmarch I. Zopiclone: Cyclopyrrolone hydrate. J New Dev Clin Med 1992;10:1–10.
17. Wadworth AN, McTavish D. Zopiclone: A review of its pharmacological properties and therapeutic efficacy as an hypnotic. Drugs Aging 1993;3:441–459.
18. Kuitunen T, Mattila MJ, Seppala T, et al. Actions of zopiclone and carbamazepine alone and in combination on human skilled performance in laboratory and clinical tests. Br J Clin Pharmacol 1990;30:453–461.
19. Tyrer P. Zopiclone. Br J Hosp Med 1990;44:264–265.
20. Blanchard JC, Boireau A, Garret C, Julou L. In vitro and in vivo inhibition by zopiclone of benzodiazepine binding in rodent brain receptors. Life Sci 1979;24:2417–2420.
21. Julou L, Bardone MC, Blanchard JC, et al. Pharmacological studies on zopiclone. Pharmacology 1983;27(suppl. 2):46–58.
22. Rendle MA. Zopiclone (Imovane®): Evaluation in general practice. NZ Med J 1990;103:225.
23. Billiard M, Besset A, de Lustrac C, Brussaud L. Dose–response effect of zopiclone on night sleep and in nighttime and daytime functioning. Sleep 1982;10(suppl. 1):27–34.
24. Anderson A. Imovane (zopiclone). NZ Med J 1989;102:647.
25. Dorian P, Sellers EM, Kaplan H, Hamilton C. Evaluation of zopiclone physical dependence liability in normal volunteers. Pharmacology 1983;27(suppl. 2):228–234.
26. Thakore J, Dinan TG. Physical dependence following zopiclone usage: A case report. Hum Psychopharmacol 1992;7:143–145.
27. Sutherland JC. Imovan and narcotic addiction. NZ Med J 1991;104:103.
28. Vertraete A, Deros M, Buysse A-M. Measurement of serum zopiclone concentration by HPLC in cases of acute poisoning. Clin Chem 1990;36:1047.
29. Regouby Y, Delomez G, Tisserant A. First degree atrioventricular block in self poisoning with zopiclone. Therapie 1990; 45:161–166.
30. Guerault E, Garnier R, Efthymiou ML. Intoxication aigue volontaire par la zopiclone: 239 cas. Therapie 1992;47:223. Abstract.
31. Ahmad Z, Herepath M, Ebden P. Diagnostic utility of flumazenil in coma with suspected poisoning. Br Med J 1991;302: 292.
32. Lariviere L. Personal communication. Rhone–Poulenc Pharmaceuticals, October 23, 1992.

Chapter 42

Endocrine Drugs

DANAZOL

Danazol (Fig. 42–1) is a synthetic attenuated androgen that can interfere with normal interactions between the pituitary hypothalamic axis and the gonads.[1] It is used in the treatment of endometriosis, benign breast disease, hereditary angioedema, idiopathic thrombocytopenic purpura, and myelodysplastic syndromes.[1–5] By its inhibition of gonadotropin-releasing hormone and gonadotropin secretion, it suppresses menstruation, inhibits ovulation, and causes regressive changes in the vaginal smear and atrophic changes in the endometrium. It is not estrogenic or progestogenic. Danazol is available for oral use in capsules of 50, 100, and 200 mg. Total daily doses range from 100 to 400 mg. (See also Chapter 19.)

Toxicokinetics

Danazol is rapidly absorbed from the upper gastrointestinal tract into the enterohepatic circulation. Plasma levels reach a maximum of 80 ng/mL about 2 hours after a dose of 400 mg. The half-life is about 2 to 4 hours. It is metabolized in the liver to an inactive metabolite.[1,6,7] In the peripheral circulation it binds to the sex hormone-binding globulin, displacing testosterone and estradiol. Free testosterone in the peripheral circulation increases. Danazol exhibits weak androgenic activity. It has been abused by athletes because of its presumed influence on athletic performance[8] (see Chapter 19). Fetal virilization occurs when danazol usage by the mother continues up to 12 weeks' gestation.[9] It has been observed both at low doses (200 – 400 mg daily) and at high doses.[10]

Clinical Presentation

The most frequent adverse effects include mild hirsutism, decreased breast size, weight gain, menometrorrhagia, amenorrhea, altered libido, deepened voice, flushing, and acne. Like other 17-alkylated steroids, danazol induces cholestatic jaundice, peliosis of the liver, and benign hepatic adenoma.[11–14] Other toxic effects include benign intracranial hypertension, headaches, dizziness, myalgias, and nausea.[15] Few cases of overdose have been reported. It is unlikely that serious immediate reactions will occur from a single excessive dose.

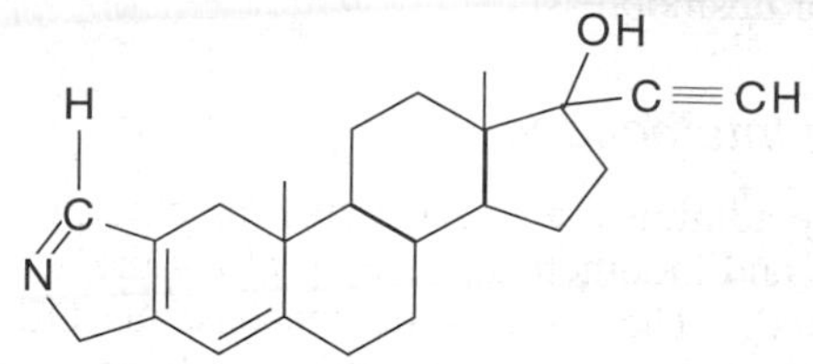

Figure 42-1 Structures of danazol and stanazolol. (From de Boer D, de Jong EG, Maes RA. The detection of danazol and its significance in doping analysis. J Anal Toxicol 1992;16(1):14–18.)

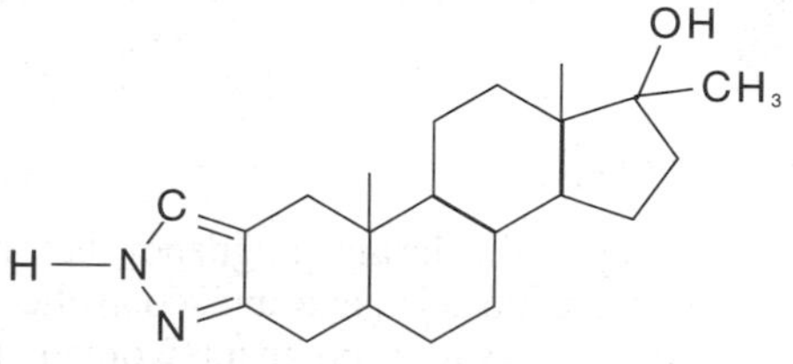

Laboratory

Hepatic enzymes (alkaline phosphatase, transaminases) may be elevated after doses of 400 mg or more daily. A radioimmunoassay method can detect levels of 1.4 to 2.8 ng/mL in human plasma.[16]

Treatment

Emesis induction and gastric lavage may be effective in removing the drug if patients are seen within 2 to 4 hours of ingestion. Supportive and symptomatic therapy is the mainstay of management. Diabetic patients should be monitored for possible insulin resistance.[17] Increases in prothrombin time may occur after simultaneous use of anticoagulants. An anecdotal report suggests that intravenous *S*-adenosylmethionine (800–1600 mg daily) may be useful in patients with severe drug-induced cholestasis.[18]

REFERENCES—DANAZOL

1. Donaldson VH. Danazol. Am J Med 1989;87:3-49N–3-50N.
2. Dmowski WP. Danazol: Steroid derivative with multiple and diverse biological effects. Br J Clin Pract 1988;24:343–347.
3. Mylvaganam R, Ahn YS, Garcia RO, et al. Very low dose danazol in idiopathic thrombocytopenic purpura and its role as an immune modulator. Am J Med Sci 1989;298:215–220.
4. Stadlmauer EA, Cassileth PA, Edelstein M, et al. Danazol treatment of myelodysplastic syndrome. Br J Haematol 1991; 77:502–505.
5. Noel P, Solberg LA Jr. Myelodysplastic syndromes: Pathogenesis, diagnosis and treatment. Crit Rev Oncol/Hematol 1992;12:193–215.
6. Potts GO, Schane HP, Edelson J. Pharmacology and pharmacokinetics of danazol. Drugs 1980;19:321–331.
7. Davison C, Banks W, Fritz A. The absorption, distribution and metabolic fate of danazol in rats, monkeys and human volunteers. Arch Int Pharmacodyn 1976;221:294–310.
8. Marshall E. The drug of champions. Science 1988;242:183–184.
9. Brunskill PJ. The effects of fetal exposure to danazol. Br J Obstet Gyenecol 1992;99:212–215.
10. Kingsbury AC. Danazol and fetal masculinization: A warning. Med J Aust 1985;143:410–411.
11. Silva MO, Reddy KP, McDonald T, et al. Danazol-induced cholestasis. Am J Gastroenterol 1989;84:426–428.
12. Middleton C, McCaughan GW, Pointer DM, et al. Danazol and hepatic neoplasm: A case report. Aust NZ J Med 1989; 19:733–735.
13. Fermand JP, Levy Y, Bouscary D, et al. Danazol-induced hepatocellular adenoma. Am J Med 1990;88:529–530.
14. Qaseen T, Jafri W, Khurshod M, Kahn H. Cholestatic jaundice associated with danazol therapy. Postgrad Med J 1992; 68:984–986.
15. Spooner JB. Classification of side-effects to danazol therapy. J Int Med Res 1977;5(suppl. 3):15–17.
16. Peterson JE, King ME, Banks WF, et al. Radioimmunoassay for danazol in human and monkey plasma. J Pharm Sci 1978;67:1425–1432.
17. Seifer DB, Freedman LN, Cavender JR, Baker RA. Insulin-dependent diabetes mellitus associated with danazol. Am J Obstet Gynecol 1990;162:474–475.
18. Bray GP, Tredger JM, Williams R. Resolution of danazol-induced cholestasis with *S*-adenosylmethionine. Postgrad Med J 1993;69:237–239.

DESMOPRESSIN

Desmopressin is a potent antidiuretic agent. It may induce severe hypotonic hyponatremia with convulsions, especially in children. There is no antidote.

Structure and Classification

Desmopressin is a synthetic polypeptide structurally related to arginine vasopressin (antidiuretic hormone), the natural human posterior pituitary hormone.[1] Its structural name is 1-desamino-8-D-arginine vasopressin (DDAVP).[2,3]

Use

Desmopressin is used similarly to vasopressin in the diagnosis and treatment of central (hypothalamic or neurogenic) diabetes insipidus.[2,4] By itself it has little effect on polyuria or polydipsia in patients with nephrogenic (vasopressin-resistant) diabetes insipidus.[5] Preliminary data suggest a role for DDAVP, together with indomethacin, in the treatment of resistant lithium-induced nephrogenic diabetes insipidus.[6] DDAVP raises the circulating levels of factor VIII coagulant activity and von Willebrand's factor and shortens the prolonged bleeding time. Therefore, it has been useful as a nontransfusional form of treatment for mild and moderate hemophilia and von Willebrand's disease.[7,8] It may also be useful in other conditions with a prolonged bleeding time such as uremia, congenital platelet defects, cirrhosis of the liver,[7,9] and hereditary hemorrhagic telangiectasia.[10] DDAVP can (in a nasal spray at bedtime) decrease bedwetting in some children with primary nocturnal enuresis.[11,12] It may be helpful in decreasing the macrohematuria associated with sickle tract hemoglobinopathy.[13] DDAVP may decrease the severity of spinal headaches after lumbar puncture.[2]

Product Formulation

Desmopressin acetate is available as a nasal solution containing 10 μg/0.1 mL metered dose (0.01%) and 100 μg/mL (0.01%), both with chlorobutanol. It is also available in a parenteral injection of 4 μg/mL with chlorobutanol 5 mg/ml and sodium chloride 9 mg/mL. DDAVP ampoules should be stored at 4°C and protected from light. The maximum shelf-life is 2 years.[14]

Source

Desmopressin is a synthetic analog of arginine vasopressin.

Therapeutic Dose

For the management of neurohypophyseal diabetes mellitus, the usual adult maintenance dose of desmopressin acetate recommended by the manufacturer is 10 to 40 ug (0.1–0.4 mL of 0.01% solution or 1–4 sprays from the spray pump) given in one to three divided doses daily. In children 3 months to 12 years of age the usual intranasal dosage is 5 to 30 μg (0.05–0.3 mL of 0.1% solution) daily in a single evening dose or divided in two doses.[1] For primary nocturnal enuresis, the initial recommended dosage of the nasal spray for children is 20 μg at bedtime.[12]

Toxic Dose

Doses of 0.3 μg/kg intravenously to 2.4 μg/kg intranasally have induced hyponatremia and seizures in children and adults.[15] Young children, especially under the age of 2 years, may be at increased risk of developing hyponatremia and seizures following DDAVP.[15]

Fatal Dose

No fatal dose has been established.

Toxicokinetics

Absorption

The bioavailability following a subcutaneous dose of 0.4 μg/kg in adults ranges from 94 to 112%; following a 300-μg intranasal dose, it is 2%.[16] A maximum plasma concentration of 568 pg/mL is reached 87 minutes after a subcutaneous dose in adults; a maximal plasma concentration of 98 pg/mL is reached 54 minutes after an intranasal dose.[16]

Distribution

It is not known if desmopressin crosses the placenta. It is distributed into breast milk in low concentrations, less than 2 ng/L.[1,17]

Elimination

The metabolic fate of DDAVP is unknown. Following a dose of 0.4 μg/kg subcutaneously in adults, the elimination half-life ranges from 2.7 to 4.6 hours. After 300 μg is administered intranasally to adults, the elimination half-life is 3.62 hours.[16] The liver and kidneys are the chief sites of metabolic inactivation of arginine vasopressin and probably that of desmopressin.[2]

Drug Interactions

Orally administered agents such as chlorpropamide, clofibrate, and indomethacin may prolong the action of desmopressin.[1,2] The antidiuretic response to DDAVP may be decreased in patients receiving lithium, large doses of epinephrine, demeclocycline, heparin, or alcohol. Carbamazepine may decrease the duration of action of desmopressin.[1]

Pregnancy/Lactation

Safe use of desmopressin during pregnancy has not been established. There are no adequate and controlled studies to date using desmopressin in pregnant women. It is not known whether desmopressin is distributed into breast milk and therefore the drug should be used with caution by nursing mothers. Fluid balance and plasma osmolality should be monitored. During pregnancy there is a normal decrease in plasma osmolality (about 10 mmol/kg).[18] Desmopressin has, however, been used during pregnancy and lactation without reports of adverse effects either on the pregnant or lactating mother or on the fetus or nursing infant.[1]

Mechanism of Action

Desmopressin is an analog of antidiuretic hormone, whose principal action is antidiuresis or oliguria. DDAVP binds to V_2 receptors, which activate adenylate cyclase in the distal medullary nephron and which exert their effect by elevating cyclic AMP in those cells.[2] It has little or no effect on V_1 vasopressin receptors of smooth muscle and, therefore, has little vasoconstrictive effect; it does not increase blood pressure or contract the uterus or gastrointestinal tract. All of these effects are related to the stimulation of V_1 receptors.[7]

Clinical Presentation

Excessive administration of desmopressin may lead to development of hypotonic hyponatremia. Doses of DDAVP not considered high have been associated with the development of arterial thromboses (myocardial infarction) in adults[19–21] and hyponatremia with convulsions in both children and adults.[15,22–25] Reactions to the preservative, chlorbutanol, are discussed in Chapter 52. Adverse effects following either the intranasal or parenteral route of administration of DDAVP have generally been infrequent and mild (parenteral: transient headache, nausea, mild abdominal cramps, vulval pain; intranasal: conjunctivitis, ocular edema, lacrimation, transient headache, dizziness, rhinitis, vulval pain, abdominal cramps).[1] Hyponatremic seizures and pulmonary edema[26] have been observed.[27]

Risk factors for the development of hyponatremia in patients receiving DDAVP include young age, frequent dosing, administration of hypotonic intravenous fluids, and administration of DDAVP in the postoperative period.[28]

Patients with a primary thirst abnormality may be misdiagnosed as having diabetes insipidus. If they are given DDAVP and continue drinking they may develop a profound hypotonic hyponatremia due to water retention. Excess DDAVP in the treatment of hemophilia or von Willebrand's disease may also lead to a state of hypotonic hyponatremia with possible increase in severity of any preexisting angina or hypertension.

Laboratory

Analytical Methods

A radioimmunoassay, both sensitive and specific, is available to determine plasma levels.[29]

Blood Levels

A plasma level of about 98 pg/ml is reached after intranasal administration; a level of about 550 pg/mL is attained after subcutaneous use. It can be expected that 0.3 µg/kg DDAVP would result in peak DDAVP levels of approximately 400 to 500 pg/mL.[16]

Ancillary Tests

Desmopressin causes a 40-fold increase in factor VIII after intravenous use; a 2.9-fold increase after subcutaneous use; and a 1.2-fold increase after intranasal administration. Subcutaneous DDAVP and intravenous DDAVP induce a 1.4- to 1.6-fold increase in the leukocyte count.[16]

Treatment

Guidelines have been suggested for the use of DDAVP in young children.[15]

- Prior to administration, obtain baseline electrolytes and a serum osmolality.
- Restrict fluids to three-fourths maintenance or less.
- Avoid large amounts of oral or intravenous hyponatremic fluids.
- If anesthesia is required, discuss the side effect of DDAVP with the anesthesiologist and request that a minimum of fluids be given.
- After use of DDAVP, follow serum Na^+, osmolality, and urine output closely for at least 20 to 24 hours, as experience suggests that the nadir of hyponatremia occurs 9 to 20 hours after DDAVP administration.
- Avoid repeat doses of DDAVP if at all possible.

Similar precautions may be advisable in older children and adults in the postoperative period, if multiple doses of DDAVP are given, or if other risk factors are present (narcotics for pain relief, liver disease, renal tubular acidosis).[15]

If hypotonic hyponatremia develops after administration of excess DDAVP, restriction of fluids to 500 to 1000 mL per 24 hours usually permits plasma sodium levels to return to normal within a few days. If the hyponatremia is severe, furosemide with oral salt supplementation may be useful.

There is no antidote to desmopressin and no V_2 receptor antagonists are available.

REFERENCES—DESMOPRESSIN

1. McEvoy GK, ed. *AHFS Drug Information 94.* Bethesda, MD: American Hospital Formulary Service, 1994:2083–2086.
2. Richardson DW, Robinson AG. Desmopressin. Ann Intern Med 1985;103:228–239.
3. Reynolds JEF, ed. *Martindale: The Extra Pharmacopoeia.* 30th ed. London: Pharmaceutical Press, 1993:952–953.
4. Ziai F, Walter F, Rosenthal IM. Treatment of central diabetes insipidus in adults and children with desmopressin: A synthetic analogue of vasopressin. Arch Intern Med 1978; 138:1382–1385.
5. Robertson GL, Harris A. Clinical use of vasopressin analogues. Hosp Pract 1989; 24(10):114–139.
6. Stasior D, Kikeri D, Duel B, Seifter JL. Nephrogenic diabetes insipidus responsive to indomethacin plus DDAVP. N Engl J Med 1991;324:850–851.
7. Mannucci PM. Desmopressin: A nontransfusional form of treatment for congenital and acquired bleeding disorder. Blood 1988;72:1449–1455.
8. Rose EH, Aledort LM. Nasal spray desmopressin (DDAVP) for mild hemophilia A and von Willebrand's disease. Ann Intern Med 1991;114:563-568.
9. Soslau G, Schwartz AB, Putatunda B, et al. Desmopressin-induced improvement in bleeding times in chronic renal failure patients correlates with platelet serotonin uptake and ATP release. Am J Med Sci 1990;300:372–379.
10. Quitt M, Froom P, Veisler A, et al. The effect of desmopressin on massive gastrointestinal bleeding in hereditary telangiectasia unresponsive to treatment with cryoprecipitate. Arch Intern Med 1990;150:1744–1746.
11. Meadow SR, Evans JHC. Desmopressin for enuresis: Useful in the short term. Br Med J 1989;298:1596–1597.
12. Desmopressin for nocturnal enuresis. Med Lett Drugs Ther 1990;32(816):38–39.
13. Baldrie LA, Ault BH, Chesney CM, Stapleton FB. Intravenous desmopressin acetate in children with sickle tract and persistent macroscopic hematuria. Pediatrics 1990;86:238–243.
14. Desmopressin acetate. In Dollery C, ed. *Therapeutic Drugs.* Edinburgh: Churchill Livingstone, 1991:D37–D40.
15. Smith TJ, Gill JC, Ambruso DR, Hathaway WE. Hyponatremia and seizures in young children given DDAVP. Am J Hematol 1989;31:199–202.
16. Kohler M, Harris A. Pharmacokinetics and haematological effects of desmopressin. Eur J Clin Pharmacol 1988;35:281–285.
17. Anderson K-E, Arner B, Furst E, Hedner P. Antidiuretic responses to hypertonic saline infusion, water deprivation, and a synthetic analogue of vasopressin in patients with hereditary, hypothalamic diabetes insipidus. Acta Med Scand 1974; 195:17–23.
18. Davison JM, Gilmore EA, Durr J, et al. Altered osmotic thresholds for vasopressin secretion and thirst in human pregnancy. Am J Physiol 1984;246:F105–F109.
19. Desmopressin and arterial thrombosis. Lancet 1989;1:938–939. Editorial.
20. Bond L, Bevan D. Myocardial infarction in a patient with hemophilia treated with DDAVP. N Engl J Med 1988;318:121.
21. McLeod BC. Myocardial infarction in a blood donor after administration of desmopressin. Lancet 1990;336:1137–1138.
22. Weinstein RE, Bona RD, Altman AJ, et al. Severe hyponatremia after repeated intravenous administration of desmopressin. Am J Hematol 1989;32:258–261.
23. Bamford MFM, Cruickshank G. Dangers of intranasal desmopressin for nocturnal enuresis. J R Coll Gen Pract 1989;39: 345–346.
24. Simmonds EJ, Mahony MJ, Littlewood JM. Convulsions and coma after intranasal desmopressin in cystic fibrosis. Br Med J 1988;297:1614.
25. Shepherd LL, Hutchinson RJ, Worden EK, et al. Hyponatremia and seizures after intravenous administration of des-

mopressin acetate for surgical hemostasis. J Pediatr 1989; 114:470–472.
26. Cone A, Riley R. DDAVP and pulmonary edema. Anaesthesia Intens Care 1994;22:502–503.
27. Beach BS, Beach RE, Smith LR. Hyponatremic seizures in a child treated with desmopressin to control enuresis: A rational approach to fluid intake. Clin Pediatr 1992;31: 566–570.
28. Humphries JE, Siragy H. Significant hyponatremia following DDAVP administration in a healthy adult. Am J Hematol 1993;44:12–15.
29. Harris AH, Nilsson IM, Wagner ZG, Alkner U. Intranasal administration of peptides: Nasal disposition, biological response and absorption of desmopressin. J Pharm Sci 1986; 75:1085–1088.

FERTILITY DRUGS

Ovulation induction agents include clomifene, bromocriptine, gonadotropin preparations, and gonadotropin-releasing hormone (GnRH) and its analogs (Table 42–1). Each agent is associated with its own specific adverse effects. Although many of these adverse effects are benign and self-limited, some, in particular those effects associated with gonadotropins, may be life-threatening.[1]

Clomifene has been associated with hot flashes, multiple gestation, visual disturbances, cervical mucus abnormalities, and luteal phase deficiency. Most of the adverse symptoms associated with bromocriptine, such as nausea and postural hypotension, are short-lived. Gonadotropin therapy, even when used appropriately, may lead to the ovarian hyperstimulation syndrome (which is occasionally life-threatening) and a high incidence of multiple gestation. Pulsatile GnRH therapy may be accompanied by adverse effects similar to those of gonadotropins, but at a far lower incidence.[1]

OVARIAN HYPERSTIMULATION SYNDROME

Ovarian hyperstimulation syndrome is the most severe acute confirmed adverse effect related to the pharmacologic therapy of infertility. The symptoms of ovarian hyperstimulation syndrome are noted from 5 to 7 days after administration of human chorionic gonadotropin. Severe ovarian hyperstimulation is relatively uncommon (<2%). Body weight gain, dyspnea, hypotension, oliguria, electrolyte imbalance, hemoconcentration, and increased coagulability are commonly noted in these patients.[1]

Many of the adverse effects related to ovulation induction agents can be predicted based on their mechanisms of action. Clomifene is an antiestrogen, and thus its adverse effects may include hot flashes and disruption of the cervical mucus and proper endometrial maturation. As a dopamine agonist, bromocriptine often results in postural hypotension, a result of increased dopaminergic tone with exogenous gonadotropins. Its major adverse effects (eg, multiple gestation and ovarian hyperstimulation syndrome) are related to the development of multiple follicles and exaggerated estradiol levels. Pulsatile GnRH therapy has adverse effects that are related primarily to its route of administration (indwelling catheters).[1]

Table 42–1
Dosages of Fertility Drugs

Clomifene	50–250 mg/d for 5–12 d
Bromocriptine	2.5 mg orally bid (range, 1.25–20 mg/d; can be used vaginally
Gonadotropins	5000–10,000 IU IM

Patients are admitted to the hospital, where fluid intake and output are monitored. Intake should be restricted to maintain adequate output and electrolyte balance, but avoid excessive ascites or hydrothorax. Intravenous fluids and plasma expanders, but preferably not diuretics, should be used judiciously to maintain urine output. Because of the increased risk of ovarian hemorrhage, given the friability of the ovaries in ovarian hyperstimulation syndrome, heparin therapy should be reserved for those in whom there is evidence of thrombosis.

If rupture occurs, surgical measures should also be conservative when possible. Rarely, oophorectomy may be required to control hemorrhage. If pregnancy does not ensue, the symptoms of ovarian hyperstimulation syndrome often regress spontaneously and rapidly, within 7 days (ie, when menses ensue). In contrast, when conception occurs, the symptoms may persist for weeks.[1]

The most significant acute adverse effects are multiple gestation and the ovarian hyperstimulation syndrome.[1]

DIETHYLSTILBESTROL

An estimated 5 to 10 million Americans received diethylstilbestrol (DES) during pregnancy or were exposed to the drug in utero. Exposure to DES has been associated with an increased risk for breast cancer in DES mothers (relative risk, <2.0) and with a lifetime risk for clear cell cervicovaginal cancer in DES daughters of 1/1000 to 1/10,000. The association between DES exposure and testicular cancer in DES sons remains controversial. Exposure to DES has also been linked to reproductive tract abnormalities in DES sons and daughters that consist of immune system disorders and psychosexual effects (Table 42–2).[2]

Diethylstilbestrol is a synthesized stilbene whose biological properties are similar to those of naturally occurring estrogens such as estrone and estradiol-17β. In 1970, vaginal clear cell adenocarcinoma was reported in young women aged 14 to 21 years. In November 1971, the Food and Drug Administration issued a drug bulletin that brought attention to the potential adverse effects of DES and banned its use during pregnancy.[2]

On the basis of current knowledge, the American College of Obstetricians and Gynecologists proposed the following guidelines for the follow-up of women exposed to DES:

1. *DES mothers:* In light of the slight increased risk for breast cancer, the committee recommends that women who received DES during pregnancy be encouraged to do monthly breast self-examinations, have an annual breast physical examination, and follow established recommendations for screening mammography.
2. *DES daughters:* Careful inspection of the cervix and vagina using one-half strength aqueous Lugol (iodine) solution and palpation of the entire wall is recommended because most cancers in women under surveil-

Table 42–2
Summary of Known and Suspected Health Effects of Diethylstilbestrol (DES) Exposure

Well-established	Probable	Possible	Speculative*
Cervicovaginal clear cell adenocarcinoma (DES daughters) Vaginal epithelial changes (DES daughters) Reproductive tract anomalies (DES daughters) Premature births (DES daughters) Breast cancer (DES mothers)	Ectopic pregnancies (DES daughters) Infertility (DES daughters) Reproductive tract anomalies (DES sons)	Cervical dysplasia, carcinoma in situ (DES daughters) Autoimmune disorders (DES daughters) Infertility (DES sons) Testicular cancer (DES sons)	Breast cancer (DES daughters) Psychosexual effects (DES daughters and sons) Prostatic hyperplasia, cancer (DES sons) Third-generation effects (DES grandchildren)

*Based primarily on animal models.
From Giusti RM, Iwamoto K, Hatch EE. Diethylstilbestrol revisited: A review of the long-term health effects. Ann Intern Med 1995;122:778–788.

lance are detected in this manner. The Committee recommends that in addition to an annual Papanicolaou test done on the cervix, women exposed in utero to DES should also have vaginal cytologic tests and colposcopy if the results are suspicious. Biopsies should be done as indicated. Noller has reviewed in detail the appropriate examination of these women and the role of colposcopy.[3]

Because of the increased risk for spontaneous abortions, ectopic pregnancies, early cervical effacement, and premature labor, DES daughters should be followed as obstetric high-risk patients. Most women can be conservatively managed during pregnancy with good outcome.[4]

REFERENCES—FERTILITY DRUGS

1. Derman SG, Adashi EY. Adverse effects of fertility drugs. Drug Saf 1994;11:408–421.
2. Giusti RM, Iwamoto K, Hatch EE. Diethylstilbestrol revisited: A review of the long-term health effects. Ann Intern Med 1995;122:778-788.
3. Noller KL. Role of colposcopy in the examination of diethylstilbestrol-exposed women. Obstet Gynecol Clin North Am 1993;20:165–176.
4. Levine RU, Berkowitz KM. Conservative management and pregnancy outcome in diethylstilbestrol-exposed women with and without gross genital tract abnormalities. Am J Obstet Gynecol 1993;169:1125–1129.

HYPOGLYCEMIC AGENTS AND INSULIN

A clinical classification of hypoglycemic disorders associated with drugs appears in Table 42–3.

Table 42–3
Clinical Classification of Hypoglycemic Disorders: Causes or Predisposing Conditions

Healthy-Appearing Patient
- No coexisting disease
  - Drugs
    - Ethanol
    - Salicylates
    - Quinine
    - Haloperidol
  - Insulinoma
  - Factitious hypoglycemia induced by insulin
  - Intense exercise
  - Ketotic hypoglycemia
- Coexisting disease under treatment
  - Drugs
    - Dispensing error
    - Disopyramide
    - Beta-adrenergic blocking agents
    - Drugs containing sulfhydryl or thiol and autoimmune insulin syndrome
    - Ackee fruit poisoning and undernutrition

Ill-Appearing Patient
- Pentamidine for *Pneumocystis* pneumonia
- Trimethoprim–sulfamethoxazole and renal failure
- Propoxyphene and renal failure
- Quinine for cerebral malaria
- Quinidine for malaria
- Topical salicylates and renal failure

From Service FJ. Hypoglycemic disorders. N Engl J Med 1995;332:1144–1152.

INSULIN

Clinical clues to intentional insulin overdose include a history of depression, hypoglycemia unresponsive or minimally responsive to concentrated glucose infusions, significantly elevated plasma insulin levels, low or normal C-peptide levels (with elevated insulin levels), positive insulin antibody assays (unless human insulin is abused), erythematous or boggy injection sites, and acute transient hepatomegaly (in children).[1]

Although exogenous hyperinsulinism frequently occurs after accidental injection, it may occur after surreptitious self-injection and occult malicious[2] or factitious[3] administration; in addition, many cases of insulin overdose are self-inflicted, often by depressed individuals intent on suicide.[4–9] Serious complications after insulin overdose were observed the first year after insulin was introduced.[10]

The incidence of hypoglycemia due to insulin overdose may be more common than is generally appreciated.[11] Reported cases are probably only a fraction of the number of suicide attempts actually occurring.[7] Some cases of insulin overdose may be unrecognized in the absence of severe hypoglycemia, or they may be considered accidental hypoglycemic episodes in patients with unstable diabetes.[11] Four of 204 severe hypoglycemic episodes in 1 year in a casualty department were intentional overdoses[12]; over a 2-year period, 18 cases of self-poisoning with insulin were reported to one agency, of whom 4 with diabetes died and 3 others sustained irreversible brain damage.[13] In another center, 20 episodes of self-poisoning were observed within 3 years; 2 of the patients died. The 2 who died had a history of either alcohol intake or decreased food intake.[14] Munck and Quaade reported a mortality of 25% in 16 published cases of attempted suicide with insulin.[15]

Medications can influence plasma glucose levels to induce hypoglycemia or hyperglycemia (Table 42–4).[16]

Hypoglycemia and Human Insulin

In the United Kingdom, some patients who have transferred to human insulin from bovine insulin have experienced an increased frequency of hypoglycemia and a loss of premonitory symptoms.[17] Bovine insulin is known to be more immunogenic than porcine or human insulin.[18] A dose reduction of 10% (or even more) has been proposed for patients previously taking less than 100 U of bovine insulin daily, and a reduction of 25% for those on greater than 100 U a day.[18] Fewer deaths and no increase in asymptomatic hyperglycemia have followed use of human insulin as compared with nonhuman insulin in the United States.[19,20]

Table 42–4
Medications Influencing Plasma Glucose Levels

Hyperglycemia	Hypoglycemia
Thiazide and loop diuretics	Salicylates
Beta blockers	Beta blockers
Calcium channel blockers	β_2 agonists
Central alpha blockers	Pentamidine
Minoxidil	Quinine and quinidine
Diazoxide	ACE inhibitors
Corticosteroids and ACTH	Disopyramide
Oral contraceptive	Fibric acid derivatives
Nicotinic acid	Streptozotocin
β_2 agonists	MAOIs
Cyclosporine	Acetaminophen
Thyroid hormones	Tricyclic antidepressants
Pentamidine	Trimethoprim–sulfamethoxazole
Isoniazid	Propoxyphene
Phenytoin	Octreotide
Phenothiazines	Tetracycline
Nalidixic acid	Mebendazole
Asparaginase	Cibenzoline
Dapsone	Stanozolol
Morphine	Fluoxetine
Encainide	Ethanol
Lithium	Sertaline
L-Dopa	Tromethamine
Theophylline	Ganciclovir
Acetazolamide	Lithium
Rifampicin	Temafloxacillin
Indomethacin	
Dopamine	
Chlordiazepoxide	
Amoxapine	
Droperidol	
Doxapram	
Octreotide	
Quinathazone	
Ethanol	
Amiodarone (?)	

ACE, angiotensin-converting enzyme; ACTH, adrenocorticotropic hormone; MAOI, monoamine oxidase inhibitor.
From Pandit MK, Burke J, Gustafson AB, et al. Drug-induced disorders of glucose tolerance. Ann Intern Med 1993;118:529–539.

Therapeutic Dose

Dosage is expressed in USP units. For example, U-100 contains 100 U/mL. Therapy is initiated with small doses of regular insulin (5–10 U in adults, 2–4 U in children). All insulins are administered subcutaneously for usual diabetic care, but regular insulin can be given intravenously for severe diabetic ketoacidosis and coma.

Toxicokinetics

Distribution

Insulin is distributed throughout the extracellular fluids. Commercial insulin preparations differ in onset, peak, and duration of action after subcutaneous administration (Table 42–5).

Elimination

Insulin is metabolized to the extent of 50% in the liver.[21] It then undergoes a reduction cleavage of the two intrachain disulfide bonds by glutathione with the enzyme glutathione–insulin transhydrogenase.[22]

The half-life of regular insulin administered intravenously is 20 minutes[23]; if administered by the subcutaneous or intramuscular route, it is 2 hours. Isophane insulin is reduced to one third of its peak value in 9 hours.[4]

Insulin is reabsorbed in the proximal tubules (98%); 60% is returned to the venous blood, and 50 to 60% is metabolized. Less than 2% is excreted unchanged.[24]

Table 42–5
Insulin Pharmacokinetics

	Onset (h)	Peak (h)	Duration (h)
Rapid Acting			
Insulin (regular)	½–1	2–3	5–7
Prompt insulin zinc (Semilente)	½–1	4–7	12–16
Intermediate Acting			
Insulin zinc (Lente)	1–2	8–12	18–24
Isophane insulin (NPH)	1–2	8–12	18–24
Long Acting			
Extended insulin zinc (Ultralente)	4–8	16–18	36
Protamine zinc insulin (PZI)	4–8	14–20	36
Mixtard (Isophane insulin, 70 μ/mL; regular insulin, μ/mL)	30 min	4–8	24

From Ellenhorn MJ, Barceloux DG. *Medical Toxicology.* New York: Elsevier, 1988:457.

Table 42–6
Signs and Symptoms of Hypoglycemia After Insulin Administration

Time After Insulin Administration	Symptoms
30 min	Perspiration; salivation; somnolence; excitement and restlessness; tachycardia if stimulated (bradycardia if somnolent)
2–5 h	Loss of contact with environment; myoclonus; primitive reflexes (grasping, sucking); reactive, dilated pupils
4–5 h	Comatose; depressed response to pain; roving eye movements; tonic and torsion muscular spasms; extensor plantar response
5–6 h	Decerebrate rigidity
6–7 h	Small pupils; bradycardia; flaccid tone; depressed reflexes

Modified from Simon R. Management of prolonged coma and determination of brain death. In: *Symposium on Poisonings and Toxicological Emergencies, San Francisco Bay Regional Poison Center, June 24, 1983*:33–47.

Drug Interactions

The hypoglycemic action of insulin appears to be increased by fasting,[8,25] alcohol,[11,25] barbiturates,[11,15] and possibly salicylates and benzodiazepines.[11] It is decreased by epinephrine,[10] glucagon, thyroxine, estrogens, adrenocortical hormones, and somatotropin.[21,24]

Pregnancy/Lactation

Insulin requirements may increase in pregnancy; insulin may concentrate in the placenta.[21] No systematic studies are available in relation to its concentration in breast milk.[26]

Clinical Presentation

The typical patient with an insulin overdose is often found in an unconscious state. Patients with intermediate or extended insulin overdose may not develop symptoms for 18 to 38 hours (coma, vomiting).[7,15] Table 42–6 delineates symptoms of hypoglycemia after insulin administration.[27]

General Observations

With longer-acting insulin,[7] in the first 24 hours there is a compensatory mechanism to maintain normoglycemia as glycogen stores are mobilized. Later, this is exhausted; hypoglycemia becomes very severe. This may lead to irreversible brain and myocardial damage.[7] Abolition of cerebral circulation (a situation similar to severe hypoglycemia) for 4 minutes in animals results in coma for 24 hours, and probably also in irreversible brain damage.[15] Hypoglycemia for 15 to 30 minutes after coma, hyporeflexia, and shallow respirations have developed is likely to lead to brain damage.[15] Prolonged hypoglycemia may result in behavior disturbances, seizures, coma, and death. Serious sequelae are often related to the duration of hypoglycemia.[24] Focal neurologic deficits may occur as a result of hypoglycemia.[28] It is the duration of hypoglycemic encephalopathy or of successive hypoglycemic periods that causes posthypoglycemic encephalopathy, rather than the quantity of insulin ingested.

Hypoglycemia may develop much later[14] than predicted for the conventional duration of action of various insulin preparations. Nondiabetics are more likely to present with decreased blood sugar and develop recurrent hypoglycemia.[14]

After insulin administration, the blood sugar may continue to decrease despite large, repeated doses of glucose. The most prolonged hypoglycemias occur with delayed-action insulins and with larger doses.[11] A rapid decline from hyperglycemic to normal blood sugar levels may produce symptoms.[29] Severe hypoglycemia may be mistaken for an intracerebral disorder.[28]

Long-acting insulins are often used in self-poisoning.[28] Mortality in attempted suicidal overdose with insulin is 25%.[10] Five of 20 diabetics who took 800 to 3200 U of insulin died.[11] Patients who attempt suicide with insulin may repeat the attempt using the same method. Recovery may occur even after there is a period with no measurable blood sugar.[15] There is little correlation between insulin dose and severity of hypoglycemia.[11] Hypoglycemia of less than 40 mg/dL is usually associated with symptoms.[29] Sequelae are worse when insulin overdose is combined with other agents (eg, barbiturates).[15] One of four patients who had also ingested alcohol and barbiturates recovered but with residual brain damage.[11] The period from injection of an overdose of insulin to irreversible brain damage is frequently about 7 hours.[27]

Diabetic coma may be misdiagnosed as overdose of insulin.[13] After an insulin overdose, 12 days of treatment may be required before insulin needs return to normal.[7]

Systemic Effects

Head, Ears, Eyes, Nose, and Throat. The face may be flushed.[5] Pupils may show no reaction to light[10] or may be dilated.[8] External ocular movement may be sluggish, with dysconjugate gaze.[28]

Nervous System. The patient may present with headaches, hysterical behavior, or depression.[5] Drowsiness, confused behavior, violent action, and restlessness may be present even with a blood sugar that is brought to above-normal levels by therapy.[6] The gag reflex may be absent.[28] The patient may have no deep tendon reflex response, may have a normal response, or may be hyperreflexic.[30] Extensor spasms may be observed. The doll's-eye test is positive.[31] Extensor plantar reflexes may be present.[31] Twelve weeks after a "large dose" of NPH, a 41-year-old woman was demented.[15] After recovery, patients may be amnesic, withdrawn, and confused for an extended period.[8] Patients may present with blood glucose levels of 22 and 28 mg/dL and a history of generalized seizure and have no evidence of acute poisoning on examination.[32]

Skin. The skin may be cold, clammy, and pale, with profuse sweating.[5] There may be elevation of temperature[8] or hypothermia.[5]

Table 42–7
Factitious Hypoglycemia (Serum Levels)

	Glucose	Immunoreactive Insulin (IRI)	C-Peptide Immunoreactivity
Sulfonylureas	Decreased	Increased	Increased
Insulinoma	Decreased	Increased	Increased
Insulin (exogenous)	Decreased	Increased	Decreased

From Ellenhorn MJ, Barceloux DG. *Medical Toxicology.* New York: Elsevier, 1988:459.

Respiratory System. Breathing may be deep and heavy, with periods of apnea.[10] Pulmonary edema[7] and aspiration pneumonitis have been observed.[8]

Cardiovascular System. Tachycardia is most often observed.

Extremities. Pain, cramps,[5,10] fibrillary spasms,[10] and twitching[15] may be noted in the leg muscles and other skeletal muscles.

Factitious Hypoglycemia: Exogenous Insulin Administration

C-peptide and insulin are secreted from the beta cells of the pancreas in equimolar concentration. Exogenous insulin administration can now be more easily diagnosed by the simultaneous demonstration of low concentrations of blood glucose, high concentrations of immunoreactive insulin, and suppressed C-peptide immunoreactivity.[3] This triad can distinguish such patients from those with insulinoma (hyperinsulinism due to an islet cell insulin-producing tumor), in whom a hypoglycemic episode is accompanied by high blood levels of both immunoreactive insulin and C-peptide immunoreactivity[33] (Table 42–7). Surreptitious insulin administration may be a symptom of serious underlying psychiatric dysfunction in adolescents with insulin-dependent diabetes mellitus.[34]

Chronic Overtreatment with Insulin

Wilson has reviewed the problem of excessive insulin therapy[35] in patients with insulin-dependent (type I) diabetes. Chronic overtreatment can present either as intermittent episodic hypoglycemia after mildly excessive insulin doses or as frequent and recurrent hypoglycemia with grossly excessive doses.

Clues to the diagnosis of overtreatment with insulin as delineated by Wilson include those derived from the history and physical findings, such as symptoms of neuroglycopenia (pallor, restlessness, stertorous respirations, depression, inattentiveness, marital discord), symptoms or signs of autonomic discharge (sweating, peripheral vasodilatation), nocturnal distress (nightmares, night sweats, difficulty in awakening), large insulin doses (>0.75 U/kg body weight), failure to decrease insulin doses after stress, good regulation on lower doses, glycogen-laden hepatomegaly, and morning hypothermia. Additional clues come from laboratory findings, including highly variable glucose values, alternating heavy glycosuria and aglycosuria, and documented hypoglycemia.

Management involves treatment of the underlying psychological issues and reduction by one third to one half of the daily dose in type II (non-insulin-dependent) diabetics or by 10% daily in type I diabetics to avoid severe hypoglycemia.

Laboratory

Analytical Methods

Insulin assays and fractionation (free, bound) tests are available, but their usefulness in an acute hypoglycemic episode is limited.

Blood Levels

Plasma insulin levels are not correlated with the severity of hypoglycemia.[11] Maximum immunoreactive insulin (IRI) concentrations in the plasma are correlated with the alleged insulin dose. Plasma glucose before therapy for an overdose is begun does not correlate with IRI plasma concentration.[14] There is no correlation between plasma potassium and plasma glucose levels in these cases.

Ancillary Tests

Blood Tests. Leukocytosis may frequently be observed.[8] Potassium levels usually are within normal limits, but may be depressed. Blood urea nitrogen, sodium, and bicarbonate levels are usually normal.[14] Immunoreactive insulin levels and C-peptide immunoreactivity levels may aid in the differential diagnosis of hypoglycemia due to insulin administration from an insulinoma (see Factitious Hypoglycemia: Exogenous Insulin Administration).

Electrocardiogram. Sinus tachycardia, occasional premature ventricular beats, and elevated ST segments may be seen.[7] Frequently, the electrocardiogram is normal.

Electroencephalogram. The electroencephalogram may be normal[10] or display slow diffuse waves without lateralizing discharges.[8,31]

Urinalysis. Albuminuria and hyaline casts may be present.[5]

Treatment

Treatment is supportive, with glucose administration playing the pivotal role.

Stabilization

Airway, breathing, and circulation must be quickly established. Where required, endotracheal intubation and assisted mechanical ventilation should be immediately instituted.

The comatose patient should be given an intravenous bolus of 50 mL 50% dextrose on admission with little delay. In an undiagnosed coma, naloxone and thiamine should also be given on admission (see Section I of this text). This should be immediately followed by continuous glucose infusion of

5 or 10% dextrose in water (D_5W or $D_{10}W$) sufficient to maintain slight hyperglycemia. Glucose administration may be required for more than 5 days before the effect of insulin dosage is overcome (as demonstrated by a glucose concentration > 100 mg/dL on two successive occasions).[9]

Elimination Enhancement

No substantive studies are available to support the use of extracorporeal procedures to remove insulin. Hemodialysis does not affect the rate of elimination of insulin.[36] Insulin has been absorbed from the peritoneal dialysis fluid in dog studies, but no studies have been reported in humans.[36]

Antidote

Glucose is the specific agent to counteract the effects of excess insulin (see Supportive Measures).

Supportive Measures

The basal level of glucose utilization and production is 125 mg/kg/h.[37] In the normal individual, an intravenous bolus of regular insulin provokes a rise in serum insulin. This provokes an increase in glucose utilization and a fall in glucose production. Thirty minutes later, the plasma insulin falls back to the physiologic range (100–200 mU/L), and glucose utilization returns to its basal rate, but glucose production is increased for a short period.[9] In large overdoses of insulin, serum insulin ranges up to 32,000 mU/L,[14] and these increases may last several days.[11] In the nondiabetic adult, an intravenous infusion rate of 375 mg/kg/h glucose (or 25 g/h in a 70-kg adult) should compensate for the maximal hypoglycemic effect of insulin and prevent hypoglycemia.[9] Frequent monitoring of serum glucose is essential. Diabetics have lower maximum glucose utilization rates in response to insulin than nondiabetics.[9]

Oral glucose cannot be relied on to maintain euglycemia, as 70 to 75% of oral glucose is absorbed after 150 to 180 minutes, and even in the presence of normal postprandial insulin concentrations, about 60% of ingested glucose is stored in the liver as glycogen, 15% is stored in tissues that are insulin dependent, and only 15% is left for the brain, which is non-insulin dependent.[9]

Intramuscular glucagon 1 to 2 mg has a fast onset of action and mobilizes hepatic glycogen stores; however, once hepatic glycogen stores are exhausted (prolonged hypoglycemia, fasting, alcohol abuse), the effect may be variable or nil.

Epinephrine (1:1000) 1 mg subcutaneously was dramatically effective in one case[10] in relieving cramps, restoring respirations to normal, returning normal skin color, and permitting the patient to talk. This effect was short-lived; the epinephrine was administered again with similar effects.

Excision of a boggy, swollen, visible insulin injection site depot was effective in the hands of Campbell and Ratcliffe[25] and Levine and Bulstrode.[38] Skin, subcutaneous tissue, and fat were removed in a block down to the muscle layer. The ease of intravenous glucose use usually obviates this procedure. An artificial pancreas[30] may serve to maintain a normal desired blood glucose concentration while adequate glucose is administered intravenously; however, it is not essential to treatment of an overdose.[14]

Cerebral edema may be managed with mannitol and dexamethasone. Potassium supplements may be useful for any clinically important hypokalemic states. Diazoxide has not been studied in insulin overdose (see Sulfonylureas). Psychiatric follow-up is important in the care of the suicidal patient. Repeat attempts are not uncommon. The patient should not be discharged until there is reasonable assurance the original act will not be repeated.

ORAL HYPOGLYCEMIC AGENTS

There are currently two main groups of oral hypoglycemic drugs, the sulfonylureas and the biguanides.[39,40]

SULFONYLUREAS

Deliberate overdose with oral hypoglycemics in diabetics appears to occur more often than self-poisoning with insulin.[13] There are, in addition, factitious hypoglycemics,[41,42] who are often medical or paramedical personnel. In a few instances, inadvertent name confusion leads to an unpredicted and unwanted hypoglycemic response.[43–46] Finally, there are the extremes of age in which therapeutic dosage can produce a severe hypoglycemic response with its associated neurologic adversities, from which the individual may partially recover euglycemic, but in disabling neurodeficit, that is, if death does not prevail.[46]

Overdoses of oral hypoglycemic drugs and insulin in both diabetics and nondiabetics probably occur more frequently than reported, as poison centers may not be contacted after an overdose. The fact that the patient was a diabetic may not be mentioned, and suicide attempts may not be recognized as such by family, friends, and physicians.

The hypoglycemic patient in coma may resemble the patient with a cerebrovascular accident, uremia, or trauma and may, indeed, also have these other diagnoses.[47] In addition, simultaneous overdose with such other drugs as alcohol, salicylates, and insulin must be considered. Salicylate[48] and alcohol overdose may be a cause of or contributing factor to hypoglycemia in a child, as alcohol may be in an adolescent.

Therapeutic Dose

Therapeutic doses of sulfonylureas are summarized in Table 42–8.

Table 42–8
Therapeutic Doses of Sulfonylureas

Sulfonylurea	Usual Initial Dose (mg)	Dose Range
Tolbutamide	500	500–3000
Acetohexamide	250	250–1000
Tolazamide	100	100–500
Chlorpropamide	100	100–500
Glipizide	5	2.5–30
Glyburide	2.5	1.25–20

Sources: Gerich JE. Sulfonylureas in the treatment of diabetes mellitus. Mayo Clin Proc 1985;60:439–443. McEvoy HK, ed. *Drug Information 94.* Bethesda, MD: American Society of Hospital Pharmacists, 1994:2056–2075.

Table 42–9
Sulfonylurea Pharmacokinetics

	Tolbutamide	Acetohexamide	Tolazamide	Chlorpropamide	Glipizide	Glyburide
Duration of action (h)	6–12	8–12	12–18	24–72	12–24	16–24
Half-life (h)	3–25	3.5–11	7	24–48	2–4	1.36–1.59
Volume of distribution (L/kg)	0.1–0.15	0.21	—	0.09–0.27	0.16	0.13–0.57
Protein binding (%)	95–97	65–88	94	88–96	92–99	99
Metabolism	Hepatic	Hepatic	Hepatic	Hepatic	Hepatic	Hepatic
Metabolites	Inactive	1 Active 1 Inactive	3 Inactive 3 Weakly active	Active and inactive	Inactive	Weakly active
Excreted unchanged (%)	—	10	—	6–20	3–15	None
Excreted (%)	100	60	85–95	60	68–89	50
Oral bioavailability	Complete	Complete	Complete	Complete	Complete	Complete
Peak plasma levels (h)	3–6	—	6–8	2–4	1–3	2–8
Clearance (L/h)	—	—	—	—	3.1	—

From Ellenhorn MJ, Barceloux DG. *Medical Toxicology.* New York: Elsevier, 1988:444.

Table 42–10
Drug Interactions With Sulfonylurea Drugs*

Interactions	Hypoglycemic Effect
Pharmacokinetic	Increased
Displacement From Plasma Protein Binding Sites	
Aspirin	
Clofibrate	
Coumarin anticoagulants (eg, warfarin)	
Phenylbutazone	
Sulfonamide	
Hepatic Microsomal Enzyme Inhibition	Increased
Monoamine oxidase inhibitors	
Possibly coumarins, chloramphenicol, phenylbutazone	
Cimetidine	
Hepatic Enzyme Induction	Decreased
Alcohol	
Barbiturates	
Phenytoin	
Rifampicin	
Decrease in Urinary Excretion of Sulfonylureas	Increased
Phenylbutazone	
Probenecid	
Salicylates	
Sulfonamide	
Pharmacodynamic	
Drugs That Inhibit Insulin Release and Action and Increase Blood Glucose Levels	Decreased
Estrogens	
Glucocorticoid steroids	
Loop diuretics (furosemide)	
Nicotinic acid	
Phenytoin	
Sympathomimetic drugs	
Thiazides	
Drugs Blocking Physiologic Response to Hypoglycemia	Increased
β-adrenoreceptor blockers	
Monoamine oxidase inhibitors	
Salicylates in high doses	

*Sulfonylureas in the presence of alcohol may induce a disulfiram–ethanol-like reaction. See Clinical Presentation.

Adapted from Paice BJ, Paterson KR, Lawson DH. Undesired effects of the sulphonylurea drugs. Adverse Drug React Acute Poison Rev 1985;1:23–26.

Toxic Dose

Prolonged hypoglycemic reactions may be observed after relatively low doses of sulfonylureas in patients with defective metabolism or excretion of the sulfonylureas or decreased glycogen storage or in conditions of prolonged and excessive insulin secretion. These conditions may be exacerbated following (1) liver damage, which may predispose to both diminished glycogen storage (cirrhosis, malnutrition) and slow metabolic inactivation of drugs; (2) renal damage, in which impaired sulfonylurea excretion may become critical; (3) insulinomas; (4) other drug intake (salicylates, alcohol); (5) diarrhea; (6) prior strokes; and (7) prior cardiac disorders.[49–51]

It is not uncommon for patients who have been maintained on a set dose for months to develop severe hypoglycemic symptoms requiring hospitalization.

Toxicokinetics

Sulfonylureas are rapidly absorbed from the gastrointestinal tract, transported in the blood in highly protein-bound complexes, and subjected to extensive hepatic metabolism (except for chlorpropamide).[52–58] Wide variation exists among the sulfonylureas in hepatic metabolism and renal clearance, factors that tend to alter the steady-state serum levels. Metabolites may be active, so there may be a variation between the plasma half-life of the parent drug and the degree of hypoglycemia encountered.

Table 42–9 summarizes the pharmacokinetics of both first- and second-generation sulfonylureas.

Drug Interactions

Drug interactions with sulfonylureas occur after either pharmacokinetic interactions (alterations in drug absorption, protein binding, and renal elimination) or pharmacodynamic interactions (alteration of blood glucose levels by changing insulin release or action).[59]

Table 42–10 summarizes drug interactions with sulfonylureas.

The binding sites on albumin for glyburide and glipizide are different from those of the first-generation agents.

Therefore, displacement by such drugs as coumarins, heparin, or phenylbutazone is less likely.[39,60,61] Alcohol interactions (chlorpropamide alcohol flush) may resemble those that occur following disulfiram (see Chapter 16), but they are not a problem with second-generation sulfonylureas.[39]

Pregnancy/Lactation

Severe hypoglycemia in the newborn may develop in the first days after delivery.[62,63] Sulfonylureas cross the placenta and stimulate insulin release from the fetal pancreas; however, hypoglycemia develops only after delivery, when the ability of maternal glucose to cross the placenta and ameliorate such hypoglycemia is halted by birth.[64]

Mechanism of Action

Sulfonylureas are now generally thought to act by a number of different mechanisms.[40]

1. Sulfonylureas produce a depolarization of the pancreatic islet beta cell membrane mediated by enhancement of calcium flux and cell membrane potassium ion permeability.[57] This results in release of preformed insulin into the circulation and occurs mostly in non-insulin-dependent diabetics.
2. Sulfonylureas may reduce basal glucose output from the liver; evidence is inconclusive.[56]
3. Sulfonylureas may increase insulin receptor binding. According to a current view, insulin resistance is distal to the bonding site of insulin with its receptor.[65] Evidence for this remains inconclusive.[56] Pancreatic effects are more preponderant in the acute use of sulfonylureas, and they depend on the presence of functioning pancreatic beta cells for their effect. In chronic doses or overdoses, sulfonylureas may have pronounced effects outside the pancreas, including potentiation of the effects of insulin on the liver, inhibition of hepatic gluconeogenesis in response to glucagon, stimulation of glucose uptake by muscle, and possibly an effect on insulin disposal.[39]
4. Sulfonylureas may act by increasing intracellular levels of AMP; sulfonylureas are known to potentiate adenylate cyclase and to inhibit phosphodiesterase in the pancreatic islet cell.[66,67]
5. Indirectly, sulfonylureas may increase insulin secretion by suppressing the release of glucagon and somatostatin from alpha and delta pancreatic cells.[68]

Clinical Presentation

Coma or altered mental status is generally the most important presenting sign in the majority (90%) of patients who have ingested excessive doses of the sulfonylureas. The comatose state may be unresponsive to glucose or glucagon for many hours. Blood sugars may rise to normal or above-normal levels while the patient is still comatose. Conversely, consciousness may be associated with severe hypoglycemic levels.

Paice and colleagues consider undesirable effects of the sulfonylurea drugs as either predictable or unpredictable.[64] Predictable effects include hypoglycemia due to either an exaggerated physiologic effect or a severe accidental hypoglycemia. Severe accidental hypoglycemia in diabetic patients may be affected by age (more in old patients), impaired renal function, impaired hepatic function, reduced food intake, weight reduction (reduces insulin resistance), drug interactions, consumption of sulfonylureas in late pregnancy by the mother (in babies), and inadvertent errors in medication dispensed. Other predictable effects include deliberate self-induced hypoglycemia (factitious), more common among medical and paramedical personnel.

Unpredictable adverse effects include dermatologic, hematologic, hepatic, endocrine, fluid and electrolyte, cardiovascular, gastrointestinal, and other adverse effects.

Overdoses similar in nature to those involving the first-generation products have been reported with the second-generation hypoglycemic sulfonylureas.[69–71]

Overdose

Head, Ears, Eyes, Nose, and Throat. Pupils may be normal, 3 mm in diameter, or fixed and dilated.[49] They may react sluggishly to light.

Nervous System. The patient may be combative or trembling[72] or exhibit fatigue, confusion,[73] and slurring of speech and loss of concentration as hypoglycemia becomes apparent. Irritability, delirium, and fainting may supervene.[74] A child may have screaming episodes and be difficult to feed.[75] Neurologic defects may simulate a stroke in the elderly patient. Dysarthria, monoplegia, hemiplegia, ataxia, athetoid movements, flaccidity, absence of deep tendon reflexes, bilateral ankle clonus, and bilateral Babinski reflexes (extensor plantar responses) are often observed. Diabetes insipidus,[76] cranial nerve III palsy,[75] motor aphasia, right hemiparesis, mental retardation,[77] and diminished visual acuity[75] may be present. Tonic–clonic seizures with or without alterations in consciousness, opisthotonos,[73] decerebrate posture, semicoma, and then death may supervene.[78] If the patient lives, residual brain death may be present.

Skin. The skin may be hot and diaphoretic.[79] Peripheral vein thrombophlebitis may be observed after continued use of high glucose concentration solutions intravenously. Sensitivity responses may rarely (1–2%) include pruritic rash, urticaria, acute toxic erythema, erythema multiforme, Stevens–Johnson syndrome, and exfoliative dermatitis.[64]

Gastrointestinal Tract. The patient may have a poor appetite, history of limited food intake, nausea, vomiting, abdominal pain, and/or dyspepsia.

Respiratory System. Apnea,[48] acute pulmonary edema,[80] and dyspnea[72] have been observed.

Renal System. Patients with prior renal disease may present with proteinuria, hyaline or granular casts in the urine, oliguria, or anuria.

Cardiovascular System. Hypotension, tachycardia, and/or cardiac arrest may occur.[80] An increase in myocardial infarction with long-term tolbutamide treatment has been studied[81,82] and remains a controversial observation.[83]

Blood. Aplastic anemia, agranulocytosis, pancytopenia, leukopenia, and thrombocytopenia have been described.[62] In overdoses, a leukocytosis (> 20,000/μL) may be observed.

Liver. Jaundice is the most frequent hepatic adverse effect; it is usually cholestatic, and recedes on removal of the drug.[64]

Endocrine System. Hypothyroidism has rarely been observed, though not after short-term use.[84]

Fluids and Electrolytes. Dilutional hyponatremia and water intoxication due to inappropriate antidiuretic hormone secretion are observed with chlorpropamide and tolbutamide.[64]

Disulfiram-like Reactions

An unusual phenomenon associated with the ingestion of alcohol during chlorpropamide therapy was observed by Signorelli in 1959.[85] It is characterized by flushing and an intense feeling of facial warmth spreading from the face occasionally to the trunk, with nausea, giddiness, occasional tachycardia, conjunctival injection, a pounding headache, and a feeling of breathlessness, occurring about 3 to 10 minutes after ingestion of even a small amount of ethyl alcohol.[86,87] It reaches maximum intensity in 20 minutes and lasts an hour. No change in the electrocardiographic pattern has been observed.[85] High blood acetaldehyde levels have been implicated by some,[85,88] but neither this nor increased excretion of 5-hydroxyindoleacetic acid has been confirmed.[87] Flushing also occurs rarely with tolbutamide.[87] The reaction may be dose dependent.[88] It has also been associated with the second-generation sulfonylureas (glipizide, glyburide).[89]

Errors by staff members involved in preparation and distribution of drugs to nondiabetic pregnant patients may occur (Table 42–8).[60]

Factitious Hypoglycemia Induced by Sulfonylureas

Sulfonylurea-induced factitious hypoglycemia can masquerade as an insulinoma both clinically and biochemically (these drugs stimulate beta cell secretion) and can be reliably excluded only by analysis of the patient's blood for sulfonylurea drugs.[41,90] (See Table 42–7.)

Laboratory

Analytical Methods

Plasma assays of the oral hypoglycemic agents are now available, generally with high-performance liquid chromatography, but they are clinically useful only to confirm the history of ingestion. Management of an overdose does not rely on blood levels of the offending agent, and the clinical state is not correlated closely with such levels. Further, availability of these assays in many hospitals is limited.

Blood Levels

Frequent measurement of blood sugar levels is important. Reliance on clinical appearance and alertness alone may not reflect the seriousness of the hypoglycemia simultaneously present. Serious hypoglycemia (blood sugar < 40 mg/dL) may be present in an asymptomatic individual.[74] Coma may be present with a normal blood sugar.

Blood levels of sulfonylurea drugs do not always correlate with the toxic clinical response. For example, therapeutic serum levels of chlorpropamide are generally reported to be 4 to 16 mg/dL; however, toxic effects were observed at 2.5 mg/dL in a child.[91] Normal doses of tolbutamide in the aged have resulted in severe hypoglycemia and death.[92]

Ancillary Tests

Arterial blood gases and serum potassium levels may reflect a hypokalemic metabolic acidosis.[72] Other blood electrolyte levels (sodium, calcium) should be obtained, but are not usually altered. Serum insulin and nonesterified fatty acids are frequently inversely correlated. Hypokalemic metabolic acidosis may be present.[72] The electrocardiogram may be normal, reflect prior cardiac problems, or exhibit sinus tachycardias,[72] T-wave inversion, or changes reflecting low cellular potassium levels. Atrial dysrhythmias and ST elevations may occur.[47] The electroencephalogram and brain scan aid in localizing any concomitant intracranial pathology that may be present in the hypoglycemic comatose patient who does not clinically respond to intravenous glucose. Cerebrospinal fluid glucose levels may be depressed for hours after the blood glucose level has been returned to normal with intravenous or oral glucose.[93] A complete blood count may reveal a moderate leukocytosis (about 20,000/uL).

Treatment

The hypoglycemic patient in coma known to have overdosed on an oral hypoglycemic agent must be subjected to the same thorough clinical and laboratory examinations as the patient who arrives in coma from any undetermined source. Immediate establishment of vital life support systems and use of intravenous glucose are paramount, however, as delay for careful examinations may expose the patient to unnecessary brain damage. The patient must be admitted to an intensive care facility and monitored for at least 24 hours. Naloxone and thiamine, in addition to glucose, should be given to the comatose patient.

Stabilization

Respirations must be established. Endotracheal intubation, or an oropharyngeal airway, attached to a mechanical source of assisted ventilation, may be required.

Hypoglycemia

Glucose. Fifty milliliters of 50% glucose is given as an intravenous bolus immediately after blood is withdrawn for analysis. At the same time, an intravenous infusion of 10% glucose in water is started. Such infusions may require a central venous line for long-term (24–48 hours) usage (eg, chlorpropamide overdose). Lilien and colleagues suggest that symptomatic neonatal hypoglycemia be treated with 200 mg/kg glucose (2 mL/kg 10% glucose in water) administered over 1 minute, followed by a constant glucose infusion by a variable-speed pump (IVAC) at a rate of 8 mg/kg/min, all intravenously.[94]

Frequent blood glucose determinations are required even after the patient has regained consciousness, as the onset of symptoms may be delayed more than 12 hours.[74]

Glucagon. Glucagon hydrochloride may aid in producing an increase in blood sugar.[95,96] Glucagon induces an increase in blood sugar and ketones, both of which are utilizable energy substrates for the central nervous system.[97] Doses of 1 to 2 mg, preferably intramuscular[98] (can be given subcutaneously or intravenously), have been useful in raising the blood sugar level from 46 to 320 mg/100 mL in 30 minutes.[96] Glucagon administration must follow the use of glucose; however, repeated doses every few hours may be necessary, its effect may be less striking on repeated use, and it may induce nausea and vomiting. The efficacy of glucagon depends on the presence of adequate glucose stores, which are often absent in an alcoholic. Glucagon has been approved by the Food and Drug Administration for the treatment of hypoglycemia. Its usefulness still remains controversial,[99] as it may also increase insulin release.

Diazoxide. Diazoxide is a direct inhibitor of insulin secretion[97]; it also increases hepatic glucose output and decreases cellular glucose uptake.[100] It has been effective in the treatment of hypoglycemia when used in doses of 200 mg orally (Proglycem capsules) every 4 hours.[99] Orally, it has been approved by the Food and Drug Administration (FDA) for hypoglycemia due to hyperinsulinism after inoperable islet cell adenoma or carcinoma or extrapancreatic malignancy in adults and for leucine sensitivity, islet cell hyperplasia, nesidioblastosis, extrapancreatic malignancy, islet cell adenoma, or adenomatosis when surgery or other therapy is unsuccessful.[101] When used intravenously in doses of 300 mg over a 30-minute period every 4 hours, it has been useful as an aid to glucose infusion in countering hypoglycemia.[97] The intravenous preparation has not yet been approved for this use by the FDA.[102]

Diazoxide should be considered for patients with marked hypoglycemia unresponsive to glucose administration.[103] Patients often rapidly respond to intravenous diazoxide, which may be required for several days.[103] The clinician should test for glucose, insulin, and C-peptide before using corrective medication. Oral hypoglycemic overdose may respond poorly to intravenous 50% glucose and negligibly to glucagon or steroids.

Alkalinization. Sodium bicarbonate, used to alkalinize the urine, appears to reduce the half-life of chlorpropamide from about 49 to about 13 hours. Conversely, acidification of the urine with ammonium chloride prolonged the half-life to about 68.5 hours.[104] If urine pH can be brought up to 8 with an adequate urine flow, more than 80% of the chlorpropamide can be eliminated in 24 hours instead of 4 to 5 days. Use of alkalinization procedures with other sulfonylureas remains to be established.

A multicenter prospective study of sulfonylurea exposure was carried out in children. Neither seizures, coma, nor sequelae were observed in the children, some of whom had a blood glucose level less than 60 mg/dL. Close monitoring of blood glucose without intravenous glucose infusion for the first 8 hours postingestion may be useful in predicting which children will become hypoglycemic.[105]

Gut Decontamination

In the presence of a history of sulfonylurea overdose within the previous 4 to 8 hours and if the patient is alert, has an intact gag reflex, is not obtunded, and is not convulsing, emesis may be induced with syrup of ipecac. If the patient is not alert, has convulsed, or is in coma, gastric lavage with prior placement of an endotracheal tube is required.

A cathartic may be administered (magnesium sulfate, magnesium citrate, sodium sulfate, or sorbitol 70%), although there are few clinical reports to substantiate their usefulness. Activated charcoal administered either 1 hour after emesis or through the gastric lavage tube (50–100 g in adults, 15–30 g in children) should be useful in reducing absorption of the drug when it is given within the first few hours of ingestion.[104,106] In an acidic medium in vitro (below pH 7.5), the oral hypoglycemic agents seem to be absorbed better onto activated charcoal.[107] Multiple 6-hour-interval doses of activated charcoal did not appear to shorten chlorpropamide's half-life.[104]

Elimination Enhancement

The sulfonylureas are highly protein bound. Experience with extracorporeal removal (peritoneal dialysis)[48] has been limited and ineffective. There are no substantive data on the use of charcoal hemoperfusion, hemodialysis, exchange transfusion, plasmapheresis, or forced diuresis in the management of oral hypoglycemic overdose.[102]

Antidote

There is no antidote to oral hypoglycemic overdose, except for glucose.

Supportive Measures

Blood glucose, arterial blood gases, serum electrolytes, liver and kidney function, and glucose balance should be monitored at frequent intervals dependent on the clinical status. Plasma insulin levels may guide the effectiveness of treatment. Blood should also be analyzed on admission for salicylates and alcohol. Urine may be analyzed for sedative–hypnotic drugs. Vital signs (pulse, respiration, blood pressure, state of consciousness) should be measured and recorded hourly during the period of intensive care. Patients may go quickly from coma into an alert state and then back into a coma throughout the course of treatment until the blood sugar level finally stabilizes. This may take several days.[102,108,109] The patient should be kept in the hospital under intensive observation until a sufficient period of clinical and biochemical stability has been reached (at least 24 hours). There is little correlation between the amount of drug allegedly ingested and the depth of hypoglycemia or length of coma experienced.

Steroid use has been proposed for severe hypoglycemia.[108] Data to support this use are not convincing. Hypotension may be managed by placing the patient in Trendelenburg position, infusing fluid intravenously (with care not to promote fluid overload), and using pressor amines (dopamine or norepinephrine) as required. Seizures may be treated with intravenous diazepam. Phenytoin may be used as required. Mannitol and/or dexamethasone may be used as indicated for cerebral edema.

Octreotide

Octreotide 50 μg every 12 hours subcutaneously may be useful in sulfonylurea overdose[110] (see Octreotide Acetate).[111] It suppresses plasma insulin and C-peptide levels, permitting the plasma glucose concentration to remain above 5.0 mmol/L without additional dextrose support.

REFERENCES—HYPOGLYCEMIC AGENTS AND INSULIN

1. Roberge RJ, Martin TG, Delbridge TR. Intentional massive insulin overdose. Ann Emerg Med 1993;22:228–234.
2. Birkinshaw VJ, Gurd MR, Randall SS. Investigations in a case of murder by insulin poisoning. Br Med J 1958;2:463–468.
3. Scarlett JA, Makoi ME, Robenstein AH, et al. Factitious hypoglycemia: Diagnosis by measurement of serum C-peptide immunoreactivity and insulin binding antibodies. N Engl J Med 1977;297:1029–1032.
4. Bauman WA, Yalow RS. Insulin as a lethal weapon. J Forens Sci 1981;26:594–598.
5. Beardwood JT. A case of attempted suicide with insulin. JAMA 1934;102:765–766.
6. Jordan H. Unusual sequel of a large overdose of insulin. Br Med J 1946;1:276.
7. Vogl A, Youngwirth SH. The effects of a single dose of 2,000 units of Protamine Zinc Insulin taken by a diabetic patient with suicidal intent. N Engl J Med 1949;241:606–609.
8. Nicholson WA. Attempted suicide with insulin. Practitioner 1965;195:790–793.
9. Stapczynski JS, Haskell RJ. Duration of hypoglycemia and need for intravenous glucose following intentional overdoses of insulin. Ann Emerg Med 1984;13:505–511.
10. Lindgren L. Enormous dose of insulin with suicidal intent. Acta Med Scand 1960;167:297–300.
11. Martin FIR, Hansen N, Warne GL. Attempted suicide by insulin overdose in insulin requiring diabetics. Med J Aust 1977; 1:58-60.
12. Gale E. Hypoglycemia. Clin Endocrinol Metab 1980;9:461–475.
13. Jefferys DB, Volans GN. Self poisoning in diabetic patients. Hum Toxicol 1983;2:345–348.
14. Critchley JAJH, Proudfoot AT, Boyd SG, et al. Deaths and paradoxes after intentional insulin overdosage. Br Med J 1984;289:225.
15. Munck O, Quaade F. Suicide attempted with insulin. Dan Med Bull 1963;10:139–141.
16. Service FJ. Hyperglycemic disorders. N Engl J Med 1995; 332:1144–1152.
17. Transferring diabetic patients to human insulin. Lancet 1989; 1:762–763. Editorial.
18. Peacock I, Tattersall RD, Taylor A, et al. Effects of new insulins on insulin and C-peptide antibodies, insulin dose and diabetic control. Lancet 1983;1:149–152.
19. Gorden P. Human insulin and hypoglycemia. N Engl J Med 1990;322:1007–1008.
20. Jick SS, Derby LE, Gross KM, Jick H. Hospitalizations because of hypoglycemia in uses of animal and human insulins: 2. Experience in the United States. Pharmacotherapy 1990;10:398–399.
21. Williams RH, Porte D Jr. The pancreas. In: Williams RH, ed. *Textbook of Endocrinology.* 5th ed. Philadelphia: WB Saunders, 1974:523–527, 591–597, 627–659.
22. Katzen HM, Tietze F, Stetten D Jr. Further studies on the properties of hepatic glutathione insulin transhydrogenase. J Biol Chem 1973;238:1006–1011.
23. Berson SA, Yalow RS. Insulin in blood and insulin antibody. Am J Med 1966;40:676–690.
24. McEvoy GK, ed. *Drug Information 94.* Bethesda, MD: American Society of Hospital Pharmacists, 1994:2046–2056.
25. Campbell IW, Ratcliffe JG. Suicidal insulin overdose managed by excision of insulin injection site. Br Med J 1982;285: 408–409.
26. Chaplin S, Sanders GL, Smith JM. Drug excretion in human breast milk. Adverse Drug React Acute Poison Rev 1982; 1:255–287.
27. Simon R. Management of prolonged coma and determination of brain death: Symposium on poisonings and toxicological emergencies. Presented at San Francisco Bay Area Regional Poison Center, June 24, 1983:33–47.
28. Bobzien WF III. Suicidal overdoses with hypoglycemic agents. JACEP J Am Coll Emerg Physicians 1979;8:467–470.
29. Baruh S, Sherman L, Kolodny HD, et al: Fasting hypoglycemia. Med Clin North Am 1973;57:1441–1462.
30. Gin H, Larnaudie B, Aubertin J. Attempted suicide by insulin injection treated with artificial pancreas. Br Med J 1983; 287:249–250.
31. Sturner WQ, Putnam RS. Suicidal insulin poisoning with nine day survival: Recovery in bile at autopsy by radioimmunoassay. J Forens Sci 1972;17:514–521.
32. Colsky LC, Campo AE, Gonzalez-Blanco M. Insulin and the suicidal patient. West J Med 1985;143:679.
33. Levy WJ, Gardner D, Moseley J, et al. Unusual problems for the physician in managing a hospital patient who received a malicious insulin overdose. Neurosurgery 1985;17:992–996.
34. Orr DP, Eccles T, Lawlor R, et al. Surreptitious insulin administration in adolescents with insulin-dependent diabetes mellitus. JAMA 1986;256:3227–3230.
35. Wilson DE. Excessive insulin therapy: Biochemical effects and clinical repercussions: Current concepts of counterregulation in type I diabetes. Ann Intern Med 1983;98:219–227.
36. Shapiro DJ, Blumenkrantz MJ, Levin SR, et al. Absorption and action of insulin added to peritoneal dialysate in dogs. Nephron 1979;23:174–180.
37. Christensen NJ, Orskov H. The relationship between endogenous serum insulin concentration and glucose uptake in the forearm muscles of nondiabetics. J Clin Invest 1986;47: 1262–1268.
38. Levine DF, Bulstrode C. Managing suicidal insulin overdose. Br Med J 1982;285:974–975.
39. Peden N, Newton RW, Feely J. Oral hypoglycaemic agents. Br Med J 1983;286:1564–1567.
40. Gerich JE. Sulfonylureas in the treatment of diabetes mellitus. 1985. Mayo Clin Proc 1985;60:439–443.
41. Jordan RM, Kanmer H, Riddle MR. Sulfonylurea induced factitious hypoglycemia. Arch Intern Med 1977;137:390–393.
42. Scarlett JA, Mako ME, Rubenstein AH, et al. Factitious hypoglycemia: Diagnosis by measurement of serum C-peptide immunoreactivity and insulin binding antibodies. N Engl J Med 1977;297:1029–1032.
43. Crowson TW, Kriel RL. Hypoglycemia from inadvertent use of hypoglycemic agents. Ann Intern Med 1980;92:134.
44. Aderka D, Pinkhas J. Inadvertently induced hypoglycemia. JAMA 1978;240:1140.
45. Ahlquist DA, Nelson RL, Callaway CW. Pseudoinsulinoma syndrome from inadvertent tolazamide ingestion. Ann Intern Med 1980;93:281–282.
46. Berger W. 88 Schwere Hypoglykamiezwischenfalle unter der Behandlung mit Sulphonylharnstoffen. Schweiz Med Wochenschr 1971;71:1013–1022.
47. Lacouture PG. Oral hypoglycemics. Clin Toxicol Rev 1984; 7(3):1–2.
48. Graw RG, Clarke RR. Chlorpropamide intoxication: Treatment with peritoneal dialysis. Pediatrics 1970;45:106–109.

49. Alexander RW. Prolonged hypoglycemia following acetohexamide administration: Report of two cases with impaired renal function. Diabetes 1966;15:362–364.
50. Asplund K, Wiholm BE, Lithner F. Glibenclamide associated hypoglycaemia: A report on 57 cases. Diabetologia 1983; 24:412–417.
51. Blohme G, Branegard B, Fahler M, et al. Glipizide induced severe hypoglycemia. Acta Endocrinol 1981;98 (suppl. 245): 13.
52. Shen S, Bressler R. Clinical pharmacology of oral antidiabetic agents. N Engl J Med 1977;296:493–497.
53. Jackson JE, Bressler R. Clinical pharmacology of sulphonylurea hypoglycaemic agents. Drugs 1981;22:211–245, 295–320.
54. Skillman TG, Feldman JM. The pharmacology of sulfonylureas. Am J Med 1981;70:361–372.
55. Balant L. Clinical pharmacokinetics of sulphonylurea hypoglycaemic drugs. Clin Pharmacokinet 1981;6:215–241.
56. Asmal AC, Marble A. Oral hypoglycaemic agents: An update. Drugs 1984;28:62–78.
57. Campbell RK, Hansten PD. Metabolism of chlorpropamide, correspondence. Diabetes Care 1981;4:332.
58. Ings RMJ, Lawrence JR, McDonald A, et al. Glibenclamide pharmacokinetics in healthy volunteers: Evidence for zero order drug absorption. Br J Clin Pharmacol 1982;13:264P–265P.
59. Sartor G. Melander A, Schersten B, et al. Comparative single dose kinetics and effects of four sulfonylureas in healthy volunteers. Acta Med Scand 1980;208:301–307.
60. Brown KF, Crooks MJ. Displacement of tolbutamide, glibenclamide and chlorpropamide from serum albumin by anionic drugs. Biochem Pharmacol 1976;25:1175–1178.
61. McKillop G, Fallon M, Slater SD. Possible interaction between heparin and a sulphonylurea a cause of prolonged hypoglycaemia. Br Med J 1986;293:1073.
62. Harris EL. Adverse reactions to oral antidiabetic agents. Br Med J 1971;3:29–30.
63. Seltzer HS. Severe drug induced hypoglycemia: A review. Compr Ther 1979;5:21–29.
64. Paice BJ, Paterson KR, Lawson DH. Undesired effects of the sulphonylurea drugs. Adverse Drug React Acute Poison Rev 1985;1:23–26.
65. Mandario LJ, Campbell PJ, Gottesman IS, Gerich JE. Abnormal coupling of insulin receptor binding in non-insulin dependent diabetes. Am J Physiol 1984;247:E688–E692.
66. Prendergast BD. Glyburide and glipizide: Second generation oral sulfonylurea hypoglycemic agents. Clin Pharm 1984; 31:473–485.
67. Sharpe GWG. The adenylate-cyclase–cyclic AMP system in islets of Langerhans and its roles in the control of insulin release. Diabetologia 1979;16:196–289.
68. Melander A, Wahlin-Boll E. Clinical pharmacology of glipizide. Am J Med 1983;75(5B):41–45.
69. Shuman CR. Glipizide: An overview. Am J Med 1983;75(5B): 55–59.
70. Kullavanijaya P. Recovery from overdose with glibenclamide. Br Med J 1970;4:53–54.
71. Sturgess NC, Ashford MLJ, Cook DL, et al. The sulphonyl receptor may be an ATP-sensitive potassium channel. Lancet 1985;2:474–475.
72. Meatherall RC, Green PT, Kennick S, et al. Diazoxide in the management of chlorpropamide overdose. J Anal Toxicol 1981;5:287–291.
73. Cowen DL, Burtis B, Youmans J. Prolonged coma after acetohexamide ingestion. JAMA 1967;201:155–156.
74. Greenberg B, Weihl C, Hug G. Chlorpropamide poisoning. Pediatrics 1968;41:145–147.
75. Sillence DO, Court JM. Glibenclamide induced hypoglycaemia. Br Med J 1975;3:490–491.
76. De Troyer A, Ectors M, Hubert JP. Chlorpropamide poisoning and diabetes insipidus. Lancet 1975;2:514.
77. Pavone L, Mollica F, Musumeci S, et al. Accidental glibenclamide ingestion in an infant: Clinical and electroencephalographic aspects. Dev Med Child Neurol 1980;22:366–371.
78. Scala-Barnett DM, Donoghue ER. Dispensing error causing fatal chlorpropamide intoxication in a non-diabetic. J Forens Sci 1986;31:293–295.
79. Dall JLC, Conway H, McAlpine SG. Hypoglycaemia due to chlorpropamide. Scott Med J 1967;12:403–404.
80. Dowell RC, Mirie AH. Chlorpropamide poisoning in non-diabetics. Scott Med J 1972;17:305–309.
81. University Group Diabetes Program. A study of the effects of hypoglycemic agents in vascular complications in patients with adult onset diabetes: II. Mortality results. Diabetes 1970; 19(suppl. 2):785–830.
82. Feinstein AR. Clinical biostatistics: XXXV. The persistent clinical failures and fallacies of the UGPD study. Clin Pharmacol Ther 1976;19:78–93.
83. Shen S, Bressler R. Clinical pharmacology of oral antidiabetic agents. N Engl J Med 1977;296:787–793.
84. Hunton RB, Wells MV, Skipper EW. Hypothyroidism in diabetics treated with sulphonylurea. Lancet 1965;2:449–451.
85. Signorelli S. Tolerance for alcohol in patients on chlorpropamide. Ann NY Acad Sci 1959;74:900–903.
86. Singer DL, Hurwitz D. Long term experience with sulfonylureas and placebo. N Engl J Med 1967;277:450–456.
87. Fitzgerald MG, Gaddie R, Malins JM, O'Sullivan DJ. Alcohol sensitivity in diabetics receiving chlorpropamide. Diabetes 1962;11:40–43.
88. Jerntorp P, Almer L-O, Ohlin H, et al. Plasma chlorpropamide: A critical factor in chlorpropamide alcohol flush. Eur J Clin Pharmacol 1983;24:237–242.
89. Glyburide and glipizide. Med Lett Drugs Ther 1984;26(669): 79–80.
90. Ludman B, Mason P, Joplin GF. Dangerous misuse of sulphonylureas. Br Med J 1986;293:1287–1288.
91. Parker CE, Tisdell EJ. Chlorpropamide poisoning: A case report of accidental ingestion in a two year old child. Clin Pediatr 1963;2:185–186.
92. Cosnett JE. Tolbutamide overdosage and irreversible cerebral damage. S Afr Med J 1961;35:43–44.
93. Kaplinsky N, Frankl O. The significance of cerebrospinal fluid examination in the management of chlorpropamide induced hypoglycemia. Diabetes Care 1980;3:248–249.
94. Lilien LD, Pildes RS, Srinivasan G, et al. Treatment of neonatal hypoglycemia with minibolus and intravenous glucose infusion. J Pediatr 1980;97:295–298.
95. Davies DM, MacIntyre A, Millar EJ, et al. Need for glucagon in severe hypoglycaemia induced by sulphonylurea drugs. Lancet 1967;1:363-364.
96. Davies DM. Glucagon in sulphonylurea hypoglycaemia. Lancet 1968;1:1154.
97. Johnson SF, Schade DS, Peake GT. Chlorpropamide induced hypoglycemia: Successful treatment with diazoxide. Am J Med 1977;63:699–803.
98. Taylor JR, Sherratt HSA, Davies DM. Intramuscular or intravenous glucagon for sulphonylurea hypoglycaemia. Eur J Clin Pharmacol 1978;14:125–127.
99. Marri G, Cozzolino G, Palumbo R. Glucagon in sulphonylurea hypoglycaemia? Lancet 1968;1:303–304.
100. Altszuler N, Hampshire J, Moraru E. On the mechanism of diazoxide induced hyperglycemia. Diabetes 1977;26: 931–935.
101. Huff BB, ed. *Physicians' Desk Reference.* 49th ed. Montvale, NJ: Medical Economics, 1995:2261–2263.
102. Bobzien SF III. Author's reply: Treatment of drug induced hypoglycemia. Ann Emerg Med 1980;9:233.
103. Palatnick W, Meatherall RC, Tenenbein M. Clinical spectrum of sulfonylurea overdose and experience with diazoxide therapy. Arch Intern Med 1991;151:1859–1862.
104. Neuvonen PJ, Karkkainen S. Effects of charcoal, sodium bicarbonate and ammonium chloride on chlorpropamide kinetics. Clin Pharmacol Ther 1983;33:386–393.
105. Spiller HA, Villalobos D, Krenzelok EP, et al. Prospective multicenter study of sulfonylurea ingestion in children. Clin Toxicol 1995;33:475–485 (Abstract 60).
106. Neuvonen PJ, Kannisto H, Hirvisalo EL. Effect of activated charcoal on absorption of tolbutamide and valproate in man. Eur J Clin Pharmacol 1983;24:243–246.
107. Kannisto H, Neuvonen PJ. Adsorption of sulfonylureas onto activated charcoal in vitro. J Pharm Sci 1984;73:253–256.
108. Forrest JAH. Chlorpropamide overdosage: Delayed and prolonged hypoglycemia. Clin Toxicol 1974;7(1):19–24.

109. Forman BH, Feeney E, Boas L. Drug induced hypoglycemia. JAMA 1974;229:522.
110. Vukmir RB, Yealy DM. Glucagon: Prehospital therapy for hypoglycemia. Ann Emerg Med 1989;18:479.
111. Boyle PJ, Justice K, Krentz AJ, et al. Octreotide reverses hyperinsulinemia and prevents hypoglycemia induced by sulfonylurea overdose. J Clin Endocrinol Metab 1993;76:752–756.

BIGUANIDES

Phenformin and its related biguanides (metformin, buformin) are sold in Europe and other countries throughout the world.[1–5]

Source

The biguanides are synthetic chemicals.

Use

Biguanides are employed for oral use in the management of mild to moderately severe stable, non-insulin-dependent (type II) diabetes mellitus in patients who are usually over the age of 40 years and obese and most often have an adult onset of their illness.

Mechanism of Action

The biguanides exert their pharmacologic effects by a similar basic mechanism.[2] They induce an increase in peripheral glucose utilization,[7] a decrease in hepatic gluconeogenesis,[8] and a decrease in intestinal absorption of glucose,[9,10] vitamin B,[11–13] and bile acids. The biguanides do not usually lower the blood sugar in a normal individual unless ethanol or another hypoglycemic agent is simultaneously ingested[14] or there is severe hepatic insufficiency.[15] Phenformin generally lowers the blood sugar only in the diabetic patient; it also depresses the blood sugar level in a nutritionally starved individual but not in one who is well fed.[16] In its usual dose administered to a healthy individual, phenformin does not induce lactic acidosis.[17] Phenformin requires insulin for its action, but does not induce an elevation in plasma insulin levels.

Clinical Presentation

Head, Ears, Eyes, Nose, and Throat. Absent corneal reflexes[14] and fixed dilated pupils[9] have been observed.

Gastrointestinal Tract. Nausea, vomiting, diarrhea,[18] abdominal cramps,[19] anorexia, weight loss, epigastric discomfort and pain, and hematemesis[20] have been seen in patients with phenformin poisoning.

Nervous System. Agitation, confusion, lethargy, seizures,[14] extensor plantar reflexes, coma,[21] and death have occurred.

Respiratory System. The patient may have rapid, deep respiratory efforts. Pulmonary hypertension has been observed.[22]

Cardiovascular System. Tachycardia, hypotension,[21] and myocardial infarction have been seen.[23,24] Rare leukocytoclastic vasculitis has been induced by metformin.[25]

Skin. The skin may be dry and hot; the patient may be dehydrated.[18] Hypothermia has been observed.

Lactic Acidosis

Lactic acidosis was first clearly defined and classified by Huckabee.[26] Lactic acidosis has been produced by all three biguanides.[27] The incidence, however, is by far the greatest after phenformin use.[5]

Diagnosis of lactic acidosis is usually made by excluding other causes of metabolic acidosis while considering the clinical state of the patient (acute onset, change in state of consciousness, hyperventilation, diarrhea, vomiting) as well as laboratory findings (anion gap metabolic acidosis, low serum bicarbonate and pH, elevated serum potassium, normal or depressed serum chloride, increased blood lactate and lactate/pyruvate ratio).[18]

Lactic acidosis may be either primary, secondary to diseases associated with hypoxemia, or idiopathic in onset.[18] Metabolic acidosis with a high anion gap must include, in the differential diagnosis, diabetic ketoacidosis (usually elevated serum β-hydroxybutyrate and acetoacetate), uremic acidosis, drug ingestions (salicylates, paraldehyde, methanol, ethanol, ethylene glycol, isoniazid), and lactic acidosis.

The origins of lactic acidosis are still the subject of investigation; however, phenformin may act on the cell membranes to decrease oxidative phosphorylation, produce tissue anoxia, increase peripheral glucose uptake (Pasteur effect), and lead to lactic acidosis and hypoglycemia.[28–30]

Biguanide-induced lactic acidosis has a 50 to 75% mortality; this is lessened if patients are not over 60 years of age, do not have cardiovascular, hepatic, renal, or infectious disease, and do not suffer from other conditions leading to increased lactate production such as shock, diabetic ketoacidosis, surgery, pulmonary insufficiency, alcoholism,[31] weight reduction, or fasting. An excellent summary of biguanide toxicity is available.[32]

Laboratory *Abnormalities*

Biguanides may induce elevations in the lactate/pyruvate ratio (normally 10:1), the hydroxybutyrate/acetoacetate ratio, the concentration of 3-β-hydroxybutyrate, the alanine/pyruvate ratio, and free fatty acids.[33] Blood glucose concentrations may be depressed,[14] normal,[19] or elevated. Some children and adults have had severe acidosis with normal blood sugar levels[34]; early reports indicated that phenformin could produce acidosis without warning in adult patients whose blood glucose concentrations were within normal limits and who had no glycosuria.[35] A leukocytosis (20,000–60,000/μL) is frequently observed. Thrombocytopenia may be present.[22] Plasma insulin levels are usually not elevated.

Death may occur even after serum bicarbonate and pH levels have been corrected, if the serum lactate level is still elevated.[26]

Ancillary Tests

Arterial blood gases and electrolyte levels may reflect a high-anion-gap metabolic acidosis. Renal function tests may reflect abnormalities (elevated serum creatinine, albuminuria).

REFERENCES—BIGUANIDES

1. Bosisio E, Kienle MG, Galli G, et al. Defective hydroxylation of phenformin as a determinant of drug toxicity. Diabetes 1981;30:644–649.
2. Asmal AC, Marble A. Oral hypoglycaemic agents: An update. Drugs 1984;28:62–78.
3. Peden N, Newton RW, Feely J. Oral hypoglycaemic agents. Br Med J 1983;286:1564–1567.
4. Korhoner T, Idanpaan-Heikkila J, Aro A. Biguanide induced lactic acidosis in Finland. Eur J Clin Pharmacol 1979;15:407–410.
5. Biron P. Metformin monitoring. Can Med Assoc J 1980;123: 11–12.
6. Reynolds JEF, ed. *Martindale: The Extra Pharmacopoeia.* 30th ed. London: Pharmaceutical Press, 1993:289–290.
7. Butterfield WJH, Whichelow MJ. The hypoglycemic action of phenformin: Effect of phenformin on glucose metabolism in peripheral tissues. Diabetes 1962;11:281–286.
8. Haeckel R, Haeckel H. Inhibition of gluconeogenesis from lactate by phenylethylbiguanide in the perfused guinea pig liver. Diabetologia 1972;8:117–124.
9. Czyzyk A, Tawecki J, Sadowski J, et al. Effect of biguanides on intestinal absorption of glucose. Diabetes 1968;17:492–498.
10. Schafer G. Some new aspects on the interaction of hypoglycemia producing biguanides with biological membranes. Biochem Pharmacol 1976;25:2015–2034.
11. Jefferys DB, Volans GN. Self poisoning in diabetic patients. Hum Toxicol 1983;2:345–348.
12. Tomkin GH, Hadden DR, Weaver JA, et al. Vitamin B_{12} status of patients on long term metformin therapy. Br Med J 1971; 2:685–687.
13. Tomkin GH. Malabsorption of vitamin B_{12} in diabetes patients treated with phenformin: A comparison with metformin. Br Med J 1973;3:673–675.
14. Davidson MB, Bozarth WR, Challoner DR, et al. Phenformin hypoglycemia and lactic acidosis: Report of attempted suicide. N Engl J Med 1966;275:886–888.
15. Fajans SS, Moorhouse JA, Doorenbos H, et al. Metabolic effects of phenethylbiguanide in normal subjects and in diabetic patients. Diabetes 1960;9:194–201.
16. Lyngsoe J, Trap-Jensen J. Phenformin induced hypoglycaemia in normal subjects. Br Med J 1969;2:224–226.
17. Guttler F, Petersen FB, Kjeldsen K. Influence of phenformin on blood lactic acid in normal and diabetic subjects during exercise. Diabetes 1973;12:420–423.
18. Medical Staff Conference. Lactic acidosis. Calif Med 1969; 110:330–336.
19. Dobson HL. Attempted suicide with phenformin. Diabetes 1965;14:811–812.
20. Pashley NRT, Felix RH. Phenformin overdose. Br Med J 1972;1:112–113.
21. Bingle JP, Storey GW, Winter JM. Fatal self poisoning with phenformin. Br Med J 1970;3:752.
22. Bergman U, Boman G, Wiholm B-E. Epidemiology of adverse drug reactions to phenformin and metformin. Br Med J 1978;2:464–466.
23. Sirtori CR, Franceschini G, Galli-Kienle M, et al. Disposition of metformin (*N,N*-demethyl-biguanide) in man. Clin Pharmacol Ther 1978;24:683–693.
24. UGDP: A study of the effects of hypoglycemic agents on vascular complications in patients with adult onset diabetes: V. Evaluation of phenformin therapy. Diabetes 1975; 24(suppl. 1):65–184.
25. Klapholz L, Leitersdorf E, Weinrauch L. Leucocytoclastic vasculitis and pneumonitis induced by metformin. Br Med J 1986;293:483.
26. Huckabee WE. Lactic acidosis. Am J Cardiol 1963;12:663 666.
27. Luft D, Schmulling RM, Eggstein M. Lactic acidosis in biguanide treated diabetes: A review of 330 cases. Diabetologia 1978;14:75–78.
28. Steiner DF, Williams RH. Actions of phenethylbiguanide and related compounds. Diabetes 1959;8:154–157.
29. Bernier GM, Miller M, Sporingate CS. Lactic acid and phenformin hydrochloride. JAMA 1963;184:43–46.
30. Tranquada RE, Bernstein S, Martin HE. Irreversible lactic acidosis associated with phenformin therapy. JAMA 1963;184: 37–42.
31. Tucker GT, Casey C, Philips PJ, et al. Metformin kinetics in healthy subjects and in patients with diabetes mellitus. Br J Clin Pharmacol 1981;12:235–246.
32. Paterson KR, Paice BJ, Lawson DH. Undesired effects of biguanide therapy. Adverse Drug React Acute Poison Rev 1984;3:173–182.
33. Wittman P, Haslbeck M, Bachmann W, et al. Lactacidosen bei Diabetikern unter Biguanidbehandlung. Dtsch Med Wochenschr 1977;102:5–10.
34. Walker RS, Lindon AL. Phenethyldiguanide: A dangerous side effect. Br Med J 1959;2:1005–1006.
35. McGavack TH. Discussion. Diabetes 1958;7:91–92.

METFORMIN

Metformin (dimethylbiguanide) is an antihyperglycemic drug used to treat non-insulin-dependent diabetes mellitus. It acts in the presence of insulin to increase glucose utilization and reduce glucose production, thereby countering insulin resistance. The effects of metformin include increased glucose uptake, oxidation and glycogenesis by muscle, increased metabolism of glucose to lactate by the intestine, reduced hepatic gluconeogenesis, and possibly a reduced rate of intestinal action. Metformin may exert effects that are independent of insulin. In muscle, metformin increases translocation into the plasma membrane of certain isoforms of the glucose transporter.[1]

Structure and Classification

Metformin is *N*-1,1-dimethylbiguanide hydrochloride.[2] Its molecular weight (free base) is 165.6 (129.2). It is prepared by chemical synthesis: $(CH_3)NC(=NH_2^+)NHC(=NH)NH_2$.

Use

Metformin is used in the treatment of type II diabetes (non-insulin-dependent diabetes [NIDDM]); as a lipid-lowering agent; and in the treatment of obesity in patients with non-insulin-dependent diabetes mellitus.

Product Formulation

Metformin hydrochloride (LA 6023, 1,1-dimethylbiguanide hydrochloride) is sold as 500- and 850-mg oral tablets (Glucophage) in the United Kingdom, Canada, Australia, South Africa, and Europe.

Therapeutic Dose

The therapeutic dose is 500 mg twice daily.

Toxic Dose

Overdoses (7 and 20 g) induce lactic acidosis. One patient recovered from an overdose of 25 g.[3]

Toxicokinetics

Absorption

Oral bioavailability is 50 to 60%. Absorption is completed within 6 hours. The plasma concentration is about 1 to 2 μg/mL 1 to 2 hours after an oral dose of 500 to 1000 mg. Metformin is negligibly bound to plasma proteins.

Distribution

The mean apparent volume of distribution ranges from 63 to 276 L/kg.

Elimination

The plasma elimination half-life ranges from 1.5 to 1.8 hours.[4] It is prolonged in patients with renal impairment and is correlated with creatinine clearance. Metformin is rapidly eliminated by renal excretion. More than 80% is excreted unchanged.

Drug Interactions

Alcohol potentiates the antihyperglycemic and hyperlactatemic effects of metformin.[5] Cationic drugs (eg, amiloride, digoxin, morphine, procainamide, quinidine, quinine, ranitidine, traimterene, trimethoprim, and vancomycin) that are eliminated by renal tubular secretion theoretically have the potential to interact with metformin by competing for common renal tubular transport systems. Certain drugs tend to produce hyperglycemia and may lead to loss of glycemic control: oral contraceptives, phenytoin, nicotinic acid, sympathomimetics, calcium channel blocking drugs, and isoniazid.

Mechanism of Action

Metformin is believed to work by inhibiting hepatic glucose production and increasing the sensitivity of peripheral tissue to insulin. It does not stimulate insulin secretion, which explains the absence of hypoglycemia. Metformin also has beneficial effects on plasma lipid concentrations and promotes weight loss.[6] In virtually all reports, the major side effects of metformin treatment are decreased appetite, nausea, and diarrhea.[7]

Clinical Presentation

Metformin can provoke lactic acidosis, which may be fatal.[8] The estimated incidence of metformin-related lactic acidosis is about 1/10th to 1/20th that reported with phenformin, or 0.03 case per 1000 patient-years.[6] Impaired renal function is the predominant condition associated with the development of lactic acidosis. Other predisposing conditions are hepatic dysfunction, cardiac failure, and alcohol abuse. Early symptoms of lactic acidosis are nausea, vomiting, diarrhea, and lower abdominal pain. The diagnosis of nonketotic metabolic acidosis may be an early indication of lactic acidosis. The diagnosis of lactic acidosis should be confirmed by plasma or blood lactate concentrations. Measurement of the anion gap may be useful. Treatment includes bicarbonate, glucose, and insulin. Acute hemodialysis may be required.

Gastrointestinal symptoms are seen in about 20% of patients and include a metallic taste, abdominal distension, nausea, vomiting, diarrhea, and anorexia.

Laboratory

Analytical Methods

Gas–liquid chromatography,[9] high-pressure liquid chromatography,[10] and mass fragmentography[4] are highly specific and sensitive. The limit of detection is 50 μg/L.

Blood Levels

Therapeutic plasma concentrations average about 1 to 2 mg/L. Monitoring has little clinical value.[8] There is no correlation between plasma lactate concentration and plasma metformin concentration at therapeutic drug levels.[4]

Abnormalities

Hypoglycemia does not occur when metformin is given alone, but may be observed when the drug is given in combination with sulfonylurea and/or alcohol.[11]

Treatment

Stabilization

An airway must be established and assisted ventilation initiated with positive end-expiratory pressure if required after endotracheal intubation. Circulatory competence must be maintained. (Blood pressure must be carefully monitored.)

Gut Decontamination

Emesis induction with syrup of ipecac may be less frequently indicated (because of biguanide-induced gastric mucosal irritation); gastric lavage may be preferred after endotracheal intubation. Activated charcoal and cathartics placed through the lavage tube may be useful but have not been systematically studied.

Elimination Enhancement

Forcing fluids may be counterproductive and result in fluid overload. Hemodialysis has been used by two investigators.[12,13] Althoff and colleagues dialyzed nine diabetic patients under treatment for biguanide-induced lactic acidosis, five of whom had had no prior renal disease; seven lived. They observed that hemodialysis, in addition to rapid removal of biguanide and excess lactate, permitted adequate amounts of sodium bicarbonate to be given without risking fluid overload or hypernatremia.[13] The use of hemoperfusion has not been evaluated in the treatment of biguanide-induced lactic acidosis.

Antidote

Hypoglycemia is treated immediately with 50 mL of 50% glucose intravenously in adults or 0.5 g/kg per dose in children.

Glucagon 1 mg intravenously had no effect on increasing blood sugar in one study.[14] Toxic doses of phenformin may depress hepatic gluconeogenesis,[15,16] and glucagon-induced hepatic glycogenolysis to raise blood glucose levels may not occur.[16]

Supportive Measures

Acidosis may be treated with intravenous sodium bicarbonate (1–2 mEq/kg). Doses of 44 to 50 mEq every 15 minutes may be required.[17] Monitoring of arterial blood gases, serum sodium chloride and potassium, and the electrocardiogram is important when administering bicarbonate. The patient may require 200 to 400 mEq of sodium bicarbonate.[18] Dehydration and hypovolemia may require placement of a central venous line.

Hypotension may be treated by placing the patient in the Trendelenburg position and cautiously using intravenous fluids. Fluids containing lactate should be avoided. Pressor amines (dopamine, norepinephrine) may increase lactic acid production by producing a relative hypoxemia of the skeletal muscles and should be used cautiously, with blood lactate monitoring.

Serum potassium levels and the electrocardiogram may reflect a tendency to hypokalemia as the alkalinization process is instituted. Serum potassium must be monitored.

REFERENCES—METFORMIN

1. Bailey CJ. Metformin—An update. Gen Pharmacol 1993;14:1299–1309.
2. Product Information: Glucophage (metformin hydrochloride). Bristol-Myers-Squibb, F5-K001, May 1995.
3. McLellan J. Recovery from metformin overdose. Diabetic Med 1985;2:410–411.
4. Sirtori CR, Franceschini G, Galli-Kienle M, et al. Disposition of metformin (*N,N*-demethyl-biguanide) in man. Clin Pharmacol Ther 1978;24:683–693.
5. Schaffalitsky de Muckadell OB, Mortensen H, Lyngsoe J. Metabolic effects of glucocorticoid and ethanol administration in phenformin and metformin-treated obese diabetics. Acta Med Scand 1979;206:269–273.
6. DeFronzo RA, Goodman AM, Multicenter Metformin Study Group. Efficacy of metformin in patients with non-insulin-dependent diabetes mellitus. N Engl J Med 1995;333:541–549.
7. Crofford OB. Metformin. N Engl J Med 1995;333:588–589.
8. Dollery C, ed. *Therapeutic Drugs.* Vol 2. Edinburgh: Churchill Livingstone, 1991:M84–M88.
9. Tucker GT, Casey C, Phillips PJ, et al. Metformin kinetics in healthy subjects and in patients with diabetes mellitus. Br J Clin Pharmacol 1981;12:235–246.
10. Charles BG, Jacobsen NW, Ravencroft PJ. Rapid liquid chromatographic determination of metformin P in plasma and urine. Clin Chem 1981;27:434–436.
11. Campbell IW. Metformin and the sulphonylureas: The comparative risk. Horm Metab Res Suppl Ser 1984;15:105–111.
12. Ewy GA, Pabico RC, Maher JF, et al. Lactic acidosis associated with phenformin therapy and localized tissue hypoxia. Ann Intern Med 1963;59:878–883.
13. Althoff P-H, Fassbinder W, Neubauer M, et al. Hamodialyse bei der Behandlung der Biguanid-induzierten Lactacidose. Dtsch Med Wochenschr 1978;103:61–68.
14. Marri G, Cozzolino G, Palumbo R. Glucagon in sulphonylurea hypoglycemia. Lancet 1000,1.303–304.
15. Schafer G. Some new aspects on the interaction of hypoglycemia producing biguanides with biological membranes. Biochem Pharmacol 1976;25:2015–2034.
16. Taylor JR, Sherratt HSA, Davies DM. Intramuscular or intravenous glucagon for sulphonylurea hypoglycaemia. Eur J Clin Pharmacol 1978;14:125–127.
17. Johnson HK, Waterhouse C. Lactic acidosis and phenformin. Arch Intern Med 1968;122:367–370.
18. Medical Staff Conference: Lactic acidosis. Calif Med 1969;110:330–336.

HYPOTHALAMIC AND PITUITARY HORMONES

Gonad-regulating hormones such as goserelin, leuprorelin, and buserelin are gonadotropin-releasing hormone analogs useful for the suppression of testosterone in the treatment of endometriosis and of advanced breast cancer in pre- and perimenopausal women; in the diagnosis of hypothalamic–pituitary–gonadal dysfunction; and in the treatment of amenorrhea and infertility associated with hypogonadotropic hypogonadism and multifollicular ovaries.[1–5]

The initial rise in circulating hormone levels can cause a disease flare (eg, increased bone pain), which settles as testosterone levels fall.

CYPROTERONE

Cyproterone, a synthetic progestogen, is an androgen inhibitor that also suppresses gonadotropin secretion and has been associated with hepatitis. An initial study[7] that is somewhat controversial[8] suggests its association with hepatocellular carcinoma.[6,7]

Disease flare at the start of treatment with a GnRH analog can be minimized by cessation of treatment and use of an antiandrogen such as cyproterone acetate (300 mg daily divided into two or three doses) or flutamide (250 mg three times daily). (See also Chapter 61.)

REFERENCES—HYPOTHALAMIC AND PITUITARY HORMONES

1. Gonadotrophin-releasing hormone analogues for advanced prostate cancer. Drug Ther Bull 1992;30(17):65–67.
2. Veronesi A, Re GL, Bo VD, et al. Buserelin treatment of advanced prostatic carcinoma: Prognostic factor analysis. Eur Urol 1992;21:274–279.
3. Herman A, Ron-El R, Golan A, et al. Impaired corpus luteum function and other undesired results of pregnancies associated with inadvertent administration of a long-acting agonist of gonadotrophic-releasing hormone. Hum Reprod 1992;7:465–468.
4. Reichel RP, Schweppe K-N. Goserlin (Zoladex[R]) depot in the treatment of endometriosis. Fertil Steril 1992;57:1197–1202.
5. Dowsett M, Mehta A, Mansi J, Smith IE. A dose-comparative endocrine clinical study of leuprorelin in premenopausal breast cancer patients. Br J Cancer 1990;62:834–837.
6. Derman SG, Adashi EY. Adverse effects of fertility drug. Drug Saf 1994;11:408–421.
7. Rabe T, Feldmann K, Grunwald K, Runnebaum B. Three cases of hepatocellular carcinoma among cyproterone users. Lancet 1994;344:1567–1568.
8. Rabe T, Feldmann K, Grunwald K, Runnebaum B. Liver tumours in women on oral contraceptives. Lancet 1994;344:1868–1869.

METYRAPONE

Metyrapone (Metopirone) is an inhibitor of 11β-hydroxylase, a cytochrome P450 enzyme involved in the biosynthesis of cortisol and aldosterone. It also inhibits phenobarbital-induced cytochromes P450.[1–3] In overdose it may induce gastrointestinal symptoms and signs of adrenocortical insufficiency. Fatalities may occur.

Structure and Classification

Metyrapone has an empirical formula of $C_{14}H_{14}N_2O$. Its chemical formula is 2-methyl-1,2-di-3-pyridyl-1-propanone.

Use

Metyrapone is used in the investigation of anterior pituitary function in patients with suspected hypopituitarism,[4] in the differential diagnosis and management of patients with Cushing's syndrome, and in the treatment of resistant edema associated with secondary hyperaldosteronism where it is used together with glucocorticoid.

Product Formulation

Metyrapone is available in 250-mg capsules and tablets. Ampoules of 10 mL containing 1 g of active substance (in the form of the ditartrate, 1 g ditartrate equals 0.438 g base) are also available.

Source

Metyrapone is a synthetic chemical product.

Therapeutic Dose

Six capsules (1.5 g) are given daily in three to four fractional doses. In the metyrapone test, either 500 to 700 mg (average, 15 mg/kg by mouth every 4 hours for 24 hours; total dose, 3–4.5 g) or 1 to 2 mg of the ditartrate (average, 30 mg/kg intravenously over 4 hours) is administered.[2]

Fatal Dose

A 6-year-old child was given 2000 mg daily for 2 days. She died in cardiac arrest.[2]

Toxicokinetics

Absorption

The drug is absorbed after oral ingestion, producing a peak plasma level of 2.7 μg/mL at 1 hour.[4,5] Plasma levels of metyrapone exceed 0.3 μg/mL after doses of 750 mg every 4 hours.[6]

Elimination

The plasma half-life following 600 mg metyrapone ditartrate intravenously ranges from 20 to 26 minutes. Metyrapone is metabolized in the liver. Less than 1% of a dose is excreted unchanged.[2]

Drug Interactions

In patients under treatment with insulin or oral antidiabetic agents, the signs and symptoms of acute poisoning with metyrapone may be aggravated.[2]

Mechanism of Action

Plasma concentrations greater than 0.3 μg/mL during a 24-hour period are associated with inhibition of cortisol biosynthesis and elevation of plasma 11-deoxycortisol levels, demonstrating 11β-hydroxylase inhibition.[6]

Clinical Presentation

The clinical picture of poisoning with metyrapone is characterized by gastrointestinal symptoms and signs of acute adrenocortical insufficiency. Cardiac arrhythmias, hypotension, dehydration, anxiety, confusion, weakness, impairment of consciousness, nausea, repeated vomiting, and epigastric pain may also be observed.[2]

Metyrapone administration to long-term methadone-maintained patients and to patients undergoing slow dose reduction to drug-free status following chronic treatment may induce a narcotic withdrawal-like syndrome.[7] Alopecia has been reported in several patients following long-term metyrapone therapy.[8]

Laboratory

A high-performance liquid chromatography method with ultraviolet detection at 254 nm is available.[9] The method is sensitive to 4.4 nmol/L.

Treatment

Treatment of an overdose following early (within a few hours of ingestion) gastric lavage centers on intravenous hydrocortisone, saline, and glucose, repeated as required. Patients should be monitored for several days with special attention to blood pressure, fluids, and electrolyte balance.[2,10]

REFERENCES—METYRAPONE

1. Product Labeling: Metyrapone. C86-6. Summit, NJ: Ciba Pharmaceutical, March 1986.
2. Signs, symptoms and treatment of acute poisoning. Basel: Ciba-Geigy, 1976:94–95.
3. Reynolds JEF, ed. *Martindale: The Extra Pharmacopoeia.* 30th ed. London: Pharmaceutical Press, 1993:776.
4. Leisti S. Evaluation of 3 hour metyrapone test in children and adolescents. Clin Endocrinol 1977;6:305–320.
5. Sprunt JG, Browning MCK, Hannah DM. Some aspects of the pharmacology of metyrapone: Mem Soc Endocrinol 1968;17:193–203.
6. Jubiz W, Matsukura S, Meikle AW, et al. Plasma metyrapone, adrenocorticotropic hormone and deoxycortisol levels sequential changes during oral and intravenous metyrapone administration. Arch Intern Med 1987;125:468–471.
7. Kennedy JA, Hartman N, Sbriglio R, et al. Metyrapone-induced withdrawal symptoms. Br J Addict 1990;85:1133–1140.
8. Harries-Jones R, Overstall P. Metyrapone-induced alopecia. Postgrad Med J 1990;66:584.

9. Usansky JI, Damani LA, Houston JB. The pharmacokinetics of metyrapone in the rat. J Pharm Pharmcol 1984;36(suppl.):280.
10. Metopirone. ABPI. Data Sheet Compendium 1989–1990. London: Datapharm Publications, 1989:317–318.

MIFEPRISTONE (RU-486)

Mifepristone is an antiprogestogen with abortifacient properties. In overdose it may be expected to induce vaginal bleeding.

Structure and Classification

Mifepristone is 17β-hydroxy-11β-(dimethylaminophenyl)-17α-(1-propynyl)estra-4,9-dien-3-one). It is a derivative of norethisterone and is chemically related to progesterone.[1] Mifepristone has a molecular weight of 429.6. Mifepristone is available commercially in France as Mifegyne.

Use

Mifepristone, when used together with a prostaglandin in the first 35 days of pregnancy, is an effective abortifacient.[2,3] Its use in second-trimester abortion is being evaluated. It is effective in inducing labor in the presence of intrauterine death. Preliminary data suggest its use in Cushing's syndrome, adrenal cancer, and even glaucoma because of glucorticoid receptor blocking.[3] Anecdotal data also suggest its use in the treatment of meningioma. Mifepristone has also been used alone as a cervical ripening agent before transcervical operative procedures.[4]

Therapeutic Dose

Most centers use a single dose of 600 mg of mifepristone followed 36 to 48 hours later by either 0.25 mg of sulprostace by injection or a single vaginal pessary of 1 mg of gemeprost.[5]

Toxicokinetics

Absorption

The bioavailability of mifepristone is about 70%. Plasma concentration peaks in 1 to 2 hours. Mifepristone is about 98% bound to plasma protein, mostly α_1-acid glycoprotein.[6–9]

For termination of early pregnancy a single dose of 200 mg mifepristone is as effective as 600 mg when used in combination with a vaginal pessary of 1 mg gemeprost.[10]

Distribution

The apparent volume of distribution at steady state after intravenous administration is about 26 L.[8]

Elimination

The elimination half-life is 12 to 24 hours. Total plasma clearance is about 3 L/h.[6]

Pregnancy/Lactation

Mifepristone crosses the placenta.[6] A study of three pregnant patients who received mifepristone in the first 8 to 9 weeks of gestation indicates that the pregnancy progressed satisfactorily. Labor began at 39 to 41 weeks and the infants were born without obvious defects.[4] Mifepristone may have been associated with a malformed fetus aborted in the second trimester after the mother took the drug to terminate an early pregnancy.[11]

Mechanism of Action

Mifepristone competes with progesterone for its specific receptors and thereby antagonizes its action.[2] It has almost no agonist activity and almost no effect on estrogen receptors in the uterus or mineralocorticoid receptors in the kidney. It has slight antiglucocorticoid activity. Mifepristone increases the sensitivity of the uterus to prostaglandins. The combination of these agents induced effective abortion.

Clinical Presentation

Some patients experience excessive blood loss with or without complete expulsion of the products of conception.[12] Other undesirable effects may include fatigue, hot flashes, gynecomastia, partial alopecia,[13] nausea, vomiting, and abdominal pain. Cardiovascular complications may follow mifepristone use.[14]

Laboratory

Analytical Methods

A radioimmunoassay for plasma mifepristone concentrations is sensitive to 72.5 nmol/L.[9]

Abnormalities

Cortisol and thyroid-stimulating hormone levels appear to rise, with a decrease in T_4 thyroxine level.[12]

Treatment

Management of an overdose is symptomatic and supportive. An obstetric consultation should be obtained. Clinicians should be prepared for excessive bleeding. Patients should be hospitalized in an intensive care unit where airway, breathing, and circulatory integrity can be monitored.

General Review Articles

- French abortion pill reinstated. Lancet 1988;2:1153. Editorial.
- Haak HP, de Keizer RJW, Hagenouw-Taal JCW, et al. Successful mifepristone treatment of recurrent inoperable meningioma. Lancet 1990;336:124–125.
- Hill NCW, Ferguson J, MacKenzie IZ. The efficacy of oral mifepristone (RU-38, 486) with a prostaglandin E_1 analog vaginal pessary for the termination of early pregnancy: Complications and patient acceptability. Am J Obstet Gynecol 1990;162:414–417.

- Lamberts SWJ, Tanghe SLJ, Avezaat CJJ, et al. Mifepristone (RU486) treatment of meningiomas. J Neurol Neurosurg Psychiatry 1992;55:486–490.
- Mifepristone: Application for UK license. Lancet 1990; 336:240. Editorial.
- Segal SJ. Mifepristone (RU-486). N Engl J Med 1990;322:691–693.
- Silvestre L, Dubois C, Renault M, et al. Voluntary interception of pregnancy with mifepristone (Ru-486) as a prostaglandin analogue: A large-scale French experience. N Engl J Med 1990;322:645–648.
- Urquhart DR, Templeton AA. Mifepristone (RU-486) and second trimester termination. Lancet 1987;2:1405.
- Van der Lely A-J, Foeken K, Van der Mast RC, Lamberts SWJ. Rapid reversal of acute psychosis in the Cushing's syndrome with the cortisol-receptor antagonist mifepristone (RU-486). Ann Intern Med 1991; 114:143–144.

REFERENCES—MIFEPRISTONE (RU-486)

1. Baulieu EE. RU-486 as an antiprogesterone steroid: From receptor to contragestion and beyond. JAMA 1989;262: 1808–1814.
2. Paeyron R, Aubeny E, Targosz V, et al. Early termination of pregnancy with mifepristone (RU 486) and the orally active prostaglandin misoprostol. N Engl J Med 1993; 328:1503–1513.
3. Reproductive health and mifepristone. Lancet 1990;336: 1480–1481. Editorial.
4. Lim RH, Lees PAR, Bjornsson S, et al. Normal development after exposure to mifepristone in early pregnancy. Lancet 1990;336:257–258.
5. Guillebaud J. Medical termination of pregnancy combined with prostaglandin RU-486 is effective. Br Med J 1990;301: 352–354.
6. Brogden RN, Goa KL, Faulds D. Mifepristone: A review of its pharmacodynamic and pharmacokinetic properties, and therapeutic potential. Drugs 1993;45:384–409.
7. Norman J. Antiprogesterones. Br J Hosp Med 1991;45:372–375.
8. Deraedt R, Bonnat C, Busigny M, et al. Pharmacokinetics of RU 486. In: Beaulieu EE, Egal SD, eds. *The Antiprogestin Steroid RU 486 and Human Fertility Control.* New York: Plenum, 1985:103–132.
9. Swabor HL, Wang G, Aaedo AR, et al. Plasma levels of antiprogestin RU 486 following oral administration in nonpregnant and early pregnant women. Contraception 1986;34: 469–481.
10. World Health Organization Task Force on Post-ovulatory Method of Fertility Regulation. Termination of pregnancy with reduced doses of mifepristone. Br Med J 1993;307:532–537.
11. Henrion R. RU-486 abortions. Nature 1989;338:110.
12. Herrmann W. The clinical use of RU-486 (mifepristone). Res Reprod 1989;21(4):3.
13. Grunberg S, Weiss M, Spitz I, Dubois C. Effects of long term oral treatment with RU-486 on unresectable meningioma. Eur J Cancer 1990;172.
14. Spitz IM, Bardin CW. Mifepristone (RU486): A modulator of progestin and glucocorticoid action. N Engl J Med 1993;329:404–412.

OCTREOTIDE ACETATE

Octreotide (Sandostatin) is a somatostatin analog (Fig. 42–2); it is a synthetic eight-amino-acid peptide (octapeptide).[1,2] It is administered in a dose of 100 μg subcutaneously three times daily.[3] Higher doses are needed in about 10% of patients. (See also Hypoglycemic Agents and Insulin.)

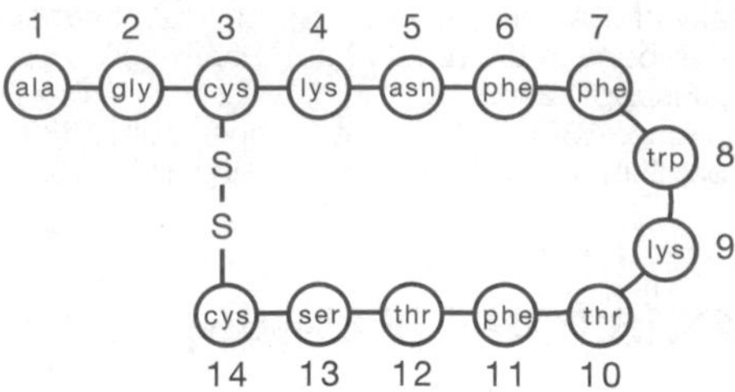

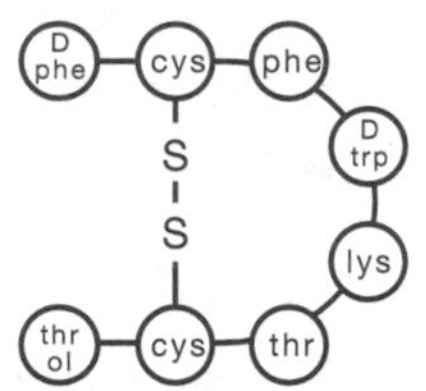

Figure 42-2 Amino acid sequences of somatostatin and octreotide. (From Chanson P, Timsit J, Harris AG. Clinical pharmacokinetics of octreotide: Therapeutic applications in patients with pituitary tumours. Clin Pharmacokinet 1993;25:375–391.)

Use

In acromegaly the main indication is after pituitary surgery if the growth hormone concentration remains above 5 ng/L or if insulin-like growth factor 1 is raised or growth hormone is not suppressed by an oral glucose level. It is also indicated for patients unfit for surgery or preoperatively in those with large pituitary adenomas to induce tumor shrinkage. Octreotide inhibits endocrine and exocrine gastrointestinal secretion and may be useful in treatment of gastroenteric pancreatic tumors. It may be useful in carcinoid tumors, vasoactive intestinal peptidoma, glucagonoma and acromegaly.[4] Octreotide also inhibits intestinal transplant and mobility and gallbladder motility. Octreotide reduces gastrointestinal fistula output (eg, external pancreatic fistulas)[5] and inhibits splanchnic blood flow (use in variceal bleeding). It may be of use in the treatment of refractory diarrhea associated with AIDS; reduces complications of pancreatectomy or pancreatic transplantation, such as fistula formation and acute pancreatitis; improves visual acuity in patients with preproliferative diabetic retinopathy and macular edema; reduces the raised luteinizing hormone and androgen concentrations characteristic of patients with polycystic ovaries; and inhibits growth of implanted pancreatic tumor cells in animals.[2]

Ocreotide may also be potentially useful as an antidote for the hyperinsulinemia induced by a large sulfonylurea overdose.[6] Octreotide is useful in treatment of thyroid-stimulating hormone-secretory adenomas.[7] An anecdotal report suggests it may have value in the treatment of benign intracranial hypertension based on the central nervous system effects of somatostatin.[8]

Toxicokinetics

After subcutaneous injection of 100 μg, a peak serum concentration of about 2 μg/mL is reached in 20 to 30 minutes.[2]

Distribution

Serum distribution half-life is about 75 to 100 minutes. The volume of distribution is about 0.4 L/kg. In blood, octreotide is distributed mainly in the plasma. About 65% is bound to plasma proteins.

Elimination

The serum elimination half-life is 90 to 110 minutes. Total body clearance is 160 mL/min. Ten to twenty percent of the drug is eliminated unchanged in the urine.

Drug Interactions

Octreotide prevents the basal and meal-stimulated increases in serum gastrin caused by omeprazole.[9]

Pregnancy

Transplacental passage of octreotide may occur by passive diffusion. Octreotide does not seem to affect the fetus. The apparent half-life of octreotide in the infant is approximately 350 minutes, instead of 90 to 110 minutes in adults.[10]

Clinical Presentation

Chronic Use

The most important complications of octreotide treatment are gallstone formation and gastritis. Diarrhea is not troublesome. Nausea, vomiting, abdominal pain, flatulence, and steatorrhea may be minimized by avoiding administration at mealtime.[11] Congestive heart failure may worsen[12,13] because of growth hormone inhibition (diminished inotropic effect). Hepatotoxicity has been reported in an anecdotal case report.[14] Hair loss has been observed.[15] Acute pancreatitis may be induced.[16]

Overdose

One patient was given 250 μg/h instead of 25 μg/h intravenously for 48 hours without any side effects.[1]

Withdrawal

Withdrawal of octreotide may induce recovery of gallbladder function and asymptomatic resolution of gallstones after the induction of gallstones by octreotide.[17] Biliary colic,[18] acute cholecystitis,[19] and acute pancreatitis[20] have followed withdrawal.

Laboratory

A specific radioimmunoassay measures plasma octreotide concentrations with a sensitivity of 10 to 20 ng/L.[20]

Treatment

Management of overdose is symptomatic. No antagonists are available. Patients should be observed for development of hyperkalemia.[21]

REFERENCES—OCTREOTIDE ACETATE

1. Dollery CT, ed. *Therapeutic Drugs.* Edinburgh: Churchill Livingstone, 1991:O1–O4.
2. Chanson P, Timsit J, Harris AG. Clinical pharmacokinetics of octreotide: Therapeutic applications in patients with pituitary tumors. Clin Pharmacokinet 1993;25:375–391.
3. Octreotide steaming ahead. Lancet 1992;339:837–839. Editorial.
4. Octreotide for endocrine tumours. Drug Ther Bull 1991;29(5): 19–20.
5. Tulassay Z, Flautner L, Vadasz A, Fehervari I. Octreotide in the treatment of external pancreatic fistulas. Aliment Pharmacol Ther 1993;7:323–325. Short Report.
6. Boyle PJ, Justice K, Krentz AJ, et al. Octreotide reverses hyperinsulinemia and prevents hypoglycemia induced by sulfonylurea overdoses. J Clin Endocrinol Metab 1993;76: 752–756.
7. Chanson P, Weintraub BD, Harris AG. Octreotide therapy for thyroid-stimulating-hormone-secretory pituitary adenomas: A follow-up of 52 patients. Ann Intern Med 1993;119:236–240.
8. Antaraki A, Piadites G, Vergados J, et al. Octreotide benign intracranial hypertension. Lancet 1993;342:1170.
9. Meijer JL, Jansen JBMJ, Crobach LFSJ, et al. Inhibition of omeprazole induced hypergastrinemia by SMS201-995, a long acting somatostatin analogue in man. Gut 1993;34: 1186–1190.
10. Caron P, Gerbeau C, Pradayrol L. Maternal–fetal transfer of octreotide. N Engl J Med 1995;333:601–602.
11. Sadoul J-L, Benchimol D, Thyss A, Freychet R. Side effects of octreotide withdrawal. Lancet 1992;339:376.
12. Leclerq F, Fille A, Albat R, et al. Congestive heart failure worsening with octreotide in acromegalic patient. Lancet 1991;338:1272–1273.
13. Chanson P, Timsit J, Harris AG. Heart failure and octreotide in acromegaly. Lancet 1992;339:242–243.
14. Minocha A, Dean HA Jr. Octreotide-induced acute hepatic toxicity. Am J Gastroenterol 1991;86:526.
15. Jonsson A, Manhem P. Octreotide and loss of scalp hair. Ann Intern Med 1991;115:913.
16. Gradon JD: Schulman RH, Chapnick EK, Sepkowitz DL. Octreotide-induced acute pancreatitis in a patient with acquired immunodeficiency syndrome. South Med J 1991; 81:1410–1411.
17. Bigg-Wither GW, Kok KY, Greenstein RR, et al. Effects of long term octreotide on gallstone formation and gallbladder function. Br Med J 1992;304:1611–1612.
18. James RA, Rhodes M, Rose P, Kendall-Taylor P. Biliary colic in abrupt withdrawal of octreotide. Lancet 1991;338:1527.
19. Sadoul J-L, Benchomal D, Thyss A, Freychet R. Acute pancreatitis following octreotide withdrawal. Am J Med 1991; 90:763–784.
20. Kutz K, Nuesch E, Rosenthaler J. Pharmacokinetics of SMS 201-995 in healthy subjects. Scand J Gastroenterol 1986; 21(suppl. 119):65–72.
21. Sargent AI, Overton CC, Kuwik RJ, et al. Octreotide-induced hyperkalemia. Pharmacotherapy 1994;14:497–501.

OXYTOCIN

Oxytocin is available as a synthetic octopeptide used for the induction of labor. It may lead to significant uterine dysfunction in the mother as well as fetal or maternal death. Its antidiuretic properties can lead to water intoxication. An overdose of oxytocin in the mother may lead to hepatic and central nervous system damage and death in the fetus. Treatment of an overdose is largely symptomatic and supportive.

Source

Oxytocin is a cyclic nonapeptide produced by the supraoptic and periventricular nuclei in the hypothalamus. It is stored in the posterior pituitary. For clinical use, it is available as a synthetic chemical compound. Its molecular weight is 1007.2. Oxytocin is structurally and functionally related to vasopressin/antidiuretic hormone.[1] The two hormones store six amino acids: asparagine, glutamine, tyrosine, cystine, proline, and glycinamide. Oxytocin also contains leucine and isoleucine, whereas vasopressin/antidiuretic hormone contains arginine and phenylalanine. Synthetic oxytocin is marketed as Pitocin and Syntocinon.

Use

Oxytocin is used to induce or stimulate labor, control postpartum uterine bleeding, and treat incomplete or inevitable abortion.[2] Oxytocin antagonists may inhibit myometrial contractility. These agents need to be studied in controlled clinical trials to determine their efficacy and safety.[3]

Product Formulation

Oxytocin is available in an injectable form and as a nasal spray. Oxytocin (Syntocinon) is available in ampoules of 1 mL (10 USP U) and as a nasal spray containing 2 or 5 mL of oxytocin solution. Each milliliter of synthetic preparations of oxytocin is expressed in USP units. Each milliliter of synthetic oxytocin is equivalent to 10 USP U. Each unit is approximately equal to 2 μg of the pure hormone.[1]

Therapeutic Dose

A 1-mL ampoule is combined aseptically with 1000 mL of nonhydrating diluent and rotated in the infusion bottle to ensure a concentration of 10 mU/mL. The initial dose is 1 to 2 mU/min gradually increased in increments of no more than 1 to 2 mU/min, until a contraction pattern similar to normal labor has been established. To control postoperative bleeding, 10 to 40 U of oxytocin is added to 1000 mL of a nonhydrating diluent and run at the rate necessary to control uterine atony. One milliliter (10 U) of oxytocin can be given intramuscularly after delivery of the placenta.[2]

Toxic Dose

When doses of oxytocin exceed 20 to 50 mU/min, a decrease in urinary output is observed. Maternal antidiuretic effect is probably attained at doses of 45 mU/min or above.[4] A single intravenous dose of oxytocin greater than 300 mU causes a drop in blood pressure within 1 minute, usually with subsequent recovery. A secondary rise in blood pressure may follow.

Fatal Dose

A mother received oxytocin (17,300 mU over 2 minutes) during end-stage labor. Following delivery the infant was flaccid and cyanotic. The infant died on the fourth day.[5]

Toxicokinetics

Absorption

Thirty to sixty minutes following an infusion of 132 mU/min, the plasma oxytocin concentration reaches a steady state concentration of 228 to 241 pg/mL.[6] Protein binding has not been detected.[7]

Distribution

The mean apparent volume of distribution is 0.3 L/kg.[6]

Elimination

The half-life of oxytocin is about 10 minutes.[6,7] Oxytocin is removed from the plasma by the liver, kidney, and functioning mammary glands.[8] Oxytocinase inactivates oxytocin by breaking the cystine–tyrosine bond.

Drug Interactions

The use of oxytocin after prostaglandin for midtrimester abortion mimics the situation at term. The grand multiparous patient is at considerable risk if this treatment is used.[8]

Pregnancy/Lactation

Exogenous oxytocin crosses the human placenta.[9]

Mechanism of Action

Oxytocin is a potent constrictor of uterine, placental, and umbilical cord vessels.[9,10] Water intoxication is probably due to a combination of the antidiuretic effect of oxytocin and the large volumes of water sometimes used as a vehicle for the oxytocin.[11]

Clinical Presentation

Routine oxytocin administration has been associated with uterine rupture, antepartum fetal death, and prolonged neonatal hyperbilirubinemia.[5] Water intoxication with seizures is caused by the antidiuretic effect of oxytocin and may occur if large doses (40–50 mL/min) are infused for long periods[2,11] (see Water Intoxication in Chapter 52). Oxytocin in more than physiologic doses may be followed by a rapid transient fall in blood pressure (due to peripheral vasodilation), sometimes followed by a pressor response.[4] Maternal deaths due to hypertensive episodes, subarachnoid hemorrhage, and rupture of the uterus have been reported.[2,7]

Autopsy of a term infant whose mother received a large, rapid overdose of oxytocin (17,300 mU over 20 minutes) during end-stage labor showed extensive hepatic infarction, persistent patency of the ductus venosus, diffuse alveolar damage, and periventricular leukomalacia.[5]

Laboratory

Analytical Methods

Radioimmunoassay methods are available for determination of plasma oxytocin concentrations.[12,13] Limits of detection average about 2.5 pg.[12]

Abnormalities

High serum hepatic enzyme activity and coagulopathy may be observed in the fetus after maternal oxytocin overdose.[5]

Treatment

1. Monitor fetal heart, resting uterine tone, and frequency, duration, and force of contractions. Discontinue immediately in the event of uterine hyperactivity or fetal distress. Administer oxygen to the mother. Obtain an obstetric consultation.
2. Water intoxication should be managed by discontinuation of oxytocin, restriction of fluid intake, diuresis, intravenous hypertonic saline solution, correction of elecrtrolyte imbalance, control of seizures with judicious use of a barbiturate, and special nursing care for the comatose patient.[2]
3. Monitor the blood pressure and pulse of both the mother and fetus.

REFERENCES—OXYTOCIN

1. Petrie RH. The pharmacology and use of oxytocin. Clin Perinatol 1981;8:35–47.
2. Syntocinon. In: *Physicians' Desk Reference.* 47th ed. 1993. Montvale, NJ: Medical Economics, 1993:2128–2129.
3. Higby K, Xenakis EMJ, Pauerstein CJ. Do tocolytic agents stop preterm labor? A critical and comprehensive review of efficacy and safety. Am J Obstet Gynecol 1993;168:1247–1259.
4. Pauerstein CJ. Use and abuse of oxytocic agents. Clin Obstet Gynecol 1973;16:262–277.
5. Robichaux WH, Perper JA. Massive perinatal hepatic necrosis from maternal oxytocin overdose. Pediatr Pathol 1992; 12:761–765.
6. Dawood MY, Ylikorkala O, Trivedi D, Gupta R. Oxytocin levels and disappearance rate and plasma follicle-stimulating hormone and luteinizing hormone after oxytocin infusion in man. J Clin Endocrin Metab 1980;50:397–400.
7. Fabian M, Forsling ML, Jones JJ, Pryor JS. The clearance and antidiuretic potency of neurohypophyseal hormones in man and their plasma binding and stability. J Physiol 1969;204:653–668.
8. Propping D, Stubblefield PG, Golub J, Zuckerman J. Uterine rupture following midtrimester abortion by laminaria, prostaglandin F_{2alpha}, and oxytocin: Report of two cases. Am J Obstet Gynecol 1977;128:689–690.
9. Dawood MY, Wang CF, Gupta R, Fuchs F. Fetal contribution to oxytocin in human labor. Obstet Gynecol 1978;52:205–209.
10. Seitchik J, Chatkoff ML, Hayaski RH. Intrauterine pressure waveform characteristics of spontaneous and oxytocin or prostaglandin F_{2alpha}-induced active labor. Am J Obstet Gynecol 1977;127:223–227.
11. Morgan DB, Kirway NA, Hancock KW, et al. Water intoxication and oxytocin infusion. Br J Obstet Gynecol 1977;84: 6–12.
12. Dawood MV, Raghavan KS, Pociask C. Radioimmunoassay of oxytocin. J Endocrinol 1978;76:270–271.
13. Chard T. The radioimmunoassay of oxytocin and vasopressin. J Endocrinol 1973;58:143–160.

SOMATOSTATIN

Structure and Classification

Somatostatin is a polypeptide obtained from the hypothalamus or by synthesis (Fig. 42–2). The naturally occurring form has a cyclic structure. Somatostatin is also called GH-RIF, GHRIH, growth hormone release-inhibiting hormone, and somatotropin release-inhibiting factor.

Use

Somatostatin has been tried in the management of upper gastrointestinal hemorrhage,[1,2] insulin resistance, hormone-secreting tumors, other hypersecretory disorders, and pancreatic disorders.

Mechanism of Action

Somatostatin inhibits the release of growth hormone from the anterior pituitary, thyrotropin and corticotropin from the pituitary, and glucagon and insulin from the pancreas. In addition, it appears to have a role in the regulation of duodenal and gastric secretions. It has a very short duration of action. Analogs have been produced to prolong its activity as well as to make its inhibitory effects more specific (see Octreotide Acetate).

Somatostatin inhibits the basal and stimulated hydrochloric acid output, as well as pepsin, intrinsic factor, and gastric secretion. It also reduces gastrointestinal motility and splanchnic blood flow after infusions of 250 μg/h for 120 hours.[2]

Somatostatin administered in an intravenous infusion at a rate of 250 μg/h after a loading dose of 250 μg has led to life-threatening water intoxication and hyponatremia. Hypertonic saline may be required.[3]

REFERENCES—SOMATOSTATIN

1. Jenkins SA. Somatostatin in acute bleeding oesophageal varices. Drugs 1992;44(suppl. 2):36–55.
2. Torres AJ, Landa I, Hernandez F, et al. Somatostatin in the treatment of severe upper gastrointestinal bleeding: A multicentre controlled trial. Br J Surg 1986;73:786–789.
3. Halma C, Jansen JBMJ, Janssens AP, et al. Life-threatening water intoxication during somatostatin therapy. Ann Intern Med 1987;107:518–520.

STEROIDS

Steroids fall into two major classes: (1) natural steroid hormones (progestogens, estrogens, androgens, and corticoids), and (2) synthetic derivatives of testosterone (anabolic steroids). Steroids are widely used in almost every area of medical practice. A number of areas are of special interest to the medical toxicologist. Excellent reviews of the toxicokinetics of major steroids are available.[1–13]

Toxicokinetics

The toxicokinetics of some steroids are summarized in Table 42–11.

Table 42–11
Steroid Toxicokinetics

	Dose (mg)	V_D (L/kg)	CL (L/h/kg)	$t_{1/2}$ (h)	Method	Bioavailability (%)	Protein Binding (%)	Excreted Unchanged (%)
Corticosteroids								
Prednisolone	5 mg IV	0.34	0.10	2.74	HPLC		80–90	
	20 mg IV	0.49	0.13	2.58				11–14
	40 mg IV	0.74	0.17	3.45				
	Oral			2.5–3.5		80–100		
	Intraarticular					50		
Hydrocortisone	5 mg IV	0.30	0.164	1.3	HPLC		70	
	40 mg IV	0.54	0.23	1.9				
Dexamethasone	5–10 mg IV	1.15	0.43	2.95–5	HPLC	80		
	Oral[6]	0.75	1.5	3.0				
Methylprednisolone	1000 mg IV	1.2%	0.45	2.4	HPLC		77[4]	
	PO	1.5		1.5		49–92		
Prednisolone after prednisone	5 mg PO	0.31	0.1	2.27	HPLC			
Prednisone	PO[10]				81			
Betamethasone	PO							2.5
	Intraarticular[3]			5		78		
Triamcinolone	Intraarticular[3,13]			63 d				
Declomethasone[2]						35–70	40	
Oral Contraceptives[10]			0.1		HPLC			
Norethisterone[7]	PO							
Levonorgestrel	PO			1.2		64		
	Vaginal	1.6		5.6		107		80
Ethinylestradiol[8,9]		3.8	1.0	7.7		40		
Norethindrone[9]	PO	3.6		7.8		52		63
Androgen							63	
Testosterone							98	

V_D, volume of distribution; CL, total body clearance; $t_{1/2}$, elimination half-life; HPLC, high-performance liquid chromatography.

Topical Steroids

Topical steroids are listed in Table 42–12.[14] Long-term use of topical glucocorticoids has led to Cushing's syndrome.[15]

Prodrugs

Prednisone is a prodrug and is converted to its active form prednisolone by 11β-hydroxydehydrogenase.[1] Similarly, cortisone is an inactive prodrug that is converted to its active form hydrocortisone by 11β-hydroxydehydrogenase.

Lactation

Concentrations of prednisolone in breast milk do not appear to exceed 10% of the plasma concentration. Beggs and colleagues state that no restriction to breastfeeding is necessary for doses of prednisolone up to 20 mg/d.[1] For larger doses it is recommended that the infant is nursed at least 4 hours after maternal ingestion of prednisolone.

Clinical Presentation

Liver

Exogenous estrogen therapy has been associated with a variety of infrequent epithelial liver lesions (focal nodular hyperplasia, adenoma and hepatocellular carcinoma), mesenchymal lesions (sarcomas, rhabdomyosarcomas), and mixed tumors of the liver.[16]

Heart

Older oral contraceptives containing 50 μg of estrogen have been associated with an increased risk for fatal myocardial infarctions. Additional risk factors associated with fatal myocardial infarction in women are a history of hypertension in pregnancy, non-pregnancy-associated hypertension, hyperlipidemia, diabetes, and smoking. These risks are reduced by use of newer oral contraceptive preparations containing new synthetic progestins and/or lower doses of both estrogenic and progestogenic components.[17]

Adrenal Insufficiency

Acute adrenal insufficiency (Addisonian crisis) may follow suppression of the hypothalamic–pituitary axis caused by long-term use of inhaled steroids (eg, budesonide). Sudden cessation of use may be followed by lethargy, malaise, nausea, vomiting, dizziness, headache, and varying states of consciousness. Plasma cortisol levels may be depressed. Plasma aldosterone is normal. Treatment includes the use of oral or intravenous corticosteroids (eg, hydrocortisone IV).[18,19] Adrenal insufficiency may occur in patients who develop an adrenocorticotropic hormone (ACTH)-induced bilateral adrenal hemorrhage.[20] The clinical presentation is suggested by a sudden onset of severe upper abdominal and flank pain, which may radiate to the shoulders. Peritoneal signs may occur if blood has seeped into the peritoneal cavity. There may also be vomiting, fever, profound

Table 42–12
Groups of Topical Corticosteroid Products, in Order of Decreasing Potency*

Drug	Trade Name*	Concentration (%)
Group I		
Betamethasone dipropionate	Diprolene	0.05
Halbertasol propionate	Ultravate	0.05
Clobetasol propionate	Temovate	0.05
Diflorasone diacetate	Psorcon	0.05
Group II		
Amcinonide	Cyclocort	0.1
Betamethasone dipropionate	Diprosone	0.05
Desoximetasone	Topicort	0.25
Diflorasone diacetate	Florone, Maxiflor	0.05
Fluocinolone acetonide	Synalar-HP	0.2
Fluocinonide	Lidex	0.05
Halcinonide	Halog	0.1
Triamcinolone acetonide	Aristocort, Kenalog, etc	0.5
Group III		
Betamethasone benzoate	Benisone, Uticort	0.025
Betamethasone valerate	Betatrex, Beta-Val	0.1
Desoximetasone	Topicort LP	0.05
Flurandrenolide	Cordran	0.025
Hydrocortisone valerate	Westcort	0.2
Triamcinolone acetonide	Aristocort, Kenalog, etc	0.1
Group IV		
Betamethasone valerate	Valisone, Reduced Strength	0.01
Clocortolone pivalate	Cloderm	0.1
Fluocinolone acetonide	Fluonid, Flurosyn, Synalar, etc	0.025
Flurandrenolide	Cordran SP	0.025
Triamcinolone acetonide	Aristocort, Kenalog, Triacet	0.025
Group V		
Alclometasone dipropionate	Aclovate	0.05
Desonide	DesOwen, Tridesilon	0.05
Fluocinolone acetonide	Fluonid, Synalar	0.01
Group VI		
Dexamethasone	Aeroseb-Dex, Decaderm	0.01–0.1
Hydrocortisone	(generic, over-the-counter)	0.25–2.5
Methylprednisolone acetate	Medrol	0.25–1.0

*No significant difference exists among agents in a group. These products come in various forms (ie, creams, gels, lotions, solutions, and ointments), although some products are not available in all forms.
†Use of trade names is for identification only and does not imply endorsement by the Public Health Service or the U.S. Department of Health and Human Services.
Adapted from Cornell RC, Stoughton RB. The use of topical steroids in psoriasis. Dermatol Clin 1984;2:397–409.

prostration, and changes in mental status. Diagnosis is enhanced by ultrasound and computed tomography. If the patient has no evidence of ongoing bleeding and remains hemodynamically stable, conservative management without surgery may be appropriate. Vital signs and fluid and electrolyte balance should be monitored to ensure that acute adrenal insufficiency is not developing. ACTH is discontinued and replaced with parenteral corticosteroids. If the diagnosis is in doubt or there is evidence of further bleeding or hemodynamic compromise, exploratory laparotomy must be considered. An ACTH-induced adrenal hemorrhage is often fatal within a few days to weeks of an acute episode.[21]

Psychiatric Responses

Psychiatric responses to steroids may range from mild euphoria to psychosis.[22,23] The majority of steroid psychoses have an onset within 5 days of commencing medication.[24] They may vary up to 2 to 4 weeks.[22] The frequency of steroid-induced psychiatric disorders increases with the daily dose of medication, ranging from 4.2% in those taking 40 to 80 mg prednisone or the equivalent to 18% of those taking more than 80 mg.[25] Affective schizophreniform and organic symptoms may be observed.[22] Peak plasma levels of steroid medication may be related to the development of psychiatric symptoms.[26] Mania may follow higher than recommended doses of beclomethasone dipropionate.[22] Behavioral changes may be observed in young children after steroid inhalation therapy for asthma.[27] Antidepressants may make the symptoms worse.[28] Neuroleptic medication may be preferred.

Overdose

Steroid overdose is an infrequent, if not altogether rare, finding.

Beclomethasone. Use of twice the prescribed dose of beclomethasone dipropionate spray for allergic rhinitis may induce severe behavioral changes including pressurized speech, visual and auditory hallucinations, and disorientation. Discontinuation of the spray should lead to improvement and recovery over the following 1 to 3 months.[26]

Testosterone. High-dose testosterone therapy (2% testosterone propionate) topically applied in excessive doses (up to 60 mg daily) to the vulva has led to masculinization, including deepening of the voice. Vaginal spotting and secondary amenorrhea may occur. Blood testosterone levels are increased. Discontinuation of the local medication is indicated.[29]

Estrogens

Implants. Estradiol implant overdose (200 mg estradiol by implant every 3 weeks) led to fluid retention, facial swelling, and pitting edema of the thighs. Serum estradiol levels were elevated and fell over several years after the implants were discontinued.[30] In two other patients, repeated implants of estradiol over a 1- to 2-year period led to hypertension, flushing, fatigue, and nasal congestion. Serum estradiol concentrations of 200 to 300 nmol/L or lower should guide timing for other implants.[31]

Ingestion. A 19-year-old woman ingested 80 tablets containing 2 mg of estradiol valerate each (160 mg). The next morning she underwent gastric lavage. On admission the serum estradiol level was elevated (2 nmol/L). In addition, serum cholesterol, phospholipids and triglycerides were elevated. An electroencephalogram showed findings typical of subcortical disturbance. One week later the electroencephalogram was normal. Estradiol valerate taken orally in overdose appears to be associated with low toxicity and minimal side effects.[32]

Triamcinolone. Injection of an overdose (intramuscular) of triamcinolone acetonide (1200 mg) over a 1 month period led to the clinical picture of Cushing's syndrome with associated extremely low plasma and urinary cortisol levels. Hydrocortisone was substituted to prevent adrenal insufficiency.[33] Excessive intramuscular doses of triamcinolone (400–1080 mg) led to features of Cushing's syndrome, ecchymoses, atrophy of pelvic and shoulder girdle muscle, ulceration and perforation of the sigmoid colon, overt diabetes, hypoproteinemia, hypokalemia, hyponatremia, hypophosphatemia, and osteoporosis.[34]

ANABOLIC STEROIDS

See also Chapter 19.

Clinical Presentation

Chronic Use

Behavioral changes suggested by anecdotal reports include depression (responsive to fluoxetine),[35] paranoia, obsessional thinking, euphoria, bizarre and irrational ideas, heightened self-confidence,[36,37] intracranial hypertension,[38] myocardial infarction,[39] and pulmonary embolus.[40] Steroid users share injecting equipment with amphetamine users. There remains the possibility of spread of HIV among anabolic steroid users sharing needles.[41]

Hepatotoxicity

Asymptomatic elevations in liver enzymes appear to be the most frequent manifestation of anabolic steroid hepatotoxicity. The hepatotoxicity is dose dependent and related to the duration of administration. Resolution of jaundice may take months.[42]

Dependence

Steroids may induce dependence, meeting the American Psychiatric Association's *Diagnostic and Statistical Manual* (3rd ed., revised) criteria for psychoactive substances.[43,44] The most frequent manifestations of dependency are withdrawal symptoms including acts of physical violence, feelings of anger or hostility, manic or psychotic episodes or depression, withdrawal-related fatigue, restlessness, anorexia, and insomnia.[40,44] Those who become dependent have used larger steroid dosages, had more cycles of use, were more dissatisfied with their body size, and had more aggressive symptoms than nondependent users. An increase in use of alcohol, cocaine, and amphetamines appears to be associated with steroid dependence.[44]

Laboratory

Drug testing for anabolic steroids is performed by radioimmunoassay (RIA) and gas chromatography with mass spectrometry (GC–MS). Urine is screened using RIA. The drug is subsequently identified by GC–MS.[45] Oral agents are usually detectable several weeks after discontinuation. Parenteral agents may be detectable for up to 3 months. Few laboratories offer anabolic steroid testing for individuals.

Treatment

Treatment is largely directed initially at prevention in the adolescent by education directed toward parents, teachers, and coaches. The physician may be able to direct the young athlete to alternatives to steroid use, to appropriate nutritional counseling and weight training, and to counseling sessions aimed at improving self-esteem. Treatment of the complications induced by anabolic steroid use and abuse is symptomatic and supportive. An anecdotal report suggests that clomiphene 100 mg/d may restore follicle-stimulating hormone, luteinizing hormine, and free testosterone levels in men after recreational steroid-induced pituitary–gonadal failure.[46] There is no antidote nor effective means for the enhancement of elimination.

INHALED STEROIDS

Substitution at the 17α ester portion of cortisol has resulted in a new group of very potent steroids (eg, beclomethasone dipropionate [BDP], betamethasone, and budesonide) that are effective when applied topically for skin diseases and when inhaled for asthma.[47] The antiasthmatic potency of an inhaled steroid is approximately proportional to its potency as an antiinflammatory agent. Budesonide is about twice as potent as BDP and 1000 times more potent than prednisolone.[48] Most patients get a maximal response at a dose of 400 μg of BDP per day. Several inhaled preparations are available, including BDP, triamcinolone, flunisolide, and budesonide, which has the highest topical potency but is not available in the United States.

γ-AMINOBUTYRIC ACID-ACTIVE STEROIDS

γ-Aminobutyric acid (GABA) is a chemical messenger mediating synaptic transmission at about 3% of all synapses within the nervous system.[49] This amino acid is the major inhibiting neurotransmitter in the brain. GABA interacts with two classes of neurotransmitter receptor complexes: $GABA_A$ and $GABA_B$. The $GABA_A$ receptor complex is composed of distinct membrane-spanning subunits that form an integral chloride ion channel. GABA increases the membrane conductance of chloride ions by increasing the frequency of channel opening subsequent to its reversible interaction with a specific domain on the $GABA_A$ receptor complex. A variety of modulatory sites on the complex bind benzodiazepine receptor ligands, barbiturates, and GABA-active steroids. The pharmacologic actions of many anxiolytic, sedative–hypnotic, anticonvulsant, anesthetic, and muscle relaxant medications result from their interaction with those modulatory sites. Major GABA-negative steroids (pregnenolone sulfate and dehydroepiandrosterone sulfate) appear to interact with the $GABA_A$ receptor complex in a manner analogous to those of the inverse benzodiazepine receptor agonists. $GABA_A$-positive steroids (allopregnanolone and allotetrahydrodeoxycorticosterone) and pentobarbital are synergistic with respect to their ability to potentiate chloride ion flux through the $GABA_A$ receptor complex in the absence of GABA or other GABA agonists. Muscle relaxant effects of steroids may be mediated by $GABA_A$ receptor complexes in the frontal cortex. Most of these studies have been performed in animals. Clinical confirmation is required to evaluate the importance of these concepts to patient treatment.

REFERENCES-STEROIDS

1. Beggs EJ, Atkinson HC, Gianarkis N. The pharmacokinetics of corticosteroid agents. Med J Aust 1987;146:37–41.
2. Martin LE, Tanner RJN, Clark TJH, Cochrane GM. Absorption and metabolism of orally administered beclomethasone dipropionate. Clin Pharmacol Ther 1974;15:267–275.
3. Derendorf H, Mollmann H, Gruner A, et al. Pharmacokinetics and pharmacodynamics of glucocorticoid suspensions after intraarticular administration. Clin Pharmacol Ther 1986;39: 313–317.
4. Szefler SJ, Ebling WF, Georgitis JW, Jusko WJ. Methylprednisolone versus prednisolone pharmacokinetics in relation to dose in adults. Eur J Clin Pharmacol 1986;30:323–329.
5. Al-Habet SMH, Rogers HJ. Methylprednisolone pharmacokinetics of intravenous and oral administration. Br J Clin Pharmacol 1989;27:285–290.
6. Swartz SL, Slusky RG. Corticosteroids: Clinical pharmacology and therapeutic use. Drugs 1978;16:238–255.
7. Shenfield GM, Griffin JM, Griffin JM. Clinical pharmacokinetics of contraceptive steroids: An update. Clin Pharmacokinet 1991;20:15–37.
8. Kanarkowski R, Tornatore KM, D'Ambrosia R, et al. Pharmacokinetics of single and multiple doses of ethinyl estradiol and levonorgestrel in relation to smoking. Clin Pharmacol Ther 1988;43:23–31.
9. Goebelsmann U. Pharmacokinetics of contraceptive steroids in man. In: Gregoire AT, Blye RR, eds. *Contraceptive Steroids: Pharmacology and Safety.* New York: Plenum, 1986:67–111.
10. Gambertoglio JG, Ammend WJC Jr, Benet LZ. Pharmacokinetics and bioavailability of prednisone and prednisolone in healthy volunteers and patients: A review. J Pharmacokinet Biopharm 1980;8:1–51.
11. Frey BM, Frey FJ. Clinical pharmacokinetics of prednisone and prednisolone. Clin Pharmacokinet 1990;19:126–146.
12. Bergren H, Grottum P, Rugstad HE. Pharmacokinetics and protein binding of prednisolone after oral and intravenous administration. Eur J Clin Pharmacol 1983;24:415–419.
13. Mollmann H, Rohdewald P, Schmidt EW, et al. Pharmacokinetics of triamcinolone acetonide and its phosphate ester. Eur J Clin Pharmacol 1985;29:85–89.
14. Hall AH, Hogan DJ. Skin lesions and environmental exposures: Rash decisions. Atlanta: ASTDR Case Studies in Environmental Medicine, May 28, 1993.
15. Teelucksingh S, Bahall M, Coomansingh D, et al. Cushing's syndrome from topical glucocorticoids. Wis Med J 1993; 42:77–78.
16. Cote RJ, Urmacher C. Rhabdomyosarcoma of the liver associated with long-term oral contraceptive use: Possible role of estrogens in the genesis of embryologically distinct liver tumors. Am J Surg Pathol 1990;14:784–790.
17. Thorogood M, Mann J, Murphy M, Vessey M. Is oral contraceptive use still associated with an increased risk of fatal myocardial infarction? Report of a case–control study. Br J Obstet Gynecol 1991;9:1245–1253.
18. Wong J, Black P. Acute adrenal insufficiency associated with high dose inhaled steroids. Br Med J 1992;304:1415.
19. Zwaan CM, Odink RJH, Delemarre-Van de Waal HA, et al. Acute adrenal insufficiency after discontinuation of inhaled corticosteroid therapy. Lancet 1992;340:1230–1289.
20. Rao RH, Vagmicci AH, Amino JA. Bilateral massive adrenal hemorrhage: Early recognition and treatment. Ann Intern Med 1989;110:227–236.
21. Kornbluth AA, Salomon P, Sachar DB, et al. ACTH-induced adrenal hemorrhage: A complication of therapy masquerading as an acute abdomen. J Clin Gastroenterol 1990;12: 371–377.
22. Doherty M, Garstin I, McClelland RJ, et al. A steroid stupor in a surgical ward. Br J Psychiatry 1991;158: 125–127.
23. Rome HP, Braceland FJ. Psychological response to corticotrophin, cortisone and related steroid substances. JAMA 1952;142:27–30.
24. Kaufman MW, Casadonte PE, Peslow ED. Steroid psychosis: Treatment advances. NY State J Med 1981;81: 1795–1797.
25. Boston Collaborative Drug Surveillance Program. Acute adverse reactions to prednisone in relation to dosage. Clin Pharmacol Ther 1972;13:694–698.
26. Phelan MC. Beclomethasone mania. Br J Psychiatry 1989; 155:871–872.
27. Connett G, Lenney W. Inhaled budesonide and behavioral disturbances. Lancet 1991;338:634–635.
28. Hall RC, Popkin MK, Kirkpatrick B. Tricyclic exacerbation of steroid psychosis. J Nerv Ment Dis 1978;166:738–742.
29. Punch MR, Ansbacher R. Autogenic masculinization. Am J Obstet Gynecol 1990;163:114–116.
30. Eden JA. Sustained effects of oestrogen implant overdose. Lancet 1988;2:1061.
31. Eden J. Too much of a good thing? Two cases of oestrogen overdosage associated with oestradiol implants. Med J Aust 1990;152:558.
32. Pnnonen R, Salmi T. Effects of a massive single oral dose of oestradiol valerate in a young woman. Ann Clin Res 1983; 15:134–136.
33. Girre G, Vincens M, Gompel A, Fournier PE. Iatrogenic Cushing's syndrome due to acute triamcinolone overdosage. Therapie 1987;42:317–318.
34. Mazanek-Szymanska E, Gasinska T, Starzewska H, et al. Effect of excessive doses of Kenalog given for short time periods. Pol Tyg Lek 1979;34:997–1001. [in Polish] (From Mickiewicz CW. Personal communication. Lederle Laboratories, June 29, 1989.)

35. Malone DA Jr, Dimeff RJ. The use of fluoxetine in depression associated with anabolic steroid withdrawal: A case series. J Clin Psychiatry 1992;51:130–132.
36. Dalby JT. Brief anabolic steroid use and sustained behavioral reactions. Am J Psychiatry 1992;149:271–272.
37. Uzych L. Anabolic androgenic steroids and psychiatric-related effects: A review. Can J Psychiatry 1992;37:23–28.
38. Tully MP, Cooper RG, Jayson MIV. Intracranial hypertension associated with stanozolol. DICP Am Pharmacother 1990;24:1234.
39. French GS, Adelman S. Myocardial infarction associated with anabolic steroid use in a previously healthy 31-year old weight lifter. Am Heart J 1992;124:507–508.
40. Montine TJ, Garede JT. Massive pulmonary embolus and anabolic steroid abuse. JAMA 1992;267:2238–2239.
41. Perry HM, Littlepage BNC. Misusing anabolic drugs: A drug history from well muscled patients. Br Med J 1992;305:1241–1242.
42. Forbes GM, Bramston BA, Collins BJ. Anabolic steroid hepatotoxicity: Lessons to be learned? Aust NZ J Med 1993;23:308–310.
43. Johnson MD. Anabolic steroid use in adolescent athletes. Pediatr Clin North Am 1990;37:1111–1123.
44. Goodwin FK. Anabolic steroids and dependence. JAMA 1991;266:1619.
45. Hatton CK, Catlin DN. Detection of androgenic anabolic steroids in urine. Clin Lab Med 1987;7:655–668.
46. Bickelman C, Ferries L, Eaton RP. Impotence related to anabolic steroid use in a body builder: Response to clomiphenyl citrate. West J Med 1995;162:158–160.
47. British National Formulary No. 24. September 1992:124–125.
48. Barnes PJ. Pulmonary disorders. In: Melmon KL, Morrelli HF, Hoffman BB, Nierenberg DW, eds. *Clinical Pharmacology: Basic Principles in Therapeutics.* 3rd ed. New York: McGraw Hill, 1992:198–202.
49. Deutsch SI, Mastropaolo J, Hitri A. GABA-active steroids: Endogenous modulation of GABA-gated chloride ion conductance. Clin Neuropharmacol 1992;15:352–364.

THYROID HORMONES

Clinical Presentation

Doses of levothyroxine up to 0.25 and 0.26 mg/kg (3.00–4.33 mg) are well tolerated even without gastric decontamination. In mild to moderate thyroid intoxications, excessive heat production, increased motor activity, and heightened sympathetic activity induce tachycardia, fever (to 38–40°C), and diarrhea.

Gastrointestinal Tract

Vomiting, diarrhea, abdominal pain, and increased appetite may be observed. If thyroid hormone is chronically abused, weight loss may occur.[1]

Cardiovascular System

Tachycardia, palpitations, hypertension, cutaneous vasodilation, and diaphoresis may be seen; severe angina, hypotension, congestive heart failure, and cardiovascular collapse rarely occur. Arrhythmias are usually supraventricular but may evolve into ventricular dysrhythmias. Such symptoms may occur after chronic ingestion of high doses.[2]

Central Nervous System

Anxiety, apprehension, headache, confusion, agitation, mydriasis, and diaphoresis may be observed. Occasional weakness, tremor, acute psychosis, and coma have been reported.[2] Other effects include intolerance to heat and warm, flushed, moist skin. Chronic thyroid abuse may result in angina, myocarditis, weight loss, ventricular arrhythmias, and sudden death.[2]

Table 42–13
Drugs That Influence Thyroid Function*

Drugs That Decrease TSH Secretion
Dopamine
Glucocorticoids
Ocreotide
Drugs That Alter Thyroid Hormone Secretion
Decreased thyroid hormone secretion
Lithium
Iodide
Amiodarone
Aminoglutethimide
Increased thyroid hormone secretion
Iodide
Amiodarone
Drugs That Decrease T_4 Absorption
Colestipol
Cholestyramine
Aluminum hydroxide
Ferrous sulfate
Sucralfate
Drugs That Alter T_4 and T_3 Transport in Serum
Increased serum TBG concentration
Estrogens
Tamoxifen
Heroin
Methadone
Mitotane
Fluorouracil
Decreased serum TBG concentration
Androgens
Anabolic steroids (eg, danazol)
Slow-release nicotinic acid
Glucocorticoids
Displacement from protein binding sites
Furosemide
Fenclofenac
Mefenamic acid
Salicylates
Drugs That Alter T_4 and T_3 Metabolism
Increased hepatic metabolism
Phenobarbital
Rifampin
Phenytoin
Carbamazepine
Decreased T_4 5′-deiodinase activity
Propylthiouracil
Amiodarone
Beta-adrenergic–antagonist drugs
Glucocorticoids
Cytokines
Interferon alfa
Interleukin-2

*TSH, thyrotropin; T_4, thyroxine; T, triiodothyronine; TBG, thyroxine-binding globulin.
From Surks MI, Sievert R. Drugs and thyroid function. N Engl J Med 1995;333:1688–1694.

Toxicokinetics

Table 42–13 lists drugs that influence thyroid function. In addition, (1) nonsteroidal antiinflammatory drugs rarely cause thyroid disease; anticonvulsants reduce total and free thyroxine (T_4) concentrations; and (3) propranolol decreases free triiodothyronine (T_3) concentrations.

Iodine-induced thyrotoxicosis has been reported after iodine supplementation: the most well-described case occurred in Tasmania after the iodization of bread, and lasted 5 to 6 years. Zimbabwe is experiencing a similar problem. Iodine supplements should be added at the minimum level necessary, and urinary iodine levels in target populations should be carefully monitored.[3] (See also Chapter 57.)

Treatment

Protection from toxicity after acute massive ingestion of T_4 is probably conferred by increased conversion of T_4 to reverse T_3, which blocks the thyroid hormone receptor site. Aggressive therapy of T_4 overdose with prednisolone and propranolol to block the peripheral effect of thyroxine, propylthiouracil to block endogenous T_4 production, cholestyramine to block enterohepatic circulation of thyroid hormone, and charcoal hemoperfusion to remove excess T_4 have been advocated by Lehrner and Weir.[5] Because T_4 is mostly protein bound, plasmapheresis rather than charcoal hemoperfusion could be effective but its role remains to be determined.[6]

The majority of pediatric T_4 ingestions are not severe and may be managed on an outpatient basis. Conclusions reached by Litovitz and White indicate that despite marked elevations in thyroid function assays, initial therapy of acute T_4 ingestions can be limited to gut decontamination.[7] Hospitalization or prophylactic treatment with propranolol, propylthiouracil, corticosteroids, cholestyramine, or extracorporeal detoxification is unnecessary in the early asymptomatic phase. Children can be treated initially and observed safely at home. Tenenbein and Dean agree and note that close scrutiny of a child between days 3 and 5 after ingestion is important.[8]

After ingestion of more than 4 mg or unknown quantities of T_4, an initial T_4 concentration may predict delayed onset of toxicity, fever, tachycardia, hypertension, and agitation in the absence of early clinical manifestations.[9] Admission should be considered for all symptomatic patients or those with T_4 levels greater than 75 μg/d regardless of presentation. In most cases treatment with a beta blocker and observation is all that is necessary after overdose with T_4.[10]

When more serious symptoms develop, hospitalization and other measures may be required. Signs and symptoms may be delayed for 10 to 15 days after T_4 ingestion. Patients with large overdoses, prior cardiac disease, or chronic abuse may suffer severely after thyroid poisoning. Such cases are infrequently observed. Treatment is based on dividing patients into two categories: (1) symptomatic, compromised cardiovascular status, chronic ingestion; and (2) healthy, asymptomatic, single ingestion.

Calcium Channel Blockers

Calcium channel blocking drugs may be useful as adjunctive therapy for thyrotoxicosis in the presence of angina, congestive failure, and tachyrhythmias.[11]

Six patients were admitted after erroneous massive intake of T_4 (70–1200 mg over an interval of 2–12 days). All developed the classic symptoms of thyrotoxicosis within 3 days of the first day of treatment; five patients presented in grade II to III coma and one became stuporous. Two developed left ventricular failure and three had arrhythmias (days 8–11). Total serum thyroid hormonal levels on admission ranged from 935 to 7728 nmol/L for T_4 and 23 to 399 nmol/L for T_3. All received hydrocortisone and propranolol. Propylthiouracil was also used in three cases. Charcoal hemoperfusion and/or plasmapheresis led to a substantive increase in the plasma disappearance rate of T_4 with a shortened average half-life.[12]

THYROID STORM

Thyroid storm is a rare complication of untreated or partially treated hyperthyroidism, associated with cardiovascular, hepatic, gastrointestinal, and neurologic dysfunction. Mortality is approximately 20%.[13] Because of the heightened sensitivity to adrenergic stimulation seen in thyroid storm, ingestion of stimulant medications such as pseudoephedrine may be life-threatening (intracranial hemorrhage, hypertensive crises, rhabdomyolysis, seizures).[14]

Thyroid storm following a massive ingestion of the hormone in children is thought to reflect high serum free T_4 and free T_3 levels, combined with hepatic and renal impairment.[15]

Most patients present with exaggerated signs of hyperthyroidism and extreme agitation, emotional lability, and restlessness. Neurologic complications including altered behavior, seizures, pyramidal tract disease, and choreoathetosis have been described in association with hyperthyroidism.

Cardinal manifestations include fever, a widened pulse pressure, flushing, sweating, new-onset cardiac dysrhythmias, tachycardia progressing to atrial flutter or fibrillation (similar to catecholamine excess states) with or without associated congestive heart failure, deterioration in central nervous system function (apathy, altered behavior, seizures, pyramidal tract disease, choreoathetosis, basal ganglia infarction, and coma, which can develop within 36 hours). Severe diarrhea, nausea, vomiting, or jaundice may be present.[13]

Often a precipitating factor such as surgery, radioactive iodine therapy, use of an iodinated contrast medium,[16] or intercurrent illness in a previously untreated or partially treated patient with hyperthyroidism can be identified.

Treatment of thyroid storm is pursued in an intensive care facility and is aimed at reducing both synthesis and peripheral conversion of T_4 to T_3. Beta-adrenergic blockade decreases heart rate, slows cardiac dysrhythmias, and ameliorates the hyperpyrexia. Propranolol and nadolol also inhibit conversion of T_4 to T_3 in the peripheral tissue. Propylthiouracil decreases the intrathyroid production of thyroid hormone and blocks peripheral T_4-to-T_3 conversion, an effect not found with methimazole. Other agents used for blocking T_4-to-T_3 conversion include dexamethasone and iopanoic acid. Iodide and lithium are used to block thyroidal secretion of hormone. The patient should be observed for life-threatening emergencies such as intracranial hemorrhage, hypertensive crisis, rhabdomyolysis, and seizures.[12–14] It may also be ameliorated by procedures such as exchange transfusion,[17] plasmapheresis,[18] charcoal hemoperfusion,[19] and peritoneal dialysis.[20]

THYROTOXICOSIS FACTITIA

Thyrotoxicosis resulting from the ingestion of excessive amounts of exogenous thyroid hormone may be seen in patients receiving the medication for treatment of hypothyroidism, goiter, or nodules (thyrotoxicosis medicamentosa) or in patients who ingest the hormone to reduce weight or because of personality disorders (thyrotoxicosis factitia).[21] In a study of six patients with this condition, Mariotti and associates found that serum thyroglobulin levels (elevated in many types of hyperthyroidism) were undetectable by a sensitive immunoassay.[22] Thyrotoxicosis factitia can be assumed to be present when clinical hyperthyroidism is coupled with elevated levels of serum T_4 and T_3, depressed thyroid uptake of radioiodine, and a low or undetectable serum level of thyroglobulin in the absence of, or corrected for, the uncommon serum antithyroglobulins.[23]

Catecholamine levels are low or normal with thyrotoxicosis, a condition in which the tissues have increased sensitivity to the catecholamine-like effect of thyroid hormones.

REFERENCES—THYROID HORMONES

1. Haynes RC Jr, Murad F. Thyroid and antithyroid drugs. In: Gilman AE, Goodman LS, Rall TW, et al., eds. *The Pharmacologic Basis of Therapeutics.* 7th ed. New York: MacMillan, 1985:1398–1408.
2. Bhasin S, Wallace W, Lawrence JB. Sudden death associated with thyroid hormone abuse. Am J Med 1981;71: 887–890.
3. Todd CH, Allain T, Gomo ZAR, et al. Increase in thyrotoxicosis associated with iodine supplements in Zimbabwe. Lancet 1995;346:1563–1564.
4. Quin JP, Thomson JA. Adverse effects of drugs on the thyroid gland. Adverse Drug React Toxicol Rev 1994;13:43–50.
5. Lehrer LM, Weir HR. Acute ingestions of thyroid hormones. Pediatrics 1984;73:313–317.
6. Singh GK, Winterborn MH. Massive overdose with thyroxine: Toxicity and treatment. Eur J Pediatr 1991;150:217–218.
7. Litovitz TL, White JD. Levothyroxine ingestions in children: An analysis of 78 cases. Am J Emerg Med 1985;3:297–300.
8. Tenenbein M, Dean HJ. Benign course after massive ingestion of levothyroxine. Vet Hum Toxicol 1981;23(suppl.1): 50. Abstract.
9. Lewander WJ, Lacouture PG, Silva JE, et al. Acute thyroxine ingesiton in pediatric patients. Pediatrics 1989;48:262–265.
10. Tunget CL, Turchen SG, Manoguerra AS, Clark RF. Determination of an acute safe exposure dose in overdoses for thyroid containing products. Vet Hum Toxicol 1993;35:348.
11. Roti E, Montermini M, Roti S, et al. The effect of diltiazem, a calcium channel-blocking drug on cardiac rate and rhythm in hyperthyroid patients. Arch Intern Med 1988;148: 1919–1921.
12. Binimelis J, Bassas L, Marruecos L, et al. Massive thyroxine intoxication: Evaluation of plasma extraction. Intens Care Med 1987;13:33–38.
13. Page SR, Scott AR. Thyroid storm in a young woman resulting in bilateral basal ganglia infarction. Postgrad Med J 1993;69:813–831.
14. Wilson BE, Hobbs WN. Case report: Pseudoephedrine-associated thyroid storm: Thyroid hormone – catecholamine interactions. Am J Med Sci 1993;306:317–319.
15. Matthews SJ. Acute thyroxine overdosage: Two cases of parasuicide. Ulster Med J 1993;63:170–173.
16. Shimura H, Takazawa K, Endo T, et al. Thyroid storm after CT scan with iodinated contrast media. J Endocrinol Invest 1991;13:73-76.
17. Gerard P, Malraux P, de Visscher M. Accidental poisoning with thyroid extract treated by exchange transfusion. Arch Dis Child 1972;47:980–982.
18. May ME, Mintz PD, Lowry P, et al. Plasmapheresis in thyroxine overdose: A case report. J Toxicol Clin Toxicol 1983;20: 517–520.
19. Herrmann J, Rudorff KH, Gockenjan G, et al. Charcoal haemoperfusion in thyroid storm. Lancet 1977;1:248.
20. Herrmann J, Kruskemper HL, Grosser KD, et al. Peritoneal-dialysis in der Behandlung der thyreotoxischen Krise. Dtsch Med Wochenschr 1971;96:742–745.
21. Braunstein GD, Koblin R, Sugawara M, et al. Unintentional thyrotoxicosis factitia due to a diet pill. West J Med 1986;145:388–391.
22. Mariotti S, Martino E, Cupin C, et al. Low serum thyroglobulin as a clue to the diagnosis of thyrotoxicosis factitia. N Engl J Med 1982;307:410–412.
23. Hamolsky MW. Truth is stranger than factitious. N Engl J Med 1982;307:436–437.

ANTITHYROID DRUGS

Antithyroid drugs (the thionamides) may be associated with agranulocytosis, hepatotoxicity, arthralgias, and rashes. In overdose, these symptoms and signs together with a transient decrease in T_3 concentrations may be observed, followed by full recovery. Reactive metabolites of antithyroid drugs or hypersensitivity responses may be the basis for antithyroid toxicity. The perchlorates have been associated with serious adverse effects when used as antithyroid agents and have been generally replaced by other agents.

Structure and Classification

The main antithyroid agents are the thiourea derivatives (thiocarbamides, thionamides, or thioureylenes). The thiourea compounds include the imidazole derivatives (carbimazole [Neomercazole] and methimazole [Tapazole, Strumazole, Thyrozol] and the thiouracils (benzylthiouracil, methylthiouracil, and propylthiouracil [Propycil, Procasil, Propylthyracil, Prothyram]). Carbimazole is ethyl-3-methyl-2-thioxo-4-imazoline-1-carboxylate. Methimazole is 1-methylimidazole-2-thiol. Propylthiouracil is 2,3-dihydro-6-propyl-2-thioxopyrimidine-4(1*H*)-one.[1,2]

	CAS No.	Molecular Weight	Empirical Formula
Carbimazole	222232-54-8	186.2	$C_7H_{10}H_2O_2S$
Methimazole	60-56-0	114.2	$C_4H_6N_2S$
Propylthiouracil	51-52-5	170.2	$C_7H_{10}N_2OS$

The Perchlorates

Potassium perchlorate and sodium perchlorate, also used illicitly for the preparation of explosives or fireworks, have been used as antithyroid agents. Sodium perchlorate ($NaClO_4$) has a molecular weight of 122.4; its CAS numbers are 7601-89-0 (anhydrous) and 7791-97-3 (monohydrate).[1]

Use

Antithyroid agents are used in the management of hyperthyroidism, including the treatment of Graves' disease, preparation of hyperthyroid patients for surgery, and as an adjunct to radioiodine therapy of hyperthyroid disease.[1] Potassium perchlorate 1 g in association with a thiourea has led to rapid control of hyperthyroidism induced by amiodarone.[3,4] Methimazole has also been used in the treatment of psoriasis when it may have an ameliorative effect on the immune system.[5]

Product Formulation

Methimazole is available for oral use as 5- and 10-mg tablets. Carbimazole is available only as oral 5- and 20-mg tablets. Propylthiouracil is available as a 50-mg tablet (British National Formulary).

Source

Carbimazole, methimazole, and propylthiouracil are synthetic chemical compounds.

Therapeutic Dose

Carbimazole	Oral dose: 20 to 60 mg daily
Methimazole	Initial oral dose: 15 to 60 mg daily
Propylthiouracil	Initial dose: 300 to 600 mg daily.
Potassium perchlorate (adults)	600 mg to 1 g daily.[1]

Toxic Dose

Propylthiouracil overdose (100–260 50-mg tablets [5000–13,000 mg]) was associated with a benign clinical course and recovery.[6] Acute overdose of the thionamides may be associated with minor and transient changes in thyroid hormone levels. Following 300 mg daily of propylthiouracil, an adult developed a transient hepatitis.[7]

Fatal Dose

Fatal doses for these three compounds have not been determined.

Toxicokinetics[2,8]

	Carbimazole	Methimazole	Propylthiouracil
Bioavailability (%)	90–100	90–100	50–75
Plasma half-life (h)	3–5	3–5	1–3
Volume of distribution (as methimazole) (L/kg)	0.5	0.L	~ 30 L
Plasma protein binding (as methimazole) (%)	40	40	~ 80%

Carbimazole is rapidly converted to its active metabolite, methimazole. Peak levels of methimazole of 0.2 to 2.0 μmol/L occur 1 to 2 hours after 60 mg carbimazole orally.[9]

Drug Interactions

No significant drug interactions have been reported. Increased sensitivity to warfarin has been observed in hyperthyroidism.[10]

Pregnancy/Lactation

The thiourea compounds cross the placenta and are excreted in breast milk.[1] Fetal outcome is generally satisfactory in drug-treated pregnancies.[11,12] Neonatal hepatitis has followed treatment of the mother with propylthiouracil for Graves' disease.[13]

Mechanism of Action

The thioureas block the production of thyroid hormones through inhibition of thyroid peroxidase. Propylthiouracil also inhibits the peripheral deiodination of T_4 to T_3. The perchlorates competitively inhibit the active transport mechanism of the thyroid gland for the uptake of iodide and other anions. Reactive metabolites of propylthiouracil may be generated by activated neutrophils and may be involved in hypersensitivity reactions associated with propylthiouracil, such as agranulocytosis.[14] Vasculitis and antineutrophil cytoplasmic antibodies have been observed during propylthiouracil therapy.[15]

Clinical Presentation

Overdose

Few reports of overdose with the thioureas or perchlorates are available. An oral ingestion of 5000 to 13,000 mg of propylthiouracil led to a benign clinical course with recovery.[6] There was a transient reduction in T_3 levels. Overdose of the thionamides may induce vomiting, epigastric distress, headache, fever, arthralgia, pruritus, and pancytopenia.[2]

Chronic Use

Agranulocytosis and granulocytopenia are most frequent in patients taking high doses of antithyroid drugs (40–120 mg methimazole daily and about 700 mg of propylthiouracil daily).[16] Hepatotoxicity is a rare reaction of antithyroid drugs.[11] Initial recovery may be followed by a delayed exacerbation.[7] Hanson has proposed the following criteria for diagnosing drug-induced hepatitis[17]:

- Clinical and laboratory evidence of hepatocellular dysfunction
- Onset of symptoms temporally related to drug therapy
- No serologic evidence for current hepatitis A or B, cytomegalovirus, or Epstein–Barr virus infections
- Absence of an acute hepatic insult (shock, sepsis)
- No evidence of chronic liver disease
- Absence of other concomitantly administered drugs especially known as hepatotoxins

Rashes may follow high doses of methimazole (120 mg daily).[18] Both major (agranulocytosis, hepatotoxicity) and minor (arthralgias, skin rash, gastric intolerance) adverse effects are not dose related.[19]

Laboratory

Analytical Methods

Propylthiouracil. A gas–liquid chromatographic method is sensitive to 5 mg/dL in urine and 1 μg/mL in blood.[7]

Methimazole. Methods of analysis of methimazole include high-pressure liquid chromatography (sensitivity, 5 μg/L), gas chromatography–mass spectrometry (sensitivity, 2 μg/L), and radioimmunoassay.[9]

Blood Levels

Twelve hours following an ingestion of 5000 to 13,000 mL or propylthiouracil, the blood level was 1 μg/mL, and the urine level, 90 mg/dL. Within 17 hours no propylthiouracil was detected.[7]

Abnormalities

Following an overdose with 5000 to 13,000 of propylthiouracil there was a transient decrease in T_3 concentration and an increase in thyroid-stimulating hormone concentration.[7] Liver function tests were slightly elevated.

Ancillary Tests

Peripheral lymphocyte transformation may be an indicator of drug-induced liver damage.[12]

Treatment

Treatment of an overdose is symptomatic and supportive. There is no antidote. Periodic follow-up should include neutrophil counts and laboratory evaluation for evidence of hepatotoxicity.

IODINE

Acute ingestion of iodine often results in corrosive injury of the gastrointestinal tract and renal damage. Cardiopulmonary collapse secondary to circulatory failure, edema of the epiglottis, and aspiration pneumonia may cause death. Administration of starch (25 g to 500 mL water) followed by sodium thiosulfate (to 15%) to convert iodine to relatively harmless iodide, maintenance of the airway, and circulatory stabilization are the mainstays of therapy. Milk every 15 minutes may be used to manage stomach irritation.[20] Gastric lavage is contraindicated if there is evidence of esophageal damage. Fluid and electrolyte balance must be monitored. (See also Chapter 56.)

REFERENCES—ANTITHYROID DRUGS

1. Reynolds JEF, ed. *Martindale: The Extra Pharmacopoeia.* 30th ed. London: Pharmaceutical Press, 1993:531–535.
2. Dollery CT, ed. *Therapeutic Drugs.* Edinburgh: Churchill Livingstone, 1991:(carbimazole) C66–C69; (methimazole) M95–M97; (propylthiouracil) P282–P287.
3. Reichert LJM, De Rooy HAM. Treatment of amiodarone induced hyperthyroidism with potassium perchlorate and methimazole during amiodarone treatment. Br Med J 1989; 298:1547–1548.
4. Modebe O. Experience with carbimazole in the drug treatment of the hyperthyroidism of Graves' disease in Nigerians. East Afr Med J 1992;69:153–156.
5. Elias AN, Goodman MM, Rohan MK, et al. Methimazole (2-mercaptol-methylimidazole) in psoriasis: Results of an open trial. Dermatology 1993;187:24–29.
6. Jackson GL, Flickinger FW, Wells LW. Massive overdosage of propylthiouracil. Ann Intern Med 1979;91:418–419.
7. Peter SA. Propylthiouracil-associated hepatitis. J Natl Med Assoc 1991;83:75-77.
8. Melander A, Hallengren B, Rozendal-Helgesen S, et al. Comparative in vitro effects and in vivo kinetics of antithyroid drugs. Eur J Clin Pharmacol 1980;17:295–299.
9. Skellern GG, Stenlack JB, Williams WD, McLarty DG. Plasma concentrations of methimazole, a metabolite of carbimazole, in hyperthyroid patients. Br J Clin Pharmacol 1974;1: 265–269.
10. Kellett HA, Sawers JSA, Boulton FE, et al. Problems of anticoagulating with warfarin in hyperthyroidism. Q J Med 1986;225:43–51.
11. Chatral P, Sidhu R, Joplin CF, Hawkins DF. Treatment of thyrotoxicosis in pregnancy. J Obstet Gynecol 1981;2: 11–19.
12. Ramsay I, Kaur S, Krassas G. Thyrotoxicosis in pregnancy: Results of treatment by antithyroid drugs combined with T_4. Clin Endocrinol 1983;18:73–85.
13. Hayashida CY, Durate AJS, Sato AE, Yamashiro-Kanashiro EH. Neonatal hepatitis and lymphocyte sensitization by placental transfer of propylthiouracil. J Endocrinol Invest 1990;13:937–941.
14. Waldhauser L, Uetrecht J. Oxidation of propylthiouracil to reactive metabolites by activated neutrophils: Implications for agranulocytosis. Drug Metab Dispos 1991;19:354–359.
15. Dolman KM, Grans ROB, Vervaat TJ, et al. Vasculitis and antineutrophil cytoplasmic autoantibodies associated with propylthiouracil therapy. Lancet 1993;342:651–652.
16. Romaldini JN, Werner MC, Bromberg N, Werner RS. Adverse effects related to antithyroid drugs and their dose regimen. Exp Clin Endocrinol 1991;97:261–264.
17. Hanson JJS. Propylthiouracil and hepatitis. Arch Intern Med 1982;14:994–996.
18. Wiberg JJ, Nuttall FQ. Methimazole toxicity from high doses. Ann Intern Med 1972;77:414–416.
19. Werner MC, Romeldini JH, Bromberg N, et al. Adverse effects related to thionamide drugs and their dosage regimen. Am J Med Sci 1989;297:216–219.
20. Lin T-H, Kirkland RT, Kirkland JL. Clinical features and management of overdosage with thyroid drugs. Med Toxicol 1988;3:264–272.

TRILOSTANE

Few reports of overdose with trilostane (Fig. 42–3) are available. As the drug inhibits steroidogenesis, intravenous hydrocortisone may be useful in overdose.

Structure and Classification

Trilostane is a synthetic steroid that is related structurally to testosterone but does not possess direct hormonal activity.

Figure 42-3 Structure of trilostane. (From McEvoy GK, ed. *AHFS Drug Information 94.* Bethesda, MD: American Society of Hospital Pharmacists, 1994.)

Trilostane is marketed as Modrastane and Modrenal in the United Kingdom.[1]

Use

In patients with Cushing's syndrome, trilostane generally decreases cortisol secretion rate, plasma cortisol concentration, urinary excretion of free cortisol and 17-hydroxycorticosteroids, and the adrenocortical response to stimulation by corticotropin (ACTH).[2] Some patients with Cushing's syndrome who are not candidates for or are awaiting surgery or radiation may respond to trilostane.[3] It has been effective in the palliative treatment of primary aldosteronism (Conn's syndrome) secondary to adrenal adenoma or adrenal hyperplasia. It has been used in the treatment of hormone-sensitive metastatic breast carcinoma in postmenopausal women.

Product Formulation

Trilostane is available in 30- and 60-mg oral capsules.

Source

Trilostane is a synthetic chemical compound.

Therapeutic Dose

The usual adult dose is 30 mg four times daily. The dosage may be increased every 3 to 4 days up to a maximum of 480 mg/d.

Toxic Dose

A patient ingested 3600 mg of trilostane and survived.[4]

Fatal Dose

A fatal dose has not been established.

Toxicokinetics

Absorption

Trilostane is readily absorbed from the gastrointestinal tract. Plasma concentrations are detected within 20 to 60 minutes of a single oral administration of 120 mg. After such a dose, peak plasma trilostane and 17-ketotrilostane concentrations average about 4–1 and 1.5–2.5 µg/mL, respectively.

Distribution

Trilostane is most widely distributed into the adrenal glands, liver, lungs, and kidneys.

Elimination

Plasma levels decline to negligible levels within 6 to 8 hours. Trilostane is metabolized in the liver by hydroxylation and glucuronidation. 17-Ketotrilostane is the major metabolite with enzyme velocity activity twice that of trilostane.

Drug Interactions

If trilostane is given with other drugs that suppress adrenal function (aminoglutethimide, metyrapone, mitotane), it may induce severe adrenal hypofunction. In patients with hypokalemia treated with trilostane, serum potassium concentration usually increases. Trilostane may reduce the kaliuresis observed with concomitant thiazides or loop diuretics.

Pregnancy/Lactation

Trilostane is contraindicated during pregnancy. It is not known whether trilostane or its metabolite is distributed to breast milk. Trilostane is teratogenic in animals and may result in a spontaneous abortion.

Mechanism of Action

Trilostane is an inhibitor of adrenocortical steroidogenesis. The exact mechanism of drug action has not been fully determined. It may inhibit both glucocorticoid and mineralocorticoid synthesis by inhibiting 3β-hydroxy-Δ^5-steroid dehydrase (progesterone reductase). It does not possess inherent hormonal agonist or antagonist activity.[2] Trilostane also inhibits steroidogenesis in the ovaries, placenta, and testes.

Clinical Presentation

A 29-year-old man ingested 3600 mg of trilostane. There were no changes in his pulse rate or blood pressure. The plasma potassium level was 33 mEq/L.[4] Trilostane may cause diarrhea, abdominal pain, nausea, burning of mucus membranes, flushing, headache, rhinorrhea, and suppression of gonadal function and Addison's crisis. In a woman who received 960 mg of trilostane daily for 5 days, manifestations of adrenal insufficiency included lethargy, confusion, and severe hypotension within 5 days of therapy.[1]

Laboratory

Analytical Methods

Trilostane interferes with determination of corticosteroids in plasma and urine by fluorometry.

Blood Levels

Following ingestion of 960 mg daily, the plasma cortisol concentration was 1.8 µg/dL.

Treatment

In acute overdose, gastric emptying should be performed immediately. Therapy with physiologic replacement dosages of a corticosteroid may be required. Blood pressure and serum potassium concentration should be monitored for at least 24 to 48 hours and appropriate therapy should be provided as required. Hypotension and elevated serum potassium concentrations may respond to corticosteroid therapy alone.

REFERENCES—TRILOSTANE

1. Reynolds JEF, ed. *Martindale: The Extra Pharmacopoeia.* 30th ed. London: Pharmaceutical Press, 1993:1427.
2. McEvoy GK, ed. *AHFS Drug Information 94.* Bethesda, MD: American Society of Hospital Pharmacists, 1994:2489–2490.
3. Med Lett Drugs Ther 1985;27(698):87–88.
4. Barnes N, Thomas N. Overdose of trilostane. Br Med J 1983;286:1784–1785.

THE PROSTATE GLAND

BENIGN PROSTATIC HYPERTROPHY

The first changes of benign prostatic hypertrophy (BPH) begin around age 35 years and consist of microscopic stromal nodules that occur around the periurethral glands. Acinar hyperplasia then begins around these microscopic nodules. As men age, their levels of estrogen rise. This rise is related to both an absolute decrease in the level of testosterone production and an increased conversion of serum testosterone to estrogen in the peripheral adipose tissues. The stromal hyperplasia may trigger acinar hyperplasia. The androgen critical to prostatic growth is dihydrotestosterone.[1,2]

Pathophysiology

The clinical manifestations of BPH are related primarily to obstructive and irritative phenomena caused by prostatic enlargement (prostatitis). Obstructive symptoms include hesitancy and straining to initiate urination, a diminished caliber and interrupted urinary stream, postmicturition dribbling, urinary frequency and nocturia (awakening during the night to urinate), dysuria (burning during urination), and urgency (the impending need to urinate).

Therapeutic Approaches

Current pharmacotherapy for BPH is based on agents that relax the smooth muscles of the prostatic urethra and stroma and those that deprive acinar cells of androgen. Drugs tried in the treatment of BPH affect either the smooth muscle and prostatic stroma or the glandular elements by androgen deprivation.[2]

Mechanism of Alpha-Blocker Therapy

α_{1A} subtypes are present in the human prostate. The α_{1C} subtype constitutes 70% of all α_1 adrenoceptors in the human prostate. The contractile properties of prostate smooth muscle are mediated by α_1 adrenoceptors. α_1-adrenergic antagonists are ideally suited for treatment of the dynamic component of bladder outlet obstruction because they can selectively reduce resistance along the bladder outlet without impairing detrusor contractility.

TERAZOSIN

Terazosin is one of two selective long-acting α_1-adrenoceptor antagonists that are currently approved by the Food and Drug Administration for the treatment of hypertension.[3–6]

Therapeutic Dose

Terazosin hydrochloride (Hytrin, Abbott Laboratories) is initiated with 1 mg at night; the dose may be increased to 1, 5, or 10 mg. Alpha-blocker therapy is recommended for a minimum of 6 months to a year to achieve maximal response.

Toxicokinetics

The toxicokinetics of terazosin are summarized in Table 42–14.

Clinical Presentation

Terazosin overdose is most likely to be followed by orthostatic hypotension, dizziness, syncope, lethargy, and shock.

Treatment

The patient is placed in a supine head-down position. Blood pressure, respiration, pulse, and state of consciousness are monitored. If hypotension is severe, plasma volume expanders and nonadrenergic vasopressors should be considered. Dialysis would most likely be ineffective (highly protein bound). Gastric lavage may be attempted if the patient is seen within 1 to 2 hours of ingestion.

FINASTERIDE

Selective blockade of androgen action at the prostatic cellular level includes the 5α-reductase inhibitors, enzymes required for intraprostatic conversion of testosterone to its active form, dihydrotestosterone (DHT).

Table 42–14
Toxicokinetics

	Terazosin[a–d]	Finasteride[e]
Bioavailability	90	80
Time to peak blood level (h)	1–2	2–3
Peak plasma concentration		40–800 mg/mL after dose of 5–100 mg
Protein binding	90%	90%
Elimination half-life (h)	12	4–7
Excreted in urine unchanged (%)	About 30%	0.04%

[a]Hypertension Symposium. Clinical applications of alpha$_1$-receptor blockade: Terazosin in the management of hypertension. J Clin Pharmacol 1993;33:866–899.
[b]Terazosin for benign prostatic hyperplasia. Med Lett Drugs Ther 1994; 36(916):15–16.
[c]Hill SJ, Lawrence SL, Lepor H. New use for alpha blockers: Benign prostatic hyperplasia. Am Fam Physician 1994;45:1885–1888.
[d]Lowe FC. Safety assessment of terazosin in the treatment of patients with symptomatic benign prostatic hyperplasia: A combined analysis. Urology 1994;44:46–51.
[e]Gormley GJ, Stoner E, Bruskewitz RC, et al. The effect of finasteride in men with benign prostatic hyperplasia. N Engl J Med 1992;327:1185–1191.

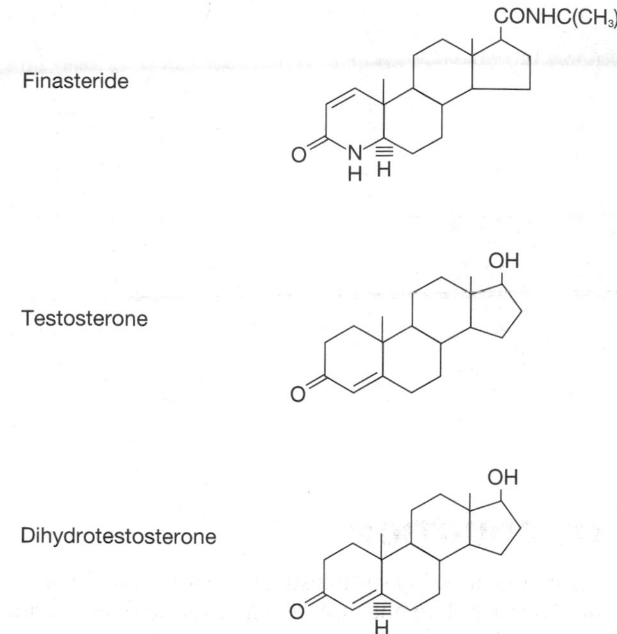

Figure 42-4 Structures of finasteride, testosterone, and dihydrotestosterone. (From Steiner JF. Finasteride: A 5 alpha-reductase inhibitor. Clin Pharm 1993;12(1):15–23.)

Finasteride (Proscar) is a competitive specific inhibitor of 5α-reductase (Fig. 42–4). After a single 5-mg oral dose, it produces a rapid reduction in serum DHT concentration within 8 hours, and this is maintained for as long as 24 hours. It does not affect the hypothalamus–pituitary–testicular axis. It is available as 5-mg tablets for oral administration. Serum DHT concentrations decrease to castration levels soon after finasteride therapy is initiated.[7] Serum testosterone and luteinizing hormone concentrations increase only slightly. A median reduction in prostate volume of 19% is noted within 3 months of the initiation of therapy. This was associated with a substantial decrease in serum prostate-specific antigen levels, indicating a decrease in prostatic epithelial cell function. There is a significant decrease in symptoms of obstruction and an increase in maximum urinary flow rates.[1,2,7–12]

Therapeutic Dose

Finasteride is used at a dose of 5 mg/d. Spouses who are of childbearing age are advised not to come in contact with the semen of men who are taking finasteride, to avoid any effects on a developing fetus.

Toxicokinetics

The toxicokinetics of finasteride are summarized in Table 42–14.

Finasteride interacts little with other medications and may be safely used in patients taking alpha blockers, beta blockers, theophylline, digoxin, sodium warfarin, diuretics, antiinflammatory agents, calcium channel blockers, and H_2 antagonists. About 40% of metabolized finasteride is excreted in urine and 59% in stool.

Clinical Presentation and Treatment

Side effects of finasteride include decreased libido, ejaculatory disorder, and impotence.

Prolonged use may lead to a reduction in libido, ejaculatory disorders, and impotence. There is no antidote. Specific drug therapy is not indicated.

REFERENCES—THE PROSTATE GLAND

1. Narayan P, Indudhara R. Pharmacotherapy for benign prostatic hyperplasia. West J Med 1994;161:495–501.
2. Smith AY. Pharmacologic management of benign prostatic hyperplasia: Changing times. West J Med 1994;161: 521–523.
3. Hypertension Symposium. Clinical applications of alpha$_1$-receptor blockade: Terazosin in the management of hypertension. J Clin Pharmacol 1993;33:866–899.
4. Terazosin for benign prostatic hyperplasia. Med Lett Drugs Ther 1994;36(916):15–16.
5. Hill SJ, Lawrence SL, Lepor H. New use for alpha blockers: Benign prostatic hyperplasia. Amer Fam Phys 1994;45:1885–1888.
6. Lowe FC. Safety assessment of terazosin in the treatment of patients with symptomatic benign prostatic hyperplasia. A combined analysis. Urology 1994;44:46–51.
7. Gormley GJ, Stoner E, Bruskewitz RC, et al. The effect of finasteride in men with benign prostatic hyperplasia. N Engl J Med 1992;327:1185–1191.
8. Winchell GA, Gregoire S, Taylor AM, et al. Finasteride: A steroid 5-alpha reductive inhibitor does not affect the oxidative metabolism of antipyrine. J Clin Pharmacol 1993;33:967–970.
9. Steiner JF. Finasteride: A 5-alpha-reductase inhibitor. Clin Pharm 1993;12:15–23.
10. Browley OW, Ford LG, Thompson I, et al. 5-Alpha-reductase inhibition and prostate cancer prevention. Cancer Epid Biomarkers Prev 1994;3:177–182.
11. Gregoretti S. Intraoperative hypotension in a patient treated with terazosin, a new alpha-adrenergic receptor antagonist. J Clin Anesth 1994;6:170–171.
12. Dollery C, ed. *Therapeutic Drugs.* Edinburgh: Churchill Livingstone, 1994:238–243.

Chapter 43

Gastrointestinal Drugs

INTRODUCTION

Drug treatment of gastrointestinal disease was for a long period restricted to the use of antacids, anticholinergics, antispasmodics, cathartics, and laxatives. In the past 10 years histamine H_2-receptor antagonists (eg, cimetidine, ranitidine, famotidine, nizatidine) have emerged as useful products for the treatment of peptic acid disorders. Muscarinic M_1-receptor antagonists (eg, pirenzepine), proton pump inhibitors (eg, omeprazole), prostaglandin analogs (eg, misoprostol), site-protective drugs (eg, colloidal bismuth subsalicylate and sucralfate), antiemetics with prokinetic properties (eg, metoclopramide, domperidone, and cisapride), antiinflammatory salicylates (eg, olsalazine and mesalazine), and nonspecific antidiarrheal agents (diphenoxylate and loperamide) are also in current use (Table 43–1). Overdose is usually not fatal, with the exception of diphenoxylate in children, although serious multisystem effects have been observed.[1,2]

ANTIINFLAMMATORY SALICYLATES: 5-AMINOSALICYLIC ACID-BASED DRUGS

Sulfasalazine, originally developed for the treatment of rheumatoid arthritis, combined one of the first sulfonamides, sulfapyridine, with an aspirin analog, 5-aminosalicylate (5-ASA).[3] Sulfasalazine became widely used in the treatment of inflammatory bowel disease.[2,4] Its use became limited by a high degree of intolerance and frequent adverse reactions, most of which were attributed to the serum sulfapyridine levels. The parent drug, sulfasalazine, may be a vehicle for delivery of the active component 5-ASA to distal disease sites. As the sulfa moiety was responsible for the toxicity of the drug and the 5-ASA moiety for its therapeutic efficacy, 5-ASA was modified to be delivered to areas of diseased bowels. Oral 5-ASA agents[3] appear to be as effective prophylactically for ulcerative colitis as topical 5-ASA and sulfasalazine.[5]

Toxic Dose

A 23-year-old man ingested 50 500-mg sulfasalazine tablets. He developed a headache and felt dizzy. He was treated with

Table 43-1
Drugs Used in the Treatment of Gastrointestinal Diseases

Antiulcer Drugs
Antacids
Histamine H_2-receptor antagonists
Cimetidine
Ranitidine
Famotidine
Nizatidine
Muscarinic M_1-receptor antagonists
Pirenzepine
Prostaglandin analogs
Proton pump inhibitors
Omeprazole
Site-protective agents
Colloidal bismuth subcitrate
Sucralfate
Antiemetic and Prokinetic Drugs
Metoclopramide
Domperidone
Cisapride
Antispasmodic Agents
Antiinflammatory Agents
Corticosteroids
Antiinflammatory salicylates
Sulfasalazine
Olsalazine
Mesalazine
Antidiarrheal Agents
Specific antidiarrheal agents
Antiinfective agents
Nonspecific antidiarrheal agents
Opioids
Diphenoxylate
Loperamide
Laxatives and Cathartics

From Lauritsen K, Laursen LS, Rask-Madsen J. Clinical pharmacokinetics of drugs used in the treatment of gastrointestinal diseases (Part I). Clin Pharmac okinet 1990;19:11–31.

gastric lavage, activated charcoal with sorbitol, and intravenous dextrose with sodium bicarbonate. He survived with few ill effects.[6]

Clinical Presentation

More adverse effects have been reported with oral 5-ASA than with topical therapy.[7]

Olsalazine

Olsalazine is a product consisting of 2 mesalazine (5-ASA) moieties bridged by an azo bond developed to deliver 5-ASA to the colon. It is administered in doses of 1 to 3 g daily.[3,8] No reports of overdose with olsalazine are available.[9] Adverse effects include diarrhea, headache, nausea, abdominal pain, rash, dizziness, and joint pain.[8]

Mesalazine

Mesalazine (5-ASA, mesalamine), the active moiety of sulfasalazine in inflammatory bowel disease, may be delivered to the colon by replacing sulfapyridine with another carrier as has been done with olsalazine.[10] It is administered orally as coated tablets in doses of 1.5 to 3.2 g daily and as retention enemas or suppositories in doses of 1 to 4 g daily. Adverse effects include headache, nausea, dizziness, indigestion, muscular ache, fever,[10] skin and cardiac hypersensitivity reactions, interstitial nephritis,[11] pancreatitis,[12] thrombocytopenia,[13] and aplastic anemia.[14] No reports of overdose with the use of rectal suppositories arc available.[15]

Sulfasalazine

Unsplit sulfasalazine inhibits prostaglandin synthesis, prostaglandin degradation, and thromboxane synthesis, as well as interfering with neutrophil chemotaxis and scavenging radicals. The therapeutic importance of these actions is unclear.[4] Sulfasalazine has rarely been associated with fulminant hepatic failure, hypersensitivity pneumonitis, and a nephrotic syndrome.

REFERENCES—5-AMINOSALICYLIC ACID-BASED DRUGS

1. Lauritsen K, Lauritsen LS, Rask-Madsen J. Clinical pharmacokinetics of drugs used in the treatment of gastrointestinal diseases (Part I). Clin Pharmacokinet 1990;119:11–31.
2. Lauritsen K, Lauritsen LS, Rask-Madsen J. Clinical pharmacokinetics of drugs used in the treatment of gastrointestinal disease (Part II). Clin Pharmacokinet 1990;19:94–125.
3. Jarnerot G. Newer 5-aminosalicylic based drugs in chronic inflammatory bowel disease. Drugs 1989;37:73–86.
4. Sulphasalazine: Drug or pro-drug. Lancet 1987;1:1299–1330. Editorial.
5. Bruckstein AH. New salicylate therapies for ulcerative colitis. Postgrad Med 1990;88:79–89.
6. Minocha A, Dean HA, Mayle JE. Acute sulfasalazine overdose. Clin Toxicol 1991;29:543–551; Am J Gastroenterol 1991;86:1358
7. Peppercorn MA. Advances in drug therapy for inflammatory bowel disease. Ann Intern Med 1990;112:50–60.
8. Wadworth AN, Fitton A. Olsalazine: A review of its pharmacodynamic and pharmacokinetic properties and therapeutic potential in inflammatory bowel disease. Drugs 1991;41:647–664.
9. Hessemer CA. Personal communication. Kabi Pharmacia, March 22, 1991.
10. Brogden RN, Sorkin EM. Mesalazine: A review of its pharmacodynamic and pharmacokinetic properties and therapeutic potential in chronic inflammatory bowel disease. Drugs 1989; 38:500–523.
11. Mehta RP. Acute interstitial nephritis due to 5-aminosalicylic acid. Can Med Assoc J 1990;143:1031–1032.
12. Isaacs KL, Murphy D. Pancreatitis after rectal administration of 5-aminosalicylic acid. J Clin Gastroenterol 1990;12:198–199.
13. Daneshmend TK. Mesalazine-associated thrombocytopenia. Lancet 1991;337:1297–1298.
14. Abbouti ZH, Marsh JCW, Smith-Laing G, Gordon-Smith EC. Fatal aplastic anemia after mesalazine. Lancet 1994;343:542.
15. Fraser D. Personal communication. Reid Powell, April 18, 1991.

NONSPECIFIC ANTIDIARRHEAL AGENTS

DIPHENOXYLATE

See Chapter 25.

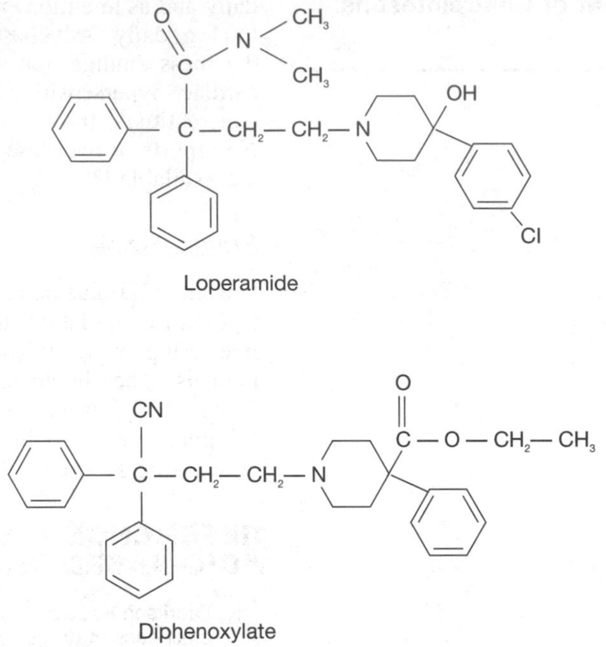

Figure 43-1 Structures of loperamide and diphenoxylate. (From Heel RC, Brogden RN, Speight TM, Avery GS. Loperamide: A review of its pharmacological properties and therapeutic efficacy in diarrhoea. Drugs 1978;15:33–52.)

LOPERAMIDE

Loperamide (Imodium) is a piperidine-derivative antidiarrheal agent (Fig 43–1).[1,2] Overdoses have occurred in infants in developing countries. There have been fatalities.[3,4] Overdose may lead to constipation, ileus, and neurologic symptoms (miosis, muscular hypotonia, somnolence, and bradypnea). Naloxone is an effective antidote. Loperamide syrup has been withdrawn by the manufacturer in those countries where the World Health Organization has a program for control of diarrheal disease.[5]

Toxicokinetics[1,2,6,7,8]

Bioavailability	About 100%
Peak plasma level	0.75 ng/mL (after 4 mg)
Time to peak plasma level	4 hours
Plasma protein binding	97%
Elimination half-life	15 hours
Excreted unchanged	About 1%

Drug Interactions

No specific studies on loperamide drug interactions are available. Concomitant use of narcotics probably increases the tendency toward bradypnea, muscular hypotonia, somnolence, and miosis.

Pregnancy/Lactation

There are no adequate studies of loperamide in pregnancy or during lactation.

Mechanism Of Action

Loperamide appears to exert its antisecretory effect via μ–opiate receptors acting distal to the adenylate cyclase–cyclic AMP system.[9] The antisecretory effects are due partly to stimulation of absorption, and are mediated by opiate receptors.[10] In animals loperamide reverses prostaglandin E_2 and cholera toxin-induced secretion to absorption.[11] Unlike diphenoxylate or codeine, loperamide does not appear to exert opiate activity in humans at normal therapeutic doses.[1]

Clinical Presentation

Overdose

Disorientation, lethargy, hallucinations, inability to walk, miotic pupils, bradypnea, toxic megacolon, and coma have been observed.[9,12]

Chronic Use

Nausea, abdominal cramping, dizziness, rash, and dry mouth have occasionally been reported.[1] A double-blind study suggests that loperamide has little abuse potential.[13]

Laboratory

Analytical Methods

A radioimmunoassay for loperamide is available. The method is sensitive to amounts in human plasma as small as 50 pg.[14] Loperamide can be accurately assayed in a range from 100 pg up to 10 ng contained in 0.5 mL of plasma. The loperamide antibody does not bind to the structurally related drugs haloperidol, diphenoxylate, and difenoxin. The *N*-dealkylate metabolites do not interfere with the assays.[11]

Blood Levels

Following a dose of 1.08 mg of loperamide, an 8-day-old infant exhibited a blood level of 1.99 mg/100 mL blood.[15] The infant responded to activated charcoal and naloxone.

Abnormalities

Hypokalemia may predispose to ileus.[9]

Treatment

Stabilization

Infants with loperamide overdose should be admitted to a pediatric intensive care facility where continuous monitoring of vital signs can be performed and where access to oxygen, intravenous fluids, and naloxone are available. Respiratory assistance (mechanical ventilation) may be required for up to 24 hours.

Gut Decontamination

Gastric lavage should be instituted in overdose. Activated charcoal slurry 100 g can be administered through the gastric tube. If vomiting has occurred spontaneously, 100 g of activated charcoal slurry can be administered orally as soon as fluids are retained. Twenty-four-hour observation may not be necessary in children with small overdoses after gastric decontamination.[16,17]

Elimination Enhancement

Forced diuresis is not expected to be effective in loperamide overdose, as relatively little drug is excreted in the urine. There have been no studies on the use of hemodialysis or hemoperfusion in loperamide overdose.

Antidote

Naloxone is an effective antidote and may be administered if central nervous system depression occurs. Because the duration of action of loperamide is greater than that of naloxone, the patient must be closely watched and additional doses of naloxone administered if required. Vital signs should be monitored for recurrence of symptoms of drug overdose for at least 24 hours after the last dose of naloxone.

Supportive Measures

Patients must be monitored for the recurrence of symptoms of drug overdose for at least 24 hours after the last dose of naloxone. The plasma potassium level should be monitored frequently in any sick infant receiving loperamide as hypokalemia may predispose to ileus in some infants.[9]

REFERENCES—LOPERAMIDE

1. McEvoy GK, ed. *AHFS Drug Information 94.* Bethesda, MD: American Society of Hospital Pharmacists 1994:1880–1881.
2. Heel RC, Brogden NN, Speight TM, Avery GS. Loperamide: A review of its pharmacological properties and therapeutic efficacy in diarrhoea. Drugs 1978;15:33–52.
3. Bhutta FL, Tahir KI. Loperamide poisoning in children. Lancet 1990;335:363.
4. Bhutta II. Anti-motility drug for infants. Lancet 1990;331:314.
5. Gussin RZ. Withdrawal of loperamide drops. Lancet 1990; 335:1603–1604.
6. Minton NA, Smith PGD. Loperamide toxicity in a child after a single dose. Br Med J 1987;294:1383.
7. Blum D, Kahn A. Poisoning and near-miss cot death. Vet Hum Toxicol 1987;29(suppl. 2):27.
8. Lauritsen K, Lauritsen LS, Rask-Madsen J. Clinical pharmacokinetics of drugs used in the treatment of gastrointestinal diseases (Part II). Clin Pharmacokinet 1990; 19:94–125.
9. Sandhu BF, Tripp JH, Candy DCA, Haries JT. Loperamide: Studies on its mechanism of action. Gut 1981;22: 658–662.
10. Sandhu BF, Tripp JH, Milla RJ, Harries JT. Loperamide in severe protracted diarrhoea. Arch Dis Child 1983; 58:39–43.
11. Walley T, Milson D. Loperamide related toxic megacolon in *Clostridium difficile* colitis. Postgrad Med J 1990;66:582–584.
12. Marcovitch H. Loperamide in 'toddler' diarrheoea. Lancet 1980;1:1413.
13. Jaffe JH, Kanzler M, Green J. Abuse potential of loperamide. Clin Pharmacol Ther 1980;28:812–819.
14. Michiels M, Hendriks R, Heykants J. Radioimmunoassay of the antidiarrhoeal loperamide. Life Sci 1977;21: 451–460.
15. Ramirez MS, Bastidas O, Berudez EL. A suspected case of loperamide toxicity. Vet Hum Toxicol 1983;25:341.
16. Hart LM, Dean BS, Krenzelok EP. Loperamide overdose in children: Is it as bad as Lomotil? Vet Hum Toxicol 1992; 34:332.
17. Litovitz TL, Clancy C, Koverly BH, et al. Surveillance of loperamide ingestions: Analysis of 216 poison center reports. Vet Hum Toxicol 1993;35:369.

PROSTAGLANDIN ANALOG: MISOPROSTOL

Nonsteroidal antiinflammatory drugs (NSAIDs) can cause acute upper gastrointestinal tract bleeding.[1] The stomach is more severely affected than the duodenum. Such bleeding may be fatal, especially in the elderly.[2–5] These life-threatening complications of NSAID-induced gastrointestinal tract bleeding may present without warning in up to 60% of patients.[1,6]

Nonsteroidal antiinflammatory drugs inhibit prostaglandin synthesis. A deficiency in prostaglandins in the gastric mucosa may contribute to the mucosal damage caused by NSAIDs by decreasing bicarbonate and mucus secretion. Prostaglandin E_1 has an antisecretory effect in gastric acid production; however, it is not effective orally, has a short duration of action, and has undesirable side effects.[2] Misoprostol (Cytotec) is a prostaglandin E_1 analog, has a greater oral activity, a longer duration of action, and a more selective effect. NSAIDs may still induce a gastric ulcer or gastrointestinal bleeding, even in a patient currently receiving misoprostol therapy.[7]

Misoprostol contains approximately equal amounts of two diasteromers with their enantiomers indicated by (+–). It is a water-soluble, viscous liquid.[8] Misoprostol overdose has induced fetal death[9] and other systemic symptoms.[10] Patients have recovered with symptomatic and supportive treatment.

Use

Misoprostol was approved by the Food and Drug Administration specifically for the prevention of NSAID-induced gastric ulcers in patients at high risk of complications from gastric ulcer, for example, the elderly and patients with concomitant debilitating disease, as well as patients at high risk of developing gastric ulceration, such as patients with a history of ulcer.[2]

Therapeutic Dose

For the prevention of NSAID-induced gastric ulcer the usual adult oral dose of misoprostol is 200 µg four times daily. Misoprostol is taken for the duration of NSAID therapy.[8]

Toxic Dose

Misoprostol 1600 µg daily has been tolerated with only mild gastrointestinal discomfort.[5] A 19-year-old woman at 31 weeks' gestation ingested about 30 200-µg tablets (6 mg) and four 2-mg trifluoperazine tablets. The fetus did not survive; the mother recovered.[9] A 71-year-old woman accidentally ingested 15 200-µg tablets of misoprostol (approximately 3 mg) and recovered with supportive care.[10]

Fatal Dose

A fatal dose in humans has not been established.

Toxicokinetics[5,11–17]

Bioavailability	88%
Peak plasma level	500 pg/mL (after 400 µg orally)
Time to peak plasma level	<30 minutes
Volume of distribution	12 L/kg
Plasma protein binding	80–90%
Elimination half-life	20–40 minutes (metabolism)
Active metabolites	Misoprostol acid

Drug Interactions

Misoprostol does not alter the toxicokinetics of concomitantly administered ibuprofen, aspirin, or diclofenac.[12,18] Misoprostol does not appear to interfere with the metabolism of drugs, including diazepam and propranolol, by the hepatic cytochrome P450 microsomal enzyme system.[18–20]

Pregnancy/Lactation

Misoprostol has abortifacient properties and is contraindicated in women who are pregnant. When administered in an overdose at 31 weeks of gestation, misoprostol resulted 2 hours later in the delivery of a dead fetus with diffuse ecchymosis.[9] Misoprostol is known to induce labor. Misoprostol is not a "safe" drug for inducing uterine bleeding or spontaneous abortion.[21] It is ineffective about half of the time and may expose the fetus to possible risk of severe malformation.[21] Ingestion of 400 to 600 µg orally and/or vaginally in the first trimester of pregnancy appeared to lead to a number of infants with a malformation consisting of a localized frontal and/or temporal skull defect—an asymmetrical, well-circumscribed defect of the cranium and overlying scalp, exposing dura through which the cerebrum could be seen.[22] Others have not seen this type of malformation.[23]

In France, 600 mg of mifepristone,[23] followed 2 days later by 400 µg of misoprostol orally, effected a complete abortion in 95 of 100 women after gestations of up to 45 days. Four had an incomplete abortion and required suction evacuation.[24] In Scotland, a similar regimen using 200 mg mifepristone followed by 200 to 1000 µg misoprostol 48 hours later led to complete abortion in 18 of 21 women.[25,26]

It is not known whether misoprostol or its acid metabolite are excreted in breast milk.

Clinical Presentation

Overdose

Patients may experience hyperthermia, chills, shortness of breath, nausea, and abdominal cramps, but are alert, oriented, and coherent.[9,10]

Chronic Use

Chronic misoprostol ingestion leads to diarrhea and cramping, abdominal pain, nausea and vomiting, delirium,[27] urinary incontinence,[28] and headache.

Laboratory

Analytical Methods

Misoprostol and its major active metabolite misoprostol acid can be estimated by radioimmunoassays with a detection limit of 23 ng/L.[12]

Treatment

Treatment of misoprostol overdose is largely symptomatic and supportive. All overdose patients, whether pregnant or not, should be seen in an emergency care facility. Patients should be afforded access to cardiac monitoring, a source of oxygen, and an intravenous line. Laboratory tests should include serum electrolytes, blood urea nitrogen, creatinine, glucose, and creatine kinase. Arterial blood gases should be drawn and followed if there is evidence of acidosis or hypoxia. Blood levels of misoprostol acid are not useful, not easy to obtain, and not predictive of the clinical course. A gynecologic examination should be performed. The rapid absorption of misoprostol and the rapid peak plasma concentrations (<30 minutes) lessen the usefulness of gastric emptying procedures. If the patient presents closer to the time of ingestion or if the history is in doubt, gastric emptying with tracheal protection may be useful. Activated charcoal may be administered but there are no data to support its effectiveness. There is no antidote. It is unlikely that dialysis procedures or hemoperfusion would be useful (high volume of distribution). Diarrhea may be ameliorated with psyllium hydrophilic colloid.[29]

REFERENCES—MISOPROSTOL

1. Graham DY. Prevention of gastrointestinal injury induced by chronic nonsteroidal antiinflammatory drug therapy. Gastroenterology 1989;96:675–681.

2. Arns PA. Misoprostol. Am J Med Sci 1991;301:133–137.
3. Stern WR. Summary of the 33rd meeting of the Food and Drug Administration's Gastrointestinal Drugs Advisory Committee, September 15–16, 1988. Am J Gastroenterol 1989; 84:951–954.
4. Feldman M. Southwestern Internal Medicine Conference: Prostaglandins and gastric ulcers: From seminal vesicle to misoprostol (Cytotec^R). Am J Med Sci 1990;300:116–132.
5. Garris RE, Kirkwood CF. Misoprostol: A prostaglandin E_1 analogue. Clin Pharm 1989;8:627–644.
6. Edelson JT, Tosteson ANA, Sax P. Cost-effectiveness of misoprostol for prophylaxis against nonsteroidal antiinflammatory drug-induced gastrointestinal tract bleeding. JAMA 1990;264:41–47.
7. Barnworth B, Schaeverbeke T, Dehais J, Doumayrou F. NSAIDs, misoprostol and gastrointestinal bleeding. Lancet 1991;337:973–974.
8. Cytotec^R (misoprostol): Product Literature. Skokie, IL: GD Searle, 1991.
9. Bond GR, Van Zee A. Intentional misoprostol (Cytotek^R) overdosage in pregnancy. Vet Hum Toxicol 1990;32:352.
10. Grober DJ, Meier KH. Acute misoprostol toxicity. Ann Emerg Med 1991;20:549–551.
11. Moran M, Mozes MF, Maddux MS, et al. Prevention of acute graft rejection by the prostaglandin E analogue misoprostol in renal transplant recipients treated with cyclosporine and prednisone. N Engl J Med 1990; 322:1183–1188.
12. Karim A. Antiulcer prostaglandin misoprostol: Single and multiple dose pharmacokinetic profile. Prostaglandins 1987; 33(suppl):40–50.
13. Karim A, Burns TS, Miller SR. Pharmacokinetics and safety of the anti-ulcer prostaglandin misoprostol in elderly male subjects. Clin Pharmacol Ther 1987;41:205.
14. Halstenson CE, Lee DR, Karim A. Misoprostol disposition in patients with various degrees of renal function. J Clin Pharmacol 1990;30:838.
15. Karim A, Rozek LF, Burns TS. Pharmacokinetic profile of antiulcer prostaglandin (misoprostol) in humans. Postgrad Med J 1988;64(suppl. 1):80. Abstract.
16. Misoprostol. In: Dollery CT, ed. *Therapeutic Drugs.* Vol 2. Edinburgh: Churchill Livingstone, 1991:M210–M214.
17. Karim A, Nicholson P. Misoprostol in elderly patients on NSAIDs: Pharmacokinetics and drug interactions: Protection from NSAID beyond stomach and duodenum. In: Cheli R, ed. *Treatments and Prevention of NSAID-Induced Gastropathy.* New York: Royal Society of Medicine Series, 1989:43–45.
18. Small RE, Wilmont-Pater MG, Mcgee BA, Willis HE. Effects of misoprostol on ranitidine or ibuprofen pharmacokinetics. Clin Pharm 1991;10:870–872.
19. Bennett PN, Fenn GC, Notarianni LJ. Potential drug interactions with misoprostol: Effects on the pharmacokinetics of antipyrine and propranolol. Postgrad Med J 1988;64(suppl. 1):21–24.
20. Bennett PN, Fenn GC, Notarianni LJ, Lee CE. Misoprostol does not alter the pharmacokinetics of propranolol. Postgrad Med J 1991; 67:455–457.
21. Schonhofer PS. Brazil: Misuse of misoprostol as an abortifacient may induce malformations. Lancet 1991;337:1534–1535.
22. Fonseca W, Alencai AJC, Mota FSB, Coelho HLL. Misoprostol and congenital malformations. Lancet 1991;338:1241–1242.
23. Schuler L, Ashton PW, Sanseverino MT. Teratogenicity of misoprostol. Lancet 1992;339:437.
24. Aubery E, Baulieu E-E. Activite contragestive de l"association au RU486 di'une prostaglandin active par voie orale. CR Acad Sci III 1991;312:539–545.
25. Norman JE, Thong KJ, Baird DT. Urine contractility and induction of abortion in early pregnancy by misoprostol and mifepristone. Lancet 1991;338:1233–1236.
26. Misoprostol and legal medical abortion. Lancet 1991;338: 1241–1242. Editorial.
27. Morton MR, Robbins ME. Delirium in an elderly woman possibly associated with administration of misoprostol. DICP Ann Pharmacother 1991;25:133–134.
28. Fossaluzza V, di Benedetto P, Zampa A, De Vita S. Misoprostol induced urinary incontinence. J Intern Med 1991;230: 463–464.
29. Bobrove AM. Misoprostol, diarrhea and psyllium mucilloid. Ann Intern Med 1990;112:386.

PROTON PUMP INHIBITORS

OMEPRAZOLE

Omeprazole (Prilosec), a synthetic substituted benzimidazole (Fig. 43–2), is a specific inhibitor of the enzyme H^+/K^+-ATPase found on the secretory surface of the parietal cell (Fig. 43–3). It is available in the United States and elsewhere. There are suggestions of possible carcinogenicity with prolonged use.

Use

Omeprazole has been approved by the Food and Drug Administration (FDA) for the treatment of gastrointestinal reflux disease (GERD), including severe erosive esophagitis and poorly responsive symptomatic GERD. It may also be useful in some pathologic hypersecretory conditions such as Zollinger–Ellison syndrome,[1] multiple endocrine adenomas, and systemic mastocytosis.[2] Omeprazole has also been used for stress-induced gastric mucosal hemorrhage.[3] It has been recommended by the FDA Advisory Committee for approval as first-line therapy in duodenal ulcer disease.[4]

Product Formulation

Omeprazole is available as 20-mg delayed-release capsules.

Therapeutic Dose

The usual therapeutic adult dose for GERD is 20 mg daily for 4 to 8 weeks; in pathologic hypersecretory conditions, up to 120 mg three times daily has been used. Doses of up to 400 mg/d have been well tolerated with no serious adverse effects.[5,6] A dose of 0.5 mg/kg/d (20 mg/d per 1.73 m^2 body surface area) has been suggested for the treatment of refractory gastroesophageal reflux in children.[7]

Toxic Dose

A pregnant woman who ingested 320 mg of enteric-coated capsules and an adult man who ingested 400 mg both survived.[6]

Fatal Dose

There have been no reports of a fatal dose.

Figure 43-2 Structure of omeprazole. (From Lauritsen K, Laursen LS, Rask-Madsen J. Clinical pharmacokinetics of drugs used in the treatment of gastrointestinal diseases (Part I). Clin Pharmacokinet 1990;19:11–31.)

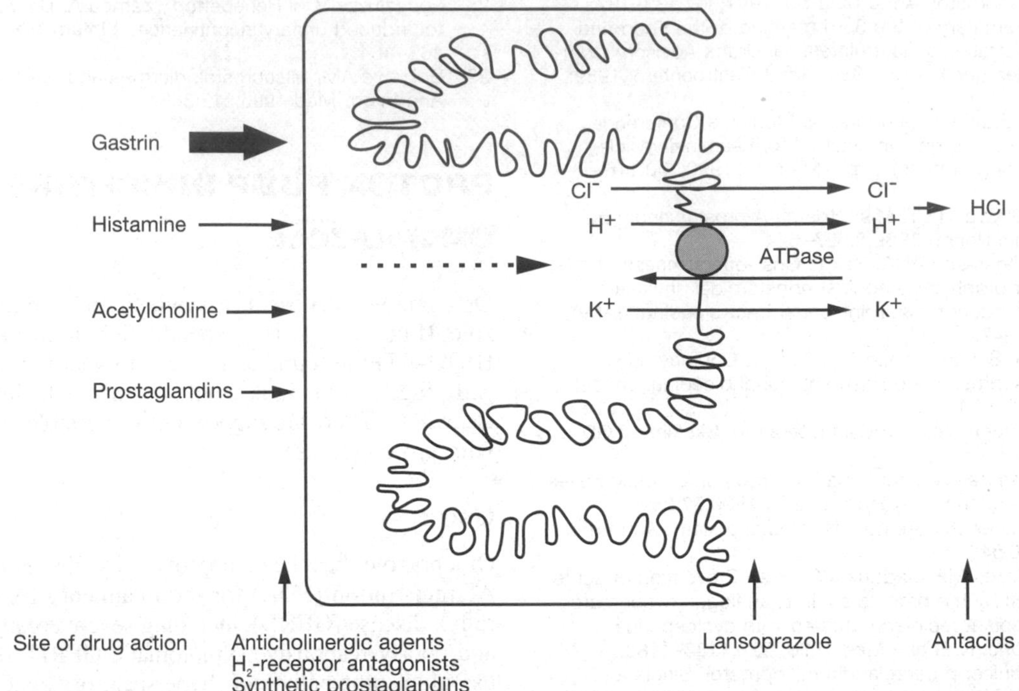

Figure 43-3 Simplified diagram of the gastric parietal cell showing the secretion of acid and the site of action of various antisecretion agents. Acid pump inhibitors block the final common pathway of acid secretion on the apical region of the parietal cell, whereas histamine H_2-receptor antagonists and anticholinergic agents block receptors on the basolateral surface of the parietal cell. (From Spencer CM, Faulds D. Lansoprazole: A reappraisal of its pharmacodynamic and pharmacokinetic properties, and its therapeutic efficacy in acid-related disorders. Drugs 1994;48:404–430.)

Toxicokinetics[8–12]

Bioavailability	30–60%
Peak plasma level	50–4,000 µg/L (after 10–60 mg orally)[13,14]
Time to peak plasma level	1.5 hours
Volume of distribution	0.3 L/kg
Plasma protein binding	95%[15]
Elimination half-life	1 hour

Drug Interactions

Omeprazole can bind to hepatic cytochrome P450 and inhibit the oxidative metabolism of a number of drugs (Table 43–2)[16] (eg, diazepam, aminophenazine [aminopyrine], and phenazone [antipyrine]), the less pharmacologically active *R* enantiomer of warfarin, and nifedipine.[17] Catatonia has been reported with concomitant disulfiram.[18] An ataxia has been described when omeprazole is used with benzodiazepines.[19]

Mechanism of Action

Omeprazole is selectively concentrated in the parietal cells, where it acts as a noncompetitive inhibitor of H^+, K^+-ATPase. Suppression of acid secretion is not correlated with plasma omeprazole concentration.[20]

Clinical Presentation

Overdose

Acute overdoses may be followed by drowsiness, sweating, headache, blurred vision, and a dry mouth. Symptoms recede within 3 hours.[6]

Chronic Use

Subacute myopathy,[21] hemolytic anemia,[22] gynecomastia,[23] headache,[24] diarrhea, abdominal pain, nausea, painful erections, headache,[25] fulminant hepatic failure,[26] gastric polyposis (after long-term therapy),[27] peripheral neuropathy,[28] and gastric carcinoid tumors in patients with Zollinger–Ellison syndrome have been reported.[29]

Carcinogenic Potential

Suppression of acid secretion may predispose to enteric infection and may increase the endogenous[30] generation of potential carcinogens such as *N*-nitroso compounds.[31–33] One study has demonstrated enterochromaffin-like cell proliferation in patients treated with omeprazole for more than 4 years.[33–35]

Treatment

Stabilization

In the event of an overdose, treatment should be largely symptomatic and supportive.[5] The stomach should be emptied if the patient is seen within 4 hours of ingestion.[36–39]

Elimination Enhancement

Omeprazole is extensively protein bound and is, therefore, not readily dialyzable.[5] When hemodialysis was used in anemic patients, however, it became apparent that omeprazole is dialyzable.[40]

Table 43–2
Omeprazole and Cytochrome P450: Implications for Drug–Drug Interactions

	Cytochrome P450				
	I	II			III
	IA IA2	IIC IIC8–10	IID IID6	IIE IIE1	IIIA IIIA3–5
Inhibitor	Cimetidine +	Cimetidine + Omeprazole ±	Cimetidine + Ranitidine ±		Cimetidine + Ranitidine ±
Main inducer	Polycyclic hydrocarbons	Phenobarbital Rifampicin		Alcohol	Glucocorticoids Rifampicin
Substrate	Theophylline (–) Caffeine (–) Phenacetin Paracetamol (acetaminophen)	Diazepam (+) Omeprazole Mephobarbital Hexobarbital Phenytoin (±) Tolbutamide	Metoprolol (–) Propranolol (–) Timolol Bufarlol Propafenone Flecainide Encainide Nortriptyline Desipramine Clomipramine Imipramine Perphenazine Dextromethorphan Codeine *N*-Propylamaline etc	Alcohol (–) Acetone Halothane *N*-Nitroso-DNA	Lidocaine (–) [lignocaine (–)] Quinidine (–) Cyclosporine (–) Nifedipine* Diltiazem Erythromycin Midazolam Triazolam Hydrocortisone Progesterone Testosterone Androstenedione Oral contraceptive pills etc

*Increased absorption with omeprazole.
+, interaction; (+), interaction with omeprazole; –, no interaction; (–), no interaction with omeprazole.
From Andersson T. Omeprazole drug interaction studies. Clin Pharmacokinet 1991;21:195–212.

Antidote

There is no antidote.

REFERENCES—OMEPRAZOLE

1. Vezzadini P, Tomassetti P, Marrano D, Labo G. Life-threatening gastrointestinal hemorrhage with omeprazole. Dig Dis Sci 1988;33:766–768.
2. Product Literature: Omeprazole (Prilosec[R]). Merck, 1990.
3. Barie PS, Harivi RJ. Therapeutic use of omeprazole for refractory stress-induced gastric mucosal hemorrhage. Crit Care Med 1992;20:899–901.
4. Holt S, Howden CW. Omeprazole: Overview and opinion. Dig Dis Sci 1991;31:385–393.
5. Shackleford RW. Personal communication. Merck Sharp and Dohme, April 1, 1991.
6. Ferner RE, Allison TR. Omeprazole overdose. Hum Exp Toxicol 1993;12:541–542.
7. Alliet P, Raes M, Gillis P, Zimmerman A. Optional dose of omeprazole in infants and children. J Pediatr 1994;125:332–333.
8. Andersson T, Cederberg C, Regardh CG, Skanberg I. Pharmacokinetics of various single intravenous and oral doses of omeprazole. Eur J Clin Pharmacol 1990;39:1971.
9. Andersson T, Andren K, Cederberg C, et al. Pharmacokinetics and bioavailability of omeprazole after single and repeated oral administration in healthy subjects. Br J Clin Pharmacol 1990;29:557–563.
10. Scott G. Omeprazole. Hosp Phys 1990;26(2):48–51.
11. Weintraub M, Evans P. Omeprazole: A long acting acid secretion inhibitor. Hosp Formul 1988;23:875–882.
12. Lampkin TA, Ouellet D, Hak LJ, Dukes GE. Omeprazole: A novel antisecretory agent for the treatment of acid peptic disorders. DICP Ann Pharmacother 1990;24:393–402.
13. Howden CW. Clinical pharmacology of omeprazole. Clin Pharmacokinet 1991;20:38–49.
14. Lauritsen K, Lauritsen LS, Rask-Madsen J. Clinical pharmacokinetics of drugs used in the treatment of gastrointestinal diseases (Part I). Clin Pharmacokinet 1990;19:11–31.
15. Regardh CG, Andersson T, Lagerstrom PA, et al. The pharmacokinetics of omeprazole in humans: A study of single intravenous and oral doses. Ther Drug Monit 1990;12:163–172.
16. Andersson T. Omeprazole drug interaction studies. Clin Pharmacokinetics 1991;21:195–212.
17. Humphries TJ. Clinical implications of drug interactions with the cytochrome P-450 enzyme system associated with omeprazole. Dig Dis Sci 1991;36:1665–1669.
18. Hajela R, Cunningham GM, Kapur BM, et al. Catatonic reaction to omeprazole and disulfiram in a patient with alcohol dependence. Can Med Assoc J 1990;145:1207–1208.
19. Marti-Masso JF, de Munain AL, Dicastillo GL. Ataxia following gastric bleeding due to omeprazole–benzodiazepine interaction. Ann Pharmacother 1992;26:429–430.
20. Ekman L, Hansson E, Haru N, et al. Toxicological studies on omeprazole. Scand J Gastroenterol 1985;20(suppl. 108):53–69.
21. Garrotte FJ, La Cambra C, de Ser T, et al. Subacute myopathy during omeprazole therapy. Lancet 1992;340:672.
22. Marks DR, Joy JV, Bonheur NA. Hemolytic anemia associated with the use of omeprazole. Am J Gastroenterol 1991;86:217–218.
23. Santucci L, Farroni F, Fiorucci S, Morelli A. Gynecomastia during omeprazole therapy. N Engl J Med 1991;324:635.
24. Convens C, Verhelst J, Mahler C. Painful gynaecomastia during omeprazole therapy. Lancet 1991;338:1153.
25. Dutertre JP, Soutif D, Jonville AP, et al. Sexual disturbances during omeprazole therapy. Lancet 1991;338:1022.
26. Jochem V, Kirkpatrick R, Greenson J, et al. Fulminant hepatic failure related to omeprazole. Am J Gastroenterol 1992;87:523–525.
27. Graham JR. Gastric polyposis: Onset during long-term therapy with omeprazole. Med J Aust 1992;157:287–288.

28. Sellapah S. An unusual side effect of omeprazole: Case report. Br J Gen Pract 1990;40:389.
29. Goldfain D, Le Bodic MF, Lavergne A, et al. Gastric carcinoid tumors in patients with Zollinger–Ellison syndrome on long-term omeprazole. Lancet 1989;1:776–777.
30. Selway SAM. Potential hazards of long-term acid suppression. Scand J Gastroenterol 1990;25(suppl. 178):85–92.
31. Omeprazole and genotoxicity. Lancet 1990;1:386–387. Editorial.
32. Burlinson B, Morriss SH, Gatehouse DG, Tweats DJ. Genotoxicity studies of gastric acid inhibiting drugs. Lancet 1990;335:419.
33. Wormsley KG. Omeprazole. Aliment Pharmacol Ther 1991;5: 670–673.
34. Jackson MP, Wood JP. Omeprazole. Br Med J 1991;303: 1200–1201.
35. Ekman L, Bolosfoldi G, Macdonald J, Nicols W. Genotoxic studies of gastric acid inhibiting drugs. Lancet 1990;335: 419–420.
36. Omeprazole. USDI Update 1990;1(4):172–174.
37. Omeprazole. Med Lett Drugs Ther 1990;32(813):19–21.
38. Adams MH, Ostrosky JD, Kirkwood CF. Therapeutic evaluation of omeprazole. Clin Pharm 1988;7:725–745.
39. First in new class of GI drugs approved. FDA Consumer 1990(March):3.
40. Roggo A, Filippini L, Colombi A. The effect of hemodialysis on omeprazole plasma concentrations in the anuric patient: A case report. Int J Clin Pharmacol Ther Toxicol 1990;28:115–117.

LANSOPRAZOLE

Lansoprazole (Prevacid-TAP), a proton pump inhibitor similar to omeprazole, has been approved by the Food and Drug Administration for short-term treatment of active duodenal ulcer and erosive reflux esophagitis and for long-term treatment of chronic hypersecretory conditions, including Zollinger–Ellison syndrome. There have been no reports of overdose.[1]

Structure and Classification

Lansoprazole is a benzimidazole derivative with a novel trifluoroethoxy group (Fig. 43–4).[2]

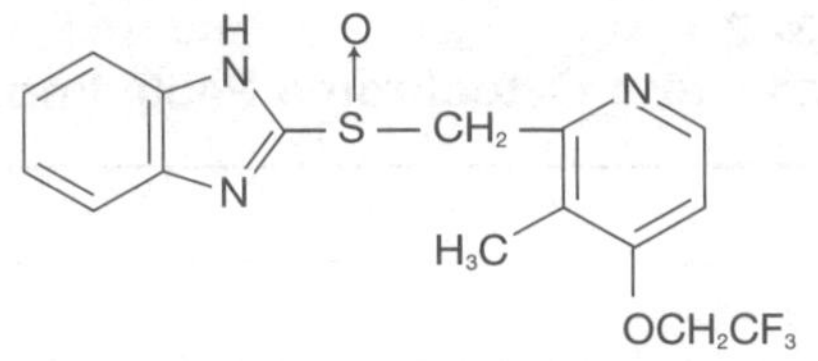

H N O S CH₂ N N H₃C OCH₂CF₃

Figure 43-4 Structure of lansoprazole. (From Spencer CM, Faulds D. Lansoprazole: A reappraisal of its pharmacodynamic and pharmacokinetic properties, and its therapeutic efficacy in acid-related disorders. Drugs 1994;48:404–430.)

Mechanism of Action

Lansoprazole, like omeprazole, is a benzimidazole derivative that binds to H^+,K^+ -ATPase at the surface of the gastric parietal cell, inhibiting the final step in secretion of hydrogen ions into the gastric lumen.[1]

Therapeutic Dose

A single dose of lansoprazole inhibits 80 to 97% of acid secretion in healthy volunteers.[2] Usual doses range from 15 to 30 mg/d.[1,2] In one reported case of overdose, the patient consumed 600 mg of lansoprazole with no adverse reactions.[3]

Abdominal pain, nausea, and diarrhea have been reported. Lansoprazole is metabolized by the CYP3A and CYP2C19 isozymes of the cytochrome P450 system.[4] Benzimidazole compounds, such as lansoprazole and omeprazole, partially inhibit the oxidative metabolism of drugs metabolized by the cytochrome P450 enzyme subfamily IIC, such as diazepam and phenytoin.[2]

There have been no reports of clinically relevant interactions between lansoprazole and diazepam, propranolol, warfarin, prednisone (or prednisolone), phenytoin, or theophylline.[2]

Headache, dizziness, skin rashes, and respiratory tract symptoms have been observed.[2]

Theophylline, which is also metabolized partly by the CYP3A isozyme, may be cleared more rapidly in patients taking lansoprazole. Sucralfate (Carafte) taken concurrently delays absorption of lansoprazole.[1]

Toxicokinetics

In the fasting state, about 80% of the dose, compared with 50% of omeprazole, reaches the systemic circulation, where it is 97% bound to plasma proteins. Plasma concentrations peak in 1 to 2 hours. The drug is metabolized in the liver to two main metabolites, lansoprazole sulfone and hydroxylansoprazole. Lansoprazole has not been recovered from the urine in an unchanged form. About 20% of a dose is excreted as conjugated and unconjugated metabolites and excreted in bile and urine, with a plasma half-life of about 1.5 hours.[1] Maximum serious lansoprazole concentrations of 0.75 to 1.15 mg/L are reached within 1.5 to 2 hours of oral administration.[2,5]

There have been few reports of lansprazole overdose.

Laboratory

Increases have been observed in serum gastrin levels, liver enzymes, hematocrit, hemoglobin, urinary protein excretion, and uric acid levels.[2]

Treatment

Treatment is similar to that for omeprazole.

REFERENCES—LANSOPRAZOLE

1. Lansoprazole. Med Lett Drugs Ther 1995;37(953): 63–64.
2. Spencer CM, Faulds D. Lansoprazole: A reappraisal of its pharmacodynamic and pharmacokinetic properties and its therapeutic efficacy in acid-related disorders. Drugs 1994; 48:404–430.
3. Clarke CB (Katia). Personal communication. Medical services, TAP Pharmaceuticals, September 14, 1995.
4. Tucker GI. The interaction of proton pump inhibitors with cytochrome PL-450. Pharmacol Ther 1994;8(suppl. 1):13–38.
5. Gladziwa V, Klotz V. Pharmacokinetic optimisation of the treatment of peptic ulcer in patients with renal failure. Clin Pharmacokinet 1994;27:29–48.

ANTACIDS

INFANTS

Use

Antacid therapy is widely used prophylactically in pediatric intensive care units to prevent stress ulcers. It has also been used in the medical management of gastric bleeding in newborn infants.[1]

Clinical Presentation

Complications of antacid therapy in the newborn infant include hypotonia, difficulty in arousing, asymptomatic hypermagnesemia without hypercalcemia, and aluminum hydroxide bezoar formation.[1] The serum magnesium level may be elevated[2] and may be accompanied by an elevated serum calcium level.[1]

Treatment

Intravenous calcium gluconate and potassium and glucose infusion may lead to a fall in magnesium concentration and stabilization within 24 hours.[2]

ADULTS

Calcium Carbonate

A 40-year-old woman with surgical hyperparathyroidism ingested up to 15 g of calcium daily (calcium carbonate). Her serum calcium level was 5.35 mmol/L (normal, 2.20–2.60 mmol/L). She experienced fatigue, anorexia, nausea and vomiting, an elevated blood pressure, hemoconcentration, leukocytosis, metabolic alkalosis, elevated body weight, and hypokalemia.

Diuresis was induced with normal saline and furosemide and also with calcitonin and hydrocortisone. The serum calcium fell to 259 mmol/L in 24 hours and her symptoms disappeared. She was given potassium chloride.[3]

Magnesium Hydroxide–Aluminum Hydroxide Simethicone (Mylanta II)

A 28-year-old ingested this preparation (1500 – 2000 mL and up to 15 tablets of the same preparation per week, giving an average daily consumption of 21 g each of magnesium hydroxide and aluminum hydroxide) and developed phosphate depletion, nephrolithiasis, and bilateral ureteric obstruction. Myalgia, weakness, and bone pain were absent. Biochemical features included hypophosphatemia, hypercalcemia, hypophosphatasia, elevated plasma 1,2-dihydroxyvitamin D level, and low plasma intact parathyroid hormone level. These abnormalities were corrected when antacid ingestion was reduced and phosphate intake supplemented.[4]

Osteomalacia and osteitis fibrosa may also follow long-term antacid ingestion. Oral inorganic phosphorus supplementation and withdrawal of antacids may result in prompt clinical and radiographic improvement of the bone disease.[5]

REFERENCES—ANTIULCER AGENTS: ANTACIDS

1. Brand JM, Greer FR. Hypermagnesemia and intestinal perforation following antacid administration in a premature infant. Pediatrics 1990;85:121–124.
2. Mofenson HC, Caraccio TR. Magnesium intoxication in a neonate from oral magnesium hydroxide laxative. J Toxicol Clin Toxicol 1981;29:215–222.
3. McAlister NH, Abrams HB, Schlosser R, Sturtridge W. Unintentional self-intoxication with inorganic calcium. J Intern Med 1990;228:193–195.
4. Harmeln DL, Martin FIR, Wark JD. Antacid induced phosphate depletion syndrome presenting as nephrolithiasis. Aust NZ J Med 1990;20:803–805.
5. Carmichael KA, Fallon MD, Dalinka M, et al. Osteomalacia and osteitis fibrosa in a man ingesting aluminum hydroxide antacid. Am J Med 1984;76:1137–1140.

H_2 RECEPTOR ANTAGONISTS

The concept of a histamine (H_2) receptor antagonist was initiated with the discovery of the H_2 receptors in 1972.[1] Since then, a plethora of articles on histamine pharmacology and peptic ulcer therapy have appeared (4500 in the first decade).[2] The Food and Drug Administration approved the use of cimetidine in 1977 for the treatment of patients with duodenal ulcer disease, Zollinger–Ellison syndrome, and other hypersecretory states. Since that time, they have become the largest selling drugs in the world; approximately 20 million people have been treated with these agents.

Conventional antihistamines antagonize certain histamine-induced responses. The receptors mediating the antihistamine action are known as H_1. Other histamine-induced responses (eg, gastric acid secretion) are blocked by other compounds, known as H_2 antagonists. Cimetidine and ranitidine are examples of the H_2 antagonist group. Overdoses with cimetidine are not common but can be serious; in one report the outcome was fatal after unknown amounts of cimetidine, diazepam, and digoxin were ingested.[3]

CIMETIDINE

Structure

Cimetidine is similar to histamine (Fig. 43–5).[4] It has an imidazole ring, like histamine, but a longer side chain. The

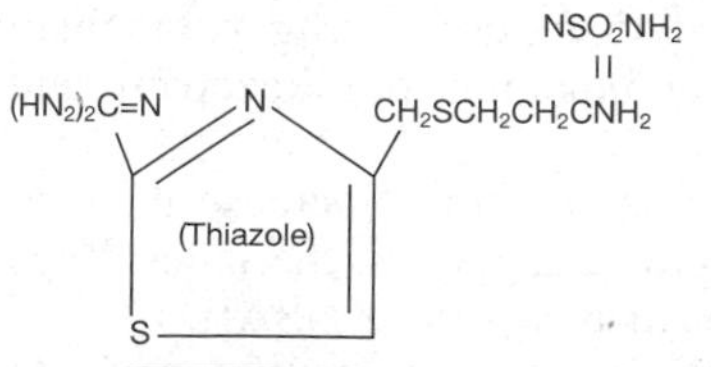

$(HN_2)_2C{=}N$ — (Thiazole) — $CH_2SCH_2CH_2CNH_2$ ($=NSO_2NH_2$), S — Famotidine

$(CH_3)_2NCH_2$ — (Thiazole) — $CH_2SCH_2CH_2NHCNHCH_3$ ($=CHNO_2$), S — Nizatidine

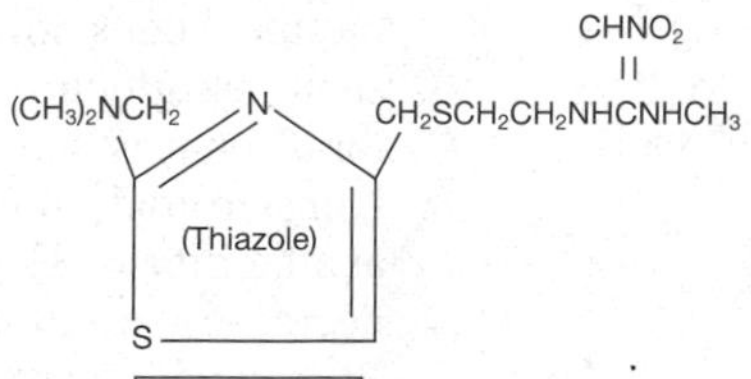

Figure 43-5 Chemical structures of histamine and four H^+-receptor antagonists. Cimetidine, like histamine, contains an imidazole ring. Ranitidine has a furan ring, whereas famotidine and nizatidine contain thiazole rings. Ranitidine and nizatidine have identical side chains. (From Feldman M. Pros and cons of over-the-counter availability of histamine 2-receptor antagonists. Arch Intern Med 1993;153:2415–2424.)

H_1 antagonists have neither an imidazole ring (as histamine and cimetidine do) nor a furan ring (as ranitidine does).

Source

Cimetidine is a synthetic chemical, marketed as Tagamet by SmithKline Beecham Laboratories, Philadelphia.

Use

Cimetidine has been approved by the Food and Drug Administration for short-term treatment of active duodenal ulcer, prophylactic use to prevent duodenal ulcer recurrences in patients likely to need surgical treatment, short-term treatment of active benign gastric ulcer (up to 8 weeks), and treatment of pathologic hypersecretory conditions (ie, Zollinger–Ellison syndrome, systemic mastocytosis, multiple endocrine adenomas).[5]

Product Formulation

Cimetidine is available as tablets—200, 300, and 400 mg; a liquid—300 mg/5 mL; and an injection—300 mg/2 mL vials (single dose) and 8-mL multiple-dose vials. The recommended oral dose is 300 mg four times each day, or 800 to 1200 mg/d.

Toxic Dose

An oral dose of 300 mg raises basal gastric pH to at least 5.0 for more than 2 hours in most patients. More than 90% inhibition of acid secretion occurs for 4 hours after administration. Serious drug reactions are relatively uncommon. Normal persons have ingested massive amounts of cimetidine and had no neurologic symptoms.[6] Three adults in a recent survey[7] remained symptom-free after ingestion of 20 g of cimetidine. In one case, the blood level was 45.8 μg/mL 3 hours after the overdose. Therapeutic blood cimetidine concentrations associated with a 50% reduction of stimulated acid secretion range from 0.25 to 1.00 μg/mL.[3,8] A 39-year-old woman ingested 24 g of cimetidine and died.[9]

Toxicokinetics

Absorption

Cimetidine can be given orally, intravenously, and intramuscularly. It is completely absorbed after oral administration. After a 300-mg dose with a meal blood levels peak in 45 to 90 minutes and remain above 0.5 μg/mL for at least 4 hours. Two peaks have been reported, the first during the first 2 hours and the second in 3 to 5 hours.[10]

Distribution

Cimetidine is widely distributed. Approximately 13 to 25% is plasma protein bound.[10] The apparent volume of distribution is 1.4 to 4.3 L/kg (mean, 2.1 L/kg).[10]

Elimination

About 15% of cimetidine is metabolized in the liver. Seventy percent is excreted unchanged in the urine, with fecal losses accounting for approximately 10%.[11] The elimination half-life in humans is 1.9 to 2.2 hours.[10,12,13]

Drug Interactions

Cimetidine, like other substituted imidazole compounds, binds strongly to and inhibits the cytochrome P450 mixed-function oxidase involved in hepatic metabolism of certain drugs.[14,15] It also reduces hepatic blood flow and may impede elimination of drugs such as propranolol that are metabolized in the liver.[16] It does not induce any significant alteration in renal blood flow or glomerular filtration rate.[14]

Cimetidine affects the hepatic oxidative metabolism of many drugs, but does not usually affect the conjugation reaction. It does not appear to affect the glucuronide conjugation of drugs such as oxazepam, phenprocoumon, and morphine. The propensity of cimetidine to inhibit hepatic drug metabolism is probably related to the imidazole ring in its structure, similar to other drugs with an imidazole structure that are known to be inhibitors of drug metabolism (ketoconazole, miconazole, itraconazole, metronidazole, omeprazole).[17]

Important interactions involving cimetidine include the following:

1. Plasma ethanol concentration increases compared with a placebo.[18]
2. High-potency antacids inhibit the absorption of cimetidine when the two are taken together, but not when taken apart.[19]
3. There is a potentially lethal interaction with morphine.[20] Morphine is highly extracted by the liver and is dependent on liver blood flow for metabolism. Cimetidine reduction of hepatic blood flow could increase potentially lethal central nervous system effects of morphine.[15]
4. Theophylline accumulated to potentially toxic serum levels in an asthmatic patient given cimetidine[21] and in cigarette smokers and nonsmokers.[22]
5. Phenytoin clearance was decreased when cimetidine was added to the regimen in normal subjects.[23]
6. Serum lidocaine levels rose[24] and the steady volume of distribution and clearance fell when cimetidine was administered simultaneously.[24,25] Increased symptoms of lidocaine toxicity may be experienced when the two are administered simultaneously.
7. Cimetidine may also prolong the effects of anticoagulants,[26] benzodiazepines,[27] many beta blockers, digoxin, procainamide, verapamil,[28] caffeine, carbamazepine, salicylates, metronidazole, quinidine, morphine, and theophylline[20,29–34] and is associated with changes in the hepatic oxidative metabolism of many of these drugs. Such interactions (eg, with benzodiazepines) may have minimal clinical importance.[27] Cimetidine does not inhibit nonoxidative drug metabolism such as glucuronide conjugation of oxazepam and lorazepam in humans.
8. Nonsteroidal antiinflammatory drugs increase the bioavailability of H_2-receptor antagonists; the latter drugs decrease the volume of distribution of NSAIDs.[35]
9. Probenecid decreases the renal clearance of cimetidine by decreasing both the filtration clearance and the net secretory clearance.[36]

Pregnancy/Lactation

Cimetidine crosses the placental barrier and is secreted in human milk. No overdose studies in pregnancy have been reported.[10] Initial unconfirmed data on the use of H_2-receptor antagonists (cimetidine and ranitidine) suggest that these compounds may not be a teratogenic risk in humans.[37]

Clinical Presentation

Side Effects

Central Nervous System. Cimetidine penetrates the blood–brain barrier and has been associated with somnolence, confusion, restlessness, lethargy, agitation, visual hallucinations, seizures, and slurred speech. Such symptoms are more frequent in the elderly and very young, those who receive high doses, and those with renal or liver disease or both. Yet, very high plasma cimetidine concentrations after overdose in otherwise normal patients have not been associated with central nervous system toxicity.[6]

Cimetidine may cause extrapyramidal problems such as parkinsonism, facial twitching, dyskinesia, chorea, and acute dystonia.[38,39] Sensory and motor peripheral neuropathies have been reported.[40,41]

Blood. Granulocytopenia (white blood cell count, ≤2000/μL) or a neutrophil count of 1000/μL or less has occasionally been observed, but has been complicated by the presence of serious underlying disease or use of other drugs.[2] One case of fatal aplastic anemia, possibly an idiosyncratic reaction, was reported after therapeutic doses.[42] Thrombocytopenia has rarely been observed.

Renal System. Transient rises in serum creatinine have been observed after therapeutic doses.[43] An acute interstitial nephritis has followed cimetidine use but may be a hypersensitivity reaction.[44] No reports are available on effects after overdose.

Endocrine System. Gynecomastia, antiandrogen effects, a decrease in plasma testosterone, and a rise in serum prolactin have been inconsistently observed.[45,46] A decrease in circulating immunoreactive parathyroid hormone has not been associated with decreases in total serum calcium levels in patients with primary hyperparathyroidism.[47] No reports are available on effects after overdose.

Cardiovascular System. The myocardium and peripheral blood vessels possess H_2 receptors. Stimulation of such receptors results in positive inotropic and chronotropic responses. Cimetidine use has been associated with bradycardia, hypotension, sinus arrest, and cardiac arrest in a few cases[2] after rapid intravenous infusion, especially when more than 200 mg was administered in less than 4 to 5 minutes to seriously ill patients. Five patients had cardiac arrests after intravenous cimetidine.[48,49] One recovered with residual cerebral dysfunction, one died after 7 days from respiratory failure (diazepam was also given to this patient), two died immediately, and one died after 14 days from renal failure. No blood levels were reported. Cardiovascular toxicity is rare.

Liver. Reactions reported in the liver reflect hypersensitivity.

Gastric Carcinoma. Cimetidine can cause partial or complete healing of a malignant gastric ulcer.[50] There is no convincing evidence to support the position that cimetidine is carcinogenic.

Salmonella Infection. Neal and colleagues suggested in an initial case–control study that current users of H_2 antagonists appear to be predisposed to *Salmonella* infections.[51]

Overdose

Overdoses may be associated with dizziness, slurred speech, confusion, dilated pupils, disorientation, and drowsiness, with or without sweating and flushing. Cardiovascular findings are described above.

A review of 881 cases of overdose with up to 15 g of cimetidine revealed an absence of symptoms in 79%. There were no major medical complications and no fatalities in both children and adults. A few patients exhibited vomiting, bradycardia, and drowsiness, all of which were minor and without sequelae.[52]

Laboratory

Plasma cimetidine values do not appear to correlate well with symptoms and are difficult to obtain from the average clinical laboratory. In eight cases of cimetidine overdose, blood concentrations ranged from 18.7 to 57 μg/mL.[11] All recovered.

A high-performance liquid chromatography method is available.[3] Clinical symptoms dictate use of liver function tests, renal function tests, electrocardiographic monitoring, electroencephalographic studies, and/or bone marrow or endocrine assays.

Treatment

In view of the occasional report of cardiac problems despite the apparent lack of toxicity of cimetidine, it would be prudent to ascertain the airway, breathing, and circulatory status of the patient on admission and observe for seizures and dysrhythmia. If not more than 4 hours have elapsed since ingestion of the drug, gastric emptying should be administered provided the patient is not experiencing seizures or in coma and has not lost the gag reflex; if the gag reflex is absent, gastric lavage, after endotracheal intubation or with continuous suction, would be preferred.[7]

There is no evidence that forced diuresis enhances excretion of cimetidine.[7] No studies support the effectiveness of hemoperfusion or hemodialysis. There is no known antidote. Seizures should be treated with intravenous diazepam. Arrhythmias may be treated with the usual antiarrhythmic medications (eg, atropine for bradycardias, lidocaine for ventricular arrhythmias). Supportive and symptomatic measures form the mainstay of treatment. Limited experience with overdose treatment precludes recommendation for use of specific agents. Hemodialysis may be useful, but experience is limited.[7,53] Peritoneal dialysis may remove a maximum of 20 to 30 mg per day.[7]

Laboratory monitoring includes the following: complete blood count including platelets, liver and kidney function tests, sperm counts, and prothrombin times (if an oral anticoagulant is also taken). Significant laboratory abnormalities after overdose with cimetidine have not been reported.

REFERENCES—CIMETIDINE

1. Black JW, Duncan WAM, Durant CJ, et al. Definition and antagonism of histamine H-2 receptors. Nature 1972;236: 385–390.
2. Freston JW. Cimetidine: I. Developments, pharmacology and efficacy. Ann Intern Med 1982;97:573–580.
3. Hiss J, Hepler BR, Falkowski AJ, et al. Fatal bradycardia after intentional overdose of cimetidine and diazepam. Lancet 1982;2:982.
4. Feldman M. Pros and cons of over-the counter availability of histamine$_2$-receptor antagonists. Arch Intern Med 1993; 153:2415–2425.
5. *Physicians' Desk Reference.* 49th ed. Oradell, NJ: Medical Economics, 1995:2401–2404.
6. Illingworth RN, Jarvie DR. Absence of toxicity in cimetidine overdosage. Br Med J 1979;1:453–454.
7. Meredith TJ, Volans GN. Management of cimetidine overdose. Lancet 1979;2:1367.
8. Gugler R, Fucho G, Dieckmann M, et al. Cimetidine plasma concentration relationship. Clin Pharmacol Ther 1981;29: 744–748.
9. Case 399. Litovitz TL, Schmitz BF, Bailey KM. 1989 Annual Report of the American Association of Poison Control Centers National Data Collection System. Am J Emerg Med 1990;8:439.
10. Abate MA, Hyneck ML, Cohen IA, et al. Cimetidine pharmacokinetics. Clin Pharm 1982;1:225–233.
11. Sawyer D, Conner, CS, Scalby R. Cimetidine: Adverse reactions and acute toxicity. Am J Hosp Pharm 1981;38:188–197.
12. Martyn JAJ, Greenblatt DJ, Abernethy DR. Increased cimetidine clearance in burn patients. JAMA 1985;253:1288–1291.
13. Bauer LA, Wareing-Tran C, Edwards WAD, et al. Cimetidine clearance in the obese. Clin Pharmacol Ther 1985;37: 425–430.
14. Jackson JE, Bentley J, Powell JR, et al. Cimetidine–gentamicin interaction. Clin Res 1986;34:400A.
15. Mangini RJ. Clinically important cimetidine drug interactions. Clin Pharm 1982;1:433–440.
16. Feely J, Wilkinson GR, Wood AJJ. Reduction of liver blood flow and propranolol metabolism by cimetidine. N Engl J Med 1981;304:992–996.
17. Hansten PD. Overview of the safety profile of the H_2 receptor antagonists. DICP Ann Pharmacother 1990;24(suppl.):S38–S41.
18. Feely J, Wood AJ. Effects of cimetidine on the elimination and actions of ethanol. JAMA 1982;247:2819–2821.
19. Steinberg W, Lewis JH, Katz DM. Antacids inhibit absorption of cimetidine. N Engl J Med 1982;307:400–404.
20. Fine A, Churchill DW. Potentially lethal interaction of cimetidine and morphine. Can Med Assoc J 1981;125:1212.
21. Weinberger MM, Smith G, Milavetz G, et al. Decreased theophylline clearance due to cimetidine. N Engl J Med 1981; 304:672.
22. Cusack BJ, Dawson GW, Mercer GD, et al. Cigarette smoking and theophylline metabolism: Effects of cimetidine. Clin Pharmacol Ther 1985;37:330–336.
23. Bartle WR, Walker SE, Shapero T. Dose dependent effects of cimetidine on phenytoin kinetics. Clin Pharmacol Ther 1983;33:649–655.
24. Knapp AB, Maguire W, Keren G, et al. The cimetidine–lidocaine interaction. Ann Intern Med 1983;98:174–177.
25. Jackson JE, Bentley JB, Glass SJ, et al. Effects of histamine-2 receptor blockade on lidocaine kinetics. Clin Pharmacol Ther 1985;37:544–548.
26. Grahnen A, von Bahr C, Lindstrom B, et al. Bioavailability and pharmacokinetics of cimetidine. Eur J Clin Pharmacol 1979;16:335–340.
27. Greenblatt DJ, Abernethy DR, Morse OS, et al. Clinical importance of the interaction of diazepam and cimetidine. N Engl J Med 1984;310:1639–1643.
28. Loi C-M, Rollins DE, Dukes GE, et al. Effect of cimetidine on verapamil disposition. Clin Pharmacol Ther 1985;37:654–657.
29. Lalonde RL, Koob RA, McLean WM, et al. The effects of cimetidine on theophylline pharmacokinetics at steady state. Chest 1983;83:221–224.
30. Serbin JH, Mossman S, Sibeon RG, et al. Cimetidine: Interaction with oral anticoagulants in man. Lancet 1979;2: 317–319.
31. Henry DA, MacDonald IA, Kitchingman G, et al. Cimetidine and ranitidine: Comparison of effect on hepatic drug metabolism. Br Med J 1980;281:775–777.
32. Reimann IW, Klotz D, Frolich JC. Effects of cimetidine and ranitidine on steady state propranolol kinetics and dynamics. Clin Pharmacol Ther 1982;32:749–757.
33. Kelly HW, Powell JR, Donohue JF. Ranitidine at very large doses does not inhibit theophylline elimination. Clin Pharmacol Ther 1986;39:577–581.
34. Powell JR, Donn KH. Histamine H_2-antagonist drug interactions in perspective: Mechanistic concepts and clinical implications. Am J Med 1984;77(suppl. 5B):57–84.
35. Delhotal-Landes B, Flouvat B, Liote F, et al. Pharmacokinetic interactions between NSAIDs (indomethacin or sulindac) and H_2-receptor antagonists (cimetidine or ranitidine) in human volunteers. Clin Pharmacol Ther 1988;44:442–452.
36. Gisclon LG, Boyd RA, Williams RL, Giacomim. The effect of probenicid on the renal elimination of cimetidine. Clin Pharmacol Ther 1989;45:444–452.
37. Koren G, Zemlickis DM. Outcome of pregnancy after first trimester exposure to H_2 receptor antagonists. Am J Perinatol 1991;8:37–38.
38. Lehmann AB. Reversible chorea due to ranitidine and cimetidine. Lancet 1988;2:158.
39. Romisher S, Felter R, Dougherty J. Tagamet^R-induced acute dystonia. Ann Emerg Med 1987;16:1162–1164.
40. Walls TJ, Pearce SJ, Venables GS. Motor neuropathy associated with cimetidine. Br Med J 1980;281:974–975.
41. Vincent D, Penicaud-Vedrine A, Rancurel G, et al. Neuropathie peripherique au cours d'un traitment par la cimetidine. Presse Med 1988;17:589–590.
42. Chang HK, Morrison SL. Bone marrow suppression associated with cimetidine. Ann Intern Med 1979;71:580.
43. Colin-Jones DG, Langman MJS, Lawson DH, et al. Safety of cimetidine. Br Med J 1985;291:1721–1722.
44. Pitone JM, Santoro JJ, Biondi RJ, et al. Cimetidine induced acute interstitial nephritis. Am J Gastroenterol 1982;77: 169–171.
45. Enzmann GD, Leonard JM, Paulsen CA. Effect of cimetidine on reproductive function in men. Clin Res 1981;29:26A. Abstract.
46. Lardinois CK, Mazzaferri EL. Cimetidine blocks testosterone synthesis. Arch Intern Med 1985;145:920–922.
47. Palmer FJ, Sawyers TM, Wierzbinski SJ. Cimetidine and hyperparathyroidism. N Engl J Med 1980;302:692.
48. Shaw RG, Mashford MI, Desmond PV. Cardiac arrest after intravenous injection of cimetidine. Med J Aust 1980;2:629–630.
49. Cohen J, Weetman AP, Dargie HJ, et al. Life-threatening arrhythmias and intravenous cimetidine. Br Med J 1979;2:768.
50. Taylor RH, Lovell D, Menzies-Gow N, et al. Misleading response of malignant gastric ulcers to cimetidine. Lancet 1978;1:686–688.
51. Neal KR, Brij S, Slack RCB, et al. Recent treatment with H_2 antagonists and antibiotics and gastric surgery as risk factors for salmonella infection. Br Med J 1994:308:176.
52. Krenzelok EP, Litovitz T, Lippold KP, McNally CF. Cimetidine toxicity: An assessment of 881 cases. Ann Emerg Med 1987; 16:1217–1221.
53. Cimetidine. In: Long JW, ed. *Clinical Management of Prescription Drugs.* Philadelphia: Harper & Row, 1984:229.

FAMOTIDINE

Famotidine (Fig. 43–5) is an H_2-receptor antagonist that has not been reported in overdoses. Except for a need to observe patients who have overdosed for cardiac, hematologic, central nervous system, and muscle dysfunction, overdose with famotidine is not likely to require strenuous intervention. Symptomatic and supportive therapy will probably be effective in most cases.

Clinical Presentation

Adverse effects following usual therapeutic doses of famotidine include thrombocytopenia,[1,2] drug-induced fever,[3] leukocytoclastic vasculitis,[4] sinus bradycardia and second-degree atrioventricular block,[5] rhabdomyolysis,[6] and mental confusion. The last effect has also been reported with cimetidine and ranitidine.[7] Decreases in stroke volume and cardiac index have been observed following the use of famotidine.[8]

Hyperprolactinemia, which has been observed with cimetidine and ranitidine, has also been observed with famotidine therapy.[9]

Treatment

Treatment of an overdose should be symptomatic and supportive. Unabsorbed material can be removed, if clinically indicated, by gastric lavage if the patient is seen within the first few hours of an oral ingestion. Patients should be monitored for about 24 hours for cardiac arrhythmias, development of rhabdomyolysis, and the possible onset of thrombocytopenia. Mental confusion may be treated symptomatically. Activated charcoal may be of some benefit in hastening excretion. Following release, the patient should have platelet counts periodically for 1 week to determine if thrombocytopenia has developed.

REFERENCES—FAMOTIDINE

1. Milander JH. Pepcid^R: Poison control monograph. Personal communication. Merck, Sharp and Dohme, May 23, 1989.
2. Humphries JE. Thrombocytopenia associated with famotidine in a hemophiliac. Ann Pharmacother 1992;26:262.
3. Norwood J, Smith TM, Stein DS. Famotidine and hyperpyrexia. Ann Intern Med 1990;112:632.
4. Andreo JA, Vivancos F, Lopez VM, Soriano J. Leucocytoclastic vasculitis and famotidine. Med Clin 1990;95:234–235. In: Reactions ADIS International, Sept 15, 1990.
5. Ahmad S. Famotidine and cardiac arrhythmia. DICP Ann Pharmacother 1991;25:315.
6. Roblin X, Becot F, Jacquot JM, et al. Acute rhabdomyolysis and famotidine. Semin Hop 1991;67:337–338.
7. Henann NE, Carpenter DV, Janda SM. Famotidine-associated mental confusion in elderly patients. Drug Intell Clin Pharm 1988;22:976–978.
8. Hinrichsen H, Halabi A, Kirch W. Hemodynamic effects of different H_2 receptor antagonists. Clin Pharmacol Ther 1990; 48:302–307.
9. Dalpre G, Lapidot M, Lipchitz A, et al. Hyperprolactinemia during famotidine therapy. Lancet 1993;342:868.

NIZATIDINE

Nizatidine (Fig. 43–5) is a specific and potent H_2-receptor antagonist in vitro and in vivo.[1] Gastric acid suppression induced by 100 mg of nizatidine is equal to that induced by 300 mg of cimetidine. The therapeutic recommended dose of nizatidine for treatment of active duodenal ulcer is 300 mg on retiring or 150 mg twice daily.[2] Nizatidine bioavailability is nearly 100%. Protein binding is about 30% and plasma clearance is 0.6 L/kg/h.[3] Nizatidine does not interfere with the hepatic metabolism of drugs such as oral anticoagulants and theophylline.

Sweating, urticaria, somnolence, and hepatic toxicity (similar to cimetidine or ranitidine) have been reported. Nizatidine, like cimetidine and ranitidine, may occasionally exhibit negative chronotropic effects.[4] Leukocytosis, mild thrombocythemia, and eosinophilia have been observed after therapeutic use.

REFERENCES—NIZATIDINE

1. Callaghan JT, Bergstrom RF, Obermayer BD, et al. Intravenous nizatidine kinetics and acid suppression. Clin Pharmacol Ther 1985;37:162–165.
2. Nizatidine (AXID). Med Lett Drugs Ther 1988;30(772):77–78.
3. Aranoff GR, Bergstrom RF, Boff RJ, et al. Nizatidine disposition in subjects with normal and impaired renal function. Clin Pharmacol Ther 1988;43:688–695.
4. Halabi A, Kirch W. Negative chronotropic effects of nizatidine. Gut 1991;32:630–634.

RANITIDINE

Ranitidine is an effective H_2-receptor antagonist that acts on the gastric parietal cell to inhibit gastric acid secretion.[1] It inhibits gastric acid secretion with a potency four to eight times that of cimetidine.[2–4] Its structure is similar to that of histamine, but it has a furan instead of an imidazole ring. (Fig. 43–5). It is 4 to 10 times more potent than cimetidine on a molar basis in its ability to inhibit acid secretion.[3,5] Unlike cimetidine, it has little affinity for androgen receptors and does not bind substantially to the hepatic cytochrome P450 mixed-function oxidase enzyme system.[4,5] Ranitidine is marketed as Zantac by Glaxo, Fort Lauderdale, Florida (oral tablets, 150 mg; parenteral injection, 25 mg/mL). It is also marketed by Hoffman–La Roche. The therapeutic dose is 150 mg twice daily.

Toxicokinetics

Absorption

Ranitidine is well absorbed after ingestion, with a bioavailability of 48%.[6] Absorption is not influenced by food ingestion.

Distribution

Peak plasma concentrations occur from 1 to 4.2 hours after ingestion. Small amounts appear in the cerebrospinal fluid.[7] The plasma concentration producing 50% inhibition of gastric acid secretion is 36 to 94 ng/mL (maintained 6 hours after ingestion of 150 mg).[8] The volume of distribution is approximately 1.5 L/kg, similar to that of cimetidine.[4] The serum half-life after oral administration is 2 to 3 hours, and after intravenous administration, it is 1.87 hours.[9] In older age groups, critically ill patients, and those with liver disease, the half-life is prolonged two- or threefold.[8,10] Ranitidine is distributed into breast milk.[11]

Elimination

Ranitidine is metabolized by the liver by "first-pass" kinetics. Up to 30% is metabolized to nitrogen oxide, sulfuric oxide, and desmethyl derivatives. After intravenous use, 50 to 70% is excreted unchanged by the kidney.[4]

Drug Interactions

Ranitidine does not inhibit drug metabolism or interfere with androgenic function.[5] Cimetidine, with an imidazole ring structure, binds and inhibits hepatic cytochrome P450, the mixed-function oxidative enzyme system whose activity is closely related to the oxidative biotransformation of many drugs. Ranitidine, with a furan ring structure instead, retains potent H_2-receptor blocking activity but binds cytochrome P450 with much less affinity.[12] Ranitidine has been reported to interact with warfarin,[13] midazolam, benzodiazepines, fentanyl, metoprolol,[14] nifedipine, and acetaminophen,[15] but may be preferred to cimetidine when warfarin is also being administered (because ranitidine does not appear to affect hepatic drug metabolism in comparison with cimetidine).[16] In contrast with cimetidine inhibition of theophylline clearance, ranitidine, in doses up to 14 times the usual recommended dose for the treatment of peptic ulcer, does not inhibit theophylline metabolism.[17]

Pregnancy/Lactation

Ranitidine is secreted into breast milk with a milk-to-serum ratio of 7.1 to 24.1.[18]

Clinical Presentation

Minor side effects include headache, malaise, dizziness, constipation, nausea, and skin rash, all of which resolve or subside despite continued therapy. Transient increases in hepatic transaminase levels have been noted, and a hypersensitivity type of hepatitis has been observed.[19–21] Ranitidine apparently produces a higher incidence of hepatic hypersensitivity reactions than cimetidine, although hepatotoxicity from either H_2 blocker is uncommon.[22] There is one report of glaucoma and several of severe bradycardia.[23] Unlike cimetidine, ranitidine does not decrease basal testosterone levels and has no antiandrogenic activity; similarly, no rise in prolactin secretion has been observed. Gynecomastia in patients with the Zollinger–Ellison syndrome on high doses of cimetidine was reversed when ranitidine was substituted; however, unilateral painful gynecomastia has been observed.[24] Less confusion and mental depression has been reported than with cimetidine,[7] and no interstitial nephritis has thus far been reported. One patient whose medication was changed from cimetidine to ranitidine developed thrombocytopenia.[25] The platelet count returned to pretreatment levels on discontinuation of the drug. At least five reports have indicated that ranitidine may be associated with thrombocytopenia. It is a relatively rare side effect.[26]

Agranulocytosis has been reported following ranitidine use. The patients recovered after the drug was stopped.[27,28] There have been additional anecdotal reports of cardiac arrest, bradycardia, granulocytopenia, bone marrow hypoplasia, mania, chest pain, confusion, and pancreatitis. An acute dystonic reaction in a 3-month-old child followed an inadvertent overdose.[29] Intramuscular injection of 1 mg/kg (6 mg) of diphenhydramine resulted in resolution of symptoms within 5 minutes.

Laboratory

A reverse-phase high-performance liquid chromatography method is available for determination of ranitidine in whole blood and plasma. The limit of detection of the method is 0.70 ng/mL for a 100-μL injection. The assay is linear between 7.0 ng/mL and 30 μg/mL.[30] Ranitidine may induce a positive result in the EMIT-d.a.u. Monoclonal Amphetamine/Methamphetamine Assay.[31]

Treatment

Treatment of overdose should be similar to that for cimetidine. Ranitidine is poorly dialyzable.[32]

REFERENCES—RANITIDINE

1. Feely J, Warmsley KG. H_2 receptor antagonists: Cimetidine and ranitidine. Br Med J 1983;286:695–697.
2. Ranitidine (Zantac). Med Lett Drugs Ther 1982;24:111–113.
3. Sewing KF, Biliam A, Malchow H. Comparative study with ranitidine and cimetidine on gastric secretion. Scand J Gastroenterol 1981;16(suppl. 69):45–48.
4. Berner BD, Conner CS, Sawyer DR, et al. Ranitidine: A new H_2 receptor antagonist. Clin Pharm 1981;1:499–509.
5. Abernethy DR, Greenblatt DJ, Eshelman FN, et al. Ranitidine does not impair oxidative or conjugative metabolism: Noninteraction with antipyrine, diazepam, and lorazepam. Clin Pharmacol Ther 1984;35:188–192.
6. Blumer JL, Rothstein FC, Kaplan BS, et al. Pharmacokinetic determination of ranitidine pharmacodynamics in pediatric ulcer disease. J Pediatr 1985;107:301–306.
7. Kagevi I, Whalby L. CSF concentrations of ranitidine. Lancet 1985;1:164–165.
8. Zeldis JB, Friedman LS, Isselbacker KJ. Ranitidine: A new H_2 receptor antagonist. N Engl J Med 1983;309:1368–1373.
9. Leiden JS, Harding L, MacLeod SM, et al. Ranitidine pharmacokinetics in children. Clin Pharmacol Ther 1985;37:201.
10. Ilett KF, Nation RL, Tjokrosetio R, et al. Pharmacokinetics of ranitidine in critically ill patients. Br J Clin Pharmacol 1986;21:279–288.
11. Kearns GL, McConnell RF Jr, Trang JM, et al. Appearance of ranitidine in breast milk following multiple dosing. Clin Pharm 1983;4:322–324.
12. Henry DA, MacDonald IA, Kitchingman G, et al. Cimetidine and ranitidine: Comparison of effect on hepatic drug metabolism. Br Med J 1980;281:775–777.
13. Fischer J. Ranitidine and warfarin interaction. Drug Intell Clin Pharm 1985;19:664–665.
14. Spahn H, Mutschler E, Krich W, et al. Influence of ranitidine on plasma metoprolol and atenolol concentration. Br Med J 1983;286:1547–1564.
15. McCarthy DM. Ranitidine or cimetidine. Ann Intern Med 1983;99:551–553.
16. McAllister RG Jr. Questions and answers. JAMA 1984;252:3253.
17. Kelly HW, Powell JR, Donohue JF. Ranitidine at very large doses does not inhibit theophylline elimination. Clin Pharmacol Ther 1986;39:577–581.
18. Kearns GL, McConnell RF Jr, Trang JM, Kluza RB. Appearance of ranitidine in breast milk following multiple dosing. Clin Pharm 1985;4:322–324.
19. Lima MA. Hepatitis associated with ranitidine. JAMA 1984;252:3253.

20. Hiesse C, Cantarovich M, Santelli C, et al. Ranitidine: Hepatotoxicity in renal transplant recipient. Lancet 1985;1:1280.
21. Karachalios GN. Ranitidine and hepatitis. Ann Intern Med 1985;103:634–635.
22. Lima MAS. Ranitidine and hepatic injury. Ann Intern Med 1986;105:140.
23. Camarri E, Chirone E, Fanteria G, et al. Ranitidine induced bradycardia. Lancet 1982;2:160.
24. Tosi S, Cagnoli M. Painful gynaecomastia with ranitidine. Lancet 1982;2:160.
25. Spychal RT, Wickham NWR. Thrombocytopenia associated with ranitidine. Br Med J 1985;291:1687.
26. Bajjoka AE. Ranitidine-induced thrombocytopenia. Arch Intern Med 1991;151:203.
27. Brenner LO. Agranulocytosis and ranitidine. Ann Intern Med 1986;104:896.
28. Shields LI, Files JA, Doll DC, et al. Ranitidine and agranulocytosis. Ann Intern Med 1986;104:128.
29. Maack DK, Spiller HA. Rare dystonic reaction from accidental overdose of ranitidine in a 3 month old. Vet Hum Toxicol 1993;35:343.
30. Rustum AM. High performance liquid chromatographic determination of ranitidine in whole blood and plasma by using a short polymeric column. J Chromatogr Biomed Appl 1987; 321:418–424.
31. Grinstead GF. Ranitidine and high concentrations of phenyl propanolamine crossreact in the EMIT Monoclonal Amphetamine/Methamphetamine Assay. Clin Chem 1989;35: 1998–1999. Technical Brief.
32. Sica DA, Harford A, Comstock T. Ranitidine pharmacokinetics in continuous ambulatory peritoneal dialysis. Clin Pharmacol Ther 1985;37:229.

HISTAMINE-H_3 RECEPTORS

Histamine H_3 receptors are located not only in the central nervous system but also in peripheral tissues where they exert inhibitory functions. This new type of histamine receptor may be added to the list of prejunctional receptors that regulate neurotransmission processes in the gastrointestinal tract. It is unclear if H_3-receptor agonists and antagonists are likely to be clinically useful.[1]

REFERENCES—HISTAMINE-H_3 RECEPTORS

1. Bertaccini G, Coruzzi G, Poli E. Review article: The histamine H_3-receptor: A novel prejunctional receptor regulating gastrointestinal function. Aliment Pharmacol Ther 1991;5:585–591.

PROKINETIC DRUGS

A group of receptors have been shown to affect gut function. New agents under study enhance gastrointestinal motor function and accelerate transit by their action on such receptors.[1] These drugs may aid patients who have various conditions that produce gut hypomotility: esophageal reflux, with inefficient clearance of gastric acid; poor gastric emptying after surgery or in diabetes; small bowel hypomotility or pseudo-obstruction; slow colonic transit in some patients with constipation.[2] (See also Chapter 61.)

BETHANECHOL

Bethanechol, a muscarinic agonist, has been used to stimulate contractions. Muscarinic agonists are contraindicated in patients with asthma, coronary artery disease, and peptic ulcer disease.[3] Bethanechol has had limited success in improving gut motility but may aid in diminishing the side effects of concurrently administered anticholinergic agents.[1] It is a quaternary amine and does not cross the blood–brain barrier. It is available as Myotonine in the United Kingdom and as Urecholine in the United States.[4]

DOMPERIDONE

Domperidone blocks the inhibitory effect of dopamine in gut motility. It has no central nervous system effects, but produces an increase in prolactin secretion (breast enlargement, nipple tenderness, galactorrhea, menstrual irregularities). It is not available in the United States but is available as Evoxin and Motilium in the United Kingdom and Europe.

Domperidone was associated with cardiac arrhythmias, seizures, and sudden death when it was used by the intravenous route. Parenteral use of this product has been discontinued.

METOCLOPRAMIDE

Metoclopramide reduces the inhibitory effect of dopamine in gut motility but it passes through the blood–brain barrier and, in about 10 to 30% of patients, may induce extrapyramidal signs (ranging from a Parkinson-like syndrome to tremors and agitation).[5] It induces prolactin secretion and is an antiemetic. Metoclopramide is commercially available in the United States (Reglan) and throughout the world (Maxolon and Primiperan in the United Kingdom). A number of reports of overdose have appeared.

CISAPRIDE

Cisapride represents the third generation of prokinetic agents. It is unique in that it does not have antidopaminergic properties, but exerts its effect by increasing the release of acetylcholine from postganglionic nerve endings of the myenteric plexus. It is not an antiemetic, nor does it increase prolactin release. Cisapride has not been approved for use in the United States but is available as Prepulsid and Alimix in the United Kingdom.[6]

PROPERTIES OF PROKINETIC DRUGS

Structure and Classification

These drugs are substituted methoxybenzamides (Fig. 43–6).[7]

Product Formulation

Metoclopromide is available in the United States and other countries as the hydrochloride salt in oral tablet, suspension (5 mg/5 mL), and injectable (5 mg/mL) forms (Reglan, Maxolen, Octamide).

Domperidone (as the maleate) is available in the United Kingdom as Evoxon in 10-mg tablets and 30-mg suppositories; and as Motilium in 10-mg tablets (as maleate), 5 mg/5 mL suspension, and 30-mg suppositories.

Cisapride is available in the United Kingdom as Prepulsid and Alimix in 10-mg tablets.

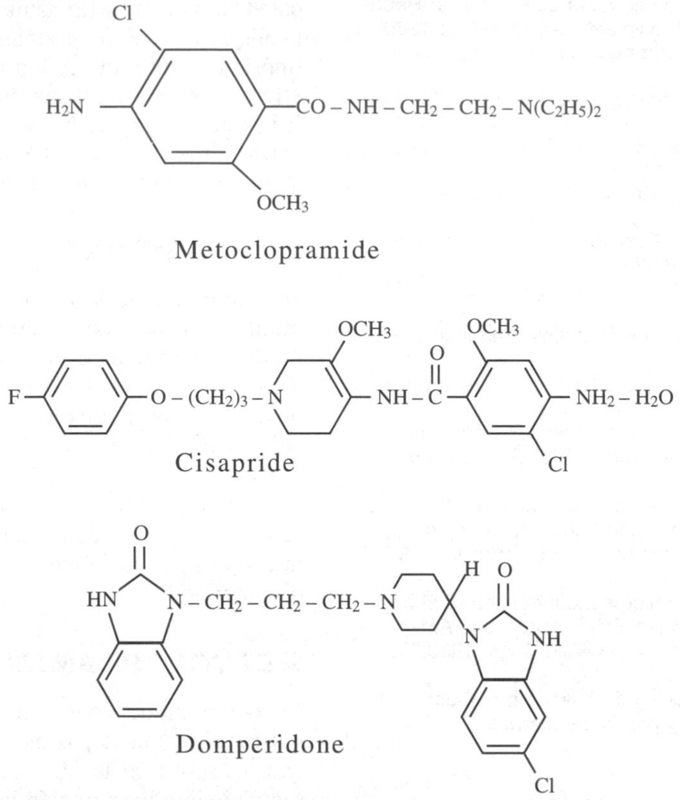

Metoclopramide

Cisapride

Domperidone

Figure 43-6 Structures of three prokinetic agents. (From Reynolds JC, Putnam PE. Prokinetic agents. Gastroenterol Clin North Am 1992;21:567–596.)

Source

Metoclopramide, domperidone, and cisapride are synthetic chemicals.

Therapeutic Dose

All the following are adult doses:

- Metoclopramide — 10 mg four times daily (orally)[6]
- Domperidone — 40 to 120 mg in three or four divided doses
- Cisapride — 10 mg four times daily, or 20 mg three times daily[5]

Toxic Dose

Nine children aged 1 month to 9 years received doses of 5 to 50 mg of metoclopramide and were hospitalized; they recovered.[6] Two children aged 10 months and 2 years 9 months received metoclopramide 0.6 mg/kg/24 h and 0.33 plus 1.66 mg/kg/24 h, respectively (manufacturer-recommended dose up to 0.5 mg/kg/14 h[9]); both recovered. Fifteen children aged 5 months to 11 years 7 months ingested doses of 0.9 to 8.3 mg/kg/d metoclopramide; they recovered.[10]

Fatal Dose

No lethal dose of metoclopramide has been reported. Doses of 360 and 800 mg have been followed by survival with minimal supportive care.[11] Death followed ventricular fibrillation in an adult administered a 200-mg intravenous dose of domperidone.[12] Another death followed multiple 60-mg intravenous domperidone injections.[13] Parenteral preparations of domperidone are no longer available.

Toxicokinetics

Table 43–3 summarizes the toxicokinetics of metoclopramide, domperidone, and cisapride.

Drug Interactions

Metoclopramide. Metoclopramide enhances gastric emptying and therefore it may be able to alter the absorption of various drugs. It has been reported to decrease the half-life of aspirin, cimetidine, cyclosporine, diazepam, digoxin, levodopa, mexiletine, morphine, acetaminophen, pivampicillin, tetracycline, and tolfenamic acid.[14] An increased maximum serum concentration occurred only with aspirin, cyclosporine, diazepam, and levodopa. With digoxin and quinidine, there may be a slight decrease in absorption.[14]

Cisapride. Cisapride 10 mg prevents the delay in gastric emptying associated with the administration of morphine.[15] It results in a decrease in plasma ranitidine levels when taken together with ranitidine.[16]

Pregnancy/Lactation

Metoclopramide crosses the placenta and is distributed into breast milk. Domperidone crosses the placenta.[17] Cisapride crosses the placenta and is found in human milk.[5]

Mechanism of Action

Metoclopramide. These substituted benzamide prokinetic agents block 5-hydroxytryptamine[4] (5-HT_3) receptors in the gastrointestinal motor system when administered in high doses. Their prokinetic action is believed to reflect their agonist effects on the putative HT_4 receptor. 5-HT_3 antagonists and 5-HT_4 agonists may affect upper and lower gastrointestinal transit (Table 43–4).[1,18]

Metoclopramide enhances acetylcholine release and sensitizes muscarinic receptors in the gastrointestinal tract.[4] It stimulates gastric emptying without increasing gastric acid secretion.[1] Metoclopramide antagonizes the inhibitory effect of dopamine receptors located in the smooth muscle of the gastrointestinal tract. It also exerts an antidopaminergic effect within the central nervous system, resulting in extrapyramidal adverse effects.[19]

Domperidone. Domperidone is a peripherally acting dopamine antagonist. It has no important effects within the central nervous system. Domperidone inhibits gastric relaxation and enhances central contractions probably through antagonism of dopamine receptors in the gastrointestinal tract.[8]

Cisapride. Cisapride increases gastric motility by enhancing the release of acetylcholine from postganglionic neurons in the gut. It does not produce dopaminergic inhibition of either the gastrointestinal tract or central nervous system.[1,8] Cisapride is a serotonin (5-HT_4) agonist and may stimulate 5-HT_4 receptors in the right atrium.[20]

This may account for the reports of tachycardia following its use.[21]

Clinical Presentation

Overdose

Metoclopramide. Doses in excess of manufacturer recommendations may, in young children, produce intermittent opisthotonos, increased muscle tone in the limbs, oculogyric crisis, torticollis, facial grimacing, agitation, diplopia, tris-

Table 43–3
Pharmacokinetic Profiles of Metoclopramide, Domperidone, and Cisapride in Healthy Volunteers

Variable	Metoclopramide (Reglan)	Domperidone (Motilium)	Cisapride (Prepulsid)
Absolute bioavailability (%)			
By mouth	30–100	13–17	40–50
Intramuscular	74–96	90	
Volume of distribution (L/kg)	2.2–3.4	5.7	2.4
Time (min) to peak plasma concentration			
Intravenous	1–3	—	—
Intramuscular	10–15	10–30	
By mouth	00–00	10–30	60–120
By rectum	—	60–120	180
Elimination half-life (h)	2.5–5	7.5	7–10
Protein binding (%)	13–22	92	98
Dosage adjustment required in patients with renal failure	Yes; 50% reduction suggested in patients with creatinine clearance <60 mL/min	No	No
Dosage adjustment required in patients with liver failure	Unknown	Unknown	Yes; 50% reduction

From Brown CK, Khanderia U. Use of metoclopramide, domperidone, and cisapride in the management of diabetic gastroparesis. Clin Pharm 1990;9:357–365.

Table 43–4
Prokinetic Agents

	Agonists	Antagonists
Muscarinic receptor	Bethanechol	
Dopamine antagonists		
Block dopamine-1 inhibitor receptors of smooth muscle cells	Domperidone Metoclopramide	
Block dopaminergic inhibition of enteric neuronal acetylcholine release via dopamine-2 receptor 5-HT_3 receptor antagonists		
Agents that stimulate excitatory myenteric receptors	Motilin Cholecystokinin (CCK) Ceruletide (CCK analog)	Loxiglumide (CCK antagonist)
Agents that enhance release of acetylcholine from enteric neurons	Cisapride	
Motilin receptor agonists	Erythromycin IV1 (and other macrolides)	

From Poeters TL. Erythromycin and other macrolides as prokinetic agents. Gastroenterology 1993;106:1886–1899.

mus, nystagmus, strabismus, crying, seizures, cyanosis of the extremities, conjugate deviation of the eyes, and cogwheel rigidity.[9,10,22] Most patients develop symptoms within 36 hours of starting treatment with metoclopramide[10]; rarely symptoms may begin as late as 120 hours.[9] Opisthotonus and torticollis are the most common extrapyramidal manifestations of overdose.[9] Two deaths related to metoclopramide have been reported since 1966. Both followed acute dystonic reactions to the drug.[11] Bradycardia and total heart block have followed intravenous use.[23]

Domperidone. Ventricular arrhythmias, hypokalemia,[24] cardiac arrest,[25] and sudden death[12,26] were reported following intravenous domperidone in high doses. In all instances patients had a malignancy for which they were also receiving cytotoxic drugs, usually cisplatin, sometimes with methylprednisolone.[27] The manufacturers have withdrawn the parenteral preparation from general use.[24] Seizures also followed high-dose intravenous domperidone in patients receiving cisplatin.[28]

Cisapride. There are no reports of acute overdose following cisapride use.

Chronic Use

Metoclopramide. Methemoglobinemia,[29] extrapyramidal symptoms,[19,30] dystonic reactions with sudden death after high-dose intravenous metoclopramide,[31,32] tardive dyskinesia following high-dose intravenous infusion,[33] and neuroleptic malignant syndrome[34] (reported after intramuscular injection and oral ingestion) have been seen with metoclopramide use. A withdrawal syndrome with oscillating akinesia (rigid) and akathisia (restless) symptoms may follow discontinuation of metoclopramide. This may persist for many months and be refractory to therapy.[35]

Domperidone. Domperidone produces few dystonic reactions as a result of its low penetration through the blood–brain barrier. Dopamine receptors in the pituitary, however, are blocked, resulting in prolactin excess with resulting breast tenderness, galactorrhea, gynecomastia, and menstrual irregularities.[13] A neuromuscular malignant syndrome has also followed domperidone use.[36]

Cisapride. Cisapride is generally well tolerated. Undesirable effects include transient abdominal cramping, borborygmi, diarrhea, somnolence and fatigue, tachycardia, palpitations, hypertension and premature beats[5,21] and aggravating parkinsonian tremors.[37] Extrapyramidal symptoms are rare but a dystonic-like reaction has been reported.[38] Cisapride has been associated with life-threatening ventricular arrhythmias, including torsade de pointes, when used in combination with ketoconazole, a potent inhibitor of the cytochrome P4503A4 enzyme system. Ketoconazole appears to inhibit the metabolism of cisapride, leading to a sharp increase in its blood level.[39] Tachycardia following its use may be a procainamide-like effect associated with prolongation of conduction time through the atrioventricular node.[21] This may reflect its similarity of structure with procainamide. Intravenous ketoconazole, itraconazole, and miconazole inhibit the metabolism of cisapride and troleandomycin. They are potent inhibitors of the cytochrome P4503A4 enzyme system and may be associated with QT prolongation and torsade de pointes in patients receiving cisapride.[39]

Laboratory

Analytical Methods

Metoclopramide. A rapid liquid chromatographic method is available for the determination of metoclopramide in human plasma. The limit of detection for metoclopramide is 3 ng/mL. The method compares favorably with high-performance liquid chromatography methods.[40]

Domperidone. Concentrations of unchanged domperidone in plasma and urine have been determined by radioimmunoassay using antibodies raised in rabbits against domperidone.[17]

Cisapride. Levels of cisapride and its major metabolite in biological fluids have been measured by high-performance liquid chromatography.[41]

Blood Levels

Low-dose-therapy plasma levels of metoclopramide are usually less than 0.2 μg/mL, but plasma concentrations of 0.5 to 1.5 μg/mL are measured after high dose intravenous therapy. Following five 1 mg/kg intravenous infusions over 10 minutes, the plasma level was 2.1 μg/mL.[11]

Ancillary Tests

Hypopotassemia was associated with serious cardiac arrhythmias and sudden death following intravenous use of domperidone. An anecdotal report suggests that the long QT syndrome, syncope, and nonsustained ventricular arrhythmia follow high doses of cisapride.[42]

Treatment

Stabilization

Maintenance of the airway, support of respirations, and cardiovascular integrity are the important factors in sustaining life following a prokinetic drug overdose. Extrapyramidal signs following metoclopramide overdose should be followed in a hospital facility where an intravenous line, cardiac monitoring, and oxygen are available. Seizures should be evaluated with a careful neurologic examination, including brain scans and electroencephalograms.

Gut Decontamination

There is no published evidence to support the use of gastric emptying procedures, activated charcoal, cathartics, or whole-bowel irrigation following overdose with this group of drugs. Absorption is rapid, and syrup of ipecac may induce emesis at the same time that the patient has seizures, predisposing the patient to an aspiration pneumonitis. If gastric emptying procedures are to be attempted, tracheal protection is advised.

Elimination Enhancement

Activated charcoal and extracorporeal procedures (hemodialysis or hemoperfusion) have not been used following overdose with prokinetic drugs. The high apparent volumes of distribution of all of the drugs in this group and their high protein binding (for domperidone and cisplatin) would tend to mitigate against the use of these elimination procedures. Toxicokinetic studies indicate that cisapride is not cleared by hemodialysis.[43]

Antidote

There is no antidote for metoclopramide, domperidone, or cisapride overdose.

Supportive Measures

Supportive and symptomatic measures are the mainstays of treatment with this group of drugs.

Repetitive Seizures. Treat with diazepam and other standard anticonvulsive procedures.

Electrolytes. Obtain and follow serial electrolytes. Watch for hypokalemia.

Cardiac Arrhythmias. Few arrhythmias have been reported with domperidone therapy since the parenteral preparation was withdrawn from distribution.

Extrapyramidal Effects. Withdrawal of metoclopramide is usually followed by amelioration of symptoms.

Methemoglobinemia. Discontinue the drug (usually metoclopramide) and give methylene blue, if clinically indicated.

Neuroleptic Malignant Syndrome. Muscle rigidity and fever following metoclopramide use have responded to intravenous dantrolene 2 mg/kg, immediate discontinuation of the causal drug, temperature reduction, and other supportive measures.[44]

REFERENCES—PROKINETIC DRUGS

1. Chaudhuri TK, Fink S. Update: Pharmaceuticals and gastric emptying. Am J Gastroenterol 1990;85:223–230.
2. Hastening drug transit. Lancet 1990;336:974–975. Editorial.
3. Boyson SJ. Bethanechol for anticholinergic side effects. Ann Neurol 19088;23:422–423.
4. Reynolds JEF, ed. *Martindale: The Extra Pharmacopoeia.* 29th ed. London: Pharmaceutical Press, 1989.
5. McCallum RW and the American College of Gastroenterology Committee on FDA Related Matters. Cisapride: A new class of prokinetic agent. Am J Gastroenterol 1991;86:135–149.
6. Cisapride: More selective than metoclopramide. Drug Ther Bull 1990;28(23):89–90.
7. Reynolds JC, Putnam PE. Prokinetic agents. Gastroenterol Clin North Am 1992;21:567–596.
8. Brown CK, Khanderia V. Use of metoclopramide, domperidone and cisapride in the management of diabetic gastroparesis. Clin Pharmacol 1990;9:357–366.
9. Sills JA, Glass EJ. Metoclopramide in young children. Br Med J 1978;2:431.
10. Low LCK, Goel KM. Metoclopramide poisoning in children. Arch Dis Child 1980;55:310–312.
11. Beno JM, Nemeth DR. Diltiazem and metoclopramide overdose. J Anal Toxicol 1991;15:285–287.
12. Joss RA, Goldhirsch A, Brunner KW, Galeazi RL. Sudden death in cancer patient on high dose domperidone. Lancet 1982;1:1019.
13. Jay GT, Chow MSS, Feldman TA. Focus on domperidone: A selective dopamine antagonist for diabetic gastroparesis and idiopathic gastric stasis. Hosp Formul 1991;26:171–183.
14. Lauritsen K, Lauritsen LS, Rask-Madsen J. Clinical pharmacokinetics of drug use in the treatment of gastrointestinal disease (Part 1). Clin Pharmacokinet 1990;19:11–31.
15. Rowbotham DJ, Nimms WS. Effect of cisapride on morphine-induced delay in gastric emptying. Br J Anaesth 1987;59:536–539.
16. Rowbotham DJ, Milligan K, McHugh P. Effects of single doses of cisapride and ranitidine administered simultaneously on plasma concentrations of cisapride and ranitidine. Br J Anaesth 1991;67:302–305.
17. Brogden RN, Carmine AA, Heel RC, et al. Domperidone: A review of its pharmacologic activity, pharmacokinetics and therapeutic efficacy in the treatment of chronic dyspepsia and as an antiemetic drug. Drugs 1982;24:360–400.
18. Talley NJ. Review article: 5-Hydroxytryptamine agonists and antagonists in the modulation of gastrointestinal mobility and sensation: Clinical implications. Aliment Pharmacol Ther 1992;6:279–289.
19. Miller LG, Jankovic J. Metoclopramide induced movement disorders: Clinical findings with a review of the literature. Arch Intern Med 1989;149:2486–2492.
20. Humphrey PPA, Bunce KT. Tachycardia during cisapride treatment. Br Med J 1992;303:1019–1020.
21. Olsson S, Edwards IR. Tachycardia during cisapride treatment. Br Med J 1992;305:748–749.
22. Fournier A, Pauli A, Ducoulombier H, Cousin J. Effets du surdosage en metoclopramide chez 1'enfant. Pediatric 1969; 24:799–805.
23. Midttun M, Oberg B. Total heart block after intravenous metoclopramide. Lancet 1994;343:182–183.
24. Osborne RJ, Slevin ML, Hunter RW, Hamer J. Cardiotoxicity of intravenous domperidone. Lancet 1985;2:385.
25. Roussak JB, Carey P, Parry H. Cardiac arrest after treatment with intravenous domperidone. Br Med J 1984;289:1579.
26. Giaccone G, Bertello O, Calciati A. Two sudden deaths during prophylactic treatment with high doses of domperidone and methylprednisolone. Lancet 1984;2:1336–1337.
27. Quinn N, Parkes D, Jackson G, Upward J. Cardiotoxicity of domperidone. Lancet 1985;2:724.
28. Weaving A, Bezwoda WR, Derman DP. Seizures after antiemetic treatment with high dose domperidone: Report of four cases. Br Med J 1984;288:1728.
29. Kearns GL, Fiser DH. Metoclopramide induced methemoglobinemia. Pediatrics 1988;82:364–366.
30. Sethi KD, Patel B, Meador KJ. Metoclopramide induced parkinsonism. South Med J 1989;82:1581–1582.
31. Pollera CF, Cognetti F, Nardi M, Maza D. Sudden death after acute dystonic reaction to high dose metoclopramide. Lancet 1984;2:440–446.
32. Reasbeckand P, Hossenbouis A. Death following dystonic reaction to oral metoclopramide. Br J Clin Pract 1979;33:31–33.
33. Breitbart W. Tardive dyskinesia associated with high dose intravenous metoclopramide. N Engl J Med 1986;315:518.
34. Robinson MB, Kennett RP, Harding AE, et al. Neuroleptic malignant syndrome associated with metoclopramide. J Neurol Neurosurg Psychiatry 1985;40:1304–1312.
35. Noll AM, Pinsky D. Withdrawal effects of metoclopramide. West J Med 1991;154:726–728.
36. Spirt AJ, Chan W, Thieberg M, Sachar DB. Neuroleptic malignant syndrome induced by domperidone. Drug Dis Sci 1992;37:946–948.

37. Sempere AP, Duarte J, Cabezax C, et al. Aggravation of Parkinson tremor by cisapride. Clin Neuropharmacol 1995;18: 76–78.
38. Bucci KK, Haverstick DE, Abercrombie SA. Dystonic-like reaction following cisapride therapy. J Fam Pract 1995;40: 86–88.
39. Ahmad SR, Wolfe SM. Cisapride and Torsade de pointes. Lancet 1995;345:508.
40. Buss DC, Hutchings AD, Scott S, Routledge PA. A rapid liquid chromatographic method for determination of metoclopramide in human plasma. Ther Drug Monit 1990;12: 293–296.
41. Woestenborghs R, Lorreyne W, Van Rompacy F, Heykants J. Determination of cisapride in plasma and animal tissues by high performance liquid chromatography. J Chromatogr 1988;424:195–200.
42. Bran S, Murray WA, Hirsch IB, Palmer JP. Long QT syndrome during high dose cisapride. Arch Intern Med 1995; 155:765–768.
43. Gladziwa V, Bares R, Klotz V, et al. Pharmacokinetics and pharmacodynamics of cisapride in patients undergoing hemodialysis. Clin Pharmacol Ther 1991;50:673–681.
44. Henderson AS, Longdon P. Fulminant metoclopramide induced neuroleptic malignant syndrome rapidly responsive to intravenous dantrolene. Aust NZ J Med 1991;21:741–743.

SITE-PROTECTIVE AGENTS

SUCRALFATE

Sucralfate is an aluminum salt used to treat duodenal ulcer. In overdose it may be associated with abdominal pain, nausea, and vomiting; in uremic patients it may induce aluminum toxicity with an encephalopathy and bone pain. Treatment of overdose includes withdrawal of the sucralfate and supportive and symptomatic management.[1] (See also Aluminum in Chapter 67.)

Toxicokinetics

Sucralfate decreases the bioavailability of digoxin, quinidine, theophylline, tetracycline, cimetidine, phenytoin, warfarin, thyroxine,[2] ciprofloxacin, and norfloxacin when taken simultaneously possibly because of chelation with the aluminum ion that is released on dissociation of the sucralfate molecule.[2–4]

Laboratory

In normal individuals increments in urinary aluminum concentrations are more sensitive indicators of sucralfate absorption than plasma levels.[5,6] Bone biopsies may show an osteomalacia after a few years of treatment.

Treatment

Treatment of an overdose includes withdrawal of sucralfate and is largely supportive and symptomatic. Use of cimetidine may increase the gastric pH and lead to an increase in aluminum absorption.

REFERENCES—SUCRALFATE

1. Anderson W, Weatherstone G, Ved C. Esophageal medication bezoar in a patient receiving enteral feedings and sucralfate. Am J Gastroenterol 1989;8:205–206.
2. Harrankova J, Lahaie R. Levothyroxine binding by sucralfate. Ann Intern Med 1992;117:445–446.
3. Bevardi RR, Kirking DM, Townsend KA, Melonakos TK. Identifying potential interactions of sucralfate with other drugs in hospitalized patients. Am J Hosp Pharm 1992;49: 1488–1490.
4. Rey AM, Gums JG. Altered absorption of digoxin, sustained-release quinidine and warfarin with sucralfate administration. DICP Ann Pharmacother 1991;25:745–746.
5. Robertson JA, Salusky IB, Goodman WG, et al. Sucralfate, intestinal aluminum absorption and aluminum toxicity in a patient on dialysis. Ann Intern Med 1989;111: 179–181.
6. Min DI, D'Elia JA. Sucralfate-associated aluminum toxicity in a patient with renal failure: Treatment with deferoxamine. Clin Pharm 1992;11:636–639.

COLLOIDAL BISMUTH SUBSALICYLATE (PEPTO-BISMOL)

Elderly patients may ingest large amounts of Pepto-Bismol daily, resulting in agitation, confusion, lethargy, disorientation, slurred speech, and acute pulmonary edema. Such patients may develop a mixed respiratory alkalosis and metabolic acidosis. Barium-like contrast densities may be seen on an abdominal plain film.[1,2] (See also Bismuth in Chapter 67.)

Sixty milliliters of Pepto-Bismol leads to a peak salicylate concentration of 40.1 μg/mL in 1.8 hours. Aspirin doses of 650 and 1000 mg lead to peak salicylate levels of 34.3 μg/mL in 1.9 hours and 59.9 μg/mL in 2.3 hours, respectively.[3] After ingestion of 30 mL of Pepto-Bismol (525 mg bismuth subsalicylate) every 30 minutes for eight doses (total daily dose, 4.2 g bismuth subsalicylate), a peak plasma salicylate level of 137 μg/mL is reached in 5 hours.[4] One adult dose of Pepto-Bismol liquid (30 mL of original strength) provides 25 mg of salicylate; one adult dose of Pepto-Bismol tablets (2 tablets) provides 204 mg of salicylate, similar to the salicylate dose delivered by one regular-strength aspirin (249 mg of salicylate). Maximum-strength Pepto-Bismol liquid contains 460 mg salicylate per dose. Ingestion of 66 tablets by a 36-kg patient resulted in a salicylate dose of 187 mg/kg; the patient died.[5] This may be compared with the recommended dosing schedule of 2 tablets four times a day, which would deliver 11.6 mg of salicylate/kg/d to a 70-kg adult.[2]

REFERENCES—COLLOIDAL BISMUTH SUBSALICYLATE

1. Steffers M, Esnard J, Meyer R, Bellucci A. Salicylate toxicity from bismuth subsalicylate overuse. Clin Res 1989;32: 336A.
2. Ching CK, Long RG, O'Hara R, Richardson J. Iatrogenic bismuth toxicity associated with inadvertent long term De-Nortab ingestion. Int J Pharm Pract 1993;2:111–113.
3. Feldman S, Chew S-L, Pickering LK, et al. Salicylate absorption from a bismuth subsalicylate preparation. Clin Pharmacol Ther 1981;29:788–792.
4. Pickering LK, Feldman S, Ericsson CD, Cleary TG. Absorption of salicylate and bismuth from a bismuth subsalicylate containing compound (Pepto-bismol). J Pediatr 1981;99: 654–656.
5. Sainsbury SJ. Fatal salicylate toxicity from bismuth subsalicylate. West J Med 1991;155:637–639.

DRUGS THAT INDUCE COLONIC TOXICITY

Cappell and Simon have provided an extensive survey of drug-induced colonic toxicity.[1] Medications associated with colonic ischemia include cocaine, ergotamine, estrogen, amphetamines, digitalis, methysergide, and vasopressin. Medications associated with colonic pseudo-obstruction include narcotics, phenothiazines, vincristine, atropine or other anticholinergics, ganglionic blocking agents, and tricyclic antidepressants. Medications promoting infectious or necrotizing enterocolitis include numerous antibiotics associated with pseudomembranous colitis, deferoxamine associated with *Yersinia* enterocolitis, chemotherapy associated with neutropenic colitis, and hyperosmolar medications or formulas in infants. Medications associated with an allergic, inflammatory or cytotoxic colitis include gold compounds, nonsteroidal antiinflammatory drugs, α-methyldopa, flucytosine, methotrexate, salicylates, and sulfasalazine. Potassium chloride, administered in slow-release wax matrices, can cause intestinal ulcers. Chronic use of cathartics leads to colonic hypomotility and abdominal distension. Methysergide can cause a colonic stricture due to retroperitoneal fibrosis. Intrarectally administered compounds that have produced a toxic colitis include powerful acids, bases, and other corrosives. Enemas using hypertonic radiographic contrast agents have been associated with colitis in patients with colonic obstruction.[1]

REFERENCE: DRUGS THAT INDUCE COLONIC TOXICITY

1. Cappell MS, Simon T. Colonic toxicity of administered medications and chemicals. Am J Gastroenterol 1993;88:1684–1699.

SOMATOSTATIN

See Chapter 42.

MUSCARINIC M_1-RECEPTOR ANTAGONIST: PIRENZEPINE

Pirenzepine (Gastrozepine) is a muscarinic cholinergic receptor antagonist (see Chapter 46). In overdose it can be expected to exhibit anticholinergic clinical effects. It acts synergistically with cimetidine to reduce gastric acid output.[1,2]

Product Formulation

Pirenzepine dihydrochloride is available in oral form in the United Kingdom. Each tablet contains about 50 mg of the anhydrous substance.

Therapeutic Dose

The dose is 50 mg twice daily up to a maximum of 150 mg (one tablet three times a day).

Fatal Dose

No deaths from pirenzepine have been reported.

Toxicokinetics

Drug Interactions

Pirenzepine and H_2 antagonists such as cimetidine and ranitidine appear to act synergistically to provide greater gastric acid inhibition than either product alone.[3]

Pregnancy/Lactation

Pirenzepine is not recommended for use during pregnancy. No controlled studies in pregnancy are available.

Pirenzepine selectively blocks muscarinic receptors controlling gastric and acid pepsin secretion.

Clinical Presentation

In overdose, anticholinergic (antimuscarinic) effects and sedation may be observed.

Laboratory

Concentrations of pirenzepine in biological fluids have been determined by high-performance liquid chromatography (sensitivity, 100 μg/mL) and radioimmunoassay.[4]

Treatment

Treatment of an overdose is symptomatic and supportive. Hemodialysis would not be expected to remove significant amounts of pirenzepine (low volume of distribution), but plasma concentrations of pirenzepine can be reduced by up to 50% during hemodialysis. There is no antidote.

REFERENCES—MUSCARINIC M_1-RECEPTOR ANTAGONISTS: PIRENZEPINE

1. Hammer R, Giachetti A. Muscarinic receptor subtypes M_1 and M_2: Biochemical and functional characterization. Life Sci 1982;31:2991–2998.
2. Tryba M, Huchzermeyer H, Torok M, et al. Single drug and combined medication with cimetidine, antacids and pirenzepine in the prophylaxis of acute upper gastrointestinal bleeding. Hepato-gastroenterol 1983;30:154–157.
3. Lauritsen K, Lauritsen LS, Rask-Madsen J. Clinical pharmacokinetics of drugs used in the treatment of gastrointestinal diseases (Part I). Clin Pharmacokinet 1990;19:11–31.
4. Meinecke I, Witsch D, Brendel E. Sensitive high performance liquid chromatographic determination of pirenzepine in plasma. J Chromatogr 1986;375:369–375.

Chapter 44
Immunotoxicology

INTRODUCTION

DEFINITION OF IMMUNOTOXICOLOGY

Immunotoxicology can be defined as the discipline concerned with the study of the interactions of foreign substances with the immune system and the assessment of their importance in terms of risk to human or animal health. Some chemicals that have produced immunologic disturbances in experimental animals and/or humans are listed in Table 44–1.[1] A detailed overview of drug-induced immune diseases and immunotoxic drugs and chemicals has been presented by Descotes.[2,3]

IMMUNE RESPONSE

Basic response steps subserved by the immune system are listed in Table 44–2. Functional components of the immune response include activities of leukocyte subsets (T lymphocytes, B lymphocytes, natural killer lymphocytes, mononuclear phagocytes).[4,5] Drugs associated with neutrophil immunotoxicity and environmental agents affecting macrophage function are listed in Table 44–3.[4] Agents leading to hematologic immunotoxicity are listed in Table 44–4.[4]

Immunotoxicity, or an immunotoxic effect, is defined as an adverse or inappropriate change in the structure or function of the immune system after exposure to a foreign substance, either of synthetic or natural origin. Such foreign substances include industrial, transportation, agricultural, and household chemicals, drugs, and food additives.[6] Conditions known to alter reactivity to substances, in addition to genetic factors, are age, presence of concurrent disease, nutritional status, hormone levels, diurnal variation in drug disposition or sensitivity, environmental factors that induce or inhibit drug metabolism, smoking, and efficiency of repair mechanism. An additional risk factor may be the occurrence of infection prior to exposure.[4] Immunotoxic effects may be caused by the direct or indirect action of a foreign substance (xenobiotic), and may also result from an immunologically mediated host response to a xenobiotic, its metabolites, or host antigens altered by such foreign substances.[7] The clinical effects of immunotoxic substances may be manifested at both ends of a spectrum—as an

Table 44–1
Examples of Xenobiotics Known or Presumed to Produce Immunologic Disturbances in Experimental Animals and/or Humans

Immunomodulation
Aflatoxin, ochratoxin, ricin, gelonin
Airborne pollutants (eg, NO_2, SO_2, O_3, asbestos, carbon, silica)
Antibiotics
Antimalarial and antileprosy agents
Benzene
Benzidine
Contraceptive steroid combinations
Diethylstilbestrol
Dimethylnitrosamine
Environmental estrogens (eg, Kepone)
Food additives and oxidants
Heavy metals (eg, Pb, Cd, Hg)
Insecticides (eg, DDT, mirex, carbaryl, lindane, aldrin)
Organometals (eg, dioctyltin, dichloride, butyltin dichloride, methylmercury)
Phenol
Phorbol esters
Polycyclic aromatic hydrocarbons (eg, 7,12-DMBA, benzo[a]pyrene, 1,2,5,6-DBA, 3-MCA, BA)
Polyhalogenated aromatic hydrocarbons (eg, TCDD, TCDF, polychlorinated biphenyls, polybrominated biphenyls, hexachlorobenzene)
Styrene
Substances of abuse (eg, cannabinoids, heroin, morphine)
Urethane
Various anesthetic gases and chemicals
Various central nervous system-active agents (eg, Li, barbiturates)

Autoimmune Syndromes
Acetazolamide
Anticonvulsants
Chlorpromazine
Elliptinium
Gold salts
Hydralazine
Isoniazid
Mercury salts
Methimazole
Nitrofurantoin
Penicillamine
Phenylvinylimidazolyldimethione
Procainamide
Propranolol
Propylthiouracil
Rifampicin
Salicylates
Sulfonamides
Vinyl chloride

Allergy/Hypersensitivity
Antibiotics
Antioxidants
Castor beans
Diisocyanates
Dusts
Enzymes
Ethylenediamide
Formaldehyde
Hexachlorophene
Insecticides
Metals
Natural resins
Phthalic anhydride
Pyrolytic products of polyvinyl chloride
Reactive dyes
Resorcinol
Trimellitic anhydride
Etc

From Spreafico F. Immunotoxicology in 1987: Problems and challenges. Fundam Clin Pharmacol 1988;2:353–367.

Table 44–2
Normal Response of the Immune System

1. Encounter of lymphocyte with antigen
2. Antigen recognition by the immune system
3. Activation of lymphocytes
4. Amplification of the immune response
5. Immune discrimination between self and nonself
6. Regulation and control over the immune response

From Sullivan JB Jr. Immunological alterations and chemical exposure. J Toxicol Clin Toxicol 1989;27:311–343.

enhanced but inappropriate immune response and as a failure to mount an appropriate immune response. The principal effects induced by immunotoxic substances are immunosuppression, autoimmunity, and hypersensitivity[5] (Table 44–1).

IMMUNOTHERAPY

Immunotherapy involves the use of antibodies or antibody fragments for therapeutic purposes.[8,9] Antibodies are complex glycoproteins synthesized by B lymphocytes and plasma cells and derived from immunoglobulin G (IgA), M (IgM), or A (IgA). IgG is the main circulating immunoglobulin and the one usually employed therapeutically. Each molecule has two class-specific heavy chains and two light chains arranged to provide two binding sites. IgG can be cleared by the enzyme pepsin to give an $F(ab)_2$ fragment containing the two binding sites and one Fc component, with a molecular weight of about 60,000, not required for antibody binding. IgG can also be cleaved by papain to yield two identical Fab fragment each with a molecular weight of about 50,000 and a single binding site and one constant

Table 44–3
Selected Environmental Agents That Affect Macrophage Function

Agent	Effect
Silica	Cytotoxicity; in small quantities, depression
Crocidolite asbestos	Enhancement
Fly ash	As particle size decreases, enhancement; also cytotoxicity
Coal mine dust	Depression
Manganese dioxide	Depression and cytotoxicity
Cigarette smoke	Depression
Carbon monoxide	Enhancement
SO_2	5–20 ppm, enhancement
NO_2	25 ppm, depression
Formaldehyde	10 ppm, enhancement 20 ppm, depression
Aflatoxin, mycotoxins	Depression and cytotoxicity

From Burrell R. Human immune toxicity. Mol Aspects Med 1993;14(1):1–81.

Table 44-4
Some Agents Leading to Hematologic Immunotoxicity

Idiopathic Thrombocytopenic Purpura	Autoimmune Hemolytic Anemia	Idiosyncratic Neutropenia
Sedormid	α-Methyldopa	Indomethacin
Quinine	Penicillin	*p*-Aminophenol derivatives
Quinidine	Quinidine	Pyrazolon derivatives
Heparin	Stibophen	Chloramphenicol
Gold salts	Chlorpromazine	Penicillins
Sulfonamides	Sulfonamides	Phenothiazines
Sulfa derivatives	Cephalothin	Phenytoins
p-Aminosalicylic acid	Procainamide	Sulfonamides
Phenytoin	Isoniazid	
Heroin		
Indomethacin and aspirin		
Toluene diisocyanate		
Vinyl chloride		

From Burrel R. Human immune toxicity. Mol Aspects Med 1993;14(1):1–81.

fraction, F_c, whose amino acid sequences determine the main functional activity of the molecule.

History

Antibodies raised in horses have frequently been associated with severe and, sometimes, fatal side effects. These risks of immunotherapy have been reduced by the production of antibodies in sheep rather than horses and the use of Fab rather than intact IgG or $F(ab)_2$. Antibodies raised against small molecules, such as drugs, by covalently coupling them to a carrier protein, have also increased the potential for immunotherapy.

Polyclonal and Monoclonal Antibodies

Antibodies raised in animals are called polyclonal because they are the product of many different clones of the B lymphocyte, each clone producing antibodies directed against different sites (epitopes) on the antigen to which they bind with different strengths (affinities). Most companies and research groups produce monoclonal antibodies using hybridomas consisting of B lymphocytes fused with cancer cells. These are bound to a single epitope with the same affinity, but may be less effective than their polyclonal counterparts.

Polyclonal Antibody Production

Polyclonal Fab fragments directed against digoxin, tricyclic antidepressants, and some snake venoms are produced as follows:

1. Obtain or synthesize the appropriate immunogen.
2. Prepare a water-in-oil emulsion of the immunogen in Freund's adjuvant.
3. Immunize sheep monthly in six sites.
4. Take samples of blood regularly, and, once suitable antibody titers (levels) have been achieved, bleed each sheep monthly (10 mL/kg body weight).
5. Separate the red cells from the antiserum (serum containing antibodies).
6. Precipitate the immunoglobulin fraction of the antiserum with sodium sulfate.
7. Cleave the antibodies with papain to give both specific and nonspecific Fab.
8. Purify to specific Fab by affinity chromatography.[8]

Toxicokinetic Criteria

- *Knowledge of the active toxin structure:* Some compounds act mainly via metabolites; antibodies should be developed to cross-react with these active metabolites. With digitalis, both the parent drug digoxin and its active metabolites are reactive. A similar approach is taken for selection of anti-tricyclic antidepressant antibodies.
- *Knowledge of molecular mechanisms of toxin action:* Anti-paraquat antibodies reduce the paraquat pool in lung cells inefficiently because of the strong binding of paraquat.
- *Appropriate pharmacokinetic parameters of the toxin:* If a toxin has a low apparent volume of distribution and a high total body clearance, immunotherapy is not indicated. Classic clearance techniques will suffice. Toxins with a low clearance and a high volume of distribution are the best candidates for immunotherapy.
- *Knowledge of the dose–lethality curve.* This curve must be known to estimate the number of antibody binding sites (ABSs) required to reach a critical dose threshold. If the lethal curve is steep, a small number of ABSs will suffice (cardiac glycosides, colchicine).[9,10] A large number of ABSs are required for drugs that are toxic at high doses (tricyclic antidepressants, chloroquine).[11]

Fab fragments are usually used in immunotherapy because of their greater diffusion in body compartments and the higher renal clearance of the toxin–ABS conjugate compared with IgG or $(Fab)_2$.

Tricyclic Antidepressants

Toxic dose levels of tricyclic antidepressants (TCAs) are higher than those of digoxin or colchicine. Therefore, reversal of TCA toxicity may require a large amount of Fab fragments. Now under development are antibodies directed predominantly against the tricyclic ring that can recognize both the TCA molecule and its active demethylated metabolite.[12] Animal studies with anti-TCAs appear to demonstrate neutralization of the TCA function in the vascular compartment with reduction of TCA distribution into the heart. This may be of interest in the management of acute TCA poisoning in humans.[13–17]

In TCA (amitriptyline) poisoning, seizures may occur during the alpha half-life phase of 1.5 to 31 hours following ingestion. The volume of distribution in the alpha phase may correlate more significantly with signs and symptoms of acute TCA poisoning.[18] The volume of distribution is small in the alpha phase, and less antidote may be required to lower plasma TCA concentrations. Addition of sodium bicarbonate to anti-TCA Fab in TCA-poisoned rats appears to reduce desipramine-induced QRS prolongation to a greater extent than either treatment alone.[19] Further animal and clinical studies remain to be done in this area over the next few years.[13–19]

Antidigoxin and Digitoxin Fab Fragments

See Chapter 32.

Colchicine

Colchicine binds to tubulin and blocks mitosis in metaphase. The binding is reversible. The half-life of the tubulin–colchicine complex is about 36 hours.[20] Colchicine exerts multiorgan toxicity. The severity and mortality rate are closely dose related. Mortality is 10 to 50% with ingested doses between 0.5 and 0.8 mg/kg and is 100% with a dose larger than 0.8 mg/kg.[21] Fatal intoxications have been reported in adults after ingestion of 7 to 12 mg or after intravenous injection of 6 mg. Treatment at present is based on decontamination by early gastric lavage and aggressive supportive measures to correct shock and hematologic and coagulation disturbances, prevent sepsis, and maintain electrolyte balance. Plasma expanders (for shock) and inotropic agents may be useful. Despite aggressive therapy, mortality is high. Anti-colchicine antibodies may be able to detach colchicine from its target organs before cellular damage has occurred (see Chapter 74). Use of anti-colchicine antibodies may ultimately be indicated in patients who have ingested more than 0.8 mg/kg and who will most likely die.[22]

Conventional therapy is not effective because of the high volume of distribution and low circulating blood concentration of colchicine. The drug has a low systemic clearance. Fab fragments (produced in goats) administered to mice and rabbits improved survival, led to a 10- to 16-fold increase in colchicine plasma concentrations, an increase in the plasma concentration–time area under the curve, a decrease in the free plasma fraction of colchicine, a 24-fold decrease in the volume of distribution, and an increase in the amount recovered in the urine.[23] Goat colchicine IgG antibodies administered to mice appeared to reduce toxic effects and lethality.[24] Studies in animals have further defined properties of colchicine binding to tubulin and to the antibody.[25] Human data remain to be obtained. The drug is absorbed rapidly from the gastrointestinal tract. Clinical trials of Fab may confirm the usefulness of Fab if administered within the first few hours of poisoning. Before such trials are undertaken, approvals (human trial committee; government agencies, eg, Food and Drug Administration) would need to be obtained.

Nerium Oleander

Preliminary studies in oleander-intoxicated dogs with anti-digoxin–Fab fragments suggest that large doses of Fab appear effective in the treatment of dysrhythmias and hyperkalemia. Further studies are required to confirm these observations and to evaluate the use of lower doses.[26]

Paraquat

Rabbit-induced antiparaquat antibodies were employed in rats prior to intravenous administration of paraquat 0.1 mg/kg. The plasma paraquat concentration increased and the amount of paraquat in the urine decreased. Immunotherapy succeeded in sequestering paraquat in the plasma compartment, but did not prevent it from accumulating in the tissues.[27] Further studies are in progress.

Phencyclidine (PCP)

There is no known specific antagonist to the actions of PCP. The drug is lipophilic and has extensive extravascular distribution, and low renal clearance. These toxicokinetic criteria render it a good candidate for immunotherapy.[28] It should be possible to use high-affinity PCP-specific Fab to produce both a redistribution and an inactivation of the drug through high-affinity binding. Animal studies[29] with high-affinity goat-produced antibodies induced an immediate increase in serum PCP concentration (11- to 56-fold), indicating that substantial amounts of the drug were being removed from, and prevented from returning to, peripheral sites. There was also a 10-fold decrease in the volume of distribution (V_D). Fab did not appear to alter the terminal elimination half-life ($t_{1/2}$) of PCP. As $t_{1/2} = 0693 V_D / Cl_s$ (Cl_s = systemic clearance) and V_D and Cls changed by an equal order of magnitude (about 10-fold) no change in $t_{1/2}$ was expected. The percentage of unbound PCP decreased from about 50% before Fab use to less than 1% after Fab use. Whether Fab will be effective in actually reversing clinical toxicity remains to be determined.

Arsenic

The low molecular weight, high volume of distribution, antigenicity, and high potency of arsenic compounds provide a model for studying the therapeutic application of antibodies. Ovalbumin–azobenzene arsenate induces antibodies in mice. Preliminary studies indicate a modest effect on arsenic-induced mortality in mice. Further purification of the antibodies may be required to decrease mortality. Additional studies are required to define the usefulness of immunotherapy for poisoning with this metal.[30]

REFERENCES—INTRODUCTION

1. Spreafico F. Immunotoxicology in 1987: problems and challenges. Fundam Clin Pharmacol 1988;2:353–367.
2. Descotes J. *Drug-Induced Human Diseases.* Amsterdam: Elsevier, 1990:222.
3. Descotes J. *Immunotoxicology of Drugs and Chemicals.* 2nd ed. Amsterdam: Elsevier, 1988:444.
4. Burrell R. Human immune toxicity. Mol Aspects Med 1993; 14:1–81.
5. Stevenson GW, Hall SC, Rudnick S, et al. The effect of anesthetic agents on the human immune response. Anesthesiology 1990;72:542–552.
6. Identifying and controlling immunotoxic substances: Background paper. Congress of the United States. Office of Technology Assessment. OTA-BP-BA-75. Washington DC: U.S. Government Printing Office, April 1991:1–93.
7. Brooks BO, Sullivan JB Jr. Immunotoxicology. In: Sullivan JB Jr, Krieger GR, eds. *Hazardous Materials Toxicology: Clinical Principles of Environmental Health.* Baltimore: Williams & Wilkins, 1991:190–214.
8. Landon J. An immunology primer: Some definitions and how to make a Fab. Personal Communication. Lyon Poison Center's 30th Anniversary and European Association of Poison Centres and Clinical Toxicologists, Technical Meeting, May 22-24, 1991.
9. Scherrmann J-M, Urtizberea M, Sabouraud A. Toxicokinetics, mechanisms and prerequisites of immunotherapy. Personal communication. In: *Proceedings, European Association of Poison Centres and Clinical Toxicologists, Technical Meeting, Lyon, May 22–24, 1991.*
10. Scherrmann J-M, Terrien N, Urtizberea M, et al. Immunotoxicotherapy: Present status and future trends. Clin Toxicol 1989;27:1–35.
11. Sabouraud A, Redureau M, Gires P, et al. Effect of colchicine-specific Fab fragments on the hepatic clearance of colchicine. Drug Metab Dispos 1993;21:997–1002.
12. Sabouraud A, Urtizberea M, Scherrmann JM. Immunotherapy of tricyclic antidepressant poisoning: Recent experimental data. Personal Communication. In: *Proceedings, European Association of Poison Centres and Clinical Toxicologists, Technical Meeting, Lyon, France, May 22–24, 1991.*
13. Pentel PR, Schoof DD, Pond SM. Redistribution into plasma of tracer doses of ^{3}H-desipramine by anti-DMI antiserum in rats. Biochem Pharmacol 1985;36:293–295.
14. Sabouraud A, Denis H, Urtizberea M, et al. The effect of nortriptyline-specific active immunization on amitriptyline toxicity and disposition in the rabbit. Toxicology 1990;62:349–360.
15. Hursting MJ, Opheim KE, Raisys VA, et al. Tricyclic antidepressant-specific Fab fragments alter the distribution and elimination of desipramine in the rabbit: A model for overdose treatment. Toxicology 1989;27:53–66.
16. Pentel PR, Keyler DE, Brunn GJ, et al. Redistribution of tricyclic antidepressants in rats using a drug-specific monoclonal antibody: Dose–response relationship. Drug Metab Dispos 1991;19:24–28.
17. Pentel PR, Brunn GJ, Pond SM, Keyler DE. Pretreatment with drug-specific antibody reduces desipramine cardiotoxicity in rats. Life Sci 1991;48:675–683.
18. Heath AJ. Immunotherapy for tricyclic antidepresant poisoning: A clinical perspective. In: *Proceedings, European Association of Poison Centres and Clinical Toxicologists, Technical Meeting, Lyon, France, May 22–24, 1991.*
19. Brunn GJ, Keyler DE, Pond SM, Pentel PR. Interaction of drug-specific antibody Fab[1] fragment and $NaHCO_3$ for reversal of desipramine cardiotoxicity in rats. Vet Hum Toxicol 1991;33:350.
20. Jaeger A, Sander PH, Kopferschmitt J, Flesch F. Clinical features and management of colchicine poisonings: Rationale for immunotherapy. In: *Proceedings, European Association of Poison Centres and Clinical Toxicologists, Technical Meeting, Lyon, France, May 22–24, 1991.*
21. Bismuth C, Gaultier M, Conso F. Aplasie medullaire apres intoxication. In: *Proceedings, Association of Poison Centres and Clinical Toxicologists, Technical Meeting, Lyon, France, May 22–24, 1991.*
22. Putterman C, Ben-Chetrit E, Caraco Y, Levy M. Colchicine intoxication: Clinical pharmacology, risk factors, features and management. Semin Arthritis Rheum 1991;21:143–155.
23. Scherrmann JM, Sabouraud A, Urtizberea M, et al. Immunotherapy of colchicine poisoning. In: *Proceedings, European Association of Poison Centres and Clinical Toxicologists, Technical Meeting, Lyon, France May 22–24, 1991.*
24. Terrien N, Urtizberea M, Scherrmann JM. Reversal of advanced colchicine toxicity in mice with goat colchicine-specific antibodies. Toxicol Appl Pharmacol 1990;104:504–510.
25. Wolff J, Capraro HG, Brossi A, Cook GH. Colchicine binding to antibodies. J Biol Chem 1980;255:7144–7148.
26. Clark RF, Selden BS, Curry SC. Antidigoxin-Fab fragments in the treatment of a canine model of oleander toxicity. Vet Hum Toxicol 1990;32:358.
27. Nagao M, Takatori T, Wu B, et al. Immunotherapy for the treatment of acute paraquat poisoning. Hum Toxicol 1989;8: 121–123.
28. MacDonald DI. New treatment for PCP toxicity? JAMA 1987; 257:3188.
29. Owens SM, Mayersohn M. Phencyclidine-specific Fab fragments alter phencyclidine disposition in dogs. Drug Metab Dispos 1986;14:52–58.
30. Leikin JB, Goldman-Leikin RE, Evans MA, et al. Immunotherapy in acute arsenic poisoning. Clin Toxicol 1991;29: 59–70.

IMMUNOSUPPRESSION

Immunosuppression reflects a generalized decrease in immune responsiveness that may result in an increased incidence of infectious disease or neoplasms such as lymphoma, cancers of the skin and lips, and leukemia.[1,2] Pharmaceuticals, abused drugs, pesticides, and other chemicals may destroy or inhibit innate and acquired resistance mechanisms in both humans and animals. For example, patients with confirmed immune alterations exposed to polybrominated biphenyls appear to have an increased tumor incidence.[3] Air pollutants such as ozone, nitrogen dioxide, and sulfur dioxide may increase susceptibility to infection.[4,5] Infectious disease have been used to study potential immunotoxicants. Finally, in vivo and in vitro tumor resistance assays are useful for detecting immunotoxicity.[6,7]

MECHANISM OF ACTION OF IMMUNOSUPPRESSANTS

The most frequently used immunosuppressive drugs (Table 44–5) fall into four basic categories: alkylating agents, glucocorticosteroids, antimetabolites, and natural products. Alkylating agents (eg, cyclophosphamide) disrupt cell functions, particularly mitosis, and are highly toxic to rapidly proliferating cells, such as lymphoid cells. Glucocorticosteroids alter phagocytosis and depress T- and B-lymphocyte function. Antimetabolites (eg, azathioprine) act chiefly by inhibiting protein synthesis. Natural products such as cyclosporine A appear to act through modulation of mechanisms regulating immune responsiveness. It suppresses T-cell function but spares B-cell function.

Table 44-5
Most Common Therapeutic Immunosuppressants Used in Humans

Immunosuppressant	Description	Effect
Corticosteroids	Isoprenoid lipids	Antiinflammatory Cytokine inhibitors Phagocytic inhibition
Azathioprine	Purine antagonist	Antiproliferation T-cell antigen receptor inhibitor Antibody-dependent cellular cytotoxicity inhibitor
Methotrexate	Aminopterin derivative	Folate metabolism inhibitor
Cyclophosphamide	Aromatic alkylating agent	Crosslinks DNA More selective for B, suppressor T cells
Cyclosporine	Cyclic polypeptide	Inhibits helper T cytokines by inhibiting mRNA translation
FK 506	Polycyclic peptide	Inhibits cytokines, interleukin-2 receptors Inhibits signal transduction

From Burrell R. Human immune toxicity. Mol Aspects Med 1993;14(1):1–81.

IMMUNOSUPPRESSANTS IN PREGNANCY

Immunosuppressive drugs (eg, azathioprine, corticosteroids) have been administered throughout pregnancy to prevent rejection of a transplanted kidney. Lymphopenia, decreased survival of lymphocytes in culture, absence of IgM, and a reduced level of IgG at birth are all evidence of suppression of thymus-dependent and thymus-independent systems in the infant and mother. Recovery of both these systems by approximately 15 weeks of age is indicated by reappearance of the thymic shadow, development of palpable lymph nodes, and near-normal concentrations of serum IgG and IgM. Absence of IgA at 1 year of age is not uncommon. The transplacental transmission of agents that suppress the immune system of the developing fetus could increase the child's susceptibility to malignancy. Management of children born to mothers receiving immunosuppressive agents should include a complete immunologic workup as well as endocrinologic and genetic studies. If immunoglobulin deficiency is severe, hepatitis-associated antigen-negative plasma could provide some passive antibody during the recovery period. As adrenal insufficiency is possible, use of hydrocortisone may be indicated in the first few months of life. Karyotype analysis should be performed to rule out chromosomal abnormalities. Some children born to mothers treated with large doses of azathioprine and prednisone are in good health years after birth.[8]

IMMUNOSUPPRESSANTS AND TRANSPLANTS

Use of immunosuppressant drugs in transplant patients may be associated with an increase in the posttransplantation incidence of neoplasms,[9,10] infections, and severe neurologic complications.[11] Despite the fact that 6% of allograft recipients develop cancers, only 1% die from them.

REFERENCES—IMMUNOSUPPRESSION

1. Penn I. Lymphomas complicating organ transplantation. Transplant Proc 1983;15:2790–2797.
2. Penn I. The occurrence of cancer in immune deficiencies. Curr Probl Cancer 1982;6:1–64.
3. Berlin A, Dean J, Draper M, et al. Synopsis, conclusions and recommendations. In: Berlin A, Dean J, Draper M (eds). *Proceedings of the International Seminar on the Immunological System as a Target for Toxic Damage: Present Status, Open Problems and Future Perspectives.* Boston: Martinus Nijhoff, 1987:XI–XXVII.
4. Bates DV. The health effects of air pollution. J Respir Dis 1980;1:29–37.
5. Graham JA, Gardner DE. Immunotoxicity of air pollutants. In: Dean J, Luster MI, Munson AE, Amos H (eds). *Immunotoxicology and Immunopharmacology.* New York: Raven Press, 1985:367–380.
6. Identifying and controlling immunotoxic substances: Background paper. Congress of the United States, Office of Technology Assessment, Landrigan PC, Chairman. Washington, DC: U.S. Government Printing Office, April 1991.
7. Rossi SJ, Schroeder TJ, Hariharan S, Finst MR. Prevention and management of the adverse effects associated with immunosuppressive therapy. Drug Saf 1993;9:104–131.
8. Cote CJ, Meuwissen WJ, Pickering RJ. Effects on the neonate of prednisone and azathioprine administered to the mother during pregnancy. J Pediatr 1974;85:324–328.
9. Wilkinson AH, Smith JL, Hunsicher LG, et al. Increased frequency of posttransplant lymphomas in patients treated with cyclosporin, azathioprine, and prednisone. Transplantation 1989;47:293–296.
10. Cancer following organ transplantation. WHO Drug Info 1991;5:56–59.
11. Walker RW, Brochstein JA. Neurologic complications of immunosuppressive agents. Neurol Clin 1988;6:261–278.

AZATHIOPRINE

Azathioprine is a synthetic purine antagonist used mainly as an immunosuppressant for the prevention of rejection of kidney allografts in conjunction with other immunosuppressive therapy including local radiation therapy, corticosteroids, and cytotoxic agents.[1] Its principal toxic effect in long-term use is bone marrow depression. Massive overdose has been associated with nausea, vomiting, diarrhea, mild leukopenia, mild abnormalities in liver function, and improved renal function in a renal transplant recipient.[2] Azathioprine is metabolized to 6-mercaptopurine (see Chapter 61).

Structure and Classification

Azathioprine is a purine. It is also known as BW 57-322, NSC 39084, azathioprimum, Imuran, Imurel, and other trade names. It is an immunosuppressant and antiinflammatory agent.[3]

Use

Azathioprine is used as an adjunct for the prevention of rejection of kidney allografts. It has also been used in the treatment of rheumatoid arthritis.

Product Formulation

Azathioprine is available for oral use as tablets, 50 mg, with povidone and parenterally for injection in doses of 100 mg.

Therapeutic Dose

The usual initial oral dosage of azathioprine for renal transplantation in children and adults is 3 to 5 mg/kg/d; later, the dosage is decreased 1 to 3 mg/kg/d. For rheumatoid arthritis the initial oral adult dosage is 1 mg/kg/d (approximately 50–100 mg). This may be increased by increments of 0.5 mg every 4 weeks to a maximum of 2.5 mg/kg/d.

Toxic Dose

A toxic overdose of 7500 mg was ingested by a renal transplant patient (see Overdose under Clinical Presentation), resulting in a number of minor transient signs and symptoms (mild vomiting, transient fall in the leukocyte count, and rise in serum bilirubin and transaminases) with ultimate recovery. The manufacturer has knowledge of one unpublished case of an overdose of 850 mg who developed no symptoms or laboratory abnormalities.[4]

Occupational Exposure

Azathioprine and its metabolite 6-mercaptopurine should be considered as cytotoxic waste requiring decontamination (see Treatment).

Toxicokinetics

Absorption

Azathioprine is well absorbed from the gastrointestinal tract and has an oral bioavailability of approximately 60%.[5] Orally administered azathioprine is rapidly divided in vivo to form 6-mercaptopurine.

Distribution

Azathioprine is rapidly cleared from the blood; both azathioprine and mercaptopurine are approximately 30% bound to serum proteins, both appear dialyzable, and both appear to cross the placenta.[1]

Elimination

6-Mercaptopurine undergoes extensive intestinal and hepatic metabolism along three major competing routes. One is thiomethylation, catalyzed by thiopurine methyltransferase (TPMT), an enzyme controlled by a common genetic polymorphism, with 0.33 to 11% of the population having very little enzyme. The second is an oxidation pathway catalyzed by xanthine oxidase, leading to the formation of 6-thiouric acid. The third pathway is catalyzed by the enzyme hypoxanthine phosphoribosyltransferase, leading to 6-thioguanine nucleotides. The cytotoxicity of azathioprine is due, in part, to the incorporation into DNA of 6-thioguanine nucleotides derived from 6-mercaptopurine.[6,7]

The metabolites are excreted in the urine, largely as 6-mercaptopurine. Less than 2% of azathioprine and 20 to 40% of 6-mercaptopurine are excreted as unchanged drugs in the urine. The elimination half-life of azathioprine is approximately 12 to 15 minutes, and that of 6-mercaptopurine is approximately 30 minutes to 4 hours. Total body clearance of azathioprine is 60 mL/min/kg, and that of 6-mercaptopurine, 10 mL/min/kg.[5]

Drug Interactions

Allopurinol inhibits the principal metabolic pathway of azathioprine, the oxidative metabolism of mercaptopurine by xanthine oxidase. This may lead to toxic accumulation of azathioprine with concomitant bone marrow depression.[8]

Pregnancy/Lactation

Azathioprine is teratogenic in animals. Wherever possible its use in pregnant women should be avoided. One retrospective analysis of the outcome of 16 pregnancies in 14 women receiving azathioprine for inflammatory bowel disease revealed no congenital abnormalities or subsequent health problems in the children. This suggests that termination of pregnancy is not mandatory for those who conceive while taking the drug.[9] Neither azathioprine nor its metabolites have been detected in appreciable quantities in breast milk.[10]

Mechanism of Action

Azathioprine inhibits DNA synthesis and, as a purine antimetabolite, exerts its effect on activated lymphocytes, which requires purines during their proliferative phase. It inhibits both cellular and humoral responses, but does not interfere with phagocytosis or interferon production. It is a nonspecific cytotoxic agent.[11] Its immunosuppressive effect is believed to be due to mercaptopurine, to which it is metabolized.

Clinical Presentation

Chronic Use

Therapeutic use may lead to bone marrow depression (leukopenia, anemia, thrombocytopenia, bleeding), hepatic dysfunction (elevated serum bilirubin, alkaline phosphatase, and transaminases, jaundice, hepatic reno-occlusive disease)[11–15] infection, drug fever, rash, urticarial eruption,[16] hypersensitivity vasculitis,[17] nausea, vomiting and diarrhea,[18] and possibly an increase in non-Hodgkin's lymphoma when used with corticosteroids in rheumatoid arthritis.[19,20]

Overdose

An overdose of 7500 mg was ingested by a 44-year-old renal transplant recipient. He vomited and had diarrhea, and his total white blood cell count decreased to 4100/m^3 on the third day after the overdose. Serum transaminase and bilirubin levels increased slightly but returned to normal within 6 days. When azathioprine 50 mg/d was reinstituted, he again experienced a drop in the white blood cell count 3 days later.[2] The manufacturer reported on a patient with an overdose of 850 mg who exhibited no unusual sequelae.[4]

Laboratory

Blood levels of azathioprine are below 1 μg/mL and are transient following ingestion. Measurement of the red blood cell concentration of 6-thioguanine nucleotides may predict bone marrow toxicity.[6,7]

Treatment

The patient should be monitored for airway patency, breathing difficulties, and circulatory stability. Supportive care is the mainstay for management of azathioprine overdose. It is unlikely that early gastric emptying will reduce the rapidly absorbed 6-mercaptopurine metabolite. There is no evidence for the usefulness of gastric emptying, activated charcoal, or whole-bowel irrigation; however, if an attempt is made within the first 30 minutes to 1 hour, gastric emptying may reduce the likelihood of bone marrow depression or hepatotoxicity following an overdose. There are no published experiences to confirm the use of hemodialysis. Treatment is symptomatic.

Occupational Exposure

An area of the body that has been exposed should be thoroughly washed with soap and water, and the soap and water placed in a separate container, properly labeled to distinguish it from other trash. Protective clothing should be worn by personnel involved in a spill and special care taken to decontaminate a spill area and remove the drug from the site of spillage to an approved disposal site.

Supportive Measures

Patients should be periodically monitored for the development of hepatotoxicity (serum bilirubin, alkaline phosphatase, transaminases) and bone marrow depression (including red blood cell, platelet, and white cell counts and red cell 6-thioguanine nucleotide level, if possible).

REFERENCES—AZATHIOPRINE

1. McEvoy GK, ed. *AHFS Drug Information 94.* Bethesda, MD: American Society of Hospital Pharmacists, 1994:2428–2431.
2. Carney DM, Zukoski CF, Ogden DA. Massive azathioprine overdose: Case report and review of the literature. Am J Med 1974;56:133–136.
3. Reynolds JEF, ed. *Martindale: The Extra Pharmacopoeia.* 30th ed. London: Pharmaceutical Press, 1993:457–458.
4. Rocky Mountain Poison Center Staff. Azathioprine/mercaptopurine. Poisindex 1982, 1987, 1989.
5. Dorr RT, Fritz WL. *Cancer Chemotherapy Handbook.* New York: Elsevier, 1980:246–250, 513–518.
6. Lennard L, Van Loon JA, Weinshilboum RM. Pharmacogenetics of acute azathioprine toxicity: Relationship to thiopurine methyl transferase genetic polymorphism. Clin Pharmacol Ther 1989;46:149–154.
7. Klemetsdal B, Tollefsen E, Loennechen T, et al. Interethnic differences in thiopurine methyltransferase activity. Clin Pharmacol Ther 1992;51:24–31.
8. Raman GV, Sharman VL, Lee HA. Azathioprine and allopurinol: A potentially dangerous combination. J Int Med 1990;228:69–71.
9. Alstead EM, Ritchie JK, Lennard-Jones JE, et al. Safety of azathioprine in pregnancy in inflammatory bowel disease. Gastroenterology 1990;99:443–446.
10. Beeley L. Drugs and breast feeding. Clin Obstet Gynecol 1986;13:247–251.
11. James DG. Which immunomodulator? Br J Clin Pract 1991; 45:53–56.
12. Small P, Lichter M. Probable azathioprine hepatotoxicity: A case report. Ann Allergy 1989;62:518–520.
13. Perini GP, Bonadiman C, Fraccaroli GP, Vantini I. Azathioprine-related cholestatic jaundice in heart transplant patients. J Heart Transplant 1990;9:577–578.
14. Katzka DA, Saul SH, Jorkasky D, et al. Azathioprine and hepatic veno-occlusive disease in renal transplant patients. Gastroenterology 1986;90:446–454.
15. Mion F, Napolean B, Berger F, et al. Azathioprine induced liver disease: Nodular regenerative hyperplasia of the liver and perivenous fibrosis in a patient treated for multiple sclerosis. Gut 1991;32:715–717.
16. Wijnands MJ, Perret CM, van Riel PL, van de Putte LB. Generalized urticarial eruption during azathioprine treatment for rheumatoid arthritis. Scand J Rheumatol 1990;19:167–169.
17. Bergman SM, Krane NK, Leonard G, et al. Azathioprine and hypersensitivity vasculitis. Ann Intern Med 1988;109:83–84.
18. Vanderpitte K, Vanrenterghem Y, Michielsen P. Azathioprine hypersensitivity in a renal transplant recipient. Transplant Int 1990;3:47–48.
19. Pitt PI, Sultan AH, Malone M, et al. Association between azathioprine therapy and lymphoma in rheumatoid disease. J R Soc Med 1987;80:428–429.
20. Lawson DH, Lovatt GE, Gurton CS, Hennings RC. Adverse effects of azathioprine. Adverse Drug React Acute Poison Rev 1984;3:161–171.

CYCLOSPORINE

Cyclosporine (Cyclosporin A) is an immunosuppressive medication that is frequently used before and after organ transplants, where it has been effective in suppressing an undesirable immune response.[1,2] Overdose with cyclosporine has been reported following suicidal attempts or inadvertent errors. Oral overdoses of up to 150 mg/kg (10–30 times the recommended values) have led to few overt signs and symptoms (vomiting, drowsiness, headache, and episodic hypertension). Parenteral overdoses may lead to fatalities with renal failure, especially in neonates.[3] All patients except for one premature neonate have survived with the aid of symptomatic and supportive therapy.[3]

Structure and Classification

Cyclosporine is a neutral, lipophilic undecapeptide with a molecular weight of 1203.[2]

Use

Cyclosporine is used for the prevention of rejection of kidney, liver, or heart allografts. Other uses for which cyclosporine is being investigated include plague-type psoriasis, refractory atopic dermatitis, uveitis, rheumatoid arthritis, nephrotic syndrome, Crohn's disease, aplastic anemia, primary biliary cirrhosis, lichen planus, allergic asthma, autoimmune hemolytic anemia, and myasthenia gravis.

Product Formulation

Cyclosporine (Sandimmune) is available as oral, liquid-filled, 25- and 100-mg capsules (with dehydrated alcohol 12.7% v/v) and as a 100 mg/mL solution (with alcohol 12.5%, olive oil, and polyethylene glygol 5-oleate). A parenteral concentrate for injection and intravenous infusion (Sandimmune IV) contains 50 mg/mL (with alcohol 32.9% and polyoxyl 35 castor oil 650 mg/mL).[4] To avoid drug interactions with plasticizers in intravenous solution bags, cyclosporine is dispensed from glass bottles.[2]

Source

Cyclosporine is produced by *Tolypocladinum inflatum* Gams or *Cylindrocarpon lucidum* Booth. It is one of several biologically active antibiotics produced by these fungi.

Therapeutic Dose

For prevention of allograft rejection in adults and children the usual initial dosage of cyclosporine is 15 mg/kg (14–18 mg/kg) administered as a single dose 4 to 12 hours before transplantation. The usual postoperative dosage of 15 mg/kg (range, 14–18 mg/kg) daily administered as a single dose is continued for 1 to 2 weeks and then tapered by 5% per week (over 6–8 weeks) to a maintenance dosage of 5 to 10 mg/kg daily. For those unable to take cyclosporine orally, the usual intravenous dosage for adults and children is 5 to 6 mg/kg administered 4 to 12 hours before transplantation. The usual postoperative intravenous dosage of 5 to 6 mg/kg/d is continued until the patient is able to tolerate the drug orally. Corticosteroids are often used with cyclosporine to prevent an allograft rejection.[4]

Toxic Dose

An adult ingested 25,000 mg over 8 days and survived.[5] Two adults and one child received 5000 mg of cyclosporine each by error and lived.[6–8] A 37-year-old woman took 7500 mg in a suicide attempt and exhibited few symptoms.[9] A 2-year-old received 240 mg, developed hypotension, wheezing, pallor, and tachycardia, and lived.[3] A neonate received 400 mg/kg, developed cyanosis, metabolic acidosis, respiratory depression, and renal failure, and survived.[3] Oral overdoses from 10 to 150 mg/kg were reported with only mild signs of toxicity.[3] An adult received, by error, a 250-mg dose of intravenous cyclosporine in 30 minutes with ornithine–vasopressin and, within 15 minutes, developed anxiety and an irregular weak pulse.[10] An adult accidentally received 30 mg/kg/d (1.1 mg/kg/h) for 33 hours by intravenous infusion; he survived.[11] The highest recorded total dose is approximately 10 g.[3]

Fatal Dose

A premature neonate received 178 mg/kg intramuscularly, developed metabolic acidosis, and renal failure, and subsequently died.[3]

Toxicokinetics

Absorption

Cyclosporine exhibits a two- to three-fold interindividual variation in its absorption and elimination.[12–14] Peak blood and plasma concentrations occur at about 2.5 hours.[15] Following oral administration, cyclosporine is metabolized on first pass through the liver. The absolute bioavailability of orally administered drug is about 35%.[16] Part of this relatively poor oral bioavailability may be due to substantial cyclosporine metabolism by cytochrome P450IIIA found in enterocysts lining the gut. Erythromycin, a known inhibitor of P450IIIA, leads to a steady increase in maximum blood concentrations of oral but not intravenous cyclosporine.[17] Following oral administration of cyclosporine 600 mg a mean peak plasma concentration of 540 ng/mL is reached in 3 to 4 hours.[4] The peak plasma or blood concentration of cyclosporine (high-performance liquid chromatography [HPLC]) is about 1.4 to 2.7 ng/mL/mg of an orally administered dose. The unbound fraction varies between 1 and 2.4% (99 and 97.6% protein bound, mainly to lipoproteins).[13] About 50% of cyclosporine in whole blood is bound to erythrocytes.[18]

Distribution

Clinicians can administer cyclosporine by continuous intravenous infusion during the first few days after transplantation, then orally by twice-daily doses, to achieve plasma cyclosporine concentrations (measured by HPLC) of 75 to 150 ng/mL (equivalent to whole blood cyclosporine concentrations of 300–600 ng/mL measured by radioimmunoassay). It appears safe to maintain a trough plasma cyclosporine concentration of about 75 to 150 ng/mL[19]; however, this does not necessarily guarantee safety from nephrotoxicity.[20] Because of preferential distribution of cyclosporine and its metabolites into red blood cells, blood levels are generally higher than plasma levels. When blood cyclosporine levels are 300 to 600 ng/mL by radioimmunoassay, cerebrospinal fluid levels range from 10 to 50 ng/mL.[21] The apparent volume of distribution in children under 10 years of age is about 35 L/kg, and in adults, 4.7 L/kg.

Elimination

The elimination half-life after an oral cyclosporine dose of 350 mg is 8.9 hours; after a 1400-mg dose, the half-life is 11.9 hours.[22] Elimination occurs predominantly by metabolism in the liver to form 18 to 25 metabolites.[18] Metabolites of cyclosporine possess little immunosuppressive activity.[15,23] Cyclosporine is extensively metabolized in the liver by cytochrome P450IIIA oxidase[24]; however, neurotoxicity and possibly nephrotoxicity usually correlate with raised blood levels of cyclosporine metabolites.[25,26] Only 0.1% of a dose is excreted unchanged.

Table 44-6
Drugs With Clinically Established Effects on Cyclosporine Metabolism

Decrease Metabolism (Increase Blood Cyclosporine Levels)		Increase Metabolism (Decrease Blood Cyclosporine Levels)
Calcium channel blockers		Sulfadimidine
Diltiazem	Sulindac	Phenytoin
Nlfedipine	Sex hormones	Phenobarbital
Verapamil	Corticosteroids	Primidone
Ceftriaxone	Metolazone	Carbamazepine
Erythromycin	Acetazolamide	Rifampin
Norfloxacin	Alcohol	Ethambutol
Ketoconazole	Cimetidine	Isoniazid
Fluconazole	Danazol	Quinine
Ciprofloxacin	Imipenem/cilastin	Griseofulvin
Josamycin	Itraconazole	Rifamycin
Methyltestosterone	Oral contraceptives	Warfarin
Omeprazole	Pristinamycin	Chlorambucil

Drug Interactions

Cyclosporine increases the volume of distribution, half-life, and renally eliminated fraction of digoxin. Cyclosporine potentiates vecuronium blockade and prolongs recovery time.[27] Drugs with clinically established effects on cyclosporine metabolism are listed in Table 44–6.

Pregnancy/Lactation

Cyclosporine crosses the placenta and is distributed into milk.

Mechanism of Action

The predominant immunologic effect of cyclosporine is the inhibition of T-lymphocyte proliferation. Cyclosporine reversibly inhibits activation of the primary helper T cell and the subsequent release of many of its lymphokines. Its use is not associated with myelosuppression. The production and secretion of interleukin-2 are decreased. Cyclosporine also inhibits the production of interferon gamma by lymphocytes. It is able to suppress the delayed-type hypersensitivity reaction.[1]

Clinical Presentation

Clinical responses to cyclosporine overdose vary widely. An adult was given 5000 mg of cyclosporine by error and suffered few toxic effects.[6] Other patients have had headache, nausea, feeling of drunkenness[7]; burning sensation in the mouth, altered taste, hyperesthesia of the hands, burning sensation in the feet, sore gums, flushing of the face, sensation of increased abdominal girth, foot swelling, mild stomach upset[5]; abdominal pain with mild hepatotoxicity[11]; anxiety, diarrhea, vomiting, perspiration[10]; sinus tachycardia[9]; hypertension and headache[28]; vomiting and drowsiness[8]; and transient rise in blood pressure.[29] Premature infants and neonates have developed hypotension, wheezing, pallor, tachycardia, cyanosis, metabolic acidosis, respiratory depression, and renal failure, which ended, in one case, with death[3] (Table 44–7).

Table 44-7
Adverse Effects of Cyclosporine

Adverse Effect	Prevention/Management
Hypertension	1. Dietary sodium restriction 2. Calcium channel blocker* 3. Second agent such as a beta blocker, angiotensin-converting enzyme inhibitor, alpha agonist, peripheral vasodilators
Hyperuricemia	1. Dietary restrictions 2. Urinary alkalinization 3. Allopurinol† or probenecid‡ 4. Colchicine (acute gout attacks)§
Hyperkalemia	1. Dietary restrictions 2. Loop diuretics 3. Sodium polystyrene sulphonate (if serum potassium >6 mmol/L)
Hyperlipidemia	1. Dietary restrictions 2. Steroid reduction or withdrawal 3. HMG-CoA inhibitors 4. Second-line agents (gemfibrozil, nicotinic acid, binding resins)‖
Neurotoxicity	1. Correct electrolyte abnormalities 2. Use oral formulation if possible
Hypertrichosis	1. Avoid agents with similar toxicity (eg, minoxidil)
Gingival hyperplasia	1. Oral hygiene 2. Avoid other agents with similar toxicity (eg, phenytoin, nifedipine)

HMG-CoA, 3-hydroxy-3-methylglutaryl-coenzyme A reductase.
*Diltiazem, verapamil, and nicardipine inhibit the metabolism of cyclosporine.
†Reduce dose of concomitant azathioprine by 50 to 75% and monitor white blood cell count.
‡Probenecid is effective only in patients with a creatinine clearance >50 mL/min (3.0 L/h).
§Closely monitor white blood cell count in patients on colchicine and azathioprine.
‖Toxicity of specific antilipid agents may be compounded in transplant patients.
From Rossi SJ, Schroeder TJ, Hariharan S, First MR. Prevention and management of the adverse effects associated with immunosuppressive therapy. Drug Saf 1993;9:104–131.

Oral Overdose

Healthy persons or those with stable renal function exhibit little or no signs of toxicity. In those with previously impaired renal function, there is a moderate decrease in renal function.

Parenteral Overdose

Premature neonates are apparently at high risk of sustaining serious toxicity, especially metabolic acidosis and renal failure.[3]

Chronic Use

Neurologic Effects. Tremor, burning palmar and plantar paresthesias, headache, flushing, depression, confusion, and somnolence may occur. Seizures of new onset may be triggered by hypocholesterolemia, hypertension (particularly in children), intravenous methylprednisolone therapy, hypomagnesemia, infection, hemorrhage, or cerebral infarction. Visual disorders (including optic disk edema and visual hallucinations), paresis, disorientation, and coma improve when cyclosporine treatment is discontinued. Cyclosporine use in patients undergoing transplantation may induce fever, seizures, altered mental status, cortical blindness, and speech and motor disturbances. Reversible changes in the cerebral white matter may be observed on magnetic resonance imaging.[30] Severe neurotoxicity is observed in transplant patients with elevated serum cyclosporine levels or in patients receiving more than 10 mg/kg/d.[31]

Dermal Effects. Hypertrichosis of the face, arms, shoulders, and back develops in at least 50% of renal transplant recipients given cyclosporine.

Gastrointestinal Effects. Anorexia, bloating, nausea, or vomiting may follow ingestion of the unpalatable suspension of oral cyclosporine. Acute pancreatitis has been reported.

Endocrine Effects. Hyperglycemia, increased serum prolactin, decreased testosterone levels, and gynecomastia in men have been observed.

Hepatotoxicity. Cholestasis with hyperbilirubinemia and elevated transaminase levels are frequently observed.

Nephrotoxicity. Cyclosporine causes at least a 20% reduction in renal function in almost all patients, usually reversed in 2 weeks on discontinuation of therapy. Other drugs may enhance cyclosporine-induced nephrotoxicity (Table 44–8). The risk of nephropathy in patients with autoimmune diseases who are treated with cyclosporine can be minimized by allowing a dose no higher than 5 mg/kg/d and avoiding increases in serum creatinine more than 30% above the patient's baseline value.[32] Acute nephrotoxicity may occur within 7 days of initiation of therapy; subacute toxicity appears at 7 to 60 days with evidence of tubular and glomerular dysfunction; chronic toxicity appears after 30 days (irreversible renal insufficiency).[33]

Myopathy. Cyclosporine may induce myopathies with abnormal electromyograms. Colchicine and lovastatin added to a cyclosporine regimen may enhance such muscular toxicity.[34]

Table 44–8
Drugs Enhancing Cyclosporine-Induced Nephrotoxicity

Drug
Enhancement of Nephrotoxicity Clearly Demonstrated
Aminoglycosides
Amphotericin B
Sulfonamides/trimethoprim
Furosemide (frusemide)
Indomethacin
Mannitol
Ketoconazole
Enhancement of Nephrotoxicity Possible
Cephalosporines (cefotaxime, cefuroxime, cephradine)
Acyclovir
Vancomycin
Etoposide
Captopril

From Scott JP, Higenbottam TW. Adverse reactions and interactions of cyclosporin. Med Toxicol Adverse Drug Experience 1988;3:107–127.

Laboratory

Analytical Methods

Cyclosporine can be measured in the blood by either HPLC or radioimmunoassay.[35] HPLC has been the only specific method available to measure the parent drug, whereas radioimmunoassay measures the parent drug and some of its metabolites. Concentrations of cyclosporine measured by radioimmunoassay in blood are usually about two- to fourfold higher than the corresponding HPLC results. Most medical centers nevertheless prefer to monitor cyclosporine by radioimmunoassay, despite the lack of specificity, because it is more easily performed.[35] A specific radioimmunoassay has been developed that may be used instead of HPLC to measure the parent drug in blood; its limit of detection is about 12 μg/L, and the sample volume required is 50 μgL of blood.[35] Problems may still require confirmation of the usefulness of this assay. An HPLC method has been proposed that measures cyclosporine and its metabolites.[36] A method has been developed to monitor the free fraction of cyclosporine in plasma.[12] The data suggest a decrease in the free fraction of cyclosporine during episodes of acute transplant rejection, but stable free fractions during episodes of acute nephrotoxicity and infection in renal transplant recipients.[12] A radioimmunoassay kit specific for the parent drug has been developed by Sandoz (East Hanover, NJ). Cyclosporine concentrations measured by radioimmunoassay appear to correlate better with nephrotoxicity than those measured by HPLC.[37]

Blood Levels

Reported blood cyclosporine concentrations vary widely due to the heterogenicity of patients, analytical methods, and extraction times, and no direct correlation with clinical symptoms can easily be found. Assuming a therapeutic range of 200 to 800 ng/mL, a neonate with reversible, severe acute renal failure and oliguria was exposed to blood concentrations ranging from 4360 to 13,045 ng/mL and survived.[3] Other neonates with similar symptomatology had peak blood values of 520, 2040, and 2540 ng/mL.[3] The adult who ingested 25,000 mg in 8 days had a whole blood value of 1778 ng/mL.[5] The half-life of the parent compound ranged from 2.5 to 51 hours. These data include the neonates; if they are excluded, the half-life varies from 2.5 to 235 hours after an overdose. An intravenous infusion of 1 mg/kg/h led to a plasma level greater than 4000 ng/mL continuously for 33 hours with a serum half-life of about 30 hours. This was associated with abdominal pain and mild evidence of hepatotoxicity.[11] A 45-year-old ingested 3000 mg (170 mg/kg) of cyclosporine, developed a blood concentration of 190 ng/mL, and recovered.[38]

The report of the American Association for Clinical Chemistry Task Force on Cyclosporine Monitoring recommends whole blood as the preferred assay material and also that the assay method ought to be specific for unchanged drug.[18]

Abnormalities

Renal function is usually not affected by the overdose but is more closely related to the underlying condition of the patient. Serum creatinine exceeding 130% of a patient's pretreatment values may be a useful indicator of incipient cyclosporine nephropathy.[4] Magnetic resonance imaging and computed tomography scans demonstrate symmetric, nonenhancing cortical and/or white matter changes; both clinical and imaging changes are reversible.[39]

Treatment

Stabilization

Oral Overdose. Cyclosporine overdose patients should be admitted to a health care facility where blood pressure, pulse and respiration, and renal function can be monitored. Apparently healthy subjects or patients with stable renal function usually exhibit minor or no signs of toxicity and can be discharged within about 24 hours of disappearance of all symptoms and signs such as hypertension, headache, and diarrhea, and after return to baseline of renal function tests such as serum creatinine, creatinine clearance, and urinalysis.[40]

Parenteral Overdose. Premature neonates have been subject to the few overdoses of cyclosporine reported in the infant age group. They appear to be at high risk of sustaining metabolic acidosis and renal failure. Therefore, on admission to a newborn intensive care facility, preparations must be made to treat metabolic acidosis (arterial blood gases), depressed respiratory function (oxygen, assisted ventilation, intubation), renal failure, and hyponatremia.

Gut Decontamination

The relatively minor clinical picture of toxicity following oral cyclosporine overdose and the absence of a definite correlation between blood levels and clinical severity mitigate against dependence on the blood level for guidance and for the use of strenuous decontamination methods. Cyclosporine has a molecular weight of 1202, only about 30% of the oral dose is absorbed from the gut, and its volume of distribution can be as large as 13.8 L/kg. It is doubtful whether activated charcoal, single or multiple doses, will be useful, but a controlled clinical trial has not been performed. In patients with preexisting altered renal function it may be worthwhile to take measures to reduce the absorption of the drug, such as emesis induction and gastric lavage, although there are few data to support their usefulness.

Prolonged vomiting following induction of emesis may precariously alter fluid balance in a renally compromised patient. Peak serum concentrations in patients who have received an overdose may be delayed to as late as 6 hours after ingestion of the drug.[29] Therefore, an attempt can be made to decrease absorption even if a considerable period has passed since the intake. Multiple-dose oral activated charcoal was associated with a reduction in blood cyclosporine level and half-life in a patient who overdosed with 5000 mg.[6] There is no evidence that cathartics are useful.

Elimination Enhancement

Cyclosporine is highly protein bound and has a high volume of distribution. It is therefore unlikely that extracorporeal methods such as hemodialysis, plasmapheresis, and charcoal hemoperfusion will be effective.[5] Total blood exchange was used to reduce the blood concentration of the parent cyclosporine from 13,045 to 9200 ng/mL in one neonate. The procedure eliminated only 3.25% of the dose ingested.[3] Renal failure in a neonate should be managed by a neonatal nephrology group according to current standards of treatment.

Antidote

There is no antidote for cyclosporine overdose.

Supportive Measures

Serial renal function tests, evaluation of fluid balance and electrolytes, and measurement of arterial blood gases assist in indicating renal status and base balance, especially in an infant who has inadvertently been given an overdose of cyclosporine. Patients with stable renal function can be treated symptomatically and supportively. Hypertension can be evaluated by serial blood pressure measurements, chest x-ray for heart size, evaluation of retinal blood vessels, and urinary catecholamines.

IMMUNOTHERAPEUTIC DRUGS AND BIOLOGICALS

Immunotherapeutic drugs (Table 44–9) and biologicals (Table 44–10) are in clinical use in Europe and Japan.[41] Thymic hormones may increase T-cell number, function, and receptor display and certain aspects of cell-mediated immunity. Lymphokines play a central regulatory role in the cellular immune response. Interferons in high doses inhibit both B- and T-cell proliferation and can decrease humoral and cellular immune responses. At lower doses they stimulate the immune system principally by increasing the cytocidal activity of natural killer cells, macrophages, and T lymphocytes. They may activate microbicidal function. Interferons produce a "flulike" syndrome with fever, malaise, and myalgias. Monoclonal antibodies can fix complement, and can kill human and murine tumors in vivo.

Table 44-9
Immunotherapeutic Drugs

Azimexon
Bestatin
Inosine pranobex
Levamisole hydrochloride
Maleic anhydride, divinyl ether copolymer
Muramyl dipeptides
Pyrimidones
Tuftsin

From Hadden JW. Immunopharmacology: Immunomodulation and immunotherapy. JAMA 1987;258:3005–3010.

Table 44-10
Immunotherapeutic Biologicals

Interferons
Leukocyte extracts/transfer factor
Lymphokines
Interleukin-2
Tumor necrosis factor
Monoclonal antibodies
Thymic hormones
Thymopoietin
Thymosin α_1
Thymulin

From Hadden JW. Immunopharmacology: Immunomodulation and immunotherapy. JAMA 1987;258:3005–3010.

LEVAMISOLE HYDROCHLORIDE

Levamisole hydrochloride appears to reverse anergy in some human cancer patients. It potentiates the stimulation of lymphocytes, granulocytes, and macrophages by such stimuli as antigens, mitogens, lymphokines, and chemotactic factors. Cell-mediated immunity is enhanced more than humoral immunity. Side effects include nausea and vomiting, rash, a flulike syndrome, and a reversible agranulocytosis.

H_2 ANTAGONISTS

H_2 receptor antagonists exhibit immunostimulatory effects (increases in IgM, IgG and interleukin-2 beginning on day 21),[42,43] inhibit suppressor T lymphocytes,[44,45] enhance cell-mediated immunity (increased response to skin test antigens), restore sensitivity following development of acquired tolerance,[45] increase responses of lymphocytes to mutagen stimulation,[46] induce IgE-mediated fever,[47] and enhance deposition of C_3 and IgA in small vessels (vasculitis rash).[48] Inhibition of activity of suppressor T cells or increase in interleukin-2 production in helper T cells may be of sufficient assistance to increase survival in human cancer.[49] Cimetidine, which blocks histamine receptors on the lymphocyte surface, may restore immunoglobulin secretion in patients with common variable immunodeficiency.[50] Complete regression of melanoma modules was observed an a patient treated with ranitidine.[51]

IMMUNOMODULATORS

Immunomodulators may diminish adverse immune reactions, but they may also depress immunity and lower

Table 44-11
Immunomodulators

Name	Manufacturer's Name	Preparation	Dose	Remarks
Azathioprine	Imuran	Tablet 25 mg/50 mg Powder for injection	2 mg/kg	Bone marrow depression
Cyclophosphamide	Endoxana	Tablet 100 mg/200 mg 500 mg Powder for injection	1 mg/kg	Bone marrow depression Hemorrhagic cystitis Azoospermia
Chlorambucil	Leukeran	Tablet 2 mg/5 mg		Bone marrow depression
Cyclosporine	Sandimmune	Capsule 25 mg/100 mg Oral solution 100 mg/mL IV 50 mg/mL	5–10 mg/kg	In combination with steroids Azathioprine and possibly FK 506
FK 506 (tacrolimus)	FK 506 (Japanese)	Oral/intravenous	0.15 mg/kg	In combination with steroids and possibly cyclosporine
Interferons	Intron-A	Solution and powder in vials of 3–30 MU	MU 100 µg/m² body surface or 3–6 MU 3 times weekly	During administration patient suffers "flulike ill health" but it may well be lifesaving
Immunoglobulin	Sandoglobulin Gammabulin Gamimune-N Humotet Intraglobin Gammagard SNBTS IV IgG	Intravenous Intramuscular	0.02–0.12 mL/kg monthly 300 mg/kg monthly	Lifelong monthly replacement therapy keeps at-risk patients free from bacterial infections and back at work

From James DG. Which immunomodulator? Br J Clin Pract 1991;45(1):53–56.

resistance against infection. Some immunomodulators are listed in Table 44–11.[52]

REFERENCES—CYCLOSPORINE AND IMMUNOTHERAPEUTIC DRUGS

1. De Groen PC. Cyclosporin: A review and its specific use in liver transplantation. Mayo Clin Proc 1989;64:680–689.
2. Kahan BD. Cyclosporins. N Engl J Med 1989;321:1725–1738.
3. Avellano F, Monka C, Krupp PF. Acute cyclosporin overdose: A review of present clinical experience. Drug Saf 1991;6:226–276.
4. Cyclosporin. In: McEvoy G, ed. *AHFS Drug Information 94.* Bethesda, MD: American Society of Hospital Pharmacists, 1994:2443–2449.
5. Baumhefner RW, Myers LW, Ellison GW, et al. Huge cyclosporin overdose with favourable outcome. Lancet 1987;2:332.
6. Honcharik N, Anthone S. Activated charcoal in acute cyclosporin overdose. Lancet 1985;1:1051.
7. Schroeder TJ, Wadhawa NK, Pesce AJ, First MR. An acute overdose of cyclosporin. Transplantation 1986;41:406–409.
8. Kruger H-V, Bross-Back V, Proksch B, et al. A case of accidental cyclosporin overdose with pharmacokinetic analysis. Bone Marrow Transplant 1988;3:167–169.
9. Cantineau A, Breurec JY, Baert A, et al. Intoxication aigue volontaire par la ciclosporine. Presse Med 1987;16:589.
10. Wallemacq PE, Lesne ML. Accidental massive IV administration of cyclosporin in man. Drug Intell Clin Pharm 1985;19:29–30.
11. Kokado Y, Takahara S, Ishibashi M, Sonoda T. An acute overdose of cyclosporin. Transplantation 1989;47:1096–1097.
12. Lindholm A. Monitoring of the free concentration of cyclosporin in plasma in man. Eur J Clin Pharmacol 1991;40:571–575.
13. Lindholm A, Henricsson S. Intra- and interindividual variability in the free fraction of cyclosporin in plasma in recipients of renal transplants. Ther Drug Monit 1989;11:230–623.
14. Clandy CW, Schroeder TJ, Myre SA, et al. Clinical variability of cyclosporin pharmacokinetics in adult and pediatric patients after renal, cardiac, hepatic and bone-marrow transplants. Clin Chem 1988;34:2012–2015.
15. Frey FJ, Horber FF, Frey BM. Trough levels and concentration time curves of cyclosporin in patients undergoing renal transplantation. Clin Pharmacol Ther 1988;43:550–562.
16. Wandstrat TL, Schroeder TJ, Myre SA. Cyclosporin pharmacokinetics in pediatric transplant recipients. Ther Drug Monit 1989;11:493–496.
17. Kolars JC, Awni WM, Merior RM, Watkins PG. First-pass metabolism of cyclosporin by the gut. Lancet 1991;338:1488–1490.
18. Grevel J. Significance of cyclosporin pharmacokinetics. Transplant Proc 1988;20(suppl. 2) :428–434.
19. Lui SF, Varghese Z, Sweny P, et al. Blood cyclosporin concentrations and renal allograft dysfunction. Br Med J 1986;293:1435.
20. Henry ML, Bowers VD, Fanning WJ, et al. Cyclosporin levels are not helpful. Transplant Proc 1988;20(suppl. 2):419–421.
21. Scharan HF, Hassell AE, Baumhefner RW, et al. Distribution of cyclosporin in cerebrospinal fluid. Neurology 1988;38(suppl. 1):99.
22. Reymond J-P, Steimer J-L, Niederberger W. On the dose dependency of cyclosporin A absorption and disposition in healthy volunteers. J Pharmacokinet Biopharm 1988;16:331–351.
23. Copeland KR, Yatscoff RW, McKenna RM. Immunosuppressive activity of cyclosporin metabolites compared and characterized by mass spectroscopy and nuclear magnetic resonance. Clin Chem 1990;36:225–229.
24. Lucey MR, Kolars JC, Merion RM, et al. Cyclosporin toxicity at therapeutic blood levels and cytochrome P-450 III A. Lancet 1990;335:11–15.
25. Kunzendorg V, Brocmoller J, Jochimsen F, et al. Cyclosporin metabolites and central nervous system toxicity. Lancet 1988;1:1223.
26. Leunissen KML, Beuman G-H, Bosman F, Van Hooff JP. Cyclosporin metabolites and nephrotoxicity. Lancet 1986;2:1398.
27. Sharpe MD, Gelb AW. Cyclosporin potentiates vecuronium blockade and prolonged recovery time in humans. Can J Anaesth 1992;39(5,pt II):A126.
28. De Ligny BH, Camsonne R, Ryckelynck JP, et al. Intoxication aigue par la ciclosporine. Presse Med 1987;16:830.
29. De Meer K, Houwen RHJ, Bijleveld CMA, et al. Blood concentrations after accidental cyclosporin overdose. Eur J Pediatr 1989;149:219–220.
30. Truwitt CL, Denaro CP, Lake JR, DeMarco T. MR imaging of reversible cyclosporin A-induced neurotoxicity. Am J Radiol 1991;157:857–859.
31. Humphreys TR, Leyden JJ. Acute reversible central nervous system toxicity associated with low-dose oral cyclosporin therapy. J Am Acad Dermatol 1993;29:490–492.
32. Feutren G, Mihatsch MJ. Risk factors for cyclosporin-induced nephropathy in patients with autoimmune diseases. N Engl J Med 1992;326:1654–1660.
33. Shannon M. Cyclosporin. Clin Toxicol Rev 1993;15(1):1–2.
34. Goy J-J, Deruaz JP, Avellano F, Krupp P. Cyclosporin and muscle. Lancet 1992;339:254.
35. Ball PE, Munzer H, Keller HP, et al. Specific ^3H radioimmunoassay with a monoclonal antibody for monitoring cyclosporin in blood. Clin Chem 1988;34:257–260.
36. Christians U, Schlitt HJ, Bleck JS, et al. Measurement of cyclosporin and 18 metabolites in blood, bile, and urine by high performance liquid chromatography. Transplant Proc 1988;20(suppl. 2):609–613.
37. Yee GC, Rosano T, Ptachcinski R. Pharmacology: Profiles, parameters, interpretations and drug interactions. Transplant Proc 1988;20(suppl. 2):715–721.
38. Anderson AB, Primack W. Treatment of a child with acute cyclosporin overdose. Pediatr Nephrol 1992;6:222–223.
39. Pace MT, Slovins TL, Kelly JK, Abella SD. Cyclosporin A toxicity: MRI appearance of the brain. Pediatr Radiol 1995;25:180–183.
40. Feutren G, Mason J. Serum creatinine or glomerular filtration rate for monitoring cyclosporin therapy. Lancet 1991;338:1017.
41. Hadden JW. Immunopharmacology: Immunomodulation and immunotherapy. JAMA 1987;258:3005–3010.
42. Aweeka F, Amend W, Garavoy M, et al. The effects of H_2 antagonists in immunological function. Clin Pharmacol Ther 1988;43:128.
43. Gifford RRM, Tilberg AF. Histamine type-2 receptor antagonist immune modulation: II. Cimetidine and ranitidine increase interleukin-2 production. Surgery 1987;102:242–247.
44. Sahasrabudhe DM, McCuine CS, O'Donnell RW, Henshaw EC. Inhibition of suppressor T lymphocytes by cimetidine. J Immunol 1987;138:2760–2763.
45. Mavligit GM. Immunologic effects of cimetidine: Potential uses. Pharmacotherapy 1987;7 (6, pt 2):120S–124S.
46. Kumar A. Cimetidine: An immunomodulator. DICP Ann Pharmacother 1990;24:289–295.
47. Hiraide A, Yoshioka T, Ohshima S. IgE-mediated drug fever due to histamine H_2-receptor blockers. Drug Saf 1990;5:455–457.
48. Haboubi N, Asquith P. Rash mediated by immune complexes associated with ranitidine treatment. Br Med J 1988;296:897.
49. Tonnessen H, Bulow S, Fischerman K, et al. Effect of cimetidine on survival after gastric cancer. Lancet 1988;2:990–992.
50. White WB, Ballow M. Modulation of suppressor-cell activity by cimetidine in patients with common variable hypogamma globulinuria. N Engl J Med 1985;312:198–202.
51. Smith T, Clark JW, Popp MB. Regression of melanoma nodules in a patient treated with ranitidine. Arch Intern Med 1987;1815–1816.
52. James DG. Which immunomodulator? Br J Clin Pract 1991;45:52–56.

TACROLIMUS

Tacrolimus (FK 506) is a macrolide immunosuppressant used in transplant surgery. It was entered into clinical trials in the United States in human liver transplantation in February 1989.[1] It is currently under investigation in the United States, Europe, and Japan for prevention of organ transplant rejection.[2] Excessively high plasma levels of tacrolimus may be associated with renal dysfunction and neurotoxicity.

Structure and Classification

Tacrolimus belongs to the macrolide group of compounds, which includes erythromycin, spiramycin, and rapamycin.[3]

Use

Tacrolimus is an immunosuppressive agent used to prevent organ transplant rejection. It has also been used effectively in some autoimmune diseases such as cyclosporine-induced hemolytic–uremic syndrome,[4] severe recalcitrant psoriasis,[5] refractory uveitis including Behcet's disease,[6] and type I diabetes mellitus.[7]

Source

Tacrolimus is a macrolide compound produced by *Streptomyces tsukubaensis.*

Therapeutic Dose

For human organ transplantation tacrolimus has been used as a primary immunosuppressive agent in a single intravenous dose of 0.15 mg/kg over 1 to 2 hours on the first day, and 0.075 mg/kg intravenously at 12-hour intervals on the second or third day.[8] Other dosage schedules call for 0.05 mg/kg infused over each 12-hour period for the first 3 days, followed by oral doses of 0.15 mg/kg every 12 hours thereafter.[9] A dose of 2 to 24 mg/d is required to maintain therapeutic plasma trough concentrations (0.5–2.0 ng/mL).[10] Oral therapy is started on the fourth day with a dose of 0.15 mg/kg twice daily. The dosage should be altered according to trough plasma levels.[8] Good cardiac allograft function and quality of life in adults and children have followed maintenance doses of 0.2 to 0.4 mg/kg/d tacrolimus as primary immunosuppressive.[11]

Toxicokinetics

Absorption

Following oral administration tacrolimus is poorly absorbed.[12] An oral dose of 0.15 mg/kg results in a peak plasma concentration of 0.4 to 3.7 ng/mL, which is reached in 0.5 to 4 hours.[10] Trough levels of tacrolimus range from less than 0.1 ng/mL to nearly 5 ng/mL after an oral dose of 0.15 mg/kg/d.[8] The mean bioavailability is 25%.[8,13] After intravenous administration of 0.15 mg/kg over 2 hours, the peak plasma level reached is 10 to 24 ng/mL. Desired plasma concentrations are 0.5 to 1.5 ng/mL.[10,13]

Distribution

The mean apparent volume of distribution is about 19 L/kg, indicating extensive tissue distribution of tacrolimus.[10,12] Erythrocytes concentrate tacrolimus so that whole blood values are higher than plasma values (whole blood:plasma ratio, 11:50).[9] α_1-Acid glycoprotein is the main circulating binding protein for tacrolimus.[14]

Elimination

The intravenous elimination half-life varies from 3.5 to 40.5 hours.[8,13] Less than 1% of an intravenous or oral dose of tacrolimus is excreted in the urine. The drug is completely metabolized before elimination.[13] Tacrolimus, like cyclosporine, is eliminated mainly by hepatic cytochrome P450IIIA metabolism.[15] The total body clearance ranges from 7 to 103 mL/min/kg. Renal clearance is less than 1 mL/min.[10]

Drug Interactions

An increase in tacrolimus concentration has also been observed with inhibitors such as ketoconazole, fluconazole, erythromycin, diltiazem, and cimetidine.[16]

Cyclosporine. When tacrolimus is added to cyclosporine therapy, the half-life of oral cyclosporine may increase.[12] Tacrolimus and cyclosporine exhibit a synergistic nephrotoxic effect.[10]

Methylprednisolone. Methylprednisolone induces an increase in plasma tacrolimus concentration in some patients. The exact mechanism of interaction is not known.[10,12] Erythromycin, fluconazole, clotrimazole, and danazol can raise the plasma tacrolimus level.[13,17] Inhibitors of hepatic metabolism require a decrease in the dose of tacrolimus with careful monitoring of blood concentration.

Mechanism of Action

Tacrolimus suppresses cell-mediated and humoral responses.[15] In vivo assays show that tacrolimus is a more potent inhibitor of lymphoproliferation than cyclosporine: it takes 24 mg/kg cyclosporine to induce the same suppression as 3 mg/kg tacrolimus.[18]

Tacrolimus, unlike cyclosporine, does not inhibit the activity of peptidyl-prolyl *cis–trans* isomerase or the phosphate-mediated release of calcium from the mitochondria.[19] In vitro, tacrolimus suppresses the immune response by interfering with the synthesis of interleukin-2 and other lymphokines.[20] It prevents the activation of T lymphocytes in response to antigenic or mitogenic stimulation.[21]

Tacrolimus may ameliorate cyclosporine-induced hypertension, possibly through a reduction in peripheral vascular resistance.[22] In a group of liver transplant patients there appeared to be a significantly lower incidence of overall infection following use of tacrolimus than in a similar group treated with cyclosporine.[23] Nevertheless, 23 of 110 consecutive liver transplant recipients acquired cytomegalovirus infection, and infection remains a common cause of death.[15] No acute hemodynamic disturbance or dysrhythmia has followed intravenous infusion of the drug in human liver transplant recipients.[24]

Clinical Presentation

Chronic Use

Most adverse effects following tacrolimus use are associated with intravenous therapy; few symptoms occur with oral tacrolimus.[25]

In humans the primary toxic effects of tacrolimus are, in order of decreasing frequency, insomnia, tremors, headaches, tingling sensations, muscle achiness, itching, fatigue, visual sensitivity to light, and gastrointestinal symptoms.[15,26] These symptoms usually disappear on conversion from intravenous to oral therapy. Few patients on oral therapy experience these symptoms. When intravenous tacrolimus is used as rescue therapy (eg, liver grafts undergoing rejection despite conventional treatment) intravenous cyclosporine has usually been given. These patients tend to experience a higher incidence of headache, nausea, and hyperesthesia than the primary treatment group. Flushing, itching, tremor, anorexia, shortness of breath, abdominal cramps, night sweats, photophobia, and blurred vision may be observed. The frequency and severity of these effects decline when cyclosporine is eliminated and tacrolimus is converted to oral use.[25] Hypertrophic cardiomyopathy has been observed in children and adults.[27]

The principal adverse effects of tacrolimus—nephrotoxicity (often the dose-limiting factor), infectious complications such as Epstein–Barr virus,[28] neurotoxicity (Table 44–12), and diabetes—are similar to those of cyclosporine.[13] Posttransplant lymphoproliferation disorders have been reported in liver transplant patients given tacrolimus alone or with other immunosuppressants.[2,13,29,30] Most lymphoproliferative disorders occur during the first year posttransplantation.[22]

Large cell malignant lymphoma that developed at a trough plasma tacrolimus concentration of 0.4 to 1 ng/mL regressed at a reduced dosage of tacrolimus sufficient to maintain trough plasma concentrations of 0.1 to 0.25 ng/mL.[28] Toxic blood tacrolimus levels (4.4, 5.2, and 2.1 ng/mL) were associated with cerebral infarction in three of four children who had developed this complication following tacrolimus use after organ transplantation.[31]

Table 44–12
Neurologic Side Effects of Tacrolimus

Major	Minor
Akinetic mutism	Tremors
Seizures	Headache
Psychosis	Sleep disturbances
Encephalopathy	Nightmares
Focal deficits	Vertigo
Movement disorder	Dysesthesia
	Mood changes
	Photophobia

From Eidelman BH, Abu-Elmagd K, Wilson J, et al. Neurologic complications of FK 506. Transplant Proc 1991;23:3175–3178.

Overdose

Overdose leading to profound immunosuppression and severe infection remains a serious hazard. Infections have often contributed to deaths.[13] Tacrolimus in its initial experiences appeared to cause less hypertension, less hypercholesterolemia, use of less steroid, relative absence of hirsutism and gum hyperplasia, and better quality of life when compared with cyclosporine.[13] Ingestion of up to 375 mg of tacrolimus produced minimal signs and symptoms in one series of four patients.[32]

Neurologic complications (Table 44–12) following tacrolimus appear to be correlated with blood levels.[33] Mild tremulousness is the most common finding, but akinetic mutism is prominent. Cerebral infarctions following tacrolimus use in patients receiving organ transplantation may present with headache and seizures, less often with seizures alone, or with the sudden onset of agitation, confusion, and right gaze preference.[31]

Laboratory

Analytical Methods

Plasma tacrolimus levels are quantitated by an enzyme immunoassay using a mouse monoclonal anti-tacrolimus antibody (Fujisawa Pharmaceuticals, Osaka, Japan).[34] The sensitivity of the enzyme immunoassay is 0.1 ng/mL. This assay may measure both tacrolimus and its metabolites.[35] An enzyme-linked immunosorbent assay method attempts to minimize cross-sensitivities.[14] A whole blood assay sensitive to 3.3 ng/mL is available.[36]

Blood Levels

Monitoring of whole blood is considered preferable to monitoring of plasma because of the rapid distribution of tacrolimus to red cells.[37] Elevated blood levels may be correlated with nephrotoxicity.[38] Peak trough tacrolimus plasma levels greater than 3 ng/mL have been associated with neurotoxic effects.[33] Blood levels of tacrolimus were considered toxic in three of four patients with cerebral infarctions (4.4, 5.2, and 2.1 ng/mL).[31]

Abnormalities

Tacrolimus is a nephrotoxin; cyclosporine may also cause a deterioration of renal function.

Ancillary Tests

Hyperkalemia may be observed during tacrolimus therapy and is usually associated with low or low-normal renin and aldosterone levels (hyporeninemic hypoaldosteronism).[8] Hyperkalemic patients may have associated elevated serum creatinine levels. Impaired glucose tolerance has been observed.[39] Serum uric acid levels tend to be elevated.[40] Similar to cyclosporine, tacrolimus induces a significant decline in total serum cholesterol levels.[40] A dose-related rise in serum creatinine may be observed. Computed tomography scans or magnetic resonance imaging may be used to demonstrate focal cerebral infarctions.[31]

Treatment

Stabilization

Toxic effects of tacrolimus requiring treatment include alterations in kidney function, alterations in glucose metabolism, neurotoxicity, and susceptibility to infection or malignancy. Toxicity generally improves with reduction of the dose of tacrolimus. Treatment is largely symptomatic and supportive.

Elimination Enhancement

As tacrolimus is highly lipid soluble with a high apparent volume of distribution, it is unlikely to be dialyzable.[10] There is no evidence to support the use of whole-bowel irrigation or cathartics after an inadvertent overdose of tacrolimus.

Antidote

There is no antidote for tacrolimus overdose.

Supportive Measures

Hyperkalemia has responded to treatment with fludrocortisone acetate.[25,26]

REFERENCES—TACROLIMUS (FK 506)

1. Starzl TE, Todo S, Fung J. FK 506 for liver, kidney and pancreas transplantation. Lancet 1989;2:1000–1004.
2. FK 506: An investigation immunosuppressant. Med Lett Drugs Ther 1991;33(854):94.
3. Goto T, Kino T, Hatanaka H, et al. FK 506: Historical perspectives. Transplant Proc 1991;23:2713–2717.
4. McCauley J, Bronsther O, Fung J, et al. Treatment of cyclosporin-induced haemolytic uremic syndrome with FK 506. Lancet 1989;2:1516.
5. Abu-Elmagd K, Van Thiel D, Jegasothy BV, et al. FK 506: A new therapeutic agent for severe recalcitrant psoriasis. Transplant Proc 1991;23:3322–3324.
6. Japanese FK 506 Study Group on Refractory Uveitis. A multicenter clinical open trial of FK 506 in refractory uveitis following Behcet's disease. Transplant Proc 1991;23:3343–3346.
7. Carroll PB, Tzakis AG, Ricordi C, et al. The use of FK 506 in new-onset type 1 diabetes in man. Transplant Proc 1991; 23:3351–3353.
8. Li PKT, Nicholls MG, Lai KN. The complications of newer transplant antirejection drugs: Treatment with cyclosporin A, OKT3 and FK 506. Adverse Drug React Acute Poison Rev 1990;9:123–155.
9. Jusko WJ, D'Ambrosio R. Monitoring FK 506 concentrations in plasma and whole blood. Transplant Proc 1991;23: 2732–2735.
10. Venkataramanan R, Jain A, Warty VS, et al. Pharmacokinetics of FK 506 in transplant patients. Transplant Proc 1991;23: 2736–2740.
11. Thomson AW, Woo J. Immunosuppressive properties of FK 506 and rapamycin. Lancet 1989;2:443–444.
12. Venkataramanan R, Jain A, Codoff E, et al. Pharmacokinetics of FK 506: Preclinical and clinical studies. Transplant Proc 1990;22(No. 1, suppl. 1):52–56.
13. Nossal GJV. Summary of the First International FK 506 Congress: Perspectives and prospects. Transplant Proc 1991;23:3371–3375.
14. Kobayashi M, Tamura K, Katayama N, et al. FK 506 assay past and present: Characteristics of FK 506. Elisa Transplant Proc 1991;23:2725–2729.
15. Macleod AM, Thomson AW. FK 506: An immunosuppressant for the 1990's? Lancet 1991;337:25–27.
16. Wallemacq PE, Reding R. FK 506 (tacrolimus). Clin Chem 1993;39:2219–2228.
17. Shapiro R, Venkatataramanan R, Warty US, et al. FK 506 interaction with danazol. Lancet 1993;341:1344–1345.
18. Morris RE, Wu J, Shorthouse R. Comparative immunopharmacologic effects of FK 506 and CyA in in vivo models of organ transplantation. Transplant Proc 1990;22(No. 1, suppl. 1):110–112.
19. Fischer G, Wittman-Liebold B, Lang K, et al. Cyclosphilin and peptidyl-prolyl *cis–trans* isomerase are probably identical proteins. Nature 1981;337:476–478.
20. Thomson AW. FK 506: How much potential? Immunol Today 1989;10:6–9.
21. Sawada S, Suziki G, Kawase Y, Takakre F. Novel immunosuppressive agent FK 506: In vitro effects on the cloned T cell activation. J Immunol 1987;139:1797–1803.
22. McCauley J, Fung J, Jain A, et al. The effects of FK 506 on renal function after liver transplantation. Transplant Proc 1990;22(No. 1, suppl. 1):17–20.
23. Alessiani M, Kusne S, Martin FM, et al. Infections with FK 506 immunosuppression: Preliminary results with primary therapy. Transplant Proc 1990;22(No. 1, suppl. 1): 44–46.
24. Lai KN. Adverse effects of immunosuppressant agents. Adverse Drug React Bull 1991(December):No. 151:510.
25. Shapiro R, Fung JJ, Jain AB, et al. The side effects of FK 506 in humans. Transplant Proc 1990;22(No. 1, suppl. 1): 35–36.
26. Fung JJ, Alessiani M, Abu-Elmagd K, et al. Adverse effects associated with the use of FK 506. Transplant Proc 1991;23: 3105–3108.
27. Brand PLD, Brus F. Immunosuppressive drugs and hypertrophic cardiomyopathy. Lancet 1995;345:1644.
28. Cox KL, Lawrence-Miyasaki LS, Garcia-Kennedy R, et al. An increased incidence of Epstein–Barr virus infection and lymphoproliferative disorder in young children on FK 506 after liver transplantation. Transplantation 1995;59:524–529.
29. Kitahara S, Makuuchi M, Kawasaki S, et al. Lymphoproliferative disorders after FK 506. Lancet 1991;337:1234.
30. Nalensnik MA, Demetris AJ, Fung JJ, Strazel TE. Lymphoproliferative disorders arising under immunosuppression with FK 506: Initial observations in a large transplant population. Transplant Proc 1991;23:1108–1110.
31. Barabas RE, Painter MJ. Cerebral vasculopathy in patients receiving organ transplantation who are treated with FK 506. Ann Neurol 1991;30:472. Abstract.
32. Mrvos R, Hodgman M, Dean B, Krenzelok E. FK 404 overdose: A report of four cases. Clin Toxicol 1995;33:475–486. Abstract.
33. Eidelman BH, Abu-Elmagd K, Wilson J, et al. Neurologic complications of FK 506. Transplant Proc 1991;23: 3175–3178.
34. Cadoff EM, Venkataramanan R, Krajack A, et al. Assay of FK 506 in plasma. Transplant Proc 1990;22(No. 1, suppl. 1): 50–51.
35. Sewing K-F, Christians U. FK 506. Lancet 1991;337:499.
36. Grenier FC, Luczkiw J, Bergmann M, et al. A whole blood FK 506 assay for the IMx[R] analyzer. Transplant Proc 1991;23: 2748–2749.
37. Beysens AJ, Wijnen RMH, Beuman GH, et al. FK 506 monitoring in plasma or in whole blood? Transplant Proc 1991;23: 2745–2747.
38. Winkler M, Jost V, Ringe B, et al. Association of elevated FK 506 plasma levels with nephrotoxicity in liver-grafted patients. Transplant Proc 1991;23:3153–3155.
39. Mieles L, Todo S, Fung JJ, et al. Oral glucose tolerance test in liver recipients treated with FK506. Transplant Proc 1990;22(No. 1, suppl. 1):41–43.
40. Van Thiel DH, Iqbal M, Jain A, et al. Gastrointestinal and metabolic problems associated with immunosuppression with either CyA or FK 506 in liver transplantation. Transplant Proc 1990;22(No. 1, suppl. 1):37–40.

MUROMONAB-CD3

Muromonab-CD3 (Orthoclone OKT3) is a potent immunosuppressive agent which provokes a severe systemic reaction after a first dose that can be fatal. Toxic effects may relate to dose. Long-term effects include posttransplantation lymphoproliferative disorders, neoplasms, and infections.

Structure and Classification

Muromonab-CD3 is a biochemically purified IgG_{2a} consisting of a heavy chain of approximately 50,000 daltons and a light chain of approximately 25,000 daltons. It is manufactured by a process involving the fusion of mouse myeloma cells to lymphocytes from immunized animals to produce a hybridoma that secretes antigen-specific antibodies to the T_3 antigen of human T lymphocytes. Trivial names used to identify the preparation include murine monoclonal antibody, anti-CD3, and human T-cell inhibitor. Commercially it is available as Orthoclone OKT3.[1]

Use

Muromonab-CD3 is useful as an effective immunosuppressive agent in acute allograft rejection (eg, kidney, heart, and liver) and in graft-versus-host disease.[2] It is used as salvage therapy in patients with steroid-resistant or anti-lymphocyte globulin-resistant organ rejections.[3,4] The prophylactic use of muromonab-CD3 alone in transplant recipients has resulted in the rapid production of IgG anti-OKT_3 antibodies, which can neutralize OKT3 and allow acute rejection to develop. When muromonab-CD3 is combined with azathioprine, steroid, and cyclosporine, there may be fewer rejection episodes.[5]

Product Formulation

Muromonab-CD3 (Orthoclone OKT_3) is available as a solution (1 mg/mL). The solution is filtered before use and is injected intravenously as a bolus.

Therapeutic Dose

The currently recommended dose of muromonab-CD3 in the treatment of acute allograft reaction is 5 mg/d for 10 to 14 days.[6] A sample protocol with precautions is provided in Table 44–13.

Toxicokinetics

Absorption

Over the first 4 hours after initial intravenous administration, serum levels of muromonab-CD3 decline approximately 60% from a peak level of about 1 μg/mL due to the rapid binding of muromonab-CD3 to the T-cell pool.[7] Subsequent dosing of muromonab-CD3 gives rise to an apparent steady-state 24-hour trough level of approximately 1000 ng/mL.[8] In vitro, plasma muromonab-CD3 levels of 1000 ng/mL can block the killing of specific targets by cytotoxic T cells.[9] Anti-OKT_3 antibodies may prevent a serum level of OKT_3 from developing.[8]

Table 44–13
Sample Protocol for the Administration of Muromonab-CD3

Protocol	Comment
Daily dose	
>30 kg IBW	5.0 mg IV
<30 kg IBW	2.5 mg IV
Premedication	1 g methylprednisolone IV 6–12 h before first dose of muromonab-CD3 **or** 1 g hydrocortisone IV 1 h prior to first dose
	Acetaminophen 10 gr PO or PR and diphenhydramine 50 mg PO or IV 30 min prior to first dose
Precautions	Have emergency crash cart outside the patient's room for first two doses
	After first two doses, assess vital signs every 15 min for first 2 h; then every 20 min for next 2 h; then per routine monitoring procedures
	After subsequent doses monitor vital signs after routine procedures
	Evaluate chest radiograph after first doses

IBW, ideal body weight.
From Hooks MA, Wade CS, Millikan WJ Jr. Muromonab CD 3: A review of its pharmacology, pharmacokinetics, and clinical use in transplantation. Pharmacotherapy 1991;11:26–37.

Distribution

The apparent volume of distribution is approximately 0.93 L/kg.[7]

Elimination

Muromonab-CD3 is eliminated mostly by binding to the T-cell population and forming complexes with the antigen CD3. The elimination half-life of muromonab-CD3 has been estimated to be 18 hours.[7]

Mechanism of Action

Muromonab-CD3 is a murine monoantibody (mAb) directed to lymphocytes with CD3 antigen on the T-cell surface.[9] It reacts specifically with the CD3 antigen recognition structure and modulates the CD3 complex, deleting it from the membrane of T lymphocytes, thus rendering the cells immunologically impotent.[10] In vivo it efficiently clears circulatory T cells; within minutes of muromonab-CD3 infusion they become undetectable.[11] The therapeutic effectiveness of muromonab-CD3 in reversing acute organ rejection appears related to its ability to block killing of the allograft by host cytotoxic T cells. Initially, after the first dose, however, muromonab-CD3 actually activates lymph node production of T cells.[12]

First-Dose Reaction

Within 1 hour of administration, there is a rise in plasma and serum levels of interleukin-2, interferon gamma, and tumor necrosis factor α, a "cytokine release syndrome" which may reflect T-cell stimulation.[10,11,13] In addition, T cells expressing antigens CD3, CD4, CD8, CD38, and CD58 disappear from the circulation within 2 hours of muromonab-CD3 administration.[10] Interleukin-2 may induce an increase in endothelial permeability leading to a vascular leak syndrome and focal edema by its production of other cytokines (interleukin-1, tumor necrosis factor α, lymphotoxins, and interferon gamma).[2,14]

Aseptic Meningitis

The etiology of aseptic meningitis is uncertain. Destruction of circulatory T cells may cause release of substances that attract lymphocytes into the cerebrospinal fluid and induce inflammation.[15]

Clinical Presentation

First-Dose Systemic Reactions

The first dose of muromonab-CD3 and, to a lesser extent, the second injection induce in 50 to 80% of patients a symptom complex that does not occur with subsequent injections.[6] Within 45 minutes to 2 hours of the first injection, symptoms, lasting several hours, begin, with responses ranging in severity from very mild to life-threatening.[10,13] Deaths have been reported during this period.[13] Typically, the symptom complex includes some combination of fever, chills, dyspnea/wheezing, tachycardia, hypotension, and nausea and vomiting. Hypertension may be associated with a state of relative fluid overload at the time of initial muromonab-CD3 treatment.[8] Hypertensive emergencies may require treatment.[16] A second dose may induce periorbital edema, a petechial rash, and severe dyspnea.[8,17]

Days 2 to 5

On the second to fifth days of treatment, symptoms referable to the gastrointestinal tract (nausea, vomiting, diarrhea) and the central nervous system (headache, rarely aseptic meningitis, seizures) may manifest. These are self-limited and resolve in 2 to 4 days.[8] Neurotoxicity does not recur with subsequent treatment.[18]

Aseptic Meningitis

Aseptic meningitis may begin within 72 hours of starting muromonab-CD3 treatment and resolves over a few days without treatment even if muromonab-CD3 is continued for the standard 10- to 14-day protocol.[8,18–22] Fever is often present, and meningeal signs may be absent[23]; symmetric hyperreflexia and mental status changes may be the only signs.[23]

Seizures

Generalized seizures occur in about 6% of patients receiving muromonab-CD3. Encephalopathy can be distinguished from aseptic meningitis.[24] Aseptic meningitis, encephalopathy, and seizures are the most common neurologic complications associated with muromonab-CD3. Fever and hypocalcemia may be risk factors for muromonab-CD3-induced seizures. Additional risk factors include acute tubular necrosis, hyponatremia, fluid overload (2-kg gain), hypertension and hypoglycemia,[8] cerebritis,[2] photophobia,[19] encephalopathy (obtundation, quadriparesis),[25] and cerebral edema.[26]

Pulmonary Edema

Pulmonary edema may be related to left ventricular failure due to increased afterload.[13] Hypervolemic patients are at risk for developing both pulmonary edema and hypertension.[17] Two deaths have occurred due to anoxic sequelae of pulmonary edema after the initial injection of muromonab-CD3.[13] Cardiac arrest has been reported.[3]

Infections

Patients on muromonab-CD3 may develop fungal, bacterial, and viral infections (cytomegalovirus, herpes simplex virus, Epstein–Barr virus) within weeks of use.[6]

Anti-OKT3 Antibodies

Immunoglobulin G anti-OKT3 antibodies may develop during or after muromonab-CD3 (a xenogeneic protein) therapy. Such antibodies have a neutralizing effect on the immunosuppressive capacity of muromonab-CD3.[6]

Posttransplantation Lymphoproliferative Disorder

Posttransplantation lymphoproliferative (PTLP) disorder is a well-recognized, frequently fatal complication of immunosuppression. The risk of PTLP disorder rises sharply after cumulative doses above 75 mg of muromonab-CD3 have been added to a multiple-immunosuppressive-drug regimen.[27–29] The Epstein–Barr virus may have an important role in the pathogenesis of PTLP disorder.[27,29,30] Lymphomas may constitute up to 64% of neoplasms occurring when muromonab-CD3 is added to a multiple-immunosuppressive-agent regimen.[31] Most occur within 4 months of therapy.

Intraoperative Muromonab-CD3

Muromonab-CD3 administered intraoperatively may lead to severe bradycardia, atrioventricular block, hypotension, and a decrease in arterial hemoglobin saturation.[32] Risk factors include a high dose (on a mg/kg basis), concomitant administration of drugs that decrease cardiac contractility (eg, phenytoin, beta blockers, calcium channel blockers, volatile anesthetic agents), and hypovolemia.

Anaphylactic Reactions

Dyspnea, hypotension, urticarial rash, wheezing, and diaphoresis may follow an intravenous bolus.[33]

Laboratory

Analytical Methods

Plasma muromonab-CD3 levels can be measured by a sandwich enzyme-linked immunosorbent assay.[34] Anti-OKT3 antibodies can be detected by immunofluorescence or immunochemical assays.[6]

Ancillary Tests

Pleocytosis (predominantly lymphocytes)[35] of the cerebrospinal fluid (CSF) is observed in patients who develop aseptic meningitis following use of muromonab-CD3. Bacterial, fungal, and viral cultures of the CSF are negative.[19,35] Computed tomography may disclose brain edema.[25] In aseptic meningitis patients, the total leukocyte counts, neutrophil counts, and protein levels of CSF decrease over 1 to 3 days.[36] Graft rejection may be diagnosed on the basis of an increase in serum creatinine concentrations. A noninvasive double-isotope assessment of pulmonary microvascular permeability to transferrin may indicate extravascular pulmonary transferrin accumulation, indicating increased capillary permeability.[17]

Treatment

Stabilization

Patients should be placed in an intensive care facility where oxygen and intubation equipment are available. Cardiorespiratory monitoring should be available.

Blood pressure and heart rate should be closely monitored during the first 3 days of treatment with muromonab-CD3 to prevent hypertensive emergencies.

Prophylactic ultrafiltration and dialysis may lessen the risk of development of pulmonary edema and hypertension.[16,17] Development of pulmonary edema may require temporary cessation of muromonab-CD3 and urgent hemodialysis.[19] Resolution of the pulmonary edema may be followed by resumption of treatment.[17]

To avoid potentially fatal pulmonary edema, a chest radiograph and careful assessment of fluid status should be evaluated for evidence of fluid overload before muromonab-CD3 is used.[17] Muromonab-CD3 should be given only if there has been less than 3% gain in body weight over the previous 7 days.

Antidote

No antidote is available for muromonab-CD3 overdose. The possible use of anti-OKT3 antibodies for this condition has not been investigated.

Supportive Measures

1. Corticosteroid premedication (methylprednisolone 1 mg/kg intravenously followed by hydrocortisone 100 mg 30 minutes after muromonab-CD3) has been used in an attempt to reduce the likelihood of first-dose reactions.[6,10,37] Acetaminophen (650 mg) and antihistamine premedication (diphenhydramine 50 mg) may also be given.[6,10] Even though premedication with corticosteroids is used and tumor necrosis factor α, interleukin-2, and interferon gamma levels are reduced, first-dose reaction still may occur.[10]
2. Patients with high CSF pressure may improve rapidly after CSF removal.[26]
3. Close follow-up for early indications of PTLP disorder may improve its prognosis.[27]
4. Intraoperative administration of muromonab-CD3 may result in bradycardia, hypotension, and atrioventricular block.[32] Negative inotropic agents should be discontinued. Intravenous fluid resuscitation, positive-pressure mechanical ventilation with positive end-expiratory pressure, and, in extreme cases, inotropic and vasopressor agents may be required.[32]
5. Anaphylactic response to reactions to intravenous muromonab-CD3 should respond to intravenous epinephrine and diphenhydramine. Rapid intravenous desensitization with muromonab-CD3 may be followed by resumption of treatment.[33]
6. Patients receiving muromonab-CD3 should be monitored at intervals for the appearance of anti-idiotypic OKT3 antibodies.
7. Indomethacin administration during the first 48 hours of muromonab-CD3 therapy ameliorates clinical symptoms resulting from cytokine release.[38]

REFERENCES—MUROMONAB-CD3

1. USAN Council. Muromonab-CD3. Clin Pharmacol Ther 1989; 45:579.
2. Capone PM, Cohen ME. Seizures and cerebritis associated with administration of OKT3. Pediatr Neurol 1991;7:299–301.
3. D'Allesanro AM, Pirsch JD, Stratta RJ, et al. OKT3 salvage therapy in a quadruple immunosuppressive protocol in cadaveric renal transplantation. Transplantation 1989;47:297–300.
4. Shennib H, Mercado M, Nguyen D, et al. Successful treatment of steroid-resistant double lung allograft rejection with Orthoclone[R] OKT3. Am Rev Respir Dis 1991;144:224–226.
5. Konertz W, Weyand M, Friedl A. Prophylactic use of OKT3 in cardiac transplantation. Transplant Proc 1989;21:2494–2496.
6. Li PKT, Nicholls MG, Lai KN. The complications of newer transplant antirejection drugs: Treatment with cyclosporin A, OKT3 and FK 506. Adverse Drug React Acute Poison Rev 1990;9:123–155.
7. Goldstein G, Norman DJ, Henell KR, Smith IL. Pharmacokinetic study of Orthoclone OKT3 serum levels during treatment of acute renal allograft rejection. Transplantation 1988; 46:587–589.
8. Thistlethwaite JR Jr, Stuart JK, Mayes JT, et al. Monitoring and complications of monoclonal therapy: Complications and monitoring of OKT3 therapy. Am J Kidney Dis 1988;9: 112–119.
9. Chang TW, Kung PC, Gingras SP, Goldstein G. Does OKT3 monoclonal antibody react with an antigen recognition structure on human T-cells? Proc Natl Acad Sci USA 1981;78: 1805–1808.
10. Gaston RS, Deierhoi MH, Patterson T, et al. OKT3 first-dose reaction: Association with T-cell subsets and cytokine release. Kidney Int 1991;39:141–148.
11. Cosimi AB, Burton RC, Colvin RB, et al. Treatment of acute renal allograft rejection with OKT3 monoclonal antibody. Transplantation 1981;32:535–539.
12. Ellenhorn JDI, Woodle ES, Thistlethwaite JR, Bluestone JA. T-lymphocyte activation following OKT3 treatment. Curr Surg 1990;47:458–459.
13. Orthomulticenter Transplant Study Group. A randomized clinical trial of OKT3 monoclonal antibody for acute rejection of cadaveric renal transplants. N Engl J Med 1985;313: 337–342.
14. Chatenoud L, Ferran C, Reuter A, et al. Systemic reaction to the anti-T-cell monoclonal antibody OKT3 in relation to serum levels of tumor necrosis factor and interferon-alpha. N Engl J Med 1989;320:420–421.
15. Miller RA, Maloney DG, McKillop J, et al. In vivo effects of murine monoclonal antibody in a patient with T-cell leukemia. Blood 1981;58:78–86.
16. Spieker C, Zidek W, Barenbrock M, et al. Acute hypertension after renal allograft rejection therapy with OKT3 monoclonal antibody. J Int Med Res 1991;19:419–423.

17. Rome PA, Rocher GM, Morgan Ag, Shale DJ. OKT3 and pulmonary capillary permeability. Br Med J 1987;295:1099–1100.
18. Richards JM, Vogelzang NJ, Bluestone JA. Neurotoxicity after treatment with muromonab-CD3. N Engl J Med 1990;323:487–488.
19. Emmons C, Smith J, Flanigan M. Cerebrospinal fluid inflammation during OKT3 therapy. Lancet 1986;2:510–511.
20. Rello J, Vallaverdu I, Coll P, et al. Aseptic meningitis associated with muromonab-CD3. DICP Ann Pharmacother 1990;24:1233.
21. Joy ME, Michals ML, Canafax DM. Aseptic meningitis associated with muromonab-CD3 therapy. Clin Pharm 1988;7:721.
22. Figg WD. Aseptic meningitis associated with muromonab-CD3. DICP Ann Pharmacother 1991;25:1395.
23. Adair JC, Woodley SL, O'Connell JB, et al. Immunosuppression with OKT3 monoclonal antibody: A cause of fever and neurologic dysfunction after cardiac transplantation. Neurology 1990:40(suppl. 1):252.
24. Min DI, Fallo SA. Encephalopathy associated with muromonab-CD3. Clin Pharm 1993;12:610–612.
25. Coleman AE, Norman DJ. OKT3 encephalopathy. Ann Neurol 1990;28:837–838.
26. Thomas DM, Nicholls AJ, Feest TG, Riad H. OKT3 and cerebral edema. Br Med J 1987;295:1486.
27. Swinnen LJ, Costanzo-Nordin MR, Fisher SG, et al. Increased incidence of lymphoproliferative disorder after immunosuppression with the monoclonal antibody OKT3 in cardiac transplant recipients. N Engl J Med 1990;323:1723–1728.
28. Emery RW, Lake KD. Post-transplantation lymphoproliferative disorder and OKT3. N Engl J Med 1991;324:1437.
29. Brouwer RML, Balk AHMM, Weimar W. Post-transplantation lymphoproliferative disorder and OKT3. N Engl J Med 1991;324:1437.
30. Cohen JI. Post-transplantation lymphoproliferative disorder and OKT3. N Engl J Med 1991;324:1438.
31. Penn I. Cancers complicating organ transplantation. N Engl J Med 1990;323:1767–1769.
32. Roth S, Kupferberg JP. Adverse responses following intraoperative administration of orthoclone OKT3. Anesth Analg 1989;69:822–825.
33. Georgitis JW, Browning MC, Steiner D, Lorentz WB. Anaphylaxis and desensitization to the murine monoclonal antibody used for renal graft rejection. Ann Allergy 1991;66:343–347.
34. Goldstein G, Fuccello AJ, Norman DJ, et al. OKT3 monoclonal antibody plasma levels during therapy and the subsequent development of host antibodies to OKT3. Transplantation 1986;42:507–511.
35. Sutton JD, Prioleau MH, Wordell CJ, Francos GC. Aseptic meningitis associated with muromonab-CD3 administration. DICP Ann Pharmacother 1989;23:257–258.
36. Martin MA, Massanari M, Nghien DD, et al. Nosocomial aseptic meningitis associated with administration of OKT3. JAMA 1988;259:2002–2005.
37. Goldman M, Abramowicz D, De Pauw L, et al. OKT3 induced cytokine release attenuation by high dose methylprednisolone. Lancet 1989;2:802–803.
38. Gaughan WJ, Francos BB, Dunn SR, et al. A retrospective analysis of the effect of indomethacin on adverse reactions to Orthoclone OKT3 in the therapy of acute renal allograft rejection. Am J Kidney Dis 1994;24:486–490.

INTRAVENOUS IMMUNE GLOBULIN

The ideal intravenous immune globulin (IVIG) preparation should contain structurally and functionally intact immunoglobulin molecules with normal biologic half-lives and a normal proportion of immunoglobulin subclasses. The preparation should contain high levels of the antibody(ies) relevant to its proposed use. There should be no contamination with vasomotor peptides, endotoxin, or infectious agents, particularly viruses.[1–3] Doctors should know if the IVIG they are using has been subjected to viral inactivation procedures (so-called third-generation IVIGs).[4]

Structure and Classification

Intravenous immune globulin consists primarily of IgG, although trace quantities of IgA, IgM, IgE, and other serum proteins are also present.[5] The World Health Organization has established the following guidelines for preparation of IVIG[6]:

1. The preparation should be obtained from a group of at least 1000 donors.
2. At least 90% of the IVIG should consist of intact monomeric IgG molecules.
3. IgA should be present in very low concentrations.
4. Antibody activity against at least two bacterial species (or toxins) and two viruses should be determined.
5. Opsonic, complement-activating, and other biologic activities should be maintained.
6. All IgG subclasses should be present in a distribution similar to that of normal pooled plasma.
7. The preparation should be as free as possible from potentially harmful contaminants, such as prekallikrein activator, kinins, and plasmins.

Use

In symptomatic HIV-infected children, the prophylactic use of IVIG appears to be safe and significantly increases the time free from serious bacterial infections for those entering treatment with CD4+ lymphocyte counts greater than $0.2 \times 10^9/L$.[7,8] IVIG may be useful in pyridoxine-dependent seizures.[9] Table 44–14 lists recognized indications for use of IVIG.

Product Formulation

Intravenous immune globulin is prepared from plasma derived from many donors. All IVIG preparations in the United States (Table 44–15) are manufactured with stabilizing agents, are acidified, and are recommended for infusion over several hours.[10] Subcutaneous[11] and intramuscular administration may be useful.

Therapeutic Dose

The recommended dosage for Sandoglobulin and Gamimune N in the treatment of idiopathic thrombocytopenic purpura[12] is 400 mg/kg/d for 2 to 5 days.[5] Induction with 500 mg/kg is recommended when using Venoglobulin-I. The recommended dosage of Gammagard in idiopathic thrombocytopenic purpura is 1 g/kg/d, plus two repeated infusions given on alternate days if necessary. Immunologic reactions can be modified, often dramatically, by the intravenous administration of large amounts of immune globulin (400–2000 mg/kg body weight over 2–5 days).[13]

Table 44–14
Recognized Indications for Intravenous Immune Globulin

Replacement Therapy	Immunomodulatory
Primary Antibody Deficiencies X-linked agammaglobulinemia X-linked immunodeficiency with hyperimmunoglobulin M Common variable immunodeficiency Immunoglobulin G subclass deficiencies with infections Severe combined immunodeficiency (SCID) prior to bone marrow transplantation Failure of B-cell engraftment after bone marrow transplantation for SCID **Selective Cases of Secondary Antibody Deficiency** Intestinal lymphangiectasia Chronic lymphocytic leukemia and B-cell lymphoma with hypogammaglobulinemia Myeloma with specific antibody deficiency Low-birth-weight babies at risk of sepsis Infants and children with HIV infection	Immune thrombocytopenia purpura (ITP) Kawasaki's disease Guillain–Barré syndrome Chronic inflammatory demyelinating neuropathy Acquired hemophilia

From Misbah SA, Chapel HM. Adverse effects of intravenous immunoglobulin. Drug Saf 1993;9:254–262.

Toxicokinetics

Peak serum immunoglobulin levels measured immediately after intravenous administration correlate with the dose.[1] A dose of 100 mg/kg body weight results in an average increment of about 200 mg/dL.[14,15] A dose of 500 mg/dL results in an average increment of about 1 g/dL.[16] By 24 hours, serum immunoglobulin levels are 70 to 80% of peak levels and decrease to about 50% by 72 hours.[10,17] Baseline levels are usually reached by 21 to 28 days after infusion. In most studies, 150 mg/kg body weight is regarded as the minimal effective dose. Immunologic reaction can be modified by using 400 to 2000 mg/kg body weight over 2 to 5 days.[7] In hypogammaglobulinemia, the dose is titrated to achieve a postinfusion serum concentration in the low range (800 mg/dL) and to maintain a minimum IgG serum concentration of 200 to 500 mg/dL between doses.[13]

Elimination

The elimination half-life of most immunoglobulin preparations is 18 to 32 days, similar to that of native IgG.[12] The half-life in neonates is similar to that in adults.[18,19] The half-life of IgG is dependent on the half-lives of the individual IgG subclasses. The half-lives of IgG1 and IgG2 are 4 and 23 to 25 days. IgG3 has a half-life of 9 days.[5]

Pregnancy/Lactation

Administration of IVIG throughout pregnancy resulted in the birth of a healthy 3500-g infant with 1- and 5-minute Apgar scores of 9 and 9, respectively.[20] A live healthy infant was delivered from a mother with severe idiopathic thrombocy-

Table 44–15
Characteristics of the Preparations of Intravenous Immune Globulin Available in the United States

Brand Name	Manufacturing Process	Additives	Approximate IgA Content* (µg/mL)	Form Supplied	Manufacturer
Gamimune N	pH 4.25, diafiltration	10% maltose	270	5% liquid, pH 4.25	Cutter Biological, Miles Laboratories
Gammagard†	Polyethylene glycol, DEAE–Sephadex, ultrafiltration	2% maltose, 0.2% polyethylene glycol, 0.3 M glycine, 0.15 M sodium chloride, 3% albumin	0.4–1.9‡	Lyophilized, 5%, pH 6.8	Hyland Division, Baxter Healthcare
Gammar-IV	Low-ionic-strength ethanol	5% sucrose, 2.5% albumin, 0.5% sodium chloride	20‡	Lyophilized, 5%, pH 7.0	Armour Pharmaceutical
IVEEGAM	Immobilized trypsin, polyethylene glycol	5% glucose, 0.3% sodium chloride, 0.5 polyethylene glycol	5‡	Lyophilized, 5%, pH 6.8	Immuno-US
Sandoglobulin	pH 4.0, 1:10,000 trypsin	5% or 10% sucrose (sodium chloride in diluent)	720	Lyophilized, 3% or 6%, pH 6.6	Sandoz Pharmaceutical
Venoglobulin-1	Polyethylene glycol, DEAE-Sephadex	2% D-mannitol, 1% albumin, 0.5% sodium chloride, <0.6% polyethylene glycol	24‡	Lyophilized, 5%, pH 6.8	Alpha Therapeutics

*Values are approximate; there is a great deal of lot-to-lot variability.
†Another preparation, marketed by the American Red Cross, is prepared by Baxter Hyland with plasma from Red Cross volunteer donors.
‡Data provided by manufacturer.
From Buckley RH, Schiff RI. The use of intravenous immune globulin in immunodeficiency diseases. N Engl J Med 1991;325:110–117.

topenic purpura who had responded to IVIG 400 mg/kg/d for 5 days.[21] High doses of IVIG can be given to preterm very-low-birth-weight newborn infants with little risk of interference with natural killer cell activity.[22]

Mechanism of Action

In immune deficiency, the major effects seems to be replacement of deficient immunoglobulins. In immune regulatory disorders, either reticuloendothelial blockade, an increase in suppressor T cells or natural killer cells, or a decrease in antibody synthesis may be mediated by anti-idiotype antibodies in the immunoglobulin preparation. Treatment with immunoglobulin preparations containing anti-idiotype antibodies may decrease the synthesis of autoantibodies.[1] The mode of action of IVIG in bacterial and viral infections is not known but most likely involves antibacterial or antiviral antibodies in the preparation. Infused antibodies may also block recognition of infected cells by cytotoxic T lymphocytes, thus preventing immune-mediated cell damage.[1]

Clinical Presentation

Allergic Reaction

Two persons with immune complexes that developed after IVIG administration complained of abdominal pain and chest tightness.[21] Individuals with IgA deficiency often have IgG antibodies to IgA and may develop an anaphylactic reaction to IVIG.[23,24] Prekallikrein activator, β-lipoprotein, and IgA are present in IVIG preparations and may provoke allergic reaction. If the IVIG preparation contains aggregates with anticomplementary activity, vasomotor symptoms may develop including chills, nausea, flushing, chest tightness, and wheezing. No convincing correlation with complement levels has been found. Stabilizing agents such as maltose may reduce immunoglobulin aggregates in the IVIG preparation. Hemolysis and thrombosis have been rarely reported.[25]

Hepatitis

Symptomatic non-A, non-B hepatitis[26,27] and elevated hepatic transaminase levels[28,29] probably reflect contaminated lots of IVIG. The current consensus is that IVIG preparations do not transmit non-A, non-B hepatitis. Similarly, no cases of hepatitis B have followed use of IVIG.

A recent report of hepatitis in a small cluster of patients in Italy receiving an IVIG preparation with a previously established safety record suggests that very little margin for safety exists in some of the current manufacturing techniques.[4] The major outbreaks in the last 10 years have been associated with patients who developed relatively rapid (within 7 years) deterioration in liver function and cirrhosis. The hepatitis C virus apparently follows an aggressive course in patients with hypogammaglobulinemia.

In 1994 the IVIG preparation Gammagard was withdrawn worldwide by the manufacturers because of a possible association with hepatitis C virus. This product has been replaced with Gammagard-SD treated with a solvent as a detergent to inactive hepatitis viruses.[30]

Neurologic Effects

Transient headaches, vomiting, altered consciousness with chills and fever, meningitis, and aseptic meningitis have been reported following use of IVIG.[31] IVIG appeared to induce thrombogenesis and a cerebral infarction in an 84-year-old man with polyneuritis cranialis.[32]

Dermal Effects

Three patients developed alopecia within 1 to 4 weeks of IVIG treatment. The alopecia resolved within 4 months.[33]

Hematologic Effects

Two cases of hemolysis induced by IVIG were the result of passively acquired anti-A or anti-D antibodies. A crossmatch procedure prior to the IVIG would have avoided this.[34]

Overrapid Self-Induced Infusion: IVIG Abuse

Overrapid infusion of IVIG produced an intense tingling, electric "buzz" sensation, lasting up to 5 minutes followed by shivering, sweating, myalgia, and bronchospasm.[35]

Pulmonary Effects

Hypotension with respiratory failure is very rare after IVIG use.

Renal Effects

Renal dysfunction has followed the use of IVIG in three patients, in all of whom renal function returned to normal after the drug was stopped.[36] Acute renal failure can follow use of IVIG in patients with prior evidence of impaired renal function.[37]

Laboratory

Abnormalities

Reversible neutropenia followed use of IVIG in a 6-year-old boy with idiopathic autoimmune hemolytic anemia.[38]

Ancillary Tests

Use of IVIG 400 mg/kg/d for 5 days resulted in a reversible rise in serum creatinine when IVIG was administered to nephrotic patients.[39] High catecholamine levels may be observed after a severe reaction.[40]

Treatment

Adverse reactions can often be alleviated by reducing the rate or the volume of infusion. For patients with repeated severe reactions unresponsive to these measures, hydrocortisone 1 to 2 mg/kg intravenously can be given 30 minutes before IVIG infusion.[3] Corticosteroids may decrease adverse reactions to IVIG in persons with previous side effects such as fever, chills, headache, hypertension, and chest pain.[41] IVIG was used to treat a patient who had severe reactions to intramuscular immune-globulin.[42] Patients who experience an anaphylactic reaction to IVIG should be given symptomatic and supportive treatment with epinephrine, assurance of an airway and adequate respiration, cardiac monitoring, and oxygen as required.

Selected References

- Misbah SA, Chapel HM. Adverse effects of intravenous immunoglobulin. Drug Saf 1993;9:254–262.
- Stiehm ER. New developments: Recent progress on the use of intravenous immunoglobulin. Curr Prob Pediatr 1992;22:335–349.

REFERENCES—INTRAVENOUS IMMUNE GLOBULIN

1. Berkman SA, Lee ML, Gale RP. Clinical uses of intravenous immunoglobulin. Ann Intern Med 1990;112:278–292.
2. Buckley RH, Schiff RI. The use of intravenous immune globulin in immunodeficiency diseases. N Engl J Med 1991; 325:110–117.
3. NIH Consensus Conference. Intravenous immunoglobulin: Prevention and treatment of disease. JAMA 1990;264:3189–3193.
4. Webster ADB. Intravenous immunoglobulins of benefit in primary hypogammaglobulinemia. Br Med J 1991;303:375–376.
5. Knapp MJ, Colburn PA. Clinical uses of intravenous immune globulin. Clin Pharm 1990;9:509–529.
6. Appropriate use of human immunoglobulin in clinical practice: Memorandum from an IVIS/WHO meeting. Bull WHO 1982;60:43–47.
7. Dwyer JM. Manipulating the immune system with immune globulin. N Engl J Med 1992;326:107–116.
8. National Institute of Child Health and Human Development Intravenous Immunoglobulin Study Group. Intravenous immune globulin for the prevention of bacterial infections in children with symptomatic human immunodeficiency virus infection. N Engl J Med 1991;325:73–80.
9. Connolly MB, Jan JE, Junker AK. Intravenous immunoglobulin and pyridoxine-dependent seizures. Neurology 1991;41: 1524.
10. Pirofsky B. Intravenous immune globulin therapy in hypogammaglobulinemia: A review. Am J Med 1984;76:53–60.
11. Gardulf A, Hammarstrom L, Edvard Smith CI. Treatment of hypogammaglobulinemia with subcutaneous gamma globulin by rapid infusion. Lancet 1991;338:162–166.
12. Smith EL, Hill RL, Lehman IR, et al. *Principles of Biochemistry: Mammalian Biochemistry.* 7th ed. Tokyo: McGraw-Hill, 1983:40.
13. Wordell CJ. Use of intravenous immune globulin therapy: An overview. DICP Ann Pharmacother 1991;25:805–817.
14. Buckley RH. Long term use of intravenous immune globulin patients with primary immunodeficiency disease: Inadequacy of current dosage practices and approaches to the problem. J Clin Immunol 1982;2:15S–21S.
15. Ochs HD, Fisher SH, Wedgwood RJ. Modified immune-globulin: Its use in the prophylactic treatment of patients with immune deficiency. J Clin Immunol 1982;2:22S–30S.
16. Montanaro A, Pirofsky B. Prolonged interval high-dose intravenous immunoglobulin in patients with primary immunodeficiency states. Am J Med 1984;76:67–72.
17. Nolte MT, Pirofsky B, Gerritz GA, Golding B. Intravenous immunoglobulin therapy for antibody deficiency. Clin Exp Immunol 1979;36:237–243.
18. Potter M, Stockley R, Storry J, Slade R. ABO alloimmunisation after intravenous immunoglobulin infusion. Lancet 1988;1:932–933.
19. Noya FJD, Rench MA, Courtney JT, et al. Pharmacokinetics of intravenous immunoglobulin in very low birth weight neonates. Pediatr Infect Dis J 1989;8:759–763.
20. Parke A, Maier D, Wilson D, et al. Intravenous gamma globulin, antiphospholipid antibodies and pregnancy. Ann Intern Med 1989;110:495–496.
21. Gibson J, Laird PP, Joshua DE, et al. Very high dose intravenous gamma globulin in thrombocytopenia of pregnancy. Aust NZ J Med 1989;19:151–153.
22. Chirico G, Maccario R, Montagna D, et al. Natural killer cell activity in preterm infants: Effect of intravenous Immune globulin administration. J Pediatr 1990;117:465–466.
23. Day NK, Good RA, Wahn V. Adverse reactions in selected patients following intravenous infusions of gamma globulin. Am J Med 1984;76:25–32.
24. Branigan EF, Stevenson MM, Charles D. Blood transfusion reaction in a patient with immunoglobulin A deficiency. Obstet Gynecol 1983;61(suppl. 3):47S–49S.
25. Woodruff RK, Grigg AP, Firkin FC, Smith IL. Fatal thrombotic events during treatment of autoimmune thrombocytopenia with intravenous immunoglobulin in elderly patients. Lancet 1986;2:217–218.
26. Lane RS. Non-A, non-B hepatitis from intravenous immunoglobulin. Lancet 1983;2:974–975.
27. Lever AM, Brown D, Webster AD, Thomas HC. Non-A, non-B hepatitis occurring in agammaglobulinemia patients after intravenous immunoglobulin. Lancet 1984;2:1062–1064.
28. Ochs HD, Fischer SH, Vivant FS, et al. Non-A, non-B hepatitis and intravenous immunoglobulin. Lancet 1985;1:404–405.
29. Webster AD, Lever AM. Non-A, non-B hepatitis after intravenous immunoglobulin. Lancet 1986;1:323.
30. Schiff RI. Transmission of viral infections through intravenous immune globulin. N Engl J Med 1994;331:1649–1650.
31. Kato E, Shindo S, Eto Y, et al. Administration of immune globulin associated with aseptic meningitis. JAMA 1988;259: 3269–3270.
32. Silbert PL, Knezevic WV, Bridge DT. Cerebral infarction complicating intravenous immunoglobulin therapy for polyneuritis cranialis. Neurology 1992;42:257–258.
33. Chan-Lan D, Fitzsimons EJ, Douglas WS. Alopecia after immunoglobulin infusion. Lancet 1987;1:1436.
34. Nicholls MD, Cummins JC, Davies VJ, Greenwood JK. Haemolysis induced by intravenously-administered immunoglobulin. Med J Aust 1989;150:404–406.
35. Cochrane S, Haeney MR. Self-induced "buzz" achieved by rapid infusion of immunoglobulin. Lancet 1990;336: 123–124.
36. Rault R, Piraino B, Johnston JR, Oral A. Pulmonary and renal toxicity of intravenous immunoglobulin. Clin Nephrol 1991; 36:83–86.
37. Tan E, Hajnazarian M, Bay W, et al. Acute renal failure resulting from intravenous immunoglobulin therapy. Arch Neurol 1993;50:137–139.
38. Majer RV, Green PJ. Neutropenia caused by intravenous immunoglobulin. Br Med J 1988;296:1262.
39. Schifferli J, Leski M, Favre H, et al. High-dose intravenous IgG treatment and renal function. Lancet 1991;337:457–458.
40. Biasi D, Corrocher R, Bambara LM, et al. Increased secretion of norepinephrine after intravenous gamma globulin therapy in a patient with rheumatoid arthritis. Br J Rheumatol 1993;32:1026–1027.
41. Lederman HM, Roifman CM, Lavi S, Gelfand EW. Corticosteroids for prevention of adverse reactions to intravenous immune serum globulin infusions in hypogammaglobulinemic patients. Am J Med 1986;81:443–446.
42. Frame WD, Crawford RJ. Thrombotic events after intravenous immunoglobulin. Lancet 1986;2:468.

AUTOIMMUNITY

Autoimmunity results from a breakdown in the immune system's ability to distinguish "self" and "nonself." In the autoimmune reaction, the body mounts an immune response against some of its own normal components. These immune responses are mounted by antigens of self (autoantigens) and may be humoral responses (ie, production of antibodies directed against one autoantigen—autoantibodies) and/or cell-mediated immune responses (ie, development of delayed-type hypersensitivity reactions to that autoantigen that are mediated by "self"-reacting T lymphocytes).

DEFINITION OF AUTOIMMUNE DISEASE

Autoimmune diseases are defined as diseases secondary to autoimmune antibody or T-cell mediated phenomena. Autoimmune disease appear to be exclusively mediated by autoantibodies. Anti-receptor antibodies can induce a number of autoimmune diseases either by depressing (myasthenia gravis, insulin-resistant diabetes) or stimulating (Graves' disease) the receptor function. Autoantibodies also are involved through the deposition of circulating or in situ-formed immune complexes (systemic lupus erythematosus, glomerulonephritis, and a number of connective tissue diseases [periarteritis nodosa, Wegener's granulomatosis, mixed connective tissue disease]). These diseases are relatively resistant to cyclosporine, but are sensitive to corticosteroids and alkylating agents (cyclophosphamide).

T cell-mediated autoimmune diseases include insulin-dependent diabetes mellitus, uveitis, psoriasis, atopic dermatitis, primary biliary cirrhosis, and rheumatoid arthritis. These diseases are very sensitive to cyclosporine and relatively resistant to alkylating agents. They usually respond to corticosteroids.

Some diseases are sensitive to immunosuppressive agents but there are no immunoglobulin deposits in glomeruli and no clear immunologic abnormalities. This group includes the idiopathic nephrotic syndrome, inflammatory bowel disease including Crohn's disease and ulcerative colitis, aplastic anemia, lichen planus, and polymyositis.[1]

IMMUNOSUPPRESSIVE THERAPY IN AUTOIMMUNE DISEASE

Agents

Six classes of agents have been widely used as immunosuppressive agents in autoimmune disease: (1) corticosteroids; (2) antimetabolites (azathioprine, methotrexate); (3) alkylating agents (cyclophosphamide, chlorambucil); (4) cyclosporine; (5) other agents such as intravenous gamma globulins and anti-lymphocyte globulins (used occasionally); and (6) newer agents such as tacrolimus (FK 506) and anti-CD3 antibodies.

Problems With Use

Several problems are related to the use of immunosuppressive agents in autoimmune disease: insufficient rate of response; occurrence of relapse at cessation of treatment; and persistent risk of direct drug toxicity or of overimmunosuppression (tumors, infections).[1]

AUTOIMMUNITY INDUCED BY CHEMICALS

Mechanisms of chemical-induced autoimmunity are summarized in Table 44–16.

Table 44–16
Mechanisms of Chemical-Induced Autoimmunity

Suggested Mechanism	Chemicals
Complex with autoantigen	Hydralazine
Release of autoantigen	Gold, cadmium
Cross-reaction with autoantigen	Hydralazine
Immunogen or hapten	Penicillamine
Inhibition of suppressor T cells	Methyldopa, practolol and procainamide, mercury
Stimulation of helper T cells	Procainamide, beta blockers and phenytoin, mercury
Stimulation of B cells	Mercury, beta blockers and phenytoin, penicillamine, iodine
Stimulation of macrophages	Penicillamine and propylthiouracil, iodine
Changes in production of cytokines and lymphokines	?
Altered major histocompatibility complex expression	?
Alteration of idiotype–antiidiotype network	?

Adapted from Bigazzi PE. Autoimmunity induced by chemicals. Clin Toxicol 1988;26:125–156.

Table 44–17
Drugs and Systemic Lupus Erythematosus

Definite Proof of Association: Controlled Prospective Studies
Chlorpromazine
Hydralazine
Isoniazid
Methyldopa
Procainamide
Quinidine

Probable Association
Anticonvulsant agents
Antithyroid drugs
Beta blockers
Lithium
Penicillamine
Sulfasalazine

Anecdotal Reports
p-Aminosalicylic acid
Estrogens
Gold salts
Griseofulvin
Penicillin
Reserpine
Tetracycline

Adapted from Hess E. Drug-related lupus. N Engl J Med 1988;318:1460–1462.

Systemic Lupus Erythematosus

Drugs associated with systemic lupus erythematosus (SLE) are listed in Table 44–17. Criteria for diagnosis of drug-induced lupus are listed in Table 44–18.[2,3]

- Penicillamine
  Response ranges from no or mild symptoms to severe multisystem disease. Hydralazine- and procainamide-induced lupus erythematosus is usually milder than

SLE, and has little renal or central nervous system involvement; antinuclear antibodies (ANA) are present, but antibodies to native (double stranded) DNA are seldom detected (the rim or peripheral immunofluorescence pattern). Antibodies (ANA) are histone dependent and are induced by both chemicals. Slow acetylators have an enhanced tendency to develop ANA. HLA-DR4 phenotype and/or the C4 null allele may predispose to the development of hydralazine-induced SLE.[4] Penicillamine induces lupus in up to 2% of patients; ANA, anti-DNA antibodies, and a lupus band test (deposition of immunoglobulins and complement along the dermal–epidermal junction of the skin) may be present. Penicillamine acts as an immunomodulator capable of potentiating and initiating anti-DNA antibody synthesis as well as suppressing it.[5]

- Other chemicals
  Circulating ANA and immune complexes are found in subjects exposed to vinyl chloride, asbestos, and silica.[6] The HLA type of human adjuvant disease may follow implantation of paraffin/silicone and silicone polymers for cosmetic reasons.[7] The major evidence that other drugs such as aminosalicylic acid, penicillin, tetracycline, streptomycin, griseofulvin, phenylbutazone, methylthiouracil, and propylthiouracil can produce SLE is resolution of signs and symptoms after these drugs are discontinued.
- Tienilic acid

Scleroderma

Progressive systemic sclerosis (scleroderma) is a collagen–vascular disease with antinuclear antibodies formed to extractable nuclear antigens, the nucleolus, the centromere, and ScI-70. Scleroderma has a number of occupational and drug associations (Table 44–19).[8]

Pemphigus

- Penicillamine
  Immunoglobulin deposited at intercellular levels of skin or at basement zone level. Circulating autoantibodies to the basement zone in penicillamine-induced bullous pemphigoid. Termination of treatment is followed by a decrease in autoantibody titers and clinical improvement.
- Pyrithioxine

Table 44–18
Drug-Related Lupus: Diagnosis

- Abrupt onset of fever, myalgias, arthralgias, pleurisy, pericarditis
- Absence of central nervous system and renal involvement
- Absence of classic malar rash, alopecia, discoid lesions, mucosal ulcers
- Very severe anemia, leukopenia, or thrombocytopenia unusual
- Many positive lupus erythematosus cells
- Diffusely positive antinuclear activity
- Normal levels of complement
- Absence of antibody to active DNA

- α-Mercaptopropionyl glycine
- Captopril[10]

Autoimmune Hemolytic Anemia

- Red Cell Antibodies
- Methyldopa
  Positive direct antiglobulin test (IgG): the antibody develops after several weeks of exposure to methyldopa; the titer and incidence of positive tests are dose dependent; withdrawal of the drug leaves a positive antiglobulin test for weeks or months before gradually becoming negative.
- Procainamide
- Chlorpropamide

Antiplatelet Antibodies: Autoimmune Thrombocytopenia

- Carbamazepine
- Gold therapy
- Interferon[9]

Myasthenia Gravis

- Penicillamine
  Long term (months to years). Improves after drug withdrawal; autoantibodies appear to acetylcholine receptors. Disease is similar but less severe than idiopathic myasthenia gravis. Presents more frequently with ocular manifestations (ptosis, diplopia). No good correlation between antibody titers and severity of myasthenia gravis or dosages of D-penicillamine.

Mediated by Autoantibodies to Renal Antigens

- Penicillamine—Goodpasture's syndrome?
- Hydrocarbon solvent

Table 44–19
Classification of Scleroderma

Generalized scleroderma
- Diffuse skin involvement
- Limited skin involvement (CREST syndrome: calcinosis, Raynaud's phenomenon, esophageal hypomotility, sclerodactyly, telangiectasia)

Localized scleroderma
- Morphea
- Linear

Scleroderma-like syndromes
- Occupational and environmental
  - Vinyl chloride associated
  - Vibratory associated
  - Silicosis associated
  - Toxic oil syndrome
- Fasciitis with eosinophilia
- Graft-vs-host reaction
- Drug-induced
  - Bleomycin-induced
  - Tryptophan- and carbidopa-induced

From Condemi JJ. The autoimmune diseases. JAMA 1987;258:2920–2929.

- Toxic oil syndrome (rapeseed oil adulterated with aniline)
- Antibodies against renal glomerular basement membrane.[15]

Glomerulonephritis

- Mediated by immune complexes
- Penicillamine
  Membranous nephropathy. Granular deposits of IgG and complement along capillary walls.[11–13] IgM nephropathy may be observed.[14]
- Chronic mercury intoxication
  Membranous nephropathy. Deposits of immunoglobulins and complement at level of the glomerular basement membrane.[4] Mechanism unknown.
- Cadmium
- Gold

Autoimmune Thyroid Disease (Hashimoto's Disease, Graves' Disease)

- Dietary iodine
- Polybrominated biphenyls[16]
- Polychlorinated biphenyls[16]
- Lithium
- Anticonvulsant therapy[17]
- Penicillamine[11]
- Amiodarone
  Antibodies to thyroglobulin and thyroid microsomal antigen. Thyroid-stimulating immunoglobulins.

Hepatitis

- Methyldopa
  Acute viral hepatitis-like syndrome. Chronic active hepatitis-like syndrome.
- Oxyphenisatin
  Chronic active hepatitis. Circulating ANA and/or anti-smooth muscle antibodies.
- Halothane
  Eosinophilia. Humoral and cellular immune responses to kidney and liver microsomal antigens. Normal liver membrane components
- Isoniazid
- Nitrofurantoin
- Fenofibrate
- Papaverine

REFERENCES—AUTOIMMUNITY

1. Back J-F. The new era of immunosuppressive therapy in autoimmune disease. Transplant Proc 1991;23:3319–3321.
2. Hess E. Drug-related lupus. N Engl J Med 1988;318:1460–1462.
3. Bigazzi PE. Autoimmunity induced by chemicals. Clin Toxicol 1988;26:125–156.
4. Spears CJ, Batchelor JR. Drug-induced autoimmune disease. Adv Nephrol 1987;16:219–230.
5. Mach PS, Brouilhet H, Amor B. D-Penicillamine, a modulator of anti-DNA antibodies production. Clin Exp Immunol 1986;63:414–418.
6. Descotes J. *Immunotoxicology of Drugs and Chemicals.* Amsterdam: Elsevier, 1986:359.
7. Sergott TJ, Limoli JP, Baldwin CM Jr, Laub DR. Human adjuvant disease, possible autoimmune disease after silicone implantation: A review of the literature, case studies and speculation for the future. Plast Reconstr Surg 1986;78: 104–114.
8. Comdemi JJ. The autoimmune diseases. JAMA 1987;258: 2920–2929.
9. Abdi EA, Brien W, Venne PM. Auto-immune thrombocytopenia related to interferon therapy. Scand J Haematol 1986; 36:515–519.
10. Jaffe W. Adverse effects profile of sulfhydryl compounds in man. Am J Med 1986;80:471–476.
11. Smith CIE, Hammarstrom L. Immunologic abnormalities induced by D-penicillamine. PAR Pseudo-allergic Reactions 1985;4:138–180.
12. Howard-Lock HE, Lock CJL, Mewa A, Kean WF. D-Penicillamine: Chemistry and clinical use in rheumatic disease. Semin Arthritis Rheum 1986;15:261–281.
13. Jaffe IA. Induction of auto-immune syndromes by penicillamine therapy in rheumatoid arthritis and other diseases. Spring Semin Immunopathol 1981;4:193–207.
14. Rehan A, Johnson K. IgM nephropathy associated with penicillamine. Am J Nephrol 1986;6:71–74.
15. Arnaiz-Villena A, Vicario JL, Serrano-Rios M, et al. Glomerular basement-membrane antibodies and HLA-DR2 in Spanish rapeseed oil disease. N Engl J Med 1982;307:1404–1405.
16. Safran M, Paul TL, Roti E, Braverman E. Environmental factors affecting autoimmune thyroid diseases. Endocrinol Metab Clin North Am 1987;16:327–342.
17. Nishiyama S, Matsukura M, Fujimoto S, Matsuda I. Reports of two cases of autoimmune thyroiditis while receiving anticonvulsant therapy. Eur J Pediatr 1983;140:116–117.

IMMUNOTOXICANTS AND RELATED DISEASE

CIPROFLOXACIN

Ciprofloxacin administration was associated with a serum sickness type of reaction in an adult, classified as a leukocytoclastic vasculitis. Tests for antinuclear antibodies, rheumatoid factor, and cryoglobulins and Coombs' test were negative. C3 was normal; C4 was depressed. A low C4 value is a sensitive indication of a low level of activation of the complement system. Tests for circulatory immunocomplexes were positive. Skin biopsy showed a small cell vasculitis. This can be considered an immune complex-mediated disease.[1]

CONTRAST MEDIA

The lymphocyte transformation test exhibits a positive response to amidotrizoate. Lymphocytes from patients sensitive to amidotrizoate cross-react to structurally related ionic contrast media. Nonionic contrast agents do not induce proliferation of the lymphocytes. Ionic radiographic contrast agents may be antigenic in humans.[2] (See Chapter 60.)

FORMALDEHYDE

Anti-formaldehyde human serum albumin antibodies (IgE, IgM, IgG), analyses of helper/suppressor T ratios, and an increase in Tal cells (antigen memory cells) suggest that formaldehyde may induce chronic antigenic stimulation in patients who have multiple subjective health complaints.[3,4]

HALOGENATED POLYAROMATIC HYDROCARBONS

Polychlorinated biphenyls (PCBs), phenols, chlorinated dibenzo-*p*-dioxins, dibenzofurans, hexachlorobenzene, pentachlorophenol, and polybrominated biphenyls are included in this group. Human studies have not disclosed any significant immunologic health effects. Exposure to PCBs in Taiwan indicated that a population of T cells may have been diseased. Further work is required to confirm these findings.

HYDRALAZINE

Hydralazine-associated nephritis in humans is associated with antinuclear antibody, but not with antibodies to DNA. Antibodies to myeloperoxidase and neutrophil cytoplasm antigen may be present.[5] Hydralazine may facilitate induction of serious nephritic or systemic reactions with autoantibody production.

INSULIN

In diabetic patients, abnormal antibody responses have been associated with syndromes of insulin hypersensitivity. Routine administration of insulin results in the production of insulin antibodies of the IgG1, IgG3, and IgG4 isotypes. Patients with local hypersensitivity to insulin appear to have an elevated IgG response.[6]

Insulin and Automimmune Syndrome

The combination of a high serum concentration of total immunoreactive insulin, the presence of insulin autoantibodies, and a fasting hypoglycemia is known as the *insulin autoimmune syndrome*[7] or *insulin autoimmune hypoglycemia*.[8] HLA typing indicates that most patients have the DR4 antigen. More than half of patients with this syndrome have previously received methimazole, α-mercaptopropionyl glycine, gold thioglucose, glutathione, D--penicillamine, or tolbutamide. All these drugs are sulfhydryl compounds.

INTRAVENOUS DRUG ABUSERS (IVDA)

Studies on intravenous drug abusers (IVDAs) must also consider the possible presence of AIDS. Immunologic abnormalities observed in IVDAs are summarized by Sobel.[9] Active parenteral heroin users have shown depressed natural killer cell activities with higher absolute number of CD2-, CD3-, CD4-, and CD8-positive cells.[10] Methadone does not appear to have any effect on natural killer cell activity.[11] Changes in the humoral immune system, cell-mediated immune system, and neutrophil–monocyte functions in IVDAs are listed in Table 44–20.[12]

Table 44–20
Changes in the Immune System of Intravenous Drug Abusers

Parameter Studied	Result
Changes in the Humoral Immune System	
Immunoglobulin levels	
IgM	Increased
IgG	Increased
	Normal
IgA	Normal
False-positive VDRL	Increased
Antibodies to *Brucella,* Q fever, lymphogranuloma venereum, *Salmonella, Proteus*	Increased
Rheumatoid factor	Increased
Antibody response to novel antigen	Normal
Changes in Cell-Mediated Immune System	
Mitogenic response	Diminished
Skin tests	Anergic
	Nonanergic
T-cell rosettes	Decreased
T_4 lymphocytes	Normal
	Decreased*
Changes in Neutrophil–Monocyte Function	
Phagocytosis	Normal or decreased
Superoxide production	Decreased
Bactericidal capacity	Normal or decreased
Chemotaxis, migration	Normal
Adherence	Normal

*These studies did not exclude possible HIV-infected patients.
Adapted from Kauffman CA, Bradley SF. Host defense mechanisms in intravenous drug abusers. In: Levine DP, Sobel JD, eds. *Infections in Intravenous Drug Abusers.* New York: Oxford Universtiy Press, 1991:27–33.

METALS

Exposure to metals has been shown to modulate the immune response.[13]

Lead

Lead modulates the immune response in vivo,[14] inhibiting macrophage development, activating B cells, and both inhibiting and enhancing T-cell subsets.[13,15] Lead involvement in immune-mediated nephritis has been suggested.[16] Data directly implicating lead in autoimmune disease are not available; however, lead can promote immune dysfunctions characteristic of automimmune disease dysfunction.

Children with measurable blood lead concentrations showed no associated significant effects on major immunoglobulin concentrations, total complement, C3 component of complement, or antigenic response to tetanus toxoid.[17,18] Helper/inducer T cells (CD4) tended to decrease in workers after a 30-day exposure to lead accompanied by elevated blood lead levels; suppressor/cytotoxic T cells were not decreased.[19]

Mercury

T cell-dependent autoimmune phenomena are induced by mercuric chloride in animals. [20] IgG autoantibodies may be induced against the glomerular basement membrane[21,22]; this may be the first step in the formation of an autoimmune glomerulonephritis. Membranous nephropathy with immunofluorescent deposits of finely granular IgG/IgM and C3 complement has followed use of skin-lightening creams containing inorganic mercury.[23]

Nickel

Nickel and nickel compounds (nickel, nickel carbonyl, nickel carbonate, nickel hydroxide, nickel sulfate) can induce both dermal and pulmonary disease. Lung and nasal cancer,[24,25] asthma, and nasal septal necrosis have followed nickel exposure.[25] Nickel subsulfide administered to cynomolgus monkeys induced a decrease in macrophage phagocytic activity. Nickel may enhance tumor progression by inhibiting natural killer cell activity.[26] Nickel may also be a cause of allergic contact dermatitis.[27]

Cadmium

Glomerulonephritis and renal tubular lesions may follow cadmium use.[22,28] IgG glomerular deposits in the basement membrane,[22] suppression of antibody formation in animals,[29] as well as both impairment and enhancement of growth of animal tumors indicate that cadmium can deter certain segments of the immune system but augment others.

Aluminum

Exposure to aluminum produced abnormal T4/T8 ratios due to a disproportionate increase in the T8 cells. This was associated with B-cell lymphoma in adult workers. Immunodeficiency is a known risk factor for B-cell lymphoma.[30]

Other Metals

Beryllium, zinc, arsenic, manganese, selenium, chromium, and calcium may have profound clinical effects on the skin, lungs, peripheral nervous system, and hematologic system. A lymphocyte transformation test (blood and lung lavage lymphocytes) may be used as a beryllium screening test for occupationally exposed workers.[31,32] In chronic beryllium disease, beryllium acts as an antigen, stimulating local proliferation and accumulation in the lungs of beryllium-specific CD4-positive (helper/inducer) T cells.[32]

PESTICIDES

There is little evidence that occupational or environmental exposure to pesticides has led to clinically significant immunosuppression and, therefore, to an increased risk of developing infections or cancer. Hypersensitivity reactions to pesticides are generally low.[33]

Phenobarbital Hypersensitivity

A 5-year-old child treated with phenobarbital for 3 weeks developed a high fever, generalized erythematous rash, and edematous swelling of the face and limbs. Serum transaminase levels were elevated. Immunoglobulins (IgG, IgA, IgM) were decreased. Total complement activity (CH50) was low. Antinuclear antibody titer was not elevated. Renal biopsy demonstrated a tubulointerstitial nephritis. In this patient phenobarbital had induced a hypersensitivity state consisting of tubulointerstitial nephritis, an exfoliative dermatitis, and hepatitis.[34]

Toluene Diisocyanate

Preliminary studies suggest that pulmonary hypersensitivity and contact sensitivity to toluene diisocyanate may be diagnosed by determination of toluene diisocyanate-specific antibodies and by a rat mast cell degranulation test, respectively.[1] These initial studies should be confirmed by additional studies on exposed individuals.[35]

REFERENCES—IMMUNOTOXICANTS AND RELATED DISEASE

1. Tomas S, Pedro-Botet J, Auguet T. Ciprofloxacin and immunocomplex-mediated disease. J Intern Med 1991;23: 550–551.
2. Stejskal V, Nilsson R, Crepe A. Immunologic basis for adverse reactions to radiographic contrast media. Acta Radiol 1990;31:605–612.
3. Thrasher JD, Broughton A, Micovich P. Antibodies and immune profile of individuals occupationally exposed to formaldehyde: Six case reports. Am J Ind Med 1988;14:479–488.
4. Thrasher JD, Broughton A, Madison R. Human activation and autoantibodies in humans with long-term inhalation exposure to formaldehyde. Arch Environ Health 1990;45: 217–223.
5. Almroth G, Enestrom S, Hed J, et al. Autoantibodies to leucocyte antigens in hydralazine-associated nephritis. J Intern Med 1992;231:37–42.
6. Soto-Aguilar MC, de Shazo RD, Morgan JE et al. Total IgG and IgG subclass specific antibody responses to insulin in diabetic patients. Ann Allergy 1991;67:499–503.
7. Uchigata Y, Kawata S, Tokunaga K, et al. Strong association of insulin autoimmune syndrome with HLA-DR4. Lancet 1992;339:393–394.
8. Meschi F, Dozio N, Bognetti E, et al. An unusual case of recurrent hypoglycemia: 10 year follow-up of a child with insulin autoimmunity. Eur J Pediatr 1992;151:32–34.
9. Sobel JD. Acquired immunodeficiency syndrome in intravenous drug abusers. In: Levine DP, Sobel JD, eds. *Infections in Intravenous Drug Abusers.* New York: Oxford University Press, 1991:342–379.
10. Novick DM, Ochsharn M, Ghali V, et al. Natural killer call activity and lymphocyte subsets in parenteral heroin users and long term methadone maintenance patients. J Pharmacol Exp Ther 1989;250:606–610.
11. Novick DM, Kreek MJ. Methadone and immune function. Am J Med 1992;92:113–114.
12. Kauffman CA, Bradley SF. Host defense mechanisms in intravenous drug abusers. In: Levine DP, Sobel JD, eds. *Infections in Intravenous Drug Abusers.* New York: Oxford University Press, 1991:27–33.
13. Koller LD. Immunotoxicology of heavy metals. Int J Immunopharmacol 1980;2:269–279.
14. Warner GL, Lawrence DA. The effect of metals on IL-2 related lymphocyte proliferation. Int J Immunopharmacol 1988; 10:629–637.
15. McCabe MJ Jr, Lawrence DA. Lead, a major environmental pollutant, is immunomodulatory by its differential effects on CD4+ T-cell subsets. Toxicol Appl Pharmacol 1991;111: 13–23.
16. Wedeen RP. Occupational renal disease. Am J Kidney Dis 1984;3:241–258.
17. Reigart JR, Graber CD. Evaluation of the humoral immune response of children with low level lead exposure. Bull Environ Contam Toxicol 1976;16:112–117.
18. Sachs HK. Intercurrent infections in lead poisoning. Am J Dis Child 1978;132:315–316.
19. Pospischil E, Wolf C, Meisinger V, Jahn O. Immunological parameters in occupational lead poisoning: Trace elements in human health and disease. In: *Proceedings, Second Nordic Symposium. WHO/CEC/EPA.* Geneva: World Health Organization, 1987:110–114.
20. Inorganic mercury. Environmental Health Criteria 118 Geneva: World Health Organization, 1991.
21. Druet P, Hirsch F, Pelletier L, et al. Mechanisms of chemical-induced glomerulonephritis. In: Fowler BA, ed. *Mechanisms of Cell Injury: Complications for Human Health.* Dahlein Konferenzen. Chichester: John Wiley & Sons, 1987: 153–173.

22. Druet P, Bernard A, Hirsch F, et al. Immunologically mediated glomerulonephritis induced by heavy metals. Arch Toxicol 1982;50:187–194.
23. Kibukamusoke JW, Daires DR, Hutt MSR. Membranous nephropathy due to skin-lightening cream. Br Med J 1974;2: 646–647.
24. Sunderman FW. A review of the metabolism and toxicity of nickel. Ann Clin Lab Sci 1977;7:377–398.
25. Sunderman FW Jr. Mechanisms of nickel carcinogenesis. Scand J Work Environ Health 1989;15:1–12.
26. Haley PJ, Bice DE, Muggenburg BA, et al. Immunopathology: Effects of nickel subsulfide on the primate pulmonary immune system. Toxicol Appl Pharmacol 1987; 88:1–12.
27. Fisher AA. Unusual reaction associated with allergic reactions to nickel. Cutis 1991;47:86–88.
28. Buchet JP, Lauwerys R, Roels H, et al. Renal effects of cadmium body burden of the general population. Lancet 1990; 336:699–702.
29. Koller LD, Exon JH, Roan JG. Antibody suppression by cadmium. Arch Environ Health 1975;30:598–601.
30. Davis RL, Milham S Jr. Altered immune status in aluminum reduction plant workers. Am J Ind Med 1990;18:79–85.
31. Kreiss K, Newman LS, Mroz MM, Campbell PN. Screening blood test identified subclinical berryllium disease. J Occup Med 1989;31:602–608.
32. Saltini C, Winestock K, Kirby M, et al. Manitenance of alveolitis in patients with chronic beryllium disease by beryllium-specific helper T cells. N Engl J Med 1989;320:1103–1109.
33. Botham PA. Are pesticides immunotoxic? Adverse Drug React Acute Poison Rev 1990;9:91–101.
34. Sawaishi Y, Komatsu K, Takeda O, et al. A case of tubulointerstitial nephritis with exfoliative dermatitis and hepatitis due to phenobarbital hypersensitivity. Eur J Pediatr 1992;151: 69–72.
35. Huang J, Wang X-p, Chen B-m, et al. Immunologic effects of toluence diisocyante exposure on painters. Arch Environ Contam Toxicol 1991;21:607–611.
36. Gleichmann E, Kimber I, Purchase IFH. Immunotoxicology: Suppressive and stimulatory effects of drugs and environmental chemicals on the immune system. Arch Toxicol 1989;63:257–273.

HYPERSENSITIVITY

Immunologic hypersensitivity is an overreaction of the immune system to a substance and is probably the most prominent form of immunotoxicity seen in patients. This reaction is an exaggerated response to antigenic stimulus in which there is a reduced threshold to antigen. Terms used to describe hypersensitivity include anaphylaxis, atrophy, and allergy.

CONTACT SENSITIVITY AND SKIN DISORDERS

Occupational exposure to chemicals and other xenobiotics (see Chapters 65 and 66) is an important cause of hypersensitivity reactions. Some common contact sensitizers are listed in Table 44–21.

Table 44–21
Common Contact Sensitizers

Plants	Minerals
Poison ivy	Beryllium
European primrose	Nickel
Synthetic compounds	Cadmium
Benzocaine	Chromates
Epoxy resins	Silver
Mercaptan	Zirconium
Picric acid derivatives	Cutting oils
C-1 hydrocarbons	
Ethylenediamine	
p-Phenylenediamine	
Thimerosol	

Source: Office of Technology Assessment, 1991.

OCCUPATIONAL ASTHMA

Many chemicals can induce asthma. Large-molecular-weight substances, usually proteins, can cause classic IgE-mediated asthma. Low-molecular-weight materials can cause non-IgE-mediated, longer-lasting types of asthma. Occupational asthma is often of the non-IgE-mediated type. Workers can become sensitized after exposure to concentrations of chemicals well below the statutory exposure limits. Some common industrial chemicals associated with occupational asthma are listed in Table 44–22.[1]

Table 44–22
Industrial Chemicals Associated With Occupational Asthma

Platinum salts	Ethylenediamine
Nickel salts	Phthalic anhydrides
Pyrethrum	Colophony resins
Diisocyanates	Exotic wood dusts

Source: Office of Technology Assessment, 1991.

Table 44–23 summarizes some drugs that may induce adverse pulmonary effects, among which are those associated with hypersensitivity pneumonitis (see also Chapter 66).

HYPERSENSITIVITY MYOCARDITIS

The diagnosis of hypersensitivity myocarditis (Table 44–24) should be considered when new electrocardiographic changes, mildly elevated enzyme levels, cardiomegaly, or unexplained tachycardia is noted in a patient who has an ongoing allergy reaction to a drug, usually with eosinophils. Percutaneous transverse biopsy of the myocardium may yield tissue for confirmation of the diagnosis, which consists of histologic demonstration of a diffuse interstitial infiltrate rich in eosinophils, with or without cellular necrosis. Most cases of hypersensitivity myocarditis due to drugs have been caused by methyldopa, the sulfonamides, and penicillin.[2]

GELL AND COOMBS CATEGORIES OF IMMUNOPATHOLOGY

Immunopathologic mechanisms involved in hypersensitivity disorders have been classified according to Gell and Coombs as types I through IV[3] (Table 44–25). More than one mechanism can operate simultaneously in a patient.

Table 44-23
Some Drugs That Cause Adverse Pulmonary Effects

Drug	Reaction	Estimated Frequency	Risk Factors
Amiodarone (Cordarone)	Acute pneumonitis, fibrosis, hypersensitivity pneumonitis	Occasional	High doses
Aspirin	See Salicylates		
Atracurium (Tracrium)	See Neuromuscular blockers		
Azathioprine (Imuran)	Hypersensitivity pneumonitis	Rare	Not known
Beta-adrenergic blockers	Bronchospasm	Occasional	High doses, nonselective, asthma, atopy
Bleomycin (Blenoxane)	Acute pneumonitis, fibrosis, bronchiolitis obliterans, hypersensitivity pneumonitis	Occasional	Total dose, age, oxygen, radiotherapy, multiple drugs
Bromocriptine (Parlodel)	Pleuritis, fibrosis	Occasional	Age, male, smoker
Busulfan (Myleran)	Fibrosis	Occasional	Duration of treatment
Captopril (Capoten)	Cough	Occasional	Not known
Carbamazepine (Tegretol, others)	Hypersensitivity pneumonitis	Rare	Not known
Carmustine (BiCNU)	Acute pneumonitis, fibrosis (may be delayed for years)	Frequent in long-term survivors	Dosage, duration, multiple drugs in short-term
Chlorambucil (Leukeran)	Acute pneumonitis, fibrosis	Rare	Not known
Cocaine	Edema, hemorrhage	Occasional	Inhaled or IV cocaine
Cyclophosphamide (Cytoxan, others)	Hypersensitivity pneumonitis, edema, fibrosis	Rare	Multiple drugs
Cytarabine (Cytosar-U)	Edema	Frequent	Total dose
Dantrolene (Dantrium)	Pleuritis, pneumonitis	Rare	Not known
Diclofenac (Voltaren)	See NSAIDs		
Enalapril (Vasotec)	Cough	Occasional	Not known
Ethchlorvynol (Placidyl, others)	Edema	Rare	Overdose only
Gold salts (Myochrysine, Solganal, others)	Hypersensitivity pneumonitis, fibrosis, bronchiolitis obliterans	Rare	Not known
Hydrochlorothiazide (Esidrix, others)	Edema	Rare	Not known
Ibuprofen (Motrin, others)	See NSAIDs		
Indomethacin (Indocin, others)	See NSAIDs		
Interleukin-2 (Proleukin)	Edema	Occasional	Increased capillary permeability
Lidocaine (Xylocaine, others)	Edema	One report	Not known
Lisinopril (Prinivil, Zestril)	Cough	Occasional	Not known
Lomustine (CeeNu)	Fibrosis	Rare	Not known
Melphalan (Alkeran)	Fibrosis	Rare	Not known
Methadone (Dolophine, others)	See Opiates		
Methotrexate (Folex, others)	Pleuritis, hypersensitivity pneumonitis, edema, fibrosis	Occasional	Cancer, frequent doses, multiple drugs, withdrawal from corticosteroids, adrenalectomy
Methysergide (Sansert)	Pleuritis	Rare	Not known
Mitomycin (Mutamycin)	Acute pneumonitis, fibrosis	Occasional	Frequent doses, concurrent or consecutive vinblastine or vindestine
Naloxone (Narcan)	Edema	Rare	Not known
Naproxen (Naprosyn)	See NSAIDs		
Neuromuscular blockers	Bronchospasm	Rare	Not known
Nitrofurantoin (Furadantin, others)	Hypersensitivity pneumonitis, fibrosis	Rare	Acute or long-term use
NSAIDs	Bronchospasm, hypersensitivity pneumonitis, edema, fibrosis	Occasional	Asthma, aspirin intolerance
Opiates	Edema	Rare	Overdose
Pancuronium (Pavulon)	See Neuromuscular Blockers		
Penicillamine (Cuprimine, Depen)	Bronchiolitis obliterans, hypersensitivity pneumonitis, fibrosis	Rare	Not known
	Pulmonary–renal syndrome	Rare	Duration of treatment
Phenylbutazone (Butazolidin, others)	See NSAIDs		
Phenytoin (Dilantin, others)	Hypersensitivity pneumonitis	Rare	Not known
Pilocarpine	Bronchospasm	Rare	Asthma
Pindolol (Visken)	See Beta-adrenergic Blockers		
Piroxicam (Feldene)	See NSAIDs		
Procarbazine (Matulane)	Hypersensitivity pneumonitis	Rare	Not known

NSAIDs, nonsteroidal antiinflammatory drugs.
From Drugs that cause pulmonary toxicity. Med Lett Drugs Ther 1990;32(827):88–90.

Table 44–23 *(Continued)*

Drug	Reaction	Estimated Frequency	Risk Factors
Propafenone (Rythmol)	Bronchospasm	Rare	Asthma
Propoxyphene (Darvon, others)	See Opiates		
Propranolol (Inderal, others)	See Beta-adrenergic Blockers		
Protamine	Edema	Rare	Previous exposure
Pyrimethamine–chloroquine (Daraclor)	Hypersensitivity pneumonitis	Rare	Not known
Pyrimethamine–dapsone (Maloprim)	Hypersensitivity pneumonitis	Rare	Not known
Pyrimethamine–sulfadoxine (Fansidar)	Hypersensitivity pneumonitis	Rare	Not known
Ritodrine (Yutopar)	Edema	Rare	Not known
Salicylates	Edema	Occasional	Overdosage only
	Bronchospasm	Occasional	Asthma, NSAID sensitivity
Semustine	Fibrosis	Rare	Not known
Sulfasalazine (Azulfidine, others)	Hypersensitivity pneumonitis, bronchiolitis obliterans, fibrosis	Rare	Not known
Sulindac (Clinoril)	See NSAIDs		
Suxamethonium	See Neuromuscular Blockers		
Terbutaline (Brethine)	Edema	Rare	Not known
Timolol (Blocadren, others)	See Beta-adrenergic Blockers		
Tocainide (Tonocard)	Pneumonitis, fibrosis	Rare	Not known
Tryptophan	Pneumonitis	Rare	Not known
Tubocurarine (Metubine, others)	See Neuromuscular Blockers		
Vecuronium	See Neuromuscular Blockers		
Vinblastine (Velban, others)	Acute pneumonitis, bronchospasm	Frequent	Concurrent or consecutive mitomycin only
Vindesine (Eldisine)	Acute pneumonitis, bronchospasm	Frequent	Concurrent or consecutive mitomycin only

Table 44–24
Drugs Reported to Be Associated With Hypersensitivity Myocarditis

Acetazolamide	Oxyphenbutazone
p-Aminosalicylic acid	Penicillin
Amitriptyline hydrochloride	Phenindione
Amphotericin B	Phenylbutazone
Ampicillin	Phenytoin
Carbamazepine	Spironolactone
Chloramphenicol	Streptomycin
Chlorthalidone	Sulfadiazine
Hydrochlorothiazide	Sulfisoxazole
Indomethacin	Sulfonylureas
Isoniazid	Tetracycline
Methyldopa	

From Taliercio CP, Olney BA, Lie JT. Myocarditis related to drug hypersensitivity. Mayo Clin Proc 1985;60:463–468.

Table 44–25
Allergic and Pseudoallergic Reactions to Drugs: Immune Mechanism

Drug Allergy (Immunologic Adverse Reactions)
Type I: IgE-mediated hypersensitivity (eg, penicillin, chymopapain, and insulin anaphylaxis)
Type II: Cytotoxic antibodies, often with participation of complement (eg, penicillin-induced hemolytic anemia)
Type III: Antigen-antibody immune complex and complement-amplified reactions (eg, serum sickness from any drug, drug fever, and pituitary snuff allergic alveolitis)
Type IV: Cell-mediated hypersensitivity (eg, neomycin and paraben contact dermatitis)

Possible Drug Allergy (Reactions Involving Suspected Immune Mechanisms)
Many drug-associated skin reactions (eg, erythema, erythema multiforme, maculopapular rash, and fixed drug reaction)
Febrile mucocutaneous syndrome (erythema multiforme, Stevens–Johnson syndrome, toxic epidermal necrolysis, or Lyell's syndrome)
Drug fever
Eosinophillic pneumonitis
Drug-induced cholestasis and hepatitis
Interstitial nephritis
Lymphadenopathy

Pseudoallergic Drug Reaction (Drug Idiosyncrasy)
Anaphylactoid (anaphylaxis-like) reaction (eg, radiocontrast media)
Salicylate intolerance (in some cases due to modification of mediator production or release)
Sulfite preservative sensitivity
Ampicillin rash

From Anderson JA, Adkinson NF Jr. Allergic reactions to drugs and biologic agents. JAMA 1987;258:2891–2899.

REFERENCES—HYPERSENSITIVITY

1. Salvaggio GE. Overview of occupational immunologic lung disease. J Allergy Clin Immunol 1982;70:5–10.
2. Taliercio CP, Olney BA, Lie JT: Myocarditis related to drug hypersensitivity. Mayo Clin Proc 1985;60:463–468.
3. Anderson JA, Adkinson NF Jr. Allergic reactions to drugs and biologic agents. JAMA 1987;258:2891–2899.

HUMAN ADJUVANT DISEASE AND SILICONE IMPLANTS

Approximately 100,000 breast implants are performed each year in the United States,[1] and more than half a million augmentation mammoplasties using silicone implants were estimated to have been performed between 1959 and 1979.[2,3] Connective tissue disease may have followed the use of various implant materials including silicone, often after an interval of many years,[4–14] but there have been no controlled clinical trials to support this. The term *human adjuvant disease* was proposed to describe such connective tissue disorders.[5]

DEFINITION OF ADJUVANT

The term *adjuvant* means assistance or help. An *immunologic adjuvant* is a substance that nonspecifically increases or changes the characteristics of the immune response to an antigenically unrelated antigen.[7,14] Freund's complete adjuvant is an example. It is prepared by adding killed mycobacteria to a water-in-oil emulsion containing an antigen in the water phase. The adjuvant-killed mycobacteria increase the humoral response (antibodies) and induce a cellular immunity to the antigen.[15]

DEFINITION OF AUTOIMMUNE DISORDERS

An *autoimmune disorder* is one in which the immune system reacts to an endogenous antigen with subsequent injury to the tissues. The course is characterized by abnormalities of the immune response, chronic inflammation, and autoantibody formation. These disorders are often associated with human leukocyte antigens (HLA) related to a complex of genes known as the *major histocompatibility complex* and of major importance in graft rejection after organ transplantation.[7]

CHARACTERISTICS OF HUMAN ADJUVANT DISEASE

Characteristics of human adjuvant disease have been proposed[5,6]:

1. Autoimmune disease-like symptoms that develop in a woman usually several years after a plastic surgery with foreign substance injection
2. Injection into the breasts or other areas of silicone, paraffin, or related substances that possibly have adjuvant effects
3. Histopathological observation of foreign-body granulomas in the injected areas and their draining lymph nodes
4. Some serologic abnormality such as autoantibodies
5. Improvement in the symptoms of some patients after removal of the foreign substance
6. No infection or malignancy in the operated region

Table 44-26
Adjuvants

Nonbacterial Compounds
Mineral compounds
Aluminum (used with human vaccines), silicone, beryllium, and calcium compounds
Liposomes
Synthetic polymers
Nonionic block polymer surfactants, eg, Pluronic polyols, Tween 80, and muramyl dipeptide
Synthetic ionic polymers
Polyadenylic–polyuridylic acid complexes
Host mediators
Other interleukin-1 and interleukin-2 compounds: colchicine, saponins, bestatin (phenylbutyryl leucine)
Bacterial immunostimulants
Bordetella pertussis, Corynebacterium parvum, lipopolysaccharides from *Escherichia coli,* muramyl peptides

Examples of Adjuvants

Adjuvants are listed in Table 44–26.

Silicone

Early use of paraffin, processed petroleum, and liquid silicone often induced severe local inflammatory and general immunologic tissue responses.[4–8] After 1950 these materials were supplanted by organosilicone polymers, which can be synthesized as liquids, gels, or rubberlike (elastomer) products. Subsequently, silicone was largely used in either saline or gel-filled elastomer envelopes.[8]

Silicone Polymers

Silicone polymers (polydimethylsiloxane) as used in implant surgery are compounds of polymer, filler, and catalyst.

Dimethylpolysiloxane is polymerized into long chains as an elastomer.

Silicone Shells

Silicone mammary implant shells for both gel- and saline-filled implants consist of the dimethylpolysiloxane polymer with 30% silicone dioxide filler. The silicone dioxide is fused to the silicone polymer by a chemical process. It is possible that silicone dioxide projections may be sheared off from the surface.

Silicone Gel

The elastomer polymer is crosslinked to produce the gel.

Liquid Silicone

Glucose-like dimethylpolysiloxane polymer chains without filler have been used as liquid silicone.

Elastomeric silicone is also used in the production of heart valves, prosthetic finger joints, arteriovenous shunts for dialysis patients, and ventricular shunts for hydrocephalus control. No connective tissue diseases (CTDs) have been reported following these uses.[8] Such diseases have been reported only following breast implants. The form (gel-filled implant) or the amount of silicone used may be a contributing factor.

Other Adjuvants

Other adjuvants used to encourage greater persistence of antigenic stimulation experimentally and clinically (eg, vaccines) are listed in Table 44–26.[7,9,16] These compounds may enhance helper T cells, block suppressor T cells, and stimulate B cells.

Adjuvants may potentiate the immune response by enhancing antigen localization (aluminum compounds, liposomes, water-and-oil emulsion [Freund's incomplete adjuvant]); enhancing antigen presentation (interferon gamma interferon inducers, beryllium, muramyl dipeptide, Freund's complete adjuvant); and activating lymphocytes (interleukins-1 and -2).[16]

Mechanism of Action

An exact mechanism explaining the relationship between adjuvant use and the induction of connective tissue diseases remains obscure. Silicone is known to be converted to silica. Silicone has been found outside the breast prosthesis, even when there has been no apparent defect in the envelope. Therefore, silica may be exposed to circulating macrophages, which then could release factors that increase collagen synthesis by fibroblasts.[17] Silica has been reported to induce the development of autoantibodies and connective tissue diseases including systemic lupus erythematosus and scleroderma.[12,14] In addition, silicone itself may act as an adjuvant leading to autoimmune disease.

Complications occur after silicone implants. Silicone gel may diffuse through the silicone elastomer membrane (gel bleed), and can migrate through lymphatic or hematogenous pathways to involve multiple organ systems. Silicone granulomas have been found in the abdominal wall, breasts, neck, penis, sacrum, thighs, and upper extremity.[14]

Clinical Presentation

Acute Injury

Three patients were accidentally exposed to Freund's adjuvant.[18–20] In two of the patients injection was into a finger[18–20]; in one, into the hand.[19] There were delays in the onset of illness of 3 weeks (herpesvirus infection of the eye),[18] 25 days (headache, fever, meningeal signs, lateral rectus palsy),[19] and 3 days (swelling of finger, pleural pain, fever),[20] respectively. In each case, a granuloma formed at the site of injury. All recovered.

Chronic Delayed Hypersensitivity (Silicone Implant-Associated Syndrome)

Connective tissue diseases (systemic lupus erythematosus, progressive systemic sclerosis [scleroderma], mixed connective tissue disease, rheumatoid arthritis, Hashimoto's thyroiditis, Sjögren's syndrome, and morphea) have been reported following use of silicone or paraffin for breast augmentation.[5–14] Such disease may arise from 0.2 to 18 years after the original injection or implant.[10] Raynaud's phenomenon, arthralgia, liver dysfunction, and jaundice may be observed.[11] Dry mouth and swollen stiff fingers are often experienced by the patient early in the course of the connective tissue disease. One clinical study found no association between silicone breast implants and connective tissue diseases.[21]

Laboratory

Elevations in the erythrocyte sedimentation rate, hypergammaglobulinemia, and leukopenia may be observed.[10] Autoantibodies such as rheumatoid factor (RF), antithyroglobulin antibody, antinuclear antibody, anti-DNA, anti-ribonucleoprotein, and anti-Sm have been observed. Positive lupus erythematosus preparations can occasionally be found.

Treatment

Treatment is symptomatic and supportive. Mild discomfort may respond to nonsteroidal antiinflammatory drugs. Steroids may be of value depending on clinical judgment. Surgical consultation should be obtained if there are obvious tumor excrescences, which should be surgically removed. If connective tissue disease or human adjuvant disease begins consideration should be given to removal of the silicone breast implants, although this procedure may not be effective in lessening evidence of the connective tissue disease. Patients should have a full immunohematologic workup including erythrocyte sedimentation rate, immunoglobulin levels (IgG, A, E, and M), complement C_3 and C_4 levels, fluorescent antinuclear antibody levels, and, if positive, tests for extractable nuclear antigen, followed by ribonucleoprotein and Smith and rheumatoid factors. HLA typing could then be obtained, including HLA-A, -B, -Dr, and -DQ.[14]

Histopathologic and immunopathologic examinations should be done from biopsied tissue. Histologic examination should include a hematoxylin and eosin stain for evidence of inflammation, fragmentation, plasma cells, lymphocytes and histiocytes, including macrophages, and immunofluorescence studies, including IgM, IgG, light-chain immunoglobulins, complement, and fibrinogen. Special stains for class II transplantation antigens may be useful.[14]

FDA Panel Recommendations

On February 20, 1992, the Food and Drug Administration's General and Plastic Surgery Devices Panel recommended that silicone gel-filled breast implants be available only to women enrolled in clinical protocols. They recommended that any woman who requires breast reconstruction, for example, after mastectomy or injury to the breast, be allowed to participate in the clinical protocols if alternative reconstruction methods are not suitable. They further recommended that women who already have silicone breast implants should not consider having them removed unless there are problems. Women should be alert to symptoms that may signal implant rupture, capsular contracture, or autoimmune or connective tissue disorders. Symptoms may include changes in the firmness, size, shape, or color of the breasts as well as any pain or tenderness. Symptoms related to autoimmune disorders include joint swelling and pain, skin redness or swelling, swollen glands, unusual fatigue, and swelling of the hands and feet.

Periodic medical examinations are also recommended to detect breast cancer or probable implant rupture.

Women with implants should have regular mammography examinations to detect breast cancer, if recommended for their age group. Mammography screening facilities (preferably those accredited by the American College of Radiology) should use special techniques to detect cancer in patients with implants. The panel recommended against routine mammograms to detect "silent" ruptures of the implants, and noted that other methods to detect ruptures are still considered experimental.

Until the Food and Drug Administration makes its final decision, it recommends to physicians that:

1. Surgeons should not implant silicone gel breast implants.
2. Saline-filled implants can be used when breast implants are medically necessary.
3. Physicians should evaluate patients' problems with the possible link between immune-related disorders and the implants in mind.[22]

REFERENCES—HUMAN ADJUVANT DISEASE AND SILICONE IMPLANTS

1. Spiera H. Scleroderma after silicone augmentation mammoplasty. JAMA 1988;260:236–238.
2. Uretsky BF, O'Brien JJ, Courtisi EH, et al. Augmentation mammoplasty with a severe systemic illness. Ann Plast Surg 1979;3:445–447.
3. Walsh FW, Solomon DA, Espinoza LR, et al. Human adjuvant disease: A new cause of chylous effusions. Arch Intern Med 1989;149:1194–1196.
4. Miyoshi K, Miyamura T, Kobayashi Y, et al. Hypergammaglobulinemia by prolonged adjuvanticity in men: Disorders developed after augmentation mammaplasty. Jpn Med J 1964;2122:9–14.
5. Miyoshi K, Shiragami H, Yoshida K. Adjuvant disease of man. Clin Immunol (Tokyo) 1973:785–794.
6. Kumagai Y, Abe C, Shiokawa Y. Scleroderma after cosmetic surgery: Four cases of human adjuvant disease. Arthritis Rheum 1979;22:532–537.
7. Osebold JW. Mechanisms of action by immunologic adjuvants. JAMA 1982;181:983–987.
8. Van Nunen SA, Gatenby PA, Basten A. Post-mammoplasty connective tissue disease. Arthritis Rheum 1982;25:694–697.
9. Baldwin CM Jr, Kaplan EN. Silicone-induced human adjuvant disease? Ann Plast Surg 1983;10:270–273.
10. Kumagai Y, Shiokawa Y, Medsger TA Jr, Rodman GP. Clinical spectrum of connective tissue disease after cosmetic surgery: Observations on eighteen patients and a review of the Japanese literature. Arthritis Rheum 1984;27:1–12.
11. Okano Y, Nishikai M, Sato A. Scleroderma, primary biliary cirrhosis and Sjogren's syndrome after cosmetic breast augmentation with silicone injection: A case report of possible human adjuvant disease. Ann Rheum Dis 1984;43:520–522.
12. Fock KM, Feng PH, Tey BH. Autoimmune disease developing after augmentation mammoplasty: Report of 3 cases. J Rheumatol 1984;11:98–100.
13. Byron MA, Venning VA, Mowat AG. Post-mammoplasty human adjuvant disease. Br J Rheumatol 1984;23:227–229.
14. Sergott TJ, Limoli JP, Baldwin CM Jr, Laub DR. Human adjuvant disease, possible autoimmune disease after silicone implantation: A review of the literature, case studies and speculation for the future. Plast Reconstr Surg 1986;78:104–114.
15. Freund J, McDermott K. Sensitization to horse serum by means of adjuvants. Proc Soc Exp Biol Med 1942;49:548–553.
16. Lise LD, Audibert F. Immunoadjuvants and analogs of immunomodulatory bacterial structures. Curr Opin Immunol 1989;2:269–274.
17. Vargas A. Shedding of silicone particles from infected breast implants. Plast Reconstr Surg 1979;64:252–253.
18. Conklin HB, Curtis RM, Ben-Efraim S. Koch's phenomenon involving the flexor tendon sheath: Adjuvant-induced tenosynovitis in man. J Bone Joint Surg 1964;51A:1413–1419.
19. Drachman DA, Paterson P, Bornstein MB. Experimental allergic encephalomyelitis in man: A laboratory accident. Neurology 1974;24:364.
20. Berry EM, Geltner D, Chajek T. Accidental injection of Freund's adjuvant. Lancet 1975;1:863–864.
21. Sanchez-Guerrero J, Colditz GA, Karlson EW, Silicone breast implants and the risk of connective tissue diseases and symptoms. N Engl J Med 1995;332:1666–1670.
22. Recommendations on Silicone Breast Implants. FDA Med Bull 1992;22(1):3–4.

INITIAL SCREENING OF IMMUNOLOGIC FUNCTION

The World Health Organization's Immunology Section has recommended eight immunologic tests as an initial screening for patients with suspected immune dysfunction: (1) a complete blood count with differential cell count; (2) quantitative protein electrophoresis; (3) humoral mediated immunity immunoelectrophoresis; (4) quantitation of IgG, IgM, IgA, and IgE; (5) isoantibody titers; (6) cell-mediated immunity; delayed hypersensitivity skin testing; (7) autoimmunity, autoantibody titers; and (8) C3, and C4 levels (Table 44–27).

IMMUNOLOGIC LABORATORY FORMAT

A clinical immunologic investigation should involve parameters suggested by the World Health Organization.[1,2]

ALTERNATIVE ANTIBODIES

Practitioners of alternative medical approaches to diagnosis and treatment may use the laboratory to support therapeutic regimens based on unique and often unproven ecology concepts. Tests such as those for antimyelin antibodies and antibenzene antibodies frequently have not been subjected to careful prospective studies involving determinations of sensitivity and specificity when correlated with definitive diseases.

Table 44–27
Initial Screening Tests of Immune Function

Test	Comment
A. Humoral Immunity	
1. Quantitative immunoglobulin levels	Serum concentration
Proteins carrying antibody activity	
Antibodies (the secreted products of plasma cells)	
IgG	8.00–15.00 g/L (800–1500 mg/dL)
Most prevalent Ig	
IgM	0.45–1.50 g/L (45–250 mg/dL)
IgA (Principal Ig in secretory fluids)	0.90–3.25 g/L (90–325 mg/dL)
IgD represented on B-cell surface	30 mg/L (30 μg/mL)
IgE (lowest Ig in serum, associated with reaginic hypersensitivity reactions in humans)	100 μg/L (100 ng/mL)
2. Tests of specific antibody formation	
3. Isohemagglutinin titer	Measures IgM response
Antistreptolysin O: antibodies to measles, mumps, polio	
B. Cell-Mediated Immunity	
1. White blood cell count with differential	Measures total lymphocyte levels
2. Delayed hypersensitivity skin tests: *Trichophyton, Candida albicans,* PPD, mumps antigen	Measures specific T-cell and macrophage response to antigens; indicates intact and normally functioning cell-mediated immune system
C. Phagocytosis	
1. White blood cell count with differential	Measures total neutrophils
2. Nitroblue tetrazolium (NBT) test, superoxide production	Measures metabolic function
3. Chemotaxis	Measures cell motility
4. Quantitative measurement of intracellular bacterial killing	
D. Autoimmunity	
1. Complement	Monitors immune complex disease (eg, systemic lupus erythematosus, glomerulonephritis)
Total hemolytic complement (CH_{50})	
Total complement activity	
Assay of individual complement components	Defines complement component deficiency
C3	Alternate complement pathway (0.55–1.2 g/L)
C4	Classic complement pathway
2. Autoantibody titers	
Against nuclei, smooth muscle DNA, and thyroid tissue	

ORGAN DONORS

An increase in the need for organ donors has recently brought attention to the possibility of organ donation by victims of toxin exposures.[3,4] Donor organs may contain a significant store of a toxin that preferentially accumulates in donated organs (see Table 6–15).[3,4] Leikin and colleagues suggest that death from poisoning does not seem to be an absolute contraindication to liver or kidney donation. Organs from victims of cyanide and carbon monoxide poisoning have been transplanted with success. Meperidine neurotoxicity (recurrent seizures, myoclonus, and asterixis) was diagnosed in an organ transplant recipient. Drug interactions, deranged drug metabolism, or impaired drug elimination can occur in transplant recipients.[5]

REFERENCES—INITIAL SCREENING OF IMMUNOLOGIC FUNCTION

1. Report of an IUIS/WHO Working Group. Use and abuse of laboratory tests in clinical immunology: Critical considerations of eight widely used diagnostic procedures. Clin Exp Immunol 1981;46:662–674.
2. De Shazo RD, Lopez M, Salvaggio JE. Use and interpretation of diagnostic immunologic laboratory tests. JAMA 1987;258:3011–3031.
3. Leikin JB, Heyn-Lamb R, Aks S, et al. The toxic patient as a potential organ donor. Am J Emerg Med 1994;12:151–154.
4. Baselt RC, Carvey RH. *Disposition of Toxic Doses and Chemicals in Man.* 3rd ed. Chicago: Year Book Medical, 1989.
5. Adair JC, Gilmore RL. Meperidine neurotoxicity after organ transplantations. Clin Toxicol 1994;32:325–328.

Chapter 45
Respiratory Drugs

ALMITRINE DIMESYLATE (BISMESYLATE)

Almitrine dismesylate (Vectarion, Duxil) is used in Europe as a respiratory stimulant in patients with the hypoxemic form of chronic respiratory insufficiency caused by chronic bronchitis and emphysema.[1] Prolonged use may lead to a severe and disabling peripheral neuropathy, which may have a pharmacogenetic association. Acute overdose may result in abdominal discomfort, headaches, and flushing, hyperventilation, or hypercapnia. Few overdoses have been reported. This drug has not been approved by the Food and Drug Administration.

Use

Almitrine, an agonist of peripheral chemoreceptors, is used in the treatment of hypoxemia and hypercapnia associated with chronic respiratory disease.[1]

Product Formulation

Almitrine bismesylate is prescribed as white oral film-coated tablets of 50 mg. An intravenous form (pH 2–3) contains lyophilized almitrine bismesylate (15 mg) with methanesulfuric acid and mannitol as excipients and malic acid as a solvent for injection.

Therapeutic Dose

Oral almitrine 100 to 200 mg daily improves arterial blood gas tension in patients with stable hypoxemic chronic obstructive airway disease.[2,3]

Toxic Dose

At doses of 100 to 200 mg daily, some patients attain plasma concentrations well above the optimal therapeutic plasma concentration of 200 to 300 ng/mL. Such raised almitrine levels are related to the incidence of peripheral paresthesias.[4]

Toxicokinetics

Absorption

The bioavailability of oral almitrine is about 70% of an intravenous dose because it undergoes hepatic first-pass metabolism.[5] After a single dose of 50 mg, a plasma almitrine concentration of 18.5 ng/mL is reached in 0.6 hour. A dose of 1.5 mg/kg leads to a peak plasma level of 300 ng/mL.[6] Following 50 mg twice daily for 14 days, the plasma level is 172 ng/mL. Peak steady-state plasma levels reach 480 ng/mL in 270 days.[7] After 100 mg twice daily, blood levels were less than 200 to 300 ng/mL (optimum therapeutic range) until day 14. Following 50 mg orally twice daily, maximum plasma loading almitrine levels of 150 to 200 ng/mL were reached in 2 to 3 hours. Toxicokinetics in patients with chronic obstructive lung disease are similar to those in healthy subjects.[2,3] Almitrine is 99% protein bound, mostly to albumin.[8] The volume of distribution is relatively high (14 L/kg).[6,8]

Metabolism

Almitrine undergoes hepatic oxidation to several hydroxylated metabolites.[9]

Elimination

Almitrine is metabolized in the liver followed by rapid excretion of the metabolites in the bile. Elimination half-life is 40 to 60 hours. Steady-state elimination is 11 to 15 days.[6] About 10% of a dose appears in the urine.[10] Plasma clearance is comparatively low.[8]

Mechanism of Action

Almitrine bismesylate acts directly on peripheral chemoreceptors to stimulate ventilation and improve arterial blood gas tensions.[11] Almitrine appears to be effective in increasing Pao_2 in patients with hypoxemic chronic bronchitis and emphysema.[12,13] Almitrine reduced the ventilation/perfusion inequalities present in acute respiratory distress syndrome through a reduction in the shunt present in those patients.[14] The effect is transient, ending as soon as administration of the drug ceases.[14] Almitrine causes a 60% decrease in the distensibility of the right pulmonary artery.[15]

Herve and colleagues suggest the following as a working hypothesis: Almitrine decreases arterial wall distensibility, and increased pulmonary vascular resistance levels, leading to redistribution of pulmonary blood flow. This induces recruitment of gas-exchange vessels, which in turn leads to improvement of arterial blood gas levels.[15] Susceptibility to development of almitrine neuropathy is not related to a poor metabolizer phenotype with regard to the isoenzyme involved in the oxidation of dextromethorphan and debrisoquin.[15]

Clinical Presentation

Doses greater than 100 mg/d are associated with nausea, abdominal discomfort, headache, and flushing.[3] Sensory neuropathy may develop after 2 to 12 months of treatment with almitrine.[16] In patients with chronic obstructive airway disease, neuropathies have been observed. Weight loss is a reliable criterion for the diagnosis of almitrine neuropathy.[16] Weight loss occurs more in overweight patients.[17]

Laboratory

Analytical Methods

A sensitive high-pressure liquid chromatography method has a detection limit of 5 ng/mL for almitrine and 10 to 25 mg/mL for its metabolites.[5,10]

Blood Levels

Increased plasma levels (> 30 ng/mL) are related to the incidence of symptoms (peripheral paresthesias),[12] but plasma level monitoring cannot circumvent the occurrence of such peripheral paresthesias. There is no correlation between arterial blood gas and plasma almitrine concentrations.[13,17]

Suggested Review Articles

- Alani SM, Twomey JA, Peak MD. Almitrine and peripheral neuropathy. Lancet 1985;2:1251.
- Barre J, Didey F, Urien S, et al. In vitro studies on the blood distribution of almitrine. Pharmacology 1989;38: 381–387.
- Belu L, Larry D, de Cremoux H, et al. Extensive oxidative metabolism of dextromethorphan in patients with almitrine neuropathy. Br J Clin Pharmacol 1989; 27:387–390.
- Bouche P, Lacomblez L, Leger JM, et al. Peripheral neuropathies during treatment with almitrine: Report of 46 cases. J Neurol 1989;236:29–33.
- Bromet N, Courte S, Anbut Y, et al. Pharmacokinetics of almitrine bismesylate: Studies in patients. Eur J Respir Dis 1983;64(suppl. 126):363–375.
- Lerebours G, Moore N, Senant J. Almitrine and peripheral nerve function. Lancet 1988;2:799–800.
- Racine A, Bromet N, Courte S, Voisin C. Dosage de l'almitrine dans les milieux biologiques. J Chromatogr Biomed Appl 1981;223:219–224.
- Touaty E, Viau F, Pariente R. A therapeutic trial of intravenous almitrine and exacerbation of chronic respiratory failure. Rev Fr Mal Respir 1980;8:621–628.

REFERENCES—ALMITRINE DIMESYLATE (BIMESYLATE)

1. Bakran I, Vrhovac B, Stangl B, et al. Double blind placebo controlled clinical trial of almitrine bismesylate in patients with chronic respiratory insufficiency. Eur J Clin Pharmacol 1990;38:249–253.
2. Bardsley PA, Howard P, De Bache W, et al. Two years treatment with almitrine bismesylate in patients with hypoxic chronic obstructive airways disease. Eur Respir J 1991;4: 308–310.
3. Bardsley PA, Tweney J, Morgan N, Howard P. Oral almitrine in treatment of acute respiratory failure and cor pulmonale in patients with an exacerbation of chronic obstructive airway disease. Thorax 1991;46:493–498.
4. Howard P. Hypoxia, almitrine and peripheral neuropathy. Thorax 1989;44:247–250.
5. Vidon N, Chaussade S, Jeanniot P, et al. Almitrine bismesylate disposition in the human digestive tract. Eur J Clin Pharmacol 1989;37:487–491.

6. Bromet N, Singla E. Pharmacokinetique clinique de bismesylate d'almitrine. Presse Med 1984;13:2071–2077.
7. Watanabe S, Kauner RE, Cutillo AG, et al. Long term effect of almitrine bismesylate in patients with hypoxemic chronic obstructive pulmonary disease. Am Rev Respir Dis 1989;140:1269–1273.
8. Campbell OB, Gordon B, Taylor D, Williams J. The biodisposition of almitrine bismesylate in man: A review. Eur J Respir Dis 1983;64:337–348.
9. Belic L, Laurray D, De Cremoux H, et al. Extensive oxidative metabolism of dextromethorphan patients with almitrine neuropathy. Br J Clin Pharmacol 1989;27:387–390.
10. Herchuelz A, Gangji D, Derenne F, et al. Metabolism of almitrine in extensive and poor metabolizers of debrisoquine/sparteine. Br J Clin Pharmacol 1991;31:73–76.
11. Wouters EFM, Greve LH, Steenhuis ES, Gimeno F. Almitrine and peripheral neuropathy. Lancet 1988;2:336.
12. Voisin C, Howard P, Ansquard C. Almitrine bimesylate: A long-term placebo controlled double-blind study in COAD-Vectarian International Multicentre Study Group. Bull Eur Physiopathol Respir 1987;23(suppl. 11):1695–1825.
13. Allen MB. Almitrine and peripheral neuropathy. Lancet 1988; 2:571.
14. Reyes A, Roca J, Rodriguez-Roisin R, et al. Effect of almitrine in ventricular perfusion distribution in adult respiratory distress syndrome. Am Rev Respir Dis 1989;137:1062–1067.
15. Herve J, Musset D, Simmoneau G, et al. Almitrine decreases the distensibility of the large pulmonary arteries in man. Chest 1989;96:572–577.
16. Ghirardi R, Belec L, Louarn F. Almitrine-induced peripheral neuropathy and weight loss. J Neurol 1989;236:374.
17. Tweney J. Almitrine bismesylate: Current status. Bull Eur Physiopathol Respir 1987;23(suppl. 1):156–163.

BAMIFYLLINE HYDROCHLORIDE

Bamifylline (benzatomofylline) is a theophylline derivative (a methylxanthine) used as a bronchodilator, similar to theophylline. It is easily absorbed from the gastrointestinal tract but does not liberate theophylline in the body. Bamifylline is available as a suppository by intramuscular or slow intravenous injection.[1]

Bamifylline is marketed as Briofil, Bamfin, Famimed, and Trendahl.

Use

Bamifylline is used in the treatment of asthma and obstructive bronchopneumonopathies.[2]

Therapeutic Dose

The usual dose is 600 mg twice daily.

Fatal Dose

Ingestion of about 20 tablets was fatal in an adult.[3]

Toxicokinetics

Absorption

Peak plasma levels of 400 to 1700 ng/mL are reached within 1 hour.[4]

Distribution

The apparent volume of distribution is about 18 L/kg. The concentration of bamifylline is higher in the lung than in the plasma.[2]

Elimination

The terminal half-life of bamifylline is about 20 hours.[4]

Clinical Presentation

Death may follow a catecholamine-induced dysrhythmia. There are no myocardial pathologic changes.

Laboratory

Analytical Methods

A gas chromatography–mass spectrometry method is available for confirmation of bamifylline in body fluids. It has a detection limit of 20 μg/mL.[4]

Blood Levels

Following ingestion of about 20 tablets of Bamifix, a blood bamifylline level of 205 μg/mL was measured. In animals, bamifylline exhibits a broad interval between minimum active and maximum tolerated plasma levels (0.18–20 μg/mL). Clinical efficacy is observed at levels of about 0.18 μg/mL, whereas clinical efficacy of theophylline is observed at more than 6 μg/mL. The toxicity threshold for both compounds is 20 μg/mL.[2]

Treatment

Treatment of bamifylline overdose is guided largely by the therapeutic approach to theophylline poisoning (see Theophylline). There is no antidote. It is unlikely that hemodialysis or hemoperfusion would be effective in removing significant quantities of bamifylline because of its high volume of distribution.

REFERENCES—BAMIFYLLINE

1. Berti F, Magni F, Rossoni G, et al. New pharmacological data on the bronchospasmolytic activity of bamifylline. Arzneimittelforschung 1988;38:40–44.
2. Schiantarelli P, Acerbi D, Botta GC, et al. Evidence of pulmonary tropism of bamifylline and its main active metabolite. Arzneimittelforschung 1989;39:215–219.
3. Offidani C, Ottaviano V, Chiarotti M. Fatal case of bamifylline intoxication. Am J Forens Med Pathol 1993;14:244–245.
4. Segre G, Cerretani D, Moltoni L, et al. Pharmacokinetics of bamifylline during chronic therapy. Arzneimittelforschung 1990;40:450–452.

β_2 ADRENOCEPTOR AGONISTS

Isoprenaline (isoproterenol) was the first selective beta-adrenoceptor agonist and was developed in the 1940s before the concept of alpha and beta subgroups had been developed by Ahlquist in 1948.[1] Metaproterenol (orciprenaline sulfate) was later developed as an orally active agent.[2] Marked cardiac stimulation with these products remained a problem. In the mid-1960s beta adrenoceptors were further classified as β_1 or β_2.[3] The force and rate of contraction of cardiac muscle were considered to be mediated by β_1 receptors, and relaxation of the bronchial and uterine smooth muscle appeared to be mediated by β_2 receptors.[4] This stimulated the search for more selective β_2-adrenoceptor agonists, which led to isoetharine, salbutamol (albuterol), and terbutaline. Some of these β_2-agonist drugs are useful in the treatment of asthma (salbutamol, terbutaline, fenoterol), and others are used as tocolytic agents in the treatment of premature labor (ritodrine, isoxsuprine) (see also Tocolytic Drugs in Chapter 8). At high doses, however, skeletal muscle tremor and cardiac stimulation limit the use of all these drugs. Prodrugs (ibuterol, bambuterol, bitolterol) have been developed that are converted to the active drug in a target organ.

Mortality

An increase in the death rate from asthma in the United Kingdom during the 1960s was associated with the use of inhalers delivering high-potency isoproterenol, a relatively nonselective beta agonist.[5,6] Similar association with death after increasing the number of cannisters or metered-dose inhalations per month has been observed with other beta agonists (salbutamol).[5] In the 1970s, an increase in the mortality rate from asthma in New Zealand was associated with increased use of fenoterol, a long-acting selective β_2 agonist never released for use in the United States.[7,8] Factors considered as possible causes of such deaths included regular use versus use for acute attacks only,[7,9,10] production of hypokalemia,[11,12] unsupervised use,[13–15] increased potency of fenoterol compared with other beta agonists,[16] the unique fenoterol formulation as a bromide,[17] and the induction of paradoxical bronchospasm by products that may contain propellants, emulsifying agents, preservatives (benzalkonium chloride, sulfites), or even contaminants.[18] Fenoterol use has since been considerably restricted in New Zealand[19,20]; it is available in Australia for use in mild to moderate asthma.[21] Guidelines for the management of asthma have been issued in the United Kingdom[22] and the United States.[23] About 20 asthma patients have died because of the possible use of salmeterol xinafoate.[24]

Structure and Classification

The β_2-adrenoceptor agonists are synthetic compounds comprising a molecule containing a catechol ring or closely related group and an ethanolamine side chain. The catechol ring is used primarily for potency and the side chain primarily for selectivity. The most potent drugs (eg, terbutaline, fenoterol, salbutamol) have two hydroxyl groups on the benzene ring. *N*-Alkyl substitution on the side chain depresses beta-adrenoceptor activity and enhances β_2 activity[2] (Figs. 45–1, 45–2).

Use

The primary therapeutic effect of most β_2-adrenoceptor drugs is related to their use as bronchodilators in the treatment of bronchial asthma, chronic bronchitis, and bronchospastic states. Many of the β_2-adrenoceptor agonists have been used to inhibit uterine contractions in premature labor.

Product Formulation

Table 45–1 lists β_2-adrenoceptor agonists available in the United States. Table 45–2 lists those agents available in the United Kingdom. Some other similar drugs are listed in Table 45–3.

Therapeutic Dose

Formulations and initial dosages of some β_2-adrenoceptor agonists are listed in Table 45–4. β_2 agonists such as salbutamol (albuterol) 100 to 200 µg and terbutaline 250 to 500 µg are used as required, rather than regularly. Inhalation is the preferred means of administration in asthma. The drug is delivered direct to the airways, doses are small, and side effects are minimized. In patients with normal lung function who have only infrequent symptoms, this may be the only treatment required.[22] In acute severe asthma an inhaled β_2 agonist may be used (salbutamol 2.5–5 mg or terbutaline 5–10 mg). This may be nebulized with oxygen (in hospital and during transport by ambulance) or, if both methods are unavailable, given by multiple actuations of a metered-dose inhaler to a larger space device (2 × 5 mg, ie, 20–50 puffs,

Table 45–1
Commercial β_2 Bronchodilator Agonists Available in the United States

Generic Name	Brand Name	Manufacturer	Use: Oral	Use: Inhalation
Albuterol (salbutamol)	Ventolin	Allen & Hanbury	+	+
(salbutamol sulfate)	Proventil	Schering	+	+
Bitolterol mesylate*	Tornalate	Sanofi Winthrop	–	+
Isoetharine hydrochloride	Bronkosol	Sanofi Winthrop	–	+
Isoproterenol	Duo-Medihaler Aerosol	3M	–	+
hydrochloride	Isuprel	Sanofi Winthrop	+	+
Metaproterenol sulfate	Alupent	Boehringer Ingelheim	+	+
(orciprenaline)	Metaprel	Sandoz	+	+
Arbuterol acetate	Maxair	3M	–	+
Terbutaline sulfate	Brethaine	Geigy	+	+

*Prodrug hydrolyzed to colerol.

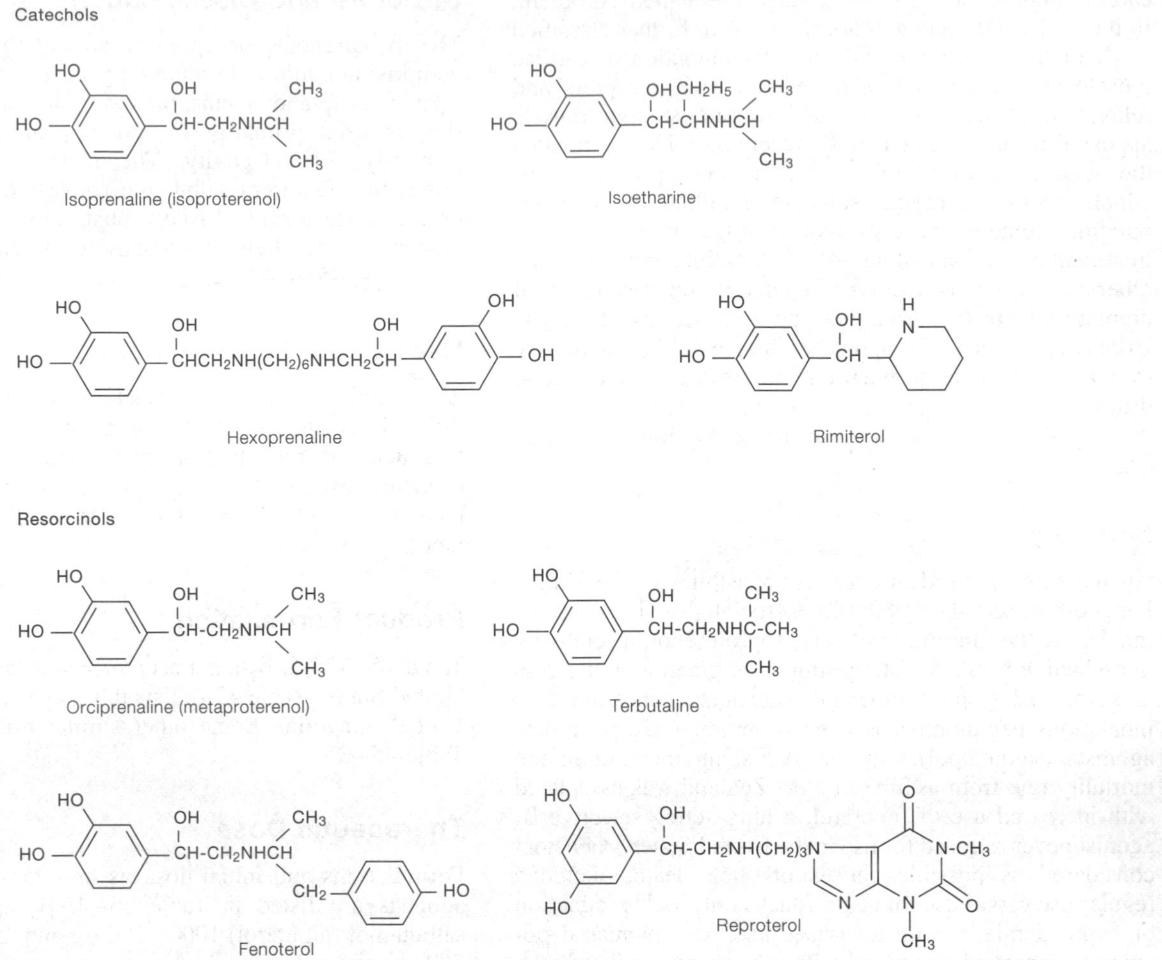

Catechols

Isoprenaline (isoproterenol)

Isoetharine

Hexoprenaline

Rimiterol

Resorcinols

Orciprenaline (metaproterenol)

Terbutaline

Fenoterol

Reproterol

Figure 45–1 Structures of β_2-selective agonists. (From Morgan DJ. Clinical pharmacokinetics of beta-agonists. Clin Pharmacokinet 1990;18:270–294.)

Table 45–2
β_2 Bronchodilator Agonists Available in the United Kingdom

Generic Name	Brand Name	Manufacturer	Use	
			Oral	Inhalation
Fenoterol hydrobromide	Berotec	Boehringer-Ingelheim	–	+
	Duovent	Boehringer-Ingelheim	–	+
Pirbuterol hydrochloride	Exival	Pfizer	+	+
Reproterol hydrochloride	Bronchodil	Schering	+	+
Rimiterol hydrobromide	Pulmadil	Riker	–	+
Salmeterol xinafoate	Serevent	Allen & Hanbury	–	+
Xamoterol	Corwin	ICI	+	–

5 puffs at a time).[22] β_2 agonists are given as part of a total program of treatment (oxygen, steroids, intravenous bronchodilators).

Toxic Dose

Salbutamol (Albuterol)

Adults. A 44-year-old woman ingested 100 2-mg salbutamol tablets (therapeutic dose, 2- to 4-mg three or four times daily), was admitted to the hospital, developed some features of overdose with β_2-adrenergic stimulating drugs (tachycardia, skeletal muscle irritability, agitation), and survived.[25] A 76-year-old woman ingested 40 salbutamol (4-mg) tablets, developed similar symptoms plus hypokalemia, and responded to supportive therapy.[26]

A 17-year-old woman developed symptoms of overdose after ingesting an unspecified quantity of 2-mg tablets of salbutamol. She responded to supportive therapy.[27] A 26-year-old man ingested both salbutamol and theophylline, developed seizures and a bezoar of tablets in the stomach,

Table 45-3
Other β_2 Bronchodilator Selective Drugs

Generic Name	Use: Oral	Use: IV	Use: Inhalation
Clenbuterol	+	+	+
Mabuterol (investigational)	+	−	+
Salmefamol			
Tulobuterol hydrochloride	+	−	−
Prodrugs			
Ibuterol hydrochloride*	+		
Bambuterol†	+	−	−

*Hydrolyzed to terbutaline.
†Prodrug of terbutaline.

and subsequently died.[28] A 35-year-old woman with asthma who was accidentally administered salbutamol 10 mg intravenously developed symptoms of overdose and recovered within 1 day.[29] Five adult patients with salbutamol overdose (ingestions) recovered satisfactorily.[30]

Children. A survey of 40 patients revealed ingestions of salbutamol between 5 to 100 mg (< 10 years of age) and 14 to 240 mg (> 10 years of age). All made an uneventful recovery.[31]

One hundred twelve children under the age of 12 years who ingested up to 96 mg of albuterol and (salbutamol) were observed either at home (<0.6 mg/kg ingested) or in a health care facility (0.3–6.3 mg/kg); all recovered with minimal intervention.[32] A 14-year-old asthmatic ingested 40 mg of

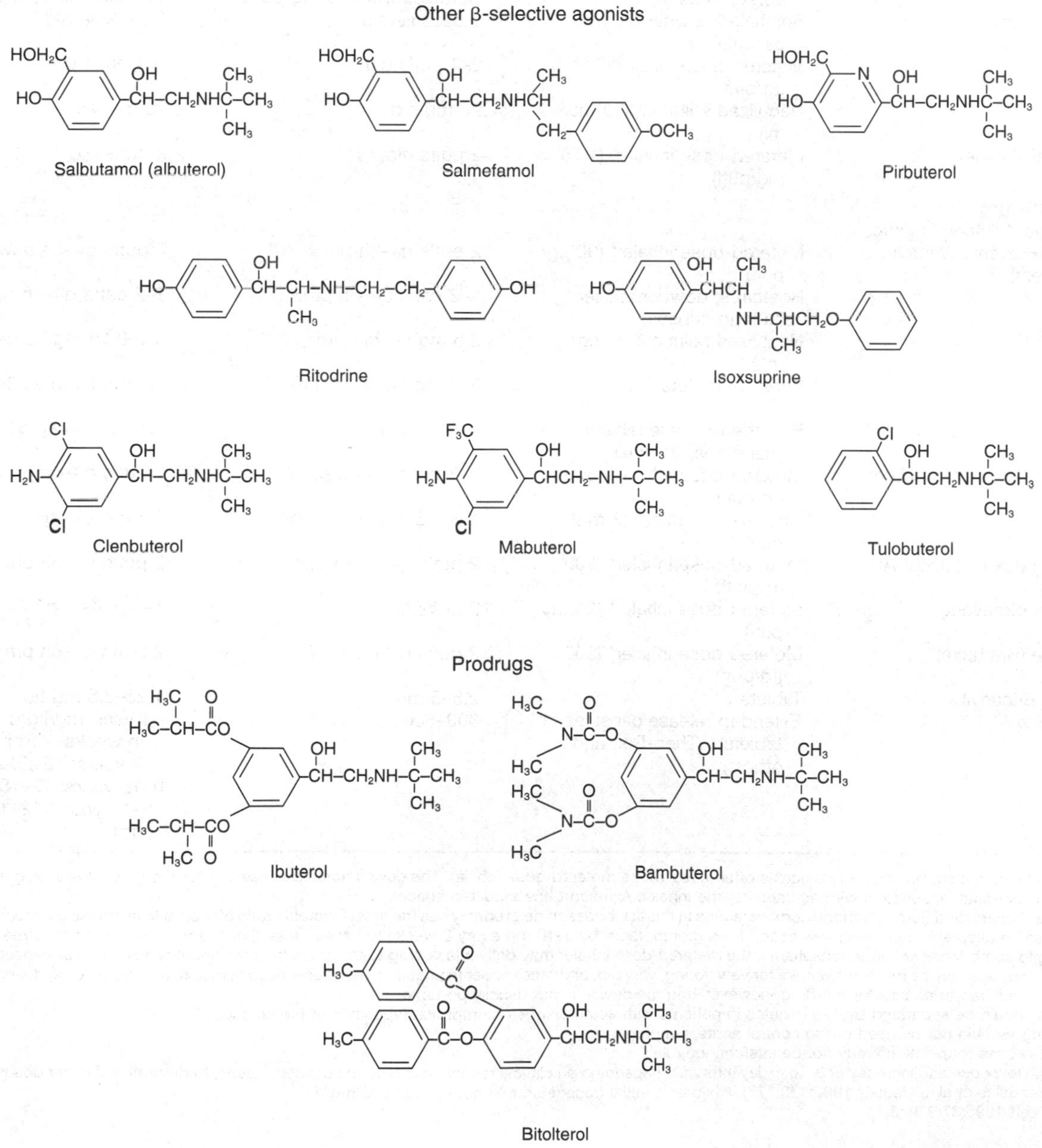

Other β-selective agonists

Salbutamol (albuterol) Salmefamol Pirbuterol

Ritodrine Isoxsuprine

Clenbuterol Mabuterol Tulobuterol

Prodrugs

Ibuterol Bambuterol

Bitolterol

Figure 45-2 Structures of other β_2-selective agonists and prodrugs. (From Morgan DJ. Clinical pharmacokinetics of beta-agonists. Clin Pharmacokinet 1990;18:270–294.)

Table 45-4
Some Drugs for Ambulatory Asthma

Drug	Formulation	Initial Dosage	
		Adult	Child (≤40 kg)
Antiinflammatory Drugs			
Corticosteroids			
Beclomethasone dipropionate (Beclovent, Vanceril)	Metered-dose inhaler* (42 µg/puff)	2–4 puffs bid–qid	2 puffs qid or 4 puffs bid
Budesonide (Pulmicort)†	Metered-dose inhaler* (50, 200 µg/puff) or Tubuhaler (100, 200, 400 µg/puff)	400–2400 µg divided bid–qid	200–400 µg bid
Flunisolide (Aerobid)	Metered-dose inhaler* (250 µg/puff)	2–4 puffs bid	2 puffs bid
Triamcinolone acetonide (Azmacort)	Metered-dose inhaler* (100 µg/puff)	2 puffs tid–qid or 4 puffs bid	1–2 puffs tid–qid or 4 puffs bid
Prednisone or prednisolone	Oral tablets (5, 10, 20 mg) Oral liquid (Liquid Pred, Pediapred, Prelone)	Acute: up to 50 mg/d × 5–14 d Chronic: up to 40 mg qod‡	Acute: 10–40 mg bid × 5–14 d Chronic: 20–40 mg qod‡
Cromolyn (Intal)	Spinhaler, powder (20 mg/capsule)	1 capsule qid	1 capsule qid
	Metered-dose inhaler*,§ (800 µg/puff)	2–4 puffs qid	2–4 puffs qid
	Nebulized solution‖ (10 mg/ml)	20 mg qid	20 mg qid
Nedocromil (Tilade)	Metered-dose inhaler* (1.75 mg/puff)	2 puffs qid	2 puffs qid
Bronchodilators			
β₂-Selective Adrenergic Drugs			
Albuterol (Proventil, Ventolin, and others)	Metered-dose inhaler* (90 µg/puff)	2 puffs q4–6h prn#	2 puffs q4–6h prn#
	Rotacaps, powder inhaler (200 µg/capsule)	1–2 caps q4–6h prn#	1–2 caps q4–6h prn#
	Nebulized solution‖ (5 mg/mL)	2.5 mg tid–qid prn	0.1–0.15 mg/kg q4–6h prn
	Syrup or tablets	2–4 mg tid or qid prn	0.1 mg/kg (max 2 mg) q6–8h prn
	Extended-release tablets (Repetabs, Volmax)	4–8 mg q12h	0.1–0.2 mg/kg q12h
Bitolterol mesylate (Tornalate)	Metered-dose inhaler* (370 µg/puff)	2–3 puffs q4–6h prn#	2 puffs q4–6h prn#
	Nebulized solution‖ (2 mg/mL)	1.5–3.5 mg bid–qid prn	1.5 mg bid–qid prn
Pirbuterol (Maxair, Maxair Autohaler)	Metered-dose inhaler* (200 µg/puff)	2 puffs q4–6h PRN#	2 puffs q4–6h prn#
Salmeterol (Serevent)	Metered-dose inhaler* (21 µg/puff)	2 puffs bid¶	1–2 puffs bid¶
Terbutaline (Brethaire)	Metered-dose inhaler* (200 µg/puff)	2 puffs q4–6h prn#	2 puffs q4–6h prn#
(Brethine, Bricanyl)	Tablets	2.5–5 mg tid	1.25–2.5 mg tid
Theophylline	Extended-release capsules or tablets** (Theo-Dur, and others)	300–600 mg/day††	<1 year: mg/kg/d = (0.2) (age in weeks) + 5†† 1–9 years: 12–20 mg/kg/d†† 9–12 years: 12–18 mg/kg/d†† 12–16 years: 12–16 mg/kg/d††

*An aerosol-holding chamber (spacer device) is often used with a metered-dose inhaler. The device acts as a reservoir for the aerosolized drug and decreases the need to coordinate inspiration with actuation of the inhaler. Azmacort has a built-in spacer.
†Available in Canada and Europe; among corticosteroids in this list, budesonide probably has the most favorable ratio of topical to systemic glucocorticoid activity.
‡Single dose on alternate days; when controlled for a month, taper by 5–10 mg every 2 weeks to lowest dose that keeps patient symptom-free.
§According to some *Medical Letter* consultants, the metered-dose inhaler may deliver less drug to the lungs than the nebulized solution or capsule formulation.
‖Nebulized solutions may be more convenient for very young, very old, and other patients unable to use pressurized aerosols, and higher drug doses can be used. More time is required to administer the drug, however, and the device is not usually portable.
#Each puff should be separated by 1–3 minutes in patients with acute distress to improve deposition of the aerosol.
¶Long-acting. Should not be used prn to control acute symptoms.
**Extended-release formulations may not be interchangeable.
††Begin with low dose and increase at 3- to 4-day intervals, depending on clinical response and serum concentrations, to determine if larger doses can be given safely (L. Hendeles et al, J Pediatr 1992;120:177). Children's initial dosage should not exceed 600 mg/d.
From Med Lett 1995;37(939):3.

albuterol, developed a similar clinical response, and recovered.[33] A 22-month-old child ingested about 30 mg of albuterol (up to 3 mg/kg); developed tremor, hyperglycemia, and a mild hypokalemia; and recovered with supportive care only.[34]

Terbutaline

A 67-year-old woman with bronchospasm and a theophylline blood level of 7 μg/mL 18 hours previously received terbutaline 2.5 mg instead of the recommended dose of 0.25 mg subcutaneously. Symptoms of palpitations, chest pain, tremor, tachycardia, and hypertension developed with electrocardiographic changes reflecting myocardial ischemia. The tremor abated over the next 24 hours.[35] A 77-year-old man ingested 20 2.5-mg tablets of terbutaline with 9 15-mg tablets of flurazepam. Tremor and tachycardia persisted for 24 hours.[36] A 35-year-old diabetic woman suspected of premature labor was inadvertently given a subcutaneous dose of 2.5 mg of terbutaline instead of 0.25 mg. This was followed by chest pain, tachycardia, and electrocardiographic changes of myocardial ischemia, which reverted to normal in 2 days.[37] The terbutaline was successful in preventing the premature labor, which resulted in a spontaneous abortion. Two other pregnant patients, following inadvertently given doses 10 times the normal dose (2.5 mg vs 0.25 mg) developed similar symptoms (tachycardia, rise in pulse pressure); the fetus of one patient survived.[36]

A 3-year-old child ingested 45 mg of terbutaline, developed symptoms of tachycardia, tremor, nausea, and vomiting, was treated with a beta-adrenergic blocker, and recovered.[38,39] A 22-year-old asthmatic woman on two occasions ingested 100 5-mg tablets of terbutaline, developed characteristic features of β_2-adrenoceptor poisoning, was treated supportively with gastric lavage and activated charcoal, and recovered.[40] A 22-year-old woman ingested 30 7.5-mg sustained-action terbutaline tablets, developed bronchospasm, tachycardia, tremor, hypotension, rhabodomyolysis, and acute renal failure, and recovered.[41]

Toxicokinetics

Beta agonists are administered orally, by inhalation, and by subcutaneous, intramuscular, and intravenous injection. Their bioavailability is dependent on their mode of administration.

Absorption

Oral Administration. Following oral administration, most β_2 agonists (salbutamol, bitolterol) are well absorbed, with the exception of xamoterol, rimiterol, orciprenaline, and terbutaline. Despite extensive absorption, the systemic bioavailability of oral beta agonists is very low due to extensive sulfation of the drugs in the liver and possibly in the wall of the small intestine. As a result, the oral dose of beta agonists needs to be 5 to 10 times greater than the parenteral dose.[2]

Pulmonary Administration. For relief of bronchospasm, β_2 agonists can be administered directly to the lung by inhalation via a pressurized metered-dose inhaler or as a spray generated by a nebulizer. After aerosol administration the proportion of an administered dose recovered in the urine as unchanged drug and metabolites is up to 80% for salbutamol and salmefamol,[42] 69% for isoprenaline,[43] about 50% for terbutaline,[44] and 12% for fenoterol.[45] Most of an inhaled dose is deposited on the pharynx after inhalation and is then swallowed. First-pass metabolism is avoided with oral inhalation. After aerosol administration, the time to maximum plasma drug concentration is approximately 2 to 4 hours, comparable to that following oral administration and consistent with swallowing most of an inhaled dose. Maximum bronchodilation occurs within 15 to 30 minutes.[2] On direct bronchial instillation, plasma concentration peaks in about 10 minutes.[46] About 3% of an oral inhaled dose reaches the lungs.[44] With a nebulizer, about 10 to 20% is absorbed[47]; more of the dose is absorbed by the lungs and less is swallowed.

Subcutaneous and Intramuscular Administration. Plasma concentrations of terbutaline peak more rapidly (within 15 to 30 minutes) after subcutaneous administration than after oral use.[48] Systemic bioavailability of subcutaneous terbutaline is about 100%.[49] The plasma concentration of ritodrine peaks rapidly, within 15 minutes.[50]

Distribution

The plasma protein binding of most beta agonists is about 10% (Table 45–5). Tissue distribution is large (from 1 to 29 L/kg).[2]

Elimination

Systemic clearance of beta agonists ranges from low (terbutaline, mabuterol) to relatively high (eg, prenalterol, ritodrine). Beta agonists are eliminated by metabolism and renal excretion of unchanged drug (Table 45–5). Metabolism of the resorcinol derivatives (terbutaline, salbutamol, fenoterol, xamoterol, prenalterol, pirbuterol, orciprenaline) is by sulfate conjugation as the only significant metabolite. Ritodrine is metabolized to a glucuronide. The sulfate and glucuronide conjugates of beta agonists do not appear to possess pharmacologic activity.[51] After direct intrabronchial administration in humans, drugs that are substrates for catechol-*o*-methyltransferase may undergo a first-pass pulmonary effect.[43] Renal excretion is the major route of elimination of parenterally administered beta agonists.

Drug Interactions

Treatment with diuretics augments the hypokalemia that occurs with β_2 agonists.[52] Use of orally inhaled β_2 agonists with other oral sympathomimetics produces additive sympathomimetic effects. Administration of a beta agonist by any route other than oral inhalation (eg, intravenous, oral, subcutaneous) together with theophylline, may lead to deleterious cardiovascular effects. β_2 agonists should be administered with caution to patients being treated with monoamine oxidase inhibitors or tricyclic antidepressants because the action of the β_2 agonist on the vascular system may be potentiated. Beta-receptor agonists are inhibited by beta-receptor antagonists, especially those without β_1-receptor selectivity.[2,53–55]

Table 45–5
Toxicokinetics of Beta Agonists

Drug	Plasma Protein Binding (%)	CL (L/h/kg)	CL_R (L/h/kg)	V_Z (L/kg)	$t_{1/2}$ (h)	D_f (%)	Unchanged Drug in Plasma* (%)		Excreted Unchanged in Urine†	
							IV	PO	IV	PO
(±)-Bitolterol								<1, 3‡		0.4‡
(±)-Clenbuterol	97				34, 35			75		20, 43
(±)-Fenoterol	55					15		<10	60	3
(±)-Isoetharine									10	10
(±)-Isoprenaline (isoprotefenol)					0.05		>80	Very small	43	14
(+)-Isoprenaline			0.16							
(±)-Mabuterol		0.198		6.4	20, 23			50		24, 64
(±)-Orciprenaline	10	0.84§	0.08§ 0.13§	7.6§	2.1, 6.3					4, 11, 20
(±)-Pirbuterol					2.5					17
(−)-Prenalterol	<5	1.14, 1.14§	0.72	3.4, 3.9§	2.0				60	20
(±)-Rimiterol					0.05	1.0, 4.6	10–73	<10	25	2
(±)-Ritodrine	32, 36	1.38§		29§	15					
(±)-Salbutamol (albuterol)	8	0.41, 0.38, 0.46	0.28	1.9, 2.2, 2.5	3.2, 3.9, 4.0, 5.0, 6.0	4	>50	25, 25	64, 65	20, 32
(±)-Salmefamol							7		7	
(±)-Salmeterol	94–98	0.14			360					
(±)-Terbutaline	15	0.198, 0.2, 0.26	0.1, 0.13	1.3, 1.6, 4.0	3.6, 4.3, 5.3, 13.7, 20, 20	3.3	50, 85	13, 15	55, 55, 56, 60	12, 12, 14, 20
(+)-Terbutaline		0.192	0.16	3.5	12.7				58	12
(−)-Terbutaline		0.13	0.09	2.6	15.3				53	14
(±)Tulobuterol					2.4					
(±)-Xamoterol	3	0.18, 0.3	0.11, 0.14	1.1, 2.0	2.6, 7.7	5	≈100	50	62, 81, 90	40, 60

CL, total plasma clearance; CL_R, renal clearance, V_Z, apparent volume of distribution during the terminal phase; $t_{1/2}$, elimination half-life, D_f, intravenous dose excreted in feces.
*Percentage of total drug and metabolites.
†Percentage of absorbed dose.
‡*N*-t-Butylarterenol.
§Adjusted for total body weight of 70 kg.
From Morgan DJ. Clinical pharmacokinetics of beta-agonists. Clin Pharmacokinet 1990;18:270–294.

Pregnancy

Pregnancy does not appear to influence significantly the toxicokinetics of β_2 agonists. A 30% greater systemic clearance of terbutaline with a correspondingly lower systemic availability of orally administered drug is observed during pregnancy.[2] Schatz and colleagues suggest that any of the inhaled beta-agonist bronchodilators are useful for the management of asthma during pregnancy.[56]

A woman suspected of premature labor in the 21st week of pregnancy inadvertently received 2.5 mg of terbutaline (recommended starting oral dose) subcutaneously instead of 0.25 mg. She developed substernal chest pressure, tachycardia, and an electrocardiographic indication of inferolateral ischemia. Within 2 days the electrocardiogram reverted to normal. She subsequently had a spontaneous abortion.[37] An anecdotal report describes the death of a 25-week-pregnant woman from cardiac arrhythmia after she received terbutaline subcutaneously.[57]

Placental Transfer

When β_2 agonists are administered for the treatment of premature labor, fetal tachycardia is seen, with hyperglycemia, hypotension, and a respiratory distress syndrome in infants delivered after the failure of tocolytic therapy. Placental transfer is rapid. The Food and Drug Administration has placed albuterol in Pregnancy Category C.

Lactation

After oral terbutaline administration to the mother, milk concentrations of the drug may be similar to or greater than plasma concentrations. The calculated intake of terbutaline in milk is 0.4 to 0.7 μg/kg/d, less than 1% of the adult dose. Nursing infants exhibit no clinical signs of beta-adrenoceptor stimulation. Few data are available on other beta-adrenoceptor drugs.[58]

Perinatal Effects and Infancy

The rates of perinatal mortality, congenital malformations, and preterm delivery or delivery of low-birth-weight infants, the mean birth weight, and the number of small-for-gestational-age infants are not increased in pregnant women using β_2-adrenergic agonists for asthma. There are no differences in Apgar scores, rates of complications of labor or delivery, or postpartum bleeding.[56,59]

Mechanism of Action

β_2-Adrenoceptor agonists (Table 45–6) produce effects on smooth muscle and skeletal muscle. These include bronchodilatation, relaxation of uterine muscle, and some vasodilating effect on peripheral vasculature (acute reduction of diastolic blood pressure), resulting in flushing and tremor probably due to the increased contractility of skeletal muscle caused by β_2 stimulation. Smooth muscle relaxation may occur when the drug binds to the beta-adrenergic receptor site in the cell membrane, resulting in conversion of ATP to cyclic AMP; this activates protein kinase, leading to phosphorylation of proteins which increase bound intracellular calcium. The reduced availability of intracellular ionized calcium inhibits actin–myosin linkage, leading to relaxation of smooth muscle.

β_2 agonists also have an antiallergic effect on mast cells, causing inhibition of release of bronchoconstriction mediators including histamine, neutrophil chemotactic factor, and prostaglandin D_2. The cyclic AMP system probably acts as the second messenger in regulating the mast cell response.

β_2-Adrenergic stimulation also promotes an intracellular shift of potassium from serum, possibly via stimulation of Na^+, K^+ATPase; this may lead to a temporary decrease in both elevated and normal potassium concentrations. Both intravenous and orally inhaled β_2-adrenergic agonist drugs may cause a decrease in serum potassium concentrations.[60,61]

Stimulation of nonpulmonary β_2 receptors may lead to an increase in heart rate, prolongation of the QT_c interval, nonspecific T-wave changes, skeletal muscle tremor (β_2 receptors on skeletal muscle), and slight increases in blood glucose and nonesterified fatty acids.[62,63] Selective β_2 agonists such as terbutaline at high concentration may have β_1 stimulant effects.[35]

Table 45–6
Properties of Beta-Adrenergic Agonists Used in Asthma

Drug	Relative Stimulation of Adrenergic Receptors: β_2	β_1	α	Duration of Action When Given by Inhalation (h)
Albuterol	+++	+	0	4–6
Bitolterol*	+++	+	0	4–6
Ephedrine	++	++	+++	3–5
Epinephrine	+++	+++	+++	1–2
Isoetharine	+++	++	0	2–3
Isoproterenol	+++	+++	0	2–3
Metaproterenol	+++	++	0	3–5
Pirbuterol	+++	+	0	5
Terbutaline	+++	+	0	4–6

+++, high; ++, medium; +, low; 0, none.
*Prodrug hydrolyzed to colterol in vivo.
From Murphy CM, Coonce SL, Simon PA. Treatment of asthma in children. Clin Pharm 1991;10:685–703.

Clinical Presentation

Overdose

Characteristic features of β_2-adrenoceptor agonist poisoning include nausea, tachycardia, tremor, hyperglycemia, and hypokalemia.[40] The skin may be warm and pink with evidence of diaphoresis.[25] General symptoms may include agitation,[30] a coarse hand tremor (probably the most common sign observed), apprehension, dizziness, nausea, vomiting,[39] headaches,[30] and dilated pupils.[31] Rarely, rhabdomyolysis, lactic acidosis, acute renal failure, a leukemoid reaction, and hypoglycemia[64] have been observed.[41] In children, albuterol overdoses result in prominent cardiovascular and metabolic findings.[65]

Cardiovascular effects of overdose often include precordial pressure or chest pain,[35] angina pectoris,[66] and hypotension,[26] together with electrocardiographic changes (see Laboratory). β_2-Adrenoceptor agonists can provoke myocardial ischemia by acute reduction of diastolic blood pressure or by precipitation of cardiac rhythm disturbances.

Chronic Poisoning: Drug Abuse

Continued dependence on salbutamol tablets taken in high doses (30–40 tablets daily[67] and 48–64 mg/d)[68] has led to symptoms of toxic psychosis[67] in one elderly woman and paranoid psychosis in a 52-year-old man.[68] Up to 60 to 90 100-μg inhalations of salbutamol daily has been used by asthmatics who increased doses not because of increased symptoms of asthma, but because they "needed it" and wanted to "feel good."[69–72] Long-term tolerance (subsensitivity) develops to bronchodilator action, tremor, tachycardia, prolongation of the QT_c interval, hyperglycemia, hypokalemia, and vasodilator response.[59]

Laboratory

Analytical Methods

Fenoterol. Plasma concentrations of fenoterol can be assayed by high-pressure liquid chromatography separation with ultraviolet spectrum monitoring at 275 or 295 nm.[73]

Formoterol. Gas chromatography–mass spectrometry and radioimmunoassay systems, with lower detection limits of 5 and 0.1 μg/mL, respectively, have been developed.[74–76]

Salbutamol. Salbutamol can be assayed by a gas chromatography–mass spectrometry method.[77] A method combining immunoaffinity chromatography with high-performance liquid chromatography is now available and is sensitive to a plasma concentration of 0.79 ng/mL.[78]

Terbutaline. Terbutaline has been determined in the serum and plasma by thin-layer fluorometry,[79] liquid chromatography with electrochemical detection (lower limit of detection, <0.5 ng/mL plasma),[48] and gas chromatography–mass spectrometry.[80]

Blood Levels

Lung function improvement, plasma cyclic AMP concentration, and increases in skeletal muscle tremor and heart rate appear to correlate with plasma concentrations of salbutamol, terbutaline, ritodrine, and rimiterol.[2] Peak pharmacologic effects occur later than peak plasma drug concentration. For a given plasma concentration of B_2 agonist, there is a large interpatient variation in bronchodilation, tremor, and heart rate responses.[2,81] There is also considerable intrapatient variability reflecting the development of tolerance during continuous treatment.[2]

Salbutamol (Albuterol). Six hours after admission, an adult man who had ingested both sustained-release aminophylline and salbutamol exhibited a salbutamol plasma concentration of about 160 ng/mL and a theophylline concentration of nearly 80 μg/mL. Following multiple seizures, he died.[29] Five patients who overdosed on salbutamol developed maximum plasma concentrations of 50 to 76 ng/mL 1.5 to 8 hours after ingestion. All exhibited sinus tachycardia, four had tremor, four had dilated pupils, and three had a depressed plasma potassium level.[31] A 14-year-old asthmatic who ingested 40 mg of albuterol developed a blood albuterol level of 91 ng/dL (therapeutic range, 5.3–6.8 ng/dL).[33] Following a course characterized by palpitations and tremor and depressed serum potassium concentration, she received propranolol and recovered.[33] High plasma concentrations of salbutamol appear to be tolerated without serious cardiac arrhythmias or any fatalities.[82]

Terbutaline. The approximate serum terbutaline concentration required to produce bronchial muscle relaxation is 2 ng/mL.[81,83] Bronchodilator effects correlate with plasma levels[83] when measured by forced expiratory volume[81] and cyclic cAMP.[84] The normal therapeutic concentration of terbutaline is 2 to 6 ng/mL.[40] Following ingestion of 45 mg of terbutaline, a 3-year-old girl subsequently developed tremor, tachycardia, nausea, and vomiting; her plasma terbutaline concentration 3 hours after ingestion was 33.9 ng/mL.[39] Three adults who overdosed with terbutaline developed maximum plasma concentrations of 41 to 88 ng/mL 1.5 to 5 hours after ingestion. Sinus tachycardia was present in all three patients and tremor in two.[31] A 22-year-old who ingested 500 mg of terbutaline with 10 g of acetaminophen developed a peak plasma terbutaline concentration of about 200 ng/mL concomitant with characteristic features of β_2-adrenoceptor agonist poisoning; the blood concentration fell to therapeutic levels within 36 hours.[40]

Abnormalities

Hypokalemia. The hypokalemia seen in β_2-adrenoceptor agonist overdose may be caused by redistribution of potassium from the plasma and extracellular fluid into the cells mediated by an increase in intracellular cyclic AMP concentration and activation of Na^+, K^+ATPase.[31,60,61,85] Reduction of plasma potassium concentrations due to fenoterol appears to be more than double that of salbutamol.[62] Hypokalemia following β_2-agonist therapy has been associated with cardiac arrhythmias.[86]

Hyperglycemia. Hyperglycemia may be due to the glycolytic effect of β_2-adrenoceptor agonists on hepatic glycogen stores.[87]

Electrocardiographic Changes. β_2-adrenoceptor agonists in overdose may induce prolongation of the QT_c interval,[63] atrial fibrillation,[88] atrial premature beats, right bundle-branch block, and nonspecific ST–T wave changes.[80] Sinus tachycardia is the most frequent electrocardiographic abnormality seen and may be a reflex reaction secondary to peripheral vasodilation.[27] Ventricular tachycardias may be precipitated by aerosolized terbutaline in patients with preexisting coronary artery disease.[89] Cardiac arrest followed inhalation exposure to the equivalent of 675 doses of fenoterol.[90]

Ancillary Tests

There is one report of rhabdomyolysis after a β_2-adrenoceptor overdose (terbutaline) with subsequent acute renal failure, lactic acidosis, hyperglycemia, hypokalemia, and a leukemoid reaction.[41]

Terbutaline induces skeletal muscle uptake of phosphorus, which may result in hypophosphatemia.[91]

Urinalysis demonstrates ketonuria, proteinuria, and hematuria, and blood studies show leukocytosis, metabolic acidosis with high anion gap, and hypoxemia. Blood creatine kinase and lactate dehydrogenase levels may rise. *ortho*-Toludine dipsticks may be positive for myoglobinuria, but many red blood cells in the urine can interfere with this test.[41]

Treatment

Stabilization

Treatment of β_2-adrenoceptor overdose is largely symptomatic and supportive. Selective β_2-adrenoceptor drugs may be relatively innocuous in overdose in the younger age groups. In the middle-aged and the elderly with preexisting cardiovascular disease and coronary artery insufficiency, these drugs may induce signs and symptoms of acute myocardial ischemia. In the younger overdosed patient, observation in the emergency department for 4 to 6 hours and attention to presence of a normal heart rate, absence of tremor, presence of a normal blood sugar, and presence of a normal serum potassium level are sufficient for discharge if the patient is otherwise asymptomatic. Patients who are in older age groups or who present with symptoms of chest pressure, chest pain, or unusual arrhythmias should be placed on a cardiac monitor with a source of oxygen available. Airway, respirations, and circulatory status should be monitored carefully. Usually such evidence of acute cardiovascular response regresses within 48 hours without any additional specific therapy.

Gut Decontamination

When the patient is seen within the first 4 to 6 hours, gastric lavage may be useful, although patients with little evidence of cardiovascular abnormality, tremor, hyperglycemia, or hypokalemia will probably do well with observation only, after which they can be discharged. There are no data to support the use of activated charcoal in these patients.

Elimination Enhancement

A high apparent volume of distribution and often high plasma protein binding make the use of extracorporeal techniques (hemodialysis, hemoperfusion) of little potential value. In the rare instance of rhabdomyolysis with acute renal failure,[41] hemodialysis may be required.

Antidote

There is no specific antidote for β_2-adrenoceptor agonist overdoses although various authors[92] have suggested the use of beta-adrenoceptor blocking agents (eg, propranolol 0.01 mg/kg) to symptomatically improve the tremor, tachycardia, and hypokalemia.[85] Although there is danger in the use of such drugs (eg, propranolol) in the presence of asthma, and some have advocated a more cardioselective blocking agent (eg, metoprolol),[40] there is scant evidence that this group of drugs materially enhances recovery.

Supportive Measures

1. For chest pain, monitor oxygen status, and obtain serial arterial blood gases and creatine kinase levels with cardiac enzyme fractions. Watch electrolytes, especially potassium, with serial determinations. Treat as a potential myocardial infarction. Provide a central line. Monitor QT_c intervals with serum potassium levels.[93]
2. Hypokalemia usually reverts to normal spontaneously. Beta blockers may speed this return to normality, but must be used with great care in the asthmatic patient. If the serum potassium level, as also reflected on the electrocardiogram, is seriously depressed, consider slow administration of potassium chloride, with repeat serum potassium levels and serial electrocardiograms. More often, added potassium chloride is probably unnecessary.
3. If an overdose has been administered to a pregnant patient in labor, pulmonary edema may be precipitated. Oxygen, intravenous diuretics, and possibly fluid restriction may be required.
4. In children with large overdoses of beta-sympathomimetic agents, monitor blood glucose levels for several hours. If marked hyperglycemia is observed, extend monitoring until blood glucose levels normalize.[93]
5. A retrospective study of accidental albuterol ingestion in children suggests that for ingestions of 0.6 mg/kg or less, treatment at home with observation may be sufficient. For ingestions greater than 0.6 mg/kg, consideration should be given to direct medical evaluation and gastrointestinal decontamination. Dosages ranged from 1 to 27 mg in children 1 to 11 years of age. Symptoms and signs observed included irritability, nausea, vomiting, tachycardia, tremors, and a widened pulse pressure. Albuterol levels do not peak for 3 to 4 hours after administration, but peak therapeutic effects do not correlate well with serum levels. Methodologic limitations of this study include the small number of patients in each dosage category, its retrospective nature, and the selection bias (only patients reported to a regional poison center). Even though no child in the study, when treated with ipecac or activated charcoal, experienced symptoms after an ingestion less than 0.9 mg/kg, the clinical presentation would tend to indicate immediate medical attention in a health care facility.[94]

REFERENCES—β_2-ADRENOCEPTOR AGONISTS

1. Ahlquist RP. A study of adrenotropic receptors. Am J Physiol 1948;153:586–600.
2. Morgan DJ. Clinical pharmacokinetics of beta-agonists. Clin Pharmacokinet 1990;18:270–294.
3. Lands AM, Arnold A, McAuliff JP, et al. Differentiation of receptor systems activated by sympathomimetic amines. Nature 1967;214:597–598.
4. Ahrens RC, Smith GD. Albuterol: An adrenergic agent for use in the treatment of asthma: Pharmacology, pharmacokinetics and clinical use. Pharmacotherapy 1984;4:105–121.
5. Woolcock AJ. Beta-agonists and asthma mortality: What have we learned? What questions remain? Drugs 1990;40: 653–656.
6. Speizer FE, Doll R, Heaf P. Observations on recent increase in mortality from asthma. Br Med J 1968;1:335–339.
7. Burrows B, Lebowitz MD. The beta-agonist dilemma. N Engl J Med 1992;326:560–561.
8. Spitzer WO, Suissa S, Ernst P, et al. The use of beta-agonists and the risk of death and near death from asthma. N Engl J Med 1992;326:501–506.
9. Sears MR. $Beta_2$ agonists and asthma. Br Med J 1991;303: 123.
10. Sears MR, Taylor DR, Print CG, et al. Regular inhaled beta-agonist treatment in bronchial asthma. Lancet 1990;336: 1391–1396.
11. Lipworth BJ. Risks versus benefits of inhaled $beta_2$-agonists in the management of asthma. Drug Saf 1992;7:54–70.
12. Haalbom JRE, Deenstra M, Struyvenberg A. Effect of fenoterol on plasma potassium and cardiac ectopic activity. Lancet 1989;2:45.
13. Crane J, Pearce N, Flatt A, et al. Prescribed fenoterol and death from asthma in New Zealand 1981–1983: Case control study. Lancet 1989;1:917–922.
14. Pearce N, Crane J, Burgess C, et al. Fenoterol and asthma mortality. Lancet 1989;1:1196–1197.
15. Pearce N, Grainger J, Atkinson M, et al. Case–control study of prescribed Venoterol and death from asthma in New Zealand, 1977–81. Thorax 1990;45:170–175.
16. Grand IWB. Fenoterol and asthma deaths in New Zealand. NZ Med J 1990;April 11:160–161.
17. Green WF. Fenoterol and its bromide. Lancet 1991;337:1613.
18. Nicklas RA. Paradoxical bronchospasm associated with the use of inhaled beta agonists. J Allergy Clin Immunol 1990;85: 959–964.
19. Fenoterol. Lancet 1989;1:971.
20. Elwood JM. Fenoterol: The evidence leading to restriction of its use. NZ Med J 1990;103:395–397.
21. Revised indications for fenoterol. Aust Adverse Drug React Bull, May 1990.
22. British Thoracic Society Research Unit of the Royal College of Physicians of London, King's Fund Centre, National Asthma Campaign. Guidelines for management of asthma in adults: I. Chronic persistent asthma. Br Med J 1990;301: 651–653; II. Acute severe asthma. Br Med J 1990;301:797–800.
23. National Asthma Education Program. *Guidelines for the Diagnosis and Management of Asthma.* Publication No. 91-3042. Bethesda, MD: Department of Health and Human Services, 1991.
24. Bone RC. Another word of caution regarding a new long-acting bronchodilator. JAMA 1995;273:967–968.
25. Morrison GW, Farebrother MJB. Overdose of salbutamol. Lancet 1973;2:681.

26. O'Brien IAD, Fitzgerald-Fraser J, Lewin IG, Corrall RJM. Hypokalaemia due to salbutamol overdosage. Br Med J 1981;282:1515–1516.
27. Connell JMC, Cook GM, McInnes GT. Metabolic consequences of salbutamol poisoning reversed by propranolol. Br Med J 1982;285:779.
28. Whyte KF, Addis GJ. Toxicity of salbutamol and theophylline together. Lancet 1983;2:618–619.
29. MacKay MJ. Overdose of salbutamol during an asthma attack. Br Med J 1985;290:286.
30. Jarvie DR, Thompson AM, Dyson EH. Laboratory and clinical features of self-poisoning with salbutamol and terbutaline. Clin Chim Acta 1987;168:313–322.
31. Prior JG, Cochrane GM, Raper SM, et al. Self-poisoning with oral salbumatomol. Br Med J 1981;282:1932.
32. Spiller HA, Henvetig FM, Ramoska E, Jaffe M. Two year retrospective study of pediatric albuterol ingestions. Vet Hum Toxicol 1990;32:352.
33. Jaffe M, Ramoska E, Schwartz S, et al. Severe albuterol poisoning treated with propranolol. Vet Hum Toxicol 1990;32:351.
34. King W, Holloway M, Palmisano P. Albuterol overdose in a preschooler: A case report. Vet Hum Toxicol 1991;33:357.
35. Lawyer C, Pond A. Problems with terbutaline. N Engl J Med 1977;296:821.
36. Gomolin I, Ingelfinger JA. Terbutaline overdose. N Engl J Med 1979;300:143.
37. Brandstetter RD, Gotz V. Inadvertent overdose of parenteral terbutaline. Lancet 1980;1:485–486.
38. Kaul AF, Stubblefield PG. Terbutaline sulfate overdosage. Drug Intell Clin Pharm 1980;14:866.
39. Host A, Foged N. Terbutaline intoxication in a three-year-old child. Ugeskr Laeger 1983;145:1450.
40. Heath A, Hulten B-A. Terbutaline concentrations in self-poisoning: A case report. Hum Toxicol 1987;6:525–526.
41. Blake PG, Ryan F. Rhabdomyolysis and acute renal failure after terbutaline overdose. Nephron 1989;53:76–77.
42. Evans ME, Shenfield GM, Paterson JW. The clinical pharmacology of salmefamol. Br J Clin Pharmacol 1974;1:391–397.
43. Blackwell E, Briant RH, Conolly ME, et al. Metabolism of isoprenaline after aerosol and direct intrabronchial administration in man and dog. Br J Pharmacol 1974;50:597–601.
44. Nilsson HT, Simonsson BG, Strom B. The fate of ^{3}H-terbutaline sulphate administered to man as an aerosol. Eur J Clin Pharmacol 1976;10:1–7.
45. Laros CD, Van Urk P, Rominger KL. Absorption, distribution and excretion of the tritium-labelled beta$_2$-stimulator fenoterol hydrobromide following aerosol administration and instillation into the bronchial tree. Respiration 1977;34:131–134.
46. Shenfield GM, Evans ME, Paterson JW. Absorption of drugs by the lung. Br J Clin Pharmacol 1976;3:583–589.
47. Shenfield GM, Evans ME, Paterson JW. The effect of different nebulizers with and without intermittent positive pressure breathing on the absorption and metabolism of salbutamol. Br J Clin Pharmacol 1974;1:295–300.
48. Oosterhuis B, Braat P, Ross CM, et al. Pharmacokinetic-pharmacodynamic modeling of terbutaline bronchodilator in asthma. Clin Pharmacol Ther 1986;40:469–475.
49. Leferink JG, Lamont H, Wagemaker-Engles I, et al. Pharmacokinetics of terbutaline after subcutaneous administration. Int J Clin Pharmacol Biopharm 1979;17:181–185.
50. Gandar R, de Zoeten LW, Der Schoot JB. Serum levels of ritodrine in man. Eur J Clin Pharmacol 1980;17:117–122.
51. Evans ME, Walker SR, Brittain RT, Paterson JW. The metabolism of salbutamol in man. Xenobiotica 1973;3:113–120.
52. Salbutamol. In: Dollery CT, ed. *Therapeutic Drugs.* Edinburgh: Churchill Livingstone, 1991:S1–S4.
53. Salbutamol. In: Reynolds JEF, ed. *Martindale: The Extra Pharmacopoeia.* 30th ed. London: Pharmaceutical Press, 1993:1255–1257.
54. Albuterol. In: McEvoy GK, ed. *AHFS Drug Information 94.* Bethesda, MD: American Society of Hospital Pharmacists, 1994:757–760.
55. Ventolin. In: *Physicians' Desk Reference.* 49th ed. Montvale, NJ: Medical Economics, 1995:485–488.
56. Schatz M, Zeiger RS, Harden KM, et al. The safety of inhaled beta-agonist bronchodilators during pregnancy. J Allergy Clin Immunol 1988;82:686–695.
57. Hudgens DR, Conradi SE. Sudden death associated with terbutaline sulfate administration. Am J Obstet Gynecol 1993;169:120–121.
58. Boreus L, de Chateau P, Lindberg C, Nyberg L. Terbutaline in breast milk. Br J Clin Pharmacol 1982;13:731–732.
59. Nelson HS. Beta-adrenergic bronchodilators. N Engl J Med 1995;333:499–506.
60. Whyte KF, Addis GJ, Whitesmith R, Reid JL. The mechanism of salbutamol-induced hypokalaemia. Br J Clin Pharmacol 1987;23:65–71.
61. Montoliu J, Lens XM, Revert L. Potassium-lowering effect of albuterol for hyperkalemia in renal failure. Arch Intern Med 1987;147:713–717.
62. Crane J, Burgess C, Beasley R. Cardiovascular and hypokalaemic effects of inhaled salbutamol, fenoterol, and isoprenaline. Thorax 1989;44:136–140.
63. Windom HH, Burgess CD, Siebers RWL, et al. The pulmonary and extrapulmonary effects of inhaled beta-agonists in patients with asthma. Clin Pharmacol Ther 1990;48:296–301.
64. Wasserman D, Amitai Y. Hypoglycemia following albuterol overdose in a child. Am J Emerg Med 1992;10:556–557.
65. Spiller HA, Wiley JF, Krenzelok EP, Bory D. Accidental albuterol ingestion in children. Vet Hum Toxicol 1992;34:325.
66. Tye K-H, Desser KB, Benchimol A. Angina pectoris associated with use of terbutaline for premature labor. JAMA 1980;244:692–693.
67. Gluckman L. Ventolin psychosis. NZ Med J 1974;80:411.
68. Whitehouse AM, Novosel S. Salbutamol psychosis. Biol Psychiatry 1989;26:631–633.
69. Gaultier M, Gervais P, Lagier G, Danan L. Pharmacodependence psychique au salbutamol en aerosol chez une asthmatique. Therapie 1976;31:465–470.
70. Brennan PO. Inhaled salbutamol: A new form of drug abuse? Lancet 1983;2:1030–1031.
71. Edwards JG, Holgate ST. Dependency upon salbutamol inhalers. Br J Psychiat 1979;134:624–626.
72. Thompson PJ, Dhillon P, Cole P. Addiction to aerosol treatment: The asthmatic alternative to glue sniffing. Br Med J 1983;287:1515–1516.
73. Formoterol. In: Dollery CT, ed. *Therapeutic Drugs.* Edinburgh: Churchill Livingstone, 1991:F23–F25.
74. Faulds D, Hollingshead LM, Goa KL. Formoterol: A review of its pharmacological properties and therapeutic potential in reversible obstructive airways disease. Drugs 1991;42:115–137.
75. Kamura H, Sasaki H, Higuchi S, Shiobara Y. Quantitative determination of the beta-adrenoceptor formoterol in urine by gas chromatography–mass spectrometry. J Chromatogr 1982;229:337–345.
76. Yokoi K, Murase K, Shiobara Y. The development of a radioimmunoassay for formoterol. Life Sci 1983;33:1665–1672.
77. Tanner RJN, Martin LE, Oxford J. An automatic GCMS assay for salbutamol in plasma. Anal Proc 1983;20:38–47.
78. Ong H, Adam A, Perreault S, et al. Monitoring of salbutamol (albuterol) in humans: Application of an immunoaffinity clean up procedure combined with HPLC with fluorometric detection. Drug Saf 1990;5(suppl. 2):164.
79. Tripp SL, Williams E, Roth WJ, et al. Analysis of terbutaline in human serum by thin layer fluorometry. Anal Lett 1978; BII:727–740.
80. Jacobson SE, Jonsson S, Lindberg C, Svensson LA. Determination of terbutaline in plasma by gas chromatography chemical ionization mass spectrometry. Biomed Mass Spectrom 1980;7:265–268.
81. Billing B, Dahlqvist R, Garles M, et al. Separate and combined use of terbutaline and theophylline in asthmatics. Eur J Respir Dis 1982;63:399–409.
82. Lewis LD, Essex E, Volans GN, Cochrane GM. A study of self-poisoning with oral salbutamol: Laboratory and clinical features. Hum Exp Toxicol 1993;12:39–41.

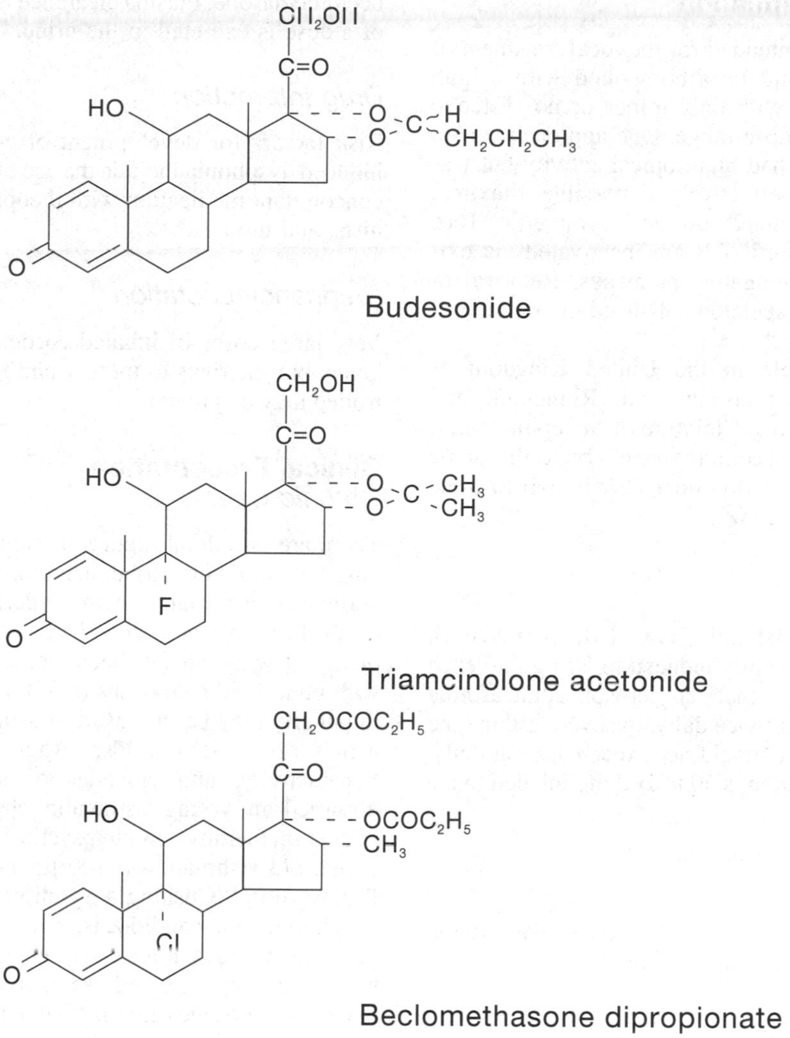

Budesonide

Triamcinolone acetonide

Beclomethasone dipropionate

Figure 45–3 Structures of three glucocorticoids. (From Ryrfeldt A, Anderson P, Edsbacker S, et al. Pharmacokinetics and metabolism of budesonide, a selective glucocorticoid. Eur J Respir Dis 1982;62(suppl. 22):86-95.)

83. Hornblad Y, Ripe E, Magnusson PO, Tegner K. The metabolism and clinical activity of terbutaline and its prodrug ibuterol. Eur J Clin Pharmacol 1976;10:9–18
84. Van den Berg W, Leferink JG, Maes RAA, Kreukniet J, Bruynzeel PLR. Correlation between terbutaline serum levels, c-AMP plasma levels and FEV_1 in normals and asthmatics after subcutaneous administration. Ann Allergy 1980;44:235–239.
85. Ramoska EA, Henretig F, Joffe M, Spiller HA. Propranolol treatment of albuterol poisoning in two asthmatic patients. Ann Emerg Med 1993;22:1474–1476.
86. Hoffner CA, Kendall MJ. Metabolic effects of $beta_2$-agonists. J Clin Pharm Ther 1992;17:155–164.
87. Waller DG. Beta-adrenoceptor partial agonists, a renaissance in cardiovascular therapy? Br J Clin Pharmacol 1990;30:157–171.
88. Breeden CC, Safirstein BH. Albuterol and spacer-induced atrial fibrillation. Chest 1990;98:762–763.
89. Kinney EL, Trautlein JJ, Harbaugh CV, et al. Ventricular tachycardia after terbutaline. JAMA 1978;240:2247.
90. McQueen ZG. New Zealand Committee on Adverse Drug Reactions. 14th Annual Report, 1979. NZ Med J 1980; 91:226–229.
91. Dachman WD, Ford GA, Hoffman BB, Blaschke RF. Terbutaline-induced hypophosphatemia. Clin Pharmacol Ther 1991;49:201. Abstract.
92. Minton NA, Baird AR, Henry JA. Modulation of the effects of salbutamol by propranolol and atenolol. Eur J Clin Pharmacol 1989;36:449–453.
93. Robin ED, McCauley R. Sudden cardiac death in bronchial asthma and inhaled beta-adrenergic agonists. Chest 1992;101:1699–1702.
94. Spiller HA, Ramoska EA, Henretig FM, Joffe M. A two-year retrospective study of accidental pediatric albuterol ingestions. Pediatr Emerg Care 1993;9:338–340.

BUDESONIDE

Drugs such as budesonide beclomethasone, triamcinolone and flunisolide may be used for the topical treatment of asthma by inhalation (Fig. 45–3).[1,2] At low dosage the corticosteroids are largely free of adverse effects. For more severe asthma, where higher doses are required, there may be a greater suppression of the hypothalamus–pituitary–adrenal axis. Behavior changes may be observed in young children.[3] Treatment of excessive dosage requires cessation of use of the inhaled corticosteroid. Otherwise, treatment is symptomatic and supportive. No fatalities have been reported.

Structure and Classification

The ideal glucocorticoid intended for the local treatment of respiratory disorders should be a compound with a high activity in the lungs, but with only minor or no systemic effects in the therapeutic dose range. One approach was to develop a compound that had high topical activity but was inactivated as rapidly and effectively as possible. Maximal topical activity was obtained by an asymmetric 16α, 17α-acetal group. Glucocorticoids are inactivated via oxidative, reductive, and conjugative pathways. Removal of halogens from the steroid skeleton enhanced the rapidity of metabolism of budesonide.[4]

Budesonide is available in the United Kingdom as Pulmicort[5] and in Europe as Preferid, Rhinocort, and Spirocort.[6] Budesonide is a 1/1 mixture of the epimers 22*R* and 22*S*, both of which seem to have about the same pharmacodynamic effects, but epimer 22*R* is two to three times as potent as epimer 22*S*.[7]

Therapeutic Dose

Budesonide is used in a usual initial dose of 100 μg into each nostril twice daily, subsequently reduced to 50 μg into each nostril twice daily. From a metered aerosol, adult asthma patients may inhale 300 μg twice daily. In severe asthma the dose may be increased but should not exceed 1.2 mg daily. A suggested dose for children is 50 to 200 mg inhaled twice daily.[6]

Toxic Dose

At inhaled doses of 200 to 400 μg of budesonide, young children develop adverse behavior problems.[3]

Fatal Dose

No dose associated with fatality has been reported.

Toxicokinetics

Absorption

Systemic availability is 10.7% after oral administration and 72.8% after inhalation, which points to an extensive first-pass metabolism of budesonide, probably in the liver. Two metabolites are formed that have 1/10th to 1/100th the activity of the original compound. Plasma protein binding is 88.3%, similar to that reported for other glucocorticosteroids. Inhalation of 5 puffs (260 μg) led to a peak plasma level of about 6 nmol/L in 4 hours.[4]

Distribution

Budesonide has an apparent volume of distribution of 4.2 L/kg.[6]

Elimination

The plasma elimination half-life is about 2 hours in adults and 1.5 hours in children.[2] This can be compared with half-lives of 1.5 to 2 hours for flunisolide and 15 hours for beclomethasone. Plasma clearance is 1.2 L/kg/h. About 70% of a dose is excreted in the urine.

Drug Interactions

Risk factors for development of corticosteroid inhalation-induced dysphonia include the use of oral corticosteroids and concomitant medication with theophylline, calcium antagonists, and nitrates.[8]

Pregnancy/Lactation

Very large doses of inhaled corticosteroids may be teratogenic, but the risks to mother and fetus if asthma is uncontrolled may be greater.[2]

Clinical Presentation

Chronic Use

There are anecdotal reports of skin thinning and spontaneous, easy bruising, striae, acneiform eruptions, and contact dermatitis, especially in the elderly who have used high doses for long periods.[9,10] Growth retardation has been observed with inhaled beclomethasone dipropionate[11] and with budesonide[8] in doses of 200 and 800 μg/d. Any delay in puberty may be the result of asthma itself rather than the action of corticosteroids.[2] Aggressiveness, bed wetting, hyperactivity, and episodes of severe temper may be observed in young asthmatic children after budesonide inhalation therapy.[3] Acute psychosis has been described in a 5-year-old asthmatic on 100 μg budesonide twice daily.[12] Rarely, florid Cushing's syndrome, adrenal suppression, dysphoria, oral candidiasis, nausea, headache, dry throat, gas, pruritus, rash, impaired taste, diarrhea, constipation, and heartburn have followed use of inhaled corticosteroid. At a budesonide dosage (2.4 mg/d) that affected the cortisol level there appeared to be no effect on calcium, phosphorus, and vitamin D levels and bone metabolism.[2]

Overdoses

No cases of acute overdose after ingestion have been reported. Following excessive doses by inhalation, enhancement of the chronic effects of budesonide may be expected.

Laboratory

Analytical Methods

A sensitive specific radioimmunoassay has been developed for detection of budesonide in plasma. It can detect concentrations down to 0.5 ng/mL.[13]

Blood Levels

Inhalation of 1 mg of budesonide has led to a peak plasma budesonide level of 2.3 ng/mL in about 1 hour.[13]

Abnormalities

A slight transient depression of plasma cortisol levels has been observed, together with an increase in neutrophils, decrease in lymphocytes,[4] and fall in eosinophils.[14]

Ancillary Tests

An increase in serum cholesterol and insulin levels has been reported.[2] This has not been associated with overt hypoglycemic symptoms.

Treatment

Treatment is largely symptomatic and supportive. Cessation of use of the inhaled corticosteroid is indicated. Oral preparations may be useful in its place. There is no antidote.

REFERENCES—BUDESONIDE

1. Haahtela T, Jarvinen M, Kava T, et al. Comparison of a beta$_2$-agonist, terbutaline, with an inhaled corticosteroid, budesonide, in newly detected asthma. N Engl J Med 1991; 325:388–392.
2. Toogood JH. Complication of topical steroid therapy for asthma. Am Rev Respir Dis 1990;141(suppl.):89–96.
3. Connett G, Lenney W. Inhaled budesonide and behavioral disturbances. Lancet 1991;338:634–635.
4. Ryrfeldt A, Andersson P, Edsbacker S, et al. Pharmacokinetics and metabolism of budesonide, a selective glucocorticoid. Eur J Respir Dis 1982;62(suppl. 22):86–95.
5. Barnes PJ. Pulmonary disorders. In: Melmon KL, Morrelli HF, Hoffman BB, Nierenberg DW, eds. *Clinical Pharmacology: Basic Principles in Therapeutics.* 3rd ed. New York: McGraw Hill, 1992:198–202.
6. Reynolds JEF, ed. *Martindale: The Extra Pharmacopoeia.* 30th ed. London: Pharmaceutical Press, 1993:726.
7. Ryrfeldt A, Edsbacker S, Pauwels R. Kinetics of the epimeric glucocorticoid budesonide. Clin Pharmacol Ther 1984;35: 525–530.
8. Wolthers OD, Pedersen S. Growth of asthmatic children during treatment with budesonide: A double blind trial. Br Med J 1991;303:163–165.
9. Boe J, Skoogh BE. Is long term treatment with inhaled steroids in adults hazardous? Eur Respir J 1992;5:1037–1039.
10. Holmes P, Cowen P. Spongiotic (eczematous-type) dermatitis after inhaled budesonide. Aust NZ J Med 1992;22:511.
11. Balfour-Lynn L. Growth retardation in asthmatic children treated with inhaled beclomethasone dipropionate. Lancet 1988;1:475–476.
12. Lewis LD, Cochrane GM. Psychosis in a child inhaling budesonide. Lancet 1983;2:634.
13. Aherne W, Littleton P, Marks V. A sensitive radioimmunoassay for budesonide in plasma. Eur J Respir Dis 1982; 63(suppl. 122):254–256.
14. Evan MM, O'Connor BJ, Fulder RW, et al. Effect of inhaled budesonide on eosinophil density in asthma. Br J Clin Pharmacol 1991;31:616P.

CLENBUTEROL

Clenbuterol, 4-amino-α-[(*tert*-butylamino)methyl]-3,5-dichlorobenzyl alcohol,[1] is a sympathomimetic bronchodilator[2–4] that can affect muscle mass and function.[5,6] Clenbuterol stimulates protein deposition in striated muscle (20% increase) and simultaneously, by its thermogenic properties, increases energy expenditure and hence reduces muscle glycogen and body fat deposition (20% decrease).[2] These properties are often seen with other classic beta-adrenoceptor agonists. The effects on cardiac muscle are propranolol sensitive and probably β_1 adrenoceptor mediated; skeletal muscle may respond with β_2 adrenoceptor-, atypical adrenoceptor-, or even non-receptor-mediated pathways. Clenbuterol induces a true hypertrophy of muscle (type II fibers) and an increase in the 1-glycolytic capacity of the muscle as a whole, giving rise to an increase in force and a reduction in relaxation time. Clenbuterol and similar beta agonists taken in large doses can induce a protein anabolic response that may be performance enhancing.[2] Athletes feel that they can derive 10 to 25% of the effect of anabolic steroids by taking between 60 and 100 μg of clenbuterol per day. Some take as much as 600 μg per day. Clenbuterol has also been used as a uterine relaxant without noticeable side effects on the fetus.[7] Its half-life is 29 hours.[7] The Sports Council has considered β_2 agonists to be related to androgenic anabolic steroids.[8] (See also Chapter 19.)

Therapeutic Dose

Clenbuterol is used as a β_2 receptor agonist in obstructive lung disease,[9,10] where it is administered in doses of 20 to 40 μg twice daily.[10] It may improve pulmonary function equal to the action of terbutaline.

Toxicokinetics

About 34 to 43% of an administered dose is excreted in the urine as unchanged drug.[10]

Laboratory

Clenbuterol can be quantitated in the urine using high-performance thin-layer chromatography and capillary gas chromatography with electron-capture detection. The detection limit is 0.2 ppb.

Clinical Presentation

Clenbuterol is a self-limiting compound because headaches can be disturbing. Clenbuterol may lead to a dose-dependent tremor and palpitations.[1,9,10] Tardive dyskinesia has been described after long-term treatment.[3] At high doses it is associated with headaches, nervousness, lightheadedness,[3] an increase in heart rate, and a slight rise in systolic blood pressure.[1] A decrease in T-wave amplitude may be seen on the electrocardiogram.[1] Symptoms appear between 30 minutes and 6 hours after exposure and normally cease spontaneously after about 40 hours.[11]

REFERENCES—CLENBUTEROL

1. Whitsett TL, Manion CV, Wilson MF. Cardiac, pulmonary and neuromuscular effects of clenbuterol and terbutaline compared with placebo. Br J Clin Pharmacol 1981;12:195–200.
2. Muscling in on clenbuterol. Lancet 1992;340:403. Editorial.
3. Reynolds JEF, ed. *Martindale: The Extra Pharmacopoeia.* 30th ed. London: Pharmaceutical Press, 1993:1241.
4. Whitsett TL, Manion CV, Wilson MF. Cardiac, pulmonary and neuromuscular effects of clenbuterol, terbutaline and placebo. Clin Pharmacol Ther 1980;27:294–295.
5. MacLennan PA, Edward RHT. Effect of clenbuterol and propranolol on muscle mass: Evidence that clenbuterol stimulates muscle beta-adrenoceptors to induce hypertrophy. Biochem J 1989;264:573–579.
6. Delday MI, Williams PE, Maltin CA. Effect of clenbuterol on immobilized muscle. J Neurol Sci 1990;98:376.

7. Zahn V, Krumbacher G. Clenbuterol: A long term uterine relaxant. J Perinat Med 1981;9:96–100.
8. Beckett AH. Clenbuterol and sports. Lancet 1992;340:1165.
9. Blom-Bulow P, Boe J, Bulow K, Hagelqvist I. A comparison of oral $beta_2$-agonists clenbuterol and salbutamol in obstructive lung disease: A double blind cross-over study. Curr Ther Res 1985;37:51–57.
10. Michel F, Gatto E, Gene R, Pardal MF. Clenbuterol-induced tardive dyskinesia. Clin Neuropharmacol 1991;14:427–431.
11. World Health Organization. Wkly Epidemiol Rec 1992;67:273–280.

CLOBUTINOL HYDROCHLORIDE

Clobutinol (KAT-256) is a non-opioid antitussive agent that can induce muscle rigidity, fasciculations, and grand mal seizures in overdose.

Product Formulation

Clobutinol is available in the Venezuelan pharmaceutical market in drop form (20 drops = 40 mg) and in syrup form (1mL = 4 mg).[1]

Source

Clobutinol is a synthetic chemical.

Therapeutic Dose

As a centrally active cough suppressant, clobutinol is given by mouth in doses of 40 to 80 mg three times daily. Doses of 20 mg have been given by subcutaneous, intramuscular, or intravenous injection. The recommended pediatric dose in Venezuela is 30 mg.[1]

Toxic Dose

A 5-mL dose containing 200 mg clobutinol was given to a 5-year-old child; the child survived.[1]

Toxicokinetics

Absorption

Absorption is rapid. Maximum plasma levels of 160 to 220 ng/mL are reached in about 2 hours. The absorption half-life is 15 to 30 minutes.[2]

Elimination

About 80 to 90% of a dose is eliminated in the urine, of which 17% is unchanged clobutinol. Elimination half-life is 1.5 to 3 hours with a slower total elimination of 23 to 32 hours.[2]

Clinical Presentation

Overdose of clobutinol has been followed by stupor, muscle rigidity, fasciculations, and seizures. Animal studies of clobutinol at doses of 15 to 20 mg/kg have reported an association with an irreversible bradycardia and hypotension.[3]

Laboratory

An ion-selective electrode with a membrane of polyvinyl chloride matrix sensitive to clobutinol has been used to detect clobutinol.[4]

Treatment

Treatment is largely supportive and symptomatic.

REFERENCES—CLOBUTINOL HYDROCHLORIDE

1. Ramirez MS, Rojas AM, Perez LA, et al. Grand mal seizures and clobutinol overdose. Vet Hum Toxicol 1993;35:444.
2. Zimmer A, Bucheler A, Kascke S. Pharmacokinetic comparison of clobutinol-HCl (with and without orciprenaline-SO_4), as solution, juice and syrup in man. Arzneimittelforschung 1977;27:2012–2017.
3. Salonen RO. Comparison of the effects of two opioid antitussives, vadocaine hydrochloride, clobutinol and lidocaine on lung-mechanics in guinea pigs. Arzneimittelforschung 1988;38:609–612.
4. Fukamachi K, Ishibashi N. Clobutinol-sensitive electrode. J Pharm Soc Jpn 1979;9:126–130.

IODINATED GLYCEROL

Iodinated glycerol may induce hypothyroidism, hyperthyroidism, and arrhythmias. Few reports of overdose are available in the medical literature. Treatment is symptomatic and supportive and requires cessation of use.

Structure and Classification

Iodinated glycerol is a stable complex represented mainly by isomers of iodopropylidene glycerol. The drug contains 50% organically bound iodine and virtually no inorganic iodide or free iodine.[1,2] The molecular weight is 288.1.[2] Iodinated glycerol is marketed as Organidin, Iotuss, Iotuss DM, and Iophen.

Use

Iodinated glycerol is used as a mucolytic expectorant in the therapy of chronic obstructive pulmonary disease.[1,2] Its effectiveness for this indication has yet to be demonstrated by controlled clinical studies. It may have use in the symptomatic treatment of chronic bronchitis.[3]

Product Formulation

Iodinated glycerol is a viscous, tasteless, straw-colored liquid. The product is available alone as an oral solution containing 60 mg/5 mL or 50 mg/mL and in tablets of 30 mg. It is available in combination with theophylline (10 mg/5 mL with theophylline anhydrous 40 mg/mL) and codeine (30 mg/5 mL with codeine phosphate 10 mg/5 mL) and as 30 mg/5 mL iodinated glycerol with dextromethorphan hydrobromide 10 mg/5 mL.[2]

Source

Iodinated glycerol is a synthetic chemical product.

Therapeutic Dose

Iodinated glycerol is used by adults in doses of 60 mg four times daily with fluids. Children have received up to one-half the adult dosage.[1,2]

Toxicokinetics

The toxicokinetics of iodinated glycerol have not been studied. Once absorbed in the bloodstream, iodinated glycerol appears to be slowly metabolized into free iodide and glycerol.[3]

Iodinated glycerol is contraindicated in pregnant or nursing women and in neonates.[2]

Clinical Presentation

Iodism may manifest as skin eruptions; burning of the mouth and throat; coryza; eye irritation and swelling of the eyelids; frontal headache; pulmonary edema; gastric disturbances; and inflammation of the pharynx, larynx, tonsils, and parotid and submaxillary glands. Hyperthyroidism,[4] central nervous system depression, fever, vasculitis, flareup of adolescent acne, glomerulonephritis, and a parkinsonian syndrome have been described in anecdotal reports. In hyperthyroid patients, increasing dyspnea, fatigue, weight loss, and proximal muscle weakness are prominent symptoms after iodinated glycerol use.[3] Arrhythmias such as atrial fibrillation and irregular tachycardias have been observed.[4]

Laboratory

In the usual dosage, iodinated glycerol does not elevate the protein-bound iodine concentration.

Treatment

1. Discontinue iodinated glycerol therapy.
2. If a woman becomes pregnant while receiving iodinated glycerol, discontinue the drug and inform her of the potential risks to the fetus[2] (eg, fetal goiter with or without hypothyroidism and with the potential for airway obstruction).
3. Watch for symptoms of hyperthyroidism such as tremor, tachycardia, and anxiety.[4]
4. Monitor thyroid function tests.
5. Admit if severe hyperthyroidism, hypothyroidism, or arrhythmias are present.[5]

REFERENCES—IODINATED GLYCEROL

1. McEvoy GK, ed. *AHFS Drug Information 94.* Bethesda: American Society of Hospital Pharmacists, 1994:1759–1760.
2. Reynolds JEF, Ed. *Martindale: The Extra Pharmacopoeia.* 30th ed. London: Pharmaceutical Press, 1993:970.
3. Becker CB, Gordon JM. Iodinated glycerol and thyroid function: Four cases: A review of the literature. Chest 1993; 103:188–192.
4. Huseby JS, Bennett SW, Hagensee ME. Hyperthyroidism induced by iodinated glycerol. Am Rev Respir Dis 1991;144: 1403.
5. Gomolin IH. Iodinated glycerol-induced hypothyroidism. Drug Intell Clin Pharm 1987;21:726–727.

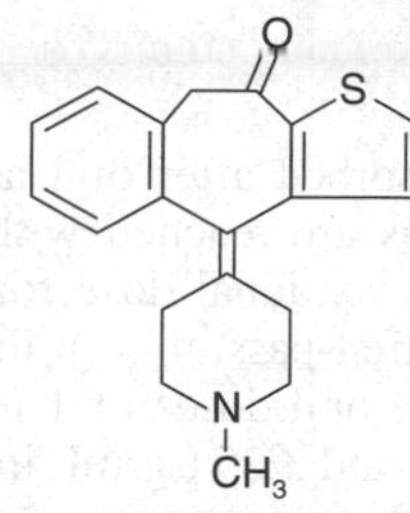

Figure 45–4 Structure of ketotifen, a benzocycloheptathiophene compound. (From Grant SM, Goa KL, Fitton A, Sorkin EM. Ketotifen: A review of its pharmacokinetic properties and therapeutic use in asthma and allergic disorders. Drugs 1990;40:412–448.)

KETOTIFEN

Ketotifen (Fig. 45–4) is a prophylactic, nonbronchodilator, antiasthmatic drug with marked antianaphylactic properties and a specific antihistaminic effect.[1,2] The manufacturer is aware of 21 cases of acute overdose; all recovered.[3]

Structure and Classification

Ketotifen is a benzocycloheptathiophene compound with a molecular weight of 425.5.[1]

Use

Ketotifen is an orally active prophylactic agent for the management of bronchial asthma and allergic disorders.[1]

Product Formulation

Ketotifen is formulated in 1-mg capsules and 1-mg tablets (Zaditen) containing 1.38 mg of ketotifen hydrogen fumarate equivalent to 1 mg of ketotifen base.

Source

Ketotifen is a synthetic chemical.

Therapeutic Dose

For adult patients with bronchial asthma and allergic responses, the dosage of ketotifen is 1 mg orally twice daily with meals. There is also a 2-mg slow-release tablet, permitting once-daily administration. A maximum of 2 mg twice daily may be reached slowly. Children aged 6 months to 3 years are administered ketotifen in doses of 0.5 mg (half-tablet or 2.5 mL syrup) twice daily. Children over 3 years of age receive the adult dose.[1–3]

Toxic Dose

Ingestion of 20 mg of ketotifen produced no serious signs or symptoms as reported to the manufacturer.[2] All patients, including adults who ingested up to 120 mg, made a full recovery.

Fatal Dose

No lethal dose has been established.[2]

Toxicokinetics

Absorption

Ketotifen is well absorbed after oral administration. Peak plasma concentrations are reached within 2 to 4 hours of administration of conventional dose forms. Bioavailability of the drug is 50% (first-pass effect). Peak plasma concentrations after multiple oral doses of 1 mg twice daily were 1.92 μg/mL in adults and 3.25 μg/mL in children. Ketotifen is 75% protein bound.[2]

Distribution

The volume of distribution is high (56 L/kg).[2]

Elimination

Ketotifen is extensively metabolized to the inactive ketotifen-*N*-glucuronide and the active norketotifen. Only 1% of a dose is excreted in the urine unchanged. Clearance is biphasic, with a half-life of distribution of 3 hours and a half-life of elimination of 22 hours.[1]

Drug Interactions

The sedative effects of ketotifen can be potentiated by other central nervous system depressants including alcohol, hypnotics, and antihistamines. A reversible fall in platelet counts has been reported when oral antidiabetic agents are used concomitantly.[4]

Pregnancy/Lactation

There have been no controlled studies in pregnant or lactating women.

Mechanism of Action

Ketotifen is a nonbronchodilator mast cell stabilizer with many features of an antihistamine. Its action resembles that of disodium cromoglycate (cromolyn sodium).

Clinical Presentation

Overdose

Ingestion of an overdose produces drowsiness, confusion, dyspnea, cyanosis, tachycardia, hyperexcitability, and seizures.[5]

Chronic Use

The most frequent adverse effects are sedation, dizziness, dry mouth, nausea, and headache.[1–8] Symptoms of overdose are similar in children and adults.[2]

Laboratory

Analytical Methods

Ketotifen can be quantitated by mass spectrometry and gas chromatographic separation with a limit of sensitivity of 50 ng/L.[3,4]

Blood Levels

Therapeutic plasma concentrations of ketotifen range from 1 to 4 μg/mL.[5] Twenty hours after ingestion of 120 mg, the plasma concentration of ketotifen base was 122 μg/mL. Two hours after ingestion of 40 mg, the plasma concentration was 5 μg/mL. Three hours after ingestion of 50 mg, the plasma concentration was 54 μg/mL. Patients exhibited headache, drowsiness, bradycardia, confusion, and loss of consciousness.

Gut Decontamination

Gastric lavage should be performed within 2 to 4 hours of ingestion. Activated charcoal may be administered even after 4 hours, as ketotifen metabolism is mainly hepatic and biphasic (alpha elimination half-life, 4 hours; beta elimination half-life, 21 hours).

Elimination Enhancement

Hemodialysis and hemoperfusion are not likely to be of value because of the high volume of distribution.

Antidote

There is no antidote.[2]

Supportive Measures

Central nervous system depression should be treated symptomatically; seizures can be controlled with diazepam. Hypotension can be treated supportively with fluid administration if required. The role of vasopressor agents (dopamine, phenylephrine, norepinephrine) has not been established. Grant et al. state that adrenaline (epinephrine) is contraindicated. Patients should be monitored for at least 6 to 8 hours after an overdose.[1]

REFERENCES—KETOTIFEN

1. Grant SM, Goa KL, Fitton A, Sorkin EM. Ketotifen: A review of its pharmacodynamic and pharmacokinetic properties and therapeutic use in asthma and allergic disorders. Drugs 1990;40:412–448.
2. Le Blaye I, Donatini B, Hall M, Krupp P. Acute ketotifen overdosage: A review of present clinical experience. Drug Saf 1992;7:387–392.
3. Perhaj Z, Laplanche R. Documenta Sandoz. Basle: Sandoz, March 1979.
4. Ketotifen. In: Dollery CT, ed. *Therapeutic Drugs.* Edinburgh: Churchill Livingstone, 1991:K28–K31.
5. Jefferys DR, Volans GN. Ketotifen overdose: Surveillance of the toxicity of a new drug. Br Med J 1981;282:1755–1756.
6. Maclay WP, Crowder D, Spiro S, Turner P. Postmarketing surveillance: Practical experience with ketotifen. Br Med J 1984;288:911–914.
7. Rackham A, Brown CA, Chardra RK, et al. A Canadian multicenter study with Zaditen (ketotifen) in the treatment of bronchial asthma in children aged 5 to 17 years. J Allergy Clin Immunol 1989;84:286–296.
8. MacDonald GF. An overview of ketotifen. Chest 1982;82(suppl.):30A–32S.

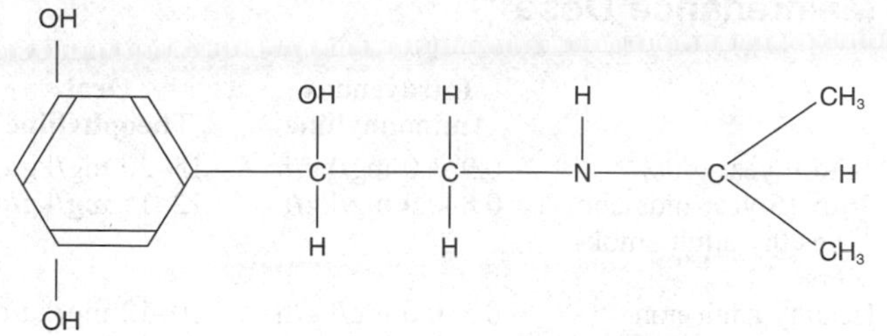

Orciprenaline

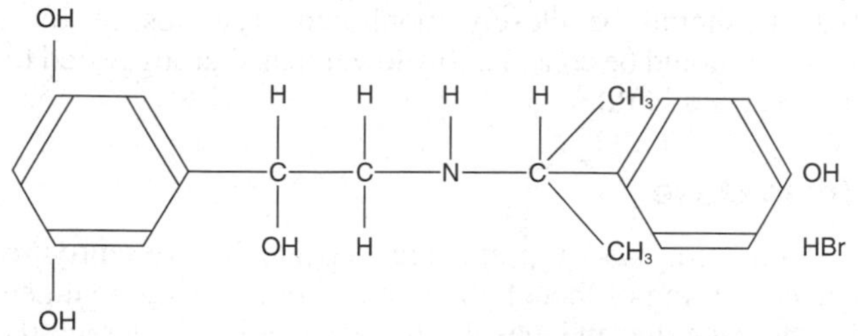

Hydroxyphenylorciprenaline

Figure 45–5 Structures of orciprenaline (metaproterenol) and hydroxyphenylorciprenaline. (From Beardshaw J, MacLean L, Chan-Yeung M. Comparison of the bronchodilation and cardiac effects of hydroxyphenylorciprenaline and orciprenaline. Chest 1974;65: 507–511.)

METAPROTERENOL (ORCIPRENALINE SULFATE)

Metaproterenol (orciprenaline sulfate) overdoses may produce hypokalemia, hyperglycemia, and hyperlactatemia similar to the toxic effects of theophylline and other β_2-adrenergic agonists.[1]

Structure and Classification

Metaproterenol (Fig. 45–5) has an empirical formula of $(C_{11}H_{17}NO_3)_2 \cdot H_2SO_4$ and a molecular weight of 220.6. It is a synthetic β_2-adrenoceptor agonist.[2–4]

Use

Metaproterenol is used in the treatment of asthma, bronchitis, and other types of reversible airway obstruction.

Product Formulation

Orciprenaline is available in tablet form (Alupent) and as a 5% solution from a hand nebulizer.

Therapeutic Dose

In bronchial asthma, orciprenaline sulfate is given by mouth in a dose of 20 mg four times daily. The following doses are suggested for children: up to 1 year, 5 to 10 mg three times daily; 1 to 3 years, 5 to 10 mg four times daily; 3 to 12 years, 10 mg four times daily to 20 mg three times daily.[3] Use of a nebulizer solution of 0.3 mL 5% solution diluted with 2.5 mL of sterile water or physiologic saline may require up to 10 inhalations.[3]

Toxic Dose

A 14 year old ingested 80 mg of metaproterenol and survived.[4]

Fatal Dose

No fatal dose has been reported.

Toxicokinetics

Absorption

About 40% of the drug is absorbed orally. Enzymes in the gut contribute to its presystemic metabolism.

Distribution

The apparent volume of distribution is about 10 L/kg.

Elimination

The elimination half-life is 5 to 6 hours. A hydroxyphenyl derivative of orciprenaline appears to have similar β_2-adrenoceptor agonist properties.[2]

Drug Interactions

Tricyclic antidepressants may enhance the bronchodilator effects of beta agonists and also exacerbate their serious cardiovascular effects. Beta-adrenoceptor blockers antagonize the bronchodilation produced by orciprenaline. Orciprenaline given with adrenalin or other sympathomimetics may exhibit additive effects in stimulating beta adrenoceptors. Anesthetics (eg, halothane, trichlorethylene, enflurane) may sensitize the myocardium to the arrhythmogenic properties of the beta agonists. Beta-agonist bronchodilators may enhance the risk of serious cardiac arrhythmias in patients receiving digitalis. The effects of theophylline may be enhanced by beta agonists.[5]

Pregnancy/Lactation

Use of metaproterenol by pregnant or lactating women has not been systematically evaluated.

Mechanism of Action

Although orciprenaline is selective for β_2 adrenoceptors, it is less β_2 selective than albutamol, terbutaline, or fenoterol.[6]

Clinical Presentation

Symptoms of beta-agonist overadministration may include marked tachycardia, tremor, excitement, restlessness, anxiety, headache, nausea, and changes in blood pressure. Cardiac arrhythmias may be a potential problem in some patients with cardiac problems. After ingesting 8 mg of orciprenaline, a 14-year-old developed hypokalemia, hyperglycemia, and hyperlactatemia, a triad similar to that seen in acute theophylline toxicity and with other beta-adrenergic agonists.[4]

Laboratory

Analytical Methods

A high-performance liquid chromatographic assay using fluorescence detection may be sensitive to a level of 0.5 mg/mL.[7]

Abnormalities

Hypokalemia, hyperglycemia, and hyperlactatemia may be produced by an overdose of orciprenaline.[4] The electrocardiogram may show sinus tachycardia.

Treatment

Treatment of overdose is largely symptomatic and supportive and guided by the treatment suggestions in the section on β_2-Adrenoceptor Agonists. There is no antidote.

REFERENCES—METAPROTERENOL (ORCIPRENALINE SULFATE)

1. Edwards G. Orciprenaline in treatment of airways obstruction in chronic bronchitis. Br Med J 1964;1:1015–1017.
2. Beardshaw J, MacLean L, Chan-Yeung M. Comparison of the bronchodilation and cardiac effects of hydroxyphenyl-orciprenaline and orciprenaline. Chest 1974;65:507–511.
3. Reynolds JEF, 30th ed. *Martindale: The Extra Pharmacopoeia.* 30th ed. London: Pharmaceutical Press, 1993:1950.
4. Barnewolt BA, Walter FG. Metabolic effects of metaproterenol orciprenaline overdose: Hypokalemia, hyperglycemia and hyperlactatemia. Vet Hum Toxicol 1990;32:346.
5. Orciprenaline. In: Dollery CT, ed. *Therapeutic Drugs.* Edinburgh: Churchill Livingstone, 1991:O29–O34.
6. McFadden ER. Beta$_2$ receptor agonist metabolism and pharmacology. J Allergy Clin Immunol 1981;68:91–97.
7. Macgregor TR, Nastasi L, Farine PR, Keirns JJ. Isolation and characterization of metaproterenol-*O*-sulfate: A conjugate of metaproterenol in human urine. Drug Metab Dispos 1983;11:568–573.

THEOPHYLLINE

Theophylline and beta-adrenergic agonists induce similar clinical (vomiting, tachycardia, tremulousness, agitation, wide pulse pressure, and hypotension) and laboratory (hypokalemia, hyperglycemia, lactic acidosis) effects after overdose. Hypophosphatemia, hypomagnesemia, respiratory alkalosis, hypercalcemia, and leukocytosis have been associated with both types of overdoses but are more prevalent after a theophylline overdose.[1] In low doses, theophylline toxicity is similar to beta-adrenergic agonist toxicity.

Therapeutic Dose

Guidelines for intravenous aminophylline and theophylline maintenance doses are based on lean body weight. The standard intravenous loading dose of aminophylline in adults is 5 to 6 mg/kg given over 20 to 30 minutes.

Maintenance Dose

	Intravenous Aminophylline	Oral Theophylline
1- to 9-year-olds	0.9–1.0 mg/kg/h	15–20 mg/kg/d
9- to 16-year-olds and healthy adult smokers	0.8–0.9 mg/kg/h	12–15 mg/kg/d
Healthy adult non-smokers	0.5–0.6 mg/kg/h	10–12 mg/kg/d
Adults with cardiac or liver dysfunction	0.2–0.3 mg/kg/h	5–6 mg/kg/d

Patients with decreased albumin levels (50% protein bound) should be closely monitored. The dosage for a neonate should be considerably lower than that suggested for a 1-year-old child.[2]

Toxic Dose

A 5-day-old, 1.3-kg premature neonate inadvertently received 180 mg of theophylline in 26 hours during treatment for bradycardia and developed tachycardia, hyperventilation, increased diuresis, central nervous system excitation, an increase in blood glucose concentration followed by a prolonged decrease, and hypercalcemia. Seizures, arrhythmias, and vomiting did not occur. The child survived.[3]

Toxicokinetics

Distribution

The apparent volume of distribution remains relatively constant, ranging from 0.2 to 0.7 L/kg (mean, 0.5 L/kg). Liver cirrhosis increases and obesity decreases the volume of distribution at therapeutic doses, whereas age, sex, chronic pulmonary disease, and smoking have little effect. In plasma, protein binding of theophylline at therapeutic concentrations is approximately 50%. The elderly have a slightly smaller volume of distribution than do young adults.

Elimination

Metabolism. The compound 1-methylxanthine appears in much smaller quantities.[4] Cytochrome P1A2 is responsible for the major part of theophylline metabolism in humans.[5] In adults, about 10% of a dose of theophylline is excreted unchanged in the urine. In the neonate, 50% is excreted unchanged.

At therapeutic doses, blood levels follow first-order kinetics, but in overdose, mixed first- and zero-order (Michaelis–Menten) kinetics prevail. Overdose may produce a biphasic elimination pattern with a slow initial phase due either to continued absorption or to saturation of metabolic pathways.[6] The kidney excretes 5 to 10% of a therapeutic dose unchanged.

Factors Affecting Metabolism. In the neonate, all the metabolic pathways of theophylline observed in adults are only partially developed. In premature infants, theophylline has a half-life nine times that of children 1 to 4 years old. The clearance in premature infants is one-seventh that of children 1 to 4 years old, presumably due to immaturity of the mixed-function oxidase system. The unique dif-

Table 45–7
Drug Interaction of Theophylline

Drugs That Decrease Theophylline Clearance (may increase plasma theophylline concentration)	**Drugs That Increase Theophylline Clearance (may decrease plasma theophylline concentration)**
Verapamil	Isoproterenol
Erythromycin	Terbutaline
Troleandomycin	Corticosteroids
Roxithromycin	Phenytoin
Enoxacin	Phenobarbital
Ciprofloxacin	Activated charcoal
Pefloxacin	Felodipine
Norfloxacin	Moricizine
Ofloxacin	Benzodiazpines
Cimetidine	Sulfinpyrazone
Famotidine	**Drugs That Have No Effect on Theophylline Disposition Kinetics**
Fametidine	Ephedrine
Propranolol	Metaproterenol
Diltiazem	Prednisone
Nifedipine	Prednisolone
Furosemide	Terfenadine
Viloxazine	Amoxicilin
Allopurinol	Ampicillin
Ticlopidine	Cephalexin
Thiabendazole	Trimethoprim–sulfamethoxazole
Disulfiram	Tetradyne
Interferon	Doxycycline
Caffeine	Nalidixic acid
Influenza vaccination	Metronidazole
Bacillus Calmette–Guerin vaccination	Antacids
Rifampicin	Metoclopramide
Isoniazid	Metoprolol
Pirantel pamoate	Atenolol
Oral contraceptives	Nadolol
Ranitidine	
Fluvoxamine	
Mexiletine	
Propafenone	

Source: Upton[8]; Skinner[9]; Dal Negro et al.[10]

ference in theophylline disposition between adults and neonates is the formation of caffeine in the neonate. Although the major metabolic pathways in the adult involve demethylation and oxidation, producing more methylxanthine and methyluric acids, in premature infants theophylline can also be methylated to caffeine, which can itself be toxic.[7] Theophylline and its metabolites are eliminated more slowly in infants than in older children and adults.[3] Phenytoin, phenobarbital, diazepam, chloramphenicol, and other drugs eliminated following metabolic degradation also undergo slower elimination in the newborn period. Unlike theophylline and caffeine, most metabolites appear to reach adult values by a month of age.

Drug Interactions

Theophylline may be particularly susceptible to alteration of its clearance because the particular form of the P450 system involved (CyPIA2), because of its metabolism is saturable, and/or because 90% of its elimination is via metabolism. Its clearance has been found to increase or decrease (typically by around 25%, but often up to 80%) when other drugs are administered (Table 45–7).

Pregnancy/Lactation

The Collaborative Perinatal Project of the National Institute of Neurological Communicative Disorder and Stroke studied 59,931 pregnancies and concluded that theophylline use during pregnancy is not associated with any increase in risk of stillbirth.[11] Association of some rare cardiovascular anomalies (aortic anomalies, double-outlet right ventricle, transposition of the great arteries, anomalous pulmonary venous connection, hypoplasia of the left ventricle) with theophylline exposure both in animals and in an initial human study suggests that theophylline may be a cardiovascular teratogen in a susceptible human fetus. For the fetus with prenatal exposure to theophylline, fetal echocardiography may be useful in detecting any possible severe cardiac defect. Additional studies are required to confirm the validity of these observations.[12]

Theophylline levels in breast milk and maternal blood concentrations follow similar kinetics, with a milk: serum ratio of 0.67.[13] Pregnancy reduces theophylline protein binding (11% vs 23%) and increases the volume of distribution (31 L vs 37 L) and elimination half-life (262 minutes vs 389 minutes).[14] Increased clearance of unbound drug, however, offsets these effects.

Mechanism of Action

Theophylline, in addition to promoting diaphragmatic contractility, promotes mucociliary clearance, aids cardiac function, lowers pulmonary artery pressure, and exhibits antiinflammatory effects.[15] This product can reduce asthmatic symptoms, alleviate dyspnea, and relieve nocturnal asthma when added to a regimen of beta agonists and corticosteroids.[15]

Clinical Presentation

Metabolic Effects

In acute theophylline poisoning, β_2-adrenergic stimulation appears to be an important mediator of hypokalemia and hyperglycemia.[16]

Potassium. Hypokalemia may be due to potassium loss following protracted vomiting, but it may occur in the absence of vomiting. Potassium diuresis is observed in patients with metabolic acidosis. Following hyperglycemia and hyperinsulinemia potassium may shift from the extracellular compartment. An intracellular shift of potassium follows the catecholamine-induced stimulation of membrane-bound sodium–potassium ATP. These factors may be contributory mechanisms in the production of hypokalemia. Remember that potassium shifts and not potassium depletion are usually the cause of the hypokalemia. As the serum theophylline level decreases, potassium returns from the cells. Overzealous replacement of potassium may produce hyperkalemia.

Catecholamines. Increased circulatory catecholamines (epinephrine and norepinephrine) are observed after both therapeutic use of theophylline and theophylline intoxication. The hypercatecholamine effects of theophylline intoxication include possible mediation of hyperglycemia, hypercalcemia, metabolic acidosis, and prolongation of the QT

Table 45–8
Theophylline: Acute and Chronic Poisonings

Acute	Chronic
Hypotension	
Hypokalemia: dysrhythmias, seizures (severe, more frequent, correlated with serum theophylline concentrations)	
Low serum bicarbonate level	
Serious complications at levels >100 µg/mL	Serious complications at lower levels, 40–70 µg/mL
Hypophosphatemia	Hypercalcemia
Hyperglycemia	Less hyperglycemia, metabolic acidosis, leukocytosis
Hypomagnesemia	
Metabolic acidosis, (Lactic acidosis?), Leukocytosis } Excess sympathetic effect	
Nausea, vomiting, abdominal pain	Gastrointestinal symptoms less common
Seizures, tremulousness, agitation	Seizures may be initial sign of toxicity
Sinus tachycardia, supraventricular tachycardia, hypotension	Sinus and/or supraventricular tachycardia and atrial fibrillation
(all correlated with blood levels >19 µg/mL)	Hypotension infrequent
Toxic symptoms correlate better with blood levels	Toxic signs and symptoms may not correlate well with blood levels
Young adults	Very young or elderly
Minimal toxicity at peak levels, 20–40 µg/mL	Poisoning at lower serum levels
Moderate toxicity, 40–100 µg/mL	Seizures, serious dysrhythmias at 40–70 µg/mL
Severe toxicity, >100 µ/mL	
Activated charcoal useful (blood levels 40–100 µg/mL)	
Hemoperfusion useful at levels >100 µg/mL	Hemoperfusion useful at levels >60 µg/mL
Endpoint of hemoperfusion: serum levels <60 µg/mL	Endpoint of hemoperfusion: serum level <40 µg/mL
High incidence of vomiting of charcoal	Lower incidence of vomiting
Sustained-release preparations	Uncoated tablets and liquids
Serious toxicity develops hours after initial presentation	
Serum levels may peak in 12 h	Serum levels peak in 1–2 h
Bezoars	
Secondary elevation in serum levels; toxicity	
High-fat meals increase absorption	

Source: Skopnik et al.[3]

interval on the electrocardiogram and may be a cause of theophylline-induced tachyrhythmias.[17] The exact etiology of the metabolic acidosis is unclear, but it may result from a lactic acidosis secondary to catecholamine-induced glycolysis.[18,19] The clinical effects of xanthine-induced increases in circulating catecholamine and cyclic AMP effects appear synergistic. Theophylline apparently causes hypercalcemia by a mechanism subject to beta-adrenergic regulation, because propranolol can reduce serum calcium levels in theophylline-poisoned patients.[20]

Hyperglycemia. Hyperglycemia may aid in supporting a diagnosis of theophylline poisoning in the absence of a serum theophylline level if it is present together with tachycardia, seizures, and/or hypokalemia.

Definition of Intoxication

Acute intoxication in the absence of theophylline therapy has been defined as ingestion or intravenous administration of a toxic dose of theophylline in a patient not currently receiving the medication. Intoxication due to chronic overmedication is defined as repeated administration of theophylline without the ingestion of a single toxic dose (> 10 mg/kg body weight). Acute intoxication while receiving therapy is defined as the ingestion or administration of a toxic quantity of theophylline in a patient who has been receiving theophylline in appropriate doses.[21]

Shannon and co-workers consider overdoses as acute (single exposure), chronic (long-term exposure), or acute-on-therapeutic (single toxic exposure superimposed on maintenance therapy).[22,23] In a prospective study, 125 pediatric patients with theophylline intoxication exhibited about a 10% frequency of life-threatening events (seizures, arrhythmias). Three factors were found to influence this rate: manner of intoxication, peak theophylline concentration, and patient age. In acute intoxication, theophylline concentration was significantly elevated in patients with seizures or arrhythmias. Patient age was not a factor. Patients with acute intoxication had lower serum potassium (3.04 mmol/L vs 3.8 mmol/L) and higher serum glucose (10.8 mmol/L vs 7.0 mmol/L, 194 mg/dL vs 127 mg/dL) levels than did children with chronic intoxication (Table 45–8).

In chronic or acute-on-therapeutic intoxication, theophylline levels were not different between the two groups. Children who experienced life-threatening events were young (1.6 years vs 8 years). Peak theophylline concentration does not identify high-risk patients after acute-on-therapeutic or chronic intoxication. Aggressive management should be considered for young children in these groups.[22] In a further study, major theophylline toxicity (seizures, arrhythmias) was associated with peak theophylline levels greater than 555 µmol/L (100 mg/L) in patients with acute intoxication and in those 60 or older (regardless of peak serum theophylline concentration) with chronic intoxication. Despite lower theophylline levels, major theophylline toxicity was more common with chronic intoxication. Major toxicity after theophylline overdose can be predicted in most patients, permitting rapid identification of those patients who will benefit from hemoperfusion or dialysis.[23]

Central Nervous System Effects

Seizures may result in status epilepticus, rhabdomyolysis, hypothermia, and hypoxic injury.[24,25] Patients with a preexisting seizure disorder or other neurologic conditions such as meningitis, head trauma, and cerebrovascular accident are vulnerable. In chronic overmedication, seizures may be the initial sign of toxicity. Theophylline-induced seizures are associated with a significant morbidity. Theophylline induces cerebral vasoconstriction and relative ischemia. Cardiac arrhythmias result in cerebral hypoperfusion. Theophylline, a phosphodiesterase inhibitor, increases tissue levels of cyclic AMP, a potentially epileptogenic substance. Theophylline is also an adenosine receptor antagonist and may cause seizures by antagonizing the depressant effect of adenosine in the cerebral cortex. Diazepam and phenobarbital appear to potentiate the effect of adenosine.[26] Seizures in both children and adults may occur at therapeutic or mildly toxic levels. Elderly patients have a poor prognosis following theophylline-induced seizures. Other risk factors for serious outcome in theophylline-associated seizures are previous brain injury or disease, severe pulmonary disease, and possibly a low serum albumin level.[27] Coma is an uncommon sign of theophylline intoxication. Ataxia and visual hallucinations have been reported in a series of pediatric theophylline overdose cases.[28]

Cardiovascular Effects

Theophylline-induced cardiotoxicity may be due to its direct action on cardiac membrane depolarization, antagonism of the cardioprotective effects of endogenous adenosine, stimulation of plasma catecholamine activity, and the resultant increase in myocardial oxygen demand. Cardiotoxic effects may occur not only in patients with theophylline intoxication but also in patients whose levels are within the therapeutic range.[29]

In patients with serum theophylline concentrations greater than 30 μg/mL (about 150 μmol/L) followed with continuous electrocardiographic recordings, sinus tachycardia and complex atrial and ventricular ectopy are common, but sustained supraventricular and ventricular tachyrhythmias are uncommon.[30,31] Potentially life-threatening cardiac arrhythmias are rare. Ventricular tachycardia appears to be a rare complication of toxicity that tends to occur in the setting of advanced age, underlying heart disease, and/or very high serum theophylline concentrations due to oral or intravenous medication. In contrast to ventricular tachycardia, ventricular fibrillation and cardiac arrest typically follow intentional and self-poisoning with a single ingestion of a quantity of theophylline tablets sufficient to result in a serum theophylline concentration greater than 100 μg/mL (about 500 μmol/L) or it may follow the rapid central venous infusion of theophylline. These life-threatening arrhythmias often develop in young or middle-aged patients with no known underlying heart disease.[31]

Sustained-Release Overdose

Overdose with sustained-release theophylline preparations can lead to hypokalemia, hypomagnesemia, hypophosphatemia, hyperglycemia, metabolic acidosis, neutrophil leukocytosis, nausea, vomiting, sinus tachycardia, and seizures. Gastric emptying followed by activated charcoal reduces theophylline absorption from the gut, reduces the serum theophylline concentration and elimination half-life, and may result in a reduced hospital stay.[32] An acute myocardial infarction followed by severe heart failure occurred in a 26-year-old woman after ingestion of 25 tablets of controlled-release theophylline (270 mg theophylline tablets). Her serum theophylline concentration was 32 μg/mL. She recovered after aggressive therapy.[33]

Muscle Effects

Acute compartment syndrome rarely occurs in theophylline poisoning[34,35] and may follow the rhabdomyolysis that has been reported in theophylline poisoning. It also can follow repeated seizures, exacerbated by hypokalemia, hypotension, and limb compression. These complications can relate to the severity of theophylline intoxication. To reduce the likelihood of the development of rhabdomyolysis, Valc and colleagues prophylactically ventilate all patients who have repeated convulsions despite the use of intravenous diazepam and the correction of electrolyte and acid–base disturbances. If these measure fail, compartment pressure monitoring is indicated.

Hypersensitivity

Asthmatic patients may experience a delayed hypersensitivity reaction to the ethylenediamine component of theophylline (aminophylline). Cross-reactivity may occur with chemically related agents including ethanolamine antihistamines (diphenhydramine, carbinoxamine, clemastine), triethanolamine-containing creams (Aspercreme, Myoflex, Sportscreme), and the piperazine antihistamine hydroxyzine.[36]

Laboratory

Analytical Methods

High-performance liquid chromatography is the standard of measurement but requires a high capital expense. Initial studies suggest that a commercially available theophylline assay obtained by fingerstick is able to measure theophylline concentrations within the range 0.4 to 30 μg/mL. Multiple drug concentrations may be determined simultaneously with results in about 15 minutes. The method correlates well with high-performance liquid chromatography. Additional clinical studies should be performed to determine its clinical usefulness in theophylline intoxication.[37,38] Rapid tests for theophylline appear to be well suited to the emergency department setting and may be cost effective.

Serum Levels

Acute Versus Chronic Poisoning. Generally, after acute single ingestions, minimal toxicity occurs between peak theophylline levels of 20 and 40 μg/mL, moderate toxicity at 40 to 100 μg/mL, and severe toxicity at more than 100 μg/mL. A blood concentration of 5 to 10 mg/L provides a useful therapeutic level.[15]

Infants and Neonates. Seizures have been reported in neonates 7 to 8 hours after acute intoxication with concentrations of 51 and 54 μg/mL.[39] Older infants have developed seizures at concentrations in the range 40 to 50 μg/mL.[40]

Some individual variation appears, and the severity of intoxication should not be judged by laboratory values alone. Typically, chronic overmedication, which usually develops in the very young or the elderly, causes poisoning at lower serum theophylline levels than acute overdoses, which occur primarily in young adults. Seizures and serious dysrhythmias frequently appear in those chronic overmedication cases at theophylline levels between 40 and 70 μg/mL.[41,42] Patients under 40 years of age tend to develop serious dysrhythmias when theophylline levels exceed 50 μg/mL; older patients can display serious rhythm disturbances at levels above 35 μg/mL.[43] Clinical evidence of toxicity from theophylline in children is variable and cannot be used to screen those who should have their serum levels monitored.[44]

Sustained-Release Preparations. As toxicity depends in part on peak theophylline levels, the increasing use of sustained-release preparations complicates the initial evaluation of overdosed patients. Peak levels after the ingestion of sustained-release preparations occur within 1 to 24 hours (mean, 11 hours); regular formulations produce peak levels 2 to 8 hours (mean, 5 hours) postingestion.[41] Bezoar formation can produce secondary peaks in theophylline levels.[45] Two serial theophylline levels 3 to 4 hours apart should be drawn in all significant ingestions to confirm elimination. Peak serum theophylline levels cannot predict which elderly patients with chronic theophylline intoxication will have a life-threatening effect.[46]

Serum Theophylline Predictors. Shannon and colleagues, in a retrospective and prospective study, found that serum potassium [K] and glucose [Glu] concentrations correlated with admission serum theophylline levels and appeared to correlate with increased plasma catecholamine activity.[15] The following formula is used to predict actual serum theophylline levels as less than 60 μg/mL, 61 to 80 μg/mL, or more than 80 μg/mL: theophylline level = 14.9 + 0.3215[Glu] − 44.95[K]. This may be useful in anticipating management of patients with acute theophylline intoxication when measurement of theophylline concentration is delayed. The feasibility of use of this formula in a busy emergency center remains to be seen.[47] A nomogram using the formula may ultimately enhance the ease of use.

Abnormalities

An increased-anion-gap metabolic acidosis is often observed following theophylline overdose. Serum lactate levels can be elevated. Early hemoperfusion can reverse the acidosis, the elevated serum theophylline level, and the hyperadrenergic state.[48] Hypermagnesemia may follow treatment of theophylline intoxication with multiple-dose oral activated charcoal with magnesium-containing cathartics.[49] Similarly, multiple-dose oral activated charcoal and sorbitol may lead to hypernatremia and dehydration in the theophylline-intoxicated patient.[50] In both instances, patients must be closely monitored for the possible development of fluid and electrolyte abnormalities.[51]

Predictors of Major Toxicity

Shannon and co-workers conducted a prospective study of theophylline intoxication (defined as a peak serum theophylline concentration of 167 μmol/L [30 mg/L] or greater) over a 5-year period and concluded that (1) the risk for major toxicity is influenced by the method of intoxication; (2) patients with chronic theophylline intoxication have a greater risk for major toxicity (seizures or cardiac arrhythmias associated with hemodynamic instability) at lower serum theophylline concentrations than those with acute intoxication; (3) the risk for major toxicity in cases of acute theophylline intoxication is best predicted by peak serum theophylline concentration; (4) the risk for major toxicity in cases of chronic overmedication cannot be predicted by the peak serum theophylline concentration; (5) age provides the best prediction of major toxicity in cases of chronic theophylline overmedication. Age greater than 60 years has the greatest diagnostic accuracy in identifying patients at highest risk, but age does not provide the same degree of prognostic accuracy in cases of chronic overmedication as the peak serum theophylline concentration does in cases of acute intoxication.[22]

Treatment

Stabilization

Henderson and colleagues identified 38 patients with acute theophylline poisoning, 35 of whom had taken a sustained-release preparation. The vomiting in 17 patients was controlled by intravenous metoclopramide (10 mg), but the remaining patients required mechanical ventilation with sedation and muscle relaxation for effective delivery of nasogastric charcoal. In 9 patients, the serum theophylline concentration continued to rise despite enteral charcoal. Charcoal hemoperfusion was used in 7 patients. Figure 45–6 is an algorithm including gastrointestinal decontamination with tracheal protection of all patients, particularly those with intractable vomiting.[41,52] Hemoperfusion has been used in patients with life-threatening complications (seizures, arrhythmias) or with serum theophylline concentrations greater than 550 μmol/L (100 mg/L). Parr and colleagues emphasize that charcoal hemoperfusion should be reserved for patients when vigorous supportive measures fail to control toxicity.[32]

Day and colleagues use aggressive potassium replacement aimed to achieve a serum potassium concentration greater than 5 mmol/L,[53] whereas Henderson et al. use cautious potassium supplementation if the initial serum potassium concentration is less than 3 mmol/L.[52] Serum electrolytes are monitored every 4 hours.[52] These criteria follow experience with one series of 38 patients[52] and another series of 64 patients.[41] Care must be exercised to avoid hyperkalemia (> 5 mmol/L) within the first 24 hours of admission.

Cardiac Problems. Propranolol and verapamil have been successfully administered to theophylline-poisoned patients with supraventricular tachycardia and multifocal

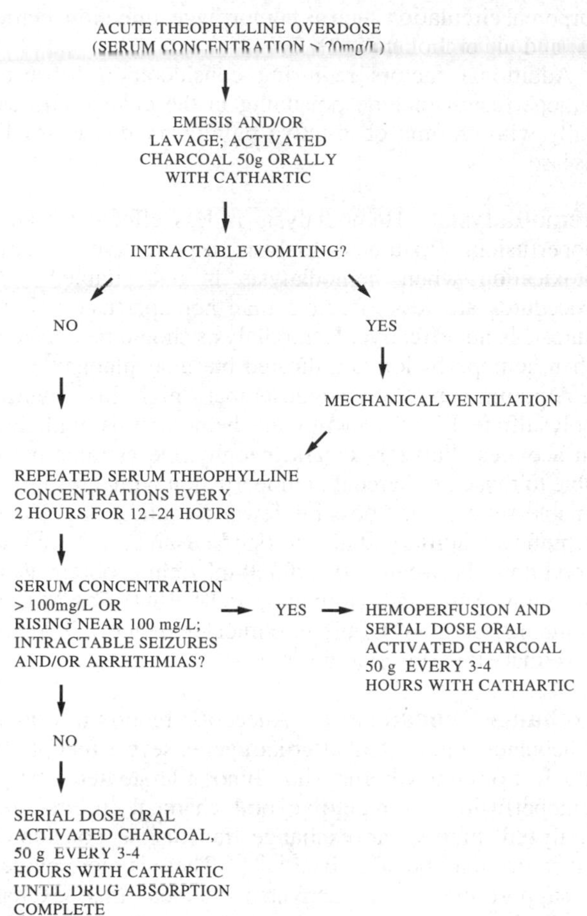

Figure 45-6 Algorithm for the treatment of acute theophylline overdose, modified from that of Olson et al.[41] to include gastrointestinal decontamination for all patients, particularly those with intractable vomiting. (From Henderson A, Wright DM, Pond SM. Management of theophylline overdose patients in the intensive care unit. Anaesth Intens Care 1992;20:56–62.)

atrial tachycardia, respectively.[4] Hypotension may be refractory to fluids and vasopressors such as dopamine, which has primarily beta-adrenergic specificity at lower doses. Hence, vasopressors with strong alpha-adrenergic properties, such as levarterenol, may be needed. Propranolol may block the vasodilator properties of theophylline and, particularly, may improve diastolic hypotension.[54] Although some authors have not encountered bronchospasm with the use of propranolol in the acute toxicity setting,[54,55] the administration of propranolol to poisoned asthmatics requires careful evaluation of risks and benefits.

An anecdotal report suggests that esmolol with its relative cardioselectivity and short duration of activity may be useful to reduce tachycardia and hypotension in a patient with theophylline intoxication. Limited data are available regarding the safety and efficacy of esmolol for this use.[56]

Seizures. Convulsions are a hallmark of serious toxicity and may not respond to the usual treatment measures (diazepam, phenytoin). General anesthesia (eg, with thiopental) should be considered when continuous seizures last more than 1 hour in adults or 0.5 hour in children. Consider the early use of hemoperfusion, especially if serum theophylline levels are expected to rise into the serious toxicity range. Theophylline administration should be stopped immediately, and the theophylline concentration should be decreased as soon as possible.

Gut Decontamination

Emesis should be induced in all patients suspected of ingesting more than 10 mg/kg of theophylline compounds, unless contraindicated by coma, seizures, or an absent gag reflex. Activated charcoal binds theophylline and should be administered in doses of 1 g/kg.

Vomiting in acute sustained-release theophylline toxicity may be protracted. This can limit the use of activated charcoal in patients with severe acute theophylline poisoning.[57] Activated charcoal has been used in infants as young as 1 week.[58] An anecdotal report describes a single total dose of 0.6 g/kg (1 g) aqueous activated charcoal not containing sorbitol which was employed to treat theophylline toxicity in a premature infant on the second day of life. This was diluted with sterile water 1:1, which was followed by sterile water every 6 hours via a nasogastric tube to facilitate passage of charcoal stool.[58] This led to a decrease in the half-life theophylline concentration with clinical improvement.[58]

Elimination Enhancement

Serial Activated Charcoal. Activated charcoal should be continued to bind the drug subjected to an enterohepatic recirculation as well as the drug still in the gut and should continue throughout the course of toxicity when hemoperfusion is initiated.

The Boston group recommend that enhancement of drug elimination in patients with acute theophylline intoxication and a peak serum theophylline level less than 555 μmol/L (100 mg/L) be restricted to the administration of multiple-dose activated charcoal.[22] In patients with a peak serum theophylline concentration of 555 μmol/L or greater or with a serum theophylline concentration less than 555 μmol/L (100 mg/L) and intractable vomiting, hemoperfusion (or hemodialysis) should be performed immediately. Antiemetic therapy should be used to ensure the successful administration of activated charcoal. Patients with chronic theophylline intoxication should initially receive multiple-dose activated charcoal not containing sorbitol. Hemoperfusion should be done in all patients over age 60 who have a peak serum theophylline concentration of 167 μmol/L (30 mg/L) or greater. There are risks with hemoperfusion at the extremes of age (the elderly and neonates).

Sustained-Release Overdose. Oral activated charcoal may be considered to be the treatment of choice in acute theophylline overdose with sustained-release theophylline tablets and in infants, although even this therapy might not be feasible in neonates with absent bowel sounds or potential risk factors for necrotizing enterocolitis.[22] In about 25% of patients who have taken overdoses of sustained-release theophylline, a further rise in serum theophylline concentration may occur despite conventional therapy with gastric lavage followed by the administration of activated charcoal. one dose of activated charcoal (50 mg in 150 mL of 70% sorbitol), may be followed by a second dose of charcoal not containing sorbital 4 hours after the first. If vomiting is resistant to an antiemetic and the delivery of activated charcoal by nasogastric tube, the patient is paralyzed and ventilated before further charcoal is administered. Serum theophylline levels, measured at two-hourly intervals for the first 12 to 24 hours, are used as a guide to further therapy.[59]

Hemoperfusion. Hemoperfusion effectively enhances theophylline clearance (1.88–5.84 mL/kg/min)[43] and, on the basis of case studies, is the elimination procedure of choice[19] when indicated.

Indications for hemoperfusion include intractable seizures with a duration longer than 30 minutes, persistent hypotension unresponsive to fluids and vasopressors, uncontrollable dysrhythmias, chronic overmedication with serum theophylline levels greater than 60 µg/mL, and single acute ingestions with theophylline levels exceeding 100 µg/mL.[60] With chronic theophylline intoxication, hemoperfusion has been recommended if (1) otherwise healthy patients have a peak serum theophylline intoxication exceeding 333 µmol/L (66 µg/mL), (2) patients with cardiac or hepatic disease have peak serum concentrations greater than 222 µmol/L (44 µg/mL), or (3) peak serum theophylline concentration is greater than 110 µmol/L (22 µg/mL) and the patient has active seizures or arrhythmias.[61]

The early use of hemoperfusion is necessary if serum theophylline levels in the moderately toxic range are rising quickly after the ingestion of sustained-release preparations. Shannon and colleagues studied cases of acute, chronic, and acute-on-therapeutic theophylline poisoning in which the mean peak serum concentration was 110 µg/mL (555 µmol/L) and observed that extracorporeal drug removal (hemoperfusion/hemodialysis) performed prior to the onset of major toxic effects (seizures/arrhythmia) may alter the clinical course of the intoxication.[62]

Charcoal hemoperfusion probably is more effective than resin hemoperfusion[63]; however, it is not universally available, it has not been shown to reduce morbidity or mortality in late severe toxicity, and its prophylactic role before severe manifestations is yet to be assessed. Hemoperfusion is not without morbidity.[32] Endpoints of hemoperfusion are serum theophylline levels below 60 µg/mL in acute overdose and 40 µg/mL in chronic overmedication *plus* the resolution of serious symptoms (seizures, dysrhythmias, hypotension).

The Massachusetts Poison Control System protocol for hemoperfusion includes a serum theophylline concentration greater than 444 µmol/L (80 mg/L) in cases of acute intoxication; a serum theophylline concentration greater than 222 to 278 µmol/L (40–50 mg/L) in cases of chronic intoxication; and intractable seizures or cardiac arrhythmias, regardless of serum theophylline concentration. All interventions continue until the serum theophylline concentration decreases to below 100 µmol/L (20 mg/L).[22] The exact role of hemoperfusion after theophylline poisoning remains to be determined by a randomized clinical trial. The patient should be observed for hypotension, hypocalcemia, platelet consumption, and a bleeding diathesis. The data do not support the prophylactic use of these procedures solely because the theophylline level is high. They favor a more conservative approach using oral charcoal therapy in all patients with high serum theophylline levels. Hemoperfusion or hemodialysis could be reserved for those patients who are unable to tolerate oral medication or who manifest serious toxic effects (seizures, major arrhythmias).

Charcoal hemoperfusion may cause thrombocytopenia, hypoglycemia, and complications associated with the extracorporeal circulation such as hemorrhage, infection, hemolysis, and air embolism.[64,65]

Additional factors requiring consideration for use of hemoperfusion include poisoning in the elderly and especially with chronic obstructive pulmonary disease or liver disease.

Hemodialysis. Hemodialysis is less effective than hemoperfusion. Peritoneal dialysis is effective in severe intoxication when hemodialysis is unavailable.[66] Both procedures are less effective than hemoperfusion. Forced diuresis is not effective. Hemodialysis should be considered when hemoperfusion is indicated but unavailable.[67]

A preliminary study suggests that "high-flux" synthetic (polysulfone PS600) membrane hemodialysis with large-surface-area dialyzers clears theophylline at rates comparable to those of charcoal hemoperfusion with a faster setup time, lesser cost, and possibly fewer complications. The P80 Hemoflow capillary dialyzer (surface area, 1.8 m^2) with blood flows between 250 and 300 mL/min is obtained from Fresonius AG (Bad Homburg, POB 1800 D-6380, Bad Homburg, Germany). Further clinical experience is required to validate this observation.[68]

Exchange Transfusion. Anecdotal reports in critically ill neonates suggest that after iatrogenic severe theophylline intoxication in newborns who cannot tolerate hemodialysis, hemoperfusion, or repetitive oral charcoal (premature or paralyzed infants), an exchange transfusion, considered a last resort, may be effective.[58,69–71] There is more evidence to support the use of activated charcoal than exchange transfusion for the treatment of theophylline toxicity in premature infants.[58]

Neonates. Iatrogenic overdose due to inadvertent administration of theophylline or miscalculation of dose in the neonatal period has followed its use in the treatment of apnea of the newborn. Toxic effects include tachycardia, jitteriness, clonic posturing, emesis, diarrhea, generalized seizures, and intracranial hemorrhage. Toxicity is enhanced by the delayed elimination of theophylline in the premature infant presumably due to immaturity of the mixed-function overdose system. This results in a half-life that can be nine times that and a clearance one-seventh that of children 1 to 4 years old. Hemodialysis and hemoperfusion may not be effective options due to hemodynamic instability, small size, and a concern about anticoagulation. Multiple-dose activated charcoal in the neonate may possibly increase the risk for necrotizing enterocolitis and may be impeded by vomiting or ileus. A simple volume exchange transfusion described in one anecdotal study resulted in a 19% decrease in plasma theophylline and removal of 13.5% of the whole-body theophylline. Multiple volume exchanges could further reduce the body burden, but no controlled clinical experiences have been published to support this.[72] The procedure has also been used effectively in a young child (1½ years old) who received an overdose of theophylline.[73]

Whole-Bowel Irrigation. Whole-bowel irrigation has been used successfully in patients who have ingested both sustained-release[74] and conventional preparations.[75] It may be useful in patients with rapidly increasing serum theophylline concentrations that persist even after multiple doses of activated charcoal or extracorporeal removal. It can be used in combination with activated charcoal (eg, 50 g of activated charcoal added to each liter of polyethylene glycol solution). Current recommendations are for administration of nonabsorbable isosmolar fluid containing polyethylene glycol by way of a nasogastric tube at a rate of 1-2 L/m 2 L/h in adults and 500 mL/h in children until the rectal effluent is clear and the abdominal x-ray is clear of sustained release on and radiopaque tablets. The mean time for this to be achieved is usually about 4 hours.[75] There is, however, no clinical evidence that whole-bowel irrigation provides additional benefit over activated charcoal alone in sustained-release theophylline poisoning.[76,77] There is also the possibility that the lavage solution used with whole-bowel irrigation may displace theophylline from activated charcoal, which may be used simultaneously.[78,79]

Antidote

No medication antagonizes all the adverse effects of a theophylline overdose. Adenosine is experimental.[80] There is no clinical evidence to support the use of pyridoxine for theophylline-induced seizures.[81]

Supportive Measures

1. Supportive care is an important part of treatment, as recovery has occurred following single acute ingestions with serum theophylline levels as high as 204 μg/mL.[82]
2. Monitor cardiac rhythm.
3. Only mild repletion of extracellular potassium is necessary (5–10 mEq KC1 per hour).
4. Monitor serum magnesium, phosphate, calcium, and potassium levels, acid–base balance, and blood theophylline levels in moderate-to-severe theophylline intoxication, at least until peak theophylline levels are confirmed.
5. Monitor urine myoglobin and serum creatinine and creatine kinase levels to detect evidence of rhabdomyolysis.
6. Persistent vomiting after a theophylline overdose may preclude the ability to administer activated charcoal. A slow infusion of ondansetron, 8 mg in 100 mL of normal saline, controlled vomiting in a 14-year-old.[83] A further report has confirmed its usefulness (8 mg intravenously over a 20-minute period) in three patients.[84] Metoclopramide ranitidine and ondansetron may be useful.
7. Dantrolene 1 mg/kg over 20 minutes and then 2 mg/kg/h for 4 hours appeared useful for one patient with severe theophylline poisoning with hyperthermia and rhabdomyolysis. Further study of dantrolene in theophylline poisoning seems justified.[85]
8. Beta-adrenergic blockade (propranolol, esmolol) may be of benefit in the management of theophylline overdose, especially in the nonasthmatic patient and also, possibly, in the asthmatic patient with severe hypokalemia or cardiac arrhythmias. If the situation is life-threatening and mechanical ventilation is available, the potential risk of bronchospasm may be justified. Nevertheless, treatment with a nonselective beta-blocking agent is potentially hazardous in asthmatic patients.[86] A preliminary anecdotal report suggests that esmolol, a relatively cardioselective β_1 blocker, provided prompt resolution of theophylline-induced tachycardia and hypotension.[56,87,88] The initial dosage of intravenous esmolol administered was a 500 μg/kg bolus over 1 minute, followed by a 50 μg/kg/min continuous infusion.[56] Prolonged hypotension following theophylline overdose may require higher than conventionally recommended doses of vasopressors to prevent the development of serious sequelae.[89] Both supraventricular and ventricular arrhythmias may produce hemodynamic compromise. Ventricular arrhythmias should be controlled using cardiac life support protocols.
9. Diazepam and phenobarbital are the drugs of choice for treatment of theophylline-induced seizures.[26] Suction and secure the airway. Set up an intravenous drip.

Duration of Seizure	Treatment
0 minutes	Diazepam 5–10 mg intravenously or lorazepam; may be repeated once after 10 minutes
15 minutes	Phenobarbital 10 mg/kg IV intravenously
45 minutes	Thiopental anesthesia; paralysis may be required.

10. Where available, arrange transfer to a hospital with facilities for hemoperfusion.[90]
11. Treatment of rhabdomyolysis and myoglobinuria requires hydration and maintenance of a high urine output.

Admission Criteria

Serum theophylline concentrations should be drawn and repeated hourly while they are increasing. Dawson and colleagues in Australia have suggested as criteria for admission to an intensive care unit the presence of one or more of the following[86]:

- Moderate or severe clinical toxicity
- Theophylline concentration greater than 50 mg/L (275 μmol/L) in acute poisoning
- Theophylline concentration greater than 40 mg/L (220 μmol/L) in chronic overmedication
- Theophylline concentration greater than 40 mg/L (220 μmol/L) in patients less than 6 months of age or more than 60 years of age
- Theophylline concentration greater than 40 mg/L (220 μmol/L) in patients with chronic illness

REFERENCES—THEOPHYLLINE

1. Stark CM, Howland MA, Goldfrank LR. Concepts and controversies of bronchodilator overdose. Emerg Med Clin North Am 1994;12:415–436.
2. Baker MD. Theophylline toxicity in children. J Pediatr 1986; 109:538–542.
3. Skopnik H, Bertl U, Heimann G. Neonatal theophylline intoxication: Pharmacokinetics and clinical evaluation. Eur J Pediatr 1992;151:221–224.
4. Jenne JW, Nagasawa HT, Thompson RD. Relationship of urinary metabolites of theophylline to serum theophylline levels. Clin Pharmacol Ther 1976;19:375–381.
5. Fuhr U, Woodcock BG, Siewert M. Verapamil and drug metabolism by the cytochrome P450 isoform CYPIA2. Eur J Clin Pharmacol 1992;42:463–464.

6. Greenburg A, Piraino BH, Kroboth PD, et al. Severe theophylline toxicity: Role of conservative measures, antiarrhythmic agents and charcoal hemoperfusion. Am J Med 1984; 76:854–860.
7. Bory C, Baltassat P, Porthault M, et al. Metabolism of theophylline to caffeine in premature newborn infants. J Pediatr 1979;94:988–993.
8. Upton RA. Pharmacokinetic interactions between theophylline and other medications (Part I). Clin Pharmacokinetics 1991;20:66–80.
9. Skinner NH. Adverse reactions and interactions with theophylline. Drug Saf 1990;5:275–285.
10. Dal Negro R, Pomari C, Turco P. Famotidine and theophylline pharmacokinetics: An unexpected cimetidine-like interaction in patients with chronic obstructive pulmonary disease. Clin Pharmacokinet 1993;24:255–258.
11. Neff RK, Leviton A. Maternal theophylline consumption and the risk of stillbirth. Chest 1990;97:1266–1267.
12. Park JM, Schmer V, Myers TL. Cardiovascular anomalies associated with prenatal exposure to theophylline. South Med J 1990;83:1487–1488.
13. Stec GP, Greenberger P, Ruo TI, et al. Kinetics of theophylline transfer to breast milk. Clin Pharmacol Ther 1980;28: 404–408.
14. Frederiksen MC, Ruo TI, Chow MJ, et al. Theophylline pharmacokinetics in pregnancy. Clin Pharmacol Ther 1986;40: 321–328.
15. Banner AS. Theophylline: Should we discard an old friend? Lancet 1993;343:618.
16. Shannon M. Hypokalemia, hyperglycemia and plasma catecholamine activity after severe theophylline intoxication. Clin Toxicol 1994;32:41–47.
17. Shannon M, Lovejoy FH Jr. Hypokalemia after theophylline intoxication: The effects of acute vs chronic poisoning. Arch Intern Med 1989;149:2725–2729.
18. Sawyer WT, Caravati EM, Ellison MJ, et al. Hypokalemia, hyperglycemia and acidosis after intentional theophylline overdose. Am J Emerg Med 1985;3:408–411.
19. Park GD, Spector R, Roberts RJ, et al. Use of hemoperfusion for treatment of theophylline intoxication. Am J Med 1983;74:961–966.
20. McPherson ML, Prince SR, Atamer ER, et al. Theophylline-induced hypercalcemia. Ann Intern Med 1986;105: 52–54.
21. Shannon M. Predictors of major toxicity after theophylline overdose. Ann Intern Med 1993;119:1161–1167.
22. Shannon M, Lovejoy FH Jr. Effect of acute versus chronic intoxication on clinical features of theophylline poisoning in children. J Pediatr 1992;121:125–130.
23. Shannon MW, Lovejoy FH, Woolf A. Acute complications and predictions of major toxicity after theophylline overdose. Vet Hum Toxicol 1992;34:328.
24. Modi KB, Horn EH, Bryson SM. Theophylline poisoning and rhabdomyolysis. Lancet 1985;2:160–161.
25. MacDonald JB, Jones HM, Cowan RA. Rhabdomyolysis and acute renal failure after theophylline overdose. Lancet 1985;1:932–933.
26. McGuigan MA. AACT Clin Toxicol Update 1989;2(2):3.
27. Bahls FH, Mak K, Bird TD. Theophylline-associated seizures with "therapeutic" or low toxic serum concentrations: Risk factors for serious outcome in adults. Neurology 1991; 41:1309–1312.
28. Baker MD. Theophylline toxicity in children. J Pediatr 1986; 109:538–542.
29. Shannon M. Therapeutic theophylline levels and adverse cardiac events. Ann Intern Med 1994;120:891.
30. Levine JH, Michael JR, Guarnieri T. Multifocal atrial tachycardia: A toxic effect of theophylline. Lancet 1985;1: 12–14.
31. Sessler CN, Cohen MD. Cardiac arrhythmias during theophylline toxicity: A prospective continuous electrocardiographic study. Chest 1990;98:672–678.
32. Parr MJ, Anaes FC, Day AC, et al. Theophylline poisoning: A review of 64 cases. Intens Care Med 1990;16:394–398.
33. Hantson P, Gautier P, Vekemans MC, et al. Acute myocardial infarction in a young woman: Possible relationship with sustained-release theophylline acute overdose. Intens Care Med 1992;18:496.
34. Lloyd DM, Payne SPK, Tomson CRV, et al. Acute compartment syndrome secondary to theophylline overdose. Lancet 1990;2:312.
35. Ryan MF, Vale JA. Acute compartment syndrome secondary to theophylline poisoning. Lancet 1990;2:882.
36. Terzian CG, Simon PA. Aminophylline hypersensitivity apparently due to ethylenediamine. Ann Emerg Med 1992;21: 312–317.
37. Poklis A, Saady JJ, Edinboro LE. Evaluation of the Abbott Vision Analyzer[R] for determination of theophylline and implementation of a program for on-site emergency room testing. Clin Chem 1990;36:1040.
38. Jones LA, Gonzalez ER, Venitz J, et al. Evaluation of the Vision[R] theophylline assays in the emergency department setting. Ann Emerg Med 1992;21:777–781.
39. Gal P, Roop C, Robinson H, Erkan NV. Theophylline-induced seizures in accidentally overdosed neonates. Pediatrics 1980;65:547–549.
40. Augenstein WL, Kulig KW, Riggs BS. Theophylline toxicity in infants treated for bronchiolitis or asthma. In: *Proceedings, AACT/AAPCC/ABMT/CAPCC Annual Scientific Meeting, Vancouver, 1987:* Abstract 68.
41. Olson KR, Benowitz NL, Woo OF, Pond SM. Theophylline overdose: Acute single ingestion versus chronic repeated overmedication. Am J Emerg Med 1985;3:386–394.
42. Zwililich CW, Sutton FD Jr, Neff TA, et al. Theophylline induced seizures in adults: Correlation with serum concentration. Ann Intern Med 1975;82:784–787.
43. Gaudreault P, Guay J. Theophylline poisoning: Pharmacological considerations and clinical management. Med Toxicol 1986;1:169–191.
44. Powell EC, Reynolds SL, Rubenstein JS. Theophylline toxicity in children: A retrospective review. Pediatr Emerg Care 1993;9:129–133.
45. Coupe M. Self-poisoning with sustained-release aminophylline: A mechanism for observed secondary rise in serum theophylline. Hum Toxicol 1986;5:341–342.
46. Shannon M, Lovejoy FH Jr. The influence of age vs peak serum concentration on life-threatening events after chronic theophylline intoxication. Arch Intern Med 1990;150: 2045–2048.
47. Shannon AW, Lovejoy FH Jr, Woolf A. Prediction of serum theophylline concentration after acute theophylline intoxication. Ann Emerg Med 1990;19:627.
48. Leventhal LJ, Kochan G, Feldman NH, et al. Lactic acidosis in theophylline overdose. Am J Emerg Med 1989;7:417–418.
49. Weber CA, Santiago RM. Hypermagnesemia: A potential complication during treatment of theophylline intoxication with oral activated charcoal and magnesium-containing cathartics. Chest 1989;95:56–59.
50. Gazda-Smith E, Synhavsky A. Hypernatremia following treatment of theophylline toxicity with activated charcoal and sorbitol. Arch Intern Med 1990;150:689–690.
51. Garrelts JG, Watson WA, Holloway KD, Sweet DE. Magnesium toxicity secondary to catharsis during management of theophylline poisoning. Am J Emerg Med 1989;7:34–37.
52. Henderson A, Wright DM, Pond SM. Management of theophylline overdose patients in the intensive care unit. Anaesth Intens Care 1992;20:56–62.
53. Day C, Crone D, Rankin N. Theophylline poisoning. Anaesth Intens Care 1992;20:531–532.
54. Biberstein MP, Ziegler MG, Ward DM. Use of beta-blockade and hemoperfusion for acute theophylline poisoning. West J Med 1984;141:485–490.
55. Renton KW, Gray JD, Hall RI. Decreased elimination of theophylline after influenza vaccination. Can Med Assoc J 1980; 123:288–290.
56. Seneff M, Scott J, Friedman B, Smith M. Acute theophylline toxicity and the use of esmolol to reverse cardiovascular irritability. Ann Emerg Med 1990;19:671–673.
57. Amitai Y, Lovejoy FH Jr. Characteristics of vomiting associated with acute release theophylline poisoning: Implications for management with oral activated charcoal. Clin Toxicol 1987;27:539–554.

58. Jain R, Tholl DA. Activated charcoal for theophylline toxicity in a premature infant on the second day of life. Dev Pharmacol Ther 1992;19:106–110.
59. Henderson A, Salin P, Pond SM. Rapid rise in serum theophylline concentration after overdose with sustained release theophylline. Med J Aust 1992;157:354–355.
60. Woo OF, Pond SM, Benowitz NL, et al. Benefit of hemoperfusion in acute theophylline intoxication. Clin Toxicol 1984;22:411–424.
61. Shannon M, Amitai Y, Lovejoy FH Jr. Multiple dose activated charcoal for theophylline poisoning in young infants. Pediatrics 1987;80:368–370.
62. Shannon MW, Woolf A. Does extracorporeal removal alter the course of major toxicity after theophylline intoxication? Vet Hum Toxicol 1992;34:320.
63. Jefferys DB, Raper SM, Helliwell M, et al. Haemoperfusion for theophylline overdose. Br Med J 1980;280:1167.
64. Laussen P, Shann F, Butt W, Tibballs J: Use of plasmapheresis in acute theophylline toxicity. Crit Care Med 1991;19: 288–290.
65. Bania TC, Hoffmann RS, Howland MA, Goldfrank LR. Plasmapheresis for theophylline intoxication. Vet Hum Toxicol 1992;34:330.
66. Miceli JN, Clay B, Fleischmann LE, et al. Pharmacokinetics of severe theophylline intoxication managed by peritoneal dialysis. Dev Pharmacol Ther 1980;1:16–25.
67. Cooling OS. Theophylline toxicity. J Emerg Med 1993;11: 415–425.
68. Agnone F, Gorkin D, Curry S. 'High flux' hemodialysis for theophylline intoxication. Vet Hum Toxicol 1993; 35:336.
69. Shannon MW, Wernovsky G, Morris C. Exchange transfusion in the treatment of severe theophylline intoxication. Vet Hum Toxicol 1991;33:354.
70. Shannon M, Wernovsky G, Morris C. Exchange transfusion in the treatment of severe theophylline poisoning. Pediatrics 1992;89:145–147.
71. Henry GC, Wax PM, Howland MA, et al. Exchange transfusion for the treatment of a theophylline overdose in a premature neonate. Vet Hum Toxicol 1991;33:356.
72. Osborn HN, Henry G, Wax P, et al. Theophylline toxicity in a premature neonate: Elimination kinetics of exchange transfusion. Clin Toxicol 1993;31:639–644.
73. Barazarte V, Rodriguez Z, Caballos S, et al. Exchange transfusion in a case of severe theophylline poisoning. Vet Hum Toxicol 1992;34:526.
74. Laggner AN, Kaik G, Lenz K, et al. Treatment of severe poisoning with slow release theophylline. Br Med J 1985;288: 1497.
75. Tenenbein M, Cohen S, Sitar DS. Whole bowel irrigation as a decontamination procedure after acute drug overdose. Arch Intern Med 1987;147:905–907.
76. Burkhart KK, Wuerz RC, Donovan JW. Whole bowel irrigation as adjunctive treatment for sustained-release theophylline poisoning. Vet Hum Toxicol 1991;33:353.
77. Burkhart KK, Wuerz RC, Donovan JW. Whole bowel irrigation as adjunctive treatment for sustained-release theophylline overdose. Ann Emerg Med 1992;21:1316–1320.
78. Hoffman RS, Chiang WR, Howland MA, et al. Drug desorption from activated charcoal caused by whole bowel irrigating solution. Vet Hum Toxicol 1989;31:336.
79. Hoffman RS, Chiang WH, Howland MA, et al. Theophylline desorption from activated charcoal caused by whole bowel irrigation solution. Clin Toxicol 1991;29:191–201.
80. Henry JA, Minton NA. Adenosine as a theophylline antidote? In: *Proceedings, Meeting of European Association of Poison Centres and Clinical Toxicologists, Lyon, France, May 22, 1991.*
81. Glenn GM, Krober MS, Kelly P, et al. Pyridoxine as therapy in theophylline-induced seizures. Vet Hum Toxicol 1995;37: 342–343.
82. Dean LS, Brown JW. Massive theophylline overdose: Survival without hemoperfusion. JAMA 1982;248:1742.
83. Brown SGA, Prentice DA. Ondansetron in the treatment of theophylline overdose. Med J Aust 1992;156:512.
84. Roberts JR, Carney S, Boyle SM, Lee DC. Ondansetron quells drug-resistant emesis in theophylline poisoning. Am J Emerg Med 1993;11:609–610.
85. Parr MJA, Willatts SM. Fatal theophylline poisoning with rhabdomyolysis: A potential role for dantrolene treatment. Anaesthesia 1991;46:557–559.
86. Amin DN, Henry JA. Propranolol administration in theophylline overdose. Lancet 1985;1:520–521.
87. Dawson AH, Whyte IM. The assessment and treatment of theophylline poisoning. Med J Aust 1989;151:689–693.
88. Britt A, Burkhart KK. Theophylline toxicity. Top Emerg Med 1992;15:72–77.
89. Detleff RW, Touchette MA, Zarowltz BJ. Vasopressor-resistant hypotension following a massive ingestion of theophylline. Ann Pharmacother 1993;27:781–784.
90. McGuigan MA, Tenenbein M, Goldman B. Planning an effective strategy for theophylline poisoning in adults. Emerg Med Rep 1987;8(6):41–48.

THE PIPERAZINES: ZIPEPROL HYDROCHLORIDE

From 1975 to 1982, 199 cases of accidental or intentional acute poisoning with zipeprol, eprazinone, and eprazinol (related drugs) were collected by the Poison Control Centre of Paris. In 7 cases seizures were observed that resolved rapidly and without recurrence after symptomatic treatment. The piperazine nucleus is common to all three drugs and may be a factor in the seizure production.[1]

The piperazine nucleus can be found in H_1-histamine antagonists (hydroxyzine, cyclizine, meclizine), nonopiate antitussive agents (zipeprol, eprazinone, eprazinol), antidepressants (trazodone), and antipsychotic drugs (fluphenazine, perphenazine, trifluoperazine, thiothixene).[3]

Zipeprol (Fig. 45–7) is a synthetic enterally absorbed piperazine derivative without structural similarities to known drugs of addiction.[2] The piperazine group of drugs should be considered a possible cause of transient encephalopathy and nonepileptic seizures in previously healthy individuals.[3] Piperazine-derived antihistamines and antipsychotic medications can either lower the seizure threshold in epileptic patients or precipitate de novo seizures.[3] Because of its molecular structure, zipeprol is a mild antihistamine and shows anticholinergic effects.[4] Fatalities are relatively infrequent. In Italy zipeprol has been documented as a drug of abuse, frequently among individuals addicted to opiates.[5,6] Treatment of overdose is symptomatic and supportive.

Zipeprol is not legally available in the United States but is available in Europe.

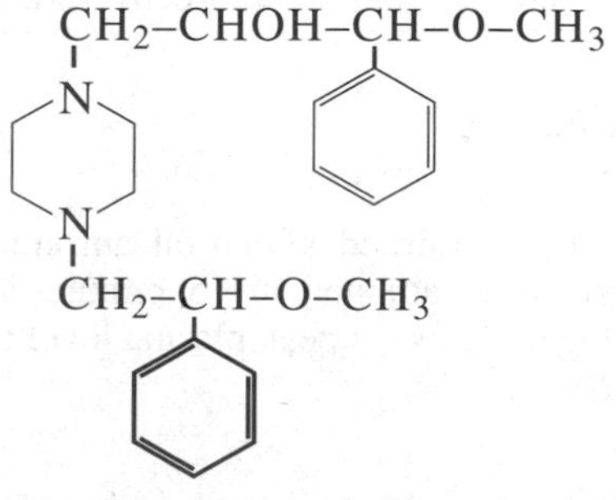

$CH_2–CHOH–CH–O–CH_3$

N

N

$CH_2–CH–O–CH_3$

Figure 45–7 Structure of zipeprol. (From Jouglard J. Zipeprol abuse: An opportunity for assessment of its neurotoxicity. Eur Assoc Pois Control Centres Toxicol Newslett 1991:5–13. Oslo, Norway.)

Use

Piperazines in different forms (hexahydrate, phosphate, tartrate, and adipate) are widely used in Germany for the treatment of ascarides and threadworms.[7] Zipeprol hydrochloride is a cough suppressant that may have a peripheral action on bronchial spasm[6] where it may have bronchospasmolytic and mucolytic activity. Zipeprol has been used for heroin withdrawal.[1]

Product Formulation

Zipeprol is commercially available in Italy as 75-mg coated tablets, 9.3 and 0.5% syrups, and 50- and 150-mg suppositories.

Therapeutic Dose

Doses of 150 to 300 mg may be given daily by mouth in divided doses.[4] In children under 14 years of age the recommended daily dose is 3 to 5 mg/kg.[4]

Toxic Dose

Toxic doses of 800 mg (adults) and 10 to 20 mg/kg (children) have been reported by French Poison Centres. Convulsant doses are 1.50 g (adults) and more than 25 mg/kg (children). Somnolence, narrow fixed pupils, cyanosis, bradycardia, depressed respiration, and flaccid paralysis of the legs were reported after doses of 11.6 g. All symptoms cleared in 1 to 2 days.[7]

Abuse

Zipeprol has been abused by drug addicts. The dose taken for recreational purpose has varied from 11 to 28 mg/kg.[5] The psychotoxic syndrome manifests itself after oral ingestion of doses not less than 300 mg. Some abusers take zipeprol rectally using even higher doses (up to 2250 mg or more).[4] Doses of 27, 154, and 1.2 mg/kg daily in young children have been associated with restlessness, seizures, and abnormalities of posture and gait.

Fatal Dose

A 17-year-old woman ingested 975 mg of zipeprol and experienced a confusional state and seizures; she recovered.[6] A 17-year-old man ingested 750 mg of zipeprol, developed seizures and cerebral edema, and recovered.[6]

Toxiconkinetics

Absorption

Zipeprol is well absorbed after oral administration. Peak plasma levels were attained in 15 minutes.[8] Following a single 175-mg oral dose, a peak plasma level of 0.75 μg/mL was reached.[8]

Distribution

Zipeprol freely passes the blood–brain barrier.[5]

Elimination

Excretion of unchanged drug and its metabolites peaks about 1 hour after ingestion. About 1 to 5% of zipeprol is excreted unchanged. Two main *N*-dealkylated metabolites have been identified.[4] The elimination half-life is about 6 hours.[1]

Pregnancy/Lactation

A 27-year-old pregnant woman ingested 1 to 2 g of zipeprol daily and went into active labor at 32 weeks of pregnancy. The infant delivered had Apgar scores at 1 and 5 minutes of 5 and 8, respectively. The child was irritable within hours of birth. A sonogram of the head on the third day showed bilateral echogenic rales thought to be consistent with leukoencephalitic malaria. The child was discharged after a 6-week stay in the intermediate care nursery. At 6 months of age, there was no irritability, hypertonicity, and possible hyperreflexia.[2]

Mechanism of Action

Zipeprol is an antitussive possessing bronchospasmolytic and mucolytic activity. It lacks opiate-like side effects. It is a mild antihistamine and exhibits anticholinergic effects.[4] Seizures may be due to inhibition of the γ-aminobutyric acid system (GABA).

Clinical Presentation

At the end of the last century, when piperazine was used in the treatment of gout, the following side effects were observed: clonic spasms, tremor of the upper extremities, muscular weakness, impaired coordination, inability to think clearly, and hallucinations.[7] Use of zipeprol for recreational purposes has led to seizures and coma.[3,4] Seizures generally resolve rapidly and without recurrence after symptomatic treatment.[9] Although drowsiness is usually the only manifestation of drug overdose, seizures have been described.[4,5] Abusers describe zipeprol effects as hallucinations and a series of euphoric episodes that diminish rapidly about 1.5 to 2 hours after ingestion. This is followed by depressive rebound associated with retrograde anemia. Piperazine-derived antihistamines and antipsychotic medication can either lower the seizure threshold in epileptic patients or precipitate seizures. Piperazine-related compounds should be considered a possible cause of encephalopathy, incoordination, and nonepileptic seizures, particularly in patients not native to the United States.[3] Three patients of average age 19 years ingested 11 to 28 mg/kg as a single dose or as repeated doses for 3 to 25 days; they presented with seizures followed by coma. In childhood, restlessness, abnormalities of posture and gait, and choreic movements have been observed. The clinical picture appears to be more severe in adults than in children.[5] Withdrawal from zipeprol use has resulted in abdominal pain, irritability, and insomnia.[10]

Laboratory

Analytical Methods

Thin-layer chromatography and gas chromatography methods are available for zipeprol analysis.[4]

Blood Levels

Blood levels of zipeprol in two drug addicts found dead were 10.6 and 5.8 μg/mL, respectively.[4]

Abnormalities

The electroencephalogram exhibits generalized 2- to 4-Hz activity in up to 70% of neurologically normal children taking therapeutic doses of piperazine salt.[3] No epileptic electroencephalographic changes have been observed in this group. Split-wave inverts and slow theta wave activity have been experienced after an overdose of zipeprol.[5]

Ancillary Tests

Computed tomography screening revealed areas of hypotonicity in the corpus callosum and the left cerebellar hemisphere. These changes have disappeared in 3 to 6 months.[5]

Treatment

Treatment is largely symptomatic and supportive. Immediate gastric decontamination (gastric lavage) with endotracheal intubation is preferred to syrup of ipecac (tendency toward seizures, with risk of aspiration pneumonitis). The usual precautions for coma patients should be instituted with special protection of respiration and cardiovascular monitoring. Glucose, naloxone, and oxygen should be available.

Pyridoxine (2–4 g intravenously) may be useful in treating seizures, but no controlled studies using this drug are available.

Use of elimination enhancement techniques (hemodialysis, hemoperfusion) has not been reported after a zipeprol overdose.

Supportive measures with careful serial neurologic follow-up include electroencephalograms and computed tomography scans. Patients should not be discharged until at least 24 hours after there is no evidence of seizure activity (clinically, electroencephalogram).

REFERENCES—ZIPEPROL

1. Jouglard J. Zipeprol abuse: An opportunity for assessment of its neurotoxicity. Eur Assoc Pois Control Centres Toxicol Newslett 1991:5–13. Oslo, Norway.
2. Slobodkin D, Thompson D, Levin G, Jesurun CA. Habituation to zipeprol hydrochloride during pregnancy. J Subst Abuse Treat 1992;9:129–131.
3. Yohai D, Barnett SH. Absence and atonic seizures induced by piperazine. Pediatr Neurol 1989;5:393–394.
4. Crippa O, Polettini A, Avat FM. Lethal poisoning by zipeprol in drug addicts. J Forens Sci 1990;35:992–997.
5. Moroni C, Cerchiari EL, Gasparin M, Roter E. Overdosage of zipeprol, an non-opioid antitussive agent. Lancet 1984;1: 45.
6. Perroro F, Bearchi A. Convulsions and cerebral oedema associated with zipeprol abuse. Lancet 1984;1:45–46.
7. Schuch P, Stephan U, Jacobi F. Neurotoxic side effects of piperazines. Lancet 1966;1:1218.
8. Beckett AH, Achar R. Plasma concentrations and excretion of zipeprol in man under acidic urine conditions. J Pharm Pharmacol 1977;29:589–592.
9. Merigot PH, Garnier R, Efthymious ML. Seizure with three piperazine compounds used as antitussive agents (zipeprol, eprazinone and eprozinol). Ann Pediatr (Paris) 1985;32: 504–511.
10. Roche J, Hamici R, Danel T, et al. Zipeprol addiction: A report of three cases. Semin Hop Paris 1991;67:1725–1727.

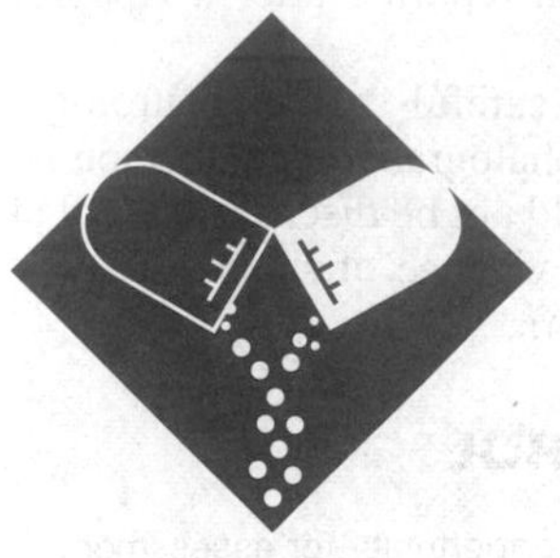

Part E
Receptor Toxicology

Chapter 46
Antimuscarinic Drugs

INTRODUCTION

Antimuscarinic drugs competitively inhibit the muscarinic effects of acetylcholine. They are also known as parasympatholytic, atropinic, atropine-like, or anticholinergic agents. Atropine is the prototype antimuscarinic agent. Antimuscarinic agents can be classified on the basis of their source (natural, semisynthetic, or synthetic) and/or their cationic structure (tertiary amine or quaternary ammonium compounds). Atropine, hyoscyamine, and scopolamine are naturally occurring tertiary amines (Table 46–1).[1]

Use

Antimuscarinic agents are used mainly in the treatment of peptic ulcer disease and irritable bowel syndrome. Atropine is used in the diagnosis of sinus node dysfunction (see Atropine). Atropine, scopolamine, and glycopyrrolate are used as preoperative medications to inhibit salivation and diminish excessive secretions of the respiratory tract. Genitourinary tract disorders such as uninhibited contractions and reflex neurogenic bladder have been treated with atropine, oxybutynin, and propantheline. The antimuscarinic agents are potent bronchodilators. Benztropine and benzhexol (trihexyphenidyl) are used in the management of Parkinson's disease and drug-induced extrapyramidal reactions.

Clinical Presentation

Peripheral symptoms of overdose may include dilated and unreactive pupils; blurred vision; hot, dry, and flushed skin; dry mucous membranes; difficulty in swallowing; diminished or absent bowel sounds; urinary retention; tachycardia; hyperthermia; hypertension; and increased respiratory rate. Central nervous system manifestations may resemble acute psychosis (disorientation, incoherence, confusion, hallucinations, delusions, paranoia, disturbed speech, periods of hyperactivity, anxiety, abnormal motor behavior, and restlessness). In severe overdose, central nervous system depression, circulatory collapse, and hypotension have been observed. Coma and skeletal muscle paralysis may be

Table 46–1
Classification of Antimuscarinic Agents

Tertiary	Quaternary	Selective
atropine	atropine methobromide	pirenzepine hydrochloride
atropine sulfate	atropine methonitrate	telenzepine
benzhexol hydrochloride	clidinium bromide	
benztropine mesylate	diphemanil methylsulfate	
biperiden hydrochloride	emepronium bromide	
biperiden lactate	glycopyrronium bromide	
cyclopentolate hydrochloride	homatropine methobromide	
dicyclomine hydrochloride	hyoscine butylbromide	
homatropine	hyoscine methonitrate	
homatropine hydrobromide	ipratropium bromide	
hyosceine	isopropamide iodide	
hyosceine hydrobromide	mepenzolate bromide	
hyosceyamine	octatropine methylbromide	
methixene hydrochloride	otilonium bromide	
oxybutynin hydrochloride	oxitropium bromide	
oxyphencyclimine hydrochloride	pipenzolate bromide	
procyclidine hydrochloride	prifinium bromide	
tropicamide	poldine methylsulphate	
	propantheline bromide	
	tiemonium iodide	
	tiemonium methylsulfate	
	timepidium bromide	
	valethamate bromide	

From Reynolds JEF, ed. *Martindale: The Extra Pharmacopoeia.* 30th ed. London: Pharmaceutical Press, 1993:418.

followed by death from respiratory failure, hyperthermia (especially in children), or cardiac depression or from environmental exposure or drowning by patients who were delirious. Electrocardiographic abnormalities include widening of the QRS complex, prolongation of the QT interval, ST segment depression, ventricular arrhythmias, and premature beats and sinus tachycardia and supraventricular tachycardia.

Treatment

Treatment of overdose is largely symptomatic and supportive. Patients should be hospitalized and closely monitored with a continuous electrocardiographic monitoring. Gastric lavage with a cuffed endotracheal tube, activated charcoal, and saline cathartics have been used. Hemodialysis or peritoneal dialysis is not useful. Fluid therapy is administered and shock treated as required. Hyperthermia is treated with cold packs, mechanical cooling devices, or sponging with tepid water. Diazepam may be useful to control excitement, delirium, or manifestations of acute psychosis. Phenothiazines should not be used because they may also have anticholinergic effects. Maintenance of an adequate airway, respiratory assistance, and urinary catheterization are important aspects of patient management. Physostigmine use is controversial. It may induce seizures, bronchospasm, or asystole. It has been used in patients with extensive delirium or agitation, repetitive or long-lasting seizures, severe sinus tachycardia or supraventricular tachycardia, or extensive hyperthermia unresponsive to mechanical cooling. The usual therapeutic adult dose is 2 mg intravenously. If there is no response, 1 to 2 mg may can be given every 20 minutes until reversal of toxic antimuscarinic effects occurs or adverse cholinergic effects develop. The usual pediatric intravenous dose of physostigmine salicylate recommended by the manufacturer is 0.02 mg/kg. Physostigmine should not be used to treat cardiac conduction defects or ventricular tachyrrhythmias. Excessive doses of physostigmine may produce cholinergic toxicity (eg, bradycardia, increased salivation, diarrhea, seizures, or respiratory arrest). Physostigmine-induced life-threatening bronchoconstriction, bradycardia, and seizures may respond to intravenous administration of 0.5 to 1 mg of atropine sulfate. (See also Chapter 38 [section on Antihistamines] and Chapter 40.)

REFERENCE—INTRODUCTION

1. Reynolds JEF, ed. *Martindale: The Extra Pharmacopoeia.* 30th ed. London: Pharmaceutical Press, 1993:418.

ATROPINE, HOMATROPINE HYDROBROMIDE, AND ATROPINE METHYL NITRATE

ATROPINE

Atropine is the prototype of those anticholinergic drugs (eg, cyclic antidepressants, phenothiazines, antihistamines) and plants that can induce a similar set of toxic signs and symptoms including dryness of the mouth; flushed, hot, and dry skin; dilated and nonreactive pupils; tachycardia; hallucinations; and restlessness.

Atropine toxicity is seen clinically (1) as a manifestation of an unusual sensitivity to a therapeutic dose[1–26]; (2) after erroneous or excessive amounts have been administered by medical personnel, prescribed by pharmacy error, or voluntarily administered[27–41]; (3) after covert use (a factitious atropine syndrome)[42]; (4) after excessive use of eyedrops by

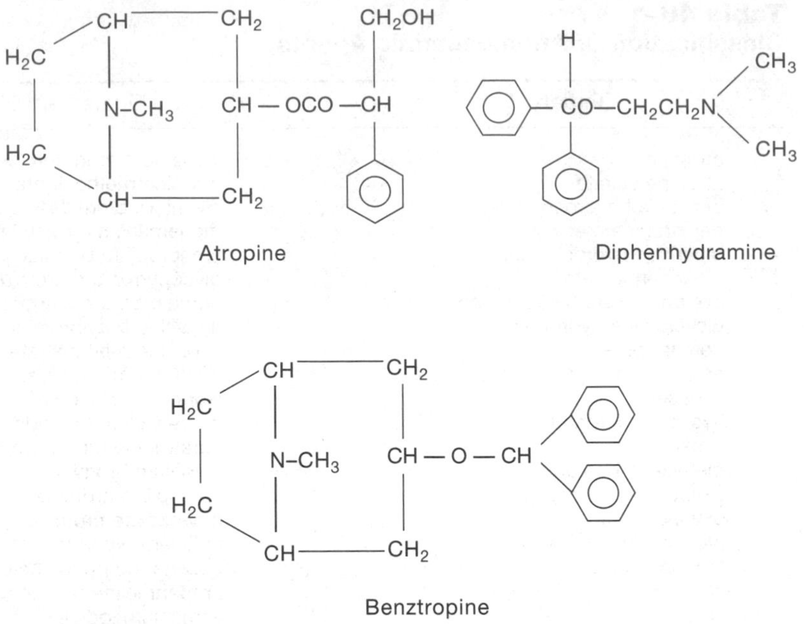

Atropine

Diphenhydramine

Benztropine

Figure 46–1 Structures of atropine, diphenhydramine, and benztropine (From Howrie DL, Rowley AH, Krenzelok EP. Benztropine-induced acute dystonic reaction. Ann Emerg Med 1986;15:594–596.)

a confused older patient; and (5) occasionally after overexuberant use in the treatment of organophosphate or carbamate poisonings, especially when there is no significant depression of red cell cholinesterase levels.

Atropine toxicity may follow oral ingestion; applications of eyedrops or eye ointment; subcutaneous, intramuscular, or intravenous injections; and inhalation. The clinical responses to both therapeutic doses and overdoses may be similar. Fatalities have followed doses far lower than those that have been tolerated by other individuals.[43–46] Clinical symptoms correlate poorly with dosage; however, a general correlation of dosage with effects has been suggested.

Structure/Classification

Atropine is an antimuscarinic anticholinergic compound[47,48] (Fig. 46–1). It is a mixture of two isomers, *d*(+) and *l*(–) hyoscyamine. Only the *l*(–) +hyoscyamine is pharmacologically active.

In clinical preparations, 0.6 mg of the racemic atropine contains 250 μg/mg of the active base. One drop of 1% atropine sulfate eyedrops contains approximately 0.6 to 0.75 mg of atropine.

Source

Atropine and hyoscine are alkaloids that are produced by the roots, leaves, and beans of plants of the Solanaceae family, of which the deadly nightshade *(Atropa belladonna)* is the best known. Hyoscyamine is another solanaceous alkaloid. These alkaloids can be synthesized, but plant extraction is less expensive. *Duboisia myoporoides* is now the main source, in addition to *Atropa belladonna* and *Datura stramonium* (jimsonweed).[48]

These plants have been regarded as poisonous for centuries. Linnaeus named the deadly nightshade shrub *Atropo belladonna* after Atropos, eldest of the three fates, the one whose duty it was to cut the thread of life.[16]

Use

Atropine sulfate is used in ophthalmic preparations to induce mydriasis and cycloplegia for examination of the retina and optic disk and for measurement of refractive error.[48] Atropine is used often in older people before and after glaucoma surgery (trabeculectomy with peripheral iridectomy) to maintain a dilated pupil and prevent posterior synechiae.[49]

Atropine is also used in the diagnosis of sinus node dysfunction; in evaluation of coronary artery disease during atrial pacing; in sinus bradycardia-induced by drugs with cholinergic effects (pilocarpine, organophosphate pesticides, *Clitocybe* and *Inocybe* mushroom species); in advanced cardiac life support during cardiopulmonary resuscitation for sinus bradycardia accompanied by severe hypotension or frequent ventricular ectopic beats; by oral inhalation in short-term treatment and prevention of bronchospasm associated with chronic bronchial asthma, bronchitis, and chronic obstructive pulmonary disease[48]; and for symptomatic relief in parkinsonism. It has been used to treat spider *(Latrodectus mactans)* bites,[50] but other drugs are more effective.

An automatic injection device for administration of atropine (Atropen, Survival Technology, Bethesda, MD) contains 1.67 mg of atropine base (equivalent to atropine sulfate 2 mg) and is available in Israel for use in nerve gas poisoning. Its use by women against potential rapists may lead the attacker to suffer a rapid heartbeat, palpitations, marked dryness of the mouth, dilated pupils, and some blurring of near vision. This use is at present illegal and probably ineffective in preventing violent assault.[51]

Therapeutic Dose

The usual therapeutic dose of atropine is 0.6 mg (approximately one drop of 1% atropine sulfate). In a normal subject, three drops is sufficient to produce parasympathetic paralysis. Intoxication after eyedrop use may result from the swallowing of atropine-laden tears.

Toxic Dose

Atropine in toxic amounts leads to drowsiness, stupor, convulsions, and coma.[19] A fatal dose may be as low as 1.6 mg[45] and as high as 100 mg in children.[46] Recovery in an adult has followed ingestion of 1 g.[31]

Ketchum et al. observed that 175 µg/mg/kg (12.15 mg intramuscularly) produced initial peripheral autonomic effects such as tachycardia and dryness of mouth.[52] Concomitant with these effects were central disturbances: somnolence, restlessness, ataxia, incoordination, hyperreflexia, hyperthermia and hypertension, disruption of awareness, and incoherent speech or inability to carry out instructions lasting 10 to 12 hours. Atropine sulfate 0.5 mg via nebulizer every 4 hours led to central anticholinergic intoxication; the patient recovered.[53]

Toxicokinetics[54–61]

Bioavailability	About 95%
Presystemic metabolism	860 ng/mL (after 40 µg 1% atropine in cul-de-sac of eye
Peak plasma level	(patient can't read)
Time to peak plasma level	13 minutes (IM)[62]
	1 hour (oral)[63]
	1.5–4 hours (aerosol)[64,65]
Volume of distribution	2–4 L/kg[66]
Plasma protein binding	50%[67]
Elimination half-life	2–4 hours[65,68]
Excreted unchanged	20–50%[68,69]

Pharmacologic effects are observed at blood levels of 2 to 3 ng/mL.[68]

Drug Interactions

Anticholinergic Agents. Atropine may exert additive effects when used with other drugs that have anticholinergic effects such as anti-Parkinson's drugs and methixene hydrochloride—Benztropine (Cogentin): Biperiden (Akineton): Chlorphenoximine (Phenoxene): Cycrimine (Pagitane): Orphenadrine (Disipal, Norflex): Procyclidine (Kemadrin): Trihexyphenidyl (Artane) (the latter three compounds are not available in the United States); phenothiazines; amantadine; meperidine; tricyclic antidepressants; glutethimide; quinidine; disopyramide; and some antihistamines.[48,70]

Succinylcholine. This combination though commonly used in children has been observed to increase the occurrence of skeletal muscle rigidity with malignant hyperthermia.[71]

Pralidoxime Chloride. When atropine (1 mg/mL) was mixed with pralidoxime chloride (300 mg/mL) or sodium chloride (8.5%) and administered intramuscularly, there appeared to be a significant delay in the time course of atropine effects on heart rate (tachycardia).[72] In another study,[73] however, no delay was induced by atropine 2 mg/mL on the rate of uptake of pralidoxime mesylate; nor was there any delay in the absorption of atropine as judged by its effect on heart rate when 500 or 700 mg of pralidoxime mesylate was given alone or mixed with the atropine.

Pilocarpine. Atropine may decrease the effects of pilocarpine eyedrops, reducing their ability to lower intraocular pressure in the treatment of glaucoma.[74]

Monoamine Oxidase Inhibitors. This interaction may result in an exaggerated response to normal doses of atropine or atropine-like drugs.[74]

Pregnancy/Lactation

Atropine has been used as a premedication in obstetric anesthesia, as a test of fetoplacental insufficiency,[75–77] and in the diagnosis of fetal asphyxia (atropine given to the mother produces changes in the fetal heart rate: first bradycardia, then tachycardia).[78,79] There is evidence of rapid placental transfer of atropine.[77]

No data are available on atropine concentrations in breast milk.[80,81] Some infants, however, are known to be extremely sensitive to atropine.

Studies in mice indicate that atropine is associated with a low incidence of skeletal anomalies; no malformations were observed in dogs.[82] Injection of 0.6 to 1.5 mg of atropine into chick eggs during the fourth to twelfth days of incubation did not lead to any defects in the newborn chicks.[83]

Mechanism of Action

Atropine competitively inhibits the muscarinic effects of acetylcholine;[48] it is an antimuscarinic anticholinergic agent. Atropine prevents acetylcholine from exerting its usual action on effector cells but does not diminish the production of acetylcholine. Its sites of action are at the autonomic effectors innervated by postganglionic cholinergic nerves or on smooth muscles that do not contain cholinergic innervation. Central nervous system effects of atropine and related drugs result from their central antimuscarinic actions (in usual doses, mild vagal stimulation and decrease in heart rate).[47,84]

Clinical Presentation

Adverse Reactions

Toxic antimuscarinic anticholinergic responses to both therapeutic doses and overdoses of atropine have been remarkably similar. The more prominent and commonly observed signs and symptoms of "atropinism" may follow use of atropine by any route (eye, oral, intramuscular, intravenous, or inhalation). Slow cerebration, inattention, somnolence, and restlessness are frequently observed in patients older than 60 with myocardial infarction whose sinus bradycardia has been treated with atropine.[31]

Down Syndrome

Those with Down syndrome have an increased sensitivity to atropine.[85] One drop of 1% atropine into the right eye induces a tendency for the pupil to dilate more quickly and for the reaction to be sustained longer in those with than in those without Down syndrome. The increased pupillary reactivity was attributed to hypoplasia of the peripheral stroma of the iris, a structural anomaly present in 95% of such cases.[86] The increased sensitivity to atropine in Down subjects may result from the genetic imbalance imposed by the extra chromosome 21 in this syndrome.[87]

Seizures

Seizures without prior evidence of hallucinations or delirium have followed the use of atropine in an adult and in children.

Overdose

The lethal dose of atropine in children has varied between 1.6 and 100 mg. Up to 1000 mg of atropine sulfate has been ingested with ultimate recovery.[31] The overdose patient[4,7,9,28,35] frequently exhibits thirst, parched throat and lips, slurred speech, dilated pupils with no reaction to light or accommodation, blurred vision, visual hallucinations, restlessness, delusions of place and identity, agitation and amnesia for episodes, delirium, incoherence, flushed and hot cheeks and skin, rapid pulse, bladder distension, ataxic gait, temperature to 105°F, hyperreflexia, and convulsions.[88,89] A respiratory therapist who administered atropine sulfate via aerosol ten times during the preceding 24 hours developed an anticholinergic syndrome that responded to symptomatic treatment.[90]

Mortality

Deaths reported after atropine administration have usually been in children and are frequently associated with high fevers, which may be due to the inhibition of sweating produced by atropine.[16]

Withdrawal

One day after cessation of long-term use of atropine eyedrops for the management of amblyopia, nausea, vomiting, and perspiration were observed. All symptoms disappeared in 24 hours.[91]

Laboratory

Analytical Methods

A gas chromatography–mass spectrometry method for the rapid quantitation of atropine in blood has a limit of detection of atropine to about 10 ng/mL.[1]

Ancillary Tests

Plasma levels confirm a clinical diagnosis but do not guide management, which must be based on clinical evaluations. There is little correlation between the dose of atropine, the plasma or serum concentration,[64] and observed clinical effects.[69] Blood studies may show a leukocytosis[34] to 15,000/m^3 with a predominance of neutrophils.[17] The fasting blood sugar is usually normal[34] but may be decreased.[45] The blood urea nitrogen was normal in one case[34] and elevated in a child who died.[45] Urinalysis has generally remained within normal limits unless there were complications (eg, convulsions, hyperthermia). An electroencephalogram and computer tomography scan were normal in one study.[42] The cerebrospinal fluid has usually been found to be within normal limits.[31,42] Sinus tachycardia,[14] S-segment elevations, diphasic T waves,[14] prolonged QT interval, ventricular tachycardia, and ventricular fibrillation[92] have been described after therapeutic doses.

Test in Cats. For the differential diagnosis of postepileptic delirium or belladonna poisoning, Coates[93] cites Dr. Hughlings Jackson's advice to instill a few drops of the patient's urine into the eye of a cat.[94] This may result in rapid dilation of the cat's pupil.[95]

Atropine as a Cause of Dilated Fixed Pupils. Two to three drops of 1% pilocarpine are instilled in the affected eye. If the pupil does not constrict in 15 to 30 minutes it is dilated because of atropine or other anticholinergic drugs. Pilocarpine 1% usually constricts a neuropathologically induced dilation.[96]

Blood Levels

Death following ingestion of atropine tablets is associated with an atropine blood level of 200 ng/mL and a urine level of 1.5 μg/mL. A healthy adult ingested 1 g of atropine and developed an anticholinergic syndrome. The blood atropine level several hours later was 129 ng/mL.[97] Inadvertent injection of atropine 2 mg into Israeli children during the Gulf Crisis led to relatively mild symptoms of atropinization. Serum atropine levels ranged from 7.5 to 69 ng/mL.[97–99]

Treatment

Patients may be conscious on admission but may quickly lapse into coma with profound respiratory depression. Treatment should be provided in a hospital intensive care facility with adequate respiratory assistance available. A quiet dark room, with avoidance of unnecessary stimuli and padding of bedsides, may be useful for agitated subjects. The clinician must rule out other causative factors for dilated pupils such as angle-closure glaucoma, cerebral aneurysm, brain tumor, and subdural or subarachnoid hemorrhage. Appropriate consultations (eg, ophthalmology, neurology) should be obtained where feasible. Such care may be required for several days before unassisted ventilation is resumed by the patient. Cooling measures should be available. Use of drugs with strong anticholinergic properties (phenothiazines, antihistamines, tricyclic antidepressants), quinidine, disopyramide, and procainamide should be avoided.

Stabilization

Prehospital care may require use of an Ambu bag in the ambulance for assisted ventilation with 40% oxygen by inhalation.

The airway should be maintained by endotracheal intubation where necessary. Tidal volume should be at least 10 to 15 mL/kg.

Electrocardiogram, pulse (bradycardia, tachycardia), respiration, and temperature (hyperthermia frequent in overdose) should be continuously monitored. Periodic evaluation of renal function, hepatic function, and electroencephalograms is useful during coma and after return of consciousness.

Gut Decontamination

Emesis may be useful after substantial ingestions if initiated within 30 minutes of ingestion (peak blood level at 1 hour) and if there is no evidence of present or impending obtundation, coma, or convulsions, or gastric lavage with endotracheal intubation should be performed early if the patient is obtunded and is unable to protect the airway. Toxicity from ingested doses may not correlate well with the suspected amount ingested.

Activated charcoal (50–100 g, adults; 15–30 g, children) may be administered as an aqueous slurry, 30 g/240 mL, as a mixture with saline cathartics, or with sorbitol for the first dose only.

The safety and efficacy of cathartics have not been established in the treatment of atropine toxicity.

Elimination Enhancement

Enhancement of elimination of atropine by extracorporeal means (peritoneal dialysis, hemoperfusion) has not been evaluated but is not likely to be effective in view of the large volume of distribution. In cases of overdose reported to date, recovery has been achieved without use of these procedures.

Antidote

Physostigmine may be useful after either oral or parenteral (intramuscular, intravenous, ocular, inhalation) exposure to atropine sufficient to result in coma,[100] arrhythmias, hallucinations, severe hypertension, or seizures. Reversal of coma, arrhythmias, hallucinations, and other findings can be expected within minutes if there has not been any other central nervous system damage or exposure to a combination of drugs. Patients should be observed carefully for evidence of physostigmine toxicity (seizures, asystole, hypotension, hypersalivation, bradyrhythmics). Physostigmine must be used with great caution in the presence of asthma, gangrene, or mechanical obstruction of the gastrointestinal or urogenital tract.

The pediatric physostigmine dose is 0.5 mg intravenously slowly. The patient must be observed for development of cholinergic effects. If there is no improvement, the dose is repeated at 5-minute intervals to a maximum of 2 mg.

The adolescent or adult is administered 2 mg intravenously slowly. This is repeated, if required, in 20 minutes and if life-threatening symptoms recur. Physostigmine should not be administered as a continuous intravenous drip. The patient must be observed for evidence of bronchial constriction. Continuous cardiac monitoring must accompany the use of physostigmine.

Neostigmine and pyridostigmine are cholinesterase inhibitors. They are quaternary ammonium compounds that do not traverse the blood–brain barrier and, therefore, are not useful in treating atropine-induced central nervous system toxicity. Physostigmine is a tertiary amine and does pass the blood–brain barrier.[101]

Supportive Measures

Supportive care is the mainstay of treatment.

Hyperthermia. Hydration, cooling measures.

Hydration. Intravenous fluids. Watch and chart intake and output and renal function.

Seizures. Diazepam intravenously may result in further central nervous system depression and must be given with concern for maintenance of respiration.

Agitation. Avoid promethazine, an antihistamine with anticholinergic properties. Phenothiazines are strongly anticholinergic and should not be used.[101] Reassurance and diazepam can be employed as indicated. Pilocarpine antagonizes only the peripheral actions of atropine,[102] but does not antagonize central nervous system effects and, therefore, is of little use.[17] Morphine further depresses the respiratory center and should not be used.[19]

Urinary Retention. Bladder catheterization may be required.

HOMATROPINE HYDROBROMIDE

Homatropine hydrobromide is a tertiary amine antimuscarinic agent used as eyedrops to produce mydriasis and cycloplegia for refraction and in the management of acute inflammatory conditions in the uveal tract. It is available as a 2% solution (homatropine hydrobromide ophthalmic solution, Isopto [homatropine with benzalkonium chloride, viscous]) or as a 5% solution (AK-Homatropine, homatropine hydrobromide ophthalmic solution, Isopto homatropine [with benzalkonium chloride, viscous]).[48] It is a short-acting mydriatic and cycloplegic agent. Mydriasis reaches a maximum in 10 to 30 minutes and lasts 6 hours to 4 days; cycloplegia reaches a maximum in 30 to 90 minutes and lasts 10 to 48 hours.

Confusion, hallucinations, disorientation, restlessness, photophobia, incoherent speech, and abnormal gait combined with rapid respirations and pulse, a flushed face, and dilated pupils were observed in a young woman who had used 1% homatropine drops in one eye; she recovered.[101] Similar symptoms were reported by Whittemore after a 2% solution was used by an 11-year-old boy; he recovered in 7 hours.[102]

Hoefnagel reported four reactions involving the central nervous system after the use of 2% homatropine eyedrops in children.[17] Treatment is supportive. No fatalities have been reported. Prognosis is good for complete recovery.

ATROPINE METHYL NITRATE (ATROPINE METHONITRATE)

Atropine methyl nitrate is a quaternary ammonium congener of atropine that has poor mucosal absorption compared with atropine sulfate and may cause fewer systemic side effects when inhaled.[103] or when taken orally.[50] It is under clinical trials in North America and Europe[103] and is sold in the United Kingdom, Australia, and South Africa as Eumydrin (0.6% atropine methyl nitrate in 90% alcohol) for oral use. Each drop contains 0.2 mg.

Reports of its toxicity appeared in 1966 when Purcell described a 2-month-old boy with an upper respiratory infection who received 2 drops orally (0.4 mg), a therapeutic dose, with each feeding for 1 week. He presented with coma, a rectal temperature of 107.4°F (41.9°C), respirations of 70/min, and a pulse rate of 160/min. His pupils were widely dilated. His white blood cell count was 17,300. The abdomen was distended. He responded to cooling measures.[104]

Stephenson cited a 2-year 7-month-old girl who received atropine methonitrate drops up to 8 mg/d orally for the treatment of convulsive breath-holding attacks. After 5 days, her lips began to crack and her pulse rate increased. The dose was reduced to 4.8 mg/d. She continued treatment. Pupils were normally reactive and not dilated.[105]

Meerstadt described eight cases of atropine methonitrate toxicity in infants aged 1 to 27 weeks who received overdoses of 0.8 to 16 mg (0.39–3.55 mg/kg). Central nervous system signs (dilated pupils, irritability, restlessness) were apparent, indicating an effect on the central nervous system similar to that of atropine sulfate. Symptoms in these infants lasted 24 to 60 hours. None was treated with physostigmine salicylate. Supportive treatment was rendered. All recovered. Meerstadt feels that atropine methonitrate is not indicated in whooping cough and has a doubtful place in the management of congenital hypertrophic pyloric stenosis.[106] Comparable doses of atropine sulfate that have led to convulsions and coma in infants averaged approximately 0.09 mg/kg[23]; death has resulted from as little as 0.2 mg/kg.[45]

Gross and Skorodin accidentally administered an overdose of 32 mg atropine methonitrate by inhalation to a 65-year-old man with a long history of cigarette smoking and chronic airway obstruction. The planned dose was 2.25 mg nebulized over 1 hour. He had no symptoms other than a transient headache. This may indicate that quaternary ammonium congeners of atropine have a wider therapeutic margin than atropine sulfate in adults when inhaled.[103]

REFERENCES—ATROPINE, HOMATROPINE HYDROBROMIDE, AND ATROPINE METHYL NITRATE

1. Tyson WJ. Toxic effects of atropine drops. Br Med J 1889;2:921.
2. Owens SM. Notes on two cases of atropine poisoning. Lancet 1890;2:443–444.
3. Kelynack TN. Atropine poisoning by absorption from the conjunctiva. Br Med J 1890;1:421.
4. Harris WJ. A case of rapid development of symptoms of belladonna poisoning from use of sulphate of atropine eye drops. Lancet 1898;1:98.
5. Rodger WG. Case of acute poisoning after instillation of a small dose of atropine into the eye. Glasgow Med J 1903;60:102–105.
6. Wise CH. Case of poisoning from atropine eye drops. Br Med J 1904;1:189–190.
7. Spurgin PB. Two cases of poisoning from the application of atropine to the eyes. Lancet 1905;2:964.
8. White PJ. Atropine fever in early infancy. Am J Dis Child 1929;37:745–750.
9. Munns GF. Atropine hyperpyrexia in early infancy. JAMA 1929;93:171–173.
10. Metivier VM. A case of atropine poisoning. Lancet 1935;2:1232.
11. Scally CM. Poisoning after one instillation of atropine drops. Br Med J 1936;1:311.
12. Hopkins F, Robyns-Jones J. Psychosis associated with atropine administration. Br Med J 1937;1:663.
13. Duggan PJ. Mental disturbance following atropine administration. Br Med J 1937;1:918.
14. Baker JP, Farley JD. Toxic psychosis following atropine eye drops. Br Med J 1958;2:1390–1392.
15. Hill DW. Toxic psychosis after atropine eye drops. Br Med J 1958;2:1594.
16. Garlington LN, Bailey PJ. Is atropine a poison? Anesth Analg 1959;38:254–258.
17. Hoefnagel D. Toxic effects of atropine and homatropine eyedrops in children. N Engl J Med 1961;264:168–171.
18. Karliner W. Accidental convulsion induced by atropine. Am J Psychiatry 1965;122:578–579.
19. Shah PM. Toxic effects of atropine eye drops. Indian J Pediatr 1966;33:13–17.
20. Erikssen J. Atropine psychosis. Lancet 1969;1:53–54.
21. German E, Siddiqui N. Atropine toxicity from eyedrops. N Engl J Med 1970;282:689.
22. Weinstock FJ. Dilated fixed pupils from atropine. JAMA 1974;229:267–268.
23. Gillick JS. Atropine toxicity in a neonate. Br J Anaesth 1974;46:793–794.
24. Gooding JM, Holcomb MC. Transient blindness following intravenous administration of atropine. Anesth Analg 1977;56:872–873.
25. Berman KR, Pearson C, Waltz GW, et al. Atropine-induced psychosis. Chest 1980;78:891–893.
26. Lacouture PB, Lovejoy FH Jr, Mitchell AA. Acute hypothermia associated with atropine. Am J Dis Child 1983;137:291–292.
27. Jones LW. An adventure in atropism. JAMA 1921;76:813–814.
28. Heller G. Atropine poisoning in a child. JAMA 1929;92:800.
29. Comroe BI. Atropine poisoning: Recovery after 7 grains of atropine sulfate by mouth. JAMA 1933;101:446–447.
30. Carter AB. Atropine poisoning: Description of an unusual case. Br Med J 1940;2:664–665.
31. Alexander E Jr, Morris DP, Eslick RL. Atropine poisoning: Report of a case with recovery after ingestion of one gram. N Engl J Med 1946;234:258–259.
32. Hamilton M, Sclare AB. Belladonna poisoning. Br Med J 1947;2:611–612.
33. Welbourn RB, Buxton JD. Acute atropine poisoning: Review of eight cases. Lancet 1948;2:211–213.
34. Hoffman GM, Gay JR. Accidental atropine poisoning. Pa Med J 1959;62:1340–1341.
35. Leczycka F, Trembla K. The course and consequences of coma after huge doses of atropine. Pol Med J 1969;8:381–383.
36. Mackenzie AL, Pigott JFG. Atropine overdose in three children. Br J Anesth 1971;43:1088–1090.
37. Arthurs GJ, Davison R. Atropine: A safe drug. Anaesthesia 1980;35:1077–1079.
38. Worth DP, Davison AM, Roberts TG, et al. Ineffectiveness of haemodialysis in atropine poisoning. Br Med J 1983;286:2023–2024.
39. Forrer GR. Atropine toxicity in the treatment of mental disease. Am J Psychiatry 1951;108:107–117.
40. Forrer GR. Symposium on atropine toxicity therapy: History and future research. J Nerv Ment Dis 1956;124:256–259.
41. Miller JJ. Symposium on atropine toxicity therapy. J Nerv Ment Dis 1956;124:260–264.
42. O'Connor PS, Mumma JV. Atropine toxicity. Am J Ophthalmol 1985;99:613–614.
43. Rockliffe W. Notes on a death supposed to be from atropine drops applied to the eye. Trans Ophthalmol Soc UK 1902;22:302–305.
44. Morton HG. Atropine intoxication: Its manifestations in infants and children. J Pediatr 1939;14:755–760.
45. Heath WE. Death from atropine poisoning. Br Med J 1950;2:608.
46. Legroux P. A propos d'un cas d'intoxication mortelle par un collyre a l'atropine. Ann Ocul 1962;195:48–52.
47. Weiner N. Atropine, scopolamine and related antimuscarinic drugs. In: Gilman A, Goodman LS, Rall TW, et al., eds. *Goodman and Gilman's the Pharmacological Basis of Therapeutics.* 7th ed. New York: Macmillan, 1985:138.
48. McEvoy GK, ed. *Drug Information 94.* Bethesda, MD: American Society of Hospital Pharmacists, 1994:516–519, 741–744, 1827–1829.

49. Merli GJ, Weitz H, Martin JH, et al. Cardiac dysrhythmias associated with ophthalmic atropine. Arch Intern Med 1986; 146:45–47.
50. Gotlieb A. Spider bites. Lancet 1970;2:246.
51. Seidman DS. Atropine for self-defence. Ann Emerg Med 1987;16:732–734.
52. Ketchum JS, Sidell FR, Crowell EB Jr, et al. Atropine, scopolamine and ditran: Comparative pharmacology and antagonists in man. Psychopharmacologia 1973;28:121–145.
53. Hirschman ZJ, Silverstein J, Blumberg G, Lehrfield J. Central nervous system toxicity from nebulized atropine sulfate. Clin Toxicol 1991;29:273–277.
54. Cullumbine H, McKee WHE, Creasey NH: The effects of atropine sulphate upon healthy male subjects. Q J Exp Physiol 1955;40:309–319.
55. Janes RG, Stiles JF. The penetration of C^{14} labeled atropine into the eye. Arch Ophthalmol 1959;67:97–102.
56. Davies DS. Pharmacokinetics of inhaled substances. Postgrad Med J 1975;51(suppl. 7):69–75.
57. Moller J, Rosen A. Comparative studies on intramuscular and oral effective doses of some anticholinergic drugs. Acta Med Scand 1968;184:201–209.
58. Adams RG, Verma P, Jackson AJ, et al. Plasma pharmacokinetics of intravenously administered atropine in normal human subjects. J Clin Pharmacol 1982;22:477–481.
59. Lahdes K, Kaila T, Hunponen R, et al. Systemic absorption of topically applied ocular atropine. Clin Pharmacol Ther 1988; 44:310–314.
60. Kalser SC. The fate of atropine in man. Ann NY Acad Sci 1971;179:667–683.
61. Kalser SC, McClain PL. Atropine metabolism in man. Clin Pharmacol Ther 1970;11:214–227.
62. Kentala E, Kaila T, Kanto J. Intramuscular atropine in elderly people: Pharmacokinetic studies using the radioreceptors assay and some pharmacodynamic responses. Pharmacol Toxicol 1989;65:110–113.
63. Beermann B, Hellstrom, Rosen A. The gastrointestinal absorption of atropine in man. Clin Sci 1971;40:95–106.
64. Kradjan WA, Smallridge RC, David R, et al. Atropine serum concentrations after multiple inhaled doses of atropine sulfate. Clin Pharmacol Ther 1985;38:12–15.
65. Kradjan WA, Lakshminarayan S, Hayden PW, et al. Serum atropine concentrations after inhalation of atropine sulfate. Am Rev Respir Dis 1981;123:471–472.
66. Hayden PW, Larson SM, Lakshminarayan S. Atropine clearance from human plasma. J Nucl Med 1979;20:366–367.
67. Shutt LE, Bowes JB. Atropine and hyoscine. Anesthesia 1979;34:476–490.
68. Gosselin RE, Gabourel JD, Wills JH: The fate of atropine in man. Clin Pharmacol Ther 1960;1:597–603.
69. Berghem L, Bergman U, Schildt B, et al. Plasma atropine concentrations determined by radioimmunoassay after single dose I.V. and I.M. administration. Br J Anaesth 1980;52: 597–601.
70. Reynolds JEF, ed. *Martindale: The Extra Pharmacopoeia.* 30th ed. London: Pharmaceutical Press, 1993:419–421.
71. Kalow W, Britt BA. Drugs causing rigidity in malignant hyperthermia. Lancet 1973;2:390–391.
72. Sidell FR. Modification by diluents of effects of intramuscular atropine on heart rate in man. Clin Pharmacol Ther 1974; 16:711–715.
73. Holland P, Parkes DC, White RG. Pralidoxime mesylate absorption and heart rate response to atropine sulphate following intramuscular administration of solution mixtures. Br J Clin Pharmacol 1975;2:333–338.
74. Atropine. In: Long JW, ed. *Clinical Management of Prescription Drugs.* Philadelphia: Harper & Row, 1984:110–119.
75. Hellman LM, Fillisti LP. Analysis of the atropine test for placental transfer in gravidas with toxemia and diabetes. Am J Obstet Gynecol 1965;91:797–808.
76. Barrier G, Olive G, Onnen I, et al. La pharmacocinetique de l'atropine chez la femme enceinte et la foetus en fin de grossesse. Anesth Analg Reanimat 1976;33:795–800.
77. Onnen I, Barrier G, d'Athis P, et al. Placental transfer of atropine at the end of pregnancy. Eur J Clin Pharmacol 1979; 15:443–446.
78. Kivalo I, Saarikoski S. Quantitative measurements of placental transfer and distribution of radioactive atropine in human fetus. Ann Chir Gynaecol Fem 1970;59:80–81.
79. Kivalo I, Saarikoski S. Placental transmission of atropine at full-term pregnancy. Br J Anaesth 1977;49:1017–1021.
80. Chaplin S, Sanders GL, Smith JM. Drug excretion in human breast milk. Adverse Drug React Acute Poison Rev 1982; 1:255–287.
81. O'Brien TE. Excretion of drugs in human milk. Am J Hosp Pharm 1974;31:844–854.
82. Arcuri PA, Gautieri RF. Morphine induced fetal malformations: 3. Possible mechanisms of action. J Pharm Sci 1973;62: 1626–1634.
83. Beuker ED, Platner WS. Effect of cholinergic drugs on development of chick embryo. Proc Soc Exp Biol Med 1956;91: 539–543.
84. Gross NJ, Skorodin MS. Anticholinergic, antimuscarinic bronchodilators. Am Rev Respir Dis 1984;129:856–870.
85. Walsh FB. *Clinical Neuro-ophthalmology.* 2nd ed. Baltimore: Williams & Wilkins, 1957:1192.
86. Lowe RF. Eyes in mongolism. Br J Ophthalmol 1949;33:131–174.
87. Harris WS, Goodman RM. Hyper-reactivity to atropine in Down's syndrome. N Engl J Med 1968;279:407–410.
88. Jahnke W. Atropinvergiftigungen im heiszen Klima. Arch Toxikol 1957;16:243–247.
89. Horne GD. Sensitivity to atropine in anhydrotic heat exhaustion. Trans R Soc Trop Med Hyg 1984;48:153–155.
90. Larkin GL. Occupational atropine poisoning via aerosol. Lancet 1991;337:917.
91. Schafer WD, Sauerland H-J. Observations after long term atropine administration [Beobachtungen nach atropine-Langzeit verordnung]. Klin Monatsblaetter Augenheilkunde 1976;68:421–423.
92. Cooper MJ, Abinader EG. Atropine induced ventricular fibrillation: Case report and review of the literature. Am Heart J 1979;97:225–228.
93. Coates W. Belladonna poisoning. Br Med J 1947;2:886.
94. Seelye HH. Atropia poisoning from eating turkey. Med Rec 1894;45:14.
95. Winslow RL, Pecora JL. Atropine pupils. JAMA 1974;229: 1863–1864.
96. Lapan D, Smith JW. Atropine coma: Physostigmine reversal. Ariz Med 1977;34:159–160.
97. Michelson EA, Schneider SM, Martin TG. Adult inadvertent massive oral atropine overdose. Vet Hum Toxicol 1991;33:360.
98. Corbett BW, McBay AJ. Atropine poisoning. Bull Int Assoc Forens Toxicol 1978;14(1):37–38.
99. Amitai Y, Singer R, Almog S, Bentur Y. Atropine poisoning in children from automatic injectors during the Gulf Crisis. Vet Hum Toxicol 1991;33:360.
100. Greenblatt DJ, Shader RI. Atropine overdose in three children. Br J Anaesth 1972;44:750.
101. Listwan IA, Whealy NG. Mental symptoms in poisoning with atropine and its derivatives. Med J Aust 1953;1:581–583.
102. Whittemore JB. Mental symptoms in poisoning with atropine and its derivatives. Med J Aust 1952;1:752.
103. Gross NJ, Skorodin MS. Massive overdose of atropine methonitrate with only slight untoward effects. Lancet 1985;2:386.
104. Purcell MJ. Atropine poisoning in infancy. Br Med J 1966;1: 738.
105. Stephenson JBP. Atropine methonitrate in management of near fatal reflex anoxic seizures. Lancet 1979;2:955.
106. Meerstadt PWD. Atropine poisoning in early infancy due to eumydrin drops. Br Med J 1982;285:196–197.

BENZTROPINE

Benztropine mesylate, a synthetic tertiary amine antimuscarinic antiparkinsonian agent that resembles both atropine and diphenhydramine in chemical structure (Fig. 46–1),[1,2] exhibits anticholinergic, antihistaminic, and local anesthetic properties. Overdose may produce an anticholinergic poisoning syndrome, which can be present for at least 9 days[3] and may end fatally.[4] Benztropine mesylate is also known as benzatropine methanesulfonate.[5]

Use

Benztropine mesylate is used for the symptomatic treatment of parkinsonism (postencephalitic, idiopathic, and arteriosclerotic types). It is also used for the treatment of drug-induced extrapyramidal symptoms except for tardive dyskinesia, which may be exacerbated. It has been investigated for use in the control of bedwetting by schizophrenic patients.[6]

Product Formulation

Benztropine mesylate is available in oral form as tablets of 0.5, 1, and 2 mg, and for parenteral injection as 1 mg/mL with sodium chloride 9 mg/mL (Cogentin, Benzylate, Cogentine, Congentinol).[1]

Therapeutic Dose

Benztropine mesylate is administered orally or by intramuscular injection. It may also be given intravenously. For parkinsonian syndrome the usual adult dose is 1 to 2 mg daily (0.5–6 mg daily).[1] For symptomatic relief of antipsychotic agent-induced extrapyramidal reactions (except tardive dyskinesia), the dose is usually 1 to 4 mg once or twice daily. If it is used for an acute dystonic reaction, benztropine mesylate may be given intravenously at a dose of 1 to 2 mg.

Toxic Dose

A 17-year-old who had ingested an unknown quantity of benztropine mesylate was found wandering, incoherent, disoriented, and confused with hot flushed skin, dilated pupils, and dry mouth; symptoms diminished after 32 hours.[7] A 20-year-old ingested 70 mg of benztropine mesylate plus an unknown amount of amitriptyline; she recovered.[8] A 35-year-old man received 12 mg of benztropine daily for 3 weeks and recovered.[9] A 20-month-old ingested an unknown number of tablets of benztropine, developed an acute dystonic reaction, and recovered.[2]

Fatal Dose

Two fatal cases have been reported: a 30-year-old man observed taking a handful of benztropine tablets 1.5 hours before death, and a patient found dead.[4]

Toxicokinetics

The toxicokinetics of benztropine have not been systematically studied. Data on its bioavailability, half-life, apparent volume of distribution, and clearance are not available. Therapeutic serum levels have not been established. Patients receiving 4 mg/d exhibited plasma levels of 19 to 125 ng/mL.[10]

Elimination

Urine levels of 5.3 to 123 ng/mL were observed after 4 mg/d was ingested by four patients.[10]

Drug Interactions

Administration of benztropine with other drugs having anticholinergic effects may increase the risk of adverse anticholinergic effects. If benztropine is administered with phenothiazines or tricyclic antidepressants, paralytic ileus, hyperthermia, or heat intolerance may occur and may be fatal.[5]

Pregnancy/Lactation

Safe use of benztropine during pregnancy and lactation has not been established.

Mechanism of Action

Benztropine exerts its effects by blocking central and peripheral muscarinic cholinergic receptor sites. Overdose is followed by an anticholinergic syndrome.

Clinical Presentation

Adverse Effects

Adverse reactions to benztropine include dryness of the mouth, blurred vision, mydriasis, nausea, nervousness, tachycardia, and skin rash (see also Chapter 19).

Toxic Effects

In high doses or in particularly susceptible patients, benztropine may produce mental confusion or excitement, weakness, inability to move muscle groups, urinary retention, constipation, numbness of the extremities, listlessness, depression, vomiting, paralytic ileus, hyperthermia, fever, heat stroke, and visual hallucinations.[1] Choreoathetoid movements of the fingers, agitation, repetitive picking at bed sheets, rapid incoherent speech, and auditory and visual hallucinations may occur.[8] Rectal temperature may reach 108°F.[9] Coma may be observed.[9] Acute dystonic reaction (buccolingual, torticollic, and tortipelvic forms of muscle involvement) and signs of acute dyskinesias (lip smacking and chewing) may not be accompanied by other signs of acute anticholinergic poisoning such as tachycardia, flushing, mydriasis, and mania.[2] A suicide attempt with benztropine led to a severe anticholinergic poisoning syndrome that lasted 9 days.[3] Anticholinergic toxicity may last 8 days[8] to 9 days.[3] Acute psychosis characterized by confusion and bizarre behavior has been reported.[11,12]

Laboratory

Analytical Methods

A quantitative gas chromatography–mass spectrometry (GC–MS) assay is available for determination of benztropine in human urine and plasma. The assay can measure 5 ng/mL benztropine with about 6% precision.[10] The assay is sensitive (to 2 ng/mL) and specific when high-performance liquid chromatography, gas chromatography, or thin-layer chromatography methods is used; cross-reactions of benztropine, phenothiazines, and butyrophenones may occur.[2] Benztropine is not detected during GC–MS because the energization produced during mass spectroscopy causes cleavage of benztropine into diphenhydramine and "a tropic compound" detected by the tropic acid nucleus of the compound.[2] Gas chromatography with a combination of electron impact and chemical ionization mass spectrometry was useful in determing the concentration of benztropine in blood and urine (7.123 μg/L).[13]

Blood Levels

An adult with acute anticholinergic poisoning syndrome (agitation, active hallucinations, and combativeness) had a serum benztropine level of 100 ng/mL.[3] It decreased in an erratic course until it reached 9 ng/mL, at which time there was no further evidence of anticholinergic toxicity. Postmortem blood benztropine concentrations of 700 ng/mL have been reported after ingestion of an unknown amount of benztropine.[14]

Ancillary Tests

The electrocardiogram may indicate a sinus tachycardia without evidence of QRS or QT_c prolongation.[8] The patient should be observed for evidence of rhabdomyolysis (urine myoglobin, serum creatine kinase).

Treatment

Stabilization

Patients should be evaluated for intact airway, respiration (including tidal volume), and circulatory status. Although there have been no reports of sudden hemodynamic irritability, fatalities have occurred within 1.5 hours of ingestion. Patients should be carefully treated with oxygen, naloxone, glucose, and, if indicated, thiamine if there is evidence of altered mental status. Arterial blood gases are determined and electrocardiographic monitoring instituted. Patients should be treated as if a cyclic antidepressant has been ingested in overdose (see Chapter 37) and are initially treated in an intensive care facility.

Gut Decontamination

The time to reach peak blood levels is not available. In view of an early fatal response, an attempt should be made to empty the stomach and introduce activated charcoal. Such measures may be taken at least as late as 12 hours after ingestion in those symptomatic patients who have ingested a large quantity of drug, in view of its strong anticholinergic properties. Syrup of ipecac must be used cautiously, if at all, and within the very first hour of the ingestion, in view of the possibility of seizures and obtundation. There is no evidence that activated charcoal adsorbs benztropine.

Elimination Enhancement

There are no data on the apparent volume of distribution of benztropine. It may be assumed to be large, similar to other anticholinergic products such as cyclic antidepressants. There has been no experience with active elimination methods such as forced diuresis, peritoneal dialysis, hemodialysis, and hemoperfusion.

Antidote

Physostigmine use (see Chapter 37) should be carefully reserved as most patients with benztropine overdose require only supportive care while it is being cleared from the body. If there is a serious danger to agitation and hallucinations without a history of gangrene, asthma, ulcerative colitis, cardiovascular disease, or history of seizures, then physostigmine may be considered.

Supportive Measures

Patients who are admitted should receive cardiac monitoring until they are symptom free for 24 hours. No drugs with significant anticholinergic activity should be administered. The bladder should be catheterized, if necessary. Hyperthermia usually resolves with conservative measures (cooling blankets, ice bags). Patients usually require observation for a number of days. Serum benztropine levels, if they can be obtained, may have some correlation with the clinical course. Hypertension may appear early in the course of poisoning; it is usually mild and requires no special treatment.

REFERENCES—BENZTROPINE

1. McEvoy GK, ed. *AHFS Drug Information 94.* Bethesda, MD: American Society of Hospital Pharmacists, 1994:730–731.
2. Howrie DL, Rowley AH, Krenzelok EP. Benztropine-induced acute dystonic reaction. Ann Emerg Med 1986;15:594–596.
3. Fahy P, Arnold P, Curry SC, Bond R. Serial serum drug concentrations and prolonged anticholinergic toxicity after benztropine (Cogentin) overdose. Am J Emerg Med 1989;7:199–202.
4. Baselt RC, Cravey RH. *Disposition of Toxic Drugs and Chemicals in Man.* 3rd ed. Chicago: Year Book Medical, 1989:84–85.
5. Reynolds JEF, ed. *Martindale: The Extra Pharmacopoeia.* 30th ed. London: Pharmaceutical Press, 1993:421–422.
6. Costa JF, Sramek J, Bera RB, et al. Control of bedwetting with benztropine. Am J Psychiatry 1990;147:674.
7. Perry PJ, Wilding DC, Juhl RP. Anticholinergic psychosis. Am J Hosp Pharm 1978;35:725–727.
8. Stern TA. Continuous infusion of physostigmine in anticholinergic delirium. J Clin Psychiatry 1983;44:463–464. Case Report.
9. Goldstein MR, Kasper R. Hyperpyrexia and coma due to overdose of benztropine. South Med J 1968;61:988–989.
10. Jindal SP, Lutz T, Hallstrom C, Vestergaard P. A stable isotope dilution assay for the antiparkinsonian drug benztropine in biological fluids. Clin Chim Acta 1981;112:267–273.
11. Ananthy JV, Jain RC. Benztropine psychosis. Can Psychiatr Assoc J 1973;18:409–414.
12. Woody GE, O'Brien CP. Anticholinergic toxic psychosis in drug abusers treated with benztropine. Compr Psychiatry 1974;15:439–442.
13. Rosano TG, Meola JM, Jindal SP, et al. Benztropine indentification and quantitation in a suicidal overdose case. In: *Proceedings, California Association of Toxicologists, October 1993.*
14. Moffat AC, Jackson JV, Moss MS, et al. *Clarke's Isolation and Identification of Drugs.* 2nd ed. London: Pharmaceutical Press, 1986:388.

DICYCLOMINE HYDROCHLORIDE

Dicyclomine overdose has been reported mainly in young children who have ingested products usually containing dicyclomine together with other drugs. Blood concentrations of dicyclomine may be roughly correlated with toxic symptoms, but are not correlated with dose ingested in children and can be used only as an indication of ingestion and not necessarily as a guide to severity of disease. Signs and symptoms of overdose should be treated as an anticholinergic poisoning with symptomatic and supportive treatment. Sudden death has been observed.

Use

Dicyclomine hydrochloride is used in functional disturbances of the gastrointestinal tract such as irritable bowel syndrome. Although not approved by the Food and Drug Administration for other uses, dicyclomine has been used for infantile colic[1] and to increase bladder capacity in patients with uninhibited bladder contractions that result in incontinence.[2]

Product Formulation

Dicyclomine hydrochloride is available in oral capsules of 10 and 20 mg (Bentyl); as a solution of 10 mg/5 mL with parabens and propylene glycol (Bentyl); and as an injection for intramuscular use only, 10 mg/mL (with or without chlorobutanol, different sources). Dicyclomine hydrochloride is also marketed as Merbentyl (United Kingdom), Ametil (Italy), Bentylol (Canada), Benacol (United States), and Procyclomin (Australia).

Dicyclomine hydrochloride is a constituent of some multiingredient preparations such as Kolanticon gel (United Kingdom), which contains dicyclomine 2.5 mg with aluminum hydroxide 200 mg and magnesium oxide 100 mg in 5 mL; it also contains dimethylsiloxane 20 mg in 5 mL. Debendox (United Kingdom)/Bendectin (United States) was withdrawn by the manufacturer in 1983 from both the U.K. and U.S. markets; it contained dicyclomine hydrochloride 10 mg, doxylamine succinate 10 mg, and pyridoxine hydrochloride 10 mg.[3–6]

Source

Dicyclomine hydrochloride is a synthetic chemical.

Therapeutic Dose

Oral

Oral dicyclomine hydrochloride therapy is initiated with 80 mg daily divided in four equal doses for 1 week. If additional therapy is required, the dosage can be raised to 160 mg/d in four equal doses for a maximum of 1 week.[4]

Intramuscular

The intramuscular dose of dicyclomine hydrochloride is 80 mg daily in four equally divided doses administered for no longer than 1 to 2 days.[3–5]

Toxic Dose

A 2½-year-old child ingested 90 mg, exhibited slightly dilated pupils, and appeared to be slightly intoxicated; she survived.[7] A 2-year-old ingested 20 Bendectin tablets (dicyclomine hydrochloride dose, 200 mg) and survived.[8] A 15-month-old boy ingested 30 Debendox tablets containing 300 mg dicyclomine and survived.[9] A 1-year 8-month-old child ingested dicyclomine 200 mg, experienced a toxic delirium, and was discharged in 1 day.[10] A 3½-year-old boy ingested an unknown quantity of Debendox and became agitated, restless, and hallucinative with dilated pupils, dry mouth, hot dry skin, and tachycardia; he responded to treatment and was discharged in 1 day.[11] Administration of 10 mg of dicyclomine to two infants aged 5 and 6 weeks resulted in apnea and cyanosis in one case and rigidity and apnea in the second case; both recovered.[12] Other infants have experienced similar symptoms[13] including, in one case, respiratory arrest.[14] The maximum human doses of dicyclomine hydrochloride recorded were 600 mg by mouth in a 10-month-old child and approximately 1500 mg in an adult, each of whom survived.[5]

Fatal Dose

An 18-month-old ate a bottle full of Debendox tablets; he developed signs of anticholinergic toxicity and respiratory and cardiac arrest, and died.[9] A 3-year-old ingested 100 Bendectin tablets, developed signs of restlessness, disorientation, and ataxia and tonic–clonic seizures, and later died in cardiorespiratory arrest.[15]

Toxicokinetics

Absorption

Dicyclomine is rapidly absorbed after oral administration, with a peak plasma dicyclomine concentration of about 20 ng/mL observed in one subject 1.5 hours after a single 20-mg oral dose. Oral administration of a single 40-mg sustained-release tablet resulted in a peak plasma concentration of approximately 80 ng/mL in 2 hours. Within the next 2 hours the level dropped to about 25 ng/mL.[16]

Distribution

The apparent volume of distribution of dicyclomine is about 3.65 L/kg.[4]

Elimination

Approximately 80% of a dose is eliminated in the urine and 10% in the feces.[17] The half-life of the drug in the initial distribution phase is about 1.8 hours and the half-life in the terminal elimination phase is about 9 to 10 hours.[4]

Drug Interactions

Dicyclomine is an anticholinergic drug and will probably interact in an additive manner with other drugs whose site of action is the muscarinic cholinergic receptor. Agents that may increase certain actions or side effects of anticholinergic drugs include amantadine, class I antiarrhythmic agents of (eg, quinidine), antihistamines, antipsychotic agents (eg, phenothiazines), benzodiazepines, monoamine oxidase inhibitors, narcotic analgesics (eg, meperidine), nitrates and nitrites, sympathomimetic agents, and tricyclic antidepressants.

Pregnancy/Lactation

Bendectin has not been demonstrated to be associated with a significant increase in teratogenic congenital limb defects.[18–20] The Food and Drug Administration has placed dicyclomine in Pregnancy Category B (no evidence of risk in humans).[21] A prospective study on 22,977 pregnant women, 620 of whom were given Debendox during pregnancy, disclosed a normal outcome in 95%, a malformed infant in 1.3%, and other outcomes in 3.7%. In the same series, 2.0% of patients not given Debendox produced infants with malformations.[22]

Mechanism of Action

Dicyclomine hydrochloride is a competitive antagonist at muscarinic cholinergic neurons.

Clinical Presentation

Serious toxicity has been described in very young children, although there are few reports of ingestion of dicyclomine alone. Signs and symptoms of overdose cases that terminated fatally include restlessness, disorientation, ataxia, myoclonic seizures, tonic–clonic seizures, flushed facies, fever, agitation, dilated pupils, rolling of eyes, coarse nystagmus, vomiting, and cardiac and respiratory arrest.[9,15,23] Survivors of overdose have exhibited dilated pupils, an intoxicated appearance,[7] dry mouth, smacking of the lips, agitation, confusion, nervousness,[8] vomiting, drowsiness, flushed facies,[9] toxic delirium,[10] hallucinations, hot dry skin, tachycardia, apnea, cyanosis, and rigidity.[12] Reported cases of apnea, seizures, and coma following dicyclomine use all occurred within 30 minutes of administration.[12–14]

Laboratory

Analytical Methods

Dicyclomine has been determined in blood by gas chromatography using nitrogen-selective (limit of detection in plasma, 1 μg/mL)[16] or flame ionization detection.[24] A capillary gas chromatography method using nitrogen-selective detection is adequate for analyzing plasma concentrations as low as 5 ng/mL.[25]

Blood Levels

A 2½-year-old found unresponsive in a crib had a blood dicyclomine concentration of 505 ng/mL. Another 2½-month-old child was discovered apneic and died with a blood dicyclomine concentration of 221 ng/mL. The concentrations measured in these infants represented 10 and 4 times adult therapeutic concentrations, respectively.[23] A 9½-week-old infant who apparently died of sudden infant death syndrome had a postmortem blood dicyclomine level of 200 ng/mL; he had received two 5-mg doses of dicyclomine on the day of death.[24]

Treatment

Treatment of dicyclomine overdose is largely symptomatic and supportive and should follow the guidelines for treatment of poisoning with other anticholinergic agents.

REFERENCES—DICYCLOMINE HYDROCHLORIDE

1. Weissbluth M, Christoffel KK, Todd Davis A. Treatment of infantile colic with dicyclomine hydrochloride. J Pediatr 1984;104:951–955.
2. Fischer CP, Dioko A, Lapides J. The anticholinergic effects of dicyclomine hydrochloride in uninhibited neurogenic bladder dysfunction. J Urol 1978;120:328–329.
3. Reynolds JEF, ed. *Martindale: The Extra Pharmacopoeia.* 30th ed. London: Pharmaceutical Press, 1993:423.
4. McEvoy GK, ed. *AHFS Drug Information 94,* Bethesda, MD: American Society of Hospital Pharmacists, 1994:747–748.
5. *Physicians' Desk Reference.* 46th ed. Montvale, NJ: Medical Economics, 1992:1322–1324.
6. Dicyclomine (hydrochloride). In: Dollery C, ed. *Therapeutic Drugs.* Edinburgh: Churchill Livingstone, 1991:D103–D105.
7. Pittman AR Jr. Accidental administration of dicyclomine (Bentyl[R]) hydrochloride in overdosage. NC Med J 1952;13:486.
8. Wise GW, Green VA. Toxicant cases: Bendectin ingestion. Aaction 1974;2:5.
9. Meadow SR, Leeson GA. Poisoning with delayed release tablets: Treatment of Debendox poisoning with purgation and dialysis. Arch Dis Child 1974;49:310–312.
10. Greenblatt DJ, Allen MD, Koch-Weser J, Shader RI. Accidental poisoning with psychotropic drugs in children. Am J Dis Child 1976;130:507–511.
11. Clarkson SG, Glanvill. Debendox overdosage in children. Br Med J 1977;2:459–460.
12. Williams J, Watkin-Jones R. Dicyclomine: Worrying symptoms associated with its use in some small babies. Br Med J 1984;288:901.
13. Edwards PDL. Dicyclomine in babies. Br Med J 1984;288:1230.
14. Spoudeas H, Shribman S. Dicyclomine in babies. Br Med J 1984;288:1230.
15. Bayley M, Walsh FM, Valaske MJ. Fatal overdose from Bendectin. Clin Pediatr 1975;14:507–514.
16. Meffin PJ, Moore G, Thomas J. Determinations of dicyclomine in plasma by gas chromatography. Anal Chem 1973;45:1964–1966.
17. Danhof IE, Schreiber EC, Wiggans DS, Leyland HM. Metabolic dynamics of dicyclomine hydrochloride in man as influenced by various dose schedules and formulations. Toxicol Appl Pharmacol 1968;13:16–23.
18. Kalter H, Warkary J. Congenital malformations (second of two parts). N Engl J Med 1983;308:491–497.
19. Holmes LB. Teratogen update: Bendectin. Teratology 1983;27:277–281.
20. McCredie J, Kricher A, Elliott J, Forrest J. The innocent bystander: Doxylamine/dicyclomine/pyridoxime and congenital limb defects. Med J Aust 1984;140:525–527.
21. Friedman JM, Little BB, Brent RL, et al. Potential human teratogenicity of frequently prescribed drugs. Obstet Gynecol 1990;75:594–599.
22. Fleming DM, Knox JDE, Crombie DL. Debendox in early pregnancy and fetal malformation. Br Med J 1981;283:99–101.
23. Garriott JC, Rodriguez R, Norton LE. Two cases of death involving dicyclomine in infants: Measurement of therapeutic and toxic concentrations in blood. Clin Toxicol 1984;22:455–462.
24. Death syndrome (SIDS): A cause of death or an incidental finding? J Forens Sci 1986;31:1470–1474.
25. Walker BJ, Lang JF, Okerholm RA. Quantitative analysis of dicyclomine in human plasma by capillary gas chromatography and nitrogen-selective detection. J Chromatogr Biomed Appl 1987;416:150–153.

IPRATROPIUM BROMIDE

Ipratropium bromide overdose often follows excessive use of metered-dose inhalers for bronchospasm. Symptoms are short-lived and often remit spontaneously without any measures other than symptomatic and supportive treatment. One possible fatality has been described.[1]

Use

Ipratropium bromide is used as a bronchodilator for maintenance treatment of bronchospasm associated with chronic obstructive pulmonary disease, including chronic bronchitis and emphysema.[2–8] Ipratropium has been useful in organophosphate insecticide poisoning when given intratracheally.[9]

Product Formulation

In the United Kingdom, the aerosol (Atrovent) is supplied as a metered-dose inhaler with a mouthpiece. A 14-g vial provides sufficient medication for 200 inhalations.[3] Each actuation of the valve delivers 18 μg of ipratropium bromide from the mouthpiece. The inert ingredients are dichlordifluoromethane, dichlorotetrafluoroethane, and trichloromonofluoromethane as propellants. In the United Kingdom, each metered-dose inhaler contains 10 mL of ipratropium bromide and carrier freons. Each metered dose contains 20 μg of ipratropium bromide (Atrovent). Duovent is a 10-mL vial (20 metered doses) containing carrier freons, fenotenol hydrobromide 0.1 mg, and ipratropium bromide 40 μg per inhalation. It is also available in the United Kingdom as a nebulizer solution comprising an isotonic solution of ipratropium 0.5 mg/mL in normal saline in a 20-mL glass bottle.[10] Atrovent in the United Kingdom may be formulated with benzalkonium chloride (0.25 g/L) and edetic acid (EDTA) (0.5 g/L), both of which may have bronchoconstrictive properties.[11]

Source

Ipratropium bromide is prepared by chemical synthesis.

Therapeutic Dose

The usual starting dose of Atrovent is 2 inhalations (36 μg) four times daily with a maximum of 12 inhalations in 24 hours. It produces its maximal effect in adults at a dose of 40 to 80 μg delivered by 2 to 4 activations of the inhaler.[4] With the nebulized solution the optimal dose is between 50 and 125 μg for both adults and children.[4]

Toxic Dose

A 64-year-old patient with chronic obstructive pulmonary disease became agitated after taking "puff after puff."[1] She recovered in 24 hours. One elderly patient used the product 6 or more times per day, developed shortness of breath and increased bronchospasm, and recovered.[1]

Fatal Dose

A 66-year-old woman suspected of overusing Atrovent developed hypoxia secondary to status asthmaticus and apparently went into cardiac arrest. No further information is available.[1]

Toxicokinetics

Absorption

After it is inhaled ipratropium starts to act within 15 minutes. Activity peaks after 30 minutes to 2 hours, and is sustained for 3 to 4 hours. Ninety percent of the inhaled drug remains in the upper airways.[5] After inhalation or oral use, plasma concentration peaks in 2 hours.[6] After inhalation of 3 sniffs of 0.555 mg, a peak plasma concentration of 60 pg/mL was measured at 3 hours.[12]

Distribution

The volume of distribution of ipratropium bromide is approximately 5 L/kg.[13] Ipratropium does not cross the blood–brain barrier.[5]

Elimination

Most of a dose of ipratropium is excreted unchanged in the feces. Its half-life in the circulation is of the same order as that of atropine, about 3 to 2.8 hours.[4,12–16] Ipratropium bromide is partially metabolized. One metabolite is *N*-isopropylnoratrpropine bromomethylate.[12] Fifty percent appears unchanged in the urine after intravenous administration. Total clearance is 2325 mL/mg.[13]

Drug Interactions

Acute angle-closure glaucoma has been reported in elderly patients receiving combined nebulized ipratropium bromide and salbutamol.[17,18] Use with terbutaline sulfate inhalers has led to pharyngeal blistering.[19] The concurrent use of ipratropium and terbutaline does not result in a greater improvement in the (FEV_1) at 60 and 90 minutes, over inhaled terbutaline alone.[20] It may have an additive effect on bronchodilation when used with albuterol for the emergency treatment of acute severe asthma.[21–23]

Pregnancy/Lactation

It is unknown whether placental transfer or excretion into human milk occurs.[5] No adequately controlled studies have been conducted in pregnant women.[5]

Mechanism of Action

The predominantly central distribution of cholinergic nerves and muscarinic receptors in the airways contrasts with the more peripheral distribution of beta-adrenergic receptors.[4,7] Ipratropium is a competitive antagonist of the muscarinic acetylcholine receptor. By blocking the cholinergic receptor present on the surface of most cells, it inhibits the release of cyclic guanosine monophosphate, which in turn inhibits the release of bronchoconstrictive mediators, such as antihistamine.[15]

Clinical Presentation

Large doses of ipratropium can lead to cough, a metallic or bitter taste, dry mouth, buccal ulceration,[19,24] blurred vision, paralytic ileus,[25,26] and bladder neck obstruction.[27] Paradoxical bronchoconstriction may occur.[7,27,28]

One case of drug abuse and five possible cases of overdose (with Atropent inhalation aerosol) have been reported to the manufacturer since the product was marketed in 1987.[1] A 64-year-old woman was admitted to the hospital with flushed skin, adynamic ileus, distended bladder, pulse of 120 beats/min, and orthostatic hypotension. The symptoms spontaneously subsided within 24 hours. Several elderly patients developed shortness of breath and increased bronchospasm after several weeks of therapy. The product was withdrawn and the patients recovered without any treatment.[1] A 66-year-old woman developed hypoxia secondary to status asthmaticus and went into cardiac arrest; she was suspected of overusing Atrovent.[1]

Laboratory

Analytical Methods

There is no reliable method for measurement of ipratropium in body fluids.[12,16] Pharmacokinetic studies have been performed using labeled drug.[10] Few clinical laboratories have the facilities to measure blood ipratropium levels. There is little evidence that blood level studies would be clinically useful. A radioreceptor assay can detect urine levels to 5 ng/mL and plasma levels to 500 ng/mL.[13]

Blood Levels

Blood levels have not been studied in overdose.

Abnormalities

Intraocular pressure may increase after ipratropium bromide use.[17,18]

Treatment

Stabilization

Patients developing side effects after excessive use often recover within 24 hours of cessation of ipratropium use.[1]

Elimination Enhancement

Measures to enhance elimination of ipratropium have not been used in patients with suspected overdose. Hemodialysis and hemoperfusion would probably be ineffective in view of the extensive volume of distribution.

Antidote

There is no antidote.

Supportive Measures

Patients who have used ipratropium excessively will probably respond to symptomatic and supportive care combined with cessation of drug use.

REFERENCES—IPRATROPIUM BROMIDE

1. Chin TH. Personal correspondence. Boehringer Ingleheim Pharmaceuticals, June 19, 1989; March 21, 1991.
2. Reynolds JEF, ed. *Martindale: The Extra Pharmacopoeia.* 30th ed. London: Pharmaceutical Press, 1993:427–428.
3. Atrovent. In: *Physicians' Desk Reference.* Montvale, NJ: Medical Economics, 1992:675–676.
4. Gross MJ. Ipratropium bromide. N Engl J Med 1988;319: 486–494.
5. Atsman J. Topics in clinical pharmacology: Ipratropium bromide in COPD and asthma. Am J Med Sci 1988;296:140–142.
6. Ipratropium. Med Lett Drugs Ther 1087;29(745):71–72.
7. Gross MJ, Skorodin MS. Anticholinergic, antimuscarinic bronchodilators. Am Rev Respir Dis 1984;129:8566–8700.
8. Wood M. Anticholinergic drugs: Anesthetic predmedication. In: Wood M, Wood AJJ, eds. *Drugs and Anesthesia.* 2nd ed. Baltimore: Williams & Wilkins, 1990:120–121.
9. Shemesh I, Bourvin A, Gold D, Kutscherowsky M. Chlorpyrifos poisoning treated with ipratropium and dantrolene: A case report. Clin Toxicol 1988;26:495–498.
10. Ipratropium bromide. In: Dollery C, ed. *Therapeutic Drugs.* Edinburgh: Churchill Livingstone, 1991:168–170.
11. Beasley CRW, Rafferty P, Holgate ST. Bronchoconstriction properties of preservatives in ipratropium bromide (Atrovent) nebuliser solution. Br Med J 1987;29:1197–1198.
12. Adlung VJ, Hohlen KD, Zeren S, Wahl D. Studies on the pharmacokinetics and biotransformation of ipratropium bromide in man. Arzneimittelforschung 1976;26:1005–1010.
13. Ensing K, de Zeeuw RA, Nossent GD, et al. Pharmacokinetics of ipratropium bromide after single dose inhalation and oral and intravenous administration. Eur J Clin Pharmacol 1989;36:189–194.
14. Engelhardt A, Klupp H. The pharmacology and toxicology of a new tropane alkaloid derivative. Postgrad Med J 1975; 51(suppl. 7):82–94.
15. Cugell DW. Chemical pharmacology and toxicology of ipratropium bromide. Am J Med 1986;8(suppl. 5A):18–22.
16. Rominger KL. Chemistry and pharmacokinetics of ipratropium bromide. Scand J Respir Dis 1979;suppl. 130:116–126.
17. Shah P, Dharjon L, Metcalfe T, Gibson JM. Acute angle closure glaucoma associated with nebulised ipratropium bromide and salbutamol. Br Med J 1992;304:40–41.
18. Humphreys DM. Acute angle closure glaucoma association with nebulised ipratropium bromide and salbutamol. Br Med J 1992;264:320.
19. High AS. Pharangeal blistering with combined inhalation therapy. Br Med J 1986;292:380.
20. Tiernan SM, Cellucci PP, Dire DJ. Adjunctive use of ipratropium bromide in the emergency treatment of acute asthma. Ann Emerg Med 1989;18:466–467.
21. Higgins RM, Stradling JR, Lane DJ. Should ipratropium bromide be added to beta-agonists in treatment of acute severe asthma? Chest 1988;94:718–722.
22. O'Driscoll BR, Taylor RJ, Horsley MG, et al. Nebulised salbutamol with and without ipratropium bromide in acute air flow obstruction. Lancet 1989;1:1418–1420.
23. Henry RL. Ipratropium bromide: An additive effect? J Paediatr Child Health 1990;26:124–125.
24. Spencer PA. Buccal ulceration with ipratropium bromide. Br Med J 1986;292:380.
25. Mulherin D, Fitzgerald MV. Meconium ileus equivalent in association with nebulised ipratropium bromide in cystic fibrosis. Lancet 1990;1:552.
26. Markus HS. Paralytic ileus associated with ipratropium. Lancet 1990;335:1224.
27. Lozewicz S. Blood outflow obstruction induced by ipratropium bromide. Postgrad Med J 1989;65:260–261.
28. O'Callaghan C, Milner AD, Swarbrick A. Paradoxical bronchoconstriction in wheezing infants after nebulised preservative free iso-osmolar ipratropium bronchitis. Br Med J 1989;299:1433–1434.

OXYBUTYNIN HYDROCHLORIDE

Oxybutynin hydrochloride is a smooth muscle antispasmodic agent used mainly in patients with urinary incontinence due to detrusion irritability or detrusion hyperreflexia.[1] Following an overdose, it may lead to a series of anticholinergic effects involving primarily the central nervous system, eyes, skin, and heart. There have been no fatalities.

Structure and Classification

Oxybutynin chloride is a synthetic tertiary amine that is chemically and pharmacologically similar to some anticholinergic antispasmodic local anesthetic and antihistamine components.[1–3]

Use

Oxybutynin is used in the treatment of urinary frequency, incontinence, and nocturnal enuresis; in uninhibited vesical hyperactivity after bladder surgery and prostatectomy; and in association with acute and chronic cystitis.[4–8]

Product Formulation

Oxybutynin chloride is available in 5-mg tablets and as a syrup (5 mg/5 mL).[1]

Source

Oxybutynin is a synthetic chemical product.

Therapeutic Dose

The usual adult dose of oxybutynin chloride is 5 mg two or three times daily to a maximum of 5 mg four times daily. In children older than 5 years of age, 5 mg twice daily to a maximum of 5 mg three times daily is the recommended dose.[1,2,6]

Toxic Dose

A 100-mg oral dose (20 5-mg tablets) were ingested by a 34-year-old woman. She became drowsy, hallucinated, and later becoming comatose. She recovered by the third day.[4]

Fatal Dose

Fatalities following overdose have not been reported.

Toxicokinetics

Absorption

Oxybutynin is rapidly absorbed in the gastrointestinal tract. The absolute systemic availability is about 6%. An average plasma concentration of about 8 ng/mL is reached less than 1 hour after oral ingestion of 5 mg.[3] Levels of 20 to 50 ng/mL have been reached following a 5-mg dose.

Distribution

The apparent volume of distribution is 0.5 to 1.2 L/kg.[3,9]

Elimination

Oxybutynin is rapidly metabolized in the liver to *N*-desethyloxybutinin and oxybutynin-*N*-oxide.[10] The elimination half-life is 2 hours. Very little oxybutynin is excreted unchanged in the urine (0.017% of a dose in 12 hours).

Drug Interactions

Alcohol or other sedatives may increase the drowsiness observed with oxybutynin. Antihistamines, tricyclic antidepressants, phenothiazines, and atropine may enhance the anticholinergic effects of oxybutynin.

Pregnancy/Lactation

Oxybutynin has not been studied in either pregnant or lactating women. The Food and Drug Administration has assigned the drug to Pregnancy Category B.[6]

Mechanism of Action

Oxybutynin is a direct smooth muscle relaxant with weak antimuscarinic properties. It exerts atropine-like anticholinergic action.[9] In addition, it possesses a local anesthetic/analgesic effect.[4,7] Oxybutynin has no antinicotinic effects at skeletal neuromuscular junctions or autonomic ganglia.[4]

Clinical Presentation

Overdose

Oxybutynin overdose may produce central nervous system disturbances such as restlessness, tremor, irritability, disorientation, seizures, delirium, hallucinatory excitement or psychotic behavior, widely dilated pupils, dry skin and mouth, and urinary retention, and cardiovascular symptoms including flushing, tachycardia, hypertension, hypotension, and circulatory failure. Fever, nausea, and vomiting may also occur. Severe overdose may lead to paralysis, respiratory failure, coma, and death.[1,4,11]

Adverse Effects

After a therapeutic dose of oxybutynin chloride, adverse effects are similar to those produced by other antimuscarinic agents and may include dry mouth, decreased sweating, urinary hesitancy and/or retention, hot flashes, fever, tachycardia, palpitations, vasodilation, amblyopia, transient blurred vision, mydriasis, cycloplegia, decreased lacrimation, and increased ocular tension. Other effects include drowsiness, weakness, dizziness, hallucinations, restlessness, insomnia, nausea, vomiting, decreased gastrointestinal motility, constipation, impotence, and suppression of lactation. Oxybutynin may aggravate signs and symptoms of hyperthyroidism, coronary heart disease, congestive heart failure, cardiac arrhythmias, hiatal hernia, hypertension, tachycardia, and prostatic hypertrophy. In patients with ulcerative colitis, it may enhance induction of paralytic ileus or toxic megacolon. In areas of high environmental temperature, oxybutynin may decrease sweating and induce fever and heat stroke.[5,6]

Laboratory

Analytical Methods

A radioreceptor assay is available.[9] The product and its metabolites have been studied by gas chromatography and mass spectrometry.[10] A preferred method comprises reverse-phase high-performance liquid chromatography with coulometric detection. The human detectable concentration is 0.1 ng.[3]

Blood Levels

Following a dose of 10 mg, the maximum plasma level is 16 ng/mL (about 38 nmol/L). Blood levels after an overdose have not been reported. Plasma analysis may be useful to confirm presence but not to guide treatment of oxybutynin after an overdose. With higher doses, the elimination half-life of 2 hours is probably increased, due to a dose-related increase in the apparent volume of distribution.[3]

Abnormalities

The electrocardiogram showed evidence of sinus tachycardia lasting 3 hours following an overdose of 100 mg of oxybutyinin. Ventricular premature beats lasted 30 hours. Full recovery followed in 3 days.[4]

Treatment

Overdose with oxybutynin may be treated with gastric lavage if the patient is seen with 2 hours. Treatment is largely symptomatic and supportive. Emesis induction is not advised in patients who are precomatose, having seizures, or in a psychotic state. Activated charcoal may be useful. Fever is treated with cooling measures. Airway patency should be ascertained at all times. Assisted ventilation may be required if paralysis of respiratory muscles occurs.[1] In patients with severe intoxication, slow carefully titrated intravenous administration of a 2% solution of thiopental sodium or rectal infusion of 100 × 200 mL of a 2% solution of chloral hydrate may be necessary to combat extreme excitement. Physostigmine salicylate may be considered to counteract central nervous system disturbances; however, this product may enhance a tendency toward seizures, bronchospasm, or asystole (see Chapter 38). Restlessness and delirium can be treated with diazepam. Phenothiazines can lead to additive anticholinergic effects. Intravenous fluids may be necessary because of the vomiting.[1,4]

REFERENCES—OXYBUTYNIN HYDROCHLORIDE

1. Thuroff JW, Bunke B, Ebner A, et al. Randomized double-blind multi-center trial on treatment of frequency, urgency and incontinence related to detrusion hyperactivity: Oxybutinin versus propantheline versus placebo. J Urol 1991;125:813–817.
2. Reynolds JEF, ed. *Martindale: The Extra Pharmacopoeia.* 30th ed. London: Pharmaceutical Press, 1993:429.
3. Douchamps J, Derenne F, Stockis A, et al. The pharmacokinetics of oxybutynin in man. Eur J Clin Pharmacol 1988; 35:515–520.
4. Banerjee S, Routledge PA, Pugh S, Smith PM. Poisoning with oxybutynin. Hum Exp Toxicol 1991;10:222–226.
5. Malone-Lee J, Lubel D, Szonyi G. Low dose oxybutynin for the unstable bladder. Br Med J 1992;304:1053.
6. *Physicians' Desk Reference.* 46th ed. Montvale NJ: Medical Economics, 1992:1332–1333.
7. Diokno AC, Lapides J. Oxybutynin: A new drug with analgesic and anticholinergic properties. J Urol 1972;108:307–309.
8. Moisey CU, Stephenson TP, Brendler OB. The urodynamic and subjective results of treatment of detrusion Instability with oxybutinin chloride. Br J Urol 1980;52:472–475.
9. Aaltonen L, Allonen H, Iisalo E, et al. Antimuscarinic activity of oxybutynin in the human plasma quantitated by a radioreceptor assay. Acta Pharmacol Toxicol 1984;55: 100–103.
10. Lindeke D, Brotell H, Karlen B, et al. Determination of oxybutynin (4-diethylamino but-2-ynyl-2-cyclohexyl-2-phenylglycolate) in serum and urine by gas chromatography/mass spectrometry with single ion detection. Acta Pharma Suec 1981;18:25–34.
11. Mozer CH. Personal communication. Marion Merrell Dow, November 15, 1993.

PIRENZEPINE: A MUSCARINIC M_1-RECEPTOR ANTAGONIST

Pirenzepine is a muscarinic cholinergic receptor antagonist. In overdose, it can be expected to exhibit anticholinergic clinical effects. It acts synergistically with cimetidine to reduce gastric acid output.[1,2]

Product Formulation

Pirenzepine dihydrochloride (Gastrozepine) is available in the United Kingdom in oral form. Each tablet contains about 50 mg of the anhydrous substance.

Therapeutic Dose

The dose is 50 mg given twice daily up to a maximum of 150 mg (one tablet three times a day).

Fatal Dose

No deaths from pirenzepine have been reported.

Toxicokinetics

Bioavailability	20–30%
Peak plasma level	20–30 μg/L (after 25 mg)
Time to peak plasma level	2–3 hours
Volume of distribution	0.2 L/kg
Plasma protein binding	12%
Elimination half-life	11 hours
Excreted unchanged	7–12%

Pirenzepine selectively blocks muscarinic receptors controlling gastric and acid pepsin secretion.

Clinical Presentation

In overdose, anticholinergic (antimuscarinic) effects and sedation may be observed.

Laboratory

Concentrations of pirenzepine in biological fluids have been determined by high-performance liquid chromatography (sensitivity of 100 μg/mL) and radioimmunoassay.[4]

Treatment

Treatment of overdose is symptomatic and supportive. Hemodialysis would not be expected to remove significant amounts of pirenzepine (low volume of distribution), but plasma concentrations of pirenzepine can be reduced by up to 50% during hemodialysis. There is no antidote.

REFERENCES—PIRENZEPINE

1. Hammer R, Giachetti A. Muscarinic receptor subtypes M_1 and M_2: Biochemical and functional characterization. Life Sci 1982;31:291–298.
2. Tryba M, Huchzermeyer H, Torok M, et al. Single drug and combined medication with cimetidine, antacids and pirenzepine in the prophylaxis of acute upper gastrointestinal bleeding. Hepto-gastroenterology 1983;30:154–157.
3. Lauritsen K, Laursen LS, Rask-Madsen J. Clinical pharmacokinetics of drugs used in the treatment of gastrointestinal diseases (Part I). Clin Pharmacokinet 1990;19:11–31.
4. Meinecke I, Witsch D, Brendel E. Sensitive high performance liquid chromatographic determination of pirenzepine in plasma. J Chromatogr 1986;375:369–375.

PROCYCLIDINE

Procyclidine is a synthetic antimuscarinic agent with actions and uses similar to those of trihexiphenidyl. Reports of overdose are rare[1] and usually reflect the presence of other drugs.[2]

Structure and Classification

Procyclidine is a synthetic tertiary amine structurally and pharmacologically related to trihexyphenidyl. It has an atropine-like action.[3,4]

Use

Procyclidine is used for the symptomatic treatment of parkinsonism and to alleviate the extrapyramidal syndrome induced by drugs such as the phenothiazine derivatives, but it is of no value against tardive dyskinesia.

Product Formulation

Procyclidine hydrochloride is available as 5-mg oral tablets (Kemadrin) in the United States. It is also available as a liquid oral preparation, 2.5 to 5 mg (Arpicolin), and as an intravenous injection, 10 mg in 2 mL (Komadra), in the United Kingdom.[4,5]

Source

Procyclidine is a synthetic chemical.

Therapeutic Dose

The usual initial dosage for symptomatic treatment of Parkinson's syndrome is 2.5 mg three times daily. Increments of 2.5 mg are added until symptoms are controlled.

Toxicokinetics

Absorption

Procyclidine is rapidly and completely absorbed after oral administration. Systemic bioavailability is 75% due to presystemic metabolism. After a 10-mg oral dose, plasma procyclidine concentration peaks in 2 hours. Steady-state plasma concentrations following daily use of 10 to 30 mg average about 0.15 mg/L.[2]

Distribution

The apparent volume of distribution is 0.7 to 1.3 L/kg.[2]

Elimination

The elimination half-life is 8 to 18 hours.[2,6] A *para*-hydroxylated metabolite was isolated from the blood in a patient with a fatal overdose.[1]

Pregnancy/Lactation

Safe use during pregnancy or lactation has not been established.

Clinical Presentation

Reports of overdose are rare.[1] Symptoms are due to its anticholinergic action (dry mouth, blurred vision, constipation, urinary retention, agitation, restlessness, confusion). Severe sleeplessness, visual hallucinations, auditory hallucinations, seizures, and death have been reported.[1,5] Worsening of mental symptoms or toxic psychosis may occur in patients with mental disorders who are being treated for extrapyramidal symptoms. High doses may cause vertigo and possible confusion or hallucinations, especially in the elderly. Other symptoms are similar to those observed with use of other antimuscarinic (anticholinergic) agents.

Laboratory

Analytical Methods

Plasma procyclidine can be determined by gas–liquid chromatography, a method that detects plasma levels down to 10 μg/L.[7]

Blood Levels

In overdose blood concentrations of procyclidine have averaged 2.7 μg/mL.[2]

Treatment

The patient should be placed in a controlled hospital setting after ascertaining airway, breathing, and circulatory status. Electrocardiographic monitoring should be instituted and access to intravenous fluids and oxygen provided. Seizures are treated with intravenous diazepam. Supportive therapy is the mainstay of management.

REFERENCES—PROCYCLIDINE

1. Ashton PG. Two fatalities involving procyclidine and the identification of a procyclidine metabolite. Bull Int Assoc Forens Toxicol 1980;15:9–11.
2. Baselt RC, Cravey RH. *Disposition of Toxic Drugs and Chemicals in Man.* 3rd ed. Chicago: Year Book Medical, 1989:720–721.
3. Reynolds JEF, ed. *Martindale: The Extra Pharmacopoeia.* 30th ed. London: Pharmaceutical Press, 1993:431.
4. Procyclidine hydrochloride. In: McEvoy GK, ed. *AHFS Drug Information 94.* Bethesda, MD: American Society of Hospital Pharmacists, 1994:732–733.
5. Procyclidine. In: Dollery CT, ed. *Therapeutic Drugs.* Edinburgh: Churchill Livingstone, 1991:240–245.
6. Whiteman PD, Fowbe ASE, Hamilton MJ, et al. Pharmacokinetics and pharmacodynamics of procyclidine in man. Eur J Clin Pharmacol 1985;28:73–78.
7. Dean K, Land G, Bye A. Analysis of procyclidine in human plasma and urine by gas–liquid chromatography. J Chromatogr 1980;221:408–413.

SCOPOLAMINE

Scopolamine (hyoscine) is a naturally occurring belladonna alkaloid and anticholinergic agent. Its peripheral action resembles that of atropine. It antagonizes the action of acetylcholine at cholinergic postganglionic nerve endings. Scopolamine is a tertiary amine and therefore may cross the blood–brain barrier and enter the central nervous system. Scopolamine is generally used by anesthesiologists as a premedicant when its central sedative effects and smaller rise in heart rate are desired.[1] The transdermal patch is available over-the-counter in Europe.[2]

Reports of accidental poisoning with transdermal scopolamine have resulted from a misinterpretation of the prescribing information: patients either applied subsequent transdermal patches at intervals more frequent than the recommended 3 days or applied multiple transdermal systems.[3] Side effects with increased blood levels of scopolamine have included hallucinations, fever, confusion, and disorientation.[3–5] Treatment of scopolamine overdose is largely symptomatic and supportive.

Structure and Classification

Scopolamine is composed of a tropic acid residue attached to a complex organic base, scopine.[6,7] The different scopolamine compounds are known by the following names:

Scopolamine butyl bromide	Hyoscine *N*-butyl bromide
Scopolamine hydrobromide	Hyoscine hydrobromide
Scopolamine methyl bromide	Hyoscine methobromide
Scopolamine methyl nitrate	Hyoscine methonitrate

Use

Scopolamine is used by anesthesiologists as a premedicant and to control postoperative nausea and vomiting.[1] It is also administered by the transdermal route to treat motion sickness.[8–10]

Product Formulation

Each transdermal scopolamine patch contains 1.5 mg of scopolamine and is programmed to deliver 0.5 mg scopolamine over 3 days.[4] Buccal scopolamine is available in the United Kingdom as an over-the-counter preparation (Kwells). Scopolamine hydrobromide for parenteral injection is available in strengths of 0.3, 0.4, 0.86, and 1 mg/mL.[11]

Source

Scopolamine is a synthetic chemical product.

Therapeutic Dose

The adult parenteral dose of scopolamine is 0.2 to 0.6 mg. It is often given in combination with a narcotic analgesic because in some patients, particularly the elderly and the young, scopolamine produces confusion and restlessness.[1] The transdermal patch contains a drug reservoir of 1.5 mg of scopolamine and is designed to deliver 0.5 mg of the drug over a 72-hour period.

Toxicokinetics

Absorption

When the transdermal patch is applied, an initial primary dose of 140 μg is provided. The remainder is released at 5 μg/h.[1] Plasma concentrations in normal adults with a transdermal patch in place for 12 hours averaged 118 pg/mL, and the urinary scopolamine excretion rate was 0.6 μg/h.[12] Following ingestion of 0.6 mg scopolamine or use of buccal scopolamine 0.6 mg, peak levels of about 1.2 nmol/L scopolamine are obtained in about 1 hour.[13]

Distribution

The apparent volume of distribution in animals is 1.6 to 3.7 L/kg.[1]

Elimination

Following a 1-hour intravenous infusion of scopolamine 1.4 mg administered to a 16-year-old patient, the half-life was 46.8 minutes.[14] Systemic clearance varies between 0.4 and 0.9 L/kg/h.[1] The percentage of administered dose excreted as unchanged scopolamine is 1.7 to 5.9%.[1]

Pregnancy/Lactation

The Food and Drug Administration has placed the transdermal scopolamine patch in Pregnancy Category C. Controlled studies have not been performed in pregnant women or during lactation. Scopolamine crosses the placenta.[1]

Mechanism of Action

Scopolamine acts by antagonizing acetylcholine competitively at the neuroreceptor site. It also has an antimuscarinic action. Its action on the iris, ciliary body, and certain secretory glands (salivary, bronchial, sweat) is more potent than that of other belladonna alkaloids. Cardiac muscle, exocrine glands, and smooth muscles of the gastrointestinal tract are also affected. Therefore, the blood pressure increases, pulse rate may decrease, pupils become dilated, and hallucinations may occur.

Clinical Presentation

Acute Transdermal Use

Symptoms following transdermal use have included drowsiness, dry mouth, reduced concentration, confusion, and hallucinations.[3,5] The problems in three patients began 12 to 30 hours after the disk was placed. A 14-year-old girl developed hallucinations, visual problems, and anxiety 12 hours after use; she remained restless and confused for about 15 hours. A 5-year-old boy to whom 2 disks were attached became hyperactive and had hallucinations within 2 to 3 hours. A 28-year-old man experienced fatigue and dizziness one day after a transdermal dose was removed.[5]

Parenteral Use

Severe scopolamine toxicity presents with flushed, hot skin, dilated fixed pupils, cardiac arrhythmias, and convulsions. Without treatment, these conditions may terminate fatally.[15]

Adverse Reactions

The most frequent reaction to transdermal scopolamine is dryness of the mouth.[16,17] Drowsiness, blurred vision, and dilated pupils may be observed. Disorientation, memory disturbances, dizziness, restlessness, hallucinations, confusion, difficulty urinating, rashes, erythema, acute narrow-angle glaucoma, and dry, itchy, or red eyes have been seen less frequently.[5] A toxic psychosis was described in a 6-year-old child who wore the patch for 12 hours; The child was symptom free 14 hours after the patch was removed.[2] Seizures may follow transdermal scopolamine use. Such patients may have had prior seizures.[18,19]

Withdrawal

When transdermal scopolamine has been used longer than 3 days, withdrawal of its use has occasionally been followed by dizziness, nausea, vomiting, headache, and disturbance of equilibrium.[4,5,15]

Central Anticholinergic Syndrome

Occasionally, restlessness, hallucinations, and delirium may follow the use of scopolamine in the elderly.[1,20] Headache may accompany use of transdermal scopolamine. Repeat use of the patch every 72 hours without a 24-hour interval between patches led to scopolamine intoxication and migraine attacks in a 20-year-old man.[21]

Pupillary Reactions

Bilateral mydriasis was observed in a 46-year-old woman who used two patches every 72 hours and "rubbed" them to heighten the effect; symptoms cleared within 3 hours.[22] More than 90% of unilateral dilated pupils occur on the same side as the patch. The diagnosis of scopolamine contamination can be confirmed by prompt and extensive constriction of the pupil on instillation of 0.5 to 1.0% pilocarpine hydrochloride in the affected eye.[23]

Laboratory

Analytical Methods

A radioreceptor assay has been described for analysis of blood scopolamine levels.[14] The lower detection limit is 0.08 nmol/L in plasma.[13]

Blood Levels

Scopolamine intoxication in a 6-year-old child was confirmed by free scopolamine levels of 890 pg/mL (2.93 nmol/L) in plasma and 113 ng/mL (0.37 μmol/L) in urine.[2] Both samples were taken 5 hours after the patch was removed.

Treatment

Stabilization

Treatment of overdose with scopolamine is largely symptomatic and supportive. Symptoms associated with the use of the transdermal patch largely subside within 24 to 36 hours. The patch should be removed.

Gut Decontamination

After the patch is in place, the hands should be washed to remove any scopolamine. Any adhesive remaining on the hands after application or removal of the patch contains scopolamine. Subsequent touching of the eye may produce mydriatic effects.[16]

Elimination Enhancement

There are no data to support use of hemodialysis or hemoperfusion, which are, in any case, not likely to be useful in enhancing elimination of scopolamine because of its extensive volume of distribution.

Antidote

There is no antidote. Physostigmine may rarely need to be considered. Precautions must be observed. (see Benztropine in this chapter).

Supportive Measures

Patients infrequently require admission to a hospital (see Atropine in this chapter).

REFERENCES—SCOPOLAMINE

1. Wood M. Anticholinergic drugs: Anesthetic premedication. In: Wood M, Wood AJJ, eds. *Drugs and Anesthesia: Pharmacology for Anesthesiologists.* Baltimore: Williams & Wilkins, 1991:111–127.

2. Sennhauser FH, Schwarz HP. Toxic psychosis from transdermal scopolamine in a child. Lancet 1986;2:1033.
3. Kriegman AG. Personal communication. Ciba-Geigy, July 10, 1989.
4. Transdermal scopolamine: Product literature. Ciba-Geigy, February 1988.
5. Kjeldaas L. Scopderm reservoir plaster: State of confusion and hallucinations. Tidsskr Nor Laegeforen 1986: No. 5.
6. Van der Willigram AH, Oranje AP, Stolz E, van Joost T. Delayed hypersensitivity to scopolamine in transdermal therapeutic systems. J Am Acad Dermatol 1988;18:146–147.
7. Trozak D. Delayed hypersensitivity to scopolamine delivered by a transdermal device. J Am Acad Dermatol 1985;13: 247–251.
8. McCauley ME, Royal JW, Shaw JE, Schmitt LG. Effect of transdermally administered scopolamine in preventing motion sickness. Aviat Space Environ Med 1979;50:1108–1111.
9. Price NM, Schmitt LG, McGuire J, et al. Transdermal scopolamine in the prevention of motion sickness at sea. Clin Pharmacol Ther 1981;29:414–419.
10. Lebuisson DA, Risvegliato M. La mydriase unilaterale du voyageur. Presse Med 1983;12:2214.
11. McEvoy GK, ed. *AHFS Drug Information 94.* Bethesda, MD: American Society of Hospital Pharmacists, 1994:754–757.
12. Muir C, Metcalfe R. A comparison of plasma levels of hyoscine after oral and transdermal administration. J Pharm Biomed Anal 1983;1:363–367.
13. Golding JF, Gosden E, Gerrell J. Scopolamine blood levels following buccal versus ingested tablets. Aviat Space Environ Med 1991;62:521–526.
14. Schnabel J, Ray M, Sandy J, et al. Applications of a scopolamine radioreceptor assay to pharmacokinetic studies in rats and humans. Clin Chem 1990;36:1045.
15. Saxena K, Saxena S. Scopolamine withdrawal syndrome. Postgrad Med 1990;87:63–66.
16. Simpson A. Bilateral scopolamine mydriasis in a traveller. Br Med J 1987;194:775.
17. Wilkinson JA. Side effects of transdermal scopolamine. J Emerg Med 1987;5:389–392.
18. Strom BL, Carson JL, Schinnar R, et al. Seizures from transdermal scopolamine. Clin Pharmacol Ther 1989;45:155.
19. Strom BL, Carson JL, Schinnar R, et al. No causal relationship between transdermal scopolamine and seizures: Methodologic lesson for pharmacoepidemiology. Clin Pharmacol Ther 1991;50:107–113.
20. Rozzini M, Inzoli M, Trabucchi. Delirium from transdermal scopolamine in an elderly women. JAMA 1988;260:478.
21. Gordon CR, Mankuta D, Shupak A, et al. Recurrent classic migraine attacks following transdermal scopolamine intoxication. Headache 1991;31:172–174.
22. Marcon GM, Schiavo F. Bilateral scopolamine mydriasis in a traveller. Br Med J 1987;294:250.
23. Price BH. Anisocoria from scopolamine patch. JAMA 1985;253:1561.

TERODILINE

Terodiline hydrochloride (*N-tert*-butyl-1-methyl-3, 3-diphenylpropylticlopidineamine),[1] an inhibitor of bladder and muscle contractions, has been marketed in the United Kingdom (Micturine) as a treatment for urinary incontinence. It is usually prescribed as the hydrochloride in 12.5-mg tablets, with one to two taken twice daily. Doses are not expected to exceed two tablets per day.

Toxicokinetics

At a dose level of 12.5 mg, the distribution half-life is 0.31 hour.[2] The apparent volume of distribution ranges from 4 to 12 L/kg.[2] The bioavailability of oral terodiline ranges from 78 to about 108%.[1,2] At dose levels of 50 mg/d, serum terodiline concentrations averaging 0.5 μg/mL have been reported after 10 to 15 days, with maximum levels being reached 1 to 2 hours after an oral dose; the elimination half-life is 60 hours.[2,3] Serum clearance ranges from 2.2 to 8.4 L/h. Less than 10% is excreted unchanged in the urine.[2]

Fatal Dose

About 140 tablets of terodiline were probably ingested in one fatal case.[4]

Mechanism of Action

Terodiline has both anticholinergic and calcium antagonist properties and effectively reduces abnormal bladder contractions caused by detrusor irritability.[1]

Clinical Presentation

Overdose

A 20-year-old man was found dead after taking at least 10 terodiline tablets. Blood and urine were analyzed by thin-layer chromatography and gas chromatography. The quantities of terodiline found in both the blood and urine were greater than 100 μg/mL (therapeutic serum level, up to 1 μg/mL). Blood terodiline levels averaged 20 μg/mL, and urine levels, 108 μg/mL.[3]

Chronic Use

The most common adverse effects are dry mouth, abnormal ocular accommodation, tremor, and nausea.[1]

Torsade de Pointes

Terodiline was associated in four cases with atrioventricular dissociation and polymorphic ventricular tachycardia (Torsade de pointes). There was, after 1 week of treatment, prolongation of the QT and QT_c intervals with a significant reduction in heart rate.[5]

In August 1991, the U.K. Committee on Safety of Medicine warned of reports of ventricular tachycardia (Torsade de pointes), heart block, and bradycardia developing 1 week to 2 years after initiation of therapy. Predisposing factors were age (>75 years)[6]; ischemic heart disease; concomitant administration of diuretics, tricyclic antidepressants, antipsychotic agents, and cardioactive agents; and hypokalemia.[7,8] In October 1991, the manufacturer withdrew terodiline worldwide after a number of life-threatening cardiovascular disorders (Torsade de pointes) were reported.[7–13]

REFERENCES—TERODILINE

1. Langtry HD, McTavish D. Terodiline: A review of its pharmacological properties and therapeutic use in the treatment of urinary incontinence. Drugs 1990;40:748–761.
2. Karlen B, Andersson K-E, Ekman G, et al. Pharmacokinetics of terodiline in human volunteers. Eur J Clin Pharmacol 1982; 23:267–270.
3. Terodiline (Micturine) and adverse cardiac reactions. London: Committee on Safety of Medicines, 1991.
4. Boyd G. A correction to "An apparent fatal overdose of terodiline." J Anal Toxicol 1990;14:194.

5. Cattini RAP, Makin HLD, Trafford DJH, Vanezis P. An apparent fatal overdose of terodiline. J Anal Toxicol 1989;13: 110–112.
6. Stewart DA, Taylor J, Ghosh S, et al. Terodiline causes polymorphic ventricular tachycardia due to reduced heart rate and prolongation of QT interval. Eur J Clin Pharmacol 1992; 42:577–580.
7. Walt AH. Terodiline and Torsades de pointes. Br Med J 1991; 303:519.
8. UK doctors and pharmacists reactivate a warning about terodiline reaction. August 10, 1991. Editorial.
9. Connolly MJ, Astridge PS, White EG, et al. Torsade de pointes ventricular tachycardia and terodiline. Lancet 1991; 338:344–345.
10. Worldwide withdrawal of terodiline. Reactions, October 5, 199●●● p.2.
11. Triazolam and terodiline withdrawn in Britain. NZ Med J 1991;101.
12. Geraint M. Terodiline and Torsade de pointes. Br Med J 1991;303:519–520.
13. Dans SW, Brecker SJ, Stevenson RN. Terodiline for treating detrusion instability in elderly patients. Br Med J 1991;302:1276.

TRIHEXYPHENIDYL

The effects of overdose with trihexyphenidyl hydrochloride (benzhexol hydrochloride) are typical of anticholinergic drug toxicity. Complete recovery usually occurs in 3 to 4 days, but symptoms and signs may continue for 1 month. Treatment in a hospital is symptomatic and supportive.

Use

Trihexyphenidyl is used in the treatment of parkinsonian syndrome and to ameliorate drug-induced extrapyramidal effects.[1] It may be useful in the prevention or treatment of nerve gas poisoning in chemical warfare.[2]

Product Formulation

Trihexyphenidyl hydrochloride is available as oral extended-release capsules of 5 mg, tablets of 2 and 5 mg, and an elixir of 2 mg/5 mL.

Source

Trihexyphenidyl is a synthetic tertiary amine antimuscarinic agent.

Therapeutic Dose

For the symptomatic relief of parkinsonian syndrome, the usual initial dose is 1 mg on the first day, increased in incremental doses up to 12 to 15 mg daily as required. For the relief of antipsychotic extrapyramidal disorders, the dose ranges from 5 to 15 mg daily. Doses of 30 to 40 mg daily may produce an anxiolytic and euphoriant effect.[3] A controlled trial of trihexyphenidyl at a dose of 30 mg daily appeared to be effective in lessening torsion dystonia.[1]

Toxic Dose

Ingestion of 180 mg of trihexyphenidyl hydrochloride resulted in symptoms of anticholinergic overdose; the patient recovered within several weeks.[4] Another patient ingested 300 mg of trihexyphenidyl hydrochloride with suicidal intent, developed evidence of anticholinergic toxicity, and recovered in 1 week.[5] An adult ingestion of 150 mg led to lip smacking and tasty movements of the tongue, disorientation, delusions, and visual hallucinations; The patient recovered in 3 to 4 days.[6]

Fatal Dose

No deaths following overdose with trihexyphenidyl hydrochloride have been described.

Toxicokinetics

Absorption

Trihexyphenidyl hydrochloride is almost completely absorbed from the gastrointestinal tract. Peak plasma levels are reached about 1 hour after an oral dose.[7,8]

Elimination

Trihexyphenidyl hydrochloride is eliminated by first-order kinetics with a half-life of about 4 hours.[7,8] About one half of an oral dose is excreted in the urine as hydroxylated metabolites within 72 hours.[9]

Mechanism of Action

Trihexyphenidyl hydrochloride is an antimuscarinic agent with anticholinergic toxic effects after an overdose.

Clinical Presentation

Overdose

Confusion, hallucinations, dry mouth, dilated pupils, blurring of vision, tachycardia, and fever may be observed in addition to other symptoms and signs of anticholinergic overdose (see Introduction to this chapter). Patients over 60 years of age with arteriosclerotic changes and a previous history of confusion induced by sedatives, who receive 7.5 mg or more of the drug, may develop a mental disorder such as paranoid psychosis.[10] Cognitive impairment may persist after acute intoxication.[11]

Chronic Use

Long-term abuse (6–20 mg/d) can lead to memory and cognitive impairments.[12] Complete recovery usually occurs in 1 week to 1 month.[13]

Drug Abuse

Antiparkinsonian drugs can be abused by some patients to achieve pleasurable effects ranging from mild euphoria with increased sociability at lower doses to a toxic anticholinergic psychosis with disorientation and hallucinations at higher doses.[14]

Withdrawal Syndrome

Following prolonged use of trihexyphenidyl hydrochloride 20 mg daily, withdrawal can lead to anxiety, irritability, persecutory ideas, insomnia, headache, excessive perspiration, and tachycardia.[12]

Recovery

Most patients have recovered after 2 to 4 days, although symptoms may persist for 1 week to 1 month.

Laboratory

Gas–liquid chromatography is used to assay trihexyphenidyl hydrochloride in body fluid.[15] The minimum detectable level is 0.4 ng.

Treatment

Stabilization

Patients should be admitted to a hospital for continuous electrocardiographic and cardiac monitoring for at least 24 hours[13] (see Introduction to this chapter).

Supportive Measures

Withdrawal symptoms may respond to cessation of drug use and flunitrazepam.[12]

TRIHEXYPHENIDYL—REFERENCES

1. Burke RE, Fahn S, Marsden CD. Torsion dystonia: A double-blind prospective trial of high dosage trihexyphenidyl. Neurology 1986;36:160–164.
2. Lennox WJ, Harris LW, Anderson DR, et al. Successful pretreatment therapy of soman, sarin and VX intoxication. Drug Chem Toxicol 1992;15:271–283.
3. Kammer Y, Munitz H, Wijsenbeek H. Trihexyphenidyl (Artane) abuse: Euphoriant and anxiolytic. Br J Psychiatry 1982; 140:473–474.
4. Morgenstorn GF. Trihexyphenidyl (Artane) intoxication due to overdosage with suicidal intent. Can Med Assoc J 1962; 87:79–80.
5. Ananth JV, Lehman HE, Ban TA. Toxic psychosis caused by benzhexol hydrochloride. Can Med Assoc J 1970;103:771.
6. Stephens DA. Psychotoxic effects of benzhexol hydrochloride (Artane). Br J Psychiatry 1967;113:213–218.
7. Burke RE, Fahn S. Pharmacokinetics of trihexyphenidyl after short-term and long-term administration to dystonic patients. Ann Neurol 1985;18:35–40.
8. Burke RE, Fahn S. Serum trihexyphenidyl levels in the treatment of torsion dysphonia. Neurology 1985;35:1066–1069.
9. Nation RL, Triggs EJ, Vine J. Metabolism and urinary excretion of benzhexol in humans. Xenobiotica 1978;8:165–169.
10. Mengech HNKA. Psychiatric manifestations of benzhexol toxicity. East Afr Med J 1984;61:78–81.
11. Crawshaw JA, Mullen RC. A study of benzhexol abuse. Br J Psychiatry 1984;145:300–303.
12. Kajimura N, Mizuki Y, Kai S, et al. Memory and cognitive impairment in a case of long-term trihexyphenidyl abuse. Pharmacopsychiatry 1993;26:59–62.
13. Enchava D. Trihexyphenidyl overdose: Clinical presentation and management. Vet Hum Toxicol 1993;35:370.
14. Smith JM. Abuse of antiparkinson drugs: A review of the literature. J Clin Psychiatry 1980;41:351–354.
15. Bargo E. GLC determination of trihexyphenidyl hydrochloride dosage forms. J Pharm Sci 1978;68:503–505.

Chapter 47

Dopamine Receptor Drugs

INTRODUCTION

DOPAMINE RECEPTORS

D_1 Receptors

D_1 receptors activate adenyl cyclase and increase intracellular levels of cyclic AMP; D_2 receptors exert an inhibitory effect on adenyl cyclase (Table 47–1). D_2 receptors may also be linked to additional second messenger systems including inhibition of phosphatidyl inositol turnover, activation of K^+ channels, and inhibition of Ca^{2+} channel activity. Eight pharmacologically distinct dopamine receptors have now been identified through molecular cloning techniques (D_1, D_{1A}, D_{1B}, D_{2A}, D_{2B}, D_{2C}, D_3, D_4).[1–9] Dopamine receptor agonists and antagonists are summarized in Table 47–2. Catecholamine receptor activities of the dopaminergic agonists are summarized in Table 47–3.[10]

Anatomic Location

The substantia nigra and ventral tegmental nuclei are composed of dopaminergic neurons with branches distributed to the corpus striatum, limbic nuclei, and frontal cortex (Fig. 47–1).[11]

DA_2 Receptors

In the early 1980s two distinct receptor subtypes (DA_1 and DA_2) were identified as involved in regulating the cardiovascular system.[12–14] Stimulation of the postsynaptic DA_2 receptor leads to vasodilation preferentially in renal, mesenteric, coronary, and cerebral blood vessels. DA_1 receptors are also found in the central nervous system, some vascular beds, the kidney, and sympathetic ganglia. Agonists at the DA_2 receptor located presynaptically diminish the release of noradrenaline at sympathetic nerve endings, resulting in a reduction of vascular resistance. DA_2 receptors are also present in sympathetic ganglia, where activation also inhibits neurotransmission. Other DA_2 receptors are found in the central nervous system and adrenal cortex.

Mechanism of Action

At the terminal regions of the peripheral adrenergic nerves, there are a number of presynaptic receptors some of which,

Table 47–1
Peripheral Actions of Dopamine

Receptor	Location	Response
Alpha	Blood vessels	Vasoconstriction
Beta	Heart	Cardiac stimulation; ↑ rate and force
	Blood vessels	Vasodilation (minor)
DA_2 (prejunctional)	Sympathetic ganglia and prejunctional sympathetic nervous system nerve terminal	Inhibition of norepinephrine release; ↓ rate; passive vasodilation
DA_1 (postjunctional)	Blood vessels, renal tubules	Vasodilation; ↑ renal flow; diuresis; natriuresis

From Rosenkranz RP, McClelland DL. An historical perspective of dopamine and its analogs. Proc West Pharmacol Soc 1990;33:15–19.

Table 47–2
Dopamine Receptor Agonists and Antagonists

	Agonists	Antagonists
D_1	Bromocriptine	Chlorpromazine
	Dihydroergotamine	Haloperidol
	Dopamine	Metoclopramide
	Dopexamine	Sulpiride
	Epinine	
	Ibopamine	
	Pergolide	
	Propylbutyl dopamine	
D_2	Apomorphine	Chlorpromazine
	Bromocriptine	Doniperidine
	Carmoxirole	Fluphenazine
	Dopamine	Haloperidol
	Dopexamine	Metoclopramide
	Lisuride	Prochlorperazine
	Pergolide	Remoxipride
	Pimozide	Reserpine
	Propylbutyl dopamine	Sulpiride
	Quinapiral	Tiapride
		Triethylperazine

on stimulation, reduce release of noradrenaline (inhibitory) presynaptic receptors and others that augment its release. Inhibitory presynaptic receptors include adenosine, muscarinic, opiate, prostaglandin, and dopamine receptors of the dopamine-2 receptor subtype.[14]

DOPAMINE

Dopamine is a catecholamine and the immediate precursor of norepinephrine. The effects that dopamine produces in the body are directly related to its actions on alpha, beta, and dopaminergic receptor sites.[14,15] When these receptors are stimulated cyclic AMP levels increase, permitting an increase in calcium transport into the cell.[1,2,6–9]

The amount of dopamine determines which receptors are predominantly stimulated. Low-dose dopamine (0.5–1.5 μg/kg/min) results mainly in stimulation of dopaminergic receptors. At moderate doses of 2 to 4 μg/kg/min, β_1 effects on the myocardium predominate. Myocardial contractility increases together with heart rate, with a resultant increase in cardiac output. At infusion rates greater than 5 to 10 μg/kg/min, alpha-receptor stimulation predominates, resulting in peripheral vasoconstriction, with a rise in blood pressure. At infusion rates greater than 20 μg/kg/min, the vasoconstrictive alpha effect can be greater than the β_1 effect.[16]

DOPAMINE AGONISTS

Dopamine agonists directly stimulate dopamine receptors. By acting at the postsynaptic dopamine receptors of the striatum, agonists bypass the degenerating presynaptic neuron from the substantia nigra and act independently of the synthetic dopaminergic enzyme system. Agonists have long half-lives. They do not increase the level of dopamine itself and are specific to subpopulations of dopamine receptors. They are devoid of properties related to norepinephrine and serotonin. Only bromocriptine and pergolide are available in the United States.

Toxicokinetics

Drug Interactions

Sodium bicarbonate inactivates both dopamine and dobutamine. Proper flushing between intravenous administrations can avoid this problem. Recent administration of beta blockers may render dopamine ineffective.[15]

Pregnancy

None of these drugs in table 47-2 is recommended for use during pregnancy unless the potential benefits justify the possible risk to the fetus.

Clinical Presentation

Hypovolemia

Hypovolemia may be a primary cause of a low-cardiac-output state. Vigorous diuretic therapy may predispose patients to this condition. Fluid resuscitation must precede the use of dopamine.

Acute Myocardial Infarction

Dopamine may increase myocardial contractility and increase myocardial oxygen consumption. This, in turn, may lead to an increase in infarct size.[17]

Use With Valvular Heart Disease

In patients with severe pulmonic or aortic valve disease, the increase in contractility produced by dopamie may impede blood flow across the disease valves.

Extravasation of Dopamine

Extravasation of dopamine into surrounding tissue can lead to necrosis and sloughing. A central or larger vein is the

Table 47-3
Adrenergic Receptor Specificity of Sympathomimetic Amines

Drug/Dose	Dopaminergic	$Beta_1$	$Beta_2$	Alpha
Epinephrine				
0.01–0.1 μg/kg/min	0	+++	++	+
>0.1 μg/kg/min	0	++	0	+++
Norepinephrine 2–10 μg/min	0	++	0	++++
Dopamine				
1–3 μg/kg/min	+	++	+	0
5–15 μg/kg/min	0	++	+	+
15–20 μg/kg/min	0	++	0	+++
Dobutamine 2.5–15 μg/kg/min	0	+++	+	+
Isoproterenol 2–10 μg/min	0	++++	+++	0
Phenylephrine 20–200 μg/min	0	0	0	+++

0, No effect; +, effect.
From Whipple JK, Medicus-Bringa MA, Schimel BA, et al. Selected vasoactive drugs: A readily available chart reference. Crit Care Nurs 1992;12:23–29.

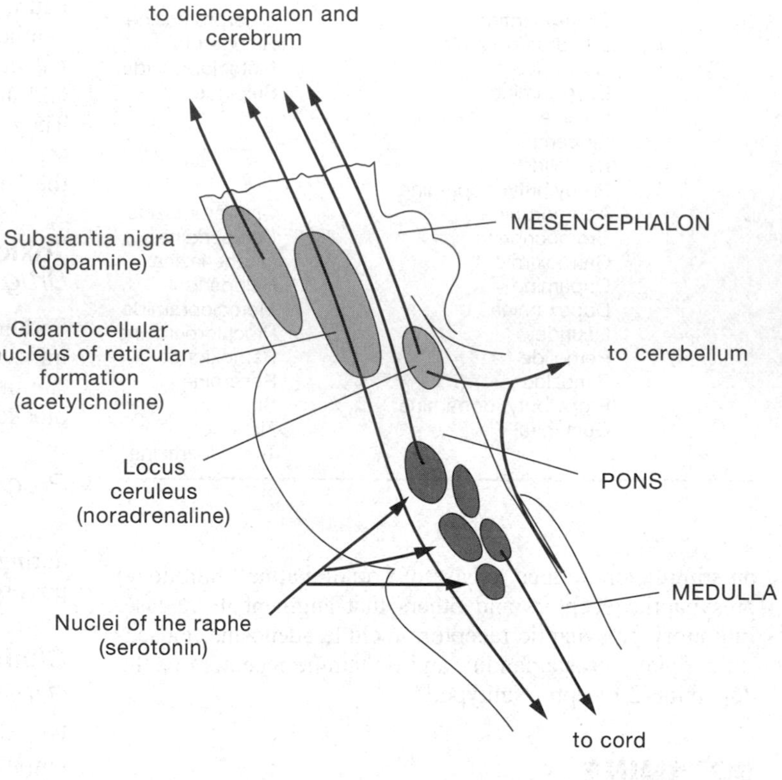

Figure 47-1 Brainstem reticular activating system showing nuclei that secrete different neurotransmitters. From Ashton CH, Teoh R, Davies DM. Drug-induced stupor and coma: Some physical signs and their pharmacological basis. Adverse Drug React Acute Poison Rev 1989;8(1):1–59.

preferred site for infusion. If extravasation occurs, phentolamine (Regitin) should be injected subcutaneously in the affected area within 12 hours of the extravasation.

Occlusive Vascular Disease

Patients should be carefully monitored for changes in skin color, sensation, and temperature in the extremities. The infusion should be decreased or discontinued as required.

Pheochromocytoma

Dopamine is contraindicated in patients diagnosed or suspected to have a pheochromocytoma because of the potential for severe hypertension.

Iron and Dopamine D_2 Receptors

Iron modulates dopamine D_2-receptor function and constitutes a part of this receptor. Low serum iron levels, through an induced D_2-receptor hypofunction, may increase the susceptibility to akathisias of patients taking antipsychotic medication.[18]

Dopamine Agonists for Parkinson's Disease

Bromocriptine (Parlodel), lysergide, and pergolide (Permax) are dopamine agonists derived from ergot, rapidly absorbed from the gut, and extensively metabolized in the liver. Bromocriptine has a plasma half-life of 7 hours, lysergide 2 hours, and pergolide more than 7 hours. Bromocriptine, lysergide, and pergolide stimulate D_2 receptors; pergolide acts additionally on D_1 sites. The clinical relevance of this difference is uncertain.[19] All three drugs can cause confusion, hallucinations, paranoia, nausea, and vomiting. Ergot derivatives can also cause peripheral ischemia. Bromocriptine may rarely cause pleural, pulmonary, or retroperitoneal fibrosis. A similar syndrome may be expected with other ergot derivatives in high doses. All three may result in postural hypotension.[1,2]

Pleuropulmonary Disease

Pleuropulmonary disease (PPD) may occur during treatment with bromocriptine, mesulergine, lisuride, and cabergoline, all dopamine agonists. Other ergot derivatives with a similar molecular structure—methysergide, ergotamine, and bromocriptine—have been associated with PPD and retroperitoneal fibrosis. All these drugs are tetracyclic compounds.[18,20] The majority of patients who were reported to develop PPD during bromocriptine therapy were receiving high doses (>20 mg) for a prolonged time (>6 months). Dyspnea, pleuritic pain, and nonproductive cough are frequent symptoms of PPD.

IBOPAMINE AND EPININE

Ibopamine is an oral adrenergic and dopaminergic agent that produces beneficial responses in patients with congestive heart failure.[21] The compound, a diisobutyric ester of *N*-methyldopamine (epinine), is absorbed orally and diesterified primarily in the gastrointestinal tract and liver, releasing the active drug epinine into the circulation.[22] Oral ibopamine can permit a reduction in intravenous dopamine dosage.[23] Epinine stimulates adrenergic and dopaminergic receptors. Ibopamine exhibits adrenergic and dopaminergic properties.[24] It has been associated with abdominal pain, tachycardia, extrasystoles, nausea, vomiting, and headache.[25] A high-performance liquid chromatography method with fluorometric detection is available for determination of epinine concentrations at limits of detection of 6 ng/mL in plasma and 15 ng/mL in urine.[26]

CARMOXIROLE

Carmoxirole is a dopamine agonist selective for peripheral presynaptic DA_2 receptors. It has been developed as an antihypertensive agent. Carmoxirole is 3-[4-(4-phenyl-1,2,3,4-tetrahydro-1-pyridinyl)butyl]indole-5-carboxylic acid hydrochloride. It is absorbed rapidly and nearly completely (about 80%) and reaches a peak plasma concentration of 8 ng/mL in about 2 to 3 hours. The principal metabolite is an ester-type glucuronide. The elimination half-life is about 5 hours. Clearance is 25 L/h. A specific high-performance liquid chromatography method with fluorometric detection is available for determination of carmoxirole and its metabolites. Its limit of detection is 0.5 ng/mL. Ingestion of 0.5 and 1 mg has led to orthostatic reactions (relieved by position change) without a compensatory increase in heart rate. There is a dose-dependent increase in reports of adverse events after oral doses of 0.7 to 1.5 mg. The most frequent side effects are headache, dizziness, fatigue, nausea, and nasal congestion, all of which disappear with continued treatment.[14] Carmoxirole exerts dopaminergic inhibition of norepinephrine release by activating peripheral DA_2 receptors.[27] Other compounds that can inhibit adrenergic neurotransmission and eventually lower blood pressure by stimulation of postsynaptic dopamine receptors are pergolide, dihydroergotamine, and bromocriptine.

MOVEMENT DISORDERS

Movement disorders include hypokinetic disorders (various forms of parkinsonism), hyperkinetic disorders (Huntington's chorea, tardive dyskinesia, etc), and dystonias.

Hypokinetic disorders	Blockers of dopaminergic transmission
Hyperkinetic disorders	Enhancers of dopamine stimulation
Dystonias	Dopamine antagonists (acute or chronic)

Drugs that cause parkinsonism are summarized in Table 47–4.[28] Neuroleptic drugs can be ranked by potency of antipsychotic effects which correlate with the potency of D_2-receptor antagonism. High-potency drugs are haloperidol and fluphenazine (dystonic reactions); intermediate-potency drugs are perphenazine and loxapine; and low-potency drugs are chlorpromazine and thioridazine.

Table 47–4
Drugs That Cause Parkinsonism

Drug	Indication	Mechanism
All antipsychotics (except clozapine)	Treatment of psychosis and agitated behavior	D_2-receptor blockade
Metoclopramide (Reglan)	Gastroparesis	D_2-receptor blockade
Prochlorperazine (Compazine)	Antiemetic	D_2-receptor blockade
Droperidol (Inapsine)	Antiemetic	D_2-receptor blockade
Methyldopa (Aldomet)	Hypertension	Competitive inhibition of dopa decarboxylase, an enzyme necessary for the conversion of dopa to dopamine, plus formation of a false neurotransmitter that may compete with dopamine for receptors in the striatum
Rauwolfia alkaloids, eg, reserpine	Hypertension, psychosis	Presynaptic depletion of dopamine
Tetrabenazine	Hyperkinetic movement disorders	Presynaptic depletion of dopamine
Amoxapine	Depression	D_2-receptor blockade

From Rich SS. Drug-induced movement disorders. Rhode Island Med 1993;76(11):556–562.

Table 47-5
Antiparkinsonian Drugs

Drug	Mechanism of Action
Levodopa	Decarboxylated to dopamine in the brain or peripheral tissue
Carbidopa	Blocks action in peripheral tissues (a peripheral decarboxylase inhibitor)
Selegiline	Inhibits catabolism of dopamine in brain; MAO-B inhibitor
Ergot-derived dopamine agonists	Cause postural hypotension
Bromocriptine, lisuride	Can potentiate dyskinesias or toxic psychosis caused by levodopa
Pergolide	Peripheral dopaminergic effects (cardiac arrhythmias, nausea); blocked by dopamine antagonist domperidone
Ropinirole	Investigational; available in Canada, not United States
Anticholinergic drugs	In Parkinson's disease, decrease dopamine activity; increase excitatory effects of acetylcholine
Trihexiphenidyl (Artane, others)	
Benztropine (Cogentin, others)	
Procyclidine (Kemadrin)	
Biperiden (Akineton)	
Antihistamine	
Diphenhydramine (Benadryl)	
Antiviral drugs	
Amantadine	Increases dopamine release in the brain
Antidepressants	
Tricyclics	
Trazodone (Desyrel)	
Selective serotonin uptake inhibitors	
Fluoxetine (Prozac)	May worsen signs and symptoms of parkinsonism
Bupropion (Wellbutrin)	
MAO-A inhibitors	Do not use: cause wide swings in blood pressure in patients taking levodopa
Clozapine	For psychosis associated with levodopa or dopamine agonists
Fetal brain tissue	Dopaminergic cell transplantation

MAO, monoamine oxidase.

Antiparkinsonian Drugs

Antiparkinsonian drugs are listed in Table 47-5.[29]

NEUROLEPTIC-INDUCED DEFICIT SYNDROME

Classic antipsychotic drugs that induce a blockade of central dopamine (D_2) receptors are often associated with a deficit syndrome (impairment of cognitive, social, and affective function) when administered to schizophrenic patients. Symptoms include sedation, indifference to internal and external stimuli, passivity, and reduced initiation. Use of newer drugs such as clozapine, sulpiride, remoxipride, and risperidone can lead to an "awakening" characterized by the lifting of a "physical straitjacket" (probably extrapyramidal in nature) followed by a physical and physiologic stimulation associated with akathisia, a decreased need for sleep, and an intellectual and emotional arousal.[30,31]

REFERENCES—INTRODUCTION

1. Creese I, Sibley DR, Leff S, Hamblin M. Dopamine receptors: Subtypes, localization and regulation. Fed Proc 1981;40: 147–152.
2. Waddington JL, O'Boyle KM. Dogs acting on brain dopamine receptors: A conceptual re-evaluation five years after the first selective D_1 antagonist. Pharmacol Ther 1989;43:1–52.
3. Sibley DR, Monsma FJ Jr. Molecular biology of dopamine receptors. Trends Pharmacol Sci 1992;13:61–69.
4. Rosenkrantz RP, McClelland DL. An historical perspective of dopamine and its analogs. Proc West Pharmacol Soc 1990;33:15–19.
5. Cooper JR, Bloom FE, Roth RH. *The Biochemical Basis of Neuropharmacology.* 6th ed. New York: Oxford University Press, 1991:285–337.
6. Strange PG. D_1/D_2 dopamine receptor interaction at the biochemical level. Trends Pharmacol Sci 1991;12:48–49.
7. Strange PG. Aspects of the structure of the D_2 dopamine receptor. Trends Neurol Sci 1990;13:373–378.
8. Sokoloff P, Girus B, Martres M-P, et al. Molecular cloning and characterization of a novel dopamine receptor (D_3) as a target for neuroleptics. Nature 1990;347:146–151.
9. Mercuri NB, Calabresi P, Bernardi G. Physiology and pharmacology of dopamine D_2-receptors: Their implications in dopamine-substitute therapy for Parkinson's disease. Neurology 1989;39:1106–1108.
10. Horn PT, Murphy MB. New dopamine receptor agonists in heart failure and hypertension: Implications for further therapy. Drugs 1990;40:487–492.
11. Ashton CH, Teoh R, Davies DM. Drug-induced stupor and coma: Some physical signs and their pharmacological basis. Adverse Drug React Acute Poison Rev 1989;8: 1–59.
12. Stoof JC, Kebabian JW. Two dopamine receptors: Biochemistry, physiology and pharmacology. Life Sci 1984;34: 2281–2286.
13. Goldberg LI, Rajkes SI. Dopamine receptors: Applications in clinical cardiology. Circulation 1985;72:245–248.
14. Haeusler G, Lues I, Minck K-O, et al. Pharmacological basis for antihypertensive therapy with a novel dopamine agonist. Eur Heart J 1992;13(supp. D):129–135.
15. Budny J, Anderson-Drews K. IV inotropic agents: Dopamine, dobutamine and amrinone. Crit Care Nurse 1991;10:54–62.
16. Whipple JK, Medicus-Bringa MA, Schimel BA, et al. Selected vasoactive drugs: A readily available chart reference. Crit Care Nurs 1992;12:23–29.
17. Cohen JN. Recognition and management of shock and acute failure. In Hurst JW, ed. *The Heart.* 5th ed. New York: McGraw-Hill, 1982:463–476.
18. White T, Brown K. Low serum iron levels and neuroleptic malignant syndrome. Am J Psychol 1991;148:148.
19. Dopamine agonists for Parkinson's disease. Drug Ther Bull 1991;29(2):7–8.

20. Bhatt MP, Keenan SP, Fletthan JA, Calme DB. Pleuropulmonary disease associated with dopamine agonist therapy. Ann Neurol 1991;30:613–616.
21. Ren JH, Unverferth DV, Leier CV. The dopamine congener, ibopamine, in congestive heart failure. J Cardiovasc Pharmacol 1985;6:748–755.
22. Harvey JN, Worth DR, Brown J, Lee MR. Lack of effect of ibopamine, a dopamine pro-drug, on renal function in normal subjects. Br J Clin Pharmacol 1984;17:671–677.
23. Milner AR, Zwaveling JH, Girbes ARJ. Ibopamine substitution in a dopamine-dependent patient. Lancet 1993;342:1555.
24. De Mey C, Enterling D, Brendel E, Wesche H. Pharmacokinetics and pharmacodynamics of single oral doses of ibopamine, quinidine and their combination in normal man. Eur J Clin Pharmacol 1988;34:415–418.
25. Henwood JM, Todd PA. Ibopamine: A preliminary review of its pharmacodynamic and pharmacokinetic properties and therapeutic efficacy. Drugs 1988;36:11–31.
26. Boomsma F, Alberts G, Van der Hoorn FAJ, et al. Simultaneous determination of free catecholamines and epinine and estimation of total epinine and dopamine in plasma and urine by high performance liquid chromatography with fluorometric detection. J Chromatogr Biomed Appl 1992;574: 109–117.
27. Meyer W, Buhrmy K-U, Steiner K, et al. Pharmacokinetics and first clinical experiences with an antihypertensive dopamine (DA_2) agonist. Eur Heart J 1992;13(suppl. D):121–128.
28. Rich SS. Drug-induced movement disorders. Rhode Island Med 1993;76:556–562.
29. Med Lett Drugs Ther 1993;35(894):31–34.
30. Lader MH. Neuroleptic-induced deficit syndrome. J Clin Psychiatry 1993;54:493–500.
31. Weller MPI. Neuroleptic-induced deficit syndrome. Postgrad Med J 1993;69:957–958.

BROMOCRIPTINE

Bromocriptine (Parlodel, Pravidel) is an ergot derivative with a potent dopaminergic agonist action. Few reports of overdose are available. Drug interactions and use after pregnancy can induce life-threatening responses.[1–8]

Structure and Classification

The ergot alkaloids are indole alkaloids. They have a four-ringed structure known as ergoline of which there are two types: the lysergic acid derivatives and the clavines. The lysergic acid derivatives are usually either amides or cyclic peptides. Bromocriptine (2-bromo-α-ergocryptine maleate) belongs to the cyclic peptide group of lysergic acid derivatives. Addition of the bromine atom in position 2 gives bromocriptine its property of inhibiting prolactin secretion.[3]

Use

Bromocriptine is used for the treatment of hyperprolactinemia-associated dysfunctions, suppression of puerperal lactation, cyclic benign breast disease, acromegaly,[9] parkinsonism, and neuroleptic malignant syndrome.[10] Bromocriptine has been used to treat the manic phase of manic–depressive psychosis[11] in patients in whom the use of phenothiazines or lithium carbonate is contraindicated. It has been used to reverse cocaine craving.[12]

The Italian Health Ministry requested the withdrawal of bromocriptine for cocaine craving last year following reports of adverse reactions including syncope, vomiting, convulsions, rigidity, respiratory disorders, precordial pain, and myocardial infarction associated with the agent.

Sandoz withdrew the lactation suppression indication for bromocriptine in the United States and Canada in August last year after the Food and Drug Administration indicated its intention to remove the indication; however, the company continued to promote this indication in other countries.

Sereno has also withdrawn the lactation suppression indication for their bromocriptine product (Serocryptin) in Italy at the request of the Health Ministry.[13]

Product Formulation

Bromocriptine is commercially available as the methanesulfonate[3] in 2.5- and 5-mg tablets.

Source

Bromocriptine is chemically synthesized from the ergotoxin group of alkaloids.

Therapeutic Dose

The dose for suppression of lactation is one 2.5-mg tablet twice daily. The usual dosage range is 2.5 to 7.5 mg daily.[2] Dosages for other indications are similar but may range up to 100 mg/d in acromegaly.[3,9]

Toxic Dose

Toxic effects may be seen after ingestion of 50 mg, although nausea and orthostatic hypotension are commonly observed at the initiation of treatment.[14] Most side effects are dose related and can occur at doses exceeding 10 mg.[3] No dangerous effects have been reported in adults taking up to 225 mg or infants taking up to 7.5 mg as an acute overdose.[1] Involuntary movements, chorea, orofacial dyskinesias, and dystonic posture of the trunk and limbs may appear after doses of 90 to 180 mg.[15] Withdrawal of bromocriptine therapy is associated in most patients with reversal of the beneficial effects: return of hyperprolactinemia, return of excess growth hormone secretion, exacerbation of Parkinson's disease,[14] and hyperthermia.[1,6]

Fatal Dose

No fatal dose has been determined.

Toxicokinetics

Absorption

Between 40 and 90% of the drug is absorbed from the gastrointestinal tract. Peak plasma levels of 8 to 12 ng/mL are observed about 100 minutes after doses up to 100 mg.[15]

Distribution

The volume of distribution is 1 to 4 L/kg.[6] Following a dose of 50 mg, plasma levels peak in 2 to 3 hours. This peak–time relationship correlates well with the peak antiparkinsonism action as well as the maximum severity of dyskinesias.[3] Bromocriptine penetrates the brain readily. Plasma protein binding is 96%.

Elimination

The main site of bromocriptine metabolism is the liver. The main route of elimination of its metabolites is biliary. Less than 0.1% is excreted unchanged. The plasma half-life is about 15 hours.[3]

Drug Interactions

The bioavailability of bromocriptine is increased by the concomitant intake of erythromycin.[16] Interaction of bromocriptine with other prolactin secretagogues (eg, neuroleptics, tricyclic antidepressants, rauwolfia alkaloids, estrogens) (Table 47–6) may be observed. Alcohol may reduce tolerance to bromocriptine, and the drug may likewise decrease tolerance to alcohol.[1] Lack of efficacy may occur when patients are treated with dopamine antagonists (eg, phenothiazines, butyrophenones, metoclopramide, prochlorperazine, α-methyldopa, reserpine).

Pregnancy/Lactation

Bromocriptine is a Pregnancy Category B drug.[2] No adverse effects of bromocriptine secreted in breast milk have been reported.[1] There does not appear to be an increased incidence of spontaneous abortion or birth defects. A possible early identifying symptom in patients who are at risk for severe reaction to bromocriptine in the postpartum period is headache, which may occur hours to days before the development of hypertension, seizures, stroke, or myocardial infarction.[5,6]

Mechanism of Action

Bromocriptine is a dopamine (D_2)-receptor agonist that activates postsynaptic dopamine receptors. It inhibits prolactin secretion at both the pituitary and the hypothalamus.[3] In acromegaly it inhibits growth hormone release. Bromocriptine has central effects like L-dopa and the amphetamines, induces arterial and venous relaxation, increases gastric acid output, and inhibits furosemide-induced plasma aldosterone increase.[3]

Clinical Presentation

Chronic Use

The most commonly reported side effects of bromocriptine during clinical use are nausea, vomiting, dizziness, postural hypotension, nasal congestion, constipation, and mood changes.[3] With doses in excess of 20 mg, hallucinations, fatigue, erythromelalgia (tender red edematous foot), digital vasospasm, bladder disturbances, and alcohol intolerance have been reported. Dyskinesia, diplopia, ergotism, and aggravation of angina have been reported.[3] Pleural effusions have been seen in Parkinson's patients after long-term treatment.[17] Hyperthermia may follow discontinuation of therapy.[18]

Overdose

Symptoms of overdose include drowsiness,[19] dizziness, postural hypotension, sweating, hallucinations, nausea, and vomiting as a result of overstimulation of dopaminergic receptors.[1]

Table 47–6
Drugs That Induce Increases in Serum Prolactin Levels

Neuroleptics
Phenothiazines
Thioxanthenes
Butyrophenones
Antihypertensive agents
Reserpine
Methyldopa
Dopamine receptor antagonist
Metoclopramide
Antidepressant
Amoxapine

Laboratory

Analytical Methods

Radioimmunoassay methods have a detection limit of about 0.2 μg/L.[1]

Blood Levels

The plasma concentration of bromocriptine that inhibits prolactin excretion is about 0.7 μg/L.[20]

Abnormalities

Bromocriptine has been associated with transient increases in levels of serum transaminases, creatine kinase, alkaline phosphatase, uric acid, and blood urea nitrogen.[7,8] Drugs that induce increases in serum prolactin levels are listed in Table 47–6.

Treatment

Patients should be observed for development of hypertension or shock and treated symptomatically. Patients seen within 1 to 2 hours of ingestion should receive gastric lavage. There is no evidence that activated charcoal, antidotes, or extracorporeal methods of elimination enhancement are useful in treating an overdose.

REFERENCES—BROMOCRIPTINE

1. Dollery C, ed. *Therapeutic Drugs.* Edinburgh: Churchill Livingstone, 1991:B-109–B113.
2. *Physicians' Desk Reference.* 49th ed. Montvale, NJ: Medical Economics, 1995:2178–2180.
3. Mehta AE, Tolis G. Pharmacology of bromocriptine in health and disease. Drugs 1979;17:313–325.
4. Tukali I, Brown P, Krupp P. Surveillance of bromocriptine in pregnancy. JAMA 1982;247:2589–2591.
5. Kulig K, Moore LL, Kirk M, et al. Bromocriptine-associated headache: Possible life-threatening sympathomimetic interaction. Obstet Gynecol 1991;78:941–943.
6. Miller LG, Bakht FR, Baker T, Kirshon B. Possible cocaine predisposition to adverse cerebrovascular and cardiovascular sequelae of bromocriptine administered postpartum. J Clin Pharmacol 1989;29:781–785.

7. Thorner MO, Flackiger E, Calne DB. *Bromocriptine: A Clinical and Pharmacological Review.* New York: Raven Press, 1989.
8. McEvoy GK, ed. *AHFS Drug Information 94.* Bethesda, MD: American Society of Hospital Pharmacists, 1974:2431–2435.
9. Wass JAH, Thorner MO, Morris DV, et al. Long-term treatment of acromegaly with bromocriptine. Br Med J 1977; 1:875–878.
10. Guerrero RW, Shifrar KA. Diagnosis and treatment of neuroleptic malignant syndrome. Clin Pharm 1988;7:697–701.
11. Dorr C, Sathananthan K. Treatment of mania with bromocriptine. Br Med J 1976;1:1342–1343.
12. Dackis CA, Gold MS, Sweeney DR, et al. Single-dose bromocriptine reverses cocaine craving. Psychiatry Res 1987;20:261–264.
13. Parlodel indication withdrawn in Italy. Scrip 1995;2022:23.
14. Vance ML, Evans WS, Thormer MO. Bromocriptine. Ann Intern Med 1984;100:78–91.
15. Price P, Debono A, Parkes JD, et al. Plasma bromocriptine levels, clinical and growth hormone response in parkinsonism. Br J Clin Pharmacol 1978;6:303–309.
16. Nelson MV, Berchov RC, Kareti D, Le Witt PA. Pharmacokinetic evaluation of erythrocin and caffeine administered with bromocriptine. Clin Pharmacol Ther 1990;47:694–697.
17. Figa-Talamanca L, Gualandi C, Di Meo L, et al. Hyperthermia after discontinuation of levodopa and bromocriptine therapy: Impaired dopamine receptors a possible cause. Neurology 1985;35:258–261.
18. Schmid PA, Suter T, Speich R, et al. Pleuropulmonary changes during bromocriptine treatment. Dtsch Med Wochnschr 1994;119:1542–1546.
19. Tunca Z, Alkin T, Guven H. A case of bromocriptine poisoning that resembles Pickwick syndrome. Pharmacol Toxicol 1993;73(suppl.):78.
20. Griffiths RW. Toxicity studies with 2-bromo-alpha-ergocryptine mesylate (CB154) effect of prolonged oral administration in rats. IRSS Med Sci 1974;2:1661.

BUPROPION

Bupropion is an antidepressant chemically distinct from previous agents. Originally introduced in 1985, it was withdrawn from the market in 1986 after clinical experience indicated an approximately 6% incidence of seizures in bulimic patients taking a maximum of 450 mg bupropion daily.[1] Subsequently, after an extensive survey indicated a convulsion rate of 0.4%, it was released to the market in 1989. Bupropion has resulted in deaths after an overdose. In overdose, bupropion seems to lack cardiovascular toxicity but it does manifest significant neurologic toxicity.[2]

Structure and Classification

Bupropion (amfebutamon) is an antidepressant phenylbutamine of the amino ketone class chemically unrelated to tricyclic, tetracyclic, or other known antidepressant agents. Chemically it is 2-*tert*-butylamino-3′-chloropropophenone hydrochloride.[1] The molecular weight is 276.2. The powder is white, crystalline, and highly soluble in water. Bupropion has a bitter taste and produces the sensation of local anesthesia on the oral mucosa.[3,4]

Use

Bupropion hydrochloride is indicated for the treatment of depression.[4] Other potential uses (not yet approved by the Food and Drug Administration) include attention-deficit hyperactivity disorder in adults[5] and children,[6] reduction of cocaine use,[7] rapid cycling predominantly depressed bipolar patients,[8] and chocolate craving.[9]

Product Formulation

Bupropion is available in 75- and 100-mg tablets (Wellbutrin).

Source

Bupropion is a synthetic chemical.

Therapeutic Dose

The initial dosage ranges up to 200 mg/d in divided amounts.[1] After a 3-day period of treatment, the dosage of bupropion in adults may be increased to 100 mg three times daily. After several weeks of treatment at 300 mg/d and in patients in whom no clinical improvement is seen, the dosage may be increased gradually to 450 mg/d given in divided doses of no more than 150 mg each, provided that there is clinical improvement at this level. If not, bupropion is then discontinued.

Toxic Dose

See Overdose under Clinical Presentation.

Fatal Dose

Ingestion of 16,500 mg of bupropion was fatal in one patient.[10] Lethal doses may be less than 10 g.[11]

Toxicokinetics

Absorption

Absorption of bupropion from the gastrointestinal tract is rapid.[12] Following a 200-mg dose of bupropion, maximal plasma concentrations of 156 to 429 ng/mL were obtained within 3 hours (mean $t_{max} = 1.5$ hour).[12] The optional therapeutic range is 50 to 100 ng/mL.[13] First-pass metabolism and enterohepatic circulation may also occur.[3] In vitro studies show that about 80% of bupropion is bound to plasma protein.[14]

Distribution

The mean half-life for the rapid distribution phase (alpha) ranges from 1.2 to 1.4 hours. Bupropion cerebrospinal fluid/plasma ratios average approximately 0.43/1. The volume of distribution is 1.4 to 3.2 L/kg.[14]

Elimination

The elimination half-life (beta) of bupropion is 10 to 14 hours. Bupropion is metabolized mostly by side-chain oxidative cleavage in the liver. Less than 1% of a bupropion dose is excreted unchanged.[12,15] The major metabolites of bupropion have substantially longer half-lives (up to 43 hours)[16,17] than the parent compound.[18,19] Hydroxybupropion (HB), *threo*-hydrobupropion, and *erythro*-hydrobupropion predominate over the parent compound in the plasma. The renal clearance of bupropion is 1.5 to 1.6 L/h.[20]

Drug Interactions

Bupropion can lower the seizure threshold. Precautions are indicated when bupropion is prescribed concurrently with neuroleptics, xanthines, and other epileptogenic compounds because ictal thresholds may be depressed even further, increasing the likelihood of convulsions.[1] Abrupt discontinuation of ethanol, benzodiazepines, and sedatives during bupropion therapy may precipitate seizure activity. Bupropion should be avoided in physiologic states associated with lowering of the ictal thresholds, for example, hyponatremia. Carbamazepine, cimetidine, phenobarbital, and phenytoin are hepatic drug-metabolizing enzyme inducers and may affect the clinical activity of bupropion when administered together. Monoamine oxidase inhibitors, such as phenelzine, may enhance bupropion toxicity. Bupropion has dopamine reuptake-blocking activity. When bupropion is used with amantadine, which facilitates release of presynaptic dopamine, dopaminergic overdrive may be associated with delirium.[21,22] Caution is advised with concomitant use of L-dopa.[23]

Pregnancy/Lactation

There have been no adequate and well-controlled clinical studies in pregnant or lactating women. Safe use during pregnancy and lactation has not been established. Bupropion accumulates in human breast milk in concentrations much higher than in maternal plasma.[24]

Mechanism of Action

Bupropion is not a monoamine oxidase inhibitor,[3] exerts no effect on 5-hydroxytryptamine uptake, and minimally alters the reuptake of norepinephrine at presynaptic sites. It is a weak inhibitor of dopamine reuptake,[18] but its mechanism of action has not been clarified.

Clinical Presentation

Overdose

Healthy volunteers used doses of 375 mg/d and experienced dizziness, nausea, vomiting, and miosis. At overdoses of 850 to 4200 mg during the clinical development of bupropion, 3 of 12 patients had a mild sinus tachycardia, and 3 patients experienced hypokalemia, one of whom was treated with intravenous fluids containing potassium. No electrocardiographic or electroencephalographic abnormalities were observed. A 57-year-old woman ingested 9000 mg of bupropion (92 mg/kg), 300 mg tranylcypromine, and an unspecified amount of aspirin. She experienced a tonic–clonic seizure and was treated with intravenous diazepam 10 mg, recovering without further sequelae.[4]

Overdoses with 900 to 3000 mg of bupropion in five patients led to vomiting, confusion, hypokalemia, and nonspecific ST–T changes. All survived.[25]

Thirty-two cases of bupropion hydrochloride overdose have been reported to the manufacturer during the postmarketing period. All recovered without lasting sequelae. After doses of 500 mg to an unconfirmed 25,000 mg, one patient became comatose after ingesting bupropion and a phenothiazine. Nine patients experienced grand mal seizures after ingesting 600 to 6500 mg of bupropion hydrochloride. Sinus tachycardia was observed in one patient after an overdose of bupropion 3800-mg together with temazepam and in two patients following bupropion overdoses of 1200 and 1000 to 2000 mg, respectively. Ingestion of 10 tablets of bupropion hydrochloride plus other psychotropic drugs (strength unknown) by one patient resulted in fever, muscle rigidity, hypotension, tachycardia, and a serum creatine phosphokinase level of approximately 1800. The patient was treated symptomatically and survived.[10]

Table 47–7
Factors That May Be Related to Bupropion-Induced Seizures

- History of presence of bulimia/anorexia nervosa
- Doses in excess of 450 mg/d
- Past history of seizures (including febrile convulsions), head injury, or loss of consciousness
- Overdose
- Recent withdrawal from alcoholism or anxiolytic drugs, especially short-acting benzodiazepines
- Concomitant therapy with other drugs that lower seizure threshold (eg, lithium, neuroleptics)
- Recent or rapid dose escalation of bupropion
- Known electroencephalographic abnormality
- Past history or current presence of organic brain disease
- High plasma levels of parent drug or metabolites
- Once-daily administration of full 45-mg dose

Source: Davidson.[26]

One patient ingested 3000 mg of bupropion hydrochloride, 3000 mg of trazodone, an unknown quantity of a tablet containing butalbital, aspirin, caffeine, and an unspecified benzodiazepine, became comatose, and developed respiratory failure. Another patient ingested approximately 17,500 mg of bupropion, 25 mg of alprazolam, and 200 mg of clonazepam, became confused, developed slurred speech, and recovered in 3 days. One patient ingested 16,500 mg and developed bradycardia, left bundle-branch block, cardiac failure, and cardiac arrest.[10]

Bupropion in doses of up to 450 mg did not adversely affect ejection fraction or other indices of left ventricular function.[26] Overdoses of up to 16,500 mg, however, have led to uncontrolled seizures, bradycardia, reduction in ejection fraction, congestive heart failure, and cardiac arrest prior to death in these patients.[10]

Bupropion can lower the seizure threshold. In overdose, seizures have been noted in approximately one third of patients.[10] Table 47–7 lists those factors that may be related to bupropion-induced seizures.[26] The estimated seizure incidence for bupropion increases about tenfold between 450 and 600 mg/d. The risk of seizure appears to be strongly associated with dose and the presence of predisposing factors such as a history of head trauma or prior seizure, central nervous system tremor, concomitant medication that lowers the seizure threshold, and so on.

Chronic Use

Frequent (occurring in at least 100 patients during its preapproval association) adverse effects include edema, nonspecific rashes, nocturia, ataxia/incoordination, seizures, myoclonus,[22] dyskinesia, dystonia, mania/hypomania, increased libido, hallucinations, decrease in sexual function and depression, stomatitis, and flulike symptoms. The depressant effect on cardiac conduction tissue is minimal.[3,27] Menstrual irregularities have been described.[28]

Laboratory

Analytical Methods

A specific radioimmunoassay with a sensitivity limit of 1 ng/mL is available.[12] A liquid chromatography method with dual-wavelength ultraviolet detection has been developed.[29]

Blood Levels

High plasma concentrations of bupropion metabolites may be associated with a poorer outcome.[18,19] There are, however, insufficient data available to relate blood levels of bupropion to the clinical course after ingestion. In two fatal cases, blood levels of 4.0 and 4.2 mg/L were reported.[11]

Abnormalities

Hypokalemia and elevated creatine kinase and transaminase levels have been observed following overdoses of bupropion.[4,10,30] Electrocardiographic abnormalities including a left bundle-branch block have followed extensive overdoses.[10]

Ancillary Tests

There may be a trend toward a reduction in cerebrospinal fluid 3-methoxy-4-hydroxyphenylglycol and homovanillic acid concentrations following bupropion treatment.[18,19]

Treatment

Stabilization

Patients should be hospitalized after a bupropion overdose. Modalities for seizure treatment should be prepared and available, as should an intravenous line, oxygen, and cardiac monitoring. Initial attention should be directed to the adequacy of ventilation (arterial blood gases, tidal volume, cyanosis). If the patient is stuporous or in coma, oxygen, naloxone, glucose, and, if necessary, thiamine should be administered. Protection of the airway (endotracheal intubation), if necessary and mechanical ventilation should have top priority.

Gut Decontamination

The usual measures for gut decontamination should be employed. Syrup of ipecac should not be used in view of the possibility of seizures or myoclonus following an overdose of bupropion. Activated charcoal, after tracheal protection, may be useful administered every 6 hours during the first 12 hours after ingestion to impede absorption of the drug from the gastrointestinal tract and perhaps interfere with its enterohepatic circulation. If the patient is stuporous or comatose, airway intubation, followed by gastric lavage, may be of value in the first 12 hours after ingestion.

Elimination Enhancement

The usefulness of diuresis, dialysis, or hemoperfusion would tend to be minimal in view of the large volume of distribution. No clinical experience with these modalities in bupropion overdose has been published.

Antidote

There is no available antidote.

Supportive Measures

1. Recurrent seizures indicate the need to monitor urine myoglobin and serum creatinine and creatine kinase levels to detect evidence of rhabdomyolysis.
2. Hypokalemia usually results from the intracellular transport of potassium rather than depletion of body stores. Therefore, only mild repletion of extracellular potassium is necessary (5–10 mEq KCl/h).
3. Seizures usually respond to intravenous diazepam; phenytoin is a second-line drug; phenobarbital may be used or, if necessary, intubation and neuromuscular blockade with a nondepolarizing neuromuscular blocking agent and thiopental general anesthesia to prevent complications such as permanent neurologic sequelae, rhabdomyolysis, paralysis, and acute renal failure. Continuous electroencephalographic and hemodynamic monitoring is helpful in determining the effectiveness of therapy.
4. Baseline laboratory values include serum electrolytes, arterial blood gases, creatinine, creatine kinase, myoglobin, and complete blood count. Urine studies are obtained for myoglobin. Electrocardiographic and electroencephalographic monitoring should be continued for at least 48 hours.

REFERENCES—BUPROPION

1. James WA, Lippmann S. Bupropion: Overview and prescribing guidelines in depression. South Med J 1991;84:222–224.
2. Spiller HA, Ramoska EA, Krenzelok EP, et al.: Bupropion overdose: A 3 year multicenter retrospective analysis. Am J Emerg Med 1994;12:43–45.
3. Bryant SG, Guernsey BG, Ingrim NB. Review of bupropion. Clin Pharm 1983;2:525–537.
4. Storrow AB. Bupropion overdose and seizures. Am J Emerg Med 1994;12:183–184.
5. Wender PH, Reimherr FW. Bupropion treatment of attention-deficit hyperactivity disorder in adults. Am J Psychiatry 1990;147:1018–1020.
6. Bloomingdale LM. Change from Mg-pemoline to bupropion in a 12 year old boy with attention deficit hyperactivity disorder. J Clin Psychopharmacol 1990;10:382–383.
7. Margolin A, Kosten T, Petrakis I, et al. Bupropion reduces cocaine abuse in methadone-maintained patients. Arch Gen Psychiatry 1991;48:87.
8. Haykal RF, Akiskal HS. Bupropion as a promising approach to rapid cycling bipolar II patients. J Clin Psychiatry 1990;51:450–455.
9. Michell GF, Mebane AH, Billings CK. Effect of bupropion on chocolate craving. Am J Psychiatry 1989;146:119–120.
10. Collins GE, McConnell B. Personal communications. Burroughs–Wellcome, March 7, 1991; August 12, 1991.
11. Friel PN, Logan BK, Fligner CL. Three fatal overdoses involving bupropion. J Anal Toxicol 1993;17:436–438.

12. Findlay JWA, Fleet JVW, Smith PG, et al. Pharmacokinetics of bupropion, a novel antidepressant agent following oral administration to healthy subjects. Eur J Clin Pharmacol 1981; 21:127–135.
13. Ramcharitar V, Levine BS, Golderberger BA, Caplan IH. Bupropion and alcohol fatal intoxication. Forens Sci Int 1992; 56:151. Case report.
14. Lai AA, Schroeder DH. Clinical pharmacokinetics of bupropion: A review. J Clin Psychiatry 1983;44:5(sect. 2):82–84.
15. Schroeder DH. Metabolism and kinetics of bupropion. J Clin Psychiatry 1983;44:79–81.
16. Preskorn SH, Fleck RJ, Schroeder DH. Therapeutic drug monitoring of bupropion. Am J Psychiatry 1990;147:1690–1691.
17. Preskorn SH, Katz SE. Bupropion plasma levels: Intraindividual and interindividual variability. Ann Clin Psychiatry 1989;1:59–61.
18. Golden RN, DeVane CL, Laizure SC, et al. Bupropion in depression: II. The role of metabolites in clinical outcome. Arch Gen Psychiatry 1988;45:145–149.
19. Golden RN, Rudorfer WV, Sherer MA, et al. Bupropion in depression: I. Biochemical effects and clinical response. Arch Gen Psychiatry 1988;45:139–143.
20. De Vane CL, Laizure SC, Stewart JT, et al. Disposition of bupropion in healthy volunteers and subjects with alcoholic liver disease. J Clin Psychopharmacol 1990;10:328–332.
21. Dager SR, Heritch AJ. A case of bupropion-associated delirium. J Clin Psychiatry 1990;51:307–308.
22. Van Putten T, Shaffer I. Delirium associated with bupropion. J Clin Psychopharmacol 1990;10:234.
23. Liberzon I, Dequardo JR, Silk KR. Bupropion and delirium. Am J Psychiatry 1990;147:1689–1690.
24. Briggs GG, Samson JH, Ambrose PJ, Schroeder DH. Excretion of bupropion in breast milk. Ann Pharmacother 1993; 27:431–437.
25. Wenger TL, Stern WC. The cardiovascular profile of bupropion. J Clin Psychiatry 1983;44(5, sect. 2):176–182.
26. Davidson J. Seizures and bupropion: A review. J Clin Psychiatry 1989;50:256–261.
27. Roose SP, Glassman AH, Giardina EGV, et al. Cardiovascular effects of imipramine and bupropion in depressed patients with congestive heart failure. J Clin Psychopharmacol 1987; 7:247–251.
28. Halbreich U, Rojansky N, Bakhai Y, Wang K. Menstrual irregularities associated with bupropion treatment. J Clin Psychiatry 1991;52:15–16.
29. Cooper TB, Suckow RF, Glassman A. Determination of bupropion and its basic metabolites in plasma by liquid chromatography with dual wavelength UV detection. J Pharm Sci 1984;73:1104–1107.
30. Oslin DW, Duffy K. The rise of serum aminotransferases in a patient treated with bupropion. J Clin Psychopharmacol 1993;13:364–365.

CLEBOPRIDE

Clebopride is a derivative of the orthoprumide group with central dopaminergic activity and an affinity for dopamine D_2 receptors. It is used in Spain and Italy for the treatment of gastrointestinal distress.[1] Chronic use of 1 to 1.5 mg/d has resulted in a reversible parkinsonian syndrome and tardive dyskinesia.[1,2] There are few reports of overdose. Treatment of clebopride overdose should be symptomatic and supportive.

REFERENCES—CLEBOPRIDE

1. Sempere AP, Duarte J, Palomares JM, et al. Parkinsonism and tardive dyskinesias after chronic use of clebopride. Mov Disord 1994;9:114–115.
2. Martinez-Martin P. Transient dyskinesia induced by clebopride. Mov Disord 1993;8:125–126.

DOBUTAMINE HYDROCHLORIDE

Few patients with dobutamine overdose have been reported.[1–5] Toxic symptoms and signs are usually related to excessive cardiac beta-receptor stimulation. There have been no reported fatalities due to an overdose. Dobutamine is primarily an inotropic agent with modest peripheral vasodilating properties.[6]

Structure and Classification

Dobutamine hydrochloride has a molecular weight of 337.8. Its freebase molecular weight is 301.4. Dobutamine, a synthetic product, is structurally related to dopamine. The hydrochloride occurs as a white to off-white crystalline powder sparingly soluble in water and in alcohol. Dobutamine hydrochloride is a synthetic catecholamine.

Use

Dobutamine hydrochloride injections are used when parenteral therapy is necessary for inotropic support in the *short-term* treatment of adults with cardiac decompensation due to depressed contractility resulting either from organic heart disease or from cardiac surgical procedures.[7,8] In doses that produce similar increases in cardiac output, dobutamine may produce a smaller increase in heart rate, a smaller decrease in peripheral resistance, and a smaller decrease in diastolic blood pressure than isoproterenol.[9,10] The relative value of dobutamine and dopamine in patients with congestive heart failure remains to be established.[9] Controlled trials of dobutamine in acute heart failure or cardiogenic shock have not been conducted. Dobutamine infused at 15 μg/kg/min may be useful in reversing the hemodynamic collapse produced by early administration of beta-adrenergic blocking agents in patients with myocardial infarction.[11]

Product Formulation

Dobutamine hydrochloride is available as a parenteral concentrate for injection and for intravenous infusion containing 12.5 mg (of dobutamine) per milliliter, with sodium bisulfite 0.24 mg/mL and water for injection (Dobutrex). The 20-mL sterile solution vial should be diluted in 5% dextrose or 9% sodium chloride 100 to 500 mL prior to administration. Dobutamine hydrochloride should not be added to an alkaline diluent.[9]

Therapeutic Dose

The concentration of dobutamine administered depends on the dosage and fluid requirements of the patient but should not exceed 5000 μg/mL.[9] The rate and duration of infusion should be adjusted according to the patient's response as indicated by heart rate, blood pressure, urine flow, presence of ectopic heart beats, and, whenever possible, measurement of central venous pressure or pulmonary wedge pressure and cardiac output. The rate of infusion usually required to increase cardiac output is 2.5 to 15 μg/kg/min following an adequate fluid resuscitation. Up to 40 μg/kg/min has rarely been required.

Toxic Dose

A patient with an acute myocardial infarction received 40 μg/kg/min and survived.[2] Dobutamine 50 mg was administered as a bolus injection to a 36-year-old patient in cardiogenic shock. There were no significant immediate sequelae.[4] One 56-year-old patient accidentally received 70 μg/kg/min dobutamine and survived but died 10 days later of an arterial embolus.[1] A 47-year-old inadvertently received 130 μg/kg/min for 30 minutes; there were no sequelae.[3] A 2-hour infusion of 30 μg/kg/min in one patient and a 5-minute infusion of 80 μg/kg/min did not produce any life-threatening reactions.[2]

Fatal Dose

A fatal dose of dobutamine has not been determined.

Toxicokinetics

Absorption

Dobutamine is inactive after oral administration because of extensive presystemic metabolism in the gastrointestinal mucosa and the liver.[12] Infusion of 2 μg/kg/min produces a serum dobutamine level of approximately 20 ng/mL in about 10 minutes.[9,13] The duration of action is less than 10 minutes.[14] In children, infusions of dobutamine ranging from 2 to 15 mg/kg/min result in plasma levels of 6.4 to 347 ng/mL.[15] Dobutamine toxicokinetics in children follow a first-order kinetic model.[16] The threshold plasma level for increasing cardiac output in children is about 8 ng/mL, and that for an increase in systolic blood pressure, about 34 ng/mL.[17]

Distribution

Dobutamine has an apparent volume of distribution of 0.20 to 0.08 L/kg in patients with low-output cardiac failure.[14] In children post-open heart surgery the volume of distribution is 3.2 L/kg.[18]

Elimination

The plasma half-life of dobutamine is about 2 minutes. Dobutamine is metabolized in the liver and other tissues by catechol-*O*-methyltransferase to an inactive compound, 3-*O*-methyldobutamine, and by conjugation with glucuronic acid. Conjugates of dobutamine and 3-*O*-methyldobutamine are excreted mainly in the urine.[19] Total body clearance values in children vary from 32 to 625 mL/kg/min.[15] Plasma clearance in children averages about 15 mL/kg/min.[17]

Drug Interactions

Beta-adrenergic Blocking Agents. In animals the cardiac effects of dobutamine may be antagonized by beta-adrenergic blocking agents such as propranolol and metoprolol, resulting in unopposed alpha-adrenergic effects and increased peripheral resistance.[9]

General Anesthesia. Ventricular arrhythmias have occurred in animals receiving dobutamine during halothane or cyclopropane anesthesia. There is preliminary evidence that nitroprusside and organic nitrates may be additive to dobutamine, resulting in a higher cardiac output and a lower pulmonary wedge pressure than use of either drug alone.[13] There is no evidence of drug interaction in clinical use when dobutamine is administered concurrently with digitalis preparations, furosemide, spironolactone, lidocaine, glyceryl trinitrate, isosorbide dinitrate, morphine, atropine, heparin, protamine, potassium chloride, folic acid, and acetaminophen.[7]

Pregnancy/Lactation

Safe use of dobutamine during pregnancy has not been established. It is not known whether dobutamine crosses the placenta.

Mechanism of Action

Dobutamine exerts its cardiovascular action through its β_1-adrenergic agonist activity. It also induces α_1-adrenoceptor-mediated vasoconstriction and β_2-adrenoceptor-mediated vasodilation. In animals, this results in an increase in cardiac output but little change in blood pressure. The (*d*) enantiomer acts on β_1 adrenoceptors to increase cardiac contractility and on β_2 adrenoceptors to cause vasodilation.[20] The (*l*) enantiomer acts on α_1 adrenoceptors to increase vascular resistance.[21,22] Dobutamine has no action on dopamine receptors. Unlike dopamine, dobutamine does not cause release of endogenous norepinephrine.

Clinical Presentation

Overdose

Dobutamine excess induces a decrease in systemic vascular resistance with hypotension and oliguria; supraventricular tachycardia; stuffy nose, hoarseness, red warm skin[1]; feelings of anxiousness, jitteriness, tachypnea; palpitations, anginal or chest pain, paresthesias of the upper extremities, enuresis, and urinary incontinence.[3] Signs and symptoms usually clear within 2 hours.[4] The commercial dobutamine solution contains sodium bisulfite, which can induce allergic-type reactions including anaphylaxis or a life-threatening clinical state. Sulfite sensitivity is frequently seen in asthmatics. Hypersensitivity-type local erythema and pruritus develop 4 to 12 days after dobutamine use at the site of intravenous administration.[23] Positive inotropic and chronotropic effects of dobutamine on the myocardium may cause hypertension, tachyrhythmias, myocardial ischemia, and ventricular fibrillation.[7,24,25]

Withdrawal

Many patients with severe decompensated ventricular failure who have been hemodynamically stabilized with dobutamine develop an intolerance to dobutamine withdrawal with a worsening of symptoms of dyspnea, systemic hypertension, or a deterioration of renal function. Hemodynamic intolerance to dobutamine withdrawal is defined as (1) a decrease in cardiac index to less than 2.2 L/min/m^2 or, if the baseline measure was less than this, a 10% decrease in cardiac index; (2) an increase in pulmonary wedge pressure to 20 mm Hg or an increase of 10% over the baseline value; and (3) a decrease in systolic blood pressure to less than 70 mm Hg.[26]

Laboratory

Analytical Methods

A high-performance liquid chromatography method with electrochemical detection is available for quantitative dobutamine assays. The limit of sensitivity is 0.1 μg/L.[14] A radioenzymatic assay also has been developed.[17]

Ancillary Tests

Dobutamine, like other β_2 agonists, may produce a mild reduction in serum potassium concentrations, rarely to hypokalemic levels.[7] Ischemia induced by dobutamine stress testing at doses up to 40 μg/kg/min given to post-myocardial infarction patients induced a decrease in stroke volume with no change in pulmonary artery wedge pressure.[27]

Treatment

Stabilization

Dobutamine should be stopped after an overdose until the condition of the patient stabilizes, at which time it may be reintroduced at a lower dose. An airway should be established, a supply of oxygen ensured, and respirations monitored and supported. Vital signs, blood pressure, and, where possible, central venous pressure and pulmonary wedge pressure must be monitored.

Gut Decontamination

If an overdose has been ingested orally, consider use of activated charcoal. There has been no clinical evidence for the safety or effectiveness of syrup of ipecac, gastric lavage, activated charcoal, or cathartics after an oral dobutamine overdose.

Elimination Enhancement

Forced diuresis, peritoneal dialysis, hemodialysis, and charcoal hemoperfusion have not been evaluated in the treatment of an overdose of dobutamine hydrochloride.

Antidote

There is no antidote.

Supportive Measures

1. Monitor the patient's vital signs, arterial blood gases, and serum electrolytes and maintain within acceptable limits.
2. Monitor the patient in an intensive care unit for 24 hours after an overdose.
3. Do not discharge or transfer the patient until serial electrocardiograms and cardiac enzymes show no evidence of myocardial damage.[3]
4. Dobutamine withdrawal symptoms and signs may be ameliorated by hydralazine 25 mg immediately before the first reduction in the dobutamine infusion, and every 4 hours thereafter to a maximal dose of 150 mg.[26]

REFERENCES—DOBUTAMINE HYDROCHLORIDE

1. Goethals M, Demey H. Massive dobutamine overdose in a cardiovascular compromised patient. Acta Cardiol 1984; 39:373–378.
2. Gillespie TA, Ambos HD, Sobel BE, Roberts R. Effects of dobutamine in patients with acute myocardial infarction. Am J Cardiol 1977;39:588–593.
3. Paulman PM, Cantral K, Meade JG, et al. Dobutamine overdose. JAMA 1990;264:2386–2387.
4. Gabry AL, Pourriat J-L, Hoang The Dan Ph, et al. Choc cardiogenique au cours d'une intoxication neuroleptique: Reversibilite par bolus de dobutamine. Presse 1982;11: 2225–2226.
5. Leier CV, Webel J, Bush CA. The cardiovascular effects of the continuous infusion of dobutamine in patients with severe cardiac failure. Circulation 1977;56:468–472.
6. Wood M. Drugs and the sympathetic nervous system. In: Wood M, Wood AJJ, eds. *Drugs and Anesthesia: Pharmacology for Anesthesiologists.* Baltimore: Williams & Wilkins, 1990:395.
7. *Physicians' Desk Reference.* 46th ed. Montvale, NJ: Medical Economics, 1992:1259–1260.
8. Mueller HS. Inotropic agents in the treatment of cardiogenic shock. World J Surg 1985;9:3–10.
9. McEvoy GK, ed. *AHFS Drug Information 92.* Bethesda, MD: American Society of Hospital Pharmacists, 1992:669–670.
10. Parmley WW, Chatterjee K, Francis GS, et al. Congestive heart failure: New frontiers. West J Med 1991;154:427–441.
11. Waagstein F, Malek I, Hjalmarson AC. The use of dobutamine in myocardial infarction for reversal of the cardiodepressive effect of metoprolol. Br J Clin Pharmacol 1978;5:515–521.
12. Dollery C, ed. *Therapeutic Drugs.* Edinburgh: Churchill Livingstone, 1991:D196–D201.
13. Leiser CV, Unverferth DV, Kates RE. The relationship between plasma dobutamine concentrations and cardiovascular responses in cardiac failure. Am J Med 1979;66:238–242.
14. Kates RE, Leier CV. Dobutamine pharmacokinetics in severe heart failure. Clin Pharmacol Ther 1978;24:537–541.
15. Banner W, Vernon DD, Minton SD, Dean JM. Nonlinear dobutamine pharmacokinetics in a pediatric population. Crit Care Med 1991;19:871–873.
16. Habil DM, Padbury JF, Anas NG, et al. Dobutamine pharmacokinetics and pharmacodynamics in pediatric intensive care patients. Crit Care Med 1992;20:601–608.
17. Padbury JF, Perkin RM, Anas NG, et al. Dobutamine pharmacokinetics in pediatric intensive care patients. Clin Res 1989;37:176A.
18. Blumer JL, Ruggerie DP, Witte WK, et al. Polymorphic clearance (l) of dopamine (DA) and dobutamine (DB) in children (K). Clin Pharmacol Ther 1989;45:140.
19. Murphy PJ, Williams TL, Kare DLK. Disposition of dobutamine in the dog. J Pharmacol Exp Ther 1976;199:423–431.
20. Broadley KJ. Cardiac adrenoceptors. J Auton Pharmacol 1982;2:119.
21. Ruffalo RR Jr, Spradlin TA, Pollock GD, et al. Alpha- and beta-adrenergic effects of the stereoisomers of dobutamine. J Pharmacol Exp Ther 1981;219:447–452.
22. Ruffalo RR Jr, Yaden EL. Vascular effects of the stereoisomers of dobutamine. J Pharmacol Exp Ther 1983;224:46–50.
23. Wu C-C, Chen W-J, Cheng J-J, et al. Local dermal hypersensitivity from dobutamine hydrochloride (Dobutrex solution) injection. Chest 1991;99:1547–1548.
24. Majerus TC, Dasta JF, Bauman JL, et al. Dobutamine: Ten years later. Pharmacotherapy 1989;9:245–249.
25. Mutnick AH, Szymusiak-Mutnick B, Drea EJ. Dopamine versus dobutamine: Are all the facts there? Pharmacotherapy 1990;10:224–229.

26. Binkley PF, Starling RC, Hammer DF, Leier CV. Usefulness of hydralazine to withdraw from dobutamine in severe congestive heart failure. Am J Cardiol 1991;68:1103–1106.
27. Pierard LA, Berthe C, Albert A, et al. Haemodynamic alterations during ischaemia induced by dobutamine stress testing. Eur Heart J 1989;10:783–790.

DOPAMINE HYDROCHLORIDE

Dopamine hydrochloride is a commonly used pressor agent. When administered intravenously it stimulates alpha-adrenergic receptor sites to induce peripheral vasoconstriction, which may become so severe that it compromises the peripheral arterial circulation and can lead to gangrene. Few cases of accidental overdose have been reported, but tissue extravasations have required infiltration of an antidote, phentolamine mesylate. Fatalities have occurred in association with dopamine overdose.

Structure and Classification

Dopamine hydrochloride is an endogenous catecholamine. The conversion factor is 5.27: μg/mL × 5.27 = μmol/L; umol/L ÷ 5.27 = μg/mL.

Use

Dopamine hydrochloride is indicated for the correction of hemodynamic imbalances present in the shock syndrome due to myocardial infarctions, trauma, endotoxic septicemia, open heart surgery, renal failure, and chronic cardiac decompensation as in congestive failure. It is useful in conditions caused by poor perfusion of vital organs, low cardiac output, and hypotension.

Product Formulation

Dopamine hydrochloride (Intropin) contains, in each milliliter, either 40, 80, or 160 mg as a concentrate for injection for intravenous infusion (equivalent to 323, 64.6, and 129.2 mg dopamine base), respectively, in water for injection, containing 1% sodium metabisulfite as an antioxidant. The solution is sterile and nonpyrogenic with a pH of 2.5 to 4.5. Dopamine hydrochloride in dextrose is available for intravenous infusion containing 0.8 mg/mL (200 or 400 mg), 1.6 mg/mL (400 or 800 mg), or 32 mg/mL (800 m) as 0.08, 0.16, or 32%, respectively of dopamine hydrochloride in dextrose 5% injection (with sulfites). Dopamine hydrochloride in dextrose injection has a pH of 3 to 5; it is incompatible with iron salts, oxidizing agents, and sodium bicarbonate and other alkaline solutions. Dopamine hydrochloride is sensitive to and should be protected from light. Yellow, brown, or pink to purple discoloration of solutions indicates decomposition of the drug. Such solutions should not be used.

Source

Dopamine hydrochloride used commercially is a synthetic chemical. It is also a naturally occurring catecholamine.

Therapeutic Dose

One suggested solution for infusion may be prepared by diluting 5 mL of the injection containing 40 mg/mL dopamine hydrochloride (a total of 200 mg of dopamine hydrochloride) with either 250 or 500 mL of a solution such as 0.9% sodium chloride, 5% dextrose, 5% dextrose with 0.9% sodium chloride, 5% dextrose with 0.45% sodium chloride, lactated Ringer's, 5% dextrose in lactated Ringer's. Dilution with 250 mL of solution yields a concentration of 800 μg/mL. Dopamine infusion is usually begun at a rate of 1 to 5 μg/kg/min. The infusion rate may be increased by 1 to 4 μg/kg/min at 10- to 30-minute intervals until optimal response is reached. Most patients can be maintained at 20 μg/kg/min or smaller dosages.

Toxic Dose

Intravenous dopamine in dosages greater than 10 μg/kg/min may induce sufficient alpha-adrenergic stimulation to cause excessive peripheral vasoconstriction and gangrene, often requiring amputation. Patients have lived after such doses. A similar result followed 1.5 μg/kg/min.[1] Infiltration of dopamine into the tissues following extravasation has occurred following 5.9 and 7 μg/kg/min.[2,3] In both patients, amputation was required.

Fatal Dose

A 30-year-old woman received daily doses of dopamine ranging from 14 to 115 μg/kg/min and doses of dobutamine from 9 to 54 μg/kg/min; she died.[4] A 1-day-old 29-week premature infant received an overdose of 125 μg/kg/min during a 1-hour period and died within 1 hour.[5]

Toxicokinetics

Absorption

Dopamine is inactivated after oral administration and therefore is administered only by the intravenous route. Dopamine administered in dosages of 1, 3, 6, 9, and 14 μg/kg/min leads to plasma levels that correlate with the infusion rate, increasing from 0.04 μg/L to 208 μg/L during the highest infusion rates. The so-called renal dose of dopamine (3 μg/kg/min) corresponds to a plasma level of 57 μg/L. This is higher than the plasma level, which affects most metabolic (glucose, nonesterified fatty acids) and cardiovascular (systolic, diastolic, blood pressure, heart rate) variables.[6–8] As a normal constituent of plasma most dopamine (99%) is conjugated to sulfate.[8]

Distribution

Following intravenous administration dopamine is rapidly distributed with a volume of distribution of 0.89 L/kg. In newborns the average apparent volume of distribution is 1.81 L/kg.[9] Steady-state plasma concentrations are achieved in 5 to 10 minutes. In infants such steady-state concentrations ranged from 0.013 to 0.3 μg/mL.[10] Infants and young children appear to require larger weight-normalized dosages of dopamine to achieve effects comparable to those in adults.[11] Clearance may be more rapid in infants. Dopamine does not cross the blood–brain barrier and therefore does not affect D_1 and D_2 receptors in the central nervous system.

Elimination

After termination of an infusion dopamine is eliminated from the plasma with a half-life of about 9 minutes. The pharmacologic half-life of an intravenous bolus dose is about 2 minutes, and the duration of action is about 10 minutes. Total body clearance of dopamine is approximately 73 $mL/kg/min^3$ and averages 115 mL/kg/min in newborns.[9] Dopamine is extensively metabolized in the liver. Less than 10% of a dose is recovered unchanged in the urine.[11] The principal means of elimination appears to be *O*-methylation by catechol-*O*-methyltransferase to form 3-methoxytyramine, followed either by sulfoconjugation (by phenosulfotransferase) or by deamination (by monoamine oxidase) to homovanillic acid.[12] About 20% of dopamine is also cleared by the lungs, especially when plasma dopamine levels are elevated.[13]

Drug Interactions

Monoamine Oxidase Inhibitors. Monoamine oxidase inhibitors may prolong and intensify the effects of dopamine as dopamine is metabolized by monoamine oxidase. In patients who have received monoamine oxidase inhibitors in the previous 2 to 3 weeks, the initial dose of dopamine should be no greater than 10% of the usual dose.

Alpha- and Beta-adrenergic Receptors. The cardiac effects of dopamine are antagonized by beta-adrenergic blocking drugs such as propranolol and metoprolol. The peripheral vasoconstriction caused by high doses of dopamine is antagonized by alpha-adrenergic blocking agents.

General Anesthetics. Ventricular arrhythmias and hypertension may occur when therapeutic doses of dopamine are administered during halothane or cyclopropane anesthesia.

Phenytoin. Intravenous phenytoin infused into patients receiving dopamine may result in hypotension and bradycardia.

Other Drugs. Ergot alkaloids, tricyclic antidepressants, and guanethidine may potentiate pressor responses to dopamine.

Pregnancy/Lactation

Dopamine hydrochloride has been placed in Pregnancy Category C. There are no adequate and well-controlled studies in pregnant women. Dopamine is unlikely to be excreted in breast milk. Any that is excreted would probably be inactivated by the neonate before reaching the systemic circulation. Animal studies indicate that dopamine interferes with vitamin B_1 metabolism.[14]

Mechanism of Action

At low dosages (0.5–2 μg/kg/min), D_1 and D_2 receptors are activated.

D_1 receptors are located on vascular smooth muscle and participate in renal, mesenteric, cerebral, and coronary vascular dilation.[15]

D_2 receptors are located on postganglionic sympathetic neuron endings and autonomic ganglia. D_2 receptor activation inhibits noradrenaline release from sympathetic nerve endings. Blood pressure remains stable or may decrease.[16] Renal plasma flow, glomerular filtration rate, and sodium excretion usually increase.[17–19]

At higher dosages (2–5 μg/kg/min), beta adrenoceptors are activated leading to increased cardiac contractility, heart rate, and atrioventricular conduction. Dopamine acts on β_1 receptors to release noradrenaline from myocardial storage sites; cardiac output and systolic blood pressure increase.

After an increase in dosage (>5 μg/kg/min), α_1 and α_2 receptors are activated.[20] These are located on vascular effector cells and, when activated by dopamine, cause vasoconstriction. Activation of α_2 adrenoceptors on the prejunctional sympathetic nerve terminals leads to inhibition of noradrenaline release. Systolic and diastolic pressures increase.

Clinical Presentation

Patients with prior vascular disease may be subject to excess ischemic effects from the alpha-adrenergic stimulated vasoconstriction induced by dopamine.[20–24] Such ischemic effects often begin after 24 hours of dopamine use and may progress to gangrene of an extremity (often requiring amputation); they are more likely to occur at dopamine infusion levels of 10 μg/kg/min or above. One patient developed bilateral retinal infarctions after dopamine infusion at a rate of 14 to 115 μg/kg/min.[4] A newborn died within 1 hour of receiving an overdose of 125 μg/kg/min.[5] Extravasation and infiltration of dopamine may lead to ischemia, gangrene, and amputation of an extremity.[2,3]

Laboratory

Analytical Methods

Dopamine in plasma may be measured by high-performance liquid chromatography using electrochemical detection with a carbon paste electrode; this method is sensitive to 1 μg/L. A radioenzymatic assay is also available.[25]

Abnormalities

Dopamine or its metabolites may interfere with urine tests for catecholamines, amino acids, uric acid, or urobilinogen.

Treatment

Stabilization

Patients receiving dopamine should be under careful observation in a health care facility with continued cardiac monitoring of cardiac rate and blood pressure. Patients should be under electrocardiographic surveillance. Urine flow and fluid balance should be measured. Determinations of cardiac output and pulmonary wedge pressure are useful. In case of an accidental dopamine overdose, as evidenced by an excessive blood pressure elevation, the rate of administration should be reduced or the dopamine infusion temporarily discontinued until the patient's condition stabilizes. Additional remedial measures are usually not necessary. If these measures fail to stabilize the patient's condition, phentolamine should be considered (see Antidote).

Antidote

To prevent sloughing and necrosis in ischemic areas, the area should be infiltrated as soon as possible with 10 to 15 mL of saline solution containing from 5 to 10 mg of Regitine (brand of phentolamine mesylate), and adrenergic blocking agent. A syringe with a fine hypodermic needle should be used, and the solution liberally infiltrated throughout the ischemic area. Sympathetic blockade with phentolamine causes immediate and conspicuous local hyperemic changes if the area is infiltrated within 12 hours. Therefore, phentolamine should be given as soon as possible after the extravasation is noted.[26] Blood pressure should be monitored for hypotension following phentolamine use, and the patient observed for development of arrhythmias or tachycardias.

Phentolamine mesylate 50 mg, diluted to 1 mg/mL with 0.9% sodium chloride injection, has been administered in multiple subcutaneous injections of 0.5 mg each to cover an entire area of extravasation. No apparent adverse reactions were observed and the blood pressure did not decrease. The half-life of phentolamine is about 20 minutes. The possible risk of phentolamine-induced hypotension may be minimized by giving multiple small doses over a period of 1 to 2 hours.[27,28]

Supportive Measures

1. Continuously monitor the peripheral extremity arterial pulses and observe the color of the extremities during a dopamine infusion, especially in elderly patients with preexisting vascular damage from arteriosclerosis, diabetes mellitus, Raynaud's disease, or frostbite.
2. In such cases, reduce the starting dose of dopamine to 1 μg/kg/min or less and frequently examine the extremities.[1]
3. If discoloration appears, stop the infusion, give phentolamine 5 to 10 mg intravenously, and repeat as required.
4. Intravenous chlorpromazine 10 mg as a loading dose and 0.6 mg/min drip has been used for digital ischemia following dopamine use.[21] In one patient use of chlorpromazine permitted continued use of dopamine without recurrence of ischemia.[21] Further clinical trials with this medication are indicated.
5. Before pharmacologic intervention, carefully evaluate intravascular volume and institute adequate fluid replacement if hypovolemia is present.[20]
6. Even in patients without vascular disease, exercise great care when infusing dopamine, especially in a peripheral vein.[2]
7. Consider administration of dopamine through indwelling venous catheters.[2,3]
8. For any child receiving dopamine by a peripheral infusion, perform careful serial examinations of the extremities throughout the period of dopamine administration.[23]

REFERENCES—DOPAMINE HYDROCHLORIDE

1. Greene SI, Smith JW. Dopamine gangrene. N Engl J Med 1976;294:114.
2. Ebels TJ, Homan van der Heide JN. Dopamine-induced ischaemia. Lancet 1977;2:762.
3. Boltax RS, Dineen JP, Scarpa FJ. Gangrene resulting from infiltrated dopamine solution. N Engl J Med 1977;296:823.
4. Opremcak EM, Davidorf FH. Bilateral retinal infarction associated with high dose dopamine. Ann Ophthalmol 1985; 17:141–144.
5. Curel HE. Personal communication. DuPont Pharmaceuticals, January 30, 1992.
6. Ensinger H, Schulich S, Grunert A, Ahnefeld FW. Dopamine: Cardiovascular and metabolic effects in relation to plasma levels. Crit Care Med 1990;18:S179.
7. Padbury JF, Agata Y, Baylen BG, et al. Pharmacokinetics of dopamine in critically ill newborn infants. J Pediatr 1990; 17:472–476.
8. Eldrup E, Hagen C, Christensen NJ, Olgaard K. Plasma free and sulfoconjugated dopamine in man: Relationship to sympathetic activity, adrenal function and meals. Dan Med Bull 1988;35:291–294.
9. Bhatt-Mehta V, Nahata MC, McClead RE, Menke JA. Dopamine pharmacokinetics in critically ill newborn infants. Eur J Clin Pharmacol 1991;40:593–597.
10. Eldadah MK, Schwartz PH, Harrison R, Newth CJL. Pharmacokinetics of dopamine in infants and children. Crit Care Med 1991;19:1008–1011.
11. Notterman DA, Greenwald BM, Moran F, et al. Dopamine clearance in critically ill infants and children: Effect of age and organ system dysfunction. Clin Pharmacol Ther 1990;48:138–147.
12. Kopin IJ. Catecholamine metabolism: Basic aspects and clinical significance. Pharmacol Rev 1985;37:333–363.
13. Sumikawa K, Hayashi Y, Yamatodani A, Yoshiya I. Contribution of the lungs to the clearance of exogenous dopamine in humans. Anesth Analg 1991;72:622–626.
14. Weir MR, Keniston RC, Enriquez JI Sr, McNamee GA. Depression of vitamin B_6 levels due to dopamine. Vet Hum Toxicol 1991;33:118–121.
15. Frederickson Ed, Bradley TJ, Goldberg LI. Block of the renal effects of dopamine in the dog by the DA_1 antagonist, SCH 23390. Am J Physiol 1985;249:F236–F240.
16. Levinson PD, Goldstein PS, Mundson PJ, et al. Endocrine, renal and hemodynamic responses to graded dopamine infusions in normal men. J Clin Endocrinol Metab 1985;60:821–826.
17. McDonald RH, Goldberg LI, McNay JL. Effects of dopamine in man: Augmentation of sodium excretion, glomerular filtration rate and renal plasma flow. J Clin Invest 1964; 43:1116–1124.
18. Goldberg LI. Cardiovascular and renal actions of dopamine: Potential clinical applications. Pharmacol Rev 1972;24:1–29.
19. Parker S, Carlon GC, Isaacs M, et al. Dopamine administration in oliguria and oliguric renal failure. Crit Care Med 1981;9:630–632.
20. Greenlaw CW, Null LW II. Dopamine-induced ischemia. Lancet 1977;2:555.
21. Alexander CS, Sako Y, Mikulic E. Pedal gangrene associated with the use of dopamine. N Engl J Med 1975;293:591.
22. Valdes ME. Post-dopamine ischemia treated with chlorpromazine. N Engl J Med 1976;295:1081–1082.
23. Goldbranson FL, Lurie L, Vance RM, Vondell RF. Multiple extremity amputations in hypotensive patients treated with dopamine. JAMA 1980;243:1145–1146.
24. Maggi JC, Angelats J, Scott JP. Gangrene in a neonate following dopamine therapy. J Pediatr 1982;100:323–325.
25. Prada M, Zurcher G. Simultaneous radioenzymatic determination of plasma and tissue adrenaline, noradrenaline, and dopamine within the femtomole range. Life Sci 1976;19: 1161–1174.
26. Intropin[R] (dopamine HCl injection, USP): Product Literature. 6227-1/Rev. Du Pont Pharmaceuticals, January 1991.

27. Cooper BE. High-dose phentolamine for extravasation of pressors. Clin Pharm 1989;8:689.
28. Siwy BK, Sadove AM. Acute management of dopamine infiltration injury with Regitine. Plast Reconstruct Surg 1987; 80:610–612.

DOPEXAMINE HYDROCHLORIDE

Dopexamine hydrochloride (Dopacard, United Kingdom) is a synthetic dopamine receptor agonist designed for use in low-cardiac-output states. Dopamine itself exhibits strong alpha-adrenoceptor stimulant effects (vasoconstriction) and strong β_1-adrenoceptor stimulation (tachycardia, arrhythmias). This may limit its therapeutic value. Dopexamine reduces systemic vascular resistance and afterload. This is followed by an increase in cardiac output. It has specific renal vasodilating properties but little direct and indirect positive inotropic and chronotropic effects, properties that suggest that it may be superior to dopamine in treatment of low-cardiac-output states without any attendant vasoconstriction, excess tachycardia, and arrhythmias.[1–4] Overdoses and fatalities have not been reported.[5]

Structure and Classification

Dopexamine is a derivative of dopamine.[6]

Therapeutic Dose

Dopexamine hydrochloride infused by the intravenous route at a rate of 0.5 to 6.0 μg/kg/min produces therapeutically useful systemic and renal vasodilation, enhanced diuresis, and improvement in indices of myocardial function in patients with acute heart failure. An initial dose of 0.5 μg/kg/min can be titrated upward in increments of 1.0 μg/kg/min based on hemodynamic response to a maximum of 6.0 μg/kg/min.[2]

Toxicokinetics

Absorption

Dopexamine hydrochloride infused at a rate of 1 to 4 μg/kg/min results in peak plasma concentrations of 124 μg/mL after 1 hour.[2]

Elimination

The elimination half-life is 7 minutes (11 minutes in patients with low cardiac output). Dopexamine is cleared from the plasma at the rate of 36 mL/min/kg (vs 17 mL/min/kg in patients following cardiac surgery.)[2] Dopexamine hydrochloride is metabolized by *O*-methylation and subsequent sulfate conjugation. The 2-methoxy-1-sulfate metabolite accounts for more than 90% of the excreted drug recovered from the urine.[2]

Mechanism of Action

DA_1 Receptors

Dopexamine is an agonist at DA_1 receptors with a potency 33% that of dopamine.[3]

DA_2 Receptors

Dopexamine is a four to five times less potent agonist at the DA_2 receptor site than dopamine.[3]

Alpha Adrenoceptors

Postjunctional alpha adrenoceptors mediate vasoconstriction and belong to both α_1 and α_2 subtypes. The vasoconstrictive effects of dopamine are thought to be mediated predominantly by α_2 adrenoceptors. Dopexamine has little, if any, alpha-adrenoceptor stimulant properties.[3]

β_1 Adrenoceptors

β_1 receptors, found predominantly in the heart, are responsible for the positive chronotropic and inotropic effects produced by sympathetic nerve stimulation and by catecholamines. They are also involved in the arrhythmogenic actions of catecholamines. Dopexamine has weak β_1-agonism activity.[1,3]

β_2 Adrenoceptors

β_2 adrenoceptors are located in the arterial smooth muscle (particularly in the skeletal muscle bed) and mediate vasodilation. They may also exist in the heart. Dopexamine is a stronger agonist of β_2-adrenoceptor activity than dopamine.[1,3]

Clinical Presentation

Dopexamine overdose has not been reported. Effects of an overdose are likely to be related to the pharmacologic actions and include tachycardia, tremulousness, tremor, nausea, vomiting, and anginal pain.[8] Treatment should be symptomatic and supportive.

The most frequently encountered adverse effects—nausea, vomiting, tachycardia, angina/chest pain, ventricular extrasystole, and tremor—are related to the drug's agonist effect on dopamine DA_2 receptors in the chemoreceptor trigger zone and beta adrenoceptors. These adverse effects usually respond rapidly to dose reduction and discontinuation of the infusion.[2]

Treatment

Treatment of an overdose requires immediate cessation of the infusion and cardiac monitoring including electrocardiogram, pulse, and blood pressure. A central venous line should be placed and oxygen made available; serial pulmonary wedge pressures will be useful if required based on clinical judgment. There is no antidote. Treatment guidelines follow, in general, those for dopamine and dobutamine overdoses.

REFERENCES—DOPEXAMINE HYDROCHLORIDE

1. Smith GW, O'Connor SE. An introduction to the pharmacologic properties of Dopacard (dopexamine hydrochloride). Am J Cardiol 1988;62:9C–17C.

2. Fitton A, Benfield P. Dopexamine hydrochloride: A review of its pharmacodynamic and pharmacokinetic properties and therapeutic potential in acute cardiac insufficiency. Drugs 1990;39:308–330.
3. Stephan H, Sonntag H, Henning H, Yoshimine K. Cardiovascular and renal haemodynamic effects of dopexamine comparison with dopamine. Br J Anaesth 1990;65:380–387.
4. Tan L-B, Littler WA, Murray RG. Comparison of the haemodynamic effects of dopexamine and dobutamine in patients with severe congestive heart failure. Int J Cardiol 1991; 30:203–208.
5. Hoff R. Personal communication. Fisons Pharmaceuticals, January 28, 1992.
6. Reynolds JEF, ed. *Martindale: The Extra Pharmacopoeia.* London: Pharmaceutical Press, 1989:1462.

LEVODOPA AND CARBIDOPA–LEVODOPA

LEVODOPA

Levodopa is an indirect dopamine agonist by virtue of its peripheral and central conversion to dopamine. Dopaminergic toxic effects include nausea, vomiting, hypotension, cardiac arrhythmias, behavioral changes, and abnormal involuntary movements. Acute overdose was reported in a 61-year-oid man following ingestion of 100g of levodopa. He experienced hypertension initially, followed by hypotension for a few hours, mild nausea, and severe anorexia that gradually resolved over 1 week. He had insomnia for about 1 week, confusion for 2 days, and agitation for 3 to 4 days.[1]

CARBIDOPA–LEVODOPA

Carbidopa–levodopa (Sinemet) in overdose may lead to convulsions, agitation, paranoia, or mania.[2] Carbidopa is a decarboxylase inhibitor that prevents peripheral destruction of levodopa. A 57-year-old woman ingested 15 to 17 tablets of carbidopa–levodopa 10/100 tablets (carbidopa 150 mg and levodopa 1500 mg) together with carisoprodol, ibuprofen, and hydrocodone–acetaminophen. She became obtunded and developed choreiform movements, hypoventilation, myoglobinuria, and an increase in the creatine kinase level. She was treated supportively with pancuronium and was discharged without symptoms after the eighth day.[3] Withdrawal of levodopa or carbidopa–levodopa may result in a neuroleptic malignant syndrome with hyperpyrexia, which may be fatal.[4]

The decarboxylation of levodopa to dopamine is catalyzed by the pyridoxine-dependent enzyme L-amino acid decarboxylase. Pyridoxine has been used to reverse the dyskinesias and choreoathetosis of levodopa.[5]

Levodopa levels in urine after an overdose show elevations in free and total levels of levodopa, dopamine, dihydroxyphenylacetic acid, norepinephrine, and homovanillic acid.[1]

LEVODOPA–CARBIDOPA—REFERENCES

1. Hoehn MM, Rutledge CO. Acute overdose with levodopa. Neurology 1975;25:792–794.
2. Nausieda PA. Sinemet "abusers." Clin Neuropharmacol 1985;8:318:327.
3. Sporer KA. Carbidopa–levodopa overdose. Am J Emerg Med 1991;9:47–48.
4. Sechi GP, Tanda F, Mutani R. Fatal hyperpyrexia after withdrawal of levodopa. Neurology 1984;34:249–251.
5. Jameson HD. Pyridoxine for levodopa induced dystonia. JAMA 1970;211:1700.

LISURIDE HYDROGEN MALEATE

Lisuride hydrogen maleate is a semisynthetic ergot derivative with dopaminergic activity and antiserotoninergic activity. It reduces thyroid-releasing hormone. Lisuride induces hypoprolactinemia in healthy women and reduces plasma prolactin concentrations in patients with pituitary tumors or functional hyperprolactinemia. Lisuride inhibits lactation and suppresses serum prolactin levels, effects that are dose related.[1] Lisuride is a prototype of the dopaminergic ergot alkaloids known as ergolines. It has not been approved by the Food and Drug Administration, but a related drug, pergolide, is now marketed in the United States. Lisuride is marketed outside the United States as Dopergic, Revanil, and Curvolet.

Use

See the preceding paragraph. Lisuride also has been used alone or in combination with levodopa for the treatment of parkinsonism. Lisuride has been used in the prophylaxis of migraine, hyperprolactinemia, and acromegaly.[2] Intravenous treatment may be indicated for neuroleptic malignant syndrome.[2]

Product Formulation

Lisuride hydrogen maleate is available in tablets of 0.025, 0.2, and 0.5 mg for oral use.

Source

Lisuride hydrogen maleate is a semisynthetic ergot derivative belonging the the 8-α-aminoergoline group.

Therapeutic Dose

Lisuride is administered in doses of between 1.5 and 4.5 mg daily to a maximum recommended dose of 10 mg daily.

Toxicokinetics

Absorption

Oral administration of 300 μg of lisuride hydrogen maleate results in a peak concentration of 0.3 to 3.30 ng/mL in about 40 minutes. Systemic availability after oral administration is 10 to 15%. Most of a dose is metabolized on first passage through the liver. Protein binding is about 80%. Parenteral use exhibits the following toxicokinetics.[2]

	Intravenous	Subcutaneous	Intramuscular
Plasma concentration	307 gg/mL	180 pg/mL	184 ng/mL
Total clearance	13 mL/min/kg		
Half-life		Biphasic 25 min 1.9 hours	Biphasic 19 min 1.5 hours
Systemic bioavailability		94%	90%
Apparent volume of distribution		2 L/kg	

Elimination

About 0.01 to 0.08% of a dose of lisuride is excreted unchanged.[3] Plasma clearance is 0.81/min (total clearance, 10–20 mL/min/kg).[4] The elimination half-life is 2 hours. Lisuride is eliminated almost entirely by the liver. Metabolites are not active. Lisuride with a plasma half-life of about 2 hours compares with bromocriptine (5 hours) and pergolide (>7 hours).

Drug Interactions

Synergism or antagonism follows interaction with other drugs acting on dopamine receptors.

Pregnancy/Lactation

Safe use of lisuride during pregnancy has not been established.

Mechanism of Action

Lisuride interacts with serotonin, dopamine, and noradrenergic receptors. It is a potent antagonist at peripheral serotonin receptors and is a potent agonist at central dopamine receptors. Its major effect is a long-lasting decrease in the plasma level of prolactin.[3] The effectiveness of lisuride in parkinsonism is enhanced when combined with a low dose of levodopa, a combination that stimulates both D_1 and D_2 receptors.[4] Dopamine agonists such as the ergot-derived bromocriptine, pergolide, and lisuride can cause postural hypotension and potentiate dyskinesias or toxic psychosis caused by levodopa. They may induce dopaminergic effects such as cardiac arrhythmias and nausea.

Clinical Presentation

Chronic Use

Lisuride may be associated with lightheadedness, drowsiness, vivid dreams, and abdominal discomfort.[5] There have been no significant changes in cardiovascular hemodynamics.[2] Nausea and orthostatic hypotension have been observed.[6] Symptoms include memory disturbances[7] and confusion, delirium, and visual hallucinations, which are often dose related. Cold extremities, digital vasospasm, burning of the skin, and chest pain may be ergotism-like symptoms. Headache, bradycardia, constipation, and diarrhea have been experienced.[8]

Overdose

A bolus subcutaneous injection of about 3 mg resulted in deep sedation with spontaneous recovery in 24 hours.[8] Ergotism and dopaminergic hyperstimulation may be observed.

Laboratory

A radioimmunoassay method for measuring lisuride hydrogen maleate in body fluids is highly sensitive and is relatively specific.[9]

Treatment

Stabilization

Patients should be placed on a cardiac monitor. A rapid increase in blood pressure and a left bundle-branch block have followed intravenous use of lisuride.[10]

Supportive Measures

Nausea and vomiting may be ameliorated by use of domperidone, a dopamine receptor antagonist[11] available in Canada but not in the United States.

REFERENCES—LISURIDE HYDROGEN MALEATE

1. De Cecco L, Venturini PL, Ragni N, et al. Effect of lisuride on inhibition of lactation and serum prolactin. Br J Obstet Gynecol 1979;86:905–908.
2. Krause W, Magen T, Kuhne G, Duka T, Voet B. The pharmacokinetics and pharmacodynamics of lisuride in healthy volunteers after intravenous, intramuscular and subcutaneous injection. Eur J Clin Pharmacol 1991;40:399–403.
3. Burns RS, Gopinatham G, Humpel M, et al. Disposition of oral lisuride in Parkinson's disease. Clin Pharmacol Ther 1984;35:548–556.
4. Rinne UK. Lisuride, a dopamine agonist in the treatment of early Parkinson's disease. Neurology 1989;39:336–339.
5. Ulm G. Experiences with lisuride in the treatment of Parkinson's disease. In: Calme DB, et al., ed. *Lisuride and Other Dopamine Agonists.* New York: Raven Press, 1983:463–472.
6. Bassi S, Ferrarese C, Frattola L, et al. Lisuride in generalized dystonia and spasmodic torticollis. Lancet 1982;1:1514–1515.
7. Liebermann AN, Leibowitz M, Gopinthan G, et al. Review: The use of pergolide and lisuride, two experimental dopamine agonists, in patients with advanced Parkinson's disease. Am J Med Sci 1985;290:102–106.
8. Dollery CT, ed. *Therapeutic Drugs.* Vol 2. Edinburgh: Churchill Livingstone, 1992:L43–L46.
9. Humpel M. The pharmacokinetics of lisuride in animal species and humans. In: Calme DB, Horowski R, McDonald RJ, Wuttke W, eds. *Lisuride and Other Dopamine Agonists.* New York: Raven Press, 1983.
10. Capria A, Attanasio A, Frongillo D, et al. Transient left bundle branch block following intravenous lisuride bolus. Fundam Clin Pharmacol 1993;7:115–117.
11. Dopamine agonists for Parkinson's disease. Drug Ther Bull 1991;29:7–8.

PERGOLIDE MESYLATE

Pergolide mesylate (Permax, Celance) is a synthetic ergoline derivative that acts as a dopamine agonist useful in the treatment of Parkinson's disease and hyperprolactinemia.

Dosage begins with oral tablets of 0.05 mg every day. This is titrated up to a maximum dose of 3 mg/d. A fatal dose has not been established. Oral absorption is more than 60%. The plasma half-life is 15 to 42 hours. Pergolide has an extensive volume of distribution (about 20 L/kg) and exhibits plasma protein binding of 90%. Overdoses of up to 19 mg/d have resulted in hallucinations, involuntary movements, palpitations, hypotension, and ventricular premature beats. Management of an overdose is largely symptomatic and supportive. The patient's airway is protected and cardiac function monitored. Activated charcoal may be useful. There is no experience with hemodialysis or hemoperfusion, and there is no antidote. Nausea may respond to an antiemetic (eg, domperidone). Prognosis for recovery is good.

REFERENCES—PERGOLIDE MESYLATE

1. Dollery C, ed. *Therapeutic Drugs.* Edinburgh: Churchill Livingstone, 1992:162–166.
2. Langtry HD, Clissold SP. Pergolide: A review of its pharmacological properties and therapeutic potential in Parkinson's disease. Drugs 1990;39:491–501.
3. Malcolm R, Hutto BR, Phillips JD, Ballenger JC. Pergolide mesylate: Treatment of cocaine withdrawal. J Clin Psychiatry 1991;52:39–40.
4. Bouckoms A, Mangini L. Pergolide: An antidepressant adjuvant for mood disorders? Psychopharmacol Bull 1993;29: 207–211.
5. Fuller RW, Clemens JA. Pergolide: A dopamine agonist at both D_1 and D_2 receptors. Life Sci 1982;49:925–930.
6. Arky RT, Medical Consultant. In: *Physicians' Desk Reference.* 48th ed. Montvale, NJ: Medical Economics, 1994.
7. British National Formulary, No. 24. September 1992:195.

QUINAGULIDE

Quinagulide (CV205-502) is an octahydrobenzol-[*g*]-quinoline that stimulates D_2 receptors with only weak D_1 activity and is used for hyperprolactinemia. An overdose of 225 mg resulted in nausea and mild hypotension. Treatment is symptomatic and supportive. The prognosis is good for recovery.[1]

REFERENCE—QUINAGULIDE

1. Tauveron I, Gesta J-M, Jalenques I, Thieblot P. Acute overdose of a new dopamine agonist (CV205-502). Clin Endocrinol 1994;40:551–553.

SULPIRIDE

Sulpiride is a substituted benzamide. Its molecular weight is 341.4.[1] It exerts its antipsychotic action via a selective blockade of central dopamine D_2 receptors. Although this mechanism of action was believed to preclude its association with extrapyramidal side effects (seen with classic neuroleptic drugs), drug-induced parkinsonism, tardive dystonia, akathisia, and tardive dyskinesia have followed its use.[2–4] It has also been used to treat tardive dyskinesias.[5] No significant binding occurs at adenylate cyclase-dependent (D_1), histaminergic (H_1), serotonergic (5-HT), adrenergic (α_1 and α_2), cholinergic (muscarinic), or γ-aminobutyric acidergic receptors. It is available in the United Kingdom as Dolmatil and Sulpitil tablets 200 mg. Intravenous preparations (100 mg/2 mL) and a syrup are also available.

Toxicokinetics

Sulpiride is absorbed from the gastrointestinal tract but has a low bioavailability (about 37%). Following oral administration of 100 mg, peak serum concentrations of up to 180 ng/mL are observed in 3 to 6 hours.[6] There is very little first-pass metabolism by the liver after oral administration. Sulpiride has an apparent volume of distribution (after intravenous use) of 2.7 L/kg.[7] About 70% of the dose is recovered as unchanged drug in the urine.[7] The renal clearance values are 223 mL/min (oral) and 310 mL/min (intravenous). The total systemic clearance is 115 mL/min. The elimination half-life is about 7 hours.[8] A high-performance liquid chromatography assay is available.[9] The lower detection limit is 2.7 ng.[10,11] Little sulpiride passes into the cerebrospinal fluid.[7]

Clinical Presentation

Therapeutic doses range between 200 and 1800 mg daily.[12] Coma has followed ingestion of sulpiride, but patients have survived doses up to 20 g. Overdoses may result in restlessness, extrapyramidal symptoms, agitation, confusion, and hypertension. Symptoms may last several hours. No special hematologic, biochemical, or electrocardiographic abnormalities have been observed. In a study of 20 patients who overdosed, there were no deaths.[13] One fatality involving sulpiride has been reported.[14] A 67-year-old woman died after ingesting theophylline and sulpiride. Both drugs exhibited blood concentrations of 75 μg/mL.[15] Tardive akathisia has been described.[16]

Treatment

Management of sulpiride overdose is largely symptomatic and supportive with appropriate care of coma (glucose, naloxone, thiamine, oxygen, endotracheal intubation) in an intensive care unit. Parkinsonism symptoms may be managed with appropriate medication as indicated. Blood levels may be useful in confirmation of drug presence, but will not likely be used in gauging the severity of poisoning or guiding the management of patients.

REFERENCES—SULPIRIDE

1. Mielke DH, Gallant DM, Roniger JJ, et al. Sulpiride: Evaluation of antipsychotic activity in schizophrenic patients. Dis Nerv Syst 1977;38:569–571.
2. Linazasoro G, Masso JFM, Olasagasti B. Acute dystonia induced by sulpiride. Clin Neuropharmacol 1991;14:463–464.
3. Miller LG, Jankovic J. Sulpiride induced tardive dyskinesia. Mov Disord 1990;5:83–84.
4. Achiron A, Zoldom Y, Melamd E. Tardive dyskinesia induced by sulpiride. Clin Neuropharmacol 1990;13:248–252.
5. Zarebinski JM, Royds JNA. Sulpiride in tardive dyskinesia. South Afr Med J 1990;78:374–375.
6. Alfredsson G, Bjerkenstedt L, Edman G, et al. Relationships between drug concentrations in serum and CSF, clinical effects and monoaminergic variables in schizophrenic patients treated with sulpiride or chlorpromazine. Acta Psychiatr Scand 1984;69:49–74.

7. Wiesel FA, Alfredsson G, Ehrenebo M, Sedvall G. The pharmacokinetics of intravenous and oral sulpiride in healthy human subjects. Eur J Clin Pharmacol 1980;17:385–391.
8. Bressolle F, Bres J, Nourad G. Pharmacokinetics of sulpiride after intravenous administration in patients with impaired renal function. Clin Pharmacokinet 1989;17:367–373.
9. Alfredsson G, Sedvall G, Wiesel FA. Quantitative analysis of sulpiride in body fluids by high performance liquid chromatography with fluorescence detection. J Chromatogr 1979;164:187–193.
10. Lenhard G, Kieferndir FU, Berner G, et al. The importance of pharmacokinetic data on sulpiride 200 mg preparations following oral administration. Int J Clin Pharmacol Ther Toxicol 1991;29:231–237.
11. Imondi AR, Alam AS, Brennan JJ, Hagerman LM. Metabolism of sulpiride in man and rhesus monkeys. Arch Int Pharmacol Ther 1978;232:799.
12. Rees DM. Analysis of sulpiride in body fluids. In: *Proceedings, 25th International Meeting, International Association of Forensic Toxicologists, Groningen, June 27–30, 1988.*
13. Gaultier M, Frejaville JP. A propos de 20 surdosages en sulpiride. Eur J Toxicol Hyg Environ 1979;6:42–44.
14. Kintz P, Tracqui A, Parent Y, et al. Fatal sulpiride intoxication. Bull Int Assoc Forens Toxicol 1994;24:37.
15. Duffield AD, Kemmenol AV. A fatality involving theophylline and sulpiride. Bull Int Assoc Forens Toxicol 1990;20(3):9–12.
16. Lopez de Minian A, Poza JJ, Gorospe A, et al. Tardive akathisia due to sulpiride. Clin Neuropharmacol 1994;17: 481–483.

TIAPRIDE

Tiapride, an atypical neuroleptic agent, is a selective dopamine D_2-receptor antagonist with little propensity for causing catalepsy and sedation. Tiapride demonstrates antidyskinetic activity reflecting antidopaminergic actions and also anxiolytic activity mediated by mechanisms that are poorly understood.[1]

Use

Tiapride facilitates management of alcohol withdrawal. Tiapride ameliorates psychological distress, improves abstinence, reduces drinking behavior, and, in the short-term, facilitates reintegration within society. These benefits were associated with reduced consumption of health care resources; however, the potential risk of tardive dyskinesia at the dosage employed (300 mg/d) requires evaluation and necessitates medical supervision.[1]

Mechanism of Action

Tiapride is a selective adenyl cyclase-independent dopamine D_2-receptor antagonist that lacks affinity for dopamine D_1 receptors. Tiapride does not appear to cause physical or psychological dependence. It does not possess antiepileptic properties, but does not lower the epileptogenic threshold. In common with other dopaminergic antagonists, tiapride causes hyperprolactinemia, although the effects of prolonged tiapride administration on circulating prolactin levels have not been assessed.[1]

Toxicokinetics

Bioavailability of tiapride is about 75% following oral or intramuscular administration. Peak plasma tiapride concentrations are achieved within about 0.4 to 1.5 hours when given by either route, and steady state occurs 24 to 48 hours after initiating three-times-daily administration. The drug is rapidly distributed and does not bind appreciably to plasma proteins. Tiapride is eliminated mainly by renal excretion, principally in the unchanged form. The elimination half-life is approximately 3 to 4 hours.

Clinical Presentation

The most frequently reported adverse events (>1%) are drowsiness and extrapyramidal syndromes, dizziness, and orthostatic hypotension. There have been four reports of tardive dyskinesia, and these were in elderly patients undergoing long-term therapy. For patients undergoing acute alcohol withdrawal with tiapride, the most worrisome serious event appears to be malignant neuroleptic syndrome.

Therapeutic Dose

For the treatment of delirium or predelirium during alcohol withdrawal, intravenous or intramuscular tiapride 400 to 1200 mg/d given every 4 or 6 hours is recommended, increased to 1800 mg/d if required. Recommended dosages for the treatment of agitation and aggressiveness are 200 to 300 mg/d for 1 to 2 months, or longer with medical supervision. Higher dosages are recommended for the treatment of abnormal movements (300–800 mg/d) and may be necessary for alleviation of tremor during alcohol withdrawal.[1]

REFERENCE—TIAPRIDE

1. Peters DH, Faulds D. Tiapride: A review of its pharmacology and therapeutic potential in the management of alcohol dependence syndrome. Drugs 1994;47:1010–1073.

Chapter 48

H_1-Receptor Drugs

INTRODUCTION

Toxicokinetics and dosages of H_1-receptor antagonists are listed in Tables 48–1 and 48–2, respectively.[1] Table 48–3 is a pharmacologic profile of nonsedating antihistamines as compared with classic antihistamines. Structural formulas are found in Figure 48–1.

Table 48–1
Toxicokinetics of Representative H_1-Receptor Antagonists*

H_1-Receptor Antagonist	Time to Peak Level† (h)	Half-life‡ (h)	Clearance Rate (mL/min/kg)
First generation			
Chlorpheniramine	2.8 ± 0.8	27.9 ± 8.7	1.8 ± 0.1
Hydroxyzine	2.1 ± 0.4	20.0 ± 4.1	9.8 ± 3.2
Diphenhydramine	1.7 ± 1.0	9.2 ± 2.5	23.3 ± 9.4
Second generation			
Terfenadine	0.78 – 1.1	16–23	NA
Terfenadine carboxylate§	3	17	598–697 mL/min
Astemizole	0.5 ± 0.2 to 0.7 ± 0.3	1.1 d	1500 mL/min
N-Desmethyl-astemizole§	NA	9.5 d	NA
Loratadine	1.0 ± 0.3	11.0 ± 9.4	202
Descarboethoxyloratadine§	1.5 ± 0.7	17.3 ± 6.9	NA
Cetirizine¶	1.0 ± 0.5	7.4 ± 1.6	1.0 ± 0.2
Acrivastine	0.85 – 1.4	1.4 – 2.1	4.56
Ketotifen¶	3.6 ± 1.6	18.3 ± 6.7	NA
Azelastine	5.3 ± 1.6	22 ± 4	8.5 ± 3.2
Demethyl-azelastine¶	20.5	54 ± 15	NA

*Values are those for healthy young adults; plus–minus values are means ± SD.
†Time from oral intake to peak plasma concentration.
‡Plasma elimination half-life.
§Metabolite of the parent compound.
¶Not approved for use in the United States at this time.
From Simons FE, Simons KJ. The pharmacology and use of H_1-receptor-antagonist drugs. N Engl J Med 1994;330:1663–1670.

Table 48–2
Formulations and Dosage of Representative H_1-Receptor Antagonists

H_1-Receptor Antagonist	Formulation	Recommended Dose*
First generation		
Chlorpheniramine maleate (Chlor-Trimeton)	Tablets: 4 mg, 8 mg,† 12 mg† Syrup: 2.5 mg/5 mL Parenteral solution: 10 mg/mL	Adult: 8–12 mg bid‡ Child: 0.35 mg/kg/24 h
Hydroxyzine hydrochloride (Atarax)	Capsules: 10 mg, 25 mg, 50 mg Syrup: 10 mg/5 mL	Adult: 25–50 mg bid (or once a day, at bedtime) Child: 2 mg/kg/24 h
Diphenhydramine hydrochloride (Benadryl)	Capsules: 25 mg, 50 mg Elixir: 12.5 mg/5 mL Syrup: 6.25 mg/5 mL Parenteral solution: 50 mg/mL	Adult: 25–50 mg tid Child: 5 mg/kg/24 h
Second generation		
Terfenadine (Seldane)	Tablets: 60 mg, 120 mg§ Suspension: 30 mg/5 mL§	Adult: 60 mg bid or 120 mg/d Child: 3–6 y, 15 mg bid; 7–12 y, 30 mg bid
Astemizole (Hismanal)	Tablets: 10 mg Suspension: 10 mg/5 mL§	Adult: 10 mg/d Child: 0.2 mg/kg/d
Loratadine (Claritin)	Tablets: 10 mg Syrup: 1 mg/mL§	Adult: 10 mg/d Child: 2–12 y, 5 mg/d; >12 y and >30 kg, 10 mg/d
Cetirizine hydrochloride (Reactine)§	Tablets: 10 mg	Adult: 5–10 mg/d
Acrivastine (Semprex)	Tablets: 8 mg	Adult: 8 mg tid
Ketotifen fumarate (Zaditen)§	Tablets: 1 mg, 2 mg† Syrup: 1 mg/5 mL	Adult with urticaria: 4 mg/d Child >3 y: 1 mg bid or 2 mg/d‡
Azelastine hydrochloride (Astelin)§	0.1% Nasal solution: 0.137 mg/spray	Topical: 2 sprays/nostril/d or bid
Levocabastine hydrochloride (Livostin)	Microsuspension: 0.5 mg/mL	Topical: 2 sprays (50 μg each)/nostril bid–qid or 1 drop (0.15 μg) in each eye bid–qid

*The dose for a child should be given if the patient weighs 40 kg (90 lb) or less.
†A tablet of this size is a timed-release formulation.
‡The timed-release formulation should be given.
§Not approved for use in the United States at this time.
From Simons FER, Simons KJ. The pharmacology and use of H_1-receptor-antagonist drugs. N Engl J Med 1994;330:1663–1670.

Table 48–3
Pharmacologic Profile of Nonsedating Antihistamines Compared With Classic Antihistamines

	Antihistaminic Activity	Sedative Activity	Anticholinergic Activity	Activity on Other Receptors					
				H_2	5-HT	α_1	β_1	β_2	D_2
Nonsedating									
Terfenadine	+++	0	0	0	0	0	0	0	0
Astemizole	+++	0	0	+	+	+	0	0	0
Loratadine	+++	0/+*	0	NA	NA	0	NA	NA	NA
Mequitazine	+++	0/++*	+/++	NA	NA	NA	NA	NA	NA
Classic									
Chlorpheniramine	+++	+/++*	0/++*	NA	NA	+	NA	NA	NA
Diphenhydramine	+++	+++	++	NA	NA	NA	NA	NA	NA
Promethazine	+++	+++	++	NA	NA	++	NA	NA	NA
Clemastine	+++	++	+/++	NA	NA	NA	NA	NA	NA
Triprolidine	+++	+/++*	++	NA	NA	NA	NA	NA	NA

0, none; +, slight; ++, moderate; +++, marked; NA, information not available.
*Dose-dependent.
From Woodward JK. Pharmacology and toxicology of nonclassical antihistamines. Cutis 1988;42(4A):5–9.

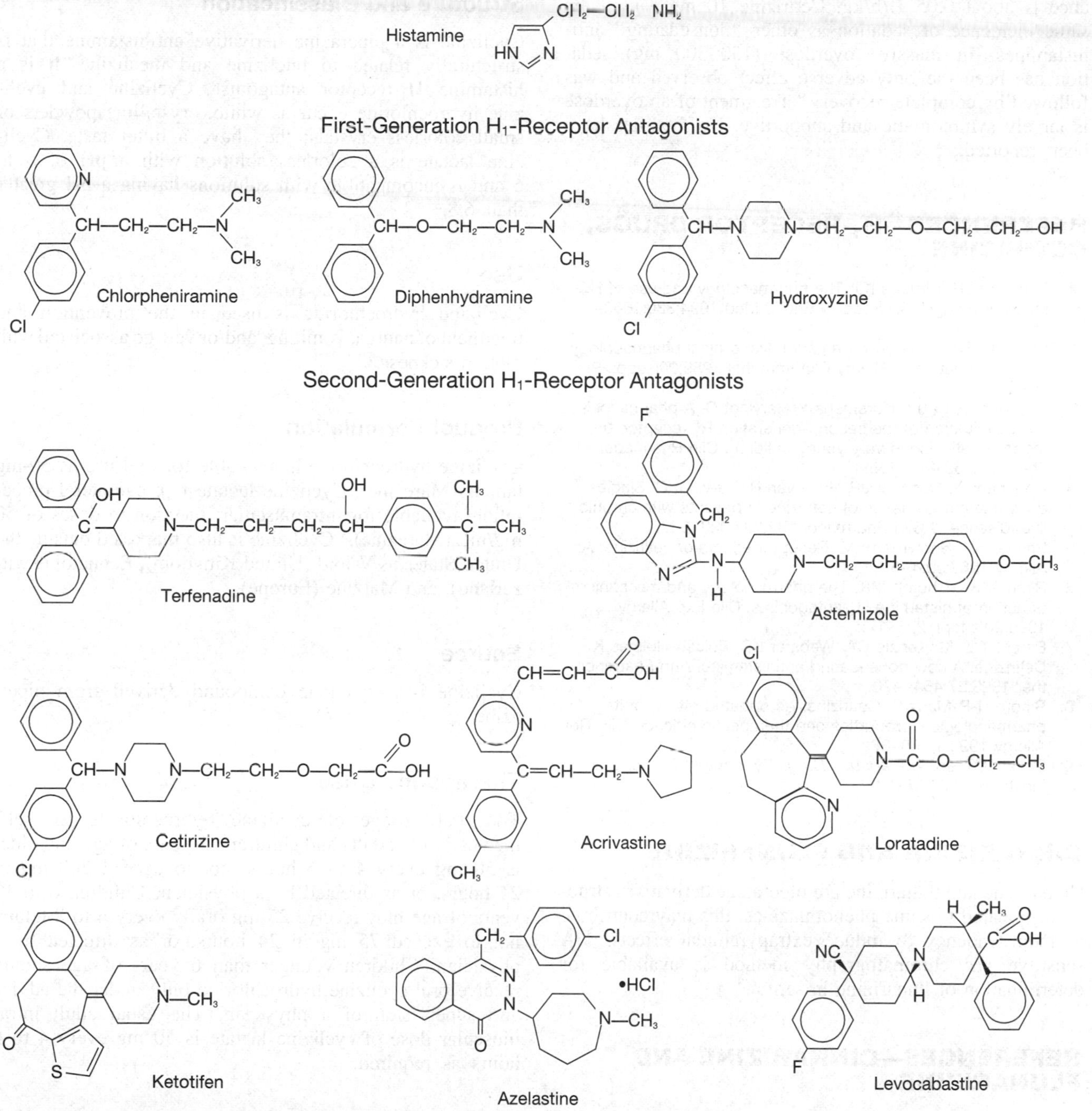

Histamine

First-Generation H_1-Receptor Antagonists

Chlorpheniramine Diphenhydramine Hydroxyzine

Second-Generation H_1-Receptor Antagonists

Terfenadine Astemizole

Cetirizine Acrivastine Loratadine

Ketotifen Azelastine Levocabastine

Figure 48-1 Chemical structures of histamine and representative H_1-receptor antagonist drugs. For practical purposes, H_1 antagonists are now often divided into first-generation, relatively sedating medications and second-generation, relatively nonsedating medications. The latter group includes most H_1 antagonists introduced since 1981, of which terfenadine, astemizole, loratadine, and cetirizine are the best known. Some second-generation H_1 antagonists do not fit readily into any of the traditional classes: alkylamines (eg, chlorpheniramine), ethanolamines (eg, diphenhydramine), piperazines (eg, hydroxyzine), piperidines, ethylenediamines, and phenothiazines. For example, although terfenadine, astemizole, loratadine, ketotifen, and levocabastine all contain a piperidine ring, they have diverse chemical structures. Cetirizine, ketotifen, and azelastine are not approved for use in the United States at this time. (From Simons FER, Simons KJ. The pharmacology and use of H_1-receptor-antagonist drugs. N Engl J Med 1994;330:1663–1670.

PIPERAZINE DERIVATIVES

CETIRIZINE

Cetirizine, a second-generation H_1-receptor antagonist, is a piperazine derivative (Fig. 48–1)[2] and is the principal human metabolite of hydroxyzine. It lacks affinity for muscarinic, cholinergic, alpha-adrenergic, 5-hydroxytryptamine (serotonin), dopamine D_2, and calcium channel receptors.[3–6] The recommended daily dose is 10 mg. Cetirizine is rapidly absorbed (about 100%), reaching mean peak plasma concentrations of about 250 to 500 mg/mL within 1 hour of oral doses of 10 and 20 mg (Table 48–2).[5] The volume of distribution is about 0.6 L/kg. Approximately 93% is protein bound. The terminal half-life is 7 hours.[2,7,8] Cetirizine is excreted mainly unchanged by the kidneys. Total body clearance is about 0.05 L/h/kg. Cetirizine 10 mg causes the same incidence of sedation as other "nonsedating" antihistamines. In massive overdose (150–300 mg) sedation has been the only adverse effect observed and was followed by complete recovery.[9] Treatment of an overdose is largely symptomatic and supportive. No fatalities have been reported.

REFERENCES—H_1-RECEPTOR DRUGS, CETIRIZINE

1. Simons FER, Simons KJ: The pharmacology and use of H_1-receptor-antagonist drugs. N Engl J Med 1994;330:1663–1670.
2. Simons FER. H_1-receptor antagonists: clinical pharmacology and therapeutics. J Allergy Clin Immunol 1989;20(suppl. 2): 19–24.
3. Desager JP, Dab I, Horsmans Y, Harvingt C. A pharmacokinetic evaluation of the second-generation H_1-receptor antagonist cetirizine in very young children. Clin Pharmacol Ther 1993;53:431–435.
4. Horsmans Y, Oesager JP, Hulhoven R, Harvingt C. Single-dose pharmacokinetics of cetirizine in patients with chronic liver disease. J Clin Pharmacol 1993;33:929–932.
5. Snyder SH, Snowman AM. Receptor effects of cetirizine. Ann Allergy 1987;59:4–8.
6. Rimmer SJ, Church MK. The pharmacology and mechanism of action of histamine H_1-antagonists. Clin Exp Allergy 1990;20(suppl. 2):3–17.
7. Barnes CL, McKenzie CA, Webster KD, Poisett-Holmes K. Cetirizine: A new nonsedating antihistamine. Ann Pharmacother 1993;27:464–470.
8. Rihoux J-P, Mariz S. Cetirizine: An updated review of its pharmacological properties and therapeutic efficacy. Clin Rev Allergy 1993;11:65–88.
9. Dollery CT, ed. *Therapeutic Drugs.* Edinburgh: Churchill Livingstone, 1992:57–61.

CINNARIZINE AND FLUNARIZINE

Cinnarizine and flunarizine are piperazine derivatives structurally related to some phenothiazines; this may contribute to their tendency to induce extrapyramidal effects.[1,2] A sensitive gas chromatography method is available for determination of flunarizine in serum.[3]

REFERENCES—CINNARIZINE AND FLUNARIZINE

1. Capella D, Laporte J-P, Castell J-M, et al. Parkinsonism, tremor and depression induced by cinnarizine and flunarizine. Br Med J 1988;29:722–723.
2. Benvenuti F, Baroni A, Bandinelli S, et al. Flunarizine-induced parkinsonism in the elderly. J Clin Pharmacol 1988;28:600–608.
3. Yamaji A, Kataoko K, Oiski M, et al. Simple method for determination of flunarizine in serum by gas chromatography. J Chromatogr Biomed Appl 1987;421:372–376.

CYCLIZINE

Cyclizine, an antihistamine antiemetic, may lead to anticholinergic signs, seizures, extrapyramidal effects, hypertension, aspiration pneumonia, respiratory depression, coma, and death. Seizures are more often observed in children than adults.[1,2]

Structure and Classification

Cyclizine is a piperazine derivative antihistamine that is structurally related to buclizine and meclizine. It is a histamine H_1-receptor antagonist. Cyclizine and cyclizine hydrochloride occur as white, crystalline powders or small colorless crystals; they have a bitter taste. Cyclizine lactate is a colorless solution with a pH of 5 to 6 and is incompatible with solutions having a pH greater than 6.8.[3–5]

Use

Cyclizine hydrochloride is used in the prevention and treatment of nausea, vomiting, and/or vertigo associated with motion sickness.[5]

Product Formulation

Cyclizine hydrochloride is available for oral use as 50-mg tablets (Marezine). Cyclizine lactate is a parenteral preparation available for intramuscular injection in doses of 50 mg/mL (Marezine).[5] Cyclizine is also marketed outside the United States as Valoid (United Kingdom), Echnatol (Switzerland), and Marzine (Europe).

Source

Cyclizine is a synthetic compound derived from piperazine.

Therapeutic Dose

The oral dosage of cyclizine hydrochloride for self-medication in adults and children 12 years of age and older is 50 mg every 4 to 6 hours, not to exceed 200 mg in 24 hours, or as directed by a physician. Children 6 to 12 years of age may receive 25 mg orally every 6 to 8 hours, not to exceed 75 mg in 24 hours, or as directed by a physician. Children younger than 6 years of age should receive oral cyclizine hydrochloride only under the advice and supervision of a physician. The usual adult intramuscular dose of cyclizine lactate is 50 mg every 4 to 6 hours as required.[5]

Toxic Dose

At 5 mg/kg body weight, toxic effects have been observed in children and adults including malaise, tremor, athetoid movement, ataxia, rigidity, and other extrapyramidal signs.[2] Hyperkinesias may lead to tonic–clonic seizures in children. At 40 mg/kg, about 60% of children experience seizures.[2] Similarly, in most children, 40 mg/kg cyclizine may induce atropine-like effects (hallucination, disorientation, flushed dry skin, mydriasis, and tachycardia).[2]

A minimum lethal cyclizine dose of about 80 mg/kg was observed in one series.[2] One child died following aspiration pneumonia, status epilepticus, and respiratory arrest 5 days after a cyclizine ingestion of 88.8 mg/kg body weight.[2] Ingestion of 800 mg of cyclizine by a 2-year-old child ended fatally.[6]

Toxicokinetics

Absorption

Intravenous administration of 50 mg of cyclizine to a normal adult induces a plasma concentration of about 300 μg/L in 20 minutes. Two hours later, the plasma concentration is about 50 μg/L.[7] Approximately 2 hours after administration of an oral dose of 50 mg of cyclizine to an adult, the blood concentration peaked at 69 μg/L.[8] One day after discontinuing daily oral doses of 150 mg in volunteers, the mean plasma concentration of norcyclizine was 14 μg/L (range, 4–22 μg/L).[9]

Distribution

In animal studies cyclizine and norcyclizine are 75% protein bound.[2]

Elimination

Cyclizine is metabolized by *N*-demethylation to form norcyclizine,[9] a weak antihistamine.[10] About 0.01% of a dose is excreted unchanged in a 24-hour urine.[8] The half-life of norcyclizine after a therapeutic dose of cyclizine is less than 24 hours.[2]

Mechanism of Action

Cyclizine is an antihistamine and antiemetic; it also exhibits antimuscarinic activity but has little sedative effect.[3]

Clinical Presentation

Massive overdoses with cyclizine may result in convulsions, hallucinations, respiratory depression, and coma, with the subsequent development of aspiration pneumonitis and death.[2,6,11] Seizures have been observed frequently in children but not in adults.[2]

Laboratory

Analytical Methods

Gas–liquid chromatography with nitrogen–phosphorus detection[7,8,12] and liquid chromatography[12] have been employed in the analysis of cyclizine and its metabolites.

Blood Levels

Cyclizine was found in postmortem specimens of blood at levels of 15 μg/mL following an overdose.[13] Following a suicide by injection of cyclizine and dipipanone, the postmortem blood concentration of cyclizine was 15 μg/mL.[14] Postmortem tissue levels of a 2-year-old child who died 5 days after an overdose of cyclizine measured 3 to 37 mg/kg.[6] A 17-year-old girl experienced seizures and died with a blood cyclizine level of 80 μg/mL.[11]

Abnormalities

Intravenous administration of cyclizine 50 mg to patients in heart failure was followed by an increase in the heart rate and the right atrial, pulmonary arterial, pulmonary artery wedge, and systemic arterial pressures.[15]

Ancillary Tests

Hypersensitivity hepatitis has followed cyclizine use in an 8-year-old child.[16]

Treatment

See Diphenhydramine in this chapter.

REFERENCES—CYCLIZINE

1. Gott PH. Cyclizine toxicity: Intentional drug abuse of a proprietary antihistamine. N Engl J Med 1968;279:596.
2. Resch F, Bachner I, Hruby K, Lenz K. Die intoxikation mit cyclizin in kindes und envachenenalter (Erfahrungen einer Vergiftungs Informations Zentrale). Klin Padiatr 1982;191:42–45.
3. Reynolds JEF, ed. *Martindale: The Extra Pharmacopoeia.* 29th ed. London: Pharmaceutical Press, 1989:450–451.
4. Gilman AG, Rall TW, Nies AS, Taylor P, eds. *Goodman and Gilman's the Pharmacological Basis of Therapeutics.* 8th ed. New York: Pergamon Press, 1991:585.
5. McEvoy GK, ed. *AHFS Drug Information 91.* Bethesda, MD: American Society of Hospital Pharmacists, 1991:1743–1744.
6. Battista HJ, Henn R, Schnabel F. Verlauf, morphologische and toxikologische befunde eine todlichen cyclizin-vergiftung in kindesalter. Beitr Gerichtl Med 1978;36:429–431.
7. Land G, Dean K, Bye A. Determination of cyclizine and norcyclizine in plasma and urine using gas–liquid chromatography with nitrogen selective detection. J Chromatogr 1981; 222:235–240.
8. Griffin DS, Baselt RC. Blood and urine concentrations of cyclizine by nitrogen–phosphorus gas–liquid chromatography. J Anal Toxicol 1984;8:97–99.
9. Kuntzman R, Tsai I, Burns JJ. Importance of tissue and plasma binding in determining the retention of norchlorcyclizine and norcyclizine in man, dog and rat. J Pharmacol Exp Ther 1967;158:332–339.
10. Kuntzman R, Kutch A, Tsai I, Burns JJ. Physiological distribution and metabolic inactivation of chlorcyclizine and cyclizine. J Pharmacol Exp Ther 1965;149:29–35.
11. Backer RC, McFeeley P, Wohlenberg N. Fatality resulting from cyclizine overdose. J Anal Toxicol 1989;13:308–309.
12. Patterson SC, Smith GT, Fieldstead K. Plasma levels of cyclizine and dipipanone as measured by HPLC and GLC after a single oral dose. In: *Proceedings, International Association of Forensic Toxicologists, TIAFT, Newmarket, England, 1984.*
13. Lewin JF. Personal communication, 1981. In: Baselt RC, Cravey RH. *Disposition of Toxic Drugs and Chemicals in Man.* 3rd ed. Chicago: Year Book Medical, 1989:229–230.
14. Sengupta A. Personal communication, 1976. In Baselt RC, Cravey RH. *Disposition of Toxic Drugs and Chemicals in Man.* 3rd ed. Chicago: Year Book Medical, 1989.
15. Tan LB, Bryant S, Murray RG. Detrimental haemodynamic effects of cyclizine in heart failure. Lancet 1988;1:560–561.
16. Kew MC, Segel J, Zoutendyk A. "Hypersensitivity hepatitis" associated with administration of cyclizine. Br Med J 1973;2:307.

DIMENHYDRINATE

Dimenhydrinate (Dramamine) is an H_1 antagonist composed of equimolar concentrations of diphenhydramine and 8-chlorotheophylline. An anecdotal report describes an adult who presented with status epilepticus and ventricular dysrhythmias less than 1 hour after ingesting 5000 mg dimenhydrinate and died.[1] Dimenhydrinate may be subject to drug abuse and withdrawal symptoms (nausea, vomiting, diarrhea).[2] An overdose in a 4-month-old infant resulted in status epilepticus, coma, and life-threatening ventricular arrhythmias. Dimenhydramine 40 μg/mL was present in the serum. Intravenous sodium bicarbonate led to resolution of the dysrhythmias. The infant recovered.[3]

REFERENCES—DIMENHYDRINATE

1. Winn RE, McDonnell KP. Fatality secondary to massive overdose of dimenhydrinate. Ann Emerg Med 1993;22:1481–1484.
2. Craig DF, Mellor SS. Dimenhydrinate dependence and withdrawal. Can Med Assoc J 1990;142:970–973.
3. Farrell M, Heinrichs M, Tilelli JA. Response of life threatening dimenhydrinate intoxication to sodium bicarbonate administration. Clin Toxicol 1991;29:527–535.

DIPHENHYDRAMINE

Toxic Dose

An adult ingested 100 50-mg tablets (5 g) of diphenhydramine (80 mg/kg) and developed hyperpyrexia, status epilepticus, coma, and cardiac arrhythmias. The patient survived with supportive treatment.[1]

A 17-year-old woman who ingested 30 25-mg capsules of diphenhydramine became lethargic with signs of anticholinergic poisoning and seizures. A wide-complex tachycardia resolved after 1 ampule of intravenous sodium bicarbonate.[2]

Toxicokinetics

Paton and Webster discuss the clinical pharmacokinetics of H_1-receptor antagonists.[3]

Clinical Presentation

Koppel and colleagues reviewed 136 cases of diphenhydramine overdose.[3,4] Diphenhydramine plasma levels ranged from (0.1 to 4.7 μg/mL). Impaired consciousness was the most common symptom. Psychotic behavior similar to catatonic stupor was observed. Treatment included gastric lavage, activated charcoal, and cathartics. Hemodialysis and hemoperfusion was of limited assistance.[4] Topical antihistamine lotions may induce acute anticholinergic toxicity in young children.[5] A 15-month-old boy who ingested about 495 mg of diphenhydramine developed tonic–clonic seizures with a blood diphenhydramine level of 1.0 mg% (lethal, 0.5 mg%). The child died in 7 days.[6]

Adults usually present with central nervous system depression leading to coma. Seizures may occur. Death may occur as a result of respiratory failure or circulatory collapse. Signs of peripheral anticholinergic toxicity may include arrhythmias, tachycardia, urinary retention, decreased gastrointestinal motility, dryness of mouth, thickening of bronchial secretions, and blurry vision.

Allergies have been reported and other members of the ethanolamine group (eg, carbinoxamine [Clistin, Twiston], clemastin [Tavist], dimenhydrinate [Dramamine], doxylamine [Decapryn]) may cross-react.

Laboratory

Electrocardiographic changes may include a wandering pacemaker, prolonged QT interval, nonspecific ST–T changes, and left bundle-branch block that clear with recovery.[7,8] Electroencephalographic changes may include a general cerebral dysrhythmia and diffuse delta wave activity.[8]

Treatment

Antihistamine toxicity may induce conduction disturbances or dysrhythmia. Rarely, an antihistamine overdose may produce clinically significant myocardial pump failure. If such cardiogenic shock is refractory to vasopressor support, use of an intraaortic balloon pump may be useful until normal cardiac function is regained. Though not diphenhydramine this treatment was effective in a similar antihistamine in a 46-year-old woman who ingested 10 g of pyrilamine maleate and developed a serum pyrilamine level of 121 ng/mL, with a severe cardiogenic shock refractory to vasopressors.[9]

REFERENCES—DIPHENHYDRAMINE

1. Rinder CS, D'Amato SL, Rinder HM, Cox PM. Survival in complicated diphenhydramine overdose. Crit Care Med 1988;16:1161–1162.
2. Clark BF, Vance MR. Diphenhydramine poisoning resulting in a wide complex tachycardia: Treated with sodium bicarbonate. Vet Hum Toxicol 1991;3:356.
3. Paton DM, Webster DR. Clinical pharmacokinetics of H_1-receptor antagonists (the antihistamines). Clin Pharmacokinet 1985;10:477–497.
4. Koppel C, Ibe K, Tenczer J. Clinical symptomatology of diphenhydramine overdose: An evaluation of 136 cases in 1982 to 1985. Clin Toxicol 1987;25:53–70.
5. Reilly JF Jr, Weisse ME. Topically induced diphenhydramine toxicity. J Emerg Med 1990;8:59–61.
6. Goetz CM, Lopez G, Dean BS, Krenzelok EP. Accidental childhood death from diphenhydramine overdosage. Am J Emerg Med 1990;8:321–322.
7. Hestand HE, Tesky DW. Diphenhydramine hydrochloride intoxication. J Pediatr 1977;90:1017–1018.
8. Huxtable RF, Landwirth J. Diphenhydramine poisoning treated by exchange transfusion. Am J Dis Child 1963;106: 496–500.
9. Freedberg RS, Friedman GR, Palu PN, Feit F. Cardiogenic shock due to antihistamine overdose: Reversed with intraaortic balloon counter pulsation. JAMA 1987;257:660–661.

DOXYLAMINE SUCCINATE

Doxylamine succinate is an antihistamine used as a sleeping aid that produces signs and symptoms of anticholinergic toxicity in overdose. Fatalities and rhabdomyolysis have been reported. Most cases recover with symptomatic and supportive treatment.

Structure and Classification

Doxylamine (histadoxylamine succinate and doxylamine succinate) is not structurally related to the cyclic antidepressants. It is marketed as Unisom Nighttime Sleep Aid, Sleep 2-nite, and doxylamine succinate tablets.[1,2]

As Bendectin (tablets containing 10 mg doxylamine succinate, 10 mg dicyclomine hydrochloride, and 10 mg pyridoxine) doxylamine was prescribed for many years for the treatment of nausea and vomiting associated with pregnancy.

Use

Doxylamine succinate is an antihistamine that is also used as a nighttime sleep aid. In combination with antitussives and decongestants, it may provide temporary relief of cough and cold symptoms.

Product Formulation

Doxylamine succinate is available as an oral 2.5-mg tablet.

Source

Doxylamine succinate is a synthetic chemical product.

Therapeutic Dose

The usual dosage of doxylamine succinate for self-medication in adults and children 12 years of age or older is 25 mg taken 25 minutes before retiring. As an antihistamine the usual dosage of doxylamine succinate for self-medication in adults and children 12 years of age or older is 7.5 to 12.5 mg every 4 to 6 hours, not to exceed 75 mg in 24 hours.[3]

Toxic Dose

A toxic dose for children of more than 1.8 mg/kg has been reported.[4] Rhabdomyolysis was observed in an adult after ingestion of doxylamine 2.25 g.[5]

Fatal Dose

A 3-year-old died 18 hours after ingesting 1000 mg doxylamine succinate.[6]

Toxicokinetics

Absorption

Doxylamine is easily absorbed from the gastrointestinal tract. Following an oral dose of 25 mg the mean peak plasma level is 99 ng/mL 2.4 hours after ingestion.[2,5,7] This level declines to 28 μg/L at 24 hours and 10 μg/mL at 36 hours.[8]

Distribution

The apparent volume of distribution is 2.5 L/kg.[7]

Elimination

The elimination half-life is 10.1 hours. Oral plasma clearance is 217 mL/min.[2] The drug is excreted in the urine as unchanged doxylamine (60%),[9] nordoxylamine, and dinordoxylamine.[9] The major metabolic pathways are *N*-demethylation, *N*-oxidation, hydroxylation, *N*-acetylation, *N*-desalkylation, and ether cleavage.[5]

Pregnancy/Lactation

Bendectin was introduced in 1956 as a formulation of doxylamine, dicyclomine, and pyridoxine. The dicyclomine was removed from the formulation by the United States in 1976 because of a lack of demonstrated effectiveness. Controversial and unproved association with teratogenic effects led to numerous lawsuits and antagonism in the lay press. In 1983, the company decided to cease production.[10]

Mechanism of Action

Doxylamine is an antihistamine drug with hypnotic, anticholinergic, and local anesthetic properties.

Clinical Presentation

Overdose

Acute doxylamine overdose may be followed by impaired consciousness, seizures, tachycardia, mydriasis, and a "psychosis" similar to that in catatonic stupor.[5,11] Rhabdomyolysis with impairment of renal function and acute renal failure has been observed.[5,12,13] In one series 39% of patients studied had no symptoms.[5]

Fatalities

Fatal doxylamine intoxication has been characterized by coma, grand mal seizures and cardiorespiratory arrest.[6,14,15] Children appear to be at a high risk for cardiorespiratory arrest.[5]

Laboratory

Analytical Methods

Doxylamine may be analyzed in biological specimens by gas chromatography using flame ionization[16] and nitrogen–phosphorus detection.[2] Liquid chromatography has been used for analysis of doxylamine in plasma and serum. Sensitive and specific doxylamine detection and quantitation may be achieved with gas chromatography–mass spectrometry.[17]

Blood Levels

A 3-year-old died 18 hours after taking 100 tablets of Bendectin. The postmortem doxylamine blood concentration was 12 μg/mL blood.[6] There is no correlation between the amount of doxylamine ingested, the doxylamine plasma level, and clinical symptomatology.[5] A suicide involving doxylamine in an adult was associated with a blood level of 0.7 mg/L.[17]

Ancillary Tests

A suicide involving doxylamine was associated with a urine level of 17 mg/L, higher than the level found in the blood.[17]

Treatment

Stabilization

Doxylamine overdose may lead to a life-threatening emergency with severe cardiovascular or central nervous system reactions. Patients who exhibit any abnormalities of vital signs should receive an intravenous line, cardiac monitor, oxygen, and assisted ventilation as required. Adequacy of ventilation and blood pressure should be assessed and abnormalities corrected if present. The patient should be observed for evidence of rhabdomyolysis. Most patients recover with symptomatic and supportive care.

Gut Decontamination

Doxylamine was identified in the gastric rinsing fluid of an overdose patient even as late as 7 hours after ingestion.[8] Gastric lavage may be useful in the first 12 hours after ingestion.

Elimination Enhancement

Hemodialysis, hemofiltration, and peritoneal dialysis have not been studied in the treatment of doxylamine overdose. These modalities are unlikely to be effective in view of the high volume of distribution. The efficacy of forced diuresis has not been established.

Antidote

There is no antidote.

Supportive Measures

In all suspected cases of doxylamine overdose, the patient should be observed for evidence of rhabdomyolysis. Laboratory tests on admission should include a determination of creatine kinase. If this enzyme is elevated, a test for myoglobin in the urine should be done. The presence of myoglobinuria is a contraindication to acid diuresis. Adequate fluid replacement must be provided and good urine output maintained.

REFERENCES—DOXYLAMINE SUCCINATE

1. Reynolds JEF, ed. *Martindale: The Extra Pharmacopoeia.* 30th ed. London: Pharmaceutical Press, 1993:938–939.
2. Friedman H, Greenblatt DJ. The pharmacokinetics of doxylamine: Use of automated gas chromatography with nitrogen–phosphorus detection. J Clin Pharmacol 1985;25: 448–451.
3. McEvoy GK, ed. *AHFS Drug Information 92.* Bethesda, MD: American Society of Hospital Pharmacists, 1992:20.
4. Wurmli K. Vergiftungen mit antihistaminica. Pharm Acta Helv 1973;4:200–205.
5. Koppel C, Tenczer J, Ibe K. Poisoning with over the counter doxylamine preparations: An evaluation of 109 cases. Hum Toxicol 1987;6:355–359.
6. Bayley M, Walsh FM, Valaske MJ. Fatal overdose from Bendectin. Clin Pediatr 1975;14:507–509.
7. Friedman H, Greenblatt DJ, Scavone JM, et al. Clearance of the antihistamine doxylamine reduced in elderly men but not in elderly women. Clin Pharmacokinet 1989;16: 312–316.
8. Kohlhof KJ, Stump D, Zizzamia JA. Analysis of doxylamine in plasma by high performance liquid chromatography. J Pharm Sci 1983;72:961–962.
9. Gieldorf W, Schubert K. Biotransformation of doxylamine: Isolation, identification and synthesis of some metabolites. J Clin Chem Clin Biochem 1981;19:485–490.
10. Leeder JS, Spielberg SP. Teratogenicity and litigation. In: Koren G, ed. *Maternal–fetal Toxicology: A Clinician's Guide.* New York: Marcel Dekker, 1990:415–425.
11. Mendoza FS, Atiba JO, Krensky AM, Scannell LM. Rhabdomyolysis complicating doxylamine overdose. Clin Pediatr 1987;26:595–597.
12. Wax PM. Fulminant rhabdomyolysis without renal compromise from doxylamine overdose. In: *Proceedings, European Association of Poison Centres and Clinical Toxicologists, Scientific Meeting: Metabolic complications of poisoning. Birmingham, UK, May 26, 1993.*
13. Koppel C, Ibe K, Oberdisse U. Rhabdomyolysis in doxylamine overdose. Lancet 1987;1:442–443.
14. Clarkson SG, Glanville AP. Debendox overdosage in children. Br Med J 1977;2:459–460.
15. Meadow SR. Poisoning from delayed release tablets. Br Med J 1972;1:512.
16. Fontan CR, Smith WC, Kirk PL. Gas chromatography of the antihistamines. Anal Chem 1963;35:591–593.
17. Wu Chen NB, Schaffer MI, Liu R-L, et al. The general toxicology unknown: II. A case report: Doxylamine and pyrilamine intoxication. J Forens Sci 1989;28:398–403.

HYDROXYZINE

Hydroxyzine is an antihistaminic drug with anxiolytic properties, which, in overdose, produces anticholinergic effects including sinus tachycardia, seizures, and flushing of the skin. Reports of poisoning with hydroxyzine include coma and death. Blood levels confirm the presence of hydroxyzine but do not guide medical treatment. Treatment is symptomatic and supportive.

Structure and Classification

Hydroxyzine is a piperazine-derivative antihistamine structurally similar to buclizine, cyclizine, and meclizine. It is commercially available as the hydrochloride and pamoate salts. Hydroxyzine hydrochloride is a white odorless powder very soluble in water and freely soluble in alcohol. Hydroxyzine pamoate is a light yellow, almost odorless powder insoluble in water and in alcohol.[1]

Hydroxyzine hydrochloride has a molecular weight of 447.8; the pamoate salt has a molecular weight of 763.3.[2]

The conversion factors are 2.23 for hydroxyzine hydrochloride:

$$\mu g/mL \times 2.23 = \mu mol/L$$
$$\mu mol/L \div 2.23 = \mu g/mL$$

and 1.31 for hydroxyzine pamoate:

$$\mu g/mL \times 1.31 = \mu mol/L$$
$$\mu mol/L \div 1.31 = \mu g/mL$$

The molecular formula of the hydrochloride is $C_{21}H_{27}ClN_2O_2 \cdot 2HCl$ and that for the pamoate is $C_{21}H_{27}ClN_2O_2 \cdot C_{23}H_{16}O_6$.

Use

Hydroxyzine has the actions and uses of the antihistamines. Its main uses are in the symptomatic management of anxiety and tension associated with psychoneuroses, and as an adjunct in organic disease states in which anxiety is manifested; for the management of pruritus due to allergic conditions such as chronic urticaria and atopic and contact dermatoses, and in histamine-mediated pruritus; and as a sedative before and after general anesthesia.[1]

Product Formulation

Hydroxyzine hydrochloride is available as an oral solution (10 mg/5 mL) containing alcohol 0.5% (Ararax Syrup); as oral tablets of 10, 25, 50, and 100 mg (Atarax); as film-coated tablets of 25 and 50 mg (Anxanil); and as a parenteral injection for intramuscular use only: 25 mg/mL (Vistaril [with benzyl alcohol 0.9%], Vistaject-25 [with benzyl alcohol 0.9%]) and 50 mg/mL (Vistaril [with benzyl alcohol 0.9%]), and other similar generic formulations. The injections have a pH of 3.5 to 6.

Hydroxyzine pamoate is available in oral capsules equivalent to hydroxyzine hydrochloride 25 mg (Hy-Pam, Vistaril), 50 mg (Hy-Pam, Vistaril), and 200 mg (Vistaril). It is also available as a suspension equivalent to hydroxyzine hydrochloride 25 mg/5 mL (Vistaril with propylene glycol). The oral suspension has a pH of 4.5 to 7.[1]

Source

Hydroxyzine hydrochloride and hydroxyzine pamoate are synthetic commercial products.

Therapeutic Dose

The usual oral dosages of hydroxyzine are for adults, 50 to 100 mg four times daily; for children 6 years of age or older, 50 to 100 mg daily in divided doses; and for children younger than 6 years of age, 50 mg daily in divided doses. For pruritus, the oral dose for adults is 25 mg three or four times daily; for children 6 years of age or older, 50 to 100 mg/d in divided doses; and for children less than 6 years, 50 mg/d in divided doses.

For sedation before and after general anesthesia, the usual adult dose of hydroxyzine is 50 to 100 mg orally or 25 to 100 mg intramuscularly. In children for the same use the usual dose of hydroxyzine is 0.6 mg/kg orally or 1.1 mg/kg intramuscularly.[2] For control of emesis, the usual adult intramuscular dose is 25 to 100 mg. For control of acutely disturbed or hysterical patients and for agitation caused by alcohol withdrawal, the usual adult intramuscular dose of hydroxyzine is 50 to 100 mg, repeated as required every 4 to 6 hours.

Toxic Dose

The manufacturer states that 1 to 2 g of hydroxyzine pamoate in adults produces drowsiness and lethargy, which may progress to coma.[3] A 13-month-old child ingested between 500 and 625 mg of hydroxyzine, developed seizures and coma, and recovered. The plasma level was 102.7 μg/ml (see clinical presentation and blood levels on this patient which follow).[4]

Fatal Dose

Two adults were found dead: one had ingested hydroxyzine, chlordiazepoxide, and cimetidine,[5] and the other had 20 25-mg tablets left in the stomach.[6]

Toxicokinetics

Absorption

The absorption of hydroxyzine by the gastrointestinal tract is rapid following oral administration. The plasma absorption half-life is about 1 hour.[7] An oral dose of 100 mg led to a mean peak plasma level of 78 ng/mL in 4 hours[7]; following a mean dose of 49 mg, the peak plasma level in young adults reached 72.5 ng/mL in 2.1 hours,[8] and in those aged 65 years or over the peak plasma level reached 77 ng/mL in 2.3 hours.[9] Sedative effects may persist 2 to 6 hours following administration of a single dose. The mean peak cetirizine (metabolite) level following 49 mg orally is 462 ng/mL, reached in 3.8 hours.[9] Another group of young adults were given 25 mg of hydroxyzine and 36 hours later were found to have mean serum hydroxyzine and cetirizine concentrations of 3 and 120 ng/mL, respectively.[10]

Distribution

The apparent volume of distribution in young adults in one study was 16.0 L/kg,[8] and in those over 65 years of age, 22.5 L/kg.[10]

Elimination

The mean hydroxyzine elimination half-life in one study was 3 hours[7]; in another study of young adults, values of 14.0 and 20 hours were obtained.[8] The mean elimination half-life of hydroxyzine in older adults was 29.3 hours; the cetirizine half-life was 24.8 hours.[9] Hydroxyzine is eliminated by hepatic metabolism. There is at least one pharmacologically active metabolite, cetirizine, 70% of which is excreted unchanged via the kidney.[9,10] The mean oral clearance of hydroxyzine is 9.7 mL/min/kg in young adults[8] and 9.6 mL/min/kg in older adults.[9]

Drug Interactions

Central Nervous System Depressants. Hydroxyzine may be additive with or may potentiate the action of other central nervous system depressants such as opiates or other analgesics, barbiturates or other sedatives, anesthetics, and alcohol.

Anticholinergic Agents. Additive anticholinergic effects may occur when hydroxyzine is administered with other anticholinergic agents.[7]

Epinephrine. Hydroxyzine may inhibit and reverse the vasopressor effects of epinephrine. Norepinephrine or metaraminol should be used if a vasopressor is needed in patients receiving hydroxyzine. Epinephrine should not be used.[1]

Pregnancy/Lactation

There are no adequate studies on the effects of hydroxyzine in pregnancy. The drug is therefore contraindicated in early pregnancy. There is one report of hydroxyzine toxicity associated with neonatal drug withdrawal.[11] Following high-dose maternal ingestion of hydroxyzine hydrochloride, the infant experienced involuntary jerking movements, clonic seizures, and irritability.

Mechanism of Action

Hydroxyzine has central nervous system-depressant, anticholinergic, antispasmodic, local anesthetic, antihistaminic, sedative, and antiemetic effects.

Clinical Presentation

Hydroxyzine toxicity, manifested by increased motor activity, central nervous system irritability, tremor, and generalized seizures, appears to be rare.[4] A 13-month-old child who ingested between 500 and 625 mg of hydroxyzine hydrochloride developed generalized seizures, sinus tachycardia, mydriasis, intermittent apnea, flushed skin, and decreased bowel sounds; following symptomatic and supportive therapy the child recovered in 3 days.[4] An adult aged 43 years was found dead after ingesting hydroxyzine; twenty 25-mg hydroxyzine tablets were found in the stomach.[6] Another 46-year-old adult with a history of alcohol abuse was found dead after ingesting hydroxyzine, chlordiazepoxide, and cimetidine.[5] An 18-year-old was found dead with containers of hydroxyzine nearby; postmortem examination revealed edematous lungs.[12] Inadvertent intraarterial administration of hydroxyzine has led to necrosis of extremities and fingers.[13]

Laboratory

Analytical Methods

Hydroxyzine may be analyzed by electron-capture gas chromatography after conversion to a benzophenone,[14] or by gas chromatography–mass spectrometry of the acetyl derivative,[7] or by gas chromatography with nitrogen–phosphorus detection.[12] Hydroxyzine and cetirizine are also assayed by high-performance liquid chromatography (HPLC).[8,15] The lower limits of sensitivity for hydroxyzine and cetirizine assayed by HPLC are 1.0 and 2.0 ng/mL, respectively.[9]

Blood Levels

Eight hours after an overdose of 20 25-mg hydroxyzine hydrochloride capsules in a 13-month old-child, the plasma hydroxyzine concentration was 102.7 μg/mL (102,700 ng/mL).[4] An adult found dead with 20 25-mg tablets of hydroxyzine in the stomach had a blood level of 39 μg/mL (39,000 ng/mL).[6] Another adult who had probably overdosed on hydroxyzine hydrochloride, chlordiazepoxide, and cimetidine was found dead with a blood level of 1.1 μg/mL (1100 ng/mL).[5] A hydroxyzine blood level of 4.18 μg/mL (4100 ng/mL) was measured in a suicide victim.[12]

Treatment

Stabilization

Treatment of hydroxyzine overdose generally involves symptomatic and supportive care. Following an acute ingestion, the airway, breathing, and circulatory status must be closely monitored. These patients may become rapidly obtunded and develop seizures. After endotracheal intubation, mechanical ventilation may be required. The patient should be monitored with a continuous electrocardiographic recording, and should have an adequate oxygen supply available. Cardiac monitoring with frequent pulse and blood pressure determinations should be available. An intravenous line should be established. Those with altered mental status should receive oxygen, naloxone, glucose, and thiamine. Initial attention should be directed toward the adequacy of ventilation (ie, tidal volume, arterial blood gases, cyanosis). Serious toxicity may result from seizures or respiratory insufficiency.

Gut Decontamination

Syrup of ipecac should not be administered because seizures may intervene and lead to serious aspiration pneumonitis. Gastric lavage with prior endotracheal intubation may be performed if a clinically significant ingestion has occurred. Activated charcoal may be left in the stomach, but there are scant data to support its efficacy.

Elimination Enhancement

The large volume of distribution of hydroxyzine precludes the probable efficacy of hemodialysis or hemoperfusion.

Antidote

There is no specific antidote for hydroxyzine intoxication.

Supportive Measures

1. Observe all patients with hydroxyzine ingestion for at least 12 hours postingestion in a medical facility. Admit any patient with a sign of a major toxicity (eg, depressed consciousness or respirations, hypotension, conduction disturbances or seizures) for intensive emergency care.
2. Admission laboratory and monitoring procedures should include electrocardiograms, electrolytes, arterial blood gases, serial vital signs, complete blood count, and cardiac monitoring. Check the urine for myoglobin in patients who have repeated seizures. Draw serum for blood levels to confirm overdose. Do not delay treatment until blood level reports are received.
3. If there are few anticholinergic symptoms (eg, heart rate less than 110), no skin flushing, normal active bowel sounds, and the patient is awake without seizures or muscle jerks, then consider discharge after 12 hours, provided there is no evidence of major toxicity. Give the patient an additional dose of activated charcoal and provide psychiatric counseling prior to discharge.

4. Maintain cardiac monitoring for all admitted patients until they are symptom free for 24 hours. Watch for late development of serious arrhythmias.
5. For hypothermia, institute passive rewarming measures. For hyperthermia, institute cooling measures provided seizures are controlled.
6. In comatose patients, place a urinary catheter to check urine output and prevent urinary retention.
7. Obtain chest x-rays if there has been a gastric lavage, any respiratory difficulties, or seizures.

REFERENCES—HYDROXYZINE

1. McEvoy GK, ed. *AHFS Drug Information 92.* Bethesda, MD: American Society of Hospital Pharmacists, 1992:1368–1370.
2. Reynolds JEF, ed. *Martindale: The Extra Pharmacopoeia.* 29th ed. London: Pharmaceutical Press, 1989:455–456.
3. *Recognition and Management of Acute Toxicity From Overdosage With Selected Pfizer Laboratories Drugs.* New York: Pfizer, 1978.
4. Magera BE, Betlach CJ, Sweatt AP, Derrick CW Jr. Hydroxyzine intoxication in a 13-month-old child. Pediatrics 1981; 67:280–283.
5. Spiehler VR, Fukumoto RI. Another fatal case involving hydroxyzine. J Anal Toxicol 1984;8:242–243.
6. Johnson GR. A fatal case involving hydroxyzine. J Anal Toxicol 1982;6:69–70.
7. Fouda HG, Hobbs DC, Stambaugh JE. Sensitive assay for determination of hydroxyzine and plasma and its human pharmacokinetics. J Pharm Sci 1979;68:1456–1458.
8. Simons FER, Simons KJ, Frith EM. The pharmacokinetics and antihistaminic effects of H_1-receptor antagonist hydroxyzine. J Allergy Clin Immunol 1984;73:69–75.
9. Simons KJ, Watson WTA, Chen XY, Simons FER. Pharmacokinetic and pharmacodynamic studies of the H_1-receptor antagonist hydroxyzine in the elderly. Clin Pharmacol Ther 1989;45:9–14.
10. Gengo FM, Dabronzo J, Yurchak A, et al. The relative antihistaminic and psychomotor effects of hydroxyzine and cetirizine. Clin Pharmacol Ther 1987;42:265–272.
11. Prenner BM. Neonatal withdrawal syndrome associated with hydroxyzine hydrochloride. Am J Dis Child 1977;131:529.
12. Kintz P, Godelare B, Mangin P. Gas chromatographic identification and quantification of hydroxyzine: Application in a fatal self-poisoning. Forens Sci Int 1990;48:139–143.
13. Hardesty WH. Inadvertent intra-arterial injection. JAMA 1970; 213:872.
14. Hartvig P, Handl W. Gas chromatography and electron-capture detection of benzophenones. Acta Pharm Suec 1975;12:349–360.
15. Wood SG, John BA, Chasseaud LF, et al. The metabolism and pharmacokinetics of ^{14}C cetirizine in humans. Ann Allergy 1987;59:31–34.

METHYPYRILENE

Analysis of the postmortem blood for methypyrilene in a suicide victim revealed a level of 10.1 mg%.[1]

PHENIRAMINE

A 23-year-old man ingested 3,750 mg of pheniramine aminosalicylate over 2.5 hours, developed seizures, became unconscious, and died in 2 hours. Gas–liquid chromatography analysis with a flame ionization detection disclosed a blood pheniramine level of 10.7 μg/L.[2]

Ingestion of 500 to 1000 mg of pheniramine *p*-aminosalicylate resulted in apparent hallucinogenic effects.[3]

PYRILAMINE

A 25-year-old woman was found dead with a blood pyrilamine concentration of 11 μg/L.[4]

REFERENCES—METHYPYRILENE, PHENIRAMINE, PYRILAMINE

1. Singh KD, Rho YM, Galante L, Bastas ML. Fatal use of methypyrilene and salicylamide poisoning. Bull Int Assoc Forens Toxicol 1987;14:35–36.
2. Chan LFT, Allender MW. A fatal case involving an overdose of pheniramine. Bull Int Assoc Forens Toxicol 1983;17(2):25–26.
3. Csillag ER, Landauer AA. Alleged hallucinogenic effects of a toxic overdose of an antihistamine preparation. Med J Aust 1973;1:653–657.
4. Johnson GR. A fatal case involving pyrilamine. Clin Toxicol 1981;18:907–909.

NONSEDATING HISTAMINE H_1-RECEPTOR ANTAGONISTS

Nonsedating histamine H_1-receptor antagonists include terfenadine (Seldane), astemizole (Hismanal^R), loratidine (Claritin), and acrivastine (in combination with pseudoephedrine, DuAct). Terfenadine and astemizole are approved for marketing in the United States.

In overdose, this group of drugs, chemically related to tricyclic antidepressants, may induce life-threatening ventricular arrhythmias including Torsade de pointes. Treatment is symptomatic and supportive and may respond to magnesium sulfate followed by overdrive pacing.

H_1 antagonist-induced Torsade de pointes usually results from increased drug concentration. Three major reasons are intentional overdose (900–3360 mg), a decrease in metabolism due to liver disease (cirrhosis because of alcohol abuse), or a drug–drug interaction.

The increased levels of parent terfenadine, astemizole, or its metabolite desmethylastemizole caused by overdose or impairment of metabolism block the potassium current by a mechanism similar to that of quinidine-induced arrhythmia. This block delays repolarization and causes the characteristically prolonged QT interval and morphologic changes in the TU complex that define Torsade de pointes.[1]

Structure and Classification

The chemical structures of terfenadine, astemizole, loratidine, and acrivastine are shown in Figure 48–1.[2] Terfenadine is structurally related to haloperidol. The butanol moiety of the terfenadine molecule is considered to be responsible for the lack of central nervous system-depressant effects associated with terfenadine. The antihistamine properties are most likely related to the α-diphenyl-4-piperidine methanol moiety. The molecular weight is 471.7.

Astemizole contains a piperidino-2-aminobenzimidazole core that is necessary for its antihistaminic activity. Its molecular weight is 458.6.

Loratidine is a piperidine and is structurally related to azetadine (Optimin) and cyproheptadine (Periactin). It is also chemically similar to imipramine (Tofranil), nortriptyline (Pamelor), and doxepin (Jinequane). Its molecular weight is 392.9.

Acrivastine is a side chain reduced metabolite of triprolidine (Actidil). Its molecular weight is 348.4.

Use

Terfenadine, astemizole, loratidine, and acrivastine have found use in the systematic treatment of allergic rhinitis, chronic rhinitis, and chronic urticaria.[2]

Product Formulation

Terfenadine (Seldane) is available as a 60-mg tablet. Terfenadine (60 mg) and pseudoephedrine (10 mg in an outer press-coat for immediate release, 100 mg in an extended-release core) (Seldane-D) are available in combination. In the United Kingdom, terfenadine is available in 60-mg tablets and as a suspension of 6 mg/mL. Astemizole is available in scored white 10-mg tablets (Hismanal). In the United Kingdom, it is available in scored white round 10-mg tablets and a fruit-flavored suspension (1 and 2 mg/mL).

Source

The H_1-receptor antagonists are synthetic chemicals.

Therapeutic Dose

See Table 48–1.

Astemizole. QT prolongation, ventricular arrhythmias, serious drug reactions, and death may occur in children who ingest more than 10 mg (1 tablet) a day.

Terfenadine. Terfenadine is reported to be a new antihistamine without sedating or anticholinergic properties. The therapeutic dose for children 3 to 6 years is 15 mg twice daily; for those age 7 and older (Europe, Canada), it is 30 mg twice daily. Terfenadine is only approved for adults in the United States.[3]

Toxic Dose

A patient ingested 60 mg of terfenadine twice daily with ketoconazole, developed severe Torsade de pointes, and survived.[4] A 26-year-old ingested 900 to 1200 mg of terfenadine, developed Torsade de pointes, and survived.[5] Terfenadine 360 mg/d may lead to prolongation of the QT interval.[6] Children receiving 60 to 600 mg of terfenadine exhibited fatigue, flushing, drowsiness, and tachycardia.[7] One patient ingested terfenadine 3360 mg, cephalexin 7 g, and ibuprofen 1200 mg, and developed Torsade de pointes 15 hours postingestion.[8] Small doses, up to 170 mg, do not appear to induce toxicity in small children. Loratidine 160 mg was well tolerated.[9]

Fatal Dose

A fatal dose for the nonsedating antihistamines has not been established.

Toxicokinetics

Absorption

Toxicokinetic values for the nonsedating histamine H_1-receptor antagonists are summarized in Table 48–2.[2] All of these compounds are well absorbed. Terfenadine and astemizole are highly protein bound.

Terfenadine. Serum levels after ingestion of 60 mg twice daily are 10 ng/mL for terfenadine and 215 to 250 ng/mL for its main metabolite.[3] The mean maximum blood level after a single 120-mg dose is 501 ng/mL, occurring in 2.3 hours.[10]

Astemizole. The mean steady-state serum concentrations of astemizole plus hydroxylated metabolites are 3.8 ng/mL in adolescents and 2.72 to 3.63 ng/mL in adults after 10 mg/d. Protein binding is 97%. The volume of distribution is 250 L/kg.[11]

Loratidine. See Table 48–2.[2,12] Peak plasma concentrations of 5, 11, and 26 ng/mL occur 1 to 1.5 hours after ingestion of 10-, 20-, and 40-mg capsules, respectively. Loratidine is 97 to 99% bound to plasma proteins.[12]

Distribution

Acrivastine. Acrivastine has a volume of distribution of 0.64 L/kg.

Terfenadine. Neither the parent drug nor the metabolites penetrate the blood–brain barrier. A volume of distribution has not been determined.

Elimination

Terfenadine. More than 99% of an absorbed dose is metabolized. It is eliminated through hepatic metabolism by cytochrome P4503A4 into two metabolites: a carboxylic acid analog (some antihistaminic activity) and a piperidine carbinol derivative (no antihistaminic activity). The alpha (distribution) half-life is 3 to 4 hours, and the beta (elimination) half-life, 20.3 hours. Elimination occurs via the fecal route (60%) and in the urine.

Astemizole. Astemizole is extensively metabolized by aromatic hydroxylation, oxidative dealkylation, and glucuronidation. Desmethylastemizole is an active metabolite. The apparent half-life of astemizole is about 20 to 60 hours, and that of the metabolite is 18 to 20 days. In overdose, the serum elimination half-life was 13.5 days.[13]

Loratidine. Loratidine is extensively metabolized in the liver to a minor active metabolite.[2,9,12] The elimination half-life is 7.8 to 15 hours.

Acrivastine. The half-life is about 1.7 hours. Total body clearance is 4.4 mL/min/kg.[2] Mean peak plasma concentrations of 7 μg/L (parent drug) and 179 μg/L (metabolites) are reached about 1.4 hours after single doses of 4-mg capsules of 17-mg oral solutions. About 15 to 17% of a dose is recovered in the urine.[14]

Drug Interactions

Symptomatic life-threatening ventricular arrhythmias have been reported from concomitant use of terfenadine (Seldane) or astemizole[15] and ketoconazole (Nizoral), an antifungal agent.[4,16–19] Ketoconazole can be associated with prolongation of the QT interval in healthy individuals or when used with terfenadine. Ketoconazole and itraconazole inhibit the metabolism of terfenadine, resulting in reduced clearance of terfenadine and its active metabolite.[12] Any drug that inhibits hepatic metabolism such as erythromycin,[20] ciprofloxacin, cimetidine, or disulfiram may impair clearance of terfenadine.[21]

Patients with impaired hepatic function, or who are receiving ketoconazole, troleandomycin, or macrolide antibiotics including erythromycin,[20] or who have conditions that may lead to QT prolongation (eg, hypokalemia, congenital QT syndrome, procainamide, quinidine, disopyramide) may experience QT prolongation, Torsade de pointes, and/or ventricular tachycardia in addition to cardiac arrest and death at recommended terfenadine and astemizole doses.[4] Astemizole is contraindicated in patients with hepatic dysfunction or electrolyte abnormalities such as hypokalemia and hypomagnesemia or in those ingesting diuretics with potential for the induction of electrolyte abnormalities. Chronic astemizole therapy, in combination with propoxyphene, may produce profound QT_c prolongation and life-threatening ventricular arrhythmias despite therapeutic astemizole levels.[22]

Pregnancy/Lactation

Terfenadine and astemizole are classified as Pregnancy Category C drugs. Controlled clinical studies in pregnant or lactating women are not available for terfenadine, astemizole, lopatidine, and acrivastine. Loratidine is excreted into breast milk.[12,23]

Mechanism of Action

The antihistamines competitively block H_1- and H_3- receptor sites. Table 48-3 contrasts the pharmacologic profiles of the classic and nonsedating antihistamines. Terfenadine (Seldane) and astemizole (Hismanal) are available in the United States.

Terfenadine. Terfenadine is a selective histamine H_1-receptor antagonist that does not exhibit substantial anticholinergic alpha-adrenergic, beta-adrenergic, or antiserotonin effects.[24–27] It preferentially binds to peripheral rather than central histamine H_1 receptors.

Astemizole. Astemizole is a long-acting selective histamine H_1-receptor antagonist without substantial central and autonomic nervous system effects. Binding at the H_1 receptors persists for 3 days. Such inhibition of histamine H_1 receptors occurs predominantly in the periphery. There is little cerebellar binding. Astemizole penetrates the central nervous system poorly, which may account for its lack of sedative effects.

Loratidine. Loratidine is a selective peripheral histamine H_1- receptor antagonist that has no substantial cerebral and autonomic nervous system effects.

Acrivastine. Acrivastine is a potent competitive histamine H_1- receptor antagonist. The potency and duration of action of acrivastine are similar to those of triprolidine.

H_1- receptor antagonists such as astemizole are structurally related to tricyclic antidepressants, known provokers of Torsade de pointes.[13] Stimulation of cardiac histamine receptors (H_1 and H_2) increases cyclic AMP via activation of adenylate cyclase and phosphorylase, producing both increased inotropic and chronotropic effects.[13]

Clinical Presentation

Overdose

Terfenadine. One case of Torsade de pointes was reported in a patient who ingested 3360 mg of terfenadine with 7 g of cephalexin and 1200 mg of ibuprofen; another patient ingested 1500 mg of terfenadine with no ill effects after gastric lavage.[8] Serious reactions may be preceded by episodes of syncope.[3]

Central Nervous System. Headache, nausea, confusion and seizures have followed overdoses with terfenadine.[8,28]

Cardiovascular System. Mild hypotension, Torsade de pointes, QT_c prolongation, and ventricular arrhythmias have been reported.[4]

Astemizole. One 15-year-old girl who took 10 mg of astemizole daily for 10 weeks had recurrent syncope for 3 days, then collapsed with premature ventricular contractions, a prolonged QT interval and first-degree atrioventricular block, followed by two episodes of Torsade de pointes.[13] An adolescent who overdosed with 200 mg of astemizole exhibited QT prolongation.[8] Another adolescent overdosed with 200 mg of astemizole but had no cardiac problems.[29] Six cases of accidental overdose in children who took 2.5 to 16.7 mg/kg of astemizole exhibited prolonged QT_c intervals. Nineteen hours after discharge, one child developed serious ventricular arrhythmias and one episode required cardioconversion.[16] A 3-year-old took 100 mg of astemizole and developed second-degree heart block, multiple conduction abnormalities, and a prolonged QT interval which became normal after about 8 hours without any treatment.[30] A 26-year-old woman ingested astemizole 700 mg with terfenadine 900 to 1200 mg and developed Torsade de pointes and ventricular fibrillation; cardioversion was used; she recovered on the third day.[5] A 26-year-old woman ingested 200 mg of astemizole with 750 mg of hydroxyzine and alcohol; she developed Torsade de pointes 13 hours later.[4,31] Following an overdose, gastrointestinal symptoms and lethargy may develop within 1 hour. Symptoms may not develop until the onset of coma or arrhythmias 4 to 20 hours after an overdose. Arrhythmias may last several days.[32]

Children. Accidental astemizole ingestion in young children is dangerous because (1) a few tablets can cause toxicity, (2) routine measures to prevent absorption seem to have limited effect, perhaps because of rapid astemizole absorption, and (3) the worst cardiac effects can appear late and last long, probably because of the slow elimination of astemizole and metabolites. QT_c intervals should be monitored and the patient should not be discharged from hospital until the QT_c interval is normal. Repeated oral activated charcoal may be useful. In ventricular arrhythmias, class IA and III antiarrhythmic agents should be avoided, whereas electrolytes need to be normalized, lidocaine, mexiletine, magnesium sulfate, and isoprenaline may be tried. Temporary cardiac pacing to 100 to 120/min is suggested in serious intoxication and repeated direct-current cardioversion may be necessary.[11,30,33]

Chronic Use

A 2-year-old boy took an unknown dose of terfenadine and developed apnea, hypoxia, seizures, hypotonia, and sinus tachycardia.[7] A 21-year-old woman developed seizures after an overdose; the electrocardiogram showed prolonged QT_c intervals; she survived.[28]

Somnolence, depression, apathy, confusion, agitation, anxiety, paresthesia, tremor, insomnia, and depersonalization have been reported after use of astemizole and terfenadine.[34] Syncope may precede the onset of severe arrhythmias.

Laboratory

Analytical Methods

Terfenadine. A gas chromatography method is sensitive to 10 ng/mL.[9] A radioimmunoassay with a limit of detection of less than 1 μg/L is also available.[35]

Astemizole. A high-performance liquid chromatography method on a reversed-phase column with ultraviolet detection can estimate astemizole and its metabolite to 1 mg/L.[36] Thirteen hours following ingestion of 200 mg of astemizole, the plasma level of astemizole plus desmethyl astemizole (active metabolites) was 61.3 ng/mL.[33] At a maintenance dose of 10 mg/d, the mean therapeutic level of astemizole plus hydroxylated metabolites is 2 to 5 ng/mL.[37]

Blood Levels

Terfenadine. After an acute overdose with seizures, the terfenadine concentration was 43 ng/mL; the acid metabolite level was 1504 ng/mL.[28] Blood terfenadine levels with concomitant administration of ketoconazole reached 57 ng/mL; the acid metabolite level was 385 ng/mL.[4] A warning has been issued by the manufacturers and the Food and Drug Administration[38] that rare cases of serious cardiovascular adverse effects including death, cardiac arrest, Torsade de pointes,[39] and ventricular arrhythmias have occurred in the following clinical settings, frequently in association with increased terfenadine levels, which lead to electrocardiographic QT prolongation: (1) concomitant administration of ketoconazole; (2) overdose, including single doses as low as 6 mg twice daily; (3) concomitant use of erythromycin in significant hepatic dysfunction.[15,38]

Astemizole. A 15-year-old girl who developed Torsade de pointes had a serum concentration of astemizole with hydroxylated astemizole metabolite 38 hours after the last astemizole dose totaling 44.6 ng/mL; this decreased to 1.8 ng/mL 6 weeks later.[13] A 14-year-old overdosed with 200 mg and exhibited serum astemizole plus hydroxylated metabolite concentrations of 79.9 ng/mL 10 hours later.[40] Following an overdose of 200 mg, a 14-year-old exhibited a plasma half-life of 31 hours for astemizole plus metabolites.[29]

Abnormalities

Significant QT prolongation, Torsade de pointes, ventricular arrhythmias, and cardiac arrest with use of terfenadine may follow concomitant use of ketoconazole; overdose, including single doses as low as 360 mg twice daily; concomitant administration of erythromycin; and significant hepatic dysfunction.[17] The electrocardiogram following an astemizole overdose usually shows a prolonged QT_c interval, which may be associated with large U waves.[20] Patients should immediately be brought to the nearest emergency department in the hospital.

Treatment

Stabilization

Children with any electrocardiographic abnormalities after an astemizole overdose should be admitted to a unit capable of continuous cardiac monitoring and treatment of potential dysrhythmias.[41]

Gut Decontamination

Decontamination of the gastrointestinal tract is achieved with gastric lavage and activated charcoal.

Supportive Measures

Astemizole. For asymptomatic patients, an electrocardiogram is done to determine the QT_c interval. Electrocardiographic monitoring is continued until the QT_c returns to normal.

For symptomatic patients, standard life support measures and treatment of arrhythmias are instituted as required. Supportive care and electrocardiographic monitoring are continued until the QT_c interval returns to normal. Rao and colleagues suggest the following[42]:

1. Consider astemizole-induced toxicity in the differential diagnoses of prolonged QT_c interval, ventricular tachyarrhythmias, syncope, and seizures. If dizziness, palpitations, syncope, or seizures occur, use of the drug should be discontinued immediately and the patient should be hospitalized for cardiac monitoring.
2. Do not prescribe astemizole for patients known to be taking medications or to have conditions associated with a prolonged QT_c interval.
3. Avoid concomitant administration of erythromycin (and other macrolide antibiotics), ketoconazole, and itraconazole, metronidazole, fluconazole, and miconazole nitrate (the last four drugs are chemically similar to ketoconazole).

4. Advise patients to adhere to the recommended dosage of 10 mg/d and not increase it. Ask them to seek advice about concurrent use of any other medication with astemizole.
5. Administer astemizole to patients with hepatic impairment with caution.
6. For all patients who have taken an overdose of astemizole institute early treatment consisting of gastric lavage and oral administration of charcoal. Admit to the hospital for at least 2 to 3 days for cardiac monitoring. Electrocardiographic abnormalities are an absolute indication for admission to the intensive care unit. Do not discharge patients until the arrhythmias have abated or the QT_c interval has returned to baseline (or both).
7. Immediately treat astemizole-induced ventricular arrhythmias by intravenous administration of magnesium sulfate or isoproterenol, temporary atrial or ventricular pacing, and, if necessary, direct-current cardioversion.
8. Prevent electrolyte abnormalities and avoid drugs that prolong the QT_c interval.

In ventricular arrhythmias following astemizole overdose or overdose of other related drugs, it appears logical to avoid drugs known to prolong the QT_c interval or to cause torsade de pointes (eg, amiodarone, quinidine, procainamide, disopyramide and sotalol). Lidocaine, isoprenaline, and propranolol have been effective in reversing astemizole-induced ventricular arrhythmias and cardioversion has also been used.[30]

Terfenadine. Children who ingest more than 10 mg or who are less than 1 year old should be referred to a health care facility.[3] Electrocardiographic monitoring for at least 24 hours postingestion should be considered for as long as the QT_c interval is prolonged. There is limited experience with hemodialysis and hemoperfusion.[8]

If torsade de pointes develops, magnesium sulfate 20% solution, 2 g every 2 to 3 minutes, is administered. If there is no response in 10 minutes, the preceding is repeated, then followed by a continuous infusion of 5 to 10 mg/min or 50 mg/min for 2 hours followed by 30 mg/min for 90 minutes, twice daily for several days. In children, the dose is 25 to 50 mg/kg initially; maintenance is 30 to 60 mg/kg/24 h (0.25–0.50 mEq/kg/24 h) up to 1000 mg/24 h. The serum magnesium level must be monitored. The magnesium is given slowly with electrocardiographic monitoring and calcium gluconate available.

Diazepam 0.3 mg/kg is administered every 5 minutes to a total dose of 10 mg in children; adults received 10 mg every 15 minutes up to 30 mg. This is followed by intravenous phenytoin 15 mg/kg in children slowly over at least 20 minutes or in adults 1 g at 50 mg/min. The electrocardiogram and blood pressure are monitored. (See also Chapter 38.)

Antidote

There is no antidote. Astemizole is not removed by hemodialysis.[37] Children poisoned with astemizole need emergency medical evaluation, a 12-lead electrocardiogram with calculation of the corrected QT intervals, and continuous cardiac monitoring for at least 24 hours[11] until the QT_c interval has returned to normal. This may last 3 days.[27]

Children with any electrocardiographic abnormalities after an astemizole overdose should be admitted to a unit capable of continuous cardiac monitoring and treatment of potential dysrhythmias.[41] Ventricular tachycardia has been effectively treated with intravenous magnesium.[20] The toll-free number for the manufacturer of terfenadine (Marion Merrell Dow in the United States) is 1–800–395–6825; the number for the manufacturer of astemizole (Janssen) is 1–800–JANSSEN.

HISTAMINE H_3 RECEPTORS

Histamine H_3 receptors are located not only in the central nervous system but also in peripheral tissues, where they exert inhibitory functions. This new type of histamine receptor may be added to the list of prejunctional receptors that regulate neurotransmission processes in the gastrointestinal tract. It is unclear if H_3-receptor agonists and antagonists are likely to be clinically useful.[43]

REFERENCES—NONSEDATING HISTAMINE H_1-RECEPTOR ANTAGONISTS

1. Kelloway JS, Pongowski MA, Schoenwetter WF. Additional causes of Torsade de pointes. Mayo Clin Proc 1995;70:197–200.
2. Mann KV, Crowe JP, Tietze KJ. Non-edative histamine H_1-receptor antagonists. Clin Pharm 1989;8:331–344.
3. Woodward JK. Pharmacology and toxicology of nonclassical antihistamines. Cutis 1988;42:5–9.
4. Monahan BP, Ferguson CL, Killearny ES, et al. Torsade de pointes occurring in association with terfenadine use. JAMA 1990;264:2788–2790.
5. Bastocky J, Krasnicka J, Vortel J, et al. Severe intoxication with antihistamines complicated by ventricular tachycardia. Vnitrni Lekarstri 1990;36:266–269.
6. MacConnell TJ, Stanneis AJ. Torsade de pointes: Complication of treatment with terfenadine. Br Med J 1991;30:1469.
7. Roney JE. Personal communication. Marion Merrell Dow, May 15, 1991.
8. Spiller HA, Picciotti M, Perez E. Accidental terfenadine ingestion in children. Vet Hum Toxicol 1989;31:154–156.
9. Barenholtz HA, McLeod DC. Loratidine: A nonsedating antihistamine with once daily dosing. DICP Ann Pharmacother 1989;23:445–450.
10. Eller MG, Walker BJ, Westmark PA, et al. Pharmacokinetics of terfenadine in healthy elderly subjects. J Clin Pharmacol 1992;32:267–277.
11. Wiley JF II, Gelber ML, Henretig FM, et al. Cardiotoxic effects of astemizole overdose in children. J Pediatr 1992;120: 799–802.
12. Clissold SP, Sorkin EM, Goa KL. Loratidine: A preliminary review of its pharmacodynamic properties and therapeutic efficacy. Drugs 1989;27:42–57.
13. Simons FER, Kesselman MS, Giddins NG, et al. Astemizole induced Torsade de pointes. Lancet 1988;2:624.
14. Brogden RN, McTavish D. Acrivastine: A review of its pharmacological properties and therapeutic efficacy in allergic rhinitis, urticaria and related disorders. Drugs 1991;41:927–940.
15. Honig PK, Woosley RL, Zamani K, et al. Changes in the pharmacokinetics and electrocardiographic pharmacodynamics of terfenadine with concomitant administration of erythromycin. Clin Pharmacol Ther 1992;52:231–238.
16. Safety of terfenadine and astemizole. Med Lett Drugs Ther 1992;34(863):9–10.

17. Dear Health Care Professional Letter. Marion Merrell Dow, 1991.
18. Labelling changes to reflect drug interaction between terfenadine and ketoconazole. FDA Med Bull 1991;21(2):4.
19. Eller MG, Okerholm RA. Pharmacokinetic interaction between terfenadine and ketoconazole. Clin Pharmacol Ther 1991;49:130.
20. Leor J, Harman M, Rabinowitz B, Mozes B. Giant U-waves and associated ventricular tachycardia complicating astemizole overdose: Successful therapy with intravenous magnesium. Am J Med 1991;91:94–97.
21. Mathews DR, McNutt B, Okerholm R, et al. Torsade de pointes occurring in association with terfenadine use. JAMA 1991;266:2375–2376.
22. Cuttin T, Bogart T, Horowitz RS, et al. Refractory Torsade de pointes (TdP) associated with therapeutic levels of astemizole (Hismanal[R]). Vet Hum Toxicol 1993;35:344.
23. Hilbert J, Radwanski E, Affrime MP, et al. Excretion of loratidine in human breast milk. J Clin Pharmacol 1988;28:234–239.
24. McTavish D, Goa KL, Ferrill M. Terfenadine: An update review of its pharmacological properties and therapeutic efficacy. Drugs 1990;39:552–574.
25. Okerholm RA, Weiner DL, Hook RH, et al. Bioavailability of terfenadine in man. Biopharm Drug Dispos 1981;2:185–190.
26. Sorkin EM, Heal RC. Terfenadine: A review of its pharmacodynamic properties and therapeutic efficacy. Drugs 1985; 29:34–56.
27. Garteiz DA, Hook RH, Walker RJ, Okerholm RA. Pharmacokinetic and biotransformation studies of terfenadine in man. Arzneimittelforschung 1982;32:1185–1190.
28. Davies AJ, Harinadra V, McEvan A, Ghose RR. Cardiotoxic effect with convulsions in terfenadine overdoses. Br Med J 1989;298:325.
29. Kingwood JC, Routledge PA, Lazarus JH. A report of overdose with astemizole. Hum Toxicol 1986;5:43–44.
30. Hoppu K, Tikanoja T, Tapanainen P, et al. Accidental astemizole overdose in young children. Lancet 1991;338:538–540.
31. Burke TG, Mutnick AH. Ventricular fibrillation and anoxic encephalopathy secondary to astemizole overdose. Ann Pharmacother 1993;27:239–241.
32. Huebner GD. Piscataway, NJ: Personal communication. Janssen Research Foundation, February 28, 1989.
33. Tobin JR, Doyle TP, Ackerman AD, Brenne JI. Astemizole-induced cardiac conduction disturbances in a child. JAMA 1991;266:2737–2740.
34. Non-sedating antihistamines. Aust Adverse Drug React Bull, May 1991;10.
35. Cook CE, Williams DL, Myers M, et al. Bioavailability of terfenadine in man. Biopharm Drug Dispos 1981;2: 185–190.
36. Woestenborghs R, Embrects LL, Heykants J. Simultaneous determination of astemizole and its demethylated metabolites in animal plasma and tissues by high performance liquid chromatography. J Chromatogr 1983;278: 359–366.
37. Saviuc P, Danel V, Dixmerias F. Prolonged QT interval and Torsade de pointes following astemizole overdose. Clin Toxicol 1993;31:121–125.
38. New boxed warnings added for seldane, hismanal. FDA Med Bull 1992;22(2):1–2.
39. Pohjola-Sintoren S, Viitasalo M, Toivonen L, Neuvonen P. Torsade de pointes after terfenadine–itraconazole interaction. Br Med J 1993;306:186.
40. Craft TM. Torsade de pointes after astemizole overdose. Br Med J 1986;292:660.
41. Nightingale SL. US Food and Drug Administration warnings issued on nonsedating antihistamines, terfenadine and astemizole. JAMA 1992;268:705.
42. Rao KA, Adlakha A, Verna-Ansil B, et al. Torsade de pointes ventricular tachycardia associated with overdose of astemizole. Mayo Clin Proc 1994;6:589–593.
43. Bertaccini G, Coruzzi G, Poli E. Review article: The histamine H3 receptor: A novel prejunctional receptor regulating gastrointestinal function. Aliment Pharmacol Ther 1991;5:585–591.

Chapter 49

5-Hydroxytryptamine (Serotonin) Receptor Drugs

INTRODUCTION

Successful treatment of depression began with the use of electroconvulsive therapy in the 1930s.[1] Heterocyclic antidepressants and monoamine oxidase inhibitors followed in the 1950s, lithium in the 1960s, and carbamazepine, a mood-stabilizing anticonvulsant, in the 1970s.[2] To find agents with fewer side effects (eg, drying up of the nasopharynx, constipation, cardiac irritation, fainting, sedation) drugs were produced that could increase the concentration of serotonin (5-hydroxytryptamine [5-HT]) at the synapse (Fig. 49–1). These included fluoxetine. Fluoxetine was rapidly followed by fluvoxamine and sertraline.[3] Subsequently, a number of 5-HT receptor agonists and antagonists were developed.[4] (Tables 49–1, 49–2, and 49–3). Each 5-HT receptor subserves a specific function.

SEROTONIN RECEPTORS

Serotonin or 5-HT is a regulatory neurotransmitter with general inhibitory effects. It is synthesized from L-tryptophan, which crosses the blood–brain barrier. Serotonin does not cross the blood–brain barrier. The central nervous system absorbs L-tryptophan and then synthesizes 5-HT in the cell. The cell bodies of the serotonergic system are concentrated primarily in the raphe or midline section of the brainstem.[5] This network is the largest chemical system in the mammalian brain.

TYPES OF SEROTONIN RECEPTORS

Four major types of serotonin receptors have been identified[6]: Types 5-HT_1, 5-HT_2, 5-HT_3, and 5-HT_4.[4] The 5-HT_1 group is further divided into subtypes A, B, C, D, and E. The 5-HT_2 group is also subdivided into subtypes A and B. The 5-HT_3 receptors are found both in the periphery and in the central nervous system. Antagonists of peripheral 5-HT_3 receptors such as ondansetron, granisetron, and zacopride are used in the treatment of nausea and vomiting.[4] The selective serotonin reuptake inhibitors (SSRIs) do not bind to any specific neuroreceptor systems but produce antidepressant effects through selective blockade of serotonin uptake[7–9] (Table 49–3).

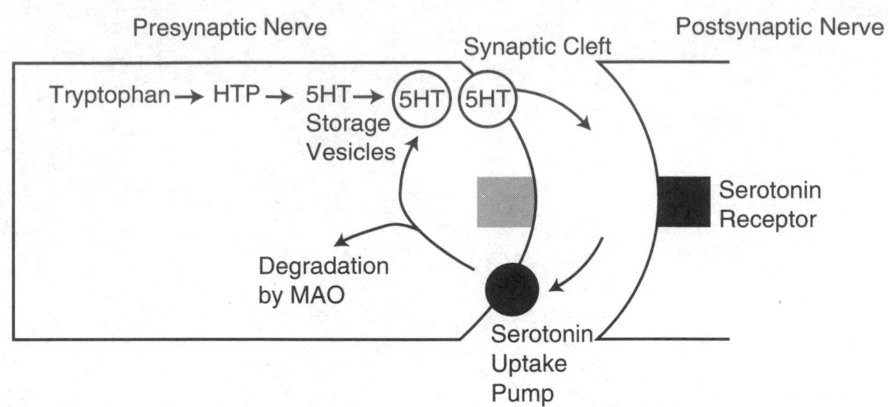

Figure 49-1 A serotonin synapse. Serotonin (5HT), synthesized from precursor tryptophan, is released by a presynaptic nerve into the synaptic cleft. From there, serotonin can act on the postsynaptic receptor and thus initiate neurotransmission or return to the presynaptic cell via a pumplike uptake mechanism. Once returned to the presynaptic cell, serotonin either is taken back into storage vesicles for future release or is degraded by monoamine oxidase (MAO). (From Stokes PE. Fluoxetine: A five-year review. Clin Ther 1993;15:216–243.)

Table 49–1
Properties of Some Serotonin (5-HT) Receptor Agonists and Antagonists

Drug	Target Receptor or System	Distribution of Target Sites	Action at Target Sites	Use
Buspirone (Buspar)	5-HT_{1A}-receptors	5-HT neuronal cell bodies in brain; postsynaptically	Presynaptic partial agonist in low doses and postsynaptic partial agonist in high doses	Anxiety; depression?
Lithium	5-HT_{1A} receptors	5-HT neuronal cell bodies in brain; postsynaptically	Agonist	Manic depression
Mianserin (Bolvidon, Norval)	5-HT_{1C} receptors	Brain	Antagonist	Depression
Sumatriptan (Imigran)	5-HT_{1D} receptors	Intracranial; pial and dural vessels; 5-HT neuron terminals	Agonist (vasoconstricts)	Migraine
LSD	5-HT_2 receptors	Brain	Partial agonist	Abuse (illegal)
Ketanserin	5-HT_2 receptors	Arteries, platelets, spinal cord, lungs	Antagonist	Hypertension? (unlicensed)
Ritanserin	5-HT_2 receptors	Gastrointestinal tract	Antagonist	Depression and anxiety? (unlicensed)
Methysergide (Deseril)	5-HT and 5-HT_2 receptors (nonselective)	Cranial vessels	Antagonist	Migraine prophylaxis
Pizotifen (Sanomigran)		Cranial vessels	Antagonist	Migraine prophylaxis
Ondansetron*† (Zofran)	5-HT_3 receptors	Vagus (gut)	Antagonist	Nausea and vomiting due to chemotherapy; irradiation*; postoperative†
Granisetron* (Kytril)	5-HT_3 receptors	Hindbrain	Antagonist	
Tropisetron (Navoban)	5-HT_3 receptors	Hindbrain	Antagonist	
Fluoxetine (Prozac)‡	5-HT uptake	Brain	Blocks reuptake	Depression; obsessive–compulsive disorder; bulimia nervosa‡
Fluvoxamine (Faverin)	5-HT uptake	Brain	Blocks reuptake	
Paroxetine (Seroxat)	5-HT uptake	Brain	Blocks reuptake	
Sertraline (Lustral)	5-HT uptake	Brain	Blocks reuptake	
Fenfluramine (Ponderax)	5-HT release	Brain	Increase release; block reuptake	Appetite suppression
Dexfenfluramine (Adifax)	5-HT release	Brain		
MDMA (Ecstasy)	5-HT release	Brain	Increases release	Abuse (illegal)

From Drugs affecting 5-hydroxytryptamine function. Drug Ther Bull 1993;31:26.

SELECTIVE SEROTONIN REUPTAKE INHIBITORS

Serotonergic dysfunction has been implicated in illnesses such as depression, anxiety, obsessive–compulsive disorder, sleep and eating disorders, schizophrenia, Alzheimer's dementia, personality disorders, alcoholism, autism, pain, aggression, and impulse disorders. Agents that modulate serotonergic activity may be useful in the treatment of these illnesses. A new class of drugs with antidepressant actions has been developed that selectively block the reuptake of serotonin into presynaptic neurons. Selective serotonin uptake inhibitors include fluoxetine, sertraline, paroxetine,

Table 49–2
Classification of Serotonin (5-HT) Receptors and Summary of Some Functional Responses Mediated by Receptor Subtypes

Receptor Subtype	Location	Functional Response
5-HT_{1A}	Neuronal, mainly in the CNS	Hypotension; neuronal hyperpolarization
5-HT_{1B}	Found in humans and rodents	Marked difference in pharmacologic activity between human and rat receptors
5-HT_{1C}	CNS (high density in choroid plexus)	Increased turnover of phosphatidylinositol
5-HT_{1D}	CNS sensory fibers	Inhibition of neurotransmitter release; inhibition of neuropeptide release
5-HT_{1E}	CNS	?
5-HT_1-"like"	Intracranial vasculature	Contraction of cephalic arteries and arteriovenous anastomoses
5-HT_1-"like"	Vascular smooth muscle; GI smooth muscle	Relaxation
5-HT_2	Vascular smooth muscle; platelets; lung; CNS; GI tract	Vasoconstriction; platelet aggregation; bronchoconstriction
5-HT_3	Peripheral and central neurons	Membrane depolarization; activation of sensory afferents
5-HT_4	GI tract; CNS; heart	Increase in cyclic AMP; activation of neurotransmitter release
5-HT_{s31}	?	?

CNS, central nervous system; GI, gastrointestinal.
From Dechart KL, Clissold SP. Sumatriptan: A review of its pharmacodynamic and pharmacokinetic properties, and therapeutic efficacy in the acute treatment of migraine and cluster headache. Drugs 1992;43:776–798.

Table 49–3
Serotonin (5-HT) Receptors: Actions and Examples

Receptor	Action	Antagonists	Agonists
5-HT_1	Close cerebral vessels Use: migraine	Methiothepin Methysergide	
5-HT_{1A}	Inhibits 5-HT neurons Induce response to anxiety, depression, hypertension	Pindolol	Buspirone (ipsapirone, urapidil, gepirone, tandospirone, 5-carboxaminidotryptamine, ergotamine, chlorophenyl piperazine (GR 43175)
5-HT_{1B}	Inhibit 5-HT release		
5-HT_{1C}	Induce slow-wave sleep		
5-HT_{1D}	Inhibit 5-HT release Induce slow-wave sleep Vasoconstrict cranial vessels (acute migraine)	Sumatriptan	
5-HT_2	Contract vascular smooth muscle Induce platelet aggregation Depolarize neurons Use: migraine, anxiety, hypertension	Ketanserin (antihypertensive) Pizotifen (antimigraine) Cyproheptadine Ritanserin Mianserin Nefazodone Buspirone (downregulator) Amitriptyline	
5-HT_3	Receptors in gastrointestinal area and posterior brain Mediate emesis 5-HT in gastrointestinal tract Depolarize peripheral neurons Stimulate adenyl cyclase in brain Regulate emesis	Ondansetron Granisetron Metoclopramide (high dose) Renzapride Zacopride Cisapride (high dose)	5-Methyl-5-hydroxytryptamine
5-HT_4		ICS 205930 (tropisetron) Ondansetron Metoclopramide (high dose)	Metoclopramide Zacopride Renzapride
	Selective serotonin reuptake inhibitors Induce response to depression Mitigate obsessive–compulsive disorders	Paroxetine Sertraline Fluoxetine Fluvoxamine Citalopram Indalpine	Cisapride Benzamides (Cisapride, renzapride, zacopride, metoclopramide), benzimidazoles, indoles

Table 49–4
Basic Pharmacokinetic Parameters of Selective Serotonin Reuptake Inhibitors

Parameter	Fluvoxamine	Fluoxetine	Paroxetine	Sertraline	Citalopram
Gastrointestinal absorption	≥94%	80%	≥64%	≥44%	≈100%
t_{max} (h)	5 (2–8)	6–8	5 (0.5–11)	6–8	2–4
F (%)	60 (dogs)	72 (dogs)	≈50		≈100
CL/F (L/h)					
Single dose	65	36	167	96	26
Multiple dose	41	11	36		26
PB (%)	77	95	95	99	50
V_D (L/kg)	>5	20–42	17		14
$t_{1/2}$					
Parent compound	15h	1.9 d	10–16 h	26 h	33 h
Active metabolite	NA	7 d	NA	62–104 h	
Urinary excretion (% of oral dose)					
Radioactivity	94	80	64	44	
Parent compound	<4	11	<2	0	12
Fecal excretion (% of oral dose)					
Radioactivity		15	36	44	
Parent compound			<1		

t_{max} = time to reach peak plasma concentration; F, absolute bioavailability; CL/F, oral clearance; PB, protein binding; V_D, volume of distribution; $t_{1/2}$, half-life following a single dose; NA, not applicable.
From Van Harten J. Clinical pharmacokinetics of selective serotonin reuptake inhibitors. Clin Pharmacokinet 1993;24:203–220.

fluvoxamine, citalopram, ifoxetine, and indalpine.[8] Of these, fluoxetine, fluvoxamine, paroxetine, and sertraline are the only agents currently marketed in the United States. Fluvoxamine, paroxetine, and sertraline are also available in the United Kingdom.[10] Zimeldine was withdrawn from clinical use in 1983 because of its association with Guillain–Barré syndrome.

Toxicokinetics

These agents undergo extensive metabolism to clinically inactive compounds, possess relatively large volumes of distribution, and are highly bound to plasma proteins. Their elimination half-lives range from 15 to 26 hours.[11] (Table 49–4).

Uses

Selective serotonin reuptake inhibitors are employed in the treatment of depression, panic attacks, obsessive–compulsive disorder, obesity, substance abuse, sleep disorders, chemotherapy-induced nausea and vomiting, migraine, and appetite suppression[12] (Table 49–1).

Special References and Reviews

Blier P, de Montigny C, Chaput Y. A role for the serotonin system in the mechanism of action of antidepressant treatments: Preclinical evidence. J Clin Psychiatry 1990;51(suppl.):14–20.

Bockaert J, Fozard JR, Dumuis A, Clarke DC. The 5-HT_4 receptor: A place in the sun. Trends Pharmacol Sci 1992;13:141–144.

Cowen PJ. A role for 5-HT in the action of antidepressant drugs. Pharmacol Ther 1990;46:43–51.

Drugs acting on 5-hydroxytryptamine receptors. Lancet 1989;2:717–719. Editorial.

Gonzalez-Heydrich J, Peroutka SJ. Serotonin receptor and reuptake sites: Pharmacologic significance. J Clin Psychiatry 1990;51(4, suppl.):5–12.

Healey D. The marketing of 5-hydroxytryptamine: Depression or anxiety. Br J Psychiatry 1991;158:737–742.

Hesketh PJ, Gandara DR. Serotonin antagonists: A new class of antiemetic agents. J Natl Cancer Inst 1991;83: 613–620.

5-HT blockers and all that. Lancet 1990;336:345–346. Editorial.

Marsden CA: The pharmacology of new anxiolytics acting on 5-HT neuroses. Postgrad Med J 1990;66 (suppl. 2):S2–S6.

Meltzer NY, Nash JF. VII. Effects of antipsychotic drugs on serotonin receptors. Pharmacol Rev 1991;43:588–604.

Montgomery SA. The benefits and risks of 5-HT uptake inhibitors in depression. Br J Psychiatry 1988;153 (suppl. 3):7–18.

Peroutka SJ. 5-hydroxytryptamine receptor subtypes. Pharmacol Toxicol 1990;67:373–383.

Peroutka SJ. VI. Serotonin receptor subtypes and neuropsychiatric diseases: Four of 5-HT^{1D} and 5-HT_3 receptor agents.

Van Heuven-Nolsen. 5-HT receptor subtype-specific drugs and the cardiovascular system. Trends Pharmacol Sci 1988;9:423–425.

Zifa E, Fillion G. 5-Hydroxytryptamine receptors. Pharmacol Rev 1992;44:402–458.

REFERENCES—INTRODUCTION

1. 5-HT blockers and all that. Lancet 1990;336:345–346. Editorial.
2. Price LH, Charney DS, Delgado DL, et al. Clinical data on the role of serotonin in the mechanism(s) of action of antidepressant drugs. J Clin Psychiatry 1990;51(suppl.):44–50.
3. If at first you do succeed. Lancet 1991;337:650–651. Editorial.

4. Talley NJ. 5-Hydroxytryptamine agonists and antagonists in the modulation of gastrointestinal motility and sensation: Clinical implications. Aliment Pharmacol Ther 1992;6:273–289. Review Article.
5. Ashton CH, Teoh R, Davies DM. Drug-induced stupor and coma: Some physical signs and their pharmacological basis. Adverse Drug React Acute Poison Rev 1989;8:1–59.
6. Cowen PJ. Serotonin receptor subtypes: Implications for psychopharmacology. Br J Psychiatry 1991;159(suppl. 12): 7–14.
7. Stokes PE. Fluoxetine: A five-year review. Clin Ther 1993;15: 216–243.
8. Grimsley SR, Jain MW. Paroxetine, sertraline and fluoxamine: New selective serotonin reuptake inhibitors. Clin Pharm 1992;11:930–957.
9. Mills KC. Serotonin toxicity: A comprehensive review for emergency medicine. Top Emerg Med 1993;15:54–73.
10. British National Formulary Number 24. London: British Medical Association, Pharmaceutical Press, September 1992.
11. Van Harten J. Clinical pharmacokinetics of selective serotonin reuptake inhibitors. Clin Pharmacokinet 1993;24: 203–220.
12. Gonzalez-Heydrich J, Peroutka SJ. Serotonin receptor and reuptake sites: Pharmacologic significance. J Clin Psychiatry 1990;51(suppl.):5–12.

THE SEROTONIN SYNDROME

Associated Illness

The serotonin syndrome has been reported in patients with unipolar and bipolar depression, obsessive–compulsive disorder, eating disorders with depression, and Parkinson's disease.[1] The syndrome was first reported by Sternbach in 1991.[1] Mills has provided a comprehensive review.[2]

Pathophysiology

The serotonin syndrome is most commonly the result of the interaction between serotonergic agents and monoamine oxidase inhibitors (MAOIs). The 5-HT receptors responsible for producing the serotonin syndrome are located in the lower brainstem or spinal cord.[3,4]

Tricyclic antidepressants, MAOIs, 5-HT reuptake inhibitors, antidepressants, electroconvulsive therapy, and 5-HT_{1A} receptor agonists appear to enhance 5-HT neurotransmission in the brainstem and spinal cord.

Clinical Presentation

The most frequent clinical features observed are changes in mental status, and behavioral changes (agitation, restlessness, confusion, incoordination, hypomania, coma, or possibly seizures) altered muscle tone or neuromuscular activites (myoclonus, hyperreflexia), shivering, rigidity, tremor,[5] autonomic instability (hypertension or hypotension, tachycardia or profuse sweating), hyperpyrexia, and diarrhea.[5,6] Death may follow the use of fluoxetine and a MAOI within hours.[7] These drugs are capable of increasing the availability of serotonin in the central nervous system. The serotonin syndrome most commonly occurs within 2 hours of the first dose of the precipitating agent and resolves within 6 to 24 hours of removal of the offending agent.[6] Similarities of the neuroleptic malignant syndrome to MDMA toxicity have been observed (Table 49–5).[7] In one patient, the serotonergic syndrome resulted in hyperthermia, rhabdomyolysis, disseminated intravascular coagulation, and myoglobinuric renal failure.[5] Di-

Table 49–5
Comparison of Serotonin Syndrome, Neuroleptic Malignant Syndrome, and Ecstasy (MDMA)

	Serotonin Syndrome	Neuroleptic Malignant Syndrome	Ecstasy (MDMA)
Cause	Drugs that enhance brain serotonin activity MAOI–tryptophan MAOI–fluoxetine Fluoxetine–tryptophan MAOI–meperidine hydrochloride Meclobemide–climipramine Fluoxetine–carbamazepine	Dopamine-blocking agents	3,4-Methylenedioxymethamphetamine
Clinical presentation	Hyperthermia, tachycardia, autonomic instability, agitation, diaphoresis, myoclonus, shivering, tremor, confusion, or delirium (± hyperthermia, disseminated intravascular coagulation, rhabdomyolysis, acute renal failure)	Hyperthermia, rigidity, fluctuating consciousness, autonomic instability	Hyperthermia, tachycardia, disseminated intravascular coagulation, rhabdomyolysis, acute renal failure
Mechanism of action	Hyperstimulation of 5-HT_{1A} receptor in brainstem and spinal cord	Acute depletion of dopamine (rigidity), Hyperthermia, tachycardia, elevated creatine phosphokinase levels, renal failure from rhabdomyolysis	Affects both dopamine- and serotonin-containing neurons Stimulates neuronal serotonin release
Treatment	Methysergide maleate; beta blocker	Discontinuation of medication, bromocriptine, dantrolene sodium, cooling blankets, hydration, respiratory support	Removal of medication, cooling or dantrolene sodium for hyperthermia, anticonvulsants for seizures; monitoring in intensive care unit; methysergide? cyproheptadine?

MAOI, monoamine oxidase inhibitor; 5-HT, serotonin.
Adapted from Ames D, Wirshing WC. Ecstasy, the serotonin syndrome and neuroleptic malignant syndrome: A possible link? JAMA 1993;269:869–870.

agnostic criteria for the serotonin syndrome are described by Sporer[8] (Table 49–5).

Drug Interactions

Drug interactions most commonly reported in connection with the serotonin syndrome are those between L-tryptophan and the MAOIs, with or without concomitant lithium. Fluoxetine in conjunction with MAOIs or L-tryptophan is the second most frequent drug combination associated with the serotonin syndrome. As a result of the long-lasting serotonergic activity of the MAOIs and serotonin uptake inhibitors, depressed patients who have been switched from fluoxetine to an MAOI without a drug interval of at least 5 weeks are susceptible to the serotonin syndrome.[9] Three deaths have occurred probably secondary to the use of tranylcypromine after withdrawal of fluoxetine.[10] Combinations of tricyclic antidepressants (eg, clomipramine, trazodone, imipramine)[11] with MAOIs may induce the syndrome.[12] The MAOI–meperidine interaction is one of central serotonergic overactivity and may include muscle twitching, fever, hyperreflexia, diaphoresis, hypotension, hypertension, coma, and death. Meperidine blocks neuronal reuptake of 5-HT. In conjunction with a MAOI it causes an increase in central nervous system 5-HT.[13] Patients receiving MAOIs who need opiates should be given morphine, which does not block serotonin reuptake.

Dextromethorphan blocks neuronal uptake of 5-HT and has been implicated in the serotonin syndrome when used with a MAOI.[14] Similarly, pentazocine 100 mg with fluoxetine 40 mg led within 30 minutes to lightheadedness, anxiety, nausea, upper extremity paresthesias, diaphoresis, flushing, ataxia, tremulousness, and hypertension.[15] Fluvoxamine alone has been implicated in the serotonin syndrome.[16] Serotonin syndrome has been induced by concomitant use of fluovoxamine and lithium.[17] Similarly, combinations of trazodone or buspirone, and paroxetine have induced the syndrome.[18]

Treatment

When the offending agents are removed, the syndrome often resolves on its own within 24 hours. Supportive measures may be helpful. Cooling blankets for hyperthermia, benzodiazepines, artificial ventilation for respiratory insufficiency, anticonvulsants for seizures, clonazepam for myoclonus, and nifedipine for hypertension are useful. If these measures are not effective, propranolol or methysergide, both 5-HT_{1A}-receptor antagonists, may be of limited benefit.[19] Groups in the United Kingdom recommend that MAOI overdose or interaction patients with a core temperature greater than 39°C should be electively paralyzed by a nondepolarizing agent and mechanically ventilated.[20] Cyproheptadine (4 mg) has been useful in terminating symptoms.[21]

REFERENCES—THE SEROTONIN SYNDROME

1. Sternbach H. The serotonin syndrome. Am J Psychiatry 1991;148:705–713.
2. Mills KC. Serotonin toxicity: A comprehensive review of emergency medicine. Top Emerg Med 1993;15:54–73.
3. Luck I, Nobler MS, Frazer A. Differential actions of serotonin antagonists on two behavioral models of serotonin receptor activation in the rat. J Pharmacol Exp Ther 1989;1:133–139.
4. Azmitia EC, Whitaker-Azmitia PM. Awakening the sleeping giant: Anatomy and plasticity of the brain serotonergic system. J Clin Psychiatry 1991;52(suppl.):4–16.
5. Miller F, Friedman R, Tanenbaum J, Griffin A. Disseminated intravascular coagulation and acute myoglobinuric renal failure: A consequence of the serotonergic syndrome. J Clin Psychopharmacol 1991;11:277–279.
6. Nierenberg DW, Semprebon M. The central nervous system serotonin syndrome. Clin Pharm Ther 1993;5:84–88.
7. Klein SS, Mauro LS, Scala-Barnett DM, Zick D. Serotonin syndrome versus neuroleptic malignant syndrome as a cause of death. Clin Pharm 1989;8:510–514.
8. Sporer KA. The serotonin syndrome: Implicated drugs, pathophysiology and management. Drug Saf 1995;13:94–104.
9. Tueth MJ. The serotonin syndrome in the emergency department. Ann Emerg Med 1993;22:1369.
10. Feighner JP, Boyes WF, Tyler DL, et al. Adverse consequences of fluoxetine–MAOI combination therapy. J Clin Psychiatry 1990;51:222–225.
11. Neuvonen PJ, Pohjoia-Sontonen S, Tacke U, Vuor L. Five fatal cases of serotonin syndrome after moclobemide–citalopram or moclobemide–clomipramine overdoses. Lancet 1993;342:1410.
12. Insel TR, Roy BF, Cohen RM, et al. Possible development of the serotonin syndrome in man. Am J Psychiatry 1982;139: 954–955.
13. Brown TCK, Cass NM. Beware: The use of MAO inhibitors is increasing again. Anaesth Intens Care 1979;7:65–68.
14. Rivers N, Hormer B. Possible lethal reaction between Nardil[R] and dextromethorphan. Can Med Assoc J 1970;103:85.
15. Hansen TE, Dieter K, Keepers GA. Interaction of fluoxetine and pentazocine. Am J Psychiatry 1990;147:949–950.
16. Lenzi A, Raffaeli S, Marazziti D. Serotonin syndrome-like symptoms in a patient with obsessive–compulsive disorder following inappropriate increase in fluvoxamine dosage. Pharmacopsychiatry 1993;26:100–101.
17. Ohman R, Spigset O. Serotonin syndrome induced by fluvoxamine–lithium interaction. Pharmacopsychiatry 1993;26: 263–264.
18. Reeves RR, Bullen JA. Serotonin syndrome produced by paroxetine and low-dose trazodone. Psychosomatics 1995;36: 159–160.
19. Dursun SM, Mathew VM, Revelrey MA. Toxic serotonin syndrome after fluoxetine plus carbamazepine. Lancet 1993;342: 442–443.
20. Henry JA. Serotonin syndrome. Lancet 1994;343:607.
21. Lappin RI, Auchincloss EL. Treatment of the serotonin syndrome with cyproheptadine. N Engl J Med 1994;331:1091–1092.

SEROTONERGIC DRUG WITHDRAWAL

Abrupt or gradual withdrawal of paroxetine, sertraline, or fluoxetine may be followed by vertigo, lightheadedness, severe nausea, emesis, fatigue, and myalgia. Symptoms lessen after cautious reintroduction of the drug and gradual tapering downward. No chronic neurologic deficits have been observed.[1–4]

REFERENCES—SEROTONERGIC DRUG WITHDRAWAL

1. Keuthen NJ, Cyr P, Ricciardi JA, et al: Medical withdrawal symptoms in obsessive–compulsive disordered patients

treated with paroxetine. J Clin Psychopharmacol 1994;14:206–207.
2. Barr LC, Goodman WK, Price LH. Physical symptoms associated with paroxetine discontinuance. Am J Psychiatry 1994;15:289.
3. Louie AK, Lannon RA, Ajari LJ. Withdrawal reaction after sertraline discontinuation. Am J Psychiatry 1994;151:450–451.
4. Lauterbach EC. Fluoxetine withdrawal and chronic pain. Neurology 1994;44:983–984.

BUSPIRONE

Buspirone hydrochloride is an anxiolytic agent that appears to have a high affininty for 5-HT_{1A} receptors and dopamine D_2 pre- and postsynaptic terminal receptors in the central nervous system. It is minimally toxic in overdose.

Structure and Classification

Buspirone hydrochloride is a member of a new class of structurally unique molecules, the azapirones[1]; it is an azaspirodecanedione derivative, but has also been referred to as an arylpiperazine derivative. Buspirone differs structurally and pharmacologically from benzodiazepines, barbiturates, and other anxiolytic agents. The heteroaryl (pyrimidinyl) piperazine moiety may be responsible for its anxiolytic and serotonergic activity.[2–5]

Use

Buspirone is used for the management of anxiety disorders (anxiety and phobic neuroses).[6,7] It may be useful in the treatment of maladaptive behavior and anxiety in developmentally disabled persons,[8,9] the premenstrual syndrome,[10,11] Tourette's syndrome,[12] and anxiety in HIV-infected drug users.[13] Preliminary observations indicate its possible usefulness in tardive dyskinesia,[14] smoking,[15] and obsessive–compulsive disorder (when used with fluoxetine).[16] Further confirmation of these additional uses is required before the drug is generally considered effective in such conditions. Buspirone may have advantages over tricyclic antidepressants in treating depression in those patients with severe heart disease, including minimal orthostatic hypotension and lack of prolongation of intraventricular conduction.[17]

Product Formulation

Buspirone hydrochloride is available as 5- and 10-mg tablets for oral use (Buspar).

Source

Buspirone is a synthetic chemical. It is very soluble in water and has a molecular weight of 422.[2] Buspirone is a heterocyclic compound with a pK_{a1} of 4.12 and pK_{a2} of 7.32.

Therapeutic Dose

The usual adult dosage of buspirone hydrochloride is 10 to 15 mg daily. The manufacturer recommends that adult dosage not exceed 60 mg daily.

Toxic Dose

Doses up to 2400 mg daily were administered during early trials.[3,18] Akathisia, tremor, and rigidity were observed. Doses of 250 mg[18] and up to 300 mg resulted in drowsiness in about one half of patients who ingested an overdose.[19]

Fatal Dose

Fatal doses have not been established.

Toxicokinetics

Absorption

After oral administration the drug is rapidly and completely absorbed in the gastrointestional tract, but first-pass metabolism reduces its mean bioavailability in humans to 4%.[5,20] Mean maximal plasma concentrations of 1 to 6 ng/mL occur within 40 to 90 minutes and appear to be dose related.[5]

Distribution

The apparent volume of distribution is approximately 5.3 L/kg after intravenous administration.[20] Buspirone is approximately 95% bound to plasma proteins, about two-thirds to albumin; the remainder is bound to α_1-acid glycoprotein.[21]

Elimination

Following extensive hepatic metabolism, less than 1% of buspirone is excreted unchanged. Its elimination half-life averages 2 to 4 hours. Buspirone is metabolized to 5-hydroxybuspirone (HB) and 1-pyrimidinylpiperazine (1-PP). HB is further oxidized to two hydroxy metabolites which undergo conjugation. 1-PP, 5-HB, and the glucuronide of 5-HB have elimination half-lives of 6.1, 4.8, and 3.2 hours, respectively.[4] Buspirone is rapidly cleared from the plasma at the rate of 2 to 3.5 L/h/kg.[5] 1-PP reaches levels four times higher than buspirone after a 20-mg dose of buspirone and may have pharmacologic activity.[2]

Drug Interactions

Buspirone given with a monoamine oxidase inhibitor may induce a rise in blood pressure. With trazodone, an elevation in alanine transaminase has been observed. Buspirone raises the plasma level of haloperidol when both are given together.[4] Buspirone with fluoxetine may have an additive effect in the treatment of obsessive–compulsive disorder.[16] Fluoxetine may antagonize the anxiolytic action of buspirone.[22] Although buspirone appears to exhibit little abuse tendency or potential and little evidence of a withdrawal syndrome,[23–27] when it is ingested with other psychotherapeutic drugs (eg, lithium), dependence or craving may be observed.[26]

Pregnancy/Lactation

There are no adequate and controlled studies using buspirone in pregnant women. The extent of distribution of buspirone and its metabolites into human milk is not known.[4]

Mechanism of Action

Buspirone may also block presynaptic and postsynaptic dopamine (D_2) receptors. Buspirone has no affinity for the γ-aminobutyric acid–benzodiazepine–chloride ionophore receptor site, no affinity for α_1-, α_2-, or β-adrenergic receptors, no effect on norepinephrine uptake, and no effect on cholinergic receptors.[4,28] It induces no euphoric effect[5] but has been subject to abuse.[29,30]

Clinical Presentation

Chronic Use

Frequent adverse effects following buspirone overdose are dizziness, drowsiness, and headache (in 10% of patients) and fatigue, nervousness, insomnia, and lightheadedness (5%).[3,4] Peripheral muscle tremors, lower motor restlessness, tardive dyskinesia, exacerbation of preexisting spasmodic torticollis, stiffness, and dystonia have been observed.[31,32] Manic states have been described following buspirone use, but the mechanism of mania development has not been elucidated.[33–37] Panic attacks, hypertension, and priapism have been rarely observed.[38–40] Buspirone metabolite 1PP is an α_2-adrenergic receptor antagonist and may induce hypertensive responses in some panic disorder patients who have a dysfunction of brain α_2 receptors.[39]

Overdose

Clinical symptoms may include nausea, gastrointestinal distress, hypotension, lightheadedness, and loss of consciousness.[3] Acute overdose with up to 300 mg of buspirone resulted in only drowsiness in approximately one half of patients studied.[19] No dizziness, headache, or nausea was observed in one patient who ingested 250 mg of buspirone.[18] One fatality followed ingestion of 450 mg of buspirone with other drugs (alprazolam, diltiazem, alcohol, and cocaine).[41]

Laboratory

Analytical Methods

A high-pressure liquid chromatography method is available for buspirone determinations. The assay is linear from 1 to 612 ng/mL.[42] An assay is available for the active metabolite, 1-PP.[43]

Blood Levels

Blood levels of 1 to 6 ng/mL are observed after a single 20-mg dose of buspirone.[4,5] Blood levels in overdose patients have not been evaluated.

Treatment

Treatment of overdose with buspirone involves symptomatic and supportive care. Conservative management of the asymptomatic patient should be considered. Blood pressure, pulse, and respiration should be monitored. The patient should be observed for development of any extrapyramidal signs or for evidence of behavior disturbances such as panic and mania.

Gut Decontamination

Clinical judgment determines whether it is necessary to initiate gastric lavage within 1 to 1.5 hours of ingestion by a buspirone overdose patient.

Elimination Enhancement

Methods to enhance elimination are probably not necessary in a buspirone overdose. Diuresis, hemodialysis, and hemoperfusion have not been used in a buspirone overdose. The extensive volume of distribution of buspirone would tend to preclude the efficacy of such therapeutic measures.

Antidote

There is no antidote.

Supportive Measures

Careful observation of the patient for 24 hours with electrocardiographic determinations and liver function tests is indicated in those depressed patients who may also have concomitantly ingested other drugs.

REFERENCES—BUSPIRONE

1. Eison AS. Azapirones: History of development. J Clin Psychopharmacol 1990;10:25–55.
2. Hatfield SM, Parenti MA. Buspirone hydrochloride. Hosp Pharm 1987;22:580–587.
3. Sathananthan GL, Sanghui I, Phillips N, Gershon S. MJ9022: Correlation between neuroleptic potential and stereotypy. Curr Ther Res 1975;18:701–705.
4. McEvoy GK, ed. *AHFS Drug Information 94.* Bethesda, MD: American Society of Hospital Pharmacists, 1994:1512–1519.
5. Goa KL, Ward A. Buspirone: A preliminary review of its pharmacological properties and therapeutic efficacy as an anxiolytic. Drugs 1986;32:114–129.
6. Bohm C, Robinson DS, Gammans RE. Buspirone therapy for elderly patients with anxiety or depressive neurosis. J Clin Psychiatry 1990;51:309.
7. Rakel RE. Long-term buspirone therapy for chronic anxiety: A multicenter international study to determine safety. South Med J 1990;83:194–198.
8. Ratey JJ, Sovner R, Mikkelsen E, Chmielinski HE. Buspirone therapy for maladaptive behavior and anxiety in developmentally disabled persons. J Clin Psychiatry 1989;50:382–384.
9. Colenda CC. Buspirone in treatment of agitated demented patient. Lancet 1988;1:1169.
10. Richels K, Freemen E, Sondheimer S. Buspirone in treatment of premenstrual syndrome. Lancet 1989;1:777.
11. Yatham LN, Barry S, Dinan TG. Serotonin receptors, buspirone and premenstrual syndrome. Lancet 1989;1:1447–1448.
12. Dersun SM, Burthe JG, Reveley MA. Buspirone treatment of Tourette's syndrome. Lancet 1995;345:1366–1367.
13. Batki SL. Buspirone in drug users with AIDS or AIDS-related complex. J Clin Psychopharmacol 1990;10:111S–115S.
14. Neppe VM. High dose buspirone in case of tardive dyskinesia. Lancet 1989;2:1458.
15. Garvin F, Compton M, Byck R. Buspirone reduces smoking. Arch Gen Psychiatry 1989;46:288–289.
16. Markovitz PJ, Stagno SJ, Calabrese JR. Buspirone augmentation of fluoxetine in obsessive–compulsive disorders. Am J Psychiatry 1990;147:798–800.
17. Roose SP, Dalack GW, Glassman AH, et al. Cardiovascular effects of bupropion in depressed patients with heart disease. Am J Psychiatry 1991;149:512–516.

18. Tiller JWG, Burrows GD, O'Sullivan BT. Buspirone overdose. Med J Aust 1989;150:54–55.
19. Goetz CM, Krenzelok EP, Lopez G, Borys D. Buspirone toxicity: A prospective study. Ann Emerg Med 1990; 19:630.
20. Mayol RF, Adamson DS, Gammans RE, La Budde JA. Pharmacokinetics and disposition of ^{14}C-buspirone HCl after intravenous and oral dosing in man. Clin Pharmacol Ther 1985;37:210.
21. Bullen WW, Bivens DL, Gammans RE, La Budde JA. The binding of buspirone to human plasma proteins. Fed Proc 1985;44:1123.
22. Bodkin JA, Teicher MH. Fluoxetine may antagonize the anxiolytic action of buspirone. J Clin Psychopharmacol 1989; 9:150.
23. Balster RL. Abuse potential of buspirone and related drugs. J Clin Psychopharmacol 1990;10:31S–37S.
24. Raleigh FR. Buspirone: Potential for abuse? DICP Ann Pharmacother 1989;23:1035.
25. Lader M. Assessing the potential for buspirone dependence or abuse and effects of its withdrawal. Am J Med 1987;82 (suppl. 5A):20–26.
26. Rock NL. Possible adverse effects of buspirone when used with other psychotropic drugs. J Clin Psychopharmacol 1990;10:380–381.
27. Yocca FD. Neurochemistry and neurophysiology of buspirone and gepirone: Interactions at presynaptic and postsynaptic 5-HT_{1A} receptors. J Clin Psychopharmacol 1990;10: 6S–12S.
28. Tan SA, Tan LG. The effects of buspirone on the peripheral beta-endorphin and norepinephrine levels. Clin Res 1989; 37:104A.
29. Cummins TK, Diamond RJ. Intranasal buspirone. J Clin Psychopharmacol 1990;10:297–298.
30. Raleigh FR. Buspirone: Potential for abuse? DICP Ann Pharmacother 1989;23:1035.
31. Boylan K. Persistent dystonia associated with buspirone. Neurology 1990;40:1904.
32. Le Witt PA, Walters A, Hening W, McHale D. Persistent movement disorders induced by buspirone. Mov Disord 1993;8:331–334.
33. McIvor RJ, Sinanan K. Buspirone-induced mania. Br J Psychiatry 1991;158:136–137.
34. Pols HJ, Griez E, Zandbergen J. Does buspirone have anxiogenic properties? Lancet 1989;2:682–683.
35. Liegghio NE, Yeragani VK. Buspirone-induced hypomania: A case report. J Clin Psychopharmacol 1988;8:226.
36. Price WA, Bielefeld M. Buspirone-induced mania. J Clin Psychopharmacol 1989;9:150–151.
37. McDaniel JS, Ninan PT, Magnuson JV. Possible induction of mania by buspirone. Am J Psychiatry 1990;140: 125–126.
38. Fuller RW. Buspirone metabolite and panic attacks. Lancet 1990;2:470.
39. Chignon JM, Lepine JP. Panic and hypertension associated with single dose of buspirone 1989;2:46–47.
40. Coates NE. Priapism associated with Buspar. South Med J 1990;83:983.
41. Napoliello MJ, Domantay AG. Buspirone: A world wide update. Br J Psychiatry 1991;159(suppl. 12):40–44.
42. Eudy SF, Conch LH, Morrow MG, et al. Analysis of buspirone, a new anxiolytic agent by high pressure liquid chromatography. AJCP 1989.
43. Kerns EH. Quantitative analysis of 1,2-(2-pyrimidinyl)piperazine in plasma by capillary gas chromatography/mass spectrometry. J Chromatogr 1986;377:195–203.

CYPROPHEPTADINE

Cyproheptadine is an H_1-receptor antagonist and a serotonin antagonist. It also may have antimuscarinic and calcium channel blocker activity.[1] It is widely used as an appetite stimulant in some countries (eg, France).[2] Central nervous system depression, hallucinations, ataxia, seizures, and death have followed an overdose. Treatment is symptomatic and supportive.[2–4]

Structure and Classification

Cyproheptadine is structurally and pharmacologically related to azatadine, another H_1-receptor antagonist.[5] Cyproheptadine is available commercially in the United States as Periactin. Its molecular weight is 350.9.

Use

Cyproheptadine hydrochloride has the actions and uses of other antihistamines. It has also been used for appetite stimulation and in anorexia nervosa, Cushing's syndrome, carcinoid syndrome, migraine, acromegaly, hyperlactinemia, and antidepressant (or fluoxetine)-induced inorgasmia.[6,7] Cyproheptadine has been used in the treatment of essential blepharospasm (depresses serotonin-enhanced excitability of facial motor neurons).[8] Anecdotal reports indicate some improvement in tardive dyskinesia and akathisia[9] and in the serotonin syndrome (see The Serotonin Syndrome). Initial studies indicate that cyproheptadine may reverse the resistance of *Plasmodium falciparum* to chloroquine.[10,11] Anecdotal reports indicate that combat nightmares persisting after antidepressant therapy appear to respond to cyproheptadine.[12]

Product Formulation

Cyproheptadine is available for oral use as a solution 2 mg/5 mL (containing alcohol 5% and sorbic acid) and as 4-mg tablets, white, round, scored, and coded MSD62.

Source

Cyproheptadine is a synthetic chemical compound.

Therapeutic Dose

For the treatment of allergic conditions, the usual adult dosage of cyproheptadine hydrochloride is 4 mg three times daily. The total dose should not exceed 0.5 mg/kg daily. Most adults require 12 to 15 mg daily. In children 2 to 6 years of age, the usual dosage is 2 mg two to three times daily; total dose should not exceed 12 mg daily. For children 7 to 14 years of age, the usual dosage is 4 mg two or three times daily; total dose should not exceed 16 mg daily. Alternatively, children may receive 0.25 mg/kg or 8 mg/m^2 daily in divided doses.[5]

Toxic Dose

A 3-year-old child ingested 12 mg of cyproheptadine and developed a staggering gait, disorientation, grimaces, and akathisia; he recovered. A 7-year-old child was inadvertently administered 16 mg and developed a toxic psychosis. No life-threatening effects were observed in children after doses of 0.3 to 6.5 mg/kg body weight.[3–4]

Fatal Dose

Fatal doses appear to range between 25 and 250 mg/kg.[7]

Toxicokinetics

Absorption

Cyproheptadine appears to be well absorbed following oral administration. Following a single dose of radiolabeled drug in fasting healthy adults in one study, plasma concentrations of radioactivity peaked 6 to 9 hours after administration.[13] The radioactivity appears to represent cyproheptadine metabolites.[5] Peak plasma levels reach 30 μg/L.

Distribution

The low plasma levels of cyproheptadine and metabolites in humans after an oral dose are consistent with extensive distribution of the drug and its metabolites.[13]

Elimination

The drug appears to be completely metabolized principally to the quaternary ammonium glucuronide conjugate. Cyproheptadine also undergoes aromatic ring hydroxylation, *N*-demethylation, and heterocyclic injury oxidation. Most of the metabolites are conjugated with glucoronic acid or sulfate. Cyproheptadine is not excreted unchanged in the urine, but is excreted as the metabolites within 24 hours (30%), 48 hours (50%), or 6 days (65–75%).[5]

Drug Interactions

Monoamine oxidase inhibitors prolong and intensify the anticholinergic effects of antihistamines, including cyproheptadine.[1]

Pregnancy/Lactation

Controlled studies with cyproheptadine have not been performed during pregnancy or lactation.[5]

Mechanism of Action

Cyproheptadine has 5-HT_2 antagonist properties. It is an H_1-receptor antagonist, and has antimuscarinic, anticholinergic, and calcium channel blocking properties.[8]

Clinical Presentation

At therapeutic doses cyproheptadine has a sedative effect.[2] Following an overdose, the major clinical problem is central nervous system depression or stimulation with hallucinations, ataxia, and seizures. About 20 deaths have been reported in infants or children. Fatal doses appear to range between 25 and 250 mg/kg.[1–4]

Symptoms in 113 children who accidentally ingested excessive doses of cyproheptadine included somnolence, excitation, hallucinations, ataxia, tachycardia, muscle twitching, gastric distress, mydriasis, and facial erythema. Symptoms appeared rapidly after ingestion and did not last longer than 6 to 12 hours.[4]

Laboratory

Analysis in plasma serum and urine has been performed by a gas–liquid chromatographic method sensitive to 3 ng/mL. A high-performance liquid chromatography method with nitrogen-sensitive detection distinguishes cyproheptadine from its desmethyl metabolite with an assay sensitivity of 20 ng/L.[14,15]

Treatment

Stabilization

Treatment of cyproheptadine overdose is largely symptomatic and supportive and is similar to the treatment given to patients who have been poisoned with other H_1-receptor antagonist antihistamines.

Gut Decontamination

Vomiting usually occurs spontaneously, but cyproheptadine may also be removed by gastric lavage.

Elimination Enhancement

There is no clinical evidence for the use of hemodialysis or hemoperfusion after cyproheptadine overdose. It is not likely that these measures would be useful for this drug in view of its probable extensive volume of distribution.

Antidote

There is no antidote. Physostigmine has not been evaluated after a cyproheptadine overdose.

Supportive Measures

Patients with hypotension, hallucinations, and seizures should be admitted to a hospital intensive care unit after emergency treatment of seizures (diazepam, phenytoin, phenobarbital). Hypotension may require treatment with pressor agents. Patients should be observed for at least 24 hours until there is no further evidence of ataxia, seizures, and hallucinations and there is no evidence of electrocardiographic abnormality.

REFERENCES—CYPROHEPTADINE

1. Reynolds JEF, ed. *Martindale: The Extra Pharmacopoeia.* 30th ed. London: Pharmaceutical Press, 1993:935–937.
2. Hakkou F, Jaouven C, Iraki L. A comparative study of cyproheptadine and DL-carnitine on psychomotor performance and memory in healthy volunteers. Fundam Clin Pharmacol 1990;4:191–200.
3. Bharucha BA, Kalawala TY, Pandya AL, et al. Cyproheptadine poisoning. Indian Pediatr 1987;24:165–169.
4. Muhlendahl KE, Krienke EG. The toxicity of cyproheptadine, side effects and accidental poisoning. Monatsschr Kinderheilkd 1978;126:123–126.
5. McEvoy GK, ed. *AHFS Drug Information 94.* Bethesda, MD: American Society of Hospital Pharmacists, 1994:16–17.
6. McCormick S, Olin J, Brotman AW. Reversal of fluoxetine in induced inorgasmia by cyproheptadine in two patients. J Clin Psychiatry 1990;51:383–384.
7. Dollery CT, ed. *Therapeutic Drugs.* Edinburgh: Churchill Livingstone, 1991:C377–C380.

8. Fasanella RM, Aghajanian GK. Treatment of benign essential blepharospasm with cyproheptadine. N Engl J Med 1990; 322:778.
9. Bacher NM, Lewis HA, Field PB. Cyproheptadine in movement disorders. Am J Psychiatry 1989;146:557–558.
10. Bjorkman A, Willcox M, Kihamia CM, et al. Field study of cyproheptadine/chloroquine synergism in falciparum malaria. Lancet 1990;336:59–60.
11. Peters W, Ekong R, Robinson BL, et al. Antihistamine drugs that reverse chloroquine resistance in *Plasmodium falciparum.* Lancet 1989;2:334–335.
12. Brophy MH. Cyproheptadine for combat nightmare in post-traumatic Shers disorder and dream anxiety disorder. Milit Med 1991;156:100–101.
13. Hintze KL, Wold JC, Fischer LJ. Disposition of cyproheptadine and DL-carnitine on psychomotor performance and memory in healthy volunteers. Fundam Clin Pharmacol 1990; 4:191–200.
14. Hucker HB, Hutt JE. Determination of cyproheptadine in plasma and urine by GLC with a nitrogen-sensitive detector. J Pharmacol Sci 1983;72:1069–1070.
15. Novak EA, Stanley M, McIntyre IM, Hryhorczuk L. High performance liquid chromatographic method for quantification of cyproheptadine in serum or plasma. J Chromatogr 1985;339:457–461.

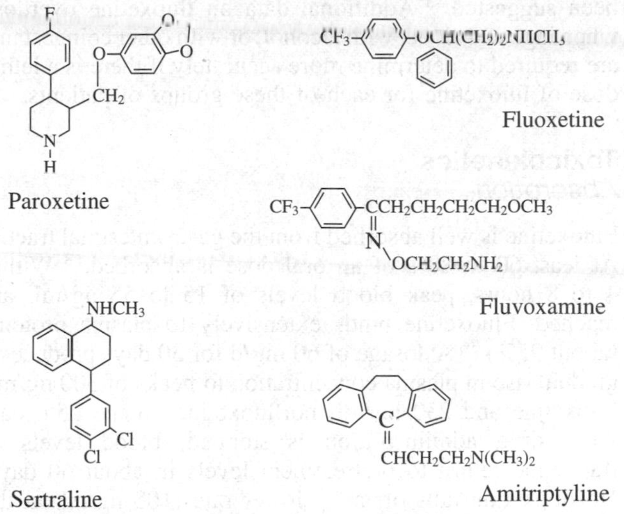

Figure 49-2 Structures of five antidepressants. (From Tulloch IF, Johnson AM. The pharmacologic profile of paroxetine, a new selective serotonin reuptake inhibitor. J Clin Psychiatry 1992;53(2, suppl.):7–12.

FLUOXETINE

Fluoxetine ingested alone in overdose appears to be minimally toxic in doses up to 1500 mg. Symptoms may include drowsiness, tremor, nausea, vomiting, and tachycardia. When fluoxetine is ingested with alcohol, tachycardia, an increase in blood pressure, and a decreased level of consciousness may be observed. With other coingestants, a fluoxetine overdose may lead to serious symptomatology and occasionally death.[1] The incidence of overdose has been low in relation to the extensive worldwide use of the product. About half of overdose patients are asymptomatic. Asymptomatic patients can be discharged within 4 hours depending on clinical judgment. Other patients may require medical observation, intensive care, or psychiatric follow-up.

Structure and Classification

Fluoxetine is an aromatic ring phenylpropylamine derivative and a bicyclic antidepressant.[2] Fluoxetine hydrochloride has a molecular weight of 345.8. The free base (fluoxetine) has a molecular weight of 308.3. To convert to SI units, μg/mL × 3.24 = μmol/L. To convert from SI units, μmol/L ÷ 3.24 = μg/mL (Fig. 49–2).

Use

Fluoxetine is approved by the Food and Drug Administration for the treatment of depression.[3–5] Limited numbers of patients have shown evidence of effectiveness (some with low doses of fluoxetine starting at 5 mg) in the treatment of obsessive–compulsive disorders,[6–11] eating disorders including bulimia,[12–14] anorexia nervosa, [15,16] obesity,[17] bipolar disorders,[18] cataplexy,[19] panic disorders,[20] agitated dementia,[21] and other conditions such as premenstrual syndrome,[22] fetishes,[23] trichotillomania,[24] pathologic jealousy,[25] and some problematic behaviors associated with autism.[26] Fluoxetine may have some ameliorative effect in diabetic neuropathy.[27]

Product Formulation

Fluoxetine hydrochloride is available in oral capsules containing 20 mg of fluoxetine (Prozac Pulvules) and as an oral solution containing 20 mg of fluoxetine per 5 mL (Prozac, with alcohol 0.23%).[18,28]

Source

Fluoxetine hydrochloride is a synthetic chemical product.

Therapeutic Dose

For the management of major depression, the recommended initial and maintenance dosage of fluoxetine in adults is 20 mg daily.[18] Dosage may be increased over several weeks to a maximum of 80 mg/d. Many patients respond to 20 mg or less daily. Some centers have used 100 mg/d or more.[29]

Toxic Dose

Serious toxic effects do not usually appear until fluoxetine doses greater than 1500 mg have been ingested.[1] Dose ingested and blood concentrations of fluoxetine and norfluoxetine appear to be linearly related.[30] When fluoxetine is ingested in doses greater than 500 mg together with ethanol, tachycardia, a rise in blood pressure and a decrease in the level of consciousness are usually observed.[1] Ingestion of 1200 mg of fluoxetine was asymptomatic in one patient.[1] Mean overdose in asymptomatic patients in one study was 341 mg; symptomatic patients had ingested a mean dose of 544 mg.[1] Children who ingested an average of 1.76 mg/kg fluoxetine had minor symptomatology (sleepiness, hyperactivity, diarrhea); all recovered.[1]

Fatal Dose

Deaths have usually followed ingestion of varying amounts of fluoxetine together with coingestants (see Clinical Presentation).[1,31–34] An estimated lethal dose of 1 to 2 g has been suggested.[33] Additional data on fluoxetine overdose when ingested alone, with alcohol, or with other coingestants are required to determine more accurately if there is a lethal dose of fluoxetine for each of these groups of patients.

Toxicokinetics

Absorption

Fluoxetine is well absorbed from the gastrointestinal tract.[35] At least 60 to 80% of an oral dose is absorbed.[18] Within 4 to 8 hours, peak blood levels of 15 to 55 ng/mL are reached. Fluoxetine binds extensively to plasma proteins (about 95%).[36] A dosage of 60 mg/d for 30 days produces a gradual rise in plasma concentration to peaks of 300 ng/mL fluoxetine and 250 ng/mL norfluoxetine on the 25th day. After drug administration is stopped, blood levels of fluoxetine return to pretreatment levels in about 60 days. Norfluoxetine falls off at a slower rate (100 ng/mL at the 60th day).[35,37] Chronic therapeutic dosing results in serum fluoxetine concentrations ranging from 47 to 469 ng/mL and norfluoxetine concentrations ranging from 52 to 446 ng/mL.[38]

Elimination

Fluoxetine is metabolized largely by *N*-demethylation to the active metabolite, norfluoxetine. Less than 5% of fluoxetine is excreted in the urine unchanged.[36] About 10% of norfluoxetine is excreted in the urine unchanged; approximately 73% is excreted as unidentified metabolites.[39] Fluoxetine has elimination half-lives of 1 to 4 days after a single dose and 2 to 7 days after multiple doses.[35] Norfluoxetine has an elimination half-life of 7 to 15 days following either single or multiple doses.[39] Plasma clearance of fluoxetine ranges from 94 to 703 mL/min. The rate of norfluoxetine elimination is generally slower than that of the parent compound.

Pregnancy/Lactation

A survey of women receiving fluoxetine while pregnant revealed no significant increase in spontaneous abortions or major malformations.[40,41] Further studies are indicated to validate these observations.

In one patient, 20 mg daily ingested by the mother led to ingestion of 15 to 20 µg/kg/d by the nursing infant, who thrived and developed normally.[42]

Drug Interactions

Fluoxetine may induce toxic drug interactions by several mechanisms[43–45] (Table 49–6).

Mechanism of Action

Fluoxetine is a selective inhibitor of serotonin uptake at the presynaptic neuronal membrane. It appears to have minimal or no effect on the reuptake of norepinephrine or dopamine

Table 49–6
Fluoxetine Drug Interactions

1. Inhibition of hepatic metabolism (inhibition of cytochrome P450IID6)[43] by fluoxetine and norfluoxetine increases plasma levels and toxicity of the following drugs administered concomitantly:
   - Tricyclic antidepressants[15–42,46–53]: seizures, delirium, hypotension
   - Trazodone[54,55]
   - Haloperidol[56,57]: extrapyramidal symptoms
   - Diazepam[58,59]: increase in half-life, decrease in plasma clearance
   - L-Tryptophan[60]: serotonin syndrome
   - Morphine[61] meperidine[32]
   - Carbamazepine[62–64]: ataxia, myoclonus, slurred speech
   - Barbiturates[44,46]
   - Warfarin: spontaneous bleeding[65]
2. Serotonin syndrome[43]: coma, cyanosis, acidosis, hypotension, renal failure
   - Monoamine oxidase inhibitors such as phenelzine and tranylcypromine, which inhibit catabolism of serotonin, interact with fluoxetine, which prevents reuptake of serotonin (5-HT)[66–70]
   - L-Tryptophan (a precursor of 5-HT)[60]
3. Serotonin uptake blockers:
   - Counteracts 5 HT_{1A} agonist effects of buspirone.[71–73]
   - May decrease alcohol intake[74] without affecting ethanol metabolism.[75]
4. Fenfluramine potentiates response to fluoxetine by releasing serotonin.[44,46]
5. Lithium blood levels may be increased or decreased when fluoxetine is added. Lithium toxicity (encephalopathy, mania) may be observed. When both compounds are used together, frequent monitoring of lithium levels is indicated.[76–81]
6. With selegiline, mania.[82]
7. Central nervous system active drugs: Many drugs have not been studied in patients who are simultaneously ingesting fluoxetine.
8. The tightly protein-bound fluoxetine displaces protein-bound drugs such as warfarin and digitoxin.
9. Fluoxetine plus marijuana have induced mania. Fluoxetine and 9-tetrahydrocannabinol are both potent inhibitors of serotonin reuptake.[83]
10. Fluoxetine may reduce cocaine use in animals.[84]
11. Cyproheptadine, a serotonin antagonist, reverses antidepressant effect of fluoxetine.[85,86]
12. Pentazocine, when used with fluoxetine, may induce lightheadedness, nausea, anxiety, diaphoresis, ataxia, and paresthesias of the extremities.[87]
13. Use of haloperidol and fluoxetine together leads to tardive dyskinesia.[88]
14. Fluoxetine may reduce an elevated plasma phenytoin concentration with signs and symptoms of phenytoin toxicity when both compounds are administered simultaneously.[89]

and does not exhibit clinically important anticholinergic, antihistaminic, or α_1-adrenergic blocking activity at the usual therapeutic dosage. The potency and selectivity of serotonin reuptake inhibition of the principal metabolite, norfluoxetine, are similar to those of the parent drug.[90]

Clinical Presentation

Fluoxetine, compared with other antidepressants, is a relatively nontoxic compound. Reviews of overdose studies may be grouped into overdoses with fluoxetine alone, fluoxetine with alcohol, and fluoxetine with other congestants.

Fluoxetine Alone

Fluoxetine ingested by itself in overdose produces minor symptoms, which are usually not serious or life threatening.[1,30,91–97] Common symptoms and signs include drowsiness, tachycardia, nausea, vomiting, and tremor. Infrequent effects include euphoria, headache, sore throat, agitation,[92] lightheadedness, seizures,[98] and dry mouth.[69] One patient developed flulike symptoms including pruritus, rashes, malaise, urticaria, cough, and swelling of the fingers.[91] About 50% of patients reported to have taken an overdose remained asymptomatic.[1] Patients generally recover quickly without sequelae. Reversible hair loss has been reported in patients receiving fluoxetine 20 mg daily.[99] Fluoxetine does not induce hepatotoxicity.[100]

Fluoxetine With Alcohol

When fluoxetine is ingested with alcohol, more toxic effects are observed. Only 2 of 26 patients studied were asymptomatic in one report.[1] Common findings include depressed consciousness, tachycardia,[92] drowsiness, tremor, nausea, vomiting, inebriation, and gastrointestinal symptoms. Patients usually recover without sequelae.[30,92–96]

Fluoxetine With Coingestants

Fluoxetine ingestion has been reported in overdose patients who have also ingested benzodiazepines, tricyclic antidepressants, phenothiazines, acetaminophen, opiates, diphenhydramine, clonazepam, haloperidol, methamphetamine, meprobamate, and lithium.[1] In most of these cases signs and symptoms reflect the coingestant. More serious toxic efects (with methamphetamine, diphenhydramine, and meprobamate) include seizures,[6] respiratory arrest (with tricyclic antidepressants), dystonic reactions (with haloperidol), and unresponsiveness (tricyclic antidepressants).[86] Most patients recover. Dyskinesias and akathisia with fluoxetine use may follow enhancement of serotonergic neurotransmission, which, in turn, enhances serotonergically mediated inhibition of dopamine neurotransmission.[101]

Fatalities

Fatalities following overdose with fluoxetine have generally been associated with a coingestant (diphenhydramine and carbon monoxide,[34] meperidine,[32] clonidine, acetaminophen, pargyline, fluphenazine, lorazepam, diphenhydramine,[102] propranolol,[33] ethanol,[32] and maprotiline[1]). Kincald believes that the lethal dose of fluoxetine is between 1 and 2 g, and considers its toxicity rating to be similar to that of tricyclic antidepressants and monoamine oxidase inhibitors.[33] This conclusion, however, requires further study of patients who have ingested fluoxetine alone at doses greater than 1500 mg and fluoxetine together with coingestants, and correlation of fluoxetine plasma levels with clinical toxicity.[103]

Suicide Ideation

Several initial studies comprised patients who appeared to develop suicidal ideation while on fluoxetine therapy.[104–107] Consideration of risk factors that may serve to increase the possibility of suicidal ideation or behavior include (1) the possibility of a "therapeutic window" of plasma fluoxetine concentration above and below which unusual suicidal thoughts may evolve[108]; (2) limbic system dysfunction[109]; (3) presence of hypersomnia, poor concentration, anorexia, blurred vision, hallucinations, and a feeling of "being stoned," which may indicate a predisposition to suicidal ideation or behavior[107]; (4) prior suicidal ideation[110]; (5) preliminary induction of anxiety, insomnia, agitation, or akathisia[111,112] by fluoxetine; (6) unmasking of a bipolar disorder[113]; (7) induction of mania[113]; and (8) an increase in dose of fluoxetine or an unusually strong depression in serotonin transmission by the drug.[114] The Food and Drug Administration and the UK Committee on Safety of Medicine reviewed all the data on suicide and fluoxetine[115] including an extensive review of controlled studies on 3065 patients[116] (1765 of whom received fluoxetine) treated for depression (meta-analysis indicated no fluoxetine-induced increase in suicidal acts or emergence of substantial suicidal thoughts) and concluded that fluoxetine does not cause suicidal ideation or violent behavior in depressed patients.[117] The report suggests that patients treated with fluoxetine should be monitored closely in the early stages of treatment during which time the risk of suicide is highest. Whether the drug increases hostility or aggression remains an open question.

Emergency Adverse Effects

Conditions that may cause the fluoxetine patient to seek emergency medical attention include serum sickness (fever, rash, arthralgia, lymphadenopathy, skin eruptions), which generally resolves spontaneously in 1 to 2 weeks (antihistamines for urticarial symptoms, corticosteroids for severe symptoms)[118]; seizures beginning 3 to 5 days after initiation of fluoxetine (resolve with symptomatic treatment—diazepam, phenytoin, immediate discontinuation of fluoxetine)[119,120]; narrow-angle glaucoma, which may be associated with other anticholinergic activity (dry mouth, difficulty in urination, constipation, mydriasis) and which clears 48 hours after fluoxetine is withdrawn[121]; stuttering that interferes with speech and with sleep[122]; rhabdomyolysis following combined drug overdose with alcohol[123]; prolonged bleeding time and petechiae (see Laboratory); exacerbation of symptoms of multiple sclerosis[124]; cardiac dysrhythmias in the elderly (see Laboratory)[125]; chest discomfort (tightness, pain) with or without syncope associated with bradycardia[126]; dizziness, pressure in the throat, and shortness of breath associated with supraventricular tachycardia and hypotension[127]; eye tics with hearing impairment[128]; other extrapyramidal symptoms (dystonia, akathisia)[129]; mania or violence (observed with antidepressants such as fluoxetine and amitriptyline, which inhibit serotonin reuptake).[130,131]

Withdrawal

Agitation, inability to concentrate, and insomnia were experienced by one patient within 48 hours of discontinuation.[132] A 32-year-old man who had received fluoxetine for 6 months developed an acute dystonic reaction involving the neck, back, and upper extremities and torticollis 2 days after stopping fluoxetine therapy.[133] Diffuse diaphoresis and tremulousness, protuberant tongue movements, and increased motor tone were observed. All symptoms resolved 45 minutes after intramuscular administration of diphenhydramine 50 mg.

Abuse

Fluoxetine abuse has been reported that follows the criteria for substance dependence established by the American Psychiatric Association's *Diagnostic and Statistical Manual,* Third Edition, Revised. This is seen in patients who have abused alcohol or other drugs.[134,135]

Pregnant/Lactating Women

Of 184 pregnancies in women who received fluoxetine while pregnant, 41 were therapeutically aborted, 35 aborted spontaneously, and in one twins were stillborn. One hundred fourteen infants were liveborn: 93 were normal, 9 were premature, 9 had perinatal complications, 3 had malformations (1 hepatoblastoma, 1 major cardiac malformations [drug given in second trimester], 1 pyloric stenosis).[136]

Ingestion of fluoxetine 20 mg daily by a nursing mother for 2 months led to a plasma fluoxetine level of 100.5 ng/mL and plasma norfluoxetine level of 194.5 ng/mL; breast milk levels were 28.8 ng/mL for fluoxetine and 41.6 ng/mL for norfluoxetine. Nursing mothers should be warned that fluoxetine and its active metabolite are excreted into breast milk.[137]

Newborns

A newborn whose mother has ingested fluoxetine may exhibit nervousness, jitteriness, tremor, and occasionally seizures.[138]

Laboratory

Analytical Methods

Quantitation of fluoxetine and norfluoxetine in human plasma can be performed using gas chromatography with a ^{63}Ni electron-capture detector. The linear range of detection is 25 to 800 ng/mL for each drug.[139] A reverse-phase high-performance liquid chromatography (HPLC) method with ultraviolet detection is also available.[38] Fluoxetine or norfluoxetine may interfere with some tricyclic antidepressant assays and with their metabolites.[140] The limits of detection by an HPLC method is 50 ng/mL. The assay is linear for fluoxetine and norfluoxetine concentrations between 50 and 500 ng/mL.[141] A recent HPLC method for plasma or serum fluoxetine and norfluoxetine quantitation is linear in the range 10 to 500 ng/mL.[142]

Blood Levels

Fluoxetine levels are often not readily available in community hospitals and are of limited value in treatment of an overdose.

Fluoxetine Alone. Fluoxetine doses of 20 to 80 mg/d produce plasma concentrations of 50 to 1100 ng/mL.[30] After 30 mg/d for 7 days, combined fluoxetine and norfluoxetine levels ranged from 108 to 197 ng/mL in one study[30]; at 60 mg/d, they rose to 366 to 847 ng/mL. Patients receiving 80 mg/d reached combined levels of 1118 ng/mL.[37] Two reviews indicate that there is little evidence of toxicity unless the combined fluoxetine and norfluoxetine level is greater than 1390 ng/mL,[1] or 2,000 ng/mL.[1,30] Seizures are usually correlated with combined levels greater than 3000 ng/mL.[30] All have recovered.

Fluoxetine and Ethanol. Blood levels of fluoxetine when it is ingested with ethanol do not significantly differ from levels after ingestion of fluoxetine alone.[94]

Fluoxetine With Coingestants. When fluoxetine is ingested in overdose with coingestants, blood fluoxetine concentrations may vary widely. Drug concentrations do not correlate well with toxicity whether fluoxetine is ingested alone or with other drugs.

Fatalities. Blood fluoxetine levels of patients who have died have varied but were usually above a combined value of 1300 ng/mL, and have usually been associated with the presence of a coingestant.

Abnormalities

Syndrome of Inappropriate Secretion of Antidiuretic Hormone. Fluoxetine is a possible cause of the syndrome of inappropriate secretion of antidiuretic hormone (SIADH).[143] Within a few weeks of beginning fluoxetine treatment, some patients (usually older patients) begin to experience drowsiness, confusion, and lightheadedness. Laboratory findings include depression of serum sodium and serum chloride values with depressed serum and urine osmolality.[144,145] Hyponatremia that develops without being preceded by polydipsia in SIADH usually arises from either psychiatric illness or treatment with psychotropic medications.[146] There appears to be a relationship between serotonin uptake blockers, which include tricyclic antidepressants and monoamine oxidase inhibitors, and SIADH.[143] I the elderly patient who presents with hyponatremia, fluoxetine should be considered as a cause of SIADH.[147]

Bleeding Time. Rare prolongation of the bleeding time with petechiae may be accompanied by a normal platelet count.[148] Platelet dysfunction may not respond to platelet therapy.[149]

Ancillary Tests

Regional Cerebral Blood Flow. Central nervous system signs of a frontal lobe syndrome (increased apathy, poor attention and concentration, and occasionally perseveration and forgetfulness following chronic fluoxetine use) were associated with evidence of diminished regional cerebral blood flow when measured by single photon emission computed tomography (SPECT).[150]

Electroencephalogram. Epileptiform activity, or a slow occipital rhythm,[120] may be seen after fluoxetine-associated seizures.[119]

Serum transaminase levels may be infrequently elevated in patients who develop an acute hepatitis while receiving chronic fluoxetine treatment.[151]

Electrocardiogram. Bradycardia, supraventricular tachycardia, and atrial fibrillation may be observed on the electrocardiographic tracing in patients with no other evidence of cardiac toxicity. Infrequent reports of atrial flutter and atrioventricular block have followed fluoxetine use.[125] Rare prolongation of the PR interval, left bundle-branch block, and left anterior division block have been observed.[152] Two patients with fluoxetine overdose (1000 and 200 mg, respectively) exhibited no electrocardiographic abnormalities.[44] Electrocardiographic abnormalities are usually observed in fluoxetine overdoses with coingestants and include junctional rhythms, low-voltage and nonspecific T-wave changes,[102] ventricular tachycardia, and multiple premature ventricular contractions (with imipramine)[1]; supraventricular tachycardia (with lithium)[1]; and premature auricular contractions and trigeminy (with triazolam and caffeine), right bundle-branch block (with lithium or doxepin), and first-degree heart block (with encainimide).[1]

Treatment

Stabilization

Acute fluoxetine overdose involves primarily symptomatic and supportive care. Airway patency, an adequate source of oxygen, and careful monitoring of ventilation are paramount. Cardiac monitoring and an intravenous line should be instituted on admission. Vital signs and hemodynamic status must be closely monitored as many patients may have simultaneously ingested drugs such as tricyclic antidepressants. A 12-lead electrocardiogram provides a more accurate status of cardiac rhythm abnormalities.

Gut Decontamination

Fluoxetine reaches peak blood levels slowly (4–8 hours). In the alert patient within 4 to 6 hours of ingestion, gastric emptying should be initiated. Emesis induction should not be performed if the patient is not alert, is having seizures, or has a repressed gag reflex. Gastric lavage in such patients should be performed after prior cuffed endotracheal intubation. Activated charcoal (50–100 g in adults, 15–30 g in children) with a single dose of saline cathartic or sorbitol may be administered.

Elimination Enhancement

The large apparent volume of distribution and tight plasma protein binding of fluoxetine indicate that removing substantial amounts of fluoxetine or norfluoxetine after an acute ingestion by hemodialysis, hemoperfusion, forced diuresis, peritoneal dialysis, or exchange transfusion would most likely not be effective. Whole-bowel irrigation has not been evaluated in fluoxetine overdose. Serum alkalinization, often used for tricyclic antidepressant poisoning, has not been shown to be of value in a fluoxetine overdose.

Antidote

There is no specific antidote for fluoxetine overdose.

Supportive Measures

1. Where patients are entirely asymptomatic, have no evidence of significant electrocardiographic changes, and no cardiovascular irritability, consider discharge from the emergency department after an observation period of 6 to 8 hours.
2. Admit a depressed or suicidal patient to a psychiatric unit.
3. If a high dose (>1500 mg) of fluoxetine has been ingested, admit the patient for observation, even if asymptomatic, for 24 hours.
4. If the patient is symptomatic (seizures, altered mental status, dysrhythmias), admit to an intensive care facility for at least 24 hours.
5. If fluoxetine was ingested with alcohol or other coingestants, admit to an intensive care facility after gastric decontamination, activated charcoal, and specific treatment directed at the most lethal agent.
6. Intravenous diazepam is a drug of choice for treatment of seizures that do not remit spontaneously. If seizures recur after diazepam, use phenytoin or phenobarbital.
7. Treat cardiac dysrhythmias with standard antiarrhythmic agents. Continuous electrocardiographic monitoring is indicated. Rule out a myocardial infarction if ST depression is observed.
8. As blood levels of fluoxetine may be clearly detectable 4 weeks after an overdose or after discontinuation of therapy and those of norfluoxetine for 8 weeks, do not initiate therapy with monoamine oxidase inhibitors, tricyclic antidepressants, and other drugs known to adversely interact with fluoxetine (see Drug Interactions) for at least 5 weeks. Clinical judgment, however, determines whether and when fluoxetine or other medication should be resumed.[37,71]
9. Agitation, tremulousness, diaphoresis, insomnia, and inability to concentrate may indicate fluoxetine withdrawal symptoms, and may be accompanied by a dystonic reaction within 48 hours of an overdose. Intravenous diphenhydramine 50 mg often relieves such symptoms.

10. Monitor suicidal patients closely, especially in the early stages of treatment. Assess clinical evidence of severity of depression, suicidal ideation, aggressive ideation or behavior, agitation, or akathisia. Those patients who have intense suicidal thoughts, or who describe violent behavior or act in such a manner, or who appear agitated and who have started fluoxetine recently or have had a dose increase 2 to 6 weeks prior to presentation may be at increased risk for suicide and should be admitted to a psychiatric unit for observation.
11. As fluoxetine blocks serotonin reuptake in platelets, observe patients for platelet dysfunction and bleeding.

Extrapyramidal Symptoms

Akathisia. Discontinue fluoxetine. Akathisia can be treated with propranolol 60 mg/d. If beta blockers are contraindicated, treat with oral diphenhydramine 50 mg twice daily.

Parkinsonian Symptoms. Discontinue fluoxetine. Administer antiparkinsonian drugs as indicated if symptoms are severe.

Acute Dystonic Reaction. Discontinue fluoxetine. For a mild reaction, give 50 mg diphenhydramine by mouth three times a day for 1 week. For a severe reaction, give 50 mg diphenhydramine intravenously. Hospitalize and observe. Fluoxetine has a long half-life.

Syndrome of Inappropriate Secretion of Antidiuretic Hormone. Within 48 hours of discontinuation of fluoxetine, serum sodium and serum chloride levels usually return to normal. If the hyponatremia is mild and attributable to the drug, discontinuation of the drug and restriction of total fluid intake to at least 500 mL/d below the sum of urinary insensible losses will prevent a further fall in plasma sodium and may slowly restore it to normal. This may be combined with oral sodium chloride supplementation if required. If the hyponatremia is symptomatic or sufficiently severe to pose the threat of seizures (usually less than 120 mEq/L), hypertonic (3%) saline should be infused to raise the plasma sodium to asymptomatic levels (usually 125 mEq/L). Greater or more rapid correction may carry a risk of neurologic complications.

General Review Articles

- Messrha FS. Fluoxetine: Adverse effects and drug–drug interactions. Clin Toxicol 1993;31:603–630.
- Stokes PE. Fluoxetine: A five year review. Clin Therap 1993;15:216–243.

REFERENCES—FLUOXETINE

1. Borys DJ, Setzer SC, Ling LJ, et al. Acute fluoxetine overdose: A report of 235 cases. Am J Emerg Med 1992;10:115–120.
2. Dollery CT, ed. *Therapeutic Drugs.* Edinburgh: Churchill Livingstone, 1991:F74–F78.
3. Byerley WF, Reimhert FW, Wood DR, Grosser BI. Fluoxetine, a selective serotonin uptake inhibitor for the treatment of outpatients with major depression. J Clin Psychopharmacol 1988;8:112–115.
4. Chouinard G. A double blind controlled trial of fluoxetine and amitriptyline in the treatment of outpatients with major depressive disorders. J Clin Psychiatry 1985;46(3, sect. 2): 32–37.
5. Feighner JP, Cohn JB. Double blind comparative trials of fluoxetine and doxepin in geriatric patients with major depressive disorder. J Clin Psychiatry 1985;46(3, sect. 2): 20–25.
6. Leibowitz MR, Hollander E, Schneier F, et al. Fluoxetine treatment of obsessive–compulsive disorder: An open clinical trial. J Clin Psychopharmacol 1989;9:423–427.
7. Debus JR, Rush AJ, Hummel C, et al. Fluoxetine versus trazodone in the treatment of outpatients with major depression. J Clin Psychiatry 1988;49:422–426.
8. Kinney-Parker JL, Smith D, Ingle SF. Fluoxetine and weight: Something lost and something gained? Clin Pharm 1989; 8:727–733.
9. Pigott TA, Pato MT, Bernstein SE, et al. Controlled comparison of clomipramine and fluoxetine in the treatment of obsessive–compulsive disorder. Arch Gen Psychiatry 1990; 47:926–932.
10. Liebowitz MR, Hollander E, Fairbanks J, Campeas R. Fluoxetine for adolescents with obsessive–compulsive disorder. Am J Psychiatry 1990;147:370–371.
11. Como PG, Kurlan R. An open-label trial of fluoxetine for obsessive–compulsive disorder in Gilles de la Tourette's syndrome. Neurology 1991;41:872–874.
12. Fava M, Herzog DB, Hamburg P, et al. Long-term use of fluoxetine in bulimia nervosa: A retrospective study. Ann Clin Psychiatry 1990;2:53–56.
13. Ramirez LC, Rosenstock J, Strowig S, et al. Effective treatment of bulimia with fluoxetine in a patient with type 1 diabetes mellitus. Am J Med 1990;88:540–541.
14. Fluoxetine Bulimia Nervosa Collaborative Study Group. Fluoxetine in the treatment of bulimia nervosa: A multicenter placebo-controlled double-blind trial. Arch Gen Psychiatry 1992;49:139–147.
15. Gwirtsman HE, Guze BH, Yager J, Gainsley B. Fluoxetine treatment of anorexia nervosa: An open clinical trial. J Clin Psychiatry 1990;51:378–382.
16. Lee S. Fluoxetine in anorexia nervosa. J Clin Psychiatry 1991;52:240–241.
17. Darga LL, Carroll-Michals L, Botsford SJ, Lucas CP. Fluoxetine effect on weight loss in obese subjects. Am J Clin Nutr 1991;54:321–325.
18. McEvoy GK, ed. *AHFS Drug Information 92.* Bethesda, MD: American Society of Hospital Pharmacists, 1992:1236–1246.
19. Frey J. Fluoxetine suppresses human cataplexy: A pilot study. Neurology 1990;40(suppl. 1):13T.
20. Schneier FR, Liebowitz MR, Davies SO, et al. Fluoxetine in panic disorder. J Clin Psychopharmacol 1990;10:119–121.
21. Sobin P, Schneider L, McDermott H. Fluoxetine in the treatment of agitated dementia. Am J Psychiatry 1989;146:1636.
22. Metz A. Fluoxetine treatment of premenstrual syndrome. J Clin Psychiatry 1990;51:260.
23. Lorefice LS. Fluoxetine treatment of a fetish. J Clin Psychiatry 1991;52:41.
24. Alexander RC. Fluoxetine treatment of trichotillomania. J Clin Psychiatry 1991;52:88.
25. Gross MD. Treatment of pathological jealousy by fluoxetine. Am J Psychiatry 1991;148:683–684.
26. Todd RD. Fluoxetine in autism. Am J Psychiatry 1991;1118: 1089.
27. Theesen KA, Marsh WR. Relief of diabetic neuropathy with fluoxetine. DICP Ann Pharmacother 1989;23:572–576.
28. *Physicians' Desk Reference,* 46th ed. 1992. Montvale, NJ: Medical Economics, 1992:920–923.
29. Stoll AL, Pope HG Jr, McElroy SL. High dose fluoxetine: Safety and efficacy in 27 cases. J Clin Psychopharmacol 1991;11:225–226.
30. Beasley CM Jr. Personal communication. Lilly Research Laboratories, September 30, 1991.
31. Rohrig TP, Prouty RW. Fluoxetine overdose: A case report. J Anal Toxicol 1989;13:305–307.
32. Fraser AD, Isner AF, Susnik E. A fluoxetine related fatality. Bull Int Assoc Forens Toxicol 1991;21(3):23–25.

33. Kincaid RL, McMullin MM, Crookham SB, Riedero F. Report of a fluoxetine fatality. J Anal Toxicol 1990;14:327–329.
34. Roettger JR. The importance of blood collection site for determination of basic drugs: A case with fluoxetine and diphenhydramine overdose. J Anal Toxicol 1990;14:191–192.
35. Benfield P, Heel RC, Lewis SP. Fluoxetine: A review of its pharmacodynamics and pharmacokinetic properties and therapeutic efficacy in depressive illness. Drugs 1986;32: 481–508.
36. Aronoff GR, Bergstrom RF, Pottratz ST, et al. Fluoxetine kinetics and protein binding in normal and impaired renal function. Clin Pharmacol Ther 1984;36:238–244.
37. Pato MT, Murphy DL, DeVane CL. Sustained plasma concentrations of fluoxetine and/or norfluoxetine four and eight weeks after fluoxetine discontinuation. J Clin Psychopharmacol 1991;11:224–225.
38. Orsulak PJ, Kenney JT, Debas JR, et al. Determination of the antidepressant fluoxetine and its metabolite norfluoxetine in serum by reverse-phase HPLC with ultraviolet detection. Clin Chem 1988;34:1875–1878.
39. Lemberger L, Bergstrom RF, Wolen RL, et al. Fluoxetine: Clinical pharmacology and physiologic disposition. J Clin Psychiatry 1985;46(3, sect. 2):14–19.
40. Goldstein DJ, Williams ML. Fluoxetine exposed pregnancies. Clin Res 1992;40:168A.
41. Pastuszak A, Schick-Boschetto B, Zuber C, et al. Pregnancy outcome following first trimester exposure to fluoxetine (Prozac[R]). JAMA 1993;269:2246–2248.
42. Burch KJ, Wells GB. Fluoxetine/norfluoxetine concentrations in human milk. Pediatrics 1991;89(pt I):676–677.
43. Levinson ML, Lipsy RJ, Fuller DK. Adverse effects and drug interactions associated with fluoxetine therapy. DICP Ann Pharmacother 1991;25:657–661.
44. Ciraulo DA, Shader RI. Fluoxetine drug–drug interactions: I. Antidepressants and antipsychotics. J Clin Psychopharmacol 1990;10:48–50.
45. Goodnick PJ. Pharmacokinetics of second generation antidepressants: Fluoxetine. Psychopharmacol Bull 1991;27: 503–512.
46. Bronson K, Skjelbo E. Fluoxetine and norfluoxetine are potent inhibitors of P450IID6: The source of the sparteine/debrisoquine oxidation polymorphism. Br J Clin Pharmacol 1991;32:136–137.
47. Bell IR, Cole JO. Fluoxetine induces elevation of desipramine level and exacerbation of geriatric nonpsychotic depression. J Clin Psychopharmacol 1988;8:447–448.
48. Vaughan DA. Interaction of fluoxetine with tricyclic antidepressants. Am J Psychiatry 1988;145:1478.
49. Westermeyer J. Fluoxetine-induced tricyclic toxicity: Extent and duration. J Clin Pharmacol 1991;31:388–392.
50. Kahn DG. Increased plasma concentration in a patient cotreated with fluoxetine. J Clin Psychiatry 1990;51:36.
51. Aranow RB, Hudson JI, Pope HG Jr, et al. Elevated antidepressant plasma levels after addition of fluoxetine. Am J Psychiatry 1989;146:911–913.
52. Cavanaugh SVA. Drug–drug interactions of fluoxetine with tricyclics. Psychosomatics 1990;31:273–276.
53. Preskorn SH, Beber JH, Faul JC, Hirschfield RMA. Serious adverse effects of combining fluoxetine and tricyclic antidepressants. Am J Psychiatry 1990;147:532.
54. Swerdlow NR, Andia AM. Trazodone–fluoxetine combination for treatment of obsessive–compulsive disorder. Am J Psychiatry 1989;146:1637.
55. Metz A, Shader RI. Adverse interactions encountered when using trazodone to treat insomnia associated with fluoxetine. Int Clin Psychopharmacol 1990;5:191–194.
56. Tate JL. Extrapyramidol symptoms in a patient taking haloperidol and fluoxetine. Am J Psychiatry 1989;146: 399–400.
57. Goff DC, Midha KK, Brotman AW, et al. Elevation of plasma concentrations of haloperidol after the addition of fluoxetine. Am J Psychiatry 1991;148:790–792.
58. Lemberger L, Rowe H, Bosomworth JC, et al. The effect of fluoxetine on the pharmacokinetics and psychomotor responses of diazepam. Clin Pharmacol Ther 1988;43: 412–419.
59. Lock JD, Gwirtsman HE, Targ EF. Possible adverse drug reactions between fluoxetine and other psychotropics. J Clin Pharmacol 1990;10:383–384.
60. Steiner W, Fontaine R. Toxic reaction following the combined administration of fluoxetine and L-tryptophan: Five case reports. Biol Psychiatry 1986;21:1067–1071.
61. Hynes MD, Lochner MA, Bemis KG, Hymson DL. Fluoxetine, a selective inhibitor of serotonin uptake, potentiates morphine analgesia without altering its discriminative stimulus properties or affinity for opioid receptors. Life Sci 1985; 36:2317–2323.
62. Grimsley SR, Jann MW, D'Mello AP, et al. Pharmacodynamics and pharmacokinetics of fluoxetine/carbamazepine interaction. Clin Pharmacol Ther 1991;49:135.
63. Pearson HJ. Interaction of fluoxetine with carbamazepine. J Clin Psychiatry 1990;51:126.
64. Grimsley SR, Jann MW, Carter HG, et al. Increased carbamazepine plasma concentrations after fluoxetine coadministration. Clin Pharmacol Ther 1991;50:10–15.
65. Hunger HC, Thomas F. Fluoxetine and warfarin interactions. NZ Med J 1995;108:157.
66. Graham PM, Ilett KF. Danger of MAOI therapy after fluoxetine withdrawal. Lancet 1988;2:1255–1256.
67. Feighner JP, Bayer WF, Tyler DL, Neborsky RJ. Adverse consequences of fluoxetine–MAOI combination therapy. J Clin Psychiatry 1990;51:222–225.
68. Chiang WK, Smilkstein MJ. Fluoxetine–monoamine oxidase inhibitor interaction. Vet Hum Toxicol 1989;31:369.
69. Ooi TK. The serotonin syndrome. Anaesthesia 1991;46: 507–508.
70. Sternbach H. Danger of MAOI therapy after fluoxetine withdrawal. Lancet 1988;2:850–851.
71. Bodkin JA, Teicher MH. Fluoxetine may antagonize the anxiolytic buspirone. J Clin Psychopharmacol 1989;9:150.
72. Tanquary J, Masand P. Paradoxical reaction to buspirone augmentation of fluoxetine. J Clin Psychopharmacol 1990; 10:377.
73. Metz A. Interaction between fluoxetine and buspirone. Can J Psychiatry 1990;35:722–723.
74. Naranjo CA, Kadlec KE, Sanhueza P, et al. Fluoxetine differentially alters alcohol intake and other consumatory behaviors in problem drinkers. Clin Pharmacol Ther 1990;47: 490–498.
75. Lemberger L, Rowe H, Bergstrom RF, et al. Effect of fluoxetine on psychomotor performance, physiologic response and kinetics of ethanol. Clin Pharmacol Ther 1985;37: 658–664.
76. Noveske FG, Hahn KR, Flynn RJ. Possible toxicity of combined fluoxetine and lithium. Am J Psychiatry 1989;146: 1515.
77. Pope HG Jr, McElroy SL, Nixon RA. Possible synergism between fluoxetine and lithium in refractory depression. Am J Psychiatry 1988;145:1292–1294.
78. Hadley A, Cason MP. Mania resulting from lithium–fluoxetine combination. Am J Psychiatry 1989;146:1637–1638.
79. Sacristan JA, Iglesias C, Arellano F, Lequerica J. Absence seizures induced by lithium: Possible interaction with fluoxetine. Am J Psychiatry 1991;148:146–147.
80. Salana AA, Shafey M. A case of severe lithium toxicity induced by combined fluoxetine and lithium carbonate. Am J Psychiatry 1989;146:278.
81. Wright R, Ram S. Lithium toxicity, hypomania and leucocytosis with fluoxetine. Ir J Psychol Med 1992;9:59–60.
82. Suchowersky O, Devries J. Possible interactions between Deprenyl and Prozac. Can J Neurol Sci 1990;17:352–353.
83. Stoll AL, Cole JO, Lukas SE. A case of mania as a result of fluoxetine–marijuana interaction. J Can Psychiatry 1991;32: 280–281.
84. Goodwin FK. Fluoxetine lowers rat cocaine use. JAMA 1990; 263:1610.
85. Goldbloom DS, Kennedy SH. Adverse interaction of fluoxetine and cyproheptadine in two patients with bulimia nervosa. J Clin Psychiatry 1991;52:261–262.
86. Feder R. Reversal of antidepressant activity of fluoxetine by cyproheptadine in three patients. J Clin Psychiatry 1991;52: 163–164.

87. Hansen TE, Dieter K, Keepers GA. Interaction of fluoxetine and pentazocine. Am J Psychiatry 1990;147:949–950.
88. Stein MH. Tardive dyskinesia in a patient taking haloperidol and fluoxetine. Am J Psychiatry 1991;148:683.
89. Nightingale LL. Fluoxetine labeling revised to identify phenytoin interaction and to recommend against use in nursing mothers. JAMA 1994;271:1067.
90. Stark P, Fuller RW, Wong DT. The pharmacologic profile of fluoxetine. J Clin Psychiatry 1985;46(3, sect. 2]:7–13.
91. Chiang WK, Ford M, Wax P, et al. Prospective evaluation of fluoxetine ingestions. Vet Hum Toxicol 1990;32:348.
92. Spiller HA, Morse S, Muir C. Fluoxetine ingestion: A one year retrospective study. Vet Hum Toxicol 1990;32:153–155.
93. Jenkins J, Shannon MW, Woolf A. Fluoxetine intoxication: Clinical course and serum concentrations. Vet Hum Toxicol 1990;32:348.
94. Moore JL, Rodriguez R. Toxicity of fluoxetine in overdose. Am J Psychiatry 1990;147:1089.
95. Borys DJ, Seltzer SC, Ling LJ, et al. Acute fluoxetine overdose. Vet Hum Toxicol 1990;32:348.
96. Borys DJ, Seltzer SC, Ling LJ, et al. The effects of fluoxetine in the overdose patient. J Toxicol Clin Toxicol 1990;28:331–340.
97. Kim SW, Pentel PR. Flu-like symptoms associated with fluoxetine overdose: A case report. Clin Toxicol 1989;27:389–393.
98. Braitberg G, Curry S. Fluoxetine-induced seizure after overdose. Vet Hum Toxicol 1994;36:372.
99. Ogilvie AD. Hair loss during fluoxetine treatment. Lancet 1993;342:1423.
100. Gram LF. Fluoxetine. N Engl J Med 1995;332:960–961.
101. Fishbain DA, Dominguez M, Goldberg M, et al. Dyskinesia associated with fluoxetine use. Neuropsychiatry Neuropsychol Behav Neurol 1992;5:97–100. Case report.
102. Litovitz TL, Schmitz BF, Bailey KM. 1989 annual report of the American Association of Poison Control Centers National Data Collection System. Am J Emerg Med 1990;8:438.
103. Chiang WK, Ford M, Wax P, et al. Prospective evaluation of fluoxetine ingestions. Ann Emerg Med 1991;20:1084.
104. Teicher MH, Glod C, Cole JO. Emergency of intense suicidal preoccupation during fluoxetine treatment. Am J Psychiatry 1990;147:207–210.
105. Papp LA, Gorman JM. Suicidal preoccupation during fluoxetine treatment. Am J Psychiatry 1990;147:1380.
106. Teicher MH, Glod C, Gole JO. Suicidal preoccupation during fluoxetine treatment. Am J Psychiatry 1990;147:1380–1381.
107. Dasgupta K. Additional cases of suicidal ideation associated with fluoxetine. Am J Psychiatry 1990;147:1570.
108. Fichtner CG, Jobe TH, Braun BG. Does fluoxetine have a therapeutic window? Lancet 1991;338:520–521.
109. Downs J, Ward J, Farmer R. Preoccupation with suicide in patients treated with fluoxetine. Am J Psychiatry 1991;148:1090–1091.
110. Tollefson GD. Fluoxetine and suicidal ideation. Am J Psychiatry 1990;147:1691–1692.
111. Healy D, Creasey W. Fluoxetine and suicide. Br Med J 1991;303:1058–1059.
112. Rothschild AJ, Locke CA. Reexposure to fluoxetine after serious suicide attempts by three patients: The role of akathisia. J Clin Psychiatry 1991;52:491–493.
113. Ahmad SR. USA: Fluoxetine "not linked to suicide." Lancet 1991;338:875–876.
114. Mann JJ, Kapur S. The emergency of suicidal ideation and behavior during antidepressant pharmacotherapy. Arch Gen Psychiatry 1991;48:1027–1033.
115. Fava M, Rosenbaum JF: Suicidality and fluoxetine: Is there a relationship? J Clin Psychiatry 1991;52:108–111.
116. Beasley CM Jr, Dornseif BE, Bosomworth JC, et al. Fluoxetine and suicide: A meta-analysis of controlled trials of treatment for depression. Br Med J 1991;303:685–692.
117. Fluoxetine, suicide and aggression. Drug Ther Bull 1992;30:5–6.
118. Miller LG, Bowman RC, Mann D, Tripathy A. A case of fluoxetine-induced serum sickness. Am J Psychiatry 1989;146:1616–1617.
119. Ware MR, Stewart RB. Seizures associated with fluoxetine therapy. DICP Ann Pharmacother 1989;23:428.
120. Weber JJ. Seizure activity associated with fluoxetine therapy. Clin Pharm 1989;8:296–298.
121. Ahmad S. Fluoxetine and glaucoma. DICP Ann Pharmacother 1991;25:436.
122. Guthrie S, Greenhaus L. Fluoxetine-induced stuttering. J Clin Psychiatry 1990;51:85.
123. Lazarus A. Rhabdomyolysis in a depressed patient following overdose with combined drug therapy and alcohol. J Clin Psychopharmacol 1990;10:154–155.
124. Browning WN. Exacerbation of symptoms of multiple sclerosis in a patient taking fluoxetine. Am J Psychiatry 1990;147:1089.
125. Buff DD, Bremmer R, Kirtane SS, Gilboa R. Dysrhythmia associated with fluoxetine treatment in an elderly patient with cardiac disease. J Clin Psychiatry 1991;52:174–176.
126. Ellison JM, Milofsky JE, Ely E. Fluoxetine-induced bradycardia and syncope in two patients. J Clin Psychiatry 1990;51:385–386.
127. Gardner SF, Rutherford WF, Munger MA, Panacek EA. Drug-induced supraventricular tachycardia: A case report of fluoxetine. Ann Emerg Med 1991;20:194–197.
128. Cunningham M, Cunningham K, Lydiard RB. Eye tics and subjective hearing impairment during fluoxetine therapy. Am J Psychiatry 1990;147:947–948.
129. Reccoppa L, Welch WA, Ware MR. Acute dystonia and fluoxetine. J Clin Psychiatry 1990;51:487.
130. Hughes T, Sugarman P. Assault after ingestion of antidepressant. Br Med J 1991;303:1552.
131. Lensgarf SJ, Favazza AR. Antidepressant induced mania. Am J Psychiatry 1990;147:1569.
132. Cooper GL. The safety of fluoxetine: An update. Br J Psychiatry 1988;153(suppl. 3):77–86.
133. Stoukides JA, Stoukides CA. Extrapyramidal symptoms upon discontinuation of fluoxetine. Am J Psychiatry 1991;148:1263.
134. Tinsley JA, Olsen MW, Laroche PR, Palmen MA. Fluoxetine abuse. Mayo Clin Proc 1994;69:166–168.
135. Pagliano LA, Pagliaro AM. Fluoxetine abuse by an intravenous drug use. Am J Psychiatry 1993;150:1818.
136. Goldstein DJ, Williams ML, Pearson DK. Fluoxetine-exposed pregnancies. Clin Res 1991;39:768A.
137. Isenberg KE. Excretion of fluoxetine in human breast milk. J Clin Psychiatry 1990;51:169.
138. Spencer MJ. Fluoxetine hydrochloride (Prozac) toxicity in a neonate. Pediatrics 1994;92:721–722.
139. Nash JF, Bopp RJ, Carmichael RH, et al. Determination of fluoxetine and norfluoxetine in plasma by gas chromatography with electron-capture detection. Clin Chem 1982;28:2100–2102.
140. Column CN. Liquid-chromatographic assays of tricyclic antidepressants and metabolites. Clin Chem 1991;37:1304–1305.
141. Kelly MW, Perry PJ, Holstad SG, Gravey JJ. Serum fluoxetine and norfluoxetine concentrations and antidepressant response. Ther Drug Monit 1989;11:165–170.
142. Natasimhachari N, Silverman J, Landa B. Quantitation of fluoxetine and norfluoxetine in serum samples by HPLC. Clin Pharmacol Ther 1990;47:192.
143. Hoover CE. Fluoxetine as a cause of SIADH. Am J Psychiatry 1991;148:542–543.
144. Gommans JH, Edwards RA. Fluoxetine and hyponatraemia. NZ Med J 1990;103:106.
145. Hwang AS, Magraw RM. Syndrome of inappropriate secretion of antidiuretic hormone due to fluoxetine. Am J Psychiatry 1989;146:399.
146. Brown RP, Kocis JH, Cohen SK. Delusional depression and inappropriate antidiuretic hormone secretion. Biol Psychiatry 1983;18:1059–1063.
147. Staab JP, Yerkes SA, Cheney AM, Clayton AH. Transient SIADH associated with fluoxetine. Am J Psychiatry 1990;147:1569–1570.
148. Humphries JE, Wheby MS, Vanden Berg SR. Fluoxetine and the bleeding time. Arch Pathol Lab Med 1990;114:727–728.

149. Evans TG, Buys SS, Rodgers GM. Acquired abnormalities of platelet dysfunction. N Engl J Med 1991;324:1671.
150. Hoehn-Saric R, Harris GJ, Pearlson GD, et al. A fluoxetine-induced frontal lobe syndrome in an obsessive–compulsive patient. J Clin Psychiatry 1991;52:131–133.
151. Mars F, Dumas de la Roque G, Goissen P. Acute hepatitis during treatment with fluoxetine. Gastroenterol Clin Biol 1991;15:270–271.
152. Fisch C. Effect of fluoxetine on the electrocardiogram. J Clin Psychiatry 1985;46(3, sect. 2):42–44.

FLUVOXAMINE

Fluvoxamine is a monocyclic antidepressant drug that has been ingested in overdose by more than 300 patients; 13 patients, all of whom ingested multiple drugs, have died.[1] Although fluvoxamine has been relatively benign in overdose when compared with the tricyclic antidepressants,[2,3] evidence of cardiac dysfunction in these patients is sufficiently serious to warrant close observation during the first 48 hours, at least, or longer after an ingestion. Experience in Europe continues to be accumulated. The drug is not available in the United States.

Structure and Classification

Fluvoxamine is an antidepressant drug that is a novel monocyclic selective inhibitor of neuronal uptake of 5-hydroxytryptamine.[3–6] It is similar in structure and action to fluoxetine[7] (Fig. 49–2). It has a molecular weight of 434.4.[8] The conversion factor is 2.30. To convert to SI units, μg/mL × 2.30 = μmol/L. To convert from SI units, μmol/L ÷ 2.30 = μg/mL. Fluvoxamine maleate is marketed under the names Faverin (United Kingdom), Fevarin, Floxyfral, LUVOX, and Dumyrox.[8]

Use

Fluvoxamine has been reported to be an effective treatment for major depression[5,9,10] and obsessive–compulsive disorder.[11] Preliminary data suggest that it may also be effective in alcohol amnestic disorder (Korsakoff's psychosis or Wernicke–Korsakoff syndrome).[11,12]

Product Formulation

Fluvoxamine maleate is available in the United Kingdom as oral enteric-coated tablets that contain 50 or 100 mg. The 50-mg tablet is circular, yellow, and marked "DUPHAR" and "219." The 100-mg tablet is oval, yellow, and marked "DUPHAR" and "313."

Source

Fluvoxamine maleate is a synthetic chemical product.

Therapeutic Dose

Published efficacy studies of fluvoxamine have employed an initial dose of 50 to 100 mg daily. An eventual daily dose of 150 to 300 mg may be most effective in the treatment of depression.[3]

Toxic Dose

A 74-year-old woman ingested 3 g of fluvoxamine (60 tablets of 50 mg each); she recovered.[13] Two patients ingested 4.8 and 3.0 g, respectively, and recovered.[14] Another ingested 5.0 g of fluvoxamine plus bromazepam, and whiskey and recovered. A 31-year-old woman ingested 4.8 g of fluvoxamine with 0.75 g of amitriptyline and 7 g of naproxen; she recovered.[14] The highest documented dose of fluvoxamine taken is 9 g; the patient recovered.[1] Doses up to 1000 mg in several patients have been asymptomatic.[15] Suicidal ideation occurred in a 32-year-old woman with obsessive–compulsive disorder when the fluvoxamine dose was increased from 200 to 250 mg/d; these symptoms lessened when the fluvoxamine dose was reduced to 200 mg/d.[16]

Fatal Dose

Thirteen patients have died following a fluvoxamine overdose (all with multiple drugs). A 50-year-old woman ingested 50 to 100 tablets each of fluvoxamine (50 mg), desipramine, clozapine (25 mg), ethylephrine, promethazine, propranolol and L-tryptophan and died.[1] A 71-year-old woman ingested 57 tablets of fluvoxamine and 80 tablets of thioridazine and died.[1]

Toxicokinetics

Absorption

At oral doses of 100 mg/d fluvoxamine is almost totally absorbed, with peak concentrations reached 2 to 8 hours after ingestion. The mean steady-state plasma concentration is about 0.4 μg/mL.[13] Steady-state plasma concentrations are usually achieved within 10 days.[5,17] Plasma protein binding is 77%.

Distribution

Animal data suggest an apparent volume of distribution of 5 L/kg.[8] The drug crosses the blood–brain barrier.

Elimination

Fluvoxamine is extensively metabolized by hepatic oxidative demethylation to about nine metabolites, which are excreted by the kidney.[18] The metabolites appear to be inactive.[18] The mean plasma half-life is biphasic with a mean of 15 hours[13]; an initial elimination half-life averages 12.3 hours and a final half-life is 30 hours.[15] Renal clearance in one case was 19.6 mL/min in the first 7 hours after admission and 16.6 mL/min during the next 16.5 hours.[15]

Drug Interactions

Fluvoxamine can prolong the elimination of drugs metabolized by hepatic oxidation. Plasma levels of warfarin, propranolol, and theophylline[19] rise when these drugs are used with fluvoxamine.[5] Fluvoxamine raises the serum levels of tricyclic antidepressants, probably due to an inhibition of the first stage of demethylation of tricyclic antidepressants.[20] As fluvoxamine relies on hepatic oxidative metabolism for its elimination, its time course in the body may be affected by metabolic enzyme inhibitors and inducers. The serotonin syndrome (hyperthermia, neuromuscular irritability, altered mental state) that follows the interaction between fluoxetine and MAOIs, lithium, or tryptophan may occur when fluvoxamine and MAOIs, lithium, or tryptophan are used together.[21]

Pregnancy/Lactation

Fluvoxamine should not be administered to pregnant patients until controlled studies in pregnant patients are undertaken. A 31-year-old woman receiving 100 mg of fluvoxamine (2.09 mg/kg/d) twice a day had a plasma fluvoxamine base concentration of 0.31 μg/mL and a milk concentration of 90 ng/mL. The dose to the baby was calculated at 0.0104 mg/kg/d. The baby ingested about 0.5% of the maternal intake.[17] Fluvoxamine is not recommended for nursing mothers or children.

Mechanism of Action

Fluvoxamine is specific as a serotonin reuptake inhibitor. It has almost no effect on norepinephrine or dopamine reuptake, does not inhibit monoamine oxidase, and does not appear to bind to serotonergic, dopaminergic, alpha- or beta-adrenergic, or muscarinic receptors.[3,4,7]

Clinical Presentation

Overdose

Fluvoxamine overdoses smaller than 1000 mg are usually relatively benign. Drowsiness, tremors, nausea, vomiting, abdominal pain, sinus bradycardia, diarrhea, headache, anxiety, a rash, and mild anticholinergic symptoms have been observed.[15,22] Serotonin syndrome has followed an increase in fluvoxamine dosage.[23] At higher doses, seizures and coma may be seen. Fluvoxamine may be associated with extrapyramidal symptoms, especially in patients with preexisting neurologic disease or already compromised extrapyramidal function due to neuroleptic medication.[24] In many cases bradycardia has been the only sign of cardiac toxicity; in some patients depolarization abnormalities, atrioventricular conduction disturbances, bundle-branch block, and ventricular premature beats are evident on the electrocardiogram.[15] Hypotension and tachycardia may be present. A patient recovered after a prolonged (5-day) coma.[13] Thirteen deaths have occurred following fluvoxamine overdose with multiple-drug ingestions.[1] Aspiration pneumonitis has been observed.

Withdrawal

Following withdrawal, patients experience dizziness, headache, weakness, memory problems, confusion, poor appetite, and tightness in the chest.[25]

Laboratory

Analytical Methods

Determination of plasma fluvoxamine concentrations employs a reverse-phase high-performance liquid chromatography method sensitive to 2 ng/mL.[26]

Blood Levels

One patient recovered from prolonged coma when the plasma fluvoxamine concentration fell below 0.7 μg/mL.[13] Peak plasma concentrations after overdose are often attained 6 to 24 hours after ingestion.[15] Fluvoxamine plasma concentrations below 2 μg/mL have usually not been reported to be associated with toxicity.[1]

Ancillary Tests

A moderate elevation in hepatic enzymes may be observed after overdose.[15] Hypokalemia has been observed in almost 1 of 10 patients with fluvoxamine overdose.[1] Electrocardiographic abnormalities frequently observed include atrioventricular block, repolarization disturbances, bundle-branch block, premature ventricular beats, bradycardia, and tachycardia.[1] Chest x-rays may indicate evidence of aspiration pneumonitis.

Treatment

Stabilization

Fluvoxamine is a monocyclic antidepressant but shares many effects of overdose with tricyclic antidepressants. All patients who have ingested more than 10 to 15 mg/kg fluvoxamine should immediately receive an intravenous line and cardiac monitoring. Those with altered mental status should receive oxygen, naloxone, glucose, and, if indicated, thiamine. Tidal volume and arterial blood gases should be determined and the patient checked for cyanosis to ascertain the adequacy of ventilation. Hypotension and seizures require supportive and symptomatic therapy.

Gut Decontamination

Activated charcoal may be useful. Enterohepatic recycling of fluvoxamine has not been adequately studied. No controlled studies have used single- or multiple-dose activated charcoal or cathartics. Gastric lavage with tracheal protection within the first 24 hours should aid in removing a sufficient number of potentially dangerous tablets and lessen the tissue distribution of fluvoxamine. As absorption may be delayed, gastric lavage up to 24 hours is recommended. The possible agglomeration (bezoar formation) of the enteric-coated tablets may require removal under direct gastroscopic observation.

Elimination Enhancement

The large volume of distribution and high degree of protein binding are likely to preclude removal (hemodialysis, hemoperfusion) of any substantial quantities of fluvoxamine or its metabolites.

Antidote

There is no antidote.

Supportive Measures

1. Observe patients with a history of fluvoxamine ingestion for the first 48 hours. If signs of depressed consciousness, hypotension, dysrhythmias, serious conduc-

tion disturbances, or seizures occur, admit the patient immediately. If no abnormal signs appear within 48 hours (tachycardia, bradycardia, absent bowel sounds) and there is no indication of a multiple-drug overdose, the patient may be discharged. The long elimination half-life precludes discharge before 48 hours.

2. Laboratory and monitoring procedures should include electrocardiograms, electrolytes, serial vital signs, arterial blood gases, and cardiac monitoring. Seizures may require diazepam intravenously. Plasma drug levels confirm overdose and may be of some predictive value on the clinical course.
3. For admitted patients, institute cardiac monitoring until they are symptom free after an initial 48-hour observation period.
4. For comatose patients, place a urinary catheter to check urine output and prevent urinary retention.
5. Sudden withdrawal of fluvoxamine in patients treated with 100 to 300 mg/d over 6 months may lead to dizziness, incoordination, headache, irritability, and nausea. Symptoms peak by day 5 but may last up to 14 days. Continue outpatient follow-up for at least 14 days.[27]
6. An anecdotal report suggests that cyproheptadine, useful in the serotonin syndrome, has also reversed fluvoxamine-induced anorgasmia.[28]

REFERENCES—FLUVOXAMINE

1. Van der Velden JW. Overview of overdose cases with fluvoxamine. Personal communication. The Netherlands: Duphar BV, July 19, 1989 and March 2, 1991.
2. Henry JA. Overdose and safety with fluvoxamine. Int Clin Psychopharmacol 1991;6(suppl. 3):41–47.
3. Claassen V, Davies JE, Hertting G, Placheta P. Fluvoxamine, a specific 5-hydroxytryptamine uptake inhibitor. Br J Pharmacol 1977;60:505–516.
4. Claassen V. Review of the animal pharmacology and pharmacokinetics of fluvoxamine. Br J Clin Pharmacol 1983; 15: 349S–355S.
5. Benfield P, Ward A. Fluvoxamine: A review of its pharmacodynamic and pharmacokinetic properties and therapeutic efficacy in depressive illness. Drugs 1986;32:313–334.
6. Flett SR, Szabadi E, Bradshaw CM. Comparison of fluvoxamine and amitriptyline on autonomic functions in healthy volunteers. Br J Clin Pharmacol 1991;31:6044.
7. Stimmel GL, Skowron DM, Chameides WA. Focus on fluvoxamine: A serotonin reuptake inhibitor for major depression and obsessive–compulsive disorder. Hosp Formul 1991;26:635–643.
8. Dollery CT, ed. *Therapeutic Drugs.* Edinburgh: Churchill Livingstone, 1991;1:F99–F101.
9. Mullin J, Pandita-Gunawardena VR, Whitehead AM. A double blind comparison of fluvoxamine and dothepin in the treatment of major affective disorder. Br J Clin Pract 1988;42: 51–55.
10. March JS, Kobak KA, Jefferson JW, et al. A double-blind placebo-controlled trial of fluvoxamine versus imipramine in outpatients with major depression. J Clin Psychiatry 1990; 51:200–202.
11. Goodman WK, Price LH, Delgado PL, et al. Specificity of serotonin reuptake inhibitors in the treatment of obsessive–compulsive disorder: Comparison of fluvoxamine and desipramine. Arch Gen Psychiatry 1990;47:577–585.
12. Marin PR, Adinoff B, Eckardt MJ, et al. Effective pharmacotherapy of alcoholic amnestic disorder with fluvoxamine. Arch Gen Psychiatry 1989;46:617–621.
13. Banerjee AK. Recovery from prolonged cerebral depression after fluvoxamine overdose. Br Med J 1988;296:1774.
14. Lebeque B. Survivable fluvoxamine overdose. Am J Psychiatry 1990;147:1689.
15. Azoyan PH, Garnier R, Chalaignor D, Efthymiou MI. Toxicokinetics of fluvoxamine in overdose. In: *Proceedings, Fourteenth International Congress of the European Association of Poison Centres, Milan, Italy, September 25–29, 1990.*
16. Pitchot W, Gonzalez-Moreno A, Ansseau M. Therapeutic window for 5-HT reuptake inhibitors. Lancet 1992;32:689.
17. Wright S, Dawling S, Ashford JJ. Excretion of fluvoxamine in breast milk. Br J Clin Pharmacol 1991;31:209.
18. Overmars H, Scherpenisse PM, Post LC. Fluvoxamine maleate: Metabolism in man. Eur J Drug Metab Pharmacokinet 1987;1:269–280.
19. Sperber AD. Toxic interaction between fluvoxamine and sustained release theophylline in an 11 year old boy. Drug Saf 1991;6:460–462.
20. Bertschy G, Vandel S, Vandel B, et al. Fluvoxamine–tricyclic antidepressant interaction: An accidental finding. Eur J Clin Pharmacol 1991;40:119–120.
21. Warnings from the Committee on Safety of Medicine: Fluvoxamine and fluoxetine interactions with MAOIs, lithium and tryptophan. Int Pharm J 1989;3:137.
22. Deahl M, Trimble M. Serotonin reuptake inhibitors, epilepsy and myoclonus. Br J Psychiatry 1991;159:433–435.
23. Lenzi A, Raffaeli S, Marazzit D. Serotonin syndrome-like symptoms in patients with obsessive–compulsive disorder following inappropriate increase in fluvoxamine dosage. Pharmacopsychiatry 1993;26:100–101.
24. Wills V. Extrapyramidal symptoms in a patient treated with fluvoxamine. J Neurol Neurosurg Psychiatry 1992;55: 330–331.
25. Mallya G, White K, Gunderson C. Is there a serotonergic withdrawal syndrome? Biol Psychiatry 1993;33:851–852.
26. Foglia JP, Perel JM, Nathan RS, et al. Therapeutic drug monitoring (TDM) of fluvoxamine: A selective antidepressant. Clin Chem 1990;36:1043.
27. Black DW, Wesner R, Gabel J. The abrupt discontinuation of fluvoxamine in patients with panic disorder. J Clin Psychiatry 1993;34:146–149.
28. Arnott S, Nutt D. Successful treatment of fluvoxamine-induced anorgasmia by cyproheptadine. Br J Psychiatry 1994;164:833–836.

KETANSERIN

Ketanserin is a 5-HT_1 receptor antagonist that appears to be useful in the treatment of hypertension and peripheral vascular disease. In overdose it may induce hypotension and drowsiness, which are reversible with symptomatic and supportive treatment. When used in doses of 20 to 40 mg one to three times daily together with potassium-losing diuretics, it may result in ventricular arrhythmias and death.

Structure and Classification

Ketanserin (R-41468, R-49945 [tartrate]) is 3-{2-[4(4-fluorobenzoyl)piperidino]ethyl}quinazoline-2,4-(1*H*,3*H*)-dione. It has a molecular weight of 395.4 as the free base and 545.52 as the tartrate. Ketanserin is marketed in Europe and elsewhere as Suprexal.[1]

Use

Ketanserin may be useful in the management of mild, moderate, or severe hypertension,[2] Raynaud's disease, and peripheral vascular disease.[3]

Product Formulation

Ketanserin (Serefrex, United Kingdom) is available in ampules containing 5 mg ketanserin/mL and tablets containing 20 or 40 mg ketanserin. The tablets are oblong, white, scored, and film-coated inscribed with "Ke20" or "Ke40" on one side and "Janssen" on the other. Twenty-milligram tablets contain 27.6 mg ketanserin tartrate (equivalent to 20 mg ketanserin); 40-mg tablets contain 55.2 mg ketanserin tartrate (equivalent to 40 mg ketanserin).[2]

Source

Ketanserin is a synthetic chemical.

Therapeutic Dose

Oral therapy begins with 20 mg twice daily.[4,5]

Toxic Dose

Initial oral doses of 40 mg may (within 50 minutes) induce profound hypotension, bradycardia, persistent drowsiness, nausea, and dizziness.[6] Following ingestion of 3200 mg, hypotension, bradycardia, drowsiness, and flushing were observed; the patient recovered within 24 hours.[3] Severe hypotension may follow an intravenous dose of 10 mg or an oral dose of 60 mg.[7]

Fatal Dose

A fatal dose has not been established.

Toxicokinetics

Absorption

Following oral administration ketanserin is almost completely (>98%) and rapidly absorbed. Plasma concentrations peak in 0.8 to 2 hours (ketanserin) and 1.6 hours (ketanserinol). Peak plasma concentrations average 127 ng/mL (ketanserin) and 119 ng/mL (ketanserinol).[8] Plasma protein binding is 95%, mainly to albumin.[5]

Distribution

Ketanserin is extensively distributed to tissues with a volume of distribution of 3 to 6 L/kg.[5,9]

Elimination

Ketanserin undergoes presystemic metabolism in the liver involving the reduction of ketanserin to ketanserinol (an inactive metabolite).[5] Urinary excretion of ketanserin is negligible. Ketanserinol excretion accounts for 13 to 17% of the ketanserin dose. Ketanserinol partially and slowly reconverts to ketanserin. This may account for the half-life of 15 to 19 hours for ketanserin and that of 25 hours for ketanserinol.[4,9] Total plasma clearance is 410 mL/min (after intravenous use) and 829 mL/min (after oral administration).[10,11]

Drug Interactions

Pretreatment with cimetidine (which reduced gastric acidity) and antacids in combination results in decreased oral absorption of ketanserin.[5] Ketanserin has no effect on indices of hepatic enzyme induction.[6] Ketanserin tends to impair the oral clearance of propranolol, leading to a higher serum propranolol C_{max}.[5] Ketanserin has no significant effect on the toxicokinetics of digoxin or digitoxin. Ketanserin taken with potassium-losing diuretics has resulted in an increase in sudden deaths.[12,13] Combinations of ketanserin and potassium-losing diuretics may induce an additional prolongation of the QT_c interval and an increase in Torsade de pointes ventricular arrhythmias.[14–16] Use of ketanserin with drugs that prolong repolarization or markedly depress conduction and affect repolarization should be avoided.[16–18]

Pregnancy/Lactation

There are few studies of the effect of ketanserin on pregnant women, the fetus, or lactation.[19]

Mechanism of Action

Ketanserin is a selective antagonist at 5-HT_2 receptors. It also has α_2-adrenoceptor antagonist activity,[6] H_1-histaminergic antagonist properties, and weak dopamine-blocking activity. It selectively inhibits serotonin-induced vasoconstriction but not vasodilation and inhibits serotonin-induced platelet aggregation. The fall in blood pressure following ketanserin use results mainly from its ability to block α_1 adrenoceptors.[10,17,19–22] Ketanserin appears to protect against adenosine-induced, but not histamine-induced, bronchoconstriction.[23]

Clinical Presentation

A 16-year-old girl with a history of Raynaud's disease ingested 3200 mg of ketanserin and became somnolent and uncooperative, but easily arousable and fully oriented. Blood pressure, pulse, and temperature were normal. Extremities were warm. No nausea, headaches, or blurred vision were experienced. The blood pressure remained at 90/50 for 12 hours with a bradycardia of 70/min. By 18 hours after admission, the blood pressure was 120/80, and heart rate was 90/min. She was still flushed 24 hours after admission. There were no ventricular arrhythmias. She recovered with symptomatic treatment (gastric lavage, elevation of legs, intravenous normal saline).[3]

A patient was treated with ketanserin for neuralgia. He suffered from depression for which he was treated with carbamazepine. The patient died after taking an overdose of ketanserin and an unspecified tricyclic antidepressant. The patient was suspected of having taken 20 20-mg tablets of ketanserin and an unknown quantity of an unspecified tricyclic antidepressant. He was admitted to the hospital comatose with a blood pressure of 60/30; an electrocardiogram showed no evidence of ventricular tachycardia. He exhibited high levels of carbamazepine and ketanserin; it was not possible to implicate one drug alone.[24]

A 15-year-old girl took her mother's ketanserin trial supplies—three bottles containing 26 40-mg tablets of ketanserin. All were empty but it is not clear how much was taken. In the hospital the blood pressure was 100/25, QT_c interval 0.76 second, and serum potassium 3.0 mEq/L. The patient was drowsy but had no arrhythmias. She was monitored. No fluids or pressor agents were given. The ketanserin/ketanserinol ratio (2/1) suggested intake of a very high dose of ketanserin. The level was found to be 15 times higher than the expected ketanserin and ketanserinol plasma level after one oral 40-mg dose. These plasma level findings suggested that this patient probably ingested at least 20 40-mg tablets (800 mg). On the other hand, if we assume a vomitus weight of 100 mL, the amount of measured ketanserin is approximately 700 mg, suggesting an intake of 15 to 20 40-mg tablets. In conclusion, this patient may have taken a total of 36 tablets.[24]

Laboratory

Analytical Methods

Plasma levels of ketanserin are measured by high-performance liquid chromatography with ultraviolet[24] or fluorescence[25] detection. The limits of sensitivity are 1 to 10 ng/mL for the ultraviolet method.[25,26]

Blood Levels

Ingestion of 3200 mg of ketanserin was followed (in 3 hours) by a plasma ketanserin level of 2873 ng/mL. The plasma level dropped to 151 ng/mL 18 hours after ingestion. Ketanserinol concentrations were 1155 ng/mL at 3 hours and 1117 ng/mL at 18 hours.[3]

Abnormalities

There have been no effects of ketanserin on routine hematology or biochemistry (liver function, urea, electrolytes, creatinine studies).[3,10,12] The serum potassium level may be depressed.[24]

Ancillary Tests

The electrocardiogram may show an increase in the QT interval when ketanserin is given alone. This is further increased when potassium-sparing diuretics are added.[12] Following an overdose of 3200 mg of ketanserin, the QT_c interval was 0.53 second (prolonged) and the potassium level was low at 3.3 mmol/L. The electrocardiogram showed atrial fibrillation with a short QRS in addition to prolonged QT complexes.

Treatment

Stabilization

Treatment of an overdose is largely symptomatic and supportive. Patients should be admitted to an intensive care facility where oxygen, cardiac monitoring, and an intravenous line are available. Initial attention should be directed toward evaluation of the adequacy of ventilation (ie, tidal volume, arterial blood gases, cyanosis). Serious toxicity may result from ventricular dysrhythmia or hypotension. Patients with altered mental status should receive oxygen, naloxone, glucose, and, if indicated, thiamine. Seizures have not been described following ketanserin overdose.

Gut Dcoontamination

Gut decontamination (emesis or lavage, activated charcoal, cathartics) may be used within the first few hours of ingestion of an overdose. Tracheal protection should be provided as rapid drowsiness may ensue.

Elimination Enhancement

Measures such as hemodialysis and hemoperfusion are unlikely to be effective in view of the strong degree of protein binding and extensive volume of distribution.

Antidote

There is no antidote.

Supportive Measures

Patients with a ketanserin overdose should be admitted to an intensive care facility where cardiac monitoring, oxygen, and overdrive pacing are available. All patients with a plasma potassium level less than 3.0 mmol/L, a second- or third-degree heart block, or a prolonged QT_c interval with or without Torsade de pointes or a ventricular arrhythmia should be admitted. Hypertension may be managed with elevation of legs, intravenous fluids, and pressor amines as indicated. Ventricular arrhythmias may be treated with discontinuation of ketanserin and overdrive pacing.[27] Serum potassium, calcium, and magnesium concentrations obtained periodically may be useful.[14]

Blood levels of ketanserin and ketanserinol will probably not be easily available to the hospital laboratory. Such levels confirm the presence of the product and may generally relate to the clinical status of the patient, but cannot be relied on to guide treatment.

An initial electrocardiogram and further electrocardiographic tracings should be obtained in patients who have a plasma potassium concentration less than 3.0 mmol/L, a second- or third-degree heart block, or a corrected QT interval longer than 500 milliseconds or who were being treated electively with an antiarrhythmic drug.[12–14]

REFERENCES—KETANSERIN

1. Reynolds JEF, ed. *Martindale: The Extra Pharmacopoeia.* 30th ed. London: Pharmaceutical Press, 1993:366–367.
2. Dollery CT, ed. *Therapeutic Drugs.* Edinburgh: Churchill Livingstone, 1991;2:K13–K18.
3. Roffe C, Tidmarsh M, Howlett TA. Ketanserin overdose: A case report. Postgrad Med J 1991;67:857.
4. Waller PC, Tucker GT, Ramsay LE. The pharmacokinetics of ketanserin after a single dose and at steady-state in hypertensive subjects. Eur J Clin Pharmacol 1887;33:423–426.
5. Persson B, Heykants J, Hedner T. Clinical pharmacokinetics of ketanserin. Clin Pharmacokinet 1991;2:263–279.
6. Waller PC, Cameron HA, Ramsay LE. Profound hypotension after the first dose of ketanserin. Postgrad Med J 1987;63: 305–307.
7. Andren L, Svensson A, Dahlof B, et al. Ketanserin in hypertension. Acta Med Scand 1983;210:125–130.
8. Barendregt JNM, Van Peer A, Van der Hoeven JG, et al. Ketanserin pharmacokinetics in patients with renal failure. Br J Clin Pharmacol 1990;29:715–727.
9. Reimann IV, Okonkwo PO, Klotz U. Pharmacokinetics of ketanserin in man. Eur J Clin Pharmacol 1983;25:73–76.

10. Brogden RN, Sorkin EM. Ketanserin: A review of its pharmacodynamic and pharmacokinetic properties and therapeutic potential in hypertension and peripheral vascular disease. Drugs 1990;40:903–949.
11. Lebrec D, Hadengue A, Gaudin C, et al. Pharmacokinetics of ketanserin in patients with cirrhosis. Clin Pharmacokinet 1990;19:160–166.
12. Ketanserin Trial Group. Prevention of atherosclerotic complications: Controlled trial of ketanserin. Br Med J 1989; 298:424–430.
13. Kirkendall WM. Prolonged QT_c, thiazides and sudden death. Arch Intern Med 1991;151:398–399.
14. Vandermotten M, Verhaeghe R, de Geest H. Ventricular arrhythmias and QT prolongation during therapy with ketanserin: Report of a case. Acta Cardiol 1989;44:431–437.
15. Vanhoutte P, Amery A, Birkenhager W, et al. Serotonergic mechanisms in hypertension: Focus on the effects of ketanserin. Hypertension 1988;11:1113–1133.
16. Singh B, Nademanee K, Symoens J, Janssens M. Ketanserin and Qt_c prolongation. Eur Heart J 1987;8:667–668.
17. Donnelly R, Elliott HL, Meredith PA, et al. Ketanserin concentration–effect relationship in individual hypertension patients. Br J Clin Pharmacol 1988;26:61–62.
18. Nademanee K, Lockhart E, Pruitt C, Singh BN. Cardiac electrophysiologic effects of intravenous ketanserin in humans. J Cardiovasc Pharmacol 1987;10(suppl. 3):581–585.
19. Weiner CP, Socol ML, Vaisrab N. Control of preeclamptic hypertension by ketanserin, a new serotonin receptor antagonist. Am J Obstet Gynecol 1984;149:496–500.
20. Bogle RG. Ketanserin for hypertension after upper gastrointestinal surgery. Lancet 1991;337:1219–1220.
21. Blauw GJ, Van Brummelen P, Doorenbos CJ, et al. The acute and chronic antihypertensive effects of ketanserin cannot be explained by blockade of vascular serotonin, type 2, receptors or alpha$_1$ adrenergic receptors. Clin Pharmacol Ther 1991;49:377–384.
22. O'Rangero EA, White WB, Chow MSS. Focus on ketanserin: A serotonin antagonist for the treatment of mild to moderate essential hypertension. Hosp Formul 1991;26:99–106.
23. Cazzola M, Matera MG, Santangelo G, et al. Effect of the selective $5HT_2$ antagonist ketanserin on adenosine-induced bronchoconstriction in asthmatic subjects. Immunopharmacology 1992;23:21–28.
24. Van Gool N. Personal communication. Janssen Research Foundation, September 8, 1992.
25. Okonkwo PO, Reimans IV, Woestenborghs R, Klotz U. High performance liquid chromatography assay with fluorometric detection of ketanserin, a new antihypertensive agent and serotonin S_2 antagonist in human plasma. J Chromatogr 1983;272:411–416.
26. Lindelauf F. Determination of ketanserin and its major metabolite (reduced ketanserin) in human plasma by high performance liquid chromatography. J Chromatogr 1983; 277:396–400.
27. Van Camp G, Dereppe H, Renard M, Bernard R. Ketanserin and syncope. Acta Cardiol 1989;44:429–430.

ONDANSETRON

Ondansetron (Zofran) is useful in the prevention of emesis during cytotoxic chemotherapy (eg, cisplatin). Ondansetron was approved in the United States for clinical use in January 1991.[1] Few reports of overdose have been published. Treatment of an overdose is symptomatic and supportive. No fatalities have been reported following overdose.

Structure and Classification

Chemically, ondansetron (GR 38032F) is 1,2,3,9-tetrahydro-9-methyl-3-[(3-methyl-1*H*-imidazol-l-yl)methyl]carazol-4-one hydrochloride dihydrate. The drug is a racemic mixture with a molecular weight of 366.

Table 49–7
Drugs Incompatible With Ondansetron When Administered Through the Same Set (Y-Site)

Chemotherapeutic Agents	Antiinfective Agents	Miscellaneous Agents
Amsacrine	Acyclovir sodium	Aminophylline
5-Fluorouracil*	Amphotericin B	Furosemide
	Ampicillin sodium	Lorazepam
	Ampicillin sodium, sulbactam sodium	Methylprednisolone
	Cefoperazone sodium	Sodium succinate
	Ganciclovir sodium	
	Mezlocillin disodium	
	Piperacillin sodium	

*Concentrations of 5-fluorouracil greater than 0.8 mg/mL may result in precipitation of ondansetron.
From Burnette PK, Perkins J. Parenteral ondansetron for the treatment of chemotherapy- and radiation-induced nausea and vomiting. Pharmacotherapy 1992;12(2):120–131.

Use

Ondansetron is indicated for the prevention of nausea and vomiting associated with initial and repeat courses of emetogenic cancer chemotherapy including high-dose cisplatin.[2–5] It appears to be less effective with moderately emetic chemotherapy such as cyclophosphamide, 5-fluorouracil, and adriamycin,[6] but is effective in ifosfamide-induced nausea and vomiting.[7] Ondansetron appears to be effective in decreasing postoperative nausea and vomiting,[8] following radiation-induced emesis,[9] and in the nausea and vomiting occurring during the terminal stage of cancer.[10,11] It is not effective as an anti-motion sickness drug,[12] but has been useful in ameliorating the symptoms of carcinoid[13] and in diminishing the symptoms associated with diarrhea-predominant irritable bowel syndrome.[14] Ondansetron has been useful in the treatment of vomiting associated with a theophylline overdose.[15,16] An anecdotal report indicates a potential use in hyperemesis gravidarum.[17] It appears to be effective in intoxication-associated emesis[5] (Table 49–1).

Product Formulation

Ondansetron is available as an injection of 2 mg/mL.[2] The injectable formulation should be diluted in 50 mL of 5% dextrose injection or 0.9% sodium chloride injection before administration.[18] Ondansetron is unstable in an alkaline environment.[19] To prevent precipitation of ondansetron in the intravenous tubing of a patient receiving an alkaline solution, the access line should be flushed both before and after the infusion. Drugs incompatible with ondansetron when administered through the same set (Y-site) are listed in Table 49–7. Although the subcutaneous route is not recommended for ondansetron administration by the manufacturer because of the acidic pH of the injection form (pH 3.5), continuous subcutaneous infusion appears to be well tolerated in patients with advanced cancer.[20]

Source

Ondansetron is a synthetic chemical product.

Therapeutic Dose

The recommended intravenous dosage of ondansetron is three 0.15 mg/kg doses. The first dose is infused over 15 minutes beginning 30 minutes before the start of emetic chemotherapy.

Anaphylactoid–anaphylactic reactions occur after the first ondansetron dose during the second or third course of chemotherapy and are characterized by urticaria, angioedema, hypotension, bronchospasm, and dyspnea.[21]

Toxic Dose

Individual doses as large as 145 mg (1.5 mg/kg) and a total daily dose of 252 have been administered intravenously. Another patient received three individual 84-mg doses (1.5 mg/kg at 2-hour intervals, 10 times the intended dose) and survived. A third patient received a single dose of 40 mg with no adverse effects.[22] No serious effects occurred.[23–25]

A patient who received 145 mg (1.5 mg/kg) experienced hot flashes and a feeling that the skin was hot where it touched the bed linen. The patient also experienced a transient, mild increase in serum lactate dehydrogenase. There were no electrocardiographic changes or extrapyramidal events.[26] A patient who received 252 mg (1.5 mg/kg every 2 hours) experienced itchy nose, vague restlessness, and hot flashes. These patients recovered with no sequelae.

Fatal Dose

A fatal dose has not been established.

Toxicokinetics

Absorption

The oral bioavailability of ondansetron is 60%.[27] Peak plasma concentrations averaging about 30 ng/mL follow an oral dose of 8 mg and are reached in 1 hour.[27] The protein binding of ondansetron is about 70 to 76%.[28]

Distribution

The apparent volume of distribution of ondansetron is large, about 1.8 L/kg.[29,30]

Elimination

Ondansetron is cleared from the body almost entirely by metabolism, with 5 to 10% of a dose excreted unchanged in the urine.[28] Hydroxylation followed by glucuronide or sulfate conjugation is the major route of metabolism.[31] Ondansetron has a terminal plasma half-life of 3.0 to 3.5 hours[30] and a plasma clearance of 600 mL/min.[27] Renal clearance is approximately 20 mL/min.[27] There is no evidence of accumulation at the steady state.

Drug Interactions

Ondansetron does not appear to induce or inhibit the cytochrome P450 drug-metabolizing enzyme system of the liver. Ondansetron itself is metabolized by hepatic cytochrome P450 drug-metabolizing enzymes. Inducers or inhibitors of these enzymes may change the clearance and half-life of ondansetron. In humans, carmustine, etopoxide, and cisplatin do not affect the toxicokinetics of ondansetron.[22] Drugs incompatible with ondansetron when administered through the same set (Y-site) are listed in Table 49–7.[32]

Pregnancy/Lactation

Safe use of ondansetron during pregnancy or lactation has not been established. The Food and Drug Administration has placed ondansetron in Pregnancy Category B.

Clinical Presentation

Clinical presentation following suspected overdoses of ondansetron have included fever (hot flashes), rash, pruritus, and restlessness, which were treated with diphenhydramine and resolved within 12 hours.[22,24,25] Adverse effects may include extrapyramidal symptoms, head jerking, and akathisia.[33,34] Headaches, diarrhea, anaphylactic reactions, and seizures have been reported.[1,35]

Laboratory

Analytical Methods

Plasma concentrations can be assayed using high-performance liquid chromatography produced with solid-phase extraction and ultraviolet detection.[29] The limit of sensitivity of the assay is 1 ng/mL.[28]

Blood Levels

A relationship between serum concentrations and efficacy has not been clearly established.[29] Plasma levels may not necessarily reflect drug activity at the target receptors.

Abnormalities

Mild transient elevations of the serum lactate dehydrogenase level occur.[22,24]

Treatment

Treatment of ondansetron overdose is largely symptomatic and supportive. There is no antidote. Methods to enhance elimination (hemodialysis, hemoperfusion) are unlikely to be of value because of its high protein binding and large volume of distribution.

General Review Article

- Markham A, Sorkin EM. Ondansetron: An update of its therapeutic use in chemotherapy-induced and postoperative nausea and vomiting. Drugs 1993;45:934–952.

GRANISETRON

Granisetron is a 5-HT_3 receptor antagonist used in the treatment of cancer chemotherapy emesis. Side effects are mild and include headache and constipation. No extrapyramidal effects have been reported.[36]

TROPISETRON

Tropisetron, a 5-HT_3 receptor antagonist, has been used in the prevention of radiation-induced nausea, vomiting, and diarrhea. Headaches and abdominal cramps have been observed in less than 10% of patients. The drug has a terminal half-life of 11 hours after a single intravenous dose, which is divided into 10 mg before and 10 mg after chemotherapy. Mild sedation, hypotension, hypertension, and transient elevation of serum transaminase levels have been observed. No extrapyramidal effects have been seen.[37,38]

REFERENCES—ONDANSETRON, GRANISETRON, AND TROPISETRON

1. Ondansetron granted marketing approval. Clin Pharmacol 1991;10:249.
2. *Physicians' Desk Reference.* 49th ed. Montvale, NJ: Medical Economics, 1995:858–862.
3. Drugs recently released in Belgium: Ondansetron. Acta Clin Belg 1991;46:58–60.
4. Grunberg SM, Stevenson LL, Russell CA, McDermed JE. Dose ranging phase I study of the serotonin antagonist GR38032F for prevention of cisplatin-induced nausea and vomiting. J Clin Oncol 1989;7:137–141.
5. Reed MD, Marx CM. Ondansetron: Optimal antiemetic therapy for the poisoned patient. Vet Hum Toxicol 1992; 34:336.
6. Dundee JW, McMillan CM, Yang J, Wright MMC. Is ondansetron a less effective antiemetic against moderately emetic as compared with highly emetic chemotherapy. Br J Clin Pharmacol 1992;33:200–201.
7. Green JA, Watkin SW, Hammond P, et al. The efficacy and safety of GR38032F in the prophylaxis of ifosfamide-induced nausea and vomiting. Cancer Chemother Pharmacol 1989; 24:137–139.
8. Derswitz M, Rosow CE, Di Biase PM, et al. Ondansetron is effective in decreasing postoperative nausea and vomiting. Clin Pharmacol Ther 1992;52:96–101.
9. Rosenthal SA, Marquez CM, Hourigan HP, Ryce JH. Ondansetron for patients given abdominal radiotherapy. Lancet 1992;339:490.
10. Vohra S. High-dose and long-term use of ondansetron. Ann Pharmacother 1992;26:128–129.
11. Nicholson S, Evans C, Mansi J. Ondansetron in intractable nausea and vomiting. Lancet 1992;339:490.
12. Stott JRR, Barner GR, Wright RJ, Ruddock CJS. The effect on motion sickness and oculomotor function of GR 38032F, a $5HT_3$-receptor antagonist with anti-emetic properties. Br J Clin Pharmacol 1989;27:147–157.
13. Platt AJ, Heddle RM, Rake MO, Smedley H. Ondansetron in carcinoid syndrome. Lancet 1992;339:1416–1417.
14. Steadman SJ, Talley NJ, Phillips SF, Zinsmeister AR. Selective 5-hydroxytryptamine type 3 receptor antagonism with ondansetron as treatment for diarrhea-predominant irritable bowel syndrome: A pilot study. Mayo Clin Proc 1992;67: 732–738.
15. Brown SGA, Prentice DA. Ondansetron in the treatment of theophylline overdose. Med J Aust 1992;156:512.
16. Dollery CT, ed. *Therapeutic Drugs.* Edinburgh: Churchill Livingstone, 1991:O20–O23.
17. World M. Ondansetron and hyperemesis gravidarum. Lancet 1993;341:185.
18. Zofran[R] (ondansetron hydrochloride) Injection Product Monograph. Glaxo Pharmaceuticals, May 1991.
19. Jarosinski PF, Hirschfeld S. Precipitation of ondansetron in alkaline solutions. N Engl J Med 1991;325:1315–1316.
20. Mulvenna PM, Reynard CFB. Subcutaneous ondansetron. Lancet 1992;339:1059.
21. Chen M, Tanner A, Gallo-Torres H. Anaphylactoid–anaphylactic reactions associated with ondansetron. Ann Intern Med 1993;119:862.
22. Finn AL. Toxicity and side effects of ondansetron. Semin Oncol 1992;19(4, suppl. 10):53–60.
23. Pritchard JF, Wells CD. The relationships between systemic exposure and efficacy of ondansetron. Clin Pharmacol Ther 1990;47:206(Abstract 111).
24. Davidson JS. Personal communication. Glaxo Pharmaceuticals, August 12, 1992.
25. Hainsworth J, Harvey W, Pendergross K, et al. A single-blind comparison of intravenous ondansetron, a selective serotonin antagonist, with intravenous metoclopramide in the prevention of nausea and vomiting associated with high-dose cisplatin chemotherapy. J Clin Oncol 1991;9:721–728.
26. Bryson JC. Clinical safety of ondansetron. Semin Oncol 1992;19(suppl. 15):26–32.
27. Blackwell CP, Harding SM. The clinical pharmacology of ondansetron. Eur J Cancer Clin Oncol 1989;25(suppl. 1): S21–S24.
28. Colthup PV, Palmer JL. The determination in plasma and pharmacokinetics of ondansetron. Eur J Cancer Clin Oncol 1989;25(suppl. 1):S71–S74.
29. Pritchard JF, Bryson JC, Kernadle NE, et al. Age and gender effects on ondansetron pharmacokinetics: Evaluation of healthy aged volunteers. Clin Pharmacol Ther 1992;51:51–55.
30. Lazarus HM, Bryson JC, Lemon E, et al. Antiemetic efficacy and pharmacokinetic analyses of the serotonin antagonist ondansetron (GR 38032F) during multiple-drug chemotherapy with cisplatin prior to autologous bone marrow transplantation. J Natl Cancer Inst 1990;82:1776–1778.
31. Saynor DA, Dixon CM. The metabolism of ondansetron. Eur J Cancer Clin Oncol 1989;25(suppl. 1):S75–S77.
32. Burnett PK, Perkins J. Parenteral ondansetron for the treatment of chemotherapy and radiation-induced nausea and vomiting. Pharmacotherapy 1992;12:120–131.
33. Halperin JR, Murphy B. Extrapyramidal reaction to ondansetron. Cancer 1992;69:1275.
34. Smith RN. Safety of ondansetron. Eur J Cancer Clin Oncol 1989;25(suppl. 1):S47–S50.
35. Sargent AI, Deppe SA, Chan FA. Seizure associated with ondansetron. Clin Pharm 1993;14:613–615.
36. Joss RA, Dott CS, Granisteron Study Group. Clinical studies with granisetron, a new 5-HT_3 receptor antagonist for the treatment of cancer chemotherapy-induced emesis. Eur J Cancer 1993;29A(suppl. 1):S22–S29.
37. Sorbe B, Berlind A-M. Tropisetron, a new 5-HT_3-receptor antagonist, in the prevention of radiation-induced nausea, vomiting and diarrhea. Drugs 1992;43(suppl. 3):33–39.
38. Kris MG, Tyson LB. Tropisetron (ICS 205-930): A selective 5-hydroxytryptamine antagonist. Eur J Cancer 1993;29A (suppl. 1):S30–S32.

OXAFLOZANE

Oxaflozane is a nontricyclic antidepressant sold in France as Conflictan. Its molecular weight is 272.3. Oxaflozane belongs to the group of phenyl-2 tetrahydroaxins-1,4 agents Some of them are serotonergic partial agonists and others are agonists stronger than serotonin. It has little anticholinergic or sympatholytic effects.

Toxicokinetics

After oral administration of oxaflozane 20 mg, three metabolites have been identified: the main metabolite *N*-dealkyloxaflozane and two minor metabolites. No unmetabolized oxaflozane has been detected in human urine.[1] The plasma concentration of *N*-dealkyloxaflozane peaks at 30 ng/mL after a therapeutic dose.

Clinical Presentation

A 2-year-old child ingested 150 mg of oxaflozane, lost consciousness, and developed opisthotonus. Treatment was conservative. The child recovered in 3 hours.[2] Serum oxaflozane concentrations 2 hours after ingestion averaged 63 ng/mL; 3 hours after, they were undetectable. The peak plasma concentration was 890 ng/mL and the elimination half-life of *N*-dealkyloxaflozane was 4.8 hours.

REFERENCES—OXAFLOZANE

1. Constantin M, Pognat JF. Comparative study of oxaflozane urinary metabolism in man, the dog and the rat. Arzneimittelforschung 1979;29:107–114.
2. Dutertre JP, Barbier P, Suc AL, et al. Oxaflozane overdose in a child. Clin Toxicol 1992;30:1231–1236.

OXETORONE FUMARATE

Oxetorone fumarate is a tetracyclic antiserotonergic agent marketed in Europe as Nourtone for maintenance treatment of migraine in daily doses of 180 ng orally.[1–3] The toxicity of oxetorone in overdose is similar to that observed during tricyclic and tetracyclic antidepressant overdose. Treatment is based on careful supportive care.

Clinical Presentation

Three and a half hours after ingestion of about 2.4 g of oxetorone, a 37-year-old woman was admitted in coma with a heart rate of 120 beats/min. Thirty minutes after admission she entered into cardiac arrest with progressive widening of the QRS complexes and a bradycardia preceding asystole. Within a few minutes she exhibited generalized seizures. She awoke 72 hours after arrival following vigorous treatment. The electrocardiographic disturbances regressed over 48 hours. The myocardial toxicity of oxetorone probably results from quinidine-like effects.[2]

Laboratory

Analytic Methods

Plasma concentrations of oxetorone may be measured by high-performance liquid chromatography using a reverse-phase column.

Blood Levels

Following ingestion of 2.4 g, the plasma concentration was 1.6 to 1.8 μg/mL.[2] After a single 60-mg dose of oxetorone the plasma level peaks at 0.44 ng/mL in 4 hours. Oxetorone has a plasma half-life of about 24 hours. The steady-state plasma level of about 1.2 ng/mL is attained after 3 days of three daily 60-mg doses.[4]

Treatment

Management may require cardiopulmonary resuscitation, sodium lactate (11.2%) 500 mL, with intravenous potassium chloride 4 g (serum potassium, 2.9 mg/L), intravenous clonazepam 2 mg (for seizures), repeat gastric lavage (to 24 hours after ingestion), and assisted ventilation.[2]

REFERENCES—OXETORONE FUMARATE

1. Aussems G, Bauthier J, Chaillet F, et al. Research on a series of benzofurans: XLV. Pharmacologic profile of oxetorone. Therapie 1971;261:1135–1155.
2. Bismuth C, Baud FJ, Conso F, et al. *Toxicologie Clinique.* 4th ed. Paris: Medecine-Sciences, Flammarion, 1987:198.
3. Galerneau V, Petit J, Deghmani M, et al. Severe self-poisoning with oxetorone: Report of one case. Clin Toxicol 1990; 28:111–116.
4. Rascol A, Fanchamps A. Antimigraineux. Semin Hop Paris 1984;4445:3137–3160.

PAROXETINE

Paroxetine is a selective serotonin reuptake inhibitor (SSRI) that has few anticholinergic side effects. Overdoses have been relatively nontoxic. Patients should respond to symptomatic and supportive treatment.

Structure and Classification

Paroxetine hydrochloride is a phenylpiperidine derivative that is structurally distinct from other selective serotonin reuptake inhibitors (Fig. 49–2).[1,2]

Use

Paroxetine is used in the treatment of depression, including severe depression and depression with associated symptoms of anxiety.[3]

Product Formulation

Paroxetine is available in the United States as Paxil in 10-mg tablets.

Source

Paroxetine is a synthetic chemical.

Therapeutic Doses

The therapeutic dose is 20 to 50 mg daily. In the elderly, the therapeutic dose range is 20 to 40 mg daily.[4]

Toxic Dose

The maximum overdose with paroxetine was 850 mg. Patients have recovered fully without seizures or loss of consciousness.[2,4] In one series of pediatric exposures, ingestion of 120 mg or less by children less than 5 years of age led to favorable outcomes with gastrointestinal decontamination and minimal symptomatic care.[5]

Fatal Dose

No fatalities have been reported after overdose.

Toxicokinetics

See Table 49–4.

Absorption

When ingested orally, paroxetine is readily absorbed from the gastrointestinal tract.[6] There is a marked first-pass effect both in the gut wall and in the liver. Plasma concentrations peak at 0.8 to 65 ng/mL in approximately 5 hours.[7] Paroxetine is 95% protein bound. Serum levels at steady state are 10 to 110 ng/mL.[8] There is no evidence of a relationship between serum levels and antidepressant effect.

Distribution

The apparent volume of distribution of paroxetine is 13 L/kg, indicating a large volume of distribution.[8]

Elimination

Paroxetine is eliminated primarily by hepatic metabolism to glucuronide and sulfate conjugated metabolites that are inactive.[8] The urinary excretion of unchanged paroxetine is less than 2% of a daily dose.[7] Plasma clearance is 0.76 L/h/kg. There are no active metabolites.[4] The elimination half-life is 24 hours.[4,7]

Drug Interactions

Paroxetine appears to have a low potential to cause toxicokinetic interactions with other drugs (Table 49–8).[7] Paroxetine has shown little effect on the kinetics of diazepam, digoxin, phenytoin, propranolol, tranylcypromine, or warfarin.[9] Phenobarbital has no effect on paroxetine kinetics. Experience with other SSRIs suggests that a clinical serotonin syndrome may occur in combination with MAOIs.[8] There are no reported interactions with lithium.[2,4,8] Paroxetine is an inhibitor of an isozyme of cytochrome P450, CYP2D6.[10,11]

Pregnancy/Lactation

There have been no controlled clinical trials of paroxetine during pregnancy or lactation. All offspring have been reported to be healthy in cases in which the pregnancies proceeded to term.[12]

Mechanism of Action

Paroxetine acts through the selective inhibition of the reuptake of the neurotransmitter serotonin in brain neurons.

Table 49–8
Paroxetine Drug Interactions

Alcohol	Paroxetine does not potentiate the psychomotor effects of alcohol.
Analgesics	Aspirin and other nonsteroidal antiinflammatory drugs have been coadministered safely in clinical studies of depressed patients.
Anticonvulsants	Coadministration of paroxetine and phenytoin, a known metabolizing enzyme inducer, is associated with decreased plasma concentrations of paroxetine. Clinical experience with concomitant administration of other anticonvulsants such as carbamazepine and valproate is limited.
Barbiturates	Coadministration of the barbiturates amobarbital and phenobarbital is associated with increased adverse experiences. Careful titration of paroxetine dose should be undertaken in depressed patients requiring barbiturate treatment.
Benzodiazpines	No pharmacokinetic or pharmacodynamic interaction with benzodiazepines has been demonstrated. As with any medication with CNS action, caution should be exercised in the use of multiple CNS-active medications.
Cimetidine	Coadministration of cimetidine and paroxetine is associated with increased paroxetine plasma concentrations. The clinical significance of this increase is unknown. Consideration should be given to keeping doses of paroxetine toward the lower end of its recommended dosage range.
Digoxin	Pharmacokinetic studies have indicated that there is no interaction between paroxetine and digoxin.
Monoamine oxidase inhibitors	Animal studies indicate that interaction between paroxetine and MAOIs may occur. Given the fatal interactions reported with fluoxetine and MAOI, combined use of paroxetine and MAOI should be avoided. At least 14 days should elapse between discontinuation of paroxetine and initiation of therapy with a MAOI.
Oral contraceptives	Coadministration of birth control medication has not been associated with pharmacokinetic or pharmacodynamic interactions.
Tryptophan	As tryptophan can be metabolized to serotonin, the use of paroxetine together with tryptophan may result in adverse experiences including agitation, restlessness, and gastrointestinal distress, as has been noted with fluoxetine. Although clinical experience with patients on concomitant paroxetine and tryptophan is limited, increased adverse experiences were indeed observed.
Warfarin	In a pharmacokinetic study an increased bleeding tendency in the face of unaltered prothrombin time was found in a small number of volunteers ($N = 27$). Whether this was due to the paroxetine–warfarin combination or warfarin alone is unclear. Clinical experience with combined use of warfarin and paroxetine in depressed patients is extremely limited; however, no clinically significant bleeding episodes have been reported in clinical trials.

CNS, central nervous system; MAOI, monoamine oxidase inhibitor.
From Boyer WF, Blumhardt CL. The safety profile of paroxetine. J Clin Psychiatry 1992;53(suppl.):61–66.

It exerts its antidepressant action through an increased concentration of the neurotransmitter at the synaptic cleft, thereby enhancing serotonergic transmission.[8] Paroxetine in normal doses shows little affinity for the catecholaminergic or histaminergic systems. At higher concentrations, the SSRIs also inhibit the reuptake of norepinephrine and, to a lesser degree, dopamine. Paroxetine has a low affinity for alpha adrenoceptors and dopamine D_2, histamine H_1, and 5-HT_2 receptors and therefore has a little ability to cause central and autonomic side effects. It is less likely to exhibit anticholinergic effects than tricyclic antidepressants.[8]

Clinical Presentation

Adverse Effects

Adverse effects during clinical trials included nausea, headache, somnolence, dry mouth, asthenia, insomnia, sweating, constipation, dizziness, tremor,[2,4] and akathisia (also seen with fluoxetine and sertraline, other SSRIs).[13] In patients with bipolar disorders, paroxetine may be associated with a 2% rate of mania.[4]

The Committee on Safety of Medicines in the United Kingdom observed that extrapyramidal reactions are more common with paroxetine than with other SSRIs.[14] Dizziness, sweating, nausea, insomnia, tremor, and confusion appeared to be more common with withdrawal from paroxetine than with withdrawal from other SSRIs.[15]

Overdose

Nine patients overdosed with paroxetine alone and six in combination with another drug. The maximum overdose with paroxetine was 850 mg. Five of the patients who overdosed with paroxetine were hospitalized. There was no loss of consciousness or seizure. One patient had sinus tachycardia. Electrocardiograms were otherwise normal. All recovered.[4]

Laboratory

Analytical Methods

A high-performance liquid chromatography method for quantitation is available.[9]

Blood Levels

There is little correlation between paroxetine plasma concentrations and clinical or adverse effects.[7,16] Hyponatremia has followed its use in the elderly, in whom it may be due to the syndrome of inappropriate secretion of antidiuretic hormone.[15]

Abnormalities

Paroxetine causes a small decrease in hemoglobin level, hematocrit, and white blood cell level.[4]

Ancillary Tests

Paroxetine at 30 to 40 mg/d has not induced significant changes in heart rate, blood pressure, or electrocardiographic parameters.[17] No significant effects have been observed on the electroencephalogram.[4]

Treatment

Treatment of a paroxetine overdose is symptomatic and supportive. Few anticholinergic symptoms are observed. Patients should be hospitalized and provided with access to a cardiac monitor. Most do not experience a loss of consciousness. Few changes in heart rate (except for an occasional sinus tachycardia), blood pressure, or electrocardiographic parameters should be expected.[18]

Gut Decontamination

There are no data to substantiate the use of activated charcoal in paroxetine overdose. If the patient is seen within 5 hours of ingestion, gastric emptying may lessen the peak blood levels.

Elimination Enhancement

The high degree of protein binding and large volume of distribution suggest that hemodialysis or other extracorporeal methods of treating overdose would be inefficient in removing a significant amount of drug from the body.

Antidote

There is no antidote.

Supportive Measures

All overdose patients should be observed for about 6 hours. Special attention should be given to other drugs ingested simultaneously. If the patient is symptom free, has no evidence of seizures or cardiac abnormalities (normal electrocardiogram) has normal vital signs and is alert, consideration can be given to discharge within 12 hours after psychiatric counseling.

General Review Articles

- Caley CF, Weber SS. Paroxetine: A selective serotonin reuptake inhibiting antidepressant. Ann Pharmacother 1993;27:1212–1222.
- Meltzer HY. Paroxetine: A safe and effective once-daily oral antidepressant agent. Hosp Formul 1993;28:4–13.

REFERENCES—PAROXETINE

1. Reynolds JEF, ed. *Martindale: The Extra Pharmacopoeia.* 30th ed. London: Pharmaceutical Press, 1993:267.
2. Boyer WF, Feighner JP. An overview of paroxetine. J Clin Psychiatry 1992;53(2,suppl.):3–6.
3. Dunner DL, Dunbar GC. Optimal dose regimen for paroxetine. J Clin Psychiatry 1992;53(2, suppl.):21–26.
4. Boyer WF, Blumhardt CL. The safety profile of paroxetine. J Clin Psychiatry 1992;53(suppl.):61–66.
5. Myers LB, Dean BS, Krenzelok ER. A pediatric focus: Paroxetine (PAXL) overdose. Clin Toxicol 1995;33:475–486 (Abstract 172).
6. De Vane CL. Pharmacokinetics of the selective serotonin reuptake inhibitor. J Clin Psychiatry 1992;52(2, suppl.):13–20.
7. Tulloch IF, Johnson AM. The pharmacological profile of paroxetine, a new selective serotonin reuptake inhibitor. J Clin Psychiatry 1992;52(2, suppl.):7–12.
8. Jambon L. Analysis of two new antidepressants, paroxetine and sertraline. Cal Assoc Toxicol Newslett, Spring 1992: 19–20.

9. Kaye CM, Hadock RT, Langley PF, et al. A review of the metabolism and pharmacokinetics of paroxetine in man. Acta Psychiatr Scand 1989;8(suppl. 350):60–75.
10. Sindrup SH, Brosen K, Gram LF, et al. The relationship between paroxetine and sparteine oxidation polymorphism. Clin Pharmacol Ther 1992;51:278–287.
11. Sindrup SH, Brosen K, Gram LF. Pharmacokinetics of the selective serotonin reuptake inhibitor paroxetine: Nonlinearity and relation to the sparteine oxidation polymorphism. Clin Pharmacol Ther 1992;51:288–295.
12. Baldwin JA, Davidson EJ, Pritchard AL, et al. The reproductive toxicology of paroxetine. Acta Psychiatr Scand 1989; 8(suppl. 350):37–39.
13. Adler LA, Angrist BM. Paroxetine and akathisia. Biol Psychiatry 1995;37:336–337.
14. Paroxetine and extrapyramidal reactions. Lancet 1993;341: 624. Editorial.
15. Van Harten J. Clinical pharmacokinetics of selective serotonin reuptake inhibitors. Clin Pharmacokinet 1993;24: 203–241.
16. Tasler TCG, Kaye CM, Zussnam BD, et al. Paroxetine plasma levels: Lack of correlation with efficacy or adverse events. Acta Psychiatr Scand 1989;80(suppl. 350):152–155.
17. Edwards JG, Goldie A, Papayanni-Papasthatis S. Effect of paroxetine on the electrocardiogram. Psychopharmacology 1989;95:96–98.
18. Jenner PN. Paroxetine: An overview of dosage, tolerability and safety. Int Clin Psychopharmacol 1992;6(suppl. 14): 69–80.

PIZOTIFEN

Pizotifen malate (pizotyline malate) is a benzocycloheptathiaphene that is structurally related to the tricyclic antidepressant drugs and to cyproheptadine.[1–3] It has strong antiserotonergic (5-HT_2 antagonist) and antihistaminic effects, but also possesses weak anticholinergic and antidepressant activity.[1–3] The product is sold as Sandomigran, Sandomigrin, Sanomogran, and Sannigran in Europe.[1] It is not available in the United States. Pizotifen is used for the treatment of vascular headaches of the migraine type (classic migraine, common migraine, cluster headache) in an initial dose of 0.5-mg tablets three times daily (1.5 mg/d), which is gradually increased 0.5 mg per week up to a maximum of 3 to 4.5 mg daily.[4–6] Its molecular weight is 429.5.[1]

Toxicokinetics

Pizotifen is readily absorbed (80%) in the gastrointestinal tract, reaching peak plasma concentrations after 5 to 7 hours of about 9 ng/mL (mostly its *N*-glucuronide metabolite). It is extensively protein bound in the plasma (91%) and has a large apparent volume of distribution (approximately >7 L/kg).[7,8] Gas chromatography methods are available for its measurement in body fluids.[9] Pizotifen has a plasma half-life of 26 hours. Less than 1% is excreted unchanged in the urine. Pizotifen has not been studied in pregnancy or during lactation.[10]

Tolerance to alcohol may be lowered.[5] Increased and prolonged sedative effects may occur when pizotifen is used concurrently with tranquilizers, sedatives, narcotics, or some tricyclic antidepressants. It should not be used in patients receiving monoamine oxidase inhibitors. Pizotifen may antagonize the adrenergic nerve blockade induced by bethanidine, debrisoquin or guanethidine.[7]

Clinical Presentation

Chronic Use

Chronic use may lead to drowsiness, weight gain (excessive appetite), and anticholinergic effects such as tachycardia, dry mouth, and blurred vision.[7] Fever has not been reported after therapeutic use.[7]

Overdose

A 16-year-old girl ingested 60 0.5-mg tablets and then began to complain of blurred vision and colicky abdominal pain. Four hours later she was drowsy and flushed, with an elevated temperature of 38°C. Physical examination revealed dilated pupils, a sinus tachycardia, and blood pressure of 110/60. Gastric lavage did not reveal any tablets. In 12 hours she felt uncomfortably hot. The skin was dry and the temperature had risen to 39°C. The fever and tachycardia persisted for about 10 hours before remitting spontaneously.[3]

Mechanism of Action

It appears more likely that the anticholinergic properties of pizotifen were responsible for most of the clinical manifestations of the overdose. An increase in serotonergic activity may result in elevation of body temperature,[11] in which case hypothermia might be expected to follow an overdose of a serotonin inhibitor. Pizotifen increases the levels of 5-hydroxyindoleacetic acid (HIAA) and homovanillic acid in the urine.[12]

Treatment

Treatment is largely symptomatic and supportive and directed to ameliorating the anticholinergic effects. In the case described, tepid sponging and a cooling fan appeared to be sufficient. There is no antidote. Intravenous physostigmine is not a drug of first choice (see Chapter 38). Hemodialysis and hemoperfusion are not likely to be of value in view of the strong protein binding and extensive volume of distribution.

REFERENCES—PIZOTIFEN

1. Reynolds JEF, ed. *Martindale: The Extra Pharmacopoeia.* 30th ed. London: Pharmaceutical Press, 1993:416–417.
2. Dollery CT, ed. *Therapeutic Drugs.* Edinburgh: Churchill Livingstone, 1991;2:144–146.
3. Griffiths AP, Penn ND, Tindall H. A report of acute overdosage of the anti-serotonergic drug pizotifen. Postgrad Med J 1987;63:59–60.
4. Gillies D, Sills M, Forsythe I. Pizotifen (Sanoragran) in childhood migraine: A double-blind controlled trial. Eur Neurol 1886;25:32–35.
5. Peet BMS. Use of pizotifen in severe migraine: A long term study. Curr Med Res Opin 1977;5:192–199.
6. Behan PO. Prophylactic treatments for migraine: A comparison of pizotifen as clonidine. Cephalalgia 1975;5(suppl. 3): 524–527.
7. Speight TM, Avery GS. Pizotifen: A review of its pharmacological properties and its therapeutic efficacy in vascular headaches. Drugs 1972;3:159–203.
8. Meier J, Schreier E. Human plasma levels of some antimigraine drugs. Headache 1976;16:96–104.
9. Laplanche R. Determination of BC105 (pizotifen) in body fluids by gas chromatography–mass spectrometry. In: Usdin E, Eckert H, Forrest IS, eds. *Phenothiazines and Structurally*

Related Drugs: Basic and Clinical Studies. Developments in Neurosciences, Vol 7. Amsterdam: Elsevier, 137–140.
10. Drife JO. Answer. Br Med J 1984;288:375.
11. Myers RD. Serotonin and thermoregulation: Old and new views. J Physiol (Paris) 1981;77:505–513.
12. Elghczi JL, Laude D, Duprat P, Mignot E. Pizotifen increases 5-HIAA urinary excretion in male healthy volunteers. Eur J Clin Pharmacol 1984;27:191–196.

RISPERIDONE

Risperidone is an antipsychotic agent with antagonist action on dopamine (D_2) and serotonin (5-HT_2) receptors. Overdose induces electrolyte changes (hyponatremia, hypokalemia) and reversible changes in the QT_c and QRS intervals on the electrocardiogram and follows a benign course.

Structure and Classification

Risperidone (R 64766, RIS) is a benzisoxazole derivative with a molecular weight of 410.5.[1]

Use

Risperidone appears to be a useful antipsychotic drug in the treatment of "negative" symptoms of chronic schizophrenia (emotional withdrawal, scarcity of speech, affective blunting).[2]

Product Formulation

Risperidone is available in 2-mg tablets. It is marketed in the United States as Risperdal.

Source

Risperidone is a synthetic chemical.

Therapeutic Dose

In human trials, oral doses generally averaged about 2 mg/d.[2,3] The therapeutic dose range is 3 to 8 mg twice daily.[1,4,5]

Toxic Dose

An adult ingested 240 mg (120 2-mg tablets) of risperidone; he was treated symptomatically and recovered in 24 hours.[6] High doses of risperidone (16 mg/d) cause extrapyramidal effects at a frequency similar to that reported during treatment with haloperidol 20 mg/d.[7]

Toxicokinetics

Absorption

Risperidone is rapidly absorbed after oral administration. Plasma risperidone concentration peaks in 2 hours.[1] Absorption is consistent with some first-pass metabolism.[8]

Distribution

Risperidone is rapidly distributed and has an apparent volume of distribution of 1 to 2 L/kg. Risperidone is 88% bound to plasma proteins (albumin and α_1-acid glycoprotein). 9-Hydroxyrisperidone is 77% bound to plasma protein.

Elimination

About 4 to 30% of risperidone is excreted in the urine unchanged.[1] The terminal half-life is about 34 hours for 9-hydroxyrisperidone and 2 to 4 hours for risperidone in extensive metabolizers. The metabolite, 9-hydroxyrisperidone, is active.

Drug Interactions

Difficulties may be expected with concurrent administration of dopamine agonists (eg, for parkinsonism) or with drugs that produce postural hypotension (eg, many tricyclic antidepressants, other antipsychotic agents, alcohol). Excess sedation may occur with concomitant administration of antihistamines.[9]

Pregnancy/Lactation

Safe use during pregnancy or lactation has not been established.

Mechanism of Action

Risperidone is a centrally acting potent serotonin 5-HT_2 and catecholamine antagonist. It also exhibits dopamine D_2 antagonism.[3] Risperidone has an affinity for the cholinergic muscarinic receptors. It is a potent LSD antagonist. Classic antidopamine antipsychotic compounds treat the positive active symptoms of schizophrenia (hallucinations, delusions, thought disorders) effectively, but not the negative inactive symptoms (emotional withdrawal, blunted affect, poverty of speech, avolition).[2,8] Risperidone, perhaps because of its serotonin antagonism, seems to treat the positive and the negative symptoms simultaneously while lessening extrapyramidal symptoms.[6] Risperidone also has α_1- and α_2-noradrenergic activity and is antihistaminic.[9]

Clinical Presentation

Overdose

Few cases of risperidone overdose have been reported. An anecdotal case report described auditory hallucinations, electrocardiogram changes (QRS and QT_c prolongation), hyponatremia, and hypokalemia.[6] Abnormalities appear to resolve over a 12-hour period. Heather and Vicas reviewed six patients with risperidone overdose, five of whom had ingested from 5 to 270 mg. Tachycardia, drowsiness, slurred speech, a changed level of consciousness, hypertension, tremors, agitation/hypomania, and extrapyramidal effects (noted in one patient) were observed. Symptoms lasted 6 hours.[10] Neuroleptic malignant syndrome, which may be fatal, has been described.[11,12]

Chronic Use

Chronic use leads to blurred vision, vertigo, postural dizziness, impaired concentration, decreased appetite, and erection and ejaculation disturbances.[5] Risperidone, like clozapine, can precipitate or exacerbate obsessive–compulsive symptoms in patients with schizophrenia.[13]

Laboratory

Analytical Methods

Radioimmunoassays and high-performance liquid chromatography are preferred for the analysis of risperidone and its metabolites in blood and urine. Sensitivity is 0.1 ng/mL.[1]

Abnormalities

Prolongation of QTc and QRS intervals was observed after an overdose of 240 mg.[6] These returned to normal within 24 hours in one anecdotal case report. No clinically significant electrocardiographic changes have been seen after doses of up to 25 mg/d.[3,6] Low blood levels of potassium and sodium have been measured. Risperidone induces an increase in prolactin levels that is reversed on drug withdrawal.[7]

Treatment

Treatment of hypotension and circulatory collapse is largely symptomatic and supportive. Use of risperidone is discontinued. Early gastric lavage (within 2 to 3 hours of ingestion) followed by activated charcoal and a cathartic may lessen absorption and decrease both time and severity of toxic symptoms. Management is similar to that for tricyclic antidepressant overdose. Gastric lavage, activated charcoal, and oral magnesium citrate, in addition to intravenous normal saline and a 40-mEq increment of potassium chloride, appeared to be sufficient to maintain a hemodynamically stable state. Cardiac and electrolyte monitoring is indicated in an intensive care setting for at least 24 hours. There is no specific antidote.[14] Anticholinergic agents can be used to treat extrapyramidal symptoms.

REFERENCES—RISPERIDONE

1. Mannens G, Huang M-L, Meuldermans W, et al. Absorption, metabolism and excretion of risperidone in humans. Drug Metab Dispos 1993;21:1134–1141.
2. Meco G, Bedini L, Bonifati V, et al. Risperidone in the treatment of chronic schizophrenia with tardive dyskinesia. Curr Ther Res 1989;46:876–883.
3. Mesotten F, Suy E, Pietquin M, et al. Therapeutic effect and safety of increasing doses of risperidone (R64766) in psychotic patients. Psychopharmacology 1992;99:445–449.
4. Kane JM. Newer antipsychotic drugs: A review of their pharmacology and therapeutic potential. Drugs 1993; 46:585–593.
5. Claus A, Bollen J, De Coyper H, et al. Risperidone versus haloperidol in the treatment of chronic schizophrenic inpatients: A multicentre double-blind comparative study. Acta Psychiatr Scand 1992;85:295–305.
6. Brown K, Levy H, Brenner C, et al. Overdose of risperidone. Ann Emerg Med 1993;22:1908–1910.
7. Edwards JG. Risperidone for schizophrenia: Encouraging results await further research. Br Med J 1994;308: 1311–1312.
8. Janssen RAJ, Niemegeers CJE, Awouters F, et al. Pharmacology of risperidone (R 64766), a new antipsychotic with serotonin-C2 and dopamine-D2 antagonistic properties. J Pharmacol Exp Ther 1988;244:685–693.
9. Livingston MG. Risperidone. Lancet 1994;343:457–460.
10. Heather GS, Vicas IMO. Risperidone overdose: A case series. Vet Hum Toxicol 1994;36:371.
11. Webston P, Wijeratne C. Risperidone-induced neuroleptic malignant syndrome. Lancet 1994;344:1228–1229.
12. Lee H, Ryan J, Mullett G, Lawlor PA. Neuroleptic malignant syndrome associated with the use of risperidone, an atypical antipsychotic agent. Hum Psychopharmacol 1994; 9:303–305.
13. Kopala L, Homer WG. Risperidone, serotonergic mechanisms and obsessive–compulsive symptoms in schizophrenia. Am J Psychiatry 1994;151:1714–1715.
14. Cohen LJ. Risperidone. Pharmacopsychotherapy 1994; 14:253–265.

SERTRALINE

Sertraline is a selective 5-HT reuptake inhibitor antidepressant that, in overdose, appears to have a low risk of toxicity. There is no antidote. Patients are largely treated symptomatically and supportively.

Structure and Classification

Sertraline is a naphthylamino compound and is structurally dissimilar to other antidepressants[1,2] (Fig. 49–2).

Use

Studies with sertraline suggest that it is effective in the treatment of depression and obsessive–compulsive disorder. Animal studies suggest that sertraline might be helpful in the pharmacologic treatment of obesity and reduction of alcohol craving.[1]

Product Formulation

Zoloft (sertraline) is available as capsule-shaped scored tablets containing sertraline hydrochloride equivalent to 50 and 100 mg of sertraline.[3]

Source

Sertraline is a synthetic chemical product.

Therapeutic Dose

The initial dose for depression is 50 mg/d with gradual upward titration based on clinical response.[1]

Toxic Dose

The manufacturer is aware of four patients who have taken an overdose. Doses taken were 750 to 1000 mg in one case, 2100 mg in the second case, and 1400 mg in the third case. Up to a maximum of 2.6 g was ingested alone or in combination with other medications or alcohol.[4] All survived. Up to 4500 mg may be tolerated without profound toxicity.[5]

Fatal Dose

A fatal dose has not been established.

Toxicokinetics

Absorption

Sertraline is absorbed readily through the gastrointestinal tract.[6] Its absolute bioavailability has not been determined in humans. It displays first-order kinetics. Maximum plasma concentrations following doses of 50 and 200 mg are 22 to 29 μg/L (ng/mL). These concentrations are reached in 4.5 to 8.4 hours.[1] Serum levels at steady state are 10 to 120 ng/mL of sertraline and its desmethyl metabolites.[7] Plasma protein binding is extensive (approximately 98%) to both albumin and α_1-acid glycoprotein.[2] At concentrations up to 300 and 200 μg/mL, respectively, sertraline and *N*-desmethylsertraline do not appear to alter the plasma protein binding of two other highly protein-bound drugs, warfarin and propranolol.[3]

Distribution

Distribution following oral administration of sertraline is biphasic with a prolonged absorption phase. The elimination phase begins 12 to 16 hours following the dose.[1] The volume of distribution has not been determined in humans but is more than 20 L/kg in rats and dogs.[8] Both sertraline and its metabolites exhibit extensive distribution into tissues outside the blood.[1]

Elimination

Sertraline undergoes extensive metabolism. The parent drug is *N*-demethylated, followed by glucuronidation, deamination, or both. Most metabolites in the urine are α-hydroxyketone glucuronides. The elimination half-life (beta) of sertraline in humans is 24 to 25 hours. The clinically active desmethyl metabolite is eliminated more slowly than the parent drug with a half-life of approximately 66 hours.[9,10] Unchanged sertraline is not detected in the urine.[3,11]

Drug Interactions

Because of its extensive protein binding, sertraline may cause a shift in plasma concentrations of other drugs similarly tightly protein bound (eg, warfarin, propranolol). The risk of using sertraline in combination with other central nervous system adrenergic drugs has not been systematically evaluated. Sertraline appears to induce hepatic microsomal enzymes. Patients receiving a sertraline reuptake inhibitor drug in combination with a monoamine oxidase inhibitor may develop serious, sometimes fatal, reactions including hyperthermia, rigidity, myoclonus, autonomic instability, and mental changes (extreme agitation, delirium, coma) (see The Serotonin Syndrome earlier in this chapter). At least 14 days should be allowed after starting sertraline before starting a MAOI.[3]

Pregnancy/Lactation

Sertraline has not been subject to controlled studies during human pregnancy or lactation.

Mechanism of Action

Sertraline is a selective 5-HT reuptake inhibitor. It does not have cardiovascular, anticholinergic, antidopaminergic, convulsant, or monoamine oxidase-inhibiting effects.[12,13] Most antidepressants are associated with either norepinephrine reuptake inhibition, 5-HT reuptake inhibition, and monoamine oxidase inhibition. Sertraline does not cause significant reuptake blockade of dopamine or norepinephrine. Sertraline, through inhibition of 5-HT release, may cause beta-adrenoceptor downregulation.[1]

Clinical Presentation

Adverse Effects

Sertraline may induce nausea, dry mouth, diarrhea, male sexual dysfunction (primary ejaculatory delay), tremor, akathisia, dyspepsia, and chest pain (see also Sumatriptan).[14] Amitriptyline produced more somnolence, fatigue, dry mouth, dizziness, constipation, urinary retention, and amnesia than sertraline in one study.[15] Systolic blood pressure may rise within 8 hours of a dose. Sertraline has been associated with an abrupt change in mood from depression to hypomania, a reaction that is seen with other effective antidepressants.[16] Paradoxical sedation has been described.[17] Sertraline has been associated with hypernatremia and the syndrome of inappropriate antidiuretic hormone secretion[18] and the sertraline syndrome.[19] Extrapyramidal effects, similar to those seen with other sertraline reuptake inhibitors, have been observed after sertraline use.[20] Tachycardia, hypertension, hallucinations, coma, hyperthermia, tremors, and skin flushing have been reported in a 9-year-old child following ingestion of 50 sertraline tablets; the child recovered.[19]

Overdose

A 23-year-old woman with a past history of depression ingested an overdose of 700 to 1000 mg; a 28-year-old man took an overdose of 2100 mg. Both received gastric lavage and recovered fully with no sequelae. A 43-year-old woman with a past history of depression took an overdose of 1400 mg together with unsuspected amounts of mefenamic acid, temazepam, and alcohol; the patient was discharged the next day with no sequelae. None of the four cases of overdose reported to the manufacturer with a maximum ingestion of 2.6 g of sertraline (equivalent to 13 times the maximum daily dose) required intensive monitoring and there were no significant changes in vital signs, cardiovascular function, or level of consciousness. There were no known sequelae.[4,21] Up to 4500 mg may be tolerated without profound toxicity.

In a U.S. series of six cases of overdose, all experienced lethargy and four had sinus tachycardia. All recovered within 24 hours of gastric lavage, activated charcoal, and supportive care. The quantity of sertraline ingested and the time before symptoms were noted were not provided in the report.[22] Sertraline does produce the classic toxic syndrome associated with cyclic antidepressants.

Laboratory

Analytical Methods

A gas chromatography–mass spectrometry method is available for quantitation of plasma concentrations. This analytical procedure may not be available in hospital clinical laboratories. Sensitivity is 10 ng/mL. The method is linear from 10 to 150 ng.[7]

Blood Levels

Ingestion of approximately 1000 mg led to a plasma concentration of about 245 mg/mL. Toxic plasma levels are greater than 200 ng/mL.[23] There is no indication that blood levels are clinically useful in guiding treatment or that they correlate with the severity of overdoses.

Abnormalities

Sertraline may rarely cause a transient elevation in hepatic transaminase levels.[1]

Ancillary Tests

Sertraline at doses of 50 to 400 ng/d has had no effect on the QT_c, PR, or PR interval.[24]

Treatment

Stabilization

Treatment of overdose is largely symptomatic and supportive. Patients should be hospitalized where adequate oxygen, cardiac monitoring, and a central line are available. An airway should be established and maintained, and adequate oxygenation and ventilation ensured. Cardiac function and vital signs must be monitored. The possibility of multiple-drug involvement should be considered.

Gut Decontamination

Activated charcoal, used with sorbitol, may be as or more effective than emesis. No controlled studies have compared these measures in sertraline overdose.

Elimination Enhancement

Because of the large volume of distribution and extensive protein binding of sertraline, forced diuresis, dialysis, hemoperfusion, and exchange transfusion are not likely to be of benefit.

Antidote

There is no specific antidote.

Supportive Measures

Patients should remain under observation for at least 48 hours after an overdose (the metabolite has a half-life of several days).

REFERENCES—SERTRALINE

1. Guthrie SK. Sertraline: A new specific reuptake blocker. DICP Ann Pharmacother 1991;25:952–961.
2. De Vane CL. Pharmacokinetics of the selective serotonin reuptake inhibitors. J Clin Psychiatry 1992;53(suppl.):12–30.
3. Package Insert: Zoloft[R] (sertraline hydrochloride) tablets. New York: Roerig, Division of Pfizer. January 1992.
4. Doogan DR. Tolerance and safety of sertraline: Experience. worldwide. Int Clin Psychopharmacol 1991;6(suppl. 2):47–56.
5. Myer LB, Dean BS, Krenzelok EP. Sertraline (Zoloft[R]): Overdose assessment of a new antidepressant. Vet Hum Toxicol 1993;34:341.
6. Jambor L. Analysis of two new antidepressants: Paroxetine and sertraline. Calif Assoc Toxicol Newslett, Spring 1992: 19–20.
7. Ostrosky DD. Personal communication. Roerig-Pfizer, April 21, 1992.
8. Tremaine LM, Welch WM, Romfeld RA. Metabolism and disposition of 5-hydroxytryptamine uptake blocker sertraline in the rat and dog. Drug Metab Dispos 1989;17:542–550.
9. Fouda HG, Ronfeld RA. Gas chromatographic–mass spectrometric analysis and preliminary pharmacokinetics of sertraline, a new antidepressant drug. J Chromatogr 1987;417: 197–207.
10. Koe PK, Weissman A, Welch WM, et al. Sertraline, 1*S*, 4*S*-*N*-methyl-4-(3,4 dichlorophenyl)-1,2,3,4-tetrahydro-1-naphthylamine, a new uptake inhibitor with selectivity for serotonin. J Pharmacol Exp Ther 1983;226:686–700.
11. Waalinder J, Feighnner JP. Novel selective serotonin reuptake inhibitors: Part I. J Clin Psychiatr 1992;53:107–117.
12. Doogan DP, Caillard V. Sertraline: A new antidepressant. J Clin Psychiatry 1988;49(suppl. 9):461.
13. If at first you do succeed. Lancet 1991;337:650–651. Editorial.
14. Iruela LM. Sudden chest pain with sertraline. Lancet 1994; 343:1106.
15. Reinherr FW, Chauminard G, Cohm CK, et al. Antidepressant efficacy of sertraline: A double-blind, placebo and amitriptyline-controlled, multicenter comparison study in patients with major depression. J Clin Psychiatry 1990;51(12, suppl. B):28–33.
16. La Porta M, Chouinard G, Goldbloom D, Beauclair L. Hypomania induced by sertraline, a new serotonin reuptake inhibitor. Am J Psychiatry 1987;144:1513–1514.
17. Gupta S, Freimer M, Popli A. Paradoxical sedation with sertraline. Am J Psychiatry 1993;150:1427–1428.
18. Crews JR, Potts NLS, Schreiber J, Lippe S. Hyponatremia in a patient with sertraline. Am J Psychiatry 1993;150:1564.
19. Kaminski CA, Robbins MS, Weibley RE. Sertraline intoxication in a child. Ann Emerg Med 1994;23:1371–1374.
20. Shihabuddin L, Rapport D. Sertraline and extrapyramidal side effects. Am J Psychiatry 1994;151:288.
21. Murdock D, McTavish D. Sertraline: A review of its pharmacodynamic and pharmacokinetic properties and therapeutic potential in depression and obsessive–compulsive disorder. Drugs 1992;44:604–624.
22. Kassner J, Woolf A. Sertraline HCl: A new antidepressant. Vet Hum Toxicol 1992;34:343.
23. Myers LB, Dean BS, Krenzelok ER. Sertraline (Zoloft[R]): Overdose assessment of a new antidepressant. Vet Hum Toxicol 1993;35:341.
24. Guy S, Silke B. The electrocardiogram as a tool for therapeutic monitoring: A critical analysis. J Clin Psychiatry 1990; 51(12, suppl. B):37–39.

SUMATRIPTAN

Sumatriptan (GR 43175), an antimigraine drug, is usually used subcutaneously. Few overdoses have been reported, but symptoms have been minimized. Nevertheless, it has been associated with coronary vasospasm, chest pain, hypertension, ventricular arrhythmias, and ST wave changes on the electrocardiogram. No fatalities have been reported after an overdose. Treatment is symptomatic.

Structure and Classification

Sumatriptan chemically resembles 5-hydroxytryptamine (Fig. 49–3).[1] Sumatriptan is available in the United States as Imitrex.[2] Its molecular weight is 295.4.[3]

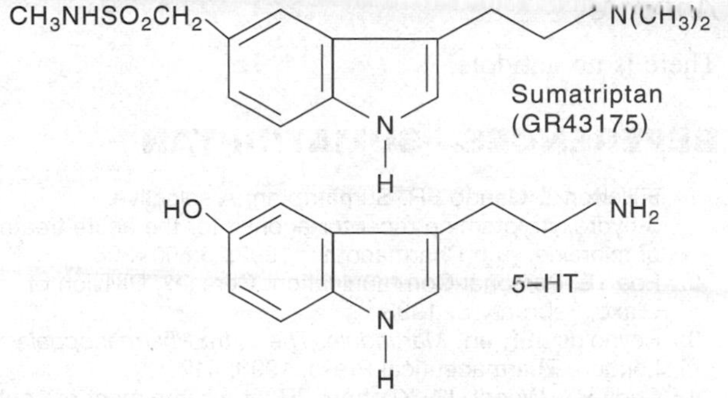

$CH_3NHSO_2CH_2$ $N(CH_3)_2$
Sumatriptan (GR43175)
N–H
HO NH_2
5–HT
N–H

Figure 49-3 Structures of sumatriptan (GR 43175) and serotonin (5-hydroxytryptamine [5-HT]). (From Fullerton T, Gengo FM. Sumatriptan: A selective 5-hydroxytryptamine receptor agonist for the acute treatment of migraine. Ann Pharmacother 1992;26:800-808. Erratum: 1992;26:1160E.)

Use

Sumatriptan is used in the acute treatment of migraine and cluster headaches.[4–7]

Product Formulation

Sumatriptan is available as oral 100-mg tablets or as the succinate salt. Injectable doses of 6 mg of sumatriptan are available for subcutaneous use.

Source

Sumatriptan is a synthetic chemical product.

Therapeutic Dose

The maximum recommended adult dose of sumatriptan is 6 mg injected subcutaneously. A second 6-mg injection after 1 hour may be administered if symptoms of migraine return. The maximum recommended dose in 24 hours is two 6-mg injections separated by at least 1 hour.[2]

Toxic Dose

Doses of 100 to 200 mg/kg in animals resulted in seizures, tremor, inactivity, erythema of the extremities, reduced respiratory rate, cyanosis, ataxia, mydriasis, injection site reactions, and paralysis[2] (see Clinical Presentation).

Fatal Dose

A fatal dose has not been determined.

Toxicokinetics

Absorption

Plasma concentrations in volunteers are 75% of maximum plasma levels (about 70 ng/mL) within 45 minutes of a subcutaneous ingestion. The plasma concentrations after intravenous use (3 mg, 15-minute infusion) peaks at 76.8 ng/mL. After an oral 100-mg dose, the plasma level peaks at 53.8 ng/mL in 1.5 hours. Bioavailability after subcutaneous injection is 96%; after oral administration, it is 14%.[8]

Distribution

The apparent volume of distribution is about 2.4 L/kg. Plasma protein binding of sumatriptan is low (14–20%). Sumatriptan does not cross the blood–brain barrier.[9]

Elimination

Most of the drug is eliminated as metabolites (80%). The principal one is an indoleacetic analog, which appears to have no activity. The half-life is about 2 hours with single dosing, but longer after repeat oral dosing. Following intravenous administration, clearance is about 1.2 mL/min. Renal clearance of sumatriptan is greater than the glomerular filtration rate (250 mL/min).[8]

Drug Interactions

Sumatriptan should not be used in patients receiving MAOIs, lithium, or 5-HT reuptake inhibitor antidepressants.[8] Its vasoconstrictive effects may be additive to those of ergotamine and the catecholamines.[10]

Pregnancy/Lactation

Experience in pregnancy is limited. Safe use of sumatriptan has not been established. There are no data on its excretion in breast milk.

Mechanism of Action

Vasodilation within the cerebral circulation contributes to the severity of migraine headaches. 5-HT receptors on blood vessels are vasoconstrictive. Sumatriptan has induced stroke after a 6-mg subcutaneous injection in a patient with sagittal sinus thrombosis.[11] Receptors on the cerebral arteries are predominantly subclass 5-HT_1. Those on the temporal arteries are $5\ \text{HT}_2$.[8,9] Sumatriptan, a 5-HT antagonist, was developed to stimulate 5-HT receptors on the blood vessels, redistribute blood flow within the brain, and reduce headaches.[12,13] Sumatriptan is a highly selective agonist at 5-HT receptors of the 5-HT_{1D} or 5-HT_1-like subtype. It is almost devoid of activity at 5-HT_2 and 5-HT_3 receptors.[9,14]

Clinical Presentation

There are few reports of overdose with sumatriptan. An anecdotal report indicated severe burning on the forehead, which resolved spontaneously in 90 months.

Therapeutic Use

The most common adverse effect is an unpleasant taste or an injection site reaction.[15] Most side effects are minor and resolve within 30 minutes. Tingling, a warm or hot sensation, dizziness, malaise, and fatigue may occur in up to 10% of patients. Chest tightness and pressure were observed in 5% of patients. The Committee on Safety of Medicine reviewed 34 reports of chest pain by June 1992.[8]

The Netherlands Centre for Monitoring of Adverse Reactions to drugs also received reports of 12 similar cases, mostly after oral intake.[16] The Drug Data Sheet in the United Kingdom warns against use of sumatriptan in patients with ischemic heart disease. There have also been reports of asthma and ventricular arrhythmias.[17,18] Sumatriptan is contraindicated in Prinzmetal's angina. It may cause a rise in blood pressure. Coronary vasoconstriction has been observed.[19]

Sumatriptan may cause flow-limiting coronary artery stenosis resulting in myocardial ischemia and infarction.[20–22] The drug is contraindicated in patients with symptomatic ischemic heart disease when either angina or an earlier myocardial infarction or silent ischemia has been documented previously.[20,21] No association between chest complaints and electrocardiographic changes has been observed.[23] Sumatriptan probably potentiates alpha-adrenoceptor-mediated vasoconstriction.[10,19] Controlled pharmacodynamic studies are indicated.

Overdose

Three cases of accidental overdose with sumatriptan (up to twice the recommended daily dose) led to few symptoms except for severe burning on the forehead of one patient.[24] During clinical trials, volunteers received single doses as high as 16 mg without serious adverse effects.[2] A single subcutaneous dose of 16 mg produced dysphonic effects and subjective apathetic sedation.[25]

Laboratory

Analytical Methods

Sumatriptan and its principal metabolites are determined in plasma, urine, and other biological fluids by reverse-phase high-performance liquid chromatography with either electrochemical detection (sumatriptan) or ultraviolet detection (metabolite). The lower limit of sensitivity using plasma samples is 1 ng/mL.

Abnormalities

In occasional patients, T-wave abnormalities may be observed. ST elevations have been seen.[26]

Treatment

Stabilization

Following a significant overdose, supportive and symptomatic treatment should be provided. The blood pressure and electrocardiogram should be monitored for at least 12 hours. Vasodilation therapy may be required. If sumatriptan induces symptoms suggestive of angina, nitrites should be used.[21]

Elimination Enhancement

There are no data on the use of hemodialysis, hemoperfusion, or peritoneal dialysis in relation to the serum concentrations of sumatriptan.[2]

Antidote

There is no antidote.

REFERENCES—SUMATRIPTAN

1. Fullerton T, Gengo FR. Sumatriptan: A selective 5-hydroxytryptamine receptor agonist for the acute treatment of migraine. Ann Pharmacother 1992;26:800–808.
2. Poe TE. Personal Communication. Cerenex, Division of Glaxo, February 8, 1993.
3. Reynolds JEF, ed. *Martindale: The Extra Pharmacopoeia.* London: Pharmaceutical Press, 1993: 417.
4. Cady RK, Wendt JK, Kirchner JR, et al. Treatment of acute migraine with subcutaneous sumatriptan. JAMA 1991; 265:2831–2835.
5. Sumatriptan Auto-injection Study Group. Self-treatment of acute migraine with subcutaneous sumatriptan using an auto injection device. Eur Neurol 1991;31:323–331.
6. Sumatriptan Cluster Headache Study Group. Treatment of acute cluster headache with sumatriptan. N Engl J Med 1991;325:322–326.
7. Subcutaneous Sumatriptan International Study Group. Treatment of migraine attacks with sumatriptan. N Engl J Med 1991;325:316–321.
8. Bateman DN. Sumatriptan. Lancet 1993;3241:221–224.
9. Edvinsson L, Jansen I. Characterization of 5-HT receptors mediating contraction of human cerebral, meningeal and temporal arteries: Target for GR 43175 in acute treatment of migraine? Cephalgia 1989;9 (suppl. 10):49–55.
10. Buikena H, Grandjean JG. Potentiation of alpha-adrenoceptor-mediated vasoconstriction by sumatriptan. Lancet 1993;342:1121.
11. Cavazos JE, Caress JB, Chilukuri VL, et al. Sumatriptan-induced stroke in sagittal sinus thrombosis. Lancet 1994;334:1105–1106.
12. Lance JW. 5-Hydroxytryptamine and its role in migraine. Eur Neurol 1991;31:279–281.
13. Friberg L, Olesen J, Iversen HK, Sperling B. Migraine pain associated with middle cerebral artery dilatation: Reversal by sumatriptan. Lancet 1991;338:13–17.
14. Yaskowitz MA. Neurogenic versus vascular mechanisms of sumatriptan and ergot alkaloids in migraine. Trends Pharmacol Sci 1992;13:307–311.
15. Brown EG, Endersby CA, Smith RN, Talbot JCC. The safety and tolerability of sumatriptan: An overview. Eru Neurol 1991; 31:339–344.
16. Stricker BHC. Coronary vasospasm and sumatriptan. Br Med J 1992;305:118.
17. Inmana W, Kubota K. Cardiorespiratory distress after sumatriptan given by injection. Br Med J 1992;305:714.
18. Curtin T, Brooks AP, Roberts JA. Cardiorespiratory distress after sumatriptan given by injection. Br Med J 1992;305:713–714.
19. McIntyre P, Gemmill J, Hogg K, et al. The effect of subcutaneous sumatriptan (GR 43175) on central haemodynamics and the coronary circulation. Clin Pharmacol Ther 1992; 51:152.
20. Chester AH, O'Neil GS, Yacoub MH. Sumatriptan and ischaemic heart disease. Lancet 1993;341:1419–1420.
21. Hillis WS, MacIntyre PD. Sumatriptan and chest pain. Lancet 1993;341:1564–1565.
22. Ottervanger JP, van Witsen PB, Valkenburg HA, Stricker BHC. Postmarketing study of cardiovascular adverse reactions associated with sumatriptan. Br Med J 1993;307:1185.
23. Neighbor ML. Sumatriptan: A new treatment of migraine. West J Med 1993;159:597–598.
24. Dollery C, ed. *Therapeutic Drugs.* Edinburgh: Churchill Livingstone, 1991:S153–S157.
25. Fowler PA, Lacey LF, Thomas M, et al. The clinical pharmacology, pharmacokinetics and metabolism of sumatriptan. Eur Neurol 1991;31:323–331.
26. Willett F, Curzen N, Adams J, Armitage M. Coronary vasospasm induced by subcutaneous sumatriptan. Br Med J 1992;304:1415.

ZIMELDINE

Zimeldine (Zelmid, Zelmidine, Normud) was the first antidepressant that selectively inhibited neuronal serotonin (5-HT) reuptake and it soon came into general use in many Western European countries. It was withdrawn from common use in September 1983, however, because of an acute flulike syndrome comprising fever, signs of liver function disturbance, and myalgia and/or arthralgia and tentatively termed a hypersensitivity syndrome. The withdrawal followed reports of peripheral neuropathy, with a Guillain–Barré syndrome that followed the hypersensitivity syndrome in a few of these patients.[1]

Zimeldine is still in use and prescribed on license in Sweden.[1]

REFERENCE—ZIMELDINE

1. Bengtsson B-O, Wiholm B-E, Myrhed M, Walinder J. Adverse experience during treatment with zimeldine on special licence in Sweden. Int Clin Psychopharmacol 1994; 9:55–61.

IBOGAINE

Ibogaine, an alkaloid, is an investigational drug being developed as a possible addiction interrupter for heroin, cocaine, amphetamine, nicotine, and alcohol. The product is used in Gabanese villages to induce visions during initiation rites. It has not been approved for general use by the Food and Drug Administration. The concept of a hallucinogen disrupting addictive behavior has not been clinically tested. Ibogaine exerts stimulatory, hallucinogenic, and tremorigenic properties. Its major effects appear to be inhibition of cholinesterase, resulting in hypertension; central nervous system stimulation, leading to seizures, paralysis, and respiratory arrest at high doses in animals; and visual and other hallucinations often associated clinically with severe anxiety and apprehension. It may have a profound effect on the serotonergic system.

Structure and Classification

The molecular formula of ibogaine is $C_{20}H_{26}N_2O$. Ibogaine hydrochloride is an indole alkaloid.[1]

Ibogaine (Endabuse) is a Schedule I controlled substance in the United States, similar to other hallucinogenic substances such as LSD and mescaline-like heroin.

Source

One of the main alkaloids extracted from the roots of *Tabernanthe iboga,* a shrub indigenous to French equatorial Africa, is ibogaine. It may also be synthesized. The plant belongs to the Apocynaceae family. The powdered bark is cultivated by West Africans.

Therapeutic Dose

Doses of 500 mg (7.7 mg/kg) to 1000 mg have been used in clinical investigations. The usual regimen by individuals who choose to use this chemical involves one or two test doses (50 100 mg orally), followed the next day by a therapeutic dose (9–25 mg/kg). Data in humans are limited.[2]

Toxic Dose

At 150 mg, some difficulty in sleeping and perception of colored lights may be experienced. Doses of 20 mg or higher lead to dilation of the pupils and an increase in systolic blood pressure, but no effects on temperature, pulse rate, or respiratory rate.[3] At 300 mg of the dried root bark powder, slight nausea, dizziness, and a lack of muscular control or coordination may be experienced. Visual imagery and heightened empathy have been observed. At 1 g, ibogaine is a type of hallucinogen. In humans, single oral doses of 5 to 25 mg/kg lead to the onset of central nervous system and cardiovascular effects in 15 to 40 minutes.

Toxicokinetics

Many of the toxicokinetic studies have been performed on animals.

Distribution

The volume of distribution is estimated at about 5 L/kg.

Elimination

The 24-hour recovery of unchanged ibogaine in the urine is less than 5% of the dose. An indole metabolite accounts for about 15% of the dose.[4] The elimination half-life is about 38 hours.

Drug Interactions

Ibogaine prevents the rise in brain dopamine levels usually observed after a morphine injection.[5] Ibogaine antagonizes adrenaline, acetylcholine, yohimbine, and atropine.[2] In animals ibogaine enhances amphetamine- and cocaine-induced increases in brain dopamine levels.

Mechanism of Action

In animal studies a negative chronotropic effect on the heart has been observed. Both a decrease (vasodilatory) and increase in blood pressure have been seen. This is caused by an excitatory action of ibogaine on the reticular activating system.[1] Negative chronotropic and inotropic effects are reported.[6] This alkaloid has distinct central stimulating properties and exhibits weak but definite anticonvulsant properties.[2] Ibogaine and its primary metabolite 12-hydroxyibogamine inhibit the oxidation of serotonin and catalyze that of catecholamine by a monoamine oxidase, ceruloplasmin.[7] Ibogaine does not possess opiate-like pharmacologic properties. It does not produce physical dependence. It is not a substitute for morphine and it has no analgesic properties. Ibogaine does not modulate the effects of norepinephrine, serotonin, acetylcholine, and histamine in the heart. Ibogaine produces selective degeneration of Purkinje cells in the cerebellum.[8] This may be related to its putative antiaddictive effects, suggesting that the cerebellum may be involved in addictive behavior.[9]

Clinical Presentation

Crude extracts of *Tabernanthe iboga* have been associated with a feeling of excitement, drunkenness, mental confusion, and hallucinations in high doses.[1] The effect of ibogaine lasts about 30 hours, during which time ibogaine exerts a stimulant effect. Effects are noticed 15 to 20 minutes after oral administration. Initially, a numbing of the skin is accompanied by an auditory buzzing and oscillating sounds. In 25 to 30 minutes, objects appear to vibrate. Nausea may follow. The visions end abruptly and the numbness of the skin begins to abate, followed by 6 to 8 hours of a high-energy state with "lighting" or flashes of light dancing about the subjects. Between 26 and 36 hours, stimulation diminishes and the subject falls asleep. Ibogaine results in the complete elimination of narcotic withdrawal sequelae.[2] Postural tremor, vertigo, and nystagmus have been observed clinically. There are few controlled clinical data to support its use in treating opiate addiction.[9]

Acute effects have included photophobia, ataxia, oscillating vision, dizziness, out-of-body experiences, vertigo, nystagmus, nausea, and hallucinations. Peak cardiovascular and central nervous system effects occur 1.5 to 2 hours after ingestion of about 20 mg/kg. Most patients recover from tremor and ataxia in 4 to 8 hours. Animal studies indicate that clinical signs of toxicity include tremors, abnormal breathing, spasticity of the legs, and seizures. Parasympathetic findings include diarrhea, lacrimation, salivation, and nasal discharge. The increase in body temperature is dose-related.

REFERENCES—IBOGAINE

1. Schneider JA, Sigg EB. Neuropharmacological studies on ibogaine, an indole alkaloid with central stimulant properties. Ann NY Acad Sci 1956;66:766–776.
2. Endabuse[R] (ibogaine hydrochloride). Staten Island, NY: NDA International.
3. Isbell H. Preliminary trials with ibogaine. Personal communication to Ciba. USPHS Hospital, Addiction Research Center, Lexington, KY. November 1956.
4. Dhahir HI. A comparative study on the toxicity of serotonin. Doctoral dissertation, Indiana University, University Microfilms International 71–25–34. 1971:pharmacology, p. 151.
5. Maissoneuve IM, Keller RW, Glick SD. Interactions between ibogaine, a potential anti-addictive agent, and morphine: An in vivo microdialysis study. Eur J Pharmacol 1991;199: 35–42.
6. Schneider JA, Rinhart RR. Analysis of the cardiovascular action of ibogaine hydrochloride. Arch Int Pharmacodyn 1957;110:92–102.
7. Mash DC, Staley JK, Baumann MH, et al. Identification of a primary metabolite of ibogaine that targets serotonin transporters and elevates serotonin. Life Sci 1995;57:45–50.
8. Clouet NH. Personal communication.
9. O'Hearn EO, Molliver ME. Degeneration of Purkinje cells in parasagittal zones of cerebellar vermis after treatment with ibogaine or harmaline. Neuroscience 1993;55:363–370.

Chapter 50
Muscle Relaxants

INTRODUCTION

Skeletal muscle relaxants used to relieve spasticity include baclofen, diazepam (and other benzodiazepines), chlormezanone, methocarbamol, carisoprodol, cyclobenzaprine, orphenadrine, and dantrolene.[1] Chlormezanone is a tranquilizer with muscle relaxant properties.[2] Carisoprodol has skeletal muscle relaxant properties, which may be largely secondary to its related sedation. Overdose with baclofen may be more common than heretofore presumed and is discussed in this section.[3–9] Diazepam is discussed in detail in Chapter 36. Dantrolene has rarely been reported in overdose. Chlormezanone has been the subject of a few reports of poisoning,[2] and methocarbamol has been involved in a few fatalities associated with overdose.[10] Carisoprodol is discussed in a later section. Symptoms of overdose with antispasticity agents appear to be an exaggeration of therapeutically desired effects; generally, there is diminished consciousness or coma, profound muscle hypotonia, absent limb reflexes, and respiratory depression. Laboratory studies are usually normal. Patients given good supportive care usually survive.[11]

BACLOFEN, DIAZEPAM, DANTROLENE, CHLORMEZANONE, AND METHOCARBAMOL

Structure and Classification

Baclofen is the β-(*p*-chlorophenyl) derivative of the inhibitory neurotransmitter γ-aminobutyric acid (GABA).[12] As GABA itself is a strongly polar and hydrophilic substance, and cannot penetrate the blood–brain barrier, a lipophilic substance was added to the molecule.[13]

Dantrolene sodium is a hydantoin derivative, 1-([5-(*p*-nitrophenyl)furfurylidene]amino) hydantoin sodium salt hydrate.[13] Diazepam is a benzodiazepine; chlormezanone is a substituted metathiazonone[14]; methocarbamol is a carbamate derivative (guaiphenesin carbamate).[15]

Source

Baclofen, diazepam, dantrolene, chlormezanone, and methocarbamol are synthetic chemicals.

Use

Baclofen, diazepam, and dantrolene are used to alleviate spasticity, clonus, spinal automatic movements, flexor spasms, and associated pain in patients with multiple sclerosis and spinal disorders.[1,16,17] Intrathecal baclofen is available in the United States for amelioration of spasticity caused by multiple sclerosis or spinal cord injury in patients unresponsive to oral baclofen under a Treatment Investigational New Drug Application granted March 1990 by the Food and Drug Administration. (manufacturer's telephone number: 1–800–328–0810).[18] Respiratory depression, somnolence, and coma have been observed with this route of administration.[19] Chlormezanone is mainly a tranquilizer that may have some muscle relaxant qualities.[20] Methocarbamol is used for the symptomatic relief of muscle spasm.[15] Dantrolene may also have a use in treating malignant hyperthermia[21] and possibly neuroleptic malignant syndrome.[22] Dantrolene appears to diminish hyperthermic states and muscle rigidity associated with amphetamine overdose,[23] carbon monoxide poisoning,[24] monoamine oxidase overdose,[25] and organophosphate poisoning.[26] Confirmation of its usefulness for these indications requires further controlled studies. Dantrolene was not effective in a controlled study of heat stroke.[27,28] Dantrolene appears to be useful in controlling the hypermetabolic state associated with the rhabdomyolysis secondary to theophylline poisoning.[29]

Baclofen is probably used more often as an antispasticity drug of choice, because it is often effective at doses that are free of undesired side effects.[1] Baclofen has been effective in relieving intractable hiccups. This effect may be due to its action in mimicking the inhibitory neurotransmitter GABA.[30,31] Diazepam and chlormezanone cause more sedation, and dantrolene is associated with hepatotoxicity.[32]

Product Formulation

Baclofen	Oral scored tablets, 10 and 20 mg: Lioresal (Geigy); available throughout the world (Ciba, Geigy).
Diazepam	See Benzodiazepines in Chapter 36.
Dantrolene sodium	Oral capsules, 25 mg, 50 and 100 mg: Dantrium (Norwich Eaton); Procter & Gamble, Dantamacrin; parenteral for injection, 20 mg: Dantrium Intravenous (with mannitol 3 g, Norwich Eaton), Procter & Gamble.
Chlormezanone (chlormethazonone)	Oral scored tablets, 100 and 200 mg: Trancopal Caplets (Winthrop–Breon); Trancopal throughout the world; Supotran (France); Muskel (Germany); Rexan (Italy); Chlormedinon (Japan).
Methocarbamol	Oral scored tablets, 500 mg: Delaxin, Robaxin, Robomol-500; 750 mg: Marbaxin-750, Robasin-750, Robomol-750; Lumirelax (France); Miowas (Italy); Traumacut (Germany); parenteral, 100 mg/mL: Robaxin (with 50% polyethylene glycol 300). Combination oral 400-mg tablets with aspirin 325 mg: Robaxisal, Robaxical-Forte (United Kingdom).[14,15]

Therapeutic Dose (Adult)

Baclofen	40–80 mg/d
Dantrolene	150–225 mg/d
Chlormezanone	100–200 mg three to four times daily
Methocarbamol	4–4.5 g daily

After administration of baclofen 40 to 80 mg/d orally, 50 to 500 μg has been used intrathecally during the investigation phase for treatment of severe spasticity. The solution of baclofen was injected directly into the subarachnoid space by a programmable pump. Continuous infusion over 24 hours for each patient was calculated on the basis of toxicokinetic parameters after administration of a single dose.[33]

Toxic Dose

Adult patients have ingested up to 1125 mg of baclofen and survived.[34] Ingestion of 1250 to 2500 mg by one patient led to a fatality.[8] Serious poisoning has occurred with doses of 150 and 300 mg in adults. Ingestion of 4 g of chlormezanone with 1500 mg of diclofenac sodium led to some transient confusion and hypotonia; the patient recovered.[35]

Toxicokinetics

Absorption

Baclofen is almost completely absorbed from the gastrointestinal tract.[12] Its bioavailability is considered to be 70 to 80% complete.[36] A single oral dose of 40 mg begins to act in 30 to 45 minutes.[37] Plasma levels for the unchanged drug peak within 2 hours (approximately 0.3–0.6 μg/mL). A metabolite formed by deamination and oxidation (β-[*p*-chlorophenyl])-γ-hydroxybutyric acid) peaks at 4 hours (< 0.2 μg/mL). The activity of the metabolite has not been clinically evaluated. Total peak drug levels (drug and metabolites) for a 10-mg oral dose average about 0.3 μg/mL; for 20 mg, 0.4 μg/mL; and for 40 mg, 0.6 μg/mL.[12]

Following oral administration of 50 mg of dantrolene, plasma concentrations of dantrolene (0.5–0.95 μg/mL) and 5-hydroxydantrolene (0.11–0.3 μg/mL) peak in 4 to 8 hours and 6 to 8 hours, respectively.[13] Peak blood concentrations of 4.3 to 6.5 μg/mL were found in subjects with suspected or proven malignant hyperthermia who received 2.5 mg/kg intravenously before surgery.[38] Dantrolene 2.4 mg/kg administered intravenously to children resulted in blood dantrolene concentrations of 6 μg/mL within 1 minute of the end of infusion. The whole blood concentration of 5-hydroxydantrolene reached a maximum of 0.60 μg/mL approximately 7 hours after the dantrolene. When malignant hyperthermia susceptible patients were given 5 mg/kg oral dantrolene in up to four doses every 6 hours prior to surgery (last dose, 4 hours before surgery), plasma dantrolene levels averaged 2.8 μg/mL at induction of anesthesia and remained at this level for 6 hours and, in some patients, for 18 hours.[39,40] Baclofen is 30% bound to plasma proteins.

Methocarbamol 1.5 g orally induces a peak blood level of about 23 μg/mL in 1.1 hours. Protein binding ranges between 46 and 50%.[41] Therapeutic blood levels are reported to range from 16 to 41 μg/mL.[42]

Distribution

Baclofen has a distribution time of 1.29 ± 0.7 hours (alpha half-life, 0.54 hour).[36] The apparent volume of distribution is about 0.8 L/kg.[36] Tissue studies have not been performed in humans. Animal studies indicate a wide tissue distribution[12] (liver, kidneys) with slow release from brain and nervous tissue.[16] Approximately 30% of baclofen is bound to blood proteins in humans.[12]

The apparent volume of distribution of dantrolene is 0.65 L/kg.[43] Dantrolene interacts with human serum albumin in vitro but its binding to serum proteins has not been reported. Methocarbamol exhibits a half-life of 1.14 hours in normal control subjects.[41]

Elimination

Approximately 85 to 90%[12,16] of an oral dose of baclofen is excreted unchanged in the urine; 10% is excreted in the feces. In the first 6 hours, two thirds of the drug is excreted, by 24 hours, 80% has been excreted; and by 72 hours, all has been excreted. Prior to excretion, perhaps 15% is deaminated in the liver, where it also undergoes oxidation (see Absorption) and enters the Krebs cycle.[9] The elimination half-life averages about 3.6 hours[36] and ranges from 2 to 6 hours.[12] Baclofen half-life in overdose may rise to 34.6 hours[5] or longer. The intrathecal baclofen elimination half-life ranged from 0.9 to 5 hours, and the clearance, from 13 to 8 mL/h[29] suggesting that baclofen remains longer in the cerebrospinal fluid than in the plasma. Chlormezanone, after a single oral dose of 400 mg,[44] exhibited a mean half-life of 24 hours; this value rose to 29 hours after a 6-g overdose in another patient.[2]

After intravenous dantrolene administration in children, the elimination half-life of dantrolene was approximately 10.0 hours[39]; the elimination half-life of hydroxydantrolene was 9.0 hours. In a study of patients with malignant hypertension the mean elimination half-life was 12 hours.[38] Hydroxydantrolene appears to be active as a muscle antispasmodic agent in animals.[45] Approximately 15 to 25% of an orally administered dose of dantrolene is excreted renally, almost 80% appears as 5-hydroxydantrolene, and 4% is excreted as unchanged drug. The renal clearance of 5-hydroxydantrolene is 1.8 to 7.8 L/h.[3]

Drug Interactions

As baclofen is a neuronal depressant in the central nervous system, it may potentiate other sedative drugs such as diazepam and alcohol.[3] Ibuprofen-induced renal insufficiency led to baclofen toxicity in one 64-year-old man under treatment for spinal cord injury.[44] Animal studies demonstrate an increase in lethality with a concomitant decrease in seizures when dantrolene is added to theophylline.[46] Complete heart block developed in animals pretreated with verapamil who were than given dantrolene.[47] Ethanol and methocarbamol (a carbamate) taken together can lead to severe central nervous system depression and death.[42]

Pregnancy/Lactation

Insufficient data are available regarding the passage of baclofen, chlormezanone, or methocarbamol through the placenta or into breast milk. Dantrolene is known to cross the placental barrier.[48]

Mechanism of Action

Baclofen acts mainly as a mimetic of GABA in the spinal cord, blocking the excitatory effects of the sensory input from limb muscles. It inhibits both monosynaptic (H reflex) and polysynaptic flexor transmissions, but has no effect on neuromuscular transmission.[16] Baclofen is not a GABA receptor agonist, but appears to act at a novel site on the nerve terminal[49]; however, it is as active as GABA in reducing evoked transmitter output.[49] Baclofen is also thought to inhibit substance P, which normally acts to stimulate monoaminergic neurons in the brainstem.[50] In animals, baclofen produces a diminution of norepinephrine and epinephrine content in heart muscle.[3] In humans, baclofen produces a deep coma and respiratory depression. The mechanisms of action for these effects have not been elucidated.[3]

Diazepam probably acts by enhancing the response to locally released GABA. Its action on the spinal cord is independent of an action in the brain.[1] Dantrolene acts peripherally on the muscle itself by interfering with release of calcium from the sarcoplasmic reticulum, thus preventing membrane excitation leading to contraction.[1]

Dantrolene sodium acts in the treatment of hypercatabolic syndromes such as malignant hyperthermia and neuroleptic malignant syndrome by affecting calcium flux across the sarcoplasmic reticulum of skeletal muscle cells, resulting in rapid resolution of hyperthermia, dysrhythmias, muscle rigidity, tachycardia, hypercapnia, and metabolic acidosis.[51]

Clinical Presentation

The clinical features of baclofen overdose in both adults and children include coma, muscle flaccidity, hyporeflexia, and respiratory depression.[52]

Baclofen

Overdose

Neurologic Effects. On admission, the severely poisoned patient may be tearful and agitated,[6] but within 3 to 5 hours, patients become flaccid, have absent limb reflexes, develop a deep coma, become unresponsive to pain stimuli, have no spontaneous respirations, and exhibit absence of the ciliospinal reflex, doll's-eyes response, and ice-water caloric response.[3,53] Involuntary movements may be observed[3] initially, with grand mal seizures[3,4] developing 6 hours after ingestion.[3] In 12 published cases of intrathecal overdose, seizures were not reported.[54] Inadvertent intrathecal administration of 10 mg of baclofen into a brain-injured patient led to somnolence, flaccidity, nystagmus, and respiratory depression, all of which did not respond to physostigmine. Status epilepticus responded to removal of 30 mL of cerebrospinal fluid.[55]

Muscle twitching and jerking are often noted throughout the course of treatment until recovery. Behavior disturbances and delirium have been observed.[8] Akinetic mutism followed one 10-mg dose of baclofen in an adult with end-stage renal failure.[56]

In another study, seven events of intrathecal baclofen overdose (sedation, coma, respiratory depression) occurred in five patients. The doses resulting in coma ranged from 50 μg administered as a bolus to 1500 μg/24 h infused continuously. Physostigmine was not always effective in reversing these symptoms. Lumbar puncture drainage (eg, 30 mL) was useful in such cases. This approach together with symptomatic treatment (cardiac respiratory monitoring, airway patency, ventilating adequacy, oxygen) in an intensive care environment probably offers a safer alternative than physostigmine used alone as an antidote.[57]

A 30-year-old man probably ingested between 1000 and 1800 mg of baclofen, became comatose, and died in 5 days.[58]

Cardiovascular Effects. Hypotension and hypertension have been observed after baclofen overdose[8]; normal sinus rhythm, sinus bradycardia, and supraventricular tachyarrhythmia have also been seen.[59]

Other Effects. Hypothermia[4,6] or normal temperature may be seen. Extremities may become blue and mottled.[4] Consciousness and muscle and neurologic function may not return for several days. This may be due to the slow elimination rate of baclofen from nerve tissue[12] or the use of diazepam to control convulsions.[5] Evidence of cerebral edema at autopsy was reported in one fatal case.[8] A 10-mg bolus of baclofen was inadvertently delivered into the intrathecal space. Within 80 minutes the patient developed nystagmus, flaccidity, absence of tendon jerks, and coma.[60] The patient recovered after 6 days of symptomatic therapy.

Chronic Use

Neurologic Effects. Fatigue, lassitude, giddiness, mental confusion, depression, headaches, euphoria, and muscle weakness may be observed.[16] In two patients with epilepsy, electroencephalographic deterioration was observed.[16]

Gastrointestinal Effects. Nausea, vomiting, and diarrhea have been observed.

Withdrawal. Abrupt cessation of baclofen after its use for many months[61] may lead within 12 to 96 hours[37,53] to grand mal seizures, auditory and visual hallucinations, paranoid ideas, insomnia, confusion, buccolingual dyskinesias, sleeplessness, agitation, belligerence, hyperactivity, and grandiose ideas. Such symptoms may last up to 8 days.[61] This experience is similar to that seen after similar withdrawal from the benzodiazepines, chlormezanone, and many sedative–hypnotic drugs.[50,53,61,62] As there may be a "rebound" effect from the rapid release of inhibition of substance, restoring baclofen in normal dosage with gradual tapering may be an effective approach to management.[62] An acute withdrawal syndrome may follow cessation of intrathecal baclofen in a patient with spasticity.[63]

Anecdotal case reports suggest that patients with preexisting brain dysfunction or a family history of seizures may be at increased risk of baclofen withdrawal seizures, even after short-term administration.[64]

Chlormezanone

Therapeutic dosages may be associated with a hypersensitivity type of hepatitis whose onset is 1 to 2 months after ingestion. Overdose (12 g) has been followed by an abrupt elevation of liver enzymes.[65]

Dantrolene

Overdose

General Effects. Use of dantrolene as emergency therapy in acute anesthetic or neuroleptic-induced malignant hyperthermia or as a prophylactic measure in patients with known susceptibility to these syndromes is short term; few adverse effects are observed, except for a possible local inflammatory phlebitis at the injection site.[45] Use of oral dantrolene as a prophylactic drug in patients suspected to be susceptible to malignant hyperthermia may induce nausea, vomiting, dizziness, and diarrhea.

Cardiovascular Effects. An adult patient given gradually increasing daily doses of dantrolene to 250 mg developed acute pulmonary edema and severe cardiac insufficiency after 11 days of therapy. Myocardial function returned to normal when drug treatment was stopped.[66]

Overdoses of dantrolene in three patients (20-month-old child, 25-year-old adult, and 23-year-old second-trimester pregnant woman) were reported following doses of 10 to 12 mg/kg, comparable to maximal intravenous recommendations. The child and pregnant woman exhibited no symptoms; only lethargy was noted in the 25-year-old. All routine chemistry, hematology, and urinary laboratory tests were normal. The patients were treated supportively and recovered uneventfully. The pregnant woman delivered a healthy child at term.[67]

Chronic Use. After at least 2 months of therapy with oral dantrolene, patients may develop hepatotoxicity, which can be fatal.[68–71]

Laboratory

Analytic Methods

Accurate plasma levels of baclofen are available with use of a gas–liquid chromatography method.[72] Dantrolene and its reduced and oxidized metabolites in plasma may be determined by high-performance liquid chromatography (HPLC). This method uses a small amount of plasma (50 μL) and has a sensitivity of 1.0 μg/mL.[73] A HPLC method has a limit of detection of 0.8 μg/mL.[58] Plasma methocarbamol concentrations are fluorometrically determined by HPLC with a sensitivity to 200 ng/mL.[41]

A reverse-phase HPLC method can detect quantities of baclofen in plasma and urine to 5 ng.[58,74] HPLC with ultraviolet detection can rapidly quantitate baclofen and its γ-hydroxy metabolite in urine.[75]

Blood Levels

Plasma baclofen levels are confirmatory of a clinical diagnosis but do not function to dictate management, which must remain supportive and based on clinical evaluations. A secondary blood level peak is observed after recovery of consciousness[4,5] and may reflect either a release of the lipophilic drug from lipid stores or evidence of enterohepatic recycling of baclofen. Toxic blood levels have been reported to range from 1100 to 3500 ng/mL (therapeutic plasma trough concentrations after baclofen 15–90 mg range from 100–400 ng/mL).[58] Blood levels following a baclofen ingestion of probably between 1000 and 1800 mg averaged 17 μg/mL (17,000 ng/mL). The urine baclofen concentration was 760 μg/mL.[58] Ingestions of baclofen 1 to 1.8 g led to coma and death in 5 days with serum and urine baclofen concentrations of 17 and 760 μg/mL, respectively.[58]

Ancillary Tests

The electrocardiogram is usually within normal limits; occasional transient elevations of lactic dehydrogenase and aspartate transaminase levels have been observed.[3] The chest x-ray and liver and kidney function tests are usually within normal limits.[8]

Treatment

Patients may be conscious on admission but may quickly lapse into a deep coma with profound respiratory and generalized flaccidity. Treatment of severe overdose should be provided in a hospital intensive care facility with adequate respiratory assistance available. Such care may be required for several days before unassisted ventilation is resumed by the patient.

Stabilization

The airway should be maintained by endotracheal intubation if respiratory depression or obstruction occurs. Assisted ventilation is frequently required early after an overdose because of the severe respiratory depression that quickly supervenes.[7,9] The tidal volume should be at least 10 to 15 mL/kg.

Continuous monitoring of electrocardiogram, pulse (bradycardia), respiration, and temperature (hypothermia frequent in overdose), periodic evaluation of renal and hepatic function, and encephalographic evaluation are useful during coma and after return of consciousness.

Gut Decontamination

Syrup of ipecac should be used with caution, as absorption of baclofen is rapid and obtundation and coma develop rapidly. Gastric lavage with endotracheal intubation should be performed as early as possible after ingestion of an overdose (>100–400 mg, adult; 5 mg/kg, child)[7] of baclofen.

Activated charcoal can be introduced through the gastric lavage tube; cathartics have not been evaluated in the treatment of baclofen overdose.

Elimination Enhancement

Forced diuresis may be useful in view of the excretion of baclofen (largely unchanged) in the urine.[7,8,12,16] NaCl 0.45% in 5% dextrose in water and a diuretic such as furosemide 1 mg/kg to a maximum of 40 mg in a single dose can be administered to obtain a urine flow of 3 to 6 mL/kg/h. Careful attention should be given to central nervous system signs (pupils, doll's eyes, ice-water calorics, electroencephalogram), state of consciousness, renal function, electrolytes, fluid balance, and arterial blood gases while fluids are administered.

Enhancement of elimination of baclofen by extracorporeal means (peritoneal dialysis, hemodialysis) has not been evaluated; however, the low degree of protein binding and the excretion of almost all baclofen as unchanged drug may favor such measures in the treatment of overdose of this product. Patients with overdoses reported to date have all recovered without use of these procedures.

Antidote

No specific antidote is available for the treatment of overdose with baclofen, chlormezanone, methocarbamol, or dantrolene. Anecdotal reports suggest that intravenous flumazenil 0.3 mg followed by 0.1 mg/h may counteract coma and respiratory depression associated with intrathecal baclofen administration[76]; however, preliminary data in three patients who experienced an intrathecal baclofen overdose (80-, 150-, and 80-μg boluses, respectively) suggest a role for intravenous physostigmine in treatment. Respiratory depression, somnolence, coma, pinpoint pupils, and areflexia appeared to respond to a dose of 1 to 2 mg of physostigmine. Physostigmine was prepared by diluting 4 mg of the commercial physostigmine salicylate solution (2 ampules of 2 mg/2 ml in the United States) in a 100-mL bag of sterile saline for injection, yielding a concentration of approximately 0.04 mg/mL. This was placed in an intravenous infusion pump and dispensed at a flow rate of 5 mL/min (0.2 mg/min) for 5 to 10 minutes, yielding a total dose of 1 to 2 mg. Repeat doses of 1 to 2 mg were administered if there was improvement in respiration and alertness. Intubation should be instituted to provide adequate respiration as required. Precautions and dangers associated with physostigmine use (lacrimation, miosis, salivation, bradycardia, heart block, gut and bladder spasms, diarrhea, seizures, asystole, bronchospasm) are discussed elsewhere in this volume. In any event, physostigmine should not be administered to patients with cardiorespiratory depression.[54]

Supportive Measures

Patients with signs and symptoms of overdose following baclofen ingestion should be hospitalized in an intensive care unit. Children who have ingested more than 5 mg/kg or adults who have ingested more than 100 mg should also be admitted to the unit.

Supportive management is the mainstay of care for overdose with the antispasticity drugs. Coma with baclofen may continue for several days after an overdose despite its therapeutic half-life of 3 to 4 hours.

Seizures following baclofen overdose should be managed with intravenous diazepam. If there is an inadequate response to diazepam (0.25 mg/kg up to 10 mg/dose intravenously for adults, repeated every 15 minutes as necessary; 0.25–0.4 mg/kg/dose up to 10 mg/dose for a child), then intravenous phenytoin may be required.

Hypotension can be managed by placing the patient in Trendelenburg position, starting an infusion of intravenous fluids, and, if required, administering pressor amines (dopamine or norepinephrine). Intravenous atropine 600 μg was temporarily effective in elevating depressed body temperature, increasing respiratory tidal volume, and restoring depressed heart rate and blood pressure.[6] Sinus tachycardia may be responsive to propranolol.[5] Baclofen withdrawal hallucinations can be managed by reintroducing the drug and tapering it gradually. Withdrawal reactions occur after use of baclofen for many months and have not been reported after acute poisonings.[77]

Monitoring of central nervous system function, renal function, complete blood counts, electrolytes, arterial blood gases, and hepatic function provides guidelines for determination of time of discharge from the intensive care unit.[78]

REFERENCES—INTRODUCTION; BACLOFEN, DANTROLENE, CHLORMEZANONE, AND METHOCARBAMOL

1. Drugs to relieve spasticity. Drugs Ther Bull 1983;21(1):1–3.
2. Armstrong D, Braithwaite RA, Vale JA. Chlormezanone poisoning. Br Med J 1983;286:846–847.
3. Paulson GW. Overdose of Lioresal. Neurology 1976;26:1105–1106.
4. Lipscomb DJ, Meredith TJ. Baclofen overdose. Postgrad Med J 1980;56:108–109.
5. Ghose K, Holmes KM, Matthewson K. Complications of baclofen overdosage. Postgrad Med J 1980;56:865–867.
6. Ferner RE. Atropine treatment for baclofen overdose. Postgrad Med J 1981;57:580–581.
7. Blankenship JMK, Moses ES. Baclofen overdose in a child resulting in respiratory arrest. Vet Hum Toxicol 1983;25 (suppl. 1):45–46.
8. Haubenstock A, Aruby K, Jager U, et al. Baclofen (Lioresal[R]) intoxication: Report of 4 cases and review of the literature. Clin Toxicol 1983;20(1):59–68.
9. May CR. Baclofen overdose. Ann Emerg Med 1983;12: 171–173.
10. Kemal M, Imami R, Poklis A. A fatal methocarbamol intoxication. J Forensic Sci 1982;27:217–222.
11. Lebby TI, Dugger K, Lipscomb JW, Leikin JB. Skeletal muscle relaxant ingestion. Vet Hum Toxicol 1990;32: 133–135.
12. Faigle JW, Keberle H. The chemistry and kinetics of Lioresal. Postgrad Med J 1972;October suppl.:9–13.
13. Katogi Y, Tamaki N, Adachi M, et al. Simultaneous determination of dantrolene and its metabolite, 5-hydroxydantrolene, in human plasma by high-performance liquid chromatography. J Chromatogr 1982;228:404–408.
14. Chlormezanone. In: McEvoy GK, ed. *AHFS Drug Information 94.* Bethesda, MD: American Society of Hospital Pharmacists, 1994:1521.
15. Reynolds JEF, ed. *Martindale: The Extra Pharmacopoeia.* 30th ed. London: Pharmaceutical Press, 1993:1205–1206.
16. Brogden RN, Speight TM, Avery GS. Baclofen: A preliminary report of its pharmacological properties and therapeutic efficacy in spasticity. Drugs 1974;8:1–14.
17. Muller H, Borner V, Zierski J, Hempelmann G. Intrathecal baclofen in tetanus. Lancet 1986;1:317–318.
18. Promising drugs available under treatment IND. FDA Drug Bull 1990(April);20(1):10.
19. Penn RD, Kroin JS. Intrathecal baclofen. N Engl J Med 1989; 321:1414–1415.
20. Baldessarini RJ. Drugs and the treatment of psychiatric disorders. In: Gilman AG, Goodman LS, Rall TW, et al., eds. *The Pharmacological Basis of Therapeutics.* 7th ed. New York: Macmillan, 1985:437.
21. Waterman PM. Malignant hyperthermia syndrome. Am J Ophthalmol 1981;92:461–465.
22. Bismuth C, de Rohan-Chabot P, Goulon M, et al. Dantroline: A new therapeutic approach to the neuroleptic malignant syndrome. Acta Neurol Scand 1984;70(suppl. 100):193–198.
23. Barone JA, Peppers MP. Use of dantrolene in the management of amphetamine-induced hyperthermia. Clin Pharm 1989;8:324–325.
24. Ten Holter JBM, Schellens RLLAM. Dantrolene sodium for treatment of carbon monoxide poisoning. Br Med J 1988; 296;1772–1773.
25. Kaplan RF, Feinglass NG, Webster W, Mudra S. Phenelzine overdose treated with dantrolene sodium. JAMA 1986; 255:642–644.
26. Shemesh I, Bourvin A, Gold D, Kutscherowsky M. Chlorpyrifos poisoning treated with ipratropium and dantrolene: A case report. Clin Toxicol 1988;26:495–498.
27. Bouchama A, Cafege A, Devol EB, et al. Ineffectiveness of dantrolene sodium in the treatment of heat stroke. Crit Care Med 1991;19:176–180.
28. Channa AB, Seraj MA, Saddique AA, et al. Is dantrolene effective in heat stroke patients? Crit Care Med 1990;18: 290–293.
29. Parr MJA, Willatts SM. Fatal theophylline poisoning with rhabdomyolysis: A potential role for dantrolene treatment. Anaesthesia 1991;46:557–559.
30. Bhalotra R. Baclofen therapy for intractable hiccoughs. J Clin Gastroenterol 1990;12:122.
31. Intractable hiccup: Baclofen and nifedipine are worth trying. Drug Ther Bull 1990;12(9):36.
32. Durham JA, Gandolfi AJ, Bentley JB. Hepatotoxicological evaluation of dantrolene sodium. Drug Chem Toxicol 1984; 7(1):23–40.
33. Sallerin-Caute B, Lazorthes Y, Monsarrat B, et al. CSF baclofen levels after intrathecal administration in severe spasticity. Eur J Clin Pharmacol 1991;40:363–365.
34. Andersen P, Noher H, Swahn CG. Pharmacokinetics in baclofen overdose. Clin Toxicol 1984;22:11–20.
35. Netter P, Lambert H, Larcan A, et al. Diclofenac sodium–chlormezanone poisoning. Eur J Clin Pharmacol 1984; 26:535–536.
36. Kochak GM, Rakhit A, Wagner WE, et al. The pharmacokinetics of baclofen derived from intestinal infusion. Clin Pharmacol Ther 1985;38:251–257.
37. Garabedian-Ruffalo SM, Ruffalo RL. Adverse effects secondary to baclofen withdrawal. Drug Intell Clin Pharm 1985;19: 304–306.
38. Flewellyn EH, Nelson TE. Intravenous dantrolene pharmacokinetics in malignant hyperthermia suspect patients. Anesthesiology 1985;63(suppl. 3A):300.
39. Lerman J, McLeod ME, Strong HA. Pharmacokinetics of intravenous dantrolene in children. Anesthesiology 1989;70: 625–629.
40. Allen GC, Cattran CB, Peterson RG, Lalande M. Plasma levels of dantrolene following oral administration in malignant hyperthermia susceptible patients. Anesthesiology 1988;69: 900–904.
41. Sica DA, Comstock TJ, Davis J, et al. Pharmacokinetics and protein binding of methocarbamol in renal insufficiency and normals. Eur J Clin Pharmacol 1990;39:193–194.
42. Ferslew KE, Hagardorn AN, McCormick WF. A fatal interaction of methocarbamol and ethanol in an accidental poisoning. J Forens Sci 1990;35:477–482.
43. Comunale ME, DiNardo JA, Schwartz MJ. Pharmacokinetics of dantrolene in an adult patient undergoing cardiopulmonary bypass. J Cardiothor Vasc Anesth 1991;5:153–155.
44. McChesney EW, Banks WF Jr, Portmann GA, et al. Metabolism of chlormezanone in man and laboratory animals. Biochem Pharmacol 1967;16:813–826.
45. Ward A, Chaffman MO, Sorkin EM. Dantrolene: A review of its pharmacodynamic and pharmacokinetic properties and therapeutic use in malignant hyperthermia, the neuroleptic malignant syndrome and an update of its use in muscle spasticity. Drugs 1986;32:130–168.
46. Tayeb OS. A serious interaction of dantrolene and theophylline. Vet Hum Toxicol 1990;32:442–443.
47. Salzman LS, Kates RA, Corke GC, et al. Hyperkalemia and cardiovascular collapse after verapamil and dantrolene administration in swine. Anesth Analg 1984;63:473–478.

48. Dahlin PA, George J. Baclofen toxicity associated with declining renal clearing after ibuprofen. Drug Intell Clin Pharm 1984;18:805–808.
49. Morison DH. Placental transfer of dantrolene. Anesthesiology 1983;59:265.
50. Bowery NG, Hill DR, Hudson AL, et al. (–) Baclofen decreases neurotransmitter release in the mammalian CNS by an action at a novel GABA receptor. Nature 1980;283:92–94.
51. Van de Kelft E, de Hert M, Heytens L, et al. Management of lethal catatonia with dantrolene sodium. Crit Care Med 1991; 19:1449–1451.
52. Cooke DEM, Glasstone MA. Baclofen poisoning in children. Vet Hum Toxicol 1994;35:448–450.
53. Arnold ES, Rudd SM, Kirshner H. Manic psychosis following rapid withdrawal from baclofen. Am J Psychiatry 1980;137: 1466–1467.
54. Muller-Schwefer G, Penn RD. Physostigmine in the treatment of intrathecal baclofen overdose. J Neurosurg 1989;71: 273–275.
55. Saltuari L, Marosi MJ, Kopler M, Bauer G. Status epilepticus complicating intrathecal overdose. Lancet 1992;339: 373–374.
56. Parmar MS. Akinetic mutism after baclofen. Ann Intern Med 1991;115:499–500.
57. Delhaas EM, Brouwers JRBJ. Intrathecal baclofen overdose: Report of 7 events in 5 patients and review of the literature. Int J Clin Pharmacol Ther Toxicol 1991;29:274–280.
58. Fraser AD, MacNeil W, Isner AF. Toxicological analysis of a fatal baclofen (Lioresal[R]) ingestion. J Forens Sci 1991;36: 1596–1602.
59. Roberge RJ, Marton TG, Hodgman M, et al. Supraventricular tachyarrhythmia associated with baclofen overdose. Clin Toxicol 1994;32:291–297.
60. Kofler M, Saltuari L, Schumatzhard E, et al. Electrophysiological findings in a case of severe intrathecal baclofen overdose. Electroencephalogr Clin Neurophysiol 1992;83:83–86.
61. Nugent S, Katz MD, Little TE. Baclofen overdose with cardiac conduction abnormalities: Case report and review of the literature. Clin Toxicol 1986;24:321–328.
62. Lees AJ, Clarke CRA, Harrison MJ. Hallucinations after withdrawal of baclofen. Lancet 1977;1:858.
63. Siegfried RN, Jacobson L, Chabal C. Development of an acute withdrawal syndrome following the cessation of intrathecal baclofen in a patient with spasticity. Anesthesiology 1992;77:1048–1050.
64. Kofler M, Leis AA. Prolonged seizure activity after baclofen withdrawal. Neurology 1992;42:697–698.
65. Sheu B-S, Lin C-Y, Chen K-W, Chi C-H, et al. Severe hepatocellular damage induced by chlormezanone overdose. Am J Gastroenterol 1995;90:833–835.
66. Paloucek FP, Erickson TE, Lundquist S, Ferraro C. Oral dantrolene ingestion: A case series. Vet Hum Toxicol 1991;33:362.
67. Robillart A, Bopp P, Vailly B, Dupeyron JP. Cardiac failure due to dantrolene overdose. Ann Fr Anesth Reanim 1986; 5:617–619.
68. Chan CH. Dantrolene sodium and hepatic injury. Neurology 1990;40:1427–1432.
69. Utili R, Boitnott JK, Zimmerman HJ. Dantrolene-associated hepatic injury. Gastroenterology 1977;72:610–616.
70. Wilkinson SP, Portmann B, Williams R. Hepatitis from dantrolene sodium. Gut 1979;20:33–36.
71. Cornette M, Gillard C, Borlee-Hermans G. Hepatite toxique mortelle associee a l'usage du dantrolene. Acta Neurol Belg 1980;80:336–347.
72. White WB. Aggravated CNS depression with urinary retention secondary to baclofen administration. Arch Intern Med 1984;145:1717–1718.
73. Lalande M, Mills P, Peterson RG. Determination of dantrolene and its reduced and oxidized metabolites in plasma by high-performance liquid chromatography. J Chromatogr 1988;430:187–191.
74. Wuis EW, Dirks RJM, Vree TB, Van den Kleyn E. High performance liquid chromatographic analysis of baclofen in plasma and urine of man after precolumn extraction and derivitization with o-phthaldialdehyde. J Chromatogr Biomed Appl 1985;337:341–350.
75. Wuis EW, Van Beijsterveldt LEC, Dirks RJM, et al. Rapid simultaneous determination of baclofen and its gamma-hydroxy metabolite in urine by high-performance liquid chromatography with ultraviolet detection. J Chromatogr 1987; 420:212–216.
76. Saissy JM, Vitris M, Demaziere J, et al. Flumazenil counteracts intrathecal and baclofen-induced central nervous system depression in tetanus. Anesthesiology 1992;76: 1051–1053.
77. Terrence CF, Fromm GH. Complications of baclofen withdrawal. Arch Neurol 1981;38:588–589.
78. Kochak G, Honc F. An unproved gas–liquid chromatographic method for the determination of baclofen in plasma and urine. J Chromatogr 1984;310:319–326.

CARISOPRODOL

Carisoprodol, a centrally acting skeletal muscle relaxant, is both structurally and pharmacologically related to meprobamate (Fig. 50–1), mebutamate, and tybamate.[1] Its skeletal muscle relaxant effects are minimal and are probably secondary to its sedative effect. It is not a neuromuscular blocking agent. It also has weak anticholinergic, antipyretic, and analgesic properties.[2,3] Poisoning with carisoprodol is reported infrequently, in part because it is relatively ineffective as a muscle relaxant. Overdose, however, can be fatal,[4] and similarities to meprobamate intoxication should be noted. Overdose patients who are symptomatic should be admitted for intensive observation.

Structure and Classification

Carisoprodol is *N*-isopropyl meprobamate (2-methyl-2-propyl-1-3-propanediol dicarbamate). It is a white odorless crystalline powder with a bitter taste. It is freely soluble in alcohol.[1,3]

Carisoprodol is also known as carisoprodate, isobamate, and isopropyl meprobamate. It is marketed as Caprodat (Sweden); Somadril (Denmark, Norway, Sweden); Carisoma (United Kingdom); Carisoma Compound (United Kingdom, containing carisoprodol, 175 mg, and acetaminophen, 350 mg); Flexartal (France); and Mioxom (Italy).

Source

Carisoprodol is a synthetic chemical related to meprobamate.

Use

Carisoprodol is used as an adjunct to analgesics, rest, and physical therapy for the relief of pain in acute musculoskeletal conditions. Its efficacy has not been established. Its relaxant effects may be related to its sedative properties.

Product Formulation

Oral tablets, 350 mg	Rela (with tartrazine); Sodol; Soma; Soprodol; Soridol
Oral tablets, 200 mg, with aspirin, 325 mg	Carisoprodol Compound; Sodol Compound; Soma Compound
Oral tablets, 200 mg, with aspirin, 325 mg, and codeine phosphate, 16 mg	Soma Compound with codeine[1]

Meprobamate

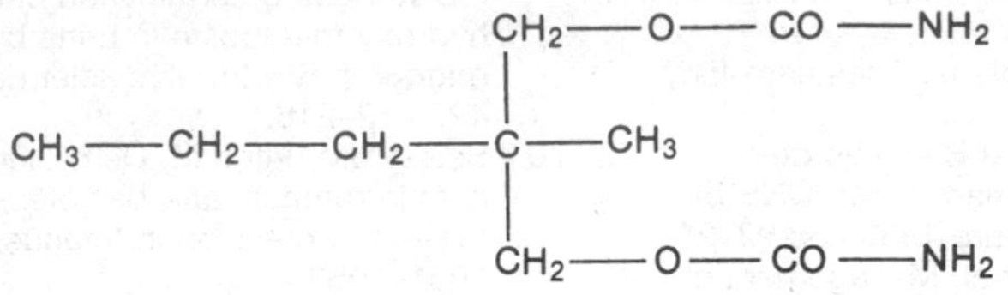

$$CH_3—CH_2—CH_2—C(CH_3)(CH_2—O—CO—NH_2)_2$$

2-Methyl-2-propyl-1,3-propanediol dicarbamate

Carisoprodol

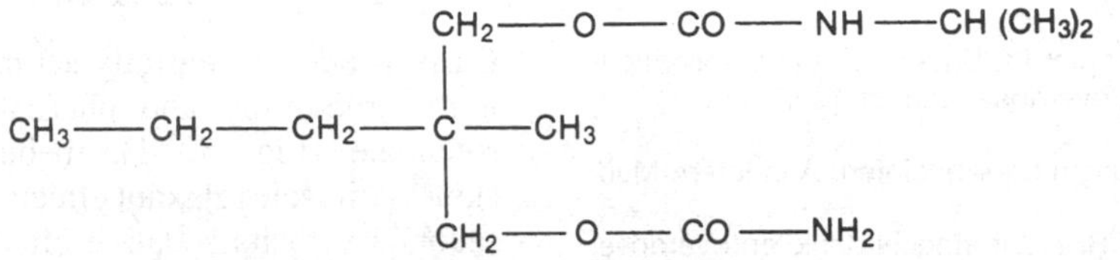

$$CH_3—CH_2—CH_2—C(CH_3)(CH_2—O—CO—NH—CH(CH_3)_2)(CH_2—O—CO—NH_2)$$

N-Isopropyl-2-methyl-2-propyl-1,3-propanediol dicarbamate

Figure 50–1 Structures of meprobamate and carisoprodol. (Adapted from Maes R, Bouche R, Laruelle L. Determination quantitative de meprobamate et de carisoprodol par chromatographie en phase gazeuse, dans different cas d'intoxications. Eur J Toxicol 1970;3:140–143.)

Therapeutic Dose

Carisoprodol is usually administered orally, 350 mg four times daily. Safe doses in children have not been established.

Toxic Dose

Severe toxic overdoses (central nervous system stimulation, depression, and death) have followed ingestion of 9.45 g, 8.40 g,[2] 3.5 g (in a child), and 14.7 g.[5]

Toxicokinetics

Absorption

Carisoprodol has a pK_a of 4.2. Two tablets (700 mg) of carisoprodol given to a normal individual produced peak serum levels of 9.3 μg/mL (carisoprodol) and 2.9 μg/mL (meprobamate) in 1 hour; the carisoprodol level decreased to 4.3 μg/mL in 2 hours, whereas the meprobamate level increased to 4.1 μg/mL. In another normal subject, levels were 0.7 and 5.4 μg/mL for carisoprodol and meprobamate 9 hours after ingestion.[5]

Distribution

Carisoprodol is rapidly distributed into the central nervous system.[6] Its apparent volume of distribution and protein binding in humans are not available.

Elimination

The drug is rapidly metabolized by dealkylation, hydroxylation, and conjugation in the liver. The rate of metabolite formation is greater than the absorption rate after normal doses.[6] Meprobamate is the major metabolite. Approximately 7.5% of carisoprodol is recoverable in the urine of the rat in 48 hours, and 0.3% in the feces.[7] In Goldberg's first patient, 5 g was excreted in the urine within the first 20 hours; but in patient 2, only 637 mg was excreted in the first 20 hours.[2] The assay method, however, measured both carisoprodol and meprobamate together.[8] Adams et al. found meprobamate to be the major metabolite excreted after overdose, with hydroxymeprobamate present in small quantities.[4]

Drug Interactions

Additive effects in relation to central nervous system depression with carisoprodol may follow concomitant use of alcohol, other central nervous system depressants, antihistamines, and/or anesthetics.

Pregnancy/Lactation

Carisoprodol is excreted in human milk in a concentration two to four times that in maternal plasma.[9] Its distribution through the placenta in humans has not been evaluated; however, animal data indicate penetration through the placenta.[6]

Mechanism of Action

Carisoprodol produces prolonged symptoms of central nervous system depression resulting from its metabolism to meprobamate.

Clinical Presentation

Overdose

Massive overdose has been implicated in the death of one patient,[2] but no details are available. Goldberg described two patients. An 18-year-old man took about 27 350 mg carisoprodol tablets (9.45 g).[2] In 2 hours he was drowsy and lethargic. After ipecac-induced emesis, he exhibited few signs except for a tachycardia and nystagmus on lateral gaze. He became uncooperative and required restraints. By 6 hours he was less drowsy, but had headache, dizziness, and double vision. At 8 hours he was awake and normal. Treatment was entirely supportive with intravenous fluids. He had amnesia for these events the next day. The second patient, a 20-year-old man, took 24 350-mg carisoprodol tablets (8.40 g). Three hours later his stomach was lavaged. He was then given syrup of ipecac and vomited. He was drowsy and complained of intermittent occipital headache, vertigo, objects floating before his eyes, and drowsiness. He had nystagmus on lateral gaze, diplopia, ataxia, slow speech, and tachycardia. He was treated supportively with intravenous fluids, and 12 hours after ingestion he was alert and neurologically normal. He had amnesia for these events the next day.

A boy 4 years and 10 months old ingested 10 350-mg tablets (3500 mg) of carisoprodol. He became stuporous and semicomatose. A cuffed endotracheal tube was inserted and the stomach lavaged. Blood count, urinalysis, serum glucose, serum calcium, electrolytes, and blood gases were within normal limits. He was comatose for 11 hours, then vomited, developed bilateral diffuse infiltrates and cardiac arrest, and died 36 hours after admission. The serum level of carisoprodol 4 hours after ingestion was 36.4 μg/mL, with a meprobamate level of 15 μg/mL. In the urine, meprobamate concentration was present in a ratio of about 7:1 to that of carisoprodol.[4]

A 19-year-old woman ingested 14.7 g of carisoprodol, had convulsions for 17 hours, and was unconscious for 33 hours. Tachycardia was present throughout. When she awoke the blood concentration of carisoprodol was 4.7 μg/mL, but the meprobamate concentration was 53.8 μg/mL.[5]

Chronic Use

Chronic adverse effects include skin rash, drowsiness, nausea, vomiting, vertigo, facial flush, fatigue, pruritus, ataxia, tremor, headache, irritability, epigastric distress, and fixed drug eruption.[2] Cross-reaction to meprobamate may occur. Carisoprodol may, like other skeletal muscle relaxants, become a drug of abuse.[10,11]

Laboratory

Analytical Methods

A colorimetric assay for carbamates is available,[8] and a more specific gas chromatography method for carisoprodol appears useful.[12]

Blood Levels

There appears to be a correlation of plasma levels of carisoprodol and meprobamate with sedation and toxic effects. Mild poisoning with slight stupor was observed in a patient with a blood carisoprodol level of 31 μg/mL.[12] Symptoms appeared at serum levels above 33 μg/mL in the case reported by Goldberg (see Overdose under Clinical Presentation). These levels decreased 70% in 20 hours, falling 92% in 48 hours.[2] Brandslung et al. measured levels of 13.4 μg/mL (carisoprodol) and 63.4 μg/mL (meprobamate) in an adult in coma, 19 hours after ingestion.[5]

Treatment

Stabilization

Patients with any symptoms of overdose should be carefully observed in a hospital care facility for at least 24 hours. If there is no evidence of overdose or other unexplained clinical signs or symptoms in the first 8 hours after ingestion, consideration may be given to discharge from intensive observation. Airway, breathing, and circulatory status should be monitored until the patient is awake and breathing normally. Assisted ventilation is probably not required in most cases.

Gut Decontamination

Emesis induction with syrup of ipecac or gastric lavage with prior tracheal protection may be useful within the first 3 to 4 hours. Drowsiness may occur within several hours of ingestion. Activated charcoal and cathartics may be of assistance, but there are no studies to establish their value. Following a carisoprodol overdose there is no evidence for the formation of gastric masses similar to those following meprobamate overdoses.

Elimination Enhancement

Intravenous fluids (5% dextrose in water or 5% dextrose in normal saline) should be administered only in sufficient quantity to maintain a normal urine flow. There are no data substantiating the use of forced diuresis, hemodialysis, peritoneal dialysis, exchange transfusion, charcoal or resin hemoperfusion, plasmapheresis, or whole-bowel irrigation. Meprobamate bezoar formation can usually be treated with gastric lavage and high dose activated charcoal.

Antidote

There is no antidote.

Supportive Measures

Supportive care is the mainstay of management for a carisoprodol overdose. Intravenous fluids to maintain normal urine flow for at least 24 hours are required until consciousness is restored, oral intake commences, and most of the drug and its metabolites has been excreted.

REFERENCES—CARISOPRODOL

1. McEvoy GK, ed. *AHFS Drug Information 86.* Bethesda, MD: American Society of Hospital Pharmacists, 1986:617–618.
2. Goldberg D. Carisoprodol toxicity. Milit Med 1969;134: 597–601.
3. Reynolds JEF, ed. *Martindale: The Extra Pharmacopoeia.* 30th ed. London: Pharmaceutical Press, 1993:1202.
4. Adams HR, Kerzee T, Morehead CD. Carisoprodol related death in a child. J Forens Sci 1975;20:200–202.
5. Brandslung I, Klitgaard NA, Kristensen O. A case of acute intoxication with carisoprodol: Symptoms and metabolism. Ugeskr Laeg 1976;138:281–283.

6. Van der Kleijn E. Kinetics of distribution and metabolism of ataractics of the meprobamate group in mice. Arch Int Pharmacodyn 1969;178:457–480.
7. Kato R, Vasanelli P, Frontino G, et al. Metabolism and distribution of carisoprodol in tissues and organs of the rats. Med Exp 1962;6:149–157.
8. Hoffman AJ, Ludwig BJ. An improved colorimetric method for the determination of meprobamate in biological fluids. J Am Pharm Assoc 1959;48:740–742.
9. O'Brien TE. Excretion of drugs in human milk. Am J Hosp Pharm 1974;31:844–854.
10. Elder NC. Abuse of skeletal muscle relaxants. Am Fam Physician 1991;44:1223–1226.
11. Luehr JG, Meyerle KA, Larson EU. Mail order (veterinary) drug dependence. JAMA 1990;263:657.
12. Maes R, Bouche R, Laruelle L. Determination quantitative de meprobamate et de carisoprodol par chromatographie en phase gazeuse, dans differents cas d'intoxications. Eur J Toxicol 1970;3:140–143.

CYCLOBENZAPRINE

Cyclobenzaprine (Flexeril, proheptatriene, MK-130), 3-(5*H*-dibenzo[*a,d*]cyclohepten-5-ylidene)-*N,N*-dimethyl-1-propanamine hydrochloride, is a synthetic chemical prescribed as an adjunct to rest and physical therapy for the relief of muscle spasm associated with acute, painful musculoskeletal conditions.[1–5] Its efficacy for this condition is controversial.[6–10] No fatalities have been described. There have been three reports[11–13] of overdose, although one poison center reported 35 consultations during 1 year for possible overdose.[11]

Cyclobenzaprine is a tricyclic amine similar in structure and pharmacologic action to amitriptyline (Fig. 50–2). Originally studied during the 1960s as an antidepressant[14,15] in doses of 75 to 250 mg daily (maximal dose, 400 mg/d),[14] it was subsequently evaluated for use in chronic tension headache[16] (30–60 mg/d) and for rigidity in Parkinson's disease (≤60 mg/d).[17] There is no evidence of its effectiveness in the treatment of spasticity associated with cerebral or spinal cord disease or in children with cerebral palsy.[18] It is available as oral film-coated, butterscotch-yellow "D"-shaped 10-mg tablets, coded "MSD 931."[18]

The therapeutic dosage for acute skeletal muscle spasm is usually 10 mg three times daily to a maximum of 60 mg/d.[18,19] At these doses, manifestations of both peripheral and central anticholinergic blockade are frequently observed. Prominent side effects include dry mouth,[8,20,21] drowsiness,[8,20,21] dizziness,[10] nausea,[3] and unpleasant taste sensations.[4] Less frequent undesirable effects have included rash,[9] ataxia and weakness,[3,5] headache,[5] fatigue, and nervousness.[20] Occasional patients (<1%) have reported tachycardia, disorientation, hallucination, cardiac arrhythmias, and seizures (see Mechanism of Action below).[20,21] Beeber and Manning reported a patient who developed a manic psychosis after cyclobenzaprine use; the patient had a history of a prior manic episode.[6]

Poisoning has followed overdoses of cyclobenzaprine when taken alone in quantities of 600 mg[11] to approximately 1000 mg,[13] and after a dose of 260 mg in one patient who also ingested 9000 mg of acetaminophen and 1800 mg of codeine.[11] There were no fatalities.

A 15-year-old ingested about 800 mg (80 tablets) of cyclobenzaprine and died on the eighth day.[22] A 45-year-old adult ingested 900 mg (90 tablets), became comatose, developed cardiac arrest in 4 days, and died.[23]

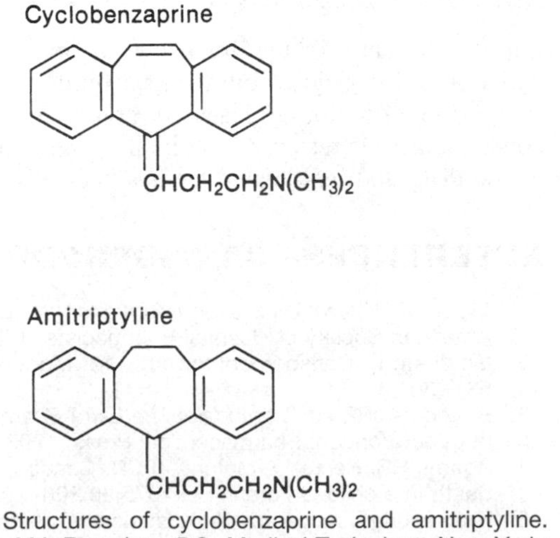

Cyclobenzaprine

$CHCH_2CH_2N(CH_3)_2$

Amitriptyline

$CHCH_2CH_2N(CH_3)_2$

Figure 50–2 Structures of cyclobenzaprine and amitriptyline. (From Ellenhorn MJ, Barceloux DG. *Medical Toxicology.* New York: Elsevier, 1988:470.)

Toxicokinetics

Cyclobenzaprine is completely but slowly absorbed from the intestine. Average plasma levels increase with increasing daily dosage. A 10-mg oral dose (three times daily for 3 days) led to a peak plasma level of 22 ng/mL.[24] After a single 10-mg dose orally, plasma levels may vary from 15 to 25 ng/mL.[19] Oral ingestion of 40 mg in humans resulted in a peak plasma level of about 30 ng/mL at 6 hours (time to peak plasma level varies from 3 to 8 hours); a similar dose given intravenously produced a peak plasma level of 51 ng/mL 0.5 and 2 hours after administration.[24,25] Eight hours after injection, the plasma level was about 27 ng/mL. Such data suggest that cyclobenzaprine is rapidly taken up by tissues, from which sites the drug is slowly released into the blood. In view of the fact that plasma levels after the intravenous dose were considerably higher during the first 4 hours than those attained following the oral dose, first-pass hepatic metabolism may be important in cyclobenzaprine metabolism.[24] Enterohepatic recirculation has been postulated.[24]

The drug is almost completely metabolized. Very little unchanged drug is excreted in the urine (0.2–1.5% of administered doses)[25]; the *N*-desmethyl metabolite (inactive) is the most prominent metabolite found in the urine. The half-life of cyclobenzaprine is approximately 1 to 3 days.

It is not known whether cyclobenzaprine crosses the placenta or is distributed into breast milk. About 93% is bound to plasma proteins.[11]

Mechanism of Action

Cyclobenzaprine toxicity is related to its ability to produce central and peripheral antimuscarinic anticholinergic blockade. In animals,[26] it blocks muscarinic cholinergic receptors[27]; augments the activity of exogenously administered norepinephrine, releasing endogenous catecholamines from presynaptic neurons (probably by reducing reuptake at high doses); and acts as an antihistamine.

In animal experiments intravenous administration of cyclobenzaprine abolished the rigidity of both intercollicular decerebration (gamma rigidity) and anemic decerebration (alpha rigidity) and lessened the rigidity after spinal cord ischemia.[9]

Clinical Presentation

Although only five patients with overdose have been reported to date,[11–13] one poison center was consulted during one year regarding 35 cases.[11] Thirty-two patients developed only mild symptoms, which were similar to those reported as adverse effects of therapeutic dosages.

Linden et al. found that symptoms and signs of central cholinergic blockade (eg, agitation, confusion, and hallucinations) were the most striking features of overdose in three patients aged 18 to 33 years.[11] Peripheral anticholinergic findings (eg, dry skin and mucous membranes, tachycardia, decreased gastrointestinal motility, and urinary retention) were present in all three cases. None of the patients developed the coma, convulsions, hypotension, arrhythmias, or impaired cardiac conduction and contractility seen after tricyclic antidepressant poisoning.[28] The pupils were midposition, equal, and reactive in the two patients who ingested cyclobenzaprine without other drugs. All recovered. Physostigmine was used in two cases. Heckerling and Bartow described a 22-year-old man who took an unknown quantity of cyclobenzaprine in a suicide attempt. Tachycardia, lethargy, and later agitation and confusion were observed. The skin was profusely diaphoretic and of normal color and temperature. The pupils were midposition and sluggishly reactive. Bowel sounds were normal, and the bladder was not enlarged. There was a sinus tachycardia. The mucous membranes were moist. Pyrilamine (an antihistamine) was also found in the urine drug screen. The patient recovered with supportive treatment.[12]

O'Riordan et al. reported a 31-year-old woman who may have ingested up to 1000 mg of cyclobenzaprine. Twenty-four hours later she was observed to be disoriented as to time, place, and person, and exhibited slurred speech. There was a supraventricular tachycardia on admission. The white blood cell count was 18,300 with 82% polymorphonuclear leukocytes. The patient was treated supportively and subsequently recovered after an episode of renal failure. Induced emesis (syrup of ipecac), gastric lavage (36 Ewald tube—multiple pill fragments recovered), activated charcoal, and Fleet's phosphate were used.[13]

A 28-year-old man ingested about 16 tablets (1600 mg) of cyclobenzaprine and became confused, agitated, and disoriented. He was treated with gastric lavage and activated charcoal via a nasogastric tube. Midazolam, lorazepam, and haloperidol intravenously did not significantly change his level of agitation. Physostigmine 1 mg intravenously over 2 to 3 minutes was followed by an immediate dramatic reversal of confusion and a return to normal orientation. Repeat physostigmine doses (1 mg) over the next 2 hours kept him calm.[29] Two octogenarians ingested therapeutic doses of cyclobenzaprine over a period of 3 to 4 days and developed sleeplessness, agitation, delusions, and confusion; they recovered.[30]

Laboratory

Gas–liquid chromatography methods are available for quantitative analysis of cyclobenzaprine in the plasma and urine.[24,25] These procedures are not performed routinely in clinical laboratories and have not been correlated either with side effects after therapeutic dosage or with toxicity associated with overdose.[11–13] Toxicology urine screens may also include a qualitative test for cyclobenzaprine.[13]

Because of its structural similarity to amitriptyline (see Fig. 50–2), cyclobenzaprine is not distinguished from amitriptyline by conventional thin-layer chromatography, gas chromatography, high-performance liquid chromatography, EMIT enzyme immunoassay, or gas chromatography–mass spectrometry. This reinforces the necessity of obtaining a careful clinical history in conjunction with analytical techniques.[31]

Treatment

Treatment of cyclobenzaprine overdose should follow the steps recommended for overdose of tricyclic antidepressant drugs (see Chapter 38). As anticholinergic effects may delay gastric emptying, gastric lavage may be effective for many hours after an overdose ingestion.[13] Ventricular arrhythmias, QRS widening, or intraventricular conduction defects can be treated with sodium bicarbonate (1 mEq/kg intravenously) sufficient to increase the arterial pH to 7.5.[13] Physostigmine use (see Chapter 37 for details) in cyclobenzaprine poisoning must be reserved for patients with very serious symptoms (agitation, delirium, hypertension, coma, or life-threatening supraventricular tachyarrhythmias).[11,32] Supportive care continues to be the mainstay of treatment for a cyclobenzaprine overdose. With such treatment most patients should recover.

Cyclobenzaprine, baclofen, and orphenadrine induce, in high doses, a "buzz" (baclofen), "euphoria" (carisoprodol), and "mood enhancement and pleasant disperception." Skeletal muscle relaxants are frequently used in combination with alcohol, benzodiazepines, or narcotics either to prolong the effect of alcohol or a narcotic drug, to increase the efficacy of the primary drug of abuse, or to achieve the same effects with a smaller amount of alcohol or narcotic.[33]

REFERENCES—CYCLOBENZAPRINE

1. Share NN, McFarlane CS. Cyclobenzaprine: A novel centrally acting skeletal muscle relaxant. Neuropharmacology 1975; 14:675–684.
2. Molina-Negro P, Illingworth RH. MK-130: Une nouvelle drogue pour le traitement de hypertonie musculaire: Essai preliminaire chez dix patients avec spasticitae d'origine spinale. Union Med Can 1971;100:1947–1951.
3. Bercel NA. Cyclobenzaprine in the treatment of skeletal muscle spasm in osteoarthritis of the cervical and lumbar spine. Curr Ther Res 1977;22:462–468.
4. Nibbelink DW, Strickland SC, McLean LF, et al. Cyclobenzaprine, diazepam and placebo in the treatment of skeletal muscle spasm of local origin. Clin Ther 1978;1:409–424.
5. Azoury FJ. Double-blind comparison of Parafon Forte^R and Flexeril^R in the treatment of acute musculoskeletal disorders. Curr Ther Res 1979;26:189–197.
6. Beeber AR, Manning JM Jr. Psychosis following cyclobenzaprine use. J Clin Psychiatry 1983;44:151–152.

7. Elenbaas JK. Centrally acting oral skeletal muscle relaxants. Am J Hosp Pharm 1980;37:1313–1323.
8. Basmajian JV. Cyclobenzaprine hydrochloride effects on skeletal muscle spasm in the lumbar region and neck: Two double-blind controlled clinical and laboratory studies. Arch Phys Med Rehabil 1978;59:58–163.
9. Ashby P, Burke D, Rao S, et al. Assessment of cyclobenzaprine in the treatment of spasticity. J Neurol Neurosurg Psychiatry 1979;35:599–605.
10. Brown BR, Womble J. Cyclobenzaprine in intractable pain syndromes with muscle spasm. JAMA 1978;240: 1151–1152.
11. Linden CH, Mitchiner JC, Lindzon RD, et al. Cyclobenzaprine overdosage. J Toxicol Clin Toxicol 1983;20:281–288.
12. Heckerling PS, Bartow TJ. Paradoxical diaphoresis in cyclobenzaprine poisoning. Ann Intern Med 1984;101:881.
13. O'Riordan W, Gillette P, Calderon J, et al. Overdose of cyclobenzaprine, the tricyclic muscle relaxant. Ann Emerg Med 1986;15:592–593.
14. Vinar O, Grof P. Proheptatriene in depression (extensive study). Activ Nerv Super 1965;7:290.
15. Nahunek K, Misurec J, Rodova A, et al. Some clinical and experimental experience with proheptatrien. Activ Nerv Super 1965;7:291.
16. Lance JW, Anthony M. Cyclobenzaprine in the treatment of chronic headache. Med J Aust 1972;2:1409–1411.
17. Tourtellotte WW, Potvin AR, Costanza AM, et al. Cyclobenzaprine: A new type of anti-Parkinsonian drug. Prog Neuropsychopharmacol 1978;2:553–578.
18. *Physicians' Desk Reference.* 49th ed. Montvale, NJ: Medical Economics, 1995:1550–1551.
19. McEvoy GK, ed. *AHFS Drug Information 94.* Bethesda, MD: American Society of Hospital Pharmacists, 1994: 844–846.
20. Nibbelink DW, Strickland SC. Cyclobenzaprine (Flexeril[R]) postmarketing surveillance program: Preliminary report. Curr Ther Res 1979;25:564–570.
21. Nibbelink DW, Strickland SC. Cyclobenzaprine (Flexeril™): Report of postmarketing surveillance program. Curr Ther Res 1980;28:894–903.
22. Litovitz TL, Normann SA, Veltri JC. Case 260: 1985 Annual Report of the American Association of Poison Control Centers National Data Collection System. Am J Emerg Med 1986;4:457.
23. Litovitz TL, Bailey KM, Schmitz BF, et al. Case 539: 1990 Annual Report of the American Association of Poison Control Centers National Data Collection System. Am J Emerg Med 1991;9:539.
24. Hucker HB, Stauffer SC, Albert KS, et al. Plasma levels and bioavailability of cyclobenzaprine in human subjects. J Clin Pharmacol 1977;17:719–727.
25. Hucker HB, Stauffer SC. GLC determination of cyclobenzaprine in plasma and urine. J Pharm Sci 1976;65: 1253–1255.
26. Benesova O, Nahunek K. Correlation between the experimental data from animal studies and therapeutical effects of antidepressant drugs. Psychopharmacologia 1971;20: 337-347.
27. Hughes MJ, Lemons S, Barles C. Cyclobenzaprine: Some pharmacological cardiac actions. Life Sci 1978;23:2779–2786.
28. Biggs JT, Spiker DA, Petit JM, et al. Tricyclic antidepressant overdose: Incidence of symptoms. JAMA 1977;238: 135–138.
29. Stephen JM, Ghezzi KT, Bailey K, Shesser R. Post-triathalon delirium. J Emerg Med 1991;9:265–269.
30. Engel PA, Chapron D. Cyclobenzaprine-induced delirium in two octogenarians. J Clin Psychiatry 1993;51:39.
31. Tasset JJ, Schroeder TJ, Pesce AJ. Cyclobenzaprine overdose: The importance of a clinical history in analytical toxicology. J Anal Toxicol 1985;10:258.
32. Newton RW. Physostigmine salicylate in the treatment of tricyclic antidepressant overdosage. JAMA 1975;231: 941–943.
33. Elder NC. Abuse of skeletal muscle relaxants. Am Fam Physician 1991;40:1223–1226.

ORPHENADRINE

Orphenadrine is an anticholinergic drug that has been used as a skeletal muscle relaxant and has also been prescribed to combat the parkinsonian effects of phenothiazines.[1] In children it has produced severe poisoning and death after ingestion. In adults who are emotionally disturbed, its ingestion often starts as a suicidal "gesture"[1] and may end fatally. Between 1977 and 1980, 12 deaths due to orphenadrine were recorded by the National Poisons Unit at Guy's Hospital.[2] Serious symptoms (convulsions, cardiac arrest) may lead to death within a few hours. Treatment must be aggressive and supportive. Physostigmine may be a useful antidote.

Structure and Classification

Orphenadrine (*N,N*-dimethyl-2-(*o*-methyl-α-phenylbenzyloxy)ethylamine) is a tertiary amine antimuscarinic agent closely related to the antihistamine diphenhydramine, from which it differs only in the presence of a methyl group attached in an *ortho* position to a benzene ring[3,4] (Fig. 50–3). This difference is sufficient to reduce its antihistaminic activity, increase its anticholinergic activity, and permit it to have certain central effects mainly on muscle tone.[5,6]

Source/Use

Orphenadrine is a synthetic chemical used as an adjunct to rest and to physical and other measures for the relief of discomfort associated with acute painful muscular conditions.[7] It has also been used for symptomatic treatment of Parkinson's disease[8] and drug-induced parkinsonism and as an antidepressant.[3]

According to one report up to 50% of patients receiving neuroleptic drugs (eg, phenothiazines) have also been given prophylactic anticholinergic agents.[9] Treatment with orphenadrine in many of these patients where there is a risk of self-poisoning may carry a greater risk than the drugs whose side effects it was deemed to control.[2]

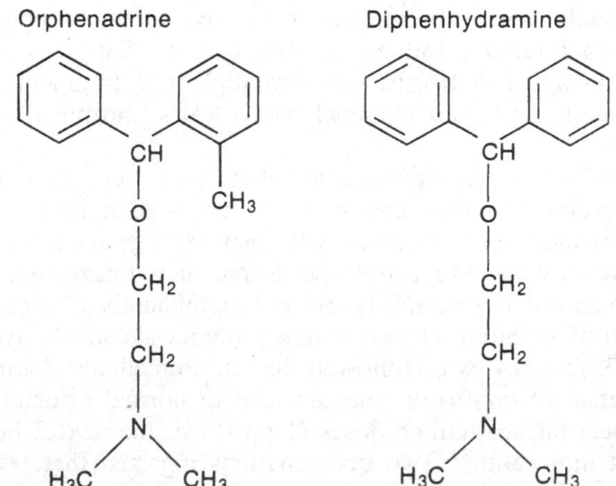

Figure 50–3 Structures of orphenadrine and diphenhydramine. (From Ellenhorn MJ, Barceloux DG. *Medical Toxicology.* New York: Elsevier, 1988:473.)

Product Formulation

Orphenadrine citrate (United States)	Oral tablets, 100 mg: Norflex, Marflex, Novadex, Orflagen, X-Otag, S.R. Parenteral injection, 30 mg/mL: Banflex Flexoject; Marflex; Myolin, Orphenate, X-Otag (all with benzethonium chloride and sodium bisulfite); Flexon
Orphenadrine citrate combinations (United States)	Oral tablets 25 mg with aspirin 385 mg, caffeine 30 mg: Norgesic; 50 mg with aspirin 770 mg, caffeine 60 mg: Norgesic Forte (scored)
Overseas	Injection, 20 mg/mL; tablets, 50 mg: Disipal (United Kingdom, Australia, Belgium, Canada, France, Italy, Netherlands, Norway, South Africa, Switzerland)[10,11]

Therapeutic Dose

For symptomatic relief of acute skeletal muscle conditions in adults, the usual oral dosage of orphenadrine citrate tablets is 100 mg twice daily.[10]

Toxic Dose

The acute oral LD_{50} in mice is 219 mg/kg,[6] and in rats, 400 mg/kg.[12] In one 2-year-old child a dose of 650 to 700 mg resulted in severe toxicity and death.[13] Another 2-year-old boy ingested 1400 mg and recovered.[14] An overdose of 2000 to 3000 mg ingested by a 59-year-old woman led to her death[15]; a 19-year-old woman recovered after ingesting 7500 mg[6] (Table 50–1). Bozza-Marrubini et al. reviewed a series of fatal cases, which indicated that death occurred in adults after ingestion of 22 mg/kg and in children after 72 mg/kg.[3] Recoveries after intensive supportive treatment followed ingestions of 51 mg/kg (adults) and 220 mg/kg (children).

Fatal Dose

The lethal dose in adults can be considered to be about 2 to 3 g (20–30 tablets of 100 mg, 40–60 tablets of 50 mg).[16–18]

Table 50–1
Toxic Doses: Orphenadrine

Age	Sex	Dose (mg)	Blood Level (μg/mL)	Outcome
2	M	650–700		Death
2	M	1400		Recovery
59	F	2000–3000		Death
24	M	5000	2.64 (12-h level)	Recovery
30	M	1000		Recovery
25	M	1200–1500		Recovery
24	F	2250		Recovery
3	M	3000		Recovery
62	F	3900		Recovery
23	F	4500		Recovery
40	M	?	16.2	Recovery
33	M	5000		Recovery
19	F	7500		Recovery
(18 cases—postmortem)			1.1–55	

From Ellenhorn MJ, Barcelou DG. *Medical Toxicology.* New York: Elsevier, 1988:473.

This may be associated with a lethal blood level of 4 to 8 μg/mL[19] (see Laboratory). Death is rapid and occurs within 2 to 5 hours.[20–22]

Toxicokinetics

Absorption

Orphenadrine is rapidly and completely absorbed from the stomach and intestines[23]; 50% of an oral dose is absorbed within 30 minutes.[14] Following a single oral dose of 100 mg in normal volunteers, plasma levels peaked between 2 and 4 hours and ranged from 107 to 213 ng/mL.[24] Peak blood levels are reached 1 hour after an intramuscular dose.[25] Plasma levels tend to increase in proportion to the dose administered. A daily dose of 300 mg was associated with a mean plasma value of 426 to 572 ng/mL.[24] After chronic orphenadrine use, plasma levels of the major metabolite, *N*-demethylorphenadrine (NDO), were approximately the same as for the parent compound. Competition of NDO with orphenadrine for biotransformation may account for the elevated plasma concentration of the parent drug after chronic administration.[24] Orphenadrine has a pK_a of 8.4 and is about 20% protein bound.[26]

Distribution

High concentrations are found in the liver and lungs.[23,27,28] Orphenadrine may undergo an enterohepatic cycle in its path from the intestine to the liver and then into the bile.[3]

Elimination

Orphenadrine is almost completely metabolized by a first-order kinetic process[29] to at least eight metabolites.[23,27] The clinical activity of the metabolites has not been clinically evaluated. The major metabolite, NDO, appears to compete for biotransformation with orphenadrine[24] and may be active.[12]

The elimination half-life of orphenadrine is about 15 hours (13–20 hours) after a single oral dose and 30 to 40 hours after chronic dosage.[24] In humans, the half-life of NDO is slightly longer than that of orphenadrine.[25] Approximately 50 to 60% is excreted in the urine as metabolites; small amounts (about 8%) are excreted unchanged.[23] Large amounts are excreted in the bile and feces.[27]

Drug Interactions

Orphenadrine may be additive with other anticholinergic agents (eg, phenothiazines, antiparkinsonian drugs, atropine, antihistamines, tricyclic antidepressants). Additive effects with propoxyphene may result in mental confusion, anxiety, and tremors.[10]

Pregnancy/Lactation

Data from the manufacturer indicate that orphenadrine may appear in breast milk.[30] Beall reported that orphenadrine produces enlarged, darkened urinary bladders in rat offspring when given to mothers in doses of 15 to 30 mg/kg.[31]

Mechanism of Action

Orphenadrine may exert a direct depressant effect on myocardial contraction and cardiac conduction.[3] Sangster et al. conclude that there is a significant cardiotoxic effect from orphenadrine in overdose.[17] Orphenadrine produces mainly a peripheral cholinergic block but has central effects, which may also account for its ability to reduce skeletal muscle spasm; it does not have direct skeletal muscle relaxant activity.[23] It also has some antihistaminic and local anesthetic action.

Clinical Presentation

Overdose

Within 2 hours of ingestion of an overdose, convulsions, coma, mydriasis, and tachycardia may occur. These effects are similar to those following tricyclic antidepressant overdose. Athetoid movements, cardiac arrest, shock, and hypothermia have been described.[3,13] Occasional hypoglycemia, increases in hepatic transaminase levels, fall in prothrombin time, disseminated intravascular coagulation, hepatomegaly, pulmonary hemorrhage, and hypokalemia may be seen. Death is often due to cardiac or respiratory arrest and may also follow status epilepticus.

Pathologic changes include severe diffuse brain edema, hemorrhagic pulmonary edema, central and hepatic necrosis, and renal congestion.[3]

Chronic Use

Anticholinergic effects are most evident following long-term use of higher-than-therapeutic doses. Dry mouth, urinary retention, tachycardia, blurred vision, pupillary dilation, nausea, vomiting, headache, dizziness, agitation, drowsiness, tremors, and mental confusion may be observed. Rare cases of aplastic anemia, urticaria, and anaphylactic reaction have been reported.[7] Reduction in dosage eliminates undesirable side effects.

Case Studies

Between 1972 and 1975 eight cases of severe orphenadrine poisoning were observed by the Poison Control Center of Milan.[3] All had rapid onset of coma with mydriasis and loss of pupillary reactivity, convulsions or athetoid movements, tachycardia, urinary retention, and hot dry skin. This lasted 1 to 48 hours. Six recovered. One 6-year-old boy had a cardiac arrest but survived with brain damage. One 18-month-old man took an unknown dose and developed hypoglycemia, hepatic insufficiency, disseminated intravascular coagulation, and pulmonary hemorrhages, resulting in cardiac arrest and death within 36 hours of ingestion. Orphenadrine was detected in the urine (100 μg/mL) and in the blood (4 μg/mL). Postmortem examination revealed brain edema, right-sided heart dilation, hemorrhagic pulmonary edema, and central hepatic necrosis. A 62-year-old woman developed hypothermia and severe hypokalemia and cardiac arrest; she recovered. By 1977, Bozza-Marrubini had collected 21 cases of severe orphenadrine poisoning with 15 deaths. Death usually occurred within a few hours.[3]

Two women died after an overdose of orphenadrine taken as a suicidal "gesture."[1] They may have been given the drugs to control the parkinsonian effects of phenothiazines.[1] Dr. A.T. Proudfoot of the Regional Poisoning Treatment Centre, Edinburgh Royal Infirmary, reported 11 patients admitted to his unit, with one death, in the first 6 months of 1977.[1]

Sangster et al. studied 158 cases of poisoning by orphenadrine alone and in combination with other drugs. There were 25 deaths. Coma, seizures, shock, and cardiac dysrhythmias were described; these were often unresponsive to usual methods of treatment. In dogs the intravenous lethal dose was found to be 15 to 20 mg/kg; the cause of death was cardiac in origin.[16]

Bosche and Mallach describe a 2-year-old boy who swallowed 650 to 700 mg of orphenadrine hydrochloride. He died 23 hours later. At postmortem there was considerable cerebral edema. The highest concentration of orphenadrine was found in the liver, which exhibited centrilobular fatty degeneration.[13]

Heinonen et al. reported a 19-year-old woman who took about 150 tablets of Disipal (7500 mg of orphenadrine chloride). She was in respiratory arrest on arrival at the hospital. She had clonic convulsions and was deeply comatose. The pupils were dilated and unresponsive to light. In the intensive care unit she received intermittent positive-pressure ventilation. Convulsions were controlled by *d*-tubocurarine chloride. Some fluids and tablets were aspirated through a nasogastric tube. Metaraminol (Aramine) 3 mg intravenously kept the systolic blood pressure above 100 mm Hg. Hypokalemia, metabolic acidosis, arrhythmias, and conduction disturbances continued for 2 days. On the second day she reacted to painful stimuli and opened her eyes. Convulsions ceased by day 4, after which the endotracheal tube was removed. The patient recovered.[6]

Deceuninck et al. reported a woman aged 59 years who took 40 to 50 tablets of orphenadrine 50 mg with suicidal intent. She was found in a coma and later became semicomatose, developed delirium, and was found to have dilated nonreactive pupils, hypertension, fever, tachycardia, urinary retention, and loss of salivation and perspiration. Convulsions continued and led to death.[15]

A 2-year-old boy ingested about 28 orphenadrine tablets (>100 mg/kg). He developed status epilepticus, cyanosis, and widely dilated pupils. After conservative treatment in the hospital for 18 days, he recovered.[14]

Robinson et al. studied data in 10 fatal cases of orphenadrine poisoning (used alone) and 8 cases in which orphenadrine was present in combination with alcohol or another drug. Unchanged drug was found in the bile and urine. The concentration of unchanged drug was similar in the liver and lungs.[20]

Bennet and Kohn described a 33-year-old man who had allegedly ingested 5000 mg of Norflex. Initially hyperreflexic, with extensor plantar responses, widely dilated pupils, and a sinus tachycardia, he was treated conservatively and awoke in 6 hours. He was disoriented, vomiting, and hallucinating. Within 2 minutes of receiving physostigmine 2 mg intravenously, he was rational and talkative. This dose was repeated 1 hour later. He recovered in 3 days.[21]

Snyder et al. reported a 5-year-old boy who ingested 1200 to 1500 mg of orphenadrine. Within 2 hours he exhibited delirium, tachycardia (50/min), dilated pupils, and combative behavior. Sweating and blood pressure were normal.

Physostigmine 1 mg intravenously reduced his heart rate to 75 in 1 minute. He became alert, oriented, and cooperative.[22]

An anecdotal report indicates that abuse of orphenadrine to doses of 1500 mg/d may be accompanied by dizziness, tremor, euphoria, and visual hallucinations.[32] All the skeletal muscle relaxants possess sedative properties and are abused mainly for this effect. They have been described as producing a "buzz" (baclofen), "euphoria" (carisoprodol), and "mood enhancement and pleasant disperceptions" (orphenadrine). Skeletal muscle relaxants are frequently used in combination with other central nervous system depressants, such as alcohol, benzodiazepines, and narcotics. They are used to prolong the effect of alcohol or narcotics, increase the effect of the primary drug of abuse, or achieve the same effect with a smaller dose of alcohol or narcotic.[33]

Orphenadrine, like other antiparkinsonian drugs with anticholinergic properties, may be subject to drug abuse.[32]

Laboratory

Analytical Methods

A gas chromatographic procedure that is specific with a sensitivity down to 1 ng/mL has been described for orphenadrine and its major metabolite NDO.[29] A high-performance liquid chromatography method can also be employed.[34]

Blood Levels

After ingestion of 100 tablets (about 5 g) of orphenadrine hydrochloride by a 24-year-old man, impairment of consciousness and hallucinations disappeared at concentrations less than 1.77 μg/mL, and mydriasis and tachycardia at concentrations less than 2.19 μg/mL. Furlanut et al. suggest that at serum concentrations less than 3 μg/mL 12 hours after ingestion, there is a reduced risk of death.[8] Further studies are necessary to corroborate these observations.

Toxicity appears to begin at a blood level of about 2 μg/mL. Concentrations of 4 to 8 μg/mL may be fatal.[19] Blood levels up to 55 μg/mL were reported in one series of orphenadrine-related deaths.[21]

A 48-year-old woman who had possibly ingested 1400 mg of orphenadrine hydrochloride together with haloperidol 210 mg developed a wide-complex polymorphous tachycardia (Torsade de pointes) which responded to atrial overdrive pacing. The serum orphenadrine level was 9.5 μg/mL. She recovered.[35]

Use of laboratory studies (blood, urine levels) is not available in many community hospitals. When used, they can confirm the presence of orphenadrine. Treatment, which frequently must be immediate and aggressive, should be guided by clinical evaluations and should not be delayed while laboratory studies of blood levels are being obtained.

Treatment

Stabilization

Electrocardiographic monitoring should be instituted on arrival. Continuous monitoring of pulse, respiration, temperature, and renal and hepatic function is necessary. Equipment for cardiac resuscitation should be immediately available. The orphenadrine-depressed heart is responsive to the positive inotropic and chronotropic actions of catecholamines.[3] Convulsive seizures may begin within 20 minutes of ingestion or en route to the hospital.

Gut Decontamination

Orphenadrine may be retained in the stomach for several hours because of its anticholinergic properties.[28] Therefore evacuation of gastric contents by emesis (syrup of ipecac, if patient is not convulsing, obtunded, or in coma and has not lost the gag reflex) or gastric lavage with tracheal protection can be instituted within the first 4 hours of ingestion. Emesis induction should be avoided because of the rapid onset of symptoms such as seizures in the first few hours after an ingestion. Activated charcoal (adults, 50–100 g; children, 15–50 g) can be given orally or introduced through the gastric lavage tube. As a slurry, 240 mL of diluent is given per 30 g of charcoal. Cathartics (magnesium or sodium sulfate, magnesium citrate, sorbitol) have not been evaluated in the treatment of orphenadrine overdose but may be useful in preventing additional absorption (magnesium or sodium sulfate [10% solution]: adult, 20 g/dose; child, 250 mg/kg/dose; magnesium citrate: adult, 250–300 mL; child, 4 mL/kg; sorbitol (70%): adult, 50–150 mL; child, 2 mL/kg).

Elimination Enhancement

No reports are available on the use of forced diuresis or extracorporeal methods of drug removal (hemodialysis, peritoneal dialysis, hemoperfusion).

Antidote

Physostigmine (see Chapter 37) can be of use in the treatment of hallucinations, arrhythmias, hypertension, coma, myoclonic seizures, and life-threatening supraventricular tachycardia when anticholinergic signs and symptoms are present. When gangrene, asthma, serious cardiovascular disease, or mechanical obstruction of the gastrointestinal or urogenital tract is present, physostigmine can be used only if there is a life-threatening emergency. Sangster et al., however, warn that orphenadrine in overdose is cardiotoxic, that the anticholinergic properties are of relatively minor importance, and that ventilatory therapy and gastric lavage should be instituted with careful cardiovascular evaluation before physostigmine is used.[17] The pediatric dose is 0.5 mg intravenously, slowly. The patient is observed for evidence of cholinergic effects. If there is no improvement, the dose is repeated at 5-minute intervals to a maximum of 2 mg. The dose for adolescents and adults is 2 mg intravenously, slowly, repeated if required in 20 minutes and if life-threatening symptoms recur. A continuous drip should not be used. The patient should be observed for evidence of bronchial constriction.

A 3-year-old, who may have ingested 1000 to 5000 mg of orphenadrine, developed a wide-complex (probably) ventricular tachycardia. The arrhythmia did not respond to precordial thumps, cardioversion, and repeated doses of intravenous lidocaine. The patient converted to a sinus tachycardia after several doses of physostigmine intravenously (0.02 mg/kg). He recovered.[36]

Supportive Measures

Supportive care is the mainstay of treatment after an orphenadrine overdose.

Convulsions. Avoid barbiturates or other central nervous system depressants. Intravenous diazepam may be effective (adult, 0.25 mg/kg up to 10 mg/dose, repeated every 15 minutes as required; child, 0.25–0.4 mg/kg/dose up to 10 mg/dose administered over 3 minutes).

Hypoxia. Institute endotracheal intubation with assisted ventilation.

Laboratory Studies. Closely follow hepatic transaminases, prothrombin time, blood sugar, acid–base balance, and electrolytes. Hypokalemia may require replacement with potassium under careful electrocardiographic monitoring.

REFERENCES—ORPHENADRINE

1. Millar WM. Deaths after overdoses of orphenadrine. Lancet 1977;2:566.
2. Clarke B, Mair J, Rudolf M. Acute poisoning with orphenadrine. Lancet 1985;1:1386.
3. Bozza-Marrubini M, Frigerio A, Ghezzi R, et al. Two cases of severe orphenadrine poisoning with atypical features. Acta Pharmacol Toxicol 1977;41(suppl. 2):137–152.
4. Bassett JR, Story M, Cairncross KD. The influence of orphenadrine upon the actions of a series of sympathicomimetic drugs. Eur J Pharmacol 1968;4:198.
5. Ginzel KH. The blockade of reticular and spinal facilitation of motor-function by orphenadrine. J Pharmacol Exp Ther 1966;154:128–141.
6. Heinonen J, Heikkila J, Mattila MJ, et al. Orphenadrine poisoning: A case report supplemented with animal experiments. Arch Toxicol 1968;23:264–272.
7. *Physicians' Desk Reference.* 49th ed. Montvale, NJ: Medical Economics, 1995:1386–1387.
8. Furlanut M, Bettio D, Bertin I, et al. Orphenadrine serum levels in a poisoned patient. Hum Toxicol 1985;4:331–333.
9. Edwards SE, Kumar V. A survey of prescribing of psychotropic drugs in a Birmingham psychiatric hospital. Br J Psychiatry 1984;145:502–507.
10. McEvoy GK, ed. *AHFS Drug Information 94.* Bethesda, MD: American Society of Hospital Pharmacists, 1994:851–852.
11. Reynolds JEF, ed. *Martindale: The Extra Pharmacopoeia.* 30th ed. London: Pharmaceutical Press, 1993:428–429.
12. Blomquist M, Bonnichsen R, Schubert B. Lethal orphenadrine intoxications: A report of five cases. Z Rechtsmed 1971;68:111.
13. Bosche J, Mallach HJ. Uber anatomische und chemisch toxikologische Befunde bei einer todlichen Vergiftung durch Orphenadrin. Arch Toxikol 1969;25:76–82.
14. Stoddard JC, Parkin JH, Wynne NA. Orphenadrine: A case report. Br J Anaesth 1968;40:789–790.
15. Deceuninck F, Silverman RM, Veltman JGJ. A patient with psychosis following orphenadrine poisoning. Ned Tijdschr Geneesk 1973;117:25–27.
16. Sangster B, Van Heijst ANP, Zimmerman ANE, et al. Intoxication by orphenadrine HCl: Mechanism and therapy. Acta Pharmacol Toxicol 1977;41(suppl. 2):129–136.
17. Sangster B, Van Heijst ANP, Zimmerman ANE. Treatment of orphenadrine overdose. N Engl J Med 1977;296:1006.
18. Sangster B, van Heijst ANP, Zimmerman ANE. Vergiftiging door orphenadrine (Disipal). Ned Tijdschr Geneesk 1978; 122:988–992.
19. Wineck CL. Tabulation of therapeutic, toxic and lethal concentrations of drugs and chemicals in blood. Clin Chem 1976;22:832.
20. Robinson AE, Holder AT, McDowall RD, et al. Forensic toxicology of some orphenadrine-related deaths. Forens Sci 1977;9:53–62.
21. Bennet MB, Kohn J. Orphenadrine overdose: Cerebral manifestations treated with physostigmine. Anaesth Intens Care 1976;4:67. Case Report.
22. Snyder BD, Kane M, Plocher D. Orphenadrine overdose treatment with physostigmine. N Engl J Med 1976;295:1435.
23. Ellison T, Snyder A, Bolger J, et al. Metabolism of orphenadrine citrate in man. J Pharmacol Exp Ther 1971;176: 284–295.
24. Labout JJM, Thijssen CT, Keijser GGJ, et al. Difference between single and multiple dose pharmacokinetics of orphenadrine hydrochloride in man. Eur J Clin Pharmacol 1982;21:343–350.
25. Rutigliano G, Labout JJM. The bioavailability of orphenadrine hydrochloride after intramuscular and oral administration. J Int Med Res 1982;10:447–450.
26. Heel RC, Avery GS. Appendix A. In: Avery G, ed. *Drug Data Information in Drug Treatment.* Sydney: ADIS Press, 1980: 1222.
27. Hespe W, De Roos AM, Nauta WT. Investigation into the metabolic fate of orphenadrine hydrochloride after oral administration to male rats. Arch Int Pharmacodyn 1965; 156:180–200.
28. Prins H, Hespe W. Autoradiographic study of the distribution of radioactivity in mice after oral administration of tritium-labelled orphenadrine hydrochloride. Arch Int Pharmacodyn 1968;171:47–57.
29. Labout JJM, Thijssen CT, Hespe W. Sensitivity and specific gas chromatographic and extraction method for the determination of orphenadrine in human body fluids. J Chromatogr 1977;144:201–208.
30. Chaplin S, Sanders GL, Smith JM. Drug excretion in human breast milk. Adverse Drug React Acute Poison Rev 1982; 1:255–287.
31. Beall JR. A teratogenic study of chlorpromazine, orphenadrine, perphenazine and LSD-25 in rats. Toxicol Appl Pharmacol 1972;21:230–236.
32. Schifano F, Marra R, Magni G. Orphenadrine abuse. South Med J 1988;8:546–547.
33. Elder NC. Abuse of skeletal muscle relaxants. AFHJ 1991; 44:1223–1227.
34. Suckow RF, Cooper TB. Simultaneous determination of amitriptyline, nortriptyline and their respective isomeric 10-hydroxy metabolites in plasma by liquid chromatography. J Chromatogr 1982;230:391–400.
35. Henderson RA, Lane S, Henry JA. Life-threatening ventricular arrhythmia (Torsade de pointes) after haloperidol overdose. Hum Exp Toxicol 1991;10:59–62.
36. Danze LK, Langdorf MI. Reversal of orphenadrine induced ventricular tachycardia with physostigmine. J Emerg Med 1991;9:453–457.

PILOCARPINE

Pilocarpine is a direct-acting parasympathomimetic agent that exerts its effects primarily on muscarinic receptors.

Structure and Classification

Pilocarpine hydrochloride is 3-ethyldihydro-4-[(1-methyl-1*H*-imidazol-5-yl)methyl]-2(3*H*)-furanone monohydrochloride) and has a molecular weight of 244.72.[1]

Product Formulation

Pilocarpine hydrochloride ophthalmic solutions are available in 0.35, 0.8, 1, 2, 3, 4, 5, 6, 8, and 10% concentrations. Benzalkonium chloride 0.01% is used as a preservative. Solutions are available with epinephrine bitartrate 1% (with pilocarpine 2, 4, or 6%). Salagen tablets contain 5 mg pilocarpine hydrochloride for oral administration.[1]

Therapeutic Dose

Although used topically, systemically absorbed pilocarpine is considered safe in doses below 20 mg.[2] The ophthalmic dosage is usually 2 to 3 drops in the eye up to three to four times daily.

Toxic Dose

One hundred milligrams is considered dangerous and may potentially be fatal.[1,3] Ten to fifteen milligrams causes marked diaphoresis when administered hypodermically.[4]

Fatal Dose

A systemically absorbed dose as low as 60 mg is considered to be lethal, although in the few fatal cases no unequivocal relationship between dosage and outcome could be established.[5,6]

Toxicokinetics

Absorption

Blood levels peak 0.9 to 1.25 hours after ingestion of 5- or 10-mg tablets.[7]

Elimination

Pilocarpine is excreted in the urine.

Lactation

It is not known whether pilocarpine is excreted in human breast milk.

Mechanism of Action

Pilocarpine is a muscarinic drug with no nicotinic properties.

Clinical Presentation

Symptoms of pilocarpine overdose begin with flushing of the face and neck followed shortly by diaphoresis, salivation, nausea, vomiting, diarrhea, and pupillary constriction. Breathing may be difficult because of bronchiolar spasm. Pulmonary edema may occur in patients with preexisting circulatory disturbances and can be fatal.[2] Following intravenous atropine, tremor and sweating cease in a few minutes, blood pressure and pulse return to normal within 1 hour, and accommodation of the eye returns to normal within 2 hours.[5]

The safety and effectiveness of pilocarpine in children have not been established.

Laboratory

Analytical Methods

Gas chromatography after chemical derivatization is confirmed by gas chromatography–mass spectrometry. The detection limit is 0.1 μg/mL (0.48 μmol/L).[3,7]

Blood Levels

Few studies have correlated blood levels with the clinical course. Following 5 or 10 mg, maximum serum concentrations are 15 ng/mL and 41 mg/mL.[1]

Ancillary Tests

Serum cholinesterase values are usually normal.[3]

Treatment

Overdose should be treated with atropine titration (0.5–1.0 mg given subcutaneously or intravenously) and supportive measures to maintain respiration and circulation. Epinephrine (0.5–1.0 mg subcutaneously or intramuscularly) may be of value in the presence of severe cardiovascular depression or bronchoconstriction.[1,5]

Gut Decontamination

Emesis induction may be useful after an oral overdose.

Elimination Enhancement

It is not known if pilocarpine is dialysable.

REFERENCES—PILOCARPINE

1. Salagen Tablets. In: *Physicians' Desk Reference*. 49th ed. Montvale, NJ: Medical Economics, 1995:1378–1379.
2. Kastl RR. Inadvertent systemic injection of pilocarpine. Arch Ophthalmol 1987;105:28–29.
3. Cordner SM, Fysh RR, Gordon H, Whitaker SJ. Deaths of two hospital inpatients poisoned by pilocarpine. Br Med J 1986;293:1285–1287.
4. Epstein E, Kaufman I. Systemic pilocarpine toxicity from overdosage. Am J Ophthalmol 1965;59:109–110.
5. Pfliegler GP, Palatka K. Attempted suicide with pilocarpine drops. Am J Ophthalmol 1995;120:399–400.
6. Clarke EGC. Isolation and identification of drugs. Lond Pharm Press 1969;1:500–501.
7. Bayne WF, Chu LC, Tao FT. Subnanogram assay for pilocarpine in biological fluids. J Pharm Sci 1976;65:1724–1727.

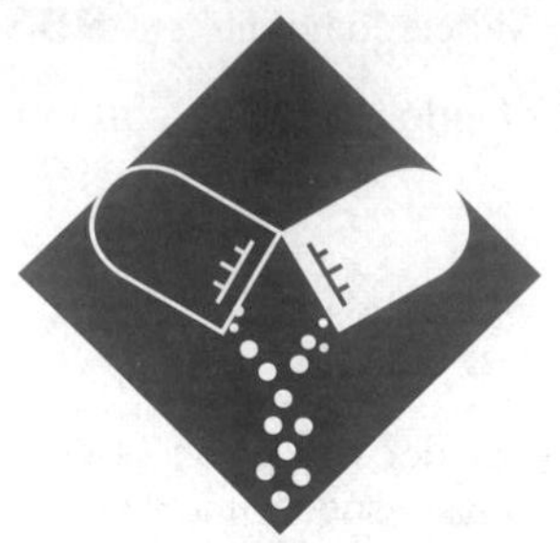

Part F
Unclassified Drugs

Chapter 51
Unclassified Drugs

ALLOPURINOL

Allupurinol is a xanthine oxidase inhibitor used in the regulation of uric acid production and the correction of hyperuricemia associated with gout (primary hyperuricemia), blood dyscrasias such as polycythemia vera and myeloid metaplasia (secondary hyperuricemia), and antineoplastic chemotherapy (secondary hyperuricemia). It is often reserved for uric acid overproducers, stone formers, patients intolerant of uricosuric agents, and patients with impaired renal function. Allopurinol administration has also been used as a simple reliable test for identification of women who are heterozygous for X-linked ornithine carbamoyl transferase deficiency.[1] Preliminary studies indicate that allopurinol, combined with a sulfhydryl-based free radical scavenger such as *N*-acetylcysteine, may have a potential use in diminishing or limiting neuropsychiatric damage after carbon monoxide poisoning.[2–4] Uncontrolled studies suggest that seizure frequency appears to decrease in epileptics maintained with antiepileptic drugs in the therapeutic range when allopurinol is added to the regimen.[5,6] Status epilepticus has followed withdrawal of allopurinol in a seizure-free patient.[7] Controlled clinical trials suggest its usefulness in the treatment of cutaneous leishmaniasis[8] and Chagas' disease (*Trypanosoma cruzi*).[9,10]

Overdoses are rare and in one report did not cause any symptoms or signs of illness in the patient following a massive ingestion (22 g).[5] Others have observed nausea, vomiting, abdominal pain, diarrhea, headache and somnolence, renal insufficiency in an adult after an acute ingestion of 9.9 g, and hepatitis in a child.[7]

Therapeutic Dose

Therapeutic doses in adults range from 200 to 300 mg daily. Doses up to 800 mg daily may be required. With renal impairment, recommended doses have been modified depending on the creatinine clearance.[11]

Toxic Dose

A massive overdose of 22 g did not produce evidence of toxicity in a 15-year-old girl.[5] Renal insufficiency has been reported after ingestion of 9.9 g.[7]

Fatal Dose

Fatalities after overdose have not been reported.

Toxicokinetics

Absorption

Oral allopurinol is readily absorbed (80–90%) from the gastrointestinal tract.[12] Levels of both allopurinol and oxipurinol peak in 2 to 3 hours.[12] A single dose of allopurinol may achieve therapeutic concentrations of its main metabolite, oxipurinol (40–60 μmol/L), in the plasma for a week or longer. Net reabsorption of oxipurinol is increased in states of volume contraction and hypovolemia, including those induced by diuretics.[13] Net reabsorption is decreased in states of volume expansion.[11]

Distribution

Allopurinol and oxipurinol are not bound to plasma proteins. The approximate estimated volumes of distribution of allopurinol and oxipurinol are approximately 2 L/kg.[5,12]

Metabolism

From 60 to 70% of allopurinol is metabolized to its active metabolite, oxipurinol, which is excreted through the kidney together with allopurinol itself and allopurinol riboside, the second major metabolite.[14] Allopurinol and its riboside are rapidly cleared, but oxipurinol is reabsorbed in the renal tubule, just like urate itself.[12]

Elimination

The serum half-life of allopurinol is about 40 to 50 minutes, and that of oxipurinol is approximately 14 to 28 hours.[12] Renal clearance of allopurinol is 13.6 to 18.9 mL/min; that of oxipurinol was 23.2 and 30.6 mL/min in two patients studied.[12,15] Oxipurinol may accumulate in patients with renal failure or gout or in patients treated with thiazide. Approximately 10% is excreted in the urine unchanged and 70% is excreted as allopurinol.[16] After a massive overdose (<22 g) the half-life of allopurinol was 3.6 hours, and that of oxipurinol, 26 hours.[5]

Drug Interactions

Allopurinol may increase the effects of azathioprine,[17] oral anticoagulants, theophylline, cyclophosphamide, iron, and ampicillin.[18,19] The effects of allopurinol may be decreased by chlorthalidone, ethacrynic acid, furosemide, metolazone, pyrazinamide, quinethazone, and thiazide diuretics.[18] Increased blood cyclosporine levels and cyclosporine toxicity have been observed with simultaneous ingestion of allopurinol.[20,21]

Pregnancy/Lactation

Few clinical studies have been performed with allopurinol in pregnant women. Allopurinol and oxipurinol are distributed into breast milk.

Mechanism of Action

Allopurinol diminishes uric acid production primarily by inhibiting the conversion of hypoxanthine to xanthine, but it also acts to depress purine synthesis through feedback inhibition of amidophosphoribosytransferase and by depletion of the essential substrate, phosphoribosyl pyrophosphate.[12,22]

Clinical Presentation

Overdose

Few symptoms or signs may be expected in the overdose patient unless there is significant underlying renal insufficiency.

Chronic Use: Allopurinol Hypersensitivity Syndrome

Approximately 2% of patients develop itching and rashes when they ingest therapeutic doses. They may develop life-threatening toxic syndrome characterized by a diffuse erythematous, desquamative skin rash, exfoliative dermatitis or toxic epidermolysis, fever, leukocytosis, eosinophilia with interstitial nephritis or vasculitis, hepatotoxicity, bone marrow depression, and worsening renal function.[11,15] Elevation of serum concentrations of oxipurinol appears to correlate with the development of this syndrome.[15] Allopurinol is photobound in the lens in the presence of ultraviolet radiation.[16] Aplastic anemia has followed use of allopurinol.[23–25]

Laboratory

Analytical Methods

Plasma oxipurinol assays are not readily available.[11] Blood allopurinol and oxipurinol levels after a 300-mg oral dose are approximately 3 to 9 μg/mL[26] and 4 to 8 μg/mL,[27] respectively.

Blood Levels

After a massive allopurinol overdose (> 10 g),[1] the concentration of allopurinol plus oxipurinol was 720 μmol/L, with a subsequent concentration of oxipurinol of more than 100 μmol/L, the upper limit of the therapeutic range.[28] Centrilobular hepatic necrosis in a 79-year-old alcoholic patient was associated with a blood allopurinol level of 230.8 μg/mL, about 50 times normal; the patient died.[26]

Ancillary Tests

Allopurinol may increase blood levels of alanine transaminase, aspartate transaminase, alkaline phosphatase, bilirubin, eosinophils, blood urea nitrogen, and serum creatinine. It may lead to decreased levels of cholesterol, glucose, hematocrit, uric acid, hemoglobin, leukocytes, and platelets.

Treatment

Stabilization

General symptomatic and supportive care should suffice to treat the patient with allopurinol overdose.

Gut Decontamination

Gut decontamination may be indicated, especially when details of renal function testing have not yet been obtained. Syrup of ipecac administered within the first hour or activated charcoal administered orally on admission to a hospital may lessen the total absorbed dose. Studies have not confirmed the usefulness of either procedure.

Elimination Enhancement

Insufficient data have been accumulated to recommend forced diuresis, dialysis procedures, hemoperfusion, or exchange transfusion. Hemodialysis would not appear to be a potentially useful procedure in view of the large apparent volume of distribution of allopurinol.

Antidote

No antidote is available.

Supportive Measures

Persons with allopurinol overdoses, if massive, should be admitted to a hospital for evaluation. Such patients should not be released until a careful evaluation of renal and hepatic function indicates that there is no evidence of significant renal or hepatic insufficiency. When normal renal and hepatic function has been confirmed and there are no other significant signs or symptoms, the patient may be discharged. Patients should be observed for the development of allopurinol hypersensitivity syndrome (see Clinical Presentation).

REFERENCES—ALLOPURINOL

1. Ferner RE, Simmonds HA, Bateman DN. Allopurinol kinetics after massive overdosage. Hum Toxicol 1988;7:293–294.
2. Bismuth C, Baud FJ, Conso F, et al. *Toxicologie Clinique.* 4th ed. Paris: Medicine-Sciences, Flammarion, 1987:115.
3. Hauser ER, Finkelstein JE, Valle D, Brusilow SW. Allopurinol-induced orotidinuria: A test for mutations at the ornithine carbamoyltransferase focus in women. N Engl J Med 1990; 322:1641–1645.
4. Howard RJMW, Blake DR, Pall H, et al. Allopurinol/*N*-acetylcysteine for carbon monoxide poisoning. Lancet 1987;2:628–629.
5. De Marco P, Zagnoni P. Allopurinol and severe epilepsy. Neurology 1986;36:1538–1539.
6. Tada H, Morooka K, Arimoto K, Matsuo T. Clinical effects of allopurinol on intractable epilepsy. Epilepsia 1991;32: 279–283.
7. Kramer LD, Loche GE, Nelson LG, Ogunyemi AO. Status epilepticus following withdrawal of allopurinol. Ann Neurol 1990;27:691.
8. Martinez S, Marr JJ. Allopurinol in the treatment of cutaneous leishmaniasis. N Engl J Med 1992;326:741–744.
9. Marr JJ, Berous RL, Nelson PJ. Antitrypanosomal effect of allopurinol: Conversion in vivo to aminopyrazolopyrimidine nucleotides by *Trypanosoma cruzi.* Science 1978; 201:1018–1020.
10. Shapiro TA, Were JBO, Danso K, et al. Pharmacokinetics and metabolism of allopurinol riboside. Clin Pharmacol Ther 1991;49:506–514.
11. Cameron JS, Simmonds HA. Use and abuse of allopurinol. Br Med J 1987;294:1504–1505.
12. Hande K, Reed E, Chabner B. Allopurinol kinetics. Clin Pharmacol Ther 1978;23:598–605.
13. Wood MH, Sebel E, O'Sullivan WJ. Allopurinol and thiazide. Lancet 1972;1:751.
14. Reiter S, Simmonds HA, Webster DR, Watson AR. On the metabolism of allopurinol: Formation of allopurinol-1-riboside in purine nucleoside phosphorylase deficiency. Biochem Pharmacol 1983;32:2167–2174.
15. Hande KR, Noone RM, Stone WJ. Severe allopurinol toxicity: Description and guidelines for prevention in patients with renal insufficiency. Am J Med 1984;76:47–56.
16. Frauenfelder F, Lerman S. Allopurinol therapy. Am J Ophthalmol 1985;99:215–216.
17. Raman GV, Sharman VL, Lee HA. Azathioprine and allopurinol: A potentially dangerous combination. J Intern Med 1990;228:69–71.
18. McEvoy GK, ed. *AHFS Drug Information 94.* Bethesda, MD: American Society of Hospital Pharmacists, 1994:2423–2426.
19. Barry M, Feely J. Allopurinol influences aminophenazone elimination. Clin Pharmacokinet 1990;19:167–169.
20. Gorrie M, Beaman M, Nicholls A, Backwell P. Allopurinol interaction with cyclosporine. Br Med J 1984;308:113.
21. Stevens SL, Goldman MH. Cyclosporine toxicity associated with allopurinol. South Med J 19092;85:1265–1266.
22. McCollister RJ, Gilbert WR, Ashton DM, Wyngaarden JB. Pseudofeedback inhibition of purine synthesis by 6-mercaptopurine ribonucleotide and other purine analogues. J Biol Chem 1977;239:1560–1563.
23. Hanger HC, Pillans PI. Death following allopurinol hypersensitivity syndrome. N Z Med J 1994;107:229.
24. Conrad ME. Fatal aplastic anemia associated with allopurinol therapy. Am J Hematol 1986;22:107–108.
25. Shinohara K, Okafuji K, Ayame H, Tanaka M. Aplastic anemia caused by allopurinol in renal insufficiency. Am J Hematol 1990;35:68.
26. Tain S, Carroll W. Allopurinol therapy. Am J Ophthalmol 1985; 99:215–216.
27. Middleberg R, Fossum PM, Sanders DE, Brown SL. An acute death involving allopurinol. In: *Proceedings, Annual Meeting of American Academy of Forensic Sciences, San Antonio, February 14, 1994:* Abstract G61.
28. Elion GB, Benezra FM, Beardmore TD, Kelley WN. Studies with allopurinol in patients with impaired renal function. Adv Exp Med Biol 1980;122A:263–267.

4-AMINOPYRIDINE AND 3,4-DIAMINOPYRIDINE

4-Aminopyridine (Fig. 51–1) has been used as a bird repellent in Europe.[1] Although not approved for sale in the United States by the Food and Drug Administration, it is being used in a number of medical centers for the treatment of multiple sclerosis and after spinal cord trauma.[2] Its use has been restricted by its tendency to induce seizures.[3] 3,4-Diaminopyridine (3, 4-DAP) given alone (in oral doses of 60 mg per day) or combined with pyridostigmine is also useful in the Eaton–Lambert myasthenic syndrome. Seizures have also been reported with this product at doses of 60 mg/d (Table 51–1).[4,5] 4-Aminopyridine (4-AP) has been tried in verapamil overdose (see Chapter 32) and to

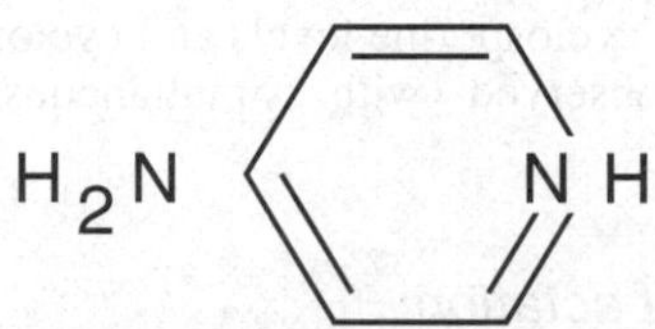

Figure 51-1 Structure of 4-aminopyridine. (From Morgan D. *Recognition and Management of Pesticide Poisonings.* EPA-540/9-88-001. Washington, DC: U.S. Environmental Protection Agency, March 1989:148–149.

Table 51–1
Side Effects of 3,4-Diaminopyridine

Central Nervous System Effects	Adrenergic Peripheral Effects
Nausea	Palpitations
Unsteadiness	Ventricular extrasystoles
Increased wakefulness	Peripheral coldness
Anxiety	Raynaud's phenomenon
Sleep problems	**Other Effects**
Chorea	Perioral paresthesia
Epileptic fits	Peripheral paresthesia
Cholinergic Peripheral Effects	
Blurred vision	
Diarrhea	
Cough	
Bronchial hypersecretion	
Provocation of bronchial asthma	

From Lundh H, Nilsson O, Rosen I, Johansson S. Practical aspects of 3,4-diaminopyridine treatment of the Lambert–Eaton myasthenic syndrome. Acta Neurol Scand 1993;88(2):136–140.

reverse neuromuscular blockade. Overdose has led to seizures and gastrointestinal symptoms. (See also Chapter 5.)

Structure

4-Aminopyridine has a molecular weight of 94.2. 4-AP is marketed as Avitrol and Pymadine.

Use

4-Aminopyridine has been used intravenously to reverse the effects of nondepolarizing muscle relaxants. In addition, it has been used orally and intravenously in the management of Eaton–Lambert syndrome,[6,7] multiple sclerosis,[7] myasthenia gravis, Huntington's chorea,[8,9] and Alzheimer's disease[10]; in the reversal of neuromuscular blockade in patients with botulism[2]; and in the treatment of patients with incomplete spinal cord injury.[11]

4-Aminopyridine has also been used as a bird repellent at concentrations of 0.5 to 3% added to grain baits, but concentrates of 25 and 50% in powdered sugar are available.[7] 4-AP enhances the rate of recovery of patients anesthetized with ketamine and diazepam.[12] 4-AP antagonizes the neuromuscular block produced by most antibiotics.

Product Formulation

4-Aminopyridine has been available as 2-mL ampules of 0.5% solutions in Bulgaria.[13]

Therapeutic Doses

The therapeutic dose is 0.02 g intravenously. In multiple sclerosis, an intravenous dosage of 1 to 5 mg in separate doses have been administered every 10 to 60 minutes over 1.5 to 3.5 hours.[8]

Toxic Dose

Toxicity has followed ingestion or injection of 10 to 100 mg of 4-AP; all patients have recovered.[1] Doses of 0.5 to 3.5 mg/kg induce nausea and vomiting, increased perspiration, flickering of the eyelids, ataxia, confusion, hyperventilation, and seizures.[14] In the treatment of multiple sclerosis, intravenous use was not associated with significant side effects below doses of 30 to 35 mg.[6] No side effects are observed up to doses of 25 mg after oral administration.[9] Doses of 1 mg/kg result in restlessness, confusion, and excitement.[15] Seizures may follow doses of 80 to 100 mg daily.[16]

Fatal Dose

No fatalities have been reported.

Toxicokinetics

Absorption

The bioavailability of 4-AP is about 95%. Protein binding is negligible. The estimated peak serum concentration following a 60-mg dose is greater than 2 μg/mL.[1,16]

Distribution

The apparent volume of distribution is 2.6 L/kg.

Elimination

No metabolites have been demonstrated. About 87% of an administered dose of 4-AP is excreted unchanged. The terminal half-life is about 4 hours. Total serum clearance is 0.6 L/h/kg.[17]

Drug Interactions

4-Aminopyridine potentiates the antagonist activity of neostigmine and pyridostigmine and decreases the dose of anticholinesterase needed. The requirement of atropine is reduced by 60 to 70%.[15] The dose of 4-AP necessary for complete antagonism of neuromuscular blockades (including antibiotics) is greater than 1 mg/kg, sufficient to stimulate the central nervous system and induce restlessness and confusion.[15,18]

Mechanism of Action

4-Aminopyridine probably inhibits the passage of potassium ions through excitable membranes. This is associated with an increase in the inward current of sodium and calcium ions during depolarization of presynaptic nerve endings, resulting in an evoked and spontaneous increase in acetylcholine from motor nerve terminals. 4-AP enhances the release of acetylcholine presynaptically, increasing the force of muscle contraction.[2,18] It antagonizes the neuromuscular blockade produced by many antibiotics. 4-AP is relatively free of muscarinic side effects.[18] 4-AP readily crosses the blood–brain barrier. It may be useful as an antagonist of nondepolarizing neuromuscular blocking agents such as *d*-tubocurarine,[19] gallamine, pancuronium, atracurium, vecuronium, doxacurium, and pipecuronium[20] (see Chapter 56). 4-AP acts on demyelinated axons to restore or improve conduction.[8]

Clinical Presentation

Acute poisoning has been followed by "metallic" tastes in the mouth, muscle spasms, abdominal cramps, paresthesias of the lower extremities, hyperventilation, anxiety, increased muscle tone, and confusion. The patient is alert and oriented to person, place and time. Hyperexcitability, tremors, seizures, depressed mental state,[21] muscle fasciculations, cardiac abnormalities, and respiratory arrest have been reported.[10,13] Recovery occurs within 24 hours, but weakness and lightheadedness may last 3 to 4 days.

Ingestion of about 60 mg each by two individuals led to immediate abdominal discomfort, nausea and vomiting, weakness, dizziness, and profuse diaphoresis. One patient suffered a tonic–clonic seizure and respiratory arrest. Both recovered in 3 days. Recovery after 4-AP poisoning usually occurs within 24 hours, but weakness and lightheadedness may last 3 to 4 days.[1,14] After ingestion of a high dose of 4-AP, severe vomiting, with a high risk of esophageal damage, diarrhea, intestinal spasm, and even ileus may develop.[14]

Laboratory

Analytical Methods

A gas–liquid chromatographic assay has a lower limit of sensitivity of 10 ng/mL.[16]

Blood Levels

Ingestion of 6 mg of 4-AP led to a blood concentration of 136.3 ng/mL.[21] Patients should be monitored with complete blood counts, electrolytes, creatine kinase (if seizures), blood glucose, blood urea nitrogen, creatinine, liver enzymes, and alkaline phosphatase. During continuous administration of 4-AP 15 mg/h, seizure activity was associated with serum 4-AP concentrations of 35 to 190 ng/mL.[21]

Abnormalities

Electrocardiographic evidence of sinus tachycardia and moderate ST wave changes follow exposure. There is a slight elevation of the blood glucose.[13]

Treatment

Stabilization

Establish and maintain vital functions (respirations, airway, cardiac function). Obtain a 12-lead electrocardiogram and monitor for cardiac disturbances. The tidal volume should be 10 to 15 cc/kg. Employ cardiopulmonary resuscitation as required.

If ingestion has occurred less than several hours before treatment, empty the stomach by intubation, aspiration, and lavage with a slurry of activated charcoal following placement of an endotracheal tube. Avoid ipecac-induced emesis. There is a risk of aspiration of gastric contents if seizures, depressed consciousness, or depressed reflexes occur before emesis. Seizures may occur within 5 to 15 minutes of exposure. If treatment is delayed, immediate oral administration of charcoal and sorbitol may represent optimal management. Treat dehydration with intravenous fluids if oral fluids cannot be retained.[10]

Elimination Enhancement

Consider hemoperfusion after an intake of more than 0.5 to 1 g (based on serum concentrations).[14] Provide sufficient infusion of fluids to maintain a diuresis of about 200 to 250 mL/h and to avoid dehydration.[14]

Supportive Measures

Control anxiety by sedation with diazepam. Control seizures with diazepam 0.1 mg/kg (maximum, 10 mg/dose); and phenytoin as required. If seizures persist, consider the use of neuromuscular blockers, intubation, and assisted ventilation. Nondepolarizing agents (eg, tubocurarine, dimethyltubocurarine) can be used to counteract the skeletal muscle effects of prolonged and refractory 4-AP-induced seizures. Atracuronium and vecuronium may be used, but there are few data to support their efficacy. Pancuronium is not usually recommended because of its cardiovascular effects. If the above treatment is unsuccessful, tubocurarine can be administered under assisted ventilation. Monitor with an electrocardiogram. Use sodium bicarbonate if metabolic acidosis is present. Atropine can be used to control abdominal cramps and diarrhea. Long-term anticonvulsant therapy is not indicated in patients who have had a single seizures from 4-AP. Obtain a neurology consult. Propranolol may block some of the cardiac toxicity of 4-AP and should be considered in treatment of severe arrhythmias.[1]

REFERENCES—4-AMINOPYRIDINE AND 3,4-DIAMINOPYRIDINE

1. Spyker DA, Lynch C, Shabanowitz J, Sinn JA. Poisoning with 4-aminopyridine: Report of three cases. Clin Toxicol 1980; 16:487–497.
2. Van Diemen HAM, Polman CH, Van Dongen MMMM, et al. 4-Aminopyridine induced functional improvement in multiple sclerosis patients: A neurophysiological study. J Neurol Sci 1993;116:220–226.
3. Morgan D. *Recognition and Management of Pesticide Poisonings.* EPA-540/9-88-001. Washington, DC: U.S. Environmental Protection Agency, March 1989:148–149.
4. Lundh H, Nilsson O, Rosen I, Johansson S. Practical aspects of 3,4-diaminopyridine treatment of the Lambert–Eaton myasthenic syndrome. Acta Neurol Scand 1993;88:136–140.
5. Rosen I, Lundh H, Nilsson O. Improvement of neuromuscular transmission by 3,4-diaminopyridine in the Lambert–Eaton myasthenic syndrome and in myasthenia gravis. Ann NY Acad Sci 1987;505:776–779.
6. Murray NMF, Newson-Davis J. Treatment with oral 4-aminopyridine in disorders of neuromuscular transmission. Neurology 1981;31:265–271.
7. Agoston S, Van Weeden T, Westra P, Brockert A. Effects of 4-aminopyridine in Eaton–Lambert syndrome. Br J Anaesth 1978;50:383–389.
8. Stefoski D, Davis FA, Faut M, Schauf CL. 4-Aminopyridine improves clinical signs in multiple sclerosis. Ann Neurol 1987;21:71–77.
9. Davis FA, Stefoski D, Rush J. Orally administered 4-aminopyridine improves clinical signs in multiple sclerosis. Ann Neurol 1990;27:186–192.
10. Wesseling H, Agoston S, Van Dam GBP, et al. Effects of 4-aminopyridine in elderly patients with Alzheimer's disease. N Engl J Med 1984;310:988–989.
11. Hansebout RR, Blight AR, Fawcett S, Reddy K. 4-Aminopyridine in chronic spinal cord injury: A controlled double-blind crossover study in eight patients. J Neurotrauma 1993;10:1–18.

12. Agoston S, Salt PJ, Erdmann W, et al. Antagonism of ketamine–diazepam anaesthesia by 4-aminopyridine in human volunteers. Br J Anaesth 1980;52:367–370.
13. Mofenson HC, Caraccio TR, Brody G, et al. Poison perspectives for health professionals. LI Regional Poison Control Center at Winthrop University Hospital. 1993;12(9):37–41.
14. Uges DRA, Buirs B, Sangster B. Treatment of 4-aminopyridine poisoning after oral overdose: A proposal. Pharm Acta Helv 1984;59:172–176.
15. Miller RD, Booij LHDJ, Agoston S, Crui JF. 4-Aminopyridine potentiates neostigmine and pyridostigmine in man. Anesthesiology 1979;50:416–420.
16. Evenhuis J, Agoston S, Salt PJ, et al. Pharmacokinetics of 4-aminopyridine in human volunteers. Br J Anaesth 1981; 53:567–570.
17. Uges DRA, Sohn YJ, Greijdanus B, et al. 4-Aminopyridine kinetics. Clin Pharmacol Ther 1982;31:587–593.
18. Wood M. Cholinergic and parasympathomimetic drugs: Cholinesterases and anticholinesterases. In: Wood M, Wood AJJ, eds. *Drugs and Anesthesia: Pharmacology for Anesthesiologists.* 2nd ed. Baltimore: Williams & Wilkins, 1990:104.
19. Mitzov V, Vlaskovska M. Effects of anticurare agents produced in Bulgaria on the smooth muscles of the gastrointestinal tract. Acta Physiol Pharmacol Bulg 1987;13:56–65.
20. Carlesson C, Rosen I, Nilsson E. Can 4-aminopyridine be used to reverse anaesthesia and muscle relaxation? Acta Anaesthesiol Scand 1983;27:87–90.
21. Stork CM, Howland MA, Hoffman RS. 4-Aminopyridine overdose. Vet Hum Toxicol 1994;36:375.

GLYCINE

Glycine is used as a component of irrigating solutions during transurethral prostatic surgery and may be partially responsible for production of the transurethral resection of the prostate (TURP) syndrome. Symptoms are referable to excess ammonia production (a glycine metabolite), excess fluid absorption (hyponatremia, hypervolemia), or both (water intoxication). Excess absorption of glycine irrigating solution may result in serious circulatory and central nervous system toxicity and may terminate in death. The surgeon and anesthetist are usually the first to observe these toxic effects if glycine is used as part of an irrigating solution.

Structure and Classification

Glycine (aminoacetic acid, Gly) is a nonessential amino acid normally present in the circulation.[1] Its formula is NH_2CH_2COOH and its molecular weight is 75.07; the CAS number is 56-40-6. Glycine is a white odorless crystalline powder that is soluble 1 in 4 in water and very slightly soluble in alcohol and ether.[2] Glycine is marketed as Glycocoll and Sucre de Gelatine. The conversion factor is 13.33.

Use

Glycine is used as a dietary supplement, and is sometimes used with antacids for the treatment of gastric hyperacidity.[2] It is widely used as a component of irrigation solutions during urogenital surgical procedures.

Product Formulation

Glycine for urogenital irrigation is used as a sterile 1.5% solution in water for injection. Glycine irrigation has a pH of 4.5 to 6.5 and the 1.5% irrigation has a calculated osmolarity of approximately 200 mOsm/L.[3] The formulation is packaged in 1500- to 5000-mL quantities.

The ideal transurethral irrigation fluid should be isotonic, nonhemolytic, nonelectrolytic, nontoxic when absorbed, not metabolized, provide clear visibility during an operation, not influence the osmolality of the blood, be rapidly excreted, be an osmotic diuretic, and not crystallize on instruments. Finally, the expansion of plasma or extracellular fluid volume from absorption of the fluid should be low and transient.[4] Glycine irrigation fluid is nonhemolytic and nonconductive and has a refractive index close to that of water.

Toxic Dose

Mild symptoms of TUR syndrome may occur after absorption of about 1000 mL of irrigant.[5] Severe signs and symptoms of TURP syndrome after a TURP develop when absorption of irrigating solution exceeds 2000 mL.[6] With greater absorption volumes, symptoms become more frequent and more severe.

Toxicokinetics

Plasma Glycine

Plasma glycine is normally present in concentrations of 120 to 386 μmol/L[7,8] (8.5–24.9 μg/mL).[9] After 20 g of oral glycine and 10 g every 2 hours for 10 hours, the plasma glycine level in one study was 56.2 μg/mL (746 μmol/L).[9] Plasma glycine rises immediately after glycine irrigation is used in a TURP, but usually returns to normal within 24 to 48 hours.[4] There may be a simultaneous increase in plasma serine (a metabolite of glycine) and plasma alanine within 2.5 hours.[10] Plasma glycine following a TURP may rise to more than 50 times normal values, decreasing rapidly to normal.[4]

Metabolism

Three routes of metabolism of glycine are clinically important.

1. The main route for glycine metabolism following a reversible oxidative cleavage with glycine synthase to carbon dioxide, ammonia, and N^5- and N^{10}-methylenetetrahydrofolate (ammonia is produced largely by the liver, some by the kidney).[11]
2. Conversion of glycine to serine by serine hydroxymethyltransferase with pyridoxal phosphate as coenzyme. Serine is then dehydrated and deaminated by serine dehydratase to pyruvate with pyridoxal phosphate as coenzyme. Serine may also be metabolized with the aid of serine hydroxymethyltransferase to glycine and N^5- and N^{10}-methylenetetrahydrofolate, a process that is reversible intracellularly.[4]
3. Conversion of glycine in the liver to glyoxalate, which is further metabolized into oxalate, which is excreted in the urine.[12]

Elimination

The elimination half-life of glycine is 85 minutes.[4]

Drug Interactions

Exogenous glycine increases the rate of formation of salicyluric acid in salicylate overdose. Plasma glycine is usually depressed in patients with aspirin overdose.[9]

Mechanism of Action

Glycine irrigation and absorption during TURP may lead to ammonia toxicity with concomitant central nervous system-depressive effects. Absorption of large volumes of irrigating fluid may also induce dilutional hyponatremia and hypervolemia. In such patients the serum osmolality may be depressed but the serum ammonia level may be normal. Where ammonia toxicity and hypervolemia are present, evidence of water intoxication may become apparent.[1] Visual abnormalities may reflect the role of glycine as a putative neurotransmitter between amacrine inhibitory cells of the retina.[13–15] Glycine exhibits an excitatory property that potentiates one of the glutaminergic receptors, the *N*-methyl-D-aspartate (NMDA) receptor, considered to play a role in excitotoxicity.

Clinical Presentation

Transurethral Resection of the Prostate Syndrome

Absorption of the irrigating solution used during TURP is the probable cause of TURP syndrome. Symptoms of TURP syndrome depend on the volume of irrigant absorbed into the systemic circulation either through the prostatic plexus of veins or indirectly via the periprostatic and retroperitoneal space if there is extravasation of fluid due to a breach in the capsule.[12,16]

Ammonia Toxicity

Ammonia, a metabolite of glycine, may accumulate in the blood following intravascular absorption of glycine during TURP. Ammonia toxicity should be suspected in patients undergoing a TURP who experience predominantly a central nervous system depression with smaller degrees of systemic symptoms.[1] Encephalopathy may be manifested as a delayed awakening in the postoperative period that persists despite correction of intravascular fluid volume and electrolyte balance.[1,2] Nausea and vomiting for 0.5 to 1 hour after surgery may follow absorption of 1 to 2 L of glycine-containing irrigation fluid and may be associated with a rise in blood ammonia concentration to more than three times its normal level.[16] Persistent nausea and vomiting may follow large-volume absorption concomitant with a moderately severe glycine toxicity and a blood ammonia concentration more than six times normal. Severe glycine intoxication is reflected in blood ammonia levels 15 times higher than normal concentrations together with either somnolence, marked alteration in consciousness,[10] seizures (rarely),[12] or coma.[17] Patients may develop convulsions and/or oliguria up to 24 hours after the operation.[12] The practice of irrigating the bladder with 1.5% glycine after the operation may be contributory.

Hyponatremia–Hypervolemia

A second group of patients may develop symptoms due to dilutional hyponatremia and hypervolemia with a decrease in osmolality in the absence of excessive blood concentrations of ammonia. These patients are likely to develop systemic symptoms. Such symptoms may include an initial hypertension followed by hypotension,[12] bradycardia,[12] headache, visual disturbance, restlessness, chest pain, agitation, confusion, and lethargy.[18,19]

Water Intoxication

Symptoms of excessive glycine-containing irrigation fluid absorption may be due to both ammonia toxicity and hypervolemia and can be reflected in hyponatremia, cerebral edema, hemolysis, and even death.[12,20] Signs and symptoms of excessive fluid absorption are usually evident during or immediately after the surgery but may be delayed for some hours.

Visual Loss

Loss of vision occurs within 20 minutes of a TURP when 1.5% glycine irrigation fluid has been used.[13,14] Pupillary response to light may be absent. The pupils may be dilated. Complete blindness may be experienced.[17] Vision generally returns to normal within 30 minutes[17] to 14 hours.[8,14] Visual difficulties may not be accompanied by a change in the blood ammonia concentration.[19] Transient blindness has followed glycine solution absorption ranging from 1000 to 3200 mL, corresponding to glycine absorption of 300 to 600 mg/kg, well into the toxic range for glycine in humans.[17] Visual changes may be accompanied by alterations in visual evoked potentials.[19]

Laboratory

Analytical Methods

Methods available for quantitation of plasma glycine include the amino acid analyzer[4] and a high-performance liquid chromatography method with fluorescence or electrochemical detection, which provides linearity between 0.2 and 40 μg/mL.[7,9] One percent ethanol added to the 1.5% glycine used in irrigating fluids may be reflected by measurement of breath ethanol concentrations sufficient to detect fluid absorption greater than 2000 mL.[6]

Blood Levels

Blood glycine volumes immediately following glycine 1.5% irrigation at surgery may rise to 20,000 to 25,000 μmol/L,[7,8] levels that are about 1000 times normal plasma glycine values.[17] Absorption of 15 mL of fluid into the extracellular fluid can increase plasma glycine concentrations to twice the normal value.[17]

Abnormalities

Glycine absorption may lead to hyperoxaluria and an increase in urine glycolate.[21] An increase in absorption of irrigation fluid may also lead to an acute dilutional hyponatremia with an accompanying decrease in serum albumin and hemoglobin.[12] A decrease in serum sodium tends to correlate with the absorption of irrigating fluid and, therefore, may be an indicator of glycine absorption.[4] Blood ammonia levels may rise to 15 times normal.[12] Deterioration in cerebral function may be associated with blood ammonia concentrations greater than 150 μmol/L.[1] Low serum osmolality is also a common feature.[12]

Following use of 2.2% glycine intravenously an increase in plasma vasopressin was observed, indicating the water retention may depend, in part, on an increase in vasopressin secretion.[22] If 300 mL of 1.5% glycine irrigation fluid is absorbed, there is usually no change in serum potassium concentration.[23] When more than 300 mL is absorbed, serum potassium may rise by 0.5 mmol/L, decreasing within 6 to 48 hours of surgery.[24]

The TURP syndrome may be reflected by electrocardiographic changes including depression in the ST segment, widening of the QRS, and disappearance of the P wave, probably associated with the hyponatremia.[12]

Treatment

1. Stop surgery if excessive fluid absorption is suspected. Continuing the resection will only lead to further absorption of fluid.
2. In mild to moderate cases spontaneous diuresis occurs, the fluid and electrolyte abnormalities are automatically corrected, and the blood chemistry often returns to normal within 24 hours.
3. Diuresis may be induced by intravenous furosemide. Mannitol 10 or 20% may also be used, because, unlike furosemide, it does induce sodium loss through the kidney, and it also may assist in reducing cerebral edema.
4. Treat hyponatremia if the serum sodium concentration falls below 120 mmol/L (see Water Intoxication under Clinical Presentation). Infusions of saline or hypertonic saline should be performed cautiously and slowly titrated against serum sodium levels. Reserve hypertonic saline for severe or refractory cases (eg, seizures, coma). Central pontine myelinosis, congestive heart failure, and cerebral hemorrhage may result from too rapid administration of hypertonic salt. Symptomatic patients with hyponatremia may tolerate an increase of 2 mEq (2 mmol) per liter per hour in the serum sodium concentration up to a level of 120 to 130 mEq/L.[25] "Masterly inactivity," fluid restriction, or loop diuretics may be sufficient depending on clinical judgment. Saline infusion may resolve mild to moderate central nervous system and electrolyte disturbances.
5. In extreme cases of fluid absorption not responding to therapy, hemodialysis may be required.
6. When hyperammonemia is present with associated symptomatology, consideration should be given to an infusion of L-arginine, which may inhibit the conversion of glycine to ammonia.[1,11,26]
7. Monitoring serum sodium concentrations, central venous pressure, and pulmonary arterial pressures may be useful, but invasive procedures are probably of little help in preventing absorption during a TURP. Monitoring fluid entering and leaving the bladder while measuring a rise in bladder pressure when the former exceeds the latter may one day be useful, but is probably not feasible.[12] Breath ethanol measurements may reflect use of 1% ethanol together with 1.5% glycine as an irrigating fluid. This may become a more generally accepted method for monitoring fluid absorption.[5,6]

REFERENCES—GLYCINE

1. Roesch RP, Stelting RK, Lingeman JE, et al. Ammonia toxicity resulting from glycine absorption during a transurethral resection of the prostate. Anesthesiology 1983;58:577–579.
2. Reynolds JEF, ed. *Martindale: The Extra Pharmacopoeia.* 30th ed. London: Pharmaceutical Press, 1993:1043.
3. McEvoy GK, ed. *AHFS Drug Information 94.* Bethesda, MD: American Society of Hospital Pharmacists, 1994:1728–1730.
4. Norlen H, Allgen L-G, Vinnars E, Bedrelidou-Classon G. Glycine solution as an irrigating agent during transurethral prostatic resection: Glycine concentrations in blood plasma. Scand J Urol Nephrol 1986;20:19–26.
5. Hahn RG. Early detection of the TURP syndrome by making the irrigating fluid with 1% ethanol. Acta Anaesthesiol Scand 1989;23:146–151.
6. Hahn RG. Prevention of TURP syndrome by detection of trace ethanol in the expired breath. Anaesthesia 1990;45:577–581.
7. Sherwood RA, Bayliss EM, Chappatte O. Assay of plasma glycine by HPLC with electrochemical detection in patients undergoing glycine irrigation during gynaecological surgery. Clin Chim Acta 1991;203:275–284.
8. Brady AY, Chyka PA. Glycine toxicity during hysteroscopic resection of the endometrium. Vet Hum Toxicol 1991;33:365.
9. Patel DK, Ogunbona A, Notarianni LJ, Bennett PN. Depletion of plasma glycine and effect of glycine by mouth on salicylate metabolism during aspirin overdose. Hum Exp Toxicol 1990;9:389–395.
10. Hutchesson ACJ, Wilkinson PA, Rattenbury JM, Manning N. Transient hyperglycinemia after transurethral surgery: Are metabolites of glycine significant? Clin Chem 1990;36:704–705.
11. Nathans D, Fahey JL, Ship AG. Sites of origin and removal of blood ammonia formed during glycine infusion: Effect of L-arginine. J Lab Clin Med 1958;51:124–133.
12. Rao PN. Fluid absorption during urological endoscopy. Br J Urol 1987;60:93–99.
13. Ovassapian A, Voshi CW, Brunner MD. Visual disturbances: An unusual symptom, a transurethral prostate resection reaction. Anesthesiology 1982;57:332–334.
14. Wright N, Seggie J. Glycine associated blindness: A case report and animal data. Vet Hum Toxicol 1987;29:478.
15. Hahn RG, Stalberg HP, Ekengren J, Rundgren M. Effects of 1.5% glycine solution with and without 1% ethanol on the fluid balance in elderly men. Acta Anaesthesiol Scand 1991;35:725–730.
16. Hahn RG. Blood ammonia concentrations resulting from absorption of irrigating fluid containing glycine and ethanol during transurethral resection of the prostate. Scand J Urol Nephrol 1991;25:115–119.
17. Burkhart SS, Barnett CR, Snyder SJ. Transient postoperative blindness as a possible effect of glycine toxicity. Arthroscopy 1990;6:112–114.
18. Bernstein GT, Loughlin KR, Gittes RF. The physiologic basis of the TURP Syndrome. J Surg Res 1989;46:135–141.
19. Hahn RG. Glycine absorption and visually evoked potentials. Anaesthesia 1992;47:78.
20. Baumann R, Magos AL, Kay JDS, Turnbull AC. Absorption of glycine irrigating solution during transcervical resection of endometrium. Br Med J 1990;300:304–305.
21. Fitzpatrick JM, Kasidar GP, Rose GA. Hyperoxaluria following glycine irrigation for transurethral prostatectomy. Br J Urol 1981;53:250–252.
22. Hahn RG, Stalberg HP, Gustafsson SA. Vasopressin and cortisol levels in response to glycine infusion. Scand J Urol Nephrol 1991;25:121–123.

23. Hirse M, Tanaka Y. Serum potassium change during the TURP syndrome by cell volume regulation. Can J Anaesth 1992;39:300–301.
24. Jensen V. Serum potassium change during the TURP syndrome by cell volume regulation. Can J Anaesth 1992; 39:300.
25. Nairns RG. Therapy of hyponatremia: Does haste make waste? N Engl J Med 1986;314:1573–1575.
26. Fahey JL. Toxicity and blood ammonia rise resulting from intravenous amino acid administration in man: The protective effect of L-arginine. J Clin Invest 1957;36:1647–1655.

PILOCARPINE

In acute poisoning with pilocarpine, a muscarinic agent, the lethal dose in a healthy adult has been estimated to be as low as 60 mg.[1] There are few reports of the disposition, metabolism, and excretion of pilocarpine after oral consumption or of its detection in the blood and urine.[2] Poisoning with ophthalmic solutions presents a potential hazard as they are usually stored in household refrigerators and are readily accessible.[3]

Clinical Presentation

Two elderly patients developed bronchoconstriction and an increase in bronchial mucous secretion leading to death. Coughing, salivation, and dyspnea was observed after every meal at a hospital. Two of 24 patients recovered. Serum cholinesterase levels were normal. Hourly administration of pilocarpine eyedrops to an 89-year-old man with chronic glaucoma led to symptomatic atrioventricular block.[4]

Clinical symptoms of acute overdose with pilocarpine eyedrops may include nausea, vomiting, diarrhea, abdominal pain, and intestinal cramps. Frequent urination, excessive salivation, lacrimation, sweating, pallor, cyanosis, bronchoconstriction, or an increase in nasal secretion may occur. Severe toxicity may induce vertigo, tremor, muscle weakness, paresthesias, bradycardia, cardiac arrhythmias, hypotension, syncope, increased systemic vascular resistance, and central nervous system excitation followed by depression, confusion, ataxia, seizures, and coma.[5,6]

Laboratory

Pilocarpine was identified in the urine[7] by gas chromatography and mass spectrometry with a detection limit of 0.1 μg/mL.[2] A high-performance liquid chromatography method is sensitive to 10 ng/mL.[8]

Treatment

When systemic reactions follow administration of pilocarpine, its use should be immediately discontinued. Tracheostomy, bronchial aspiration, and potential drainage may be required to maintain an adequate airway. Oxygen and assisted ventilation may be required. Atropine sulfate is an antidote (1–4 mg given intravenously, intravascularly, or subcutaneously). Muscarinic symptom control may require administration of atropine every 30 to 60 minutes; treatment may be required for 24 to 48 hours. In children the dose of atropine sulfate is 0.04 to 0.08 mg/kg up to 4 mg intramuscularly or intravenously. Atropine should be administered with caution in the presence of cyanosis because of the risk of ventricular fibrillation.

REFERENCES—PILOCARPINE

1. Clarke GFC. *Isolation and Identification of Drugs.* London: Pharmaceutical Press, 1995:500–501.
2. Cordner SM, Fysh RP, Gordon H, Whitaker SJ. Deaths of two hospital inpatients poisoned by pilocarpine. Br Med J 1986; 293:1285–1287.
3. Pfliegler GP, Palatka K. Attempted suicide with pilocarpine eyedrops. Am J Ophthalmol 1995;120:398–400.
4. Littmann L, Kempler P, Rohla M, Fenyresi T. Severe symptomatic atrioventricular block induced by pilocarpine eye drops. Arch Intern Med 1987;147:586–587.
5. Elis IP. Pilocarpine therapy. Surv Ophthalmol 1971;16: 165–169.
6. Havener WH. *Ocular Pharmacology.* St. Louis: Mosby, 1983: 319–347.
7. Bayne WF, Shu IC, Tao FT. Subnanogram assay for pilocarpine in biological fluids. J Pharm Sci 1976;65:1724–1727.
8. Weaver ML, Tanzer JM, Kramer PA. High-performance liquid chromatographic determination of pilocarpine in plasma. J Chromatogr Biomed Appl 1992;581:293–296.

PROBENECID

Probenecid, *p*-(dipropylsulfomoyl) benzoic acid, is widely used as an uricosuric agent and as an adjunct to therapy with penicillin and other antibiotics to enhance plasma antibacterial concentrations. It is also a competitive inhibitor of active transport processes in the brain,[1] kidney, liver, and eye.[2]

Toxicokinetics

Absorption

Absorption of probenecid after oral administration (0.5–2 g) is rapid, with concentrations peaking in 1 to 2 hours. Plasma probenecid concentration following an oral dose of 2 g peaks at 149 μg/mL between 3 and 4 hours.[3] Probenecid is 83 to 95% bound to plasma proteins (albumin) and diffuses freely across the blood–brain barrier.[2]

Elimination

Probenecid is metabolized by oxidation of the alkyl side chains (about 70%) and by glucuronide conjugation (about 20%).[4] The elimination half-life following a 2-g dose (oral or intravenous) ranges from 6 to 12 hours. About 5 to 11% of the drug is excreted in the urine unchanged.[5]

Drug Interactions

Probenecid increases the renal clearance of cimetidine.[5] Probenecid decreases the plasma protein binding of ceftriaxone and increases the free fraction of ceftriaxone in the plasma.[5,6]

Mechanism of Action

Probenecid has the ability to impair renal tubule excretion of other drugs and may also be an inducer of the mixed function oxidase system.[7]

Clinical Presentation

A 49-year-old man ingested 47 g of probenecid, developed coma and status epilepticus, and subsequently recovered. Therapeutic doses may cause anorexia, nausea, vomiting, and headache. Hypersensitivity occurs rarely.[8] A 36-year-old male alcoholic consumed 75 g of probenecid, lapsed into coma, suffered seizures, hypertension, and cardiac arrest, and died.[9]

Laboratory

Analytical Methods

High-performance liquid chromatographic assays are available for simultaneous measurement of probenecid and some of its metabolites.[1]

Blood Levels

Serum levels following ingestion of 75 g of probenecid averaged 7 μg/mL.[9]

Treatment

Treatment should be symptomatic and supportive. There is no antidote. Syrup of ipecac is inadvisable as an antiemetic in view of the tendency to early seizures and the possibility of aspiration pneumonia. Gastric lavage should be performed after endotracheal intubation. Hypotension can be treated with position change, intravenous fluids, and pressor amines.

REFERENCES—PROBENECID

1. Perel JM, Levitt HM, Dunner DL. Plasma and cerebrospinal fluid probenecid concentrations as related to accumulation of acidic biogenic amine metabolites in man. Psychopharmacologia 1974;35:83–90.
2. Cunningham RF, Israili ZH, Dayton PG. Clinical pharmacokinetics of probenecid. Clin Pharmacokinet 1981;6:135–151.
3. Israili ZH, Peril JM, Cunningham RF, et al. Metabolites of probenecid, chemical, physical and pharmacological studies. J Med Chem 1972;13:709–713.
4. Gisclon LG, Boyd RA, Williams RL, Giacomini AM. Effect of probenecid on the renal elimination of cimetidine. Clin Pharmacol Ther 1989;45:404–412.
5. Perel JM, Cunningham RF, Fales HM, Dayton PG. Identification and renal excretion of probenecid metabolites in man. Life Sci 1970;9:1337–1343.
6. Probenecid–ceftriaxone: An unusual interaction. Perspect Clin Pharm 1988;6:91–93. Editorial.
7. Bammel A, Monig H, Zuborn KH, et al. Enzyme-inducing properties of probenecid in man. Br J Clin Pharmacol 1991; 31:41.
8. Rizzuto VJ, Inglesby TV, Grace WJ. Probenecid (Benemid) intoxication with status epilepticus. Am J Med 1965;38: 646–648.
9. McIntyre IM, Crump K, Roberts AM, Drummer OH. A death involving probenecid. J Forens Sci 1992;37:1190–1193.

TACRINE HYDROCHLORIDE

The Food and Drug Administration approved tacrine hydrochloride (Cognex) for the treatment of mild to moderate Alzheimer's disease in 1993.[1–8] Reversible hepatic toxicity, nausea, vomiting, diarrhea, and rash have been observed with its use.[2,3] Its efficacy has been questioned in controlled clinical studies.[9–11] Overdoses may include a cholinergic crisis responsive to atropine.[12]

Structure and Classification

Tacrine is 9-amino-1,2,3,4-tetrahydroacridine (THA). It has a molecular weight of 252.74.[13]

Use

Tacrine is available for the treatment of mild to moderate Alzheimer's disease. It has also been potentially promising in the treatment of the acute anticholinergic syndrome associated with tricyclic antidepressant overdose.[14] Tacrine has been used in the management of the pain of terminal cancer, myasthenia gravis, and tardive dyskinesia and has also been used as a decurarizing agent.[15] It prolongs the muscle relaxation caused by succinylcholine.[16] A preliminary study of senile dementia of the Lewy body type (fluctuating cognitive impairment with delusions and/or hallucinations) suggests a possible association between the presence of Lewy bodies and a response to the drug.[17] Animal studies suggest that tacrine is not useful as a pretreatment for nerve agent intoxication.[18] Tacrine was originally developed as a partial antagonist of morphine and has been used with morphine in the treatment of intractable terminal cancer pain.[19]

Product Formulation

Tacrine is formulated as the hydrochloride. Each 10-, 20-, 30-, (and 40-mg capsule for oral administration) contains 12.75, 25.50, 38.25, and 51.00 mg of tacrine hydrochloride, respectively.[13]

Therapeutic Dose

The dosage of tacrine usually begins at 40 mg/d and is titrated in 6-week intervals to a maximum of 160 mg/d.[4,20]

Fatal Dose

The estimated lethal dose in animals is 40 mg/kg.[12,13]

Toxicokinetics

Absorption

Plasma concentrations peak (60 ng/mL) about 2 hours after oral administration and reach a steady state within 24 hours.[20,21] Tacrine is about 55% bound to plasma proteins.[22]

Distribution

The volume of distribution at steady state is 5 L/kg.[21]

Elimination

The drug is extensively metabolized in the liver to an active metabolite, 1-hydroxy-THA.[21] Negligible amounts of the drug are found in the urine.[15] The elimination half-life is about 2 hours after oral administration.[20] The elimination half-life of the metabolite is about 2.5 to 3 hours.[23] Plasma clearance ranges from 1 to 4 L/min.[21]

Drug Interactions

Tacrine inhibits cimetidine and theophylline metabolism by the cytochrome P450IA2 pathway.[20,24] The patient's theophylline concentration must be monitored. Other interactions may occur with drugs also metabolized by this pathway. Additive or synergistic effects with cholinergic agents and cholinesterase inhibitors may occur.[20] Smokers exhibit an increase in P450IA2 catalytic activity. These patients tend to have lower blood levels of tacrine.[23] Increases in blood pressure and heart rate have been reported with other cholinomimetics when coadministered with quaternary anticholinergic agents such as glycopyrrolate.[12]

Pregnancy/Lactation

Controlled studies have not been performed in pregnancy. It is not known whether the drug is excreted in human milk.

Mechanism of Action

The symptoms of Alzheimer's disease may be partially due to a decrease in acetylcholine levels within the Alzheimer brain.[4] Tacrine is a centrally active, noncompetitive reversible cholinesterase inhibitor that also acts as a partial agonist at muscarinic receptors, blocks reuptake of dopamine, serotonin, and norepinephrine, inhibits monoamine oxidase activity, and can block sodium and potassium channels.[16,20] It is a potent inhibitor of butyryl- and acetylcholinesterase, both of which appear to be sequestered in the pathologic plaques and tangles observed in the brain of Alzheimer's disease patients.[16] It is a longer-acting anticholinesterase than physostigmine.[16] Tacrine produces dose-dependent inhibition of human platelet aggregation.[19]

Clinical Presentation
Chronic Use

An increase in serum alanine transaminase activity is observed within 4 to 12 weeks of the first dose in about 50% of patients who take the drug,[20] but no clinical signs of hepatitis or jaundice have been observed.[5] Hepatic function returns to normal a few weeks after discontinuation of the drug. It is not clear whether this effect is dose related. Nausea, vomiting, diarrhea, headache, myalgia, and ataxia have also been observed.[22] Exacerbation of Parkinsonism has been seen.[25]

Overdose

Overdose with tacrine and other cholinesterase inhibitors may cause a cholinergic crisis characterized by severe nausea and vomiting, salivation, sweating, bradycardia, hypotension, collapse, and seizures. Increasing muscle weakness may result in death if respiratory muscles are involved.[12]

Laboratory
Analytical Methods

Plasma concentrations of tacrine are determined by high-performance liquid chromatography with ultraviolet detection. The detection limit is about 0.3 ng/mL for the drug and its metabolites.[21]

Blood Levels

Measurement of blood concentrations of tacrine and its metabolites appears to provide a better prediction of the risk of adverse effects than dose alone.[26] The tacrine:metabolite ratio is also higher in patients with adverse effects.[26] Serum concentrations above 20 ng/mL are associated with a high risk of symptomatic adverse effects.[26] A therapeutic window of between 7.5 μg/L (associated with improvement in cognitive rating scale) and 20 μg/L has been proposed.[27]

Abnormalities

An absolute neutrophil count less than 500 μL has been observed.[13]

Treatment
Stabilization

General symptomatic and supportive treatment is indicated after an overdose of tacrine (see Antidote).

Elimination Enhancement

As a result of its high volume of distribution it is unlikely that tacrine or its metabolites will be eliminated by dialysis (hemodialysis, peritoneal dialysis or hemofiltration).[12]

Antidote

Tertiary anticholinergic agents such as atropine may be used as an antidote for tacrine poisoning. The initial intravenous dose of atropine sulfate is 1.0 to 2.0 mg, with subsequent doses based on clinical response.[12]

Supportive Measures

Monitor aminotransferase activity weekly for at least the first 18 weeks of therapy and for the 6 weeks following each further increase in dosage.[28]

General Review Articles

- Crismon ML. Tacrine: First drug approved for Alzheimer's disease. Ann Pharmacother 1994;28:744–751.
- Wagstaff AJ, McTavish D. Tacrine: A review of its pharmacodynamic and pharmacokinetic properties and therapeutic efficacy in Alzheimer's disease. Drugs Aging 1994;4:510–540.

REFERENCES—TACRINE HYDROCHLORIDE

1. Relman AS. Tacrine as a treatment for Alzheimer's dementia. N Engl J Med 1991;324:349–352. Editor's Note.

2. New Product Approvals: First Alzheimer's drug. FDA Med Bull 1993;23(3):5–46.
3. First Alzheimer's drug approval. FDA Consumer 1992; 27:2.
4. Wilcock GK, Surmon DJ, Scott M, et al. An evaluation of the efficacy and safety of tetrahydroaminoacridine (THA) without lecithin in the treatment of Alzheimer's disease. Age Aging 1993;22:316–324.
5. Farlow M, Gracon SL, Hershey LA, et al. A controlled trial of tacrine in Alzheimer's disease. JAMA 1992;268:2523–2529.
6. Knapp MJ, Knopman DS, Solomon PR, et al. A 30-week randomized controlled trial of high-dose tacrine in patients with Alzheimer's disease. JAMA 1994;271:985–991.
7. Eagger SA, Morant N, Levy R, Sahakian BJ. Tacrine in Alzheimer's disease: Time course of changes in cognitive function and practice effects. Br J Psychiatry 1992;160: 36–40.
8. Eagger SA, Levy R, Sahakian BJ. Tacrine in Alzheimer's disease. Lancet 1991;337:989–992.
9. Maltby N, Broe GA, Creasey H, et al. Efficacy of tacrine and lecithin in mild to moderate Alzheimer's disease: Double blind trials. Br Med J 1994;309:879–883.
10. Byrne EJ, Arieg T. Tetrahydroaminoacridine and Alzheimer's disease: For the few but we don't know which few. Br Med J 1994;308:868–869.
11. Molloy DW, Guyatt GH, Wilson DB, et al. Effect of tetrahydroaminoacridine on cognition, function and behavior in Alzheimer's disease. Can Med Assoc J 1991;144:29–34.
12. Benezra DA. Personal communication. Parke-Davis, April 27, 1994.
13. Product Literature: Cognex[R] (Tacrine HCl capsules). Parke-Davis (PD-102-JA-8622-A0093-310039).
14. Sumners WK, Kaufman KR, Altman F Jr, Fischer JM. THA: A review of the literature and its use in treatment of five overdose patients. Clin Toxlcol 1980;16:269–281.
15. Forsyth DR, Wilcock GK, Morgan RA, et al. Pharmacokinetics of tacrine hydrochloride in Alzheimer's disease. Clin Pharmacol Ther 1989;46:634–641.
16. Freeman SE, Dawson RM. Tacrine: A pharmacological review. Progress Neurobiol 1991;36:257–277.
17. Levy R, Eagger SA, Griffiths M, et al. Lewy bodies and response to tacrine in Alzheimer's disease. Lancet 1994; 343:176.
18. Fricke RF, Koplowitz I, Scharf BA, Rockwood GA. Efficacy of tacrine as a nerve agent pretreatment. Drug Chem Toxicol 1994;17:15–34.
19. Liu S, Sylvester DM. The inhibitory effect of 9-amino-1,2,3,4-tetrahydroacridine (THA) on platelet function. Thromb Res 1992;67:533–544.
20. Tacrine for Alzheimer's disease. Med Lett Drugs Ther 1993; 35(905):87–88.
21. Hartvig P, Askmark H, Aquilonius SM, et al. Clinical pharmacokinetics of intravenous and oral 9-amino-1,2,3,4-tetrahydroacridine, tacrine. Eur J Clin Pharmacol 1990;38: 259–263.
22. Davis KL, Powchik P. Tacrine. Lancet 1995;345:625–630.
23. Sitar DS, Lou GL, Montgomery PR. Bioavailability and pharmacokinetic disposition of tacrine hydrochloride in elderly patients with Alzheimer's disease. Clin Pharmacol Ther 1995; 57:Abstract PIII-17.
24. Watkins PB, Zimmerman HJ, Knapp MJ, et al. Hepatotoxic effects of tacrine administration in patients with Alzheimer's disease. JAMA 1994;271:992–998.
25. Ott BR, Lannon MC. Exacerbation of parkinsonism by Tacrine. Clin Neuropharmacol 1992;15:322–325.
26. Ford JM, Truman CA, Wilcock GK, Roberts CJ. Serum concentrations of tacrine hydrochloride predict its adverse effects in Alzheimer's disease. Clin Pharmacol Ther 1993; 53:691–695.
27. Roberts C, Ford J, Makela P, Truman C. Serum tacrine concentrations too low. Br Med J 1994;308:1501.
28. Wagstaff AJ, McTavish D. Tacrine: A review of its pharmacodynamic and pharmacokinetic properties and therapeutic efficacy in Alzheimer's disease. Drugs Aging 1994; 4:510–540.

MULTIPLE CHEMICAL SENSITIVITY

Environmental illnesses have been referred to by a number of different terms[1] (Table 51–2).

Definition

Cullen has provided a definition of multiple chemical sensitivity (MCS) (Table 51–3).[2]

Diagnostic Testing

There is no established or widely available test used to diagnose MCS. Testing is requiring to rule out the presence of other environmental or nonenvironmental illnesses or treatable diseases in the differential diagnosis.

Risk Exposures

Examples of factors associated with onset on MCS are summarized in Table 51–4.[3]

Multiple Chemical Sensitivity by Proxy

Robertson has defined this syndrome.[4] Criteria for such a diagnosis include a parent's seemingly being very concerned about the effects of environmental chemicals on his, her, or their child, who on examination appears not to be ill. No

Table 51–2
Terms for Environmental Illness

- Environmentally-induced disease
- Chemical hypersensitivity syndrome
- Multiple chemical sensitivities
- Cerebral allergy
- Chemically induced immune disregulation
- Twentieth-century disease
- Total allergy syndrome
- Ecologic illness
- Food and chemical sensitivities

Adapted from Terr AI. American College of Physicians: Clinical ecology. Ann Intern Med 1989;111(2):168–178.

Table 51–3
Cullen's Definition of the Multiple Chemical Sensitivity Syndrome

1. Syndrome is acquired in relation to documentable environmental exposure(s), insult(s), or illness(es).
2. Symptoms involve more than one organ system.
3. Symptoms recur and abate in response to predictable stimuli.
4. Symptoms are elicited by exposure to chemicals or diverse structural classes and toxicologic modes of action.
5. Symptoms are elicited by exposures that are demonstrable (albeit of low level).
6. Exposures that elicit symptoms must be very low (several standard deviations below levels known to cause adverse human responses).
7. No single widely available test of organ system function can explain symptoms.

Adapted from Cullen MP. The worker with multiple chemical sensitivities: An overview. In: Cullen MP, ed. *Occupational Medicine: State of the Art Reviews.* Philadelphia: Hanley & Belfus, 1987;655–666.

Table 51–4
Factors Associated with the Onset of Multiple Chemical Sensitivity

Factor
Solvents
Paint or lacquer thinner, printing ink/press cleaners, xylene, methylene chloride, paints, petroleum distillates, glycol ethers
Paint thinner, xylene, trichlorethane, kerosene, methylene chloride
Pesticides
Chlordane
Formaldehyde
Hydrogen sulfide
Formaldehyde, germicide, nitric acid, freon, toluene diisocyanate, argon
Workplace
Copy machines, new carpets
Smoke, new building, hairsprays, dry air, heat at work
Metals
Nickel, lead
Dusts
Woods
Scabies
Viral infection
food poisoning
Drug reactions
Stress
Fall at work

Adapted from Nethercott JA, Davidoff LL, Curbow B, Abbey H. Multiple chemical sensitivities syndrome: Toward a working case definition. Arch Environ Health 1993;48:19–26.

specific physical finding or laboratory test is available to confirm or refute such a diagnosis with certainty.

Clinical Presentation

Symptoms reported to be associated with the onset of MCS include the following[5,6]:

Head/ears/eyes/neck/throat	Headaches, sore throat, sinus, eye irritation, nasal stuffiness, eye focus difficulties, nasal soreness
Respiratory	Shortness of breath, cough, wheeze, chest tightness
Gastrointestinal	Nausea, abdominal pain, gas, vomiting, constipation, bloating, decreased appetite
Vestibular	Dizziness, intoxication
Neurologic/Psychological	Memory concentration loss, numbness, tremors, palpitation, body pain
Skin	Urticaria

In most cases awareness of an odor is the triggering factor.[7]

Clinical Perspectives

1. The syndrome may be severely distressing and functionally disabling, even as patients increasingly avoid universally present chemical exposures.
2. The fact that there is no agreement on any one etiology for most patients with MCS does not prevent clinicians from helping affected patients with their symptoms.
3. Reinforcement of illness behavior by unjustifiably giving a patient the diagnosis of a disease due to toxic, immunologic, or neurologic mechanisms based on diagnostic testing that is clinically unsubstantiated or invalid may actually perpetuate illness, prolong disability, and delay effective therapy.
4. Even if the etiologies of the symptoms in those diagnosed with MCS are controversial and unknown in most patients, these patients can still be helped with their symptoms.

Neurologic Testing

No form of neurologic testing has been shown to be diagnostic of either exposure to specific chemicals or illness due to exposure in patients with MCS.[7] Neuropsychological testing does not reveal consistent or specific findings in MCS.[8–9]

Treatment

Approaches to the drug stress include massage, physical therapy, prayer, meditation, and regular exercise. Odors and exposure to volatile organic compounds in the workplace that are perceived as irritating or noxious by the symptomatic person should be reduced and controlled as much as possible. Recommendation for long-term avoidance of chemical exposures is contraindicated because there is no evidence for a cumulative toxic injury underlying MCS. Engineering controls, personal protective equipment, work practices and job modification or removal may lessen exposure to toxic levels of any chemical. Firm recommendations for specific treatment modalities must await the results of definitive clinical trials.

Kurt suggests the following treatment guideline modalities[7]:

- Acute medical care
- Avoidance of adrenergic inhalants if at all possible, as they tend to increase anxiety and panic symptoms.
- Use of anxiety/panic attack approach with antidepressants and behavioral modification to "deprogram" fear of toxic exposures by using properly educated caution in exposures without improper exaggeration (long-term strategy)

Community resources and providers helpful in evaluating MCS include industrial hygienists; clinical neurologists; neuropsychologists (for testing: anxiety/depression vs organicity); psychiatrists; and information sources such as poison control centers, Medline, Toxline, Occupational Safety and Health Administration, Environmental Protection Agency, National Institute of Occupational Safety and Health, and the Food and Drug Administration.

Spyker and Sparks has extensively reviewed MCS.[10,11]

REFERENCES—MULTIPLE CHEMICAL SENSITIVITY

1. Terr AI. American College of Physicians: Clinical ecology. Ann Intern Med 1989;111:168–178.
2. Cullen MP. The worker with multiple chemical sensitivities: An overview. In: Cullen MP, ed. *Occupational Medicine: State of the Art Reviews.* Philadelphia: Hanley & Belfus 1987: 655–666.
3. Nethercott JR, Davidoff LL, Curbow B, Abbey H. Multiple chemical sensitivities syndrome: Toward a working case definition. Arch Environ Health 1993;48:19–26.

4. Robertson WO. MCS (multiple chemical sensitivity) by proxy. Vet Hum Toxicol 1994;36:579–580.
5. Cone JE, Harrison R, Reiter R. Patients with multiple chemical sensitivities: Clinical diagnostic subsets among an occupational health clinic population. Occup Med State of the Art Reviews. 1987;2:721–738.
6. Kilburn KH. Symptoms, syndrome and semantics: Multiple chemical sensitivity and chronic fatigue syndrome. Arch Environ Health 1993;48:368–369.
7. Kurt TL. Multiple chemical sensitivities. Presented at the American Academy of Clinical Toxicology Meeting, Salt Lake City, September 24, 1994.
8. Sparks PJ, Daniell W, Black DW, et al. Multiple chemical sensitivity syndrome: A clinical perspective: I. Case definition, theories of pathogenesis, and research needs. J Occup Med 1994;36:718–730.
9. Simon GE, Daniell W, Stockbridge H, et al. Immunologic, psychological and neuropsychological factors in multiple chemical sensitivity. Ann Intern Med 1993;119:97–108.
10. Sparks PJ, Daniell W, Black DW, Kipen HM, Altman LC, Simon: Multiple chemical sensitivity syndrome: A clinical perspective: II. Evaluation, diagnostic testing, treatment and social considerations. J Occup Med 1994;36:731–737.
11. Spyker DA. Multiple chemical sensitivities. Presented at the American Academy of Clinical Toxicology Meeting, Salt Lake City, September 24, 1994.

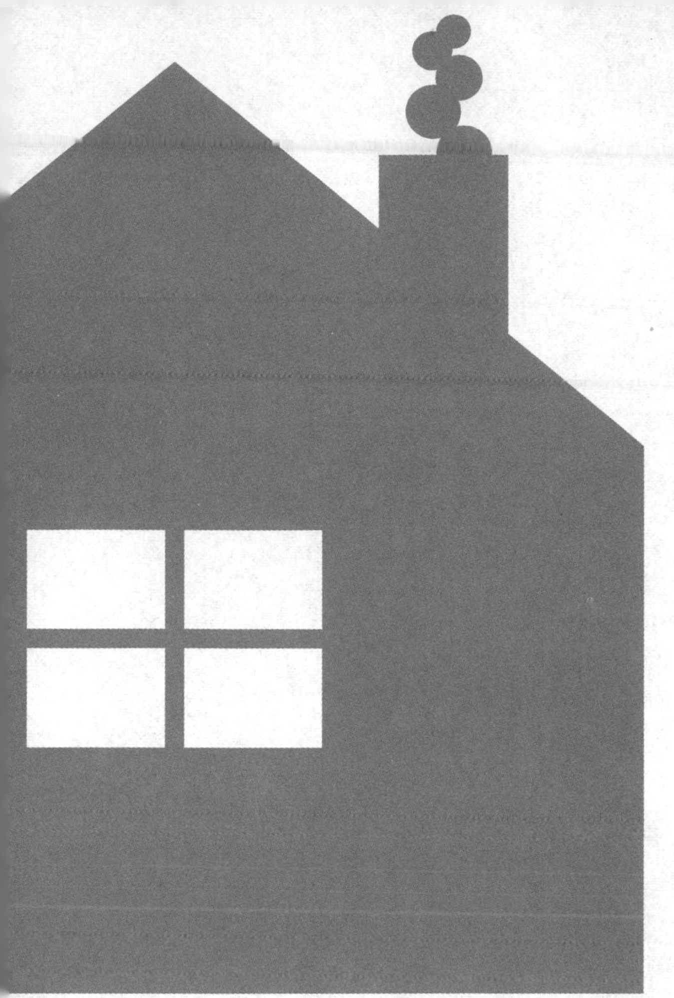

Section III
THE HOME

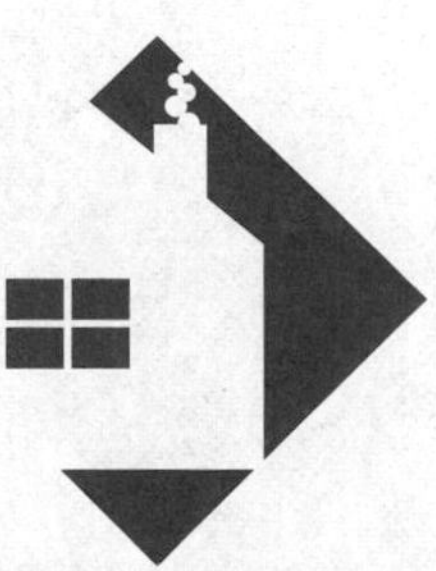

Chapter **52**

Over-The-Counter Products Drug Interactions

COLD MEDICATIONS

EPHEDRINE AND PSEUDOEPHEDRINE

CLINICAL PRESENTATION

A 64-year-old hemodialysis patient developed myoclonic jerking and bizarre behavior after ingesting conventional doses (60 mg four times daily) of pseudoephrine.[2] Pseudoephrine overdoses can be as severe as other sympathomimetic ingestions and may include tachycardia, hypertension, intracranial hemorrhage, agitation, rhabdomyolysis, hyperthermia, and seizures.[3] Chronic overuse of ephedrine may induce a vasculitis of the central nervous system.[4] Pseudoephedrine's adverse effects may present as recurrent toxic shock syndrome.[5]

Phenylephrine (10%), total dose 20 mg, was administered by drops into the eyes during surgery. The patient developed severe acute hypertension to 260/120 mm Hg, cardiac arrhythmias, and a non–Q-wave anterolateral myocardial infarction and survived.[6]

Inadvertent splashing of phenylephrine (Neosynephrine) nose spray (0.5%) into the eye of a comatose patient produced a fixed dilated left pupil, resulting in a misdiagnosis of cerebral herniation.[7]

An adult ingested 22,500 mg of ephedrine and developed a tachycardia and agitation. Recovery within 24 hours followed gastric lavage, activated charcoal, and propranolol.[8] Propranolol, 1 mg intravenously (IV), has also been used effectively in the treatment of hypertension following a pseudoephedrine dose of 4500 mg and an ephedrine dose of 17,500 mg. Remember that unopposed alpha agonists such as propranolol may aggravate hypertension.[9] Ephedrine has a high-abuse potential. Following ingestion of excess ephedrine both ischemic and hemorrhagic stroke have been observed.[10] A retrospective study of 17 cases of pure pseudoephedrine effects in children who ingested from 30 to 1050 mg of pseudoephedrine revealed frequent drowsiness, especially in doses over 120 mg. Despite therapy (syrup of ipecac, activated charcoal), children who ingested 120 mg or less developed no significant symptoms, regardless of any treatment. Therapy may be unnecessary in these children.[11] A prospective study appears to confirm these results.[12]

Table 52-1
Some Common Over-the-Counter Drugs That May Increase Blood Pressure[a]

Ephedrine
Amesec Capsules
Asthmalixir
Azma Aid Tablets
Bronitin Tablets
Bronkaid Mist and Tablets
Bronkolixir
Bronkotabs
Efed II
Efedron Nasal
Ephedrine Sulfate
Guiaphed Elixir
Phedral C.T. Tablets
Primatene Tablets (M, P, and Regular Formula)
Quelidrine Cough Syrup
Tedral Tablets, Suspension, and Elixir
Tedrigen Tablets
Theodrine Tablets
Theoral Tablets
Vicks Vatronol Nose Drops
Epinephrine
Adrenalin Chloride
AsthmaHaler
Bronitin Mist
Bronkaid Mist and Mist Suspension
Medihaler-Epi
Primatene Mist and Suspension
Ibuprofen
Aches-N-Pain
Advil Caplets and Tablets
Haltran Tablets
Ibuprin
Ibuprofen
Medipren Caplets and Tablets
Midol 200 Advanced Pain Formula
Nuprin Caplets and Tablets
Pamprin-IB
Trendar Tablets
Phenylephrine
Alamine Liquid
AL-AY Modified Tablets
Alconefrin 12, 25, and 50
Cerose-DM
Codimal DM Syrup
Colrex Cough Syrup
Conar Syrup and Conar-A Tablets
Covangesic Tablets
Dallergy-D Syrup
Decohist Syrup
Dexafed Cough Syrup
Dihistine Elixir
Dimetane Decongestant Caplets and Elixir
Dondril Tablets
Dristan Advanced Formula Tablets, Caplets, and Nasal Spray
Duphrene Tablets
Duration 4 Hour Decongestant Nasal Spray
Father John's Medicine Plus Liquid
4-Way Fast Acting Nasal Spray
Guistrey Fortis Tablets
Histagesic Modified Tablets
Histatab Plus Tablets
Hista-Vadrin Syrup
Kolephrin Capsules
Myhistine Elixir
Neo-Synephrine
Nor-Lief Tablets
Phenylephrine (continued)
Nostril Nasal Decongestant
Novahistine Elixir
Phenhist Elixir
Quelidrine Cough Syrup
Rhinall and Rhinall-10
Rhinogesic Tablets
Robitussin Night Relief
Ru-Tuss Liquid
Salphenyl Capsules
Sinophen
Spec-T Sore Throat/Decongestant Lozenges
Trimedine Liquid
Tussar DM Cough Syrup
Tussex Cough Syrup
Vicks Sinex Spray and Mist
Phenylpropanolamine
Acutrim Late Day and 16 Hour Appetite Suppressant
Acutrim II Maximum Strength Appetite Suppressant
Alka-Seltzer Plus and Night-Time Cold Medicine
Allerest Headache Strength Tablets and Sinus Pain Formula
Allerest Tablets or 12 Hour Caplets
Allergy Relief Medicine
Allergy Tablets
Anatuss Syrup
Appedrine Appetite Suppressant
Appetite Control Tablets
A.R.M. Allergy Relief Medicine Caplets
Bowman Cold Tablets
BQ Cold Tablets
Bromanate DC Cough Syrup
Bromatap Elixir
Cheracol Plus Head Cold/Cough Formula
Chexit Tablets
Chlor-Rest Tablets
Codimal Expectorant
Cold and Allergy Relief Tablets
Combat Cold Capsules
Comtrex Multi-Symptom Cold Reliever Tablets/Caplets/Liquid
Conex Plus and D.A. Tablets and Syrup
Congespirin Liquid Cold Medicine
Contac Caplets, Capsules, and Severe Cold Formula Caplets
Control Appetite Suppressant
Coricidin "D" and Extra Strength Sinus Headache Tablets
Coryban-D Caplets (Tablets)
Covangesic Tablets
Demazin Nasal Decongestant/ Antihistamine Repetabs
Dex-a-diet and Dex-a-diet plus Vitamin C
Dexatrim
Diadax
Dimetapp Elixir, Extentabs, Plus Caplets, and Tablets
Drinophen Capsules
Duadacin Capsules
Endecon Tablets
Fendol Tablets
Fiogesic Tablets
4-Way Cold Tablets
Genamin Syrup
Genatap Elixir
Phenylpropanolamine (continued)
Genex Capsules
Grapefruit Diet Plan with Diadex
Halls Menthol-Lyptus Decongestant Liquid
Head and Chest Liquid
Hista-Vadrin Syrup
Histosal Tablets
Hungrex Plus
Kleer Comp Tablets
Kolephrin DM Capsules and NN Liquid
Kophane Cough and Cold Formula Syrup
Lanatuss Expectorant
My-K Formula 77D Liquid
Myminic Syrup and Expectorant
Myminicol Liquid
Myphetapp Elixir
Naldecon DX or DX Adult Liquid
Nasal Decongestant Antihistamine Tablets and Elixirs
Noraminic Syrup
Ornacol Cough and Cold Tablets
Permathene-12
Pertussin AM Liquid
Phenapap and No. 2 Tablets
Poly-Histine Expectorant Syrup
Primatuss Cough Mixture 4D Liquid
Prolamine
Propagest
Pyrroxate Capsules
Remcol Cold Capsules
Rhinocaps Capsules
Robitussin-CF
Saleto D Capsules
Sinal Sinus Tablet
Sinapils Tablets
Sinarest Regular and Extra Strength Tablets
Sine-Off Sinus Medicine Tablets—Aspirin Formula
Sinulin Tablets
Sinus Headache Tablets
Slimtime
Spec-T Sore Throat/Decongestant Lozenges
Stay Trim Diet Gum
Sucrets Cold Decongestant Formula
Syracol Liquid
Threamine DM
Triminol Cough Syrup
Triaminic Tablets, Chewables, Cold Syrup, Cough Formula, and Expectorant
Triaminic Tablets
Triaminocol Multi-Symptom Cold Syrup and Tablets
Tricodene Forte Liquid
Tricodene NN Cough and Cold Medication Syrup
Trind or Trind-DM
Tri-Nefrin Extra Strength Tablets
Triphenyl Syrup
Tussagesic Tablets
Tussin CF
12 Hour Cold Capsules
12-Timed
Unitrol
Pseudoephedrine
Actacin Tablets
Actagen Tablets and Syrup
Actamine Tablets and Syrup

[a]Adapted from Prisant LM, Carr AA. Postgrad Med 1989;86:205–208.

Table 52–1 *(Continued)*

Pseudoephedrine (continued)	**Pseudoephedrine (continued)**	**Pseudoephedrine (continued)**
Actifed Capsules, Tablets, and Syrup	Entafed Capsules	T-Dry Capsules
Afrinol Repetabs Tablets	Extreme Cold Formula Caplets	T.P.I. Tablets
AllerAct Tablets and Caplets	Fedahist Decongestant Syrup, Expectorant Syrup, and Tablets	Triofed Syrup
Allerest No Drowsiness Tablets	Fedrazil Tablets	Tripodrine Tablets
Allerfed Capsules and Syrup	Genac Tablets	Triposed Tablets and Syrup
Allerfrin OTC Tablets and Syrup	Genaphed	Tussin Ephedrine
All-Nite Cold Formula Liquid	Genite Liquid	Tussin PE
Alpha-Phed Capsules	Glycofed Tablets	12 Hour Antihistamine Nasal Decongestant
Ambenyl-D Decongestant Cough Formula Liquid	Halofed and Halofed Syrup	Ty-Cold Tablets
Anahist Decongestant	Head and Chest Caplets	Tylenol Maximum Strength Sinus Tablets and Caplets
Aphedrid	Isoclor Tablets and Timesules (Capsules)	Ursinus Inlay-Tabs
Aprodine Tablets and Syrup	Mediquell Decongestant Formula	Vicks Daycare Daytime Colds Medicine Caplets
Aprofed	Myfed Syrup	Vicks Daycare Multi-Symptom Colds Medicine Liquid
Benadryl Decongestant Elixir, Kapseals, and Tablets	Myfedrine and Myfedrine Plus Liquid	Vicks Formula 44D Decongestant Cough Mixture
Benylin Decongestant	Naldegesic Tablets	Vicks Formula 44M Multisymptom Cough Mixture
Beta-Phed Capsules	Napril Tablets	Vicks Nyquil Nighttime Colds Medicine
Bromfed Syrup	Neofed	Viro-Med Tablets
Cenafed, Cenafed Plus, and Cenafed Syrup	Nite Time Cold Formula	**Racinephrine**
Chlorafed Liquid	Noratuss II Expectorant	AsthmaNefrin and AsthmaNefrin Solution "A" Bronchodilator
Chlor-Trimeton Decongestant and Long-Acting Decongestant Repetab Tablets	Novahistine DMX	Dey-Dose Epinephrine
Co-Apap Tablets	NyQuil Nighttime Cold Medicine Liquid	microNefrin
Codimal Capsules and Tablets	Nytime Cold Medicine Liquid	S-2 Inhalant
Cold and Allergy Medicine Tablets	Ornex Caplets	Vaponefrin
Cold Capsules	Pertussin PM	Vaponephrine Solution
Coldrine Tablets	Phenapap Sinus Headache and Congestant Tablets	**Theophylline**
Comtrex A/S Multi-Symptom Allergy-Sinus Formula Tablets and Caplets	Pseudo Syrup	Amesec Capsules
Congestac Caplets	Pseudo-gest and Pseudo-gest Plus Tablets	Asthmalixir
Contac Nighttime Cold Medicine	Pseudo-Hist Liquid and Tablets	Azma Aid Tablets
Contac Severe Cold Formula Liquid	Quiet Night Liquid	Bronitin Tablets
Co-Pyronil 2 Pulvules (capsules)	Robitussin-PE	Bronkaid Tablets
CoTylenol Cold Medication Liquid, Caplets, and Tablets	Rymed Liquid	Bronkolixir
Cremacoat 3 and 4	Ryna, Ryna-C, Ryna-CX Liquid	Bronkotabs
Dallergy-D Capsules	St Joseph Nighttime Cold Medicine	Guiaphed Elixir
Decofed Syrup	Sinarest No Drowsiness Tablets	Phedral C.T. Tablets
Dimacol Caplets and Liquid	Sine-Aid	Primatene Tablets (M, P or Regular Formula)
Disophrol Tablets and Chronotab Sustained-Action Tablets	Sine-Off	Tedral Tablets, Suspension, and Elixir
Dristan Maximum Strength Decongestant/Analgesic Coated Caplets	Singlet Tablets	Tedrigen Tablets
Drixoral and Drixoral Plus Tablets and Syrup	Sinus Excedrin Analgesic, Decongestant Tablets and Caplets	Theodrin Tablets
Duration Long Acting Nasal Decongestant Tablets	Sinus Headache Tablets	Theoral Tablets
	Sinus Tablets	
	Sinus Tab2	
	Sinutab	
	Sudafed	
	Sudrin	
	Super Anahist Tablets	
	Su-phedrine and Su-phedrine Plus	

Many over-the-counter drugs may increase blood pressure (Table 52–1).

LABORATORY

Blood Levels

After prolonged ingestion of 240 mg/day, blood levels of pseudoephedrine were 1425 ng/mL.

Abnormalities

The ephedrine concentrations in three fatalities with caffeine/ephedrine combinations were 3.49, 7.85, and 20.5 mg/L.[13] Pseudoephedrine blood concentrations in a case of fatal overdosage were 19 mg/L.[14]

TREATMENT

Hemodynamic (hypertension, tachyarrhythmias, palpitation) dysfunction and central nervous system dysfunction (tremors, agitation) respond to careful propranolol administration. Propranolol, 1 mg IV, rapidly (within 5 minutes) corrected severe hypertension in two patients who had ingested pseudoephedrine 4500 mg and ephedrine 17,500 mg, respectively. The patients survived.[9]

An anecdotal report of two patients with an overdose of pseudoephedrine (one patient) and ephedrine respectively suggests a potential therapeutic benefit from intravenous propranolol administered in intravenous doses of 1 mg. In the treatment of severe hypertension, sodium nitroprusside remains a first-line agent.[9] Further experience with propranolol in the treatment of sympathomimetic-

Table 52–2
Sympathomimetic Amine-Induced Responses of Effector Organs Subserved by α, β-1, and β-2 Adrenoceptors[a]

Subserved by the α Adrenoceptor		Subserved by the β-1 Adrenoceptor		Subserved by the β-2 Adrenoceptor	
Effector Organ	Response	Effector Organ	Response	Effector Organ	Response
Vascular smooth muscle	Vasoconstriction	Heart	Augmented pacemaker Augmented contractility	Vascular smooth muscle	Vasodilatation
Liver	Glycogenolysis	Vascular smooth muscle		Tracheal and bronchial smooth muscle	Relaxation
		coronary	Relaxation		
		intestine	Relaxation		
Intestinal smooth muscle	Relaxation	Adipose tissue (white)		Skeletal muscle	
			Lipolysis Lipogenesis		Contraction Glycogenolysis
				Potassium uptake	Hypokalemia

Adapted from Paradis NA, Koscove EM. Epinephrine in cardiac arrest: a critical review. Ann Emerg Med 1990 Nov, 19(11):1288–1301. Pub type: Journal Article; Review; Review, Tutorial.

induced hypertension is indicated. Propranolol is a beta-blocker. Watch for aggravation of hypertension due to unopposed alpha agonist effects from the sympathomimetic.[9,15]

TOXICOKINETICS

The normal apparent total body clearance and volume of distribution for pseudoephedrine is approximately 250 to 300 mL/min and 2.0 to 2.0 L/kg, respectively. Hemodialysis does not appear to be useful in removal of pseudoephrine (high V_D).[1]

REFERENCES—EPHEDRINE AND PSEUDOEPHEDRINE

1. Sica DA, Comstock TJ. Case report. Pseudoephedrine accumulation in renal failure. Am J Med Sci 1989;29:261–263.
2. Clark RF, Curry SS. Pseudoephedrine dangers. Pediatrics 1990;85:389–391.
3. Salmon J, Nicholson D. DIC and rhabdomyolysis following pseudoephedrine overdoses. Am J Emerg Med 1988;6:545–546.
4. Vin PA. Ephedrine-induced intracerebral hemorrhage and central nervous system vasculitis. Stroke 1990;21:1641.
5. Cavanah DK, Ballas ZK. Pseudoephedrine reaction presenting as recurrent toxic shock syndrome. Ann Intern Med 1993; 119:302–303.
6. Lai Y-K. Adverse effects of intraoperative phenylephrine 10%: case report. Br J Ophthalmol 1989;73:468–469.
7. Roberts JR. Pseudocerebral herniation due to phenylephrine nasal spray. N Engl J Med 1989;320:1757.
8. Snook C, Otten M, Hassan M. Massive ephedrine overdose: case report and toxicokinetic analysis. Vet Hum Toxicol 1992;34:335.
9. Burkhart KK. Intravenous propranolol reverse hypertension after sympathomimetic overdose. J Toxicol Clin Toxicol 1992; 30:109–114.
10. Bruno A, Nolte KB, Chapin J. Stroke associated with ephedrine use. Neurology 1993;43:1313–1316.
11. Wezorek C, Kurta D, Dean B, Krenzelok E. Pediatric pseudoephedrine ingestions. A retrospective study. Vet Hum Toxicol 1991;33:362.
12. Rose SR, Gorman RL, Oderda GM, Klein-Schwartz W. Prospective evaluation of pseudoephedrine ingestion. Vet Hum Toxicol 1988;3:359.
13. Garriott JC, Simmons LM, Poklis A et al. Five cases of fatal overdose from caffeine-containing "look-alike" drugs. J Anal Toxicol 1985;9:141–143.
14. Registry of Human Toxicology. American Academy of Forensic Sciences, 1978.
15. Snook C, Otten M, Hasan M. Massive ephedrine overdose: case report and toxicokinetic analysis. Vet Hum Toxicol 1992;34:335.

EPINEPHRINE

Epinephrine and norepinephrine are relatively nonselective and stimulate alpha-1 and alpha-2 receptors with roughly similar potency. Epinephrine, in addition to its alpha effects, also stimulates beta-1 and beta-2 receptors (Table 52–2).[1] Some epinephrine preparations are listed in Table 52–3.

CLINICAL PRESENTATION

Local Injection

Accidental injection of epinephrine into a finger may induce severe ischemia with a painful, pale, and cool finger demonstrating poor capillary refill that can last for several hours. Digital blocks with 1% lidocaine or topical nitroglycerine may not restore perfusion. Phentolamine 1.5 mg (0.3 mL Regitine) locally infiltrated may lead to hyperemia, a warm digit, and normal capillary refill within 5 minutes.[2] Others have found the local injection of a mixture of 0.5 mg pentolamine (in 1-mL solution) with 1 mL 2% locaine to be effective in restoring circulation.[3,4] Accidental intraarterial injection of 3 mg of epinephrine led to unconsciousness, hypotension, and ventricular tachycardia with marked pallor of the arm. Phentolamine 5 mg injected through the same arterial catheter led to rapid return of perfusion to the arm.[4,5] Intravenous epinephrine in doses of 1333 μg/min (80 mg/hour) was required to restore blood

Table 52 3
Various Preparations of Epinephrine[a]

Preparation of Epinephrine	Route of Administration	Clinical Use	Concentration
1:100	Inhalation	Aerosolized for croup	1GM in 100 ml (1%)
■ Very concentrated; not for parenteral use. ■ May use for inhalation; 0.25–0/5 ml in saline nebulizer. ■ L-isomer only.			
1:1,000	Subcu	Asthma, anaphylaxis	1GM in 1000 ml (0.1%)
■ This is L-isomer only. ■ Can be used for inhalation for croup in dose 3–5 ml(mg).			
1:10,000	IV	"Cardiac" epinephrine for codes; small doses IV for anaphylaxis	1GM in 10,000 ml (0.01%)
■ L-isomer, in prefilled 10 ml syringe in crash cart.			
1:100,000	Infiltration Subcu	Combined with local anesthetics for subcu use	1GM in 100,000 ml (0.001%)
■ Also comes in 1:200,000.			
Racemic epinephrine	Inhalation	Aerosolized for croup	2.25% Equal parts of D- and L-isomers = 1.125% L-epinephrine
■ Dose for child with croup is 0.25–0.5 ml in saline nebulizer. ■ Basically equivalent to 1:100 L-epinephrine.			
Primatene (mist and mist suspension)	Inhalation	Asthma	Mist: 0.22 mg/puff. Mist suspension = 0.16 mg/puff
■ Available OTC. ■ Tablet contains no epinephrine (theophylline, epinephrine ± phenobarbital and antihistamine.			
Sus-Phrine	Subcu	Asthma allergic reactions (not anaphylaxis)	0.5% or 1:200 20% solution (immediate) and 80% suspension (slow release)
■ Not for anaphylaxis. ■ Last 4–6 hours. ■ Not "in oil." ■ Contains only L-isomer. ■ Has both immediate and delayed bioavailability.			

[a]Adapted from Roberts JR. Emerg Med News November 1993, p. 28.

pressure after an overdose of 5600 to 7000 mg of labetalol.[6]

Epinephrine Overdose[7]

Symptoms of pallor, cyanosis, headache, diaphoresis, hypertension, tachycardia, ECG evidence of myocardial ischemia, premature ventricular contractions (PVCs), bigeminal rhythmic, precordial chest discomfort, palpitations, numbness and paresthesias of the hands and feet, and abdominal pain commonly develop within seconds to minutes after injection of excessive amounts of epinephrine, depending on the route.[8] Metabolic acidosis, hypotension, and pulmonary edema[9] have a delayed onset.[10,11] Recovery of ventricular function may follow supportive care (IV saline, sodium nitroprusside, dobutamine, balloon pump, and noradrenaline).[11,12]

Cardiac Arrest

ACLS (advanced cardiac life support) standards recommend 7.5 to 15 μg/kg of epinephrine (0.5 to 1 mg in an adult) in cardiac arrest.[13] Higher doses of epinephrine (over 0.2 mg/kg), 1 to 15 mg (bolus doses), may improve initial resuscitation rates in children but has been disappointing in adults.[14,15]

Formulation

ACLS guidelines recommend epinephrine doses equivalent to a maximum of 2.8 μg/kg/minute. Others recommend 40 μg/kg per minute. An intravenous bolus dose of 50 μg/kg or more is considered a high-dose epinephrine therapy.[16] Others report a minimum lethal dose of 5 μg/mg and a maximum tolerated dose of 114 μg/kg.[17] High-dose epinephrine (15 mg) is being used increasingly in cardiac arrest.[14]

Doses of 0.1 to 0.2 mg/kg are favored by some centers.[14,18] The optimal doses of epinephrine in cardiac arrest is not known.[19] An IV dose of 3 mg has been reported as fatal, while other patients have survived IV doses as large as 30 mg.[20]

Two controlled clinical studies suggest that there does not appear to be any difference in the overall rate of return by spontaneous circulation, survival to hospital admission, survival to hospital discharge, or neurologic outcome between patients treated with a standard dose of epinephrine (0.2 mg/kg body weight) and those treated with a high dose.[21,22]

The Adrenergic Agonist Panel concluded that the standard IV bolus dosage of epinephrine should be simplified to 1.0 mg every 3 to 5 minutes. The endotracheal dosing of epinephrine should be at least 2 to 2.5 times larger than the peripheral IV dosage.[22] Roberts has summarized situations where epinephrine should be avoided in wheezing patients (Table 52–4).[23]

Table 52-4
Situations Where Epinephrine Should Be Avoided in Wheezing Patients [a]

Scenario	Reason
Hydrocarbon aspiration	Hydrocarbons sensitize the myocardium to catecholamines and even small doses of epinephrine can precipitate ventricular dysrhythmias
Patients taking non-selective beta-blockers	With the beta receptors blocked, unopposed alpha agonism results in exaggerated hypertension
Pregnancy	Epinephrine, in high doses, constricts uterine blood flow (relative contraindication only)
Wheezing due to pulmonary edema	This condition is often misdiagnosed as primary bronchoconstriction (bronchitis, asthma), and epinephrine therapy is not indicated
Pheochromocytoma/ MAO-inhibitor use	Exaggerated catecholamine response can be seen

Source: James R. Roberts, MD.
[a]Adapted from Roberts JR. Emerg Med News, October 1993, p. 12.

TREATMENT

Intravenous phentolamine (Regitine) is useful in the treatment of epinephrine-induced hypertension. A short-acting beta-blocker such as esmolol can be useful for a severe tachycardia. Labetalol has been effective, but there is the potential for an incomplete alpha-blockade in the face of a more complete beta-blockade. Rebound brochospasm must be prevented by extreme caution and titration of the dose.[24] Adrenergic blocking agents and vasodilators should be used with caution because of the frequent biphasic hypertensive-hypotensive nature of epinephrine overdose. Fluids should be given with caution and with careful monitoring because of the possible late development of pulmonary edema. Cardiac monitoring for arrhythmias should be in place. Serial ECGs and cardiac enzymes should be obtained to rule out myocardial infarction.[12] Labetalol (5 mg IV) may be used cautiously to reduce hypertension.[24]

REFERENCES—EPINEPHRINE

1. Paradis MA, Koscove EM. Epinephrine in cardiac arrest: a critical review. Ann Emerg Med 1990;19:1288–1301.
2. McCauley WA, Gerace RV, Scilley C. Treatment of accidental injection of epinephrine with an auto-injector. Vet Hum Toxicol 1990;33:375.
3. Maguire WA, Reisdorff EJ, Smith D, Wiegenstein JG. Epinephrine-induced vasospasm reversed by phentolamine digital block. Am J Emerg Med 1990;8:46–47.
4. Deshmukh N, Tollard JT. Treatment of accidental epinephrine injection in a finger. J Emerg Med 1989;7:408.
5. Roberts JR, Krisanda TJ. Accidental intra-arterial injection of epinephrine treated with phentolamine. Ann Emerg Med 1989;18:424–453.
6. Hicks PR, Rankin APN. Massive adrenaline doses in labetalol overdose. Anaesth Intensive Care 1991;19:447–450.
7. Karch SB. Coronary artery spasm induced by intravenous epinephrine overdose. Am J Emerg Med 1989;7:485–488.
8. Kurachek SS, Rochoff MA. Inadvertent intravenous administration of racemic epinephrine. JAMA 1985:253:1441–1442.
9. Egoz N, Firestone SC. Adrenaline-induced pulmonary edema and its treatment. A report of two cases. Br J Anaesth 1971;43:709–712.
10. Novey HS, Meleyco IN. Alarming reaction after intravenous administration of 30 mL of epinephrine. JAMA 1969;209: 2435–2441.
11. Fyke AI, Daly PA, Dorian P, Tough J. Reversible "cardiomyopathy" after accidental adrenalin overdose. Am J Cardiol 1991;67:318–319.
12. Hall AH, Kulig NN, Rumack BH. Intravenous epinephrine abuse. Ann J Emerg Med 1987;5:64–65.
13. Callaham M. High-dose epinephrine in cardiac arrest. West J Med 1991;155:289–292.
14. Barton C, Callaham M. High-dose epinephrine improves the return of spontaneous circulation rates in human victims of cardiac arrest. Ann Emerg Med 1991;20:722–725.
15. Martin D, Werman HA, Brown CG. Four case studies: high dose epinephrine in cardiac arrest. Ann Emerg Med 1990;19: 232–236.
16. Callaham M, Barton CW, Kayser S. Potential complications of high-dose epinephrine therapy in patients resuscitating from cardiac arrest. JAMA 1991;265:1117–1122.
17. Friedman B. Accidental adrenaline overdose and its treatment with piperoxan. Lancet 1955;266:575–578.
18. Hebert P, Weitzman BN, Stiell G, Stark RM. Epinephrine in cardiopulmonary resuscitation. J Emerg Med 1991;9: 487–495.
19. Brown CG, Martin DR, Peper PE, Stueven H, Cummins RO, Gonzalez E et al. A comparison of standard dose and high dose epinephrine in cardiac arrest outside the hospital. N Engl J Med 1992;327:1051–1055.
20. Paradio NA, Kossone EM. Epinephrine in cardiac arrest: a critical review. Ann Emerg Med 1990;19:1288–1301.
21. Stiell IG, Hebert PC, Weitzman BN, Wells GA, Raman S, Stark RM et al. High-dose epinephrine in adult cardiac arrest. N Engl J Med 1992;327:1045–1050.
22. Ornato JP. Members of the Use of Adrenergic Agonists During CPR Panel. Use of adrenergic agonists during CPR in adults. Ann Emerg Med 1993;22:411–416.
23. Roberts JR. Emergency Med News, October 1993, p. 12.
24. Larsen LS, Larsen A. Labetalol in the treatment of epinephrine overdose. Ann Emerg Med 1990;19:680–682.

PHENYLPROPANOLAMINE

Serious toxic effects are usually induced at doses considerably in excess of those used therapeutically.[1]

DRUG INTERACTIONS

Phenylpropanolamine (PPA) and caffeine administered together may lead to severe life-threatening and occasionally fatal hypertensive reactions. PPA with caffeine results in significantly elevated caffeine levels (Table 52–5).[2]

CENTRAL NERVOUS SYSTEM

Abuse of excessively high doses of Vicks Formula 44-D (phenylpropanolamine 12.5 mg, dextromethorphan 15 mg, and guanifenesin 100 mg per 5 mL) has led to chronic behavioral abnormalities and hypertension. Cessation of use led to recovery in one patient.[3]

Of the many well-documented intracerebral hemorrhages caused by phenylpropanolamine (PPA) there seems to be no correlation of dose or blood pressure with incidents of hemorrhage. Some patients have had strokes after one or two tablets; the measured blood pressure, though usually elevated, is often not dramatically high.[4]

Table 52–5
Drug Interactions With Over-the Counter Preparations[a]

OTC Drug	Prescription Drug	Interaction
Sympathomimetics (**phenylpropanolamine,** pseudoephedrine, ephedrine, phenylephrine)	MAO inhibitors	Hypertensive crisis
	Bethanidine, debrisoquine, guanethidine	Poor blood pressure control
	Bronchodilators	Increased side effects
Theophylline	Cimetidine, erythromycin, ciprofloxacin, omeprazole, allopurinol, vaccinations, frusemide, hydrocortisone	Increased theophylline levels and side-effects
Antihistamines (brompheniramine, chlorpheniramine, cyproheptadine, diphenhydramine, phenindamine, pheniramine, promethazine, triprolidine)	Benzodiazepines and other sedatives	Additive effects to cause increased sedation or anticholinergic effects
	Narcotic analgesics	
	Anticholinergics (benzhexol, orphenadrine, tricyclic antidepressants)	
Aspirin	Sulphinpyrazone, probenecid	Blocks uricosuric effects
	Warfarin	Potentiates by blocking platelet action
	Corticosteroids	Decreased aspirin levels. Ulcerogenic
	Sulphonylureas	Hypoglycemia
	Valproate	Increased valproate levels and toxicity
Ibuprofen	Diuretics	Antagonism of diuretic and antihypertensive effect
Antacids	Tetracyclines, cimetidine, phenytoin, digoxin, warfarin, phenothiazines	Chelation in the GIT with decreased absorption
Ferrous salts	Tetracycline	Chelation
Iodine-containing drugs	Lithium	Hypothyroidism
Pyridoxine	Levodopa	Decreased anti-Parkinsonian effect
Liquorice	Antihypertensives, diuretics	Fluid retention, antagonizing diuretic or antihypertensive effects
Sodium salts, eg sodium bicarbonate	Lithium	Decreased lithium concentration
Vitamin K-containing herbal preparation	Warfarin	Antagonizes anticoagulant effect
Potassium citrate	Potassium-sparing diuretic or ACE inhibitor	Hyperkalemia

[a]Adapted from Walley T. Practitioner 1991;235:171–172.

Table 52–2 lists phenylpropanolamine and other over-the-counter drugs that may increase blood pressure.[5] In one study 25 mg of immediate-release PPA administered at 4-hour intervals did not cause significant increases in blood pressure in stable hypertensive patients.[6] Another controlled study indicates that single (75 mg) or double (150 mg) doses of PPA may cause a significant increase in blood pressure (from 148 to 173 mm Hg).[7]

LABORATORY

Analytic Methods

A stereospecific high-performance liquid chromatography assay for the enantiomers of phenylpropanolamine in human plasma has been developed which is sensitive to as little as 10 μg/L of each enantiomer. Following 75 mg of dL-PPA a peak level of about 200 μg/L is obtained for both L- and D-PPA.[8]

TREATMENT

Supportive Care

1. Obtain a CT scan immediately in any patient with sudden onset of severe headache, headache associated with vomiting, neurologic deficits, abnormal mental status, or headache which persists after blood pressure lowering.
2. Treat severe hypertension with intravenous nitroprusside or phentolamine.
3. Tachycardia: propranolol IV.
4. Bradycardia: atropine.
5. Ventricular tachycardia, premature ventricular contacts with lidocaine.
6. CNS toxic effects: Treat symptomatically.
7. Seizures: diazepam.

REFERENCES—PHENYLPROPANOLAMINE

1. Veltri JC, Bradford DC, Dring T, Kassner S, McEwee NE et al. Acute exposure to phenylpropanolamine: an analysis of 5447 cases reported to poison control centers from 1984-1987. Postmarket Surveill 1992;6:95–106.
2. Lake CR, Rosenberg DB, Gallant S, Zaloga G, Chernow R. Phenylpropanolamine increases plasma caffeine levels. Clin Pharmacol Ther 1990;47:675–685.
3. Craig DF. Psychosis and Vicks Formula 44-D abuse. Can Med Assoc J 1992;146:1199–1200.
4. Brown CR. Phenylpropanolamine—an ongoing problem. Clin Toxicol Update 1987;9(2):5–8.
5. Prisant LM, Carr AA. Over-the-counter drugs that may increase blood pressure. Postgrad Med 1989;86:205–208.
6. Kroenke K, Omori DM, Simons JO, Wood DR, Meier NJ. The safety of phenylpropanolamine in patients with stable hypertension. Ann Intern Med 1989;111:1043–1044.
7. Lake CR, Zaloga G, Bray J, Rosenberg D, Chernow B. Transient hypertension after two phenylpropanolamine diet aids and the effects of caffeine. A placebo-controlled follow-up study. Am J Med 1989;86:427–432.
8. Stockley CS, Wing LMH, Miners JO. Stereospecific high-performance liquid chromatographic assay for the enantiomers of phenylpropanolamine in human plasma. Ther Drug Monit 1991;13:322–338.

BAKING SODA

GASTRIC RUPTURE[1-9]

Gastric rupture can follow ingestion of sodium bicarbonate. The lesser curvature of the stomach is the usual site of rupture.

MECHANISM OF ACTION

The approximate volume of gas produced from the chemical reaction of 12 g of sodium bicarbonate (1 full teaspoon) using Avogadro's and Charles' Laws is 3.4 liters, which, with a large meal and aerophagy (while attempting to belch), readily approaches the 4 liters that has been calculated as necessary for gastric rupture.[1] The rapidity of pressure buildup probably also plays a large part.[1] The usual recommended dose of baking soda is 1/2 teaspoon, which, if accurately measured, contains about 1.6 g of sodium bicarbonate. A 1.8-g measure of baking soda contains 21.4 mEq of sodium bicarbonate; its ingestion could produce 21.4 mmol of CO_2, assuming that the stomach contained at least 21.4 mEq of HCl. If this 21.4 mmol of CO_2 remained in solution, gastric volume would not be expanded, but if the 21.4 mmol of CO_2 evolved suddenly into the gas phase, gastric volume could be suddenly increased by 475 mL, a contributing factor to spontaneous gastric rupture.[7]

People with a full feeling after overeating would be well advised not to ingest anything, regardless of whether it has the potential for gas production, to avoid air swallowing, and to avoid attempts to vomit. If, in spite of this admonition, sodium bicarbonate is ingested under these conditions, it would be advisable to use the recommended dose of one-half of one level teaspoon, rather than a large dose.[7]

CLINICAL PRESENTATION

The maximum recommended dose of baking soda for an adult is 8 half-teaspoons over a 24-hour period. A child was given 8 to 10 tablespoons of baking soda a day for 10 days for mild abdominal pain. The child developed a hypernatremia, became lethargic, and developed a gout imbalance. Following correcting the hypernatremia (5% dextrose and 0.9% saline) the neurologic status improved. She continued to have some cognitive problems.[10]

DIAGNOSIS

The diagnostic triad for spontaneous rupture of the stomach includes surgical emphysema of the neck and a distended abdomen following sudden abdominal pain.[1] Radiography is often unhelpful. A perforated peptic ulcer is rarely bigger than 1.5 cm, whereas most ruptures are about 5 cm long.[9]

TREATMENT

Early surgery is important with thorough peritoneal lavage. Post-operative intraabdominal sepsis is a real danger.[11]

SODIUM BICARBONATE ABUSE

Sodium bicarbonate (3 to 4 tablespoons per day) may be ingested by patients with anorexia nervosa to dampen the appetite. This may be associated with recurrent hypokalemic metabolic alkalosis.[12] Such abuse (50 to 150 g per day) may be accompanied by features of Munchausen's syndrome.[13-15] An infant was given baking soda ("two pinches"/day with water) by the mother to treat the infant's "gas." The child developed an inability to sleep and was "fussy." Laboratory examination indicated a serum sodium of 160 mEq/L and potassium of 3.9 mEq/L. The child was 10% dehydrated. Treatment included IV fluids (saline, glucose, potassium chloride), and the child recovered. Hypernatremia with metabolic alkalosis in a child may be caused by dietary indiscretion (see Salt Poisoning). An adult "pinch" is approximately a quarter teaspoon; the child received ½ teaspoon of sodium bicarbonate in 6 ounces of water for a final concentration of 116 mEq/L of each, or 1½ to 2½ times the sodium concentration and 3½ times the bases (bicarbonate) concentration of commercially available oral glucose electrolyte solution.[12]

BAKING SODA POISONING[16]

Inadvertent substitution of baking soda for powdered formula may lead to obtundation, convulsions, persistent neurologic abnormalities, or cardiorespiratory arrest, associated with a hypernatremia. Either table salt or sodium bicarbonate may be causal in producing hypernatremia when serum Na exceeds 150 mEq/L.

	mEq Na
One teaspoon baking soda	55
One teaspoon table salt	80
One formula scoop $NAHCO_3$	165
One formula scoop NaCl	240
One scoop of formula powder	1
(One formula scoop = 1 tablespoonful)	

CLINICAL PRESENTATION

Baking powder is composed of 30% sodium bicarbonate with cornstarch, sodium aluminum sulfate, calcium acid phosphate, and calcium sulfate. The main effect of ingestion and chronic abuse is hypokalemic hypochloremic metabolic alkalosis.[17] Other metabolic abnormalities, including hypernatremia and hypocalcemia, are possible. Transient albuminuria, neuromuscular irritability, including hyperreflexia, and elevations in blood urea nitrogen have been observed. Acute withdrawal from baking powder may induce a hyperaldosterone-like state. An elevated urine pH value may induce a false-positive urine protein determination. The presence of hypernatremia with metabolic alkalosis and an elevated urine pH suggests the possibility of ingestion of exogenous alkali. Hyperglycemia is present in about half the patients with hypernatremia dehydrates.[10,18]

A 23-year-old pregnant woman consumed large (7 ounces) quantities of baking powder daily and developed hypertension, hypokalemia, and elevated liver function tests.[19] Absence seizures have been induced in a 2½-year-old child receiving orally 4 mEq/kg of sodium bicarbonate per day.[19] The blood pH level was raised from 7.33 (prior renal tubular acidosis) to 7.43.[20]

A 6-week-old girl was given a "pinch" of baking soda to "help the baby to burp after feeds." On admission she was lethargic and dehydrated with sunken eyes, dry mucous membranes, and a sunken fontanelle. The baby had a poor respiratory effort and nystagmus. The blood gases were pH 7.34, pCO_2 82, pO_2 170, and bicarbonate 7, with a base excess of 18. The sodium soda was 180 mEq/L, potassium 5.3 mEq/L, chloride 91 mEq/L, bicarbonate over 40 mEq/L, creatinine 1.8 mg/dL, and BUN 23 MEq. She had a generalized tonic-clonic seizure. ACT scan indicated loss of grey-white matter differentiation, indicating hypoxic injury. A magnetic resonance examination showed a choroid plexus hemorrhage. Treatment included 25% dextrose, 60 mL/kg of isotonic fluids, IV lorazepam, and phenobarbital. She recovered and at 6 months was developing normally.[21]

TREATMENT[22]

1. Intravenous saline, electrolytes. In infants rehydration with oral electrolyte solutions may be useful in cases of mild metabolic alkalosis from bicarbonate ingestion.
2. Watch potassium levels for "rebound hyperkalemia," which may require up to 3 weeks to normalize.
3. Acetazolamide promotes renal excretion of both sodium and bicarbonate. There is a risk of volume depletion.
4. Follow and monitor serum sodium, electrolytes, pH, and volume status.

REFERENCES—BAKING SODA

1. Downs NM, Stonebridge PA. Gastric rupture due to excessive sodium bicarbonate ingestion. Scott Med J 1989;34:534–535.
2. Murdfield P. Rupture of stomach from sodium bicarbonate. Klin Wochenschr 1926;5:1612–1615.
3. Tonetti F, Gorini P. Un caso di rottura dello stomaco dopo ingestiore du bicarbonato di sodio. A case of stomach rupture following ingestion of bicarbonate of soda. Minerva Chir 1988;43:1737–1739.
4. Mastrangelo MR, Moore EW. Spontaneous rupture of the stomach in a healthy adult man after sodium bicarbonate ingestion. Ann Intern Med 1984;101:649–650.
5. Lemmon WT, Paschal Glu Jr. Rupture of the stomach following ingestion of sodium bicarbonate. Ann Surg 1941;114: 997–1003.
6. Glassman O. Subcutaneous rupture of the stomach is traumatic and spontaneous. Ann Surg 1929;89:247–263.
7. Fordtran JS, Morawski SG, Santa Ana CA, Rector FC Jr. Gas production after reaction of sodium bicarbonate and hydrochloric acid. Gastroenterology 1984;87:1014–1021.
8. Zer M, Chaimoff C, Dintsman M. Spontaneous rupture of the stomach following ingestion of sodium bicarbonate. Arch Surg 1970;101:522–533.
9. Lazebnik N, Iellin A, Michowitz M. Spontaneous rupture of the normal stomach after sodium bicarbonate ingestion. J Clin Gastroenterol 1986;8:454–456.
10. Puczynski MS, Cunningham DG, Mortimer JC. Sodium intoxication caused by use of baking soda as a home remedy. Can Med Assoc J 1983;128:821–822.
11. Revilloid E. Rupture l'estomec. Rev Med Suisse Romande 1885;5:5.
12. Kennedy S. Sodium bicarbonate abuse in anorexia nervosa. J Clin Psychiatry 1988;49:18.
13. Linford SMJ, Janey HD. Sodium bicarbonate abuse. A case report.
14. Mennen M, Slovis CM. Severe metabolic alkalosis in the emergency department. Ann Emerg Med 1988;17:354–357.
15. Fuchs S, Listernich R. Hypernatremia and metabolic alkalosis as a consequence of the therapeutic misuse of baking soda. Pediatr Emerg Care 1987;3:242–243.
16. Del Beccaro M, Robertson WO. Baking soda poisoning. Vet Hum Toxicol 1988;30:164–165.
17. Wechsler D, Ibsen L, Focarelli P. Apparent proteinuria as a consequence of sodium bicarbonate ingestion. Pediatrics 1990;86:318–319.
18. Finberg L. Hypernatremia (hypertonic) dehydration in infants. N Engl J Med 1973;289:196–198.
19. Barton JR, Riely CA, Sibai BM. Baby powder pica mimicking preeclampsia. Am J Obstet Gynecol 1992;167:98–99.
20. Reif S, Holzman M, Barak S, Spirer Z. Absence seizures associated with bicarbonate therapy and normal serum pH. JAMA 1989;262:1328–1329.
21. Holloway M, Wason S. Baking soda: a potentially fatal home remedy. Vet Hum Toxicol 1990;32:371.
22. Thomas SH, Stone CK. Acute toxicity from baking soda ingestion. Am J Emerg Med 1994;12:57–59.

BROMIDES

Bromide ion is found in some over-the-counter preparations such as dextromethorphan hydrobromide and in drugs (Table 52–6).[1–7]

Halothane releases bromide ions, which peak in 2 to 3 days postanesthesia.[8]

Drugs that contain bromides are listed in Table 52–7.[9] Methyl bromide is a fumigant insecticide in some fire extinguishers and refrigerants. Ethylene dibromide is a scavenger of lead in leaded fuels and a fumigant insecticide. Bromide intoxication has followed pyridostigmine bromide intoxication.[9]

Table 52–6
Bromide Ion in Over-The-Counter Products

Product	Generic	Percent Bromide
Bromoquinine	Quinine hydrobromide	17
Bromo-seltzer	Potassium bromide	67 (not available)
Carbitral	Carbromal	34
Dimetane	Brompheniramine	25
Nervene	Ammonium bromide	80 (not available)
Romilar DM	Dextromethorphan	23
Bromocriptine	Parodel	

Table 52–7
Drugs With Bromide Ions

Drug	% Bromide
Acecarbromal	29
Ammonium bromide	80
Bromodiphenhydramine	24
Bromisovalum	36
Brompheniramine maleate	25
Calcium bromogalactogluconate	16.7
Carbromal	34
Dexbrompheniramine	25
Dextromethorphan hydrobromide	43
Halothane hydrobromide	81
Homatropine methylbromide	29
Neostigmine bromide	38
Pamabrom	23
Pancuronium bromide	37
Potassium bromide	67
Propantheline bromide	17.8
Pyridostigmine bromide	30.6
Quinine hydrobromide	17
Scopolamine hydrobromide	28.8
Vecuronium bromide	25

Table 52-8
Toxicity and Blood Bromide Levels[10,11]

Bromide blood concentration		
mg/dL	mEq/L = mmol/L	Toxicity
below 50	6.3	Therapeutic
50 to 100	6.3 to 12.5	Possible toxicity
100 to 200	12.5 to 25	Usually serious toxicity
200 to 300	25 to 31	Possible coma
300 or more	37.5	Possibly fatal

LABORATORY[10,11]
Blood Levels

$$8\ \text{mg/dL} = 80\ \text{mg/L} = 1\ \text{mEq/L}$$

Therefore the fatal dose is 300 mg/ml or 3000 mg/L or 37.5 mEq/L. Correlation of toxicity with blood bromide levels is found in Table 52–8.

TREATMENT

1. Stop bromide ingestion.
2. Give sodium chloride orally. Watch until blood bromide level falls about 50 to 100 mg/d.
3. Supportive and symptomatic care.

REFERENCES—BROMIDES

1. Eisenga B, Saxema K, Anthony SL et al. Discussion of case of the month bromism. Vet Hum Toxicol 1985;27:57–58.
2. Iberti TJ, Patterson BK, Fisher CJ Jr. Prolonged bromide intoxication resulting from a gastric bezoar. Arch Intern Med 1984;144:402–403.
3. Trump DL, Hochberg MC. Bromide intoxication. Johns Hopkins Med J 1976;138:119–123.
4. Hanes F, Yates A. An analysis of four hundred instances of chronic bromide intoxication. South Med J 1938;31:667–671.
5. Raskind MA, Kitchell M, Alvarez C. Bromide intoxication in the elderly. J Am Geriat Soc 1978;26:222–224.
6. Brenner I. Bromism: Alive and well. Am J Psychiatry 1978; 857–858.
7. Carney MWP. Five cases of bromism. Lancet 1971;2:523–524.
8. Mofenson HC, Caraccio TR, Brody G, Greensher J, Leggiadro R, Mancini R, Sherman J. PP/T News. NC Regional Poison Control Center. 1989;8(9–10):167–169.
9. Rothenberg DM, Berns AS, Barkin R, Glantz RN. Bromide intoxication secondary to pyridostigmine bromide therapy. JAMA 1990;263:1121–1122.
10. Palatucci DM. Paradoxical halide levels in bromide intoxication. Neurology 1978;28:1189–1191.
11. Elin RJ, Robertson EA, Johnson F. Bromide interferes with determination of chloride by each of four methods. Clin Chem 1981;27:778–779.

CENTRAL NERVOUS SYSTEM STIMULANTS

CAFFEINE (TABLE 52-9)

In South America caffeine is ingested during "mate-drinking" or the habit of consuming the herbal infusion of *Ilex Paraguayensis.* In a typical mate-round 80 to 350 mg of caffeine may be ingested in 1 to 3 hours.[1] Caffeine metabolism is dose-dependent, resulting in accumulation of methylxanthines in the body. This may explain why people who drink large amounts of coffee appear to be at greater risk for cardiovascular disease.[2] Ingestion of 6 to 8 grams of caffeine by a 16-year-old male led to a 16-hour half-life with maximum serum levels of 470 μmol/L (91 μg/mL). He survived.[4]

Table 52-9
Typical Caffeine Content of Foods and Medications[a]

Substance	Caffeine Content
Coffee	
Brewed	100 mg/cup (177 ml)
Instant	70 mg/cup (177 ml)
Decaffeinated	4 mg/cup (177 ml)
Tea	40 mg/cup (177 ml)
Caffeinated soda	45 mg/can (355 ml)
Cocoa beverage	5 mg/cup (177 ml)
Chocolate	
Chocolate milk	4 mg/cup (177 ml)
Dark chocolate	20 mg/bar (29 g)
Milk chocolate	6 mg/bar (29 g)
Medications	
Caffeine-containing cold remedies	25–50 mg/tablet
Caffeine-containing analgesics	25–65 mg/tablet
Stimulants	100–350 mg/tablet
Weight-loss aids	75–200 mg/tablet

[a]Strain EC, Griffiths RR. Caffeine dependence—fact or fiction. J Roy Soc Med 1995;88:437–440.

DRUG INTERACTIONS

Coadministration of caffeine and phenylpropanolamine appears to produce an additive increase on the blood pressure.[5] Verapamil may inhibit caffeine elimination.[6] Carbamazepine and valproic acid have no effect on caffeine metabolism. Phenytoin appears to increase the clearance of caffeine and reduce its half-life.[7] Animal studies suggest that caffeine potentiates the acute toxicity of both cocaine and amphetamine.[8]

PREGNANCY/LACTATION

The weight of evidence indicates that high levels of caffeine intake (over 300 mg/day) during pregnancy are potentially harmful (intrauterine growth retardation, possibly spontaneous abortion), but no conclusion can be made regarding the safety of lower levels.[9–11]

Infants exposed to high maternal levels of caffeine for the majority of the pregnancy may develop irritability, jitteriness, and vomiting in the immediate newborn period.[12] Over three maternal servings of coffee or cola per day (or over 300 mg/day of caffeine from all sources) may be associated with a decrease in birthweight.[13,14] Studies of coffee consumption and increased rates of spontaneous abortion and delayed time to conception are inconsistent. Conclusions cannot yet be drawn.[15]

In babies the enzyme or enzymes necessary to metabolize caffeine are absent until several days after birth. Disturbances in the baby's heart rate caused by an excessive intake of caffeine by the mother should stop several days after birth.[16]

Most women consume less than 300 mg/day of caffeine during pregnancy. Few adverse pregnancy outcomes have been reported in women who consume less than 300 mg/day of caffeine during pregnancy.[17]

CAFFEINE DEPENDENCE SYNDROME

Caffeine tends to produce a pattern of subjective effects that varies as a function of dose. Although low doses, in the range of 20 to 200 mg, generally produce mild, positive, subjective effects (e.g., increased feelings of well-being, alertness, energy), higher doses, in the range of 200 to 800 mg, can produce negative effects (e.g., nervousness, anxiety), especially in volunteers who are usually caffeine abstinent. Previous studies have shown that subjects can be intoxicated with the excessive use of caffeine and that caffeine can produce a withdrawal syndrome when subjects stop habitual use.[18]

The existence of a caffeine withdrawal syndrome seems to be established, even though this diagnosis was put in an appendix in DSM-IV along with other categories in need of further study. The new report by Strain et al[18] provides preliminary evidence for the occurrence of a syndrome of caffeine dependence, although this will require further characterization. The most common symptom of caffeine withdrawal is headache. Caffeine withdrawal headache generally occurs 12 to 24 hours after the last dose of caffeine and usually resolves with 2 to 4 days. Other features of caffeine withdrawal include sleepiness/drowsiness, impaired concentration/lassitude/work difficulty, anxiety/depression, and flulike symptoms (including headache, fatigue, muscle aches and stiffness, hot or cold spells, nausea and vomiting). Caffeine withdrawal can include impairments in psychomotor performance, irritability, rhinorrhea, confusion, diaphoresis, blurred vision, and craving for caffeine. The severity of caffeine withdrawal appears to be a function of the dose of caffeine. Caffeine withdrawal has been shown to occur with doses as low as 100 mg per day, the equivalent of about 1 cup of brewed coffee or two to three caffeinated sodas per day.[3] Physicians should advise patients who experience adverse effects from caffeine (such as anxiety, palpitations, sleep disturbance, gastrointestinal symptoms, or compulsive use) to taper off their consumption.[19]

DOSAGE

There is little evidence that a modest dose of coffee (200 mg caffeine or 3 to 7 caffeine-containing lozenges daily)[20] is arrhythmogenic even among patients with known life-threatening arrhythmia.[21] A prospective study in 51,529 men in the United States aged 40 to 75 years of age does not support the hypothesis that either coffee or caffeine consumption increases the risk of coronary heart disease or stroke.[22]

A 23-year-old female ingested 40 "speed" capsules, developed ventricular fibrillation, and died with a caffeine blood level of 189 μg/mL.[23] Following an ingestion of 35 g of caffeine by a 58-year-old woman, multiple runs of supraventricular tachycardia with ventricular bigeminy with a blood pressure of 150/110 mm Hg were observed together and a blood caffeine concentration of 194 μg/mL. The patient was treated supportively (gastric lavage, activated charcoal, sorbital, lidocaine, esmolol) and recovered.[24] Ingestion of 1.45 g of caffeine by a 29-year-old male led to blood caffeine levels of 23.1 μg/mL (1) (normals 0.2 to 1.3 μg/mL; 0.001 to 0.065 mmol/L).[25] Child abuse by administration of caffeine capsules to a 14-month-old girl led to death with a blood caffeine level of 117.3 μg/mL and a blood theophylline level of 35.9 μg/mL.[26]

OVERDOSE

Adults

Caffeine appears to increase urinary calcium output and has been implicated as a risk factor for osteoporosis. Ingestion of over 2.5 cups of coffee/day may be associated with an increased risk of hip fracture.[27]

LABORATORY

Analytic Methods

A high-performance liquid chromatography method is available for determination of dimethylxanthine metabolites of caffeine in human plasma.[28] Measurement of theophylline concentration in the management of caffeine overdose is not usually indicated and may be misleading unless a highly specific assay is used.[29]

Blood Levels

A 2-year-old ingested 6 g of caffeine and developed caffeine blood levels of 170 μg/mL (with an admission theophylline level of 7 μg/mL), agitation, diaphoresis, hematemesis, seizures, and an elevation of intracranial pressure. The child survived.[30]

Some correlations of caffeine blood levels and clinical effects appear to exist. Seizures occur with caffeine levels ranging from 79 to 199 μg/mL. Arrhythmias other than sinus tachycardia may be seen with levels greater than 180 μg/mL. Deaths have occurred with caffeine levels from 106 to 180 μg/mL.[30] Cardiac arrest following caffeine ingestion was associated with a blood level of 1560 μg/mL.[31] Patients with levels from 190 to 200 μg/mL have survived.

Ancillary Tests

Controlled trials appear to suggest that filtered coffee does not affect serum lipid levels.[32,33] However, coffee may affect mortality from coronary heart disease over and above its effect in raising cholesterol concentrations.[34]

TREATMENT

1. Charcoal hemoperfusion may be useful in patients with a potentially lethal ingestion who are exhibiting life-threatening complications (cardiac arrhythmias, severe central nervous system toxicity).[35]

2. IV glucose may lead to quick recovery in children with acute caffeine poisoning. Glucose is known to antagonize the excitatory effect of caffeine and theobromine in the nervous system.[36] Beta-blockers (e.g., esmolol) may be useful in caffeine-induced arrhythmias.[37]

REFERENCES—CAFFEINE

1. Pronczuk J, Laborde A, Heukes L, Moyna P et al. Mate-drinking. Another source of caffeine. Vet Hum Toxicol 1987; 29(Suppl 2):70–71.
2. Denaro CP, Brown CR, Wilson M, Jacob P III, Benowitz NL. Dose-dependency of caffeine metabolism with repeated dosing. Clin Pharmacol Ther 1990;48:277–285.
3. Strain EC, Griffiths RR. Caffeine dependency: fact or fiction? J Roy Soc Med 1995;88:437–440.
4. Leson CL, McGuigan MA, Bryson SM. Caffeine overdose in an adolescent male. Clin Toxicol 1988;26:407–415.
5. Brown NJ, Ryder D, Branch RA. A pharmacodynamic interaction between caffeine and phenylpropanolamine. Clin Pharmacol Ther 1991;50:363–371.
6. Nawoot S, Wong D, Mays DC, Gerber W. Inhibitor of caffeine elimination by verapamil. Clin Pharmacol Ther 1986; 43:148.
7. Wiethholz H, Zysset T, Kreiten K, Kohl D, Buchsel R, Matern S. Effect of phenytoin, carbamazepine, and valproic acid on caffeine metabolism. Eur J Clin Pharmacol 1989;3:401–406.
8. Derlet RW, Tseng JC, Albertson TE. Potentiation of cocaine and d-amphetamine toxicity with caffeine. Am J Emerg Med 1992;10:211–216.
9. Mills JL, Holms LB, Aarons JH et al. Moderate caffeine use and the risk of spontaneous abortion and intrauterine growth retardation. JAMA 1993;269:593–597.
10. Eskenazi B. Caffeine during pregnancy: grounds for concern? JAMA 1993;270:2973–2974.
11. Infante-Rivard C, Fernandez A, Gauthier R, David M, Rivard GE. Fetal loss associated with caffeine intake before and during pregnancy. JAMA 1993;270:2940–2943.
12. McGowan JD, Altman RE, Kanto WP Jr. Neonatal withdrawal symptoms after chronic maternal ingestion of caffeine. South Med J 1988;8:1092–1094.
13. Caan BJ, Goldhaber MK. Caffeinated beverages and low birthweight: a case-control study. Am J Public Health 1989; 29:1299–1300.
14. Fenster L, Eskenazi B, Windham GC, Swan SM. Caffeine consumption during pregnancy and fetal growth. AM J Public Health, 1991;8:458–461.
15. Narod SA, de Sanjose S, Victoria C. Coffee during pregnancy: a reproductive hazard? AM J Obstet Gynecol 1991;161:1109–1114.
16. Oei SG, Vusters RPL, van der Hagen NLJ. Fetal arrhythmia caused by excessive intake of caffeine by pregnant women. Br Med J 1989;298:568.
17. Mills JL, Conley MR, Graubard BI, Brown ZA, Simpson JL, Holmer LP. Caffeine use during pregnancy: how much is safe? JAMA 1993;270:45–46.
18. Strain EC, Mumford GK, Silverman K, Griffiths RR. Caffeine dependency syndrome. Evidence for case histories and experimental evaluations. JAMA 1994;272:1043–1048.
19. Glass RM. Caffeine dependence. What are the implications? JAMA 1994;272:1065–1066.
20. Graboys TB, Blatt CM, Lown B. The effect of caffeine on ventricular ectopic activity in patients with malignant ventricular arrhythmia. Arch Intern Med 1989;149:637–638.
21. Myers MG. Caffeine and cardiac arrhythmia. Chest 1988; 94:4–5.
22. Grobbee DE, Rimn EB, Giovannucci E, Colditz G, Stumpfer M, Willett W. Coffee, caffeine and cardiovascular disease in man. N Engl J Med 1990;323:1026–1032.
23. Rejent T, Michalek R, Krajewski M. Caffeine fatality with coincident ephedrine. Bull Int Assoc Forensic Toxicol 1981; 16(1):18–19.
24. Price KP, Fligner DJ. Treatment of caffeine toxicity with esmolol. Ann Emerg Med 1990;19:44–46.
25. Michaelis HC, Sharifi S, Schoed G. Rhabdomyolysis after suicidal ingestion of an overdose of caffeine, acetaminophen and phenazone as a fixed-dose combination (Spalt N). Clin Toxicol 1991;29:521–526.
26. Morrow PL. Caffeine toxicity: a case of child abuse by drug ingestion. J Forensic Sci 1987;32:1801–1805.
27. Kiel DP, Felson DT, Hannan MT, Anderson JJ, Wilson DWF. Caffeine and the risk of hip fracture: the Framingham Study. Am J Epidemiol 1990;132:675–684.
28. Wahllander A, Renner E, Kanlaganis G. J Chromatograph (Biomed Appln) 1985;338:369-375 in Bull Intern Assoc for Tox J 1981;19(2):59.
29. Fligner CL, Opheim KE. Caffeine and its phenethylxanthine metabolites in two cases of caffeine overdose: a case of falsely elevated theophylline concentrations in serum. J Anal Toxicol 1988;12:339–343.
30. Walsh I, Wasserman GS, Mestad P, Lanman RC. Near-fatal caffeine intoxication treated with peritoneal dialysis. Pediatr Emerg Care 1987;3:244–249.
31. Mrvos RM, Reilly PI, Dean BS, Krenzelok EP. Massive caffeine ingestion resulting in death. Vet Hum Toxicol 1989; 31:571–572.
32. Bak AAA, Groobbee DE. The effect on serum cholesterol levels of coffee brewed by filtering or boiling. N Engl J Med 1989;321:1432–1437.
33. Ahola I, Jauhiainen M, Aro A. The hypercholesterolaemic factor in boiled coffee is retained by a paper filter. J Intern Med 1991;230:392–397.
34. Tverdal A, Stensvold I, Solvoll K, Foss OP, Lund-larsen P, Bjartveit K. Coffee consumption and death from coronary heart disease in middle-aged Norwegian men and women. Br Med J 1990;300:566–569.
35. Dietrich AM, Mortensen ME. Presentation and management of an acute caffeine overdose. Pediatr Emerg Care 1990; 6:296–298.
36. Jorens DG, Van Hauwaert JM, Selala M, Schepens PJC. Acute caffeine poisoning in a child. Eur J Pediatr 1991;150: 860.
37. Price KP, Fligner DJ. Treatment of caffeine toxicity with esmolol. Ann Emerg Med 1990;19:44–46.

CAMPHOR

Progressive symptomatology is depicted in Table 52–10.[1] A list of camphor-containing products is found in Table 52–11.

Table 52–10
Progressive Symptomatology of Severe Camphor Intoxication[a]

1. Nausea and vomiting
2. Feeling of warmth, headache
3. Confusion, vertigo, excitement, restlessness, delirium and hallucinations
4. Increased muscular excitability, tremors, and jerky movements
5. Tremors, progressing to epileptiform convulsions, followed by depression
6. Coma, CNS depression
7. Death from respiratory failure or from status epilepticus
8. Slow convalescence

[a]Adapted from Koppel C, et al. Arch Toxicol 1982;51:101–106.

Table 52–11
List of Camphor-Containing Products[a]

Product	% of Camphor
Absorbine Arthritic Pain Lotion	10
Act-On Rub Lotion	1.5
Anabalm Lotion	3
Aveeno Anti-Itch Conc. Lotion	0.3
Avalgesic	†
Banalg Muscle Pain Reliever	2
Bangesic	†
Ben Gay Children's Vaporizing Rub	5
Betuline Lotion	†
Campho-phenique First Aid Gel	10.8
Campho-phenique Liquid	10.85
Campho-phenique Powder	4.375
Counterpain Rub	†
Deep Down Rub	0.5
Dencorub Cream	1
Dermal Rub	†
Dermolin Liniment	†
Emul-O-Balm	1.1
Heet Lotion	3
Heet Spray	3.6
Minit-Rub	3.5
Mollifene Ear Drops	†
Musterole Regular	4
Panalgesic	3
Pronto-Gel	1
Save the Baby	6
Sloan's Liniment	3.35
Soltice Quick Rub	5
Suring Ointment	0.475
ThermoRub Lotion	†
Vicks VapoRub	4.75
Vicks Vaposteam	6.2
Vicks Throat Drops	<0.5
Yager's Liniment	†

†These agents list camphor as an ingredient, but the concentrations are not specified.
[a]Kauffman RE. Committee on Drugs. Pediatrics 1994;94:127–128.

ACUTE POISONING

In 1983 the US Food and Drug Administration (FDA) ruled that the concentration of camphor in medicinal products must not exceed 11%. Camphorated oil in concentrations of up to 20% is still stocked in many Canadian drug stores.[2]

Camphor is rapidly absorbed when taken orally, but a considerable amount can also be absorbed via inhalation or through intact skin. Typically, symptoms begin 5 to 90 minutes after ingestion of a toxic dose. The onset of seizures can be sudden and may be followed by postconvulsive depression and coma. Death may result from respiratory depression or complications of status epilepticus. Other neurologic symptoms include confusion, vertigo, restlessness, delirium, and hallucinations. Increased muscular activity, tremors, and jerky movements often progress to epileptiform convulsions. Gastrointestinal symptoms occur in most patients and consist of oral and intestinal burning, nausea, and vomiting. Other clinical manifestations that have been reported are tachycardia, mydriasis, visual disturbances, urinary retention, albuminuria, mild transient elevations of the aspartate dehydrogenase and lactic dehydrogenase concentrations, and, rarely, hepatic failure.[2]

CHRONIC INTOXICATION

A 74-year-old chronically ingested Vicks Vaporub over a 5-year period and presented with weakness, fever, intensive pruritus, anorexia and weight loss. Liver biopsy showed a granulomatous hepatitis. The patient improved thereafter.[3]

LABORATORY

Blood Levels

In one study serum camphor was undetectable in 7 asymptomatic patients. One patient with seizures had a serum concentration of 14.5 ng/L (14.5 μg/mL).[4]

TREATMENT

1. Intensive supportive therapy. Watch airway, breathing, and circulation.
2. Elimination enhancement procedures are of little value.[5,6]

Severe symptoms may arise very rapidly. Emergency transportation to a medical facility is warranted. Siegel and Wason[7] suggest that ipecac be used to try to prevent absorption if more than 1 g is ingested, if the patient is seen within 2 hours, and no symptoms are present. If symptoms are present and the patient is seen within 2 hours, they recommend the use of gastric lavage, charcoal, and cathartics; if the patient is seen later, they recommend the use of only charcoal and cathartics. This approach, however, is not supported by experimental data. Others have recommended that the use of ipecac be abandoned and that gastric lavage be used with caution. Activated charcoal has been given, but no study has demonstrated its effectiveness as a decontaminant in cases of camphor poisoning.[2]

SUPPORTIVE CARE

Special attention must be provided for elderly, pregnant, and chronically ill patients. Recovery is usually complete within 24 to 48 hours following ingestion, but more prolonged recovery periods have been reported.[8] One death occurred 4 days following ingestion.[9] An excellent review of this subject is availables.[10]

A study of 82 ingestions of camphor suggests that minor "taste" or "swallow" ingestions of camphor-containing products cause only minor symptoms of oral and gastrointestinal irritation and can be safely handled at home.[11]

A protocol for camphor management has been proposed by Siegel and Wason and is found in Figure 52–1.[7] This group concludes that the vast majority of accidental camphor ingestions will remain asymptomatic and can be observed at home if the amount ingested is known to be less than 1 g. If the ingestion exceeds 1 g, observation in a health care facility is recommended.[12]

Respiratory support may be necessary. An EEG may be of value in patients who have had seizures. Liver function tests are indicated after chronic camphor exposure.

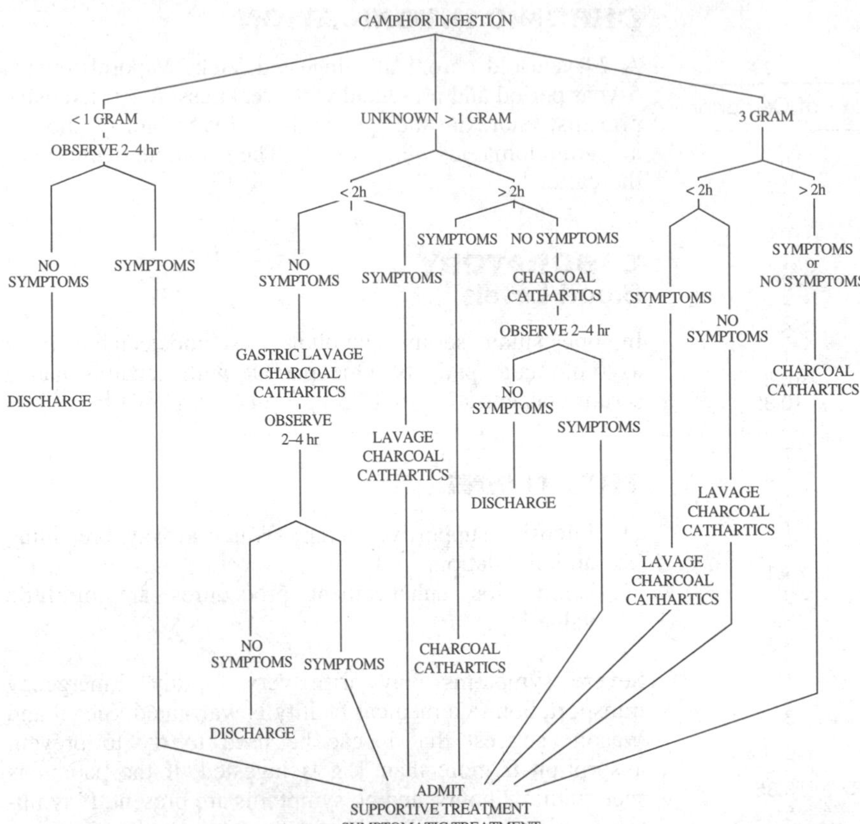

Figure 52–1 Camphor ingestion protocol (Children's Hospital Medical Center, Cincinnati). (Adapted from Siegel E, Wason S. Pediatr Clin North Am 1986;33:376–379.)

REFERENCES—CAMPHOR

1. Committee on Drugs, American Academy of Pediatrics. Camphor revisited: focus on toxicity. Pediatrics 1994;94:127–128.
2. Theis JGW, Koren G. Camphorated oil: still endangering the lives of Canadian children. Can Med Assoc J 1995;152:1821–1824.
3. McCollam A, Blick R, Lipscomb JW, Pompei P. Chronic camphor ingestion. A case report of granulomatous hepatitis. Hum Toxicol 1989;31:337.
4. Winter ML, Rice BS, Snodgrass WR. Seizures and serum camphor concentration in man. Vet Hum Toxicol 1991;33:375.
5. Koppel C, Martens F, Schirop T, Ibe K. Hemoperfusion in acute camphor poisoning. Intensive Care Med 1988;14:431–433.
6. Chung HM, Tsai WJ, Yang GY, Ger J, Tominack R. Camphor intoxication treated with lipid hemodialysis. Vet Hum Toxicol 1988;30:346–347.
7. Siegel E, Wason S. Camphor toxicity. Ped Clin North Am 1986;33:376–379.
8. Skoglund RR, Ware LL Jr, Schanberger JE. Prolonged seizures due to contact and inhalation exposure to camphor. Clin Pediatr 1977;16:901–902.
9. Jacobziner H, Raybin HW. Camphor poisoning. Arch Pediatr 1962;79:28–30.
10. Skoutakis VA, Koumbourlis TC. Camphor intoxication: diagnosis and management. Clin Toxicol Consult 1981;4:131–136.
11. Alsop JA. Camphor toxicity from accidental ingestions. Vet Hum Toxicol 1993;35:346.
12. Gonzalez de Rey J, Baker R, Holloway M, Wason S. Pediatric camphor ingestion. Hum Toxicol 1990;32:371.

CARBONLESS COPY PAPER

Carbonless copy paper (CCP) was developed and introduced in the early 1950s. Over one million tons of CCP are produced and used annually. In the 1960s medical complaints began to be reported, which were published in the 1970s and sporadically thereafter. These have consisted of case reports, case series, cross-sectional surveys, and skin tests and other challenges with various types of CCP or paper components.[1]

PHYSICAL PROPERTIES

This system involved special coatings on either the front or the back of the paper.[2] The top paper (CB) is coated on the undersurface with a suspension of microcapsules containing a colorless dye. The receiving paper (CF) is coated on the front surface with a color-developing material. When pressure is applied to the top sheet, the microcapsules are broken, allowing the colorless dye to react chemically with the color-developing material on the bottom sheet, resulting in visualization of the type. If there are several sheets of paper, the middle sheets are coated on the front and back (CFB). The papers may differ from different manufacturing sources in their use of solvent color formers, capsule wall, coreactive surface, and paper. One chemical color former is a paratoluene sulfinate of Michler's hydrol.[2]

CLINICAL

Allergic contact dermatitis has occasionally been reported. More commonly hoarseness, fatigue, headache, nausea, itching and redness of the skin, and burning of the eyes, nose, mouth, and chest are described.[1–3]

LABORATORY

Patch testing and prick and photo testing with components have been unrewarding in elucidating a mechanism for these clinical symptoms.[1,2,4] No single specific chemical or paper type has been consistently identified as the responsible factor. The vast majority of skin tests have been negative.

CONCLUSIONS

There does not appear to be a scientific basis on which to conclude that there is a valid statistical association between occupational exposure to CCP and various health effects.[1,5] The United States continues to collect data.[6]

REFERENCES—CARBONLESS COPY PAPER

1. Buring JE, Hennekens CH. Carbonless copy paper: a review of published epidemiologic studies. J Occup Med 1991;33: 486–495.
2. Marks JG Jr, Trautlein JJ, Zwillich CW, Demers LM. Contact urticaria and airway obstruction from carbonless copy paper. JAMA 1984;252:1038–1040.
3. Morgan MS, Camp JE. Upper respiratory irritation from controlled exposure to vapor from carbonless copy forms. J Occup Med 1986;28:415–419.
4. La Marte FP, Merchant JA, Casale TB. Acute systemic reactions to carbonless copy paper associated with histamine release. JAMA 1988;260:242–243.
5. Jeansson I, Lofstrom A, Lidblom A. Complaints relating to the handling of carbonless copy paper in Sweden. Am Ind Hyg Assoc J 1984;45:B24–B25.
6. National Institute for Occupational Safety and Health. Request for comments and secondary data on the toxicity of carbonless copy paper. Fed Reg 1987;52:2534–2535.

DEXTROMETHORPHAN

STRUCTURE AND CLASSIFICATION

Dextromethorphan (DM) has a molecular weight of 271.4.[1] Its conversion factor (CF) (to or from SI units) is 3.6. To convert to SI units µg/mL × CF = umol/L. To convert from SI units: umol/L divided by CF = µg/mL.

O- and *N*-demethylation followed by subsequent conjugation are the main metabolic pathways. Less than 2.5% of a dose is excreted unchanged in the urine within 24 hours. Besides these metabolic processes, 15 previously unknown metabolites and derivatives of dextromethorphan give evidence for additional metabolic degradation processes. It is not known whether these metabolic steps are also subject to genetic enzyme polymorphism as described for *o*-methylation.[2]

DRUG INTERACTIONS

DM is a high-affinity substrate for the debrisoquin hydroxylase enzyme (P450IIDC) and competitively inhibits P450IIID6-mediated metabolism. Over 30 drugs are substrates for the same enzyme. Their disposition can be altered by dextromethorphan. Monoamine oxidase inhibitors increase CNS levels of serotonin through blockade of oxidative deamination. DM is also a specific inhibitor of serotonin uptake and increases CNS serotonin levels. Combined use of DM and MAOIs may result in the "serotonin syndrome" (see 5-HT Drug Section).[3,4]

PATHOPHYSIOLOGY

Neurotoxicity by endogenous excitatory amino acids such as glutamate has been implicated as a mechanism for central neuronal cell loss after hypoxia and ischemia. Blockage of synaptic transmission and antagonism of specific postsynaptic glutamate receptors (especially the N-methyl-D-aspartate [NMDA] subclass) can be protective. Dextromethorphan (DM) is a potent NMDA receptor antagonist and appears to protect against hypoxic-ischemic damage in animal models of brain injury (e.g., retinal ischemia).[5] DM has been initially studied clinically in patients at risk for brain ischemia (dose 60 mg 4 times daily). Studies are ongoing.[6] Physical dependence on and tolerance to opiates may depend on blockade by opiates of the aspartatergic and glutamatergic receptors, especially NMDA. Dextromethorphan is known to decrease responsiveness of NMDA receptors and may be useful in the treatment of heroin addicts.[7]

CLINICAL PRESENTATION

Acute Toxicity

Symptoms of acute dextromethorphan toxicity induce central nervous system effects (hyperexcitability and restlessness, lethargy, ataxia, slurred speech, and tremors); ophthalmologic effects, including nystagmus and variable pupillary changes; diaphoresis; and hypertension. The drug has been subjected to abuse by teenagers who describe an acute euphoria after consumption, with intense craving and dysphoria on withdrawal. Many of the effects of intoxication are probably caused by its active metabolite, dextrophan.[8] Dextromethorphan hydrobromide can cause bromide poisoning (headache, apathy, irritation, slurred speech, psychosis, tremulousness, ataxia, hallucinations, coma, weight loss, and acneiform rash) (see page 980).[9]

Long-Acting Dextromethorphan

A controlled clinical study suggests that the frequency of complex partial seizures appears to increase after a long-acting dextromethorphan (120 mg/day) is used.[10]

LABORATORY

Analytic Method

A high-performance liquid chromatography assay is available for the simultaneous determination of dextromethorphan, dextrorphan, 3-hydroxymorphinone, and 3-methoxymorphine in plasma and urine. The lowest detectable concentrations were 0.5 ng/mL for 3-hydroxymorphinone and 3-methoxymorphinan and 1 ng/mL for dextromethorphan and dextrorphan in plasma.[11] Although dextromethorphan is structurally similar to opioids, the ingestion of a single normal, or twice normal, dose of dextromethorphan is not likely to produce a falsely positive 6-hour urine opioid EMIT screen.[12]

Blood Levels

Postmortem examination of two fatalities following ingestion of an unknown quantity of dextromethorphan (DM) revealed serum dextromethorphan levels of 9.2 and 3.3 ng/mg, respectively. The gas chromatography method has a detection limit of about 50 ng for DM and about 25 ng/mL for dextrorphan.[13,14] Debrisoquin oxidative phenotypes may be determined for poor metabolizers and extensive metabolizers by a dextromethorphan/dextrorphan metabolic ratio (MR) based on a saliva measurement.[15]

Dextromethorphan 30 mg and caffeine (25 to 40 mg) can be given together to children to determine Debrisoquin oxidative urine/dextrorphan metabolic ratios and *N*-acetylation (caffeine metabolites) phenotypes, a noninvasive method for the assessment of polymorphic drug metabolism in various pediatric populations.

TREATMENT

Gut Decontamination

Gastric decontamination should be considered after acute ingestions of over 10 mg/kg.[16] Activated charcoal and/or gastric lavage may be preferable to syrup of ipecac in drowsy patients or if the time from ingestion is greater than 15 minutes.[16] There are no controlled clinical data to support the usefulness of either activated charcoal or cathartics.

Antidotes

Some authors recommend administration of naloxone 0.4 to 2.0 mg IV in an adult with repetition of the dose every 2 to 3 minutes as needed to a total dose of 10 mg. Symptomatic patients who respond to naloxone should be observed for at least 4 to 6 hours. Continuous IV infusion of naloxone may be required when long-acting preparations of dextromethorphan have been involved.[16]

Three children who were overdosed with 5 to 21 mg/kg of dextromethorphan developed neurologic symptoms, including coma, nystagmus, mydriasis, ataxia, and dystonia. All responded dramatically to naloxone at total bolus doses of 0.03 to 0.36 mg/kg. In two patients naloxone infusions of 0.03 and 0.13 mg/kg/hr were given for 9 to 10 hours after an initial naloxone reversal by 0.03 and 0.22 mg/kg, respectively.[17]

Supportive Care

It appears prudent to admit and observe patients with persistent cardiovascular or neurologic signs. Those who intentionally abuse dextromethorphan should receive the appropriate psychosocial support.[18] Treatment with naloxone has produced mixed results.

REFERENCES—DEXTROMETHORPHAN

1. Reynolds JEF, ed. *Martindale: the extra pharmacopoeia.* 13th ed. London: Pharmaceutical Press, 1993.
2. Koppel C, Tenczer J, Ibe K. Urinary metabolism of dextromethorphan in men. Azzneimittel-Forsch/Drug Des 1987; 37:1304–1306.
3. Sauter D, MacNeil P, Weinstein E, Azar A. Phenelzine sulfate-dextromethorphan interaction: a case report. Vet Hum Toxicol 1991;133:365.
4. Sovner R, Wolfe J. Interaction between dextromethorphan an monoamine oxidase inhibitor therapy with isocarboxazid. N Engl J Med 1988;319:1671.
5. Yoon YH, Marmor MF. Dextromethorphan protects retinal against ischemic injury in vivo. Arch Ophthalmol 1989; 10:409–411.
6. Albers GW, Saenz RE, Noses JA Jr, Chai DW. Pilot study of oral dextromethorphan patients at risk for brain ischemia. Neurology 1990;40(Suppl 1):193.
7. Koyuncuoglu H, Saydam B. The treatment of heroin addicts with dextromethorphan. A double-blind comparison of dextromethorphan with chlorpromazine. Int J Clin Pharmacol Ther Toxicol 1990;28:147–152.
8. Wolfe TR, Caravati EM. Massive dextromethorphan ingestion and abuse. Am J Emerg Med 1995;13:174–176.
9. NG YY, Lin WL, Chen TW et al. Spurious hyperchloremia and decreased anion gap in a patient with dextromethorphan bromide. Am J Nephrol 1992;12:268–270.
10. Fisher RS, Cysyk BJ, Lesser RP, Pontecorvo MJ, Ferkany JT, Schwerdt PR et al. Dextromethorphan for treatment of complex partial seizures. Neurology 1990;40:547–548.
11. Chen ZR, Somogyi AA, Bachner F. Simultaneous determination of dextromethorphan and the metabolites in plasma and urine using high-performance liquid chromatography with application to their disposition in man. Ther Drug Monit 1990;12:97–108.
12. Storrow AB, Magoon MR, Norton J. The dextromethorphan defense: dextromethorphan and the opioid screen. Acad Emerg Med 1995;2:791–794.
13. Rammer L, Holmgren P, Sandler H. Fatal intoxication by dextromethorphan: a report on two cases. Forensic Sci Int 1988;37:233–236.
14. East T, Dye D. Determination of dextromethorphan metabolites in human plasma and urine by high-performance liquid chromatography with fluorescence detection. J Chromatogr 1985;338:99–112.
15. Houz Y, Pickle L, Meyer PS, Woosley RL. Salivary analyses for determination of dextromethorphan metabolic phenotype. Clin Pharmacol Ther 1990;47:150.
16. Schneider SM, Michelson EA, Baucek CD, Ilkhanipour K. Dextromethorphan poisoning reversed by naloxone. Am J Emerg Med 1991;9:237–238.
17. Henretig F, Cugini D, Durbin D, Kearney T, Insley BV, Torrey S et al. Dextromethorphan (DM) overdose in children. Vet Hum Toxicol 1988;3:364.
18. Fisher DD: Dextromethorphan. Clin Toxicol Rev 1991;13(4):1–2.

EXCIPIENTS

Drug dosage forms contain many substances in addition to the active drug. Such substances are known as excipients. Excipients may include diluents, binders, lubricants, disintegrators, colors, flavors, and sweetening agents. Excipients may provide hidden hazards in many drug products.[1] Extensive reviews of such hidden hazards produced by excipients are available.[2–4] A detailed update of the literature has been published by Golightly and colleagues.[5]

COLORING AGENTS

Reports of allergic reactions to coloring agents confirm the importance of full disclosure of information on the labeling: (a) FD&C Red 40 in carbamazepine (Tegretol[6]); (b) carmine, an alimentary or cosmetic coloring agent (allergic alveolitis[7]); (c) quinolone yellow (E104), a dye banned in Australia, Japan, Norway, and the United States (urticarial reaction).[8]

REFERENCES—EXCIPIENTS

1. Smith JM, Dodd TRP. Adverse reactions to pharmaceutical excipients. Adverse Drug React Acute Poisoning Rev 1982;1: 93–142.
2. Federal Register, August 8, 1991, Vol 56 No 153, p. 37797.
3. Napke E, Stevens DGH. Excipients and additives. Hidden hazards in drug products and in product substitution. CMA J 1984;131:1449–1452.
4. Smolinske SC. Toxicity of drug excipients. Rocky Mountain Poison Center General Syllabus. Poisoning Symposium:

Legal Issues/Toxicology Controversies for the Clinician. Cooper Mountain, CO, March 4–8, 1985, pp. 181–191.
5. Golightly LK, Smolinske SS, Bennett ML, Sutherland EW III, Rumack BH. Pharmaceutical excipients adverse drug effects associated with "inactive" ingredients in drug products. Parts I and II. Med Toxicol 1988;3:128–135; 209–240.
6. Koppel BS, Harden CL, Daras M. Tegretol excipient-induced allergy. Arch Neurol 1991;48:789.
7. Dietemann-Molard A, Braun JJ, Solier PJ, Pauli G. Extrinsic allergic alveolitis secondary to carmine. Lancet 1991;338:460.
8. Bell T. Colourants and drug reactions. Lancet 1991;338:55–56.

RHODAMINE B

Rhodamine B is a red-colored dye. It is not allowed to be used in food in the United States, but its use is permitted in cosmetics. Occupational exposure may cause considerable skin and mucous membrane irritation. Folowing ingestion the urine fluoresces intensely. Recovery from acute symptoms is complete within 24 hours. Treatment is symptomatic and supportive.

STRUCTURE AND CLASSIFICATION

Rhodamine B is tetraethyl-3′,6′-diaminofluoran and is also known as "FD & C Red No. 19," "Basic violet 10," and "Food Red 15".[1,2] The empirical formula is $C_{28}H_{31}ClN_2O_3$, and the molecular weight is 479.0. It is very soluble in water with a bluish red color. Rhodamine B presents as green crystals or a reddish violet powder.[3]

USES

Rhodamine B is commonly used as a coloring in lipsticks (although the US Food and Drug Administration restricts its concentration to less than 6%). It is also used to check for fuel leaks in M-1 tanks and other military vehicles by adding a small quantity of it into the diesel fuel and observing for the appearance of any red coloring on the outside of the fuel tank. Oral ingestion is limited to 0.75 mg per day.[4] Other uses include a dye for fabrics, analytical reagent for metals, a tracing agent in water pollution studies, and a color marker in herbicidal sprays.[5]

SOURCES

Rhodamine B may be found in food products.[2]

OCCUPATIONAL EXPOSURE

Seventeen patients were exposed to aerosolized rhodamine B inside a maintenance shop for a mean duration of 26 minutes. They developed transient skin and mucous membrane irritation that resolved within 24 hours.[1]

ELIMINATION

Other major compounds found in the urine include a metabolite of rhodamine B, triethylrhodamine, and diethylated metabolites.[6,7]

CLINICAL PRESENTATION

Acute exposure to aerosolized rhodamine can lead to burning of the eyes, excessive tearing, nasal burning, nasal itching, chest pain/tightness, rhinorrhea, cough, dyspnea, burning of the throat, headache, and nausea. Symptoms resolve in 4 to 24 hours without evidence of serious sequellae.[1]

Rhodamine B is considered to be a possible carcinogen.[4] It shows mutagenic activity in the Ames test and causes DNA damage in hamster ovary cells.[2] Two patients who had purchased "pink-colored" cookies were found to have intensely fluorescent compounds in the urine.[2] Both recovered.

LABORATORY

Analytical Methods

A high-performance liquid chromatography method is available for analysis of human plasma. The detection limit is 2 ng of rhodamine B, corresponding to a plasma concentration of 25 ng/mL.[5]

Abnormalities

Ingestion may result in urine that fluoresces intensely under long-wave ultraviolet light.[2]

TREATMENT

Stabilization

Treatment of exposure after either ingestion or occupational exposure is largely symptomatic and supportive. Following occupational exposure patients should be treated and evaluated in a decontamination facility set up outside the emergency department entrance.[1] Occupational exposure should be followed by removal of clothing and vigorous washing of the skin and hair with Phisohex soap and water. Chest x-rays, visual acuities, and forced expiratory volumes (FEV_1) should be measured in the emergency department. FEV_1 should be repeated in 3 to 5 days.

REFERENCES—RHODAMINE

1. Dine DJ, Wilkinson JA. Acute exposure to rhodamine B. Clin Toxicol 1987;25:603–607.
2. Kelner MJ. Rhodamine ingestion as a cause of fluorescent red urine. West J Med 1985;143:523–534.
3. Windholz M, ed. The Merck Index. 9th ed. Rahway, NJ: Merck & Co, 1976, p. 1061.
4. International Agency for Research on Cancer. IARC Monographs on the Evaluation of the Carcinogenesis Risk of Chemical to Man, 1978;16:221–231.
5. Mason RW, Edwards IR. High-performance liquid chromatographic determination of rhodamine B in rabbit and human plasma. J Chromatograph Biomed Applic 1989;491:468–472.
6. Webb JM, Hansen WH. Studies on the metabolism of rhodamine B. Toxicol Appl Pharmacol 1961;3:86–95.
7. Webb JM, Hansen WH, Desmond A et al. Biochemical and toxicologic studies of rhodamine band 3,6-diaminofluran. Toxicol Appl Pharmacol 1961;3:696–706.

SWEETENING AND FLAVORING AGENTS

SYNTHETIC SWEETENING AGENTS

Tables 52–12A, 52–12B, and 52–12C list sucrose, sorbitol, and saccharin contents of common liquid pediatric antibiotic, antifungal, respiratory, anticonvulsant, and miscella-

Table 52-12A
Sweetener Content of Common Liquid Pediatric Antibiotic and Antifungal Preparations

Drug Product	Manufacturer	Sweetener Concentration in g/5 mL (Percent Concentration in w/v%)		
		Sucrose	Sorbitol	Saccharin
Ampicillin 125 mg/5 mL				
Amcill oral suspension	Warner-Chilcott	0.9(18)		0.0045(.09)
Ampicillin oral suspension	Biocraft	. . .[a]		. . .[a]
Ampicillin trihydrate oral suspension	Lederle	2.07(41)		
Ampicillin trihydrate oral suspension	Schein	2.4(48)[b]		. . .[c]
Omnipen oral suspension	Wyeth	4.0(80)		
Polycillin oral suspensoin	Bristol	1.7(34)[b]		
Principen oral suspension	Squibb	. . .[d]		. . .[d]
Totacillin oral suspension	Beecham	1.64(33)		
Ampicillin 250 mg/5 mL				
Amcill oral suspension	Warner-Chilcott	1.8(36)		0.009(0.18)
Ampicillin oral suspension	Biocraft	. . .[a]		. . .[a]
Ampicillin trihydrate oral suspension	Lederle	1.91(38)		
Ampicillin trihydrate oral suspension	Schein	2.25(45)[b]		. . .[c]
Omnipen oral suspension	Wyeth	4.0(80)		
Polycillin oral suspension	Bristol	1.8(36)[b]		
Principen oral suspension	Squibb	. . .[d]		. . .[d]
Totacillin oral suspension	Beecham	1.79(36)		
Ampicillin 500 mg/5 mL				
Omnipen pediatric drops	Wyeth	3.5(70)		
Polycillin oral suspension	Bristol	1.5(30)[b]		
Polycillin pediatric drops	Bristol	1.5(30)[b]		
Amoxicillin 125 mg/5 mL				
Amoxil oral suspension	Beecham	1.67(33)		
Amoxicillin oral suspension	Biocraft	. . .[a]		. . .[a]
Amoxicillin oral suspension	Schein	2.4(48)[b]		. . .[c]
Larotid oral suspension	Beecham	1.67(33)		
Polymox oral suspension	Bristol	2.5(50)[b]		
Trimox oral suspension	Squibb	. . .[d]		
Utimox oral suspension	Warner-Chilcott	0.85(17)		
Wymox oral suspension	Wyeth	2.1(42)		
Amoxicillin 250 mg/5 ml				
Amoxil oral suspension	Beecham	1.84(37)		
Amoxil pediatric drops	Beecham	2.03(41)		
Amoxicillin oral suspension	Biocraft	. . .[a]		. . .[a]
Amoxicillin oral suspension	Schein	2.25(45)[b]		. . .[c]
Larotid oral suspension	Beecham	1.84(37)		
Polymox oral suspension	Bristol	2.4(48)[b]		
Polymox pediatric drops	Bristol	2.5(50)[b]		
Trimox oral suspension	Squibb	. . .[d]		
Ultimox oral suspension	Warner–Chilcott	1.7(34)		
Wymox oral suspension	Wyeth	1.9(38)		
Amoxicillin–Clavulanic Acid Combination				
Augmentin oral suspension 125 mg/5 mL[e]	Beecham			0.0325(0.65)
Augmentin oral suspension 250 mg/5 mL[f]	Beecham			0.0325(0.65)
Cefaclor				
Ceclor oral suspension 125 mg/5 mL	Lilly	2.9(58)		
Ceclor oral suspension 250 mg/5 mL	Lilly	2.8(56)		
Cefadroxil 250 mg/5 mL				
Ultracef oral suspension	Bristol	2.1(42)[b]		
Cephalexin 125 mg/5 mL				
Cephalexin oral suspension	Biocraft	. . .[a]		
Keflex oral suspension	Dista	3.1(62)		

[a]For exact amounts of sweeteners, call Biocraft at 201-796-3434.
[b]Not confirmed in 1987.
[c]Amount not disclosed by manufacturer.
[d]For exact amounts of sweeteners, call Squibb at 609-921-4006.
[e]Also contains mannitol 0.51 g/5 mL (10.2% w/v).
[f]Also contains mannitol 0.63 g/5 mL (12.6% w/v).
[g]For exact amount of sweetener, call Abbott Scientific Affair at 312-937-7302.
[h]For exact amount of sweeteners, call Upjohn at 616-323-6615.
[i]For exact amount of sweetener, call Ross at 614-227-3333.
[j]Also contains aspartame 0.008 g/5 mL (0.16% w/v).
[k]For the exact amounts of sweeteners, call Burroughs Wellcome at 919-248-3000.
[l]Source: Physicians' Desk Reference, 41st ed. Oradell, NJ: Medical Company Economics, Inc.; 1987.

Table 52–12A *(Continued)*

Drug Product	Manufacturer	Sweetener Concentration in g/5 mL (Percent Concentration in w/v%)		
		Sucrose	Sorbitol	Saccharin
Cephalexin 250 mg/5 mL				
Cephalexin oral suspension	Biocraft	. . .[a]		
Keflex oral suspension	Dista	2.9(58)		
Cephalexin 500 mg/5 mL				
Keflex pediatric drops	Dista	3.1(62)		
Cephradine 125 mg/5 mL				
Anspor oral suspension	SmithKline Beecham	3.1(62)		
Velosef oral suspension	Squibb	. . .[d]		
Cephradine 250 mg/5 mL				
Anspor oral suspension	SmithKline Beecham	2.9(58)		
Velosef oral suspension	Squibb	. . .[d]		
Dicloxacillin 62.5 mg/5 mL				
Dynapen oral suspension	Bristol	2.3(46)[b]		. . .[c]
Pathocil oral suspension	Wyeth	3.1(62)		. . .[c]
Erythromycin Ethylsuccinate 200 mg/5 mL				
E.E.S. drops	Abbott	. . .[g]		
E.E.S. granules	Abbott	. . .[g]		
E.E.S. 200 liquid	Abbott	. . .[g]		
E-Mycin E liquid	Upjohn	. . .[h]	. . .[h]	
Erythromycin ethylsuccinate oral suspension	Lederle	2.25(45)		0.02(0.4)
Pediamycin drops	Ross	. . .[i]		
Pediamycin liquid	Ross	. . .[i]		
Pediamycin oral suspension	Ross	. . .[i]		
Wyamycin E liquid	Wyeth	3.25(65)		
Erythromycin Ethylsuccinate 400 mg/5 mL				
E.E.S. 400 liquid	Abbott	. . .[g]		
E-Mycin E liquid	Upjohn	. . .[h]	. . .[h]	
Eryped oral suspension	Abbott	. . .[g]		
Erythromycin ethylsuccinate oral suspension	Lederle	2.25(45)		0.03(0.6)
Pediamycin 400	Ross	. . .[i]		
Wyamycin E liquid	Wyeth	3.25(65)		
Erythromycin Estolate 125 mg/5 mL				
Erythromycin estolate oral suspension	Lederle	2.25(45)		
Ilosone liquid	Dista	1.85(37)		
Erythromycin Estolate 250 mg/5 mL				
Erythromycin estolate oral suspension	Lederle	2.25(45)		
Ilosone liquid	Dista	1.8(36)		0.0025(0.05)
Erythromycin Estolate 500 mg/5 mL				
Ilosone ready-mixed drops	Dista	1.8(36)		
Erythromycin Ethysuccinate 200 mg-Sulfisoxazole 600 mg Combination				
Pediazole oral suspension	Ross	. . .[i]		
Oxacillin 250 mg/5 mL				
Oxacillin oral suspension	Biocraft	. . .[a]		. . .[a]
Oxacillin sodium oral solution	Schein	2.25(45)[b]		. . .[c]
Prostaphlin oral suspension	Bristol	2.3(46)[b]		. . .[c]
Penicillin G				
Pentids oral syrup 125 mg/5 mL	Squibb	. . .[d]		. . .[d]
Pentids oral syrup 250 mg/5 mL	Squibb	. . .[d]		. . .[d]
Penicillin VK 125 mg/5 mL				
Beepen-VK oral suspension	Beecham	2.87(57)		0.005(0.1)
Betapen-VK oral suspension	Bristol	2.8(56)[b]		. . .[c]
Ledercillin VK oral suspension	Lederle	3.5(70)		0.0134(0.27)
Penapar VK oral suspension[j]	Warner-Chilcott	2.5(50)		0.0125(0.25)
Penicillin VK oral suspension	Schein	2.2(44)[b]		. . .[c]
Penicillin V potassium solution	Biocraft	. . .[a]		. . .[a]
Pen-Vee K oral suspension	Wyeth	2.5(50)		. . .[c]
V-Cillin oral suspension	Lilly	2.9(58)		
Veetids oral suspension	Squibb	. . .[d]		. . .[d]
Penicillin VK 250 mg/5 mL				
Beepen-VK oral suspension	Beecham	3.18(64)		0.005(0.1)
Betapen-VK oral suspension	Bristol	2.8(56)[b]		. . .[c]
Ledercillin VK oral suspension	Lederle	3.5(70)		0.027(0.53)
Penapar VK oral suspension[j]	Warner-Chilcott	2.5(50)		0.0175(0.35)
Penicillin VK oral suspension	Schein	2.0(40)[b]		. . .[c]

(continued)

Table 52-12A *(Continued)*

Drug Product	Manufacturer	Sweetener Concentration in g/5 mL (Percent Concentration in w/v%)		
		Sucrose	Sorbitol	Saccharin
Penicillin VK 250 mg/5 mL (continued)				
Penicillin V potassium solution	Biocraft	. . .		. . .
Pen-Vee K oral suspension	Wyeth	3.3(66)		. . .
V-Cillin oral suspension	Lilly	3.2(64)		0.033(0.66)
Veetids oral suspension	Squibb	. . .		. . .
Sulfisoxazole 500 mg/5 mL				
Gantrisin syrup	Roche	3.5(70)		
Gantrisin pediatric suspension	Roche	2.7(54)		
Sulfamethoxazole 500 mg/5 mL				
Gantanol suspension	Roche	2.5(50)		0.0125(0.25)
Sulfamethoxazole 200 mg-Trimethoprim 40 mg/5 mL Combination				
Bactrim pediatric suspension	Roche	2.5(50)	0.35(7)	0.005(0.1)
Bactrim suspension	Roche	2.5(50)	0.35(7)	0.005(0.1)
Septra suspension	Burroughs Wellcome		. . .	. . .
Sulfamethoxazole & trimethoprim pediatric suspension	Biocraft		. . .	. . .
Sulfamethoxazole & trimethoprim pediatric suspension	Lederle	2.8(56)	0.5(10)	0.005(0.1)
Nystatin 500,000 Units/5 mL				
Mycostatin oral suspension	Squibb	2.5(50)[i]		. . .
Nilstat oral suspension	Lederle	3.05(61)		
Nystex oral suspension	Savage	2.5(50)[i]		

Table 52-12B
Sweetener Content of Common Liquid Pediatric Respiratory, Anticonvulsant, and Miscellaneous Agents[a]

Drug Product	Manufacturer	Sweetener Concentration in g/5 mL (Percent Concentration in w/v%)		
		Sucrose	Sorbitol	Saccharin
Aminophylline 105 mg/5 mL				
Aminophylline oral liquid	Barre-National			. . .
Aminophylline oral liquid	Roxane		1.0(20)	0.0075(0.15)
Aminophylline oral liquid	Schein			. . .
Somophyllin oral liquid	Fisons			. . .
Somophyllin-DF oral liquid	Fisons			. . .
Diphenhydramine 12.5 mg/5 mL				
Benadryl elixir	Parke-Davis	1.5(30)		
Benylin cough syrup[d]	Parke-Davis	3.0(60)		0.0185(0.37)
Diphenhydramine hydrochloride cough syrup	Lederle	3.84(77)		
Diphenhydramine Hydrochloride Elixir, USP	Lederle	1.5(30)		
Diphenhydramine Hydrochloride Elixir, USP	Roxane	1.5(30)		
Hydroxyzine Hydrochloride 10 mg/5 mL				
Atarax syrup	Roerig	5.9(108)		
Hydroxyzine hydrochloride syrup	Schein	0.6(12)		
Hydroxyzine Pamoate 25 mg/5 mL				
Vistaril oral suspension	Pfizer		. . .	
Hydroxyzine 2.5 mg-Ephedrine 6.25 mg-Theophylline 32.5 mg/5 mL Combination				
Marax DF syrup	Roerig	5.0(100)		
Metaproterenol 10 mg/5 mL				
Alupent syrup	Boehringer Ingelheim		1.4(28)	0.0035(0.07)
Metaprel syrup	Sandoz		. . .	. . .
Oxtriphylline				
Choledyl elixir 100 mg/5 mL	Parke-Davis	1.0(20)	0.965(19.3)	
Choledyl pediatric syrup 50 mg/5 mL[h]	Parke-Davis		0.525(10.5)	0.006(0.12)
Theophylline 80 mg/15 mL				
Aquaphyllin syrup	Ferndale	. . .		
Elixophyllin elixir	Forest			0.005(0.1)
Slo-Phyllin 80 mg syrup	Rorer		2.02(40)	. . .
Theoclear-80 syrup	Central Pharmaceuticals		1.3(26)	0.01(0.2)
Theolair liquid	Riker	2.4(48)	0.75(15)	

Adapted from Hill EM, et al. Am J Hosp Pharm 1988;45:135-142.
American Journal of Hospital Pharmacy, 1988 Jun, 45(6):1346-9.
Hill EM; Flaitz CM; Frost GR. Sweetener content of common pediatric oral liquid medications. Am J Hosp Pharm 1988;45(1):135-142.

Table 52–12B *(Continued)*

Drug Product	Manufacturer	Sweetener Concentration in g/5 mL (Percent Concentration in w/v%)		
		Sucrose	Sorbitol	Saccharin
Theophylline 80 mg/15 mL (continued)				
Theophylline elixir	Barre–National			. . .
Theophylline oral solution	Roxane		3.25(65)	0.0037(0.075)
Theostat 80 syrup	Laser	2.4(48)		
Theophylline 150 mg/5 mL				
Accurbron liquid[k]	Merrell Dow		0.40(8)	. . .
Aerolate liquid	Fleming		1.19(24)	
Synophylate elixir	Central Pharmaceuticals	1.25(25)		0.004(0.08)
Theon syrup	Bock		. . .	. . .
Theophylline–Guaifenesin Combinations				
Elixophyllin GG	Forest		2.3(46)	
Quibron	Mead Johnson	2.75(55)	0.208(4.2)	
Slo-Phyllin GG syrup	Rorer		0.62(12.4)	. . .
Synophylate GG syrup	Central Pharmaceuticals	1.0(20)	1.05(21)	0.0067(0.13)
Theolair-Plus liquid	Riker	2.5(50)		
Theophylline–Ephedrine–Phenobarbital Combinations				
Tedral elixir	Parke–Davis		0.42(8.4)	0.010(0.2)
Tedral suspension[m]	Parke–Davis			0.018(0.36)
Ethosuximide 250 mg/5 mL				
Zarontin syrup	Parke–Davis	3.0(60)		0.0075(0.15)
Phenobarbital 20 mg/5 mL				
Phenobarbital Elixir, USP	Lilly	0.64(13)		
Phenobarbital Elixir, USP	Roxane	0.64(13)		
Phenobarbital #2 liquid	Pharmaceutical Associates	0.65(13)		
Phenobarbital 15 mg/5 mL				
Phenobarbital liquid	Pharmaceutical Associates	0.65(13)		
Phenytoin				
Dilantin-30 suspension 30 mg/5 mL	Parke–Davis	1.0(20)		
Dilantin-125 suspension 125 mg/5 mL	Parke–Davis	1.0(20)		
Primidone 250 mg/5 mL				
Mysoline suspenson	Ayerst			0.00375(0.075)
Valproic Acid 250 mg/5 mL				
Depakene syrup	Abbott	. . .	. . .	
Ferrous Sulfate				
Feosol elixir 220 mg/5 mL[o]	SmithKline Beecham	0.822(16.4)		. . .
Fer-In-Sol drops 75 mg/0.6 mL	Mead Johnson	1.9(38)	1.6(32)	
Fer-In-Sol syrup 90 mg/5 mL	Mead Johnson	3.0(60)	.35(7)	
Ferrous sulfate elixir 220 mg/5 mL	Lederle	1.8(36)		0.0024(0.048)
Ferrous sulfate liquid 300 mg/5 mL	Roxane	2.0(40)		0.00125(0.025)
Cimetidine 300 mg/5 mL				
Tagamet liquid	SmithKline Beecham		2.8(56)	0.02(0.4)

Table 52–12C
Sweetener Content of Common Chewable Pediatric Medications

Drug Product	Manufacturer	Sweetener (mg/tablet)		
		Sucrose	Mannitol	Saccharin
Antibiotics				
Amoxil (amoxicillin) chewable tablet 125 mg	Beecham	96.6	76	0.45
Amoxil (amoxicillin) chewable tablet 250 mg	Beecham	193.3	152	0.9
Augmentin (amoxicillin–clavulanic acid) chewable tablet 125 mg	Beecham		171	1.0
Augmentin (amoxicillin–clavulanic acid) chewable tablet 250 mg	Beecham		341	2.0
E.E.S. (erythromycin ethylsuccinate) 200 mg chewable tablet	Abbott	. . .[a]		
Ilosone (erythromycin estolate) chewable tablet 125 mg	Dista	25	292	4.0
Ilosone (erythromycin estolate) chewable tablet 250 mg	Dista	50	585	8.0
Antifungal Agents				
Clotrimazole 10 mg Troches[b]	Miles	903.5		
Anticonvulsants				
Dilantin (phenytoin) Infatab 50 mg	Parke–Davis	463		1.2
Tegretol (carbamazepine) chewable tablet 100 mg	Geigy	249.95		

[a]For exact amount of sucrose, call Abbott Laboratories at 312-937-7302.
[b]Not chewable.

Table 52–13
Sweeteners, Flavorings, Dyes, and Preservatives in Antidiarrheal Preparations

Brand Name	Manufacturer	Sweeteners*	Flavorings	Dyes/Colors	Preservatives
Prescription products					
Coly-Mycin Oral Suspension	Parke-Davis	Sa, So, Su, Co	Imitation chocolate Imitation vanilla	Unspecified	Methylparaben Propylparaben
Donnagel-PG	Robins	F	Unspecified	Yellow 10	Sodium benzoate
Lomotil Liquid	GD Searle	So	Cherry	Yellow 6	Unspecified
Parepectolin Liquid	Rover	Sa	Peppermint oil	Unspecified	Ethylparaben, propylparaben
Over-the-counter products					
Disasorb Antidiarrheal	Columbia	Sa, So	Unspecified	Unspecified	Benzoic acid, propylparaben, methylparaben
Donnagel	Robins	So	Unspecified	Yellow 10 Blue 1	Sodium benzoate
Imodium A-D Caplets	McNeil	La	Unspecified	Blue 1 Yellow 10	Methylparaben, propylparaben
Imodium A-D Anti-Diarrheal Liquid	McNeil	Unspecified	Unspecified	Unspecified	Propylparaben
Kaopectate concentrated antidiarrheal	Upjohn	Su	Vanilla	Red 40 Titanium dioxide	Methylparaben
Pepto-Bismol Liquid	Proctor & Gamble	Sa	Wintergreen	Red 22, red 28	Benzoic acid
St Joseph Anti-Diarrheal	Schering-Plough	So, Sa	Cola	None	Benzoic acid, methylparaben, propylparaben

*Abbreviations used for sweeteners in all tables: As, aspartame; Ca, caramel; Co, cocoa; F, fructose; G, glucose; In, invert sugar; La, lactose; Ma, mannitol; Sa, saccharin; So, sorbitol; Su, sucrose; V, vanillin.

Table 52–14
Sweeteners, Flavorings, Dyes, and Preservatives in Analgesic/Antipyretic Preparations (Prescription Products)[a]

Brand Name	Manufacturer	Sweeteners[b]	Flavorings	Dyes/Colors	Preservatives
Roxicet Oral Solution	Roxane	F, Sa	Vanilla Creme de menthe	Red 40	Unspecified
Tylenol with Codeine Elixir	McNeil	Sa, Su	Unspecified	Yellow 6	Sodium benzoate
Demerol HCl Syrup	Winthrop	G, Sa	Artificial banana	Not specified	Benzoic acid
MSIR Oral Solution	Purdue-Frederick	In, Su	Chocolate	Red 40	Sodium benzoate
Methadone HCl, Oral Solution	Roxane	So	Lemon	Red 40 Yellow 6	Benzoic acid
Trilisate Liquid	Purdue-Frederick	F	Artificial cherry	Yellow 6 Caramel color	Potassium sorbate

[a]Adapted from Kumar A et al. Pediatrics 1993;91:927–933.
[b]Abbreviations are explained in the footnote to Table 52–13.

Table 52–15
Sweeteners, Flavorings, Dyes, and Preservatives in Cold and Cough Preparations (Over-the-Counter Products)[a]

Brand Name	Manufacturer	Sweeteners[b]	Flavorings	Dyes/Colors	Preservatives
Antitussives and combinations					
Children's Bayer Cough Syrup	Glenbrook Labs	G, Sa, So	Cherry Black F-8900	None	Parabens
Benylin Cough Syrup	Parke-Davis	Ca, G, Sa, Su	Unspecified	Red 33 Red 40	Unspecified
Benylin DM	Parke-Davis	Ca, G, Su	Unspecified	Red 33	Unspecified
Benylin Decongestant	Parke-Davis	Sa, Su, G	Unspecified	Yellow 6	Unspecified
Cerose-DM	Wyeth-Ayerst	Sa	Artificial black currant Artificial cherry morello Artificial fritzboro fruit essence	Yellow 6	Sodium benzoate
Cheracol-D Cough Formula	Roberts	F, Su	Wild cherry Imitation grenadine	Red 40	Benzoic acid Methylparaben Propylparaben

[a]Adapted from Kumar A et al. Pediatrics 1993;91:927–933.
[b]Abbreviations are explained in the footnote to Table 52–13.

Table 52–15 *(Continued)*

Brand Name	Manufacturer	Sweeteners[b]	Flavorings	Dyes/Colors	Preservatives
Contac Cough Formula Cough Suppressant and Expectorant	SmithKline Beecham	Sa, Su	Natural & artificial cherry punch (#715)	Red 40	Methylparaben, propylparaben, sodium benzoate
Delsym	McNeil	F, Su	Unspecified	Yellow 6	Methylparaben, propylparaben
Dorcol Children's Cough Syrup	Sandoz	Su	Unspecified	Blue 1 Red 40	Benzoic acid
Naldecon Dx Children's Syrup	Bristol-Myers Squibb	So	Raspberry Strawberry	Yellow 10 Red 33	Sodium benzoate
Novahistine DMX	Marion Merrell Dow	Sa, So, In	Cherry Black currant	Red 40 Yellow 6	Unspecified
Robitussin	Robins	Ca, G, F, Sa	Unspecified	Red 40	Sodium benzoate
Robitussin-DM	Robins	F, Sa, G	Unspecified	Red 40	Sodium benzoate
Ryna-C	Wallace	Sa, So	Artificial cinnamon	Unspecified	Sodium benzoate
Sudafed Cough Syrup	Burroughs Wellcome	Sa, Su	Unspecified	Yellow 10 Blue 1	Sodium benzoate, methylparaben
Triaminic-DM Cough Formula	Sandoz	So, Su	Unspecified	Blue 1 Red 40	Benzoic acid
Vicks Children's Cough Syrup	Richardson-Vicks	Sa, Su	Cherry	Green 3 Red 40	Methylparaben
Vicks Formula 44 Cough Mixture	Richardson-Vicks	Ca, In	Cherry Licorice	Red 40	Sodium benzoate
Expectorants and combinations					
Benylin Expectorant	Parke-Davis	Sa, Su	Unspecified	Red 40	Sodium benzoate
FedaHist Expectorant	Schwarz	Sa, So	Artificial apricot	Red 40	Benzoic acid
Triaminic Expectorant	Sandoz	Sa, So, Su	Grapefruit (WONF #24082) Spearmint oil Clove oil Artificial cinnamon oil	Yellow 6 Yellow 10	Benzoic acid
Vicks Daycare Liquid	Richardson-Vicks	Sa, Su	Fruit	Yellow 6	Sodium benzoate
Vicks Formula 44M	Richardson-Vicks	Sa, Su	Fruit	Blue 1 Red 40	Sodium benzoate
Vicks Children's Nyquil	Richardson-Vicks	So, Su	Cherry	Red 40	Unspecified
Vicks Nyquil	Richardson-Vicks	Su	Licorice	Blue 1 Yellow 5	Sodium benzoate

[a]Adapted from Kumar A et al. Pediatrics 1993;91:927–933.
[b]Abbreviations are explained in the footnote to Table 52–13.

Table 52–16
Sweetener's Flavorings, Dyes, and Preservatives in Analgesic/Antipyretic Preparations (Over-the-Counter Products)[a]

Brand Name	Manufacturer	Sweeteners[b]	Flavorings	Dyes/Colors	Preservatives
Children's Anacin-3 (acetaminophen)	Whitehall Labs	As, Ma, Su	Cherry	Red 40, lake	Unspecified
Children's Anacin-3 Liquid (acetaminophen)	Whitehall	So, Su	Cherry	Red 33 Red 40	Sodium benzoate, methylparaben
Children's Anacin-3 Infants' Drops (acetaminophen)	Whitehall	So, Sa	Tutti-frutti	Red 40 Yellow 6	Sodium benzoate
St Joseph Aspirin-Free Fever Reducer Chewable Tablets (acetaminophen)	Schering-Plough	Ma, Sa	Fruit	Red 7 Calcium lake Red 30 Aluminum lake	Unspecified
St Joseph Aspirin-Free Fever Reducer Liquid (acetaminophen)	Schering-Plough	Sa, So	Artificial cherry	Red 40 Aluminum lake Blue 2	Sodium benzoate, methylparaben, propylparaben
St Joseph Aspirin-Free Fever Reducer Infant Drops (acetaminophen)	Schering-Plough	Sa	Artificial cherry Casia flavor	Yellow 6	Sodium benzoate

[a]Adapted from Kumar A et al. Pediatrics 1993;91:927–933.
[b]Abbreviations are explained in the footnote to Table 52–13.

(continued)

Table 52–16 *(Continued)*

Brand Name	Manufacturer	Sweeteners[b]	Flavorings	Dyes/Colors	Preservatives
Children's Bayer Chewable Aspirin (acetylsalicylic acid)	Glenbrook Labs	G, Sa	Orange	Yellow 6 Aluminum lake Dye B-3015	Unspecified
Children's Panadol Chewable Tablets (acetaminophen)	Glenbrook	Ma, Sa	Cherry (Trusil 5–9098)	Red 40 Red 28	Unspecified
Children's Panadol Liquid (acetaminophen)	Glenbrook	Sa, So	Unspecified	Red 40	Benzoic Acid, potassium sorbate
Infants' Panadol Drops (acetaminophen)	Glenbrook	Sa	Raspberry (21820) Cherry, vanilla (21146)	Red 40	Parabens
Congespirin for Children Aspirin-Free Chewable Cold Tablets (acetaminophen)	Bristol-Myers	Ma, Sa, Su	Unspecified	Yellow 6, red 30 Aluminum lake	Unspecified
Dorcol Children's Fever & Pain Reducer	Sandoz	Su	Artificial Strawberry (13418251)	Red 40	Benzoic acid
Liquiprin Infant Drops (acetaminophen)	Menley & James	G, F, In	Raspberry (13518251)	Red 33 Red 40	Methylparaben, propylparaben
Liquiprin Children's Elixir (acetaminophen)	Menley & James	G, F, In	Cherry (135–37121)	Red 33 Red 40	Methylparaben, propylparaben
Children's Tylenol Chewable Tablets (acetaminophen)	McNeil	As, Ma	Unspecified	Red 7 Blue 1 (for grape only)	Unspecified
Children's Tylenol Elixir (acetaminophen)	McNeil	So, Su	Cherry	Red 40 Blue 1 (for grape only)	Sodium benzoate
Children's Tylenol Drops (acetaminophen)	McNeil	Sa	Unspecified	Yellow 6	Unspecified

[a]Adapted from Kumar A et al. Pediatrics 1993;91:927–933.
[b]Abbreviations are explained in the footnote to Table 52–13.

Table 52–17
Sweeteners, Flavorings, Dyes, and Preservatives in Cough Medications (Prescription Products)[a]

Brand Name	Manufacturer	Sweeteners[b]	Flavorings	Dyes/Colors	Preservatives
Codimal DH	Central	Su	Pineapple Vanilla Apricot	Red 40	Unspecified
Phenergan Syrup Plain	Wyeth-Ayerst	Sa, G	Artificial black currant	Red 33 Yellow 10 Blue 1 Yellow 6	Sodium benzoate
Polaramine Syrup	Schering-Plough	So, Su	Unspecified	Red 40 Yellow 6	Propylparaben, methylparaben
Tussi-Organidin Liquid	Wallace	Sa, So	Raspberry	Red 40	Sodium benzoate
Ambenyl Cough Syrup	Forest	G, Su	Cherry	Red 33	Unspecified
Calcidrine Syrup	Abbott	G, Su	Menthol Apricot Cherry	Yellow 6	Unspecified
Dilaudid Cough Syrup	Knoll	Sa, So, Su	Peach	Red 40 Yellow lemon Shade	Sodium benzoate
Hycodan Syrup	DuPont-Merck	Su, So	Wild cherry	Red 40 Caramel color	Methylparaben, propylparaben
Nucofed Pediatric Expectorant	SmithKline Beecham	Sa, Su	Artificial strawberry	Red 40	Unspecified
Robitussin A-C	Robins	Sa, F	Unspecified	Red 40	Sodium benzoate
Tussar-2	Rhone-Poulenc Rorer	G, Sa, Su	Peppermint oil Spearmint oil	Blue 1 Yellow 10	Methylparaben
Entex Liquid	Norwich-Eaton	Sa, So, Su	Mixed fruit	Yellow 6	Sodium benzoate

[a]Adapted from Kumar A et al. Pediatrics 1993;91:927–933.
[b]Abbreviations are explained in the footnote to Table 52–13.

Table 52–18
Sweeteners, Flavorings, Dyes, and Preservatives in Antihistamine/Decongestant Preparations (Over-the-Counter Products)[a]

Brand Name	Manufacturer	Sweeteners[b]	Flavorings	Dyes/Colors	Preservatives
Actifed Syrup	Burroughs-Wellcome	So	Unspecified	Yellow 10	Sodium benzoate, methylparaben
Benadryl Decongestant Elixir	Parke-Davis	G, Sa, Su	Unspecified	Yellow 6	Unspecified
Bromfed Syrup	Muro	Sa, So, Su	Orange Lemon	Yellow 6	Methylparaben, sodium benzoate
Dimetane Decongestant Elixir	Robins	So	Unspecified	Blue 1 Red 40	Sodium benzoate
Dimetapp Elixir	Robins	Sa, So	Unspecified	Blue 1 Red 40	Sodium benzoate
Dorcol Children's Decongestant Liquid	Sandoz	So, Su	Unspecified	Yellow 6 Yellow 10	Benzoic acid
Fedahist Decongestant Syrup	Schwarz Pharma	So, Sa, Su	Artificial grape	Blue 1 Red 40	Methylparaben, sodium benzoate
Pediacare Infants' Oral Decongestant Drops	McNeil	So, Su	Unspecified	Red 40	Benzoic acid, sodium benzoate
Sudafed Children's Liquid	Burroughs Wellcome	So, Su	Unspecified	Red 40	Methylparaben, sodium benzoate
Triaminic Chewables	Sandoz	Ma, Sa, Su	Artificial vanilla Lemon juice	Yellow 6 Yellow 10	Unspecified
Actidil Syrup	Burroughs Wellcome	So	Unspecified	Yellow 6	Methylparaben, sodium benzoate
Chlor-Trimeton Allergy Syrup	Schering-Plough	Su, V	Unspecified	Green 3 Yellow 6	Benzaldehyde, methylparaben, propylparaben
Drixoral Antihistamine/ Nasal Decongestant Syrup	Schering-Plough	So, Su	Unspecified	Red 33 Yellow 6	Sodium benzoate

[a]Adapted from Kumar A et al. Pediatrics 1993;91:927–933.
[b]Abbreviations are explained in the footnote to Table 52–13.

Table 52–19
Sweeteners, Flavorings, Dyes, and Preservatives in Antihistamines/Decongestants (Prescription Products)[a]

Brand Name	Manufacturer	Sweeteners[b]	Flavorings	Dyes/Colors	Preservatives
Deconamine Syrup	Berlex	Su, So	Artificial grape	None	Sodium benzoate
Naldecon Cough Adult Liquid	Bristol	G, Sa	Raspberry Strawberry	Blue 1 Red 40	Sodium benzoate
Rondec DM Oral Drops	Ross	So	Natural & artificial grape	Red 33 Blue 1	Sodium benzoate
Actifed With Codeine	Burroughs Wellcome	So	Unspecified	Unspecified	Sodium benzoate, methylparaben
Atarax Syrup	Pfizer-Roerig	Su	Spearmint oil Peppermint oil	Unspecified	Sodium benzoate
Extendryl Syrup	Fleming	Su	Root beer (5820)	Caramel	Sodium benzoate
PBZ Elixir USP	Geigy	Su	Unspecified	Green 5	Unspecified
Periactin Syrup	MSD	Su, Sa, La	Unspecified	Yellow 10	Unspecified
Tacaryl Syrup	Westwood-Squibb	So, Su	Cherry chocolate Ethyl vanillin Menthol	None	Benzoic acid
Tavist Syrup	Sandoz	Sa, So	Artificial peach (F9770) Lemon (5–9738)	Unspecified	Methylparaben, propylparaben
Vistaril Oral Suspension	Pfizer	So	Lemon No. 78	Unspecified	Unspecified

[a]Adapted from Kumar A et al. Pediatrics 1993;91:927–933.
[b]Abbreviations are explained in the footnote to Table 52–13.

Table 52–20
Sweeteners, Flavorings, Dyes, and Preservatives in Liquid Preparations of Theophylline[a]

Brand Name	Manufacturer	Sweeteners[b]	Flavorings	Dyes/Colors	Preservatives
Marax Syrup	Roerig	Su	Cherry Others	Unspecified	Sodium benzoate
Theolair Liquid	3M Riker	So, Su	Berry citrus	None	Methylparabens, propylparabens
Theostat 80 Syrup	Laser	Sa, So, Su	Artificial cherry Vanilla	None	Unspecified
Elixophyllin Elixir	Forest	Sa	Artificial guarana	Red 40	Unspecified
Slo-Phyllin Syrup	Rorer	Sa, So	Lemon Vanilla	Red 3 Yellow 6	Sodium benzoate, methylparabens
Theolear 80 Syrup	Central	Sa, So	Cherry Anise	None	Benzoic acid
Theon Syrup	Blaine	Unspecified	Unspecified	None	Unspecified

[a]Adapted from Kumar A et al. Pediatrics 1993;91:927–933.
[b]Abbreviations are explained in the footnote to Table 52–13.

Table 52–21
The Regulatory Status of Sweeteners in the United States[a]

Type of Sweetener	Regulatory Status
Common Sugars	
Monosaccharides	
glucose (also called dextrose)	GRAS (generally recognized as safe)
fructose (also called levulose) fruit sugar	GRAS
galactose	none; cannot be directly added to food
Disaccharides	
sucrose (glucose + fructose) white table sugar, beet sugar, turbinado sugar, raw sugar	GRAS
lactose (glucose + galactose) milk sugar	GRAS petition under consideration
maltose (glucose + glucose) malt sugar	GRAS
Sugar Alcohols	
sorbitol	GRAS
xylitol	limited FDA approval for special uses, removed from GRAS; regulated as "interim food additive"
mannitol	
Nonnutritive and High-Intensity Sweeteners	
aspartame	approved
acesulfame K	approved
cyclamate	banned
saccharin	remains on market through congressional moratorium

[a]Adapted from Greeley A. FDA Consumer 1992;26(3):17–27.

Table 52–22
Adverse Effects Reported in Literature: Sweeteners[a]

Sweetener	Adverse Effects
Sucrose	Cariogenecity, increased degradation of active drug
Sorbitol	Osmotic diarrhea, poor absorption of active drug, flatulence, abdominal pain
Lactose	Diarrhea and malabsorption in lactose-intolerant population, vomiting, flatulence
Saccharin	Urticaria, pruritis, nausea, diarrhea, tachycardia, papular skin eruptions, gait disturbances, wheezing, cross-reactivity with sulfonamides
Aspartame	Urticaria, angioedema, granulomatous panniculitis, cross-reactivity with sulfonamides, renal tubular acidosis (with large amounts)
Cyclamates[b]	Photosensitization, eczema, dermatitis, pruritus

[a]Adapted from Kumar A et al. Pediatrics 1993;91:927–933.
[b]Not used in the United States (banned by the Food and Drug Administration in 1970).

neous agents.[1] Kumar surveyed adverse effects of sweeteners, dyes, flavorings, and preservatives (Tables 52–13 through 52–20).[2] The regulatory status of sweeteners in the United States is summarized in Table 52–21.[3] Adverse effects caused by sweeteners are summarized in Table 52–22.

Cyclamate

Cyclohexylamine is an indirectly acting sympathomimetic amine. Cyclamate ingestion (1.0 g/day) may result in plasma concentrations of cyclohexylamine in excess of 0.7 μg/mL sufficient to induce an increase in mean arterial blood pressure.[4,5] Cyclohexylamine, a metabolite of cyclamate, appears to interfere with the TDX amphetamine assay.[5]

An 18-year-old male with bulimia nervosa ingested up to 22.0 g of cyclamate daily. He developed diarrhea, dilatation of the proximal small bowel, and loss of the normal mucosal pattern. These findings reverted to normal after cessation of cyclamate ingestion.[6]

Aspartame (Fig. 52–2)

Data accumulated to date appear to indicate that the majority of individuals—including pregnant women and children—who consume less than 50 mg/kg/d of aspartame should not experience any adverse effects.[7] A double-blind controlled study in 40 volunteers found that the incidence of headaches after aspartame use was no different from that after placebo use.[8] The study has been subject to criticism.[8,9] A double-blind randomized cross-over study indicates that migraine sufferers may experience a significant increase in frequency of migraines after aspartame ingestion.[10] A randomized double-blind crossover study in healthy adults who received a single dose of aspartame (15 mg/kg body weight) showed no significant differences with placebo in measures of sedation, hunger, headache, reaction time, cognition, or memory, although plasma phenylalanine levels were significantly higher in the aspartame group at 1 and 6 hours following dosage when compared with placebo.[11] A similar study using 75 mg/kg/day of aspartame revealed insignificant increases in blood methanol, blood formate, and 24-hour urinary excretion of formate.[12]

Ingestion of aspartame (34 mg/kg) led to blood methanol concentrations of 0.5 mg/dL.[13] Following 200 mg/kg of aspartame the blood methanol levels were 2.58 mg/dL. Ophthalmologic examination disclosed no change following aspartame loading. Since May 1983, the NutraSweet Company had received 9 anecdotal reports of accidental ingestion of large numbers of Equal tablets (25 to 100) by small children without adverse effects. The NutraSweet Company has a toll-free number for physicians: 800-321-7254.[14]

Ingestion of aspartame 34 mg/kg by healthy 9- and 10-year-old children involved in a double-blind crossover study appeared to exert no detrimental effects on learning, behavior, or mood.[15] A double-blind controlled study has associated aspartame with seizures.[16]

Acesulfame

Acesulfame, also known as acesulfame K, has been approved for use in chewing gum, dry drink mixes, gelatine, puddings, and nondairy creamers. It is about 200 times sweeter than sugar and is not metabolized or broken down for use by the body. Tumors found in some rats were not considered significant by the FDA.[17,18] Acesulfame has some structural resemblance to saccharin and may bind to the same receptor.[19]

Licorice

Aldosterone secretion rates and plasma renin concentrations are low. Long-term ingestion of 1 g or more daily of glycyrrhizic acid can result in severe metabolic disturbances. Hypokalemia may be severe and require potassium chloride by central venous catheter.[20,21]

Mechanism of Action

The mineralocorticoid activity of licorice results from the inhibition of 11 beta-hydroxysteroid dehydrogenase (an enzyme that normally inactivates cortisol by converting its C11 alcohol to a ketone) by glycyrrhetininic acid, the active ingredient in licorice (Fig. 52–3). By preventing the inactivation of cortisol, licorice increases the glucocorticoid concentration in mineralocorticoid responsive tissues. As a result, glucocorticoids occupy the mineralocorticoid receptors and produce a mineralocorticoid response, as evidenced by increased sodium retention and hypertension.[22] Glycyrrhetinic acid also inhibits 15-hydroxyprostaglandin dehydrogenase and ^{13}-prostaglandin reductase, two enzymes important in the metabolism of prostaglandin E and F2.[23]

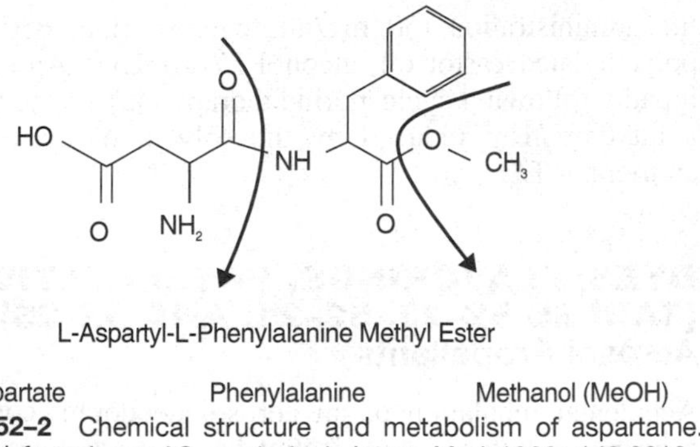

HO, NH, O, CH3, NH2

L-Aspartyl-L-Phenylalanine Methyl Ester

Aspartate Phenylalanine Methanol (MeOH)

Figure 52–2 Chemical structure and metabolism of aspartame. (Adapted from Leon AS et al. Arch Intern Med 1989; 149:2318–2324.)

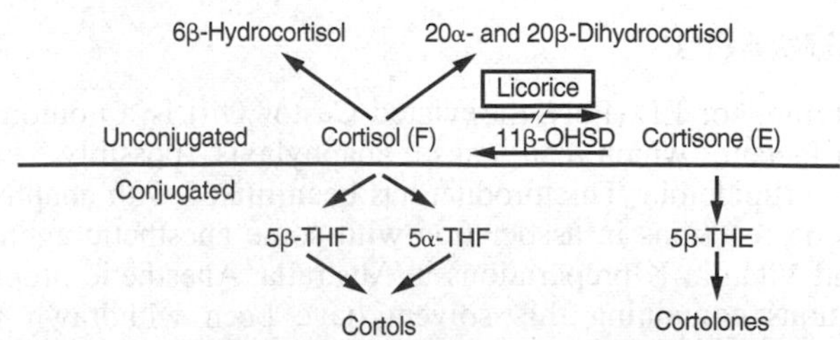

Figure 52–3 Overview of Cortisol Metabolism. Licorice inhibits 11 β-hydroxysteroid dehydrogenase (11 β-OHSD) activity, resulting in a relative increase in cortisol *(F)* metabolites, such as 5α- and 5β-tetrahydrocortisol *(THF)* and cortols, and a relative decrease in cortisone *(E)* metabolites, such as 5β-tetrahydrocortisone *(THE)* and cortolones. (Adapted from Farese RV et al. N Engl J Med 1991;325: 1223–1227.)

Table 52-23
Adverse Effects Reported in Literature: Dyes[a]

Dye	Adverse Effects
Azo dyes	
Tartrazine (FD&C Yellow 5)	Anaphylactoid reactions, angioedema, asthma, urticaria, contact dermatitis, rhinitis, hyperkinesis in hyperactive patients, eosinophilia, cross-reactivity with aspirin, sodium benzoate, and indomethacin
Sunset Yellow (FD&C Yellow 6)	Anaphylactoid reactions, angioedema, anaphylactic shock, vasculitis, retching, abdominal pain, purpura, vomiting, belching, cross-reactivity with aspirin, acetaminophen, sodium benzoate, and other azo dyes
FD&C 4 (Ponceau Sx)	Bronchoconstriction
FD&C Red 36	Contact dermatitis
FD&C 17	Contact dermatitis
Quinoline dyes	
Quinoline Yellow (FD&C Yellow 10)	Contact sensitization
Quinoline Yellow SS (FD&C 11)	Contact sensitization
Triphenylmethane dyes	
FD&C Blue 1	Bronchoconstriction in asthmatic patients
FD&C Blue 2 (Brilliant blue)	Weak sensitizer
FD&C Green 3 (Fast green)	Erythema multiforme-like skin rash
Xanthene dyes (fluran dyes)	In general, photosensitizer, anaphylactoid and asthmatic reactions
FD&C 3 (erythrosine)	Potent photosensitizer, elevation of protein-bound iodine
FD&C Orange 5	None reported
FD&C Yellow 7 (fluorescein)	Urticaria, angioedema, syncopy, shock, anaphylaxis
FD&C Orange 10	None reported
FD&C Red 19 (rhodamine)	None reported
FD&C Red 21 (tetrabromo fluorescein)	None reported
FD&C Red 22 (eosin)	Potent photosensitizer
FD&C Red 27 (tetrabromo tetrachloro-fluorescein)	None reported
Others	
Carmine	Allergic cheilitis, asthma

[a]Adapted from Kumar A et al. Pediatrics 1993;91:927–933.

Table 52-24
Adverse Effects Reported in Literature: Flavorings[a]

Flavoring	Adverse Effects
Cocoa or chocolate	Sympathomimetic; tachycardia, insomnia
Essential oils	Cheilitis, burning sensation
Oil of Peppermint	Atrial fibrillation, muscle pain, cooling sensation, burning sensation
Lemon oil	Contact dermatitis
Menthol	Hypersensitivity reactions, systemic allergic reaction

[a]Adapted from Kumar A et al. Pediatrics 1993;91:927–933.

Table 52-25
Adverse Effects Reported in Literature: Preservatives[a]

Preservatives	Adverse Effects
Benzoic acids and benzoates	Displacement of bile from albumin binding sites in neonates
Parabens	Skin sensitization and cross-sensitization with each other
Ethylenediamine	Irritant to skin and mucous membranes
Propyl gallate	Methemoglobinemia

[a]Adapted from Kumar A et al. Pediatrics 1993;91:927–933.

SUGARS

Cremophor EL (Polyethoxylated Castor Oil) is a nonionic surfactant, which can cause anaphylaxis, possibly, and hyperlipidemia. This product has been linked with anaphylactic reactions in association with some anesthetic agents and Vitamin K preparations in Australia. Anesthetic preparations containing this solvent have been withdrawn in Australia.[24] Sweating, pallor, nausea, chest pain, breathlessness, wheezing, urticaria, and pyrexia have been observed in the UK when teniposide infusions (which contain cremophor EL) have been used.[25]

Nervous system complications (disorder of central white matter and peripheral neuropathy) may follow IV cyclosporine administration (50 mg/mL cyclosporine; 650 ng/mL polyethylated castor oil, alcohol 27 g/mL).[26] An encephalopathy following cyclosporine therapy may be the result of a fat embolism induced by the solvent of cyclosporine, cremophor EL.[27]

DYES, FLAVORINGS, PRESERVATIVES (TABLES 52-23, 52-24, AND 52-25)

Aerosol Propellants

Accidental inhalation of an aerosol deodorant containing propane, *n*-butane, and isobutane was associated with ventricular tachycardia and seizures in a child.[28]

Thickening, Suspending, and Binding Agents

Ethylenediamine

An ethylenediamine-induced delayed hypersensitivity reaction was described in a 46-year-old woman who received parenteral aminophylline for an acute asthma exacerbation. Patch test for ethylenediamine was positive. Products containing ethylenediamine include many brands of rubber gloves and other rubber products, shellacs, insecticides, waxes, and dyes. Cross-reactivity may occur with chemically related agents, including the ethanolamine antihistamines (diphenhydramine, carbinoxamine, clemastine); triethanolamine-containing creams, including Aspercreme, Myoflex, and Sportscreme; and the piperazine antihistamine, hydroxyzine.[29]

Benzothiazoles

Large amounts of 2-(carboxymethylthio) benzothiazole have been found in the serum of premature babies receiving prolonged intravenous therapy. This compound is derived from the oxidation of 2-(hydroxyethylthio) benzothiazole, which is leached out of rubber components of intravenous administration sets and syringes. The potential displacement by CMB of bilirubin from albumin could increase the risk of kernicterus. Toxic effects directly attributable to benzothiazole have not been described in these babies.[30]

The Committee on Drugs of the American Medical Association endorses the 1985 recommendation made by the American Academy of Pediatrics Committee on Drugs that the labeling of pharmaceutical agents should include qualitative listings of all inactive ingredients.[31]

REFERENCES—EXCIPIENTS

1. Hill EM, Flaitz CM, Frost GR. Sweetener content of common pediatric oral liquid medications. Am J Hosp Pharm 1988; 41:135–142.
2. Kumar A, Rawlings RD, Beaman DC. The mystery ingredients: sweeteners, flavorings, dyes, preservatives in analgesic/antipyretic, antihistamine/decongestants, cough and colds, antidiarrhea and liquid theophylline preparations. Pediatrics 1993;91:927–933.
3. Greeley A. Not only sugar is sweet. FDA Consumer 1992; 26(3):17–21.
4. Buss NE, Renwick AG, Donaldson K, George CE. Cyclamate (CHS), cyclohexylamine (CHA) and cardiovascular (CV) toxicity in man. An initial population study. Hum Exp Toxicol 1990;9:359–360.
5. Martz W, Schutz HW. Synthetic sweetener cyclamate as a potential source of false-positive amphetamine results in the TDx system. Clin Chem 1991;37:2016–2017.
6. Derfler K, Meryn S, Herold C, Neuhold N, Mostbeck G, Gangl A. Reversible malabsorption caused by high doses of cyclamate. Am J Med 1988;85:446–447.
7. Shaban HM, Albert ML. Aspartame. An evaluation of adverse effects. Hosp Formul 1988;23:543–546.
8. Schiffman SS, Buckley CE, Campsor HA, Massey EW, Baranjuk JM et al. Aspartame and susceptibility to headache. N Engl J Med 1987;317:1181–1185.
9. Letters. N Engl J Med 1988;318:1200–1202.
10. Kochler SM, Glaros A. The effect of aspartame on migraine headache. Headache 1988;28:10–13.
11. Lapierre KA, Greenblatt DJ, Goddard JE, Harmatz JS, Shader RI. The neuropsychiatric effects of aspartame in normal volunteers. J Clin Pharmacol 1990;30:454–460.
12. Leon GG, Hunninghake DB, Bell C, Rassin DK, Tephley TR. Safety in long-term large doses of aspartame. Arch Intern Med 1989;149:2318–2324.
13. Stegink LD, Brummel MC, McMartin K, Martin-Amat G, Filer LJ Jr, Baker GL, Tephly TR. Blood methanol concentrations in normal adult subjects administered abuse doses of aspartame. J Toxicol Environ Health 1981;7: 281–290.
14. Butchko HH, Strathman I. Nutrasweet overdosage. Pediatrics 1989;8:750.
15. Saravis S, Schachar R, Zlotkin S, Leiter LA, Anderson GH. Aspartame: effects on learning, behavior and mood. Pediatrics 1990;86:75–83.
16. Camfield PR, Camfield CS, Dooley JM, Gordon K, Jollyman S, Weaver DF. Aspartame exacerbated EEG spike-wave discharge in children with generalized absence epilepsy: a double-blinded controlled study. Neurology 1992;42: 1000–1003.
17. New sweetener approved. FDA Consumer 1988;28 (6):4.
18. Van der Heijden A, Van der Wel H, Peer HG. Structure-activity relationships in sweeteners. II. Saccharins, acesulfames, chlorosugars, tryptophans and ureas. Chem Senses (IRL Press Ltd, Oxford, England) 1985; 10:73–88.
19. Acesulfame—a new artificial sweetener. Med Lett Drug Ther 1988;30(Issue 781):116.
20. Nielsen I, Pedersen RS. Life-threatening hypokalaemia caused by liquorice ingestion. Lancet 1984;1:1305.
21. Haberer JP, Jouve P, Bedock B et al. Severe hypokalaemia secondary to overindulgence in alcohol-free "Pastis!" Lancet 1984;1:575.
22. Baker ME, Fanestil DD. Liquorice as a regulator of steroid and prostaglandin metabolism. Lancet 1991;337:428–429.
23. Farese RV Jr, Biglieri EG, Schakleton CHL, Irony I, Gomez-Fontes R. Licorice-induced hypermineralocorticoidism. N Engl J Med 1991;325:1223–1227.
24. Martin JC. Anaphylactoid reactions and vitamin K. Med J Austral 1991;155:851.
25. Siddall SJ, Martin J, Nunn AJ. Anaphylactoid reactions to teniposide. Lancet 1989;1:394.
26. Blexrud MD, Windebank AJ, de Groen PC. Potential neurotoxicity of the solvent vehicle in which intravenous cyclosporine is formulated. Neurology 1990;40(Suppl 1): 344.
27. Hoefnagels WAJ, Gerritsen EJA, Brouwer OF, Souverijn JHM. Cyclosporine encephalopathy associated with fat embolism induced by the drug's solvent. Lancet 1988;2:901.
28. Wason S, Gibler R, Hassan M. Ventricular tachycardia associated with non-freon aerosol propellants. JAMA 1986;256: 78–80.
29. Terzian CG, Simon PA. Aminophylline hypersensitivity apparently due to ethylenediamine. Ann Emerg Med 1992;21: 312–317.
30. Meek JH, Pettit BR. Avoidable accumulation of potentially toxic levels of benzothiazoles in babies receiving intravenous therapy. Lancet 1985;2:1090–1092.
31. American Academy of Pediatrics Committee on Drugs. "Inactive" ingredients in pharmaceutical products. Pediatrics 1985;76:635–645.

EYE AND NOSE DROPS: THE IMIDAZOLINES

Over-the-counter eye and nasal preparations available in the United States are listed in Table 52–26. Imidazoline derivatives include naphazoline, tetrahydrozoline, oxymetazoline, and xylometazoline. These drugs act peripherally and centrally as alpha$_2$-adrenergic agonists. Clinically, patients may exhibit miosis, mydriasis, palpitations, hypertension or hypotension, bradycardia, pallor, cyanosis, diaphoresis,

Table 52–26
Imidazoline Decongestants—Over-the-Counter Eye and Nasal Preparations[a]

Active Ingredient and Concentration (%)	Products	Available Container Sizes (mL)	Maximum Container Dose (mg)
Eye Preparations			
Tetrahydrozoline (.05)	Collyrium Fresh Eye Drops®	15	7.5
	Mallazine Drops®	15	7.5
	Murine Plus®	15, 30	15.0
	Optigene III®	15	7.5
	Soothe Eye Drops®	15	7.5
	Visine®	15, 22.5, 30	15.0
	Visine AC®	15, 30	15.0
	Visine Extra®	30	15.0
Naphazoline (.012)	Allerest Eye Drops®	15, 30	3.6
	Allergy Drops® (Bausch & Lomb)	15	1.8
	Clear Eyes®	15, 30	3.6
	Degest 2®	15	1.8
	Naphcon®	15	1.8
	20/20 Eye Drops®	15	1.8
(.02)	VasoClear®	15	3.0
	VasoClear A® (Includes $ZnSO_4$ 0.25%)	15	3.0
(.03)	Comfort Eye Drops®	15	4.5
Oxymetazoline (.025)	OcuClear®	15, 30	7.5
	Visine LR®	30	7.5
Nasal Preparations			
Naphazoline (.05)	4-Way Nasal Spray®	15	7.5
	Privine Nasal Solution®	20	10.0
	Privine Nasal Spray®	15	7.5
Oxymetazoline (.05)	Afrin Cherry Nasal Spray®	15	7.5
	Afrin Menthol Nasal Spray®	15	7.5
	Afrin Nasal Spray/Pump®	15, 30	15.0
	Afrin Nose Drops®	20	10.0
	Allerest 12-Hour®	15	7.5
	Chlorphed-LA®	15	7.5
	Dristan Long Acting Spray® (regular & menthol)	15, 30	15.0
	Duramist Plus®	15	7.5
	Duration 12 Hour® (regular & menthol)	15, 30	15.0
	4-Way LA Nasal Spray®	15	7.5
	Genasal®	15, 30	15.0
	Neo-Synephrine 12 Hour® (Adult dose drops)	30	15.0
	Neo-Synephrine 12 Hour Spray®	15	7.5
	Nostrilla LA Nasal Spray®	15	7.5
	NTZ Long Acting Spray®	15	7.5
	Sinarest 12 Hour®	15	7.5
	Sinex Long Acting®	15, 30	15.0
	Twice-a-Day®	15, 30	15.0
(.025)	Afrin Children's Strength Nose Drops®	20	5.0
	St Joseph's Nose Drops®	15	3.8
Xylometazoline (.1)	Otrivin Nasal Spray/Drops®	15, 20	20.0
	Neo-Synephrine II®	*	
	Sine Off Once-a-Day®	*	
	Sinutab Nasal Spray®	*	
(.05)	Otrivin Pediatric Nasal®	20	10.0

*Volume data unavailable.
[a]Adapted from Higgins GL III et al. Ann Emerg Med 1991;20:655–658.

anxiety, insomnia, tremor, agitation, hallucinations, seizures, lethargy, obtundation, and coma.[1] Treatment is symptomatic and supportive.

EYE DROPS

Some systemic effects following use of eye drops include those listed in Table 52–27.[2]

DOSAGE

A detailed review of systemic reactions to ophthalmic drug preparations is available.[6]

INTERACTIONS

Table 52–28 summarizes a number of interactions between topical glaucoma medications and systemic drugs.[7]

Table 52–27
Eye Drops—Systemic Effects

Phenylephrine hydrochloride (1%)	Myocardial infarction, severe hypertensive reaction, coronary artery spasm
Epinephrine drops	Ventricular extrasystole, palpitations, hypertension, tachycardia, anxiety
Topical pilocarpine	Nausea, vomiting, abdominal cramps, diarrhea, sweating, rhinorrhea, respiratory distress, muscular fasciculations, weakness
Ethothiopate	Cardiac arrest, bronchospasm, diarrhea, hyperhidrosis, fatigue, muscle weakness
Anticholinergic drugs	Confusion, hallucinations, ataxia, dysarthria, restlessness, convulsions, fever, coma, death in small infants
Atropine	Atrial fibrillation, supraventricular tachycardia
Propanidone isethionate (0.1%)	Toxic keratopathy
Proparacaine hydrochloride (0.5%)	Seizures
Beta-blockers	Bradycardia, hypotension, wheezing

Cyclopentolate (Prescription Products)

Cyclopentolate is a mydriatic and cycloplegic topical preparation resembling atropine in clinical structure. Use of the eye drop 1.0% or 2.0% solution in children may induce facial flushing, seizures, tachycardia, delirium, disorientation, delirium, disorientation, hallucinations, agitation, hyperactivity, urinary retention, and hypothermia.[8–11] This anticholinergic syndrome appears to follow absorption from the nasal and gastrointestinal mucosa after passage down the nasolacrimal ducts. The use of 0.5% eye drops appears preferable and potential absorption may be minimized with punctal occlusion.[8]

NASAL DROPS

Continuous alpha adrenergic stimulation after overuse (abuse) of nasal decongestants, including oxymetazoline hydrochloride (20 mg/d), phenylephrine hydrochloride (100 mg/day), and ephedrine hydrochloride (330 mg/day), has

Table 52–28
Summary of Nonocular Interactions Between Topical Glaucoma Medications and Systemic Drugs[a]

Topical Glaucoma Medication	Systemic Drug	Interaction: Additive	Interaction: Antagonistic	Potential Result
Beta-adrenergic antagonist	Anesthetic agents (inhalational)	X		Systemic hypotension
	Hypoglycemia agents		X	a) Retard hypoglycemic rebound b) Mask hypoglycemic symptoms c) Produce hypoglycemia
	Beta-adrenergic antagonists	X		Increased toxic effects of beta-antagonists
	Calcium channel blockers	X		Cardiac depression
	Cholinesterase inhibitors	X		Weakness of striated muscle
	Clonidine	X		Systemic hypertensive rebound following clonidine withdrawal
	Digitalis glycosides	X		Cardiac depression
	Fentanyl derivatives	X		Increased toxic effects of fentanyl
	Phenothiazines	X		Increased serum levels of beta-blockers and phenothiazines with potential for toxic side effects
	Quinidine	X		Cardiac depression
	Reserpine	X		Cardiac depression
	Sympathomimetic amines			
	1) Subcutaneous epi		X	Abrupt systemic hypertension
	2) Xanthines		X	a) Bronchoconstriction b) Reduced theophylline clearance
	3) Beta-adrenergic agonists for the treatment of:			
	a) Heart failure		X	Cardiac depression
	b) Bronchoconstriction		X	Bronchoconstriction
Adrenergic agonist	Anesthetic agents (inhalational)	X		Cardiac arrhythmias
	Digitalis glycosides	X		Cardiac arrhythmias
	Monoamine oxidase (MAO) inhibitors	X		Hypertensive crises refuted by literature
	Sympathomimetic amines	X		Systemic hypertension and cardiac arrhythmias
	Tri- and tetracyclic antidepressants	X		Cardiac arrhythmias
Cholinesterase inhibitors	Anesthetic agents (local: ester-type)	X		Prolonged anesthetic action with cardio-pulmonary depression
	Cholinesterase inhibitors	X		Cholinergic toxicity
	Succinylcholine	X		Prolonged neuromuscular blockade

[a]Adapted from Gerber SL et al. Surv Ophthalmol 1990;35:205–218.

led to hypertension, cardiomegaly, and congestive heart failure.[12]

The clinical picture may be confusing with periods of hyperactivity alternating with episodes of cardiopulmonary and central nervous system depression. Signs and symptoms depend on whether peripheral or central $alpha_2$ adrenergic receptor stimulation predominates. Drug screening and specific drug analytic methods are not helpful.

Neosynephrine (phenylephrine) is an alpha adrenergic sympathomimetic receptor stimulant structurally similar to ephedrine and epinephrine. After topical ocular instillation systemic absorption may occur. A 2.5% solution of neosynephrine contains 1.2 to 2.0 mg per drop. Cardiovascular effects (acute hypertension) are more likely to follow use of the 10% ocular solution of Neo-synephrine, but have occurred within 30 minutes after the topical administration of 2.5% of Neo-synephrine.[13]

Treatment is mainly supportive. No specific antidote exists. Complications such as hemodynamic instability, respiratory insufficiency, and seizures respond to traditional measures.[1]

TREATMENT

Rapid onset of depressed consciousness following use of the topical imidazolines makes use of ipecac inadvisable. Activated charcoal may be useful if administered shortly after an ingestion; efficacy data is not available. If CNS depressant symptoms are present (e.g., change in consciousness, bradycardia, hypotension); 5 to 10 mL/kg of crystalloid boluses may be given over 15 minutes to treat hypotension. Atropine sulfate or isoproterenol may be used to treat bradycardia. Provide airways protection and ventilatory support to the patient with depressed consciousness. Diazepam may be used for seizures. Naloxone 0.01 to 0.1 mg/kg IV in children or up to 2 mg in adults has been suggested because the imidazoline derivatives show central alpha-receptor stimulation properties with the antihypertensive agent. Naloxone has been useful in reversing CNS depression in some instances of clonidine overdose. Additional data are required to confirm the usefulness of naloxone.[1,14]

Timolol and Betaxolol (Table 52–29)

About 80% of a topical dose of timolol is absorbed from the conjunctiva and nasal mucosa and enters the systemic circulation, bypassing the "first pass" hepatic metabolism, which normally accounts for 75% of the oral dose. A fairly small dose administered topically may result in systemic beta adrenoceptor blocking effects. Timolol eye drops interacted with verapamil to cause some node dysfunction with severe bradycardia.[15] Patients with obstructive airways disease may be critically dependent on beta-adrenergic stimulation for the maintenance of airway patency and thus be susceptible to severe and potentially fatal bronchospasm following administration of timolol solution. Patients with clinical evidence of increased airway reactivity should receive the usual dose of timolol ophthalmic solution under medical observation. Personal aid facilities should be available to perform resuscitation if needed. Such patients should have close medical follow-up throughout the course of timolol therapy.[16]

Table 52–29
Dosage of Ophthalmic Beta-Blockers

Drug	Usual Daily Dosage
Betaxolol: Betoptic (Alcon) 0.25%	
suspension	1 drop twice
0.5% solution	1 drop twice
Levobunolol: Betagan (Allergan) 0.25%	
solution	1 drop twice
0.5% solution	1 drop once or twice
Metapranolol: OptiPranolol (Bausch & Lomb)	
solution	1 drop twice
Timolol: Timoptic (MSD) 0.25% solution	1 drop once or twice
0.5% solution	1 drop once or twice

Metapranolol for ophthalmic use has been withdrawn from the market in the UK[17] because of reports of anterior uveitis with all strengths of the ophthalmic drug.

LABORATORY

A high-performance liquid chromatography method is available for identification and quantification in plasma and urine of beta-adrenergic receptor antagonists (betaxadol, carteolol, metapranolol, and timolol) commonly prescribed in ophthalmology. The lower detection of the beta blockers were found to be 4 to 27 ng/mL.[18]

Phospholine Iodide (Echothiophate Iodide)

Echothiophate iodide is a strong irreversible inhibitor of cholinesterase used in the treatment of glaucoma and strabismus. There is sufficient absorption from the ophthalmic preparations to produce a decrease of cholinesterase activity within several days after initiation of therapy. The maximum depression occurs in the fifth to seventh week of treatment. When the drug is discontinued, plasma cholinesterase activity returns to normal within 3 to 6 weeks, while red cell cholinesterase activity requires about 120 days to return to normal.[19] Chronic phospholine intoxication can mimic myasthenia gravis.[20] Symptoms improve on withdrawal of eye drops.

Errors

A 32-year-old female nurse accidentally splashed 1 or 2 drops of undiluted dopamine into her left eye. She developed a supraventricular tachycardia, diffuse nonspecific ST-T wave abnormalities on the ECG, a pulse of 160 beats/minute and blood pressure of 152/100 mm of mercury. There were additional periods of paroxysmal supraventricular tachycardia and intermittent sinus tachycardia. Assuming 10 drops per mL, 1 drop of undiluted dopamine (40 mg/mL) contains 4000 mg. This patient received a bolus of 60 mg/kg. She survived.[21]

Cyanoacrylate Glue (See Also Plastics)

Cyanoacrylate nail glue (Superglue), may be mistaken for prescribed eye drops. Many bottles used for nail glue appear identical to those used for ophthalmic solutions. Poorly sighted individuals, careless persons, and children are at risk for this error. Treatment of the resultant upper to lower lid adhesion and transient keratoconjunctivitis may require use of scissors[22–25] or eye pads saturated with tap water.[26] Eye drops may be misused due to interchanged caps.[27] Other preparations (e.g., Hemoccult) with confusing bottle cap colors have also been instilled in the eye when they were mistaken for an ophthalmic drop.[28]

REFERENCES—EYE AND NOSE DROPS ADRENERGIC AGENTS

1. Higgins GL III, Campbell B, Wallace K, Talbot S. Pediatric poisoning from over-the-counter imidazoline-containing products. Ann Emerg Med 1991;20:655–658.
2. Adler AG, McElwain GE, Merli GJ, Martin JH. Systemic effects of eye drops. Arch Intern Med 1982;142:2293–2294.
3. Fraunfelder FT, Meyer SM. Systemic reactions to ophthalmic drug preparations. Med Toxicol 1987;2:287–293.
4. Merli GJ, Weitz H, Martin JH, McKay EF, Adler AG et al. Cardiac dysrhythmias associated with ophthalmic atropine. Arch Intern Med 1986;146:45–47.
5. Johns KJ, Head WS, O'Day DM. Corneal toxicity of propamidine. Arch Ophthalmol 1988;106:68–69.
6. Cydulka RK, Betzelos S. Seizures following the use of proparacaine hydrochloride eye drops. J Emerg Med 1990;8:131–133.
7. Gerber SL, Cantor LB, Brater DC. Systemic drug interactions with topical glaucoma medications. Survey Ophthalmol 1990;35:205–218.
8. Fitzgerald DA, Hanson RM, West C, Martin F, Brown J, Kilham HA. Seizures associated with 1% cyclopentolate eye drops. J Paediatr Child Health 1990;26:106–107.
9. Adcock EW III. Cyclopentolate (Cyclogyl) toxicity in pediatric patients. J Pediatr 1971;79:127–129.
10. Kennerdell JS, Wucher FR. Cyclopentolate associated with two cases of grand mal seizures. Arch Ophthalmol 1972; 87:6374–6375.
11. Simcoe CW. Cyclopentolate (Cyclogyl) toxicity. Arch Ophthalmol 1962;67:406–408.
12. Heyman SN, Mevorach D, Ghanem J. Hypertension crisis from chronic intoxication with nasal decongestant and cough medications. DICP 1991;26:1068–1070.
13. Weisberg LA. Intracerebral hemorrhage after topical administration of mydriatic agents. South Med J 1993;86:1064–1066.
14. Knauerhase TP. Topical imidazoles. Clin Toxicol Rev 1990; 12(12):1–2.
15. Pringle SD, MacEwen CJ. Severe bradycardia due to interaction of timolol eye drops and verapamil. Br Med J 1987; 294:155–156.
16. Prince DS, Carliner NH. Respiratory arrest following first dose of timolol ophthalmic solution. Chest 1983;84:640–641.
17. Glauline withdrawn. Br Med J 1991;302:132.
18. Tracqui A, Kintz P, Hinber J, Lugnier AAJ, Mangin P. A specific HPLS method for determination of beta-blockers topically used in ophthalmological diseases. Forensic Sci Int 1988;38:37–41.
19. Chairelli D. Phospholine iodide ophthalmic drops and skeletal muscle relaxants. Can J Hosp Pharm 1985;38:58.
20. Turchen SG, Whitney C, Clark PF, Manoguerra AS. Chronic phospholine intoxication mimicking myasthenia gravis. Vet Hum Toxicol 1993;35:347.
21. Strauss R. Accidental dopamine in the eye. West J Med 1985;142:397–398.
22. Margo CE, Trobe JD. Tarsorrhaphy from accidental instillation of cyanoacrylate adhesive in the eye. JAMA 1982;24:660–661.
23. Morgan SJ, Astbury NJ. Inadvertent self-administration of Superglue: a consumer hazard. Br Med J 1984;289: 226–227.
24. De Respiris RA. Cyanoacrylate nail glue mistaken for eye drops. JAMA 1990;263:2301.
25. Cromie BW. Superglue inadvertently used as eye drops. Br Med J 1990;300:680.
26. Raynor LA. Treatment for inadvertent cyanoacrylate tarsorrhaphy. Arch Ophthalmol 1988;106:1033–1084.
27. Frenkel REP, Honig YJ, Shin DH. Misuse of eye drops due to interchanged caps. Arch Ophthalmol 1988;106:17.
28. Ling RTK, Villalobos R, Latina M. Inadvertent instillation of hemoccult developer in the eyes. Arch Ophthalmol 1988;106:1033–1034.

FLUORIDES

TOXIC DOSAGE

Eighty-four children ages 9 months to 6 years ingested dental fluoride products. One died (after a sodium fluoride ingestion), 26 of 87 became symptomatic with GI symptoms (nausea, vomiting, diarrhea, abdominal pain). Only three patients developed symptoms later than 1 hour after ingestion. All patients who ingested 4 to 8.4 mg/kg of elemental fluoride developed mild and self-limited symptoms, but only 8% who ingested less than 1 mg/kg developed symptoms.[1]

A 25-year-old man ingested 120 g of roach powder (97% sodium fluoride). He developed immediate nausea, vomiting, excessive salivation, respiratory and metabolic acidosis, tetanic contractions, respiratory arrest, ventricular fibrillation, and cardiac asystole. He was treated with gastric lavage (with 0.15% calcium hydroxide), calcium gluconate 1 gm IV, endotracheal intubation, external cardiac massage, further IV calcium gluconate (2 g) and magnesium sulfate (8 mEq), direct current countershock, IV lidocaine, a transvenous pacemaker, IV fluids, and diuretics. He survived.[2]

A 2½-year-old girl ingested sodium silicofluoride ($Na_2S_1F_6$), developed acute respiratory failure, a prolonged AT interval, ventricular tachycardia and fibrillation, hypokalemia, hypocalcemia (3 to 4 mg/100 mL), and aspiration pneumonia. She was treated with IV lidocaine, direct current cardioversion, 0.3 g IV 10% calcium chloride (X3) followed by a continuous infusion of calcium gluconate, oral 0.1% calcium hydrazide by G tube, antibiotics, and peritoneal dialysis, which was not effective in fluoride removal.[3] She recovered.

Ingestion of as little as a spoonful of glass etching cream (ammonium bifluoride 20% and sodium bifluoride 13%) can lead to life-threatening risk of injury.[4] See Tables 52–30A and 52–30B.

CLINICAL PRESENTATION

Acute Toxicity

Sulfur hexafluoride (SF_6). Two women were rapidly rendered unconscious when exposed to SF_6. One developed an acute pulmonary edema.[5] Both recovered. SF_6 degrades to a variety of sulphur oxyfluorides during electrical arcing in the presence of oxygen. SF_4 (sulfur tetrafluoride) is highly reactive and forms thionyl fluoride (SOF_2) (odor similar to

Table 52–30A
Recommended Emergency Treatment for Persons Who Ingest Dry Fluoride Chemicals (NaF and Na_2SiF_6)[a]

Milligrams Fluoride Ion (mg) Ingested per Body Weight (kg)[b]	Treatment
<5.0 mg of fluoride ion/kg†[c]	1. Give calcium (milk) orally to relieve gastrointestinal symptoms. Observe for 2–4 hours. (A can of evaporated milk should be available at all times to use for emergency treatment.) 2. Induced vomiting is not necessary.
≥5.0 mg of fluoride ion/kg	1. Move the person away from any contact with fluoride and keep him or her warm. 2. Call the Poison Control Center. 3. If the person is conscious, induce vomiting by rubbing the back of the person's throat with either a spoon or your finger or giving the person syrup of ipecac. To prevent aspiration of vomitus, the person should be placed face down with the head lower than the body. 4. Give the person a glass of milk or any source of soluble calcium (i.e., 5% calcium gluconate or calcium lactate solution). 5. Take the person to the hospital as quickly as possible

[a]CDC, MMWR 1995;44(RR-13):1–40.
[b]Average weight/age: 0–15 kg/0–2 years; 15–20 kg/3–5 years; 20–23 kg/6–8 years; 23–45 kg/9–15 years; 45–70 kg and higher/15–21 years and older.
[c]5 mg of fluoride (F) equals 11 mg of sodium fluoride (8 mg of sodium fluorosilicate). Ingesting 5 mg F/kg is equivalent to a 154-lb. (70 kg) person consuming 0.8 grams of sodium fluoride (0.6 grams of sodium fluorosilicate).

Table 52–30B
Recommended Emergency Treatment for Persons Who Ingest Fluorosilicic Acid (H_2SiF_6)[a]

Milligrams Fluoride Ion (mg) Ingested per Body Weight (kg)[b]	Treatment
<5.0 mg of fluoride/kg[c]	1. Give calcium (milk) orally to relieve gastrointestinal symptoms. Observe for 2–4 hours. (A can of evaporated milk should be available at all times to use for emergency treatment.) 2. Induced vomiting is not necessary.
≥5.0 mg of fluoride/kg	1. Move the person away from any contact with fluoride and keep him or her warm. 2. Call the Poison Control Center. 3. If advised by the Poison Control Center and if the person is conscious, induce vomiting by rubbing the back of the person's throat with a spoon or your finger or use syrup of ipecac. To prevent aspiration of vomitus, the person should be placed face down with the head lower than the body. 4. Give the person a glass of milk or any source of soluble calcium (i.e., 5% calcium gluconate or calcium lactate solution). 5. Take the person to the hospital as quickly as possible. **It is important that whoever takes the person to the hospital notify physicians that the person is at risk for pulmonary edema as late as 48 hours afterward.**

[a]CDC, MMWR 1995;44(RR-13):1–40.
[b]Average weight/age: 0–15 kg/0–2 years; 15–20 kg/3–5 years; 20–23 kg/6–8 years; 23–45 kg/9–15 years; 45–70 kg and higher/15–21 years and older.
[c]5 mg of fluoride (F) equals 27 mg of 23% fluorosilicic acid. Ingesting 5 mg F/kg is equivalent to a 154-lb. (70 kg) person consuming 2 grams of fluorosilicic acid.

hydrogen sulfide) and hydrogen fluoride (HF) in the presence of water. It has an odor similar to sulfur dioxide. The toxicity of SF_4 has been compared with that of phosgene. Shortness of breath, chest tightness, productive cough, nose and eye irritation, headache, nausea, and vomiting may follow exposure to the degradation products of SF_6.[6]

Chronic Toxicity (Chronic Fluorosis)

An ecologic cohort study suggests that fluoridation of the water supply to 1 ppm is associated with an increase in the rate of hip fracture in men and women.[7]

Osteoporosis

Sodium fluoride increases spinal bone mass, but does not appear to prevent vertebral fractures in patients who have already had vertebral fractures. The US Food and Drug Administration has not approved sodium fluoride for osteoporosis. There is still little evidence that sodium fluoride increases cortical bone mass. Bone in which fluoride ions are incorporated is more resistant to bone remodeling, and this may lead to a more brittle skeleton as it ages. Bone that forms with fluoride therapy does not appear to have normal strength and appears to be qualitatively inferior.[8] Sodium fluoride does not appear to be an effective or safe treatment for postmenopausal osteoporosis.[9,10] In one study sodium fluoride appeared to increase the risk of hip fracture in osteoporotic women.[11] A UK study suggests that water fluoridation to levels that protect against dental caries (1 mg/liter) does not also help to prevent hip fractures.[12] The recommended optimal level of fluoride set by the Environmental Protection Agency for municipal water systems is 0.17 to 1.2 parts per million (ppm). The maximum acceptable level is 4 ppm. Fluoride contents in some bottled water are shown in Table 52–31.[13,14]

LABORATORY

Acute Poisoning

Analytic Methods

A fluoride-specific, ion-specific potentiometer electrode method is available for measurement of fluoride ion.[15]

A 61-year-old male ingested sodium fluoride and developed serum fluoride levels of 3.4 ng/L (lethal serum fluoride level 3 mg/L), normal serum calcium, and potassium concentration. N urine fluoride level 24 hours after ingestion was 21.2 μg/mL. He survived.[16] Urine fluoride values as high as 320 μg/mL have been reported in cases of fatal ingestion.

Leukocytosis and fever may be secondary to the known ability of fluoride to activate superoxide production and arachidonic acid release from neutrophils.[17]

TREATMENT FOR ACUTE POISONING

Augenstein and colleagues[18] suggest the following treatment protocol for fluoride poisonings.

Fluoride Insecticide Ingestions

Gastric lavage (if recent ingestion) followed by milk, and refer immediately to health care facility.

Noninsecticide Fluoride Ingestions

Less Than 8 mg/kg of Elemental Fluoride Ingested

Give milk. Observe at home for at least 6 hours. Refer to health care facility immediately if any symptoms develop. (Usual symptoms are gastrointestinal—nausea, vomiting, diarrhea, abdominal pain. Other symptoms may include lethargy, fatigue, weakness, or pale appearance.) Whether to induce emesis with syrup of ipecac in this group of patients is somewhat controversial. Symptoms of fluoride toxicity almost always include nausea, vomiting, or diarrhea, which are the same symptoms resulting from the administration of ipecac. Thus giving ipecac may confuse the clinical picture. Inasmuch as children in our study who ingested less than 8 mg/kg of elemental fluoride had benign, self-limited clinical courses, we believe it is safe to withhold the administration of syrup of ipecac in this group, provided that symptomatic patients are referred immediately to a health care facility for proper evaluation.

More Than 8 mg/kg of Elemental Fluoride Ingested

Gastic lavage (if recent ingestion) and milk, and refer immediately to health care facility.

Unknown Amount Ingested

If asymptomatic, give milk, observe at home for at least 6 hours, and refer to health care facility if any symptoms develop. If symptomatic, give milk and refer immediately to health care facility.

Treatment in Health Care Facility:

1. Monitor and support vital signs, including cardiac monitoring.
2. Gastric lavage, if emesis has not occurred. Charcoal is probably not of benefit.
3. Monitor serum electrolyte, calcium, and magnesium levels, being prepared to treat hypocalcemia, hypomagnesemia, and hyperkalemia or hypokalemia.
4. Administer milk, oral calcium salts, or aluminum- or magnesium-based antacids to bind fluoride.
5. Consider hemodialysis in patients with significant toxicity.
6. Consider quinidine treatment for arrhythmias, especially in the presence of refractory hyperkalemia.
7. Consult a regional poison center for the latest treatment recommendations.

Table 52–31
Fluoride Content of Bottled Water[a,b]

Type of Water	Source	Fluoride Level ppm
Drinking water		
Ice Mountain Spring Water	Maine	0.1
Poland Springs Carbonated Spring Water	Maine	<0.1
Evian Spring Water	France	0.1
Star Natural Spring Water	Massachusetts	0.2
Poland Springs Distilled Water	Maine	<0.1
Triton Spring Water	North Carolina	0.1
Belmont Springs Distilled Water	Massachusetts	0.1
Granite State Spring Water	New Hampshire	0.25
Mineral water		
Perrier Naturally Sparkling Mineral Water	France	1.9
Saratoga Naturally Sparkling Mineral Water	New York	<0.1
S. Pellegrino Sparkling Natural Mineral Water	Italy	0.65
Apollinaris Naturally Sparkling Mineral Water	West Germany	0.65

[a]Adapted from McGuire S. N Engl J Med 1989;321:836–837.
[b]Analyses by the State of Iowa Hygienic Laboratory, Des Moines.

REFERENCES—FLUORIDES

1. Augenstein WL, Spoerke DG, Hall, AH, Hall PK, El Saadi MS, et al. Fluoride ingestion in children—a review of 87 cases. Vet Hum Toxicol 1987;29:471–472.
2. Abukurah AR, Moser AM Jr, Baerd SL, Randall RE Jr, Selter JG, Blanke RV. Acute sodium fluoride poisoning. JAMA 1972;222:816–817.
3. Yolken R, Konecny P, McCarty P. Acute fluoride poisoning. Pediatrics 1976;50:90–93.
4. Swanson L, Filandrinos DT, Shevlin JM, Willett JR. Death from accidental ingestion of an ammonium and sodium bifluoride glass etching compound. Vet Hum Toxicol 1993; 35:351.
5. Pilling KJ, Jones HW. Inhalation of degraded sulphur hexafluoride resulting in pulmonary edema. J Soc Occup Med 1988;38:82–84.
6. Kraut A, Lilis R. Pulmonary effects of acute exposure to degradation products of sulphur hexafluoride during electrical cable repair work. Br J Indust Med 1990;47:829–832.
7. Danielson C, Lyon JL, Egger M, Goodenough GK. Hip fractures and fluoridation in Utah's elderly population. JAMA 1992;268:746–748.

8. Skolnick A. New doubts about benefits of sodium fluoride. JAMA 1990;263:1752–1753.
9. Riggs BL, Hodgson SF, O'Fallon WM, Chao EYS, Wahner HW, Muhs JM et al. Effect of fluoride treatment on the fracture rate in postmenopausal women with osteoporosis. N Engl J Med 1990;232:802–809.
10. Mamelle N, Dusan R, Martin JL, Prost A, Meuxier DJ, Guillaume M et al. Risk-benefit ratio of sodium fluoride treatment in primary vertebral osteoporosis. Lancet 1988;2: 361–365.
11. Hedlund LR, Gallagher JC. Increased incidence of hip fracture in osteoporotic woman treated with sodium fluoride. J Bone Miner Res 1989;4:223–225.
12. Cooper C, Wickham C, Lacey RF, Barker DJP. Water fluoride concentration and fracture of the proximal femur. J Epidemiol Commun Health 1990;44:17–19.
13. Environmental Protection Agency. National primary and secondary drinking water regulation: fluoride. Fed Reg 1986; 51:11396–11412.
14. McGuire S. Fluoride content of bottled water. N Engl J Med 1989;321:836–837.
15. Ohlson G, Sheridan F. Blood fluoride by ion-specific potentiometer. Bull Int Assoc Forensic Toxicol 1991;21(4):36–78.
16. Saadi JJ, Rose SS. A case of nonfatal sodium fluoride ingestion. J Anal Toxicol 1988;2:270–271.
17. Harchelroad F, Goetz C. Systemic fluoride intoxication with leucocytosis and pyrexia. Vet Hum Toxicol 1993;35:351.
18. Augenstein WL, Spoerke DG, Kulig KW, Hall AH, Hall PK, Rigs BS et al. Fluoride ingestion in children: a review of 87 cases. Pediatrics 1991;88:907–912.

HOLIDAY HAZARDS

HALLOWEEN[1]

1. If a parent suspects a tampering (torn wrapper, seal broken, etc.) and there has been no ingestion, discard the product.
2. If tampering is suspected and there has been an ingestion, seek emergency room evaluation.
3. If the product has obviously been tampered with (glass, foreign objects, razor blades) and no ingestion has occurred, the parent should report this immediately to the local police department (see Tampering).

The American Association of Poison Control Centers and the Rocky Mountain Poison Center discourage hospitals from offering free x-ray screening of Halloween candy. While some x-rays may show adulteration with some substances of a metallic nature, it offers no true screening to assure product safety. Negative x-rays may contribute a false sense of security that the candy is fit to eat. They do not rule out contamination and are not substitutes for careful visual examination by parents.

Poison Center and emergency room personnel are often asked about exposures to other common Halloween items:

1. *Dry Ice:* When ingested in solid form, oral burns may occur. Therefore immediate dilution is recommended. It is not a problem in punch as long as no ice is ingested. Direct contact with the skin can also cause tissue damage. Irrigate immediately with lukewarm water.
2. *Light sticks:* Necklaces and bracelets that glow in the dark contain cyalume, a higher alcohol, which is usually not found in amounts large enough to be harmful if swallowed.
3. *Makeup:* Many are nontoxic or contain small amounts of emollient laxatives, talc, or hydrocarbons. Treatment should depend on the amount ingested, the ingredients of the specific product and the symptoms present.

As Halloween approaches, medical personnel may receive questions from parents concerning safety. The Rocky Mountain Poison and Drug Center offers the following suggestions to parents to help reduce the possibility that their child may be harmed.

1. Hold a block party or private party in the neighborhood.
2. If children do trick-or-treat, it should only be to familiar homes and preferably before dark. Avoid dark or deserted looking homes.
3. A full meal before trick-or-treating decreases a child's urge to eat treats along the way.
4. Parents should carefully inspect all candies before allowing children to eat them. Discard any treat that appears opened, torn, or out of the original wrapper. Eat homemade treats only if the parent knows the giver.
5. All children should be accompanied by an adult. If they must be out after dark, each child should have a flashlight. Reflective tape placed on costumes can facilitate children being seen on dark streets.

A parents' newsletter has been prepared by Marilyn Marsh on "Keeping Halloween Safe" by the L.I. Regional Poison Control Center at Winthrop-University Hospital.

CHRISTMAS (TABLE 52–32)

Potentials for harm during Christmas are summarized in Table 52–32.

The inventory of potential hazards should at least include: toys, food, beverages, decorations, and plants.

I. TOYS: Children look forward to the holiday toys they will be receiving. Watch out for the tiny button batteries that are easily swallowed by curious infants. Battery-operated toys are usually safer than electrical plug-in toys. Think twice about passing on older toys to youngsters since some of these may contain harmful lead paint. The following guide: "Christmas Toys—Good and Bad" (from the publication, "For Kids' Sake," published by the Medical Center, University of Virginia, Winter, 1985) may help in purchasing gifts for children.
   A. *For Infants Under 1 Year:*
      Good: Wooden blocks, float and squeeze toys, soft animals without buttons.
      Bad: Small toys that can be swallowed, toys with strings longer than 12 inches. (These can strangle.)
   B. *For 1- to 2-year-olds:*
      Good: Plastic books, kiddy cars, nesting blocks, large puzzles.
      Bad: Toys with buttons or small parts that can be swallowed, toys that can be dismantled by persistent fingers.

Table 52-32
Christmas Hazards

Product	Ingredients	Hazard
Artificial Christmas Tree	Aluminum, plastic	Mechanical obstruction, mucous membrane irritation
Christmas Tree Decoration		
Angel hair	Spun glass	Considered nontoxic in small amounts but may be irritating to mucous membranes
Icicles or tinsel	Polyvinyl chloride (metalized) aluminum coloring, some may be tin, lead, and plastic	Nontoxic but possibly may cause mechanical obstruction
Glitter or sparkle	Small pieces of plastic or glass	Nontoxic
Christmas tree ornaments	Metal, plastic, wood, glass	Nontoxic, but may cause lacerations
Christmas tree lights	Glass	Nontoxic, but may cause lacerations
Christmas tree bubble lights	Methylene chloride	Toxicity unlikely if small amount ingested
Christmas tree hook hanger	Metal	Possibility for choking, if lodged in throat or esophagus
Homemade Christmas ornaments	Shellac, paint polyurethane spray	Small amounts are not a problem.
Snow spray/snow flock	Propellant—methylene chloride	Dry snow—nontoxic prolonged inhalation of spray—dizziness and headache may occur
Under the Christmas Tree		
Crayons	Wax	Nontoxic
Candles	Wax	Nontoxic
Snow scene globes	Plastic or calcium carbonate	Potential for salmonella enteritis if water is not sterile.
After shave, perfume, toilet water, colognes	Can be up to 90% ethanol	Doubtful will see symptoms from this exposure as children typically do not ingest more than a swallow of these products. If large ingestion does occur, may see drowsiness, ataxia, and hypoglycemia.
Sachets	Talc powder & essential oils	Small amounts not serious. May cause respiratory irritation or obstruction from powder.
Airplane glue	Toluene, benzene, zylene	Mucous membrane irritation. Inhalation can produce headache, dizziness, excitement.
Disc battery	Various heavy metals, alkaline corrosive	If lodged in the gastrointestinal tract can cause erosion. Location by x-ray is needed with follow-up to ensure passage.
Battery	Acid or alkaline corrosive	Mucous membrane irritation or burns.
Bubble bath soaps	Detergent	Vomiting
Silly putty	Silicones, glycerin, borates	Small amounts not serious. Mechanical obstruction may occur with large amounts.
Gift Wrapping		
Ribbon and wrapping paper		Nontoxic
Scotch tape		Nontoxic, possibility of obstruction
Ballpoint pens, felt tip pens		Not serious in small amounts
Watercolor paints		Nontoxic
Others		
Fireplace colors	Salt of metals such as copper, selenium & lead	Gastrointestinal irritation. Treatment will depend on amount and type of salt ingested.
Fireplace ashes		Nontoxic
Matches	Chlorates	20 wooden matches (not fireplace matches) or two books of paper matches not serious
Salt to melt ice	Sodium chloride	Hypernatremia

C. *For over 2-year-olds:*
Good: Developmental toys that encourage the imagination to expand.
Bad: Projectile type toys: guns, weapons, etc.; toys with sharp edges or points.

D. *Gift suggestions for the nursery set:*
Infant carrier with crotch seat and easy to use safety belt.
Crib toys that fasten securely to the side of the crib.
Gates that do not accordion but have straight tops.
Pacifiers with shields that cannot fit into a child's mouth and do not have strings or ribbons attached.
Rattles that will not break or cause choking.
Toy chest with soft closing, ventilation holes, and latches to prevent a child from being trapped inside.

II. FOODS: What's a holiday without food? Because there is so much work to be done, "cooks" often take shortcuts that may help to spread germs and may result in food poisoning. Here are some suggestions for a safe holiday turkey:

1. Before the bird is purchased, make sure it can be safely refrigerated before and after cooking.
2. Keep frozen birds frozen until ready for defrosting. Once defrosted, it should be kept refrigerated no more than one day before roasting.
3. Refuse a bird that was defrosted and refrozen.

4. Remove giblets and store separately immediately after purchase.
5. Keep work areas, utensils, and hands soap-and-hot-water clean at all times to reduce chances for bacterial contamination.
6. Thaw turkey by refrigeration in original wrapper for 3 to 4 days or by running cold water or emersing in cold water and changing the water every 60 minutes. May keep fresh or thawed turkey in refrigerator 2 to 3 days. It is suggested that turkey and stuffing be *cooked separately.* Cook turkey until thermometer in breast is 170°F and the drumstick moves easily. Let stand 10 to 15 minutes after cooking for easier carving.
7. Carve turkey immediately after roasting and store leftovers in small airtight packages in the refrigerator or freezer.
8. Leftover turkey can safely be refrigerated for 3 to 5 days. Gravy and stuffing should be eaten in 1 or 2 days.
9. If you are uncertain about whether a food is safe to eat follow this rule: WHEN IN DOUBT, THROW IT OUT.

Salmonella in Turkeys, Chickens, and Eggs

Salmonella is frequently found in turkeys, chickens, and their eggs. Handle raw and cooked fowl carefully. Keep work areas, utensils, and hands clean to reduce chances for bacterial infection. Soap and hot water are important in preventing salmonella germs from spreading.

Eggs may be infected with salmonella from infected fowl. The germ may penetrate the shell from the bird's ovary and enter the yolk. Therefore it is important that the following preventive measures in egg preparation be taken:

1. PASTEURIZING all eggs used in processed foods (mayonnaise, etc.)
2. RECOGNIZING DISHES OF HIGH RISK for potential salmonella contamination (stuffing for seafood, Hollandaise sauce, homemade eggnog, Caesar salad [with raw eggs], gefilte fish, potato salad, egg salad, homemade ice cream, cake fillings.)
3. EGG PREPARATION. Do not eat raw eggs. Boil the eggs (salmonella can be killed by temperatures of 130°F for 1 hour or 140°F for 15 minutes). If salmonella is in the yolk, it can resist boiling for 2 to 3 minutes. It is recommended that hard-boiled eggs should be boiled at least 7 minutes; scrambled eggs be cooked thoroughly, leaving no runny, undercooked egg; fried eggs be fried for at least 3 minutes on each side and do not eat "sunnyside up"; and poached eggs be cooked for 5 minutes.
4. COLD EGG DISHES should be kept below 40°F, HOT EGG DISHES kept above 140°F, and never leave EGG DISHES AT ROOM TEMPERATURE for more than 1 hour.
5. DO NOT USE cracked eggs; do not wash the surface of eggs until ready to use; check expiration date before purchasing eggs.

III. BEVERAGES: Alcoholic beverages are often part of the holiday celebrations. Children often imitate adults and they will drain partially filled glasses regardless of the contents. Small amounts of alcohol can be harmful or fatal to children by causing hypoglycemia and coma. Empty beverage glasses and place them out of the reach of curious children. Run a careful check of all rooms for partially consumed beverages before going to bed at night to prevent early rising children from exploring and drinking them the following morning. REMINDER; DON'T DRINK AND DRIVE!!

IV. PERFUMES, COLOGNES, AFTER-SHAVE PREPARATIONS: Contain alcohol; therefore these items should be placed out of the reach of young children.

V. CHRISTMAS DECORATIONS: By their own nature, youngsters are attached to decorations. They will touch, taste, and manipulate these items. Be alert to the hazards associated with some of these:

A. Angel Hair: This is made of spun glass, which can cause irritations of the eyes, skin, and digestive tract. Observe children for evidence of irritations and/or bleeding caused by angel hair.
B. Candles: Consist of wax and synthetic materials, which are inert and are not toxic. Coloring and scents are added in such small quantities that they do not present toxic problems. However, small chunks of candles may lodge in the respiratory passages.
C. Christmas Tree Ornaments: Often made of metal, plastic, or foam, can be hazardous because they can obstruct air passages and can cut the skin, digestive tract, or air passages.
D. Christmas Tree Lights with Bubbling Fluid: The fluid in a single bulb contains a nontoxic amount of methylene chloride. If the contents of several bulbs are consumed, convulsions, coma, liver, and kidney damage may occur. The glass may cause internal cuts.
E. Fireplace Colors/Log Colors: Colors are produced by metallic salts, which may be toxic if ingested in large quantities.
F. Gift Wrapping: Often contain toxic metals; therefore do not allow children to chew them. Do not burn them in fireplaces.
G. Metallic Icicles/Tinsel: Ingestions of these can cause intestinal irritation and obstruction and choking. Since they usually contain lead and tin, they may be toxic with repeated ingestion.
H. Styrofoam: If swallowed, may produce irritation. Otherwise, it is not toxic.
I. Artificial Trees: The plastic or metallic portions of these may cause digestive tract irritations. Otherwise they are not toxic.
J. Check all electrical connections for proper insertion into outlets and contacts.
K. Turn out tree lights when no adult is at home. Electrical fires can quickly consume trees, decorations, and packages. Be alert for fire hazards.

VI. HOLIDAY PLANTS: Leaves, stems, flowers, and berries found on holiday plants are attractive nuisances for children. Some of the more toxic plants used at holiday time are MISTLETOE, JERUSALEM CHERRY, HOLLY, and RHODODENDRON. Consider whether you want to have these plants at home when young children are present. If you do have them, keep them out of the reach of curious youngsters.

REFERENCES—HOLIDAY HAZARDS

1. Janco N. Seasonal topics. Halloween hazards. Rocky Mountain Poison Center Bulletin 1988;7(3):6–7.
2. Rocky Mountain Poison Center Bulletin 1990;9(2) and 1988;(7):4.
3. Long Island Regional Poison Control Center. Holiday Hazard Prevention for Parents, November/December, 1991.

TYPES OF LAXATIVES

Laxatives are now available over-the-counter in liquid, tablets, gum, powder, granule, suppository, and enema dosage forms. They work in different ways to promote stool evacuation.

STIMULANT LAXATIVES

Stimulant laxatives agitate or excite intestinal walls, causing waves of muscular contractions that expel fecal matter. Product names include *Carter's Little Pills, Caster Oil, Dulcolax, Ex-Lax, Feen-A-Mint, Fletcher's Castoria,* and *Modane.* The FDA has banned the following stimulant-laxative ingredients beginning in May 1991: calomel, colocynth, elaterin resin, gamboge, ipomea, jalap, podophyllum resin, aloin, bile salts, bile acids, calcium pantothenate, frangula, ox bile, prune concentrate, prune powder, rhubarb-Chinese, and sodium oleate.

LUBRICANTS

Lubricant laxatives "grease" stools, facilitating excretion. Mineral oil and mineral-oil emulsion are the most common forms of lubricants. Among them are *Agoral Plain* and *Fleet Mineral Oil Enema.*

SALINE LAXATIVES

Saline laxatives act like a sponge to draw water into the bowel, thereby promoting easier passage of stools. Loss of body salts is a key risk of long-term use of these products. Among laxatives in this group are *Milk of Magnesia, Citrate of Magnesia,* and *Epsom Salts.* The recent ban forbids the use of tartaric acid as a saline-laxative ingredient.

STOOL SOFTENERS

Stool softeners or emollients soften hard stools by enabling them to absorb more liquids. They are often given to women after childbirth and to patients recovering from surgery. Brands include *Colace, Dialose, Regutol,* and *Surfak.* Stool softeners should never be taken within 2 hours of a mineral oil dose because the combination can result in excessive buildup of mineral oil in body tissues. *Polaxamer 188* is now banned as a stool-softener ingredient.

HYPEROSMOTICS

Hyperosmotic laxatives mimic the action of saline laxatives, but pose less risk of salt depletion. Over-the-counter hyperosmotics such as glycerin are available for rectal use only. Oral hyperosmotics must be prescribed by a physician. Overuse of hyperosmotics can cause continuing diarrhea.

CARBON DIOXIDE–RELEASING AGENTS

Carbon dioxide–releasing suppositories produce carbon dioxide in the bowels. The gas pushes stubborn stools toward excretion. The suppositories are available over-the-counter under the brand name *Ceo-Two.*

BULK LAXATIVES

Bulk-forming laxatives absorb water in the intestine and swell the stool into an easily passed soft mass. Each dose should be taken with an 8-ounce glass of liquid. Although bulk agents are generally regarded as the safest form of laxative, users should be aware that the products can interfere with absorption of certain drugs, including aspirin, digitalis, antibiotics, and anticoagulants. People with the genetic disorder phenylketonuria should not take any sugar-free bulk laxative containing phenylalanine because it can damage brain tissue.

Bulk laxatives include *FiberCon, Metamucil,* and *Serutan.* Although bran is considered a bulk agent, the FDA has said that bran cereals marketed solely as food products will not be subject to laxative regulations. However, any bran product marketed as a laxative will be regarded as a drug and therefore must conform with FDA rules.

The following bulk-laxative ingredients are now banned: carrageenan (degraded, agar, carrageenan [native], and guar gum). Many bulk-laxative products contain water-soluble gums as their active ingredients—for example, karaya, methylcellulose, plantago seed, psyllium, and polycarbophil. Recognizing that water-soluble gums taken without adequate water can cause problems, the FDA proposed in the *Federal Register* of October 30, 1990, that products containing water-soluble gums have the following warning on their labels:

"Warning: (Select one of the following, as appropriate: Take or Mix) this produce with at least 8 ounces (a full glass) of water or other fluid. Taking this product without adequate fluid may cause it to swell and block your throat or esophagus and may cause choking. Do not take this product if you have ever had difficulty in swallowing or have any throat problems. If you experience chest pain, vomiting, or difficulty in swallowing or breathing after taking this product, seek immediate medical attention."

COMBINATION LAXATIVES AND BOWEL-CLEANSING SYSTEMS

Some products contain a combination of laxatives that act together to promote evacuation. These drugs may carry a higher risk of side effects. A combination laxative drug with more than two active ingredients will be permitted only if it can be shown that the combination is equal to or better than each of the active ingredients used alone at its therapeutic dose and presents no additional safety risk.

Although bowel-cleansing systems contain a number of ingredients used sequentially at specified intervals, they are not true combination drug products. Bowel-cleansing systems are used to evacuate the bowel before surgery or diagnostic exams, but such products are not intended for general laxative use and will be labeled for use only as directed by a physician.

SENNA

Tetany (associated with hypokalemia and hypocalcemia with finger clubbing) has been associated with chronic ingestion of excessive quantities of senna. Similarly osteomalacia and arthropathy have also followed Senna (3 to 8 tablets of *Senokot* daily) abuse. The clubbing may be reversible. A 26-year-old woman ingested 10 times the recommended dose of sennoside laxative and developed hepatitis, which was reversible on discontinuation of the sennoside abuse. Pericentral vein hepatic necrosis may follow senna abuse. Sennoside, the major substrates of senna leaf and fruit are split to rhein anthron in the intestine by *E.* coli and other intestinal bacteria. Rhein anthron is structurally similar to danthron, a known hepatotoxic laxative. Anthraquinones such as rhein anthron in rhubarb have been incriminated by liver disease.

These patients undergo extensive diagnostic workups, including sigmoidoscopy, barium enema studies, rectal biopsies, upper gastrointestinal series, and CT scans. Laxative abuse (e.g., phenolphthalein, senna) may result in interstitial nephritis or ammonium urate renal calculi. Hypomagnesemia, hypocalcemia, hypokalemia, hypophosphatemia, and muscle weakness have been observed in laxative abusers.

Severe systemic anaphylaxis may occur among nurses and pharmaceutical workers who handle psyllium-containing laxatives. Eating psyllium-containing foods may provoke an IgE mediated Type I hypersensitivity reaction.

LAXATIVE PHOSPHATE POISONING (SEE ALSO DRUGS OF ABUSE)

Adult-sized sodium phosphate enemas administered to a 4-year-old boy with long-term constipation led to an episode of hypocalcemic tetany (elevated serum phosphate, decreased serum calcium). He received IV calcium gluconate with resolution of symptoms within minutes. He later received oral calcium supplementation and hydration.[1]

Hazards of phosphate enemas administered rectally include hypocalcemia, hyperphosphatemia, hypokalemia, tetany, rectal necrosis, perforation, and death.[2]

DIFFERENTIAL DIAGNOSIS

The differential diagnosis of tetany includes two toxic syndromes associated with normocalcemia, strychnine poisoning, and tetanus. The muscle spasm of clostridial tetanus usually begins in the head and neck area. Trismus is an early symptom in tetanus and uncommon in tetany. In strychnine poisoning the spasms are clonic, are not tetanic, and involve the entire body. In tetany the upper extremities are characteristically involved first, followed by the lower extremities. Usually the patient exhibits elbow extension and metacarpophalangeal flexion. The lower extremities are held in extension at the knees with the ankle plantar and the toes flexed.

CLINICAL PRESENTATION

Clinical features of hypocalcemia other than tetany include weakness and fatigue with psychiatric manifestations of anxiety, depression, and irritability. Extrapyramidal movement disorders, abdominal pain, urinary frequency, and muscle cramps may be seen early. Arrhythmias with QT and ST prolongation are early cardiac manifestations. As hypocalcemia progresses, tetany, seizures, psychosis, bronchospasm, laryngospasm, heart failure, or hypotension may develop.[3] Sodium phosphate enemas may lead to fatal poisoning, especially in infants.[4] Shock and metabolic acidosis may be observed in infants.

TREATMENT

Calcium

Correct the underlying pathology. Calcium replacement is indicated in any patient with hypocalcemia (less than 5 mg/dL) or any patient exhibiting hypocalcemic symptoms. Monitor for signs of cardiac toxicity, including heart block or arrhythmias; these are more prevalent in patients taking digoxin because digoxin potentiates the effects of the drug. The initial pediatric dose is 100 mg/kg of 10% calcium gluconate (100 mg = 1 mL) up to 1 g (2 to 3 g in adults) given in 50 to 100 mL of 5% dextrose in water over 10 minutes. The dilution is often necessary to prevent vein irritation. This can be followed by oral or IV supplementation as required.

Electrolytes

Monitor serum electrolyte levels (calcium, magnesium, phosphate, and potassium) and renal function. Hyperkalemia and hypomagnesemia potentiate the cardiac toxicity of hypocalcemia. Hypokalemia reduces the neuromuscular irritability caused by hypocalcemia.

Children with gastrointestinal anomalies such as Hirschsprung's disease and chronic renal failure are at high risk for complications after the use of hypertonic phosphate enemas.[5]

LABORATORY

Following use of a Fleet enema in acutely ill elderly patients or children, serum inorganic phosphorus may rise and serum calcium fall. Hypovolemia and hypernatremia may be observed. Findings may be severe in patients with diminished renal capacity.[6]

REFERENCES—LAXATIVE PHOSPHATE POISONING

1. Edmondson S, Almquist TD. Iatrogenic hypocalcemic tetany. Ann Emerg Med 1990;19:938–940.
2. Hunter MF, Ashton MR, Griffiths DM, Ilangovan P, Roberts JP, Walker V. Hyperphosphatemia after enemas in childhood: prevention and treatment. Arch Dis Childh 1993;68:233–234.
3. Edmonson S, Almquist TD. Iatrogenic hypocalcemic tetany. Ann Emerg Med 1990;19:938–940.
4. Martin RR, Lisehora GR, Braxton M Jr, Barcfia RJ. Fatal poisoning from sodium phosphate enema. Case report and experimental study. JAMA 1987;257:2190–2192.
5. Wason S, Tiller T, Curra G. Severe hyperphosphatemia, hypocalcemia, acidosis and shock in a 5-month-old child following the administration of adult Fleet enema. Ann Emerg Med 1989;8:696–700.

6. Grosskopf I, Graff E, Charach G, Binyamin G, Spinrad S, Blum I. Hyperphosphatemia and hypocalcemia induced by hypertonic phosphate enema. An experimental study and review of the literature. Hum Exper Toxicol 1991;10: 351–355.

PHENOLPHTHALEIN

Phenolphthalein is a stimulant laxative similar in many respects to bisacodyl, another diphenyl methane derivative. Child abuse may lead to multiple "illnesses" associated with diarrhea and multiple hospitalizations.[1] Children who acutely ingest 1 gram or less of a phenolphthalein-containing product are at minimal if any risk for developing dehydration caused by excess diarrhea and fluid loss.[2] Hypersensitivity reactions may lead to death.[3–6] Treatment is largely symptomatic and supportive.

STRUCTURE AND CLASSIFICATION

Phenolphthalein, like bisacodyl, is a diphenyl methane derivative. The molecular weight is 318.3.

USES

Phenolphthalein (white) is available as an oral tablet, 60 mg (Alophen Pills), 120 mg (Medilax), 130 mg (Modane); chewable tablets (60 mg Prulet, 64.8 mg Phenolax wafers, 120 mg Medilax; tablets of 65 mg (Feen-a-mint). It is also available in combination with docusate sodium (Colax, Modane Plus, Agoral, Disolan). Phenolphthalein yellow is available in an oral chewing form (97.2 mg)—Feen-A-Mint, chewable tablets (80 mg)—Evac-U-Lax, (90 mg)—Ex-Lax, Lax-Pills, and (97.2 mg)—Es opotabs. Combinations of yellow phenolphthalein are also available with docusate sodium or docusate colon. A kit containing 2 tablets of phenolphthalein 130 mg is available.[8]

SOURCES

Phenolphthalein is a synthetic chemical compound.

THERAPEUTIC DOSES

The usual dose is 30 to 200 mg for adults and 15 to 60 mg for children.

TOXIC DOSE

Toxic doses range from 400 mg to 130 g.

FATAL DOSE

Doses associated with fatalities have been 1.8 g,[3] and 0.65 to 1.3 g.[4] Ingestion of a box of Ex-Lax[6] and ingestion by a laxative abuser[5] led to fatalities.

TOXICOKINETICS

Absorption

Up to 15% of a therapeutic dose of phenolphthalein is absorbed and eliminated by the kidney, most of it in conjugated form.[7]

Elimination

The urine becomes pink or red if it is sufficiently alkaline (pH 7 or more).[1] Some absorbed drug is also excreted in the bile, and the resulting enterohepatic cycle may contribute to prolongation of the laxative effect.

MECHANISM OF ACTION

Stimulant drugs alter fluid and electrolyte absorption, producing net intestinal fluid accumulation and laxation. Increased concentrations of cyclic 3′-5′-adenosine monophosphate (CAMP) occurring in colonic mucosal cells may alter the permeability of these cells leading to net fluid accumulation and laxative action. Phenolphthalein also acts directly or reflexly to increase the activity of the small intestine.[8] Phenolphthalein acts mainly on the colon about 6 hours after ingestion.

CLINICAL PRESENTATION

The major dangers of overdosage of the diphenyl methane derivative are fluid and electrolyte deficits resulting from excessive laxative effect. A fixed-drug eruption, Stevens-Johnson syndrome, a syndrome that resembles lupus erythematosus, osteomalacia, and protein-losing enteropathy has been reported to follow the use of phenolphthalein. In therapeutic oral doses, all stimulant laxatives may produce some degree of abdominal discomfort, nausea, mild cramps, griping, and/or faintness. Stimulant laxatives are habit-forming. Excess use may induce electrolyte disturbances such as hypokalemia, hypocalcemia, metabolic acidosis or alkalosis, abdominal pain, diarrhea, malabsorption, weight loss, and protein-losing enteropathy. Electrolyte disturbance may produce vomiting and muscle weakness; rarely osteomalacia, secondary aldosteronism, and tetany may occur. "Cathartic colon" with atony and dilatation of the colon, especially the right side, may follow habitual use (several years) and may resemble ulcerative colitis. Children subject to drug abuse by parents have multiple illnesses and hospitalizations for diarrhea.[1] Other side effects have included encephalitis,[4] epidermal necrolysis,[9] and erythema multiforme.[10]

Phenolphthalein sensitization may be manifested by three types of reactions[3]: (a) cutaneous type with rash, pruritus, palpebral edema, fever, and joint pains; (b) general type with severe diarrhea, colic, and hypotension; and (c) encephalitic type, with seizures, paresis, coma, and death.[4]

A 32-year-old woman ingested an unknown quantity of Nylax tablets (thiamine hydrochloride 30 mg, phenolphthalein 60 mg, cascara dry extract 30 mg, aloin 2 mg, powdered Senna leaf 15 mg, bisacodyl 2 mg). She developed multiple organ failure, coma, pulmonary edema, muscle and myocardial damage, acute tubular necrosis, predominant massive liver necrosis, and disseminated intravascular coagulation that ended fatally despite vigorous supportive therapy. The serum phenolphthalein level was 0.4 µg/L.[5] A 3-year-old ingested 1.8 g of phenolphthalein and died of pulmonary and cerebral edema. No serum level was obtained. There was no liver involvement.[3] The encephalitis was thought to be a hypersensitivity reaction.[4] A 10-year-old boy ate the contents of a box of Ex-Lax. Autopsy showed hemorrhagic areas throughout the intestine, brain, kidneys, and liver.[6] A 35-year-old man ingested 2 g of phenolphthalein and developed shock, pulmonary edema, hypothermia, renal failure, and acidosis with no evidence of liver dysfunction. He survived.[11]

A retrospective study of 172 phenolphthalein ingestions, ranging from 32.5 to 1620 mg (average 558.9 mg) in children indicated that about 20% had no symptoms. Most had minor symptoms that resolved within 24 hours. The authors conclude that children ages 5 years and under who acutely ingest 1 gram or less of a phenolphthalein-containing laxative need no specific treatment other than fluid replacement and supportive care. They appear to be at minimal risk for developing dehydration caused by excessive diarrhea and resulting fluid loss. Table 52–1 presents some over-the-counter products containing phenolphthalein.[2]

LABORATORY

Analytical Methods

Phenolphthalein concentration in the serum may be determined by thin layer chromatography detected under ultraviolet light,[5] and by a red color in the urine and feces[1] (Table 52–33).

Blood Levels

Serum phenolphthalein levels of 0.4 ug/L were observed in a chronic laxative abuser who developed coma and fever.[5]

Abnormalities

J-waves, typical of hypothermia may be seen on electrocardiogram.[11] Metabolic acidosis may be present with a lactic acidosis.[11] Myoglobin in serum and urine, increased in creatine phosphokinase, hypoglycemia elevated aminotransferases.[3]

Ancillary Tests

In one patient with an apparent hypersensitivity reaction to phenolphthalein long induced a generalized pruritus within 15 minutes.[9] Cerebrospinal fluid has shown a lymphocytosis in one patient,[6] and a few red cells and white cells in another patient.[4]

TREATMENT

Stabilization

Treatment is largely symptomatic and supportive.

Table 52–33
Some Causes of Red Urine or Feces

Blood
Hemoglobin
Ingestion of red foods or beverages
Ingestion of eosin dye
Congenital erythropoietic porphyria
Phenolphthalein

Decontamination

Children will usually not require gastric decontamination.[13] They should be encouraged to consume extra fluids.[2]

Elimination Enhancement

There is little indication for the use of activated charcoal or cathartics. Peritoneal dialysis was employed in an adult with a lactic acidosis and pulmonary edema. The patient recovered.[11] There is little clinical data on the use of extracorporeal methods to hasten elimination of phenolphthalein.

Antidotes

There are no antidotes.

REFERENCES—PHENOLPHTHALEIN

1. Fleisher D, Ament ME. Diarrhea, red diapers and child abuse. Clinical alertness needed for recognition: clinical skill needed for success in management. Clin Pediatr 1977;16: 820–821.
2. Mrvos R, Swanson-Bierman B, Dean BS, Krenzelok AP. Acute phenolphthalein ingestion in children. A retrospective review. J Pediatr Health Care 1981;5:147–151.
3. Sarcinelli L, Signore L, Malizia. Lethal phenolphthalein poisoning in a child. Proc Eur Soc Study Drug Tox 1970, XI, Venice March-April 1979; Amsterdam Exerpta Med 1970.
4. Kendall AC. Fatal case of encephalitis after phenolphthalein ingestion. Br Med J 1954;2:1461–1462.
5. Sidhu PS, Wilkenson ML, Sladen GE, Filipe MI, Toseland PA. Fatal phenolphthalein poisoning with fulminant hepatic failure and disseminated intravascular coagulation. Hum Toxicol 1989;8:381–384.
6. Cleeves M. Poisoning by "Ex-Lax" tablets. JAMA 1932;99: 657.
7. Brunton LL. Agents affecting gastrointestinal water flux and mobility digestants and bile acids. In: Gilman AG, Rall TW, Nies AS, Taylor P, eds. Goodman and Gilman's the pharmacological basis of therapeutics. 8th ed. New York: Pergamon Press, 1991.
8. McEvoy GK, ed. AHFS Drug Information 92. Bethesda. Am Soc Hosp Pharm 1992;1728–1731.
9. Kar PK, Dutta RK, Shah BH. Toxic epidermal necrolysis in a patient induced by phenolphthalein. J Ind Med Assoc 1986;84:189–190.
10. Baer RL, Harris H. Types of cutaneous reactions to drugs. JAMA 1967;202–210.
11. Buchanan N, Cane RD, Glantz R, Hunt JA. Phenolphthalein poisoning. S Afr Med J 1976;50:1060–1061.
12. Lambrianidis AL, Rosin RD. Acute pancreatitis complicating excess intake of phenolphthalein. Postgrad Med J 1984; 60:491–492.
13. Blatt ML, Steigmann F, Dyniewica JM. Phenolphthalein tolerance in childhood. J Pediatr 1943;22:719–725.

POLYSTYRENE SODIUM IN SORBITAL ENEMAS

Sodium polystyrene (Kayexalate) in sorbitol enemas may lead to catastrophic colonic complications such as extensive transneural necrosis and infarction.[1] Kayexalate crystals may be found adherent to the mucosa. All patients have been uremic.[1,2] In both studies patients apparently were not administered cleansing enemas. Experimental data suggest that sorbitol should not be included in Kayexalate enemas given for hyperkalemia in renal transplant patients.[3] Further data will be required to clarify these findings.

REFERENCES—POLYSTYRENE SODIUM IN SORBITAL ENEMAS

1. Lillemore KD, Romolo JL, Hamilton SR, Pennington LR, Burdick JF, Williams GM. Intestinal necrosis due to sodium polystyrene (Kayexalate) in sorbital enemas—clinical and experimental support for the hypothesis. Surgery 1987;101:267–372.
2. Wootton FT, Rhodes DF, Lec WM, Fitts CT. Colonic necrosis with Kayexalate-sorbital enemas after renal transplantation. Ann Intern Med 1989;111:947–954.
3. Shepard KV. Cleansing enemas after sodium polystyrene sulfonate enemas. Ann Intern Med 1990;112:711.

PSYLLIUM

Psyllium hydrophilic mucilloid, a nonproteinaceous gum composed of a mixture of polysaccharides, is derived from the seeds or husk of the plant, *Plantago ovata* (also called ispaghula).[1] Psyllium seed hypersensitivity (asthma, allergic rhinitis, anaphylaxis) has been observed in nurses dispensing the product or pharmaceutical workers[2] involved in its manufacture.[3] IgE is a factor in its pathogenesis.[1] Anaphylaxis has followed oral ingestion of a psyllium-containing cereal.[1]

REFERENCES—PSYLLIUM

1. Lantner RR, Esplritu BP, Zumerchik P, Tobin MS. Anaphylaxis following ingestion of a psyllium-containing cereal. JAMA 1990;264:2534–2536.
2. Malo J-L, Carter A, L'Archeveque J, Ghezzo H, Lagier F, Trudeau C, Dolovich J. Prevalence of occupational asthma and immunologic sensitization to psyllium among health personnel in chronic care hospitals. Am Rev Respir Dis 1990;142:1359–1366.
3. Nelson WL. Allergic events among health care workers exposed to psyllium laxatives in the workplace. J Occup Med 1987;29:497–499.

HYPERMAGNESEMIA

CLINICAL

Magnesium Excess

Hypermagnesemia may follow excessive intake, impaired excretion, or parenteral administration of magnesium.[1,2]

Excessive Intake

Excessive oral intake of magnesium in the absence of either intestinal or renal disease infrequently occurs.[3,4] It has been observed in neonates receiving Mylanta (containing 56 mg of elemental Mg in 4 mL) or following Philips Milk of Magnesia (8 teaspoonsful per day—381.6 mg/kg/day).[3] Patients treated for overdose of drugs with frequent oral dosage of magnesium-containing cathartics may develop signs and symptoms of hypermagnesemia[5–7]; excessive oral intake of magnesium may induce diarrhea with increased levels of fecal magnesium.[8] Fatal hypermagnesemia from rectal administration of magnesium preparations has followed in cases of megacolon and bowel obstruction.[1]

Impaired Excretion

Hypermagnesemia is seen in patients with chronic renal failure who have been receiving magnesium-containing antacids, enemas, or infusions. Excessive dialysate magnesium may also cause symptomatic hypermagnesemia. In acute renal failure serum magnesium values are 2.6 to 3.8 mEq/L (1.3 to 1.9 mmol/L).[2] Azotemia, acidosis, rhabdomyolysis, and continued magnesium intake are contributing factors.

Parenteral Administration

Symptoms of excess magnesium may be induced by parenteral magnesium therapy. A 250-ml bolus containing 20 g of magnesium sulfate administered to an adult over 15 minutes induced respiratory arrest, hypotension, bradycardia, and QRS and QT prolongation.[9] Errors in administration of IV magnesium (50-ml vial of 50% magnesium sulfate instead of 2 ml of 50% solution) may rapidly induce signs and symptoms associated with hypermagnesemia.[10]

Clinical Manifestations

Biochemical

The plasma magnesium concentration usually exceeds 4 mEq/liter (2 mmol/L) before any signs or symptoms of magnesium excess appear. Parenteral administration of magnesium lowers plasma calcium concentrations in both normal and hypoparathyroid patients. The anion gap may be unchanged.[11] The osmolal gap can be increased.[12]

Neuromuscular

Excess magnesium decreases impulse transmission across the neuromuscular junction. At blood levels of 4 mEq/liter (2 mmol/L) a decrease or disappearance of deep tendon reflexes appears. Somnolence is observed at levels of 4 to 7 mEq/liter (2 to 3.5 mmol/L) and flaccid paralysis of voluntary muscles at 10 mEq/liter (5 mmol/L) or greater. This may lead to impairment of respiratory function and apnea, an effect that is antagonized by calcium. When the deep tendon reflexes are absent, respiration must be closely monitored.

Cardiovascular

Bradycardia and hypotension due to the direct vasodilator and ganglionic blocker effect of magnesium on peripheral arteries and arterioles may be observed at plasma levels of 4 to 5 mEq/liter (2 to 2.5 mmol/L). At plasma magnesium concentrations of 5 to 10 mEq/liter (2.5 to 5 mmol/L) the PR, QRS, and QT intervals may increase. Complete heart block and cardiac arrest in asystole may occur at levels of 15 mEq/liter (7.5 mmol/L) or greater.[2]

Cardiopulmonary arrest with coma, nonreactive pupils, flaccid extremities, loss of deep tendon reflexes, and no response to painful stimulus may be observed early after magnesium overdose.[13]

In normal humans 4 g of magnesium sulfate diluted in 20 mL of 5% glucose given intravenously appears to increase cardiac output and heart rate and produce a decrease in systolic arterial pressure and systemic vascular resistance. This is accompanied by a vasodilation of the coronary arteriolar bed.[14] Parenteral magnesium sulfate appears to prolong conduction through the sinoatrial and atrioventricular nodal tissues; it also increases AV nodal refractoriness in normal humans and may be useful in the treatment of paroxysmal atrial fibrillation with a rapid response.[14,15]

For torsades de pointes—single or multiple doses of magnesium sulfate 2 g IV over 1 to 2 minutes followed by a continuous IV infusion of 3 to 20 mg Mg/minute have been useful in terminating this arrhythmia.[16,17] For preeclampsia (as an anticonvulsant): 4.0 g IV loading dose and 1.0 to 2.0 g/hour has been used.

TREATMENT

1. Discontinue administration of magnesium.
2. Eliminate magnesium by enema if it is in the bowel.
3. Activated charcoal does not absorb magnesium salts.
4. Monitor serum electrolytes, calcium, phosphorus, renal function, fluid intake, urinary output, and electrocardiogram.
5. Intravenous lines, oxygen, and cardiac monitor must be available.
6. If patient is symptomatic (hypotonic, central nervous system depression) and has electrocardiographic changes and a serum magnesium level over 2.9 mg/dL (2.3 mEq/L or 1.1 mmol/L), begin therapy.[18]
7. Therapy with calcium gluconate 10% is administered intravenously, 10 to 20 ml in adults; 100 mg/kg in infants and children up to a maximum of 1 g slowly over 5 to 10 minutes with electrocardiographic monitoring. This may reverse hypotension and paralysis. Give calcium in the presence of severe hypermagnesemia even if total serum calcium levels are normal.
8. If renal function is normal, intravenous furosemide (40 mg, adults, 1 mg/kg infants and children) may be administered as alternate therapy with replacement of urine volume by 0.89% to 0.90% saline. Forced diuresis with mannitol (25 g by rapid IV infusion) has also been useful.[9]
9. Dialysis may be useful and exchange transfusion has been instituted in a neonate with severe magnesium intoxication.
10. Aminoglycosides should not be used since they may potentiate the neuromuscular blockade of magnesium.[19]
11. Pacemaker therapy may be useful.

REFERENCES—HYPERMAGNESEMIA

1. Mordes JP, Wacker WEC. Excess magnesium. Pharmacological Reviews 1978;29:273–300.
2. Rude RK, Singer FR. Magnesium deficiency and excess. Ann Rev Med 1981;32:245–259.
3. Humphrey M, Kennon S, Pramanik AK. Hypermagnesemia from antacid administration in a newborn infant. J Pediatr 1981;98:313–314.
4. Mofenson HC, Caraccio TR. Magnesium intoxication in a neonate from oral magnesium hydroxide laxative. Clin Toxicol 1991;29:215–222.
5. Jones J, Heiselman D, Dougherty J, Eddy A. Cathartic-induced magnesium toxicity during overdose management. Ann Emerg Med 1986;15:1214–1218.
6. Smilkstein MJ, Smolinske SC, Kulig KW, Rumack BH. Severe hypermagnesemia due to multiple dose cathartic therapy. West J Med 1988;148:208–211.
7. Woodard JA, Shannon M, LaCouture PG, Woolf A. Serum magnesium concentrations after repetitive magnesium cathartic administration. Am J Emerg Med 1990;297–300.
8. Fine KD, Santa Ana CA, Fordtran JS. Diagnosis of magnesium induced diarrhea. N Engl J Med 1991;324:1012–1017.
9. Bohman VR, Cotton DB. Supralethal magnesemia with patient survival. Obstet Gynecol 1990;76:984–986.
10. Hoffman RS, Smilkstein MJ, Rubenstein F. An "amp" by any other name. The hazards of intravenous magnesium dosing. JAMA 1989;261:557.
11. Ortiz-Interian CJ, Schlessinger FB, Oster JR. Severe hypermagnesemia without reduction in the anion gap. Magnesium Trace Elem 1991;9:110–114.
12. Gerard SK, Hernandez C, Khayam-Bashi H. Extreme hypermagnesemia caused by an overdose of magnesium-containing cathartics. Ann Emerg Med 1988;17:728–731.
13. McCubbin JH, Sibai BM, Abdella TN, Anderson GD. Cardiopulmonary arrest due to acute maternal hypermagnesemia. Lancet 1981;1:1058.
14. Vigorito C, Giordano A, Ferraro P, Acanfora D, Ce Caprio L, Naddes C et al. Hemodynamic effects of magnesium sulfate on the normal human heart. Am J Cardiol 1991;67:1435–1437.
15. Kulick DL, Hong R, Ryzen E, Rude RK, Rubin JN, Elkayan U et al. Electrophysiologic effects of intravenous magnesium in patients with normal conduction system and no clinical evidence of significant cardiac disease. Am Heart J 1988;115:367–373.
16. Tsivoni D, Banai S, Schuger C et al. Treatment of torsades de pointes with magnesium sulfate. Circulation 1988;77:392–397.
17. Tsivoni D, Keren A, Cohen AM et al. Magnesium therapy for torsade de pointes. Am J Cardiol 1984;53:528–530.
18. Tsang RC. Neonatal magnesium disturbances. Am J Dis Child 1972;124:282.
19. L'Hommedieu CS, Nicholas N, Armes DA. Potentiation of magnesium sulfate-induced neuromuscular weakness by gentamicin, tobramycin and amikacin. J Pediatr 1983;102:629–631.

SALT (SODIUM CHLORIDE)

CAUSES OF SALT POISONING

Hypernatremia may follow amniotic fluid embolism during a saline-induced abortion.[1,2] The most severe hypernatremia in adults has been seen as a result of salt emetics,[3] bicarbonate administration during cardiac arrest,[4] saline abortion,[2] and accidental or voluntary ingestion of salt[5–7] (Table 52–34).

A relatively small quantity of salt (1 or 2 tablespoons) may produce a profound hypernatremia and rapidly progressive and fatal clinical course in the pediatric population. Prior case reports of salt poisoning in the literature have demonstrated lethal dosages as low as 0.75 g/kg body weight,[5] but have generally been estimated to be 3 g/kg body weight.[8]

PATHOPHYSIOLOGY

Survival Risk Factors

A review of published reports on hypernatremia from exogenous sodium[12] revealed improved chances of survival were associated with (a) younger age and (b) lower initial serum sodium levels (severe—160 to 179 mEq/L; very

Table 52-34
Causes of Hypernatremia [a]

Loss of water in excess of sodium
- through the gastrointestinal tract
  - infantile diarrhea and vomiting
- through the kidney
  - chronic renal failure
  - diabetes insipidus
- through the skin
  - fever
  - heat stroke—environmental heat loss
- through the lungs
  - overventilation
  - fever
- iatrogenic
  - excessive removal of water by peritoneal dialysis or hemodialysis, by the infusion of hyperosmolar solutions, e.g., urea, mannitol.

Failure to replace water loss
- interference with water intake by nausea, vomiting
- stuporose or comatose patients
- physical disability, e.g. stroke, fracture, old age or infancy
- inability to swallow
- adipsia

Administration of excess solute
- high intake of protein supplements
- "salt poisoning," accidental substitution of salt for sugar in infants' feeds
- infusion of mannitol, urea

Steroid excess
- cortisol
  - Cushing's syndrome
- aldosterone
  - Conn's syndrome

[a]Adapted from Ross EJ, Christie SB. Medicine 1969;48:441–473.

severe—180 to 199 mEq/L; extreme—more than 200 mEq/L). Factors such as the type of fluid therapy (5% dextrose in water, 0.09% sodium chloride) and the rate of correction of the hypernatremia did not influence mortality. The use of peritoneal dialysis also did not seem to improve survival.[9]

LABORATORY

In a study of elderly patients with hypernatremia, patients with a peak serum sodium >100 mEq/L were rarely alert (10%), although only 31% were alert with severe sodium concentrations of 148 to 160 mEq/L. In diabetic patients without ketoacidosis, symptoms generally appeared when the plasma osmolality exceeded 330 to 340 mOsm/kg, while coma occurred at >380 mOsm/kg.[10]

In most reports of severe hypernatremia due to salt or hypertonic saline intake, no patients with serum sodium levels over 170 mmol/L have survived.[11] The mortality rate among adult patients with serum sodium levels over 160 mmol/L is 60%.[12] Even in those who survived, severe central nervous system sequelae occurred. An 85-year-old man who ingested salt presented with an initial serum sodium level of 193 mmol/liter and survived without major sequelae.[11] He was treated with 5% dextrose intravenously (at 150 mL/hr) for 48 hours with furosemide 20 mg. Death can be expected from severe osmolality values between 400 and 500 mOsm/kg.[13]

A mother estimates that her 3-year-old, 30 pound (13.6-kg) child ingested a tablespoon of salt (14.5 to 21.75 grams). (A teaspoon of salt weighs 7.25 grams); a teaspoon of sodium bicarbonate contains 41.8 mg of sodium; a tablespoon contains 125.4 mEq sodium; molecular weight of sodium bicarbonate is 84. Then the serum sodium may increase by

$$\frac{\text{Ingested dose (mg)}}{\text{m.w. NaCl}} = \frac{21{,}750\ \text{mg}}{58} = 375\ \text{mEq sodium}$$

$$\frac{\text{mEq sodium}}{\text{Wt (kg)} \times V_D} = \frac{375}{13.6\ \text{kg} \times V_D} (= 0.6\ \text{L/kg}) = 45\ \text{mEq/liter}$$

This child's serum sodium can potentially increase by 45 mEq/L. The serum sodium can then be elevated to 180 to 190 mEq/L. At 185 mEq/L death may ensue.

TREATMENT

The exact rate at which hypernatremia should be corrected is unknown.[14] Star[14] recounts that plasma sodium be lowered to normal gradually over 48 to 72 hours. Typically, half the deficit is replaced over the first 12 to 24 hours. The remaining deficit is replaced over the second 24- to 48-hour period. Slower rates are recommended in elderly patients: half the deficit should be replaced over 24 hours.[11] Suggested rates of decrease of plasma Na range from 0.5 mEq/hr in chronic hypernatremia to 2 mEq/hr in acute hypernatremia, but many suggest ≤ 1 mEq/hr.[13,14] Faster may be tolerated in hyperacute hypernatremia but cannot be recommended.[14] Thc amount of water that needs to be replaced can be approximated by using the formula:

$$\text{Water deficit} = 0.5\ \text{body weight}\ \frac{(1-140)^9}{\text{Na}}$$

Hemofilters have been developed that are suitable for use in infants and children. Continuous arteriovenous hemodiafiltration may be a useful alternative in the management of hypernatremia, particularly in the presence of renal failure. The rate of fall in plasma sodium concentration is regulated by the judicious selection of the sodium concentration of dialysate and maintenance and replacement fluids.[15]

REFERENCES—SALT POISONING

1. Mirchandani HG, Mirchandani IH, Parith SR. Hypernatremia due to amniotic fluid embolism during a saline-induced abortion. Am J Forensic Med Pathol 1988;9:48–50.
2. De Villota EJ, Cavamilles JM, Stein L, Shubin H, Weil MH. Hyperosmolar crisis following infusion of hypertonic sodium chloride. Am J Med 1973;55:116–122.
3. Winter M, Taylor DJ. Danger of saline emetics in first aid for poisoning. Br Med J 1974;3:802.
4. Mattar JA, Weil MH, Shubin H, Stein L. Cardiac arrest in the critically ill. II. Hyperosmolar states following cardiac arrest. Am J Med 1974;56:162–168.
5. Johnston GG, Robertson WW. Fatal ingestion of table salt by an adult. West J Med 1977;126:141–143.
6. Addleman M, Pollard A, Grossman RF. Survival after severe hypernatremia due to salt ingestion by an adult. Am J Med 1985;78:176–178.

7. Raya A, Giner P, Aranequi P, Guerrero F, Vazquez G. Fatal acute hypernatremia caused by massive intake of salt. Arch Intern Med 1992;152:640–646.
8. Smith EJ, Palevsky S. Salt poisoning in a 2-year-old child. Am J Emerg Med 1990;8:571–582.
9. Moder KG. Fatal hypernatremia from exogenous salt intake: report on a case and review of the literature. Mayo Clin Proc 1990;65:1581–1594.
10. Aerif AP, Carroll HJ. Cerebral edema and depression of sensorium in nonketotic hyperosmolar coma. Diabetes 1974; 23:525–531.
11. Snyder NA, Feigal NW, Arreff AI. Hypernatremia in elderly patients. A heterogenous morbid and iatrogenic entity. Ann Intern Med 1987;107:309–319.
12. Elisaf M, Litou H, Siamopoulos KS. Survival after severe iatrogenic hypernatremia. Am J Kidney Dis 1989;14:230–231.
13. Cassorla FG, Gill JR Jr, Gold PW, Rosen SW. Nosocomial hypernatremia. N Engl J Med 1985;313:229.
14. Star MA. Southwestern Internal Medicine Conference. Hyperosmolar states. Am J Med Sci 1990;300:402–420.
15. Moss GD, Primavesi RJ, McGraw ME, Chambers TL. Correction of hypernatremia with continuous arteriovenous haemodiafiltration. Arch Dis Child 1990;65:628–630.

TAMPERING (TABLES 52–35 AND 52–36)

The deliberate introduction of dangerous substances into medicines and other consumer products has led to a number of deaths.

Table 52–35
Tampering Cases—Summary

Date	Chemical Introduced	Product Involved	Injury
1982	Cyanide	Extra-Strength Tylenol	7 deaths[1,2,3]
2/1986	Cyanide	Extra-Strength Tylenol	1 death[4]
	(or CardoEl)	Tylenol capsules	——[4]
6/1986	Cyanide (Seattle)	Extra-Strength Excedrin	2 deaths[4]
1/1989	Cyanide	Breyers Black Cherry Yogurt	17 yr F, Coma
1989	Cyanide?	Chilean fruit	?Hoax[5]
1/91	Cyanide	Sudafed	2 deaths[6,7,8]
1991	Glass slivers	Baby food	none[9]
1991	PCP	Nestle's Sweetened Condensed Milk (La Lechera)	2 children hospitalized[10]
1991	Cyanide	Sudafed—12 hour capsule	1 wan -ill[11,12]
1991	Beta-propiolactone	Nasal Spray	Local pain, stinging (recovery)[13]

[1]Logan B. Product tampering crime: a review. J Forensic Sci 1993;38:918–927.
[2]Wolnik KA, Riche FL, Bonnin E, Gastron CM, Satzger RD. The tylenol tampering incident—tracing the source. Anal Chem 1984;56:466A–474A.
[3]Gates TN. McNeil Consumer Products Co. Dear Doctor Letter. October 8, 1982.
[4]CDC. Cyanide poisoning associated with over-the-counter medication—Washington State, 1991. MMWR 1991;40:161–168.
[5]Lifshultz BD, Donoghue ER. The tylenol cyanide poisoning. Am Acad Forensic Sci, Las Vegas, Nev. February 15, 1989.
[6]Tracy PR. Burroughs Wellcome Co. Dear Doctor Letter. March, 1990.
[7]Modeland V. Ninety-year prison term in tampering deaths. FDA Consumer 1988;22(8):34–35.
[8]Brahams D. "Sudafed" capsules poisoned with cyanide. Lancet 1991;337:968.
[9]Cyanide yogurt case still puzzles officials. New York Times, January 5, 1989.
[10]Tamperer sentenced. FDA Consumer 1991;25(7):4.
[11]Tainted milk prompts a recall. New York Times, March 15, 1991.
[12]Grigg B, Modeland V. The cyanide scare. A tale of two grapes. FDA Consumer 1989;23(6):7–11.
[13]Drug tampering suspected in illness of Hawaiian. New York Times, March 11, 1991.

Table 52–36
Things To Remember

1. In multiple deaths, search for a common denominator.
2. As a general rule, if two or more individuals are found sick or dead, in a house or motor vehicle, without signs of violence, the most probable cause is carbon monoxide intoxication.
3. Only two commonly available ingestible poisons are capable of causing very rapid collapse and death: cyanide and nicotine.
4. Cyanide exerts its toxic effect by blocking the action of the enzyme cytochrome oxidase, which prevents the utilization of oxygen by cells. Cyanide is a chemical asphyxiant.
5. Cyanide has a characteristic pungent, bitter-almond aroma. Unfortunately, a large percentage of the population cannot smell cyanide.
6. Important clinical signs facilitating the rapid diagnosis of cyanide poisoning include a bitter-almond odor on the breath of the victim, alkaline gastric contents, metabolic acidosis, and elevated oxygen partial pressure in venous blood.
7. Autopsy findings in cyanide poisoning by ingestion include red lividity in the skin, bitter-almond odor over body and organs, hemorrhagic gastritis, and congestive organs.
8. All autopsy findings may not be present in an individual case. Cases of cyanide ingestion without hemorrhagic gastritis have been reported. The most reliable and specific finding is probably the bitter-almond odor.
9. Large volume testing of recalled drugs for cyanide contamination may be accomplished using Cyantesmo strips manufactured by Machery-Nagel in West Germany. This method of examination requires opening of tamper-resistant packaging and allows possible destruction of fingerprint evidence.
10. Certain types of cyanide are radioopaque. If capsule contamination by these types of cyanide is suspected, recall testing may be done by x-ray or fluoroscopic examination. X-ray and fluoroscopic examination leave tamper-resistant packaging intact and allow preservation of fingerprint evidence.
11. The combination of capsules and off-the-shelf marketing made the product-tampering cases discussed here possible. Tamper-resistant packaging has proven to be no safeguard. As long as capsules are available, the potential for further tampering cases exists.

Publications advocating the use of product tampering and other poisoning methods as techniques for exacting revenge against individuals and corporations, as methods of committing murder, and for other criminal purposes have been reviewed by Dietz.[1] An attempt to monitor the integrity of pediatric parenteral nutrient solutions for controlled substances has been proposed.[2]

Packaging methods recognized by the US Food and Drug Administration provide a barrier to entry or leave an indication when opened.[3]

PREVENTION[4-16]

Suggestions on alerting the public for signs of tampering have been proposed.[17,18] Lifshultz and Donoghue of the Cook County, Illinois Medical Examiner's office have offered suggestions for consideration of cyanide contamination in tampering cases.[10]

REFERENCES—TAMPERING

1. Dietz PE. Dangerous information. Product tampering and poisoning advice on revenge and murder manuals. J Forensic Sci 1988;33:1201-1217.
2. Cheung JF, Chong S, Kitrenos GG, Fung HL. Use of refractometers to detect control substances tampering. Am J Hosp Pharm 1991;48:1488-1492.
3. Logan B. Product tampering crime: A review. J Forens Sci 1993;38:918-927.
4. Wolnik KA, Riche FL, Bonnin E, Gastron CM, Satzger RD. The tylenol tampering incident - tracing the source. Anal Chem 1984;56:466A-474A.
5. Gates TN. McNeil Consumer Products Company Dear Doctor Letter. October 8, 1982.
6. Tracy PR. Burroughs Wellcome Company Dear Doctor Letter. March, 1990.
7. Modeland V. Ninety year prison term in tampering deaths. FDA Consumer 1988;22(8):34-35.
8. Brahams D. "Sudafed" capsules poisoned with cyanide. Lancet 1991;337:968.
9. CDC. Cyanide poisoning associated with over-the-counter medication—Washington State, 1991. MMWR 1991;40:161-168.
10. Lifshultz BD, Donoghue ER. The tylenol cyanide poisoning. Am Acad Sci, Las Vegas, NV. February 15, 1989.
11. Cyanide yogurt case still puzzles officials. New York Times, January 5, 1989.
12. Tamperer sentenced. FDA Consumer 1991;25(7):4.
13. Tainted milk prompts a recall. New York Times, March 15, 1991.
14. Grigg B, Modeland V. The cyanide scare. A tale of two grapes. FDA Consumer 1989;23(6):7-11.
15. Drug tampering suspected in illness of Hawaiian. New York Times, March 11, 1991.
16. Scientist accused of spiking spray in attempt to kill Texas colleague. New York Times, May 4, 1991.
17. Cramer T. Look twice. How to protect yourself against drug tampering. FDA Consumer 1991;25(8):20-23.
18. Tips against tampering. Office of Public Affairs. The Proprietary Association, Washington, DC 20056.

L-TRYPTOPHAN AND THE EOSINOPHILIA–MYALGIA SYNDROME

Tryptophan has been available in the United States since about 1974 as a dietary supplement without prescription. It was a popular remedy for insomnia, the premenstrual syndrome, depression, or loss of weight. Average patient dose of tryptophan ranged from 1 to 5 grams/day. In comparison single servings of meat, fish, poultry and some cheeses contain more than 200 mg of tryptophan.[1]

HISTORY

In 1974 diffuse fasciitis with eosinophilia was first described.[2] Some patients may have had the eosinophilia-myalgia syndrome before 1989.[3]

In October 1989 three patients presented with an unexplained acute illness characterized by intense myalgia and eosinophilia. A nationwide outbreak of the disease, termed the eosinophilia–myalgia syndrome, was subsequently recognized. Case-control studies confirmed an unequivocal epidemiologic association between the eosinophilia-myalgia syndrome and the use of L-tryptophan-containing products. Despite the discontinuation of L-tryptophan use, a substantial proportion of patients developed a protracted course dominated by

Table 52-37
Clinical Features of Patients With the Eosinophilia Myalgia Syndrome[7-18]

Symptoms	
Myalgias	Paresthesias
Fatigue	Hair loss
Edema	Muscle cramping
Extremities	Cough
Facial	Diarrhea
Dysesthesias, peripheral	Arthralgia
Dyspnea on exertion	Acute respiratory failure due to pulmonary vasculitis[19-21]
Weight loss	
Low-grade fever	
Signs	
Muscle tenderness	Scleroderma-like skin changes
Skin rashes (diffuse reticular)	Flexion contractures of joints
Edema of extremities	Decreased vibratory perception
Muscle atrophy	Cognitive deficits
Muscle weakness	Malaise
Repeated coronary artery spasm[22]	Fever
Acute eosinophilic pulmonary disease[21,23-25]	Raynaud's phenomenon
	Itching
Occasional hepatomegaly[13]	Peripheral neuropathy[26-31]
Cardiomyopathy	Pancreatitis[32]
Laboratory	
Eosinophilia	Elevated serum aldolase
(Creatine kinase normal) or slightly elevated	Arterial blood gas hypoxia
Chest x-ray	
Pleural effusions[21,25]	Diffuse interstitial infiltrates
Unilateral lower lobe interstitial infiltrates	
Electrocardiogram	
Minor ventricular conduction delays	
Electromyogram	
Myopathy	Peripheral neuropathy
Muscle biopsy[32]	
Minor myositic changes	Perivascular lymphocytes, monocytes, and eosinophil infiltrate
Pulmonary function test abnormalities[32-34]	
MRI scan	Multiple white matter lesions[27]
Chronic long-term disability due to polyneuropathy, scleroderma	

Table 52-38
CDC Diagnostic Criteria for EMS Syndrome

1. Eosinophil count equal to or greater than 1000 cells/mm^3.
2. Generalized myalgias of severity sufficient to affect a patient's ability to pursue his or her daily activities.
3. Plus one or more of the following:
   a. Exclusion of trichinosis by serologic tests performed at an appropriate interval after onset of symptoms (no longer required).
   b. A muscle biopsy specimen that does not show Trichinella larva but does show an inflammatory infiltrate including eosinophil.
   c. Absence of any infection or neoplasm that could account for eosinophilia or generalized myalgias.[16]

Table 52-39
Clinical Stages of the Eosinophilia Myalgia Syndrome[5]

Early (1–2 months)	Intermediate (2–6 months)	Late (>6 months)
Myalgia	Mylagia	Myalgia
Fever	Eosinophilic fasciitis	Sclerodermatous induration
Weight loss	Mucinous papules	Myopathy
Edema	Myopathy	Neuropathy
Pulmonary infiltrates	Neuropathy	Cytopenia
Hyperesthesia	Myocarditis	Pulmonary hypertension
Paresthesia	Xerostomia	Arthralgia
Xerostomia	Alopecia	Fatigue
Arthralgia	Arthralgia	
Arthritis	Fatigue	
Fatigue		

manifestations of cutaneous and neuromuscular involvement. By August 1992, 1571 cases of the eosinophilia–myalgia syndrome had been reported to the Centers for Disease Control (CDC), and it was suggested that the actual number may be considerably higher. Eighty-five percent of the affected patients developed symptoms between July 1989 and February 1990. One-third of the patients required hospitalization, and 38 deaths from neurologic, cardiac, and pulmonary complications, in addition to secondary infection attributable to the eosinophilia–myalgia syndrome, have been reported (Table 52–37).

The CDC diagnostic criteria for the eosinophilia–myalgia syndrome are summarized in Table 52–38.

Leukocytosis, thrombocytosis, eosinophilia, mild basophilia, and absent stainable neutrophil alkaline phosphatase suggesting a diagnosis of chronic myelogenous leukemia have been observed in the eosinophilia–myalgia syndrome.[4]

Clinical stages of the eosinophilia–myalgia syndrome are summarized in Table 52–39.[5]

Eighteen to 24 months after the onset of illness most symptoms and physical findings in most patients with eosinophilia–myalgia syndrome resolve or improve. Cognitive changes were reported to be worse in 32% of patients. Prednisone was helpful in the acute phase of illness. No treatment was clearly valuable in the management of the later phase of the syndrome.[6]

TOXIC OIL SYNDROME AND EOSINOPHILIA–MYALGIA SYNDROME

Similarities between the toxic oil syndrome (TOS) and the eosinophilia–myalgia syndrome (EMS) have been summarized by the WHO.[35]

CLINICAL ASPECTS

Similarities

1. The organs affected by TOS and EMS are similar: skin, muscles, lungs, nervous system, and fasciae. The early constitutional symptoms (such as malaise, fatigue, and fever) are also similar.
2. These two syndromes share special features: alopecia, pruritus, xerostomia, pulmonary hypertension, and cutaneous papules.
3. Similarities in laboratory results include marked eosinophilia, elevated aldolase with normal creatine phosphokinase, and x-ray findings of pulmonary interstitial infiltrates.
4. The two syndromes have evolved, to date, similarly over time. In addition, the differences between TOS and EMS in the early stages tend to disappear in the later stages.
5. Both syndromes show a similar pattern of cutaneous and deep tissue involvement, although the severity may vary.
6. The thromboembolic phenomena described in TOS have not been commonly reported in EMS, although unpublished data from a cohort study conducted in South Carolina suggest a similar prevalence in both syndromes.

Differences

1. Early and often severe lung involvement is virtually universal in TOS, but is less prevalent and/or less severe in EMS.
2. The early elevation of immunoglobulin E (IgE) levels in about 50% of TOS cases is generally not seen in EMS cases.
3. The two syndromes affected different populations. This reflects different exposure patterns to the toxic agents, particularly in relation to socioeconomic class, gender, and age.
4. The hyperglycemia and elevated levels of tryglyceride found in the intermediate state of TOS have not been reported in EMS.

PATHOLOGY

1. The syndromes have major similarities: vascular changes, pulmonary changes, skin pathology, skeletal muscular lesions, peripheral nerve changes, and cardiac abnormalities.
2. The pathologic lesions in TOS, however, are much more severe than in EMS, which may indicate that the etiologic agent in TOS was more potent or that its cation was more extensive and/or intensive than that of EMS.
3. Over time and with further examination, the more chronic changes seen in TOS may be found in EMS.

4. The volume and type of material available for pathologic study are currently much greater for TOS than for EMS. This difference is related to the relative size of the epidemics, the distribution of affected people, the greater availability of autopsy material for TOS, and the longer period of observation of TOS patients.

IMMUNOLOGY

1. Two significant points of similarity were noted: eosinophilia was a prominent component in both syndromes; and blood levels of eosinophil granule major basic proteins were elevated in both syndromes.
2. The following important differences were reported: IgE levels were elevated early in the development of TOS, but not in EMS; several types of autoantibodies were common in TOS, but an elevated prevalence has not been reported in EMS, basophils were decreased in TOS, but not in EMS, a modest elevation of complement components was reported in some TOS patients, but not in EMS patients; decreased numbers of $CD8^+$ T cells were found in TOS patients, but have not been reported in EMS patients; and possible human leucocyte antigen predisposition was described in late manifestations of TOS, but comparable data on EMS are not available.

DIFFERENTIAL DIAGNOSIS

Drugs and chemicals associated with the production of eosinophilia, fibrosing disorders, and scleroderma-like syndromes are summarized in Tables 52–40, 52–41, and 52–42. The differential diagnosis of the combination of eosinophilia and musculoskeletal pain is found in Table 52–43.

Table 52–40
Fibrosing Disorders Induced by Chemical Agents and Drugs[36]

Tryptophan metabolites
5-Hydroxytryptamine
Kynurenine
Anilides
Polyvinyl chloride
Methysergide (a 5-hydroxytryptophan antagonist)
Bleomycin
Practolol

Table 52–41
Causes of Scleroderma-like Syndromes[37,38]

Vinyl chloride
Pentazocine
Bleomycin
5-Hydroxytryptophan
Trichlorethylene
Toxic oil syndrome
Breast augmentation neoplasm (silicone leakage)

PREGNANCY

In pregnant women, hypersensitivity or toxicity to prescription or nonprescription medications, including L-tryptophan, should be considered in the differential diagnosis of maternal eosinophilia. This may result in eosinophilia in their newborns.[39] In one patient who had ingested two 500 mg tablets of L-tryptophan daily from the fourth month of gestation until delivery, a full-term live infant was delivered with an eosinophilia and no other remarkable symptoms.[40]

PEAK "E"

A single high-performance liquid chromatographic peak was most predictive of L-tryptophan lots associated with eosinophilia–myalgia syndrome cases.[41–43] The contaminant present in "peak E" was isolated, purified, and shown to be 1,1'-ethylidenebis [tryptophan], a novel amino acid comprising two L-tryptophan molecules joined into a dimeric compound by an ethylidene bridge between the two indole ring nitrogens.[3] This product may be involved in the pathogenesis of EMS through an interleukin-5 mediated mechanism.[44,45]

Up to 5% of EMS cases have not been definitely linked to Showa Denka's product. At least 10 cases of EMS-like illnesses have been related to L-5-hydroxytryptophan, a related compound produced from botanical sources.

PEAK UV-5 (PAA)

In 1991 investigators in Japan reported the discovery of a second trace contaminant in L-tryptophan; peak UV-5.[46] Mayeno and associates found a peak for UV-5-3 (phenylamine) alanine (PAA).[47] There is a structural similarity between PAA and the 3-phenylamino 1,2 propanediol impurity that was found in implicated rapeseed oil from Spain and that was isolated from samples of oil consumed by persons in whom the toxic oil syndrome developed. This raises the possibility that eosinophilia–myalgia syndrome and toxic oil syndrome have a common etiologic trigger.[48]

Table 52–42
Drug-Induced Eosinophilia[36]

Antiinflammatory Agents	Opiates
Arsenicals	Gold Salts
Tricyclics	Hydralazine
Antibiotics	Chlorpropamide
Phenothiazines	Phenytoin
Sulfa drugs	Quinidine

Table 52–43
Eosinophilia and Musculoskeletal Pain[4]

Trichinosis
Eosinophilic fasciitis
Chung-Strauss Syndrome
Eosinophilic myositis
Hypereosinophilic syndrome
Toxic oil syndrome

TREATMENT

Some patients experience a gradual spontaneous improvement of symptoms. Corticosteroids have been used (with the return of eosinophils to normal being controversial[49] and with some clinical recovery in the resolution of pulmonary symptoms).[31] Plasma exchange, IV methotrexate, and hydroxychloroquine have been used in a limited number of severely ill patients, and conclusions cannot be made on their efficacy. Nonsteroidal antiinflammatory drugs (cyclosporine, azathioprine, and penicillamine)[50] and steroids have not been associated with long-term improvement in symptoms.[48] Prednisone 10 to 100 mg/d may relieve myalgia, pulmonary manifestation, and cutaneous involvement in some patients. Exacerbation of myalgia may occur when prednisone therapy is tapered or discontinued. Cyproheptadine has been successful in relieving muscle cramps in some patients.

REFERENCES—TRYPTOPHAN

1. Broide DH. Eosinophilia-myalgia syndrome. West J Med 1991;154:459.
2. Shulman LE. Diffuse fasciitis with eosinophilia: a new syndrome? Trans Assoc Am Physicians 1975;88:70–86.
3. Varga J, Uitto J, Jimenez SA. The cause and pathogenesis of the eosinophilia-myalgia syndrome. Ann Intern Med 1992; 116:140–147.
4. Jaffe I, Kopelman R, Baird R, Grossman M, Hays A. Eosinophilic fasciitis associated with the eosinophilia-myalgia syndrome. Am J Med 1990;88:542–546.
5. Kaufman LD, Gruber BL, Gregersen PK. Clinical follow-up and immunogenetic studies of 32 patients with eosinophilia-myalgia syndrome. Lancet 1991;337:1071–1074.
6. Hertzman PA, Clauw DJ, Kaufman LD, Varga J, Silver RM, Thacker HL et al. The eosinophilia-myalgia syndrome: status of 205 patients and results of treatment 2 years after onset. Ann Intern Med 1995;122:851–855.
7. Naeyaert JM, Cuelenaere C, De Bersaques J, Platevoet D, Kint A. A Belgian case of the eosinophilia-myalgia syndrome. Br J Dermatol 1991;124:303–305.
8. Martin R et al. Eosinophilia-myalgia syndrome associated with L-tryptophan ingestion. Clin Res 1990;38:318.
9. Silver RM, Heyes MP, Maize JC, Quearry B, Vionnet-Fuasset M, Sternberg EM. Scleroderma, fasciitis and eosinophilia associated with the ingestion of tryptophan. N Engl J Med 1990;322:874–881.
10. Troy JL. Eosinophilia-myalgia syndrome. Mayo Clin Proc 1991;66:535–538.
11. Saag KG, Goldschmidt R, Vernof H, Golbus J. An eosinophilia-myalgia syndrome associated with an L-tryptophan–containing product. J Rheumatol 1990;17:1551–1553.
12. Kilbourne EM, Swygert LA, Philen RM, Sun RK, Auerbach SB et al. Interim guidance on the eosinophilia-myalgia syndrome. Ann Intern Med 1990;112:85–87.
13. Montanaro A, Wakefield D. Eosinophilia-myalgia syndrome associated with L-tryptophan use. Med J Austral 1990; 153:491–493.
14. Gibbons RB, Metzger JR. Eosinophilia-myalgia syndrome. Arch Intern Med 1990;150:2175–2177.
15. Hertzman P, Falk H, Kilbourne EM, Page S, Shulman LE. The eosinophilia myalgia syndrome: the Los Alamos Conference. J Rheumatol 1991;18:867–873.
16. Update. Analysis of L-tryptophan for the etiology of eosinophilia-myalgia syndrome. MMWR 1990;39(43):789–790.
17. Lewkonia RM. Myalgia and eosinophilia associated with ingestion of tryptophan. An intriguing new syndrome. Arch Intern Med 1990;150:2005–2007.
18. Hedberg K, Urbach D, Slutsker L, Matson P, Fleming D. Eosinophilia-myalgia syndrome. Natural history in a population-based cohort. Arch Intern Med 1992;152:1889–1892.
19. Banner AS, Borochovitz D. Acute respiratory failure caused by pulmonary vasculitis after L-tryptophan ingestion. Am Rev Respir Dis 1991;143:661–664.
20. Strumpf IJ, Drucker RD, Anders KH, Cohen S, Fajolu O. Acute eosinophilic pulmonary disease associated with ingestion of L-tryptophan–containing products. Chest 1991;99: 8–13.
21. Campagna AC, Blanc PD, Criswell LA, Clarke D, Sach A-E, Gold WM, Golden JA. Pulmonary manifestations of the eosinophilia-myalgia syndrome associated with tryptophan ingestion. Chest 1992;101:1274–1278.
22. Hertzman PA, Maddoux GL, Sternberg EM, Heyes MP, Mefford IN, Kephart GM, Gleich GJ. Repeated coronary artery spasm in a young woman with the eosinophilia-myalgia syndrome. JAMA 1992;267:2932–2934.
23. Ivey M, Eichenhorn MS, Glasberg MR, Hyzy RC. Hypercapnic respiratory failure due to L-tryptophan–induced eosinophilic polymyositis. Chest 1991;99:756–757.
24. Tazelaar HD, Myers JL, Drage CW, King TE Jr, Aguayo S, Colby TV. Pulmonary disease associated with L-tryptophan–induced eosinophilic myalgia syndrome. Clinical and pathologic features. Chest 1990;97:1032–1036.
25. Read CA, Clauw D, Weir C, Da Silva AT, Katz P. Dyspnea and pulmonary function in the L-tryptophan–associated eosinophilia-myalgia syndrome. Chest 1992;101:1282–1286.
26. Tolander LM, Bamford CR, Yoshino MT, Downing S, Bryan G. Neurologic complications of the tryptophan-associated eosinophilia-myalgia syndrome. Arch Neurol 1991;48:436–438.
27. Tolander LM, Bamford CR. Central and peripheral nervous system involvement in the L-tryptophan–associated eosinophilia-myalgia syndrome. Intern J Neurosci 1991;61: 69–75.
28. Smith BE, Dyke PJ. Peripheral neuropathy in the eosinophilia-myalgia syndrome associated with L-tryptophan ingestion. Neurology 1990;40:1035–1040.
29. Dicker RM, James N, Cunha BA. The eosinophilia-myalgia syndrome with neuritis associated with L-tryptophan use. Ann Intern Med 1990;112:957–958.
30. Selwa JF, Feldman EL, Blaivas M. Mononeuropathy multiplex in tryptophan-associated eosinophilia-myalgia syndrome. Neurology 1990;40:1632–1633.
31. Heiman-Patterson TD, Bird SJ, Parry GJ, Varga J, Shy ME, Culligan NW, Edelsohn L et al. Peripheral neuropathy associated with eosinophilia-myalgia syndrome. Ann Neurol 1990; 28:269–270.
32. Chiba S, Miyagawa K, Tanaka T, Moriya K, Takahashi K, Hirai H, Takaku F. Tryptophan-associated eosinophilia-myalgia syndrome and pancreatitis. Lancet 1990;336:121.
33. Yakovlevitch M, Siegel M, Hoch DH, Rutlen DL. Pulmonary hypertension in a patient with tryptophan-induced eosinophilia-myalgia syndrome. Am J Med 1991;90:272–273.
34. Andre M, Canon JL, Levecque P, Dermine P, Mortiar C, Leveau F. Eosinophilia-myalgia syndrome associated with L-tryptophan. A case report with pulmonary manifestations and review of the literature. Acta Clin Belg 1991;46:278–282.
35. WHO. Toxic oil syndrome and eosinophilia-myalgia syndrome. Pursuing parallels in pathogenesis. Report on WHO meeting. Washington, DC, May 8-10, 1991.
36. Katz JD, Wakem CJ, Parke AL. L-tryptophan–associated eosinophilia-myalgia syndrome. J Rheumatol 1990;17:1559–1561.
37. Varga J, Peltonen J, Uitto J, Jimenez S. Development of diffuse fasciitis with eosinophilia during L-tryptophan treatment: demonstration of elevated type I collagen gene expression in affected tissues. A clinicopathologic study of four patients. Ann Intern Med 1990;112:344–351.
38. Sagman DL, Melamed JC. L-tryptophan–induced eosinophilia-myalgia syndrome and myopathy. Neurology 1990;40:1629–1630.
39. Hatch DL, Garona JE, Goldman LR, Waller KO. Persistent eosinophilia in an infant with probable intrauterine exposure to L-tryptophan–containing supplements. Pediatrics 1991; 88:810–813.

40. Winkelman RK, Connolly SM, Quimby SR, Griffing WL, Lie JT. Histopathologic features of the L-tryptophan-related eosinophilia-myalgia (fasciitis) syndrome. Mayo Clin Proc 1991;66:457–463.
41. Belongia EA, Hedberg CW, Gleich GJ, White KE, Mayeno AN, Loegering DA, Dunnette SL et al. An investigation of the cause of the eosinophilia-myalgia syndrome associated with tryptophan use. N Engl J Med 1990;323:357–365.
42. Werner-Felmayer G, Werner ER, Weiss G, Wachter H. Peak E contaminated L-tryptophan and immune activation. Lancet 1991;338:511.
43. Slutsker L, Hoesly FC, Miller L, Williams LP, Watson C, Fleming DW. Eosinophilia-myalgia syndrome associated with exposure to tryptophan from a single manufacturer. JAMA 1990;264:213–217.
44. Yamaoka KA, Miyasaka N, Kashiwazaki S. L-tryptophan contaminant "peak E" and interleukin-5 production from T cells. Lancet 1991;338:168.
45. Mayeno AN, Lin F, Foote CS et al. Characterization of "Peak E" a novel amino acid associated with eosinophilia-myalgia syndrome. Science 1990;150:1707–1708.
46. Duffy J. Eosinophilia-myalgia syndrome. Mayo Clin Proc 1992;67:1201–1202.
47. Mayeno AN, Belongia EA, Lin F, Lundy SK, Gleich GJ. 3-(phenylamino) alanine, a novel amiline-derived amino acid associated with the eosinophilia-myalgia syndrome. A link to the toxic oil syndrome? Mayo Clin Proc 1992;67: 1134–1139.
48. Milburn DS, Myers CW. Tryptophan toxicity: a pharmacoepidemiologic review of eosinophilia-myalgia syndrome. DICP Ann Pharmacother 1991;25:1259–1262.
49. Culpepper RC, Williams RG, Mease PJ, Koepsell TD, Kobayashi JM. Natural history of eosinophilia-myalgia syndrome. Ann Intern Med 1991;115:437–442.
50. Martinez-Osuna P, Espinoza LR. On the treatment of the eosinophilia-myalgia syndrome. Arch Intern Med 1991;151: 1239.

VITAMINS

Large overdoses of most water-soluble vitamins (pyridoxine, vitamin B_6, vitamin C, niacin, nicotinic acid) are readily excreted in the urine, yet have been associated with potentially toxic problems when taken for long periods.[1] Fat-soluble vitamins (A, D, E, and K) are stored in the tissues and therefore most likely to cause adverse effects when taken in excess.[2] There are no antidotes for vitamin overdosages.

REFERENCES—VITAMINS

1. Rudman D, William PJ. Megadose vitamins. Use and misuse. N Engl J Med 1983;309:488–489.
2. Toxic effects of vitamin overdosages. Med Lett Drugs Ther 1984;26(issue 667):73–74.

FAT-SOLUBLE VITAMINS
VITAMIN A (1,2)
CLINICAL PRESENTATION

A 28-year-old woman ingested 1.3 million units of vitamin A as a remedy for sunburn. She experienced nausea, vomiting, intense headache, and blurring of vision. Papilledema was noted on the physical examination. The symptoms gradually subsided over the next 3 days. Exfoliation began on the fourth day and lasted 2 weeks. The patient recovered.[3]

A 62-year-old male ingested 8 mL of a veterinary preparation containing 500,000 units/mL of vitamin A. Symptoms included nausea, severe headache, and blurring of vision. Exfoliation of the skin began on day 3. The patient recovered completely.[4]

CHRONIC TOXICITY

The lowest reported intakes causing toxicity have occurred in persons with liver function compromised by drugs, viral hepatitis, or protein-energy malnutrition. Especially vulnerable groups include children with adverse effects occurring with intakes as low as 1500 IU/kg/day and pregnant women with birth defects associated with maternal intakes as low as about 25,000 IU/day.[5]

Signs and symptoms of acute and chronic vitamin A toxicity are found in Tables 52–44 and 52–45.[6]

PREGNANCY

The association between vitamin A itself (as retinol or retinyl esters) and human teratogenicity is unclear.[7] The Teratology Society[8] has recommended the following actions:

Table 52–44
Signs and Symptoms of Acute Vitamin A Toxicity[a]

Children	Adults
Anorexia	Abdominal pain
Bulging fontanelles	Anorexia
Drowsiness	Blurred vision
Increased intracranial pressure	Drowsiness
Irritability	Headache
Vomiting	Hypercalcemia
	Irritability
	Muscle weakness
	Nausea, vomiting
	Peripheral neuritis
	Skin desquamation

[a]Adapted from Hathcock JN et al. Am J Clin Nutr 1990;52:183–202.

Table 52–45
Signs and Symptoms of Chronic Vitamin A Toxicity[a]

Children
Alopecia, anorexia, bone pain and tenderness, bulging of fontanelles, craniotabes, fissuring at lip corners, hepatomegaly, hyperostosis, premature epiphyseal closure, photophobia, pruritis, pseudotumor cerebri, skin desquamation, skin erythema
Adults
Alopecia, anemia, anorexia, ataxia, bone pain, bone abnormalities, brittle nails, cheilitis, conjunctivitis, diarrhea, diplopia, dryness of mucous membranes, dysuria, edema, elevated CSF pressure, epistaxis, exanthema, facial dermatitis, fatigue, fever, headache, hepatomegaly, hepatotoxicity, hyperostosis, insomnia, irritability, menstrual abnormalities, muscular stiffness and pain, nausea, negative nitrogen balance, nervous abnormalities, papilledema, petechiae, polydypsia, pruritis, pseudotumor cerebri, skin desquamation, skin erythema, skin rash, skin scaliness, splenomegaly, vomiting, weight loss

[a]Adapted from Hathcock JN et al. Am J Clin Nutr 1990;52:183–202.

1. Women in their reproductive years should be informed that the excessive use of vitamin A shortly before and during pregnancy could be harmful to their babies. (A bioaccumulation of vitamin A from continuous high doses is also a concern).
2. Manufacturers of vitamin A (as retinol or retinyl esters) should lower the maximum amount of vitamin A per unit dosage to 5000 and 8000 IU (1500 and 2400 retinol equivalents) and identify the source of the vitamin A.
3. The labeling of products containing vitamin A supplements (as retinol or retinyl esters) should indicate that consuming excessive amounts of vitamin A may be hazardous to the embryo or fetus when taken during pregnancy and that women of childbearing potential should consult with their physicians concerning birth control before consuming these products. Doses lower than 10,000 IU do not appear to be teratogenic.[9]

TREATMENT

Stop all vitamin A supplements. The current vitamin A protocol at the Maryland Poison Center requires GI emptying with syrup of ipecac when the amount ingested is ≥12,000 units/kg. This corresponds to an ingestion of 180,000 units in a 15-kg child, and an ingestion of 840,000 units in a 70-kg adult.[10]

REFERENCES—VITAMIN A

1. Wason S. Vitamin A. Clin Toxicol Rev 1982;5(3):1–2.
2. Wason S, Lovejoy FH. Vitamin A toxicity. Am J Dis Child 1982;136:174.
3. Fairman II. Acute hypervitaminosis A in an adult. Am J Clin Nutr 1973;26:575–577.
4. La Mantia RS, Andrews CE. Acute vitamin A intoxication. South Med J 1981;74:1012–1114.
5. Hathcock JN, Hattan DG, Jenkins MY, McDonald JT, Sundaresen PR, Wilkening VL. Evaluation of vitamin A toxicity. Am J Clin Nutr 1990;52:183–202.
6. Hathcock JN, Hattan DG, Jenkins MY, McDonald JT, Sundaresea PR, Wilkening VL. Evaluation of vitamin A toxicity. Am J Clin Nutr 1990;52:183–202.
7. Kizer KW, Fan AM, Bankowska J, Jackson RJ, Lyman DO. Vitamin A—a pregnancy hazard alert. West J Med 1990;152: 78–81.
8. Teratology Society position paper. Recommendations for Vitamin A use during pregnancy. Teratology 1987;35:269–277.
9. Martinez-Frias, ML, Salvador J. Megadose vitamin A and teratogenicity. Lancet 1988;1:236.
10. Fossler MJ. The acute toxicity of vitamin A. Toxalert. Maryland Poison Center 1991;8:(3):1.

THE RETINOIDS

Retinoids are vitamin A derivatives (Table 52–46) that have therapeutic benefit in the treatment of hyperkeratotic geodermatosis, psoriasis, and acne.[1–8] In the early 1960s synthetic derivatives of vitamin A were synthesized. There are now more than 1500 synthetic retinoids and three major oral retinoids marked in the United States and Europe[8]: retinol (vitamin A), isotretinoin, and etretinate.[9,10] Systemic administration of these compounds is frequently associated with mucocutaneous side effects, ocular toxicity,[11–14] liver toxicity,[15] and abnormalities of serum lipid profiles.[1] The teratogenic effects of all retinoids limit their use in women of childbearing potential.[2,10,16–42] Chronic toxic effects include skeletal abnormalities (diffuse idiopathic hyperostosis and premature epiphygeal closure.[8,42–45] Overdose with isotretinoin has been reported[46–50] followed by minor symptoms and no deaths. All patients have recovered with supportive and symptomatic treatment.

Table 52–46
Retinoids[a]

Nonaromatic retinoids (first generation)
Tretinoin (retinoic acid).
Isotretinoin (13-cis retinoic acid)
Monoaromatic retinoids (second generation)
Etretinate
Acitretin (USA), Etretin (Europe)
Polyaromatic retinoids (third generation)
Arotinoid ethyl ester (Ro 13-6298)
Arotinoid ethyl sulphone (Ro 15-1570)

[a]Adapted from David M et al. Med Toxicol 1988;3:273–288.

Synthetic derivatives[9] of vitamin A are marketed in Europe and the United States, including isotretinoid (13-cis-retinoic acid, RO Accutane), and etrotinate (Tigason, Tegison).[9,51] These have been used mainly for the treatment of a wide variety of skin disease, but are useful in lymphoproliferative conditions, certain forms of leukemia, and extracutaneous malignancies.[9]

CHRONIC TOXICITY

Adverse effects of isotretinoin are observed in the eyes and the mucocutaneous, central nervous, musculoskeletal,[1,46] and gastrointestinal systems. Teratogenicity has been reported when retinoids are used during the first trimester.[10,46]

STRUCTURE AND CLASSIFICATION

Isotretinoin was released in the United States in September 1982 (Accutane) and is now available in Europe (Roaccutan). Etretinate is available in the United States and Europe (Tegison).[51] Carotinoids are under clinical investigation. Tretinoin is applied topically.

Tretinoin

(Vitamin A acid, Retin HA gel, Retin A, Retin HA Lotion). Molecular weight is 300.4. Slightly soluble in alcohol, insoluble in water. $C_{20}H_{28}O_2$.[4]

Isotretinoin

(13-cis-retinoic acid, Roaccutane, Accutane, Accuton). Molecular weight 300.4. Slightly soluble in alcohol, insoluble in water. $C_{20}H_{28}O_2$.

Etretinate (Tigason, Tegison)

Molecular weight 354.5. $C_{23}H_{30}O_3$. Soluble in alcohol. Insoluble in water.

Acitretin

(Under clinical investigation)—derivative of etretinate.[9]

USES[7]

Isotretinoin

Severe nodulocystic acne, milder acne, excessive oiliness, and seborrhea; acne rosacea, gram-negative folliculation; hidradenitis suppurativa; genodermatoses; Darier's disease; pityriasis rubra piloris, saccoidosis, psoriasis.[3,5,8] Myelodysplastic syndrome.[52] Skin cancer;[53–55] photo-aged skin.[56,57]

Etretinate

Major use: psoriasis. Also used in genodermatosis, pustular bacterioids, hyperkeratotic eczema of palms and soles, cutaneous lupus erythematosus.

Tretinoin

Acne vulgaris; senile comedones.[58,59]

PRODUCT FORMULATION

Isotretinoin

Available orally. Capsules containing 5 mg and 20 mg of isotretinoin (UK). Accutane (US) capsules 10 mg, 20 mg, 40 mg.

Etretinate

Capsules 10 mg, 25 mg.[5]

Tretinoin (Retin-A)

Cream and Gel 25 g (0.025% cream) to 45 g (0.0025% gel).[5] Tretinoin is all-*trans*-retinoic acid.

SOURCES

Retinoids are synthetic chemical products.

THERAPEUTIC DOSES

Isotretinoin

Recommended dosage is 1 mg/kg/day for at least 4 months.[1]

Etretinate

About 80% of patients have good to excellent results with a daily dose of 0.5 to 1.0 mg/kg.[3]

TOXIC DOSE

A 15-year-old female ingested 350 mg of isotretinoin, developed mild abdominal symptoms, and recovered.[50] An 18-year-old male ingested 800 mg of isotretinoin and was asymptomatic.[46] A 15-year-old male ingested 440 mg of isotretinoin on one day and 1600 mg the next day. He recovered with few symptoms.[47] A 21-month-old male was given 1220 g (63.3 mg/kg) and recovered.[48]

FATAL DOSE

A fatal dose for the retinoids in humans has not been established.

TOXICOKINETICS

Absorption

Etretinate

Peak plasma concentrations occur about 4 hours after intake of a single dose. On oral administration about 40% of a dose is absorbed from the gut.[9] About 98% of a dose is bound to plasma proteins. Etretinate is predominantly bound to lipoproteins. As isotretinoin levels in the general circulation decrease, there is a concomitant increase in levels of the 4 oxo-metabolite.[60,61]

Isotretinoin

Peak blood concentrations occur in 2 to 4 hours. It is transported largely bound to albumin.

Acitretin

Acitretin is bound primarily to albumin.[9] After oral administration peak serum concentrations are noted in 3 to 5 hours.

Distribution (V_D)

Isotretinoin

The apparent volume of distribution of isotretinoin is 1.54 L/kg.[7]

Elimination

Isotretinoin

Isotretinoin has a half-life of only 1 day (10.4-29.5 hours).[3] The major metabolite of isotretinoin following oral administration is 4-oxo-isotretinoin.[60,61] Tretinoin has also been isolated. The 4-oxo-metabolite is eliminated with a half-life of 20 to 50 hours. About 53 to 74% of a dose is recovered in the feces.[62]

Etretinate

Etretinate is lipophilic and has a half-life of about 10 hours (both the parent compound and its active metabolite acitretine—RO1620).[9] After multiple doses during long-term treatment the terminal elimination half-life in plasma reaches a value of about 100 days.[63] It can be detected in the serum in low levels for more than 2 years after a course of therapy has been discontinued.[3]

Acitretin

Acitretin has a half-life of 50 hours. It cannot be detected in serum 3 weeks after discontinuation of treatment.[3]

Drug Interactions

Isotretinoin

In the presence of raised concentrations of liver enzymes, abstinence from alcohol is advised.

Etretinate

Simultaneous administration with vitamin A may increase toxic effects. Concomitant treatment with tetracycline and corticosteroids may increase the risk of intraarterial hypertension.[2] Drugs that increase serum lipids should be used with caution in patients receiving etretinate. Phenytoin or barbiturate blood levels may be altered. Special care should be used in epileptics receiving both drugs.[7]

Pregnancy/Lactation[2,10,16–43]

Isotretinoin

Since isotretinoin has a half-life of only 1 day, it is possible that after 1 month off therapy and the completion of one full menstrual cycle, women may safely become pregnant.[3] This must be confirmed by controlled clinical studies.

Isotretinoin was first marketed in the United States in 1982. Within a year of the manufacture reports of birth defects and spontaneous abortions were received by the FDA after exposure to isotretinoin during the first trimester of pregnancy.[37] By 1983 and in 1984 case reports of affected infants began to appear in the literature. These publications established isotretinoin as a potent human teratogen. Warnings were sent to physicians in 1984. Infants with defects have been reported in 1986, 1988, 1989, and 1990.[36] Teratogenicity has been associated with both isotretinoin (oral, cream)[22,26] and etretinate.[3,17,39] Defects have included external ear malformations, cleft palate, micrognathia, heart defects, ventricular septal defects, aortic arch malformations, and some brain malformations.[4] Babies have been born with a syndrome similar to retinoid[4] embryopathy but with no prenatal history of exposure to isotretinoin.[64] Fetal malformation has followed 4 months to 1 year after the last dose of etretinate.[38,39,65] Limb reduction defects have followed maternal use of isotretinoin in the first trimester of pregnancy.[18] Both isotretinoin and etretinate carry category X labeling.

Current guidelines[27] include the following:

1. Isotretinoin and etretinate should not be used by women who are pregnant or who may become pregnant while taking the drug.
2. Pregnancy should be ruled out before treatment begins. This precaution may best be accomplished by obtaining a negative pregnancy test no more than 2 weeks prior to the beginning of therapy and starting therapy on the second or third day of the patient's next menstrual period.
3. An effective form of contraception should be used for at least 1 month before therapy begins.
4. Women who have received isotretinoin should continue using an effective form of contraception for 1 month after discontinuing treatment.
5. The period during which pregnancy must be avoided after treatment is discontinued has not been determined for women who have received etretinate.
6. Female patients should be counseled on the risk of major birth defects associated with first-trimester exposure to isotretinoin or etretinate. Should a pregnancy occur during treatment (or after treatme.., in the case of etretinate), the woman should consult her physician about the management of her pregnancy.

In addition, patients should be counseled not to share prescription drugs with friends or family members.

CONTRAINDICATIONS

Isotretinoin is contraindicated in women of childbearing potential unless *all* of the following conditions apply:[36]

1. The patient has severe, disfiguring cystic acne that is recalcitrant to standard therapies.
2. The patient is reliable in understanding and carrying out instructions.
3. The patient is capable of complying with the mandatory contraceptive measures.
4. The patient has received both oral and written warnings of the hazards of pregnancy and the risks of contraceptive failure and has acknowledged these in writing.
5. The patient has had a pregnancy test with a negative result within 2 weeks of initiating therapy. The test must be performed in the physician's office or by a licensed laboratory. Therapy must not be initiated until the second or third day after the start of the next normal menstrual period. (Monthly pregnancy tests are also recommended).

In addition, the new measures include provision for signed informed consent; extensive education initiatives aimed at physicians, patients and pharmacists; further studies (e.g., to evaluate alternative dosage regimens); and a follow-up survey ascertaining patient awareness, disease status, contraception use, and any pregnancy that occurs and the outcome, etc.

Etretinate

Etretinate is a potent teratogen. Women of childbearing potential who receive this drug must avoid pregnancy for an as yet undetermined period after treatment.[39,39]

Acitretin

Acitretin is also a potent teratogen.[42] Its half-life is shorter than etretinate. Therefore women may possibly conceive sooner after discontinuing therapy than after discontinuing therapy with etretinate. Careful controlled studies are required to confirm this possibility.

MECHANISM OF ACTION

The actions of retinoids on the skin are similar to those of Retin A and include inhibition of inflammation, keratinization, and cell growth.[3]

CLINICAL PRESENTATION

Acute

Overdose of oral isotretinoin has led to vague abdominal discomfort,[50] transient headaches, irritability, vomiting, mild tachycardia, tachypnea, hypertension, facial flushing, cheilosis, abdominal pain, dizziness, and ataxia.[5] All symptoms have resolved quickly without apparent residual effects.[46,48,50] No fatalities have been reported following an overdose.

Chronic

Chronic use of isotretinoin has been associated with a number of undesired effects that are generally mucocutaneous, dose-dependent, and reversible with discontinuation of the drug.[2] Depression has followed etretinate use (100 mg/day). This resolved after the drug was discontinued.[66] The two most serious potential ocular side effects are corneal deposits and papilledema secondary to pseudotumor cerebri.[12–15] Dry eye has been observed.[13] Immune complex vasculitis has followed isotretinoin and etretinate therapy.[67] Isotretinoin and etretinate have been associated with skeletal abnormalities after both long-term and short-term therapy.

Retinal function disturbances have followed long-term use of the synthetic retinoids.[14] Olfactory and taste disturbances may persist after isotretinoin therapy ceases.[68]

Hepatotoxicity

Chronic use of Retin A may be hepatotoxic. Etretinate has been implicated in reversible serum aminotransferase elevations, acute hepatitis, and chronic active hepatitis. The main metabolite of etretinate, acitretin, may induce a severe hepatotoxic reaction with progression to liver cirrhosis.[69]

LABORATORY

Analytic Methods

A reversed-phase high-performance liquid chromatography method is available for retinoic acid and its metabolites.[61]

Blood Levels

Seven and 20 days following ingestion of 350 mg of isotretinoin, only insignificant levels of isotretinoin have been found. However, 5 ng/mL and 2 ng/mL, respectively, of R022-6595, the 4-oxo metabolite of isotretinoin, were found.[50]

Abnormalities

No lipid or hepatic enzyme abnormalities were observed following isotretinoin overdose.[46–50] The infrequent elevation of liver function values after chronic use is transient and totally reversible on withdrawal of the drug.

Ancillary Tests

Thrombocytopenia may follow use of retinoids.[70] Monitoring of the platelet count during therapy may be advisable. Hypertriglyceridemia has been observed.[71]

TREATMENT

Stabilization

Treatment of retinoid overdose is largely supportive and symptomatic.

Antidote

There are no antidotes.

Supportive Measures

Ophthalmic examination of patients on long-term etretinate should be done with special attention to color vision and dark adaptation.[7] Patients on chronic long-term therapy with retinoids should be evaluated by x-ray for any retinoid induced bone change. Strict contraception should probably continue for 2 years after etretinate therapy.[72]

REFERENCES—THE RETINOIDS

1. Roenigk HH Jr. Retinoids. Cutis 1987;39:301–308.
2. Millan SB, Flowers FP, Sherertz EF. Isotretinoin. South Med J 1987;80:494–499.
3. Goldfarb MT, Ellis SM, Voorhees JJ. Retinoids in dermatology. Mayo Clin Proc 1987;62:1161–1164.
4. Reynolds JEF, ed. *Martindale: The extra pharmacopoeia.* 29th ed. London: Pharmaceutical Press, 1989.
5. Physicians Desk Reference 1992. Accutane. Mountvale, NJ: Medical Economics, 1992.
6. McEvoy GK, ed. AHFS Drug Information 92. Bethesda, MD: Soc Hosp Pharm 1992;2175–2180.
7. Dollery CF, ed. Therapeutic drugs. Edinburgh. Churchill Livingstone, 1991.
8. Strauss JS, Ropini RP, Shalita AR et al. Isotretinoin therapy for acne: results of a multicenter dose-response study. J Am Acad Dermatol 1984;10:490–496.
9. David M, Hodak E, Lowe NJ. Adverse effects of retinoids. Med Toxicol 1988;3:273–288.
10. Teelmann K. Retinoids: toxicology and teratogenicity to date. Pharm Ther 1989;40:29–43.
11. Bigby M, Stern RS. Adverse reactions to isotretinoin. A report from the Adverse Drug Reaction Reporting System. J Ann Acad Dermatol 1988;18:543–552.
12. Lebowitz MA, Berson DS. Ocular effects of oral retinoids. J Am Acad Dermatol 1988;19:209–211.
13. Brown RD, Grattan CEH. Visual toxicity of synthetic retinoids. Br J Ophthalmol 1989;73:286–288.
14. Fraunfelder FT. Ocular side effects of isotretinoin therapy. JAMA 1983;250:2545.
15. Roenigk HH Jr. Liver Toxicity of retinoid therapy. Pharm Ther 1989;40:145–155.
16. Dai WS, La Braico JM, Stern RS. Epidemiology of isotretinoin exposure during pregnancy. J Am Acad Dermatol 1992;26:599–606.
17. Mitchell AA. Oral retinoids. What should the prescriber know about their teratogenic hazards among women of childbearing potential. Drug Safety 1992;7:79–85.
18. Rizzo R, Lammer EJ, Parano E, Pavone L, Argyle JC. Limb reduction deficits in humans associated with prenatal isotretinoin exposure. Teratology 1991;44:599–604.
19. McBride WG. Limb reduction deformities in child exposed to isotretinoin in utero on gestation days 26–40 only. Lancet 1985;1:1276.
20. Rosa E. Isotretinoin dose and teratogenicity. Lancet 1987;2:1154.
21. Ayne S, Julian S, Gambarelli D, Mariotti B, Movrin N. Isotretinoin dose and teratogenicity. Lancet 1988;1:655.
22. Kligman AM. Is topical tretinoin teratogenic JAMA 1988;259:291–318.
23. Camera G, Pergliasco P. Malformation in baby born to mother using tretinoin cream. Lancet 1992;339:687.
24. Saich G, Rosa F. When a uniquely effective drug is teratogenic: the case of isotretinoin. N Engl J Med 1989;321:756–757.
25. Rappaport EB, Knapp M. Isotretinoin embryopathy—a continuing problem. J Clin Pharmacol 1989;29:463–465.
26. Accutane risks evaluated. Strong precautions needed. FDA Drug Bull 1990;20(2):5–6.
27. The Teratology Society Public Affairs Committee. Recommendations for isotretinoin use in women of childbearing potential. Teratology 1991;4:1.
28. CDC: Birth defects caused by isotretinoin—New Jersey. JAMA 1988;239:2362–2365.

29. Cordero J, Kochbar D, Fantel A. Teratology Society. Recommendations of isotretinoin use in women of childbearing potential. Teratology 1991;44:1–6.
30. FDA panels urge Accutane labeling changes. FDA Med Bull; 1991;21(2):4.
31. Continued reports of birth defects with isotretinoin engender labeling packaging changes. FDA Drug Bull 1988;18(3):27–28.
32. Accutane. Med Economics. Dec 19, 1988. Roche Dermatologics. PI 1088.
33. Howard WB, Willhite CC. Toxicity of retinoids in humans and animals. J Toxicol (Toxic Reviews) 1986;5:55–94.
34. Dear Doctor Letter. Roche Dermatologics, September, 1988.
35. Nightingale SL (FDA): Isotretinoin restrictions. JAMA 1988; 260:315.
36. Willis J: New warning about Accutane and birth defects. FDA Consumer 1988;22(8):25–29.
37. Stern RS. When a uniquely effective drug is teratogenic. The case of isotretinoin. N Engl J Med 1989;320:1007–1009.
38. Blake KD, Wyse RKH. Embryopathy of infant conceived one year after termination of maternal etretinate. A reappraisal. Lancet 1988;2:1254.
39. Lammer EJ. Embryopathy in infant conceived one year after termination of maternal etretinate. Lancet 1988;2:1080–1081.
40. Hopf G, Mathias P. Teratogenicity of isotretinoin and etretinate. Lancet 1988;2:1143.
41. Vahlquist A, Rollman O. Etretinate and the risk for teratogenicity: drug monitoring in a pregnant woman for 9 months after stopping treatment. Br J Dermatol 1990; 123:131.
42. Kistler A, Hummler H. Teratogenesis and reproductive safety evaluation of the retinoid etretin (RO10-1670). Arch Toxicol 1985;58:50–56.
43. Pittsley RA, Yoder FW. Retinoid hyperostosis: skeletal toxicity associated with long-term administration of 13-cis-retinoic acid for refractory ichthyosis. N Engl J Med 1983;308:1012–1014.
44. Ellis CN, Madison KC, Pennes DR et al. Isotretinoin therapy is associated with early skeletal radiographic changes. J Am Acad Dermatol 1984;10:1024–1029.
45. White SI, McKie RM. Bone changes associated with oral retinoid therapy. Pharm Ther 1989;40:137–144.
46. Lindemayr H. Isotretinoin intoxication in attempted suicide. Acta Derm Venereol 1986;66:452–453.
47. Sutton JD: Overdose of isotretinoin. J Am Acad Dermatol 1983;9:600.
48. Munter DW, Wilkinson JA. Isotretinoin ingestion in a pediatric patient. J Emerg Med 1988;6:273–275.
49. Dwyer MA. Rose dermatologics. Personal Correspondence, May 3, 1989.
50. Hepburn NC. Deliberate self-poisoning with isotretinoin. Br J Dermatol 1990;122:840–841.
51. Physicians Desk Reference 1992. Tegison. Mountvale, NJ. Medical Economics, 1992.
52. Tricot G. Effect of isotretinoin on survival of patients with myelodysplastic syndrome. Lancet 1987;1:1271.
53. Lippman SM, Meyskens Jr. Treatment of advanced squamous cell carcinoma of the skin with isotretinoin. Ann Intern Med 1987;107:499–501.
54. Kraemer KH, Di Giovanna JJ, Moshell AM, Tarone RE, Peck GL. Prevention of skin cancer in xeroderma pigmentosum with the use of oral isotretinoin. N Engl J Med 1988;318: 1633–1637.
55. Hang WV, Lippman SM, Itri LM, Karp DD, Lee JS, Byers RM et al. Prevention of second primary tumors with isotretinoin in squamous cell carcinoma of the head and neck. N Engl J Med 1990;323:795–901.
56. Weiss JS, Ellis SN, Headington JT, Tincoff T, Hamilton TN, Voorhees JJ. Topical tretinoin improves photo-aged skin. A double-blind vehicle-controlled study. JAMA 1988; 259:527–532.
57. Warren EW, Khanderia U. Use of retinoids in the treatment of psoriasis. Clin Pharm 1989;8:344–351.
58. Tretinoin for photodamaged skin. Med Lett Drugs Ther 1992; 34(Issue 866):28–29.
59. Rafal ES, Griffiths SEM, Ditre CM, Finkel LJ, Hamilton TA, Ellis CM, Voorhees JJ. Topical tretinoin (retinoic acid) treatment for liver spots associated with photodamage. N Engl J Med 1992;326:368–374.
60. Vane FM, Rugge CJL. Identification of 4-oxo-12-cis-retinoic acid as a major metabolite of 13-cis-retinoic acid in human blood. Drug Metab Dispos 1981;9:515–550.
61. Vane FM, Stoltenborg JK, Bugge CJL. Determination of 13-cis-retinoic acid, its major metabolite 4-oxo-13-cis-retinoic acid in human blood by reversed-phase high-performance liquid chromatography. J Chromat 1982;227: 471–487.
62. Allen JG, Bloxham DP. The pharmacology and pharmacokinetics of the retinoids. Pharm Ther 1989;40:1–27.
63. Ellis CN, Voorhees JJ. Etretinate therapy. J Am Acad Dermatol 1987;123:55–58.
64. Kawashima H, Ohno I, Veno Y, Nakaya S, Kato E, Taniguchi N. Syndrome of microtia and aortic arch anomalies resembling isotretinoin embryopathy. J Pediatr 1987;111:738–740.
65. Grote W, Harms D, Janig V, Kietzmann H, Ravens V, Schwarz I. Malformations of fetus conceived 4 months after termination of etretinate treatment. Lancet 1985;2:1276.
66. Henderson CA, Highet AS. Depression induced by etretinate. Br Med J 1989;298:964.
67. Dwyer JM, Kenicer K, Thompson BT, Chen D, LaBraico J et al. Vasculitis and retinoids. Lancet 1989;1:494–496.
68. Herse E, Schnuch A. Taste and olfactory disturbance after treatment for acne with isotretinoin, a 13-cis-isomer of retinoic acid. Eur Arch Otolaryngol 1990;247:382–383.
69. Van Ditzhuijsen TJM, Van Haelst JJGM, Van Dooren-Greebe RJ, Van de Kerkhof DCM, Yag SH. Severe hepatotoxic reaction with progression to cirrhosis after use of a novel retinoid (acitretin). J Hepatol 1990;11:185–188.
70. Naldi L, Rozzoni M, Finazzi G, Pini P, Marchesi L et al. Etretinate therapy and thrombocytopenia. Br J Dermatol 1991; 124:295.
71. Flynn WJ, Freeman PG, Wickboldt LG. Pancreatitis associated with isotretinoin-induced hypertriglyceridemia. Ann Intern Med 1987;63:65.
72. Weber V, Melnik B, Goerz G, Michaelis L. Abnormal retinal function associated with long-term etretinate. Lancet 1988;1:235–236.

VITAMIN D

CLINICAL PRESENTATION

A 6-month-old boy with a short history of vomiting, constipation, and increasing apathy presented as a drowsy, listless child with 5 to 10% dehydration. The plasma calcium concentration was raised to 5.86 mmol/L. There was an increase in vitamin D concentration (25-hydroxycholecalciferol) at 2226 mmol/L (normal 10 to 120 mmol/L) and undetectable parathyroid hormone. The parents had been giving the child compound preparations of vitamin A, C, and D since the age of 4 months. After receiving IV fluids for 5 days and a low-calcium, low–vitamin D diet, the calcium returned to normal by day 19. The vitamin D concentration remained elevated for over 6 months. At 1 year the child showed moderate global developmental delay.[1]

In one study infants given more than 1800 units of vitamin D daily did not grow as well as infants given 340 units daily.[2] In adults it is estimated that continued ingestion of 60,000 units per day caused intoxication.[3] Adults who had ingested 1/3 to 3 cups of vitamin D fortified milk daily (with cholecalciferol vitamin D_3: concentration is up to 232,565 IU per quart—245,840 IU per liter) developed elevated serum 25 hydroxyvitamin D concentration (293 ng/mL, 731 mmol/L) (normal 22 to 200 mmol/liter). Most had hypercalcemia, and one had hypercalciuria. When vitamin D intoxication is found in a patient who is not taking a pharmaceutical preparation of vitamin D, a careful search for another exogenous source is warranted.[4]

LABORATORY

Peak serum vitamin D concentration occurs approximately 12 hours after a single oral dose and returns to basal levels within 72 hours; the serum half-life of 25(OH)D is 2×2 weeks. Serum 25(OH)D measurements are a good indicator of exposure to vitamin D from dietary sources and synthesis of the vitamin by the skin.[4]

TREATMENT

Stop vitamin D in any form. Insure kidney function.

REFERENCES—VITAMIN D

1. Ko MLB, Liberman MM, Salzmann M. Chronic vitamin D overdosage: a reminder. Arch Dis Child 1991;66:1002.
2. Jean PC, Sterns G. The effect of vitamin D on linear growth in infancy. II. The effect of intakes above 1,800 USP units daily. J Pediatr 1938;13:730–740.
3. Haynes RC Jr. Agents affecting calcification, calcium, parathyroid hormone, calcitonin, vitamin D, and other compounds. In: Gilman AG, Rall TW, Nies AS, Taylor P, eds. Goodman and Gilman's The pharmacological basis of therapeutics. 8th Ed. New York. Pergamon, 1990.
4. Jacobs CH, Holick MF, Shao Q, Chen TC, Holm IA, Kolodney JM et al. Hypervitaminosis D associated with drinking milk. N Engl J Med 1992;326:1173–1177.

NIACIN (NICOTINIC ACID)

RECOMMENDED DAILY ALLOWANCE (USRDA)[1]

US RDAs as of 1991 are as follows:

Infants 0–12 mo	8 mg
Children 1–3 years	9 mg
Adults and children 4 years+	20 mg
Pregnant or nursing women	20 mg

CLINICAL PRESENTATION[2–4]

High doses of niacin (over 4 g/day) may be associated with a lactic acidosis,[5] a cystoid maculopathy,[6] a myopathy (leg cramps and painful muscles after 1 to 2 g/day),[7] and fulminant hepatic failure (after 2 g to 3 g daily).[8,9] Hepatic toxicity may be more severe following sustained release nicotinic acid than after an unmodified nicotinic acid preparation in equivalent therapeutic doses.[10] An anecdotal report describes an atrioventricular block in an adult that followed ingestion of 15 niacin 500 mg tablets (7500 mg), which responded to symptomatic treatment.[11] Severe life-threatening hyperglycemia has been described following 3 grams per day doses of niacin.[12]

TREATMENT

Stop use immediately.

REFERENCES—NIACIN

1. Kurtzweil P, Young TA. FDA Consumer 1991;25(4):36.
2. Coronary Drug Project Research Group. Clofibrate and niacin. Coronary heart disease. JAMA 1975;231:360–381.
3. Centers for Disease Control. Niacin intoxication from pumpernickel bagels—New York. MMWR 1983;32:305.
4. Toxic effects of vitamin overdosage. Med Lett Drug Ther 1984;26(667):73–74.
5. Earthman TP, Odom L, Mullins CA. Lactic acidosis associated with high-dose niacin therapy.
6. Millay RH, Klein ML, Illingworth DR. Niacin maculopathy. Ophthalmology 1988;95:930–936.
7. Litin SC, Anderson CF. Nicotinic acid–associated myopathy. A report of three cases. Am J Med 1989;86:481–483.
8. Clementz GL, Holmes AW. Nicotinic acid–induced fulminant hepatic failure. J Clin Gastroenterol 1987;9:582–587.
9. Fischer DJ, Knight LL, Vestal RE. Fulminant hepatic failure following low-dose sustained-release niacin therapy in hospital. West J Med 1991;155:410–412.
10. Rader JI, Colvert RJ, Hathcock JM. Hepatic toxicity of unmodified and time-release preparations of niacin. Am J Med 1992;92:77–81.
11. Kim S, Sporer K. Acute niacin ingestion associated with third-degree atrioventricular block. Vet Hum Toxicol 1993;35: 347.
12. Schwartz ML. Severe reversible hyperglycemia as a consequence of niacin therapy. Arch Intern Med 1993;153:2050–2052.

VITAMIN C (ASCORBIC ACID)

In vitro studies suggest that ascorbic acid therapy places the erythrocytes of premature infants at risk of oxidative damage. The significance of these findings to the routine management of premature infants remains to be determined.[1] An anedcotal report of a diet with glucose-6-phosphate dehydrogenase deficiency suggests that high doses of intravenous ascorbic acid may lead to an acute hemolysis.[2]

LABORATORY

High doses of ascorbic acid may interfere with tests that check for blood in the stool (which will be falsely negative) and tests for urine sugar (results in Tes-Tape and ChemStrip G) can be falsely lowered, whereas Clintest gives a falsely high result.[3]

TREATMENT

Stop the vitamin use.

REFERENCES—VITAMIN C

1. Ballin A, Brown EJ, Koren G, Zipursky A. Vitamin C–induced erythrocyte damage in premature infants. J Pediatr 1988; 113:114–120.
2. Rees DC, Kelsey H, Richards JDM. Acute haemolysis induced by high-dose ascorbic acid in glucose-6-phosphate dehydrogenase deficiency. Br Med J 1993;306:842.
3. Harvard Med School Health Letter 1987;12(3):8.

WATER INTOXICATION

CAUSES

Water intoxication is an infrequent clinical event that follows excessive parenteral or enteral water administration by medical personnel, malicious forcing of water on a child, repeated immersion (infant swimming lessons), and voluntary ingestion of ice water to control toothache. It may occur during marathon runs, after drug testing (individuals drink massive quantities of water to dilute the urine enough to drive drug levels down), or as a manifestation of psychosis.[1] In the infant hunger is the most important factor combined with unavailability of formula. Mechanisms of hyponatremia are summarized in Table 52–47.[2]

TREATMENT

Swales has provided a treatment approach for acute and chronic hyponatremia as follows:

Chronic hyponatremia (e.g., hyponatremia secondary to diuretic therapy, or syndrome of inappropriate secretion of ADH). When the condition is asymptomatic, there is no indication for acute emergency treatment. Treatment should be directed primarily at the underlying cause. When the condition is symptomatic, treatment should be designed in relation to the severity of the clinical manifestations. If these are mild (e.g., lethargy, confusion), treatment should consist of removal of the primary cause and water restriction. Oral potassium loading (when the serum concentration of potassium is decreased or low normal) also increases the serum concentration of sodium through an increase in predominantly intracellular osmolality.[2]

Acute hyponatremia usually occurs secondary to iatrogenic fluid overload in the postoperative period or excessive ingestion of fluids as a result of psychiatric disturbance. Within 24 hours of onset, the danger of acute correction is probably small. In contrast, the dangers of severe hyponatremia *per se* are relatively great. Acute correction to a target concentration of sodium 120 to 130 mmol liter $^{-1}$ by means of water restriction and infusion of calculated amounts of saline should be carried out. Increase in serum concentration of sodium should be limited to 10 mmol liter $^{-1}$ per day^{-1}. Twice-normal saline would seem adequate and should avoid the major acute changes in serum osmolality induced by greater concentrations. Serum electrolytes should be measured at 2- to 3-hour intervals. Where hyponatremia is associated with fluid overload, infusion should be accompanied by IV furosemide.[2]

Table 52–47
Mechanisms of Hyponatremia[a]

Decreased free water clearance caused by ADH:
- Administration of vasopressin or its analogues
- Inappropriate secretion of ADH (malignant neoplasms, central nervous system lesions, pulmonary tuberculosis, pneumonia and IPPV)
- Appropriate secretion in response to extracellular fluid volume contraction
- Secretion in response to "effective extracellular volume contraction" (e.g., congestive cardiac failure, cirrhosis and nephrotic syndrome)
- Secretion in response to increased sympathetic nervous system activity
- Baroreceptor stimulation
- "Stress"

Decreased free water clearance caused by other agents (e.g., oxytocin, diuretics)

Retention of water caused by renal disease

Decreased free water clearance caused by local reversible renal causes:
- Decreased delivery of solute load to diluting segment as a result of decreased renal blood flow and glomerular filtration rate and increased proximal tubular sodium reabsorption
- Change in water permeability of loop of Henlé and collecting ducts not caused by ADH (e.g., steroid deficit)

Movement of water from intra- to extracellular compartments:
- Potassium depletion
- Infusions (e.g., mannitol and dextran)
- Hyperglycemia

[a]Adapted from Swales JD. Br J Anaesth 1991;67:146–153.

NEAR DROWNING—HIGH SALINITY WATER

Drowning in fresh water is characterized by hypoxia, pulmonary edema, hemodilution, and hemolysis associated with hypoosmolarity. Drowning in sea water is accompanied by hemoconcentration with marked elevation of serum sodium and hemoglobin concentration.[3] Lakes with high salinity are located east of the crest of the Andes and Cordilleras in South and North America (e.g., Great Salt Lake in Utah, Basque Lake in British Columbia, Canada) and along the east rift in Ethiopia, Kenya, and Tanzania.[4]

THE DEAD SEA SYNDROME (TABLE 52–48)

The Dead Sea, an inland lake that lies 1286 feet below sea level in the arid area of the Syria-Africa fault in Israel, has a high specific gravity of 1.175 to 1.05 permitting one to float on the surface with little possibility of submersion. Momentary submersion is still possible and may lead to ingestion, aspiration, or both. Extreme hypercalcemia, hypermagnesemia, and hyperchloremia may be present with a syndrome similar to the acute respiratory distress syndrome,[5] tachyarrhythmias, and conduction disturbances. The fatality rate may be high. An obtunded sensorium or adenosa is a strong predictor for ultimate fatality. Metabolic acidosis, sometimes coupled with respiratory acidosis, and tachyarrhythmias are ominous signs. A serum calcium over 15.5 mg/dL appears to predict mortality. Therapy may require mechanical ventilation, hemodialysis, intravenous fluids, and forced diuresis with isotonic saline and diuretics under central venous or wedge-pressure monitoring. Gastrointestinal lavage with hypotonic fluids and peritoneal lavage have been used.[4] Serial serum electrolyte analysis to include calcium and magnesium should be performed. Initial normal levels of serum electrolytes may continue to rise after admission as a result of delayed absorption from the gastrointestinal tract. Patients in whom electrolyte abnormalities are found on admission should be observed for 24 to 48 hours and discharged only if no further electrolyte abnormalities or respiratory complications develop. If 100 mL of Dead Sea water is swallowed, a rise in serum magnesium levels of 33.6

Table 52–48
Solute Content of the Dead Sea, Basque Lake, Great Salt Lake, and Mediterranean Sea[a]

Solute (mg/dL)	Dead Sea, Israel–Jordan	Basque Lake, British Columbia	Great Salt Lake, Utah	Mediterranean Sea
Sodium	387	137	820	117
Potassium	67	16	42	4
Chloride	2,050	17	1,390	210
Calcium	157	9	3	5
Magnesium	394	424	72	14
Bromide	48	NA	NA	Trace
Sulphate	6	1,960	164	Trace

[a]Adapted from Porath A et al. Ann Emerg Med 1989;18:187–191.

mmol/L would be expected, as opposed to 0.6 mmol/L from the Mediterranean Sea. Similarly, ingestion of 100 mL of Dead Sea water would be expected to increase the serum calcium by 17 mmol/L as opposed to 0.47 mmol/L for ordinary sea water. Hypermagnesemia may lead to neuromuscular blockade, respiratory muscle paralysis, sympathetic blockade, central nervous system depression, hypotension, and cardiac dysrhythmias. Hypercalcemia may similarly result in central nervous system disturbance, neuromuscular dysfunction, and cardiac arrhythmias.[6,7]

WATER INTAKE

Contaminants

Under the authority of the Safe Drinking Water Act (PL 93-523), the Environmental Protection Agency (EPA) has had national authority since 1974 over drinking water quality and the regulation of public drinking water systems, but states may create and administer their own safe drinking water programs if they meet minimum EPA standards. The California Safe Drinking Water Act states that water delivered by public water systems in the state shall "be at all times pure, wholesome and potable." Table 52–49 represents industrial and other contaminants that may be found in ground water and polluted surface water.[8,9]

Bottled Water

There are various classes of bottled water.[10] Figure 52–4 summarizes the types of bottled water now available. In the United States the quality of bottled water sold across state lines is under the jurisdiction of the U.S. Food and Drug Administration. The standards of chemical content are identical to the drinking water criteria of the Environmental Protection Agency. Comparative data of water with statistically high concentrations of chemicals is found in Table 52–50.

The clinical significance of chemical contaminants in drinking water has not yet been subjected to long-term prospective controlled epidemiologic studies.[11]

INFANTS

In an infant the excessive water has usually been ingested as tap water from an 8 oz baby bottle. The rate of water intake is about 7.5 L/m^2/day, and the period during which it was taken is usually from 2 to 8 hours. Caregivers may mix formula with three or four times the usual amount of water rather than offer water alone. Such water substitution may be explained as follows: ran out of formula, gave water for diarrhea, and gave water because of irritability or fussiness. The infant is often fed by more than one person, with poor communication about the contents of the previous bottles.[1]

ACUTE SYMPTOMATIC HYPONATREMIA

Acute symptomatic hyponatremia in infants includes generalized tonic-clonic seizures, hypothermia, and respiratory insufficiency. Hyponatremic seizures are prolonged and respond poorly to usual anticonvulsant doses. Hyponatremic seizures typically occur at serum sodium concentrations lower than the 125-mmol/L cutoff level. Hyponatremia should be strongly considered in infants presenting with their first seizures in whom evidence of another cause is lacking. Patients experiencing hyponatremic seizures are at high risk of status epilepticus, have poor response to anticonvulsant medications, and have increased risk of respiratory failure.[12]

PSYCHOGENIC WATER INTOXICATION

In 1938 Barabal documented the first case of water intoxication in a patient with schizophrenia.[13] In 1974 Raskind reported a fatality from self-induced water intoxication.[14] Self-induced water intoxication is a condition found almost exclusively (80%) in patients with psychiatric disorders.[15,16] Between 7 and 18% of inmates in state mental hospitals in the United States experience compulsive water drinking; half of these suffer from the complications of water intoxication.[15] Self-induced water intoxication is associated with a mortality of 10% over 2 years.[15,17] The two most important pathogenic factors are primary polydipsia (also referred to as compulsive water drinking or psychogenic polydipsia) and an inappropriate antidiuretic state.[18]

Compulsive Water Drinking (Synonyms: Psychogenic Polydipsia, Primary Polydipsia)

Compulsive water drinking (CWD) usually refers to continuous or habitual drinking of greater than normal quantities of water, and psychogenic polydipsia refers to the consumption of excessive quantities in a relatively short period; the latter is more likely to lead to intoxication.[19]

Table 52–49
Industrial and Other Contaminants in Drinking Water[a]

Chemical Name	Use	MCL or Action Level	Health Concern	Status
Trichloroethane	Industrial solvent	200 ppb, Calif action level; proposed US MCL, 200 ppb	Carcinogen in one mouse study, not in four other studies; no evidence in exposed workers; data inadequate to assess; no significant effects but showed delayed development that was reversible	Common contaminant in groundwater
Trichloroethylene	Industrial solvent	5 ppb, Calif action level; proposed US MCL, 5 ppb	Probable human carcinogen with low potency; no teratogenicity in animal studies‡	Common contaminant in groundwater
Tetrachloroethylene (1,1-dichloroethylene)	Industrial solvent	4 ppb action level	Carcinogen in mice and rats; some evidence in exposed workers; no teratogenicity; possible fetotoxicity at high doses§	Common contaminant in groundwater
Vinylidene chloride	Plastics manufacture	6 ppb action level	Evidence of carcinogenicity equivocal; weak, if at all‖	Common contaminant in groundwater
Total trihalomethanes	Water disinfectant by-product	100 ppb MCL	Cancer	Under review by EPA
Fluoride	Naturally occurring element	1.4 to 2.4 ppm, Calif; 4 ppm US	Teeth mottling, skeletal fluorosis	Recent change in US MCL under legal challenge
Asbestos	Naturally occurring element	None	Cancer	Widespread in drinking water systems
Arsenic	Naturally occurring element	5 ppb MCL	Cancer	Elevated in some mineral waters
Selenium	Naturally occurring element	10 ppb MCL	Causes deformities in avian and livestock offspring; high levels in humans cause gastrointestinal problems, hair and nail loss	Main concern is environmental contamination

[a]Adapted from Russell HH et al. West J Med 1987;147:615–622.
EPA, Environmental Protection Agency; MCL, maximum contaminant level; ppb, parts per billion; ppm, parts per million.

Suggested Causes of the Disorder

CWD usually occurs among psychiatric inpatients. The suggested causes of the disorder include polydipsia as an inherent part of psychosis (dopaminergic aberration); a neuroleptic driven thirst; a neuroleptic hypersensitivity phenomenon; a response to medication-induced xerostomia; a response to delusions of poisoning, possession, etc.; and also boredom and accessibility of fluids in a psychiatric hospital where polydipsia may be a cheap source of pleasure.[19] Patients can be divided into four groups based on severity. Those in the first and most severe group have a history of severe cerebral impairment (seizures, delirium, and coma) with morning and afternoon urine specific gravities (SG) at 1.003 or less, and they probably consume over 10 liters per day. Those in the second group generally show milder disturbances of water homeostasis and cerebral functioning and have afternoon urine SGs of 1.005 or less. These patients probably consume 5 to 10 liters per day. Those in the third group have mild polydipsia (3 to 5 liters per day) and only very rarely show laboratory abnormalities. Those in the fourth group have only mild polydipsia, without complications or laboratory abnormalities.[19]

SYNDROME OF INAPPROPRIATE ANTIDIURETIC HORMONE (SIADH)[20] (TABLE 52–51)

Barrter and Schwartz[21] (1967) described the essential features of SIADH as the following:

1. Hyponatremia with hypoosmolality of serum.
2. Continued renal excretion of sodium despite hyponatremia.
3. Absence of clinical evidence of dehydration.
4. Urine less than maximally dilute; that is, urine is hypertonic relative to plasma.
5. Normal renal and adrenal function.

Among the factors reported to be associated with SIADH are: stress, smoking, head injury, psychotropic drugs (e.g., amitriptyline, fluphenazine, haloperidol, chlorpromazine, and thiothixene), anticonvulsants (e.g., carbamazepine), diuretics, anticancer drugs, and various medical disorders (notably malignant tumors).[19–21]

SIADH is similar to psychogenic polydipsia in that serum sodium, osmolality, and blood urea nitrogen are low, due to the extracellular fluid expansion that is secondary to excess renal water retention. Consequently, the urine of SIADH patients is concentrated, with high osmolality, while that of patients with psychogenic polydipsia is dilute, due to the high volume throughout.[20]

SELF-INDUCED WATER INTOXICATION

With respect to self-induced water intoxication, cases are defined by neurologic symptoms in association with low serum sodium and/or osmolality, and a history of recent polydipsia, with no other cause for the neurologic symptoms or hyponatremia being apparent.[22]

Clinical Presentation[16,20]

Early features of water intoxication include headache, blurred vision, polyuria, vomiting, tremor, and worsening of psychosis. More severe features include muscle cramps, ataxia, delirium, stupor, coma, and convulsions. Major motor seizures are the most common present feature of self-induced water intoxication in patients with psychiatric illness and have been reported in about 80% of the reported cases. Self-induced water intoxication should therefore be included in the differential diagnosis of seizures of recent onset, especially in psychiatric patients in hospitals.[16]

Treatment

Treatment of self-induced water intoxication depends on recognition, restriction of fluids in the early stages, and furosemide. The SIADH associated with polydipsia can be treated with the antidiuretic hormone, demeclocycline[16] (600 to 1200 mg/day) or lithium carbonate 900 to 1200 mg/day. An initial controlled study suggests that naloxone injections appeared to attenuate compulsive drinking in psychiatric patients with psychosis, intermittent hyponatremia, and polydipsia.[23]

CLINICAL PRESENTATION[24]

Diagnosis

Arieff has proposed an outline for the treatment of symptomatic hyponatremia.[25] The treatment of hyponatremia is controversial because of the risk of causing central or extrapontine myelinolysis (Table 52–52). Some proposed rapid correction with hypertonic saline to a low-normal sodium level. Others feel that slow correction to below-normal sodium values is preventative. Most investigators feel that overcorrection should be avoided. It is not known whether the magnitude of serum sodium change is more important than the actual rate of correction. Harris and colleagues suggest that water restriction alone combined with cessation of diuretic therapy and observation may lead to a more salutary outcome in patients with symptomatic hyponatremia and normal renal function.[26]

Water intoxication is diagnosed after obtaining an adequate history of excessive water intake accompanied by a low serum sodium and low urine sodium and specific gravity. If seizures occur, other more ominous causes should be excluded before concluding hyponatremia as a

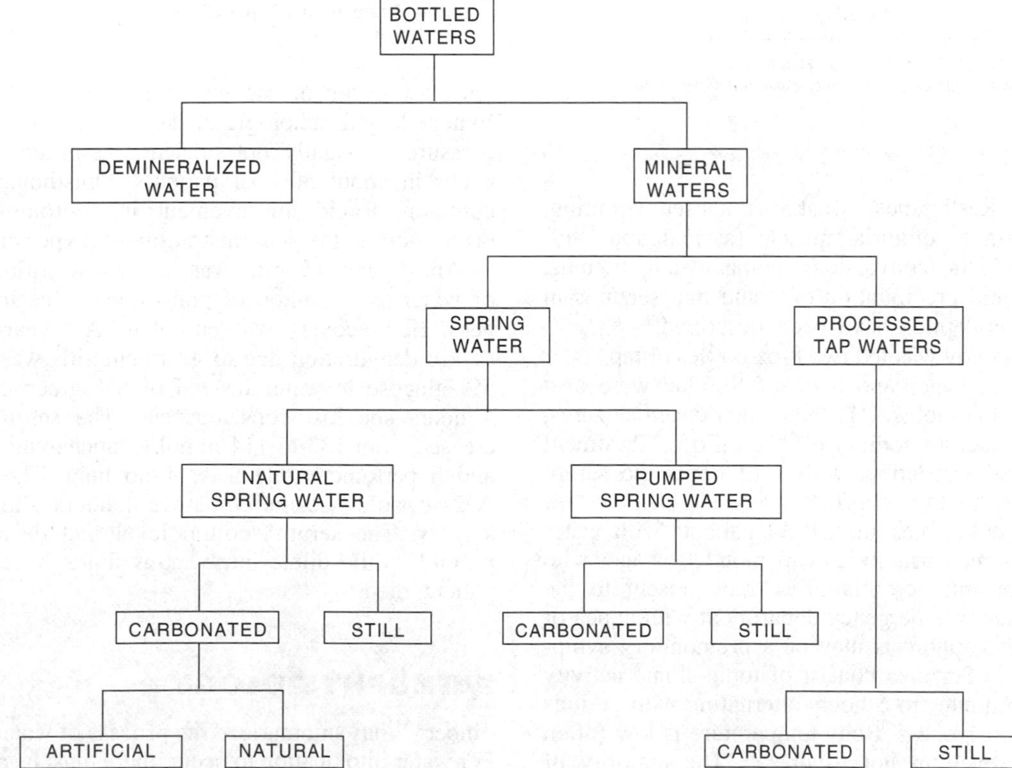

Figure 52–4 Classification of bottled waters. (Adapted from Allen HE et al. Arch Environ Health 1989;44:102–116.)

Table 52–50
Waters With Statistically High Concentrations[a,b]

Water	Determinand
Apollinaris	alkalinity, B, Cl, K, Li, Mg, Na, SO_4
Aqui	B, Cl, F, Na, SO_4
Badoit	alkalinity, Cl, K, Li, Mg, Na, NO_3, SO_4
Black Forest	alkalinity, B, F, K, Li, Mg, Mn, Na
Calso	alkalinity, Cd, Na, PO_4
Carola	B, Cl, Fe, K, Li, Mg, Na, NO_3, V
Contrexeville	B, Fe, Mg, SO_4, V
Crodo Lisiel	SO_4
Ferrarelle	alkalinity, B, K, Mg, V
Fiuggi	NO_3
Germaniabrunnen	alkalinity, B, Cd, Cl, K, Li, Mg, Na, SO_4
Gerolsteiner Sprudel	alkalinity, Cl, Fe, Hg, K, Li, Mg, Mn, Na
Glamis	Cl, Na
Health Valley	B, Cl, Hg, Na, SO_4
Hessen Quelle	alkalinity, B, Cl, Hg, K, Li, Mg
Hinckley & Schmitt	B, K, Mg
Imperator	alkalinity, B, F, K, Li, Mg, Na
Knjazmilos	alkalinity, B, F, Li, Na
Lanjaron	Cu
Le-Nature's	Hg
Mountain Valley	Hg
Perrier	Hg, SO_4
Poland Spring-sparkling	Hg
Poland Spring-still	Hg
Radenska	alkalinity, B, Cl, Hg, K, Li, Mg, Na, SO_4
a Sante	B, Cl, Li, Na, PO_4
San Pellegrino	B, Cl, Li, Mg, Mo, SO_4
Source Verniere	alkalinity, B, Hg, K, Li, Mg, Na, SO_4
Staatl	alkalinity, B, Cl, F, K, Li, Mg, Na
Vichy Celestins	alkalinity, B, F, K, Li, Na, SO_4
Vichy St. Yorre Royal	Al, alkalinity, B, Cd, F, K, Li, Na, Pb, PO_4, SO_4
Vittel	Hg, Mg
Voslau	Mg, SO_4

[a]Adapted from Allen HE et al. Arch Environ Health 1989;44:102–116.
[b]No statistical analysis of pH or conductivity data was carried out.

causative factor. Restlessness, weakness, nausea, vomiting, diarrhea, polyuria or oliguria, muscle fasciculations, hypotonia, hyporeflexia, convulsions, coma, death, trismus, opisthotonus,[27] and precipitation of grand mal seizures in well-controlled epileptics have been described.[2]

A 4-month-old boy was fed two 8-oz bottles of tap water mixed with 7-Up; sugar and 8 oz of Similac were also administered by his mother. He then experienced seizures, and developed a serum sodium of 112 mEq/L. Treatment consisted of fluid restriction; within 12 hours the serum sodium level rose to 147 mEq/L.[28]

Keating and colleagues studied 34 patients with water intoxication.[1] Infants, usually 3 to 6 months of age, who come from poor inner-city families may present to the ambulance service or emergency department with apnea or seizure. Marked diaphoresis may be a premonitory symptom to seizures.[29] Seizures consist of tonic-clonic activity and last for 15 minutes to 6 hours alternating with periods of reduced responsiveness. Body temperature is low (often less than 36°C even in hot weather.[30] The majority of

Table 52–51
Drugs Known to Induce Syndrome of Inappropriate Antidiuretic Hormone or Hyponatremia[a]

Captopril	Monoamine oxidase inhibitors
Carbamazepine	Miconazole
Chlorpropamide	Neuroleptics
Chlorthalidone	Oxytocin
Clofibrate	Polymixin B
Clonidine	Propafenone
Cyclobenzaprine	Selective serotonin reuptake inhibitors
Cyclophosphamide	Silver nitrate
Diuretics	Tricyclic antidepressants
Lorcainide	Vasopressin
Mannitol	Vincristine

[a]Rider JM, Mauger TF, Jameson P, Notman DD. Ann Pharmacother 1995;29: 663–666.

Table 52–52
Central Pontine Myelinolysis: Clinical Features[a]

- Tetraparesis: usually spastic although flaccidity has been described especially soon after onset
- Pseudobulbar palsy: dysarthria, dysphagia, weakness of tongue and palatal movement, exaggerated jaw jerk and emotional lability
- Early depression of conscious level
- Progression to "locked-in" state
- Other brainstem features according to extent of myelinolysis; failure of ocular movement, absence of pupil reactions
- Cerebellar ataxia if cerebellar peduncles or cerebellar hemispheres are involved
- Seizures may occur if associated with hyponatremic encephalopathy

[a]Martin PJ, Young CA. Central pontine myelinolysis: clinical and MRI correlates. Postgrad Med J 1995;7:430–442.

episodes occur in the summer months. Bulging of the fontanelle and radiologic evidence of increased intracranial pressure is usually not present. Respiratory failure may occur in about 50% of patients. Opisthotonic posting is common. Rapid improvement in neurologic signs may occur during the administration of hypertonic saline.[1]

An 8-year-old girl was forced to drink 12 glasses of water as a method of punishment. She lost consciousness. Her recovery was complete. A 3-year-old girl with severe dehydration due to gastroenteritis was administered 5% glucose in water instead of 5% glucose in saline. In 4 hours she lost consciousness. The serum sodium decreased from 133 to 114 mmol/L, apnea and coma ensued, and hypertonic saline was of no help. The patient died. A 2-year-old became comatose 4 hours after elective hip surgery. The serum sodium level had decreased to 112 mmol/L while dilute intravenous fluids were infused. The patient died.[1]

PATHOPHYSIOLOGY

Finberg[31] has summarized the process of water intoxication. For water intoxication to occur, there must be a rapid decline in extracellular solute concentrations (osmolality) creating a concentration gradient between extracellular fluid and cell water generally and a gradient between the vascular fluid of the brain and the rest of the brain fluids in particular. The brain is affected differently because, unlike other tissues, the endothelial cells of the cerebral blood vessels are bound by tight junctions (the so-called blood-brain barrier). When an osmolal gradient is produced, relief of the gradient in the brain cannot be quickly achieved by rapid diffusion of sodium and chloride ions from the extracellular fluid of the brain, but must be equilibrated by movement of water molecules into both the extracellular fluid and cells of the brain. The brain picks up disproportionately more water than other organs. Such swelling causes the convulsion but only if the dilution occurs over a few hours. If the change is gradual (a few millimoles every 12 hours or so), enough sodium chloride diffusion occurs, keeping the respective volumes constant and preventing a convulsion. This rate of change in the clinical picture of convulsions or hyponatremic status is more important than the degree of hyponatremia.

LABORATORY

The serum sodium is usually rapidly reduced within a few hours to less than 125 mmol/L. Urine specific gravity is usually about 1.004; serum urea nitrogen may be about 1.4 mmol/L, serum calcium 240 mmol/L, serum magnesium 0.88 mmol/L, and serum glucose 5.5 mmol/L. Cerebrospinal fluid is sterile and usually contains a nucleated cell count of less than 8×10^6/L. The serum and serum ammonia levels are within the normal reference range. Urine toxic screen will usually fail to reveal substances capable of causing seizures, respiratory failure, or hyponatremia. The platelet count is about 600×10^9/L. Imaging studies of the brain (computer tomography ultrasound, skull roentgenography) usually show no evidence of trauma, structural abnormalities, or gross cerebral edema. Neurologic and development examination Eisbruch[27] and Cosgray[32] have identified the signs for water intoxication as follows: restlessness, weakness, nausea, vomiting, diarrhea, polyuria, muscle fasciculations, hypotonia, seizures and coma.

Stabilization

Respiratory depression must be vigorously checked with endotracheal intubation, mechanical ventilation with a pressure cycle respirator, and frequent blood gas determinations. Circulation must be maintained by use of hypertonic solutions.

Fluid restriction must include restriction of free water and dilute solute sources.

Saline infusion may result in resolution of central nervous system and electrolyte disturbances. Hypertonic saline and diuretics (furosemide) should be reserved for severe or refractory cases (e.g., seizures, coma). Serious problems, for example, central pontine myelinolysis, congestive heart failure, and cerebral hemorrhage, may result from too rapid administration of hypertonic salt.[34] When the prime abnormality leading to hyponatremia is excess of water rather than deficit of salt, there is an illogicality in hypertonic saline treatment. "Masterly inactivity," fluid restriction, or loop diuretics may be more appropriate.[35] Though very rapid correction of severe hyponatremia may be dangerous, Nairns[36] indicates that an increase of 2 mEq (2 mmol) per liter per hour in the serum sodium concentration up to a level of 120 to 130 mEq/L would not be excessive in symptomatic patients with hyponatremia.[37] Use of automatic infusion systems can keep infused fluids to a minimum volume.

Where adrenal insufficiency or hypothyroidism should be treated with appropriate hormone replacement, any drugs associated with hyponatremia should be discontinued. Water restriction is usually impractical because of thirst and is not appropriate if the patient has central nervous system symptoms. When a fluid restriction of <0.8 L/day can be maintained, a negative water balance will occur. The serum sodium will be corrected but usually not more than 2 mmol/L/day. This is not useful for extended therapy where demeclocycline is a better alternative. In patients with severe symptomatic hyponatremia, water restriction is not sufficient to relieve symptoms. Mortality and morbidity of correction by water restriction alone may be high. Any form of administration of hypertonic sodium chloride can be continued as "rapid." The controversy is not so much between "rapid" versus "slow" therapy as between active therapy versus no therapy at all (25). Frequent monitoring of serum sodium is essential.[38]

Soupart[39] suggests the rates of correction of serum sodium in acute symptomatic hyponatremia, especially in the presence of seizures, may be life-saving without harmful effects. A rise of 10% in serum sodium (10 to 13 mEq/L) or an osmotic gradient of 20 to 30 mOsm/kg H_2O should be sufficient to reduce brain edema significantly. Infusion of 1 to 2 mL/kg/hour of 3% (0.513 mEq/mL) saline will raise the serum sodium about 1 to 2 mEq/L/hour (total body water $0.6 \times$ body weight) $\times$ desired correction = amount of sodium needed in mEq/hour.[38]

Children

In children with hyponatremic seizures (symptomatic, recent onset) anticonvulsants are not always effective, may induce respiratory depression, and may require mechanical ventilation. Treatment with a rapid IV bolus of 4 to 6 mL/kg body weight of 3% saline may quickly control seizures and respiratory depression with 0.6 L/kg body weight as the apparent volume of distribution of sodium. This will lead to immediate increase of 3 to 5 mmol/L serum sodium concentration. Chronic asymptomatic hyponatremia is encountered when the CNI osmoregulator mechanism has already normalized brain water content, and in these situations a rapid increase in serum sodium could be hazardous.[40]

CENTRAL PONTINE MYELINOLYSIS (CPM)

The clinical manifestation may be a decreasing level of consciousness, behavioral changes without focal findings, spastic quadriplegia, and pseudobulbar palsy associated with an increase in serum sodium of over 0.5 mmol/L/hour. Patients with hyponatremia less than 105 mmol/L appear to be at greater risk to develop the complication associated with rapid correction of hyponatremia than are patients with higher sodium concentrations.[41]

Finally, Arieff and associates[42] suggest that CPM is rarely associated with hyponatremia. The condition is often misdiagnosed by inaccurate evaluation of the radiologic examination.

The available data are insufficient to link any of the therapeutic approaches for hyponatremia firmly to CPM. More data are required.[43]

Remove the patient from diets that encourage excess water ingestion.

Infants

A single infusion of hypertonic 3% saline over 30 to 90 minutes is administered. Dose is calculated as follows: (body weight in kilograms) × (125 mEq-initial serum sodium level × 0.6) or about 10 mL of 3% saline per kilogram of body weight.[1] Ventilatory support is seldom needed for more than 12 hours. Recovery usually appears complete within a few days. There is a minimal but definite risk of death or hypoxic organ damage. For symptomatic patients with acute hyponatremia the rate of hypertonic saline administration of at least 1 mmol/L/hour should suffice. In adults, rapid correction with hypertonic saline (500 mmol/L) has been associated with pontine myelinolysis. When a pediatric patient receiving hypotonic fluid saline begins to have headache, emesis, nausea, or lethargy, a serum sodium concentration should be measured. Hypertonic saline should be administered such that the serum sodium concentration is increased to about 125 to 130 mmol/L but by no more than 25 mmol in the initial 24 hours.[44] Permanent neurologic damage is not common after water intoxication.[30]

Having hypertonic solution in the same cabinet with others may lead to erroneous administration of the solution to a different patient. Patients who do not have renal damage will also recover by expenditure of insensible water while being given higher than usual amounts of sodium (100 to 150 mol/L) in fluids. Some may need definite replacement if they are dehydrated despite water intoxication. Hypertonic solutions should only be used for this purpose when a renal or pediatric consultant is available to direct the therapy.[31]

REFERENCES—WATER INTOXICATION

1. Keating JP, Schears GJ, Dodge PR. Oral water intoxication in infants. American epidemic. Am J Dis Child 1991;145:985–990.
2. Swales JD. Management of hyponatremia. Br J Anaesth 1991;67:146–153.
3. Alkan ML, Gegztes T, Koter S, Ben-Ari J. Near drowning in the Dead Sea. Isr J Med Sci 1977;13:290–294.
4. Porath A, Mosseri M, Harman I, Orsyshcher I, Keynan A. Dead Sea water poisoning. Ann Emerg Med 1989;18:187–191.
5. Cohen DS, Matthay A, Cogan NG, Murray JF. Pulmonary edema associated with salt water near-drowning: new insights. Am Rev Respir Dis 1992;146:794–796.
6. Yagi Y, Stalnikowciz R, Michaeli J, Mogle P. Near drowning in the Dead Sea. Electrolyte imbalances and therapeutic implications. Arch Intern Med 1985;145:50–53.
7. Neale TJ, Dewar JM, Parr R, Kimber J, Hatfield PJ, Dixon P. Acute renal failure following near drowning in salt water. N Z Med J 1984;97:319–322.
8. Russell HH, Jackson RJ, Spath DP, Book SA. Chemical contamination of California drinking water. West J Med 1987; 147:615–622.
9. California Safe Drinking Water Act of 1986. Cal Health and Safety Code, Div 5, Chap 7, p. 4010.
10. Allen HE, Halley-Henderson MA, Hass CN. Chemical composition of bottled mineral water. Arch Environ Health 1989; 44:102–116.
11. Medical Staff Conference. The clinical significance of water pollution. West J Med 1988;148:192–196.
12. Farrar HC, Chande VT, Fitzpatrick DF, Shema SJ. Hyponatremia as the cause of seizures in infants: a retrospective analysis of incidence, severity and clinical predictors. Ann Emerg Med 1995;26:42–48.
13. Barabal HS. Water intoxication in a mental case. Psychiatr Q 1938;12:767–771.
14. Raskind M. Psychosis, polydipsia and water intoxication. Report of a fatal case. Arch Gen Psychiatry 1974;30:112–114.
15. Ferrier IM. Water intoxication in patients with psychiatric illness. Br Med J 1985;291:1594–1595.
16. Emsley RA, Taljaard JJF. Self-induced water intoxication. A case report. S Afr Med J 1988;74:80–81.
17. Vieweg WVK, David JJ, Rowe WT, Wampler GJ, Burns WJ, Spradlin WW. Death from self-induced water intoxication among patients with schizophrenic disorders. J Nerv Ment Dis 1985;173:161–165.
18. Cooney JA. Compulsive water drinking, water intoxication and alcohol abuse. Irish J Psycholog Med 1991;8:22–25.
19. Singh S, Padi MH, Bullard H, Freeman N. Water intoxication in psychiatric patients. Br J Psychiatry 1985;146:127–131.
20. Friedman AL, Segar WF. Antidiuretic hormone excess. J Pediatr 1979;94:521–526.
21. Barrter FC, Schwartz WB. The syndrome of inappropriate secretion of antidiuretic hormones. Am J Med 1967;42:790–800.
22. Bremner AJ, Regan A. Intoxicated by water. Polydypsia and water intoxication in a mental handicap hospital. Br J Psychiatry 1991;158:244–250.
23. Nishikawa T, Tsuda A, Tanaka M, Nishikawa M, Koga I, Uchida Y. Naloxone attenuates drinking behavior in psychiatric patients displaying self-induced water intoxication. Prog Neuropsychopharmacol Biol Psychiatry 1994;18:149–153.
24. Arieff A. Managing hyponatremia. Br Med J 1993;307:305–308.
25. Arieff AI, Ayus JC. Treatment of symptomatic hyponatremia: neither haste nor water. Crit Care Med 1991;19:748–751.
26. Harris CP, Townsend JJ, Baringer JR. Symptomatic hyponatraemia: can myelinolysis be prevented by treatment? J Neur Neurosurg Psych 1993;56:626–632.
27. Eisbruch A, Lewinski U, Djaldett M. Severe opisthotonus and trismus associated with water intoxication. J Roy Soc Med 1984;77:158.
28. Gold I, Koenigsberg M. Infantile seizures caused by voluntary water intoxication. Am J Emerg Med 1986;4:21–23.
29. Medani CR. Seizures and hypothermia due to dietary water intoxication in infants. South Med J 1987;8:421–425.
30. Vercammen M, Ramet Sacre L. Water intoxication in infants: report of twin brother case and review of the literature. Vet Human Toxicol 1987;29(Suppl 2):28–30.
31. Finberg L. Water intoxication. A prevalent problem in the inner city. Am J Dis Child 1991;145:981–982.
32. Cosgray R, Davidhizar R, Giger JM, Kreisl R. A program for water-intoxication patients at a state hospital. Clin Nurse Spec 1993;7:55–61.
33. Harris CP, Towsend JJ, Baringer JR. Symptomatic hyponatraemia: can myelinolysis be prevented by treatment? J Neur Neurosurg Psych 1993;56:626–632.
34. Thompson PD, Gldehill RF, Quinn NP et al. Neurological complication associated with parenteral treatment: central pontine myelinolysis and Wernicke's encephalopathy. Br Med J 1986;292:684–685.

35. Gill G. Treatment of hyponatraemic seizures with intravenous 29.2% saline. Br Med J 1986;292:925.
36. Nairns RG. Therapy of hyponatremia. Does haste make waste? N Engl J Med 1986;314:1573–1575.
37. Ohya Y, Ochi N, Mizutani N, Hayakawa C, Watanabe K. Nonketotic hyperglycinemia: treatment with NMDA antagonist and consideration of neuropathogenesis. Pediatr Neurol 1991;7:65–68.
38. Laurence RL, Karp BI. Pontine and expontine myelinolysis following rapid correction of hyponatremia. Lancet 1988; 1:1439–1441.
39. Soupart A. Optimal management of severe hyponatremia: a therapeutic dilemma. Acta Clin Belg 1991;46:277–282.
40. Sarnaik AP, Meert K, Hachbarth R, Fleishman L. Management of hyponatremia seizures in children with hypertonic saline. A safe and effective strategy. Crit Care Med 1991;19:758–762.
41. Brunner JE, Redmonds JM, Haggar AM, Kruger DF, Elias SB. Central pontine myelinolysis and pontine lesions after rapid correction of hyponatremia. A prospective magnetic resonance imaging study. Ann Neurol 1990;27: 61–66.
42. Arieff AI, Tien R, Kucharczyk J. Central pontine myelinolysis is not a complication of hyponatremia or its therapy. Kidney Int 1990;37:212.
43. Haibach H, Ansbacher LE, Dix JD. Central pontine myelinolysis a complication of hyponatremia or therapeutic intervention? J Forensic Sci 1987;32:444–451.
44. Arieff AL, Ayus JC, Fraser CL. Hyponatraemia and death or permanent brain damage in healthy children. Br Med J 1992;304:1218–1222.

Chapter 53

Food Poisonings

Foodborne illness may follow ingestion of foods contaminated with microbial toxins (bacteria, parasites, viruses), marine biotoxins (envenomation contact), or chemical additives. Bacterial food poisoning (with the exception of botulism and cholera) exhibits a short incubation period (1 to 3 days) and is usually mild and self-limited, lasting for 1 to 3 days. These illnesses may occur in epidemics and lead to a fatal outcome, especially in infants and young children, the elderly, and in the immunologically compromised patients with preexisting severe illness.

ACUTE DIARRHEA

Diarrhea kills about four million people in developing countries each year. It remains a problem in developed countries as well. In the United States children <5 years of age experience >20 million episodes of diarrhea each year, leading to several million doctor visits, 200,000 hospitalizations, and approximately 400 deaths. Over 10,000 children worldwide die each day from associated diarrhea. Much of this morbidity is the result of the dehydration associated with acute watery diarrhea. The current epidemic of cholera in South and Central America serves as a conspicuous reminder of the morbidity and mortality associated with diarrheal diseases.

Most hospitalizations and deaths due to diarrhea occur in the first year of life. In the United States, despite the many improvements in water treatment, sanitation, education, and medical care, diarrhea remains one of the most common pediatric illnesses.

Guerrant and Bobak have suggested an approach to the diagnosis and management of infective diarrhea (Fig. 53–1).[1] Information relevant to outbreaks of bacterial, parasitic, and viral gastroenteritis are summarized in Tables 53–1, 53–2, and 53–3.

AIDS AND INTESTINAL INFECTIONS

Etiology

In HIV-infected patients diarrhea can be a presenting manifestation of AIDS or a life-threatening complication.

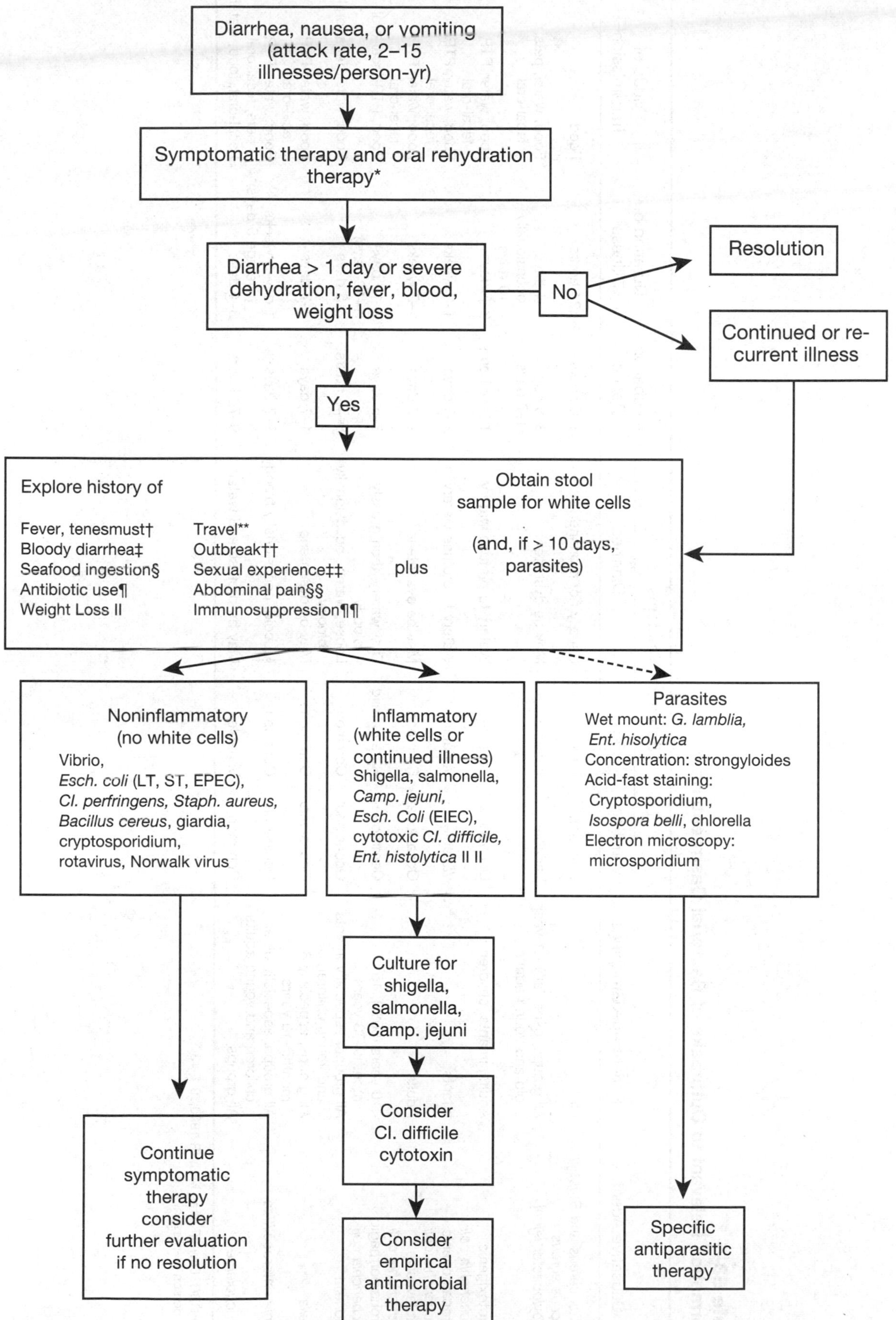

Figure 53–1 Approach to the diagnosis and management of infectious diarrhea.

Table 53–1
Information Relevant to Outbreaks of Bacterial Gastroenteritis[a]

Causative Agent	Patient Age Groupings	Selected Symptoms			Incubation Period	Duration of Illness	Mode of Transmission[b]
		Vomiting	Fever	Diarrhea			
Bacillus cereus and *Staphylococcus aureus*	All	Common	Rare	Usually not prominent	1–6 hours	<24 hours	Food
Campylobacter jejuni	All groups, especially <1 year old and young adults	Variable	Variable	May be dysenteric	3–5 days (1–7 days)	1–4 days, occasionally 10 days	Food, water, pets, fecal-oral
Enterotoxigenic *Escherichia coli*	Adults, infants, children	Occasional	Variable	Watery to profuse watery	12–72 hours	3–5 days	Food, water, PTP, fecal-oral
Enteropathogenic *Escherichia coli*	Infants	Variable	Variable	Watery to profuse watery	2–6 days	1–3 weeks	Food, water, PTP, fecal-oral
Enteroinvasive *Escherichia coli*	Adults	Occasional	Common	May be dysenteric	2–3 days	1–2 weeks	Food, water, PTP, fecal-oral
Enterohemorrhagic *Escherichia coli*	<10 years (50%), 15 months–73 years	Common	Rare or mild	First watery, then grossly bloody	3–5 days	7–10 days (1–12 days)	Food, PTP, fecal-oral
Salmonella	All groups, especially infants and young children	Occasional	Common	Loose, watery, occasionally bloody	8–48 hours	3–5 days	Food, water, fecal-oral
Shigella	All groups, especially 6 months–10 years	Occasional	Common	May be dysenteric	1–7 days	4–7 days	Food, water, PTP, fecal-oral
Yersinia enterocolitica	All groups, especially older children and young adults	Occasional	Common	Mucoid, occasionally bloody	2–7 days	1 day–3 weeks (average 9 days)	Food, water, PTP, pets, fecal-oral
Vibrio cholerae	All groups	Common	Variable	May be profuse and watery	9–72 hours	3–4 days	Fecal-oral, food, water

[a]From CDC. Lew JF et al. MMWR 1990;39:1–13.
[b]*PTP*, person-to-person.

Table 53–2
Information Relevant to Outbreaks of Parasitic Gastroenteritis[a]

Causative Agent	Patient Age Groupings	Selected Symptoms			Incubation Period	Duration of Illness	Mode of Transmission[b]
		Fever	Diarrhea	Abdominal			
Balantidium coli	Unknown	Rare	Occasional mucous or blood	Mild to severe pain	Unknown	Unknown	food, water, fecal-oral
Cryptosporidium	Children, adults with AIDS	Occasional	Profuse, watery	Occasional cramping	1–2 weeks	4 days–3 weeks	Food, water, PTP, pets, fecal-oral
Entamoeba histolytica	All groups, adults	Variable	Occasional mucous or blood	Colicky pain	2–4 weeks	Weeks–months	Food, water, fecal-oral
Giardia lamblia	All groups, children	Rare	Loose, pale, greasy stools	Cramps, bloating, flatulence	5–25 days	1–2 weeks to months and years	Food, water, fecal-oral
Isospora belli	Adults with AIDS	Unknown	Loose stools	Unknown	9–15 days	2–3 weeks	Fecal-oral

[a]From CDC. Lew JF et al. MMWR 1990;39:1–13.
[b]*PTP*, person-to-person.

Table 53-3
Information Relevant to Outbreaks of Viral Gastroenteritis[a]

Causative Agent	Patient Age Groupings	Selected Symptoms: Vomiting	Selected Symptoms: Fever	Incubation Period	Duration of Illness	Mode of Transmission[b,c]
Astrovirus	Young children and elderly people	Occasional	Occasional	1–4 days	2–3 days; occasionally 1–14 days	Food, water, fecal-oral
Calicivirus	Infants, young children, and adults	Common for infants; variable for adults	Occasional	1–3 days	1–3 days	Food, water, nosocomial, fecal-oral
Enteric adenovirus	Young children	Common	Common	7–8 days	8–12 days	Nosocomial, fecal-oral
Norwalk virus	Older children and adults	Common	Rare or mild	18–48 hours	12–48 hours	Food, water, PTP, ?air, fecal-oral
Rotavirus, group A	Infants and toddlers	Common	Common	1–3 days	5–7 days	Water, PTP, ?food, ?air, nosocomial, fecal-oral
Rotavirus, group B	Children and adults	Variable	Rare	56 hours (average)	3–7 days	Water, PTP, fecal-oral
Rotavirus, group C	Infants, children, and adults	Unknown	Unknown	24–48 hours	3–7 days	Fecal-oral

[a]From CDC. Lew JF et al. MMWR 1990;39:1–13.
[b]Diarrhea is common and is usually loose, watery, and nonbloody when associated with gastroenteritis.
[c]*PTP*, person-to-person.
? = not confirmed.

The diarrhea may be accompanied by fever, malaise, and marked weight loss and may be severely disabling.[2] Such diarrhea may be present in HIV-infected patients who have no other clinical evidence of the acquired immunodeficiency syndrome (AIDS).[3,4] Infections are often so difficult to treat that they may be fatal. Etiologies vary as follows: (a) cytomegalovirus, *Endamoeba histolytica* and Cryptosporidium in one series[2]; (b) Campylobacter species, herpes simplex virus, and *Neisseria gonorrhoeae* in another study[3]; (c) *Campylobacter jejuni* was isolated in a series of four patients[4]; and (d) *Campylobacter jejuni, Salmonella* and *Listeria monocytogenes,* in that order of frequency, were especially noted to be associated with the AIDS-patients diarrhea group.[5]

Patients with AIDS and diarrhea have lower numbers of OKT4 cells and a higher incidence of enteric pathogens and extraintestinal opportunistic infections.[2] Direct HIV infection of mucosa epithelial cells may be a possible cause of diarrhea. HIV-positive patients often harbor more than one pathogen.[3]

Treatment

These patients may require prolonged antimicrobial therapy.[6] Even with this, specific therapy may be no more effective in reducing the diarrhea than symptomatic treatment with diphenoxylate hydrochloride.[6] Weight loss and malabsorption may persist and even progress despite the elimination of potential pathogenic organisms. Since the onset of diarrhea in patients with AIDS may be a forerunner of deteriorating immune function, restoration of normal immune function would appear to be an obvious solution to address this problem. Until such a solution presents itself, control of the diarrhea with symptomatic therapy may be the most cost-conscious approach that will add the least to the suffering of the patient.[6]

AIDS OR HIV ENTEROPATHY

AIDS enteropathy is a chronic, well-established diarrhea (over 1 month's duration) for which no infectious cause can be determined after complete evaluation, including duodenal biopsy with electron microscopy of the small bowel, and is found in patients with advanced HIV infection. Occult enteric pathogens *(Mycobacterium avium-intracellulare* and Microsporida may be found. Villous atrophy and crupt hyperplasia may be related to T-cell dysfunction.[7,8]

Anecdotal case reports suggest that immune serum globulin,[9] somatostatin,[10] spiramycin,[11] and hyperimmune bovine colostrum[12] may be useful in long-standing chronic cryptosporidiosis.

Cyanobacteria-like bodies (CLBS)

CLBS are found in immunocompromised patients and travelers to tropical regions following ingestion of contaminated water. Symptoms include fatigue, malaise, and low-grade fever followed by explosive, watery diarrhea. Treatment is supportive. Diarrhea usually resolves even in patients with AIDS.[13]

Anaerobiospirillum spp.

This organism, a genus of spiral bacterial with bipolar tufts of flagella, may produce a chronic diarrhea in man.[14–17] Transfer from pets may occur.[18] The organism can be cultured under anaerobic conditions. It has a potential for invasiveness and pathogenicity, especially in compromised hosts.[19,20]

NEUROLOGIC SYMPTOMS

Seizures (shigella), blurred vision, diplopia, dysarthria, dysphagia, descending paralysis *(Clostridium botulinum),* headache, dizziness (scombroid fish), paresthesias and hot-cold sensation reversal (ciguatera), respiratory paralysis (paralytic shellfish poisoning), fatalities, and respiratory depression (tetrodotoxin from puffer fish) are important neurologic components of food poisoning.

NEPHROTOXICITY

Nephrotoxicity from ingested foods is uncommon and is usually only seen in patients with aberrant behavior. In the case of Vichy water, Worcestershire sauce, milk, licorice, and rhubarb such high quantities of food are ingested that one component reaches nephrotoxic levels (Table 53–4).[21]

STOOL SPECIMENS

Instructions for collection of stool specimens are listed in Table 53–5.[22]

Stool Osmolality[23]

Diarrhea caused by defective electrolyte absorption or by excessive electrolyte secretion by intestinal epithelial cells is called secretory diarrhea. In secretory diarrhea the fecal fluid should be rich in electrolytes because secretion of electrolytes or failure to absorb electrolytes is the primary cause of the diarrhea. By contrast, osmotic diarrhea is caused by the osmotic effect of poorly absorbed solutes that are ingested in the diet or as medications. Secretory and osmotic diarrhea can be differentiated by measurement of fecal electrolytes. The monovalent electrolyte composition of fecal fluid can be estimated by the sum of the sodium and potassium concentrations, multiplied by a factor of 2 to account for associated anions. When this value is subtracted from fecal osmolality, the "osmotic gap" is derived; the osmotic gap should be large in osmotic diarrhea and small in secretory diarrhea. The osmotic gap is calculated using the theoretic osmolality of fecal fluid as it exits the rectum, which is the same as plasma osmolality of 290 mOsm/kg.[23]

In phenolphthalein-induced secretory diarrhea an osmotic gap is less than 50 mOsm/kg. In osmotic diarrhea caused by polyethylene glycol (PEG), magnesium hydroxide, lactulose, or sorbitol the osmotic gap is usually greater than 50 mOsm/kg. The osmotic gaps are more often over 140 mOsm/kg and often over 200 mOsm/kg.[23]

Table 53–4
Nephrotoxic Foods

Probable Renal Lesion	Food	Toxic Component
Chronic interstitial nephritis	Vichy water[36]	Fluoride
	Worcestershire sauce[77]	Unknown
Hypercalcemia (milk-alkali syndrome)	Milk[78]	Calcium
Hemoglobinuric tubular necrosis	Fava or broad beans (*Vicia faba* L)[79]	Divicine and isouramil
Myoglobinuric tubular necrosis	Licorice[80]	Glycyrrhizic acid (hypokalemia)
	Wild birds (chaffinch,[81] quail,[82,83] or European robin[81])	? Cicutoxin
Nephrotoxic tubular necrosis	Djenkol beans (*Pithecolabium lobatum*)[84]	? Djenkolic acid
	Bile of the grass carp (*Clenopharyngodon idellus*)[84,85]	?Cyprinol
Oxalosis	Rhubarb (*Rheum rhaponticum*)	Oxalic acid

[a]Adapted from Abuelo JG. Arch Intern Med 1990;150:505–510.

THE MANAGEMENT OF ACUTE DIARRHEA IN CHILDREN: ORAL REHYDRATION, MAINTENANCE, AND NUTRITIONAL THERAPY[24]

Oral therapy has now become the mainstay of the World Health Organization's efforts to decrease diarrhea morbidity and mortality, and diarrheal disease control programs have been established in more than 100 countries worldwide. (Tables 53–6, 53–7, and 53–8).

Development of Oral Therapy

Proper nutrition for children with diarrhea is viewed as an important adjunct to therapy, whereas antibiotics and other drugs play only a limited role. Intravenous therapy remains essential for diarrheal episodes associated with severe dehydration.

ORT (ORAL REHYDRATION THERAPY)

The treatment of acute diarrhea rather than persistent diarrhea lasting 2 weeks or longer is aimed primarily at watery diarrhea rather than bloody diarrhea (dysentery). Oral rehydration therapy (ORT) encompasses two phases of treatment: (a) the rehydration phase in which water and electrolytes are given as oral rehydration solution (ORS) to replace exiting losses and (b) the maintenance phase, which includes both replacement of ongoing fluid and electrolyte losses and adequate dietary intake. Although ORT implies rehydration alone, the definition has been broadened to include maintenance fluid therapy and nutrition.

Etiology

A causative agent for diarrhea is found in 60 to 80% of cases. Rotavirus is the most common cause of acute diarrhea among children, accounting for one-fourth of all cases, but many other viruses can cause childhood diarrhea as well, including Norwalk-like viruses, enteric adenoviruses, astroviruses, and calciviruses. Important bacterial pathogens include *Salmonella, Shigella, Yersinia, Campylobacter,* and certain strains of *Escherichia coli.* Common parasitic causes of diarrhea include *Giardia, Cryptosporidium,* and *Entamoeba histolytica.*

ORAL REHYDRATING SOLUTIONS

ORS can be used to treat diarrhea regardless of the patient's age, causative pathogen, or initial sodium values. Many physicians continue to prescribe a variety of "clear liquids" to treat patients with diarrhea instead of an appropriately composed ORS.

Table 53-5
General Instructions for Collection of Stool Specimens[a,b]

Instructions for Collecting Specimens	Type of Agent To Be Tested: Virus	Bacterium	Parasite
When to collect	Within 48–72 hours after onset of illness	During period of active diarrhea (preferably as soon after onset of illness as possible).	Any time after onset of illness (preferably as soon after onset of illness as possible).
How much to collect	As much stool sample from each of 10 ill persons as possible (at least 10 cc each person); samples from 10 controls may also be submitted.	Two rectal swabs or swabs of fresh stool from each of 10 ill persons; samples from 10 controls may also be submitted.	A fresh stool sample from each of 10 ill persons; samples from 10 controls may also be submitted.
Method of collection	Place fresh stool specimens (liquid preferable), unmixed with urine, in clean, dry containers, (e.g., urine specimen cups).	For rectal swabs, moisten each of two swabs in Cary-Blair medium first, then insert sequentially 1–1.5 inches in rectum and gently rotate. Place both swabs into the same Cary-Blair medium tube. Break off top portions of swab sticks and discard.	Collect a bulk stool specimen, unmixed with urine, in a clean container. Place a portion of each stool sample into 10% formalin and polyvinyl alcohol preservatives at a ratio of 1 part stool to 3 parts preservative. Mix well.
Storage of specimen after collection	Immediately refrigerate at 4 C. DO NOT FREEZE if electron microscopy is anticipated.	Immediately refrigerate at 4 C if testing is to be done within 48 hours after collection; otherwise freeze samples at –70 C.	Store at room temperature, or refrigerate at 4 C. DO NOT FREEZE.
Transportation	Keep refrigerated. Place bagged and sealed specimens on ice or with frozen refrigerant packs in an insulated box. Send by overnight mail. DO NOT FREEZE.	Refrigerate as directed for viral specimens. For frozen samples: place bagged and sealed samples on dry ice. Mail in insulated box by overnight mail.	Refrigerate as directed for viral specimens. For room-temperature samples: mail in waterproof containers. DO NOT FREEZE.

[a]From CDC. Lew JF et al. MMWR 1990;39:1–13.
[b]Label each specimen container with a waterproof marker. Put samples in sealed, waterproof containers (e.g., plastic bags). Batch collection and send by overnight mail, scheduled to arrive at destination on a weekday during business hours.

Table 53-6
Comparison of Electrolyte-Glucose Concentrations of Solutions Commonly Administered at Home[a]

Clear Liquids	Na (mEq/L)	K (mEq/L)	HCO_3 (mEq/L)	Glucose (g/L)	Osmolarity (mM/L)
Cola	2	0.1	13	50–150 g glucose & fructose	550
Ginger ale	3	1	4	50–150 g glucose & fructose	540
Apple juice	3	20	0	100–150 g glucose & fructose	700
Chicken broth	250	5	0	0	450
Tea	0	0	0	0	5
Gatorade	20	3	3	45 g glucose & other sugars	330

[a]Adapted from CDC. MMWR 1992;41:6.

Studies in Dhaka and Calcutta have confirmed that the addition of glucose to sodium-containing solutions results in net movement of salt and water from the intestinal lumen to the bloodstream of patients with severe cholera. These studies suggest that the use of a glucose-electrolyte solution provides safe, effective, and practical maintenance therapy for severely dehydrated patients who typically required IV rehydration to correct shock. Providing additional drinking water at the bedside of rehydrated patients allows for excretion of any excess salt intake. More importantly, oral therapy allows fluid losses to be replaced in a timely manner and on a volume-for-volume basis with rehydration solution.

"Clear fluids" can cause osmotic diarrhea and electrolyte imbalance, and they often contain inadequate sodium bicarbonate and excess sugar for appropriate replacement of stool losses.

Guidelines

A key factor in the excellent therapeutic and safety record of ORT has been the development of simple rules that can be successfully taught by hospital and community clinical medical staff. Several approaches are effective, but all guidelines include communicating to the parent or guardian rules enabling him or her to mix the solution appropriately. These guidelines also permit the amount of oral solution administered to be related to the condition of the child and the frequency of stools. In addition, all rules encourage the parent or guardian to begin appropriate dietary liquids and foods early in the maintenance phase.

Availability of ORS in the United States

When caretakers are asked to mix ORS from packets at home, detailed written and oral instructions should be given. With premixed solutions, the concentration can be ensured, but cost can limit access.

Recently, the bicarbonate component of the WHO-ORS has been replaced with the bicarbonate precursor, citrate, because it has a longer shelf life. In the past 5 years, United States manufacturers of ORS have altered their formulations to contain lower, more appropriate concentrations of carbohydrate. The sodium concentrations of the fluids have also increased compared with previously available ORS.

When fluids with >60 mEq/L of sodium are used for maintenance, other low-sodium fluids such as breast milk, diluted or undiluted infant formula, or water need to be administered as well to prevent sodium overload.

The most widely used solutions in the United States, Pedialyte and Ricelyte, contain 45 and 50 mEq/L of sodium, respectively. These fluids are intended for maintenance of hydration and prevention of dehydration in clinical practice. Pedialyte, Ricelyte, and other similar low-sodium solutions can be used for rehydration when the alternative is physiologically inappropriate liquids or IV fluids. When the rate of purging is very high (e.g., >10 mL/kg/hour), solutions with 75 to 90 mEq/L are recommended for rehydration.

Other Forms of ORS

Glucose-based ORS does not reduce the duration of illness or the volume of stool output. Early feeding, however, can reduce the severity, duration, and nutritional consequences of diarrhea.

One advantage of cereal-based ORS, at least in developing countries, is that these solutions can be easily prepared at home. The solutions require time and effort to prepare, and

Table 53–7
Comparison of Electrolyte and Carbohydrate Concentrations of Commercial Oral Rehydration Solution (ORS) and Solutions Commonly Administered at Home[a]

	Commercial ORS (manufacturer)			
Component of Solution[b]	WHO[c]	Pedialyte[d] (Ross)	Rehydralyte[d] (Ross)	Ricelyte[d] (Mead Johnson)
Sodium (mEq/L)	90	45	75	50
Potassium (mEq/L)	20	20	20	25
Chloride (mEq/L)	80	35	65	45
Citrate (mEq/L)	30	30	30	34
Glucose (g/L)	20	25	25	
Rice-syrup solids (g/L)				30

[a]Adapted from CDC. MMWR 1992;41:7.
[b]Composition of solutions taken from package inserts.
[c]WHO-ORS is dispensed in packets. This product is considered the optimal. Manufactured and distributed in the United States by Jianas Brothers, Kansas City, Missouri.
[d]Pedialyte, Rehydralyte, and Ricelyte are dispensed in premixed liquid form.

Table 53–8
Diarrhea Treatment Chart[a]

Degree of Dehydration	Signs[b]	Rehydration Therapy (within 4 hrs)	Replacement of Stool Fluid Losses	Dietary Therapy[c]
Mild (3%–5%)	Slightly dry buccal mucous membranes, increased thirst	ORS 50 mL/kg	10 mL/kg or 1/2–1 cup of ORS for each diarrheal stool	Human milk feeding, or half- or full-strength lactose-containing milk or undiluted lactose-free formula
Moderate (6%–9%)	Sunken eyes, sunken fontanelle, loss of skin turgor, dry buccal mucous membranes	ORS 100 mL/kg	Same as above	Same as above
Severe (≥10%)	Signs of moderate dehydration with one of the following: rapid thready pulse, cyanosis, cold extremities, rapid breathing, lethargy, coma	Intravenous fluids (Ringer's lactate), 20 mL/kg/hr until pulse, perfusion, and mental status return to normal; then 50–100 mL/kg of ORS	Same as above	Same as above

[a]Adapted from CDC. MMWR 1992;41:14.
[b]If no signs of dehydration are present, rehydration therapy is not required. Proceed with maintenance therapy and replacement of stool losses.
[c]Infants and children who receive solid food can continue their usual diet, but foods high in simple sugars and fats should be avoided.

they can become contaminated if left unrefrigerated. Standardization of cereal-based solutions may prove difficult. The practice of early feeding reduces the severity, duration, and nutritional consequences of diarrhea.

Home Use of Oral Rehydration and Maintenance Solutions (Tables 53–6 and 53–7)

Management of acute diarrhea should begin at home. Families with infants and small children should be encouraged to keep a supply of ORS at home at all times and use the solution when diarrhea first occurs in the child. Regardless of the type of fluid used, an appropriate diet should be administered as well.

The most crucial aspect underlying home management of diarrhea is the need to administer increased volumes of appropriate fluids, as well as to maintain adequate caloric intake. Medications, other treatments, or inappropriate home remedies should be avoided. Infants should be offered more frequent feedings at the breast or bottle, and children should also be given more fluids.

Limitations and Advantages of ORS

Bloody Diarrhea

ORT is not sufficient therapy for some cases of bloody diarrhea (dysentery), since patients with bloody diarrhea may have a bacterial or parasitic infection requiring treatment with an antimicrobial agent. These patients need to seek medical care immediately.

Severe Dehydration (Table 53–8)

Patients in shock or near shock should be treated initially with IV solutions. Also, patients with intestinal ileus should not be given oral fluids until bowel sounds are audible.

Intractable Vomiting

Many patients with clinical significant acute diarrhea have concomitant vomiting. Nevertheless, >90% can be successfully rehydrated or maintained with oral fluids when small volumes of ORS (4 to 10 mL) are administered every 1 to 2 minutes, with a gradual increase in the amount consumed. A frequent mistake is to allow a thirsty child to drink large volumes of ORS fluids (ad libitum) from a cup or a bottle; the caretaker should be instructed to administer ORS in small amounts via a spoon, syringe, cup, or feeding bottle. Continuous, slow nasogastric infusion of ORS via a feeding tube can be helpful for the child who is vomiting.

High Stool Output

Stool output >10 mL/kg/hour is associated with a lower rate of success of oral rehydration, although these data are derived from a study performed among patients who had cholera. In general, no patient should be denied ORT simply because of a high purging rate, since most patients will respond well when administered adequate replacement fluid. In severely purging patients, subtle differences in substrate and electrolyte composition of oral solutions play a critical role in the success of therapy.

Monosaccharide Malabsorption

The presence of glucose or reducing substances in the stools, accompanied by a dramatic increase in stool output with the administration of ORS, is an indication of glucose malabsorption. The presence of stool-reducing substances alone is not sufficient to make the diagnosis, since this is a common finding among patients with diarrhea and does not indicate failure of oral therapy. Patients with true glucose malabsorption will show an immediate reduction in stool output when IV therapy is begun instead of oral therapy. Malabsorption of lactose, maltose, and sucrose can also occur because of deficiencies of their respective enzymes or starvation associated with the lack of enzyme induction.

Lactose Intolerance

Breast-fed infants should continue nursing on demand. For bottle-fed infants, full-strength, lactose-free, or lactose-reduced formulas should be administered immediately on rehydration in amounts sufficient to satisfy energy and nutrient requirements. Patients with true lactose intolerance will have exacerbation of diarrhea when a lactose-containing formula is introduced. The presence of low pH (<6.0) or reducing substances (>5%) in the stool in the absence of clinical symptoms is not diagnostic of lactose intolerance; this diagnosis is indicated by more severe diarrhea on introduction of lactose-containing foods. If lactose intolerance occurs, appropriate therapy includes temporary reduction or removal of lactose from the diet.

Excess fluid losses via vomiting or diarrhea must be replaced with ORS as outlined above.

Dietary Therapy of Acute Diarrhea

Although dehydration is the most serious direct effect of diarrhea, adverse nutritional consequences also can occur when nutritional management is not appropriate.

Acute diarrhea can endanger the nutritional status of affected children for the following reasons: (a) anorexia and food withdrawal interfere with adequate intake; (b) carbohydrates, fats, proteins, and micronutrients are often malabsorbed; (c) excess urinary and stool nitrogen losses are likely, even with subclinical infections; and (d) metabolic demands are generally higher with fever and systemic illness.

Continuation of Regular Diet

Older children accustomed to eating a variety of table foods should continue receiving a regular diet; cereal-milk and cereal-legume diets have been used successfully for the dietary management of these children. Other recommended foods include starches (e.g., rice, potatoes, noodles, crackers, and bananas), cereals (e.g., rice, wheat, and oat cereals), soup, yogurt, vegetables, and fresh fruits. Foods to be avoided are those that are high in simple sugars, which can exacerbate diarrhea by osmotic effects. These foods include soft drinks, undiluted apple juice, Jell-O, and presweetened cereals. In addition, foods high in fat may not be tolerated because of their tendency to delay gastric emptying. Although there have been no controlled trials concerning its efficacy, the "BRAT" diet (bananas, rice, applesauce, and toast) has long been used as a dietary-management tool among pediatric practices in the United States. To the extent that it included starches and fruits, it is a reasonable dietary recommendation. Prolonged use of the BRAT diet or a protracted course of diluted formulas can result in inadequate energy and protein content in the recovering child's diet.

Drug Therapy

Antibiotics should be considered when dysentery or a high fever is present, when watery diarrhea lasts for >5 days, or when stool cultures, microscopy, or epidemic setting indicate an agent for which specific treatment is required.

Pharmacologic Therapy of Acute Diarrhea

Antimicrobial agents (Table 53–9) and other drugs have limited usefulness in the management of acute diarrhea. Viral agents are the predominant cause of acute diarrhea. Bloody diarrhea or the presence of white blood cells on methylene blue stain of the stool specimen suggests a bacterial agent causing invasive mucosal damage and indicates that stool cultures should be performed to identify the organism. Other clinical clues suggesting infectious diarrhea amenable to antimicrobial therapy include a history of recent antibiotic use (in which case *Clostridium difficile* should be suspected), exposure to children in day-care centers where *Giardia* or *Shigella* is prevalent, recent foreign travel, and an immunodeficiency, and the infectious cause of the diarrhea should be diligently evaluated. Watery diarrhea and vomiting in a child <2 years of age most likely represent viral gastroenteritis and therefore do not require antimicrobial therapy.

Table 53–9
Role of Antibiotics in Specific Causes of Bacterial Gastroenteritis[a]

Role of Antibiotics	Enteropathogen
Always indicated	*Shigella* Enteroinvasive *Escherichia coli*[b] Cholera
Indicated in certain clinical settings or hosts	*Salmonella* *Campylobacter* Enteropathogenic *Escherichia coli* Enterotoxigenic *Escherichia coli* *Clostridium difficile*
Unclear	Enterohemorrhagic *Escherichia coli* Enteroadherent *Escherichia coli* *Aeromonas* spp. *Plesiomonas shigelloides* Noncholera *Vibrio* spp.

[a]Adapted from Ashkenazi S, Cleary TG. Pediatr Infect Dis J 1991;10:140–148.
[b]Based on the microbiologic and clinical similarity to *Shigella;* controlled studies not available.

Nonspecific Antidiarrheal Agents

Use of adsorbents (e.g., kaolin-pectin), antimotility agents (e.g., loperamide), antisecretory drugs, or toxin binders (e.g., cholestyramine) is a common practice in many developed and developing countries. Available data do not demonstrate their effectiveness in reducing diarrhea volume or duration. Stool water losses are unchanged, and electrolyte losses may increase. Side effects of these drugs are well known, including opiate-induced ileus, drowsiness and nausea due to atropine effects, and binding of nutrients and other drugs. Reliance on antidiarrheal agents shifts the therapeutic focus away from appropriate fluid, electrolyte, and nutritional therapy; can interfere with oral therapy; and can unnecessarily add to the economic cost of the illness. Little evidence exists to support the use of nonspecific drug therapy in children, and much information exists to the contrary.

CLINICAL ASSESSMENT

A detailed history and physical examination are important in identifying acute gastroenteritis as a likely diagnosis when symptoms and signs are nonspecific and for ruling out other serious illnesses. An accurate body weight must be obtained. Auscultation for adequate bowel sounds is important before oral therapy is initiated. Visual examination of the stool can confirm abnormal consistency and determine the presence of blood or mucus.

Infants with acute diarrhea are more apt to dehydrate than are older children because they have a higher body surface-to-weight ratio (i.e., somewhat high insensible loss/kg of body weight), have a higher metabolic rate, and are dependent on others for fluid. The most accurate assessment of fluid status is acute weight change, but the patient's premorbid weight often is not known. The clinical signs and symptoms of mild dehydration (3 to 5% fluid deficit) include increased thirst and slightly dry mucous membranes, whereas moderate dehydration (6 to 9% fluid deficit) is associated with loss of skin turgor, tenting of skin when pinched, and dry mucous membranes. Signs and symptoms of severe dehydration (10% fluid deficit) are severe lethargy or altered state of consciousness, prolonged skin tenting and skin retraction time (>2 seconds), cool and poorly perfused extremities, and decreased capillary refill. Rapid, deep breathing (a sign of acidosis), prolonged skin retraction time, and decreased perfusion are more reliably predictive of dehydration than sunken fontanelle or absence of tears. A good correlation has been reported between time of capillary refill and fluid deficit. However, fever, ambient temperature, and age can affect capillary refill time as well.

LABORATORY

Supplementary laboratory studies in the assessment of the patient with acute diarrhea are rarely needed. However, serum electrolytes can be measured when the physician recognizes clinical signs or symptoms suggesting abnormal sodium or potassium concentrations. Stool cultures are indicated for dysentery (bloody diarrhea), but are not needed to initiate treatment in the usual case of acute watery diarrhea in the immunocompetent patient.

TREATMENT

Rehydration (Table 53–8)

Rehydration therapy is based on the degree of dehydration. For the mildly dehydrated patient (3 to 5% fluid deficit), oral rehydration should commence with a fluid containing 50 to 90 mEq/L of sodium. The amount of fluid administered should be 50 mL/kg over a period of 2 to 4 hours. Using a teaspoon, syringe, or medicine dropper, the caregiver should initially provide small volumes of fluid (e.g., one teaspoon) and then gradually increase the amount as tolerated. After 2 to 4 hours, hydration status should be reassessed. If the patient is rehydrated, treatment should progress to the maintenance phase of therapy. If the patient is still dehydrated, the fluid deficit should be reestimated and rehydration therapy should begin again.

For the moderately dehydrated patient (6 to 9% fluid deficit) ORS should be administered by the same procedures as used for the mildly dehydrated patient. The initial amount of fluid administered for rehydration should be increased to 100 mL/kg, administered over 2 to 4 hours.

Severe dehydration (≥10% fluid deficit, shock, or near shock) constitutes a medical emergency. IV rehydration should begin immediately. Boluses (20 mL/kg) of Ringer's lactate solution, normal saline, or a similar solution should be administered until pulse, perfusion, and mental status return to normal. This treatment may require two IV lines or even alternate access sites (e.g., venous cutdown, femoral vein, intraosseous infusion). When the patient's level of consciousness returns to normal, he or she can take the remaining estimated deficit by mouth.

Maintenance

For patients with acute diarrhea, but without signs of dehydration, the rehydration phase of therapy should be omitted and maintenance therapy started immediately.

Replacement of Ongoing Fluid Losses

One mL of ORS should be administered for each gram of diarrheal stool. Alternatively, stool losses can be approximated by administering 10 mL/kg for each watery or loose stool passed, and 2 mL/kg of fluid should be administered for each episode of emesis. Excess fluid losses during maintenance therapy can be replaced either with low-sodium ORS (containing 40 to 60 mEq/L of sodium) or with ORS containing 75 to 90 mEq/L of sodium. When the latter type of fluid is used, an additional source of low-sodium fluid is recommended (e.g., breast milk, formula, or water).

Vomiting

In the child with vomiting, oral rehydration should proceed with small, frequent volumes at first (e.g., 5 mL every minute). Administration via a spoon or syringe—with close observation—helps guarantee a gradual progression in the amount taken. Often, simultaneous correction of dehydration lessens the frequency of vomiting.

Pepto-Bismol (Bismuth subsalicylate)

A typical 30 mL dose of bismuth subsalicylate (Pepto Bismol) yields 303 mg of bismuth, 258 mg of salicylate, and 10.2 mg of sodium. Two Pepto-Bismol tablets contain 303 mg of bismuth, 204 mg of salicylate, 0.6 mg of sodium, and 280 mg of calcium.[25] Reye's Syndrome has been reported in patients whose only exposure to salicylates was to bismuth subsalicylate.[26] The Centers for Disease Control and Prevention states that it is prudent to avoid all compounds containing salicylate for presumed viral illnesses (including most cases of gastroenteritis) in children.[27] The routine use of bismuth subsalicylate as adjunctive therapy for gastroenteritis with three or more watery stools in a 24-hour period may be unsafe.[28] Hypercalcemia also develops after large doses of Pepto-Bismol tablets.[29, 30]

Doses of 30 to 90 ml of Pepto-Bismol providing a total ingestion of 5.2 to 9.4 g/d of bismuth every 2 hours were ingested by a 45-year-old man with watery diarrhea. After 7 days of therapy the patient developed lethargy, dysarthria, and myoclonic jerking of the facial and axial muscles. The clinical course progressed from stupor to coma and death. Blood and urinary bismuth concentrations were 95 nmol/L (normal <48 nmol/L) and 14,164 nmol/L (normal <479 nmol/L), respectively.[31] Daily doses of 2.1 g and 4.2 g of bismuth subsalicylate for 3 weeks resulted in dark tongues, dark stools, and mild tinnitus.[32] A patient with a blood bismuth concentrations of 344.5 nmol/L developed encephalopathy after bismuth subsalicylate ingestion.[33]

PREVENTION

Prevention is especially important for HIV positive patients.[34] Some food storage guidelines are summarized in Table 53–10. The U.S. Food and Drug Administration has suggested some guidelines for food selection and preparation, especially for those with HIV to lessen the hazard of infection with contaminated food:

Check displays, labels, and containers

1. Look for cleanliness at meat and seafood counters and salad bars. For example, cooked shrimp lying on the same bed of ice as raw fish could be contaminated.
2. Buy only Grade A or better eggs. Avoid eggs that are cracked or leaking.
3. Do not buy any foods whose "sell by" or "best used by" date has passed. Read the label to see whether a food contains raw or undercooked animal-derived ingredients. Caesar salad dressing, for instance, traditionally uses raw eggs.
4. Buy only milk and cheeses labeled "pasteurized." (Firms may sell cheese made of raw milk provided it has been aged for over 60 days. To be safe, AIDS patients should avoid this as well.)

Keep groceries safe

5. Put raw seafood, poultry, and meat in plastic bags so drippings cannot contaminate other foods in the shopping cart or bag.

Table 53–10
Storage Guidelines for Some Foods That Are Regulars on America's Dinner Tables[a]

Product	Storage Period	
	In Refrigerator	In Freezer
Fresh Meat:		
Beef: ground	1–2 days	3–4 months
Steaks and roasts	3–5 days	6–12 months
Pork: chops	3–5 days	3–4 months
Ground	1–2 days	1–2 months
Roasts	3–5 days	4–8 months
Cured meats:		
Lunch meat	3–5 days	1–2 months
Sausage	1–2 days	1–2 months
Gravy	1–2 days	3 months
Fish:		
Lean (such as cod)	1–2 days	up to 6 months
Fatty (such as blue, perch, salmon)	1–2 days	2–3 months
Chicken:		
Whole	1–2 days	12 months
Parts	1–2 days	9 months
Giblets	1–2 days	3–4 months
Dairy Products:		
Swiss, brick, processed cheese	3–4 weeks	[b]
Milk	5 days	1 month
Eggs:		
Fresh in shell	3–5 weeks	—
Hard-boiled	1 week	—

[a]Adapted from FDA Consumer 1991;25:20–21.
[b]Cheese can be frozen, but freezing will affect the texture and taste.
(Sources: Food Marketing Institute for fish and dairy products, USDA for all other foods.)

6. Take groceries directly home and refrigerate cold foods. Hot foods from the deli should be eaten, kept hotter than 60°C (140°F), or refrigerated right away. Leaving foods unrefrigerated for even a few hours fosters bacterial growth.
7. Store eggs in their original carton in the main section of the refrigerator. Do not put them in the egg section of the door because the temperature there is higher.

Be meticulously clean

8. Wash hands, utensils, counters, and cutting surfaces with hot soapy water between preparation of different foods, particularly after handling raw eggs, meat, poultry, or fish. In other words, wash repeatedly during meal preparation to avoid cross-contamination.
9. Use plastic or glass cutting boards rather than wooden ones, which are difficult or impossible to clean adequately.
10. Be sure to disassemble and thoroughly wash the meat grinder and blender after grinding raw meat or poultry or blending eggs or vegetables.
11. Wash fresh fruits and vegetables with water, using a brush if appropriate.
12. Protect yourself with a plastic sealing bandage or plastic gloves if a hand has a cut or open sore, for wounds are easy entry points to the body for bacteria when handling raw meat, poultry, or fish.

Use thermometers

13. Promptly refrigerate or cook foods, including vegetables, after you cut them up. Bacteria can grow at temperatures above 4°C (40°F) and below 60°C (140°F), so temperature is vital in keeping food safe.
14. Using a thermometer, periodically check to be sure the temperature of the refrigerator is below 4°C (40°F) and the freezer is no higher than minus 18°C (zero F).
15. Use a meat thermometer to ensure complete cooking. Follow the recipe for seafood, but do not overcook it. Avoid lightly steamed mussels and snails, for instance. Fish should be flaky, not rubbery, when cut. Never eat oysters on the half shell, raw clams, sushi, or sashimi.
16. Cook eggs thoroughly until both the yolk and white are firm, not runny. Researchers at Cornell University recommend these cooking times; scrambled— 1 minute at medium stovetop setting (121°C [250°F] for electric frying pan). Sunny side—7 minutes at medium stovetop setting (121°C [250°F] for electric frying pan) or cook covered 4 minutes at medium. Fried, over easy—3 minutes at medium stovetop setting (121°C [250°F]for electric frying pan) on one side, then turn the egg and fry for another minute on the other side. Poached—5 minutes in boiling water. Boiled—7 minutes in boiling water.
17. Consider using pasteurized eggs instead of shell eggs whenever possible.
18. Reheat food or heat partially cooked foods all the way through to at least 74°C (165°F). Follow recipe's time and temperature requirements, and check with a meat thermometer. When using a microwave, observe the recipe's standing time and directions about turning the dish. When using a barbecue grill, precook meat and poultry.
19. Refrigerate leftovers in covered containers to avoid cross-contamination. Divide hot foods into small portions for quick cooling, and allow room for circulation around containers to prevent the refrigerator or freezer temperature from rising. If food looks or smells suspicious, throw it out.

Take charge when dining out

20. As at home, do not eat uncooked animal-derived dishes such as steak tartare, sushi, raw oysters, Hollandaise sauce, and homemade mayonnaise, eggnog, or ice cream. If you do not know what is in a particular dish, ask.
21. Send back undercooked food—poultry, for instance, that is even slightly pink.
22. When ordering eggs, specify that scrambled eggs be "dry" and that fried eggs be well cooked on both sides. The runnier the yolk, the higher the risk.

Be extra careful during foreign travel

23. Check with your doctor before traveling to a foreign country.
24. Do not buy food from street vendors.

25. Avoid salads and raw vegetables, peel your own fruit, and only eat cooked food that is still hot.
26. Drink only boiled or bottled water and only use ice cubes made from boiled water.
27. A consumer or physician who believes an episode of diarrhea is related to a particular food or restaurant should tell the local health department or nearest FDA office. Such reporting can help others avoid the illness.

TRAVELER'S DIARRHEA

Sources of information for travel medicine are summarized in Table 53–11.

ETIOLOGY (TABLE 53–12)

Although a heat-labile enterotoxin derived from *Escherichia coli* (see Section below) is the most common cause of traveler's diarrhea, site and season may predispose the traveler to diarrhea associated with other causative bacteria.[35] These infections are most commonly acquired through ingestion of contaminated food and water, but may be transmitted by person-to-person contact. Many beaches around the world are now contaminated with sewage and fecal microorganisms.

CLINICAL PRESENTATION

Most episodes of traveler's diarrhea are self-limiting and do not require specific treatment. Usually, the illness can be allowed to run its course with symptomatic treatment alone and no need to isolate the pathogen. Exceptions are bloody diarrhea (dysentery) and diarrhea lasting over 7 days.

Table 53–11
Sources of Information for Travel Medicine[a]

References

Centers for Disease Control (CDC): *Health Information for International Travel.* Superintendent of Documents, Government Printing Office, Washington, DC 20402, telephone (202) 783-3238

CDC: Weekly Summary: Countries With Areas Infected With Quarantinable Diseases ("Blue Sheet"). CDC Center for Prevention Services, Division of Quarantine, Atlanta, GA 30333

American Society of Tropical Medicine and Hygiene: *Health Hints for the Tropics,* Karl A. Western MD (ed): Tropical Medicine and Hygiene News, 6436 31st St, NW, Washington, DC 20015-2342

Goldsmith R, Heyneman D (Eds): *Tropical Medicine and Parasitology.* Norwalk, Conn, Appleton & Lange, 1989

Telephone Sources

Public Health Service Quarantine station: Chicago (312) 686-2150, Honolulu (808) 541-2552, Los Angeles (213) 215-2365, Miami (305) 526-2910, New York (718) 917-1685, San Francisco (415) 876-2872, Seattle (206) 442-4519

CDC, travel recommendations: (404) 332-4559

Information Sources for Patients

Bezruchka S: *The Pocket Doctor.* Seattle, Wash, The Mountaineers, 1988. Gives practical medical advice for laypersons

United States Department of State, Bureau of Consular Affairs: "Your Trip Abroad," "Travel Tips for Senior Citizens," "Tips for Travelers to . . . (different countries)"

[a]Adapted from Studemeister A. West J Med 1991;154:418–422.

TREATMENT

Therapy of traveler's diarrhea based on clinical features is listed in Tables 53–13 and 53–14.[36]

For watery diarrhea the cornerstone of treatment is the replacement of lost fluid and electrolytes either by formal oral rehydration therapy with glucose-electrolyte solutions (very important for infants and young children and probably for the elderly patient) or informally by encouraging a high fluid intake, including salty soups (sodium), fruit juices or bananas (potassium), and a source of complex carbohydrates to promote active glucose-sodium cotransport.[37]

BACTERIAL FOODBORNE ILLNESS

BACILLUS CEREUS[38]

B. cereus, a ubiquitous, spore-forming bacteria, causes two recognized forms of foodborne gastroenteritis: an emetic syndrome resembling that caused by *Staphylococcus aureus* and characterized by an incubation period of 1 to 6 hours and a diarrheal illness characterized by an incubation period of 6 to 24 hours. Fever is uncommon with either syndrome. The emetic syndrome is mediated by a highly stable toxin that survives high temperatures and exposure to trypsin, pepsin, and pH extremes; the diarrheal syndrome is mediated by a heat- and acid-labile enterotoxin that is sensitive to proteolytic enzymes.

Treatment

This mild, self-limited disease requires supportive treatment only.

STAPHYLOCOCCUS AUREUS

Pathophysiology

Preformed heat-stable enterotoxins (A–E) produce the gastroenteritis. Recently, an *S. aureus* strain producing enterotoxin F was isolated during an outbreak of suspected food poisoning. There is a strong correlation between *S. aureus* strains producing enterotoxin F and toxic shock syndrome. Enterotoxin A is now the most common type.

Source

This organism probably is the most common cause of bacterial foodborne illnesses. All previously cooked, proteinaceous food (e.g., ham, shrimp, potato and egg salads, and natural cream–containing baked goods) may be reservoirs.

Imitation cheeses and synthetic cream filling can support the growth of *Staphylococcus* organisms at room temperatures. The staphylococcal toxin forms at temperatures between 68°F and 112°F; the optimum temperature is 95 to

Table 53–12
Causative Organisms, Epidemiologic Aspects, and Current Methods of Detection in Travelers' Diarrhea[a]

Causative Organism	Epidemiologic Features (Geographic and Seasonal Distribution)	Detection Methods[b]
Enterotoxigenic *Escherichia coli*	Worldwide, summer	Research laboratory
Invasive *E. coli*	Unusual cause of foodborne illness	Research laboratory
Shigella spp.	Worldwide, summer	Stool culture
Salmonella spp.	Worldwide, summer	Stool culture
Aeromonas spp.	Worldwide, summer	Stool culture
Plesiomonas shigelloides	Worldwide, summer, fish source	Stool culture
Campylobacter jejuni	Worldwide, all year, especially winter	Stool culture
Vibrio cholerae	Indian subcontinent and South America	Stool culture using TCBS media
Vibrio parahemolyticus	Coastal areas, summer	Stool culture using TCBS media
Viral agents (e.g., rotavirus)	Worldwide, all year, especially winter	Rotavirus antigen test
Cryptosporidium spp.	Waterborne disease, particularly in Russia	Stool parasite examination
Giardia lamblia	Mountainous areas, Russia	Stool parasite examination
Entamoeba histolytica	Areas with markedly reduced hygienic standards	Stool parasite examination

Adapted from DuPont HL. Drugs 1993;45:917–927.

Table 53–13
Agents for Teatment of Travelers' Diarrhea in Adults[a]

Agent	Dosage	Comments
Attapulgite	3 g initially, then 3 g after each loose stool or every 2 h (whichever comes first) for a total of 9 g/d	Nonabsorbed; use should be safe during pregnancy.
Bismuth subsalicylate	1 oz every 30 min for a total of 8 oz/d	Salicylate is absorbed.
Loperamide	4 mg initially, then 2 mg after each loose stool (not to exceed 16 mg/d)	Avoid use in cases of dysentery.
Trimethoprim-sulfamethoxazole	320/1,600 mg once *or* 160/800 mg twice a day for 3 d	Use of loading dose followed by standard doses for 3 d is most effective.
Fluoroquinolone		Efficacy of administration of fluoroquinolones as a loading dose followed by 3 days of therapy has not been studied.
Norfloxacin	800 mg once *or* 400 mg twice a day for 3 d	
Ciprofloxacin	1,000 mg once *or* 500 mg twice a day for 3 d	
Ofloxacin	600 mg once *or* 300 mg twice a day for 3 d	

[a]Adapted from Ericsson CD, HL. Clin Infect Dis 1993;16:616–626.

Table 53–14
Approach to Treatment of Travelers' Diarrhea in Adults[a]

Severity of diarrhea	Preferred treatment[b]	Comments
Mild (1–2 loose stools/24 h. tolerable symptoms)	None	Attapulgite, bismuth subsalicylate, or loperamide could be used.
Moderate (≥3 loose stools/24 h. tolerable symptoms)	Loperamide	Attapulgite or bismuth subsalicylate could be used: 3-day antimicrobial therapy is necessary if symptoms persist for >2 d.
Moderate to severe (≥3 loose stools/24 h. distressing symptoms)	Loperamide plus single-dose antimicrobial therapy	Continue standard dosing of antimicrobial agent for 3 d if symptoms clearly are no better after 12 h.
Severe (≥3 loose stools/24 h [incapacitating symptoms] *or* fever *or* bloody stools)	Loading dose of antimicrobial agent plus standard doses for 3 d	Avoid use of loperamide.

[a]Adapted from Ericsson CD, DuPont HL. Clin Infect Dis 1993;16:616–626.
[b]Rehydration is assumed.

99°F. The toxin is detectable within 4 to 8 hours after the incubation begins.

Signs/Symptoms

The illness has a short incubation period (average, 4 hours), with a range of 1 to 6 hours and a mean duration of 20 hours. Vomiting, nausea, diarrhea, and abdominal pain are present in descending order of frequency. Vomiting frequently is severe whereas diarrhea is mild. The subjective feeling of fever occasionally occurs, but fever usually is absent.

Diagnosis

About 1 μg toxin/100 g of food will induce clinical symptoms. A diagnostic test must be able to detect 1 ng toxin/g of food.[39] A radioimmunoassay and enzyme-linked immunosorbent assay can detect as little as 0.1 to 1.0 ng toxin/g of food,[40] but may not be able to distinguish between biologically active (animal tests useful) and inactive toxin.

Treatment

The illness is a mild, self-limited disease that requires supportive treatment only.

CLOSTRIDIUM PERFRINGENS

A protein-losing enteropathy[41] and a total intravascular hemolysis (hematocrit <5% usually associated with an underlying malignancy)[42] have been reported in *Clostridium perfringens* infections. Systemic distribution of *Clostridium perfringens* type A and its cytotoxins-enterotoxins has been suggested as a possible cause of sudden infant death syndrome in the immunologically vulnerable infant.[43]

Source

This ubiquitous organism commonly contaminates meat, meat products, gravy, and poultry. Two to five percent of normal subjects harbor this organism.

Signs/Symptoms

The incubation period is approximately 12 hours (range, 6 to 24 hours), and the duration approximately 24 hours (range, 12 to 48 hours). Vomiting and fever are uncommon. Characteristically, watery diarrhea occurs with occasional abdominal pain and nausea.

Treatment

Treatment is supportive, since this organism usually causes a mild illness lasting 24 to 36 hours.

SHIGELLA

Source

These organisms can contaminate fruits, vegetables, and milk. In addition, person-to-person transmission through the oral-anal route occurs commonly in homosexuals.

Signs/Symptoms

Classically, this organism requires an incubation period of 1 to 3 days before the onset of large, watery stools. This is followed in 24 hours by bloody diarrhea and constitutional complaints. Children may have seizures, but the role of a neurotoxin is unclear. Fatality rates in a large Bangladesh trial were highest in *Shigella sonnei*–infected patients, and lowest in *Shigella dysenteriae* type 1–infected patients. Predictive risk factors were age <1 year, lack of breast feeding in patients 1 to 2 years of age, hypothermia, severe malnutrition, severe dehydration, altered consciousness, abdominal distension, thrombocytopenia, hypoproteinemia, hyponatremia, hypoglycemia, renal failure, and bacteremia.[44] Additionally, intestinal perforation, toxic megacolon, seizures and encephalopathy, hemolytic uremic syndrome (Table 53–15), and pneumonia are complications that can lead to death during shigellosis.[45]

Diagnosis

Fecal leukocytes are present in up to 90% of *Shigella* cases. Stool cultures are important in determining sensitivities.

Treatment

In developing countries resistance among *Shigella dysenteriae* type isolates is developing to both ampicillin and trimethoprim-sulfamethoxazole. Nalidixic acid, the newer quinolones, and amnidocillin pivoxil show evidence of effectiveness. There is a need for more data on the safety of quinolones before they can be routinely administered to children.[46]

SALMONELLA

Source

Salmonella arizonae, an opportunistic pathogen in compromised patients (e.g., AIDS), is commonly found in reptiles.[47] Rattlesnake powder or meat is a common Mexican folk remedy used to treat cancer, diabetes, arthritis, skin disorders, or other ailments. The capsules are sold without prescription in *farmacias* in Hispanic neighborhoods in Los Angeles and Mexico.[48]

In the Latin-American community such capsules are known as polvo de vibora, carne de vibora, and vibora de cascabel. Ingestion of dried rattlesnake powder or capsules of dried rattlesnake meat powder by patients with acquired immunodeficiency syndrome may lead to a *Salmonella* bacteremia that can be fatal.[49] Pet iguanas may transmit *Salmonella* to humans.[50] A high proportion of iguanas and other reptiles are asymptomatic carriers of *Salmonella.* Guidelines have been suggested by CDC for prevention of transmission of Salmonella from reptiles to humans (Table 53–15A).[51]

Eggs

Salmonella enteritis infection has been associated with the consumption of raw shell eggs.[52, 53]

Table 53–15
Etiology of Hemolytic Uremic Syndrome[a]

Infectious Causes	Sporadic, Noninfectious Causes
E. coli diarrhea–associated	Idiopathic
Shigella-associated	Familial
Neuraminidase-associated	Drugs
HIV infection	Tumors
Others	Pregnancy
	Systemic lupus erythematosus
	Transplantation
	Scleroderma
	Malignant/accelerated hypertension superimposed on glomerulonephritis

[a]Neild GH. Lancet 1994;343:398.

Table 53–15A
Recommendations for Preventing Transmission of *Salmonella* From Reptiles to Humans[a]

- Persons at increased risk for infection or serious complications of salmonellosis (e.g., pregnant women, children aged <5 years, and immunocompromised persons such as persons with AIDS) should avoid contact with reptiles.
- Reptiles should not be kept in child-care centers and may not be appropriate pets in households in which persons at increased risk for infection reside.
- Veterinarians and pet store owners should provide information to potential purchasers and owners of reptiles about the increased risk of acquiring salmonellosis from reptiles.
- Veterinarians and operators of pet stores should advise reptile owners always to wash their hands after handling reptiles and reptile cages.
- To prevent contamination of food-preparation areas (e.g., kitchens) and other selected sites, reptiles should be kept out of these areas—in particular, kitchen sinks should not be used to bathe reptiles or to wash reptile dishes, cages, or aquariums.

[a]CDC. MMWR 1995;44:347–350.

A U.K. Advisory Committee recommends marking packs of eggs with a use-by-date of 3 weeks from lay, storage at no more than 20°C during retailing, storage in a refrigerator below 8°C after purchase, and increased use of pasteurized eggs both by caterers and in the home.[54]

Phage type 4 (PT_4) in Europe and Phage type 13A (PT_{13A}) in the United States have been associated both with food poisoning due to eggs and egg products and concurrent infection of commercial poultry flocks.[55] Gastroenteritis is the most common symptom.

Unpasteurized Milk Products

Raw milk products (e.g., unpasteurized goat's milk cheese) have been associated with outbreaks of *Salmonella enterica* infection in France.[55a]

Signs/Symptoms

Four clinical syndromes characterize *Salmonella* infections.

1. *Gastroenteritis.* The incubation period of 8 to 48 hours is followed by 2 to 5 days of large, loose, watery diarrhea, which may contain blood or mucus.
2. *Bacteremia with focal extraintestinal infection.* This form is seen in infants, sickle cell disease patients, the elderly, and immunosuppressed patients (AIDS). Patients with AIDS are especially susceptible. Watery diarrhea may precede septic arthritis by 5 to 15 days, thus making the diagnosis difficult.
3. *Enteric fever.* This subacute disease is characterized by an incubation period of about 1 week, active invasion of gut lymphoid tissue during the second week, and establishment of foci of bacteremia in the gut over the third week.
4. *Asymptomatic carrier state.* Indiscriminate use of antibiotics encourages this state, and antibiotics lengthen the course of intestinal shedding.

Clinical Presentation

Gastroenteritis caused by *Salmonella* is characterized by abdominal cramps and diarrhea, vomiting, fever and headache. Antimicrobial therapy is not indicated in uncomplicated gastroenteritis, which typically resolves within 1 week. Persons at increased risk for infection or more severe disease include infants; the elderly; persons with achlorhydria; those receiving immunosuppressive therapy; persons who may have received antimicrobials for another illness; and those persons with sickle-cell anemia, cancer, or acquired immunodeficiency syndrome. Complications include meningitis, septicemia, Reiter's syndrome, and death.[56]

Treatment

Antibiotics are given selectively to bacteremic and high-risk individuals (sickle cell disease and AIDS patients, the elderly, infants). Chloramphenicol is the drug of choice if no sensitivity test is available. Either ampicillin or trimethoprim-sulfamethoxazole is indicated if sensitivity on culture confirms their effectiveness.

YERSINIA ENTEROCOLITICA

Y. enterocolitica 0:3 is emerging as an important pathogen in the United States particularly among black infants and children who consume chitterlings, an ethnic food often prepared by blacks for holiday meals. Raw chitterlings are an important vehicle for transmitting *Y. enterocolitica* infections.[57]

Pathophysiology

Yersinia enterocolitica is an invasive gram-negative coccobacillary organism that may produce mesenteric lymphadenitis, septicemia, and peritonitis. *Yersinia* infections result in three clinical types of response, depending on the age of the patient.

Source

Both wild and domestic animals harbor this organism. It contaminates the food chain because of its frequency in farm animals. Outbreaks follow ingestion of tofu and both unpasteurized and pasteurized milk. The organism can replicate at refrigerator temperatures.

Signs/Symptoms

Patients under 5 years of age generally develop a self-limited gastroenteritis with variable amounts of diarrhea and fever. In a recent outbreak, the dysentery-like picture was characterized by fever (93%), abdominal pain (86%), diarrhea (83%), vomiting (41%), sore throat (22%), rash (22%), bloody stools (20%), and joint pain (15%). Older children often develop mesenteric adenitis and ileitis, which mimics appendicitis. In 10% of confirmed cases in the above outbreak, patients underwent laparotomy for suspected appendicitis.[58] Adults may develop bacteremia, hepatic abscess, Reiter's syndrome, glomerulonephritis, polyarthritis, arthralgias, or erythema nodosum. Intestinal perforation,

Table 53–16
Features of Vibrios Causing Infections in the United States[a]

Vibrio Species	Source of Infection	Clinical Disease	Comments
V. cholerae	Water or food	Gastroenteritis	Profuse watery diarrhea caused by an enterotoxin. Need to replace fluids, electrolytes, and glucose; tetracycline may shorten the clinical course.
V. cholerae (non-group 01)	Shellfish[b]	Gastroenteritis	Self-limited gastroenteritis. Bacteremia occurs; sepsis is rare.
V. parahaemolyticus	Shellfish[b]	Gastroenteritis	Self-limited gastroenteritis.
V. alginolyticus	Fish Seawater	External otitis, soft-tissue infection	Soft-tissue, wound, or external otitis infections. Bacteremia occurs in immunosuppressed patients. Uncommon infection.
V. hollisae	Shellfish[b]	Gastroenteritis	Self-limited gastroenteritis. Uncommon infection.
V. damsela	Seawater	Soft-tissue infection	Wound infection versus colonization. Uncommon infection.
V. mimicus	Shellfish[b] Seawater	Gastroenteritis External otitis	Mild gastroenteritis. External otitis. Uncommon infection.
V. vulnificus	Shellfish[b] Seawater	Cellulitis[c]	Clinical syndromes: 1. Primary bacteremia with secondary cellulitis. 2. Primary wound infection and cellulitis with bullae; secondary bacteremia and sepsis.

[a]Adapted from Case 41-1989. N Engl J Med 1989;321:1029–1038.
[b]Raw or poorly cooked.
[c]May be associated with bullae, fasciitis, and local necrosis.

peritonitis, and gangrene of the small bowel have been reported after *Y. enterocolitica* infections.

Y. enterocolitica, using deferoxamine produced by *Streptomyces pilosis,* as a siderophore, can transfer iron across its membranes for its metabolic needs. Iron loading increases the virulence of *Y. enterocolitica.* Iron overload and deferoxamine therapy are independent predisposing factors for systemic infections with *Y. enterocolitica.*[59] Iron enrichment may similarly have been a factor in *Y. enterocolitica* bacteremia cases and endotoxic shock associated with red blood cell transfusions in the United States[60] and Australia.[61]

Diagnosis

Diagnosis by stool culture requires the special culture technique of cold enrichment. Serologic examination of paired sera also helps establish the diagnosis.

Treatment

This disease is usually self-limiting. Tetracycline is reserved for severe, protracted cases. Trimethoprim-sulfamethoxazole is also effective. Little medical literature is available to guide antibiotic therapy.

VIBRIO PARAHAEMOLYTICUS AND OTHER MARINE *VIBRIO* SPECIES (TABLE 53–16)[62]

Pathophysiology

Vibrio vulnificus infections resulting in septicemia are more often found in diseases in which serum iron is increased. The bacteria can produce siderophores that bind iron and transport it across the bacterial cell membrane, making it available for metabolic needs.[63] Chronic iron overload may enhance susceptibility to infection with *V. vulnificus.*[64]

Shellfish-associated outbreaks of gastroenteritis may be associated with *Vibrio* species, *Salmonella typhi, Campylobacter* species, hepatitis A, and Norwalk-like viruses. For most reported outbreaks an etiologic agent is not identified. Such outbreaks may be of viral origin. Illness following virally contaminated oysters is self-limited and not life-threatening except for immunocompromised individuals or those with other chronic medical problems.[65] (See Viral Gastroenteritis.)

Source

Shellfish-borne *Vibrio* infections can be prevented by cooking seafoods thoroughly, keeping from cross-contamination after cooking, and eating them promptly. Cooked seafood is best stored at 60°C (140°F) or greater, or 4°C (39.2°F) or below. Patients with liver disease and those who are in any way immunocompromised (including AIDS) should be warned of the dangers of eating raw seafood.[66]

Signs/Symptoms

Healthy persons are unlikely to develop septicemia after ingesting food contaminated with *V. vulnificus.*[67] High-risk factors include liver disease, hematopoietic disorder, malignancies, or immunosuppressive disorders. Any person with a risk factor for septicemia should never eat raw seafood, especially raw oysters.[67]

Diagnosis (Table 53–16)

Diagnosis is confirmed by stool culture. *V. vulnificus* is a marine organism that causes either wound infection in healthy persons or septicemia in immunosuppressed patients. Risk factors for septicemia include underlying liver disease, hematopoietic disorders, chronic renal insufficiency, immunosuppressive agents, and alcoholism.[67] Patients who develop sepsis secondary to *V. vulnificus* frequently do not demonstrate gastrointestinal symptoms. A recent review of *V. vulnificus* sepsis cases revealed the following symptoms: fever (94%), chills (91%), skin lesions (64%), nausea (58%), vomiting (16%), diarrhea (40%), and hypotension (37%).[68]

Treatment

V. parahaemolyticus infections require only supportive treatment and no antibiotics. There are limited in vivo data on the treatment of *V. vulnificus* septicemia, but tetracycline appears efficacious.[69]

VIBRIO CHOLERAE

In October 1992 an epidemic of cholera-like illness began in Madras, India, associated with an atypical strain of *V. cholerae.* In early 1993 similar epidemics began in Calcutta (with more than 13,000 cases) and in Bangladesh (with more than 100,000 cases and 1500 deaths) caused by similarly atypical strains of *V. cholerae.* These strains could not be identified as any of the 138 known types of *V. cholerae* and have been designated as a new serogroup, 0139 or Bengal. Although the extent of the ongoing epidemic in southern Asia is unclear, this strain is now associated with epidemic cholera-like illness along a 100-mile coastline of the Bay of Bengal (from Madras, India, to Bangladesh) and appears to have largely replaced *V. cholerae* 01 strains in affected areas.

Epidemiology

An epidemic of cholera that began in Peru in January 1991 led to over 533,000 cases of cholera and 7400 deaths in 19 countries in South America. Cholera cases have been reported in 14 states in the United States.[70, 71]

The emergence of this new cause of epidemic cholera represents an important shift in the epidemiology of this infections disease. Until 1993 the only recognized causes of epidemic cholerae were *V. cholerae* strains that were part of serogroup 01.

Prevention

Persons traveling in cholera-affected areas should not eat food that has not been cooked and is not hot (particularly fish and shellfish) and should drink only beverages that are carbonated or made from boiled or chlorinated water.[72] Travelers should also be advised not to transport food from cholera-affected areas.

Descriptions of the symptoms associated with *V. cholerae* 0139 infection suggest it is indistinguishable from cholera caused by *V. cholerae* 01 and should be treated with the same rapid fluid replacement. The diagnosis of cholera should be considered in patients with watery diarrhea who have recently (i.e., within 7 days) returned from cholera-affected countries.[72]

The rapid spread of the *V. cholerae* 0139 epidemic in southern Asia, even among adults previously exposed to cholera caused by *V. cholerae* 01, suggests that preexisting immunity to toxigenic *V. cholerae* 01, whether the result of natural infection or cholera vaccine, offers little or no protective benefit.[73,74]

Source

Two types of *V. cholera* are pathogenic: the classical biotype that causes the most severe disease is found currently only in Bangladesh; the *Vibrio cholerae* 01, Inaba, El Tor biotype is responsible for some current epidemics.[75]

Raw oysters and crabs are the most common sources of foodborne epidemics. Infections are most common during the summer and early fall.

Diagnosis

Diagnosis is confirmed by stool culture. *V. vulnificus* is a marine organism that causes either wound infection in healthy persons or septicemia in immunosuppressed patients. Risk factors for septicemia include underlying liver disease, hematopoietic disorders, chronic renal insufficiency, immunosuppressive agents, and alcoholism. Patients who develop sepsis secondary to *V. vulnificus* frequently do not demonstrate gastrointestinal symptoms. A recent review of *V. vulnificus* sepsis cases revealed the following symptoms: fever (94%), chills (91%), skin lesions (64%), nausea (58%), vomiting (16%), diarrhea (40%), and hypotension (37%).

Treatment

The 0139 serotype is sensitive to tetracycline but resistant to co-trimexazole and furazolidone.[75] Antibiotic treatment decreases the duration of illness, the requirements for fluid replacement, and the period of *Vibrio* excretion. Tetracycline and doxycycline are the drugs of choice.[75] Treatment of cholera includes rapid fluid and electrolyte replacement with adjunctive antibiotic therapy. Stool specimens should be cultured on thiosulfate-citrate bile salts-sucrose (TCBS) agar. Clinical isolates of non-01 *V. cholerae* should be referred to a state public health laboratory for testing for 0139 if the patient traveled in an 0139-affected area, has life-threatening dehydration typical of severe cholera, or has been linked to an outbreak of diarrhea.[72]

Prevention

Crabs must be boiled 10 to 14 minutes or steamed 30 minutes to kill *Vibrio* organisms. Avoid contaminated water, ice, fruit, vegetables, and raw or undercooked seafood.

ESCHERICHIA COLI

Pathophysiology

Pathogenic *E. coli* strains include the following:

1. Enterotoxigenic *E. coli* (ETEC) (traveler's diarrhea)—a cholera-like illness.
2. Infantile enteropathogenic *E. coli* (EDEC).
3. Enteroinvasive strains (EITC) that result in a dysentery-like picture.

4. Enterohemorrhagic strains (hemorrhagic colitis, hemolytic uremic syndrome [Table 53–15]).
5. Enteroadherent *E. coli* (EAEC) is a less well defined category that is associated with traveler's diarrhea.[77] O serogroups have not yet been defined. The bacteria adhere in tight clusters on the surfaces of Hep-2 cells. Further data will determine if these strains will be fully accepted as diarrheagenic *E. coli*.[78]
6. Diffuse adherent *E. coli* (DAEC) bind to the entire surface of He La or HEP-2 cells as well-separated, distinct bacteria. Their pathogenic capability and epidemiologic significance are at present controversial.[79]
7. Enteroaggregative *E. coli* (EAggEC): Clumps of bacteria exhibit a "stacked brick" appearance when attached to the surface of cultural epithelial cells.
8. These strains have been associated with acute and chronic diarrhea.[79] The dysentery-like syndrome resembles *Campylobacter, Yersinia,* and *Shigella* infections; the cholera type mimics *Vibrio-* and *Bacillus cereus*–induced diarrheas.

Source

An outbreak of food poisoning in January 1993 sent scores of children who required dialysis because of the hemolytic uremic syndrome to the hospital. This was linked to the deaths of three infants. The bacteria was traced to contaminated frozen beef patties served by a fast-food hamburger chain in Washington State. *E. coli* 0157:157 produces two shigalike toxins similar to the shiga toxin produced by *Shigella dysenteriae.* Poultry, pork, dairy, and other food products have also been implicated.[80] Another large outbreak of *E. coli* 0157-H7 in Missouri in 1989 and 1990 (243 patients) led to bloody diarrhea or diarrhea and abdominal pain. There were four deaths, and two patients developed the hemolytic uremic syndrome.[81]

Signs/Symptoms

A hemolytic uremic syndrome (Table 53–15) can develop after *E. coli* 0157:H7 enteric infections and is characterized by microangiopathic hemolytic anemia, thrombocytopenia, and renal dysfunction. The diarrheal phase of illness usually precedes the appearance of hemolysis. Shigellalike toxin producing *E. coli* (SLTEC) (e.g., E. coli:0111) are a cause of postdiarrheal hemolytic uremic syndrome and thrombocytopenia purpura.[82]

Diagnosis

Stool culture identifies the presence of *E. coli* strains, but differentiation between invasive and toxigenic strains requires expensive animal testing, which is not routinely cost-effective. The sorbitol fermentation reaction is an effective screening procedure for patients with hemorrhagic colitis or hemolytic uremic syndrome, since the *E. coli* 0157:H7 is a sorbitol-negative strain compared with the other *E. coli* organisms.

Prevention

Travelers can protect themselves by drinking only bottled beverages or purified water. Boiling is the most reliable way to purify water. Bring the water to a boil and keep boiling for several minutes. Alternatively 5 drops of Tincture of Iodine can be added per quart (or liter) of clear water 30 minutes before drinking. Cold or turbid water requires 10 drops and a delay preferably of several hours before it is drunk. Portable water filters may offer some protection, but they have not been extensively tested and the Centers for Disease Control makes no specific recommendations regarding their use. Travelers should not consume ice, uncooked food, unpasteurized milk, and fruit that cannot be peeled.

Treatment

Prophylactic antibiotic treatment for travelers' diarrhea is reserved for the medically compromised patient. Either trimethoprim (160 mg)–sulfamethoxazole (800 mg) daily or doxycycline (200 mg) twice daily is effective.

Pepto-Bismol, 60 mL four times daily, reduces the incidence of travelers' diarrhea by 60%. Some travelers substitute Pepto-Bismol tablets, which contain 350 mg of calcium carbonate in addition to the 300 mg of bismuth subsalicylate. The recommended dose of 14 tablets per day corresponds to 4.9 g of calcium carbonate per day. Subsequent hypercalcemia is a potential risk under certain conditions (dehydration, renal insufficiency, use of vitamin D preparations or thiazide diuretics, asymptomatic primary hyperparathyroidism). These tablets also contain 130 mg of absorbable salicylate each; consequently, 14 Pepto-Bismol tablets contain the equivalent of 38 grains of salicylate (5.6 regular adult salicylate tablets). Lower doses (4 to 8 tablets/day) of bismuth subsalicylate may help prevent travelers' diarrhea.

CLOSTRIDIUM BOTULINUM

FOODBORNE BOTULISM

Pathophysiology

Table 53–17 summarizes the relative lethality of a number of toxins. A differential diagnosis of botulism has been suggested by Mofenson and colleagues in Table 53–18.

ADULT BOTULISM TOXIN (TYPES A, B, AND E)[82A]

Incidence

In one series, type A toxin caused illness in 48% of patients, type B in 29%, and type E in 23%. The median incubation period for all patients was 1 day (ranges: 0 to 7 days, type A; 0 to 5 days, type B; 0 to 2 days, type E).

Stool Specimens

The inability to detect toxin in most stool specimens obtained more or less than 3 days after toxin ingestion indicates that toxin is absorbed, degraded, or excreted by this time. It is not known if intravenous antitoxin administration affects disappearance of intraluminal toxin.

Table 53–17
Relative Lethality of Selected Toxins[a]

Toxin	Source	MLD (μg/kg Mouse)	# Molecules Causing Death
Botulinum toxin	bacteria	0.0003	2×10^{7}
Tetanus toxin	bacteria	0.001	8×10^{7}
Diphtheria toxin	bacteria	0.03	6×10^{9}
Batrachotoxin	frog	2.0	5×10^{13}
Taipoxin	snake	2.0	6×10^{11}
Ricin	plant	3.0	6×10^{11}
Conotoxin	snail	5.0	4×10^{13}
Tetrodotoxin	fish	8.0	3×10^{14}
Saxitoxin	dinoflagellate	9.0	3×10^{14}
Alpha-latrotoxin	spider	10.0	9×10^{11}
Beta-bungarotoxin	snake	14.0	8×10^{12}
Cobrotoxin	snake	75.0	1×10^{14}
Curare	plant	500	2×10^{16}
DFP	synthetic nerve gas	1,000	7×10^{16}
Sodium cyanide	chemical	10,000	2×10^{18}

[a]Adapted from Middlebrook JL. J Toxicol-Toxin Rev 1980;5:177–190.

Laboratory

Every patient with suspected botulism should have serum, stool, and, when possible, gastric aspirate specimens submitted for toxin assay and anaerobic culture. However, botulism may be incorrectly excluded if the diagnostic process depends too heavily on laboratory testing.

Treatment

Most outbreaks of foodborne botulism in the United States result from eating improperly preserved home-canned foods; vegetables (especially asparagus, green beans, and peppers) account for most outbreaks caused by home-canning (CDC, unpublished data, 1995). A pressure cooker must be used to home-can vegetables safely because it can reach temperatures necessary to kill botulism spores (substantially >212°F [>100°C] for 10 minutes); however, specific times and pressures needed vary for different foods. Jams and jellies can be safely home-canned without a pressure cooker because their high sugar content will not support the growth of *C. botulinum.* Instructions for home-canning are available from county extension offices. Cooked foods should not be held at temperatures 40°F to 149°F (4°C to 60°C) for >4 hours. Boiling food for 10 minutes before eating destroys any toxin present.[83]

3,4-Diaminopyridine used in a double-blind placebo-controlled study in type A botulism did not improve muscle strength, respiratory function, or electromyographic compound muscle action potentials.[84]

Human-derived botulism immune globulin (BIG) was to be available in California as of January 1, 1991,[85] but because of the Gulf War should have commenced on February 1, 1992. The clinical trial of BIG is an efficacy (Phase II) study sponsored by the Orphan Drug Program of the U.S. Food and Drug Administration and the California Department of Health. Available experience with foodborne botulism suggests that prompt treatment of botulism yields the best outcome. Physicians who suspect infant botulism may obtain BIG for their patients by calling a 24-hour number (510) 540 2646.[86] It is hoped that treatment with BIG will substantially shorten both the duration of illness and the cost of hospital stay for affected infants.

WOUND BOTULISM

Wound botulism is a rare, life-threatening complication of trauma and IV drug abuse.[87] Wound botulism, first described in association with traumatic injury, is a rare illness that occurs after spores of *C. botulinum* have germinated in a wound and produced botulinal toxin, resulting in flaccid paralysis (87a). Patients present with cranial nerve weakness and descending paralysis without sensory involvement. Symptoms can lead to respiratory failure and last for months.[88]

Clinical Manifestations

The most commonly reported symptoms include the following: shortness of breath, dysphagia, dysphonia or dysarthria, diplopia, poor accommodation, and dry or sore throat. The most common signs on physical examination include descending paralysis, respiratory insufficiency, and diplopia. Temperature elevation above 38°C is an inconsistent finding.

Botulism should be suspected in patients with acute onset of flaccid paralysis with ophthalmoplegia, ptosis, or other cranial nerve dysfunction, particularly when the paralysis is descending, symmetric, and associated with a normal cerebrospinal fluid protein level. A history of drug injection or a food history that does not identify a probable source for foodborne botulism should prompt consideration of wound botulism and elicitation of a thorough history and physical examination for evidence of cellulitis or abscess.

A meticulous physical examination is necessary because wounds containing *C. botulinum* may be small and initially unnoticed. Inspection of the intranasal septum and paranasal sinuses also may disclose a focus of *C. botulinum* infection in persons who snort cocaine.[88a]

Diagnosis

The diagnosis is supported by either conventional electromyography showing potentiation after supramaximal stimulation at 20 to 50 Hz, or single-fiber electromyography showing increased jitter and blocking. A diagnosis of myasthenia gravis would be supported by improvement in muscle function after the administration of edrophonium bromide (Tensilon). Initial treatment decisions should not necessarily await neurologic test results.[88a]

Laboratory

A detailed history and physical examination are the main keys to diagnosing wound botulism and initiating treatment. Wound cultures and serum assays for botulinum toxin are confirmatory. Other laboratory findings are nonspecific.

Differential Diagnosis

Rule out foodborne botulism, infant botulism, and classification undetermined botulism. Consider the Eaton-Lambert

Table 53–18
Differential Diagnosis of Botulism[a]

Disease	Fever	Eye Signs	Ascend Descend	Symmetric Asymmetric	Motor Sensory Autonomic	Comment
Botulism	–	Yes	Descend Bulbar	Symmetric	Motor > Autonomic	DTR absent late Ptosis late
Guillain Barré	+	No	Ascend Bulbar	Symmetric	Motor > Sensory Autonomic	Abnormal CSF DTR absent early
Fisher type		Yes				Previous URI
Poliomyelitis	+	No	Ascend Bulbar	Asymmetric Focal	Motor	Abnormal CSF DTR absent early
Paralytic Shellfish	–	No	Ascend	Symmetric	Motor = Sensory	History, onset within 30–60 min
Tick Paralysis	–	No	Ascend	Symmetric	Motor > Sensory	Presence of tick
Diphtheria	+	No	Ascend	Symmetric	Motor	Membrane in pharynx
Myasthenia Gravis	–	Yes	Descend Bulbar	Symmetric	Motor Autonomic	Ptosis early, fatigue
Lead	–	No	Ascend	Symmetric	Motor	History
Arsenic	–	No	Ascend	Symmetric Distal	Sensory > Motor	History
Periodic Familial Paralysis	–	No	Ascend	Symmetric	Motor	Family history
			Does not effect muscles of respiration			

[a]Adapted from Mofenson HC et al, eds. PP/T News MMWC Poison Control Center 1989;8:139.

syndrome, hypermagnesemia, and aminoglycoside toxicity, especially when associated with compatible electromyographic data.

INFANT BOTULISM[90]

Clinical Presentation

Look for a decrease in general activity level, decrease in feeding activity, and a history of decreased stool frequency in the parents' history, which may be accompanied by subtle changes in motor tone and strength, deep tendon reflexes, and cranial nerve findings on physical exam. The infants are usually not febrile.

A positive edrophonium test in a weak infant neither excludes infant botulism nor diagnoses congenital myasthenia gravis.[89]

Treatment

Treatment is supportive. Although testing is important in confirming the diagnosis and identifying the toxin type, the delay in obtaining the results and the relative insensitivity of laboratory tests dictate that treatment decisions be made on the basis of other data such as medical history, signs, symptoms, food consumption history, other epidemiologic data, and other diagnostic tests, especially electromyography.[82a] Botulinum antitoxin and respiratory support are the mainstay of treatment of foodborne botulism. Nutritional supplementation and respiratory support are the principal methods of supportive treatment. Oral feeding should not be resumed until a gag reflex is present and swallowing is normal. Botulism antitoxin is not recommended in infants because of its substantial side effects and lack of effect on the toxin-producing organisms in the gut. Studies have shown a high rate of complications among infants, but few long-term problems. Hospitalizations often are prolonged because of respiratory depression and the need for tube feedings.

Antibiotics have not been shown to be effective in treating or preventing wound botulism.[91] Surgical debridement of the wound and intensive respiratory care are the most important aspects of therapy. The appearance of the wound may not be clinically helpful. The efficacy of the use of botulism antitoxin in the treatment of wound infection has not been firmly established.[92]

Botulinum Toxin—Therapeutic Uses

Botulinum toxin type A has been of therapeutic value in the treatment of a variety of neurologic and ophthalmologic disorders (Table 53–19). The U.S. Food and Drug Administration recently approved botulinum toxin (Oculinum) as a therapeutic agent in patients with strabismus, blepharospasm, and other facial nerve disorders, including hemifacial spasm.[93] The toxin exerts its paralytic action by rapidly and strongly binding to presynaptic cholinergic terminals. It becomes internalized and inhibits the exocytosis of acetylcholine and decreases the frequency of acetylcholine release. The treatment of muscle with botulinum toxin results in an accelerated loss of junctional acetylcholine receptors. The toxin available in the United Kingdom (Dysport) is much more potent than that available in the United States. One nanogram of the British toxin contains 40 mouse units; 1 mg of the American toxin contains 2.5 mouse units. Side effects have included skin rash, fever, malaise, backache, and polyradiculoneuritis.[94,95] Other adverse effects have included ptosis, excessive tearing, and dry eye symptoms.[96] Well-controlled studies will be required for many suggested indications. Initial studies with botulinum toxin suggest side effects, although the duration of action with type F is somewhat shorter.[97]

If local and state officials are not available, CDC can be contacted directly (telephone: 404-639-2206, Monday through Friday, 8 A.M.–4:30 P.M. eastern time or 404-639-2888 at other times). In California, health-care workers should contact CDHS (telephone: 510-540-2308) where consultation is available at all times for suspected botulism cases.[88a]

CAMPYLOBACTER

Campylobacter is one of the three most common causes of diarrhea in the world; the other two are rotavirus and *Shigella.* (*E. coli* is more common in underdeveloped countries.)

Source

Campylobacter species are found in a large number of animals, including chicken, turkeys, pigs, cattle, sheep, goats, dogs, cats, horses, and rodents. Unchlorinated water, as well as raw cow and goat milk, transmits *Campylobacter* diarrheal disease. Human-to-human transmission is rare, although an asymptomatic carrier state dose exist. Recent evidence of its presence in homosexual men may provide a basis for gastrointestinal symptoms found in this group.

Signs/Symptoms

C. jejuni infection has been increasingly associated with immune-mediated disorders, including Guillain-Barré syndrome, reactive arthritis, Reiter's syndrome, and acute glomerulonephritis.[98] The onset of symptoms ranges from 1 to 8 days (mean, 3 days). Patients develop watery or bloody diarrhea together with fever, malaise, abdominal pain, and headache. In adults *Campylobacter* illness may be clinically indistinguishable from shigellosis, but children under 5 years of age with shigellosis frequently have higher fevers (over 38°C). *Campylobacter* illness may resemble the inflammatory bowel diseases. Rarely, acute anterior uveitis, mild reactive arthritis (HLA-B27) positive), myalgias, hemolytic uremic syndrome, erythema nodosum, and urticaria have been reported after *Campylobacter* infections. The average duration is 3 to 4 days (range, 5 hours to 12 days), but symptoms of illness may persist in an immunocompromised patient. Neurologic complications of *Campylobacter* enteritis include seizures, meningoencephalitis, subarachnoid hemorrhage, stroke, subdural empyema, and encephalopathy. *C. jejuni* septicemia affects patients at the extremes of life, as well as immunocompromised patients, although mortality occurs primarily in the latter group. Up to 30% of these septic patients have no symptoms of gastroenteritis.

Table 53–19
Uses for Botulism Toxin

- Clinical Uses
  - Strabismus—ocular motility (85% effective)
  - Less effective
    - Infantile esotropia
    - Lateral rectus palsy
    - Nystagmus
    - Dysthyroid myopathy
  - Dystonias
    - Facial dystonus
    - Segmental dystonus (if unresponsive to drug therapy)
    - Blepharospasm
    - Cervical dystonia (spasmodic torticollis)
    - Oromandibular dystonia
    - Spasmodic dysphonia (laryngeal dystonia)
    - Tash-specific dystonias
      - Writer's cramp, musicians, athletes
  - Tremor (moderate to marked improvement)
    - Hemifacial spasm and other movement disorders

Diagnosis

Graded compression ultrasonography of the right lower abdominal region may show mural thickening of the terminal ileum and cecum.[99] Dark-field microscopy of the stool may reveal the characteristic curved gram-negative nonsporing, thin, motile rod (*Campylobacter:* "curved rod" [Greek]). Gram stains should be counterstained with carbolfuchsin. Blood cultures are appropriate in immunocompromised or toxic patients. Sigmoidoscopy demonstrates an edematous, hyperemic mucosa with shallow gray-based aphthous ulcers.

Treatment

Without treatment, *Campylobacter* enterocolitis usually resolves in 7 to 10 days. Avoid opiates and anticholinergics that can lengthen intestinal transit time or worsen the disease. Fluids alone are often the only treatment necessary. Erythromycin ethyl succinate is the drug of choice; 400 mg four times a day often shortens the excretion of the organism. Its effectiveness in reducing symptoms when administered over the first 5 days of the illness is questionable.

LISTERIA MONOCYTOGENES

Pathophysiology

L. monocytogenes, a facultative, intracellular bacterium, causes disease primarily in pregnant women, neonates, and immunocompromised patients.

Source

L. monocytogenes is ubiquitous, appearing in streams, sewage, soil, domestic and wild animals, fowl, and humans. Carrier rates in man approximate 5% in healthy adults and are higher in special risk groups. Listeria can penetrate the placenta and produce intrauterine infections. *L. monocytogenes* organisms can remain in pasteurized milk even after proper processing. Recent epidemics of listeriosis resulted from the consumption of cabbage, cheese, pasteurized milk, and raw vegetables.

Signs/Symptoms

In healthy adults and children, *L. monocytogenes* produces a mild flulike syndrome, with gastrointestinal symptoms and myalgias resolving in several days. A meningitis and/or sepsis characterized by nausea, vomiting, headache, and fever develops in immunocompromised patients. Perinatal infections can cause either perinatal meningitis or intrauterine fetal demise.

Table 53–20
Intravenous Antibiotics Suggested for Treating Listeria: Dosages and Dosage Intervals[a]

Antibiotic	Dosage per Day	Interval
Ampicillin	200–300 mg/kg	Every 4 hr
Penicillin G	240,000–48,000 U/kg	Every 4 hr
Gentamicin	5–6 mg/kg	Every 6–8 hr
Tobramycin	5–6 mg/kg	Every 6–8 hr
Erythromycin	40–60 mg/kg	Every 6 hr
Tetracycline	15 mg/kg	Every 6 hr
Doxycycline	3 mg/kg intravenous load, then 1.5 mg/kg	Every 12 hr
Sulfmethoxazole and trimethoprim	15 and 75 mg/kg	Every 8 hr
Vancomycin	2 g	Every 12 hr

[a]Adapted from Gellin BG, Broome CV. JAMA 1989;261:1313–1318.

Diagnosis

An initial study of human listeriosis suggests that detection of antibodies against listeriolysin O (LLO), an extracellular hemolysin, may aid in the diagnosis of listeriosis, especially when bacteria have not been isolated.[100] LLO appears to be produced by all pathogenic strains of *L. monocytogenes.* Prior agglutination tests and complement fraction tests have been non-specific. Immunosuppression increases the risk of listeriosis. Total rise is 33%.[101]

Treatment

Intravenous antibiotics suggested for listeriosis treatment are found in Table 53–20.

REFERENCES—BACTERIAL FOODBORNE ILLNESS

1. Guerrant RL, Bobak DA. Bacterial and protozoal gastroenteritis. N Engl J Med 1991;325:327–340.
2. Smith PD, Lane HC, Gill VJ, Manischewitz JF, Quinnan GV, Fauci AS, Masur H. Intestinal infections in patients with acquired immunodeficiency syndrome (AIDS). Etiology and response to therapy. Ann Intern Med 1988;108:328–333.
3. Laughon BE, Druckman DA, Vernon A, Quinn TC, Polk BF, Modlin JF et al: Prevalence of enteric pathogens in homosexual men with and without acquired immunodeficiency syndrome. Gastroenterology 1988;94:984–993.
4. Perlman DM, Ampell NM, Schifman RB, Cohn DL, Patton CM, Aquirre ML et al. Persistent *Campylobacter jejuni* infections in patients infected with human immunodeficiency virus (HIV). Ann Intern Med 1988;109:540–546.
5. Farley D. Food safety crucial for people with lowered immunity. FDA Consumer 1990;24:7–9.
6. Johanson JF, Sonnenberg A. Efficient management of diarrhea in the acquired immunodeficiency syndrome (AIDS). Ann Intern Med 1990;112:942–948.
7. Greenson JK, Belitsos PC, Yardley JH, Bartlett JG: AIDS enteropathy: occult enteric infections and duodenal mucosal alterations in chronic diarrhea. Ann Intern Med 1991;114: 366–372.
8. Archer DL. Food counseling should be given to all persons infected with the human deficiency virus. J Infect Dis 1990;161:358–359.
9. Borowitz SM, Saulsbury FT. Treatment of chronic cryptosporidial infection with orally administered human serum immune globulin. J Pediatr 1991;119:593–595.
10. Cook DJ, Kelton JG, Stanisz A, Collins SM. Somatostatin treatment for cryptosporidial diarrhea in a patient with the acquired immunodeficiency syndrome (AIDS). Ann Intern Med 1988;108:708–709.
11. Fafard J, Lalonde R. Long-standing cryptosporidiosis in a normal man: clinical response to spiramycin. J Clin Gastroenterol 1990;12:190–191.
12. Ungar BLP, Ward DJ, Fayer R, Quinn CA. Cessation of cryptosporidium-associated diarrhea in an acquired immunodeficiency syndrome patient after treatment with hyperimmune bovine colostrum. Gastroenterology 1990;98: 486–488.
13. Hale D, Aldeen W, Carroll K. Diarrhea associated with cyanobacteria-like bodies in an immunocompetent host. An unusual epidemiological source. JAMA 1994;271:144–145.
14. Shera AG. Specific granular lesions associated with intestinal Spirochaetosis. Br J Surg 1962;50:68–77.
15. Harland WA, Lee FD. Intestinal spirochaetosis. Br Med J 1967;3:718–719.
16. Kaplan LR, Takeuchi A. Purulent rectal discharge associated with a non-turponemal discharge. JAMA 1979;241:52–53.
17. Malnick H, Thomas M, Lotay H, Robbins M. Anaerobiospirillum species isolated from humans with diarrhea. J Clin Pathol 1983;36:1097–1101.
18. Malnick H, Jones A, Vickers JC. Anaerobiospirillum: cause of a "new" Zoonosis? Lancet 1989;1:1145–1146.
19. Rifkin GD, Opdyke JE. *Anaerobiospirillum succinicproducens* septicemia. J Clin Microbiol 1981;13:811–813.
20. Shlaes DM, Dul MJ, Lerner PI. *Anaerobiospirillum* bacteremia. Am Intern Med 1982;97:63–64.
21. Abuelo JF. Renal failure caused by chemicals, foods, plants, animal venoms, and misuse of drugs. An overview. Arch Intern Med 1990;150:505–510.
22. CDC. Bacterial enteritis. MMWR 1990;39:3.
23. Eherer AJ, Fordtran JS. Fecal osmotic gap and pH in experimental diarrhea of various causes. Gastroenterology 1992; 103:545–551.
24. CDC. The management of acute diarrhea in children: oral rehydration, maintenance and nutritional therapy. MMWR 1992;41:1–20.
25. DuPont HL. Bismuth subsalicylate in the treatment and prevention of diarrheal disease. Drug Intell Clin Pharm 1987;221: 687–693.
26. Horwitz ES, Barrett MJ, Bregman D et al: Public Health Service Study of Reye's syndrome and medications: report of the main study. JAMA 1987;257:1905–1911.
27. Barrett MJ. Association of Reye's syndrome with use of Pepto-Bismol (bismuth subsalicylate). Pediatr Infect Dis 1986;5:611.
28. Abramson JS, Givner LB, Woods CR Jr. Bismuth in infants with watery diarrhea. N Engl J Med 193;329:1762.
29. Pickering LK, Feldman S, Ericsson CD et al: Absorption of salicylate and bismuth from a bismuth subsalicylate-containing compound (Pepto-Bismol). J Pediatr 1981;99: 654–656.
30. Levine RA. Risk of hypercalcemia from prophylaxis of traveler's diarrhea. JAMA 1983;249:1151–1152.
31. Mendelowitz PC, Hoffman RS, Wacher S. Bismuth absorption and myoclonic encephalopathy during bismuth subsalicylate therapy. Ann Intern Med 1990;112:140–141.
32. Du Pont HL, Ericsson CD, Johnson PC, Javier de la Caboda F. Use of bismuth subsalicylate for the prevention of traveler's diarrhea. Rev Infect Dis 1990;12(Suppl 1):564–567.
33. Hasking GJ, Duggan JM. Encephalopathy from bismuth salicylate. Med J Aust 1982;2:167.
34. Farley D. Food safety crucial for people with lowered immunity. FDA Consumer July-August 1990;24:7–9.
35. DuPont HL. Traveller's diarrhoea. Which antimicrobial? Drugs 1993;4:917.
36. DuPont HL, Ericsson CD. Prevention and treatment of traveler's diarrhea. N Engl J Med 1993;328:1821–1827.
37. Farthing MJG. Traveller's diarrhoea. Mostly due to bacteria and difficult to prevent. Br Med J 1993;303:1425–1426.
38. Bacillus cereus food poisoning associated with fried rice at two child day care centers—Virginia 1993. MMWR 1994; 43:177–178.
39. Ericsson CD, DuPont HL. Traveler's diarrhea: approaches to prevention and treatment. Clin Infect Dis 1993;16:616–626.

40. Fey H. Staphylococcal enterotoxins. In Kohler RB, ed. Antigen to diagnose bacterial infection, Vol 2, Boca Raton, FL: CRC Press, 1986.
41. Ehringhaus C Dominick H-C, Schuller M. Protein-losing enteropathy associated with *Clostridium perfringens* infection. Lancet 1989;2:268–269.
42. Abdominal pain, total intravascular hemolysis and death in a 53-year-old woman. Clinicopathologic conference. Am J Med 1990;88:667–674.
43. Lindsay VA, Mach AS, Wiulkinson MA, Martin LM, Wallace FM, Keller A. *Clostridum perfringens* type A cytotoxin-enterotoxin(s) as triggers for death in the sudden infant death syndrome. Development of a toxico-infection hypothesis. Curr Microbiol 1993;27:51–59.
44. Bennish ML, Harris JR, Wojtyniak BJ, Struelens M. Death in Shigellosis: incidence and risk factors in hospitalized patients. J Infect Dis 1990;161:500–506.
45. Bennish ML. Potentially lethal complications of Shigellosis. Rev Infect Dis 1991;13(Suppl 4):S319–S324.
46. Salam MA, Bennish ML. Antimicrobial therapy for Shigellosis. Rev Infect Dis 1991;13(Suppl 4):S332–S341.
47. Babu K, Sonnenberg M, Kathpalia S, Ortego P, Swiatlo AL, Kocka FE. Isolation of Salmonellae from dried rattlesnake preparations. J Clin Microbiol 1990;28;361–362.
48. Cone LA, Boughton WH, Leliu LH. Rattlesnake capsule-induced *Salmonella arizonae* bacteremia. West J Med 1990; 153:315–316.
49. Noskin GA, Clarke JT. *Salmonella arizonae* bacteremia as the presenting manifestation of human immunodeficiency virus infection following rattlesnake meat ingestion. Rev Infect Dis 1990;12:514–517.
50. Iguana-associated salmonellosis–Indiana 1990. MMWR 1992; 41:38–39.
51. CDC. Reptile-associated salmonellosis. Selected states, 1994–1995. MMWR 1995;44:347–350.
52. CDC. Outbreak of *Salmonella enteritidis* infection associated with consumption of raw shell eggs. MMWR 1992;41:369–372.
53. Blumenthal D. From the chicken to the egg. FDA Consumer 1990;24(3):7–8.
54 Advisory Committee on the Microbiological Safety of Food. Report on Salmonella in Eggs. London: HM Stationery Office, 1993.
55. Rampling A. Salmonella enteritis five years on. Lancet 1993; 324:317–318.
55a. Desenclos J-C, Bouvet P, Benz-Lemoine E, Grimont F et al. Large outbreak of *Salmonella enterica* serotype *paratyphin B* infection caused by a goat's milk cheese, France, 1993: a case finding and epidemiologic study Br Med J 1996;12: 91–94.
56. CDC. Outbreak of *Salmonella enteritidis* associated with nationally distributed ice cream products—Minnesota, South Dakota and Wisconsin, 1994. MMWR 1994;43: 740–741.
57. Lee LA, Taylor J, Carter GP, Quinn B, Farmer JJ III, Tauxe RV, and the *Yersinia enterocolitica* Colloborative Study Group. *Yersinia enterocolitica* 0:3: an emerging cause of pediatric gastroenteritis in the United States, J Infect Dis 1991;163: 660–663.
58. Tacket CO, Narain JP, Sattin R, et al. A multistate outbreak of infection caused by *Yersinia enterocolitica* transmitted by pasteurized milk. JAMA 1984;251:483–486.
59. Cover TL, Aber RC. *Yersinia enterocolitica.* N Engl J Med 1989;321:16–24.
60. CDC. *Yersinia enterocolitica* bacteremia and endotoxic shock associated with red blood cell transfusions—United States, 1991. MMWR 1991;40;176–178.
61. Munro R, Lye A. *Yersinia enterocolitica* bacteraemia after blood transfusion. Med J Aust 1990;152:280.
62. Case 41-1989. Case records of Massachusetts General Hospital. 1989;321:1029–1038.
63. Ali MB, Raff MJ. Primary *Vibrio vulnificus* sepsis in Kentucky. South Med J 1990;83:356–357.
64. Bullen JJ, Spalding PB, Ward CG, Gutteridge JMC. Hemochromatosis, iron and septicemia caused by *Vibrio vulnificus.* Arch Intern Med 1991;151:1606–1609.
65. CDC. Multistate outbreak of viral gastroenteritis related to consumption of oysters—Louisiana, Maryland, Mississippi and North Carolina, 1993. MMWR 1993;42:945–948.
66. Concern continues about *Vibrio vulnificus.* FDA Drug Bulletin 1988;18(1):3.
67. Johnston JM, Becker SF, McFarland FM. *Vibrio vulnificus:* man and the sea. JAMA 1985;253:2850–2853.
68. Tacket CO, Brenner F Blake PA. Clinical features and an epidemiologic study of *Vibrio vulnificus* infection. J Infect Dis 1984;149:558–561.
69. Morris JG. Antibiotic therapy for *Vibrio vulnificus* infection. JAMA 1985;253:1121–1122.
70. CDC. Update: cholera—Western Hemisphere, 1992. MMWR 1993;42:89–91.
71. Swerdlow DL, Ries AA. Cholera in the Americas. Guidelines for the clinical. JAMA 1992;267:1495–1499.
72. CDC. Update. *Vibrio cholerae* 01—Western hemisphere, 1991–1994, and *V. cholerae* 0139—Asia, 1994. JAMA 1995; 273:1169.
73. CDC. Imported cholera associated with a newly described toxigenic *Vibrio cholerae* 0139 strain—California, 1993. MMWR 1993;42:501–503.
74. Cholera Working Group, International Centre for Diarrhoeal Diseases Research, Bangladesh. Large epidemic of cholera-like disease in Bangladesh caused by *Vibrio cholerae* 0139 synonym Bengal. Lancet 1993;342:387–390.
75. CDC. Cholera—Peru 1991. MMWR 1991;40:108–110.
76. Swerdlow DL, Ries AA. *Vibrio cholerae* non–01—the eighth pandemic? Lancet 1993;324:382–383.
77. Mathewson JJ, Johnson PC, Du Pont HL, Morgan DR, Thornton SA, Wood LV, Ericsson CD. A newly recognized cause of traveler's diarrhea: enteroadherent *Escherichia coli.* J Infect Dis 1985;151:471–475.
78. Giron JA, Jones T, Millan-Velasco F, Catro-Munoz E, Zarate L, Fry J et al. Diffuse adhereing *Escherichia coll* (DAEC) as a putative cause of diarrhea in Mayan children in Mexico. J Infect Dis 1991;163:507–513.
79. Borczyzk AA, Karmali MA, Lior H, et al. Bovine reservoir for verotoxin-producing *Escherichia coli* 0157:H7. Lancet 1987; 1:98.
80. McCarty M. US seeks to rid beef of *E. Coli.* Lancet 1993; 341:687.
81. Swerdlow DL, Woodruff BA, Brady RC, Griffen PM, Tiffen S, Donnell HD et al: A waterborne outbreak in Missouri of *Escherichia coli* 0157-H7 associated with bloody diarrhea and death. Ann Intern Med 1992;117:812–819.
82. CDC. Community outbreak of hemolytic uremia syndrome attributable to *Escherichia coli*:0111:NM–South Australia, 1995. MMWR 1995;44:550–558.
82a. Woodruff BA, Griffin PM, McCroskey, Smart JF, Wainwright RB, Bryant RG et al: Clinical and laboratory comparison of botulism from toxin types A, B, and E in the United States, 1975–1988. J Infect Dis 1992;166:1281–1286.
83. CDC. Foodborne botulism—Oklahoma, 1994. MMWR 1995; 44:200–201.
84. Davis LE, Johnson JK, Bichnell JM, Levy H, McEvoy KM. Human type A botulism and treatment with 3,4-diamino pyridine. Neurology 1991;41(Suppl 1):142.
85. Frankovich TL, Arnon SS. Clinical trial of botulism immune globulin for infant botulism. West J Med 1991;154:103.
86. Schwartz PJ, Arnon SS. Botulism immune globulin for infant botulism arrives—one year and a Gulf War later. West J Med 1991;156:197–198.
87. Mechen CC, Walter FG. Wound botulism. Vet Hum Toxicol 1994;36:233–237.
87a. Weber JT, Goodpasture HC, Alexander H, Werner SB, Hatheway CL, Tauxe RV. Wound botulism in a patient with a tooth abscess: case report and review. Clin Infect Dis 1993;16:635–639.
88. Burmingham MD, Water FG, Mecham C. Wound botulism. Ann Emerg Med 1994;24:1184.
88a. CDC. Wound botulism—California, 1995. JAMA 1996;275: 95–96.
89. Donley DK, Knight P, Tenoro G, Oh SJ. A patient with infant botulism improving with edrophonium. Neurology 1991; 41(Suppl 1):201.

90. Schmidt RD, Schmidt TW. Infant botulism. A case series and review of the literature. J Emerg Med 1992;10:713–718.
91. Hikes DC, Manoli A II. Wound botulism. J Trauma 1981;21: 68–71.
92. Swedberg J, Wendel TH, Deiss F. Wound botulism. West J Med 1987;147:335–338.
93. Corridan P, Nightingale S, Mashoudi H, Williams AC. Acute angle closure glaucoma following botulinum toxin injection for Blepharospasm. Br J Ophthalmol 1990;74: 309–310.
94. Haug BA, Fresler D, Prange NCI. Polyradiculoneuritis following botulinum toxin therapy. J Neurol 1990;237:62–63.
95. Glanzman RL, Gelb DJ, Drury I, Bromberg MB, Truong DD. Bracheal plexopathy after botulinum toxin injections. Neurology 1990;41:1143.
96. Botulinum toxin for ocular muscle disorders. Med Lett Drugs Ther 1990;32(830):100–101.
97. Janovic J, Brin MF. N Engl J Med 1991;324:1186–1194.
98. Andrew PI, Kainer G, Yong LCJ, Tobias VH, Rosenberg AR. Glomerulonephritis, pulmonary hemorrhage and anemia associated with *Campylobacter jejuni* infection. Austral NZ J Med 1989;19:721–723.
99. de Bois MHW, Schoemaker MC, van der Werf SDJ, Puylaert JBCM. Pancreatitis associated with *Campylobacter jejuni* infection: diagnosis by ultrasonography. Br Med J 1989;298: 1004.
100. Berche P, Reich KA, Bonnichon M, Beretti J-L, Geoffrey C, Raveneau J et al. Detection of anti-listeriolysin 0 for serodiagnosis of human listeriosis. Lancet 1990;335:624–627.
101. Pigrau C, almiran B, Pahissa A, Gasser I, Vazquez JMM. Clinical presentation and outcome in cases of listeriosis. Clin Infect Dis 1993;17:143–146.
102. Gellin BG, Broome CV. Listeriosis. JAMA 1989;261(9):1313–1318.
103. Blatt SP, Zajac RA. Treatment of listeria bacteremia with vancomycin. Rev Infect Dis 1991;13:181–182.

VIRAL GASTROENTERITIS

Table 53–3 summarizes information relevant to an outbreak of viral gastroenteritis.

PATHOPHYSIOLOGY

Diminished absorption of Na^+ and glucose (plus water) related to decreased Na^+, K^+ - ATPase activity causes a loss of significant amounts of Na^+ and $C1^-$ (but not K^+) in the stools of infants with rotavirus diarrhea who do not receive electrolyte solutions.[1]

SOURCE

Astroviruses are a common cause of viral gastroenteritis in children, producing clinical findings similar to those caused by rotavirus infection. They appear to be associated with illness more frequently than the enteric adenoviruses and are associated with almost half as many illnesses as rotavirus infection.[2,3]

SIGNS/SYMPTOMS

Two classic types of presentation of viral gastroenteritis occur.

Rotavirus/Adenovirus

Rotavirus and adenovirus produce intestinal disease, often in an epidemic setting, with a 24- and 72-hour incubation period. Vomiting begins abruptly and then resolves. Four to 7 days of watery, foul-smelling diarrhea follow.

Parvovirus

Parvovirus gastroenteritis is the adult variety with a 24- to 36-hour incubation period followed by the abrupt onset of diarrhea, nausea, malaise, and mild abdominal cramps. Nonspecific symptoms (e.g., myalgias) often accompany the illness. No blood appears in the stools.

TREATMENT

Treatment is supportive. Every child should be evaluated for signs of dehydration. Small children should be placed on a clear, caffeine-free, hypotonic fluid diet devoid of milk (e.g., cola, ginger ale, apple juice) and supplemented with a balanced electrolyte solution (Pedialyte RD, Infalyte, Lytren). Older children and adults may benefit from the BRATT diet (*B*ananas, *R*ice, *A*pples, *T*ea, *T*oast). The severity of symptoms and dehydration determines the need for hospitalization.

REFERENCES—VIRAL GASTROENTERITIS

1. Haffejee IE. The pathophysiology, clinical features and management of rotavirus diarrhea. Q J Med 1991;79:289–299.
2. Herrmann JE, Taylor DN, Echeverria P, Blacklow NR. Astroviruses as a cause of gastroenteritis in children. N Engl J Med 1991;324:1757–1760.
3. CDC. Viral gastroenteritis. 1990;39:6.

PROTOZOA AND OTHER GASTROINTESTINAL PARASITES (TABLE 53–2)

Table 53–2 lists less common parasitic infections. Table 53–21 summarizes protozoa parasites many of which are transmissible by water or food.

CRYPTOSPORIDIOSIS

The protozoan *Cryptosporidiosis parvum* has emerged in the past decade as a cause of severe diarrhea in immunodeficient patients and as a cause of failure to thrive or malnutrition, persistent diarrhea, and impaired delayed skin hypersensitivity in immunocompetent patients, particularly children in developing countries.[1]

Signs/Symptoms

Studies with HIV-positive patients suggest that pulmonary cryptosporidiosis with respiratory symptoms may be present and that cryptosporidiosis should be considered in all immunoincompetent patients with lung symptoms.[2] Toxic megacolon may also be found in the AIDS patient.[3] Cryptosporidiosis is often fatal in patients in AIDS.[4]

Table 53–21
Protozoa Parasitic for Man Transmissible by Water or Food[a]

Parasite	Pathogenicity for Man	Stage Transmitted
Balantidium coli	+	Cyst
Blastocystis hominis	–/+	Not known
Cryptosporidium parvum	+	Oocyst
Other *Cryptosporidium* spp	–*	Oocyst
Chilomastix mesnili	–/+	Cyst
Dientamoeba fragilis	–/+	Trophozoite
Endolimax nana	–/+	Cyst
Entamoeba coli	–	Cyst
Entamoeba histolytica	+	Cyst
Microsporidia (e.g., *Enterocytozoom*)	–/+	Spore
Enteromonas hominis	–	Cyst
Giardia intestinalis	+	Cyst
Iodamoeba butschlii	–	Cyst
Isospora belli	–/+	Oocyst
Retortamonas intestinalis	–	Cyst
Sarcocystis spp	+	Oocyst/tissue stages
Toxoplasma gondii	+	Oocyst/tissue stages
Trichomonas hominis	–	Trophozoite
Trichomonas tenax	–	Trophozoite

[a]Adapted from Casemore DR. Lancet 1990;336:1428.
–/+ = low or doubtful for immunocompetent individuals; pathogenicity for the immunocompromised individual may differ.
*Transmission to man not yet documented but probably occurs.

Diagnosis

Biopsy of the large or small bowel reveals hemotoxylin-and-eosin darkly stained structures 4 to 5 micrometers in diameter at the tips of intestinal microvilli of the epithelial brush border. Contrast radiographic studies and other routine laboratory tests such as complete blood count and liver function are not helpful in establishing the diagnosis.[5]

Treatment

There is no specific therapy for cryptosporidiosis. Symptomatic patients are treated with intravenous fluids, electrolyte management, and nonspecific antidiarrheal agents.[6]

Cryptosporidium oocysts are present in 65 to 95% of surface water (i.e., rivers, lakes, and streams) tested throughout the United States. Risk of transmission can be reduced by water filtration.[7] Treating water before bottling by distillation or reverse osmosis filtration ensures removal of oocysts if they are present.

MICROSPORIDIOSIS

Microsporidia are now being increasingly recognized as important opportunistic pathogens in human immunodeficiency virus (HIV) infection. Microsporidiosis has also been described in immunocompetent hosts. Diseases caused by the different microsporidia that infect humans include diarrhea, keratoconjunctivitis, disseminated disease, hepatitis, myositis, kidney and urogenital infection, ascites, cholangitis, and asymptomatic carriage. Knowledge of the epidemiology of microsporidiosis in humans is limited, but as with cryptosporidiosis, microsporidiosis is probably a common, self-limited or asymptomatic infection in immunocompetent hosts.[8]

Epidemiology

The epidemiology of microsporidiosis is poorly understood. Most likely, these are waterborne pathogens, and the environmental reservoirs need to be identified.

Life Cycle

Microsporidia have a life cycle consisting of three phases: a proliferative phase, the spore production phase (sporogonial phase), and the spore or infective phase. Although spores are environmentally resistant, they may be killed by exposure for 30 minutes to 70% ethanol, 1% formaldehyde, or 1% hydrogen peroxide or by placing them in an autoclave at 120°C for 10 minutes.

Genera Associated with Human Disease

Six microsporidian genera have been associated with human disease: *Nosema (N. corneum* has been recently renamed *Vittaforma corneae,* generally found in insects; *Pleistophora,* a pathogen of fish and insects; *Encephalitozoon,* found in many mammals; *Enterocytozoon,* found in many mammals; *Enterocytozoon,* found in patients with AIDS and several species of fish; and *Septata (Encephalitozoon),* also in patients with AIDS. A seventh genus, *Microsporidium,* has been used to designate microsporidia of uncertain taxonomic status. *Pleistophora* has been associated with myositis. *Encephalitozoon hellem* has been associated with superficial keratoconjunctivitis in patients with HIV infection, and these infections reportedly respond to topical fumagillin. *Encephalitozoon hellem* has also been associated with sinusitis, respiratory disease, prostatic abscesses, and disseminated infection, and these infections may respond to albendazole. *Nosema, Vittaforma,* and *Microsporidium* have been associated with stromal keratitis, which is seen with trauma in immunocompetent hosts. *Enterocytozoon bieneusi,* first described in 1985, is associated with malabsorption and diarrhea and has been described only in humans. *Encephalitozoon (Septata) intestinalis* causes enteric and disseminated infections in patients with AIDS and is found in enterocytes and cells of the lamina propria and urinary tract. On morphologic analysis *Septat intestinalis* was most closely aligned with the family *Encephalitozoonidae,* but its unique structure led to the establishment of a new genus for this organism. Because recent studies on small subunit rRNA have shown that *Septata intestinalis* is closely related to *Encephalitozoon hellem* and *Encephalitozoon cuniculi,* its status as a separate genus has been challenged, and it has been renamed *Encephalitozoon intestinalis.*

Laboratory

The small intestine has provided the highest diagnostic yield, but organisms have been seen in colon biopsy specimens.

Table 53-22
Marine Toxins[a]

Toxin	Produced By	Found In	Sequelae
Tetrodotoxin	Bacteria	Pufferfish, Newts	Neurotoxicity "Locked-In" Syndrome
Brevetoxin	Dinoflagellate (Ptychodiscus brevis)	Florida's red tides	Neurotoxic shellfish poisoning, death of fish
Palytoxin	Marine coelenterates (Palythora Spp.)	Philippine crabs, mackerel, triggerfish (Mariana Island)	May be fatal
Okadaic Acid	Marine dinoflagellates Sponges		Diarrhetic shellfish poisoning (DSP)
Ciguatera	Gambierdiscus toxicus (a marine dinoflagellate)	Reef fishes (throughout Pacific) Amberjack	Ciguatera
Maitotoxin	Toxic dinoflagellates	Tropical fish	Ciguatera (associated with Ciguatera)

[a]Adapted from Hokama Y. J Toxicol-Toxin Rev 1991;10:1–35; Alcala AC et al. Toxicon 1988;26:105–107; and Naharashi T. In: Bolans GN et al. Basic science in toxicology. Proceedings of the 5th International Congress of Toxicology, Brighton, England, July 16–21, 1988. London: Taylor and Francis, 1990.

Clinical Presentation

The major syndrome associated with microsporidiosis is diarrhea and wasting. This condition is usually caused by *Enterocytozoon bieneusi* (more than 90% of cases in the United States) and occasionally by *Septata intestinalis* (although in Europe this organism may be a more frequent cause of diarrhea than is *Enterocytozoon bieneusi*). Several studies have been done on the association between microsporidiosis and diarrhea. In HIV-infected patients evaluated for diarrhea, the prevalence of microsporidiosis has ranged from 10 to 40%.

Treatment

Therapy with albendazole (400 mg twice daily) eliminates *Encephalitzoon (Septata) intestinalis* infection and its symptoms. Diarrhea is markedly reduced in patients with *Enterocytozoon bieneusi* infection who received albendazole treatment. In such treated patients, however, the organism can still be seen in biopsy specimens, and relapse is common when treatment is stopped.

MARINE TOXINS

Properties of marine toxins are delineated in Table 53–22.

REFERENCES—PROTOZOA AND OTHER GASTROINTESTINAL PARASITES

1. Molbak K, Hojlyng N, Gottschau A, Correia SJC, Ingholt L, da Silva APJ, Aaby P. Cryptosporidiosis in infancy and childhood mortality in Guinea Bissau, West Africa. Br Med J 1993;307:417–420.
2. Hojlyng N, Jensen BN. Respiratory cryptosporidiosis in HIV-positive patients. Lancet 1988;1:590–591.
3. Connolly GM, Gazzard BG. Toxic megacolon in cryptosporidiosis. Postgrad Med J 1987;63:1103–1104.
4. Current VL, Carcia LS. Cryptosporidiosis. Clin Microbiol Rev 1991;4:325–358.
5. Wofsy C. Cryptosporidiosis and isosporiasis. AIDS Clin Care 1991;3(4):25–27.
6. Peterson C. Cryptosporidium and the food supply. Lancet 1995;345:1128–1129.
7. CDC. Assessing the public health threat associated with waterborne cryptosporidiosis: report of a workshop. MMWR 1995;44(RR-6):1–19.
8. Weiss LM . . . And now microsporidiosis. Ann Intern Med 1995;123:954–956.

MARINE FOODBORNE ILLNESS[1]

MARINE BIOTOXINS (TABLE 53-22)

Marine biotoxins are classified as orally acquired parenteral toxins (injected by teeth or spines), or crinotoxins (secreted directly into the water). Subclassification of fish containing oral toxins includes (a) ichthyosarcotoxic fish, which contain a poison within their flesh (e.g., scombroid, ciguatera fish poisoning); (b) ichthyohemotoxic fish, which have poisonous blood; and (c) ichthyootoxic fish, which contain a poison specifically in their gonads.[2]

Three conditions that may occur after consumption of seafoods (puffer fish poisoning, ciguatera, and paralytic shellfish poisoning) are caused by a group of poisons that block voltage-gated sodium channels in myelinated and nonmyelinated nerves. These conditions cannot easily be distinguished clinically.[3] Neurotoxins acting on the sodium channel are listed in Table 53–23[4]. Food neurotoxins are summarized in Table 53–23. Temporal sequence of clinical symptoms among seafood neurotoxins is summarized in Table 53–23A. Characteristics of toxins and poisons that occur naturally in seafood are presented in Table 53–24.

FISH ROE POISONING

Ichthyootoxic fresh and saltwater fish are numerous, but the exact nature of the toxin or toxins is unknown. Some of the toxins are heat resistant, so cooking may not prevent poisoning. Symptoms usually develop within several hours of ingestion and include abdominal pain, nausea, vomiting, dizziness, bitter taste, pallor, tachycardia, hypotension, and tinnitus. Recovery usually occurs within several days. Severe cases have progressed to seizures, coma, and death. Treatment is entirely supportive.[5]

CIGUATERA

Pathophysiology

At least three toxins may be responsible for ciguatera intoxication: ciguatoxin, maitotoxin, and scaritoxin and perhaps palytoxin and okadaic acid (Table 53–25).[7] Small reef fish ingest the dinoflagellate *Gambierdiscus toxicus,* which probably produces the toxic agents.[8] Gambiertoxins

Table 53–23
Food Neurotoxins

Toxin	Source	Chemistry	Mode of Action
Na^+ channel			
Guanidinium toxins			
Tetrodotoxin (TTX)	Japanese puffer fish: *Fugu* sp. Globe fish: *Spheroides rupripes* (Tetraodontidae), [identical with tarichatoxin of salamander *(Taricha torosa),* and maculotoxin from blue-ringed octopus *(Hapalochlaena maculosa)*]	Heterocyclic	Paralytic, blockade of nerve and muscle action potentials
Saxitoxin (STX)	Dinoflagellates: *Gonyaulax* spp.	Heterocyclic	Paralytic, blockade of nerve and muscle action potentials
Lipophilic toxins			
Brevetoxins (PbTx-1, PbTX-2, PbTX-3, PbTX-9)	Dinoflagellate: *Ptychodiscus brevis*	Cyclic polyether	Excitatory agent; repetitive firing in axons
Ciguatoxin	Dinoflagellate: *Gambierdiscus toxicus*	Cyclic polyether	Excitatory agent; repetitive firing in axons
Ca^+ channels			
Polypeptide toxins			
Maitotoxin	Dinoflagellate: *Gambierdiscus toxicus*	Water-soluble polyether	Contributes to ciguatera poisoning involving parasthesia; gastrointestinal and neurological distress
Presynaptic toxins			
Bacterial toxins			
Botulinum toxins (seven immunological types: A, B, C1, C2, D, E, F, G)	Bacterium: *Clostridium botulinum*	150 kDa polypeptides, proteolytically processed to form heavy chain (100 kDa) and light chain (50 kDa)	Flaccid paralysis resulting from inhibition of depolarization-induced transmitter release
Tetanus toxin	Bacterium: *Clostridium tetani*	140 kDa polypeptide	Similar to botulinum toxin; spastic paralysis; possibly different target neurons involved
Protein phosphatase			
Okadaic acid	Marine dinoflagellates: accumulates in sponges and mussels	Polyether derivative of 38-carbon fatty acid	Smooth and cardiac muscle contracture; tumor promoter; causative agent in diarrhetic shellfish poisoning
Ionophores			
Palytoxin	Marine coelenterates of genus *Palythoa:* (e.g., *P. caribaeorum*)	Polycyclic hemiketal	Depolarization, contracture, vasoconstriction; cytotoxic at picomolar concentrations; induces histamine release

[a]Adapted from Adams ME, Swanson G. Trends Neurosci 1994;(Suppl).

Table 53–23A
Temporal Sequence of Clinical Symptoms Among Seafood Neurotoxins Ciguatoxin (CTX), Saxitoxin (STX), Tetrodotoxin (TTX), Neurotoxic Shellfish Poison (NSP), and Domoic Acid (DA)[a]

	CTX	STX	TTX	NSP	DA
GI	0–8 hr	0–1 hr	0–1 hr	0–3 hr	1–24 hr
Paresthesia	12–24 hr	0–8 hr	0–3 hr	1–3 hr	24–28 hr
Sens paradox	2–5 days	—	1–3 hr	1–3 hr	—
Bulbar	—	1–12 hr	1–4 hr	—	—
Motor	10–18 hr	Flaccid	Flaccid	—	Neuropathy
Respiratory	—	Apnea	Apnea	—	—
Other	—	Neuropathy	DIC	Rhinorrhea Bronchospasm	Seizure Coma Amnesia
Mortality	0.1%	8–10%	50–80%	1%	3%

[a]Watters MR. Clin Neurol Neurosurg 1995;97:119–125.

produced in *Gambierdiscus toxus* probably are precursors that are oxidized to ciguatoxins (CTX-1, 2, and 3)[9,10]

Maitotoxin exerts an arrhythmogenic effect by increasing Ca^{++} membrane permeability.[11] In animal models, ciguatoxin partially inhibits the action potential,[12] perhaps by blockade of calcium sites that regulate passive sodium permeability. Ciguatoxin causes persistent sodium channel opening in the nerve membranes. Permeability of the sodium

Table 53–24
Characteristics of Toxins and Poisons That Occur Naturally in Seafood[a]

Type of Toxin or Poison	Seafood Involved	Cause	Signs and Symptoms	Onset	Duration	Treatment
Scombroid fish poisoning	Mahimahi, tuna, bluefish, mackerel, skipjack	Histidine in flesh decarboxylated by action of *Proteus* species or other bacteria	Metallic or peppery taste; intense headache, dizziness, nausea, vomiting, facial swelling and flushing, throbbing of carotid and temporal vessels, rapid and weak pulse, burning of throat, itching of skin, generalized erythema and urticarial eruptions	Few minutes to 4 hr	Up to 24 hr	Administering antihistamines results in immediate improvement of condition
Ciguatera poisoning	Tends to be fish from coral reefs (>400 species)	Ciguatoxin; lipid-soluble, polyether multicomponent	Abdominal pain, diarrhea, vomiting, paresthesia, vertigo, ataxia, cold-to-hot sensory reversal, mylagia, itching	3 to 5 hr, up to 24 hr	24 hr usually, but neurologic effects up to 6 mo	No effective antidote; mannitol may be effective in acute cases
Paralytic shellfish poisoning	Mussels, clams, other shellfish; some finfish	Saxitoxin or related compounds; purine base, water soluble	Tingling or burning and numbness around lips and fingertips; respiratory paralysis within 12 hr; patients often report feeling of lightness or floating on air	<1 hr	Prognosis good after 24 hr	No antidote; artificial respiration; rest
Neurotoxic shellfish poisoning	Bivalves and most plankton feeders	Neurotoxin from *Ptychodiscus;* lipid-soluble polyether	Similar to mild case of ciguatera or paralytic shellfish poisoning	<3 hr	<48 hr	No specific treatment
Amnesic shellfish poisoning	Mussels, clams, crabs, anchovies	Domoic acid	Vomiting, cramps, diarrhea, short-term memory loss, disorientation, facial grimace or chewing motion; memory loss can be long term and in severe cases can cause brain damage or death	24 to 48 hr	Unknown	No known antidote

[a]Adapted from Gellert GR et al. West J Med 1992;15:645–647.

Table 53-25
Toxins Involved in the Pathogenesis of Ciguatera

	Chemical	M.W. (daltons)	Action
Ciguatoxin ($C_6G_{86}I_{19}$)	Polyether	1111.7	Increase in sodium passage intracellularly Increase intracellular calcium, fluid secretion, diarrhea
Maitotoxin ($C_{160}H_{225}S_2O_{74}$)	Polyether	3402	Mobilizes intracellular calcium
Scaritoxin	Polyether		
Okadaic Acid ($C_{44}H_{66}O_{12}$)	Polyether	787.01	Sodium ionophore
Palytoxin ($C_{129}H_{223}N_3O_{54}$)	Polyether	2781	Causes severe muscle tonic contractions

Table 53-26
Toxins Specific to Voltage-Gated Sodium Channels

1. Tetrodotoxin, saxitoxin	Sodium channel antagonists
2. Veratridine, batrachotoxin, grayanatoxin	Lipid-soluble toxins that cause activation of sodium channels
3. Polypeptide toxins (sea anemone toxins, scorpion toxins)	Slow sodium current inactivation
4. Scorpion toxins	Shift voltage dependence of sodium channel activator
5. Pyrethroids	Transform fast sodium channels into slow ones
6. Ciguatoxin	Increased binding affinity during sodium channel activation

ion is thereby increased (Table 53–26).[13] Paradoxical sensory discomfort is probably due to an exaggerated and intense nerve depolarization occurring in peripheral myelinated and nociceptor fibers.[14]

Diagnosis

A test kit is being developed by Hawaii Chentect International of Pasadena, California. At present there is no available blood test that will confirm ciguatera poisoning in man.[15]

Clinical Presentation

Ciguatera produces characteristic gastrointestinal, neurologic, and to a lesser extent, cardiovascular symptoms.[16]

Gastrointestinal symptoms are often the first to appear with abdominal pain, nausea, painful defecation, diarrhea, and vomiting. Though dehydration by vomiting and diarrhea may prove serious, gastrointestinal symptoms usually last only 1 or 2 days. Vomiting is less common with second attacks. It is unknown if a central or gastrointestinal action of the toxin causes vomiting.

Neurologic symptoms are usually the most bothersome and lingering complaints. Paresthesias, described as uncomfortable tingling sensations, most often develop in the extremities, oral cavity (sensation of loose tooth), and pharynx. Perhaps the most characteristic hallmark is paradoxical dysesthesias, often labeled as temperature reversal, which most often manifests as cold objects feeling hot, burning, or painful to the touch.[16] Neurologic complaints persist as long as 6 months.[7]

Treatment

Based on a suspected cerebral edema in two patients who were comatose from ciguatera fish poisoning, administration of a mannitol infusion was administered and resulted in dramatic improvement of symptoms.[18] Subsequently use of 0.5 g to 1.0 g/kg of 20% mannitol IV given over a 30-minute to 1-hour period has appeared to shorten morbidity and shorten hospital stays[1] by inducing improvement in headache, malaise, pruritus, irritability, and other manifestations of acute ciguatoxin poisoning.[19,20] A 23-month-old child responded to 50 mL of a 20% mannitol solution (1.1 g/kg) administered over 10 minutes with diminished irritability within minutes and less carpopedal spasm. Thirty-six hours after admission, the carpopedal spasm totally resolved and the neurologic examination was normal.[21] Dopamine, plasma expanders, and calcium gluconate may be useful for shock.[22]

Mannitol is a strong diuretic and may present a potential hazard to a patient dehydrated from vomiting and diarrhea. Assess and correct fluid and electrolyte balance before mannitol is given. If the patient has been symptomatic for 24 hours or more, mannitol may be less effective.

Steroids, opiates, and barbiturates are not effective on ciguatera. Alcohol consumption may exacerbate symptoms.[16] Similar case reports suggest that tocainide may improve the chronic neurologic symptoms.[23]

The mechanism of action of amitriptyline is not clear, but it is likely through sodium channel modulation.[24] Trials with tocainide and mexiletine were undertaken because of their more specific pharmacologic action-blocking sodium channels.[25] The rationale for phenytoin and carbamazepine also relate to their pharmacologic effect on sodium channels. Since maitotoxin opens calcium channels, another approach has used amitriptyline in conjunction with a calcium channel blocking agent such as nifedipine.

Prevention

Preventive measures that may reduce the incidence of poisoning outbreaks following seafood ingestion include the following[26]:

1. Avoidance of eating raw seafood.
2. Avoidance of eating mollusks that have been partially cooked (steamed for 1 minute, just to open the shell).

Table 53–27
Recommended Treatment of Scombroid Poisoning[a]

Degree of Poisoning	Clinical Features	Treatment
Mild poisoning	Rash only or brief flushing Tachycardia	• Observe for 2 hours • Consider parenteral antihistamines if condition fails to improve or worsens
Moderate poisoning	Rash and persistent flushing Tachycardia Headache and/or gastrointestinal symptoms	• Basic life support ABC, O_2 • Intravenous access • Parenteral antihistamines (H_1 and H_2 antagonists). Repeat if necessary • Oral activated charcoal without gastric emptying • Overnight admission if symptoms slow to resolve
Severe poisoning	Any of the above and/or bronchospasm and/or hypotension and/or airway compromise and/or angio-edema	• Basic life support ABC, O_2 and/or advanced life support • Intravenous fluids • Adrenaline • Parenteral antihistamine (H_1 and H_2 antagonists). Repeat as necessary • Orogastric lavage • Activated charcoal • Nebulized bronchodilators • Hospital admission

[a]Adapted from Smart DR. Med J Aust 1992;157:748–751.

3. Adherence to the state, local, or federal guidelines regarding the safety of the waters for harvesting shellfish.
4. Prompt refrigeration of the catch by sport fishermen.
5. Avoidance of eating the usually implicated species in ciguatera poisoning, especially barracuda.
6. Avoidance of eating fish liver.
7. Prompt reporting of the suspected outbreaks of seafood poisoning to local health departments.

SCOMBROID FISH (TABLE 53–27)

Sources

Scombroid families may include the saurie, needlefish, kingfish, wahoo, and albacore in addition to the tuna, bonita, skipjack, and mackerel. Other dark meat fish not belonging to the scombridae also implicated include the amberjack (yellowtail or Kahala, mahi mahi (dolphin fish), bluefish *(Pomatomus saltatrix),*[27] kahawai, anchovy, herring, and Australian ocean salmon. In Hawaii the fish most frequently implicated is mahi mahi *(Coryphaena hippurus).*[28] If scombroid are inadequately preserved, bacteria breakdown endogenous histidine in the fish tissue to form high levels of histamine and of a toxic substance, saurine.

Signs/Symptoms

Within minutes to hours after ingesting the fish, the patient develops signs and symptoms of a severe histamine-mediated reaction: a diffuse erythema of the face resembling sunburn, giant urticaria, pruritis or a hot burning sensation, dizziness, throbbing headache, nausea, vomiting, abdominal cramps and diarrhea, and, in severe cases, bronchospasm, respiratory distress, and hypotension. The symptoms generally are self-limited subsiding in 8 to 10 hours.

Diagnosis

Diagnosis is based on the clinical presentation.

Histamine levels in normal fresh fish should be less than 1 mg%, (1 mg/100 mg). Levels of 20 mg/100 g in some species have been reported to produce symptoms.[29] The FDA has established 50 mg% as the hazard action level for histamine in tuna.[30,31] Demonstration of levels greater than 100 mg% is diagnostic for histamine fish poisoning. Isoniazid inhibits the diamine oxidase that oxidizes histamine. Individuals accumulate high concentrations of histamine following a histamine challenge. Levels of histamine and its metabolite, *N*-methylhistamine, in the urine were 9 to 20 times, and 15 to 20 times normal, respectively, in one series of poisoned patients.[32]

Treatment

Chronic persistent symptoms such as headache, abdominal cramps, and diarrhea may respond to oral cimetidine 300 mg every 6 hours. Symptoms have resolved within 48 hours.[33] Fluids and bronchodilators should be administered as needed. Smart from Australia has summarized a recommended treatment of scombroid poisoning (Table 53–27).[34] Cimetidine (Tagamet) 300 mg (adult dose; pediatric dose 20 mg/kg) administered intravenously over 5 to 30 minutes gives immediate and complete resolution of the symptoms.[35]

Prevention

The scombrotoxins are heat stable, so cooking (drying, heating, smoking) will not alter the poisoned fish, nor will freezing, salting, or marinating fish that are already contaminated. Effective prevention of scombroid poisoning requires proper handling and storage of fish (rapid refrigeration).[36] Histamine formation usually appears negligible in fish stored at 0°C.[37]

PARALYTIC SHELLFISH TOXINS

Sources

Crabs found on the coral reefs of the Capricorn group in the southern region of the Great Barrier Reef, Queensland, Australia *(Atergatis floridus)* contain saxitoxin, neosaxitoxin, and gonyautoxin 1 and 2.[38] Mussels present the greatest hazard.[39]

A marine bacteria, *Moraxella sp.*, produces saxitoxin and has been associated with paralytic shellfish toxins (PSP toxins) in marine bivalves found in known toxic dinoflagellate-free water.[40]

Symptoms

Man who subsequently ingests the toxic mollusks may develop gastrointestinal, allergic, or paralytic symptoms. The most common type of poisoning is gastrointestinal characterized by nausea, vomiting, diarrhea, abdominal pain, and weakness, occurring 8 to 12 hours after ingestion and lasting up to 48 hours. It is believed that the symptoms are due to bacterial pathogens rather than to toxic tisues.[41]

Symptoms occur 30 minutes after eating a mollusk or crab. Paresthesia is noted first. The tingling, numbing, or burning sensations begin over the lips and tongue and spread over the face, scalp, and neck to the fingertips and toes. Sensory and proprioception are distorted, and the patient becomes ataxic and incoordinated. Speech is incoherent and aphasia may develop. The patient feels faint and weak and often complains of headache and "tightness" in the throat and chest. Salivation and perspiration are profuse. Nausea and vomiting may occur. The pulse becomes weak and thready. The deep-tendon reflexes are markedly diminished, and the superficial reflexes are absent. The symptoms grow progressively worse and may culminate in respiratory paralysis and death. The first 12 hours are critical, but if the patient survives this period, the prognosis is favorable.[40]

Treatment

No antidote is available. Treatment is supportive and includes gastric lavage or induced emesis to remove ingested toxins and careful monitoring of vital signs and fluid and electrolyte balance.[40]

Diarrhetic Shellfish Poisoning

Diarrhetic shellfish poisoning (DSP) has led to severe gastroenteritis among the Japanese. Gastrointestinal symptoms start within 4 hours after ingestion and may last up to 3 days. This has been traced to another genus of dinoflagellates, *Dinophysis* sp., common in Japan. The *Dinophysis* sp. elaborate pectenotoxin, dinophysistoxin, and okadaic acid, a potent tumor promoter.[42,43]

Amnestic Shellfish Poisoning (ASP)

ASP may be associated with a severe loss of memory.[44] Domoic acid is the parent structure of marine toxins produced by phytoplankton responsible for ASP.[45] (See Domoic Acid.)

Diagnosis

A capillary electrophoresis (CE) method with ultraviolet (UV) detection has been described for the separation and determination of underivatized toxins associated with paralytic shellfish poisoning. This permits detection of levels of 15 and 18 pg for underivatized saxitoxin (STX) and neosaxitoxin (NEO). Gonyautoxins (GTX), often found in toxic shellfish and dinoflagellates, can also be identified in a single CE-UV study together with NEO and STX.[46] Creatine kinase MB elevation has been found in four of five patients with PSP.[47]

Treatment

Decontaminate the gut (syrup of ipecac, charcoal, cathartics) if spontaneous vomiting does not occur within several hours of exposure. Watch carefully for signs of respiratory depression and admit symptomatic patients for observation for 24 hours.

Prevention

The California shellfish monitoring program has detected early toxic dinoflagellate blooms and enabled health agencies to issue special guidelines, close commercial harvesting areas, alert the sport shellfishing public, and take other public health measures.[48]

TETRODOTOXIN (PUFFER FISH)

Pathophysiology

Serial nerve conduction studies in a patient with tetrodotoxication caused by ingesting puffer fish indicated that tetrodotoxin equally and reversibly affects myelinated nerve fibers throughout the entire length of the axon by lowering the conduction of sodium currents at nodes of Ranvier.[49]

Signs/Symptoms

Patients with preexisting hypertension may respond to relatively small doses of tetrodotoxin with a dramatic rise in blood pressure that may be fatal.[50] Death may occur within the first 12 hours.[51] A rare "locked-in" syndrome has been described in which the patient appears completely flaccid but remains conscious. Symptoms generally resolve over a period of days. The prognosis is good if the patient survives 18 to 24 hours.[52] A recent sociologic investigation implicated the use of tetrodotoxin as the cause of zombiism in Haitian voodoo culture,[53] but this observation has been challenged.[54]

Treatment

Hypotension may be reversible by catecholamines.[55] Decontamination and endoscopic removal of the fish, if feasible, are important. Admit all patients. Intravenous edrophonium

(10 mg) or intramuscular neostigmine (0.5 mg) has been effective in restoring motor strength.[56]

REFERENCES—MARINE FOODBORNE ILLNESS

1. Halstead BW. Current status of marine biotoxicology—an overview. Clin Toxicol 1981;18:1–24.
2. Mills AR, Passamo R. Pelagic paralysis. Lancet 1988;1:161–163.
3. Mills AR, Passmore R. Pelagic paralysis. Lancet 1988;1:161–162.
4. Lombet A, Didard JN, Ladzunski M. Ciguatoxin and brevetoxins share a common receptor site on the neuronal voltage-dependent NA+ channel. FEBS Lett 1987;219:355–359.
5. Listernick R. Fish-roe poisoning childhood. J Pediatr 1987; 111:729–731.
6. Gellert GA, Ralls J, Brown C, Huston J, Merryman R. Scombroid fish poisoning underreporting and prevention among non-commercial recreational fishers. West J Med 1992;157: 645–647.
7. Ho AMH, Fraser IM, Todd EDC. Ciguatera poisoning: a report of three cases. Ann Emerg Med 1986;15:1225–1228.
8. Bagnis R, Chanteau S, Chungue E et al. Origins of ciguatera fish poisoning: a new dinoflagellate, *Gambierdiscus toxicus* Adachi and Fukuyo, definitely involved as the causal agent. Toxicon 1980;18:199–208.
9. Lewis RJ, Sellin M, Poli MA, Norton RS, Macleod JK, Sheil MM. Purification and characterization of ciguatoxins from Moray eel *(Lycodontus Javanicus, Muraenidae).* Toxicon 1991;29:1115–1127.
10. Juranovic LR, Park IL. Foodborne toxins of marine origin. Ciguatera. Rev Environ Contam Toxicol 1991;117:51–52.
11. Chanfour B, Longjon B, Lionet Ph, Jaeger A. Cardiovascular disturbances in 27 cases of ciguatera fish poisoning. Proc Eur Assoc Pois Cont Center, 1988, p. 29.
12. Setliff J, Rayner MD, Hong SK. Effect of ciguatoxin on sodium transport across the frog skin. Toxicol Appl Pharmacol 1971;18:676–684.
13. Swift AEB, Swift TR. Ciguatera. Clin Toxicol 1993;31:1–29.
14. Cameron J, Caupra MF. The basis of the paradoxical disturbance of temperature perception in ciguatera poisoning. Clin Toxicol 1993;31:571–579.
15. Adams MJ. An outbreak of ciguatera poisoning in a group of scuba divers. J Wilderness Med 1993;4:304–311.
16. Swift AEB, Swift TR. Ciguatera. Clin Toxicol 1993;31(1): 1–29.
17. Di Nuble MJ, Kohami Y. Ciguatera poisoning syndrome from farm-raised salmon. Ann Intern Med 1995;122:113–114.
18. Palafox NA, Jain LG, Pinano AZ, Gulick TM, Williams RK, Schatz IJ. Successful treatment of ciguatera fish poisoning with intravenous mannitol. JAMA 1988;259: 2740–2742.
19. Pearn JH, Lewis RJ, Ruff T, Tait M, Quinn J, Murtha W et al. Ciguatera and mannitol: experience with a new treatment regimen. Med J Aust 1989;151:77–80.
20. Williamson J. Ciguatera and mannitol: a successful treatment. Med J Aust 1990;153:306–307.
21. Williams RK, Palafox NA. Treatment of pediatric ciguatera fish poisoning. Am J Dis Child 1990;144:747–848.
22. Eastaugh J, Shepherd S. Infectious and toxic syndromes from fish and shellfish consumption. A Review. Arch Intern Med 1989;149:1735–1740.
23. Lange WR, Kreider SD, Hattwick M, Hobbs J. Potential benefit of tocainide in the treatment of ciguatoxin: report of three cases. Am J Med 1988;84:1087–1988.
24. Lange WR, Snyder RF, Fudala PJ. Travel and ciguatera fish poisoning. Arch Intern Med 1992;152:2049–2053.
25. Lange WR, Kneider SD, Hattwich M, Hobbs J. Potential benefit of tocainide in the treatment of ciguatera: report of three cases. Am J Med 1988;84:1087–1088.
26. Saavedra-Delgado AM, Metcalfe DD. Seafood toxins. Clin Rev Allergy 1993;11:241–260.
27. Etkind P, Wilson ME, Gallagher K, Cournoyer J. The working group on foodborne illness control. JAMA 1987;258:3409–3410.
28. Withers NW. Personal communication. Marine Medicine Symposium, University of California at San Diego, July 10–14, 1989.
29. CDC. Scombroid: fish poisoning—Illinois, South Carolina. MMWR 1989;39:140–147.
30. Kow-Tong C, Malison MD. Outbreak of scombroid fish poisoning, Taiwan. Am J Public Health 1987;77: 1335–1336.
31. U.S. Food and Drug Administration. Defect action levels for histamine in tuna: availability of guide. Fed Reg 1982;47: 40487
32. Morrow JD, Margolies GR, Rowland J, Roberts LJ. Evidence that histamine is the causative toxin of scombroid fish poisoning. N Engl J Med 1991;324:716–720.
33. Auerbach PS. Persistent headache associated with scombroid poisoning: resolution with oral cimetidine. J. Wilderness Med 1990;1:279–283.
34. Smart DR. Scombroid poisoning. A report of seven cases involving the Western Australian salmon, *Arripis truttaceus.* Med J Aust 1992;157:748–751.
35. Wingert W. Poisoning by marine animals. Personal communication.
36. Eastaugh J, Shepherd S. Infectious and toxic syndromes from fish and shellfish consumption. A review. Arch Intern Med 1989;149:1735–1740.
37. Taylor SL. Histamine food poisoning: toxicology and clinical aspects. CRC Crit Rev Toxicol 1987;17(2):91–128.
38. Llewellyn LE, Endean R. Paralytic shellfish toxins in the xanthid crab *(Atergatis floridus)* collected from Australian coral reefs. J Wilderness Med 1991;2:118–126.
39. Paralytic shellfish poisoning. LA County Public Health Lett 1983;5:26.
40. Ogata T, Sato S, Kodama M. Paralytic shellfish toxins in bivalves which are not associated with dinoflagellates. Toxicon 1989;27:1241–1244.
41. Wingert W. Paralytic shellfish poisoning. Personal communication on poisoning of marine animals.
42. Watters D, Lavin M. Toxins '89 Symposium. Toxicon 1990;28: 245–260.
43. Stabell OR, Hormazabal V, Steffenak I, Pedersen K. Diarrhetic shellfish toxins: improvement of sample clean-up for HPLC determinations. Toxicon 1991;29:21–29.
44. Fenicol W. Personal communication. Proc Marin Medicone Symposium. University of California San Diego, July 10–14, 1989, pp. 331–333.
45. Dickey RW, Rynell GA, Granade HR, Roelke D. Detection of the marine toxins okadaic acid and domoic acid in shellfish and phytoplankton in the Gulf of Mexico. Toxicon 1992; 30:355–359.
46. Thibault P, Pleasance S, Laycock MV. Analysis of paralytic shellfish poisons by capillary electrophoresis. J Chromatogr 1991; 542:483–501.
47. Cheng H-S, Chua SO, Hung J-S, Yip K-K. Creatine kinase MB elevation in paralytic shellfish poisoning. Chest 1991;99: 1032–1033.
48. Price DW, Kizer KW. California's paralytic shellfish poisoning prevention program 1927–1989. California Department of Health Services, 1990, pp. 1–36.
49. Oda K, Araki K, Totoki T, Shibasaki H. Nerve conduction study of human tetrodotoxication. Neurology 1989;39:743–745.
50. Deng J-F, Tominack RL, Chung H-M, Tsai W-J. Hypertension as an unusual feature in an outbreak of tetrodotoxin poisoning. Clin Toxicol 1991;29:71–79.
51. Habermetil GG, Krebs HC, Rasormaivo P, Ramishaliharisо A. Severe ciguatera poisoning in Madagascar. A case report. Toxicon 1994;1539–1541.
52. Bower DJ, Hart RJ, Matthew PA et al. Nonprotein neurotoxins. Clin Toxicol 1981;18:813–863.
53. Rivier L, Benedek C. Evidence for the presence of tetrodotoxin in a powder used in Haiti for zombification. Toxicon 1989;27:473–480.
54. Kao CY, Yasumoto T. Tetrodotoxin in "Zombie Powder." Toxicon 1990;28:129–132.
55. Kao CY. Pharmacology of tetrodotoxin and saxitoxin. Fed Proc 1972;31:1117–1123.

56. Chew SK, Chew LS, Wang KW et al. Anticholinesterase drugs in the treatment of tetrodotoxin poisoning. Lancet 1984;2:108.

DOMOIC ACID

Okadaic acid and domoic acid are the parent structure of marine toxins produced by the phytoplankton that are responsible for diarrhea, shellfish poisoning, and amnesic shellfish poisoning, respectively.[1,2]

Another outbreak followed ingestion of shellfish on the Pacific Northwest Coast in 1991.

STRUCTURE

Domoic acid[3] is a natural, heat-stable, water-soluble neuroexitatory amino acid produced by microscopic algae (photoplankton) known as *Nitzschia* pseudoserita.

MECHANISM OF ACTION

Domoic acid impersonates the normal neurotransmitter glutamic acid, resulting in neuronal damage. It is considered to be a natural "excitatotoxin," an agent that overstimulates but does not destroy cells.

CLINICAL PRESENTATION

Risk

Immunocompromised individuals appear to be most susceptible, including patients with hepatic gastric or hematologic diarrhea. In the 1987 Canada outbreak (107 cases studied) an acute illness followed ingestion of mussels contaminated with domoic acid.[4,5] Gastrointestinal symptoms (vomiting, abdominal cramps, diarrhea) within the first 24 hours were followed in 48 hours by unusual neurologic abnormalities (headache, loss of short-term memory, confusion, disorientation, disordered eye movements, mutism, purposeless chewing and grimacing, seizures, myoclonus, coma).[4,5] Additional signs included profuse respiratory secretions, hemodynamic instability, hiccups, cardiac arrhythmias, and piloerection. Chronic manifestations included an amnesic syndrome with relative preservation of other cognitive functions.[6] Three patients died. Two to four days after mussel ingestion fever developed in some patients.[5]

SOURCES

The source of domoic acid in the Canadian outbreak appears to have been *Nitzschia pungens,* a pennate phytoplanktonic diatom present in extensive blooms in the Cardigan River estuary in November and December 1987.[7] Contaminated mussels harvested from these waters contained *N. pungens. N. pungens* produces domoic acid in cell culture. Domoic acid has also been isolated from the internal organs of Dungeness crabs harvested off the coasts of California, Oregon, and Washington.[8] Extracts of seaweed containing domoic acid have been used as an ascaricidal agent in Japan for many years, but no adverse effects have been reported. The dose (20 mg) of domoic acid ingested in Japanese seaweed extract was much lower than the doses ingested in the Canadian mussel poisoning outbreak (60 to 290 mg).[7]

LABORATORY

CT scans may be normal. Electroencephalogram may demonstrate generalized, slow wave activity. Mussels can be tested for the presence of domoic acid by a mouse bioassay and high-performance liquid chromatography.[4] The relative preservation of intellect and higher cortical functions distinguishes the mussel-induced intoxication syndrome from Alzheimer's disease. The absence of confabulation, together with the relatively well-preserved frontal lobe function, is atypical of the amnestic syndrome associated with alcohol-induced Korsakoff's syndrome.[5]

DIAGNOSIS

Diagnosis is based on the abrupt onset (median 5.5 hours) of gastrointestinal symptoms and the later development of neurologic symptoms following ingestion of mussels or related marine animals.

Neuropathologic studies show neuronal necrosis and loss, most pronounced in the hippocampus, amygdalin, and parts of the thalamus.[6]

TREATMENT

Treatment is supportive and symptomatic. Patients should be hospitalized in an intensive care unit where neurologic dysfunction may be immediately evaluated and treated. Respiratory intubation and mechanical ventilation may be required. Tachycardia and pulmonary edema should be treated appropriately. Kynurenic acid administered prior to domoic acid in animals has provided protection against convulsions and lethality.[9] Further clinical and animal studies may determine its ultimate usefulness in man.

PREVENTION

Sacks of mussels are labeled with respect to time and place of harvesting. Before commercial distribution mussels are tested for the presence of domoic acid.

NEUROTOXIC SHELLFISH POISONING

BREVETOXIN

Neurotoxic shellfish poisoning is characterized by paresthesia, reversal of hot and cold temperature sensation, myalgia, vertigo, and ataxia. In addition abdominal pain, nausea, diarrhea, burning pain in the rectum, headache, bradycardia, and dilated pupils have been reported. It is caused by eating filter-feeding shellfish (oysters, clams, coquinas, and other bivalve molluscs) containing neurotoxins (brevetoxins) produced by the marine dinoflagellate *Ptychodiscus brevis.* Accumulation of the neurotoxins in fish probably does not occur. The health problems caused by *P. brevis* are associated with a red tide bloom seen along the Florida, Texas, and North Carolina coasts. Proliferation of the dinoflagellate occurs mostly in October and November and results in massive fish kills. Treatment is symptomatic and supportive.[10]

ICHTHYOCRINOTOXICATION

Ichthyocrinotoxication occurs after ingestion of secretions from fish skin of lampreys, hagfish, moray eels, toadfish, puffer fish, porcupine fish, and trunkfish. Abdominal pain, nausea, vomiting, diarrhea, and weakness may follow. Treatment is supportive.

Ichthyohepatotoxication

The syndrome follows ingestion of fish liver, usually from tropical sharks, and is probably due to an excessive dose of vitamin A. Severe headaches, neurologic symptoms, nausea, vomiting, and diarrhea may follow. Treatment is supportive.[11]

Clupeotoxin fish poisoning

This syndrome is caused by ingestion of plankton-eating fish (herrings, sardines). Vomiting, diarrhea, abdominal cramps, dizziness, hypotension, heart failure, and death have been described. Treatment is supportive.

Hallucinatory fish poisoning

Hallucination and nightmares may follow the ingestion of fish brain and spinal cord. Treatment is supportive.

SEA HARES

Sea hares are a group of marine gastropod mollusks belonging to the order Aplysiomorpha. In Fiji the animal is known as "veata" *(Dolabella auricularia).* Poisoning may lead to vomiting, tachypnea, tremor, diarrhea, limb pain, tingling, restlessness, muscle fasciculations, disturbed coordination, fever, and hallucinations, but normal sensation. Recovery occurred in one patient after 6 days with some residual perioral muscle twitching. The sea hares are known to concentrate bromine. Fractions of the sea hare digestive glands have been characterized as brominated susquiterpenes. Sea-hare poisoning in man may be a form of subacute organic bromine intoxication. Treatment is symptomatic and supportive. Sodium or ammonium chloride therapy may have a theoretic basis for use, but has not been tried.[12]

SEAFOOD PRECAUTIONS[13]

1. Bacteria survive well in seafood and can double in number every 15 minutes between temperatures of 40 and 120°F. Seafood should be bought from a source that maintains high standards and should be kept cold. Groceries should not be left on the car seat on a hot day. Fish that have been caught should be packed in ice before being transported home. At home the fish should be refrigerated immediately. Fresh seafood should be stored in "cling wrap" or in airtight containers at 35 to 40°F. Fresh fish or shellfish should not be held more than 1 or 2 days before being cooked.
2. Live clams and oysters survive in the refrigerator for a week or longer. Store live shellfish in open containers covered with a damp cloth. Storage in salt water shortens their shelf life; storage in fresh water kills them.
3. Frozen seafood requires storage at 0°F or lower. Frozen lean fish (sole, rockfish) can be stored for 9 to 12 months. Shellfish and fatty fish (salmon, mackerel) should be held in frozen storage only 3 to 4 months before cooking.
4. The rule on eating shellfish in months whose names contain the letter *R* applies only to cooler climates of the northern hemisphere. It does not apply in the tropics or the southern hemisphere.
5. Cooking or placing shellfish in clean, running water greatly reduces, but does not eliminate, the chance of poisoning.
6. The broth remaining after cooking shellfish should not be ingested. Marine toxin is water soluble.
7. Travelers should eat fish weighing less than 5 pounds, especially those from tropical waters. The larger the fish, the more concentrated the ciguatera toxin. Watch: barracuda, grouper, red snapper, eel, and jack.

REFERENCES—DOMOIC ACID

1. Lee W. Seafood leader 1992;12(3):1, Lambert A et al: FEBS Lett 1987;219:355–359.
2. Dickey RW, Fryxell GA, Granada HP, Roelka D. Detection of marine toxins okadaic acid and domoic acid in shellfish and phytoplankton in the Gulf of Mexico. Toxicon 1992;30: 355–359.
3. Stone R. Hot field: neurotoxicology. Science 1993;259:1397.
4. Perl TM, Bedard L, Kosatsky T, Hockin JC, Todd ECD, Remis RS. An outbreak of toxic encephalopathy caused by eating mussels contaminated with domoic acid. N Engl J Med 1990;322:1775–1780.
5. Teitelbaum JS, Zatorre RJ, Carpenter S, Gendron D, Evans AC, Gjedde A, Cashman NR. Neurologic sequelae of domoic acid intoxication due to the ingestion of contaminated mussels. N Engl J Med 1990; 322:1781–1787.
6. Neurological complications of domoic acid intoxication. Lancet 1990;336:601 (editorial).
7. Glavin GB, Bose R, Pinsky C. Infections and toxic syndromes from fish and shellfish consumption. Arch Intern Med 1990;150:2425.
8. FDA warns against eating organs of Dungeness crab. Los Angeles Times, December 28, 1991, p. A19.
9. Glavin GB, Pinsky C, Bose R. Mussel poisoning and excitatory amino acid receptors. Trends Pharm Sci 1989;10:15–16.
10. Morris PD, Campbell DS, Taylor TJ, Freeman JI. Clinical and epidemiological features of neurotoxic shellfish poisoning in North Carolina. Am J Public Health 1991;81:471–474.
11. Holliman CJ. Something fishy. Prehospital management of toxic seafood ingestions. Emerg Med Services January 1994, pp. 32–37.
12. Sorokin M. Human poisoning by ingestion of a sea hare. *(Dolabella auricularia).* Toxicon 1988;26:1095–1097.
13. Price RJ. Safe handling and storing of seafoods. Leaflet 21119. California Sea Grant Marine Advisory Publication, Division of Agricultural Science, University of California, 1979.

BLUE-GREEN ALGAE

SOURCE

The majority of algal poisonings occur in lakes, rivers, and ponds of the great plains of North America and Australia. Hot weather encourages algal blooms and light winds concentrate the algae in slimy, blue-green masses. Human exposures are uncommon because of the distasteful appearance of the water, but exposures have occurred as a result of consumption of contaminated water while swimming in contaminated lakes.

TOXINS

Cyanobacterial toxins are classified as neuro- and hepatotoxins according to their toxicity type. Anatoxin-a is an alkaloid neurotoxin and is by far the most often detected neurotoxin associated with cyanobacteria. Cyanobacterial hepatotoxins are cyclid hepta- and pentapeptides called microcystins and nodularins.[1]

SIGNS/SYMPTOMS

Local irritant effects (swelling, conjunctivitis, earache), as well as allergic reactions (rhinitis, pruritic maculopapular rash), can develop after both blue-green and marine algal exposures. A gastroenteritis beginning within 3 to 5 hours (diarrhea, abdominal cramps, nausea, vomiting) of the ingestion of contaminated water may appear, similar to amoebic dysentery, but resolves within 1 to 2 days. Consumption of water contaminated by *M. aeruginosa* produced significant γ-glutamyltranspeptidase elevations and smaller alanine aminotransferase elevations in one Australian epidemiologic study.

LABORATORY

An analytic method using gas chromatography with electron capture detection is available to analyze anatoxin-a. It is sensitive to 5 ng. This has not been used clinically.[2]

No human deaths have been definitely linked to blue-green algal toxins. Workers at risk include teachers of water sports, cleaners and maintainers of canals and rivers, water quality testers, and fish farmers. Workers at risk should be monitored for eye, skin, pulmonary, and gastrointestinal (especially liver) problems.[3]

TREATMENT

Treatment is supportive. Chronic copper poisoning may result from treatment of the local water supply with copper sulfate, an algicide. Symptoms related to this may be ascribed to blue-green algae.[4]

REFERENCES—BLUE-GREEN ALGAE

1. Pelander A, Ojanpera I, Vouri E. Cyanobacterial toxins. Bull Int Assoc Forensic Toxicol 1995;25:6–10.
2. Stevens DH, Krieger RI. Analysis of anatoxin-a by GC/ECD. J Anal Toxicol 1988;17:126–131.
3. Baxter IJ. Toxic marine and freshwater algae: an occupational hazard? Br J Indust Med 1991;49:505–506.
4. Proci VP. Blue-green algae: fact or fantasy? Med J Aust 1992;156:366–377.

PROTOTHECOSIS

Protothecosis is a chronic infection in man caused by the achloric algae of the genus *Prototheca.* In one report it was isolated from the skin of a farmer.[1] Protothecosis has been associated with malignancy, diabetes mellitus, continuous ambulatory peritoneal dialysis, renal transplantation, steroid use, and specific immunologic defects associated with Hodgkin's disease, severe malnutrition, and breaking of the skin by the Hickman catheter. Amphotericin B has been used therapeutically, but there have been no controlled studies.[2]

FOOD ADDITIVES

Acceptable daily intake values of a number of food additives and contaminants have been proposed by the Joint FAO/WHO Expert Committee on Food Additives (Table 53–28).[3]

TARTRAZINE (FD&C YELLOW NO. 5)

Pathophysiology

A prospective double-blind trial in children using 125 mg of a combination of artificial colors (tartrazine, sunset yellow, carmoisine, and amaranth) appeared to induce hyperactivity in children who had previously been observed to improve on an artificial food additive free diet.[4] A partial pharmacologic mechanism suggested for food additive intolerance may involve the ability of the dyes to cause histamine release from basophils.[4]

In January 1990 the U.S. Food and Drug Administration banned about one-fifth of the uses of the color additive FD+C Red No. 3 because it caused cancer in high doses in laboratory rats.[5] FD+C Yellow No. 6, an azodye related to yellow No. 5 (tartrazine) induced an allergic gastroenteritis in a 43-year-old physician.[6]

MONOSODIUM GLUTAMATE (MSG)—THE CHINESE RESTAURANT SYNDROME

Possible etiologic factors for the Chinese Restaurant Syndrome have been suggested, but have not been supported by clinical studies (e.g., aspartame, alcohol, high sodium intake, deficiency of Vitamin B_6).[7] Additional causes have been postulated without substantive clinical supportive data: coffee, high sodium content of some Chinese dishes, histamine, sulfites, reflux esophagitis, and bacterial contamination.[7]

Pathophysiology

Glutamate fed to immature animals appears to destroy CNS neurons in the hypothalamus.[8,9] The significance of this data to humans has not been evaluated. Glutamates and protein hydrolysates (rich in MSG) are present in many foods.[8]

A panel of experts, convened by the Federation of American Society for Experimental Biology under contract with the U.S. Food and Drug Administration, found no evidence linking MSG to any serious long-term medical problems in the general population. The report suggests that some individuals can develop short-term reactions after consumption of about 3 grams or more per meal of MSG or related "free glutamates." When glutamate that has been bound within a protein is released during breakdown of the protein molecule "free glutamate" is formed. Some foods such as ripe tomatoes and parmesan cheese contain high levels of naturally occurring free glutamate.[10]

Table 53–28
Acceptable Daily Intakes, Other Toxicologic Information, and Information on Specifications[a]

Substance	Specifications[1]	Acceptable Daily Intake (ADI) for Humans and Other Toxicological Recommendations
A. Food additives		
Antioxidant		
Butylated hydroxyanisole	R	0–0.5 mg/kg of body weight
Flavoring agents		
trans-Anethole	R	0–1.2 mg/kg of body weight[2]
d- & *l*-Carvone	R	0–1.0 mg/kg of body weight[2, 3]
Flour-treatment agent		
Potassium bromate	S	0–60 mg bromate/kg of flour[4]
Food color		
Erythrosine	R	0–0.05 mg/kg of body weight[2]
Sweetening agents		
Maltitol	N_6	ADI not specified[6]
Maltitol syrup	R[7]	ADI not specified[6, 8]
Trichlorogalactosucrose[9]	N, T	0–3.5 mg/kg of body weight[2]
Thickening agent		
Karaya gum	S	ADI not specified[6]
Miscellaneous food additives		
Glycerol ester of wood rosin	R, T	No ADI allocated[10]
Mineral oil	R	ADI not specified[2, 6, 11]
Paraffin wax	R, T	No ADI allocated[10]
Petroleum jelly	S, T	No ADI allocated[10]
Sodium, potassium, and calcium salts of oleic acid	R	ADI not specified[6]

Substance	Provisional Tolerable Weekly Intake (PTWI) for Humans and Other Toxicological Recommendations
B. Contaminants	
Aluminum	7 mg/kg of body weight[12]
Arsenic (inorganic)	0.015 mg/kg of body weight
Cadmium	0.007 mg/kg of body weight
Bis(2-ethylhexyl) phthalate	Provisional acceptance[13]
Iodine	[0.017 mg/kg of body weight[14]]
Methylmercury	0.0033 mg/kg of body weight[16]
Tin	14 mg/kg of body weight[16]

Specifications Only[1]	
Bone phosphate	R
Insoluble polyvinylpyrrolidone	R
Isomalt	R

[a]WHO. Technical Reprod Series 776. Geneva: WHO, 1989.

1. *N*, new specifications prepared; *R*, existing specifications revised; *S*, specifications exist, revision not considered or not required; and *T*, the existing, new, or revised specifications are tentative and comments are invited (see Annex 3).
2. Temporary acceptance (see Annex 3).
3. ADI applies to the two listed compounds, alone or in combination.
4. Acceptable level for treatment of flours for bread-making.
5. New specifications were developed for 98% pure maltitol separately from maltitol syrup.
6. ADI "not specified" means that, on the basis of the available data (chemical, biochemical, toxicological, and other), the total daily intake of the substance, arising from its use at the levels necessary to achieve the desired effect and from its acceptable background in food, does not, in the opinion of the Committee, represent a hazard to health. For that reason, and for the reasons stated in the individual evaluations, the establishment of an ADI expressed in numerical form is not deemed necessary.
7. Designated as "hydrogenated glucose syrups" at previous meetings.
8. The ADI previously allocated to hydrogenated glucose syrups applies to maltitol syrup meeting the revised specifications.
9. This compound was on the agenda under the name "sucralose."
10. Insufficient information available on the toxicology and/or chemical composition of the substance(s) to establish an ADI.
11. Applies only to those mineral oils currently in use as releasing agents and lubricants.
12. The PTWI includes food additive uses of aluminum salts.
13. The use of food-contact materials from which bis(2-ethylhexyl) phthalate may migrate is provisionally accepted, on condition that the quantity of the substance migrating into the food is reduced to the lowest level technically attainable.
14. Provisional maximum tolerable daily intake. The nutritional requirement for iodine is currently considered by WHO to be in the range of 0.10 to 0.14 mg per person per day for adults. The nutritional requirement for iodine is under review by WHO.
15. Applies to methylmercury. New data were not available on inorganic mercury.
16. Includes tin resulting from food additive uses. Efforts should be made to keep tin levels in canned foods as low as practicable, because of the possibility of gastric irritation.

(continued)

Table 53–28 *(Continued)*

	Specifications Only[1]
Lactitol	R, T
Mannitol	R
Modified starches	R, T[17, 18]
Potassium iodate	R
Saccharin	R
Sorbitan monooleate	R
Sorbitol	R
Sorbitol syrup	R
Xanthan gum	R, T
Xylitol	R

17. Separate specifications for enzyme-treated starches were published in FAO Food and Nutrition Paper, No. 4, 1978.
18. The "tentative" qualification applies to oxidized starch and acetylated distarch adipate.

Clinical Presentation

Pulce and colleagues, after an exhaustive survey, have concluded that Chinese Restaurant Syndrome (CRS) may occur in at least a small fraction of the population.[11] Burning sensation, facial pressure, and chest pain are the most constant findings. Whether all case reports of CRS fit into this definition is not yet certain. There is still a paucity of evidence to support the involvement of MSG. Most provocative tests using MSG have failed to reproduce symptoms of CRS. Typical CRS has only been reported at a Chinese meal. Although the reality of CRS is not widely doubted, the causative agent has yet to be defined.

Additional controlled clinical challenge studies suggest a relationship between ingestion of monosodium glutamate, angioedema of the face and extremities (16 hours after ingestion of 250 mg)[12], and asthma (together with symptoms of the Chinese Restaurant Syndrome) 6 to 12 hours after MSG doses of 0.5 to 5.0 g.[3] Anecdotal reports of supraventricular and ventricular tachycardia have followed ingestion of Chinese food.[14,15] The patients recovered with symptomatic treatment. Provocative MSG tests (1 to 2 g) were administered to two patients who experienced either headaches or attacks of severe upper abdominal pain and pressure, diaphoresis, and a burning sensation in the chest within 1 to 2 hours after eating MSG-containing food. In each case the MSG provocative test (with 1 to 2 g of MSG) elicited symptoms: in one patient a severe generalized headache followed in 10 minutes. In another patient shortness of breath, palpitations, numbness of the legs, and a feeling of heat in the face and chest followed within 30 minutes after ingesting 2 g MSG.[16]

Treatment[17]

The U.S. Food and Drug Administration is planning to require the phrase "contains glutamate" be added to the label as part of the common or usual name for those hydrolyzed protein products that contain significant amounts of glutamate.[18] Some precautions for those possibly sensitive to MSG have been suggested by Swan[19]:

1. Shop carefully and read labels! Never buy or use Accent, soy sauce, bouillon cubes, or dried or canned soups. Dried foods, processed meats, canned foods other than plain vegetables and fruit, frozen dinners, and "gourmet" specialties are all suspect.
2. Avoid catered food, including airline meals.
3. If you plan to dine out at a restaurant:
   a. Phone ahead and request food without MSG.
   b. Eat a snack before you go: cottage cheese or a glass of milk.
   c. Go easy on alcoholic beverages.
   d. Do not eat hors d'oeuvres (with the exception of olives, fresh vegetable sticks, etc.) or soup.
   e. Be aware that many food items that are prepared in advance contain MSG. Your meal may be assembled from this pool of prepared items—sauces, vegetables, and so on.
   f. Avoid casserole dishes, oriental foods, or marinated meats, and beware of the "chef's special" (generally a dish prepared in quantity in advance and containing MSG).
   g. Again, specifically request that your meal be prepared without MSG. Eat freshly prepared, broiled or sauteed meats or fish without sauces or seasonings.
   h. Avoid salad dressings or request oil and vinegar.
   i. Be sure to drink a cup of coffee with the meal, or at least before you leave the restaurant.
   j. When you get home write a letter to the Food and Drug Administration complaining that you have to go through all this and request the removal of MSG from the GRAS listing.

REFERENCES—FOOD SENSITIVITY

1. Davies RC, Spencer H,. Wakelin PO. A case of human protothecosis. Trans R Soc Trop Med Hyg 1964;58:448–451.
2. Heney C, Greeff M, Davis V. Hickman catheter-related protothecal algaemia in an uncompromised child. J Infect Dis 1991;163:930–931.
3. Evaluation of certain food additives and contaminants. Thirty-third Report of the Joint FAO/WHO Expert Committee on Food Additives. World Health Organization Technical Report Series 776. Geneva: WHO, 1989.
4. Pollock I, Warner JO. Effect of artificial food colours on childhood behavior. Arch Dis Child 1990;65:74–77.
5. Blumenthal D. Red No. 3 and other colorful controversies. FDA Consumer May 1990, pp. 18 –21.
6. Gross PA, Lance K, Whitlock RJ, Blume RE. Additive allergy: allergic gastroenteritis due to yellow dye #6. Ann Intern Med 1989;111:87–88.
7. Zautcke JL, Schwartz JA, Mueller EJ. Chinese restaurant syndrome: a review. Ann Emerg Med 1986;15:1210–1213.
8. Olney JW. Excitatory neurotoxins as food additives: an evaluation of risk. Neurotoxicology 1980;2:163–192.

9. Olney JW. Excitatoxicity and neuropsychiatric disorders. In: Ascher P, Choi DW, Cristen Y, eds. Glutamate, cell death and memory. Berlin: Springer Verlag, 1991.
10. MSG judged safe for most people. FDA Consumer 1995; 29:2.
11. Pulce C, Vial T, Verdier F, Testud F, Nicolas B, Descotes J. The Chinese restaurant syndrome: a reappraisal of monosodium glutamate's causative role. Adverse Drug React Toxicol Rev 1992;11:19–39.
12. Squire EN Jr. Angioedema and monosodium glutamate. Lancet 1987;1:988.
13. Allen DH, Deloheny J, Baker G. Monosodium L-glutamate–induced asthma. J Allergy Clin Immunol 1987;80:530–537.
14. Goldberg LH. Supraventricular tachyrhythmia in association with the Chinese restaurant syndrome. Ann Emerg Med 1982;11:333.
15. Gann D. Ventricular tachycardia in a patient with the "Chinese restaurant syndrome." South Med J 1977;70:874–881.
16. Ratner D, Ethel E, Shoshani E. Adverse effects of monosodium glutamate: a diagnostic problem. Isr J Med Sci 1984;20:252–253.
17. Swan GF. Management of monosodium glutamate toxicity. J Asthma 1982;19:105–110.
18. FDA Background. Monosodium glutamate (MSG). HF1-40, October 1991.
19. Swan GF. Management of monosodium glutamate toxicity. J Asthma 1982;19:105–110.

A monosodium glutamate adverse reactions report is available. "Analysis of Adverse Reactions to Monosodium Glutamate (MSG)" was prepared for the U.S. Food and Drug Administration by the Life Sciences Research Office, Federation of American Societies for Experimental Biology. Single copies cost $50 and may be purchased from the Life Sciences Research Office, 9650 Rockville Pike, Bethesda, MD 20814; telephone (301) 530-7030.

Expert Committee on Food Additives.[1]

Information sources for food safety are listed in Table 53–28.[2]

Table 53–28 Resources for Further Information

Resource	Telephone No.
U.S. Food and Drug Administration	301-433-3170
U.S. Environmental Protection Agency	202-382-2090
American Institute for Cancer Research Nutrition Hotline	800-843-8114
National Cancer Institute Cancer Information Hotline	800-4CANCER
National Pesticide Telecommunications Network Hotline	800-858-PEST
U.S. Department of Agriculture Meat and Poultry Hotline	800-535-4555

REFERENCES

1. Evaluation of certain food additives and contaminants. Thirty-third Report of the Joint FAO/WHO Expert Committee on Food Additives. World Health Organization Technical Report Series 776. Geneva: WHO, 1989.
2. Frazier L, Darcely DJ, Langley RL. Food safety. Lead pesticides, antibiotics, hormones and Irradiation. NC Med J 1992;53:372.

FOOD PRESERVATIVES [1,2]

When 0.5 mg/kg butylated hydroxyanisole was ingested for 120 days, it did not induce changes in clinical plasma parameters (aminotransferases, gamma-glutamyl transpeptidase, creatine phosphokinase, lactate dehydrogenase, total protein, albumin, urea, creatinine, or Na^+ or Cl^{1-}).[3]

SULFITES

Sulfiting agents are effective antioxidants and are used in beverages, foods, and medications. Approximately 450,000 (5%) of the 9 million asthmatics in the United States may be sulfite sensitive.[4] The FDA has withdrawn approval for use of sulfites with fresh vegetables.[5] In addition, packaged sulfited foods are required to be labeled if sulfites are present at 10 ppm or more. That regulation went into effect on January 1, 1987.[6] Prescription drugs containing sulfites must be labeled. Sulfite food preservatives include sulfur dioxide, potassium metabisulfite, sodium sulfite, sodium metabisulfite, sodium bisulfite, and potassium bisulfite.

Sulfites appear in parenteral steroid and antibiotic preparations, parenteral cardiovascular drugs, intravenous infusions, peritoneal dialysis solutions, local anesthetics, radioconstrast dyes, and other medications.[7] Although ingestion of food containing sulfiting agents can result in type-I, immediate-hypersensitivity reactions in normal, nonasthmatic individuals, reactions have occurred without evidence for an IgE-mediated mechanism in asthmatics.

Clinical Presentation

Symptoms may include sudden generalized flush, faintness, syncope, sneezing, shortness of breath, cyanosis, rapid pulse, and cold, clammy skin. Urticaria, angioedema, and abdominal distress may be seen within minutes after exposure. Acute asthma attacks and respiratory arrest may occur. Patients develop sensitization to sodium sulfite from previous contact with topical preparations containing it.

Supportive Care

The usual therapy for anaphylactic and bronchoconstriction reactions is applicable with special care to avoid epinephrine suspended in a sulfiting agent.

REFERENCES—FOOD PRESERVATIVES

1. Lecos C. Food preservatives: a fresh report. FDA Consumer 1984; 18(3):23–25.
2. Levine AS, Labuza TP, Morley JE. Food technology. A primer for physicians. N Engl J Med 1985;312:628–634.
3. Verhagen H, Maas LM, Beckers RHG, Thijssen HHW, Ten Hoor F, Handerson P Th, Kleinjans JCS. Effect of subacute oral intake of the food antioxidant butylated hydroxyanisole on clinical parameters and phase-I and -II biotransformation capacity in man. Hum Toxicol 1989;8:451–459.
4. Simon RA, Green L, Stevenson DD. The incidence of ingested metabisulfite sensitivity in an asthmatic population. J Allergy Clin Immunol 1982;69:118.
5. Sulfiting agents: revocation of GRAS status for use on fruits and vegetables intended to be served or sold raw to consumers. Fed Reg 1986;51 (131):25021–25026.
6. Food labeling: declaration of sulfiting agents. Fed Reg 1986; 51(131):25012–25020.
7. Sogn D. The ubiquitous sulfites. JAMA 1984;251:2986–2987.

CANTHAXANTHIN

Canthaxanthin is a carotenoid pigment with an orange-red color, but unlike beta-carotene it possesses no vitamin A activity.[1]

STRUCTURE AND CLASSIFICATION

Canthaxanthin is a $beta_1$ beta-carotene-4,4′-dione; 4,4′-dioxo-beta-carotene; Roxanthin Red 10. Canthaxanthin is a synthetic carotenoid,[2] but may be made by certain bacteria and algae[2]; beta-carotene is a natural carotenoid.

USES

Listed as "Generally Recognized as Safe" (GRAS), canthaxanthin is used as a food coloring and is added to animal feed to enhance the color of egg yolks and skin of chicken and flesh of rainbow trout.[3] It has also been taken orally by humans to produce a sun tan. It is also used in cosmetics, but has not been approved for this use in the United States, and is used as a yellow-orange colorant in soft drinks, candy, fruit, lemonade, and yogurt.[4]

PRODUCT FORMULATION

Canthaxanthin has been marked in the United States as a tablet for tanning skin under such names as Orobronze, Darker Tan, Bronze Glo, and Carotinoid-N (25 mg beta-carotene and 35 mg canthaxanthin). In Europe a combination of beta-carotene and canthaxanthin (Phenoro: 10 mg beta-carotene and 15 mg canthaxanthin per capsule) is used in doses of up to 150 mg/d.[5]

DOSAGE

An average daily intake of canthaxanthin is approximately 5.6 mg (mostly from foods such as salad dressing and ketchup).[2] The FAO (Food and Agriculture Organization of the United Nations) has assessed canthaxanthin as harmless, and the approved maximum daily intake (for the EEC—European Economic Community) was set at 25 mg/kg.[4]

TOXICOKINETICS

Absorption

The bioavailability of canthaxanthin is 9 to 34%.[2,6] Steady-state plasma concentrations of canthaxanthin after daily ingestion of 6 mg (6 times/ng) or 48 mg (6 times 8 ng) were 1843 or 10,346 μg/L, respectively.[2] An intake of 30 mg of canthaxanthin/day would lead to steady-state blood concentrations of approximately 6 mg/L; 3.5 mg/day would lead to a concentration of 1.1 mg/L. [6]

Distribution

About 6% of the absorbed dose is transferred to lipid deposits.[6] Concentrations of canthaxanthin found in the omentum of three patients after ingestion of 67 g were 270 μg/g; after 6 g—49 μg/g, and after 16 g—34; μg/g, respectively.[7]

Elimination

Canthaxanthin is cleared from the serum with a half-life of 4.5 to 5.3 days.[3,6]

CLINICAL PRESENTATION

Retinopathy[8]

A gold dust retinopathy consisting of fine dust-like golden particles is found in the layer of nerve fibers close to the maculae and also in the paramacular region. These are about 30 μm in diameter.[9] These particles appear in the eyes of about 12 to 14% of patients who have ingested total doses of from 37 g to 60 g.[9] The retinopathy may appear at lower doses (12 to 14 g)[10] in those who have focal disease of the pigment epithelium, ocular hypertension, or have used beta-carotene concurrently.[9] Two of six patients with these crystalline depositions had visual loss, but a history of canthaxanthin intake was not clear[4]; a decrease in visual acuity has been described in another case.[11] A prolonged darkness adaptation curve has been described.[12,13] Electroretinogram tests have indicated some abnormalities.[14] There does not appear to be a close relationship between appearance of crystalline deposits and dose level or duration.[10]

Further controlled studies will be required to define these observations.

Aplastic Anemia[15]

A 20-year-old woman ingested "tanning" pills containing an unknown amount of canthaxanthin. Her skin became deep orange. She developed an aplastic anemia and died. Definite canthaxanthin causation of the aplastic anemia has not been established, but it was implicated by association.

Hepatitis and generalized urticaria have also been described following canthaxanthin use.[16,17]

REFERENCES—CANTHAXANTHIN

1. Reynolds JEF. *Martindale: The extra pharmacopoeia*. 13th ed. London: Pharmaceutical Press, 1993.
2. "French bronze" fades away. FDA Consumer 1990;24(1):34–35.
3. Herbert V. Canthaxanthin toxicity. Am J Clin Nutr 1991;53: 573.
4. Oosterhuis JA, Nijman NM, de Wolff FA, Remky H. Canthaxanthin retinopathy with and without intake of canthaxanthin as a drug. Hum Toxicol 1988;7:45–47.
5. Mathews, Roth MM. Reply to V Herbert. Am J Clin Nutr 1991;53:573–574.
6. Kubler W. Biokinetic evaluation of canthaxanthin plasma levels after multiple doses of 1 mg and 8 mg canthaxanthin. Unpublished report submitted to WHO by F. Hoffmann-La Roche and Co., Basle, Switzerland. In: Toxicological evaluation of certain food additives and contaminants. Geneva: WHO Food Additive Series 76, 1990; pp. 45–73.
7. Schalch W. Biokinetic evaluation of canthaxanthin in humans. Unpublished Research Report. No. B-107, 134 submitted to WHO by Hoffmann-La Roche & Co, Basle, Switzerland. In: Toxicological evaluation of certain food additives and contaminants. Geneva: WHO Food Additives Series 26, 1990; pp. 45–73.
8. Hoffmann-La Roche. Canthaxanthin. Unpublished Research Report. No. B-107, 134 submitted to WHO by F. Hoffmann-La Roche & Co, Basle, Switzerland. In: Toxicological evaluation of certain food additives and contaminants. Geneva: WHO Food Additives Series 26, 1990; pp. 45–73.

9. Harnois C, Samson J, Malenfant M, Rousseau A. Canthaxanthin retinopathy. Anatomic and functional reversibility. Arch Ophthalmol 1989;107:538–540.
10. Canthaxanthin. Toxicological evaluation of certain food additives and contaminants. Geneva: WHO Food Additives Series 26, 1990; pp. 45–73.
11. Lonn LI. Canthaxanthin retinopathy. Arch Ophthalmol 1987; 105:1590–1591.
12. McGuiness R, Beaumont P. Gold dust retinopathy after the ingestion of canthaxanthin to produce skin-bronzing. Med J Aust 1985;143:622–623.
13. Weber U, Goerz G. Ophthalmological disorders through carotenoid ingestion. Dtsch Artzeblatt 1985;41:181–182.
14. Arden GB, Oluwole JOA, Polkinhorne P, Bird AC, Barker FM, Norris PG et al. Monitoring of patients taking canthaxanthin and carotene: an electroretinographic and ophthalmological survey. Hum Toxicol 1989;8:439–450.
15. Bluhm R, Branch R, Johnston P, Stein R. Aplastic anemia associated with canthaxanthin ingested for "tanning" purposes. JAMA 1990;264:1141–1142.
16. Boudreault G, Cortin P, Corriveau LA, Rousseau AP, Tardif Y, Malenfant M. Canthaxanthin retinopathy. I. Clinical study in 51 consumers. Can J Ophthalmol 1983;18:325–328.
17. Hart L, Mowers RM. DIAS rounds—drug information analysis service. Drug Intell Clin Pharmacol 1987;21:173–174.

SEAWEED POISONING

Seaweed is frequently served as a side dish at meals in the Pacific Islands and is a common component in the diet of many persons living in the Pacific Rim. Seaweed is often harvested at beaches, gathered in nearshore waters, or purchased at local markets. It is served either raw or cooked and is commonly prepared with salt and/or other spices and herbs (e.g., chili pepper, ginger, and garlic). A case is defined as the onset of a burning sensation in the mouth or throat or two or more of the following symptoms: vomiting, diarrhea, nausea, or lethargy within 2 hours after ingestion. The seaweed has been identified as *Gracilaria coronopifolia.* The first reported episode of seaweed-related illness in Hawaii was identified as *Gracilaria tsudai,* and manifestations included gastrointestinal illness, fever, wheezing, muscle fasciculations, and hypotension. In 1992 three persons had onset of illness after eating seaweed harvested on a beach in California; the seaweed species implicated in that epidose was *Gracilariopsis lemanaeformis.* In 1993 two persons became ill, and one of them died after eating *Gracilaria verrucosa* seaweed in Japan.[1]

REFERENCES—SEAWEED POISONING

1. CDC. Outbreak of gastrointestinal illness associated with consumption of seaweed—Hawaii, 1994. MMWR 1995;44: 724–727.

OSTRICH FERN POISONING

Fiddleheads (crosiers) of the ostrich fern *(Matteuccia struthiopteris)* are a seasonal delicacy harvested commercially in the northeastern United States and in coastal provinces of Canada. This species has been considered to be nontoxic. In May 1994 outbreaks of food poisoning were associated with eating raw or lightly cooked fiddlehead ferns in New York and western Canada.

CLINICAL PRESENTATION

Patients complain of nausea, vomiting, and diarrhea shortly after eating. Some attributed their illness to the fiddlehead ferns served with their entree. The mean incubation period was 6.7 hours (range: 0.5 to 11.5 hours). Symptoms last a mean of 1.3 days (range: 3 hours to 3 days).

The ostrich fern was a spring vegetable for American Indians of eastern North America and became part of the regular diet of settlers to New Brunswick in the late 1700s. The ferns are available commercially either canned or frozen. Heating and boiling may either inactivate or leach the toxin from the plant. Fresh fiddlehead ferns only recently have become widely available in restaurants. In addition, many vegetables now are lightly cooked rather than steamed or boiled. Fiddleheads must be cooked thoroughly (e.g., boiling for 10 minutes) before eating.[1]

REFERENCES—OSTRICH FERN POISONING

1. CDC. MMWR 1994;43:677, 683–684: Ostrich fern poisoning—New York and Western Canada, 1994, JAMA 1995;273:912–913.

FAT OVERLOAD SYNDROME

Sterile fat emulsions (such as Intralipid) are administered intravenously as a source of calories and essential fatty acids to patients requiring parenteral nutrition.[1] The emulsions are made predominantly of soybean oil with egg yolk phospholipids, glycerin, and water. The emulsified particles are approximately 0.5 μm in size. Clearance of such fat emulsions is catalyzed by lipoprotein lipase, the rate limiting step, at the capillary epithelial cells.[2] The maximum clearance rate has been calculated to be 3.8 g fat/kg body weight per 24 hours in healthy adults. When these levels are exceeded, the blood triglyceride level increases.[3] Treatment with fat emulsions is monitored by triglyceride levels or plasma turbidity.[1]

COMPLICATIONS

Complications of intravenous fat emulsion therapy are uncommon and usually result from contamination of the intravenous catheter. The fat overload syndrome is a relatively infrequent but serious complication.[4,5]

PATHOPHYSIOLOGY

The fat overload syndrome appears to follow fat sludging within the microvasculature of the spleen, liver, kidney, retina, lungs, and brain.[6] It is hypothesized that observed hyperlipidemia and lipid deposits in pulmonary capillaries may result in compromise of pulmonary gas exchange.[7]

CLINICAL PRESENTATION

The fat overload syndrome is characterized by the acute onset of fever, jaundice, irritability, spontaneous hemorrhage,[8] and hyperlipemia. Other symptoms and signs include lethargy, tachycardia, tachypnea, headache, nausea, vomiting, abdominal pain, hepatosplenomegaly, and cough occasionally accompanied by hemoptysis.[9–11] Seizures,[1] cardiac failure, and respiratory difficulties have been observed.[10] Untreated, the condition may terminate in death.[1,12]

LABORATORY

Anemia, leucocytosis, vacuolated granulocytes, and burr cells[13] on a peripheral smear; a normal platelet count but giant platelets on a smear; elevated serum aminotransferases, alkaline phosphatase, and bilirubin (conjugated); elevated levels of fibrin degradation products; normal to decreased fibrinogen levels; prolonged activated partial thromboplastin time; prolonged thrombin time; normal to prolonged prothrombin time; and normal to low serum sodium levels may be observed.[11] The serum has a thick, creamy, burgundy colored appearance. Serum triglyceride levels may be as high as 10,000 mg/dL (113 mmol/L).[6] Pulmonary vascular resistance may be observed.[14,15] At autopsy fat depositions and fat emboli may be found in the heart, lungs, liver, spleen, and kidneys.[16,17]

TREATMENT

Removal of the fat emulsion infusion and supportive care have been the mainstays of treatment. A complete plasma exchange (5.6 L removed and replaced with fresh frozen plasma and albumin) has resulted in definitive improvement within 18 hours in one patient.[6]

REFERENCES—FAT OVERLOAD SYNDROME

1. Haber LM, Hawkins EP, Seilheimer DK, Saleem A. Fat overload syndrome. An autopsy study with evaluation of the coagulopathy. Am J Clin Pathol 1988;89:223–227.
2. Halberg D. Elimination of exogenous lipids from the blood stream. Acta Physiol Scand 1965;65 (Suppl 254):1–23.
3. Adamkin DH, Gelke KN, Andrews BF. Fat emulsions and hypertriglyceridemia. J Parenter Enteral Nutr 1984;8:563–567.
4. Johnson WA, Freeman S, Meyer KA. Some effects of intravenous fat emulsions on human subjects. J Lab Clin Med 1952;39:176–183.
5. Watkin DM. Clinical, chemical, hematologic and anatomic changes accompanying the repeated intravenous administration of fat emulsion in man. Metabolism 1957;6:785–806.
6. Kollef MH, McCormack MT, Caras WE, Reddy VVB, Bacon D. The fat overload syndrome: successful treatment with plasma exchange. Ann Intern Med 1990;112:545–546.
7. Stolee B, Purssell R, Ashbourne JF, Vicas IMO. Intralipid overdose in a neonate. Vet Hum Toxicol 1994;34:375.
8. Campbell AN, Freedman MH, Pencharz PB, Zlotkin SH. Bleeding disorders from the fat overload syndrome. J Parenter Enteral Nutr 1984;8:447–449.
9. Meng HC, Kaley JS. Effects of multiple infusions of a fat emulsion on blood coagulation, liver function and urinary excretion of steroids in schizophrenic patients. Am J Clin Nutr 1965;16:156–164.
10. Belin RP, Bivins BA, Jona JZ, Young VL. Fat overload with a 10% soybean oil emulsion. Arch Surg 1976;111:1391–1393.
11. Heyman MB, Storch S, Ament ME. The fat overload syndrome. Report of a case and literature review. Am J Dis Child 1981;135:628–630.
12. Levene MI, Wigglesworth JS, Desai R. Pulmonary fat accumulation after interlipid infusion in the preterm infant. Lancet 1990;2:815–819.
13. Taylor RF, Buckner CD. Fat overload from 10 percent soybean oil emulsion in a marrow transplant recipient. West J Med 1982;136:345–349.
14. Zakinthinos S, Baltopoulos G, Roussos CH. Fat emulsion and ARDS. Chest 1990;98:509–510.
15. Venus B. Fat emulsion and ARDS. Chest 1990;98:510.
16. Hesson I, Melsen F, Haug A. Postmortem findings in three patients treated with intravenous fat emulsions. Arch Surg 1979;114:66–68.
17. Levene MI, Batisti O, Wigglesworth JS, Desai R, Meek JH, Bulusu S, Hughes E. A prospective study of intrapulmonary fat accumulation in the newborn baby following intralipid infusion. Acta Paediatr Scand 1984;73:454–460.

Chapter 54
Household Poisonings

NONTOXIC INGESTIONS (TABLE 54–1)

In 1970 Mofenson and Greensher[1] defined a nontoxic ingestion as that which occurs after an individual consumes a nonedible product that usually does not produce symptoms. Table 54–1 details some of the most frequently ingested household items considered "usually nontoxic." Qualifications exist for many categories, so the extent of symptoms may depend on actual circumstances (e.g., specific product, quantity, host).

Consulting lists such as that in Table 54–1 may not be sufficient without careful investigation:

1. The name—spelled out carefully—of the item.
2. Details of the package labeling, if any.
3. Name and address of the manufacturer.
4. Date on the label.
5. Date purchased.
6. Consultation with a current reference source or the manufacturer to determine *current* ingredients in the preparations.

Problems also may result from inaccurate historical information about the ingestion. Some questions that might be considered in responding include the following:

1. How certain are you that only a single dose was ingested?
2. Were any other substances ingested simultaneously?
3. Have there been any symptoms?
4. Is there a history of repeated ingestions of "nontoxic" substances?
5. Does the patient have any significant medical history: allergies, liver or kidney problems, adverse drug reactions?

Factors that mitigate against an oversimplified evaluation by the poison information professional include the following:

1. The information obtained may be incorrect and misleading. Repetitive questioning and insistence on details may minimize such errors.

Table 54-1
Criteria for Nontoxic Ingestions[a]

1. Absolute identification
2. Time and amount of ingestion is known
3. Amount ingested relative to patient's weight—is less than smallest amount known or predicted to induce toxicity.
4. Time elapsed since ingestion—greater than the longest predicted interval between ingestion and peak toxicity.
5. Detailed history—no symptoms or signs of toxicity.

The Usually Nontoxic Ingestion (unless ingested in very large quantities)

Abrasives
Adhesives
A&D ointment
Ajax cleaner
Air fresheners
Aluminum foil
Antacids
Antibiotic ointments
Antiperspirants
Ashes (wood, fireplace)

Baby products cosmetics
Baby wipes
Ballpoint pen pinks
Bathtub floating toys
Battery (convention if bitten)
Bath oil (castor oil and perfume)
Bleach less than 5%
Body conditioners
Bubble bath soaps (detergents)

Calamine lotion
Candles
Cat food
Caulk
Caps (for toy pistols)
Chalk (calcium carbonate)
Charcoal and charcoal briquettes
Cigarettes (less than one)
Cigarette ashes
Clay (modelling)
Colognes[b]
Contraceptive pills (without iron)
Comet Cleanser
Corticosteroids & their ointments
Cold packs (a swallow)
Crayons (marked AP, CP, CS-140)
Crayola Markers
Crazy glue (cyanoacrylate)
Cyclamate

Dehumidifying packets (silica or charcoal)
Deodorants Detergents (phosphate type, anionic)
Deodorants (spray and refrigerator)
Disposable diapers—not aspirated
Dishwashing liquid soap (not automatic electric dishwasher: Mr. Clean, Dawn, Joy, Tide, Wisk)

Erasers
Etch-A-Sketch
Eye Makeup

Fabric softener
Felt tip markers and pens
Fertilizer (nitrogen, phosphoric acid, and potash)
Fingernail polish
Fish bowl additives
Fluoride-caries preventive

Glade plug in
Glitter Glues & pastes
Glowstick/jewelry
Golf ball core (may cause mechanical injury)
Grease
Gypsum

Hair products (conditioner, shampoos, not Lindane)
Hand lotions and creams

Indelible markers
Ink (blue, black)
Iodophor disinfectant

Kaolin
Kitty litter

Lanolin
Latex paint
Laxatives
Lipstick
Lotrimin cream
Lubricants
Lysol Disinfectant Spray (70% ethanol)

Magic marker
Makeup (eye, liquid facial)
Mascara (domestic)
Matches (book type, 3 books)
Massengil disposable douches
Miracle Gro Plant Food
Mineral oil

Newspaper
Nutrasweet

PAAS Easter egg dyes (after 1980)
Paints (indoor latex acrylic)
Preparation H suppository/ointment
Pencil lead (graphite)
Perfumes[b]
Petroleum jelly (vaseline)
Photographs
Plastics
Plaster (non-lead containing)
Play-doh
Polaroid picture coating
Porous tip ink marking pens
Prussian blue (ferricyanide)
Putty

Rouge
Rust
Rubber cements
Most rug cleaners/shampoos (Glory, Resolve, Woolite)

Saccharin
Sachets (essential oils)
Shampoo (liquid)
Shaving creams
Shoe polish
Silica gel
Silly putty
Soaps and soap products
Soil Shackles

[a]Mofenson HF et al. Poison perspectives. Long Island Poison Control Center at Winthrop-University Hospital, 1995;14:2–3.
[b]Depends on the alcohol content.

(continued)

Table 54—1 *(Continued)*

Starch	Vaseline
Sunscreen and tan preparations	Vitamins (even fluoride); excludes iron
Sweetening agents	
	Warfarin (single dose)
Teething rings (fluid may have bacteria)	Watercolors paint
Thermometers (mercury, phthalate alcohol)	Windex Glass Cleaner with ammonia D
Toilet water[b]	
Toothpaste (even fluoride)	Zinc oxide
	Zirconium oxide

2. The constantly changing chemical composition of items.
3. Agents formerly thought to be "nontoxic" may cause damage.
4. The litigious climate in which we live can be chilling to the "off-the-cuff" answer.

HOUSEHOLD CLEANING PRODUCTS

SOAPS

CLINICAL PRESENTATION

Soaps are mild gastrointestinal and mucous membrane irritants that occasionally produce nausea, vomiting, diarrhea, and abdominal pain. Deodorant bars contain some photosensitizing agents (e.g., biocides, perfumes, detergents). Most other ingredients (e.g., hexachlorophene) are present in concentrations too low to produce toxicity.

TREATMENT

1. Ipecac-induced emesis is not required.
2. Irrigate all symptomatic ocular exposure with saline (water is an acceptable alternative if saline is unavailable). Minor ocular irritation may benefit from a soothing agent (e.g., a vasoconstrictor solution containing naphazoline). Local ophthalmic anesthetic agents (e.g., tetracaine) should not be prescribed for outpatient use.
3. Administer clear liquids and antiemetic if needed for gastrointestinal symptoms.
4. Cases usually can be managed at home with symptomatic treatment.

DETERGENTS

Surfactants

Detergents contain synthetic, organic, surface-active agents called *surfactants,* which are derived from petroleum product precursors.

Anionic Surfactants

Examples include alkyl sodium sulfate, sodium lauryl sulfate, sodium aryl-alkyl sulfate, dioctyl sodium sulfosuccinate, sodium oleate, linear alkyl benzene, and tetrapropylene benzene sulfonates. Anionic surfactants possess irritant properties with the major exception of electric dishwasher products in which builders enhance alkalinity.

Nonionic Surfactants

Electrically neutral medium- to long-chain polyether sulfates, alcohols, or sulfonates (e.g., alkyl-aryl polyether sulfates, alkyl ethoxylate, alkyl phenoxy polyethoxy ethanols, polyethylene glycol stearate). Nonionic surfactants produce less local irritation than anionic ones.

Cationic Surfactants

Benzalkonium chloride—Zephiran, benzethonium chloride—Phemerol, cetylpyridinium—Ceepryn, alkyl dimethyl 3,4-dichlorobenzene ammonium chloride. Concentrated cationic solutions (10 to 15%) are caustic and even dilute solutions (0.1 to 0.5%) produce significant mucosal irritation. Large ingestions may produce central nervous system symptoms.

Amphoteric Surfactants

These compounds contain both anionic and cationic surface-active molecules and occur more commonly in industrial cleaning products.

Builders

Manufacturers add inorganic "builder" to detergents to improve their wetting and emulsifying properties, which are inhibited by hard-water minerals such as calcium. Most heavy-duty detergents contain builders and include inorganic salts such as phosphates, carbonates, silicate, sodium citrate, and aluminosilicates.

Death has occurred after intentional ingestion of a low-phosphate detergent.

Additives

Detergents contain a variety of additives (e.g., bleaches, bactericidal agents, enzymes, perfumes, colorants, whitening agents, softeners), but their concentrations are too low to produce primary irritation. However, these additives may cause a contact dermatitis by sensitizing certain individuals.

Liquid Detergents

In a dose of 3 tablespoons, liquid dishwashing detergent products (not laundry or electric dishwashing detergents) have been recommended as a substitute emetic when syrup of ipecac is unavailable.

CLINICAL PRESENTATION

Systemic Complaints

Most exposures to household cleaning products reported to poison control centers do not result in symptoms. Symptomatic patients most often exhibit gastrointestinal symptoms (nausea, vomiting, diarrhea). Granular laundry detergents, liquid laundry detergents, and liquid dishwashing agents produce more nausea, vomiting, and diarrhea than other laundry products (e.g., fabric softener, bar soap). Symptoms resolve within 24 hours. Cationic detergents produce systemic toxicity and, in rare circumstances, death (fatal adult dose estimated between 1 and 3 grams).

Local Complaints

Cationic detergents are more potent irritants than anionic or nonionic detergents.

TREATMENT

1. Most detergents and soap ingestions require only dilution with water or milk. Patients should be observed at home several hours in the upright position for spontaneous vomiting.
2. Cationic detergent (quaternary ammonium compounds; e.g., Zephiran chloride—benzalkonium chloride; Ceepryn chloride—cetylpyridinium chloride; Phemerol chloride—benzethonium chloride) ingestions require gut decontamination except when a small amount has been ingested (less than a swallow), the concentration is less than 1%, or the time since ingestion exceeds several hours. Ingestion of agents containing greater than 5 to 10% cationic detergent should be treated as caustic ingestions (immediate dilution plus esophagoscopy as needed). Transient contact with cationic detergent requires only dilution.
3. Copiously irrigate all eye exposures with saline for 20 minutes. Be sure to retract the eyelids to search for granules in the fornices of the conjunctiva. Each patient should receive an eye examination, including fluorescein staining to detect corneal abrasions.
4. Cationic detergent ingestion that requires emesis also may be given charcoal and cathartics, although no clinical studies demonstrate their effectiveness in detergent ingestions.
5. Hypocalcemia and tetany are rare complications of ingestion of phosphate-containing detergents.
6. Published evidence that weak soap solutions bind quaternary ammonia compounds to prevent absorption is lacking. Since most soaps now contain anionic surfactants, the recommended use of soap for these ingestions is not practical.

GENERAL-PURPOSE CLEANERS

PRODUCT FORMULATIONS/USES

Pine oil is a mixture of highly lipophilic unsaturated cyclic hydrocarbons (cylic terpene alcohols, monoterpenes) that is one-fifth as toxic as turpentine in animals. Turpentine is a natural solvent composed of pine oils, camphenes, and terpenes. The volatile components of turpentine (alpha-pinene, beta-pinene, gamma-3-carene) are significant pulmonary aspiration hazards. Abrasive cleaners contain pumice or silica, which have minimal toxicity.

CLINICAL PRESENTATION

Pine Oil

The suggested adult lethal dose of pine oil is 60 to 120 g, although survival without sequelae after an ingestion of 400 to 500 g has been reported. Pine oil produces primarily gastrointestinal irritation and central nervous system depression. Renal failure may occur, but death is rare.

Turpentine

Quantities in excess of 2 mL/kg should be considered toxic and removed by gut decontamination. As little as 15 mL of turpentine may produce symptoms in children: 120 to 180 mL is a potentially lethal adult dose. This compound is a local irritant, central nervous system depressant, and pulmonary aspiration hazard, similar to other volatile oils such as camphor, sassafras, eucalyptus, and wintergreen; however, acute turpentine toxicity is less severe than that of these volatile oils. Casual exposures may produce mucosal irritation, mild respiratory tract inflammation, and urinary tract irritation. In large intentional doses, coma and convulsions may occur. Pulmonary aspiration of turpentine produces a hemorrhagic pulmonary edema.

TREATMENT

Most accidental ingestions of household cleaners (including hydrocarbons) require only dilution with milk or water to reduce mucosal irritant properties. Turpentine ingestions should be treated like toluene exposures and gut decontamination measures should be used only when the ingestion exceeds approximately 2 mL/kg. Patients who ingest more than several swallows of concentrated pine oil products (e.g., Pine Sol, which contains 20 to 35% pine oil) should receive either syrup of ipecac or lavage as indicated by the ability of the patient to handle secretions. Be sure to check product contents to determine the appropriateness of decontamination measures.

SHAMPOOS

PRODUCT FORMULATIONS/USES

Some liquid shampoos contain alkyl sodium sulfate, which has more mucosal irritant properties than nonionic surfactants. Dry shampoos may contain methanol or isopropanol. Industrial-strength rug shampoos and carpet-cleaning products may contain potentially toxic compounds, especially when the products are not properly diluted. Potentially toxic compounds include sodium carbonate, sodium perborate, sodium phosphate, ammonia compounds, borax, pine oil, trichloroethylene, tetrachloroethylene, naphtha, naphthalene, kerosene, petroleum solvents, alkyl benzene sulfonate, and alkyl-aryl sodium sulfonate.

CLINICAL PRESENTATION

Household shampoos usually produce only mild gastrointestinal tract irritation. A rug shampoo caused a respiratory illness characterized by cough, headache, sore throat, awareness of unusual odor, dyspnea, fatigue, nausea, and other gastrointestinal complaints. The duration of illness was 2 to 17 days with a 5-day average.

TREATMENT

Symptomatic treatment, including milk or water dilution and several hours of observation for spontaneous vomiting, usually suffices in most household shampoo exposures. Heavy-duty or industrial-strength solution exposures may require further treatment (i.e., emesis) if highly toxic substances are involved (see specific treatment sections). Respiratory symptoms in rug shampoo exposures respond to improved ventilation and removal from the source.

BLEACHES

PRODUCT FORMULATION/USES

Most household bleaches (e.g., Clorox) contain less than 5% sodium hypochlorite, which causes a moderate mucosal irritation. Granular bleaches are considered more toxic because the granules prolong mucosal contact and because solid bleaches tend to be more concentrated. Commercial bleaches contain other bleaching agents (e.g., sodium peroxide, sodium perborate, sodium carbonate, oxalic acid), and proper therapy requires accurate identification.

CLINICAL PRESENTATION

Local Toxicity

Household bleaches are mild to moderate mucosal irritants. Products with a pH below 12.5 do not cause serious burns, but failure to remove moderately alkaline liquids (e.g., bleaches with a pH of 11 to 12) from these areas may produce deep, partial-thickness chemical burns, especially after large, intentional ingestions.

Systemic Toxicity

Of all household cleaning products, bleaches produce the highest percentage of nausea, vomiting, and abdominal pain. Industrial-strength hypochlorite bleaches (15 to 20% solutions) may induce caustic injuries. Massive suicidal ingestions may produce fatal hyperchloremic metabolic acidosis or aspiration pneumonitis. Sodium peroxide decomposes in the stomach by releasing oxygen and may cause a gastritis. Sodium perborate is metabolized to peroxide and borate, which has moderate mucosal irritating properties and systemic effects.

Pulmonary Toxicity

Sodium hypochlorite solutions may release small amounts of hypochlorous acid and chlorine gas, but usually the concentrations of these toxic gases are too low to cause damage. Mixing solutions of ammonia and sodium hypochlorite produces monochloramine (NH_2C1) and dichloramine ($NHC1_2$) fumes. Chloramine fumes in a confined bathroom resulted in a chemical pneumonitis. Prolonged inhalation of chloramine fumes can produce obstructive pulmonary deficits, chest infiltrates, and acute pulmonary edema.

TREATMENT

1. Immediate dilution with water or milk is the first-aid procedure of choice for suspected caustic ingestion. Exposure to products such as industrial-strength hypochlorite solution and perborate should be evaluated as a potential caustic exposure.
2. Decontaminate both skin and eyes with copious saline irrigation. Be sure to remove all contaminated clothing (e.g., diapers in chlorine bleach exposure). Check all exposed eyes for corneal abrasions with fluorescein staining.
3. Emesis or lavage and cathartics are indicated for all except minor boric acid exposures. Activated charcoal does not adsorb boric acid.
4. Chlorine exposures require evaluation of acid-base and respiratory status.

DISINFECTANTS AND DEODORIZERS

PRODUCT FORMULATIONS/USES

Liquid Disinfectants

These products may contain acids, alkali, alcohol, pine oil, phenol, or cationic detergents such as quaternary compounds (e.g., Zephiran). Combination cleaners with pine oil and phenol are the most toxic compounds in this group.

Cake Deodorizers (See *P*-dichlorobenzene naphthalene)

TREATMENT

1. Immediately administer water or milk to any symptomatic patients or to any patient who ingests disinfectants. Treat as a caustic ingestion if the solution pH exceeds 12.
2. Irrigate exposed skin or eyes copiously with saline and check for corneal abrasions with fluorescein staining.
3. Determine the product contents to search for toxic constituents (e.g., nitrites, naphthalene, pine oil).
4. Emesis or lavage is indicated for ingestion of nitrites, cationic surfactants, substantial amounts of pine oil (more than several swallows of 30% concentrate), and large amounts of *p*-dichlorobenzene (several mothballs or a whole cake). The presence of low-viscosity hydrocarbon and turpentines dictates caution to prevent aspiration pneumonitis. Ingestion of a single naphthalene mothball requires gut decontamination in a small child presenting within 2 hours of exposure.
5. Antiemetics and demulcents such as antacids may be necessary.

ACIDS

PRODUCT FORMULATIONS

Household Use[2]

Toilet Bowl Cleaners

Sulfuric acid (8 to 10%), hydrochloric acid (10–25%), oxalic acid (2%), sodium bisulfate (70–100%).

Drain Cleaners

Sulfuric acid (95–99%).

Metal Cleaners and Antirust Compounds

Phosphoric acid (5–80%), oxalic acid (1%), hydrochloric acid (5–25%), sulfuric acid (10–20%), chromic acid (5–20%). Gun-bluing products contain selenious acid.

Soldering Fluxes

Zinc chloride (10–35%), hydrochloric acid (up to 40%).

Automobile Battery Fluid

Sulfuric acid (25–30%).

Swimming Pool Sanitizers

Calcium or sodium hypochlorite (70%).

Bleaches

Household products usually contain 3 to 6% sodium hypochlorite, which seldom causes more than minor mucosal erosion in contrast to the highly concentrated swimming pool sanitizers. Commercial household bleach solutions are formed by adding 12 to 15% sodium hydroxide to gaseous chlorine until the solution is neutralized and then diluting the hypochlorite concentration to 3 to 6%. Since acidic hypochlorite solutions are unstable, some poorly controlled hypochlorite processes add too little chlorine, leading to the production of an alkaline but stable hypochlorite product. All hypochlorite products (especially acidic ones) decompose slowly to nontoxic constituents.

Industrial Uses

Chromic Acid

Chromic anhydride (99.9%) is a strong inorganic acid. Commerical uses include plating, chemical and dyestuff manufacturing, photography, cement manufacturing, and leather tanning.

Hydrochloric Acid (Muriatic Acid)

Bleaching agents contain dilute (less than 10%) hydrochloric acid. Concentrated solutions (36%) are involved in dye and chemical synthesis, metal refining, and the plumbing industry.

Nitric Acid

Engraver's acid is 63% nitric acid. Other commercial users include soda makers, metal refiners, electroplaters, and fertilizer manufacturers.

Phosphoric Acid

The 85 to 90% solution is involved in metal cleaning, rustproofing, and superphosphate production. The dilute 10% solution is a disinfectant.

Hydrofluoric Acid

The concentrated (90%) solution is used as an anhydrous catalyst for high-octane gasoline, removal of sand from metal casing, petroleum refining, antimony fluoride extraction, and synthesis of pharmaceutics and germicides. Dilute solutions (10–20%) are used in tanning, frosting, and metal etching processes. Hydrogen fluoride burns now are a hazard in the semiconductor industry in which this acid is used as an "etchant" for chip manufacturing.

Sulfuric Acid

Chemical, munitions, and fertilizer manufacturers use the 95 to 98% solution. The more dilute 25 to 30% solution is used in machinery and batteries. Toilet bowl cleaners contain an 8 to 10% solution.

Acetic Acid

The more concentrated 60% solution appears in hat making, printing, dyeing, and rayon manufacturing. Dilute solutions (6–40%) are disinfectants and hair wave neutralizers.

Formic Acid

Airplane glue makers, cellulose formate workers, and tanning workers are exposed to a 60% solution.

Oxalic Acid

Tanning, blueprint paper, chemical synthesis, cleaning iron, leather.

Carbolic Acid (Phenol)

Disinfectant, dye, pharmaceuticals, plastics manufacturing.

PATHOPHYSIOLOGY

Determinants of Toxicity

1. *Type of substance ingested.*[2] Generally, substances with a pH below 2 are strong corrosives; however, pH alone is not the only determinant of severity since lemon juice has a pH around 2 and is not irritating. Important factors increasing the corrosive properties of an acid include concentration, molarity, and complexing affinity for hydroxyl ions. The more concentrated the solution, the greater the probability of serious injury regardless of other factors. Higher-molarity sulfuric acid (18 *M*) produces more damage compared with the stronger hydrochloric acid at lower molarity (12 *M*). In addition, the greater the amount of base required to neutralize the acid, the greater the tissue damage.
2. *Volume ingested.* Large volumes increase the area of injury, as well as predispose to emesis, which reexposes gastrointestinal tissue to damage.
3. *Contact Time.* Areas of slowing in the gastrointestinal tract (e.g., cricopharyngeus, pyloric sphincter, diaphragmatic hiatus, aortic arch) increase contact time and therefore predispose the area to corrosive damage. Increased viscosity and higher specific gravity reduce esophageal contact time, but speed the acid to the stomach, where prolonged contact occurs. Crystals tend to produce intense localized upper esophageal lesions, whereas liquid preparations produce severe, circumferential, and more distal lesions.
4. *Volume of liquid and material in stomach.* Fluid dilutes the corrosive and washes crystals off the mucosa. A full stomach is less susceptible to injury and the corrosive effect is more diffuse and superficial.
5. *Toxicity of the pyloric sphincter.* Pyloric spasm prevents gastric emptying and prolongs contact time.

Mechanism of Action

Strong acids produce a coagulation necrosis characterized by the formation of a coagulum (eschar) as a result of the desiccating action of the acid on proteins in superficial tissue. The coagulum limits the penetrating ability of acids compared with the liquefaction necrosis of alkali ingestions where continuing penetration produces injury after exposure ceases. Hydrofluoric acid exposure is the major exception: the fluoride anion (not the hydrogen ion) produces a liquefaction necrosis by combining with calcium and magnesium in the tissues. Sulfuric, sulfurous, and chromic acids have limited penetrating ability, but perforation is much more common with sulfuric acid than with hydrochloric acid.

Phases of Injury

Three pathophysiologic phases characterize both acid and alkali ingestions.[3]

1. *Acute inflammatory phase (first 4 to 7 days).* Vascular thrombosis and cellular necrosis reach a maximum in the first 24 to 48 hours, with destruction of the columnar epithelium, submucosa, and muscularis. The necrotic mucosa sloughs by the third or fourth day, and an ulcer forms.
2. *Latent granulation phase.* Fibroplasia begins about the middle of the first week, and fresh granulation tissue fills the sloughed area of mucosa. Collagen starts to replace the granulation tissue by the end of the first week. Perforation is most likely during this phase, which lasts 2 weeks after injury.
3. *Chronic cicatrization phase.* The formation of excessive scar tissue around the submucosa and the muscularis produces contractures. This dense fibrous tissue begins to form 2 to 4 weeks after injury, at a rate that may be either rapid or slowly progressive. The primary goal of management is to prevent this relentless complication.

Location of Injury

The distal stomach (antrum and pylorus) is the most frequently injured gastrointestinal site. Fluid propulsion physiology in the esophagus predicts the location of major damage. A common pathway (Magenstrasse) directs the rapid transit of fluid along the stomach's lesser curvature to the pylorus. Stomachs that contain food prior to ingestion have predominantly pyloric damage and lesser curvature damage, although the hydrophilic nature of acid tends to produce a diffuse damage. In empty stomachs the lesser curvature is more upright and contracted so that prolonged acid contact occurs in the antrum and midgastric regions. Chronic stricture formation may result in pyloric obstruction, antral stenosis, or an hourglass-type deformity.

Esophageal injury occurs in 6 to 20% of acid ingestions and almost always in association with major gastric damage. Esophageal injury usually is mild and responds to supportive care. No esophageal perforations have been reported to date. The limited esophageal damage in acid ingestion probably results from rapid esophageal transit and limited penetrating ability rather than from any special protective properties of the columnar epithelium. Relaxation of the pyloric sphincter allows the antegrade progression of acid contents and the production of small-bowel perforations.

CLINICAL PRESENTATION

Initial Effects

Initial symptoms reflect the corrosive properties of strong acids: severe pain on tissue contact associated with dysphagia, drooling (for esophageal involvement), vomiting, hematemesis, substernal and abdominal pain, and melena. The presence of oropharyngeal burns suggests, but does not confirm, gastric involvement.

TREATMENT

Stabilization

Airway problems may arise from laryngeal edema and inhalation exposure. Treat with 100% oxygen initially. Respiratory distress may require cricothyroidotomy if endotracheal intubation is contraindicated by excessive swelling. Intravenous lines should be established immediately in all cases where there is evidence of circulatory compromise.

Immediate dilution (milk or water) within 30 minutes postingestion is widely recommended for oral ingestions despite the fact that tissue injury occurs rapidly, especially with liquids. Do not attempt to neutralize the acid with weak bases since the exothermic reaction may extend the corrosive injury. In vitro studies indicate that water dilution is ineffective in reducing pH and that buffering agents (e.g., antacids) produce significant exothermic reactions without significantly altering the pH.[4] Since reexposure of the mucosa to acid is harmful, be careful to avoid further vomiting and limit fluids to one or two glasses in an adult. Grade 1 to 2 burns usually can be admitted to a general medical ward. Grade 2 to 3 burns should be admitted to an intensive care unit.

Decontamination

Emesis by syrup of ipecac is contraindicated because of reexposure of the esophagus to corrosive material. Charcoal has no place in acid management because it is ineffective and obscures the endoscopic field. Most authors advise against lavage with a soft rubber catheter, and no clinical trials support its use; however, some authors[2] recommend the use of lavage within 1 hour of ingestion (pylorospasm may prolong injury after initial contact) because most esophageal acid injuries are superficial and gastric intubations have not caused complications. The removal of ingested acids such as hydrogen fluoride may outweigh the risk of perforation. Remove all contaminated clothes and irrigate exposed skin copiously with saline. Copiously irrigate caustic eye injuries immediately for at least 20 to 30 minutes.

Supportive Care

1. Patients should not be fed orally until endoscopy has confirmed the extent of injury.
2. The administration of steroids is highly questionable in humans since no clinical study supports their use. Although steroid therapy delays stricture formation in animals when given within 48 hours of injury, steroids have been implicated in the obscuration of developing peritoneal signs after an acid ingestion.[5,6]
3. Antibiotics should be reserved for documented infections.
4. Initial observation should be directed toward detecting gastrointestinal perforation by serial abdominal examinations, complete blood counts, and, if indicated, radiographs and water-soluble contrast studies.
5. Follow fluid and electrolyte balance carefully (including calcium, phosphorus, and protein levels in hydrogen fluoride and oxalic acid poisoning).
6. Skin lesions require copious saline irrigation and removal of any contaminating fragments. Hydrogen fluoride burns may benefit from cool benzalkonium chloride (Zephiran) or 25% magnesium sulfate (Epsom Salts) soaks. Do not add ice to a basin in which human tissue is soaking. Prolonged exposure to hydrogen fluoride concentrations greater than 20% often requires intradermal 10% calcium gluconate infiltrated with a 27- to 30-gauge needle into subcutaneous skin at the rate of 0.5 mL/cm^2 of skin area. Kunkel has used intraarterial calcium gluconate via an intraarterial line and infusion pump for resistant hydrogen fluoride burn cases with good results.[7] Consider nail debridement if subungual injury occurs. (See Hydrofluoric Acid for complete details.)
7. Treat chemical burns as thermal burns with nonadherent gauze and wrapping. Deep second-degree burns may benefit from topical silver sulfadiazine.
8. Hospitalized patients should be followed after discharge for the development of gastric-outlet obstruction. Patients should return if signs of obstruction develop (progressive anorexia, weight loss, early satiety, nausea). A routine upper gastrointestinal series 3 to 4 weeks after exposure detects early contractures.

Eye Care

Copious irrigation of acid injuries requires retraction of the eyelids so that the conjunctival cul-de-sacs are well washed. Use anesthetic agents (proparacaine, tetracaine) and retractors as necessary. Be sure to remove all particulate matter. Irrigation should last at least 20 to 30 minutes. Do not use neutralizing solutions or any other additives. Several liters of saline are required. As long as the lids are retracted, simple intravenous tubing is all that is required to adequately decontaminate the eye. Caustic injuries require a complete eye examination, preferably with a slit lamp, to detect the extent of corneal injury after decontamination. The examination should include the following:

1. Visual acuity and extraocular motility.
2. Examination of eyelids, conjunctiva, and sclera.
3. Pupillary reactions.
4. Anterior chamber depth.
5. Staining of corneal surfaces with fluorescein to detect abrasions and ulcerations. Do not use fluorescein if a corneal perforation is suspected. In such cases shield the eye and contact an ophthalmologist.
6. Examination of the retina and posterior chamber with an ophthalmoscope.

Cycloplegic drops (1% cyclopentolate for short-term use or 5% homatropine for longer use), antibiotic drops, vasoconstrictive agents, or artificial tears may be indicated depending on the severity of symptoms. Steroid eye drops should be given only with the approval of the consulting ophthalmologist. Although most acid exposures are less severe than alkali exposures, hydrogen fluoride exposure is an exception. All such exposures should be treated as alkali exposures and an ophthalmologist should be consulted immediately after decontamination.

ACETIC ACID—ACETATES

Acetic acid ingestion may result in pharyngeal, esophageal, and gastrointestinal burns, bleeding, and volume depletion.

USE

Acetic acid is widely used as a chemical feedstock for the products of vinyl plastics, acetic anhydride, acetone, acetanilide, acetylchloride, ethyl alcohol, ketone, methyl ethyl ketone, acetate esters, and cellulose acetates. It is also used alone in the dye, rubber, pharmaceutical, food preserving, textile, and laundry industries and is used in the manufacture of Paris green, white lead, tint rinse, photographic chemicals, stain removers, insecticides, and plastics.[8]

PHYSICAL PROPERTIES

CH_3COOH, acetic acid, is a colorless liquid with a pungent vinegar-like odor. Glacial acetic acid contains 99% acid. Synonyms include ethanoic acid, ethylic acid, methane carboxylic acid, vinegar acid, and pyroligneous acid. Acetic acid has a CAS no: 64-19-7. The OSHA standard is a time-weighted average of 10 ppm (25 mg/m^3). Short-term exposure limits are 15 ppm (37 mg/m^3). Immediate damage to life and health follows exposure to 1000 ppm.[3,9]

CLINICAL PRESENTATION

Local

Acetic acid vapor may produce irritation and damage of the eyes, nose, throat, and lungs. Contact with concentrated acetic acid may lead to severe skin damage and eye damage sufficient to cause a loss of sight. Repeated or prolonged exposure to acetic acid may cause skin darkening, erosion of the exposed front teeth, and chronic inflammation of the nose, throat, and bronchi.[3]

Systemic[2]

Acute Exposure

Bronchopneumonia, pulmonary edema, and reactive airways dysfunction syndrome[10] (see Airborne chapter) may follow acute inhalation overexposure.

Chronic Exposure

Chronic exposure may result in pharyngitis and bronchitis.

Ingestion

Ingestion may result in penetration of the esophagus, hematemesis, hemolysis, diarrhea, shock, disseminated intravascular coagulation, and hemoglobinemia followed by anuria.[3,4,11]

TREATMENT

Assess local injury (mouth, pharynx) following ingestion. Consider replacement of intravascular volume and coagulation factors, diuretics, and prompt correction of the acidosis. Exchange transfusion should be considered in the face of significant intravascular hemolysis.[6]

PERSONAL PROTECTIVE METHOD

Workers who work with glacial acetic acid should have personal protective equipment; protective clothing, gloves, and goggles should be worn. Eye fountains and showers should be available in areas of potential exposure.[3]

FORMIC ACID

Formic acid ingestions are unique by their ability in many patients to cause death after a prolonged (several weeks) course of classical acid-induced gastrointestinal damage. Other complications include severe metabolic acidosis, intravascular hemolysis, and disseminated intravascular coagulation.[12–18] Accidental ingestions in children ordinarily do not lead to fatalities since the pungent taste of the chemical usually precludes an ingestion of a lethal dose. It is nevertheless a problem when used deliberately for suicide. In South India formic acid seems to be the favorite agent for self-destruction, especially among low-income families and laborers.[9] In Europe it is a well-known, if relatively infrequent, vehicle for suicide.[7,8,10–13] Formic acid skin burns may result in systemic toxicity.[19]

STRUCTURE AND CLASSIFICATION

Formic acid is HCOOH and has a molecular weight of 46. The conversion factor (CF) is 21.7. To convert to SI units: $\mu g/mL \times 21.7 = \mu mol/L$; to convert from SI units: $\mu mol/L$ divided by $21.7 = \mu g/mL$. CAS 64-18-6. The melting point of formic acid is 8°C; its boiling point is 100°C. It is completely soluble in water. It is a colorless liquid with a pungent penetrating odor.[20] The IDLH (immediately dangerous to life and health) level is 30 ppm.[14]

Synonyms

Methanoic acid, formylic acid, hydrogen carboxylic acid.[21]

Standards[22]

USA (NIOSH/OSHA)	TWA	9 mg/m^3
(ACGIH)	TWA	5 ppm
		9.4 mg/m^3

UK	TWA	5 ppm 9.4 mg/m^3	
Germany	TWA	5 ppm 9 mg/m^3	local irritant
France	STEL	5 ppm 9 mg/m^3	
Australia	TWA	5 ppm 9 mg/m^3	

USES

Formic acid is used as a component of proprietary descaling agents and in stain-removing fluids. It is also used in dyeing colorfast wool, in electroplating, coagulating latex rubber, regenerating old rubber, and dehairing and tanning leather; for the manufacture of acetic acid, airplane dope, allyl alcohol, cellulose formate, phenolic resins, and oxalate used in laundry; and in the textile, insecticide, refrigeration, and paper industries.[16] In the UK it has been marketed as "Kleenoff" (55%); "Ataka" (44%); Descale (55%); Kilrock (60%).[12]

SOURCES

Formic acid is a synthetic chemical.

TOXIC DOSES

Less than 10 grams[12]

Ingestions of less than 10 grams in children have led to superficial oropharyngeal burns; the children recovered.

5 to 30 grams

Ingestions of 5 to 30 grams in adults may cause minor superficial oropharyngeal burns, some abdominal pain, dyspnea, and dysphagia; a few patients may exhibit hematemesis, pneumonitis, or esophageal stricture. No fatalities are usually seen in this group.

30 to 45 grams

Ingestions of 30 to 45 grams of formic acid usually lead to hematemesis, hepatotoxicity, ulcerations, hemorrhage, and perforation in the gastrointestinal tract. Some patients may experience a reversible disseminated intravascular coagulation or acute renal failure; many will develop esophageal strictures. Occasional deaths have been reported.

45 to 200 grams

Reversible disseminated intravascular coagulation, pneumonitis, acute renal failure, and esophageal stricture may be observed in the few who recover. Most develop corrosive perforations of the abdominal viscera, gastrointestinal hemorrhage, and in some cases acute renal failure. Death occurs at this dose level in the majority of patients within 36 hours after ingestion. Ingestion of 50 mL of formic acid led to a reversible acute renal failure and, following a gastrointestinal hemorrhage, the patient recovered.[10]

TOXICOKINETICS

Absorption

Formic acid blood levels of 348 μg/mL (7.6 mmol/L) were obtained about 2 hours after ingestion of approximately 100 g of formic acid.[13]

Elimination

The elimination half-life of formic acid in one case was approximately 2.5 hours.[13]

MECHANISM OF ACTION

Formic acid directly damages clotting factors leading to an increase in bleeding time and hemorrhage. It has a direct coagulative necrosis type of corrosive action on the gastrointestinal tract and destroys the normal histology down to the muscularis mucosa. Hematemesis may lead to hypovolemia. Formic acid has a direct hemolytic effect on red blood cells.[13] Hemolysis plus the effect of formic acid on the renal parenchyma may lead to acute renal failure.[23] Necrotic tissue fragments probably trigger the disseminated intravascular coagulation.

CLINICAL PRESENTATION

Depending on the dose ingested, direct effects can be observed:

Oral

Burning pain in the mouth and pharynx; salivation; hyperemic, edematous mucosae; ulcerations of the buccal mucosa and pharynx.

Eyes

Mydriasis; hyperemic conjunctivae.

Gastrointestinal

Nausea, vomiting, abdominal pain; upper gastrointestinal bleeding; abdominal rigidity; pancreatitis.

Esophagus

Hemorrhagic esophagitis; slough of mucosa.

Stomach

Sloughing ulcerations of the stomach.

Skin

Erythema, blisters; cutaneous purpura, bruising around venepuncture sites (usually after the first few days).[7]

CNS

Depression, drowsiness, weakness, coma, death.

Respiratory

Shortness of breath, aspiration pneumonitis, bilateral coarse rhonchi, "shock lungs"; acute respiratory distress syndrome; respiratory arrest; alveolar-capillary leak on the fourth day.[12]

Urinary

Diuresis; anuria after 2 or more days.

Muscle

Muscle contractions in severe cases.

Cardiovascular

Tachycardia, bradycardia, hypertension, hypotension; often beginning on the tenth day or later—central cyanosis, asystole.

Hematologic

Methemoglobinemia; intravascular hemolysis; disseminated intravascular coagulation.

Metabolic

Metabolic acidosis, respiratory acidosis. Complications include severe gastrointestinal bleeding, pneumonia, acute tubular necrosis, acute respiratory distress syndrome, peritonitis, sepsis, disseminated intravascular coagulation, hemolysis, abscesses of the liver, metabolic acidosis, shock, and death.

LABORATORY

Analytic Methods

Formic acid serum concentrations are quantitated enzymatically using formate dehydrogenase (formic acid UV method) with spectrophotometric measurements.[13]

Blood Levels

Formic acid concentrations 2 hours following ingestion of about 100 grams of formic acid (200 mL 50% formic acid) were 348 μg/mL (7.6 mmol/L) and declined exponentially with an elimination half-life of approximately 2.5 hours. Ingestion of 50 mL of formic acid led to a serum formic acid level of 180 μg/mL in 6 hours.[10]

Abnormalities

Gastroscopy may (in the first 24 hours) discern severe lesions of the esophagus, stomach, and duodenum. Coagulation parameters exhibit an increase in the prothrombin time, accelerated partial thromboplastin time, and fibrin degradation products. Other laboratory abnormalities encountered include elevations in the lactic acid dehydrogenase, aminotransferases, amylase, glucose, lactate, and creatinine. There may be an increase in free hemoglobin, methemoglobin, and the white blood cell and platelet counts. The hematocrit and fibrinogen levels may be within normal limits. The urine will be red. Arterial blood gases will often reflect a severe metabolic acidosis. The chest x-ray may be normal[13] or exhibit bilateral patchy consolidation or a "shock lung" picture.[1] Formic acid poisoning is one of the few chemicals that can bring the bicarbonate level to zero.[24]

TREATMENT

Stabilization

Patients who have ingested formic acid should be hospitalized for treatment in an intensive care facility. Airway problems may arise from laryngeal edema. The patient should be monitored for cardiorespiratory function. A supply of 100% oxygen should be available. Intravenous lines should be inserted and central venous pressure measurements should be taken periodically to ensure circulatory stability. Immediate dilution with milk but not with alkalis, which may cause a local exothermic reaction, may be useful.

Decontamination

Emesis with syrup of ipecac or gastric lavage or use of a nasogastric tube is contraindicated. Activated charcoal has not been used and could enhance mucosal irritation in addition to its possible penetration through a mucosal perforation. It has no place in acid management and obscures the endoscopic field.

Supportive Care

1. Renal failure may require dialysis. Peritoneal dialysis may be preferable to hemodialysis since heparin used with hemodialysis may increase gastrointestinal bleeding.[7]
2. Intravascular hemolysis may respond to an exchange transfusion.
3. Respiratory distress may respond to intubation and ventilatory support with intermittent positive pressure breathing and oxygen.
4. Anuria may respond to IV mannitol.
5. Special attention should be given to the condition of the eyes, the skin, clotting parameters, arterial blood gases, and the lungs (periodic chest x-rays).
6. The role of cimetidine and steroids is not clear.
7. Diazepam may be used for sedation provided tracheal protection is in place.
8. Lidocaine irrigation may be useful for mouth lesions.
9. Blood loss may require transfusions.
10. Follow fluid intake and output and electrolytes, especially potassium, in the presence of hemolysis. Provide required fluids according to clinical judgment.
11. Sodium bicarbonate to maintain urine pH at about 1.5 may be indicated for severe metabolic acidosis. Correction of acidemia and urinary alkalinization is used to decrease lipophilicity of formic acid and enhance urinary elimination of formate. Urinary alkalinization may increase hemoglobin solubility and decrease the rate of acute tubular necrosis.
12. IV furosemide 20 mg every 4 hours to block the formate chloride exchanges, preventing renal tubular reabsorption of formate in the urine.

High-dose IV folinic acid (1 mg/kg bolus IV followed by 6 doses of 1 mg/kg IV at 4-hour intervals until clinical improvement) may enhance formate degradation by the liver.[25]

HYDROFLUORIC ACID

ORAL

Ingestion of hydrofluoric acid may lead to death within 1 to 7 hours.[26–29] Ingestions of relatively dilute solutions of hydrofluoric acid may be rapidly fatal. One mouthful of rust remover led to severe hypocalcemia, acidosis, and fatal asystole in 90 minutes.[30] Following ingestion patients may present with hematemesis, hypovolemic tetanic convulsions, upper airway obstruction, severe hypocalcemia, acidosis, shock, and coma.[31] Myocardial irritability and subsequent life-threatening cardiac arrhythmias may be due to binding of potassium, magnesium, and calcium ions.

A significant hypocalcemic risk (general guidelines) may follow (a) a dermal exposure to 50% or greater hydrofluoric acid concentration to 1% of the body surface area (e.g., one complete hand); (b) any dermal exposure of more than 5% body surface area; (c) an inhalation of vapors from 60% or greater concentration of acid solution; or (d) ingestion of hydrofluoric acid solutions.[26]

Fluoride ions may have a direct toxic effect on the central nervous system leading to stupor, coma, and respiratory failure. Hemorrhagic gastritis, hypocalcemia, pulmonary edema, and metabolic acidosis may supervene.[32] Survival has been reported in one case following ingestion of 2 ounces of a rust-removal agent containing 12% hydrofluoric acid. Lidocaine-resistant ventricular fibrillation developed in this patient with an associated hypocalcemia and hypomagnesemia.[33]

TOPICAL

Hydrofluoric acid burns of the skin require immediate and copious irrigation with water, preferably under a shower or faucet for at least 15 to 30 minutes. Cleansing and debridement follows. For exposures to hydrofluoric acid concentrations less than 20%, liberal and frequent application of a 2.5% calcium gluconate gel may be the topical therapy of choice. A 2.5% calcium gluconate gel is formulated by mixing 3.5 g of calcium gluconate powder USP with 150 mL (5 oz.) of a water-soluble lubricant such as K-Y Jelly.[22,26] The gel may be secured by an occlusive barrier (e.g., vinyl gloves or plastic wrap), and repeated application may be administered as often as necessary to eliminate pain. Calcium gluconate gel has not been approved by the U.S. Food and Drug Administration.

INFILTRATION THERAPY

Skin lesions resulting from exposure to hydrogen fluoride concentrations over 20% usually require intradermal injection of 10% calcium gluconate (0.5 mL/cm^2 of skin, with a 30-gauge needle).[34] The use of 10% magnesium salts was effective in some but not all animal models.[35] Recommendations for the use of magnesium salts in hydrofluoric acid burns await further clinical trials. Do not use calcium chloride for infiltrations; it is corrosive and may cause further tissue damage.

INTRAARTERIAL INFUSION OF CALCIUM

Frequently, hydrofluoric acid burns occur on the fingers, where intradermal calcium injections are hazardous. For these areas, the intraarterial infusion of 10 mL of 20% calcium gluconate (180 mg calcium) in 40 mL of normal saline over 4 hours has been recommended.[28] A preinjection arteriogram will document blood flow to the affected area. Calcium chloride infusion (10 mL of a 10% solution mixed in 40 to 50 mL 5% dextrose) is also an effective treatment for concentrated hydrofluoric acid burns of the fingers. In animal models, the application of calcium gluconate ointment after a hydrofluoric acid burn reduces the subsequent necrosis.

An intraarterial infusion protocol has been suggested by Siegel and Heard[36]:

1. Minimum baseline laboratory includes calcium, magnesium, phosphorus, prothrombin time (PT), and partial thromboplastin time (PTT).
2. The appropriate artery is cannulated with a 20-gauge, 4 French or 5 French arterial catheter.
3. If thumb and index fingers only are involved, the brachial artery is cannulated, and if the leg or foot are involved, the femoral artery is cannulated.
4. The patient is admitted to the Intensive Care Unit (ICU) for arterial pressure wave monitoring.
5. An intraarterial infusion is given over 4 hours using a mixture of 10 mL of 10% calcium chloride diluted with 40 mL of normal saline.
6. The arterial wave form is checked every hour and the arterial line is flushed with heparinized saline.
7. After infusion of the calcium chloride mixture, the infusion tubing is flushed with another 10 mL of normal saline over a 15-minute period.
8. With the addition of 500 units of heparin to the infusion mixture, catheter clotting has been significantly reduced.
9. Catheter clots (manifested by a flattened waveform or difficulty withdrawing blood by a flattened waveform or difficulty withdrawing blood from the catheter) are lysed with 5000 units of urokinase.
10. After infusion is complete, the waveform is monitored continuously and the line flushed with heparinized saline every hour and as needed.
11. The patient is observed for 48 hours.
12. The injured extremity is checked for residual pain and tenderness at the end of 4 hours. If tenderness persists, then another infusion is given.
13. Serum calcium, magnesium, phosphorus, PT, and PTT are obtained 1 hour after completion of the infusion.
14. If the serum magnesium falls by 0.3 mg/dL or falls below 1.7 mg/dL, an IV infusion of magnesium sulfate is begun using 1.015 mEq/hour to 4.06 mEq/hour, adjusting the rate according to the subsequent serum magnesium levels and number of calcium infusions being delivered.

15. The process of 4 hours of infusion followed by 4 hours of rest is repeated until there is no residual tenderness to gentle pressure.
16. After tenderness has resolved, the catheter is removed and the patient is transferred to the surgical floor for an observation period of 16 to 24 hours before being discharged.

INTRAVENOUS REGIONAL CALCIUM GLUCONATE PERFUSION

Henry[37] has observed immediate relief of pain in an extremity after regional perfusion with 5 mL of 10% calcium gluconate added to 20 mL normal saline injected intravenously.[32]

Consider admitting all symptomatic patients (persistent cough, dyspnea), since the onset of pulmonary edema may be delayed 24 hours.

Burns

All patients should be admitted to a burn unit or intensive care unit if the total extent of the burns is greater than 2 to 3% body surface area, or if there is significant respiratory distress. Administer 1 gram (10 mL) 10% calcium gluconate IV if immediate serum calcium levels are not available and exposure was extensive—greater than 5% body surface area.[26,30]

Acidosis

Correct systemic acidosis with sodium bicarbonate guided by arterial blood gas measurements. Cardiac arrhythmias secondary to electrolyte imbalance, acidosis, or hypoxia should be identified and corrected. Obtain frequent calcium, magnesium, phosphorus, and potassium levels. Watch for electrocardiographic evidence of hypocalcemia—a prolonged QT interval. Watch for fluoride-induced hyperkalemia as a cause of arrhythmias. Dialysis may be required to remove excess serum potassium and fluoride. Hypotension should be managed with volume expansion and vasopressors as required.

Eye

Eye exposures should be treated by immediate and copious irrigation of the exposed eye for at least 30 minutes after exposure. Local ophthalmic anesthetic drops will increase patient comfort and compliance with prolonged irrigation. The pH of the eye fluid should be periodically checked with litmus paper and irrigation continued until it is normal. Assess visual acuity after the eye irrigation is completed. Obtain an ophthalmologic consultation. Repeated instillation of 1% calcium gluconate eye drops combined with conventional treatment of acid eye burns is effective in hastening recovery from a hydrofluoric acid–induced corneal erosion.[38]

Inhalation

Inhalation exposure and injury are treated by removing the victim from the source and into fresh air, accompanied by decontamination of the clothes and skin. Monitor the patient for laryngeal edema, pneumonitis, pulmonary edema, pulmonary hemorrhage, and systemic toxicity.

Ingestion

Ingestion at home may be treated immediately with milk to dilute the acid and perhaps bind some of the fluoride ion. If spontaneous vomiting has not occurred and the time between ingestion and treatment is less than 90 minutes, consider gastric lavage. Addition of 10% calcium gluconate to the lavage fluid may provide some free calcium to bind the fluoride. There are no data or guidelines for the amount of lavage fluid used for decontamination of the stomach. Syrup of ipecac is not advised. After decontamination, monitor the patient for signs of airway compromise, gastric perforation, gastric hemorrhage, and systemic toxicity.

Calcium and Magnesium

Ingestions that induce hypocalcemia (prolonged QT interval, positive Trousseau's or Chvostek's sign) and hypomagnesemia may require multiple intravenous doses of calcium gluconate (e.g., 9 and 10 ampules in one patient with two ingestions) and magnesium sulfate (2 grams and 5 grams) over a period of 6 to 7 hours together with repeated cardioversions (for ventricular fibrillation) until normal blood calcium and magnesium levels and cardiac stability are achieved.[28]

MONOCHLOROACETIC ACID (MCA)

Monochloroacetic acid (MCA) is corrosive and stronger than acetic acid.[39] MCA is extremely toxic both via the dermal and inhalation routes.[40]

USES

Monochloroacetic acid is used in the production of carboxymethyl cellulose, phenoxyacetates, pigments, and drugs.[34] It is also used as a wart remover and herbicide.[35]

OCCUPATIONAL EXPOSURE

The toxic effect of ethylene chlorhydrin may be related to its metabolites, chloroacetaldehyde and chloroacetic acid.[41]

TOXICOKINETICS

Absorption

MCA is readily absorbed after ingestion and after skin contact.[34,35]

MECHANISM OF ACTION

MCA reacts with the sulfhydryl groups of essential enzymes.[37] MCA can produce severe local reactions of the skin, eye, or respiratory tract as might be expected from its ionization constant.[37] MCA inhibits the tricarboxylic acid cycle and prevents the conversion of citrate to isocitrate.[35]

CLINICAL PRESENTATION

Splashes of 80% MCA solution on the skin can lead to epidermal and superficial skin burns. Within a few hours features of systemic poisoning occur, including disorientation, agitation, cardiac failure, and coma. Severe metabolic acidosis, rhabdomyolysis, renal insufficiency, and cerebral edema with uncal herniation can lead to death.[34] Oral exposure led to refractory ventricular tachycardia, pulmonary edema, acidemia, and death in 8 hours.[35] Other manifestations of poisoning include malaise, vomiting, cardiovascular shock, and seizures.[42] Vomiting and diarrhea are common early signs. CNS features include excitability with disorientation, delirium, and seizures followed by CNS depression and coma with cerebral edema. Severe myocardial depression with shock and electrocardiographic changes of nonspecific myocardial danger are observed. Progressive renal failure, hypokalemia, and severe metabolic acidosis are observed. Hypocalcemia may be delayed for 1 to 2 days. Acetylating agents such as glacial acetic acid, acetic anhydride, monochloroacetic acid, and dichloroacetic acid cause a bullous dermatitis or delayed onset with extensive desquamation.[43]

LABORATORY

Analytical Methods

A gas chromatography–mass spectrometry method for determining MCA in plasma was developed from a gas chromatography method used for measuring MCA in industrial waste water.[34] It is sensitive to 0.22 μg/mL.

Blood Levels

Four hours after a skin splash of 80% MCA on 25 to 30% of the body surface an adult exhibited an MCA concentration of 33 μg/mL.[34] Following an inadvertent administration of 5 to 6 mL of an 8% MCA wart remover (Verzone) a 5-year-old died and exhibited a postmortem MCA level of 100 μg/mL.[35]

Abnormalities

Hypokalemia and high creatine kinase, aspartic aminotransferase, and amine aminotransferase concentrations may be observed.[34] Hypocalcemia may be delayed for 1 to 2 days. Myoglobinuria can appear due to rhabdomyolysis.[35]

TREATMENT

Stabilization

After exposure to liquid MCA, urgent skin decontamination and removal of contaminated clothing are indicated.

Decontamination

After ingestion, emesis should be induced at the accident site, despite the risk of corrosive damage, to lessen the inception of severe systemic poisoning.

Elimination Enhancement

MCA is found in plasma in fairly high concentrations. Hemodialysis may be of benefit if commenced at an early stage.[34]

Antidote

Ethanol and glyceryl monoacetate have been advocated both for fluoroacetate poisoning and for MCA poisoning, but there is little clinical evidence to support its use.[34] MCA is bound to glutathione and other sulfhydryl-containing substances. *N*-acetylcysteine could be tried as a sulfhydryl donor. No clinical experience is available with this product in MCA poisoning.

Supportive Measures

If more than 1% of body surface is exposed to liquid MCA, hospitalize the patient for supportive therapy, including fluids, correction of acid-base and electrolyte disturbances (hypokalemia and hypercalcemia), alkalinization of the urine to prevent myoglobin deposition in the renal tubules, inotropic support (dopamine or dobutamine) as indicated for hemodynamic compromise, and controlled hyperventilation to prevent and treat cerebral edema.[34]

OXALIC ACID

Ingestion of oxalic acid from sorrel or rhubarb may lead to extensive renal damage and death.

HYPOCALCEMIA[44–46]

Lethal Dose

The lethal dose of oxalic acid for adults is 15 to 30 g, although amounts as low as 5 g have been fatal.[40]

USES

Oxalic acid is used as an analgesic reagent and in the manufacture of dyes, inks, bleaches, paint removers, varnishes, wood and metal cleaners, dextrin, cream of tartar, celluloid, oxalates, tartaric acid, purified methyl alcohol, glycerol, and stable hydrogen cyanide. It is also used in the photographic, ceramic, metallurgic, rubber, leather, engraving, pharmaceutical, paper, and lithographic industries.[41]

Synonyms

Ethanedioic acid, oxalic acid (aqueous, oxalic acid dihydrate).

PHYSICAL PROPERTIES

Oxalic acid is a colorless odorless powder or granular solid. Oxalates are present in sorrel *(Rurex Crispus)* and rhubarb, where its content is high in the leaves and low in the stalk. It occurs in plants in a partly insoluble form as acid oxalate and free oxalic acid and partly in insoluble form as calcium oxalate. The OSHA TWA standard is 1 mg/m^3 with a short-term exposure limit of 2 mg/m^3. Immediate danger to life and health follows an exposure of 500 mg/m^3.[47]

PATHOPHYSIOLOGY

Target organs for oxalic acid poisoning include the skin, eyes, respiratory system, and kidneys. Oxalic acid has a corrosive effect on the digestive tract. Once absorbed it reacts with calcium in plasma, and insoluble calcium oxalate tends to precipitate in organs such as the kidneys, blood vessels, heart, lungs, and liver. This reaction may also lead to hypocalcemia.[40]

An estimated 66% of renal calculi and 75% of bladder calculi are composed of calcium oxalate. Such stones may be caused by hypercalciuria (free hyperparathyroidism, sarcoidosis, renal tubular acidosis, hypervitaminosis DP, or hyperoxaluria).[48]

CLINICAL PRESENTATION

Local

Liquid oxalic acid has a corrosive action on the skin, eyes, and mucous membranes that may result in irritation. Local prolonged contact with extremities may result in localized pain, cyanosis, and possibly gangrenous changes secondary to localized vascular damage.

Systemic

Chronic exposure may lead to chronic inflammation of the upper respiratory tract.

Ingestion

A 53-year-old man ingested soup containing 500 g of sorrel *(Rurex crispus)*. The ingested dose of oxalic acid was about 6 to 8 g. He developed vomiting, diarrhea, coma, respiratory depression, kidney and liver failure, severe metabolic acidosis, and hypocalcemia. Within 2 hours he developed ventricular fibrillation and died.[40] A 4-year-old child ate rhubarb leaves, became drowsy, vomited, and lapsed into a coma. An oxalic acid test of the urine was strongly positive. The child died in 1½ hours. No typical oxalate crystals were observed in the urine.[41]

LABORATORY

The presence of increased urinary oxalate crystals may be useful in evaluation of oral poisoning. Serum calcium and oxalate levels may also be considered.[39]

TREATMENT

Management of a patient with acute oxalic acid poisoning consists of gastric lavage with calcium gluconate (10 mL, 10% IV) or lactate solutions, intravenous calcium gluconate, and dialysis or exchange transfusions as required for renal failure.[40,41] Electrocardiographic monitoring and serum calcium determinations should be initiated.

Local

Eyes—irrigate immediately for 15 minutes with copious amounts of water. Skin—flush with water promptly. Large renal calculi may require surgical removal or lithotripsy and a brisk diuresis (urine output of 1 to 2 liters/day).[43]

PERSONAL PROTECTIVE METHOD

Protective clothing and goggles should be worn when working in areas where direct contact is possible. Respiratory protection from mist or dust may be necessary.

REFERENCES—ACIDS

1. Mofenson HC, Greensher J. The non-toxic ingestion. Pediatr Clin North Am 1970;17:583–590.
2. Klein-Schwartz W, Oderda GM. Management of corrosive ingestions. Clin Toxicol Consult 1983;5:39–55.
3. Friedman EM, Lovejoy FH. The emergency management of caustic ingestions. Emerg Med Clin North Am 1984;2:77–80.
4. Maull KI. Liquid caustic ingestions: an in vitro study of the effects of buffer, neutralization, and dilution. Ann Emerg Med 1985;14:1160–1162.
5. Nicosia JR, Thornton JP, Folk FA. Surgical management of corrosive gastric injuries. Ann Surg 1974;180:139–143.
6. Kirsh MM, Ritter F. Caustic ingestion and subsequent damage to the oropharyngeal and digestive passages. Ann Thorac Surg 1976;21:74–82.
7. Kunkel DB. Burning issues: acids and alkalis. II. Skin and eye exposures. Emerg Med 1984;16(11):165–171.
8. Occupational Disease. A Guide to their Recognition. Revised edition. Publication No. DHEW (NIOSH) 77-181. National Institute for Occupational Safety and Health. Washington, DC. US Government Printing Office, June 1977, pp. 178–180.
9. NIOSH Pocket Guide to Chemical Hazards. NIOSH Publication No. 90-117. US Department of Health and Human Services. Washington, DC. US Government Printing Office, June 1990, pp. 30–31.
10. Kern DG. Outbreak of the reactive airways dysfunction syndrome after a spill of glacial acetic acid. Am Rev Respir Dis 1991;144:1058–1064.
11. Hall S, Saliares R, Arrigoni J, Flynn T. Systemic acidosis, hemolysis and hemoglobinuria renal failure from acetic acid ingestion. Vet Hum Toxicol 1985;28:291.
12. Naik RB, Stephens WP, Wilson DJ, Walker A, Lee HA. Ingestion of formic acid-containing agents—report of three fatal cases. Postgrad Med J 1980;56:451–456.
13. Rosewarne FA. Self-poisoning with formic acid. Anaesthesia 1983;38:1104–1105.
14. Rajan N, Rabim R, Kumar SK. Formic acid poisoning with suicidal intent: a report of 53 cases. Postgrad Med J 1985; 61:35–36.
15. Wiernikowski A, Guzik E. Ostre zatrucie Kwasem mrowkowyn. (Acute poisoning from formic acid). Przeglad Lekarski 1973;30:395–396.
16. Malizia E, Reale C, Pietropaoli P, De Ritis GC. Formic acid intoxications. Acta Pharmacol Toxicol 1977; 41(Suppl): 342–347.
17. Jeffrys DB, Wiseman HM. Formic acid poisoning. Postgrad Med J 1980;56:761–762.
18. Verstraetz AG, Vogelaers DP, Van den Bogaerde JF, Colardyn FA, Ackerman CM, Buylaert WA. Formic acid poisoning. Case report and in vitro study of the hemolytic activity. Ann J Emerg Med 1989;7:286–290.
19. Chan TC, Williams SR, Clark RF. Formic acid skin burns resulting in systemic toxicity. Ann Emerg Med 1995;26:383–386.

20. NIOSH. Pocket Guide to Chemical Hazards. DHHS (NIOSH). Publication No. 90-117. Washington, DC. US Government Printing Office, June 1990, pp. 118–119.
21. Key MM, Henschel AF, Butler J, Ligo RN, Tabershaw IR. Occupational Diseases. A Guide to their Recognition. Revised Edition. DHEW (NIOSH). Publication No. 77-181. Washington, DC. US Government Printing Office, Revised June 1977, pp. 180–181.
22. Occupational Exposure Limits for Airborne Toxic Substances. Occupational Safety and Health Series 37. Geneva. International Labour Office, 1991, pp. 206–207.
23. Penner GE. Acid ingestion: toxicology and treatment. Ann Emerg Med 1980;9:374–379.
24. Tintinalli JE. Of anions, osmols and methanol poisoning. JACEP 1977;6:417.
25. Moore DF, Bentley AM, Dawling S, Hoare AM, Henry JA. Folinic acid and enhanced renal elimination in formic acid intoxication. Clin Toxicol 1994;32:199–204.
26. Menchel SM, Dunn WA. Hydrofluoric acid poisoning. Am J Forensic Med Pathol 1984;5:245–248.
27. Curry AS. Twenty-one uncommon causes of poisoning. Br Med J 1962;1:687–689.
28. Degawa K. A fatal case of hydrogen fluoride poisoning. Bull Int Assoc Forensic Toxicol 1984;17(3):35.
29. Rieders MF, Morrow PL, Rieders F, Crookham S, Zelonis S. A case of suicidal ingestion of a hydrofluoric acid/ammonium bifluoride rust remover solution with fatal outcome during antidepressant treatment with fluoxetine. Abst K36. Proc Am Acad Sci, February 18–23, 1991.
30. Manoguerra AS, Neuman TS. Fatal poisoning from acute hydrofluoric acid ingestion. Am J Emerg Med 1986;4:362–363.
31. Upfal M, Doyle C. Medical management of hydrofluoric acid exposure. J Occup Med 1990;32:726–731.
32. Caravati EM. Acute hydrofluoric acid exposure. Am J Emerg Med 1988;6:143–150.
33. Stremski ES, Grande GA, Ling LJ. Survival following hydrofluoric acid ingestion. Vet Hum Toxicol 1991;33:363.
34. El Saadi MS, Hall AH, Hall PK, Riggs BS, Augenstein WL, Rumack BH. Hydrofluoric acid dermal exposure. Vet Hum Toxicol 1989;31:243–247.
35. Sadove R, Hainsworth D, Van Meter W. Total body conversion hydrofluoric acid. South Med J 1990;83:698–700.
36. Siegel DC, Heard JM. Intra-arterial calcium infusion for hydrofluoric acid burns. Aviat Space Environ Med 1992;63: 206–211.
37. Henry JA. Intravenous regional calcium gluconate perfusion for hydrofluoric acid burns. Clin Toxicol 1992;30:203–207.
38. Bentur Y, Tannenbaum S, Yaffe Y, Halpert M. The role of calcium gluconate is the treatment of hydrofluoric and eye burns. Ann Emerg Med 1993;22:1488–1490.
39. Kulling P, Andersson H, Bostrom K, Johansson LA, Lindstrom B, Nystrom B. Fatal systemic poisoning after skin exposure to monochloracetic acid. Clin Toxicol 1992;30: 643–652.
40. Feldhaus K, Hudson D, Rogers D, Horowitz RS, Brent J, Dart RC, Gomez H. Pediatric fatality associated with accidental oral administration of monochloroacetic acid (MCA). Vet Hum Toxicol 1993;35:344.
41. Key MM, Henschel AF, Butler J, Ligo RN, Tabershaw IR, eds. Occupational diseases. A guide to their recognition. National Institute for Occupational Safety and Health, Washington, DC. US Government Printing Office. DHEW (NIOSH). Publication No 77-181, Revised Edition June 1977, p. 156.
42. Fassett DW. Organic acid, anhydrides, lactones, acid halides and amides, thioacids. In Patty FA, ed. Industrial hygiene and toxicology. Second Revised Edition. Vol 2 (Fassett DW, Irish DD, eds), New York. Interscience, 1963, pp. 1795–1796.
43. Hunter D. The Diseases of Occupations. London. Hodder and Stoughton. 1975 p. 1121.
44. Tallqvist H, Vaananen. Death of a child from oxalic acid poisoning due to eating rhubarb leaves. Ann Paediatr Fenn 1960;60:144–147.
45. Farre M, Xirgu J, Salgado A, Penacaula R, Reig M, Sanz P. Fatal oxalic acid poisoning from sorrel soup. Lancet 1989;2: 1524.
46. Occupational Disease. A Guide to their Recognition. Revised edition. Publication No. DHEW (NIOSH) 77-181. National Institute for Occupational Safety and Health. Washington, DC. US Government Printing Office, June 1977, pp. 182–184.
47. NIOSH Pocket Guide to Chemical Hazards. NIOSH Publication No. 90-117. US Department of Health and Human Services. Washington, DC. US Government Printing Office, June 1990, pp. 1701–1771.
48. Woolf A. Oxalates. Clin Toxicol Rev 1993;16:1–2.

ALKALIS

EPIDEMIOLOGY

Product Formulations

Drain Cleaner

Sodium or potassium hydroxide clears plugged drains and cuts grease buildup. Red Devil Drain Opener and Lye (96 to 100% sodium hydroxide) has a pH of 14. Crystalline Drano (57% sodium hydroxide) has a pH of 14. Both Liquid Drano (10% sodium hydroxide) and Liquid Plumber (5% sodium hydroxide) also have a pH of 14. Some drain cleaners have been reformulated to contain 1,1,1-trichloroethane, which is a hydrocarbon rather than a caustic.

Household Ammonia

The ammonium hydroxide concentration ranges from 3 to 10%. Weaker 3% solutions are mild irritants, but higher concentrations may be significantly corrosive.[1] Volatile ammonia solutions can produce inhalation injuries and systemic symptoms. An 8.8% ammonia solution has a pH of 12.5.[2]

Automatic Dishwasher Detergents

These products contain builders (e.g., sodium tripolyphosphate, sodium metasilicate, sodium silicate, sodium carbonate), which produce corrosive lesions (pH 10.5 to 13).[3]

Clinitest Tablets

These formulations contain copper sulfate (20 mg), citric acid (300 mg), sodium hydroxide (232.5 mg), and sodium carbonate (80 mg). Injury occurs both by direct corrosive action and by an exothermic heat reaction. Commonly damaged sites include the proximal esophageal mucosa and, occasionally, the gastric and duodenal mucosa.[4]

Oven Cleaners

These products contain sodium hydroxide.

Bleaches

Sodium hypochlorite (e.g., Clorox) household bleach products usually contain 3 to 6% concentrations and have a pH up to 11. Some bleaches (e.g., Purex) contain silicate (15 to 17%) and sodium carbonate (60%) and have a pH around 10.5. Household bleaches may produce erosions, but rarely penetrate the submucosa to cause esophageal strictures. Granular and commercial bleaches may contain higher concentrations of hypochlorite or carbonate, leading to greater tissue destruction.

Hair Relaxers

Hair relaxers are alkaline and produce caustic injury, which usually does not induce severe esophageal injury but can produce extensive superficial burns of the pharynx and larynx.

Other Alkaline Corrosives

Potassium permanganate, nonphosphate detergents (sodium carbonate), metal cleaners (but usually not metal polishes, which are ammonia compounds), paint removers, washing powders, and some home concoctions used to determine the sex of the fetus from the mother's urine[5] can produce alkali injuries. Cement can produce full-thickness chemical burns after prolonged skin contact (e.g., cement spilled inside a boot).[6]

Malfunctioning automobile air-bag inflation systems may release sodium hydroxide powder, a byproduct in the chemical conversion of sodium azide to nitrogen gas that inflates the auto air bags. Chemical surface burns will require symptomatic treatment.[7]

MECHANISM OF ACTION

Alkali agents create injury to tissue by the mechanism of liquefaction necrosis. Alkalis, unlike acids, produce extensive penetrating damage. This pathogenesis of injury is rapidly progressive. The observed pathophysiologic course of alkali injury extends for several weeks after onset. Severe esophageal damage is caused by alkali agents with a pH as low as 11.8. This pathophysiologic process is quite dependent on the pH of the offending alkali. Other factors include volume ingested, viscosity, and contact time.[8,9]

Alkali corrosives damage the gastrointestinal tract by liquefaction necrosis whereby the saponification of fats and solubilization of proteins allow deep penetration into tissues.

Liquid Lye Ingestion[10]

Potent liquid lye, commonly available as drain cleaner, has increased the severity and number of potential injuries due to caustic ingestion. These agents produce a more severe injury than that produced by powder or granular alkaline agents or by nonalkaline corrosive liquids. Solid lye tends to stick to the mucosa and rarely injures the gastrointestinal tract beyond the proximal esophagus unless ingested as a tablet or put in a capsule in a suicide attempt. Nonalkaline liquids cause a coagulation necrosis. Liquid alkaline agents quickly cover the surface of the esophagus and move on to the stomach producing a liquefaction necrosis.

CLINICAL PRESENTATION

Clinical Effects

Symptoms of esophageal chemical burns include dysphagia, odynophagia, spontaneous vomiting, and abdominal pain. Most patients with esophageal injury complain of pain, but the symptoms do not localize the area of greatest mucosal injury,[5] perhaps because of the loss of nerve endings. Whether all patients with significant esophageal injury have symptoms has not been resolved. Although Gaudreault et al.[11] found no significant relationship between the presence of any symptom and injury, Crain et al. found a positive correlation between the presence of two of three symptoms (drooling, vomiting, stridor) and esophageal damage in a small series.[12]

Signs of chemical injury include drooling, inability to swallow, erythema/ulceration of oropharynx, hematemesis, and occasionally shock and respiratory distress. Severe signs indicate severe injury, but not all patients with significant esophageal damage have external signs of injury. Extensive alkali mucosal burns present as gray or gray-black pseudomembranes covering the buccal mucosa or palate. Approximately one-third of patients with oral burns have significant esophageal injury, whereas 2 to 15% of patients with esophageal injuries have no oral burns.[13] Automatic dishwasher detergents often produce esophageal and gastric erosion without evidence of oral burns, although esophageal strictures are rare.[14] Clinitest tablet ingestions differ from liquid alkali ingestions in the higher frequency of accidental adult ingestions. Compared with other alkali exposures, esophageal strictures are relatively more proximal and less severe. Gastric erosion and even duodenal erosion are more common, but oropharyngeal burns are rare.[15] Complications of alkali burns represent the greatest hazard to the patient, and each patient should be examined carefully for adverse consequences of alkali exposure.

The emergency risks of alkali injury primarily include acute and subacute airway compromise from upper airway edema and acute and subacute micro- and macroperforation of the esophagus and the stomach. In addition, the risks of delayed stricture formation and very delayed esophageal malignancy are well known.[9]

LABORATORY

Endoscopy

Liquid lye made from powdered Drano is a common manner of attempted suicide. If liquid lye has been ingested, first do an oropharyngeal examination. If the back of the throat is burned badly, do not insert a nasogastric tube. Do an esophagoscopy quickly. If circumferential second-degree burns are observed, the patient may require a laparotomy and may need to have the stomach removed. If the oropharynx is not burned, place a nasogastric tube, measure the pH of the fluid contents and begin a lavage. Patients who try to eat the powder rarely swallow very much and will usually not suffer circumferential second-degree esophageal burns. The granules will usually stick to the mucosa. Such patients should have a nasogastric tube placed. If the oropharynx is not significantly burned, pass a nasogastric tube and empty the stomach.[16] Signs and symptoms do not correlate well with the location or severity of injury. When flexible fiberoptic scopes are used within the first 48 hours, the risk of perforation is small. The exact timing of esophagoscopy within the first 48 hours depends on availability, edema, and the patient's general condition. The issue of whether to pass the first site of injury is controversial. The risk of potential perforation versus the necessity of finding more serious lesions, which would indicate the use of steroids, must be considered.[17] Esophageal findings can be classified into three categories (superficial, transmucosal, transmural), which have therapeutic significance.[18]

Indications

1. The presence of oral burns.
2. Symptomatic patients.
3. The use of esophagoscopy for asymptomatic patients without symptoms is controversial and requires consideration of time lapsed since ingestion, type of corrosive involved, and extent of exposure. Accidental ingestion of household bleach does not require endoscopy, but intentional, symptomatic ingestion of more than 1 mL/kg may benefit from endoscopy.
4. The presence or absence of oropharyngeal burns does not correlate well with the presence or absence of esophageal lesions. In children drooling, vomiting, or stridor may assist in determining the need for endoscopy.[19]

Contraindications

1. Upper airway obstruction.
2. Signs and symptoms of perforation.
3. More than 48 hours since exposure (relative).

Barium Swallow

A routine 3-week postinjury barium swallow is suggested for evaluation of stricture formation unless symptoms dictate an earlier study. An upper gastrointestinal series is useful for evaluating the pylorus and duodenum when endoscopy is not helpful. The routine series is necessary to identify complications such as scarring and outlet obstruction at the end of the first month. Water-soluble contrast media should be used whenever perforation is a possibility.

Ancillary Tests

The chest x-ray is usually unremarkable. Search for signs of perforation (free subdiaphragmatic air, mediastinal emphysema), and examine lung parenchyma for signs of aspiration.

Hospitalized patients should receive a complete blood count, electrolytes, creatinine, type and cross for several units of blood, and a Hemoccult test for blood in stool. Metabolic acidosis is rare without the concomitant presence of shock, but has been reported.[20]

Titratable Acid/Alkali Reserve (TAR)

TAR is defined as the number of mL of a 0.1-M solution of HC1 or NaOH required to titrate 100 mL of a 1% solution test product to pH 8.00, expressed as the mean of three determinations. An animal study suggests that the TAR correlated better than pH with the production of caustic esophageal injury. Determining the usefulness of this procedure in prognosticating the danger of potentially caustic household agents requires additional clinical confirmation.[21]

TREATMENT

Literature reports are confounded by uncertainty about the amounts ingested, grouping acid and alkali injections together, differing or absence of burn classification, grouping of adults and children together, and the use of different regimens for corticosteroids, antibiotics, and dilates.

Stabilization

Respiratory distress is uncommon, but presents occasionally because of soft-tissue edema. Unless endotracheal intubation can be accomplished under direct vision, a cricothyroidotomy or tracheostomy may be necessary (blind nasotracheal intubation in this setting is contraindicated). Oxygen is given as indicated.

The presence of shock suggests perforation and mandates an intravenous line and fluid administration.

Decontamination

Milk and water are the preferred diluents, especially for solid lye particles from which the diluent washes off adherent particles. Although diluents are commonly recommended, their value in liquid ingestions is less clear since vomiting may reexpose the esophagus to alkali. No more than one to two glasses of water should be given to an adult. Some authors now do not recommend the routine use of diluents as a first aid measure because of the lack of proven efficacy and the potential harm of inducing vomiting.[22] Dilution more than 1 hour after injury probably is not efficacious. Neutralizing agents should never be given since the exothermic heat reaction may enhance injury.[23] Homan et al.[8] conclude that pH neutralization using a weak acid reduces alkali-induced injury. Any dilution or neutralizations must be done rapidly if it is to have any beneficial impact. Homan et al. suggest that the window of opportunity may be as brief as 5 minutes.[8]

Catharsis and emesis are absolutely contraindicated. It is believed that emesis increases the risk of upper airway compromise and esophageal injury by reexposing these tissues to the offending agent. In addition, the increased intraluminal pressure generated by emesis is speculated to increase the risk of perforation when tissue is markedly weakened.[9] Activated charcoal does not absorb alkali and obscures the endoscopic visual field. Gastric lavage should not be used in alkali ingestions.

Alkali injuries to the eye and skin should be irrigated copiously for at least 20 to 30 minutes. Alkali injuries to the eye are ophthalmologic emergencies and require ophthalmologic consultation after copious irrigation with saline.

Antidotes

Do not use neutralizing agents.

Supportive Care

1. Withhold all oral feedings initially.
2. Carefully assess fluid and electrolyte balance.
3. Watch for development of complications such as

esophageal perforation, sepsis, mediastinitis, and upper gastrointestinal hemorrhage in severe ingestions by serial physical examinations and vital signs.

4. The use of a nasogastric tube as a stent and for nutrition is controversial, and such a tube should be passed only during endoscopy. Some authors recommend early surgical intervention and use of an intraluminal stent in patients with second- or third-degree esophageal burns because perforations that require surgical repair may be missed.[24] With liquid lye ingestion, there must be immediate treatment of drug life-threatening, full-thickness aerodigestive tract injuries. Meredith and colleagues recommend early pharyngolaryngoscopy, bronchoscopy, and esophagoscopy of the entire esophagus or to the point of circumferential confluent second-degree or third-degree burns of the esophagus; exploratory laparotomy if circumferential second-degree or third-degree burns of the esophagus are seen; gastric resection and esophagectomy if gastric necrosis is seen at laparoscopy; and for patients with serious injuries not undergoing gastrectomy and esophagectomy, gastrostomy with placement of a string to guide subsequent dilatation.[16]
5. The use of steroids is based on studies in animals that show that corticosteroids given within the first 48 hours reduce subsequent stricture formation.[25] High-dose corticosteroid therapy predisposes the patient to infection and perforation, as well as masks symptoms of developing peritonitis or mediastinitis. Steroids should be avoided if perforation is likely or there is a history of peptic ulcer disease or active infection. A prospective, controlled, randomized trial evaluated the efficacy of corticosteroids in the treatment of endoscopically graded esophageal burns following caustic ingestion. The study concluded that the development of stricture was related to the severity of injury and was not influenced by treatment with steroids.[26,27] Steroids do not appear to be needed for first- and second-degree injuries and are ineffective and possibly dangerous for third-degree injury.[28] Steroids should not be used routinely in caustic ingestions, but may be effective in patients with dyspnea, stridor, hoarseness, or other evidence of respiratory compromise. Steroids in such cases may decrease laryngotracheal edema and may lessen respiratory dysfunction.[28] A controlled, long-term, prospective study suggests that there is no benefit from the use of steroids to treat children who have ingested a caustic substance. The development of esophageal stricture appears to be related only to the severity of the corrosive injury.[28,29] Most patients with third-degree burns develop esophageal strictures regardless of therapy.[29]
6. Although data on animals suggest the need for prophylactic antibiotics in steroid-treated animals, no controlled human studies confirm the effectiveness of antibiotics in reducing the infectious complications of steroid therapy. Several authors recommend withholding antibiotics until signs of perforation or secondary infection exist.[13,19]
7. Total parenteral nutrition may be useful in preventing esophageal trauma.[30] Studies have contained inadequate numbers of severely injured patients to evaluate its effectiveness.
8. The use of early surgical intervention (esophagogastrectomy with colonic disposition) to prevent subsequent fistulas, abscesses, and strictures requires careful evaluation of the amount of tissue necrosis.
9. Intraluminal splinting with Silastic tubes, penicillamine, and lathyrogens (which prevent formation of covalent collagen crosslinks) to reduce stricture formation are under investigation.
10. An esophagram is recommended at 3 weeks to evaluate the formation of strictures. Patients should be instructed to seek medical attention immediately whenever they develop dysphagia.[31]

REFERENCES—ALKALIS

1. Ernst RW, Leventhal M, Luva R et al. Total esophagogastric replacement after ingestion of household ammonia. N Engl J Med 1963;208:815–816.
2. Vancura EM, Clinton JE, Ruiz E et al. Toxicity of alkaline solutions. Ann Emerg Med 1980;9:118–122.
3. Muhlendal KE, Oberoisse V, Krienke EG. Local injuries by accidental ingestion of corrosive substances by children. Arch Toxicol 1978;39:299–314.
4. Warren JB, Griffin DJ, Olson RC. Urine sugar reagent tablet ingestion causing gastric and duodenal ulceration. Arch Intern Med 1984;144:161–162.
5. Grenga TE. A new risk of lye ingestion by children. N Engl J Med 1983;308:156–157.
6. Early SH, Simpson RL. Caustic burns from contact with wet cement. JAMA 1985;254:528–529.
7. Hadley CM, Laubacher MA, Watson PD. Dermal and inhalation burns caused by the automotive air bag inflation system. Vet Hum Toxicol 1993;35:358.
8. Homan CS, Maitra SR, Lane BP, Thode HC, Finkelshteyn J, Davidson L. Effective treatment for acute alkali injury to the esophagus using weak-acid neutralization therapy: an ex-vivo study. Acad Emerg Med 1995;2:952–958.
9. Smilkstein MJ. Should we add an acid to an alkali injury? For now, let's remain neutral! Acad Emerg Med 1995;2:945–946.
10. Meredith JW, Kon ND, Thompson JN. Management of injuries from liquid lye ingestion. J Trauma 1988;28:1173–1180.
11. Gaudreault P, Parent M, McGuigan M et al. Predictability of esophageal injury from signs and symptoms: a study of caustic ingestions in 378 children. Pediatrics 1983;71:767–770.
12. Crain EF, Gershel JC, Mezey AP. Caustic ingestions: symptoms as predictors of esophageal injury. Am J Dis Child 1984;138:863–865.
13. Knopp R. Caustic ingestions. JACEP 1979;8:329–336.
14. Krenzelok EP, Clinton JE. Caustic esophageal and gastric erosion without evidence of oral burns following detergent ingestion. JACEP 1979;8:194–196.
15. Mallory A, Schaefer JW. Clinitest ingestion. Br Med J 1977;2:105–107.
16. Meredith JW. Personal communication, May 11, 1993.
17. Thompson JN. Corrosive esophageal injuries. I. A study of nine cases of concurrent accidental caustic ingestion. Laryngoscope 1987;97:1060–1068.
18. Friedman EM, Lovejoy FH. The emergency management of caustic ingestions. Emerg Med Clin North Am 1984;2:77–86.
19. Crain EF, Gershel JC, Mezey AP. Caustic ingestion. Am J Dis Child 1984;138:863–865.
20. Okonek S, Bierbach H, Atzpodien W. Unexpected metabolic acidosis in severe lye ingestion. Clin Toxicol 1981;18:225–230.
21. Hoffman RS, Howland MA, Kamerow HN, Goldfrank LR. Comparison of titratable acid/alkaline reserve and pH in

potentially caustic household products. Clin Toxicol 1989;27: 241–261.
22. Wasserman RC, Ginsburg CM. Caustic substance injuries. J Pediatr 1984;107:169–174.
23. Rumack BH, Burrington JD. Caustic ingestion: a rational look at diluents. Clin Toxicol 1977;11:27–34.
24. Estrera A, Taylor W, Mills LJ et al. Corrosive burns of the esophagus and stomach. A recommendation for an aggressive surgical approach. Ann Thorac Surg 1986;41:276–283.
25. Webb WR, Koutras P, Ecker RR et al. An evaluation of steroids and antibiotics in caustic burns of the esophagus. Ann Thorac Surg 1970;9:95–102.
26. Anderson KD, Rouse TM, Randolph JG. A controlled trial of corticosteroids in children with corrosive injury of the esophagus. N Engl J Med 1990;323:637–640.
27. Lovejoy FH Jr. Corrosive injury of the esophagus in children. Failure of corticosteroid treatment reemphasizes prevention. N Engl J Med 1990;323:668–670.
28. Wijburg FA, Heymans HSA, Urbanus NAM. Caustic esophageal lesions in childhood: prevention of stricture formation. J Pediatr Surg 1989;24:171–173.
29. Howell JM, Dalsey WC, Hartsell FW, Batzin CA. Steroids for the treatment of corrosive esophageal injury. A statistical analysis of past studies. Am J Emerg Med 1992;10:421–425.
30. Di Costanzo J, Nouclere M, Jougland J et al. New therapeutic approach to corrosive burns of the upper gastrointestinal tract. Gut 1980;2:370–375.
31. Moore WR. Caustic ingestions: pathophysiology, diagnosis, and treatment. Clin Pediatr 1986;25:192–196.

AVERSIVES

DENATONIUM BENZOATE

A number of aversive agents (quassin, brucine, bitter aloes, sucrose octaacetate sucrose benzoate) have been used in the past to deter ingestions of dangerous substances. Denatonium benzoate, which may be the bitterest substance available, was discovered in 1958 when a series of *N*-substituted lidocaine-derivatives were prepared in a search for new local anesthetics. Its chemical name is benzyl diethyl [(2,6 xylyl carbamoyl) methyl] ammonium benzoate and is marketed as Bitrex. It is an inert odorless material that can be detected by taste at 10 ppb and is recognizably bitter at 50 ppb. The product is now used as an alcohol denaturant, in windscreen washes, for oil and tallow denaturing, as an animal repellent, in antinailbiting formulations, in finger-paints (Germany), as a bird-repellent seed dressing, and in rodenticides. It is used in liquid detergents in the United States by Procter and Gamble (Bold, Solo) and in Sterno fuel. It is being considered as an additive to toxic household and other commercial products to aid in limiting the amount of such substances ingested by young children.[1–6] The role of denatonium benzoate in preventing serious poisoning has yet to be defined.[7–10]

REFERENCES—AVERSIVES

1. Engen T. The potential usefulness of sensations of odor and taste in keeping children away from harmful substances. Ann NY Acad Sci 1974;237:224–228.
2. Berning CK, Griffith JF, Wild JE. Research on the effectiveness of denatonium benzoate as a deterrent to liquid detergent ingestion in children. Fundam Appl Toxicol 1982;2:44–48.
3. Lawless HT, Hammer LD, Corina MD. Aversions to bitterness and accidental poisonings among preschool children. J Toxicol Clin Toxicol 1982–83;19:951–964.
4. Robertson WO. American Association of Poison Control Centers Resolution. Vet Hum Toxicol 1989;31:479.
5. Hinds M de C. Mother fights to ruin the taste of poison. New York Times, May 20, 1989.
6. Schumer CE. Denatonium benzoate. News release. June 21, 1989; Clin Toxicol 1989;27:395.
7. Klein-Schwartz W. Denatonium benzoate. Review of efficacy and safety. Vet Hum Toxicol 1991;33:545–547.
8. Rich V. Poland: curbing ethylene glycol abuse. Lancet 1993; 341:169.
9. Sibert JR, Frude N. Bittering agents in the prevention of accidental poisoning: children's reaction to denatonium benzoate (Bitrex). Arch Emerg Med 1991;8:1–7.
10. Hansen SR, Janssen C, Beasley VR. Denatonium benzoate as a deterrent to ingestion of toxic substance: toxicity and efficacy. Vet Hum Toxicol 1993;234–236.

BEZOARS

The word bezoar means antidote, and it is believed to derive either from the Hebrew word Beluzaar, the Arabic word Bedzehr, or the Persian word Padzahr.[1] They were, at various times, thought to cure a variety of ailments, neutralize poisons, and rejuvenate the aged.[2]

TYPES

Phytobezoar

Phytobezoars consist of vegetable products or concretions of citrus fruit. Persimmons, fruit stones, raisins, grape skins, oranges, peaches, apples, bran, figs, husks of oats or psyllium, and peanuts are the foods most commonly found.[3] This group constitutes as many as 40% of all bezoars. They are largely afflictions of adult males and are more frequent since the increased incidence of gastric resection and vagotomy for peptic ulcer disease.[4]

Trichobezoars—Hair Balls

The second most common type are concretions of human and/or animal hairs, synthetic or natural fibers, and are found usually in the stomach or small intestine. Patients frequently are young women between the ages of 15 and 20 years with long hair who are either mentally retarded, have psychiatric problems, or engage in trichotillomania.[2]

Mixed Bezoars

These are combinations of hair and vegetable matter.

Concretions

Concretions are industrial exposures or ingested medications forming a gastric mass. Medications may include Vitamin C or antacid tablets, liquid antacid gels, cholestyramine, hydroscopic bulk laxatives, aspirin, iron, glutethimide, meprobamate, and sucralfate.[5]

Lactobezoars

These are undigested milk concretions that are reported usually within the first year of life and follow feedings of

Table 54–2
Contributing Factors to Bezoar Formation[a]

Bizarre dietary habits
Lack of teeth
Inadequate chewing
Dehydration
Gastric outlet obstruction
Vagotomy
Altered gastric mucosa and secretion
Anticholinergic or narcotic drugs (reduce peristalsis)

[a]From Delpre G et al. J Clin Gastroenterol 1984;16:231–237.

incorrectly prepared powdered formula, ingestion of undiluted concentrated formula, and ingestion of 24 calories/ounce low-birth-weight infant formulas.[6–8]

Contributing factors that accelerate bezoar formation are found in Table 54–2.

CLINICAL

Patients often present with an epigastric mass and/or pain, nausea and vomiting, hematemesis, weight loss, lethargy, diarrhea, or constipation (also anemia, halitosis, anorexia, flatulence, and presence of foreign material in the vomitus). There may be no symptoms.[1]

COMPLICATIONS

Complications include massive bleeding, obstruction with metabolic abnormalities, perforation complicated by peritonitis, and gastrocutaneous or colocutaneous fistulas.[1]

DIAGNOSIS

Gastric dilatation and an intraluminal gastric mass with irregular surface contours separate from the gastric mucosa may be seen on a contrast study of the upper gastrointestinal tract. Gastroscopy with biopsy, echography, and an analysis of stool contents are also useful. Esophageal bezoars may be visualized by endoscopy.

TREATMENT

1. Esophageal Bezoars
   Bougienage, endoscopic manipulation.[5,10]
2. Gastric Bezoars
   Endoscopy. Irrigation of stomach with 0.9% sodium chloride solution; irrigation with papain (e.g., Adolph's Meat Tenderizer, Cheseborough-Pond, Inc.) 1 to 3 teaspoonfuls in 8 ounces of water before each meal.[11]

   Caution must be exercised in using Adolph's Meat Tenderizer in view of a report of hypernatremia and confusion in a 65-year-old patient following its use for treatment of a phytobezoar.[12]

   Cellulase (Kanulase, Dorsey Laboratories) in capsules to prevent bezoar formation or as an irrigant (instillation of 1 liter of a 0.5 g/100 ml solution over 24 hours).[13] Metoclopramide up to 10 mg three or four times daily may be useful. Limited experience suggests that acetylcysteine may enhance dissolution of gastric mucous, which may encase cellulose bezoars.[14]
3. Small bowel bezoars.
   Enterotomy may be necessary.[15]
4. Rectal bezoars.
   Dilate rectum, if necessary, under anesthesia. Anoscopy, proctoscopy.
5. Surgery can be useful when bleeding, obstruction, or perforation has occurred. If a large bezoar is present, gastrotomy, enterotomy, or bowel resection may be the treatment of choice.

REFERENCES—BEZOARS

1. Yelin G, Taff ML, Sadowski GE. Copper toxicity following massive ingestion of coins. Am J Forensic Med Pathol 1987; 8:78–85.
2. DeBakey M, Ochsner A. Bezoars and concretions. A comprehensive review of the literature with an analysis of 303 collected cases and a presentation of 8 additional cases. Surgery 1938;4:934–963;1939;5:132–160.
3. Eshel G, Broide E, Azizi E. Phytobezoar following raisin ingestion in children. Pediatr Emerg Care 1988;4:192–193.
4. Deal DR, Vitale Q, Raffin SB. Dissolution of a postgastrectomy bezoar by cellulose. Gastroenterology 1973;64: 467–470.
5. Carrougher JG, Barrilleaux CN. Esophageal bezoars: the sucralith. Crit Care Med 1991;19:837–839.
6. Singer JI. Lactobezoar causing an abdominal triad of colicky pain, emesis and mass. Pediatr Emerg Care 1988;4:194–196.
7. Schreiner RL, Brady MS, Franken EA. Increased incidence of lactobezoars in low birth weight infants. Am J Dis Child 1979;133:936–940.
8. Reddy ER, Joseph S. Lactobezoars in the low birth weight neonate. CMAJ 1985;133:297.
9. Delpre G, Glanz I, Neeman A, Aridor I, Kadish V. New therapeutic approach in postoperative phytobezoars. J Clin Gastroenterol 1984;16:231–237.
10. Schneider RP. Perdiem causes esophageal impaction and bezoars. South Med J 1989;82:1449–1450.
11. DePiro JT, Bowden TA Jr. Treatment of gastric bezoars. Clin Pharm 1989;8:181–182.
12. Zarling EJ, Moeller DD. Bezoar therapy. Complication using Adolph's Meat Tenderizer and alternatives from literature review. Arch Intern Med 1981;141:1669–1670.
13. Andrus CH, Ponsky JL. Bezoars: classification, pathophysiology and treatment. Am J Gastroenterol 1988;83:476–478.
14. Schlang HA. Acetylcysteine in removal of bezoar. JAMA 1970;214:1329.
15. Cooper SG, Tracey EJ. Small-bowel obstruction caused by oat bran bezoar. N Engl J Med 1989;320:1148–1149.

BORON COMPOUNDS

Poisoning has followed ingestion, parenteral injection, enemas, and lavage of cavities. Toxicity has been produced by excessive topical use in surgical wounds, burns, ulcers, and diaper dermatitis. Fatalities have resulted from accidental administration of boric acid to infants.[1]

SOURCES/PRODUCT FORMULATIONS

Sodium borate, sodium biborate, sodium pyroborate, and sodium tetraborate (in borax cleaners) contain 21.50% boron by weight. A teaspoon of 100% boric acid crystals contains approximately 2.9 to 4.4 g of boric acid. Sodium borate solution (Dobell's solution) contains 1.5 g of sodium borate, 1.5 g of sodium bicarbonate, and 0.3 mL of liquified phenol. Boric anhydride, boron oxide, boron trioxide, boric oxide, boron sesquioxide, borax, tincal, and tinkal are 33% boron by weight. Sodium perborate (oxidizer in tooth powders and toothpastes) is 7.03% boron by weight, sodium metaborate is 16.44% boron, and magnesium perborate is 14% boron. Saturated solutions of boric acid contain 5.55% boron.

Other sources include Harris Famous Roach Tablets, Roach-Pruf, Boraxo Powdered Hand Soap, and contact lens solutions.

TOXIC DOSAGE

Acute

Single acute ingestions frequently are asymptomatic. Linden and colleagues [2] documented several acute ingestions that produced minimal systemic toxicity. A 14-month-old child ingested 20 g but developed no signs. A 2-year-old ingested 10 g and had only spontaneous emesis for 3 hours. A 28-year-old ingested 297 g in a suicide attempt. The only toxicity was spontaneous emesis 1 hour after ingestion. The fatal dose in 5 infants was 4.5 to 14 g.[1] As little as 1 g has been fatal.[1] Systemic poisoning in humans has resulted from the ingestion of as little as 0.2 g/kg of boric acid.[3,4] Infants have survived ingestions of 1.95 g to 20 g.[1,2,5] Fatalities have been reported in adults after use of 15 to 30 g.[6]

Chronic

Chronic poisoning occurred after ingestion of 4 to 5 g of boric acid per day for 3 to 4 weeks or 6 to 20 g of borax ($Na_2B_4O_7 \cdot 10H_2O$) daily for several months.[7] This is equivalent to 2.12 g of boron per day. (See Clinical Presentation.)

CLINICAL PRESENTATION

Acute Boron Poisoning

Gastrointestinal

Persistent nausea, vomiting, and diarrhea in children leads to acute dehydration, shock, and coma. Death resulting from circulatory collapse occurs rarely after boric acid ingestion. Nausea, vomiting, diarrhea and epigastric pain, hematemesis, and blue-green discoloration of both feces and vomitus characterize adult boron intoxication.

Skin

Erythema, desquamation in 1 to 2 days, and exfoliation (generalized or localized to the hands, feet, or face) may occur (the "boiled lobster" syndrome).[2,8] Erythema may be prominent on the buttocks and scrotum. Acute skin changes may develop after boric acid ingestion or applications of a boric acid powder.[9]

Central Nervous System

Hyperexcitability, irritability, restlessness, opisthotonus, tremors, convulsions,[10] delirium, coma, weakness, lethargy, headaches, excitement, and depression have been reported.

Chronic Boron Poisoning

This syndrome usually is seen in children who have been treated in the past with a boric acid preparation for diaper rash. Cutaneous findings develop regardless of the route of poisoning. Renal toxicity includes oliguria, anuria, and renal tubular necrosis, which may supervene after several days. Hypothermia and hyperthermia may occur. Death is more common in infants than adults.[1,3,7,11,12]

Pentaborane Poisoning

Poisoning from pentaborane gas (B_5H_9) was manifested by three patients who, within 15 to 20 minutes of exposure, developed respiratory irritation and, within 15 to 45 minutes, displayed convulsions. Blood pH was 6.4 and serum bicarbonate was 5 mEq/L in two patients. Blood pressure and ventilation required support in two patients. All had elevated aminotransferase levels and rhabdomyolysis with an elevation in creatine kinase. One died and one remained unconscious for over 2 weeks.[13] Psychiatric symptoms of stress reaction and minimal brain dysfunction may persist for at least 4 to 12 weeks.[14]

LABORATORY

Boron Levels

Serum and urine borate levels reflect the fact that exposure has occurred, but they do not correlate well with the clinical state. Symptoms of toxicity generally occur when blood levels exceed 20 to 150 μg/mL, although blood levels of 56 and 147 μg/mL produced only mild irritability, diarrhea, and perianal erythema in two neonates.[1,5] In one series with a median age of 2 years, blood borate concentrations as high as 340 μg/mL were not associated with significant toxicity.[12]

Urine and whole blood boric acid concentrations 52 hours after the ingestion of about 280 g of boric acid were 160 and 42 mg/dL, respectively, equivalent to urine and blood boron concentrations of 28 and 7 mg/dL, respectively. The patient died.[15]

Most laboratories are not equipped to do accurate blood boron or boric acid levels. Their usefulness in the treatment of poisoning is limited. Blood samples can be analyzed at no charge by the U.S. Borax and Chemical Corporation. Send 10 mL heparinized blood (in a polyethylene bottle) and a case summary, by air mail, to U.S. Borax Laboratories, 412 Crescent Way, Anaheim, California 92803.

Specific urine tests (turmeric paper; one drop of the patient's urine is acidified with HC1 and applied to turmeric paper; the paper may turn brownish red if boric acid is present) are unreliable.

Litovitz concluded that minimal toxicity occurs at blood levels of 34 mg/dL.[12]

Abnormalities

Dehydration may lead to electrolyte (Na, K, Ca, Mg) abnormalities. Elevated blood urea nitrogen and serum creatinine levels reflect renal damage. Liver function tests (aspartate and alanine aminotransferases) may be elevated.

TREATMENT

A protocol for acute boric acid ingestions suggests that for patients weighing less than 30 kg, observation alone is adequate. For ingestions less than 200 mg/kg, 400 mg/kg, lavage in an emergency department after a boric acid level is obtained and 2 to 3 hours have elapsed postingestion. For patients weighing 30 kg or more, observation only is recommended for ingestions of less than 6.0 g; for ingestions of 6.0 to 12.0 g lavage in an emergency department. A boric acid level is obtained 2 to 3 hours postingestion for ingestions of greater than 12.0 g.[12]

Stabilization

Assess and correct any abnormalities found in airway, breathing, and circulation. A tidal volume of 10 to 15 mL/kg should be maintained.

Gut Decontamination

Emesis should be induced unless the patient is in coma, is experiencing seizures, or has lost the gag reflex. If any of these are present, gastric lavage should be performed with a large-bore tube after endotracheal intubation or in the presence of continuous respiratory suction.

Activated charcoal has not been shown to be of value and probably does not absorb boron well. When the patient is brought in within a few hours after ingestion, activated charcoal (adults, 60 to 100 g; children, 30 to 60 g) may follow gastric evacuation, but its value is still not defined.[16]

A cathartic should help eliminate any boric acid remaining in the gastrointestinal tract (magnesium sulfate: adults, 30 g; children, 250 mg/kg).

Elimination Enhancement

Diuresis may be useful if the kidneys are able to excrete the borates before they have irreversibly damaged the renal tubular epithelium. Administration of 0.45% saline in D_5W intravenously with a diuretic (furosemide, 1 mg/kg to 40 mg per dose) may be useful; urine flow should be maintained at 3 to 6 mL/kg body weight per hour.

Peritoneal dialysis and hemodialysis remove some borates.[17] Hemodialysis may be preferable. There have been no systematic studies documenting the clinical effectiveness of these modalities. Presence of some clinical symptoms and serum boric acid levels exceeding 185 to 200 μg/mL are indications for hemodialysis.[8,18]

Antidotes

There are no known antidotes.

Supportive Care

Shock

Administer isotonic fluids initially. Pressor agents may be useful, but have not been studied.

Seizures

Administer diazepam intravenously (adult, slowly up to 10 mg, repeat if necessary; children, 0.1 to 0.3 mg/kg slowly).

Skin

Prevent secondary infection. Wash exposed areas several times with mild soap and water.

Eye

Irrigate copiously with water for at least 20 minutes. If irritation or pain persists, obtain an ophthalmologic consultation. Otherwise treat as above.

Respiratory

Remove to fresh air. Check for respiratory distress, bronchitis, or pneumonia.

REFERENCES—BORON COMPOUNDS

1. Wong IC, Heimbach MD, Truscott DR et al. Boric acid poisoning: report of 11 cases. Can Med Assoc J 1964;90: 1018–1023.
2. Linden CH, Hall AH, Kulig KW et al. Acute ingestions of boric acid. Clin Toxicol 1986;24:269–279.
3. Martin Gl. Asymptomatic boric acid intoxication. NY Stat J Med 1971;71:1842–1844.
4. Schillinger BM, Berstein M, Goldberg LA et al. Boric acid poisoning. J Am Acad Dermatol 1982;7:667–673.
5. Baker MD, Bogema SC. Ingestion of boric acid by infants. Am J Emerg Med 1986;4:358–361.
6. Ross CA, Conway JF. The dangers of boric acid: its use as an irrigant and report of a case. Am J Surg 1943;60:386–395.
7. Valdes-Dapena MA, Arey JB. Boric acid poisoning: three fatal cases with pancreatic inclusions and a review of the literature. J Pediatr 1962;61:534–546.
8. Balaih T, MacLeish H, Drummond KN. Acute boric acid poisoning: report of an infant successfully treated by peritoneal dialysis. Can Med Assoc J 1969;101:166–168.
9. Stein KM, Odom RB, Justice GR et al. Toxic alopecia from ingestion of boric acid. Arch Dermatol 1973;108:95–97.
10. Gordon AS, Prichard JS, Freeman MH. Seizure disorders and anemia associated with chronic borax intoxication. Can Med Assoc J 1973;108:719–722.
11. Rubenstein AD, Musher DM. Epidemic boric acid poisoning simulating staphylococcal toxic epidermal necrolysis of the newborn infant: Ritter's disease. J Pediatr 1970;77:884–887.
12. Litovitz TL, Klein-Schwartz W, Oderda GM, Schmitz BP. Clinical manifestations of toxicity in a series of 784 boric acid ingestions. Am J Emerg Med 1988;6:209–213.
13. Zolet DI, Miller T, Yarborough B et al. Pentaborane poisoning causing extreme acidosis and death. Vet Hum Toxicol 1982;24:277–278 (abstract).
14. Silverman JJ, Hart RP, Garrettson LK et al. Posttraumatic stress disorder from pentaborane intoxication. Neuropsychiatric evaluation and short-term follow-up. JAMA 1985;254: 2603–2608.
15. Restuccio A, Mortensen ME, Kelley MT. Fatal ingestion of boric acid in an adult. Am J Emerg Med 1992;10:545–547.
16. Oderda GM, Klein-Schwartz W, Insley BM. In vitro study of boric acid and activated charcoal. Vet Hum Toxicol 1985; 28(4):314 (abstract).
17. Goldbloom RB, Goldbloom A. Boric acid poisoning: report of four cases and a review of 109 cases from the world literature. J Pediatr 1953;43:631–643.
18. Litovitz TL et al. Clinical manifestations of toxicity in a series of 784 boric acid ingestions. Vet Hum Toxicol 1986;28:505 (abstract).

COSMETICS

The cosmetic industry selects from more than 5000 different ingredients (Table 54–3).

PRODUCT FORMULATIONS/USES

Hair Coloration

Permanent hair colors contain an oxidizer, which usually is 6% hydrogen peroxide, and a dye intermediate (*p*-phenylenediamine, resorcinol, aminophenols along with water, ammonia glycerin, isopropanol, and propylene glycol). Semipermanent hair colors (for covering gray) contain propylene glycol, isopropanol, fatty acids, fragrance, alkanolamines, and dyes. Some formulations (e.g., Grecian Hair Formula) contain lead.

Hair Waving

Waving lotions possess thioglycolic acids and ammonia sulfides, whereas most wave neutralizer solutions contain hydrogen peroxide, sodium bromate, or perborate in mildly acidic solutions. Some permanent wave fixatives contain 2 to 8% (w/v) mercuric chloride, and the accidental ingestion of 125 mL of a 2% mercuric chloride solution caused severe mercury poisoning in an adult. Bromate salts (e.g., potassium) are extremely toxic and are capable of causing serious poisonings (deafness, renal failure) at doses between 240 and 500 mg/kg.

Hair Straighteners

The sodium hydroxide used in the 1 to 3% solution is highly caustic (pH 13). Ingestion by children results in drooling, vomiting, lip swelling and redness, and skin blisters. Most remain asymptomatic. Esophagoscopies are noncontributory.[1]

Hair Sprays

These products contain ethanol solvents with resin polymers (e.g., vinyl acetate, acrylamide, methyl vinyl ether).

Conditioners

Synthetic cationic surfactants, perfumes, alcohols.

Bath Preparations

Bubble bath usually contains the mildly toxic anionic and nonionic surfactants along with alcohols and preservatives. The presence of trisodium phosphate builders enhances causticity. Bath salts may contain borax, which causes boric acid poisoning in large ingestions in addition to mucosal irritation. Bath oils contain vegetable and mineral oils. The

Table 54–3
Cosmetic Ingredients[a]

Moisturizers function as a moisture barrier or to attract moisture from the environment:
- cetyl alcohol (fatty alcohol)—keeps oil and water from separating, also a foam booster
- dimethicone—silicone skin conditioner and anti-foam ingredient
- isopropyl lanolate, myristate, and palmitate
- lanolin and lanolin alcohols and oil (used in skin and hair conditioners)
- octyl dodecanol—skin conditioner
- oleic acid (olive oil)
- panthenol (vitamin B-complex derivative)—hair conditioner
- stearic acid and stearyl alcohol

Preservatives and antioxidants (including vitamins) to prevent product deterioration:
- trisodium and tetrasodium edetate (EDTA)
- tocopherol (vitamin E)

Antimicrobials fight bacteria
- butyl, propyl, ethyl, and methyl parabens
- DMDM hydantoin
- methylisothiazolinone
- phenoxyethanol (also rose ether fragrance component)
- quaternium-15

Thickeners and waxes used in stick products such as lipsticks and blushers:
- candelilla, carnauba, and microcrystalline waxes
- carbomer and polyethylene—thickeners

Solvents used to dilute:
- butylene glycol and propylene glycol
- cyclomethicone (volatile silicone)
- ethanol (alcohol)
- glycerin

Emulsifiers break up and refine:
- glyceryl monostearate (also pearlescent agent)
- lauramide DEA (also foam booster)
- polysorbates

Color additives—synthetic organic colors derived from coal and petroleum sources (not permitted for use around the eye):
- D&C Red No. 7 Calcium Lake (lakes are dyes that do not dissolve in water)

Inorganic pigments—approved for general use in cosmetics, including for the area of the eye:
- iron oxides
- mica (iridescent)

Hair dyes—phenol derivatives used in combination with other chemicals in permanent (two-step) hair dyes:
- aminophenols

pH adjusters stabilize or adjust acids and bases:
- ammonium hydroxide—in skin peels and hair waving and straightening
- citric acid—adjusts pH
- triethanolamine—pH adjuster used mostly in transparent soap

Others:
- magnesium aluminum silicate—absorbent, anti-caking agent
- silica (silicon dioxide)—absorbent, anti-caking, abrasive
- sodium lauryl sulfate—detergent
- stearic acid—cleansing, emulsifier
- talc (powdered magnesium silicate)—absorbent, anti-caking
- zinc stearate—used in powder to improve texture, lubricates

[a]From Foulke JE. FDA Consumer 1994;28:21.

volatile essential oils may produce systemic complaints after large ingestions of concentrated solutions.

Makeup Products

Because they contain innocuous ingredients and are sold in small packages, these compounds are essentially nontoxic, except for local hypersensitivity reactions.

Nail Polish and Removers

Nail polish contains hydrocarbon solvents (xylene, toluene, acetone), alcohol solvents (methanol, ethanol), plasticizers, and resins such as nitrocellulose. The chief ingredients of nail polish remover are solvents such as acetone or ethanol. On a weight basis, nail polish and nail polish remover are similar in toxicity, but the smaller volumes of nail polish bottles limit their toxicity.

Colognes, Perfumes, Toilet Waters

Toxicity depends on the ethanol concentration, which may range from 50 to 95%.

Dental Products

Toothpastes, tooth powders, and tooth liquids contain nontoxic constituents such as calcium phosphates, alumina, abradants, and anionic surfactants. Fluoride concentrations are too small to contribute to acute toxicity. Mouthwashes and breath fresheners usually contain alcohol, flavoring, and sweeteners. Toxicity depends on the ethanol content. Denture cleaners contain bicarbonates, borates, phosphates, and carbonates, some of which may be caustic. The methyl methacrylate constituent of acrylic denture material may produce a contact dermatitis in health care professionals who mix this substance, even when gloves are worn.

Deodorants

The aluminum and zinc included in deodorants for their antiperspirant properties have limited toxicity because of packaging and formulations.

CLINICAL PRESENTATION

Most accidental exposures result in no symptoms or, at worst, minor gastrointestinal upset. Systemic symptoms are unusual. In clinical studies, hair dyes produce no evidence of systemic effect or teratogenesis. Skin care products, hair preparations (including colors), and facial makeup are the cosmetic products most often associated with contact dermatitis. Fragrances, preservatives (quaternium-15, formaldehyde, imidazolidinyl urea, parabens), *p*-phenylenediamine, and glycerol monothioglycolate are the most frequent skin sensitizers. Triethanolamine and diethanolamine produce mild skin irritation only in concentrations above 5%; little skin sensitization develops.

Hydrogen Peroxide

In household dilutions up to 9%, ingestions usually are nontoxic. Large ingestions may produce a mild gastritis from the decomposition of peroxide, which releases large volumes of oxygen and causes gastric distension.

Sodium Perborate

This compound decomposes to sodium borate and peroxide and produces less toxicity than potassium bromate. Potentially fatal doses of boric acid range from 3 to 6 g in children and from 15 to 30 g in adults. Cutaneous manifestations are characterized by a "boiled lobster look" (i.e., toxic epidermal necrolysis) with a desquamating, erythematous rash commonly over the buttocks, scrotum, palms, and soles. This lesion may progress to exfoliation. Central nervous system symptoms range from irritability, restlessness, and headache to coma and convulsions in severe cases. Gastrointestinal symptoms (anorexia, nausea, vomiting, diarrhea) are common, and severe cases may display hematochezia. Acute renal tubular necrosis occurs in moderate to severe cases and may result in renal failure.

Potassium Bromate

This clear odorless, tasteless compound ($KBrO_3$) is an extremely toxic agent that produces nausea, vomiting, diarrhea, deafness, acute renal failure, hypotension, central nervous system depression, and hemolysis. Gastrointestinal symptoms usually begin within one-half hour of ingestion. Both the otic symptoms and renal impairment may be permanent. Renal biopsies indicate primarily tubular damage, which can progress to interstitial fibrosis and glomerular sclerosis.

Volatile or Essential Oils

Sage, eucalyptus, turpentine, pine, pennyroyal, and cinnamon are colorless liquids that contain cyclic hydrocarbons, ethers, alcohols, esters, and ketones. Essential oils are moderate mucosal irritants leading to gastrointestinal distress and salivation. Concentrated formulations of essential oils produced convulsions in adults and central nervous system depression in doses as low as 10 mL. Chemical pneumonitis results from aspiration, but high viscosity limits toxicity to a chemical lipoid pneumonia. Perfumes, colognes, mouthwashes, and toilet water may contain substantial amounts of ethanol and produce intoxication. Hypoglycemia may complicate ethanol intoxication, especially in children.

TREATMENT

1. Since most cosmetics ingested are nontoxic, only supportive care and perhaps dilution are required. The decision to induce emesis depends on the product toxicity, quantity ingested, time since exposure, patient's weight, and presence of symptoms. Most ingestions of cosmetics do not require emesis. Cationic surfactants, perborates, and substantial essential oil ingestions that exceed one to two swallows of pure solution may benefit from emesis. The risk of ethanol exposures that produce serum ethanol levels higher than 50 mg/dL may be reduced if the patient receives syrup of ipecac within 1 hour. The use of syrup of

ipecac should be considered in ingestions of hydrocarbons containing glues (e.g., toluene, xylene) only when the total dose of hydrocarbon exceeds 1 to 2 mL/kg.

2. Potassium bromate exposures are potentially serious. Toxicity does not correlate with serum bromide levels. The usual gut decontamination measures (ipecac or lavage) should be administered if the patient presents within the first several hours after ingestion. Lavage with 2% sodium bicarbonate solution and the intravenous administration of 10 to 50 mL of 10% sodium thiosulfate solution (1.5 to 3 mL/kg) at a maximum rate of 3 mL/min theoretically is advantageous to reduce the bromate to the less toxic bromide ion. An alternative intravenous solution is 100 to 500 mL of 1% sodium thiosulfate. All symptomatic patients should be observed in the hospital for the development of renal and otic damage. The role of early dialysis in the prevention of nephrotoxicity and ototoxicity remains unproven, and its use depends on clinical judgment of the severity of toxicity.
3. The acute exposure setting provides a good opportunity to counsel patients about poison prevention.

GAMMA-BUTYROLACTONE

Gamma-butyrolactone is a chemical solvent used in nail polish removers. It may increase the sensitivity of gamma aminobutyric acid (GABA) receptors in the central nervous system. Ingestion leads to rapid loss of consciousness. There have been no fatalities.

Butyrolactone (dihydro-2(3H)-furanoneγ-butyrolactone; 1,2-butanolide) is an intermediate used in the synthesis of polyvinylpyrrolidone, D-L methionine, piperidine, phenylbutyric acid, and thiobutyric acids. It is also used as a solvent for polymers such as polyacrylonitrile, cellulose acetate, methyl methacrylate polymers, and polystyrene. It is a constituent of paint removers, textile aids, and drilling oils.[2]

PHYSICAL PROPERTIES

Gamma-butyrolactone is a viscous fluid that is miscible with water and soluble in methanol, ethanol, acetone, ether, and benzene. It can be hydrolyzed by hot alkaline solutions.

STRUCTURE AND CLASSIFICATION

Synonyms include dihydro-2[2H]-furanone; 1,2 butanolide, 1,4-butanolide, gamma hydroxybutyric acid lactone, 3-hydroxybutyric acid lactone, 4-hydroxybutanoic, and lactone.

USES

In the past few years, gamma-butyrolactone (GBL) has been used in glue removers, especially for cyanoacrylate glue, and for nail polish removers. Such products are commonly found in homes. Poisoning with gamma-butyrolactone has been experienced in Scandinavia.[3,4]

SOURCES

Gamma-butyrolactone can be prepared from gamma-hydroxlybutyric acid.[1]

MECHANISM OF ACTION

Gamma-butyrolactone (GBL) in animal studies is rapidly converted to gamma hydroxybutyrate. This may account for the subsequent central nervous system depressant.[5] GBL is an anesthetic that causes a selective increase in brain dopamine by antagonizing transmitter release from nerve terminals. It is also an endogenous brain metabolite that may be derived from glutamate through gamma-aminobutyrate.[6] GBL induces hyperthermia in animals during anesthesia.[6] GBL increases the sensitivity of gamma amino butyric acid (GABA) receptors to GABA mimetics.[7]

CLINICAL PRESENTATION

Clinical Pharmacology

Gamma-butyrolactone 2.5 g orally given to normal volunteers produced sleep (behavior and electroencephalogram) beginning an average of 20 minutes after dosing and lasting 1 hour.[5,8] Two adults ingested 50 mL of GBL, lost consciousness, and developed a bradycardia. They recovered in a few hours.[9]

Animal studies indicate that gamma-butyrolactone is rapidly converted to gamma-hydroxybutyrate, which may account for the subsequent depression of the central nervous system.[5]

Fogh and colleagues in Scandinavia have described poisoning from gamma-butyrolactone in children 1 to 5 years old. Amounts ingested were 2 to 8 mL. This was followed by dizziness, a rapid loss of consciousness within 15 minutes, and, in one case, respiratory depression following ingestion of 5 mL. All the children recovered.[4]

Cyanosis, seizures, and sinus arrhythmia were observed in one patient; nodal rhythm was observed in another patient. Mydriasis was present in one patient. Electroencephalogram, computer tomography scanning, arterial blood gases, and electrolytes were normal. X-rays of the chest showed minimal changes. Patients were treated variously with oxygen, atropine, intravenous fluids, gastric lavage, activated charcoal, sodium bicarbonate, and methylprednisolone.

Nail Polish Remover (30% gamma-butyrolactone)

A 1½-year-old girl who ingested an unknown quantity of nail polish remover became comatose in 30 minutes; intubation was performed and sodium bicarbonate was given IV. A chest x-ray showed signs of pulmonary aspiration; the body temperature was slightly elevated. Within a few hours, the child regained consciousness and was sent home after 1 day.

TREATMENT

Stabilization

Treatment is symptomatic and supportive. All patients should be hospitalized and observed in an intensive care facility with access to oxygen, intravenous fluids, and cardiac monitoring. Airway patency, respirations, and circulatory stability must be insured. Aspiration pneumonitis may be present. Aggressive therapeutic and investigational procedures will depend on clinical judgement. All patients have recovered within 24 hours with conservative treatment.

REFERENCES—GAMMA-BUTYROLACTONE

1. Mrvos R, Dean B, Krenzelok E. Hair relaxers: lack of morbidity despite high pH. Clin Toxicol 1995;33:475–481 (abstract).
2. Fassett DW. Gamma-butyrolactone. In Fassett DW, Irish DD, eds. Toxicology. In Patty FA. Industrial hygiene and toxicology. New York. Interscience Division of John Wiley and Sons, 1962; pp 1824–1825.
3. Windholz M, ed. Merck Index. 9th ed. Rahway Merchant, 1976; p. 1590.
4. Fogh A, Ihnestedt B, Wickstrom E. Gamma-butyrolactone poisonings in children. Experiences in Scandinavia. Proc Eur Assoc Pois Cont Centers Toxicol 1988;55.
5. Roth RH, Giarman NJ. Preliminary report on the metabolism of gamma-butyrolactone and gamma-hydroxybutyric acid. Biochem Pharmacol 1965;14:177–178.
6. Borbely AA, Huston JP. Gamma-butyrolactone. An anaesthetic with hypothermic action in the rat. Experientia 1972;28:1455–1456.
7. Tatsuta M, Iishi H, Baba M, Nakaizui A, Euhara H, Tanegushi H. Effect of gamma-butyrolactone on baclofen inhibition of gastric carcinogenesis induced by *N*-methyl-*N'*-nitro-*N*-nitrosoguanidine in wistar rats. Oncology 1992;49:123–126.
8. Jenney EH, Murphree HB, Goldstein L, Pfeiffer CC. Behavioral and EEG effects of gamma-butyrolactone and gamma hydroxbutyric acid in man. Pharmacologist 1962;4: 166.
9. Inderson M, Wetterstrom B. Loss of consciousness after ingestion of nail varnish remover. Ugeskr Laeger 1992;154: 3064.

DISC BATTERIES

CONTENT (TABLE 54–4)

Mercuric oxide enhances longevity and improves performance, but increases the potential toxicity of mercury poisoning. A typical mercury button battery contains 15 to 50% mercuric oxide, which suggests that ingestible amounts of mercury range from 0.09 to 21 g with the average 1 to 5 g.[1] The electrolyte solution contains 40 to 45% potassium or sodium hydroxide, but generally amounts only to 1 to 13% of the weight of the battery.

Battery formulations contain varying amounts of heavy metals (lithium hydroxide, nickel hydroxide, manganese dioxide, oxides of mercury, zinc, silver, and cadmium), as well as alkaline corrosives.

Disc batteries range from 8 to 25 mm (a dime is 17 mm and a quarter is 23 mm). Size is an important determinant of esophageal impaction since most esophageal perforation case studies to date involved disc batteries larger than 18 mm (the size of an American penny).[2] Batteries with diameters of 15 to 23 mm have been reported to arrest in the esophagus,[3] and batteries as small as 7.9 mm have stopped at least transiently in the esophagus.[4] Neither battery diameters nor symptoms are predictive of the esophageal battery position.[3]

PATHOPHYSIOLOGY

Histopathology

All severe complications to date involved disc battery impaction with subsequent tissue necrosis.[5] A 22 × 5–mm alkaline camera battery trapped for 4 days in the esophagus of a 16-month-old infant produced a fatal esophageal perforation characterized by liquefaction necrosis. A 25 × 5–mm movie camera disc battery produced a fatal tracheoesophageal fistula after more than 24 hours of esophageal impaction and steroid treatment.[6] Votteler et al. reported a nonfatal case of tracheoesophageal fistula after a disc battery impaction in the esophagus that was reported to have the appearance of a coagulation necrosis surrounded by a black precipitate.[7] A 15 × 8–mm hearing aid battery lodged in a Meckel's diverticulum, producing necrosis, hemorrhage, and perforation after 2 days and necessitating small-bowel resection.[8]

Mechanism

The mechanism of mucosal erosion probably is multifactorial.[5] The alkaline electrolyte material (40 to 45% potassium hydroxide) approximates an 8N solution, which has caused liquefaction necrosis in animal models. Spontaneous leakage from the seal area of the battery can occur, especially after the corrosive effects of gastric acid on the casing. Impaction would produce a cumulative local effect in contrast to a free-floating battery, in which intestinal juices dilute the caustic electrolyte solution.

The generation of hydroxide at the anode surface may contribute to the subsequent necrosis, and studies in animal models indicate that the area of maximum burn appears at the anode near the plastic seal connecting the two poles.[9] The electrolyte-rich fluids of the gastrointestinal tract provide a suitable medium for the passage of current between the anode and cathode. Within 10 seconds in a 1N NaCl solution, the pH of a pH indicator paper strip connecting the positive and negative button battery terminals reached 11.[10]

Pressure necrosis from impaction may contribute to the above two mechanisms, but the presence of liquefaction necrosis on autopsy indicates that pressure necrosis is not the only pathophysiologic mechanism.

Heavy Metal Toxicity

Mercury toxicity has been a concern because of the amount of inorganic mercury present in disc batteries.[1] Despite the fact that at least 17 disc batteries retrieved from patients were corroded, pitted, or split, only one case of slightly elevated mercury levels has been reported in an asymptomatic patient. The serum mercury level was 19 μg/dL (normal, below 5

Table 54–4
Typical Composition of Button Batteries[a,b]

Mercury cell				%
Mercuric oxide				40.0
Manganese dioxide				5.0
Graphite				1.5
Potassium hydroxide (as 45% aqueous solution)				7.0
Zinc oxide (as aqueous solution)				0.5
Zinc powder amalgam:	Zn	12.2%		
	Hg	1.4%		
	Gel	0.4%	Total	14.0
Total inert constituents				32.0
Silver cell				%
Silver oxide				39.0
Manganese dioxide				3.0
Potassium hydroxide (as 45% aqueous solution)				8.0
Zinc oxide (as aqueous solution)				0.15
Sodium aluminate				0.05
Zinc powder amalgam:	Zn	11.2%		
	Hg	1.3%		
	Gel	0.5%	Total	13.0
Total inert constituents				37.0
Alkaline manganese cell				%
Manganese dioxide				16.0
Graphite				3.0
Potassium hydroxide (as 45% aqueous solution)				12.0
Cement				1.5
Zinc oxide (as aqueous solution)				0.5
Zinc powder amalgam:	Zn	5.8%		
	Hg	1.0%		
	Gel	0.2%	Total	7.0
Total inert constituents				60.0
Lithium/manganese cell				%
Manganese dioxide				24.8
Graphite				1.8
Ethylene glycol dimethyl ether				4.3
Propylene carbonate				6.0
Lithium perchlorate				1.0
Lithium metal anode				2.0
Total inert constituents				60.1
Zinc/air cell				%
Zinc metal				32.0
Carbon black				2.0
Potassium hydroxide (as 45% aqueous solution)				10.0
Manganese dioxide				0.3
Mercury metal				1.0
Total inert constituents				54.5

[a]Adapted from Thompson N et al. Adv Drug React 1990;9:157–182.
[b]Constituents are of typical cells, listed by percentage of the total weight of the battery. The exact composition will vary considerably according to both the manufacturer and the particular type of cell, and these figures should therefore be taken as a rough guide rather than a precise description. It should also be noted that the chemical composition of cells changes as they discharge (see text).
Source: Duracell Batteries Ltd, quoted with permission.

μg/dL), and the urine mercury level, 98 μg/L (normal, below 50 μg/L).[11] The toxic and lethal levels of mercury oxide in humans are not known, although Lewis reported that the oral lethal dose (LD_{50}) in rats is 18 mg/kg. Despite several split disc batteries, mercury screens have been negative.[12,13] Mercuric oxide has corrosive effects, but is poorly soluble and slowly absorbed. Gastric acid may further limit absorption by reducing inorganic mercury to metallic mercury, which has minimal potential for absorption. Iron corrosion of disc battery cases apparently catalyzes the virtually complete reduction of mercuric oxide to the insoluble elemental mercury.[14]

CLINICAL PRESENTATION

The presence of gastrointestinal signs and symptoms suggests necrosis and perforation, since most free-floating disc batteries pass spontaneously without symptoms.[5] Patients with impacted esophageal batteries present with fever, dysphagia, vomiting, tachypnea, odynophagia, and tenderness. Intermittent abdominal pain, guarding, tenderness, and vomiting occurred after perforation of a Meckel's diverticulum.[8] Split disc batteries produced asymptomatic black, nonmelanotic stool[12]; mild gastrointestinal tract bleeding[5]; and mild vomiting, anorexia, and lassitude.[15] Symptoms of mercury toxicity have not been reported after disc battery ingestions. Black stools most often reflect elemental mercury precipitate rather than gastrointestinal bleeding. Vital sign instability occurred in two cases of aortic arch perforation with subsequent exsanguination. The transit time of an ingested battery ranges from 14 hours to 7 days.[5] Ingestion of batteries may interfere with the ability to obtain electrocardiographic tracings.[16,17]

The report by Litovitz and Schmitz on over 2000 cases of button battery and 62 cases of cylinder type ingestions concluded the following:[18]

1. The vast majority of patients did well; less than 10% developed any symptoms, and only 2 patients had a major complication (both of these were strictures requiring dilatation).
2. Disc batteries from hearing aids were a particular problem: 44.6% of cases involved hearing aid batteries, and 32.8% of these were from the child's own hearing aid.
3. The size of the battery or lack of symptoms did not reliably predict that the battery had passed through the esophagus; x-rays are required to confirm passage.
4. A battery held in the mouth while the hands were busy was a common scenario of accidental ingestion in adults.
5. Mercuric oxide cells were more likely than other types to break apart in the GI tract; zinc/air cells were especially resistant to breakage.
6. Lithium cells, perhaps because of their larger size and higher voltage, may be more likely to cause injury.
7. Ipecac was useless; it produced only one battery in 37 cases in which it was used, and in one patient it caused a battery to move from the stomach and lodge in the esophagus.
8. Endoscopy was successful in removing batteries 90% of the time if they were in the esophagus, but only 42.5% of the time if they were in the stomach. Endoscopy is probably indicated only in cases where the battery is in the esophagus or fails to pass through the pylorus after a long observation period. Seven of 16 batteries seen in the esophagus on initial x-rays passed into the stomach spontaneously; thus repeat films should be done just prior to endoscopy to see if the procedure is still indicated.
9. Surgery is rarely if ever justified just to remove a battery.
10. Most ingested batteries were already discharged: 52.5% were ingested immediately after removal from the device they had powered, and 41.4% were loose or discarded; only 5.4% were known to be new. However, it is not clear from the data if new batteries are more dangerous than spent ones.
11. Small cylindrical batteries appear to be of no greater concern than disc batteries regarding clinical outcome.

TREATMENT

1. An initial roentgenogram should be obtained promptly to determine battery location. Despite growing complacency with cases of button cell ingestion, battery size and symptom occurrence cannot be used reliably to detect every patient with a button cell lodged in the esophagus. Glucagon 0.05 mg/kg intravenously may be used to relax the esophagus. The usual side effects of glucagon are diarrhea, nausea, and vomiting, which could lead to risk of aspiration when a distal esophageal foreign body is present. These effects can be minimized by administering the glucagon slowly, over 1 minute. A prospective randomized trial of IV glucagon versus observation is indicated to determine the efficacy of this method of managing coin ingestions lodged in the distal esophagus.[19]
2. Batteries lodged in the esophagus should be removed immediately. Burns due to esophageal lodgment have occurred as early as 4 hours after ingestion, and perforation has occurred as soon as 6 hours after ingestion. Removal should be done under direct visualization (endoscopy). Neither Foley nor magnetized catheter removal of batteries lodged in the esophagus is highly successful, unlike endoscopic removal from more distal sites.
3. An attempt should be made to identify the battery diameter and chemical system by determining the imprint code of a duplicate battery, by measuring the battery compartment within the product, or by checking product or battery instructions and packaging. Most button cells are 7.9 mm or 11.6 mm in diameter. If the battery can be determined to be one of these sizes, identification of the chemical system is rarely necessary (unless fragmentation or free radiopaque material is documented on roentgenogram). However, if the battery is more or less 15 mm in diameter, it will be beneficial to know whether the cell contains mercuric oxide. If the chemical system cannot be identified from packaging or product instructions, it can be determined from the imprint code by calling the National Button Battery Ingestion Hotline at 202-625-3333.
4. Batteries that have passed beyond the esophagus need not be retrieved unless:
   a. The patient manifests signs or symptoms indicative of injury to the gastrointestinal tract (hematochezia, abdominal pain with tenderness, etc.). Minor gastrointestinal symptoms such as a few episodes of vomiting generally do not necessitate battery removal. Stool discoloration alone, in the absence of evidence of gastrointestinal blood or other signs or symptoms, should *not* prompt battery retrieval.
   b. A large diameter cell fails to negotiate the pylorus (see item 5b below). Instead, patients with batteries beyond the esophagus can continue normal activity and diet, with outpatient observation.
5. If the patient remains asymptomatic, follow-up roentgenograms are necessary only to confirm battery passage so that patient monitoring and parental consternation can cease. Preferably, battery passage can be confirmed by inspection of all stools. More frequent follow-up roentgenograms should be *considered,* but are by no means mandatory, if:
   a. A 15.6-mm diameter mercuric oxide cell is ingested (due to the greater likelihood that these cells will split in the gastrointestinal tract). Roentgenograms may be obtained on these patients once or twice weekly.

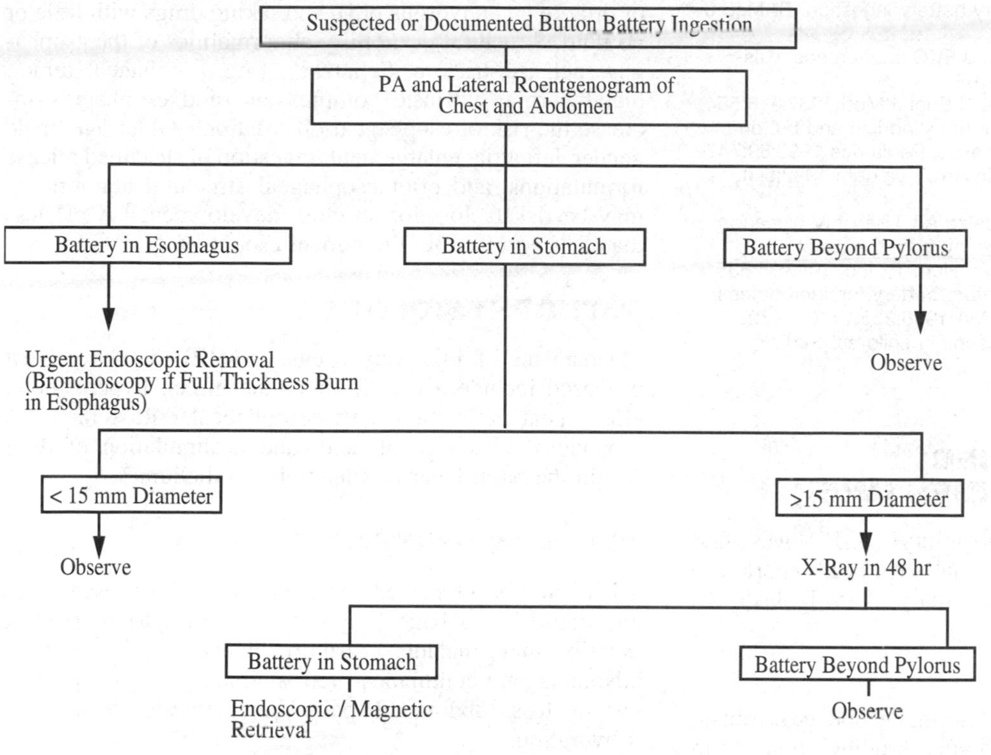

Figure 54–1. Flow diagram of suggested management of button battery ingestions in children. (Adapted from Sheikh A. Pediatr Emerg Care 1993;9:224–229.)

b. A battery with a diameter of 15 mm or greater is ingested by a child less than 6 years of age, due to the delayed transit through the stomach. If these batteries do not pass within 48 hours, they are unlikely to pass. Thus a roentgenogram at this point may identify those cases that might benefit from early endoscopic retrieval. If the battery diameter is unknown, we do *not* recommend routine roentgenograms at 48 hours, as ingestion of these larger cells is infrequent (3% of ingestion cases) and the potential adverse consequences are limited.

6. When mercuric oxide cells are ingested, blood and urine mercury levels are necessary only if the cell is observed to split in the gastrointestinal tract or radiopaque droplets are evident in the gut. Chelation therapy need not be initiated in asymptomatic patients until toxic mercury levels are documented.
7. Button batteries lodged in the external auditory canal or nasal cavity must be removed promptly because of their potential to produce dermal necrosis, nasal perforation, and destruction of the ossicles.[20] Saline solutions and drops should be avoided prior to removal since these liquids may increase local currents. After removal, the area may be irrigated to remove debris. A flow diagram of suggested management of button battery ingestions in children has been suggested by Sheikh (Fig. 54–1).[21]
8. Syrup of ipecac or other emetic is ineffective and unsafe (battery may become lodged in the esophagus). There does not appear to be any indication for use of activated charcoal.

Conservative treatment of foreign body ingestion usually results in a favorable outcome. In the absence of symptoms, non-radiopaque objects may not require any medical intervention. Location of metallic objects and coins by x-ray will determine uncomplicated passage into the stomach.

REFERENCES—DISC BATTERIES

1. Temple DM, McNeese MC. Hazards of battery ingestions. Pediatrics 1983;71:100–103.
2. Rumack BH, Rumack CM. Disc battery ingestions. JAMA 1983;249:2509–2510.
3. Litovitz TL, Schmitz BF, Soloway RA. Ghost blasting with button batteries. Pediatrics 1990;85:384–385.
4. Rumack CM, Rumack BH. Battery ingestion. Pediatrics 1992;89:771–772.
5. Litovitz TL. Button battery ingestions: a review of 56 cases. JAMA 1983;249:2495–2500.
6. Blatnick BS, Toohill RJ, Lehman RH. Fatal complications from an alkaline battery foreign body in the esophagus. Ann Otol Rhinol Laryngol 1977;86:611–615.
7. Votteler TP, Nash JC, Rutledge JC. The hazards of ingested alkaline disc batteries in children. JAMA 1983;249:2504–2506.
8. Willis GA, Ho WC. Perforation of Meckel's diverticulum by an alkaline hearing aid battery. Can Med Assoc J 1982;126:497–498.
9. Maves MD, Carithers JS, Birck HG. Esophageal burns secondary to disc battery ingestions. Ann Otol Rhinol Laryngol 1984;93:364–369.
10. Langkau JF, Noesges RA. Esophageal burns from battery ingestion. Am J Emerg Med 1985;3:265.
11. Kulig K, Rumack CM, Rumack BH et al. Disc battery ingestion: elevated urine mercury levels and enema removal of battery fragments. JAMA 1983;249:2502–2504.
12. Reilly DT. Mercury battery ingestion. Br Med J 1979;1:859.
13. Lewis RJ, Tatken RL. Registry of Toxic Effects of Chemical Substances. Cincinnati, Ohio. US Department of Health and Human Services, 1980, vol 2.
14. Barber TE, Manke RD. The relationship of ingested iron to the absorption of mercuric oxide. Am J Emerg Med 1984;2:500–503.

15. Barros EA, Banos AAB. Mercury battery ingestion. Br Med J 1979;1:218.
16. Kaplan DS. Battery ingestion and EKG interference. Gastrointest Endosc 1990;36:162–163.
17. Proctor MH. Assault by battery. N Engl J Med 1987;316:554.
18. Litovitz T, Schmitz BF. Ingestion of cylindrical and button batteries: an analysis of 2382 cases. Pediatrics 1992;89:747–757. Commentary by K. Kulig in AACT Update 1992;5(4): 1–2.
19. Blume CM, Thompson MW, Scalzo AJ. Use of IV glucagon to facilitate the passage of a penny from the distal esophagus into the stomach. Vet Hum Toxicol 1993;35:335.
20. Kavanaugh KT, Litovitz T. Miniature battery foreign bodies in auditory and nasal cavities. JAMA 1986;255:1470–1472.
21. Sheikh A. Button battery ingestions in children. Pediatr Emerg Care 1993;9:224–229.

MEDICATION-INDUCED ESOPHAGEAL INJURIES (MIEI)

Medication-induced esophageal injury (MIEI) was first described in 1970.[1] Medications that have been reported to induce esophageal injury are summarized in Table 54–5.

RISK FACTORS

Risk factors for MIEI include abnormal esophageal transit, habit of drug ingestion (reclining after drug ingestion), form of drug (e.g., anhydrous pill), and taking drugs with little or no fluid. Structural or motility abnormalities of the esophagus such as stricture, Schatzki's ring, esophageal tumor, hiatal hernia, extrinsic compression, and esophagitis increase the risk of esophageal obstruction.[2] Older age, male gender, left atrial enlargement, ingestion of sustained release formulations, and prior esophageal structural abnormality may be risk factors for stricture development.[3] A pH less than 3 is corrosive in the human esophagus.[4]

Table 54–5
Medication-Induced Esophageal Injury (MIEI)

Ampicillin
Anhydrous pills
Apocillin
Aspirin
Centrum Jr tablets
Clindamycin
Cloxacillin
Cocaine
Decagesic (dexamethasone, aspirin, aluminum hydroxide gel)
Dextropropoxyphene/acetaminophen
Dicloxacillin
Dietary fiber
Doxycycline
Emepronium bromide
Erythromycin
Indomethacin
Iron
Lincomycin
Mexiletine
Minocycline
Oxytetracycline
Paraflex (aspirin, dextropropoxyphene, chlorzoxazone)
Percogesic (phenyl toloxamine citrate 30 mg, acetaminophen 325 mg)
Per diem (82% Psyllium, 18% senna)
Phenoxymethylpenicillin
Piroxicam
Pivmecillinam
Potassium chloride (slow-release, enteric coated)
Quinidine
Sodium meclofenamate
Sulindac
Tetracycline
Tinidazole
Trimethoprim-Sulfamethoxazole
Zidovudine

PATHOPHYSIOLOGY

Mechanisms of injury by drugs in MIEI that have been proposed include a caustic or acidic effect, hyperosmotic effect, heat production, gastroesophageal reflux, impaired esophageal clearance of acid, and accumulation of drug within the basal layer of squamous epithelium.[5]

CLINICAL PRESENTATION

MIEI must be suspected in all patients who present with unexplained esophageal symptoms.[6] Symptoms present initially may include heartburn, nausea and vomiting, odynophagia, continuous retrosternal pain, dysphagia, weight loss, abdominal pain, hematemesis, fever, and dehydration.

SITE

The most common site of MIEI is the mid-esophagus at the level of the aortic arch or the area adjacent to the left atrium.[6] The proximal third of esophagus is involved in 26% of pill-induced esophageal strictures; 52% are found in the middle third, and 22% of patients experience distal-third pill-induced strictures in the esophagus.[3]

COMPLICATIONS[7](TABLE 54–6)

DIAGNOSIS

The diagnosis of MIEI can often be suspected by the clinical history alone.[6] Flexible fiberoptic endoscopy is probably the most reliable method for diagnosing MIEI, but endoscopic findings are not by themselves diagnostic. Multiple ulcers at the mid-esophageal region are an important clue to MIEI. Definitive endoscopic evidence of MIEI must include debris of the drug at the ulcer base, but this is not common.[7] Single contrast barium swallow is not sufficiently sensitive in detecting esophageal ulcers,[7] but double contrast barium swallows may be more useful.[9]

Esophagoscopy findings may include:

Discrete ulcers (pinpoint to circumferential lesions 6 cm in length). Some patients have inflammation without ulcerations: antibiotics, antiinflammatory drugs, Emepronium bromide; smooth or ulcerated strictures, mucosal edema, nodularity, profuse exudate: potassium chloride, quinidine.

TREATMENT

Patient Instruction

Patients should remain standing at least 90 seconds after taking medication. Tablets should be swallowed with at least

Table 54-6
MIEI—Effect of Drugs[a]

Indirect
Stevens-Johnson syndrome: sulfa drugs
  Esophageal stricture
Candida esophagitis
  Antibiotic therapy
  Immunosuppressive drugs
  Cancer chemotherapeutic agents
Drugs may lower esophageal sphincter pressure and promote gastroesophageal reflux disease
Direct
Mucosal injury: after prolonged contact; pH may play some role
Local vascular injury, thrombosis: ulcerogenic lesions produced by potassium chloride in the small bowel
Aspirin may disrupt the normal cytoprotective barrier in the mucosa of the esophagus and stomach
Obstruction or delayed esophageal transit:
  Slow-release or metric formulations of drugs enhance likelihood of esophageal injury
Adherence to esophageal mucosa: drugs that are hygroscopic

[a]Adapted from Bott S et al. Am J Gastroenterol 1987;82:758–763.

100 mL of fluid. Large tablets should preferably be oval and not round. Capsules of a high density are easier to swallow than light ones. Patients who are bedridden or have difficulty in swallowing should be given liquid medication.[10] Material may be removed with normal saline irrigation, suction, and optical peanut forceps.[11] Repeat esophagoscopy 7 to 10 days later.[11] Symptoms resolve and endoscopic healing is evident in 3 days to 6 weeks. Continuation of the medication may result in worsening of symptoms and even death.

REFERENCES—MEDICATION-INDUCED ESOPHAGEAL INJURIES (MIEI)

1. Pemberton J. Oesophageal obstruction and ulceration caused by oral potassium therapy. Br Heart J 1970;32:267–268.
2. Nandi P, Ong GR. Foreign body in the oesophagus. Review of 2394 cases. Br J Surg 1978;65:5–9.
3. McCord GS, Clouse RE. Pill-induced esophageal strictures: clinical features and risk factors for development. Am J Med 1990;88:512–518.
4. Minocha A, Greenbaum DS. Pill-esophagitis caused by nonsteroidal antiinflammatory drugs. Am J Gastroenterol 1991; 86:1086–1089.
5. Ovartlarnporn B, Kulwichit W, Hiranniramol S. Medication-induced esophageal injury. Report of 17 cases with endoscopic documentation. Am J Gastroenterol 1991;86:748–750.
6. Bott S, Prokash C, McCallum RW. Medication-induced esophageal injury. Survey of the literature. Am J Gastroenterol 1987;82:758–763.
7. Kikendall JW, Friedman AC, Oyewole MA, Fleischer D, Johnson LF. Pill-induced esophageal injury. Case reports and review of the medical literature. Dig Dis Sci 1983;28:174–182.
8. Shirazi SS, Zike WL, Brubacker M et al. Effect of aspirin, alcohol and pepsin on mucosal permeability of esophageal mucosa. Gastroenterology 1974;66:A-123/777.
9. Amendola MA, Spera TD. Doxycycline-induced esophagitis. JAMA 1985;253:1009–1011.
10. Hey H, Jorgensen F, Sorensen K, Hasselbalch H, Wamberg T. Oesophageal transit of six commonly used tablets and capsules. Br Med J 1982;285:1717–1719.
11. Perry PA, Dean BS, Krenzelok EP. Drug-induced esophageal injury. Vet Hum Toxicol 1988;30:349.

MOTH BALLS

NAPHTHALENE

TOXICOKINETICS

Humans absorb naphthalene by pulmonary, gastrointestinal, and cutaneous routes. Naphthalene is found in the urine within a few days of ingestion. Naphthalene and its metabolites may be retained in adipose tissue. Naphthalene is more frequently a precipitator of acute hemolysis in children with glucose-6-phosphate dehydrogenase (G-6-PD) deficiency. Naphthalene mothballs put such children at risk for life-threatening anemia.

CLINICAL PRESENTATION

Nausea, vomiting, abdominal pain, headache, confusion, and hemolytic anemia[1] may follow inhalation. Renal toxicity, vertigo, listlessness, lethargy, vertigo, and death may follow ingestion.[2,3]

LABORATORY

1-Naphthol is found in the urine of industrial workers exposed to naphthalene.[4] It is analyzed by spectrophotometry, thin-layer chromatography, and gas chromatography. Elevated plasma levels of hepatic enzymes may be observed.

TREATMENT

Reduce exposure. Activated charcoal may be useful. Protect the respiratory tract. Hemolysis may require blood transfusion, packed red blood cell transfusions, or exchange transfusion, particularly in infants.

REFERENCES—NAPHTHALENE

1. Chusid E, Fried CT. Acute hemolytic anemia due to naphthalene ingestion. Am J Dis Child 1955;86:612–614.
2. Ojwang PJ, Ahmed-Jushuf IH, Abdullah MS. Naphthalene poisoning following ingestion of moth balls. Case report. East Afr Med J 1985;62:72–73.
3. Hibbs BF, Donahue JM, Normandy MJ. Naphthalene. Toxicological profile. Draft Agency for Toxic Substances Disease Registry, October, 1993.
4. Bieniek G. The presence of 1-naphthol in the urine of industrial workers exposed to naphthalene. Occup Environ Med 1994;5:357–359.

P-DICHLOROBENZENE

Mothballs contain either paradichlorobenzene or naphthalene compressed into a solid ball, occasionally with added essential oils and fragrances. Naphthalene is more toxic than paradichlorbenzene, exhibiting more hematologic (hemolytic anemia, methemoglobinemia) and nervous system effects. An abdominal radiograph indicates that paradichlorobenzene is strongly radiopaque, but products containing naphthalene are radiolucent. Other products also containing halogens may also be radiopaque.[1]

REFERENCES—*P*-DICHLOROBENZENE

1. Woolf AD, Saperstein A, Zauvin J, Cappock R, Sue Y-J. Radiopacity of household deodorants, air fresheners and moth repellents. Clin Toxicol 1993;31:418–428.

TOBACCO PRODUCTS

Major toxic agents in the particulate matter of cigarette smoke are listed in Tables 54–7 and 54–8. Tobacco, its substitutes and flavorings, and other plant sources are summarized in Table 54–9.

NICOTINE DEPENDENCE

The American Psychiatric Association has proposed criteria for nicotine dependence disorders (Table 54–10).[1] Nicotine withdrawal disorders have also been defined (Table 54–11). The Fagerstrom test (Table 54–12) also scores degrees of nicotine dependency.[2] These scores are based on data obtained by Heatherton and colleagues.[3]

PASSIVE SMOKING

The association of medical problems with passive smoking has been reported for adults (lung cancer, small airway damage, worsened angina, increased blood pressure), children (bronchitis, pneumonia, worsened asthma, middle ear effusions, decreased height, sudden infant death syndrome), and in utero exposure (low birth weight, increased risks of prematurity and neonatal death). Further, nicotine is found in the breast milk of lactating women and may be associated with colic.[4]

Table 54-7
Major Toxic Agents in the Particulate Matter of Cigarette Smoke (Unaged)[a,b]

Agent	Biologic Activity[c]	Concentration/Cigarette			
		Range Reported		US Cigarettes[d]	
Benzo[a]pyrene	TI	8–50	ng	20	ng
5-Methylchrysene	TI	0.5–2	ng	0.6	ng
Benzo[*j*]fluoranthene	TI	5–40	ng	10	ng
Benz[*a*]anthracene	TI	5–80	ng	40	ng
Other polynuclear aromatic hydrocarbons (>20 compounds)	TI	?		?	
Dibenz[*a,j*]acridine	TI	3–10	ng	8	ng
Dibenz[*a,h*]acridine	TI	?		?	
Dibenzo[*c,g*]carbazole	T1	0.7	ng	0.7	ng
Pyrene	CoC	50–200	ng	150	ng
Fluranthene	CoC	50–250	ng	170	ng
Benzo[*g,h,i*]perylene	CoC	10–60	ng	30	ng
Other polynuclear aromatic hydrocarbons (>10 compounds)	CoC	?		?	
Naphthalenes	CoC	1–10	μg	6	μg
1-Methylindoles	CoC	0.3–0.9	μg	0.8	μg
9-Methylcarbazoles	CoC	0.005–0.2	μg	0.1	μg
Other neutral compounds	CoC	?		?	
Catechol	CoC	40–460	μg	270	μg
3- and 4-methylcatechols	CoC	30–40	μg	32	μg
Other catechols (>4 compounds)	CoC	?		?	
Unknown phenols and acids	CoC	?		?	
N-Nitrosonornicotine	C	100–250	ng	250	ng
Other nonvolatile nitrosamines	C	?		?	
β-Naphthylamine	BC	0–25	ng	20	ng
Other aromatic amines	BC	?		?	
Unknown nitro compounds	BC	?		?	
Polonium 210	C	0.03–1.3	pCi	?	
Nickel compounds	C	10–600	ng	?	
Cadmium compounds	C	9–70	ng	?	
Arsenic	C	1–25	μg	?	
Nicotine	T	0.1–2.0	mg	1.5	mg
Minor tobacco alkaloids	T	0.01–0.2	mg	0.1	mg
Phenol	CT	10–200	μg	85	μg
Cresols (3 compounds)	CT	10–150	μg	70	μg

[a]Adapted from Jaffe JH, Kanzler M. In Lowinson JH, Ruiz P, eds. Substance abuse: clinical problems and perspectives. Baltimore, MD: Williams & Wilkins, 1981.
[b]Incomplete list.
[c]*C*, Carcinogen; *BC*, bladder carcinogen; *TI*, tumor initiator; *CoC*, cocarcinogen; *CT*, cilia toxic agent; *T*, toxic agent.
[d]85-mm cigarettes without filter tips bought on the open market 1973–1976.

Table 54–8
Major Toxic Agents in the Gas Phase of Cigarette Smoke (Unaged)[a,b]

Agent	Biologic Activity[c]	Concentration/Cigarette: Range Reported		Concentration/Cigarette: US Cigarettes[d]	
Dimethylnitrosamine	C	1–200	ng	13	ng
Ethylmethylnitrosamine	C	0.1–10	ng	1.8	ng
Diethylnitrosamine	C	0–10	ng	1.5	ng
Nitrosopyrrolidine	C	2–42	ng	11	ng
Other nitrosamines (4 compounds)	C	0–20	ng	?	
Hydrazine	C	24–43	ng	32	ng
Vinyl chloride	C	1–16	ng	12	ng
Urethane	TI	10–35	ng	30	ng
Formaldehyde	CT, CoC	20–90	μg	30	μg
Hydrogen cyanide	CT, T	30–200	μg	110	μg
Acrolein	CT	25–140	μg	70	μg
Acetaldehyde	CT	18–1400	μg	800	μg
Nitrogen oxides (NO_x)[e]	T	10–600	μg	350	μg
Ammonia	T[f]	10–150	μg	60	μg
Pyridine	T[f]	9–93	μg	10	μg
Carbon monoxide	T	2–20	mg	17	mg

[a]Adapted from Jaffe JH, Kanzler M. In Lowinson JH, Ruiz P, eds. Substance abuse: clinical problems and perspectives. Baltimore, MD: Williams & Wilkins, 1981.
[b]Cigarettes may also contain such carcinogens as arsine, nickel carbonyl, and possibly volatile chlorinated olefins and nitro-olefins.
[c]*C*, Carcinogen; *BC*, bladder carcinogen; *TI*, tumor initiator; *CoC*, cocarcinogen; *CT*, cilia toxic agent; *T*, toxic agent.
[d]85-mm cigarettes without filter tips bought on the open market 1973–1976.
[e]NO_x > 95% NO; remainder, NO_2.
[f]Not toxic in smoke of blended US cigarettes because pH < 6.5, and, therefore, ammonia and pyridines are present only in protonated form.

Table 54–9
Smoking: Tobacco, Its Substitutes and Flavorings, and Other Plants[a,b]

Angiosperm Family and Species	Vernacular Name	Remarks
Anacardiaceae		
Rhus glabra, R. triloba, R. sempervirens, R. virens	Sumac	Dried leaves mixed with tobacco or alone smoked by eastern and central North American Indians and occasionally by early settlers
Apiaceae		
Angelica archangelica	Angelica	Root used to flavor cigarette tobacco (source of volatile oil of angelica)
A. atropurpurea	Purple angelica	Root mixed with tobacco for smoking by Arkansas Indians
Coriandrum sativum	Coriander	Fruit for flavoring cigarette tobacco (source of aromatic volatile oil of coriander)
Asteraceae		
Matricaria chamomilla	Chamomile	Dried flowering heads contain a volatile oil for flavoring cigarette tobacco
Trilisa odoratissima	Deer's tongue	Leaves containing coumarin added to cigarette tobacco to give a sweet taste (southeastern United States)
Betulaceae		
Corylus avellana	European hazel	Leaves smoked in Eurasia
Boraginaceae		
Tournefortia argentea		Leaves smoked in the Seychelles
Campanulaceae		
Lobelia excelsa		Leaves smoked in India
L. inflata	Indian tobacco	Contains an alkaloid lobeline allied to nicotine; leaves often smoked by North American Indians with or without tobacco; lobeline is substituted for nicotine in commercial products to help stop smoking (Bantron, Lobidan, Nikoban)
L. tupa	Tobaco del diablo	Contains lobeline and other piperidine alkaloids, smoked by Mapuches of Chile
Cornaceae		
Cornus stolonifera	Red-osier dogwood	Inner bark smoked by eastern North American Indians with or without tobacco
Daphniphyllaceae		
Daphniphyllum humile		In Japan, the Ainu smoke its leaves in place of tobacco
Ericaceae		
Arctostaphylos uva-ursi	Bearberry	Eastern North American Indians and colonists mixed leaves with tobacco for smoking

[a]Adapted from Lewis WH, Elvin-Lewis MPF. Medical botany. Plants affecting man's health. New York: John Wiley, 1977. Used with permission.
[b]Cigarettes are often smoked in India and southeastern Asia as "beedi" or "bidi," which is sundried, uncured tobacco wrapped in a dried leaf of temburni *(Diospyros melanoxylon)* or banana *(Musa sapientum)* and secured at one end by a thin string. Other domestic wrappings for cigarettes include young leaves of the palms of *Licuala pumila* and *Nypa fruticans*.
[c]Nicotine content may be as high as 9%, and these species are the source of the widely used natural-contact insecticide obtained from tobacco leaves.

(continued)

Table 54–9 *(Continued)*

Angiosperm Family and Species	Vernacular Name	Remarks
Euphorbiaceae		
Sauropus quadrangularis		Leaves smoked for tonsillitis in Hindu medicine
Fabaceae		
Dipteryx odorata	Tonka tree	Fermented tonka beans produce coumarin and are used for flavoring cigarette tobacco; also supposed to be narcotic and stimulant
Lamiaceae		
Mentha arvensis	Mint	Mint oil containing 90% menthol for flavoring mentholated cigarettes
Moraceae		
Dorstenia contrajerva		Dried rhizomes for flavoring cigarettes (from tropical America)
Myristicaceae		
Myristica fragrans	Nutmeg and mace	Mace containing volatile aromatic oil used for flavoring cigarettes
Poaceae		
Zea mays	Corn	Dried silks are a traditional tobacco substitute in the New World
Rosaceae		
Crataegus oxyacantha	Hawthorn	Young leaves substituted for tobacco
Prunus spp.		Essences of prune or peach added to flavor cigarettes
Solanaceae		
Datura fastuosa		Leaves smoked in Africa to relieve asthma
D. metel	Hindu datura	Leaves smoked in India and elsewhere to relieve asthma
D. stramonium	Jimson weed	Leaves at one time widely smoked to relieve respiratory complaints
Nicotiana tabacum	Common tobacco	
N. alata		Leaves smoked in South America and also chewed
N. attenuata		Dried leaves smoked in pipes and as cigarettes by New Mexican Indians
N. glauca	Tree tobacco	Contains an alkaloid anabasin[c]
N. quadrivalvis		Leaves smoked by Indians in western United States
N. rustica	Aztec tobacco, yellow henbane	Leaves smoked by Mexican and North American Indians, also cultivated in Old World[c]
N. trigonophylla		Smoked by Indians of southwestern United States and Mexico
Solanum inaequilaterale		Leaves smoked in the Philippines
Tiliaceae		
Tilia cordata	Linden	Leaves used to adulterate tobacco

Table 54–10
Criteria of the American Psychiatric Association for Nicotine Dependence Disorder[a]

Nicotine dependence disorder is a maladaptive pattern of substance use, leading to clinically important impairment or distress, as manifested by three or more of the following at any time in a 12-month period:

1. Tolerance, as defined by either of the following, occurs: a need for markedly increased amounts of the substance to achieve intoxication or the desired effect, or a markedly diminished effect with continued use of the same amount of the substance.
2. Withdrawal, as manifested by either of the following, occurs: the characteristic withdrawal syndrome for the substance, or the taking of the same (or a closely related) substance to relieve or avoid withdrawal symptoms.
3. The substance is often taken in larger amounts or for a longer period than was intended.
4. There is a persistent desire or unsuccessful effort to cut down or control substance use.
5. A great deal of time is spent in activities necessary to obtain the substance (e.g., visiting multiple doctors or driving long distances), use the substance (e.g., chain-smoking), or recover from its effects.
6. Important social, occupational, or recreational activities are given up or reduced because of substance use.
7. The substance use is continued despite the knowledge that there is a persistent or recurrent physical or psychological problem likely to have been caused or exacerbated by the substance (e.g., current cocaine use despite the recognition of cocaine-induced depression, or continued drinking despite the recognition that an ulcer was made worse by alcohol consumption).

[a]Data were obtained from the *Diagnostic and statistical manual of mental disorders.* 4th ed. Washington, DC: American Psychiatric Association, 1994.

Table 54–11
Criteria of the American Psychiatric Association for Nicotine Withdrawal Disorder[a]

1. Nicotine is used daily for at least several weeks.
2. There is abrupt cessation of nicotine use, or reduction in the amount of nicotine used, followed within 24 hours by four or more of the following symptoms:
   Dysphoric or depressed mood;
   Insomnia;
   Irritability, frustration, or anger;
   Anxiety;
   Difficulty in concentrating;
   Restlessness;
   Decreased heart rate; and
   Increased appetite or weight gain.
3. The symptoms cause clinically important distress or impairment in social, occupational, or other important areas of functioning.
4. The symptoms are not due to a general medical condition and are not better accounted for by another mental disorder.

[a]Data were obtained from the *Diagnostic and Statistical Manual of Mental Disorders.* Adapted from Henningfield JE. N Engl J Med 1995;333:1196–1203.

ENVIRONMENTAL TOBACCO SMOKE

Benowitz has studied the human pharmacology of nicotine (Table 54–13) and has compared its addictive properties to other drugs of abuse (Table 54–14).[5] Environmental tobacco smoke consists of mainstream smoke, sidestream smoke, and vapor-phase components that diffuse through cigarette paper into the environment. Byrd has summarized the present status of environmental tobacco smoke.[6] Exposure to ETS by nonsmokers occurs frequently in the home, in the workplace, and in other public areas where smoking is allowed.

Although smoking is declining in the United States,[7] aids for the prevention of smoking cessation withdrawal symptoms (transdermal nicotine,[8,9] nicotine gum, nicotine spray)[10] have not been evaluated in controlled studies that address their usefulness in diminishing the undesirable effects (lung disease, cancer) of smoking. Data on transdermal nicotine systems (Table 54–15) include its effect on plasma nicotine concentration (Figs. 54–2, 54–3, and 54–4). Positive urine cotinine levels are an indication of active or passive exposure to tobacco smoke.[11] Smoking cessation materials are available (Table 54–16).

Table 54–12
The Fagerström Test for Nicotine Dependence

Questions and Answers	Score
How soon after you wake up do you smoke your first cigarette?	
≤5 min	3
6–30 min	2
31–60 min	1
≥61 min	0
Do you find it difficult to refrain from smoking in places where it is forbidden—e.g., in church, at the library, in a cinema?	
Yes	1
No	0
Which cigarette would you hate most to give up?	
The first in the morning	1
Any other	0
How many cigarettes per day do you smoke?	
≤10	0
11–20	1
21–30	2
≥31	3
Do you smoke more frequently during the first hours after waking than during the rest of the day?	
Yes	1
No	0
Do you smoke if you are so ill that you are in bed most of the day?	
Yes	1
No	0

[a]Data were obtained from Heatherton et al. Scores of more than 6 are generally interpreted as indicating a high degree of dependence, with more severe withdrawal symptoms, greater difficulty in quitting, and possibly the need for higher doses of medication.
Adapted from Henningfield JE. N Engl J Med 1995;333:1196–1203.

Table 54–13
Human Pharmacology of Nicotine[a]

Primary Effects[b]	Withdrawal
Pleasure	Irritability, restlessness
Arousal, enhanced vigilance	Drowsiness
Improved task performance	Difficulty concentrating; impaired task performance
Relief of anxiety	Anxiety
Reduced hunger	Hunger
Body weight reduction	Weight gain
	Sleep disturbance
	Cravings or strong urge for nicotine
EEG desynchronization	Decreased catecholamine excretion
Increased circulating levels of catecholamines, vasopressin, growth hormone, ACTH, cortisol, prolactin, beta-endorphin	
Increased metabolic rate	
Lipolysis, increased free fatty acids	
Heart rate acceleration	Heart rate slowing[c]
Cutaneous and coronary vasoconstriction	
Increased cardiac output	
Increased blood pressure	
Skeletal muscle relaxation	

[a]Adapted from Benowitz NL. Med Clin North Am 1992;76:415–537.
[b]Some of these effects are due in part to relief of withdrawal symptoms.
[c]May represent a return to baseline rather than true withdrawal.

Table 54–14
Attributes of Drug Addiction: Comparison of Drugs of Abuse[a]

	Nicotine	Heroin	Cocaine	Alcohol	Caffeine
Psychoactive effects	+	+	+	+	+
Drug-reinforced behavior	+	+	+	+	+
Compulsive use	+	+	+	+	–/+
Use despite harmful effects	+	+	+	+	–/+
Relapse after abstinence	+	+	+	+	–
Recurrent drug cravings	+	+	+	+	+
Tolerance	+	+	+	+	+
Physical dependence	+	+	+	+	+
Agonist useful in treating dependence	+	+	–	+	–

[a]Adapted from Benowitz NL. Med Clin North Am 1992;76:415–437.

Table 54-15
Profiles of Currently Available Transdermal Nicotine Systems (Data Obtained From Manufacturers' Prescribing Information Sheets)[a]

Manufacturer	Delivery Control Method	Application Period (Hours)	Size (cm^2)	Total Nicotine Content (mg)	Nicotine Absorbed (mg/Application Period)	Nicotine Remaining in System After Application Period (% of Total Content)	Dose Absorbed (% of Total Released)
CIBA-Geigy	Polymer	24	30	52.5	21	60	98
			20	35.0	14		
			10	17.5	7		
Elan/Cyanamid/ Lederle	Gel matrix	24	7	30	22	27	98
			3.5	15	11		
Marion Merrell Dow/Alza	Rate controlling membrane	24	22	114	21	73	68
			15	78	14		
			7	36	7		
Kabi Pharmacia/ Cygnus	Adhesive	16	30	24.9	15	40	95
			20	16.6	10		
			10	8.3	5		

[a]Adapted from Palmer KJ et al. Drugs 1992;44:498–529.

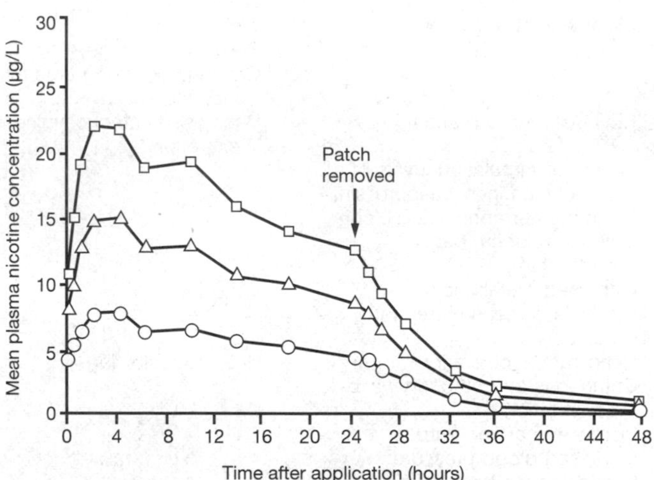

Figure 54–2. Mean plasma nicotine concentrations in 24 smokers following 24-hour application of a transdermal nicotine system delivering 7 (○), 14 (△) or 21 (□ mg/24h) (unpublished data on file, Marion Merrell Dow). (Adapted from Palmer KJ, Buckley MM, Faulds D. Drugs 1992;44:498–529.)

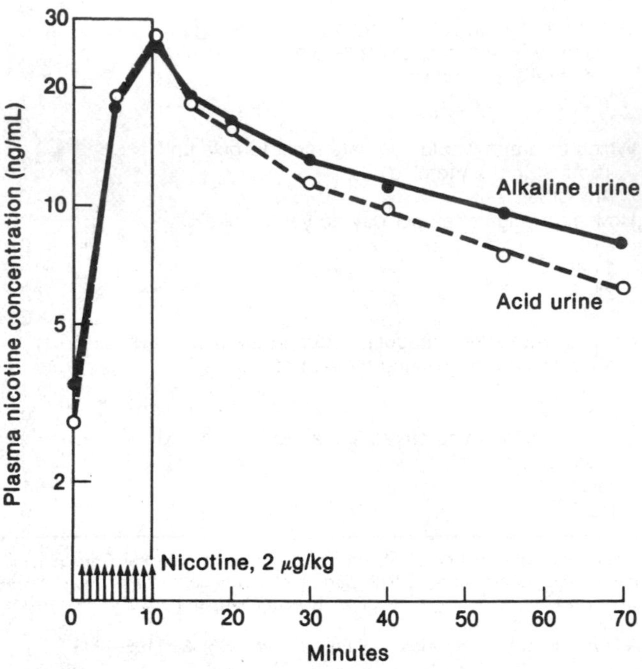

Figure 54–3. Mean plasma nicotine concentrations for single series of injections of nicotine with alkaline and acid urine. Data are plotted on semilogarithmic coordinates to demonstrate log-linearity of terminal decline phase. Hatched area indicates 10-minute interval during which intravenous injections of nicotine, 2µg/kg/min, were given. Data represent mean values for six subjects. (Adapted from Rosenberg J, Benowitz NL, Jacob P et al. Clin Pharmacol Ther 1980;28:518.)

CLONIDINE

For smoking cessation, clonidine dosage of 200 to 400 µg/day may be useful. Its high incidence of side effects (sedation, postural hypotension) preclude its use as first-line treatment for most patients.[12]

Recent nonnicotinic pharmacologic interventions in smoking cessation and abstinence include buspirone, serotonin uptake inhibitors, doxepin, ascorbic acid aerosol, and mecamylamine combined with a nicotine patch.[13] Moclobemide appeared to facilitate smoking cessation in high-dependent smokers enrolled in a randomized, double-blind, placebo-controlled study.

Sachs reports a controlled clinical study that suggests that Nicotine polacrilex, 4 mg, may be useful in the initial phase of tobacco dependence in high-dependent smokers. This observation should be validated by further clinical trials.[13a]

NICOTINE POISONING

Nicotine is a highly toxic alkaloid that causes stimulation of the autonomic ganglia and central nervous system and is the principal pharmacologically active component in cigarettes and cigars. Poisoning occurs in children who ingest cigarettes, snuff, and nicotine gum and less often industrially in the tobacco and insecticide industries.

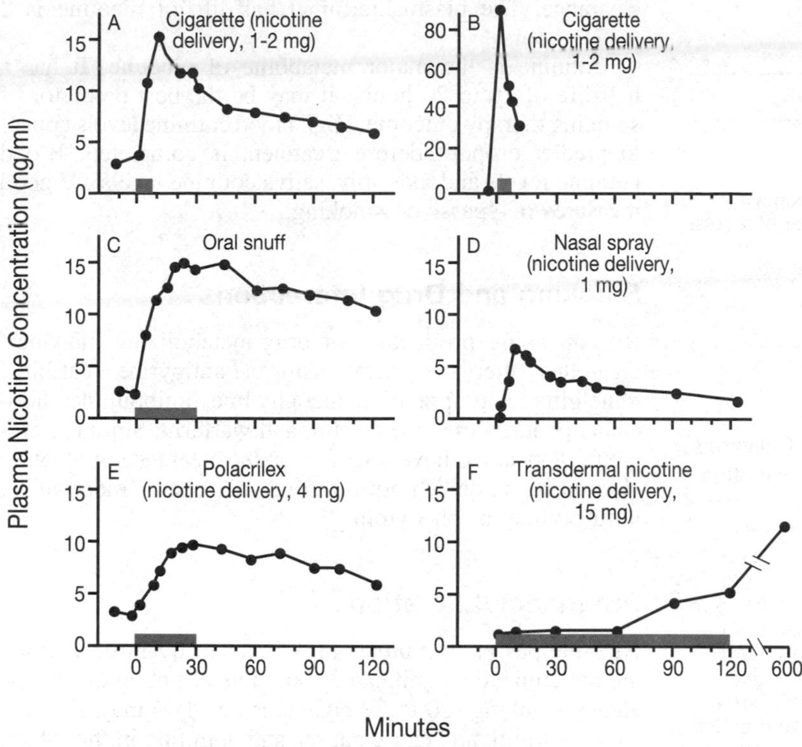

Figure 54–4. Plasma nicotine concentrations before and after the administration of a single dose of nicotine in several forms. The shaded bar in each panel indicates the period of nicotine delivery. The amount of nicotine delivered from the subjects' standard cigarettes was assumed to be 1 to 2 mg. The data on oral snuff were obtained in 10 subjects after each used 2.5 g of commercially available moist snuff with no nicotine dose specified.[17] All plasma nicotine values are based on samples of venous blood, except those in Panel B, which are based on arterial blood collected in one subject while he smoked a cigarette (data replotted from Henningfield et al.[16]). The data on transdermal nicotine (11 subjects) are replotted from Benowitz;[18] the data in Panel A on cigarettes (10 subjects) and on nicotine polacrilex (10 subjects) are from Benowitz et al.;[17] and the data on nasal spray (8 subjects) are from Johansson et al.[19] (From Henningfield JE. N Engl J Med 1995;333:1196–1203.)

Table 54–16
Smoking Cessation Materials Available[a]

American Cancer Society (local office)
American Heart Association (local office)
  7320 Greenville Ave, Dallas, TX 75231
American Lung Association (local office)
American Dental Association
  211 E Chicago, Chicago, IL 60611
National Cancer Institute
  Office of Cancer Communications,
  National Institutes of Health,
  Bldg 31, Room 4B-43,
  Bethesda, MD 20892
  (800) 4-CANCER
National Heart, Lung, and Blood Institute
  Smoking Education Program,
  National Institutes of Health,
  Bldg 31, Room 4A-18, Dept A-1,
  Bethesda, MD 20892
  (202) 783-3238
National Audio Visual Center
  Customers Services Section,
  8700 Edgeworth Dr,
  Capital Heights, MD 20743-3701
Health Promotion Group Inc
  PO Box 59687, Homewood, AL 35259
Warner Brothers
  Attn: Lorimar Home Video,
  4000 Warner Blvd,
  Burbank, CA 91522
  (800) 323-5275
Office on Smoking and Health
  5600 Fishers Ln, Park Bldg, Room 110,
  Rockville, MD 20857

[a]Adapted from Lee EW, D'Alonzo GE. Arch Int Med 1993;153:34–48.

STRUCTURE AND CLASSIFICATION

Nicotine is a liquid alkaloid with the structure (S)-3-(1-methyl-2-pyrrolidinyl) pyridine. It is water soluble and has a pK_a of 8.5. It is a colorless, bitter-tasting liquid that is strongly alkaline in reaction. Nicotine is the major pharmacologically active constituent of tobacco.

USES/SOURCES/PRODUCT FORMULATIONS[14]

Table 54–9 lists the variety of plants used for smoking. Blending of tobacco results in a tobacco nicotine content of 1 to 2%. A cigarette contains 13 to 19 mg of nicotine; a cigar contains 15 to 40 mg (Table 54–17). Smoke from nonfiltered ciagrettes possesses 1 to 2.5 mg; that from filtered cigarettes contains 0.2 to 1.0 mg. About one-fourth of original total nicotine is recovered from cigarette butts.

Of the available nicotine, 10 to 50% is absorbed during mouth puffing and 80 to 100% during deep lung inhalation. Nicotine can be found in the urine of most nonsmokers. A single cigarette puff delivers approximately 0.05 to 0.15 mg of nicotine.

Poisoning may occur in adults who smoke or chew tobacco. Toxicity also occurs in those who are involved in processing and extracting tobacco (green tobacco sickness), as well as mixing, storing, and applying certain insecticides. Children are most commonly exposed through ingestion of cigarettes or cigars. Nicotine gum toxicity has been reported in adults and children.

Tobacco pouches introduced between the lip and gum may release varying amounts of nicotinic acid. They are

Table 54–17
Sources of Nicotine[a]

Sources	Nicotine Content	
Cigarette	13–19 mg	
Cigarette butt	5–7 mg	
Clove cigarette	70% tobacco; thought to contain 2× amount of nicotine as that of regular cigarettes	
Cigar	15–40 mg	
Snuff	12–15 mg/g dry snuff 5–30 mg/g wet snuff	
Chewing tobacco	2–8 mg/g	
Nicorette gum	2–4 mg/piece	
Tobacco leaf	1–6% nicotine per leaf	
Insecticides	Up to 40%	
Transdermal Nicotine Patches:	Total Nicotine	Delivered Nicotine
Habitrol	17.5 mg	7 mg/d
	35 mg	14 mg/d
	52.5 mg	21 mg/d
Prostep	15–30 mg	10–21 mg/d
Nicoderm	114 mg	21 mg/d
	78	14 mg/d
	35	7 mg/d
Nicotrol	24.9	15 mg/16 h
	16.6	10 mg/16 h
	8.3	5 mg/16 h

[a]Adapted from Blanchard J. Clin Toxicol Rev 1993;15(1):1–2.

mistakenly considered to be a "safe" alternative to more conventional tobacco products, even though there is cumulative evidence of production of oral cancer.

DOSAGE

Nicotine is highly toxic: 2 to 5 mg may cause nausea; 40 to 60 mg may be lethal. Survival has followed ingestions of 1 to 4 g.

TOXICOKINETICS (FIGS. 54–2, 54–3, AND 54–4)

The oral mucosa, respiratory tract, gastrointestinal tract (except stomach), and skin absorb nicotine readily. In an alkaline medium there is an increase in the small amount of nicotine absorbed in the stomach.

Distribution

Nicotine undergoes a large first-pass effect during which the liver metabolizes 80 to 90%. Smaller amounts are metabolized in the lung and kidney.

Elimination

Nicotine and its metabolites (cotinine and nicotine-1′-*N*-oxide) are excreted in the urine. At a pH of 5.5 or less, 23% is excreted unchanged. At a pH of 8, only 2% is excreted in the urine (Fig. 54–3). The effect of urinary pH on total clearance is due entirely to changes in renal clearance. The plasma terminal half-life of nicotine is 2 to 2.2 hours.

Cotinine is the major metabolite of nicotine. It has a half-life of 10 to 20 hours. It may be the best predictor of smoking therapy outcome. High blood cotinine levels appear to predict dropout before treatment is completed. Blood cotinine levels and, possibly, saliva cotinine levels are good measures of "passive" smoking.

Smoking and Drug Interactions

By enhancing production of drug-metabolizing enzymes, cigarettes alter the metabolism of antipyrine, caffeine, glutethimide, propranolol, theophylline, imipramine, lidocaine, pentazocine, phenacetin, and warfarin. Smoking cigarettes appears to have no effect on the clearance of alcohol, chlordiazepoxide, chlorpromazine, diazepam, meperidine, nortriptyline, or phenytoin.

Pregnancy/Lactation

Nicotine passes into breast milk in small quantities, which are not clinically significant, averaging 91 ppb in one study. Heavy smoking (20 to 30 cigarettes per day) may alter the supply of milk and cause nausea and vomiting in the infant. There is a greater danger to the infant from "second-hand smoking" (i.e., inhaling smoke from others). Cigarettes increase the risk of pneumonia, bronchitis, and sudden infant death syndrome.

PATHOPHYSIOLOGY

Initially, and only briefly, nicotine is stimulating to the autonomic nervous system ganglia and neuromuscular junction. The most prominent effects relate to stimulation of the adrenal medulla, central nervous system, cardiovascular system (release of catecholamines), gastrointestinal tract (parasympathetic stimulation), salivary and bronchial glands, and the medullary vomiting center.

There is subsequent blockade of autonomic ganglia and the neuromuscular junction transmission, inhibition of catecholamine release from the adrenal medulla, and central nervous system depression.

CLINICAL PRESENTATION

Nicotine is an exceedingly lethal poison, but few deaths have been reported from its use. Serious toxicity resulting from ingestion of cigarette tobacco is rare.

Symptoms of nicotine alkaloid poisoning may develop within 15 minutes. The onset of symptoms is much more rapid after the ingestion of liquid nicotine (e.g., insecticides, teas) compared with nicotine-containing organic material (plant parts). Death may occur within 5 minutes of ingestion of concentrated nicotine insecticides. Four to eight milligrams orally[15] may produce serious symptoms in nonhabituated individuals. Gastrointestinal signs and symptoms occur first and include mouth and throat burning followed by profuse salivation, nausea, vomiting, abdominal pain, and occasionally diarrhea.

Cigarette Ingestions

Children ingesting less than 2 cigarettes or less than 6 cigarette butts may experience vomiting within 20 minutes. Lethargy or irritability is observed infrequently and completely resolves. Initially, asymptomatic patients do not usually develop symptoms. Symptomatic patients improve without sequelae. Seizures are not observed. The absence of vomiting predicts a favorable outcome. Cigarette ingestions in children rarely require specific treatment. Ingestions of greater than two whole cigarettes or six butts are potentially toxic and should be referred to the emergency department regardless of symptoms. Decontamination of the mouth with water and administration of syrup of ipecac are recommended before transport to the emergency department.[16]

Central Nervous System

Headache, confusion, dizziness, agitation, restlessness, and incoordination develop initially after serious nicotine overdoses. Later, within 30 minutes, in a severe poisoning, convulsions and coma occur. Other cholinergic signs often observed are, initially, diaphoresis, salivation, lacrimation, increased bronchial secretions, and miosis and, later, mydriasis.

Neuromuscular symptoms include hypotonia, decreased deep tendon reflexes, weakness, fasciculations, and paralysis of muscles (including respiratory muscles).

Respiratory System

Initial tachypnea, but later dyspnea, decreased respiratory rate, and cyanosis may be seen. Respiratory arrest may occur within minutes, and resultant death within 1 hour.

Cardiovascular System

A transient increase in blood pressure followed by hypotension, bradycardia, paroxysmal atrial fibrillation, or cardiac standstill is observed.

Malizia and colleagues[15] described four children who ingested two cigarettes each and developed salivation, vomiting, diarrhea, tachypnea, tachycardia, and hypertension within 30 minutes and depressed respiration and cardiac arrhythmias within 40 minutes. Convulsions occurred within 60 minutes of ingestion. All recovered after gastric lavage, activated charcoal, intermittent positive pressure ventilation, and 5 mg diazepam intravenously for convulsions.

Green tobacco sickness occurs in young workers who do not smoke but who work with wet, uncured tobacco. They experience nausea, vomiting, and prostration.[17]

Addiction

Dependence on nicotine is still controversial. Tolerance may occur, but data on these phenomena and withdrawal symptoms after cessation of cigarette smoking are far from established. Need for oral gratification and other psychologic problems may result in the production of symptoms of withdrawal, including anxiety, impaired concentration and memory, depression, hostility, sleep disturbances, and increased appetite. Correlations between smoking and alcoholism have been observed (Table 54–10).

Psychologic habituation to smoking is a complex and so far largely insoluble problem for most smokers. Commercial preparations to cure smoking (containing lobeline) are of marginal value. Corticotropin therapy (180 IU of corticotropin gelatin—Acthar Gel—intramuscularly) has been shown to reduce or abolish the smoking withdrawal syndrome. This work is of a preliminary nature.[18] Nicotine gum and transdermal nicotine may reduce cigarette craving.

LABORATORY

Overdose

Nicotine concentrations in the urine are not useful in management of overdosage since they fluctuate greatly with changes in pH and urine flow. The plasma nicotine level correlates well with absorbed dose and can provide a means of evaluating occupational exposure to nicotine, but the short half-life of nicotine in plasma requires that blood be drawn shortly after exposure. Prior smoking may affect levels. A rapid high-pressure liquid chromatography assay is now available. Cotinine in plasma, saliva, and urine appears to have a clear dose-response relationship to passive smoke exposure. Urine cotinine is used as an index to nicotine exposure in tobacco harvesters.

Polymorphonuclear leukocytosis and glycosuria occur after nicotine overdose.

Smoking

Smoking induces elevations in the serum thiocyanate levels. This may be an indication of its effect on drug metabolism induction and may also be useful as a measure of the effect of passive smoking on children.

Plasma Levels of Nicotine	
After pipe smoking	4–6 ng/mL
After cigarette smoking	18.3–22 ng/mL (mean plasma nicotine trough level after hourly smoking)
After chewing 2 mg nicotine gum	11.8 ng/mL
After chewing 4 mg nicotine gum	23.2 ng/mL
After transdermal patch (Fig. 54–2)	

A study of 306 male pipe and cigar smokers revealed that serum thiocyanate levels were significantly higher than those of nonsmokers.[19] Thiocyanate, formed from the cyanide in tobacco, is an indicator of exposure to both the particulate and gas phases of tobacco smoke; however, it does not appear to be as useful as other markers such as nicotine, cotinine, and carbon monoxide. Carboxyhemoglobin levels are good indicators of gas-phase absorption by cigarette smokers.

TREATMENT

Stabilization

1. Immediate establishment of an airway, monitoring of breathing patterns, and maintenance of circulation are essential in serious overdose cases.
2. Preparations for possible seizures or rapid progression to coma must be initiated in serious overdose cases by

establishment of an intravenous line, supplemental oxygen, cardiac monitoring, and direct observation.
3. Artificial ventilation procedures should be kept ready; oxygen may be required.

Decontamination

1. If vomiting has not occurred following liquid nicotine (insecticide) ingestion, remove stomach contents by gastric lavage. Induction of emesis is less preferable than lavage since convulsions or coma may intervene. Children who ingest more than one cigarette should receive activated charcoal and medical observation for at least several hours.
2. Single or multiple doses of activated charcoal may be used, but its use in acute poisoning has not been established.
3. Wash exposed skin with nonabrasive, nonalkaline soaps and cool water.

Elimination Enhancement

Hemodialysis and hemoperfusion have not been evaluated in acute nicotine poisoning.

Antidotes

There are no known antidotes.

Supportive Care

1. Seizure activity and agitation can be controlled with diazepam or barbiturates.
2. Bronchial secretions, excess salivation, and diarrhea may be ameliorated by atropine.
3. Acidification of urine may increase excretion of nicotine. Although pharmacologically sound, its clinical value remains to be established.
4. Mechanically assisted ventilation should be readily available for respiratory depression.
5. Preventive measures for occupational exposure to nicotine include adequate ventilation, chemical goggles, mechanical filter respirator, rubber gloves, aprons, and boots.

NICOTINE GUM

Nicotine gum has been approved by the FDA for prescription use as an aid to cessation of smoking. Each piece of gum contains nicotine (2 mg) bound to an ion-exchange resin in a sugar-free, flavored gum base, with a bicarbonate buffer. Chewing one piece for 20 to 30 minutes releases 90% of the nicotine. Its efficacy remains to be shown.

DOSE

Two mg of Nicorette gum produces blood levels equivalent to smoking half a cigarette per hour. A patient had signs and symptoms of nicotine overdose after briefly chewing a single piece of Nicorette gum. The minimum lethal oral dose for nicotine in human adults is 40 to 60 mg.[20]

Children ingesting more than one cigarette or three cigarette butts develop signs or symptoms. Severe symptoms (e.g., limb jerking and unresponsiveness) are only seen with the large amounts. Nicotine resin gum produces toxicity in children who chew ½ to 4 pieces. Agitation, lethargy, tachycardia, hypotension, abdominal pain, and vomiting are seen within 30 minutes of exposure to the gum.[21]

TOXICOKINETICS

Nicotine from the gum is absorbed through the buccal mucosa. Peak serum levels of nicotine are attained in 15 to 30 minutes, much longer than the time to peak after smoking a cigarette (2 minutes). The nicotine is metabolized in the liver to nicotine-1′-*N*-oxide and cotinine. The metabolites are excreted by the kidneys (72.1%) in 96 hours. Usual use is 10 to 12 sticks per day. A 2-mg stick of nicotine gum produces blood levels of nicotine equivalent to smoking one-half cigarette in 1 hour.

CLINICAL PRESENTATION

The gum may aggravate coronary heart disease, vasospastic disease, hypertension, peptic ulcers, diabetes, hyperthyroidism, and esophagitis. It is contraindicated in smokers who have had a recent myocardial infarction; who have life-threatening arrhythmias, severe or worsening angina, or active temporomandibular joint disease; or who are pregnant (Table 54–18).

Case Studies

Saxena and Scheman describe a depressed patient who planned his suicide using nicotine as the lethal drug: he extracted the nicotine from chewing tobacco. He remained asymptomatic for the next 24 hours, then was transferred to a psychiatric care facility.[22]

Ingestion of 7.5 to 15 g of snuff by two children was followed by gastrointestinal symptoms, agitation, and unre-

Table 54–18
Nicotine Gum[a]

Proper Use	Exclusion Criteria
Chew slowly	Active temporomandibular joint disease
Chew intermittently	Postmyocardial infarction
About 15 chews to release	Serious cardiac dysrhythmias
Park the gum	Systemic hypertension
One piece lasts 20–30 minutes	Vasospastic disease
Do not swallow immediately	Active peptic ulcer disease
Use enough	Active esophagitis
Use steadily	Oral or pharyngeal inflammation
Use for relief of discomfort	Pheochromocytoma
Use for urges to smoke	Hyperthyroidism
Avoid drinking liquids	Pregnancy
Gradually wean	Lactation
	Insulin-dependent diabetes mellitus[b]
	Extensive dental work[b]

[a]Adapted from Sees KL. West J Med 1990;152:578–584.
[b]Although not absolute exclusion criteria, exercise caution when prescribing nicotine gum for these patients.

sponsiveness. Ingestion of 1 pinch of snuff elicited no symptoms in the five children who partook of this tobacco. In severe cases, symptoms begin in 30 to 90 minutes and last 2 to 4 hours.

Nicorette gum produced toxicity within 15 to 30 minutes in four of five children who chewed up to 4 pieces and included agitation or lethargy in two children and one case each of tachycardia, hypotension, abdominal pain, vomiting, and salivation. The nicotine content of a whole cigarette is 13 to 29 mg; a cigarette butt, 3 to 7 mg; a pinch of snuff, 35 to 41 mg; and nicorette gum, 2 mg.

A 23-year-old woman who had smoked two packs per day for several years chewed a single piece of nicotine gum (2 mg nicotine) after which she developed nausea, tremulousness, flushing, palpitations, paresthesias, pruritus, vomiting, diarrhea, confusion, and abdominal pain. She recovered after treatment with compazine, morphine, and atropine.[20]

An FDA expert panel indicated that the following ingredients are not safe and effective smoking deterrents: ground cloves, ground coriander, eucalyptus oil, ground Jamaica ginger, terpeneless lemon oil, licorice root extract, menthol, methyl salicylates, quinine ascorbate, silver nitrate, and thymol. Povidone-silver nitrate is also not considered safe and effective by the FDA.[23]

CHRONIC HEALTH EFFECTS OF SMOKING[24]

EPIDEMIOLOGY

Cigarette smoking is the number one public health problem in the United States and is the single largest preventable cause of disease and death in the United States. Each year, more than 350,000 premature deaths are attributed to smoking, including 170,000 deaths from coronary heart disease, 130,000 deaths from cancer, and 50,000 deaths from obstructive lung disease. These figures do not include fetal and neonatal deaths caused by smoking during pregnancy nor do they include more than 2300 deaths caused by fires attributed to cigarette smoking.

Cancer

Cigarette smoking is a major cause of cancer of the lung, larynx, esophagus, and oral cavity and a contributing factor in causing cancer of the urinary bladder, kidney, and pancreas in both men and women. Approximately 30% of deaths from cancer have been attributed to smoking.

Lung Cancer

Since the 1950s the most common cause of death from cancer in American men has been lung cancer. In 1986 women reached a similar state. A person who smokes two packs per day is 15 to 25 times more likely to develop lung cancer than a nonsmoker.

Cancer of the Larynx

Cigarette smoking is the major causative factor for laryngeal cancer (20 to 30 : 1 smokers versus nonsmokers).

Oral Cancer

Cigarette smoking is the major cause of cancer of the lips, tongue, salivary glands, oral cavity, and middle and lower pharynx. The AMAs Council on Scientific Affairs concluded that the use of snuff or chewing tobacco is associated with an increased incidence of oral cancers.[25]

Esophageal Cancer

As with oral and laryngeal cancer, alcohol abuse acts synergistically to increase the likelihood of developing this cancer.

Urinary Bladder Cancer

Cigarette smoking increases the chance of development (3 : 1 smokers versus nonsmokers).

Kidney Cancer

The outlook is similar to that for urinary bladder cancer.

Pancreatic Cancer

Smoking is a contributory factor.

Cervical Cancer

Cigarette smoking increases the risk of developing cancer of the uterine cervix between 8 and 17 times that of the nonsmoking population. This is independent of sexual activity.[26] Risk increases with intensity and duration of smoking.[27]

Cardiovascular Disease[28]

Filter-tipped, low-tar, low-nicotine cigarettes do not appear to protect a smoker from the development of tobacco-related cardiovascular diseases. Total number of cigarettes smoked correlated significantly with severity of coronary artery disease and with the number of coronary arteries with 50% or greater stenosis.[29] After a myocardial infarction, a person who continues smoking has a greater chance of a second heart attack and sudden cardiac death. Within a few days of the cessation of smoking, carboxyhemoglobin levels, catecholamine levels, platelet adhesiveness, rapid heart rate, and myocardial irritability return toward normal. Cerebral perfusion then improves.[30] Sudden cardiac death occurs more frequently in smokers than in nonsmokers. The incidence of peripheral vascular disease and cerebral thrombosis also increases in smokers.[31] Two-pack-a-day cigarette smokers have an eight times greater risk of developing and dying from atherosclerotic aortic aneurysm than nonsmokers. In a short-term study (3 years), smoking acted to enhance vulnerability to cardiac arrest.[32]

Pulmonary Disease

Cigarette smoking is the major cause of chronic obstructive lung disease in the United States in both men and women. Cigarette smoking induces an alteration in the usual balance between alpha-antiproteases (deficient) and elastase. These alterations lead to an average 3 to 4% decline in FEV_1 per 10-pack-year history of smoking[33]; however, such an average decline does not explain the severe respiratory impairment seen in patients with disabling chronic lung disease. Atopy and childhood respiratory illness appear to increase the risk of chronic lung disease in those patients who smoke.

Neonatal Effects

Pregnant smokers deliver babies who are lighter and smaller. The risk of spontaneous abortion, fetal death, and neonatal death increases as does the frequency of abruptio placentae, placenta previa, early- or late-bleeding pregnancy, premature and prolonged rupture of membranes, and preterm delivery. Sudden infant death syndrome is more common among infants of smoking mothers. Children born to smoking mothers develop more slowly physically and mentally through the teen years.

Nieburg and colleagues[34] suggest that the term *fetal tobacco syndrome* be applied to an infant when (a) the mother smoked five or more cigarettes per day throughout the pregnancy; (b) the mother had no evidence of hypertension during pregnancy (specifically, no preeclampsia occurred and normal blood pressure was documented at least once after the first trimester); (c) the newborn had symmetrical growth retardation at term (37 weeks or more). The parameters of retardation are defined by a birth weight less than 2500 g and a ponderal index (weight in grams/length in centimeters) greater than 2.32.

Women Who Smoke

A case-control study from Sweden indicates an increased cancer risk (non-Hodgkin's lymphoma, acute lymphoblastic leukemia, Wilms' tumor) in children whose mothers smoked during pregnancy. A dose-response relationship was found between the number of cigarettes smoked per day by the mother during pregnancy and cancer risk in the offspring.[25]

Subarachnoid hemorrhage is 5.7 times more common in smokers than in nonsmokers. It is 6.5 times more common in smokers who use oral contraceptives than in smokers who do not use oral contraceptives. The risk of subarachnoid hemorrhage in women who smoke and take oral contraceptives is 22 times that in women who do not smoke and do not use oral contraceptives.

There is also an increased risk of myocardial infarction in women who smoke and use oral contraceptives.[35] Mortality of female smokers versus nonsmokers is 1.25. For women who smoke two packs per day, the ratio is 1.63. More days off work, more respiratory disease, more episodes of hospital admission, and more severe cough after lower respiratory disease occur in women who smoke. In addition, increased incidence of peptic ulcer disease (also in male smokers) and reduced fertility[36] associated with reduction in urinary estrogens are seen.[37]

REFERENCES—TOBACCO PRODUCTS

1. Diagnosis and Statistical Manual of Mental Disorders. 4th ed. DSM-IV. Washington, DC. American Psychiatric Association, 1994.
2. Henningfield JE. Nicotine medications for smoking cessation. N Engl J Med 1995;333:1196–1203.
3. Heatherton TF, Kozlowski LT, Frecker RC, Fagerstrom KO. The Fagerstrom Test for nicotine dependence: a revision of the Fagerstrom Tolerance Questionnaire. Br J Addict 1991; 86:1119–1127.
4. Lavoie FW, Harris TM. Fatal nicotine ingestion. J Emerg Med 1991;9:133–136.
5. Benowitz NL. Cigarette smoking and nicotine addiction. Med Clin North Am 1992;76:415–537.
6. Byrd JC. Environmental tobacco smoke: medical and legal issues. Med Clin North Am 1992;76:377–386.
7. Fisher EB, Jr, Haire-Joshu D, Morgan GD, Rehberg H, Post K. Smoking and smoking cessation. Am Rev Respir Dis 1990;142:702–720.
8. Tonnesen P, Norregaard J, Simonsen K, Sama V. A double-blind trial of a 16-hour transdermal nicotine patch in smoking cessation. N Engl J Med 1991;325:311–315.
9. Daughton DM, Heatley SA, Brendergast JJ, Causey D, Knowles M, Rolf CN et al. Effect of transdermal nicotine delivery as an adjunct to low-intervention smoking cessation therapy. A randomized, placebo-controlled, double-blind study. Arch Intern Med 1991;151:749–752.
10. Hjalmarson A, Franzon M, Westin A, Wiklind O. Effect of nicotine nasal spray on smoking cessation. A randomized, placebo-controlled, double-blind study. Arch Intern Med 1994;154:2567–2572.
11. Aspseloff G, Ashton HM, Friedman H, Gerber N. The importance of measuring cotinine levels to identify smokers in clinical trials. Clin Pharmacol Ther 1994;56:460–462.
12. Gourlay SG, Benowitz ML. Is clonidine an effective smoking cessation therapy? Drugs 1995;50:197–207.
13. Berlin I, Said S, Spreux-Varoquaux O, Launay J-M, Olivares R, Millet V et al. A reversible monoamine oxidase A inhibitor (moclobemide) facilitates smoking cessation and abstinence in heavy, dependent smokers. Clin Pharmacol Ther 1995;58:444–452.

13a. Sachs DPL. Effectiveness of the 4-mg dose of nicotine polacrilex for the initial treatment of high-dependent smokers. Arch Intern Med 1995;155:1973–1980.

14. Blanchard J. Nicotine. I. Clin Toxicol Rev 1993;15(1):1–2.
15. Malizia E, Andreucci G, Alfani F et al. Acute intoxication with nicotine alkaloids and cannabinoids in children from ingestion of cigarettes. Hum Toxicol 1983;2:315–316.
16. McGee D, Brabson T, McCarthy J, Picciotti M. Four-year review of cigarette ingestions in children. Pediatr Emerg Care 1995;11:13–16.
17. Gehlbach SH, Williams WA, Freeman JI. Protective clothing as a means of reducing nicotine absorption in tobacco harvests. Arch Environ Health 1979;34:111–114.
18. West R. Corticotrophin injections to treat cigarette withdrawal symptoms. J R Soc Med 1985;78:1065–1066.
19. Pechacek RF, Folsom AR, de Gaudermaris R et al. Smoke exposure in pipe and cigar smokers. Serum thiocyanate measures. JAMA 1985;254:3330–3332.
20. Mensch AR, Holden M. Nicotine overdose after a single piece of nicotine gum. Chest 1984;86:801–802.
21. Smolinske SC, Spoerke DG, Spiller SK, Wruk KM, Kulig K, Rumach BH. Cigarette and nicotine chewing gum toxicity in children. Hum Toxicol 1988;7:21–31.
22. Saxena K, Scheman A. Suicide plan by nicotine poisoning. Vet Hum Toxicol 1985;28:299 (abstract).
23. No smoking deterrents. FDA Consumer 1985;19(8):2–3.
24. Steinfeld JL. Smoking and health. West J Med 1984;141: 878–883.
25. Council on Scientific Affairs. Health effects of smokeless tobacco. JAMA 1986;255:1038–1044.
26. Lyon JD. Cancer in situ of the uterus and cigarette smoking. West J Med 1985;143:659.
27. Brinton LA, Schairer C, Haenszel W et al. Cigarette smoking and invasive cervical cancer. JAMA 1986;255:3265–3269.
28. Office on Smoking and Health. The health consequences of smoking: cardiovascular disease. A report of the Surgeon General. Rockville, MD: US Public Health Service, US Department of Health and Human Services, 1983.

29. Ramsdale DR, Faragher EB, Bray CL et al. Smoking and coronary artery disease assessed by routine coronary arteriography. Br Med J 1985;290:197–200.
30. Rogers RL, Meyer JS, Judd BW et al. Abstention from cigarette smoking improves cerebral perfusion among elderly chronic smokers. JAMA 1985;253:2970–2974.
31. Doll DC, Greenberg BR. Cerebral thrombosis in smoker's polycythemia. Ann Intern Med 1985;102:786–787.
32. Hallstrom AP, Cobb LA, Ray R. Smoking as a risk factor for recurrence of sudden cardiac arrest. N Engl J Med 1986;314: 271–275.
33. Burrows B, Knudson RJ, Cline MG et al. Qualitative relationships between cigarette smoking and ventilatory function. Am Rev Respir Dis 1977;115:195–205.
34. Nieburg P, Marks JS, McLaren NM et al. The fetal tobacco syndrome. JAMA 1985;253:2998–2999.
35. Rosenberg L, Kaufman DW, Helmirch SP et al. Myocardial infarction and cigarette smoking in women younger than 50 years of age. JAMA 1985;253:2965–2969.
36. Baird DD, Wilcox AJ. Cigarette smoking associated with delayed conception. JAMA 1985;253:2979–2983.
37. MacMahon B, Trichopoulos D, Cole P et al. Cigarette smoking and urinary estrogens. N Engl J Med 1982;307:1062–1065.

CLOVE CIGARETTES[1]

Clove cigarettes are imported from Southeast Asia, principally from Indonesia, and are composed of approximately one-third shredded cloves and two-thirds tobacco. The type of tobacco in a clove cigarette delivers approximately twice as much tars, nicotine, and carbon monoxide as does tobacco in ordinary American cigarettes.[2]

In addition, substantial amounts of eugenol, an anesthetic agent, are found in cloves and in the smoke of clove cigarettes. The typical clove cigarette smoker inhales approximately 7 mg of eugenol per clove cigarette.[2]

CLINICAL PRESENTATION

In 1984 and 1985 the U.S. Centers for Disease Control received 11 case reports of acute respiratory system injury in adolescents and young adults, including two deaths that occurred in close temporal association with smoking clove cigarettes. The acute pulmonary effects included hemoptysis, bronchospasm, hemorrhagic and nonhemorrhagic pulmonary edema, pleural effusion, respiratory insufficiency, respiratory infection, and aspiration of foreign material. The long-term dangers from the inhalation of eugenol and other chemicals in the cloves are simply not known. Another area of concern is the possible association of clove cigarette smoking and subsequent marijuana use. Because the eugenol in the clove cigarette acts as a topical anesthetic to the posterior oropharynx, it reduces the noxious elements of smoking. Thus it may facilitate the learning of smoking techniques.[2]

REFERENCES—CLOVE CIGARETTES

1. Land BW, Ellenhorn MJ, Hulbent TV, McCarron M. Clove oil ingestion in an infant. Hum Exp Toxicol 1991;10:291–294.
2. Pruitt AW, Jacobs EA, Schydlower M, Stands BO, Sutton JM, Tenenbein M et al. for the Committee on Substance Abuse. Hazards of clove cigarettes. Pediatrics 1991;88:395–396.

PARAPHENYLENEDIAMINE (PPD)

Paraphenylenediamine (Table 54–19) is used as an oxidizable hair dye, in the dyeing of furs and in the photochemical and tire vulcanizing industries. The most frequently used types of hair dyes are the oxidized "para-dyes" such as PPD. In Africa, the Middle East, and some African countries PPD is often used as a poisoning agent.

SOURCE

PPD is a derivative of paranitroaniline. It is an aromatic diamine related to aniline. The dyeing action of PPD depends on its oxidation by the addition of hydrogen peroxide forming a base that is allergenic, mutagenic, and highly toxic. The metabolic products are oxidized to a quinone structure that may be nephrotoxic. Methemoglobinuria and hemolysis probably result in the acute renal failure observed.

CLINICAL PRESENTATION

An oral dose of about 7 g is followed within 4 to 6 hours by edema of the head and neck, respiratory difficulty, drowsiness, vomiting, and dysplasia.[1] Acute renal failure, shock, increased muscle tone, rhabdomyolysis, and death may follow within 24 hours.[2] Permanent blindness may be observed. Anemia, leucocytosis, hemoglobinuria, and hemoglobinemia are common.

Table 54–19
Paraphenylenediamine Compared With Glyceryl Monothioglycolate[a]

	Use	Dermatitis	Protective Gloves	Treated Hair	Cross-Reactions
Paraphenylene-diamine (PPDA)	Most common hair dye	Allergic	All types protective vinyl recommended	PPDA-treated hair not sensitizing	Local anesthetics (procaine, novocaine), sulfonamides PPDA sunscreens
Glyceryl monothioglycolate (GMTG)	Most common permanent wave chemical	Irritant and allergic	Thick, heavy rubber gloves that are not practical investigative "4H" Danish glove	GMTG-treated hair sensitizing for three months	Very rarely cross-reacts to ammonium thioglycolate

[a]Adapted from Fisher AA. Cutis 1989;43:316–318.

TREATMENT

Treatment is mainly supportive. Early asphyxia followed by renal failure require an early tracheostomy. Renal dialysis is required when oliguria develops. Most such cases survive and make a full recovery. Intravenous corticosteroids and antihistamines have an as yet indeterminate role.

REFERENCES—PARAPHENYLENEDIAMINE

1. Ashraf W, Dawling S, Farrow LJ. Systemic paraphenylenediamine poisoning: a case report and review. Hum Exp Toxicol 1994;13:167–170.
2. Averbuch A, Modai D, Leonov Y. Rhabdomyolysis and acute renal failure induced by paraphenylenediamine. Hum Toxicol 1989;8:345–348.

PICA

DEFINITION

Pica derives from the Latin for magpie, a bird of fickle appetite that will steal and consume almost anything. The term encompasses the eating of clay, laundry starch, ashes, sand, coffee grounds, oyster shells, matches, ice, newspapers, and cigarette butts.[1] It may occur in half of patients with iron deficiency.[2–4] Patients usually conceal the problem from the physician. Oral iron therapy may lead to remission of the pica.[3,5] It is especially prevalent in Africa, Australia (among the aborigines), and in the southern states of the United States.[6,7] Controversy surrounds the cause or effect relationship with both iron and zinc.[8] Some risk factors for pica development are found in Table 54–20. Examples of pica are found in Table 54–21. Cissa is a craving for unusual or unwholesome articles of food, for example, the unusual longings of pregnancy.

FOOD PICA

Food pica is a common symptom of iron deficiency. The patient compulsively eats one kind of food. Celery, potato chips, carrots, peanut butter, sunflower seeds, parsley, soda crackers, pickles, orange juice, chocolate ice cream, lettuce, Life Savers, chewing gum, and pretzels have been ingested. It is rarely a good source of iron, but is often brittle and crunched by the teeth.[2] Food pica may terminate fatally.[6]

PAPER PICA

Pica for paper is not uncommon, especially in the mentally retarded, and can cause intestinal obstruction, intestinal perforation, and lead poisoning.[9] Glossy paper is produced by the addition of varnish, commonly ethyl cellulose, during manufacture, and may lead to a paper bezoar.[10] Mercurial compounds used as antifungal agents in the pulp and paper industry may lead to mercury poisoning in paper pica (Kleenex box, cigarette package, paperback books) devotees.[5]

Table 54-20
Risk Factors for Pica[a]

Risk Factors
Family disorganization
Poor nutrition (including iron deficiency)
Poverty
Cultural trait
Mental retardation

[a]Adapted from Sheahan K et al. Am J Forensic Med Pathol 1988;9:51–53.

Table 54–21
Pica

Cause	Effect
Starch eaters (14, 15)	Iron deficiency anemia
Magnesium carbonate (16)	Iron deficiency anemia (iron absorption interference)
Clay ingestion (geophagy) (14, 17, 18)	Hypokalemia, hyperkalemia (in chronic renal failure) (19); diminished iron absorption (20)
Paint chips from old walls or cribs	Lead poisoning (infants, children)
Ice eating (pagophagia) metabolism (21)	Disorder of iron
Food pica	Symptoms of iron deficiency? parasitic infestation
Sand, stones	Anemia, possible celiac disease

GEOPHAGY

Geophagy is the deliberate consumption of earth substances, and is classified as a form of pica. It groups together aberrant behaviors such as the consumption of starch, ice, paint, cigarette butts, and burnt matches.[11] Geophagy is widespread in the animal kingdom and is common among primates, including chimpanzees.[12] It has been implicated both as a cause and a result of particular nutritional deficiencies in man[13] and is practiced all over the world, especially in developing nations among poor blacks, the pregnant, and children.[1] It is not restricted to disadvantaged people.[2] Australian aborigines have used clay for stomach discomfort and diarrhea.[1] An abdominal x-ray may show clay opacities. The children of clay-eating, starch-eating women eat dirt, pieces of paper, flakes of paint and plaster, or whatever comes to hand.[2]

TREATMENT

Geophagy or pica for ice (pagophagia) in some patients may rapidly resolve after iron therapy.[2] Parenteral iron can stop pagophagia and food pica in some patients in a week; oral iron stops it in 2 weeks.[8]

REFERENCES—PICA

1. Editorial. Clay eating. Lancet 1978;2:614–615.
2. Crosby WH. Pica. JAMA 1976;235:2765.
3. Crosby WH. Pica: a compulsion caused by iron deficiency. Br J Hematol 1976;34:341–342.
4. Callinan V, O'Hare JA. Cardboard chewing: cause and effect of iron deficiency anemia. Am J Med 1988;85:449.

5. Olynyk F, Sharpe DH. Mercury poisoning in paper pica. N Engl J Med 1982;306:1056–1057.
6. Sheahan K, Page DV, Kemper T, Suarez R. Childhood sudden death secondary to accidental aspiration of black pepper. Am J Forensic Med Pathol 1988;9:51–53.
7. Vermeer DE, Frate DA. Geophagia in rural Mississippi: environmental and cultural contexts and nutritional implications. Am J Clin Nutr 1979;32:2129–2135.
8. Korman SH. Pica as a presenting symptom in celiac disease. Am J Clin Nutr 1990;51:139–141.
9. Keeling PJ, Ransay J, Shand WS. Pica, paper and pseudoporphyria. Lancet 1987;2:1095.
10. Uretsky BF. Paper bezoar causing intestinal obstruction. Arch Surg 1974;109:123.
11. Johns T, Duquette M. Detoxification mineral supplementation as function of geophagy. Am J Clin Nutr 1991;53:448–456.
12. Hladik CM, Gueguen L. Geophagy and mineral nutrition in wild primates. C R Acad Sci 1974;279:1393–1396 (in French).
13. Halstead JA. Geophagia in man: its nature and nutritional effects. Am J Clin Nutr 1968;21:1384–1393.
14. Roselle HA. Association of laundry starch and clay ingestion with anemia in New York City. Arch Intern Med 1970;125:57–61.
15. Warshauer SE. Starch eater's anemia. South Med J 1966;59:538–540.
16. Leming PD, Reed DC, Martello DJ. Magnesium carbonate pica: an unusual case of iron deficiency. Ann Intern Med 1981;94:660.
17. Gonzalez JJ, Owens W, Ungaro PC, Werk EE Jr, Wentz PW. Clay ingestion. A rare cause of hypokalemia. Ann Intern Med 1982;97:65–66.
18. Severance HW Jr, Holt T, Patrone NA, Chapman L. Profound muscle weakness and hypokalemia due to clay ingestion. South Med J 1988;81:272–274.
19. Gelfand MC, Zarate A, Knepshield JH. Geophagia: a cause of life-threatening hyperkalemia in patients with chronic renal failure. JAMA 1975;234:738.
20. Minnich V, Okcuoglu A, Tarcon Y, Arcasoy A, Cin S, Yorukoglu O et al. Pica in Turkey. II. Effect of clay upon iron absorption. Am J Clin Nutr 1968;21:78–86.
21. Coltman CAJ. Pagophagia and iron lack. JAMA 1969;207:513–516.

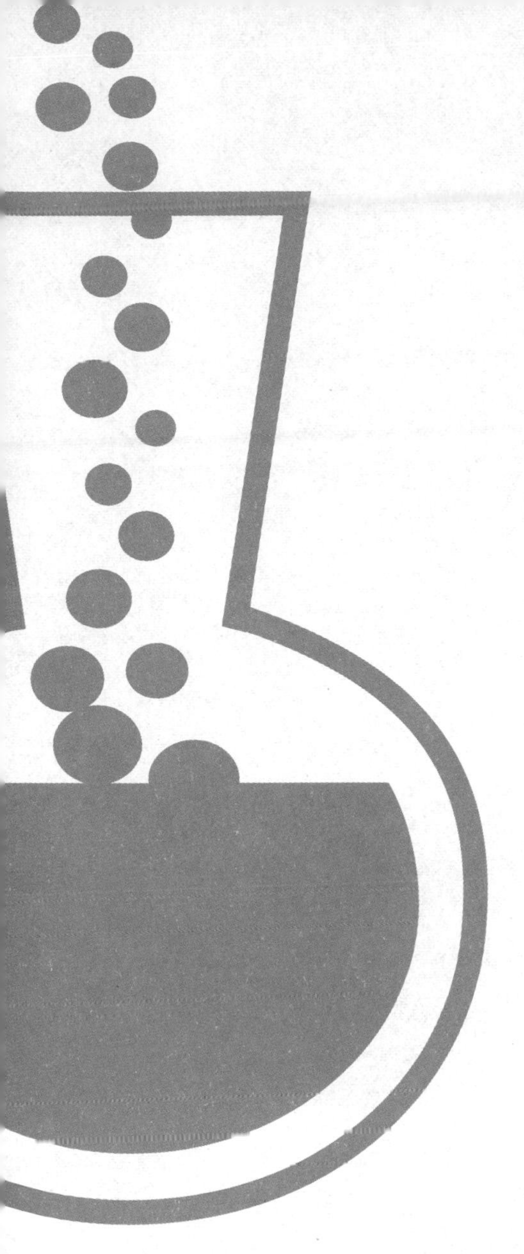

Section IV
CHEMICALS

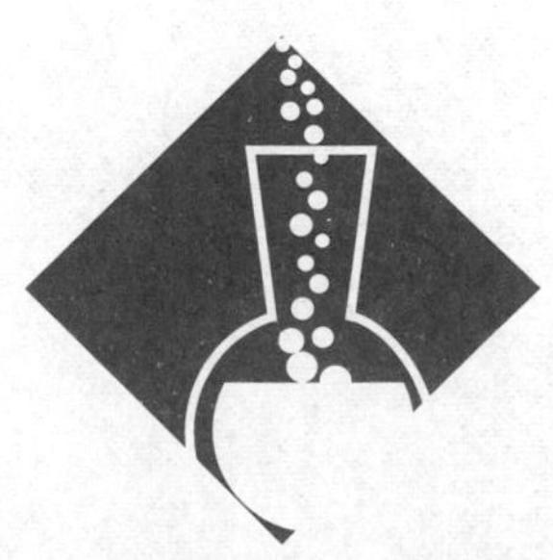

Chapter 55
Alcohols and Glycols

ETHANOL

ACUTE TOXICITY

Clinical toxicities related to ethanol use are summarized in Table 55–1. A survey of clinical and laboratory manifestations seen in the critical care setting with the alcohols is seen in Table 55–2.[1]

Figure 55-1 presents a summary of statutory limits for alcohol while driving in Europe. Similar levels are applicable for the United States. Although lower BACs (0.01 to 0.09 g/dL) can cause driving impairment associated with an increased risk for fatal crash involvement, the risk is substantially greater for high levels of alcohol (BACs more or less than 0.10 g/dL).[2] In the UK there is some support for changing the legal drinking-driving limit from 17.4 mmol/L (0.8 g/L) to 10.9 mmol/L.[3,4]

TRAUMA

An increase in blood alcohol has been associated with fatal aircraft accidents,[5] fatal aqauatic activity,[6,7] pedestrian deaths,[7] and fatal[5] motor vehicle crashes.[8] Interestingly, a prospective cohort study suggests that chronic but not acute alcohol abuse adversely affects outcome from blunt or penetrating trauma (increase in complications, particularly pneumonia, and longer hospital stays). Screening trauma patients for chronic alcohol abuse may help to confirm this observation.[9]

OVER-THE-COUNTER FORMULATIONS WITH ETHANOL

Tables 55–3 and 55–4 summarize ethanol content in some common products.

URETHANE

Urethane, a carcinogen in animals, forms naturally during the fermentation process (Table 55–5).[10] The U.S. Food and Drug Administration does not at present have recommendations limiting urethane in alcoholic beverages.

Table 55-1
Acute Toxicity of the Alcohols[a]

	Ethanol	Methanol	Ethylene Glycol	Isopropanol
CNS depressant	+	+	+	+
Convulsion	+	+	+	+
Odor	+	–	–	+ (acetone)
Blood gases	Respiratory Acidosis Ketoacidosis	Severe Metabolic Acidosis	Severe Metabolic Acidosis	Mild Metabolic Acidosis
Anion gap	+	+++	+++	+
Osmolar gap	+	+	+	+
Oxalate crystaluria	–	–	++	–
Symptom onset	30 min	12–48 hr	30 min–12 hr	Rapid
Lethal dose	5–8 g/kg	1–5 g/kg	1.5 g/kg	3–4 g/kg
Lethal blood level (mg/dL)	350–500	80	200	400
Special treatment	HD	ETOH; HD	ETOH; HCO_3; HD	HD; HCO_3

HD, hemodialysis.
[a]Adapted from Ellenhorn MJ. In: Hall JB et al, eds. Principles of critical care. New York: McGraw-Hill, 1992, 2080–2093.

Table 55-2
Ethanol Toxicity in the Critical Care Setting[a]

- Suicides/Trauma
  - Traffic accidents
  - Suicide attempts
  - Cervical and cerebral trauma
  - Subdural hematoma
- Gastrointestinal
  - Acute and chronic recurrent pancreatitis
  - Mallory-Weiss syndrome
  - Hematemesis—ruptured esophageal varices
  - Hepatic failure with encephalopathy
- Respiratory
  - Aspiration pneumonia
  - Atelectasis
  - Pneumothorax
  - Fractured ribs
- Muscular
  - Rhabdomyolysis
  - Myoglobinuria
- Neurologic
  - Seizures
  - Central pontine myelinosis
  - Polyradiculoneuropathy
  - Wernicke's encephalopathy
  - Korsakoff's psychosis
  - Pellagra encephalopathy
  - Coma
- Cardiovascular
  - Hypertension
  - Subarachnoid hemorrhage
  - Depressed left ventricular function
  - Supraventricular arrhythmias
  - Cardiomyopathy
- Endocrine/Metabolic
  - Hypoglycemia, especially young children
  - Acidosis, metabolic and respiratory
  - Hypokalemia, hypomagnesemia
- Ethanol Withdrawal Syndromes
- Coingested Alcohols
  - Methanol, ethylene glycol, isopropyl alcohol

[a]Adapted from Ellenhorn MJ. In: Hall JB et al, eds. Principles of critical care. New York: McGraw-Hill, 1992, 2080–2093.

TOXICOKINETICS

Absorption

Gastric Alcohol Dehydrogenase

Alcohol dehydrogenase in the gastric mucosa contributes substantially to alcohol metabolism (gastric first-pass metabolism). Studies of alcohol dehydrogenase activity in gastric biopsies of women suggest a significant decrease in such gastric alcohol dehydrogenase activity in women when compared with men. This can explain the findings in women of higher peak blood alcohol concentrations, smaller volumes of distribution, higher bioavailability of alcohol, and the presence of liver damage after consumption of relatively smaller quantities of alcohol when compared with men.[11,12] This finding is reversed in men over age 50 years.[13]

Elimination/Drug Interactions (Table 55-6)

P450IIE1 Induction

P450IIE1 is an ethanol-inducible form of cytochrome P-450 that may, after long-term consumption of alcohol, be capable of metabolically activating some other compounds to metabolites or to compounds known to be hepatotoxic. Susceptible compounds include carbon tetrachloride, bromobenzene, and anesthetic agents, aflatoxin B–induced necrosis and steatosis, isoniazid, phenylbutazone, acetaminophen, cocaine, nitrosodimethylamine, and methadone. Short-term alcohol use, on the other hand, inhibits microsomal demethylation of methadone, thus enhancing brain and liver concentrations of the drug by direct competition for cytochrome P-450. Ethanol can inhibit metabolism of tranquilizers and barbiturates, enhancing their concentration in the blood.[14]

Both aspirin and H_2 receptor antagonists inhibit the action of gastric alcohol dehydrogenase and thereby increase the blood levels of alcohol.[15,16] Cigarette smoking appears to slow gastric emptying and thereby delays alcohol absorption with resultant reductions in peak blood alcohol concentrations after ingestions of 0.5 g/kg of ethanol (from 13.5 mML/L [63.1 mg/dL] to 11.4 mML/L [511 mg/dL]).[17]

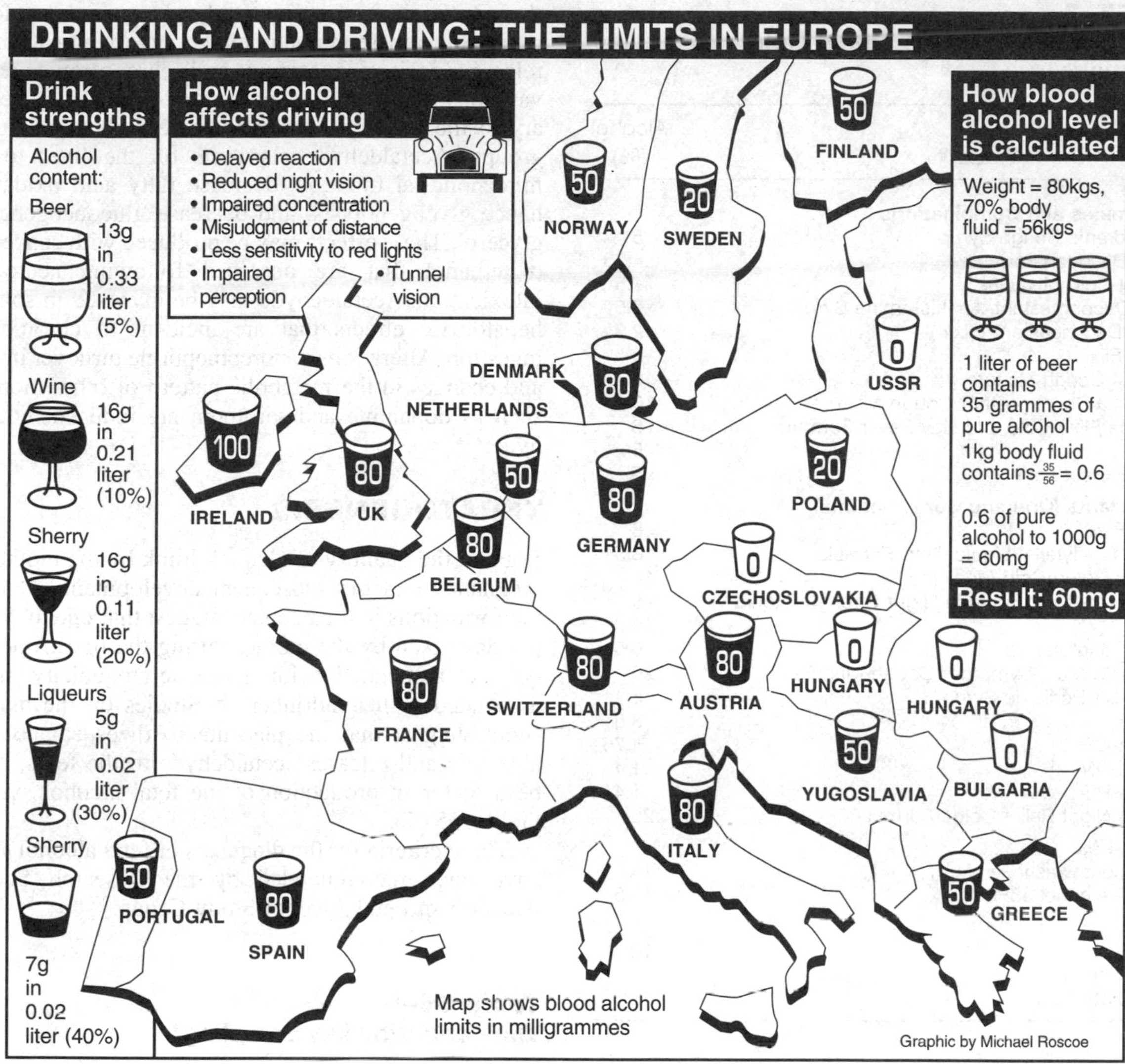

Figure 55–1. One for the road: holidaymakers driving in Europe this summer will find widely differing limits on drink-driving. In some countries, such as Bulgaria, Romania and Turkey, drivers must be teetotal. Those who like a tipple will discover that the rules are most relaxed in Republic of Ireland. (From The European. May 24, 1991.)

Cocaethylene (See Cocaine Chapter)/ Cocapropylene

Cocapropylene (propylcocaine) is formed by transesterification of cocaine with *n*-propanol in whole human liver homogenates in vitro.[18] This product appears to have strong topical anesthetic activity.[19] Its importance in clinical cocaine toxicity has yet to be determined.[19]

ACETALDEHYDE

Clinical Presentation

Acetaldehyde, produced by all known oxidative pathways of ethanol metabolism, is in turn converted to acetate by aldehyde dehydrogenase. Asians often harbor an inactive aldehyde dehydrogenase variant that causes them to experience high blood acetaldehyde levels when they drink, with subsequent development of ethanol intolerance and flushing.[20] Disulfiram, an inhibitor of acetaldehyde dehydrogenase, raises the acetaldehyde levels similarly in most subjects after drinking and causes flushing and other adverse effects. Similar elevations of plasma acetaldehyde and facial flushing follow ingestions of calcium carbamide.[21] Other inhibitors of acetaldehyde dehydrogenase include metronidazole, sulfonylurea antidiabetic drugs, the fungicide thiram, and the ink cap mushroom, *Coprinus atramentarius.* Acetaldehyde is also a metabolite of paraldehyde. Pathologic findings in deaths from acetaldehyde poisoning include pulmonary edema, nausea, narcosis, respiratory failure, cardiac dilatation, cardiovascular collapse, congestive heart failure, seizures, and sudden death.[22,23] Death of a 17-year-old boy after ethanol ingestion was associated with a blood acetaldehyde level of 1 mg/mL and an ethanol level of 110 mg/dL.[23]

Mechanism of Action

Acetaldehyde in blood is decreased by reactions with compounds containing sulfhydryl and amino groups (e.g.,

Table 55-3
Alcohol Content of Some Liquid Cold Preparations

Product	Alcohol (%)
Antihistamines and Combinations	
Vicks Children's Cough Syrup	5
Cheracol D Cough Formula	4.75
Co-Tylenol Cold Medicine	7.5
Demazin Decongtestant–Antihistamine Syrup	7.5
Dimetane Decongestant Elixir	2.3
Dimetane Elixir	3
Formula 44 Cough Mixture	10
Formula 44D Decongestant Cough Mixture	10
Novahistine Elixir Cold and Hay Fever Formula	5
Nyquil	25
Triaminic Expectorant	5
Decongestants (Oral and Combinations)	
Cheracol Plus	8
Children's Co-Tylenol Liquid Cold Formula	8.5
Cogespirin Liquid Cold Medicine	10
Contac Severe Cold Formula Night Strength Liquid	25
Contac Jr	10
Coricidin Cough Syrup	0.5
Formula 44M Multi-Symptom Cough Mixture	20
Naldecon-DX Pediatric Syrup	5
Robitussin	3.5
Robitussin-CF	4.75
Robitussin-DM	1.4
Robitussin-PE	1.4
Robitussin Night Relief Colds Formula	25
Mouthwashes	
Cepacol Mouthwash/Gargle	14
Scope (SD Alcohol 38F)	18.5
Other	
Geritol	12
Paregoric tincture	45
Terpin hydrate elixir	42

Table 55-4
Approximate Percent Ethanol Content of Some Common Products[a]

Product	Percent EtOH
Ale	3–6%
After-shaves	15–80%
Brady	40–50%
Beer	4–6%
Bourbon	40–50%
Colognes	40–60%
Cough medicine	5–70%
Elixirs	2–10%
Gasohol	10%
Medications	0.3–68%
Nyquil	25%
Mouthwash	15–25% up to 75%
Perfumes	25–95%
Rum	40–50%
Scotch	40–50%
Vodka	40–50%
Wine	10–20%

[a]From Vogel C et al. Clin Toxicol 1995;33:25–33.

d-penicillamine). Cardiovascular sequelae develop as a result of sympathomimetic effects involving catecholamine release (positive inotropic and chronotropic responses, vasoconstriction and hypertension), which may be secondary to the reaction of acetaldehyde with tissue sulfhydryl groups. Acetaldehyde also acts on the liver to depress mitochondrial function, decrease fatty acid oxidation, enhance glycogenolysis, and decrease gluconeogenesis from glycerol. These effects may be produced with concentrations of ethanol that are observed following acute ethanol intoxication. Acetaldehyde may be involved in some of the hepatotoxic effects that are incident to chronic ethanol ingestion. Alterations in norepinephrine turnover in the brain and changes in the metabolic pattern of other monoamines such as dopamine and serotonin are induced by acetaldehyde.[22]

TERATOGENESIS

Data on the quantity of alcohol drunk by the mother during pregnancy and the subsequent development of congenital malformations in the neonate suggest that one to two drinks per day taken by the mother during the first trimester may not be associated with more teratogenicity than that associated with nondrinkers.[24] Studies on the human placenta suggest that the placenta oxidizes ethanol to acetaldehyde and releases acetaldehyde to the fetus. This may be a factor in production of the fetal alcohol syndrome[25] (Table 55–7).

Three criteria for the diagnosis of fetal alcohol syndrome have been recommended by the Research Society on Alcoholism Fetal Alcohol Study Group.[26]

Table 55-5
Wine and Whiskey Sampling[a]

FDA and the U.S. Bureau of Alcohol, Tobacco and Firearms has sampled wines and whiskeys from domestic and foreign producers to determine urethane levels.

The following are the results of two samplings measuring average urethane levels in parts per billion (ppb). The 1987 figures represent the FDA-ATF initial survey of domestic and imported alcoholic beverages, collected from January 1986 through August 1987. This compares with an ATF sampling done in 1991 that shows urethane levels decreasing in most instances.

	Average Urethane Level (ppb)		
	1987	1991	
Product		Domestic	Imported
Brandy (grape)	40	10	45
Brandy (fruit)	1,200	5	255
Bourbon (retail)	150	70	55
Rum	20	2	5
Liqueur	100	10	25
Scotch	50	[b]	55
Sherry	130	10	40
Port	60	23	26
Grape wine	13	10	15
Sake	300	55	60

[a]Adapted from Foulke FL. FDA Consumer. 1993;27(1):23.
[b]Scotch is not manufactured domestically.

Table 55-6
Adverse Interactions With Alcohol[a]

Interacting Drug	Adverse Effect	Probable Mechanisms
Acetaminophen (Tylenol, others)	Increased acute hepatotoxicity	Increased production of toxic metabolites
Anesthetics	Decreased effectiveness for induction of anesthesia	Increased tolerance to anesthetics
	Increased level of anesthesia	Additive
Anticoagulants, oral	Decreased anticoagulant effect with chronic alcohol abuse	Increased metabolism
	Increased anticoagulant effect with acute intoxication	Decreased metabolism
Antihistamines	Increased CNS depression with acute intoxication	Additive
Barbiturates	Decreased sedative effect with chronic alcohol abuse	Increased metabolism
	Increased CNS depression with acute intoxication	Additive; decreased metabolism
Benzodiazepines	Increased CNS depression	Additive
Bromocriptine (Parlodel)	Nausea, abdominal pain	Possible increased dopamine receptor sensitivity
Chloral hydrate (Noctec, others)	Prolonged hypnotic effect	Synergism
Chloramphenicol (Chloromycetin, others)	Minor Antabuselike symptoms	Inhibition of intermediary metabolism of alcohol
Cycloserine (Seromycin)	Increased convulsions with chronic abuse	Not established
Disulfiram (Antabuse)	Abdominal cramps, flushing, vomiting, psychotic episodes, confusion	Inhibition of intermediary metabolism of alcohol
Hypoglycemics, oral, sulfonylureas	Decreased hypoglycemic effect with chronic alcohol abuse	Increased metabolism
	Increased hypoglycemic effect with ingestion of alcohol, particularly in fasting patients	Suppression of gluconeogenesis
	Minor Antabuselike symptoms	Inhibition of intermediary metabolism of alcohol
	Flushing with chlorpropamide (Diabinese)	Not established
Isoniazid (INH, others)	Increased incidence of hepatitis	Not established
	Decreased isoniazid effect in some patients with chronic alcohol abuse	Increased metabolism
Meprobamate (Equanil, Miltown, others)	Decreased sedative effect with chronic alcohol abuse	Increased metabolism
	Increased CNS depression with acute intoxication	Additive; decreased metabolism
Methisazone (Marboran)	Increased methisazone toxicity	Not established
Metronidazole (Flagyl)	Mild Antabuselike symptoms	Possible inhibition of intermediary metabolism of alcohol
Narcotics	Increased CNS depression with acute intoxication	Additive
Phenformin	Lactic acidosis	Synergism
Phenothiazines	Increased CNS depression	Additive
Phenytoin (Dilantin, others)	Decreased anticonvulsant effect with chronic alcohol abuse	Increased metabolism
	Increased anticonvulsant effect wtih acute intoxication	Decreased metabolism
Propranolol (Inderal)	Masks tachycardia and tremor of alcoholic hypoglycemia	β-Receptor blockade
Quinacrine (Atabrine)	Minor Antabuselike symptoms	Inhibition of intermediary metabolism of alcohol
Salicylates	Gastrointestinal bleeding	Additive

[a]Adapted from Interactions of drugs with alcohol. Med Lett Drugs Ther 1981;23:34. Used by special permission from The Medical Letter.

1. Prenatal growth retardation of length, weight, or head circumference (≤2 SD) or postnatal growth retardation of length, head circumference (≤2 SD), or relative weight (≤10%) or both.
2. Dysfunction of central nervous system indicated (a) by performance below −2 SD on the Bayley Mental Scale or in the Reynell Verbal Comprehension Test or (b) by performance better than −2 SD in the developmental tests used, but with difficulties in active speech, fine motor development, or perception needing further follow-up.
3. Craniofacial criteria with at least two of the following: (a) head circumference ≤2 SD, (b) palpebral fissure ≤2 SD, and (c) hypoplastic philtrum and thin upper lip.

The diagnosis of fetal alcohol effects is made when only two of the criteria are present.[27]

Table 55-7
Features Observed in Fetal Alcohol Syndrome/ Fetal Alcohol Effects[a]

Growth
- Prenatal and postnatal growth deficiency†
- Decreased adipose tissue‡

Performance
- Mental retardation†
- Developmental delay
- Fine-motor dysfunction
- Infant irritability†, child hyperactivity‡, and poor attention span
- Speech problems
- Poor coordination, hypotonia‡
- Cognitive, behavioral, and psychosocial problems

Craniofacial
- Microcephaly†
- Short palpebral fissures†
- Ptosis§
- Retrognathia in infancy†
- Maxillary hypoplasia‡
- Hypoplastic long or smooth philtrum†
- Thin vermillion of upper lip†
- Short upturned nose‡
- Micrognathia in adolescence‡

Skeletal
- Joint alterations including camptodactyly, flexion contractures at elbows, congenital hip dislocations
- Foot position defects
- Radioulnar synostosis
- Tapering terminal phalanges, hypoplastic finger- and toenails||
- Cervical spine abnormalities
- Altered palm crease pattern§
- Pectus excavatum§

Cardiac
- Ventricular septal defect||
- Atrial septal defect§
- Tetralogy of Fallot, great vessel anomalies||

Other
- Cleft lip and/or cleft palate||
- Myopia||, strabismus§
- Epicanthal folds§
- Dental malocclusion
- Hearing loss, protuberant ears
- Abnormal thoracic cage
- Strawberry hemangiomata§
- Hypoplastic labia majora§
- Microophthalmia, blepharophimosis||
- Small teeth with faulty enamel||
- Hypospadias, small rotated kidneys, hydronephrosis||
- Hirsutism in infancy||
- Hernias of diaphragm, umbilicus or groin, diastasis recti||

[a]From Committee on Substance Abuse. American Academy of Pediatrics. Pediatrics 1993;91:1004–1006.
Principle (†,‡) and associated (§,||) features observed in 245 affected individuals.[15] † >80%; ‡>50%; § 26% to 50%; || 1% to 25% of patients.

Fetal alcohol syndrome (FAS) is difficult to recognize in newborns because facial stigmata of FAS are often subtle. Some types of central nervous system deficits in infants are difficult to detect and the birth weight of some affected infants is normal.[28]

The National Institute on Alcohol Abuse and Alcoholism (NIAAA)—which joined the National Institutes of Health (NIH) on October 1, 1992—has the major responsibility for research on FAS and ARBD. At NIAAA's Fetal Alcohol Research Center at Wayne State University, Detroit, Michigan, Robert J. Sokol, M.D., and associates Susan S. Martier, MSSA, and Joel W. Ager, PhD, have developed a four-question test (T-ACE) that takes less than 1 minute to administer. The quiz circumvents the problems of denial and underreporting that historically make self-reporting, the only other screening technique available, of limited value.

Known as T-ACE, the test has the further advantage of not seeming to pry into current drinking habits, which might prompt untruthful answers. The key question concerns *tolerance,* one of the best predictors of continued drinking throughout pregnancy: "How many drinks does it take to make you feel high?"

A woman who replies "more than two," Sokol's team found, is more likely to drink enough alcohol to bear an infant with alcohol-related birth defects or fetal alcohol syndrome. That risk is amplified by positive responses to at least one of T-ACE's other queries about whether she has been *annoyed* by criticism of her drinking, has felt she should *cut down,* and has ever had a drink first thing in the morning to steady her or get rid of a hangover *(eye-opener).*

Lactation

Following ingestion of ethanol by the lactating mother, breast milk samples will contain alcohol that can be perceived by odor. Studies of infant behavior suggest that alcohol in breast milk will lead to a reduced consumption of milk by the infant.[29]

PATHOPHYSIOLOGY

Abuse

A positive association between the A1 allele of the D2R dopamine receptor gene and alcoholism has been reported, suggesting that a mutation that confers susceptibility to this clinical condition is present in the vicinity of the restriction site of the Taq 1 enzymes, located in the DRD2 gene. The number of DRD2 sites is reduced in human alcoholics. Further data to validate the significance of these observations are indicated.[30–32]

Alcohol Dependency

Diagnostic tests have been devised to identify problem drinkers or alcohol dependence. Alcohol dependence represents a syndrome diagnosed by DSM-III-R (Diagnostic and Statistical Manual of Mental Disorders, Revised, Third Edition—American Psychiatric Association) and the International Statistical Classification of Diseases, Tenth Revision (ICD-10) (Table 55–8).

Several questionnaires have been developed for the detection of alcohol disorders, including the CAGE (cut down, annoyed by criticism, guilty about drinking, eye-opener drinks) questionnaire, the Michigan Alcoholism Screening Test (MAST) (Table 55–9), and the AUDIT (Table 55–10), and they are summarized by Allen and Colleagues (Table 55–11).[33] The most widely used are the CAGE questionnaire and the MAST. Of these the MAST has been more thoroughly studied in terms of reliability and accuracy. However, the MAST and its shortened versions are more complicated than the CAGE questionnaire. The CAGE questionnaire is short, easily memorized, and reasonably accurate, making it the screening test of choice for busy house officers and practitioners.

Some authors contend that ingestion of four or more drinks per day in man and two or more drinks per day in women constitute a "hazardous" consumption level that increases the risk of alcohol dependence and medical problems. A "drink" is defined as equivalent volume amounts that have an ethanol content of 0.6 oz. Twelve ounces of beer, 5 oz of wine, and 1.5 oz of liquor all contain 0.6 oz of ethanol.

The CAGE questionnaire can be a useful tool in the diagnosis of DSM-III-R–defined abuse and dependence and very heavy drinking (>8 drinks per day). Scores of 3 or 4 strongly support the diagnosis of alcohol abuse. The CAGE questionnaire has not been tested as a tool for identifying persons who may be engaged in hazardous drinking of lesser amounts of alcohol, for example, 4 drinks per day. The AUDIT was recently developed to identify hazardous drinkers.[34]

Table 55-8
DSM III-R and ICD-10 Diagnostic Criteria for Substance Abuse, Harmful Use, and Substance Dependence[a]

DMM-III-R Dependence (3 Items Required)
1. Substance often taken in larger amounts or over a longer period than the person intended.
2. Persistent desire or one or more unsuccessful efforts to cut down or control substance use.
3. A great deal of time spent in activities necessary to get substance, taking substance, or recovering from its effects.
4. a. Recurrent use when substance use is physically hazardous (eg, drives while intoxicated) or
b. Frequent intoxication or withdrawal symptoms when expected to perform major role obligations at work, school, or home.
5. Important social, occupational, or recreational activities given up or reduced because of substance use.
6. Continued substance use despite knowledge of having persistent or recurrent social, psychological, or physical problem that is caused or exacerbated by the use of substance.
7. Marked tolerance: need for markedly increased amounts of substance (at least a 50% increase) to achieve intoxication or desired effect, or markedly diminished effect with continued use of the same amount.
8. Characteristic withdrawal symptoms.
9. Substance often taken to relieve or avoid withdrawal symptoms.
DSM-III-R Abuse
1. Continued use despite knowledge of having persistent or recurrent social, occupational, psychological, or physical problem that is caused or exacerbated by the use of substance.
2. Recurrent use in situations in which use is physically hazardous.
ICD-10 Dependence (3 Items Required)
1. A strong desire or sense of compulsion to use a substance.
2. Evidence of impaired capacity to control the use of a substance. This may relate to difficulties in avoiding initial use, difficulties in terminating use, or problems controlling levels of use.
3. A withdrawal state or use of the substance to relieve or avoid withdrawal symptoms, and subjective awareness of the effectiveness of such behavior.
4. Evidence of ??? of the effects of the substance.
5. Progressive neglect of alternative pleasures, behaviors, or interests in favor of substance use.
6. Persisting with substance use despite clear evidence of harmful consequences.
ICD-10 Harmful Use
1. Clear evidence that the use of a substance was responsible for causing actual psychological or physical harm to the user.

[a]DSM-III-R indicates Diagnostic and Statistical Manual of Mental Disorders, Revised Third Edition; ICD-10, International Statistical Classification of Diseases, 10th Revision.

Wernicke's Encephalopathy

Acute pancreatitis, hyperemesis gravidarum, anorexia nervosa, prolonged fasting, malnutrition in infancy, gastric plication, prolonged feeding (including total parenteral nutrition), leukemia, lymphoma, chronic renal failure, thyrotoxicosis, and acquired immunodeficiency syndrome, in addition to ethanol, have been associated with the development of Wernicke's encephalopathy and Korsakoff's syndrome.[35,36]

CLINICAL PRESENTATION

Acute Intoxication

Children

Percutaneous alcohol intoxication has been described in young children after use of alcohol-soaked gauze pads.[37] Chemical burns of the skin in neonates can follow applications of alcoholic skin preparations.[38] In juvenile alcohol intoxication, metabolic acidosis and decreased blood pH may be correlated with the blood alcohol concentration and loss of consciousness. Hypoglycemia is the most common reported symptom in children under 5 years of age. The hypoglycemic effects of ethanol are not dose dependent. The fasting state may predispose a child to ethanol-induced hypoglycemia.[39] Hypokalemia is an important concomitant finding. Alcohol abuse occurs in very young children.[40,41]

Adults

Ethanol is a selective CNS depressant in low doses and a generalized depressant in high doses. Comparison of cognitive and psychomotor skills at blood ethanol levels of 90 and 135 mg/dL indicates that attention, concentration, motor coordination, and reaction time are significantly more affected at the higher level. At these same levels no difference was observed in visual and verbal memory.[42] Initially, ethanol produces exhilaration, which progresses to loss of restraint, behavioral abnormalities, loquaciousness, slurred speech, ataxia, gait disturbances, irritability, drowsiness, and finally stupor and coma. A flushed face, dilated pupils, excessive sweating, and gastrointestinal distress may accompany CNS symptoms. Rarely, alcohol-induced urticaria occurs, which is partially mediated by histamine.[43] Ethanol can produce dysrhythmias (e.g., atrial fibrillation) in nontolerant binge drinkers, as well as in chronic alcoholics.[44] Ethanol is a venodilator that produces decreased preload, afterload, and systemic vascular resistance in healthy adults after acute ingestion. When these factors are corrected, acute ingestion also has a myocardial depressant effect.[45] Toler-

Table 55-9
Life-style Risk Assessment Instrument, Northeastern Vermont Regional Hospital, St Johnsbury[a]

	Score
Name	
Date of birth	
Sex	
Medical record No.	
Date	
Time	
I. Trauma history (from Skinner et al[26])	
Since your 18th birthday, have you	
had any fractures or dislocations to your bones or joints?	____
been injured in a road traffic accident?	____
injured your head?	____
been injured in an assault or fight (excluding sports)?	____
been injured after drinking?	____
Total ____	
Do you wear seat belts while riding in a car?	____
II. Exercise and physical fitness	
Do you exercise regularly each week? How many times per week	____
Do you feel you haven't enough time for exercising?	____
Do you feel more exercise would be better for your health?	____
III. CAGE questions (from Mayfield et al[11])	
Have you ever felt you should Cut down on your drinking?	____
Have people Annoyed you by criticizing your drinking?	____
Have you ever felt bad or Guilty about your drinking?	____
Have you ever had a drink first thing in the morning to steady your nerves or get rid of a hangover (*E*ye-opener)?	____
Total ____	
IV. Smoking	
How much do you smoke each day?	____
Have you tried to stop smoking? How many times?	____
What is the longest time you were able to stop?	____
V. Stress management	
Are you a nervous person?	____
Do you feel discouraged much of the time?	____
Do you manage your nerves effectively?	____
Have you taken a vacation this year?	____
VI. Diet	
Do you control your diet for	
cholesterol?	____
salt (sodium)?	____
total calories?	____
VII. Michigan Alcoholism Screening Test (MAST; from Selzer et al[9]; see below for questions)	
Total score	____
Yes to questions 8, 19, or 20	____
VIII. Laboratory data[b]	
MCV	____
GGT	____
AST	____
Admitting BAC	____
IX. Miscellaneous observations during interview; previous alcohol, drug, or psychiatric care	
X. Reason for admission	
XI. Conclusion and interpretation	
XII. Has this interview been a positive experience for you?	
NO 1 2 3 4 5 Yes	

MAST questions[c]	Score
1. Do you feel you are a normal drinker (by normal we mean you drink less than or as much as most other people)?	N 2
2. Have you ever awakened the morning after some drinking the night before and found that you could not remember a part of the evening?	Y 2
3. Does your wife, husband, a parent, or other near relative ever worry or complain about your drinking?	Y 1
4. Can you stop drinking without a struggle after 1 or 2 drinks?	N 2
5. Do you ever feel guilty about your drinking?	Y 1
6. Do friends or relatives think you are a normal drinker?	N 2
7. Are you always able to stop drinking when you want to?	N 2
8. Have you ever attended a meeting of Alcoholics Anonymous?	Y 5
9. Have you gotten into physical fights when drinking?	Y 1
10. Has drinking ever created problems between you and your wife, husband, a parent, or other near relative?	Y 2
11. Has your wife, husband, a parent, or other near relative ever gone to anyone for help about your drinking?	Y 2
12. Have you ever lost boyfriends or girlfriends because of your drinking?	Y 2
13. Have you ever gotten into trouble at work because of your drinking?	Y 2
14. Have you ever lost a job because of drinking?	Y 2
15. Have you ever neglected your obligations, your family, or your work for 2 or more days in a row because you were drinking?	Y 2
16. Do you drink before noon fairly often?	Y 1
17. Have you ever been told you have liver trouble? Cirrhosis?	Y 2
18. After heavy drinking, have you ever had delirium tremens (DTs) or severe shaking, or heard voices or seen things that weren't really there?	Y 2
19. Have you ever gone to anyone for help about your drinking?	Y 5
20. Have you ever been in a hospital because of drinking?	Y 5
21. Have you ever been a patient in a psychiatric hospital or a psychiatric ward where drinking was part of the problem that resulted in hospitalization?	Y 2
22. Have you ever been seen at a psychiatric or mental health clinic, or gone to any doctor, social worker, or clergyman for help with any emotional problem where drinking was part of the problem?	Y 2
23. Have you ever been arrested for drunken driving, driving while intoxicated, or driving under the influence of alcoholic beverages?	Y 2
24. Have you ever been arrested, even for a few hours, because of drunken behavior?	Y 2
Total Score	____

[a]Adapted from Graham AW. Arch Intern Med 1991;151:958–964.
[b]MCV indicates mean corpuscular volume; GGT, γ-glutamyltransferase; AST, aspartate aminotransferase; and BAC, blood alcohol concentration.
[c]Revised 1975. Scores of 0 to 4 indicate nonalcoholic; 5 or 6, suggestive of alcoholism; and over 7, alcoholism. These are the more conservative screening values of Selzer et al, with reduced false positives but reduced sensitivity.

Table 55-10
Alcohol Use Disorders Identification Test (AUDIT) Questions[a]

1. How often do you have a drink containing alcohol?
   Never | Monthly or less | 2 to 4 times a month | 2 or 3 times a week | 4 or more times a week
2. How many drinks containing alcohol do you have on a typical day when you are drinking?
   1 or 2 | 3 or 4 | 5 or 6 | 7 to 9 | 10 or more
3. How often do you have 6 or more drinks on one occasion?
   Never | Less than monthly | Monthly | Weekly | Daily or almost daily
4. How often during the last year have you found that you were not able to stop drinking once you had started?
   Never | Less than monthly | Monthly | Weekly | Daily or almost daily
5. How often during the last year have you failed to do what was expected from you because of drinking?
   Never | Less than monthly | Monthly | Weekly | Daily or almost daily
6. How often during the last year have you needed a first drink in the morning to get yourself going after a heavy drinking session?
   Never | Less than monthly | Monthly | Weekly | Daily or almost daily
7. How often in the last year have you had a feeling of guilt or remorse after drinking?
   Never | Less than monthly | Monthly | Weekly | Daily or almost daily
8. How often during the last year have you been unable to remember what happened the night before because you had been drinking?
   Never | Less than monthly | Monthly | Weekly | Daily or almost daily
9. Have you or someone else been injured as a result of your drinking?
   No | Yes, but not in the last year | Yes, during the last year
10. Has a relative or friend or a doctor or other health worker been concerned about your drinking or suggested you cut down?
   No | Yes, but not in the last year | Yes, during the last year

[a]From Kitchens JA. JAMA 1994;272:1782–1787.

Table 55-11
Characteristics of Self-report Alcoholism Screening Tests[a]

Test	No. of Items	Administration Scoring Time, min	Notes
Michigan Alcoholism Screening Test (MAST)	25	10 (5)	Does not include quantity or frequency items. Asks about lifetime symptoms. Focus on late-stage symptoms of alcoholism. Differential weighting of items.
Brief MAST	10	5 (3)	See MAST.
Veterans Alcoholism Screening Test	25	15 (5)	Similar to MAST, but distinguishes recent from past symptoms.
Malmo Modification of MAST	9	5 (3)	Similar to MAST, but focuses on drinking attitudes and customs rather than consequences of drinking.
Short Michigan Alcoholism Screening Test	13	7 (4)	Abbreviated MAST. Eliminates complaints of physical symptoms of drinking.
Self-administered Alcoholism Screening Test[b]	35	10 (5)	Differs from MAST by using unit-item weights and adding early-stage symptoms. Also available in short form. Copyrighted.
CAGE[c]	4	1 (1)	Brief. Can be integrated into clinical interview. Does not include quantity or frequency items. Inquires about lifetime symptoms.
TWEAK	5	2 (1)	See CAGE. Recommended for pregnant women.
MacAndrew Alcoholism Scale[d]	49	10 (5)	Derived from Minnesota Multiphasic Personality Inventory. Items do not allude to drinking. May be helpful for patients who would deny problems on direct inquiry about drinking. Copyrighted.
Mortimer-Filkins Questionnaire	58	15 (5)	Nonobvious items that distinguish alcoholics from nonproblem drinkers.
Alcohol Use Disorders Identification Test	10	2 (1)	Asks about symptoms in last year. Includes quantity and frequency and alcohol-dependence items.
Adolescent Drinking Index[e]	24	5 (5)	Can be used with patients aged 12 through 17 years. Distinguishes self-medicational and rebellious drinking styles. Copyrighted.

[a]Adapted from Allen et al. Arch Intern Med 1995;155:1726–1730.
[b]Department of Psychiatry and Psychology, Mayo Clinic, Rochester, MN 55905.
[c]CAGE indicates an acronym for questions about cutting down on drinking, annoyance at others' concern about drinking, feeling guilty about drinking, and using alcohol as an eye-opener in the morning.
[d]NCS Inc, Professional Assessment Services, 5605 Green Circle Dr, Minnetonka, MN 55343.
[e]Psychological Assessment Resources, PO Box 998, Odessa, FL 33556.

ance lessens acute ethanol effects, but may exacerbate chronic metabolic effects. In all acutely inebriated patients, search for concurrent trauma (e.g., subdural hematoma), underlying disease, and coingestion of drugs and toxic alcohol substitutes (i.e., methanol, ethylene glycol).

Chronic Ethanolism (Alcoholism)

In 1972 the Criteria Committee of the National Council on Alcoholism proposed criteria for the diagnosis of alcohol.[46] This has been recently modified.[47]

Alcoholism is a primary, chronic disease with genetic, psychosocial, and environmental factors influencing its development and manifestations. The disease is often progressive and fatal. It is characterized by impaired control over drinking, preoccupation with the drug alcohol, use of alcohol despite adverse consequences, and distortions in thinking, most notably denial. Each of these symptoms may be continuous or periodic.

Clinical Presentation

Nervous System

Diminished fine motor skills, diminished cognition, peripheral motor/sensory neuropathy, and Wernicke's-Korsakoff's syndrome have been observed. Movement disorders are summarized in Table 55–12.[48] Data on alcohol consumption suggests that low levels of alcohol consumption (below 390 g weekly) may have some protective effect on the cerebral vasculature, but heavy consumption (over 400 g weekly) appears to predispose to both hemorrhagic and nonhemorrhagic stroke.[49]

Table 55–12
Movement Disorders Associated With Alcoholism[a,b,c]

1. Acute/transient movement disorders in alcoholism:
   - Postural tremor[d]
   - Parkinsonism[d]
   - Chorea/orolingual dyskinesias[d]
   - Akathisia[d]
2. Variable movement disorders associated with decompensated (alcoholic) liver disease:
   - "Metabolic tremor"
   - Asterixis
   - Myoclonus
3. Movement disorders associated with alcoholic cerebellar degeneration:
   - Cerebellar ataxia
   - 3-Hz leg tremor
   - Parkinsonian tremor
4. Movement disorders (usually persistent) with portosystemic shunts (acquired hepatocerebral degeneration):
   - Tremor
   - Chorea
   - Dystonia
   - Parkinsonism
   - Myoclonus
   - Cerebellar ataxia
5. Movement disorders responsive to alcohol occasionally resulting in alcoholism:
   - Essential tremor
   - Essential myoclonus
   - Autosomal dominant myoclonic dystonia
   - (Spasmodic torticollis, postanoxic action myoclonus)[e]

[a]Adapted from Neiman J et al. Neurology 1990;40:741–746.
[b]Consider the possibility that an underlying neurologic disease associated with a movement disorder may be the cause of aberrant behavior resulting in alcoholism (eg, Huntington's disease).
[c]Consider the possibility of additional other substance abuse.
[d]Occurring during alcohol withdrawal. Occurring during alcohol abuse.
[e]Response to alcohol usually mild, alcoholism rarely if ever results.

Gastrointestinal Tract

Acute pancreatitis may be associated with a retinopathy characterized by multiple cotton-wool patches. Vision may be impaired.[50]

Liver

A prospective multicenter study suggests that in alcoholic cirrhosis with or without alcoholic hepatitis, progression to cirrhosis from alcoholic hepatitis occurs in about half of proven chronic alcoholics. The presence or absence of Mallory bodies does not correlate with either the severity or mortality of patients with alcoholic hepatitis and cirrhosis. There is still controversy relating to the reversibility of cirrhosis and to whether abstinence from alcohol improves survival. Risk factors for survival include the patient's age, race, prothrombin time, ALT levels, AST:ALT ratio, ascites, histologic severity score, alcohol intake prior to admission, and clinical disease severity.[51] Professor Sheila Sherlock estimates that the minimum alcohol intake associated with appreciable liver damage is 16 units of alcohol daily for 5 years (1 unit, 10 g of alcohol is contained in 28 mL [1 fluid ounce] of whiskey or similar spirits, 85 mL of wine, or 230 mL of beer).[52]

Muscle

Patients may develop proximal-muscle weakness with elevated serum creatine kinase levels and myoglobinuria. Myopathy generally appears in middle-aged alcoholics after many years of drinking. It is estimated that myopathy is more likely to occur in a 70 kg man who drinks more than 12 oz of 86 proof whiskey (120 g of ethanol) a day for 20 years—a lifetime dose of 876 kg.[53,54]

Movement Disorders

Movement disorders associated with alcoholism are summarized in Table 55–12.

Hematologic Abnormalities

Hematologic effects of alcoholism on the platelets, red cells, and neutrophils are presented in Tables 55–13 and 55–14.

Table 55–13
Hematologic Abnormalities

Decreased platelets
- On withdrawal
- Reticulocytosis
- Rise in white cell count
- Fall in serum iron

Table 55–14
Alcohol Effects on Neutrophil Function[a]

		Production	Delivery	Phagocytosis/Killing
In Vivo				
	Acute	No effect	↓ Delivery ↓ Adherence Normal chemotaxis	Normal
	Chronic	Neutropenia Marrow suppression	↓ Chemotaxis ↓ Delivery, adherence only with high blood levels	Normal
In Vitro		↓ Marrow colonies ↓ Colony stimulating factor production	↓ Adherence Normal chemotaxis	Normal

[a]Adapted from MacGregor RR. JAMA 1986;256:1474–1479.

Table 55–15
Initial Electrocardiographic Findings in Alcoholic Cardiomyopathy[a]

Rhythm disturbance
- Premature ventricular contractions
- Ventricular tachycardia
- Premature atrial contractions
- Atrial fibrillation or flutter

Conduction disturbance
- First-degree atrioventricular block
- Left anterior hemiblock
- Left posterior hemiblock
- Left bundle-branch block
- Right bundle-branch block
- Intraventricular conduction defect

Atrial abnormality
- Left atrial enlargement
- Biatrial enlargement

Ventricular abnormality
- Left ventricular hypertrophy
- Right ventricular hypertrophy
- Biventricular hypertrophy

Other abnormality
- ST-T changes

[a]Adapted from Moushmoush B, Abi-Mansour P. Arch Intern Med 1991;151:38.

Cardiac Dysfunction

The "Holiday Heart Syndrome" reflects a supraventricular arrhythmia induced by drinking binges (over 6 drinks a day). Atrial fibrillation is the most common arrhythmia, but atrial flutter, atrial tachycardia, junction tachycardia, and multiple atrial premature beats have also been observed.

An isolated episode of atrial fibrillation is often the first complaint. About 10 to 20 years of high alcohol use (about 200 mL—7 oz of 86 proof whiskey a day) may be required before cardiac decompensation becomes apparent.[53,55] Right- and left-sided heart failure then become more apparent.[56] Early electrocardiographic changes include left ventricular hypertrophy with abnormal T-waves and non-specific ST-T–wave changes. There are few specific changes found on myocardial biopsy. Therapy should include abstinence from alcohol, dietary salt restriction, diuretics, digoxin, vasodilator drugs, possibly angiotensin-converting enzyme inhibitors, and thiamine.

Primary ventricular arrhythmias culminating in fibrillation may partially explain why alcoholics die suddenly and unexpectedly.[56] Decreased variability of heart rate—a sign of cardiac vagal neuropathy and a factor notorious for increase in the risk of death after myocardial infarction—is a relatively common finding among men dependent on alcohol. Most episodes of cardiac arrhythmias terminate within 24 to 48 hours either spontaneously or after treatment with beta-blockers combined with adequate sedation, rehydration, and treatment of any potassium and magnesium depletion. Standard alcoholism questionnaire (Tables 55–6 and 55–7) should be administered to all patients presenting with otherwise unexplained tachyrhythmias.[57]

Alcoholic Cardiomyopathy (Table 55–15)

Alcoholic cardiomyopathy shares certain features with the Beriberi heart failure found in malnourished, vitamin-deficient alcoholics: cardiac chamber dilatation, tachycardia, elevated venous pressure, and peripheral edema. However, the thiamine-deficient patient exhibits a high cardiac output state and warm extremities, while the chronic alcoholic patient has depressed cardiac output and ventricular hypocontractility.[56] Concomitant toxic substances such as cobalt chloride (additive used as a beer-foam stabilizer resulting in death),[58] features of chronic arsenic intoxication in some wine drinks,[59] and lead contamination in some moonshiners[60] may have been contributing factors affecting the development of cardiomyopathy in particular groups of chronic alcoholics. Hypokalemia, hypophosphatemia, and hypomagnesemia are contributory factors in some patients with alcoholic cardiomyopathy.[56] A controlled study suggests that susceptibility to alcoholic cardiomyopathy and myopathy appears to be more pronounced in women than in men.[61]

Cardiac Conduction

Cardiovascular death is the most important cause of mortality in alcoholics, yet alcohol may protect against ischemic heart disease. QT-interval prolongation in some patients with alcoholic liver disease is associated with an adverse prognosis, especially sudden cardiac death.[62]

Hypertension

Acutely, alcohol causes a modest fall in blood pressure.[63] Continued consumption of more than the amount contained in two usual portions a day (one portion contains 10 to 12 g of ethanol) results in a dose-dependent rise in blood pressure.[64,65]

Bone

Hip fractures[66]. Osteopenia and fractures, especially of the spine and ribs, are associated with osteoporosis rather than osteomalacia; circulatory levels of Vitamin D metabolites are observed. The role of parathyroid hormone and calcitonin has yet to be established.[67,68]

Immune Defense

Tables 55–16 and 55–17 summarize the effects of alcohol on cell-mediated and humoral immunity.[69]

Transient Hypoparathyroidism

Short-term alcohol administration causes a decline in the secretion of parathyroid hormone and this may account at least in part for the transient hypocalcemia, hypercalciuria, and hypermagnesemia that follow alcohol ingestion.[70]

Magnesium Deficiency

Alcoholism is probably the most important cause of magnesium deficiency (see Table 55–18). Alcoholics ingest low levels of magnesium in their diet, excrete more in their urine, and have decreased albumin (with cirrhosis of the liver) for binding magnesium. The serum magnesium level may not reflect this deficit.[71] Hypomagnesemia may be present, but serum levels of magnesium do not predict body deficits accurately. Magnesium deficiency interferes with thiamine action. Thiamine should be administered with magnesium to prevent Wernicke-Korsakoff syndrome. Administer the 30% solution slowly when given intravenously to avoid pain and sclerosis. The chronic alcoholic has a mean magnesium deficit of about 1.2 mEq/hour. For life-threatening states (e.g., dysrhythmia) $MgSO_4$ may be administered in a dosage of up to 4 g over 3 to 4 minutes.[72]

Renal

Patients with chronic alcoholism have a variety of renal tubular abnormalities that are independent of chronic liver disease, pancreatitis, and rhabdomyolysis and that occur in the presence of normal glomerular filtration. These abnormalities are reversible, disappearing after 4 weeks of abstinence despite many years of alcohol abuse.[73]

Table 55–16
Alcohol Effects on Cell-Mediated Immunity[a]

	Lymphocytes	Macrophages/ Monocytes	Reticuloendothelial System Clearance
In Vivo			
Acute	Normal delayed hypersensitivity	↓ Pulmonary macrophage mobilization	↓ Peritoneal, hepatic, pulmonary
Chronic	↓ Delayed hypersensitivity with liver disease ↓ Delayed hypersensitivity sensitization Lymphopenia ↓ T and natural killer cells with liver disease	Unknown	↓ Hepatic
In Vitro	↓ Lymphocyte transformation ↓ Lymphocyte migration ↓ Natural killer cell activity ↓ Antibody-dependent cellular cytotoxicity	↓ Alveolar macrophage adhesion, phagocytosis and bactericidal activity ↓ Monocyte Fc-receptors, phagocytosis	. . .

[a]Adapted from MacGregor RR. JAMA 1986;256:1474–1479.

Table 55–17
Alcohol Effects on Humoral Immunity

	Immunoglobulins	Complement
In Vivo		
Acute	Unknown	? ↓ Bactericidal activity No change in total serum hemolytic complement
Chronic	↓ Primary antigen response Normal anamnestic response Nondrinking cirrhotics have ↑ serum levels, ↑ spontaneous B-cell production, normal primary antigen response	No change in total serum hemolytic complement

[a]Adated from MacGregor RR. JAMA 1986;256:1474–1479.

Table 55–18
Symptoms and Signs of Magnesium Deficiency Syndrome[a]

Behavioral	Organic
Apathy	Muscular twitching and tremor
Depression	Muscular wasting and weakness
Poor memory	Chvostek's sign
Somnolence	Numbness and tingling
Confusion	Diaphoresis
Disorientation	Tachycardia
Hallucinations	Ventricular premature contractions
Paranoia	Ventricular tachycardia
Apprehensiveness	Ventricular fibrillation
Anxiety	Convulsions
Hyperactivity	Coma
Delusions	Death
Other personality changes	Athetoid, choreiform movements (rare)
	Vertigo (rare)
	Ataxia (rare)
	Nystagmus (rare)
	Trousseau's sign (rare)
	Spontaneous carpopedal spasm, tetany (rare)

[a]Adapted from Miller G. Compr Ther 1985;11:58–64.

Alcoholic Pellagra Encephalopathy[1]

Recent studies indicate that some alcoholic patients who have received thiamine and pyridoxine but not niacin have developed a secondary pellagra consisting of confusion or an altered state of consciousness, oppositional hypertonia, and myoclonus. Such findings may develop over a period of weeks or during hospitalization several days after admission and apparent recovery from Wernicke's encephalopathy. Treatment with niacin may result in dramatic improvement. Stimulation of metabolic pathways by pyridoxine and thiamine may increase the relative deficit of niacin.

ALCOHOLIC KETOACIDOSIS[1]

Clinical Presentation

Alcoholic ketoacidosis (AKA) follows withdrawal from alcohol and develops in chronic alcoholics with a recent history of heavy episodes.[1,74,75] Such patients have often experienced symptoms of nausea, vomiting, abdominal pain,[76] and decreased food intake often due to gastritis, hepatitis, or pancreatitis or related to alcohol withdrawal, fatty liver infiltration, or aspiration pneumonia. They become volume depleted and usually have abruptly stopped or markedly decreased their alcohol intake 24 to 72 hours before presentation. The patient becomes confused, drowsy, and occasionally comatose. Tachypnea and tachycardia are common signs, and the patient may present with breathlessness in a Kussmaul breathing pattern compensatory for the ketoacidosis. These patients often have no measurable blood alcohol levels when first seen in a health care facility. The blood glucose level is usually normal to slightly elevated. Most patients will respond to glucose-containing intravenous fluids without insulin. In some areas alcoholic ketoacidosis is the causative factor in up to 20% of patients presenting with ketoacidosis. Patients are usually conscious and able to give a good history.

The moderate-to-severe ketoacidosis is due to the formation of beta hydroxybutyrate (BOHB) and acetoacetate (AcAc). The BOHB usually predominates and therefore testing with Ketostix and Acetest (which are most sensitive to acetoacetate, less so to acetone, and not at all to beta hydroxybutyrate) may show only a weakly positive reaction when levels of BOHB are highest. The finding of ketonuria without glycosuria suggests the diagnosis. Serum lactate levels are only moderately elevated. Severe lactic acidosis would suggest another serious disorder such as hypoxemia or hypoperfusion.

Metabolic effects associated with alcoholic ketoacidosis include hormonal changes (increased levels of cortisol, growth hormone, glucagon, free fatty acids, catecholamines, decreased levels of insulin, and ADH) and effects secondary to any increase in the NADH/NAD ratio (increase in the BOHB/AcAc ratio and lactate production; decreased gluconeogenesis and citric acid cycle activity).

Electrolyte, glucose, and arterial blood gas measurements are essential in making a diagnosis. The basic acid-base abnormality in alcoholic ketoacidosis is an elevated anion-gap metabolic acidosis. Hypokalemia and hypochloremia are often seen due to the bouts of prolonged vomiting. Serum potassium must be carefully monitored during treatment. The blood pH may vary from 6.96 to 7.61. A significant respiratory alkalosis may be seen as a compensatory response to the metabolic acidosis or due to alcohol withdrawal or other associated illnesses. The protracted vomiting can lead to a primary metabolic alkalosis. The initial blood pH and bicarbonate levels are not good indicators of eventual outcome.

Serum ketones are markedly elevated. AcAc levels over 2 mEq/L (normal:<0.05) and BOHB levels over 10 mEq/L (normal:<0.05) may be present. The BOHB/AcAc ratio (normally 1:1) rises to 4:10.1. When alcoholics with ketoacidosis are treated, the BOHB is oxidized to AcAc and later to acetone. Thus the nitroprusside test may worsen when the patient is actually improving. Remember that when severe elevations of the anion gap (>30 mEq/L) are found in ketoacidosis, hyperosmolar coma, lactic acidosis, and ingestion of ethylene glycol or methanol, an osmolal gap is present.[77,78]

Treatment

Management of these patients requires correction of volume depletion and administration of glucose.[1,71–75] The volume depletion is usually amenable to infusion of solutions of normal saline with dextrose. When the volume deficit is corrected (normal orthostatic blood pressure and pulse), 0.5 N saline with dextrose may be continued. Such intravenous therapy is continued until the serum bicarbonate level reaches 18 to 20 mEq/L, signs of orthostasis have resolved, and oral fluids are well tolerated. Patients will respond to therapy within 12 hours. Close monitoring (every 4 to 6 hours) of serum potassium and phosphorus levels during treatment is important because hypokalemia and hypophosphatemia may ensue quickly. Potassium supplementation may be required. Sodium bicarbonate administration is usually not necessary except in severe cases of acidosis (pH <7.1). Insulin therapy is not required. Thiamine (50 to 100 mg) should be given to prevent development of the Wernicke-Korsakoff syndrome. Magnesium and multivitamins may be considered.

LABORATORY

Markers may assist in the diagnosis of alcoholism (Table 55–19).[79]

Analytic Methods

Two methods provide rapid quantitative determination of blood alcohol concentrations (BAC). One uses an electrochemical method and the other, saliva.[80,81] Limitation to the saliva test may include cross-reactivity with other congeners such as methanol. Mouthwash, phenol-containing lozenges, tobacco products, and patient cooperation may affect these determinations. Vomitus containing alcohol may produce a falsely elevated test result. Further data is required before clinical usefulness of these procedures can be defined.

Blood Levels (Table 55–20)

Ethanol doses calculated to achieve and maintain blood ethanol concentrations of 100 mg/dL in a 70-kg adult are presented in Table 55–21. A 30-month-old 13-kg child became comatose after ingesting up to 16 ounces of wine containing 20% ethanol. Despite the initial blood ethanol level of 98.78 mmol/L (455 mg/dL), the child recovered following prompt gastric decontamination and maintenance of adequate hydration and euglycemia.[82] In spite of intensive investigation, there is still no satisfactory useful clinical laboratory marker for surreptitious alcohol ingestion. Inges-

Table 55–19
Markers for Alcoholism[a]

Markers of proven value
- Gamma glutamyl transferase
- Aspartate aminotransferase
- mAST and mAST/tAST ratio
- Mean corpuscular volume

Markers of limited, disputed value
- Alanine aminotransferase
- Alkaline phosphatase
- Lactate dehydrogenase
- Glutamate dehydrogenase
- Ornithine carbamoyltransferase
- Sorbitol dehydrogenase
- Isocitrate dehydrogenase
- Guanine deaminase
- 5′-Nucleotidase
- Albumin
- γ-Globulin
- Bilirubin
- Serum bile acids
- Blood ethanol
- α-Amino-*N*-butyric acid/leucine ratio
- Creatine phosphokinase
- D-Glucaric acid
- Serum amylase
- Uric acid
- Linoleic acid
- 2,3-Butanediol
- Plasma steroids
- Blood lactate/pyruvate ratio
- Urinary salsolinol
- Serum Indole-3-acetic acid

Markers of limited, disputed value
- Urinary biogenic amine metabolites
- Serum osmolality
- Urinary zinc
- Urinary coproporphyrin
- Galactose tolerance test
- Aminopyrine breath test

Markers currently under evaluation
- Acetaldehyde adducts
- High density lipoproteins
- Blood acetate
- Urinary dolichol
- Erythrocyte γ-aminolevulinic acid dehydrase
- Erythrocyte aldehyde dehydrogenase
- Erythrocyte superoxide dismutase
- Erythrocyte neuron-specific enolase
- Erythrocyte hemolysis resistance
- Platelet adenylate cyclase
- Platelet serotonin uptake
- PGA index (prothrombin, gamma glutamyl transferase, apolipoprotein)

Newer markers
- Carbohydrate-deficient transferrin

[a]Adapted from Mihas AA, Tavassoli M. Am J Med Sci 1992;303:415–428.

Table 55–20
Stages of Acute Alcoholic Influence/Intoxication in Nontolerant Individuals[a]

Blood Alcohol Concentration (% w/v)	Stage of Alcohol Influence	Clinical Sign/Symptom
0.01–0.05	Sobriety	No apparent influence Behavior nearly normal by ordinary observation Slight changes detectable by special tests
0.03–0.12	Euphoria	Mild euphoria, sociability, talkativeness Increased self-confidence; decreased inhibitions Diminution of attention, judgment, and control Loss of efficiency in finer performance tests
0.09–0.25	Excitement	Emotional instability; decreased inhibitions Loss of critical judgment Impairment of memory and comprehension Decreased sensory response; increased reaction time Some muscular incoordination
0.18–0.30	Confusion	Disorientation, mental confusion; dizziness Exaggerated emotional states (fear, anger, grief, etc.) Disturbance of sensation (diplopia, etc.) and of perception of color, form, motion, dimensions Decreased pain sense Impaired balance; muscular incoordination; staggering gait, slurred speech
0.27–0.40	Stupor	Apathy; general inertia, approaching paralysis Markedly decreased response to stimuli Marked muscular incoordination; inability to stand or walk Vomiting; incontinence of urine and feces Impaired consciousness; sleep or stupor
0.35–0.50	Coma	Complete unconsciousness; coma; anesthesia Depressed or abolished reflexes Subnormal temperature Incontinence of urine and feces Embarrassment of circulation and respiration Possible death
0.45+	Death	Death from respiratory paralysis

[a]Adapted from Dubowski KM. Am J Clin Pathol 1980;74:747–750.

Table 55–21
Ethanol Doses Calculated to Achieve and Maintain Blood Ethanol Concentrations of 100 mg/dL in a 70-kg Adult[a]

		Loading Dose	Infusion Rate During Dialysis[b]	Infusion Rate After Dialysis	Total Over 36 h[c]
Amount of ethanol	Chronic drinker[d]	42 g	18.0 g/h	10.8 g/h	474 g
	Nondrinker[e]	42 g	11.8 g/h	4.6 g/h	251 g
Volume of 10% intravenous	Chronic drinker	530 mL	228 mL/h	137 mL/h	6,010 mL
	Nondrinker	530 mL	149 mL/h	58 mL/h	3,180 mL
Volume of 43% oral	Chronic drinker	125 mL	54 mL/h	32 mL/h	1,410 mL
	Nondrinker	125 mL	35 mL/h	14 mL/h	749 mL
Volume of 90% oral	Chronic drinker	60 mL	26 mL/h	15 mL/h	666 mL
	Nondrinker	60 mL	17 mL/h	7 mL/h	359 mL

[a]Adapted from McCoy HG, Cipolle RJ, Ehlers SM et al. Am J Med 1979;67:806.
[b]Assuming ethanol dialysance of 120 mL/min.
[c]Assuming a 6-hour dialysis period.
[d]Assuming $V_m = 175$ mg/kg/h, $K_m = 13.8$ mg/dL.
[e]Assuming $V_m = 75$ mg/kg/h, $K_m = 13.8$ mg/dL.

Table 55–22
Effect of Some Solutes on Serum Osmolality[a]

For Each 1 mg/dL of:	Serum Osmolality Will Increase (mO/kg H_2O):
Methanol	0.34
Ethanol	0.22
Ethylene glycol	0.20
Acetone	0.18
Isopropyl alcohol	0.17

[a]Adapted from Ellenhorn MJ. In: Hall JB et al, eds. Principles of critical care. New York: McGraw-Hill, 1992, 2080–2093.

tion of 80 g of ethanol over 30 minutes by heavy drinkers (720 to 2000 g/week) may produce a significant rise in plasma glutathione-S-transferase with peak values 60 minutes after alcohol ingestion, suggestive of mild subclinical acute liver damage.[83] Further work is required to determine clinical usefulness of this test. Additional important prognostic abnormalities of alcoholic liver disease include serum albumin levels less than 2.5 g/dL and serum bilirubin values over 136 μmol/L (7.5 mg/dL).[84,85]

Abnormalities

Serum Osmolality (Table 55–22)

Geller and colleagues found that the osmolal gap (mOsm/kg) was related to the serum ethanol concentration (nmol/L) by the formula:

$$\text{Ethanol} = 0.83 \times \text{osmolal gap}$$ [86]

Hypophosphatemia

Hypophosphatemia may be observed in alcoholics and is often found in malnourished individuals. Reduced phosphate reabsorption capacity in alcoholics is probably the result of a proximal tubular dysfunction related to brush border damage. Data suggest that liver-function impairment is not required for this proximal tubular dysfunction.[87] Associated neurologic deficits have varied from anisocoria, ballismus, paresthesia, hyporeflexia, ataxia, convulsions, coma, and even death. Coma is usually accompanied by seizures.[88] Management includes intravenous phosphate, thiamine, and potassium and magnesium replacement as required.

Lactic Acidosis

The most common cause of elevated blood lactate, in general, is circulatory shock. Acute or chronic alcohol abuse predisposes to sepsis, gastrointestinal hemorrhage, pancreatitis, and other disorders that can lead to shock. Other causes of lactic acidosis encountered in emergency departments include seizures, liver disease, alcoholic ketoacidosis, thiamine deficiency, and poisoning with methanol, ethylene glycol, acetaminophen, cyanide, and carbon monoxide. Lactic acidosis solely attributable to ethanol is uncommon. Look for an underlying pathophysiologic process.[89]

Acetone

Abnormally high concentrations of acetone in the blood might occur if a person drinks 2-propanol, undertakes a prolonged fast, has diabetes mellitus, or engages in strenuous exercise. The highest recorded concentration of acetone (61.9 μg/mL) was observed in the blood of a drunk driver (blood alcohol concentration 0.11 g %). This suggests that in a population of motorists an individual with an abnormally high concentration of acetone in the blood or breath is unlikely to be observed. The risk of acetone interfering with breath-alcohol analyzers may be exaggerated.[90]

Carbohydrate-Deficient Transferrin

A new and potentially useful diagnostic marker of alcohol abuse utilizes carbohydrate-deficient transferrin in the serum.[91] This transferrin abnormality measures an accumulated effect of alcohol consumption, appearing after regular intake of 50 to 80 g of ethanol/day for at least 1 week and normalizing slowly during abstinence (half-life = about 15 days). Koppel considers this to be a specific marker for alcohol abuse patients admitted to the intensive care unit. This test is not yet widely used.[92]

Selenium

A controlled clinical study suggests that chronic alcohol abuse may be associated with a decreased serum selenium level. The significance of this finding must be validated by further study.[92a]

TREATMENT

Flumazenil

Flumazenil (3 mg IV) may aid in reversing the respiratory depression associated with ethanol ingestion, but this observation has not been clinically validated.[93] Analeptic agents should not be used.

RO 15-4513

RO 15-4513 is a synthetic chemical closely related to the benzodiazepine antagonist flumazenil. It is an antagonist of the action of ethanol in animals[94] and specifically is antagonistic to ethanol-induced depression of the central nervous system, where it inhibits the neurochemical and behavioral effects of ethanol.[95] RO 15-4513 may be valuable in attenuating drunkenness, but is useless in life-threatening, ethanol-overdosage–induced coma.

Since it can reverse the central nervous system effects of ethanol while allowing the peripheral effects of the drug to remain, RO 15-4513 would probably lead to an increase in the incidence of alcohol-related disease of the liver, cardiovascular system, and gastrointestinal tract. The manufacturer has decided not to market the product.[91,92]

Antagonists

Calcium Carbamide

This investigational drug inhibits the enzyme aldehyde dehydrogenase, which metabolizes acetaldehyde to acetic acid. Ingestion of alcohol causes an accumulation of acetaldehyde and brings on nausea and vomiting. Optimum dose and dosage schedule have not been established; adverse reactions and deleterious drug interactions preclude its use at present.[96]

Carbamazepine

Studies with carbamazepine suggest that it is effective in treating alcohol withdrawal, including delirium tremens.[97] It appears to be effective without adjunctive medication.[98] Carbamazepine may offer the advantage of rapid return to work or early induction into an alcoholism treatment program.[99]

Chlormethiazole

(Sold in Great Britain as Heminevrin.) Chlormethiazole has hypnotic, anxiolytic, and anticonvulsant properties. In Britain, where it is given in a rapidly reducing dosage over 6 days it is the most popular drug used for alcohol withdrawal. However, alcoholics rapidly become dependent on this drug. Chlormethiazole abuse may lead to serious self-poisoning with deep coma and centrally mediated respiratory depression that may be fatal.

Preliminary reports suggest the use of clonidine[100] (60 to 180 μg/hour IV) and gamma-hydroxybutyric acid[101,102] (50 mg/kg orally) for the treatment of withdrawal symptoms. Confirmatory controlled clinical studies will be required to evaluate these findings.

Disulfiram

(See Disulfiram chapter.)

Lithium Carbonate

Maintenance of therapeutic serum levels of lithium appears to assist in maintenance of sobriety.[103] Further studies are required to substantiate the dose and efficacy of this drug in alcoholism.[103–105]

4-Methylpyrazole

Initial studies suggest that a dose of 7 mg/kg of intravenous 4-methylpyrazole appears to decrease the rate of elimination of ethanol and to suppress typical manifestations of ethanol ingestion in humans.[106]

Naltrexone

In 1994 the Food and Drug Administration approved naltrexone (Revia) as a treatment for alcoholism. Research indicates that the drug appears to reduce the craving for alcohol. Naltrexone should not be used in patients receiving opioids or currently dependent on them, those in acute opioid withdrawal, those who have a history of sensitivity to naltrexone, or those patients with acute hepatitis or liver failure. Patients with alcohol-induced liver dysfunction may be poor candidates for naltrexone therapy. The recommended dose of naltrexone for treatment of alcohol dependence is 50 mg once a day for 12 weeks. Long-term trials are lacking. There is no evidence that the drug is effective without regular counseling.[107]

Ritanserin

A potent and specific $5HT_2$-receptor antagonist that may act to decrease alcohol intake in chronic alcoholics without harmful side effects. It remains in the investigational phase at present.[108]

Tiapride

Tiapride, an atypical neuroleptic agent, is a selective dopamine D_2-receptor antagonist. It facilitates management of alcohol withdrawal, but its use in patients at risk of severe reactions in acute withdrawal should be accompanied by adjunct therapy for hallucinosis and seizures. The usefulness of tiapride in this setting is likely to be limited. Tiapride ameliorates psychologic distress, improves abstinence, reduces drinking behavior, and in the short-term facilitates reintegration within society. The potential risk of tardive dyskinesia at the dosage employed (300 mg/day) requires evaluation and necessitates medical supervision. Tiapride does not appear to cause physical or psychologic dependence.

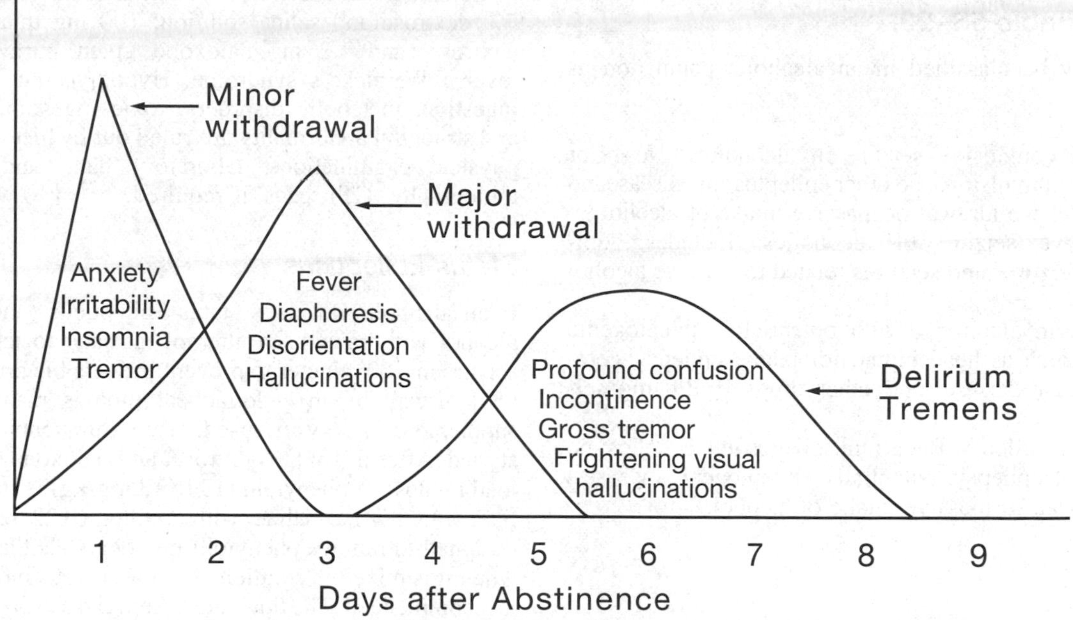

Figure 55-2. Severity of signs and symptoms of alcohol withdrawal. (From Freedland ES, McMicken DB. J Emerg Med 1993;11:605–618.)

Table 55-23
Ethanol Withdrawal Syndromes Times of Onset after Cessation of Drinking[a]

Common abstinence syndrome	6–8 hr
Alcoholic hallucinations	24–36 hr
Seizures (rum fits)	7–48 hr (peak 24 hr)
DTs	3–5 days (up to 14 days)
Alcoholic ketoacidosis (AKA)	24–72 hr

[a]Adapted from Ellenhorn MJ. In: Hall JB et al, eds. Principles of critical care. New York: McGraw-Hill, 1992, 2080–2093.

Toxicokinetics. Bioavailability of tiapride is about 75% following oral or intramuscular administration. Peak plasma tiapride concentrations are achieved within about 0.4 to 1.5 hours. The drug is rapidly distributed and does not bind appreciably to plasma proteins. Tiapride is mainly eliminated by renal excretion, principally in the unchanged form. The elimination half-life is approximately 3 to 4 hours and may increase with age and declining renal function ($V_D = 1.436$ L/kg).

Clinical presentation. The most frequently reported adverse events (>1%) are drowsiness, extrapyramidal syndromes, dizziness, and orthostatic hypotension.

Dosage. For the treatment of delirium or predelirium during alcohol withdrawal, intravenous or intramuscular tiapride 400 to 1200 mg/day given every 4 to 6 hours is recommended, increased to 1800 mg/day if required.[109]

Zimeldine

Blocks serotonin uptake, possibly leading to a decrease in daily intake of alcohol and an increase in days of abstinence in chronic alcoholics. Zimeldine was withdrawn worldwide because of reports of hepatitis and Guillain-Barré syndrome.[93]

Table 55-24
Equivalent, Potential Initial Doses of Benzodiazepines Frequently Used for Treatment of Alcohol Withdrawal[a]

	Administration	
Drug	Oral (mg)	Intravenous (mg)
Chlordiazepoxide	100	. . .
Oxazepam[b]	120	. . .
Lorazepam[b]	4	1–2
Diazepam	20	5–10

[a]Adapted from Lohr MH. Mayo Clin Proc 1995;70:777–782.
[b]Shorter-acting formulations with fewer active metabolites.

WITHDRAWAL SYNDROMES (FIG. 55-2) (SEE TABLE 55-23)

Abstinence[110]

The majority of patients (over 95%) experiencing acute alcohol withdrawal probably do not require psychotropic drug therapy. Studies with clonidine 0.2 mg orally given several times daily over a 4-day period suggest that it is effective in reducing some of the adrenergic manifestations of alcohol withdrawal.[111]

Additional studies with other drugs have suggested potential uses for dexamethasone,[112] phenobarbital,[113] chlormethiazole, beta-blockers (for mild symptoms),[114] subanalgesic doses of nitrous oxide,[115] clorazepate,[116] haloperidol,[111] and hydroxybutyric acid[101] in ameliorating some of the symptoms associated with alcohol withdrawal. They may be useful as supplements to benzodiazepine therapy or for patients resistant to benzodiazepines (Table 55-24). Additional work is required with each group of drugs before specific recommendations can be made.

ALCOHOLIC SEIZURES

Seizures (Table 55–23)

Seizures may be classified in an alcoholic population as follows:

1. Solitary, convulsive seizure in alcoholics. No prior epileptic convulsions, no other epileptogenic disease, no relation to withdrawal or massive intake of alcohol.
2. Convulsive seizure of alcoholics. Includes withdrawal seizures and seizures related to massive alcohol intake.
3. Seizures in alcoholics with potentially epileptogenic disease such as head injury, idiopathic epilepsy, cerebrovascular disease, and other drugs facilitating seizures.
4. Alcoholic epilepsy. Recurrent seizures in alcoholics; no history of epilepsy, potentially epileptogenic diseases, withdrawal, or massive intake of alcohol.

Risk Factors

Factors associated with alcohol withdrawal and considered most likely to precipitate seizures are hypoglycemia, hypomagnesemia, and respiratory alkalosis. Alcohol withdrawal also heightens photic sensitivity and can lead to television-induced seizures.

Clinical Presentation

A history of seizures before age 18 years or before the onset of heavy drinking is usually due to idiopathic epilepsy. Alcohol withdrawal seizures appear 6 to 48 hours after either cessation or precipitous decline of alcohol intake. The true alcohol withdrawal seizure will be manifest prior to the onset of delirium tremens (DT). It is a generalized seizure and does not manifest an aura, a focal onset, or a significant period (e.g., more than 30 minutes) of postictal confusion, agitation, or aggression. Persons who differ from this pattern (i.e., have an aura, begin the seizure with a focal presentation, have onset during DT, have an extended period of postictal confusion, suffer a second seizure) should be carefully evaluated for other conditions. Alcohol withdrawal may exacerbate partial (focal) seizures common with posttraumatic epilepsy. Partial seizures must be considered indicative of a mass lesion until proven otherwise. Seizures in a setting of alcohol consumption or withdrawal will usually not require long-term anticonvulsant therapy since the seizures are self-limited.[1]

Any patient arriving at an emergency department with seizures should be questioned about alcohol intake. It is involved in up to 40% of adults with seizures admitted to a hospital and in about 15% of patients with status epilepticus.

Seizures with alcohol use are dose-dependent and may be causal, independent of alcohol withdrawal. Alcohol contributes to seizure frequency in the general epileptic population. This may be enhanced by sleep deprivation, enhanced photic sensitivity, and accelerated metabolism of antiepileptic drugs due to drinking alcohol. Sudden withdrawal of phenytoin may enhance the convulsive effects of alcohol withdrawal.

Seizure treatment should include an intravenous line with 5% dextrose and saline solution; 100 mg thiamine, 25 g dextrose, and 1.2 mg naloxone given intravenously to reverse Wernicke's syndrome. Hypoglycemia or narcotic ingestion, metabolic disorders, toxic ingestion, infection, and structural abnormality are ruled out by history, repeated physical examinations, laboratory data, and computed tomography (CT) scans, if required.

Status Epilepticus

If an alcoholic develops status epilepticus (uncommon in alcohol withdrawal), an attempt is made to terminate the seizure in <60 minutes to prevent irreversible brain damage. Oral airway or an endotracheal tube is maintained and supplementary oxygen used. Two intravenous lines are started. After thiamine, dextrose, and naloxone are given, a loading dose of phenytoin (13 to 18 mg/kg) is started in one line with normal saline with a filter (0.22 or 0.45 μm) designed to remove phenytoin microcrystals that may form when it is mixed in solution. An intravenous infusion pump is recommended. The flow rate is kept at 40 to 50 mg/minute, with caution in patients with preexisting heart disease. In a second line, diazepam is given at 2 to 4 mg/minute up to 20 mg. Diazepam has a short duration of action (20 to 30 minutes) and is given for immediate seizure control with caution in the elderly who are more vulnerable to respiratory depression and hypotension; here, lorazepam may be useful. If seizures persist, a diazepam drip is begun, with 50 to 100 mg diazepam diluted in 500 mL of 5% dextrose in water (D_5W) and run at 40 mL/hour. If there is no response to phenytoin or diazepam, or if cardiac disease or phenytoin allergy preclude its use, intravenous phenobarbital is given at 15 to 50 mg/minute after a loading dose of 7 to 20 mg/kg. Phenobarbital should not be administered together with an intravenous diazepam drip because of their potential incompatibilities in solution. By the time that phenobarbital is added, endotracheal intubation and mechanical ventilation are invariably helpful.

For the alcoholic in withdrawal with no present seizure but a past history of withdrawal give either an intravenous loading dose to those admitted or an oral loading dose of 19 to 20 mg/kg in two to three divided doses over 6 hours with no more than 6000 mg/dose to outpatients. For withdrawal seizures, the patient is maintained on phenytoin 300 mg/day for 5 days, but a prospective, randomized, placebo-controlled study suggests that phenytoin is not effective in preventing withdrawal seizures.[117] The alcoholic who has already had a single or short burst of seizures and is now alert may only need treatment for alcohol withdrawal. Further seizures will be rare if adequately treated with a benzodiazepine. The patient should be observed for at least 6 hours after the seizures before discharge. Possible causes of a decreased level of consciousness following seizures in the obtunded patient include postictal state, occult head trauma, unrecognized metabolic disorder, or poisoning.

Wernicke's-Korsakoff's Syndrome

Even when a Korsakoff's state is evident, use of thiamine may assist about 25 to 50% of patients in making at least a partial recovery.[118]

Treatment

Patients suspected of having Wernicke's encephalopathy should be treated immediately with 100 mg thiamine daily, infused slowly in 500 mL fluid for at least 5 days. At the same time, deficiencies of other vitamins, including niacin, minerals, electrolytes, and especially magnesium, should be corrected. Intravenous glucose should be given only in conjunction with thiamine since the glucose alone can precipitate Wernicke's encephalopathy in thiamine-deficient patients. Fortification of alcoholic beverages with thiamine has been suggested.[1]

Transplantation

An extensive discussion of alcoholic liver disease (cirrhosis, hepatitis, encephalopathy) is outside the scope of this book. Alcohol-associated progressive impairment of the liver may, however, develop despite abstaining from alcohol ingestion. Hematemesis, advanced portal hypertension, hepatocellular carcinoma, intractable ascites, or encephalopathy may provide reasons for transplantation, especially in patients who have no serious disease of other organs, no history of alcohol dependence, excellent family and social support, and an estimated length of survival of less than 1 year.[119] This remains a controversial area of interest,[120,121] but tends to favor serious consideration of employing this procedure in selected alcoholic patients.[118,122]

Children

Once a poisoning has occurred, the blood ethanol and glucose should be monitored and the child should be treated with glucose if necessary.[123] A retrospective study of 102 cases suggests that children who by history have ingested up to 105 mL of cologne, perfume, or after-shave (containing 15 to 99% ethanol) and who remain asymptomatic can be observed at home if parents refuse to bring their asymptomatic children to the emergency department. Home assessment must include extremely close hourly observation for symptoms of central nervous system depression and hypoglycemia for at least 3 to 6 hours postingestion.[12,14]

The Toxic Dose

In small children a blood ethanol concentration greater than 20 mg/dL may produce hypoglycemia.[124] The average lethal concentration in adults is quoted as being 450 mg/dL.[125] The most common lethal dose of ethanol reported in patients not receiving supportive therapy is 5 to 8 g/kg in adults and 3 g/kg in children.[126]

Unlike in adults, poor nutritional status or a prolonged fast does not appear to be a prerequisite for hypoglycemia to occur in children. Serious ethanol poisoning with hypoglycemia also results from children ingesting mouthwash products. If a child consumes a volume of an ethanol-containing product that can produce a blood ethanol concentration of 50 mg/dL, evaluate for immediate and delayed hypoglycemia.[123]

The expected BEC can be calculated by the following formula:

$$\text{BEC (mg/dL)} = \frac{\text{Amt Ingested} \times \text{\%EtOH} \times \text{SpG (0.79)}}{V_D \text{ (0.6 L/kg)} \times \text{Body Weight (kg)}}$$

$$(V_D = \text{Volume of distribution})$$

$$(\text{BEC} = \text{Blood ethanol concentration})$$

Rearrangement of the above equation allows calculations of the amount ingested if the BEC and the preparation's percent ethanol concentration is known.[123]

$$\text{Amt ingested (mL)} = \frac{\text{BEC (mg/dL} \times V_D \text{ (0.6 L/kg)} \times \text{wt (kg)}}{\text{\%EtOH} \times \text{Specific Gravity (0.79)}}$$

REFERENCES—ETHANOL

1. Ellenhorn MJ. The alcohols. In: Hall JB, Schmidt GA, Wood LDH eds. Principles of critical care. New York: McGraw-Hill, 1992, 2080–2093.
2. MMWR. Update. Alcohol-related traffic fatalities—United States 1982–1993. JAMA 1994;272:1892.
3. Guppy A. At whole blood concentration should drunk-driving be illegal? Something lower than 17.4 mmol/L (0.8 g/L). Br Med J 1994;308:1055–1056.
4. Bradley KA, Donovan DM, Larson EB. How much is too much? Advising parents about safe levels of alcohol consumption. Arch Intern Med 1993;153:2734–2740.
5. Canfield DV, Kupiec T, Huffine E. Postmortem alcohol production in fatal aircraft accidents. J Forensic Sci 1993; 38:914–917.
6. CDC. Alcohol use and aquatic activities—United States, 1991. MMWR 1993;42:675–682.
7. CDC. Alcohol involvement in pedestrian fatalities—United States, 1982–1992. MMWR 1993;42:716–719.
8. CDC. Quarterly table reporting alcohol involvement in fatal motor vehicle crashes. MMWR 1993;42:729.
9. Jurkovich GJ, Rivara FP, Gurney JG, Fligner C, Ries R, Mueller BA, Copass M. The effect of acute alcohol intoxication and chronic alcohol abuse on outcome for trauma. JAMA 1993;270:51–66.
10. Foulke FL. Alcohol beverages under investigation. FDA Consumer 1993;27(1):23.
11. Frezza M, di Padova C, Pozzato G, Terpin M, Baraona E, Lieber CS. Higher blood alcohol levels in women. The role of decreased gastric alcohol dehydrogenase activity and first-pass metabolism. N Engl J Med 1990;322:95–99.
12. Schenker S, Speeg KV. The risk of alcohol intake in men and women. All may not be equal. N Engl J Med 1990;322:127–129.
13. Seitz HK, Egerer G, Simanowski UA. High blood alcohol levels in women. N Engl J Med 1990;323:58.
14. Lieber CS. Biochemical and molecular basis of alcohol-induced injury to liver and other tissues. N Engl J Med 1988; 319:1639–1650.
15. Holt S. Alcohol and H_2 receptor antagonist: over the counter, under the table? Am J Gastroenterol 190;185:516–517.
16. Roine R, Gentry T, Hernandez-Munoz R, Baraona E, Lieber CS. Aspirin increases blood alcohol concentrations in humans after ingestion of ethanol. JAMA 1990;264: 2406–2408.
17. Reference Deleted.
18. Bailey DN. Cocapropylene (propylcocaine) formation by human liver in vitro. J Anal Toxicol 1995;19:1–4.
19. Novy FG. Some higher analogues of cocaine. Am Chem J 1988;10:145–148.

20. Harada S, Misawa S, Agarwal DP, Goedde HW. Liver alcohol and aldehyde dehydrogenase in the Japanese: isozyme variation and its possible role in alcohol intoxications. Am J Hum Genet 1980;32:8–15.
21. Jones AW, Neiman J, Hillbom M. Concentration-time profiles of ethanol and acetaldehyde in human volunteers treated with the alcohol-sensitizing drug calcium carbamide. Br J Clin Pharmacol 1988;25:213–221.
22. Brien JF, Loomis CW. Pharmacology of acetaldehyde. Can J Physiol Pharmacol 1983;61:1–22.
23. Schootstra R, Bloemhof H, Bouma P, Uges DRA. An unusual case of acetaldehyde intoxication. In: Uges DRA, de Zeeuw RA, eds. Proc Int Assoc Forensic Toxicol. 25th Meeting, Groningen, Netherlands: June 1988, pp. 85–91.
24. Mills JL, Graubard BI. Is moderate drinking during pregnancy associated with an increased risk for malformations? Pediatrics 1987;80:309–314.
25. Karl PI, Gordon BHJ, Lieber CS, Fisher SE. Acetaldehyde production and transfer by the perfused human placental cotyledon. Science 1988;242:273–275.
26. Rosett HL. A clinical perspective of the fetal alcohol syndrome. Alcohol Clin Exp Res 1980;4:119–122.
27. Autti-Ramo I, Korkman M, Hilakivi-Clarke L, Lehtonen M, Halmesmaki E, Granstrom M-L. Mental development of 2-year-old children exposed to alcohol in utero. J Pediatr 1992;120:740–746.
28. CDC. Fetal alcohol syndrome—United States 1979–1992. MMWR 1993;42:339–341.
29. Mennella JA, Beauchamp GK. The transfer of alcohol to human milk. Effects on flavor and the infant's behavior. N Engl J Med 1991;325:981–985.
30. Amadeno S, Abbou M, Fourcade ML, Waksman G, Leroux MG, Madec A et al. DZ dopamine receptor genes and alcoholism. J Psychiatr Res 1993;27:173–179.
31. Noble EP, Blum K. Alcoholism and the D_2 dopamine receptor gene. JAMA 1993;270:1547.
32. Gelernter J, Risch N, Goldman D. Alcoholism and the D_2 dopamine receptor gene. JAMA 1993;270:1547–1548.
33. Allen JP, Maisto Connors GJ. Self-report screening tests for alcohol problems in primary care. Arch Intern Med 1995;155:1726–1730.
34. Kitchens JM. Does this patient have an alcohol problem? JAMA 1994;272:1782–1787.
35. Engel PA, Grunnet M, Jacobs B. Wernicke-Korsakoff syndrome complicating T-cell lymphoma: unusual or unrecognized. South Med J 1991;84:253–256.
36. Fried RT, Levy M, Leibowitz AB, Bronster DJ, Iberti TJ. Wernicke's encephalopathy in the intensive care patient. Crit Care Med 1990;18:779–780.
37. Da Dalt L, Dall'Amico R, Lawerda AM, Chemollo C, Chiandelti L. Percutaneous ethyl alcohol intoxication in a one-month-old infant. Pediatr Emerg Care 1991;7:343–344.
38. Watkins AMC, Keogh EJ. Alcohol burns in the neonate. J Paediatr Child Health 1992;28:306–308.
39. Hornfeldt CS. A report of acute ethanol poisoning in a child: mouthwash versus cologne, perfume and after-shave. Clin Toxicol 1992;30:115–121.
40. Lammingoa A, Vilska J. Acute alcohol intoxications in children treated in hospital. Acta Paediatr Scand 1990;79:847–854.
41. Kingston R, Saxona K, Sioris LJ, Lelwica T. Alcohol abuse in a 47-month-old child. Vet Hum Toxicol 1991;33:385.
42. Minocha A, Roberson DG, Herold DA et al. Impairment of cognitive and neuromuscular function by ethanol in social drinkers. Vet Hum Toxicol 1985;28:319.
43. Elphinstone PE, Black AK, Greaves MW. Alcohol-induced urticaria. J Roy Soc Med 1985;78:340–341.
44. Thorton JR. Atrial fibrillation in healthy non-alcoholic people after an alcoholic binge. Lancet 1984;2:1013–1014.
45. Lang RM, Borow KM, Neumann A et al. Adverse cardiac effects of acute alcohol ingestion in young adults. Ann Intern Med 1985;102:742–743.
46. Criteria Committee, National Council on Alcoholism. Criteria for the diagnosis of alcoholism. Am J Psychiatry 1972;129:129.
47. Morse RM, Flavin DK. Joint Committee of the National Council on Alcoholism. JAMA 1992;268:1012–1014.
48. Neiman J, Lang AE, Fornazzari L, Carlen PL. Movement disorders in alcoholism: a review. Neurology 1990;40:741–746.
49. Gill JS, Shipley MJ, Tsementzis SA, Hornby RS, Gill SK, Hitchcock ER et al. Alcohol consumption—a risk factor for hemorrhagic and non-hemorrhagic stroke. Am J Med 1991;90:489–497.
50. Steel JK, Cockcroft JR, Ritter JM. Blind drunk: alcoholic pancreatitis and loss of vision. Postgrad Med J 1993;69:151–152.
51. Chedid A, Mendenhall CL, Gartside P, French SW, Chen T, Rubin L, VA Cooperative Study Group. Am J Gastroenterol 1991;86:210–216.
52. Sherlock S. Alcoholic liver disease. Lancet 1995;345:227–229.
53. Diamond I. Alcoholic myopathy and cardiomyopathy. N Engl J Med 1989;320:458–460.
54. Urbano-Marquez A, Estruch R, Navarro-Lopez F, Grau JM, Mont L, Rubin E. The effects of alcoholism on skeletal and cardiac muscle. N Engl J Med 1989;220:409–415.
55. Alderman LE, Coltart DJ. Alcohol and the heart. Br Med Bull 1982;38:77–80.
56. Moushmoush B, Abi-Mansour P. Alcohol and the heart. The long-term effects of alcohol on the cardiovascular system. Arch Intern Med 1991;151:36–42.
57. Reference Deleted.
58. Knieriem HJ, Herbertz G. Electron-microscopic findings and photometric activation analytical results in experimental cardiac insufficiency caused by cobaltous chloride. Virchows Arch B Cell Pathol 1969;2:32–46.
59. Munzinge W. Cardiomyopathy and arsenic intoxication. Arch Klin Med 1987;19:444.
60. Asokan SK, Witham AC. Myocardial malfunction of unknown cause. Cardiovasc Clin 1972;4:113–132.
61. Urbano-Marquez A, Estruch R, Fernandez-Sola J, Nicolas JM, Parc JC, Rubin E. The greater risk of alcoholic cardiomyopathy and myopathy in women compared with men. JAMA 1995;274:149–153.
62. Day CP, James OFW, Butler TJ, Campbell RWF. QT prolongation and sudden cardiac death in patients with alcoholic liver disease. Lancet 1993;341:1423–1428.
63. Abe H, Kawano Y, Jojima S et al. Biphasic effects of repeated alcohol intake on 24-hour blood pressure in hypertensive patients. Circulation 1994;89:2626–2633.
64. Kei N, Swales JD, Grobbee DE. Alcohol intake and its relation to hypertension. Cardiovasc Risk Factors 1993;33:189–200.
65. Kaplan NM. Alcohol and hypertension. Lancet 1995;345:1588–1589.
66. Felson DT, Kiel DP, Anderson JJ, Kannel WB. Alcohol consumption and hip fractures. The Framingham Study. Am J Epidemiol 1988;128:102–110.
67. Bikle DD, Stesin A, Halloran B, Steinbach L, Recher D. Alcohol-induced bone disease: relationship to age and parathyroid hormone levels. Alcohol Clin Exp Res 1993;17:690–695.
68. Rico H. Alcohol and bone mineral density. Br Med J 1993;307:939.
69. MacGregor RR. Alcohol and immune defense. JAMA 1986;256:1474–1479.
70. Laitinen K, Lamberg-Allardt C, Tunninen R, Karonen S-L, Tahtela R, Ylikahri R et al. Transient hypoparathyroidism during acute alcohol intoxication. N Engl J Med 1991;324:721–727.
71. Miller G. Magnesium deficiency syndrome. Compr Ther 1985;11:58–64.
72. Freedland ES, McMichen DB. Alcohol-related seizures. II. Clinical presentation and management. J Emerg Med 1993;11:605–618.
73. De Marchi S, Cecchin E, Basile A, Bertotti A, Nardini R, Bartoli E. Renal tubular dysfunction in chronic alcohol abuse—effects of abstinence. N Engl J Med 1993;329:1927–1934.

74. Adams SL, Mathews JJ, Flaherty JJ. Alcoholic ketoacidosis. Ann Emerg Med 1987;16:90–97.
75. Thompson CJ, Johnston DG, Baylis PH, Anderson J. Alcoholic ketoacidosis: an underdiagnosed condition? Br Med J 1986;292:463–465.
76. Duffens K, Marx JA. Alcoholic ketoacidosis—a review. J Emerg Med 1987;5:399–406.
77. Wrenn KD, Slovis CM, Minion GE, Rutkowski R. The syndrome of alcoholic ketoacidosis. Am J Med 1991;91:119–128.
78. Schelling JR, Howard RL, Winter SD, Linas SI. Increased osmolal gap in alcoholic ketoacidosis and lactic acidosis. Ann Intern Med 1990;113:580–582.
79. Milas AA, Tavassoli M. Laboratory markers of ethanol intake and abuse: a critical appraisal. Am J Med Sci 1992;303: 425–428.
80. Wax PM, Hoffman RS, Goldfrank LR. Rapid quantitative determination of blood alcohol concentration in the emergency department using an electrochemical method. Ann Emerg Med 1992;21:254–259.
81. Christopher TA, Zeccardi JA. Evaluation of the QED saliva alcohol test: a new rapid accurate device for measuring ethanol in saliva. Ann Emerg Med 1992;21:1135–1136.
82. Lopez GP, Yealy DM, Krenzelok EP. Survival of a child despite unusually high blood ethanol levels. Am J Emerg Med 1989;7:283–285.
83. Beckett GJ, Hayes JD. Plasma glutathion-S-transferase measurements and liver disease in man. J Clin Biochem Nutr 1987;2:1–24.
84. Blake J, Orrego H. Monitoring treatment of alcoholic liver disease: evaluation of various severity indices. Clin Chem 1991;37:5–13.
85. Chedid A, Mendenhall CL, Gartside P, French SW, Chen T, Rabin L et al. Prognostic factors in alcoholic liver disease. Am J Gastroenterol 1991;86:210–216.
86. Geller RJ, Spyler PA, Herold DA, Bruns DE. Serum osmolal gap and ethanol concentration: a simple and accurate formula. Clin Toxicol 1986;24:77–84.
87. Angeli P, Gatta A, Caregaro L, Luisetto G, Menon F, Merkel C et al. Hypophosphatemia and renal tubular dysfunction in alcoholics. Are they related to liver function impairment? Gastroenterology 1991;100:502–512.
88. Naughton M, Grand J. Hypophosphatemia in a comatose alcoholic. Med J Aust 1991;155:723–724.
89. MacDonald L, Kruse JA, Levy D, Marulendra S, Sweeny PJ. Lactic acidosis and acute alcohol intoxication. Am J Emerg Med 1994;12:32–35.
90. Jones AW. Update on the concentration of acetone in blood from drinking drivers, Type-1 diabetes, out-patients and healthy blood donors. Proc Am Acad Forensic Sci, 44th Annual Meeting, New Orleans: February 17–22, 1992; p 193.
91. Stibler W. Carbohydrate-deficient transferrin in serum: a new marker of potentially harmful alcohol consumption reviewed. Clin Chem 1991;37:2029–2093.
92. Koppel C, Muller C, Wrobel N. Diagnostic value of carbohydrate-deficient transferring for identifying patients with drug overdose at risk of developing an alcohol withdrawal syndrome (Personal communication).
92a. Koppel C, Rosick U, Bratter P. Influence of chronic alcohol abuse on selenium status in ICU patients. Ann Emerg Med 1995;26:723.
93. Donnelly A, Paloucek F, Leikin J. Possible reversal of ethanol-induced respiratory depression of flumazenil. Vet Hum Toxicol 1991;33:389.
94. Koch HP. The story of the anti-alcohol drug RO 15-4513. Int Pharmacol J 1988;2:85–86.
95. Littleton J. Alcohol intoxication and physical dependence. A molecular mystery tour. Br J Addict 1989;84:267–276.
96. Naranjo CA, Sellers EM, Wu PH, Lawrin MO. Moderation of ethanol drinking: role of enhanced serotonergic neurotransmission. In : Naranjo CA, Sellers EM, eds. Research advances in new psychopharmacological treatments for alcoholism. Amsterdam: Elsevier, 1985.
97. Cook C, Lipsedge M. Chlormethiazole and alcohol: a lethal cocktail. Br Med J 1987;294:1099.
98. Agricola R, Mazarino M, Urani R. Treatment of acute alcohol withdrawal syndrome with carbamazepine: a double-blind comparison with tiapride. J Int Med Res 1982;10: 100–105.
99. Ballenger JC, Post RM. Carbamazepine in alcohol withdrawal syndromes and schizophrenia psychoses. Psychopharmacol Bull 1984;20:572–584.
100. Yam PCI, Forbes A, Kox WJ. Clonidine in the treatment of alcohol withdrawal in the intensive care unit. Br J Anaesth 1992;68:106–108.
101. Gallimberti L, Canton G, Gentile N, Ferri M, Cibin M, Ferrara SD et al. Gamma-hydroxybutyric acid for treatment of alcohol withdrawal syndrome. Lancet 1989;2:787–789.
102. Reference Deleted.
103. Flemenbaum A. Affective disorders and "chemical dependence": lithium for alcohol and drug addiction? Dis Nerv Syst 1974;35:281–289.
104. Flemenbaum A. Lithium carbonate prophylaxis of alcoholism: its time has come. Arch Gen Psychiatry 1989;46:290.
105. Fawcett J, Aagesen CA, Tilkin JM, McGuire M, Clark DC, Pisani VD et al. Lithium carbonate prophylaxis of alcoholism. Its time has come. Arch Gen Psychiatry 1989;46:290–291.
106. Baud FJ, Galliott M, Astier A, VuBien D, Garnier R, Likforman J, Bismuth C. Treatment of ethylene glycol poisoning with intravenous 4-methylpyrazole. N Engl J Med 1988;319:97–100.
107. Naltrexone for alcohol dependence. Med Lett Drug Ther 1995;37(Issue 953):64–66.
108. Monti J, Alterwain P. Ritanserin decreases alcohol intake in chronic alcoholics. Lancet 1991;337:60.
109. Peters DH, Vaulds D. Tiapride. A review of its pharmacology and therapeutic potential in the management of alcohol dependence syndrome. Drugs 1994;47:1010–1032.
110. Lewis DC, Femind J. Management of alcohol withdrawal. Pharmacol Physicians 1982;16:1.
111. Baumgartner GR, Rowen RC. Clonidine vs chlordiazepoxide in the management of acute alcohol withdrawal syndrome. Arch Intern Med 1987;147:1223–1226.
112. Pol S, Nalpas B, Berthelot P. Dexamethasone for alcohol withdrawal. Ann Intern Med 1991;114:705–706.
113. Ives TJ, Mooney AJ III, Gwyther RE. Pharmacokinetic dosing of phenobarbital in the treatment of alcohol withdrawal syndrome. South Med J 1991;84:18–21.
114. Rosenbloom A. Emerging treatment options with alcohol withdrawal syndrome. J Clin Psychiatry 1988;49 (Suppl 12): 28–31.
115. Gillman MA, Lichtigfeld FJ. Analgesic nitrous oxide for alcohol withdrawal: a critical appraisal after 10 years' use. Postgrad Med J 1990;66:543–546.
116. Haddox VG, Bidder TG, Waldron LE, Derby P, Achen SMW. Clorazepate use may prevent alcohol withdrawal convulsions. West J Med 1987;146:695–696.
117. Fish SS, Heeren T. Does phenytoin prevent alcohol withdrawal seizures: a meta analysis. Vet Hum Toxicol 1993;35:366.
118. Korsakoff's syndrome. Lancet 1990;336:912–913.
119. Neuberger JM. Transplantation for alcoholic liver disease contraindicated by alcohol dependence or extrahepatic disease. Br Med J 1989;299:693.
120. Moss AH, Siegler M. Should alcoholics compete equally for liver transplantation? JAMA 1991;265:1295–1298.
121. Cohen C, Benjamin M, and the Ethics and Social Impact Committee of the Transplant and Health Policy Center. Ann Arbor, MI: JAMA 1991;205:1299–1301.
122. Bird GLA, O'Grady JG, Harvey FAH, Calne RY, Williams R. Liver transplantation in patients with alcoholic cirrhosis: selection criteria and rates of survival and relapse. Br Med J 1990;301:15–17.
123. Vogel C, Caraccio T, Mofenson H, Hart S. Alcohol intoxication in young children. Clin Toxicol 1995;33:25–33.
124. Leung AK. Ethyl alcohol ingestion in children. A 15-year review. Clin Pediatr 1986;25:617–619.
125. Gibson PJ, Cant AJ, Mant TG. Ethanol poisoning. Acta Paediatr Scand 1985;74:977–978.
126. Redetzki HM. Ethanol (Management Treatment Protocol): Poisindex Information System. Rumack BH, ed. Colorado: Micromedex, Inc. Edition expires 8/30/92.

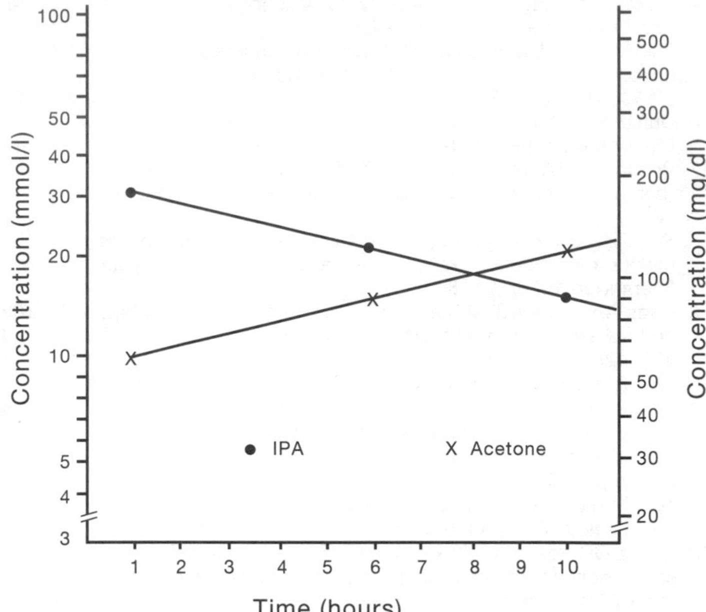

Figure 55–3. Pharmacokinetics of IPA and acetone (semilogarithmic scale). (From Vicas IMO, Beck R. Clin Toxicol 1993;31:473–481.)

ISOPROPYL ALCOHOL

In hospitals isopropyl alcohol (IPA) is often colored with blue dye to distinguish it from many other clear and colorless liquids; this has led to the designation *blue heaven* by abusers.[1]

TOXICOKINETICS

Absorption

Ingestion of 1 oz of 70% isopropyl alcohol (0.4 mL/kg) by volunteers led to peak serum isopropyl alcohol concentrations of about 28 mg/dL in 30 minutes; peak serum acetone concentrations of about 34 mg/dL were not observed until approximately 4 hours after ingestion. Urine tests positive for acetone are measurable by 3 hours postingestion. A positive urine test for acetone may still be present at 24 hours postingestion. Serum acetone is measurable within 30 minutes postingestion (Fig. 55–3). If no acetone is quantified by 30 minutes postexposure, exposure to isopropyl alcohol is unlikely.[2] A large overdose may delay absorption. Skin absorption is probably relatively small, but contributes to toxicity with prolonged contact.

LABORATORY

Blood Levels

A given isopropanol blood level is roughly twice as toxic as the same blood ethanol level.

Endogenous Isopropanol Formation

Isopropanol may be found in type I insulin-dependent acetonemic diabetes mellitus patients not exposed to isopropyl alcohol who are hyperglycemic and usually acidotic, indicating that acetone may be converted to isopropanol in physiologic conditions in which reduced nicotinamide adenine dinucleotide is elevated. Isopropanol serum levels up to 29.7 mg/dL have been observed in such patients with acetone levels up to 32.1 mg/dL.[3] Chronic alcoholics, who also are known to produce elevated NADH concentrations, may develop acetonemia (e.g., through starvation ketosis) and theoretically could produce detectable concentrations of isopropyl alcohol. This remains to be confirmed.

Acetone (Fig. 55–3)

Endogenous concentrations of acetone in the blood of healthy individuals range from about 0.1 to 0.5 mg/dL.[4] The highest concentration of acetone from 500 randomly selected blood specimens in one series was 6 mg/dL.[5] Levels of 20 to 30 mg/dL are considered toxic. A lethal concentration of 55 mg/dL has been reported.[6] Others have reported acetone blood concentrations of over 200 mg/dL in nonfatal cases of isopropanol ingestion.[5,7]

CLINICAL CASE REPORT

Inhalation of 70% isopropyl alcohol by a neonate led to sedation, hypotension, cyanosis, bradycardia, asystole, and death.[8] The isopropyl alcohol elimination half-life was 9.6 hours.

ABNORMALITIES

Osmolal Gap

Elevations of endogenous glycerol, acetone, and acetone metabolite levels may also be causes for an increased osmolal gap in the alcoholic patient. Before alcohol therapy and/or hemodialysis is instituted in patients with both an increased anion gap metabolic acidosis (Table 55–22) and increased osmolar gap, alcoholic acidosis and lactic acidosis should be excluded. Any contribution of ethyl alcohol to the increased osmolal and anion gap can be evaluated from an initial serum ethyl alcohol level. Each 10 mg/dL of ethanol adds 2.3 mOsm/kg H_2O to the serum osmolality. Isopropyl alcohol may increase the osmolal gap and induce ketosis since it is metabolized to acetone, but metabolic acidosis is rare.[9]

TREATMENT

Large doses of activated charcoal can absorb significant amounts of isopropanol and acetone.[10]

REFERENCES—ISOPROPYL ALCOHOL

1. Rich J, Scheife RT, Katz N, Caplan LR. Isopropyl alcohol intoxication. Arch Neurol 1970;417:322–324.
2. Lacoutre PG, Heldreth DD, Shannon M, Lovejoy FH Jr. The generation of acetonemia/acetonuria following ingestion of a subtoxic dose of isopropyl alcohol. Am J Emerg Med 1989;7:38–40.
3. Bailey DN. Detection of isopropanol in acetonemic patients not exposed to isopropanol. Clin Toxicol 1990;28:459–466.
4. Levey S, Balchun OJ, Medrano V, Jung R. Studies of metabolic products in expired air. II. Acetone. J Lab Clin Med 1964;63:574–584.
5. Jones AW. Driving under the influence of isopropanol. Clin Toxicol 1992;30:153–155.
6. Stead AN, Moffat AC. A collection of therapeutic, toxic and fatal blood drug concentrations in man. Hum Toxicol 1983;3: 437–464.
7. Kelner M, Beuley DN. Isopropanol ingestion: interpretation of blood concentrations and clinical findings. J Toxicol Clin Toxicol 1983;20:497–507.
8. Vicas IMO, Beck R. Fatal inhalational isopropyl alcohol poisoning in a neonate. Clin Toxicol 1993;31:473–481.
9. Braden GL, Strayhorn CH, Germain MJ, Mulhern JG, Skutcher CL. Increased osmolal gap in alcoholic acidosis. Arch Intern Med 1993;153: 2377–2380.
10. Burkhart KK, Martinez MA. The absorption of isopropanol and acetone by activated charcoal. Clin Toxicol 1992; 30:371–375.

METHANOL

USES

An anecdotal report suggest that methanol poisoning may follow intentional "sniffing."[1]

CLINICAL PRESENTATION

Initial Presentation

Clinical Effects

A patient survived a serum methanol level of 493 mg/dL without loss of eyesight following aggressive therapy with an ethanol drip, bicarbonate, and hemodialysis.[2]

Gastrointestinal Tract

Methanol is a mucosal irritant and produces nausea, vomiting, and abdominal pain in over one half of cases. Absence of gastrointestinal symptoms does not rule out serious toxicity. Pancreatitis, as defined by elevated serum amylase, occurs commonly,[3] appearing in two-thirds of a recent series of cases.[4] Hemorrhagic pancreatitis may appear on autopsy. Elevation of hepatic aminotransferases usually is mild and transient.

LABORATORY

Analytic Methods

A modified headspace gas chromatographic method for analysis of formate in blood has a limit of detection of 2.5 mg/dL. Ocular toxicity may correlate better with formate concentration than with methanol concentration.[5]

Abnormalities

Acidosis.

Blood Levels

Serum and urine formate levels do not appear to be good biologic markers of methanol intoxication.[6]

A patient fell into a vat of furniture finish stripping solution. Three hours later his peak methanol level was 247 mg/dL. With intravenous ethanol, bicarbonate, folate, gastric lavage, and hemodialysis the blood methanol dropped to 4 mg/dL 43 hours later. The patient survived.[7]

A 6-week-old infant was fed Similac infant formula accidentally diluted with a methanol-containing windshield washer fluid. The infant, who appeared normal, was treated with activated charcoal and folic acid and developed a serum methanol level of 45.6 mg/dL (14.2 mmol/L) on the third day. No abnormal ophthalmologic fundus optic changes or severe metabolic acidosis developed, and no ethanol therapy was instituted. The long half-life of methanol in this case (28 hours) was probably due to the relative inactivity of alcohol dehydrogenase in this age group. Formate levels were not measured.[8]

Urine Levels

There is a correlation between occupational exposure to methanol vapor and levels of methanol measured in shift-end urine samples. Levels of about 42 mg methanol/liter of urine are excreted in a shift-end urine sample following 8 hours of exposure to methanol at 200 ppm (current permissible limit).[9]

Formate Levels—Predictive Value

Criteria predictive of severe methanol poisoning possibly leading to permanent sequelae can include: (a) an interval between ingestion and treatment exceeding 10 hours and (b) blood formate levels about 0.5 g/L (or 11.1 mmol/L)[7,10] (Fig. 55–4).

Ancillary Tests

Hypomagnesemia occurs following ethyl alcohol and methanol ingestion, diuretic therapy, and sympathomimetic use.[11] Hypokalemia may be due to the formation of potassium formate. In the presence of a metabolic acidosis associated with hypokalemia, methanol poisoning should be considered.[12]

Reduction in pH will not begin to occur before 6 hours after ingestion. Plasma bicarbonate levels and percent change in plasma bicarbonate levels correlate poorly with the time after ingestion.[12a]

An anecdotal study suggests that magnetic resonance imaging was useful in the evaluation of a patient with methanol-induced toxic optic neuropathy.[13]

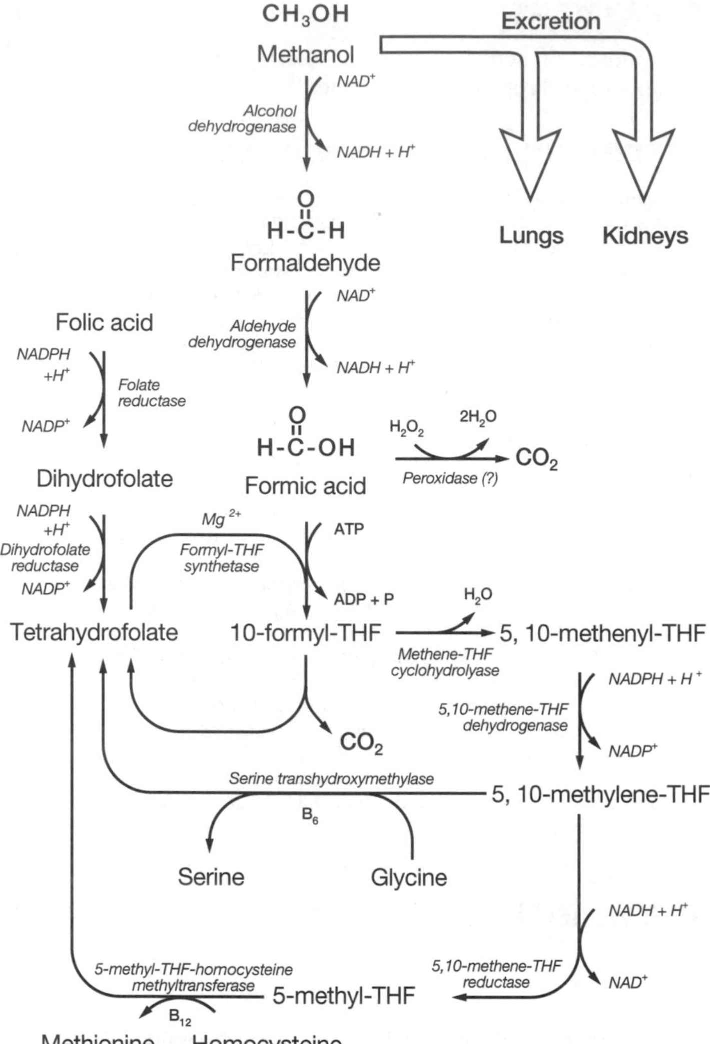

Figure 55–4. Metabolic pathways involved in methanol metabolism and relationship with folate metabolism. *THF,* tetrahydrofolate. (Adapted from Kruse JA. Intensive Care Med 1992;18:292–297.)

TREATMENT

Stabilization

If the patient is asymptomatic and methyl alcohol ingestion is suspected, perform gastric lavage with activated charcoal. Obtain serum methanol and arterial blood gas.

Chronic Alcoholics

Chronic alcoholics on drinking bouts may often drink solutions containing both methanol and ethanol and exhibit no signs of a formate-induced metabolic acidosis on admission in spite of high methanol and ethanol blood levels. The methanol content of 20 commercial wines ranged from 5.0 to 32.5 mg/dL,[14] and the level in 24 distilled liquors ranged from 1.3 to 10.6 mg/dL. Therefore consumption of large amounts of wine or liquor theoretically can result in detectable levels of serum methanol.[15,16]

Such patients may not require hemodialysis. The diagnosis and treatment of combined methanol and ethanol poisoning should be based on the case history, clinical signs, and the presence of a metabolic acidosis, not on blood methanol concentrations alone.[17]

Elimination Enhancement

Consideration should be given to the reduction of hemorrhage complicating brain necrosis by performing hemodialysis without heparinization, using an artificial kidney with a biocompatible membrane such as polymethylmethacrylate and an albumin coating.[18]

Forced diuresis is not effective, but hemodialysis effectively removes methanol (100 to 200 mL/min clearance), as well as formaldehyde and formic acid.[19] Hemoperfusion removes neither methanol nor formate well.[20] Although peritoneal dialysis increases methanol clearance, hemodialysis is about eight times more effective.[21] Indications for dialysis procedures include the following:

1. A peak methanol level over 50 mg/dL is recommended in the medical literature,[22] but the exact level is debatable. Dialysis does reduce the prolonged intensive care time required for ethanol therapy at methanol levels above 50 mg/dL.
2. Metabolic acidosis is not immediately correctable with bicarbonate therapy. High formate levels (i.e., over 20 mg/dL) suggest the need for hemodialysis.

3. Any visual impairment.
4. Renal failure.

Dialysis may be stopped when the methanol level falls below 25 mg/dL. Remember that ethanol also is dialyzed and therefore maintenance levels must be increased during dialysis.

Antidotes

Administration of ethanol blocks the formation of formaldehyde and formic acid because of the preferential affinity of ethanol for alcohol dehydrogenase. Ethanol levels should be maintained between 100 and 150 mg/dL to completely inhibit toxic metabolite formation. Average dosages necessary to maintain a blood ethanol concentration of 100 mg/dL in a 70-kg patient are listed in Table 55–21.

4-MP (4-methyl-pyrazole) exhibits nonlinear elimination kinetics and probably induces its own metabolism. This may make it difficult to establish a safe dosage regimen with the drug. Multiple dosing with 4-MP may cause transient hepatotoxicity. Further work will be required to determine the safe use of 4-MP.[23]

Ethanol Administration

Intravenous administration is more reliable than oral administration, but ethyl alcohol is irritating to veins. An intravenous solution of 10% ethanol in D_5W is optimal. Note that maintenance infusion must be increased during dialysis. Blood must be drawn frequently before, during, and after dialysis until a steady-state ethanol level is confirmed. Continue ethanol infusion until the methanol level falls below the range of 20 to 25 mg/dL. Ethanol prolongs the elimination half-life of methanol to 24 to 30 hours; hence several days may be required to reduce the methanol level below 25 mg/dL when hemodialysis is not used.

Ethanol Indications

1. Peak methanol level over 20 mg/dL.
2. Any patient with a history of ingestion of 0.4 mL/kg or any symptomatic patient should receive ethanol pending confirmatory blood methanol levels.
3. Acidosis.
4. Any patient considered for hemodialysis.
5. Palatnick and colleagues suggest that ethanol may prolong the risk for toxicity and potential complications. Hemodialysis should be considered for methanol poisoned patients who are treated with ethanol infusions.[24]

Supportive Care

1. If the methyl alcohol level is below 40 mg/dL and the blood pH is normal, further alcohol administration or hemodialysis is usually not necessary.
2. If the methyl alcohol level is about 40 to 50 mg/dL and the blood pH is normal, use either a continuous IV alcohol infusion with frequent monitoring of both methanol and ethanol serum levels (requires prolonged hospitalization) or use IV alcohol and hemodialysis, which will usually remove the methanol in about 5 hours and decrease hospitalization.
3. If the methyl alcohol level is above 50 mg/dL and the blood pH is normal, use IV alcohol and begin hemodialysis.
4. If the blood pH supports a metabolic acidosis with normal lactic acid levels, the concentration of methanol is not a determining factor, and the patient should be treated with IV ethyl alcohol and hemodialysis to remove formaldehyde and formic acid from the blood.[25]
5. Frequent assessment of vital signs (hourly) until stable. Watch for variations in blood pressure, hypothermia, tachycardia, arrhythmias, cyanosis, and dyspnea.
6. Measurements of ethanol and methanol levels and calculation of anion and osmolar gaps provide an estimate of the elimination rate.[26]
7. Folic acid probably accelerates the detoxification of the toxic metabolite, formic acid.

REFERENCES—METHANOL

1. McCormick MJ, Mogabgab E, Adams SL. Methanol poisoning as a result of inhalational solvent abuse. Ann Emerg Med 1990;19:639–642.
2. Pamies RJ, Sugar D, Rives L, Herold AH. Methanol intoxication. Case report. J Fla Med Assoc 1993;80:465–467.
3. Bennett JL, Cary FH, Mitchell GL et al. Acute methyl alcohol poisoning: a review based on experiences in an outbreak of 323 cases. Medicine 1953;32:431–463.
4. Swartz RD, Millman RP, Billi JE et al. Epidemic methanol poisoning: clinical and biochemical analysis of a recent episode. Medicine 1981;60:373–382.
5. Fraser AD, MacNeil W. Gas chromatographic analysis of methyl formate and application in methanol poisoning cases. J Anal Toxicol 1989;13:73–76.
6. D'Alessandro A, Osterloh J, Chumers P, Quinlan P, Kell T, Becker C. Formate in serum acid urine following controlled methanol exposure at the threshold limit value. Vet Hum Toxicol 1993;35:358.
7. Keller K, Pearigen PD, Olsen KR. Severe methanol poisoning and chemical burn after submersion in a furniture stripping solution. Vet Hum Toxicol 1991;33:366.
8. Brent J, Lucas M, Kulig K, Rumack BH. Methanol poisoning in a 6-week-old infant. J Pediatr 1991;118:644–646.
9. Kawai T, Yasugi T, Mizunama K, Horiguchi S, Hirase Y, Uchida Y, Ikeda M. Methanol in urine as a biological indicator of occupational exposure to methanol vapor. Int Arch Occup Environ Health 1991;63:311–318.
10. Mahieu P, Hassoun A, Lauwerys R. Predictors of methanol intoxication with unfavourable outcome. Hum Toxicol 1989;8: 135–137.
11. Harchelroad F. Hypomagnesemia during methanol intoxication. Vet Hum Toxicol 1993;35:364.
12. Hassoun A, Mahieu P, Lauwerys P. Hypokalemia in acute methanol poisoning. Proc Eur Assoc Pois Cont Clin Toxicol, Birmingham, UK: May 1993.

12a. McGuigan MA. Analysis of the temporal development of acidosis in uncomplicated methanol poisoning. Ann Emerg Med 1995;26:725.

13. Bernstein JM, McNally J, Boyer L. Magnetic resonance imaging of methanol-induced optic nerve toxicity. Vet Hum Toxicol 1993;35:365.
14. Carroll RB. Analysis of alcoholic beverages by gas-liquid chromatography. QJ Stud Alcohol 1970; 5(Suppl)6–19.
15. Tintinalli JE. Serum methanol in the absence of methanol ingestion. Ann Emerg Med 1995;26:393.
16. Lee CY. Acree TE, Butts RM. Determination of methyl alcohol in wine by gas chromatography. Anal Chem 1975;47:747–748.
17. Martensson E, Olofsson U, Heath A. Clinical and metabolic features of ethanol-methanol poisoning in chronic alcoholics. Lancet 1988;1:327–328.

18. Phang PT, Passerini L, Mialke B, Berendt R, King EG. Brain hemorrhage associated with methanol poisoning. Crit Care Med 1988;16:137–140.
19. McCoy HG, Cipolle RJ, Ehlers SM et al. Severe methanol poisoning: application of a pharmacokinetic model for ethanol therapy and hemodialysis. Am J Med 1979;67:804–807.
20. Whalen JE, Richards CJ, Ambre J. Inadequate removal of methanol and formate using the sorgent based regeneration hemodialysis delivery system. Clin Nephrol 1979;11:318–321.
21. Settler JG, Singh R, Brackett NC et al. Studies on the dialysis of methanol. Trans Am Soc Artif Intern Organis 1967; 13:179–182.
22. Gonda A, Gault H, Churchill D et al. Hemodialysis for methanol intoxication. Am J Med 1978;64:749–758.
23. Jacobsen D, McMartin KE. Methanol and ethylene glycol poisoning: 4-methylpyrazole or ethanol. Proc Intern Cong Eur Assoc Poison Control Centres, Milan, Italy: September 25–29, 1990; p. 142.
24. Palatnick W, Redman LW, Sitar DS, Tenenbein M. Methanol half-life during ethanol administration: implications for management of ethanol poisoning. Ann Emerg Med 1995;26: 202–207.
25. McCarron MM. Methyl alcohol. September, 1993 (Personal communication).
26. King ML. Acute methanol poisoning: a case study. Heart Lung 1992;21:260–264.

ETHYLENE GLYCOL

CLINICAL PRESENTATION

Toxic Dosage

The approximate minimum lethal dose is 1 to 1.5 mL/kg or approximately 100 mL in an adult. Persons who attempted suicide by ingesting 1 and 2 L and who were treated within 1 hour have survived.[1,2]

TOXICOKINETICS

Absorption

Ethylene glycol is rapidly absorbed orally but not by lung or dermal routes. Peak levels occur 1 to 4 hours postingestion.

Distribution

Since ethylene glycol is highly water soluble, it distributes evenly throughout body tissue.

Elimination

The renal glomeruli filter and then passively reabsorb most of the absorbed ethylene glycol dose.[3] Approximately 20% of a dose of 1 mg/kg is excreted unchanged; less than 1% of the ethylene glycol is metabolized to oxalic acid at this dose. The liver oxidizes ethylene glycol primarily to glycoaldehyde, glycolate, and then glyoxylate.

The metabolism of glyoxylate follows several pathways that depend on the cofactors thiamine and pyridoxine. The oxidation of ethylene glycol to glyoxylate and subsequently to oxalate requires the conversion of NAD to NADH. The altered NAD/NADH ratio shifts pyruvate to lactate and thereby helps produce lactic acidosis. The acidic metabolites are more toxic than the parent compound. The order of toxicity appears to be glyoxylate > glycoaldehyde > ethylene glycol.[4]

The plasma half-life of ethylene glycol is approximately 3 to 5 hours. At ethanol levels of 100 to 200 mg/dL, the half-life of ethylene glycol is prolonged to 17 hours because of the 100-times-greater affinity of ethanol for alcohol dehydrogenase.[5]

PATHOPHYSIOLOGY

Ethylene glycol produces roughly the same CNS depression as ethanol, but ethylene glycol produces toxic metabolites. The metabolic acidosis and anion gap result primarily from glycolic acid formation and some lactic acid formation.[6] The inhibition of the citric acid cycle resulting from reduced NAD/NADH ratios and formation of oxalic acid contribute, to a limited extent, to the metabolic acidosis. Oxalate formation produces myocardial depression and acute tubular necrosis, although the exact mechanism is unclear since only a small amount of oxalate is formed. Glycoaldehydes, glycolic acid, and glyoxylic acid may contribute to CNS depression and may contribute to renal toxicity by producing renal edema; however, McChesney and colleagues[7] and Clay and Murphy[8] have shown that little oxalic acid, glycoxylic acid, glycoaldehyde, or formic acid is found during ethylene glycol intoxication. Hypocalcemia may result from chelation of oxalate,[1] although there are scant data available to support this hypothesis.

CLINICAL PRESENTATION

The classic three-stage presentation depends on the amount of severity of ingestion.[9] Hepatic damage usually is minimal.

Stage 1: CNS Depression (1 to 12 Hours Postingestion)

Transient exhilaration occurs without the odor of ethanol. Gastrointestinal complaints include primarily nausea and vomiting. Acidosis, coma, convulsions, and myoclonic jerks also may be present. The optic fundus is usually normal, although the occasional presence of papilledema may confuse the clinical presentation with that of methanol. Nystagmus and ophthalmoplegias may appear. Cerebral edema secondary to cytotoxic damage and calcium oxalate deposition synergistically depress CNS activity in severe poisoning.

Stage 2: Cardiopulmonary Symptoms (12 to 24 Hours Postingestion)

Tachycardia, tachypnea, and mild hypertension often occur. Congestive heart failure and circulatory collapse are seen in severe ingestions.

Stage 3: Renal Stage (24 to 72 Hours Postingestion)

This stage is characterized by oliguria, flank pain, acute tubular necrosis, renal failure, and rarely bone marrow arrest.[10] Renal damage may be permanent.

Ethylene glycol toxicity is suggested by the following: ethanol-like intoxication with no odor, large-anion-gap acidosis and coma, osmolal gap, calcium oxalate crystals, and mental status changes.

ACUTE INTOXICATION (SEE TABLE 55-1)

CHRONIC INTOXICATION

Cranial Nerve Deficit and Peripheral Nerve Deficits

Multiple cranial nerve deficits can develop 1 to 2 weeks after ethylene glycol ingestion.[11] Cranial nerve deficits may follow within 1 to 3 weeks the ingestion of generally over 100 mL of ethylene glycol in spite of aggressive therapy (hemodialysis with correction of fluid and acid-base abnormalities) of the underlying acute poisoning.[11] Most patients exhibit a bilateral facial nerve (VII) paralysis, although hearing loss, dysarthria, dysphagia, anisocoria, and blurred vision may also be present.[12] The deficit may be permanent.[3] Several weeks after the cranial nerve deficits have been established, a demyelinating sensorimotor peripheral neuropathy may develop with proximal muscle weakness, stocking-glove sensory loss, and areflexia.[13]

LABORATORY

Abnormalities

Urine

Although oxalate normally is a minor metabolic product of ethylene glycol metabolism, urinary oxalate crystals are a common, but not invariable, feature of ethylene glycol intoxication (Figs. 55–5 and 55–6).[14] There are two forms of urinary calcium oxalate crystals: the octahedral or tent-shaped form of the dihydrate crystals, and the prism or dumbell-shaped monohydrate form.[15] The latter form is stable under normal physiologic conditions; the dihydrate form appears only during high urinary calcium and oxalate concentrations, as seen in ethylene glycol poisoning. The dihydrate form can transform into the monohydrate form.[16]

Analytic Methods

2,3-Butanediol

Ethylene glycol determinations frequently are performed by precipitation of plasma proteins with acetonitrile, formation of the cyclic phenylboronate ester derivative of ethylene glycol, and analysis of gas chromatography with OV-17 as the stationary phase. Alcoholics may drink industrial alcohol preparations that contain 2-butanone. This ketone may be converted in the liver to 2,3-butanediol, which has an identical retention time to ethylene glycol and may be mistakenly reported as ethylene glycol. This problem may be easily corrected by changing the stationary phase from OV-17 to, for example, SE-30.[17]

Propylene Glycol

Propylene glycol (PG) has been used as an internal standard for quantifying ethylene glycol by gas chromatography in serum. Intravenous administration of drug formulations containing PG (e.g., phenytoin—Dilantin, diazepam—Valium) may lead to potentially serious underestimations of ethylene glycol concentrations in serum.[18]

Urine

Check the urine each hour for at least 5 hours after ingestion before ethylene glycol intoxication is ruled out for consideration. If urine oxidate crystals are seen and a second 1-hour urine specimen also shows calcium oxalate crystals, begin IV alcohol and hemodialyze (Fig. 55–6).

Some commercial ethylene glycol antifreeze products contain sodium fluorescein as a colorant to aid in the detection of automobile cooling system leaks. The urine of a patient suspected of an antifreeze ingestion may disclose visually detectable fluorescein under a Wood's lamp in the first several hours after ingestion. This observation must be confirmed by appropriate quantitative tests.[19]

In anuric patients, irrigation of the urinary bladder with 50 to 100 mL of saline, centrifugation of the irrigant, and examination of the sediment for calcium oxalate crystals may increase the chances of detection of calcium oxalate crystalluria in a suspected ethylene glycol ingestion.[20]

Blood

Hypocalcemia may occur and is manifested by QT prolongation on the ECG; tetany may result. Myalgias, elevated serum creatinine levels, and increased serum creatine phosphokinase levels may be seen.[6] Anion-gap metabolic acidosis indicates the production of organic acids. Toxicity may occur without significant elevation of the osmolal gap. Serious ethylene glucol toxicity (50 mg/dL) produces an approximate rise in the osmolal gap of 10 mOsm. The osmolal and anion gaps may remain elevated in spite of low serum ethylene glycol levels because of the accumulation of the blood glycolate.[21]

Serum Levels

Quantitative levels require gas chromatography and are not routinely included on toxicology screens. Serum levels exceeding 50 mg/dL suggest the need for hemodialysis. Recovery has occurred with aggressive treatment in the presence of ethylene glycol levels of 145 mg/dL (8-hour level) and 560 mg/dL (1-hour level).[2,22] Reported serum ethylene glycol levels in survivors ranged up to 650 mg/dL, whereas levels between 98 and 775 mg/dL were reported in fatalities.[2,5,23,24] Glycolic acid and bicarbonate levels correlated better than serum ethylene glycol levels with the clinical picture, since the former two levels reflect the action of the toxic metabolites.

TREATMENT

Stabilization

Do not wait for symptoms to appear before treatment. Time elapsed between ingestion (fatalities reported if longer than 12 hours) and treatment and the dose ingested are major predictive factors of morbidity fatality.[25]

Elimination Enhancement

A primary indicator for hemodialysis (HD) is a significant metabolic acidosis with a pH less than 7.15. Patients with very high concentrations of ethylene glycol (EG) (over 60 mmol/L or 373 mg/dL) without acidosis may also be

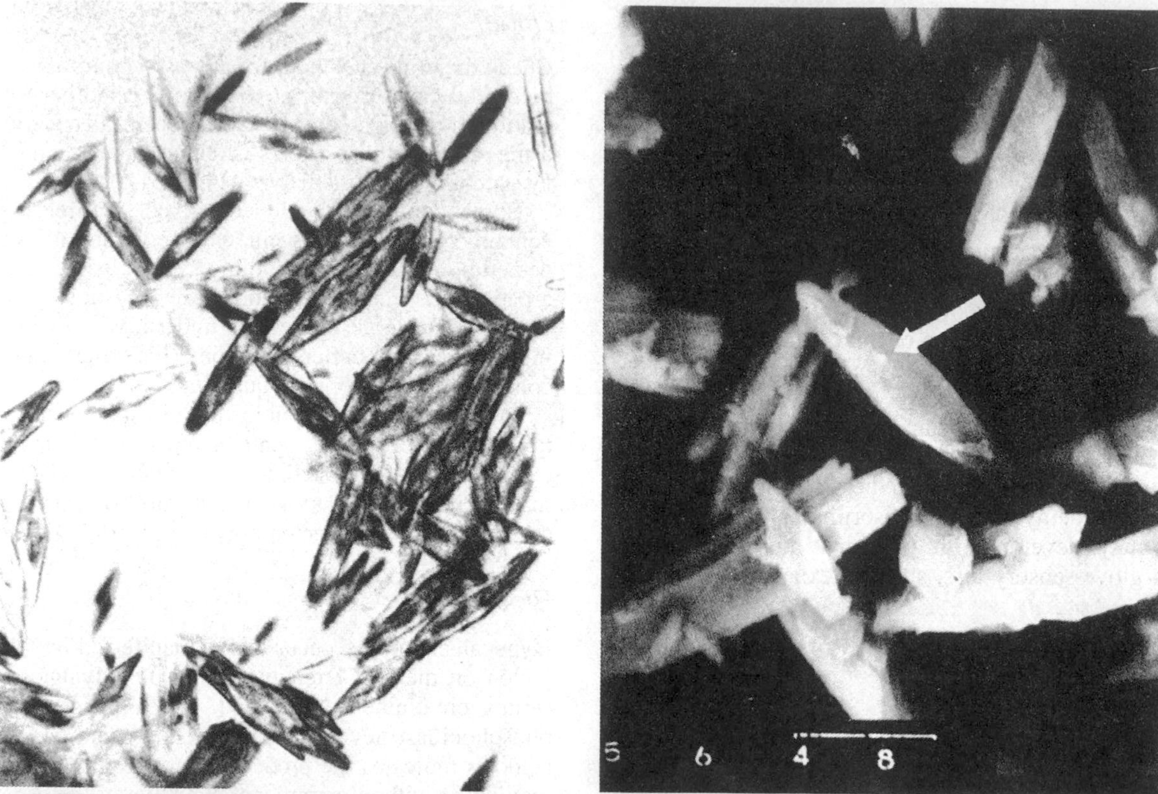

Figure 55–5. Calcium monohydrate crystals. Left, × 400; right, scanning electron micrograph, × 1,200; white arrow indicates a point of x-ray fluorescence. (From Terlinsky AS, Grochowski J, Geoly KL et al. Am J Clin Pathol 1981;76:224–225.)

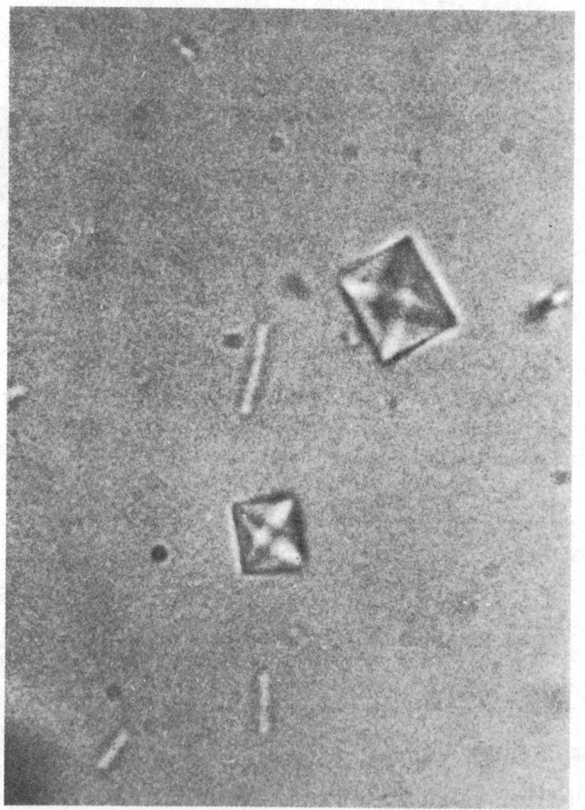

Figure 55–6. Calcium dihydrate crystals, × 400. (From Terlinsky AS, Grochowski J, Geoly KL et al. Am J Clin Pathol 1981;76: 224–225.)

candidates for HD to shorten the course of treatment and reduce the risk of renal complications. HD should be carried out at EG levels as low as 50 mg/dL (10 mmol/L) if the patient is anuric. During HD there is no need for ethanol administration intravenously or in the dialysate since glycolate is effectively eliminated. After termination of HD ethanol may be administered (IV boluses of 500 mL 5% glucose with 10% ethanol over 20 to 30 minutes, followed by a continuous infusion of 70 to 100 mL/hour). Monitor serum ethanol every hour until a constant level of 20 to 30 mmol/L (92 to 135 mg/dL) is obtained. Ethanol is continued until the serum concentration of EG is less than 10 mmol/L (about 60 mg/dL).[26]

Glycolate

Glycolate has a low volume of distribution (0.5 to 0.6 L/kg) and a low molecular weight and is rapidly cleared by hemodialysis. Careful monitoring can proceed with hourly acid-base balance without ethanol administration since glycolate assays are often not easily available.[26,27] Glycolate appears to be the causative factor for acidosis in ethylene glycol poisoning. It is effectively reversed by hemodialysis.[28]

Antidotes

Ethanol

If the urine fluoresces under a Wood's lamp, begin intravenous alcohol and hemodialyze the patient. However, if the serum concentration of ethylene glycol (EG) is high (over 30 mmol/L to 180 mg/dL) without metabolic acidosis, there is no immediate indication for hemodialysis. Ethanol will effectively inhibit the metabolism of EG, so that HD may be deferred until staff and equipment are available. During HD glycolate (low volume of distribution—0.5 to 0.6 L/kg, low molecular weight) is effectively eliminated. If the patient is admitted with metabolic acidosis, ethanol treatment and HD on an emergency basis is indicated to remove glycolate as soon as possible.[26]

Supportive Management

Margaret McCarron has presented a useful regimen for the management of ethylene glycol poisoning:

1. Ethylene glycol serum concentrations are not performed in most hospital laboratories; a specimen should be taken and sent to a contract lab.
   Results will be obtained in 3 to 5 days; therefore ETHYLENE GLYCOL SERUM LEVELS are NOT USEFUL IN DETERMINING ACUTE TOXICITY. They should be obtained for later confirmation of the diagnosis.
2. Gastric lavage with charcoal for any suspected case. The diagnosis of ethylene glycol poisoning should be made by the history and examination of the urine.
   a. *Waiting for symptoms to appear before treatment is too late,* because the symptoms are due to the metabolic abnormalities that often cannot be adequately treated.
   b. Examination of the urine is used to substantiate the diagnosis. Recommend that urine be checked every hour if negative, for at least 3 hours after the ingestion, before ethylene glycol intoxication is ruled out.
      1) *Check urine for calcium oxalate crystals.* If next specimen in 1 hour shows more crystals: IV ALCOHOL AND HEMODIALYZE.
      2) *Check urine under Wood's lamp.* If antifreeze has been taken, the urine will fluoresce from the fluorescent dye in the product. If urine fluoresces: IV ALCOHOL AND HEMODIALYZE.
3. If the patient enters the emergency room with metabolic acidosis and is in coma:
   1) Treat with bicarbonate for pH 7.20 or less.
   2) IV alcohol infusion.
   3) *Hemodialysis.* Note: Addition of 95% ethanol to dialysate is necessary to replace the ethanol lost during the procedure.
   4) Pyridoxine 50 mg and Thiamine 100 mg IM q.i.d. × 2 days.
   5) Monitor fluid and electrolytes, especially calcium and magnesium.

4-Methylpyrazole

4-Methylpyrazole has been shown to reduce blood glycolate levels after ethylene glycol ingestion and appears to be effective after both oral and intravenous administration. The product has not yet received FDA approval in the United States.[29–31]

Continuous arteriovenous hemofiltration dialysis may be an alternative when hemodialysis and 4-methylpyrazole therapy are not available. This observation has not been validated by controlled clinical trials.[32]

Supportive Care

1. Follow electrolyte fluid balance carefully. Renal clearance of ethylene glycol is inversely related to water absorption; therefore maintenance of good urine volumes is necessary to enhance urinary elimination.
2. Monitor serum calcium level and replace as indicated with 10% calcium gluconate intravenously.
3. Follow arterial pH and correct pH below 7.2 with intravenous bicarbonate.

REFERENCES—ETHYLENE GLYCOL

1. Scully R, Galdabini J, McNealy B. Case records of the Massachusetts General Hospital. Discussion of Levinsky NG. Case 38:1979. N Engl J Med 1979;301:650–657.
2. Stokes JB, Averon F. Prevention of organ damage in massive ethylene glycol ingestion. JAMA 1980;243:2065–2066.
3. Von Oettinggen VF. Ethylene glycol. US Public Health Bull 1943;281:166–174.
4. Beasley VR, Buck WB. Acute ethylene glycol toxicoses: a review. Vet Hum Toxicol 1980;22:255–263.
5. Peterson DC, Collins AJ, Himes JM et al. Ethylene glycol poisoning: pharmacokinetics during therapy with ethanol and hemodialysis. N Engl J Med 1981;304:21–23.
6. Gabow PA, Clay K, Sullivan JB et al. Organic acids in ethylene glycol intoxication. Ann Intern Med 1986;105:16–20.
7. McChesney EW, Goldberg L, Parekh CK et al. Re-appraisal of the toxicology of ethylene glycol. II. Metabolism studies in laboratory animals. Food Cosmet Toxicol 1971;9:21–38.
8. Clay KL, Murphy RC. On the metabolic acidosis of ethylene glycol intoxication. Toxicol Appl Pharmacol 1977;39:39–49.
9. Brown CG, Trumbull D, Klein-Schwartz W et al. Ethylene glycol poisoning. Ann Emerg Med 1983;12:501–506.
10. Bobbit WH, Williams RM, Freed CR. Severe ethylene glycol intoxication with multisystemic failure. West J Med 1986;144: 225–228.
11. Spillane L, Roberts JR, Meyer AE. Multiple cranial nerve deficits after ethylene glycol poisoning. Ann Emerg Med 1991; 20:208–210.
12. Factor SA, Lava NS. Ethylene glycol intoxication: a new stage in the clinical syndrome. NY State J Med 1987;87:179–180.
13. Thomas D, Claussen G, Suggs S, Oh SJ, Joy JL. Ethylene glycol-induced peripheral neuropathy. Neurology 1990; 40(Suppl 1):344.
14. Turk J, Morrell L, Avioli LV. Ethylene glycol intoxication. Arch Intern Med 1986;146:1601–1603.
15. Terlinsky AS, Grochowski J, Geoly KL et al. Identification of atypical calcium oxalate crystalluria following ethylene glycol ingestion. Am J Clin Pathol 1981;76:223–226.
16. Burns JR, Finalyson B. Changes in calcium oxalate crystal morphology as a function of concentration. Invest Urol 1980; 18:174–177.
17. Jones AW, Nilsson L, Gladh SA, Karlsson K, Beck-Friis J. 2,3-Butanediol in plasma from an alcoholic mistakenly identified as ethylene glycol by gas-chromatographic analysis. Clin Chem 1991;37:1453–1455.
18. LeGatt DF, Tisdell RH. Ethylene glycol quantifications. Avoid propylene glycol as an internal standard. Clin Chem 1990;36: 1860–1861.
19. Winter ML, Ellis MD, Snodgrass WR. Urine fluorescence using a Wood's lamp to detect the antifreeze additive sodium fluorescein: a qualitative adjunctive test in suspected ethylene glycol ingestion. Ann Emerg Med 1990;19:663–667.
20. Goodkin DA. Ethylene glycol poisoning. Am J Med 1990;88: 201.

21. Hewlett TP, McMartin KE. Ethylene glycol poisoning: the value of glycolic acid determinations for diagnosis and treatment. Clin Toxicol 1986;24:389–402.
22. Underwood F, Bennett WM. Ethylene glycol intoxication. JAMA 1973;57:143–150.
23. Parry MF, Wallach R. Ethylene glycol poisoning. Am J Med 1974;57:143–150.
24. Godolphin W, Meagher EP, Sanders HD et al. Unusual calcium oxalate crystals in ethylene glycol poisoning. Clin Toxicol 1980;16:479–486.
25. Groszek B. Ethylene glycol poisoning: why so high mortality? Proc Eur Assoc Pois Cont Clin Toxicol, Birmingham, UK: May 26–28, 1993.
26. Malmlund H-O, Berg A, Korlman G, Magnusson A, Lillman B. Considerations for the treatment of ethylene glycol poisoning based on analysis of two cases. Clin Toxicol 1991;29: 231–240.
27. Curtin L, Kramer J, Wine H, Savitt D, Abuelo JG. Complete recovery after massive ethylene glycol ingestion. Arch Intern Med 1992;152:1311–1313.
28. Jacobsen D, Orrebo S, Ostborg J, Sejerst OM. Glycolate causes the acidosis in ethylene glycol poisoning and is effectively removed by hemodialysis. Acta Med Scand 1994;216:409–416.
29. Baud FJ, Galliott M, Astier A, VuBien D, Garnier R, Likforman J, Bismuth C. Treatment of ethylene glycol poisoning with intravenous 4-methylpyrazole. N Engl J Med 1988;319:97–100.
30. Baud F, Bismuth C, Garnier R, Galliott M, Astier A, Maistre G et al. 4-Methylpyrazole may be an alternative to ethanol therapy for ethylene glycol intoxication in man. J Toxicol Clin Toxicol 1986–87;24:463–483.
31. Saladino R, Shannon M. Accidental and intentional poisoning with ethylene glycol in infancy: diagnostic clues and management. Pediatr Emerg Care 1991;7:93–96.
32. Christiansson KK, Kapersson KB, Kulling PEJ, Orrebo S. Treatment of severe ethylene glycol intoxication with continuous arterio-venous hemofiltration dialysis. J Toxicol Clin Toxicol 1995;33:267–270.

PROPYLENE GLYCOL

USES

Propylene glycol has been used as a nontoxic antifreeze in dairies and breweries, as a component of automotive brake fluids and antifreeze preparations, in the production of varnishes and synthetic resins, as a flavoring agent in baking and candy production, and as an emulsifier and nontoxic preservative in the foods industry.[1] Among prescription medications it can be found in several oral antibiotics, and it is a major ingredient in the formulation of several parenteral preparations, including diazepam (Valium) and phenytoin (Dilantin) in which its concentration may be as high as 40%.[1]

Propylene glycol is used in commercially available IV nitroglycerin solutions in quantities of 30 to 96% or more (Table 55–25).[2,3] It is also present in other parenteral medications (Table 55–26).[3]

TOXICOKINETICS

Intravenous administration of propylene glycol (PG) in amounts from 3 to 15 g/m^2 is followed by a maximum plasma concentration of 60 to 425 µg/mL, respectively, with a half-life of 1.8 to 3.3 hours, a volume of distribution of 0.51 to 0.88 L/kg, and a clearance rate of about 300 mL/min/1.73 m^2.[4] Cerebrospinal fluid concentrations are as high as 85% of the serum concentrations.[5]

CLINICAL PRESENTATION

Propylene glycol may cause hemolysis, deafness, a high anion-gap acidosis due to elevated lactate levels, sudden collapse, cardiac arrhythmias and asystole, hepatic damage, renal damage, hemolysis and serum hyperosmolarity with a marked osmolar gap.[2] There appears to be a significant increase in seizures among infants who have received a multivitamin preparation (MVI-12 with propylene glycol 3 g/day) when compared with infants receiving MVI concentrate (propylene glycol 300 mg/d).[6]

In experimental animals, propylene glycol possesses one-third the central nervous system depressant properties of ethanol.[7] A 15-month-old child had several episodes of hypoglycemia while ingesting 7.5 mL of propylene glycol per day.[8] Seizures developed in an 11-year-old boy with multiple endocrine problems and systemic candidiasis who ingested a medication containing propylene glycol.[9] A patient who presented with a propylene glycol blood level of 70 mg/dL developed stupor and lactic acidosis.[10] Hemolysis, hemoglobinuria, skin irritation, deafness, and other neurologic disturbances may be observed after propylene glycol administration.[11] The FDA considers propylene glycol safe in small doses for pharmaceutical preparations.

A patient was admitted with a plasma propylene glycol (PG) concentration of 4 mg/mL derived from drinking fruit juice (PG 0.6 mg/mL). She developed intractable epilepsy, respiratory depression, plasma hyperosmolality, and a metabolic acidosis, and she recovered rapidly (PG plasma level fell to less than 100 µg/ml within 6 hours).[12]

LABORATORY

Propylene glycol is osmotically active and produces a concentration-dependent increase in serum osmolality. Propylene glycol contained in enoximone was infused intravenously into an infant with heart failure at the rate of 2.4 mg/kg/min. Serum osmolality rose from 304 mmol/kg before the start of the infusion to 385 mmol/kg. Estimations of the serum propylene glycol concentration were 10,000 µg/mL.[11] A rapid gas-liquid chromatographic assay has been described with a detection limit of 1 µg/mL.

Data suggests that serum PG concentrations greater than 177 µg/mL are required to increase the lactate concentration by 6 µg/mL and to result in an elevated "anion gap."[5] A serum PG concentration in excess of 1520 µg/mL is required to yield an increase in osmolality of 20 mOsm/kg.[5] A method for the gas chromatographic–mass spectrometric identification and quantification of ethylene glycol and diethylene glycol in plasma is available. The detection limit is less than 10 mg/liter.[13]

A theoretical formula for the estimation of propylene glycol concentration from the osmolal gap is: propylene glycol (mg/dL) = osmolal gap × 7.6, or 47.5 + (osmolal gap × 9.2).[14,15]

TREATMENT

Infusion rates of over 1 mL/minute of products containing propylene glycol (PG) should be avoided. PG-containing products should not be administered through the same

Table 55-25
Composition of Intravenous Nitroglycerin Solutions Available in Different Countries[a]

Name	Manufacturer	Location	Available Ampules (ml)	Nitroglycerin Dose (mg/ml)	Content (%)
			Belgium		
Nosconitrine	Biothera-Asperal	Brussels	2 and 10	1.5	Ethanol (4) Propylene glycol (96)
			1.5	3.33	Ethanol (7) Propylene glycol (93)
			France		
Penitral	Labs. Besins-Iscovesco	Paris	2 and 10	1.5	Ethanol (4) Propylene glycol (96)
			1.5	3.33	Ethanol (7) Propylene glycol (93)
			Netherlands		
Nitroglycerine "Pohl"	Tramedico	Weesp	5	1	Ethanol (100)
			10	5	Ethanol (100)
Nitro "Pohl" Infusion	Tramedico	Weesp	25 and 50	1	Isotonic aqueous solution, glucose (5)
Nitroglycerine "Bipharma"	Bipharma	Amsterdam	1.6 and 8	0.625	Propylene glycol (100)
			West Germany		
Nitro Pohl infus	Pohl-Boskamp	Hohenlockstedt	5, 25, and 50	1	Isotonic aqueous solution, glucose (5)
Nitrolingual	Pohl-Boskamp	Hohenlockstedt	5	1	Ethanol (99)
			1 and 10 ml	5	Ethanol (99)
Nitro Mack	Mack	Illertissen	5	1	Ethanol (99)
Trinitrosan	Merck	Darmstadt	1	5	Ethanol (63)
			10	5	Ethanol (63)
Perlinganit-Losung	Pharma-Schwarz	Monheim	10	1	Propylene glycol (0.1) Glucose (5)
			50	1	Propylene glycol (0.1) Glucose (5)
			England		
Nitrocine	Sanol Schwarz	Chesham	10 and 50	1	Propylene glycol (0.1) Glucose (5)
Nitrolingual	Lipha	West Drayton	5	1	Ethanol (100)
			1 and 10 ml	5	Ethanol (100)
Nitronal	Lipha	West Drayton	5, 25, and 50	1	Isotonic aqueous solution, glucose (5)
Tridil	American Hospital Supply Ltd.	Compton (Newbury)	10	0.5	Ethanol (10)
			10	5	Ethanol (30) Propylene glycol (30)
			USA		
Nitrol IV	Kremers-Urban	Milwaukee	0.8, 1, 10 and 30	0.8	Lactose (0.7) NaCl (0.9)
Nitrostat	Parke-Davis	Morris Plains	10	0.8	Ethanol (5)
			10	5	Ethanol (30) Propylene glycol (30)
Nitroglycerin	Abbott Labs.	N. Chicago	5	5	Ethanol (50) Propylene glycol (50)
Nitro Bid	Marion Labs.	Kansas City	1, 5 and 10	5	Ethanol (70) Propylene glycol (4.5)
Tridil	American Critical Care	McGaw Park	5 and 10	5	Ethanol (30) Propylene glycol (30)

[a]Adapted from Demey HE et al. Intensive Care Med 1988;14:221–226.

intravenous line as packed red cells. When amounts of PG exceeding 300 mg per day are used, serum PG levels and serum osmolality should be monitored.[16]

DIETHYLENE GLYCOL

HISTORY

The Elixir Sulfanilamide disaster of 1937 was one of the most consequential mass poisonings of the 20th century. This tragedy occurred shortly after the introduction of sulfanilamide, the first sulfa antimicrobial drug, when diethylene glycol was used as the diluent in the formulation of a liquid preparation of sulfanilamide known as Elixir Sulfanilamide. One hundred and five patients died from its therapeutic use.[17]

USES

Diethylene glycol is used in industrial solvents and antifreeze.

Table 55-26
Parenteral Drug Products[a]

Trade Name	Manufacturer	Dosage	Route	Amount of PG		Alternative
				v/v (%)	w/v (mg/ml)	
Amidate	Abbott	2 mg/ml	i.v.	35	362.6	None
Apresoline	Ciba	20 mg/ml	i.m., i.v.	10	103.6	None
Ativan	Wyeth-Ayerst	2 mg/ml	i.m., i.v.	80	828.8	None
Ativan	Wyeth-Ayerst	4 mg/ml	i.m., i.v.		828.8	None
Bactrim	Roche	TMP 16 mg/ml SMX 80 mg/ml	i.v.	40	414.4	None
Berocca PN	Roche	2 ml	i.v.	25	259	MVI Pediatric MVI-12 lyophilized
Brevibloc	DuPont	250 mg/ml	i.v.	25	259	None
Dilantin	Parke-Davis	50 mg/ml	i.m., i.v.	40	414.4	None
Dramamine	Searle	50 mg/ml	i.m., i.v.	50	518	None
Dramocen	Central	50 mg/ml	i.m., i.v.	50	518	None
Embolex	Sandoz	0.7 ml	s.c.	44	460	None
Konakion	Roche	10 mg/ml	i.m.	20	207	Aqua-Mephyton
Konakion	Rohce	2 mg/ml	i.m.	20	207	Aqua-Mephyton
Lanoxin	Burroughs Wellcome	0.25 mg/ml	i.m., i.v.	40	414.4	None
Lanoxin	Burroughs Wellcome	0.1 mg/ml	i.m., i.v.	40	414.4	None
Pediatric						
Librium	Roche	50 mg/ml	i.m., i.v.	20	207	None
Loxitane	Lederle	50 mg/ml	i.m.	70	725.2	None
Luminal Sod	Winthrop	130 mg/ml	i.v.	67.8	702.4	Phenobarbital Sodium (Lilly)
MCV9 Plus	Lyphomed	10 ml	i.v.	30	310.8	MVI Pediatric MVI-12 lyophilized
MVI-12	Armour	10 ml	i.v.	30	310.8	MVI Pediatric MVI-12 lyophilized
Nitro-BID	Marion	5 mg/ml	i.v.	4.3	45	Nitrol
Nembutal	Abbott	50 mg/ml	i.m., i.v.	40	414.4	None
Nitrostat	Parke-Davis	5 mg/ml	i.v.	30	310.8	Nitrol
Nitroglycerin	Abbott	5 mg/ml	i.v.	50	518	Nitrol
Pentobarbital	Wyeth	50 mg/ml	i.m., i.v.	40	414.4	None
Phenobarbital	Elkin-Sinns	130 mg/ml	i.m., i.v.	67.8	702.4	Phenobarbital Sodium (Lilly)
Phenobarbital	Wyeth	130 mg/ml	i.m., i.v.	67.8	702.4	Phenobarbital Sodium (Lilly)
Phenytoin	Lyphomed	50 mg/ml	i.m., i.v.	30	310.8	None
Phenytoin	Elkin-Sinns	50 mg/ml	i.m., i.v.	40	414.4	None
Septra	Burroughs Wellcome	TMP 16 mg/ml SMX 80 mg/ml	i.v.	40	414.4	None
Tridil	American Critical Care	0.5 mg/ml	i.v.	30	310.8	Nitrol
Valium	Roche	5 mg/ml	i.m., i.v.	40	414.4	None

[a]Adapted from Smolinske SC. Handbook of food, drug and cosmetic excipients. Boca Raton, FL: CRC Press, 1992.

CLINICAL PRESENTATION

A single fatal oral dose of diethylene glycol in humans is about 1.2 mL/kg (1 to 2 g/kg).

Epidemiology

Children (seven) admitted with diethylene glycol poisoning presented with a prodromal febrile illness leading to vomiting, anuria, and diarrhea. In addition, dehydration, tachypnea, hepatomegaly, depressed consciousness, irritability, palpable kidneys, papillitis, and meningeal signs were observed. The serum alanine aminotransferase (SGPT) is elevated usually in all children studied. Death may occur despite rehydration and apparent improvement.[18]

Adulteration of some wines with up to 10 to 20 g/L of diethylene glycol was observed in 1985 in the Netherlands. Elevated serum creatinine levels were observed in some patients. Further health data are not available.[19] A number of wines adulterated with diethylene glycol were imported from Austria, West Germany, and Italy.[20] Polyethylene glycol solutions may contain quantities of diethylene glycol as a contaminant.[21]

Topical application of a 1% silver sulfadiazine formulation used in Spain for application to second- or third-degree burns (500 to 4000 g/day) contained 6.2 to 7.1 g/kg of diethylene glycol stearate and free diethylene glycol.[22] These substances are not present in the United States' silver sulfadiazine product (Silvadene).[23] After 3 to 6 days of topical treatment with the formulation, oliguria, metabolic and lactic acidosis, a increased anion gap, and irreversible coma developed. All patients died despite bicarbonate replacement. No calcium oxalate crystals were observed.[18] Fourteen patients ingested glycerine contaminated with diethylene glycol. They developed severe gastrointestinal symptoms, a metabolic acidosis, and renal failure. All died. Autopsy revealed acute renal cortical necrosis, centrilobular hepatic necrosis, and extensive hemorrhages in the adrenal medullae.[24] Paracetamol elixirs with diethylene glycol as a diluent led to 51 deaths and an epidemic of acute renal failure in early 1990 in Bangladesh.[25]

Symptoms of oral diethylene glycol poisoning occur within 24 hours of ingestion and include nausea, anorexia, vomiting, abdominal pain, and diarrhea. Neurologic effects include headache, dizziness, and narcosis. Renal involvement include polyuria and oliguria. Jaundice and ascites indicate liver pathology. Near death at 2 to 22 days postingestion, the patient may exhibit seizures, coma, anuria, edema, fluid and electrolyte imbalance, and acidosis. At autopsy renal tubular damage and centrilobular liver necrosis are observed.

LABORATORY

The patient exhibits elevated serum osmolality, abnormal electrolytes, low blood glucose, elevated BUN and creatinine, an abnormal urinalysis with cells and casts, and elevated liver function test.

TREATMENT

Decontamination is recommended within 1 to 2 hours of an acute oral ingestion. Ipecac is not advised because of the potential for early seizures. Ethanol therapy has not been subjected to controlled clinical studies. Hepatitis is treated with lactulose and a low-protein diet. Comatose patients need ventilatory support. Seizures are treated with standard anticonvulsants. Monitor fluid status. Repeat hemodialysis may be indicated.[26]

2-MERCAPTOETHANOL

STRUCTURE

$SH\text{-}CH_2\text{-}CH_2\text{-}OH$

USES

2-Mercaptoethanol is a colorless liquid with a strong unpleasant odor used in laboratories for reduction of protein disulfide bonds and for protection of sulfhydryl enzymes.[27] It also has industrial uses.[28]

CLINICAL PRESENTATION

2-Mercaptoethanol is irritating to the skin, eyes, and mucous membranes. In man ingestion of about 10 to 20 mL may induce emesis and end fatally with extensive subendocardial ventricular hemorrhages. The toxicity of 2-mercaptoethanol may be due to the thiol group in the molecule, which is known to inhibit cytochrome oxidase. 2-Mercaptoacetate, a metabolite, is found in the urine and may be secreted into the gastric contents.[25]

TREATMENT

Treatment is symptomatic and supportive.

ETHYLENE GLYCOL DERIVATIVES

ETHYLENE GLYCOL MONOMETHYL ETHER

Ethylene Glycol Monomethyl Ether (EGME) and Acetate (EGMEA)

Ethylene Glycol Monoethyl Ether (EGEE) and Acetate (EGEEA)

NIOSH has recommended an occupational standard: 0.2 ppm EGME or EGMEA as a TWA for up to a 10-hour day during a 40-hour work week, and 0.5 ppm for EGEE or EGEEA as a 10-hour TWA. NIOSH also recommends that dermal contact be prohibited for all four of these glycol ethers.[29]

Synonyms

2-Ethoxyethanol	Cellosolve CG monoethyl ether
2-Butyoxyethanol	EGBE (Butyl cellosolve)
2-Methoxyethanol	EGME (Methyl cellosolve)

USES

These derivatives are used as solvents for resins and paints and as constituents of cellulose inks, industrial coatings (wood stains, epoxies, varnish, paints), and cleaning compounds (Tables 55–27 and 55–28).

PATHOPHYSIOLOGY

The alkoxyacetic acid metabolite, or its glycine conjugate, has been found in the urine from man or animals after the administration of 2-methoxy-, 2-ethoxy-2-isopropoxy-, and 2-butoxyethanol. It appears that many of the toxic effects of the short-chained alkoxyethanols can be attributed to their acid metabolites.[30]

CLINICAL PRESENTATION

Ethylene Glycol Monodiethyl Ether

An adult ingested 1 liter of an ethyl glycol monobutyl ether (EGBE)–containing window cleaner over 3 days and became comatose with hyperventilation. Treatment with hemodialysis led to recovery. Marked metabolic acidosis after the ingestion of a large amount of EGBE remains the main symptom caused by the oxidating of EGBE to butoxyacetic acid (Fig. 55–7).[31,32] Less than 1 mL of a commercial glass/window cleaner containing less than 17% EGBE does not appear to require specific therapy.[33] Bone marrow aspirates of seven lithograph workers exposed to glycol ethers, among other hydrocarbons, revealed myeloid hypo-

Table 55–27
Chemical Names, Chemical Structures, Trade Names, and Synonyms for Monoalkyl Ethers of Ethylene Glycol[a]

2-Methoxyethanol $CH_3OCH_2CH_2OH$	2-Ethoxyethanol $C_2H_5OCH_2CH_2OH$	2-Butoxyethanol $C_4H_9OCH_2CH_2OH$
CAS No. 109-86-4	CAS No. 110-80-5	CAS No. 111-76-2
Ethylene glycol monomethyl ether	Ethylene glycol monoethyl ether	Ethylene glycol monobutyl ether
Methyl cellosolve	Cellosolve	Butyl cellosolve
Dowanol EM	Dowanol EE	Dowanol EB
Methyl oxitol	Oxitol	Butyl oxitol
Ektasolve EM	Ektasolve EE	Ektasolve EB
Jeffersol EE	Jeffersol EB	

[a]Adapted from Browning RG, Curry SC. Hum Exp Toxicol 1994;13:325–335.

Table 55–28
Common Household Products Containing Glycol Ethers[a]

Acrylic polymers
Automobile brake fluid
Automobile injector cleaner
Automobile wax
Carpet steam cleaners and shampoos
Degreasing agents
Fabric cleaners
Floor finishes
Floor waxes
Ink removers
Leather dyes
Shoe polishes and savers
Shoe shampoo
Stain removers
Surface cleaning solutions and detergents
Metal cleaners
Reducing agents
Vinyl cleaners
Window cleaning solutions
Wood finishes and preps

[a]Adapted from Browning RG, Curry SC. Hum Exp Toxicol 1994;13:325–335.

plasia and stromal injury in three that could not be explained by known risk factors.[34] Studies in animals indicate that the glycol ethers Cellosolve and methyl Cellosolve (but not butyl Cellosolve) cause birth defects and testicular damage at levels near legal exposure limits (100 ppm). A consistent pattern of embryotoxic and teratogenic effects occurs with lower-molecular-weight glycol ethers perhaps acting as tumor-promoting agents.[35]

Ethylene Glycol Monomethyl Ether (EGME)

Blood seems to be the main target of toxicity in cases of chronic EGME exposure (macrocytic anemia, leukopenia, increased proportion of lymphocytes).[36] Hematologic changes are reversible after exposure is discontinued.

Following a symptom-free interval of 8 to 18 hours, two patients who had ingested 100 mL of EGME became confused and complained of nausea and weakness.[37] The subsequent course included a profound metabolic acidosis, tachypnea, rise in serum creatinine, and a marked oxaluria, from which they recovered. Treatment included intravenous sodium bicarbonate and ethyl alcohol.[38] Cutaneous occupational exposure to EGME for about 6 months led to an encephalopathy in factory workers. This was accompanied by an anemia, leukopenia, and thrombocytopenia.[39]

Monoethyl Ether (EGEE)

About 23% of absorbed EGEE is recovered in the urine.[40] Exposure to EGME and EGEE at work has led to some decrease in testicular size but no apparent alteration in fertility.[41,42]

Monobutyl Ether (EGBE)

Ethylene glycol butyl ether (EGBE) is an ingredient in commercial window glass cleaners (Table 55–29).[43] Children aged 7 months to 9 years who have ingested 5 to 300 mL of liquid products containing EGBE (0.5 to 9.9%) have all recovered.

EGBE ingestion may lead to coma, hypotension, metabolic acidosis, renal injury, hematuria, hemolysis, oxaluria, and noncardiogenic pulmonary edema.[36,44] Patients have recovered with symptomatic and supportive therapy.

EGBE is absorbed through the skin, lungs, and gastrointestinal tract. The elimination half-time is brief (40 minutes). It is oxidized by alcohol dehydrogenase in the liver. Its principal metabolite is butoxyacetic acid responsible for the metabolic acidosis[49] and possibly hemolysis.[45] Ethanol therapy or 4-methylpyrazole administration may be useful because it competitively inhibits alcohol dehydrogenase.

Ingestion of 5 to 10 mL of EGBE-containing glass/window cleaners (0.5 to 9.9%) by children aged 7 months to 9 years was treated with oral fluids at home. The patients were asymptomatic. Two children ingested amounts over 15 mL and were treated with gastric emptying and admission to a health care facility for 24 hours. No hemolysis, CNS depression, acidosis, or renal compromise was noted. Data suggest that ingestions of less than 10 mL of a commercial liquid glass/window cleaner containing less than 10% EGBE can be safely treated with simple dilution in the home setting.[50] An adult ingested about 500 mL of a window cleaning agent containing 12.7% v/v EGBE and 3.2% v/v ethanol. About 200 to 250 mL were absorbed corresponding to a total dose of 25 to 30 g of EGBE. Butoxyacetic acid, the main metabolite of EGBE, peaked in the urine about 24 hours after ingestion. The half-life of EGBE was 210 minutes. Clinically, the patient was admitted in coma with

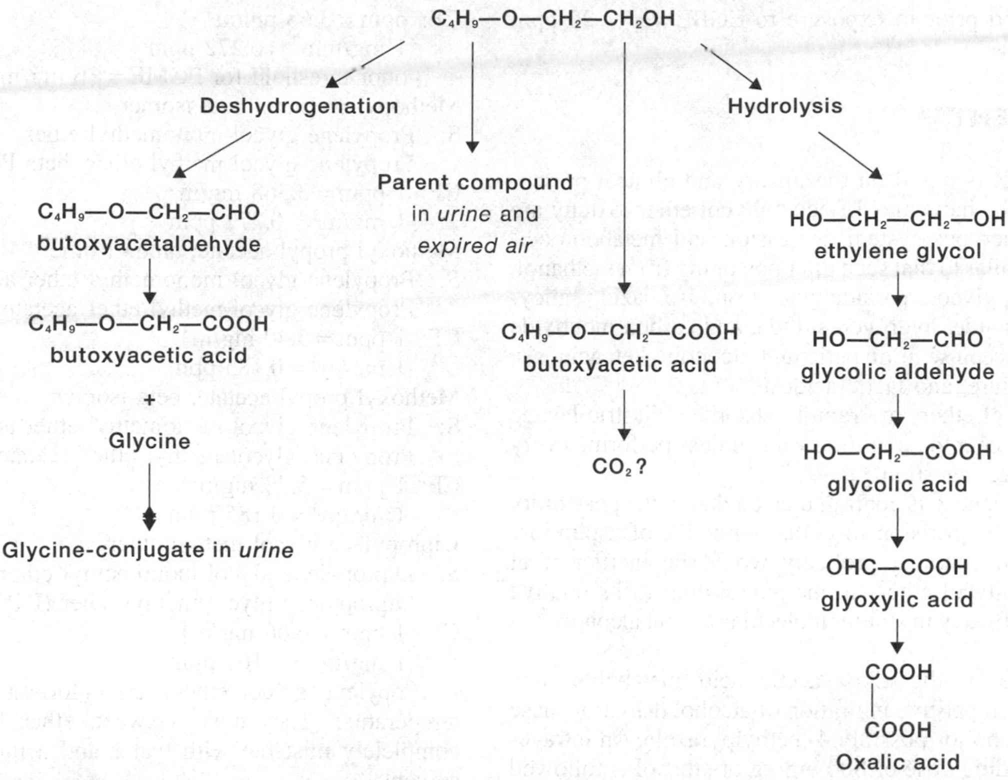

Figure 55-7. Suggested metabolic patterns of EGBE. (Adapted from Rambourg-Schepens MO et al. Hum Toxicol 1988;7:187–189.)

Table 55-29
Common Commercial EGBE-Containing Glass Cleaners[a]

Product	% EGBE	Manufacturer
Window Kleen	<3%	State Chemical
Sears Window Cleaner	15%	Brulin and Company
Tektor Window Cleaner	16%	Ridgeway Chemical
Windex with Ammonia-D	5%	Drackett Products
Windex with Vinegar-D	9%	Drackett Products
Lemon Fresh Windex with Ammonia-D	<2%	Drackett Products
Windex Professional Strength Multi-Surface	4%	Drackett Products
SOS Glass Works	5–10%	Miles Laboratories
Sparkle Glass	9.9%	A.J. Funk Inc.
Glass Plus	<10%	Dow Brands
Glance Glass Cleaner	2–5%	S.C. Johnson

[a]Adapted from Dean BS, Krenzelok EP. J Toxicol Clin Toxicol 1992;30: 557–563.

mydriasis, bradycardia, hypotension, and metabolic acidosis with a high anion gap. The patient developed anemia and hematuria on the second day, concurrent with maximum levels of butoxyacetic acid but with no oxaluria. Treatment was supportive (intubation, assisted ventilation, activated charcoal, gastric lavage, forced diuresis, dopamine), and hemodialysis was required to control the metabolic acidosis and to remove the toxic agent and its metabolites.[46]

An adult ingested 250 to 500 mL of a window cleaner containing 12% EGBE. The patient became comatose, developed a metabolic acidosis, hypokalemia, a rise in serum creatinine, a marked increase in urinary excretion of oxalate crystals, anemia, and a hemoglobinuria.

Monophenyl Ether (EGPE)

Percutaneous absorption after exposure to about 500 mL of 2-phenoxyethanol (EGPE) per day may induce headache, lightheadedness, slurred speech, euphoria, grogginess, diminished strength and sensation in the hands and fingers, forgetfulness and irritability. Alcohol intolerance may be observed.[47]

LABORATORY

Monitoring of the urinary excretion of the alkoxyacetic acid metabolites may be a useful indicator of human exposure to ethylene glycol ethers. In ten male workers exposed to ethylene glycol monoethyl ether, the maximal urinary excretion of ethoxyacetic acid occurred in 3 to 4 hours, and the urine biologic half-life was 21 to 24 hours.

Analytic Method

A sensitive method for butoxyacetic acid (BAA) and other alkoxyacetic acids in use is based on ion-pair extract with a capillary gas chromatograph and electron captive detection (GC-ECD). This method has a detection limit and a practical quantification limit of about 0.05 and 7 μmol/L, respectively. A single urine sample of 0.2 mL is sufficient to measure BAA.[35] A marked increase of EGBE in blood and urine and a marked decrease of BAA excretion follows administration of ethanol corresponding to above

0.3% in blood prior to exposure to EGBE vapor 20 ppm for 2 hours.

TREATMENT[48]

1. Diagnosis is based on the history and clinical presentation. The hallmarks of acute glycol ether toxicity are central nervous system depression and metabolic acidosis similar to that seen after poisoning from methanol, ethylene glycol, paraldehyde, iron, isoniazid, salicylates, cyanide, hydrogen sulfide, and carbon monoxide and that seen with diabetic and alcoholic ketoacidosis, renal failure, and lactic acidosis.
2. The glycol ethers are rapidly absorbed. Gastric lavage would appear to be of little value unless performed very early after ingestion.
3. Syrup of ipecac is contraindicated due to the possibility of rapid progression to coma, with risk of aspiration.
4. Activated charcoal probably would be inefficient at binding glycol ethers in the gut, similar to its relative lack of efficacy in similar molecular weight alcohols and glycols.
5. Blockade of the alkoxyacetic acid metabolite may follow competitive inhibition of alcohol dehydrogenase with alcohol or possibly 4-methylpyrazole. An intravenous loading dose of 800 mg/kg of ethanol is followed by a continuous drip of 80 to 150 mg/kg with adjustments to maintain a plasma ethanol level of 100 to 150 mg/dL.
6. Support measures, if required, include airway control, ventilatory assistance, and cardiovascular support with fluids and vasopressors.
7. Hemodialysis may be useful for severe, refractory acidosis or renal insufficiency. There have been no controlled studies to validate this theory.
8. The likelihood of fatality is low. Delayed toxicity may result from toxic metabolites of EGBE after it is metabolized by alcohol dehydrogenase. Alcohol should be given early to patients with a significant ingestion of EGBE. This could be ceased later if no toxicity develops and anion and osmolar gaps remain normal. The osmolar gap is mainly within the normal range with EGBE poisoning.[49] It would take extremely high and clinically unlikely concentrations of glycol ethers to produce a detectable increase in the osmolal gap.[50]

PROPYLENE GLYCOL ETHERS

STRUCTURE

Propylene glycol ethers commonly used include methoxypropanol, methoxypropylacetate, and dipropylene glycol monomethyl ether. Both alpha and beta isomers are present in commercial methoxypropanol and methoxypropyl acetate. The isomers differ in toxicity.

Synonyms (S) and conversion factors (CF)

Methoxypropanol, alpha isomer

S: Propylene glycol monomethyl ether
Propylene glycol methyl ether (PGME)

CF: ppm = 3.68 pm/m^3
1 mg/mm^3 = 0.272 ppm
odor threshold for PGME = 36 mg/m^3

Methopyl propanol beta isomer

S: Propylene glycol monomethyl ether
Propylene glycol methyl ether: beta PCME

CF: 1 ppm = 3.368 mg/m^3
1 mg/m^3 = 0.272 ppm

Methoxyl propyl acetate, alpha isomer

S: Propylene glycol monomethyl ether acetate
Propylene glycol methyl ether acetate PGMEA

CF: 1 ppm = 5.40 mg/m^3
1 mg/m^3 = 0.185 ppm

Methoxyl propyl acetate, beta isomer

S: Propylene glycol monomethyl ether acetate
Propylene glycol methyl ether acetate (beta PGMEA)

CF: 1 ppm = 5.40 mg/m^3
1 mg/m^3 = 0.185 ppm

Dipropylene glycol methyl ether

S: Dipropylene glycol monomethyl ether
Dipropylene glycol methyl ether (DPGME)

CF: 1 ppm = 6.06 mg/m^3
1 mg/m^3 = 0.165 ppm

Propylene glycol ethers are colorless liquids at room temperature. They have a sweet, etherlike odor and are completely miscible with water and a number of organic solvents.

USES

Propylene glycol ethers are used industrially as solvents for paints, lacquers, resins, oils, and fat. Propylene glycol ethers have increased in use in the past 10 years. One reason for the increase is probably the replacement of ethylene glycol ethers by propylene glycol ethers because of the reproductive toxicity associated with the former group of solvents.[51]

TOXICOKINETICS

The major metabolic pathways of propylene glycol ethers can be summarized as follows: (a) acetate esters are rapidly hydrolyzed to the corresponding either alcohol; (b) ether alcohols, both alpha and beta isomers, are conjugated with sulfite and glucuronic acid; (c) beta isomers, being primary alcohols, are oxidized to carboxylic acid; (d) alpha isomers, being secondary alcohols, are also oxidized to carbon dioxide after cleavage of the ether bond.

CLINICAL PRESENTATION

PGME

Exposure at 300 ppm for 5 minutes produces mild irritation of the eyes, nose, and throat. At 750 ppm the PGME vapor is extremely irritating. At concentrations of 47 to 1000 ppm for 1 to 7 hours no abnormalities in liver enzymes are observed. At exposure levels of 100 ppm to 400 ppm light-headedness, a negative Romberg test, and eye, nose, and throat irritation may be observed.

DPGME

The irritating concentration of DPGME in man is 74 ppm (450 mg/m^3) or about twice the odor threshold. Exposure to 0.6 to 6.4 ppm have resulted in bone marrow injury. There are no reports of any effects on the peripheral nervous system. There are no signs of subacute or chronic organ-specific damage at levels below 1500 ppm PGME, 1000 ppm PGMEA, and 300 to 400 ppm DPGME. There are no present indications of mutagenicity or genotoxicity.

POLYETHYLENE GLYCOL

STRUCTURE

$OH\text{-}CH_2\text{-}O\text{-}(CH_2\text{-}CH_2\text{-}O)_n\text{-}CH_2\text{-}CH_2OH$

Table 55–30 summarizes some species of polyethylene glycol used clinically.[52]

Polyethylene glycols have been used as a component of suppositories where they serve as an "inert" base and carrier for various "active" drugs. Preliminary animal data suggest that polyethylene glycol suppositories may predispose cells in the rectal or vaginal mucosa to malignant change. Further data is required on this subject.[53]

Polyethylene glycol (PEG) is used for preoperative bowel cleaning, as a medicinal to treat constipation, and as a purgative in the management of poisoning. Diethylene glycol may be a contaminant of commercial polyethylene glycol (PEG) solutions.[26]

CLINICAL PRESENTATION

Metabolic acidosis, renal insufficiency, and cardiorespiratory arrest have followed topical use in a 2½-year-old infant.[54]

LABORATORY

Polyethylene glycol may be present in temazepam, a drug often abused orally and by the intravenous route. Detection of polyethylene glycol in the urine may aid in detection and clinical treatment of drug abusers.[55]

Table 55–30
Range of Molecular Weights and Polymer Lengths for Polyethylene Glycols Used in These Studies[a]

Species	Range of Molecular Weight	n
PEG 400	380–420	8.2–9.1
PEG 600	570–630	12.5–13.9
PEG 1450	1300–1600	29–36
PEG 3350	3000–3700	68–84

[a]Adapted from Schiller LR et al. Gastroenterology 1988;94:933–941.
n, Average number of ethylene glycol units in polyethylene glycol, $H(OCH_2CH_2)_nOH$.

TREATMENT

Treatment consists of supportive care. Hemodialysis and ethanol administration have not been protective.

BENZYL ALCOHOL

(SEE ALSO ANESTHETIC DRUG CHAPTER)

PARENTERAL MEDICATIONS

Parenteral medications formulated with benzyl alcohol include atropine sulfate, glycopyrrolate, physostigmine, pyridostigmine, heparin, crystalloid solutions, succinylcholine, atracrurium, pancuronium, tubocurarine, doxapram, and metoclopramide.[56]

With dosages of benzyl alcohol ranging from 99 to 234 mg/kg/day, hypotension, severe metabolic acidosis with an increased anion gap secondary to increased blood concentrations of benzoic acid, changes in consciousness, leukopenia, thrombopenia, hyperammonemia, and respiratory gasping are observed with high mortality rates. Diazepam 1 mL contains 5 mg of diazepam, 0.5 mmol of sodium, and 15.7 mg of benzyl alcohol. When a continuous intravenous diazepam infusion is administered for status epilepticus, no dosage of more than 1 mg/kg/hour should be used. With this dosage, benzyl alcohol 75 mg/kg/day and sodium 2.4 mmol/kg/day are administered. When using dosages between 0.5 and 1 mg/kg/hour, frequent cardiovascular and respiratory monitoring are required, and serum electrolytes, blood gases, and anion gap must be measured every 6 to 12 hours. Serum and urine benzoic acid concentrations must be determined at least every 24 hours.[57]

CLINICAL PRESENTATION

The term *gasping syndrome* describes the progressive neurologic deterioration of premature infants suffering from benzyl alcohol poisoning.[58] Retrospective studies of neonates revealed a substantial decline in both mortality and major intraventricular hemorrhage among infants weighing less than 1 kg after the use of benzyl alcohol–containing solutions was discontinued.[59]

UNAPPROVED DRUGS (UNITED STATES)

CALCIUM 2-AMINOETHANOL PHOSPHATE

Calcium-2-aminoethanol phosphate is claimed to inhibit autoimmune processes and to be useful in the treatment of osteoporosis.[60,61] It is brought into the United States from Europe and may be in use by practitioners in the United States for the treatment of multiple sclerosis.

CLINICAL PRESENTATION

A 53-year-old female with a history of multiple sclerosis was given an intravenous infusion of calcium 2-aminoethanol phosphate and developed a cardiopulmonary arrest, followed by massive hemolysis, renal failure, adult respiratory distress syndrome, shock liver, and disseminated intravascular coagulation.[62]

TREATMENT

Treatment of overdose/or adverse reactions is supportive and symptomatic.

REFERENCES—OTHER GLYCOLS AND ALCOHOLS

1. Catanzaro JM, Smith JG Jr. Propylene glycol dermatitis. J Am Acad Dermatol 1991;24:90–95.
2. Demey HE, Daelemans RA, Verpooten GA, de Broe ME, Van Campenhout CM, Lakiene FV et al. Propylene glycol–induced side effects during intravenous nitroglycerin therapy. Intensive Care Med 1988;14:221–226.
3. Smolinske SC. Handbook of food, drug and cosmetic excipients. Boca Raton, FL: CRC Press, 1992.
4. Speth PAJ, Vree TB, Neilen NFM, de Mulder PHM, Newell DR, Gore ME et al. Propylene glycol pharmacokinetics and effects after intravenous infusion in humans. Ther Drug Monitor 1987;9:255–258.
5. Kelner MJ, Bailey DN. Propylene glycol as a cause of lactic acidosis. J Anal Toxicol 1985;9:40–42.
6. MacDonald MG, Getson PR, Glasgow AM, Miller MK, Boeckx RL, Johnson EL. Propylene glycol: increased incidence of seizures in low birth weight infants. Pediatrics 1987;79:622–625.
7. Lehman AJ, Newman HW. Propylene glycol: rate of metabolism, absorption and excretion with a method for estimation in body fluids. J Pharmacol Exp Ther 1937;60:312–322.
8. Martin G, Finberg L. Propylene glycol: a potentially toxic vehicle in liquid dosage. J Pediatr 1970;77:877–878.
9. Arulanantham K, Genel M. Central nervous system toxicity associated with ingestion of propylene glycol. J Pediatr 1978;93:515–516.
10. Cate JC, Hendricks R. Propylene glycol intoxication and lactic acidosis. N Engl J Med 1980;303:1237.
11. Huggon I, James I, Macrae D. Hyperosmolarity related to propylene glycol in an infant treated with enoximone infusion. Br Med J 1990;301:19–20.
12. Lolin Y, Francis DA, Flanagan RJ, Little P, Lascelles PT. Cerebral depression due to propylene glycol in a patient with chronic epilepsy—the value of the plasma osmolal gap in diagnosis. Postgrad Med J 1988;64:610–613.
13. Maurer H, Kessler C. Identification and quantification of ethylene glycol and diethylene glycol in plasma using gas chromatography–mass spectrometry. Arch Toxicol 1988;62:66–69.
14. Glasgow AM, Boeckx RL, Miller MK, MacDonald MG, August GP, Goodman SI. Propylene glycol plasma level. Pediatrics 1985;76:654.
15. Hall AH, Bronstein AC, Smolinske SC, Doutre WH, Kulig KW, Rauch BH, Spoerke DG. Propylene glycol plasma levels. Pediatrics 1985;76:656.
16. Smolinske SC, Vandenberg SA, Spoerke DG, Rumack BH. Propylene glycol content of parenteral medications. Vet Hum Toxicol 1987;29:491.
17. Wax PM. Elixirs, diluents and the passage of the 1938 Federal Food, Drug and Cosmetic Act. Ann Intern Med 1995; 122:456–461.
18. Bowie MD, McKenzie D. Diethylene glycol poisoning in children. S Afr Med J 1972;46:931.
19. Van der Linden-Cremers PMA, Sangster B. Diethylene glycol in wine: experiences in the Netherlands. Summer 1985. Vet Hum Toxicol 1987;29(Suppl 2):12–13.
20. U.S. finds traces of poison chemical in 10 more wines. Los Angeles Herald-Examiner, April 16, 1986.
21. Woolf A, Pearson K. Presence of diethylene glycol in commercial polyethylene glycol (PEG) solutions. Clin Toxicol 1995;33:475–486 (abstract 10).
22. Cantarell MC, Fort J, Camps J, Sans M, Piera L, Rodamilans M. Acute intoxication due to topical application of diethylene glycol. Ann Intern Med 1987;106:478–479.
23. McAlinney PG. Silver sulfadiazine and oliguric renal failure. Ann Intern Med 1987;107:264.
24. Pandya SK. An unmitigated tragedy. Br Med J 1988;297: 117–119.
25. Hanif M, Mobarak MR, Ronan A, Rahman D, Donovan JJ Jr, Bennish ML. Fatal renal failure caused by diethylene glycol in paracetamol elixir: the Bangladesh epidemic. Br Med J 1995;33:88–91.
26. Woolf AD. Diethylene glycol. Clin Toxicol Rev 1994; 17(3):1–2.
27. White FH Jr. Reduction and reoxidation of sulfide bonds. Methods Enzymol 1972;25(Part B):387–392.
28. Erikson A, Mohlin L, Nilsson L, Sorbo B. Mercaptoethanol poisoning. Report of a fatal case and analytical determinations. J Anal Toxicol 1989;13:60–62.
29. Wess JA. Reproductive toxicity of ethylene glycol monomethylether, ethylene glycol monoethyl ether and their acetates. Scand J Work Environ Health 1992;18(Suppl 2): 43–45.
30. Johanson G. Urine butoxyacetic acid as a therapeutic guide. Clin Toxicol 1993;31:501–552.
31. Rambourg-Schepens MO, Buffet M, Bertlaut R, Jaussaud M, Journe B, Fay R et al. Severe ethylene glycol butyl ether poisoning. Kinetics and metabolic pattern. Hum Toxicol 1988;7:187–189.
32. Felgenahuer N, Zilker T, Clarmann M. A case of severe ethylene glycol monobutyl ether poisoning. Proc Eur Assoc Pois Cont Clin Toxicol, Birmingham, UK: May, 1993.
33. Dean BS, Krenzelok E. 10 mL of 10% solution is not "significant." Clin Toxicol 1993;31:503–504.
34. Cullen MR, Rado T, Waldron JA et al. Bone marrow injury in lithographers exposed to glycol ethers and organic solvents used in multicolor offset and ultraviolet curing printing processes. Arch Environ Health 1983;38: 347–354.
35. Hardin BD, Lyon JP. Summary and overview: NIOSH symposium on toxic effects of glycol ethers. Environ Health Perspect 1984;57:273–275.
36. Larese F, Fiorito A, de Zotti R. The possible haematological effects of glycol monomethyl ether in a frame factory. Br J Ind Med 1992;49:131–133.
37. Johanson G, Kronborg H, Naslund PH, Nordqvist MB. Toxicokinetics of inhaled 2-butoxyethanol (ethylene glycol monobutyl ether) in man. Scand J Work Environ Health 1986; 12:594–602.
38. Nitter-Hauge S. Poisoning with ethylene glycol monomethyl ether. Acta Med Scand 1970;188:277–280.
39. Ohi G, Wegman DH. Transcutaneous ethylene glycol monomethyl ether poisoning in the work setting. J Occup Med 1978;20:675–676.
40. Groeseneken D, Veulemans H, Maaschelein R, Van Vlem E. Ethoxyacetic acid: a metabolite as ethylene glycol monoethyl ether acetate in man. Br J Ind Med 1987;44:488–493.
41. Welch LS, Plotkin E, Schrader S. Indirect fertility analysis in painters exposed to ethylene glycol ethers. Sensitivity and specificity. Am J Ind Med 1991;20:229–290.
42. Cook RR, Bodner KM, Kolesar RC, Utilmanu CS, Van Peenen PFD, Dickson GS et al. A cross-sectional study of ethylene glycol monomethyl ether process employees. Arch Environ Health 1982;37:346–351.
43. Dean BS, Krenzelok EP. Clinical evaluation of pediatric ethylene glycol monobutyl ether poisonings. Clin Toxicol 1992; 30:557–563.
44. Bauer P, Weber M, Mur JM, Protois JC, Bollaert PE, Condi A et al. Transient non-cardiogenic pulmonary edema following massive ingestion of ethylene glycol butyl ether. Intensive Care Med 1992;18:250–251.

45. Dean BS, Krenzelok EP. Clinical evaluation of pediatric ethylene glycol monobutyl ether poisonings. Vet Hum Toxicol 1991;33:362.
46. Gijsenbergh FP, Jenco M, Veulemans H, Groeseneken D, Verberckmoes R, Delooz HH. Acute butylglycol intoxication. A case report. Hum Toxicol 1989;8:243–245.
47. Morton WE. Occupational phenoxyethanol neurotoxicity: a report of three cases. J Occup Med 1990;32:42–45.
48. Browning RG, Curry SC. Clinical toxicology of ethylene glycol monalkyl ethers. Hum Exp Toxicol 1994;13:325–335.
49. Buckley N, Whyte IM, Dawson AH. Letters to the Editor: EGBE. Clin Toxicol 1993;31:499–500.
50. Browning RG, Curry SC. Effect of glycol ethers on plasma osmolality. Hum Exp Toxicol 1992;11:488–490.
51. NEG and NIOSH basis for an occupational health standard: propylene glycol ethers and their acetates. Center for Disease Control USDHHS. DHHS (NIOSH) Publication No. 91-103.
52. Schiller LR, Emmett M, Santa Ana CA, Fordtran JS. Osmotic effects of polyethylene glycol. Gastroenterology 1988;94:933–941.
53. Greene MH, Young TI, Eisenbarth GS. Polyethylene glycol in suppositories: cardinogenic? Ann Intern Med 1980;93:781.
54. Rodriguez ZM, Gutierrez JCL, Jimenez JMT, Mor ZR. Metabolic acidosis, intoxication caused by polyethylene glycol. Proc Eur Assoc Pois Cent Clin Toxicol, Birmingham, UK: May 26–28, 1993.
55. Farrell M, Herrod J, Smith B, Strang J. Detection of intravenous drug use. Br Med J 1990;300:612–613.
56. Weissman DB, Jackson SH, Heicher DA, Rockoff MA. Benzyl alcohol administration in neonates. Anesth Analg 1990;70:673.
57. Lopez-Herce J, Bonet C, Meana A, Albajara L. Benzyl alcohol poisoning following diazepam intravenous infusion. Ann Pharmacother 1995;29:632.
58. Gershanik J, Boecler B, Ensley H et al. The gasping syndrome and benzyl alcohol poisoning. N Engl J Med 1982;307:1384–1388.
59. Hiller JL, Benda GI, Rahatzad M et al. Benzyl alcohol toxicity: impact on mortality and intraventricular hemorrhage among very low birth weight infants. Pediatrics 1986;77:500–506.
60. Nieper HA. A comparative study of the clinical effect of CA-1-dl-aspartate (Calciretard) of Ca-2-aminoethanol phosphate (Ca—EAP) and of the cortisones. Aggressologie 1968;9:471–475.
61. Nieper HA. A clinical study of the calcium transport substances Ca 1-dl-aspartate and CA-2-amino ethanol phosphate as potent agents against autoimmunity and other anticytological aggressions. 2nd communication. Aggressologie 1967;8:395–406.
62. Sauter D, Goldfrank L, Charash BD. Cardiopulmonary arrest following an infusion of calcium-2-amino-ethanol phosphate. J Emerg Med 1990;8:711–720.

Chapter 56
Anesthetics

This chapter will survey aspects of anesthetic drug use as they relate to problems encountered following overdose or inadvertent misuse. Excellent texts are available that cover practical approaches to the clinical practice of anesthesiology.[1–3] Opioid agonists and antagonists are reviewed in the Opiate chapter.

ANESTHETIC ACCIDENTS AND DEATH

Anesthesia has been associated with a low mortality in recent years, but it is still associated with a significant morbidity[4,5] (Table 56–1).[6] The risk of death due to anesthesia decreased in the United States from 1 in 2680[1,7] to 1 in 10,000 in the period from 1954 to 1982.[8] Human error remains an important factor in the causation of anesthesia faults, near accidents, and accidents (Tables 56–2 through 56–5).[9,10]

The University Hospital, Leiden, has established a Faults, Accidents and Near Accidents Committee (FONA), which collects and analyzes reported faults, accidents, near accidents, and complications that occur in the hospital. These data also include anesthetic procedures. Definitions used by the committee include the following:[1]

Fault: A procedure that has resulted (or could have resulted) in injury or harm to a patient, while this injury or harm (or chance thereof) could have been prevented by another procedure.

Accident: Any event, except a fault or a complication, that has resulted in harm or injury to a patient.

Near Accident: An event that could have developed into a fault, a complication, or an accident but that was prevented from so developing either by chance or by a previously unplanned intervention.

Complication: Harm or injury to a patient occurring as a result of a known risk of a treatment or a diagnostic procedure.

DENTAL ANESTHESIA AND DEATHS

Prolonged anesthesia and complex techniques carry considerable risks. General anesthesia given by the operating dentist alone increases risks of death. Local anesthetics are

Table 56–1
Causative Factors Concerning Anesthetic Cardiac Arrest and Death[a]

Aspiration of gastric contents
Overdose of anesthetic drugs
Hypoxia
Airway problems
Polypharmacy
Untoward cardiac reflexes
Error in choice of anesthesia, technique, or judgment
Error in prospective evaluation or preparation of patient
Poor anesthetic management
Inadequate monitoring of the patient's condition; inadequate observation of patient or supervision of trainee
Inadequate pulmonary ventilation
Physical status and type of surgery

[a]From Kubota Y et al. J Clin Anesth 1994;6:227–238.

Table 56–2
Faults in Drug Administration[a]

100% nitrous oxide instead of 100% oxygen at the end of anesthesia.
Intramuscular suxamethonium instead of ketamine to a child.
Isoprenaline instead of atropine during an episode of bradycardia.
Intravenous sodium citrate instead of potassium chloride.
Intravenous sufentanil instead of alfentanil during general anesthesia.
Intravenous administration of saline solution which was not intended for intravenous use.
Adrenaline given instead of atropine.
Wrong premedication given.
Overdose of fentanyl during neuroleptic anestheisa.
Wrong concentration of lignocaine during cardiorespiratory resuscitation.
Wrong dose of antibiotics to a child.
Interchange of inlet and outlet of halothane (Fluotec) vaporizer leading to overdose.
Rapid intravenous injection of potassium chloride during general anesthesia.
Ketamine overdose as a result of calculation based on wrong weight of a child.

[a]Adapted from Chopra V, Borill JG, Spierdijk J. Anaesthesia 1990;45:3–6.

Table 56–3
1000 Deaths Associated With Anesthesia—Anesthesia Implicated in 589[a]

Incidence	Main Factors Reviewed
110	Regurgitation and vomiting
107	Overdose of intravenous barbiturate
49	Obvious undertransfusion
33	Postoperative respiratory obstruction
41	Mishaps associated with intubation
26	Gross underventilation
25	Spinal and epidural analgesia
17	Induced hypotension
14	Sudden death in children
12	Trichlorethylene
6	Chloroform

[a]Adapted from Dinnick OP. Anaesthesia 1964;19:536–556.

Table 56–4
600 Deaths Associated With Anesthesia—Anesthesia Implicated in 400 Approximately[a]

Incidence	Main Factors Reviewed
209	Low blood volume
74	Underventilation
48	Regurgitation and vomiting
38+	Collapse after IVB + relaxant
26	Mishaps associated with intubation
25	Death during bronchoscopy
16	Anoxia (nonspecific)
14	Overdose (not barbiturate) in adults
12	Epidural and spinal
11	Sudden death in children
10	Induced hypotension
10	Trichlorethylene

[a]Adapted from Dinnick OP. Anaesthesia 1964;19:536–556.

Table 56–5
Causes of Death and Cerebral Damage Classified Into Those Apparently Due to Misadventure and Those Apparently Due to Error[a]

Mainly Misadventure (%)		Mainly Error (%)	
Coexisting disease	10.6	Faulty technique	46.8
Unknown	10.3	Failure postoperative care	9.5
Drug sensitivity	4.6	Drug overdose	5.2
Halothane hepatic failure (?)	3.4	Failure of preoperative assessment	1.4
Hyperthermia	2.9	Drug error	1.4
Blood loss	1.7	Anesthesiologist failure	1.4
Embolism	0.9		
Clot in by-pass	0.3		
Total	34.7	Total	65.7

[a]Adapted from Utting JE, Gray TC, Shelley FC. Can Anaesth Soc J 1979;26:472–478.

not a serious risk factor.[11] Low blood volume, underventilation, regurgitation and vomiting, and a collapse after intravenous block are the main factors in deaths.[12]

PREDICTORS OF PERIOPERATIVE ADVERSE OUTCOMES

Predictors of severe perioperative adverse outcomes include a history of cardiac failure or myocardial infarction less than 1 year previously, age over 50 years, and cardiovascular, thoracic, abdominal, or neurologic surgery.[13]

REFERENCES

1. Barash PG, Cullen BF, Stoelting RK, eds. Handbook of clinical anesthesia. Philadelphia: JB Lippincott, 1991.
2. Barash PG, Cullen BF, Stoelting RK, eds. Clinical anesthesia. Philadelphia: JB Lippincott, 1989.
3. Wood M, Wood AJJ. Drugs and anesthesia. Pharmacology for anesthesiologists. 2nd ed. Baltimore: Williams & Wilkins, 1990.

4. Chopra V, Borill JG, Spierdijk J. Accidents, near accidents and complications during anaesthesia. Anaesthesia 1990;45:3–6.
5. Cohen MM, Duncan PG, Pope WDB, Wolkenstein C. A survey of 112,000 anaesthetics at one teaching hospital (1975–1983). Can Anaesth Soc J 1986;33:22–31.
6. Kubota Y, Toyoda Y, Kubota H, Yeda Y, Asada A, Okamoto T et al. Frequency of anesthesia cardiac arrest and death in the operating room at a single general hospital over a 30-year period. J Clin Anesth 1994;6:227–238.
7. Beecher HK, Todd DP. A study of the deaths associated with anaesthesia and surgery based on a study of 599,548 anaesthesias in 10 institutions 1948–1952 inclusive. Ann Surg 1954;140:2–35.
8. Lunn HN, Mushin WW. Mortality associated with anaesthesia. London: The Nuffield Provincial Hospital Trust, 1962.
9. Craig J, Wilson ME. A survey of anaesthetic misadventures. Anaesthesia 1981;36:933–936.
10. Cooper JB, Newbower RS, Kitz RJ. An analysis of major errors and equipment failure in anaesthesia management: consideration for prevention and detection. Anaesthesiology 1984;60:34–42.
11. Lewis B. Deaths and dental anaesthetics. Br Med J 1983; 286:3–4.
12. Dinnick OP. Deaths associated with anaesthesia. Anaesthesia 1964;19:536–556.
13. Forrest JB, Rehden K, Cahalan MK, Goldsmith CH. Multicenter study of general anesthesia. III. Predictors of severe perioperative adverse outcomes. Anesthesiology 1992;76:3–16.

ANESTHETIC DRUG ABUSE

Drug abuse among hospital personnel and especially anesthesia personnel is a major problem.[1–7] About 26 anesthesia personnel in the United States died of drug overdose in 1991 and 1992.[8] Alcohol, narcotics, barbiturates, tranquilizers, and nitrous oxide[9] have been implicated. Drugs that tempt the abuser can be stolen readily from anesthesia services: inhalation anesthesia (nitrous oxide, halogenated anesthetics), opiates, barbiturates, tranquilizers, or ketamine (see Intravenous Anesthetics) can easily be concealed and be undiscovered for months or years.[2] Death may follow accidental overdose or suicide.[1,7,8,10–14] Abuse of nitrous oxide may lead to a reversible neuropathy similar to that seen with Vitamin B_{12} deficiency.

Management

Everyone associated with the clinical use of these agents must be made aware of their potential for abuse and the occurrence of sudden death during abuse. Access to these drugs should be restricted to anesthetists for their immediate use. Cylinders and containers should be labeled to indicate that a suffocation hazard may exist.

TOPICAL OCULAR ANESTHETIC ABUSE

Topical ocular anesthetic abuse may result in keratitis and persistent epithelial defects with possibly permanent corneal damage and visual loss.[15–17] The physical appearance, lack of response to antimicrobials, and disproportionate pain are similar to *Acanthamoeba* keratitis.

Management

The management of patients with suspected or known use or abuse of topical ocular anesthetic agents revolves initially around discontinuation of the anesthetic agent. Counseling, confiscation of the anesthetic, a trial of patching of the eye, temporary tarsorrhaphy, or admission for observation may be useful. Supportive treatment may permit healing of the epithelial defects.

REFERENCES

1. Yamashita M, Matsuhi A, Oyama T. Illicit use of modern volatile anesthetics. Can Anaesth Soc J 1984;31:76–79.
2. Gravenstein JS, Kory WP, Marks RG. Drug abuse by anesthesia personnel. Anesth Analg 1983;62:467–472.
3. AMA Council on Mental Health. The sick physician—impairment by psychiatric disorders, including alcoholism and drug dependence. JAMA 1973;223:684–687.
4. Hughes PH, Conard SE, Baldwin DC Jr, Storr CL, Sheehan DV. Resident physician substance use in the United States. JAMA 1991;265:2069–2073.
5. Kamerow DB, Pincus HA, Macdonald DI. Alcohol abuse, other drug abuse, and mental disorders in medical practice. Prevalence, costs, recognition and treatment. JAMA 1986; 255:2054–2057.
6. Wood PR, Soni H. Anaesthesia and substance abuse. Anaesthesia 1989;44:672–680.
7. Spencer JD, Raasch FO, Trefny FA. Halothane abuse in hospital personnel. JAMA 1976;235:1034–1035.
8. Silverstein JH, Silva DA, Iberti TJ. Opioid addiction in anesthesiology. Anesthesiology 1993;79:354–375.
9. Paulson GW. "Recreational" misuse of nitrous oxide. J Am Dent Assoc 1979;98:410–411.
10. Hiroki T, Terauchi T, Kurosa T, Kagiwara M. On the fatal cases of poisoning due to abuse of Fluothane. Jpn J Legal Med 1973;27:243–247.
11. Lingenfelter RW. Fatal misuse of enflurane. Anesthesiology 1981;55:603.
12. Walker FB, Morano RA. Fatal recreational inhalation of enflurane. J Forensic Sci 1990;35:197–198.
13. Berman P, Tattersall M. Self-poisoning with intravenous halothane. Lancet 1982;1:340.
14. Suruda AJ, McGlothlin. Fatal abuse of nitrous oxide in the workplace. J Occup Med 1990;32:682–684.
15. Rosenwasser GOD, Holland S, Pfugfelder SC, Lugo M, Heidemann DG, Culbertson WW et al. Topical anesthetic abuse. Ophthalmology 1990;97:967–972.
16. Kintner JC, Grossniklaus HE, Lass JH, Jacobs G. Infectious crystalline keratopathy association with topical anesthetic abuse. Cornea 1990;9:77–80.
17. Reiser HJ, Laibson PR. Anesthetic abuse of the cornea. Ophthalmic Surg 1989;20:72–73.

PRO AND ANTICONVULSANT EFFECTS

Many anesthetic drugs have been reported to cause and/or suppress seizure activity clinically[1] (Table 56–6). Some of these drugs also have anticonvulsant properties. Variations in drug dosages, methods of drug administration, and electroencephalographic (EEG) documentation contribute to the contrasting effects recorded of these drugs on central nervous system activity.[1] For some anesthetic drugs, for example, methohexital, epileptiform activity will be produced only in patients with known seizure disorders.[2,3] EEG evaluation during administration will, for many drugs, clarify whether the drug is truly epileptogenic. Ketamine, however, induces epileptiform activity by involving subcortical neuronal pathways, and these subcortical seizures can only be detected with implanted EEG depth electrodes.[4]

Table 56–6
Anesthetics and Analgesics Reported to Cause and/or Suppress Seizure Activity in Humans[a]

Proconvulsants	Anticonvulsants
Nitrous oxide	Halothane
Halothane	Enflurane
Enflurane	Isoflurane
Isoflurane	Thiopental
Morphine	Etomidate
Meperidine	Diazepam
Fentanyl	Lorazepam
Sufentanil	Midazolam
Methohexital	Ketamine
Etomidate	Propofol
Diazepam	Local anesthetics
Ketamine	
Propotol	
Local anesthetics	

[a]Adapted from Modica PA, Tempelhoff R, White PF. Anesth Analg 1990;70: 303–315.

REFERENCES—PRO AND ANTICONVULSANT EFFECTS

1. Modica PA, Tempelhoff R, White PF. Pro and anticonvulsant effects of anesthetics. I. Anesth Analg 1990;70:303–315; II. ibid 70:443–444.
2. Gumpert J, Paul R. Activation of the electroencephalogram with intravenous Brietal (methohexitone): the findings in 100 cases. J Neurol Neurosurg Psychiatry 1971;34:646–648.
3. Paul R, Harris R. A comparison of methohexitone and thiopentone in electrocorticography. J Neurol Neurosurg Psychiatry 1970;33:100–104.
4. Ferrer-Allado T, Brechner VL, Dymond A, Cozen H, Crandall P. Ketamine-induced electroconvulsive phenomena in the human limbic and thalamic regions. Anesthesiology 1973;318: 333–311.

NIOSH has recommended exposure limits for the following anesthetic gases:

Chloroform 2 ppm (9.76 mg/m^3) ceiling (1 hour)
Trichlorethylene 2 ppm (10.75 mg/m^3) ceiling (1 hour) (Potential occupational carcinogen)
Halothane 2 ppm (16.15 mg/m^3) ceiling (1 hour)
Methoxyflurane 2 ppm (13.5 mg/m^3) ceiling (1 hour)
Enflurane 1 ppm (15.1 mg/m^3) ceiling (1 hour)
Fluoroxine 2 ppm (10.31 mg/m^3) ceiling (1 hour)
Nitrous oxide 25 ppm (30 mg/m^3) as a Time-weighted Average (TWA) over period of use.

ENVIRONMENTAL MONITORING

The vapors of anesthetic gases such as enflurane, halothane, and isoflurane can be monitored with charcoal tubes. Nitrous oxide can be monitored with a direct-reading infrared analyzer or by passive dosimeters. Records of all collected air samples should be kept, and results should be noted in the medical records of the corresponding workers.

WORK PRACTICES

Operating room workers can protect themselves from excess exposure by properly connecting the scavenging equipment, turning the gas off when the breathing system is disconnected from the patient, and ensuring that all patients have properly fitting masks.

MEDICAL MONITORING

Workers exposed to anesthetic gas should have complete medical histories on file. These should include family, genetic, and occupational histories and the outcome of all pregnancies of female workers or of the wives of male workers. Baseline data should be obtained on the hepatic, renal, and hematopoietic systems. Exposed workers should be monitored periodically for liver and kidney function.

Conclusions regarding congenital abnormalities must be judged with caution, since all reported anomalies in the Canadian study[2,3] were counted whether trivial or serious and it is possible that exposed individuals may have reported trivial anomalies ignored by unexposed respondents. A majority of studies suggest that there is no increase in spontaneous abortion among wives of exposed personnel.[4]

CANCER/IMMUNOLOGY

A relation between exposure to anesthetics and the incidence of chronic disease (cancer, leukemia, and liver and kidney disease) has not been demonstrated. Immunologic disturbances may be found in anesthetic personnel chronically exposed to high occupational concentrations of nitrous oxide and halothane.[5]

BLOOD CONTAMINATION OF ANESTHETIC AND RELATED STAFF[6]

Blood from patients may cause skin contamination to the anesthetic staff. Such staff may already have cuts on their hands. Contamination incidents may occur during oral or nasal tracheal intubations, peripheral venous cannulation, arterial cannulation, or central line insertions. Many anesthetists do not wear gloves during these procedures.

Needlestick[7] injury is similarly common among anesthetists. Many anesthetists have not received hepatitis B immunization.

Management

1. Efforts should be made to control nitrous oxide exposure in operating room areas.
2. An operating room nurse or female anesthetist becoming pregnant or wishing to become pregnant should be advised to avoid working in an environment contaminated with anesthetic gases such as an operating room without an effective scavenging system.
3. There does not appear to be sufficient evidence to recommend therapeutic abortion for operating room nurses or anesthetists who become pregnant.
4. Anesthetists should wear gloves routinely, and, in areas where there is a high incidence of HIV positivity, they should attempt to use precautionary measures now employed by surgeons.
5. Immunization against hepatitis B virus should be seriously considered by all operating room personnel.

REFERENCES—OCCUPATIONAL HAZARDS

1. Guidelines for protecting the safety and health of health care workers. US Department of Health and Human Services. September 1988. Comments abstracted and modified from DHHS (NIOSH) Publication No. 88-119.
2. Guirghuis Ss, Pelmear PL, Roy ML, Wong L. Health effects associated with exposure to anaesthetic gases in Ontario hospital personnel. Br J Ind Med 1990;47:490–497.
3. Rajhans GS, Brown Da, Whaley DA, Wong L, Guirghuis SS. Evaluation of occupational exposure to waste anesthetic gases in Ontario hospitals. Ann Occup Hyg 1989;33: 27–45.
4. Tannenbaum TN, Goldberg RJ. Exposure to anesthetic gases and reproductive outcome. A review of the epidemiological literature. J Occup Med 1985;27:659–668.
5. Peric M, Vranes Z, Marusic M. Immunological disturbances in anaesthetic personnel chronically exposed to high occupational concentrations of nitrous oxide and halothane. Anaesthesia 1991;46:531–537.
6. Harrison CA, Rogers DW, Rosen M. Blood contamination of anaesthetic and related staff. Anaesthesia 1990;45: 831–833.
7. Maz S, Lyons G. Needlestick injuries in anaesthetists. Anaesthesia 1990;45:677–678.

PREGNANCY

Mortality during anesthesia does not appear to be different in pregnant women from that of women who are not pregnant. There is also no good evidence to suggest that any particular anesthetic technique will induce preterm labor. Ketamine in a dose of more than 1 mg/kg in the first trimester may increase myometrial tone.[1] Sendak suggests that any drug that readily passes into the central nervous system can also reach the fetus.[1] Intravenous sedatives that have an effect on the central nervous system can pass the placenta. Water-soluble drugs that are highly ionized such as the muscle relaxants do not cross the placenta to any great extent. Bupivacaine is highly protein bound; very little is available to cross the placenta. Drugs with a molecular weight greater than 60 or 700 do not easily cross the placenta.[1]

Friedman[2] has reviewed anesthetics and congenital anomalies. Table 56–7 summarizes the conclusions of this study in women who were administered the anesthetic early in pregnancy.

A U.S. Center for Disease Control study suggests an increased risk for hydrocephalus and eye defects in babies born to mothers exposed to first-trimester general anesthesia.[3] One large prospective study has shown the safety of nitrous oxide in early pregnancy.[4]

NITROUS OXIDE

Nitrous oxide is used by 35 to 50% of all dentists in the United States. There are more than 175,000 dental assistants, 80,000 dental hygienists, and 15,000 female dentists in the United States. Most are women of reproductive age. Scavenging equipment that can reduce levels of exposure 90% or more is still not used in all dental offices. The Occupational Safety and Health Administration has never adopted a mandatory standard for nitrous oxide. It has therefore gone virtually unregulated. Although the National Institute for Occupational Safety and Health proposed a recommended standard of 25 ppm for nitrous oxide in 1977, many dental offices continue to have exposure to 100 ppm (using scavenging equipment) and over 1000 ppm (without scavenging equipment). Exposure to high levels of unscavenged nitrous oxide possibly impairs fertility.[5]

REGIONAL ANESTHESIA

The advantages of regional analgesia/anesthesia for labor and delivery include provision of good analgesia, decreased catecholamine secretion, stabilization of the cardiovascular system, prevention of the hypo/hyperventilation cycle, and lack of depression of the fetus and newborn. Provision of this involves insertion of a needle into a site containing the epidural plexus of veins. Epidural hematomas are rare. Therapeutic hepatitis in association with epidural anesthesia enhances the risk of epidural hematoma formation, and such regional techniques should be avoided in the parturient.

Regional anesthesias commonly used for labor and delivery include paracervical, pudendal, epidural, and spinal blockade. Contraindications to regional anesthesia include patient refusal, infection at the planned site of needle insertion, sepsis, active neurologic disease, and inherited or acquired bleeding diathesis. Relative contraindications include intravascular volume depletion, severe anemia, fetal distress, previous difficulty with regional anesthesia, and emotional or psychiatric aberration.

Deaths can follow paracervical anesthesia in first-trimester abortions and have occurred after lidocaine overdose produced seizures and cardiopulmonary arrest. Postmortem blood levels of lidocaine have been within toxic ranges.

Table 56–7
Anesthetics Congenital Risk

	Risk of Congenital Anomalies Less Likely	Spontaneous Abortion More Likely
Thiopental		
Methohexital		
Etomidate	ND	
Ketamine	ND	
General Anesthetics administered by inhalation		
Nitrous Oxide	+	
Halothane	ID	
Ether (diethyl ether)	ID	
Enflurane	ID	
Isoflurane	ID	
Methoxyflurane	ND	
Occupational Exposure to Anesthetic Gases	+	Slight increase
Local anesthetics		
Procaine	+	
Lidocaine	+	
Benzocaine	+	
Propoxycaine	+	
Tetracaine	ID	

ND, No data; *ID*, inadequate data.

MANAGEMENT OF TOXIC REACTIONS IN THE PREGNANT PATIENT

The smallest effective volume and lowest concentration of anesthetic should be employed. Recommended maximal doses should not be exceeded. Anesthetic doses should be adjusted to the patient's weight. Aspiration of a local anesthesia should be performed before injection although this does not preclude inadvertent intravascular injection. Vasoconstrictors such as epinephrine may assist in localizing the anesthetic. Patients should be questioned about previous adverse reactions or a family history suggesting pseudocholinesterase deficiency. Those with severe liver disease should be considered to have a higher risk of toxicity.

INDUCTION AGENTS

Thiopental is transferred from the human maternal circulation into placental tissue during the first trimester of pregnancy and at term. There may be a reduction in urinary blood flow.

Ketamine

Placental transfer is rapid.

Etomidate

Safe and effective induction during cesarean section.

Propofol

Crosses placenta. No adverse effects on infant. More study required.

Benzodiazepines

Cross placenta.

INHALATION AGENTS

Nitrous oxide

Crosses placenta. No apparent teratogenicity.

Halothane

Animal studies only.

Fentanyl, Sufentanyl

Maternal delay in gastric emptying, rigidity of the chest wall, difficulty with ventilation during anesthesia induction. Neonatal rigidity of the chest wall. No teratogenic abnormalities seen with use of narcotics.

Succinylcholine hydrochloride and pancuronium cross the placenta. Vecuronium bromide does not cross the placenta as readily as pancuronium. Atracurium and curare cross the placenta poorly.

LACTATION

Inhalation anesthetics usually present no hazard to the nursing infant. Lactating mothers who need surgery usually tolerate well not nursing for 12 to 24 hours, by which time virtually all anesthetic agents are gone from maternal blood.

SPINAL ANESTHETIC

Spinal anesthesia in obstetrics differs from spinal anesthesia in nonpregnant patients. Smaller doses of local anesthetic are needed in pregnancy. The spread in cerebrospinal fluid is less predictable. Hypotension, spinal headache, and spinal opioid side effects (e.g., respiratory depression) are more common in pregnant patients than in general surgical patients. The fetus may be affected adversely by maternal hypotension or inappropriate vasopressors. Technical difficulty in finding the subarachnoid space may be greater in pregnancy because of the increased lumbar lordosis.

REFERENCES—PREGNANCY

1. Sendak MJ. Getting the patient to surgery—and back. Anesthesia in pregnancy. Emerg Med 1986;18(13):111–132.
2. Friedman JM. Teratogen update: anesthetic agents. Teratology 1988;37:69–77.
3. Sylvester GC, Khoury MJ, Lu X, Erickson JD. First-trimester anesthesia exposure and the risk of central nervous system defects. A population-based case-control study. Am J Public Health 1994;84:1757–1760.
4. Crawford JS, Lewis M. Nitrous oxide in early human pregnancy. Anaesthesia 1986;41:900–905.
5. Rowland AS, Baird DD, Weinberg CR, Shore DL, Sky CM, Wilcox AJ. Reduced fertility among women employed as dental assistants exposed to high levels of nitrous oxide. N Engl J Med 1992;327:993–997.

ACID ASPIRATION SYNDROME (MENDELSON SYNDROME)

CAUSE

Aspiration of gastric contents with a pH of 3.5 or less[1] into the lungs may follow vomiting and regurgitation during general anesthesia used for obstetric patients.[2–6] Pulmonary inflammation, destruction of the alveolar lining, and transudation of fluid into the alveolar space occurs rapidly. This syndrome continues to be a cause of maternal mortality after cesarean section.[6]

CLINICAL

The patient becomes tachypneic, hypoxic, and febrile. The leukocyte count may rise, and the chest x-ray may suddenly change from normal to a complete white out within 8 to 24 hours. Pulmonary edema and bronchospasm are concomitants. There may be a fatal conclusion.

TREATMENT

Before induction of anesthesia, women in active labor receive nothing by mouth. Acid aspiration prophylaxis consisting of an H_2 receptor antagonist such as ranitidine and sodium citrate[3,4] has been used in Europe, though this is not a universal practice.[6]

REFERENCES—ACID ASPIRATION SYNDROME

1. Taylor G. Acid pulmonary aspiration syndrome after antacids. A case report. Br J Anaesth 1975;47:615–617.
2. Mendelson CL. The aspiration of stomach contents into the lungs during obstetric anesthesia. Am J Obstet Gynecol 1946;52:191–205.
3. Evans J, Rout CC, Roche DA. Acid aspiration prophylaxis. Anaesthesia 1991;46:73.
4. Sweeney B, Wright I. The use of antacids as a prophylaxis against Mendelson's syndrome in the United Kingdom. A survey. Anaesthesia 1986;41:419–422.
5. Taylor G, Pryse-Davies J. The prophylactic use of antacids in the prevention of the acid-pulmonary-aspiration syndrome (Mendelson's Syndrome). Lancet 1916;1:288–291.
6. Tordoff SG, Sweeney BP. Acid aspiration prophylaxis in 288 obstetric anaesthetic departments in the United Kingdom. Anaesthesia 1990;45:776–780.

INHALATION ANESTHETICS

Inhalation anesthetics are widely used because of their ability to induce anesthesia rapidly, their relative ease of control, and their ease and safety of recovery. The most widely used inhalation anesthetics are nitrous oxide (N_2O), halothane, enflurane, sevflurane, and isoflurane. Their anesthetic action is related to their partial pressure in the brain, which is more directly reflected by their alveolar partial pressure (P_A). By measuring and monitoring the P_A (mass spectrometry) the anesthesiologist is able to control the depth of anesthesia (partial pressure in the brain, P_{Br}).[1]

The uptake and distribution of an inhalation anesthetic depends on the inhaled concentration, pulmonary ventilation, solubility in blood, cardiac output, and tissue uptake.[2] Concentration gradients developed during general anesthesia in descending order are delivered, inspired, alveolar, arterial, and brain.[1]

Formulas for the inhalation agents are shown in Figure 56–1.[3]

Toxicity of inhalation anesthetics is most likely to be caused by pharmacologically active products of biotransformation.[2] Other mechanisms for toxicity include anesthetic protein interactions and anesthetic tissue interaction (see nitrous oxide and Vitamin B_{12}). Halothane, enflurane, and isoflurane have all been involved in serious and often fatal overdose reactions.

TOXIC DOSE

Halothane

A 2.5-mL dose of halothane was inadvertently administered IV. The patient survived.[4] Ingestion of 150 to 200 ml of halothane by an adult led to coma. The patient survived.[5] A 48-year-old patient survived an ingestion of 250 mL of halothane after a coma of 36 hours.[6]

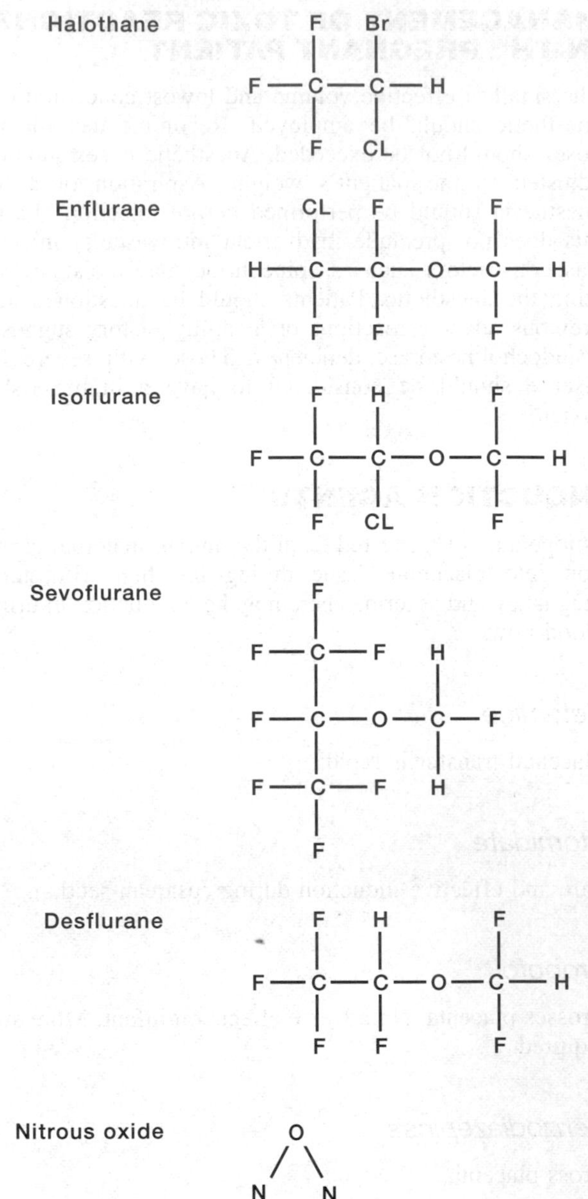

Figure 56–1 Formulas of the inhalational agents under review. (Adapted from Wrigley SR, Jones RM. Eur J Anesthesiol 1992;9: 185–201.)

Isoflurane

Inhalation of 10.2% isoflurane led to cyanosis and shock. The patient recovered.[7] Ingestion of 80 mL of isoflurane by a 37-year-old man terminated fatally.[8]

FATAL DOSE

Enflurane

Inhalation of 250 mL of enflurane led to death of a 29-year-old female.[9]

Halothane

A 3-ml mixture of halothane and methohexital given intravenously was fatal to a 20-year-old woman who died with an acute pulmonary edema.[10] Ingestion of 35 mL of halothane by an adult ended fatally.[11]

Nitrous Oxide

Exposure to 50 to 70% nitrous oxide for 3 hours may decrease hepatic methionine synthase activity and may result in aplastic anemia and death.[12]

OCCUPATIONAL EXPOSURE

There is little evidence that enflurane, halothane, or isoflurane represents a hazard to the staff of operating areas that are well ventilated with scavenging devices.[2] High occupational exposure may lead to hepatic microsomal drug metabolizing enzyme induction.

TOXICOKINETICS[2]

Cardiotoxic Effects

Ventricular irritability has been observed in adults undergoing halothane-induced anesthesia when 2.0 to 4.0 µg/kg of epinephrine in saline or 0.5% lidocaine has also been administered.[13] Halothane administered to children with up to 10 µg/mL of epinephrine by infiltration appears to be a relatively safe combination in normocarbic and hypocarbic pediatric patients without congenital heart disease.[14] Children appear less susceptible to the more serious ventricular arrhythmogenic effects of epinephrine. However, premature auricular contractions and tachycardia may still occur in children and emphasize the need for continuous electrocardiographic monitoring and caution during halothane anesthesia with epinephrine injection.[14,15] Nitrous oxide added to a steady-state halogen-oxygen anesthesia may increase mean arterial pressure, right atrial pressure, and systemic vascular resistance.[16] Cardiac arrest followed halothane use with verapamil and fenfluramine.[17] Halothane may potentiate neuromuscular blocking drugs.[18] Trichlorethane exposure may result in cardiac toxicity after halothane anesthesia.

Isoflurane

Isoflurane has caused a significant increase in action of atracurium and vecuronium. Nalbuphine reduces isoflurane requirements. Isoflurane appears to inhibit enflurane metabolism in man.[19]

Nitrous Oxide

Nitrous oxide may reduce the therapeutic benefits and increase the side effects of methotrexate therapy.[20] AV dissociation is observed when epinephrine with lidocaine is used in a patient receiving nitrous oxide.[21]

PREGNANCY/LACTATION

Enflurane

The uterine muscle is relaxed by enflurane. Uterine response to oxytocin is maintained provided that high inspired concentrations (over 2.5 to 3.0%) are not employed.[3]

Halothane

Halothane produces dose-dependent relaxation of uterine muscle in both pregnant and nonpregnant women.[3] During labor and delivery it may cause uterine atony accompanied by increased blood loss.[3]

Isoflurane

Isoflurane induces uterine relaxation.[17]

Nitrous Oxide

Administration of nitrous oxide during the second trimester of pregnancy did not result in adverse effects to the fetus.[17]

MECHANISM OF ACTION

Dose-related respiratory depression follows direct effects on the medullary respiratory centers, thoracic respiratory muscles, and diaphragm.

CLINICAL PRESENTATION

Cyclopropane

An adult was found dead as a result of the fatal ingestion of cyclopropane. This report (1989) is the first fatality report since the introduction of cyclopropane into clinical anesthesia in 1933.[22]

Desflurane

As is the case with isoflurane, use of desflurane may result in increases in brain volume or intracranial pressure. Its use in the neurosurgical patient should be carefully considered.[23,24]

Enflurane

Cardiovascular

Enflurane prolongs the QT_c interval without altering the QRS, PR, or QT intervals.[25]

Liver

Rare fatal hepatic necrosis may follow repeated enflurane anesthesia.[26,27] Clinical, biochemical, and histologic features of enflurane anesthesia–associated hepatitis injury are similar to those seen with halothane-related hepatitis.[24,28] Exposure to isoflurane can induce a fulminant hepatotoxic reaction.[29]

HALOTHANE HEPATITIS

Elliott and Strum[30] have described a halothane-associated hepatitis that presents as one of two clinical syndromes occurring most often in adult patients. These syndromes may develop after uneventful anesthesia and surgery, with no apparent time-dose relationship. One syndrome is characterized by moderate increases in the aminotransferase concentration and occasional transient jaundice. There is a low morbidity. It may also occur after an initial exposure to halothane, and its incidence may be up to 20%. The second syndrome occurs in one of 35,000 anesthetics, is associated with repeated exposure to the drug administered frequently at short intervals, and is associated with the development of fulminant hepatic failure with high mortality.

Neurologic

Prolonged halothane and enflurane used as bronchodilators in refractory status asthmaticus appeared to induce a tetraplegia and sensory disturbance in an adult who improved with cessation of both drugs.[31] Seizures without loss of consciousness may follow enflurane use.[32]

Cardiovascular

Halothane administered to adults does not appear to significantly alter the PR or QRS intervals, but does increase the QT and QT_c intervals.[24]

Acute Poisoning

The extreme toxicity of intravenous halothane (pulmonary edema, seizures) contrasts with the almost total lack of toxicity when it is given by inhalation.

DESFLURANE

Desflurane with controlled ventilation and constant P_aCO_2 causes cardiovascular depression. Cardiac output is well maintained.[33]

ISOFLURANE

Isoflurane anesthesia does not appear to significantly change the QRS, PR, or QT intervals, but significantly prolongs the QT_c interval.[25] Isoflurane may rarely be associated with malignant hyperthermia.[34]

NITROUS OXIDE

Problems

Nitrous oxide cannot be used effectively without decreasing the concentration of oxygen delivered. Its kinetic properties may expand internal gas spaces, distending the intestine, impairing operating conditions, and prolonging hospitalization. It may depress respiration and circulation and increase muscle tone, resulting in increasing dose requirements for muscle relaxants. It supports combustion. It may inactivate the vitamin B_{12} component of the enzyme methionine synthase.[35,36] Nitrous oxide also helps to break down ozone in the upper atmosphere and traps heat in the lower atmosphere (greenhouse gas).[37]

Chronic Use

The prolonged use of nitrous oxide (i.e., for days) may result in aplastic anemia, neuronal degeneration, megaloblastic changes, and death.[38–40]

Acute Use

Nitrous oxide (the minimum alveolar concentration or MAC is 104% or 1.04 atmospheres absolute [ATA]) is used as an adjunctive anesthetic agent in most people. Anesthesia with N_2O as the sole anesthetic in normal humans for periods of 2 to 4 hours has induced tachypnea, tachycardia, increased systemic blood pressure, atrioventricular junctional rhythm, acute cardiovascular failure, mydriasis, diaphoresis, and occasional clonus and opisthotonus.[41–43]

ANCILLARY TESTS

Enflurane[2]

High levels of inorganic fluoride have not been toxic.

Isoflurane

Hepatotoxicity is usually not seen in isoflurane anesthesia unless there is severe hypoxia present.[3]

Nitrous Oxide Abuse

Repeated abuse of nitrous oxide will often induce a bone marrow depression. Careful hematologic evaluation, including folate and vitamin B_{12} blood levels, may be indicated.[44] Signs of severe vitamin B_{12} and folic acid deficiency after a single operative exposure to nitrous oxide are rare.[35]

TREATMENT

Stabilization

Following the discovery of an overdose of an inhalation anesthetic, immediate measures should include discontinuation of the anesthetic, applying principles of cardiopulmonary resuscitation as indicated, and flushing the anesthetic circuit with 100% oxygen. Continuous cardiac monitoring, a supply of oxygen, and intravenous lines should be established. If the patient has not been provided an endotracheal tube, this should be put in place immediately. Mechanical ventilation should be provided as indicated. Blood is drawn for arterial blood gases, liver enzymes, B_{12} blood level, and creatinine, as well as electrolytes.

Vaporizer Failure

The wrong vaporizer for a given agent or vaporizer connected in series, rather than parallel, can produce overdosage. Accidental overdosage can also result from confusion of ON/OFF rotation direction of controls or different equipment and inappropriate exchange of equipment. Vaporizers may be left on by operating room personnel illicitly abusing halothane.[45] Awareness of unusual causes of vaporizer failure mitigate an overdose in progress.

Antidote

There is no antidote for these inhalation agents.

Supportive Measures

1. For bronchospasm: $beta_2$ adrenergic antagonists (e.g., salbutamol), oxygen, and mechanical ventilation should be administered in accordance with clinical judgment.
2. Seizures can be treated with intravenous diazepam and phenytoin if required.
3. Hypoxia may be ameliorated by oxygen and positive end-expiratory pressure ventilation.
4. Pulmonary edema may respond to oxygen, digitalis, and furosemide.
5. Continuous cardiac monitoring and serial arterial blood gases will be indicated.
6. Avoid central nervous system or respiratory depressants.
7. Frequently, a surgical procedure must be discontinued. If the anesthesiologist and surgeon agree, a procedure may proceed with another anesthetic. This should be carefully weighed with the risk of enhancing hemodynamic stability in an already compromised patient.
8. Follow-up may require careful and periodic hematologic evaluations, including bone marrow studies, complete blood counts, red cell indices, serum folate, and B_{12} levels.

A retrospective study among women employed as dental assistants exposed to high levels of nitrous oxide suggests an association with prolongation of time to conception.[46]

REFERENCES—INHALATION ANESTHETICS

1. Barash PG, Cullen BF, Stoelting RK. Handbook of clinical anesthesia. Philadelphia: JB Lippincott, 1991, pp. 148–158.
2. Dale O, Brown BR Jr. Clinical pharmacokinetics of the inhalational anaesthetics. Clin Pharmacokinet 1987;12:145–167.
3. Wrigley SR, Jones RM. Inhalational agents—an update. Eur J Anaesthesiol 1992;9:185–201.
4. Sutton J, Harrison GA, Hickie JB. Accidental intravenous injection of halothane. Case report. Br J Anaesth 1971;43:513–520.
5. Wig J, Chakravarty S, Krishnamurthy K, Mehta D. Coma following ingestion of halothane. Its successful management. Anaesthesia 1983;38:552–555.
6. Curelaru I, Stanciu S, Nicolau V, Fuhrer H, Iliescu M. A case of recovery from coma produced by the ingestion of 250 mL of halothane. Br J Anaesth 1968;40:283–288.
7. Martin ST. Hazards of agent-specific vaporizers: a case report of successful resuscitation after massive isoflurane overdose. Anesthesiology 1985;62:830–831.
8. Dooper PMM, Beerens J, Brenninkmeijer VJ, Gerlag PGF. Fatal intoxication after ingestion of isoflurane. Netherlands J Med 1988;33:74–77.
9. Lingenfelter RW. Fatal misuse of enflurane. Anesthesiology 1981;55:603.
10. Franks CR, Hudson PM, Rees AJ, Searle JF. Accidental intravenous halothane. Guy's Hosp Rep 1974;123:89–94.
11. Spencer JAE, Green NM. Suicide by ingestion of halothane. JAMA 1968;205:112–113.
12. Lampe GH, Wauk LZ, Donegan JH, Pitts LH, Jackler RK, Litt LL et al. Effect on outcome of prolonged exposure of patients to nitrous oxide. Anesth Analg 1990;71:586–590.
13. Jarnberg PO, Estrand J, Irestedt L. Renal fluoride excretion and plasma fluoride levels during and after enflurane anesthesia are dependent on urinary pH. Anesthesiology 1981; 54:48–52.
14. Karl HW, Swerdlow DB, Lee KW, Downes JJ. Epinephrine-halothane interactions in children. Anesthesiology 1983; 58:142–145.
15. Bosnjak ZJ, Turner LA. Halothane, catecholamines and cardiac conduction. Anything new? Anesth Analg 1991;72:1–4.
16. Smith NT, Eger EI II, Stoelting RK, Whayne TF, Cullen D, Kadis LB. The cardiovascular and sympathomimetic responses to the addition of nitrous oxide to halothane in man. Anesthesiology 1970;32:410–420.
17. Frank EJ Jr, Ghantous H, Malan TP, Morgan S, Fernando J, Gandolfi AJ et al. Plasma inorganic fluoride with sevoflurane anesthesia: correlation with indices of hepatic and renal function. Anesth Analg 1992;74:231–235.
18. Halsey MJ. Drug interactions in anaesthesia. Br J Anaesth 1987;59:112–123.
19. Oikkonen MP. Isoflurane inhibits enflurane metabolism in man. Anaesthesia 1989;44:763–764.
20. Ueland PM, Refsun H, Wesenberg F, Kvinnsland S. Methotrexate therapy and nitrous oxide anesthesia. N Engl J Med 1986;314:1514.
21. Lampe GH, Donegan JH, Rupp SM, Wauk LZ, Whitendale P, Fouts KE et al. Nitrous oxide and epinephrine-induces arrhythmias. Anesth Analg 1990;71:602–605.
22. Krause JG, McCarthy WB. Sudden death by inhalation of cyclopropane. J Forensic Sci 1989;34:1011–1012.
23. Young WL. Effects of desflurane on the central nervous system. Anesth Analg 1992;75:S32–S37.
24. Muzzi DA, Losasso TJ, Dietz NM, Faust RJ, Cucchiara RF, Milde LN. The effect of desflurane and isoflurane on cerebrospinal fluid pressure in humans with supratentorial mass lesions. Anesthesiology 1992;76:720–724.
25. Schmeling WT, Warltier DC, McDonald DJ, Madsen KE, Atlee JL, Kampine JP. Prolongation of the QT interval by enflurane, isoflurane, and halothane in humans. Anesth Analg 1991;72: 137–144.
26. Denlinger JK, Lecky JH, Nahrwold ML. Hepatocellular dysfunction without jaundice after enflurane anesthesia. Anesthesiology 1974;41:86–87.
27. Ona FV, Patanella H, Ayub A. Hepatitis associated with enflurane anesthesia. Anesth Analg 1980;59:146–149.
28. Lewis JH, Zimmerman HJ, Ishak KG, Mullick FG. Enflurane hepatotoxicity. A clinicopathologic study of 24 cases. Ann Intern Med 1983;98:984–992.
29. Brune EM, White H, Marsh JW, Holtmann B, Peters MG. Fulminant hepatic failure after repeated exposure to isoflurane anesthesia: a case report. Hepatology 1991;13:1017–1021.
30. Elliott RH, Strum L. Hepatotoxicity of volatile anaesthetics. Br J Anaesthesia 1993;70:339–348.
31. Tanigaki T, Kondo T, Ohta Y, Yamabayashi H. Transient neuromuscular impairment resulting from prolonged inhalation of halothane and enflurane. Chest 1990;98:1012–1013.
32. Parke TJ, Jags RH. Focal seizure following enflurane. Anaesthesia 1992;67:79–80.
33. Weiskopf RB, Cahalan MK, Eger EI II, Yasuda N, Rampil J, Ionescu P et al. Cardiovascular actions of desflurane in normocarbic volunteers. Anesth Analg 1991;73:143–151.
34. Thomas DW, Dev VJ, Whitehead MJ. Malignant hyperpyrexia and isoflurane. A case report. Br J Anaesth 1987;54:1196–1198.
35. Koblin DD, Tomerson BW, Waldman FM, Lampe GH, Wauke LZ, Eger EI II. Effect of nitrous oxide on folate and vitamin B_{12} metabolism in patients. Anesth Analg 1990;71:610–617.
36. Kones R. Folic acid 1991: an update with new recommended daily allowances. South Med J 1990;83:1454–1458.
37. No laughing matter. Harvard Med Sch Health Letter 1991; 16(7).
38. Lassen HCA, Henriksen E, Neukirch F, Kristensen HS. Treatment of tetanus. Severe bone-marrow depression after prolonged nitrous oxide anaesthesia. Lancet 1956;1:527–530.
39. Layzer RB. Myeloneuropathy after prolonged exposure to nitrous oxide. Lancet 1978;2:1227–1230.
40. Amos RJ, Amess JAL, Hinds CJ, Mollin DL. Incidence and pathogenesis of acute megaloblastic bone marrow change in patients receiving intensive care. Lancet 1982;2:835–839.

41. Russell GB, Snider MT, Richard RB, Loomis JL. Hyperbaric nitrous oxide as a sole anesthetic agent in humans. Anesth Analg 1990;70:289–295.
42. Roizen MF, Plummer GO, Lichtor JL. Nitrous oxide and dysrhythmias. Anesthesiology 1987;66:427–431.
43. Davidson JR, Chinyanga HM. Cardiovascular collapse associated with nitrous oxide anaesthetic. A case report. Can Anaesth Soc J 1982;29:484–488.
44. Van Achterbergh SM, Vorster BJ, Heyns ADP. The effect of sepsis and short-term exposure to nitrous oxide on the bone marrow and the metabolism of vitamin B_{12} and folate. So Afr Med J 1990;78:260–263.
45. Randall B, Corbett B. Fatal halothane poisoning during anesthesia with other agents. J Forensic Sci 1982;27: 225–230.
46. Rowland AS, Baird DD, Weinberg CR, Shore DL, Shy CM, Wilcox AJ. Reduced fertility among women employed as dental assistants exposed to high levels of nitrous oxide. N Engl J Med 1992;327:993–997.

INTRAVENOUS ANESTHETICS

The first effective intravenous anesthetic induction agent, hexobarbital, was introduced into clinical practice in Germany in 1932.[1] Thiopental, introduced in 1934 in the United States, remains the most widely used intravenous induction agent. Details on barbiturates, benzodiazepines, and opioids (e.g., fentanyl, alfentanil) are discussed in their respective chapters.

COMPATIBILITIES[2]

1. Barbiturate solutions are alkaline (pH 10 to 11). Mixing barbiturates with acidic solutions (lactated Ringer's solution) or other drugs may result in the precipitation of barbiturates as free acids.
2. Diazepam in solution contains propylene glycol and will precipitate when mixed with other solutions.
3. Midazolam is water soluble (pH 3.5) and compatible with other solutions.
4. Etomidate is formulated with propylene glycol.
5. Ketamine (pH 3.5 to 5.5) and propofol should not be mixed with other drugs.

Categories of intravenous anesthetics are listed in Table 56–8.

DOSAGE

Doses of nonopioid drugs can be either injected as a bolus intravenously to induce anesthesia or administered by continuous infusion for partial or complete maintenance of anesthesia.[2] A summary of comparative properties of intravenous anesthetics is found in Table 56–9.

FENTANYL DERIVATIVES

Alfentanil

Alfentanil is a structural analogue of fentanyl that is about one-fourth as potent as fentanyl and has one-third the duration of action. It appears to have a relative lack of adverse cardiovascular effects. Alfentanil used for rapid sequence intubation produces less muscular rigidity than fentanyl.[3] Age influences its elimination half-life: elderly—longer; children—shorter; liver insufficiency and obesity prolong the half-life. Cardiopulmonary bypass causes the $alpha_1$-acid glycoprotein level to decrease, increasing the free fraction that enters the extravascular space, increasing the volume of distribution, and prolonging the half-life.[3]

Fentanyl

Fentanyl is about 50 to 100 times more potent than injectable morphine. For every 30 mg of oral or 15 mg of intramuscular morphine, a starting dose of transdermal fentanyl can be 6.25 to 12.5 µg/hour.[4]

Table 56–8
Categories of Intravenous Anesthetics

Barbiturates	Thiopental
	Thiamylal
	Methohexital
Imidazoles	Etomidate
Benzodiazepines	Diazepam
	Lorazepam
	Midazolam
Arylcyclohexylamines	Ketamine
Alkylphenols	Propofol
Fentanyl analogues	Fentanyl
	Alfentanil
	Sufentanil
	Lofentanil

Table 56–9
Summary of Comparative Pharmacologic Properties of Intravenous Anesthetics[a]

Drug Group	Drug Name	Dose (mg/kg)	Onset (sec)	Duration (min)
Barbiturates	Thiopental	3.0–6.0	<30	5–10
	Thiamylal	3.0–5.0	<30	5–10
	Methohexital	1.0–2.0	<30	5–10
Imidazoles	Etomidate	0.2–0.4	15–45	5–10
Benzodiazepines	Diazepam	0.3–0.6	45–60	15–30
	Lorazepam	0.03–0.06	60–120	60–120
	Midazolam	0.2–0.4	30–60	15–30
Arylcyclohexylamines	Ketamine	1.0–2.0	45–60	10–20
Alkylphenols	Propofol	1.5–3.0	15–45	5–10

[a]Adapted from Landow L. J Intensive Care Med 1991;6:12–25.

Sufentanil

Sufentanil is highly lipophilic and distributes rapidly and extensively. Respiratory depression, delayed gastric emptying, and increased intrabiliary pressure may occur. Physical dependence occurs with prolonged usage. Muscle rigidity may follow intravenous infusion.

Lofentanil

Lofentanil is approximately 20 times more potent than fentanyl and has a duration of action about 20 times that of fentanyl.

CLINICAL TOXICITY[5]

Induction Complications

Excitatory Complications

Involuntary movements and hypertonus are seen with all IV agents when given to the unpremedicated patient. The incidence varies: thiopental has an incidence of about 8%; muscle movements following etomidate may occur in as many as 95% of patients, after methohexital in 30 to 35%, and following propofol in 14%. The incidence depends on the dose of drug administered and whether premedication was used.

Respiratory Upsets

Cough, hiccup, and laryngospasm are seen in high frequency (40 to 45%) mainly with methohexital. Barbiturates may, however, cause respiratory depression in up to 70% of patients. Hyperventilation may occur after induction with etomidate and methohexital and may be followed by apnea in 30% of patients receiving etomidate.[6] Apnea is also seen with propofol.

Tissue Irritation

All of the IV hypnotic agents used for the induction of anesthesia can cause pain on injection and postoperative venous sequelae. Incidences of such sequelae are low when veins of the antecubital fossa are employed, but rise to four to five times that level when injections are made into the dorsum of the hand.

Accidental Intraarterial Injection

Accidental injection of IV agents directly into an artery may result in marked sequelae.[6] Thiopental and methohexital both precipitate out of solution when injected into an artery, as a result of the decrease in pH. Red cell hemolysis and platelet aggregation may occur, leading to intravascular thrombosis. Severe tissue necrosis may result in amputation of affected tissue.

REFERENCES—INTRAVENOUS ANESTHETICS

1. Wood M. Intravenous anesthetic agents. In: Wood M, Wood AJJ, eds. Drugs and anesthesia. Pharmacology for anesthesiologists. 2nd ed. Baltimore: Williams & Wilkins, 1990.
2. Barash PG, Cullen BF, Stoelting RK. Handbook of clinical anesthesia. Philadelphia: JB Lippincott, 1991.
3. Simon B, Young GP. Emergency airway management. Acad Emerg Med 1994;1:154–157.
4. Cote D. Dosage of transdermal fentanyl. Clin Pharm 1993;12:718.
5. Swerdlow BN, Holley FO. Intravenous anaesthetic agents. Pharmacokinetic-pharmacodynamic relationships. Clin Pharmacokinet 1987;12:79–110.
6. Sear JW. Toxicity of IV anaesthetics. Br J Anaesth 1987;59:24–45.

DROPERIDOL

Droperidol is a synthetic butyrophenone derivative similar in chemical structure to haloperidol. It is frequently administered together with fentanyl as a neuroleptic.[1–4] Droperidol is a powerful antiemetic often used to treat opiate-induced vomiting. It exhibits extrapyramidal side effects and may cause hypotension due to its central nervous system and alpha-adrenergic blocking properties. In patients who are hypovolemic or who are receiving vasodilator therapy, droperidol can induce a profound hypotension. Arrhythmias and respiratory side effects are minimal. Droperidol has no analgesic effect. Overdose may lead to reversible parkinsonism.[5]

SUPPORTIVE MEASURES

Akathisia can be treated with anticholinergics (benztropine or diphenhydramine), dopamine agonists (such as amantadine), or with beta-blockers (such as propranolol). Discontinuation of droperidol may lead to reversal of akathisia within 72 hours.

REFERENCES—DROPERIDOL

1. Wood M. Intravenous anesthetic agents in Wood M, Wood AJJ: Drugs and Anesthesia. Pharmacology for Anesthesiologists. Baltimore: Williams and Wilkins 1990;206–207.
2. McEvoy GK, ed. AHFS Drug Information 92. Bethesda: American Society of Hospital Pharmacists, 1992; pp. 1281–1283.
3. Reynolds JEF, ed. *Martindale: The extra pharmacopoeia.* 29th ed. London: The Pharmaceutical Press, 1989.
4. Barash RG, Cullen BF, Stoelting RK. Handbook of clinical anesthesia. New York: JB Lippincott, 1991.
5. Bach V, Carl P, Rallo O, Crawford ME, Werner M. Potentiation of epidural opioids with epidural droperidol. Anaesthesia 1986;41:1116–1119.

ETOMIDATE

Etomidate is a synthetic carboxylate imidazole—a GABA-mimetic (gamma-aminobutyric acid), short-acting, nonbarbiturate sedative-hypnotic agent that lacks analgesic properties, and is used largely for induction.[1] Overdose may result in prolonged deep unconsciousness.

REFERENCES—ETOMIDATE

1. Davis PJ, Cook DR. Clinical pharmacokinetics of the newer intravenous anaesthetic agents. Clin Pharmacokinet 1986;11:18–35.

FENTANYL-INTRAVENOUS AND FENTANYL TRANSDERMAL SYSTEM (FTS) (TRANSDERMAL ANESTHESIA)

Transdermal drug delivery is an alternative to conventional oral or parenteral therapy. Excess absorption of fentanyl from this system may result in increased serum fentanyl concentration associated with symptoms of an opioid overdose.[1] (For abuse of fentanyl derivatives, see Opiate chapter—Designer Drugs.)

STRUCTURE AND CLASSIFICATION

Fentanyl Transdermal System (FTS, Duragesic) was approved by the U.S. Food and Drug Administration in 1991. FTS can provide up to 72 hours of analgesia with each application and can maintain predictable plasma concentrations with chronic dosage,[2,3] or fentanyl delivery may increase during fever.[4] Fentanyl is a schedule II controlled substance and can produce drug dependence similar to that of morphine. A comparison of intravenous and transdermal fentanyl toxicokinetics is summarized in Table 56–10.

A 10-mg IV or 60-mg oral dose of morphine every 4 hours for 24 hours (total of 60 mg/day IV or 360 mg/day orally) is about equivalent to an FTS dose of 100 μg/hour.[4]

TOXIC DOSE

Two hours after a heating pad was applied to an FTS, providing a dose of 100 μg/hour obtundation, pinpoint pupils and shallow respirations were observed, all of which responded rapidly to IV naloxone.[1]

TOXICOKINETICS[5–11]

Drug Interactions

Muscle relaxants (e.g., atracurium, vecuronium), other anesthetic agents, opiates, and benzodiazepines enhance the respiratory depression and hypotension following use of fentanyl.

Table 56–10
Fentanyl Toxicokinetics

	Intravenous	Transdermal
Bioavailability	100%	92%
Peak serum level		24–72 hours
Volume of distribution	3–7 L/kg	-
Half-life	6–9 hours	16 hours
Mean serum concentration (therapeutic range)	1–3 ng/mL	1.5–2.0 ng/mL
Loss of consciousness (plasma levels)	34 ng/mL	-
Excreted unchanged	6%	-
Blood levels at death	4 ng/mL–14 ng/mL	-
Metabolites	Inactive	-
Clearance	700–1000 mL/min	400–650 mL/min
Plasma protein binding	80%	-

Pregnancy/Lactation

Fentanyl has been placed in Pregnancy Category C by the U.S. Food and Drug Administration. Fentanyl is excreted in human milk and therefore is not recommended for use in nursing women.[4,12]

Mechanism of Action

Fentanyl is a potent opioid analgesic that interacts with the opioid μ-receptor.

CLINICAL PRESENTATION

Most adverse effects reported with the use of the transdermal system are common to opioid analgesics.[2–4] Other effects include localized itching and erythema, which usually subside within 6 hours after patch removal.[6] Serum concentration of fentanyl may increase in patients with increased body temperatures.[4] The use of heating pads by patients wearing fentanyl patches have the potential for causing serious drug overdoses (mental confusion, immediate hemodynamic collapse[12] pinpoint pupils, and shallow respirations all reversed rapidly with naloxone).[1,13,14] Fentanyl is often given therapeutically in doses that may result in death by respiratory depression.[15]

DEATHS—WARNING

The drug is not to be given at doses higher than 25 μg/hour at the start of opioid therapy and is not to be used in children under the age of 12 years or by patients under the age of 18 years who weigh less than 50 kg except in an FDA approved research setting.[16] Adverse reactions include nausea, vomiting, constipation, dry mouth, somnolence, confusion, and sweating. Seizures, hypotension, and death have followed fentanyl use.[17]

LABORATORY

Analytic Methods

A radioimmunoassay method is sensitive (60 ng/liter) and specific.[7,18]

Blood Levels

Following use of a 125-μg/hr patch, fentanyl concentration plateaus in the range of 2.5 to 3.5 ng/mL.[19]

TREATMENT

Ensure that a patent airway is established and maintained and administer oxygen. Use assisted or controlled ventilation as indicated with an oropharyngeal airway or endotracheal tube as required. Maintain an adequate body temperature and fluid intake. Remove any external source of heat. Use cooling measures for hyperthermia. Remove the transdermal patch. Instruct patients not to use heating pads at home. Naloxone is indicated for signs and symptoms suggestive of an opioid overdose. The duration of hypoventilation following an overdose may be longer than the effects of the narcotic antagonist's action. Additional treatment is symptomatic. For severe and persistent hypotension, consider hypovolemia and manage with appropriate parenteral fluid therapy.[4]

Antidote

Naloxone specifically counteracts fentanyl-induced hypoventilation. However, because of its short half-life (30 to 80 minutes) compared with fentanyl, repeated administration of naloxone may be required with careful monitoring for a recurrence in the onset of pain and release of catecholamines.

REFERENCES—FENTANYL

1. Rose PG, Macfee MS, Boswell MV. Fentanyl transdermal system overdose secondary to cutaneous hyperthermia. Anesth Analg 1993;77:390–391.
2. Miser AV, Narang PK, Dothage JA et al. Transdermal fentanyl for pain control in patients with cancer. Pain 1989;37:15–21.
3. Zech DFJ, Grand SUA, Lynch J et al. Transdermal fentanyl and initial dose finding with patient controlled analgesia in cancer pain. A pilot study with 20 terminally ill cancer patients. Pain 1992;50:293–301.
4. Physicians desk reference. 49th ed. Montvale, NJ: Medical Economics, 1995; pp. 1175–1178.
5. Hudson RJ, Thomson IR, Cannon JE, Friesen RM, Meatherall RC. Pharmacokinetics of fentanyl in patients undergoing abdominal aortic surgery. Anesthesiology 1986;64:334–338.
6. Singleton MA, Rosen JI, Fisher DM. Pharmacokinetics of fentanyl in the elderly. Br J Anaesth 1988;60:619–622.
7. Gauntlett IS, Fisher DM, Hertzka RE, Kuhls E, Spellman MJ, Rudolph C. Pharmacokinetics of fentanyl in neonatal humans and lambs: effects of age. Anesthesiology 1988;69:683–687.
8. Duthie DJR, McLaren AD, Nimmo WS. Pharmacokinetics of fentanyl during constant rate IV infusion for the relief of pain after surgery. Br J Anaesth 1986;58:950–951.
9. Duthie DJR, Rowbotham DJ, Wyld R, Henderson PD, Nimmo WS. Plasma fentanyl concentrations during transdermal delivery of fentanyl to surgical patients. Br J Anaesth 1988; 60:614–618.
10. Rowbotham DJ, Wyld R, Peacock JE, Duthie DJR, Mimmo WS. Transdermal fentanyl for the relief of pain after upper abdominal surgery. Br J Anaesth 1989;65:56–59.
11. Stoeckel H, Hengstmann JH, Schuttler J. Pharmacokinetics of fentanyl as a possible explanation for recurrence of respiratory depression. Br J Anaesth 1979;51:741–745.
12. Craft JB Jr, Coaldrake LA, Bolan JC, Mondino M, Mazel P, Gilman RM et al. Placental passage and uterine effects of fentanyl. Anesth Analg 1983;62:894–898.
13. Gourlay GK, Kowalski SR, Plumer JL et al. The transdermal administration of fentahyl in the treatment of postoperative pain: pharmacokinetics and pharmacodynamic effects. Pain 1989;37:192–202.
14. Varvel JR, Shafer SL, Hwang SS, Coen PA, Stanski DR. Absorption characteristic of transdermally administered fentanyl. Anesthesiology 1989;70:928–934.
15. Marquardt KA, Tharratt S. Inhalation abuse of fentanyl patch. Clin Toxicol 1994;32:75–78.
16. Baselt RC, Cravey RH. Disposition of toxic drugs and chemicals in man. 3rd ed. Chicago: Year Book, pp. 350–352.
17. De Sio JM, Bacon DR, Peer G, Lema MJ. Intravenous abuse of transdermal fentanyl therapy in a chronic pain patient. Anesthesiology 1993;79:1139–1141.
18. McCarthy M. Fentanyl patch misuse. Lancet 1994;343:351.
19. Goromaru T, Matsuura H, Yoshimura N, Miyawaki T, Sameshima T, Miyao J et al. Identification and quantitative determination of fentanyl metabolites in patients by gas chromatography–mass spectrometry. Anesthesiology 1984; 61:73–77.
20. Payne R, Moran K, Southan M. The role of transdermal fentanyl in the management of cancer pain. In: Estafanous FG, ed. Opioids in anesthesia II. Boston: Butterworth-Heinemann, 1991; pp. 215–222.

KETAMINE

In the 1976 film *Family Plot* Alfred Hitchcock depicted a kidnap victim sedated with a little-known drug called ketamine. Ketamine was developed because of dissatisfaction with the clinical experience of phencyclidine as a surgical anesthetic drug (duration of action and emergency excitement were too great). Street use of ketamine hydrochloride injection was first observed in San Francisco and Los Angeles in 1971.[1]

Ketamine, a synthetic chemical, is used as a general anesthetic during surgery. It induces sedation, immobility, amnesia, and analgesia. Ketamine produces an unusual trancelike cataleptic state, whereby the patient appears to be "dissociated" from his environment but not necessarily asleep. The patient can have profound analgesia and be awake with his eyes open or unconscious.[2–5] Ketamine maintains anesthesia and analgesia while preserving pharyngeal reflexes and respiratory function. Ketamine is used for anesthesia in the Third World and in military campaigns where extensive anesthetic equipment is unavailable. It is subject to drug abuse and may result in death.[3] Ketamine possesses a unique problem when assessing the level of sedation or anesthesia because of an inability to use eye signs, degree of muscle pain, or patient movement as indications.[6]

STRUCTURE AND CLASSIFICATION

Ketamine is a phencyclidine derivative chemically related to cyclohexamine. Ketamine lipid solubility is ten times that of thiopental.[7] Two enantiomers of the ketamine molecule exist: s(+)ketamine and r(−)ketamine. Commercially available racemic ketamine preparations contain equal concentrations of the two enantiomers, which may differ in anesthetic potency, in effect on the electroencephalograph, in effects in catecholamine reuptake, and possibly in the incidence of emergency reactions. The analgesic and hypnotic potency of s(+)ketamine is about four times greater than that of the r(−)isomer, which is only a partial agonist.[8]

Synonyms

Ketalar, Ketajed, Ketaret. Street names include "K," "Kay," "Super Acid," "Green" (color of ketamine in the crystalline form), "purple" or "mauve" (when mixed with vitamin B_{12}), "special LA coke," "Super C."[1,4]

Product Formulation

Ketamine is available in vials containing 10 or 50 mg of ketamine per mL.[6,9]

DOSAGE

Therapeutic Doses (Table 56–11)[2]

Fatal

A total dose of 900 mg led to a fatality in an adult.[10]

Table 56–11
Ketamine Dosage

Route	Dose	Unconscious	Peak Plasma Concentration
IV	1–2 mg/kg	5–15 minutes	1 minute
IM	5–10 mg/kg	10–30 minutes	5–15 minutes
Oral	4–5 mg/kg		30 minutes (norketamine plasma levels high)
Rectal			45 minutes

TOXICOKINETICS[2,6,10,11]

Peak plasma levels	30,000 ng/mL (highest recorded); 150 ng/mL (analgesia), 600–1000 ng/mL on awakening
Volume of distribution (L/kg)	4 L/kg
Plasma protein binding (%)	12%
Elimination half-life	2 hours
Excreted unchanged (%)	<5%

Drug Interactions

Ketamine potentiates the effect of neuromuscular blocking agents in a dose-dependent manner.[6] The elimination half-life and blood levels of ketamine are increased by the concomitant administration of diazepam and halothane.[4–7] Alcoholics tend to be resistant to ketamine anesthesia. Concurrent use of ketamine with aminophylline may decrease the seizure threshold.[12]

MECHANISM OF ACTION

The analgesia is mediated partially by the opioid μ-receptor. Ketamine interacts with sigma/phencyclidine binding sites. The sigma/phencyclidine component may mediate the dysphoria induced by ketamine. Ketamine's site of action involves the *N*-methyl-d-aspartate (NMDA) receptors, which play a major role in the transmission of sensory information and may mediate the excitation of neurons in the central nervous system secondary to interactions with excitatory amino acid neurotransmitters (EAA).

EAA (Excitatory Amino Acid Neurotransmitters)

EAAs are the most prevalent excitatory neurotransmitters in the brain and are particularly important in corticocortical and cortical-subcortical interactions. NMDA inhibition produced catalepsy. Ketamine potentiates the effect of neuromuscular blocking drugs.[6]

Phencyclidine and ketamine are noncompetitive NMDA antagonists. They bind to a site that is distinct from NMDA within the ion channel and block calcium influx. Ketamine is 10 to 50 times less potent than phencyclidine in blocking NMDA-mediated neurotoxicity, seizures, and physiologic effects and in substituting for phencyclidine in drug discrimination paradigms. The r-isomer of ketamine has an approximately sevenfold greater affinity for the σ-receptor than the S-isomer. The small contribution of the μ-receptor to the behavioral effects of ketamine is consistent with the limited capacity of naloxone hydrochloride to reverse the analgesic and behavioral effects of ketamine.

CLINICAL PRESENTATION

Central Nervous System

Ketamine produces a "dissociated anesthesia" characterized by profound analgesia, amnesia, and catalepsy. The eyes may remain open with slow nystagmus and intact corneal reflexes. Patients are usually noncommunicative though they may appear to be awake. Skeletal muscle spasm may be present.[13] It is often difficult to assess a clear endpoint where ketamine is administered. Eye signs, muscle tone, or patient movement cannot be used as indicators. Emergence phenomena are the most frequently reported adverse effects of ketamine and include a feeling of floating, vivid dreams, hallucinations, and delirium[4] in 5 to 30% of patients and are related to the dose and rate of drug administration. Ketamine vasodilates cerebral blood vessels, increasing cerebral blood flow by up to 80% and leading to increases in intracranial pressure. Seizures may result from massive overdose.[14] Acute dystonic reactions may follow intravenous use.

Cardiovascular

An acute hypertensive crisis, pulmonary hypertension, and pulmonary edema may be triggered by the use of intravenous ketamine in a patient with a history of cocaine abuse.[15] Ketamine induces an increase in heart rate, cardiac output, and blood pressure. Cardiac dysrhythmias are uncommon.

Respiratory

Ketamine maintains functional residual capacity, induces bronchodilation, stimulates salivary and tracheobronchial secretions, and causes a mild respiratory depression.[6] Laryngospasm and stridor have been reported in children. Apnea may be observed.[16,17]

Ketamine Abuse

Recreational users of ketamine are motivated by the experience of dissociative hallucinatory states. Cocaine, amphetamine, caffeine, lactose, flour, talc, and vitamins have been used as adulterants.[1,4] Mild memory impairment, flashbacks, attentional dysfunction, and decreased sociability may result from ketamine abuse.[1,18] No withdrawal reactions to ketamine have been reported. Recreational injection users employ dosages of about 1.0 to 2.0 mg/kg (0.5 to 1 mg/lb) for both intramuscular and intravenous administration. Intranasal doses range from 60 to 100 mg.[1]

LABORATORY

Blood Levels

A blood level of about 27 μg/mL (27,000 ng/mL) was found in a patient who had self-administered about 1 g by the intramuscular route.[2] Following the fatal administration of 900 mg of ketamine a blood level of 7 μg/mL was observed.[11] Blood levels in cases of overdose are not significantly different from control cases and are not helpful in management of ketamine intoxications.[6]

Ancillary Tests

Ketamine produces consistent changes in the electroencephalogram, including a reduction in alpha-wave activity, while beta-, delta-, and theta-wave activity are increased.[7]

TREATMENT

Stabilization

Ketamine adverse reactions or overdosage treatment is largely symptomatic and supportive. If respiratory depression, depressed level of consciousness, or stridor is present, establish prompt airway control and ventilatory support. Assess blood sugar by finger stick. Give naloxone intravenously. Treat seizures with usual medications. Watch for polydrug abuse.

Decontamination

Consider gastric decontamination if large amounts of ketamine have been ingested or if there is a history of coingestion of other substances.

Elimination Enhancement

Ketamine elimination cannot be enhanced because of its high lipid solubility and extensive volume of distribution.

Antidotes

There are no antidotes. Preliminary evidence suggests that 4-aminopyridine reverses the effects of both ketamine and the benzodiazepines.[7] Pulmonary hypertension and pulmonary edema may be reversed by fentanyl.[19]

Supportive Measures

Discharge from the Emergency Department after treatment with benzodiazepines and a short period of observation. Persistent alterations in mental status require assessments for other causes of central nervous system impairment. Treat dystonic reactions with intravenous diphenhydramine or benztropine. Treat emergence reactions with reassurance, a quiet dimly lit room, and benzodiazepines orally for mild reactions and intravenously for severe reactions (useful to decrease the severity of dreams, hallucinations, and illusions). Perform routine toxicologic screening in a suspected attempted suicide overdose. Use glycopyrrolate or atropine to reduce tracheobronchial secretions. Serious cardiovascular stimulation can be blocked by alpha- and beta-adrenoceptor antagonists, as well as by verapamil. Benzodiazepines may also be useful.[6]

REFERENCES—KETAMINE

1. Siegel RK. Phencyclidine and ketamine intoxication. A study of four populations of recreational users. National Institute of Drug Abuse Research Monograph series. 1978;21: 119–147.
2. Wood M: Intravenous anesthetic agents. In: Wood M, Wood AJJ, eds. Drugs and anesthesia. Pharmacology for anesthesiologists. Baltimore: Williams & Wilkins, 1990; pp. 193–196.
3. Licata M, Pierini G, Popo I. A fatal ketamine poisoning. J Forensic Sci 1994;39:1314–1320.
4. Grandins A. Ketamine. Clin Toxicol Rev 1994;16(1):1–2.
5. Committee on Drugs. American Academy of Pediatrics. Guidelines for monitoring and management of pediatric patients during and after sedation for diagnostic and therapeutic procedures. Pediatrics 1992;89:1110–1115.
6. Haas DA, Harper DG: Ketamine. A review of its pharmacologic properties and use in ambulatory anesthesia. Anesth Prog 1992;39:61–68.
7. Reich DL, Silvay G. Ketamine. An update on the first twenty-five years of clinical experience. Can J Anaesth 1989;36: 186–197.
8. Kharasch EDR. Metabolism of ketamine sterioisomers by human liver microsomes. Anesthesiology 1992;77:1201–1207.
9. Swerdlow BW, Holley FO. Intravenous anaesthetic agents. Clin Pharmacokinet 1987;12:79–110.
10. Peyton SH, Couch AT, Bost RO. Tissue distribution of ketamine: two case reports. J Anal Toxicol 1988;12:268–269.
11. Domino EF, Domino SE, Smith RE, Domino LE, Goulet JR, Domino KE, Zsigmond EK. Ketamine kinetics in unmedicated and diazepam-premediated subjects. Clin Pharmacol Ther 1984;36:645–653.
12. Hirshman CA, Krieger W, Littlejohn G, Lee R, Julien R. Ketamine-aminophylline induced decrease in seizures threshold. Anesthesiology 1982;56:464–467.
13. Richard BM, Donaldson MDJ. Ketamine and muscle spasm. Br J Anaesth 1994;73:432.
14. Burmeister-Rother R, Streatfield KA, Yoo MC. Convulsions following ketamine and atropine. Anesthesia 1993;48:82.
15. Murphy JL Jr. Hypertension and pulmonary oedema associated with ketamine administration in a patient with a history of substance abuse. Can J Anaesth 1993;40:160–164.
16. Schultz CH. Intramuscular ketamine and apnea. Ann Emerg Med 1994;23:139.
17. Smith JA, Santer J. Intramuscular ketamine and apnea. Ann Emerg Med 1994;23:140–141.
18. Jansen KLR: Ketamine—can chronic use impair memory? Int J Addict 1990;25:133–139.
19. Tarnow J, Hess W. Pulmonary hypertension and pulmonary edema caused by intravenous ketamine. Anesthetist 1978;22:486–487.

PROPOFOL

Propofol is a synthetic intravenous sedative-hypnotic anesthetic that may, in overdose, or after inadvertent intraarterial injection, induce cardiovascular and respiratory depression. A study of propofol use in patients with susceptibility to malignant hyperthermia (MH) suggests that propofol is safe in those who are susceptible to MH.[1,2] Propofol has successfully controlled seizures in status epilepticus.[3]

TREATMENT

1. Signs of potential toxicity may include apnea, bradycardia, hypotension, hypertension, and perioperative myoclonia. Oxygen, intravenous fluids, and cardiac monitoring should be available.
2. Patients should be continuously monitored for early signs of significant hypotension and/or bradycardia and for respiratory depression.
3. For cardiovascular depression: increase the rate of intravenous fluid administration; elevate lower extremi-

ties; use pressor agents and administration of atropine as required.

4. For overdose: discontinue the propofol. If there is respiratory depression, maintain artificial ventilation with oxygen and mechanical ventilation as required.
5. Maintain and handle propofol (Diprivan) with an aseptic technique.
6. There are no antidotes.

REFERENCES—PROPOFOL

1. Gallen JS. Propofol does not trigger malignant hyperthermia. Anesth Analg 1991;72:413–414.
2. Harrison GG. Propofol in malignant hyperthermia. Lancet 1991;337:503.
3. MacKenzie SJ, Kapadia F, Grant IS. Propofol infusion for control of status epilepticus. Anaesthesia 1990;45:1043–1045.

ALTHESIN

Althesin is a mixture of two steroids: alphaxalone (3α-hydroxy-5α-pregnane-11,20,dione), 9 mg/ml and alphadolone acetate (21-acetoxy-3α-hydroxy-5α-pregnane-11,20, dione), 3 mg/ml. It also contains the solubilizing agent cremophor EL (polyoxyethylated castor oil).

Eight times the required dose of althesin was accidentally administered to a 4-kg infant. The only notable effect was a delayed awakening, necessitating assisted ventilation.[1]

CHRONIC EFFECTS

Muscle tremors, cardiovascular effects similar to those produced by thiopental and methohexital, respiratory, cough, hiccough, laryngospasm, and apnea have been observed.[2] Hypersensitivity reactions (severe circulatory collapse, bronchospasm, edema, and a generalized erythematous reaction) may be caused by histamine release or may be due to the solubilizing agent. Althesin is not available in the United States, and concern over its anaphylactoid reactions have led to its withdrawal from the United States.[3]

REFERENCES—ALTHESIN

1. Boulard G, Miet G, Guerin J, Sabathie M. Surdosage accidentel en alfatesine chez un enfant polymalforme. Can Anaesth Soc J 1980;27:576–577.
2. Wood M. Intravenous anesthetic agents. In Wood M. Wood AJJ, eds. Drugs and anesthesia. Pharmacology for anesthesiologists. 2nd ed. Baltimore: Williams & Wilkins, 1990; pp. 216–217.
3. Reynolds JEF. *Martindale: The extra pharmacopoeia.* 29th ed. London: Pharmaceutical Press, 1989; p. 1114.

LOCAL ANESTHETICS

Local anesthetic overdose may follow excess anesthetic dosage administered intravenously, inadvertent spinal or epidural administration, or inadvertent intraarterial injection. Toxic reactions include cardiovascular collapse, respiratory depression or arrest, seizures, arrhythmias, and death. Treatment is largely supportive and symptomatic. Methemoglobinemia may be treated with methylene blue.

Table 56–12
Toxic Dose of Local Anesthetics: Systemic Circulation Versus Cerebral Circulation [a]

Local Anesthetic	Min IV Toxic Dose in Humans (mg/kg)	Estimated Intravertebral Artery Toxic Dose (μg/kg)[b]	Estimated Intracarotid Artery Toxic Dose (mg/kg)[a]
Procaine	19.2	288	2.592
Chloroprocaine	22.8	342	3.078
Tetracaine	2.5	37.5	0.337
Lidocaine	6.4	96	0.864
Mepivacaine	9.8	147	1.323
Bupivacaine	1.6	24	0.216
Etidocaine	3.4	51	0.459

Min IV, Minimum intravenous.
[a]Adapted from Durrani Z, Winnie AP. Anesth Analg 1991;72:249–252.
[b]Based on the cerebral circulation being 15% of the total cardiac output and vertebral basilar circulation being 10% of the total cerebral circulation.

DOSE

Toxic doses of local anesthetics are listed in Table 56–12.

TOXICOKINETICS (TABLES 56–13 AND 56–14)

PREGNANCY

The Parturient

Regional anesthesia is being used with increasing frequency in the parturient population.[1] This group of patients may be at increased risk for development of local anesthetic toxicity. Physiologic changes in pregnancy include increased cardiac output, increased blood volume, aortocaval compression, decreased functional residual capacity, increased oxygen consumption, and reduced plasma proteins. These factors may increase the volume of distribution, alter the metabolic state, and reduce the cardiopulmonary reserve of the parturient. Venous engorgement increases the risk of inadvertent IV injection, especially in the case of epidural anesthesia. Hypoglycemia and a relative plasma cholinesterase deficiency state, both found in the pregnant patient, may predispose the patient to toxicity from ester anesthetics. Hypomagnesemia in the pregnant patient may disrupt the sodium potassium exchange pump.

The Fetus

Local anesthetics may reduce sympathetic tone, decrease maternal blood pressure and cardiac output, and reduce placental perfusion. Secondly, they may directly vasoconstrict placental vessels. Finally, they may cross the placenta and act on fetal cardiac and neural tissue directly.

MECHANISM OF ACTION

Local anesthetics reversibly block the generation and conduction of impulses through sensory, motor, and autonomic fibers. The blockade of peripheral nerves usually progresses in the following order: peripheral vasodilation

Table 56–13
Actions and Plasma Levels of Local Anesthetics[a]

	Onset	Duration	Peak Plasma Levels	Time for Peak Blood Levels
Bupivacaine hydrochloride				
(Dental) 0.5%	2–10 min	7 hr	0.45–1.25 μg/mL	30–45 min
(Epidural) 0.25–0.5%	4–17 min	3–7 hr	(after 125–150 mg)	
Caudal peripheral block				
(Epidural) 0.75%	3–16 min	6–9 hr		
(Spinal) 0.75% in 8.25% dextrose	1 min (sensory blockade)	2 hr		
	15 min (motor blockade)	3.5 hr		
Chloroprocaine	6–12 min	30–60 min	3.5–4.3 μg/mL of 2-chloro-4-aminobenzoic acid after 250 mg chloroprocaine	
		90 min (with epinephrine)		
Etidocaine hydrochloride	2–8 min	4.5–13 hr	0.5–0.64 μg/mL (after 100–200 mg)	5–30 min
Lidocaine hydrochloride (0.5–1.0%)		0.5–2 hr (without epinephrine)		
		1–3 hr (with epinephrine)	0.28–0.53 μg/mL	30–60 min
Mepivacaine hydrochloride (0.5–1.0%)	0.5–2 hr (without epinephrine)			
Prilocaine hydrochloride (4%)	2 min	1–2 hr	0.5–1.0 μg/mL	10–20 min
Procaine hydrochloride (0.5–1%)	2–5 min	0.25–0.5 hr (without epinephrine)		
		0.5–1.5 hr (with epinephrine)		
Propoxycaine hydrochloride	2–5 min	2–3 hr		
Tetracaine hydrochloride	15 min	1.5–3 hr		

[a]Adapted from Dershowitz M. In: Firestone LL, Lebowitz PW, Cook CE, eds. Clinical anesthesia procedures of the Massachusetts General Hospital. 3rd ed. Boston: Little, Brown, 1988.

Table 56–14
Metabolism of Local Anesthetics[1–4]

Distribution Drug	Protein Bound	V_D
Bupivacaine	82–96%	0.4–1.0 L/mg
Etiodocaine	94–96%	1.9 L/kg
Lidocaine	62%[1,2]	2.16 L/kg[1]
Mepivacaine	60–85%	1.2 L/kg
Prilocaine	68.8[3]	–
Procaine		0.79 L/kg[4]

Elimination Drug	Half-Life (Hours—Adult)	Metabolism	Unchanged Drug Excreted
Bupivacaine	1.5–5.5 (8.1 hr—neonates)	L	5%
Chloroprocaine	Fast hydrolysis	P	(as metabolites)
Etiodocaine	1.2 hr	L	(as metabolites)
Lidocaine	0.7–1.8 hr	L	7% (in acid urine)
Mepivacaine	1.9 hr	L	Metabolites
Prilocaine hydrochloride	–	L	<1%
Procaine hydrochloride	Fast hydrolysis (7.69 min)	P	80% as aminobenzoic and
Propoxycaine hydrochloride	Fast hydrolysis	P	Renal excretion
Tetracaine		P	Metabolites

P, Plasma; *L*, liver.
[1]Denson DD et al. J Clin Pharmacol 1988;28:995–1000.
[2]Barry M et al. Clin Pharmacol Ther 1990;47:366–370.
[3]Bachmann B et al. Acta Anaesthesiol Scand 1990;34:311–314.
[4]Seifen AB et al. Anesth Analg 1979;58:382–386.

and skin temperature elevation, loss of pain and temperature sensation, loss of proprioception, loss of touch and pressure sensation, and motor paralysis.[2]

CLINICAL PRESENTATION

Local Anesthetic Toxicity—Common Complications

Complications common to many local blocks include local anesthetic toxicity, neurologic complications, block failures, total spinal anesthesia, and medication errors.[3]

A mnemonic useful when discussing local anesthetic toxicity is AILS: *A*llergy, *I*diosyncrasy, *L*ocal, *S*ystemic.

Allergic reactions to local anesthetics are rare and usually associated with the ester compounds. *Idiosyncrasies,* for example, vasovagal attack or hysterical reactions, are unusual and unpredictable. *Local* effects refer to effects on local tissue, for example, nerve or muscle. 2-Chloroprocaine causes venous thrombosis when used for intravenous regional anesthesia.[4] Accidental subarachnoid injection of large quantities of 2-chloroprocaine has been linked to adhesive arachnoiditis and cauda equina syndrome.[5] It has been reformulated. *Systemic* effects account for the majority of toxic effects of local anesthetics. They most frequently occur following accidental intravascular injection of local anesthetics.

Clinical

Perioral numbness, tingling, auditory and visual disturbances, twitching, grand mal seizures, coma, and death have been observed.

Neurologic Complications

Permanent neurologic injury in regional anesthesia[3] may be secondary to trauma, chemicals, infection, ischemia, or compression or may be idiopathic in origin. Using a marking pencil to determine landmarks, warning the patient in advance about injection, conversing with the patient, and using small gauge needles may limit toxic reactions.

Total Spinal Anesthesia

Total spinal anesthesia may follow when a large quantity of local anesthetic drug intended for the epidural space reaches the subarachnoid space or when an excessive quantity of local anesthetic drug is given during spinal anesthesia. It may follow retrobulbar blocks, brachial plexus anesthesia, and sympathetic blocks.[3]

Clinical

There is a rapid onset of flaccidity, apnea, unconsciousness, and circulatory collapse.

Medication Errors

Errors may involve overdose, injection of the wrong solution, or injection into the wrong site.

Systemic Toxicity

Cardiovascular

High serum levels of local anesthetics may decrease impulse generation in the nodal pacemaker tissue, alter conduction, and reduce myocardial contractility. Some agents may also produce ventricular arrhythmias. Higher serum levels can also cause profound vasodilation. Myocardial depression and peripheral vasodilation can lead to cardiovascular collapse.[1] Many of the cases were parturients. Fatalities have been high. Cardiovascular collapse has been resistant to conventional methods of resuscitation.[6–14]

Bupivacaine is a strong sodium channel blocker, causes QRS prolongation at much lower doses than lidocaine, and is eliminated from the myocardium more slowly than lidocaine.[15] Lidocaine 1 gram intravenously has induced apnea and asystole.[16]

Peripheral Vascular

Most local anesthetics will cause vasodilation at toxic serum levels, reducing systemic vascular resistance and venous return.

Methemoglobinemia

Prilocaine is an aniline derivative. One of its metabolic products, orthotoludine, is able to oxidize hemoglobin to methemoglobin.[17] It is also related to lidocaine, which is also known as a precipitator of methemoglobinemia.[18]

Comparative Toxicity

The more potent, lipid-soluble, larger-acting local anesthetics (bupivacaine and etidocaine) may be more cardiotoxic than less potent agents such as lidocaine. The serum concentration that induces cardiovascular collapse, compared with the production of seizures, is narrower for the potent local anesthetics.

Central Nervous System—Adverse Effects After Inadvertent IV Injection

A general pattern of increasing central nervous system signs and symptoms are discernible when local anesthetics are given by IV infusion. In ascending order they are as follows:

1. Numbness of the tongue and mouth. The drug leaves the vascular space and affects the sensory nerve endings in the extravascular space.
2. Lightheadedness
3. Tinnitus
4. Visual disturbance. Objects in the visual fields appear to oscillate either from side to side or up and down or both.
5. Slurring of speech
6. Muscular twitching
7. Irrational conversation
8. Unconsciousness
9. Grand mal convulsion
10. Coma
11. Apnea

LABORATORY

Analytic Methods

Bupivacaine, chloroprocaine, etidocaine, lidocaine, mepivacaine, prilocaine, and procaine are analyzed by gas chromatography.

Blood Levels

Bupivacaine

High blood levels may be associated with dizziness, ringing in the ears, hypotension, seizures, and ventricular tachycardia.[19,20] Toxic reactions to bupivacaine usually do not occur at plasma levels below 4 μg/mL. However, a 28-year-old woman developed convulsions with a blood level of 1.1 μg/mL.[21]

Chloroprocaine

Ten minutes after an inadvertent intravenous administration of chloroprocaine to a 23-year-old 60-kg male, a chloroprocaine plasma concentration of 17 μg/mL was detected. No adverse effects were observed.[22]

Lidocaine

Ten μg/mL appears to be the minimum blood concentration of lidocaine at which toxic manifestations, including seizures, may occur.[23] Ingestion of lidocaine solutions intended for topical anesthesia has led to serum levels of 7.3 to 12 μg/mL with toxic signs and symptoms.[24,25] A serum level of 19 μg/mL followed an accidental intravenous injection of 1200 mg of lidocaine. Asystole and grand mal seizures were observed.[26] A one-month-old child inadvertently received an intravenous bolus of 50 mg of lidocaine and developed respiratory arrest, convulsions, and coma with a blood lidocaine level of 5.39 μg/mL. The child recovered.[27]

Mepivacaine

Plasma mepivacaine concentrations of 4.4 to 8.6 μg/mL following caudal administration of 5.5 to 9.4 mg/kg are associated with apprehension, confusion, muscular twitching, nausea, and vomiting when used perinatally.[28] Neonates experiencing blood levels of up to 75 μg/mL require respiratory support and exchange transfusion. Toxic signs disappear when blood levels fall to about 8 μg/mL.[29] The toxic threshold for blood mepivacaine is about 6.3 μg/mL.[56]

Prilocaine

Following a dose of 864 mg of prilocaine, postmortem prilocaine concentrations of 13 μg/mL in blood, 69 μg/mL in urine, and 49 mg/kg in the liver were obtained. The patient died in the dentist's chair within 1 hour.[30]

Procaine

Peak plasma concentrations of 21 to 86 μg/mL followed 18 to 55 mg/kg of procaine hydrochloride by intravenous infusion. Within 17 to 44 minutes the plasma levels had recovered with plasma levels of 1 to 13 μg/mL.[31] An adult inadvertently received 4000 mg of procaine. Mydriasis, pupils unreactive to light, arterial hypertension, sinus tachycardia, and deepening and widening of the S wave on the electrocardiogram appeared. The blood procaine level reached 96 μg/mL. The patient recovered after supportive treatment.[32] Plasma procaine concentrations after intramuscular administration of 4.8 million units of procaine penicillin G ranged from 3.6 to 11 μg/mL.[33]

TREATMENT

Stabilization

Preparation for Local Anesthetic Use

Resuscitation equipment to manage changes in ventilatory and cardiac status must be available. Continuous monitoring of neurologic and cardiac systems will provide early warning of an inadvertent intravenous injection of a local anesthetic, or of elevated blood levels. Fetal heart rate monitoring of parturients is suggested when any anesthesia is being administered. Be certain that the patient has been NPO (nothing by mouth) prior to anesthesia to minimize the risk of aspiration. Give the patient oxygen by face mask. If significant vasodilation is expected, have sympathomimetic agents available. Check that intravascular volume is sufficient to accommodate any decrease in vascular tone. Use the proper test dose and the minimal concentration and total dose necessary. Communicate with the awake patient.

Mnemonic

A mnemonic may be used to recall the treatment of local anesthetic toxicity SAVED:

*S*top injection
*A*irway
*V*entilation
*E*valuation of circulation
*D*rugs

Elimination Enhancement

Use of diuresis, hemodialysis, or hemoperfusion in local anesthetic overdose cannot be recommended.

Antidote

There are no antidotes for local anesthetics. Methemoglobinemia is treated with methylene blue.

Supportive Measures

1. Seizures: Most seizures caused by local anesthetics are self-limited, unless a massive IV overdose is given. Maintain an adequate airway. Ventilate the patient with 100% oxygen. Maintain a normal acid-base balance. Acidosis decreases the protein binding of local anesthetics, increasing levels of free drug and therefore toxicity.[1] If seizures persist, thiopental (50 to 100 mg), diazepam (10 mg), or midazolam (2 mg) may be useful. It may be necessary to administer succinylcholine if

manual ventilation is to be effective in a seizure patient. (See Topical Anesthesia for cautions.)

2. Hypotension: Pressors (e.g., dopamine); intravenous fluids; position change.
3. Bradycardia: Atropine.
4. Ventricular tachycardia or fibrillation: Electrical cardioversion; bretylium (5 mg/kg IV up to a maximum of 10 mg/kg) for bupivacaine-induced PVCs[34] or ventricular tachycardia.
5. Hemodynamic instability: Elevate legs; left uterine displacement in the parturient; advanced cardiac life support; consider open-chest massage or cardiopulmonary bypass.
6. Total spinal anesthesia is managed with ventilation and circulator support.
7. When bupivacaine is used epidermally, it should always be injected slowly, there should be a high suspicion of the possibility of accidental intravenous injection, and the drugs, equipment, and knowledge required for resuscitation should be immediately available.
8. Cardiopulmonary bypass has been effective in resuscitation of a patient with bupivacaine-induced cardiac arrest.[14]
9. Extracorporeal pump assistance, an experimental procedure in dogs, suggests potential usefulness in acute overdoses of lidocaine.[35]
10. Atrioventricular cardiac pacing was successful in treatment of a cardiac arrest following a 2000-mg accidental administration of lidocaine into a cardiopulmonary bypass circuit. This procedure followed an unsuccessful use of calcium chloride and isoprenaline.[36]
11. *Lidocaine:* Acute lidocaine toxicity is best managed with nonspecific supportive therapy. (See Antiarrhythmic chapter.)

REFERENCES—LOCAL ANESTHETICS

1. Voulgaropoulos DS, Johnson MD, Covina BG. Local anesthetic toxicity. Sem Anesth 1990;9:8–15.
2. Dershowitz M. Local anesthetics. In: Firestone LL, Lebowitz PW, Cook CE, eds. Clinical anesthesia procedures of the Massachusetts General Hospital. 3rd ed. Boston: Little, Brown, 1988; pp. 185–198.
3. Finucane BT. Regional anaesthesia: complications and techniques. Can J Anaesth 1991;38:R3–R10.
4. Covino BG, Vassallo J. Local anesthetics. Mechanisms of action and clinical use. New York: Grune & Stratton, 1976; pp. 67–78.
5. Ravindran RS, Bond VK, Tasch MD, Gupta CD, Luerssen TG. Prolonged neural blockade following regional analgesia with 2-chloroprocaine. Anesth Analg 1980;59:447–451.
6. Atlee JL III, Bosnjak ZJ. Mechanisms for dysrhythmias during anesthesia. Anesthesiology 1990;72:347–374.
7. Albright GA. Cardiac arrest following regional anesthesia with Etidocaine or bupivacaine. Anesthesiology 1979;51:285–287.
8. Davis NL, de Jong RH. Successful resuscitation following massive bupivacaine overdose. Anesth Analg 1982;61: 62–64.
9. Edde RR, Deutsch S. Cardiac arrest after interscalene brachial plexus block. Anesth Analg 1977;56:446–447.
10. Prentiss JE. Cardiac arrest following caudal anesthesia. Anesthesiology 1979;50:51–53.
11. Gould DB, Aldrete JA. Bupivacaine cardiotoxicity in a patient with renal failure. Acta Anaesthesiol Scand 1983;27: 18–21.
12. Conklin KA, Ziadlou-Rad F. Bupivacaine cardiotoxicity in a pregnant patient with mitral valve prolapse. Anesthesiology 1983;58:596.
13. Bota A. Bupivacaine induced cardiac arrest. Anesth Analg 1990;70:464–465.
14. Long WB, Rosenblum S, Grady IP. Successful resuscitation of bupivacaine induced cardiac arrest using cardiopulmonary bypass. Anesth Analg 1989;69:403–406.
15. Cardiotoxicity of local anaesthetic drugs. Lancet 1986;2: 1192–1194 (editorial).
16. Finkelstein F, Kraft J. Massive lidocaine poisoning. N Engl J Med 1979;301:50.
17. Arens JF, Carrera AE. Methemoglobin levels following peridural anesthesia with prilocaine for vaginal deliveries. Anesth Analg 1970;49:219–222.
18. Weiss LD, Generalovich T, Heller MB, Paris PM, Stewart RD, Kaplan RM, Thompson DR. Methemoglobin levels following intravenous lidocaine administration. Ann Emerg Med 1987;16:323–325.
19. Hollmen H, Korhonen M, Ojala A. Bupivacaine in paracervical block plasma levels and changes in maternal and foetal acid base balance. Br J Anaesth 1969;41:603–608.
20. Moore DC, Balfour RI, Fitzgibbons D. Convulsive arterial plasma levels of bupivacaine and the response to diazepam therapy. Anesthesiology 1979;50:454–456.
21. Hasselstrom LJ, Mogensen T. Toxic reaction of bupivacaine at low plasma concentrations. Anesthesiology 1984;61: 99–100.
22. Gross TL, Kuhnert PM, Kuhnert BR. Plasma levels of 2-chloroprocaine and lack of sequelae following an apparent inadvertent intravenous injection. Anesthesiology 1981;54: 173–174.
23. Bromage PR, Robson JG. Concentrations of lignocaine in the blood after intravenous, intramuscular, epidermal and endotracheal administration. Anaesthesia 1961;16:461–478.
24. Gorman RL, King JD, Oderda GM. Ingestion of topical lidocaine. It's time to stop the pain. Vet Hum Toxicol 1984; 26:413.
25. Fruncillo RJ, Gibbons W, Bourman SM. CNS toxicity after ingestion of topical lidocaine. N Engl J Med 1982;306:426–427.
26. Edgren B, Tilelli J, Gehrz R. Intravenous lidocaine overdosage in a child. Clin Toxicol 1986;24:51–58.
27. Jonville AP, Barbier P, Blond MH, Boscq M, Autret E, Breteau M. Accidental lidocaine overdosage in an infant. Clin Toxicol 1990;28:101–106.
28. Morishima HO, Daniel SS, Finster M, Poppers PJ, James LS. Transmission of mepivacaine hydrochloride (Carbocaine) across the human placenta. Anesthesiology 1966;27:147–154.
29. Finster M, Popper PJ, Sinclair JC, Morishima HO, Daniel SS. Accidental intoxication of the fetus with local anesthetic drug during caudal anesthesia. Am J Obstet Gynecol 1965; 92:922–924.
30. Kaliciak HA, Chan SC. Distribution of prilocaine in body fluids and tissues in lethal overdose. J Anal Toxicol 1986;10: 75–76.
31. Usubiaga JE, Wikinski J, Ferrero R, Usubiaga LE, Wikinski R. Local anesthetic induced convulsions in man. An electroencephalographic study. Anesth Analg 1966;45:611–620.
32. Wikinski JA, Usubiaga JE, Wikinski RW. Cardiovascular a neurological effect of 400 mg of procaine. JAMA 1970;213: 621–623.
33. Green RL, Lewis JE, Kraus SJ, Frederickson EL. Elevated plasma procaine concentrations after administration of procaine penicillin G. N Engl J Med 1979;91:223–226.
34. Kasten GW, Martin ST. Bupivacaine cardiovascular toxicity. Comparison of treatment with bretylium and lidocaine. Anesth Analg 1985;64:911–916.
35. Freedman MD, Gal J, Freed CR. Extracorporeal pump assistance—novel treatment for lidocaine poisoning. Eur J Clin Pharmacol 1982;22:129–135.
36. Noble J, Kennedy DJ, Latimer RD, Hardy I, Bethune DW, Collis JM et al. Massive lignocaine overdose during cardiopulmonary bypass. Successful treatment with cardiac pacing. Br J Anaesth 1984;56:1439–1441.

MALIGNANT HYPERTHERMIA (MH)

Malignant hyperthermia (MH) is a rare, inherited, life-threatening disorder of skeletal muscle calcium regulation associated with a hypermetabolic state and most often initiated by volatile anesthetic agents.[1–4] It is estimated to occur in approximately 1 in 15,000 general anesthetics. The prevalence of susceptible individuals is estimated at between 1 in 20 and 1 in 5000 of the general population.[5] Children (less than 5 years of age) have comprised about half of all MH cases. Males account for about three-fourths of all reported MH fatalities. The Malignant Hyperthermia Association of the United States is located at 32 South Main Street, P.O. Box 1019, Sherbourne, New York 13460. Telephone: 607-674-2420. FAX: 607-674-2060.

ETIOLOGY

Genetically predisposed individuals may suffer from MH after being exposed to drugs such as skeletal muscle relaxants (succinylcholine chloride, decamethonium, gallamine, *d*-tubocurarine), all inhalation anesthetics, and local anesthetics (mainly amide-type such as lidocaine, mepivacaine, and bupivacaine). A wide variety of other drugs have been implicated, but data suggest they rarely precipitate an MH crisis but rather exacerbate a preexisting one.[1] Stress, high environmental temperatures, emotional excitement, severe muscle exercise, and infections have been associated with MH.[1–4,6–8]

GENETIC SUSCEPTIBILITY

Susceptibility to MH is probably due to a mutation of the ryanodine receptor gene (RYR). This receptor is the Ca^{++}-release channel of the sarcoplasmic reticulum. The RYR gene is in the region of 12-13.2 of chromosome 19.[9–11]

PATHOPHYSIOLOGY

The sarcoplasmic reticulum of the muscle cell normally takes up Ca^{++} during muscle relaxation and releases Ca^{++} to the myoplasm during contraction. Although not entirely elucidated, MH is believed to occur following a decrease in Ca^{++} uptake by the sarcoplasmic reticulum. The subsequent increase in myoplasmic Ca^{++} brought about by a number of triggering agents initiates a number of aerobic and anaerobic metabolic processes resulting in excessive heat and CO_2 and lactic acid production and causing MH.[1,2,12,13]

SUSCEPTIBILITY TESTS

Several invasive screening tests for MH susceptibility have been developed and standardized in both the United States and the United Kingdom.[14–21] Muscle biopsy specimens are exposed to halothane alone, caffeine alone, or halothane and caffeine together. A number of noninvasive tests using red blood cells (fragility), platelets (nucleotide depletion test), and mononuclear cells have not exhibited sufficient sensitivity and specificity to be clinically useful.[15] The halothane and caffeine contracture tests appear more indicative of MH susceptibility, but in view of the relative rarity of the MH reaction (1 in 15,000 in children; 1 in 50,000 in adults) the practicability of these tests as a screening method is questionable.[8] Further refinements of MH tests are required before general acceptance and routine use can be validated.[22] Detection of clinical episodes of MH continue to remain the responsibility of the anesthetist during a surgical procedure. The Malignant Hyperthermia Association of the United States has a list of muscle-biopsy centers for the caffeine-halothane test.

DIAGNOSIS—EARLY WARNING

The management of MH depends largely on early recognition of the reactions by careful and routine monitoring during anesthesia. The anesthesiologist should entertain the diagnosis if any of the following occurs:[12]

1. Unexplained tachycardia.
2. Unexplained cyanosis and tachypnea.
3. Rigidity after succinycholine administration, or failure of the masseters to relax for intubation. The rigidity may present at any time or may never occur.
4. *Later Indications.* Later indications include marked hyperthermia, increased end-tidal CO_2, and increased mixed venous CO_2. The normal anesthetized patient does not become hyperthermic if the room temperature is below 25.5°C. Any rise in temperature of the patient of more than 0.5°C in 15 minutes should be regarded as possible malignant hyperthermia. Fever is a late sign and carries a poor prognosis if therapy has not yet been started. Other signs include hypotension, complex arrhythmias, metabolic acidosis, electrolyte disturbances, hyperkalemia, hypercalcemia, rhabdomyolysis, disseminated intravascular coagulation, renal failure, and pulmonary edema.[23]

MH also can lead to hypoxemia and severe respiratory and metabolic acidosis. The anesthesiologist should obtain arterial blood gases and electrolytes. A venous PCO_2 may be diagnostic even earlier. Oximetry or end-tidal CO_2 measurements are valuable tools.

DIFFERENTIAL DIAGNOSIS FROM NEUROLEPTIC MALIGNANT SYNDROME (NMS)

MH occurs within minutes of starting anesthesia; NMS usually develops over a longer period. MH is a genetic disorder; NMS has no specific genetic component. Succinylcholine and general anesthetics may be a triggering factor for MH; patients with NMS have been given succinylcholine and general anesthesia generally without toxic effects. Patients who have had MH have not been reported to have neuroleptic-induced NMS. Neuroleptic analgesia has been used successfully in patients who are susceptible to MH. Curare and pancuronium will cause flaccidity in individuals with NMS, but will not have the same effect in patients with MH.[24–32]

Rule out other causes of sinus tachycardia such as anticholinergic drugs, hypovolemia, hypoventilation, hypoxemia, light general anesthesia, thyroid storm, porphyria, and unrecognized pheochromocytoma. Arrhythmias can include bigeminy, premature ventricular contraction, and ventricular tachycardia; all may result from the effects of hyperkalemia, acidosis, hypoxemia, hyperpyrexemia, and increased catecholamines in the myocardium. Ventricular fibrillation is a terminal event.[33]

DEATH[1,34]

Death may follow conversion of an ectopic ventricular arrhythmia into ventricular fibrillation, acute disseminated intravascular coagulopathy, acute pulmonary edema, acute myoglobinemia, renal failure, or cerebral edema with brain death.[1]

PREVENTION

Questions that may be used in identifying persons who may need further counseling and/or muscle biopsy testing for the presence of the MH trait include the following[2]:

1. Is there a history of family members who have died suspiciously during or immediately following surgery, or who had a very high fever during surgery?
2. Does the individual have a history of recurring fevers?
3. Has he had abnormal muscle rigidity or has he been told by an oral surgeon, dentist, or surgeon that he had an odd response to an anesthetic?
4. Does he have a history of muscle cramps or has he become extensively fatigued after brief periods of strenuous exercise?
5. Does he have muscle weakness following an illness or fever, or muscle pain that seems to unrelated to the illness?
6. Has he had any red-, pink-, or rose-colored urine, and when did that occur?
7. Is there a history of exercise intolerance or heat intolerance?
8. Does he avoid fluids containing caffeine such as coffee, tea, and cola because of previous adverse reactions to them?
9. Is there a family history of a sudden unexplained death of a family member?
10. Is there a history of orthopedic, muscle, or eye disorders that require treatment such as strabismus in a child or a hernia?
11. Is there a history of Raynaud's phenomenon, or autonomic dysfunction such as difficulty in regulating heat or adjusting to heat and cold, or marked flushing?
12. Is there a history of elevated CPK?
13. Is there a history of difficulty with joint abnormalities, especially of the jaw, or cardiac problems such as arrhythmia or trouble with the heart muscle?

TREATMENT

Specific Treatment[12,13,28–30,35]

Dantrolene (see Muscle Relaxant Chapter) appears to decrease Ca^{++} release from the sarcoplasmic reticulum and lowers intracellular Ca^{++} levels. A starting dose of 2.5 mg/kg is given intravenously. Dantrolene must be mixed with sterile distilled water. A 70-kg male patient will require 9 to 10 vials (20 mg in each vial) immediately. Remember each vial of dantrolene also contains mannitol. Dantrolene may be repeated every 5 to 10 minutes until a total dose of 10 mg/kg is given if symptoms persist. Continue dantrolene for 3 days after the episode to prevent recurrence. The oral dosage is 1 to 2 mg/kg/day in divided doses. Administration of dantrolene early in a MH episode generally halts progression of the syndrome. Controlled trials of dantrolene would clearly be unethical.[5] Many hospitals and free-standing surgery centers do not stock enough dantrolene to treat one fulminant episode of MH.[36]

Acute-Phase Treatment[12–18,23]

1. Immediately discontinue all volatile inhalation anesthetics and succinylcholine. Hyperventilate with 100% oxygen at high gas flows; at least 10 L/min. The circle system and CO_2 absorbent need not be changed.
2. Administer dantrolene sodium 2 to 3 mg/kg initial bolus rapidly with increments up to 10 mg/kg total. Continue to administer dantrolene until signs of MH (e.g., tachycardia, rigidity, increased end-tidal CO_2, and temperature elevation) are controlled. Occasionally, a total dose greater than 10 mg/kg may be needed. Each vial of dantrolene contains 20 mg of dantrolene and 3 grams mannitol. Each vial should be mixed with 60 mL of sterile water for injection USP without a bacteriostatic agent.
3. Administer bicarbonate to correct metabolic acidosis as guided by blood gas analysis. In the absence of blood gas analysis, 1 to 2 mEq/kg should be administered.
4. Simultaneous with the above, actively cool the hyperthermic patient. Use IV iced saline (not Ringer's lactate) 15 mL/kg q 15 min × 3.
   a. lavage stomach, bladder, rectum, and open cavities with iced saline as appropriate.
   b. Surface cool with ice and hyperthermia blanket.
   c. Monitor closely since overvigorous treatment may lead to hypothermia.
5. Dysrhythmias will usually respond to treatment of acidosis and hyperkalemia. If they persist or are life threatening, standard antiarrhythmic agents may be used, with the exception of calcium channel blockers (may cause hyperkalemia and CV collapse).
6. Determine and monitor end-tidal CO_2, arterial, central, or femoral venous blood gases, serum potassium, calcium, clotting studies, and urine output.
7. Hyperkalemia is common and should be treated with hyperventilation, bicarbonate, intravenous glucose, and insulin (10 units regular insulin in 50 mL 50% glucose titrated to potassium level). Life-threatening hyperkalemia may also be treated with calcium administration (e.g., 2 to 5 mg/kg of $CaCl_2$).
8. Ensure urine output of greater than 2 mL/kg/hr. Consider central venous or PA monitoring because of fluid shifts and hemodynamic instability that may occur.
9. Boys less than 9 years of age who experience sudden cardiac arrest after succinylcholine in the absence of hypoxemia should be treated for acute hyperkalemia first. In this situation calcium chloride should be administered along with other means to reduce serum potassium. They should be presumed to have subclinical muscular dystrophy.

Post Acute Phase

1. Observe the patient in an ICU setting for at least 24 hours since recrudescence of MH may occur, particularly following a fulminant case resistant to treatment.
2. Administer dantrolene 1 mg/kg IV q 6 hours for 24 to 48 hours post episode. After that, oral dantrolene 1 mg/kg q 6 hours may be used for 24 hours as necessary.
3. Follow ABG, CK, potassium, calcium, urine and serum myoglobin, clotting studies, and core body temperature until such time as they return to normal values (e.g., q 6 hours). Central temperature (e.g., rectal, esophageal) should be continuously monitored until stable.
4. Counsel the patient and family regarding MH and further precautions. Refer the patient for MHAUS. Fill out an Adverse Metabolic Reaction to Anesthesia (AMRA) report available through the North American Malignant Hyperthermia Registry (717) 531-6936.

CAUTION: This protocol may not apply to every patient and must of necessity be altered according to specific patient needs.

Anesthesia for Susceptible Patients[30]

1. Avoid stress and anxiety in preoperative period.
2. Pretreat a patient who has experienced a life-threatening triggering reaction and fears a repetition.[30] Give dantrolene (6 mg/kg) orally in divided doses the day before surgery or 1 mg/kg IV prior to anesthesia.
3. Premedicate with fentanyl, droperidol, or both.
4. Local or regional anesthesia is preferred. Propofol may be safe for induction.[26]
5. If general anesthesia is necessary, consider thiopental, fentanyl, droperidol, and pancuronium. Consult with anesthetists, drug information specialists, and medical toxicologists.

Mnemonic

A mnemonic has been suggested for the treatment of malignant hyperthermia[37]:

Some	STOP all triggering agents, go to 100% O_2
Hot	HYPERVENTILATE
Dude	DANTROLENE: 2.5 mg/kg immediately
Better	BICARBONATE, sodium, 1 mEq/kg to start
Give	GLUCOSE, 0.5 g/kg; INSULIN, 0.15 U/kg
Iced	IVFG fluids, cooling blanket
Fluids	Fluid output: FUROSEMIDE, mannitol prn
FAST	TACHYCARDIA: be prepared to treat V-tach

REFERENCES—MALIGNANT HYPERTHERMIA (MH)

1. Tomarken JL, Britt BA. Malignant hypothermia. Ann Emerg Med 1987;16:1253–1265.
2. Glisson SN. Malignant hyperthermia. Comprehens Ther 1988;14:33–41.
3. Petersdorf RG. Hypothermia and hyperthermia. In: Wilson JD, Braunwald E, Isselbacher KJ, Petersdorf RG, Martin JB, Fauci AS, Root RK, eds. Harrison's principles of internal medicine. 12th ed. New York: McGraw-Hill, p. 2197–2198.
4. Gronert GA. Malignant hypothermia. Anesthesiology 1980;53: 395–423.
5. Strazis KP, Fox AW. Malignant hyperthermia. A review of published cases. Anesth Analg 1993;77:297–304.
6. Lucke JN, Denny HR. The role of the sympathetic nervous system in the pathogenesis of halothane-induced malignant hyperthermia in the Pietran pig. Br J Anaesth 1978;50:75–76.
7. Wingard DW. Malignant hyperthermia. A human stress syndrome? Lancet 1974;2:1450–1451.
8. Drug reactions during anaesthesia. Lancet 1985;1:1195–1197 (editorial).
9. Scholz J, Troll U, Schulte AM, Esch J, Hartung E, Patten M, Sandig P et al. Inosital-1,4,5-triphosphate and malignant hyperthermia. Lancet 1991;337:1361.
10. MacLennan DH, Duff C, Zorato F et al. Ryanodine receptor gene is a candidate for predisposition to malignant hypothermia. Nature 1990;343:559–561.
11. McCarthy TV, Healy JMS, Hefferon WA et al. Localization of the malignant hyperthermia susceptibility locus to human chromosome 19 q 12-13.2. Nature 1990;343:562–564.
12. Firestone LL, Lebowitz PW, Cook CE, ed. Clinical anesthesia procedures of the Massachusetts General Hospital. 3rd ed. Boston: Little, Brown, 1990; pp. 476–479.
13. Barash PG, Cullen BF, Stoelting RK. Handbook of clinical anesthesia. Appendix D. Malignant hyperthermia protocol. Philadelphia: JB Lippincott, 1991.
14. The European Malignant Hyperpyrexia Group. A protocol for the investigation of malignant hyperpyrexia (MH) susceptibility. Br J Anaesth 1984;56:1267–1269.
15. Fletcher JE, Rosenberg H. Laboratory methods for malignant hyperpyrexia diagnosis. In: Williams CH, ed. Experimental malignant hyperthermia. Berlin: Springer-Verlag, 1988; pp. 121–140.
16. Melton AT, Marticci RW, Kien ND, Gronert GA. Malignant hyperthermia in humans—standardization of contracture testing protocol. Anesth Analg 1989;69:437–443.
17. Larach MG for the North American Malignant Hyperthermia Group. Standardization of the caffeine halothane muscle contracture test. Anesth Analg 1989;69:511–515.
18. Rosenberg H. Standards for halothane/caffeine contracture test. Anesth Analg 1989;69:429–430.
19. Fletcher JE, Huggins FJ, Rosenberg H. The importance of calcium ions for in vitro malignant hyperthermia testing. Can J Anaesth 1990;37:695–698.
20. Urwyler A, Ellis FR, Halsall PJ, Hopkins PM. Muscle relaxation rates in individuals susceptible to malignant hyperthermia. Br J Anaesth 1990;65:421–423.
21. Fletcher JE, Rosenberg H. In vitro muscle contractures induced by halothane and suxamethonium. Br J Anaesth 1986; 58:1433–1439.
22. Larach MG, Landis JR, Bunn JS, Diaz M, The North American Malignant Hyperthermia Registry. Prediction of malignant hyperthermia susceptibility in low-risk subjects. An epidemiologic investigation of caffeine halothane contracture responses. Anesthesiology 1992;76:16–27.
23. Emergency Therapy for Malignant Hyperthermia. Revised 1993. Malignant Hyperthermia Association of the United States.
24. Addonizio G, Susman VL, Roth SD. Neuroleptic malignant syndrome. Review and analysis of 115 cases. Biol Psychiatry 1987;22:1004–1020.
25. Caroff SN, Mann SC, Rosenberg H, Fletcher JE, Heiman-Patterson ID. The relationship between malignant hyperthermia and neuroleptic malignant syndrome. Anesthesiology 1989;70:172–173.
26. Hermesh H, Aizenberg D, Lapidot M, Munitz H. The relationship between malignant hyperthermia and neuroleptic malignant syndrome. Anesthesiology 1989;70:171–172.
27. Hermesh H, Aizenberg D, Lapidot M, Munitz H. Risk of malignant hyperthermia among patients with neuroleptic malignant syndrome and their families. Am J Psychiatry 1988;145:1431–1434.
28. Flewellen EH, Nelson TE, Jones WP, Arens JF, Wagner DL. Dantrolene dose response in awake man. Implications for management of malignant hyperthermia. Anesthesiology 1983;59:275–280.

29. Allen GC, Cattran CB, Peterson RG, Lalande M. Plasma levels of dantrolene following oral administration in malignant hyperthermia in susceptible patients. Anesthesiology 1988;69:900–904.
30. Communale ME, DiNardo JA, Schwartz MJ. Pharmacokinetics of dantrolene in an adult patient undergoing cardiopulmonary bypass. J Cardiother Vasc Anesth 1991;5:153–155.
31. Harrison GG. Propofal in malignant hyperthermia. Lancet 1991;337:503.
32. Douglas MJ, McMorland GH. The anaesthetic management of the malignant hyperthermia susceptible parturient. Can Anaesth Soc J 1986;33:371–378.
33. Bristow G, Patel L. Hyperthermia. In: Hall J, Schmidt GA, Wood LDH, eds. Principles of critical care. New York: McGraw-Hill, 1992; pp. 858–868.
34. Pamukeoglu T. Sudden death due to malignant hyperthermia. Am J Forensic Med Pathol 1988;9:161–162.
35. Cain AG, Bell AD. How much dantrolene? A case of fulminant malignant hyperthermia. Anaesth Intensive Care 1989;117:500–509.
36. Hill LW. MH Association of the United States. Professional letter, November, 1944.
37. Zuckerberg AL. A hot mnemonic for the treatment of malignant hyperthermia. Anesth Analg 1993;77:1077–1086.

SPINAL AND EPIDURAL ANESTHESIA

Spinal and epidural anesthesia both cause major conduction blockade with local anesthetic agents. Physiologic effects include production of a sympathetic blockade with venous pooling and decreased venous return, causing decreased cardiac output and hypotension. Complications include bradycardia, heart block, and, rarely, cardiac arrest. Nonphysiologic complications include high or total block from extensive spread of the local anesthetic agent or toxic reactions from inadvertent intravenous injection of local anesthetic during epidural administration. Neurologic complications include paraplegia from either hematoma or abscess, arachnoiditis, or trauma. Postdural headache is seen more often in younger patients. Cranial nerve lesions are rarely seen with spinal anesthesia.[1]

Errors in which various drugs have been inadvertently injected into the spinal or epidural space result primarily from either a mislabeled or unlabeled syringe or inadequately marked tubing. Such incidents may occur late in a shift or at the end of a busy week.

Approaches to assist in decreasing the toxicity of accidental epidural injections include (a) introducing a second epidural catheter at a higher interspace and lavaging with saline and (b) dilution of the injectate with saline, steroids, or local anesthetics. Personal communication should be emphasized between anesthesia personnel and nursing staff. Color-coding of tubing or adding water-soluble dye to the injectate may be useful. Injecting epidural drugs slowly in small, incremental doses while maintaining conversation with the patient may minimize errors.

SUBDURAL INJECTION

Subdural injection of a local anesthetic may be followed by unduly prolonged blockade.[2,3] While the subarachnoid injection of large volumes of an inappropriate formulation of a local anesthetic with a low pH or containing preservative or antioxidant, may account for neurologic sequelae of accidental total spinal blockade, as may profound hypotension, an alternative cause may be inadvertent subdural administration.[2,3]

REFERENCES—SUBDURAL INJECTION

1. Parnass SM, Schmidt KJ. Adverse effects of spinal and epidural anaesthesia. Drug Safety 1990;5:179–194.
2. Williamson JA. Inadvertent spinal subdural injection during attempted spinal epidural steroid therapy. Anaesth Intens Car 1990;18:406–408.
3. Reynolds F, Speedy HM. The subdural space: the third place to go astray. Anaesthesia 1990;45:120–123.

INTRATHECAL DRUGS

Inadvertent intrathecal drug administration results in hypotension, metabolic acidosis, hyperkalemia, seizures, contrast media in cerebral ventricular and subarachnoid space, loss of lower extremity function, cyanosis, and coma. Treatment includes mechanical ventilation, pressor amines, and intrathecal lavage.[1–6]

REFERENCES—INADVERTENT INTRATHECAL DRUG ADMINISTRATION

1. Nakazawa K, Yoshinari M, Kinefuchi S, Amaha K. Inadvertent intrathecal administration of amidetrizoate. Intensive Care Med 1988;15:55–57.
2. Reisner LS, Hochman BN, Plumer MH. Persistent neurologic deficit and adhesive arachnoiditis following intrathecal 2-chlorprocaine injection. Anesth Analg 1980;59:452–454.
3. Goonewardene TW, Sentheshanmuganathan S, Kamalanathan S, Kanagasunderam R. Accidental subarachnoid injection of gallamine. Br J Anaesth 1975;47:889–893.
4. Mesry S, Baradaran J. Accidental intrathecal injection of gallamine triethiodide. Anaesthesia 1974;29:301–304.
5. Peduto VA, Gungui P, diMartino MR, Napoleone M. Accidental subarachnoid injection of pancuronium. Anesth Analg 1989;69:516–517.
6. Katz Y, Markovits R, Rosenberg B. Pneumoencephalos after inadvertent air injection during epidural block. Anesthesiology 1990;73:1277–1279.

NEUROMUSCULAR BLOCKERS (TABLE 56–15)

Neuromuscular blockers, both depolarizing and nondepolarizing (Table 56–16), when administered in overdose, may lead to prolonged skeletal muscle paralysis, hyperkalemia, histamine release, hypotension, cardiac arrest, and death.

STRUCTURE AND CLASSIFICATION

Muscle relaxants are classified according to the mechanism by which they decrease the effects of acetylcholine. They are either depolarizing or nondepolarizing (competitive) neuromuscular blocking agents. Succinylcholine consists of 2 molecules of acetylcholine linked through the acetate methyl groups. Pancuronium and vecuronium are steroidal neuromuscular blocking agents that are structurally similar to corticosteroids.

Table 56-15
Some Currently Used Neuromuscular Blockers[a]

Drug	Dose (mg/kg)	Time to Onset (min)	Time to 25% Recovery (min)	Comment
Nondepolarizing				
Atracurium—*Tracrium* (Burroughs-Wellcome)	0.4 to 0.5	2 to 2.5	35 to 45	Not affected by renal or hepatic dysfunction; histamine release may cause hypotension
Mivacurium—*Mivacron* (Burroughs-Wellcome)	0.15 to 0.25	1.5 to 2	16 to 23	Some histamine release; duration of block may increase with renal or hepatic dysfunction
Rocuronium—*Zemuron* (Organon)	0.6 to 1.2	0.7 to 1	31 to 67	Usually no histamine release; primarily hepatic metabolism
Vecuronium—*Norcuron* (Organon)	0.08 to 0.1	2.5 to 3	25 to 40	Virtually no histamine release; primarily hepatic metabolism
Depolarizing				
Succinylcholine—*Anectine* (Burroughs-Wellcome, others)	0.6 to 1	0.5 to 1	4 to 10	Increased intragastric and intraocular pressure; potassium release; tachyphylaxis, prolonged recovery with continuous infusion or atypical plasma cholinesterase; rarely, malignant hyperthermia and cardiac arrest (especially in children)

[a]Adapted from Med Lett Drugs Ther 1994;36:71–72.

SOURCES

Atracurium, gallamine, pancuronium, succinylcholine, and vecuronium are synthetic products. Metocurine is a semisynthetic, and tubocurarine is extracted from plants of the genus Chonododendron.[1]

TOXIC DOSES

Atracurium Besylate

Intravenous dosages of 34 mg and 1.3 mg/kg were followed by survival.[1–3] There have been no fatalities reported from overdose.

Gallamine Triethiodide

Gallamine 1.4 mL (30 mg) was inadvertently administered into the subarachnoid space of an adult. The patient survived.[4]

Pancuronium Bromide

An adult self-injected 10 mL (1 mg/mL) of pancuronium bromide intravenously in addition to sodium thiopental. The patient was found dead.[5] A 79-year-old patient with renal failure was administered 105 mg of pancuronium IV within 4 days. The patient died 6 days later in circulatory shock.[6]

Tubocurarine Chloride

Inadvertent intraarterial injection of tubocurarine in the left antecubital fossa results in pain and weakness of the extremity. Full recovery occurs in 45 minutes.[7] An intravenous dose of 30 mg of tubocurarine stops breathing in most adults within 2 to 3 minutes.[8] Two cases of accidental overdose were given 80 mg and 100 mg respectively and recovered.[9]

Vecuronium Bromide

A 9.7-kg child with Down's syndrome, aged 23 months, was administered vecuronium 37 mg (3.83 mg/kg/hour) intravenously over 1 hour. The child died 5 days later of overwhelming sepsis. The dose represented a five-fold overdose of the manufacturer's recommended infusion rate (0.5 to 0.8 mg/kg/hour). There were no hemodynamic changes during the infusion and over the next 24 hours.[10]

FATAL DOSES

A fatal dose of pancuronium was 10 mg IV,[6] and fatality followed within 6 days of an administration of 105 mg of pancuronium IV over a period of 4 days.[11] Death followed within 5 days (of sepsis) after an overdose of vecuronium (37 mg).[15]

TOXICOKINETICS

A review of the toxicokinetics of the nondepolarizing muscle relaxants reveals that they are moderately protein bound, rapidly distributed within minutes, have a low apparent volume of distribution, and have an elimination half-life of several hours.

Metabolism

Succinylcholine is rapidly metabolized, mainly by plasma pseudocholinesterase to succinylmonocholine and choline. Succinylmonocholine has about one-twentieth the activity of succinylcholine and is a nondepolarizing blocking agent. Succinylmonocholine may accumulate and cause prolonged apnea in patients with impaired renal function.[1] Approximately 2 to 10% is excreted unchanged in the urine.[11–13]

Toxicity

Prolonged periods of apnea may follow succinylcholine use in those patients with genetically determined atypical pseudocholinesterase or in those who have received cholinesterase inhibitors.[11,14,15]

PRODUCT LABELING

The product labeling for Burroughs-Wellcome's suxamethonium chloride (Anectine) was recently revised following reports of hyperkalemia and cardiac arrest in apparently healthy pediatric patients. The package insert for the product now reads: "except when used for emergency tracheal intubation or in instances where immediate securing of the airway is necessary, succinylcholine (suxamethonium chloride) is contraindicated in children and adolescent patients." However, the labeling supports the use of this agent in "other circumstances where (in the opinion of the practitioner) immediate securing of the airway is necessary," for example patients with a full stomach.[16]

DRUG INTERACTIONS (TABLE 56–17)

Drugs that interfere with the action of muscle relaxants may exert their action proximal to the neuromuscular junction in the central nervous system or in the bloodstream, at the neuromuscular junction, or distal to the

Table 56–16
Clinical Variables Affecting Pharmacodynamics of Nondepolarizing Neuromuscular Blocking Agents[a,b]

Clinical Variable	Possible Effect
Pathophysiologic Variables	
Hypothermia	Potentiate blockade
Acid-base balance[c]	
Acidosis	Potentiate blockade: tubocurarine and vecuronium; no effect or antagonism: metocurine and pancuronium
Alkalosis	Antagonize blockade: tubocurarine and vecuronium; no effect or potentiation: metocurine and pancuronium
Electrolyte status	
Increased potassium	Decreased sensitivity to blockade
Increased calcium	Decreased sensitivity to blockade
Increased magnesium	Potentiate blockade
Decreased blood flow to muscles	Delay in onset
Neuromuscular disease (e.g., myasthenia gravis)	Increased sensitivity
Collagen diseases (e.g., polymyositis)	Increased sensitivity
Cardiovascular disease	Effect on heart rate and blood pressure
Pregnancy	Increased drug clearance; potential for decreased blockade
Burns	Increased drug clearance
Drug Interactions	
Other nondepolarizing neuromuscular blocking agents	Additive or possible synergistic effect
Antimicrobial agents	
Aminoglycosides	Potentiate blockade
Polymyxin	Potentiate blockade
Tetracyclines	Potentiate blockade
Clindamycin, lincomycin	Potentiate blockade
Vancomycin	Potentiate blockade
Sedative-anesthetics	
Midazolam	May potentiate blockade
Ketamine	May potentiate blockade
Cardiovascular drugs	
Furosemide[d]	Antagonize blockade of pancuronium; potentiate blockade of tubocurarine
Beta-blocking agents	Potentiate blockade
Procainamide	Potentiate blockade
Quinidine	Potentiate blockade
Calcium-channel blockers	Potentiate blockade
Methylxanthines	Antagonize blockade
Antiepileptic drugs	
Phenytoin	Increased resistance to blockade; no effect with atracurium
Carbamazepine	Increased resistance to blockade
Psychotropic drugs	
Lithium carbonate	Potentiate blockade of pancuronium
Immunosuppressive agents	
Azathioprine	Mild antagonism
Cyclosporine	Potentiate blockade
Corticosteroids	Antagonize blockade

[a]Adapted from Buck ML, Reed MD. Clin Pharm 1991;10:32–48.
[b]The use of nondepolarizing neuromuscular blocking agents in the presence of these clinical variables is not contraindicated, but it may require closer patient monitoring and adjustment of the dose necessary to achieve paralysis.
[c]The effect may depend on the chemical structure: tubocurarine and vecuronium are monoquaternary compounds, whereas the others are bisquaternary compounds. The effect on atracurium has not been reported.
[d]Antagonism of pancuronium has been reported in patients with normal renal function. Potentiation of tubocurarine has been reported in anephric patients.

Table 56–17
Plasma Cholinesterases—Drugs That May Interact With the Effects of Succinylcholine[a]

Drugs	Effect of Succinylcholine Neuromuscular Block
Local anesthetics	
Lidocaine	I
Procaine	I
Inhalation anesthetics	
Isoflurane	I
Halothane	I
Cardiovascular drugs	
Diuretics	
Furosemide—<10 mg/kg	I
Furosemide—1.4 mg/kg	D
Quinidine	I
Calcium channel blockers	I
Magnesium sulfate	I
Psychotropic drugs	
Lithium carbonate	Delayed onset—I
Phenelzine	I
Cimetidine	I
Nondepolarizing relaxants	
Pretreatment	
Gallamine	D
d-Tubocurarine	D
Pancuronium	I
Succinylcholine prolongs the effects of *d*-tubocurarine, pancuronium, and vecuronium blockade.	
Neostigmine	I if given within 1.5 hours of neostigmine
Edrophonium	I Inhibit plasma
Neostigmine	I cholinesterase
Pyridostigmine	I activity
Plasma cholinesterase (D = decreased activity; prolonged reaction to succinylcholine rarely exceeds 20 minutes).	
Corticosteroids	D—apnea, rarely
Contraceptive pills	D
Cyclophosphamide	D (35–70% of normal)
Echothiophate	D (70–100%)
Thio-TEPA	D (35–70%)
Organosphosphorus insecticides	D

I, Increased; *D*, decreased.
[a]Adapted from Kent RS. Anesthesiology 1994;80:244–245.

junction at the muscle cell membrane.[17] At the neuromuscular junction interactions may take place at the nerve terminal, in the synaptic cleft, or at the postsynaptic membrane.

Drugs That May Interact With Effect of Nondepolarizing Relaxants

Antibiotics

Antibiotics such as the aminoglycosides (amikacin, dihydrostreptomycin, gentamicin, kanamycin, streptomycin, and tobramycin) and the polypeptides (Polymyxins A, B, and C) not only potentiate nondepolarizing relaxants, but produce neuromuscular blockade on their own. The tetracyclines have weak neuromuscular blocking properties alone, but also potentiate nondepolarizing relaxants.[17]

Intravenous Anesthetic Agents

Ketamine potentiates alpha-tubocurarine but not pancuronium.[18] Midazolam potentiates vercuronium-induced blockage.[19] Otherwise, few important interactions are seen with the other intravenous anesthetic agents. Chronic tricyclic antidepressant administration may predispose a patient given pancuronium to ventricular tachycardia.[20]

Cardiovascular Drugs

Diuretics

In man furosemide 1 mg/kg facilitates recovery of pancuronium-induced blockade.[21] Large doses of furosemide may antagonize pancuronium-induced blockade in neurosurgical patients.[22]

Beta-Blocking Drugs

Beta-blockers block the acetylcholine binding site at the postsynaptic membrane. They may aggravate or unmask myasthenia gravis and induce a myasthenic syndrome.[23]

Antiarrhythmics

In man procainamide aggravates myasthenia gravis and induces weakness in healthy subjects. *d*-Tubocurarine neuromuscular blockade in cats may increase this interaction by up to 25%. Quinidine augments the block caused by nondepolarizing relaxants.[24]

Calcium Channel Blockers

Verapamil and nifedipine potentiate the neuromuscular blocking effect of *d*-tubocurarine, pancuronium, atracurium, and vecuronium.[17]

Magnesium Sulfate

Magnesium potentiates the neuromuscular blockade of pancuronium and vecuronium.[17] The dose of vecuronium should be reduced in patients receiving magnesium sulfate infusions. Magnesium decreases the presynaptic release of acetylcholine, reduces the sensitivity to acetylcholine of the postsynaptic membrane, and decreases the excitability of the muscle fiber membrane.[25]

Methylxanthines

Pancuronium is antagonized by both aminophylline and theophylline. A constant infusion of aminophylline may inhibit the ability of pancuronium to induce neuromuscular blockade.[26] This may follow the aminophylline-induced inhibition of phosphodiesterase, resulting in increased levels of cyclic adenosine monophosphate and possibly of acetylcholine.

Antiepileptic Drugs

Phenytoin

Patients on long-term phenytoin therapy may be resistant to metocurine, pancuronium, and vecuronium but not to atracurium. Phenytoin may cause a 50% reduction in the duration of neuromuscular blockade.[27] Phenytoin appears to have prejunctional effects similar to the nondepolarizing relaxants.

Carbamazepine

Patients receiving carbamazepine may be resistant to pancuronium. Recovery times from pancuronium and vecuronium may be 65% shorter in patients receiving carbamazepine.[17]

Psychotropic Drugs
Lithium Carbonate

Lithium may potentiate pancuronium blockade and may induce a myasthenic reaction.[28] Lithium reduces synthesis and release of acetylcholine at the nerve terminal.

Drugs Used in Renal Transplantation
Azathioprine

Azathioprine produces only a relatively small and transient antagonizing effect on neuromuscular blockade.[29]

Cyclosporine

Cyclosporine in its solvent cremophor and cremophor alone may potentiate the neuromuscular blocking effect of vecuronium and atracurium.[30]

Corticosteroids

Pancuronium-induced blockade may be diminished in patients on long-term steroid therapy.[31] Corticosteroids may also enhance the potential for paresis when administered with a steroidal neuromuscular blocking agent such as pancuronium and vecuronium.

PREGNANCY (TABLE 56–18)

Table 56–18
Placental Transfer of Neuromuscular Blocking Agents

Alcuronium[32]
Atracurium[33]
Fazadinium
Gallamine
Metocurine[34]
Pancuronium[35]
d-Tubocurarine[36]
Succinylcholine

MECHANISM OF ACTION

Depolarizing Muscle Relaxants
Succinylcholine

The natural transmitter acetylcholine acts not only on the nicotinic receptors at the neuromuscular junction and in autonomic ganglia, but also on muscarinic receptors located in smooth muscles, cardiac muscles, and exocrine glands.[17] Succinylcholine, which has a structural similarity to acetylcholine, exerts its effect at the neuromuscular junction, at the muscarinic receptors, and in autonomic ganglia.

Cardiac

The bradycardia on first injection of succinylcholine may be caused by stimulation of parasympathetic ganglia or cardiac muscarinic receptors in the SA node.

Histamine Release

All basic compounds may disrupt mast cells and cause release of histamine. Flushing, bronchospasm, hypotension, and other anaphylactoid reactions may follow a normal dose of 1 mg/kg.

Hyperkalemia

Following succinylcholine depolarization a slight increase in plasma potassium ion concentration (about 0.5 mmol/L, 0.5 mEq/L) may be observed. If the plasma potassium increases to 7 to 8 mmol/L, ventricular fibrillation and cardiac arrest may occur.

Neuromuscular Effects

Fasciculations, muscle pain, myoglobinuria, increased intragastric pressure, and increased intraocular pressure may be observed.[17]

Nondepolarizing Muscle Relaxants
Autonomic Effect

Most nondepolarizing muscle relaxants have two positively charged quaternary ammonium groups that attach to the negatively charged cholinergic receptor where they produce a block of competitive antagonism at the receptor site.[17]

Histamine Release

Muscle relaxants usually act directly on tissue mast cells and release histamine without antibody or complement activation (an anaphylactoid response). The histamine release is related to dose and rate of administration of the muscle relaxant. Histamine release is characterized by erythema of the upper chest and face, a transient decrease in blood pressure, and an increase in heart rate; bronchospasm may occur. Severe reactions may lead to circulatory collapse.

CLINICAL PRESENTATION

Atracurium

Atracurium may result in an increase in mean arterial pressure and heart rate that does not require treatment.[3] Overdosage with atracurium may increase the risk of histamine release.[37]

Gallamine Triethiodide

Accidental subarachnoid injection of gallamine in an adult is followed by muscle spasms of the lower limbs and anxiety; by 3 hours the arterial pressure and pulse rate increases followed by hyperthermia, profuse sweating, intense hyperesthesia, loss of consciousness, and pinpoint pupils. Within twenty-four hours the muscle spasms lessen. Treatment includes (a) dark room; (b) patient left undisturbed; (c) diazepam; (d) hydrocortisone; and (e) dexamethasone.[4] Two patients who received intrathecal gallamine developed convulsions and died.

Pancuronium

Pancuronium 105 mg was administered to a 79-year-old man without monitoring neuromuscular function. The patient died of circulating shock. There was a concomitant postoperative renal failure.[6] An adult committed suicide by self-injection of pancuronium bromide (1 mg/mL). Bromide plasma levels decline rapidly; peak plasma concentrations range from 1.0 to 1.5 μg/mL, but decline 60% within 5 minutes.[5,38]

Pipecuronium Bromide

A patient accidentally received pipecuronium bromide 520 μg/kg (about 11 times the effective dose) resulting in paralysis for 70 hours. Neostigmine and pyridostigmine administration failed to reverse the blockade. Pipecuronium is poorly dialyzable.[39]

Tubocurarine

Tubocurarine 4 mg was inadvertently given intraarterially to a 20-year-old man. The patient complained of intense pain, then weakness after hyaluronidase and 8% lidocaine were injected intraarterially. Full power returned to the arm 45 minutes later.[7]

Vecuronium

A 9.7-kg 23-month-old child with Down's Syndrome and congential heart disease received 37 mg of vecuronium (383 mg/kg/hour) in 1 hour intravenously. Hemodynamic studies remained unchanged over the next 24 hours. The child died of sepsis 5 days later. The dose given was a fiftyfold overdose of the manufacturer's recommended infusion rate (0.5 to 0.8 mg/kg/hour).[10]

CLINICAL COURSE

Poisoning by curariform blocking agents is characterized by complete paralysis of skeletal muscles beginning with the small, rapidly moving muscles of the ears, fingers, and toes, followed by those of the face and neck, then spreading to the extremities and finally the diaphragm and intercoital muscles. Consciousness may be unaffected. Death is caused by hypoxia secondary to respiratory paralysis.[5]

Anaphylactoid Reactions

Depolarizing and nondepolarizing neuromuscular blockers may rarely be associated with life-threatening anesthetic reactions manifested by circulatory collapse, bronchospasm, and skin flushing. Skin tests are positive in about one-third of cases. Evidence appears to suggest a direct action of succinylcholine on susceptible mast cells without IgE mediation. Succinylcholine and tubocurarine may lead to an increase in plasma histamine levels in normal patients during anesthesia. Anaphylactoid reactions have been reported with vecuronium.[40]

Myasthenia Gravis

An abnormal sensitivity to nondepolarizing muscle relaxants is a feature of myasthenia gravis and is manifested by prolonged neuromuscular block.[41]

Hyperkalemia

Succinylcholine-induced hyperkalemia may be seen in the following circumstances[42]:

1. Massive burns.
2. Massive muscle trauma.
3. Lower motor neuron disease, including traumatic degeneration, demyelinating disease (e.g., Guillain-Barré) and poliomyelitis.
4. Upper motor neuron disease, including spinal cord transection, cerebrovascular accidents, and encephalitis.
5. Tetanus.

Increased intraocular pressure, malignant hyperthermia (see Malignant Hyperthermia section), and muscular pain have occurred in 20 to 50% of patients receiving succinylcholine.[40]

LABORATORY

Analytic Methods

Atracurium

A high performance liquid chromatography assay is available with a sensitivity of 0.2 μg/mL for atracurium and 0.01 μg/mL for laudanosine.

Gallamine

Total (free plus bound) concentrations in plasma are measured by a fluorometric assay that has a lower limit of sensitivity of 0.05 μg/mL.[43]

Pancuronium

Analysis on blood, serum, and urine is performed by ion-pair extraction and fluorometry.[36]

Succinylcholine

Analysis in urine has been accomplished in the form of its ion-pair complex with bromothymol blue followed by thin-layer chromatography, hydrolysis of the isolated drug to succinic acid, esterification of the liberated into one or more derivatives, and quantitation gas chromatography.[44]

Tubocurarine

A sensitive radioimmunoassay employs a tritium label, requires only 10 µl of serum or urine, and is sensitive to as little as 5 ng of DTC per mL. Patients given 0.3 mg/kg of DTC IV had 25 to 83 ng/ml in the serum after 24 hours.[45] A liquid chromatography assay with ultraviolet detection has been described.[46]

Blood Levels

An adult who committed suicide by intravenous injection of 10 mg of pancuronium exhibited postmortem blood and urine levels of 1.6 and 1.5 µg/mL respectively. Thioridazine 0.7 µg/mL was also present; this is in the therapeutic range.[5]

TREATMENT

Stabilization

1. Immediately ascertain that a patent airway exists and administer assisted ventilation as required.
2. Maintain a supply of 100% oxygen to the patient, as well as a cardiac monitor and intravenous lines.
3. Consider the possibility that drugs such as the general anesthetic, opiate agonists, or barbiturates used during a surgical procedure may enhance and prolong the degree of respiratory depression.
4. If signs of malignant hyperthermia develop, prompt treatment is required (see Malignant Hyperthermia Section). Therapy will include dantrolene 1 to 2 mg/kg IV and cooling measures.
5. Since there is no agent available to reverse the activity of succinylcholine, continue ventilatory support until the muscular paralysis subsides.
6. Where cardiovascular support is required consider proper patient positioning, fluid administration, and the use of vasopressors as required.
7. A longer duration of neuromuscular blockade may result from an overdosage. Monitoring muscle twitch response to a peripheral nerve stimulator will be useful in estimating recovery.

REVERSAL OF NEUROMUSCULAR BLOCKADE (TABLES 56–19 AND 56–20)

Neuromuscular blockade spontaneously reverses when the relaxants diffuse away from their sites of action.[47] Depolarizing agents (succinylcholine) are noncompetitive and therefore cannot be reversed pharmacologically in most cases. Agents that inhibit the enzyme acetylcholinesterase (edrophonium, neostigmine, and pyridostigmine) increase the acetylcholine available to compete with the relaxants for their binding site and may accelerate recovery. All of these agents, like acetylcholine, have nicotinic and muscarinic effects. Muscarinic stimulation, which may lead to salivation, bradycardia, tearing, miosis, and bronchoconstriction, can be minimized by prior administration of an anticholinergic drug such as atropine or glycopyrrolate. 4-Aminopyridine increases the release of acetylcholine presynaptically. Antagonists are generally not administered prior to the demonstration of some spontaneous recovery from the neuromuscular block.

If reversal of neuromuscular blockade is inadequate because of severe debilitation, extensive carcinomatosis, drugs that have depressed respiration, or the presence of other drugs that may affect neuromuscular blocking ability, symptomatic treatment is indicated and manual or mechanical assisted ventilation should be instituted until there is adequate recovery.

Chemical Structure of Reversal Agents

Edrophonium	Synthetic quaternary ammonium
Neostigmine	Synthetic quaternary ammonium (derivative)
Pyridostigmine	Synthetic quaternary ammonium
Atropine	Alkaloid—tertiary amine
Glycopyrrolate	Synthetic quaternary ammonium derivative
4-Aminopyridine	Pyridine derivative

Table 56–19
Toxicokinetics of Reversal Agents[a]

	Daily Dose (mg/kg)	Peak Plasma Concentration (µg/L)	Time to Peak (hr)	Bioavailability (%)	V_D (L/kg)	CL (L/hr/kg)	T½ Alpha (hr)	T½ Beta (hr)
Neostigmine	0.06–0.07				0.52	0.57	0.09	0.44
Edrophonium					1.10	0.54	0.12	1.83
Pyridostigmine	120	40–60	2.0–3 hr	7–18	1.03	0.63	0.14	1.51

	Volume of Distribution (V_D L/kg)	Distribution Half-Life (T½ alpha min)	Elimination Half-Life (T½ beta min)	Clearance (Cl) (mL/kg/min)	Excretion of Unchanged Drug (%)
Neostigmine 5.0 mg	0.7	3.5	80	9.0	
Edrophonium 0.5–1.0 mg/kg	1.1	7.2	110	9.6	
Pyridostigmine (0.35 mg/kg)	1.1	6.8	112	8.6	
4-Aminopiridine	2.6		3.6	0.61	90

[a]Adapted from Aquilonius S-M, Hartvig P. Clin Pharmacokinet 1986;11:236–249; Cronnely R, Morris RB. Br J Anaesth 1982;54:183–184; Uges DRA et al. Clin Pharmacol Ther 1982;31:587–593; and Uges DRA. PhD Thesis. State University, Groningen, The Netherlands, 1982.

Table 56–20
Clinical Action of Neuromuscular Blockade Reversal Agents[a]

	Dose	Onset	Duration	Metabolized	Metabolized	Excreted
Neostigmine	For reversal of neuromuscular blockade—IV: 0.06–0.07 mg/kg (cautiously with an anticholinergic agent)	IV: 1–5 min IM SQ: 10–39 min	IV: 2.5–4 hr	May cause bradycardia, hypotension, CNS stimulation or depression, GI cramps, or cholinergic crisis. Cautious use with fragile bowel or anastomoses.	Liver	Kidney
Pyridostigmine	IV: 0.24 mg/kg (cautiously with an anticholinergic agent)	IV: 2–5 min IM: 15 min PO: 30–45 min	IV: 1–3 hr PO: 3–6 hr	See Neostigmine. Does not cross blood–brain barrier in significant amounts.	Tissue and liver cholinesterases	Liver Kidney (75%)
Edrophonium	IV: 0.3–1.0 mg/kg (cautiously with atropine)	IV: 1–5 min	IV: 1.1 hr	See Neostigmine.		
Glycopyrrolate	As adjunct to neostigmine and pyridostigmine reversal of neuromuscular blockade—IV: 0.01–0.02 mg/kg	IV: 1–4 min IM SQ: 20–40 min PO: 1 hr	IV: 2–4 hr IM SQ: 4–6 hr PO: 6 hr	See Atropine.	Probably minimal	Probably kidney
Atropine	As adjunct to neostigmine and pyridostigmine for reversal of neuromuscular blockade—IV: 0.02–0.03 mg/kg	IV: rapid IM/SQ/PO: 1–2 hr	IM SQ PO: 4 hr	May cause AV dissociation, premature ventricular contractions, bradycardia (low dose, dry mouth), urinary retention. Crosses blood–brain barrier and placenta.	Minimal	Kidney (77–94%) Liver

[a]Adapted from Kofke WA, Firestone LL. In: Firestone LL, Lebowitz PW, Cook C, eds. Anesthesia procedures of the Massachusetts General Hospital. Boston: Little, Brown, 1988.

PROLONGED PARALYSIS

Long-term use of nondepolarizing neuromuscular blocking agents (NMBA), especially vecuronium and pancuronium, may produce prolonged weakness.[48–54] Two patterns of neuromuscular dysfunction are observed, including a prolonged neuromuscular blockade (for hours to weeks) after termination of treatment, resulting in weakness lasting several hours to several days—likely caused by accumulation of neuromuscular blocking agents' metabolites, and myopathy, resulting in weakness lasting several weeks to several months.

The Myopathy

The clinical picture may include flaccid paralysis, mild to severe weakness, proximal muscles often weaker than distal muscles, difficulty weaning from ventilator, cognition and sensation normal, cranial nerves normal or facial weakness, ophthalmoplegia and aspiration in severe cases, and recovery over weeks to months. Electrodiagnosis indicates decreased motor-evoked response amplitudes, conduction velocities and sensory responses normal, repetitive stimulation decrement or normal, mild positive waves/fibrillations, and short-duration, low-amplitude, polyphasic motor units on needle exam. The creatine phosphokinase is normal or elevated. Muscle biopsy reveals atrophy of type I and type II fibers, myofiber necrosis, and no inflammation.[55,56]

The syndrome may be due to prolonged use of NMBA alone, prolonged use of NMBA in combination with corticosteroids, or prolonged use of NMBA in combination with other agents or disorders (acidosis, elevated serum magnesium, hepatic insufficiency, renal insufficiency, or aminoglycoside antibiotics); for example, clindamycin (in high doses),[57] lithium, tetracyclines, and polymyxin/lincomycin derivatives.[58] The differential diagnosis includes critical illness polyneuropathy,[56] disuse atrophy, [59–61] CNS disorder, Guillain-Barré Syndrome, botulism, and myasthenia gravis.

Vecuronium

Vecuronium-induced prolonged paralysis was associated with renal failure and higher plasma concentrations of a potentially active metabolite, 3-desactyneoronium.[49] Liver function is usually normal.[52]

Treatment

Supportive and symptomatic care is the mainstay of treatment. The usual outcome is one of complete recovery.[50]

REFERENCES—NEUROMUSCULAR BLOCKERS

1. Duncan J, Carter JA. Overdose of atracurium. Anaesthesia 1986;41:767.

2. Charlton AJ, Harper NJN, Edwards D, Wilson AC. Atracurium overdose in a small infant. Anaesthesia 1989;44:485–486.
3. Product literature. Atracurium besylate (Tracrium Injection). Burroughs Wellcome, December 1989.
4. Goonewardene TW, Sentheshanmuganathan S, Kamalanathan S, Kanagasunderain R. Accidental subarachnoid injection of gallamine. A case report. Br J Anaesth 1975;47: 889–893.
5. Poklis A, Melanson EG. A suicide by pancuronium bromide injection. Evaluation of the fluorometric determination of pancuronium in post-mortem blood, serum and urine. J Anal Toxicol 1980;4:275–280.
6. Vandenbrom RHG, Wierda JMKH. Pancuronium bromide in the intensive care unit. A case of overdose. Anesthesiology 1988;69:996–997.
7. Devlin E, Bali I. Accidental intraarterial injection of tubocurarine. Anaesthesia 1991;416:75–76.
8. Siegel H, Rieders F, Holmstedt B. The medical and scientific evidence in alleged tubocurarine poisonings. A review of the so-called Dr K case. Forensic Sci Int 1985;29:29–76.
9. Constantini D. In tema di iperdosaggio da tubocurarina: considerazioni su due casi. Acta Anaesthesiol 1966;17:253–258.
10. Forrest ETS, Vanner RG. "Overdose" of vecuronium. Anaesthesia 1990;45:997.
11. Foldes FF. Distribution and biotransformation of succinylcholine. Int Anesth Clin 1975;13:101–115.
12. Cook DR, Wingard LB Jr, Taylor FH. Pharmacokinetics of succinylcholine in infants, children and adults. Clin Pharmacol Ther 1976;20:493–498.
13. Chestnut RJ, Healy TEJ, Harper NJN, Faragher ER. Suxamethonium—the relation between dose and response. Anaesthesia 1989;44:14–18.
14. Viby-Mogensen J, Hanel HK. Prolonged apnoea after suxamethonium. An analysis of the first 225 cases reported to the Danish Cholinesterase Research Unit. Acta Anaesth Scand 1978;22:371–380.
15. Evans RT. Cholinesterase phenotyping: clinical aspects and laboratory applications. Crit Rev Clin Lab Sci 1986;23: 350–364.
16. Kent RS. Revised label regarding use of succinylcholine in children and adolescents. II. Reply. Anesthesiology 1994;80: 244–245.
17. Ostergaard D, Engbaek J, Viby-Mogensen J. Adverse reactions and interactions of the neuromuscular blocking drugs. Med Toxicol Adverse Drug Exp 1989;4:351–368.
18. Miller RD. Neuromuscular blocking agents. In: Smith et al, eds. Drug interactions in anesthesia. Philadelphia: Lea & Febiger, 1981; pp. 249–269.
19. Driessen JJ, Crul JF, Vree TB et al. Benzodiazepines and neuromuscular blocking drugs in patients. Acta Anaesth Scand 1986;30:642–646.
20. Roizen MF, Feeley TW. Pancuronium bromide. Ann Intern Med 1978;88:64–68.
21. Azar I, Cottrell J, Gupta B, Turndorf F. Furosemide facilitates recovery of evoked twitch response after pancuronium. Anesth Analg 1980;59:55–57.
22. Wood M. Neuromuscular blocking agents. In: Wood M, Wood AJJ, eds. Drugs and anesthesia. Pharmacology for anesthesiologists. 2nd ed. Baltimore: Williams & Wilkins, 1990; pp. 271–318.
23. Argov Z, Mastaglia FF. Disorders of neuromuscular transmission caused by drugs. N Engl J Med 1979;301:409–413.
24. Miller RD, Way WL, Katzung BG. The potentiation of neuromuscular blocking agents by quinidine. Anesthesiology 1967; 28:1036–1041.
25. Baraha A, Yazigi A. Neuromuscular interaction of magnesium with succinylcholine-vecuronium sequence in the eclamptic parturient. Anesthesiology 1987;67:806–808.
26. Doll DC, Rosenberg H. Antagonism of neuromuscular blockade by theophylline. Anesth Analg 1979;58:139–140.
27. Ornstein E, Matteo RS, Schwarts AE et al. The effect of phenytoin on the magnitude and duration of neuromuscular block following atracurium or vecuronium. Anesthesiology 1987;67:191–196.
28. Voetmann C, Jest P. A myasthenic reaction provoked by treatment with lithium carbonate. Ugestk Laeger 1978;140: 2375–2376.
29. Gramstod L. Atracurium, vecuronium and pancuronium in end-stage renal failure. Br J Anaesth 1987;59:995–1003.
30. Gramstod K, Gjerlov JA, Hysing ES et al. Interaction of cyclosporin and its solvent, cremophor with atracurium and vecuronium. Br J Anaesth 1986;58:1149–1155.
31. Laflin MJ. Interaction of pancuronium and corticosteroids. Anesthesiology 1986;65:93–94.
32. Thomas J, Climie CR, Mather LE. The placental transfer of plucuronium. A preliminary report. Br J Anaesth 1969;41: 297–302.
33. Shearer ES, Fahy LT, O'Sullivan EP, Hunter JM. Transplacental distribution of atracurium, laudanosine and monoquaternary alcohol during elective caesarean section. Br J Anaesth 1991;66:551–556.
34. Kivalo I, Saarikoski S. Placental transfer of 14C-Dimethyltubocurarine during caesarean section. Br J Anaesth 1976;48:239–242.
35. Duvaldestin P, Demetriou M, Henzel D, Desmonts JM. The placental transfer of pancuronium and its pharmacokinetics during caesarian section. Acta Anaesth Scand 1978; 22:327–333.
36. Ramzan MI, Somogyi AA, Walker JS, Shanks CA, Triggs EJ. Clinical pharmacokinetics of the non-depolarizing muscle relaxants. Clin Pharmacokinet 1981;6:25–60.
37. Mirakhur RK. Side effects of atracurium. Br J Anaesth 1990; 64:124–126.
38. Agoston S, Vermeer GA, Kersten UW, Meijer DKF. The fate of pancuronium bromide in man. Acta Anaesth Scand 1973; 17:267–275.
39. Caballero PA, Johnstone RE. Long-lasting neuromuscular blockade for pipecuronium. Anesthesiology 1992;76: 154–155.
40. Youngman PR, Taylor KM, Wilson JD. Anaphylactoid reactions to neuromuscular blocking agents: a commonly undiagnosed condition? Lancet 1983;2:597–599.
41. Lumb AB, Calder I. "Cured" myasthenia gravis and neuromuscular blockade. Anaesthesia 1989;44:828–830.
42. Yentis SM. Suxamethonium and hyperkalaemia. Anaesth Intensive Care 1990;18:92–101.
43. Ramzan IM, Shanks CA, Triggs EJ. Relationship between gallamine plasma concentration and neuromuscular paralysis in surgical patients. J Clin Pharmacol 1983;23:243–251.
44. Stevens HM, Moffat AC. A rapid screening procedure for quaternary ammonium compounds in fluids and tissues with special reference to suxamethonium (succinylcholine). J Forensic Sci Soc 1974;14:141–148.
45. Horowitz PE, Spector S. Determination of serum *d*-tubocurarine concentration by radioimmunoassay. J Pharm Exp Ther 1973;185:94–100.
46. Meulemans A, Mohler J, Henzel D, Duvaldestin P. Quantitation of *d*-tubocurarine in plasma using high performance liquid chromatography. J Chromatogr 1981;226:255–258.
47. Bitetti J. Neuromuscular blockade. In: Firestone LL, Lebowitz PW, Cook CE, eds. Clinical anesthesia procedures of the Massachusetts General Hospital. Boston: Little, Brown, 1988, pp. 167–184.
48. Gooch JL. Neuromuscular junction blocking agents in the ICU. Complications of long term use. Salt Lake City, UT: North American Congress of Clinical Toxicology—94. September 23–26, 1994.
49. Segneno V, Caldwell JE, Matthay MA, Sharma ML, Gruenke LD, Miller RD. Persistent paralysis in critically ill patients after long-term administration of vecuronium. N Engl J Med 1992;327:524–528.
50. Gooch JL, Moore MH, Ryser DK. Prolonged paralysis after neuromuscular junction blockade: case reports and electrodiagnostic findings. Arch Phys Med Rehabil 1993;74: 1007–1011.
51. Barohn RJ, Jackson CE, Rogers SJ, Ridings LW, McVey AL. Prolonged paralysis due to nondepolarizing neuromuscular blocking agents and corticosteroids. Muscle Nerve 1994;12: 647–654.

52. Partridge BL, Abrams JH, Bazemore C, Rubin R. Prolonged meuromuscular blockade after long-term infusion of vecuronium bromide in the intensive care unit. Crit Care Med 1990;18:1177–1179.
53. Kupfer Y, Namba T, Kaldawi E, Tessler S. Prolonged weakness after long-term infusion of vecuronium bromide. Ann Intern Med 1992;117:484–486.
54. Vanderheuden BA, Reynolds HM, Gerold KB, Emanuele T. Prolonged paralysis after long-term vecuronium infusion. Crit Care Med 1992;20:304–307.
55. Hirano M, Ott BR, Raps EC, Minetti C, Lennihan L, Libbey NP et al. Acute quadriplegic myopathy: a complication of treatment with steroids, nondepolarizing blocking agents, or both. Neurology 1992;42:2082–2087.
56. Ramsay DA, Zochodne DW, Robertson DM, Nag S, Ludwin SK. A syndrome of acute severe muscle necrosis in intensive care unit patients. J Neuropath Exp Neurol 1993;52:387–398.
57. Al Ahdal O, Bevan DR. Clindamycin-induced neuromuscular blockade. Can J Anaesth 1995;42:617.
58. Gooch JL. Prolonged paralysis after neuromuscular blockade. Clin Toxicol 1995;33:419–426.
59. Gooch JL, Suchyta DO, Balbierz JM, Petajan JH, Clammer TP. Prolonged paralysis after treatment with neuromuscular junctive blocking agents. Crit Care Med 1991;19: 1125–1131.
60. Kupfer Y, Okrent DG, Twersky RA, Tessler S. Disuse atrophy in a ventilated patients with status asthmaticus receiving neuromuscular blockade. Crit Care Med 1987;15:795–796.
61. Zochodnu DW, Ramsay DA, Saly V, Sheppy S, Moffatt S. Acute necrotizing myopathy of intensive care: electrophysiological studies. Muscle Nerve 1994;17:285–292.

TOPICAL ANESTHETICS (TABLES 56–21 AND 56–22) (BENZOCAINE)

Topical anesthetics applied in excess to the skin where normal barriers have been disrupted (injury, burns) or to mucous membranes (bronchoscopy) may induce seizures, cardiovascular and respiratory depression, bronchospasm, visual abnormalities, hemodynamic instability, and death. Treatment is largely supportive and symptomatic. Methemoglobinemia is treated with methylene blue. Obtain computer tomography scans and electroencephalograms following seizures according to clinical judgement.

TOXIC DOSAGE

TAC

Use of topical anesthetics on mucosal or denuded surfaces may predispose in some cases (TAC) to serious adverse reactions.[1,2] For example, TAC in amounts greater than 5 mL applied repeatedly or to contraindicated areas of the body (mucosal surfaces, burned skin) has resulted in seizures and fatality.[3,4] The maximum safe dose of tetracaine has been estimated to be 50 to 100 mg.[4] If the cocaine in TAC is completely and rapidly absorbed, 590 mg may be lethal.[4] Because TAC is exempt from FDA regulations,[5] the usual drug-testing regimens have not been performed. Recommended maximum dose for orotracheal topical use for cocaine in a 70-kg healthy adult is 100 mg (maximum dose 1.43 mg/kg) and for tetracaine 50 mg (0.71 mg/kg).[6,7] Two mL of TAC solution (236 mg of cocaine, 10 mg tetracaine/mg of adrenalin) used on the buccal mucosa led to grand mal seizures in a 5-year-old 20-kg boy. This was over 10 times the recommended maximum adult dose of cocaine.[7] As little as 20 mg of cocaine applied to mucous membranes have produced a severe toxic reaction.[8] Fatalities have followed one TAC application to the mucosal lip in a 7-month-old. Ten mL of TAC applied to multiple surface burn areas led to seizures in 2 or 3 minutes.[3]

Table 56–21
Common Over-the-Counter Products Containing Benzocaine[a]

Product	Content %
Baby Orajel	7.5
Baby Orajel Nighttime Formula	10.0
Baby Anbesol Gel	7.5
Anbesol Regular Strength	6.3
Anbesol Maximum Strength	20.0
Lanacane Spray	20.0
Americaine Topical Anesthetic First Aid Ointment	20.0
Vagisil Creme	20.0

[a]Adapted from Liebelt EL, Shannon MW. Pediatr Emerg Care 1993;9:292–297.

Tetracaine

Two patients gargled several times with 4 to 5 mL of tetracaine 5% and survived. One 75-year-old patient gargled with 4 mL of 0.5% solution and died.[9] Tetracaine 0.5% ophthalmic ointment applied every 30 to 90 minutes for 2 months produced corneal damage.[10]

Lidocaine

Suggested maximum doses of lidocaine for topical anesthesia of the pharynx, larynx, and trachea in a healthy 70-kg adult is 200 mg.[7] Doses of lidocaine of up to 8.5 mg/kg proved safe when administered over longer than 15 minutes and resulted in a therapeutic level of lidocaine when administered topically to the airways of young children.[11]

Topical application of 25 g of lidocaine base twice daily led to death from cardiorespiratory arrest.[12] A 5-month-old boy developed status epilepticus after 7.5 mg/kg/dose administered as a 2% solution over 5 days.[13] Manual application of 2% viscous lidocaine to the gums of an 11-month-old led to seizures.[2]

TOXICOKINETICS[14–17]

Volume of distribution (L/kg)	1.6 L/kg
Plasma protein binding (%)	60%
Elimination half-life	2 - 10 hours +
Active metabolites	Niomoethylglycinexylidide (MEGX) Glycine exylidide (GX)[22]

Peak blood levels of lidocaine after a 7.5-mg/kg dose as given to a 5-month-old boy reached 20 μg/mL. The elimination half-life was about 2 hours and apparent volume of distribution 0.14 L/kg. Lidocaine when introduced rectally is readily absorbed and when administered to a baby may induce convulsions.[18] When lidocaine is applied to the mucous membranes, blood levels may simulate those

Table 56–22
Topical Anesthetic Uses[a]

Anesthetic Ingredient	Concentration (%)	Pharmaceutical Application Form	Intended Area of Use
Estertype			
Benzocaine	1–5	Cream	Skin and mucous membrane
	20	Ointment	Skin and mucous membrane
	20	Aerosol	Skin and mucous membrane
	2.5–20	Solution	Ear, dental, mouth
Butacaine	4	Ointment	Denture
Cocaine	4–10%	Solution	Ear, nose, throat
	1–4%	Solution	Ophthalmic
Proparacaine	0.5%	Solution	Ophthalmic
Tetracaine	0.5–1	Ointment	Skin, rectum, mucous membrane
	0.5–1	Cream	Skin, rectum, mucous membrane
	0.25–1	Solution	Nose, tracheobronchial tree
Amide type			
Dibucaine	0.25–1	Cream	Skin
	0.25–1	Olntment	Skin
	0.25–1	Aerosol	Skin
	0.25	Solution	Ear
	0.5–1	Suppositories	Rectum
Lidocaine	2–4	Solution	Oropharynx, Tracehobronchial Tree, Nose
	2	Jelly	Urethra
	2.5–5	Ointment	Skin, mucous membranes, rectum
	2	Viscous	Oropharynx
	10	Suppositories	Rectum
	10	Aerosol	Gingival mucosa
Othera types			
Dyclonine	0.1–1	Solution	Skin, oropharynx, tracheobronchial tree, urethra, rectum
Ethyl chloride		Topical	Skin
Pramoxine	1%	Ointment	Skin, anus
	1%	Aerosol	
	1%	Cream	
	1%	Gel	
Pramoxine hydrochloride	1%	Lotion	

[a]Adapted from Saverese JJ, Covino BG. In: Miller RD, ed. Anesthesia. 2nd ed. New York: Churchill Livingstone, 1985; and from McEvoy GK, ed. AHFS Drug Information 91. Bethesda: American Society of Hospital Pharmacists, 1991.

resulting from intravenous injections.[19,20] Similarly, peak blood levels are attained quickly after application to mucous membranes of the tracheobronchial tree.

MECHANISM OF ACTION

Blood levels of a local anesthetic arising from topical anesthesia of the trachea may equal those obtained by intravenous injection. Systemic toxic reactions may occur. Salivary secretions may dilute the anesthetic and prevent adequate contact with mucous membranes. Atropine is given for the drying effect, and appropriate sedation is provided to diminish discomfort. Most topical drugs require 3 to 5 minutes before anesthesia begins, and the anesthetic action lasts 20 to 30 minutes.

CLINICAL PRESENTATION

Local anesthetics have little penetration through intact skin. This property may be misinterpreted when such preparations are administered to the mucous membrane. Numerous fatalities have been associated with use of cocaine or tetracaine for endoscopic procedures.[21] Death in such cases resulted as a consequence of overdosage due to rapid absorption. Blood concentrations may approach those following direct intravenous injection.[19]

Dibucaine

A 2-year-old child apparently ingested dibucaine hydrochloride (0.5% Nupercainal Cream), acted strangely, staggered, then seized, became cyanotic, vomited, developed a cardiorespiratory arrest, and died.[22]

Hexylcaine

A child aged 32 months received an adult dose (3.5 mL) of hexylcaine 5% to facilitate bronchoscope. Five minutes later the child developed apnea, dilated pupils, and seizures. Supportive treatment was successful for recovery.[23] An adult also became apneic and experienced seizures after swallowing 10 ml of hexylcaine (cyclaine).[24]

Lidocaine

Topical cutaneous lidocaine cream application to 60% of the body (25 g of lidocaine base) twice daily induced visual disturbances, dizziness, confusion, seizures, and a cardiorespiratory arrest.[12] Severe and even lethal intoxications have followed local application to mucous membranes.

TAC

Misuse of TAC may result in serious (grand mal seizures) or fatal results. Absolute contraindications for TAC utilization include lacerations of mucosal surfaces, digits, glans of penis, nasal alae, ear lobes, and extensively abraded skin (pain control of burned or abraded skin); relative contraindications include underlying convulsive or cardiac dysrhythmic disorders.[1]

Tetracaine

Dizziness, difficulty in speaking, tonic-clonic seizures, and a transient facial paresis have been observed. The patients recovered.

METHEMOGLOBINEMIA

Benzocaine

Methemoglobinemia has followed the topical use of benzocaine and cetacaine.[25–27] A co-oximeter may be more useful in establishing the diagnosis than a pulsed oximeter.[28] The methemoglobinemia is frequently not described in the drug package inserts, on the containers, or in the *Physician's Desk Reference*. Topical sprays and ointments containing 14 to 20% benzocaine often cause dose-dependent methemoglobinemia. This is probably a direct toxic action of the drug. Benzocaine absorbed from mucous or pulmonary membranes oxidizes blood hemoglobin in proportion to the absorbed dose.

Infants and children are more susceptible than adults to methemoglobinemia because (a) fetal hemoglobin is more easily oxidized to methemoglobin; (b) newborns have lower levels of NADH-methemoglobin reductase, catalase, and glutathione peroxidase; and (c) dosage usually is greater per kilogram body weight.[29]

Preparations containing over 8% benzocaine are listed under Product Formulation.

Lidocaine

Following topical administration of lidocaine to the nasal mucosa, severe methemoglobinemia may result in patients who have the heterozygous form of NADH-methemoglobin reductase deficiency.[30] Death is rare following a hypersensitivity reaction to topical lidocaine 10% spray prior to fiberoptic bronchoscopy.[31]

Lidocaine lowers the seizure threshold. Oral lidocaine in children is followed with a delay of minutes to hours by sedation, agitation, and seizures requiring adequate resuscitation. Aspiration of viscous lidocaine in children is followed by seizures that begin within 10 to 15 seconds.[32]

LABORATORY

Dibucaine

A 2-year-old child ingested dibucaine hydrochloride 0.5% (Nupercainal) ointment and died with a dibucaine blood level of 1.3 μg/mL.[22]

Lidocaine

Therapeutic serum concentrations for use as an antiarrhythmic are 1 to 5 μg/ml.[12] Toxic manifestations first appear at a serum lidocaine concentration of 5 μg/mL. Early symptoms (5 to 10 μg/ml) are dizziness, drowsiness, tinnitus, and perioral paresthesias. More severe symptoms (at concentrations of 10 to 20 μg/mL) include disorientation, delirium, convulsions, and coma; cardiorespiratory arrest supervenes above 20 μg/mL.[33]

When 3 mg/kg of lidocaine in a 1% gel was applied to split-skin donor sites (3 cm^2/kg), a maximum serum concentration of 0.51 μg/ml was observed.[34] Topical application of 5% lidocaine applied to 60% of the body produced serum levels of lidocaine 21.2 μg/mL, monoethylglycine xylidine (MEGX) 6.1 μg/mL, and glycine xylidide 2.1 μg/mL.[12] The patient died. In six other patients serum lidocaine concentrations of 5.4 μg/mL or less were not associated with symptoms. Two percent viscous xylocaine applied to the gums resulted in a serum level of 10 μg/mL consistent with the seizure activity observed.[16] Following a total lidocaine dose of 3.2 to 8.5 mg/kg given to children age 3 months to 9.5 years and administered to the nose, larynx, and bronchial tree, peak serum lidocaine concentration was 1 to 3.5 μg/mL.[11] Seizures and cardiopulmonary arrest followed an ingestion of 1.6 g and 0.8 g of lidocaine 2%, respectively.[35] Blood concentrations of 12.0 and 7.3 μg/mL were observed, respectively.

TAC

Following TAC use in a 7-month-old infant, the postmortem plasma cocaine level was 11.9 μg/mL and the blood tetracaine level 1 μg/mL.[4] Blood levels in 11 patients lethally overdosed with cocaine ranged from 0.1 to 20.9 μg/ml.[36]

TREATMENT

Stabilization

Evaluate airway, breathing, and circulation in all patients. Topical anesthetics (skin, mucous membranes) can, in sufficient quantities, induce seizures, cardiovascular depression, respiratory depression, or bronchospasm. Treatment will be symptomatic and supportive. Cardiac monitoring, intravenous lines and oxygen should be available. Give naloxone, glucose, and thiamine to all obtunded patients.

Decontamination

Systemic levels of oral or topical (mucous membrane) lidocaine and its metabolites MEGX and GX rapidly decrease after the use of oral charcoal.[37] Topical anesthetics on the skin can be washed off briskly with repeated soap and water washings. Gastric lavage is performed after endotracheal intubation. The possibility of seizures should alert the clinician to use gastric lavage only if the benefit outweighs the risk (e.g., aspiration pneumonitis).

Elimination Enhancement

There is little evidence to support the use of diuresis, hemodialysis, or hemoperfusion after a toxic reaction induced by a topical anesthetic.

Antidote

Severe methemoglobinemia following topical anesthetic use (lidocaine, benzocaine) is rapidly reversed by intravenous methylene blue (1 to 2 mg/kg in a 1% solution administered over 5 minutes). Bronchoscopists may consider maintaining a stock of methylene blue in the bronchoscopy area.

There are no antidotes for other topical anesthetic toxicities (depression, seizures).

Supportive Measures

1. Succinylcholine should be used with caution because it will stop peripheral muscular signs of seizure but will mask ongoing CNS seizure activity.[37] In addition, hypotension, neuromuscular block, apnea, and seizure activity may be worsened or prolonged, especially when the ester type of anesthesia is responsible for toxicity, because both the ester anesthetics and succinylcholine use pseudocholinesterase for metabolism.
2. Dopamine is the drug of choice for cardiovascular collapse in topical anesthetic toxicity because of its inotropic effect on the heart and on total peripheral vascular resistance, both of which may be markedly impaired by an absorbed anesthetic.
3. Seizures following lidocaine use may be treated with a benzodiazepine (e.g., lorazepam, diazepam, or similar anticonvulsant agents).
4. Respiratory support with intubation.
5. Cardiovascular depression may require chronotropic agents and IV fluids.[37]
6. Preventive measures are of great importance in diminishing the toxicity of topical anesthetics. When topical anesthetics are applied to the oral mucosa, an attempt should be made to have the patient expectorate any excess to diminish absorption. Since children under 7 years of age are unable to expectorate unless taught to do so, topical anesthetics pose a special hazard to them.[3]
7. Xylocaine viscous 2% is not recommended by the manufacturer for teething discomfort.
8. To diminish benzocaine methemoglobinemia[38]:
   a. The FDA must reconsider labeling changes, standards limiting concentrations, and over-the-counter availability.
   b. All products containing benzocaine in concentrations over 8% should carry suitable warning of the probability that methemoglobinemia will occur in proportion to dosage and of the possible need for methylene blue treatment and its recommended dosage.
   c. All general references used by physicians should add a warning regarding methemoglobinemia for each product containing over 8% benzocaine and should note that methylene blue should be available for prompt administration with recommended dosage.
   d. Benzocaine sprays, gels, and ointment should be avoided in infants and in patients with anemia or other diseases in which reduced oxygen transport may be of special concern. Benzocaine use should be avoided on skin or mucosa surfaces where normal tissue barriers to absorption are impaired. Pulse oximetry detects methemoglobinemia, though it underestimates its magnitude by about half in low concentrations and may only indicate a saturation decrease to 80 to 85% when there is 70% methemoglobinemia.[38] It would be prudent to administer oxygen to patients at risk of hypoxia after using benzocaine topical anesthetics.
9. *TAC*—Recommendations have been made to avoid use of TAC on mucosal or denuded surfaces.[2] Authoritative bodies such as the Food and Drug Administration and/or the Committee on Drugs of the American Academy of Pediatrics should evaluate the data on the combination product and issue a statement about its use.
10. Blood levels may be of value in following the course of lidocaine toxicity. Methodology for determination of cocaine and tetracaine blood levels (e.g., in TAC) is available. Treatment will be guided largely by clinical judgment and confirmed by laboratory studies if available.

REFERENCES—TOPICAL ANESTHETICS

1. Bonadio WA. TAC: a review. Pediatr Emerg Care 1989;5:128–130.
2. Mofenson HC, Caraccio TR. Tack up a warning on TAC. Am J Dis Child 1989;143:519–520.
3. Wehner D, Hamilton GD. Seizures following topical application of local anesthetics to burn patients. Ann Emerg Med 1984;13:456–458.
4. Dailey RH. Fatality secondary to misuse of TAC solution. Ann Emerg Med 1988;17:159–160.
5. United States Code 1982. Title 21, Subchapter V, Section 360 (g), p. 783.
6. Doya MR, Burton BT, Schleiss MR, DiLiberti JH. Recurrent seizures following mucosal applications of TAC. Ann Emerg Med 1988;17:646–648.
7. DiFazio C. Local anesthetics. Action, metabolism and toxicity. Otolaryngol Clin North Am 1981;14:515–518.
8. Meyers EF. Cocaine toxicity during dacryocystorhinostomy. Arch Ophthalmol 1980;98:842–843.
9. Patel D, Chopra S, Berman MD. Serious systemic toxicity resulting from use of tetracaine for pharyngeal anesthesia in upper endoscopic procedures. Digest Dis Sci 1989;34:882–884.
10. Duffin RM, Olson RJ. Tetracaine toxicity. Ann Ophthalmol 1984;16:836–837.
11. Amitai Y, Zylber-Katz E, Avital A, Zangen D, Noviski N. Serum lidocaine concentrations in children during bronchoscopy with topical anesthesia. Chest 1990;98:1370–1373.
12. Lie RL, Vermeer BJ, Edelbroek PM. Severe lidocaine intoxication by cutaneous absorption. J Am Acad Dermatol 1990;23:1026–1028.
13. Wason S, del Rey JG, Druckenbrod R. Avoiding lidocaine toxicity in the treatment of acute herpetic gingivostomatitis. Vet Hum Toxicol 1989;31:361.
14. Benowitz N, Forsyth RP, Melmon KL et al. Lidocaine disposition kinetics in monkey and man. I. Predication by a perfusion model. Clin Pharmacol Ther 1974;16:87–98.
15. Boyes RN, Scott DB, Jebson PJ et al. Pharmacokinetics of lidocaine in man. Clin Pharmacol Ther 1971;12:105–116.
16. Baselt RC, Cravey RH, eds. Lidocaine. In: Disposition of toxic drugs and chemicals in man. Chicago: Year Book, 1989, pp. 455–460.

17. Strong JM, Mayfield DE, Atkinson AJ et al. Pharmacological activity, metabolism and pharmacokinetics of glycinexylidide. Clin Pharmacol Ther 1975;17:184–194.
18. Pottage A, Scott DB. Safety of "topical" lignocaine. Lancet 1988;1:1003.
19. Adriani J, Zepernick R. Clinical effectiveness of drugs used for topical anesthesia. JAMA 1964;188:711–716.
20. Mofenson HC, Caraccio TR, Miller H, Greensher J. Lidocaine toxicity from topical mucosal application with a review of the clinical pharmacology of lidocaine. Clin Pediatr 1983;22:190–192.
21. Adriani J, Campbell D. Fatalities following topical application of local anesthetics to mucous membranes. JAMA 1956;162:1527–1530.
22. Vuignier BI, Henretig F, Kearney T, Clark M, Hicks M, Vaicious T. Death in a child ingesting dibucaine hydrochloride. Vet Hum Toxicol 1988;30:345–346.
23. Goldberg G, Goodman DH. Case report of a hexylcaine reaction. Anesthesiology 1957;18:652–653.
24. Spellberg MA. Hexylcaine (Cyclaine) as topical anesthetic in gastroscopy and esophagoscopy. Gastroenterology 1959;36:120–121.
25. Ferraro L, Zeichner S, Greenblott G, Groeger JS. Cetacaine-induced acute methemoglobinemia. Anesthesiology 1988;69:614–615.
26. Collins JF. Methemoglobinemia as a complication of 20% benzocaine spray for endoscopy. Gastroenterology 1990;98:211–213.
27. Gentile DA. Severe methemoglobinemia induced by a topical teething preparation. Pediatr Emerg Care 1987;3:176–178.
28. Anderson ST, Hajduczek J, Barker SJ. Benzocaine-induced methemoglobinemia in an adult. Accuracy of pulse oximetry with methemoglobinemia. Anesth Analg 1988;7:1099–1101.
29. Curry S. Methemoglobinemia. Ann Emerg Med 1982;11:214–221.
30. Hansen-Flaschen J. Methemoglobinemia after lidocaine administration. Chest 1990;98:519–520.
31. Ruffles SP, Ayres JG. Fatal bronchospasm after topical lidocaine before bronchoscopy. Br Med J 1987;294:1658–1659.
32. Garrettson KF, McGee EB. Rapid onset of seizures following aspiration of viscous lidocaine. Clin Toxicol 1992;30:413–422.
33. Mather LE, Cousins MJ. Local anesthetics and their current clinical use. Drugs 1979;18:185–205.
34. Bulmer NJ, Duchett AC. Absorption of lignocaine through split skin donor sites. Anaesthesia 1985;40:808–809.
35. Gorman RL, Kin JC, Oderda GM. Ingestion of topical lidocaine. It's time to stop the pain. Vet Hum Toxicol 1984;26:413.
36. Mittlemen RE, Wetli CV. Death caused by recreational cocaine use. JAMA 1984;252:1889–1893.
37. Hess GP, Walson PD. Seizures secondary to oral viscous lidocaine. Ann Emerg Med 1988;725–727.
38. Severinghaus JW, Xu F-D, Spellman MJ Jr. Benzocaine and methemoglobin. Recommended actions. Anesthesiology 1991;74:385–386.

Waste Inhalation, Anesthetic Gases, and Vapors

Waste inhalation, anesthetic gases, and vapors are those that are released into work areas (operating room, recovery room, delivery room, or other areas where workers may be subject to job-related exposure) associated with, and adjacent to, the administration of a gas for anesthetic purposes, and includes both gaseous and volatile liquid agents.[1]

REFERENCES

1. Criteria for recommended standard occupational exposure to waste anesthetic gases and vapors. US Department of Health Education and Welfare. NIOSH DHEW (NIOSH). Publication No. 77-140.

Day Care Anesthesia[1]

Many patients are admitted and discharged from the hospital on the day of the operation. Complications may arise after discharge from the hospital.

Impaired Psychomotor Function

Inability to retain new information within a few hours of even short procedures. Instructions should be written. Drowsiness and impaired performance may persist for 48 hours. Patients should be given written instructions not to drive a car, operate machinery, drink alcohol, or make any important decision for at least 24 hours after a general anesthetic.

Anorexia, malaise, fatigue, dizziness, headache.

Psychologic Problems

Anxiety, irritability, sleep disturbance. Rare, but may occur if patient becomes aware during a general anesthetic.

Nausea With or Without Vomiting

May persist for 1 to 2 days.

Minor Trauma to the Airway

Sore throat or hoarseness may last for several days.

Nerve Injury

Rare. Common peroneal nerve (lithotomy), brachial plexus (arms abducted).

Muscle Pain

Mild, brief. May occur after succinylcholine, affecting shoulder and neck muscles.

REFERENCES

1. Following up day care anaesthesia in general practice. Drug Ther Bull 1990;28(21):81–82.

Chapter **57**

Antiseptics And Disinfectants

DEFINITIONS[1]

ANTISEPTIC

An antiseptic refers to a chemical agent that destroys or inhibits microorganisms on living tissue and has the effect of limiting or preventing the harmful results of infection.

DISINFECTANT

A disinfectant is a chemical agent that destroys microorganisms, but not usually bacterial spores; it does not necessarily kill all microorganisms, but reduces them to a level that is harmful neither to health nor the quality of perishable goods.

STERILIZATION

Sterilization refers to the total removal or destruction of all living microorganisms; sterility is usually produced by heat or radiation methods.

PRESERVATIVES (SEE ALSO OVER-THE-COUNTER PRODUCTS CHAPTER—SURFACTANTS)

Preservatives are used to prevent microbial spoilage of preparations. (See Food Preservatives in Food Poisoning chapter.)

Types of Disinfectants

Alcohols

Alcohol, isopropyl alcohol, ethyl alcohol-methyl alcohol mixture.

Aldehydes

Formaldehyde, glutaraldehyde.

Cationic Surfactants

Benzalkonium chloride, cetrimide, cetylpyridinium chloride, domiphen bromide.

Chlorhexidine

Chlorine and Chlorine-Releasing Substances

Sodium hypochlorite, chloramine, chlorinated lime, bichlordimethylhydantoin, halazone, oxychlorosene, sodium dichloroisocyanurate.

Dyes

Acridine derivatives—acriflavine, aminacrine hydrochloride, proflavine hemisulfate; triphenylmethane derivatives—brilliant green, crystal violet, magenta, malachite green.

Gases and Vapors

Ethylene oxide, propiolactone.

Hydrogen Peroxide

Iodine

Mercurials

Thimerosal, hydrargaphen, mercurochrome, nitromersol.

Phenols

Cresol, phenol, thymol; chlorinated phenols—chlorocresol, chloroxylenol, hexachlorophene, triclosan.

PRESERVATIVES AND ANTIBACTERIALS

These compounds are added to products to maintain sterility in sterile products and to prevent spoilage by bacteria or fungi in nonsterile medications.

QUATERNARY AMMONIUM ANTISEPTICS

Preservatives in ophthalmic solutions, topical lotions, and others. Allergic contact dermatitis and hypersensitivity occur.

Benzalkonium Chloride

Used in eye drops, contact lens solutions. Allergic dermatitis, stomatitis, allergic conjunctivitis. Patch tests may be positive.

Cetrimide (Atrimonium Bromide)

Cationic surfactant, antiseptic. Contact dermatitis. Sterile chemical peritonitis.

Dequalinium

Allergic reactions, genital ulcerations, necrosis.

OTHER COMPOUNDS

Sorbic Acid

Antimicrobial in topical preparations. Weak sensitizer, contact sensitivity, eczema.

Chlorocresol

Phenolic antibacterial. Preservative. Contact dermatitis, eczema.

Triclosan

Chlorinated phenol. Antimicrobial in cosmetic products. Contact sensitivity.

Formaldehyde Polymers

Preservatives in cosmetics and topical pharmaceuticals. Antibacterial, antifungal. May release formaldehyde. May be sensitive to the polymer or formaldehyde.

BENZALKONIUM CHLORIDE

Benzalkonium chloride is a mixture of alkyldimethylbenzyl ammonium chlorides.[2] It is the preservative most commonly present in nebulizer solutions.[3] It is used for its bactericidal properties and is present in commercially available salbutamol (albuterol), beclomethasone dipropionate, metaproterenol sulfate and ipratropium bromide nebulizer solutions.[4–6] Ingestion may lead to fatalities.[7,8]

STRUCTURE AND CLASSIFICATION

Benzalkonium chloride is a quaternary ammonium disinfectant that is very soluble in water and alcohol and is slightly alkaline in water. Its molecular weight is 360.[1,3]

DOSAGE

Therapeutic Doses

Benzalkonium chloride is used as a disinfectant clinically in strengths from 0.0025 to 1.2%. It is available commercially in strengths up to 10%.[1]

The human use of benzalkonium chloride for antisepsis of the skin should be limited to dilution of at least 1:1000 or 1:750. Caustic action of the agent may occur with a preparation diluted 1:2000 or 1:5000, with dilutions of at least 1:20,000 suggested by some for use in mucous membranes.[9]

Suggested dilutions for specific application of BAC solutions include the following:[9a]

Preoperative disinfection of the skin: 1:750 tincture, aqueous solution or spray.
Surgeon's hand and arm soaks: 1:750 aqueous solution.
Minor wounds and lacerations: 1:750 tincture or spray.
Deep infected wounds: 1:3,000 to 1:20,000 aqueous solution.
Denuded skin and mucous membranes: 1:5,000 to 1:10,000 aqueous solution.
Vaginal douche and irrigation: 1:2,000 to 1:5,000 aqueous solution.
Postepisiotomy care: 1:5,000 to 1:10,000 aqueous solution.
Breast and nipple hygiene: 1:1,000 to 1:2,000 aqueous solution.
Bladder and urethral irrigation: 1:5,000 to 1:20,000 aqueous solution.

Bladder retention lavage: 1:20,000 to 1:40,000 aqueous solution.
Oozing and open infections: 1:2,000 to 1:5,000 aqueous solution.
Wet dressings: 1:5,000 aqueous solution.
Eye irrigation: 1:5,000 to 1:10,000 aqueous solution.
Preservation of ophthalmic solutions: 1:5,000 to 1:7,500 aqueous solution.
Catheters and other adsorbent articles: 1:500 aqueous solution (replenish frequently).
Metallic instruments, ampules and thermometers: 1:750 aqueous solution (replenish frequently).

Toxic Dose

A 77-year-old male swallowed 50 mL of a 10% (5 g) aqueous solution of benzalkonium chloride. He did not survive.[7] A 70-year-old woman ingested approximately 40 mL of a 33.3% aqueous solution of benzalkonium chloride. She survived.[8] The oral dose was about 13 g (200 mg/kg). A 17% solution of benzalkonium chloride was inadvertently applied to the mouth of two children. After several days of symptoms they survived.[10]

Fatal Dose

Human fatalities are described following an oral dose of 100 to 400 mg/kg,[9,11,12] or a parenteral dose of 5 to 15 mg/kg.[8]

DRUG INTERACTIONS

Incompatible drugs with BAC solutions include iodine, silver nitrate, fluorescein, nitrates, peroxide, lanolin, potassium permanganate, aluminum, caramel, kaolin, pine oil, zinc sulfate, zinc oxide, and yellow oxide of mercury.

CLINICAL PRESENTATION

Chronic Dose Related

Oral

Ingestion of benzalkonium chloride in concentrations of 10% or more may produce corrosive lesions of all mucous membranes with which it comes into contact: palate, hypopharynx, esophagus, and stomach. Nausea, vomiting, diarrhea, dyspnea, confusion, hypotension, hypoxemia, renal insufficiency, restlessness, seizures, coma, muscle weakness, pulmonary edema, and methemoglobinemia have been observed.[8] Greyish white membranes may form in the mouth, hypopharynx, and stomach. Death may follow within minutes to hours and may be due to circulatory failure, respiratory insufficiency, muscle weakness, and central nervous system depression.[7,8]

Inhalation

Benzalkonium chloride may cause bronchoconstriction by releasing spasmogenic mediators from mast cells within the bronchial wall and stimulating cholinergic and noncholinergic nerves to produce bronchoconstriction.[13] Bronchoconstriction appears in patients with reactive airway disease such as bronchial asthma and may appear to be dose related over a concentration range of 0.13 to 2.0 mg/mL that persists for over 60 minutes.[4–6] Responses to benzalkonium, although rapid in onset, are prolonged and may continue to affect the airway after lung function has returned to baseline.[5] Zhang and colleagues suggest that benzalkonium appears to act in asthmatic airways primarily by a non–IgE-dependent release of mediators.[5]

LABORATORY

Ancillary Tests

Serum creatinine levels rise; oliguria and renal failure may intervene. Heparin-bonded umbilical catheters use benzalkonium chloride during the bonding process. As the benzalkonium chloride is released, it causes a false elevation of serum sodium and potassium as measured with some ion-selective electrodes. This leads to clinical errors in management.[14] A leucocytosis and elevations in serum uric acid and serum aminotransferases are apparent for several days after local use.[10]

TREATMENT

Stabilization

Treatment of benzalkonium chloride ingestion is mainly symptomatic and supportive and follows guidelines for the treatment of caustic products (see Household Products chapter), including early esophagoscopy. Asthmatic patients should be hospitalized in an intensive care facility with access to intravenous lines, cardiac monitoring, and oxygen. Endotracheal intubation and esophagoduodenoscopy is performed if required prior to gastric lavage under appropriate anesthesia. Following esophagoscopy in the case of second-degree burns, a large bore nasogastric tube may be inserted in an attempt to prevent strictures and to lavage the stomach. In the case of more extensive burns, esophagogastrectomy is life-saving.[8] Further treatment must be directed toward rehydration, parenteral nutrition, and supplemental oxygen. The nasogastric tube may, depending on clinical and surgical judgment, be left in situ and used for enteral feeding. Local treatment for mouth and hypopharynx burns includes tepid water sponging around the mouth, acetaminophen orally, antibiotics, and intravenous fluids until oral intake is resumed.

Antidote

There are no antidotes.

Supportive Measures

When clinically indicated, expansion of circulatory blood volume, vasoactive drugs, supplemental oxygen, mechanical ventilation and treatment of seizures should be promptly instituted.

A complete blood count (hemoglobin, red blood cells packed all volume, leukocytes with differential count), methemoglobin determination, glucose, creatinine, lactic acid dehydrogenase, bilirubin, aminotransferases, and arterial blood gases should be performed periodically. Chest x-ray and electrocardiograph should be obtained early. If solutions stronger than 1:3000 enter the eyes, irrigate the eyes immediately with water for 15 to 20 minutes.

BENZYL ALCOHOL

Benzyl alcohol is a preservative and local anesthetic. It is used as a preservative in newborn medications such as bacteriostatic saline, heparin, phenobarbital injection, pancuronium, aquamephyton, and neonatal trace metal solutions. Five infants, preterm, received multiple injections of heparinized bacteriostatic sodium chloride for flushing the catheters and medications reconstituted with bacteriostatic water, both containing 0.9% benzyl alcohol. Daily quantities of benzyl alcohol equaled 99 to 234 mg/kg of body weight. They then developed gradual neurologic deterioration, severe metabolic acidosis, a striking onset of gasping respirations, hematologic abnormalities, skin breakdown, hepatic and renal failure, hypotension, and cardiovascular collapse. These products were discontinued in that hospital in June 1981. No further cases of gasping syndrome have been observed.[15] A similar episode was recorded several years later[16] (Table 57–1).

CETRIMIDE

Cetrimide orally leads to irritation of the gastrointestinal mucosa, vomiting, and generalized depolarization at cholinergic neuromuscular junctions; respiratory paralysis may cause death.[17–20] In 1974 an adult died from hypostatic pneumonia 10 days after ingesting 1 pint of cetrimide

Table 57–1
List of Parenteral Medications Frequently Used by Anesthesiologists for Which at Least One Formulation Contains Benzyl Alcohol[a]

Pharmacologic Action	Generic Name	BA-free Formulations	Formulations With BA	BA Content (mg/ml Medication)	Alternatives Without BA
Anticholinergic antisialogogue	Atropine sulfate	Abbott LyphoMed	Astra Elkins	15	
	Glycopyrrolate	–	American Regent LyphoMed Quad Schein Robins	9	
Anticholinesterase	Physostigmine	–	Forest Quad	20	Neostigmine Edrophonium
	Pyridostigmine	ICN	Organon	10	
Anticoagulants	Heparin[b]	LyphoMed Squibb Abbott Winthrop	Organon Wyeth Upjohn Elkins	10	
Anxiolytics	Diazepam	–	Legere Roche Hauck	15	
	Midazolam		Roche	10	
Crystalloid solutions	Bacteriostatic saline, water	Abbott Baxter Kendall Elkins	Elkins	9	Preservative-free saline, water
Muscle relaxants					
Short-acting	Succinylcholine	Squibb Abbott Burroughs	Organon	10	
Intermediate-acting	Atracurium	Ampules, 5-ml vial	10-mL multidose vial	9	Vecuronium when dissolved in BA-free solution
Long-acting	Pancuronium	–	Astra Elkins Quad Organon	10	Metocurine Gallamine
	Tubocurarine	Lilly	Abbott Squibb	9	
Respiratory stimulant	Doxapram	–	Robins	9	Naloxone—if narcotic being antagonized
Miscellaneous	Metoclopramide	Quad LympoMed SoloPak Robins	Robins	9	

BA, Benzyl alcohol.
[a]Adapted from Weissman DB et al. Anesth Analg 1990;70:673.
[b]Preparations contain from 1000 to 10,000 U/mL depending on manufacturer.
[c]Other nonproprietary preparations may be available.

solution of unknown strength. Necropsy disclosed esophageal damage.[17] In 1966 another patient died 24 hours after ingesting an unknown quantity of 40% cetrimide, and the postmortem revealed gastric ulceration.[17]

ACUTE

The acute systemic effects of cetrimide appear to be dose related and include: (a) a curare-like paralysis, (b) CNS depression (possibly preceded by excitement initially), (c) dyspnea and cyanosis from respiratory paralysis, and (d) hypotension and coma.

TREATMENT

Treat cetrimide ingestion as if it were a caustic agent: avoid gastric lavage; give milk. There is no specific antidote to cetrimide. (See Caustics section.)

CHLORBUTOL (CHLOROBUTANOL)

Chlorbutol, used as a preservative in some European preparations of heparin (benzyl alcohol is more often used in the United States), has significant hypotensive, respiratory depressant, sedative,[21] and cumulative effects.[22]

Chlorobutanol is structurally related to trichloroethanol, the active metabolite of the hypnotic sedative chloral hydrate. In Australia it is available commercially as an over-the-counter sleep aid (Sedu-Caps) in doses of 150 mg for oral administration. Inadvertent epidural injection of morphine sulfate 750 mg from a commercial solution containing morphine sulfate 15 mg/mL, with 0.5% chlorobutanol and 0.1% sodium bisulfite, resulted in prolonged (48 hours) somnolence.[23] A total dose of 250 mg of chlorobutanol was infused into the epidural space. The somnolence disappeared after naloxone administration.

Preservatives such as sulfites and benzalkonium chloride can cause bronchoconstriction when inhaled by asthmatic subjects.[24] A bronchial provocation study suggests that in most asthmatic subjects, chlorbutol, in the dose present in terbutaline nebulizer solution (5 mg/mL), has no significant effect on airway caliber.[24]

Death after ingestion of chlorbutol by an adult was associated with whole blood chlorbutanol concentrations of 64 μg/mL analyzed by gas chromatography.[25] An adult ingested 6 to 10 capsules of chlorbutol 150 mg daily, became drowsy, and was unable to be aroused. His speech was slow. Hepatic enzymes were elevated. The patient gradually returned to normal over 2 weeks during which time irregular clonic jerks were observed. An electroencephalogram showed diffuse slow activity. He died in 4 months of adenocarcinoma of the liver. Plasma chlorbutanol concentrations on admission were 100 μg/mL. The elimination half-life was 13.2 days.[26]

CHLORHEXIDINE

Chlorhexidine is a disinfectant that is generally used topically.[27] It has been associated with methemoglobinemia,[28] and skin, gastric,[9] eye,[30] hepatic, neurologic, and cardiac reactions when ingested, inhaled, or used topically. There have been no fatalities.

STRUCTURE AND CLASSIFICATION

Chlorhexidine is hexamethylene bis [5-(4-chlorophenyl)-biguanide].[27] It is a bisbiguanide that may decompose spontaneously at room temperature to yield parachloraniline.[28]

USES

Chlorhexidine may be effective against some Gram-positive and Gram-negative bacteria, some viruses, and some fungi. It is inactive against bacterial spores.[27]

PRODUCT FORMULATION

Chlorhexidine is commercially available as the acetate, the gluconate, and the hydrochloride.[27] A 0.5% solution of the gluconate or acetate in alcohol (70%) is used for preoperative skin disinfection and for emergency disinfection of clean instruments. A 0.05% aqueous solution is used as a wound disinfectant, as an eye irrigation, and for storage and disinfection (30 minutes immersion) of clean instruments. Solutions of 0.02% and 0.01% are also used. The gluconate may be combined with cetrimide as a disinfectant. It is available as a cream, lozenge, in dusting powder, ear drops, mouth wash, swab, spray, solution, gel, and irrigant. Trade names include Bacticlens, Chlorsept 2000, Hibiclens, and Hibitane.[27] It is most active at a neutral or slightly acidic pH.[29] Chlorhexidine gluconate in a 0.005% concentration is sometimes used as a preservative for soft and gas-permeable contact lens solutions.[30] Two percent chlorhexidine seemed the most effective antiseptic to prevent cutaneous infection prior to insertion of an intravascular device in a prospective randomized comparative trial.[31,32]

SOURCES

Chlorhexidine is a synthetic chemical.

TOXIC DOSE

Acute

Chlorhexidine gluconate 4% was used by an adult as a mouthwash and then swallowed. The patient recovered.[29] A newborn ingested chlorhexidine sprayed onto the breasts of the mother. She survived.[29] Chlorhexidine gluconate (0.025 g/100 mL) was inadvertently heated in a newborn incubator; parachloroaniline, a decomposition product, was inhaled. The babies were then moved and recovered.[28] An 89-year-old inadvertently ingested 30 mL of chlorhexidine gluconate 4%, remained asymptomatic, and survived. The chlorhexidine dose was 15.18 mg/kg of body weight.[33] Accidental feeding of newborn breast-fed babies with a solution of chlorhexidine 0.05% and cetrimide 1% in place of sterile water resulted in severe symptoms (see Clinical). All survived.[17] Ingestion of 30 g (150 mL) of chlorhexidine gluconate led to hepatotoxicity. The patient survived.[34] Accidental intravenous administration of chlorhexidine was followed by survival. Administration of 2000 mg of chlorhexidine hydrochloride daily for 7 days was not associated with any adverse effects.[35] One patient developed hemolysis and required exchange transfusion.[35]

TOXICOKINETICS

Chlorhexidine gluconate 4% is strongly adsorbed on the skin surface and may not be removed by 70% isopropyl alcohol wash.[36] Neonates exhibited blood levels of 53 to 607 ng/mL 1 hour after a chlorhexidine wash.[36] A newborn who ingested chlorhexidine sprayed on the mother's breast had a serum chlorhexidine concentration of 11 pg/L at 120 hours.[31] Parachloraniline, a decomposition product, has not been detected in the urine of animals or man.[35]

PREGNANCY/LACTATION

The dose of chlorhexidine sprayed on the mother's breast as a mastitis preventative was 430 µg. Over 24 hours (assuming six feeds) 2.5 mg was delivered to the breast and could be ingested by the baby.[31]

CLINICAL PRESENTATION

Chronic Toxicity

Gastrointestinal

Repeated ingestion of chlorhexidine gluconate 4% by an adult led to repeated episodes of vomiting. Fiberoptic gastroscopy showed multiple erosions in the stomach and duodenum with an active atrophic gastritis.[29] The patient recovered.[29]

Cardiac

A newborn ingested chlorhexidine that was used on the mother to prevent possible mastitis. This was followed by cyanotic spells and sinus bradycardia (by electrocardiogram), which responded to atropine. Chlorhexidine spray was withdrawn, and the neonate improved with cessation of bradycardia after 6 days.[31]

Hepatic

Ingestion of chlorhexidine gluconate 150 mL (30 g) by an adult was followed by pharyngeal edema, high aminotransferase blood levels, and a diffuse fatty degeneration and lobular hepatitis of the liver.[34]

Pulmonary

Babies accidentally fed chlorhexidine 0.05% with cetrimide 1% developed superficial erythema and edema of the lips, mouth, and tongue that appeared to be due to caustic burns. They were fretful and restless. One baby developed an acute pulmonary edema with prominent oral frothing. All survived without sequelae.[17]

Allergic Reactions

Urticaria, pruritus, rash, occupational asthma, dyspnea, and anaphylactic shock have followed topical use of chlorhexidine.[37–40] About 0.1% of patients exhibit a cell-mediated immunity response by intradermal testing.[41]

Eyes

Chlorhexidine gluconate 4% may produce corneal damage (bullous keratopathy, epithelial defects, corneal opacification) when applied to the eyes.[30,42]

Ears

Chlorhexidine gluconate may cause progressive sensorineural deafness when it enters the middle ear through a perforated tympanic membrane.[43]

LABORATORY

Analytic Methods

Serum chlorhexidine may be analyzed by gas-liquid chromatography after solvent extraction, acid hydrolysis, diazotisation, and iodination.[36] A high-performance liquid chromatography method is available.[44]

Blood Levels

Serum concentrations of chlorhexidine in a newborn 120 hours after oral exposure to chlorhexidine breast spray were 11 pg/L.[31]

Methemoglobinemia

When chlorhexidine gluconate (0.025 g/100 mL) was inadvertently used as a humidifying fluid for premature baby incubators, parachloraniline, known to be a chlorhexidine spontaneous decomposition product, induced methemoglobinemia in the infants. Methemoglobinemia may follow percutaneous absorption or inhalation of the parachloraniline-containing vapor.[28]

TREATMENT

Stabilization

Treatment is largely symptomatic and supportive. Ingestions should be treated as caustics. Avoid gastric lavage for fear of rupturing ulcerated areas; administer milk feedings.

Antidotes

There are no antidotes.

Elimination Enhancement

There is no data to support the use of elimination enhancement procedures (activated charcoal, cathartics, whole bowel irrigation, hemodialysis, or hemoperfusion) for chlorhexidine poisoning.

Supportive Treatment

Methemoglobinemia may be ameliorated with methylene blue if clinically indicated. Corneal defects should be treated symptomatically. Corneal transplantation may be required.[30]

Occupational

Airway hyperresponsiveness should be treated by removal from the offending site and pulmonary function evaluation with appropriate symptomatic treatment.

CHLOROACETAMIDE

Chloroacetamide is a preservative in cosmetic creams. Toxic effects include contact dermatitis and allergic contact eczema.

CHLOROXYLENOL

Chloroxylenol (Para-chlorometaxylenol; PCMX; 4-chloro-3,5-dimethylphenol) is a common constituent of proprietary disinfectants (e.g., Dettol: 4.8% chloroxylenol with isopropyl alcohol and pine oil) and is regarded to have low or moderate toxicity. Ingestion of 16.8 g of chloroxylenol by an adult led to the rapid development of a profound central nervous system and cardiovascular depression. Treatment included an intravenous line, oxygen, gastric lavage, dopamine for the hypotension, and verapamil for a nodal tachycardia. Consciousness began to return in 6 hours. The patient recovered. Minute amounts of free chloroxylenol were present in the urine, but no chloroxylenol was found in the blood. Large amounts of conjugated chloroxylenols were present in the urine.[45] Respiratory failure (ARDS), laryngeal edema, bronchospasm, gastrointestinal hemorrhage,[46] and skin sensitizing effects have been reported.[47]

CRESOL (LYSOL)—CRESYLIC ACID, CRESOL (ALL ISOMERS)

CHEMICAL AND PHYSICAL CHARACTERISTICS[48]

Cresols have a CAS number of 119-97-3, 95-48-7, 10-39-4, and 106-44-5. The chemical formula is $CH_3C_6H_4OH$. The OSHA permissible exposure limits are 5 ppm (33 mg/m^3) on skin. Synonyms include cresylic acid, tricresol, methylphenol, o-cresol, m-cresol and p-cresol.[49–51] The cresols are alkyl (derivatives of phenol).[52] The para isomer is a liquid; the orthdal meta isomers are crystalline. The odor of cresol is recognized at concentrations of 5 ppm. Lysol is an approximately 50% (v/v) solution of mixed cresols in soap solution.

ORAL

Ingestion of cresols leads to extensive corrosive effects and widespread systemic toxicity to the vascular system, liver, kidneys, and pancreas.

A 74-year-old woman was found unconscious and died in 1 hour. Postmortem examination revealed extensive mucosal desquamation of the lower third of the esophagus and stomach, both of which were bleached white. A strong odor of Lysol was detected. A 76-year-old woman swallowed an unknown quantity of Lysol, was found in a coma, and died in 2 hours. Mixed cresol concentration in the blood in both fatal cases were 190 μg/mL and 71 μg/mL, respectively.[53]

A 62-year-old woman ingested about 150 mL of Lysol solution. She became drowsy and confused. The total blood phenol concentration was 950 μg/199 mL. She was treated with gastric lavage, peritoneal dialysis, 500 mL of 5% sodium bicarbonate solution, hydrocortisone, potassium supplements, and ampicillin. The patient recovered.[54]

A 32-year-old man ingested 50 mL of a solution containing 90% cresols (1.035 g/vol). He remained conscious, became dyspneic, and developed a tachycardia, systolic hypotension and respiratory failure, myocardial failure, and pulmonary edema. He died on the fourth day after he had been hemodialyzed and had been given sodium bicarbonate, intravenous potassium, dextrose and insulin, a dopamine drip, and a forced diuresis with furosemide. Total serum phenols were 90 μg/mL.[55] (A total phenol level of 10 μg/mL has been suggested to be of serious prognostic significance.)[55]

A 2½-year-old child splashed cresol over his face and forehead, his upper chest, and back of his left hand and wrist. He recovered after scrubbing with propylene glycol.[52]

Lysol disinfectant is a mixture of cresol (50%) in saponified linseed oil, potassium hydroxide, and water. It is a yellowish or brownish liquid of syrup consistency and is strongly alkaline. The cresols are the most important alkyl derivatives of phenol. There are three isomers—orthocresol, metacresol, and paracresol, which differ a little in their antiseptic properties. Their bactericidal potency is about three times that of phenol. Like phenol, cresol is a derivative of coal tar.

DOSAGE

About 20 mL of a 90% cresol solution accidentally poured over an infant's head resulted in chemical burns, cyanosis, unconsciousness, and death within 4 hours. Pathologic examination of the tissues revealed a hepatic necrosis, cerebral edema, acute tubular necrosis of the kidneys, and hemorrhagic effusions from the peritoneum, pleura, and pericardium. The blood cresol concentration was 120 μg/mL.[56] All organs had the strong odor of cresol.

USES

Cresols are used as antiseptics, disinfectants, insecticides, resins, and plasticizers. Their bactericidal potency is about three times that of phenol.[52]

SKIN

Following skin contact a burning sensation, erythema, skin peeling, localized anesthesia, and occasionally ochronosis, darkening of the skin, have been seen. A hypersensitivity response may be observed.

CLINICAL PRESENTATION

All isomers of cresol cause skin and eye burns. Renal impairment, hepatotoxicity, and central nervous system and cardiovascular disturbances have also been observed.

Cresols may be converted to gluconol and catechol, which give a characteristic dark color to the urine.[52]

Ingestions of 4 to 120 mL of 25 to 50% cresol result, immediately or within 10 minutes, in a feeling of nausea; within 15 minutes, a burning sensation is felt in the mouth, throat, esophagus, and epigastrium. On the skin cresol leaves a red burn. Burns and scalding with cresol are potentially lethal.[52,57] Burns are seen on the lips, gums, tongue, cheeks, pharynx, and tonsils. Blisters may form followed by a painful sloughing of the mucous membrane. Hoarseness or aphonia may develop. Coma comes on quickly and may last for over 12 hours, accompanied by hypothermia. Stricture rarely forms in the gastrointestinal tract.[58] Acute pancreatitis may be seen.[59]

Renal Failure

Death after some days may follow acute renal failure.[60,61]

Attempted Intrauterine Abortions

Intrauterine injection of lysol as an abortifacient has led to shock, coma, and death within 2 hours due to pulmonary oil embolism.[62] Lysol poisoning has been associated with incomplete abortions, shock, tachycardia, leukocytosis, hemolysis, fever, central nervous system irritability, respiratory embarrassment associated with pulmonary edema and/or oil emboli, local tissue necrosis with uterine hemorrhage, and anemia.[63]

Hematologic

Methemoglobinemia, decrease in red cell glutathione, Heinz body formation, and massive intravascular hemolysis may follow ingestion of 100 to 250 mL of lysol.[64] One patient survived after an erythrocytoapheresis.[65]

Inhalation

Following a cresylic acid, methylene chloride, and phenol spill, workers experienced headache, nausea, diarrhea, dizziness, weakness, shortness of breath, blurred vision, abdominal pain, vomiting, and rash. Liver function tests were elevated in many workers. They all survived.[66]

LABORATORY

Analytic

A thin-layer chromatography method is able to identify the phenols and cresol isomers.[67] A high-performance liquid chromatography method with UV detection is able to analyze phenols, cresol, and xylenols in workplace air.[68]

Blood Levels

Cresol blood concentrations of 120 μg/mL followed the rapid death (4 hours) of a 12-month-old infant, which followed the spilling of a 90% cresol solution on the baby's head.[69] An ingestion by an adult of 25 g of cresol led to dyspnea, tachycardia, and hypotension. In 24 hours the serum total phenols were 90 μg/mL (over 10 μg/mL may have serious prognostic significance).[54] Hemodialysis for 8 hours did not significantly alter the phenol concentrations (8 mg/100 mL). The patient developed a hyperpotassemia, chest opacities, and myocardial failure and died.[70] Oxidation may cause cresol to convert to quinol and catechol, which give a characteristic dark color to the urine.

Lethal Dose

The lethal dose of Lysol is about 60 to 120 mL, although lesser amounts have been associated with death.[71]

Abuse

Lysol Disinfectant Spray contains the relatively harmless component o-phenyl-phenol (0.1%) and ethyl alcohol (79%—158 proof). Consumption has become a problem on Indian reservations where the product is mixed with orange juice and drunk by children. The user becomes quite intoxicated.[72]

TREATMENT

Treatment is supportive and symptomatic. There are no antidotes. Skin contact should be immediately washed with large volumes of water, then bathed with polyethylene glycol, propylene glycol or glycerol, vegetable oil, or soap and water. Patients may require resuscitation procedures, ventilatory support, and volume replacement.

ETHYLENE OXIDE

Ethylene oxide is used to chemically sterilize heat-sensitive materials in the hospital setting.[73–75] It is also used in the production of ethylene glycol, polyesters, and detergents.

Ethylene oxide, which is a colorless gas with a distinctive, sweet, etherlike odor, is used to sterilize medical instruments, particularly those made of heat-labile materials. This compound is regulated by OSHA as a carcinogen. Ethylene oxide is typically supplied to United States hospitals in compressed gas cylinders that contain 88% freon and 12% ethylene oxide, or in single-dose cartridges of 100% ethylene oxide[73] (Tables 57–2 and 57–3).

Workers in central supply, dental operations, and surgical suites who use ethylene oxide are at risk of potential exposure. In 1983 OSHA estimated that approximately 62,370 workers were directly exposed to ethylene oxide and that 25,000 others may have been incidentally exposed in United States hospitals. An estimated 7700 ethylene oxide sterilizers are in operation in 6300 hospitals in the United States.[73]

The typical source of ethylene oxide exposure in the hospital environment is through the operation of sterilizing equipment. Unless good engineering controls and good work practices are used, workers may encounter relatively high concentrations of ethylene oxide over relatively brief periods. Data suggest the need to control short-term peak exposures to ethylene oxide.

OCCUPATIONAL EXPOSURE

The OSHA PEL for ethylene oxide is an 8-hour TWA of 1 ppm with an excursion limit of 5 ppm for any 15-minute period. The NIOSH REL for ethylene oxide is a ceiling of

Table 57–2
Work Practice Guidelines For Ethylene Oxide Sterilizers: Post Above Ethylene Oxide Supply Cylinders[a]

DANGER!
ETHYLENE OXIDE
CANCER AND REPRODUCTIVE HAZARD

1. Before changing cylinders, make sure the local exhaust ventilation for the cylinder is working.
2. When changing cylinders, wear a full faceshield, protective gloves, and other protective clothing as required by OSHA (29 CFR 1910.1047).
3. Before disconnecting the supply line from the cylinder valve, relieve excess pressure by venting the supply line into the ventilation system.
4. In case of an ethylene oxide leak or other emergency, evacuate the area and initiate the emergency response plan. **DO NOT RE-ENTER THE AREA WITHOUT A SUPPLIED-AIR RESPIRATOR!**

[a]Adapted from Ref. 65 of the Current Intelligence Bulletin 52, National Institute for Occupational Safety and Health, HH5, July 13, 1989.

5 ppm for no more than 10 minutes in any working day, and an 8-hour TWA less than 0.1 ppm.[73,74]

CLINICAL PRESENTATION

Acute Toxicity

Although ethylene oxide has an odor threshold of about 700 ppm, exposure at 200 ppm may cause irritation of the eyes and upper respiratory system. Exposure of humans to high levels of ethylene oxide results in skin lesions, mucous membrane irritation, nausea, vomiting, headache, convulsions, and death.[73] Contact with ethylene oxide sterilized equipment or wrapping that has not been adequately aerated to remove residual ethylene oxide may cause severe burns with large blisters and peeling skin. Healing may leave hyperpigmentation (brownish discoloration of the skin). In renal hemodialysis patients (ethylene oxide used to dry-sterilize artificial kidney), platelet-pheresis donors (ethylene oxide–sterilized kits used) and hemophiliacs, ethylene oxide–mediated hypersensitivity reactions may be potentially lethal.[76]

Chronic Toxicity

Carcinogenic Status

Ethylene oxide is a mutagen and animal carcinogen and probably a human carcinogen.[77–79] It is a highly reactive epoxide and is a direct alkylating agent.[80] A study of 18,254 workers exposed to ethylene oxide at 14 plants producing sterilized medical supplies suggests a trend toward an increase in hematopoietic cancer with increasing lengths of time since first exposure.[80]

Neurologic

Data on chronic exposure to ethylene oxide suggest an increased tendency to cognitive decline,[81] a reversible sensorimotor neuropathy of the distal axonopathy type[81,82] and certain neuropsychologic deficits[75,83] suggestive of central nervous system dysfunction. Further studies will be required to define these deficits.[84,85]

Table 57–3
Work Practice Guidelines For Ethylene Oxide Sterilizers: Post by Sterilizer[a]

DANGER!
ETHYLENE OXIDE
CANCER AND REPRODUCTIVE HAZARD

1. Be sure that the sterilizer ventilation system is operating before the sterilizer is started and while the sterilizer is operating.
2. Use in-chamber aeration when possible.
3. If a sterilizer load must be transferred to an aerator, take the following precautions:
   a. After the sterilizer completes the required number of purge/aeration cycles, keep the load in the sterilizer for as many additional purge/aeration cycles as time allows.
   b. Make sure the local exhaust ventilation above the sterilizer door is working.
   c. Open the sterilizer door to the notched position (or 2 inches if there is no notched position) and leave the area for 15 minutes.
   d. Perform the load transfer as quickly as possible and keep the load as far away from your face as possible.
4. In case of an ethylene oxide leak or other emergency, evacuate the area and initiate the emergency response plan. **DO NOT RE-ENTER THE AREA WITHOUT A SUPPLIED-AIR RESPIRATOR!**

[a]Adapted from Ref. 65 of the Current Intelligence Bulletin 52, National Institute for Occupational Safety and Health, HH5, July 13, 1989.

LABORATORY

Analytic Methods

Determination of level of 2-hydroxyethyl adducts to the *N*-terminal valines in hemoglobin serves as a suitable biomonitor.[86,87]

TREATMENT

NIOSH recommended respiratory protection for ethylene oxide is summarized in Table 57–4.[88] Work practice guidelines are presented in poster forms (Tables 57–2 and 57–3). Engineering controls are recommended by NIOSH as follows:

1. The sterilizer should be enclosed either in a mechanical access room or a cabinet, and the enclosure should be exhausted to a dedicated ventilation system. A dedicated exhaust system is one that serves the sterilizer area only and routes ethylene oxide directly to the outside of the building at a location where prevailing winds will not carry the exhaust into populated areas or into the air intakes of other buildings.
2. Sterilizing operations should be centralized and access to sterilizer rooms should be restricted.
3. The sterilizer should be checked with the infrared analyzer at least once every 3 months.
4. Floor drains should have a cover with an antisiphon air gap. The air gap, at the junction of the vacuum pump discharge line with the floor drain, should be enclosed. Dedicated exhaust ventilation should be provided for the enclosure.
5. Local exhaust ventilation sufficient to effectively remove ethylene oxide should be as close as possible to the type of the sterilizer door.

6. The number of exhaust cycles recommended by the sterilizer manufacturer should be completed before the door is opened; the door should remain only slightly open for at least 15 minutes.
7. Supply cylinders should be located in a ventilated enclosure (either a ventilated cabinet or a hood that covers the point where the cylinder is connected to the sterilizer supply line).
8. Aerators and overpressure relief valves (if present) should be vented to a dedicated exhaust system.
9. Sensors should be provided to identify a ventilation failure and to detect ethylene oxide. Both audible and visual alarms should be activated by the sensors.
10. Ventilation air from the sterilizing room should not be recirculated.
11. Exhaust gases should preferably be vented directly to the outside of the building (away from intake vents); this procedure is strongly recommended for all sterilizers.
12. Sterilized material and its packaging should be aerated in aeration cabinets, since approximately 5% of the ethylene oxide in the sterilizer remains in these items. Aeration times depend on the composition, form, and weight of the material. Refer to the recommendations from the Association for the Advancement of Medical Instrumentation and follow the manufacturer's recommendations for each type of equipment sterilized. Materials that do not absorb ethylene oxide (metal and glass) need no aeration unless they are wrapped.
13. Sterilizers that use glass ampules in a plastic bag (flash bag) have a high potential for worker exposure to ethylene oxide. If they are used, all sterilization procedures should be conducted in a ventilated enclosure.

Protective Equipment

A worker should use protective gloves and splash-proof goggles and/or a face shield when changing ethylene oxide supply cylinders. If good engineering controls are used (i.e., if the cylinder is located in a ventilated hood), a respirator should not be necessary. If a respirator is necessary or desired, the worker should use a chemical cartridge respirator with an end-of-service-life indicator that has been approved by NIOSH/NSHA. The end-of-service-life indicator is needed because the odor threshold for ethylene oxide is about 700 ppm, and failure of the adsorbent material will not be detected by the user.

Protective gloves and long-sleeved garments should be worn when removing items from the sterilizer or transferring them to the aerator.

When cleaning up liquid spills that contain ethylene oxide, workers should wear protective outer clothing and dispose of or launder it immediately afterward. If leather shoes become contaminated with ethylene oxide, they should be discarded.

A positive-pressure, self-contained breathing apparatus should be available for emergency situations and should be stored in an area away from the sterilizer and the ethylene oxide supply location.

Work Practices

Sterilizers should be operated only by personnel trained in sterilization procedures and in the health and safety hazards of ethylene oxide. If local exhaust ventilation has been provided above the sterilizer door, a worker should open the door slightly and step away for an established period. The period should be determined by monitoring and should be at least 15 minutes. The door opening should be smaller than the capture distance of the hood.

To clean the sterilizer (especially the back surfaces), a worker must often reach inside the chamber with the whole upper body. Ethylene oxide exposure during this cleaning can be controlled by (a) scheduling the cleaning activity as long as possible after processing a load, (b) leaving the sterilizer door fully open for at least 30 minutes before cleaning, and (c) wearing a respirator.

Table 57–4
NIOSH Recommended Respiratory Protection for EtO [a]

Condition	Minimum Respiratory Protection [b,c]
Airborne concentration of <0.1 ppm	No respirator required
Airborne concentration of 0.1 to 5 ppm	Any air-purifying, full-facepiece canister respirator that provides protection against EtO and is equipped with an effective end-of-service-life indicator (ESLI), or Any self-contained breathing apparatus (SCBA) equipped with a full facepiece, or Any supplied-air respirator (SAR) equipped with a full facepiece
Airborne concentration ≥5 ppm, or planned or emergency entry into unknown environments	Any SCBA equipped with a full facepiece and operated in a pressure-demand or other positive-pressure mode, or Any SAR equipped with a full facepiece and operated in a pressure-demand or other positive-pressure mode in combination with an auxiliary SCBA operated in a pressure-demand or other positive-pressure mode
Firefighting	Any SCBA equipped with a full facepiece and operated in a pressure-demand or other positive-pressure mode
Escape only	Any air-purifying, full-facepiece canister respirator that provides protection against EtO and is equipped with an effective ESLI, or Any appropriate escape-type SCBA

[a]Adapted from Ethylene Oxide Sterilizers in Health Care Facilities. Current Intelligence Bulletin 52. July 13, 1989.
[b]Only NIOSH/MSHA-approved equipment should be used.
[c]The respiratory protection listed for any given condition is the minimum required to meet the NIOSH REL of 5 ppm (9 mg/m^3) for no more than 10 min/day or <0.1 ppm (0.18 mg/m^3) as an 8-hr TWA.

Medical Monitoring

Employers should obtain preemployment baseline data on workers who will be handling ethylene oxide. This information should include data on the eyes, skin, blood, and respiratory tract. Periodic examinations thereafter should include the following organs and systems:

Organ or system	Suspicious symptoms
Skin	Rashes, cracking, burns, blisters
Eyes	Swelling or irritation
Respiratory system	Breathing difficulty, nose or throat irritation, prolonged or dry cough, chest pains, wheezing
Neurologic system	Drowsiness, numbness or tingling of hands or feet, weakness or lack of coordination, headaches
Reproductive system	Spontaneous abortions, birth defects

FORMALDEHYDE

PHYSICAL AND CHEMICAL CHARACTERISTICS

Synonyms for formaldehyde include formalin, methyl aldehyde, and methylene oxide. The chemical formula is HCHO. At room temperature formaldehyde is a colorless gas with a pungent, irritating odor detectable at about 0.5 ppm. Commercially available formalin is a 37 to 50% aqueous solution of formaldehyde that contains up to 15% methanol to inhibit polymerization.

SOURCES

This highly reactive compound with wide commercial and medical applications is a commonly used disinfectant, tissue preservative, and feedstock for synthetic chemical processes. Formaldehyde is ubiquitous in our environment as a contaminant of smoke and as photochemical smog. Industrial uses include the manufacture of urea formaldehyde foam, paint pigment, and plastic molding. The formaldehyde processes produce wrinkle-free, crease-resistant textiles.

Medical uses include a disinfectant, antiseptic, deodorant, tissue fixative, and embalming agent. In industrial hygiene surveys, mean formaldehyde levels are highest in hospital autopsy rooms compared with other commercial settings. Formaldehyde is also found in plastics, dyestuff, textiles, fertilizer, paper, and foundry and tanning industries. Particle board, gas appliances, and carpeting may release formaldehyde vapor indoors. Moisture and heat causes decomposition of formaldehyde-containing products into formaldehyde vapor. Release of these vapors in mobile homes has been associated with headache and pulmonary and dermal irritation. Except after thermal degradation in fires, polyurethane foam does not release formaldehyde vapor.[89]

Urea formaldehyde foam insulation (UFFI) consists primarily of polymers of urea and formaldehyde in combination with numerous other chemicals. Free formaldehyde may be released during the initial reaction and through decomposition depending on temperature, humidity, and acid content of the foam. UFFI contributes free formaldehyde to the indoor air (average formaldehyde level in homes with UFFI was 0.049 ppm compared with 0.034 ppm in control homes), but the level decreases over 1 to 3 years to control values.[90] The adverse health effects of UFFI remain controversial since studies demonstrating excessive symptoms in exposed patients lack methodologic criteria (e.g., temporality, strength and consistency of association) for evidence of causation.[91]

Table 57–5
Acute Human Health Effects of Formaldehyde at Various Concentrations[a]

Reported Effects	Formaldehyde Concentration (ppm)
None reported	0.0–0.5
Neurophysiologic effects[b]	0.05–1.5
Odor threshold	0.05–1.0
Eye irritation[c]	0.01–2.0
Upper airway irritation	0.10–25
Lower airway and pulmonary effects	5–30
Pulmonary edema, inflammation, pneumonia	50–100
Death	>100

[a]Adapted from Sannet JM, Marbury MC, Spengler JD. Am Rev Respir Dis 1988;137:221:242.
[b]As measured by determination of optical chronaxy, electroencephalography, and sensitivity of dark-adapted eyes to light.
[c]The low concentration (0.01 ppm) was observed in the presence of other pollutants that may have been acting synergistically.

Cigarettes

Formaldehyde is a major oxidation byproduct of combustion processes, including tobacco smoking. It is produced in both the mainstream and sidestream smoke. Formaldehyde exposure appears to be in the range of 1.5 to 1.95 ppm/puff. The cumulative daily dose is about 188 to 2400 μg.[92] Cigarettes or marijuana are dipped in formaldehyde ("amp") before smoking because of its alleged hallucinogenic effect. Encephalopathy, rhabdomyolysis, pulmonary edema, and coma has followed the ingestion of two "amp"–dipped cigarettes.[93]

ACUTE TOXIC DOSAGE (TABLE 57–5)

Ingestion

Both death and survival from 4-oz formalin ingestions have been reported in adults.[94] The probable mean lethal adult dose is 1 to 2 oz. Death may occur within 3 hours; survival past 48 hours usually means recovery.

Ingestion of formalin may lead to extensive gastrointestinal corrosive damage, circulatory shock, metabolic acidosis, respiratory insufficiency, and acute renal failure associated with high plasma levels of formic acid, the main metabolite of formaldehyde and hyperlactatemia. Methanol blood levels also increase.[95,96]

Table 57–6 summarizes dose-response relationships following the ingestion of formaldehyde by humans.

Inhalation[89]

Standards and Recommendations

The OSHA Standard for formaldehyde is 1 ppm as an 8-hour TWA with a ceiling concentration of 2 ppm as a 15-minute, short-term exposure limit.[97] The NIOSH REL for formaldehyde is 0.1 ppm as determined in any 15-minute air sample and 0.016 ppm as an 8-hour TWA. The ACGIH has designated formaldehyde as a suspected human carcinogen and has recommended a TLV of 1 ppm (1.5 mg/m^3) as an 8-hour TWA with a short-term exposure limit (STEL) of 2 ppm (3 mg/m^3). Even a short period of exposure will decrease the worker's ability to smell it. Odor is not a reliable warning for the presence of formaldehyde.[98]

Many people experience conjunctival (0.01 to 0.05 ppm) and pulmonary (0.03 to 3 ppm) irritation below 1 ppm. However, a controlled study of formaldehyde gas (3 ppm or less) in patients with suspected formaldehyde-induced asthma revealed no decrease in FEV_1 or aggravation of asthmatic symptoms.[99] Effects of chronic low-dose exposure are relatively unknown, but concern exists because formaldehyde is an animal carcinogen and potent sensitizer. Severe respiratory tract irritation and dyspnea occur after exposure to levels higher than 10 ppm.

Dermal

Concentrations of formaldehyde liquid exceeding 300 ppm may cause clinical irritation.[100] In lower concentration in certain individuals, formaldehyde can combine with proteins in the epidermis (e.g., Langerhans' cells) to produce a hapten-protein complex capable of sensitizing T lymphocytes. Subsequent exposures cause a type IV hypersensitivity reaction (i.e., allergic contact dermatitis).

CLINICAL PRESENTATION

Acute Inhalation

Formaldehyde is a mild sensory irritant and potent sensitizer to which some people are more sensitive than others. Although the concentration generally is too low to cause symptoms in home environments, some low-dose formaldehyde exposure of UFFI home inhabitants does result in headache, rhinitis, and dyspnea.[101] At exposure levels of 1 to 4 ppm, formaldehyde is a strong mucous membrane irritant, producing burning and lacrimation. For sensitive individuals, formaldehyde is a potent allergen, causing asthma and dermatitis. Cough, chest pain, dyspnea, and wheezing occur frequently in individuals exposed to 5 to 30 ppm.

Ingestion

Patients present early with severe corrosion of the gastrointestinal tract and systemic effects. Inflammation and ulceration of mouth, esophagus, and stomach result in severe abdominal pain, diarrhea, and vomiting, which may progress to strictures. Severe acidosis results from rapid conversion of formaldehyde to formic acid. Coma, hypotension, renal failure, and apnea complicate severe ingestions.

CHRONIC EFFECTS

Cancer

Formaldehyde is a mutagen and animal carcinogen, but its relationship to occupational cancer is unclear. Rats exposed to 6 to 15 ppm of formaldehyde develop squamous cell carcinomas of the nasal passages, and the inhalation of hydrogen chloride induces squamous cell nasal carcinomas in rats.[102] Formaldehyde causes intracellular DNA damage of the bronchial epithelium.[103] A 57-year-old man developed squamous cell cancer of the nasal cavity after 25 years of occupational exposure to formaldehyde.[104] Two British occupational studies failed to detect significant increases in nasal or lung cancer,[105,106] although an excess lung cancer rate did occur. The British study included 7716 men in the formaldehyde industry from 1965 to 1982. A retrospective

Table 57–6
Dose-Response Relationships Following the Ingestion of Formaldehyde by Humans[a]

Amount of HCHO Ingested (mg)	N	Time Before Treatment	Responses
10,000 (100 cc)	1	Several hr	Severe epigastric pain, passed black stool; dysphagia, stenosis, and corrosive destruction of the stomach
8800 (240 ml of 37%)	1	45 min	Severe pain, ulceration, and stenosis of stomach, dysphagia
50–8214 (Few drops to 7.5 oz)	12	Various	Gastrointestinal pain, corrosion of tissues of contact organs, respiratory burns
6000 (150 ml of 40%)	1	Immediate	Death, edema of glottis, asphyxia
2200–2400	1	45 min	Cyanosis; low temperature; shallow respiration; weak, rapid, and irregular pulse
1665 (1½ oz formalin)	1	1 hr	Cyanosis, vomiting, dry mucous membranes in mouth and throat, weak and irregular pulse, shallow respiration
1200 (120 ml of 10%)	1	?	Gastric shrinkage and contracture after 3 mo
555–600 (0.5 ml of 37–40%)	1	24 hr	Coma, recovery with treatment
555–600 (½ oz formalin)	1	?	Dry and sore throat, vomiting
100–200 daily in milk for 3 weeks	11	—	Headache, stomach pain, burning sensation in throat, rash on chest and thighs in 4 of the 11
22–200 daily	2	—	Mild gastric and pharyngeal discomfort

[a]Adapted from NIOSH Criteria for a Recommended Standard of Occupational Exposure to Formaldehyde. DHEW (NIOSH) Publication No 77-121.

American study of the deaths of 256 garment workers who were involved in the manufacture of formaldehyde-treated clothes revealed no nasal cancers, but an increased incidence of cancer of the buccal cavity and multiple myelomas.[107] A retrospective study of deaths from nasal and paranasal sinus carcinoma in Denmark revealed a slight excess (relative risk 2.3 and 2.2, respectively) of these cancers in men exposed to formaldehyde at work.[108] Concern over the irritant effects and carcinogenic potential of formaldehyde vapor led to a proposed ban on the use of urea formaldehyde foam insulation.[109,110]

Subsequently, the U.S. 5th Circuit Appeals Court (New Orleans) overturned the ban on the basis that the Consumer Product Safety Commission failed to demonstrate that formaldehyde leaching from insulation would cause an unreasonable risk of cancer.[111] Despite widespread use, epidemiologic data have not clearly demonstrated that formaldehyde is a human carcinogen.[112] Conclusions on the carcinogenicity of formaldehyde must await more definitive studies involving larger groups of patients and longer follow-up periods. Formaldehyde is capable of combining with hydrogen chloride to form the potent lung carcinogen, bis(chloromethyl) ether; however, occupational studies indicate that this compound is unlikely to form when both formaldehyde and hydrogen chloride are present in concentrations below the current TLVs.[113]

Preliminary studies of mortality in embalmers and funeral directors by the National Cancer Institute suggest an increase in malignancies of the lymphatic and hematopoietic system. Such data will need confirmation to rule out artifactual associations.[114]

Lung Disease

To date, there is no evidence that prolonged exposure to formaldehyde in the occupational setting causes irreversible chronic obstructive pulmonary disease. Formaldehyde is a respiratory irritant capable of reducing FEV_1 in individuals with hyperreactive airway disease acutely.[115] This compound is absorbed primarily in the upper respiratory tract, but smoking and obligate mouth breathing may deliver formaldehyde-laden particles into the lower respiratory tract.[116] An epidemiologic study of morticians exposed to formaldehyde did not demonstrate any significant increased incidence of chronic bronchitis or reduced pulmonary function.[117]

Sensitization

Repeated exposure to formaldehyde may cause some persons to become sensitized. Sensitization may occur days, weeks, or months after the first exposure. Sensitized individuals will experience eye or upper respiratory irritation or an asthmatic reaction at levels of exposure that are too low to cause symptoms in most people. Reactions may be quite severe with swelling, itching, wheezing, and chest tightness.

Hemodialysis[118]

Patients on maintenance hemodialysis are almost invariably anemic. Although inadequate red-cell production is the predominant mechanism responsible for the anemia, a decrease in red-cell survival is frequently found. Studies suggest that the presence of formaldehyde in the water-filtration system may induce a specific defect in red-cell metabolism leading to a rapid decline in ATP stores. Serious problems (seizures, generalized erythema, cardiac arrest, anaphylactic shock) may follow accidental introduction of formaldehyde during hemodialysis.[119,120]

Anti-N-*Like Antibodies*

Hemodialysis patients are exposed chronically to trace levels of formaldehyde (by formalin sterilization of their dialyzers to permit reuse). Erythrocytes can be characterized in terms of MN phenotypes, analogous to the AB-O system. The normal distribution of MM, NN, and MN phenotypes is about 25, 25, and 50%, respectively. Only 25% of the population would be expected to have anti-*N* antibodies. Formaldehyde exposure may be followed by the development of anti-*N*-like antibodies probably as a result of reaction with the dissolved form of formaldehyde, methylene glycol. The anti-*N*-like antibodies are also found following exposure to sodium hypochlorite.[121]

Neurobehavioral Changes

Disturbances in memory, mood, equilibrium, and sleep, in addition to headache and fatigue, have been reported in occupational and nonoccupational exposure to formaldehyde. Many of these studies have been biased by the approaches used for subject selection and data collection.[116,122]

LABORATORY

Analytic Methods

An analytic procedure has been developed that may permit the specific quantitation of formaldehyde and glutaraldehyde in one sample by HPLC separation. Detection limits for a 5-liter air sample volume are 0.05 mL/m^3 for formaldehyde and 0.02 mL/m^3 for glutaraldehyde.[123]

TREATMENT

Decontamination

Dilution with milk or water in alert patients as a first aid measure may reduce corrosive effects at the scene. If ingestion has occurred within 1 hour before presentation, gentle gastric aspiration with a soft nasogastric tube may limit systemic absorption. There is little evidence to support the use of activated charcoal to absorb formate or formaldehyde.

Engineering Controls[73]

The following engineering controls are recommended to minimize formaldehyde exposure:

1. Local exhaust ventilation should be installed over work stations using formalin or specimens preserved in formalin.
2. Small quantities of formaldehyde should be purchased in plastic containers for ease of handling and safety.

3. Traps should be placed in floor drains.
4. Spill-absorbent bags should be available for emergencies.
5. Engineering controls in hemodialysis units should include (a) isolating the main system from personnel and patients in case of inadvertent spills or (b) disconnecting the dialyzers before the sterilization process is completed. Also, formaldehyde vapors should be prevented from entering the room from the drains serving the main system and the dialysis consoles. The air should be regularly monitored for formaldehyde, and in-service education should be conducted periodically on the effects of formaldehyde.

Protective Equipment

Skin and eye contact with formaldehyde should be avoided. Goggles; face shields; aprons; NIOSH-certified, positive-pressure, air-supplied respirators; and boots should be used in situations where formaldehyde spills and splashes are likely. Appropriate protective gloves should be used whenever hand contact is possible; latex examination gloves are too fragile.

Supportive Care

Preemployment baseline data should be recorded for the respiratory tract, liver, and skin condition of any worker who will be exposed to formaldehyde. Thereafter, periodic monitoring should be conducted to detect symptoms of pulmonary or skin sensitization or effects on the liver.

Elimination Enhancement

Severe acidosis (formate, circulating formaldehyde, methanol) and deteriorating vital signs are indications for considering dialysis, but the literature does not contain adequate case studies to guide treatment. Aggressive sodium bicarbonate therapy and frequent monitoring of arterial blood gases may be useful.

Antidotes

There are no antidotes.

Supportive Care

1. Monitor electrolytes, fluids, acid-base, and kidney function closely.
2. Watch for signs of gastrointestinal hemorrhage and perforation with serial vital signs, abdominal examinations, and complete blood counts.
3. Check blood methanol levels and treat accordingly in formalin ingestions.
4. Fibrosis of stomach has required partial gastrectomy in the past.[124]

GENTIAN VIOLET

Preparations of the dye gentian violet were introduced as an antiseptic in 1890 and have been used for almost 100 years.[125] To date no serious side effects have been reported when gentian violet is used externally. When used as a vermifuge, gentian violet may act as a direct irritant of the gastrointestinal mucosa.[125] It has been added routinely at a concentration of 250 µg/mL at 4°C for 24 to 48 hours to banked blood in different countries in Latin America. No serious side effects have been observed in the more than 100,000 patients transfused with this blood.[126]

In the United Kingdom recommendations have been made that gentian violet not be used on mucous membranes or open wounds and that it be restricted to topical applications on unbroken skin.[127,128] In Australia, the matter is under review.[126] In the United Kingdom the Ministry of Agriculture has also now advised against the use of gentian violet (crystal violet) as a marker for meat and citrus fruits.[128] There have been no reports of oral or intravenous overdose.

Gentian violet has been found to be a potential carcinogen in animals. There have been no reports of cancer following human exposure to this product.

STRUCTURE AND CLASSIFICATION

Gentian violet preparations contain hexamethylpararosaniline chloride (gentian violet or crystal violet) 96%, pentamethylpararosaniline chloride (methyl violet), and tetramethylpararosaniline chloride (brilliant green) 4%. These are all triphenylmethane dyes. Molecular weight is 408.0.[129]

USES

Gentian violet is used as follows[125]:

1. Antiseptic: for the control of fungal infections, to treat the umbilical cord of newborns, for the prevention of infection in burn patients.
2. Anthelmintic.
3. Blood additive: to prevent transmission of Chagas' disease by blood transfusion.
4. Mycostatic agent in poultry feed.
5. Biologic stain (Gram reaction, nucleic acid stain).[130]
6. Dye for silk, wood, cosmetics, and food.

PRODUCT FORMULATION

Gentian violet is available in the United States as a powder and topical solution, 1 and 2%.[131] A preparation known as Bonney's Blue, which contains gentian violet, has long been used as a marker by surgeons involved in cutaneous reconstruction.[132] Bonney's blue has never been associated with a human malignancy.

SOURCES

Gentian violet is a synthetic chemical preparation.

TOXIC DOSES

Therapeutic Doses

One patient received 34 liters of gentian violet–treated blood in 74 reported transfusions within a 6-month period.[125] Another patient received 4 liters of blood at one time. No toxic effects were seen in either case. Ingestion of 6.8 mg/kg of gentian violet by a septicemic adult has led to gastrointestinal irritation.[133] Intravenous administration of 5 mg/kg in an infant with staphylococcic septicemia led to a depression in the white cell count.[133] Up to 8 mg/kg body weight in 0.5% solution was used intravenously with no side effects of bradycardia and hypotension. The patients survived.[133]

FATAL DOSE

There is no fatal dose.

TOXICOKINETICS

Chronic Low Dose

The toxicokinetics of gentian violet have not been studied, but it is known that by one pathway of oxidative metabolism gentian violet is converted by liver microsomes and peroxidase to pentamethyl pararosaniline, and with a further loss of formaldehyde to tetramethyl pararosaniline. By reductive metabolism both in liver microsomes and by *T. cruzi* gentian violet forms a carbon-centered free radical and then, with the help of strict and facultative anaerobes, it forms leucogentian violet.[125]

PREGNANCY/LACTATION

Studies have not been performed with gentian violet in pregnant women or lactating mothers.

MECHANISM OF ACTION

A photodynamic action of gentian violet, apparently mediated by a free radical mechanism, has been described in bacteria and *T. cruzi*. Gentian violet is actively demethylated by liver microsomes in animals and is reduced to leucogentian violet, which appears to be carcinogenic in rats.[131]

CLINICAL PRESENTATION

Gentian violet may cause irritation or sensitivity reactions and ulceration of mucous membranes.[131] Esophagitis, laryngitis, or tracheitis may result from swallowing a solution of gentian violet. Laryngeal obstruction has followed prolonged use of the drug in the treatment of oral candidiasis. Apple packers, wood pulp workers, and dye manufacturers may develop nose bleeds from exposure to dust from gentian violet used as markers.[134] Accidental injection of gentian violet through the urethra resulted in severe hemorrhagic cystitis.[135]

TREATMENT

Treatment of the toxic effects of gentian violet administration should be symptomatic and supportive. There are no antidotes.

GLUTARALDEHYDE

Glutaraldehyde is commonly used as a sterilizing agent in medical facilities. It is effective as a disinfectant against many microorganisms and viruses, including the HIV viruses,[136] and is usually harmless to medical equipment.[136–138] Glutaraldehyde seems to be a relatively strong irritant to the nose and a severe irritant to the eyes.[139]

STRUCTURE AND CLASSIFICATION

Glutaraldehyde is a saturated dialdehyde with the formula $CHO\text{-}CH_2\text{-}CH_2\text{-}CH_2\text{-}CHO$. It has a molecular weight of 100.12. Synonyms for glutaraldehyde include GTA, glutaral, 1,5-pentanedial, 1,5 pentanedione, glutaric dialdehyde, and Cidex (2% alkaline glutaraldehyde aqueous solution).[140]

STANDARDS

The ACGIH recommended ceiling limit for glutaraldehyde is 0.2 ppm (0.8 mg/m^3). OSHA does not have a PEL for glutaraldehyde and NIOSH has no REL.[141]

USES

Some of the uses of glutaraldehyde are summarized in Table 57–7. Although glutaraldehyde is available in 50, 25, 10, and 2% solutions, most hospitals use 2% glutaraldehyde solutions buffered to pH 7.5 to 8.5 before use. Glutaraldehyde solutions also contain surfactants to promote wetting and rinsing of surfaces, sodium nitrite to inhibit corrosion, peppermint oil as an odorant, and FD&C yellow and blue dyes to indicate activation of the solution. One disadvantage of buffered glutaraldehyde solutions is that they are stable for less than 2 weeks, so solutions must be dated and made as needed. Another disadvantage is that at 20°C (68°F), a 50% solution of glutaraldehyde has a vapor pressure of 0.015 mm Hg and thus can generate an atmosphere that contains as much as 20 ppm of glutaraldehyde. This concentration is well above that shown to cause adverse health effects in animals and humans.[133]

PRODUCT FORMULATION

Cidex is 2% alkaline glutaraldehyde solution.

Table 57–7
Uses of Glutaraldehyde[a]

Sterilizing solution for medical, dental, and barber equipment
Embalming fluid
Leather tanning
Electron microscopy
Preparation of allergy and collagen extract for injection
Photograph and radiograph developing
Preservative in
Cosmetics
Skin care products
Hair care products
Fabric softeners
Medical treatment of
Warts
Hyperhidrosis
Onychomycosis
Epidemolysis bullosa
Herpes simplex

[a]Adapted from Fowler JF Jr. J Occup Med 1989;31:852–853.

TOXIC DOSE

Glutaraldehyde has a pungent odor with a threshold recognition of 0.04 parts per million by volume in air. Eye and respiratory irritation are noted at a level of 0.3 ppm.[142]

OCCUPATIONAL EXPOSURE

Occupational contact dermatitis is frequently observed in health care personnel after exposure to glutaraldehyde.[143] Hand eczema is prevalent.[144] Rubber gloves do not appear to be protective.[145] Glutaraldehyde is both an irritant and sensitizer. It can cause irritation of the eyes, nose, and throat; nausea and headache; epistaxis; and occupational asthma. Palpitation and tachycardia are reversible on cessation of exposure.[146]

PREGNANCY/LACTATION

Glutaraldehyde may produce fetotoxicity in animals.[147]

MECHANISM OF ACTION

Cross-linking of the peptidoglycan in the bacterial cell wall with intermolecular bonding between techoic acid chains and glutaraldehyde may cause a partial sealing and contraction of the outer cell envelope.[148]

CLINICAL PRESENTATION

Glutaraldehyde-containing solutions used as a disinfectant may induce skin irritation, cracking or bleeding, eye irritation, throat discomfort, nasal discomfort, chest tightness, cough, and headache.[134,149] It is a contact irritant and sensitizer.[139] A significant number of embalmers have positive patch test reactions to glutaraldehyde.[150] Mucous membrane irritation may expose the patient to epistaxis.[151]

Proctitis has been reported after the use of glutaraldehyde as a disinfectant of flexible sigmoidoscopes. Within hours of an examination patients may have acute tenesmus and bloody diarrhea. The prognosis is good. Recovery follows in a few weeks.[152]

LABORATORY

Analytic Methods

A high-performance liquid chromatography method enables quantitation of formaldehyde and glutaraldehyde in one sample.[153]

Exposure Control Methods

Workers should avoid breathing glutaraldehyde vapors. They should also be provided with and be required to use splash-proof safety goggles where there is any possibility of contaminating the eyes with glutaraldehyde. To prevent any possibility of skin contact, workers should be provided with and be required to use protective clothing. If clothing becomes contaminated with glutaraldehyde, it should be promptly removed and not reworn until the glutaraldehyde has been removed. The worker who is laundering or cleaning such clothes should be informed of hazardous properties of glutaraldehyde. Skin that becomes contaminated with glutaraldehyde should be washed immediately or showered.[133]

HOSPITAL DISINFECTANTS (TABLE 57–8)

HEXACHLOROPHENE

Hexachlorophene (2,4,6-trichlorophenol) was developed in 1939 and quickly recognized as an effective bacteriostatic agent, particularly against Gram-positive bacteria. By the 1950s hexachlorophene was a common constituent of a variety of cosmetic products, including shaving creams, soaps, shampoos, deodorants, and feminine hygiene agents. Because hexachlorophene is poorly soluble in water and remains on the skin after rinsing, the compound became a popular germicidal agent for surgical care. By the 1960s, case studies documented dermal toxicity after chronic application to both damaged and normal skin, as well as acute toxicity from accidental ingestions. Typically, symptoms involved gastrointestinal distress, lethargy, fever, jitteriness, convulsions, and, in severe cases, coma and death.

Hexachlorophene became a popular antibacterial agent in newborn nurseries, but repeated whole-body bathing of premature infants with 3% hexachlorophene emulsion was associated with vacuolar encephalopathy of the brainstem reticular activating system.[162] Full-term infants appear less susceptible to the toxic effects, perhaps because of lower skin absorption or better metabolism.

In 1972 204 French children developed neurologic toxicity resulting in 36 deaths when a baby talc was contaminated with 6.5% hexachlorophene.[163] In September 1972 the FDA issued a regulation requiring that all hexachlorophene-containing products be sold as prescription drugs. The use of hexachlorophene on full-term newborn infants remains controversial, but there may be no justification for a total ban on hexachlorophene.[164] Powders containing 0.5% hexachlorophene appear to be effective antistaphylococcal agents and result in lower hexachlorophene blood levels than the 3% emulsion.[165]

PRODUCT FORMULATIONS/USES

Hexachlorophene is available as a 3% emulsion and a powder with concentrations ranging from 0.33 to 0.5%. This polychlorinated biphenyl compound is an effective bacteriostatic agent, particularly against Gram-positive bacteria.

TOXIC DOSAGE

Gastrointestinal disorders occur after ingestion of as little as 10 to 20 mg/kg.[166] A neonate who ingested 100 mg/kg developed lethargy, jitteriness, and exaggerated startle responses, but no long-term sequelae persisted.[167] An ingestion of 250 mg/kg by a 6-year-old retarded child resulted in hypotension, convulsions, and death.[168]

Table 57–8
Hospital Disinfectants[154]

Endoscopic equipment	*Reliable*[155]
Fibre-endoscope	Glutaraldehyde (aqueous alkaline) 2%—10 to 30 minutes (between patients)
	Ethylene oxide: not for between patient procedures; best on patients with hepatitis B, tuberculosis, typhoid fever
	Povidone-iodine 2–4 minutes between patients
	Succindialdehyde 10%—10 minutes (hepatovirucidal)
	Buffered hypochlorite—rapidly germicidal and hepatovirucidal; can damage endoscope
	Not reliable[155]
	Quaternary ammonium compounds
	Chlorhexidine
	Chlorhexidine-cetrimide mixtures
	Alcohol
	Isopropyl alcohol
	Hexachlorophane
	Cresol
Recovered permanent pacemakers	Formaldehyde
	Glutaraldehyde
	Dimethylbenzyl ammonium chloride + ethylene oxide, formaldehyde, glutaraldehyde
	Ethylene oxide alone[156]
Creutzfeldt-Jacob virus	0.5% hypochlorite
	Povidine-Iodine[157]
	Reliable
Hepatitis B virus inactivated	Boiling 1 minute
	Steam autoclaving
	Ethylene oxide gas sterilization
	Glutaraldehyde 2%
	Formaldehyde 8%
	Sodium hypochlorite 0.5%
	Not reliable
	Phenolics
	Hexachlorophene
	Quaternary ammonia compounds[123]
	Spillage of HIV blood, body fluid excretion onto surfaces[158]
Human immunodeficiency virus	Glutaraldehyde 2% (freshly activated)
	Phenolic disinfectant 2%
	Hypochlorite solution, freshly prepared with 10,000 ppm "available" chlorine
	Minor Surface Contamination[159]
	Hypochlorite solution with 1,000 ppm "available chlorine"
	Phenolic disinfectant 1% with alcohol 70%,
	Isopropyl alcohol 7%,
	Glutarldehyde 2%, as alternatives
	HIV contaminated bronchoscopes, gastroscopes[160] and other lensed instruments
	Ethylene oxide sterilization
	Glutaraldehyde 2% soak for 45 minutes[156]
Viral hemorrhage fevers	*Disinfection of materials in contact*[161]
	Phenolic disinfectants 1–5%
	Disinfection with no gross contamination
	Hypochlorite solution with 1,000 ppm "available chlorine"
	Visible blood or vomit
	Hypochlorite solution with 10,000 ppm "available chlorine"
	Activated glutaraldehyde 2%
	Internal disinfection of isolators, ambulances, residential premises
	Formaldehyde vapor fumigation

PHARMACOKINETICS

Absorption

Hexachlorophene toxicity occurs via both the dermal and gastrointestinal routes. Small (less than 1200 g), premature (under 35 weeks gestation) infants and those with damaged skin or hepatorenal dysfunction are particularly susceptible to dermal toxicity after daily 3% hexachlorophene baths. Fatalities occurred after the acute ingestion of hexachlorophene by adults and the chronic dermal application of 3% hexachlorophene emulsion to neonates with severe skin defects (burns, severe ichthyosis).[169,170] Only small amounts of hexachlorophene penetrate intact human skin of full-term neonates[171] and children.[172]

Elimination

Hexachlorophene is both metabolized by the liver to glucuronide conjugates and excreted by the kidney unchanged, but the kinetics in humans have not been well studied. The elimination half-life in neonates washed daily with 3% hexachlorophene ranged from 6.1 to 44.2 hours and followed first-order kinetics.[159] Hepatic dysfunction, low birth weight, and prematurity increased the elimination half-life.

PATHOPHYSIOLOGY

The exact mechanism of toxicity is unclear. Neurologic symptoms in neonates after acute exposure probably result from cerebral edema.[173] Pathologic lesions consist of spongiform changes confined to the myelinated white matter. Characteristic empty vacuoles formed by the splitting and separation of the myelin lamellae give this lesion the name *vacuolar encephalopathy.* The rostrocaudal distribution of the vacuolation appears age related, with the medullary portion of the reticular activating system involved primarily in premature infants and the mesencephalic portion involved primarily in full-term infants.[162] Although children display vacuolation of diffuse areas of the cerebellum and cerebrum, autopsies of adult patients revealed no cerebral lesions.[170] Vacuolization of the white matter is not a lesion unique to hexachlorophene toxicity. It is produced by a number of drugs and chemicals, including isoniazid, triethyl tin, cuprizone, and phenelzine.[174]

CLINICAL PRESENTATION

The signs and symptoms of toxicity depend on the length and type of exposure, as well as the age of the patient. Gastrointestinal distress and an encephalopathy characterize hexachlorophene toxicity.

Oral Toxicity

Within several hours of large ingestions patients develop nausea, vomiting, and diarrhea, which may progress to dehydration and hypotension.[167] Later, neurologic signs, including lethargy, facial twitching, fever, blurred vision, blindness, hyperreflexia, convulsions, and coma, appear and peak within 12 to 18 hours. Cardiac dysrhythmias, apnea, and cardiac arrest occur as the final event, 48 to 60 hours postingestion.[173] Symptoms begin to diminish by the third day.

Dermal Toxicity

Topical applications produce nausea, vomiting, irritability, diplopia, hypertonicity, anorexia, weakness, and fever. In severe cases, papilledema, retinal hemorrhages, convulsions, coma, and death occur. Infants exposed to 6.3% hexachlorophene-contaminated diaper talc developed an erythematous, ulcerative groin rash that corresponds to the skin lesion produced by high-dose hexachlorophene in rats.[163]

Teratogenesis

Hexachlorophene crosses the placenta in mice and accumulates in neural tissue.[175] An epidemiologic study of women exposed occupationally to hexachlorophene suggested an increased incidence of congenital abnormalities.[176]

LABORATORY

Full-term neonates washed daily with 3% hexachlorophene develop blood levels generally below 0.1 µg/mL (range, up to 0.65 µg/mL). An acute ingestion of 3% hexachlorophene by a 2800-g infant resulted in a 24-hour postingestion blood level of 88 µg/mL, which he survived without sequelae. Deaths have been reported in infants with blood levels of 3 to 16 µg/mL, and survival has occurred in adults with levels between 23 and 74 µg/mL. Generally, clinical effects do not correlate well with blood hexachlorophene levels, and no safe level has been determined for premature infants.[177]

TREATMENT

Stabilization

Seizures and respiratory depression are the immediate life-threatening problems. Diazepam is the drug of choice and usually controls seizures. Follow arterial blood gases and respiratory rate closely in severe poisonings. Hypotension may result from dehydration and may respond to fluid and electrolyte replacement.

Decontamination

Within the first several hours patients who ingest hexachlorophene in doses larger than 10 to 20 mg/kg should receive the usual measures of decontamination (ipecac/lavage, charcoal, cathartics). Activated charcoal does not absorb hexachlorophene.[178]

Elimination Enhancement

Peritoneal dialysis did not remove significant amounts of hexachlorophene after an accidental ingestion.[179] Both hemoperfusion and serial activated charcoal are potential therapeutic modalities, but neither has been tested clinically.

Supportive Care

Follow fluid and electrolyte status. Severely poisoned patients should be monitored for several days in an intensive care setting to watch for the development of dysrhythmias, hypotension, and apnea.

HYDROGEN PEROXIDE

In 1900 hydrogen peroxide accounted for 8177 exposures in the United States.[180] Most hydrogen peroxide exposures involve the common household strength (3%) and are usually benign. Ingestion of concentrations greater than 10% can result in disastrous sequelae.[181] Deaths following ingestion are rare.

STRUCTURE AND CLASSIFICATION

1 ppm = 1.41 mg/m^3
Molecular weight 34.0

The 1990 NIOSH/OSHA TWA 1 ppm—up to 10-hour workday during a 40-hour workweek. Seventy-five ppm is considered immediately dangerous to life and health.[182] Concentrated hydrogen peroxide is a superficially corrosive agent with a pH of 8.0.[183]

USES

Hydrogen peroxide is a useful disinfectant that has also been used for removal of inspissated meconium,[184] demonstrating rectovaginal fistulae and in the therapy of constipation or fecal impaction.[185] Radiologists have employed H_2O_2 to aid in eliminating gas from the intestine during roentgenography of abdominal viscera and as a mixture with barium to identify the exact site of gastrointestinal hemorrhage under fluoroscopy, since blood bubbles form when in contact with hydrogen peroxide. It has been recommended as a disinfectant for tonometer tips, ophthalmic instruments, and trial contact lenses to prevent the transmission of viruses, especially human immunodeficiency virus.[186]

Low concentrations of H_2O_2 (3 to 9%) have been used in the treatment of inflammatory conditions of the external auditory canal.[187] and as a mouthwash or gargle. Hydrogen peroxide has been applied in root canals of teeth or other dental pulp cavities. Topically it has been used as a vaginal douche solution. More potent solutions (20 to 30%) are used as hair bleaching and tooth bleaching agents.[188] In 90% strength it may be used in the synthesis of compounds, as a bleaching agent for textiles and paper, and in rocket fuel.[189]

The U.S. Food and Drug Administration has indicated that industrial-strength hydrogen peroxide is illegally promoted as "35% Food Grade Hydrogen Peroxide" to be diluted and used in "Hyperoxygenation Therapy" for AIDS, cancer, and other conditions. The liquid is purchased in bulk from chemical plants in Texas and Mexico and repackaged into small containers for redistribution. The products are sometimes called "Biowater" and "H_2O_2" and are sold by some "health food" outlets. This concentration is not approved by the U.S. FDA for any therapeutic purpose.[190,191]

PRODUCT FORMULATION

Topical concentrate, 30.5% w/w gel 1.5% (Peroxyl Oral Spot Treatment), and solution, 1.5% (Peroxyl mouth rinse—with alcohol 6%) and 3%.[131]

Hydrogen peroxide topical solution is a clear, colorless liquid that is odorless or has an odor resembling ozone. It contains 2.5 to 3.5 g of hydrogen peroxide per 100 mL. The concentrate contains 29 to 32% w/w hydrogen peroxide. H_2O_2 is a strong oxidant. Each 1% w/w of hydrogen peroxide is equivalent to 3.3% by volume; 100 volume hydrogen peroxide is approximately equivalent to 30% w/w, 30 volume to 9% w/w, and 10 volume to 3% w/w, respectively.[188] H_2O_2 deteriorates on standing, repeated agitation, or exposure to light. It is also available in the United Kingdom commercially as 3, 6, 27, and 30% solutions.[192]

TOXIC DOSE

Inhalation of 90% hydrogen peroxide induces lung inflammation in animals.[193] Men accidentally exposed to 90% H_2O_2 vapor experienced an increased flow of saliva, scratchy feeling of the throat, and respiratory passage inflammation.[193] Serious lung damage is not expected in humans exposed to white fumes given off by 90% H_2O_2 when it is brought into contact with a heavy metal or one of its salts.

OCCUPATIONAL EXPOSURE

An adult exposed chronically to an aerosol of H_2O_2 at a concentration of 41 mEq/m^3 (1 ppm = 1.41 mg/m^3—NIOSH/OSHA TWA) developed chronic diffuse interstitial lung disease.[155]

MECHANISM OF ACTION

Cellular Damage

At the cellular level, hydrogen peroxide–induced DNA damage appears to involve a role for transition metal ions bound to DNA, which may interact with H_2O_2 resulting in the production of a reactive radical species, most likely OH. This radical species found close to the DNA interacts with DNA forming purine and pyrimidine products characteristic of those found after the exposure of aqueous DNA solutions to ionizing radiation.[194]

Clinical

The "snow white" color change (mucosal whitening and frothy bubbles) in the colonic mucosa seen after topical application arise secondary to penetration by hydrogen peroxide into the epithelial interstices and capillaries, with the subsequent production of microbubbles of molecular oxygen causing the blanching. Blood is forced out of the intramural vasculature and replaced by oxygen in a reaction mediated by tissue catalase.[185]

CLINICAL PRESENTATION

Irrigation of Wound Under Pressure[195]

Hydrogen peroxide decomposes to water and oxygen. When used in closed spaces or under pressure (as 3% H_2O_2) liberated oxygen cannot excape. Systemic oxygen embolization.[196–199] and surgical emphysema[200] may occur. Cina and coworkers[201] have described factors that should be considered for the diagnosis of hydrogen peroxide ingestion:

- Age at Risk. Between 1 and 3 years (or older if retarded).
- History. Found with open container of hydrogen peroxide; white foam issuing from mouth, nose, and/or anus; wound cleaned with hydrogen peroxide; or recent peroxide enema.
- Amount Ingested. Probably >2 to 4 ounces of a 3% solution.
- "Clinical" Diagnoses. Shock, acute coronary insufficiency, sudden infant death syndrome, respiratory arrest, status epilepticus, cerebrovascular accident, or sepsis.
- Radiologic Findings. Gas in the mesenteric, gastric, splenic, or portal venous systems; with or without gastric and duodenal distension; or with or without gas in the inferior vena cava (IVC) and right ventricle.
- Gross Findings. Gastric distension; "frosty coating" of gastrointestinal tract; gastritis, duodenitis, and/or colitis; frothy blood in the portal veins, IVC, right ventricle, and/or neck veins; crepitus of the liver; visceral congestion; petechiae of the thymus, epicardium, and, possibly, other viscera; or cerebral edema.

- Microscopic Findings. Gastritis, duodenitis and/or colitis; acute visceral congestion; clear vacuoles in the submucosa of the gastrointestinal tract; clear vacuoles in the gastrointestinal veins, lymphatics, mesenteric lymph nodes, or mucosal-associated lymphoid tissue; or other organ vacuolization (gas emboli).
- Toxicologic Analysis. No foreign substances detected in the blood, gastric contents, and container.
- Cultures. Negative for pathogens. Pneumoretroperitoneum has been described.[202]

Irrigation of the Colon and Ileus

Oxygen embolization of the small intestinal veins and lymphatics may occur during irrigation of the ileum with 1% hydrogen peroxide. Air bubbles are seen with initiation of instillation of the hydrogen peroxide and persist for about 30 minutes.[203] Hydrogen peroxide (1%) used as lavage for meconium ileus in an infant caused mesenteric and portal vein gas embolism and death.[195] Acute ulcerative colitis may follow use of hydrogen peroxide enemas.[204,205] This colitis can mimic pseudomembranous colitis.[206] Peroxide proctitis has been observed.[207]

Oral Ulceration

Excess use of hydrogen peroxide (3%) with and without concomitant use of sodium bicarbonate and salt as a mouth rinse may be abrasive to soft tissues of the gums.[208]

Corneal Damage—Soft Lens Disinfection

Use of 3% H_2O_2 to disinfect soft contact lenses may lead to stinging, tearing, hyperemia, blepharospasm, edema, and possibly permanent corneal damage.[209] An applanation tonometer tip soaked in H_2O_2 solution may cause corneal damage.[186,210–212]

Hydrogen Peroxide in Closed Body Cavities

Swabs soaked in hydrogen peroxide, with 20 mL of H_2O_2 injected down a cannula in a total hip arthroplasty, have led to severe circulatory collapse and cardiac arrest.[213]

H_2O_2 Poisoning by Ingestion—Household Strength (3 to 9%)

Ingestion of household strength peroxides are mildly irritating to the mucous membranes and may result in spontaneous emesis or mild abdominal bloating.[181]

Industrial Strength (Over 10%)

Ingestions of industrial strength peroxides can result in severe burns of the oropharynx and gastrointestinal tract, with the possibility of rupture of the hollow viscus secondary to the liberation of oxygen. The foam may cause obstruction of the respiratory tract and may result in mechanical asphyxia. Respiratory failure has been the alleged cause of death in fatalities reported after oral ingestion of industrial-strength (over 10%) hydrogen peroxide.[214,215]

TREATMENT

Stabilization

1. Early aggressive airway management is critical because respiratory failure and arrest appear to be the proximate cause of death.
2. On admittance to any emergency facility an intravenous line oxygen and cardiac monitor should be immediately available. Arterial blood gases should be obtained. Where required, the patient should be endotracheally intubated, given oxygen, mechanically ventilated, and have cardiac massage as required.
3. Prepare for early onset of seizures.
4. Begin intravenous fluids. Watch intake and output. Do not fluid overload. These patients die of respiratory insufficiency and arrest.

Decontamination

Under endotracheal lavage, gastric lavage may be attempted with iced saline. Activated charcoal, cathartics, or other gut decontamination procedures have not been shown to be useful after ingestion of industrial-strength hydrogen peroxide.

Elimination Enhancement

There are no procedures that will enhance the elimination of hydrogen peroxide except for those surgical procedures required after vascular occlusion by the peroxide.

Antidote

There are no antidotes.

Supportive Measures

Hydrogen peroxide poisoning is generally treated with symptomatic and supportive measures.

Seizures

Diazepam IV; phenytoin, if recurrent seizures. Obtain computer tomography scan of the brain.

Coma

Usual coma therapeutic measures: naloxone, thiamine, 50% dextrose.

Metabolic Acidosis

Sodium bicarbonate IV.

Esophagogastroduodenoscopy

Perform early after admission and follow up in 48 hours. Antacids may be used for gastric burns, depending on an opinion of a gastroenterologist following endoscopy.

Laparotomy

May be required where there is evidence of air in the gastrointestinal tract.

Monitor Intracranial Pressure

Hyperventilate as required.

X-ray of Abdomen

Look for air in the liver area.

IODINE

Topical iodine-containing solutions used in excess as antiseptic agents may lead to metabolic acidosis, hyperchloremia, hypernatremia, hyperosmolarity, and renal failure with a fatal termination. Iodine may result in poisoning by (a) the oral ingestion of iodine or its alcoholic solution; (b) the oral ingestion of the salts of iodine, which occasionally result in iodism; (c) the inhalation of the fumes into the upper and lower respiratory tract; (d) absorption of the tincture from a cyst into which it has been injected; and (e) the absorption of alcoholic solutions or povidone-iodine solutions applied to the skin or to body cavities.[216]

Iodine excesses may arise from dietary supplements (infant transient hypothyroidism resulting from maternal ingestion of iodine in a prenatal supplement); iodine excess from oral drugs (e.g., potassium iodide) that have resulted in deaths in hyperthyroid patients; iodine from topical medications (antiseptics); iodine excess from injected iodinated contrast media; iodine excess during pregnancy and lactation; and intentional excess iodine ingestion, which may result in corrosive gastroenteritis, ventricular irritability, large tender salivary glands, hyperthyroidism, hemolytic anemia, metabolic acidosis, seizures, and acute renal failure, and which may end fatally.[217–220]

STRUCTURE AND CLASSIFICATION

Elemental iodine, I_2, is a topical antiseptic effective at concentrations equal to or over 0.5 ppm (50 μg/100 mL). Iodophors, solutions of complex iodine-containing anionic and nonionic detergents, contain low free-iodine levels in the range of 0.8 to 1.2 ppm (80 to 120 μg/100 mL).[221] Betadine prep solution (10% povidone-iodine) is an iodophor of iodine, polyvinylpyrrolidine (PVP), and detergent. It is considered as a povidone-iodine solution (PIS). Betadine surgical scrub[222] is 7.5 povidone-iodine. Pharmadine[223] is a 10% povidone-iodine solution (1% free iodine). Ioprep solution is an aqueous iodophor with 1% available iodine.[224]

USES

Povidone-iodine (polyvinylpyrrolidine iodine) is a water-soluble antiseptic used in various concentrations for operative site preparation, hand cleansing, and wound antisepsis. Its role in intraperitoneal lavage remains to be defined.[225]

PRODUCT FORMULATION (TABLE 57-9)

Iodine is available in the United States for topical use as a solution of iodine 2% and sodium iodide 2.4%, and as a tincture of iodine 2% and sodium iodide 2.4% with alcohol 47%.[226] Iodine is also available as iodine insufflation: iodine 0.8, potassium iodide 0.4, anesthetic ether 10, and lactose, in fine powder 98.8; non-staining iodine ointment: iodine 5% w/w; nonstaining iodine ointment with methyl salicylate: methyl salicylate 5% v/w in nonstaining iodine ointment; Lugol's solution: aqueous solution of iodine 5 g, potassium iodide 10 g in water × 100 mL; compound iodine paint: iodine 1.25 g, potassium iodide 2.5 g, water 25 mL, peppermint oil 0.4 mL, alcohol (90%) 4 mL, glycerol to 100 mL; strong iodine solution iodine: 10 g, potassium iodide by water 10 ml, alcohol (90%) to 100 mL; strong iodine tincture: iodine 7 g, potassium iodide 5 g, water 5 mL, alcohol to 100 mL; weak iodine solution: iodine 2.5 g, potassium iodine 2.5 g, water 2 to 5 mL, alcohol (90%) to 100 mL.[227]

Povidone-iodine is available as povidone-iodine 5%—(Betadine Cream); povidone-iodine 10%—Betadine Medicated Gel, Medicated Douche, Medicated Vaginal Suppositories and Medicated Ointment Solution; povidone-iodine 7.5%—Betadine Skin Cleanser, Surgical Scrub[226]; Massengill Medicated Disposable Douche, Medicated Liquid Concentrate.

Table 57-9
Iodine Content of Some Iodine-Containing Medications and Radiographic Contrast Agents[a]

Substance	Amount of Iodine
Expectorants	
Iophen	25 mg/ml
Organidin (iodinated glycerol)	15 mg/tablet
Par Glycerol	5 mg/ml
R-Gen	6 mg/ml
Iodides	
Potassium iodide (saturated solution)	~25 mg/drop
Pima syrup (potassium iodide)	255 mg/ml
Lugo's solution (potassium iodide + iodine)	~7 mg/drop
Iodo-Niacin	115 mg/tablet
Antiasthmatic drugs	
Mudrane	195 mg/tablet
Elixophyllin-KI (theophylline) elixir	6.6 mg/ml
Iophylline	2 mg/ml
Antiarrhythmic drugs	
Amiodarone	75 mg/tablet
Antiamebic drugs	
Iodoquinol	134 mg/tablet
Topical antiseptic agents	
Povidone-iodine	10 mg/ml
Clioquinol cream	12 mg/g
Douches	
Povidone-iodine	10 mg/ml
Radiographic contrast agents	
Iopanoic acid	333 mg/tablet
Ipodate sodium	308 mg/tablet
Intravenous preparations	140–380 mg/ml

[a]From Surks MI, Sievert R. N Engl J Med 1995;333:1688–1694.

SOURCES

Iodine is a nonmetallic element. Povidone-iodine is a synthetic compound.

TOXIC DOSE

A 52-year-old man was accidentally exposed to 250 mL of povidone-iodine. He later died.[228] A 74-year-old woman absorbed about 800 mL of one-quarter strength Betadine solution and developed a cardiac arrest that was fatal.[221] An 83-year-old woman had gauze packs soaked with 10% povidone-iodine solution containing 1% free iodine packed into her wounds every 4 hours for 3 to 5 weeks. She died.[219] The rectum of a 3-month-old boy was irrigated with a warmed aqueous iodophor containing 1% free iodine. The child survived.[224] A 72-year-old male had a povidone wash twice daily for 6 months for decubitus ulcers of the sacral and ankle regions and developed thyrotoxicosis.[229] Very low birth weight infants subjected to use of 10% povidone-iodine solutions for insertion of intravenous cannulae and blood gas determinations developed hypothyroidism.[230,231]

FATAL DOSE

The minimum lethal dose of iodine in humans is unknown. The fatal dose of iodine has been reported as from 2 to 4 g of free iodine or 1 to 2 ounces of strong iodine tincture.[216] An enema of 50 mL of povidone iodine delivered to a 9-week-old infant led to death.[232]

OCCUPATIONAL EXPOSURE[98]

Iodine can be found throughout the hospital. The OSHA PEL for iodine is a ceiling of 0.1 ppm (1.0 mg/m^3) (29 CFR 1910.1001). The ACGIH recommends a TLV of 0.1 ppm (1.0 mg/m^3) as a ceiling. NIOSH has no REL for iodine.

To prevent skin contact with solids or liquids containing iodine, workers should be provided with and required to use personal protective equipment such as gloves, face shields, and any other appropriate protective clothing deemed necessary.

If there is any possibility that clothing has been contaminated with solid iodine or liquids containing iodine, a worker should change into uncontaminated clothing before leaving the work area. Clothing contaminated with iodine should be stored in closed containers until provision is made to remove the iodine. The person laundering or cleaning such clothes should be informed of iodine's hazardous properties.

Skin that becomes contaminated with solids or liquids containing iodine should be immediately washed with soap or mild detergent and rinsed with water. Workers who handle solid iodine or liquids containing iodine should wash their hands thoroughly with soap or mild detergent and water before eating, smoking, or using toilet facilities.[98]

TOXICOKINETICS

Absorption

The absorption of iodine has not been associated with any particular form of povidone-iodine. The occlusive nature of an ointment or the greater absorption of a povidone-iodine solution would be expected to enhance iodine absorption.[223]

Pregnancy/Lactation

Studies on the use of iodine-containing solutions as antiseptics or disinfectants in pregnant or lactating women have not been performed. Iodides do cross the placenta and are excreted in breast milk.[227]

MECHANISM OF ACTION

Metabolic acidosis, hyperchloremia, hypernatremia, hyperosmolarity, and renal failure have been associated with elevated serum iodine concentrations.[223] The metabolic acidosis may be due to the acidic pH (2.43) of the povidone-iodine or to the consumption of bicarbonate by the combination of free iodine with serum sodium bicarbonate: $6\ NaHCO_3 + 3I_2 \rightarrow 5\ NaI + NaIO_3 + 6\ CO + 3H\ O$[233] Hyperchloremia probably represents spurious elevations in the serum chloride due to the interference with the assay by iodine. Elevations in serum osmolality may result from the osmotic effects of free iodine in the blood.

CLINICAL PRESENTATION

Metabolic acidosis, hyperchloremia, hypernatremia, hyperosmolarity, diminished anion gap, and renal failure may follow excessive absorption of iodine from topical iodine-containing preparations. Clinical hypothyroidism, hyperthyroidism, changes in sensorium (agitation, confusion, hallucinations), stomatitis, and diarrhea have been observed. Hypotension, tachycardia, cyanosis, and shock are consistent with iodine toxicity.[224]

Early clinical signs of acute systemic iodine/iodide toxicity may stem from the stimulation of exocrine gland secretions producing rhinorrhea, conjunctivitis, and a serous exudate cough that may begin within 6 hours after a povidone-iodine solution is begun.[221] In the late preterminal phase a high anion-gap metabolic acidosis (lactic acid mediated), acute respiratory distress, and congestive heart failure may intervene.[221]

LABORATORY

Analytic Methods

Serum may be analyzed for I_2 and 1^- moieties utilizing the known iodine-catalyzed reduction of ceric ammonium sulfate by arsenious oxide.[234] Serum chloride determinations made by the Technician STAT/ION autoanalyzers result in false elevations in serum chloride levels in a nonlinear fashion.[223] In the presence of elevated iodine concentrations, the silver halide precipitation assay should be used for an accurate measurement of serum chloride concentration.

Blood Levels

The extent of iodine absorption appears to be related to the size of the area of application.[235] Serum iodine concentrations ranged from 590 to 1400 μg/dL (normal 0 to 3) after application of povidone-iodine ointment to burns of 0 to 15% total body surface area (TBSA); from 910 to 2390 μg/dL in

15 to 30% TBSA burns, and from 1200 to 4900 μg/dL in over 30% TBSA burns.[235] Continuous irrigation of the hip led to serum levels of 7000 μg/dL and death.[221] Irrigation of the rectum of a 3-month-old child with an aqueous iodophor containing 1% iodine led to a serum level of 51,000 μg/dL (normal 2.5 to 9.0 μg/dL) and a cardiac arrest from which he recovered.[224] A serum level of 48,000 μg/dL was accompanied by fatal cardiopulmonary arrest.[236] There are no studies of clinical correlations with serum iodine determinations, and the actual concentration at which toxic symptoms may occur is unknown.

Abnormalities

Transient hypothyroidism (increased serum thyroid stimulating hormone [TSII], decreased T_4 levels) from iodine absorption has been reported in a newborn with omphalocele, after irrigation of ostomy sites in infants, following topical application to wound dehiscence, and after cutaneous application.[224] Elevated iodine levels have been reported following application of povidone-iodine to intact skin and umbilical cords of normal infants, during continuous mediastinal irrigation, after peritoneal irrigation, and in burn patients treated topically with povidone-iodine.[224]

Ancillary Tests

Iodine toxicity may also be associated with elevated serum aminotransferase levels, hyperbilirubinemia, neutropenia, and hypoxemia.[223] Povidone iodine added to a urine sample may be a cause of factitious hematuria (false-positive dipstick).[237]

TREATMENT

Treatment of iodine toxicity from use of iodine or iodophors as antiseptics will be largely symptomatic and supportive.

DECONTAMINATION

Skin

Skin contaminated with excess povidone-iodine should be washed with soap and water. Starch may be applied to ascertain that all of the iodine has been removed (note the blue color). If skin burns develop, observe for metabolic acidosis, renal failure, and altered mental status.[238]

Eyes

Irrigate for 15 minutes with water.

Inhalation

Treat symptomatically.

Elimination Enhancement

There are no studies on the use of modalities such as extracorporeal methods (hemodialysis, hemoperfusion) in the treatment of antiseptic iodine excess.

Table 57–10
Causes of False-Positive Dipstick Hematuria[a]

Age or condition of dipstick
Bacterial peroxidases
Delay between dipstick and sediment microscopy
Hemoglobinuria
Hypochlorite cleansing solutions
Myoglobinuria
Povidone iodine solution

[a]Adapted from Baker MD, Baldassano RN. Pediatr Emerg Care 1989;5: 240–241.

Antidote

There are no antidotes for iodine antiseptic overdosage or for iodine excess after ingestion.

Supportive Measures

Patients who have developed symptoms of antiseptic iodine overdose will be usually seen in a hospital facility where they will then be followed for evidence of metabolic acidosis (arterial blood gases, lactate levels), anion gap abnormalities, hyper- or hypothyroidism, and renal failure.[231,239]

Kidney Function

Causes of false-positive dipstick hematuria are listed in Table 57–10.[237]

ISOPROPYL ALCOHOL (SEE ALSO ALCOHOL CHAPTER)

Ethanol (80%), isopropyl alcohol (70%), and *n*-propanol (50%) preparations have been used for disinfection of hands and skin and in the disinfection of dialysis connectors. Isopropyl alcohol is also used as a solvent, especially in perfumes and cosmetics, and as a vehicle for other germicidal compounds. It is used mostly to disinfect thermometers, needles, and anesthesia equipment.[240,241]

STRUCTURE AND CLASSIFICATION

Isopropyl alcohol is Propan-2-ol; 2-Propanol. Molecular weight of isopropyl alcohol is 60.10 and of acetone 58.08. Conversion factors for isopropanol are mg/dL × 0.1664 = mmol/L; mmol/L × 6.010 = mg/dL and for acetone mg/dL × 0.172 = mmol/L; mmol/L × 5.81 = mg/dL.[225]

STANDARDS

The OSHA PEL for isopropyl alcohol is 400 ppm (980 mg/m^3) as an 8-hour TWA (29 CFR 1910, 1000). The NIOSH REL for isopropyl alcohol is 400 ppm (984 sq/m^3) for up to a 10-hour TWA with a ceiling of 800 ppm (1968 mg/m^3) for 15 minutes. The odor of isopropyl alcohol may be detected at concentrations of 40 to 200 ppm.[242]

PRODUCT FORMULATION

Isopropyl Rubbing Alcohol (USP) contains 68 to 72% v/v of isopropyl alcohol.

OCCUPATIONAL EXPOSURE[228]

Workers should be provided with and required to use appropriate protective clothing such as gloves and face shields to prevent repeated or prolonged skin contact with isopropyl alcohol. Splash-proof safety goggles should also be provided and required for use where isopropyl alcohol may contact the eyes.

Any clothing that becomes wet with isopropyl alcohol should be removed immediately and reworn only after the compound has been removed. Clothing wet with isopropyl alcohol should be stored in closed containers until it can be discarded or cleaned. The worker who is laundering or cleaning such clothes should be informed of isopropyl alcohol's hazardous properties.

Skin that becomes wet with liquid isopropyl alcohol should be promptly washed or showered.

Adequate exhaust ventilation must be supplied in the hospital to remove isopropyl alcohol vapor in the work area.

CLINICAL PRESENTATION

Isopropyl alcohol has provoked symptoms of central nervous system toxicity when used as an antiseptic rectally after anal intercourse[243] or as a suicide attempt.[244] When premature babies (weighing 750 g or less) who have suffered from severe perinatal asphyxia, hypothermia, and acidosis are exposed to 70% isopropyl alcohol applied to the umbilical area, respiratory insufficiency and death may supervene within 48 hours, despite mechanical ventilation and other supportive measures.[245,246] The use of towels soaked in rubbing isopropyl alcohol applied topically on infants to reduce fever may lead to profound central nervous system depression.[247] When isopropyl alcohol was accidentally placed on the humidifier of a 37-week gestation infant with congenital defects, cyanosis, bradycardia, and asystole followed with high blood levels of isopropyl alcohol and acetone.[248]

LABORATORY

Blood Levels

A child who had extensive second-degree body burns due to scalding was treated with isopropyl alcohol soaks. She was found dead 27 hours later. Postmortem isopropyl alcohol levels in the blood and urine were 50 mg/dL and 30 mg/dL, respectively, with acetone levels of 50 mg/dL in both blood and urine.[249]

TREATMENT

Treatment of isopropyl alcohol intoxication, when it is used topically either inadvertently or as an antiseptic, is symptomatic and supportive. There are no antidotes.

Application of cotton soaks with a total of 175 mL of rubbing alcohol (70% isopropyl alcohol) over 3 weeks to the umbilicus of a 21-day infant resulted in hypotonia, lethargy, waxing and waning of consciousness, and urine concentrations of 39 mg/dL of isopropyl alcohol and 76 mg/dL of acetone 7 hours after admission. About 17 hours after admission the isopropyl alcohol concentration was 8 mg/dL and the acetone concentration, 203 mg/dL. With cessation of application the baby recovered in 2 days.[250]

KATHON CG

Kathon (CG = cosmetic grade) is the proprietary name for a family of microbicides and preservatives containing as active ingredients a mixture of methylchlorisothiazolinone and methyl isothiazolinone in an approximate ratio of 3:1.[251] Kathons are promoted as preservatives and biocides. It appears that Kathon CG has been responsible for a high number of cosmetic-related allergic contact dermatitis cases in a number of countries.[252–254]

MERCURIALS

Phenylmercuric acetate, phenylmercuric nitrate, nitromersol, thimerosal, mercurochrome, mercurobutol, and merthiolate are used as preservatives in eye drops, eye ointments, vaccines, and other products and in skin disinfection, treatment of skin infections, contraceptive jellies, and hemorrhoidal treatments.

A thimerosal-preserved hydrophilic gel contact lens left residual mercury in the cornea and aqueous humor. The concentration was similar to that reported in systemic poisoning by organic mercurials. Pooled human immunoglobulin with thimerosal preservative has raised urine mercury concentrations. Contact sensitization may occur. Eye drops with phenylmercuric nitrate used for 6 years left a brownish melanoid pigmentation on the anterior capsule of the lens.

MERCUROCHROME

Ingested mercurochrome (a mouthful) has been associated with nausea, vomiting, abdominal pain, and dizziness. Urine and blood mercury levels are elevated.[255] Magarey[256] suggests that many exposures are only a few drops leaking from a lid, and these often look worse because of the bright red color spilt on a child's face. Nevertheless, it seems that substantial absorption can take place via the oral route and caution is needed when "mouthful" quantities have been swallowed by young children.

THIMEROSAL

Thimerosal is a sodium salt of mercury that may be incorporated as a preservative in nasal drops. Hypersensitivity reactions with erythema, papular or vesicular eruption, allergic conjunctivitis, and anosmia have followed their use.[257] The U.S. FDA has proposed barring all nonprescription antiseptic products containing mercury compounds.[258]

PARAHYDROXYBENZOATE ESTERS (PARABENS)

Methyl, ethyl, propyl, butyl, and benzoyl esters of *p*-hydroxybenzoic acids are preservatives in pharmaceuticals, 0.1 to 0.3%; in cosmetics and foods, 0.01 to 0.1%. Contact allergy, contact dermatitis, bronchospasm, pruritus, rash, nausea, and vomiting may develop following use of these compounds. Cross-reaction to benzocaine and procaine has occurred.

PHENOL

USES

Phenol has been used for "face peels" by plastic surgeons.[259,260] It is also used in the management of spasticity where neuromuscular junctions are damaged or disrupted (neurolysis) by the injection of a 50 mg/L phenol solution.[261]

Phenolics were among the first disinfectants used in hospitals. Certain detergent disinfectants belong to the phenol group, including phenol, para-tertiary butylphenol (ptBP), and para-tertiary amylphenol (PtAP) They are generally used for a wide range of bacteria, but they are not effective against spores. Phenolics are widely used on floors, walls, furnishings, glassware, and instruments.[242]

TOXICITY LEVELS

The United States exposure standard is 5 ppm (19 mg/m^3) as an 8-hour TWA (skin). The NIOSH REL for phenol is 20 mg/m^3 (5.2 ppm) for up to a 10-hour TWA with a 15-minute delay of 60 mg/m^3 (15.6 ppm). The lethal oral dose is estimated between 10 and 30 g, although an adult survived a 26.7-g ingestion after a stormy course without permanent sequelae.[262] Fatalities have occurred after ingestions with as little as 2 g of pure phenol[263,264] and 4.8 g[265]; the consumption of 0.6 g has produced no symptoms.[266]

TOXICOKINETICS

Absorption

Phenol is absorbed rapidly through the lungs and through the skin. Symptoms develop in 5 to 30 minutes. Dilution of phenol may increase absorption and does increase toxicity in the rat model.[267] The lungs of human volunteers absorbed 60 to 80% of an inhaled phenol dose.[268] Children have died after the application of 5% phenol compresses.[269] Rapid water dilution of phenol burns may increase systemic absorption by decreasing the extent of the coagulum and thus allowing greater penetration.[270]

CLINICAL PRESENTATION

Systemic Effects

Severe toxicity causes rapidly profound central nervous system depression with coma and respiratory arrest. An initial excitatory phase may be seen early. Convulsions may complicate the course of poisoning and have appeared as long as 18 hours after ingestion.[262] Symptoms resolve within 24 to 48 hours. Hypotension and ventricular tachycardia that require vasopressor and antiarrhythmic therapy, respectively, can occur. Chronic exposure to phenol from contaminated well water caused diarrhea, sore throat, pharyngeal sores, and dark urine.[271] Persons may die from oral phenol poisoning without demonstrating pathologic alterations of the gastrointestinal mucosa.[272]

An accidental epidural injection of 6 mg of phenol (30 mL 0.02% solution) did not lead to neurologic damage. When employed for intentional neurolysis a 6 to 7% concentration of phenol is used.[273] Accidental cutaneous exposure (falling into a vat) of phenol resulted in acute renal failure requiring hemodialysis. One year later the patient is still polyuric.[274,275] Renal failure, fever, hypertension, acute respiratory distress syndrome, laryngeal edema, and death can follow cutaneous absorption of phenol.[260,276,277]

Skin

Ingestion of 89% phenol produced moderate erythema and streaky hyperkeratosis but no necrosis or strictures. Some form of cardiac arrhythmias has been observed in up to 50% of cases in which phenol solution was applied to the whole face over a short time.[259,260] A 10-year-old boy developed ventricular dysrhythmias following application of 6 mL (2.5 g) phenol to a giant hairy nevus on the skin.[260] Use of throat spray (Chloraseptic) containing phenol 1.5% may induce local throat burning, acute dyspnea, lethargy, vomiting, stridor, loss of consciousness, angioedema, rash, glossitis, and contact dermatitis.[278,279]

LABORATORY

A microtechnique for quantifying phenol in plasma utilizes gas chromatography–mass spectrometry and is sensitive to 0.1 mg/L.[280] Metabolic acidosis can complicate severe phenol toxicity, but whether the acidosis is a primary or secondary event is not clear. The urine may be dark because of an oxidation product of phenol metabolism. Liver and kidney function tests were normal in a severe acute ingestion.[281] Measured blood phenol levels in those cases were 2.7 and 5.6 mg/dL.

Elimination

Injection of 4 to 10 mL of 7% aqueous phenol as a lumbar or thoracic sympathetic nerve block led to peak serum levels of 3.01 μg/mL in 18.8 minutes for unconjugated phenol. Conjugated phenol peak values were 4.15 μg/mL at 54.9 minutes, further indicating rapid conjugation of phenols in the liver.[282] The maximum steady-state body burden in exposed workers should not exceed 50 mg, and urinary phenol levels above 81 mg/L suggest excessive exposure.[283] This amount (50 mg body burden of phenol in a 10-hour period) could be exceeded when large volumes of phenol-preserved medications are administered, as in a continuous glucagon infusion for treatment of beta-blocker intoxication.[284] Currently, it is recommended that glucagon be preserved with preservative-free normal saline or dextrose 5% in water, instead of the diluent provided when continuous infusions are indicated. Blood phenol levels reached 6.8 μg/mL 1 hour after facial application of phenol 1.5 g in a 50% solution, decreasing to 1 μg/mL at 4 hours.[285] Postmortem plasma phenol concentrations after phenol poisoning have ranged from 27 to 130 mg/L.[286]

TREATMENT

Antidotes

There are no antidotes.

Exposure Control Methods

When working with phenol, workers should be provided with and required to use protective clothing, gloves, face shields, splash-proof safety goggles, and other appropriate protective clothing necessary to prevent any possibility of skin or eye contact with solid or liquid phenol or liquids containing phenol.

If there is any possibility that the clothing has been contaminated with phenol, a worker should change into uncontaminated clothing before leaving the work area and the suspect clothing should be stored in closed containers until it is discarded or until provision is made for removal of the phenol. The worker laundering or cleaning such clothes should be informed of phenol's hazardous properties.

Skin that becomes contaminated with phenol should be immediately washed with soap or mild detergent and rinsed with water. Eating and smoking should not be permitted in areas where solid or liquid phenol or liquids containing phenol are handled, processed, or stored. Workers who handle solid or liquid phenol or liquids containing phenol should wash their hands thoroughly with soap or mild detergent and water before eating, smoking, or using toilet facilities.

Additional measures to control phenol exposure include process enclosure, local exhaust ventilation, and personal protective equipment.

SILVER NITRATE

Silver nitrate may act as an antiseptic, an astringent, or a caustic, depending on the concentration and duration of action. In a concentration of 75% it may be applied by a wooden applicator as a cauterizing agent for the treatment of umbilical granulomas. Chemical burning of the skin of the abdomen may occur after such application.[287] Treatment is symptomatic and supportive (local cleaning, moisturizing agent). (See also Silver in Metals chapter.)

SODIUM HYPOCHLORITE[288]

Sodium hypochlorite (NaClO) is a disinfectant useful both as a household bleach (in a 5.25% solution that effectively inactivates human immunodeficiency virus) and as a topical antiseptic (1%-Dakin) solution. Toxic effects of orally ingested hypochlorite solution are discussed in the Household Products chapter. Parenteral injections of sodium hypochlorite may lead to cardiac rate disturbances from bradycardia to cardiac arrest, hemolysis, and hypokalemia. Treatment is symptomatic and supportive.

EUSOL

Eusol (Edinburgh University Solution of Lime) is one of several hypochlorite solutions widely used in the management of open wounds left to heal without primary closure.[289] Their value remains unproved by controlled clinical studies. Eusol is a chlorinated lime and boric acid solution containing 0.3% w/v of available chlorine and a pH between 7.5 and 8.5. Hypochlorites (including Dakin's solution) are effective for cleaning working surfaces and lavatories and for purifying water. Used topically they may delay healing. Used in full strength Eusol can be an irritant and therefore should not be placed in clean, granulating wounds. It may be useful in treating dirty, necrotic wounds. Evidence that antiseptics or disinfectants like eusol reduce superficial bacterial counts is lacking. Most antiseptics are rapidly inactivated by contact with tissues and body fluids. Only clinical trials will provide an answer to whether dilute solutions can safety retain their effectiveness as an antimicrobial and wound cleaner.[290] (For hypochlorites ingested orally see Household chapter.)

XYLENOL

Xylenol containing disinfectants are used in hospitals for routine cleaning of floors and surfaces. Xylenol poisoning is similar to poisoning with phenol. The very rapid absorption of both these compounds in significant amounts often leads to fatality.[291]

CLINICAL PRESENTATION

An adult ingested a solution containing a mixture of 6 isomeric xylenol in an alcoholic, anxoric detergent base. The patient experienced nausea and vomiting and was barely arousable on admission with constricted pupils and active bowel sounds. Metabolic acidosis, anuria, hypotension, black color in the urine, and death may supervene within 24 hours.

TREATMENT

Treatment is symptomatic and supportive. Gastric lavage may recover some of the disinfectant. Bicarbonate may be administered for a severe metabolic acidosis.

SODIUM DICHLOROISOCYANURATE

Sodium dichloroisocyanurate is used in the United Kingdom as a tablet to sterilize baby bottles. Ingestions of the tablet by children have resulted in laryngeal edema and upper airway obstruction. In the United Kingdom there were 116 and 123 cases of tablet ingestions reported during 1984 and 1985, respectively, in children under 5 years of age.[1] Symptoms mainly involved nausea and vomiting with irritation in the oropharyngeal region. Treatment is symptomatic and supportive.

STRUCTURE AND CLASSIFICATION

Synonyms: Sodium dichloro-s-triazinetrione; sodium troclosene.

USES

Sodium dichloroisocyanurate is used for disinfecting baby bottles, treatment of water in swimming pools, and in various commercial bleach detergents and scouring powders as a stable source of chlorine. As stable sources of chlorine dichloroisocyanuric acid ($C_3HCl_2N_2O_3$, molecular weight 198.0), potassium dichloroisocyanurate (potassium triclosene, trochosene potassium, $C_3Cl_2KN_3O_3$, molecular weight 236.1), and trichloroisocyanuric acid (symclosene, $C_3Cl_3N_3O_3$, molecular weight 232.4) have similar uses.[2]

MECHANISM OF ACTION

Chlorine has a rapid, potent, and brief bactericidal action. Chlorinated isocyanurates in the presence of water produce hypochlorous acid and hypochlorite ion. Lethal action on organisms is due to chlorination of all proteins or enzyme systems by nonionized hypochlorous acid. Sodium dichloroisocyanurate contains about 62% of "available chlorine" and has the actions and uses of chlorine and sodium hypochlorite.[2]

CLINICAL PRESENTATION

Causes of acute laryngeal edema other than infection include abuse of the voice, accidental or surgical trauma, irritating chemical in gaseous form, thermal injury from inhalation of hot gases, ionizing radiation, and allergic reaction. Ingestion of caustic substances may produce pharyngeal and esophageal trauma and may be potentially dangerous to the airway, especially in infants.[3]

Case #1

A 7-month-old child developed a cough, vomited, became drowsy, and developed a cyanosis, pronounced stridor, supraclavicular and subcostal recession, and a tachycardia of 180 beats/minute. The supraglottic area and hypopharynx were grossly edematous and ulcerative. Oral feeding did not resume for 8 weeks. His course was followed by serial endoscopies until he recovered. The trachea and bronchi produced greatly increased amounts of mucus probably due to inhalation of chlorine gas, which is generated when sodium dichloroisocyanurate is dissolved in water.[4]

Case #2

A 7-month-old child swallowed a sterilizing tablet used for cleaning baby bottles. His emesis had an odor of bleach. He developed acute respiratory distress, inspiratory stridor, and intercostal and sternal recession. Intravenous hydrocortisone 100 mg was administered. An endotracheal intubation was followed by a laryngoscopy showing gross edema of the soft tissues of the pharynx and epiglottis. Tracheotomy was performed. Endoscopy disclosed a sloughing ulcer covering two-thirds of the epiglottis, with another ulcer in the posterior pharyngeal wall. A nasogastric tube was passed for feeding. Oral feeding was restarted at 10 days. He was discharged 12 days after admission.[3]

TREATMENT

Treat as a caustic poisoning. Admit to a hospital. Early consultation with an anesthesiologist and otolaryngologist should be sought. Supportive care will usually lead to recovery.

REFERENCES—ANTISEPTICS

1. Reynolds JEF. *Martindale: The extra pharmacopoeia.* 13th ed. London: The Pharmaceutical Press, 1993; pp. 781–805.
2. Reynolds JEF. *Martindale: The extra pharmacopoeia.* 13th ed. London: The Pharmaceutical Press, 1993; pp. 785–786.
3. Handbook of Pharmaceutical Excipients. Washington, DC: American Pharmaceutical Association; London. The Pharmaceutical Society of Great Britain, 1986; pp. 27–28.
4. Beasley CRW, Rafferty P, Holgate ST. Bronchoconstriction properties of preservatives in ipratroopium bromide (Atrovent) nebuliser solutions. Br Med J 1987;294:1197–1198.
5. Zhang YG, Wright WJ, Tam WK, Nguyen-Dang TH, Salome CM, Woolcoch AJ. Effect of inhaled preservatives on asthmatic subjects. II. Benzalkonium chloride. Am Rev Respir Dis 1990;141:1406–1408.
6. Beasley R, Rafferty P, Holgate ST. Adverse reactions to the non-drug constituents of nebuliser solutions. Br J Clin Pharmacol 1988;25:283–287.
7. Akutsu I, Motojima S, Ogata H, Fukuda T, Ikemori R, Makino S. A case of acute benzalkonium chloride intoxication. Jpn J Med 1990;29:239–240.
8. Van Berkel M, de Wolff FA. Survival after acute benzalkonium chloride poisoning. Hum Toxicol 1988;7:191–193.
9. Stoye H, Bittersohl G. Todliche vergiftung durch das desinfecktionsmittel C_4 bei einem kleinkind. Zeitsch f Arztliche Fortbild 1968;62:436–438.
9a. Olin BR, ed. Drug facts and comparisons. St. Louis: Facts and Comparisons 1992, pp. 2307–2308.
10. Wilson JT, Burr IM. Benzalkonium chloride poisoning in infant twins. Am J Dis Child 1975;120:1208–1209.
11. Tiess D, Nagel KH. Beitrag zur morphologie und analytik der invertseifenintoxikation. Zwei todliche vergiftungen durch perorale sufnahine de desinfections mittels. Arch Toxicol 1967;22:333–348.
12. Wolff F. Todliche vergiftung durch trinken des desinfeckionsmittels C_4. Arch Toxikolog 1961;19:8–14.
13. Miezkiel KA, Beasley R, Rafferty P, Holgate ST. The contribution of histamine release for bronchoconstriction provoked by inhaled benzalkonium chloride in asthma. Br J Clin Pharmacol 1988;25:157–163.
14. Gaylord MS, Pittman PA, Bartness J, Tuinman AA, Lorch V. Release of benzalkonium chloride from a heparin-bonded umbilical catheter with resultant factitious hypernatremia and hyperkalemia. Pediatrics 1991;87:631–635.
15. Gershanik JJ, Boecler B, Ensley H et al. The gasping syndrome and benzyl alcohol poisoning. N Engl J Med 1982;307:1384–1388.
16. Anderson CW, Ng KJ, Andresen B et al. Benzyl alcohol poisoning in a premature newborn infant. Am J Obstet Gynecol 1984;148:344–346.
17. Mucklow ES. Accidental feeding of a dilute antiseptic solution (chlorhexidine 0.05% with cetrimide 1%) to five babies. Hum Toxicol 1988;7:567–569.
18. Isomaa R, Reuter J, Djupsund BM. The subacute and chronic toxicity of cetyltrimethyl ammonium bromide (CTAB), a cationic surfactant. Arch Toxicol 1976;35:91–96.
19. Arena JM. Poisoning and other health hazards associated with use of detergents. JAMA 1964;190:56.
20. Davies DM, ed. Textbook of adverse drug reactions. Oxford: Oxford University Press, 1985, p. 653.
21. De Christoforo R, Corden BJ, Hood JC et al. High-dose morphine infusion complicated by chlorbutanol induced somnolence. Ann Intern Med 1983;98:335–336.
22. Bowler GMR, Galloway DW, Meiklejohn BH et al. Sharp fall in blood pressure after injection of heparin containing chlorbutol. Lancet 1986;1:848–849.

23. Salva KM, Kuhn JG. Overdose of morphine sulfate injection during refilling of an implanted infusion pump. Clin Pharm 1987;6:577–580.
24. Windom H, Burgess C, Crane J, Beasley R. Airway effects of inhaled chlorbutol in asthmatic subjects. Thorax 1990;45: 343.
25. Valentour J, Sunshine I. Chlorbutanol poisoning. Report of a fatal case. Z Rechtsmedizn 1975;77:61-63.
26. Borody T, Chinwak PM, Graham GG, Wade DN, Williams KM. Chlorbutol toxicity and dependence. Med J Aust 1979; 1:288.
27. Reynolds JEF, ed. *Martindale: The extra pharmacopoeia.* 13th ed. London: The Pharmaceutical Press, 1993, pp. 788-791.
28. Van der Vorst MMJ, Tamminga P, Wijburg FA, Schutgens RBH. Severe methaemoglobinemia due to para-chloroaniline intoxication in premature neonates. Eur J Pediatr 1990;150: 72–73.
29. Roche S, Chinn R, Webb S. Chlorhexidine-induced gastritis. Postgrad Med J 1991;67:210-212.
30. Tabor E, Bostwich DC, Evans CC. Corneal damage due to eye contact with chlorhexidine gluconate. JAMA 1989; 261:557–558.
31. Quinn MW, Bini RM. Bradycardia associated with chlorhexidine spray. Arch Dis Child 1989;64:892–893.
32. Maki DG, Ringer M, Alvarado CJ. Prospective randomised trial for povidone-iodine, alcohol and chlorhexidine for prevention of infection associated with central venous and arterial catheters. Lancet 1991;338:339-343.
33. Emerson D, Pierce C. A case of a single ingestion of 4% Hibiclens. Vet Hum Toxicol 1988;30:583.
34. Massano G, Ciocatto E, Rosabianca C, Vercelli D, Actis GC, Verme G. Striking aminotransferase rise after chlorhexidine self-poisoning. Lancet 1982;1:289.
35. Rushton A. Safety of Hibitane. II. Human experience. J Clin Periodontal 1977;4:73–79.
36. Cowen J, Ellis SH, McAinsh J. Absorption of chlorhexidine gluconate chlorhexidine gluconate chlorhexidine gluconate chlorhexidine from the intact skin of newborn infants. Arch Dis Child 1979;54:379-383.
37. Waclawski ER, McAlpine LG, Thompson NC. Occupational asthma in nurses caused by chlorhexidine and alcohol aerosols. Br Med J 1989;298:929–930.
38. Okano M, Nomura M, Hata S, Okada N, Sato K, Kitano Y et al. Anaphylactic symptoms due to chlorhexidine gluconate. Arch Dermatol 1989;125:50–52.
39. Wong WK, Goh CL, Chan KW. Contact urticaria from chlorhexidine. Contact Dermatitis 1990;22:52.
40. Moghadam BKH, Drisko CL, Gier RE. Chlorhexidine mouthwash-induced fixed drug eruption. Oral Surg Oral Med Oral Pathol 1991;71:431-434.
41. Seal D, Ficker L, Wright P, Andrews V. The case against thiomersal. Lancet 1991;338:315–316.
42. Varley GA, Meisler DM, Benes SC, McMahon JT, Zakov ZN, Fryczkowski A. Hibiclens keratopathy. A clinicopathological case report. Cornea 1990;9:341–346.
43. Bichnell PG. Sensorineural deafness following myringoplasty operations. J Laryngol Otol 1971;85:957-961.
44. Huston CE, Wainwright P, Cooke M, Simpson R. High performance liquid chromatographic method for the determination of chlorhexidine. J Chromatog 1982;237:457-464.
45. Joubert P, Hundt H, Du Toit P. Severe Dettol (chloroxylenol and terpineol) poisoning. Br Med J 1978;1:890.
46. Chan TYK, Sung JJY, Critchley AJH. Chemical gastroesophagitis, upper gastrointestinal hemorrhage and gastroscopic findings following Dettol poisoning. Hum Exp Toxicol 1995;14:18–19.
47. Chan TYK, Lau MSW, Critcheley JAJH. Serious complications associated with Dettol poisoning. Q. J Med 1993; 86:735–738.
48. Agency for Toxic Substances and Disease Registry. Toxicological Profile for Cresols, July, 1992.
49. Hathaway GJ, Proctor NH, Hughes JP, Fischman ML, eds. Proctor and Hughes' chemical hazards of the workplace. 3rd ed. New York: Van Nostrand Reinhold, 1991; pp 189–190.
50. National Institute for Occupational Safety and Health. Criteria for a Recommended Standard. Occupational Exposure to Cresol. DHEW (NIOSH). Pub N 78-133, p. 117. Washington, DC: US Government Printing Office, 1978.
51. Key MM, Hinschel AF, Butler J, Ligo RN, Tabershaw IR, eds. Occupational Diseases. A Guide to Their Recognition. Revised Edition. Washington, DC: National Institute for Occupational Safety and Health. DHEW (NIOSH). Publication No 77-181. June 1977; pp 246–249.
52. Pegg SP, Campbell DC. Children's burning due to cresol. Burns 1985;11:294–296.
53. Bruce AM, Smith H, Watson AA. Cresol poisoning. Med Sci Law 1976;16:171–176.
54. Thomas BB. Peritoneal dialysis and lysol poisoning. Br Med J 1969;3:720.
55. Arthus GJ, Wise CC, Coles GA. Poisoning by cresol. Anaesthesia 1977;32:642–643.
56. Green MA. A household remedy: misused fatal cresol poisoning following cutaneous absorption (a case report). Med Sci Law 1975;15:65–66.
57. Herwich RR, Treweek DN. Burns form anesthesia mask sterilized in compound solution of cresol. JAMA 1933;100:407–408.
58. Isaacs R. Phenol and cresol poisoning. Ohio St Med J 1922; 18:558-561.
59. Dellal V. Acute pancreatitis following lysol poisoning. Lancet 1931;1:407.
60. Cason JS. Report on three extensive industrial chemical burns. Br Med J 1959;1:827–829.
61. Finzer KH. Lower nephron nephrosis due to concentrated lysol vaginal douche. A report of two cases. Can Med Assoc J 1961;84:549.
62. Vance BM. Intrauterine injection of lysol as an abortifacient. Report of a fatal case complicated by oil embolism and lysol poisoning. Arch Pathol 1945;40:395-398.
63. Presley JA, Brown WE. Lysol induced criminal abortions. Obstet Gynecol 1956;8:368–370.
64. Chan TK, Mak LW, Ng RP. Methemoglobinemia, heme bodies, and acute massive intravascular hemolysis in lysol poisoning. Blood 1971;38:739–744.
65. Cote M-A, Lyonnais J, Leblond PF. Acute Heinz-body anemia due to severe cresol poisoning. Successful treatment with erythrocytoapheresis. Can Med Assoc J 1984;130:1319–1322.
66. Pike S, Shanly EH. An outbreak of disease due to a spill of cresylic acid, methylene chloride, and phenol among scores of postal workers at a mail processing facility at Springfield, OR. Vet Hum Toxicol 1987;29:476.
67. Bieniek G, Wilczok T. Separation and determination of phenol, alpha-naphthol, m- and p-, o-cresols and 2,5-xylenol, and catechol in the urine after mixed exposure to phenol, naphthalene, cresol, and xylenols. Br J Ind Med 1986; 43:570-571.
68. Nieminen E, Heikkila P. Simultaneous determination of phenol, cresol and xylenols in workplace air using a polystyrene-divinyl benzene column and electrochemical detection. J Chromatogr 1986;36:271-278.
69. Green MA. A household remedy misused—fatal cresol poisoning following cutaneous absorption (a case report). Med Sci Law 1975;15:65–66.
70. Arthurs GJ, Wise CC, Coles GA. Poisoning by cresol. Anaesthesia 1977;32:642-643.
71. Pols M, Green L, eds. Clinical toxicology. 3rd ed. London: Pitman Books, 1983, p. 295–296.
72. Acetol lysol to list of abused drugs. The Forensic Drug Abuse Advisor 1991;3(3):19–20.
73. Guidelines for Protecting the Safety and Health of Health Care Workers. U.S. Department of Health and Human Services, NIOSH, Sept. 1988.
74. Ethylene oxide sterilizers in health care facilities. Engineering controls and work practices. Current Intelligence Bulletin 52. NIOSH, USA HHS, July 13, 1989.
75. Estrin WJ, Bowler RM, Lash A, Becker CE. Neurotoxicological evaluation of hospital sterilizer workers exposed to ethylene oxide. Clin Toxicol 1990;28:1–20.
76. Vermylen J, Janssens S, Ceuppens J, Vermylen C. Transfusion reactions in haemophiliac caused by sensitization to ethylene oxide. Lancet 1988;1:594.

77. Hertz-Piccioto I, Neutra RR. Ethylene oxide and leukemia. JAMA 1987;257:2290.
78. Becker CE. Ethylene oxide carcinogenicity. West J Med 1990;152:175.
79. Landrigan PJ, Meinhardt TJ, Gordon J, Lipscomb JA, Burg JR, Mazzukelli LF et al. Ethylene oxide: an overview of toxicologic and epidemiologic research. Am J Ind Med 1984; 6:103–115.
80. Steenland K, Stayner L, Greife A, Halperin W, Hayes R, Hornung R, Nowlin S. Mortality among workers exposed to ethylene oxide. N Engl J Med 1991;324:1402–1407.
81. Crystal HA, Schaumburg HH, Grober E, Fuld PA, Lipton RB. Cognitive impairment and sensory loss associated with chronic low-level ethylene oxide exposure. Neurology 1988; 38:567–569.
82. Schroder JM, Hoheneck M, Weis J, Deist H. Ethylene oxide polyneuropathy: clinical follow-up study with morphometric and electron microscopic findings in a sural nerve biopsy. J Neurol 1985;232:83–90.
83. Klees JE, Lash A, Bowler RM, Shore M, Becker CE. Neuropsychologic "impairment" in a cohort of hospital workers chronically exposed to ethylene oxide. Clin Toxicol 1990;28: 21–28.
84. Katzenstein AW. Ethylene oxide and CNS dysfunction. Clin Toxicol 1991;29:285–288.
85. Becker CE, Lash A. Ethylene oxide—author's response. Clin Toxicol 1991;29:289–292.
86. Sarto F, Tornqvist MA, Tomanin R, Bartolucci GB, Osterman-Golkai SM, Ehrenberg L. Studies of biological and chemical monitoring of low level exposure to ethylene oxide. Scand J Work Environ Health 1991;17:60–64.
87. Fost U, Hallier E, Otterwalder H, Bolt HM, Peter H. Distribution of ethylene oxide in human blood and its implications for biomonitoring. Hum Exp Toxicol 1991;10:25–31.
88. Ethylene oxide sterilizers in health care facilities. Engineering controls and work practices. NIOSH. Current Intelligence Bulletin 52. July 13, 1989.
89. Harris JC, Rumack BH, Aldrich FD. Toxicology of urea formaldehyde and polyurethane foam insulation. JAMA 1981; 245:243–246.
90. Report of the National Testing Survey on Urea Formaldehyde Foam Insulation. Ottawa, Canada: Department of Consumer and Corporate Affairs, 1981.
91. Norman GR, Newhouse MT. Health effects of urea formaldehyde foam insulation: evidence of causation. CMA J 1986; 134:733–738.
92. Godish T. Formaldehyde exposure from tobacco smoke: a review. Am J Pub Health 1989;79:1044–1045.
93. Schutz P, Jones JL, Patten BM. Encephalopathy and rhabdomyolysis from ingesting formaldehyde-dipped cigarettes. Neurology 1988;38(Suppl):207.
94. Eells JT, McMartin KE, Black K et al. Formaldehyde poisoning: rapid metabolism to formic acid. JAMA 1981;246: 1237–1238.
95. Koppel C, Baudisch H, Schneider V, Ibe K. Suicidal ingestion of formalin with fatal complications. Intensive Care Med 1990;16:212–214.
96. Burkhart K, Kulig K, Rumack BH, McMartin K. Formate and methanol levels following formalin ingestion. Vet Hum Toxicol 1989;31:375.
97. 29 CFR 1910.1048.
98. Guidelines for protecting the safety and health of health care workers. U.S. Department of Health and Human Services, NIOSH. September 1988, pp 5.23–5.25.
99. Frigas E, Filley WV, Feed CE. Bronchial challenge with formaldehyde gas: lack of bronchoconstriction in 13 patients suspected of having formaldehyde induced asthma. Mayo Clin Proc 1984;59:295–299.
100. Imbus HR. Clinical evaluation of patients' complaints related to formaldehyde exposure. J Allergy Clin Immunol 1985; 76:837–840.
101. L'abbe KA, Hoey JR. Review of the health effects of urea-formaldehyde foam insulation. Environ Res 1984;35:246–263.
102. Albert RF, Sellakumar AR, Laskin S et al. Gaseous formaldehyde and hydrogen chloride induction of nasal cancer in rats. J Natl Cancer Inst 1982;68:597–603.
103. Grafstrom RC, Fornace AJ, Autrup H et al. Formaldehyde damage to DNA and inhibition of DNA repair in human bronchial cells. Science 1983;220:216–218.
104. Halperin WE, Goodman M, Stayner L et al. Nasal cancer in a worker exposed to formaldehyde. JAMA 1983;249:510–512.
105. Wald N, Richie C. Formaldehyde process workers and lung cancer. Lancet 1984;1:1066–1067.
106. Acheson ED, Barnes HR, Gardner MJ et al. Formaldehyde in the British chemical industry. Lancet 1984;1:611–616.
107. Stayner L, Smith AB, Reeve G et al. Proportionate mortality study of workers in the garment industry exposed to formaldehyde. Am J Ind Med 1985;7:229–240.
108. Olsen JH, Asnaes S. Formaldehyde and the risk of squamous cell carcinoma of the sinonasal cavities. Br J Ind Med 1986;43:769–774.
109. Infante PF, Ulsamer AG, Groth D et al. Health hazards of formaldehyde. Lancet 1981;2:980–981.
110. Report of the Federal Panel on Formaldehyde. Environ Health Perspect 1982;43:139–168.
111. Ashford NA, Ryan CW, Caldart CC. Law and science policy in federal regulation of formaldehyde. Science 1983;222: 894–900.
112. Wartew GA. The health hazards of formaldehyde. J Appl Toxicol 1983;3:121–126.
113. Kallos GJ, Solomon RA. Formation of bis (chloromethyl) ether in simulated hydrogen chloride formaldehyde atmospheric environments. Am Ind Hyg Assoc J 1973;34: 469–473.
114. Hayes RB, Blair A, Stewart PA, Herrick RF, Mahar H. Mortality of US embalmers and funeral directors. Am J Ind Med 1990;18:641–652.
115. Alexandersson R, Kolmodin-Hedmun B, Hedenstierna G. Exposure to formaldehyde: effects on pulmonary function. Arch Environ Health 1982;37:279.
116. Kilburn KH, Warshaw R, Boylen CT et al. Pulmonary and neurobehavioral effects of formaldehyde exposure. Arch Environ Health 1985;40:254–260.
117. Levine RJ, Corso RDD, Blunden PB et al. The effects of occupational exposure on the respiratory health of West Virginia morticians. J Occup Med 1984;26:91–98.
118. Orringer EP, Mattera WD. Formaldehyde-induced hemolysis during chronic hemodialysis. N Engl J Med 1976;294: 1416–1420.
119. Meglio C, Garnier R, Castot A, El Yafi S, Efthymiou M-L. Intoxication accidentelle par le formaldehyde au cours d'une seance d'hemodialysis. Therapie 1988;43:321–323.
120. Maurice F, Rivory J-P, Larsson PH, Johansson SGO, Bousquet J. Anaphylactic shock caused by formaldehyde in a patient undergoing long-term hemodialysis. J Allergy Clin Immunol 1986;77:594–597.
121. Klein E. Effects of disinfectants in renal dialysis patients. Environ Health Perspect 1986;69:45–48.
122. Samet JM, Marbury MC, Spengler JD. Health effects and sources of indoor air pollution. II. Am Rev Respir Dis 1988; 137:221–242.
123. Binding N, Witting U. Exposure to formaldehyde and glutaraldehyde in operating theatre. Int Arch Occup Environ Health 1990;62:233–238.
124. Bartone NF, Grieca RV, Henn BS. Corrosive gastritis due to ingestion of formaldehyde. JAMA 1968;203:50–51.
125. Docampo R, Moreno SNJ. The metabolism and mode of action of gentian violet. Drug Metab Rev 1990;22:161–178.
126. Drinkwater P. Gentian violet—is it safe? Aust NZ J Obstet Gynaecol 1990;30:65–66.
127. DHSS puts restrictions on use of crystal violet. Pharm J 1987;239:655.
128. Beeley L. Any questions. Br Med J 1988;297:607.
129. Reynolds JEF. *Martindale: The extra pharmacopoeia.* 13th ed. London: The Pharmaceutical Press, 1993; p. 793.
130. Churchman JW, Russell DG. The effect of gentian violet on protozoa and on growing adult tissue. Proc Soc Exp Biol Med 1913-1914;11:120–124.
131. McEvoy GK, ed. AHFS Drug Information 94. Bethesda, MD: American Society of Hospital Pharmacists, 1994, pp. 2281–2282.

132. Jones BM, Gault DT. Blue dyes in reconstructive surgery. Lancet 1988;1:949–950.
133. Young HH, Hill JH. The treatment of septicemia and local infections by intravenous injections of Mercurochrome 220 and gentian violet. JAMA 1924;82:669–675.
134. Quinby GE. Gentian violet as a cause of epidemic occupational nosebleeds. Arch Environ Health 1968;16:485–489.
135. Walsh C, Walsh A. Haemorrhagic cystitis due to gentian violet. Br Med J 1986;293:732.
136. Hanson PJV, Gor D, Jeffries DJ, Collins JV. Chemical inactivation of HIV on surfaces. Br Med J 1989;298:862–864.
137. Fowler JF Jr. Allergic contact dermatitis from glutaraldehyde exposure. J Occup Med 1989;31:852–853.
138. Piccolo R, Berkowitz I, Sacho H, Elias D, Schmeizer B, Strimling M. Glutaraldehyde disinfection. In use testing following repeated gastroscopies. S Afr Med J 1990;78:362.
139. Stonehill AA, Krop S, Borck PM. Buffered glutaraldehyde—a new chemical sterilizing solution. Am J Hosp Pharm 1963;20: 458–465.
140. Proctor NH, Hughes JP, Fischman ML. Chemical hazards of the workplace. 2nd ed. New York: Van Nostrand Reinhold, 1989; pp. 264–265.
141. Glutaraldehyde. Guidelines for protecting the safety and health of health care workers. U.S. Department of Health and Human Services. NIOSH. September 1988, pp. 5-12–5-13. DHHS (NIOSH) Publication No. 88-119.
142. Symptoms of irritation associated with exposure to glutaraldehyde—Colorado. MMWR 1987;36:190–191.
143. Bardazzi F, Melino M, Alagna G, Veronesi S. Glutaraldehyde dermatitis in nurses. Contact Dermatitis 1986;6:319–320.
144. Nethercott JR, Holness DL, Page E. Occupational contact dermatitis due to glutaraldehyde in health care workers. Contact Dermatitis 1988;18:193–196.
145. Hansen KS. Glutaraldehyde occupational dermatitis. Contact Dermatitis 1983;9:81–82.
146. Connaughton P. Occupational exposure to glutaraldehyde associated with tachycardia and palpitations. Med J Aust 1993;159:567.
147. Marks TA, Worthy WC, Staples RE. Influence of formaldehyde and Sonacide (potentiated acid glutaraldehyde) on embryo and fetal development in mice. Teratology 1980;22: 51–58.
148. Gorman SD, Scott EM, Russell AD. Antimicrobial activity, uses and mechanism of action of glutaraldehyde. J Appl Bacteriology 1980;48:161–190.
149. Norbach D. Skin and respiratory symptoms for exposure to alkaline glutaraldehyde in medical services. Scand Work Environ Health 1988;14:366–371.
150. Holness DL, Nethercott JR. Health status of funeral service workers exposed to formaldehyde. Arch Environ Health 1989;44:222–229.
151. Wiggin P, McCurdy SA, Zeidenberg W. Epistaxis due to glutaraldehyde exposure. J Occup Med 1989;31:854–856.
152. Babb RR. Paaso BT. Glutaraldehyde proctitis. West J Med 1995;163:477–478.
153. Binding N, Witting U. Exposure to formaldehyde and glutaraldehyde in operating theatres. Int Arch Occup Environ Health 1990;62:233–238.
154. Reynolds JEF, ed. *Martindale: The extra pharmacopoeia.* 13th ed. London: The Pharmaceutical Press, 1993, p. 796.
155. Kaelin RM, Kapanci Y, Tschopp MJ. Diffuse interstitial lung disease associated with hydrogen peroxide inhalation in a dairy worker. Am Rev Respir Dis 1988;137:1233–1235.
156. Rosengarten MD, Portnoy D, Chiu R-C, Paterson AK. Reuse of permanent cardiac pacemakers. Can Med Assoc J 1985;133:279–283.
157. Patterson WB, Craven DE, Schwartz DA, Nardell EA, Kasmer J, Noble A. Occupational hazards to hospital personnel. Ann Intern Med 1985;102:658–680.
158. Advisory Committee on Dangerous Pathogens. LAV/HTLV III—the causative agent of AIDS and related conditions. Revised Guidelines. London: Department of Health and Social Security, 1986.
159. Tyrala EE, Hillman LS, Hillman RE et al. Clinical pharmacology of hexachlorophene in newborn infants. J Pediatr 1977;91:481–486.
160. Conte JE Jr. Infection with human immunodeficiency virus in the hospital. Epidemiology, infection control and biosafety considerations. Ann Intern Med 1986;105:730–736.
161. Memorandum on the control of viral haemorrhagic fevers. Department of Health and Social Security. London: HM Stationery Office, 1986.
162. Shuman RM, Leech RW, Alvord ED. Neurotoxicity of hexachlorophene in the human. I. A clinicopathologic study of 248 children. Pediatrics 1974;54:689–695.
163. Martin-Bouyer G, Toga M, Lebreton R et al. Outbreak of accidental hexachlorophene poisoning in France. Lancet 1982;1:91–95.
164. Hexachlorophene today. Lancet 1982;1:87–88 (editorial).
165. Plueckhahn VD. Hexachlorophene preparations and the newborn infant. Aust Paediatr J 1980;16:40–43.
166. Liu J, Wang C-N, Yu J-H et al. Hexachlorophene in the treatment of Clonorchiasis sinesis. China Med J 1963;82:702–711.
167. Herskowitz J, Rosman NP. Acute hexachlorophene poisoning by mouth in a neonate. J Pediatr 1979;94:495–496.
168. Lustig FW. A fatal case of hexachlorophene ("pHisoHex") poisoning. Med J Aust 1963;1:737.
169. Henry LD, DiMaio VJM. A fatal case of hexachlorophene poisoning. Military Med 1974;139:41–43.
170. Mullick FG. Hexachlorophene toxicity—human experience at the Armed Forces Institute of Pathology. Pediatrics 1973; 51:395–399.
171. Kimbrough RD. Review of recent evidence of toxic effects of hexachlorophene. Pediatrics 1973;51:391–394.
172. Ulsamer AG, Yoder PD, Marzulli FN. Determinations of hexachlorophene in human and experimental animal tissues. Toxicol Appl Pharmacol 1972;22:276–277 (abstract).
173. Martinez AJ, Boehm R, Hadfield MG. Acute hexachlorophene encephalopathy: clinico-neuropathological correlation. Acta Neuropathol 1974;28:93–103.
174. Gowdy JM, Ulsamer AG. Hexachlorophene lesions in newborn infants. Am J Dis Child 1976;130:247–250.
175. Brandt I, Denker L, Larsson Y. Transplacental passage and embryonic fetal accumulation of hexachlorophene in mice. Toxicol Appl Pharmacol 1979;49:393–401.
176. Halling H. Suspected link between exposure to hexachlorophene and malformed infants. Ann NY Acad Sci 1979;320: 426–435.
177. Anderson JM, Cockburn F, Forfar J et al. Neonatal spongioform myelinopathy after restricted application of hexachlorophene skin disinfectant. J Clin Pathol 1981;34:25–29.
178. Picchioni AC, Chin L, Laird HE. Activated charcoal preparations. Relative antidotal efficacy. Clin Toxicol 1974;7:97–108.
179. Boehm RM, Czajka PA. Hexachlorophene poisoning and the ineffectiveness of peritoneal dialysis. Clin Toxicol 1979;14: 257–262.
180. Litovitz TL, Bailey KM, Schmitz BF, Holm KC, Klein-Schwartz W. 1990 Annual Report of the American Association of Poison Control Centers National Data Collection System. Am J Emerg Med 1991;9:461–509.
181. Humberston CL, Dean BS, Krenzelok EP. Ingestion of 35% hydrogen peroxide. Clin Toxicol 1990;28:95–100.
182. NIOSH Pocket Guide to Chemical Hazards NIOSH. US Dept Health and Human Services, June 1990, p. 126. DHHS (NIOSH) Publication No. 90-117.
183. Giberson TP, Kern JD, Pettigrew DW III, Eaves CC Jr, Haynes JF Jr. Near-fatal hydrogen peroxide ingestion. Ann Emerg Med 1989;18:778–779.
184. Olim CB, Ciuti A. Meconium ileus: a new method of relieving obstruction. Ann Surg 1954;140:736–739.
185. Bilotta JJ, Waye JD. Hydrogen peroxide enteritis: the "snow white" sign. Gastrointest Endosc 1989;35:428–430.
186. Pogrebniak AE, Sugar A. Corneal toxicity from hydrogen peroxide-soaked tonometer tips. Arch Ophthalmol 1988;106: 1505.
187. Brenman AK, Milner RM, Weller CR. Use of hydrogen peroxide to clear blocked ventilation tubes. Am J Otol 1986;7: 47–50.
188. McEvoy GK, ed. AHFS Drug Information 94. Bethesda, MD: American Society of Hospital Pharmacists, 1994; pp 1840–1841.

189. Proctor NH, Hughes JP, Fischman ML. Chemical hazards of the workplace. 2nd ed. New York: Van Nostrand Reinhold, 1989, pp. 281–282.
190. Hyperoxygenation therapy. US Food and Drug Administration, April 14, 1989.
191. Thompson JD. New health food hazard—35% hydrogen peroxide. Vet Hum Toxicol 1989;31:339.
192. Reynolds JEF, ed. *Martindale: The extra pharmacopoeia.* 13th ed. 1993. London: The Pharmaceutical Press, p. 798.
193. Oberst FW, Comstock CC, Hackley EB. Inhalation toxicity of nine per cent hydrogen peroxide vapor. Acute, subacute and chronic exposures of laboratory animals. Ind Hyg Occup Med 1954;10:319-327.
194. Blakely WF, Fuciarelli AF, Wegher BJ, Dizdaroglu M. Hydrogen peroxide-induced base damage in deoxyribonucleic acid. Radiat Res 1990;121:338–343.
195. Oberg M, Lindsey D. Do not put hydrogen peroxide or povidone iodine into wounds. Am J Dis Child 1987;141:27–28.
196. Shaw A, Cooperman A, Fusco J. Gas embolism produced by hydrogen peroxide. N Engl J Med 1967;277:238–241.
197. Gerrish SP. Gas embolism due to hydrogen peroxide. Anaesthesia 1985;10:1244.
198. Bassan MM, Dudai M, Shalev O. Near-fatal systemic oxygen embolism due to wound irrigation with hydrogen peroxide. Postgrad Med J 1982;58:448–450.
199. Sleigh JW, Linter SPK. Hazards of hydrogen peroxide. Br Med J 1985;291:1706.
200. Schneider DL, Hebert LJ. Subcutaneous gas from hydrogen peroxide administration under pressure. Am J Dis Child 1987;141:10–11.
201. Cina SJ, Downs CU, Conradi SE. Hydrogen peroxide: a source of lethal oxygen embolism. Am J Forensic Med Pathol 1994;15(1):44–50.
202. Swayne LC, Ginsberg HN, Ginsburg A. Pneumoretroperitoneum secondary to hydrogen peroxide wound irrigations. Am J Radiol 1987;148:149–150.
203. Danis RK, Brodeur AE. The danger of hydrogen peroxide as a colonic irrigating solution. J Pediatr Surg 1967;2:131–133.
204. Meyer CT, Brand M, DeLuca VA, Spiro HM. Hydrogen peroxide colitis: a report of three patients. J Clin Gastroenterol 1981;3:31–35.
205. Sheehan JF, Brynjolfsson G. Ulcerative colitis following hydrogen peroxide enema: case report and experimental production with transient emphysema of colonic wall and gas embolism. Lab Invest 1960;9:150–157.
206. Jonas G, Mahoney A, Murray J, Gertler S. Chemical colitis due to endoscope cleaning solutions. A mimic of pseudomembranous colitis. Gastroenterology 1988;95:1403–1408.
207. Pumphrey RE. Hydrogen peroxide proctitis. Am J Surg 1951; 81:60–62.
208. Rees TD, Orth CF. Oral ulcerations with use of hydrogen peroxide. J Periodontol 1986;57:689–692.
209. Tripathi BJ, Tripathi RC. Hydrogen peroxide damage to human corneal epithelial cells in vitro. Implications for contact lens disinfection systems. Arch Ophthalmol 1989;107: 1516–1519.
210. Levensen JE. Corneal damage from improperly cleaned tonometer tips. Arch Ophthalmol 1989;107:1117.
211. McNally JJ. Clinical aspects of topical application of dilute hydrogen peroxide solutions. CLAO J 1990;16(Suppl): S46–S52.
212. Chandler JW. Biocompatibility of hydrogen peroxide in soft contact lens disinfection: antimicrobial activity vs biocompatibility—the balance. CLAO J 1990;16(Suppl):S43–S45.
213. Timperley AJ, Bracey DJ. Cardiac arrest following the use of hydrogen peroxide during arthroplasty. J Arthroplasty 1989;4:369–370.
214. Zecevic D, Gasparec Z. Death caused by hydrogen peroxide. Z Rechtsmed 1979;84:57–59.
215. Giusti GV. Fatal poisoning with hydrogen peroxide. Forensic Sci 1973;2:99–100.
216. Seymour WB Jr. Poisoning from cutaneous application of iodine. A rare aspect of its toxicologic properties. Arch Intern Med 1937;59:952–966.
217. Pennington JAT. A review of iodine toxicity reports. J Am Diet Assoc 1990;90:1571–1581.
218. Dyck RF, Bear RA, Goldstein MB, Halperin ML. Iodine/iodide toxic reaction: case report with emphasis on the nature of metabolic acidosis. Can Med Assoc J 1979;120:704–706.
219. Moore M. The ingestion of iodine as a method of attempted suicide. N Engl J Med 1938;219:383–388.
220. Finkelstein R, Jacobi M. Fatal iodine poisoning: a clinicopathologic and experimental study. Ann Intern Med 1937;10: 1283–1296.
221. d'Auria J, Lipson S, Garfield JM. Fatal iodine toxicity following surgical debridement of a hip wound: case report. J Trauma 1990;30:353–355.
222. Goldenheim PD. Inactivation of HIV by povidone-iodine. JAMA 1987;257:2434.
223. dela Cruz F, Brown DH, Leikin JB, Franklin C, Hryhorczuk DO. Iodine absorption after topical administration. West J Med 1987;146:43–45.
224. Means LJ, Rescorla FJ, Grosfeld JL. Iodine toxicity. An unusual cause of cardiovascular collapse during anesthesia in an infant with Hirschsprung's disease. J Pediatr Surg 1990;25:1278–1279.
225. Roslyn JJ. Peritoneal irrigation with povidone-iodine. JAMA 1988;260:
226. McEvoy GK. AHFS Drug Information 94. Bethesda, MD. American Society of Hospital Pharmacists, 1994; p. 2305.
227. Reynolds JEF. *Martindale: The extra pharmacopoeia.* 13th ed. London. The Pharmaceutical Press, 1993; pp. 970–972.
228. Litovitz TL, Martin TG, Schmitz B. 1986 annual report of the American Association of Poison Control Centers National Data Collection System. Am J Emerg Med 1987;5:405–445.
229. Shetty KR, Duthie EH Jr. Thyrotoxicosis induced by topical iodine application. Arch Intern Med 1990;150:2400–2401.
230. Smerdely P, Lim A, Boyages SC, Waite K, Wu D, Roberts V et al. Topical iodine-containing antiseptics and neonatal hypothyroidism in very low birthweight infants. Lancet 1989; 2:661–664.
231. l'Allemand D, Gruters A, Heidemann P, Schurnbrand P. Iodine-induced alterations of thyroid function in newborn infants after prenatal and perinatal exposure to povidone-iodine. J Pediatr 1983;102:935–938.
232. Kurt TL, Morgan ML, Hailica V, Bost R, Petty CS. Fatal iatrogenic iodine toxicity in a 9-week-old infant. Vet Hum Toxicol 1992;34:333.
233. Cohn BNE. Absorption of compound solution of iodine from the gastrointestinal tract. Arch Intern Med 1932;49:950–956.
234. Sandell E, Koithoff IM. Microdetermination of iodine by a catalytic method. Mikrochim Acta 1937;1:9.
235. Hunt JL, Sato R, Heck EL et al. A critical evaluation of povidone-iodine absorption in thermally injured patients. J Trauma 1980;20:127–129.
236. Pietsch J, Machins JL. Complications of povidone-iodine absorption in topically treated burn patients. Lancet 1976;1: 280–282.
237. Baker MD, Baldassano RN. Povidone iodine as a cause of factitious hematuria and abnormal urine coloration in the pediatric emergency department. Pediatr Emerg Care 1989;5: 240–241.
238. White A, Joseet M. Burns from iodine. Anaesthesia 1990;45: 75.
239. Vulisma T, Menzel D, Abbad FCB, Gons MH, De Vijlder JJM. Iodine induced hypothyroidism in infants treated with continuous cyclic peritoneal dialysis. Lancet 1990;336:812.
240. Reynolds JEF, ed. *Martindale: The extra pharmacopoeia.* 29th ed. London: The Pharmaceutical Press, 1989, pp. 964–965.
241. Scarlett MI, Furman LJ. Disease transmission in the dental office: guidelines for disinfection. JAMA 1988;259:1081.
242. Guidelines for Health Care Workers. NIOSH U.S. Department of Health and Human Services, 1988, pp. 5–7.
243. Barnett JM, Ptotnick M, Fine KC. Intoxication after an isopropyl alcohol enema. Ann Intern Med 1990;113:638–639.
244. Corbett J, Meier G. Suicide attempted by rectal administration of drug. JAMA 1968;206:2320–2321.
245. Weintraub Z, Iancu TC. Isopropyl alcohol burns. Pediatrics 1982;69:506.
246. Schich JB, Milstein JM. Burn hazard of isopropyl alcohol in the neonate. Pediatrics 1981;68:588–589.

247. Arditi M, Killner MS. Coma following use of rubbing alcohol for fever control. Am J Dis Child 1987;141:237–238.
248. Vicas I, Beck R. Fatal inhalational isopropyl alcohol poisoning in a neonate. Vet Hum Toxicol 1989;341:346.
249. Russo S, Taff ML, Mirchandani HG, Monforte JR, Spitz WV. Scald burns complicated by isopropyl alcohol intoxication. A use of fatal child abuse. Am J Forensic Med Pathol 1986;7: 81–83.
250. Vivier PM, Lewander WJ, Martin HF. Isopropyl alcohol intoxication in a neonate through chronic dermal exposure. Vet Hum Toxicol 1991;33:391.
251. Hunziker N. Theilsothiazolinone story. Dermatology 1992;184: 85–86.
252. De Groot AC, Herxheimer A. Isothiazolinone preservative: cause of a continuing epidemic of cosmetic dermatitis. Lancet 1989;1:314–316.
253. Fransway AF. Sensitivity to Kathon CG: findings in 365 consecutive patients. Contact Dermatitis 1988;19:342–347.
254. Barid EA, Greig D. Kathon CG—can New Zealand avoid the epidemic? NZ Med J 1991;104:290.
255. Magarey JA. Absorption mercurochrome. Lancet 1993;324: 1424.
256. Magarey JA. Absorption of mercurochrome. Lancet 1993; 342:1404.
257. Whittet HB, Shinkwin C, Freeland AP. Anosmia due to nasal administration of corticosteroids. Br Med J 1991;303:651.
258. FDA Consumer 1991;25(8):2–3.
259. Gross BG. Cardiac arrhythmias during phenol face peeling. Plast Reconstr Surg 1984;73:590–594.
260. Warner MA, Harper JV. Cardiac arrhythmias associated with chemical peeling with phenol. Anesthesiology 1984;62:366.
261. Easton JKM, Ozel T, Halpern D. Intramuscular neurolysis for spasticity in children. Arch Phys Med Rehabil 1979;60: 155–158.
262. Haddad LM, Dimond KA, Schweistris JE. Phenol poisoning. JACEP 1979;8:267–269.
263. Cronk JD. Phenol with glucagon in cardiotherapy. N Engl J Med 1971;784:219–220.
264. Liao JF, Oehme FW. Literature review of phenol compounds. I. Phenol. Vet Hum Toxicol 1980;22:160.
265. Anderson W. Fatal misadventure with carbolic acid. Lancet 1869;1:179.
266. Leider M, Moser HS. Toxicology of topical dermatology preparations. Arch Dermatol 1961;83:928–929.
267. Conning DM, Hayes MJ. The dermal toxicity of phenol: an investigation of the most effective first aid measures. Br J Ind Med 1970;27:155–159.
268. Piotnowski JK. Evaluation of exposure to phenol: absorption of phenol vapour in the lungs and through the skin and excretion of phenol in the urine. Br J Ind Med 1971;28:172–178.
269. Lucus RC, Lane WA. Two cases of carbolic acid coma induced by application of carbolic acid compresses to the skin. Lancet 1895;1:1362–1364.
270. Jarvis SN, Straube RC, Williams ALJ et al. Illness associated with contamination of drinking water supplies with phenol. Br Med J 1985;290:1800–1802.
271. Baker EL, Landrigan PJ, Bertozzi PE. Phenol poisoning due to contaminated drinking water. Arch Environ Health 1978; 33:89–94.
272. Stajduhar-Caric Z. Acute phenol poisoning. Singular findings in a lethal case. J Forensic Med 1968;15:41–42.
273. McGuiness JP, Cantees KK. Epidural injection of phenol-containing ranitidine preparation. Anesthesiology 1990;73: 553–555.
274. Foxall PJD, Bending M, Gartland KPR, Nicholson JK. Acute renal failure following accidental cutaneous exposure to phenol application of PMR (proton nuclear magnetic resonance spectroscopic) urinalysis to monitor the disease process. Hum Exp Toxicol 1990;9:351.
275. Foxall PJD, Nicholson JK, Bending MR, Eisinger AJ. Monitoring phenol-induced nephrotoxicity by high-resolution proton NMR spectroscopy. Renal Failure 1989;11:57–58.
276. Foxall PJD, Bending MR, Gartland KPR, Nicholson JK. Acute renal failure following accidental cutaneous absorption of phenol. Application of NMR urinalysis to monitor the disease process. Hum Toxicol 1989;9:491–496.
277. Cohen N, Modai D, Khahil A, Golik A. Acute resin phenol-formaldehyde intoxication. A life-threatening occupational hazard. Hum Toxicol 1989;8:247–250.
278. Ho S-L, Hollinrake K. Acute epiglottis and Chloraseptic. Br Med J 1989;298:1584.
279. Spiller HA, Quadroni-Kushner DA, Cleveland P. A five-year evaluation of acute exposure to phenol disinfectant (26%). Clin Toxicol 1993;31:307–313.
280. Harrison LM, Morrison JE, Fennessey PV. Microtechnique for quantifying phenol in plasma by gas chromatography-mass spectrometry. Clin Chem 1991;37:1739–1742.
281. Soares ER, Tift JP. Phenol poisoning: three fatal cases. J Forensic Sci 1982;27:729–731.
282. Nomoto Y, Fujita T, Kitani Y. Serum and urine levels of phenol following phenol blocks. Can J Anaesth 1987;34:307–310.
283. Brancato DJ. Recognizing potential toxicity of phenol. Vet Hum Toxicol 1982;24:29–30.
284. Mofenson HC, Caraccio TR, Laudano J. Glucagon for propranolol overdose. JAMA 1986;255:2025.
285. Litton C. Chemical face lifting. Plast Reconstr Surg 1962;29: 371–380.
286. Lo Dico C, Caplan YH, Levine B, Smyth DF, Smialek JE. Phenol: tissue distribution in a fatality. J Forensic Sci 1989; 34:1013–1015.
287. Chamberlain JM, Gorman PL, Young GM. Silver nitrate burns following treatment for umbilical granuloma. Pediatr Emerg Care 1992;8:29–30.
288. Marroni M, Menichetti F. Accidental intravenous infusion of sodium hypochlorite. DICP 1991;25:1008–1009.
289. Leafer DJ. Eusol. Still awaiting proper clinical trials. Br Med J 1992;304:930–931.
290. Burton JL. Eusol. The continuing controversy. Br Med J 1992;304:1636.
291. Watson ID, McBride D, Paterson KR. Fatal xylenol self-poisoning. Postgrad Med J 1986;62:411–412.
292. McGarvie MJ, Volans GN. Ingestion of sterilising tablets for baby feeding bottles. Vet Hum Toxicol 1987;29(Suppl 2):126.
293. Reynolds JEF, ed. *Martindale: The extra pharmacopoeia.* 29th ed. London: The Pharmaceutical Press, 1989, p. 969.
294. Williams DC. Acute respiratory obstruction caused by ingestion of a caustic substance. Br Med J 1985;291: 313–314.
295. Siodlak MZ, Gleeson MJ, Wengraf CL. Accidental ingestion of sterilizing tablets by children. Br Med J 1985;290:1707–1708.

Chapter 58
Chemical Disasters

Industrial disasters result from the storage, processing, and transportation of large amounts of highly flammable, explosive, and toxic chemicals. Reactive or toxic chemicals become released, explode, or catch fire. Operator error, equipment failure, or facility-related factors trigger the event.[1]

Major industrial chemical accidents cause extensive damage to human health and the environment both outside and within the site of the manufacture, formulation, or processing of chemicals. This definition must include transportation of dangerous substances and their loading and discharge at installations.[2] Perhaps 50% of hazardous material spills during transport are related to human error.[3]

CONTRIBUTING FACTORS

To have a public health impact, a release must expose individuals to the chemicals, fire, or products of a blast. Workers at the scene of an incident are at initial and greatest risk. First responders (e.g., fire fighters) and health-care workers who are improperly protected or are exposed to contaminated individuals may be the next group physically affected. Finally, the magnitude of the release, distance of residents from the incident, actions taken by residents, weather conditions, and type of housing may be critical factors in determining the effects on community residents.[1]

DISASTER DEFINITIONS

The term *chemical disaster* may be understood as a great calamity in which many people (at least 50) perish and in which a chemical causes the death or injury of so many people that the normal health and emergency services are, or threaten to become, overburdened. A *catastrophic situation* may be considered a threat to perhaps 10 persons. This is the number of individuals with which the crew of an Emergency Medical Service (EMS) ambulance can effectively cope. An event in which only one or a few persons are the victims may be considered as an *accident.* A *catastrophe* can be considered to encompass any situation in which the need for aid surpasses the normal capacity to deliver medical and technical assistance. A *hazard* exists where there is a situation that in particular circumstances could lead to harm.[4] A new discipline, disaster medicine, is devoted to the

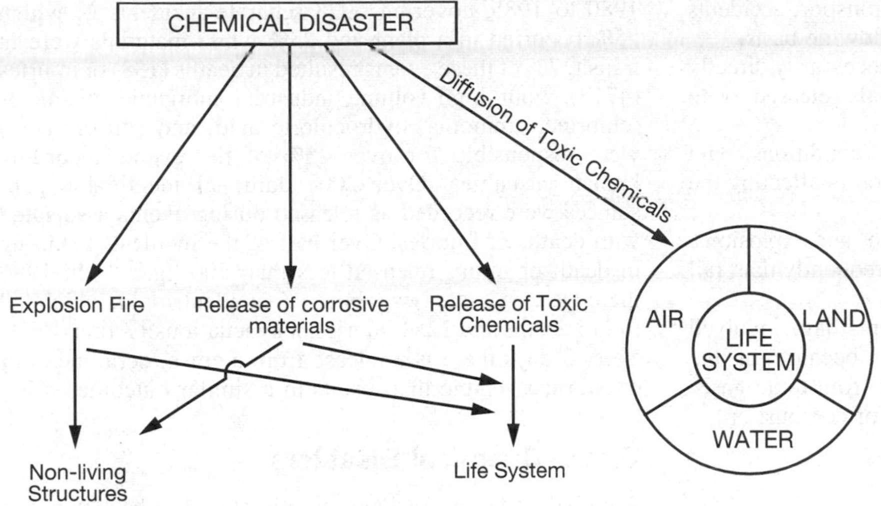

Figure 58–1 Dimensions of the sequelae of chemical disasters. (Adapted from Krishna Murti CR. In: Bourdeau P, Green G, eds. Methods for assessing and reducing injury from chemical accidents. Chichester, John Wiley, 1989.)

efficient handling of human casualties in disaster situations.[5–11]

DISASTER CLASSIFICATION

Disasters may be classified as follows:

1. According to the number of victims produced by an incident.
2. The extent of the contaminated area.
3. The population density in a contaminated area for volatile chemicals.
4. The amount of chemical involved.
5. Toxicity of the chemicals.
6. The magnitude of the measures that must be taken to counteract the accident and to limit its consequences.[6]
7. Consequences on the environment.
8. Sequelae of clinical disasters are diagrammed in Figure 58–1.[12]

EXPOSURES

Local emergency medical services should be prepared to offer medical treatment following exposure to the following chemicals: Acids, acrolein, alkalis, ammonia, arsine gas, carbon monoxide, chlorine, cyanide, formalin, formaldehyde, hydrocyanic acid, hydrofluoric acid, hydrogen sulphide gas, irritant gases, heavy metals (e.g., lead, mercury, arsenic), metallic and inorganic compounds, hydrocarbons, nitrites, nitrates methaemoglobinaemia), organophosphate and carbamate compounds (e.g., pesticides), phenols and phosphorus (both yellow and white), phosphine gas, phosgene gases, and sulphuric acid mist. Circumstances that suggest chemical contamination are outlined in Table 58–1.

COMMUNITIES AT RISK

Communities that are near a rail line or major highway are at risk for a chemical disaster.[10] Most serious Hazmat (hazardous materials) incidents occur in rural areas protected by small rural or volunteer fire departments poorly equipped to handle the accidents.[10]

Table 58–1
Circumstances That Suggest Chemical Contamination[a]

Industrial accidents (especially chemical manufacturing plants)
Explosions, fires, pipeline ruptures, spills, falls
Agricultural accidents
Transportation accidents
Trains, trucks, planes (cropdusters), ships
At the scene
Vapor clouds
Dead animals or fish
Multiple patients with same complaints
Rescue from an enclosed space
If a patient has
Unconsciousness ("found down")
Unexplained cardiac arrest
Strong odors on skin or clothing
Unidentified liquids or powders on skin or clothing
Chemical burns
Overdoses involving cleaning or agricultural chemicals
Methemoglobinemia
Irritation of skin, eyes, mucous membranes and respiratory tract
Neurologic complaints (numbness, weakness, seizures)

[a]From Kirk et al. Emerg Med Clin North Am 1994;12:461–481.

TRANSPORTATION

In the United States there are over 70,000 chemicals produced and over 180,000 daily shipments of all types of chemicals. Perhaps 6000 facilities now make hazardous chemicals in the United States.[13] In 1982 there were 100,000 transporters of hazardous materials (not including handlers of toxic wastes) and 354,000 generators of hazardous waste.[14] Inadequate industry self-regulation, too few Department of Transportation full-time inspectors, and insufficient emphasis on safety programs portend a continuation of serious Hazmat incidents and catastrophic accidents.

Transport Incidents

Study of transport incidents suggests the following observations:

1. There is no reliable information on transport accidents involving hazardous goods on a worldwide basis.
2. The number of people injured is not necessarily directly related to the amount of toxic materials released, or to the size of any fire or explosion.
3. Proximity to the public, weather conditions, and emergency response are important factors affecting the potential impact of an incident.
4. Casualties appear to follow mainly fires and explosions.
5. Road incidents seem to occur more frequently than rail incidents.
6. The largest number of serious incidents have involved flammable gas or liquids (partially because of the volume moved) with some incidents from toxic gases and toxic fumes (including products of combustion).[15]

CHEMICAL DISASTER PROCEDURES—OVERVIEW

Chemical disasters pose some unique problems. Substance identification is important prior to a massive rescue effort. On-site decontamination procedures are essential for both victims and emergency medical services personnel (Fig. 58–2). On-scene separation of hot, warm, and cold zones (Figs. 58–3 and 58–4) will facilitate safe initial responses to the injured. Protective clothing may be essential for those involved in rescue and triage procedures. Ambulances and other vehicles removing the injured require decontamination procedures. Hospitals require a triage area, a separate decontamination area, and a separate entrance. Transport vehicles may require placards to indicate the type of chemical contamination involved. Mass evacuation of the population should be considered.

With regard to the management of contaminated victims, it is essential for health-care providers to distinguish clearly between toxic chemicals that have a serious potential for contaminating the environment and emergency room and/or hospital personnel, and those that do not. Examples of the first type include known potent chemical carcinogens or radioactive substances. An example of the second is sodium hydroxide (lye). Most hazardous-material episodes fall in this latter category, and in these cases field decontamination with plenty of water (taking care to contain the run-off water) removes the risk to bystanders because the material will be rapidly diluted. In such a case there will be no need to dress up the gurneys and paper down the hospital corridors, or to gown and glove all health personnel and rope off the emergency room entry. It is important that response personnel and emergency room staff understand the difference between a "simple" contamination episode and the much more complex (but rare) situation involving highly contaminating or environmentally toxic materials such as polychlorinated biphenyls, extremely potent pesticides, or radionuclides.

ACUTE HAZARDOUS EVENTS—INCIDENCE

UNITED STATES[1]

The Acute Hazardous Events Database[16] is a partial list of releases involving toxic chemicals in the United States from 1980 to 1985, covering 6928 separate incidents of which 75% occurred in a plant and 25% while materials were in transit; 7% of these events resulted in deaths (138) or injuries (4717). Four high-volume industrial inorganic chemicals (chlorine, ammonia, hydrochloric acid, and sulfuric acid) were responsible for over 25% of the events recording human casualties. Over 200 additional identifiable substances were recorded as released during events associated with deaths or injuries. Over half of the incidents resulting in death or injury released less than 500 kg.[17–19] In 1986 there were 587 releases (about 1.6 incidents/day), which led to 115 deaths and 2254 injuries or evacuations.[1] Almost once every 3 days there is a release from a crash, derailment, or overturned vehicle that results in a similar outcome.

Global Chemical Disasters

A global survey of technologic disasters has been summarized by Dr. John A. Haines of the International Program on Chemical Safety, World Health Organization.[10]

Airborne Releases

Some air-pollution disasters are delineated in Table 58–2. Chemical disasters have been reported from pesticide food contamination (Table 58–3). Some historical chlorine and ammonia accidents are summarized in Tables 58–4 and 58–5.

Deliberate Chemical Contamination of Food

Substances used in the deliberate contamination of food have included cyanide, cannabis, caustic soda, diethylene glycol, glass, insecticides, metallic mercury, paraquat, rat poison, and thallium.[21] Food that was contaminated or allegedly contaminated included wine, fruit juices, fruit, confectionery, turkey, cole slaw, and butter.

Chemical Contamination of Drinking Water

Incidents of drinking water contamination in the United Kingdom have involved phenol contamination of the River Dee in 1984 (no apparent deaths; many consumer complaints—taste, gastrointestinal symptoms)[22] and the discharge of concentrated aluminum sulfate in water-treatment works near Camelford (many reports of nausea, vomiting, diarrhea, sore eyes, mouth ulcers, and itching, skin rashes; water aluminium concentration 10 to 50 mg/L for 1 to 3 days—no deaths).

DISASTER MEDICINE

In the United States, governmental approaches to cope with disasters include the following[23–25]:

1. National Disaster Medical Systems (NDMS) (volunteer force from the Department of Health Service/Public Health Service); Department of Defense, Federal Emergency Management Agents (FEMA); Veterans Administration.
2. Disaster medical response teams—in process of formation (NDMS and FEMA).

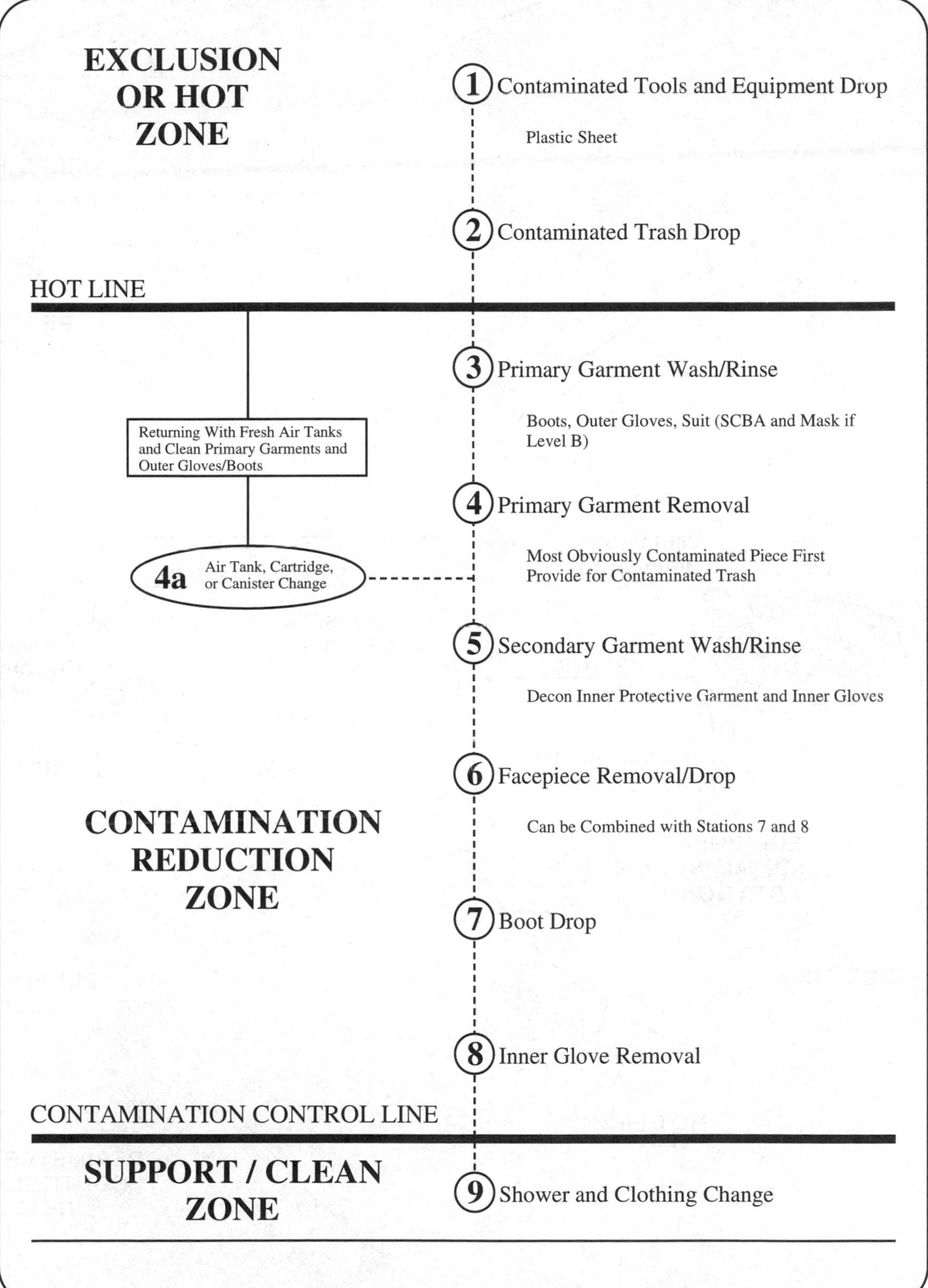

Figure 58–2 Nine-step personnel decontamination plan.

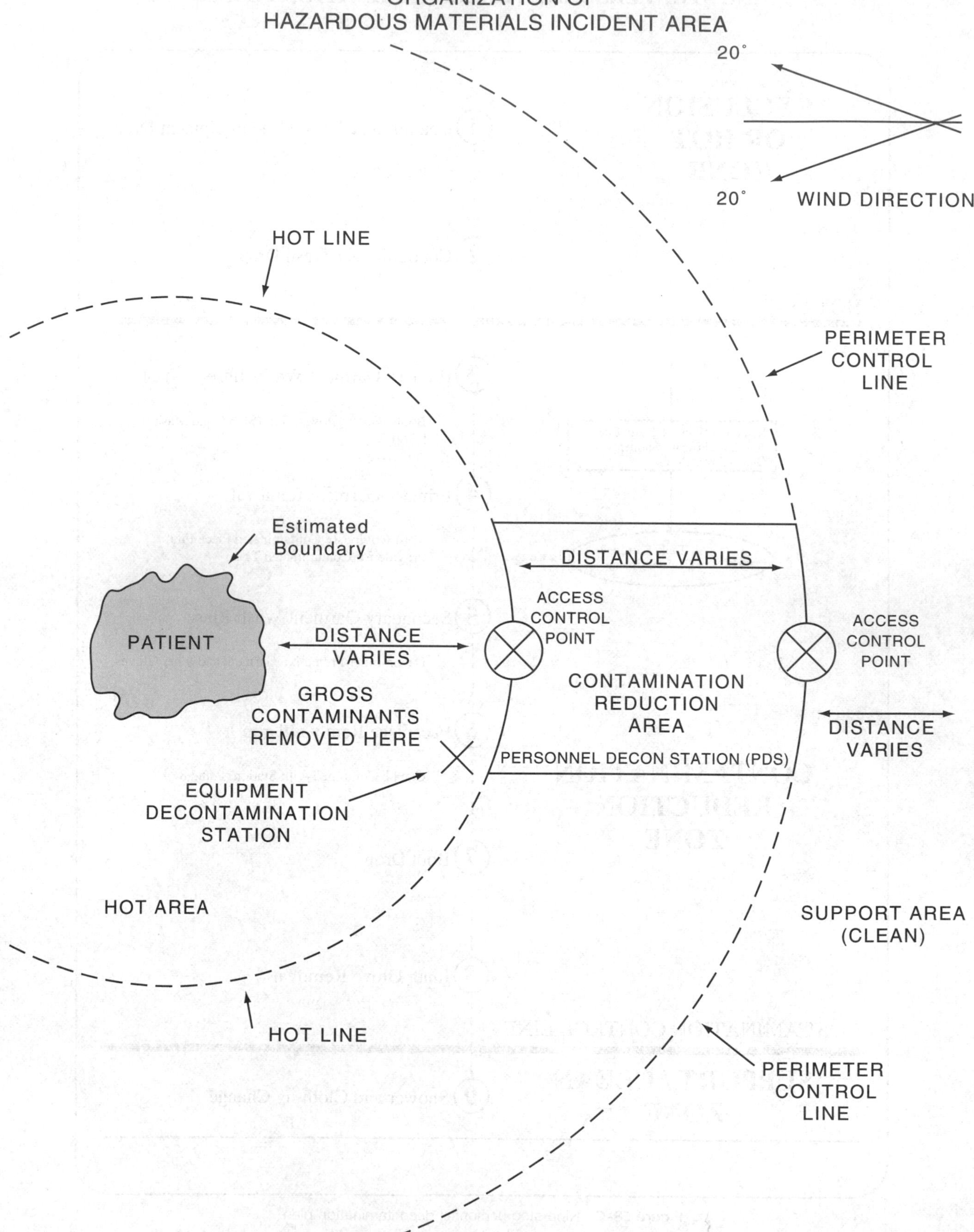

Figure 58-3 Organization of hazardous material incident area. (Adapted from Paparek PJ Jr, Karbus J, and subcommittee members. Subcommittee on Medical and Emergency Response in Managing Victims of Hazardous Materials Release. Los Angeles County Department of Health Services, 1988.)

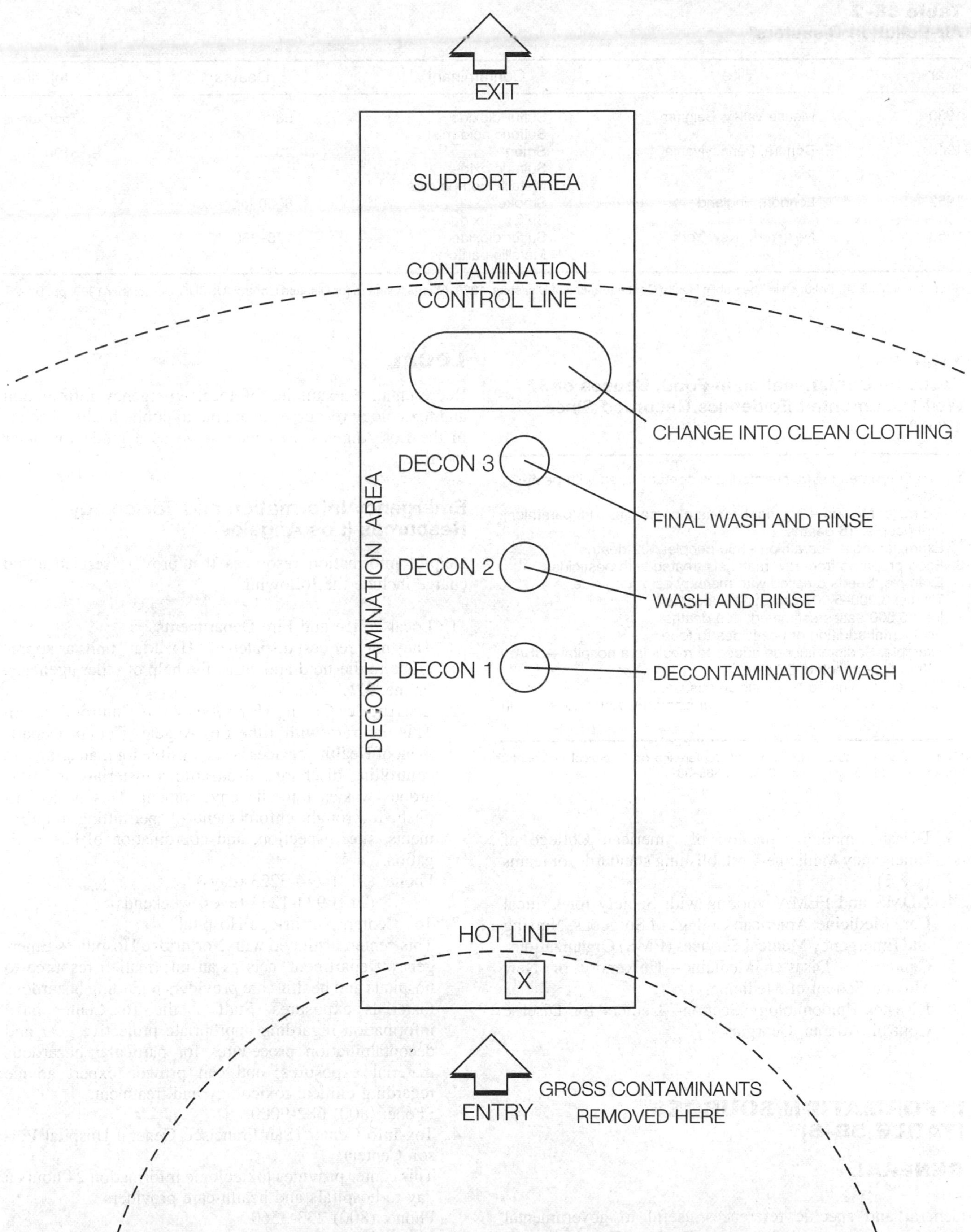

Figure 58–4 Decontamination area. (Adapted from Paparek PJ Jr, Karbus J, and subcommittee members. Subcommittee on Medical and Emergency Response in Managing Victims of Hazardous Materials Release. Los Angeles County Department of Health Services, 1988.)

Table 58–2
Air-Pollution Disasters[a]

Year	Site	Contaminant	Deaths	Injuries
1930	Meuse Valley, Belgium	Sulfur dioxide Sulfuric acid mist	63	Thousands
1948	Donora, Pennsylvania	Smog Sulfuric oxides Metallic compounds	20	5190
1952	London, England	Smoke Sulfur dioxide	8000 (approx.)	
1953	New York, New York	Sulfur dioxide Metallic particles	175–260	

[a]From French JG. Air Pollution in The Public Health Consequences of Disasters, 1989. Atlanta: Centers for Disease Control, USDHS, September 1989, pp. 91–96.

Table 58–3
Pesticide Contamination in Food. Causes of 37 Well-Documented Epidemics Recorded Since 1960[a]

1. Food prepared using intermediates contaminated with pesticides.
   Example: Mexico—Organophosphate contamination (parathion): 559 people; 16 deaths.
   Example: India—parathion—360 people; 102 deaths.
2. Food prepared from raw materials treated with pesticides.
   Example: Seeds dressed with mercury as a fungicide.
   Turkey: 3,000–5,000 cases; 11% deaths.
   Iraq: 6,500 cases estimated; 459 deaths.
3. Accidental addition of pesticides to food.
   Example: Sodium fluoride added to meals in a hospital—USA: 263 people affected; 57 died.
4. Food contaminated by pesticide misuse.
   Example: USA 1985 Aldicarb contaminated watermelons; 1,100 cases of poisoning.

[a]From Ferrer A, Cabral JRP. In: World Conference on Chemical Accidents. Edinburgh: CEP Consultants, 1985; pp. 385–387.

3. Disaster medicine section of American College of Emergency Medicine—establishing standards for teams (see 2).
4. NDMS and FEMA working with Society for Critical Care Medicine, American College of Surgeons, Nursing and Emergency Medical Services (EMS) Organizations.
5. Center for Disaster Medicine—University of New Mexico School of Medicine.
6. Disaster Epidemiology Section—Centers for Disease Control, Atlanta, Georgia.

INFORMATION SOURCES (TABLE 58–6)

GENERAL

General and specific references useful to governmental agencies, occupational physicians, Regional Poison Control Centers, members of Emergency Medical Services, and others who are involved in planning for and responding to disasters are presented in this chapter and in the OECD Environmental Monograph No. 87.[21]

LOCAL

Representative examples of local emergency information and toxicology resources available to public health officials in the Los Angeles area may serve as a guide for other localities.

Emergency Information and Toxicology Resources (Los Angeles)

Helpful information resources that provide service at no charge include the following:

1. Local Police and Fire Departments
   They may request dispatch of "Haz Mat" units as appropriate to the field and enlist the help of other agencies.
   Phone: 911.
2. Los Angeles County Hazardous Waste Control Program
   This program within the Los Angeles County Department of Health Services is responsible for managing and controlling discharge of hazardous materials and hazardous wastes into the environment. This is accomplished through enforcement of permitting requirements, site inspection, and coordination of site mitigation.
   Phone: (213) 744-3223 (days)
   (213) 974-1234 (eves, weekends)
3. Tox-Center, Northridge Hospital
   This center, affiliated with Northridge Hospital's Emergency Department, acts as an information resource to hospitals and health-care providers regarding hazardous materials exposures. Staff at the Tox-Center have information regarding appropriate protective gear and decontamination procedures for particular hazardous material exposures, and can provide expert advice regarding clinical toxicology and treatment.
   Phone: (800) 682-9000
4. Tox-Info Center (San Francisco General Hospital Poison Center)
   This center provides toxicologic information 24 hours a day to hospitals and health-care providers.
   Phone: (800) 233-3360
5. Los Angeles County Medical Association (LACMA) Regional Poison Control Center
   This center provides toxicologic information 24 hours a day to hospitals and health-care providers.
   Phone: (213) 484-5151

6. Hazardous Evaluation Service and Information System (HESIS)
   This program, administered by the California Department of Health Services, provides nonemergency information about hazardous industrial chemicals.
   Phone: (415) 540-3014 (8 AM–5 PM; Monday–Friday)
7. Federal Occupational Safety and Health Administration (OSHA)
   This agency has responsibility for protecting the health of workers in the private sector.
   Phone: (213) 861-9993—Consultation Service
   (213) 620-4036 or 620-4039—Enforcement and General Information
8. Medical Alert Center (MAC)
   This office does not provide medical or toxicologic information, but will assist with medical transportation or triage of patients in a disaster or mass casualty.
   Phone: (213) 226-6697

A helpful listing of resources for hazardous materials episodes is contained in the publication titled: Health Effects of Toxic Substances: A Directory of References and Resources, published in 1986 and available from the State of California Publications Section, P.O. Box 1015, North Highlands, CA 95660. The publication number is 7540/958/1300/3. The cost is approximately $3.95.

Table 58–4
Some Historical Chlorine Accidents[a]

Location	Year	Source	Scenario	Area	Quantity (Te)	Fatalities	Casualties	Evacuees
St Auban FR	1926	Storage	Tank burst	Urban	25	19	—	—
Zarnesti RO	1939	Storage	Tank burst	Factory	24	60	—	—
Rauma SU	1947	Storage	Overfilling/burst	Factory	30	19	—	—
Wilsum Ger.	1952	Storage	Tank failed	Factory	15	15	—	—
Los Angeles Cal. US	1976	Cylinders (14)	Fire	Urban	—	—	72	2000
Baton Rouge La. US	1976	Storage	Explosion	Factory	90	—	—	10000
Youngston Fla. US	1978	Rail tanker	Accident/puncture	—	25	8	138	—
Mississauga Ont. CND	1979	Rail tanker	Fire + puncture	Urban	70	—	—	250000
San Juan, Puerto Rico	1981	Water treatment	Valve corrosion	Urban	2	—	2000	—
Cerritos (Potosi) Mex.	1981	Rail tankers	Brake failure	Semi-urban	90–150	28	1000	>5000

First World War data

Location	Year	Source	Scenario	Area	Quantity (Te)	Fatalities	Casualties	
Yper	1915	Cylinders	6 km line release	Trenches	168	5000	15000	No masks
Total WWI	1915–1918	Chlorine + phosgene	—	—	32000	36600	100000?	Masks (probably)

[a]Adapted from Vilain J. In: Bourdeau P, Green G, eds. Methods for assessing and reducing injury from chemical accidents. Chichester: John Wiley, 1989; pp. 252–290.

Table 58–5
Some Historical Ammonia Accidents[a]

Location	Year	Source	Scenario	Area	Quantity (Te)	Fatalities	Casualties	Evacuees
Lievin FR	1968	Road tanker	Tank failed	Urban	19	6	15	—
Crete Nebr. US	1969	Rail tanker	Collision	Urban	90	8	35	—
Blair Nebr. US	1970	Storage	Overflow 2,5 Hr	Rural	160	—	—	(3 km cloud)
Potchefstroom S Afr.	1973	Storage	Embrittlement/ rupture	Urban	38	18	65	—
Houston Tex. US	1976	Road tanker	Collision	Highway/ urban	19	5	150	(Local)
Deer Park Tex, US	1976	Road tanker	Skid/crash	Highway	19	6	200	—
Cartagena, Columbia	1976	Fertilizer plant	Explosion	Urban	—	21	30	—
Cuernevaca Mex.	1977	Pipeline	Failure	Urban	—	2	90	—
Pensacola Fla. US	1977	Rail tankers (2)	Derailed	Urban	—	2	46	1000
Crestview Fla. US	1979	Rail tankers (10)	Derailed	Urban	—	—	14	5000
Los Pajaritos, Mex.	1984	Pipeline	Failure	Urban (slum)	—	4	46	—

[a]Adapted from Vilain J. In: Bourdeau P, Green G, eds. Methods for assessing and reducing injury from chemical accidents. Chichester: John Wiley, 1989; pp. 252–290.

Table 58–6
Important Resources for Emergency HAZ-MAT Response and Planning[a]

Agencies
- **Regional Poison Center**
  24-hour toxicology information
- **Health Department**
  Assist with public health and follow-up care
- **Local Emergency Planning Committee (LEPC)**
  Provide information about chemicals in community
- **Fire Department/Hazardous Materials Team**
  Assist with response and planning
- **Chemical Transportation Emergency Center (CHEMTREC)**
  24-hour information resource to manufacturers[1] product information (phone number: 1-800-424-9300)
- **Agency for Toxic Substances and Disease Registry**
  24-hour emergency assistance for health-related issues (phone number: 404-639-0615)
- **Environmental Protection Agency**
  Regional offices with technical assistance available for environmental issues
- **National Response Center**
  Provides 24-hour assistance for identifying chemicals and planning a response (phone number: 1-800-424-8802)
- **Radiation Emergency Assistance Center/Training Site (REAC/TS)**
  Provides emergency consultation for accidents involving radioactive materials (phone number: 615-481-1000)

Computer Databases
- **Chemical Hazard Response Information System (CHRIS)**
  Contains general and health hazard information (for more information: 1-800-247-8737)
- **Hazardous Substance Data Bank (HSDB)**
  Reviews toxicity information compiled by the National Library of Medicine (for more information: 301-496-6531)
- **Poisindex/Tomes**
  Contains comprehensive acute and chronic toxicity information (for more information: 1-800-525-9083)
- **Toxicology Data Network (TOXNET)**
  National Library of Medicine data bank for health effects of industrial and environmental exposures (for more information: 301-496-6531)

Publications
- Sullivan, Krieger: Hazardous Materials Toxicology: Clinical Principles of Environmental Health, Williams & Wilkins, 1992
- Borack, Callan, Abbott: Hazardous Materials Exposure: Emergency Response and Patient Care, Prentice Hall, 1991
- Agency for Toxic Substance and Disease Registry: Managing Hazardous Materials Incidents: Volume II: Hospital Emergency Departments, 1991
- 1987 Emergency Response Guidebook, ed 4. US Department of Transportation (DOT), 1987

General Toxicology Texts
- Ellenhorn, Barceloux: Medical Toxicology: Diagnosis and Treatment of Human Poisoning, Elsevier, 1988
- Goldfrank et al: Goldfrank's Toxicologic Emergencies, Appleton & Lange, 1990
- Haddad, Winchester: Clinical Management of Poisoning and Drug Overdose, WB Saunders, 1990
- Klaassen, et al: Casarett and Doull's Toxicology: The Basic Science of Poisons, MacMillan, 1986
- Rom: Environmental and Occupational Medicine, Little, Brown and Company, 1992.

Note: This is not an all inclusive list of references but has been selected as a representative list for use in an emergency department. Most Regional Poison Centers will have many of these references available.
[a]From Kirk MA, Cisek J, Rose SR. Emerg Med Clin North Am 1994;12:467.

Training Facilities

Hospitals and emergency rooms that anticipate managing hazardous materials victims on a regular basis should arrange specific training in toxicology and use of protective equipment for their medical, nursing, and other ancillary staff. Many fire and police departments are already making plans to provide such training for their staff members. It may prove helpful for hospitals to coordinate training efforts with their local emergency response agencies.

Relevant training in California and elsewhere, for example, is provided by the following resources:

1. California Specialized Training Institute (CSTI)
   CSTI in San Luis Obispo offers a number of courses for medical and nonmedical persons involved in hazardous materials management.
   Phone: (805) 544-7100
2. University of California, Los Angeles (UCLA) Extension
   UCLA Extension periodically offers classes on toxicology and hazardous materials management for health professionals and other interested persons. UCLA also offers a certification program in hazardous materials management.
   Phone: (213) 825-7093
3. UCLA Department of Industrial Safety
   The UCLA Department of Industrial Safety has developed educational materials, including films and slide-tape shows, on how to manage contamination problems.
   Phone: (213) 825-3793
4. University of California, Irvine (UCI)
   The UCI's Southern Occupational Health Center periodically offers courses and seminars on occupational and environmental toxicology.
   Phone: (714) 856-1064
5. University of California Davis (UCD)
   The UCD Medical Center offers accredited continuing

education courses on environmental and occupational medicine.
Phone: (916) 453-5390
The UCD Extension Program offers courses leading to certification in Hazardous Materials Management, including the management of contaminated victims and site management. Contact Beth Floyd.
Phone: (916) 752-6021

6. University of Southern California (USC)
The Southern California Education Resource Center has its headquarters at USC and offers courses on safety and health issues related to hazardous materials management.
Phone: (213) 743-6383
7. Oak Ridge National Laboratories, Tennessee
Oak Ridge offers in-depth training courses on radiation safety and management of radiation victims. In addition, this center has a number of excellent films and video cassette tapes available for health professionals, particularly with regard to radiation contamination problems.
Phone: (615) 576-3131
8. National Safety Council
The National Safety Council offers courses and has information material related to the safety aspects of hazardous materials management.
Phone: (213) 385-6461

Telephone Roster

A suggested telephone checklist for emergency disaster planning agencies is presented in Table 58–7.

Glossary

A glossary of frequently used terms and agencies involved in disaster planning is found in Table 58–8.

Compilation of Chemical Information

Chemical information should be available to a Poison Information Center or other government agency such as the ATSDR in the United States.

Identifying the Chemical

Kirk and colleagues have suggested some steps for identification of chemicals and obtaining health risk.

Hazardous Materials Classification Systems

A classification of hazardous substances incorporates the 704M System of the National Fire Protection Association: (Figs. 58–5 and 58–6).

PLANNING FOR A CHEMICAL DISASTER[26]

PREPLANNING

Survey of Surrounding Area

An important part of any chemical disaster preplanning involves a survey of the area surrounding receiving hospitals to determine which types of hazardous materials are used by local industries.

To obtain more detailed information on specific chemicals used by nearby industries, emergency departments can obtain from these industries copies of their Material Safety Data Sheets (MSDSs) and keep them on file. MSDSs contain basic chemical, reactivity, and toxicology data and should be kept on file by an employer for each hazardous substance used in the facility.

In an emergency in the United States, legislation requires any employer or facility to provide immediately any information contained on MSDSs to health-care providers who need the information to care for an affected patient. The information must be provided without regard for "trade secrets" and may be provided by telephone or otherwise. In a nonemergency situation such information can be provided in writing, and the health care provider or agency must then take some care to safeguard.

Regional Advisory Committees

A regional advisory committee on chemical accidents should be convened to establish and coordinate the body of expertise already available within the region. The committee should ensure that a coordinated response can be provided in an emergency and that accurate and appropriate information can be disseminated to the public.[27–29] In Los Angeles this committee includes a physician from the regional department of health, an occupational physician, and physician members of local hospital emergency departments, clinical toxicologists, public health physicians, and members of local county services.[30] In the United Kingdom the Department of Health has formed an independent health advisory group to provide advice to health officials confronted with serious chemical contamination of a water supply.[27]

Regarding toxicologic information, public health authorities have to guarantee that the following activities are started and that they are updated regularly[31]:

This information should be adapted to the "level" at which it will be given and the training and knowledge of those who will be using it.

Hospital Disaster Manual

Each hospital disaster manual should clearly delineate:

1. Who is in charge.
2. What are the emergency discharge/transfer criteria.
3. How to obtain additional supplies.
4. How to use an alternative communication system.
5. What the evacuation procedures are.[32]
6. Emergency physicians should know where to report and the role they assume.
7. Hospital supplies, clothes that identify staff (vests, jumpsuits, hard hats, jackets).

Copies of evacuation procedures should be provided to all appropriate agencies and organizations (e.g., Salvation Army, churches, schools, hospitals) and could periodically be published in the local newspaper(s).

Table 58–7
Telephone Roster[a]

Contact	Availability	Telephone
Community Assistance		
Police		
Fire		
Emergency Management Agency		
Public Health Department		
Environmental Protection Agency		
Department of Transportation		
Public Works		
Water Supply		
Sanitation		
Port Authority		
Transit Authority		
Rescue Squad		
Ambulance		
Hospitals		
Utilities:		
Gas		
Phone		
Electricity		
Community Officials		
Mayor		
City Manager		
County Executive		
Councils of Government		
Volunteer Groups		
Red Cross		
Salvation Army		
Church Groups		
Ham Radio Operators		
Off-Road Vehicle Clubs		
State Assistance		
State Emergency Response Commission (Title III of SARA)		
State Environmental Protection Agency		
Emergency Management Agency		
Department of Transportation		
Police		
Public Health Department		
Department of Agriculture		
Federal Assistance (Consult Regional offices listed in Appendix F for appropriate telephone numbers.)		
Federal On-Scene Coordinator		
U.S. Department of Transportation		
U.S. Coast Guard		
U.S. Environmental Protection Agency		
Federal Emergency Management Agency	24 hours	202-646-2400
U.S. Department of Agriculture		
Occupational Safety and Health Administration		
Agency for Toxic Substances and Disease Registry	24 hours	404-452-4100
National Response Center	24 hours	800-424-8802
	in Washington, DC area	202-426-2675
	or	202-267-2675
U.S. Army, Navy, Air Force		
Bomb Disposal and/or Explosive Ordnance Team, U.S. Army		
Nuclear Regulatory Commission	24 hours	301-951-0550
U.S. Department of Energy Radiological Assistance	24 hours	202-586-8100
U.S. Department of the Treasury Bureau of Alcohol, Tobacco, and Firearms		
Other Emergency Assistance		
CHEMTREC	24 hours	800-424-9300
CHEMNET	24 hours	800-424-9300
CHLOREP	24 hours	800-424-9300
NACA Pesticide Safety Team	24 hours	800-424-9300
Association of American Railroads/Bureau of Explosives	24 hours	202-639-2222
Poison Control Center		
Cleanup Contractor		
Response Personnel		
Incident Commander		
Agency Coordinators		
Response Team Members		
Bordering Political Regions		
Municipalities		
Counties		
States		
Countries		
River Basin Authorities		
Irrigation Districts		
Interstate Compacts		
Regional Authorities		
Bordering International Authorities		
Sanitation Authorities/Commissions		
Industry		
Transporters		
Chemical Producers/Consumers		
Spill Cooperatives		
Spill Response Teams		
Media		
Television		
Newspaper		
Radio		

[a]Adapted from Makris JL, Storch RL. Hazardous Materials Emergency Planning Guide. Washington, DC. National Response Team.

Table 58–8
Glossary[a]

CAER	—	Community Awareness and Emergency Response program developed by the Chemical Manufacturers Association. Guidance for chemical plant managers to assist them in taking the initiative in cooperating with local communities to develop integrated (community/industry) hazardous materials response plans.
CEPP	—	Chemical Emergency Preparedness Program developed by EPA to address accidental releases of acutely toxic chemicals.
CERCLA	—	Comprehensive Environmental Response, Compensation, and Liability Act regarding hazardous substance releases into the environment and the cleanup of inactive hazardous waste disposal sites.
CHEMNET	—	A mutual aid network of chemical shippers and contractors. CHEMNET has more than fifty participating companies with emergency teams, twenty-three subscribers (who receive services in an incident from a participant and then reimburse response and cleanup costs), and several emergency response contractors. CHEMNET is activated when a member shipper cannot respond promptly to an incident involving that company's product(s) and requiring the presence of a chemical expert. If a member company cannot go to the scene of the incident, the shipper will authorize a CHEMNET-contracted emergency response company to go. Communications for the network are provided by CHEMTREC, with the shipper receiving notification and details about the incident from the CHEMTREC communicator.
CHEMTREC	—	Chemical Transportation Emergency Center operated by the Chemical Manufacturers' Association. Provides information and/or assistance to emergency responders. CHEMTREC contacts the shipper or producer of the material for more detailed information, including on-scene assistance when feasible. Can be reached 24 hours a day by calling 800-424-9300. (Also see "HIT.")
CHLOREP	—	Chlorine Emergency Plan operated by the Chlorine Institute. A 24-hour mutual aid program. Response is activated by a CHEMTREC call to the designated CHLOREP contact, who notifies the appropriate team leader, based upon CHLOREP's geographical sector assignments for teams. The team leader in turn calls the emergency caller at the incident scene and determines what advice and assistance are needed. The team leader then decides whether or not to dispatch his team to the scene.
ERT	—	Environmental Response Team, a group of highly specialized experts available through EPA 24 hours a day.
EOP	—	Emergency Operations Plan developed in accord with the guidance in CPG 1–8. EOPs are multi-hazard, functional plans that treat emergency management activities generically. EOPs provide for as much generally applicable capability as possible without reference to any particular hazard; then they address the unique aspects of individual disasters in hazard-specific appendices.
FAULT-TREE ANALYSIS	—	A means of analyzing hazards. Hazardous events are first identified by other techniques such as HAZOP. Then all combinations of individual failures that can lead to that hazardous event are shown in the logical format of the fault tree. By estimating the individual failure probabilities, and then using the appropriate arithmetical expressions, the top-event frequency can be calculated.
FEMA-REP-5	—	Guidance for Developing State and Local Radiological Emergency Response Plans and Preparedness for Transportation Accidents, prepared by FEMA. Provides a basis for state and local governments to develop emergency plans and improve emergency preparedness for transportation accidents involving radio active materials.
HAZARDOUS MATERIALS	—	Refers generally to hazardous substances, petroleum, natural gas, synthetic gas, acutely toxic chemicals, and other toxic chemicals.
HAZOP	—	Hazard and operability study, a systematic technique for identifying hazards or operability problems throughout an entire facility. One examines each segment of a process and lists all possible deviations for normal operating conditions and how they might occur. The consequences on the process are assessed, and the means available to detect and correct the deviations are examined.
HIT	—	Hazard Information Transmission program provides a digital transmission of the CHEMTREC emergency chemical report to first responders at the scene of a hazardous materials incident. The report advises the responder on the hazards of the materials, the level of protective clothing required, mitigating action to take in the event of a spill, leak, or fire and first aid for victims. HIT is a free public service provided by the Chemical Manufacturers[1] Association. Reports are sent in emergency situations only to organizations that have pre-registered with HIT. Brochures and registration forms may be obtained by writing: Manager, CHEMTREC/CHEMNET, 2501 M Street, N.W., Washington, DC, 20037.
ICS	—	Incident Command System, the combination of facilities, equipment, personnel, procedures, and communications operating within a common organizational structure with responsibilty for management of assigned resources to effectively accomplish stated objectives at the scene of an incident.
IEMS	—	Integrated Emergency Management System, developed by FEMA in recognition of the economics realized in planning for all hazards on a generic functional basis as opposed to developing independent structures and resources to deal with each type of hazard.
NCP	—	National Oil and Hazardous Substances Pollution Contingency Plan (40 CFR Part 300), prepared by EPA to put into effect the response powers and responsibilities created by CERCLA and the authorities established by Section 311 of the Clean Water Act.
NFA	—	The National Fire Academy is a component of FEMA's National Emergency Training Center located in Emmitsburg, Maryland. It provides fire prevention and control training of the fire service and allied services. Courses on campus are offered in technical, management, and prevention subject areas. A growing off-campus course delivery system is operated in conjunction with State fire training program offices.
NHMIE	—	National Hazardous Materials Information Exchange, provides information on hazmat training courses, planning technqiues, events and conferences, and emergency response experiences and lessons learned. Call toll-free 1-800-752-6367 (in Illinois, 1-800-367-9592). Planners with personal computer capabilities can access NHMIE by dialing FTS 972-3275 or (312) 972-3275.

[a]Adapted from Hazardous Materials Emergency Planning Guide. NRT-1 National Response Team, Washington, DC: March 1987 (Makris JL—EPA; Storch RL—US Coast Guard).

(continued)

Table 58–8 *(Continued)*

NRC	— National Response Center, a communications center for activities related to response actions, is located at Coast Guard headquarters in Washington, DC. The NRC receives and relays notices of discharges or releases to the appropriate OSC, disseminates OSC and RRT reports to the NRT when appropriate, and provides facilities for the NRT to use in coordinating a national response action when required. The toll-free number (800-424-8802, or 202-426-2675 or 202-267-2675 in the Washington, DC area) can be rached 24 hours a day for reporting actual or potential pollution incidents.
NRT	— National Response Team, consisting of representatives of 14 government agencies (DOD, DOI, DOT/RSPA, DOT/USCG, EPA, DOC, FEMA, DOS, USDA, DOJ, HHS, DOL, Nuclear Regulatory Commission, and DOE), is the principal organization for implementing the NCP. When the NRT is not activated for a response action, it serves as a standing committee to develop and maintain preparedness, to evaluate methods of responding to discharges or releases, to recommend needed changes in the response organization, and to recommend revisions to the NCP. The NRT may consider and make recommendations to appropriate agencies on the training, equipping, and protection of response teams; and necessary research, development, demonstration, and evaluation to improve response capabilities.
NSF	— National Strike Force, made up of three Strike Teams. The USCG counterpart to the EPA ERTs.
NUREG 0654/ FEMA-REP-1	— Criteria for Preparation and Evaluation of Radiological Emergency Response Plans and Preparedness in Support of Nuclear Power Plants, prepared by NRC and FEMA. Provides a basis for state and local government and nuclear facility operators to develop radiological emergency plans and improve emergency preparedness. The criteria also will be used by Federal agency reviewers in determining the adequacy of state, local, and nuclear facility emergency plans and preparedness.
OHMTADS	— Oil and Hazardous Materials Technical Assistance Data System, a computerized data base containing chemical, biological, and toxicological information about hazardous substances. OSCs use OHMTADS to identify unknown chemicals and to learn how to best handle known chemicals.
OSC	— On-Scene Coordinator, the Federal official predesignated by EPA or USCG to coordinate and direct Federal responses and removals under the NCP; or the DOD official designated to coordinate and direct the removal actions from releases of hazardous substances, pollutants, or contaminants from DOD vessels and facilities. When the NRC receives notification of a pollution incident, the NRC Duty Officer notifies the appropriate OSC, depending on the location of an incident. Based on this initial report and any other information that can be obtained, the OSC makes a preliminary assessment of the need for a Federal response. If an on-scene response is required, the OSC will go to the scene and monitor the response of the responsible party or state or local government. If the responsible party is unknown or not taking appropriate action, and the response is beyond the capability of state and local governments, the OSC may initiate Federal actions, using funding from the FWPCA Pollution Fund for oil discharges and the CERCLA Trust Fund (Superfund) for hazardous substance releases.
PSTN	— Pesticide Safety Team Network operated by the National Agricultural Chemicals Association to minimize environmental damage and injury arising from accidental pesticide spills or leaks. PSTN area coordinators in ten regions nationwide are available 24 hours a day to receive pesticide incident notifications from CHEMTREC.
RCRA	— Resource Conservation and Recovery Act (of 1976) established a framework for the proper management and disposal of all wastes. RCRA directed EPA to identify hazardous wastes, both generically and by listing specific wastes and industrial process waste streams. Generators and transporters are required to use good management practices and to track the movement of wastes with a manifest system. Owners and operators of treatment, storage, and disposal facilities also must comply with standards, which are generally implemented through permits issued by EPA or authorized States.
RRT	— Regional Response Teams composed of representatives of Federal agencies and a representative from each state in the Federal region. During a response to a major hazardous materials incident involving transportation or a fixed facility, the OSC may request that the RRT be convened to provide advice or recommendations in specific issues requiring resolution. Under the NCP, RRTs may be convened by the chairman when a hazardous materials discharge or release exceeds the response capability available to the OSC in the place where it occurs; crosses regional boundaries; or may pose a substantial threat to the public health, welfare, or environment, or to regionally significant amounts of property. Regional contingency plans specify detailed criteria for activation of RRTs. RRTs may review plans developed in compliance with Title III, if the local emergency planning committee so requests.
SARA	— The "Superfund Amendments and Reauthorization Act of 1986." Title III of SARA includes detailed provisions for community planning.
Superfund	— The trust fund established under CERCLA to provide money the OSC can use during a cleanup.
Title III	— The "Emergency Planning and Community Right-to-Know Act of 1986." Specifies requirements for organizing the planning process at the state and local levels for specified extremely hazardous substances; minimum plan content; requirements for fixed facility owners and operators to inform officials about extremely hazardous substances present at the facilities; and mechanisms for making information about extremely hazardous substances available to citizens. (See Appendix A.)

THE RESPONSE

PREHOSPITAL MANAGEMENT

Hot Zone

Only trained and appropriately attired rescuers should enter the Hot Zone. If the proper equipment is not available, or if rescuers have not been trained to use it, call for assistance from a local or regional HAZMAT team or other properly equipped response organization.

Rescuer Protection

When a chemical is unidentified, worst-case assumptions concerning toxicity must be assumed. Both severe local

DOMESTIC LABELING

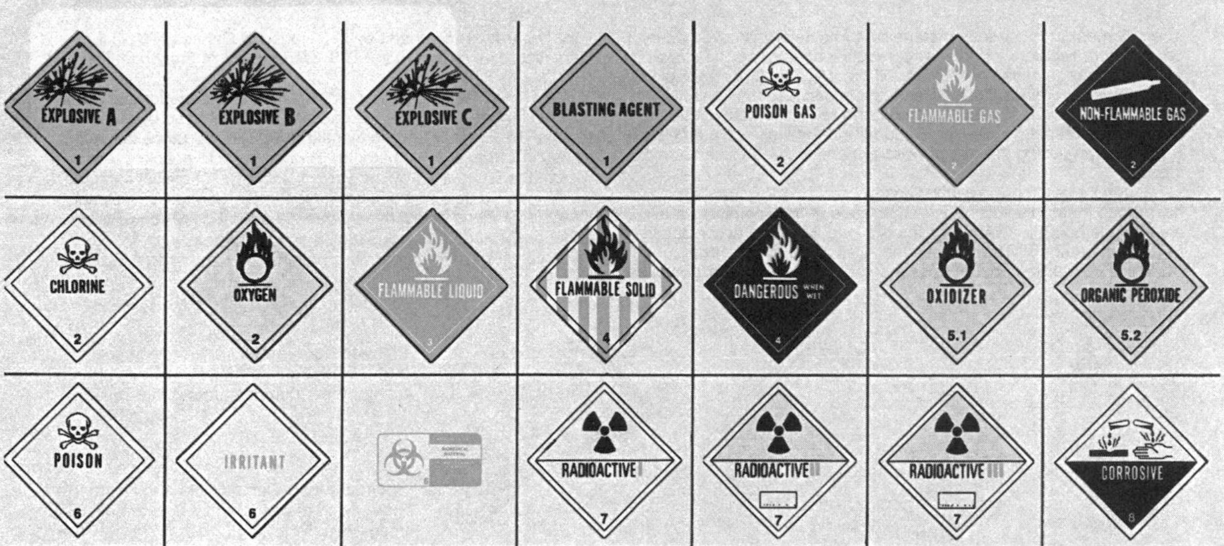

General Guidelines on Use of Labels

(CFR, Title 49, Transportation, Parts 100-177)

- Labels illustrated above are normally for *domestic shipments.* However, some air carriers *may* require the use of International Civil Aviation Organization (ICAO) labels.
- Domestic Warning Labels *may* display UN Class Number, Division Number (and Compatibility Group for Explosives only) [Sec. 172.407(g)].
- Any person who offers a hazardous material for transportation MUST label the package, if required [Sec. 172.400(a)].
- The Hazardous Materials Tables, Sec. 172.101 and 172.102, identify the proper label(s) for the hazardous materials listed.
- Label(s), when required, must be printed on or affixed to the surface of the package near the proper shipping name [Sec. 172.406(a)].
- When two or more different labels are required, display them next to each other [Sec. 172.406(c)].
- Labels may be affixed to packages (even when not required by regulations) provided each label represents a hazard of the material in the package [Sec. 172.401].

Check the Appropriate Regulations
Domestic or International Shipment

Additional Markings and Labels

HANDLING LABELS

Cargo Aircraft Only
172.402(b)

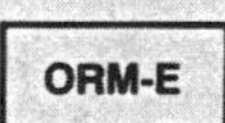

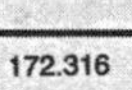

172.316

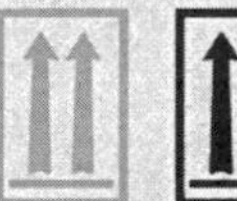

Package Orientation Markings

172.312(a)(c)

CAUTION

Bung Label
172.402(e)

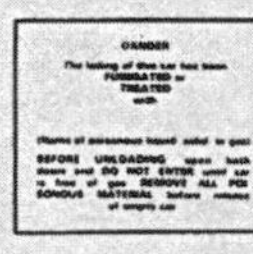

173.25(a)(4)

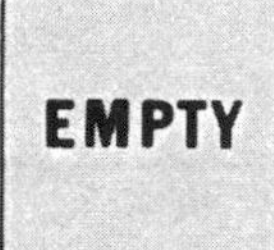

Fumigation
173.9

EMPTY

173.427

Here are a few additional markings and labels pertaining to the transport of hazardous materials. The section number shown with each item refers to the appropriate section in the HMR. The Hazardous Materials Tables, Section 172.101 and 172.102, identify the proper shipping name, hazard class, identification number, required label(s) and packaging sections.

Poisonous Materials

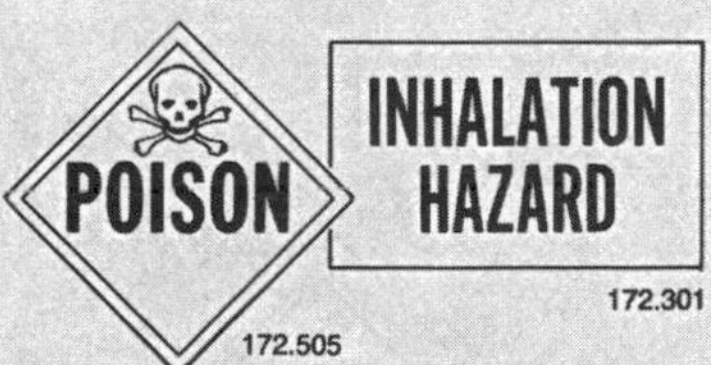

172.505

172.301

Materials which meet the inhalation toxicity criteria specified in Section 173.3a(b)(2), have additional "communication standards" prescribed by the HMR. First, the words "Poison-Inhalation Hazard" must be entered on the shipping paper, as required by Section 172.203(k)(4), for any primary capacity units with a capacity greater than one liter. Second, packages of 110 gallons or less capacity must be marked "Inhalation Hazard" in accordance with Section 172.301(a). Lastly, transport vehicles, freight containers and portable tanks subject to the shipping paper requirements contained in Section 172.203(k)(4) must be placarded with POISON placards in addition to the placards required by Section 172.504. For additional information and exceptions to these communication requirements, see the referenced sections in the HMR.

Figure 58–5

Examples of Canadian and International Placards and Labels

The shipment of hazardous materials internationally is governed by one or more regulatory bodies with regulations that may be similar to domestic regulations or radically different. Canada, for example, has adopted wordless placards and labels because their country is bilingual. Canada also requires cargo and rail tanks to use retro-reflective placarding. However, Canada and the United States have reciprocity regarding the use of wordless and worded placards and labels.

Several international organizations govern the transportation of hazardous materials according to the mode of transportation. If a shipment is going by water, the International Maritime Organization (IMO) has authority. The International Civil Aviation Organization (ICAO) is concerned about the safe shipment of dangerous goods (*i.e.,* hazardous materials) by air. Transport Canada (TC) is the Canadian counterpart to the U.S. Department of Transportation (DOT).

The United Nations publishes "Recommendations for the Transport of Dangerous Goods," a publication that is used by many nations of the world when promulgating regulations. Since the safe transport of hazardous materials is of concern to people everywhere, the work done by the United Nations is of critical importance world-wide. Labels and placards used in the Canadian, IMO, and ICAO regulations are generally based on the U.N. Recommendations, although Canada has some labels and placard designs that vary from the U.N. White borders are optional on International Placards.

Flammable Solid

Oxidizer

Non-flammable Gas

Spontaneously Combustible

Keep Away From Food

Corrosive Gas

Flammable Gas

Flammable Liquid

Dangerous When Wet

Poison

Miscellaneous Dangerous Substances

Infectious Substance

Examples of Wordless Placards and Labels

Pictured here are typical wordless placards and labels required for use in Canada and many other countries around the world.

Examples of International and Canadian Placards and Labels

Spontaneously Combustible and Keep Away From Food placards and labels are used internationally and in Canada. The Corrosive Gas placard and label are used exclusively in Canada. Most placards and labels used internationally are similar (color and symbols) to those required by DOT regulations.

UN Class Numbers

Class 1: Explosives
Class 2: Gases (compressed, liquified or dissolved under pressure
Class 3: Flammable liquids
Class 4: Flammable solids or substances
Class 5: Oxidizing substances. Division 5.1, Oxidizing substances or agents. Division 5.2, Organic peroxides.
Class 6: Poisonous and infectious substances
Class 7: Radioactive substances
Class 8: Corrosives
Class 9: Misc. dangerous substances

Examples of Explosive Labels

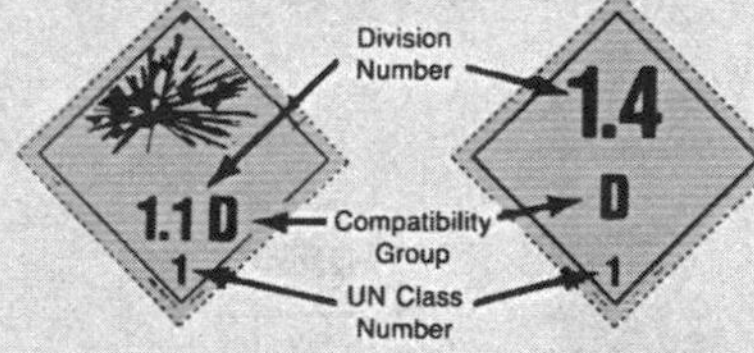

The Numerical Designation represents the Class or Division. Alphabetical Designation represents the Compatibility Group (for Explosives only). Division Numbers and Compatibility Group combinations can result in over 30 different "Explosives" labels (see IMDG Code/ICAO).

For complete details, refer to one or more of the following:

- Code of Federal Regulations, Title 49, Transportation. Parts 100-199. [All modes]
- International Civil Aviation Organization (ICAO) Technical Instructions for the Safe Transport of Dangerous Goods by Air [Air]
- International Maritime Organization (IMO) Dangerous Goods Code [Water]
- "Transportation of Dangerous Goods Regulations" of Transport Canada. [All Modes]

U.S. Department of Transportation
Research and Special Programs Administration

Available from:
American Labelmark Co.
5724 N. Pulaski Rd. • Chicago, IL 60646
Toll Free: 1-800-621-5808 • In Illinois: 312-478-0900

Figure 58–6

effects (irritation, burning) and systemic effects (organ damage, carcinogenicity) should be assumed when specific rescuer-protection equipment is selected.

Respiratory Protection

Pressure-demand, self-contained breathing apparatus should be used in all response situations that involve exposure to potentially unsafe levels.

Levels of Protection

Level A protection should be worn when the highest level of respiratory, skin, eye, and mucous membrane protection is needed. It consists of a fully encapsulating, chemical-resistant suit and self-contained breathing apparatus (SCBA).

Level B protection should be selected when the highest level of respiratory protection is needed but a lesser level of skin and eye protection is sufficient. It differs from level A only in that it provides splash protection by use of chemical-resistant clothing (overalls, long sleeves, jacket, and SCBA).

Level C protection should be selected when the type of airborne substances is known, concentration measured, criteria for using air-purifying respirators met, and skin and eye exposure unlikely. This involves a full-face-piece, air-purifying, canister-equipped respirator and chemical-resistant clothing. It provides the same level of skin protection as level B, but a lower level of respiratory protection.

Level D is primarily a work uniform. It should not be worn on any site where respiratory or skin hazards exist. It provides no respiratory protection and minimal skin protection.

Skin Protection

Chemical-protective clothing should be worn when local and systemic effects are unknown.

INITIAL RESPONSE

First responders at the site of a major disaster area are usually civilian volunteers, fire and police personnel, and Emergency Medical Services personnel. It is preferable for the first qualified medical person (as defined in a protocol) to set up an on-site command post. Communications should be established with a base hospital to mobilize the appropriate type and amount of resources. The command post is especially important in a HAZMAT situation; top priority must be given to prevent possible rescuers from become victims. Those in the command post should ensure adequate rest, food, and water for the rescue teams.

TRIAGE SITES

A minimum of two triage sites exists in any disaster: (a) on-site and (b) at the hospital. On-site triage is involved with rapid evaluation, stabilization, and evacuation. The hospital triage officer reevaluates victims to determine the most appropriate treatment for them.

ON-SITE TRIAGE

This may frequently be begun by any qualified person available (often police or fire fighters) who is later relieved by Emergency Medical Services personnel.

The ranking EMS worker to arrive first assumes the role of triage officer and is identified by a special marking on the uniform. Decisions on whether to rescue entrapped victims are made by the triage officer together with a medical liaison officer.

The field triage officer does a primary survey in a few moments and provides information about the nature of the disaster, the number of victims, special circumstances (fire, noxious gases, many children or elderly), and anticipated needs. He does not stop to treat patients.

TRIAGE/TREATMENT AREAS

On-site EMS workers triage victims to appropriate treatment and transportation areas. They are triaged and tagged where they lie and then transported to "immediate" or "delayed" transportation areas, where they are given whatever medical care is available. In a mass casualty disaster, field resuscitation is limited to airway maintenance, hemorrhage control, and correcting mechanical problems such as stabilizing suspected spinal injuries.

Immediate goals are to rescue and remove the injured and to separate potentially salvageable victims from the moribund or dead.

ABCDs

Quickly ensure a patent airway. Stabilize the cervical spine with a collar if trauma is suspected. Administer supplemental oxygen as required. Assist ventilation with a bag-valve-mask device if necessary.

Rapid classification of injury and tagging establish priorities for stabilization and evacuation of the most critically injured. Color-coded tags (attached to the great toe or wrist) indicate the severity of injury. This color-code system must remain uniform throughout all stages of triages. Special requisitions for laboratory tests and x-rays should be part of the tag. An internationally adopted system is as follows[9]:

Red — Immediate care: critically injured, requires immediate life support and first priority for hospital transport.

Yellow — Intermediate care: significant injury that is not immediately life-threatening but requires definitive care. Second priority for evacuation.

Green — Walking wounded: minor injuries (uncomplicated fractures, lacerations) or no injuries. Little or no treatment needed. Direct victims to the area for delayed hospital transportation or have them assist in the care of others.

Black (or gray) — Expectant (unsalvageable) or dead: survival is unlikely, even with the best of care. Administer analgesics but not life support, and keep these victims separated. Lowest priority of transport. Paramedics identify and label the dead and cover the remains and personal effects. The medical examiner directs removal and preservation of bodies and parts for identification.

If tags are unavailable, mark the victim's forehead as follows I = highest priority; II = second priority; III = walking wounded; 0 = unsalvageable.

Often a classification will be used producing four categories of patients[33]:

1. Victims with *life-threatening* injuries who are in immediate need of transport and/or treatment;
2. Victims with *moderate* and *severe* injuries who need treatment, but can wait for transport or treatment;
3. Patients with *mild* or *no* injuries who are not in need of any substantial treatment;
4. Severely injured victims with poor chances of survival even with adequate treatment, and primarily in need of *palliative support.*

In chemical accidents, an additional category of victims is needed: Those people who may have been exposed, and who do not experience any symptoms, but in whom delayed symptoms are to be expected. They are in need of observation, possible immediate treatment, and transport to treatment facilities.[33]

DECONTAMINATION

In a HAZMAT situation it is sometimes necessary to decontaminate prior to performing medical care. If victims can walk, lead them out of the Hot Zone to the Decontamination Zone. If victims are unable to walk, remove them on backboards or gurneys. If no other means of removal are available, carefully carry or drag victims to safety.

Frequently, it is the fire fighter personnel who bring the patient from the Hot Zone to the DECON I area (Figs. 58–2 and 58–3) where the EMS responders take over. After transfer of the patient to the EMS team, the patient is immediately stripped of all clothing and rapidly taken to the DECON 2 area (leaving all contaminated clothing in the first area). In the DECON 2 area priority care is performed following the standard ABCs of resuscitation. If possible, decontamination of the EMS personnel should also be done prior to taking the patient to the DECON 3 area. All non-essential contaminated equipment will be left in this area.

DECON 3 is the area where victims are readied for transport to the hospital. If rescuers will be accompanying the patient to the hospital, their contaminated protective clothing and equipment should remain at the scene. Victims exposed only to gas or vapors who have no skin or eye irritation do not need decontamination. They may be transferred immediately to the Support Zone. EMS personnel accompanying the victim should wear disposable clothing and gloves. EMS personnel should preferably triple-glove so that they can remove one pair at each DECON area.

THE DEAD

Prior plans should include disposition and handling of dead victims found on-site. A temporary morgue can be set up. Arrangement can be made for non-EMS personnel to transport such victims at a later time.

FIRE DEPARTMENT

The fire department may be able to identify and eliminate further dangers before the start of the rescue operations such as fires, downed power lines, and gas leaks. They will also work with search-and-rescue personnel to extricate trapped victims.

POLICE

Foremost, police must establish security at the scene and ensure that both victims and workers are safe. Rescue workers should not become victims. Entry to the area is restricted to those with authorization. Volunteers who may provide care and private transportation must be carefully managed. Injured persons should be kept within the system rather than taken to various hospitals in private vehicles without guidance. The disaster site should have traffic lanes kept open at all times for rescue vehicles.

PERSONNEL PROTECTION—SAFETY PRINCIPLES[26,34]

Personal Protective Equipment (PPE) is designed to provide personal safety for those emergency medical personnel who receive a relatively large number of contaminated victims. Levels of protection have been formulated by the Environmental Protection Agency.

DECONTAMINATION

EMERGENCY DEPARTMENT PERSONNEL

Decontamination is the process of removing or neutralizing harmful materials that have gathered on personnel and/or equipment during the response to a chemical incident. Many stories are told of seemingly successful rescue, transport, and treatment of chemically contaminated individuals by unsuspecting emergency personnel who, in the process, contaminate themselves, the equipment, and the facilities they encounter along the way. Decontamination is of the utmost importance because it does the following:

1. Protects all site personnel by sharply limiting the transfer of hazardous materials from the contaminated area into clean zones.
2. Protects the community by providing transportation of hazardous materials from the incident to other sites in the community.
3. Protects workers by reducing the contamination and resultant permeation of or degradation to their protective clothing and equipment.

THE WORKER

This section will only address the steps necessary for dealing with worker decontamination. It should be stressed that the design of the decontamination process should take into account the degree of hazard and should be appropriate for the situation. For example, a nine-station DECON process, as presented in Figure 58–2, need not be set up if only a boot wash station would suffice. Decontamination may be conducted wearing a lower level of protection than that worn in the Hot Zone if levels are determined to be safe. Quickly ensure a patent airway. Stabilize the cervical spine with a collar if trauma is suspected. Administer supplemental oxygen as required. Assist ventilation with a bag-valve-mask device if necessary.

Physical decontamination of protective clothing and equipment can be achieved in some cases by several different means. These all include the systematic removal of contaminants by washing, usually with soap and water, and then rinsing. In rare cases, the use of solvents may be necessary. There is a trend toward dry decontamination, which involves using disposable clothing (e.g., suits, boots, and gloves) and the systematic removal of these garments in a manner that precludes contact with the contaminant. The appropriate procedure will depend on the contaminant and its physical properties. A thorough work-up of the chemical involved and its properties or expert consultation is necessary to make these kinds of decisions.

Care must be taken to ensure that decontamination methods do not introduce fresh hazards into the situation due to their physical properties. In addition, the residues of the decontamination process must be treated as hazardous wastes. The decontamination stations and process should be confined to the Contamination Reduction Zone.

PREHOSPITAL[35]

The emergency medical service prehospital providers responding to a hazardous materials incient have five goals:

1. To protect themselves and other prehospital responders from any significant toxic exposure.
2. To obtain accurate information on the identity and health effects of the hazardous materials and the appropriate prehospital evaluation and medical care for victims.
3. To minimize continued exposure of the victim and secondary contamination of health-care personnel by ensuring that proper decontamination (if necessary) has been completed prior to transport to a hospital emergency department.
4. To provide appropriate prehospital emergency medical care consistent with their certification.
5. To prevent unnecessary contamination of their transport vehicle or ambulance.

PREHOSPITAL DECONTAMINATION

Unprotected EMS responders must advise on and observe the decontamination procedures from a distance to ensure that they are properly carried out. They should practice with the local HAZMAT team to become familiar with the steps involved. If there is any doubt about the potential for secondary contamination, decontaminate the victim. A contaminated appendage can be washed without wetting the whole body if that is the only part contaminated. Clothing covering the rest of the body and exposed skin should be carefully checked for contamination.

If the transport vehicle is inadvertently contaminated, advice from the local environmental health department, hazardous materials team, or local hazardous materials spill cleanup companies should be sought on how to determine the level and location of the contamination and on how to clean it up. Advice should also be sought on how to preserve evidence for law enforcement and how to dispose of or clean contaminated clothing and personal items.

PREHOSPITAL TRIAGE

Victims with obvious significant illness or injury will need rapid transport and treatment after initial stabilization and basic decontamination is carried out. In virtually all cases patients with serious trauma or medical illness can be quickly stripped and flushed with water prior to delivery to prehospital health providers outside the Hot Zone. This is true even in cold or inclement weather. If this cannot be performed because of acute life-threatening conditions or other circumstances, then the vehicle must be protected and those providing care during transport and driving the vehicle must be properly fitted and trained with the appropriate level of specialized protective gear. However, every effort should be made to decontaminate the victim at the scene if the means to do so are available. In those jurisdictions where a prehospital provider might be placed in such a situation without assistance from a properly trained HAZMAT specialist, advance arrangements for additional training and protective equipment should be made.

Victims with few or minimal symptoms are not necessarily safe from progression of illness. Many toxic substances have delayed onset effects, which may appear several hours later, after the victim has returned home. If the toxic substance is known, obtain consultation from the Regional Poison Control Center to determine if delayed effects might be seen and for guidance on triage of asymptomatic or mildly symptomatic exposure victims. Any persons suspected of being exposed should be seen and evaluated by emergency department staff.

CASUALTY COLLECTION POINTS

Casualty collection points are the second stage in the triage process and the final station for all victims at the disaster site. Such points should be established in a safe place, with easy access to both the flow of victims and traffic lanes. Before patients are evacuated, the on-scene medical officer and his staff of trained medical personnel proceed with a more definitive triage, stabilization, and treatment of injured patients. Treatment varying from first aid to lifesaving measures may need to be performed before evacuation.[8]

BASIC DECONTAMINATION

Victims who are able and cooperative may assist with their own decontamination. Remove and double-bag contaminated clothing and personal belongings. Flush exposed or irritated skin and hair with plain water or saline for 3 to 5 minutes. Remove contact lenses if present. If a corrosive material is suspected or if pain or injury is evident, continue irrigation while transferring the victim to the Support Zone.

In cases of ingestion, do not induce emesis. Administer a glass of water to dilute stomach contents if the patient is conscious and able to swallow. Obtain medical care immediately.

SUPPORT ZONE

As soon as basic decontamination is complete, move the victim to the Support Zone. Be certain that victims have been decontaminated properly. Victims who have undergone decontamination or who have been exposed only to gas or vapor—who have no evidence of skin or eye irritation—generally pose no serious risk of secondary contamination. Support Zone personnel require no specialized protective gear in such cases.

Quickly ensure a patent airway. Stabilize the cervical spine with a collar if trauma is suspected. Administer supplemental oxygen as required. Assist ventilation with a bag-valve-mask device if necessary. Evaluate the need for an intravenous line, cardiac monitor, and life support. Observe for ventricular dysrhythmias.

If skin or eyes remain irritated, continue irrigation. In cases of ingestion, do not induce emesis. Administer a glass of water to dilute stomach contents if the patient is conscious and able to swallow. Obtain medical care immediately.

Intubate the trachea in cases of respiratory compromise. When the patient's condition precludes endotracheal intubation, perform cricothyroidotomy if equipped and trained to do so. Treat patients with bronchospasm with aerosolized bronchodilators. Use these and all catecholamines with caution because of the enhanced risk of cardiac dysrhythmias after exposure to certain chemicals. Treat according to standard ALS protocol patients who have coma and ventricular dysrhythmias.

DISPATCH TO HOSPITALS[10]

The on-scene medical officer in charge should ensure that patient dispatch proceeds smoothly. Appropriate matching of individual hospital resources with the patient load to be received is critical since an overload of critically injured patients may occur at one hospital while another hospital receives minimally injured individuals. All this requires constant communication between the various hospitals and the on-scene command post.

Ambulance Transport

Guidelines for ambulances should be prepared by those involved in planning for a disaster. Supplies required for the ambulance are listed in Table 58–9.

Ambulance Departure Point[9]

The ambulance departure point, previously designated by the incident commander, is separated into "immediate" and "delayed" categories. The departure point must be accessible to traffic, such as ambulances and automobiles. Helicopters should land at least 300 feet downwind to avoid disrupting transportation and kicking up dust.

Table 58–9
Supplies Needed to Prepare the Ambulance for Care of a Hazardous Material Contaminated Patient[a]

Binoculars to assess scene from a safe distance.
Plastic (10–20 mil, preferably clear) trash bags (3 or 4 mil) to isolate and dispose of contaminated articles and toxic vomitus. Plastic sheeting to cover floor of ambulance in the rare case where a contaminated victim must be transported, or if the victim might vomit ingested toxic material.
A large supply of oxygen to treat breathing problems caused by exposure to Hazardous Materials (more than is usually carried).
A large wash basin, bucket, or plastic waste basket that can be lined with a trash bag to collect contaminated eye wash water or vomitus.
Disposable plastic-coated blankets (or "chucks") to soak up and isolate liquids from a decontaminated patient. Use these for absorbing toxic vomitus.
Disposable gowns and slippers for patients who must remove contaminated clothes at the scene and for EMS personnel (long sleeve gowns) to cover out clothes.
Disposable surgical or examination gloves.
Surgical paper masks.
Waterproof disposable shoe covers.
Splash goggles or face shields to protect EMS personnel from splashes while they work on the patient.
Inexpensive stethoscopes, blood pressure cuffs, and other gear that can be discarded if contaminated.
Isotonic saline and IV tubing for eye irrigation.
A Bag-Valve Mask (BVM) or similar device in lieu of mouth to mouth respiration. (Pocket masks are not acceptable.)
Liquid soap for washing off oil contaminants.
Epsom salts for soaking hydrofluoric acid burns.
Shears or sharp knife for removing clothing from victim.
Copy of the current "D.O.T. Emergency Response Guidebook," a copy of these protocols, and other appropriate medical management protocols.
Positive-pressure SCBA (Self-Contained Breathing Apparatus).
Full-face mask respirator with an orange and purple type cartridge (acid gas, organic vapor, highly toxic dust, mist and fumes, and radionuclides-rated cartridge).
PVC or duct tape for taping closures.
Two piece rainwear.
Rubber boots with steel toes.
Nitrile gloves with 14-inch cuffs.
Duct tape to seal suit seams if necessary.

[a]Based on a list prepared by the Contra Costa/Solano County Joint Emergency Medical Services Hazardous Materials Response Program. Additional equipment is necessary for handling radiation contamination. See Leonard RB, Ricks RC. Emergency department radiation accident protocol. Ann Emerg Med 1980;9:462–470. Also see *Medical Management of Radiation Accidents* by Mattler FA, Kelsey CA, Ricks RC. Boca Raton, FL: CRC Press, 1989.

Initial Ambulance Response[26,36,37]

1. Report to the base station and the receiving medical facility the condition of the patient, treatment given, and estimated time of arrival at the medical facility. If the victim ingested a chemical, prepare the ambulance for possible vomiting of toxic material. Cover the floor of the ambulance with plastic or other protective material and have ready several absorbent towels and opened plastic bags to quickly soak up and isolate vomitus.
2. Unless otherwise directed, park upwind and uphill from any incident where you suspect hazardous materials.
3. Do not drive or walk through any spilled materials.
4. If first-in responder, confirm that fire and police have been notified and are aware that hazardous materials might be involved.

5. If you are a first-in responder, first priority is scene isolation. KEEP OTHERS AWAY! KEEP UNNECESSARY EQUIPMENT FROM BECOMING CONTAMINATED.

Approach and Treatment of Victims

1. Do not approach any victims without first consulting with the incident commander.
2. Do not approach anyone coming from contaminated areas (particularly those potentially contaminated) until given permission by the incident commander. (NOTE: vapors can be trapped in clothing and carried out of contaminated area!)
3. Follow incident commander's instructions regarding victim decontamination. (Fire Departments will normally handle decontamination.)
   a. Ensure that all potentially contaminated patient clothing and belongings have been removed. Do not transport contaminated clothing and belongings with the patient in the ambulance unless the incident commander approves and the clothing and belongings have been adequately bagged.
   b. Ensure that skin exposures are flushed with water for a minimum of *15 minutes.* Ensure eye exposures are rinsed for a minimum of *15 minutes* (use normal saline solution if available).
   c. Depending on the nature of the hazardous materials, consider decontamination as a priority over transport.
   d. When transporting a contaminated patient by ambulance, special care should be exercised in preventing contamination of the ambulance and subsequent patients.
4. Avoid contact with contaminants. Wear protective clothing as appropriate.
5. Administer oxygen by mask for any victim with respiratory problems.
6. Continue to irrigate eye exposure with normal saline or water en route to the hospital and be alert for any respiratory distress. (NOTE: USE BASINS TO SAVE THE IRRIGATION WATER FOR PROPER DISPOSAL.)
7. Cover the entire gurney, including the pillow, with disposable (plastic) sheeting.
8. Cover the patient compartment floor with a disposable plastic sheeting. (Do this either before arriving at the scene or before you reenter the ambulance to minimize contamination from your shoes.)
9. The patient should be as clean as reasonably possible prior to transport, and further contact with contaminants should be avoided. Protective clothing should be worn by response personnel as appropriate. If decontamination cannot be performed adequately, responders should make every attempt to prevent the spread of contamination and at the very least remove patient clothing and wrap the patient in blankets followed by body bags, or plastic or rubber sheets, to lessen the likelihood of contamination to equipment and others. Considerations should be made for chemicals that present the added danger of accelerated skin absorption due to heat. In these cases, body bags and plastic or rubber sheets should not be used.
10. Write down the name of the involved chemicals, if identified, before leaving the scene.
11. Ask the incident commander for advice on decontaminating the ambulance and personnel once the patient is released to the hospital.
12. Persons exposed to toxic materials should receive oxygen by mask en route to the hospital. If fumes are detected in the patient compartment of an ambulance during transport, personnel in the patient compartment should have access to oxygen via mask.
13. Provide maximum fresh air ventilation to patient and driver compartment regardless of the presence or absence of odors.
14. Unless a Multiple Casualty Plan has been implemented, follow normal radio communication procedures with the receiving hospital, but in addition provide the name of the chemical or hazardous material involved.
15. Recontact the receiving hospital and provide an update on treatment provided or required and any other information received from the designated poison control center. Instructions for the procedure to enter the hospital with a contaminated patient should also be requested. Facilities receiving a potential hazardous material patient will need as much information as possible.
16. A checklist should be developed and made available for all vehicles and telephone or radio communication centers. Information that will aid in initiating appropriate actions includes the following:
    a. Type and nature of incident
    b. Number of victims
    c. Signs/symptoms being experienced by the victims
    d. Nature of injuries
    e. Name of chemical(s) involved
    f. Information available at the site concerning the chemical(s)
    g. Extent of victim decontamination in the field
    h. Estimated time of arrival

Support Zone

Be certain that victims have been decontaminated properly. Victims who have undergone decontamination or who have been exposed only to gas or vapor who have no evidence of skin or eye irritation generally pose no serious risk of secondary contamination. Support Zone personnel require no specialized protective gear in such cases.

Additional Decontamination

If skin or eyes remain irritated, continue irrigation. In cases of ingestion, do not induce emesis. Administer a glass of water to dilute stomach contents if the patient is conscious and able to swallow. Obtain medical care immediately.

ARRIVAL AT HOSPITAL

1. The ambulance is to park in an area away from the emergency room or go directly to a decontamination

center or area. Notify Central Coordinators on arrival at the hospital.

2. Patient(s) should not be brought into the emergency department before ambulance personnel receive permission from the hospital staff.
3. Once the patient(s) has been released to the hospital, double-bag the plastic sheeting used to cover the gurney and the floor into plastic bags. Double-bag any equipment that is believed to have become contaminated.
4. After unloading the patient from the ambulance, check with the hospital to see where the ambulance can safely be decontaminated and whether there is equipment available for this purpose. Do not begin decontamination without direction from the hospital staff.
5. Following decontamination instructions from the incident commander (or Hazardous Materials Team), decontaminate the ambulance and personnel before returning to the incident scene. If returning to the incident scene, bring bags containing contaminated materials, equipment, clothing, etc. and turn over to incident commander.
6. If not returning to the scene, keep contaminated articles sealed until given further instructions by the incident commander, County Communications, or your employing agency. Do not go back into service without rigorous decontamination of the vehicle.

AIR TRANSPORTATION OF CHEMICALLY EXPOSED PATIENTS

There is a potential danger in transporting patients in a helicopter from a hazardous materials incident. Often decontamination is not complete, and the flight crew could experience difficulty in breathing or seeing. Also the area of the incident needs to be clearly communicated to the flight crew to avoid traveling through an unsafe area. Furthermore, the downdraft from the helicopter could affect vapors or fumes on on the scene. Consideration should be given to each specific incident and chemical.

If the Fire Department's protective clothing is utilized, rainwear should be worn as an over garment. Hydrocarbons and other chemicals may permeate the "bunker clothes." NOTE: The protective equipment listed is to be utilized for patient care situations following initial decontamination. It is meant to be used when complete decontamination of the patients cannot be guaranteed or when assisting with decontamination procedures (in extreme cases positive-pressure SCBA and encapsulated suits may be required for decontamination procedures). It is not meant to be used in rescue operations of victims found in a hazardous area. Under no circumstances should this equipment be relied on for entry into hazardous environments. Protective equipment for entry must be appropriate and compatible to the products involved. This may include positive-pressure SCBA and fully encapsulated suits. There are many factors that must be taken into consideration when determining the appropriate level of protection. Consequently, selection of protective equipment must be done by a qualified individual.

NOTE: Wet plastic is slippery; stability is important.

THE HOSPITAL

A suggested procedure guide for handling patients in the Emergency Department who are thought to be contaminated with hazardous materials has been prepared by the Agency for Toxic Substances and Disease Registry.

EMERGENCY DEPARTMENTS AND HOSPITALS[8,10]

The final stage of the triage process for casualties occurs at hospitals. The first wave of victims may arrive within 30 minutes after an incident. These individuals generally have minor injuries and come of their own volition. They may easily overload the hospital facilities, interfering with the care of more severely affected patients who arrive later. On-scene triage should minimize this patient disproportion.

The hospital receiving and triage area should not be established in the emergency department. A large open area (a lobby or predesignated outer space) frees up the emergency department for use as a resuscitation area. The entry point provides rapid access to all treatment areas. Traffic is one way only: emergency vehicles unload victims and depart rapidly.

The hospital triage officer—an emergency physician or surgeon—is stationed at the entry point and reviews the triage tags of the victims. Misdiagnosis and deterioration may occur due to inaccurate field tagging. The triage officer will designate the priority in which victims will receive treatment and to which treatment area the victim is to go.

TREATMENT STATIONS[10]

A disaster may force rearrangement of the entire hospital for maximum efficiency. Treatment areas defined in a disaster manual should include a Resuscitation Area, Critical Care Treatment Area, Immediate Care Area, Ambulatory Treatment Area, and Expectant Category Area set up to care for the dying. After proper decontamination of the victim laboratory work, radiographs, and surgery may be indicated. Plans should include allocation of such resources in an emergency.

RECORDKEEPING

Planners should develop simple forms to include identification of patients and their location, a description of the patient, the patient's name, if possible, the type of injuries, triage classification, and initial disposition. When the patient arrives at the hospital, the medical records staff can generate information about the family and close relatives and more detailed assessment and classification and departure disposition.

Goals of the Hospital Provider in HAZMAT Incidents

1. Determine the potential for secondary contamination.
2. Assure that appropriate decontamination measures are carried out.
3. Obtain reliable toxicity information. Resources might include these Guidelines or a regional poison control center.

4. Provide emergency care (supportive and antidotal).
5. Perform adequate laboratory testing.
6. Determine the need for prolonged observation, hospital admission, and follow-up care.

Decontamination Area

Previously decontaminated patients and patients with exposure only to gas or vapors and with no evidence of skin or eye irritation or contamination do not need decontamination. They may be transferred immediately to the Critical Care Area. Other victims will require decontamination as described below.

ABCs

Evaluate and support airway, breathing, and circulation. Intubate the trachea in cases of respiratory compromise. If the patient's condition precludes intubation, surgically create an airway. Treat patients who have bronchospasm with aerosolized bronchodilators; use these and all catecholamines with caution because of the possible enhanced risk of cardiac dysrhythmias. Treat in the conventional manner patients who have coma, seizures, hypotension, or ventricular dysrhythmias. Establish intravenous access in seriously ill patients. Continuously monitor cardiac rhythm. Assess and treat in the conventional manner patients who have hypotension, coma, seizures, and ventricular dysrhythmias. An intravenous line should be placed as soon as possible in all patients who are unconscious, obtunded, hypotensive, or who may become so. Patients exposed to substances that may cause cardiac sensitization or intravascular hemolysis will also require intravenous access. An initial bolus of normal saline or D5W should be given as appropriate for age, typically 250 mL to 1 L in an adult. The fluid should be titrated to maintain urine output and blood pressure at acceptable levels for age. Care must be taken not to overhydrate the patient.

Basic Decontamination

Victims who are able and cooperative may assist with their own decontamination. Remove and double-bag contaminated clothing and personal belongings. Flush exposed or irritated skin and hair with plain water or saline for 3 to 5 minutes. For oily or otherwise adherent chemicals, use mild soap and shampoo on the skin and hair. Flush exposed or irritated eyes with plain water or saline for at least 5 minutes. Remove contact lenses if present. If a corrosive material is suspected or if pain or injury is evident, continue irrigation while transferring the patient to the Critical Care Area. In case of ingestion, do not induce emesis. Administer a glass of water to dilute stomach contents if the patient is conscious and able to swallow. Immediately transfer the patient to the Critical Care area.

Eye Exposure

Ensure that adequate eye irrigation has been completed. Test visual acuity. Examine the eyes for corneal damage using a magnifying device or a slit lamp and fluorescein stain. Small corneal defects may be treated with ophthalmic ointment or drops, analgesic medication, and an eye patch. Immediately consult an ophthalmologist for patients who have severe corneal injury. Be sure that contact lenses have been removed, that there is no visible residual material in the conjunctival sac, and that the pH of the conjunctival fluid is normal.

Ingestion Exposure

Do not induce emesis. Perform gastric lavage, then administer a slurry of activated charcoal. If a corrosive material is suspected, do not give a slurry of activated charcoal. Consider endoscopy to evaluate the extent of gastrointestinal-tract injury.

Laboratory Tests

Depending on the chemical exposure and the patient's symptoms and signs of toxicity, useful routine tests may include CBC, glucose, electrolytes, renal-function tests, liver enzymes, urinalysis, and ECG. Chest radiographs and measurements of arterial blood gases are recommended for severe inhalation exposure.

Disposition and Follow-up

Hospitalization should be considered for all patients with a suspected serious exposure and those with persistent or progressive symptoms.

Delayed Effects

If there is a possibility of delayed onset of serious effects, the patient should be observed for an extended period or admitted to the hospital.

Patient Release

Asymptomatic patients with minimal exposure, a normal initial examination, and no signs of toxicity after a 6- or 8-hour period of observation may be discharged with instructions to seek medical care promptly if symptoms develop (see the reverse side of Unidentified Chemical—Patient Information Sheet).

Follow-up

Provide follow-up instructions to return to the emergency department or a private physician for additional testing or to reevaluate initial findings. Patients with corneal injury should be reevaluated within 24 hours.

Reporting

If a work-related incident has occurred, you may be legally required to file a report; contact your state or local health department. Other persons may still be at risk in the setting where this incident occurred. If the incident occurred in the workplace, discussing it with company personnel may prevent future incidents. If a public health risk exists, notify an appropriate public agency. When appropriate, inform patients that they may request an evaluation of their workplace from OSHA or NIOSH.

Antidotes (Table 58–10)

Antidotes should be stored at hospitals, and some may be placed on mobile units to be brought to the scene of a major chemical accident (Table 58–10).

LABORATORY

Volans[38] has summarized the role of the analytic toxicology laboratory in chemical disasters (Table 58–11).

POISON CONTROL CENTERS

ACUTE INFORMATION DISSEMINATION

The Poison Center must plan for chemical disasters. The Poison Center should be prepared to give individuals at the site of an incident detailed information about the toxic substance used at an industrial plant. This measure must be included in the disaster checklist at chemical plants and emergency centers.

Information on chemicals frequently used in industry as components of household products is readily available. Such

Table 58–10
Antidotes To Be Stored at Hospitals and on Mobile Units To Be Brought to the Place of Accident in Case of Major Chemical Accidents. WHO/EURO Assessor Group Recommendations

Substance	Indication
Atropine	Organophosphates
Dimercaprol[a]	Arsenic, mercury
Calcium salts	Hydrofluoric acid
for injection	
tablets	
topical (Hydrofluoric acid burn jelly)	
Corticosteroids	Irritant gases
for injection	
for inhalation	
tablets	
Dicobalt edetate	Cyanide
Methylthionine (methylene blue)	Nitrobenzene and nitrites
or	
Tolonium chloride (toluidine blue)	
Obidoxime	
or	
Pralidoxime	Organophosphates
Penicillamine[b]	Arsenic, mercury
Polyethylene glycol 400	Phenol
Sodium thiosulphate	Cyanide

[a]Newer chelating agents may replace dimercaprol.
[b]Not to be stored on mobile units.

Table 58–11
Application of Analytical Toxicology in Chemical Disasters[a]

Analytical resources

Sample		*Laboratory*
Chemical	Select as appropriate to incident	Industrial
Air		Environmental
Soil		Health & Safety
Water		Water
Plant		Food
Animal		Plant science
Food		Veterinary
Human		Hospital
		Forensic
		University

Considerations in sample collection in chemical disasters

1 Agree on a general policy between all involved parties
2 Choose an agency to start/coordinate process
3 Determine appropriate samples (collection technique, size, container, preservatives)
4 Ensure samples are adequately labelled (material, place, subject, date, time, preservative)
5 Decide whether repeat samples are needed
6 Arrange appropriate storage/transport
7 Decide the time scale for analysis (urgent, routine, research?)
8 Arrange forum to report/discuss results to avoid waste of time

Assessment of analytical toxicological data

1 *Analytical interpretation:*
Use method with adequate selectivity, sensitivity and reliability ("quality control")
Compare result to those reported previously in various groups after various doses ("feasibility control")
2 *Clinical interpretation:*
Discuss analytical findings in light of other data (time course of episode, clinical chemistry, pharmacology of suspect agent, etc.)
If necessary, extrapolate from analytical results with similar compounds/groups of compounds
3 *A dialogue* between an experienced analyst and clinician is vital!

[a]Adapted from Volans GN. Medical Management of Chemical Disasters Involving Food or Water. In: Murray V, ed. Major Chemical Disasters—Medical Aspects of Management Royal Source of Medicine Services 1990; pp. 173–181.

information includes data on substance (synonyms, chemical formula and structure, molecular weight, physical data such as melting and freezing points, density), mode of action, routes of exposure, kinetics (including absorption, transport, and distribution), biotransformation, and elimination. It may also include data on toxicity (toxic doses and concentrations, lethal doses and concentrations, symptoms expected from different target organs in poisoning), measures for treatment of toxic effects, and general and specific measures such as antidotal therapy and elimination techniques.

The poison center should be prepared to provide authorities and mass media (local and national radio, TV, etc.) with information on the toxic substance: toxic effects, first aid measures, and how to avoid or minimize exposure. Finally, in the acute phase, detailed information on the toxic substance and on medical managements, where applicable, should be given to the medical rescue teams and hospitals. This should include guidelines for decontamination and how to supply and how to get access to antidotes. Poison centers should be prepared to send staff personnel to the site of an accident if requested.

CONTINGENCY PLANNING

Disaster medicine planners should establish a close collaboration with a poison center. The center should provide planners with guidelines that include decontamination, first aid, advanced medical therapy, and antidote supplies. The rescue team should be provided information about the main risks, first aid measures, and hospital treatment. Lectures and courses can be organized by the poison center personnel for medical and nonmedical rescue team members (doctors, nurses, police, ambulance services, fire department). This will include aspects of acute poisoning and organization of rescue work at the accident site, during transport, and in the hospital. Research activities relating to an incident and on-site visits should also involve poison center personnel.

COLLABORATION[39–42]

Poison centers should maintain close contact with other poison centers and with international bodies dealing with disaster medicine planning such as the World Congresses for Emergency and Disaster Medicine, the International Program on Chemical Safety (IPCS), and the World Health Organization.

RISK ASSESSMENT

A poison center's immediate aim in risk assessment is to determine the following:

1. Identity of the materials released or at risk of being released.
2. Real or estimated quantities involved.
3. Specific nature of the release or type of accident.
4. Reactions observed between released materials and the environment or any known casualty or injured.

Poison centers that aim to assist in toxic emergency responses must do the following[43]:

1. Have full-time specialists trained and proficient in the retrieval, analysis, and communication of medical toxicologic and chemical information.
2. Be accessible for information and assistance on a 24-hours-a-day 7-days-a-week basis to public safety and medical personnel; they must be similarly available to the public during incidents.
3. Have resources organized in such a manner to permit rapid access to technical and clinical information dealing with hazardous materials.
4. Have procedures and capabilities for recordkeeping and review.
5. Be located in a medical facility with ready access to consultants from various medical, laboratory, industrial, and occupational health-related clinical and scientific specialties.
6. Have interest and capability to provide training to medical and other health specialists on matters related to toxicology and hazardous substances.

During an incident the Poison Center should be able to provide the following:

1. Physician and chemical property data.
2. Reactivity and toxicity information.
3. Advice on medical management.
4. Access to a wide range of expertise—environmental and industrial toxicologists, occupational health specialists, hazardous wastes and materials specialists.

The Poison Center's role in hazardous materials emergencies has been summarized (see Tables 58–12, 58–13, and 58–14).

ON-SCENE FIELD OPERATION

The Poison Center must be in constant communication with the Base Station, Health Department, and receiving hospital emergency department by phone and by FAX. When necessary many sets of data can be distributed by FAX to all health-care facilities.

PROBLEMS—POTENTIAL AND ACTUAL[27]

1. Identification of chemicals involved in a sudden chemical release may be delayed or impossible from uncontrolled chemical reactions or fires.
2. There are over 70,000 chemicals in regular commercial use: information that hospitals can obtain from Poison Centers may therefore be limited.
3. Antidotes are available for only a few chemicals and have no role in most incidents.
4. Long-term effects from chemical injury such as carcinogenicity, teratogenicity, and other organ damage may not be fully known for many chemicals.
5. Since health professionals are more used to disaster planning for major trauma than for mass chemical exposures and their attendant medical management problems, training is important for accident and emergency personnel in the use of protective clothing, decontamination, and preparation of chemical incident protocols.

Table 58-12
The Poison Center's Role in Hazardous Materials Emergencies

1. Participate in a coordinated, community-specific response plan with clearly designated responsibilities and defined procedures when a hazardous materials emergency occurs.
2. Assist incident responders in identifying and assessing the threat to health and environment.
3. Facilitate the linkage between toxicologic expertise and information resources with incident responders and the emergency management system; the goal for such ties is to arrive at appropriate decisions dealing with health and environmental risks.
4. Assist in the mobilization of medical resources to provide rescue and emergency care of this injured or ill from exposure to toxic release.
5. Provide appropriate medical management information to medical personnel treating victims.
6. Be a mechanism by which health effects from exposures can be accurately followed up and documented post incident.
7. Be the designated toxicologic focal point for dissemination of accurate, clear, consistent, and appropriate information to the public during toxic incidents.
8. Offer educational programs and opportunities to medical and public safety personnel on control, management, and response to hazardous chemical incidents.
9. Evaluate toxicologic information and data on hazardous materials and become an accessible repository of this information and data.
10. Become involved in a surveillance role to help identify and remove undetected environmental toxic hazards from the community.

Table 58-13
Poison Control Center Collaboration

1. Other poison centers
2. World Association of Emergency and Disaster Medicine
3. International Program on Chemical Safety
4. WHO
5. Industry
   National
   International

6. Epidemiologic, laboratory, and toxicologic skills needed immediately to evaluate and advise on a chemical hazard may not be available locally and may delay an adequate medical response.
7. In the management of a comparatively small incident[44] a number of problems were observed:
   a. The failure in communication between the police, fire brigade, and ambulance and hospital services, particularly about the identification of the chemical substance and its toxicity, exemplifies the concern about communication between professional groups involved in the medical aspects of management of chemical incidents.
   b. Protective clothing is provided rarely for staff in accident and emergency departments and is not provided for the police.
   c. The accident and emergency departments (in common with many other such departments) may not have effective decontamination facilities available, and those that are available may not comply with those recommended by hospital building regulations.
   d. In addition, though a Poison Control Center may be able to provide help, it will not be able to prepare information in advance of the patient's arrival at a hospital if it is not notified by the emergency services.[45] Emergency departments need protocols for managing large numbers of casualties exposed to chemicals, particularly when they arrive without warning. Furthermore, the potential toxicity of volatile chemicals needs to be more widely appreciated; these considerations highlight the need for improved communication and closer coordination between emergency and medical services.

Table 58-14
Poison Center Resources

Chemical substance descriptions
Monographs
Chemical substituents
Drugs
Plants
Medications
Venomous animals
Case reports
Library

8. Technology transfer to Third World nations has not usually included the transfer of health and safety technology.
9. Embarrassment of unwanted material resources, including donated medical supplies that are inappropriate or unusable but consume scarce resources to ship receive, sort, and distribute.[46]
10. Outside individual volunteers whose credentials are virtually impossible to verify in a disaster situation can add to the problem instead of lessening it.

CHEMICAL DISPERSION[45]

McQuaid has summarized problems that must be considered following a chemical accident:

1. The material is, in almost all cases, stored as a liquid, so that the volume of gas involved is very large.
2. The modes of release can vary widely from a ruptured pipe to a complete tank failure, whereas pollution problems almost invariably relate to covenanted chimney emissions. The geometry of the source can take many forms and the initial momentum may be significant. The site of the accident may not be a fixed location, as in transportation and pipeline accidents.
3. The process of formation of the gaseous cloud involves the phase transformation from liquid to gas. This can occur in a number of ways, from a flashing jet entraining air to the evaporation of a pool by heat transfer from the substrate.

4. In some cases, a chemical transformation also takes place as a result of reaction with water vapor in the ambient atmosphere, for example, nitrogen tetroxide (N_2O_4), hydrogen fluoride (HF).
5. The physical properties of the materials usually result in the formation of a denser-than-air (i.e., negatively buoyant) cloud, compared with the neutrally or positively buoyant gases in pollution problems. The negative buoyancy can have a marked effect on the dispersion characteristics.
6. The release can occur over a short period, compared with the steady-state releases characteristic of most pollution problems. This gives rise to the complication of predicting dispersion for time-varying releases and to uncertainty in individual predictions resulting from variability of the ensemble mean behavior.
7. The dispersing gas, where it is denser than air, forms a low-level cloud that is sensitive to the effects of man-made and natural obstructions and of topography.

REFERENCES—CHEMICAL DISASTERS

1. Melius J, Binder S. Industrial disasters. In: Gregg MB, French J, Binder S, Sanderson LM, eds. CDC Monograph. The Public Health Consequences of Disasters 1989. Atlanta, GA: US Department of Health and Human Services, Center for Disease Control, September 1989; pp. 97–102.
2. US Congress, Office of Technology Assessment. Transportation of Hazardous Materials. Washington, DC: US Government Printing Office, 1986.
3. Bourdeau P, Green G, eds. Methods for assessing and reducing injury from chemical accidents. SCOPE 40 (Scientific Committee on Problems of the Environment) IPCS Joint Symposia 11. Scientific Group on Methodologies for the Safety Evaluation of Chemicals (SGOMSEC). Chichester: John Wiley, 1989.
4. Ferner RE. Chemical disasters. Pharmacol Ther 1993;58: 157–171.
5. Dolezal V, Pokorny J. Evaluation of exposure and hazard in chemical catastrophes. In: Bourdeau P, Green G, eds. Methods for assessing and reducing injury from chemical accidents. Chichester: John Wiley, 1989; pp. 89–104.
6. Govaerts-Lepicard M. Definition of a major incident involving chemicals. In: Murray V, ed. Major chemical disasters—medical aspects of management. London: Royal Society of Medicine Service, 1990; pp. 125–129.
7. Seliger JS, Simoneau JK. Emergency preparedness: disaster planning for health facilities. Rockville, MD: Aspen, 1988.
8. Waeckerle JF. Disaster planning and response. N Engl J Med 1991;324:815–821.
9. Dwyer BJ, Cheu D. Emergency medical response to civilian disasters. Emerg Med Rep 1990;11(8):169–176.
10. Plante DM. EMS response at a hazardous material incident: some basic guidelines. J Emerg Med 1989;7:55–64.
11. Haines JA. Technological disasters global trends. Regional Symposium on Chemical Disaster, Addis Ababa. From IPCS/WHO Geneva, Switzerland: May 30, 1991.
12. Krishna Murti CR. Biological effects of chemical disasters' human victims. In: Bourdeau P, Green G, eds. Methods for assessing and reducing injury from chemical accidents. Chichester: John Wiley, 1989.
13. Aydellote C. Bhopal tragedy focuses on change in chemical industry. Occup Health Saf 1985;54:33–59.
14. Isman SE. Emergency responders at a hazardous materials incident. JEMS 1982; :26-32.
15. Canadine IC. The possibility of major incidents in chemical distribution. In: Murray V, ed. Major chemical disasters—medical aspects of management. London: Royal Society of Medicine Service, 1990; pp. 11–43.
16. US Environmental Protection Agency, Office of Toxic Substances, Acute Hazardous Events Database, Report No. EPA 560-5-85-029, 1985.
17. McQuaid J, Vilain J, Peterson P, Sriram M, Gupta VP, Sarda PK et al. The assessment and control of chemical accidents. In: Bourdeau P, Green G, eds. Methods for assessing and reducing injury from chemical accidents. Chichester: John Wiley, 1989.
18. Green MA, Heumann MA, Wehr HM, Foster LP, Williams LP, Polder A et al. An outbreak of watermelon-borne pesticide toxicity. Am J Public Health 1987;11:1431–1434.
19. Vilain J. The nature of chemical hazards, their accident potential and consequences. In: Bourdeau P, Green G, eds. Methods for assessing and reducing injury from chemical accidents. Chichester: John Wiley, 1989; pp. 252–290.
20. Ferrer A, Cabral JRP. Epidemics due to pesticide contamination in food. In: World Conference on Chemical Accidents. Edinburgh: CEP Consultants, 1985; pp. 385–387.
21. Volans GN. Medical management of chemical disasters involving food or water. In: Murray V, ed. Major chemical disasters—medical aspects of management. London: Royal Society of Medicine Service, 1990; pp. 173–179.
22. James F, Farwell K. Lessons learnt from the River Dee pollution incident, January 1989—Public Health. In: World Conference on Chemical Accidents. Edinburgh: CEP Consultants, 1987;223–226.
23. Roth PB: Status of a national disaster medical response. JAMA 1991;266:1266.
24. Wood DR, Cowan ML. Crisis intervention following disasters: are we doing enough? (A second look). Am J Emerg Med 1991;9:598–602.
25. Facts on the National Disaster Medical System. National Disaster Medical System Implementation Task Force. Room 16A-54, Parklawn Building, 5600 Fisher's Lane, Rockville, MD 20857. Revised July, 1986. Tel: (301) 443-4893.
26. Chemical emergencies: guidance for the management of chemically contaminated patients in the prehospital setting. Washington, DC: Agency for Toxic Substances and Disease Registry.
27. Baxter PJ. Major chemical disasters. Britain's health services are poorly prepared. Br Med J 1991;302:61–62.
28. Harrison M, AW TC, Krishman C, Jones AF, Vale JA. Major chemical disasters. Br Med J 1991;302:657.
29. Koplan JP, Falk H, Green G. Public health lessons from the Bhopal chemical disaster. JAMA 1990;264:2795–2796.
30. Papanek PJ Jr, Karbus J, and Subcommittee members. Guidelines for hospital and emergency rooms in managing victims of hazardous materials release. Los Angeles County Department of Health Services, January 15, 1988.
31. Green G, Falk H, Kielling P, Levine A, McQuaid J. Disaster emergency planning. In: Bourdeau P, Green G, eds. Methods for assessing and reducing injury from chemical accidents. Chichester: John Wiley, 1989; pp. 75–81.
32. Leonard RB. Community planning for hazardous materials. Top Emerg Med 1986;7:55–64.
33. Savelkoul TJF. Triage of victims in chemical disasters. Prehospital Disast Med 1995;10 (Suppl):S81.
34. Chemical emergencies: hospital emergency department guidelines. US Department of Health and Human Services, Agency for Toxic Substances and Disease Registry.
35. Hazardous Materials Medical Management Protocols. 2nd ed. California Emergency Medical Services Authority. Hazardous Materials Advisory Committee. Koehler G, Project Manager, February 1991; pp. 21–24.
36. Guidelines for ambulance response to hazardous material spills. Health Department, County of Santa Clara, CA:1985.
37. Willis MI. Immediate response: ambulance service—the response to chemical incidents. In: Murray V, ed. Major chemical disasters—medical aspects of management. London: Royal Society of Medicine Services, 1990; pp 69–72.
38. Volans GN. Medical management of chemical disasters involving food or water. In: Murray V, ed. Major chemical disasters—medical aspects of management. London: Royal Society of Medicine Services, 1990; pp. 173–181.
39. Kulling P. Immediate response. Poison centres: their role in the management of major incidents involving chemicals.

In: Murray V, ed. Major chemical disasters—medical aspects of management. London: Royal Society of Medicine Services, 1990; pp. 79–86.
40. Kulling P. Biological effects on humans, initial management and role and responsibility of poison centres in chemical accidents. In: Bourdeau P, Green G, eds. Methods for assessing and reducing injury from chemical accidents. Chichester: John Wiley, 1989; pp. 127–140.
41. Australian Counter Disaster College Report, Toxic Chemical Incidents. Mount Macedon: Australian Counter Disaster College, October 5–9, 1981.
42. Jamsek M, Mozina M, Pance I, Krejei F. Preventive role of poison control centers in major chemical disasters. Proc Internat Congress Clin Toxicol Poison Control and Analytical Toxicology, Lux Tox '90, Luxembourg 2–5, May 1990.
43. Tong TG. Risk assessment of major chemical disasters and the role of the poison centre. In: Murray V, ed. Major chemical disasters—medical aspects of management. London: Royal Society of Medicine Services, 1990; pp. 144–148.
44. Thanabalasingham T, Beckett MW, Murray V. Hospital response to a chemical incident report on casualties of an ethyldichlorosilane spill. Br Med J 1991;302:101–102.
45. McQuaid J. Dispersal of chemicals. In: Bourdeau P, Green G, eds. Methods for assessing and reducing injury from chemical accidents. Chichester: John Wiley, 1989; pp. 157–158.
46. Musk AW, deKlerk NH, Eccles JL, Hobbs MST, Armstrong BK, Layman L, McNulty JC. Wittenoom, Western Australia: a modern industrial disaster. Am J Emerg Med 1992;21:735–747.

SUGGESTED READINGS

1. A guide to the safe handling of hazardous materials accidents. 2nd ed. ASTM Manual; 1P. ASTM, 1916 Rose Street, Philadelphia, PA 19103-1187.
2. Altenkirch H, Stoltenburg-Didinger G, Koeppel C. The neurotoxicological aspects of the toxic oil syndrome (TDS) in Spain. Toxicology 1988;25–34.
3. Auf der Heide E. Disaster response. Principles of preparation and coordination. St. Louis: CV Mosby, 1989; pp. 363.
4. Baxter PJ, Kapila M, Mfonfu D. Lake Nyas disaster, Cameroon, 1986. The medical effects of large scale emission of carbon dioxide? Br Med J 1989;298:1437–1441.
5. Borak J, Olson KR, Sublet V, Koehler G. ATSDR. US Department of Health and Human Services Medical Management Guidelines for Acute Chemical Exposures. December 1992.
6. Cheng CT. Supplementary report on perak mass poisoning. Malaysia: November 14, 1988.
7. Cheng CT, Nan Chee DW, Lyen K, Kuan CH. Report of the special team to investigate perak mass poisoning. Malaysia: October 1988.
8. Eastwood JB, Levin GE, Pazianas M, Taylor AP, Denton J, Freemont AJ. Aluminum deposition in bone after contamination of drinking water supply. Lancet 1990;336:462–464.
9. Glavin GB, Bose R, Pinsky C. Infestions and toxic syndromes from fish and shellfish consumption. Arch Intern Med 1990;150:2425.
10. Bolletta G, Bacchiocchi I, Durnati G, Maffei C. Arch Intern Med 1990;150:24–25.
11. Cassidy K. National and international legislation on major chemical hazards. In: Murray V, ed. Major chemical disasters—medical aspects of management. London: Royal Society of Medicine Service, 1990.
12. Chemical Hazard Response Information System (CHRIS), Hazardous Chemical Data, Washington, DC: Department of Transportation, US Coast Guard. Commandant Instruction M16465.12A.
13. Erlander S. An explosion, a flash fire and a Thai slum's slow poison. New York Times, March 21, 1991.
14. Leonard R. Mass evacuation in disasters. J Emerg Med 1985;2:279–286.
15. Leonard RB. Community planning for hazardous materials. Top Emerg Med 1986;7:55–64.
16. Leonard RB. Emergency evacuations in disasters. Prehosp Disast Med 1991;6:463–466.
17. Mahoney LE, Reuterschan TP. Catastrophic disasters and the design of disaster medical care systems. Ann Emerg Med 1987;16:1085–1091.
18. Managing Hazardous Materials Incidents. Vol I: Emergency Medical Services. A Planning Guide for the Management of Contaminated Patients; Vol II: Hospital Emergency Departments. A Planning Guide for the Management of Contaminated Patients. Atlanta, GA: Agency for Toxic Substances and Disease Registry.
19. Murray V, ed: Major chemical disasters—medical aspects of management. London: Royal Society of Medicine Service, 1990; pp. 1–204.
20. Occupational Safety and Health Guideline for Chemical Hazards. Cincinnati: National Institute for Occupational Safety and Health. DHHS (NIOSH) Publication No. 88-118, Supplement 1-ONG, 1988.
21. Organization for Economic Cooperation and Development Environment Monograph No. 81. UNER IE/PAC Technical Report No. 19, Health Aspects of Chemical Accidents. Guidance on Chemical Accident Awareness, Preparedness and Response for Health Professionals and Emergency Responders. Paris: 1994.
22. Simeons C. Dangerous substances—sources of information. Toxic Subst J 1988;8(1):1–5.
23. Sorensen JH. Evacuation due to off-site releases from chemical accidents. Experiences from 1980 to 1984. J Haz Mat 1987;14:247–257.
24. Van der Torn P. Health risk assessment of major accidents with toxic chemicals for disaster preparedness and response. Doctor of Environmental Science and Engineering Dissertation. Los Angeles: University of California, 1991.

TOXIC OIL SYNDROME

ACUTE PHASE

In May, 1981, the first cases of what would later be called the toxic oil syndrome occurred in Madrid, Spain, and surrounding suburbs. Hundreds and later thousands of individuals suddenly developed an acute Mycoplasma-like pneumonitis. Approximately 2 to 3% of patients died of acute respiratory insufficiency. Patients failed to respond to standard antibiotics and exhibited signs and symptoms in multiple organ systems: fever, lymphadenopathy, nausea, vomiting, arteralgias, myalgias, and pruritic exanthems.[1–3]

By mid-June 1981 it had been established that all patients with that syndrome had ingested varying quantities of an industrial oil, rapeseed oil, that had been marketed as olive oil. Rapeseed oil is required by Spanish law to be denatured with 2% aniline. Some distributors of olive oil took this rapeseed oil, removed the aniline by denaturing, and mixed it with other seed oils or olive oils. The oil was then sold as olive oil. Within 1 to 2 weeks of ingesting this oil, the patients developed the syndrome. All illegally marketed oil was removed by the Spanish government. By this time over 20,000 patients were affected and over 200 died.

By mid-August[4] many patients returned with signs and symptoms of a collagen vascular-like illness with widespread and crippling progressive myalgias. They began to lose muscle and cutaneous sensation. Their skin became diffusely or focally sclerodermoid. Their mucous membranes dried, and they began losing hair. About 10% with the initial illness developed neurologic abnormalities.[1]

ETIOLOGY

The cause of toxic oil syndrome remains obscure. Suggested causes have included the following:

1. A denaturant in the oil, either aniline or fatty acid cogeners[1,5–9]; however, the syndrome induced in animals by such substances does not match the clinical syndrome.
2. Free radicals, yet to be evaluated.
3. Gluconilate-derived isothiocyanates that may have reacted with the denaturant aniline to form phenylthiorea compounds,[10–12] including 1-phenyl-5-vinyl-2-imidazolidine-thione (PV1ZT).[12]
4. Erucic acid (cardiac and arterial lesions induced in animals fed rapeseed oil with high or low erucic acid content).[5,13,14]
5. A dual etiology: *M. pneumonia* and oleoanilides.[15–17]
6. Trichothecene mycotoxins.[18]

CLINICAL MANIFESTATIONS (FIG. 58–7)[3]

Criteria for the diagnosis are presented in Table 58–15.[19]

Acute Phase

Pulmonary

The most common manifestation in the acute phase was that of an acute pneumonitis. Patients had cough, dyspnea, fever and an x-ray film showing an interstitial pattern. This resolved quickly within 3 to 5 days or progressed into an irreversible non-cardiogenic pulmonary edema and death from respiratory insufficiency.[1] Pulmonary hypertension was observed in 1 to 3% of patients studied and accounted for 32 deaths.[20]

Gastrointestinal

Patients had vague gastrointestinal complaints: nausea, vomiting, and periumbilical pain.

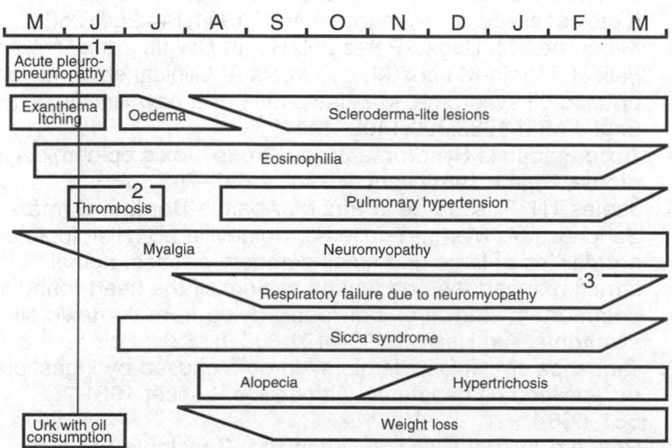

Figure 58–7 Clinical and pathologic evolution of the TES. (1) Ten deaths due to respiratory insufficiency; (2) twelve deaths due to thromboembolic accidents; (3) twelve deaths due to sepsis. (Adapted from Toxic Epidemic Study Group. Lancet 1982;2: 697–702.)

Chronic Phase

About 15% of patients developed serious late-phase symptoms about 3 months after the onset of toxic oil syndrome.[11] The most prominent manifestation of the chronic phase of the syndrome was that of neuromyopathic illness. A progressive and insidious motor and sensory neuropathy developed combined with an inflammatory myositis. Many patients lost 30 or more pounds of muscle mass. Patients became gaunt and emaciated. Other changes included pulmonary insufficiency secondary to pulmonary hypertension, xerostomia, arthralgias, and cardiac failure. Overlying the areas of neuromyopathic injury the skin became sclerodermoid.[1] Four years later, respiratory involvement (dyspnea, cough, decreased vital capacity, and reduced transfer factor for carbon monoxide) was the most common abnormality detected, followed by neurologic disorders, osteoarticular symptoms, psychiatric disorders, hepatic involvement, and sclerodermatous sequelae.[21]

Pathology

The underlying pathologic feature of toxic oil syndrome is a nonnecrotizing, nongranulomatous vasculitis.[22]

Liver

Liver biopsy specimens have disclosed both a cholestatic pattern accompanied by tissue eosinophilia and a degenerative and regenerative pattern with an inflammatory infiltrate including eosinophils.[4]

Esophagus

Esophageal monitoring has disclosed a reduction of primary waves.

Pancreas

In the first few months there was acute pancreatitis with elevated blood amylase and lipase levels observed.[4]

Table 58–15
Criteria for the Diagnosis of Toxic Oil Syndrome[a]

I	Intake of cooking oil sold in bulk, and/or other cases among relatives
II	Interstitial-alveolar pattern on chest roentgenograms during the first 4 months
III	Eosinophilia (>500 eosinophils/μL), myalgia, or rash during the first 4 months
IV	Pulmonary hypertension, hepatic disease, scleroderma, sicca syndrome, polyneuropathy, joint contractures, Raynaud disease, muscle cramps, chronic lung disease

For diagnosis, 1 of the following sets should be fulfilled:

1. At least 2 of criteria I, II, or III.
2. At least 1 of criteria I, II, or III, and 2 or more manifestations included in criterion IV

[a]From Alonso-Ruiz A et al. Medicine 1993;72:285–295.

Hematology

Increases in the prothrombin time, thrombocytopenia, and consumption coagulopathy or documented intravascular coagulation were observed early. Hypereosinophilia (over 500 cells/mL) with toxic oil syndrome permits its inclusion in hypereosinophilic syndrome. Thrombocytopenia was more often found in the chronic phase.[23]

Musculoskeletal

Crippling deformities in the upper and lower limbs were observed in at least 2% of the victims.[24,25] Carpal tunnel syndrome was observed in 5% of patients within a few months after the onset of symptoms.[26]

Pregnancy

No specific malformations have been associated with exposure to the toxic oil syndrome during pregnancy.[27,28]

Laboratory

Elevated aminotransferase and alkaline phosphatase levels were observed in almost all patients.[4] Hyperbilirubinemia was inconsistent.

Chest X-ray

Positive signs on chest radiography frequently observed after the toxic oil syndrome include A and B lines of Kerley and diffuse interstitial or alveolo-interstitial infiltrates with or without effusion.[29] Despite complete radiographic resolution of their acute bilateral interstitial pulmonary infiltrates, cardiomegaly developed in 63% of patients; 55% had pulmonary-artery pneumonia on the chest x-ray film.[30]

Immunology

Antinuclear antibody was positive in almost all patients late in the first year. Rheumatoid factor, C-reactive protein, cryoglobulins, anti-DNA, and anti-ENA (extractable nuclear antigen) were negative; C3 and C4 were normal. IgG level was high during the first 2 months.[31] No specific IgE antibodies directed against contaminants were found.[32] Granular deposits containing IgG, IgM, Clq, and C3 were found in the capillary walls of the glomeruli.[33] An increase in the frequency of HLD-Dr fractions has been observed in those with the chronic disease.[34,35]

TOXIC OIL SYNDROME AND PROGRESSIVE SYSTEMIC SCLEROSIS

Similarities

Features similar to both these conditions have been described: dermal sclerosis, dermal edema, Raynaud's syndrome, hypopigmentation, dysphagia, esophageal hypomotility, pulmonary hypertension, right-sided heart failure, and inflammatory myositis.[3]

Laboratory Abnormalities: Common Features

Eosinophilia, antinuclear antibodies, hypergammaglobulinemia, organ-specific autoantibodies, and an endovasculitis on biopsy examination.

Differences

Patients with toxic oil syndrome have an acute toxic syndrome; patients with progressive systemic sclerosis have an insidious onset. Patients with toxic oil syndrome developed pulmonary hypertension but never pulmonary fibrosis. Patients with toxic oil syndrome developed a peripheral neuropathy, rare in scleroderma. The skin changes in toxic oil syndrome developed primarily in areas of neuromuscular injury, did not involve acral sites, and were reversible with time.[1]

Other Similarities

Toxic oil syndrome contained features overlapping that of scleroderma (above), eosinophilic fasciitis, and certain rare but well-recognized conditions induced by the halogenated hydrocarbon polyvinyl chloride, trichlorethylene, and perchlorethylene.[22,36]

Treatment

Treatment has been largely symptomatic and supportive. Steroids appeared to benefit patients during the early phase of the disease. Penicillamine has been associated with some symptomatic improvement, but its role remains undefined.[2]

REFERENCES—TOXIC OIL SYNDROME

1. Phelps RG, Fleischmajor R. Clinical, pathologic and immunopathologic manifestations of the toxic oil syndrome. J Am Acad Dermatol 1988;18:313–324.
2. Gilsanz V, Alvarez JL, Serrano S, Simon J. Evaluation of the alimentary toxic oil syndrome due to ingestion of denatured rapeseed oil. Arch Intern Med 1984;144:254–256.
3. Kilbourne EM, Ragau-Perez JG, Heath CW Jr, Zack MM, Falk H, Martin-Marcos M, de Carols A. Clinical epidemiology of toxic oil syndrome. Manifestations of a new illness. N Engl J Med 1983;309:1408–1414.
4. Toxic Epidemic Syndrome Study Group. Toxic epidemic syndrome, Spain, 1981. Lancet 1982;2:697–702.
5. James TN, Posada-de la Paz M, Abaitua-Borda I, Gomez-Sanchez MA, Martinez-Tello FJ, Soldevilla LB. Histologic abnormalities of large and small coronary arteries, neural structures, and the conduction system of the heart found in postmortem studies of individuals dying from the toxic oil syndrome. Am Heart J 1991;121:803–813.
6. Tabuenca JM. Toxic allergic syndrome caused by ingestion of rapeseed oil denatured with aniline. Lancet 1981;2: 567–568.
7. Roncero AV, del Valle CJ, Duran PM, Constante EN. New aniline derivative in cooking oils associated with the toxic oil syndrome. Lancet 1983;2:1024–1025.
8. Spurzem JR, Lockey JE. Toxic oil syndrome. Arch Intern Med 1984;144:249–250.

9. Kaphalia BS, Ansari GAG. Rapid chromatographic analysis of fatty acid anilines suspected of causing toxic oil syndrome. J Anal Toxicol 1991;15:90–94.
10. Kammuller ME, Penninks AH, Seiner W. Spanish toxic oil syndrome and chemically induced graft-versus-host-like reactions. Lancet 1984;2:805–806.
11. Kammuller ME, Bloksma N, Seinen W. Chemical-induced autoimmune reactions and Spanish toxic oil syndrome. Focus on hydantoins and related compounds. Clin Toxicol 1988;26: 157–174.
12. Kammuller ME, Penninks AH, Seinen W. Spanish toxic oil syndrome is a chemically induced GVHD-like epidemic. Lancet 1984;1:1174–1175.
13. McMichael J. Erucic acid and the Spanish oil epidemic. Lancet 1981;2:1172.
14. CDC. Follow-up on toxic pneumonia—Spain. MMWR 1981; 30:436–438.
15. Rigau-Perez JG, Winkler WG. Mycoplasma pneumonias and Spanish oil syndrome. Lancet 1982;2:724.
16. Root-Bernstein R, Westall FC. Spanish toxic-allergic syndrome: an explanation. Lancet 1982;1:969–970.
17. Editorial. Toxic oil syndrome. Lancet 1983;1:1257–1258.
18. Schoental R. The toxic oil syndrome in Spain. Was it due to a combined action of trichothecene mycotoxins and of inhibition of carboxyesterase? Hum Toxicol 1988;7:365–369.
19. Alonso-Ruiz A, Calabozo M, Perez-Ruiz F, Mancebo L. Toxic oil syndrome. A long-term follow-up of a cohort of 332 patients. Medicine 1993;72:285–295.
20. Gomez-Sanchez MA, Mestre de Juan MJ, Gomez-Pajuelo C, Lopez JI, de Ataun MJD, Martinez-Tello FJ. Pulmonary hypertension due to toxic oil syndrome. A clinical pathologic study. Chest 1989;95:325–331.
21. Escribano PR, Diaz de Atauri MJ, Gamez Sanchez MA. Persistence of respiratory abnormalities. Four years after the onset of toxic oil syndrome. Chest 1991;100: 336–339.
22. Alonso-Ruiz A, Zea-Mendoza AC, Gonzalez-Lanza M, Gomez-Catalan E. Digital tuft alterations in toxic oil syndrome. Lancet 1984;2:520–521.
23. Garcia MC, Posada M, de Rojas FD, Borda IA, Oliver JMT. Hypercoagulable states and the toxic oil syndrome. Ann Intern Med 1986;104:730.
24. Bronchud MPH. Crippling deformities in Spanish toxic epidemic syndrome. Lancet 1982;2:829.
25. Bronchide MH. Toxic oil syndrome. N Engl J Med 1984;310: 1260–1261.
26. Garzon FJO, Santana CL, Ruiz AA, Meana SR. The toxic oil syndrome: a new cause of carpel-tunnel syndrome. N Engl J Med 1983;309:1455.
27. Oliver JMT, Garcia MC, Galiana JR, Alvarez-Arenas RP, de la Paz MP, Borda IA et al. Spanish toxic oil and congenital malformations. Lancet 1983;1:181.
28. Martines-Frias M-L, Salvador J, Prieto L. Spanish toxic oil and congenital malformations. Lancet 1982;2:1349.
29. Gilsanz V. Late features of toxic syndrome due to denatured rapeseed oil. Lancet 1982;1:335–336.
30. Miller DD, Chartman BR. Toxic oil syndrome. N Engl J Med 1984;310:1260–1261.
31. Gutierrez C, Gaspar L, Muro R, Kreisler M, Ferriz P. Autoimmunity in patients with Spanish toxic oil syndrome. Lancet 1983;1:644.
32. Brostoff J, Blanca M, Boulton P, Serrano S. Absence of specific IgE antibodies in toxic oil syndrome. Lancet 1982; 1:277.
33. Gutierrez-Millet V, Navas-Palacios J, Gomez-Reino J, Fernandez-Epifanio JL. Renal involvement in the toxic oil syndrome. Lancet 1982;1:1120.
34. Vicarico JL, Serrano-Rios M, San Andres F, Arnaiz-Villena A. HLA-DR3, DR4 increase in chronic stage of Spanish oil disease. Lancet 1982;1:276.
35. Pereira RS, Black CM, Arnaz-Villena A, Vicario JL, Gomez-Reino JJ. Collagen autoantibodies in toxic oil disease. Lancet 1985;1:273.
36. Bronchud MH. Toxic oil syndrome and vinyl chloride disease. Lancet 1984;2:931.

HYDROGEN CYANIDE[1]

Persons whose clothing or skin is contaminated with hydrocyanic acid or cyanide-containing solutions can secondarily contaminate response personnel by direct contact or through off-gassing vapor. Hydrogen cyanide is a volatile, flammable liquid at room temperature; as a gas, it is flammable and potentially explosive. Hydrogen cyanide is absorbed well by inhalation and can produce death within minutes. Substantial absorption can occur through intact skin if vapor concentration is high. Exposure by any route may cause systemic effects.

PREHOSPITAL MANAGEMENT

Victims whose clothing or skin is contaminated with hydrocyanic acid or cyanide-containing solutions can secondarily contaminate response personnel by direct contact or through off-gassing vapor. Avoid dermal contact with cyanide-contaminated victims or with gastric contents of victims who may have ingested cyanide-containing materials. Victims exposed only to hydrogen cyanide gas do not pose a contamination risk to rescuers. Hydrogen cyanide poisoning is marked by abrupt onset of profound toxic effects that may include syncope, seizures, coma, gasping respirations, and cardiovascular collapse, causing death within minutes. Victims exposed to hydrogen cyanide can survive with supportive care and rapid administration of specific antidotes.

EMERGENCY DEPARTMENT MANAGEMENT

Hospital personnel in an enclosed area can be secondarily contaminated by vapor off-gassing from heavily soaked clothing or skin or from toxic vomitus. Avoid dermal contact with cyanide-contaminated patients or with gastric contents of patients who may have ingested cyanide-containing materials. Patients do not pose a secondary contamination risk after contaminated clothing is removed and the skin is washed. Hydrogen cyanide poisoning is marked by abrupt onset of profound toxic effects that may include syncope, seizures, coma, gasping respirations, and cardiovascular collapse, causing death within minutes. Patients exposed to hydrogen cyanide can survive with supportive care and rapid administration of specific antidotes.

PHENOL

Persons exposed only to phenol vapor do not pose a substantial risk of secondary contamination. Persons whose clothing or skin is contaminated with liquid phenol can secondarily contaminate personnel by direct contact or through off-gassing vapor. Phenol is a flammable, highly corrosive chemical that can cause serious burns and systemic poisoning by all exposure routes. Introduced originally as an antiseptic, phenol is still used in small amounts in disinfectants and many over-the-counter products that have antiseptic qualities.

PREHOSPITAL MANAGEMENT

Victims exposed only to phenol vapor do not pose a substantial risk of secondary contamination. Victims whose clothing or skin is contaminated with liquid phenol can secondarily contaminate response personnel by direct contact or through off-gassing vapor from heavily soaked clothing or from vomitus of victims who have ingested phenol. Phenol may cause convulsions, sudden collapse, and coma. Because of its corrosivity, phenol causes severe chemical burns on contact. Rapid decontamination may greatly affect the odds of survival. There is no antidote for phenol. Treatment is supportive.

EMERGENCY DEPARTMENT MANAGEMENT

Hospital personnel in an enclosed area can be secondarily contaminated by direct contact or from vapor off-gassing from heavily soaked clothing or from the vomitus of victims who have ingested phenol. Patients do not pose a contamination risk after contaminated clothing is removed and the skin is washed. Phenol may cause convulsions, sudden collapse, and coma. Because of its corrosive nature, phenol can cause severe chemical burns on contact. There is no antidote for phenol poisoning. Treatment consists of supportive measures.

Chapter 59 Chemical Warfare (See also Chemical Disaster Chapter)

NERVE AGENTS

Nerve agents, prepared for use in chemical warfare, are organophosphate compounds similar to the organophosphates used as pesticides (see Pesticide chapter) (Fig. 59–1). Organophosphorus agents are taken up by the body (a) by inhalation (e.g., during manufacturing and processing, during application of insecticides in agriculture, or during exposure to nerve agents on the battlefield); (b) by the oral route (e.g., in suicide attempts with insecticides); and (c) percutaneously (e.g., during exposure in which the airways are protected by a gas mask). Exposure of man to very small amounts of such compounds induces severe muscarinic and nicotinic effects often leading to death.

Over the past 50 years a series of chemical countermeasures have been developed, including atropine, the oximes, and pyridostigmine. Atropine effectively ameliorates most muscarinic effects by itself, but has little effect on the nicotinic effects (muscle twitching, flaccidity); the oximes are useful as an aid in countering the nicotinic effects, but do not function well without atropine. Pyridostigmine appears to assist in protecting the body against soman toxicity when given as a preventative, but is not effective as treatment by itself; it is relatively ineffective for the treatment of poisoning with other nerve agents (tabun, sarin, VX). Diazepam may be of use in ameliorating central nervous system irritation (convulsions). Continual developments and refinements are in progress to increase the protection of the military and civilian populations exposed to these awesome weapons of human destruction.

Civilian Exposure

Unprotected civilians, in addition to military personnel, may be targets of chemical warfare. Civilians would be at risk if (a) war strategy includes chemical assault intended to produce civilian casualties on a large scale; (b) chemical weapon assault is directed against politically or strategically important installations employing civilians; or (c) they live or work within an area of military attack.[1,2] In addition, individuals living near incinerators used to dispose of chemical warfare nerve agents may have anxiety about the risk of accidental exposure to organophosphates or their combustion products.

Abbreviation	*Common Name*	*Proper Name*
GA	Tabun	Ethyl N-dimethylphosphoramidocyanidate 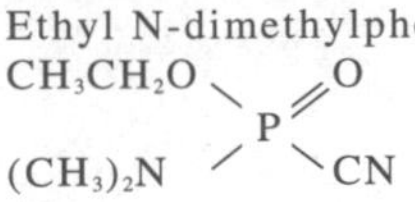 CH_3CH_2O ╲ P(=O) ╱ $(CH_3)_2N$, ╲ CN
GB	Sarin	Isopropyl methylphosphonofluoridate 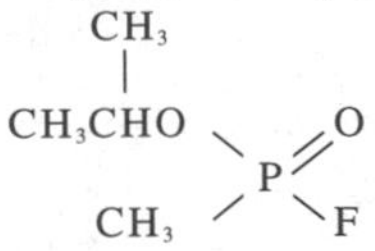 CH_3 | CH_3CHO ╲ P(=O) ╱ CH_3, ╲ F
GD	Soman	1,2,2-trimethylpropyl methylphosphonofluoridate (Pinacolyl methylphosphonofluoridate) 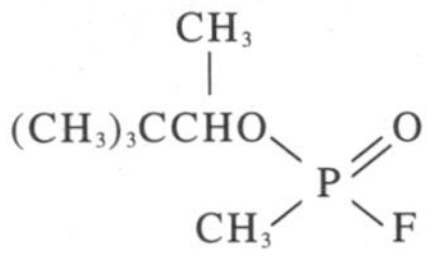 CH_3 | $(CH_3)_3CCHO$ ╲ P(=O) ╱ CH_3, ╲ F
GE	—	Isopropyl ethylphosphonofluoridate 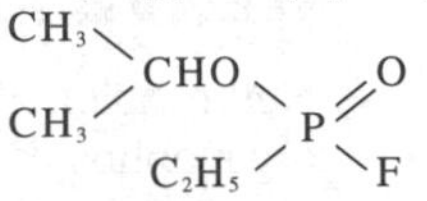 CH_3, CH_3 ╲╱ CHO ╲ P(=O) ╱ C_2H_5, ╲ F
GF	—	Cyclohexyl methylphosphonofluoridate 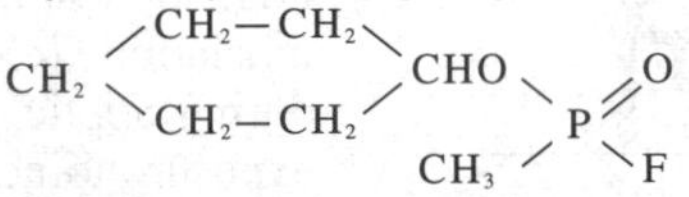 CH_2 ╱ CH_2-CH_2 ╲, ╲ CH_2-CH_2 ╱ CHO ╲ P(=O) ╱ CH_3, ╲ F
VX	—	O-Ethyl S-[2-(diisopropylamino)ethyl] methylphosphonothioate 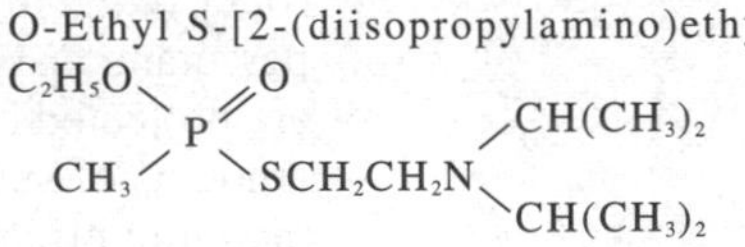 C_2H_5O ╲ P(=O) ╱ CH_3, ╲ SCH_2CH_2N ╱ $CH(CH_3)_2$, ╲ $CH(CH_3)_2$
VE	—	O-Ethyl S-[2-(diethylamino)ethyl] ethylphosphonothioate 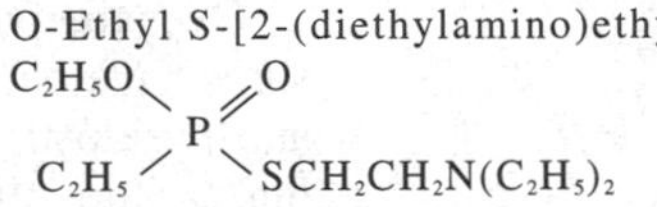 C_2H_5O ╲ P(=O) ╱ C_2H_5, ╲ $SCH_2CH_2N(C_2H_5)_2$
VG	—	O O-Diethyl S-[2-(diethylamino)ethyl] phosphorothioate 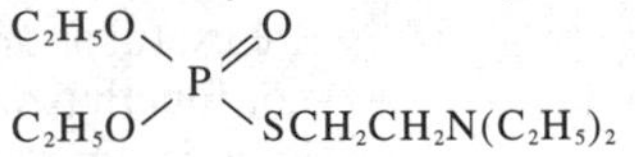 C_2H_5O ╲ P(=O) ╱ C_2H_5O, ╲ $SCH_2CH_2N(C_2H_5)_2$
VM	—	O-Ethyl S-[2-(diethylamino)ethyl] methylphosphonothioate 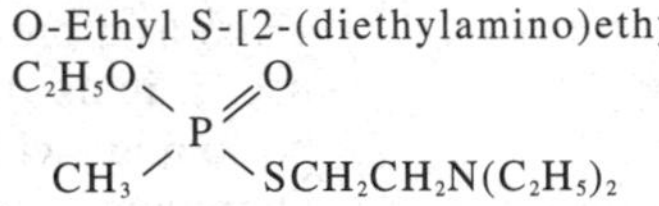 C_2H_5O ╲ P(=O) ╱ CH_3, ╲ $SCH_2CH_2N(C_2H_5)_2$

Figure 59–1 Formulas of Nerve Agents. (Adapted from Ballantyne B, Marust C, eds. Clinical and experimental toxicology of organophosphates and carbamates. Oxford: Butterworth–Heinemann, 1992.)

History

A thorough historical review of the development of the nerve gas agents and their antidotes was presented by Holmstedt in 1985[3] (see Table 59–1). A summary of the pharmacology and hormonal changes resulting from organophosphate poisoning was presented by Clement.[4] Synonyms for nerve gas agents are listed in Table 59–2.

The principal nerve agents are Tabun (GA), Sarin (GB), Soman (GD), and VX. The G agents are fluorine- or cyanide-containing organophosphates. They are colorless liquids in pure form. In field concentrations they are odorless. Clothing releases G agents for about 30 minutes after contact with vapor.

The V-agents are sulfur-containing organophosphorus compounds. They affect the body in essentially the same manner as G-agents. The nerve agents are all viscous liquids, not nerve gas per se. The vapor pressure of the G-series nerve agents are sufficiently high for the vapors to be lethal rapidly. GB is largely a vapor hazard. VX is of such low volatility that it is mainly a liquid contact hazard. G-agents spread rapidly on surfaces such as skin. VX spreads less rapidly.

Clinical

Eye Exposure

Symptoms in less than 2 to 3 minutes.

Table 59–1
Some Dates in the History of Nerve Gas Development[a]

1864	Jobst and Hesse isolate physostigmine from the seeds of the Calabar bean
1864	Kleinwachter shows that Calabar extract is an antidote for atropine poisoning
1865	Vee crystallizes the alkaloid and calls it eserine
1870	Fraser discovers atropine can prevent lethal effect of physostigmine
1873	Von Hofman synthesizes first example of C-P linkage, methylphosphoryl dichloride, an important step in the synthesis of insecticides and sarin
1903	Michaelis reports a compound with a P-CN bond which led to the synthesis of a number of insecticides and the nerve gas Tabun
1932	Lang and von Kreuger synthesize compounds with the P-F linkage
1937	Schrader patents formula for contact insecticides based on Michaelis' pupil's work. Synthesizes Sarin, Tabun
1938–1941	Schrader develops fluorine-containing compounds including DFP
1944	Schrader develops parathion
1944	Germans develop GD (Soman)
1949	Collomp develops atropine as an antidote to parasympathomimetic effects of nerve gases
1951	First account of the synthesis and pharmacology of Tabun given by Holmstedt
1951	Jandorf finds that hydroxylamine detoxifies organophosphorus inhibitors
1952	British develop VX
1955	Davies introduces oximes (PAM)
1955	Wilson reports value of 2 PAM organophophate poisoning
1956	Namba uses PAM to treat organophosphate insecticide poisoning
1958	Bispyridinium compounds introduced (obidoxime, etc.)
1961	PAM mesylate (P2S) introduced for use in U.K.
1964	Erdmann and Engelhard describe the pharmacology of obidoxime
1964	PAM licensed for use as treatment of organophosphate insecticide poisoning
1970	Oldiges and Schoene show efficacy of HI-6 in Soman poisoning in mice.

[a]Adapted from Munro NB et al. Environ Health Perspect 1990;89:205–215.

Table 59–2
Synonyms[a]

Tabun (GA): mLe-100
Sarin (GB): Zarin
Soman (GD): Zoman
Distilled Mustard (HD): HS, Kampstaff "Lost", Mustard Gas, S-Lost, Schwefel-Lost, Sulfur Mustard, Y, Yellow Cross Liquid, Yperite
Nitrogen Mustard (HN-1): Ethyl 5, NH-Lost, NOR nitrogen mustard, NSC10873
Nitrogen Mustard (HNZ): Dichloren, N methyl-Lost, Mustine, Nitrogen Mustard, NSC762, S
Mustard-T Mixture (HT): HD *Bis*[2(2 chloroethylthio) ethyl] ether
Lewisite (L): Lyvizit
Mustard Lewisite: (HL)
Phenyldichloroarsine (PD): Pfiffikus, DJ, Sternite
Ethyldichloroarsene (ED): Dick
Methyldichloroarsine (OMD): Methyl-dck, medikus
Phosgene Oxime (CX): Fosgen Oksom
Hydrogencyanide (AC): Cyclone B: Zyklon B
Cyanogenchloride (CK): Mauguinite CC Klortsian
Arsine (SA): Arthur
BZ: Oksilidin
Phosgene (CG): Collagnite; Zusatz; Green Cross; D substance
Diphosgene (DP): Difosgene, Perstoff, Surpalite, Green Cross

[a]Adapted from FM3-8-NAVFACO-467. Potential Military Chemical/Biological Agents and Compounds. Washington, DC: December 12, 1990.

Respiratory Exposure

Symptoms in 2 to 5 minutes. Lethal doses kill in less than 15 minutes.

Skin Absorption

Great enough to cause death can occur in 1 to 2 minutes.

CLINICAL PRESENTATION

Muscarinic Effects—Nicotinic Effects

Moderate Exposure

The appearance of moderate-to-severe muscarinic effects (Tables 59–3 and 59–4) is followed by involuntary muscular twitching, scattered muscular fasciculations, and occasional muscle cramps. The skin may be pale, and blood pressure may rise due to transitory vasoconstriction resulting from cholinergic stimulation of sympathetic ganglia and possibly from the release of epinephrine.[5–7] Sidell has quantitated the effects of inhalation and dermal exposure to nerve agents[8] (Tables 59–5 and 59–6).

Severe Exposure

Fascicular twitching (which usually appears first on the eyelids and in the facial and calf muscles) may then become generalized. Rippling movements are seen under the skin, and twitching movements appear in all parts of the body. This is followed by severe generalized muscular weakness, including the muscles of respiration. Respiratory movements become more labored, shallow, and rapid; they then slow and become intermittent. Later respiratory muscle weakness may become profound and contribute to respiratory depression. Central respiratory depression may be a major cause of respiratory arrest.

Central Nervous System Effects: Acute Toxicity—Animals

Pyridostigmine Pretreatment

Pyridostigmine pretreatment appears to protect guinea pigs from the lethal actions of soman and sarin. Pretreatment with

Table 59–3
Signs and Symptoms of Nerve Agent Poisoning[a]

Site of Action	Signs and Symptoms
	Following Local Exposure
1. ***Muscarinic—***	
Pupils	Miosis, marked, usually maximal (pinpoint), sometimes unequal.
Ciliary body	Frontal headache, eye pain on focusing, blurring of vision.
Nasal mucous membranes	Rhinorrhea, hyperemia.
Bronchial tree	Tightness in chest, bronchoconstriction, increased secretion, cough.
Gastrointestinal	Occasional nausea and vomiting.
	Following Systemic Absorption (depending on dose)
Bronchial tree	Tightness in chest, with prolonged wheezing expiration suggestive of bronchoconstriction or increased secretion, dyspnea, pain in chest, increased bronchial secretion, cough, cyanosis, pulmonary edema.
Gastrointestinal	Anorexia, nausea, vomiting, abdominal cramps, epigastric and substernal tightness (cardiospasm) with "heartburn" and eructation, diarrhea, tenesmus, involuntary defecation.
Sweat glands	Increased sweating.
Salivary glands	Increased salivation.
Lacrimal glands	Increased lacrimation.
Heart	Bradycardia.
Pupils	Miosis, occasionally unequal, later maximal miosis (pinpoint).
Ciliary body	Blurring of vision, headache.
Bladder	Frequency, involuntary micturition.
2. ***Nicotinic—***	
Striated muscle	Easy fatigue, mild weakness, muscular twitching, fasciculations, cramps, generalized weakness/flaccid paralysis (including muscles of respiration) with dyspnea and cyanosis.
Sympathetic ganglia	Pallor, transitory elevation of blood pressure followed by hypotension.
3. ***Central Nervous System—***	Immediate (Acute) Effects: Generalized weakness, depression of respiratory and circulatory centers with dyspnea, cyanosis and hypotension; convulsions, loss of consciousness, and coma.
	Delayed (Chronic) Effects: Giddiness, tension, anxiety, jitteriness, restlessness, emotional lability, excessive dreaming, insomnia, nightmares, headaches, tremor, withdrawal and depression, bursts of slow waves of elevated voltage in EEG (especially on hyperventilation), drowsiness, difficulty concentrating, slowness of recall, confusion, slurred speech, ataxia.

[a]Adapted from Army FM8-285, Navy NAVMED P-5041, Air Force AFM 160-11 Field Manual. The Treatment of Chemical Agent Casualties and Conventional Military Chemical Injuries. Washington, DC: Departments of the Army, the Navy, and the Air Force, February 28, 1990.

pyridostigmine alone provides little or no protection against incapacitation or lethality induced by soman or sarin.[9]

Clonidine

Clonidine appears to protect animals against soman-induced acute and chronic toxicity, including the toxic behavioral, autonomic, and cardiovascular symptoms.

Antidotes

Antidotes for nerve agents are summarized in Table 59–7.

Soman Detoxification (See Pyridostigmine)

HI-6

HI-6[10] is considered the most potent oxime antidote against soman poisoning in animals. In human muscle preparations treatment with HI-6 restored only 5% of control activity, while prophylactic use of HI-6 restored 50%.[11]

Convulsions induced by soman in rats may result from a rapid accumulation of acetylcholine in the brain after inhibition of AChE. Those neuronal processes that bear muscarinic receptors appear to be more vulnerable to convulsion-induced change than those with benzodiazepine receptors.[12]

MECHANISM OF ACTION

Figures 59–2 and 59–3 depict a two-step reaction between organophosphate compounds and acetylcholinesterase. The toxic manifestations and lethality following nerve agent exposure appear to follow the irreversible phosphorylation of the serine-containing active site of the enzyme acetylcholinesterase. A variety of proteolytic enzymes may also be inhibited by organophosphates (e.g., chymotrypsin, trypsin). Minor changes in coagulation parameters (PT, APTT, fibrinogen) are observed following soman poisoning in rabbits. Significant changes are seen in the alkaline phosphatase, calcium concentration, and CPK activity.[13]

Sarin can induce a myonecrosis. Acetylcholine accumulation is involved in the calcium flux into skeletal muscle fibers during anticholinesterase poisoning.[14] This phenomenon with OP anticholinesterases may be linked with OP-induced myopathy.[15]

In rats, treatment with atropine sulfate or HI-6 alone appears to protect against the effects of soman, but 2-PAM-Cl or atropine methyl nitrate alone did not. Addition of atropine sulfate to HI-6 enhances protection. HI-6 maintains active ChE in the periphery, and this may be important for survival of the animals after soman exposure.[16]

Table 59–4
Time Course of Effects of Nerve Agents[a]

	Types of Effects	Route of Absorption	Description of Effects	When Effects Appear After Exposure	Duration of Effects After Mild Exposure	Duration of Effects After Severe Exposure
Vapor	Local	Lungs	Rhinorrhea, nasal hyperemia, tightness in chest, wheezing.	One to several minutes	A few hours	1 to 2 days
Vapor	Local	Eyes	Miosis, conjunctival hyperemia, eye pain, frontal headache.	One to several minutes	Miosis—24 hours.	2 to 3 days.
Vapor	Systemic	Lungs or eyes.	Muscarinic, nicotinic, and central nervous system effects (see Table 2-1).	Less than 1 minute to a few minutes after moderate or severe exposure; about 30 minutes after mild exposure.	Several hours to a day.	Acute effects: 2 to 3 days. CNS effects: days to weeks.
Liquid agent	Local	Eyes	Same as vapor effects	Instantly	Similar to effects of vapor.	
Liquid agent	Local	Ingestion	Gastrointestinal (see Table 2-1)	About 30 minutes after ingestion.	Several hours to a day.	2 to 5 days.
Liquid agent	Local	Skin	Local sweating and muscular twitching.	3 minutes to 2 hours	3 days	5 days.
Liquid agent	Systemic	Lungs	See Table 2-1	Several minutes		1 to 5 days.
Liquid agent	Systemic	Eyes	Same as for vapor	Several minutes		2 to 4 days.
Liquid agent	Systemic	Skin	Generalized sweating	15 minutes to 2 hours		2 to 5 days.
Liquid agent	Systemic	Ingestion	Gastrointestinal (see Table 2-1)	15 minutes to 2 hours		3 to 5 days.

After lethal or near lethal exposures to nerve agents, the time to onset of symptoms and to maximal severity of symptoms is shorter; it may be extremely brief after overwhelming exposure. Following exposure to lethal concentrations, the time interval to death depends upon the degree, the route of exposure, and the agent. If untreated, exposure to lethal concentrations of nerve agents can result in death 5 minutes after appearance of symptoms.

[a]Adapted from Army FM8-285, Navy NAVMED P-5041, Air Force AFM 160-11 Field Manual. The Treatment of Chemical Agent Casualties and Conventional Military Chemical Injuries. Washington, DC: Departments of the Army, the Navy, and the Air Force, February 20, 1990.

Table 59–5
Effects of Vapor Exposure to Nerve Agents[a,b]

- Exposure to small amount (local effects)
  - Miosis
  - Rhinorrhea
  - Slight bronchoconstriction/secretions (slight dyspnea)
- Exposure to moderate amount (local effects)
  - Miosis
  - Rhinorrhea
  - Bronchoconstriction/secretions (moderate to marked dyspnea)
- Exposure to large amount
  - As above plus:
    - Loss of consciousness
    - Convulsions (seizures)
    - Generalized fasciculations
    - Flaccid paralysis
    - Apnea
  - Involuntary micturition/defecation

[a]Adapted from Sidell FR. In: Somani SM, ed. Chemical warfare agents. San Diego: Academic Press, 1992; pp. 155–194.
[b]Onset within seconds to several minutes after onset of exposure.

Table 59–6
Effects of Dermal Exposure to Nerve Agents[a]

- Minimal exposure
  - Increased sweating at site of exposure
  - Muscular fasciculations at site of exposure
- Moderate exposure
  - Increased sweating at site
  - Muscular fasciculations at site
  - Nausea, vomiting, and diarrhea
  - Feeling of generalized weakness
  - May be precipitant in onset after long (4–18 hr) asymptomatic interval
- Severe exposure
  - Above may be present
  - Loss of consciousness (may be precipitous in onset after asymptomatic interval)
  - Convulsions (seizures)
  - Generalized fasciculations
  - Flaccid paralysis
  - Apnea
  - Involuntary micturition/defecation

[a]Adapted from Sidell FR. In: Somani SM, ed. Chemical warfare agents. San Diego: Academic Press, 1992; pp. 155–194.

Table 59–7
Nerve Agent Antidote Summary: Actions, Dosages, Side Effects/Overdose Symptoms[a]

Antidote/Action	Dose	Overdose Symptoms/Management
Atropine (di-hyoscyamine) Anticholinergic alkaloid: used to block effects of parasympathetic nerve stimulation. Prepared from powdered roots of *Atropa belladonna* and *Datura stramonium.* In massive doses, used to treat AChE poisoning and to manage certain psychiatric states. Relieves smooth muscle constriction in lung and GI tract and reduces glandular paralysis (cleans up respiratory tract secretions). Toxicity rating 5, extremely toxic. [Probable oral lethal dose in humans of 5–50 mg/kg, or 7 drops to 1 teaspoon for 150-lb (70-kg) person].	Adult: 2–4 mg or more of atropine sulfate IM or IV. Full atropinization maintained at 2-mg doses every 3 to 8 min for several hours. Child: initial dose, 0.05 mg/kg. Maintenance doses for child range from 0.02 to 0.05 mg/kg. Mean lethal dose unknown (recovery after ingestion of 1000 mg documented); lethal estimate of 10 mg, although recovery documented at 100-mg dose in many adults; children more susceptible. For all: provide atropine until signs of atropinization occur (dry mouth and dry lungs); use until signs of improvement are seen; taper off dose.	Symptoms Dryness of mucous membranes, burning pain in throat, difficulty in swallowing, and intense thirst. Skin hot, dry, flushed. Rash over face, neck, and upper trunk, especially in infants and children. Peeling of skin may follow. Exceptionally high fever. Sinus tachycardia (rapid heartbeat), palpitations, elevated blood pressure. Uncommonly: nausea, vomiting, and abdominal distension in infants, urinary urgency and hesitancy; inability to void. Restlessness, fatigue, excitement and confusion, progressing to mania and delirium, which may persist for hours or days. Hallucinations, particularly of visual type. Patients may exhibit self-destructive acts. Management Treat symptoms with physostigmine salicylate. Onset of symptoms within 15–30 min, maximum effects at 2–3 hr and recovery within 12 hr.
2-PAM-Cl(protopam chloride; 2-pyridine aldoxime methyl chloride; pralidoxime) Treat poisoning due to organophosphate insecticides and nerve gases; anticholinesterase antagonist. Effective when given with atropine. Acts by removing organophosphate from cholinesterase and restoring normal control of skeletal muscle contraction (relieves twitching and paralysis).	Adult: 1–2 g in 100 mL saline IV over 15–30 min for initial dose. Second dose after 1 hr if symptoms indicate. Children: initial dose of 15–25 mg/kg, followed by second after 1 hr if symptoms indicate. Infants: try 15 mg/kg. Less effective after aging (when bond between organophosphate and cholinesterase becomes irreversible). Substantial aging occurs within 5 hr for GB.	Symptoms Rapid and possibly dangerous rise in blood pressure. Temporary rapid heartbeat (tachycardia). Mild weakness, dizziness. Blurred or double vision. Management Usually well tolerated with careful (slow) administration.

[a]Adapted from Munro NB et al. Environ Health Perspect 1990;89:205–215.

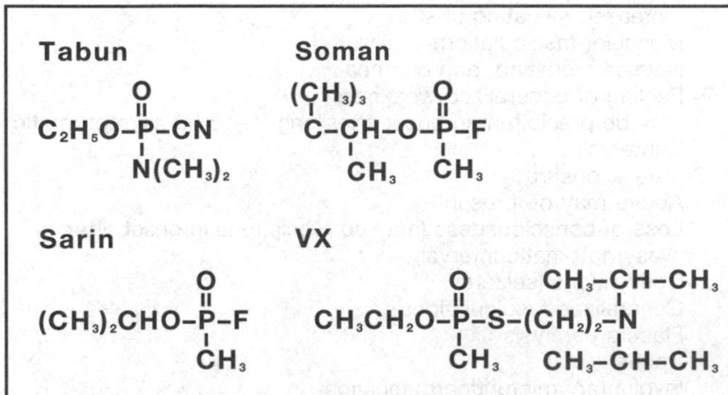

Figure 59–2 The chemical structures of nerve agents Tabun (GA), Sarin (GB), Soman (GD), and VX. (Adapted from Sidell FR, Borak J. Ann Emerg Med 1992;21:865–871.)

Step 1 $AChE{-}OH + R_1O{-}P(=O)(R_2){-}X \rightleftarrows AChE{-}OH \bullet R_1O{-}P(=O)(R_2){-}X$

Step 2 $AChE{-}OH \bullet R_1O{-}P(=O)(R_2){-}X \longrightarrow AChE{-}O{-}P(=O)(R_2){-}OR_1 + HX$

Step 3 $AChE{-}O{-}P(=O)(R_2){-}OR_1 \longrightarrow AChE{-}O{-}P(=O)(R_2){-}OH + R_1O$

Figure 59–3 The reaction between organophosphorus compounds and acetylcholinesterase occurs in a three-step process. Step 1 is the formation of a reversible enzyme-inhibitor complex. Step 2 is the phosphorylation and inactivation of the enzyme molecule. Step 3 is the "aging" reaction involving formation of a monophosphoric acid residue bound to the enzyme. (Adapted from Sidell FR, Borak J. Ann Emerg Med 1992;21:865–871.)

REFERENCES—DRUG INTERACTIONS—ORGANOPHOSPHATE INTOXICATED PATIENTS

1. Minton N, Murray SG. A review of organophosphate poisoning. Med Toxicology 1988;3:350–375.
2. World Health Organization report on the hazards to civilian health from chemical weapons. Executive Board Paper, World Health Organization, 1988.
3. Holmstedt B. The third symposium on prophylaxis and treatment of chemical poisons. April 22–24, 1985. Stockholm, Sweden. Fund Appl Toxicol 1985;5:S1–S9.
4. Clement JG. Hormonal consequences of organophosphate poisoning. Fund Appl Toxicol 1985;5:S61–S77.
5. Treatment of chemical agent casualties and conventional military chemical injuries field manual. Army FM 8-285, Navy Navmed P-5041, Air Force AFM 160-11, Departments of the Army, the Navy and the Air Force. February 1990.
6. Grob D. Anticholinesterase intoxication in man and its treatment in Ochler O, Farah A, Koelle GB, eds. Handbuch de Experimentalla Pharmacologie XV. Cholinesterase and anticholinesterase agents. Berlin: Springer-Verlag, 1963;990–1022.
7. Wills JH. Pharmacological antagonists of the anticholinesterase agents in Handbook de Experimentalla Pharmacologie XV. Cholinesterase and anticholinesterase agents. Berlin: Springer-Verlag, 1963;883–920.
8. Sidell FR. Clinical considerations in nerve agent intoxication. In: Somani SM, ed. Clinical warfare agents. San Diego: Academic Press, 1992; pp. 155–194.
9. Leadbeater L, Inns RH, Rylands JM. Treatment of poisoning by soman. Fund Appl Toxicol 1985;5:S225–S231.
10. Inns RH, Leadbeater L. The efficacy of bispyridium derivatives in the treatment of organophosphate poisoning in the guinea pig. J Pharm Pharmacol 1983;35:427–433.
11. Grubic Z, Tomazic A. Mechanism of action of HI-6 on soman Inhibition of acetylcholinesterase in preparations of rat and human skeletal muscle; comparison to SAD-128 and PAM-2. Arch Toxicol 1989;63:68–71.
12. Churchill L, Pazdërnik TL, Cross RS, Nelson SR, Samson FE. Soman- or kainic acid-induced convulsions decrease muscarinic receptors but not benzodiazepine receptors. Neurotoxicology 1990;11:57–72.
13. Lee MJ, Clement JG. Effects of soman poisoning in hematology and coagulation parameters and serum biochemistry in rabbits. Milit Med 1990;155:244–249.
14. Inns RH, Tuckwell NJ, Bright JE, Marrs TC. Histochemical demonstration of calcium accumulation in muscle fibres after experimental organophosphate poisoning. Hum Exp Toxicol 1990;9:245–250.
15. Bright JE, Inns RH, Marrs TC, Tuckwell NJ. Histochemical demonstration of sarin-induced calcium influx in mouse diaphragm. Hum Exp Toxicol 1990;9:120 (abstract).
16. Shih T-M, Whalley CE, Valdes JJ. A comparison of cholinergic effects of HI-6 and pralidoxime-2-chloride (2-PAM) in soman poisoning. Toxicol Lett 1991;55:131–147.

TREATMENT[1]

1. In intoxicated patients avoid any drug known to be or suggested to be hydrolyzed by the enzyme cholinesterase:
   Suxamethonium (succinylcholine)
   Procaine
   Amethocaine
   Chlorprocaine
   Trimethaphan
2. Use cautiously, during the cholinergic phase or during any intermediate syndromes, any drugs that produce definite and prolonged inhibition of plasma cholinesterase.
   Neostigmine
   Pyridostigmine
3. Edrophonium is probably the drug of choice for reversal. Its effects on cholinesterase are less severe.
4. During the cholinergic phase (24 to 48 hours after intoxication) motor endplates will be "soaked" with acetylcholine. Use suxamethonium cautiously. Supranormal doses of nondepolarizers may be required. Therefore the potential for histamine release can worsen existing bronchoconstriction.
5. Paralysis of muscles of respiration, proximal limb muscles, neck flexors, and muscles innervated by cranial nerves. The muscle weakness is probably due to injury to motor endplates and muscle fibers. Such patients are likely to be sensitive to nondepolarizing muscle relaxants. Benzodiazepines may be useful in stabilizing patients who are being ventilated. The muscle weakness may last up to 21 days, but diaphragmatic paralysis lasting 150 days has been reported.[2]

ATROPINE

United States soldiers carry three atropine autoinjectors, each containing 2 mg of atropine citrate. These autoinjectors permit rapid intramuscular injection of antidote through protective clothing and underlying garments. Medical aidmen carry additional atropine autoinjectors and are trained to add more atropine as required based on the end points of good control of respiratory secretions and adequate respiratory effort. Heart rate and pupil size are not reliable indicators of adequate atropinization (see Pesticides, Plants, Antimuscarinics).[3] Atropine can be given as often as every 5 minutes until secretions are minimal and respiration is adequate. Some patients require 15 to 20 mg in the first 3 minutes after exposure.[4] Atropine inhibits sweating, which could lead to hyperthermia.

Assisted Ventilation

Used alone, atropine has little influence on the mortality rates in the potentially fatal apneic cases for which assisted ventilation is much more effective. The combination of adequate atropinization plus assisted ventilation is more effective in saving life than assisted ventilation alone.[5]

Symptoms Produced by the Antidote Atropine Without Nerve Gas Exposure[5]

First Dose

Administration of a single dose of 2 mg (1 automatic injector) of atropine to an individual who has absorbed minimal or no nerve agent produces mild symptoms, including dryness of the skin, mouth, and throat, with slight difficulty in swallowing. The individual may have a feeling of warmth, slight flushing, rapid pulse, some hesitancy of urination, and an occasional desire to belch. The pupils may be dilated slightly, but react to light. In some individuals there may be mild drowsiness and slowness of memory and ability to recall. They may have a feeling that their body movements are slowed and their near vision is blurred.

Second Dose

Administration of a second dose of 2 mg of atropine within an hour without nerve agent challenge will produce moderate central nervous system symptoms (drowsiness, fatigue, slowness of memory and ability to recall, feeling that body movements are slow, and blurring of near vision for up to 24 hours), but ordinary activity can continue with some loss of efficiency. Heat injury may develop if the individual is operating in a MOPP IV posture (protective clothing) with the ability to perspire diminished by atropine.

Third Dose

A third dose (2 mg atropine) administered within 1 hour without nerve agent challenge will result in marked symptoms and possibly total incapacity. Any further administration will result in overatropinization (dry mouth, swelling of tongue and oral mucous membranes, difficulty in swallowing, thirst, hoarseness, dry and flushed skin, dilated pupils, blurring of near vision, tachycardia, urinary retention, constipation, slowing of mental and physical activity, restlessness, headache, disorientation, hallucinations, depression, increased drowsiness, extreme fatigue, rapid panting respiration, and respiratory distress).

Duration of Effect

Atropine effects without nerve agent challenge last about 3 to 5 hours after 1 or 2 injections, and 12 to 24 hours after marked atropinization.

Hot Climates

In hot climates or in heat-stressed individuals, every 2 mg of atropine can reduce efficiency. Two doses, or 4 mg, can sharply reduce combat efficiency, and 6 mg will practically incapacitate an individual for several hours.

Assessing Need

Labored breathing, including coughing, noisy breathing, wheezing, and gasping for air, indicates the need for administration of additional atropine. When adequate atropine has been given, labored breathing efforts will be relieved.

Atropine With Nerve Agent Exposure

Patients with severe symptoms due to systemic absorption of a nerve agent have an increased tolerance for atropine. Multiple doses of atropine may be required before signs of atropinization appear such as a heart rate above 90 beats per minute, diminished bronchial secretions, and dry skin. In the presence of severe nerve agent poisoning, as much as 50 mg of atropine may be required in a 24-hour period. Limited experience with nerve agent casualties indicates that 10 to 20 mg cumulative doses of atropine in the first 2 or 3 hours usually provide an adequate control of symptoms.[3]

Mark I

The nerve agent antidote kit, Mark I, is used by the U.S. Army and the Air Force in the treatment of nerve agent poisoning. Each Mark I kit consists of four separate components: an atropine autoinjector with 2 mg (0.7 mL) of atropine in solution, a pralidoxime chloride autoinjector, a plastic clip, and a foam carrying case. The atropine and the 2-PAM-Cl solution freeze at about 30°F. United States soldiers carry three pralidoxime chloride autoinjectors, each containing 600 mg of the oxime, one to be administered along with each atropine autoinjector.[3] The U.S. Navy issues 3 atropine and 2 pralidoxime chloride autoinjectors per person.[5]

Effect of Atropine

Atropine will alleviate most of the muscarinic signs, little of the central nervous system symptoms, and almost none of the nicotinic symptoms. Apneic patients require assisted ventilation. Antidotes are not very helpful.

Dose

1. Give an initial dose of 2 mg IM or IV. If severe symptoms give 6 mg. Do not administer IV until ventilation is assured to reduce risks of ventricular fibrillation. Children's dose is 0.002 to 0.08 mg/kg.
2. If hypertensive—provide endotracheal intubation. Administer atropine endotracheally.
3. Repeat atropine every 5 to 10 minutes until secretions have decreased, the skin is dry, and ventilation is adequate. The total dose in the first several hours is usually less than 20 mg.

THE OXIMES (FIG. 59–4)

The 4-µg/mL goal

In 1961 Sundwall[6] induced severe bradycardia, hypotension, respiratory failure, and death in anesthetized cats by an intravenous dose of methylisopropoxyphosphoryl thiocholine. P2S (*N*-methylpyridinium-2-aldoxime methanesulfonate) administered intramuscularly (10 mg/kg) at the first appearance of symptoms reversed most toxic symptoms within 30 minutes. When the blood pressure, heart rate, and respiration were returned to normal, plasma levels of P2S were found to be above 4 µg/mL, specifically at levels of about 8 µg/mL in several experiments. Symptoms were not reversed at oxime plasma levels of 2 to 4 µg/mL. Atropine was not used. From this one study in cats, a substantive interpolation to man has been made during the succeeding 30 years, and the plasma oxime level goal of 4 µg/mL has become ensconced in the literature of oxime countermeasures against nerve agents. Replications of this animal data have not been published in the publicly accessible literature. The level of 4 µg/mL may not be applicable to all oximes against one inhibitor or to one oxime against different inhibitors.

The Proper Oxime

Subsequently, attempts were made to establish an oxime that would be acceptable for military and civilian use (Fig.

Trivial Name	Abbreviation or trade name	Chemical Name	Structure
Pralidoxime chloride	2-PAM-CI	Pyridine-2-aldoxime methyl chloride	CH-NOH, CH_3 CI
Pralidoxime methane sulfonate	P_2S	*N*-methyl-2-pyridiniumaldoxime methanesulfonate	CH-NOH, CH_3 CH_3SO_4
Obidoxime	Toxogonin	*bis*[(4-Hydroxyiminomethyl)-pyridine-1-methyl]-ether dichloride	NOH-HC–⬡–CH_2OCH_2–⬡–CH-NOH 2CI
Trimedoxime	TMB_4	*N,N*-Trimethylene bis(pyridium-4-aldoxime) dichloride (or dibromide)	NOH-HC–⬡–$(CH_3)_2$–⬡–CH-NOH 2CI

Figure 59–4 Older Oximes: Nomenclature and Abbreviations. (Adapted from Munro NB et al. Environ Health Perspect 1990;89:205–215.)

59–4). The 4-μg/mL goal was used as a basis for determining which intramuscular dose of an oxime would be theoretically of potential use, especially to the military.

Pralidoxime Chloride

Pralidoxime chloride (2-PAM-Cl) is currently the only oxime antidote approved by the U.S. Food and Drug Administration (FDA) for clinical use in organophosphate poisoning.

Formulations

Pralidoxime Chloride Tablets (USP). 500 pralidoxime chloride. Sterile Pralidoxime Chloride (USP) for parenteral use: 1 g pralidoxime chloride and 20-mL ampule of sterile water for injection. A 5% solution has a pH of 3.5 to 4.5.

P2S—Pralidoxime mesylate (Pralidoxime methanesulfonate) M.W. 232.3. is very soluble in water.

P2S injection. U.K. License Holder: Department of Health. 1 g of P2S in 5-mL ampules (to be diluted with 5 to 10 mL sterile water before IV use).

Storage

Pralidoxime chloride (Protopam, Ayerst) stored in sterile 1-g quantities has a shelf life of more than 5 years. PAM mesylate (P2S)—20% solution, kept in a refrigerator at 5°C, has a shelf life of over 5 years. The only degradation product is cyanide, usually present in insufficient amounts to be injurious.

Uses

Pralidoxime (PAM) appears to be useful in all types of organophosphate insecticide poisoning irrespective of the route of exposure.

Pralidoxime chloride (2-PAM-Cl) is used as an adjunct to atropine, and in this role, it may increase the effectiveness of therapy in the poisoning by some, but not all, nerve agents. 2-PAM-Cl may reduce the time during which assisted ventilation is required. It is administered to all symptomatic patients after a nerve gas exposure.

Dose—for Nerve Agents

Pralidoxime as the chloride (2-PAM-Cl) or mesylate (P2S), probably will best be administered in a dose of 30 mg/kg body weight over a 30-minute period every 4 to 6 hours, preferably by intravenous injection, but it can also be given by intramuscular injection. Oxime concentrations over 4 μg/mL can be maintained for 3 to 6 hours after IM injections of 30 mg/kg body weight of either oxime (chloride or mesylate). Alternatively 2-PAM (chloride or mesylate) can be given as a continuous infusion at a rate of 550 mg/hour (8 mg/kg/hour) after the injection of 30 mg/kg/body weight on two occasions 4 hours apart.[7] PAM should be continued as long as the OP compound or its active metabolite is present in the body.

Other Suggested Doses

Mild Symptoms

At least one 600-mg IM injection of 2-PAM-Cl.

Moderate Symptoms

One or more 600-mg IV injections of 2-PAM-Cl.

Severe Symptoms

Three 600-mg IM injections of 2-PAMCl. Repeat the dose every hour if respiration has not improved. Not much more oxime benefit is usually obtained after 3 injections of 2-PAM-Cl.[5]

Induction of a positive charge on the oxime molecules appears to enhance their reactivating capacity. Pyridine 2- and 4-aldoximine methiodides are about one million times more active than the simple aldoximes.[8] Pralidoxime has modest effect on tabun poisoning in animals studies. Further study has resulted in the development of the bispyridinium dioximes, TMB-4 (Trimedoxime) and obidoxime (Toxogonin). Both appear effective in tabun poisoning in animals.[9,10]

Obidoxime

Structure and Classification

Obidoxime (Toxogonin) consists of two pyridinium rings linked by an oxygen molecule. It is about twice the size and weight of pralidoxime chloride.[11]

Table 59–8
Diagnosis, Classification and Treatment of Adult Nerve Gas Casualties[a]

Severity	Signs	Pharmacologic Treatment[b]		Supportive Treatment
		Atropine[c]	Toxogonine	
Light—casualty able to walk	Lacrimation, salivation, nasal discharge, miosis, blurring of vision, stenocardia, sweating, nausea, vomiting, abdominal pain	2 mg i.m. every 20 min until atropinization is achieved (at least 24 hr)[d]	250 mg i.m. every 2 hr totalling 2 doses (750 mg)	Follow-up
Moderate—casualty unable to walk but breathing spontaneously	In addition to the above: dyspnea, wheezing, tremor, diarrhea, urinary frequency, incontinence, coma	Start with autoinjector followed by 2 mg i.v. every 5 min until atropinization is achieved (at least 48 hr)[d]	Slow i.v. injection of 250 mg every 2 hr totalling 3 doses (750 mg); 5 additional identical doses may be given on physician's order	I.v. valium by physician's order, airway for comatose patients, suction of pulmonary secretions
Severe—casualty not breathing	In addition to the above: respiratory failure, epileptic seizures, flaccid paralysis	Same as for moderate casuality	Same as for moderate casuality	In addition to the above: artificial ventilation

[a]Adapted from Shapira Y et al. Isr J Med Sci 1991;27:616–622.
[b]Scopolamine, 0.25 mg may be administered parenterally to patients between the ages of 10 and 60 years.
[c]For patients aged >60 yr 1 mg instead of 2 mg.
[d]Signs of atropinization are dry and hot skin, and dry mucosal membranes.

Use

Obidoxime (N,N'-oxidimethylene [pyridinium-4-aldoxime] dichloride) is claimed (on the basis of in vitro studies) to be about 20 times more effective than pralidoxime in reactivating phosphorylated cholinesterase and to be capable of penetrating the blood-brain barrier.[12] In cases of organophosphate poisoning in man it appears to be about as effective as pyridinium 2-aldoxime methylchloride (2-PAM-Cl). After intramuscular injection the doses necessary to produce plasma levels above 5 μg/mL are about one-third that of 2-PAM-Cl. To obtain a plasma level of 4 μg/ml of the oxime, 250 mg IM of obidoxime is required. A second injection may be administered in 2 hours. To maintain a level of 4 μg/ml, an intravenous infusion of about 35 mg/hour may be required. Use of obidoxime (Toxigonine) by Israel during the Gulf War is summarized in Table 59–8.[13]

TOXICOKINETICS OF THE OXIMES—ABSORPTION

Oral

Pralidoxime

Oral doses of P2S (pralidoxime mesylate) (6 to 8 g) reach plasma levels of 4 μg/mL in about 20 minutes and can remain at those levels for up to 5 hours.[14] Oral 2-PAM-Cl (pralidoxime mesylate) administered as a 2-g dose reaches 4 μg/mL in about 1 hour and remains for about 4 hours.[15] An oral dose of 3 g of 2-PAM-Cl will exceed plasma levels of 5 μg/mL in about 2 hours[15] and remain for about 2 hours. Similar to P2S, a dose of 6 g of 2-PAM-Cl orally will exceed plasma levels of 6 μg/mL within ½ hour and remain at those levels for 4 hours.[16] Oral doses of the oximes would appear to be relatively slow for use in emergency situations, either military or civilian.

Obidoxime

After oral ingestion of 1 g of obidoxime, plasma concentrations of about 1 μg/mL are obtained in 1 to 2 hours. After an oral dose of 3 g, numbness of the lips and a "dry mouth" may be observed. Plasma levels of 4 μg/mL or more are reached with doses of 7 g and above, levels at which subjects often note tightness in the cheeks, faces that feel numb, a menthol taste, and coolness in the throat.[17,18]

Intramuscular (IM)

Pralidoxime Chloride

Following intramuscular doses of 30 mg/kg (of 2-PAM-Cl) plasma concentrations of 14 to 15 μg/mL are reached within 20 to 30 minutes.[15] After 7.5 to 10 mg/kg doses IM, concentrations of 4 μg/mL are reached in 5 to 10 minutes.[19,20] Blood levels over 4 μg/mL may be sustained for between 4 to 8 hours.

Pralidoxime Mesylate (P2S)

Intramuscular administration in man of 30 mg/kg body weight of P2S induces peak plasma concentrations averaging 15 μg/mL after 20 minutes. After 90 minutes concentrations are 9 μg/mL. Therapeutic plasma levels are reached in 5 to 10 minutes.[21] If these results are generally valid in man, IM injections of 20 to 30 mg P2S/kg body weight should yield therapeutic plasma concentrations after 5 to 10 minutes. P2S is effective against the neuromuscular block in animals produced by sarin, but much less effective against the block produced by tabun (dimethylamidoethoxyphosphoryl cyanide) (methyliso-propoxyphosphoryl fluoride).[6]

Intravenous Use

Pralidoxime Chloride

2-PAM-Cl IV at a dose of 35 mg/kg leads to a plasma level of 17.6 μg/mL within 30 minutes; such levels are sustained for 6 to 8 hours. At an IV dose of 45 mg/kg of P2S, oxime plasma levels of 18.7 μg/mL are attained within 30 minutes, remaining for 4 to 5 hours at about 4 μg/mL.[15]

IV Continuous Infusion

Two 30-mg/kg-bolus doses 4 hours apart may be required to cover the period before satisfactory PAM concentrations are achieved by an infusion.

Titration of Dose Method—Dose Calculations[22]

Titration of the intravenous dose of 2-PAM-Cl may be effective in patients who have breakthrough nicotinic symptoms (muscle fasciculations) secondary to OP poisoning while on IV bolus therapy. A 23-year-old healthy male arrived at the Emergency Department after ingesting several ounces of an unknown organophosphate insecticide. The patient was positive for a SLUD syndrome (salivation, lacrimation, urination, diarrhea). Pupils were 2 mm, pulse 135 beats/minute; blood pressure 150/110 mm Hg. The patient complained of being extremely weak, unable to walk, and confused. He received 2.0 mg atropine and 1 gram of 2-PAM-Cl intravenously, and gastrointestinal decontamination procedures were begun. His nicotinic symptoms appeared to abate, but muscle fasciculations were observed almost 2½ hours after the medications were administered. The medical staff considered a continuous infusion of pralidoxime, but were unsure what dose was required or for how long. The patient weighed 175 pounds. Suggested calculations were offered:

A. Concentration: Calculate the minimum effective concentration (MEC) of pralidoxime

$$\frac{\text{Loading dose (mg)}}{\text{Weight of patient (kg)}} \times \frac{1}{\text{Time break (reappearance of signs)}} \times 0.8\ (V_D) = \text{MEC}$$

Example

$$\frac{1000\text{ mg}}{79.5\text{ kg}} \times \frac{1}{2.5\text{ hours}} \times 0.8 = 4.03\text{ mcg/mL}$$

B. Infusion Rate (10% above MEC)

$$\frac{1.1\ (10\%\text{ factor}) \times \text{MEC} \times \text{clearance (mL/min)} \times 60\text{ minutes}}{1000}$$

$\text{MEC} \times 754 \times 0.06 =$

$\text{MEC} \times 50 = \text{R}$ (infusion rate of pralidoxime in mg/hr)

$4.03 \times 50 = 200$ mg/hr.

Prepare IV solution by adding 4 grams of pralidoxime to 500 mL normal saline solution; 200 mg/hr can be delivered at a rate of 25 mL/hr.

Cautions

1. Use for all symptomatic patients after a nerve gas exposure.
2. If severely dyspneic, give 4 to 6 mg atropine plus 2-PAM-Cl 1 g IV. Watch heart rate, blood pressure.
3. If moderate exposure to vapor (respiratory distress, gastrointestinal signs and symptoms, muscle twitching) give 6 mg atropine and 2-PAM-Cl. Always give diazepam (10 mg IM).
4. Seizures often respond to atropine and 2-PAM-Cl. If they do not, give diazepam (5 to 10 mg IV over 3 to 5 minutes in adults; 0.24 to 0.4 mg/kg IV (up to 10 mg) over 2 to 3 minutes in children. Watch for worsening of respiratory depression (after diazepam is used) caused by nerve agents.

Observe for recurrence of nicotinic symptoms. If they do not recur in the next 24 hours, discontinue therapy. If they recur, record time of breakthrough and estimate level of pralidoxime (MEC = minimum effective concentration) in patient at that moment. Reload immediately with 1 g of pralidoxime when breakthrough symptoms occur. Give a continuous IV infusion of pralidoxime to maintain a level approximately 10% above the estimated MEC. Weaning the patient off should be performed by set increments (e.g., 25% every 8 hours). Watch the patient for at least 1 hour after each adjustment. These guidelines may not be applicable to fat-soluble OP pesticides; they may be affected by organophosphate agent properties such as "aging," redistribution, and delayed absorption; the patient may alter the toxicokinetics of pralidoxime (renal function, serum pH); interactions with atropine effect must be considered.[22]

Doses—For Organophosphate Insecticide Poisoning—Other Methods

The usual adult dose of pralidoxime consists of 1 to 2 g for a 70-kg person (14 to 28 mg/kg) IV in 100 to 150 mL of saline given slowly over 15 to 30 minutes. A suggested initial dose for children is 15 to 25 mg/kg.[1] Sidell recommends an initial dose of 15 mg/kg for infants.

Children's Dose

Seven children were poisoned with OP insecticides and received a loading dose of 2-PAM-Cl: 15 to 50 mg/kg in 0.9% saline to yield a blood concentration of 10 to 20 mg/mL, given IV over a 30-minute period. A maintenance IV infusion of 9 to 19 mg/kg/hr was then administered. Using the toxicokinetics of 2-PAM-Cl ($T_{1/2}$ 1.14 hours; V_D 0.73 L/kg) a continuous infusion of 18 mg/kg/hr would lead to a steady-state 2-PAM serum concentration of about (as V_D) 40 μg/mL. Therefore in children a continuous infusion of 10 to 20 mg/kg/hr should provide >4-μg/mL levels.

This data suggests initiation of treatment with 25 mg/kg IV 2-PAM-Cl dose for 15 to 30 minutes and then continuous infusion of 10 to 20 mg/kg/hr. Continue for 18 hours or longer depending on the patient's clinical status and the properties of the suspected toxin.[23]

Obidoxime (Toxogonin)

In the 1950s certain nucleophiles (e.g., hydroxylamine, hydroxamine acids, and oximes) were reported capable of reactivating inhibited cholinesterase.

Plasma concentrations of 2-PAM-Cl above 4 μg/mL are elevated above controls in organophosphate-poisoned human volunteers. The maximum concentration of 2-PAM-Cl after a single IM dose of 1000 mg/3 mL is 9.9 μg/mL in patients and 7.5 μg/mL in controls and was reached in 33 to 34 minutes in both groups. The elimination half-life in patients was 174.4 minutes and in controls 148.9 minutes. Total clearance was 5.5 mL/min/kg in patients and 9.1 mL/min/kg in controls. Urinary recovery of unchanged oxime was 62.6% in patients and 80.2% in controls. The apparent volume of distribution was the same in both groups (2.8 and 2.7 L/kg). Monitoring of the plasma oxime levels, especially those with higher toxicity (e.g., trimedoxime and obidoxime), is suggested to minimize the risk of overdosing the patient.[24, 25]

Therapeutic PAM doses

IM or IV PAM or P2S: either 30 mg/kg or 8 mg/kg/hour (550 mg/hour) will produce what are considered acceptably useful oxime concentrations, but both dose regimens will require an IV bolus of PAM 30 mg/kg 4 hours apart to induce plasma levels over 4 μg/mL.[26]

P2S

Following an intravenous injection of 20 mg/kg body weight of P2S in man, plasma levels of 50 μg/mL may be reached. At these concentrations dizziness, blurred vision, and diplopia are noted, but they vanish in a few minutes. Plasma levels of P2S above 4 μg/mL (usually 8 to 12 μg/mL) were sufficient to counteract neuromuscular block, bradycardia, hypotension, and respiratory failure in the anesthetized cat.[6]

DISTRIBUTION

Pralidoxime

Pralidoxime is widely distributed in most body fluids and is not highly bound to plasma proteins. The volumes of distribution (in L/kg) of the oxime after intravenous administration are as follows[14]:

	V_1 (central compartment)	V_2 (peripheral compartment)	V_{ss} (steady state)
2-PAM-Cl	0.27	0.54	0.82
P2S	0.20	0.58	0.78

Obidoxime

The apparent volume of distribution of obidoxime is 0.173 L/kg.[14]

ELIMINATION

Pralidoxime

Pralidoxime is rapidly excreted in the urine. About 90% of 2-PAM-Cl and 87.1% of P2S are excreted unchanged following an intravenous dose of 5 mg/kg.[18] The oral elimination half-life of P2S is about 94 minutes[14]; the oral elimination half-life of 2-PAM-Cl is about 160 minutes[16] after doses of 2 to 9 g (2.9 to 128 mg/kg). The IM half-life of 2-PAM-Cl after 2.5 to 10 mg/kg IM is about 77 minutes.[15] The IV half-life of P2S is about 84 minutes; that of 2-PAM-Cl is 78 minutes.[14]

Obidoxime

About 2.2% of an oral dose is excreted in the urine over 24 hours. The elimination half-life of obidoxime after oral use is 2.64 hours.[17] After intravenous use 68% of a dose is recovered in the urine. The elimination half-life of obidoxime after IV use is 1.20 hours.[19]

INTERACTIONS

Sodium Bicarbonate—Thiamine

The total clearance is depressed when 2-PAM-Cl is given with thiamine. Thiamine chloride does not appear to increase the protective efficacy of 2-PAM-Cl.[24] Alkalinization with sodium bicarbonate appears to augment the protective efficacy of 2-PAM-Cl.[24] Pralidoxime is more likely to be excreted in an acid urine.

Pregnancy/Lactation

The safety of PAM in pregnancy and in lactation has not been established.

Aging[3]

Most nerve agent exposure (GA-tabun; GB-sarin, VX) can be effectively treated with oximes such as pralidoxime for hours after exposure (GB—5 to 6 hours, VX—48 hours), but GD-soman becomes refractory to the oximes within a few minutes. In other words GD has undergone rapid "aging." After aging has occurred, oxime therapy is ineffective. Aging of the agent-bound enzyme may result from loss of an alkyl or alkoxy group from the nerve agent moiety. The remaining enzyme-modified nerve agent complex is more stable and resistant to reactivation by oximes or similar antidotes (Table 59–9).

Table 59–9
Aging[a]

Agents	Aging Half-Life
Tabun	46 hours
Sarin	5.2–12 hours
VX	>12 days
Soman	40 sec–10 minutes
Paraxon	2.1–5.4 days

[a]Adapted from Dunn MA, Sidell RF. JAMA 1989;262:649–652.

MECHANISM OF ACTION

Like other related compounds, pralidoxime contains an oxime group RCHNOH (Fig. 59–2) that dissociates the nerve agent moiety from the acetylcholinesterase molecule, reactivating the enzyme and gradually restoring normal skeletal muscle function. Pralidoxime itself has little or no apparent central nervous system effects, because it does not appear to cross the blood-brain barrier easily. Most oximes act largely at nicotinic receptor sites to normalize skeletal muscle activity, but they have little activity at muscarinic sites. However, they may greatly enhance the effects of atropine at muscarinic sites.[4]

Pralidoxime in Summary

1. Counters the inhibited AChE.
2. Exhibits hydrolytic power against the active inhibitor.
3. Has a weak, direct, anticholinesterase effect.

Its main effect remains the reversal of cholinergic effects at peripheral nicotinic sites. Pralidoxime is probably inactive against an "aged" enzyme, but given "late" it may still be effective. No oxime appears able to prevent the development of OP-induced delayed neuropathy. 2-PAM-Cl, alone or with atropine, appears to reduce mortality following poisoning with OP insecticides.

TOXICITY

Pralidoxime

Following rapid parenteral infusions of higher doses (over 10 mg/kg) of the oximes (2-PAM-Cl, P2S) pain at the site of injection, nausea, vomiting, diarrhea, headaches, dizziness, tachycardia, rise in blood pressure, nervousness, malaise, and blurred vision may be experienced. At doses of 30 to 45 mg/kg intravenously P2S results in a marked increase in both systolic and diastolic pressure. This may be accompanied by an increase in the amplitude of T-waves and an increase in the PR interval on electrocardiographic tracings.[15] At higher than therapeutic doses pralidoxime may inhibit acetylcholinesterase and block neuromuscular transmission.[1] Oral use of 8 to 9 g of 2-PAM-Cl may induce diarrhea, anorexia, and malaise.[16] Sudden cardiac arrest was observed 2 minutes after starting 2-PAM iodide IV.[27]

Obidoxime

Obidoxime intramuscular injections are often followed by pain at the site and a symptom complex consisting of a generalized "hot feeling" over the upper part of the body within several minutes after injection. At 5 to 15 minutes this becomes localized to the face, with a feeling of "tightness" or "numbness" of the circumoral area. A hot feeling around the throat with a menthol taste is observed within 1 to 3 minutes after injection. All symptoms appear to subside within 1 to 2 hours.[19]

A 50-year-old man admitted in deep coma with miosis, hypersalivation, muscle twitching, bronchial rales, acute respiratory failure, and low serum pseudocholinesterase values did not respond to atropine alone, but improved after IV obidoxime was instituted. Obidoxime was given in a dose of 1800 mg over 5 days and atropine in a dose of 600 mg over 14 days. On the 5th day therapy-resistant ventricular arrhythmias and transient cholestatic icterus occurred, which resolved after discontinuation of obidoxime.[28]

Problems With Obidoxime

Obidoxime preparations must have a pH of 2 to 4 to attain stability. After a few months obidoxime solutions turn yellow. The acid solutions may cause the oxime moiety to split off one molecule of water to form the cyanide; a carboxamide, a carboxylic acid, and 4-pyridones may also be formed.[29]

HUMAN NERVE AGENT EXPOSURES

Published exposures of nerve agents in man are restricted to one prospective exposure study with VX and sarin[30] and to case reports of treatment of accidental exposure of one patient to soman, and one patient to sarin and of three patients exposed to sarin who developed some signs and symptoms, but required no therapy.

VX Administration

Oral4.0 µg/kg

A few symptoms (diarrhea, transient nausea) were noted within 3 to 4 hours. The RBC cholinesterase was depressed to 70% below normal values. Spontaneous recovery occurred in some subjects within 24 to 48 hours. 2-PAM-Cl IV 5 to 30 mg/kg was administered at 5 to 48 hours after VX. All subjects exhibited reactivation of 70% of the inhibited enzyme. Aging: Slow (over 24 to 48 hours).

Intravenous 1.5 µg/kg

Most subjects experienced some lightheadedness and dizziness; some had nausea and vomiting within 1 hour. An increase in heart rate and blood pressure was observed at 3 hours. RBC ChE was depressed to about 20% of normal in subjects with symptoms and to 28% of normal in asymptomatic subjects. Spontaneous recovery of RBC-ChE was observed at 1% per hour over 70 hours. 2-PAM-Cl IV 2.5 to 25 mg/kg administered at 0.5 to 24 hr after VX resulted in reactivation of 70% of the inhibited enzyme. Aging: slow (over 24 to 48 hours).

Soman Exposure

Age: 33 M. Dose: Soman 25%—1 mL. Splashed into and around mouth. Signs and symptoms: Comatose, labored respirations, miosis, injected conjunctivae, oral and nasal secretions, trismus, nucheal rigidity, muscular fasciculations, hyperactive deep tendon reflexes, and tachycardia. Treatment: Atropine (20 mg over a 2-day period); pralidoxime chloride (2-PAM-Cl) 2 mg over 30 minutes in an IV infusion; oxygen; nasopharyngeal suction, prochlorperazine for nausea. No detectable RBC-ChE was observed for 10 days. The patient recovered in about 1 week after a period

Table 59–10
Chemical Agents and Biological/Physical Characteristics Relevant to Their Toxic Activity [a]

Chemical Agent/ CAS No.	Chemical Name	Mode of Action	Special Characteristics	
			Short-Term Toxic Effects	Long-Term Toxic Effects
GA (tabun)/77-81-6	*N,N*-dimethyl phosphoroamidocyanidate, ethyl ester	Anticholinesterase	Less volatile and more persistent than GB Less toxic than GB by vapor inhalation; equally toxic by skin absorption (liquid) More effective than GB in producing miosis GB is 2–4 times as effective in terms of incapacitating dose	No information; Army has studies planned
GB (sarin)/107-44-8	Methylphosphonofluoridate isopropyl ester	Anticholinesterase	Volatile, therefore poses less of a threat by absorption through the skin either as aerosol or liquid than it does by inhalation About half as toxic as VX by inhalation Less effective than GA or VX in inducing miosis	Some information at present; studies in progress Low-dose study did not show carcinogenic activity Teratogenicity study results were negative; other reproductive parameters were unaffected Potential for a delayed neuropathy syndrome, at supralethal doses, if protection from short-term lethality is achieved with drug therapy Changes in electroencephalographic recordings after short-term exposure; consequences unknown
VX/50782-69-9	*S*-(diisopropylaminoethyl) methylphosphonothiolate o-ethyl ester	Anticholinesterase	Less volatile than G agents; very effective through skin penetration; persistent Many times as toxic in man as GB via skin absorption Head and neck areas of man are very sensitive Effective percutaneous lethal dose decreases with increasing windspeed Contaminated vegetation can cause toxic effects on ingestion VX is approximately 25 times more potent than GB in inducing miosis	Mutagenicity study results were negative Teratogenicity study results were negative; other reproductive studies in progress No delayed neuropathy induction Carcinogenic activity unknown
H/HD (mustard gas, sulfur mustard)/ 505-60-2	*Bis* (2-chloroethyl) sulfide	Blister agent	Low volatility; very persistent on earth and solid surfaces Produces skin blisters and damage to eyes and respiratory tract Toxic effects are delayed (latent period); therefore, exposed personnel do not seek immediate treatment Secondary infections of damaged tissue can occur easily Eye is most sensitive organ; instant removal of agent is required to prevent damage High doses can induce acute systemic reactions and injury to the immune system	Carcinogenic under appropriate conditions of exposure Potential increased risk of chronic bronchitis Mutagenic in a variety of test systems Teratogenicity study results were negative; one dominant lethal mutagenic study had positive results, others are in progress Potential for permanent impairment of vision if eye damage is severe Skin lesions may show permanent changes in pigmentation and be hypersensitive to mechanical injury

[a] Adapted from Carnes SA, Watson AP. JAMA 1989;262:653–659.

Table 59–10 *(Continued)*

Chemical Agent/ CAS No.	Chemical Name	Mode of Action	Special Characteristics: Short-Term Toxic Effects	Special Characteristics: Long-Term Toxic Effects
HT T/63918-89-8	60% HD and 40% T *Bis*[2(2-chloro-ethylthio)ethyl] ether	Blister agent	Very persistent on terrain Less volatile and more stable than HD More toxicologically active than HD 1% lethality dosage is half that of HD HT is more toxicologically active than HD for skin-blister development and inhalation lethality Eye is most sensitive; exposures can result in permanent eye damage	Probably carcinogenic and mutagenic due to presence of HD T is strongly mutagenic No experimental information on HT is available
L (lewisite)541-25-3	Dichloro(2-chlorovinyl) arsine	Blister agent	Intermediate persistency in soils Much greater volatility than HD; hence, it is an irritant over great distances Skin burns are more corrosive than those from HD Similar to HD on inhalation Eye very sensitive; permanent blindness may result if not decontaminated in 1 min A systemic poison when absorbed by tissue (liver and kidneys) Immediate severe pain on contact with skin or eyes	Mutagenicity experiment results were negative; other experiments planned Possible carcinogenic properties Teratogenic potential suspected Teratogenicity and reproductive toxicity studies planned

of psychologic instability (treated with scopolamine 1.2 mg orally).

Sarin Administration (Table 59–10)[31,32]

Intravenous 2 μg/kg

No subject experienced symptoms. RBC-ChE was depressed to 28% of control values. No spontaneous recovery was seen. 2-PAM-Cl 2.5 to 25 mg/kg was administered at 1 to 5 hours after sarin, resulting in reactivation of approximately 40% of the RBC-ChE. Aging: Rapid: 5 to 6 hours.

SARIN[33–35]

In March, 1995, six people were killed and about 600 injured when poison fumes believed to be Sarin overwhelmed rush-hour subway commuters in Tokyo. Passengers began coughing and complaining of headaches, diminished vision, and nausea. Several collapsed onto the floor. As trains pulled into stations, passengers staggered out onto the platforms and collapsed with bubbles coming from their mouths. In some cases blood poured from their noses.

A similar but more minor incident was reported on a subway in Yokohama where 11 passengers were hospitalized after they complained of dizziness and eye pain. In June, 1994, seven people died in a mysterious case of gas poisoning in Matsumoto, Japan. Sarin was also blamed for that outbreak. The method of gassing was unclear.

A presumed terrorist attack with sarin occurred in a residential area of the city of Matsumoto, Japan, on June 27, 1994. About 600 residents and rescue staff were poisoned; 58 were admitted to hospitals and seven died. Laboratory findings for the severely poisoned people were decreases in serum cholinesterase, red blood cell acetylcholinesterase erythrocytes, serum triglycerides, serum potassium, and chloride and increases in serum creatine kinase, leukocytes, and ketones in urine. Examination revealed no persisting abnormal physical findings in any individual. Acetylcholinesterase returned to normal within 3 months in all people examined. Although subclinical miosis and neuropathy were present 30 days after exposure, almost all symptoms of sarin exposure disappeared rapidly and left no sequelae in most people.[36]

Sarin Exposure—Case Reports[30,37]

Age: 52 yr. M. Signs and symptoms: Cyanotic, convulsing, labored respirations, miosis, muscle fasciculations, marked salivation, and rhinorrhea. Treatment: Atropine (14 mg in 1 day); pralidoxime chloride (2 mg in 150 ml normal saline IV) given three times over the first 2 hours; oxygen; assisted ventilation; nasogastric suction. The patient recovered within several days after a period of emotional lability, but died of an acute myocardial infarction 18 months later. Three adults experienced a sudden onset of rhinorrhea and slight respiratory discomfort, miosis, eye pain, increase in salivation, and scattered wheezes and rhonchi. Symptoms were mild, no treatment was given, and the RBC-ChE (lowest values 20 to 40% of normal) spontaneously recovered in 20 (plasma ChE) to 90 days (RBC-ChE).

Sarin—Inhalation

Two adults accidentally exposed to sarin vapors (0.09 mg/m^3) exhibited red cell cholinesterase levels of 19% and 84%, respectively, and developed fixed extremely miotic pupils.[38] No other signs or symptoms developed, and neither man required treatment. Recovery to normal cholinesterase activity was gradual over a 90-day period. Pupillary reflexes were not detectable 11 days after exposure. The miotic pupils dilated slowly over a 30- to 45-day period.[39] Inhibition of red cell cholinesterase activity appear to be directly related to the dose of sarin. After exposure to sarin at a concentration of 2.73 mg/m^3) for 2 minutes, one of two subjects manifested a 23% red cell cholinesterase inhibition. Pupillary contraction remained constant for 24 hours.[40] Workers exposed to sarin three or more times within the previous 6 years developed long-term brain abnormalities reflected in the electroencephalogram.[41–43]

Sarin—Oral

Oral administration of sarin in doses of 0.030 to 1.76 mg (0.0005 to 0.022 mg/kg) resulted in reduction of plasma cholinesterase and red cell cholinesterase of 69 and 72%, respectively. A single dose of 0.022 mg/kg produced mild symptoms. Symptoms began 20 to 60 minutes after oral sarin administration and lasted up to 24 hours.

TREATMENT—SUMMARY

The treatment of nerve gas exposure has developed based on one initial animal study[6] and, in the case of pretreatment with pyridostigmine for soman exposure (see Pyridostigmine), on a paucity of clinical data in man. Military and clinical recommendations for use of the oximes (both monopyridinium and bipyridinium) are, of necessity, also based on limited clinical data. The theoretical oxime plasma value of 4 µg/mL derived from one animal study has itself not been subject to a clinical test.

The Oximes

Gallagher, Kearney, and Mangione[22] have provided a treatment rationale for organophosphate poisoning based, not on a specific plasma oxime level of presumed efficacy, but on the titration of each patient with an oxime according to the nicotinic signs demonstrated by that patient. The military, faced with its need to use an intramuscular oxime preparation in the field, is constrained to treat according to the pharmacokinetics of oximes and not by the meager clinical experiences that have been accumulated with each nerve gas.

For these purposes, and with these limitations, the guidelines provided by Vale[44] seem at present to be a rational approach: PAM chloride or mesylate should be administered via a dose of 30 mg/kg body weight every 4 to 6 hours, preferably by intravenous injection. The oxime may also be given by intramuscular injection. Alternatively, PAM chloride or mesylate can be given as a continuous infusion at a rate of 550 mg/hr (8 mg/kg/hr) after the injection of PAM 30 mg/kg body weight on two occasions 4 hours apart.

Obidoxime (toxogonin), although recommended by some governments as a preferred oxime, may be hepatotoxic,[45] may be less effective alone against soman, and is associated with some minor side effects that could render it a problem in military use. Trimedoxime must be stored frozen,[46] may cause hypotension,[15] and is more toxic than most oximes,[47] all obvious problems to the military. The Hagedorn oximes (HI-6, etc.) appear to have a short half-life in aqueous solution at room temperature[48] and to exhibit some stability problems, although oral tablets have shown some possible promise in man.[49]

HLo7 (1-[4-aminocarbonyl]-pyridinio[methoxy]methyl)-2,4-*bis)* (hydroxyaminomethyl)pyridinium diiodide has shown some potential to reactivate tabun- and soman-inhibited acetylcholinesterase. However, supralethal, soman poisoning treated with HLo7 or atropine alone is insufficient, and the combination of these two compounds may be required to improve respiration.[50] In any case, atropine, in all animal experiments and in limited clinical exposures, has been a necessary therapeutic concomitant.

Based almost entirely on animal data, the following table (Table 59–11) attempts to summarize the usefulness of the oximes in nerve gas poisoning.[51]

In most cases of nerve agent exposure, even with consideration of some newer developments (see New Developments), symptomatic and supportive treatment will be critical when used with pyridostigmine pretreatment (for anticipated soman exposure), atropine, oximes, and diazepam.

Supportive Treatment[45]

A. Removal of the Toxic Compound
   1. Percutaneous Exposure: Remove clothes, wash skin with soap and water. Nerve agents are inactivated by alkalis and hypochlorite solutions, including household bleach. At field medical units a 0.5% solution of

Table 59–11
Oximes in Nerve Gas Exposure[a]

	Pralidoxime	Obidoxime	Trimedoxime	HI-6
Tabun	0	+	++	0
Sarin	+	++	++	++
Soman	0	0		+
Vx	+	+	+	+

[a]Adapted from Bismuth C et al. Proc Eur Assoc Pois Cont Center, 1988, p. 7

Table 59–12
Decontamination Materials[53,84]

Agent	Materials Used
Nerve agents	Remove contaminated clothing
Tabun	Soap and water
Soman	0.5% hypochlorite
Sarin	(1 part household bleach, 9 parts water)
VX	Ammonia
	DS2—2% sodium hydroxide
	M258A1 kit (DECON1, DECON2 wipes)
Mustard and nitrogen mustard	For liquid contamination of eyes, initially irrigate with copious amounts of water; at treatment medical facility use saline eyewash. Remove contaminated clothing. 0.5% hypochlorite solution.
Lewisite and other arsenical vesicants	Like mustards
Mustard and lewisite combinations	Like mustards
Phosgene	Remove from source
Phosgene oxime	Wash with copious amounts of water for isotonic sodium bicarbonate. Fresh air
Vomiting agents	Caustic soda, alkali solutions, DS2
Tear agents	Wash eyes with copious amounts of water; remove from source.
Incapacitating agents	For contamination of skin wash with soap and water.

calcium hypochlorite has been used for removing nerve agent from the skin of some casualties.[52]

a. Responders should protect themselves from contamination (protective mask, wearing rubber gloves, heavy rubber apron, or encapsulation).
b. Move victim from the contaminated site.
c. Start to decontaminate.
d. Administer antidote.
e. If patient is unconscious—follow ABCs of resuscitation.
f. If respiratory distress—oxygen, endotracheal intubation, assisted ventilation, frequent airway suctioning, positive end-expiratory pressure for severely hypoxic patients; improve tissue oxygenation before atropine is begun to lessen risk of ventricular fibrillation. If respiratory distress or other signs of severe exposure—begin advanced life support, including IV line placement.

2. Oral Ingestion: Cathartic, then 30 g activated charcoal. In 3 hours lavage, remove charcoal, and replace. Repeat as long as lavage fluid contains the agent. May be in lavage for over 4 days.
3. Extracorporeal Detoxification: If V_D high, not likely to be useful. Little data.

B. Decontamination (Tables 59–12 through 59–14)

Frederick R. Sidell of the U.S. Army Medical Research Institute of Chemical Defense at the Aberdeen Proving Ground in Maryland has led much of the basic and clinical research on the development of oximes as antidote against nerve agents and on the preparation of the military and civilian community for defense against chemical warfare agents, especially nerve agents. He has

Table 59–13
Military Decontamination of Nerve Agents[a]

M258A1 Kit
Each kit contains DECON-1 AND DECON-2 packets.
DECON-1
Pad prewetted with hydroxyethane 72%, phenol 10%, sodium hydroxide 5%, and ammonia 2%, and water.
DECON-2
Pad impregnated with chloramine B and sealed glass ampules filled with hydroxyethane 45%, zinc chloride 5%, and the remainder water.
Both DECON-1 and DECON-2 contain poisonous and caustic ingredients and can permanently damage the eyes. The pads must be kept out of the eyes, mouth, and open wounds.

[a]Adapted from Munro NB et al. Environ Health Perspect 1990;89:205–215.

Table 59–14
Other Decontamination Agents Available to the Military[a]

Supertropical bleach
70% diethylenetriamine pentaacetic acid, 28% ethylene glycol monoethyl ether, and 2% sodium hydroxide (DS_2)
High-test bleach
Skin irritant decontaminator
Caustic soda
Washing soda (sodium carbonate)
Monoethanolamine
Degreasing solvents
Soap and water provide adequate initial decontamination for most of the chemical warfare agents.

[a]Adapted from Barr SJ. Top Emerg Med 1985;7:62–70.

summarized some of his findings in Table 59–15.[53] Odors of chemical warfare agents are characterized in Table 59–16.

Community Emergency Response[1,53,54]

Full-scale emergency response requires (a) *localization* of the source of an agent; (b) *identification* of a chemical warfare agent (tank truck, burning warehouse, unidentified shell fragments); (c) *isolation* of the agent by a trained response team that prevents access to the area and limits spread of the agent; (d) *neutralization* (decontaminating compound, or thorough flushing with water, depending on the agent); *evacuation*—preparation of a "hot line," a clearly demarcated line—those on one side are considered "dirty" (contaminated) and those on the other are considered "clean." The line is upwind from the accident; the medical first-aid facility is further upwind. Anyone crossing the "hot line" into the "dirty" area must wear protective clothing and must undergo decontamination before returning to the "clean" area. Anyone in the "dirty" area at the time of an accident should be decontaminated before passing to the "clean" area.

Decontamination should be performed ideally by trained and protected emergency personnel, taking the utmost care to avoid self-contamination.[1]

1. Done outside at the "hot line."
2. Removal of all clothing (in winter may cause hypothermia). Any item removed from the patient should be maintained in the "dirty" area until it can

Table 59–15
Chemical Weapons, Their Effects, and Treatment for Exposure to Them[a]

Agent	Toxicity	Signs and Symptoms	Antidote	Care
Riot control agents (tear gas) CN (Mace) CS	Rarely life-threatening	Nose and eye irritation, coughing, mild dyspnea Large dose: retching, burns	None	Symptomatic treatment
Blister agents Nitrogen mustard Sulfur mustard	Delayed effects; large dose life-threatening if untreated	Erythema; vesication; burns; eye, lung, and skin damage; respiratory effects; leukopenia; thrombocytopenia; decrease in RBCs; sepsis	None; decontamination within 2 min to prevent tissue damage	Burn care, eye therapy, pulmonary support
Nerve agents GA (Tabun) GB (Sarin) GD (Soman) VX	Immediately life-threatening	Eye, nose, lung, and GI effects Large dose: almost immediate loss of consciousness, convulsions, cessation of respiration, flaccid paralysis, copious nasal and oral secretions, intense bronchoconstriction	Atropine sulfate, pralidoxime (Protopam) chloride	Administration of antidotes, ventilation, administration of diazepam (Valium)
Phosgene	Delayed effects possibly life-threatening if untreated	Eye and respiratory system irritation, dyspnea, massive pulmonary edema, hypotension, hypovolemia, bronchospasm, bronchosecretions, right ventricular failure, infection	None	Close observation for at least 4 hr, symptomatic treatment
Cyanide Hydrocyanic acid Cyanogen chloride	Immediately life-threatening	Inhalation: convulsions, death Ingestion: dizziness, nausea, vomiting, weakness, respiratory distress, loss of consciousness, convulsions, apnea, death	Amyl nitrite, sodium nitrite, sodium thiosulfate	Administration of antidotes, supplemental oxygen
Incapacitating agents				
Narcotic congeners[b] (eg, fentanyl)	Possibly life-threatening	Hypotension, paralysis, loss of consciousness	None	Observation, symptomatic treatment
Tranquilizers[b]				
BZ (QNB)	Rarely life-threatening	Sedation, confusion, hallucinations, disorientation, impaired memory, incoherent speech, manifestations of cholinolytic activity	Physostigmine salicylate (Antilirium)	Administration of antidote, observation and reassurance in quiet place

GI, gastrointestinal; *RBCs*, red blood cells.
[a]Adapted from Sidell FR. Postgrad Med 1990;88:70–84.
[b]Nonmilitary use only.

Table 59–16
Odors of Chemical Warfare Agents

Nerve agent: None or faint, sweetish, fruity or paintlike
Tear agents: Lacrimators: Irritating, pungent, pepperlike
Mustard: Garlic or horseradish, irritating
Nitrogen mustard: None or fishy, irritating
Lewisite and other arsenical vesicants: Fruity to geranium-like, very irritating
Mustard and lewisite combinations: Garliclike
Phosgene: Green corn, grass, or new-mown hay
Phosgene oxime: Unpleasant and irritating
Hydrogen cyanide: Faint bitter almonds
Cyanogen chloride: Very irritating
Vomiting agents: Burning fireworks, very irritating
Incapacitating agents: None

be properly handled. Expendable materials should be burned or buried with a quantity of bleach slurry to ensure destruction of the agent. Burning will cause toxic vapors and protection of individuals in the vicinity and downwind must be borne in mind.[55]

3. Wash and rinse at least twice with liquid soap.
4. Do not use detergents.
5. Collect, wrap, and properly discard all clothing.
6. Decontamination for most chemical warfare agents (except BZ—psychedelic agent and CS—tear gas, lacrimator) is effected with a 0.5% solution of hypochlorite (1 part household bleach to 9 parts water). Gently apply. Rinse off with water. The used solution is considered contaminated and must be disposed of accordingly (see Decontamination list). Do not rub or scrub the skin. Do not use water to wash mustard out of wounds or off the skin; mustard must be removed by thorough immediate wiping[5] (Table 59–14). Decontamination of the skin may also be carried out by using pads that release fuller's earth when dabbed and rubbed on the skin. The powder soaks up the liquid and retains it by absorption.[55]
7. Use water or saline solution only for the eyes. Do a fluorescence stain and obtain an ophthalmologic evaluation if symptoms persist over 30 minutes after thorough irrigation.[56]

Eyes

Do not use your fingers or gloved hand for holding the eyelids apart. Open the eyes as wide as possible, and pour the water or saline solution slowly while tilting the head to one side, pour the water into the eye slowly so that it will run off the side of the face to avoid spreading the contamination. This irrigation must be carried out despite the presence of toxic vapors into the atmosphere. Keep the mouth closed to prevent absorption through the mucous membranes. If skin contamination occurs while flushing the eyes, then decontaminate the face with the hypochlorite solution or other suitable solution.

8. "Dakin's" solution is chloramine T. It is an oxidizing solution. Dilute 2 parts/1000 parts of water and place as a soaked towel on any wound every 2 hours for the first day.
9. For oral exposure, use activated charcoal 40 g three times every 4 hours with cathartic of magnesium sulfate.[56]

Medical care providers should be completely encapsulated in protective gear. Those wearing the military Mission Oriental Protective Posture (MOPP) IV ensemble (protective mask and capelike hood; charcoal-impregnated two-piece suit weighing 6 pounds made of an inner-layer of cloth impregnated with charcoal and polyurethane foam and an outer layer made of a half-nylon and half-cotton mix treated with water-repellent material—the charcoal aids in preventing the absorption of nerve gas for 6 hours[11,55,56]; butyl rubber gloves and boots) are able to start intravenous lines, perform endotracheal intubation, suture wounds, and measure blood pressure. Ordinary clothing gives very little protection against nerve agents. Boots that have leather upper parts are slowly penetrated by the agent.[55] Contaminated chemical protective overgarments may be worn safely for 24 hours.[54] Agent Personnel should also wear the complete protective ensemble while decontaminating litters, ambulances, and other equipment contaminated in transporting casualties.

If the chemical is cyanide or a nerve agent or related insecticide and immediate intramuscular or intravenous administration of an antidote is required to save lives, emergency medical technicians or physician assistants may be sent into the area (properly attired) while physicians wait in the clean area to render more detailed care that cannot be done by an encapsulated individual.

Identifying the Agent—Clues to Diagnosis

1. Are people dying within minutes of exposure? If so, this indicates that the chemical agent is probably cyanide or nerve gas.
   Cyanide (short acting)—subjects begin convulsing within seconds of exposure and die within minutes; little cyanosis and few other signs.
   Nerve agent (longer to act)—copious secretions from nose and mouth; pupils are often miotic, with characteristic muscle fasciculations; cyanosis is prominent.
2. Delayed symptoms.
   Phosgene—dyspnea.
   Mustard—skin, eye, or pulmonary effects.
   Incapacitating agents—mental changes.
3. Odors (which cannot be relied on to be useful in warning of impending danger)[54] (Table 59–16).

Civilian Defense guidelines are summarized in Table 59–17.[7–13]

DS2 (Decontamination Solution 2)

DS2 is a general purpose, ready to use, reactive decontaminant with long-term storage stability and a large operating temperature range (–15 to 125°F or –26 to 52°C). This polar, nonaqueous liquid is composed, by weight, of 70% diethylenetriamine, 28% ethylene glycol monomethyl ether, and 2% sodium hydroxide.[57]

C. Artificial Ventilation
   1. Respiratory insufficiency, bronchial hypersecretion, neuromuscular paralysis and inhibition of the respiratory center require early symptomatic treatment of the resulting hypoxia by free airway maintenance, oxygen administration, and artificial ventilation.

D. Intensive Care
   1. Intravenous fluids and electrolytes: to correct acid-base and electrolyte disturbances (acidosis, hypokalemia).
   2. Antibiotics: secondary infections.

Table 59–17
Practical Guidelines for Civilian Defense Against Chemical Warfare Agents[a]

Shelter	Stay indoors. Shut all windows and doors. Move towards inner spaces, closets, etc. Seal openings with adhesive tapes. If possible, prepare ahead of time food and drinking water supply in sealed plastic containers. Cover the containers with plastic bags and seal tightly.
Protective equipment	Avoid contact with the chemical agent. Roll down sleeves. Use impermeable material such as plastic overgarments, gowns, blankets, etc., to cover exposed skin areas. Protect hands with gloves or plastic bags. If a protective chemical warfare mask is not available, use regular towels soaked with sodium bicarbonate (baking soda) solution (25 g for each 1000 ml water). Breathe through the towel, shifting it from time to time to breathe through wet areas.
Decontamination	Remove all droplets of chemical agent from the skin using clean gauze or cotton wool. Do not rub the skin. For effective skin decontamination use commercially available tubes containing Fuller's earth powder. Disperse powder over exposed skin areas. Leave powder for 1 min and remove gently with a clean gauze or cotton. Do not rub powder into the skin. If a powder is not available, use water and regular soap to remove the chemical agent from the skin. Baking soda solution can also be used for decontamination of skin including the facial area (avoid eye penetration).
After the attack	When the area is declared clean, remove all protective equipment cautiously. Use rubber gloves to protect your hands while removing contaminated material or use tweezers or similar devices. Put all contaminated material in plastic containers. Seal the containers and label them appropriately. When leaving the house or shelter (after the area is declared clean), move opposite to wind direction.

[a]Adapted from Shalit I. In: Reis ND, Dolev E, eds. Manual of disaster medicine. Civilian and military. Berlin: Springer-Verlag, 1989; p. 114.

3. Cardiovascular supportive treatment; antiarrhythmic drugs.

E. *Symptomatic Treatment*
1. Bronchial secretions, salivation—
   a. Repeat atropine injections, as required.
   b. Put patient in prone position, with foot of bed elevated.
   c. Loosen collar, pull tongue out, use syringe and catheter to clear saliva and mucous periodically from the mouth.
   d. Insert oropharyngeal airway—suction through and around the airway.
   e. If upper airway remains obstructed and adequate exchange of air does not occur and deepening cyanosis ensues, insert an endotracheal tube.
2. Seizures—seizures should be anticipated in all moderate to severe cases and expectantly treated with diazepam 10 mg intravenously; repeat as required until convulsions are controlled. Seizing is a prominent feature of GD (soman) poisoning.
3. Ocular symptoms—pain relief is obtained with local instillation of atropine sulfate ophthalmic ointment (1%) repeated every several hours as required for 1 to 3 days.
4. Gastric lavage—if water or food contaminated with a large amount of nerve agent has been ingested, colicky abdominal pain, substernal tightness, increased salivation, and possibly vomiting may occur about 1/2 hour later. Perform a gastric lavage as required.

F. *Assisted Ventilation*
For severely impaired respiration or for cessation of respiration after the administration of atropine with a potential for cyanosis and death within minutes, assisted ventilation should be begun immediately and maintained until spontaneous respiration is resumed (endotracheal intubation, mechanical ventilator, oxygen).

G. *Disposition*
1. Observe for 18 hours after a dermal exposure because of the possibility of a delayed onset of signs and symptoms.
2. Obtain a red cell cholinesterase level. If the level is low in an asymptomatic patient, no antidote may be required.

PYRIDOSTIGMINE

Pyridostigmine Pretreatment

The use of atropine and the oximes may be insufficient for protection against the toxic effects of GD (soman), even if they are administered immediately after the agent challenge GD (soman). Soman exhibits very rapid "aging" (within minutes). As Dunn and Sidell have emphasized,[3] even with good training and the ability to don a mask rapidly, some soldiers on a chemical battlefield may be at risk for absorbing up to five times the lethal dose of GD during an intense chemical attack. The *protective ratio*[1,3] is the factor by which a treatment raises the lethal dose of a toxic agent. Antidotes have not yet been devised that can raise the protective ratio sufficiently high in man to counteract the lethal effects of GD. Therefore a preexposure treatment has been sought. Pretreatment is not effective against sarin and VX challenge. When used for soman challenge, it should be followed by atropine and an oxime.

Efficacy

Pyridostigmine by itself does not provide protection without the use of the antidotes (atropine/oximes). It is an antidote "enhancer" rather than a "true" treatment. It appears to enhance the efficacy of the antidotes within 1 to 3 hours after taking the first tablet. Maximal benefit appears to develop with time and may be reached when a tablet is taken every 8 hours.[5]

Therapeutic Dose

The U.S. Army provides a pyridostigmine bromide (30 mg) pretreatment set of tablets (21 total) packaged in a blister pack, to be taken 1 every 8 hours, enough for 7 days. One tablet is taken orally with water.[5]

Toxicokinetics

After IV injection of pyridostigmine 2.5 mg, the plasma elimination half-life is 1.52 hours, the apparent volume of distribution is 1.43 L/kg and the plasma clearance is 0.65 L/kg/hr. After oral administration of 120 mg, the elimination half-life is 1.78 hr, apparent volume of distribution 1.64 L/kg and plasma clearance 0.66 L/kg/hr. The bioavailability of oral pyridostigmine is 7.6%. Peak plasma concentrations of 35 to 65 ng/ml after oral intake are reached in about 1.7 hours. From 75 to 90% of the dose is excreted in the urine unchanged.[58–61]

Drug Interactions

Antimuscarinics (atropine, glycopyrrolate, scopolamine) are antagonizers of pyridostigmine action.

Thiopental may enhance the ability of pyridostigmine to precipitate bronchospasm. It may also potentiate the bradycardia and drop in cardiac output and blood pressure occasionally observed with pyridostigmine.

Diazepam used as an anesthetic induction agent may enhance cardiovascular depressant effects in a pyridostigmine shock casualty.

Ketamine and pyridostigmine both increase the production of oropharyngeal secretion.

Pyridostigmine reverses the neuromuscular blocking effect of neuromuscular blockers. Antagonism or potentiation of neuromuscular blockers may occur.

Isoflurane use in a pyridostigmine-treated patient may decrease the requirement for succinylcholine.

Pyridostigmine inhibits the enzyme (plasma cholinesterase) that hydrolyzes ester-type local anesthetics, prolonging their action.

4-Aminopyridine potentiates the antagonism of a pancuronium-induced neuromuscular blockade by pyridostigmine.[62]

Mechanism of Action

The possible protective action of carbamates such as pyridostigmine appears to depend on the ability of the carbamate to reversibly inhibit about 20 to 40% of red blood cell acetylcholinesterase,[63] forming a semistable carbamylated enzyme that can then spontaneously break down to liberate the enzyme. The fraction of the enzyme in the tissues that is carbamylated will be protected against phosphorylation by subsequent organophosphate poisoning. The gradual decarbamylation of the enzyme in parallel with the relatively rapid removal or destruction of the organophosphate would release sufficient acetylcholinesterase to maintain life.[64] Protection against soman-induced lethality is related to the degrees of carbamylation of the AChE just prior to the challenge.[65]

Clinical Presentation—Acute Overdosage

Pyridostigmine overdosage may lead to a cholinergic crisis characterized by nausea, vomiting, diarrhea, excessive salivation and sweating, increased bronchial secretions, miosis, lacrimation, bradycardia or tachycardia, cardiospasm, bronchospasm, hypotension, incoordination, blurred vision, muscle cramps, weakness, fasciculation, and paralysis.[5] At very high doses, agitation, restlessness, confusion, visual hallucinations, and paranoid delusions may be observed. Death may result from cardiac arrest or respiratory paralysis and pulmonary edema. Weakness (in myasthenia gravis patients) that begins approximately 1 hour after drug administration suggests overdosage, whereas weakness that occurs in this group of patients 3 hours or more after drug administration is more likely to be caused by underdosage or resistance. Edrophonium can be used to distinguish cholinergic crises from myasthenic crises.

Pyridostigmine poisoning may be diagnosed by the medical history, presence of cholinergic signs, response to atropine administration, and determination of serum cholinesterase activity. Patients with cholinesterase values at preexposure in the upper normal range may exhibit a 60% inhibition of their cholinesterase activity and still have values above the lower limits of normal. Baseline values of cholinesterase in an acute pyridostigmine overdose may be determined by dilution of the sample 1:50 with saline followed by incubation at 37°C for 24 hours. This may result in a complete decarbamylation of the enzyme.[66] Plasma cholinesterase levels may be reduced by 30 to 50% before other signs or symptoms are evident. Studies in patients with pyridostigmine overdose suggest that no clear correlation exists between the extent of cholinesterase inhibition and the incidence or severity of cholinergic signs. Clinical recovery appears to precede the spontaneous recovery of the enzyme.[66]

The treatment of patients with carbamate poisoning consists of general supportive care, including establishment of an airway, stabilization of vital signs, gastric decontamination, and use of atropine as indicated. An antimuscarinic (atropine, glycopyrrolate, scopolamine) is the drug of choice for pyridostigmine overdose. In adults an initial intravenous dose of 2 mg of atropine given every 5 to 30 minutes may be required to reach atropinization. If the poisoning is moderate, one to four doses may be sufficient.[66]

Chronic Toxicity (see also Gulf War)

Pyridostigmine bromide administered in doses of either 120 mg orally four times a day or as a sustained-release dose of 180 mg orally at bedtime is sufficient to produce bromide intoxication (low or negative anion gap, falsely elevated serum chloride level, neurologic changes, headache, agitation, weakness, slurred speech, confusion, delusional ideations, hallucinations, stupor, and coma; dermatologic changes: acne from lesions on face and trunk, pyoderma gangrenosum–like lesion of bromoderma).[67]

Laboratory

Analytic

Pyridostigmine is extracted from plasma by passage through C-18–coated silica gel and quantitated by HPLC.[68]

CENTRAL NERVOUS SYSTEM DRUGS

Diazepam—Anticonvulsant Therapy

U.S. soldiers will soon carry an automatic injection containing 10 mg of diazepam to be given with the third dose of atropine.[69] Diazepam when used with atropine-oxime mixtures affords considerable anticonvulsant protection against anticholinesterases.[70] Pretreatment for nerve agent–induced brain injury with cholinolytic compounds such as benactyzine (see Benactyzine), as well as centrally active carbamate compounds such as physostigmine, carries the risk of some degree of performance impairment.[3] Physostigmine's propensity to induce bronchospasm and seizures makes this agent a less likely expedient in the presence of probable nerve agent respiratory toxicity. Currently United States medical aidmen have injectable diazepam available for nerve agent casualty care. Atropinization enhances the efficacy of nerve agent anticonvulsants. Atropine itself has antimuscarinic activity against low doses of OP-anticholinesterases and anticonvulsant properties against higher doses. Finally, diazepam and midazolam are gamma-aminobutyric acid pathway agonists, which appear effective in blocking GD-induced convulsions and incapacitation in rhesus monkeys.[3]

Benactyzine

Some oximes (bispyridiniums) in combination with atropine supported by benactyzine, will protect beagle dogs against poisoning by more than 5 times the LD50 of soman.[3,71,72] Side effects observed clinically in man, however, after intramuscular administration of about 4 mg of benactyzine may include deficits of short-term memory, concentration, and attention; reduced visual acuity; increased pupil size; reduced amplitude of accommodation; and contrast sensitivity that may last for up to 3 hours or more.[3] Central nervous system effects at present therefore preclude usefulness of this product by the military.[73] Benactyzine also has a restricted shelf-life, losing 2% of its potency after 1 year at 25°C.[74] Therefore at present diazepam, 10 mg IM, already approved in the United States and elsewhere, is preferred for counteracting seizures induced by the central nervous system effects of organophosphate poisons such as soman. Regardless of whether the patient is seizing, to ameliorate seizure activity and lessen the likelihood of subsequent brain damage, diazepam IV should be used with caution because it can worsen the respiratory depression caused by nerve agents.[75]

CHEMICAL WEAPONS DISPOSAL[76,77]

Stockpiling of Nerve Agents

The United States' stockpile of aging lethal unitary chemical weapons and agents is currently scheduled for destruction by April 30, 1997, under the Department of Defense Authorization Act (PL99-145 and PL100-456). Unitary weapons contain lethal agents at the time of assembly. Binary weapons contain agent precursors that mix on firing and react to form lethal agents.

Nerve agents

The following are organophosphate nerve agents:

GA—Tabun; *N,N*-dimethyl phosphoroamidocyanidate, ethyl ester
GB—Sarin; Methylphosphonofluoridate isopropyl ester
VX—*S*-(diisopropylamino ethyl) methylphosphono thiolate *o*-ethyl ester.

Other agents stockpiled include the vesicant blister agents H, HD sulfur mustard or di-2-chloroethylsulfide, T(*bis*[2-chlorethylthioethyl] ether), and L (Lewisite) or dichlor (2-chlorovinyl) arsine.

Recommended control limits are found in Table 59–18.

Destruction Hazards

Potential hazards for destruction of the stockpile include organophosphate-induced delayed neuropathy, electroencephalographic changes, cancer, birth defects, and keratitis.[76]

Incineration

The U.S. Army Toxic and Hazardous Materials Agency adopted incineration as the method of choice for disposal of chemical agents and munitions. Reverse assembly, incineration at temperatures up to 1370°C, and treatment of stack gases and incinerator ash by advanced pollution-abatement systems may lead to final incineration products that are not acutely lethal. The stockpile includes both organophosphate (nerve) agents and vesicant (blister) agents.

Chronic Effects

Nerve agents do not appear to cause mutations or cancer and probably do not damage fetuses or induce reproduction dysfunction. Agents GA and GB have caused delayed neuropathy in susceptible animals. Agent VX is not known to cause delayed neuropathy. Therefore acute lethality is of perhaps more immediate concern than delayed neuropathy in the evaluation of exposed persons. There is no evidence to suggest that brain dysfunction could occur on exposure to the maximum atmospheric concentrations of nerve agents that may be expected during normal operation of an incineration plant.

Vesicant Agents

No acute vesicant effects are expected at the recommended control limits in Table 59–18. There are no specific antidotes for mustard agent poisoning. Exposure to lewisite can be effectively countered by treatment with British antilewisite (BAL) after time lapses of as much as 1 hour. Further trials are required with newer analogues of BAL, meso-dimercaptosuccinic acid and the sodium salt of 2,3-dimercapto-1-propanesulfonic acid.

New Developments

Further possible improvements against the toxicity of nerve agents now under study include the following:

1. A sustained-release dose form of pyridostigmine.
2. Combined administration of two or all of three antidote elements of atropine, oxime, and anticonvulsant in a single autoinjector.
3. Other compounds to replace pralidoxime.
4. Human-based gene products that will produce sufficient excess circulating cholinesterase to permit the enzyme to serve as a scavenger that will bind the nerve agent before it can reach its critical tissue target sites.[3]
5. Human monoclonal antibodies with a long plasma half-life administered as passive protection.[78]

Table 59–18
Recommended Control Limits for Selected Chemical Agents[a]

Chemical Agent[b]	General Population (mg/m³)		Workers (mg/m³)	
Nerve Agents[c]				
GA, GB	0.000003	(3×10^{-6})	0.0001	(1×10^{-4})
VX	0.000003	(3×10^{-6})	0.00001	(1×10^{-5})
Vesicants[d]				
H, HD, HT[e]	0.0001	(1×10^{-4})	0.003	(3×10^{-3})
L	0.003	(3×10^{-3})	0.003	(3×10^{-3})
Averaging Time	72 hours		8 hours	

[a]Adapted from MMWR 1988;37:72–79.
[b]Protection against exposure to agents in aerosol and liquid form must be sufficient to prevent direct contact with the skin and eyes.
[c]*GA,* Tabun or ethyl *N,N*-dimethylphosphoramidocyanidate; *GB,* Sarin or isopropyl methylphosphonofluoridate; *VX, S*-(2-diisopropylaminoethyl) O-ethyl methyl phosphonothiolate.
[d]*H* or *HD,* Sulfur mustard or di-2-chloroethyl sulfide; *HT, Bis*(2-chloroethylthioethyl) ether (T) in a mixture with sulfur mustard; *L,* Lewisite or dichloro (2-chlorovinyl) arsine.
[e]Data supporting the ability to monitor for H at 0.0001 mg/m³ at all sites should be developed. HT is measured as HD.

6. Catalytic antibodies that bind to the transition states of small molecules such as nerve agents, thereby inactivating them.[71]
7. Circulating carboxylesterase[79] to detoxify GC from liver cytoplasm[80] and a cloned neuronal cell line.[81]

LABORATORY

Analytic Methods

A capillary column gas chromatography–mass spectrometry method is available for tabun determinations.[82] Gas chromatography retention indices have been determined for twenty-two chemical warfare agents.[83]

A summary of chemical agents and physical characteristics relative to their toxic activity is presented in Table 59–10.[77]

REFERENCES

1. Munro NB, Watson AP, Ambrose KR, Griffin GD. Treating exposure to chemical warfare agents: implications for healthy care providers and community emergency planning. Environ Health Perspect 1990;89:205–215.
2. Karalliedde L, Ganci CA, Carter M. Chemical weapons. Br Med J 1991;302:474.
3. Dunn MA, Sidell FR. Progress in medical defense against nerve agents. JAMA 1989;262:649–652.
4. Prevention and treatment of nerve gas poisoning. Med Lett Drugs Ther 1990;32(831):103–105.
5. Treatment of chemical agent casualties and conventional military chemical injuries field manual. Army FM 8-285, Navy Navmed P-5041, Air Force AFM 160-11, Departments of the Army, the Navy and the Air Force. February 1990; pp. 2-15 to 2-19.
6. Sundwall A. Minimum concentrations of N methylpyridinium-2-aldoxime methane sulphonate (P2S) which reverse neuromuscular block. Biochem Pharmacol 1961;8:413–417.
7. Vale JA, Meredith TJ, Heath A. High dose atropine in organophosphorus poisoning. Postgrad Med J 1990;66:878–881.
8. Wilson IB, Ginsburg S. A powerful reactivator of alkylphosphate-inhibited acetylcholinesterase. Biochem Biophys Acta 1955;18:168–170.
9. Christenson I. Stability of the nerve gas antidote bis (4-hydroxyiminoethyl-1-pyridinomethyl ether dichloride (toxogonin). Drug Intelligence 1968;2:234–243.
10. Vojvodic VB. Blood levels, urinary excretion and potential toxicity of N N1-trimethylenebis (pyridinium-4-aldoxime) dichloride (TMB-4) in healthy man following intramuscular injection of the oxime. Pharmacol Clin 1970;2:216–220.
11. Sidell FR, Groff WA, Kaminskis A. Toxogonin and pralidoxime: Kinetic comparison after intravenous administration to man. J Pharm Sci 1972;61:1765–1769.
12. Erdmann WD. Vergleichende untersuchungen uber das penetrations vermogen einiger esterasereaktivierender oxime in das zentrale nervensystem. Arzneimittel-forsch 1965;15:135.
13. Shapira Y, Bar Y, Berkenstadt H, Atsmon J, Damon YL. Outline of hospital organization for a chemical warfare attack. Isr J Med Sci 1991;27:616–622.
14. Sidell FR, Groff WA, Kaminskis A. Pralidoxime-methane sulfonate. Plasma levels and pharmacokinetics after oral administration to man. J Pharm Sci 1972;61:1736–1740.
15. Calesnick B, Christensen JA, Richter M. Human toxicity of oximes. 2-pyridine aldoxime methyl chloride, its methane sulfonate salt and 1,1'-trimethlyenebis-(4-formylpyridinum chloride). Arch Environ Health, 1967;15:599–608.
16. Sidell FR, Groff WA, Ellin RI. Blood levels of oxime and symptoms in human after single and multiple oral doses of 2-pyridine aldoxime methochloride. J Pharm Sci 1969;58:1093–1098.
17. Sidell FR, Groff WA. Toxogonin: oral administration to man. J Pharm Sci 1971;60:860–863.
18. Simon GA, Tirosh MS, Edery H. Administration of obidoxime tablets to man. Plasma levels and side reactions. Arch Toxicol 1976;36:83–88.
19. Sidell FR, Groff WA. Toxogonin: Blood levels and side effects after intramuscular administration in man. J Pharmaceut Sci 1970;59:793–797.
20. Sidell FR, Groff WA. Intramuscular and intravenous administration of small doses of 2-pyridinium aldoxime methochloride to man. J Pharm Sci 1971;60:1224–1228.
21. Sundwall A. Plasma concentration curves of *N*-methylpyridinum-2-aldoxime methane sulphonate (1-2S) after intravenous intramuscular and oral administration in man. Biochem Pharmacol 1960;5:225–230.
22. Gallagher K, Kerney T, Mangione A. A case report of organophosphate poisoning supporting the use of pralidoxime (2PAM) by continuous infusion (Personal communication).
23. Farrar HC, Wells TG, Kearns GL. Use of continuous infusion of pralidoxime for treatment of organophosphate poisoning in children. J Pediatr 1990;116:658–661.
24. Jeevarathinan K, Ghosh AK, Srinivasan A, Das Gupta B. Pharmacokinetics of pralidoxime chloride and its correlation to therapeutic efficacy against diisopropyl fluorophosphate intoxication in rats. Pharmazie 1988;43:114–115.
25. Jovanovic D. Pharmacokinetics of pralidoxime chloride. A comparative study in human volunteers and in organophosphate poisoning. Arch Toxicol 1989;63:416–418.
26. Vale JA, Marrs TC. Pralidoxime (Personal communication).
27. Scott RJ. Repeated asystole following PAM in organophosphate self poisoning. Anaesthesia Intensive Care 1986;14:458–468.
28. Keppens C, Maes V, Vinchen W. Severe organophosphate poisoning successfully treated by prolonged obidoxime and atropine infusion. Proc Eur Assoc Pols Cont Centers, 1988.
29. de Kort WLAM, Kienstra SH, Sangster B. The use of atropine and oximes in organophosphate intoxications: a modified approach. Clin Toxicol 1988;26:199–208.
30. Sidell FR, Groff WA. The reactivability of cholinesterase inhibited by VX and sarin in man. Toxicol Appl Pharmacol 1974;27:241–252.
31. Grob D, Harvey JC. Effects in man of the anticholinesterase compound sarin (isopropyl methyl phosphono fluoridate). J Clin Invest 1958;37:350–360.
32. Grob D. The manifestations and treatment of poisoning due to nerve gas and other organic phosphate anticholinesterase compounds. Arch Intern Med 1956;98:221–238.
33. Kristof ND. Poison gas kills 6 in Tokyo subway; sabotage is seen. New York Times, March 20, 1995; pp. A1–A2.
34. Poison fumes in Tokyo subway kill 6, hurt 900. Los Angeles Times, March 20, 1995; pp. A1 & A7.
35. Yokoyama K, Ogura Y, Kishimoton M, Hinoshita F, Hara S, Yamada A et al. Blood purification for severe sarin poisoning after the Tokyo subway attack. JAMA 1995;274:379.
36. Morita H, Yanagisawa N, Nakajima T, Shimizu M, Hirabayashi H, Okudera H et al. Sarin poisoning in Matsumoto, Japan. Lancet 1995;346:290–293.
37. Sidell FR. Soman and sarin: clinical manifestations and treatment of accidental poisoning by organophosphates. Clin Toxicol 1974;711–717.
38. Rengstorff RH. Accidental exposure to sarin: vision effects. Arch Toxicol 1985;56:201–203.
39. Oberst FW, Koon WS, Christensen MK, Crook JW, Cresthull P, Freeman G. Retention of inhaled sarin vapor and its effect on red blood cell cholinesterase in man. Clin Pharmacol Ther 1968;9:421–422.
40. Rubin LS, Goldberg MN. Effect of sarin on dark adaptation in man. Threshold change. J Appl Physiol 1957;11:439–444.
41. Duffy FH, Burchfield JL, Bartels PH, Gaon M, Sim VM. Long-term effects on organophosphate from the human electroencephalogram. Toxicol Appl Pharmacol 1979;47:161–176.
42. Burchfield JL, Duffy FH. Organophosphate neurotoxicity: chronic effects of sarin on the electroencephalogram of monkey and man. Neurobehav Toxicol Teratol 1982;4:767–778.

43. Burchfield JL, Duffy FH, Sim VM. Persistent effects of sarin and dieldrin upon the primate electroencephalogram. Toxicol Appl Pharmacol 1976;35:365–379.
44. Vale JA. Oximes-pharmacokinetic aspects. Drugs in dose and overdose. Recent advances in clinical pharmacology and toxicology abstracts. Birmingham, UK: Dudley Road Hospital, October 28–30, 1987.
45. Willems JL. Anticholinesterase poisoning. An overview of pharmacotherapy and clinical management. In: Ballantyne B, Marrs T, eds. Clinical and experimental toxicology of anticholinesterases. Guildford, UK: Butterworth, in press.
46. Ligtenstein DA. Evaluation of the pyridinium-aldoximes available for therapy of organophosphate intoxications with some remarks on the required further research for therapy of soman intoxication in humans. Proc Int Symp Protection against Chemical Warfare Agents. Stockholm, Sweden: June 6–9, 1983, pp. 129–140.
47. Marrs TC. Toxicology of oximes used in treatment of organophosphate poisoning. Adverse Drug React Toxicol Rev 1991;10:61–72.
48. Briggs CJ, Simons KJ. Treatment of organophosphorous poisoning. Pharmaceutical aspects of antidotes. Proc Internatl Assoc Forensic Toxicol, Ghent. August 24–27, 1986; pp. 514–523.
49. Jovanovic D, Maksimovic M, Koksovic D, Kovasevic V. Oral forms of the oxime H1-6: a study of pharmacokinetics and tolerance after administration to healthy volunteers. Vet Hum Toxicol 1990;32:419–421.
50. Worek FS, Scinicz L. Effect of soman, atropine and HLo7—dimethane sulfonate on respiration and circulation of anesthetized guinea pigs. Akademic Symposium 1991. Role of oximes in the treatment of anticholinesterase agent poisoning. October 7, 1991. Munich. Akademie des Sanitats und Gesundheits wesens der Bundeswehr, Nacherbergstr 11, 8000 Munchen 45, pp. 25.
51. Bismuth C, Baud FJ, Kiffer D. Potential antidotes to anticholinesterase chemical weapons. Proc Eur Assoc Pois Cont Centers, 1988, p. 7.
52. Gunderson CH, Lehmann Cr, Sidell FR, Jabbai B. Nerve agents. A review. Neurology 1992;42:946–950.
53. Sidell FR. What to do in case of an unthinkable chemical warfare attack or accident. Postgrad Med 1990;88(7):70–84.
54. Treatment of Chemical Agent Casualties and Conventional Military Chemical Injuries. Field Manual. Army FM8-285, Navy Navmed P-5041, Air Force AFM 160-11. Departments of the Army, Navy and the Air Force, February 1990.
55. JSP 312: Medical Manual of Defence Against Chemical Agents. Ministry of Defense. London: Her Majesty's Stationery Office 1987; pp. 4-2 to 4-3.
56. Mofenson HC, Caraccio TR. "War gases". Part II. PP/T News, Nassau County Medical Center Regional Poison Control Center 1991;10(2):240–245.
57. Yang Y-C, Baker JA, Ward JR. Decontamination of chemical warfare agents. Chem Rev 1992;92:1729–1734.
58. Ray R, Clark DE III, Ford KW, Knight KR, Harris LW, Broomfield CA. A novel tertiary pyridostigmine derivative [3-(*N,N-D*-methylcarbamyloxy)-1-methyl-^{3}-tetrahydropyridine]: anticholinesterase properties and efficacy against soman. Fund Appl Toxicol 1991;16:267–274.
59. Aquilonius S-M, Eckernas S-A, Hartvig P, Lindstrom B, Osterman PO: Pharmacokinetics and oral bioavailability of pyridostigmine in man. Eur J Clin Pharmacol 1980;18:423–428.
60. Brayer-Pfaff V, Schwezer A, Maier V, Brinkman A, Schumer F. Neuromuscular function and plasma drug levels in pyridostigmine treatment of myasthenia gravis. J Neurol Neurosurg Psychiatry 1990;53:502–506.
61. Keeler JR. Interaction between nerve agent pretreatment and drugs commonly used in combat anesthesia. Milit Med 1990;155:527–533.
62. Miller RD, Booij LHDJ, Agostom S, Crul JF. 4-Aminopyridine potentiates neostigmine and pyridostigmine in man. Anesthesiology 1979;50:416–420.
63. Gall D. The use of therapeutic mixtures in the treatment of cholinesterase inhibition. Fund Appl Toxicol 1981;1:214–216.
64. Gordon JJ, Leadbeater L, Maidment MP. The protection of animals against organophosphorus poisoning by pretreatment with a carbamate. Toxicol Appl Pharmacol 1978; 43:207–216.
65. Harris LW, Anderson DR, Pastelak AM, Vanderpool B. Acetylcholinesterase inhibition by (+) physostigmine and efficacy against lethality induced by soman. Drug Chem Toxicol 1990;13:241–248.
66. Almog S, Winkler E, Amitai Y, Dani S, Shefi M, Tirosh M, Sherner J. Acute pyridostigmine overdose: a report of nine cases. Isr J Med Sci 1991;27:659–663.
67. Rothenberg DM, Berns AS, Barkin R, Glantz RH. Bromide intoxication secondary to pyridostigmine bromide therapy. JAMA 1990;263:1121–1122.
68. Ellin RT, Zvirblis P, Wilson MR. Method for isolation and determination of pyridostigmine and metabolites in urine and blood. J Chromatogr 1982;228:235–244.
69. Prevention and treatment of nerve gas poisoning. Med Lett Drugs Ther 1990;32(831):103–105.
70. Green DM, Muir AW, Stratton JA, Inch TD. Dual mechanism of the antidotal action of atropine-like drugs in poisoning by organophosphorus anticholinesterases. J Pharm Pharmacol 1977;29:62–64.
71. Schenk J, Loffler W, Weger N. Therapeutic Effects of HS-3, HS-6, benactyzine and atropine in soman poisoning of dogs. Arch Toxicol 1976;36:71–81.
72. Weger N, Szinicz L. Therapeutic effects of new oximes, benactyzine and atropine in soman poisoning. I. Effects of various oximes in soman, sarin and VX poisoning in dogs. Fund Appl Toxicol 1981;1:161–163.
73. Brown B, Haegerstrom-Portnoy G, Adams AJ, Jones RT, Jampolsky A. Effects of an anticholinergic drug, benactyzine hydrochloride, on vision and vision performance. Aviat Space Environ Med 1982;53:759–765.
74. Zvirblis P, Ellin RI. Kinetics and stability of multi-component organophosphate antidote formulation in glass and plastic. J Pharm Sci 1982;71:321–325.
75. Sidell FR, Borak J. Chemical warfare agents. II. Nerve agents. Ann Emerg Med 1992;21:865–871.
76. Recommendation for protecting human health against potential adverse effects of long-term exposure to low doses of chemical warfare agents. MMWR 1988;37:72–79.
77. Carnes SA, Watson AP. Disposing of the US chemical weapons stockpile. An approaching reality. JAMA 1989;262: 653–659.
78. Lenz DE, Brimfield AA, Hunter KW Jr, Benschop HP, De Jong LPA, van Dijk C, Clow TR. Studies using a monoclonal antibody against soman. Fund Appl Toxicol 1984;4:S156–S164.
79. Maxwell DM, Brecht KM, O'Neill BL. The effect of carboxylesterase inhibition on interspecies differences in soman toxicity. Toxicol Lett 1987;39:35–42.
80. Little JS, Broomfield CA, Fox-Talbot MK, Boucher LJ, MacIver B, Lenz DE. Partial characterization of an enzyme that hydrolyzes sarin, soman, tabun and diisopropyl phosphofluoridate (DFP). Biochem Pharmacol 1989;38:23–29.
81. Ray RR, Boucher W, Broomfield CA, Lenz DE. Specific soman-hydrolyzing activity in a clonal neuronal cell culture. Biochem Biophys Acta 1988;967:373–381.
82. D'Agostino PA, Hansen AS, Lockwood PA, Provost LR. Capillary column gas chromatography-mass spectrometry of tabun. J Chromatogr 198;331:251–266.
83. D'Agostino PA, Provost LR. Gas chromatographic retention indices of chemical warfare agents and stimulants. J Chromatogr 1985;331:47–54.
84. Barr SJ. Chemical warfare agents. Top Emerg Med 1985;7(1): 62–70.

THE GULF WAR

GAS MASKS (FIG. 59–5)[1]

The Gulf War provided Israel with a national experience on the effects of preparation for a chemical warfare attack. Seven people were reported to have died of asphyxia because

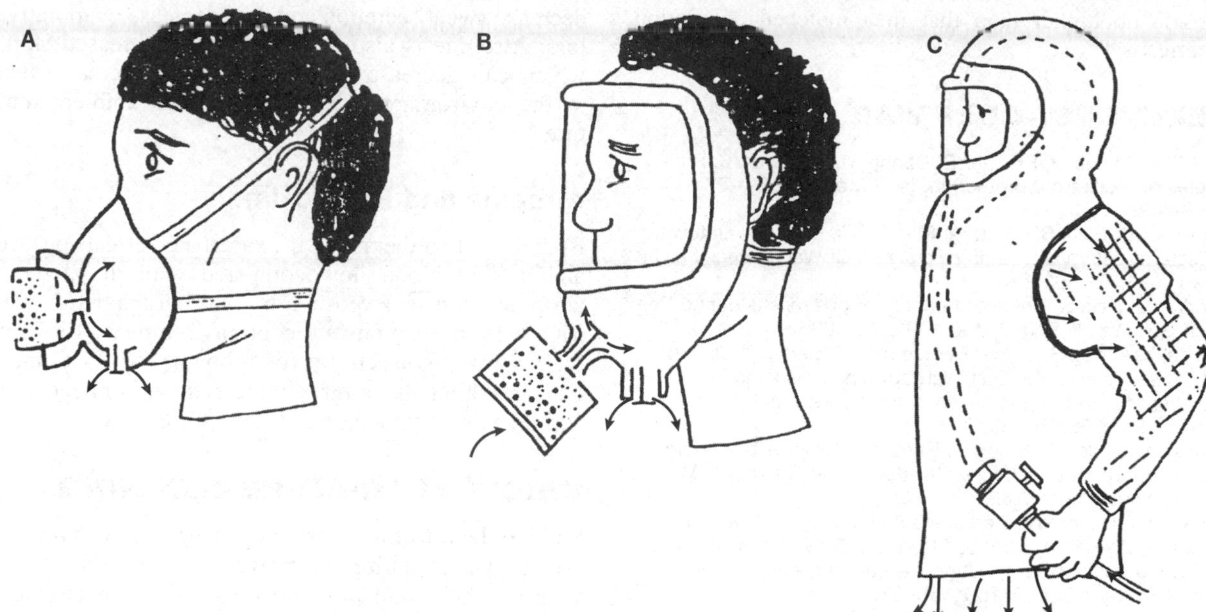

Figure 59–5 Various types of protective respirator. **A and B.** Tight-fitting systems—half-mask and full face-piece gas mask—with spontaneous breathing through an air-purifying device. Note the outflow valves for expiratory air. **C.** A loose-fitting, half-suit, airline respirator. Note the air leaking out under the loose-fitting adhesions due to overpressure inside the system. (Adapted from Arad M. et al. Isr J Med Sci 1991;27:636–642.)

of their failure to remove the protective plastic seal on the gas mask filter.[2] Transient hypoxia and syncope was observed in those with cardiopulmonary disorders. A purpuric rash, "suction purpura," facial contact urticaria, and dermatographism was transiently experienced. Other effects noted included heightened anxiety, panic attacks, claustrophobia, hyperventilation, exacerbations of asthma, and angina.[3]

ATROPINE INJECTIONS (SEE PLANT CHAPTER—ATROPINE)

Personal automatic atropine autoinjectors were distributed to the Israeli population as preparation for a potential organophosphorus nerve attack. Over 4 months 268 cases of accidental and unnecessary injections of atropine in children were administered mostly to the finger and palm, in doses up to 17-fold higher than standards for the age. Varying degrees of atropinization were observed. There were no deaths, seizures, or life-threatening arrhythmias.[4] Doses up to 0.045 mg/kg produced no signs of atropinization. Doses of 0.045 to 0.175 mg/kg and over were associated with mild and severe effects, respectively. In adults, an atropine dose of 0.032 mg/kg causes tachycardia, whereas confusion, amnesia, and hallucination occur at atropine doses of 0.13 to 0.17 mg/kg. Following a therapeutic intramuscular injection of 0.02 mg/kg to children and 1 mg to adults, peak plasma atropine levels were 2.4 and 3.0 ng/mL, respectively. In the Gulf War study in children, atropine concentrations ranged from 7.5 to 69 ng/mL[5]

Symptoms observed included mydriasis, tachycardia, drug membrane, flushed skin, hyperthermia, agitation, confusion, and ataxia. No seizures, life-threatening arrhythmias, or fatalities were noted. Serum atropine levels were 7.5 to 69 ng/mL.

PYRIDOSTIGMINE PRETREATMENT

Pyridostigmine bromide, 30 mg orally, was self-administered every 8 hours by 41,650 soldiers while under threat of nerve agent attack for 1 to 7 days in January, 1991.[6] About half of those who ingested pyridostigmine noted physiologic changes that were not incapacitating such as increased flatus, abdominal cramps, soft stools, and urinary urgency. Headaches, rhinorrhea, diaphoresis, and tingling of the extremities were occasionally observed. Fewer than 0.1% had effects sufficient to discontinue the drug. A few noted acute elevations in blood pressure. Pyridostigmine therapy was discontinued for 28 soldiers, including three with exacerbated autobronchitis, one asthmatic, two with allergic reactions, two hypertensive patients, and 20 with intolerable nausea and diarrhea. Over all, military performance was not impaired.[7]

CARDIAC DEATHS

During the first days of the Gulf War a sharp rise was observed in Israel in the incidence of acute myocardial infarctions, especially of the anterior wall of patients receiving thrombolytic therapy and of sudden death. The incidence of acute myocardial infarction reverted to normal after the initial phase of the Gulf War.[8]

THE GULF WAR SYNDROME—UNITED STATES

The United States Defense Department believes that no evidence implicates chemical or biologic weapons as causes of the illnesses suffered by veterans of the Gulf war, even though many of the illnesses cannot be diagnosed. Preliminary studies show that mortality among Gulf veterans is no higher than that in a matched population of Americans.[9]

REFERENCES—GULF WAR

1. Arad M, Epstein Y, Krasner E, Danon YL, Atsomon J. Principles of respiratory protection. Isr J Med Sci 1991;27: 634–642.
2. Huminer D, Pitlik SD, Katz A, Metzker A, David M. Untoward effects of gas masks during Persian Gulf War. N Engl J Med 1991;325:582–583.
3. Borkan J, Reis S. Untoward effects of gas masks during Persian Gulf War. N Engl J Med 1991;325:583.
4. Amitai Y, Almog S, Singer R, Hammer R, Bentur Y, Danon YL. Lessons from the Gulf War: atropine poisoning in children during the gulf crises: a national survey in Israel. JAMA 1992;268:630–632.
5. Amitai Y, Singer R, Almog S, Bentur Y. Atropine poisoning in children from automatic injector during the Gulf crisis. Vet Hum Toxicol 1991;33:36.
6. Sharabi Y, Danon YL, Berkenstadt H, Almog S, Mimouni-Block A, Zisman A, Dani S, Atsmon J. Survey of symptoms following intake of pyridostigmine during the Person Gulf War. Isr J Med Sci 1991;27:656–658.
7. Keeler JR, Hurst CG, Dunor MA. Pyridostigmine used as a nerve agent pretreatment under wartime conditions. JAMA 1991;266:693–695.
8. Meisel SR, Kutz I, Dayan KI, Pauzner H, Chetboun I, Arbel YT, David D. Effect of Iraqi missile war on the incidence of acute myocardial infarction and sudden death in Israeli civilians. Lancet 1991;338:660–661.
9. Roberts J. Chemical weapons did not cause the Gulf war syndrome. Br Med J 1995;310:692.

HEAT STRESS

VISUAL ACUITY

Visual acuity, phoria (binocular alignment of visual axes of both eyes), stereopsis (perception of apparent relative distance based on small amounts of retinal image disparity), and contrast sensitivity (ability to discern subtle brightness differences among alternating shades of grey) have been studied over 6 hours of continued exposure to combinations of atropine 2 mg, 2-PAM chloride 600 mg, severe heat (95°F—35°C), 60% relative humidity, and the wearing of either the U.S. Army battle dress uniform (BDU) or the BDU and the impermeable chemical protective clothing (MOPP-IV). (MOPP is Mission Oriented Protective Posture with increasing levels of encapsulation. MOPP (I, II, III, and IV) is used to provide greater protection.)

Subjects were able to complete 6 hours of testing under severe heat when wearing BDUs, but only for 2 hours while wearing MOPP-IV. Acuity and phoria, but not stereopsis or contrast sensitivity, are significantly impaired by the drugs in the BDU condition. Acuity, phoria, and stereopsis are all significantly impaired by heat, drug, and continued exposure under MOPP-IV conditions. Contrast sensitivity is impaired mainly by continued heat exposure in MOPP-IV.[1,2] No one was able to complete 95°F test sessions dressed in MOPP-IV gear.[2]

DRUG ACTIONS

Atropine

Cholinolytic or anticholinergic drugs, of which atropine is the classic example with an almost pure muscarinic action, decrease sweat secretion and thus decrease evaporative heat loss. Atropine is also associated with increased skin flow, which can decrease heat gain from or increase heat loss to the environment, depending on the ambient temperature.[3]

Atropine and Pralidoxime

Both drugs together result in exacerbated effects on sweating and/or skin blood flow compared with those seen with atropine alone.[2] Exposure to both drugs while wearing MOPP-IV protection in a cool environment (13°C) permit intermittent light activity for 6 hours.[3] At 35°C increased core and skin temperatures, increased rates of heat tolerance, and decreased tolerance times are observed.

CHEMICAL WARFARE CLOTHING

Soldiers tend to lose more body water and dehydrate more rapidly when wearing protective-clothing MOPP than when wearing their standard uniforms. Water discipline is an important factor and entails forced drinking in the absence of thirst, adequate rest for rehydrating, and potable water.[4]

REFERENCES—HEAT STRESS AND CHEMICAL WARFARE PROTECTION

1. Kobrick JL, Johnson RF, McMenemy DJ. Effects of atropine/2-PAM chloride, heat, and chemical protective clothing on visual performance. Aviat Space Environ Med 1990;61:722–830.
2. Kolka MA, Cadarette BJ. Heat exchange after cholinolytic and oxime therapy in protective clothing. Milit Med 1990;155:390–394.
3. Kobrick JL, Johnson RF, McMenemy DJ. Effects of nerve agent antidote and heat exposure in soldier performance in the BDU and MOPP-IV ensembles. Milit Med 1990;155:159–162.
4. Wyant KW, Walker JM. Urine specific gravity and other correlates of chemical warfare protective clothing. Milit Med 1987;152:649–652.

RECOVERY[1–3]

Patients who respond to treatment initially begin to show small skeletal muscle movements. They progress to spontaneous, random movements of the limbs and then a struggle against the ventilation. These may be alternating periods of spontaneous breathing and apnea. Weakness and obtundation may persist for 1 or more days. Miosis and subtle mental change may persist for weeks.

FUTURE STUDIES

A simple solution would be to inject extra acetylcholinesterase or butylcholinesterase to bind to a toxin, but the enzyme is a large molecule that would require massive injections to be effective. A gene-splicing antibody might be developed that could act in the bloodstream to "scavenge" a nerve toxin before it reaches acetylcholinesterase. Finally, reproducing copies of the reception of acetylcholinesterase that binds to nerve toxins may be a future development. Aerosolized atropine is absorbed systemically, but has not been subjected to clinical studies with nerve agent exposure.

REFERENCES

1. Fischetti M. Gas vaccine. Bioengineering immunication could shield against nerve gas. Sci Am April 1991;153:154.
2. Orma PS, Middleton RK. Aerosolized atropine as an antidote to nerve gas. Ann Pharmacother 1992;26:937–938.
3. Doctor BP, Blick DW, Recht KM, Castro CA, Hively HE, Murphy MP et al. Protection of rhesus monkey against soma toxicity by pretreatment with cholinesterase. Proc 4th Int Symp Protection against Chemical Warfare Agents, Stockholm, Sweden, 8–12 June, 1992; 335–340.

VESICANT AGENTS

Vesicant agents (Table 59–19) act on the eyes, mucous membranes, lungs, skin, and blood-forming organs. They incapacitate far more people than they kill.[1–33] Some vesicants have a faint odor; others are odorless. L and CX (Table 59–19) cause immediate pain on contact. Sulfur mustard and nitrogen mustards are insidious in action, with little or no pain at the time of exposure. Signs of injury may not appear for several hours.[1–3] Metabolites may be found in the urine.[34–36] Physical properties of the vesicants are delineated in U.S. Army Field Manual.[3–9]

HISTORY

Mustards got their name from their pungent mustard-garlic odor.[37–39] Mustard gas was first employed offensively by the German Army at Ypres, Belgium, on the evening of July 12, 1917.[37–39] This led to the use of nicknames: Yperite (French after Ypres), Lost (German after the name of two chemists Lommel and Steinkopf who were able to mass produce the substance), Yellow-Cross (after the markings on the mustard-containing shell cases) and HS (Hun Stuff).[37] From July, 1917, to the end of World War I British casualties from mustard gas amounted to at least 125,000 with about 1859 deaths.[37] In World War II no chemical agents were used, but from 1945 to 1948 large stockpiles of chemical weapons, including mustard gas, were dumped into the Baltic Sea. Corrosion weakened the containers, and the shells broke when they were brought on board fishing trawlers, leading to mustard-gas poisoning of 23 fishermen in 1984.[9] Finally, mustard gas appeared to have been used by Iraqi forces during the Iran-Iraq conflict.[10,11,17,18,22,23]

STRUCTURE AND CLASSIFICATION

Sulfur mustard consists of two ethyl groups bound together around an atom of sulfur. The terminal H bonds have been replaced by chlorine atoms.

MECHANISM OF ACTION (FIG. 59–6)[8]

Mustards are powerful alkylating agents and react with amino, thiol, carboxyl, hydroxyl, and primary phosphate groups.[2] As a result of its alkylating and electrophilic properties, mustard gas is able to change the structure of nucleic acids, cellular membranes, and proteins.[9] Mustard gas causes a cross-linking of the two complementary strands in the DNA molecule by a monofunctional alkylation of the nitrogenous bases. This cross-linking prevents the separation of the strands required for normal replications of the DNA molecule and so interferes with DNA syntheses and cellular division.[9] Mustard gas may induce long-term mutagenic and carcinogenic changes.[9,14,16]

Table 59–19
Vesicants or Blister Agents

Sulfur mustards	
HD	2,2′-di(chloroethyl) sulfide
Nitrogen mustards	
HN-1	2,2-dichlorotriethylamine
HN-2	2,2-dichloro-*N*-methyldiethylamine
HN-3	2,2,2-trichlorotriethylamine
Arsenicals	
MD	Methyldichloroarsine
PD	Phenyldichloroarsine
ED	Ethyldichloroarsine
L	Lewisite (dichloro [2-chlorovinyl] arsine)
Oximes	
CX	Phosgene oxime (dichloroformoxime)
Mixtures of mustards and arsenicals	
HL	Mustard-lewisite mix: 63% L and 37% HD, by weight
HT	Mustard-T(*bis*-[2-chloroethyl sulfide] monoxide) mix 60% HD and 40% T by weight—not in production

CLINICAL PRESENTATION

Mustard gas (either vapor or liquid) causes damage to the skin, eyes, respiratory system, and gastrointestinal tract, as well as having a general effect on the body similar to that of radioactive radiation.

Skin (Table 59–20)

Skin effects appear after a delay following exposure.

Eyes

Penetration of the gas causes no symptoms, but after a delay of 4 to 6 hours conjunctival irritation, lacrimation, photophobia, dryness, pain, blepharospasm, and corneal ulceration may develop. The periocular area is red and edematous. In severe cases blindness may occur. Recovery from a mild conjunctivitis may take 1 to 2 weeks, from a severe conjunctivitis, 2 to 5 weeks, and from mild corneal involvement, 2 to 3 months. A delayed keratopathy may develop decades later.[40]

Respiratory System

After a delay of 24 hours, inhalation of the gas produces initially hoarseness, which may progress to loss of voice.[1] A cough (worse at night) appears early and later becomes productive. Fever, dyspnea, and moist rhonchi and rales may develop. Bronchopneumonia frequently intervenes. Symptoms may persist for 1 or more years.

Gastrointestinal Tract

Ingestion of food or water contaminated by liquid mustard produces nausea and vomiting, pain, bloody diarrhea, and prostration resulting from dehydration.[7,9]

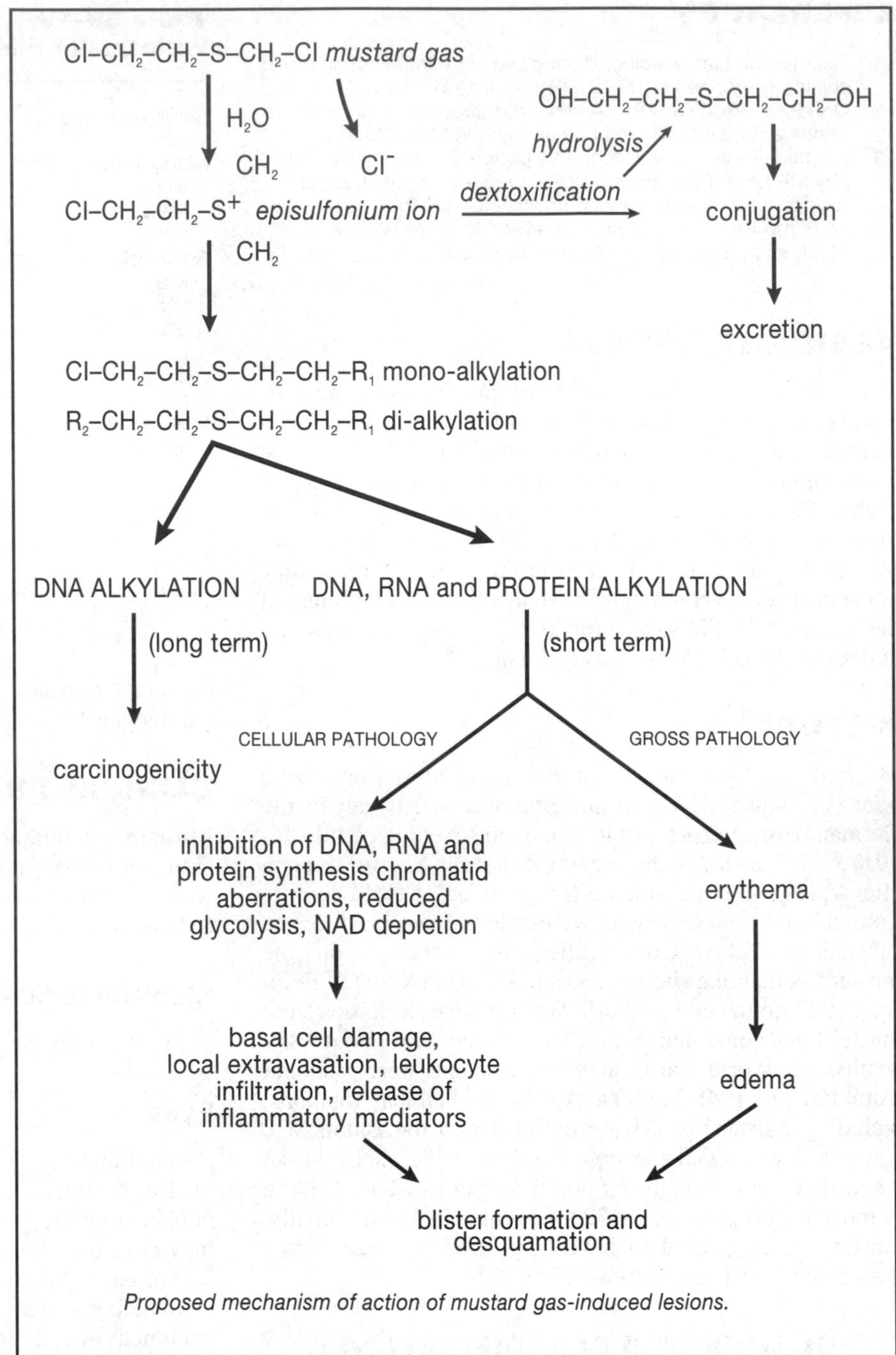

Figure 59–6 *Proposed mechanism of action of mustard gas-induced lesions.* (Adapted from Wormser U. Trends Pharmacol Sci 1991;12:164–167.)

Systemic Symptoms

Dizziness, anorexia, lethargy, and general malaise may follow exposure. Although hemoglobin values, leukocyte, differential and platelet counts, lactate dehydrogenase and aspartate aminotransferase, and serum creatinine levels are usually normal, fatalities may follow severe exposure and are largely due to respiratory complications.[8,18]

Long-Term Effects

Eye problems and recurrent bronchopneumonia may persist for many months. Exposure of human research subjects to the mustard gases during World War II has led to a number of long-term health effects identified by the Department of Veterans Affairs: asthma, chronic bronchitis, emphysema, chronic laryngitis, corneal opacities, chronic conjunctivitis, and ocular keratitis. The Institute of Medicine has cited other health problems for which a causal relationship with exposure to sulfur or nitrogen mustard exists, including respiratory cancer (especially nasopharyngeal, laryngeal and lung), skin cancer, pigmentation abnormalities of the skin, chronic skin ulceration and scar formation, recurrent ulcerative disease of the eye (including opacities), bone marrow depression, psychologic disorders, and sexual dysfunction (caused by scarring of the scrotum or penis).[41]

Table 59–20
Typical Development of Mustard Skin Lesion[a]

Effect	Time After Vapor Exposure (hr)[b]
Earliest appearance of erythema	1
Definite erythema	2–3
Raised erythema (edema)	8–12
Pinhead vesication	13–22
Vesicles coalescing into blisters	16–48
Maximum blisters or necrosis	42–72
Complete skin surface denudation	6–9 d
Removal of scab	20–28 d
Complete healing	22–29 d

[a]Adapted from Smith WJ, Dunn MA. Arch Dermatol 1991;127:1207–1213.
[b]Vapor cup exposure of forearm in healthy adult male volunteers at air temperature of 26° C with relative humidity of 51%. Exposure was 10 minutes with vapor cup containing 5- to 10-mg liquid mustard. Precise vapor concentration is not known.

Mutagenicity and Carcinogenicity

Sister chromatid exchanges, an indication of mutagenicity and carcinogenicity, were present in increased rates in the lymphocytes of fishermen exposed to leaky mustard-gas shells.[19] Follow-up studies of workers in British mustard-gas manufacture suggest an increase in the death rate from respiratory tract malignancies[16]; similarly an increased death rate from respiratory tract malignancies has been observed in Japanese and German mustard gas factories.[8,14] Only a marginal increase in lung cancer was found in exposed servicemen from the United States 46 years later.[42]

NITROGEN MUSTARD

In single exposures nitrogen mustards irritate the eyes in doses that do not significantly damage the skin or respiratory tract.

Respiratory Tract

Symptoms and signs may be similar to those following exposure to mustard gas. Residual effects may include a persistent cough and low-grade fever for a few weeks. Severe exposure may terminate in a fatal pneumonia.[1]

Gastrointestinal

In humans ingestion of 2 to 6 milligrams of a nitrogenmustard may result in nausea and vomiting. Animals develop severe hemorrhagic diarrhea.[1]

Systemic Effects

Nitrogen mustard exposure following absorption from the skin or respiratory or gastrointestinal tracts may exert profound effects on the hematopoietic and lymphoid tissue. Degenerative bone marrow changes may be detected within 12 hours and may progress to severe aplasia. There may be a transient leukocytosis for a few hours, followed by severe lymphopenia, granulocytopenia, thrombocytopenia, and a moderate anemia.

ARSENICAL VESICANTS

Arsenical vesicants are more dangerous as liquids than as vapors. The liquids will cause severe burns of the eyes and skin.

Skin

Stinging pain is usually felt in 10 to 20 seconds after contact with liquid arsenical vesicants. In a few minutes it becomes a deep, aching pain. In about 5 minutes a gray area of dead epithelium appears, resembling that seen in corrosive burns. The pain lessens in 48 to 72 hours. Erythema and blisters are similar to the other vesicants. If the arsenical vesicant burn is large and deep there may be considerable necrosis of tissue, gangrene, and slough.

Eyes

Liquid arsenical vesicants cause severe damage to the eye, including the cornea, iris, and conjunctivae; this may terminate in permanent residual damage or blindness.

Respiratory

Respiratory lesions are similar to those following mustard gas. Pulmonary edema and pleural effusion may be observed. There have been no human cases of poisoning by vapors of arsenical vesicants.

Systemic Effects

Pulmonary edema, diarrhea, restlessness, weakness, hypothermia, and hypotension has been observed in animals.

PHOSGENE OXIME (CX)

CX or dichloroformoxime has a disagreeable penetrating odor. It may be a liquid or a colorless, low-melting-point solid, soluble in water.[1,2]

CX is very irritating to the mucous membranes of the eyes and nose. Within 30 seconds, exposure to liquid or vapor can produce pain and skin necrosis at the site of contact. The original blanched area becomes brown in 24 hours, followed by eschar formation in 1 week; the eschar sloughs in about 3 weeks. Healing may be delayed for several months.

LABORATORY

Analytic Methods

A method for quantitation of exposure to mustard gas was used to test urine samples of Iranian patients, victims of an alleged mustard-gas attack in March 1984. The method analyzes thiodiglycol (2,2′-thiodiethanol) in the urine.[36] The method is sensitive to 1 ng/ml. Thiodiglycol values may also be obtained from analyses of the skin, a possible retrospective method for verifying exposure to mustard gas.[36] Unmetabolized mustard gas has been analyzed by a gas chromatography–mass spectrometry method.[34,35]

Soil, metal fragments, and wool collected from and in the vicinity of a chemical warfare spill in Northern Iraq analazyed by gas chromatography–mass spectrometry techniques (full scanning, selective ion monitoring, thermal desorption) have yielded *bis*-(2-chloroethyl) sulfide (mustard), thiodiglycol, and other sulfides and other volatile breakdown products, including 1,4-oxathiane, 1,4-dithiane, and ethene 1,1-thio-bis. Sulfur mustard may persist in the soil for weeks if the ambient temperature and rainfall are both low. 1,4,6-trinitrotoluene and tetryl suggest explosive components.[43]

Levels

Urine thiodiglycol levels found in Iranians ranged from 5 to 336 ng/ml in one study[36] and from 1 to 30 ng/ml in another.[33]

TREATMENT

Skin

Decontamination

1. If erythema has not appeared, known or likely skin areas of contamination may be decontaminated with immediate use of prewetted pad wipes (hydroxyethane 72%, phenol 10%, sodium hydroxide 5%, ammonia 0.2%, and water) and a pad impregnated with chloramine B. Cut away and discard hair contaminated with liquid mustard. If the above substances are not available, use 0.5% aqueous sodium hypochlorite solution for decontamination of the skin and hair. Wash off the decontaminating solutions within 3 to 4 minutes.
2. If erythema of the skin has appeared, soap and water is the best decontaminant.
3. Contaminated clothing should be promptly removed outside the treatment facility to prevent more severe burns and to lessen the vapor hazard to patients and attendants.

Mustard Erythema

If mild, no treatment is required. If pruritus exists, use topical steroid creams or compound calamine lotion (containing 1% each of phenol and menthol).

Mustard Blisters

If the blisters have been broken, remove the ragged roof; if not broken, drain under aseptic conditions. Clean the area with tap water or saline with application of petrolatum gauze when the areas are small. For large blisters apply ⅛-inch-thick layer of 10% mafenide acetate or silver sulfadiazine burn cream. Appropriate antibiotic drugs may be given locally or systemically as indicated.

Pain

Intense burning pain during skin healing may not be controlled by antihistamines or opioids. Considerable relief has been observed with the use of carbamazepine 200 mg three times daily.[3]

Eyes

Decontamination

Self-aid should be performed within 2 minutes after exposure. Sterile petroleum jelly is used to prevent the lid margins from sticking together.

Mustard Conjunctivitis

Mild lesions may require little treatment. A steroid antibiotic eye ointment can be applied. Ophthalmic ointment such as 5% boric acid ointment will provide lubrication and minimal antibacterial effects. If injuries are more severe, edema of the lids, photophobia, and blepharospasm may obstruct and alarm the patient. The lids may be gently forced open to provide assurance that the patient is not blinded. Pain is controlled by systemic narcotic analgesics. Severe photophobia and blepharospasm are treated with one drop of atropine sulfate solution (1%) instilled in the eye three times daily. To prevent infection a few drops of 15% solution of sodium sulfacetamide should be instilled every 4 hours. Other antibacterial ointments may be substituted. Do not bandage the eye; the lids should not be allowed to stick together. Keep the patient in a darkened room. Dark glasses or an eyeshade may be worn for photophobia.

Infected Mustard Burns of the Eye

If infection develops, start with several drops of 15% solution of sodium sulfacetamide every 2 hours. Take cultures. Apply specific antibacterial preparations. Irrigate to remove accumulated exudate. Do not use local anesthetics. Refer to an ophthalmologist.

Respiratory Tract

Mild respiratory tract injury with hoarseness and sore throat only usually requires no treatment. Cough may be relieved by codeine-containing cough syrups. Laryngitis and tracheitis may be treated symptomatically with steam or sterile cool mist inhalations. For more severe respiratory tract injury, hospitalize. Treat chemical pneumonitis initially with broad-spectrum antibiotics. Perform culture and sensitivity studies on sputum. Use appropriate specific antibiotics. Severely affected patients may need assisted ventilation and oxygen enriched air. Simple mouthwashes can be used for the oropharynx.[7]

Systemic Mustard Poisoning

Atropine subcutaneously (0.4 to 0.8 mg) may be useful in reducing gastrointestinal activity. Discomfort and restlessness may be treated with sedatives, but may also be a manifestation of hypovolemic shock from severe systemic injury. If severe systemic poisoning is present (vomiting, diarrhea, leukopenia, hemoconcentration, shock), maintain adequate nutritional status and replace loss of fluid and electrolytes. Monitor leukocytes and hemoglobin. For significant drops in the leukocyte count, isolation and appropriate antibiotics may be necessary. Sodium thiosulfate intravenously in a dose of 35 g (500 mg/kg) if given within 20 to 30 minutes of exposure may prevent or reduce damage from mustard. However, mustard gas is an alkylating agent that binds strongly to protein x, and it is unlikely that sodium thiosulfate will be very effective after a severe exposure.[44] A monoclonal antibody that binds sulfur mustard is under development.[45]

Most patients exposed to mustard gas recover completely. Only a small proportion will have long-term eye or lung damage.[3]

Nitrogen Mustard Poisoning
Skin

Liquid nitrogen mustards are absorbed through the skin slower than mustard gas. Decontamination should be performed within 2 to 3 hours of exposure even if erythema is already present and no liquid nitrogen mustard is visible on the skin.

Eyes

Treat as with mustard gas. Lesions and symptoms may be more severe than with mustard; frequent instillations of atropine may be required for pain due to spasms of ciliary and orbicular muscles.

Respiratory

Treat as for mustard gas exposure.

Systemic

Frequent hematologic evaluations (hematocrit, peripheral blood counts, and platelets) will be required. Vomiting and diarrhea will require intravenous fluids with electrolyte or volume expanders. Isolate against infection. Use antibiotics vigorously as indicated. Use sedatives, opiates, and atropine with care.

Arsenical Vesicants
Skin

If seen before actual vesication has occurred, dimercaprol (BAL) ointment should be tried, rubbed in with the fingers, allowed to remain at least 5 minutes, and then washed off with water. BAL may cause temporary stinging, itching, or urticarial wheals. Treatment of erythema, blisters, and denuded areas is similar to that for mustard lesions. For larger skin area exposure (over 20% of body surface area or less than 20% if deep lesion) hospitalization is required. Debride wound, treat with 10% mafenide acetate burn cream, or silver sulfadiazine burn cream.

Eyes

Treatment is largely symptomatic. Occlusive dressings or pressure on the globe should be avoided. Atropine sulfate ointment, sodium sulfacetamide solution, and sterile petrolatum may be applied as indicated.

Respiratory

Treatment will be similar to that following exposure to mustards.

Table 59–21
Treatment Protocol for British Anti-Lewisite (BAL) (2,3-Dimercapto-1-Propanol) (Dimercaprol)[a]

Antidote/Action	Dose	Overdose Symptoms, Management
Lifesaving in acute poisoning of arsenicals (except arsine) and solutions of organic Hg compounds. Also for chronic As or Au poisoning. Action by displacing the metal from its combination with sulfhydryl groups of enzyme proteins. Toxicity rating 4, very toxic (Probable oral lethal dose = 50–500 mg/kg or 1 teaspoon to 1 ounce for 150-lb [70-kg] person.)	IM into buttocks in dosage of 0.5 mL/25 lb body weight (commercial preparation of 10% BAL in peanut oil) up to maximum of 4.0 mL. Repeat in 4, 8, 12 hr. For severe cases, interval shortened to 2 hr.	Symptoms Consistent objective response in rise in systolic and diastolic blood pressure plus tachycardia (rapid heartbeat). Nausea and sometimes vomiting Headache Burning sensation of lips, mouth Feeling of constriction in throat, chest, hands Conjunctivitis, tearing, salivation Hand tingling Burning sensation in penis Sweating forehead and hands Abdominal pain Tremors Lower back pain Anxiety, weakness, and restlessness Tachycardia (rapid heartbeat) and elevated arterial blood pressure Persistent fever in children Occasional painful sterile abscesses at injection sites Coma and convulsions at high dose (in children, this occurs at 10, 25, and 40.5 mg/kg) (recovery prompt) Management Symptoms usually subside in 30–90 min; IM use of 1:100 solution epinephrine (HCl (0.1 to 0.5 mL) or oral ephedrine sulfate (25–50 mg)

[a]Adapted from Munro NB et al. Environ Health Perspect 1990;89:205–215.

Systemic Effects

Systemic treatment is indicated for the following: cough with dyspnea and frothy sputum, and signs of pulmonary edema; or skin covering, skin burn the size of the palm of the hand not decontaminated within 15 minutes; skin contamination by a liquid arsenical vesicant covering 5% or more of body surface with signs of grey or dead-white blanching of skin or erythema developing within 30 minutes. Treatment includes local dimercaprol (BAL) ointment and intramuscular injection of BAL in oil (10%) (Table 59–21) (see Metal and Antidote chapter—Use of BAL). Treat shock supportively.

PHOSGENE OXIME (CX)

Treatment is symptomatic and supportive. If possible flood the contaminated area as soon as possible with copious amounts of water. (See Mustard gas decontamination.)

REFERENCES—VESICANT AGENTS

1. Treatment of chemical agent casualties and conventional military chemical injuries. Field Manual. Army FM 8-285, Navy Navmed P-5041, Air Force AFM 160-11. Departments of the Army, the Navy and the Air Force. February 1990.
2. Medical Manual of Defence Against Chemical Agents. JSP 312, Ministry of Defence. D/Med (F +S) (2)/10/11. London: Her Majesty's Stationery Office, 1987.
3. Murray VSG, Volans GN. Management of injuries due to chemical weapons. Most patients exposed to mustard gas recover completely. Br Med J 1991;302:129–130.
4. Munro NB, Watson AP, Ambrose KR, Griffin DG. Treating exposure to chemical warfare agents: implications for health care providers and community emergency planning. Environ Health Perspect 1990;89:205–215.
5. Sidell FR. What to do in case of an unthinkable chemical warfare attack or accident. Postgrad Med 1990;88:70–84.
6. Shalit I. Chemical warfare and disasters: medical organization and treatment. In: Reis ND, Dolve E, eds. Manual of disaster medicine, civilian and military. Berlin: Springer Verlag, 1989; pp. 113–123.
7. Newman-Taylor AJ, Marris AJR. Experience with mustard gas casualties. Lancet 1991;337:242.
8. Wormser U. Toxicology of mustard gas. Trends Pharmaceut Sci 1991;12:164–167.
9. Aasted A, Darre E, Wolf HC. Mustard gas: clinical, toxicological and mutagenic aspects based on modern experience. Ann Plastic Surg 1987;19:330–333.
10. Balali-Mood M. Sulfur mustard poisoning in the Iran-Iraq War. Clin Pharmacol Ther 1990;47:183–184.
11. Willems JL. Clinical management of mustard gas casualties. Ann Med Mitt Belg 1989;3(Suppl 1):1–61.
12. Papirmeister B, Feister AJ, Robinson SI, Ford RD. Medical defense against mustard gas: toxic mechanisms and pharmacological implications. Boca Raton, FL: CRC Press, 1991; pp. 1–42.
13. Watson AP, Jones TD, Griffin GD. Sulfur mustard as a carcinogen: application of relative potency analyses to the chemical warfare agents H, HD and HT. Regul Toxicol Pharmacol 1989;10:1–25.
14. Yanagida J, Hozawa S, Ishioka S, Maeda H, Takahashi K, Oyana T et al. Somatic mutation in peripheral lymphocytes of former workers at the Okunojima poison gas factory. Jpn J Cancer Res 1988;79:1276–1286.
15. Requena L, Requena C, Sanchez M, Jaqueti G, Aguilar A, Sanchez-Yus E, Hernandez-Moro B. Chemical warfare. Cutaneous lesions from mustard gas. J Am Acad Dermatol 1988;19:529–536.
16. Easton DF, Peto J, Doll R. Cancers of the respiratory tract in mustard gas workers. Br J Indust Med 1988;45:652–659.
17. Somani SM, Babu SR. Toxicodynamics of sulfur mustard. Int J Clin Pharmacol Ther Toxicol 1989;27:419–435.
18. Sohrabpour H. Observation and clinical manifestations of patients injured with mustard gas. Med J Islamic Rep of Iran 1987;1:32–37.
19. Goldman M, Jacre JC. Lewisite. Its chemistry, toxicology and biological effects. Rev Environ Contam Toxicol 1989;110: 76–114.
20. Papirmeister B, Gross CL, Meier HL, Petrall JP, Johnson JB. Molecular basis for mustard induced vesication. Fund Appl Toxicol 1985;5:S134–S149.
21. Wulf HC, Aasted A, Darre E, Niebuhr E. Sister chromatid exchanges in fishermen exposed to leaking mustard gas shells. Lancet 1985;1:690–691.
22. Heyndrickx B, ed. Proceedings of the Second World Congress. New Compounds in Biological and Chemical Warfare: Toxicological Evaluation. Industrial Chemical Disasters. Civil Protection and Treatment. Ghent, The Internat Assoc For Toxicol. 23rd Eur Internat Mtg Terrorism: Analysis and Detection of Explosives, August 24–27, 1986. (See references 23 through 34.)
23. Balali-Mood M, Navaeian. Clinical paraclinical findings in 233 patients with sulfur mustard poisoning. pp. 464–473.
24. Crombez R. Medical use of mustard gas derivatives. A review. p. 474.
25. Balali-Mood M, Farhoodi M, Panjvani FK. Report of three fatal cases of war gas poisoning. pp. 475–482.
26. Dhont S, Cordonnier J, Vanheule A, Heyndrickx A. Evolution of serum and erythrocyte magnesium leads in patients attacked by the chemical warfare agent mustard gas (Yperite). pp. 483–488.
27. Balali-Mood M. First report of delayed toxic effects of Yperite poisoning in Iranian fighters. pp. 489–495.
28. Colardyn F, de Keyser K, Vogelaers D, Vandenbogaende J. The clinics and therapy of victims of war gases. pp. 506–510.
29. Vossaert K, Geerts ML, de Bersaques J, Kint A. Dermatological aspects of intoxication by mustard gas. pp. 511–513.
30. Neyrick B, Wauters A, Heyndrickx A. Treatment of intoxicated soldiers by war gases. pp. 539–541.
31. Coppens M, Roels H, Van den Heede M, Heyndrickx A. Clinical history and autopsy observations associated with the toxicological findings in an Iranian soldier exposed to Yperite (mustard gas). pp. 542–552.
32. Heyndrickx B. Report and conclusion of the biological samples of men intoxicated by war gases sent to the Department of Toxicology of the State University of Ghent for toxicological investigation. pp. 553–582.
33. Heyndrickx A, Van den Heede M. The toxicological analysis of chemical warfare agents in samples originating from Iranian soldiers. pp. 598–618.
34. Drasch G, Kretschmer E, Kauert G, Meyer L. Yperite concentrations in the tissues of a victim of a vesicant exposure. pp. 592–597.
35. Vycudilik W. Detection of bis(2-chlorethyl) sulfide lyperite in urine by high resolution gas chromatography/mass spectrometry. Forensic Sci Int 1987;35:67–71.
36. Wils ERJ, Hulst AG, Van Laar J. Analysis of thiodiglycol in urine of victims of an alleged attack with mustard gas. II. J Anal Toxicol 1988;12:15–19.
37. Harris R, Paxman J. A higher form of killing. The secret story of chemical and biological warfare. New York: Hill & Want, 1982; p. 274.
38. Douglass JD Jr, Livingstone NC. America the vulnerable. The threat of chemical/biological warfare. The new shape of terrorism and conflict. Lexington, MA: Lexington Books, 1987; p. 204.
39. Compton JAF. Military Chemical and Biological Agents. Chemical and Toxicological Properties. Caldwell, NJ: The Telford Press, 1987; p. 458.
40. Blodi FC. Mustard gas keratopathy. Internat Ophthal Clin 1971;11:1–13.
41. Pechura CM, Rall DP, ed. Veterans at risk. The health effects of mustard gas and lewisite. Committee to survey the health effects of mustard gas and lewisite. Institute of Medicine. Washington, DC: National Academy Press, 1993.

42. Norman JE Jr. Lung cancer mortality in World War I veterans with mustard-gas injury: 1919–1965. JNCI 1975;54:311–317.
43. Hay A, Roberts G. The use of poison gas against the Iraqi Kurds: analysis of bomb fragments, soil and wool samples. JAMA 1990;263:1065–1066.
44. Maynard RL, Meredith TJ, Marren TC, Vale JA. Management of chemical warfare injuries. Lancet 1991;337:122.
45. Lieske CN, Klopcic RS, Gross CL, Clark JH, Dolzine TW, Logan TP et al. Development of an antibody that binds sulfur mustard. Immunol Lett 1992;31:117–122.

BLOOD AGENTS (CYANOGENS)

The use of cyanide agents was initiated by the French in 1916 with the employment of shells filled with hydrogen cyanide (AC).[1,2] Cyanide had extreme volatility; its vapor was lighter than air. Therefore it was almost impossible to establish a lethal concentration in the field by this means of delivery. To overcome this problem, cyanogen chloride and cyanogen bromide were produced; these vapors were heavier than air. Table 59–22 lists the cyanogens of this group.[1–4]

Blood agents produce their effects by interfering with oxygen utilization at the cellular level. Inhalation is the usual route of entry. Cyanogen chloride (CK) also has a choking effect.[3]

PROTECTION

A standard protective mask with a fresh filter gives adequate protection against field concentrations of a blood agent vapor. A protective overgarment and mask are needed when exposed to or handling AC.

PATHOLOGY

AC

The clinical picture of hydrogen cyanide poisoning is discussed in the Airborne chapter.

CK

CK has systemic effects similar to AC, but it also has local irritant effects on the eyes, upper respiratory tract, and lungs.[3] It may induce severe inflammatory changes in the bronchioles and congestion and edema in the lungs.

SYMPTOMS AND SIGNS

AC—Hydrogen Cyanide

Typically, either death occurs rapidly or recovery takes place within a few minutes after removal from the toxic atmosphere. With high concentrations there is increased depth of respiration within a few seconds, violent seizures after 20 to 30 seconds, cessation of regular respiration within 1 minute, occasional shallow gasps, and asystole within a few minutes.

Table 59–22
Cyanogens

AC:	Hydrogen Cyanide
CR:	Cyanogen chloride (CNCl)
SA:	Arsine (also considered a blood agent)

With moderate exposure, vertigo, nausea, and headache appear early and are followed by seizures and coma. Long exposure to low concentrations may result in tissue anoxia and central nervous system damage. Coma and seizures may follow and persist for hours or days. There is residual damage as evidenced by irrationality, altered reflexes, and ataxia that may last for a few weeks or longer. Mild exposure may produce headache, vertigo, and nausea, but recovery is complete.

CK—Cyanogen Chloride

Signs and symptoms are a combination of those produced by AC and a lung irritant. Exposure may be followed by immediate intense irritation of the nose, throat and eyes, with coughing, tightness in the chest, and lacrimation. There may be dizziness and dyspnea. Unconsciousness, failing respiration, and death may supervene in a few minutes. Seizures, retching, involuntary urination, and defecation may occur. Pulmonary edema may develop.

DIAGNOSIS

AC

The history, odor (if detected), rapid onset of symptoms, and pink skin color suggest the diagnosis.

CK

Intense irritation and rapid onset of symptoms suggest the diagnosis.

Note: High concentrations of cyanide vapor and solutions of cyanide salts are absorbed through the skin.[1]

TREATMENT

1. Put on a mask immediately.
2. Assist ventilation with oxygen.
3. Remove from the contaminated environment.
4. Use nitrites and sodium thiosulfate as for cyanide poisoning: 10 mL 3% (300 mg) sodium nitrite IV over 3 minutes, 50 mL 25% (12.5 g) sodium thiosulfate IV over 10 minutes. A slight degree of cyanosis may indicate that the desired methemoglobin is forming.
5. The lung irritant effects of cyanogen chloride are treated as with the choking agents (e.g., phosgene).
6. Do not use amyl nitrite under an oxygen mask because of the risk of an explosion.[5]
7. Although not used in the United States, other agents such as dicobalt edetate (U.K.) and dimethylaminophenol (Germany) have been used (see Antidotes):
   a. Dicobalt edetate (toxic to liver and kidneys) directly fixes the cyanide ion: 300 mg in 20 mg of solution (kelocyanor) given IV. Repeat PRN. Follow with IV sodium thiosulfate 25 g in 50% solution slowly.
   b. Dimethylaminophenol (DMAP), a methemoglobin former: 250 mg in 5 mL IV. Repeat PRN. Follow by sodium thiosulfate 25 g in a 50% solution. (May induce a high methemoglobin value.)
8. Studies in cyanide-poisoned beagle dogs suggest that dimethylaminophenol 5 mg/kg and hydroxylamine hydrochloride 50 mg/kg were the only drugs able to reverse the lethal effects of cyanide poisoning when

administered by the intramuscular route. Sodium nitrite, amyl nitrite, and sodium thiosulfate do not appear to be effective by the intramuscular route. Further studies will be indicated to pursue this finding for military or civilian use.[5]

REFERENCES—BLOOD AGENTS (CYANOGENS)

1. Medical Manual of Defense Against Chemical Agents. JSP 312. Ministry of Defense. London: Her Majesty's Stationery Office, 1987; pp. 8-1 to 8-5.
2. Harris R, Paxman J. A higher form of killing. The secret story of chemical and biological warfare. New York: Hill & Wang, 1982.
3. Treatment of Chemical Agent Casualties and Conventional Military Chemical Injuries. Field Manual Army FM-8-285; Navy Navmed P-5041; Air Force AFM 160-11. Departments of the Army, the Navy and the Air Force. February 1990; pp. 6-1 to 6-2.
4. Compton JAF. Military chemical and biological agents. Chemical and toxicological properties. Caldwell, NJ: Telford Press, 1987; pp. 87–110.
5. Vick JA, Froehlich H. Treatment of cyanide poisoning. Milit Med 1991;156:330–339.

INCAPACITATING AGENTS

Incapacitating agents are substances that impair the subject's ability to perform duties without causing serious risk of death or permanent injury.[1] These agents are highly potent, logistically feasible, produce their effects mainly by altering or disrupting the higher regulatory activity of the central nervous system, and have a duration of effect for hours or days. This group does not include lethal agents in sublethal doses, blister agents, or riot control agents.[2] (See Lacrimators—Airborne chapter.)

PSYCHOTOMIMETIC AGENTS

Many drugs act on the central nervous system to produce incapacitation. Few are potent or safe, or possess the necessary physical and chemical properties to make them useful as potential chemical agents. Of these few, BZ, 3-quinuclidinyl benzilate (an atropine-like drug), and LSD[25] (lysergic acid diethylamide) (see chapter) are of interest.[3]

BZ

BZ appears to block the action of acetylcholine both peripherally and centrally, but unlike atropine it produces predominantly central rather than peripheral effects.[1] High doses produce a toxic delirium that renders the individual unable to perform any task.

BZ is a crystalline solid at normal temperatures, and there is no device available to detect it. Prevention is best accomplished with a protective mask.

Clinical Presentation

One to two hours after exposure BZ produces dilation of the pupils, dry mouth, and increased heart rate, which are later followed by ataxia and drowsiness. In about 6 or 7 hours these symptoms diminish to be replaced by a confused mental state with delusions, hallucinations, and aimless behavior that may last for several days. The mydriasis may last for 3 days.

Treatment

Usually symptomatic treatment will be all that is necessary. Remove dangerous objects or anything that may be swallowed. Heat stroke may occur in tropical climates. Maintain fluid intake. Reserve physostigmine use (see Cyclic Antidepressant chapter).

CANNABINOLS AND PHENOTHIAZINE-LIKE COMPOUNDS[1–4]

These act primarily as CNS depressants, which sedate and destroy motivation rather than disrupt the ability to think. They are not likely to be used in chemical warfare.

Treatment

d-Amphetamine (15 mg) can antagonize the sedation and indifference induced by marijuana-like substances.

LYSERGIC ACID DIETHYLAMIDE (LSD)

LSD is a solid at normal temperatures and is soluble in water. Since it is a difficult agent to disseminate, it most likely will be used in a clandestine manner. There is no device capable of detecting this agent in the field. Doses of 50 μg per person are capable of inducing a psychotic state. Nausea, confusion, delusions, and hallucinations are usually followed by complete relief within 12 hours.

Treatment

LSD is an indole that sometimes resembles a stimulant in its effects (anxiety, erratic behavior). Diazepam 10 to 20 mg, intravenously or intramuscularly, or sodium amytal 200 to 400 mg, intravenously, may be used to sedate the patient until spontaneous recovery results. Chlorpromazine 50 to 100 mg may be used. Effectiveness of treatment may be only partial until recovery occurs spontaneously.

OTHER DRUGS

Other psychomimetic drugs or chemicals (mescaline, psilocybin, phencyclidine [PCP]) have been considered as incapacitating agents.[5]

REFERENCES—INCAPACITATING AGENTS

1. Medical Manual of Defence Against Chemical Agents. Ministry of Defense JSP 312. London: Her Majesty's Stationery Office, 1987; pp. 7-1 to 7-4.
2. Treatment of Chemical Agent Casualties and Conventional Military Chemical Injuries. Army FM 8-285; Navy Navmed P-5041, Air Force AFM 160-11. Departments of the Army, the Navy, and the Air Force, February 1990; pp. 3-1 to 3-4.
3. Corupton JAF. Military chemical and biological agents. Clinical and toxicology properties. Caldwell, NJ: Telford Press; pp. 253–335.

4. Harris R, Paxman J. A higher form of killing. The secret study of chemical and biological warfare. New York: Hill & Wang, 1982; pp. 187–188, 206–210.
5. Douglass JD Jr, Livingston NC. America the vulnerable. The threat of chemical/biological warfare. Lexington, MA: Lexington Books, 1987. pp. 4–5.

LUNG-DAMAGING AGENTS (CHOKING AGENTS)

Chemicals that primarily attack lung tissue causing pulmonary edema are known as lung-damaging or choking agents.[1] They include the following:

CG: Phosgene (carbonyl chloride)
DP: Diphosgene (trichloromethyl chloroformate)
CL: Chlorine
PS: Chloropicrin

The best known of these agents is phosgene (CG). Agents of this group irritate the bronchi, trachea, larynx, pharynx, and nose, and this, together with acute pulmonary edema, contributes to the sensation of choking.[2–10]

Chlorine is also discussed in the Airborne chapter.

CHLOROPICRIN[11]

Chloropicrin (CCl_3NO_2) is a colorless, slightly oily liquid used as a fumigant for cereals and grains, a soil insecticide, and a chemical warfare agent. It produces a severe irritation to the eyes, mucous membranes, and lungs. A lethal exposure in humans is about 119 ppm for 30 minutes with death resulting from pulmonary edema. Residual spray may induce a dry cough.

Exposure Limits[12]

Industrial exposure limits in the United States are as follows:

	NIOSH/OSHA—TWA
Chlorine	0.15 ppm (1.5 mg/m^3)
Chloropicrin	0.1 ppm (0.7 mg/m^3)
Phosgene	0.1 ppm (0.4 mg/m^3)

History

Chlorine (CL) was the first chemical agent used as an offensive military weapon, and it initiated the age of chemical warfare on April 22, 1915, when the German army released a greenish yellow cloud and caused the death of 5000 Allied soldiers and the wounding of 10,000 more.[4] On December 22, 1915, at Ypres, the German army initiated the second major chemical, phosgene (CG), and this caused the gassing of 1069 men with 116 deaths from acute pulmonary edema. Over 80% of all chemical agent fatalities in World War I were from phosgene.[5] Diphosgene (DP), basically phosgene with chloroform grafted onto it, was created after World War I as an attempt to improve on phosgene, but by the 1930s was superseded by the nerve agents.[5] Chloropicrin (PS) was used in World War I because of its irritant action on skin and mucous membranes.[2]

PHOSGENE (CG) AND DIPHOSGENE

Physical Properties

Phosgene (carbonyl chloride) is a colorless gas at room temperature and atmospheric pressure. It has an odor of newly cut hay. The vapor is heavier than air and may remain in trenches, valleys, and woods for some time, depending on atmospheric conditions.

Protection

A standard field protective mask or a gas-particulate filter gives adequate protection against lung-damaging agents.

Doses:

1. Exposure doses below 25 ppm/min can be regarded as harmless.
2. Exposure of patients to mild doses of 50 to 150 ppm/min should receive steroids by inhalation and systemically. They should be observed for at least 8 hours and if chest x-rays are normal, they can be discharged. If no x-ray is available, continue observation for 24 hours.
3. Doses over 150 ppm/min of phosgene will induce clinical pulmonary edema. Over 300 ppm/min they are life endangering.[7–9]

MECHANISM OF ACTION

Respiratory Tract

Damage to the bronchiolar epithelium, development of patchy areas of emphysema, partial atelectasis, and edema of the perivascular connective tissue precede massive pulmonary edema.[2,3] The trachea and bronchi are usually normal in appearance following phosgene exposure. This contrasts with the findings in chlorine and chloropicrin poisoning in which both structures may show serious damage to the epithelial lining with desquamation.

CLINICAL PRESENTATION

Initial Period

Initially there may be a mild irritation of the eyes and throat with some coughing, choking, feeling of tightness in the chest, nausea and occasional vomiting, headache, and lacrimation.

Latent Period

A latent period follows during which the patient may be relatively symptom free without chest signs, lasting from 30 minutes to 48 hours.

Pulmonary Edema

Thereafter, in those developing severe pulmonary damage, progressive pulmonary edema develops rapidly with shallow rapid respiration, cyanosis, and a painful paroxysmal cough producing copious amounts of frothy white or yellowish liquid. Examination of the chest reveals increasing diminution of breath sounds with rales and rhonchi throughout the lung fields. Distress, apprehension, dyspnea, and cyanosis increase. Hypovolemia, hypoxia, and circulatory failure may then lead to death.

An x-ray of the chest during approximately half of the clinical latent period may indicate incipient toxic pulmonary edema much earlier than clinical signs and symptoms.[7] Phosgene indicator badges are used at Bayer/Germany.[7]

Diagnosis

Irritation of the nose and throat by CG may be mistaken for upper respiratory tract infection. Difficulty in breathing and complaints of tightness of the chest may suggest nerve-agent poisoning or an acute asthmatic attack. The noncardiac pulmonary edema may be confused with the edema associated with heart failure. Diagnosis depends on a definite history of exposure to CG. Arterial blood gases will confirm clinical status.

Early diagnosis of industrial phosgene overexposure is different. The sense of smell generally fails in phosgene overexposure. Significant changes in the hemoglobin, hematocrit, PaO_2, $PaCO_2$, and pH cannot be observed until near the end of the clinical latent period.[4]

TREATMENT

Supportive Therapy

1. Rest and warmth: Rest during the latent stage is very important since any activity between exposure and the onset of pulmonary symptoms and/or signs will greatly increase the likelihood of death.
2. Cough: Use codeine phosphate (30 to 60 mg).
3. Oxygen: Humidified if possible. Early use of positive airway pressure (intermittent positive pressure breathing (IPPB), positive end-expiratory pressure (PEEP), mask ("PEEP mask"), or, if necessary, intubation with or without a ventilator may delay or minimize the pulmonary edema and reduce hypoxemia.
4. Sedation: Withhold sedatives until adequate oxygenation is assured and facilities for possible respiratory assistance are available. Do *not* use atropine, barbiturates, analeptics, or antihistamines.
5. Antibiotics: Reserve for acquired bacterial bronchitis or pneumonitis. Do not use prophylactically.
6. Diuretics are largely ineffective against toxic pulmonary edema,[8,9] but they may be helpful in combination with PEEP by reducing interstitial edema.

Specific[2,3]

Steroids used soon (within 15 minutes preferably) after exposure may lessen the severity of the edema. Once preliminary edema has evolved, steroids are much less effective. The initial dose is five times that conventionally used in asthma, followed by about half the dose for 12 hours, and then standard asthma dosages for the subsequent 72 hours until the risk of pulmonary edema has passed.

Use: Betamethasone valerate, beclomethasone dipropionate, or dexamethasone sodium phosphate.

Procedures for Steroid Administration

1. Inhalation (using dexamethasone sodium phosphate): Four puffs are inhaled at once, followed by one puff every 3 minutes until any sense of irritation is overcome. Then five puffs are inhaled every 15 minutes until the entire contents of one standard inhaler are finished. Then one puff inhaled every hour by day, and five puffs every 15 minutes until 30 puffs are reached in preparation for sleep. Repeat this regimen every day for at least 5 days, or longer if there are any abnormalities, including indications of pulmonary edema or infiltrates on the chest x-ray after which treatment may be withdrawn. If recovery is slow, reduce the dose to six puffs a day until recovery is complete.
2. If beclomethasone dipropionate or betamethasone dipropionate is used, treat as soon as possible with an inhalation of 10 puffs of the steroid from an inhaler. Five puffs are given each hour for the next 10 hours. Then one puff hourly for 24 hours for at least 5 days. Systemic therapy: start with IV 20 mg of betamethasone or an equivalent; repeat IV or IM every 6 hours for 24 hours, then diminish over 5 days.
3. *Systemic Steroids*[2,3]
   Start also as soon as possible after exposure with 2 g intravenously or intramuscularly of methyl prednisolone or an equivalent, repeated after 6 and after 12 hours. Thereafter give the dose every 12 hours for 1 to 5 days dependent on the same criteria as for the steroid inhaler therapy. Antibiotic and antifungal therapy may be indicated to prevent infection and fungal suprainfections. An alternate regimen for systemic treatment includes the following:

Day 1	1000 mg prednisolone IV
Days 2 and 3	800 mg prednisolone IV
Days 4 and 5	700 mg prednisolone IV
Day 6	Begin to reduce dosage quickly provided that the chest x-ray remains clear

Adrenaline may be given in the acute stage of bronchial spasm, and oxygen may be necessary. Expectorants may be used.

Antidote

There is no antidote against phosgene.

Pepper Gas Spray

The main ingredient of pepper gas spray units is oleoresin capsicum. There have been isolated reports of severe pulmonary injury[13] and death following its use.[14] Further clinically controlled data are indicated.

LACRIMATING AGENTS

Riot control agents are aerosol-dispersed chemicals that produce eye, nose, mouth, skin, and respiratory tract irritation. Most of these symptoms resolve by 30 minutes postexposure. Both ocular and mucous membrane symptoms may persist for 24 hours. The three currently used agents are 1-chloroacetophenone (CN), 2-chlorobenzylidenemalononitrile (CS), and dibenz (b, fl-1,4-oxazepine) (CR). Serious systemic toxicity is rare.

ACUTE TOXIC DOSAGE

These lacrimators are relatively nontoxic except when dispersed in a confined, nonventilated space.

1-CHLOROACETOPHENONE

Tear gas is the most toxic lacrimator and has accounted for at least five deaths resulting from pulmonary injury and/or asphyxia.[15,16]

2-CHLOROBENZYLIDENEMALONONITRILE

This compound is a 10-times-more-potent lacrimator than 1-chloroacetophenone and is less toxic.

DIBENZ[B,FL]-1,4-OXAZEPINE

This compound is the most potent lacrimator with the least systemic toxicity.

CLINICAL PRESENTATION

Upper Respiratory Tract

Rhinorrhea, nasal irritation and congestion, bronchorrhea, sore throat, cough, sneezing, unpleasant taste, and burning of the mouth occur immediately after exposure and rapidly resolve within minutes.

Lungs

Prolonged concentrated exposures can produce an acute laryngeotracheobronchitis.[17]

Skin

Burning and sometimes erythema occur after exposure to lacrimators.

LABORATORY

A significant leukocytosis (i.e., over 20,000 WBC/cm^3 may occur after exposure to 1-chloroacetophenone and can last for several days.[17,18]

TREATMENT

Stabilization

The immediate priority is removal from exposure and establishment of an airway. Patients with respiratory distress should receive oxygen, an evaluation of airway patency and ventilation, an intravenous line, and cardiac monitoring. Obtain arterial blood gases and chest x-rays.

Decontamination

Remove all contaminated clothing, and seal it in a plastic bag. Medical personnel should use disposal rubber gloves when handling contaminated clothes. The eyes should be irrigated copiously with saline for 15 to 20 minutes. Contaminated skin should be washed thoroughly with mild liquid soap and water. Only a saline irrigation should be used over vesiculated skin.

Supportive Care

The eyes should be examined for corneal abrasions and treated with oral analgesics, topical antibiotics (sulfacetamide), and mydriatics as needed. Vesiculated skin is treated like a second-degree chemical burn. Patients with respiratory distress should be admitted if symptoms persist several hours. These patients should be observed for the development of bronchospasm and pneumonia (e.g., serial chest x-rays, arterial blood gases). Prophylactic antibiotics and steroids probably are not effective. Humidified oxygen may provide symptomatic relief.

REFERENCES—LUNG-DAMAGING AGENTS (CHOKING AGENTS)

1. Potential Military Chemical/Biological Agents and Compounds. Army Field Manual No. 3-9. Washington DC: December 12, 1990; pp. 14–17, 46–47, 71.
2. Medical Manual of Defense Against Chemical Agents. JSP 312. Ministry of Defense. London: Her Majesty's Stationery Office, 1987; pp. 5-1 to 5-4.
3. Treatment of Chemical Agent Casualties and Conventional Military Chemical Injuries. Field Manual. Army FM 8-285, Navy Navmed P-5041, Air Force AFM 160-11. Departments of the Army, the Navy, and the Air Force, February 1990; pp. 5-1 to 5-3.
4. Harris C, Paxman J. A higher form of killing. The secret story of chemical and biological warfare. New York: Hill & Want, 1982; pp. 1–3, 17–20.
5. Compton JAF. Military chemical and biological agents. Chemical and toxicological properties. Caldwell, NJ: Telford Press, 1987; pp. 111–134.
6. Wang Y-T, Lee LKH, Poh S-C. Phosgene poisoning from a smoke grenade. Eur J Respir Dis 1987;70:126–128.
7. Diller WF. Early diagnosis of phosgene overexposure. Toxicol Indust Health 1985;1:73–80.
8. Diller WF: Therapeutic strategy in phosgene poisoning. Toxicol Ind Health 1985;1:93–99.
9. Diller WF, Zantz R. A literature review: therapy for phosgene poisoning. Toxicol Ind Health 1985;1:117–128.
10. Sjogren B, Plato N, Alexandersson R, Eklund A, Falkenberg C. Pulmonary reactions caused by welding-induced decomposed trichlorethylene. Chest 1991;99:237–238.
11. Proctor NH, Hughes JP, Fischman ML. Chemical hazards of the workplace. 2nd ed. New York: Van Nostrand Rheinhold, 1989; p. 149.
12. NIOSH. Pocket Guide to Chemical Hazards. U.S. Department of Health and Human Services. June 1990.
13. Krolikowski FJ. Oleo capsicum (O.C.): the need for careful evaluation. Am J Forensic Med Pathol 1994;15:267.
14. Wiley J, Billmire D, Farina P, Freedman S, Henretig F, Panitch H et al. Severe pulmonary injury in an infant after pepper gas self defense spray exposure. Clin Toxicol 1995;33:475–486 (abstract 86).
15. Stein AA, Kirwan WE. Chloroacetophenone (tear gas) poisoning. A clinico-pathologic report. J Forensic Sci 1964;9:374–382.

16. Chapman AJ, White C. Death resulting from lacrimatory agents. J Forensic Sci 1978;23:527–530.
17. Thorburn KM. Injuries after use of the lacrimatory agent chloroacetophenone in a confined space. Arch Environ Health 1982;37:182–186.
18. Park S, Giammonia ST. Toxic effects of tear gas on an infant following prolonged exposure. Am J Dis Child 1972;123: 245–246.

SUGGESTED READINGS—CHEMICAL WARFARE

1. Medical Management of Chemical Casualties Course. Office of the Surgeon General and US Army Medical Research Institute of Chemical Defense, January 1992.
2. Field Manual. Treatment of Chemical Agent Casualties and Conventional Military Chemical Injuries. Army FM 8-285, Navy Navmed P-4051, Air Force AFM 160-11. Departments of the Army, the Navy and the Air Force, February 1990.
3. Potential Military Chemical/Biological Agents and Compounds. FM 3-9, NAVFAC P-467, AFR 355-7, Headquarters, Departments of the Army, Navy and Air Force, December 12, 1990.
4. Douglass JD Jr, Livingstone NC. America the vulnerable. The threat of chemical/biological warfare. Lexington, MA: Lexington Books, 1987; pp. 204.
5. Harris R, Paxman J. A higher form of killing. The secret story of chemical and biological warfare. New York: Hill & Wand, 1982; pp. 274.
6. Compton JAF. Military chemical and biological agents. Chemical and toxicological properties. Caldwell, NJ: Telford Press, September 1987, pp. 458.
7. Proc 4th Internat Symp on Protection against Chemical Warfare Agents. Stockholm, Sweden: 8–12 June, 1992. National Defence Research Establishment. Department of NBC Defence S-901. 82 Umea, Sweden.
8. Somani SM, ed. Chemical warfare agents. San Diego: Academic Press, 1992; pp. 443.
9. Medical Manual of Defence Against Chemical Agents. JSP 312 Ministry of Defence (UK). D/Med (Fond S) (2)/10/11. Sixth Edition, 1987. Second Impression 1990. London: Her Majesty's Stationery Office.
10. Medical Manual of Defence Against Chemical Agents. Ministry of Defence. JSP 312 A/24/Gen/4392. First published 1939, Fifth Edition, 1972. London: Her Majesty's Stationery Office, 1972.
11. Maynard RL, Beswich FW. Organophosphorus compounds as chemical warfare agents. In: Ballantyne B, Marris TC, eds. Clinical and experimental toxicology of organophosphates and carbamates. Oxford: Butterworth-Heinemann, 1992; pp. 373–385.
12. Sidell FR. What to do in case of an unthinkable chemical warfare attack or incident. Postgrad Med 1990;88:70–84.
13. NATO Handbook on the Concept of Medical Support in NBC Environments. A MED P-7(A). Unclassified. August 1982.

Chapter **60**

Contrast Media

Ten to 15 million intravascular contrast media–assisted radiologic examinations are conducted each year in North America. Although adverse side effects are infrequent (range: 5 to 12% of all intravenous injections with ionic high-osmolar contrast media or 1 to 3% with nonionic contrast media), a detailed knowledge of the variety of side effects, their likelihood in relationship to preexisting conditions, and their treatment is required to assure optimal patient care. As would be appropriate with any diagnostic procedure, preliminary considerations for the referring physician and the radiologist include the following:

1. Assessment of patient risk versus potential benefit of the contrast-assisted examination.
2. Imaging alternatives for the same or better diagnostic information.
3. Assurance of a valid clinical indication for each contrast medium administration.
4. Compliance with existing institutional informed-consent procedures and policies for administration of contrast media.

The medical toxicologist should be aware of reactions associated with the therapeutic use and overdose of radiologic contrast agents (Table 60–1)[1] and should be familiar with the prevention and treatment of the acute, possibly fatal, anaphylactoid reactions associated with their use. Useful summaries of contrast agents are available.[2–5] Overdoses and inadvertent administrations may be associated with fatalities.

STRUCTURE AND CLASSIFICATION

The basic chemical structure for iodinated contrast material is seen in Figure 60–1.[6] They are generally subdivided into ionic and nonionic groups which are compared in Table 60–2 (Fig. 60–2).[4] Structure formulas of some of these compounds are found in Figures 60–3 and 60–4.[7]

HIGHER-OSMOLALITY CONTRAST AGENTS (HOCA)

HOCA for intravenous injections have been utilized in radiologic examinations for approximately 60 years. Since

Table 60–1
Radiologic Contrast Agents[a]

Product	Chemical Structure	Anion	Cation	%Salt[b] Conc.	%Iodine[b] Conc.	%Iodine[b] (mg/mL)	Viscosity[b] 25°C (cps)	Viscosity[b] 37°C (cps)	Osmolality[+] (mOsm/kg H_2O)
Renovue®-DIP (Squibb)	ionic	iodamide	meglumine	24	≈11.1	≈111	2.0	1.8	433
Isovue®-128 (Squibb)	nonionic (iopamidol 26.1%)	none	none	none	12.8	128	2.1[c]	1.4	290
Omnipaque® 140 (Winthrop)	nonionic (iohexol 30.2%)	none	none	none	14	140	2.3[c]	1.5	322
Conray® 30 (Mallinckrodt)	ionic	iothalamate	meglumine	30	14.1	141	≈2	≈1.5	≈600
Hypaque® Meglumine 30% (Winthrop)	ionic	diatrizoate	meglumine	30	14.1	141	1.92	1.43	633
Reno-M-DIP® (Squibb)	ionic	diatrizoate	meglumine	30	14.1	141	1.9	1.4	644
Urovist® Meglumine DIU/CT (Berlex)	ionic	diatrizoate	meglumine	30	14.1	141	1.9	1.4	640
Hypaque® Sodium 25% (Winthrop)	ionic	diatrizoate	sodium	25	15	150	1.55	1.17	696
Optiray® 160 (Mallinckrodt)	nonionic (ioversol 33.9%)	none	none	none	16	160	2.7	1.9	355
Isovue®-200 (Squibb)	nonionic (iopamidol 40.8%)	none	none	none	20	200	3.3[c]	2.0	413
Conray® 43 (Mallinckrodt)	ionic	iothalamate	meglumine	43	20.2	202	≈3	≈2	≈1000
Omnipaque® 240 (Winthrop)	nonionic (iohexol 51.8%)	none	none	none	24	240	5.8[c]	3.4	520
Optiray® 240 (Mallinckrodt)	nonionic (ioversol 50.9%)	none	none	none	24	240	4.6	3.0	502
Angiovist® 282 (Berlex)	ionic	diatrizoate	meglumine	60	28.2	282	6.1	4.1	1400
Hypaque® Meglumine 60% (Winthrop)	ionic	diatrizoate	meglumine	60	28.2	282	6.16	4.10	1415
Reno-M-60® (Squibb)	ionic	diatrizoate	meglumine	60	28.2	282	6.1	4.0	1404
Conray® (Mallinckrodt)	ionic	iothalamate	meglumine	60	28.2	282	≈6	≈4	≈1400
Angiovist® 292 (Berlex)	ionic	diatrizoate	meglumine sodium	52 8	29.25	292.5	5.9	4.0	1500
MD-60® (Mallinckrodt)	ionic	diatrizoate	meglumine sodium	52 8	29.25	292.5	6.2	4.1	1557
Renografin®-60 (Squibb)	ionic	diatrizoate	meglumine sodium	52 8	29.25	292.5	5.9	4.0	1450

Hypaque® Sodium 50% (Winthrop)	ionic	diatrizoate	sodium	50	30	300	3.43	2.43	1515
Isovue®-300 (Squibb)	nonionic (iopamidol 61.2%)	none	none	none	30	300	8.8[c]	4.7	616
Omnipaque®-300 (Winthrop)	nonionic (iohexol 64.7%)	none	none	none	30	300	11.8[c]	6.3	672
Renovue®-65 (Squibb)	ionic	iodamide	meglumine	65	≈30	≈300	8.6	6.4	1558
Urovist® Sodium 300 (Berlex)	ionic	diatrizoate	sodium	50	30	300	3.3	2.4	1550
Renovist®II (Squibb)	ionic	diatrizoate	meglumine sodium	28.5 29.1	30.9	309	5.0	3.4	1517
Hexabrix (Mallinckrodt)	ionic	ioxaglate	meglumine sodium	39.3 19.6	32	320	15.7[c]	7.5	≈600
Optiray® 320 (Mallinckrodt)	nonionic (ioversol 67.8%)	none	none	none	32	320	9.9	5.8	702
Conray® 325 (Mallinckrodt)	ionic	iothalamate	sodium	54.3	32.5	325	≈4	≈3	≈1700
Omnipaque® 350 (Winthrop)	nonionic	none	none	none	35	350	20.4[c]	10.4	844
Diatrizoate Meglumine 76% (Squibb)	ionic	diatrizoate	meglumine	76	35.8	358	15	9.6	1980
Angiovist® 370 (Berlex)	ionic	diatrizoate	meglumine sodium	66 10	37	370	13.8	8.4	2100
Hypaque®-76 (Winthrop)	ionic	diatrizoate	meglumine sodium	66 10	37	370	13.34	8.32	2016
Isovue®-370 (Squibb)	nonionic (iopamidol 75.5%)	none	none	none	37	370	20.9[c]	9.4	796
MD-76® (Mallinckrodt)	ionic	diatrizoate	meglumine sodium	66 10	37	370	14.7	9.0	2179
Renografin®-76 (Squibb)	ionic	diatrizoate	meglumine sodium	66 10	37	370	13.8	8.4	1940
Renovist® (Squibb)	ionic	diatrizoate	meglumine sodium	34.3 35.0	37.05	370.5	9.1	5.7	1900
Hypaque®-M, 75% (Winthrop)	ionic	diatrizoate	meglumine sodium	50 25	38.5	385	12.69	7.99	2108
Conray® 400 (Mallinckrodt)	ionic	iothalamate	sodium	66.8	40	400	≈7	≈4.5	≈2300
Vascoray® (Mallinckrodt)	ionic	iothalamate	meglumine sodium	52 26	40	400	≈17	≈9	≈2400
Hypaque®-M, 90% (Winthrop)	ionic	diatrizoate	meglumine sodium	60 30	46.2	462	30	18.7	2938
Angio Conray® (Mallinckrodt)	ionic	iothalamate	sodium	80	48	480	≈14	≈9	≈2400

[a]Adapted from Manual on Iodinated Contrast Media, American College of Radiology, 1991; pp. 31–33.
[b]Data from product package inserts, product brochures or technical information services.
[c]Measured at 20°C.

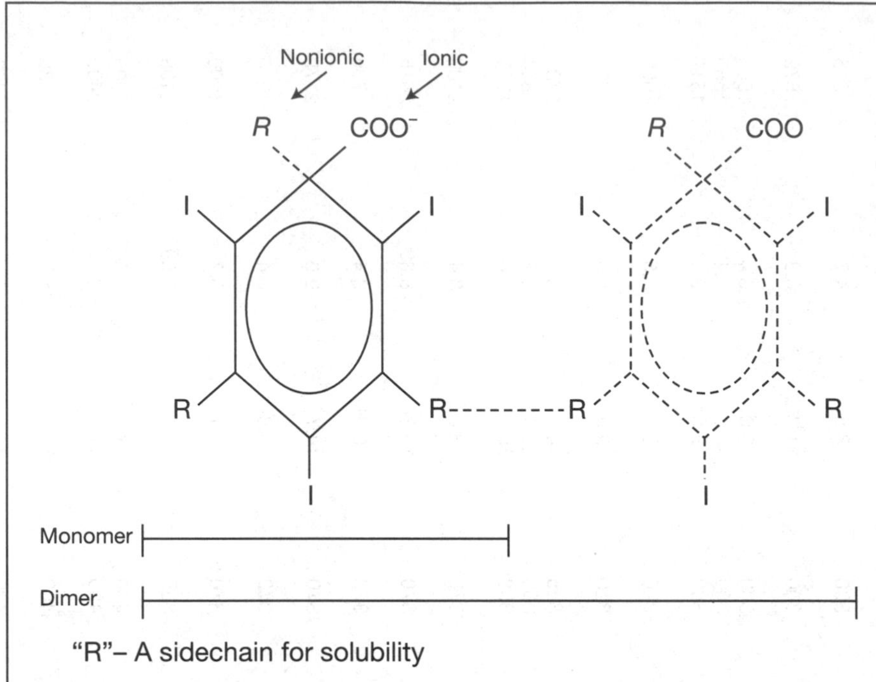

Figure 60–1 Chemical structure of iodinated contrast material. (From Siegle RL. Hosp Formul 1991;26:662–665.)

Table 60-2
Comparison of Ionic and Nonionic Agents[a]

	Ionic	Nonionic
Iodine content	28–37%	18–38%
Osmolality	1400–1700	600–1000
Percent ionized	99.9	0
Membrane permeability	Low	High
Volume of distribution	20–22%	56%
Excretion	Glomerular filtration	

Cronin RE. Renal failure following radiologic procedures. American Journal of the Medical Sciences, 1989 Nov, 298(5):342–356.

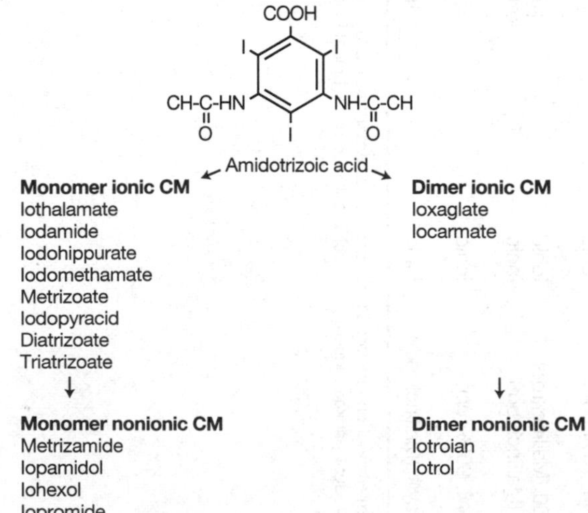

Figure 60–2 Classification of contrast media (CM). The anion structure is mentioned only for the ionic CM, which are composed either as sodium or meglumine salts. (Adapted from Westhoff-Bleck M et al. Drug Safety 1991;61:28–36.)

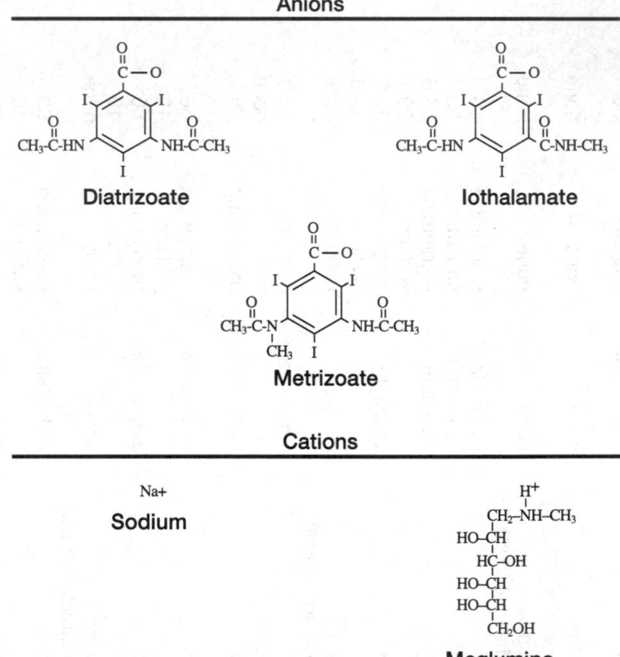

Figure 60–3 Graphic formulas of ratio 1.5 contrast media, used for cardiac angiography procedures. Diatrizoate and iothalamate are available in the US and metrizoate is available in Europe. (Adapted from Spinler SA, Goldfarb S. Ann Pharmacother 1992;26:56–64.)

first introduced, there has been progressive improvement in the quality of these agents in terms of usefulness of contrast material and safety. They are regarded by the medical community (including radiology) and the FDA as safe and effective. However, there is evidence suggesting that pretreatment with steroids (a two-dose steroid pretreatment regimen) before administering HOCA may further decrease patient risk. Subsequent reports may clarify the usefulness of steroids.

LOWER-OSMOLALITY CONTRAST AGENTS (LOCA)

Nevertheless, because of the discomfort associated with the use of HOCA and the uncommon severe adverse reactions, the search for improved contrast agents continued. This resulted in the development of lower-osmolality contrast agents, most of which are nonionic compounds.

The nonionic agents have been shown to be associated with less discomfort and have a lower incidence of severe adverse reactions.

The following guidelines for the use of LOCA are based on the currently available evidence:

1. Patients with a history of a previous adverse reaction to contrast material, with the exception of a sensation of heat, flushing, or a single episode of nausea or vomiting.
2. Patients with a history of asthma or allergy.
3. Patients with known cardiac dysfunction, including recent or potentially imminent cardiac decompensation, severe arrhythmias, unstable angina pectoris, recent myocardial infarction, and pulmonary hypertension.
4. Patients with generalized severe debilitation.

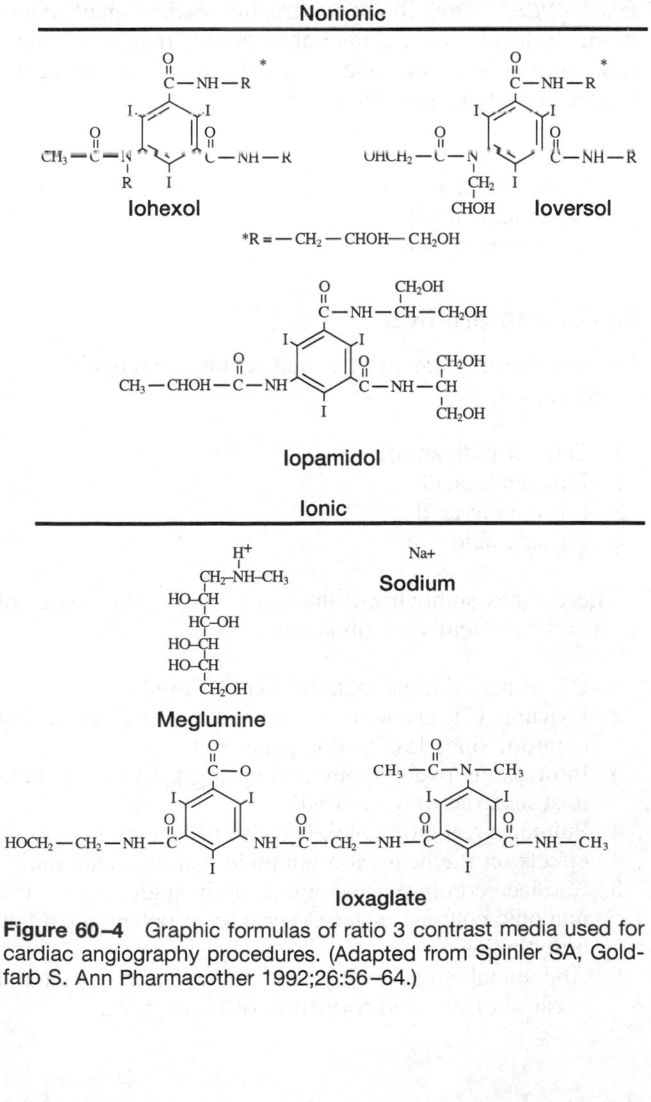

Figure 60–4 Graphic formulas of ratio 3 contrast media used for cardiac angiography procedures. (Adapted from Spinler SA, Goldfarb S. Ann Pharmacother 1992;26:56–64.)

5. Any other circumstances where, after due consideration, the radiologist believes there is a specific indication for the use of LOCA. Examples of this include but are not restricted to the following:
   a. Sickle cell disease.
   b. Patients at increased risk for aspiration.
   c. Patients who are manifestly very anxious about the contrast procedure.
   d. Patients with whom communication cannot be established to determine the presence or absence of risk factors.
   e. Patients who request or demand the use of LOCA.

Data concerning the safety of intravenous use of the ionic dimer (ioxaglate) are insufficient for these proposed guidelines. Ionic monomeric media usually have a very high osmolality and are associated with a high incidence of adverse effects. Low-osmolality contrast media are more expensive.

USES[2–7]

Indications for contrast media use are listed in Table 60–3.[2–7]

UROGRAPHY
Characteristics

Small molecule, highly water-soluble, with low protein-binding, high plasma concentrations, given IV.

Examples:

1. Ionic monomers—diatrizoates, iothalamates, metrizoates, iodamide, ioxithalamate
   Features–
   a. Monomers
   b. High osmolality
   c. High incidence of adverse effects
2. Ionic dimers—ioxaglic acid
3. Nonionic monomers (lower osmolality)—iohexol, iopamidol, iopromide, iopentol, metrizamole
4. Nonionic dimers—iotralan, iodixanol

ANGIOGRAPHY
Characteristics

Water-soluble molecule, distributed through blood vessels; low viscosity; high radiodensity.

Examples: Media low in osmolality; nonionic (e.g., iohexol), better tolerance, less pain on injection.

GASTROINTESTINAL
Characteristics

Nonabsorbable media; homogeneous coat on gastrointestinal mucosa, does not interact with gastrointestinal secretions, no radiographic artifacts.

Example: Barium sulfate.

Table 60-3
Indications for Contrast Media Use[a]

Intravascular:
Intravenous
- CT—head, body
- Digital subtraction angiography
- Intravenous urography
- Venography
  - IVC and its tributaries
  - SVC and its tributaries
- Other venous sites
  - e.g., epidural venography

Intraarterial
- Angiocardiography
- Coronary angiography
- Pulmonary angiography
- Aortography
- Visceral and peripheral arteriography
- Intraarterial digital subtraction angiography
- Central nervous system
  - cerebral, vertebral and spinal angiography

Intrathecal: (Use Nonionic CM only)
- Myelography (nonionic only)
- Cysternography (nonionic only)

Other:
- Oral—GI tract
- Body cavity use
  - Herniography
  - Peritoneography
  - Vaginography
- Hysterosalpingography
- Arthrography
- Endoscopic retrograde cholangiopancreatography (ERCP)
- Cholangiography
- Pyelography
  - retrograde and antegrade
- Urethrography
- Cystography
- Sialography
- Dacryocystography
- Miscellaneous, e.g., sinus tract injection

[a]Adapted from Manual on Iodinated Contrast Media. American College of Radiology, 1991; p. 18.

COMPUTERIZED TOMOGRAPHY OF GASTROINTESTINAL TRACT
Characteristics

Nonabsorbed, iodinated, water-soluble agents; high osmolality (less water absorption; rapid transfer through the gut).

Example: Diatrizoate.

MYELOGRAPHY
Characteristics

Nonionic; water-soluble; good tolerance; good visualization (miscible with cerebrospinal fluid); removed from subarachnoid space by normal pharmacokinetic mechanism.

Examples: Metrizamide; iotralan.

LYMPHOGRAPHY, LYMPHANGIOGRAPHY
Characteristics

High radiodensity, water-insoluble media (persist in lymphatic vessels).

Examples:

1. Iodized oil
   Not distributed throughout whole lymphatic space
   Potential for severe side effects
2. Iotasol—nonionic dimer

MAGNETIC RESONANCE IMAGING
Characteristics

Complexes that enhance magnetic resonance imaging

Examples: Gadolinium, manganese (+2), and iron (+3) as the aminopolycarboxylate chelates and gadopentetic acid.

CHOLECYSTOGRAPHY, CHOLANGIOGRAPHY
Oral Characteristics

Molecule preferentially excreted in the bile; must be sufficiently large for biliary excretions; contains free carboxy or acidic group (biliary active transfer is an ion transfer process). Molecules are large, low protein binding (protection from rapid renal excretion). Must be absorbed from gastrointestinal tract; small molecules; soluble in gastrointestinal fluids; lipophilic (to pass membranes of mucosa).

Examples: Oral cholecystographic media (small monomeric molecules to facilitate absorption); require conjugation with glucoronic acid to reach sufficient molecular weight for biliary excretion.

1. Ipodates
2. Iocetamic acid
3. Iopanoic acid
4. Sodium tyropanoate

IV Characteristics

Larger dimeric molecules; do not require conjugates.
Examples

1. Salts of iodipamide
2. Iodoxamic acid
3. Ioglycamic acid
4. Iotroxic acid

Leeds[8] has summarized the use of appropriate types of agents for particular examinations:

1. CT: either contrast material may be used.
2. Dynamic CT: use nonionic contrast material for patient comfort, since less heat is generated.
3. Intravenous pyelography and cystography: either contrast material may be used.
4. Pulmonary angiography: because of heat and potential effects on the heart, use nonionic contrast material.
5. Cardiac, coronary, and aortic arch angiography: use nonionic contrast material because of potential cardiac arrhythmias.
6. Abdominal angiography: use ionic contrast material because of reduced formation of blood clots.

7. Brachial angiography and femoral angiography to study pelvis and peripheral vessels: use nonionic contrast material because of improved patient comfort.
8. Cerebral angiography: use nonionic contrast material for patient comfort, but if a prolonged study is expected, then use ionic contrast material since a reduction in clot formation occurs.
9. In myelography, nonionic contrast material is used exclusively because of reductions in arachnoiditis and because removal is unnecessary.
10. In digital venous angiographic studies nonionics are preferred because of improved patient comfort.
11. In peripheral venous studies either contrast material may be used.
12. In pediatric patients below 1 year of age and in patients above 65 or with proven cardiac abnormality or hypertension nonionics should be used for intravenous examinations.

In most examinations, therefore, as a consequence of increased patient comfort and reduction in serious complications, nonionics would be the contrast material of choice.

NONIONIC MEDIA

Conflicting data suggest that low-osmolarity contrast media should be given to patients undergoing painful angiographic procedures and to those at high risk such as infants, the elderly, patients with diabetes, cardiac or renal impairment, hemoglobinopathies, asthma, anxieties or allergies, and those who have previously had reactions to contrast media.[9–11] Expense of these agents may be a prohibitive factor in their use.

LOW- VERSUS HIGH-OSMOLAR AGENTS

Magnetic Resonance Imaging

Intravenous gadopentate meglumine, used as a contrast agent for magnetic resonance imaging, has been associated with anaphylactoid reactions,[12] seizures,[13] headache, injection-site coldness, nausea, hypotension, and a transient increase in serum iron values within 2 to 4 hours after injection. There have been few abnormalities observed in vital signs, the electrocardiogram, the electroencephalogram, and the neurologic examination.[12] Similar experience has followed the use of gadoteridol.

TOXICOKINETICS

Water-soluble contrast media are excreted almost entirely unmetabolized by the kidneys. Only a small proportion of the agent is bound to plasma proteins.[2]

DRUG INTERACTIONS

Verapamil and contrast media exhibit a synergistic effect on the sodium:calcium ratio, important in the production of cardiac side effects.[14] The epileptogenic properties of chlorpromazine can be potentiated by intrathecal injection of contrast media.[15] Radiographic contrast agents impede the fibrinolytic effect of thrombolytic drugs.[16]

INTERLEUKIN RECALL SYNDROME

About 10% of patients who have previously received interleukin-2 therapy develop fever, chills, rash, nausea, vomiting, urticaria, diarrhea, hypotension, and dyspnea following administration of an ionic and nonionic medium.[17–20]

CLINICAL PRESENTATION

Side Effects

Contrast-media reactions vary in severity. All adverse side effects, regardless of their degree or mode of presentation, portend or progress to a worse event. Contrast-media reactions are usually evident immediately, within the first 5 to 20 minutes after administration, or, uncommonly, delayed up to 24 to 48 hours. They appear after single or multiple intravascular injections, for example, sequential or repeat injections for angiography.

Types

1. Anaphylactoid (anaphylaxis-like; allergy-like); or idiosyncratic.
2. Nonidiosyncratic.
   a. Chemotoxic, osmotoxic, direct organ toxicity (e.g., neurotoxic, cardiotoxic, nephrotoxic).
   b. Vasomotor, including vagal.
3. Combined (1 and 2) or organ specific (local; nonsystemic).

The majority of adverse side effects are mild or moderate non–life-threatening events that require only observation, reassurance, and support. However, most severe adverse side effects have a mild or moderate beginning or prodrome. The frequency and severity of contrast reactions is affected by the dose, route, and rate of delivery of contrast media.

Adverse reactions to contrast media are listed in Table 60–4.[4] Categories of reaction are listed in Table 60–5. Factors that increase risk of adverse reactions are summarized in Table 60–6. Important additional associated reactions have included pancreatitis,[21] glossitis,[22] acute hemolysis in a patient with hemoglobin SC disease,[23] and coronary artery spasm.[24]

Incidence

The true incidence of adverse side effects after the administration of intravascular contrast media is not known precisely since similar signs and symptoms may be due to concomitant medications, local anesthetics, needles, catheters, and anxiety. Underreporting or variation in this categorization or classification of reactions affects statistics regarding incidence. Most side effects are mild to moderate, do not require treatment, and are reported to occur in 5 to 12% of all patients who receive ionic, high-osmolar contrast media. Many patients will experience physiologic disturbances (i.e., warmth or heat), and this is often not recorded. Use of low-osmolar ionic and nonionic contrast media is associated with a lower overall incidence of adverse side effects, particularly serious life-threatening ones. Serious contrast reactions are rare and occur in 1 or 2 per 1000 examinations using high-osmolar contrast media.

Fatalities

The precise incidence of fatal outcome from a contrast material reaction is also unknown. In addition, resuscitative measures and treatment of adverse side effects from contrast material have improved in the past 2 decades. Comparing published incidence rates from the use of higher-osmolar contrast media, deaths are reported in between 1 per 40,000 and 1 per 170,000 intravenous administrations. In the past decade (1980s) the incidence of fatal outcomes after a contrast-medium reaction has decreased for high-osmolar contrast media to 0.9 per 100,000, essentially a rate equivalent to that observed with nonionic agents. This reflects improvements in contrast media design (LOCM and NICM), patient selection, physician awareness, and resuscitation efforts.

Delayed reactions have been reported, but are rarely serious and almost exclusively are mild in character. Delayed pain at or near the site of injection may signal impending thrombophlebitis after intravenous injection.

Table 60–4
Adverse Reactions to Contrast Media[a]

Cardiovascular
Hypotension
Bradycardias
Ventricular tachycardias/fibrillation
Decreased myocardial contractility → heart failure
Aggravation of myocardial ischemia
Electrocardiographic changes
Shock
Cardiac arrest

Respiratory
Bronchospasm
Sneezing/cough
Dyspnea
Laryngospasm
Respiratory arrest

Neurologic
Headache
Dizziness
Any focal neurologic sign
Seizures
Brown-Séquard syndrome
Transverse myelitis

Renal
Flank pain
Albuminuria
Oligo-/anuria

Gastrointestinal
Nausea
Vomiting
Paralytic ileus

Cutaneous
Urticaria
Flush
Gangrene of skin

Miscellaneous
Thrombocytopenia
Thrombosis
Swelling of salivary glands
Generalized joint pain and swelling
Chills and fever
Hyperthyroidism

[a]Adapted from Westhoff-Bleck M et al. Drug Safety 1991;6:28–36.

Anaphylactoid Reactions

Anaphylactoid reactions are observed in 5 to 20% of examinations using radiopaque agents, ranging from skin reactions to irreversible shock.[4] A history of allergy increases the likelihood of reactions at least two- to threefold.[4] Patients who have had anaphylactoid reactions to contrast material have a 35 to 60% chance of having a second reaction on rechallenge.[25] Factors that increase the risk of a chance reaction to contrast material are listed in Table 60–6.[26] Ionic contrast agents may have antigenic properties in man.[27] Additional risk factors include patients receiving adrenergic blockers.[28]

Osmotic side effects include changes in plasma volume, changes in vascular permeability, vasodilatation, local discomfort or pain, hypotension, change in the blood–brain

Table 60–5
Categories of Reactions[a]

Mild

Nausea; vomiting	Altered taste	Sweats
Cough	Itching	Rash (hives)
Warmth (heat)	Pallor	Nasal stuffiness
Headache	Flushing	Swelling—eyes; face
Dizziness	Chills	
Anxiety	Shaking	

Treatment:
Requires observation, assurance, but usually no treatment.

Moderate
Moderate degree of mild signs/symptoms (sufficient to be clinically evident) and/or systemic symptoms including:

Pulse change	Hypertension	Bronchospasm
Hypotension	Dyspnea-wheezing	Laryngospasm

Treatment:
Requires close, careful observation and often treatment but usually not hospitalization.

Severe
Potentially life-threatening, moderate or severe signs/symptoms, e.g., laryngospasm.
Plus:

Unresponsiveness	Clinically manifest arrhythmias
Convulsions	Cardiopulmonary arrest

Treatment:
Requires *prompt* recognition and treatment; almost always requires hospitalization.

[a]Manual on Iodinated Contrast Media. American College of Radiology. 1991; p. 19.

Table 60–6
Factors That Increase Risk of Adverse Reaction to Contrast Material[a]

Cerebral or renal disease in patient over age 50
Dehydration
History of allergy, including asthma
History of cardiac disease
History of reaction to contrast material
Multiple myeloma, homocystinuria, sickle cell anemia, or pheochromocytoma
Previous study in which large dose of contrast material (>20 g) was used

[a]Adapted from Gluck BS, Mitty HA. Postgrad Med 1990;88:187–194.

Table 60–7
Cardiovascular Toxicity of Ionic Contrast Agents[a]

Hemodynamic	Electrophysiologic
Myocardial depression	Sinus bradycardia
Hypotension	Heart block
Pulmonary congestion	Q-T prolongation
	Ventricular tachycardia/fibrillation
	ST segment and T wave changes

[a]Adapted from Benotti JR. Invest Radiol 1988;22(Suppl 2):S366–S372.

barrier, vasomotor instability, and vasovagal (heart rate effects) reactions.

Chemotoxic side effects include neurotoxicity, cardiac depression, arrhythmia, electrocardiogram (EKG) changes, and renal tubular or vascular injury. Chemotoxic side effects appear to relate to the cation content and the ionic nature of contrast materials that dissociate in solution. Nonionic contrast media are associated with fewer such chemotoxic side effects. This is probably related to their more hydrophilic nature.

Cardiovascular (Table 60–7)

Cardiovascular and/or pulmonary changes include cardiac ischemia resulting in pain and arrhythmia. Premature ventricular contractions with ectopy are seen after contrast medium administration. EKG changes occur in up to 33% of patients with atherosclerotic disease or coronary artery disease and in about 5% of normal patients. Tachycardia accompanies hypotension and should allow distinction from the more classic vagal reaction (hypotension and bradycardia).

Cardiac signs and symptoms are accompanied by shortness of breath (dyspnea). Hypoxia is known to predispose to cardiac arrhythmia, especially in patients with preexisting coronary artery disease or pulmonary disease. Rapid progression to ventricular tachycardia, fibrillation, and shock with cardiac arrest occur in the above-described circumstances. Increased airway resistance and decreased air flow occur after injection of ionic media, albeit usually not at clinically detectable levels. Such effects take the form of bronchoconstriction in asthmatic patients.

In coronary angiography and left ventriculography, the contrast agent reaches the coronary vessel wall almost undiluted resulting in ischemia during its presence. Patients with heart failure, pulmonary hypertension, and unstable angina pectoris are at high risk of severe hemodynamic alterations (fall in blood pressure, pulmonary edema)[4] or arrhythmias (sinus and AV nodal bradycardias, ventricular tachycardias, or ventricular fibrillation). Low-osmolar nonionic agents appear to be hemodynamically superior.[29] Such changes are usually observed within the first minutes after contrast-media injection. In patients with pulmonary hypertension, injection of contrast media causes an increase in the pulmonary artery pressure that may result in right ventricular failure. The hemodynamic changes are mainly caused by hyperosmolarity and are lessened with low-osmolar agents.

The combination of decreased blood pressure (hypotension) and bradycardia is often accompanied by apprehension, confusion, sweating, unresponsiveness, and loss of bowel or bladder control signals, a so-called vasovagal reaction. The etiology is unknown, but it can be aggravated by fear and anxiety and, if untreated, may progress to cardiopulmonary arrest. The cardiac effects of increased vagal tone include depressed sinoatrial (SA) and atrioventricular (AV) nodal activity, inhibition of AV conduction, and peripheral vasodilatation. Hypotension is out of proportion to the bradycardia and persists after the bradycardia has been corrected by treatment with atropine.

Sinus bradycardias and AV nodal conduction abnormalities are commonly observed in left ventriculography after injection into the right and left coronary artery. Slowed conduction and increased automaticity appear to be mediated by hyperosmolarity. Intracoronary thrombi may develop following administration of nonionic contrast media despite aggressive systemic heparinization.[30] Both ionic and nonionic contrast agents prolong QT intervals following intracoronary injection; ionic agents produce greater QT lengthening than nonionic agents.[31]

Gastrointestinal

Oral iohexol, 100 mL, has been followed by nausea, vomiting, abdominal pain, hypotension, and difficulty in breathing. Symptoms have subsided after IV hydrocortisone 100 mg, chlorphenamine 100 mg, and IV plasma expanders were administered.[32]

Neurologic

Neurologic signs such as headache (which may be delayed and associated with intracerebral hemorrhage),[33] visual blurring, transcortical global amnesia,[34] cortical blindness,[35] encephalopathy, meningeal reactions,[36] dizziness, sensory changes, transient paresis,[37,38] or seizures (predominantly in patients with focal brain lesions)[39–41] are observed infrequently after intravascular administration of contrast media. Patients undergoing cerebral angiography or direct opacification of the aortic arch are most at risk of irreversible neurologic damage.[4] Neurologic side effects are usually transient. Seizures require immediate treatment (IV diazepam, phenytoin, phenobarbital, intubation, intensive medical care).[4] Contrast media may enhance neuromuscular blockade in myasthenia gravis patients.[42] The extent of blood–brain barrier disruption caused by hypertonic solutions tends to rise with increasing osmolality and increasing duration of injection.[39] Use of ionic contrast media when visualizing spinal cord nerve roots may lead to an accidental intrathecal injection. Nonionic agents have been preferred in epidurography.[43] If accidental intrathecal injection is suspected the patient should not be permitted to lie down.[43,44]

Pulmonary

Noncardiogenic pulmonary edema has been reported following the intravascular administration of contrast materials.[45–47] No risk factors have been clearly identified.[48] Patients with a history of radiocontrast medium–related pulmonary edema should probably be given prophylactic

Table 60–8
Radiocontrast-Induced Acute Renal Failure[a]

Risk Factors	
Age	Hyperuricemia
Renal insufficiency	Exposure to other nephrotoxins
Diabetes mellitus	Repeated exposure to radiocontrast
Multiple myeloma	Volume of contrast
Anemia	Intraarterial vs. intravenous
Proteinuria	Male sex
Abnormal liver function	Cardiovascular disease
Volume depletion	Hypertension
Dehydration	Renal transplantation

[a]Adapted from Cronin RE. Am J Med Sci 1989;298:342–356.

Table 60–9
Risk Factors for Nonionic Contrast Media–Induced Thrombosis[a]

Antithrombin III deficiency
Protein C or protein S deficiency
Hyperfibrinogenemia
Thrombocytosis
Increased factor VIII levels
Hemoconcentration
Hyperviscosity syndrome
Paraproteinemias
Leukemias (increase in number of white cells)
Hemolysis

[a]Adapted from Fareed J et al. Radiology 1990;174:321–325.

corticosteroids, but recurrence of pulmonary edema has been described despite pretreatment with prednisone and diphenhydramine.[48] Nonionic media are probably inadvisable in patients who have developed pulmonary edema after a previous radiocontrast-media infusion. Eosinophilic pneumonia has been described after use of about 200 mL of iohexol, a low-osmolar, nonionic contrast media.[49]

Renal

Acute renal failure following injection of water-soluble contrast media has been reported with many agents currently in use.[4,50] Predisposing factors are listed in Table 60–8.[51] In any examination, a total amount of contrast media exceeding 500 to 800 mL I_2/kg body weight increases the risk of nephrotoxicity. Clinically, patients develop an acute tubular necrosis, presenting with oliguria within 24 hours after exposure to the agent. Renal function is usually restored within 2 or 3 weeks. It is controversial whether low-osmolar, nonionic agents produce less renal damage.[52–59] Katzberg[59] has observed that the majority of clinical reports of contrast medium induced–acute renal failure are anecdotal, retrospective, and confounded by multiple, uncontrolled risk factors.

A prospective controlled study[60] indicates that the nonionic contrast agent iohexol is less nephrotoxic than the ionic contrast agent diatrizoate in patients with preexisting renal insufficiency alone or combined with diabetes mellitus who undergo cardiac angiography. In contrast, in patients with normal renal function, regardless of the presence or absence of diabetes mellitus, nonionic contrast media are not less nephrotoxic compared with ionic contrast agents.

Dehydration compromises renal function. Hence, all patients undergoing examination involving contrast media should be well hydrated. One prospective study suggests that there appears to be little risk of clinically important nephrotoxicity following the use of contrast material for patients with diabetes and normal renal function or for nondiabetic patients with preexisting renal insufficiency.[61] A small fraction of patients will require dialysis. In these patients the rise in serum creatinine begins within 24 hours and is often quite rapid. A formula has been suggested for calculating the maximal amount of contrast material that can be given safely without causing a deterioration in renal function.[62]

Contrast material "limit"

$$= \frac{\text{5 mL of contrast/kg body weight (maximum 300 mL)}}{\text{Serum creatinine mg/dL}}$$

Thromboembolic Potential (Table 60–9)[63]

Serious, rarely fatal, thromboembolic events causing myocardial infarction and stroke have been reported during angiographic procedures with both ionic and nonionic contrast media. Meticulous intravascular administration technique is necessary to minimize clotting and thromboembolic events. Length of procedure, catheter and syringe material used, underlying disease state, and concomitant medications contribute to these developments. The use of plastic syringes in place of glass syringes has been reported to decrease but not eliminate the likelihood of in vitro clotting should blood enter the syringe.[64]

Thromboembolic complications have been reported in association with merely mixing of nonionic, low-osmolality contrast media with blood in a contrast-media power-injection syringe and allowing the mixture to sit undisturbed for several minutes before use.[65] Grollman and colleagues added 5 units of heparin/mL of nonionic, low-osmolality contrast media (1000 units per 200 mL).[66] The difference between ionic and nonionic contrast media and their relation to thromboembolic complication appears to be small,[67] although the incidence of thrombus formation at the site of coronary intervention is somewhat increased with both low- and high-osmolality media.[63,68,69] Caution should be exercised when using nonionic contrast media in high-risk patients such as the elderly and in those with defects in the coagulation system that may lead to thrombosis.[63] Nonionic contrast media should not be mixed with blood before intravascular injection.[65] Continuous flushing with saline solution to prevent mixing of blood and contrast media, premedication with heparin, and use of plastic syringes are important for the safe use of nonionic contrast media.[70]

Thyroid

Radiocontrast agents contain iodide atoms that are covalently bound to a phenolic ring, and these compounds cannot be metabolized in vivo by deiodinating enzymes. Contaminating free iodide is present in these preparations, and the free iodide is probably responsible for effects on the thyroid gland.[71]

In currently used radiocontrast media, the amount of inorganic iodine available to interfere with thyroid metabolism is about 0.1% of the dose administered. Westhoff-Bleck[4] suggested that patients at risk of developing hyperthyroidism should be treated prophylactically with, for example, sodium perchlorate 1.2 g administered 30 minutes before and 6 to 8 hours after exposure to the contrast media.[4] Sodium ipodate or sodium iopanoate administered to adults inhibits the extrathyroid conversion of T_4 to T_3 leading to a reduction in serum T_3 and T_4 levels. Sodium ipodate has been used to treat neonatal hyperthyroidism due to Graves' disease.[72]

Following ingestion of iodine or radiologic iodinated contrast media, diverse changes in thyroid status may occur. Iopanoic acid (Telepaque) and sodium ipodate (Biloptin) temporarily interfere with the normal extrathyroidal deiodination of iodothyronines. Using routine thyroid function tests, about one-half of patients will be suspected to be thyrotoxic. Serum T_3 assays are necessary to exclude thyrotoxicosis. Thyroid function tests should be interpreted with caution within 3 weeks of oral cholecystography.[73]

Cancer

Thorotrast, a contrast medium containing colloidal thorium dioxide 25%, has been associated with malignancies.[74]

Oxyhemoglobin Dissociation

Both ionic and nonionic contrast media may impair unloading of oxygen from hemoglobin in the capillary blood. Large volumes of such contrast media may lead to serious adverse effects in patients with leftward shifts of the oxyhemoglobin dissociation curve, such as in neonates with intracardiac shunts or adult smokers with severe coronary artery disease.[75]

Iodide Mumps

Iodide "mumps" (submandibular and parotid swelling) has been observed in patients who have had previous uncomplicated exposure to iodinated contrast agents and may recur in the same patient on repeated examination.[76]

OVERDOSE—INADVERTENT USE

Intrathecal Administration

Inadvertent administration, by the intrathecal route, of ionic contrast media (diatrizoate, iodamine, ioxitalamate) instead of iopanidol has led to fatalities.[77]

Ionic

Fatalities have followed myelography with 10 mL of diatrizoate meglumine containing 306 mg of iodine/mL corresponding to 3.06 of iodine; diatrizoate sodium and meglumine 370 mg iodine/mL corresponding to 3.7 g of iodine. With a 2.1 g dose of iodine, assuming a 70-kg body weight, the dose of iodine ranged from 0.037 to 0.053 g/kg. Two patients received diatrizoate sodium and meglumine 370 mg (iodine)/mL corresponding to 1.9 g iodine or about 0.026 g (iodine)/kg. This dose was lower than previous ones and was not fatal.

Nonionic Status

Nonionic compounds with clinical doses containing 2 to 3 times more iodine than those allowed with iothalamate or iocarmate appear to have low rates of neurotoxic reactions. With higher doses, above 4.5 g iodine, the rate of neurotoxic adverse reactions increases. In the United Kingdom and United States the recommended limit is 3 g from both iopanidol and iohexol.

Myelography

Historically the first water-soluble contrast agent used in myelography was methiodal sodium (100 mg iodine/mL). The maximum dose recommended was 10 mL, 8 g iodine, or for a subject of 70-kg body weight 0.014 g/kg. There was a high rate of neurotoxic adverse reactions. Subsequently, triiodination compounds were studied. Iothalamate exhibited lower epileptogenic activity compared with diatrizoate. Iothalamate meglumine was used at total doses of 1 to 1.5 g of iodine. Neurotoxic adverse reactions with iothalamate were lower than methiodal. Adverse reactions were still observed. An adhesive arachnoiditis was ascribed to the high osmolality of the radiopaque solutions. To reduce the osmolality, a dimeric derivative of iothalamate, iocarmate (Dimex-X), was introduced, but this also retained epileptogenic potential. Following an overdose accident Dimex-X was removed by the FDA from the market in the United States.

Inadvertent myelography with diatrizoate has led to lumbar pain, tonic–clonic seizures of the lower limbs, generalized seizures, hyperthermia, rhabdomyolysis, disseminated intravascular coagulation, renal insufficiency, pulmonary edema, and death.[77] Brain retention of contrast media in the basal ganglia has been associated with parkinsonism and has been observed following 400 mL of diatrizoate use (Renografin-76). The maximum recommended dose is 200 mL. The patient survived.[78] Treatment was largely symptomatic and supportive. Diatrizoate sodium and meglumine bind poorly to serum protein, are eliminated mainly unchanged through the kidneys, and have a half-life of about 2 hours. When accidental intrathecal accidents occur with ionic contrast agents, appropriate circulatory support, intrathecal lavage,[79] and anticonvulsant therapy will be significant in patient management.[80] Patients with injured cerebral cortex or other previously reported risk factors may need to be observed for seizures by medical personnel for up to 24 hours after intrathecal administration of these media even when there is no history of epilepsy.[81] Despite the low but still present risk of seizures after myelography, the patients should not drive or be alone for 24 hours after the procedure.[82] Factors that may decrease the incidence of side effects after myelography include elevation of the head for 6 hours after the study and avoidance of drugs that may lower the seizure threshold such as phenothiazines, monoamine oxidase inhibitors, tricyclic antidepressants, or alcohol.[82] Iothalamate salts are dialyzable.[83]

Barium Sulfate

Low-density suspensions (50 percent w/v) of barium sulfate used for bronchography have been considered relatively harmless in the bronchial tract, but aspiration of a low-density suspension (100%) in the elderly can be associated with acute pneumonia secondary to aspiration.[84] High-density (250%) aspiration in the elderly can provoke a similar response.[85] Intravenous metoclopramide may be beneficial in such patients.[86]

Iopanoic Acid—Cholecystography

Iopanoic acid (Telepaque) is an ionic monomeric contrast agent used as a cholecystographic contrast media. Doses of up to 75 g have led to nausea, vomiting, diarrhea, hypotension, coronary insufficiency, acute hepatic necrosis, renal failure, and death.[87] Oral cholecystographic agents are strongly uricosuric. Treatment is largely symptomatic and supportive. Intravenous fluids, alkalinization of the urine, and cholestyramine as a chelator of iopanoic acid have been suggested in overdose.[87] Cardiac and respiratory monitoring should be instituted in an intensive care facility.[87]

Excretory Urography

High dose (14 mL Conray 60^R – 15 mL/kg) of a high-osmolarity contrast agent (meglumine iothalamate) during excretory urography has led to cardiopulmonary failure.[83] In infants urography with diatrizoate sodium has led to fatalities.[88] Ansell[89] has observed that the weight of iodine in Urografin 60, Hypaque 45, and Conray 289 is about the same. If one of these media is used, a dose of 1 to 2 mL/lb body weight (2.2 to 4.4 mL/kg) appears adequate for high-dose urography in infants. Liver damage and cardiac disease with renal failure probably add to the risk of contrast-media administration.[89]

TREATMENT

Precontrast hydration recommendations (Table 60–10): In patients with normal renal function few precautions are necessary, and high-osmolality contrast agents can be used, unless they are contraindicated because of an increased risk of allergic or hemodynamic side effects. However, patients with preexisting renal impairment should be given 0.45% saline intravenously for 12 hours before and 12 hours after the administration of contrast agents.[90] Concomitant administration of furosemide or mannitol is not indicated, but low-osmolality contrast agents are preferable to high-osmolality agents.[91] Pretreatment protocols to prevent reaction to contrast material are summarized in Table 60–11.[26] Treatment of common adverse reactions to contrast material is present in Tables 60–12 and 60–13.[6,26] Equip-

Table 60–10
Precontrast Hydration Recommendations[a]

Composition and Rate	Duration
20% mannitol/furosemide 100 mg/mg SCr	1–6 hours
0.5% saline ± mannitol ± furosemide 75 ml/h	Before and several hours afterwards
550 ml 0.9% saline	350 ml prior to +250 ml flush per hour during arteriogram
5% dextrose in 0.45 saline	1.5 L before and 125 ml/hr after × 4 hours

[a]Adapted from Cronin RE. Am J Med Sci 1989;298:342–356.

Table 60–11
Pretreatment Protocols to Prevent Reaction to Contrast Material[a]

- Methylprednisolone (Medrol), 32 mg PO, 12 and 2 hr before administration of contrast material
- Prednisone (Deltasone, Orasone), 50 mg PO, 13, 7, and 1 hr before administration of contrast material
  plus
  Diphenhydramine (Benadryl, Diphenacen-50), 50 mg PO or IM, 1 hr before administration
- Prednisone, 50 mg PO, 13, 7, and 2 hr before administration of contrast material
  plus
  Diphenhydramine, 50 mg PO or IM, 1 hr before administration
  plus
  Ephedrine sulfate, 25 mg PO, 1 hr before administration unless contraindicated by history of angina, arrhythmia, or specific reaction
- Methylprednisolone or equivalent, 32 mg daily for 3 days before administration of contrast material, the last dose 2 hr before administration

[a]Adapted from Gluck BS. Postgrad Med 1990;88:187–194.

Table 60–12
ABCD Approach for Patient Evaluation and Treatment[a]

A. Assessment (severity and category of reaction).
Assistance (call for it).
Airway, O_2
Access (venous)—secure/improve IV line(s)—peripheral or central.

B. Breathing (begin CPR if necessary); use mouth protective barrier.
Bag—AMBU.
Begin full resuscitation efforts (CPR) if necessary; call CODE.
Beware of paradoxical responses to therapy, e.g., β-blockers.

C. Categorize reaction and patient status.
Circulatory assistance—use crystalloid, e.g., lactate; saline or colloid replenishment, infuse rapidly, may use pressure bag or forceful infusion.
Call CODE if necessary; CPR; continue to monitor.
Common denominators—assess cardiac output; capillary leak (third spacing); decreased venous return, decreased peripheral vascular resistance.

D. Drug therapies (as outlined).
Do: monitor, assess and reassure the patient; use correct dose (concentration) and route for drugs; push IV fluids and O_2.
Don't: delay (call for help); use incorrect dose(s) and drugs.

[a]Adapted from Manual on Iodinated Contrast Media. American College of Radiology, 1991; p. 22.

Table 60–13
Management of Acute Reactions[a]

Reaction:
Urticaria:
Treatment
1. No treatment needed in most cases
2. H_1-receptor blocker:
   Diphenhydramine (Benadryl) PO/IM/IV 50 mg *or*
   Hydroxyzine (Vistaril) PO/IM/IV 25–50 mg
   H_2 receptor blocker may be added:
   Cimetidine (Tagamet) 300 mg PO or IV slowly, diluted in 10 ml D5W solution *or*
   Ranitidine (Zantac) 50 mg PO or IV slowly, diluted in 10 ml D5W solution

If severely/widely disseminated:
Alpha-agonist (arteriolar and venous constriction)
Epinephrine SC (1:1000) 0.1–0.3 ml (if no cardiac contraindication)

Facial/laryngeal edema:
1. Alpha-agonist (arteriolar and venous constriction)
   Epinephrine 0.1–0.3 mL 1:1000 SC or if SC route fails or if peripheral vascular collapse then, 1.0–3.0 ml, 1:10,000 *slowly* IV
   May repeat × 3 prn up to a max. of 1.0 mg.
2. O_2 2–6 L/min

If not responsive to therapy or for obvious laryngeal edema (acute):
Call anesthesiologist/CODE team.
Consider intubation

Bronchospasm:
1. O_2 2–6 L/min
   Monitor: ECG; O_2 saturation (pulse oximeter); BP
2. Epinephrine 0.1–0.3 mL 1:1000 SC or β-agonist inhalers (bronchiolar dilators—[i.e., metaproterenol (Alupent), terbutaline (Brethaire), or albuterol (Proventil)]).
   If SC route fails or if peripheral vascular collapse, then 1.0–3.0 ml, 1:10,000 *slowly* IV
   May repeat × 3 prn up to a max. of 1.0 mg.

Alternatively
1. Aminophylline: 6.0 mg/kg IV in D5W over 10–20 minutes (loading dose); then 0.4–1.0 mg/kg/hr prn.
   or Terbutaline 0.25–0.5 mg IM/SC
2. Call CODE for severe bronchospasm (or if O_2 saturation ≤88).

Hypotension with tachycardia:
1. Legs up; Trendelenburg position. Monitor: ECG, pulse oximeter, BP.
2. O_2 2–6 L/min
3. Rapid administration of large volumes of isotonic lactated Ringer's solution. (Ringer's lactate > normal saline > D5W)

If poorly responsive:
1. Epinephrine 0.1–0.3 mL 1:1000 SC or if SC route fails or if peripheral vascular collapse then, 1.0–3.0 ml, 1:10,000 *slowly* IV
   May repeat × 3 prn up to a max. of 1.0 mg.

If still poorly responsive:
Transfer to ICU for further management

Hypotension with bradycardia—vagal reaction
1. Legs up; Trendelenburg position; secure airway; give oxygen
2. Secure IV access; give atropine 0.6–1.0 mg IV slowly
3. Monitor vital signs, repeat atropine up to 2.0 mg total dose
4. Push fluid replenishment IV (Ringer's lactate > normal saline > D5W)

Hypertension, severe:
1. Monitors in place: ECG, pulse oximeter, BP.
2. Apresoline—5.0 mg IV
3. Sodium nitroprusside—arterial line; infusion pump necessary to titrate.
4. For pheochromocytoma—phentolamine 5.0 mg (1.0 mg in children) IV

Seizures/convulsions:
1. O_2 2–6 L/min
2. Consider diazepam (Valium) 5.0 mg or midazolam (Versed) 2.5 mg IV
3. If longer effect needed, obtain consultation; consider phenytoin (Dilantin) infusion 15–18 mg/kg at 50 mg/min
4. Careful monitoring of vital signs required

Pulmonary edema:
1. Elevate torso; rotating tourniquets (venous compression)
2. O_2 2–6 L/min
3. Diuretics—furosemide (Lasix) 40 mg IV slowly
4. Consider morphine/meperidine (Demerol)
5. Corticosteroids optional

[a]Adapted from Manual on Iodinated Contrast Media. American College of Radiology, 1991; pp. 20–21.

Table 60-14
Equipment for Emergency Carts

CODE team phone number or beeper clearly posted.
- Oxygen cylinders, flow valve, nasal prongs, tubing, face masks (adult and children sizes).
- Suction—wall mounted or portable; tubing and catheters.
- Oral airways—rubber/plastic; and/or protective breathing barriers.
- AMBU bag with masks (adult and children sizes) with protective barrier.
- Endotracheal tubes—laryngoscopes (adult and children sizes).
- Stethoscope; sphygmomanometer, tourniquets, tongue depressor.
- Flashlight.
- IV solutions; IV tubing—normal saline, dextrose 5% water (D5W), dextrose 5% saline (D5S), Ringer's lactate.
- Syringes—variety of sizes; needles—variety of sizes, include cardiac needle.
- Tracheostomy set, cut down trays with sterile instruments.
- Necessary drugs and medication.

Immediately available or on emergency cart:
- Defibrillator
- ECG
- BP/pulse monitor
- Pulse oximeter (optional)

ment required for emergency carts in a radiology unit is listed in Table 60–14.[6]

Before a contrast agent is administered, a peripheral intravenous access line should be placed.[7] Glucagon may be useful for the reversal of hypotension in anaphylactoid shock due to radio contrast dye injection.[28]

REFERENCES

1. Committee on Drugs and Contrast Media, American College of Radiology. Manual on Iodinated Contrast Media. 1991.
2. Reynolds JEF, ed. *Martindale: The extra pharmacopoeia.* 30th ed. London: Pharmaceutical Press, 1993; pp. 702–711.
3. McEvoy GK, ed. AHFS Drug Information 92. Bethesda, MD: American Society of Hospital Pharmacists, 1992; pp. 1420–1474.
4. Westhoff-Bleck M, Bleck JS, Josk S. The adverse effects of angiographic radiocontrast media. Drug Safety 1991;6: 28–36.
5. Almen T. Relations between chemical structure, animal toxicity and clinical adverse effects of contrast media. In: Enge I, Edgren J, eds. Patient safety and adverse events in contrast media examinations. Amsterdam: Elsevier, 1989. Nycomed Scientific Symposium 1988. Oslo, Norway: October 18, 1988, p. 25–45.
6. Siegle RL. Treatment of contrast reactions. Hosp Formul 1991;26:662–665.
7. Spinler SA, Goldfarb S. Nephrotoxicity of contrast media following coronary angiography: pathogenesis, clinical course and preventive measures including the role of low osmolality contrast media. Ann Pharmacother 1992;26:56–64.
8. Leeds NE. The clinical application of radiopharmaceuticals. Drugs 1990;40:713–721.
9. Parfery PS, Cramer BC, McManamon PJ. Should nonionic radiographic contrast media be given to all patients? Can Med Assoc J 1988;138:497–500.
10. Katayama N, Yamaguchi K, Kozuka T, Takashima T, Seez P, Matsurra K. Adverse reactions to ionic and nonionic contrast media. A report from the Japanese Committee on the Safety of Contrast Media. Radiology 1990;175:621–628.
11. Wolf GL, Arenson RL, Cross AP. A prospective trial of ionic vs nonionic contrast agents in routine clinical practice. Comparison of adverse effects. Am J Radiol 1989;152:939–944.
12. Goldstein HA, Kashanian FK, Blumetti RF, Holyoak WL, Hugo FP, Blumenfield DM. Safety assessment of gadopenetate dimeglumine in US clinical trials. Radiology 1990;174:1723.
13. Harbury OL. Generalized seizures after IV administration of gadopenetate dimeglumine. Am J Neurol 1991;12:666.
14. Peck WW, Slutsky RA, Mancini GBJ, Higgins CB. Combined actions of verapamil and contrast media on atrioventricular conduction. Invest Radiol 1984;19:202.
15. Maley P, Olivecrona H, Almen T, Golman K. Interaction between chlorpromazine and intrathecally injected nonionic contrast media in non-anesthetized rabbits. Neuroradiology 1984;26:235.
16. Dehmer GJ, Gresalfi N, Daly D, Oberhardt B, Tate DA. Impairment of fibrinolysis by streptokinase, urokinase and recombinant tissue-type plasminogen activator in the presence of radiographic contrast agents. J Am Coll Cardiol 1995;25:1069–1075.
17. Oldham RK, Grobley J, Braud E. Contrast medium "recalls". Interleukin-2 toxicity. J Clin Oncol 1990;8:942–943.
18. Abi-Aad AS, Figlun RA, Belldegrum A, de Kernion JB. Metastatic renal cell cancer: interleukin-2 toxicity induced by contrast agent injection. J Immunother 1991;10: 292–295.
19. Zukowski AA, David CL, Coan J, Wallace S, Gutterman JV, Margalit GM. Increased incidence of hypersensitivity to iodine-containing radiographic contrast media after interleukin-2 administration. Cancer 1990;65:1521–1524.
20. Heinzer H, Huland E, Huland H. Adverse reaction to contrast material in a patient treated with local interleukin-2. Am J Roentgenol 1992;158:1407.
21. Reference Deleted.
22. Goodkin DA. Radiographic contrast medium-induced glossitis. Arch Intern Med 1985;145:171–172.
23. Rao AK, Thompson R, Durlacher L, Jones F. Angiographic contrast agents–induced acute hemolysis in a patient with hemoglobin SC disease. Arch Intern Med 1985;145: 759–760.
24. Doyama K, Kosuga K, Morikawa M, Watanabe Y. Coronary artery spasm induced by anaphylactoid reaction to a new low osmolar contrast media. Am Heart J 1990;120: 1453–1455.
25. Shehadi WH, Toniolo G. Adverse reactions to contrast media: a report from the Committee on Safety of Contrast Media of the International Society of Radiology. Radiology 1980;137:299–302.
26. Gluck BS, Mitty HA. Reactions to iodinated radiographic contrast agents. How to identify and manage patients at risk. Postgrad Med 1990;80:187–194.
27. Stejskall V, Nilsson R, Grepe A. Immunologic reactions to radiographic contrast media. Acta Radiol 1990;31:605–612.
28. Lang DM, Alperin MB, Visintainer PF, Smith ST. Increased risk for anaphylactoid reactions from contrast media in patients on beta-adrenergic blockers or with asthma. Ann Intern Med 1991;115:270–276.
29. Benotti JR. The comparative effects of ionic versus nonionic agents in cardiac catheterization. Invest Radiol 1988; 23(Suppl 2):S366–S373.
30. Steinberg EP, Moore RD, Powe NR, Gopalan R, Davidoff AJ, Litt M et al: Safety and cost effectiveness of high osmolality as compared with low osmolality contrast material in patients undergoing cardiac angiography. N Engl J Med 1992; 326:425–437.
31. Cooper MW, Reed PJ. QT prolongation with intracoronary contrast agents: significant difference between ionic and nonionic agents. Clin Res 1990;38:25A.
32. Glober JR, Thomas BM. Severe adverse reaction to oral iohexol. Clin Radiol 1991;44:137–138.
33. Martin ES. Danger of epidural use of ionic contrast media. Clin Pharm 1992;11:105.
34. Minuk J, Melancon D, Tampieri D, Ethier R. Transient global amnesia associated with cerebral angiography performed with use of iopanidol. Radiology 1990;174: 285–281.
35. Lantos G. Cortical blindness due to osmotic disruption of the blood-brain barrier by angiographic contrast material: CT and MRI studies. Neurology 1989;39:567–571.

36. Mallat Z, Vassal T, Naouri JF, Prier A, Laredo JD et al. Aseptic meningoencephalitis after iopamidol myelography. Lancet 199; 338:252.
37. Bell JA, Dowd TC, Melwaine GG, Brittain GPH. Post myelographic abducent nerve palsy in association with the contrast agent iopentol. J Clin Neuro Ophthalmol 1990;10:115–117.
38. Noda K, Miyamoto K, Beppu H, Hirose K, Tanabe H. Prolonged paraplegia after iohexol myelography. Lancet 1991;337:681.
39. Junck L, Marshall WH. Neurotoxicity of radiological contrast agents. Ann Neurol 1983;13:469–489.
40. Nelson M, Bartlett RJV, Lancet JT. Seizures after intravenous contrast media for cranial computed tomography. J Neurol Neurosurg Psychiatry 1989;52:1170–1175.
41. May P, Bach-Gan smo T, Elmquist D. Risk of seizures after myelography: comparison of iohexol and metrizamide. Am J Neuroradiol 1988;9:879–883.
42. Eliashiv S, Wirguon I, Brenner T, Argov Z. Aggravation of human and experimental myasthenia gravis by contrast media. Neurology 1990;40:1623–1625.
43. Michelis AA. Effect of intravascular contrast media on blood-brain barrier. Comparison between iothalmate, iohexol, iopentol and iodixanol. Acta Radiol 1987;28:329–333.
44. Van de Kelft E, Bosmans J, Parizel PM, Van Vyve M, Selosse P. Intracerebral hemorrhage after lumbar myelography with iohexol: report of a case and review of the literature. Neurosurgery 1991;28:570–574.
45. Bouachour G, Varache N, Szapiro N, L'Hoste P, Harry P, Alquier P. Noncardiogenic pulmonary edema resulting from intravascular administration of contrast material. Am J Radiol 1991;157:255–256.
46. Kozlowski C, Killef MM. Noncardiogenic pulmonary edema associated with intravenous radiocontrast administration. Chest 1992;102:620–621.
47. Van den Plas O, Hantson P, Dive A, Mahieu P. Fulminant pulmonary edema following intravenous administration of radiocontrast media. Acta Clin Belg 1990;45:334–339.
48. Borish L, Matloff SM, Findlay SR. Radiographic contrast media-induced noncardiogenic pulmonary edema: case report and review of the literature. J Allergy Clin Immunol 1984;74:104–107.
49. Jennings CA, Deveikis J, Azyni N, Yerager H Jr. Eosinophilic pneumonia associated with reaction to radiographic contrast media. South Med J 1991;84:92–95.
50. Berns AS. Nephrotoxicity of contrast media. Kidney Int 1989; 36:730–740.
51. Cronin RE. Southwestern Internal Medicine Conference: renal failure following radiologic procedure. Am J Med Sci 1989; 298:342–356.
52. Barrett BJ, Parfrey PS, Vavasour HM, McDonald J, Kent G, Hefferton D et al. Contrast nephropathy in patients with impaired renal function. High versus low osmolar media. Kidney Int 1992;41:1279.
53. Dawson P, Trewhella M. Intravascular contrast agents and renal failure. Clin Radiol 1990;41:373–375.
54. Harding MB, Davidson CJ, Pieper KS, Slatky M, Schwab SJ, Morris KG et al. Comparison of cardiovascular and renal toxicity after cardiac catheterization using a nonionic versus ionic radiographic contrast agent. Am J Cardiol 1991;68: 117–119.
55. Brezis M, Epstein FH. A closer look at radiocontrast-induced nephropathy. N Engl J Med 1989;320:179–181.
56. Moore RD, Steinberg EP, Powe NP, Brinker JA, Fishman EK, Graziano S et al. Nephrotoxicity of high-osmolality versus low-osmolality contrast media. Randomized clinical trial. Radiology 1992;182:649–655.
57. Cedgard S, Herlitz H, Deterud K, Attman P-O, Aurell M. Acute renal insufficiency after administration of low-osmolar contrast media. Lancet 1986;2:1281.
58. Heller CA, Knapp J, Halliday J, O'Connell D, Heller RF. Failure to demonstrate contrast nephrotoxicity. Med J Aust 1991;155:329–332.
59. Katzberg RW. What do we really know about contrast medium–induced acute renal failure? Invest Radiol 1989; 24:219–220.
60. Rucnick MR, Goldfarb S, Wexler L, Ludbrook PA, Murphy MJ, Halpern EF et al for the Iohexol Cooperative Study. Nephrotoxicity of ionic and nonionic contrast media in 1,196 patients: a randomized trial. Kidney Int 1995;47:254–261.
61. Parfrey PS, Griffiths SM, Barrett BJ, Paul MD, Genge M, Withers J et al. Contrast material-induced renal failure in patients with diabetes mellitus, renal insufficiency, or both. A prospective controlled study. N Engl J Med 1989;320: 143–149.
62. Cigarroa RG, Lange RA, Williams RH, Hillis LD. Dosing of contrast material to prevent contrast nephropathy in patients with renal disease. Am J Med 1989;86:649–652.
63. Fareed J, Walenga JM, Saravia GE, Moncada RM. Thrombogenic potential of nonionic contrast media? Radiology 1990;174:321–325.
64. Warning added to labeling of iodinated contrast agents. FDA Drug Bulletin 1989;19(2):19.
65. Robertson HJ. Thrombogenic potential of nonionic contrast media. Mayo Clin Proc 1990;65:603–604.
66. Grollman JH Jr, Liu CK, Astone RA, Lurie MD. Thromboembolic complications in coronary angiography associated with the use of nonionic contrast media. Cathet Cardiovasc Diagn 1988;14:159–164.
67. Stormarken IJ. Present state of contrast media as related to thromboembolic complications. Sem Hematol 1991; 28(Suppl 7):69–72.
68. Brinker JA. Contrast and clotting. The cardiologist's perspective. Semin Hematol 1991;28(Suppl 7):3–10.
69. Dawson P. Nonionic contrast agents and coagulation. J Invest Radiol 1988;23(Suppl 2):S310–S317.
70. Arora R, Khandelwal M, Gopal A. In vivo effects of nonionic and ionic contrast media on beta thromboglobulin and fibrinopeptide levels. J Am Coll Cardiol 1991;17:1533–1536.
71. de Bruin TWA. Iodide-induced hyperthyroidism with computed tomography contrast fluids. Lancet 1994;343: 1160–1161.
72. Karpman BA, Rapaport B, Filetti S, Fisher DA. Treatment of neonatal hyperthyroidism due to Graves' disease and sodium ipodate. J Clin Endocrinol Metab 1987;64:119–123.
73. Reiner RG, Lawson MJ, Marshall J, Read TR, Beng CG, Davies GT et al. Thyroid, renal and hepatic function tests following cholecystography with high-dose contrast agents. Dig Dis Sci 1980;25:379–383.
74. Jansen TThA, Meijer JWR, Kesselring FOHW, Mulder CJJ. Synchronous hepatic tumours 60 years after diagnostic thorotrast use. Eur J Gastroenterol Hepatol 1992;4:753–755.
75. Kim S-J, Salem MR, Joseph NJ, Madayag MA, Cavallino RP, Crystal GJ. Contrast media adversely affect oxyhemoglobin dissociation. Anesth Analg 1990;71:73–76.
76. Wylie EJ, Mitchell DB. Case report: iodide mumps following intravenous urography with iopanidol. Clin Radiol 1991;43: 135–136.
77. Rosati G, di Priolo SL, Tirone P. Serious or fatal complications after inadvertent administration of ionic water-soluble contrast media in myelography. Eur J Radiol 1992; 15:95–100.
78. May EF, Ling GSF, Geyer CA, Jabbari B. Contrast agent overdose causing brain retention of contrast, seizures and parkinsonism. Neurology 1993;43:836–838.
79. Tartiere J, Gerard J-L, Peny J, Hurpe J-M, Quesnol J. Acute treatment of accidental intrathecal injection of hypertonic contrast media. Anesthesiology 1989;71:169.
80. Nakazawa K, Yoshinari M, Kinefuchi S, Amaha K. Inadvertent intrathecal administration of amidetrizoate. Intensive Care Med 1988;15:55–57.
81. Vossler DG, Wright Jr SJ. Convulsive status epilepticus following intrathecal iopamidol administration. J Epilepsy 1994; 7:18–20.
82. Olsen J. Seizures after myelography with iopamidol. Am J Emerg Med 1994;12:329–330.
83. Harash LT. Mallinckrodt Medical. St Louis, MO. Conray (iothalamate meglumine injection USP 60%) product literature. MKP0953790. Revised 7/90. Personal communication. September 2, 1992.
84. Gray C, Sivaloganathan S, Simpkins KC. Aspiration of high density barium contrast medium causing acute pulmo-

nary aspiration. Report of two fatal cases in elderly women with disordered swallowing. Clin Radiol 1989;40:397–400.

85. Parcy JPM, Montgomery BPO, Reading N. Acute pneumonitis caused by low-density barium sulphate aspiration. J Laryngol Otol 1993;107:347–348.

86. Page B, Dallara JJ. Does Reglan (metoclopramide) prevent vomiting of oral CT contrast in stable multiple trauma patients? Acad Emerg Med 1994;1:A65.

87. Gelfand DW, Ott DJ, Klein A. Massive iopanoic acid (Telepaque) overdose without ill effects. Am J Roentgenol 1978;130:1174–1175.

88. McLennan BL, Kassner EG, Becker JA. Overdose at excretory urography. Toxic cause of death. Radiology 1972; 105:383–386.

89. Ansell G. Fatal overdose of contrast medium in infants. Br J Radiol 1970;395–396.

90. Solomon R, Werner C, Mann D, D'Elia J, Silva P. Effects of saline, mannitol and furosemide on acute decreases in renal function induced by radiocontrast agents. N Engl J Med 1994;331:1416–1420.

91. Barrett BJ, Parfrey PS: Prevention of nephrotoxicity induced by radiocontrast agents. N Engl J Med 1994;331:1449–1450.

Chapter 61

Cancer Chemotherapeutic Agents (Cytotoxic Drugs)

When cancer chemotherapeutic agents are administered in overdose (orally or by injection) or in the wrong site (intrathecally instead of intravenously), predictable (bone marrow suppression) and unpredictable (brain damage after inadvertent intrathecal use) toxic reactions may follow. Most overdoses with cytotoxic drugs are managed without antidotes, and few of these are easily available.

Clinical toxicity of antineoplastic drugs is known to be particularly centered in rapidly dividing cells: in the bone marrow, gut mucosa, hair follicles, germinal epithelium of the testes, thymus, and fetus.[1] In addition, some cytotoxic agents are photosensitizing (fluorouracil), but this is uncommon. Finally, severe toxicity has been caused by local irritation and ulceration resulting from extravasation of a cytotoxic drug into the tissues outside a vein.[1] Many antineoplastic agents have exhibited a direct irritant effect on the skin, eyes, mucous membrane, and other tissues. Protective measures for the doctor, the nurse, the patient, and other health care personnel who handle cytotoxic drugs have often been inadequate.

CLASSIFICATION

There are over 60 anticancer drugs in active general use, as well as a number of investigational drugs available for special use (Table 61–1). Anticancer drugs may be generally characterized as alkylating agents, antimetabolites, natural products, hormone inhibitors, or other miscellaneous products. Within each group of cytotoxic drugs the toxic effects exhibited by one member of the class are not easily translated to others of the same group.

DOSES

Maximally tolerated doses of some anticancer drugs in adults and children are listed in Table 61–2.[2]

Drug Interactions (see Table 61–3)

CLINICAL PRESENTATION

Table 61–4 summarizes acute and chronic toxicities of some anticancer drugs and hormones.[3]

Table 61–1
Cytotoxics-Anticancer Agents

1. Alkylating agents
   a. Nitrogen mustards
      Chlorambucil
      Cyclophosphamide
      Ifosfamide
      Mechlorethamine
      Melphalan
   b. Ethyleneimine derivatives complexes
      Thiotepa
   c. Alkyl sulfonates
      Busulfan
   d. Nitrosoureas
      Carmustine
      Lomustine
      Streptozocin
   e. Triazenes
      Dacarbazine
2. Antimetabolites
   a. Folic acid antagonists
      Methotrexate
      Trimetrexate (treatment IND)
   b. Pyrimidine analogues
      5-Fluorouracil
      Floxuridine
      Cytarabine
   c. Purine analogues
      6-Mercaptopurine
      6-Thioguanine
   d. Adenine analogue
      Fludarabine-A (treatment IND)
   e. Adenosine deaminase inhibitors
      Pentostatin (treatment IND)
   f. Interferons
      Interferon alfa 2a
      Interferon alfa 2b
3. Natural products
   a. Vinca alkaloids
      Vincristine
      Vinblastine
      Vindesine
   b. Antitumor antibiotics
      Aclarubicin
      (Actinomycin-D)
      Bleomycin
      Dactinomycin
      Mitamycin-C
      5-Azacytidine
   c. Enzymes
      6-Asparaginase
   d. Epipodophyllotoxins
      Etoposide
      Teniposide
   e. Homoharringtonine
4. Miscellaneous agents
   a. Platinum coordination
      Cisplastin
      Carboplatin
   b. Hydroxyurea
   c. Procarbazine
   d. Hexamethylmelamine
   e. Amsacrine
   f. Mitoxantrone
   g. Mitotane
   h. Leucovorin, calcium
   i. Levamisole
   j. Bacillus Calmette-Guerin (BCG)
   k. Aminoglutethimide
   l. Coumarin
   m. Estramustine
   n. Mesna
5. Androgen inhibitors
      Cyproterone acetate
      Flutamide
      Leuprolide acetate
6. Antiestrogen
      Tamoxifen citrate
7. Hormones
      Testolactone
      Investigational
      DTIC
      Esorubicin (analog of doxorubicin)
      Flavone-8-acetic acid
      Mafosfamide
      Murine monoclonal antibody vinca
      Conjugate
      Navelbine (vinca derivative)
      Suramin
      Daunorubicin
      Doxorubicin
      Epirubicin
      Plicaamycin
      Idarubicin

Table 61–2
Maximally Tolerated Doses of Some Anticancer Drugs in Adults and Children[a]

Drug	Schedule	MTD (mg/m^2) Children	MTD (mg/m^2) Adults	Ratio MTD Children: Adults
Dianhydrogalactitol	q.d. × 5 days	25	30	0.83
5-Azacytidine	q.d. × 5 days	200	225	0.89
Piperazinedione	q.d. × 5 days	3	3	1.0
Etoposide (VP-16)	Biweekly	150	125	1.20
Diglycoaldehyde	q.d. × 5 days	7500	6000	1.25
Amsacrine	q.d. × 5 days	50	40	1.25
Daunomycin (mg/kg)	q.d. × 4 days	1.0	0.8	1.25
Doxorubicin (mg/kg)	q.d. × 4 days	0.8	0.6	1.33
Teniposide (VM-26) (mg/kg)	Biweekly	4.0	3.0	1.33
3-Deazauridine (leukemia patients)	q.d. × 5 days	8.2	6.0	1.40
Azaserine (mg/kg, total dose)	Daily	156	108	1.44
Dihydroxyanthracenedione	Every 3 wks	18	12	1.5
3-Deazauridine (solid tumors)	q.d. × 5 days	2.8	1.5	1.85
Cyclocytidine	q.d. × 10 days	600	300	2.00
ICRF-187	q.d. × 3 days	>2750	1250	>2.20

[a]Adapted from Petros WP, Evans WE. Pharmacotherapy 1990;10:313–325.

Table 61–3
Drug Interactions

Anthracyclines	
+ Drugs that worsen cardiotoxicity[1]	
Etoposide	Mitomycin C
Vincristine	Cisplatin
Bleomycin	Cyclophosphamide
Busulfan	
Bleomycin	
+ Cisplatin—nephrotoxicity reduces bleomycin clearance[2]	
Carmustine	
+ Phenobarbital	Increased metabolism of chemotherapeutic agent; may reduce antitumor activity[2]
Antitumor Lomustine	
+ Misonidazole	May increase antitumor activity[3,4]
Cisplatin	
+ Furosemide	May reduce its urinary excretion, produce higher peak plasma concentrations[3]
+ Mannitol	Neutralizes cisplatin; forms platinum-thiosulfate complex[5]
+ Probenecid	
+ Sodium thiosulfate	
Cyclophosphamide	
+ Allopurinol	Increased bone marrow depression[2,6,7]
+ Phenobarbital	?Increased bone marrow depression[3]
+ Cimetidine	May depress clearance of cyclophosphamide[8]
+ Cyclophosphamide	May induce its own metabolism[9]
Cytarabine	
+ Tetrahydrouridine	Is inhibitor of cytidine deaminase; increases half-life of cytarabine[10]
Doxorubicin	
+ Increases effects of radiation; elicits radiation recall reactions[3]	
+ Cyclophosphamide: decreased doxorubicin, doxorubicinol clearance[11]	
+ Adheres to many materials—filters and tubing of administration system and to plastics; accounts for a loss of approximately 5%[12]	
+ Digoxin: Decreases gastrointestinal absorption of oral digoxin by 20%[13]	
Etoposide	
+ Phenytoin	Increased excreted metabolites of etoposide[14]
+ Vindesine & Warfarin	Displaces warfarin from its albumin binding sites[15]
Synergistic with[15]	
Carmustine	
Cisplatin	
Cyclophosphamide	
Cytosine arabinoside	
5-Fluorouracil	
Methotrexate	
Vincristine	
Potentiated by:	
Verapamil[15]	
5-Fluorouracil	
+ Methotrexate pretreatment	Increases effectiveness and toxicity of 5-fluorouracil[2,3]
+ Thymidine	Decreases renal clearance[3]
+ Cimetidine	May lead to increase in 5-FU peak concentrations[16]
+ Misonidazole	Reduces clearance of 5-fluorouracil[14,17]
Ifosfamide	
+ Disulfiram	May lessen ifosfamide-induced bladder damage[18]
+ Diethyldithiocarbamate	
6-Mercaptopurine	
+ Allopurinol	Inhibits xanthine oxidase, enhances hematotoxicity of 6-Mercaptopurine; increases plasma level[2,3]

1. Watts RG. Am J Hematol 1991;36:217–218.
2. Balis FM, Holcenberg JS, Bleyer WA. Clin Pharmacokinet 1983;8:202:232.
3. Balis FM. Clin Pharmacokinet 1986;11:223–235.
4. Lee FYF, Worhuan P. Int J Radiat Oncol Biol Phys 1984;10:1627–1630.
5. Pfeifle CE, Howell SB, Felthouse RD, Woliver BS, Andrews PA et al. J Clin Oncol 1985;3:237–244.
6. Boston Collaborative Drug Surveillance Program. JAMA 1974;227:1036–1040.
7. Witten J, Frederiksen PL, Mouridsen HT. Acta Pharm Toxicol 1980;46:392–395.
8. Dorr RT, Alberts DS. Br J Cancer 1982;45:25–43.
9. Graham MI, Shaw IC. Souhami RL, Sidau B, Harper PG et al. Cancer Chemother Pharmacol 1983;10:192–193.
10. Kreis W, Woodcock TM, Gordon CS, Krakoff IH. Cancer Treat Rep 1977;61:1347–1353.
11. Evans WE, Crow WR, Yee GC, Green AA, Hayes FA, Pratt CB, Avery TL. Proc Am Assoc Cancer Res 180;21:176.
12. Speth PAJ, Van Hoesel QGCM, Hooner C. Clin Pharmacokinet 1988;15:15–31.
13. Kuhlmann J. Dtsch Med Wochenschr 1981;106:468–470.
14. Diasio RB, Harris BE. Clin Pharmacokinet 1989;16:215–237.
15. Clark PI, Slevin ML. Clin Pharmacokinet 1987;12:223–252.
16. Harvey VJ, Slevin ML, Dilloway MR, Clark PL, Johnston A et al. Br J Clin Pharm 1984;18:421–430.
17. McDermott BJ, Van der Berg HW, Martin WMC, Murphy RF. Br J Cancer 1982;48:705–710.
18. Ishikawa M, Takayanagi Y, Sasaki K. Pharmacol Toxicol 1991;68:21–25.
19. Haim N, Kedar A, Robinson E. Cancer Chemother Pharmacol 1984;13:223–225.

(continued)

Table 61–3 *(Continued)*

Methotrexate + Salicylates Carbenicillin Cephalothin Indomethacin Ketoprofen Probenicid Sulphonamides Ticarcillin	Reduction of renal tubular methotrexate secretion; Increased blood levels of methotrexate[2, 3]
+ Cisplatin	Increased toxicities[19]
Teniposide Synergistic with: Carmustine Cytosine arabinoside Hexamethylmelamine[15] Methotrexate	

Table 61–4
Some Anticancer Drugs and Hormones[a]

Drug	Acute Toxicity[c]	Delayed Toxicity[c]
Aldesleukin (interleukin-2; *Proleukin*—Cetus Oncology)	**Fever; fluid retention; hypotension; respiratory distress;** rash; anemia; thrombocytopenia; nausea and vomiting; diarrhea; capillary leak syndrome; nephrotoxicity; myocardial toxicity; hepatotoxicity; erythema nodosum; neutrophil chemotactic defects	Neuropsychiatric disorders; hypothyroidism; nephrotic syndrome; possibly acute leukoencephalopathy; brachial plexopathy; bowel perforation
Altretamine (hexamethylmelamine; *Hexalen*—US Bioscience)	Nausea and vomiting	**Bone marrow depression;** CNS depression; peripheral neuropathy; visual hallucinations; ataxia; tremors; alopecia; rash
Aminoglutethimide (*Cytadren*—Ciba)	Drowsiness; nausea; dizziness; rash	Hypothyroidism (rare); bone marrow depression; fever; hypotension; masculinization
[b]Amsacrine (m-AMSA; amsidine; *AMSA P-D*—Parke-Davis, *Amsidyl*—Warner-Lambert)	Nausea and vomiting; diarrhea; pain or phlebitis on infusion; anaphylaxis	**Bone marrow depression;** hepatic injury; convulsions; stomatitis; ventricular fibrillation; alopecia; congestive heart failure; renal dysfunction
Asparaginase (*Elspar*—Merck; *Kidrolase* in Canada)	Nausea and vomiting; fever; chills; headache; hypersensitivity, anaphylaxis; abdominal pain; hyperglycemia leading to coma	CNS depression or hyperexcitability; acute hemorrhagic pancreatitis; coagulation defects; thrombosis; renal damage; hepatic damage
[b]Azacitidine (ladakamycin; *Mylosar*—Upjohn)	Nausea and vomiting; diarrhea; fever; rash; drowsiness	**Bone marrow depression;** hepatic damage; muscle pain and weakness; possibly cardiotoxicity
BCG (*TheraCys*—Connaught; *Tice BCG*—Organon)	Bladder irritation; nausea and vomiting; fever; sepsis	Granulomatous pyelonephritis; hepatitis; urethral obstruction; epididymitis; renal abscess
Bleomycin (*Blenoxane*—Bristol-Myers Oncology)	Nausea and vomiting; fever; anaphylaxis and other allergic reactions; phlebitis at injection site	**Pneumonitis and pulmonary fibrosis;** rash and hyperpigmentation; stomatitis; alopecia; Raynaud's phenomenon; cavitating granulomas; hemorrhagic cystitis
Busulfan (*Myleran*—Burroughs Wellcome)	Nausea and vomiting; rare diarrhea	**Bone marrow depression; pulmonary infiltrates and fibrosis;** alopecia; gynecomastia; ovarian failure; hyperpigmentation; azoospermia; leukemia; chromosome aberrations; cataracts; hepatitis; seizures and veno-occlusive disease with high doses
Carboplatin (*Paraplatin*—Bristol-Myers Oncology)	Nausea and vomiting	**Bone marrow depression;** peripheral neuropathy (uncommon); hearing loss; transient cortical blindness; hemolytic anemia

[a]Adapted from Med Lett Drugs Ther 1995;37:25–32.
[b]Available in the USA only for investigational use.
[c]Dose-limiting effects are in bold type. Cutaneous reactions (sometimes severe), hyperpigmentation, and ocular toxicity have been reported with virtually all nonhormonal anticancer drugs. For adverse interactions with other drugs, see *The Medical Letter Handbook of Adverse Drug Interactions*, 1995.

(continued)

Table 61–4 *(Continued)*

Drug	Acute Toxicity[c]	Delayed Toxicity[c]
Carmustine (BCNU; *BiCNU*—Bristol-Myers Oncology)	Nausea and vomiting; local phlebitis	**Delayed leukopenia and thrombocytopenia** (may be prolonged); pulmonary fibrosis (may be irreversible); delayed renal damage; reversible liver damage; leukemia; myocardial ischemia
Chlorambucil (*Leukeran*—Burroughs Wellcome)	Nausea and vomiting; seizures	**Bone marrow depression;** pulmonary infiltrates and fibrosis; leukemia; hepatic toxicity; sterility
[b]Chlorozotocin (DCNU—Dome)	Similar to streptozocin, but less nausea and vomiting	Similar to streptozocin, but **leukopenia** and **thrombocytopenia** are common
Cisplatin (Cis-DDP; *Platinol*—Bristol-Myers Oncology)	Nausea and vomiting; diarrhea; anaphylactic reactions	**Renal damage;** ototoxicity; bone marrow depression; hemolysis; hypomagnesemia; peripheral neuropathy; hypocalcemia; hypokalemia; Raynaud's disease; sterility; hypophosphatemia; hyperuricemia
Cladribine (2-chlorode-oxyadenosine; CdA; *Leustatin*—Ortho-Biotech)	Fever	**Bone marrow depression;** peripheral neuropathy with high doses
Cyclophosphamide (*Cytoxan*—Mead Johnson Oncology, *Procytox*—Horner, and others)	Nausea and vomiting; Type I (anaphylactoid) hypersensitivity; facial burning with IV administration; visual blurring	**Bone marrow depression;** alopecia; hemorrhagic cystitis; sterility (may be temporary); pulmonary infiltrates and fibrosis; hyponatremia; leukemia; bladder cancer; inappropriate ADH secretion; cardiac toxicity
Cytarabine HCl (*Cytosar-U*—Upjohn, and others)	Nausea and vomiting; diarrhea; anaphylaxis; sudden respiratory distress with high doses	**Bone marrow depression;** conjunctivitis; megaloblastosis; oral ulceration; hepatic damage; fever; pulmonary edema and central and peripheral neurotoxicity with high doses; rhabdomyolysis; pancreatitis when used with asparaginase; rash
Dacarbazine (*DTIC-Dome*—Miles, and others)	Nausea and vomiting; diarrhea; anaphylaxis; pain on administration	**Bone marrow depression;** alopecia; flu-like syndrome; renal impairment; hepatic necrosis; facial flushing; paresthesia; photosensitivity; urticarial rash
Dactinomycin (*Cosmegan*—Merck)	Nausea and vomiting; hepatic toxicity with ascites; diarrhea; severe local tissue damage and necrosis on extravasation; anaphylactoid reaction	**Stomatitis; oral ulceration; bone marrow depression;** alopecia; folliculitis; dermatitis in previously irradiated areas
Daunorubicin HCl (*Cerubidine*—Wyeth-Ayerst, Rhone-Poulenc Rorer in Canada)	Nausea and vomiting; diarrhea; red urine (not hematuria); severe local tissue damage and necrosis on extravasation; transient EKG changes; facial flushing; anaphylactoid reaction	**Bone marrow depression; cardiotoxicity** (may be delayed for years); alopecia; stomatitis; anorexia; diarrhea; fever and chills; dermatitis in previously irradiated areas; skin and nail pigmentation; photosensitivity
Diethylstilbestrol (Lilly; *Stilphostrol*—Miles)	Nausea and vomiting; abdominal cramps; headache	Gynecomastia in males; breast tenderness; loss of libido; thrombophlebitis and thromboembolism; hepatic injury; sodium retention with edema; hypertension; change in menstrual flow
Doxorubicin HCl (*Adriamycin*—Pharmacia, and others)	Nausea and vomiting; red urine (not hematuria); severe local tissue damage and necrosis on extravasation; diarrhea; fever; transient EKG changes; ventricular arrhythmia; anaphylactoid reaction	**Bone marrow depression; cardiotoxicity** (may be delayed for years); alopecia; stomatitis; anorexia; conjunctivitis; acral pigmentation; dermatitis in previously irradiated areas; acral erythrodysesthesia; hyperuricemia
Estramustine phosphate sodium (*Emcyt*—Kabi Pharmacia)	Nausea and vomiting; diarrhea	Mild gynecomastia; increased frequency of vascular accidents; myelosuppression (uncommon); edema; dyspnea; pulmonary infiltrates and fibrosis; decreased glucose tolerance; thrombosis; hypertension
Etoposide (VP16-213; *VePesid*—Bristol-Myers Oncology)	Nausea and vomiting; diarrhea; fever; hypotension; anaphylactoid reactions; phlebitis at infusion site	**Bone marrow depression;** rashes; alopecia; peripheral neuropathy; mucositis and hepatic damage with high doses; leukemia
Etretinate (*Tegison*—Roche)		Dryness of mucous membranes; chapped lips; hair loss; bone and joint pain; eye irritation; peeling skin; pseudotumor cerebri; premature epiphyseal closure; hepatic injury; major teratogenic effects

(continued)

Table 61–4 *(Continued)*

Drug	Acute Toxicity[c]	Delayed Toxicity[c]
Finasteride (*Proscar*—Merck)		Impotence; decreased libido; teratogenic
Floxuridine (*FUDR*—Roche, and others)	Nausea and vomiting; diarrhea	**Oral and gastrointestinal ulceration; bone marrow depression;** alopecia; dermatitis; hepatic dysfunction with hepatic infusion
Fludarabine (*Fludara*—Berlex)	Nausea and vomiting	**Bone marrow depression;** CNS effects; visual disturbances; renal damage with higher doses; pulmonary infiltrates; tumor lysis syndrome
Fluorouracil (5-FU; *Adrucil*—Pharmacia, and others)	Nausea and vomiting; diarrhea; hypersensitivity reaction (rare)	**Oral and GI ulcers; bone marrow depression;** diarrhea (especially with fluorouracil and leucovorin); neurological defects, usually cerebellar; cardiac arrhythmias; angina pectoris; alopecia; hyperpigmentation; palmar-plantar erythrodysesthesia; conjunctivitis; heart failure; seizures
Flutamide (anti-androgen; *Eulexin*—Schering, *Euflex* in Canada)	Nausea; diarrhea	Gynecomastia; hepatotoxicity
Gallium nitrate (*Ganite*—Solo Pak)	Hypocalcemia	**Hypophosphatemia;** nephrotoxicity; anemia
[b]Gemcitabine (*Gemzar*—Lilly)	Fatigue	Bone marrow depression
Goserelin (*Zoladex*—Zeneca)	Transient increase in bone pain and ureteral obstruction in patients with metastatic prostate cancer; hot flashes	Impotence; testicular atrophy; gynecomastia
Hydroxyurea (*Hydrea*—Bristol-Myers Oncology)	Nausea and vomiting; allergic reactions to tartrazine dye	**Bone marrow depression;** stomatitis; dysuria; alopecia; rare neurological disturbances; pulmonary infiltrates
Idarubicin (*Idamycin*—Pharmacia)	Nausea and vomiting; tissue damage on extravasation	**Bone marrow depression;** alopecia; stomatitis; myocardial toxicity; diarrhea
Ifosfamide (*Ifex*—Mead Johnson Oncology)	Nausea and vomiting; confusion; nephrotoxicity; metabolic acidosis and renal Fanconi's syndrome; **cardiac toxicity** with high doses	**Bone marrow depression; hemorrhagic cystitis** (prevented by concurrent mesna); alopecia; inappropriate ADH secretion; renal failure; neurotoxicity (somnolence, hallucinations, blurring of vision, coma)
Interferon alfa-2a, alfa-2b, alfa-n3 (*Roferon-A*—Roche, *Intron A*—Schering, *Alferon N*—Purdue Frederick)	Fever; chills; myalgias; fatigue; headache; arthralgias; hypotension	Bone marrow depression; anorexia; neutropenia; anemia; confusion; depression; renal toxicity; possible hepatic injury; facial and peripheral edema; cardiac arrhythmias
Isotretinoin (*Accutane*—Roche)	Fatigue; headache; nausea and vomiting; pruritis	**Teratogenicity; cheilitis;** xerostomia; rash; conjunctivitis and eye irritation; bone and joint pain; anorexia; hypertriglyceridemia; pseudotumor cerebri
Leuprolide acetate (LHRH-analog; *Lupron, Lupron Depot*—TAP)	Transient increase in bone pain and ureteral obstruction in patients with metastatic prostate cancer; hot flashes	Impotence; testicular atrophy; CNS effects; gynecomastia; peripheral edema
Levamisole (*Ergamisol*—Janssen)	Nausea and vomiting; diarrhea; flu-like symptoms; metallic taste	Agranulocytosis; arthralgias; rash; encephalopathy; hyperlipidemia; pancreatitis; fatigue; peripheral neuropathy
Lomustine (CCNU; *CeeNU*—Bristol-Myers Oncology)	Nausea and vomiting	**Delayed (4 to 6 weeks) leukopenia and thrombocytopenia** (may be prolonged); transient elevation of transaminase activity; neurological reactions; pulmonary fibrosis; renal damage; leukemia
Mechlorethamine HCl (nitrogen mustard; *Mustargen*—Merck)	**Nausea and vomiting;** local reaction and phlebitis	**Bone marrow depression;** alopecia; diarrhea; oral ulcers; leukemia; amenorrhea; sterility; hyperuricemia
Medroxyprogesterone acetate (*Provera; Depo-Provera*—Upjohn, and others)	Nausea; urticaria; headache; fatigue	Menstrual changes; gynecomastia; hot flashes; weight gain; hirsutism; insomnia; fatigue; depression; edema; thrombophlebitis and thromboembolism; sterile abscess
Megestrol acetate (*Megace*—Mead Johnson Oncology, and others)	Nausea and vomiting; headache	Menstrual changes; hot flashes; thrombophlebitis and thromboembolism; fluid retention; edema; weight gain

(continued)

Table 61–4 *(Continued)*

Drug	Acute Toxicity[c]	Delayed Toxicity[c]
Melphalan (*Alkeran*—Burroughs Wellcome)	Mild nausea; hypersensitivity reactions	**Bone marrow depression** (especially platelets); pulmonary infiltrates and fibrosis; amenorrhea; sterility; leukemia
Mercaptopurine (*Purinethol*—Burroughs Wellcome)	Nausea and vomiting; diarrhea	**Bone marrow depression;** cholestasis and rarely hepatic necrosis; oral and intestinal ulcers; pancreatitis
Mesna (*Mesnex*—Bristol-Myers Oncology; *Uromitexan* in Canada)	Nausea and vomiting; diarrhea; allergic reactions	
Methotrexate (MTX; *Folex*—Pharmacia, and others)	Nausea and vomiting; diarrhea; fever; anaphylaxis; hepatic necrosis	**Oral and gastrointestinal ulceration,** perforation may occur; **bone marrow depression;** hepatic toxicity including cirrhosis; renal toxicity; **pulmonary infiltrates and fibrosis;** osteoporosis; conjunctivitis; alopecia; depigmentation; menstrual dysfunction; encephalopathy; infertility; lymphoma
Mitomycin (*Mutamycin*—Bristol-Myers Oncology)	Nausea and vomiting; tissue necrosis; fever	**Bone marrow depression** (cumulative); stomatitis; alopecia; acute pulmonary toxicity; pulmonary fibrosis; hepatotoxicity; renal toxicity; amenorrhea; hemolytic-uremic syndrome; bladder calcification (with intravesical administration)
Mitotane (o,p′-DDD; *Lysodren*—Bristol-Myers Oncology)	Nausea and vomiting; diarrhea	**CNS depression;** rash, visual disturbances; adrenal insufficiency; hematuria; hemorrhagic cystitis; albuminuria; hypertension; orthostatic hypotension; cataracts; prolonged bleeding time
Mitoxantrone HCl (*Novantrone*—Immunex)	Blue-green pigment in urine; blue-green sclera; nausea and vomiting; stomatitis; fever; phlebitis	**Bone marrow depression;** cardiotoxicity; alopecia; white hair; skin lesions; hepatic damage; renal failure; extravasation necrosis
[b]Nilutamide (*Anandron*—Roussel Uclaf)	Nausea and vomiting; alcohol intolerance	Delayed adaptation to darkness; interstitial pneumonitis; hepatic toxicity
Octreotide (*Sandostatin*—Sandoz)	Nausea and vomiting; diarrhea	Steatorrhea; gallstones
Paclitaxel (*Taxol*—Mead Johnson Oncology)	Anaphylaxis, dyspnea, hypotension, angioedema, urticaria (probably due to vehicle)	**Bone marrow depression;** peripheral neuropathy; alopecia; arthralgias; myalgias; cardiac toxicity; mild GI disturbances; mucositis
Pegaspargase (PEG-L-asparaginase; *Oncaspar*—Rhône-Poulenc Rorer)	Similar to asparaginase	Similar to asparaginase
Pentostatin (2′-deoxycoformycin; *Nipent*—Parke-Davis)	Nausea and vomiting; rash	Nephrotoxicity; CNS depression; **bone marrow depression;** respiratory failure; hepatic toxicity; arthralgia; myalgia; photophobia; conjunctivitis
Plicamycin (*Mithracin*—Miles)	Nausea and vomiting	**Hemorrhagic diathesis;** thrombocytopenia; coagulation abnormalities; hepatic damage; hypocalcemia; renal damage
Procarbazine HCl (*Matulane*—Roche, *Natulan* in Canada)	Nausea and vomiting; CNS depression; disulfiram-like effect with alcohol; adverse interactions typical of a monoamine oxidase (MAO) inhibitor	**Bone marrow depression; stomatitis; peripheral neuropathy; pneumonitis; leukemia**
Streptozocin (*Zanosar*—Upjohn, and others)	Nausea and vomiting; local pain	**Renal damage;** hypoglycemia; hyperglycemia; liver damage; diarrhea; bone marrow depression (uncommon); fever; eosinophilia; nephrogenic diabetes insipidus
Tamoxifen citrate (*Nolvadex*—Zeneca, and others; *Tamofen* in Canada)	Hot flashes; nausea and vomiting; transient increased bone or tumor pain; hypercalcemia	Vaginal bleeding and discharge; rash; thrombocytopenia; peripheral edema; depression; dizziness; headache; decreased visual acuity; corneal changes; retinopathy; purpuric vasculitis; thromboembolism; endometrial cancer
Teniposide (VM-26; *Vumon*—Bristol-Myers Oncology)	Nausea and vomiting; diarrhea; phlebitis; anaphylactoid symptoms	**Bone marrow depression;** alopecia; peripheral neuropathy; leukemia

(continued)

Table 61–4 *(Continued)*

Drug	Acute Toxicity[c]	Delayed Toxicity[c]
Thioguanine (Burroughs Wellcome, *Lanvis* in Canada)	Occasional nausea and vomiting; diarrhea	**Bone marrow depression;** hepatic damage; stomatitis
Thiotepa (Immunex)	Nausea and vomiting; rare hypersensitivity reaction	**Bone marrow depression;** menstrual dysfunction; interference with spermatogenesis; leukemia; mucositis with high doses
[b]Tretinoin (*Vesanoid*—Roche)	**Headache; xerosis;** pruritus; "retinoic acid syndrome" (fever, dyspnea, pulmonary infiltrates, pleural effusions, peripheral edema, hypotension); arthralgias; myalgias	**Cheilitis; teratogenicity;** rashes; leukocytosis; hypertriglyceridemia; pseudotumor cerebri; thrombophlebitis
Trimetrexate (*Neutrexin*—US Bioscience)	Fever; chills; nausea and vomiting; diarrhea	**Bone marrow depression; mucositis;** peripheral neuropathy; rash; pruritis; hyperpigmentation; nephrotoxicity; hepatic injury
Vinblastine sulfate (*Velban*—Lilly, and others; *Velbe* in Canada)	Nausea and vomiting; local reaction and tissue damage with extravasation	**Bone marrow depression;** alopecia; stomatitis; loss of deep tendon reflexes; jaw pain; muscle pain; paralytic ileus
Vincristine sulfate (*Oncovin*—Lilly, and others)	Tissue damage with extravasation	**Peripheral neuropathy;** alopecia; mild bone marrow depression; constipation; paralytic ileus; jaw pain; inappropriate ADH secretion; optic atrophy
Vinorelbine tartrate (*Navelbine*—Burroughs Wellcome)	Nausea and vomiting; diarrhea; constipation; dyspnea; injection site reactions (erythema, discoloration, phlebitis, pain)	**Bone marrow depression;** alopecia; anorexia; stomatitis; asthenia; peripheral neuropathy

REFERENCES

1. Knowles RS, Virden JA. Handling of injectable antineoplastic agents. Br Med J 1981;281:589–591.
2. Petras WP, Evans WE. Pharmacokinetics and pharmacodynamics of anticancer agents: contributions to the therapy of childhood cancer. Pharmacotherapy 1990;10:313–325.
3. Drugs of choice for cancer chemotherapy. Med Lett Drugs Ther 1995;37:25–32.

PREGNANCY

The simultaneous occurrence of cancer and pregnancy is uncommon,[1,2] but cancer remains among the chief causes of maternal and fetal morbidity and mortality.[3] There is an increasing trend for women to delay childbearing. This may lead to a more frequent co-occurrence of cancer and pregnancy in the future. With progress in both curative cancer chemotherapy[4] and obstetric and neonatal care an increasing demand will be placed on the clinician to decide on the uses of chemotherapy during pregnancy.

THE PLACENTA

There are few, if any, human studies of transplacental passage of antineoplastic agents, but many antineoplastic agents have those qualities necessary to cross the placenta and enter the fetal circulation: low molecular weight, high lipid solubility, a nonionized state, and low plasma protein binding.[5]

FETAL RISKS DURING PREGNANCY

Cytotoxic drugs probably induce an all-or-none phenomenon: either a spontaneous abortion or a normal fetus, but during the first trimester chemotherapy may lead to an increase in fetal risk of congenital malformations.[6] Fetal malformation is, however, not inevitable.[3] In the second and third trimesters the drugs usually do not cause significant malformations, but they can impair fetal growth and development and result in microcephaly, mental retardation, and impaired learning behavior.[7] Other adverse effects include low birth weight, intrauterine growth retardation, premature birth, and major organ toxicity.

Late effects of maternal cytotoxic drug therapy that need further studies include physical growth, intellectual and neurologic function and development, gonadal function and reproductive capacity, transplacental mutagenesis of germline tissue, transplacental carcinogenesis, and second-generation teratogenesis.[8]

TERATOGENESIS[9–16]

In contrast to teratogenic effects from administration of cytotoxic drug treatment to the mother during the first trimester, there appears to be almost no evidence of such an increased risk of teratogenicity during the second and third trimester.

TREATMENT RECOMMENDATIONS

If the condition of the mother deteriorates and if cure or maximum amelioration of a neoplastic process is a realistic goal, then she can be treated as indicated with cytotoxic drugs regardless of the trimester. Harmful effects at any period of pregnancy are not inevitable.[17–23]

If there is no hope for cure or even significant palliation, the primary goal may become protection of the fetus from the harmful effects of antineoplastic drugs or radiation and the delivery of a healthy infant.

Throughout the decision making period, it is prudent for the clinician to interact with a team consisting of the patient's obstetrician, family physician, oncologist, pediatrician, neonatologist, and other ancillary consultants.[24]

Chemotherapy early in pregnancy may be lessened by avoiding combination therapy and use of folic acid antagonists such as methotrexate.[25–28]

Single and combination chemotherapy may be administered during the second and third trimester with a relatively low risk of teratogenicity. Delivery can be planned when maternal blood counts are optimal. Long-term follow-up of the fetus so exposed is indicated.[8]

Drugs that may be relatively safe during the first trimester include alkylating agents given alone and vinblastine alone.

REFERENCES—PREGNANCY

1. Potter JF, Schoeneman M. Metastasis of maternal cancer to the placenta and fetus. Cancer 1970;25:380–388.
2. Nieminen V, Remes N. Malignancy during pregnancy. Acta Obstet Gynecol Scand 1970;49:315–318.
3. Barber HRK. Fetal and neonatal effects of cytotoxic agents. Obstet Gynecol 1981;58:41S–47S.
4. Frei E. Curative cancer chemotherapy. Cancer Res 1985;45: 6523–6537.
5. Pons G. Anticancer drug pharmacodynamics. Cancer Chemother Pharmacol 1985;14:177–183.
6. Beely L. Adverse effects of drugs in the first trimester of pregnancy. Clin Obstet Gynecol 1986;13:177–195.
7. Doll DC, Ringenberg Q, Yarbro JW. Antineoplastic agents and pregnancy. Semin Oncol 1989;16:337–346.
8. Garber JE. Long-term follow-up of children exposed in utero to antineoplastic agents. Semin Oncol 1989;16:437–444.
9. Kalter H, Warkany J. Congenital malformations. N Engl J Med 1983;308:424–431, 491–497.
10. Malfetano JH, Goldkrand JW. Cis-platinum combination chemotherapy during pregnancy for advanced epithelial ovarian carcinoma. Obstet Gynecol 1990;75:545–547.
11. Schafer AI. Teratogenic effects of antileukemic chemotherapy. Arch Intern Med 1981;141:514–515.
12. Neubert D, Tapken S, Merker HJ. Induction of skeletal malformations in organ cultures of mammalian embryonic tissue. Naunyn Schmiedebergs Arch Pharmacol 1974;286b:271–282.
13. Lilleyman JS, Hill AS, Anderton KJ. Consequences of acute myelogenous leukemia in early pregnancy. Cancer 1977; 40:1300–1303.
14. Manson JM, Dourson ML, Smith CC. Effects of cystine arabinoside on in vivo and in vitro mouse limb development. In Vitro 1977;13:434–442.
15. Barber HRK. Fetal and neonatal effects of cytotoxic agents. Obstet Gynecol 1981;51:41S–47S.
16. Nicholson HO. Cytotoxic drugs in pregnancy. J Obstet Gynecol Br Commonw 1968;75:307–312.
17. Patel M, Dukes IAF, Hull JC. Use of hydroxyurea in chronic myeloid leukemia during pregnancy. A case report. Am J Obstet Gynecol 1991;165:565–566.
18. Doll DC. Introduction. Semin Oncol 1989;16:335–336.
19. Averette HE, Boike GM, Jarrell MA. Effects of cancer chemotherapy on gonadal function and reproductive capacity. CA Cancer J Clin 1990;40:199–209.
20. Blatt J, Mulvill J, Ziegler J, Young RC, Poplach DC. Pregnancy outcome following cancer chemotherapy. Am J Med 1980;69:828–831.
21. Ruskin GJS, Booth M, Dent J, Salt S, Rustin F, Bagshawe KD. Pregnancy after cytotoxic chemotherapy for gestational trophoblastic tumours. Br Med J 1984;288:103–105.
22. Moloney WC. Management of leukemia in pregnancy. Ann NY Academy Sci 1964;114:857–867.
23. Meador J, Armentrout S, Slater L. Third trimester chemotherapy and neonatal haemotopoiesis. Cancer Chemother Pharmacol 1987;19:177–179.
24. Zemlickis D, Loshner M, Degendorfer P, Panzarella T, Sutcliffe SB, Koren G. Fetal outcome after in utero exposure to cancer chemotherapy. Arch Intern Med 1992;152: 573–576.
25. Raffles A, Williams J, Costeloe K, Clark P. Transplacental effects of material cancer chemotherapy. Case report. Br J Obstet Gynaecol 1989; 96:1099–1100.
26. Kozlowski RD, Steinbrunner JV, MacKenzie AH, Clough JD, Wilke WS, Segal AM. Outcome of first-trimester exposure to low dose methotrexate in eight patients with rheumatic disease. Am J Med 1990;88:589–592.
27. Powell H, Ekert H. Methotrexate-induced congenital malformations. Med J Aust 1971;2:1076–1077.
28. Emerson DJ. Congenital malformations due to attempted abortion with aminopterin. Am J Obstet Gynec 1962;84:356–357.

CYTOTOXIC DRUGS AND BREAST MILK

In the newborn period, drug disposition appears to be very different from that of both adults and other children.[1,2] Such differences include a lower whole body fat content, increased extracellular fluid volume (which will affect the apparent volume of distribution), a decrease in plasma protein binding with a concomitant increase in the free drug fraction, and a decrease in renal excretory capacity (immature tubular and glomerular function). Since most drugs enter the breast milk by diffusion of the un-ionized form of the drug, the relative concentration of the drug in milk and plasma, the milk to plasma (M/P) ratio, will depend on its relative ionization in milk and plasma, the lipid solubility of the un-ionized moiety, and the relative protein binding of the drug in milk and plasma.

CLINICAL STUDIES

Methotrexate, cyclophosphamide, cisplatin, doxorubicin, and hydroxurea, readily detectable in milk and serum after use of the drug, have been assayed in breast milk.[3] Two nursing mothers received high doses of cyclophosphamide (800 mg and 900 mg). Both infants experienced bone marrow suppression.[4,5]

TREATMENT

It is at present prudent to advise lactating mothers receiving cytotoxic drugs to refrain from breast-feeding their infants.[6–11]

FERTILITY

Alkylating agents and procarbazine are especially toxic to the terminal epithelium of the testis. Single-dose alkylating agents produce dose-dependent impairment of spermatogenesis; combination chemotherapy regimens such as mechlorethamine, vincristine, procarbazine, and prednisone (MOPP) may cause permanent infertility in 90% of patients. Lower risks of permanent infertility are associated with other combinations of chemotherapy regimens such as doxorubicin, bleomycin, vinblastine, dacarbazine (ABVD) or cis-

Table 61–5
Summary of NIH Recommended Guidelines for the Handling of Parenteral Antineoplastic Drugs[a]

Preparation
1. Drug reconstitution should be done in a class II laminar-flow biologic safety cabinet.
2. Exhaust from the hood should be vented to the outside when possible.
3. Work surface in cabinet should be covered with plastic-backed paper to soak up spills. This paper should be removed after each work shift.
4. Personnel should wear surgical gloves and closed-front surgical-type gowns with knit cuffs.
5. All vials containing reconstituted drugs should be vented to reduce internal pressure.
6. A sterile, alcohol-dampened cotton pledget should be used to wrap the needle and vial top during withdrawal from the vial septum. When ejecting bubbles from the syringe, the tip of the needle should be covered with an alcohol-dampened cotton pledget.
7. External surface of syringes and IV bottles should be wiped clean of drug.
8. When breaking the top from a glass ampule, the neck should be wrapped with a sterile, alcohol-dampened cotton pledget to contain the aerosol produced.
9. Syringes and IV bottles should be labeled properly and should include a warning for appropriate disposal.
10. The safety cabinet should be cleaned with 70% alcohol and disposable towels.
11. Contaminated needles and syringes should be disposed of intact to prevent aerosol generation by clipping needles. All contaminated bottles, vials, gloves, absorbent paper, disposable gowns, gauze, and other material should be placed in a plastic bag and incinerated.
12. The hands should be washed after gloves are removed.
13. Waste antineoplastic drugs should be disposed of in accordance with the federal and state requirements applicable to toxic chemical waste.

Administration
1. Protective outer garments, such as closed-front surgical-type gowns with knit cuffs, should be worn.
2. Disposable surgical gloves should be worn when one is removing air bubbles from syringe and IV tubing, injecting drugs, disconnecting IV tubing, and fixing leaks in tubing or syringe connection.
3. When one is removing air bubbles from syringe or IV tubing, an alcohol-dampened sterile cotton pledget should be used to cover the tip of the needle, syringe, or IV tubing to collect any of the antineoplastic drug that may be discharged inadvertently.
4. Needles, syringes, bottles, and other contaminated material should be disposed of as detailed above under "Preparation."
5. In case of skin contact with the antineoplastic drug, the affected area should be thoroughly washed with soap and water. If an eye is affected, it should be flushed for at least 15 minutes with the eyelid held open.
6. The hands should be washed after administering any antineoplastic drug.

[a]Adapted from Council on Scientific Affairs. JAMA 1985;253:1590–1592.

platin, vinblastine, and bleomycin. There is no effective method to protect the testis from the effects of chemotherapy. Sperm banking prior to chemotherapy can be considered.[12]

OCCUPATIONAL EXPOSURE

Guidelines for the handling of parenteral antineoplastic drugs has been recommended by the National Institutes of Health (Table 61–5).[13]

An expanded set of guidelines has also been issued by the American Society of Hospital Pharmacists[15] (see Recommended Safe Handling Methods). Despite all these guidelines, current adherence to good practices among health care drug handlers indicates room for substantial improvement.[16–18]

NURSES HANDLING CYTOSTATIC DRUGS

Studies of nurses working with cytostatic drugs suggest a tendency toward increased mutagenicity in their urine,[19] and chromosomal changes (chromosome gaps, sister chromatid exchange).[20,21] Liver damage has been observed.[22] Finally, two studies have noted a twofold increase in the risk of spontaneous abortion among nurses exposed to antineoplastic drugs during the first trimester of pregnancy.[23,24] A promising development is the use of a urine mutagenicity test with *Salmonella typhimurium* TA98 to monitor nurses handling cytostatic drugs.[25]

PHARMACISTS

Hospital pharmacists have not exhibited any mutagenic activity[26] when their urine was tested by the Ames Salmonella system.[27]

PHYSICIANS

Few reports have evaluated risks for physicians who handle antineoplastic drugs. A Danish study suggests that there was a slightly increased risk for the development of leukemia and non-Hodgkin's lymphoma in a cohort of 21,781 physicians followed up to 33 years after initial exposure.[28]

DISPOSAL—CHEMICAL DEGRADATION OF CYTOTOXIC DRUGS

Chemical degradation and disposal of a number of antineoplastic drugs largely involves the use of potassium hydroxide, water, and a nickel-aluminum alloy.[29] Though drugs are destroyed, some of the reaction mixtures may exhibit mutagenic properties.

LABORATORY WORKERS

Studies of laboratory workers in both France and the United Kingdom suggest that past exposures have not resulted in any unusual pattern of cancer, apart from a small excess of brain and nervous system cancers and bone cancers.[30]

PATERNAL OCCUPATIONS

Odds ratios for childhood leukemia and lymphomas, childhood nervous systemic cancers, and paternal occupation are listed in Tables 61–6, 61–7, and 61–8. Specific etiologic relationships have not been clinically confirmed for many cancers by controlled studies.

CLINICAL TOXICITY

Toxic effects of anticancer drugs are presented in the following categories:

General Toxicities
  Acute and delayed toxicity—therapeutic use (Table 61–4)—See Organ-Specific Toxicities
Toxicities Related to Administration
  Extravasations
Hypersensitivity
Nausea and vomiting—antiemetics
Specific Cytotoxic-Related Toxicities
  Radiation recall—radiosensitization
Secondary malignancies
Tumor lysis syndromes
Overdoses

Table 61–6
Results of Studies of Paternal Occupation and Total Childhood Cancer[a]

Occupation	Odds Ratio[b]
Mechanic	
Motor vehicle mechanic	2.2
Mechanic, gas station attendant	1.1
Aircraft mechanics	2.3–infinity[c]
Machinist	
Machinist	1.7
Machinist	1.1
Machinist, miner, lumberman	0.5–1.8
Machine repairman	0.9
Radiation and military	
Radiation related	1.5–2.0
Radiation-exposed military	2.1–5.2[c]
Radar related	1.1–2.1
Armed forces	0.8
Electrical	
Electrician, plumber, carpenter	0.9–1.5
Electrical	1.0
Other industrial exposures	
Printer	1.8
Petroleum industry	0.7–1.6
Aircraft workers	3.1–5.2[c]
Agriculture	
Farmers	1.2[c]
Farmers	1.1
No industrial exposures	
With academic degree	1.7[c]
Professional, technical workers, artists	1.4[c]
Administrators and managers	1.7[c]
Clerical workers	1.3[c]
Sales workers	1.3[c]

[a]Adapted from Savitz DA, Chen J. Environ Health Perspect 1990;88:325–337.
[b]Range of odds ratios provided when multiple control groups were used.
[c]$p < 0.05$.

ORGAN-SPECIFIC TOXICITIES

CARDIAC TOXICITY

Cytotoxic chemotherapy, particularly with the anthracyclines (doxorubicin, daunorubicin), and less often cyclophosphamide,[32–34] may be associated with acute or delayed cardiotoxicity.[35] Heart failure from dose-related cardiomyopathy is the most clinically important manifestation of anthracycline cardiotoxicity. A higher risk is also found in patients with underlying coronary, vascular or myocardial disease, hypertension, cardiac irradiation, or a prior dose of doxorubicin >450 mg/m^2.[36]

Cardiotoxicity with doxorubicin is dose-related and usually develops after a cumulative dose of over 500 mg/m^2.[37] Hale and Lewis[38] suggest a minimum infusion time of 1 hour with electrocardiographic and echocardiogram monitoring obtained periodically thereafter. Guidelines for follow-up have been published.[39]

The cardiac changes caused by cancer therapy may progress for 1 to 15 years after treatment[33,40] and lead to functional changes (echocardiographically detectable abnormalities of left ventricular afterload and contractility) that are often initially asymptomatic.[40–42] Apparently, normal children who have received moderate doses of anthracyclines may also be shown to have changes in myocardial function that cannot be detected by resting echocardiography.[42]

Cardiac function may continue to deteriorate after doxorubicin treatment is discontinued. Only endomyocardial biopsy permits a definitive evaluation of the risk of development of congestive heart failure.[43]

PULMONARY TOXICITY[44]

Drugs representing all groups of cytotoxic agents appear to induce lung disease (Table 61–9) affecting the parenchyma or vasculature (pulmonary emboli). Factors associated with an increased risk of drug-induced pneumonitis include total dose administered, age, oxygen therapy (with bleomycin, cyclophosphamide, mitomycin, nitrosoureas), simultaneous or prior radiation therapy to the lungs, combination drug use with increased toxicity, and preexisting pulmonary disease.

Clinical

Drug-induced pulmonary toxicity most frequently produces dyspnea; nonproductive cough, fatigue, and malaise develop over a period of weeks or months. Hypersensitivity drug-induced lung disease develops within hours. Fever, chest pain, and rales are often present. Although a basilar or diffuse reticular nodular pattern is often present on radiologic examination and a restrictive ventilatory defect with diminished carbon monoxide diffusing capacity is observed, ultimately a lung biopsy is necessary for diagnosis.[45]

Bleomycin

Life-threatening bleomycin lung toxicity may be largely reversible when large doses of corticosteroids (up to 80 mg

Table 61–7
Results of Studies of Paternal Occupation and Childhood Leukemias and Lymphomas[a]

Occupation	Cancer Site	Odds Ratio [b]
Motor vehicle related		
Motor vehicle mechanic, service station attendant	Leukemia/lymphoma	2.0
Mechanic, gas station attendant	Leukemia/lymphoma	1.1
Motor vehicle driver	Leukemia/lymphoma	1.0
Motor vehicle driver	Leukemia	1.5
Motor vehicle related	Leukemia	0.8, infinity[c]
Auto mechanic, machinist, gas station attendant, miner	Acute lymphocytic leukemia	0.8
Transportation	Acute leukemia	1.4
Transportation equipment	Acute leukemia	2.5[c]
Transportation equipment operator	Leukemia	1.2
Machinst and factory worker		
Machinist, miner, lumberman	Leukemia/lymphoma	2.5[c]
Machinist	Leukemia/lymphoma	1.3
Machine repairmen	Leukemia	0.3
Factory worker, machinst, and related occupations	Leukemia	0.8, 2.5
Operators, fabricators, laborers	Leukemia	1.1
Manual and mechanical skills	Acute lymphocytic leukemia	1.0
Machinery	Acute leukemia	3.0[c]
Aircraft manufacturing	Acute leukemia	1.8
Blacksmiths, toolmakers, etc.	Leukemia	0.9
Nonauto mechanic	Acute nonlymphocytic leukemia	3.5[c]
Aggregated hydrocarbon		
Hydrocarbon related	Leukemia	0.9, 1.0
Hydrocarbon related	Leukemia	1.0, 2.5
Hydrocarbon, high	Acute leukemia	2.4–2.5[c]
Hydrocarbon, low	Acute leukemia	1.3, 3.8[c]
Hydrocarbon related	Acute lymphocytic leukemia	1.0
Paints and pigments		
Painter, dyer, cleaner	Leukemia/lymphoma	1.7
Painter	Leukemia/lymphoma	0.9
Painter	Leukemia	1.5
Painter, cleaner, dyer	Acute lymphocytic leukemia	1.6
Pigments (dyes) exposure	Acute lymphocytic leukemia	1.6
Spray paint	Acute leukemia	2.2[c]
Dyes, pigments	Acute leukemia	3.0
Painter	Acute nonlymphocytic leukemia	7.0[c]
Food related		
Baker, cook, restaurant worker	Leukemia/lymphoma	1.4
Food preparation	Leukemia	0.5
Foods and drink manufacturing	Acute leukemia	2.2
Other chemicals		
Tar or asphalt exposure	Acute lymphocytic leukemia	1.1
Petroleum chemicals manufacturing	Acute leukemia	1.0
Petroleum products	Acute nonlymphocytic leukemia	2.8[c]
Plastic or rubber exposure	Acute lymphocytic leukemia	2.0
Chemical, rubber, and plastics workers	Leukemia	1.1
Plastics	Acute nonlymphocytic leukemia	1.5
Chlorinated solvents	Acute leukemia	2.2
Solvents	Acute nonlymphocytic leukemia	2.1[c]
Other occupations		
Medical and social services	Acute lymphocytic leukemia	2.8[c]
Medical and public health workers	Leukemia	0.6

[a]Adapted from Savitz DA, Chen J. Environ Health Perspect 1990;88:325–337.
[b]Range of odds ratios provided when multiple control groups were used.
[c]$p < 0.05$.

prednisolone daily for 10 days with gradual tapering) and azathioprine (150 mg/day) are administered.[46]

VASCULAR TOXICITY

Antineoplastic agents may induce a heterogeneous group of disorders ranging from asymptomatic arterial lesions to a lethal thrombotic microangiopathic syndrome[47–49] (Table 61–10). The latter may follow treatment with cisplatin, bleomycin, or a vinca alkaloid.[49]

OCULAR COMPLICATIONS

Ocular toxic effects related to cancer chemotherapy are delineated in Table 61–11.[50]

NEUROTOXICITY

Neurologic symptoms and signs arise at some point during the treatment of many patients with malignancies (Tables 61–12 and 61–13).[51–53]

Table 61–8
Results of Studies of Paternal Occupation and Childhood Nervous System Cancers[a]

Occupation	Cancer Site	Odds Ratio[b]
Motor vehicle related		
Motor vehicle mechanic, service station attendant	Nervous system	2.8
Mechanic, gas station attendant	Nervous system	1.0
Motor vehicle driver	Nervous system	0.6
Motor vehicle driver	Brain	0.9
Transportation, utilities, communication	Neuroblastoma	0.9
Motor vehicle mechanic, service station attendant	Nervous system	0.7
Motor freight and transportation	Brain	1.6
Machinist and factory worker		
Machinist	Nervous system	0.7
Machine repairman	Brain	4.4
Factory worker, machinist, and related occupations	Brain	0.7, 25
Factory worker, machinist, and steelworker	Nervous system	1.2
Machine trades occupations	Brain	1.2
Paint		
Painter	Brain	2.6
Paint exposure	Brain	7.0
Painter	Nervous system	1.0
Painting, plastering, etc.	Brain	1.2
Chemicals		
Chemical solvent exposure	Brain	2.8
Chemical industry	Nervous system	1.4
Chemical workers	Nervous system	0.8
Chemical and petroleum refinery worker	Nervous system	3.0
Chemical and drug salesman	Nervous system	10.0
Chemical industry	CNS tumor	1.5
Petroleum industry		
Oil and gas extraction	Neuroblastoma	1.3
Petroleum refinery worker	Nervous system	2.0
Petroleum industry	CNS tumors	3.1
Aggregated hydrocarbon		
Hydrocarbon related	Brain	0.9
Hydrocarbon related	Brain	0.5, 2.3
Aromatic hydrocarbons, nonionizing radiation	Neuroblastoma	1.8
Aromatic and aliphatic hydrocarbons	Neuroblastoma	3.2
Hydrocarbon related, narrow definition	CNS tumors	1.3
Hydrocarbon related, broad definition	CNS tumors	1.4
Electrical		
Electronics workers	Neuroblastoma	11.8
Electrical assembling, installing, and repairing	Brain	2.7
Electromagnetic fields, narrow definition	CNS tumors	1.7
Electromagnetic fields, broad definition	CNS tumors	1.6
Ionizing radiation		
Industrial, less exposure	Nervous system	1.0–1.1
Occupation, less exposure	Nervous system	1.8–2.1
Industrial, more exposure	CNS tumors	2.2
Industrial, less exposure	CNS tumors	1.7
Occupation, more exposure	CNS tumors	1.0
Occupation, less exposure	CNS tumors	1.1
Metals		
Metal processors and producers	Brain	1.8
Welders, cutters	Brain	2.7
Metal working occupations	Brain	1.6
Agriculture		
Farmer	Nervous system	0.6
Farmer	Brain	1.2
Agriculture	Neuroblastoma	0.6
Farming and agricultural occupations	Brain	2.0
Construction		
Construction	Neuroblastoma	0.9
Construction industry	Brain	2.3
Construction occupations	Brain	2.0
Carpenters	Brain	1.9

[a]Adapted from Savitz DA, Chen J. Environ Health Perspect 1990;88:325–337.
[b]Range of odds ratios provided when multiple control groups were used.

(continued)

Table 61–8 *(Continued)*

Occupation	Cancer Site	Odds Ratio[b]
Paper and pulp mill		
Paper and pulp mill	Nervous system	2.8
Paper and pulp mill worker	Nervous system	4.0
Pulp and paper industry	CNS tumors	1.6
Aerospace and aircraft industries		
Aircraft industry	Brain	Infinity
Aerospace occupation	Brain	1.1
Aircraft industry worker	Nervous system	1.0
Other occupations		
Printing workers	Nervous system	4.5
Graphic arts workers	Nervous system	21.9
Glass, clay, stone industry	Brain	1.5

Table 61–9
Chemotherapeutic Agents Associated with Pulmonary Parenchymal Damage[a]

Alkylating agents	**Nitrosoureas**
Busulfan	Carmustine (BNCU)
Cyclophosphamide	Lomustine (CCNU)
Chlorambucil	**Antimetabolites**
Melphalan	Methotrexate
Antibiotics	Azathioprine
Bleomycin	Mercaptopurine
Mitomycin	Cytosine arabinoside
Miscellaneous	
Procarbazine	
Vinblastine	
Vindesine	
Teniposide	

[a]Adapted from deVita VT Jr, Hellman S, Rosenberg SA. Cancer: Principles and practice of oncology. 3rd ed. Philadelphia: JB Lippincott, 1989.

HEPATOTOXICITY

Androgen-receptor antagonists comprise two classes of anticancer drugs: the steroidal antiandrogens (cyproterone acetate, megestrol acetate) and the nonsteroidal antiandrogens (nilutamide, flutamide).[54] Reports of liver damage following use of these compounds include hepatitis (cytotoxic and cholestatic)[55–58] and fulminant hepatic failure.[59]

TOXICITIES RELATED TO ADMINISTRATION

EXTRAVASATIONS

Extravasation of cytotoxic drugs refers to the unintentional instillation or leakage of these agents into the perivascular and subcutaneous spaces during their administration.[60–68] In patients receiving IV chemotherapy, 2 to 5% of all adverse reactions consist of local tissue irritation.[61]

Vesicant Agent Administration

Guidelines for vesicant agent administration have been proposed by Doll and colleagues.[62]

Table 61–10
Vascular Complications Associated with Antineoplastic Agents[a]

Complications	Drug
Pulmonary venoocclusive disease	Bleomycin
	Mitomycin
Hepatic veno-occlusive disease	Cyclophosphamide, BCNU, cisplatin
	Cyclophosphamide, busulphan
	Cyclophosphamide, total body irradiation
	Cyclophosphamide, high-dose cytosine arabinoside
	Dacarbazine
	BCNU, VP-16-213
	Urethane
	Mitomycin
	Azathioprine
	6-Thioguanine
Budd-Chiari syndrome	Dacarbazine
	6-Thioguanine
	Cytosine arabinoside
	Methotrexate
Cerebrovascular accidents	Cisplatin-based chemotherapy
Raynaud's phenomenon	Bleomycin
	Bleomycin and vinca alkaloid
	Bleomycin, cisplatin, vinca alkaloid
Myocardial infarction	Vinca alkaloids
	VP-16-213
	Vinblastine, bleomycin
	Cisplatin, bleomycin, vinca alkaloid
	5-Fluorouracil
Thrombotic microangiopathy	Mitomycin
	Cisplatin-based chemotherapy
Venous thrombosis	Cytoxan, methotrexate, vincristine, 5-fluorouracil, prednisone
Hypotension	VP-16-213
	VM-26
	Dacarbazine
	Homoharringtonine
	Vincristine
	BCNU
Hypertension	Cisplatin
	Procarbazine
Acral erythema	Cytosine arabinoside
	Hydroxyurea
	Protracted infusion of 5-fluorouracil or doxorubicin
Retinal toxicity	BCNU (carotid infusion)
	Cisplatin (carotid infusion and intravenous high dose)

[a]Adapted from Doll DC et al. J Clin Oncol 1986;4:1405–1417.

Table 61–11
Ocular Cancer Chemotherapy Toxicity by Anatomic Site [a]

Site	Side Effect	Drugs
Orbit	AV shunts	Nitrosoureas
	Cavernous sinus syndrome	Cis-platinum
	Edema	5-FU, Methotrexate
	Exophthalmos	Corticosteroids
	Pallor	Plicamycin
	Pain	Nitrosoureas, 5-FU, and Methotrexate
Lids	Cicatricial ectropion	5-FU
	Anklyoblepharon	5-FU
	Increased lid necrosis following cryotherapy	5-FU
	Hyperpigmentation	5-FU, Busulfan
Lacrimal drainage	Tear duct fibrosis and Punctal occlusion	5-FU
Lacrimal gland	Keratoconjunctivitis sicca	Busulfan, and Cyclophosphamide
Conjunctiva	Conjunctivitis	Doxorubicin, Cyclophosphamide, Cytosine arabinoside, 5-FU, Methotrexate, and Nitrosoureas
Sclera	Discoloration	Corticosteroids
Cornea	Keratopathy	Tamoxifen, Tilorone, and Nitrosoureas
	Keratitis	Chlorambucil, Cytosine arabinoside, and 5-FU
Pupil	Pinpoint pupils	Cyclophosphamide
	Internal ophthalmoplegia	Nitrosoureas
Uvea	Uveitis	BCG, Busulfan, and Nitrogen Mustard
Trabecular meshwork and/or Ciliary Body	Increased IOP	Corticosteroids and Nitrosoureas
Lens	Cataract	Busulfan, Corticosteroids, Dibromomannitol, Methotrexate, Mitotane, and Nafoxidine
Retina	Toxic retinopathy	Chlorambucil, Cis-platinum, Mitotane, Nitrosoureas, Procarbazine, Tamoxifen, and Tilorone
Vitreous	Opacification	Nitrosoureas
Optic nerve	Disc edema, Optic neuritis, and/or Optic atrophy	Chlorambucil, Cis-platinum, Cytosine arabinoside, Fludarabine, 5-FU, Interferon, Laetrile, Methotrexate, Mitotane, Nitrosoureas, Procarbazine, and Vincristine
Cranial nerves 3, 4, 5 and 6	Ptosis, Paresis with or without Diplopia	Chlorambucil, Corticosteroids, Fludarabine, 5-FU, Laetrile, Procarbazine, and Vincristine
	Corneal hypesthesia	Vincristine
Extraocular muscles	Fibrosis	Nitrosoureas
Central nervous system	Cortical blindness	Cis-platinum, Fludarabine, and Vincristine
	Internuclear ophthalmoplegia	Nitrosoureas
	Blepharospasm	5-FU

[a]Adapted from Insler MS. Surv Ophthalmol 1989;34:201–230.

1. Administer the medication according to manufacturer's recommendations.
2. Whenever possible, administer vesicants through a central line. This is particularly important if the vesicant is ordered as a continuous infusion and a peripheral site cannot be continually monitored.
3. To ensure patency of a peripheral IV, it is best to administer a vesicant through a recently started IV. Avoid sites in the dorsum of the hand and near joints as these sites are more susceptible to permanent damage because of the close proximity to arteries and tendons.
4. Administer vesicants by slow IV push into the side-arm port of a running IV of a compatible solution.
5. Assess a peripheral site continually for signs of redness or swelling.

Table 61–12
Peripheral Neuropathy Due to Antineoplastic Drugs

Drugs
Amsacrine
Carboplatin
Cisplatin
Cytarabine
Etoposide
Procarbazine
Suramin
Taxol
Teniposide
Vincristine
Vindisine

6. Verify patency of IV site by aspirating blood return prior to vesicant infusion and 2 to 3 minutes throughout infusion.
7. Ask the patient to report any sensations of burning or pain at the infusion site. Some investigators suggest delaying the administration of antiemetics until after vesicant administration. The antiemetics often have a sedative effect and the patient is unable to report any sensations at the infusion site.
8. Never hurry. Administer medications slowly, allowing the medication to be diluted with the compatible solution and for careful assessment of the IV site.
9. Document carefully, including IV site, rate of administration, condition of site, verification of patency, and patient responses.

Drugs That Cause Local Toxicity After Extravasation

Drugs that cause local toxicity may be classified as either local irritant drugs or vesicant drugs. A *local irritant* drug may produce either pain at the site of injection or an inflammatory reaction along the vein.[60] A *vesicant* drug refers to an extravasated drug that results in blistering or frank ulceration. Doxorubicin is most frequently reported to cause tissue necrosis on extravasation.[61,69–72] Table 61–14 lists commonly used cytotoxic agents classified according to their effects when extravasated. Table 61–15 lists vesicant chemotherapeutic agents with recommended antidotes.

Table 61–13
Anticancer Drugs and Neurotoxicity [a]

Alkylating agents:
Eighth cranial nerve neuropathy
Seizures
Hemiplegia (stroke syndrome)
Myelopathy
Encephalopathy
Peripheral neuropathy

Methotrexate:
Intrathecal
- Aseptic meningitis
- Myelopathy
- Seizures
- Leukoencephalopathy
- Cortical atrophy
- Possible:
  - Cerebellar dysfunction
  - Optic atrophy

Intravenous
- Leukoencephalopathy
- Cerebral vascular accidents

5-FU:
Cerebellar dysfunction
Encephalopathy
Parkinsonism

Cytosine arabinoside:
Aseptic meningitis after intrathecal use
Cerebellar dysfunction with ataxia
Possible optic atrophy

5-Azacytidine:
Myopathy
Mental changes

Vincristine, vinblastine, and vindesine:
Peripheral neuropathy
Autonomic neuropathy
Cranial neuropathies
Myopathy
Mental changes (may be secondary to inappropriate ADH secretion)
Seizure

Nitrosoureas:
Encephalopathy (by itself in high doses intra-arterially)
Additive brain damage with radiation therapy

Cis-platinum:
Eighth cranial nerve neuropathy
Peripheral neuropathy

Hexamethylmelamine:
Encephalopathy with hallucinations
Peripheral neuropathy
Cerebellar ataxia
Tremor: parkinsonism or postural

L-asparaginase:
Encephalopathy
Seizures

[a]Adapted from Goetz CG. Neurotoxins in clinical practice. New York: SP Medical & Scientific Books, 1985.

Treatment—Reducing Complications of Extravasation[60]

1. On extravasation stop the injection of the cytotoxic drug infusion immediately. Do not remove the needle.
2. Disconnect the intravenous administration set.
3. An attempt should be made to aspirate the extravasated drug from the needle or cannula (by way of the needle). Aspiration of the surrounding tissues is usually ineffective in removing any more of the extravasated drug.
4. Instill the antidote (where appropriate) through the needle and into the surrounding tissues, infiltrating the area where the extravasation has occurred.
5. For irritant and other potentially vesicant drugs, it may be helpful to dilute the drug with 0.9% sodium chloride solution, where the extravasated volume does not preclude a further addition.
6. Remove the needle or cannula.
7. Mark the border with indelible ink and photograph to provide a baseline for later comparison and for medicolegal documentation.
8. Apply cold compresses for 20 to 40 minutes to the site of extravasation for all drugs except the vinca alkaloids.[65]
9. Apply dressings to the site.
10. Elevate the arm.
11. Apply 1% hydrocortisone cream (injections of hydrocortisone may be contraindicated in the case of

Table 61–14
Cytotoxic Agents and Extravasation[66]

Cytotoxic agents that do not usually cause local problems after extravasation
Asparaginase
Bleomycin sulfate
Cytarabine
Etoposide[a]
Methotrexate
Thioguanine

Cytotoxic drugs that cause local irritation after extravasation
Carmustine
Cyclophosphamide
Dacarbazine (DTIC)
Streptozocin
Teniposide
Thiotepa

Cytotoxic drugs that are likely to cause local ulceration after extravasation (vesicant agents)
Actinomycin D
Cisplatin[a]
Daunorubicin hydrochloride
Doxorubicin hydrochloride
Fluorouracil[a] [75]
Mitomycin[76]
Mitozantrone hydrochloride[77]
Mechlorethamine
Plicamycin (Mithramycin)
Vinblastine[75]
Vincristine sulfate[75]
Vindesine sulfate[75]

[a]Currently controversial (further data required).

vinca-alkaloid agents, and it may be appropriate to use hyaluronidase ointment instead).

12. Document the occurrence:
    a. Date of administration of the drug
    b. Time of drug administration
    c. Site of drug administration
    d. The drug or drugs thought to be extravasated
    e. Volume believed extravasated
    f. Concentration of the drug in the administered solution
    g. Appearance of the site after extravasation
    h. Information and instructions given to patient
    i. Name of person who administered the drug
13. Notify medical staff members.
14. Ask patient to return at weekly intervals unless local irritation or necrosis is not anticipated. Advise patient on follow-up care, telling patient of relevant symptoms and signs.
15. Consult with plastic surgeon as necessary.
16. Warn patient of possible inflammatory reaction. Tell patient to contact medical or nursing staff members if reactions become severe.

SPECIFIC VESICANT AGENTS—SPECIFIC TREATMENT

Doxorubicin, Daunorubicin, Actinomycin

Local corticosteroid injections, with or without sodium bicarbonate and with or without intravenous hydrocortisone, have been used for doxorubicin toxicity.[60] Dimethylsulfoxide (DMSO) has also been used to limit local doxorubicin ulceration.

Vinca Alkaloids

Hyaluronidase and normal saline have proved useful in animals in limiting the effects of the extravasation of these vesicants.[73]

Mitomycin,[74] Mechlorethamine

Sodium thiosulfate has been reported to be useful after mitomycin or mechlorethamine extravasation.[60]

LATE-COMPLICATION MANAGEMENT

After conservative measures have been initiated and there still remains a possibility of local ulceration, obtain a plastic surgery consult. Involvement of the extensor tendons or the dorsum of the hand may require surgical intervention.[66]

HYPERSENSITIVITY

Certain antineoplastic agents (L-asparaginase, cisplatin, intravenous melphalan, topical mechlorethamine, taxol, and teniposide) produce hypersensitivity reactions often enough to be a clinical problem (Table 61–16). Others (cyclophosphamide, doxorubicin, daunorubucin, methotrexate, and procarbazine) do so only occasionally.[78,79] Bleomycin induces an occasional hyperpyrexic reaction with findings similar to anaphylaxis.[80,81] Doxorubicin causes a "flare" or localized urticaria in the area of drug injection.[82] As with other medications, signs and symptoms of a severe allergic reaction or anaphylactic reaction will be evident within the first 15 minutes following the infusion or injection of the medication.[83] Treatment should include immediate cessation of an infusion, close monitoring, diphenhydramine (mild reactions) or epinephrine, and IV fluids for anaphylaxis. Aminophylline may be used to relieve bronchospasm. Rowinsky and colleagues have suggested a management program for hypersensitivity reactions with paclitoxel (Taxol).

Hypersensitivity related to cytotoxic drug use can be categorized according to the Coombs and Gell's classification. Most reported allergic reactions caused by antineoplastic agents are of the type I category (Table 61–17).[84]

CREMOPHOR EL[85,86]

Hypersensitivity reactions caused by taxol were a major concern in early studies with this agent. This may have been due to the Cremophor EL vehicle (polyoxyethylated castor oil) used in drug formulation. Other drugs formulated with this vehicle (e.g., cyclosporine, teniposide, intravenous vitamin K, didemnin) also have caused hypersensitivity reactions in humans.[85]

Table 61–15
Vesicant Chemotherapy Agents and Recommended Antidotes[1]

Drug	Antidote	Dose
Actinomycin D[a]	Sodium thiosulfate 25%	1.6 mL in 3 mL water for injection
Amsacrine[78]	None	
Dacarbazine	None	
Daunorubicin[a]	Dexamethasone 8 mg/2 mL	1 mL
Doxorubicin[a]	Hydrocortisone 100 mg/2 mL or topical dimethylsulfoxide	1 mL
Mechlorethamine[a]	Sodium thiosulfate 25% or Sodium thiosulfate 2%[77]	1.6 mL in 3 mL water for injection
Mitomycin[a]	Sodium thiosulfate 25%	1.6 mL in 3 mL water for injection
Mitoxantrone	None	
Vinblastine[b]	Sodium chloride 0.9% or topical hyaluronidase	5 mL
Vincristine[b]	Sodium chloride 0.9% or topical hyaluronidase	5 mL
Vindesine[a]	Sodium chloride 0.9% or topical hyaluronidase	5 mL

[a]Cold compresses should be used.
[b]Hot compresses should be used. However, this is controversial since different centers use hot or cold compresses. Further data are required before a firm recommendation can be made.

Table 61–16
Types of Hypersensitivity[a]

Types	Mechanisms	Major Clinical Signs
Type I IgE mediated	Crosslinking of Fc receptors for IgE on mast cells and basophils by antigen-specific IgE resulting in degranulation and release of different mediators.	Usually immediate < 30 minutes. Anaphylactic shock: hypotension, angioedema, asthma, vomiting. Urticaria.
Type II Cytotoxic	Antibodies react to antigens bound to cells or to tissue specific components resulting in cytotoxicity by activation of complement and killer cells.	Destruction of a blood cell type, e.g., hemolytic anemia or immune thrombocytopenia. Bullous skin eruption.
Type III Immune complex mediated	Deposition of antigen-antibody immune complexes in certain tissues with activation of complement and neutrophils.	Fever, chronic urticaria, arthralgia, proteinuria, vasculitis, pneumonitis or erythema multiforme depending on the site of immune complexes deposition.
Type IV Cell mediated	Antigen-specific T lymphocytes react with antigens and induce the secretion of lymphokines followed by the formation of a granuloma (inflammatory reaction).	Contact dermatitis. Chronic granuloma in certain organs.

[a]Adapted from O'Brien ME, Souberbielle BE. Ann Oncol 1992;3:605–610.

Table 61–17
Drugs and Types of Hypersensitivity Described[a]

Drug group	Chemotherapeutic agent	Type of hypersensitivity
Antimetabolites	Methotrexate	I, II, III
	5-fluorouracil	I
Alkylating agents	Cyclophosphamide	I
	Chlorambucil	I, II, IV
	Melphalan	I, anaphylactoid
	Cisplatin	I, anaphylactoid
	Carboplatin	I
Vinca alkaloids	Vinblastine	I
Anthracycline	Doxorubicin	I
	Epirubicin	I
	Mitozantrone	I, III
Antibiotic derived	Bleomycin	III
	Mitomycin	I
Epipodophyllotoxin	Etoposide	I
	Teniposide	I, II
Others	L-asparaginase	I, anaphylactoid
	Procarbazine	I, II
	Dacarbazine	III
	Deoxycoformycin	I
	Taxol	I

[a]Adapted from O'Brien MER, Souberbielle BE. Semin Oncol 1992; 3:605–610.

NAUSEA AND VOMITING

Almost every chemotherapeutic agent whether used orally or by parenteral routes has induced nausea and vomiting.[87,88] Table 61–18[87] classifies single chemotherapeutic agents according to emetogenic potential with approximate dose ranges. Chemotherapy-induced nausea and vomiting may be severe enough to prevent patients from completing curative courses of treatment.[89]

Mechanism of Action (Fig. 61–1)

Antineoplastic drugs induce vomiting through a multiafferent neural reflex arc.[90] Three major afferent limbs have now been identified, including *(a)* a humoral pathway consisting of chemical mediators that affect the chemoreceptor trigger zone (CTZ) in the brain stem; *(b)* a peripheral pathway activated by direct stimulation of nerve endings in the gastrointestinal tract; and *(c)* a cerebral cortical pathway activated by stimuli (sights, odors, or memories) associated with past episodes of emesis.[89] Disrupting this reflex arc is the key to the prevention of chemotherapy-induced vomiting. Dopaminergic, histaminergic, cholinergic, and serotonergic receptors are found both in the CTZ and gastrointestinal tract. The CTZ has no independent ability to initiate emesis and does so only through stimulation of a second area in the medulla known as the emetic center.

Treatment

Phenothiazines (prochlorperazine), butyrophenones (droperidol), and substituted benzamides (metoclopramide) all have substantial antidopaminergic activity and are widely used as antiemetic agents (Table 61–19).[91] Antiemetic regimens have usually been based on combinations that have included an antidopaminergic drug given in high doses.[92] A potent antiemetic cocktail can be prepared with metoclopramide (particularly useful in reduced emesis related to cisplatin), steroids (decadron, methylprednisolone), and lorazepam (reduces anxiety, produces sedation or amnesia). Dexamethasone is probably the most effective available agent at the present time and should be a basis of therapy (Table 61–20).[93] Extrapyramidal reactions can be managed with an intravenous antihistamine such as diphenhydramine 25 to 50 mg intravenously.

5-hydroxytryptamine[89] (serotonin) receptors appear to be principal mediators of the emetic reflex and are found in both the central nervous system and gastrointestinal tract. Ondansetron[94,95] is as effective as metoclopramide in preventing the acute nausea and vomiting that occurs within 24 hours of chemotherapy.[96–99] Guidelines for the use of ondansetron are found in Table 61–21.[100] In the delayed phase of nausea and vomiting (days 2 through 6) results with both ondansetron and metoclopramide appear less effective, although perhaps metoclopramide may be useful.[98] Ondansetron has been used in adults[98] in doses of 8 mg intravenously (acute phase) followed by 1 mg per hour for 24 hours, and in children in doses of 5 mg/m^2 once intravenously.[99] Delayed-phase doses suggested in

Table 61–18
Classification of Single Chemotherapeutic Agents According to Emetogenic Potential [a]

Class V, High (>90%)	Class IV, Moderately High (60–90%)	Class III, Moderate (30–60%)	Class II, Moderately Low (10–30%)	Class I, Low (<10%)
Cisplatin ≥ 75 mg	Cisplatin < 75 mg	Cyclophosphamide < 1 g	Methotrexate < 100 mg	Vincristine
Dacarbazine ≥ 500 mg	Dacarbazine < 500 mg	Methotrexate < 250 ≥ 100	Fluorouracil < 1000 mg	Busulfan
Cyclophosphamide > 1 g	Cyclophosphamide = 1 g	Doxorubicin < 75 > 20	Doxorubicin ≤ 20 mg	Chlorambucil
Cytarabine > 1 g	Cytarabine 250 mg–1 g	Fluorouracil ≥ 1000 mg	Cytarabine ≤ 20 mg	Thioguanine (oral)
Carmustine ≥ 200 mg	Carmustine < 200 mg	Vinblastine	Bleomycin	Cyclophosphamide (oral)
Streptozocin	Lomustine < 60 mg	Teniposide	Etoposide	Thiotepa
Pentostatin	Doxorubicin ≥ 75 mg	Azacitidine		
Mechlorethamine	Methotrexate ≥ 250 mg	Asparaginase		
Carmustine ≥ 200 mg	Mitomycin			
Lomustine ≥ 60 mg	Procarbazine			

[a]Lindley CM, Bernard S, Fields SM. J Clin Oncol 1989;7:1142–1149.

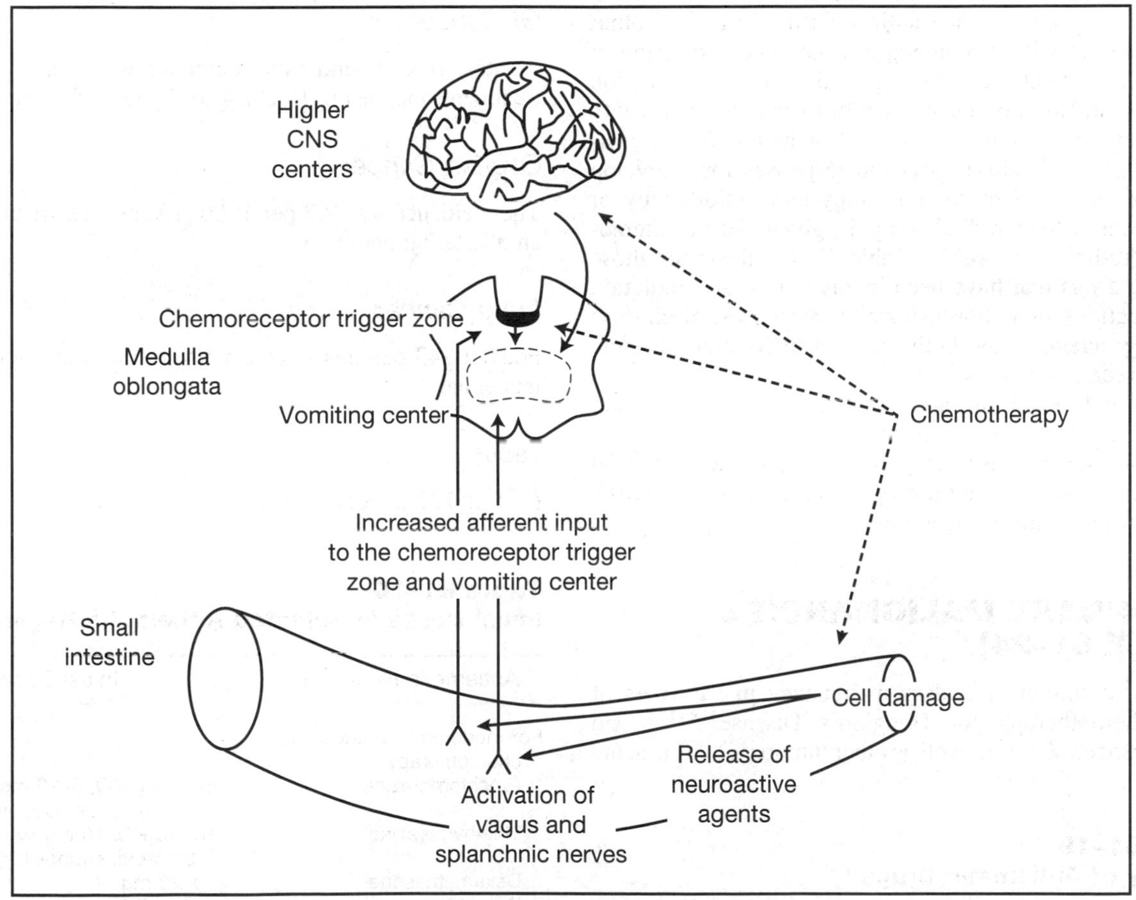

Figure 61-1 Proposed pathways of chemotherapy-induced emesis. Chemotherapeutic drugs may induce emesis through cell damage in gastrointestinal tract, direct actions on medullary centers (the vomiting center and the chemoreceptor trigger zone, which is located in the area postrema), or learned (cortical) responses. CNS denotes central nervous system. (Adapted from Grunberg SM, Hesketh PJ. N Engl J Med 1993;329:1790–1796.

adults are 8 mg three times daily;[98] children, 2 to 4 mg every 8 hours.[99]

Adverse reactions to ondansetron include headache, constipation, elevation of liver enzymes,[93] and, infrequently, anaphylactoid reaction.[101] Treatment for ondansetron overdose is largely symptomatic and supportive. Doses up to 252 mg per day intravenously do not appear to induce significant adverse effects.[94]

The efficacy and usefulness of other antiemetic modalities such as ginger root,[102,103] acupuncture,[104,105] intravenous cyclizine, and rectal thiethylperazine[105] in the prevention and treatment of chemotherapy-induced emesis remain to be established. Dronabinol (δ-9-tetrahydrocannabinol; THC; Marinol) may be effective for patients who have failed to respond adequately to conventional antiemetics. Dry mouth, sedation, orthostatic hypotension, ataxia, dizziness, and dysphoria have been observed (see Marijuana chapter).

Granisetron (Zofron, Kytril) given in a dose of 10 μg/kg intravenously over 5 minutes beginning within 30 minutes before chemotherapy is also effective. Undesirable effects include headache, ectopy, constipation, and mild elevations in liver function tests.[106] The Bristol Children's Hospital Oncology and Hematology Unit Guidelines for the Use of Antiemetics are found in Table 61–22.

SPECIFIC CYTOTOXIC-RELATED TOXICITIES

RADIATION RECALL—RADIOSENSITIZATION

Recall radiation reactions, as well as radiosensitization reactions, may occur when antineoplastic drugs and other agents interact with radiotherapy to produce a reaction at a previously sensitized area (e.g., radiation recall reaction after prior radiation of a skin area) or to enhance sensitivity of an area (e.g., skin) to doses of radiation (radiosensitization).[107–115] Radiosensitization responses may develop following concomitant chemotherapy and radiotherapy or in instances where radiotherapy is given before chemotherapy (radiation recall).[114] Table 61–23 illustrates those cytotoxic drugs that have been involved in either radiation recall reactions or radiosensitization responses. High-dose alkylating agents may both radiosensitize and promote rational recall reactions.[111,114]

The usual result of radiation–chemotherapeutic agent interactions on the skin is erythema followed by desquamation. More severe cases may be associated with painful vesicles and oozing. The most severe cases exhibit necrosis with persistent painful ulceration.[116]

SECONDARY MALIGNANCIES (TABLE 61–24)

The most common secondary malignancy in survivors of initial chemotherapy for Hodgkin's Disease[118–121] and ovarian cancer,[122–125] as well as other tumors,[126–128] is acute nonlymphocytic leukemia with two predominant subgroups: acute myelomonocytic leukemia and acute erythroleukemia. Risks of leukemia appear to be highest within the first 3 to 5 years after completing the initial therapy.[129] Risk factors for secondary neoplasia induction include the agent initially used, the cumulative dose given, the drug schedule, possibly altered immunity, a history of radiotherapy, and possibly the age of the patient. The prognosis for secondary leukemia is poor.[130] Secondary neoplastic changes in the gastrointestinal tract and other organs have also been reported.[131–134] Vaginal adenosis and clear cell carcinoma have been reported following 5-fluorouracil treatment.[135]

Breast Cancer

The relative risk of acute leukemia after alkylating agents is high.

GI Cancer

Relative risk of semustine recipients was 2.6, 2 years after treatment, increasing to 22, 4 to 7 years after treatment.

Ovarian Cancer

The incidence was 7.7 per 1000, 1 year after treatment with an alkylating agent.

Lung Cancer

Four of 243 patients treated with busulfan developed acute leukemia.

Testis Cancer

Five of 722 patients developed leukemia.

Table 61–19
Potency of Antiemetic Drugs[a]

Potency	Type of Antiemetic Drug
Active against highly emetogenic chemotherapy	Serotonin antagonist
	Substituted benzamide (high-dose)
Active against mildly or moderately emetogenic chemotherapy	Phenothiazine
	Butyrophenone
	Corticosteroid
	Cannabinoid
Minimally active	Antihistamine
	Anticholinergic agent
	Benzodiazepine

[a]Adapted from Grunberg SM, Hesketh PJ. N Engl J Med 1993;329:1790–1796.

Table 61–20
Initial Doses in Selected Antiemetic Regimens[a,b]

Antiemetic Regimen	Initial Dose
For moderately emetogenic chemotherapy	
Prochlorperazine	5–10 mg PO, 5–10 mg IV, or 25 mg by rectal suppository
Thiethylperazine	10 mg PO, 10 mg IM, or 10 mg by rectal suppository
Dexamethasone	10–20 mg IV
Dronabinol	10 mg PO
Ondansetron	8 mg PO or 10 mg IV
For highly emetogenic chemotherapy	
Dexamethasone	20 mg IV
Metoclopramide	3 mg/kg of body weight IV every 2 hr × 2
Diphenhydramine	25–50 mg IV every 2 hr × 2
Lorazepam	1–2 mg IV
Dexamethasone	20 mg IV
Ondansetron	32 mg IV (in divided doses)

[a]Adapted from Grunberg SM, Hesketh PJ. N Engl J Med 1993;329:1790–1796.
[b]Antiemetic regimens for moderately emetogenic chemotherapy consist of single drugs; regimens for highly emetogenic chemotherapy consist of drugs given in combination (denoted by brackets). PO denotes orally, IV intravenously, and IM intramuscularly.

Table 61–21
Guidelines for Ondansetron Prescribing in Adult and Pediatric Patients[a]

I. Cancer chemotherapy-induced nausea and vomiting
Ondansetron has *not been established* to be more effective than other antiemetics in the *treatment* of cancer chemotherapy-induced nausea and vomiting, even if caused by highly emetogenic agents.
  A. Ondansetron is *appropriate* in the *prevention* of nausea and vomiting if the patient is receiving chemotherapy with any of the following:
    - An agent known to cause emesis in ≥50% of patients (eg, cisplatin, dacarbazine, mechlorethamine, carmustine, cyclophosphamide, dactinomycin, plicamycin)
    - Combination chemotherapy known to cause emesis in ≥50% of patients
    - An agent with low emetic potential at standard doses, but causing emesis in ≥50% of patients at high doses (eg, cytarabine at doses >500 mg/m^2, methotrexate at doses >200 mg/m^2, and ifosfamide at doses >3 g/m^2)
    - An agent whose emetic potential increases to ≥50% of patients based on route of administration (eg, intrathecal cytarabine and intrathecal methotrexate)
    - Investigational chemotherapy known to cause emesis in ≥50 of protocol patients
  B. Ondansetron is also *appropriate* in the *prevention* of nausea and vomiting if treatment with other antiemetics (such as metoclopramide, prochlorperazine, and haloperidol) is unacceptable because such alternative agents:
    - Have caused clinically significant side effects
    - Are contraindicated (includes patients <35 yr of age in whom the risk of extrapyramidal side effects [EPSEs] caused by metoclopramide therapy is high, and patients with neurologic disorders in whom EPSEs may mask symptoms of the underlying disease)
    - Have failed to reduce the number of emetic episodes of ≤2/24 h during previous treatments

II. Postoperative nausea and vomiting (PONV)
Ondansetron is *not indicated* when anesthetic agents with low emetic potential are used (eg, propofol). Little evidence exists to demonstrate the superiority of ondansetron over *alternative antiemetic* therapy for the prevention or treatment of PONV.
  A. Ondansetron is *appropriate* in the *prevention* of nausea and vomiting in patients undergoing surgery and anesthesia associated with a *high incidence* of PONV (eg, laparoscopy, use of inhalation agents, narcotics) if the patient:
    - Has a documented history of adverse effects to other antiemetics
    - Has a history of significant PONV resistant to therapy with antiemetics other than ondansetron
    - Is to undergo a procedure in which nausea and vomiting are likely to alter the surgical outcome (eg, neck surgery)
  B. Ondansetron may be used to *treat* nausea and vomiting in patients who have undergone surgery and anesthesia only if treatment with other antiemetics has:
    - Failed to reduce the number of emetic episodes to ≤2/24 h
    - Caused clinically significant side effects

III. Other considerations
  A. Ondansetron should *not* be used in the following circumstances:
    - For the prevention or treatment of "delayed" nausea and vomiting after chemotherapy administration (nausea and vomiting occurring >24 h after the last dose of chemotherapy)
    - On an "as needed" basis
  B. There is limited information on the safety and efficacy of ondansetron in the following circumstances. Until additional information is available, the use of ondansetron for these indications should be considered investigational. If additional information becomes available to support the use of ondansetron in these conditions such use should be considered off-label rather than investigational.
    - For the prevention or treatment of nausea and vomiting caused by or associated with:
      Postoperative nausea and vomiting (in cases other than those listed previously in these guidelines)
      "Anticipatory" nausea and vomiting before the administration of chemotherapy (nausea and vomiting occurring before the administration of chemotherapy, caused by the recollection of nausea and vomiting during previous chemotherapy administration)
      The acquired immunodeficiency syndrome (AIDS) disease process or AIDS therapy
      The use of opiates
      Radiation therapy
      Hyperthermia therapy
  C. The use of ondansetron in combination with dexamethasone has been established to be more effective than therapy with either agent alone. The combination of ondansetron with an anxiolytic (eg, lorazepam) may also be appropriate in some cases. The use of other combinations of antiemetics in conjunction with ondansetron, particularly multiple-drug "cocktails," should be avoided.
  D. The dosage of ondansetron approved by the US Food and Drug Administration for chemotherapy-induced nausea and vomiting is 0.15 mg/kg administered intravenously (IV) every 4 h for three doses, with the first dose administered 30 min before chemotherapy. Other dosing regimens that have been evaluated include 32 mg administered IV once 30 min before chemotherapy administration, 8 mg administered IV 30 min before chemotherapy administration, followed by 1 mg/h infused for the following 24 h. It is not known whether other dosing options may allow dose reductions without loss of efficacy. The administration of additional ondansetron, after standard doses have failed to control nausea and vomiting, has not been established to be effective.
  E. In clinical trials conducted to support the use of ondansetron for the prevention and treatment of PONV, a single-intravenous 4-mg dose was effective.

[a]Adapted from Vermeulen LC Jr et al. Arch Intern Med 1994;154:1733–1740.

Hodgkin's Disease

The 10-year risk of developing secondary leukemia is reported as 5.6% for patients under 40 years of age and 30.9% for those aged over 40 years.

Non-Hodgkin's Lymphoma

Seven years after therapy the incidence was 6.3%.

RISK FACTORS—ALKYLATING AGENTS

Alkylating agents have been associated with the highest risk for the subsequent development of leukemia.[118–120,122,123,136] For melphalan and cyclophosphamide there is a positive relationship between the cumulative dose given and the risk of leukemia. Carcinogenicity of oncotherapeutic drugs is presented in Table 61-24.[137] Non-alkylating agents (cisplatin,[129–131,138,139] etoposide,[131,132]

Table 61–22
Bristol Children's Hospital Oncology and Haematology Unit Guidelines for Use of Antiemetics[a]

Chemotherapy Regimens	Block	Antiemetics: A Age >5 years	Antiemetics: B Age ≤5 years
	6	As below with addition of Lorazepam	As below with addition of Promethazine and Chlorpromazine
(High) Carboplatin, Cisplatin, Cyclophosphamide (high dose 60 mg/kg) ▲; Cytosine (high dose >500 mg/m²); COPADM; Ifosfamide	5	*Before chemotherapy* * Ondansetron iv and ■ Dexamethasone iv *Followed by* * Ondansetron iv/po 12 hours post ■ Dexamethasone iv/po 12 hourly +/–Metoclopramide	*Before chemotherapy* * Ondansetron iv and ■ Dexamethasone iv *Followed by* * Ondansetron iv/po 12 hours post ■ Dexamethasone iv/po 12 hourly +/–Prochlorperazine
Actinomycin D; Cyclophosphamide (intermediate dose 1 g/m²) ▲; TBI	4	*Before chemotherapy* * Ondansetron iv *Followed by* * Ondansetron iv/po 12 hours post +/–Metoclopramide	*Before chemotherapy* * Ondansetron iv *Followed by* * Ondansetron iv/po 12 hours post +/–Prochlorperazine po/pr
Adriamycin; Amsacrine; Daunorubicin; Epirubicin; Methotrexate (high dose >3 g/m²)	3	*Before chemotherapy* * Ondansetron iv *Followed by* * Ondansetron iv/po 12 hours post +/–Metoclopramide	*Before chemotherapy* Promethazine iv *Followed by* Promethazine alternating with Chlorpromazine (each 4 hourly)
CHLVPP; Cyclophosphamide (low dose <500 mg/m²); Cytosine (low dose <500 mg/m²); Methotrexate (low dose <3 g/m²); Triple IT; RADIOTHERAPY—lower chest, abdomen, spine	2	NO MEDICATION or *Before chemotherapy* Metoclopramide iv *Followed by* Metoclopramide po/iv PRN	NO MEDICATION or *Before chemotherapy* Promethazine iv *Followed by* Prochlorperazine po/pr PRN
(Low) Asparaginase; Bleomycin; Methotrexate IT; Vinblastine; Vincristine; VP-16	1	NO MEDICATION	NO MEDICATION

High → Low

- Consider moving up to next different block if recent antiemetic failure
- Consider moving sideways B → A if borderline age
- If patient suffers from anticipatory nausea and vomiting consider giving dose of Lorazepam the night before chemotherapy

* Give Ondansetron on day(s) of most emetogenic treatments only

▲ Delayed emesis risk. Give extra dose of Ondansetron at 24 hours post

■ Do NOT give Dexamethasone if:

1) Chemotherapy includes steroids
2) Brain tumors-during chemotherapy

Discuss with consultant for use in delayed emesis

ANTIEMETIC FAILURE:
4 HOURS OF NAUSEA
OR
2 VOMITS IN A 24 HOUR PERIOD

ONDANSETRON
iv: 5 mg/m² (maximum 8 mg)
Dilute in 20–50 ml of Normal Saline and give over 15 minutes
po: ≤1.2 m² 4 mg; >1.2 m² 8 mg

DEXAMETHASONE
Before chemotherapy
8 mg/m² (maximum 8 mg) iv
Followed by
8 mg/m²/day iv/po in divided doses (maximum dose 12 mg) infuse slowly in Normal Saline

LORAZEPAM
po: Age ≤10 years 0.5 mg
Age >10 years 1 mg
up to tds
Not recommended <5 years

PROMETHAZINE + CHLORPROMAZINE
iv: 0.5 mg/kg
Alternate every 2 hours for 3–4 doses
Then give on PRN basis
Dilute in 20 ml Normal Saline and infuse over 15–20 minutes

METOCLOPRAMIDE
po/iv:

Age/yrs	*Dose*	
5–9	2.5 mg	tds
10–14	5 mg	tds
≥15	10 mg	tds

Infuse slowly in Normal Saline

PROCHLORPERAZINE
po/pr: 250 mcg/kg tds

[a]Adapted from Foot AB, Hayes C. Arch Dis Child 1994;71:475–480.

hydroxyurea,[138] mitomycin,[140] doxorubicin,[129] dacarbazone,[141] interleukin-2,[142] prednimustine,[143] mitoxantrone,[144] tamoxifen,[145,150] bleomycin[146], and others) have been linked to secondary cancer development. High doses of methotrexate used for the treatment of cancer have been followed later in life by an increased incidence of other cancers.[147]

CHROMOSOMAL ABNORMALITIES

Defects in chromosomes 5 and 7, and possibly 11,[141,148,149] are associated with secondary leukemia in patients treated with chemotherapy and radiotherapy, as well as after exposure to a variety of environmental toxins such as benzene.

TREATMENT—PROGNOSIS

Few guidelines are currently available to guide the clinician in the quest for reduction or elimination of secondary cancers.

Isotretinoin

Daily treatment with high doses of isotretinoin is effective in preventing second primary tumors in patients who have been treated for squamous-cell carcinoma of the head and neck.[150]

TUMOR LYSIS SYNDROME

Tumor lysis syndrome occurs in patients who harbor rapidly growing tumors that are highly sensitive to chemotherapy or radiation.[151,152] It is characterized by the development of hyperkalemia, hyperphosphatemia, hyperuricemia, and hypocalcemia. Electrolyte imbalances lead to life-threatening complications such as cardiac dysrhythmias, severe neuromuscular dysfunction, and acute renal failure. Tumor lysis syndrome rarely follows intrathecal methotrexate[153] or prednisone.[154,155]

RISK FACTORS

Prior existence of renal insufficiency, hyperuricemia, or electrolyte imbalance place the patient at high risk of a potentially fatal outcome. Those with elevated white blood cell counts and large tumors are at additional risk.

Table 61–23
Cytotoxic Drugs That Enhance Toxic Reactions to Radiotherapy

Actinomycin D[112]
Aminoglutethimide[109, 110]
Bleomycin[114]
Cyclophosphamide[111]
Doxorubicin[107, 108, 113]
Fluorouracil[114]
Hydroxyurea[114]
Melphalan[111]
Vincristine[109]
Tamoxifen[117]

CLINICAL FEATURES

The predominant electrolyte abnormality will usually determine the clinical course. Hypocalcemia leads to muscle cramps, tetany, ventricular dysrhythmias, confusion, and convulsions. Hyperuricemia leads to nephropathy, oliguria, or hematuria. Hyperphosphatemia results in hypocalcemia and renal failure because of the production of high levels of calcium phosphate that precipitate in the kidney. Hyperkalemia is known to be associated with life-threatening ventricular arrhythmias and sudden death.[156,157]

PREVENTION AND TREATMENT

Hyperuricemia, electrolyte abnormalities, and renal function abnormalities should be aggressively treated prior to initiation of antineoplastic therapy. Allopurinol in doses up to 500 mg/m^2 body surface area is instituted for amelioration of hyperuricemia; high-flow intravenous fluids and urinary alkalinization are of value until uric acid levels are normalized. Serum electrolytes, creatinine, blood urea nitrogen, uric acid, calcium, phosphorus, and lactic acid dehydrogenase should be monitored until stable and thereafter up to 3 to 5 days.

Hemodialysis may be considered in those patients who are unresponsive to the above regimen. Suggested criteria that may be followed for initiating hemodialysis, or to reduce a rapidly rising volume overload and symptomatic hypocalcemia,[151] include the following:

Serum potassium > 6 meq/liter (6 mmol/L[9])
Serum uric acid > 10 mg/dL (590/μmol/L)
Serum creatinine > 10 mg/dL (880 μmol/L)
Serum phosphorus > 10 mg/dL (phosphate > 3.2 mmol/L)

RETINOIC ACID SYNDROME

Use of all-*trans*-retinoic acid to induce remission in promyelomonocytic leukemia can lead (within 2 to 21 days after starting treatment) to the retinoic acid syndrome characterized by hyperleucocytosis, fever, respiratory dis-

Table 61–24
Carcinogenicity of Oncotherapeutic Drugs[a]

Classification	Drugs
Group 1: Carcinogenic	Chlornaphazine, Myleran (busulfan), chlorambucil, methyl-CCNU, cyclophosphamide, melphalan, MOPP and other combined chemotherapy including alkylating agents, treosulfan
Group 2A: Probably carcinogenic	Adriamycin (doxorubicin), BCNU, CCNU, cisplatin, *N*-methyl-*N*-nitrosourea, nitrogen mustard, procarbazine hydrochloride, thiotepa
Group 2B: Possibly carcinogenic	Azaserine, bleomycins, dacarbazine, daunomycin, medroxyprogesterone acetate, merphalan, mitomycin C, streptozotocin, uracil mustard

[a]Adapted from Boivin JF. Cancer 1990; 65(suppl 3):770–775.
MOPP, Combined therapy with nitrogen mustard, vincristine, procarbazine, and prednisone; *BCNU,* carmustine; *CCNU,* lomustine.

tress, pleural and pericardial effusions, hypotension, interstitial pulmonary infiltrates, and weight gain.[158–161] Early use of corticosteroids is beneficial.[157]

HIGH-DOSE ANTINEOPLASTIC AGENTS

High-dose toxicity following antineoplastic drug use often manifests itself in signs and symptoms that frequently are not similar to those found after ordinary therapeutic use. Frequent central and peripheral nervous system manifestations, as well as hepatotoxic changes, are observed. Blood levels largely parallel dosages, but significant differences are observed within a specific drug group. Deaths occur more frequently in these dose ranges. Careful monitoring and supportive care are indicated. Specific antidotes are not generally useful, with certain exceptions such as sodium thiosulfate for cisplatin nephrotoxicity.

OVERDOSE (TABLE 61–25)

Overdoses with cytotoxic drugs must be evaluated in the light of the complexities surrounding antineoplastic treatment[162]: *(a)* the use of prior recent treatment regimens; *(b)* the use of multiple chemotherapeutic agents simultaneously; and *(c)* the presence of multiple system dysfunctions deriving from an acute or chronic disease process. Add to this the paucity of clinical experience with treatment of such overdoses and the occasional use of unusual routes (e.g., intrathecal) for instillation of what frequently are new investigational chemicals. Enough clinical experiences, however, to provide some idea of the problems of diagnosing and treating representatives of some of the classes of cytotoxic drugs are now available. Finally, it cannot be assumed that experience with one member of a chemical or biologic cytotoxic drug class provides sufficient guidelines to the diagnosis and treatment of overdose with another member of the same class.

Table 61–25
Cytotoxic Overdose Experiences

- Antitumor antibiotics
  - Actinomycin D
  - Doxorubicin
- Alkylating agents
  - Nitrogen mustards
    - Chlorambucil
    - Ifosfamide
    - Melphalan
  - Nitrosoureas
    - Lomustine
    - Mesna
- Antimetabolites
  - Folic acid antagonists
    - Methotrexate
  - Purine analogues
    - 6-Mercaptopurine
  - Pyrimidine analogues
    - Cytarabine
    - 5-Fluorouracil
- Natural products
  - Epidophyllotoxins
    - Etoposide
  - Vinca alkaloids
    - Vincristine
  - Androgen blockers
    - Flutamide
  - Immunomodulators
    - Levamisole
  - Miscellaneous
    - L-Asparaginase
    - Cisplatin
    - Hydrazine
    - Mitoxantrone
    - Procarbazine

ANTITUMOR ANTIBIOTICS

Actinomycin-D

Overdose results in seizures, hyponatremia, hypovolemia, hypocalcemia and hypomagnesemia, thrombocytopenia, oral mucositis, diarrhea, and fever.

Doxorubicin

The risk of cardiotoxicity with doxorubicin is considered to increase from 3% at 400 mg/m^2 to 7% at 550 mg/m^2 and 18% at 700 mg/m^2.[163] Doxorubicin has a large volume of distribution. In an obese individual the ideal surface area is based on ideal body weight. In a female using height and weight (50 kg + 2.3 kg/in > 5 ft),[164] the surface area would have been 30% less than the calculated surface area (based on total body weight and hence an overestimation of total body water) and therefore the dose would have been 30% less for this patient.[165] Further reduction in dose might have been made due to evidence of hepatotoxicity in this case. Cardiomyopathy may be fatal.

Acute encephalopathy, dysuria, gait disturbances, an abnormal electroencephalogram, absent tendon reflexes, coma, seizures, mydriasis, myelotoxicity mucositis,[166] and elevated cerebrospinal fluid protein levels have been observed.[167]

ALKYLATING AGENTS—NITROGEN MUSTARDS

Chlorambucil[168–177]

Therapeutic doses of chlorambucil in both adults and children range from 0.1 to 0.2 mg/kg/day. At total doses of 4 to 6 mg/kg in adults (see High Dose section) myoclonus and seizures may be induced. Dosages of 1.5 to 6.8 mg/kg may be associated with lethargy, irritability, myoclonus, vomiting, abdominal pain, ataxia, seizures, transient electroencephalographic changes, and coma.

Ifosfamide[178–180]

Therapeutic doses of ifosfamide range from 1.2 to 2.5 g/m^2/day intravenously. Doses have been given up to 5 g/m^2 by slow IV push over 30 minutes or up to 8 g/m^2 as a 24-hour continuous infusion when used with mesna.[22] The maximum tolerated dose reported has been 17 g/m^2 given by continuous intravenous infusion over 120 hours with mesna uroprotection in one study and 16 g/m^2 with mesna protection in another patient.[181] Dose limiting renal toxicity was observed at 18 g/m^2. Duration of myelosuppression, frequency and severity of mucositis, and renal tubular acidosis appear to be dose dependent.

Treatment

There are no antidotes for ifosfamide or its metabolites. Dialysis may be considered in view of the favorable toxicokinetics (low apparent volume of distribution), but no studies are yet available to confirm this.

Cyclophosphamide

Two patients received four times the lethal dose of cyclophosphamide: one died and the other has residual cardiac damage.[182]

Melphalan[183–185]

Therapeutic doses of melphalan have ranged between 0.15 to 0.25 mg/kg/day, with doses of 2.0 to 2.5 mg/kg used on occasion. Reversible bone marrow suppression (lymphocytopenia within 24 hours, neutropenia, and thrombocytopenia by the seventh day), diarrhea, a reversible nephropathy, and moderate oral ulcerations have been observed.

Symptomatic and supportive treatment appear to be the mainstay of treatment following a melphalan overdose. Colony stimulating factors (GM-CSF, G-CSF) may improve the prognosis. Hypopotassemia and hyponatremia should be appropriately managed. In view of its high protein binding and other toxicokinetic properties, hemodialysis or hemoperfusion may not be effective. There are no antidotes.

ALKYLATING AGENTS—NITROSUREAS[186–188]

Lomustine[30–31]

This nitrosurea is usually administered in doses of 100 to 130 mg/m^2 orally every 4 to 6 weeks. Overdose may lead to a pancytopenia. Treatment is symptomatic and supportive.

ALKYLATING AGENT—SUPPORTIVE

Mesna

As a uroprotectant for cyclophosphamide- and ifosfamide-induced hemorrhagic cystitis, mesna is administered in doses of 1500 mg/m^2/day (approximately 37 mg/kg/day) intravenously and orally. Toxic effects following its use may include abdominal discomfort and vomiting, both of which may tend to reflect its disagreeable taste orally. Doses of over 85 mg/kg intravenously have resulted in vomiting and diarrhea.[189]

ANTIMETABOLITES

Folic Acid Antagonist—Methotrexate[190–208]

The therapeutic use of methotrexate (MTX) as an antineoplastic agent involves doses of 20 to 80 mg/m^2 intravenously and intramuscularly or 0.5 to 2 mg/kg orally and 10 to 15 mg/m^2 intrathecally. High doses of over 20 mg/kg have been used, as well as 35 to 150 mg/kg intravenously with citrovorum factor (folinic acid) rescue. Overdose leads to a pancytopenia and severe mucositis.[209] Prompt leucovorin rescue (1000 mg/m^2 IV every 6 hours) and charcoal hemoperfusion appear useful to bring down the plasma methotrexate concentration.[210]

Intrathecal

Intrathecal methotrexate induces three types of toxic reaction[211]: the most common is a chemical arachnoiditis, generally mild, that occurs soon after intrathecal instillation of the drug and resolves within several days; occasionally the clinical and cerebrospinal fluid (CSF) findings may resemble a bacterial meningitis. A second category includes spinal cord and/or nerve damage. Paraplegia may develop and be either reversible or ascending and result in death. Finally, patients may develop encephalopathy, dementia, seizures, coma, and death. The toxicity may be partially related to preservatives (e.g., benzyl alcohol). Multiple cerebrospinal fluid exchanges after an inadvertent tenfold overdose of intrathecal methotrexate may be useful in primary signs of acute neurotoxicity.[212]

PURINE ANALOGUES

6-Mercaptopurine (6-MP)[213,214]

Overdose results in dizziness, headache, abdominal pain, and a rise in serum bilirubin. The characteristic hepatotoxic features after 6-mercaptopurine ingestion are a combination of intrahepatic cholestasis and parenchymal cell necrosis. These effects are usually reversible on discontinuation of the drug. Hepatotoxic reactions are most common when daily doses exceed 2.5 mg/kg. Elevation of serum bilirubin, in particular, may forewarn of impending cholestasis, which may prove fatal. Fatalities have been reported.[214a] Treatment is supportive. Allopurinol is not advised in treatment of an overdose since 6-MP is metabolized to thiouric acid by xanthine oxidase, which in turn is inhibited by allopurinol.[214]

5-Fluorouracil[215,216]

An overdose of 5-fluorouracil may cause nausea, vomiting, diarrhea, gastrointestinal ulceration, bleeding, and bone marrow depression.[215] Cimetidine may increase the plasma concentration[213] and would not be advised in management of an overdose. Life-threatening cardiotoxicity (atrial and ventricular arrhythmias, congestive cardiac failure, myocardial ischemia, and sudden death) following use of 5-fluorouracil has been reported. It is difficult at present to predict which patients will be affected.[217]

NATURAL PRODUCTS

Epidophyllotoxins—Etoposide[218]

Overdose may lead to a decrease in leukocyte counts, T-lymphocytes, and blast transformation.

VINCA ALKALOIDS

Vincristine[219–231] (Table 61–26)[226]

Following a vincristine overdosage[224–231] fever, nausea, and vomiting usually begins in the first 24 hours and resolves

Table 61-26
Duration of Toxicity Following Vincristine Overdose[a]

Toxic Effect	Without Leucovorin (days)	With Leucovorin (days)[b]
Nausea/vomiting	1–7	1–4
Neuropathies	3–30	3–9
Inappropriate ADH	3–16	6–10
Paresthesias	7–28	2–80
Bone marrow depression	7–21	4–16
Gastrointestinal effects	9–21	3–16
Myopathies	14–60	4–80
Cerebral dysfunction	14–50	4–25

[a]Adapted from Thomas LLM, Braat PC, Somers R, Goudsmit R. Cancer Treat Rep 1982;66:1967–1969.
[b]Starting 24 hours after vincristine overdose, 12 mg of leucovorin was given 4 times daily for 5 days.

within 1 week. There is a progressive development of peripheral neuropathies, beginning during the first week with diminished deep tendon reflexes, particularly in the lower extremities, followed by paresthesias in 10 to 14 days, and progressing to muscle weakness and disturbed gait in 2 to 3 weeks; slow recovery occurs over the subsequent 30 to 45 days. Inappropriate antidiuretic hormone secretion begins 3 to 7 days after the injection,[230] is frequently associated with seizures that do not appear to be directly related to the hyponatremia, and is resolved by the end of the second week. Sensory disturbances begin during the first week, progress to lethargy and disorientation by the second week, and resolve over the next 2 to 4 weeks. Bone marrow depression is characterized by a leukopenia with a nadir at 10 days and followed by complete recovery within 3 weeks; gastrointestinal disturbances begin in 4 to 72 hours after an injection, followed by abdominal pain, ileus, and constipation within 9 to 13 days, with clearing of these symptoms by 2 to 3 weeks; cranial nerve palsies, especially ptosis, and autonomic dysfunction occurs after 2 to 3 weeks, improving over 4 to 8 weeks; alopecia and early hypertension may be observed.

Leucovorin does not appear to significantly alter toxicity following a vincristine overdose.[228,232] Plasmapheresis was useful in treatment of a vincristine overdose in an 18-year-old patient who received ten times the intended dose of vincristine in error.[233] Vincristine is highly bound to plasma proteins (50 to 80%) and cannot be dialyzed.

Intrathecal Vincristine

Most instances of inadvertent intrathecal administration of vincristine have resulted in ascending paralysis and death in several weeks.[234]

VINDESINE (VDS) OVERDOSE

Overdose (45 mg instead of 4.5 mg) leads to generalized muscle pain, tinnitus, diarrhea, sleeplessness, burning sensation in mouth, and hiccups. Patients usually respond to supportive treatment (parenteral nutritional leucovorin, citrulline 600 mg/day, arginine 1200 mg/day, and ornithine 600 mg/day).[232]

ANDROGEN BLOCKERS

Flutamide

Clinical trials with doses up to 1500 mg per day for periods up to 36 weeks have included gynecomastia, breast tenderness, and some increases in the SGOT.[235] The dosage of flutamide associated with symptoms of overdose or considered to be life-threatening has not been established.

IMMUNE MODULATORS

Levamisole

There are no published reports on levamisole overdose.

L-asparaginase[169,234]

Central nervous system toxicity (lethargy, somnolence, and coma) has been described and appears to be associated with a fall in cerebrospinal fluid asparagine. "Asparagine rescue" infusions have been used to reverse serious drug-induced brain dysfunction syndromes,[237] but this observation must be confirmed by other studies.[236]

CISPLATIN[236–241]

Acute Overdose

Acute overdose with cisplatin results in renal failure, hepatic failure, deafness, ocular toxicity (including detachment of the retina), significant myelosuppression, intractable nausea and vomiting, and/or neuritis and death. No antidotes have been established for cisplatin overdosage. Hemodialysis is not useful in eliminating platinum from the body, but plasmapheresis lowers the plasma platinum concentration.[242] Management is based on supportive and symptomatic treatment.[243]

Three different types of errors appear to have caused overdosage: *(a)* mistaking the total dosage to be divided over several days for the daily dose; *(b)* administering cisplatin when the patient was to have received carboplatin; and *(c)* writing the wrong cisplatin dose. To minimize the possibility of error the manufacturer suggests *(a)* always write for the intended daily dose of cisplatin rather than the total dose to be administered over a period of time: for example, write "cisplatin 25 mg/gm/day for 4 days "instead of cisplatin 100 mg/sqm over 4 days," and, *(b)* institute an alert system for orders of cisplatin exceeding 120 mg/sqm per course. The present literature now states: "Caution should be exercised to prevent inadvertent overdosage with Platinol (cisplatin)." No proven antidotes have been established for Platinol (cisplatin) overdosage. Hemodialysis, even when initiated 4 hours after the overdosage, appears to have little effect on removing platinum from the body because of Platinol's (cisplatin) rapid and high degree of protein binding. Management of overdosage should include general supportive measures to sustain the patient through any period of toxicity that may occur.[244]

MISCELLANEOUS

Hydrazine[245–247]

Hydrazine overdosage leads to ataxia, lateral nystagmus, loss of vibration sense, and paresthesias. Hydrazine is also hepatotoxic in animals and may induce seizures.[248]

Mitoxantrone[244,248–250]

Mitoxantrone is an anthraquinone related chemically to the anthracyclines. Overdoses of 140 to 180 mg/m^2 have led to death with severe leukopenia, thrombocytopenia, and infection.[251]

Procarbazine

The manufacturer states the major manifestations of overdosage with procarbazine that would be anticipated are nausea, vomiting, diarrhea, hypotension, tremors, convulsions, and coma. Supportive therapy appears to be indicated.[251] Procarbazine is subject to serious hematotoxic and hepatotoxic effects.

LABORATORY

There are few indications for routine drug-level monitoring of cytotoxic drugs with the exception of high-dose methotrexate regimens.[252,253] Blood levels are not useful as a guide to the clinician who administers and guides chemotherapy. Other clinical modalities (hematology, EKG, EEG, etc.) are usually available in most health-care facilities.

Ancillary Tests

The clinical follow-up of patients who have received a cytotoxic drug will require, in most instances, careful hematologic studies frequently performed over the first 4 weeks and periodically thereafter. This may include peripheral blood counts, bone marrow analyses, and other tests related to the blood and blood-forming organs. Similarly, renal and liver function tests should be available. Since the gastrointestinal tract and central nervous system are often sites of clinical toxicity following chemotherapy, adequate use of investigative procedures for study of these organ systems (e.g., x-ray, computer tomography, nuclear magnetic resonance, endoscopy, spinal fluid studies) must be immediately available in those medical centers that are involved in care of the cancer patient.[254,255]

TREATMENT

Stabilization

Cytotoxic drugs administered in overdose by the oral route (inadvertent or self-induced) seldom result in an immediate life-threatening emergency. Caution must be exercised with those drugs known to induce early seizures. Patients who exhibit vital-sign abnormalities should receive an intravenous line, cardiac monitor, oxygen, and assisted mechanical ventilation as needed. Attention must be directed toward assessment of the adequacy of ventilation and blood pressure and correction of any abnormalities.

Gut Decontamination

Overdose with many antineoplastic drugs induces seizures at an early stage. Syrup of ipecac should not be used. If gastric lavage is contemplated, prior adequate protection of the airway must be ensured. The use of gastric emptying procedures, as well as activated charcoal and cathartics, for cytotoxic drug overdose has not been evaluated by critically controlled clinical studies; the value of these procedures will therefore depend on clinical judgement at the time of use.

ANTIDOTES

There are few antidotes useful in the amelioration of an antineoplastic drug overdose (Table 61–27). Mesna may diminish the hemorrhagic cystitis of cyclophosphamide and ifosfamide. Folinic acid (leucovorin, citrovorum factor) is used to mitigate methotrexate toxicity, but is of unproven value in vincristine toxicity. Methylene blue appears useful in reversing ifosfamide-associated encephalopathy.[256]

Doxorubicin

Dextrazoxane (Zinecard) has been approved by the U.S. Food and Drug Administration (FDA) for protection against cardiac toxicity from doxorubicin (Adriamycin and others) in women with metastatic brain cancer. Dextrazoxane is started 30 minutes before doxorubicin. They are usually given a 1:1 ratio, 500 mg/m^2 of dextrazoxane for every 40 mg/m^2 of doxorubicin[256a].

Methotrexate

Leucovorin (folinic acid or 5-formyltetrahydrofolate) can replenish and substitute for the endogenous reduced-folate cofactor (N^5, N^{10}-methylene tetrahydrofolatel) that methotrexate diminishes; thereby it replenishes intracellular reduced-folate pools and prevents methotrexate-induced cytotoxicity via blockade of thymidine synthesis. Little antidotal activity is possible unless leucovorin is administered within 48 hours of methotrexate. Other attempts at site protection (asparaginase, thymidine) are not yet clinically useful.

5-Fluorouracil (5-FU)

Chemoprotectants for 5-FU have been directed at the formation of a metabolite of 5-FU, 5-fluorouridylate triphosphate (5-FUTP), which is incorporated into RNA and interrupts further RNA synthesis. Allopurinol, through its metabolite oxipurinol, may permit doubling of the 5-FU infusion dose. This has not, however, produced significantly enhanced clinical 5-FU response rates. More active 5-FU combinations with leucovorin or levamisole are under trial.

ELIMINATION ENHANCEMENT

There is a paucity of evidence to support the use of any extracorporeal treatment methods (hemodialysis, hemoperfusion, peritoneal dialysis, or exchange transfusion) in the

Table 61-27
Antidotes—Chemoprotectants—Rescuers for Cytotoxic Drugs

Drug	Antidote	Site Specificity, Limitations
Anthracyclines (Doxorubicin)	ICRF-187	Cardiomyopathies
Asparaginase	L-Asparagine[1]	Acute brain dysfunction
Cisplatin	Fosfamycin[2] (animal data)	Ototoxicity, nephrotoxicity
	Sodium thiosulfate[3]	Nephrotoxicity, possible myelotoxicity; locoregional therapy only
	Diethyldithiocarbamate[4]	Nephrotoxicity, myelotoxicity may not be blocked; DDTC is neurotoxic
	Mesna[5] (animal data)	But neurotoxic
	WR 2721[6]	
Cyclophosphamide and Ifosfamide	Mesna	Uroprotectant: limited oral bioavailability (about 50%)
	NAC	Hematuria—incomplete protection
Methotrexate	Leucovorin[7]	Bone marrow, GI epithelium
	Thymidine[8–10]	(Investigational)
5-Fluorouracil	Allopurinol[11] (oxipurinol blocks FUTP formation and RNA synthesis inhibition)	Normal bone marrow
	FU/Leucovorin	
	FU/Levamisole[12]	

Note: Amifistine appears to be hemoprotective when nitrogen mustards are administered.[13, 14]
[1]Ohnuma T, Holland JF, Freeman A, Sinks LF. Cancer Res 1970;30:2297–2305.
[2]Dolan DF, Davidson T, Abrams GE, Snyder R. Laryngoscope 1986;97:948–958.
[3]Pfeifle CE, Howell SB, Felthouse RD, Weliver TBS, Andrews PA, Markman M et al. J Clin Oncol 1985;3:237–244.
[4]Borch RF, Katz JC, Lieder PH, Pleasants ME. Proc Natl Acad Sci 1980;77:5441–5444.
[5]Dorr RT. Semin Oncol 1991;18(Suppl 2):48–58.
[6]Mollman JE, Glover DJ, Hogan WM, Furman RE. Neurology 1985;35(Suppl 1):80.
[7]Twelves CJ. Lancet 1986;1:737.
[8]Spiegel RJ, Cooper PR, Blum RH, Speyer JL, McBride D, Mangiardi J. N Engl J Med 1984;311:386–388.
[9]Poplach DG. N Engl J Med 1984;311:400–402.
[10]Howell SB, Enxminger WD, Krishan A, Free E III. Cancer Res 1978;38:325–330.
[11]Howell SB, Wung W, Taetle R et al. Cancer 1981;48:1281–1289.
[12]Laurie JA, Moertel CG, Fleming TR et al. J Clin Oncol 1989;7:1447–1456.
[13]Van der Vijgh WJF, Peters GJ. Semin Oncol 1994;25(Suppl 11):2–7.
[14]Capizzi RL. Semin Oncol 1994:(Suppl 11):8–15.

treatment of antineoplastic drug overdose. Where it has been used (e.g., methotrexate),[257] the results have been disappointing. High volumes of distribution, high protein binding values, extensive metabolite formation, and limited clinical experience with the use of the above procedures in patients with cytotoxic agent overdose caution against use of these procedures at present.

SUPPORTIVE CARE

In the treatment of most cytotoxic drug overdoses symptomatic and supportive care remains the mainstay of therapy.

Convulsions

Intravenous diazepam remains the initial drug of choice. Airway precautions (endotracheal intubation) must be exercised if the patient has evidence of respiratory difficulty or presents in a state of diminished consciousness.

Fever and Chills

Blood, urine, sputum, or other sources of cultures should be repeatedly obtained to rule out specific bacterial or other infections. Intravenous antibiotics may be useful. Reverse isolation procedures may be indicated.

Electrolyte Depletion

Hyponatremia, hypopotassemia, hypocalcemia, and hypomagnesemia may be seen in overdose (e.g., Actinomycin D). Replacement therapy (intravenous electrolytes) should be accompanied by cardiac and respiratory monitoring, including periodic arterial blood gas determinations.

Diarrhea and Oral Mucositis

Use parenteral sources of nutrition and local therapy for oral lesions. A randomized, double-blind, placebo-controlled study suggests that topical application of 1 milliliter of vitamin E oil, 400 mg/mL, applied topically to all lesions twice a day for 5 days, is effective in the therapy of chemotherapy-induced mucositis.[258]

Conjunctivitis

Saline irrigations; ocular steroids if indicated.

Skin

Wash with soap and water. Flood with saline, especially if a vesicant drug has topically contaminated the skin (e.g., doxorubicin).

Nausea, Vomiting

(See section on Nausea and Vomiting in this chapter.)

Syndrome of Inappropriate Antidiuretic Hormone

Fluid restriction; watch fluid balance, electrolytes; if available obtain an ADH assay.

Dehydration

Intravenous fluids with careful observation of central venous pressure as indicated.

Observation

All patients suspected of ingesting toxic doses of cytotoxic drugs must have a careful hematologic analysis (red blood cells, hematocrit, white blood cells with differential counts, platelets). If the patient is asymptomatic after 8 hours, discharge may be considered. Because of delayed evidence of myelosuppression, the patient should be followed weekly with blood counts for at least 4 weeks. Similar periodic follow-up is indicated for cardiovascular evaluation following overdose (usually intravenous) with the anthracyclines. These patients should be followed weekly, then monthly in view of the frequently delayed onset of cardiotoxicity.

Severe Nephrotoxicity

May require prolonged hemodialysis.

Encephalopathy

Periodic electroencephalogram, lumbar punctures for cerebrospinal fluid analysis, computerized tomography, nuclear magnetic resonance studies, possible "CSF washout" (see section following), and rehabilitation.

Thrombocytopenia

Platelet transfusions, CSF.*

Anemia, Low Hematocrit

Red blood cell transfusions, CSF.*

Hypertension

May be treated with mannitol. If sodium nitroprusside is used in a patient with central nervous system depression, consider the possible effects of cyanide toxicity (see Antihypertensive drug chapter).

Prevention and Treatment of Cardiac Toxicity

Usefulness of prophylactic digitalis has not been evaluated. Cardiac transplantation was useful in ensuring long-term survival in a 5-year-old girl who developed doxorubicin-induced cardiomyopathy.[260]

*Use of colony stimulating factors (G-CSF, GM_2-CSF, erythropoietin) should be considered when managing undesirable effects secondary to bone marrow depression (bleeding, oral ulcerations, weakness, sepsis)[259]

Table 61–28
Amount (%) of Methotrexate Predicted To Be Recovered by CSF Removal[a, b]

Volume CSF Removed (ml)	Time After Methotrexate Injection (hr) 0.25	0.50	0.75	1.0	2.0	3.0
10	54	36	26	20	9	5
20	94	72	52	40	18	10
30	94	89	78	60	27	15
40	94	89	84	79	36	20

[a]Adapted from Addiego JE Jr et al. J Pediatr 1981;98:825–828.
[b]Assuming 10 ml of methotrexate-containing fluid was injected. Other assumptions are described in the text.

Intrathecal MTX Overdose—"Cerebral Washout" (Table 61–28)

1. *Cerebrospinal Fluid CSF drainage:* As soon as possible after an overdose or inadvertent intrathecal injection repeat the lumbar puncture. Begin CSF drainage to gravity.[202] Drainage of 30 mL of CSF within the first 15 minutes after an intralumbar overdose may remove nearly 95% of injected methotrexate.[196] Drainage 2 hours after injection may remove less than 20% of the dose.
2. *"CSF washout":* CSF drainage alone is insufficient to treat a massive methotrexate (MTX) overdose, since toxic amounts of the drug would still be present in the fluid after the procedure is completed.[197] With MTX overdoses of more than 100 mg, CSF drainage must be accompanied by ventriculolumbar perfusion.[199,200]
   a. Obtain neurosurgical consultation in a neurosurgical intensive care unit.
   b. Place a burrhole, insert a Scott ventricular cannula into the frontal horn of the right lateral ventricle.
   c. Use warmed preservative-free normal saline.
   d. Introduce 5 mL of normal saline into the ventricle through the Scott cannula; drain 5 mL of CSF from the lumbar needle.
   e. Over a period of 4 hours, up to 550 mL of normal saline is introduced through the ventricles of the patient and removed from the lumbar subarachnoid space.
   f. Leucovorin may be added to the final 100 mL of normal saline at a concentration of 0.02 mg per milliliter. However, its usefulness has not been clinically evaluated and it may be epileptogenic.[200]
   g. After the 550-mL flush the ventricular cannula is left attached to an intraventricular pressure transducer.
   h. Methotrexate levels in the CSF may be measured daily.
3. Pentobarbital and phenytoin may be given intravenously to prevent seizure.
4. Coma will require intubation with mechanical ventilating support.
5. Monitor arterial blood gases.
6. Twenty-four hours after the intrathecal overdose, rescue with thymidine. Thymidylate salvage from cytotoxic effects of methotrexate has been used[199] in a dose of 8 g/m^2/day by continuous intravenous infusion[261];

thymidine is an investigational drug for this use, and its effectiveness is unconfirmed.[200]

7. Maintain careful fluid balance to avoid any cerebral edema. Check intake and output.
8. Consider alkalinization of the urine to promote urinary excretion of MTX. There are no controlled clinical studies, however, to support this procedure in MTX overdose.
9. Leucovorin intravenously may be given at an unusually high dose (1000 mg)[197] to facilitate its passage across the blood–brain barrier; it is then continued intravenously until the MTX blood and CSF levels are within the nontoxic range. See Laboratory for methodology. Caution: see note 2f. above).
10. Cerebral edema may be ameliorated by mannitol. Steroids are not drugs of choice here; they have not been shown to prevent MTX-induced encephalopathy or myelopathy.[201]
11. Serial sampling of CSF for protein, glucose, and myelin basic protein may be useful.
12. A similar approach (cerebrospinal fluid washout) may also be of benefit if other toxic agents (e.g., vinca alkaloids, anthracyclines, cytarabine) are inadvertently instilled into the subarachnoid space. Further animal and clinical studies are indicated to confirm usefulness and safety of this procedure.[196]
13. Education of all individuals involved in the care of patients receiving intrathecal drugs is very important, including the attending physician, house officer, medical student, nursing staff, and pharmacist. Drug doses to be administered should be recalculated by each individual involved; cross-checking of proper and complete labeling of the syringe should be performed by the pharmacist, and its accuracy double-checked by the nurse and physician prior to administration.

Cytarabine Intrathecal

1. See "CSF washout" (methotrexate IT overdose) for a suggested procedure.
2. If no neurosurgical facilities are available, consider instillation of at least 10 × 5 mL exchanges of CSF over 50 minutes.
3. Monitor the patient continuously.

Cytarabine IV or subcutaneous overdose

1. Cytarabine is rapidly (half-life 10 minutes) metabolized to an inactive metabolite, uridine arabinoside.
2. Treat supportively.

Calculation methods for estimation of recovery from the spinal fluid are available.[262]

PREVENTION OF OVERDOSE

Prevention of overdose is paramount. Guidelines have been developed to preclude the danger of overdosage with any injected chemotherapeutic agent.[263]

1. All personnel involved in handling chemotherapeutic agents should be fully knowledgeable of the potential danger. Although a large number of patients in pediatric teaching hospitals may be receiving cancer chemotherapy, administration of these drugs should never be considered a routine task.
2. Charts of normal doses of chemotherapeutic agents should be available in all nursing stations and wherever drugs are prepared or administered.
3. All chemotherapeutic doses should be fully calculated and recorded in the chart by a member of the hematology-oncology service. The dose should be written in mg/kg or an equivalent SI concentration, total dose, and volume.
4. Chemotherapy should be given only by an experienced physician who can check the dose and concentration before it is administered. As with many other chemotherapy agents, drugs such as vincristine must be given intravenously. Extravasation into the skin causes severe and painful burns.
5. Stock only small dose vials of vincristine, for example, (10 mL = 1 mg) or other injectables where possible. This greatly reduces the opportunity to give a massive overdose. The maximum single dose of vincristine is usually 2 mg.

REFERENCES

1. Beeley L. Drugs and breast feeding. Clin Obstet Gynecol 1986;13:247–251.
2. Smith IJ, Wilson JT. Infant effect of drugs excreted into breast milk. Pediatr Rev Commun 1989;3;93–113.
3. Atkinson HC, Begg EJ, Darlow BA. Drugs in human milk. Clinical pharmacokinetic considerations. Clin Pharmacokinet 1988;14:217–240.
4. Amato D, Niblett JS. Neutropenia from cyclophosphamide in breast milk. Med J Aust 1977;1:383–384 (letter).
5. Duradola JI. Administration of cyclophosphamide during late pregnancy and early lactation. A case report. J Nat Med Assoc 1979;71:165–166.
6. Rieder MJ: Drugs and breastfeeding. In: Koren G, ed. Maternal-fetal toxicology. New York: Marcel Dekker, 1990, p.72.
7. Giacoia GP, Catz CS. Drugs and pollutants in breast milk. Clin Perinatol 1979;6:181–196.
8. Chaplin S, Sanders GL, Smith JM. Drug excretion in human breast milk. Adverse Drug React Acute Pois Rev 1982;1: 255–287.
9. Berlin CM Jr. Drugs and chemicals: exposure of the nursing mother. Pediatr Clin North Am 1989;36:1089–1091.
10. Committee on Drugs. American Academy of Pediatrics. The transfer of drugs and other chemicals into human breast milk. Pediatrics 1983;72:375–383.
11. La Leche League International. Breast feeding and drugs in human milk. Vet Hum Toxicol 1978;2:346–375.
12. Redman JR, Bajorunas DR, Goldstein MC et al. Semen preservation and artificial insemination for Hodgkin's disease. J Clin Oncol 1987;5:233–238.
13. Recommendations for the safe handling of parenteral antineoplastic drugs. Dept of Health and Human Service Publication. (NIH) 83-2621, Bethesda, MD: National Institutes of Health, 1982.
14. Council on Scientific Affairs. Guidelines for handling parenteral antineoplastics. JAMA 1985;253:1590–1592.
15. ASHP Technical Assistance Bulletin on Handling Cytotoxic and Hazardous Drugs. Am J Hosp Pharm 1990;47:1033–1049.
16. McDiarmid MA. Medical surveillance for antineoplastic drug handlers. Am J Hosp Pharm 1990;47:10–25.

17. Christensen CJ, Lemasters GK, Wakeman MJA. Work practices and policies of hospital pharmacists preparing antineoplastic agents. J Occup Med 1990;32:508–512.
18. Valanis B, Vollmer WM, Labuhn K, Glass A, Corelli C. Antineoplastic drug handling protection after OSHA guidelines comparison by profession, handling activity and work site. J Occup Med 1992;34:149–155.
19. Falck K, Rohn P, Sorsa M et al. Mutagenicity in urine of nurses handing cytostatic drugs. Lancet 1979;1:1250–1251.
20. Norppa H, Sorsa M, Vaino H, Grohn P, Heinonen E, Holski L et al. Increased sister chronatid exchange frequencies in lymphocytes of nurses handling cytostatic drugs. Scand J Work Environ Health 1980;6:299–301.
21. Wakvik H, Kleppo, Brogger A. Chromosome analyses of nurses handling cytostatic agents. Cancer Treat Rep 1981; 65:607–610.
22. Sotaniem EA, Sutinen S, Arranto AJ, Sutinen S, Sotaniem KA, Lehtola J et al. Liver damage in nurses handling cytostatic agents. Acta Med Scand 1983;214:181–189.
23. Selevan SG, Lindbohm M-L, Hornung RW, Hemminki K. A study of occupational exposure to antineoplastic drugs and fetal loss in nurses. N Engl J Med 1985;313:1172–1178.
24. Stucker I, Caillard J-F, Collin R, Gout M, Poyen D, Hemon D. Risk of spontaneous abortion among nurses handling antineoplastic drugs. Scand J Work Environ Health 1990;16:102–107.
25. Thiringer G, Granung G, Holmen A, Hogstadt B, Jarrholm B, Jonsson D, Persson L et al. Comparison of methods for the biomonitoring of nurses handling antitumor drugs. Scand J Work Environ Health 1991;17:133–138.
26. Staiano N, Galleli JF, Adamson RH, Thorgiersson SS. Lack of mutagenic activity in urine from hospital pharmacists admixing antitumour drugs. Lancet 1981;1:615–616.
27. Ames BN, McCann J, Yamasahi E. Methods for detecting carcinogens and mutagens with the Salmonella/mammalian-microsome mutagenicity test. Mutat Res 1975;35:347.
28. Skov T, Lynge E, Maarup B, Olsen L, Rorth M, Winthereik H. Risks for physicians handling antineoplastic drugs. Lancet 1990;2:1446.
29. Lunn G, Sansone EB, Andrews AW, Hellwig LC. Degradation and disposal of some antineoplastic drugs. J Pharm Sci 1989;78:652–659.
30. Carpenter L, Beral V, Roman E, Swerdlow AJ, Davies G. Cancer in laboratory workers. Lancet 1991;338:1080–1081.
31. Savitz DA, Chen J. Parental occupation and childhood cancer: review of epidemiologic studies. Environ Health Perspect 1990;8:325–327.
32. Von Hoff DD, Rozencweig M, Piccart M. The cardiotoxicity of anticancer agents. Semin Oncol 1982;9:23–33.
33. Makinen L, Makipernaa A, Rautonen J, Heino M, Pyrhonen S, Laitinen LA et al. Long-term cardiac sequelae after treatment of malignant tumors with radiotherapy or cytostatics in children. Cancer 1990;65:1913–1917.
34. Mills BA, Robert RW. Cyclophosphamide-induced cardiomyopathy. A report of two cases and review of the English literature. Cancer 1979;43:2223–2226.
35. Dresdale A, Bonow RO, Wesley R et al. Prospective evaluation of doxorubicin-induced cardiomyopathy resulting from post-surgical adjuvant treatment of patients with soft tissue sarcoma. Cancer 1983;52:51–60.
36. Porembka DT, Lowder JN, Orlowski JP, Bastilli J, Lockren J. Etiology and management of doxorubicin cardiotoxicity. Crit Care Med 1989;17:569–572.
37. Sriskandan S, O'Brien MER, Smith IE, Collins P, Gore ME. Aggressive management of doxorubicin-induced cardiomyopathy associated with "low" doses of doxorubicin. Postgrad Med J 1994;70:759–761.
38. Hale JP, Lewis IJ. Anthracyclines: cardiotoxicity and its prevention. Arch Dis Child 1994;74:457–462.
39. Steinherz LJ, Graham T, Hurwitz R, Sondheimer HM, Schwartz RG, Shaffer EM et al. Guidelines for cardiac monitoring of children during and after anthracycline therapy: report of the Cardiology Committee of the Childrens Cancer Study Group. Pediatrics 1992;89:942–949.
40. Lipshultz SE, Colan SD, Gelber RD, Perez-Atayde AR, Sallan SE, Sanders SP. Late cardiac effects of doxorubicin therapy for acute lymphoblastic leukemia in childhood. N Engl J Med 1991;324:808–815.
41. Doroshow JH. Doxorubicin-induced cardiac toxicity. N Engl J Med 1991;324:843–845.
42. Yeung ST, Yoong C, Spink J, Galbraith A, Smith PJ. Functional myocardial impairment in children treated with anthracyclines for cancer. Lancet 1991;337:816–818.
43. Von Hoff DD, Layard MW, Basa P et al. Risk factors for doxorubicin-induced congestive heart failure. Ann Intern Med 1979;91:710–717.
44. Stover DE. Pulmonary toxicity. Section 5 in De Vita VT Jr, Hellman S, Rosenberg SA, eds. Cancer principles and practice of oncology. 3rd ed. Philadelphia: JB Lippincott, 1989; pp. 2162–2169.
45. Weiss RB, Portero DS, Penta JS. The nitrosoureas and pulmonary toxicity. Cancer Treat Rev 1981;8:111–125.
46. Maher J, Daly PA. Severe bleomycin lung toxicity: reversal with high dose corticosteroids. Thorax 1993;48:92–94.
47. Doll DC, Ringenberg AS, Yarbro JW. Vascular toxicity associated with antineoplastic agents. J Clin Oncol 1986;4:1405–1417.
48. Fields SM, Lindley CM. Thrombotic microangiopathy associated with chemotherapy: case report and review of the literature. DICP 1989;23:582–588.
49. Jackson AM, Rose BD, Graff LG, Jacobs JB, Schwartz JH, Strauss GM et al. Thrombotic microangiopathy and renal failure associated with antineoplastic chemotherapy. Ann Intern Med 1984;101:41–44.
50. Imperia PS, Lazarus HM, Lass JH. Ocular complications of systemic cancer chemotherapy. Surv Ophthalmol 1989; 34:201–230.
51. Kaplan RS, Wiernik PH. Neurotoxicity of antineoplastic drugs. Semin Oncol 1982;9:103–130.
52. Goetz CG. Neurotoxins in clinical practice. New York: SP Medical & Scientific Books, 1985, p. 295.
53. Goldberg ID, Bloomer WD, Dawson DM. Nervous system toxic effects of cancer therapy. JAMA 1982;247:1437–1441.
54. McLeod DG. Antiandrogenic drugs. Cancer 1993;7:1046–1049.
55. Gomez J-L, DuPont A, Cusan L, Tranblay M, Tremblay M, Labre F. Simultaneous liver and lung toxicity related to the nonsteroidal antiandrogen Nilutamide (anandron). A case report. Am J Med 1992;92:563–566.
56. Gomez J-L, DuPont A, Cusan L, Tremblay M, Suburu R, LaMay M, Labrie F. Incidence of liver toxicity associated with the use of flutamide in prostate cancer patients. Am J Med 1992;92:465–470.
57. Blaker IC, Sawyer AM, Dooley JS, Sheuer PJ, McIntyre N. Severe hepatitis caused by cyproterone acetate. Gut 1990;31:556–557.
58. Parys BT, Hamid S, Thomson RGN. Severe hepatocellular dysfunction following cyproterone acetate therapy. Br J Urol 1991;67:312–313.
59. Levesque H, Trivalle C, Manchon ND et al. Fulminant hepatitis due to cypnoterone acetate. Lancet 1989;1:215–216.
60. Cox K, Stuart-Harris R, Abdini G, Grygiel J, Raghaven D. The management of cytotoxic-drug extravasation: guidelines drawn up by a working party for the Clinical Oncological Society of Australia. Med J Aust 1988;148:185–189.
61. Ignoffo RJ, Friedman MA. Therapy of local toxicities caused by extravasation of cancer chemotherapeutic drugs. Cancer Treat Rev 1980;7:17–27.
62. Doll DC, Ringenberg QS, Yarbro JW. Vascular toxicity associated with antineoplastic agents. J Clin Oncol 1986;4:1405–1417.
63. Rudolph R, Larson DL. Etiology and treatment of chemotherapeutic agent extravasation injuries: a review. J Clin Oncol 1987;5:1116–1126.
64. Larson DL. Treatment of tissue extravasation by antitumor agents. Cancer 1982;49:1796–1799.
65. Scarim SK. Treatment of doxorubicin extravasations. DICP 1989;23:386–387.

66. Loth TS. Minimal surgical debridement for the treatment of chemotherapeutic agent-induced skin extravasations. Cancer Treat Rep 1986;70:401–404.
67. Duvall E, Baumann B. An unusual accident during the administration of chemotherapy. Cancer Nursing 1980;3(4):305–306.
68. Harwood KY, Aisner J. Treatment of chemotherapy extravasation: current status. Cancer Treat Rep 1984;68: 939–945.
69. Olver IN, Schwarz MA. Use of dimethylsulfoxide in limiting tissue damage caused by extravasation of doxorubicin. Cancer Treat Rep 1983;67:407–408.
70. Olver IN, Aisner J, Hament A, Buchanan L, Bishop JF, Kaplan RS. A prospective study of topical dimethylsulfoxide for treating anthracycline extravasation. J Clin Oncol 1988;6: 1732–1735.
71. Burlock AL, Howser DM, Hubbard SM. Nursing management of adriamycin extravasation. Am J Nursing 1979;79:94–96.
72. Cox RF. Managing skin damage induced by doxorubicin hydrochloride and daunorubicin hydrochloride. Am J Hosp Pharm 1984;41:2410–2414.
73. Dorr RT, Albert DS. Vinca alkaloid skin toxicity: antidote and drug disposition studies in the mouse. JNCI 1985;74:113–120.
74. Argenta IC, Manders EK. Mitomycin C extravasation injuries. Cancer 1983;51:1080–1082.
75. Umstead GS, Fryer NL, Decker DA. Local tissue reaction to intravenous fluorouracil and leucovorin. DICP 1991;25: 249–250.
76. Tsavaris NB, Komitsopoulou P, Karagiouris P, Loukatou P, Zannou I et al. Prevention of tissue necrosis due to accidental extravasation of cytostatic drugs by a conservative approach. Cancer Chemother Pharmacol 1992;30:330–333.
77. Peters FTM, Beijnen JH, ben Bokkel Huinink WW. Mitoxantrone extravasation injury. Cancer Treat Rep 1987;71:992–993.
78. Weiss RB, Bruno S. Hypersensitivity reactions to cancer chemotherapeutic agents. Ann Intern Med 1981;94:66–72.
79. Schneider SM, Distellhorst CW. Chemotherapy-induced emergencies. Semin Oncol 1989;16:572–578.
80. Ma DDF, Isbister JP. Cytotoxic induced fulminant hyperpyrexia. Cancer 1980;45:2249–2251.
81. Blum RH, Carter SK, Agre K. A clinical review of bleomycin—a new antineoplastic agent. Cancer 1973;31:903–904.
82. Vogelzand NJ. “Adriamycin Flare”: a skin reaction resembling extravasation. Cancer Treat Rep 1979;63:2067–2069.
83. Schneider SM, Distelborst CW. Chemotherapy-induced emergencies. Semin Oncol 1989;16:572–578.
84. O'Brien MER, Souberbielle BE. Allergic reactions to cytotoxic drugs—an update. Semin Oncol 1992;3:605–610.
85. Rowinsky EK, Eisenhauer EA, Chaudhry V, Arbuck SG, Donehower. Clinical toxicities encountered with paclitaxel (TAXOL). Semin Oncol 1993;20(Suppl 2):1–15.
86. Rogers BB. Toxol: a promising new drugs of the '90s. Oncol Nurs Forum 1993;20:1483–1489.
87. Lindley CM, Bernard S, Fields SM. Incidence and duration of chemotherapy-induced nausea and vomiting in the outpatient oncology population. J Clin Oncol 1989;7:1142–1149.
88. Craig JB, Powell BL. Review: the management of nausea and vomiting in clinical oncology. Am J Med Sci 1987;293: 34–44.
89. Grunberg SM. Making chemotherapy easier. N Engl J Med 1990;322:846–848.
90. Siegel LJ, Longo DL. The control of chemotherapy-induced emesis. Ann Intern Med 1981;95:352–359.
91. Morrow GR. Chemotherapy-related nausea and vomiting: etiology and management. CA Cancer J Clin 1989;39: 89–104.
92. Graves T. Ondansetron: a new entity in emesis control. DICP 1990; 24(Suppl):S51–S54.
93. Nicolson M, Leonard RCF. Adverse effects of cancer chemotherapy. An overview of techniques for avoidance of minimisation. Drug Safety 1992;7:316–322.
94. New anti-nausea medication approved. FDA Medical Bulletin 1991;21(1):6.
95. Ondansetron hydrochloride injection (Zofran). Manufacturers' Insert. Glaxo Pharmaceuticals, January 1991.
96. Marty M, Poisillart P, Scholl S, Droz JP, Azab M, Brion N et al. Comparison of the 5-hydroxytryptamine$_3$ (serotonin) antagonist ondansetron (GR 38032F) with high-dose metoclopramide in the control of cisplatin-induced emesis. N Engl J Med 1990;322:816–821.
97. De Mulder PHM, Seynaeve C, Vermorken JB, Liessum PA, Mols-Jevdevic S, Allman EL et al. Ondansetron compared with high-dose metoclopramide in prophylaxis of acute and delayed cisplatin-induced nausea and vomiting. A multicenter randomized double-blind crossover study. Ann Intern Med 1990;113:834–840.
98. Pinkerton CR, Williams D, Wootton C, Meller ST, McElwain TJ. 5HT$_3$ antagonist ondansetron—an effective outpatient antiemetic in cancer treatment. Arch Dis Child 1990;65:822–825.
99. Cubeddu LX, Hoffmann IS, Fuenmayor NT, Finn AL. Efficacy of ondansetron (GR38032F) and the role of serotonin in cisplatin-induced nausea and vomiting. N Engl J Med 1990; 322:810–816.
100. Vermeulen LC Jr, Matuszewski KA, Ratko TA, Butler CD, Burnett DA, Vlasses PH. Evaluation of ondansetron prescribed in US Academic Medical Centers. Arch Intern Med 1994;154: 1733–1740.
101. Foot ABM, Hayes C. Audit of guidelines for effective control of chemotherapy and radiotherapy induced emesis. Arch Dis Child 1994;71:475–480.
102. Bone ME, Wilkinson DJ, Young JR, McNeil J, Charton S. Ginger root—a new antiemetic. The effect of ginger root on postoperative nausea and vomiting after major gynaecological surgery. Anaesthesia 1990;45:669–677.
103. Liu WHD. Ginger root, a new antiemetic. Anaesthesia 1990; 45:1085.
104. Dundee JW, Ghaley RG, Fitzpatrick KTJ, Abram WP, Lynch GA. Acupuncture prophylaxis of cancer chemotherapy-induced sickness. J Roy Soc Med 1989;82:268–269.
105. Dundee JW, Yang J, Ghaly RG. Vomiting and chemotherapy. Lancet 1990;535–541.
106. Jay GR, Wallace M, de Fusco P. Focus on granisetron. The second 5T$_3$-receptor antagonist approved for chemotherapy-induced emesis. Hosp Formul 1994;29:191–201.
107. Solberg LA, Wizk MR, Bruckman JE. Doxorubicin-enhanced skin reactions after whole-body radiation for leukemia cutis. Mayo Clin Proc 1980;55:711–715.
108. Shelly WB, Shelley ED, Campbell AC, Weigerberg H. Drug eruptions presenting at sites of prior radiation damage (sunlight and electron beam). Am Acad Dermatol 1984;11:53–57.
109. Vanek N, Hortobagyi GN, Buzdar AV. Radiotherapy enhances the toxicity of aminoglutethimide. Med Pediatr Oncol 1990; 18:162–164.
110. Williams DS, Leslie MD. Skin reaction following aminoglutethimide and radiotherapy. Br J Radiol 1987;60:1226–1227.
111. Kellie SJ, Plowman PN, Malpas JS. Radiation recall and radiosensitization with alkylating agents. Lancet 1987;6:1149–1150.
112. D'Angio GJ, Farber S, Maddock CL. Potentiation of x-ray effects by actinomycin D. Radiology 1959;73:175–177.
113. Donaldson SS, Glick JM, Wilbur JR. Adriamycin activating a recall phenomena after radiation therapy. Ann Intern Med 1974;8:407–408.
114. Philips TL. Radiation-drug interactions in the treatment of cancer. New York: Wiley, 1980.
115. Vassal G, Hartmann O, Habrand JL, Pico JL, Lemerle J. Radiosensitization after busulphan. Lancet 1987;1:571.
116. Nemecheck PM, Corder MC. Radiation recall associated with vinblastine in a patient treated for Kaposi Sarcoma related to Acquired Immune Deficiency Syndrome. Cancer 1992;70: 1605–1606.
117. Parry BR. Radiation recal induced by tamoxifen. Lancet 1992;340:49.
118. Kaldor JM, Day NE, Clarke EA, Van Leeuwen FE, Henry-Amar M, Fiorentino MV et al. Leukemia following Hodgkin's disease. N Engl J Med 1990;322:7–13.
119. Devereau S, Selassie TG, Hudson GV, Hudson BV, Linch DC. Leukemia complicating treatment for Hodgkin's disease:

the experience of the British National Lymphoma Investigation. Br Med J 1990;301:1077–1080.

120. Valagassa P, Santoro A, Fossati-Bellani F, Banfi A, Bonadonna G. Second acute leukemia and other malignancies following treatment for Hodgkin's disease. J Clin Oncol 1986;4:830–837.
121. Ingram L, Mott MG, Mann JR, Raafat F, Darbyshire PJ, Jones PHM. Second malignancies in children treated for non-Hodgkin's lymphoma and T-cell leukemia with the UKCCSG regimens. Br J Cancer 1987;55:463–466.
122. Glayney DW, Longo DL. Leukemia after treatment of ovarian cancer or Hodgkin's disease. N Engl J Med 1990;322:1818–1821.
123. Kaldor JM, Day NE, Petersson F, Clarke EA, Pedersen D, Mehnert W et al. Leukemia following chemotherapy for ovarian cancer. N Engl J Med 1990;322:1–6.
124. Chambers SK, Chopyk RL, Chambers JT, Schwartz PE, Duffy TP. Development of leukemia after doxorubicin and cisplatin treatment for ovarian cancer. Cancer 1989;64:2459–2461.
125. Reed E, Evans MK. Acute leukemia following cisplatin-based chemotherapy in a patient with ovarian cancer. J Natl Canc Inst 1990;82:431–432.
126. Brenez D, Devriendt J, Lenclud C, Schmerber J. Acute nonlymphocytic leukemia following chemotherapy with cisplatin and etoposide for non-small-cell carcinoma of the lung. Cancer Chemother Pharmacol 1990;26:235–236.
127. Van den Anker-Lugtenburg PJ, Sizoo W. Myelodysplastic syndrome and secondary acute leukemia after treatment of essential thrombocythermia with hydroxyurea. Am J Hematol 1990;33:152.
128. Pui C-H, Hancock ML, Raimondi SC, Head DR, Thompson E et al. Myeloid neoplasia in children treated for solid tumors. Lancet 1990;336:417–421.
129. Hawkins MM, Kingston JE, Wilson LMK. Late deaths after treatment for childhood cancer. Arch Dis Child 1990;65:1356–1363.
130. Neugat AI, Robinson E, Nieves J, Murray T, Tsai W-Y. Poor survival of treatment-related acute nonlymphocytic leukemia. JAMA 1990;264:1006–1008.
131. Hirota Y, Matsumoto I, Aso T, Kondou S, Ikematsu W et al. Hepatocellular carcinoma and bladder cancer as complications following five years of chemotherapy for acute myeloblastic leukemia. Jpn J Med 1990;29:203–207.
132. Sartori S, Nielsen I, Trevisani L, Pazzi P, Malacarne P. Barrett's esophagus after antineoplastic chemotherapy. Endoscopy 1990;22:152.
133. McKay PJ, Docherty JG, laFerla G, Lucine NP. Carcinoma of the small intestine following treated acute myeloid leukemia. Eur J Cancer 1990;26:543–544.
134. Weiss RB. Leukemia following cisplatin therapy. J Natl Cancer Inst 1990;82:795.
135. Goodman A, Zukerberg LR, Nikrui N, Scully RE. Vaginal adenosis and clear cell carcinoma after 5-fluorouracil treatment for condylomas. Cancer 1991;68:1628–1637.
136. Casciato DA, Scott JL. Acute leukemia following prolonged cytotoxic agent therapy. Medicine 1979;58:32–47.
137. Boivin J-F: Second cancers and other late side effects of cancer treatment. A review. Cancer 1990;65:770–775.
138. Chasen MR, Falkson GL. Leukemia after chemotherapy for cancer. Cancer Biotherapy 1993;8:115–122.
139. Ratain MJ, Kaminer LS, Bitran JD, Larson RA, Le Beau MM, Skosey C et al. Acute nonlymphocytic leukemia following etoposide and cisplatin combination chemotherapy for advanced non-small-cell carcinoma of the lung. Blood 1987;70:1412–1417.
140. Burde B, Haim N, Gez E, Polliack A. Acute myeloblastic leukemia following treatment with mitomycin C: a case report. Cancer Chemother Pharmacol 1989;24:71.
141. Flaherty LE, Schwert R, Redman BG. Case report: Development of Hodgkin's disease in patient receiving long-term administration of dacarbazine and interleukin-2 for metastatic melanoma. J Natl Canc Inst 1990;82:360.
142. Toh BT, Gregory SA, Knospe WH. Acute leukemia following treatment of polycythemia vera and essential thrombocythemia with uracil mustard. Am J Hematol 1988;28:58–60.
143. Andersson M, Philip P, Pedersen-Bjorgaard J. High risk of therapy-related leukemia and preleukemia after therapy with prednimustine, methotrexate, 5-fluorouracil, mitoxantrone and tamoxifen for advanced breast cancer. Cancer 1990;65:2460–2464.
144. Kreissman SG, Gelber RD, Cohen HJ, Clavell LA, Leavitt P, Sallan SE. Incidence of secondary acute myelogenous leukemia after treatment of childhood acute lymphoblastic leukemia. Cancer 1992;70:2208–2213.
145. Curtis RE, Boice JD Jr, Moloney WC, Ries LG, Flannery JT. Leukemia following chemotherapy for breast cancer. Cancer Res 1990;50:2741–2746.
146. Pedersen-Bjergaard J, Daugaard G, Hansen SW, Philips D, Larsen SO, Rorth M. Increased risk of myelodysplasia and leukaemia after etoposide, cisplatin and bleomycin for germ-cell tumors. Lancet 1991;338:359–363.
147. Potts M. Non-surgical abortion: Who's for methotrexate. Lancet 1995;346:655–656.
148. Coltman CA Jr, Dahlberg S. Treatment-related leukemia. N Engl J Med 1990;322:52–53.
149. DeVore R, Whitlock J, Hainsworth JD, Johnson DH. Therapy-related acute nonlymphocytic leukemia with monocytic features and rearrangement of chromosome 11q. Ann Intern Med 1989; 110:740–742.
150. Hong WK, Lippman SM, Itri LM, Karp DD, Lee JS, Byers RM et al. Prevention of second primary tumors with isotretinoin in squamous cell carcinoma of the head and neck. N Engl J Med 1990;323:795–801.
151. Cohen LF, Balow JE, Magrath IT, Poplack DG, Ziegler JL et al. Acute tumor lysis syndrome. A review of 37 patients with Burkitt's lymphoma. Am J Med 1980;68:486–491.
152. Baumann MA, Frick JC, Hologe PV. The tumor lysis syndrome. JAMA 1983;250:615.
153. Simmons ED, Somberg KA. Acute tumor lysis syndrome after intrathecal methotrexate administration. Cancer 1991;67:2062–2065.
154. List AF, Kummet TD, Adams JD, Chun HG. Tumor lysis syndrome complicating treatment of chronic lymphocytic leukemia with fluderabine phosphate. Am J Med 1990;89:388–390.
155. Loosveld OJL, Schouten HC, Gaillard CA, Blijham GH. Acute tumour lysis syndrome in a patient with acute lymphoblastic leukemia after a single dose of prednisone. Br J Haematol 1991;77:122–123.
156. Fields AL, Josse RG, Bergsagel DE. Oncologic emergencies, metabolic emergencies. In: DeVita VT, Jr, Hellman S, Rosenberg SA, eds. Cancer: principles and practice of oncology. Philadelphia: JB Lippincott, 1985; pp. 1866–1881.
157. Flotre M, Borenstein M, Blair TMH, eds. Evaluation and management of oncologic emergencies. Emerg Med Rep 1991; 12(2):11–16.
158. Frankel SR, Eardley A, Lauwers G, Weiss M, Warrell RP Jr. The retinoic acid syndrome in acute promyelomonocytic leukemia. Ann Intern Med 1992;117:272–296.
159. Chanarin N, Smith GB, Green A, Andrews MIJ. Retinoic acid syndrome. Lancet 1993;341:1289–1290.
160. Malinakis T, Papadimitriou CA, Koufos C, Fertakis A. A recently recognized entity associated with the treatment of acute promyelocytic leukemia: the retinoic acid syndrome. Haematologica 1993;18:192–194.
161. Frankel SR, Eardley A, Heller G, Berman E, Miller WH Jr et al. All-*trans* retinoic acid for acute promyelocytic leukemia. Results of the New York Study. Ann Intern Med 1994; 120:278–286.
162. Thomas LLM, Mertens MJF, von dem Borne AEFK, van Boxtel CJ, Veenhof CHN, Veies EP. Clinical management of cytotoxic drug overdose. Med Toxicol 1988;3:253–263.
163. Von Hoff DD, Maxwell WL et al. Risk factors for doxorubicin induced congestive heart failure. Ann Intern Med 1979;91:710–717.
164. Devine BJ. Gentamicin therapy. Drug Intell Clin Pharm 1974; 8:650–655.
165. Cox J, Penn N, Masood M, Hancock AK, Parker D. Drug overdose—a hidden hazard of obesity. J R Soc Med 1987; 80:708–709.

166. Back H, Gustavsson A, Ellsborg S et al. Accidental doxorubicin overdosage. Acta Oncol 1995;34:533–536.
167. Curran CF. Adria Laboratories. Personal communication. February 3, 1989.
168. Wolfson S, Olney MB. Accidental ingestion of a toxic dose of chlorambucil. JAMA 1957;165:239–240.
169. Galton DAG, Israels LG, Nabario JDN, Till M. Clinical trials of p-(DI-2-chloroethylamino)-phenylbutyric acid (CB 1348) in malignant lymphoma. Br Med J 1955;2:1172–1176.
170. Green AA, Naiman JL. Chlorambucil poisoning. Am J Dis Child 1968;116:190–191.
171. Amment A, Reitter B, Muller-Wiefel DE. Chlorambucil neurotoxicity. Report of two cases. Helv Paediatr Acta 1980;35: 281–287.
172. Enck RE, Bennett JM. Inadvertent chlorambucil overdose in adult. NY State J Med 1977;77:1480–1481.
173. Byrne TN Jr, Moseley TAE III, Finer MA. Myoclonic seizures following chlorambucil overdose. Ann Neurol 1981;9:191–194.
174. Blank DW, Nanji AA, Schreiber DH, Hudman C, Sanders HD. Acute renal failure and seizures associated with chlorambucil overdose. J Toxicol Clin Toxicol 1983;20:361–365.
175. Palmer RG, Denman AM. 20 cases. Malignancies induced by chlorambucil. Cancer Treat Rev 1984;11:121–129.
176. Vandenberg SA, Kulig KW, Spoerke DG, Hall AH, Bailie VJ, Rumack BH. Chlorambucil: accidental overdose of an antineoplastic. Vet Hum Toxicol 1987;29:479.
177. Vandenberg SA, Kulig K, Spoerke DG, Hall AH, Bailie VJ, Rumack BH. Chlorambucil: accidental ingestion of an antineoplastic drug. J Emerg Med 1988;6:495–498.
178. Bambarola FA. Overdosage associated with Ifex (sterile ifosfamide). Personal communication. Bristol-Myers Oncology Division, March 12, 1991, and March 21, 1991.
179. Brade WP, Herdrich K, Klein HO. Ifosfamide-dose and scheduling. Contrib Oncol 1987;26:22–52.
180. Elias AD, Eder JP, Shea T, Begg CB, Frei E III, Antman KH. High-dose ifosfamide with mesna uroprotection. A phase I study. J Clin Oncol 1990;8:170–178.
181. Antman KH, Elias A, Ryan L. Ifosfamide and mesna: response and toxicity at standard and high-dose schedules. Semin Oncol 1990;17:68–73.
182. Altman LK. Overdoses of cancer drug revealed by patient's death. New York Times, March 24, 1995.
183. Coates TD. Survival from melphalan overdose. Lancet 1984; 2:1048.
184. Ohl S, Schrader V, Gallmeier WM. Survival from melphalan overdose. J Exp Clin Hematol 1985;51:200.
185. Jost LM. Uberdosierung von melphalan (Alkeran): symptome unde behandlung. Eine Ubersicht. Onkologie 1990;13:96–101.
186. Volkin RL, Shadduck KK, Winkelstein et al. Potentiation of carmustine-cranial irradiation-induced myelosuppression by cimetidine. Arch Intern Med 1982;142:248.
187. Foon KA, Haskell CM. Inadvertent overdose with lomustine (CCNU) followed by hematologic recovery. Cancer Treat Rep 1982;66:1241–1242.
188. Hornsten P, Sundman-Engberg B, Gahrton G, Johansson B. CCNU toxicity after an overdose in a patient with Hodgkin's Disease. Scand J Haematol 1983;31:9–14.
189. Barnbarola F, Bristol-Myers Oncology Division. Mesna (Mesnex). Personal communication, April 2, 1991.
190. Schoenik SE. Ifosfamide and mesna. Clin Pharm 1990; 179–191.
191. Lampkin BC, Higgins GR, Hammond D. Absence of neurotoxicity following massive intrathecal administration of methotrexate. Case report. Cancer 1967;20:1780–1781.
192. Pruitt AW, Kinkade JM Jr, Patterson JH. Accidental ingestion of methotrexate. J Pediatr 1974;85: 686–688.
193. Winchester JF, Rahman A, Tilston WJ, Bregman H, Mortensen LM, Gelfand MC et al. Will hemoperfusion be useful for cancer chemotherapeutic drug removal? Clin Toxicol 1980;17:557–569.
194. Stoller RG, Hande KR, Jacobs SA, Rosenberg SA, Chabner BA. Use of plasma pharmacokinetics to predict and prevent methotrexate toxicity. N Engl J Med 1977;297: 630.
195. Hande KR, Balow JE, Drake JC, Rosenberg SA, Chabner BA. Methotrexate and hemodialysis. Ann Intern Med 1977; 87:496.
196. Addiego JE Jr, Ridgway D, Bleyer WA. The acute management of intrathecal methotrexate overdose: pharmacologic rationale and guidelines. J Pediatr 1981;98:825–828.
197. Ettinger LJ. Pharmacokinetics and biochemical effects of a fatal intrathecal methotrexate overdose. Cancer 1982;50: 444–450.
198. Howell SB, Enxminger WD, Krishan A, Free E III. Thymidine rescue of high-dose methotrexate in humans. Cancer Res 1978;38:325–330.
199. Spiegel RJ, Cooper PR, Blum RH, Speyer JL, McBride D, Mangiardi J. Treatment of massive intrathecal methotrexate overdose by ventriculolumbar perfusion. N Engl J Med 1984; 311:386–388.
200. Poplach DG. Massive intrathecal overdose: "Check the label twice." N Engl J Med 1984;311:400–402.
201. Williams WM, Chen TS, Huang KC. Effect of penicillin on the renal tubular secretion of methotrexate in the monkey. Cancer Res 1984;44:1913–1917.
202. Haim N, Kedar A, Robinson E. Methotrexate-related deaths in patients previously treated with cis-diamminedichloride platinum. Cancer Chemother Pharmacol 1984;13:223–225.
203. Ellison NM, Servi RJ. Acute renal failure and death following sequential intermediate dose methotrexate and 4-FU: a possible adverse effect due to concomitant indomethacin administration. Cancer Treat Rep 1985;69:342–343.
204. Thyss A, Milano G, Kubar J, Narner M, Schneider M. Clinical and pharmacokinetic evidence of a life threatening interaction between methotrexate and ketoprofen. Lancet 1986; 1:256–258.
205. Twelves CJ. Folinic acid rescue and methotrexate toxicity. Lancet 1986;1:737.
206. Yap AKL, Janmashanker JJ, Luscombe DK. Methotrexate toxicity coincident with packed red cell transfusion. Lancet 1986;2:641.
207. Bouffet E, Frappaz D, Laville M, Finaz J, Pinkerton CR, Philip T et al. Charcoal haemoperfusion and methotrexate toxicity. Lancet 1986;1:1497.
208. Frappaz D, Bouffet E, Cochat P, Laville M, de Vilaire JF, Philip T et al. Hemoperfusion sur charbon active et hemodialyse dans l'intoxication aigue au methotrexate. Presse Med 1988;17:1209–1213.
209. Brown MA, Corrigan AB. Pancytopenia after accidental overdose of methotrexate. A complication of low dose therapy for rheumatoid arthritis. Med J Aust 1991;155:493–494.
210. McIvon A. Charcoal hemoperfusion and methotrexate toxicity. Nephron 1991;58:378.
211. Ettinger LJ, Freeman AI, Creaven PJ. Intrathecal methotrexate overdose without neurotoxicity. Case report and literature review. Cancer 1978;41:1270–1273.
212. Jakobson AM, Krereger A, Mortimer O, Henningsson S, Seidel H, Moe PJ. Cerebrospinal fluid exchange after intrathecal methotrexate overdose. A report of two cases. Acta Paediatr 1992;81:359–361.
213. Hendrik D, Mirkin BL. Metabolic disposition and toxicity of 6-mercaptopurine after massive overdose. Lancet 1984; 1:277.
214. Brooks RJ, Dorr RT, Durie BGM. Interaction of allopurinol with 6-mercaptopurine and azathioprine. Biomedicine 1982; 36:217–222.
214a. Laidlaw ST, Reilly JT, Suvarna SK. Fatal hepatotoxicity associated with 6-mercaptopurine therapy. Posgrad Med J 1995;71:639.
215. Harvey VJ, Slevin MJ, Dicloway MR, Clark PI, Johnston A. The influence of cimetidine on the pharmacokinetics of 5-FU. Br J Clin Pharmacol 1984;18:421–430.
216. Product Literature. Fluorouracil injection. Roche Laboratories; July 1988.
217. McLachlan S-A, Millward MJ, Toner GC, Guiney MJ, Bishop JF. The spectrum of 5-fluorouracil cardiotoxicity. Med J Aust 1994;161:207.
218. Pawlicki M, Zuchowska-Vogelgesang B, Sliz E. The case of vespesid overdosage in a patient with Hodgkin's Disease. Cancer Chemother Pharmacol 1990;25:387.

219. Berenson MP. Recovery after inadvertent massive overdosage of vincristine (NSC-67574). Cancer Chemother Rep 1971;55:525–526.
220. FDA Reports of Suspected Adverse Reactions to Drugs. 69(3):9 (no year given).
221. Suskind RM, Brusilow SW, Zehr J. Syndrome of inappropriate secretion of antidiuretic hormone produced by vincristine toxicity (with bioassay of ADH level). J Pediatr 1972;81:90–92.
222. Kaufman IA, Kung FH, Koenig HM, Giammona ST. Overdosage with vincristine. J Pediatr 1976;89:671–674.
223. Grush OC, Morgan SK. Folinic acid rescue for vincristine toxicity. Clin Toxicol 1979;14:71–78.
224. Barna P. Vincristine overdose. Clin Pediatr 1980;19:440.
225. Wakem CJ, Bennett JM. Inappropriate ADH secretion associated with massive vincristine overdosage. Aust NZ J Med 1975;5:266.
226. Thomas LLM, Braat PC, Somers R, Goudsmit R. Massive vincristine overdose: failure of leucovorin to reduce toxicity. Cancer Treat Rep 1982;66:1967–1969.
227. Gaidys WG, Dickerman JD, Walters CL, Young PC. Intrathecal vincristine, report of a fatal case despite CNS washout. Cancer 1983;52:799–801.
228. Beer M, Cavalli F, Martz G. Vincristine overdose: Treatment with and without leucovorin rescue. Cancer Treat Rep 1983; 67:746–747.
229. Maeda K, Ueda M, Ohtaka H, Koyama Y, Ohgani M, Miyazaki A. A massive dose of vincristine. Jpn J Clin Oncol 1987;17:247–253.
230. Dyke RW. Treatment of inadvertent intrathecal injection of vincristine. N Engl J Med 1989;321:1270–1271.
231. Jackson DV, Wells HB, Atkins JN et al. Amelioration of vincristine neurotoxicity by glutamic acid. Am J Med 84: 1016–1022.
232. Fiorentin MW, Scalvagno L, Sileni VC, Paccagnella A, Ferrazzi E, Zagorel V, Fosser V. Vindesine overdose. Cancer Treat Rep 1982;66:1247–1248.
233. Pierga J-Y, Beuzebox P, Dorral T, Palangic T, Pouillart P. Favourable outcome after plasmapheresis for vincristine overdose. Lancet 1992;340:185.
234. Ohnuma T, Holland JF, Freeman A, Sinks LF. Biochemical and pharmacological studies with asparaginase in man. Cancer Res 1970;30:2297–3305.
235. Product Literature. Eulexin (flutamide). Schering Corporation 1989.
236. Pfeifle CE, Howell CB, Felthouse RD, Woliver TBS, Andrews PA et al. High dose cisplatin with sodium thiosulphate protection. J Clin Oncol 1985;3:237–244.
237. Schiller JH, Rozental J, Tutsch KD, Trump DL. Inadvertent administration of 480 mg/m^2 of cisplatin. Am J Med 1989;86: 624–625.
238. Fassoulaki A, Pavlov H. Overdose intoxication with cisplatin—a cause of acute respiratory failure. J R Soc Med 1989;82:689.
239. Borch RF, Katz JC, Lieder PH, Pleasants ME. Effects of diethyldithiocarbamate rescue on tumor response to cisplatinum in a rat model. Proc Natl Acad Sci USA 1980;77: 5441–5444.
240. Mollman JE, Glover DJ, Hogan WM et al. Cisplatin neuropathy: risk factors and a possible protective agent. Neurology 1985;35(Suppl 1):80.
241. Schweitzer VG, Dolan DF, Abrams GE et al. Amelioration of cisplatin-induced ototoxicity by fosfomycin. Laryngoscope 1986;96:948.
242. Chu G, Mantin R, Shen Y-M, Baskett G, Sussman H. Massive cisplatin overdose by accidental substitution for carboplatin. Toxicity and management. Cancer 1993;72:3707–3714.
243. Pike IM, Arbus MH, Bristol-Myers Oncology Division. Cisplatin overdosage. Am J Hosp 1992;49:1668.
244. Koppensteiner R, Minar E, Marosi L, Ehringer H. Survival following an extremely high dose of mitoxantrone in a 73-year-old female with small cell bronchial carcinoma. J Cancer Res Clin Oncol 1988;114:324.
245. Reid FJ. Hydrazine Poisoning. Br Med J 1965;2:1246.
246. Scaes MDC, Tinbrell JA. Studies on hydrazine hepatotoxicity. I. Pathological findings. J Toxicol Environ Health 1982;10: 941–953.
247. Harati Y, Niakan E. Hydrazine toxicity, pyridoxine therapy and peripheral neuropathy. Ann Intern Med 1986;104:728–729.
248. Steffen RO, Lederle Laboratories. Novantrone mitoxantrone HC1. Personal communication. March 21, 1991.
249. Hall C, Dougherty WJ, Lebish IJ, Brock PG, Man A. Warning against use of intrathecal mitoxantrone. Lancet 1989;1: 734.
250. Siegert W, Hiddemann W, Koppensteiner R, Buchner T, Essink M, Huhn D et al. Accidental overdose of mitoxantrone in three patients. Med Oncol Tumor Pharmacother 1989;6: 275–278.
251. Procarbazine. Product Information. Roche Laboratories, January 1987.
252. Chabner BA, Myers CE. Clinical pharmacology of cancer chemotherapy. In : DeVita VT Jr, Hellman S, Rosenberg SA, eds. Cancer: principles and practice of oncology. 3rd ed. Philadelphia: JB Lippincott, 1989, pp. 349–395.
253. Buice RG, Sidhu P. Reversed-phase high-pressure liquid chromatographic determination of serum methotrexate and 7-hydroxymethotrexate. J Pharm Sci 1982;71:74–77.
254. Kato Y, Matsushita T, Yokoyama T, Mohri K. Determination of 6-mercaptopurine in acute lymphoblastic leukemia patients. Plasma by high-performance liquid chromatography. Ther Drug Monit 1991;13:220–225.
255. Kato Y, Kaneko H, Matsushita T, Inamori K, Egi S, Togawa A et al. Direct injection analysis of melphalan in plasma using column-switching high-performance liquid chromatography. Ther Drug Monit 1992;14:66–71.
256. Zulian GD, Tullen E, Maton B. Methylene blue for ifosfamide-associated encephalopathy. N Engl J Med 1995;332:1239–1240.
256a. Dextrazoxane for cardiac protection against doxorubicin. Med Lett Drugs Ther 1995;37:110–111.
257. Gibson TP, Reich SD, Krumlovsky FA, Ivanorich P, Conczy C. Hemoperfusion for methotrexate removal. Clin Pharmacol Ther 1978;23:351–355.
258. Wadleigh RG, Redman RS, Graham ML, Krasnow SH, Anderson A, Cohen MH. Vitamin E in the treatment of chemotherapy-induced mucositis. Am J Med 1992;92: 481–484.
259. Mostyn G, Souza LM, Keech J, Sheridan W, Campbell L, Alton NK et al. Effect of granulocyte colony stimulating factor on neutropenia induced by cytotoxic chemotherapy. Lancet 1988;1:667–672.
260. Jenney MEM, Jones PHM. Long-term survival after heart transplantation for doxorubicin-induced cardiomyopathy. Arch Dis Child 1992;67:153.
261. Howell SB, Enxminger WD, Krishan A, Free E III. Thymidine rescue of high-dose methotrexate in humans. Cancer Res 1978;38:325–330.
262. Lafolie P, Liliemark J, Bjork O, Aman J, Wranne L, Peterson C. Exchange of cerebrospinal fluid in accidental intrathecal overdose of cytarabine. Med Toxicol 1988;3:248–252.
263. Wood JH. Physiology, pharmacology and dynamics of CSF. Neurobiology of cerebrospinal fluid. New York: Plenum, 1980, pp. 1–16.

Chapter 62
Disulfiram

Disulfiram (Fig. 62–1) is widely used all over the world as an alcohol deterrent. In spite of the large number of individuals maintained on disulfiram and the common occurrence of disulfiram (Antabuse) reactions, reports of overdose are relatively uncommon.

THERAPEUTIC DOSE

Thiuram disulfides, insecticides, and fungicides are listed in Tables 62–1 and 62–2. Synonyms of disulfiram are listed in Table 62–3.

ALCOHOL CHALLENGE TESTS

Manufacturers' Recommendations (United States):[1]

1. One to two weeks use of disulfiram orally 500 mg/d.
2. Then 15 mL (½ oz) of 100-proof whiskey taken slowly, not to exceed 30 mL (1 oz).
3. Patient should be hospitalized or have equivalent facilities available, including oxygen.

Manufacturers' Recommendations (Overseas):[2]

First day	4 tablets (800 mg) of disulfiram
Second day	3 tablets (600 mg) of disulfiram
Third day	2 tablets (400 mg) of disulfiram
Fourth day	1 tablets (200 mg) of disulfiram
Fifth day	Challenge dose, 15 to 30 mL pure ethanol

Brewer's Recommendations:[1]

Disulfiram on a consistent dose for 5 days to 2 weeks. Alcohol challenge as an outpatient procedure.

$$(C_2H_5)_2N{-}C(=S){-}S{-}S{-}C(=S){-}N(C_2H_5)_2$$

Figure 62–1 Disulfiram (tetraethylthiuram disulfide).

1. 12 mL brandy (5 mL ethanol) on an empty stomach.
2. If no reaction (flush) is observed after 20 minutes, an additional 25 mL of brandy (approximately 10 mL ethanol) is administered. This will usually produce only a noticeable flushing with tachycardia and slight fall in blood pressure. If there is still no reaction, repeat the test after 1 week with a higher Antabuse dose.

TOXIC

Toxicity in children may occur with an ingested dose of 2.5 g of disulfiram.[3]

TOXICOKINETICS

Disulfiram is metabolized in the liver to carbon disulfide (Fig. 62–2).

Table 62–1
Thiuram Disulfides (Tetramethylthiuram Disulfide)

Acetotetramethylthiuram disulfide	Tetramethylthiuram disulfide
Methylthiuram	Tetramethylthiuram (Henley Cyruan DS)
Pernasaw	Tuex
Pomarsol	Vulcacurae tetramethyl disulfide
Puralin	
Thiurad	

Table 62–2
Thiuram Insecticides and Fungicides

Arcan	Panoram
Naquets	Tersan

Table 62–3
Synonyms for Disulfiram

Antabuse
Abstensyl (Argentina)
Abstinyl (Switzerland)
Alcophobin (United States)
Antabus (Denmark, Germany, The Netherlands, Norway, Spain, Sweden, Switzerland)
Antietil (Italy)
Antivitium (Spain)
Aversan (Norway)
Esperal (France)
Refusal (The Netherlands)
Ro-Sulfram-500 (United States)

MECHANISM OF ACTION (FIGS. 62–3 AND 62–4)

1. Disulfiram inhibits enzymatic oxidation of acetaldehyde to acetate, which occurs in the liver during normal alcohol catabolism. Disulfiram competes with nicotinamide adenine dinucleotide for aldehyde dehydrogenase. When small amounts of alcohol are ingested after disulfiram administration, the acetaldehyde concentration in blood may increase to 5 to 10 times the concentration observed after the metabolism of the same amount of alcohol used alone. High blood concentrations of acetaldehyde may produce the unpleasant symptoms of the disulfiram-alcohol reaction (the acetaldehyde syndrome). Others feel that the carbon disulfide metabolite of disulfiram produces many of the disagreeable symptoms.
2. Disulfiram is metabolized in the erythrocytes and liver to DDC (Fig. 62–2). DDC inhibits the enzyme dopamine β-hydroxylase (DBH) through copper chelation and thus inhibits the reaction. This may account for the hypotension seen with the disulfiram-ethanol reaction, resulting from norepinephrine depletion. However, one clinical study did not demonstrate a drop in peripheral blood DBH.
3. Inhibition of hepatic microsomal drug metabolism.
4. Carbon disulfide, a metabolite of disulfiram, may react with pyridoxal 5-phosphate to inhibit monoamine oxidase. This may also result in depletion of pyridoxine, which can lead to a decrease in brain γ-aminobutyric acid with the subsequent increase in seizure production.

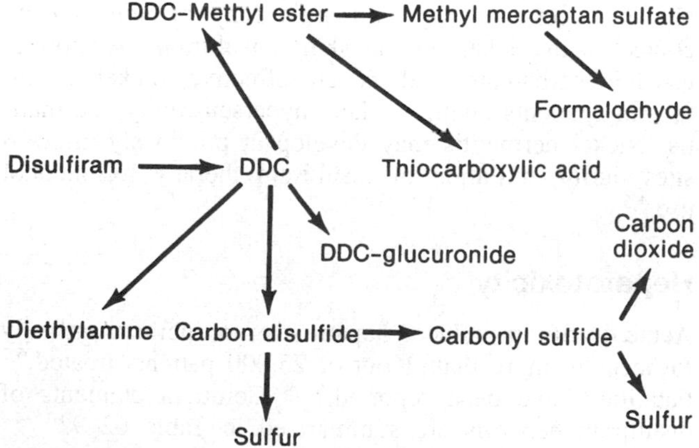

Figure 62–2 Metabolic fate of disulfiram. DDC, diethyldithiocarbamate.

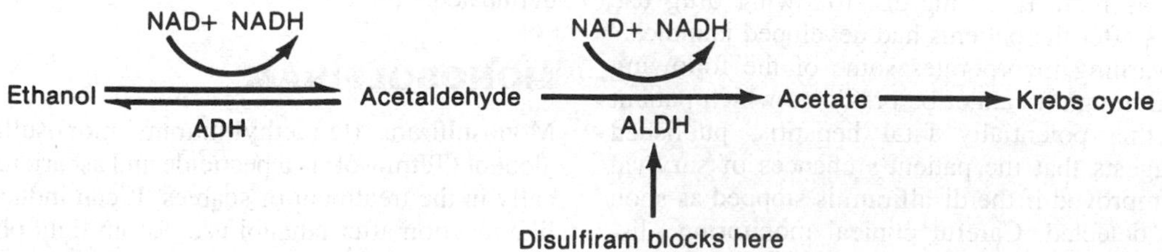

Figure 62–3 Site of disulfiram action. NAD, nicotinamide adenine dinucleotide; NADH, nicotinamide adenine dinucleotide (reduced); ADH, alcohol dehydrogenase; ALDH, aldehyde dehydrogenase.

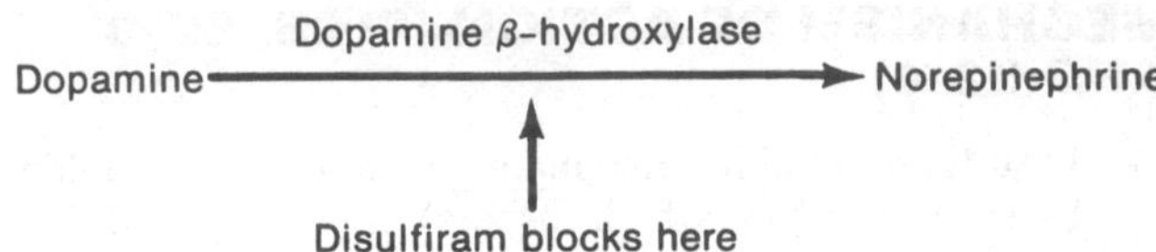

Figure 62–4 Disulfiram inhibition of dopamine-β-hydroxylase.

5. Disulfiram inhibits erythrocyte aldehyde dehydrogenase (ALDH) totally for 36 to 120 hours. Erythrocyte ALDH activity can be monitored to measure patient compliance. Because such inhibited erythrocyte ALDH activity is not regenerated until new erythrocytes are made (120 days), a significant portion of the extrahepatic acetaldehyde metabolic capacity remains inhibited for long periods after disulfiram is discontinued. Thus the recidivist may be exposed to higher ethanol-derived blood acetaldehyde levels than usual if he or she stops disulfiram and waits only several days to resume drinking.
6. Disulfiram, by its inhibition of ALDH, an enzyme required for conversion of dopamine to homovanillic acid, may lead to the low levels of homovanillic acid found in the spinal fluid. This finding augments the increase in dopamine concentration and decrease in norepinephrine concentration in the central nervous system.

CLINICAL PRESENTATION

Tables 62–4 through 62–8 summarize disulfiram toxicity.

Nickel Dermatitis Recall

Nickel hypersensitivity dermatitis may be initiated by contact with nickel on the skin. Disulfiram metabolizes to dithiocarbamate and is an effective nickel chelator in patients with nickel hypersensitivity dermatitis. Nickel dermatitis may develop at previously affected sites during initiation of disulfiram therapy for alcohol use.[4,5]

Hepatotoxicity

Acute disulfiram-induced hepatitis is rare, perhaps unlikely to occur in more than 1 out of 25,000 patients treated.[6,7] Fatalities have been reported.[6,7,8] Common elements of disulfiram hepatitis are summarized in Table 62–9.[6]

The hepatotoxicity may involve an intermediate metabolite and a Gell and Coombs Type IV immunologic reactivity. Fatalities were associated with an elevated serum bilirubin level as high as 80 mg/dL, following drug use for 1 to 21 days after the patients had developed jaundice.[9] A suggested warning incorporates some of the following comments.[10] Although it cannot be predicted which patient will develop this potentially fatal hepatitis, published experience suggests that the patient's chances of survival are markedly improved if the disulfiram is stopped as soon as jaundice is detected. Careful clinical monitoring, discontinuation of disulfiram, and laboratory determinations (bilirubin and hepatic enzyme) when hepatitis is suspected are thus recommended.[10]

Perhaps an additional "early warning system" would alert patients to the insidious symptoms of hepatitis (e.g., anorexia, fatigue, dark urine, jaundice), which they should report to their physician immediately.[8]

Basal Ganglia Lesions

Disulfiram-induced parkinsonism and catatonia is well documented.[11] Following disulfiram (in weeks to years) in doses ranging from long-term use of 500 mg daily to an acute intoxication of 37.6 g, patients have developed generalized tremor, dysphagia, dysarthria, a staggering gait, myoclonic jerks, and signs of a polyneuropathy. Marked behavioral and personality disorders have been observed. Patients recover from some of these symptoms slowly over a period of months.[12]

LABORATORY

Electroencephalogram

An EEG may exhibit diffuse symmetric slowing in the theta and delta range without focal or epileptiform abnormalities.

CT Scan

CT scans performed within 1 week to a few months after the onset of symptoms show symmetric, bilateral, low-density lesions of the basal ganglia. Such lesions may be seen within a few days after the onset of symptoms.

PATHOPHYSIOLOGY

Basal ganglia lesions that develop after disulfiram toxicity may be due to carbon disulfide, one of the disulfiram metabolites.[13] Symptoms induced by carbon disulfide, including parkinsonism and peripheral neuropathies, resemble those of disulfiram intoxication.[13,14]

A separate disruption of parallel basal ganglia thalamocortical circuits may be involved in the behavioral and motor disorders shown by patients with basal ganglia lesions.

Basal ganglia nuclei appear to be a preferential target of acute and chronic intoxication with disulfiram. This is similar to lesions produced by carbon disulfide. Patients exhibit akinesia, disturbances of posture, rigidity, and tremor. Lesions in the globus pallidus can be seen by computer tomography (CT) or magnetic resonance imaging.[15] These lesions may be mediated through carbon disulfide.[14,16] Putaminal lesions cannot be definitely delineated.[17,18]

MONOSULFIRAM

Monosulfiram (tetraethylthiuram monosulfide) (25% in alcohol (Tetmosol) is a pesticide and ascaricide applied topically in the treatment of scabies. It can induce a disulfiram-like reaction after ethanol use. Room light photochemically converts the monosulfiram to disulfiram.[19–21]

Table 62–4
Chronic Disulfiram Toxicity (Without Alcohol)

Nervous system	Drowsiness, headache, memory impairment, decreased libido, toxic psychosis, disorientation, disordered intellect, emotional lability, paranoid ideas, ataxia, dysarthria, seizures, worsening of preexisting electroencephalographic abnormalities, peripheral neuropathy (sensorimotor); distal axonopathy can develop with the recommended dose of 250 or 500 mg/d and may begin as early as 10 d of therapy or as late as 12 mo
Gastrointestinal	Garliclike aftertaste
Skin	Rashes
Eyes	Optic neuritis that improves when drug is discontinued
Other	Halitosis, reversible hypertension, impotence
Blood	Agranulocytosis, thrombocytopenic purpura, eosinophilia
Muscle	Electromyogram abnormal, evidence of motor nerve denervation, motor nerve conduction velocity depressed
Hepatotoxicity	Latent periods of 2 wk to 6 mo before symptoms appear after start of disulfiram; fibrosis, cell necrosis, cholestasis: not typical of virus hepatitis; abnormal liver function tests after alcohol ingestion has ceased may worsen or not return to normal while on disulfiram; fatal massive hepatic necrosis; extrahepatic manifestations of liver hypersensitivity (fever, arthralgia) usually do not occur if disulfiram is not discontinued, may develop chronic hepatic disease

Note: There may always be some uncertainty regarding the role of alcohol in the etiology of some of the chronic toxic effects described following disulfiram use.

Table 62–5
Disulfiram Overdose (Without Alcohol)

Adults	Children
Carbon disulfide–like symptoms	Lag period up to 12 hr; signs and symptoms (seen mostly in children)
Choreoathetosis	
Parkinson-like syndrome	
Endocrine abnormalities	Stupor
Hallucinations	Weakness
Bizarre thought processes	Hypotonia
Agitation	Coma
Coma	
Death from cardiovascular collapse	May be preceded by
	Vomiting
	Lethargy
	Dehydration
	Tachypnea
Garlic odor on breath (CS_2)	Tachycardia
Other central nervous system signs	Deep tendon reflexes decreased
Headache	Ketosis
Dysarthria	
Motor incoordination	Ammonia and aminotransferase levels in blood are normal
Flaccid paralysis	Electroencephalogram abnormal
Hypotension	Sulfur odor (garlic odor) on breath (CS_2)
	Maximal within 12–24 hr
	Recovery may take 1 wk
	Brain death and death may supervene

TREATMENT—DISULFIRAM OVERDOSE

The treatment of disulfiram poisoning is mainly supportive. All patients suspected of disulfiram overdose should be seen in an emergency medical facility and observed for the first 8 to 12 hours because of the possible later development of toxic effects (see Absorption).

Stabilization

Airway protection (endotracheal intubation) and assisted ventilation may be required in the comatose patient. Initial evaluation of the patient's physical status, including a neuromuscular examination and evaluation of mental state, should be performed. Since symptoms do not appear for 3 to 12 hours after ingestion, active measures can be instituted to eliminate tablets already ingested. After blood pressure, pulse, and respiration have been evaluated in the awakened patient, further measures can be taken.

Gut Decontamination

Since gastrointestinal absorption is very slow, gut decontamination can be started up to at least 10 hours or more after ingestion. Gastric lavage with tracheal protection is preferable to syrup of ipecac for stomach washout. Syrup of ipecac contains ethanol and may precipitate a disulfiram-ethanol reaction.

Table 62–6
Disulfiram Poisoning (Without Alcohol): Case Studies

Age (yr)	Sex	Dose (G)	Clinical Course	Disulfiram Blood Levels
Young	F	18	Headache, vomiting, diarrhea. Gastric pain for 4 days. Recovered.	—
10	F	3	Vomited, lethargic, hallucinated, motor disturbance; hypocholesterolemia, hypokalemia, urinary abnormalities. Rx: Intravenous fluids, antibiotics. Recovered.	—
5	F	20 tablets	Abdominal pain, headache, tachycardia, vomiting, lethargy. Flaccid. Impairment of gait at age 9 yr.	—
2	M	?	Coma. Diarrhea. Flaccid. Knee, ankle reflexes absent. Gait abnormal. EEG abnormal (pupils constricted). Rx: gastric lavage, intravenous fluids, mannitol, ascorbic acid. 5 mo: EEG abnormal. 3 yr: IQ-63.	9th-d blood: 17 μg/mL CSF: 7.3 μg/mL Urine: 600 μg/mL
2	M	2.5	Asymptomatic for 12 h. Vomited, lethargic, severe ataxia, hallucinations, inappropriate arm movements, irritability. Speech difficulty lasted 4 d. Recovered.	—
6	M	3.25	Lethargy, somnolence for 3 days. Vomited. Blurred vision, difficulty walking. Muscle tone decreased. Deep tendon reflexes weak. Ketonuria. Rx: intravenous fluids in hospital. Recovered on 3rd d.	—

EEG, Electroencephalogram; *CSF,* cerebrospinal fluid.

Table 62–7
Disulfiram-Ethyl Alcohol–Like Reactions: Substances With Alcohol[a]

Analgesics, Antiinflammatory Agents
Aminopyrine
Phenylbutazone (Azolid, Butazolidin)
Phenacetin (in some combination analgesics)

Antiinfective Agents
Cephalosporins
  Cefoperazone
  Cefamandole sodium
  Moxalactam disodium
  Cefmenoxime
Chloramphenicol
Furazolidone (Furoxone)
Griseofulvin (Fulvicin, Grisactin, Grifulvin, and others)
Isoniazid (INH)
Metronidazole (Flagyl)
Quinacrine hydrochloride (Atabrine)
Sulfonamides
Beta-lactams

Oral hypoglycemic agents
Acetohexamide (Dymelor)
Chlorpropamide (Diabinese)
Phenformin (DBI)
Tolazamide (Tolinase)
Tolbutamide (Orinase)
  (not seen with Glipizide)
Citrated calcium cyanamide

Industrial chemicals
4-Bromopyrazole
Carbon disulfide
Dimethyl formamide (antifreeze agent)
Hydrogen sulfide
Tetrachloroethylene
Tetraethyl lead
Tetramethyl monosulfide

Industrial chemicals (continued)
Tetraethylthiuram monosulfide
Thiuram derivatives (rubber industry, insecticides, fungicides, disinfectants)
Trichloroethylene
N-Butyraldoxime (antioxidants)
Carbamide
Cyanamide
Irgopyrine
Organic solvents
Paints
Mineral spirits

Monoamine oxidase inhibitors
Furaltadone
Furazolidone
Nifuroxime
Procarbazine hydochloride (Matulane)
Tranylcypromine (Parnate)

Alcohol-sensitizing mushrooms
Coprinus atramentarius (inky-cap mushrooms)
Clitocybe clavipes

Other
Chloral hydrate
Cyclothiazide (Anhydron)
Dimercaprol (BAL, British Anti-Lewisite)
Paraldehyde
Ethacrynic acid (Edecrine)
Nitroglycerin
Pargyline
Phentolamine (Regitine)
Procarbazine hydrochloride (Matulane)
Pyrogallol

[a]In addition to beverages, alcohol-containing products include aftershave lotions, back rubs, cough syrup, fermented foods, and sauces.

Table 62–8
Disulfiram Overdose With Ethanol: Case Studies

Age (yr)	Sex	Disulfiram Dose (g)	Clinical Course
39	F	2.0	+ 10 cans of beer + "handful" of 150-mg amitryptyline tablets Serum alcohol: 101 mg/dL. 18 hr: neurological normal. Disulfiram discontinued. Day 17: tongue numbness, dysarthria, dysphagia. 20th day: limb paresthesias, weakness, areflexia. Abnormal nerve conduction velocity (day 20). 44th day: electromyogram abnormal; hypertensive cardiovascular normal; mild limb weakness; unsteady gait
37	M	22.5	Alcoholic stupor. Cerebellar ataxia. Dysarthric speech for 6 d. Then coma. After coma, peripheral neuropathy, facial diplegia, quadriparesis. Axonal degeneration (sural nerve biopsy). Recovered from paresis in 2 yr
24	M	7	Comatose. Tachycardia, Hyperpnea. Hypotension. Hepatomegaly. Electrocardiogram: premature atrial beats. Alcoholic history. Blood alcohol: 178.5 mg/dL. Rx: intravenous fluids, oxygen, intravenous potassium. 12 hr awake. Blood pressure normal (first cases in 9 yr, where 400 patients per year are dispensed 30,000 disulfiram annually)
31	M	7.5	Alcoholic history. Hostile, combative, screaming. Hallucinations. Acetone odor on breath. Tachycardia. Leukocytosis. Hypertension. Alanine aminotransferase elevated. Urine: ketonuria. Electroencephalogram abnormal. Rx: haloperidol. Recovered on day 7. Blood levels (µg/mL):

	Patient (Hospital Day 4)	Alcoholic Volunteers[a]
Disulfiram	1.8	0.41
DDC	1.0	1.14
DDC methyl ester	3.7	1.22
CS_2	117.5	24.0
Diethylamine	103.5	3.8

DDC, Diethyldithiocarbamate.
[a]Peak plasma concentrations from sober volunteers given 250 mg/d of disulfiram for 11 days.

Table 62–9
Common Elements of Disulfiram Hepatitis Reported in the Literature

1. Normal liver biopsy or no known liver disease
2. Normal initial liver-function tests
3. No observed dose–response relationship
4. Normal serologic tests for known hepatitis-producing virus
5. Acute onset with few prodromal symptoms
6. Very rapid and high elevations of liver-function tests
7. Severe elevations of bilirubin within a few days
8. Recovery only when drug is withdrawn early
9. Relapse on rechallenge
10. Approximately 50% mortality reported in cases where substantial liver damage is sustained before drug is withdrawn

Activated charcoal through the lavage tube (children, 15 to 50 g; adults, 50 to 100 g) may be used and may be repeated (adult dose, 30 to 60 g) every 4 hours, although there are no data to substantiate its usefulness. This may be sufficient to encourage further fecal excretion of DDC glucuronide during its enterohepatic circulation.

Cathartic use has not been studied in disulfiram overdose. It may, however, be an aid in gut decontamination.

Elimination Enhancement

The high lipophilic properties of disulfiram, with its conversion to metabolites that are partially excreted through the respiratory tract, render extracorporeal procedures (hemodialysis, hemoperfusion) and forced diuresis probably ineffective. However, studies have not established the status of such procedures.

Antidotes

There are no antidotes.

Supportive Care

Pyridoxine, 1 g IV, may be useful in the treatment of patients with evidence of neurologic toxicity. Seizures may be treated with diazepam or phenytoin. If there are obvious CNS signs (coma, hallucinations, psychosis, etc.), disulfiram should be discontinued and the patient observed for any further CNS abnormalities.

Hypotensive responses may be controlled with position changes (Trendelenburg's position) and intravenous fluids. If pressor amines are required, norepinephrine is preferred. A 4-mL vial of norepinephrine (Levophed) is added to 1000 mL of D_5W to make a solution of 4 µg/mL. The intravenous drip is begun at 0.1 to 0.2 µg/kg/min and increased as required.

Exposure to any form of alcohol should be prevented for at least 2 weeks after a disulfiram poisoning.

Follow-up evaluation of renal and hepatic function and neurologic and mental status is indicated.

TREATMENT—DISULFIRAM-ETHANOL REACTION

Treatment is mainly supportive.

Stabilization

Patients with any evidence of coronary ischemia should be admitted to an intensive care unit and placed under continuous cardiac monitoring. Respiratory tract patency must be established and maintained. Assisted ventilation may be required.

Preparation should be made (respiratory protection, etc.) for immediate treatment of seizures should they occur. Seizures can be managed with endotracheal intubation, respiratory protection, and diazepam (up to 10 mg IV in an adult; 0.1 to 0.3 mg/kg IV slowly for a child). Phenytoin may also be used.

Supplemental oxygen should be administered to all patients. Hypotension and/or shock should be treated immediately with position change (Trendelenburg), intravenous fluids, norepinephrine (disulfiram induces norepinephrine depletion) as required (see Treatment of Disulfiram Overdose [Without Alcohol]), and military antishock trousers. Electrocardiographic monitoring should be continuous for evidence of myocardial ischemia and arrhythmias, both atrial and ventricular. Myocardial infarction may occur. Hypokalemia can be treated with oral or intravenous potassium supplements. Do not use phenothiazines: their alpha-blocking potential may induce or further exacerbate hypotension.

Antidotes

There is no antidote. Ferrous chloride and ascorbic acid at one time were proposed as antidotes for the treatment of a severe disulfiram-ethanol reaction, but have not demonstrated any evidence of efficacy. An experimental drug, 4-methylpyrazole, has not had sufficient testing to determine either its clinical safety or efficacy.

Elimination Enhancement

Hemodialysis or hemoperfusion has not been evaluated in the management of the disulfiram-ethanol reaction patient.

Supportive Care

Most patients will do well with supportive care only. If there are abnormal symptoms or signs or laboratory evidence of abnormalities (electrocardiogram, etc.), then the patient should be considered for admission to the hospital for further observation, treatment, and clinical evaluation. If the clinical course is, as is usually the case, mild and self-limited and if all clinical, electrocardiographic, and other laboratory evidence (see Clinical Presentation) of a disulfiram reaction indicates no residual systemic result, the patient can, after a period of at least 6 to 12 hours, be discharged.

REFERENCES—DISULFIRAM

1. Physicians Desk Reference. 49th ed. Oradell, NJ: Medical Economics, 1995, p. 264.
2. Brewer C. How effective is the standard dose of disulfiram? A review of the alcohol-disulfiram reaction in practice. Br J Psychiatry 1984;144:202–207.
3. Manoguerra AS, Kerney TE. Acute disulfiram toxicity. Vet Hum Toxicol 1982;24(4):282.
4. Klein LP, Fowler JF. Nickel dermatitis recall during disulfiram therapy for alcohol abuse. J Am Acad Dermatol 1992;26: 645–646.
5. Gamboa P, Jauregui I, Urrutia I, Antepara I, Peralta C. Disulfiram-induced recall of nickel dermatitis in chronic alcoholism. Contact Dermatitis 1993;28:255.
6. Wright C IV, Vafier JA, Lake CR. Disulfiram-induced fulminating hepatitis: guidelines for liver panel monitoring. J Clin Psychiatry 1988;49:430–434.
7. Mason NA. Disulfiram induced hepatitis: case report and review of the literature. DICP Ann Pharmacother 1989;23: 872–875.
8. Phillips M. Disulfiram-induced fulminating hepatitis and monitoring guidelines. J Clin Psychiatry 1990;51:168.
9. Wright C, Moore R, Grodin DM, Spyker DA. Disulfiram hepatotoxicity: incidence of enzyme elevation and predictors of fatal outcome. Vet Hum Toxicol 1991;33:38.
10. Spyker D. Disulfiram package insert warning? FDA/AACT Memo, September 29, 1991.
11. Fisher CM. "Catatonia" due to disulfiram toxicity. Arch Neurol 1989;46:798–804.
12. Raing JM. Disulfiram toxicity and carbon disulfide poisoning. Am J Psychiatry 1977;134:371–378.
13. Peters HA, Levine RL, Matthews CG, Chapman W. Extrapyramidal and other neurologic manifestations associated with carbon disulfide fumigant exposure. Arch Neurol 1988; 45:537–540.
14. Laplane D, Attal N, Sauron B, de Billy A, Dubois B. Lesions of basal ganglia due to disulfiram neurotoxicity. J Neurol Neurosurg Psychiatry 1992;55:925–929.
15. Mari M, de Blasi R, Lamberti P, Carella A, Ferrari E. Unilateral pallidal lesions after acute disulfiram intoxication. A clinical and magnetic resonance study. Movement Disorders 1993;8: 247–249.
16. Riley D. Pallidal and putaminal lesions resulting from disulfiram intoxication. Movement Disorders 1992;7:189–189.
17. Krauss JK, Mohadger M, Wakahloo AK, Mindinger S. Dystonia and akinesia due to pallido putaminal lesions after disulfiram intoxication. Movement Disorders 1991;6:166–170.
18. Krauss JK, Wakahloo AK. Pallidal and putaminal lesions resulting from disulfiram intoxication. Movement Disorders 1992;7:188–189.
19. Blanc D, Deperz P. Unusual adverse reaction to an acaricide. Lancet 1990;335:1291–1292.
20. Burgess I. Adverse reactions to monosulfiram. Lancet 1990; 336:873.
21. Lipsky JJ, Mays DC, Naylor S. Monosulfiram, disulfiram, and light. Lancet 1994;343:304.

Chapter 63
Explosives

Explosives are solids or liquids that can be rapidly changed to produce sudden large volumes of rapidly expanding gas and intense heat.[1]

STRUCTURE AND CLASSIFICATION

Table 63–1 contains a list of explosives, blasting agents, and detonators as prepared by the Firearms and Explosives Operations Branch, Bureau of Alcohol, Tobacco and Firearms, 1200 Pennsylvania Ave. NW, Washington, DC (202-789-3027, 202-927-7920).[2,3] A subdivision into classes of explosives is found in Table 63–2.

PRODUCT FORMULATION

A diagram of a shell is depicted in Figure 63–1.[4]

LABORATORY

Analytic Methods

The thermal energy analyzer (TEA), interfaced to both gas and high-performance liquid chromatography is sensitive to nitro-based explosives at a sensitivity of 4 to 5 pg (4 pg—TNT, RDX; 5 pg—EGDN, NG, DNT; 25 pg-Tetryl).[5] This may be solely useful for industrial needs. An explosive testing kit (ETK) is able to make determinations of trace explosives in the field and covers the vast majority of military explosives that contain the following chemical groups: polynitro aromatics (e.g., TNT); organic nitrates (nitrate esters) (e.g., nitroglycerin), and nitramines (eg., RDX). It is sensitive to as little as 10^{-7} g TNT per button and 10^{-8} g of nitroglycerin[6,7] (Table 63–3).[7]

Table 63–1
Bureau of Alcohol, Tobacco and Firearms List of Explosive Materials[a]

A
Acetylides of heavy metals.
Aluminum containing polymeric propellant.
Aluminum ophorite explosive.
Amatex.
Amatol.
Ammonal.
Ammonium nitrate explosive mixtures (cap sensitive).
*Ammonium nitrate explosive mixtures (non cap sensitive).
Aromatic nitro-compound explosive mixtures.
Ammonium perchlorate having particle size less than 15 microns.
Ammonium perchlorate composite propellant.
Ammonium picrate (picrate of ammonia. Explosive D).
Ammonium salt lattice with isomorphously substituted inorganic salts.
*ANFO (ammonium nitrate-fuel oil).

B
Baratol.
Baronol.
BEAF [1, 2-bis (2, 2-difluoro-2-nitroacetoxyethane)].
Black powder.
Black powder based explosive mixtures.
*Blasting agents, nitro-carbo-nitrates, including non cap sensitive slurry and water-gel explosives.
Blasting caps.
Blasting gelatin.
Blasting powder.
BTNEC [bis(trinitroethyl) carbonate].
BTNEN [bis(trinitroethyl) nitramine].
BTTN [1,2,4 butanetriol trinitrate].
Butyl tetryl.

C
Calcium nitrate explosive mixture.
Cellulose hexanitrate explosive mixture.
Chlorate explosive mixtures.
Composition A and variations.
Composition B and variations.
Composition C and variations.
Copper acetylide.
Cyanuric triazide.
Cyclotrimethylenetrinitramine [RDX].
Cyclotetramethylenetetranitramine [HMX].
Cyclonite [RDX].
Cyclotol.

D
DATB [diaminotrinitrobenzene].
DDNP [diazodinitrophenol].
DEGND [diethyleneglycol dinitrate].
Detonating cord.
Detonators.
Dimethylol dimethyl methane dinitrate composition.
Dinitroethyleneurea.
Dinitroglycerine [glycerol dinitrate].
Dinitrophenol.
Dinitrophenolates.
Dinitrophenyl hydrazine.
Dinitroresorcinol.
Dinitrotoluene-sodium nitrate explosive mixtures.
DIPAM.
Dipicryl sulfone.
Dipicrylamine.
DNDP [dinitropentano nitrile].
DNPA [2,2-dinitropropyl acrylate].
Dynamite.

E
EDDN [ethylene diamine dinitrate].
EDNA.
Ednatol.
EDNP [ethyl 4,4-dinitropentanoate].
Erythritol tetranitrate explosives.
Esters of nitro-substituted alcohols.
EGDN [ethylene glycol dinitrate].
Ethyl-tetryl.
Explosive conitrates.
Explosive gelatins.
Explosive mixtures containing oxygen releasing inorganic salts and hydrocarbons.
Explosive mixtures containing oxygen releasing inorganic salts and nitro bodies.
Explosive mixtures containing oxygen releasing inorganic salts and water insoluble fuels.
Explosive mixtures containing oxygen releasing inorganic salts and water soluble fuels.
Explosive mixtures containing sensitized nitromethane.
Explosive mixtures containing tetranitromethane (nitroform).
Explosive nitro compounds of aromatic hydrocarbons.
Explosive organic nitrate mixtures.
Explosive liquids.
Explosive powders.

F
Fulminate of mercury.
Fulminate of silver.
Fulminating gold.
Fulminating mercury.
Fulminating platinum.
Fulminating silver.

G
Gelatinized nitrocellulose.
Gem-dinitro aliphatic explosive mixtures.
Guanyl nitrosamino guanyl tetrazene.
Guanyl nitrosamino guanylidene hydrazine.
Guncottoen.

H
Heavy metal azides.
Hexanite.
Hexanitrodiphenylamine.
Hexanitrostilbene.
Hexogen [RDX].
Hexogene or octogene and a nitrated N-methylaniline.
Hexolites.
HMX [cyclo-1,3,5,7-tetramethylene-2,4,6,8-tetranitramine; Octogen].
Hydrazinium nitrate/hyrazine/aluminum explosive systems.
Hydrazoic acid.

I
Igniter cord.
Igniters.
Initiating tube systems.

K
KDNBF [potassium dinitrobenzo-furoxane].

L
Lead axide.
Lead mannite.
Lead mononitroresorcinate.
Lead picrate.
Lead salts, explosive.
Lead styphnate [styphnate of lead, lead trinitroresorcinate].
Liquid nitrated polyol and trimethylolethane.
Liquid oxygen explosives.

M
Magnesium ophorite explosives.
Mannitol hexanitrate.
MDNP [methyl 4,4-dinitropentonoate.].
MEAN [monoethamolamine nitrate].
Mercuric fulminate.
Mercury oxalate.
Mercury tartrate.
Metriol trinitrate.
Minol-2 [40 percent TNT, 40 percent ammonium nitrate, 20 percent aluminum].
MMAN [monoethylamine nitrate]; methylamine nitrate.
Monitrotoluene-nitroglycerin mixture.
Monopropellants.

N
NIBTN [nitroisobutametriol trinitrate].
Nitrate sensitized with gelled nitroparaffin.
Nitrated carbohydrate explosive.
Nitrated glucoside explosive.
Nitrated polyhydric alcohol explosives.
Nitrates of soda explosive mixtures.
Nitric acid and a nitroaromatic compound explosive.
Nitric acid and carboxylic fuel explosive.
Nitric acid explosive mixtures.
Nitro aromatic explosive mixtures.
Nitro compounds of furane explosive mixtures.
Nitrocellulose explosive.
Nitroderivatives of urea explosive mixture.
Nitrogelatin explosive.
Nitrogen trichloride.
Nitrogen tri-iodide.
Nitroglycerin [NG, RNG, nitro, glyceryl trinitrate, trinitroglycerine].
Nitroglycide.
Nitroglycol (ethylene glycol dinitrate, EGDN).
Nitroguanidine explosives.
Nitroparaffins Explosive Grade and ammonium nitrate mixtures.
Nitronium perchlorate propellant mixtures.
Nitrostarch.
Nitro-substituted carboxylic acids.
Nitrourea.

[a]Adapted from Higgins SE. Bureau of Alcohol, Tobacco and Firearms. Fed Reg 55:1306–1307.

(continued)

Table 63–1 *(Continued)*

O
Octogen [HMX].
Octol [75 percent HMX, 25 percent TNT].
Organic amine nitrates.
Organic nitramines.

P
PBX [RDX and plasticizer].
Pellet powder.
Penthrinite composition.
Pentolite.
PYX (2,6-bis(picrylamino)-3,5-dinitropyridine.
Perchlorate explosive mixtures.
Peroxide based explosive mixtures.
PETN [nitropentaerythrite, pentaerythrite tetranitrate, pentaerythritol tetranitrate].
Picramic acid and its salts.
Picramide.
Picrate of potassium explosive mixtures.
Picratol.
Picric acid (manufactured as an explosive.
Picryl chloride.
Picryl fluoride.
PLX [95% nitromethane, 5% ethylenediamine].
Polynitro aliphatic compounds.
Polyolpolynitrate-nitrocellulose explosive gels.
Potassium chlorate and lead sulfocyanate explosive.
Potassium nitrate explosive mixtures.
Potassium nitroaminotetrazole.

R
RDX [cyclonite,hexogen, T4, cyclo-1,3,5-trimethylene-2,4,6-trinitramine; hexahydro-1,3,5-trinitro-S-triazine].

S
Safety fuse.
Salts of organic amino sulfonic acid explosive mixture.
Silver acetylide.
Silver azide.
Silver fulminate.
Silver oxalate explosive mixtures.
Silver styphnate.
Silver tartrate explosive mixtures.
Silver tetrazene.
Slurried explosive mixtures of water, inorganic oxidizing salt, gelling agent, fuel and sensitizer (cap sensitive).
Smokeless powder.
Sodatol.
Sodium amatol.
Sodium azide explosive mixture.
Sodium dinitro-ortho-cresolate.
Sodium nitrate-potassium nitrate explosive mixture.
Sodium picramate.
Squibs.
Styphnic acid explosives.

T
Tacot [tetranitro-2,3,5,6-dibenzo-1,3a,4,6a-tetrazapentalene].
TATB [triaminotrinitrobenzene].
TEGDN [triethylene glycol dinitrate].
Tetrazene [tetracene, tetrazine, 1(5-tetrazoly)-4-guanyl tetrazene hydrate].
Tetranitrocarbazole.
Tetryl [2,4,6 tetranitro-N-methylaniline].
Tetrytol.
Thickened inorganic oxidizer salt slurried explosive mixture.
TMETN (trimethylolethane trinitrate).
TNEF [trinitroethyl formal].
TNEOC [trinitroethylorthocarbonate].
TNEOF [trinitroethyl orthoformate].
TNT [trinitrotoluene, trotyl, trilite, triton].
Torpex.
Tridite.
Trimethylol ethyl methane trinitrate composition.
Trimethylolthane trinitrate-nitrocellulose.
Trimonite.
Trinitroanisole.
Trinitrobenzene.
Trinitrobenzoic acid.
Trinitrocresol.
Trinitro-meta-cresol.
Trinitronaphthalene.
Trinitrophenetol.
Trinitrophloroglucinol.
Trinitroresorcinol.
Tritonal.

U
Urea nitrate.

W
Water bearing explosives having salts of oxidizing acids and nitrogen bases, sulfates, or sulfamates (cap sensitive).
Water-in-oil emulsion explosive compositions.

X
Xanthamonas hydrophilic colloid explosive mixture.

Table 63–2
Classes of Explosives[a]

Explosive materials
- Primary explosives
- Mercury fulminate, lead azide
- Lead styphnate, oxygen difluoride
- Ammonium nitrate & nitrite
- Ammonium picrate
- TNT
- Tetryl
- Nitroglycerin (NG)
- Dynamite
- Picric acid
- Cyclonite (RDX)
- PETN

Oxidizers & oxidizing agents
- H_2O_2
- Organic peroxides
- Benzoyl peroxide
- Peracetic acid
- Cumene hydroperoxide
- Methyl ethyl ketone peroxide

Halogenated oxidizers—halogen gas
- Perchloryl fluoride
- Oxychlorinated compounds
- Hypochlorous acid

Chromates—Cr metals
- Cr^{+6} Metallic chromates
  - Metallic dichromate
  - Cr O_3
  - Chromyl chloride
- Chromic acid
- Chromyl chloride
- Ammonium-dichromate
- CR O_3
- Permanganates
- Potassium persulfate

Reactive reducing chemicals
- Hydrazine
- Hydroxylamine
- Monomethylhydrazine
- Boron hydride
- Decaborane
- Pentaborane
- Li H
- B Br_3
- B F_3

Compressed flammable gases & cryogenic gases
- Liquid hydrogen
- Chlorous acid
- Chloric acid
- Perchlorates

Chlorates
- K^+
- Na^+
- Aluminum hydride

Perchlorates

Halogen gases
- Cl_2
- F_2
- Br_2
- I_2

Bromine pentafluoride BrF_5
Chlorine trifluoride CeF_3
Chlorine dioxide ClO_2
Liquid oxygen
Liquefied helium
Liquefied natural gas (LNG)
Liquefied ammonia gas (NH_5)
Liquefied petroleum gas (LPG)

[a]Adapted from Sullivan JB Jr. In: Sullivan JB Jr, Krieger GR, eds. Hazardous material toxicology. Clinical principles of environmental health. Baltimore: Williams & Wilkins, 1992.

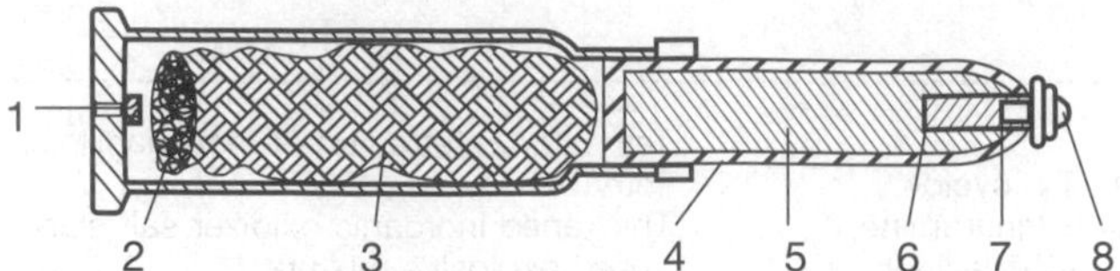

Figure 63–1 Diagram of a shell: 1. Primer (sensitive explosive). 2. Igniter—black powder. 3. Propellant charge (nitrocotton). 4. Projectile. 5. Bursting charge (TNT amatol). 6. Booster (tetryl). 7. Detonator (sensitive explosive). 8. Fuse (sensitive explosive). (Adapted from Schwartz L. JAMA 1944;125:186–190.)

Table 63–3
Limits of Detectability for Seven Explosives Using TLC [5] and HPLC[a]

Explosive	TLC, µg	HPLC, µg
NG	NA[b]	0.01[c]
EGDN	0.5	0.01[c]
HMX	0.25	0.005
RDX	0.25	0.005
Tetryl	0.25	0.0005
TNT	0.20	0.0001
PETN	0.40	0.01

[a]Adapted from Lyter AH III. J Forensic Sci 1983;28:446–450.
[b]TLC limits not available.
[c]NG and EGDN were detectable in a 1-ppm solution of dynamite that contained both compounds.

REFERENCES

1. Sullivan JB Jr. Cryogenics, oxidizers, reducing agents, and explosives. In: Sullivan JB Jr, Krieger GR, eds. Hazardous materials toxicology. Clinical principles of environmental health. Baltimore: Williams & Wilkins, 1992; pp. 1192–1201.
2. Commerce in explosives—list of explosive materials. Fed Reg 1990;55:1306–1307.
3. Higgins SE. List of explosive materials. Fed Reg 1990;55: 1306–1307.
4. Schwartz L. Dermatitis from explosives. JAMA 1944;125: 186–190.
5. Fine DH, Yu WC, Goff EU, Bender EC, Reutter DJ. Picogram analyses of explosive residues using the Thermal Energy Analyzer (TEA). J Forensic Sci 1984;29:732–746.
6. Almog J, Kraus S, Glattstein B, Bamberger Y. ETK—an operation explosive testing kits. Ghent: Proc Int Assoc Forensic Toxicology. August 24–27, 1986, pp. 332–336.
7. Lyter AH III. A high-performance liquid chromatographic (HPLC) study of seven common explosive materials. J Forensic Sci 1983;28:446–450.

AROMATIC NITRO COMPOUNDS

Aromatic nitro compounds have few direct uses other than in the formulation of explosives or as solvents. Aromatic nitro compounds are flammable and the di- and trinitro derivatives are explosive under favorable conditions (heat and shock). Contact with strong reducing agents such as sodium sulfide, zinc powder, sodium hydrosulfite, and metallic hydrides and strong oxidizing agents such as bichromates, peroxides, and chlorates must be avoided in storage and transit.[1]

CLINICAL HAZARDS

The acute hazard of aromatic nitro compounds is cyanosis (methemoglobinemia) and the chronic manifestation is anemia. The fat-soluble nitro compounds are rapidly absorbed through the intact skin. Some are excreted unchanged through the kidneys, but the major portion is reduced to cyanogenic nitroso and hydroxyalamine derivatives, which in turn are converted to the ortho- and para-aminophenol analogues and excreted in the urine.[1] In vivo animal studies suggest that the dinitrotoluenes are directly cytotoxic to hepatocytes and that this correlates with an inhibition of protein synthesis and an increase in lactate dehydrogenase.[2]

DINITROTOLUENE

Structure and Classification

Six isomers of dinitrotoluene (DNT) exist. The most important is 2,4 dinitro-l-toluene; methyl dinitrobenzene,[3] $C_6H_3CH_3\ (NO_2)$.

Description[4,5]

Exposure Limits
2,4 dinitrotoluene
CAS 121-14-2 USA TWA 1.5 mg/m^3 skin
UK TWA 1.5 mg/m^3 skin STEL 5 mg/m^3
Australia TWA 1.5 mg/m^3 skin
2,6 dinitrotoluene Denmark TWA 1.5 mg/m^3 skin
CAS 606-20-2
3,4 dinitrotoluene Denmark TWA 1.5 mg/m^3 skin
CAS 610-39-9
dinitrotoluene USA-ACGIH TWA 1.5 mg/m^3 skin
CAS 25321-14-6 Denmark TWA 1.5 mg/m^3 skin
Finland TWA 1.5 mg/m^3 skin STEL 3 mg/m^3

IDLH (Immediate danger to life and health) = 200 ng/m^3 (2,4 DNT)

Synonyms

DNT, Dinitrotoluol

Occupational Exposures

DNT is used in the manufacture of explosives and dyes and in the chemical synthesis of trinitrotoluene. A partial list of occupations in which exposure may occur includes dye makers, explosive workers, and organic chemical synthesizers. 2,4, Dinitrotoluene is used in air bags. Other chemicals used in air-bag manufacture are sodium azide, ceramic fibers, boron, potassium nitrate, cupric oxide, and nitrocellulose.

Routes Of Entry

Inhalation of vapor and percutaneous absorption of liquid.

Drug Interactions

Ingestion of alcohol may increase the toxic effect of DNT.[6]

CLINICAL PRESENTATION

Local—none

Systemic (See Airborne Chapter—Methemoglobinemia)

Acute Exposure

Dinitrotoluene exposure can induce profound methemoglobinemia with cyanosis, anoxia, and death. The onset of methemoglobinemia is often delayed up to 4 hours.[6] Symptoms begin with headache, then progress to fatigue, nausea, vomiting, chest pain, and loss of weight. Cyanosis is apparent at a methemoglobin level of about 10 to 15%. The worker is not uncomfortable until methemoglobin levels of 40% are reached. Repeated or prolonged exposure leads to a Heinz-body hemolytic anemia in normal individuals or in those with a G6PD deficiency.

In man DNT exposure has, in addition, caused dermatitis, anemia, and acute toxic hepatitis.[7–9] Cohort studies of workers suggest that exposure to 2,4 DNT leads to an increased incidence of mortality from ischemic heart disease.[8] The 2,6 isomer is thought to be largely responsible for the hepatocellular carcinomas that develop in exposed rats.[10]

Chronic Exposure

Chronic industrial exposure to organic nitro compounds may produce withdrawal symptoms in tolerant workers. Some later develop myocardial ischemia and infarction.[11,12]

LABORATORY

Analytic Methods

Spectrophotometry is required for precise methemoglobin measurements. A co-oximeter may be useful.

Blood Levels

Methemoglobin levels are elevated after exposure. Methemoglobin may be differentiated from sulfhemoglobin by the addition of a few drops of 10% potassium cyanide, which results in the rapid production of bright red cyanomethemoglobin, but has no effect on sulfhemoglobin.[13] Spectrophotometry readings for normal acid methemoglobin indicate a characteristic absorption spectrum with peaks at 502 and 632 nm, which disappear with the addition of cyanide, whereas sulfhemoglobin has a peak at 620 nm, which does not disappear with cyanide.[13]

Ancillary Tests

Urine excretion of DNT in excess of 25 ng/liter of urine indicates significant absorption[14] (see Methemoglobinemia in Airborne chapter).

Medical Surveillance

Preemployment and periodic routine bimonthly examinations for each workman should be particularly concerned with a history of blood dyscrasia, reactions to medications, alcohol intake, eye disease, skin, and cardiovascular status. Liver function, renal function, and hematologic examinations should be evaluated periodically, as well as general health (blood pressure, pulse, weight). Additional blood and urine specimens should be collected whenever unusually hazardous conditions or excessive exposures are encountered.

TREATMENT (SEE METHEMOGLOBINEMIA—AIRBORNE TOXIN CHAPTER)

Acute Exposure

Remove all dinitrotoluene on the body immediately. Remove all clothing. Wash entire body with soap and water with special attention to the hair and scalp, fingers and toenails, nostrils, and ear canals.

Stabilization

Give immediate attention to ventilation. Use assisted ventilation as required and 100% oxygen while methylene blue is prepared. Begin cardiac monitoring, especially in patients with pulmonary disease or coronary artery disease. Use Trendelenburg position and intravenous fluids for hypotension. Dopamine may be required.

Decontamination

If dinitrotoluene has been ingested, initiate gastric lavage for obtunded patients who present within 2 to 4 hours of ingestion. Provide tracheal protection. Activated charcoal and cathartics may be of some benefit after lavage.

Elimination Enhancement

Hemodialysis, forced diuresis, and hemoperfusion are theoretically not effective for pure methemoglobinemia, but may be adjunctive care for dinitrotoluene ingestion when supportive care appears inadequate. There are no data to support the use of these modalities of treatment for dinitrotoluene exposure. Hyperbaric oxygen has not been evaluated. Exchange transfusion and/or packed red blood cells may be useful for methylene blue failure or for patients with known G6PD or NADPH methemoglobin reductase deficiencies. Be aware of large blood volume changes.

Antidote

Methylene blue (tetramethylthionine chloride) is the antidote of choice for serious methemoglobinemia. Give 1 to 2 mg/kg (25.50 mg/m^2) if a 1% solution (10 mg/mL) intravenously over 5 minutes. Repeat in 1 hour if hypoxia does not subside. (For details on methylene blue toxicokinetics, mechanism of action, adverse effects, failure of therapy, indications, and contraindications see Airborne Toxin chapter.) Limit the total dose of methylene blue to 7 mg/kg. Watch for dyspnea, precordial pain, restlessness, apprehension, hemolysis, or changes in the electrocardiogram indicative of myocardial ischemia. Levels of methemoglobin above 20% in the presence of anemia, pulmonary disease, or processes that reduce coronary or cerebral perfusion should receive methylene blue. Symptomatic patients with methemoglobin levels over 30% should also received methylene blue.

Supportive Measures

1. Watch patients with preexisting pulmonary or cardiac disease with careful cardiac monitoring. Be alert for a silent myocardial infarction and congestive heart failure.
2. Repeat methemoglobin levels 1 to 2 hours after therapy to assess effectiveness of methemoglobin reduction. Large doses of methylene blue may cause a bluish skin discoloration after the methemoglobin levels have returned to normal.
3. If the patient fails to improve within 1 hour after methylene blue therapy, reconsider the diagnosis and review the causes of treatment failure (see Airborne Toxin chapter).
4. Watch for hemolysis (complete blood counts, reticulocyte counts).
5. Be prepared to administer blood transfusions as required. Evaluate the degree of cardiovascular disease present.

REFERENCES—AROMATIC NITRO COMPOUNDS

1. Linch AL. Aromatic nitrocompounds. In: Encyclopedia of occupational health and safety. Vol 2. International Labour Office. New York: McGraw-Hill, 1972;942–944.
2. Spanggord RJ, Myers CJ, Le Valley SE, Green CE, Tyson CA. Structure–activity relationship for the intrinsic hepatotoxicity of dinitrotoluenes. Chem Res Toxicol 1990;3: 551–558.
3. Key MM, Henschel AF, Butler J, Ligo RN, Taberslaw IR, eds. Occupational diseases. A guide to their recognition. Revised edition. (DHEW [NIOSH] Publication No. 77-18). Washington, DC: US Government Printing Office, pp. 278–279.
4. Occupational exposure limits for airborne toxic substances. Occupational Safety and Health Series No 37. 3rd ed. International Labour Office, Geneva: 1991; pp. 877–880.
5. NIOSH Pocket Guide to Chemical Hazards. CDC, DHHS (NIOSH) Publication No. 90-117. Washington, DC: US Government Printing Office, June 1990; pp. 100–101.
6. Proctor NH, Hughes JP, Fischman ML. Chemical hazards of the workplace. 2nd ed. New York: Van Nostrand Reinhold, 1989; pp. 218–219.
7. Levine RJ, Andjelkovoch DA, Kersteter SL, Arp EW Jr, Balogh SA, Blunden PB, Stanley JM. Heart disease in workers exposed to dinitrotoluene. J Occup Med 1986;28:811–816.
8. Data Sheet 658: Dinitrotoluene. Chicago: National Safety Council (Chemical Section), 1976.
9. McGee LC, McCausland A, Plume CA et al. Metabolic disturbances in workers exposed to dinitrotoluene. Am J Dig Dis 1942;9:329–332.
10. Richert DE, Butterworth BE, Popp JA. Dinitrotoluene: acute toxicity, oncogenicity, genotoxicity, and metabolism. CRC Crit Rev Toxicol 1984;13:217–234.
11. Hogstedt C, Andersson K. A cohort study of mortality among dynamite workers. J Occup Med 1979;21:553–556.
12. Hogstedt C, Axelson O. Nitroglycerin—nitroglycol exposure and the mortality in cardiocerebral vascular disease among dynamite workers. J Occup Med 1977;19:675–678.
13. Rieder RF. Methemoglobinemia and sulfhemoglobinemia. In: Wyngaarden JB, Smith LH, eds. Cecil. Textbook of medicine, 16th ed. Philadelphia: WB Saunders, 1989 p. 896.
14. Chemical Safety Data Sheet. SD-93. Dinitrotoluene. Washington, DC: MCA, Inc., 1960 pp. 5–6, 14–15.

CYCLOTRIMETHYLENE-TRINITRAMINE (RDX)

RDX may induce a severe convulsive state with evidence of gastrointestinal and renal dysfunction, all of which appear to be reversible after several days. Such neurologic symptoms may follow inhalation or oral ingestion during manufacturing exposure (dust inhalation); battlefront exposure (ingestion or inhalation), and nonwartime accidental exposure (ingestion). There are no specific antidotes. Treatment is symptomatic and supportive.

STRUCTURE AND CLASSIFICATION

Cyclotrimethylenetrinitramine (RDX) has a molecular weight of 222.26. In crystal form it exists as white orthothrombic crystals. RDX melts at 202°C and is insoluble in water, alcohol, ether, ethyl acetate, petroleum ether, and carbon tetrachloride; very slightly soluble in hot benzene; and soluble in acetone and in xylene. It crystallizes out in white needles from solutions in which it is soluble such as hot aniline, phenol, ethyl benzoate, and nitrobenzene.[1] It is resistant to hydrolysis.[1] RDX is a six-sided hydrocarbon containing 3 nitrite groups and 3 methylene groups.[2,3]

CYCLONITE (RDX) PERMISSIBLE LEVELS[4,5]

CAS 121-82-4

USA—	ACGIH TWA: 1.5 mg/m³	STEL 3/m³
	NIOSH/OSHA TWA: 1.5 mg/m³ (skin)	
UK—	TWA: 1.5 mg/m³ (skin)	STEL 3 mg/m³
France—	TWA: 1.5 mg/m³ (skin)	
Australia—	TWA: 1.5 mg/m³ (skin)	STEL 3 mg/m³

Molecular Formula

$C_3H_6N_6O_6$

Synonyms

Cyclonite, Hexogen, T4, Exogene, 1,3,5 trinitro trizacyclohexane, RDX, hexahydro-11,3,5 trinitro-1,3,5-triazine.

Composition C-4 contains RDX (91%), polyisobutylene (2.1%), motor oil (1.6%), and di- (2-ethylhexyl) sebacate (5.3%).[5] C-4 is not soluble in water, gastric contents, beer, bourbon, gin, vodka, or scotch,[6] but when suspended in 80% ether, it undergoes hydrolysis and reduction, producing methylamine, nitrous acid, ammonia, and formaldehyde.[2]

WATER

An ambient water quality criterion of 103 µg/liter of RDX has been proposed for ingestion of drinking water and aquatic foodstuffs; a criterion of 105 µg/L has been proposed for ingestion of drinking water alone.[7]

USES

RDX is one of the most important explosives in use. It has an explosive power much greater than that of TNT.[3] During

World War II it was used in detonators, primers, and boosters. Initially, RDX was used during World War II as a base charge for detonators and as an explosive for shells and bombs.[6] Among field troops in Vietnam it became common knowledge that ingestion of a small amount of C-4 would produce a "high" similar to that of ethanol. Now it is used as a component in mixtures with other explosives such as TNT and PETN (pentaerythritol tetranitrate) and as a plastic explosive.[3] Composition C-4 was the most common plastic explosive in use by field units in Vietnam.[7] A blasting cap was employed as a detonator. C-4 was used as a field cooking fuel when other sources of heat were unavailable. RDX is often mixed with TNT (RDX 60%; TNT 40%).[5]

SOURCES

RDX is obtained by the nitration (with nitric acid) of hexamethylenetetramine, which is formed by the reaction between ammonia and formaldehyde.[5]

TOXIC DOSE

A 3-year-old child ingested 84.82 mg/kg and survived.[8] An adult worker ingested a tablespoon of RDX and reacted with severe muscle spasms and mental confusion that was reversible.[9]

FATAL DOSE

In rats the fatal dose (MLD_{50}) is approximately 200 mg/kg when fed as a 4% solution.[1] Paper bags, used for wrapping food after having been used for packaging RDX in post–World War II Germany, apparently caused four deaths.[9]

TOXICOKINETICS

Absorption

RDX is very slowly absorbed from the gastrointestinal tract and is only very sparingly decomposed with the formation of nitrite. Nevertheless, a peak RDX blood level of 10.7 μg/ml was reached about 24 hours after the ingestion of approximately 85 mg/kg by a 3-year-old.[8] RDX was still found in the serum 120 hours after ingestion and in the feces 194 hours after ingestion.[8]

Distribution (V_D)

The apparent volume of distribution of RDX is 2.2 L/kg.[8] At 24 hours following ingestion, the cerebrospinal fluid serum ratio was 0.83, indicating passage through the blood–brain barrier.[8]

Elimination

Peak elimination in the urine occurs at about 48 hours and at approximately 96 hours for feces. The elimination half-life is 15.1 hours.[8] Absorption and elimination appear to follow first-order kinetics. About 1 to 2% of RDX is excreted unchanged in the urine.[10]

MECHANISM OF ACTION

The exact mechanism by which RDX induces a state of central nervous system irritability is not known. The chemical apparently does pass through the blood–brain barrier (cerebrospinal fluid levels) and induces electroencephalographic changes reflective of the concomitant convulsive state.

CLINICAL PRESENTATION

Animals

RDX has a typical nitrite action.[1] At RDX doses of 100 mg/kg daily, rats become aggressive and hyperirritable and have tonic clinic convulsions several hours after RDX ingestion.[1] No methemoglobinemia or alterations of the hemoglobin concentration, leukocyte count, blood glucose, blood urea nitrogen, serum calcium, chloride, carbon dioxide, or protein were observed in animals studied.[11]

Acute[7,8,12–15]

Within several hours following the presence or even absence of premonitory signs such as headache, dizziness, insomnia, restlessness, irritability, and nausea and vomiting, patients who have ingested or inhaled RDX may develop sudden multiple generalized seizures. Unconsciousness, incontinence, biting of the tongue, and defecation soon follow. The period of unconsciousness lasts for a few minutes to about 1 hour and may be followed by malaise, dizziness, muscle twitching, disorientation, nausea, vomiting, and amnesia for the episode. Seizures may recur every few minutes. Between seizures the patient appears lethargic to comatose. When awake, the patient may complain of muscle pain and bifrontal headaches and may exhibit hyperactive deep-tendon reflexes, hematuria,[13] and a low-grade fever.[6] A petechial rash presumably from the tonic phase of grand-mal seizures (Valsalva-like maneuver) is rarely observed.[16]

Chronic Exposure

Chronic RDX intoxication among workers in the munitions industry has mainly followed inhalation. RDX has no irritant action on human skin,[1] and since it is not highly lipid soluble, skin absorption is less likely.[7] Seizures may appear without warning. Symptoms are similar to those following an acute exposure.

LABORATORY

Analytic Methods

A liquid chromatography method can quantitate RDX in biologic fluids.[17] Explosives can be analyzed employing liquid chromatography, thermoscopy, and mass spectrometry.[18] A high-performance liquid chromatography method can detect RDX to levels of 5 ng.[19]

Abnormalities

Serum aminotransferases, blood urea nitrogen, and creatinine levels may be moderately elevated, but soon return to normal.[13] Gross or microscopic hematuria may be present.

Ancillary Tests

A neutrophil leukocytosis is frequently present after a severe central nervous system reaction to RDX.[3] Otherwise the complete blood count is normal. The lumbar puncture is normal.[2] An electroencephalogram may indicate bilateral synchronous symmetric spike-and-wave complexes at two to three per second maximal in the frontal areas.[2] Proteinuria and hematuria may be present, but are reversible. Liver and kidney function tests indicate mild dysfunction, but soon return to normal.[8] The serum glucose, electrolytes, coagulation parameters, and arterial blood gases are normal.[8]

TREATMENT

Stabilization

Patients must be provided an adequate airway. Endotracheal protection, cardiac monitoring, and respiratory monitoring with a supply of 100% oxygen should be available in the intensive care hospital facility where convulsive seizures are immediately treated with anticonvulsants, antiparalytic agents, and assisted ventilation as required.

Decontamination

Syrup of ipecac is not recommended because of the aspiration potential in a patient who may have sudden seizures at any time in the first 24 to 48 hours after exposure to RDX. There is no evidence to support the use of activated charcoal or cathartics, but the long half-life of RDX in the serum would tend to indicate that the compounds may be slowly absorbed from the gastrointestinal tract. In such cases gastric lavage even 4 to 5 hours after ingestion may be ameliorative, and activated charcoal may be useful.

Elimination Enhancement

There is no clinical evidence to support either the need for or efficacy of extracorporeal assistance (hemodialysis, hemoperfusion).

Antidote

There is no antidote for RDX-induced poisoning.

Supportive Measures

1. Seizures may not respond to diazepam (a first-line drug), phenytoin, or phenobarbital. Induction of paralysis with assisted ventilation may be required. Intubation and neuromuscular blockade with curare and thiopental general anesthesia can prevent complications such as permanent neurologic sequelae, rhabdomyolysis, and acute renal failure.
2. Oliguria may require a mannitol and furosemide diuresis.
3. Urine volume, fluid intake and output, and serum electrolytes should be monitored.
4. Check the urine for myoglobinuria if there have been seizures.
5. Follow muscle enzymes and potassium levels and keep external stimuli to a minimum.

REFERENCES—CYCLOTRIMETHYLENETRINITRAMINE (RDX)

1. von Oettingen WF, Donahue DD, Yagoda H, Monaco AR, Harris MR. Toxicity and potential dangers of cyclotrimethylene-trinitramine (RDX). J Indust Hyg 1949;31: 21–31.
2. Ketel WB, Hughes JR. Toxic encephalopathy with seizures secondary to ingestion of composition C-4. A clinical and electroencephalographic study. Neurology 1972;22:871–876.
3. Yinon J. Toxicity and metabolism of explosives. Boca Raton, FL: CRC Press, 1991; pp. 145–164.
4. Occupational exposure limits for airborne toxic substances. Occupational Safety and Health Series 37. Geneva: International Labour Office, 1991; pp. 120–121 (Item 599).
5. Encyclopaedia of Occupational Health and Safety. International Labour Office (Geneva). Vol 1. New York: McGraw-Hill, 1976; p. 494.
6. Stone WJ, Paletta TL, Heiman EM, Bruce JI, Knepshield JH. Toxic effects following ingestion of C-4 plastic explosive. Arch Intern Med 1969;124:726–730.
7. Etnier EL. Water quality criteria for hexahydro-1,3,5 trinitro-1,3,5-triazine (RDX). Regul Toxicol Pharmacol 1989;9: 147–157.
8. Woody RC, Kearns GL, Brewster MA, Turley CP, Sharp GB, Lake RS. The neurotoxicity of cyclotrimethylenetrinitramine (RDX) in a child: a clinical and pharmacokinetic evaluation. Clin Toxicol 1986;24:305–319.
9. Vogel W. Hexogen poisoning in human beings. Zbl Arbeitsmed 1951;1:51–54. Indust Hyg Dig 1952;16:Hem 310 (abstract).
10. Schneider NR, Bradley SL, Andersen ME. Toxicology of cyclotrimethylenetrinitramine. Distribution and metabolism in the rat and the miniature swine. Toxicol Appl Pharmacol 1977;39:531–541.
11. Kaplan AS, Berghout CF, Peczenik A. Human intoxication from RDX. Arch Environ Health 1965;10:877–883.
12. Barsott M, Crotti G. Attacchi epilettici come manifestazione di intossicazione professionale da trimetilen-trinitroamino (T4). Med Lavoro 1949;40:107–112.
13. Hollander AI, Colback EM. Composition C4 induced seizures. A report of five cases. Milit Med 1969;134:1529–1530.
14. Merrill SL. Ingestion of an explosive material, Composition C-4. A report of two cases. US Army Vietnam (USARV) Med Bull 1968;3:5–11.
15. Litovitz TL, Schmitz BF, Bailey KM. 1989 Annual Report of the American Association of Poison Control Centers. National Data Collection System. Am J Emerg Med 1990;8:431.
16. Goldberg DJ, Green ST, Nathwani D, McMenamin J, Hamlet N, Kennedy DH. RDX intoxication causing seizures and a widespread petechial rash mimicking meningococcemia. J R Soc Med 1992;85:181.
17. Turley CP, Brewster MA. Liquid chromatographic analysis of cyclotrimethylenetrinitramine in biological fluids using solid phase extraction. J Chromatogr 1987;421:430–433.
18. Berberich DW, Yost RA, Fetterolf DD. Analysis of explosives by liquid chromatography (thermospray) mass spectrometry. J Forensic Sci 1988;33:946–959.
19. Lyter AH III. A high-performance liquid chromatographic (HPLC) study of seven common explosive materials. J Forensic Sci 1983;28:446–450.

CYCLOTETRAMETHYLENETETRA-NITRAMINE (HMX)

Cyclotetramethylenetetranitramine (1,3,5,7-tetranitro-1,3,5,7-tetrazacyclooctane, octogen, HMX) has been used in military applications as burster charges for artillery shells. HMX has also been used as a component of solid-fuel rocket propellants and to implode fissionable material in nuclear devices to achieve critical mass.[1] RDX and HMX have a chemical similarity. HMX has 4 nitrite groups that can potentially be released from each molecule of HMX.[2] HPLC methods are available for testing of soil and water.[1,2]

HMX is an acronym for high melting explosive. It is a synthetic chemical. HMX explodes violently at high temperatures (534°F and above). A small amount of HMX is also formed in the synthesis of cyclotrimethylene nitramine (RDX), another explosive similar in structure to HMX. Some of the possible breakdown products of HMX are nitrites, nitrates, formaldehyde, and 1,1-dimethylhydrazine. Military personnel working at facilities that make or use HMX or RDX may be exposed by inhaling dusts containing HMX, by getting it on their skin, or by swallowing contaminated water or soil.[3]

FATAL DOSE

No deaths following inhalation exposure to HMX have been reported.[3]

TOXICOKINETICS

Absorption

HMX is poorly absorbed after it is swallowed. There have been no toxicokinetic studies on HMX.[3]

CLINICAL PRESENTATION

No evidence of hepatic or renal toxicity were observed in munitions workers exposed to HMX.[4]

A 53-year-old man who fell into a vat containing acetic acid, nitric acid, RDX, and HMX died of cardiac arrest.[5]

LABORATORY

Analytic Methods

Reverse plasma high-performance liquid chromatography methods are a available for testing soil and water.[3]

Blood Levels

Blood, urine, or stool may contain HMX.[3]

Abnormalities

No hematologic effects or adverse effects on hepatic or renal function have been observed.

TREATMENT

1. Gastric lavage, induced emesis, activated charcoal, and cathartics may reduce absorption following oral exposure.
2. Reduce dermal absorption by removing contaminated clothing and washing contaminated skin with soap and water. Do not use oils to cleanse the skin since oil may increase the dermal absorption of HMX.
3. After eye contact with HMX, remove contact lenses and flush eyes with copious amounts of water.
4. Methylene blue may be useful if nitrites or hydrazines are found.

REFERENCES—CYCLOTETRAMETHYLENETETRANITRAMINE (HMX)

1. Safire W. Object survival. New York Times, November 5, 1990, p. A19.
2. Yinon J. Toxicity and metabolism of explosives. Boca Raton, FL: CRC Press, 1991; pp. 165–170.
3. Toxicological Profile for HMX. Draft. Agency for Toxic Substances and Disease Registry, June 1994.
4. Hathaway JA, Buck CR. Absence of health hazards associated with RDX manufacture and use. J Occup Med 1977;19: 269–272.
5. Litovitz TL, Schmitz BF, Bailey KM. 1989 Annual report of the American Association of Poison Control Centers. National Data Collection System. Am J Emerg Med 1990;8: 431.

1,3-DINITROBENZENE

1-3-Dinitrobenzene (DND) and 1,3,5-trinitrobenzene (2,3,5-DNB) are substances found when trinitrotoluene is made.[1] Inhalation of these products may lead to methemoglobinemia, dyspnea, headaches, nausea, and dizziness. OSHA PEL TWA (skin designation) is 1 mg/m^3. The probable lethal oral dose in humans is estimated to be between 5 and 50 mg/kg or 7 drops to 1 teaspoonful for a 70-kg adult.[2]

REFERENCES—1,3-DINITROBENZENE

1. Garry V, Holland LM, Spanggord R. (Peer Review Panel). ATSDR. Toxicological profile for 1,3-dinitrobenzene and 1,3,5-trinitrobenzene. Draft. May 1993.
2. Von Burg R. Dinitrobenzene. J Applied Toxicol 1989;9:199–203.

ETHYLENE GLYCOL DINITRATE

Ethylene glycol dinitrate (EGDN) vapors may, in excess, affect the cardiovascular system of workers exposed to it as a component (with nitroglycerin) in the manufacture of dynamite. Dynamite manufacturing may also expose workers to ammonium nitrate, trinitrotoluene, nitrocellulose, and sawdust.[1] "Monday morning headache," angina, and sudden death appear to be associated with its acute and chronic exposure (see Nitroglycerin).

DESCRIPTION

Yellow oily liquid. Molecular weight 152.1. Boiling point 387°F.[2–4] CAS 628-96-6.

Exposure Limits[4]

USA—	ACGIH—TWA 0.05 ppm (0.31 mg/m^3) NIOSH/OSHA—STEL—0.1 mg/m^3
UK—	TWA 0.2 ppm; STEL—0.2 mg/m^3 TWA 1.2 mg/m^3; STEL—1.2 mg/m^3
Germany—	TWA 0.05 ppm; 0.3 mg/m^3
Australia—	TWA 0.05 ppm. 0.3 mg/m^3 (skin)

IDLH 500 mg/m^3

Synonyms

EGDN nitroglycol; glycoldinitrate; ethylene dinitrate; 1,2 ethanediol dinitrate; ethylene nitrate.

OCCUPATIONAL EXPOSURE

EGDN is an explosive in itself. However, it is used primarily to lower the freezing point of nitroglycerin. These compounds are the major constituents of commercial dynamite, cordite, and blasting gelatin.[5] Occupational exposure generally involves a variable mixture of the two compounds. EGDN is 160 times more volatile than nitroglycerin, is absorbed through the lungs, and is more readily absorbed through intact skin than nitroglycerin.[6] Nitroglycerin is also used as a pharmaceutical.

In most countries with a temperate to cold climate, the proportion of EGDN in dynamite varies between 10 and 80% depending on the climate and the season. However, most frequently the ratio of nitroglycerin to EGDN is 1 : 1.[1]

OCCUPATIONS

A partial list of occupations in which exposure may occur includes drug makers and explosive makers. Blasting workers are exposed to both nitroglycerin and EGDN. Propellant workers are usually exposed only to nitroglycerin.[6]

ROUTES OF ENTRY

Inhalation of dust or vapor; ingestion of dust; percutaneous absorption.[1,5]

TOXIC DOSE

Volunteers exposed to the vapor of a mixture of EGDN and nitroglycerin at a combined concentration of 2 mg/m^3 experienced headache and fall in blood pressure within 3 minutes of exposure.[7] A mean concentration of 0.7 mg/m^3 for 25 minutes also produced a lowered blood pressure and slight headache.[8]

TOXICOKINETICS

Absorption

Applications of 100 mg of an explosive containing 22% EGDN to 1 cm^2 of skin resulted in less than 6.5 $mg/cm^2/hr$ absorption.[9] Mean blood EGDN levels in exposed dynamite production factory workers rose from a mean of 63.3 ng/mL on Tuesday morning (first day of work) to 120 ng/mL on Thursday morning, dropping to 51.7 ng/mL on Thursday afternoon.[10] Urine concentrations of EGDN rose from 4.3 ng/mL on Tuesday morning to 37.7 ng/mL on Saturday afternoon.[10]

Drug Interactions

Consumption of alcohol during working hours appears to intensify acute symptoms of exposure to EGDN.[11] An intense diffuse erythema was observed in one female worker with EGDN after drinking small quantities of wine.[11]

CLINICAL PRESENTATION

Acute

Acute exposure to EGDN vapor is followed by a pulsating headache, nausea and vomiting, dizziness, and palpitations. These symptoms are most intense on Mondays. A fall in blood pressure (systolic and diastolic) may also be noted during the first days of employment.[12] Tolerance then develops and the rest of the working week is usually relatively free from effects.[13]

Chronic

Following a period of exposure to mixtures of nitroglycerin and EGDN, which varies between 6 and 10 years, workers are likely to die suddenly, normally on a Monday or Tuesday, most frequently between 4 and 7 in the morning (referred to as "Monday morning death," "Monday head,"[14] "nitrate head,"[14] "powder head," "NIG head," "Monday headache") on return from a holiday or from a weekend off work. About three-fourths of the incidents of sudden death in these workers occurs after a 1- or 2-day absence from exposure.[7,15] Signs of coronary sclerosis have not been prominent in such sudden deaths from EGDN exposure.[13,16,17]

In 1952 three cases of sudden unexpected deaths were caused by EGDN exposure in an explosives plant in the Saar.[18] Between 1952 and 1964 47 additional cases were described. Workers had been in contact with EGDN over a period of 10 years at a dynamite factory. About one-third experienced attacks of angina, usually in the summer months, usually during a Sunday night or in the early hours of Monday morning. This occurred in subjects who had finished work Friday evening.[11] Females who had worked with EGDN for an average of 9 years experienced paresthesias in the extremities. Blanching or whiteness of the toes or exposure to cold were also observed (a Raynaud's phenomenon).[11]

Dynamite workers appear to suffer a high mortality from chronic cardiovascular and cerebrovascular diseases.[19] EGDN is much more volatile than nitroglycerin and is dominant in the air surrounding the workers. Follow-up of workers in an explosives company for 16 years suggested an excess of deaths from acute myocardial infarction in younger workers exposed to both nitroglycerin and EGDN.[6]

Tolerance

Hypotensive responses in rats and dogs similarly lessen after a number of injections of EGDN. Studies of metabolites of EGDN in animals suggests that metabolic changes (ethylene glycol mononitrate, inorganic nitrate, nitrites) are not correlated with the phenomenon of tolerance.[12]

Methemoglobinemia

Acute ingestions or acute skin exposure to EGDN can lead to methemoglobinemia, cyanosis, anoxia, and the formation of Heinz bodies in erythrocytes[3] (see Airborne chapter).

LABORATORY
Analytic Methods

A spectrophotometric method for detection of 0.5 to 2.0 μg of EGDN per mL of blood is available, as well as a gas chromatographic method to separate EGDN from EGMN (the mononitrate).[20] Detection of EGDN vapors by ion mobility spectrometry using chloride reagent ions has been described as sensitive and specific.[21]

Blood Levels

Thirty explosives workers in an environment of 0.22 to 0.39 ppm EGDN were examined. In three cases about 1 μg/ml of free EGDN was observed. No significant difference in the erythrocyte count and methemoglobin content was observed between EGDN workers and controls.[22] A maximum blood level of 2 ng/ml of EGDN followed an 8-hour exposure to an environment containing about 1 mg/m^3 EGDN.[19]

Ancillary Tests

Electrocardiogram may be normal or may show a lengthening of the PQ interval immediately after an attack of angina.[2,11] Anecdotal case reports reflect atrial fibrillation returning to normal within a few hours to days after leaving work.[11]

TREATMENT
Supportive Measures

1. 22°C should not be exceeded in areas occupied by workers, and 32°C in premises where processes are remotely controlled. Vapor pressure rises rapidly with temperature:

Temperature (°C)	Vapor Pressure (mm Hg)[2] (EGDN)
0	0.0044
20	0.038
40	0.26
60	1.3
80	5.9
100	22.0

2. Skin absorption can be reduced by use of protective clothing, including polyethylene hand protection. This equipment should be washed twice per week.
3. Shower at end of each shift with sulfite indicator soap to detect any traces of nitroglycerin/EGDN mixture on the skin.
4. Separate work clothing from private clothing.
5. Respiratory protective equipment may be necessary for work in storage areas.
6. The concentration of EGDN in an explosive mixture should be reduced depending on the ambient temperature, but should not be greater than 20 to 25% EGDN. In very warm season, exclude EGDN totally.
7. Remote control (optical, mechanical, or electronic means) of the most dangerous operations (especially milling) and automation of processes such as nitration, mixing, and cartridge filling will enhance safety.
8. Monitoring of exposure to EGDN should be based on determination of EGDN in venous blood samples taken periodically and routinely from workers. An EGDN blood of 2 ng/ml appears to correspond to 1 mg/m^3 in air.
9. Methemoglobinemia should be treated according to guidelines in Airborne chapter—see also Dinitrotoluene. Methylene blue should be available.

Prevention

Potential exposure to EGDN requires a preemployment examination, periodic reexaminations, and examinations after a lengthy absence due to illness, with special attention to the cardiovascular system (electrocardiogram; blood pressure—supine, sitting, standing; pulse; auscultation).[2] Care should be exercised in accepting workers with cardiac disease, hypertension, or migraine.

REFERENCES—CYCLOTETRAMETHYLENETETRANITRAMINE (HMX)

1. Hogstedt C, Andersson K. A cohort study on mortality among dynamite workers. J Occup Med 1979;21:553–556.
2. Parmeggiani L. Ethylene glycol dinitrate. In Encyclopaedia of occupational health and safety. Vol 1. International Labour Office. New York: McGraw-Hill, 1976; pp. 483–484.
3. Proctor NH, Hughes JP, Fischman ML. Chemical hazards of the workplace. 2nd ed. New York: Van Nostrand Reinhold, 1989;247.
4. Ethylene glycol dinitrate. NIOSH Pocket guide to chemical hazards. DHHS (NIOSH) Publication No 90-117. Washington, DC: US Government Printing Office, June 1990, pp. 110–111.
5. Key MM, Henschel AF, Butler J, Ligo RN, Tabershaw IR. Occupational diseases. A guide to their recognition. DHEW (NIOSH) Publication No. 77-181. Washington, DC: US Government Printing Office, 1077, pp. 282–284.
6. Craig R, Gillis CR, Hole DJ, Paddle GM. Sixteen year follow up of workers in an explosives factory. J Soc Occup Med 1985;35:107–110.
7. Carmichael P, Lieben J. Sudden death in explosives workers. Arch Environ Health 1963;7:424–439.
8. Lund RP, Haggendal J, Johnsson G. Withdrawal symptoms in workers exposed to nitroglycerin. Br J Ind Med 1968; 25:136–138.
9. Gross E, Kiese M, Resag K. Resorption von athylene glykoldinitrat durch die haut. (Absorption of ethylene glycol dinitrate through the skin). Arch Toxicol 1960;18:194–199.
10. Fukuchi Y. Nitroglycol concentrations in blood and urine of workers engaged in dynamite production. Int Arch Occup Environ Health 1981;48:339–346.
11. Burtalini E, Cavagna G, Foa V. Epidemiological and clinical features of occupational nitroglycol poisoning in Italy. Med Lavoro 1967;58:618–623.
12. Clark DG, Litchfield MH. Metabolism of ethylene glycol dinitrate (ethylene dinitrate) in the rat following repeated administration. Br J Ind Med 1969;26:150–155.
13. Forssman S, Masreliez N, Johansson G, Sundell G, Wilander O, Bostrom G. Untersuchungen des gesundheitszustandes von nitroarbeitern bei drei schwedischen spreng stoffabriken. Arch Gewerbepath Gewerbehyg 1958;16:157–177.
14. McGuiness BW, Harris EL. "Monday Head." An interesting occupational disorder. Br Med J 1961;2:745–747.
15. Havi Hau A, Hardy HL. Industrial toxicology. 3rd ed. Acton, MA: Publishing Sciences Group, 1974; pp. 317–319.
16. Hogstedt C, Axelson O. Nitroglycerin-nitroglycol exposure and the mortality in cardio-cerebrovascular disease among dynamite workers. J Occup Med 1977;19:675–678.
17. Hogstedt C, Axelson O. Mortality from cardio-cerebrovascular diseases among dynamite workers—an extended case referent study. Am Acad Med (Singapore) 1984;23(Suppl 2):399–403.

18. Symansky H. Schere gesundheits schadigungen durch berufliche nitroglykoleinwirkung. (Serious injuries to health by occupational exposure to nitroglycol). Arch Hyg Bacteriol 1952;136:139–158.
19. Yinon J. Toxicity and metabolism of explosives. Boca Raton, FL: CRC Press, 1990; pp. 133–143.
20. Litchfield MH. The determination of di- and mononitrates of ethylene glycol and 1,2-propylene glycol in blood by colorimetric and gas chromatographic methods. Analyst 1968;93: 653.
21. Lawrence AH, Neudorfl P. Detection of ethylene glycol dinitrate vapors by ion mobility spectrometry using chloride reagent ions. Anal Chem 1988;60:104–109.
22. Trainor DC, Jones RC. Headaches in explosive magazine workers. Arch Environ Health 1966;12:231–234.

HYDRAZINE AND DERIVATIVES

Hydrazine and its derivatives (monomethylhydrazine, dimethyl hydrazine, and phenylhydrazine) are used in the explosives industry and may induce gastrointestinal, hematologic, hepatic, renal, dermal, and neurologic evidence of toxicity. Fatalities have occurred, but prognosis after inadvertent exposure is usually good. Treatment is symptomatic and supportive. Pyridoxine and methylene blue may have a role as antidotes.

STRUCTURE AND CLASSIFICATION[1–5]

Hydrazine (NH_2 NH_2)
Monomethylhydrazine (NH_2NHCH_3)
1,1-dimethylhydrazine (NH_2N $(CH_3)_2$)
Phenylhydrazine ($C_6H_5NHNH_2$)

DESCRIPTION

Hydrazine is a colorless oily liquid or white crystal.

CAS No. 302-01-2
Conversion factor 1 ppm = 1.3 mg/m^3
Molecular formula: N_2H_4
Molecular weight: 32.05
Odor: Faint, fish, ammonia-like; threshold 3 to 4 ppm, but may be lower. At lower concentrations that may occur during manufacturing or transfer processes, the warning properties of odor may not be enough to preclude low-level chronic occupational exposure in fuel handlers.[4]

Synonyms (Hydrazine and Derivatives)

Diamine; anhydrous hydrazine; methyl hydrazine; 1, 1-dimethyl hydrazine; phenyl hydrazine.

IDLH is 80 ppm (hydrazine); 295 ppm (phenylhydrazine); 50 ppm (methylhydrazine); 50 ppm (1, 1 dimethyl hydrazine).[3]

Exposure limits[3,5]

Hydrazine	CAS 302-01-2
USA (OSHA/TWA)	0.1 ppm 0.1 mg/m^3 Probable human carcinogen Skin absorption
UK TWA	0.1 ppm 0.1 mg/m^3
Germany TWA	0.1 ppm (local irritant) 0.27 mg/m^3

1,1 dimethylhydrazine is a hygroscopic mobile liquid.

CAS 57-14-7	USA (OSHA)	TWA 0.5 ppm 1.0 mg/m^3
Methylhydrazine CAS 60-34-4	USA (OSHA)	0.2 ppm (ceiling value) 0.35 mg/m^3

Phenylhydrazine is an oily colorless liquid.

CAS 100-63-0	USA (OSHA) TWA 5 ppm 20 mg/m^3	STEL 10 ppm 45 mg/m^3
	UK TWA 5 ppm 10 mg/m^3	STEL 10 ppm 45 mg/m^3
	Germany TWA 5 ppm 22 mg/m^3 (sensitizer, probably human carcinogen, absorption through skin, significant)	

Hydrazine, monomethyl hydrazine, and dimethylhydrazine are very soluble in water and ethyl alcohol. Phenylhydrazine is soluble in alcohol, slightly soluble in water.[4] Hydrazine has also been detected in cigarette smoke at levels of 31.5 ng per cigarette.[1] It is also a component of some edible mushrooms (see Gyromitrin, Group II, Mushroom chapter), as well as processed foods.

USES

Hydrazines are used in rocket propellants, as reactants in military fuel cells, as reducing agents in nickel plating, chain extenders in the polymerization of urethane, in water treatment for the removal of halogens, in photographic developers, as corrosion inhibitors in boiler feedwater, for soldering fluxes, and in the manufacture of drugs, pesticides, and agricultural chemicals. It has been used as an experimental drug for the treatment of tuberculosis, sickle cell anemia, and cancer.[1]

PRODUCT FORMULATION

The propellant grade of commercial hydrazine contains a minimum of 97.7% of the active ingredient. Other solutions of commercial hydrazine are 65, 54.4, and 35% solutions of hydrazine sulfate.[6]

TOXIC DOSE

Ingestion of a mouthful of hydrazine led to vomiting and loss of consciousness. The subject survived.[1] Ingestion of 20 to 30 mL of a 6% aqueous solution of hydrazine freebase led to immediate vomiting, somnolence, and arrhythmia. After 5 days the patient recovered.[7]

OCCUPATIONAL EXPOSURE

Inhalation

Moderate to high concentrations of hydrazine vapors are highly irritating to the eyes, nose, and respiratory system.

Concentrations of about 2% in air represent the lower explosive limit, but irritation at this level would be unbearable.[4]

Skin

Skin irritation is pronounced with the propellant hydrazines.

Ingestion

Ingestion of hydrazines produces gastrointestinal irritation, central nervous system excitability, and undesirable hematologic effects.

TOXICOKINETICS

Absorption

Hydrazines are absorbed through the skin, respiratory tract, and gastrointestinal tract.

Elimination

Acetylation of the parent compound is the principal method of metabolism. Individuals who are slow acetylators may be predisposed to the toxic effects of hydrazine or its derivatives.[8] The monoacetyl form of hydrazine appears to be more toxic than the diacetyl form.[9] Most hydrazine is excreted in the urine in the diacetyl form.[6] Approximately 20% of the dose is rapidly excreted by the lungs.[6]

Pregnancy/Lactation

No embryotoxic effects in man have been reported to be associated with occupational exposure to the hydrazines.[10] Embryotoxicity following exposure to the hydrazines has been observed in animals. There have been no prospective controlled studies of pregnancy and neonates following exposure to the hydrazines. Breast milk has not been studied.

MECHANISM OF ACTION

Hydrazine may cause liver and central nervous system dysfunction by producing a Vitamin B_6 deficiency similar to overdose with hydrazine-derived drugs such as isoniazid.[7]

CLINICAL PRESENTATION

Acute Exposure

Ingestion

Anorexia, vomiting, and hypotension may follow ingestion of the hydrazines. One patient drank a mouthful of hydrazine and immediately became confused, lethargic, and restless. Within 1 week a peripheral neuropathy developed that resolved in 6 months. Liver and central nervous system dysfunction may occur.[7] Convulsions and coma were observed after a patient accidentally drank hydrazine.[11] Temporary loss of memory, lateral nystagmus, somnolence, and arrhythmias have been observed.[1]

Inhalation

Exposure to hydrazine vapors can produce eye irritation (itching, burning), conjunctivitis, facial edema, and salivation. Bronchial mucous production, bronchial obstruction, pulmonary edema, and death may follow.[1] Severe exposure of the eyes to the vapor may cause temporary blindness lasting about 1 day.[12] Dizziness and nausea often follow inhalation.

Skin

Exposure to the hydrazines may cause strong skin irritation and produce causticlike penetrating burns.[1]

CHRONIC TOXICITY

Ingestion

Chronic oral exposure to the hydrazines has not been reported.

Inhalation

A worker who handled hydrazine once a week for 6 months developed lethargy, conjunctivitis, and tremors. Finally vomiting, fever, diarrhea, and abdominal pains ensued, leading to incoherent behavior and death 20 days after the last exposure. Autopsy revealed a tracheitis, bronchitis, evidence of liver damage, renal tubular necrosis, a lobar pneumonia, and cardiac muscle degeneration.[11]

Skin

Occupational exposures can lead to sensitization reactions. One worker experienced recurrent hand and forearm eczema within 3 weeks after handling hydrazine-treated material in a gold-plating operation. The condition completely resolved after changing jobs.[1] Another worker in the same department developed periorbital eczema after 4 months of exposure. Recovery followed a move to a new job.[13]

Immunotoxicity

Hydrazine has been associated with an occupationally induced systemic lupus erythematosus–like condition (see Immunotoxicity chapter). Macular rash, photosensitivity, antinuclear antibody, and antibody to DNA may be observed.[14]

Carcinogenicity

IARC considers the hydrazines a potential carcinogen (Category Group 2B).[15] The EPA also considers hydrazine to be a potential carcinogen.[16,17]

Hematologic Effects

Hemolytic changes with Heinz body formation appear to be dose dependent and more often follow exposure to monomethylhydrazine.[18] Hyperplastic bone marrow changes and extramedullary hematopoiesis follow exposure to phenylhydrazine.[4] Monomethylhydrazine is a strong methemoglobin former.

LABORATORY—ANALYTIC METHODS

Blood Levels

Hydrazine and dimethylhydrazine can be detected in blood.[19,20] Such methods have not been applied to human experiences with the hydrazines.

Abnormalities

Serum aminotransferase elevations may follow ingestion of hydrazine. Leukocytosis and proteinuria may follow an ingestion of hydrazine.[21]

Ancillary Tests

Muscle biopsy may slow a neurogenic atrophy.[7] Sural nerve biopsy exhibits a severe axonal degeneration. Visual evoked response may be suggestive of bilateral optic neuropathy.[7] Methemoglobinemia may follow exposure to monomethylhydrazine.[4]

TREATMENT

Stabilization

Exposure to hydrazine will generally occur at work.

Ingestion

Patients who have ingested hydrazine may become rapidly obtunded. Immediate attention to providing a patent airway and a source of oxygen should be priority. Cardiac monitoring should be started. The patient should be hospitalized in an intensive care facility where symptomatic and supportive therapy can be provided, and a neurologic, hematologic, renal, and hepatic follow-up may be required over the ensuing days.

Inhalation

Respiratory irritation will require symptomatic and supportive care. Respiratory difficulties may require endotracheal intubation and mechanical ventilation.

Skin

Contamination of the skin by hydrazines must be immediately removed with large quantities of water (e.g., shower at occupation site).

Eyes

Flushing of the affected eye or eyes should begin at once and continued for at least 20 minutes or lower depending on symptoms and appearance of the eye.

Decontamination

There is no clinical evidence that cathartics, gastric lavage, or syrup of ipecac will be of value in a hydrazine exposure. Syrup of ipecac may expose the patient to an aspiration pneumonitis and would not be recommended. Since the prognosis for acute intoxication is usually good and most changes are reversible, excessive zeal for internal decontamination is probably unnecessary. Skin and eye decontamination procedures are the most immediate needs.

Elimination Enhancement

Whole bowel irrigation, hemoperfusion, and dialysis have not been studied as an aid in the elimination of hydrazine. Extensive renal tubular failure may require hemodialysis.

Antidote

Although not specifically an antidote for hydrazine overdose, pyridoxine 10 mg by intravenous administration may be able to return altered mental status and liver function results to normal, especially following methylated hydrazine exposure.[4,7] Methemoglobinemia should respond to methylene blue.

Safety and Health Measures

1. Vinyl-coated hand protection, natural or reclaimed rubber foot protection, rubber aprons, and plastic eye and face protection should be used when working with the hydrazines. Where the possibility of gross splashing exists, full protective clothing made of rubber, neoprene, or vinyl-coated materials should be worn.[4]
2. Respiratory protection may require a self-contained breathing apparatus.
3. Exposure of workers with enzyme deficiencies such as a lack of glucose-6-phosphate dehydrogenase, 6-phosphogluconic dehydrogenase, or glutathione reductase may exaggerate hemolysis associated with exposure to monomethylhydrazine. Personnel with these enzyme deficiencies should not be exposed to monomethylhydrazine.[18]
4. Contraindications for working with hydrazine propellants should include pregnancy, anemias and hematologic disorders, history of convulsive episodes and other neurologic disorders, "slow acetylators," enzyme deficiencies (see 3), therapeutic use of tranquilizers, and the existence of "benign" tumors.[18]
5. Preemployment screening should include a complete physical examination, pulmonary function tests, chest x-rays, hematology, liver function, EEG, and kidney function tests. Tests for red cell enzymes (see 3).
6. There are no blood or urine levels of the hydrazines that can be used to monitor workers who are not suffering ill effects.[18]

REFERENCES—HYDRAZINE AND DERIVATIVES

1. Von Burg R, Stout T. Toxicology update. Hydrazine. J Appl Toxicol 1991;11:447–450.
2. Hydrazine in Proctor NH, Hughes JP, Fischman ML. Chemical hazards of the workplace. 2nd ed. New York: Van Nostrand Reinhold, 1989; pp. 272–273.
3. NIOSH Pocket Guide to Chemical Hazards. DHHS (NIOSH) Publication No. 90-117. Washington, DC: US Government Printing Office, 1990; 124–125 (Hydrazine); 152–153 (Methylhydrazine); 96–97 (1,1 dimethylhydrazine); 180–181 (phenylhydrazine).

4. Thomas AA. Hydrazine and derivatives. In: Encyclopaedia of Occupational Health and Safety, International Labour Office. Vol 1. New York: McGraw-Hill, 1976.
5. Occupational exposure limits for airborne toxic substances. 3rd ed. Occupational Safety and Health Series No. 37. Geneva, International Labour Office, 1991.
6. HSDB Hazardous Substance Data Bank. Washington, DC: National Library of Medicine, Toxicology Information Program, 1991.
7. Harati Y, Niakan E. Hydrazine toxicity, pyridoxine therapy, and peripheral neuropathy. Ann Intern Med 1986;104:728–729.
8. Reidenberg MM. Aromatic amines and the pathogenesis of lupus erythematosus. Am J Med 1983;75:1037–1042.
9. Bhide SV, Bhalerao E, Saride A, Marude GB. Mutagenicity and carcinogenicity of mono- and diacetyl hydrazine. Cancer Lett 1984;23:235–240.
10. Keller WC. Toxicity assessment of hydrazide fuels. Aviat Space Environ Med 1988;59 (Suppl 11):A100–A106.
11. Sotaniemi E, Hirvonen J, Isomaki H, Takkunen J, Kaila J. Hydrazine toxicity in the human. Report of a fatal case. Ann Clin Res 1971;3:30–33.
12. Comstock CC, Lawson LH, Greene EA, Oberst FW. Inhalation toxicity of hydrazine vapor. Arch Ind Hyg Occup Med 1954;10:476–490.
13. Wrangsjo K, Martensson A. Hydrazine contact dermatitis from gold plating. Contact Dermatitis 1986;15:244–245.
14. Reidenberg MM, Durant PJ, Harris RA, De-Baccardo G, Lahita R, Stenzel KH. Lupus erythematosus-like disease due to hydrazine. Am J Med 1983;75:365–370.
15. IARC. Monographs on the evaluation of the carcinogenic risk of chemicals to man: overall evaluations of carcinogenicity. (Geneva) World Health Organ Tech Rep Ser 1987;S7: 223–224.
16. Wald N, Boreham J, Doll R, Bonsall J. Occupational exposure to hydrazine and subsequent risk of cancer. Br J Ind Med 1984;41:31–34.
17. EPA—Methodology for Evaluating Potential Carcinogenicity in Support of Reportable Quantity Adjustments Pursuant to CEPCLA Section 102, EPA 600/8-89/053. Washington, DC. Office of Health and Environmental Assessment, 1988.
18. Back KC, Carter VL Jr, Thomas AA. Occupational hazards of missile operations with special regard to the hydrazine propellants. Aviat Space Environ Med 1978;49: 591–598.
19. Key MM, Henschel AF, Butler J, Ligo RN, Tabershaw IR. Occupational diseases. A guide to their recognition. DHEW(NIOSH) Publication No. 77-181, Washington, DC: US Government Printing Office, 1977;296–298.
20. IARC Monographs on the Evaluation of Carcinogenic Risk of Chemicals to Man. Some Aromatic Amines, Hydrazine and Related Substances, N-Nitroso Compounds and Miscellaneous Alkylating Agents. (Geneva) World Health Organ, Tech Rep Ser 1974;4:127–130.
21. Hydrazine. Environmental Health Criteria 68. (Geneva) World Health Organ Tech Rep Ser 1987;1–89.

NITROGLYCERIN

Nitroglycerin may induce a severe disabling syndrome with throbbing headaches and hypotension experienced when workers are first exposed to this chemical. Tolerance often occurs late in the work week. Relief occurs on weekends, but serious symptoms resume Monday morning. When nitroglycerin is mixed with ethylene glycol dinitrate in the manufacture of dynamite, there may be an increase in the number of sudden deaths observed in otherwise healthy young men. Preventive measures are crucial. Treatment is mainly supportive and symptomatic.

STRUCTURE AND CLASSIFICATION

Nitroglycerin is 1,2,3-propanetriol trinitrate. Molecular weight is 227.1. It is a colorless to pale-yellow viscous liquid or solid (below 56°F).[1] Nitroglycerin is slightly soluble in water and is soluble in ethyl alcohol and ethyl ether. Its chemical formula is $CH_2NO_3CHNO_3$ CH_2NO_3.[22]

CAS 55-63-0

TWA[3]	USA (OSHA)	0.1 mg/m³	(CEILING)	(skin)
	UK	0.2 ppm	2 mg/m³	(skin)
	Germany	0.05 ppm	0.5 mg/m³	(skin)
	France	0.15 ppm	1.5 mg/m³	(skin)
	Australia	0.05 ppm	0.5 mg/m³	(skin)
STEL	UK	0.02 ppm	2 mg/m³	

Synonyms

Glycerol trinitrate; nitroglycerol; trinitroglycerol; NG; trinitrin.

Nitroglycerin is a highly explosive substance that is very sensitive to mechanical shock and heat; it is readily detonated by spontaneous chemical reaction.[3,4] Defibrillation performed over a nitroglycerin skin patch may result in electrical arcing with a resultant flash of light and thermal injuries.[5,6] In commercial explosives its sensitivity is reduced by the addition of an adsorbent such as wood pulp and chemicals such as ethylene glycol dinitrate and ammonium nitrate.[2]

USES

Nitroglycerin is used in the manufacture of industrial explosives. It is also used in medicine as a coronary vasodilator for the relief of angina, for prophylaxis of angina pectoris, for the management of unstable angina pectoris, for the relief of coronary artery spasm (Prinzmetal's angina), for the management of acute cardiac pulmonary edema, for the management of chronic heart failure, acute myocardial infarction, and postoperative hypertension, and for the relief of esophageal spasm.[7]

CHRONOLOGY (TABLE 63–4)[8]

Nitroglycerin—The Headaches

Nitroglycerin was discovered in 1847 and incorporated by Alfred Nobel into a major component of dynamite in 1867, initially mixed with diatomaceous earth and later mixed with sodium nitrate (an oxidizer) and an adsorbent combustible

Table 63–4
Cardiotoxic Effects of Dynamite—A Chronology

1847	Nitroglycerin discovered.
1867	Nitroglycerin incorporated into dynamite.
1890	Severe headaches described in dynamite workers (Nitroglycerin head). Frequent reports follow. No deaths related to dynamite.
1930	Ethylene glycol dinitrate added to nitroglycerin in dynamite manufacture.
1934	Sudden deaths in United States (reported in 1978).
1950s	Reports of sudden deaths in Europe.
1963	Reports of sudden deaths in the United States.

material such as wood pulp. In 1890 a first report of occupational health hazard after exposure to nitroglycerin described severe throbbing headaches, difficulty in breathing, weak pulse, pallor, drowsiness, weakness, diaphoresis, nausea, and vomiting. Mild symptoms followed oral nitroglycerin on skin contact with dynamite.[9,10] Similar symptoms were described in 1898 as "powder headache," in 1910 as "nitroglycerin head,"[11] or "NG head" in 1914,[12] and as headaches that were enhanced by alcohol. In 1944,[13] 1946,[14] and 1949[15] descriptions were restricted to the above symptoms.

Ethylene Glycol Dinitrate (EGDN)—Sudden Death

EGDN had been discovered in 1870 and was brought into commercial use in the 1930s to lower the freezing point of nitroglycerin explosives, thereby making them safer to use.[3] The ratio of EGDN to nitroglycerin in the United States has varied from 8:2 to 9:1 (see EGDN). EGDN has a higher vapor pressure than nitroglycerin. Higher exposures to vaporized EGDN than to nitroglycerin occur among workers manufacturing or using these compounds. Both nitroglycerin and EGDN are rapidly absorbed through the skin. Beginning in 1934 sudden unexplained deaths in healthy dynamite workers were observed.[5] In the early 1950s[16,17] a survey of unexpected fatalities associated with EGDN in the United States and Europe was reported. In 1963 these deaths were summarized:[18]

1. All sudden unexpected deaths occurred after exposure to both nitroglycerin and ethylene glycol dinitrate, components of dynamite since the early 1930s.
2. All deaths occurred suddenly after a period of freedom from exposure (48 to 60 hours) before starting work again, often on a Sunday night or in the early hours of Monday morning, with some experiencing "Monday morning angina" and chest pain.[19–22]
3. Deaths occurred in young healthy men between the ages of about 25 to 50 years.
4. Deaths were attributed to coronary artery disease, but coronary atherosclerosis was minimal or absent.

TOXICOKINETICS

Absorption

Nitroglycerin is readily absorbed through the mucous membranes, lung, and intact skin. An average plasma concentration of 2.3 ng/ml was observed 1 hour after dermal application of 45 mg of nitroglycerin as an ointment.[23] Nitroglycerin is 60% bound to plasma protein at plasma concentrations between 50 and 500 ng/mL.[4]

Distribution (V_D)

The apparent volume of distribution is 2.6 to 3.3 L/kg.[4]

Elimination

Nitroglycerin is degraded in the liver by reductive hydrolysis and partially in plasma by spontaneous hydrolysis.[4] The plasma half-life of nitroglycerin has been estimated to be 1 to 3 minutes, representing the alpha distribution phase, and also at about 7.5 minutes.[24] The major urinary metabolites include glyceryl mononitrate, 1,2 glyceryl dinitrate, and 1,3 glyceryl dinitrate. The mono- and di-nitrate metabolites are glucuronidated and excreted in the urine and bile. Reactive hydrolysis in the liver by hepatic inorganic nitrate reductase leads to the formation of the free nitric oxide (NO) radical.

Route of Poisoning

When tablets are ingested or swallowed rapidly they cause little toxic effect as the drug is rapidly extracted and metabolized in the liver. Nitroglycerin poisoning is rare after oral ingestions unless very large doses are ingested. When taken sublingually or transdermally, the drug does not pass through the liver before entering the general circulation. Acute poisonings therefore usually occur from injection, inhalation, or absorption via mucous membranes or skin.[25]

Drug Interactions

Serious and prolonged hypotension may follow exposure to nitroglycerin in those who are concurrently receiving calcium channel blockers, antihypertensive agents, phenothiazines, and tricyclic antidepressants. Use of alcohol with nitroglycerin exposure may produce severe hypotension and collapse or may induce aberrant destructive behavior.[4,6–10]

MECHANISM OF ACTION

Biochemical

Nitroglycerin is devoid of action on tissues other than smooth muscle where it produces relaxation. Although it predominantly affects vascular smooth muscle, the bronchioles, gastrointestinal tract (including the biliary system), ureters, and uterus are affected.[4] Free radicals of nitric oxide (NO) may activate guanylate cyclase, resulting in increased synthesis of cyclic GMP.[26] NO may combine with sulfhydryl groups in the endothelium and produce S-nitrosothiols, which stimulate guanylate cyclase production.[27] *N*-acetylcysteine may enhance this process by providing a source of sulfhydryl groups.[28] Cyclic GMP appears to reduce stored calcium and interfere with calcium-activated smooth muscle contractions.[24]

Clinical

At low concentrations, nitroglycerin is mostly a venous dilator. Some localized arteriolar dilation of the face and trunk may produce a flush, and meningeal and cerebral vessel dilation may result in a headache. At higher concentrations, nitroglycerin produces arteriolar vasodilation with a reduction in arterial pressure. This fall in pressure associated with the reduced cardiac output secondary to venodilation is sufficient to cause hypotension. The maximum vascular effect occurs in 5 minutes. Vasodilation causes a fall in systolic, diastolic, and pulse pressure. The acute reaction and signs tend to disappear after 2 to 4 days of continuous exposure as a result of compensatory mechanisms due to an increase in vascular tone. Peripheral vasodilation leads to rapid runoff and decreased ventricular ejection time. Dilation of the coronary artery leads to increased flow in the epicardial vessels and through eccentric stenoses and collaterals; decrease in left ventricular end-diastolic pressure enhances subendocardial blood flow.[4]

CLINICAL PRESENTATION

Nitroglycerin Dynamite

Exposure to nitroglycerin among dynamite workers (and wives who have laundered and ironed their clothes, underwear, and even bedclothes)[8] has led to severe throbbing headaches, flushing, palpitations, nausea and vomiting, weakness, prostration, drowsiness, diaphoresis, and dizziness. The headache may begin in the forehead and move to the occipital region, continuing for 1 to 2 hours, or even for 3 to 4 days.[8,11,16] Restlessness and inability to lie down or lie quietly are frequently present. Sleep is difficult. Impaired vision, diarrhea, and abdominal pain may accompany the headache. Tolerance to exposure develops after 3 or 4 days of continued exposure, but is lost after 2 days away from work. Some workers have tried to avoid the Monday headache by placing nitroglycerin under their hatbands over the weekend, sucking occasionally on a piece of dynamite, or inhaling the fumes from their work clothes. Such headaches have occurred, in addition to dynamite workers, in those who make rocket propellants or nitroglycerin-containing pharmaceuticals.

Nitroglycerin Plus Ethylene Glycol Dinitrate Dynamite

A chronology of experiences is found above (Uses). Raynaud's phenomenon and peripheral neuropathy have been described. Hallucinations, depression, mania, epilepsy, paresthesias, transient hemiparesis, and aphasia have been observed. Hypoxia due to methemoglobinemia may lead to cyanosis, metabolic acidosis, coma, convulsions, and cardiovascular collapse.

Nitroglycerin may cause irritation of the skin at the site of application; eruptions of the palms and interdigital spaces and ulcers under the nails have been observed in workers handling nitroglycerin.[2]

Nitroglycerin Sprays

Use of nitroglycerin sprays by patients with cardiovascular disease for inappropriate indications such as nausea, epigastric symptoms, chest tightness, or dyspnea may lead to syncope, hypotension, and unconsciousness, which usually resolves within minutes.[29] Skin absorption continues to be an important source of toxicity.[30,31]

Nitropatch Explosions

Defibrillation performed over a nitroglycerin transdermal skin patch may result in an explosive noise, a flash of light, yellow smoke with a discoloration of the patch, superficial skin discoloration, and superficial burn injuries. The aluminized plastic in the skin patch acts as a conductor of the electrical arc between the defibrillation pad and the skin. Transdermal nitroglycerin systems should be removed before attempting defibrillation or cardioversion. Routine measures for treatment of the first- and second-degree burns will be effective.[37,38]

LABORATORY

Analytic Methods

Nitroglycerin and its dinitrate metabolites in human plasma may be quantitated by high-performance liquid chromatography with thermal energy analyzer detection.[32] The limits of sensitivity for nitroglycerin are 0.05 ng/mL and for the dinitrate metabolites 0.25 ng/mL. Skin samples containing 1,3 glyceryl dinitrate and 1,2-glyceryl dinitrate can now be analyzed with HPLC techniques.[33] Gas chromatography electron capture detection can simultaneously determine nitroglycerin and its dinitrate metabolites.[34] Limits of detection for nitroglycerin are 0.025 ng/mL, 1,2-glyceryldinitrate 0.1 ng/mL, and 1,3 glyceryl dinitrate 0.1 ng/mL.[31]

Blood Levels

The nitroglycerin blood level should not exceed 4 ng/mL corresponding to a concentration of 2 mg/m^3 in the air.[35]

Abnormalities

Methemoglobinemia up to 30% has been reported following exposure to nitroglycerin and ethylene glycol dinitrate.[36] Leukopenia and abnormal liver function tests have been observed.[33]

Ancillary Tests

Plethysmography may be a useful screening measure in the determination of abnormal pulse waves in workers at explosives factories.[37]

TREATMENT

Stabilization

Occupational Exposure

Oxygen delivery should be assured with attention to circulatory status, maintenance of an adequate airway, assisted ventilation as required, and 100% oxygen. Cardiac monitoring in a coronary care unit should continue for at least 48 hours, depending on the clinical status. Treatment is otherwise largely symptomatic and supportive. Patients with preexisting cardiovascular disease will require special consideration of cardiac and pulmonary function (see also Airborne chapter). Hypotension should be treated by elevation of legs, administration of intravenous fluids, and, if necessary, dopamine or norepinephrine; use of beta-adrenoceptor agonists should be carefully monitored. If necessary, an alpha-adrenoceptor agonist (e.g., phenylephrine) may be considered.

Decontamination

Occupational Exposure

After skin contact with nitroglycerin[38,39] thorough washing of skin with soap is necessary. Sodium thiosulfate (10% solution) has been used for this purpose.[2]

Oral Ingestion

Following ingestion, activated charcoal and cathartics may be useful, but there is scant clinical data to support this treatment.

Antidote

There is no antidote for nitroglycerin poisoning.

Supportive Measures

1. Monitor arterial blood gases and methemoglobin levels as clinically indicated. Treat methemoglobinemia with high-flow oxygen and methylene blue (1 to 2 mg/kg) intravenously.
2. Patients with preexisting pulmonary or cardiac disease should undergo cardiac monitoring carefully with special consideration to signs of a possible silent myocardial infarction or congestive heart failure.
3. Repeat methemoglobin levels 1 to 2 hours after initial therapy to assess effectiveness of methemoglobin reduction.
4. Follow with blood counts and reticulocyte counts for evidence of hemolysis (Heinz bodies), especially in patients with G6PD deficiency. Blood transfusions may be required.
5. Monitor for cerebral ischemia due to severe hypotension, especially in the older age groups, those with preexisting orthostatic dizziness, or patients with carotid artery occlusive disease.
6. Patients with normal or low pulmonary capillary wedge pressure may be particularly sensitive to the hypotensive effects of nitroglycerin.

Prevention[2,5]

1. *Engineering and dust controls*
   Process enclosure; use of dust-tight equipment; and prompt and regular cleanup procedures for equipment and work areas.[5]
2. *Explosion prevention*
   Use of explosion-proof, nonsparking dust-tight electric fixtures and wiring; prevention of smoking and the use of open sparks or flames, including welding in nonsecured areas; utilization of antifriction motor bearings; covered lighting; grounding of conductive materials; and prevention of maintenance work done without proper cleanup and entry permits. If motorized equipment is required, it must be specially designed for use in explosive atmospheres.
3. *Explosion containment*
   Detached buildings with explosion-venting systems, subdivided by fire- and pressure-resistant walls, limited personnel access and census in potential explosion areas, limited explosive accumulation in well-ventilated, bullet-resistant, dust-free storage areas; use of tightly sealed storage containers associated with planned, practiced evacuation and emergency measures.
4. *Minimizing skin contact*
   Each worker should be supplied with several complete sets of working clothes and underclothes, including headwear, which should be laundered by the employer; these clothes should be changed at the beginning of each shift; clothes should not contain cuffs or other crevices for dust accumulation; lockers, laundering, and change facilities with showers should be accessible whenever spills occur and at the end of the work shift. Natural and synthetic plastic gloves have been shown to accelerate absorption. Only cotton or cotton-lined gloves should be used by workers handling nitrate esters. Glove changes may need to be performed hourly. Skin absorption can be minimized by easy access to washrooms after spills or before breaks, meals, or toilet use. Use of handkerchiefs (which become contaminated) should be forbidden. Workers should be supplied with disposable facial tissues in a protected container.
5. Food, beverages, or tobacco should not be allowed into the workplace.
6. Where high concentrations of nitroglycerin may be suspected, workers should wear respiratory protective equipment.
7. *Employment examinations*
   Workers with cardiac disorders, hypotension, or labile emotional status should not be engaged in this type of work. Periodic examination will be performed with special regard to blood pressure, pulse rate, signs of cyanosis, edema of the lower extremities, headache, nausea, dizziness, or cough. An electrocardiogram may be of value with plethysmography for early detection of abnormalities.

REFERENCES—NITROGLYCERIN

1. Nitroglycerin. NIOSH Pocket guide to chemical hazards. DHHS (NIOSH) Publication No. 90-117. Washington, DC: US Government Printing Office, pp. 166–167.
2. Glycerol trinitrate. Occupational exposure limits in airborne toxic substances. 3rd ed. Occupational Safety and Health Series. Geneva: International Labour Office, 1991; pp. 210–211.
3. Glycerol trinitrate. Occupational exposure limits in airborne toxic substances. 3rd ed. Occupational Safety and Health Series. Geneva: International Labour Office, 1991; pp. 210–211.
4. Yamaguchi S. Nitroglycerin. In: Encyclopaedia of occupational health and safety. Vol 2. International Labour Office. New York: McGraw-Hill, 1976; pp. 942–944.
5. Panacek EA, Munger MA, Rutherford WF, Gardner SF. Report of nitropatch explosions complication defibrillation. Am J Emerg Med 1992;10:128–129.
6. Wrenn K. Hazards of defibrillation through nitroglycerin patches. Ann Emerg Med 1990;19:1327–1328.
7. Dollery C, ed. Glyceryl trinitrate. In: Therapeutic drugs. Edinburgh: Churchill Livingstone, 1991; G46–G51.
8. Daum S. Nitroglycerin and alkyl nitrates. In: Rom WN, ed. Environmental and occupational medicine. Boston: Little, Brown, 1983; pp. 639–648.
9. Darlington T. The effect of the products of high explosives, dynamite and nitroglycerin on the human system. Med Rec 1890;38:661–662.
10. Anon. The effects of nitroglycerin upon those who manufacture it. JAMA 1898;31:793–794.
11. Laws CE. Nitroglycerin head. JAMA 1910;54:793.
12. Ebright GE. The effects of nitroglycerin on those engaged in its manufacture. JAMA 1914;62:201–202.
13. Rabinowitch IM. Acute nitroglycerin poisoning. Can Med Assoc J 1944;50:199–202.
14. Schwartz AM. The cause, relief and prevention of headaches arising from contact with dynamite. N Engl J Med 1946; 235:541–544.

15. Bresler RR. Nitroglycerin reactions among pharmaceutical workers. Ind Med 1949;18:519–523.
16. Symanski H. Schwere goœundheits schadingungen durch berufliche nitroglykoleinwirkung. Arch Hyg (Berlin) 1952;136:139–158.
17. Barsotti M. Attacchi stenocardici mei lavoratori adettie alla produzione della dinamit con nitroglicole (Attacks of stenocardia in workers engaged in the production of dynamite with nitroglycol). Med Lavoro 1954;45:544–548.
18. Carmichael P, Liebgen J. Sudden death in explosives workers. Arch Environ Health 1963;7:424–439.
19. Lund RP, Haggendal J, Johnsson G. Withdrawal symptoms in workers exposed to nitroglycerin. Br J Ind Med 1968; 25:136–138.
20. Lange RL, Reid MS, Tresch DD, Keelan MH, Bernhard VM, Coolidge G. Nonatheromatous ischemic heart disease following withdrawal from chronic industrial nitroglycerin exposure. Circulation 1972;46:666–678.
21. Hogstedt C, Axelson O. Nitroglycerin-nitroglycol exposure and the mortality in cardio-cerebrovascular diseases among dynamite workers. J Occup Med 1977;19:675–678.
22. Ben-David A. Cardiac arrest in an explosives factory worker due to withdrawal from nitroglycerin exposure. Am J Ind Med 1989;15:719–722.
23. Wei JY, Reid PR. Quantitative determination of trinitroglycerin in human plasma. Circulation 1979;59:588–592.
24. Armstrong PW, Armstrong JA, Marks GS: Blood levels after sublingual nitroglycerin. Circulation 1979;59:585–588.
25. Frank SE, Snyder JT. Survival following severe overdose with mexiteline, nifedipine and nitroglycerin. Am J Emerg Med 1991;9:43–46.
26. Mittal CK, Murad F. Guanylate cyclase: regulation of cyclic GMP metabolism. In: Nathanson JA, Kebabian JW, eds. Cyclic nucleotides. Handbook of experimental pharmacology. Vol 8. Berlin: Springer-Verlag, 1982; pp. 225–260.
27. Murad F. Cyclic guanosine monophosphate as an mediator of vasodilation. J Clin Invest 1986;78:1–5.
28. Winniford MD, Kennedy PL, Wells PJ, Hillis LD. Potentiation of nitroglycerin-induced coronary dilatation by *N*-acetylcysteine. Circulation 1986;73:138–142.
29. Ranft K. Nitrate collapso. Munch Med Wochenschr 1991;133: 589–593.
30. Einert C, Adams W, Crothers R, Moore H, Ottoboni F. Exposure to mixtures of nitroglycerin and ethylene glycol dinitrate. Ind Hyg J 1963; 435–447.
31. Eherenpreis Ed, Young MA, Leikin JB. Symptomatic nitroglycerin toxicity from erroneous use of topical nitroglycerin. Vet Hum Toxicol 1990;32:138–139.
32. Woodward AJ, Lewis PA, Aylward M, Rudman R, Maddock J. Determination of nitroglycerin and its dinitrate metabolites in human plasma by high performance liquid chromatography with thermal energy analyzer detection. J Pharm Sci 1984;73:1838–1840.
33. Lloyd JBF. Glyceryl dinitrates in the detection of skin contact with explosives and related materials of forensic science interest. J Forensic Sci Soc 1986;26:341–348.
34. Lee FW, Watari N, Rigod J, Benet LZ. Simultaneous determination of nitroglycerin and its dinitrate metabolites by capillary gas chromatography with electron-capture detection. J Chromatogr Biomed Appl 1988;426:259–266.
35. Yinon J. Toxicity and metabolism of explosives. Boca Raton, FL: CRC Press, 1990; pp. 81–117.
36. National Institute for Occupational Safety and Health. Criteria for a Recommended Standard. Nitroglycerin and Ethylene Glycol Dinitrate. DHEW Publication No. (NIOSH) 78-167. Washington, DC: US Government Printing Office, 1978.
37. Morikawa Y, Muraki K, Ikoma Y, Honda T, Takamatsu H. Organic nitrate poisoning at an explosives factory. Plethysmographic study. Arch Environ Health 1967;14:614–621.
38. Lloyd JBF. Transfer of nitroglycerin from cardiovascular tablets to hands. J Forensic Sci Soc 1983;23:307–311.
39. Turibell JD, Home JM, Smalldon KW, Higgs DG. Transfer of nitroglycerin to hands during contact with commercial explosives. J Forensic Sci 1982;27:783–791.

PENTAERYTHRITOL TETRANITRATE

Pentaerythritol tetranitrate is a highly explosive chemical substance that does not produce the profound effects on vascular smooth muscle seen with other nitrate esters. Metabolites are generally inactive. Metabolites and residual decomposition products after an explosion are similar in composition. Methemoglobinemia has not been reported following exposure to PETN. Treatment following exposure is symptomatic and supportive.

STRUCTURE AND CLASSIFICATION

PETN is a white crystalline (tetragonal) solid explosive. The molecular weight is 316.2. Its melting point is 141.3°C. PETN explodes at 205 to 215°C.[1] It is particularly sensitive to shock. Its chemical formula is $C(CH_2NO_3)_4$. PETN is insoluble or slightly soluble in acetone. It has a higher chemical stability than all other nitric acid esters.[2] The decomposition products of PETN at 210°C are (wt%) 47.7% NO, 21.0% CO, 11.8% NO_2, 9.5% N_2O, 6.3% CO_2, 2.0% H_2, and 1.6% N_2.[2] As a drug PETN is used for the long-term prophylactic management of angina pectoris.[3]

Following an explosion lower nitrate esters of pentaerythritol (PE-trinitrate, PE-dinitrate) appear in the post-explosion debris as measured by mass spectrometry.[4]

Synonym

PETN.

USES

PETN is one of the most sensitive of the bursting charge explosives and is loaded as such only in detonators. It is also used as a booster charge, in plastic demolition explosives, or as bursting charges when desensitized with TNT or wax[5] to form the less sensitive pentolites.[2] It is also mixed with RDX as a plastic-bonded explosive to form Semtex.[2] PETN has been used as a base charge in antiaircraft shells and mixed with TNT (70-30) in mines, explosive bombs, and torpedoes.[1] When used in blasting caps, it is combined with lead azide and diazodinitrophenol.

OCCUPATIONAL EXPOSURE

PETN may be absorbed through the gastrointestinal tract and by inhalation,[5] but does not appear to be absorbed through the skin.[6,7] It is not a primary skin irritant or a sensitizer.[2]

TOXICOKINETICS

Absorption

About 1 hour after the ingestion of PETN, two organic nitrates are found in the blood (PE-dinitrate and PE-mononitrate). Following a 20-mg ingestion orally of PETN a peak plasma concentration of PE-mononitrate of 4.8 ng/mL is reached in about 4 hours.[8]

Elimination

The plasma half-life of PETN is about 10 minutes.[3] In man PETN is metabolized and degraded stepwise in the small intestine and liver[9] primarily to pentaerythritol trinitrate, pentaerythritol dinitrate, and pentaerythritol mononitrate.[10,11] Within 24 hours the urine excretes PE-mononitrate as the principal metabolite with lesser amounts of PE-dinitrate and PE.[11] Unchanged PETN is also excreted in the feces.[8] The metabolic pathway can be summarized as follows PETN- > PE-triN- > PE-diN- > PE-monoN- > PE.

CLINICAL PRESENTATION

Ingestion of 64 mg produced no change in systolic and diastolic pressure, pulse rate, or electrocardiogram. There was no evidence of a flushed face, headache, or chest discomfort. Patch skin testing with PETN did not induce irritation or sensitization.[6] A rare erythroderma was observed when PETN was ingested with nitroglycerin.[12] Compared with other aliphatic nitric acid esters, PETN demonstrates little toxicity.[7] Exposure to an explosion of PETN may lead to a period of mild hypotension for several hours. Symptoms will probably be minimal. The metabolites are relatively inactive.

LABORATORY

Analytic Methods

A gas chromatography method with ion monitoring can detect plasma levels of pentaerythritol mononitrate to a limit of approximately 0.5 ng/mL.[8] High-performance liquid chromatography can be employed for measuring PETN.[13] Application of liquid chromatography/thermospray/mass spectrometry (LC/TSP/MS) to the separation and identification of commercial and military explosives indicates that less than 2.5 picograms of PETN can be detected from the residues of an explosion.[14,15] Plasma levels can be quantitated by liquid chromatography with a nitrosyl-specific-detector.[16]

Abnormalities

There have been no reports of Heinz body anemia or methemoglobinemia following PETN exposure.

TREATMENT

Treatment will be symptomatic and supportive.

REFERENCES—PENTAERYTHRITOL TETRANITRATE

1. Sax NI. Dangerous properties of industrial materials. 5th ed. New York: Van Nostrand Reinhold, 1979; p. 889.
2. Yinon J. Toxicity and metabolism of explosives. Boca Raton, FL: CRC Press, 1991 pp. 123–132.
3. McEvoy GK, ed. AHFS Drug Information 92. Bethesda, MD: American Society of Hospital Pharmacists, 1992; p. 1022.
4. Basch A, Margalit Y, Abramovich-Bar S, Bamberger Y, Daphna D, Tamiri T, Zitrin S. Decomposition products of PETN in post-explosion analysis. In: Heyndrickx B, ed. Proc Int Assoc Forensic Toxicol. 23rd European International Meeting, Ghent: August 24–27, 2986; pp. 322–331.
5. Sutton WL. Aliphatic nitrocompounds, nitrates, nitrites. In: Patty FA, ed. Industrial hygiene and toxicology. Vol 2. Second Revised Edition. New York: Interscience, 1963; p. 2097.
6. von Oettingen WF. Acute toxic manifestations of PETN. US Public Health Bulletin, 1944;282:23–30.
7. Donahue DD, Monaco AR. Chronic toxic manifestations of PETN. US Public Health Bulletin 1944;282:30–38.
8. Gilbert JD, Aylott RI, Darffan GH, Sogtrop HH. A study of the plasma levels of pentaerythritol mononitrate following administration of pentaerythritol tetranitrate in combination with meprobamate and diphenhydramine. Arzneim-Forsch/Drug Res 1982;32:571–574.
9. Posadas del Rio FA, Juarez FJ, Garcia RC. Biotransformation of organic nitrate esters *in vitro* by human liver, kidney, intestine, and blood serum. Drug Metab Dispos 1988;16:477–481.
10. DiCarlo FJ, Hartigan MJ Jr, Phillips GE. Enzymatic degradation of pentaerythritol tetranitrate by human blood. Proc Soc Exp Biol Med 1975;118:514–516.
11. DiCarlo FJ, Crew MC, Sklow NJ, Coutinho CB, Nonkin P, Simon F, Bernstein A. Metabolism of pentaerythritol tetranitrate by patients with coronary artery disease. J Pharm Exp Ther 1966;153:254–258.
12. Reynolds JEF, ed. Pentaerythritol tetranitrate in *Martindale: The extra pharmacopoeia.* 29th ed. London: The Pharmaceutical Press, 1989; p. 1515.
13. Olsen CS, Scroggins HC. High performance liquid chromatographic determination of the nitrate esters isosorbide dinitrate, pentaerythritol tetranitrate and erythrityl tetranitrate in various tablet forms. J Pharm Sci 1984;73:1303–1304.
14. Berberich DW, Yost RA, Fetterolf DD. Analysis of explosives by liquid chromatography, thermospray/mass spectrometry. J Forensic Sci 1988;33:946–959.
15. Voyksner RD, Yinon J. Trace analysis of explosives by thermospray high-performance liquid chromatography-mass spectrometry. J Chromatogr 1986;354:393–405.
16. Yu WC, Goff EU. Determination of vasodilators and their metabolites in plasma by liquid chromatography with a nitrosyl-specific-detector. Anal Chem 1983;55:29–32.

PROPYLENE GLYCOL DINITRATE

Propylene glycol dinitrate (PGDN) (CAS 6423-43-4), an organic nitrate (Fig. 63–2), is a major component of a liquid torpedo propellant. PGDN is the explosive part of OTTO Fuel II.[1] OTTO Fuel II also contains dibutyl sebacate (a sensitizer) and 2-nitrodiphenylamine (a stabilizer). Defueling and refueling operations are part of a torpedoman's occupation. Angina pectoris and myocardial infarction, occasionally with death, appear to develop in healthy exposed torpedo mates exposed to PGDN with an increased frequency over control subjects.[2] USA OSHA TWA of PGDN is 0.05 ppm 0.3 mg/m^3. OTTO Fuel II experiences include headaches, dizziness, nausea, nasal congestion, dyspnea, and irritated eyes. Chemical identities of OTTO Fuel II and its components are summarized in Table 63–8. A proposed metabolic pathway for PGDN is seen in Figure 63–2.[3] Chemical structures of nitrate esters are found in Figure 63–3.

REFERENCES—PROPYLENE GLYCOL DINITRATE

1. Forman SA. A review of propylene glycol dinitrate toxicology and epidemiology. Toxicol Lett 1988;43:51–65.
2. Forman SA, Helmkamp JC, Bone CM. Cardiac morbidity and mortality associated with occupational exposure to 1, 2 propylene glycol dinitrate. J Occup Med 1987;29:445–450.
3. Godin S, Gregory A, Holland LM (Review Panel) for ATSDR. Toxicological Profile for OTTO Fuel and its Components. Draft profile. May 1993.

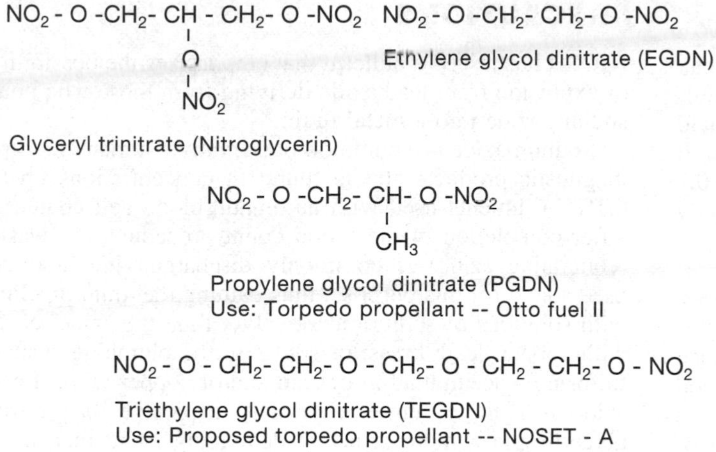

NO_2 - O -CH_2- CH - CH_2- O -NO_2 (with O-NO_2 on the central CH)

Glyceryl trinitrate (Nitroglycerin)

NO_2 - O -CH_2- CH_2- O -NO_2

Ethylene glycol dinitrate (EGDN)

NO_2 - O -CH_2- CH- O -NO_2 (with CH_3 on CH)

Propylene glycol dinitrate (PGDN)
Use: Torpedo propellant -- Otto fuel II

NO_2 - O - CH_2- CH_2- O - CH_2- O - CH_2 - CH_2- O - NO_2

Triethylene glycol dinitrate (TEGDN)
Use: Proposed torpedo propellant -- NOSET - A

Figure 63–2 Chemical structure of nitrate esters. (Adapted from Forman SA. Toxicol Lett 1988;43:51–65.)

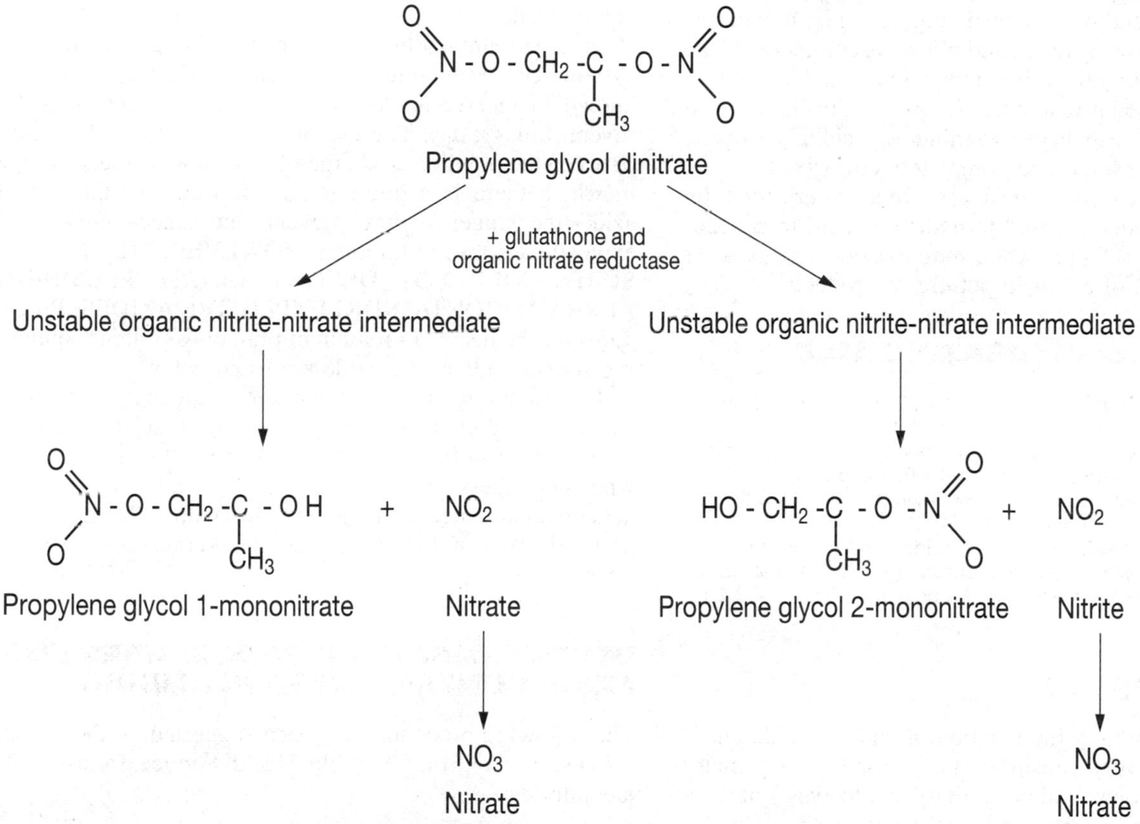

O₂N - O - CH_2 -C - O - NO₂ (with CH_3 on C)

Propylene glycol dinitrate

+ glutathione and organic nitrate reductase

Unstable organic nitrite-nitrate intermediate | Unstable organic nitrite-nitrate intermediate

O_2N - O - CH_2 -C - O H (with CH_3 on C) + NO_2

Propylene glycol 1-mononitrate | Nitrate → NO_3 Nitrate

HO - CH_2 -C - O - NO_2 (with CH_3 on C) + NO_2

Propylene glycol 2-mononitrate | Nitrite → NO_3 Nitrate

Figure 63–3 Proposed metabolic pathway for propylene glycol dinitrate. (Adapted from Agency for Toxic Substances and Disease Register

THE AZIDES

The azides can be classified into two main groups: inorganic azides and organic azides. Inorganic azides include the following:

1. Normal azide—sodium azide (NaN_3), potassium azide (KN_3), barium azide (Ba $[N_3]_2$), and lead azide (Pb $[N_3]_2$).
2. Mixed azides—azide halides, basic azides (Nickel hydroxide azide ($[OH]N_1[N_3]$).
3. Heteroazides—cyanogen azide
4. Azido complex
5. Metal organic azides—triethyl lead azide

Organic azides include ethylazides, amyl azides, azide-cAMP, azido-NAD^+, etc.

HAZARDS

Exposure of both inorganic and organic azides to concentrated sulfuric acid will lead to the production of hydrazoic acid, which can be volatile, toxic, and explosive.[1]

REFERENCES—THE AZIDES

1. Kleinhofs A, Owais WM, Nilan RA. Azide. Mutation research 1978;55:165–195.

HYDRAZOIC ACID

Hydrazoic acid (azoimide), HN_3 (CAS 7782-79-8), is a weak acid of about the same strength as acetic acid.[1] Because of its weak powers of dissociation and volatility, hydrazoic acid is liberated from aqueous solutions of the acid or its salts. It is highly explosive. In Germany the TWA for exposure is 0.1 ppm (0.27 mg/m^3). It boils at 37°C (normal human body temperature), producing a colorless pungent gas.[1]

CLINICAL PRESENTATION

Workmen exposed to hydrazoic acid fumes may experience a rapid and severe fall in both the systolic and diastolic blood pressure together with headaches.[1] Long-term (1 to 15 years) exposure of workers to hydrazoic acid in concentrations of 0.3 to 3.9 ppm failed to induce any observable pathologic change.[1] A 23-year-old chemist accidentally inhaled hydrazoic acid fumes and experienced conjunctivitis, bronchitis, swelling of both knees, fever, and bluish discoloration of the legs. He survived.[2] Intentional inhalation of a 1% solution led to a fall in blood pressure from 125/100 mm Hg to 70/50 mm Hg, collapse, recovery in 15 minutes, residual headache for about one-half hour, and complete recovery.[3]

Headaches and nasal stuffiness were experienced by laboratory personnel exposed to hydrazoic acid in concentrations as low as 0.5 ppm when sodium azide was used for the determination of sulfur in petroleum products.[4]

REFERENCES—HYDRAZOIC ACID

1. Graham JDP, Rogan JM, Robertson DG. Observations on hydrazoic acid. J Ind Hyg Toxicol 1948;30:98–102.
2. Stern R. Uber toxisches wirkungen der stickstoff wasserstoffsaure. Klin Wochenschr (Berlin) 1927;6:304–305.
3. Kocher Z. Ein fall von stickstoff wasserstoff saurevergiftung. Klin Wochenschr (Berlin) 1930;9:2160–2161.
4. Haas JM, Marsh WW Jr. Sodium azide: a potential hazard when used to eliminate interferences in the iodometric determination of sulfur. Am Ind Hyg Assoc J 1970;31:318–332.

LEAD AZIDE

Lead azide is made by the reaction of sodium azide and a lead salt.[1] It is very sensitive and is used as a primary explosive to detonate other military explosives.[1] It is a Department of Transportation Class A explosive.

STRUCTURE AND CLASSIFICATION

Lead azide is $Pb(N_3)_2$. Molecular weight: 291.258.

DESCRIPTION

Lead azide forms colorless or white crystalline needles. Breaking these crystals is believed to initiate detonation. It is very explosive, decomposes when warmed, and is sensitive to light; it is about half as sensitive a detonator as mercury fulminate. Lead azide has several advantages over mercury fulminate. It possesses a considerably higher ignition point and is completely and permanently stable at 50°C. It is unaffected by other metals. The minimum lethal injected dose of lead azide in rats is about 35 mg/kg body weight.[2]

PRECAUTIONS

NIOSH has issued a bulletin that emphasizes the possibility of explosion from lead azide deriving from those who pour sodium azide into a metal drain.[3]

Sodium azide is a common preservative in many in vitro diagnostic products and is found in concentrations up to 0.1% in diluents used with automatic blood cell counters. After completion of the blood count procedure, the waste (containing azide) is commonly discharged into a drain used solely for this purpose, thus bathing the drain pipeline with solutions of sodium azide. Over time the azide reacts with copper, lead, brass, or solder in the plumbing system to form an accumulation of lead and/or copper azide. Lead azide is a more sensitive primary explosive than nitroglycerin and a more effective detonating agent than mercury fulminate; in comparison with lead azide, copper azide is even more explosive and too sensitive to be used commercially.

Future accumulation of lead or copper azides in plumbing systems can be retarded by thoroughly flushing any drain known to receive azides with copious amounts of water several times a day. The use of copper- and lead-free lines between the point of discharge of azide and the nearest pipe in which there is a good stream of water, or the use of azide-free reagents, may prevent future accumulation of explosive azides in plumbing. HOWEVER, THESE MEASURES WILL NOT DECONTAMINATE PLUMBING ALREADY CONTAINING EXPLOSIVE AZIDES. Procedures for the decontamination of plumbing systems containing copper and/or lead azide are listed below.

Laboratory maintenance workers, especially plumbers, should be alerted to the azide hazard so that proper precautions can be taken. Violent explosions have resulted when plumbers have attempted to penetrate blocked, azide-contaminated drainage systems with a flexible metal probe (snake) or to cut or saw azide-contaminated drain lines.

DECONTAMINATION PROCEDURES FOR AZIDE CONTAMINATED PLUMBING

The following procedure has been suggested by the Center for Disease Control, US Public Health Service, for use in its laboratories:

1. Prepare 1 to 2 liters of 10% sodium hydroxide solution (100 g NaOH per liter of water).
2. Siphon all liquid from the trap and drain using a soft rubber or plastic hose. Use proper precautions against any hazardous chemicals that may be present.
3. Slowly pour the sodium hydroxide solution into the trap.
4. Tape to the sink a warning sign reading "Do Not Use Sink . . . Contains Caustic Material."
5. Allow the solution to remain in the trap for a minimum of 16 hours.
6. Flush the drain with water for a minimum of 15 minutes. If the drain will not flow, the sodium hydroxide should be removed by siphoning, if possible, then diluted with water. Maintenance personnel should be advised that the drain is potentially contaminated with explosive agents and caustic material.

The above procedure is designed to decontaminate a drain trap. Longer lengths of drain lines can be decontaminated with a similar procedure after plugging the drain below the point at which any azide contamination is likely to have occurred and then filling the entire length of pipe with 10% sodium hydroxide solution.

Where it is not possible for a drain line to remain filled with sodium hydroxide solution for at least 16 hours, Coulter Electronics, Inc. has suggested the following:

1. Pour five gallons of sodium hydroxide solution into the piping rapidly enough to simulate the flushing action of a water closet. CAUTION: The solution is caustic!
2. Allow the pipe to remain undisturbed by water or other effluents for at least 16 hours.
3. Flush with copious amounts of water.
4. Repeat steps 1, 2, and 3 two more times at intervals of a week or so.

Descriptions of several other procedures that have been suggested for the decontamination of azides are listed in the *Journal of Chemical Education.*

PRECAUTIONS

Because the possibility of residual sodium hydroxide will always exist, personnel should wear gloves and face shields when breaking the drain line or trap for maintenance. (This equipment should be worn when breaking any laboratory drain, as the presence of hazardous chemicals should always be suspected.)

Extreme caution should be exercised when plugging a drain line potentially contaminated with heavy metal azides.

The decontamination of plumbing systems containing copper or its alloys (e.g., brass) should include a supplemental treatment with nitrous acid, since the sodium hydroxide procedure may not adequately remove accumulations of copper azides. The following nitrous acid decontamination procedure[4] has been employed with success:

1. Close the exit of the drain beyond the point of potential azide accumulation.
2. Fill the drain line with nitrous acid, prepared immediately before use by mixing equal volumes of a 20% solution of acetic acid with a 20% solution of sodium nitrite. CAUTION! The area should be well ventilated, as toxic vapors (oxides of nitrogen) may be released when azide reacts with nitrous acid.
3. Allow the nitrous acid solution to remain in the drain for 24 hours.
4. Open the exit of the drain.
5. Immediately repeat procedure once.

NOTE: The decontamination of plumbing systems is complicated by a number of factors, including the possible coating of heavy metal azides by impervious materials, as well as the possible accumulation of heavy metal azides in cracks and threads of plumbing. Although the decontamination procedures do reduce the risk of explosion, even a "decontaminated" system should be treated with respect in recognition of the possibility of its being explosive. Maintenance people should be alerted so that proper precautions can be taken before working on plumbing potentially contaminated with heavy metal azides. Good work practices include shielding the person working on the plumbing, maximizing the distance between the person and the plumbing, and keeping all unnecessary personnel out of the area.

Lead azide is almost insoluble (1%) in cold water, and nearly zero in ammonium hydroxide solution, ether, acetone, or ethanol; it is quite soluble in heated, strongly acid, or strongly alkaline solutions. When dry, it does not corrode most metals; when moist, lead azide, like the azides of gold, silver, copper, mercury, tin, and zinc, forms extremely sensitive and dangerous azide compounds.[4]

REFERENCES—LEAD AZIDE

1. Winning CH. Explosives industry. In: Encyclopaedia of occupational health and safety. Vol 1. International Labour Office. New York: McGraw-Hill, 1976; pp. 493–496.
2. Fairhall LT, Henrette WV, Pritchard EA. The toxicity of lead azide. Public Health Rep (USA) 1943;58:607–617.
3. Finklea JF. Explosive azide hazard. Current Intelligence Bulletin 12. NIOSH. August 16, 1976.
4. Shaney Felt W. Complexities of lead azide. Govt Reports Announcements & Index (GR & I). Issue 23, 1985.

SODIUM AZIDE

Sodium azide is a very toxic chemical. Reports of 28 cases of illness following exposure indicate that 20 patients have survived.[1–3] Eight have died.[1,4–6] Ingestions of sodium azide have been inadvertent and intentional, and many such incidents have occurred in laboratory personnel (Table 63–5). An outbreak of epidemic hypotension occurred in a group of patients whose dialysis fluid was inadvertently contaminated during hemodialysis.[3] These patients survived. There are no effective antidotes. Treatment of sodium azide poisoning is symptomatic and supportive.

EXPLOSIVE AZIDE HAZARD

Sodium azide explosions associated with automated blood counters have occurred at hospitals. After completion of the blood count procedures, the waste (containing azide) is discharged into a drain. The azide reacts with the plumbing system to form an accumulation of lead and/or copper azide. Violent explosions have resulted when plumbers have attempted to penetrate blocked azide-contaminated drainage systems with a flexible metal probe (snake) or to cut or saw azide contaminated drain lines.[7,8]

STRUCTURE AND CLASSIFICATION

The azides, sodium azide—NaN_3; potassium azide—KN_3; and lead azide—Pb (N_3) are water-soluble crystals that form hydrazoic acid (HN_3), or azoimide, when dissolved in water. Azoimide (hydrazoic acid) has a boiling point of 37°C (normal body temperature) producing a colorless and pungent gas that is toxic when inhaled.[2]

Sodium azide is the neutral stable sodium salt of hydrazoic acid (azoimide). Hydrazoic acid forms explosive salts with heavy metals.[9]

Table 63–5
Diagnosis of Unknown Poisoning in Knowledgeable Personnel[a]

Poison	Diagnostic Clues
Barbiturates	Characteristic clinical presentation in knowledgeable personnel. Pill fragments on gastric lavage (refutes other metabolics/CNS diagnoses) Exclusion of other potential diagnoses through metabolic workup and CT scanning. Barbiturate level or toxic screen. Hypothermia. Pinpoint pupils, nystagmus.
Carbon monoxide	History of potential exposure (found unconscious in car, garage, at fire). New onset of arrhythmias/myocardial ischemia. New onset lactic acidosis, altered mental status, seizure. Equal "cherry-red" coloration of retinal arteries and veins. Oxygen saturation gap >5%.
Cyanide	Availability to victim in workplace or home. Aroma of "bitter almonds" to gastric aspirate. Unexplained "cherry-red" coloration of retinal arteries and veins. Oxygen saturation gap >5%. Anion gap metabolic acidosis (unexplained). Fire victims. New onset seizures. Pulmonary edema.
Azides	Availability to victim in workplace or home. Pungent aroma to gastric aspirate. Unexplained and severe lactic acidosis. Alternating CNS restlessness and atony. Positive ferric chloride testing of gastric aspirate (red precipitate). Headache and nausea in resuscitation team members.
Methemoglobin-inducing chemicals	Availability to victim in workplace or home. Bitter "petrochemical" smell of certain chemicals. Cyanosis refractory to oxygen. "Chocolate brown" appearance of blood.

[a]Adapted from Binder L, Fredrickson L. Am J Emerg Med 1991;9:11–15.

Sodium Azide[10]		
CAS 26628-22-8		
USA (ACGIH)		STEL 0.11 ppm (ceiling value) 0.3 mg/m^3
OSHA (as HN_3)		0.1 ppm (ceiling value)
OSHA (as NaN_3)		0.3 mg/m^3 (ceiling value)
UK	TWA 0.1 ppm 0.3 mg/m^3	STEL 0.1 ppm 0.3 mg/m^3
Germany	TWA 0.07 ppm 0.2 mg/m^3	
France	STEL -4.1 ppm; 0.3 mg/m^3	
Australia	TWA 011 ppm 0.3 mg/m^3	

USES

In the 1950s sodium azide was investigated as an antihypertensive drug.[11,12] The ability of sodium azide to degrade rapidly into nitrogen (N_2) gas makes it useful in several industries. Its main current use is in the automobile air-bag industry where it is used as a propellant and source of detonation. Additional uses include its role in the production of the explosive munition primer lead azides,[1,3] for the preservation of sera and other reagents in pathology laboratories,[13] for pressure in airplane escape chutes,[6] in the agricultural industry as a herbicide, fungicide, and menticide (but its rapid degradation limits its usefulness),[6] in the petrochemical industry for determination of the extent of sulfur contamination of oil.[14] Hospitals and laboratories use azides in automated blood cell counters as a constituent of diluting fluid,[15] in chemical reactions requiring nitrogen donors, and to poison mitochondria in physiologic experiments.[16] It may be found in a 4% concentration in a Tris buffering solution employed in screening for hepatitis antigen.[17] Hence, laboratory, pharmaceutical, and health care personnel may have access to these chemicals, as well as professionals in the munitions, automotive, petrochemical, and agricultural industries.[2]

THERAPEUTIC DOSES

Hypertensive patients have been treated with sodium azide 0.65 to 3.9 mg by mouth daily for 1 week to 2 years with few ill effects.[11] Sodium azide 1.3 mg three times daily for 10 days given to normal individuals orally did not produce a sustained effect on blood pressure. A pounding sensation in the head was felt by some subjects.[13]

TOXIC DOSE

An estimated dose of 5 to 150 mg of sodium azide was accidentally ingested. The patient survived.[13,16,18] Inadvertent contamination of dialysis fluid with sodium azide led to toxic symptoms in nine patients attending a dialysis unit who were exposed to an estimated intravenous dose of 17 to 80 μg/kg.[3] This compares with hypotensive doses following oral ingestion of approximately 300 μg/kg[17,18] and 10 to 20 μg/kg.[13]

FATAL DOSE

Fatalities have followed ingestion of 700 to 800 mg (13 to 15 mg/kg),[4,5] 1 to 2 g (20 to 40 mg/kg),[1] 10 to 20 g (200 to 400 mg/kg),[19] 15 to 20 g (300 to 400 mg/kg),[6] and 55 g (1000 mg/kg).[1]

MECHANISM OF ACTION

The azides accumulate in the mitochondria where they uncouple oxidative phosphorylation and inhibit energy transfer.[2,18,20] They strongly inhibit cytochrome oxidase and catalase[21] and increase the rate of formation of inorganic phosphate from ATP.[20] This results in lactic acid accumulation, vascular smooth muscle relaxation, increased gastrointestinal and urologic smooth muscle tone, and alternating central nervous system effects.[13,19,22] A noncardiogenic pulmonary edema may supervene.[18] A precise mechanism of action has not been determined. Although inadequate data are available on which to formulate a specific antidote, an in vitro study suggests the formation of cyanide in the presence of sodium azide.[23] Anecdotal case reports and the in vitro formation of cyanide suggest that treatment for cyanide intoxication, as well as monitoring the cyanide level in the blood, may be useful in the management of sodium azide intoxication.

CLINICAL PRESENTATION[1–24]

Azide exposure may induce cough, conjunctivitis, central nervous system depression (seizures, collapse, muscle flaccidity, hyporeflexia, coma, fixed pupils, blurred vision, headache, dizziness), gastrointestinal stimulation (nausea, vomiting, diarrhea), vascular smooth muscle relaxation (hypotension and reflex tachycardia), and a pungent odor. This may later be followed by lactic acidosis and death in a few days. Diagnosis is difficult without a history of azide exposure. If there is no history, knowledge of the patient's occupation and availability of azide may be useful. Evidence of alternating CNS restlessness and atony together with evidence of progressive cellular anoxia (clinical hypoxia, metabolic acidosis with anion gap, apnea, hypotension) and development of mild toxicity (headache, nausea) in members of the resuscitation team[6] may aid in establishing a diagnosis. In those who survive following ingestion of lower doses, and have experienced transient hypotension, headaches, and nausea,[6] recovery may be complete within hours.

LABORATORY

Analytic Methods

A high-performance liquid chromatography method is available with sensitivity to sodium azide in the nanogram range.[25] Detection limit is about 10 ng/mL.

Autopsy

Postmortem findings have demonstrated varying degrees of pulmonary, cerebral, and myocardial wall edema with foci of myocardial necrosis.[1]

Abnormalities

Sodium- and potassium azide-induced hydrazoic acid boils at 37°C and readily volatizes through the lungs, mucous membranes, and skin. The hydrazoic gas that is exhaled and also present in gastric aspirate may cause mild impairment of emergency department personnel.[6]

Elevated levels of white blood cells (leukocytes), plasma lactate, and blood glucose have been observed. A wide anion gap metabolic acidosis is probably due to lactate accumulation. The electrocardiogram may vary from a bradycardia pattern to a sinus tachycardia, with nonspecific T-wave changes.[1] Elevation in the ST-T segment ventricular tachycardias terminating in wide complex rhythm, ventricular fibrillation, and asystole have been observed.[4] Chest x-rays, coagulation parameters, cyanide levels, toxic urine screens, liver function tests, and renal function tests have usually been within normal limits.[1] A Swan-Ganz catheter may be used to measure central venous pressure, pulmonary artery pressure, and pulmonary capillary wet pressure.[19]

Ancillary Tests

A few drops of Ferrichloride added to the filtered gastric aspirate will produce a reddish precipitate due to production of ferric azide—$Fe(N^3)^3$.[13,24]

TREATMENT

Stabilization

Rapid support of respiration and circulation will require hospitalization in a unit where cardiac monitoring and an oxygen supply will be immediately available. Azide poisoning will respond to symptomatic and supportive care, including, if required, assisted ventilation, administration of 100% oxygen, and insertion of intravenous lines. Oxygen (100%) should be used routinely in moderate or severely symptomatic patients even if a normal PO_2 is present. 100% oxygen increases O_2 delivery and may reactivate azide-inhibited mitochondrial enzymes. Comatose patients should receive an initial trial of naloxone and intravenous glucose.

Decontamination

Remove contaminated clothing. Gastric lavage with tracheal protection may be useful if performed within a few hours of ingestion. Syrup of ipecac should not be used since seizures may intervene and predispose the patient to an aspiration pneumonitis. Care of a patient involved in a motor vehicle accident with an air bag should include careful examination of the eyes, as well as washing of exposed areas of skin. Emergency personnel should wear gloves and eye protection.[26]

Elimination Enhancement

There has been no clinical evidence to support the use of hemodialysis, hemoperfusion, activated charcoal, or whole bowel irrigation in azide poisoning.[19]

Antidote

There are no antidotes available. Attempts to induce methemoglobinemia with the nitrites have led to methemoglobin levels of only 15%,[13] perhaps insufficiently elevated to test the usefulness of this procedure in azide poisoning. Naloxone does not appear to be effective.[19]

Supportive Measures

Patients should be followed for at least 48 to 72 hours with cardiac monitoring. Development of aspiration pneumonia or pulmonary edema in comatose patients should be treated supportively. Metabolic acidosis should be corrected with sodium bicarbonate if the pH falls below 7.15. Hypotension may be treated with position change, intravenous fluids, or pressor amines, as required. Lidocaine and cardioversion were ineffective in one patient.[19] Cerebral edema may be responsive to hyperventilation. Intracranial pressure should be monitored where there is evidence of cerebral dysfunction. Metabolic and electrolyte abnormalities should be treated as indicated.

Special instructions have been recommended by the U.S. Food and Drug Administration for the treatment of dialysis

Table 63–6
Information Sources for Automobile Air Bags

	Phone Number
Chrysler Corporation	1-313-956-4378
Ford Motor Company	1-313-845-8301
General Motors	1-313-556-1597
National Highway Traffic Safety Admin. Office of Occupant Protection	1-202-366-2711

filters preserved with sodium azide. New sodium azide–preserved filters should be rinsed with at least 500 gallons of water, and all rinsing fluid should be discarded before beginning production of dialysis-quality water.[8] Disposal of liquid laboratory wastes containing sodium azide have been outlined by Upton and Donelson.[27]

Air Bags

Air-bag inflation involves the ignition of sodium azide through a spark detonator. Products of the combustion of sodium azide are nitrogen gas (which inflates the rubberized nylon bag), ash (black dust), and small particles of sodium hydroxide that may quickly convert by reaction with carbon dioxide and water vapor in the air to sodium carbonate and sodium bicarbonate. These products may produce ocular injuries and facial burns.[28–30] (A booklet "General Motors Answers Your Questions About Air Bags in GM Cars in Emergency Rescue Situations," dated June 1990, is available by writing ATTN: Air Bag Booklet, GM Corporation, Public Relations, N2-PR, Warren, MI 48090). Information sources for automobile air bags are listed in Table 63–6.

REFERENCES—SODIUM AZIDE

1. Klein-Schwartz W, Gorman RL, Oderda GM, Massaro BP, Kurt TL, Garriott JC. Three fatal sodium azide poisonings. Med Toxicol Adverse Drug Exp 1989;4:219–227.
2. Binder L, Frederickson L. Poisonings in laboratory personnel and health care professionals. Am J Emerg Med 1991;9:11–15.
3. Gordon SM, Crachman J, Bland LA, Reid MH, Favero M, Jarvis WR. Epidemic hypotension in a dialysis center caused by sodium azide. Kidney Int 1990;37:110–115.
4. Judge KW, Ward NE. Fatal azide-induced cardiomyopathy presenting as acute myocardial infarction. Am J Cardiol 1989;64:830–831.
5. Howard JD, Skogerbae KJ, Case GA, Raisys VA, Lacsina EQ. Death following sodium azide ingestion. J Forensic Sci 1990;35:193–196.
6. Abrams J, El-Mallakh RS, Meyer R. Suicidal sodium azide ingestion. Ann Emerg Med 1987;16:1378–1380.
7. Finklea JF. Explosive azide hazard. Current Intelligence Bulletin 13. NIOSH. August 16, 1976.
8. Precautions for hemodialysis filters. FDA Drug Bulletin 1989;19(2):18–19.
9. Graham JDP. Actions of sodium azide. Br J Pharmacol 1949;4:1–6.
10. Occupational Exposure Limits for Airborne Toxic Substances. Occupational Safety and Health Series 37. Geneva: International Labor Office, 1991.
11. Black MM, Zweifach BW, Speer FD. Comparison of hypotensive actions of sodium azide in normotensive and hypertensive patients. Proc Soc Exp Biol Med 1954:85:11–16.
12. Maher FT, Bollinan JG. Hypotensive effects of sodium nitroprusside and sodium azide in dogs. Fed Proc 1955;14:412 (abstract).
13. Edmonds OP, Bourne MS. Sodium azide poisoning in five laboratory technicians. Br J Ind Med 1982;39:308–309.
14. Haas JM, Marsh WW Jr. Sodium azide: a potential hazard when used to eliminate interferences in the iodometric determination of sulfur. Am Ind Hyg Assoc J 1970;31:318–321.
15. Richardson SGN, Giles C, Swan CHJ. Two cases of sodium azide poisoning by accidental ingestion of isoton. J Clin Pathol 1975;28:350–351.
16. Kleinhofs A, Owais WM, Nilan RA. Azide. Mutat Res 1978;55:165–195.
17. Roberts RJ, Simmons A, Barrett DA II. Accidental exposures to sodium azide. Am J Clin Pathol 1974;61:879–880.
18. Emmett EA, Ricking JA. Fatal self-administration of sodium azide. Ann Intern Med 1975;83:224–226.
19. Albertson TE, Reed S, Siefkin A. A case of fatal sodium azide ingestion. Clin Toxicol 1986;24:339–351.
20. Robertson HE, Boyer PD. The effect of azide on phosphorylation accompanying electron transport and glycolysis. J Biol Chem 1955;214:295–305.
21. Foulkes EC, Leinberg R. The azide inhibition of catalase. Enzymologia 1949;13:302–312.
22. Gobbi A. Tre casi di intossicazione da sodio-azide. Med Laboro 1967;58:297–300.
23. Kozlicka-Gajdzinska H, Brzyski J. A case of fatal intoxication with sodium azide. Archiv f Toxikolog 1966;22:160–163.
24. Lanbert W, Meyer E, De Leenheer A: Cyanide and sodium azide intoxication. Ann Emerg Med 1995;36:392.
25. Burger E, Bauer HM: Akuter vergiftungs fall durch verschentliches trinken von natriumazid losung. Archiv f Toxikolog 1965;20:279–283.
26. Swarin SJ, Waldo RA. Liquid chromatographic determination of azide as the 3,5-dinitrobenzoyl derivative. J Liq Chromatog 1982;5:597–604.
27. Lawson KS. Sodium azide. Clin Toxicol Rev 1993;15 (4):1-2.
28. Upton D, Donelson V: Proper disposal of liquid laboratory waste containing sodium azide. Am Ind Hyg Assoc J 1981; 42:A-16–A-18.
29. Ingraham HJ, Perry HD, Donnenfeld ED. Air-bag keratitis. N Engl J Med 1991;325:1599–1600.
30. Conover K. Chemical burn from automotive air bags. Ann Emerg Med 1992;21:770.
31. Steinmann B. A 40-year-old woman with an air bag–mediated injury. J Emerg Nurs 1992;18:308–310.

TETRYL

Tetryl exposure may induce a serious sensitization of the skin requiring removal from exposure. Respiratory and gastrointestinal complaints are relatively minor and respond to symptomatic and supportive treatment after removal from a tetryl source. The skin staining is easily removed and not associated with a dermatitis. Systemic effects of tetryl exposure are otherwise minimal.

STRUCTURE AND CLASSIFICATION

Tetryl (purified) is colorless when fresh, becoming yellow on exposure to light.[1] After ordinary manufacture tetryl has a pale lemon or buff color. It is odorless and forms monoclinic prisms. Pure tetryl has a melting point of 129.45°C; military tetryl melting point is 128.75°C.[1–3] It is soluble in benzene, acetone, and ethylene dichloride; slightly soluble in ethanol, ether, carbon disulfide, carbon tetrachloride, and chloroform; and almost insoluble in water.[4]

Tetryl has a molecular weight of 287.2 and explodes at a boiling point of 356 to 374°F.[5] Tetryl is blended with graphite or stearic acid and pressed into pellets.

STANDARDS[6]

CAS 479-45-8	USA—NIOSH	TWA 1.5 mg/m^3 (skin)
	UK	TWA 1.5 mg/m^3 skin, STEL 3 mg/m^3
	Germany	TWA 1.5 mg/m^3, skin, sensitizer
	France	TWA 1.5 mg/m^3, skin
	Australia	TWA 1.5 mg/m^3, sensitizer

Synonyms

"C.E." (compound, exploding); tetralite; pyrenite; 2,4,6 trinitrophenylmethylnitramine; CE powder; *N*-methyl-N,2,4,6-tetranitroaniline; nitramine; 2,4,6-tetryl.

Addition of a 13% aqueous solution of sodium sulfite to tetryl converts tetryl to a nonexplosive, water-soluble compound.[4] Tetryl is stable at room temperature for at least 20 years.[4]

USES

Tetryl is used as a booster explosive that is ignited by a detonation charge and in turn detonates the bursting charge. It is also used as a base charge in detonators.[1] Tetryl is more sensitive to impact, friction, and initiation by lead azide or mercury fulminate than TNT. It has a greater rate of detonation than TNT.[2,4]

PRODUCT FORMULATION

Tetryl is formulated with stearic acid or graphite for final use.

SOURCES

Dimethylaniline is nitrated (nitric acid) and oxidized (sulfuric acid, acetone) to form crystallized tetryl.[4]

CLINICAL PRESENTATION

Staining of Skin

Tetryl powder stains hair and the skin of the hands, face, and neck.[7–10] In industry the terms "canary" and "tetryl blood" describe this.[8] On exposure to sunlight the stain may deepen to an orange color.[7] The staining is not indicative of tetryl illness or dermatitis. Those with an oily skin or who perspire greatly appear to be most affected.[4] Fading begins as soon as the subject is removed from contact, but may not be complete for several months.

Tetryl Dermatitis

This is the most common complaint of workers with tetryl. It is found in at least 50% of those who come into close contact with the powder.[9] Within 10 to 20 days after a first exposure an erythema may appear following a few hours of exposure on the face, near the mouth, and on the cheeks appearing like a second-degree burn.[9,10] The erythema may clear spontaneously or later be accompanied by a dry, scaly rash. The skin ultimately takes on a glistening appearance. Edema of the eyelids and periorbital tissue sufficient to close the eyelids may be observed with or without conjunctivitis. Within days a serous exudate from the affected skin may be seen. Ultimately a papular patchy type of rash is found on the neck, shoulders, and forearms that may become lichenified. A true sensitization reaction affects the face, neck, forehead, ears, wrists, trunk, and legs and may cause irritation of the perineum.[10] The acute reaction may take a few hours to develop; the more chronic lesions will come on in days or weeks.

Prior presence of skin lesions such as acne vulgaris, extensive postburn scarring, pigmentary changes, or psoriasis do not appear to increase susceptibility to tetryl dermatitis. Those with seborrhea or dry scaly skin should not be in contact with tetryl. The dermatitis appears more often in male employees and more often in winter.[10] The presence of powder on workers may sensitize family members at home.

When less than 2% of the skin surface is involved, removal from contact with tetryl will often lead to skin clearing in 7 days.[4] If resumption of work leads to recurrence of the dermatitis, the patient is considered tetryl sensitive. If over 2% of the skin surface is involved, the worker is considered to be tetryl sensitive.[4]

Respiratory Tract

Burning, itching, and "dry throat," sharp tingling sensations in the nose, sneezing, and coryza may lead to repetitive rubbing of the nose and ultimately to nose bleeds. Small ulcerations of the nasal mucosa may be seen. Usually epistaxis is seen in those with a tetryl dermatitis. This may begin on the first day or as late as the third month of work. Those working in a very dusty tetryl powder environment will almost all begin to have a dry, deep cough that becomes productive within a few weeks.[4] Tracheitis and asthmalike attacks of wheezing with dyspnea on exertion may be accompanied by rhonchi, wheezes, and emphysema on a physical examination.[10,11] Removal from work will usually lead to remission of symptoms within 2 to 4 weeks.

Gastrointestinal

In the first few days at work nausea, vomiting, abdominal cramps, and diarrhea may occasionally be present. These symptoms have no relation to food intake.[7] No chronic gastrointestinal dysfunctions are observed.

Neurologic

Workers may experience irritability, easy fatigability, general malaise, headaches, lassitude, and sleeplessness, but exhibit no abnormal neurologic signs.[4] Psychologic distress may follow rumors of "power poisoning."

Hematopoietic System

No evidence of a blood disease or a hemorrhagic tendency has been seen.[4]

Circulatory System

There is no evidence of cardiovascular dysfunction.[4]

Systemic—Long-Term

No good clinical evidence exists of any chronic neurologic, hematopoietic, or cardiovascular dysfunction. Several patients followed for 5 years developed swelling of the legs and abdomen, jaundice and loss of weight, and died of cirrhosis of the liver. The role of alcohol ingestion has not been ruled out.[11]

Eyes

Conjunctivitis usually develops with a dermatitis of the face, but may persist after the rash has subsided. Iridocyclitis and keratitis may be seen.[10]

LABORATORY

Analytic Methods

Limits of detection by thin-layer chromatography (TLC) are 0.25 μg, and by high-performance liquid chromatography (HPLC), 0.0005 μg.[12,13]

Ancillary Tests

A slight decrease in hemoglobin concentrations has been observed.[9] There may be a temporary mild leukocytosis or leukopenia. Acetonuria has been observed.[11] Anemia and abnormal liver function tests have rarely been observed in patients dying of hepatic failure 5 years after exposure.[11]

TREATMENT

Staining of skin

1. Remove from source of contact.
2. Use a medicated (green soap) with an indicator (sodium sulfite). Wash until no pink color is seen in the lather. Wash at the break in work in the morning and afternoon, before lunch, and before leaving for home.

Dermatitis

1. Remove patient from tetryl exposure.
2. Calamine lotion USP without phenol or calamine ointment NF. Aluminum acetate soaks (Burow's solution) as required. Lanolin for weeping area.
3. If over 2% of body involved consider tetryl sensitivity at first examination. Do not return to work. Use of sodium thiosulfate and antihistamines are ineffective.[4]
4. For patients with over 10% of the body surface involved with a severe acute dermatitis, consider epinephrine injection and hospitalization. Patch testing may induce sensitization response.[8]
5. Nosebleeds—local nasal pressure; local epinephrine; cauterization with silver nitrate NF.[4]

Respiratory Complications

Remove patient from source of tetryl—cough, bronchitis will clear within 10 days to 3 weeks.

Gastrointestinal

For abdominal cramps, diarrhea—midmorning and mid-afternoon snacks. Milk at intervals. Aluminum hydroxide gel, antispasmodics.

Eyes

Ice packs. Ophthalmology consultation.

Prevention

1. Preemployment physical
   Do not employ if history or evidence of the following:[4]

Pulmonary	Arrested tuberculosis
	Fungous infection
	Repeated respiratory infections
	Bronchiectasis
	Pneumoconiosis
	Silicosis
	Asthma
Gastrointestinal	Peptic ulcer
	Colitis
Others	Severe anemia
	Chronic skin disorder
	Recurrent hives
	Serum sensitivity
	Drug sensitivity
	Severe food allergies

   Do chest x-ray periodically.
2. Limiting exposure
   Repeat cautions regarding personal cleanliness, washing, and clothes. Use masks where possible and protective overclothes. Employ glassed barricades for handling. Use no gloves or protective creams. Wash with indicator soap before using the lavatory, eating, or going home. Shower after each day's work. Employ separate facilities for changing clothes. Consider weekly rotation of worker's jobs.[1]
3. Ventilation
   Employ exhaust fans close to the operation. No forced air currents in room. Where possible, use respirators with masks. Take frequent air samples to test for maximal allowable concentration.
4. Utilization of affected personnel
   Do not expose tetryl-sensitive personnel to picryls. Tetryl-sensitive personnel can work with TNT, dinitrotoluene, nitroglycerin, and black powder (potassium nitrate, sulfur, carbon mixtures).[4,14]

REFERENCES—TETRYL

1. Yinon J. Toxicity and metabolism of explosives. Boca Raton, FL: CRC Press, 1990;69–80.
2. Sax NI. Dangerous properties of industrial materials. New York: Van Nostrand Reinhold, 1979;1022–1023.
3. Parmeggiam L. Tetryl. Encyclopaedia of occupational health and safety. Vol 2. Geneva: International Labour Office. New York: McGraw-Hill, 1976;1397–1398.
4. Bergman BB. Tetryl toxicity: a summary of ten years' experience. Arch Ind Hyg Occup Med 1952;5:10–20.
5. NIOSH Pocket Guide to Chemical Hazards. DHHS (NIOSH) Publication No 90-117, Washington, DC: US Government Printing Office, 1990; pp. 212–213.
6. Occupational Exposure Limits for Airborne Toxic Substances. *n*-Methyl-*n*,2,4,6-tetranitroaniline. Occupational Safety and

Health Series 37. Geneva: International Labour Office, 1991; pp. 276–277 Hem 1374.
7. Hilton J, Swanston CN. Clinical manifestations of tetryl and trinitrotoluene. Br Med J 1941;2:509–510.
8. Witkowski LJ, Fischer CN, Murdock HD. Industrial illness due to tetryl. JAMA 1942;119:1406–1409.
9. Brabham VW. Tetryl illness in munitions plants. J SC Med Assoc 1943;39:93–95.
10. Troup HB. Clinical effects of tetryl (CE powder). Br J Ind Med 1946;3:20–23.
11. Hardy HL, Maloof CC. Evidence of systemic effect of tetryl and summary of available literature. Arch Ind Hyg Occup Med 1950;1:545–550.
12. Lyter AH III. A high-performance liquid chromatographic (HPLC) study of seven common explosive materials. J Forensic Sci 1983;28:446–450.
13. Farey MG, Wilson SE. Quantitative determination of tetryl and its degradation products by high-pressure liquid chromatography. J Chromatogr 1975;114:261–265.
14. Borges T, Edwards G, Spanggord R (Peer Review Panel). ATSDR. Toxicological profile for tetryl. Draft, May 1993.

2,4,6-TRINITROTOLUENE (TNT)

The toxicity of TNT exposure in munitions workers has been reported since World War I.[1] There were 17,000 cases of TNT poisoning in the United States with 475 deaths within a period of 7½ months of the First World War. Between 1941 and 1945 there were 22 deaths (<3 occupational disease fatalities/100,000 operating employees/year). Of these twenty-two fatal cases, eight died of a toxic hepatitis and 14 of aplastic anemia.[1] In the United Kingdom there were 24 cases diagnosed as aplastic anemia due to TNT between 1939 and 1946; nine recovered and 15 died.[2] Both toxic hepatitis and aplastic anemia may have an insidious onset. A rigorous preventive medicine program should be in force at the munitions factory where workers may be exposed to TNT and where premonitory symptoms and subtle laboratory signs may enhance an early diagnosis and treatment.[3]

STRUCTURE AND CLASSIFICATION

Crystal: TNT exists as colorless orthothrombic crystal or as yellow monoclinic needles.[4,5]
Melting point: 80.65°C
Ignition temperature: 300°C
Molecular weight: 227.15
Molecular formula: $C_7H_5N_3O_6$

TNT is insoluble in water and soluble in oils, greases, ether, acetone, and alcohol.

STANDARDS[6,7]

2,4,6 trinitrotoluene

CAS 118-96-7			
	USA—OSHA	TWA 0.5 mg/m³ skin	
	UK	TWA 0.5 mg/m³ STEL 0.5 mg/m³	
	Germany	TWA 0.01 ppm: 0.1 mg/m³	Substance with systemic effects of 1 hour suspected of carcinogenic potential
	France	TWA 0.5 mg/m³ skin	
	Australia	TWA 0.5 mg/m³ skin	

Reductions in hemoglobin levels or red blood cell counts have been noted at exposures as low as 0.2 mg/m³.[7] An ambient water quality criterion for the protection of human health of 135 μg/L has been proposed when consumption of both contaminated water and fish is expected. For drinking water alone, the proposed criterion is 140 μg/L.[8] A lifetime health advisory of 2 μg/L is proposed.[9]

Synonyms

TNT, triton, trotyl, tritolo, trotol, trinol, trilite, trinitrotoluol, sym-trinitrotoluene, 1-methyl-2,4,6-trinitrobenzene.

TNT is relatively insensitive to impact, friction, shock, and electrostatic energy.[4] It requires a fall of 1.3 m for a 2-kg weight to detonate it.[3] It can be detonated by detonators and blasting caps. For full efficiency, use of a high-velocity initiator such as tetryl is required. TNT may be regarded as the equivalent of 40% dynamite and can be used under water.

USES

TNT is employed as an explosive. It is used in all types of bursting charges, including armor-piercing types.[5] TNT is used in the manufacture of a detonator fuse known as Cordeau Detonant.[5]

PRODUCT FORMULATION

TNT may be used alone or with ammonium nitrate (Amatol) or barium nitrate (Baratol).[10]

SOURCES

Toluene nitrate with a mixture of sulfuric acid and nitric acid at 100°C produces trinitrotoluene in the form of a dark yellow, oily liquid that is then washed with hot water and dried into flakes, crystalline powder, slab or biscuit, or crushed flakes.[3]

TOXICOKINETICS

TNT is absorbed through the skin, by inhalation, and by ingestion. Metabolism of TNT proceeds in the liver by two processes. The main route follows nitro reduction, leading to the excretion of the dominant urinary metabolite 2, 6-dinitro-4-aminotoluene (DNAT),[11] which can be detected at levels of 0.1 ng/ml.[12] DNAT is found at the end of the workday shift at levels of about 10 mg/L.[13] DNAT may be detected even after a worker has been away from the workplace for 17 days. About 47% of TNT metabolites are excreted as the glucuronides and 30% as aromatic amino compounds such as DNAT.[14] Control of exposure to TNT can be effectively monitored with DNAT analyses in the urine.[15] Of less importance are oxidation products of TNT (trinitrobenzyl alcohol, trinitrobenzoic acid) and simultaneous oxidation and reduction products (2, 6 dinitro-4-aminobenzyl alcohol, 2, 6-dinitro-4-amino-m-cresol).[14] DNAT remains the most clinically useful excretion product for monitoring TNT exposure.

CLINICAL PRESENTATION

Workers poisoned after TNT exposure should be hospitalized. Such patients will more likely have a prolonged period of observation and treatment.

General

Fatigue, lassitude, and dyspnea on exertion may be observed;[10] giddiness and shortness of breath on exertion are occasionally seen.

Hair, Hands

Exposure to TNT may stain the hands, face, and hair orange.[10]

Skin

A dermatitis may develop on areas of the skin exposed to direct contact with the explosive (hands, forearms, neck, wrists, ankles). On the hands it starts as a sago-grain eruption with erythema. Desquamation may follow, leading to complete exfoliation of the hands and feet.[10,16]

Cyanosis

The lips, tongue, and mucous membranes become greyish mauve (methemoglobinemia); the patient may be otherwise asymptomatic.[17,18]

Gastrointestinal, Cardiovascular

Central epigastric colicky pain, nausea with or without vomiting, anorexia, constipation, feeling of tightness in the chest. The patient often has a worried expression and a pallor over the face and cheeks. Slight epigastric tenderness may be present.[10] Arrhythmias may be evident.[7]

Hematologic

About 75% develop an anemia with depression of hemoglobin, red cell structural changes. Depression of hemoglobin to 4 g/dL and the hematocrit to 17 mm with an increase in reticulocytes to 26% has been observed following exposure of G6PD workers to TNT.[19]

Jaundice

This is a rare complication (after an average exposure to TNT of 63 days), seen first in the conjunctivae, then on the skin. It reflects severe liver damage.[10] It may also appear 2 to 3 weeks after removal from contact with TNT.[18] Often nausea, vomiting are observed; sometimes no symptoms are experienced until jaundice appears.[1]

Aplastic Anemia

A rare complication (seen after an average exposure of 216 days), nearly always fatal, sometimes preceded by jaundice.[10] Early symptoms include weakness, loss of appetite and weight, mild cough, bleeding from the nose. Occasionally no symptoms will be present except for purpuric spots.[1]

Neurologic

A peripheral neuritis has been observed.

Eyes

Cataracts.

Most cases have developed symptoms after an exposure to at least 2 to 3 mg/m^3 of TNT, although hepatitis and hematologic abnormalities have appeared at less than 1.5 mg/m^3. Decreases in hematocrit and hemoglobin have been observed at exposure levels as low as 0.2 mg/m^3 following TNT exposure.[7]

Death following TNT exposure is usually due to a severe toxic hepatitis or to aplastic anemia.

LABORATORY

Analytic Methods

An electron-capture gas-chromatography method can quantitate the TNT metabolite 2,6-dinitro-4-aminotoluene (DNAT) in urine and in sensitive levels of 1 ng/liter.[11] Thin-layer chromatography, gas chromatography, high-performance liquid chromatography, and mass spectrometry (HPLC-MS) with electron impact ionization have been used to analyze the metabolites: 4,4'azoxytoluene (4-4'A2) 4, 4,',6,6'-tetranitro-2,2'azoxytoluene (2,2'Az), 4-amino, 2,6-dinitrotoluene (4-A), and 2 amino-4,6-dinitrotoluene (2-A).[20] Liquid chromatography–mass spectrometry can quantitate urine metabolites (2-A), (4-A), and 2,4 diamino-6 nitrotoluene (2,4-A).[21] A micro-liquid chromatography–mass spectrometry method detects metabolites in urine to levels of about 0.1 ng/ml.[12] An enzyme-linked immunosorbent assay (ELISA) for TNT residue on hands can detect 50 pg of TNT.[22]

Levels

Urine levels of 1 µg/L to 1 mg/L (10^{-4} to 10^{-3}g/1) of DNAT were found in urine samples of munitions workers.[11] Levels as low as 5 ng/L have been found in human urine.[11] Hand levels of 53 to 1500 ng were recovered from the hands after contact with TNT.[22]

Abnormalities

Toxic exposure to TNT may result in depression of the hematocrit, hemoglobin concentration, and red blood cell count; an increase or decrease in the white blood cell and lymphocyte count;[18] an increase in reticulocytes, nucleated red blood cells, and eosinophils; and elevated concentrations of serum blood urea nitrogen, glucose, bilirubin, and aminotransferases.[7] Red blood cells may exhibit anisocytosis, poikilocytosis, polychromatophilia, and fragmentation. Hemoglobin is not usually found free in the blood or urine. Methemoglobin levels may be elevated. The blood may be chocolate brown. A rise in the monocyte count may precede symptoms of poisoning and return to normal 2 to 3 months after removal from TNT contact.[23]

Ancillary Tests

Webster Test

Urine that has been acidified with 20% sulfuric acid is extracted with ether, to which an alcoholic solution of potassium hydroxide is added. A purplish red color may indicate the presence of a metabolite (2,6 dinitro-4-hydroxylaminotoluene) of TNT.[23] There is no relation between the test and the severity of intoxication.[18] The test may be negative in the presence of marked cyanosis and incoordination and positive early after an intoxication and may become negative while there is continued exposure to TNT. In the presence of severe liver injury the test may be negative. The colors are unstable. A Webster test serves only to indicate that there is an excretion of TNT metabolites and not that the patient is poisoned.[23] The test has been used on the skin of workers to evaluate the adequacy of washing following exposure to TNT.[24] Subsequent analyses (HPLC, LC-MS) are more accurate, and an examination of the blood (see Clinical, Laboratory) may be a more specific indicator of poisoning.

Cumming Reaction

The Cumming reaction is a modification of the Webster test.[14] Table 63–7 indicates some color results.[14]

Mutagenicity

TNT, but not its metabolite DNAT, is positive on the Ames mutagenic assay.[15]

Table 63–7
The Cumming Reaction[a]

Compound	Color
2:4:6-Trinitrotoluene (α-T.N.T.)	Red
2:3:4-Trinitrotoluene (β-T.N.T.)	Pale yellow
2:4:5-Trinitrotoluene (γ-T.N.T.)	Yellow
2:4:6-Trinitrobenzoic acid	Dull red
2:4:6-Trinitrobenzyl alcohol	Bright red
2:4:6-Trinitrobenzyl acetate	Bright red
2:4:6-Trinitrobenzyl methyl ether	Bright red
1:3:5-Trinitrobenzene	Dull red
2:4-Dinitrotoluene	Purple
m-Dinitrobenzene	Reddish purple
2:6-Dinitro-4-hydroxyl-aminotoluene	Brownish red
N-(3:5-dinitro-4-methyl-phenyl)-*iso*benzaldoxime	No color at first, then gradually becoming pink and finally brownish red
2:6-Dinitro-4-aminotoluene	No color } Green in concentrated solutions
2:4-Dinitro-6-aminotoluene	No color } Green in concentrated solutions
2-Nitro-4:6-diaminotoluene	No color
2:2′:6:6t′-Tetranitro-4:4′-azoxytoluene	Deep blue
2:4:6-Trinitro-*m*-cresol	Yellow
2:6-Dinitro-4-amino-*m*-cresol	Orange
Trinitromesitylene	No color

[a]Adapted from Channon HJ et al. Biochen J 1944;38:70–85.

TREATMENT

Treatment of TNT intoxication is symptomatic, supportive, and preventative. Removal of the patient from a source of TNT is an immediate necessity.

Methemoglobinemia

Methemoglobinemia is treated with methylene blue (see Methemoglobinemia).

Aplastic Anemia

The diagnosis of aplastic anemia should be confirmed by a bone marrow biopsy to distinguish between myelofibrosis, metastatic tumor, marrow necrosis, hypoplastic acute leukemia, and true marrow aplasia. Bone marrow transplantation is the treatment of choice for patients with severe aplastic anemia under age 45 who have a family member with the identical human leukocyte antigen (HLA) type. In such patients, particularly if they are not transfused before transplantation, the 10-year survival rate is more than 80%. Those ineligible for bone marrow transplantation because of age or lack of an HLA-compatible donor should be considered for treatment with antilymphocyte or antithymocyte globulin.

Hepatotoxicity

TNT-induced hepatic damage should be treated symptomatically and supportively.

Prevention

1. The worker should wear overalls and cover the legs and ankles. A headdress should cover the head.
2. Gloves may induce an increase in perspiration and are removed frequently. Where used, there should be a closely woven cotton glove with a knitted top to come over the worker's sleeve. A soft washable chamois glove with a similar top can be used. No heavy seams should be present where areas of dermatitis may be initiated.[25]
3. Wash hands in sodium sulfite 10% (soap and water may be less effective). Test the hands with the Webster test for adequacy of TNT removal.
4. Eliminate air contamination.
5. Wash hands before eating.
6. Do monthly routine tests (serum bilirubin, aminotransferases, packed red cell volume, and white cell and platelet counts).[1]
7. Do hemoglobin tests every week or every other week.

Do not employ as a worker if there is a history of or a presence of the following:

1. Jaundice or gallstones.[26]
2. Severe or chronic gastric illness, including gastric ulcer, or duodenal ulcer.
3. Multiple or severe abdominal or pelvic operations.
4. Nephritis or nephrectomy.
5. Tuberculosis.
6. Moderate or severe anemia.

7. Chronic chest complaints.
8. Chronic skin lesions.
9. Previous occupational dermatitis, rheumatic fever, or Grave's disease.
10. History of glucose-6-phosphate dehydrogenase deficiency or test indicating deficiency.
11. Cataracts.[7]
12. Alcoholism or indication of excessive ethanol infarct.[27,28]

REFERENCES—2, 4, 6-TRINITROTOLUENE (TNT)

1. McConnell WJ, Flinn RH. Summary of twenty-two trinitrotoluene fatalities in World War II. Ind Hyg Toxicol 1946; 28:76–86.
2. Crawford MAD. Aplastic anemia due to trinitrotoluene intoxication. Br Med J 1954;2:430–437.
3. Paterson JD. 2,4,6-trinitrotoluene in Encyclopaedia of Occupational Health and Safety. Vol 2. Geneva, International Labour Office. New York: McGraw-Hill, 1976; p. 1436.
4. Yinon J. Toxicity and metabolism of explosives. Boca Raton, FL: CRC Press, 1991; pp. 3–67.
5. Sax NI. Dangerous properties of industrial materials. 5th ed. New York: Van Nostrand Reinhold, 1979; pp. 1065–1066.
6. Occupational exposure limits for airborne toxic substances. Occupational Safety and Health Series 37. Geneva: International Labour Office. 2,4,6-trinitrotoluene. 1991; pp. 408–409.
7. Hathaway JA. Trinitrotoluene: a review of reported dose-related effects providing documentation for a workplace standard. J Occup Med 1977;19:341–345.
8. Ryon MG, Ross RH. Water quality criteria for 2,4,6-trinitrotoluene. Regul Toxicol Pharmacol 1990;11:104–113.
9. Ross RH, Hartley WR. Comparison of water quality criteria and health advisories for 2,4,6-trinitrotoluene. Regul Toxicol Pharmacol 1990;11:114–117.
10. Hilton J, Swanston CN. Clinical manifestations of tetryl and trinitrotoluene. Br Med J 1941;2:509–510.
11. Almog J, Kraus S, Basch A. Determination of TNT metabolites in urine. Arch Toxicol 1983;(Suppl 6):351–353.
12. Yinon J, Hwang D-G. Metabolic studies of explosives. V. Detection and analysis of 2,4,6-trinitrotoluene and its metabolites in urine of munition workers by micro liquid chromatography/mass spectrometry. Biomed Chromatogr 1986;1:123–125.
13. Woollen BH, Hall MG, Craig R, Stal GT. Trinitrotoluene assessment of occupational absorption during manufacture of explosives. Br J Ind Med 1986;43:465–473.
14. Channon HJ, Mills GT, Williams RT. The metabolism of 2:4:6-trinitrotoluene (alpha-TNT). Biochem J 1944;38:70–85.
15. Ahlborg G Jr, Einisto P, Sorsa M. Mutagenic activity and metabolites in the urine of workers exposed to trinitrotoluene (TNT). Br J Ind Med 1988;45:353–358.
16. Goh CL, Rajans VS. Contact sensitivity to trinitrotoluene. Contact Dermatitis 1983;9:433–434.
17. Voegtlin C, Hooper CW, Johnson JM. Trinitrotoluene poisoning—its nature, diagnosis and prevention. J Indust Hyg 1921–22;3:239–254.
18. Voegtlin C, Hooper CW, Johnson JM. Trinitrotoluene poisoning—its nature, diagnosis and prevention (continued). J Indust Hyg 1921–22;3:280–292.
19. Djerassi LS, Vitany L. Haemolytic episode in G6PD deficient workers exposed to TNT. Br J Ind Med 1975;32:54–58.
20. Yinon J, Hwang D-G. Metabolic studies of explosives 1-EI and CI mass spectrometry of metabolites of 2,4,6-trinitrotoluene. Biomed Mass Spectrom 1984;11:594–600.
21. Yinon J, Hwang D-G. Identification of urinary metabolites of 2,4,6-trinitrotoluene in rats by liquid chromatography-mass spectrometry. Toxicol Lett 1985;26:205–209.
22. Fetterolf DD, Mudd JL, Teten K. An enzyme-linked immunosorbent assay (ELISA) for trinitrotoluene (TNT) residue on hands. J Forensic Sci 1991;36:343–349.
23. Hamilton AM. Monocytosis as an index of TNT absorption. Br J Ind Med 1946;3:24–26.
24. Webster TA. On the metabolism and excretion of 2,4,6-trinitrotoluene. Br Med Res Council. Special Rep Ser 1921; No. 58:49–52.
25. Cone TE Jr. Trinitrotoluene poisoning. US Naval Med Bull 1944;42:731–734.
26. Eddy JH Jr. Some toxic reactions of common explosives. Ind Med 1943;12:483–486.
27. Lawrence RD. Discussion on trinitrotoluene poisoning. Proc R Soc Med 1942;35:553–560.
28. Jie L, Quan-Guan J, Wei-Dong Z. Persistent ethanol drinking increases liver injury induced by trinitrotoluene exposure: an in-plant case–control study. Hum Exp Toxicol 1991;10: 405–409.
29. Holland LM, McKone T, Spanggord R (Peer Review Panel). ATSDR. Toxicological Profile for 2,4,6-Trinitrotoluene. Draft. May 1993.

ZINC CHLORIDE SMOKE

Ignition of zinc oxide/hexachloroethane (ZnHCE) mixtures results in the production of a mixture of products, including zinc oxychloride, zinc chloride, and phosgene, in addition to tetrachlorethylene, carbon tetrachloride, carbon dioxide, carbon monoxide, and unburnt hexachloroethane. Acute effects of ZnHCE smoke in humans include symptoms ranging from slight respiratory distress to pulmonary edema and acute respiratory distress syndrome (ARDS). Some of these poisonings have been fatal. Chronic effects include pulmonary fibrosis and possibly carcinogenicity. Treatment is symptomatic and supportive.[1–6]

Zinc Chloride Fume

CAS No. 7646-85-7. U STEL: 2 mg/m^3.

REFERENCES—ZINC CHLORIDE SMOKE

1. Evans EH. Casualties following exposure to zinc chloride smoke. Lancet 1945;2:368–370.
2. Blom L, Hven PE. Forgiftning med hexit-vogammunition (Poisoning with hexite smoke ammunition). Ugeskr-Laeger 1986;148:454–455.
3. Hjortso E, Bud JMI, Thomson JL, Jensen NK, Qvist J. Zinkklorid forgiftning (Zinc chloride poisoning). Ugeskr Laeger 1987;149:2381–2384.
4. Karlsson N. Poisoning from smoke grenades is not due to phosgene. Eur Respir J 1988;1:575.
5. Karlsson N, Cassel G, Fangmark I, Bergman F. A comparative study of the acute inhalation toxicity of smoke from TiO_2-hexachloroethane and Zn-hexachloroethane pyrotechnic mixtures. Arch Toxicol 1986;59:160–166.
6. Clode SA, Riley RA, Blower SD, Marrs TC, Anderson D. Studies on the mutagenicity of a zinc oxide-hexachloroethane smoke. Hum Exp Toxicol 1991;10: 49–57.

Chapter 64

Hobbies, Arts, and Crafts

Millions of people throughout the world are involved in hobbies, arts, and crafts that may subject them to health hazards of which they often may not be aware. The clinician should recognize the sources of exposure and be prepared to introduce measures to diminish the possible toxicities that may result from hazardous hobbies (Table 64–1). Hazardous exposure derives from metals, woods, dust, chemicals, and physical agents (Table 64–2). Hobbies involving chemical exposure are listed in Table 64–3. Guidelines for an industrial hygiene survey and studios used for design materials, printmaking, and metal sculpture have been proposed.[1] Southern Illinois University has developed a hazardous waste management program for the disposal of hazardous wastes.[2]

ORGANIZATION

The Center for Safety in the Arts (CSA), 5 Beekman Street, Suite 1020, New York, NY 10038, Telephone: 212-227-6220 (Michael McCann, Director) provides a comprehensive ongoing survey (Arts Hazards News) of publications devoted to problems related to chemicals used in arts and crafts (Table 64–4).[3]

THE HISTORY

Exposures

Hobby and craft exposures largely parallel those in industrial exposures. In order of frequency, the largest number of cases will be dermatologic, followed by respiratory and then general poisoning reactions. Finally, there are the smaller number of teratologic, mutagenic, and carcinogenic problems.

Questions

The patient should be asked *(a)* to list all the solids, liquids, and gases used in the activity; *(b)* what processes are used; *(c)* the number of hours per week, and the number of years of exposure to the activity; *(d)* the work environment (outdoors or indoors, small closed room or ventilated area, alone or with others); *(e)* leisure time activities; *(f)* smoking habits. Correlate these answers with the patient's complaints (e.g., weakness, numbness, and tingling in the extremities—peripheral neuropathy) (Table 64–5).

Table 64–1
Where the Hazards Lie[a]

Ingredient	Source	Toxic Effects
Lead	A wide range of arts-and-crafts materials, including ceramic glazes, stained-glass materials, and pigments—especially those used in printmaking	Abdominal pain, anemia, reproductive disorders, nephritis, central and peripheral nervous system damage, and others
Cadmium	Silver solders, pigments, ceramic glazes, and fluxes	Suspected carcinogen and teratogen; lung and kidney dysfunction, high blood pressure, nervous system disorders, and anemia
Chromium	Oil- and acrylic-paint pigments and ceramic colorants	Dermatitis, allergies, skin ulcerations, and bronchial cancer
PCBs	Contaminant of certain oil- and acrylic-paint pigments	Suspected carcinogen and possible teratogen; adverse long-term effects, including liver damage, unusual eye discharge, digestive disturbances, and chemical acne, may not appear for months after initial exposure
Manganese dioxide	Ceramic colorants and oil- and acrylic-paint pigments, such as Mars brown, raw umber, and burnt umber	With chronic poisoning, Parkinson-like symptoms and damage to lungs, liver, kidneys, and central nervous system
Cobalt	Oil- and acrylic-paint pigments, such as cerulean blue, cobalt blue, and ultramarine blue	Suspected carcinogen and neoplastigen; allergy and cardiac damage
Formaldehyde	Preservative in many acrylic paints and photographic hardeners and stabilizers	Skin, eye and mucous membrane irritation, allergy, and asthma
Asbestos	Contaminant in talc used in ceramics and lithography and in soapstone, serpentine, and greenstone	Known carcinogen
Solvents	Ubiquitous in arts and crafts and used for a multitude of purposes	
Aromatic hydrocarbons	Resin solvents, paint and varnish removers, fluorescent-dye solvent, silk-screen cleanup, lacquer thinners, aerosol sprays, and permanent markers	Toluene and xylene linked to CNS depression, dermatitis, and respiratory tract irritation; benzene associated with aplastic anemia, liver damage, and reproductive effects
Chlorinated hydrocarbons	Ink removers, lithographic solvents, rubber cements, paint strippers, aerosol sprays, and varnish removers	Liver function abnormalities, blood-clotting changes, cardiac irregularities, and dermatitis; methylene chloride suspected carcinogen and causes pulmonary edema, narcosis, CNS depression, dermatitis, and heart attack; severe liver and kidney damage with small amounts of carbon tetrachloride and large amounts may result in unconsciousness and death, especially in the presence of alcoholic beverages; may be absorbed through the skin
Petroleum distillates	Paint thinners, rubber-cement thinners, spray adhesives, silk-screen inks, and cleanup	Mild narcotic effect and lung irritation; pulmonary edema if ingested; peripheral neuropathy with chronic inhalation of n-hexane; permanent CNS damage when large amounts are inhaled
Glycol ethers and acetates	Photoresists, color photography, lacquer thinners, paints, and aerosol sprays	Anemia and kidney damage; birth defects, miscarriages, testicular atrophy, and sterility in animals

[a]Adapted from Emerg Med 1986;18(18):6.

Table 64–2
Hazardous Materials Used in Arts and Crafts

Metals	
Arsenic	Manganese
Cadmium	Mercury
Chromium	Nickel
Cobalt	Silver
Copper	Tin
Lead	Titanium
	Zinc
Woods	
Dusts	
Chemicals	
Acids, alkalis	Methyl butyl ketone
Acrylics	Methyl cellosolve acetate
Benzene	Methylene chloride
Carbon tetrachloride	Peroxide
Epoxides	Plastics
Epoxy	Styrene
Foams	Turpentine
Methanol	Vinyls
Physical hazards	
Ultraviolet radiation	
Infrared radiation	
Noise	

Table 64–3
Hobbies Involving Chemical Exposure

- Painting
- Printmaking
- Ceramics
- Stone, plaster, clay and wax sculpture
- Woodworking
- Plastic sculptures
- Metal working
- Welding
- Jewelry and enameling
- Stained glass and glassblowing
- Textile arts
- Photography
- Commercial art
- Children and art materials

Table 64-4
CSA Publications[a]

Books, Pamphlets and Articles

1. "Arsenic, Old Lace, and Stuffed Owls May Be Dangerous to Your Health: Hazards in Museum Collections," by Patricia L. Miller, *Illinois Heritage Assoc,* Technical Insert No. 50 (1991), 4 pp, $2.00
2. *Artist Beware,* by Michael McCann, Lyons & Burford, NY (fall 1992), $29.95.***
3. *Asbestos in the Home,* U.S. Consumers Product Safety Commission (1982), 12 pp, $3.00
4. *California List of Art and Craft Materials Acceptable for Grades K-6.* California State Dept of Health Services, 2nd ed. (5/1988), 40 pp, $5.00*
5. "Ceramics and Health" by Monona Rossol, article series from *Ceramic Scope* (1980-1982), 41 pp, $5.00*
6. *Health Hazards in the Arts and Crafts,* Gail Barazani and Michael McCann (Eds.). SOEH, Washington, DC (1980), 232 pp, $5.00***
7. *Health Hazards Manual for Artists,* by Michael McCann, 3rd edition, Lyons & Burford, NY (1985), 100 pp, $0.05**
8. *Kiln Safety.* Edward Orton Jr. Foundation (1990), 22 pp, free**
9. *Lights! Camera! Safety!: A Health & Safety Manual for Motion Picture and Television Production,* by Michael McCann, Center for Safety in the Arts, 98 pp, $12.00***
10. *Overexposure: Health Hazards in Photography* by Susan Shaw and Monona Rossol, Allworth Press (1991), 320 pp, $18.95***
11. *A Personal Risk Assessment for Craftsmen & Artists,* by Ted Rickard & Ronald Angus, Ontario Crafts Council & College, Univ & School Safety Council of Ontario (1986), 20 pp, $2.50*
12. *Reproductive Hazards in the Arts and Crafts,* by Jean-Ann McGrane, Center for Safety in the Arts, NY (1987), 14 pp, $3.00*
13. *Safety in the Artroom,* by Charles A. Qualley, Davis Publications (1986), 120 pp, $10.95**
14. "The Safety of Lead Frits," by Monona Rossol, from SOEH Conference on Health Hazards in the Arts and Crafts, Wash, DC (1978), 3 pp, $1.50
15. *Stage Fright: Health and Safety in the Theater,* by Monona Rossol, Allworth Press (1991), 129 pp, $12.95***
16. "Taking the Occupational History," San Diego/Imperial Counties of Amer Lung Assoc. *Annals of Internal Medicine,* 99(5) (1983), plus "Addendum on Arts and Crafts History" by Monona Rossol. 13 pp, $2.50
17. "Textile Dyes are Potential Hazards," by Catherine Jenkins, *Journal of Environmental Health,* 40(256) (1978), $2.50
18. *Ventilation,* by Nancy Clark, Thomas Cutter, and Jean-Ann McGrane, Lyons & Burford, NY (1984), 128 pp, Soft: $9.95** Hard cover: $15.95***
19. *Waste Management and Disposal for Artists and Schools,* Michael MCann and Angela Babin, Center for Safety in the Arts, NY (1992), 12 pp, $2.00*
20. *Water-based Inks: A Screenprinting Manual for Studio and Classroom,* by Lois M. Johnson and Hester Stinnett. Philadelphia College of the Arts, Printmaking Workshop, Phila, PA (1990), 40 pp. $12.00**

Postage and handling

* Plus $1.00 postage/handling
** Plus $2.00 postage/handling
***Plus $2.50 postage/handling
Foreign postage/handling: $3.00 (books under $10.00), $5.00 (books over $10.00). Additional items: add $1.00/item to highest postage/handling charge. All prices are subject to change.

General Data Sheets

Art Hazards Crossword Puzzle (3)
Art Painting and Drawing (4)
Asbestos Substitutes (4)
Bibliography (5)
Cadmium Hazards (2)
Ceramics (2)
Ceramic Glazes May Poison Food (3)
Children's Art Supplies Can Be Toxic (6)
Cleaning Up Spills and Leaks (2)
Commercial Art Hazards (1)
Electric Kiln Emissions and Ventilation (4)
Eye and Face Protection (2)
Fiber Arts Hazards (7)
Fire Prevention (5)
Flammable and Combustible Liquids Safety Checklist (3)
Formaldehyde (4)
Glove Selection (3)
Hazards in the Arts (4)
Health and Safety Resources for the Arts (7)
Health & Safety for Secondary School Arts/Industrial Arts (7)
Health and Safety Program for Arts Organizations (4)
Intro to Waste Management for Artists and Schools (2)
Labels and Labeling (2)
Lead Poisoning (4)
Material Safety Data Sheets (2)
Medical Surveillance Program for Art Schools (1)
Metal Jewelry Health and Safety (4)
Oil Painting Hazards in Classrooms (2)
OSHA Hazard Communication Standard (2)
OSHA Regs for Flammable and Combustible Spraying (2)
Paint Removers (3)
Paper Mache (3)
Peligros Laborales en Las Artes (2)
Photographic Processing Hazards in Schools (2)
Photography (2)
Plastics (see below)
Respirators (5)
Reproductive Hazards in the Arts and Crafts (4)
Silica Hazards (3)
Silk Screen Printing (3)
Solvents Used in the Arts (8)
Stained Glass (2)
Teaching Art Safely to the Disabled (8)
Traditional Sculpture/Casting (1)
Ventilation (see below)
Welding, Soldering & Brazing (1)
Woodworking Hazards (4)
Worker's Compensation for Artists (1)
Workshop Noise (4)

Conservation Hazards Data Sheets

Emergency Plans for Museum Conservation Labs (4)
Hazards of Dyes and Pigments for Museum Personnel (8)
Health and Safety for Historic Structures Preservation (8)
Health and Safety Program for Conservation Laboratories (4)
Ionizing Radiation Protection for Conservation Laboratories (8)
Nitrocellulose Film Hazards in Conservation (2)
Safe Pest Control Procedures for Museum Collections (8)
Solvents in Art Conservation Labs (8)
Storage and Disposal of Conservation Chemicals (4)
Thymol and o-Phenyl Phenol: Safe Work Practices (4)
Ventilation for Conservation Laboratories (6)

Performing Arts Hazards Data Sheets

Emergency Medical Care on Set and Location (4)
Fire/Life Safety on Location (3)
Heat Stress (3)
Hearing Loss in Musicians (4)
Intro to Theater Hazards (4)
Musculoskeletal Problems in Dancers (6)
Musculoskeletal Problems in Musicians (5)
Occupational Hazards in Music (4)
Paints in Theater Crafts (4)
Plastics in Theater Crafts (4)
Shared Theatrical Makeup (1)
Smoke and Fog Hazards (2)
Theater Health and Safety Self-evaluation Checklist (3)
Theatrical Make-up and Cosmetic Aerosol Sprays (4)
Ventilation for Theater Crafts (5)
Worker's Compensation for Performing Artists (4)

Canadian Center for Occupational Health and Safety Infograms

Abrasive Wheels (5)
Chain Saws (6)
Hand Tools (16)
Materials Handling (17)
Power Hand Tools (11)
Welding (17)
Woodworking Machines (10)

Data Sheets (number of pages)

All Data Sheets are $.50/page

Videotapes

Art Safety: Hazards and Precautions. 2-part VHS videotape describing the hazards of art & crafts materials and the necessary precautions. Includes copies of *Health Hazard Manual for Artists* and *Ventilation,* as well as a videotape outline. (50 min. each) $200.00.

Introduction to Dance Medicine: Keeping Dancers Dancing by Susan Macaluso. Describes dancer injury, including: evaluation, diagnosis, rehabilitation, prevention, and patient experiences. (50 min.) Introductory price: $150.00.

[a]Adapted from Babin A. Art Hazards News 1992;15:4-11.

(continued)

Table 64–4 *(Continued)*

Therapeutic Exercises for Musicians by Richard Norris, M.D. Videotaped lecture and demonstration on exercises beneficial to injury prevention in musicians. (60 min.) $35.00.	**Art Hazards News.** One year subscription (four 8-page issues, plus Resource Issue) $21.00, 3rd class bulk rate. For Canada & PanAm, add $2.00 for 1st class postage; other countries, add $5.00 for surface mail.	**Ordering Information** All orders must be accompanied by payment (US $) unless official purchase order is enclosed. Mailing: US—first class, or U.P.S.; Canada, Mexico—airmail under 2 lbs; other countries—surface	mail. Contact CSA for bulk orders and return policies. **Center for Safety in the Arts 5 Beekman Street, Suite 1030 New York, NY 10038 (212) 227-6220**

THE PHYSICAL EXAMINATION

Examine the patient's hands, face, and exposed chest for skin problems (industrial solvents, detergents, cutting oils, photographic chemicals, oils, solvents used in refinishing furniture). A complete neurologic examination may indicate problems related to lead or mercury exposure. Where necessary, reexamine the patient immediately after a specific period of exposure to the hobby or work (e.g., pulmonary function tests and careful chest examination after exposure to a dust-promoting material).

LABORATORY

Monitoring tests for some substances used in the arts and crafts are presented in Table 64–6.

GENERAL PRECAUTIONS*

The following are some simple precautions you can take to work safely with your art materials. More detailed information on these precautions can be found by consulting the references listed at the end of this section, especially *Artist Beware* and *Health Hazards Manual for Artists* by Michael McCann.

1. Choose the safest materials possible. Whenever possible, replace solvent-containing materials with water-based materials to eliminate solvent inhalation problems. Buy wet materials such as prepared clay, aqueous dye solutions, and water-based glazes rather than dry powders. Avoid materials that contain chemicals that can cause cancer or adverse reproductive effects.
   Individuals who are at high risk—disabled individuals, pregnant women, children, people with certain illnesses, etc.—should check to see if their art materials might be particularly dangerous to them. If so, safer substitutes, better ventilation, or other more stringent precautions might be needed. For pregnant women in particular, unless the art materials are known to be safe during pregnancy, they should be avoided.
2. Read labels carefully. Unfortunately most labels only list the acute or immediate hazards. Labels with CL (certified label) seal of the Arts and Crafts Materials Institute also have the chronic or long-term hazards listed. You should also request Material Safety Data Sheets (MSDS) on your products from the distributor or manufacturer.

*Hazards in the Arts. New York: Center for Safety in the Arts, 1986.

Table 64–5
Questionnaire for Obtaining Information About Arts, Crafts and Hobby Activities[a]

Art-Craft-Hobby History

1. List and describe your arts, crafts or hobby activities.
   ____
   ____
   ____
2. About how many hours a week do you do this work? ______
3. Do you use any protective equipment when you work?
   Gloves ______ Coverall/apron ______ Glasses/goggles ______
   Hearing protection ______ Other ______
4. When you work, are you exposed to any of the following?
   Solvents (turpentine, paint thinner, etc.) ______
   Aerosols or sprays ______
   Dusts (wood, clay, stone, etc.) ______
   Smoke ______ Metal fumes ______ Metals ______
   Other chemicals (list) ______
   ____
5. Where do you do this work?
   a. At home ? If so, how near to the kitchen or bedroom do you work? ______
   b. In an individual studio, garage or outbuilding? ______
   c. In a group studio or school? ______ If so, what other chemicals and hazards are you exposed to from other workers? ______
   ____
   d. If you have any physical ailments or health problems, do others in the school or studio have similar problems?
   Yes ______ No ______
6. Does your workspace have good ventilation? Yes ___ No ___
   Describe ______
   ____
7. Have you worked in other arts or crafts in the past?
   Yes ______ No ______
   If so, what have you done and on what approximate dates?
   ____
   ____
   ____

[a]McCunney RJ et al. Am Fam Physician 1987;36:145–153.

Children's art materials are of particular concern. The nontoxic label on children's art materials legally means that the art material passes the acute toxicity tests of the Federal Hazardous Substances Act, which do not identify possible long-term hazards. Products with the CP or AP (certified or approved product) seal of the Arts and Crafts Materials Institute are recommended. Children's art materials with these seals have had their formulations approved by a toxicologist with expertise in children's art materials.

3. Set up a studio carefully. Whenever possible, do not have a studio in the home. If the work must be done at home, set up the studio in a separate room, not in the living areas. Store art materials safely where children cannot reach them. Do not store materials in orange juice containers, soda bottles, etc. because of the danger of accidental ingestion.

4. "Use with adequate ventilation." This phrase, appearing on many product labels, needs some definition. Contrary to popular belief, it does not mean an open door or window since one has no control over wind direction or intensity. For example, the wind might blow the contaminants in the face. It also does not mean an air conditioner since air conditioners recirculate the air and

Table 64–6
Health Effects and Appropriate Monitoring Tests for Some Substances Used in the Arts and Crafts[a]

Substance	Hobby/Use	Health Effect	Test
Solvents			
Benzene	Paint remover Solvent for waxes, oils	Aplastic anemia, skin irritation and dryness, headache, nausea, vertigo, coagulopathies	Complete blood count
Methanol	Solvent in paints and varnishes	Ocular toxicity, central nervous system depression, metabolic acidosis	Urine methanol level, urine formic acid level
Methylene chloride	Paint and varnish remover Cleaning fluid	Fatigue, weakness, lightheadedness, paresthesias, eye irritation, toxic encephalopathy	Carboxyhemoglobin level
1,1,1-Trichloroethane	Paints Glues	Ataxia, lightheadedness, liver and kidney damage	Blood and urine trichloroethane levels
Toluene	Paint thinner Solvent in paints, lacquers Glues	Headache, fatigue, memory impairment, ataxia, euphoria, confusion, dilated pupils	Urine hippuric acid level
Xylene	Paints Lacquers	Dizziness, lethargy, ataxia, anorexia, mucous membrane irritation	Urine methyl hippuric acid level
Fixatives			
â-Hexane	Lacquers Solvent in quick-drying ink and cements	Central nervous system depression, peripheral neuropathy, respiratory irritation	Nerve conduction studies
Stones and clay			
Asbestos	Clays Papier-mâché Glazes Sculpture stones French chalk used in graphics	Asbestosis	Chest film, pulmonary function tests
Silica	Clays Glazes Sculpture dust Jewelry buffing compound	Silicosis	Chest film, pulmonary function tests
Metals			
Cadmium	Silver soldering alloys	Pulmonary edema, fibrosis, renal disease	Blood and urine cadmium levels
Chromates (lead and zinc)	Paint pigments	Carcinogenic (suspected), respiratory irritation	Chest film, pulmonary function tests
Lead	Solders Paints Metal alloys Enamels	Neurologic complaints, abdominal pain, fatigue, anemia	Complete blood count, blood lead level, zinc protoporphyrin
Lithium	Drying agent Metallurgy	Anorexia, nausea, tremors, central nervous system changes	Blood and urine lithium levels
Mercury	Paint preservative	Nervousness, fatigue, tremors, bleeding gums	Blood and urine mercury levels
Other chemicals			
Benzidine	Dyes Paints	Urinary tract and bladder cancer	Urinary cytology
Formaldehyde	Acrylic paints Certain glues Resins Kiln fumes	Mucous membrane irritation, cough, bronchospasm, contact dermatitis	Urine formic acid level
Pentachlorophenol (PCP)	Wood preservative	Delirium, weakness, hyperpyrexia, tachycardia, tachypnea	Blood and urine pentachlorophenol levels
Selenium	Decolorizer in ceramic glazes	Metallic taste, garlic odor of breath, headache, sore throat, fume fever, mucous membrane irritation	Urine selenium level

[a]Adapted from McCunney RJ et al. Am Fam Physician 1987;36:145–153.

whatever contaminants it contains. So what is adequate ventilation?

There are two types of ventilation for control of toxic contaminants: dilution ventilation and local exhaust ventilation. Dilution ventilation involves bringing clean air into the room where the work is performed to mix the contaminated air and diluting it to a lower—and safer—concentration, and then exhausting it to the outside with an exhaust fan. This type of ventilation is good when working with small amounts of solvents or gases that are not very toxic. For example, a window exhaust fan is adequate dilution ventilation for oil painting where a maximum of about ½ cup of turpentine per day is used. Similarly, dilution ventilation is good for black-and-white photographic darkrooms. Dilution ventilation is not good for large amounts of solvents—for example, printing with solvent-based silk screen inks, for highly toxic solvents like those in lacquer thinners, or for dusts.

Local exhaust ventilation, on the other hand, use hoods, spray booths, etc. to capture the contaminants where they are generated before they can get into the general room air. The contaminants are then exhausted to the outside through ducts. Local exhaust ventilation is preferred.

For further information on ventilation of art studios, see *Ventilation: A Practical Guide,* by Nancy Clark, Thomas Cutter, and Jean-Ann McGrane.

5. Protect against fire. Do not smoke or have open flames, sparks, or static electricity near flammable liquids or gases. Store flammable and combustible liquids in safety cans and keep only amounts on hand needed for a few days. Large amounts of flammable and combustible liquids should be stored in a flammable storage cabinet. Have smoke alarms and the right type of fire extinguisher. If ordinary combustibles, flammable liquids, and electrical equipment are used, have a Class ABC fire extinguisher. Know how to use the fire extinguisher. If flammable liquids are used, the exhaust systems must be explosion-proof.
6. Clean up carefully. Always clean up spills immediately. For dusts, wet mop or vacuum; never sweep, which stirs up dust. For clay and other highly toxic dusts, the vacuum cleaner should be equipped with a special (HEPA) filter.
7. Dispose of art materials safely. Do not pour solvents down the sink. Small amounts—less than a pint—can be disposed of safely by evaporation inside a local exhaust hood or outdoors. For large amounts, contact a waste disposal service. Nonpolluting materials dissolved in water can be poured down the sink one at a time with lots of water. Acids and alkalis should be neutralized first.
8. Have good personal work practices. Do not eat, drink, or smoke in the studio. Wash chemical splashes off the skin with lots of water. In case of eye contact, rinse with water for at least 20 minutes and call a doctor; an eyewash fountain is recommended. If concentrated acids and alkalis are used, have an emergency shower available. Do not wash hands with solvents; use soap and water. To remove oil paints, use baby oil and then soap and water. Have a first aid kit available.
9. Wear proper personal protective clothing and equipment. Wear special work clothes (smocks, hair covering, etc.) and wash separately from other clothing. Use the right type of gloves, goggles, hearing protectors, respirators, etc. Make sure they are approved for the chemicals being used and that they fit properly. Respirators in particular should be approved by NIOSH (National Institute for Occupational Safety and Health) for the particular contaminant.
10. Avoid physical and electrical hazards. Keep or put machine guards on all machinery. Do not wear loose, long hair; loose sleeves; or necklaces around machinery. Keep equipment and electrical wiring in good repair. Ground electrical equipment and do not overload the wiring.
11. Seeking medical assistance. If symptoms might be connected with an art hobby, expert medical assistance should be sought. A family physician might not have this expertise since specialized training is needed to understand both the toxic effects of chemicals and the special medical problems of performing artists. In fact the latter area is now becoming known as "arts medicine."

The Center for Safety in the Arts in New York publishes an Occupational Health Clinic list.

SUGGESTED READINGS

1. Clark N, Cutter T, McGrane J-A. Ventilation. a practical guide. New York: Center for Occupational Hazards, 1984.
2. McCann M. Artist beware: the hazards and precautions in working with art and craft materials. New York: Watson-Guptill, 1979.
3. McCann M. Health hazards manual for artists. 3rd ed. New York: Nick Lyons Books, 1985.
4. Rossol M. Ceramics and health. Compilation of articles from Ceramic Scope (1980–82).
5. Rossol M. Stage fright: health and safety in the theater. New York: Center for Occupational Hazards, 1985.
6. Seeger N. Alternatives for the artist. Revised editions. Chicago; School of the Art Institute of Chicago, 1984.
   An Introductory Guide to the Safe Use of Materials.
   A Printmaker's Guide to the Safe Use of Materials.
   A Photographer's Guide to the Safe Use of Materials.
   A Painter's Guide to the Safe Use of Materials.
   A Ceramist's Guide to the Safe Use of Materials
   A Sculptor's Guide to the Safe Use of Materials—Welding and Founding
7. Shaw S. Overexposure: health hazards in photography. California: Friends of Photography, 1983.

Most of the books listed above are available from the Center for Occupational Hazards, which also publishes the Art Hazards Newsletter. In addition, the Art Hazards Information Center distributes over 70 other books, articles, and data sheets on a variety of topics.

PREGNANCY AND LACTATION

A summary of possible adverse reproductive effects of chemical and physical agents involved in hobbies, arts, and crafts is found in Table 64–7. Many substances used by arts, crafts, and hobby enthusiasts may be mutagens (e.g., lead, formaldehyde, trichloroethane). Women in the childbearing years should be counseled regarding exposure to materials that may pass the placental barrier and possibly lead to birth defects (e.g., lead; other heavy metals such as cadmium, azo

Table 64–7
Adverse Reproductive Effects of Chemical and Physical Agents

Chemical Name	Art Process/Material	Affects Male[1]	Affects Female[2]	Fetal Death[3]	Affects Newborn[4]
Metals					
Antimony	ceramics & enameling, metal working, pewter	H/A	H/A	H/A	H/A
Arsenic	glassblowing, patinas, wood preservative	—	H/A	A	A
Cadmium	pigments, silver soldering, ceramics & enameling	H/A	A	A	H/A
Chromium	pigments, ceramics & enameling, photochemicals	A	—	—	A
Cobalt	pigments, ceramics & enameling	A	—	—	A
Copper	metalworking, ceramics & enameling	A	A	—	A
Gold Salts	photochemicals & electroplating	—	—	—	A
Lead	pigments, soft solders, ceramics & enameling, stained glass, lead casting	H/A	H/A	H/A	H/A
Lithium	ceramics & enameling	—	—	—	H/A
Manganese	pigments, metalworking, ceramics & enameling	H/A	H/A	A	A
Mercury	Pigments, photochemicals, neon sculpture	H/A	H/A	A	H/A
Nickel	electroplating, metalworking, ceramics & enameling	A	—	—	A
Selenium	pigment, photochemical	H/A	H/A	H/A	H/A
Zinc	Pigment, metalworking, solder, flux, ceramics & enameling	A	—	—	A
Solvents					
Acetone	strippers, lacquers, thinners, plastics solvent	—	—	A	A
Benzene	old paint strippers & old rubber cements, gasoline	H/A	H/A	—	H/A
Benzyl Alcohol	photochemical, solvent	—	—	—	H/A
Ethyl Alcohol	shellac denatured alcohol	H/A	H/A	H/A	H/A
Ethylene Dichloride	plastics solvent	—	H/A	A	A
Glycol Ethers	Photochemicals solvent, photo-resists, lacquers, aerosol sprays	H?[5]/A	H?[5]/A	A	A
Isopropyl alcohol	rubbing alcohol	—	—	—	A
Methyl alcohol	shellac, french dyes, duplicating fluid, paint strippers	—	—	A	A
Methyl chloroform	aerosol sprays, etching grounds, film cleaners	—	—	—	H[6]
Methylene chloride	paint strippers, aerosol sprays, plastics cement	—	—	—	A
Methyl ethyl ketone	lacquers, thinners, plastics solvent	—	—	—	H[6]
Perchloroethylene	degreasing, printmaking	—	A	—	H[6]/A
Refined Petroleum Solvents	paint thinner, lacquer, silk screen inks, aerosol sprays, rubber cements	—	H	—	—
Toluene	lacquer thinners, silk screen inks, aerosols	—	H/A	H/A	H/A
Turpentine	varnishes, painting	—	—	—	A
Xylene	lacquer thinners, printmaking, aerosol sprays	—	H	A	H/A
Organic solvents mixture	wide variety of art materials	—	H/A	H/A	H/A
Miscellaneous Chemicals					
Bromides	photochemicals	—	—	—	H
Carbon monoxide	gas-fired kilns & furnaces, carbon arcs	H/A	H/A	H/A	H/A
Cyanides	electroplating, photochemical, plastics decomposition	—	A	A	A
Fluorine & compounds	glass etching, silver solder flux & welding, ceramics & enameling	—	—	—	H/A
Formaldehyde	preservative, photochemicals, certain glues & resins, plywood, particle board	—	H	—	A
Glycidyl ethers	epoxy resins & glues	A	—	—	A
Hydrogen sulfide	decomposition of sulfide toners & sulfide metal colorants	—	A	—	A
Nitrogen dioxide	etching, arc welding, carbon arcs	—	A	A	A
Pentachlorophenol	wood preservative	A	A	H/A	H/A
Phthalate esters	plastics plasticizer, plastic resin hardener	A	—	A	A
Styrene	polyester resin	A	H/A	—	—
Textile dyes	fabric dyeing	—	—	—	A
Physical Agents					
Heat	kilns & furnaces	H/A	H/A	—	H/A
Ionizing radiation	ceramic & pottery glazes & enamels, photochemicals	H/A	H/A	—	H/A
Noise & Vibration	Wood & metalworking machinery, abrasive blasting, pneumatic tools	H/A	H/A	—	H/A

1. Includes reduced fertility, cancer of the reproductive organs, abnormal or reduced sperm, testicular damage, etc.
2. Includes reduced fertility, cancer of reproductive organs, menstrual changes & disorders, sterility, etc.
3. Includes miscarriage, stillbirth, and spontaneous abortion.
4. Includes low birth weight, birth defects, premature birth, growth retardation, etc.
5. Based on inconclusive data that is suggestive but incomplete.
6. Studies indicate appearance in breast milk after exposure of the mother.

H positive human studies
A positive animal studies
N negative test results
— no studies or insufficient data

Table 64–8
Recommendations For Pregnant And Nursing Artists

This chart lists specific recommendations for ventilation and process substitutes for pregnant and nursing artists who are working with reproductive toxins. These recommendations do not cover all potential health hazards of a particular process nor do they list all processes. *Only* those processes where potential for exposures to reproductive toxins have been commonly reported are included.

This chart should be used as a supplement to the generally recognized safety and health precautions which should be applied to all work processes. Before relying on these recommendations, every attempt should be made to substitute non-toxic materials and processes. These recommendations are advisory in nature based on current available information. It is important to maintain current information on the hazards of art materials and available substitutes.

Technique	Source of Hazards	Recommendation
Airbrush		
—water-based	Pigments, dyes	Use only with spray booth.
—solvent-based	Solvents	Do not use.
Batik	Dye powders	Use water-based liquid dyes or mix powdered dyes in box with glass top & holes in sides for arms.
Ceramics	Glazes[a]	Do not spray glazes or mix powdered glazes. Do not use lead glazes. Use prepared glazes, but avoid skin contact.
	Kilns	All kilns require canopy hoods.
Commercial art	Rubber cement	Use only with local exhaust ventilation or use wax.
	Permanent markers	Use water-based markers for substitutes.
	Aerosol sprays	Use only in explosion-proof spray booth or outdoors.
	Airbrush	See airbrush.
Computer graphics	Video display terminals	Avoid if possible due to lack of adequate scientific information on reproductive risks.
Drawing		
—pen and ink	Solvents	Use window with exhaust fan.
Enameling[a]	Powdered enamels	Do not use
Forging	Noise, vibration	Avoid.
	Carbon monoxide	Hot forging furnace requires canopy hood.
Intaglio	Photoetches	Use only with local exhaust ventilation. Use proper gloves for glycol ethers.
	Solvents	Use only with local exhaust ventilation. Avoid work scheduling which requires other solvent use without local exhaust in the work area.
Intaglio *(continued)*	Aquatint	Cans of spray paint should be used outdoors or in a spray booth.
Jewelry	Silver solders, fluxes	Do not use cadmium containing silver solders or fluoride fluxes. Requires local exhaust ventilation.
Lithography	Solvents	See intaglio.
	Dichromates	Do not use.
	Vinyl lacquers	Do not use.
Metal casting	Metals	Avoid pouring molten metals during pregnancy and nursing.
	Carbon monoxide	Gas-fired furnace requires canopy hood.
	Burnout kiln	Wax burnout kiln requires canopy hood.
Painting		
—oil	Mineral spirits Turpentine	Avoid during pregnancy. Use water-based paints instead.
—alkyds	Solvents	See painting, oils.
Pastels	Pigment dust	Avoid during pregnancy and nursing. Use oil pastels as substitutes.
	Spray fixative	Use only in explosion-proof spray booth or outdoors.
Photography		
—black and white	Developers, intensifiers	Do not mix dry chemicals.
	Toners (sulfide, selenium)	Use only with local exhaust ventilation.
—color	Solvents, formaldehyde	Use only with local exhaust ventilation.
—blue printing	Carbon arcs	Do not use carbon arcs. Use sunlight or other UV source.
Relief printing	Solvents	Use water-based inks only.

[a]Check for heavy metal accumulation prior to pregnancy.

(continued)

Table 64–8 *(Continued)*

Technique	Source of Hazards	Recommendation
Sculpture		
—clay		See Ceramics
—wood		See woodworking.
—plastic resins	Polyester, polyurethane epoxy	Do no use.
—plastics	Decomposition products	Use local exhaust if heating or burning plastics.
Silk screen	Solvents	Do not use solvent-based inks and stencils. Use water-based inks. Avoid water-based inks with solvent additives.
	Dichromates	Do not use dichromate photoemulsions. Use diazo photoemulsions.
Stained glass	Lead came and solder[a]	Avoid during pregnancy and nursing.
Weaving	See Batik	
Welding	Metal fumes	Use slot hoods for bench welding and movable exhausts for other welding. Do not use galvanized or found metals.
Woodworking	Solvents	Use only water-based paints and glues.
	Formaldehyde	Do not use formaldehyde containing glues.

dyes, benzene, and chlorinated hydrocarbon solvents; and nonchlorinated hydrocarbon solvents such as toluene and xylene). Instruct women to avoid such materials at least during the first 3 months of pregnancy; in later pregnancy ensure sufficient control over the environment to minimize or eliminate access to toxic chemicals (e.g., heavy metals, solvents, dyes, toxic dusts, and gases). Breast-feeding during use of such materials described may expose the infant to toxic substances in the mother's milk supply. Suggested recommendations for pregnant and nursing artists compiled by The Center for Safety in the Arts are presented in Table 64–8. These are general guidelines and must be supplemented by consultation with a physician for additional specific prenatal and postnatal advice. Additional references to pregnancy and lactation exposure to many of these chemicals are available.[1]

SAFETY LABELING

Public Law 100-695, 15 U.S.C. #1277, the "Labeling of Hazardous Art Materials Act" directs the U.S. Consumer Product Safety Commission to set up guidelines for determining whether arts and craft materials present chronic long-term health hazards. The law mandates a voluntary Standard—ASTM D-4236-88—as a mandatory labeling standard for art and craft materials. Artists, safety and health professionals, and the art materials industry developed this labeling standard, which took effect November 18, 1990. The law applies to many children's toy products such as crayons, chalk, paint sets, modeling clay, coloring books, pencils, and any other products used by children to produce a work or visual or graphic art. The labels must provide *(a)* a warning statement of the hazards; *(b)* identification of the hazardous ingredients; and *(c)* guidelines for safe use. The standard requires labels for all art and craft materials determined to present a chronic hazard, including solvents, spray paints, silk screen inks, adhesives, and any other substance marketed or represented as suitable for use in any phase of the creation of any work of visual or graphic art of any medium.

The Commission believes that under the broad statutory definition of "art material" three general categories can be seen:[4]

1. Those products that actually become a component of the work of visual or graphic art such as paint, canvas, inks, crayons, chalk, solder, brazing rods, flux, paper, clay, stone, thread, cloth, and photographic film.
2. Those products that are closely and intimately associated with the creation of the final work of art such as brush cleaners, solvents, ceramic kilns, brushes, silk screens, molds or mold making material, and photo developing chemicals.
3. Those tools, implements, and furniture that are used in the process of the creation of a work of art, but do not become part of the work or art. Examples are drafting tables and chairs, easels, picture frames, canvas stretchers, potter's wheels, hammers, chisels, and air pumps for air brushes.

Ideally, labels should also contain information on the type of hazard the materials present, including the following:

1. An estimate of the relative toxicity of the chemicals.
2. Precautions and detailed instructions on how to work with a chemical safely (e.g., type of ventilation, protective clothing).
3. Currently recommended first-aid instructions.

CADMIUM

A retired hobbyist began to fashion boxes from sheet metal. In 2 days he developed abdominal pain, fever to 105°F, cough, ileus, hypoxia, progressive alveolar infiltrates, and a high output failure state with low systemic vascular resistance. He died a few days after an exploratory laparotomy. His cardiac blood demonstrated very high cadmium levels. His garage shop had been unventilated.[5]

CANCER

Artists may be subject to elevated proportionate mortality ratios for arteriosclerotic heart disease, leukemias, and cancers of the bladder, colon, rectum, kidney, and brain. The significant excesses of bladder cancer and leukemia deaths in one study were limited to painters. Colon cancer deaths appear to be elevated among male painters and sculptors.[6] Data also suggest a significant elevation in prostate cancer mortality among sculptors. Known or suspected carcinogens to which artists may be exposed include 2-naphthylamine, polychlorinated biphenyls, benzidine, formaldehyde, and asbestos in art paints, and benzene, dioxane, and methylene chloride used as solvents.[7]

Table 64–9
Clay Components and Associated Pulmonary Diseases[a]

Clay Component	Disease
Alumina	Aluminosis (lung disease)
Asbestos (contaminant of talc)	Asbestosis, cancer of several sites
Diatomaceous earth (raw material for clay)	Silicosis
Feldspar	Pneumoconiosis
Iron oxide	Siderosis
Kaolin (raw material for china clay)	Kaolinosis
Talc (raw material for porcelain)	Talcosis, lung cancer
Barium carbonate	CNS disease, baritosis (benign pneumoconiosis)

[a]Adapted from Fuortes LJ. Postgrad Med 1989;85:133–136.

Table 64–10
Common Glaze Components and Associated Hazards[a]

Glaze Component	Hazards
Arsenic trioxide	Heavy metal poisoning, cancer
Antimony trioxide	Heavy metal poisoning
Beryllium	Pneumonitis, pneumoconiosis
Boric acid	Skin irritation, CNS depression
Cadmium oxide	Heavy metal poisoning
Calcium carbonate	Nonspecific
Cobalt	Sensitization of skin and lung, cardiomyopathy
Copper	Nontoxic unless in form of copper sulfate–verdigris
Chromates (nickel, iron, potassium)	Sensitization (dermatitis, asthma, pulmonary fibrosis), cancer
Lead	Heavy metal poisoning
Lithium carbonate	CNS and renal toxicities
Manganese dioxide	CNS toxicities (parkinsonism)
Nickel oxide	Sensitization, cancer
Titanium dioxide	Benign pneumoconiosis
Tin oxide	Benign pneumoconiosis
Zinc oxide	Dermatitis, metal fume fever

[a]Adapted from Fuortes LJ. Postgrad Med 1989;85:133–136.

CERAMICS[8]

1. Clays
   Many of the raw materials in clays commonly used by ceramic artists are fibrogenic and may lead to pneumoconiosis when inhaled. Little acute toxicity is experienced. Chronic exposures to fibrogenic clay compounds is associated with a number of pulmonary diseases (Table 64–9). Such diseases often go undetected until they have reached an advanced stage. Subclinical stages of these diseases can be detected by radiography, lung volume determinations, and testing of gas diffusion capacity (see Airborne chapter).
2. Glazes (Table 64–10)
   Lead poisoning from glaze materials continues to be a problem wherever there are ceramic artists and hobbyists who put themselves and others at risk. Potters in Third World countries still commonly use lead glazes. Lead poisoning and even death have been reported. Acidic foods and liquids have the greatest propensity for leaching lead from these objects.
3. Kiln emissions (Table 64–11)
   Poorly exhausted kiln emissions may cause airborne contamination because of a desire of the artist to place the kiln in a state of reduction (relative oxygen depletion), being fired under lead pressure, to bring out subtle colors of various glazes.

Table 64–11
Threshold Limit Values of Kiln Emissions[a]

Emission	Threshold Limit Value
Carbon monoxide By-product of incomplete combustion Significant exposure possible during reduction phase of firing	35 ppm
Chlorine gas By-product of salt glaze process	1 ppm
Hydrochloric acid vapor By-product of salt glaze process	5 ppm
Infrared radiation Significant exposure when cones are inspected through ports	NA
Nitrogen dioxide By-product of natural gas combustion	6 mg/m³
Nitric oxide By-product of natural gas combustion	30 mg/m³
Smoke and soot By-product of raku and smoke pit firings	NA
Sulfur dioxide By-product of bisque firing, especially of high-sulfur clay	2 ppm
Vaporized glaze constituents Various metal fumes	NA
Various hydrocarbons Aldehydes (formaldehyde) Mercaptans	1.5 mg/m³

NA, Not available.
[a]Adapted from Fuortes LJ. Postgrad Med 1989;85:133–136.

Table 64–12
Potentially Toxic Chemicals[a]

Name	Quantity Grams	Quantity Mg/Kg	Potentially Toxic Dose
Ammonium Chloride	12.73	1061	>2000 mg total
Azurite	8.36	697	>1 gm total (Cu)
	4.60 (Cu)	385 (Cu)	
Magnesium Sulfate	13.68	1140	500 mg/kg
Phenolphthalein	2.00	167	>2000 mg
Potassium Chloride	18.29	1524	238 mg/kg
Sodium Borate$_{(-H_2O)}$	5.10	425	170 mg/kg
Sodium Thiosulfate	21.82	1818	>12 gm total
Strontium Nitrate	24.85	2071	2750 mg/kg
Sulfur	10.42	868	>10 gm total
Sodium Bisulfite	16.91	1409	6.0 mg/kg

Based on Oral LD-50 (rats)
[a]Adapted from Everson GW et al. Vet Hum Toxicol 1988;30:589–592.

Table 64–13
Potentially Lethal Chemicals[a]

Name	Quantity Grams	Quantity Mg/Kg	Potentially Lethal Dose
Cobalt Chloride Hexahydrate	14.24	1187	766 mg/kg
Copper Sulfate	12.35	1030	300 mg/kg
Ferric Ammonium Sulfate	14.19		
(Elemental Fe)	(1.85)	154	60 mg/kg
Ferrous Sulfate Hexahydrate	5.72		
(Elemental Fe)	(1.14)	95	60 mg/kg
Tannic acid	8.36	697	500 mg/kg

[a]Adapted from Everson GW et al. Vet Hum Toxicol 1988;30:589–592.

4. Protective measures
   a. Glazes should be stored in liquid or slurry form to minimize dust exposure and should be applied by dipping or brushing, not spraying.
   b. Ventilation of the work area should be sufficient to exhaust away from the area all local production of toxic substances and to ensure proper functioning and exhaustion of kilns.
   c. Use personal protective clothing and devices, including gloves, overalls or aprons, and respirators.
   d. Stringent personal hygiene: frequent hand washing; no smoking, eating, or storing food in the areas used for pottery making.
   e. Do not work and live in the same quarters.
   f. Keep work clothes in the work area. Wash them often.
   g. Clean up dust in the work area with a wet vacuum or damp mop.
   h. Art materials suppliers should inform hobbyists and artisans of potential hazards. Proper labeling and storage of toxic substances should avert mishaps.
   i. Safety programs should be included in the studio arts curriculum.
   j. Replace the more toxic glaze substances (heavy metals and chromates) with nontoxic materials.[8]

Hobby Ceramicists

About two million Americans are hobby ceramicists; 95% of them are women, and 70% are between the ages of 30 and 50 years. About 80% of hobby glazing is done in educational studies run by distribution of hobby glazes. Hobby glazes are made up of frits (prefired mixtures of metal oxides, silica, aluminium, and alkalis), ceramic pigments (metal oxide–containing crystalline materials formed at high temperatures), clays, flint (fine quartz), feldspars, water, and other additives. Glazes that are certified as food safe will release less than 1 ppm lead when a standard 8-oz cup fired with such a glaze is tested by an FDA method.

Precautions[9]

1. Glazing should be done only in a room suitably equipped for the purpose.
2. Since the danger of lead poisoning is greatest where lead or its compounds are inhaled, processes that are likely to give rise to these compounds in dust form in the air should not be allowed unless there is efficient exhaust ventilation or a suitable respirator is used. Where a spray is used, there should be a separate booth with an efficient exhaust fan. These processes are normally confined to establishments of further education (trade schools).
3. Anyone who has carried out the processes should wash their hands and use a nail brush immediately afterwards.
4. All benches and work surfaces should be washed down after use, and splashes of glaze should be removed from floors and walls.
5. Food should not be eaten in any room used for pottery making.
6. Protective clothing (e.g., overalls or aprons) should be worn during all pottery classes and should be washed as necessary. An apron with bib of impervious materials should be worn by anyone while actually engaged in glaze dipping and should be washed after use.

CHEMISTRY SETS

Two children ingested an unknown substance from a chemical set. Evaluation of the urine and serum indicated an acute cobalt intoxication. Treatment with penicillamine and dimethylpropane sulfonate (DMPS) led to some increase in serum cobalt. Therapy was stopped after the cobalt urine concentration reached a normal range.[10] Three chemistry sets contained 28, 14, and 9 chemicals, respectively. Fifty-three percent of the chemicals contained quantities sufficient to be potentially toxic to a two-year-old, 12-kg child; 13% contained chemicals in potentially lethal quantities; and 18% were considered nontoxic. Only one chemistry set utilized child-resistant closures.[11] Thirty-five percent of the chemicals had incorrect or missing warning information (Tables 64–12 through 64–14). A 19-month-old who ingested about 1 ounce of a chemistry set container of cobalt chloride died within a few hours.[12] Two children were hospitalized after ingesting cobalt chloride from a chemistry set. They were given chelating agents and recovered.

Table 64–14
Potentially Caustic/Corrosive Chemicals[a]

Name	Quantity
Aluminum Sulfate	14.77 g
Ammonium Carbonate	6.97 g
Calcium Hydroxide	4.36 g
Calcium Oxide	4.90 g
Sodium Bisulfate	19.88 g
Sodium Ferrocyanide	5.53 g
Sodium Carbonate	7.90 g
Sodium Silicate	11.77 g
Calcium Chloride	6.23 g
Calcium Oxychloride	5.95 g

[a]Adapted from Everson GW et al. Vet Hum Toxicol 1988;30:589–592.

CHILDREN AND ART MATERIALS[13] (TABLE 64–15)[14]

Hazards

The common misconception that all children's products that are water-soluble are safe is not necessarily true because of the presence of preservatives. Water-soluble paints might be preserved with ammonia or formaldehyde. Fluorescent paints are toxic. Felt-tip markers have aromatic hydrocarbons. Modeling clay may contain toxic preservatives. Papier mâche is just flour and water, but if fresh newspaper is used, the color-illustrated sections may have toxic materials in the inks. Water-based glues have polyvinyl acetate emulsions. Many organic glues have solvents, and super glues have cyanoacrylate, which can cause adhesions of the conjunctiva if it gets in the eyes.[13a]

1. Swallowing paint with a high percentage of lead; ingesting lead where stained-glass work is being performed. Ingestion of turpentine, methyl alcohol, solvents (paint thinners, kerosene, lacquer thinners), acids, alkalis, photographic chemicals, dye, and pottery glaze ingredients.
2. Skin contact—burns, irritation, ulcers, allergies.

Table 64–15
Art Materials: Recommendations for Children Under 12[a]

Do Not Use	Substitutes
Dusts and Powders	
1. Clay in dry form. Powdered clay, which is easily inhaled, contains free silica and possible asbestos. Do not sand dry clay pieces or do other dust-producing activities.	1. Order talc-free, premixed clay (e.g. Amaco white clay). Wet mop or sponge surfaces thoroughly after using clay.
2. Ceramic glazes or copper enamels.	2. Use water-based paints instead of glazes. Artwork may be water-proofed with acrylic based mediums.
3. Cold water, fiber-reactive dyes or other commercial dyes.	3. Use vegetable and plant dyes (e.g. onionskins, tea, flowers) and food dyes.
4. Instant papier mâches (create inhalable dust and some may contain asbestos fibers, lead from pigments in colored printing inks, etc.).	4. Make papier mâche from black and white newspaper and library or white paste, or use approved papier mâches.
5. Powdered tempera colors (create inhalable dusts and some tempera colors contain toxic pigments, preservatives, etc.).	5. Use liquid paints or paints the teacher pre-mixes.
6. Pastels, chalks or dry markers that create dust.	6. Use crayons, oil pastels or dustless chalks.
Solvents	
1. Solvents (e.g., turpentine, shellac, toluene, rubber cement (thinner), and solvent-containing materials (solvent-based inks, ?? paints, rubber cement).	1. Use water-based products only.
2. Solvent-based silk screen and other printing inks.	2. Use water-based silk screen inks, block printing or stencil inks containing safe pigments.
3. Aerosol sprays.	3. Use water-based paints with brushes or spatter techniques.
4. Epoxy, instant glue, airplane glue or other solvent-based adhesives.	4. Use white glue, school paste, and preservative-free wheat paste.
5. Permanent felt tip markers which may contain toluene or other toxic solvents.	5. Use only water-based markers.
Toxic Metals	
1. Stained Glass projects using lead came, solder, flux, etc.	1. Use colored cellophane and black paper to simulate lead.
2. Arsenic, cadmium, chrome, mercury, lead, manganese, or other toxic metals which may occur in pigments, metal things, metal enamels, ceramic glazes, metal casting, etc.	2. Do not use these ingredients. Use approved materials only.
Miscelleneous	
1. Photographic chemicals.	1. Use blueprint paper and make sun grams, or use Polaroid cameras.
2. Casting plaster. Creates dust and casting hands and body parts have resulted in serious burns.	2. Teacher can mix plaster in a separate ventilated area or outdoors for plaster casting.
3. Acid etches and pickling baths.	3. Should not use techniques employing these chemicals.
4. Scented felt tip markers. These teach children bad habits about eating and sniffing art materials.	4. Use water-based markers.

[a]Adapted from Babo A, Peltz PA, Rossol M. Children's Art Supplies Can Be Toxic. New York: Center for Safety in the Arts, 1989.

Table 64–16
Hazards of Mordants and Dye-Assisting Chemicals[a]

Alum (potassium aluminum sulfate)
Some people may be allergic to alum, but no special precautions are needed when using it.

***Ammonia (ammonium hydroxide)**
Avoid concentrated solutions. Household strength ammonia is diluted and less hazardous. Inhalation of its vapors can cause respiratory and eye irritation.

Ammonium alum (ammonium aluminum sulfate)
Hazards are the same as those of alum (see above).

***Caustic soda (lye sodium hydroxide)**
Very corrosive to the skin, eyes, and respiratory tract.

*Clorox (household bleach, 5 percent sodium hypochlorite)
Corrosive to the skin, eyes, throat, and mucous membranes. Mixing with ammonia results in the release of poisonous nitrogen trichloride gas. Mixing with acids releases highly irritating chlorine gas.

***Copper sulfate (blue vitriol)**
May cause allergies and irritation of the skin, eyes, and upper respiratory tract. Chronic exposure to copper sulfate dust can cause ulceration and perforation of the nasal septum.

Cream ot tartar (potassium acid tartrate)
No significant hazards.

***Ferrous sulfate (copperas)**
Slightly irritating to skin, eyes, nose, and throat. No special precautions necessary.

***Formic acid (methanoic acid)**
Highly corrosive to eyes and mucous membranes. May cause mouth, throat, and nasal ulcerations.

Glauber's salt (sodium sulfate)
Slightly irritating to skin, eyes, nose, and throat.

***Oxalic acid**
Skin and eye contact may cause severe corrosion and ulceration. Inhalation can cause severe respiratory irritation and damage. Wear gloves and goggles.

***Potassium dichromate (potassium bichromate, chrome)**
Skin contact may cause allergies, irritation, and ulceration. Chronic exposure can cause respiratory allergies. A suspect carcinogen. Wear gloves and goggles.

***Salt (sodium chloride)**
Some all-purpose dyes contain enough to be toxic to children by ingestion. No other significant hazards.

***Sodium carbonate**
Corrosive to the skin, eyes, and respiratory tract.

***Sodium hydrosulfite (sodium dithionite)**
Irritating to the skin and respiratory tract. Stored solutions decompose to give irritating sulfur dioxide gas. Mixture with acids will release large amounts of sulfur dioxide gas.

***Sulfuric acid (oleum)**
Highly corrosive to skin and eyes. Vapors can damage respiratory system. Heating generates irritating sulfur dioxide gas.

***Tannin (tannic acid)**
Slight skin irritant. Causes cancer in animals. Handle with care.

***Tin chloride (tin, stannous chloride)**
Irritating to the skin, eyes, and respiratory tract.

Urea
No significant hazards.

Vinegar (dilute acetic acid)
Glacial (pure) acetic acid is highly corrosive and the vapors are irritating. Vinegar (about 5 percent acetic acid) is safer. Mildly irritating to skin and eyes.

*Can be poisonous if ingested. Keep out of reach of children.
[a]Adapted from Rossol M. New York: Center for Safety in the Arts, 1985 and 1986.

Table 64–17
Inhalation Hazards of Premixed Paints and Inks[a]

The following hazards and precautions apply to paint and ink techniques such as brushing and dipping which do not cause pigments and vehicles to become airborne. Spraying, airbrushing, and similar methods are far more hazardous and require local exhaust systems such as spray booths.

Acrylic Paints (water-based) release small amounts of formaldehyde and ammonia during drying. Can cause respiratory irritation and allergies. Formaldehyde has caused cancer in animals. Provide a small amount of dilution ventilation such as a window exhaust fan.

Acrylic Paints (solvent-based) contain solvents and are cleaned up and thinned with solvents. Provide dilution ventilation.*

Artist's Oils do not contain volatile ingredients but are thinned and cleaned up with toxic solvents such as turpentine and paint thinner. Provide dilution ventilation* such as a window exhaust fan. Some people also work thickly with paints using no thinners, cleaning brushes with baby oil followed by soap and water. No special ventilation is needed if solvents are not used.

Alkyd Paints contain solvents and must be cleaned up and thinned with solvents. Provide dilution ventilation.*

Commercial Oil Enamels and Paints contain a variety of solvents and are thinned and cleaned up with solvents. Provide dilution ventilation.*

Commercial Latex Paints. Contrary to common belief, these usually contain between 5 and 15 percent solvents—some very hazardous solvents such as the glycol ethers have been found in latex paints. Provide dilution ventilation.*

Marking Pens. Permanent markers contain solvents of varying toxicity. Watercolor markers are safer and are usually water- or water/alcohol-based. Provide dilution ventilation for solvent-containing markers.

Silk-Screen Inks (solvent-based) contain solvents and screens must be cleaned with solvents, resulting in heavy exposure to artists in unventilated studios. Provide local exhaust ventilation for printing area (e.g. slot hoods), drying racks, and screen wash area.

Silk-Screen Inks (water-based) are often specially retarded (slow drying) acrylics (see hazards above). They are an excellent alternative to more hazardous solvent-based inks. Provide some dilution ventilation.

Watercolor, caseins, tempera, poster paints, etc. often contain small amounts of preservatives such as formaldehyde, paraformaldehyde, phenol, etc. These are generally the safest types of paint. Exhaust ventilation usually is not needed.

*Ventilation rates will depend on the type and amount of solvent vaporized.
[a]Adapted from Rossol M. New York: Center for Safety in the Arts, 1985 and 1986.

3. Inhalation—solvent vapors, aerosol spray mists, metal fumes. Solvents in turpentine, paint thinner, paint and varnish removers, rubber cement, silk screen inks and solvents, lacquers and their thinners, shellac, permanent markers, cleaning solvents, aerosol spray cans, dry clay, glaze ingredients, dye powders, plaster dust, sawdust.
4. Etching gases, kiln gases, soldering fumes, gases from photographic developing.

DYES
Hazards

Acute—Caustic, skin or eye irritation.
Chronic—Chronic respiratory or skin diseases; carcinogens

Toxic Ingredients

Tables 64–16 through 64–19 contain lists of hazardous dyes and hazards of some pigments.[15,16] Most dye products are not safe for home use.[16] Precautions for use of paints, inks, and dyes are found in Table 64–20.[15,16]

ELDERLY ARTISTS

Retirement is a time for many people to pursue a favorite hobby. Some of these can involve hazardous chemical exposures. Metabolic changes in the elderly may render them less tolerant to many solvents, formaldehyde, and glycol ethers.[17,18]

ETCHING

Dutch mordant is 10% hydrochloric acid in water with potassium chlorate added. This is a reactive explosive that reacts with organic compounds, sulfur compounds, and sulfuric acid and with dirt and with clothing.[19]

FURNITURE STRIPPING—METHYLENE CHLORIDE[20–22]

Measures to Reduce Exposure

1. Ventilation system—according to design criteria of the Industrial Ventilation Manual of the American Conference of Governmental Industrial Hygienists.
2. Ambient air must comply with local, state, and federal air pollution regulations.
3. Activated charcoal filter may be required to reduce emissions of hydrocarbons.
4. Respiratory program utilizing an organic vapor cartridge respirator complying with OSHA standards.
5. Polyvinyl alcohol or butyl-rubber gloves.
6. Industrial vapors.
7. Eye rinse bath available.
8. Water available to rinse methylene chloride from skin.
9. Storage of methylene chloride in containers made of plain, galvanized, or lead-lined mild steel.
10. Clean-up of spillage.
11. Instruct all employees about the solvent used, its hazards, and emergency procedures in case of accidental ingestion, dermal contact, or unconsciousness from vapor inhalation.

Table 64–18
Hazards of Some Common Pigments [a]

Common Name	Pigment Name	
Lead Pigments—Do Not Use		
Chrome green	Pigment Green	15
Chrome yellow	Pigment Yellow	34
Flake white (white lead)	Pigment White	1
Molybdate (moly) orange	Pigment Red	104
Naples yellow	Pigment Yellow	41
Pigments associated with cancer—replace or use with caution		
Cadmium orange	Pigment Orange	20
Cadmium red	Pigment Red	108
Cadmium yellow (also other cadmium colors)	Pigment Yellow	37
Chrome yellow (also other chrome colors)	Pigment Yellow	34
Diarylide (benzidine) yellow [b]	Pigment Yellow	12
Lithol red	Pigment Red	49
Phthalocyanine (phthalo) blue [b]	Pigment Blue	15
Phthalocyanine (phthalo) green [b]	Pigment Green	7
Zinc yellow	Pigment Yellow	36
Pigments with moderate hazards—use wth caution		
Burnt and raw umber	Pigment Brown	7
Cobalt green	Pigment Green	19
Cobalt violet (cobalt phosphate)	Pigment Violet	14
Cobalt yellow	Pigment Yelow	40
Manganese blue	Pigment Blue	33
Manganese violet	Pigment Violet	16
Toluidine (hansa) red	Pigment Red	3
Pigments with no significant hazards—use with normal care		
Burnt and raw sienna	Pigment Brown	6
English red	Pigment Red	101
Ivory black	Pigment Black	9
Mars black	Pigment Black	11
Mars yellow (and all other Mars colors)	Pigment Yellow	41
Prussian blue	Pigment Blue	27
Titanium white	Pigment White	6
Ultramarine blue	Pigment Blue	29

[a]Adapted from Rossol M. New York: Center for Safety in the Arts, 1985 and 1986.
[b]Contaminated with PCBs.

GEMSTONE WORKERS[23]

Hazards

Silicosis.

Toxic Exposure

Stone sculptors in lapidaries who process tiger's eyes, rose quartz, amethyst, or quartz crystals. Seen mainly in South Africa and wherever stone sculptors work.

GLASSBLOWERS

Cough (the "usual cough"), bronchitis, hemoptysis, wheeze, and mild dyspnea is associated with diminished volume, vital capacity, and FEV, related to the total number of hours involved in glassblowing.[24]

LEAD EXPOSURE SOURCES

Sources of lead may be occupational, environmental, related to hobbies and related activities and from substance use and abuse[25] (Table 64–21). Lead exposures of parents working in pottery-producing is shared by an increase in lead exposure to children playing in these same areas.[26] Lead poisoning in the ceramics tile industry has recently been reduced due to the use of glazes with less lead.[27]

Under the Standard D4236, toxic products, including lead-based glazes, must be marked with a signal word such as "warning" or "caution," a list of ingredients, instructions for safe use of the products, and a statement that the product is inappropriate for use by children. Ceramic glaze may contain lead that can be absorbed if ingested.[28]

LEAD EXPOSURE[25–30] (TABLE 64–22)

Hazards

Acute

Not often seen in artists who usually are exposed to smaller quantities of lead chronically.

Table 64-19
Hazards of Dyes by Class[a]

Acid Dyes
Usually used on silk or wool. Often require addition of dye-assisting chemicals and/or mordants (see Table 2). Probably one of the least acutely toxic classes, but some carcinogenic food dyes and benzidine dyes belong to this class.

Azoic or Naphthol Dyes
Usually used on cellulosic fibers, acetate, triacetate and polyester. These dyes have been reported to cause severe allergies and skin reactions including depigmentation of the skin.

Basic Dyes
Usually used on wool, silk, and some synthetics. Fluorescent dyes usually belong to this class. Allergic reactions to some of these dyes have been reported and some are considered carcinogens.

Direct Dyes
Usually used on cotton, linen, and rayon applied from hot baths which contain salt. Usually present few acute hazards but the majority of cancer-causing benzidine dyes are found in this class.

Disperse Dyes
Usually used on water repellent fibers such as triacetate, nylon, polyester, and polyacrylonitrile (Dynel, Orlan, and Arlan). While other dyes have caused dermatitis on direct skin contact, only disperse dyes have caused widespread dermatitis from contact with the finished product. Use with great caution and for products other than apparel.

Fiber-Reactive Dyes
Also called "cold water," "batik," or "Procion" dyes, some forms will dye cellulosic fibers while others will dye wool, silk, and nylon. Bulk containers of these dyes are labeled with warnings about allergic respiratory reactions which some distributors fail to transfer to labels of smaller packages. Use special caution to avoid inhaling these dyes or getting them on your skin.

Vat Dyes
Most vat dyes are used for cellulosic fibers, while some are suitable for wool and acetate fibers. The dyeing process usually requires the use of lye or caustic soda either in the bath or as a pre-treatment for the dye. Pre-treated dyes are caustic to handle or inhale. Another potential hazard involves vat dye's need for oxidation after application. Air oxidizes some dyes, but others require treatment with dichromate salts which can cause allergies. Some vat dyes themselves also have been reported to cause allergies. Extreme care should be exercised if vat dyes are used; those sold as pigments are not recommended.

Other Dye Products
All-Purpose or Union Dyes
These common household dyes mix two or more classes of dye together with salt so that a wide variety of fabrics may be dyed. Only the dye which is specific for the cloth immersed is "taken" by the fabric. The number of dyes mixed obviously increases the potential hazard and some products contain the benzidine dyes. If these products must be used, liquid products should be chosen and used only occasionally with much caution.

[a]Adapted from Rossol M. New York: Center for Safety in the Arts, 1985 and 1000.

Table 64-20
Rules For Using Paints, Inks, and Dyes[a]

1. Only use dye or paint products for which C.I. names or numbers are available and obtain Material Safety Data Sheets (MSDS) on all products.
2. Use MSDS and product labels to identify the hazards of any toxic solvents, acids, or other chemicals in dyes, paints, and dye-assisting or mordanting chemicals *(see Table 2)*.
3. Use water-based products whenever possible. Generally, solvents and dyes are the most hazardous chemicals fiber artists use.
4. Buy pre-mixed paints and dyes if possible. Dyes packaged in packets which dissolve when dropped unopened into hot water also may be handled safely. Pigments and dyes are most hazardous and inhalable in the dry, powdered state.
5. Weigh out or mix dye powders or other toxic powders wth local exhaust ventilation or use a glove box *(see Figure 1)*.
6. Avoid dusty procedures. Sanding dry paints, sprinkling dry pigments or dyes on wet paint or glue, and other techniques which raise dust should be discontinued, or used only with local exhaust ventilation. If such procedures are used without ventilation, choose pigments (do not use dyes) known to be of low toxicity, wear a toxic dust respirator, and use wet mop cleaning procedures.
7. Choose brushing and dipping techniques over spray methods whenever possible.
8. Spraying paints of dyes should be done only with local exhaust ventilation such as a spray booth. Additional protection may be provided by wearing a proper respirator (dust/mist respirator for water based paints; paint, lacquer and enamel mist respirator for solvent-containing products).
9. Avoid skin contact with paints and pigments by wearing gloves or using barrier creams; use gloves with dyes. Wash off paint splashes with baby oil followed by soap and water, with non-irritating waterless hand cleaners, or with plain soap and water. Never use solvents or bleaches on skin to remove splashes.
10. Wear protective clothing including a full-length smock, special shoes and hair covering (if needed). Leave these garments in the studio to avoid bringing dusts home. Wear goggles if caustic dyes or corrosive chemicals are used.
11. Work on easy-to-clean surfaces and wipe up spills immediately. Do not cover work tables with newspapers when you use powders or dyes which will return to the powdered state when dry. Rolling up and discarding newspapers creates dust.
12. Wet mop floors and surfaces. Do not sweep.
13. Avoid ingestion of materials by eating, smoking, or drinking away from the workplace. Never point brushes with lips or hold brush handles in your teeth. Never use cooking utensils for dyeing. A pot which seems clean can be porous enough to hold hazardous amounts of residual dye. Wash hands carefully before eating or smoking, especially after handling lead weights or other lead metal items, powdered chemicals, or dusty textiles.
14. Keep containers of paint, powdered dyes and pigments, solvents, etc. closed except when you are using them.
15. Follow all solvent fire and safety rules if solvent-containing products are used. (COH has data sheet on "Common Solvents and their Hazards.")
16. Blood tests for lead should be done regularly if lead-containing paints, inks, or pigments are used.

[a]Adapted from Rossol M. New York: Center for Safety in the Arts, 1985 and 1986.

Table 64-21
Sources of Lead Exposure[a]

Occupational	Environmental	Hobbies and Related Activities	Substance Use
Plumbers, pipe fitters	Lead containing paint	Glazed pottery making	Folk remedies
Lead miners	Soil/dust near lead industries, roadways, lead-painted homes	Target shooting at firing ranges	"Health foods"
Auto repairers	Plumbing leachate	Lead soldering (e.g., electronics)	Cosmetics
Glass manufacturers	Ceramicware	Painting	Moonshine whiskey
Shipbuilders	Leaded gasoline	Preparing lead shot, fishing sinkers	Gasoline "huffing"
Printers		Stained-glass making	
Plastic manufacturers		Car or boat repair	
Lead smelters and refiners		Home remodeling	
Policemen			
Steel welders or cutters			
Construction workers			
Rubber product manufacturers			
Gas station attendants			
Battery manufacturers			
Bridge reconstruction workers			

[a]Adapted from Agency for Toxic Substances and Disease Registry. Case Studies in Environmental Medicine Lead Toxicity. September 1992.

Table 64-22
Lead Exposures[a]

Painting: oil painting, acrylics, automobile paints, boat paints, metal rust inhibiting paints; grinding pigments; sanding paints; heating paints with torching.
Ceramics: lead glazes, frits, glaze chemicals with lead, inhaling kiln fumes; eating from improperly glazed dinnerware.
Metal casting: casting lead-containing bronzes or other lead alloyed metals; finishing, chasing, or applying patinas to these metals.
Lead casting: making bullets, lead soldiers, cast and dripper lead sculpture.
Pewter work: casting of old formula (lead-containing) pewter; soldering, finishing, and sanding pewter.
Stained glass: handling, soldering (both regular and copper foil method), sanding, applying patinas to lead came; applying and firing glass enamels and paints.
Glassblowing: making and working with lead glass; using lead-containing colorants; applying gloss enamels and paints; grinding and polishing lead glass.
Art conservation and antique restoration: repairing or removing old paint and gesso, torching old paint; working with many old lead-containing metals and materials.
Welding: inhaling lead fumes from welding lead-painted metals such as old car parts.
Printmaking: using inks colored with lead pigments.
Photography: using the platinum process that employs lead oxalate.
Rubber mold making: when curing agent is lead peroxide.

Guidelines

Guidelines for reducing the risk of lead poisoning have been presented by the U.S. Food and Drug Administration. To reduce the risk of lead poisoning from ceramic dinnerware, experts advise:

- Avoid use of ceramicware for storing food. Instead, use glass or plastic containers to store foods, especially those foods with a high acid content such as orange, tomato, and other fruit juices, wines, tomato sauces, and vinegar. Acid in the food can increase the amount of lead released into the food.
- Beware of products purchased in other countries. The safety of dinnerware can vary from country to country. If you are unsure of whether products meet safety standards, it may be wise to avoid the purchase—or do not use them with foods.
- Do not use antiques or collectibles to hold food or beverages. Items bought at garage sales, craft shows, antique shops, flea markets, rummage sales, and other such places, along with family heirlooms, may have been made years before federal standards were imposed. Hence, using such items to hold food or beverages is not generally recommended.
- Be cautious of ceramic items made by amateurs or hobbyists. Glazes that are safe can be obtained by hobbyists, but there is no way of knowing if proper techniques and equipment were used to apply them. The safest course is to use such items for display purposes only.

[a]Adapted from Balin A. Lead hazards. Art Hazards News 1994;17(5):4–6.

Chronic

Exposure in air, licking paint brushes. Seen in artists, theater people, hobbyists, art conservators, children, students, and teachers.

These tips, say FDA officials, are intended as general guidelines. The fact remains there is no way of knowing for sure whether a piece is safe without having it tested. If you want further assurance, ceramic ware can be tested by a qualified commercial laboratory, though it may be expensive. Consult your local health department or the telephone book for laboratories in your area.[31–35]

Vance and colleagues have proposed recommendations for clinicians concerned with the initial management of patients who may have ingested a lead-based ceramic glaze[36] (see also Metals chapter):

1. A careful history must be obtained to determine the true extent of exposure, if possible. A history of an apparent minimal exposure (i.e., a "sip" or a "taste") should be

seriously questioned, and if any doubt exists, objective data should be obtained. All patients with more than an absolute minimal exposure should be referred to an appropriate health-care facility for evaluation.

2. An abdominal roentgenogram should be obtained in all cases in which a positive or questionable ingestion history is obtained. The presence of radiopaque material in the gastrointestinal tract is an indication for initiation of chelation therapy and decontamination of the gastrointestinal tract. However, a normal roentgenogram may be obtained if the ingestion was not discovered for some time or if any delays in referral have occurred.
3. Chelation therapy should be initiated in the presence of a roentgenogram that suggests ingestion or a definite ingestion history, even if a report of the blood lead concentration has not yet been obtained.
4. Gastrointestinal tract decontamination should be initiated in the presence of a roentgenogram that suggests ingestion or a definite ingestion history. Osmotic cathartic agents (e.g., sorbitol) and those containing magnesium should be administered cautiously, especially to young, elderly, or debilitated patients, because of the potential for fluid and electrolyte disorders secondary to excessive diarrhea or absorption of magnesium.
5. A baseline blood lead level should be obtained in cases of known or suspected exposure. Other useful laboratory studies include baseline hematologic, hepatic, and renal function tests. Serial blood lead levels should be obtained, and hepatic and renal function studies should be performed in patients who will undergo treatment.
6. A measurement of a blood lead concentration should be repeated within 2 to 3 days in a patient who does not undergo immediate treatment (because of a questionable ingestion and a normal roentgenogram) to ensure that blood lead levels are not rising markedly.

PAINTING HAZARDS[37] (TABLE 64–23)

1. Toxic pigments (Table 64–24)
   Lead, arsenic, antimony, cadmium, chromium, cobalt, manganese, and mercury can be ingested by contamination of hands, fingernails, food, cups, and cigarettes and by holding paint brushes in the mouth. When mixing paints from dry powdered pigments, airborne dust is generated.
   Toxic Ingredients: White lead or flake white (basic lead carbonate cadmium pigments), chrome yellow (lead chromate), and zinc yellow (zinc chromate) may cause lung cancer. Lamp black and carbon black may contain impurities that cause skin cancer. Chromatic pigments—chrome yellow (lead chromate) and zinc yellow (zinc chromate)—may cause skin ulcerations and allergic skin reactions.
   Precautions
   Protection is required in the form of local or exhaust ventilation, use of a glovebox or an approved respirator. The artist must wash the hands and nails

Table 64–23
Hazards to Photographers and Painters[a]

	Photographers	Painters
Metals	Borate	Arsenic
	Bromides	Barium
	Chromates	Chromates
	Iodine	Cadmium
	Lead	Lead
	Mercury	Manganese
	Silver	Mercury
	Tellurium	Magnesium
	Uranium	Titanium
	Vanadium	Zinc
Solvents	Aminophenols	Acetone
	Amylacetate	Benzene
	Benzene	Carbon Tetrachloride
	Ethylene Glycol	Methanol
	Formaldehyde	Turpentine
	Methanol	
	Trichloroethylene	
Others	Acids and Alkalis	Acids and Alkalis
	Cyanide	Carbon Disulfide
	Hydroquinone	Methylene Chloride
	Oxylate	Nitrogen Oxides
	Sodium Bisulfate	
	Sodium Hypochrome	
	Sodium Sulfide	
	Sodium Thiosulfite	

[a]Adapted from Lesser SH, Weiss SJ. Am J Emerg Med 1995;13:451–458.

Table 64–24
Toxic Pigments[a]

Known or Probable Carcinogens/Highly Toxic Pigments
Antimony white (antimony trioxide)
Barium yellow (barium chromate)
Burnt umber or raw umber (iron oxides, manganese silicates or dioxide)
Cadmium red or orange (cadmium sulfide, cadmium selenide)
Cadmium yellow (cadmium sulfide)
Cadmium barium colors (cadmium colors and barium sulfate)
Cadmium barium yellow (cadmium sulfide, cadmium selenide, barium sulfate, zinc sulfide)
Chrome green (prussian blue, lead chromate)
Chrome orange (basic lead carbonate)
Chrome yellow (lead chromate)
Cobalt violet (cobalt arsenate or cobalt phosphate)
Cobalt yellow (potassium cobaltinitrate)
Lead or flake white (basic lead carbonate)
Lithol red (sodium, barium and calcium salts of soluble azo pigment)
Manganese violet (manganese ammonium pyrophosphate)
Molybdate orange (lead chromate, lead molybdate, lead sulfate)
Naples yellow (lead antimonate)
Strontium yellow (strontium chromate)
Vermilion (mercuric sulfide)
Zinc sulfide
Zinc yellow (zinc chromate)

Moderately Toxic Pigments/Slightly Toxic Pigments
Alizarin crimson (lakes of 1,2-dihydroxyanthraquinone or insoluble anthraquinone pigment)
Carbon black (carbon)
Cerulean blue (cobalt stannate)
Cobalt blue (cobalt stannate)
Cobalt green (calcined cobalt, zinc and aluminum oxides)
Chromium oxide green (chromic oxide)
Manganese blue (barium manganate, barium sulfate)
Prussian blue (ferric ferrocyanide)
Toluidine red (insoluble azo pigment)
Toluidine yellow (insoluble azo pigment)
Viridian (hydrated chromic oxide)
Zinc white (zinc oxide)

[a]Adapted from Balin A. Art Hazards News 1991;14:3–6.

thoroughly after mixing paints and refrain from eating, drinking, or smoking in the studios.

2. Solvents—used in oil paints, as paint removers, and in varnishes. They are found in adhesives, fixatives to keep paint from smearing, permanent markers, lacquers, and thinners. Solvents include toluene, xylene, hexane, cyclohexane, methanol, methyl ethyl ketone, acetone, mineral spirits, methylene chloride, turpentine, alcohols, glycols, ethers, and others.

Precautions

Substitution with the least toxic materials, use of dilution and local exhaust ventilation, control of storage areas, disposal of solvent-soaked rags in covered containers, minimizing skin exposure, use of respirators and other personal protective equipment. Control of fire hazards.[38]

Water-Based Paints

Toxic Ingredients

Arylic paints—ammonia; formaldehyde. Casein paints—ammonium hydroxide. All water-based paints—preservatives, e.g., phenylmercuric acetate.

Non–Water-Based Paints

Toxic Ingredients

Solvents, turpentine, mineral spirits.

Airbrush, Spray Cans, Spray Guns

Toxic Ingredients

Solvents, pigments, propellants (isobutanes, propanes) that may be flammable.

Liquid Drawing Media

Toxic Ingredients

Solvent-based pen and ink and felt-tip markers: xylene, propyl alcohol.

Heavy Metal Pigments

Artists use colors such as bright yellow (arsenic, cadmium, lead), red, white, green, blue (mainly copper, cobalt, aluminum, and manganese), and violet (manganese, cobalt). Cobalt colors used by artists in the past century were often contaminated with arsenic. Earth colors such as yellow and red ochre, madder red, olive green, and brown consist of relatively harmless iron compounds. Olive green and madder red also contain lesser amounts of silicon and aluminum.

Artist colors consist of linseed oil, small amounts of aluminum stearate, and up to 80% pigment. About 8000 B.C. Egyptians used cinnabar (mercury sulfide), brilliant blues and greens (organic copper), bright yellows (arsenic sulfide), red, yellow, and brown ochre (iron compounds), and madder red (plant extract). Between the Roman Empire and the Renaissance new colors were added: white lead carbonate, yellow lead oxide, antimonate and stannate, and blue aluminum sulfosilicates and barium manganate. During the 19th century more pigment based in heavy metals began to be used: blue cobalt aluminates, yellow (cadmium sulfide and chromium oxide), red cadmium sulfide, green chromic oxide, and violets (cobalt arsenate and manganese ammonium phosphate).

Artists frequently did not wash their hands before smoking and eating; they often licked their brushes. Impoverished artists often lived, cooked, and ate in their studios. Water and food were easily contaminated by toxic heavy metals from pigments. Heat from a stove into which cloths soaked in old paint and discarded paintings were burned would have been a cheap source of heat and could have produced toxic metal fumes.

Artists today use less toxic pigments, tubes of paint carry warning labels, and artists know they should not lick brushes or burn colors indoors. Cigarettes are rarely hand-rolled, drinking water comes from taps and not buckets, and food is kept in refrigerators.

Paint Removers[39]

Hazards

Irritation to upper respiratory tract; dermatitis; renal, hepatic damage; acute CNS depression; chronic brain damage—behavioral changes, loss of memory, decreased intellectual abilities, confusion, seizures.

Toxic Ingredients

Methylene chloride, toluene, methanol, ethanol, acetone, mineral spirits.

PERFORMING ARTS

Activities

Dance studios, art rooms, classrooms, night clubs, discos, movie houses, orchestra halls, civic centers, fine arts centers, shops, arenas, lofts, big and little theater, outdoor drama structures; stages, dressing rooms, costume and fabric shops, make-up areas, amusement parks, TV and movie studios, carnivals, rock shows.

Exposure

Aerosols: methyl ethyl ketone, asbestos, acrylics, plastics for scenery, costumes, masks, armor, props. Acetone, dyes, photographic chemicals, sawdust, metal filings, gases, vapors, fiber from hemp, dust, machine oil.[40]

PHOTOGRAPHY

Many chemicals used in photographic processing can cause severe skin problems and/or lung problems through inhalations of dusts and vapors.

Simple black-and-white processing includes the mixing of chemical developers, stop bath fixing and rinsing steps. Handling concentrated stock solutions of the chemicals can be hazardous.

Developer

Hydroquinone (skin reactions, allergic reaction, eye problems) is a mutagen, a possible cancer risk. Metol (monomethyl *p*-aminophenol sulfate) may induce skin reactions and an allergic reaction. Some developers are toxic by inhalation of powders, and due to ingestion, causing methemoglobinemia and cyanosis. Developers are dissolved in a strongly alkaline solution, often containing sodium hydroxide, which can cause skin irritation and burns.

Stop Bath

Weak solution of acetic acid. Glacial acetic acid, used to make up the stop bath can induce severe skin burns; inhalation can irritate the upper and lower respiratory tract.

Stop Hardener

Potassium chrome alum—can cause skin and nasal ulceration and allergies.

Fixer

Sodium sulfate, sodium bisulfite, sodium thiosulfate (hypo), boric acid, potassium alum. Hypo and the mixture of sodium sulfite and acids can produce sulfur dioxide gas, irritating to eyes and respiratory tract, especially in asthmatics.

Hardener

Potassium alum: weak sensitizer, causes skin ulceration, dermatitis.

Hazards

Gases created during process—sulfur dioxide, chlorine, formaldehyde, ammonia, hydrogen cyanide (when reducers such as potassium cyanide and potassium ferrocyanide are heated, mixed with acids, or exposed to ultraviolet light).

Precautions

Proper handling and storage of chemicals. Use of less toxic chemical. Proper darkroom design and ventilation—10 to 20 air turnovers/hour. Materials handled with protective gloves and photographic tongs. Chemical labeled and stored individually.

ADVANCED BLACK-AND-WHITE PROCESSING

Intensification (bleaches): Potassium dichromate, hydrochloric acids—in two-component chrome intensifiers. Each component can cause burns. Together they produce chromic acid. Vapors are corrosive and may cause lung cancer. Potassium chlorochromate produces chlorine gas when heated or treated with acid.

Mercuric chloride powder can be absorbed through the skin and cause mercury poisoning. It should not be used. Reducer: "Farmer's Reducer": potassium ferrocyanide. When in contact with heat, acids, or ultraviolet radiation, hydrogen cyanide gas can be released.

Toners

May include selenium, uranium, sulfides, gold and platinum and oxalic acid.

Hardeners and Stabilizers

Often contain formaldehyde. Irritating to the eyes, skin, and upper respiratory tract, possibly carcinogenic.

COLOR PROCESSING

Same chemicals as in black-and-white processing, but in addition, dye couplers, organ solvent, formaldehyde. More sulfide dioxide fumes.[41]

PRINTMAKING

Silk Screening

Hazards

Solvent exposure by inhalation, by skin absorption, and by ingestion. Excessive solvents induce drowsiness, fatigue, and inattention. Exposure occurs when prints are dried on racks in an open studio. Xylene, toluene, and carbon blacks are contaminated with polycyclic aromatic hydrocarbons. Pigments used in paintings. Lead pigments (chrome yellow—lead chromate; chrome green—lead chromate; Milori green—lead chromate and potassium ferrocyanide; molybdate orange—lead chromate, lead molybdate, and lead sulfate). Exposure when prints are dried on racks in an open studio. Dermatitis, central nervous system damage—(dizziness, lightheadedness, fatigue, nausea, lack of coordination, headaches), eye irritation, adverse reproductive hazards.

Precaution

Ventilated drying rack enclosure, slotted table-top exhaust. Substitution and use of least hazardous materials. Proper storage of solvent-soaked rags in covered containers. Person protective equipment (selected gloves according to chemicals used). Eye protection as required.

Intaglio Hazards

Etching grounds contain asphalt in an oil or solvent. Many contain carcinogens. Rosins used in aquatinting may be allergens when inhaled. Solvents are used to clean paints. Inorganic acid as used to etch plates. Plates dipped in nitric acid and can release nitrogen oxides. Dutch mordant (hydrochloric acid, potassium chlorate, and water) can liberate chlorine gas and be explosive if mixed with organics.

Lithography (Table 64–25)[42]

Drawing is made on stone, then the stone is chemically treated with gum arabic and acid. Ink is applied. The stone and paper are run through a lithography press to create the image. Talc is used to dust the stones—possible asbestos exposure. Acids such as nitric, phosphoric, tannic are used. Dichromates—dermatitis, allergy, ulcerations of hands and nose. Precautions: Control dangling clothing, hair, and jewelry. Use guards. The following hazards are encountered:

Table 64–25
Constituents of Products Marketed for Lithography[a]

Organic Chemicals or Mixtures	Other Chemicals—Acids, Oils, Etc.
Acetone	Acetic acid
Benzene	Castor oil
Benzoyl peroxide	Flaxseed oil
Cyclohexane	Linseed oil
Ethyl benzene	Mineral oil
Ethylene dichloride	Nitric acid
Ethylene oxide	Sodium hydroxide
Heptane	Sulfuric acid
Hexane	Water
Hexylene glycol	
Isopropanol	
Kerosene	
Methyl ethyl ketone	
Methyl methacrylate	
Methanol	
Mineral spirits	
Naphtha	
Pitch	
Toluene	
1,1,1-Trichloroethane	
Turpentine	
Xylene	

[a]Adapted from Fuchs R, McCann M. Silkscreen printing. New York: Center for Safety in the Arts, 1988.

1. Improper storage of materials.
2. No metal cabinets for flammable solvent storage.
3. Working in cluttered environment.
4. Not sweeping up after sculpture or wood carving.
5. Not capping solvent cans when stored.
6. Failing to extinguish flame when not welding or soldering.
7. Little attention to label warnings.
8. No local exhaust ventilation.
9. No designated areas for curtain operations.
10. No personal protective equipment.

RELIEF PRINTING

Hazards

Caustic soda, solvents, glues, possibly methyl methacrylate.[43,44]

SCULPTURE[45,46]

Metals, plastic, and wood are commonly used.

METALS—METAL CASTING

Bronze, iron, copper, pewter, aluminium.

Hazards

Metal fumes. Lead, cadmium, chromium, beryllium.

Welding, Soldering, Brazing

Toxic fumes and gases (e.g., carbon monoxide, nitrogen oxides, ozone) generated. Metal dusts (cadmium, nickel, chromium, brass) may induce skin sensitization. Welding near chlorinated solvents can produce nickel carbonyl.

Welding Hazards

Fire, electric shock from arc welding equipments, burns. Exposure of infrared, visible, ultraviolet radiation (UVR): cataracts, conjunctivitis. UVR: skin burns, possible skin tumors.

Toxic Exposure

- Oxyacetylene torches—carbon dioxide, carbon monoxide, acetylene.
- Metal welding—nitrogen oxides, ozone.
- Near degreasing solvents—phosgene evolves from effect of ultraviolet radiation or chlorinated hydrocarbon.
- Vaporization of metals, metal alloys, electrodes—metal fumes, copper, zinc, lead, tin, cadmium, nickel, titanium, chromium.
- Welding of stainless steel—nickel plus heat produces nickel carbonyl (headaches, dizziness, neurologic disorders, pulmonary edema, possible allergic bronchial asthma; nickel fume industry may cause possible lung cancer.
- Coating—lead paint, mercury-containing anti-fouling paint, cadmium plating.

Soldering—Brazing

A third metal of lower melting point is used to join two metals.

Hazard

Zinc chloride gases, cadmium fumes, fluoride fumes. Brazing (hard or silver soldering) —higher temperature use.

PLASTICS[47] (SEE ALSO CHAPTER 69)

Polyester resins use styrene monomer, organic peroxides as catalysts (e.g., methyl ethyl ketone peroxide). Acrylic contains methyl methacrylate and peroxide catalysts. Glues contain solvents such as ethylene dichloride, methylene chloride and trichloroethane. Polyurethane may elaborate diisocyanates (e.g., toluene diisocyanate). Epoxy resin uses amines as hardeners; these are strong sensitizers and irritants. Vinyl polymers such as polyvinyl chloride can release hydrogen chloride fumes and plasticizers when heated. Styrofoam can release methyl chloride and styrene monomers when heated.

Polyester Resin

Hazards

Sensitization (allergic dermatitis, asthma); explosion and fire hazards; toxic gas inhalations.

Silicone and Natural Rubbers

Hazards

Silicone contains solvents (acetone, methylene chloride). Natural rubbers contain hexane.

Epoxy Resin

Hazards

Respiratory irritants, sensitizers, suspected carcinogens.

Polyurethane Resins

Hazards

Polyol polymers; diisocyanates; metal salts; foaming agents (freon).

Methyl Methacrylate Monomer

Hazards

Skin, eyes, respiratory tract irritant.

Polyvinyl Chloride (PVC)

Hazards

Heating PVC can release hydrogen chloride gas.

Organic Peroxides

Initiate polymerization in polyester, acrylic, some silicone resins.

Hazards

Burn vigorously; can explode.

Toxic Components

Benzoyl peroxide; methyl ethyl ketone peroxide.

WOOD (TABLES 64–26 AND 64–27)[48,49]

Methylene chloride is used as a paint stripper. Wood dust consists of small particles produced when wood is chipped, carved, milled, shaped, planed, rauted, drilled, turned, or sanded. Dust from hardwoods (mahogany, ebony and beta) produce smaller particles than that from soft woods. Most particles are larger than 2 to 10 μm. More than 90% of spherical particles with diameters of 50 μm or more are deposited in the nose. Woods may contain alkaloids, saprins, aldehydes, quinones, flavonoids, tropolones, oils, cardiotoxic steroids, stilbenes, resins, and proteins. Woods may also contain preservatives such as potassium dichromate, ethyl triethanolamine, glycol humectant, naphthenate, creosote, pentachlorophenol, arsenic compounds, and wood glues and adhesives (epoxys; urea-formaldehyde and phenol-formaldehyde resins). Nasal adenocarcinomas may be associated with exposure to wood dust.[50]

ADHESIVES[51]

Hazards

Hazardous solvents, plastics, preservatives. Possible carcinogens.

Toxic Ingredients

- Solvents—*n*-hexane, toluene, naphthas.
- Polymers—Epoxy hardeners; epoxy resins, cyanoacrylates; methyl methacrylates.
- Woodworking glues polyvinyl acetate (relatively nontoxic); resorcinol formaldehyde (releases formaldehyde); toxic phenols.
- Aerosol adhesives (sprayed)—*n*-hexane solvent.
- Wheat paste—toxic preservatives—pentachlorophenol, arsenic, or mercury derivatives.

ORGAN SYSTEM HAZARDS

Nervous System

Generalized neurotoxins include mercury, manganese, carbon disulfide, organophosphates, and plasticizers. Plasticizers are substances used to improve the working properties of resins in fiberglass sculpture. Isolated peripheral neuropathies are produced by methylbutyl ketone, aerosols, polyester resins, and lead. Central nervous system problems are caused by organic solvent intoxication (e.g., toluene and xylol). Printmakers and silk screen printers volatilize these solvents as sprays, potentiating their toxicity. Neurotrauma from the use of hammers and chisels can cause vibration syndrome and carpal tunnel syndrome.

Eyes

The eyes are a site of trauma and toxicity from almost all art forms. Ultraviolet light and heat exposure can cause cataracts, retinal damage, and a superficial punctate keratopathy ("welder's conjunctivitis").

Heart

Cardiotoxic heavy metals are contained in paints. Barium, cobalt, and many of the organic solvents (toluol, methyl chloroform, and methylene chloride) are direct cardiac toxins.

Respiratory

Respiratory tract irritants affect different sites based on particle size and solubility. Highly lipid-soluble dusts and fumes cause more systemic injury and minimally lipid-soluble substances produce more local effects. Substances that are more water-soluble will remain in the upper respiratory tract and the skin. Less water-soluble substances will affect the lower respiratory tract (see Chapter 66). Among the direct irritants are nitrogen dioxide (welding gas, carbon arc, etching, and enameling), chromium gas (from etching acid), hydrogen chromide (heating, plastics, and polyvinyl chloride), caustic dusts (lime, dichromate, soda ash, and potassium), and antiskinning agents (eugenol and clove oil). Certain substances have been associated with specific respiratory diseases. Pneumoconiosis is caused by iron oxides, aluminum, and barium sulfate. Pulmonary fibrosis is caused by silica, coal, talc, scrap stone, and asbestos. Asthma is exacerbated by wood and bone dust, fibers, reactive dyes, formaldehyde, turpentine, polyurethane, isocyanate, and freshly formed aluminum oxide ("pot room asthma"). Hypersensitivity pneumonitis is caused by wood dusts and heavy metals. Anthracosis is caused by smoke elaborated when coke is combusted.

Liver

Clinical hepatitis is caused by chlorinated hydrocarbons, phenol, ethyl alcohol, nitrobenzene, cadmium, styrene, arsenic, toluene, lead, and xylene. Manganese may cause pathologic hepatic changes.

Kidney

Direct renal toxins include oxalic acid, turpentine, ethylene glycol, and mercury. Chronic renal disease caused by cadmium is characterized by a beta$_2$-microglobulinemia and proteinuria.

Table 64–26
Toxic Woods[a]

Wood	Reaction	Site	Potency	Source	Incidence
Bald Cypress	S	R	+	D	R
Balsam Fir	S	E, S	+	LB	C
Beech	S, C	E, S, R	++	LB, D	C
Birch	S	R	++	W, D	C
Black Locust	I, N	E, S	+++	LB	C
Blackwood	S	E, S	++	D, W	C
Boxwood	S	E, S	++	D, W	C
Cashew	S	E, S	+	D, W	R
Cocobolo	I, S	E, S, R	+++	D, W	C
Dahoma	I	E, S	++	D, W	C
Ebony	I, S	E, S	++	D, W	C
Elm	I	E, S	+	D	R
Goncalo Aves	S	E, S	++	D, W	R
Greenheart (Surinam)	S	E, S	+++	D, W	C
Hemlock	C	R	?	D	U
Iroko	I, S, P	E, S, R	+++	D, W	C
Mahogany (Swietenia)	S, P	S, R	+	D	U
Mansonia	I, S,	E, S	+++	D, W	C
	N		+	D	
Maple (C. Corticale mold)	S, P	R	+++	D	C
Mimosa	N		?	LB	U
Myrtle	S	R	++	LB, D	C
Oak	S	E, S	++	LB, D	R
	C		?	D	U
Obeche	I, S	E, S, R	+++	D, W	C
Oleander	DT	N, C	++++	D, W, LB	C
Olivewood	I, S	E, S, R	+++	D, W	C
Opepe	S	R	+	D	R
Padauk	S	E, S, N	+	D, W	R
Pau Ferro	S	E, S	+	D, W	R
Peroba Rosa	I	R, N	++	D, W	U
Purpleheart		N	++	D, W	C
Quebracho	I	R, N	++	D, LB	C
	C		?	D	U
Redwood	S, P	R, E, S	++	D	R
	C		?	D	U
Rosewoods	I, S	R, E, S	++++	D, W	C
Satinwood	I	R, E, S	+++	D, W	C
Sassafras	S	R	+	D	R
	DT	N	+	D, W, LB	R
	C		?	D	U
Sequoia	I	R	+	D	R
Snakewood	I	R	++	D, W	R
Spruce	S	R	+	D, W	R
Walnut, Black	S	E, S	++	D, S	C
Wenge	S	R, E, S	++	D, W	C
Willow	S	R, N	+	D, W, LB	U
Western Red Cedar	S	R	+++	D, LB	C
Teak	S, P	E, S, R	++	D	C
Yew	I	E, S	++	D	C
	DT	N, C	++++	D, W	C
Zebrawood	S	E, S	++	D, W	

Reaction	Site	Source	Incidence
I—irritant	S—skin	D—dust	R—rare
S—sensitizer	E—eyes	W—wood LB—leaves, bark	C—common
C—nasopharyngeal cancer	R—resp.		U—unknown
P—pneumonitis, alveolitis (hypersensivity pneumonia)	C—cardiac		
DT—direct toxin	N—nausea, malaise		

[a]Adapted from Woodcock R. Toxic woods. Art Hazards News 1990;13(5):

Table 64-27
Principal Toxic Timbers[a]

Trade Name	Botanical Name	Dermatitis, Mucosal Irritation, Asthma, General Symptoms	Active Substances
Arbor vitae	*Thuja standishii*	M A	Tropolones
Ayan	*Distemonanthus benthamianus*	D	Oxyayanins
Blackwood, African	*Dalbergia melanoxylon*	D	Dalbergiones
Boxwood, Knysna	*Gonioma kamassi*	M A G	Quebrachamine ?
Cedar, Western red	*Thuja plicata*	(D) M A	Tropolones
Cocobolo	*Dalbergia retusa* et spp.	D	Dalbergiones
Cocus	*Brya ebenus*	D	Quinones ?
Dahoma	*Piptadeniastrum africanum*	M	?
Ebony	*Diospyros* spp.	D M	Quinones
Guarea	*Guarea thompsonii* et spp.	M	?
Ipé (lapacho)	*Tabebuia ipe* et spp.	D M G	Desoxylapachol
Iroko	*Chlorophora excelsa*	D (M A)	Stilbene
Katon	*Sandoricum indicum*	M G	?
Mahogany, African	*Khaya ivorensis* et spp.	D (M)	Anthothecol
Mahogany, American	*Swietenia macrophylla* et spp.	D	?
Makoré	*Tieghemella heckelii*	D M	Saponin
Mansonia	*Mansonia altissima*	(D) M G	Mansonones (quinones) Glycosides
Obeche	*Triplochiton scleroxylon*	(D) M A	?
Opepe	*Nauclea trillesii*	D M	?
Peroba rosa	*Aspidosperma peroba*	D M G	Alkaloids
Peroba, white	*Paratecoma peroba*	D M	Desoxylapachol ?
Ramin	*Gonystylus bancanus*	D	?
Rosewoods	*Dalbergia* spp., *Machaerium* spp.	D	Dalbergiones
Satinwood, Ceylon	*Chloroxylon swietenia*	D	Alkaloid ? Furocoumarins ?
Satinwood, W. Indian (and African)	*Fagara flava* et spp.	D	Alkaloid ? Furocoumarins ?
Sequoia	*Sequoia sempervirens*	M G	?
Stavewood	*Dysoxylum muelleri*	M G	?
Teak	*Tectona grandis*	D	Desoxylapachol
Liverworts and lichens on bark	*Frullania*, etc.	D	Sesquiterpene lactones

[a]Adapted from Woods B, Calnan CD. Br J Dermatol 1976;95(Suppl 13):1–97.

Skin

The grinding of fiberglass-reinforced sculptures produces particles that can cause an intensely pruritic rash. Plaster and cement contain lime, which can produce a severe dermatitis. Other causes of dermatitis include photographic developers, exotic woods, soaps, drying agents, and solvents.

Hematology

Numerous hematologic effects can be seen. Cyanosis is caused by polyvinyl chloride, nitrates, and other photographic developers. Lead, cadmium, benzene, and naphthalene can cause a hemolytic anemia.

Teratogens and Carcinogens

Teratogens and carcinogens include chromium, zinc, and arsenic. Chromium, a documented carcinogen, may be inhaled when metal sculptors grind through or weld scraps of chromium-plated steel (used in car manufacturing). Cadmium, a chronic renal toxin (see Painting), is also a carcinogen.[52]

REFERENCES—HOBBIES

1. Lucas AD, Salisbury SA. Industrial hygiene survey in a university art department. J Environ Pathol Toxicol Oncol 1992; 11:21–27.
2. Meister JF, Ogle JL. A waste disposal program for a university art department. J Environ Pathol Toxicol Oncol 1992; 11:33–37.
3. Babin A. Center for Safety in the Arts Art Hazards Information Center. Health and Safety Resources for the Arts. Hazards News 1992;15:4–7 Art.
4. Center for Safety in the Arts. Arts Hazards News 1993;16:1.
5. Fuortes L, Leo A, Ellerbeck PG, Friell LA. Acute respiratory fatality associated with exposure to sheet metal and cadmium fumes. Clin Toxicol 1991;29:279–283.
6. Miller BA, Blair A, McCann M. Mortality patterns among professional artists. A preliminary report. J Environ Pathol Toxicol Oncol 1985;6:303–313.
7. Miller BA, Silverman DT, Hoover RN, Blain A. Cancer risk among artistic painters. Am J Ind Med 1986;9:281–287.
8. McCann M. Ceramics. In: McCann M: Artists beware. New York. Lyons & Burford, 1992. See also Art Hazards News 1993;16(1):1–18.
9. Ministry of Education. Administrative Memorandum No. 517: Restrictions on the use of certain types of glazes in the teaching of pottery. London. 1973.
10. Muller C, Bertram HP, Rau W, Morandini T. Diagnosis and DMPS-treatment of accidental cobalt chloride ingestion—case report. Antidotes. Seminar on the Use of Chelating Agents in Poisoning, Munster, Germany. Eur Assoc Pois Control Center; May 31, 1989.
11. Everson GW, Normann SA, Casey JP. Chemistry set chemicals: an evaluation of their toxic potential. Vet Hum Toxicol 1988;30:589–592.
12. Jacobziner H, Raybin HW. Accidental cobalt poisoning. Arch Pediatr 1961;78:200–205.
13. McCann M. Children and arts materials. In: Health hazards manual for artists. 3rd ed. New York: Lyons & Burford, 1985.

13a. Lesser SH, Weiss SJ. Art hazards. Am J Emerg Med 1995; 13:451–458.
14. Babin A, Peltz PA, Rossol M. Children's art supplies can be toxic. New York: Center for Safety in the Arts, 1989.
15. Rossol M. Fiber art hazards and precautions. New York: Center for Safety in the Arts, 1985.
16. Rossol M. Dye hazards and precautions. New York: Center for Safety in the Arts, 1984.
17. Conklin BR. Environmental hazards to elderly artists. JAMA 1984;252:3130.
18. Glasbrenner K. Maladies may be linked to artists' materials. JAMA 1984;251:1391–1395.
19. Letts N. Dutch mordant and etching hazards. Art Hazards News 1990.
20. Anderson LA Jr, Huntebrinker T. Exposure to methylene chloride in small furniture stripping shops. In: McCann M. Health hazards manual for artists. 3rd ed. New York: Nick Lyons Books, 1985, pp. 65–74.
21. Young RJ, Infante PF. Consumer's benzene exposure during a furniture stripping operation. In McCann M. Health hazards manual for artists. 3rd ed. New York: Nick Lyons Books, 1985, pp. 75–79.
22. Health hazards manual for artists. 3rd ed. New York: Nick Lyons Books, 1985, pp. 75–79.
23. White NW, Chetty R, Bateman ED. Silicosis among gemstone workers in South Africa: tigers'-eye pneumoconiosis. Am J Ind Med 1991;19:205–213.
24. Braun SR, Tsiatis A. Pulmonary abnormalities in art glassblowers. J Occup Med 1979;21:487–489.
25. Royce SE, Needleman HL. Lead toxicity. Case studies in environmental medicine. Agency for Toxic Substances and Disease Registry. Public Health Series. June 1990.
26. Katagiri Y, Toriumi H, Kawai M. Lead exposure among 3-year-old children and their mothers living in a pottery-producing area. Int Arch Occup Environ Health 1983;52:223–229.
27. De Rosa E, Toffalo D, Sigon M, Brighenti F, Gori GP, Bartolucci GB. Evaluation of the current risk of lead poisoning in the ceramics industry. Scand J Work Environ Health 1983; 9:463–469.
28. CDC. Lead ingestion associated with ceramic glaze—Alaska, 1992. MMWR 1992;41:781–783.
29. Avila MH, Romieu I, Rios C, Rivero A, Palazuelos E. Lead-glazed ceramics are major determinants of blood lead levels in Mexican women. Environ Health Perspect 1991;91:117–120.
30. Ooi DS, Perkins SL. A ceramic glazer presenting with extremely high lead levels. Hum Toxicol 1988;7:171–174.
31. Rossol M. Lead poisoning. New York: Center for Safety in the Arts, November 1981.
32. Reducing exposure to lead from ceramic ware. FDA Backgrounder, November 1991. Arts Hazards News 1991; 14(6):1–3.
33. Bradley J, Vance M, Curry S. Environmental lead contamination in nursing homes. Vet Hum Toxicol 1988;30:361.
34. Lecos CW. Pretty poison: lead and ceramic ware. FDA Consumer 1987;21(6):6–9.
35. Fischbein A, Wallace J, Sassa S, Kappas A, Butts G, Rohl A, Kaul B. Lead poisoning from art restoration and pottery work. Unusual exposure source and household risk. J Environ Pathol Toxicol Oncol 1992;11:7–11.
36. Vance MV, Curry SC, Bradley JM, Kunkel DB, Geskin RD, Bond GR. Acute lead poisoning in nursing home and psychiatric patients from the ingestion of lead-based ceramic glazes. Arch Intern Med 1990;150:2085–2095.
37. Pederson LM, Permin H. Rheumatic disease, heavy metal pigments and the great masters. Lancet 1988;1:1267–1269.
38. Babin A. Art painting and drawing. Art Hazards News 1991; 14(6):3–6.
39. Fuchs R, Babin A, Rossol M. Paint Removers. New York: Center for Safety in the Arts, 1988.
40. Davidson R. Health hazards in the performing arts. In: McCann M. Health hazards manual for artists. 3rd ed. New York: Nick Lyons Books, 1985, pp. 23–27.
41. McCann M. Photographic processing hazard in schools. Art Hazards News 1990;13(9):1–3.
42. Fuchs R, McCann M. Silk screen printing. New York: Center for Safety in the Arts, 1988.
43. Lucas AD. Health hazards associated with the cyanotype printing process. J Environ Pathol Toxicol Oncol 1992;11:18–20.
44. McCann M, Barazeni G, ed. Proc 50EH Conference on Health Hazards in the Arts and Crafts. Society for Occup Environ Health, Washington, DC.
45. Hart C. Art hazards. An overview for sanitarians and hygienists. J Environ Health 1987;49:282–287.
46. Sidelecki JT. Potential health hazards of materials used by artists and sculptors. JAMA 1968;204:86–90.
47. Eckardt RE, Hindin R. The health hazards of plastics. J Occup Med 1973;15:808–819.
48. Woodcock R. Toxic woods. Art Hazards News 1990;13(5):
49. Woods B, Calnan CD. Toxic woods. Br J Dermatol 1976; 95(Suppl 13):1–97.
50. Wills JH. Nasal carcinoma in woodworkers: a review. J Occup Med 1982;24:526–530.
51. Babin A. Adhesives. Art Hazards News 1989;12(6):3.
52. Lesser SH, Weiss SJ. Art hazards. Am J Emerg Med 1995;13:451–458.

SUGGESTED READINGS

1. McCann M. Health hazards manual for artists. 3rd ed. New York: Lyons & Burford, 1985; pp. 100.
2. McCann M, Barazani G, eds. Health hazards in the arts and crafts. Washington, DC. Society for Occupational and Environmental Health, 1980, pp. 232.
3. Babin A. Center for Safety in the Arts. 5 Beekman Street, New York, NY 10038, 212-227-6220. Health and Safety Resources for the Arts. Art Hazards News 1992;15:4–7.
4. Thomas TL, Stewart PA. Mortality from lung cancer and respiratory disease among pottery workers exposed to silica and talc. Am J Epidemiol 1987;125:35–43.
5. Forastiere F, Lagorio S, Michelozzi P, Cavariani F, Arca M, Borgia P, Perucci C, Axelson O. Silica, silicosis and lung cancer among ceramic workers: a case-referent study. Am J Ind Med 1986;10:363–370.
6. De Rosa E, Toffolo D, Sigon M, Brighenti F, Gori GP, Bartolucci GB. Evaluation of the current risk of lead poisoning in the ceramics industry. Scand J Work Environ Health 1983; 9:463–469.
7. Annest JL, Pirkle JL, Makuc D, Neese JW, Bayse DD, Kovar MG. Chronological trend in blood lead levels between 1976 and 1980. N Engl J Med 1983;308:1373–1377.
8. Lead Toxicity. Case Studies in Environmental Medicine ATSDR, US Department of Health and Human Services, June 1990.
9. Stopford W. Safety of lead-containing hobby glazes. N C Med J 1988;49:31–34.
10. Ministry of Education. Administrative Memorandum No. 517: Restrictions on the use of certain types of glazes in the teaching of pottery. London. 1973.
11. Lecas CW. Lead and ceramic ware. FDA Consumer 1987; 21(6):6–9.
12. Bradley J, Vance M, Curry S. Environmental lead contamination in nursing homes. Vet Hum Toxicol 1988;30:361.
13. Fuortes LJ. Health hazards of working with ceramics. Recommendations for reducing risks. Postgrad Med 1989; 85:133–136.
14. Rossol M. Environmental industrial mini course: art hazards: toxic risks to artists and craftsmen. New York: Art Hazards Information Center of the Center for Occupational Hazards, December 3, 1984.
15. Pike S. Hazards from hobbies, arts and crafts. Proc Fourth Annual Southwestern Poison Symposium. Scottsdale, AZ. Arizona Poison and Drug Information Center, November 2–3, 1984, pp. 34–49.
16. Reproductive hazards in the arts and crafts. New York: Center for Occupational Hazards, 1986.
17. Miller BA, Silverman DT, Hoover RN, Blair A. Cancer risk among artistic painters. Am J Ind Med 1986;9:281–287.
18. Miller BA, Blair A, McCann M. J Environ Path Toxicol Oncol 1985;6:303–313.

19. Franklin BA. Paint use is linked to artists' cancer. New York Times, May 17, 1981.
20. Glasbrenner K. Maladies may be linked to artists' material. JAMA 1984;251:1391–1395.
21. Conklin BR. Environmental hazards to elderly artists. JAMA 1984;252:3130.
22. Consumer product safety alert. CPSC promotes safety labeling for art and craft materials. Washington, DC. US Consumer Product Safety Commission, July 1990.
23. McGill DC. Art supply makers to label hazardous items. New York Times, February 3, 1985.
24. Stover B. Toxicity of school supplies. Rocky Mountain Poison Center Bulletin 1987;6(3):5–6.
25. Pedersen LM, Permin H. Rheumatic disease, heavy metal pigments and the great masters. Lancet 1988;1:1267–1269.
26. Teitelbaum SB, Teitelbaum DT. Hobbies and hazards. Personal communication, March 1982.
27. Katagiri Y, Toriumi H, Kawai M. Lead exposure among 3-year-old children and their mothers living in a pottery-producing area. Int Arch Occup Environ Health 1983;52:223–229.
28. Jacobziner H, Raybin HW. Briefs in accidental chemical poisonings in New York City. Poisonings associated with bizarre behavior. NY State J Med 1960;60:1634–1637.
29. Lutz WK, Poetzsch J, Schlatter J, Schlatter C. The real role of risk assessment in cancer risk management. Trends Pharmacol Sci 1991;12:214–217.
30. Muller C, Bertram HP, Rau W, Morandini T. Diagnosis and DMPS—treatment of accidental cobalt chloride ingestion—Case report. Antidotes. Proc of Seminar on the use of chelating agents in poisoning. Munster, Germany. Eur Assoc Poison Control Centres, CED, IPCS, May 31, 1989.
31. Everson GW, Normann SA, Casey JP. Chemistry Set chemicals. An evaluation of their toxic potential. Vet Hum Toxicol 1988;30:589–592.
32. Everson GW, Normann SA, Casey JP. Chemistry set chemicals. An evaluation of their toxic potential. Vet Hum Toxicol 1987;29:485–486.
33. Jacobziner H, Raybin HW. Accidental cobalt poisoning. Arch Pediatr 1961;78:200–205.

Chapter 65

The Hydrocarbon Products (See also Chapter 68—Pesticides)

ALIPHATIC HYDROCARBONS—PETROLEUM DISTILLATES

EPIDEMIOLOGY

Hydrocarbon ingestions account for about 5% of all calls reported to poison control centers in the United States. Petroleum distillates represent the most common hydrocarbon exposure. In order of decreasing frequency, the most common agents involved in calls to a poison control center concerning hydrocarbons (including petroleum distillates) were gasoline (44%), lacquer thinner (12%), pine oil (e.g., Pine Sol) (6%), furniture polish (e.g., Old English Furniture Polish) (5%), kerosene (2 to 5%), and charcoal lighter fluid (2%).[1]

CLASSIFICATION

Petroleum distillates with low surface tension and viscosity are serious aspiration hazards. The most viscous by-products are higher-molecular-weight hydrocarbon mixtures, which are usually nontoxic (e.g., lubricating oil, paraffin wax, asphalt, tar, petrolatum).

Petroleum Ether

This product (benzin or benzine) consists primarily of *n*-pentane and *n*-hexane (but *not* benzene or any true ethers), which are produced at boiling points from 35 to 80°C.

Petroleum Naphtha

Various mixtures of aliphatic hydrocarbons C_5 to C_{13} produced at boiling points between 30 and 238°C; may refer to any fractionalization more volatile than kerosene. Occasionally, the term is misused as a synonym for petroleum ether.

Rubber Solvent

Consisting chiefly of C_5 to C_9 aliphatic hydrocarbons distilled between 38 and 149°C; this product is less volatile than petroleum ether.

Stoddard Solvent

A higher boiling fraction of petroleum naphtha (152 to 219°), Stoddard solvent (mineral spirits, white spirits) contains straight- and branched-chain hydrocarbons (C_9 to C_{12}), naphthalene, and higher aromatic hydrocarbons.

VM and P Naphtha

This product (varnish maker's and painter's naphtha, mineral spirits) consists chiefly of C_7 to C_{10} aliphatic hydrocarbons refined between 94 and 175°C.

Gasoline

Gasoline is a mixture of C_5 to C_{12} aliphatic hydrocarbons obtained by "cracking" heavy fractions in the boiling range 40 to 225°C. Appreciable amounts of aromatic hydrocarbons (e.g., xylene) are found in commercial fuels from California and Texas, especially those with high octane ratings. Tetraethyl lead and alcohols are added to boost the octane rating.

Kerosene

Kerosene consists chiefly of C_{10} to C_{16} aliphatic hydrocarbons obtained in the boiling range 175 to 325°C. Small amounts of unsaturated (e.g., xylene) and saturated (naphthalene) aromatics appear in these products.

Mineral Seal Oil

A light petroleum fraction obtained between boiling points 200 and 370°C, this product consists mainly of saturated, higher-molecular-weight aliphatic hydrocarbons compared with gasoline and kerosene.

Diesel Oil, Fuel Oil

Slightly less volatile but more viscous than kerosene, these products are complex mixtures of C_9 and higher hydrocarbons.

Turpentine

This liquid is an oleoresin solvent derived from the steam distillation of pine resin. Although technically not a petroleum distillate, most summary articles include turpentine with petroleum distillates because it is an aromatic hydrocarbon with similar properties, toxic effects, and uses.

COMPOSITION[2,3]

Shoe Polish

Chlorinated hydrocarbons, toluene.

Liquid Furniture Polish

Mineral seal oil (especially red-colored polish).

Solvents and Thinners

Petroleum ether, Stoddard solvent (may contain 10 to 20% aromatic hydrocarbons), and VM and P naphthas. These products also contain various concentrations of toxic aromatic hydrocarbons (benzene, toluene, xylene) or halogenated hydrocarbons (carbon tetrachloride, acetate, methylcellulose, trichloroethylene, 1,1,1-trichloroethane).

Lighter Fluid

Petroleum naphtha, kerosene.

Gasoline

This product is almost exclusively a fuel. Additives such as organic lead and cresyl phosphates usually are not acute ingestion hazards. Benzene content of American domestic gasoline is lower (0.8 to 2.0%) than that of some foreign gasolines (up to 5%).

Kerosene

Used for curing tobacco, heating, cooling, and jet fuel.

Turpentine

Solvent for oil-based paints.

RELATION OF PHYSICOCHEMICAL PROPERTIES TO TOXICITY

The physical properties of viscosity, surface tension, and volatility determine the risk for aspiration and therefore have the greatest effect on toxicity (Table 65–1).[4] Products and volatile compounds that may be abused by inhalation are summarized in Chapter 66. The metabolism of some volatile substances is summarized in Table 65–2.

Viscosity, the tendency to resist flow or change form, provides the best estimate of the aspiration potential.[5] Low viscosity allows deep penetration of the hydrocarbon into the distal airways.

Surface tension is the cohesiveness of the molecules on a liquid's surface. Reduced surface tension allows the substance to spread rapidly from the mouth to the trachea.

Volatility is the tendency of a liquid to become a gas. Highly volatile hydrocarbons displace alveolar oxygen when aspirated, leading temporarily to transient hypoxia.

ASSESSMENT OF TOXICITY

The presence of aspiration, which produces a fulminant and sometimes fatal chemical pneumonitis, is the main determinant of petroleum distillate toxicity.

Although often difficult to assess, ingestion of most petroleum distillates in concentrations below 1 to 2 mL/kg does not cause systemic toxicity. Substantially larger quantities may be necessary to produce central nervous system depression.

In general, certain hydrocarbons have higher aspiration potential than others. One empirical measure of viscosity is Saybolt Universal Seconds units (SUS). Hydrocarbons differ in viscosity (where viscosity is indicated by the rate of flow of the liquid through an orifice of standard

Table 65–1
Physical Properties and Pharmacokinetic Data of Some Volatile Compounds[a]

Compound	MWt	BPt (°C)	OEL (ppm)	Inhaled Dose Absorbed (%)	Proportion of Absorbed Dose: Eliminated Unchanged (%)	Proportion of Absorbed Dose: Metabolized (%)	$t_{1/2}$ (h)	Dist. Ratio	Part Coeff (37° C)
Acetone	58.1	56	1000				3–5		243–300
Benzene	78.1	79.5	10	46	12	80	9–24	3–6	6–9
Bromochlorodi-fluromethane	165.3	–4							
n-Butane	58.1	–0.5	1000[b]	30–45					
Isobutane	58.1	–12	1000[b]						
Butanone	72.1	80	200						
Carbon disulphide	76.1	46	10	40	8–20	50–90	<1		2.4
Carbon tetrachloride	153.8	76–78	5		?50	?50	48		1.6
Chloroform	119.4	61	10		20–70 (8h)	>30	1.5	4	8
Cyclopropane	42.1	–34.5			99	0.5		1.5–3.6	0.56
Dichloromethane	84.9	39	200		?50	<40	0.7	0.5–1	5–10
Diethyl ether	74.1	34–36	400		>90			1.1	12
Dimethyl ether	46.1	–23.6							
Enflurane	184.5	56–58		90+	>80 (5 days)	2.5	36		1.9
Ethyl acetate	88.1	77	400						
Halon 11	137.4	23.7	1000	92	89	<0.2	1.5	2.5	0.87
Halon 12	120.9	–29.8	1000	35	99	<0.2		1.4	0.15
Halon 22	86.4	–41	1000					1.9	
Halothane	197.4	50		90+	60–80 (24h)	<20	0.5	2–3	2.4
n-Hexane	86.2	69	100						
Methoxyflurane	165.0	103–108			19 (10 days)	>44		2–3	11
Methyl isobutyl ketone	100.2	117	50						
Nitrous oxide	44.0	–88.5			?>99			1.1	0.47
Propane	44.1	–42.5	1000[b]						
Styrene	104.2	146	100		1–2	>95	13		32
Tetrachloroethylene	165.9	118–122	100	60+	>90	1–2	72	9–15	9–18
Toluene	92.1	111	100	53	<20	80	7.5	1–2	8–16
1,1,1-Trichloroethane	133.4	71–81	350		60–80 (1 week)	2	10–12	2	1–3
Trichloroethylene	131.4	85–88	100	50–65	16	>80	30–38	2	9.0
Xylene	106.2	136–142	100	64	5	>90	20–30		42.1

[a]Adapted from Flanagan RJ et al. Drug Safety 1990;5:359–389.
[b]As components of liquefied petroleum gas (LPG).
MWt, Molecular weight; *BPt,* boiling point at atmospheric pressure; *OEL,* occupational exposure unit; $t_{1/2}$, terminal half-life; *Dist. ratio,* brain : blood distribution ratio from postmortem investigation; *Part. coeff.,* blood : gas partition coefficient.

Table 65–2
Summary of the Metabolism of Some Volatile Substances[a]

Compound	Principal Metabolites (% Absorbed Dose)	Notes
Acetone	Intermediary metabolites (largely excreted unchanged at higher concentrations)	Endogenous compound produced in large amounts in diabetic or fasting ketoacidosis. Acetone is also the major metabolite of propan-2-ol in humans
Benzene	Phenol 51-87, catechol (6), hydroquinone (2)	Excreted in urine as sulphate and glucuronide conjugates. Urinary phenol excretion has been used to indicate exposure but is variable and subject to interference
Carbon disulphide	2-Mercapto-2-thiazotin-5-one, 2-thiothiazolidine-4-carboxylic acid (TCCA), thiourea, inorganic sulphate, others	2-Mercapto-2-thiazolin-5-one glycine conjugates and TCCA glutathione conjugates of carbon disulphide. Urinary TCCA excretion reliable indicator of exposure
Carbon tetrachloride	Chloroform, carbon dioxide, hexachloroethane, others	Trichoromethyl free radical (reactive intermediary) probably responsible for the marked hepatorenal toxicity of this compound
Chloroform	Carbon dioxide (up to 50), diglutathionyl dithiocarbonate	Phosgene (reactive intermediate) depletes glutathione and is probably responsible for hepatorenal toxicity
Dichloromethane	Carbon monoxide	Carbon monoxide half-life 13h (5h post-inhalation). Blood carboxyhemoglobin measurement useful indicator of chronic exposure
Ethyl acetate	Alcohol, acetic acid	Rapid reaction catalyzed by plasma esterases
Halothane	Chlorotrifluoroethane, chlorodifluoroethylene, trifluoroacetic acid, inorganic bromide, others	The formation of reactive metabolites may be important in the etiology of the hepatotoxicity ("halothane hepatitis") which may occur in patients exposed to halothane
n-Hexane	2-Hexanol (as glucuronide), 2,5-hexanedione, others	2-5-Hexanedione thought to cause neurotoxicity. Methyl a-butyl ketone also neurotoxic and also metabolized to 2.5
Styrene	Mandelic acid (85), phenylglyoxylic acid (10), hippuric acid may be minor metabolite	Urinary mandelic acid excretion indicates exposure (et al. 1974), alcohol inhibits mandelic acid excretion
Tetrachloroethylene	Trichloroacetic acid (<3)	Urinary trichloroacetic acid excretion serves only as qualitative index of exposure
Toluene	Benzoic acid (80), *o*-, *m*- and *p*-cresol (1)	Benzoate largely conjugated with glycine giving hippuric acid which is excreted in urine (half-life 2-3h) Not ideal index of exposure since there are other (dietary) sources of benzoate
1,1,1-Trichloroethane	2,2,2-Trichloroethanol (2), trichloroacetic acid (0.5)	Urinary metabolites serve as qualitative index of exposure only (cf. tetrachloroethylene)
Trichloroethylene	2,2,2-Trichloroethanol (45), trichloroacetic acid (32)	Trichloroethanol (glucuronide) and trichloroacetic acid excreted in urine (half-lives ca 12 and 100h). Trichloroacetic acid excretion can indicate exposure
Xylene	Methylbenzoic acids (95), xylenols (2)	Methylbenzoic acids conjugated with glycine and urinary methylhippurate excretion used as index of exposures—no dietary sources of methylbenzoates

[a]Adapted from Flanagan RJ et al. Drug Safety 1990;5:359–389.

diameter) from less than 60 SUS (moderate aspiration potential, e.g., mineral seal oil in Old English Furniture Polish), to a range of 75.1 to 86.2 SUS (low aspiration potential, e.g., "light" mineral oil in Johnson's Baby Oil), to 35 SUS (very high aspiration potential, e.g., gasoline).[6]

Hydrocarbons are used as a vehicle for more toxic substances (e.g., camphor, pesticides, heavy metals); in these cases the particular toxic substance involved determines the severity of response. Most additives (e.g., tetraethyl lead) are present at subtoxic levels for acute ingestions. Hydrocarbons can be classified into three groups based on potential clinical effects.[7]

Group 1

High aspiration potential with little central nervous system toxicity (i.e., mineral seal oil, furniture oil polishes).

Group 2

Significant central nervous system toxicity with potential aspiration hazard (i.e., methylene chloride, carbon tetrachloride, toluene, xylene, benzene, gasoline, charcoal lighter fluid, mineral spirits, turpentine).

Group 3

Nontoxic in usual doses ingested, but may lead to lipoid pneumonias on aspiration (i.e., lubricants, motor oil, mineral and baby oils, fuel and diesel oil, suntan lotion, petrolatum).

PATHOPHYSIOLOGY

Hydrocarbon Pneumonitis

The primary target organ in a serious petroleum distillate ingestion is the lung, where toxicity occurs by aspiration rather than by hematogenous spread. Small amounts of petroleum distillates intratracheally produce several pulmonary toxicity, whereas only large intragastric quantities produce central nervous system symptoms.

Pulmonary Pathology

Aspirated hydrocarbons inhibit surfactant, leading to alveolar instability, early distal airway closure, ventilation/perfusion mismatches, and subsequent hypoxemia. Although surfactant loss probably causes the early physiologic abnormalities, direct damage to pulmonary capillaries produces pathologic findings ranging from chemical pneumonitis and hemorrhagic bronchopneumonia to gross pulmonary edema. Initially, cyanosis may result from the replacement of oxygen by vaporized hydrocarbons. Subsequent hypoxemia occurs from surfactant loss and direct alveolar injury. Bronchospasm may contribute to ventilation/perfusion defects.

Histopathologic changes of the lung include interstitial inflammation, atelectasis, hyperemia, vascular thrombosis, bronchial and bronchiolar necrosis, intraalveolar hemorrhage, edema, and polymorphonuclear exudate.

Lipoid Pneumonia

High-viscosity petroleum distillates (e.g., heavy lubricants, mineral oil, liquid paraffin) produce a lipoid pneumonia that is more localized and less inflammatory than that produced by low-viscosity petroleum distillates such as kerosene or mineral seal oil.[8]

Inhalation

Petroleum distillate inhalation abuse (e.g., gasoline sniffing) usually does not produce a chemical pneumonitis, perhaps because of alveolar concentration and duration of exposure. Neurologic abnormalities reported to be associated with chronic gasoline sniffing include behavioral changes and movement disorders (resting and action tremor, myoclonus, chorea, and ataxia), as well as pyramidal signs and seizures. An organic lead encephalopathy has been described with nausea, vomiting, excitement, irritability, hallucinations, disorientation, and a clouded conscious state. Calcium disodium edetate and dimercaprol (BAL) appear to increase urinary lead excretion. The effect on morbidity and mortality remain to be elucidated.[9]

Central Nervous System

Aspiration-induced hypoxia causes central nervous system depression in ingestions of those petroleum distillates that do not contain aromatic hydrocarbons. Poor gastrointestinal absorption limits the central nervous system toxicity of most petroleum distillate products.

CLINICAL PRESENTATION

Pulmonary System

Most low-viscosity petroleum distillates produce similar clinical effects, and deaths attributed to petroleum distillates almost always result from pulmonary damage. Symptoms of respiratory distress from aspiration usually, but not always, appear within 30 minutes of exposure. Gasping, coughing, and choking are presumptive evidence of aspiration, although transient symptoms may occur immediately after exposure because of volatilization of the petroleum distillate. Prolonged cough usually indicates aspiration. Signs and symptoms may progress over the first 24 hours, but usually resolve by the third day. Death occurs most commonly within the first 24 hours. Signs range from cough and dyspnea to retractions and cyanosis.[10]

Mild	Coughing, choking, tachypnea, irritability, drowsiness, rales, rhonchi
Moderate	Grunting, lethargy, flaccidity, bronchospasm
Severe	Tachypnea with grunting respirations, cyanosis, coma, seizures

Moderate fever (38 to 39°C) often is present and does not correlate with clinical symptoms. A majority of admitted patients have fever over 38°C on admission, but three-fourths defervesce by 24 hours postexposure.[10]

Central Nervous System

Symptoms of CNS involvement result most commonly from large intentional ingestions, toxic additives (e.g., aromatic hydrocarbons, insecticides, nitrobenzene, aniline), and aspiration-induced hypoxia. Coma is uncommon (less than 3% of hospitalized cases), and convulsions are even rarer (less than 1%). The most serious aspiration pneumonias present with depressed sensorium, and lethargy is the most common sign (91% of those with CNS symptoms).

Gastrointestinal Tract

Gastrointestinal symptoms are frequent but usually minor, especially after large ingestions. Local irritation of mouth and pharynx occurs (burning of mouth, sore throat, nausea, vomiting), but diarrhea, hematemesis, and melena are rare. Gastrointestinal symptoms are slightly more common in ingestions of furniture polish than in ingestions of other petroleum distillates.

Cardiovascular System

Myocardial involvement is rare after acute ingestions. Sudden deaths secondary to dysrhythmias occur during solvent abuse, perhaps as a result of sensitization of the myocardium to endogenous catecholamines.

Organ Dysfunction

Liver, kidney, and splenic changes are uncommon in acute ingestions and usually reversible. Death or permanent hepatic or renal sequelae have not been reported to occur as a result of acute petroleum distillate exposures, although temporary liver, spleen, or kidney dysfunction may occur.

LABORATORY ABNORMALITIES

Chest X-ray

X-ray abnormalities usually appear within 30 minutes, but may develop 12 hours after exposure. Up to 70 to 75% of patients hospitalized for suspected hydrocarbon aspiration have chest x-ray abnormalities. Most x-ray changes reach a maximum 72 hours after exposure and clear several days later, although occasionally the changes persist for several months.[11] X-ray changes tend to lag behind clinical improvement.

Chest x-ray abnormalities correlate poorly with clinical symptoms. Asymptomatic patients may have abnormal chest x-rays, but usually these x-ray changes clear without the patient developing symptoms. Symptomatic patients may have normal chest x-rays, especially within the first several hours. Most x-ray abnormalities are mild and do not progress.[10]

Arterial Blood Gases

Abnormalities reflect hypoxemia resulting from ventilation/perfusion mismatching (low P_{O2}, low P_{CO2}) rather than alveolar hypoventilation (high P_{CO2}). Rarely, after aniline or nitrobenzene exposure, methemoglobinemia may be seen.

Blood

Leukocytosis is common during the first 48 hours. Intravascular hemolysis, acute renal failure, elevated hepatic aminotransferases, and consumptive coagulopathy develop rarely in massive gasoline aspiration.[12]

Urine

The urinalysis is usually normal, and renal dysfunction is uncommon.

TREATMENT

Stabilization

The primary threat to life from pure petroleum distillate ingestion is respiratory failure. Patients should be quickly evaluated for signs of respiratory distress (e.g., cyanosis, tachypnea, intercostal retractions, obtundation) and given oxygen. Patients with inadequate tidal volumes or poor arterial blood gases (P_{O2} <50 mm Hg or P_{CO2} >50 mm Hg) should be intubated. Since arrhythmias complicate some hydrocarbon ingestions and electrocardiographic evidence of myocardial injury has been reported,[13] intravenous lines and cardiac monitors should be established in obviously symptomatic patients. A chest x-ray should be taken immediately after stabilization of breathing and circulation to document aspiration and detect the presence of pneumothorax.

Continuous positive airway pressure or positive end-expiratory pressure and intubation may be necessary in severe cases to maintain adequate oxygenation, but careful observation for the development of pneumothorax must be made during therapy. Epinephrine is not recommended for treatment of bronchospasm, because of potential myocardial sensitization to catecholamines. Inhaled cardioselective bronchodilators (e.g., Alupent, salbutamol) are the preferred bronchodilator agents, with aminophylline a second choice.

Decontamination

Gastrointestinal decontamination in accidental petroleum distillate ingestions is not recommended, because of the severe aspiration hazard. All contaminated clothing should be removed, and contaminated skin areas washed with green soap (lipophilic) and water.

Syrup of Ipecac

Ipecac-induced emesis is *not* recommended in general, and especially in the following cases:

1. Ingestion of highly viscous petroleum distillates with poor gastrointestinal absorption, including asphalt/tar, mineral oil (e.g., household and automotive oils), home fuel oils, and diesel fuel oil.
2. Ingestion of highly volatile petroleum distillates with minimal gastrointestinal absorption, including mineral seal oil, furniture polish, and signal oil.
3. Significant spontaneous vomiting.

Lavage

Lavage is indicated in those patients who require decontamination. Be sure that an endotracheal tube is in place prior to lavage; use cuffed endotracheal tubes in patients over 7 years of age.

Activated Charcoal

Although activated charcoal does not bind petroleum distillate products and may induce vomiting, in vitro studies suggest that large quantities of activated charcoal bind significant amounts of kerosene and turpentine.[14,15] However, activated charcoal may be given when the physician feels the charcoal may absorb a toxic additive.

Elimination Enhancement

There are no effective methods.

Antidotes

There are no antidotes.

Supportive Care

For serious cases of aspiration follow CBC, acid-base status, fluid and electrolyte balance, renal and liver function, and serial arterial blood gases. Keep fluid balance just at replacement to avoid precipitating pulmonary edema.

Steroid Treatment

The use of steroid therapy in mild to moderate hydrocarbon aspiration pneumonia did not improve outcome in a double-blind, controlled human study.[16]

Antibiotics

Present data do not support the use of prophylactic antibiotics. Antibiotics should be reserved for documented bacterial pneumonias (i.e., Gram stain of sputum or tracheal aspirate) or increasing infiltrates, leukocytosis, and fever after the first 24 to 48 hours. Long-term follow-up care with baseline pulmonary function tests should be established to detect the presence of obstructive pulmonary disease, which may be seen in asymptomatic children who previously developed hydrocarbon aspiration pneumonitis.[17]

Extracorporeal Membrane Oxygenation

Extracorporeal membrane oxygenation is a pulmonary bypass procedure that has been employed in adults to provide temporary treatment for reversible acute pulmonary and cardiac insufficiency. It provides a potentially lifesaving option when a patient fails to respond to conventional therapy for hydrocarbon aspiration.[6]

Hospitalization

A chest x-ray should be obtained on all patients clinically suspected of aspiration regardless and in the absence of symptoms. Admit immediately the following patients:

1. Symptomatic children who have abnormal initial chest x-rays.
2. Patients with suicidal intent or massive ingestion.
3. Hypoxic or obtunded patients regardless of x-ray.
4. Patients with a substantially abnormal chest x-ray.

Admit the following patients after an observation period as long as 6 hours:

1. Asymptomatic children with a mildly abnormal chest x-ray who develop symptoms during the observation period.
2. Asymptomatic patients who develop symptoms because of toxic additives (e.g., camphor, halogenated hydrocarbons).
3. Mildly symptomatic children who have a normal chest x-ray, but whose symptoms do not improve.
4. All patients for whom follow-up cannot be closely established.

Discharge the following patients after 6 hours of observation:

1. Asymptomatic children with a normal chest x-ray.
2. Asymptomatic children with a mildly abnormal chest x-ray who do not develop symptoms during the observation period.

REFERENCES—PETROLEUM DISTILLATES

1. McGuigan MA. The management of petroleum distillate hydrocarbon ingestions. Clin Toxicol Rev 1978;1(3):1–2.
2. Geehr E. Management of hydrocarbon ingestions. Top Emerg Med 1979;1(3):97–110.
3. Goldfrank L, Kirstein R, Bresnitz E. Gasoline and other hydrocarbons. Hosp Physician 1979;14(9):32–39.
4. Flanagan RJ, Ruprah M, Meredith TJ, Ramsey JD. An introduction to the clinical toxicology of volatile substances. Drug Safety 1990;5:359–389.
5. Gerarde HW. Toxicological studies in hydrocarbons vs kerosene. Toxicol Appl Pharmacol 1959;1:462–474.
6. Scalzo AJ, Weber TR, Jaeger RW, Connors RH, Thompson MW. Extracorporeal membrane oxygenation for hydrocarbon aspiration. AJDC 1990;144:867–871.
7. Chellino MA. Petroleum distillate hydrocarbons. San Francisco Poison Control Center Newslett 1980;2(2):2.
8. Beerman B, Christensson T, Moller P et al. Lipoid pneumonia. An occupation hazard of fire-eaters. Br J Med 1984;289:1728–1729.
9. Burns CR, Currie B. The efficacy of chelation therapy and factors influencing mortality in lead intoxicated petrol sniffers. Aust NZ J Med 1995;25:197–203.
10. Anas N, Namasonthia V, Ginsburg CM. Criteria for hospitalizing children who have ingested products containing hydrocarbons. JAMA 1981;246:840–843.
11. Eade NR, Taussig LM, Marks MI. Hydrocarbon pneumonitis. Pediatrics 1974;54:351–357.
12. Banner W, Walson PD. Systemic toxicity following gasoline aspiration. Am J Emerg Med 1983;3:292–294.
13. James FW, Kaplan S, Benzing G. Cardiac complications following hydrocarbon ingestion. Am J Dis Child 1971;121:431–433.
14. Decker WJ. Adsorption of solvents by activated charcoal, polymers and mineral sorbents. Vet Hum Toxicol 1981;23(Suppl 1):44–46.
15. Ng RC, Darwish H, Stewart PA. Emergency treatment of petroleum distillate and turpentine ingestion. CMA J 1974;111:537–538.
16. Marks MI, Chicoine L, Legere G et al. Adrenocorticosteroid treatment of hydrocarbon pneumonia in children—a cooperative study. J Pediatr 1972;81:366–369.
17. Gurwitz D, Kattan M, Levison H et al. Pulmonary function abnormalities in asymptomatic children after hydrocarbon pneumonitis. Pediatrics 1978;62:789–794.

DIBROMOCHLOROPROPANE (DBCP)

CLINICAL PRESENTATION

In July 1977 a number of pesticide production workers in California exposed to 1,2-dibromo-3-chloropropane (DCP) were found to have a marked reduction in sperm density—13% were actually azoospermic.[1] These workers had more than 100 hours of estimated exposure in production. The histologic pattern of testicular biopsies showed seminiferous tubules to be the site of damage.[2] Other men were exposed to between 10 and 90 hours. These individuals were normospermic. The outcome of pregnancies fathered by the exposed men disclosed no evidence of an increase in spontaneous abortion, infant or fetal deaths, or congenital malformations.[3] Permanent destruction of the germinal epithelium occurred in most of the DBCP-sterile persons studied 7 years after the termination of exposure.[4] Eleven years after the exposure there appeared to be a lack of spermatogenesis recovery in the DBCP-exposed oligospermic and azoospermic men. Thirteen azoospermic subjects subsequently had sperm counts over 20 million per mL. Testicular atrophy was observed with azoospermia and the testicles subsequently increased in size among those azoospermic subjects who returned to normospermic levels.[5]

REFERENCES—DIBROMOCHLOROPROPANE (DBCP)

1. Milby TH, Wharton D. Epidemiological assessment of occupationally related, chemically induced sperm count suppression. J Occup Med 1980;22:77–82.

2. Wharton D, Milby TH, Krauss RM, Stubbs NA. Testicular function in DBCP exposed pesticide workers. J Occup Med 1979;21:161–166.
3. Goldsmith JR, Potashnik G, Israeli R. Reproductive outcome in families of DBCP-exposed men. Arch Environ Health 1984;39:85–89.
4. Eaton M, Schenker M, Wharton MD, Samuels S, Perkins C, Overstreet J. Seven-year follow-up of workers exposed to 1,2-dibromo-3-chloropropane. J Occup Med 1986;28:1145–1150.
5. Olson GW, Lanham JM, Bodner KM, Hylton DB, Bond GG. Determinants of spermatogenesis recovery among workers exposed to 1,2-dibromo-3-chloropropane. J Occup Med 1990;32:979–984.

DIMETHYLAMINE

Measurement of urine levels provides an indication of body exposure to this amine. Dimethylamine is one of the short-chain aliphatic amines and is probably, like trimethylamine, a degradation product of trimethylamine *N*-oxide. Its pathophysiologic role is unclear. It is extensively absorbed (bioavailability 72%); 5% is demethylated to methylene, but 95% is secreted unchanged in the urine. The half-life is 6 to 7 hours. The plasma clearance is 190 mL/min.[1]

REFERENCE—DIMETHYLAMINE

1. Zhang AQ, Mitchell SC, Barrett T, Ayesh R, Smith RL. Fat of dimethylamine in man. Xenobiotica 1994;24:379–387.

DIMETHYL SULFATE

Dimethyl sulfate is an industrial chemical that can, on exposure to humans, produce severe ocular reactions and delayed respiratory tract reactions that frequently terminate fatally. Treatment is supportive and symptomatic.

USES

Dimethyl sulfate is widely used in industry as a methylating agent for the organic synthesis of chemicals, especially in the manufacture of pharmaceuticals, dyestuffs, perfume, and pesticides.[1]

SOURCES

There are no reported natural sources of DMS, but it may be present in the environment because of industrial processes. It may be formed during the combustion of sulfur-containing fossil fuels. It is a potential human carcinogen. Efforts should be made to use enclosed systems in processes using DMS.[2]

TOXIC DOSE

One patient licked the finger to taste DMS and suffered immediate irritation of the soft palate, laryngeal constriction, and increased salivation that improved on treatment. However, 24 hours later, there was a sudden onset of edema of the glottis, and death ensued. At autopsy, acute corrosive changes were seen in the upper gastrointestinal tract with edema of the glottis and emphysema of the lungs.[3]

MECHANISM OF ACTION

When DMS comes in contact with a moist mucosal surface, it is hydrolyzed slowly into sulfuric acid, methanol, and methyl hydrogen sulfate. The methanol may be absorbed into the circulation, leading to neurotoxic effects; the sulfuric acid and methyl hydrogen sulfate induce severe irritation and anesthetic and erosive effects on the mucosa.[1]

CLINICAL PRESENTATION

DMS can induce chemical burns on a wet epithelium; it is a strong irritant to the eyes and respiratory mucosa where it may cause desquamation and necrosis.[1] Acute exposure may be fatal.[4,5] Intoxication is usually through accidental inhalation of the vapor or contamination of skin and mucosa by liquid or vapor.

Clinically, the usual manifestations include skin burns, corneal irritation with photophobia, lacrimation and blurring of vision, oropharyngeal edema with suffocation and hoarseness of the voice, nasal septal necrosis, cough, and dyspnea.[4] Major causes of mortality in DMS intoxication include respiratory failure following mucosal inflammation, edema of major airways, and noncardiogenic pulmonary edema.[4,6] Other systemic effects include convulsions; delirium; coma; and renal, hepatic, and cardiac failure.[7,8] Irreversible loss of vision has been reported.[2]

There is usually a latent period of 20 minutes to 12 hours (mean latent period 3 hours) between exposure and onset of symptoms. This delayed effect and the absence of warning signs of exposure due to the absence of color, together with a minimal odor, make this compound particularly hazardous.

Clinical signs include a rise in body temperature (37.5 to 49°C), pulse rate (100 to 160 beats/min), and respiratory rate (22 to 40 inspirations/minute). Abnormal breath sounds, including wheezing, dry rales, and moist rales may be heard. Congestion and edema of the eyes, pharynx, and uvula are observed. After 3 to 14 days desquamation of the tracheal and bronchial mucosa occurs.

Criteria for grading the degrees of DMS intoxication have been proposed[1]:

1. Irritative reactions: A history of exposure to DMS, with appearance of symptoms and signs of mucosal irritation in the eyes, nose, and pharynx; normal chest x-ray films; no leukocytosis. No systemic signs of intoxication. These patients may be released after symptomatic treatment and medical observation for 24 to 72 hours.
2. Mild intoxication: In addition to the irritative reactions mentioned above, there are symptoms of irritative and erosive actions in the respiratory tract (congestion of pharynx, larynx, and uvula; abnormal breath sounds) and positive findings on more than one test (chest x-ray films showing peribronchitis and/or leukocytosis). With treatment, patients usually recover in 3 to 7 days and resume their ordinary work.
3. Moderate intoxication: In addition to the manifestations of mild intoxication, necrosis and desquamation of the respiratory mucosa occurs, with more than two positive clinical findings (chest x-ray films showing pneumonia or interstitial pneumonia, leukocytosis, or ECG demonstrating myocardial damage) and no other complica-

tions. After treatment and rest, these patients may recover and resume ordinary work.

4. Severe intoxication: In addition to the manifestations of moderate intoxication, the patients may exhibit significant laryngeal edema, pulmonary edema and/or toxic shock, and/or encephalopathy, and/or toxic myocardial damage. Local and systemic supportive treatment is required, with use of glucocorticoids and antibiotics.

DMS is considered to be probably carcinogenic to humans.[9]

LABORATORY

Analytic Methods

A sensitive gas chromatography/mass spectrometry technique has been developed,[10] and a fully automated gas chromatography method is available for the routine repetitive determination of DMS suitable for industrial monitoring.[11]

Ancillary Tests

Lung function tests show a restrictive pattern when forced expiratory volume in 1 second (FEV_1), forced vital capacity (FVC), FEV_1/FVC, and carbon monoxide diffusing capacity studies are performed. Periodic chest radiography indicates peribronchitis, bilateral pulmonary infiltrates, and pulmonary edema (interstitial or alveolar). The ECG shows an inversion of T waves and elevation or depression of ST segments, especially in patients with bronchopneumonia, pulmonary edema, and myocardial damage. Elevated white blood cell counts (10,500 to 24,000/mm^3) are observed.

No abnormalities are usually seen in routine urinalyses, red blood cell counts, or hemoglobin determinations. Pathologic examination of the sputum from severe cases often reveals fibrin, degenerated bronchial epithelium, and ruptured inflammatory cells. Clinical studies of blood methanol or formate levels are not available, but would be indicated within the first 24 hours if there is evidence of neurotoxicity.[1,2]

TREATMENT

Stabilization

Dimethyl sulfate can induce irritative and erosive actions on the mucosa only after its hydrolysis. Early clinical surveillance and treatment during the first 24 to 72 hours are important. Patients exposed to dimethyl sulfate should be treated as a medical emergency. At the site of injury the following may be initiated:

Eyes:	Copious irrigation should be started with water or normal saline for at least 20 to 30 minutes.
Skin:	Remove all contaminated clothes. Wash and irrigate all exposed skin thoroughly with water or saline.
Oral Ingestion:	Treat as a corrosive acid poisoning (see section on Acids).

Decontamination

Oral Ingestion

Emesis by syrup of ipecac can be dangerous because of reexposure of the esophagus to corrosive material and because of the danger of aspiration pneumonia and respiratory tract damage. Gastric lavage can be performed, preferably within 1 hour of ingestion with appropriate tracheal protection. Endoscopy will determine the extent of esophageal and gastric injury. (See Acids—Household Products Section—Chapter 53.)

Elimination Enhancement

There have been no clinical studies on procedures to accelerate the elimination of dimethyl sulfate or its hydrolysis products (sulfuric acid, methanol) after an exposure. If neurotoxic effects that may be related to methanol poisoning appear, clinical judgment must dictate whether the use of ethanol or hemodialysis is indicated.

Antidote

There are no antidotes for dimethyl sulfate exposure.

Supportive Measures

Systemic treatment will depend on the severity of exposure (see Clinical Criteria). All patients exposed to dimethyl sulfate should be admitted to a hospital for observation for at least 24 hours.

Eye

Steroid and antibiotic medication may be instilled for the prevention and treatment of inflammation. Caution must be exercised when using steroids in the presence of corneal injury. Most cases of mild corneal and conjunctival injury resolve within 24 hours.[1] Careful ophthalmologic follow-up is indicated for all patients with eye injuries.

Respiratory

Use of antibiotics and humidified oxygen has been recommended.[8] Repeated aerosol inhalations have been administered to patients with respiratory tract injury. The inhalant has been composed of dexamethasone 5 mg, aminophylline 0.25 g, and streptomycin 0.5 g or gentamicin 80,000 U in 50 ml normal saline; 10 to 20 ml/time, ½ to 6 hours/time, 2 to 8 times/day. For those who have inhaled high concentrations of DMS, early intravenous administration of hydrocortisone (300 to 1100 mg) or dexamethasone (15 to 55 mg) in short courses (2 to 6 days) may prove beneficial. In addition, antibiotics, atropine, and postural drainage have been administered. Isolation procedures may be indicated. Adult respiratory distress syndrome (ARDS) caused by chemical pneumonitis has been treated by the above measures without tracheotomy. Continuous, intermittent, positive-pressure oxygen inhalation has been given for 10 to 16 hours until hypoxia was corrected.

Follow-up

Patients who have been exposed to DMS should have periodic follow-up studies to include visual, respiratory tract, and electrocardiographic examinations. Most will resume suitable work.

Safety and Health Measures

All industrial operations using dimethyl sulfate should be carried out in fully enclosed systems with arrangements made for removing spillage. Workers should be supplied with respiratory protective equipment, chemical eye protective wear, protective clothing, and rubber gloves. Workers should be instructed not to attempt to do a hasty cleanup of massive spillages in the event of a container breakage.[7] Workers with disease of the central nervous system, lungs, kidneys, or liver should be precluded from working with dimethyl sulfate.

REFERENCES—DIMETHYL SULFATE

1. Ying W, Jing X, Qin-Wai W. Clinical report on 62 cases of acute dimethyl sulfate intoxication. Am J Ind Med 1988;13: 455–462.
2. Dimethyl sulfate. Environmental Health Criteria 48. Geneva: World Health Organization, 1985, pp. 1–55.
3. von Nida S. Fatal edema of the glottis following inflammation of the upper digestive tract due to dimethyl sulfate. Klin Wochenschr 1947;24/25:633–634.
4. Ip M, Wong K-L, Wong K-F, So S-Y. Lung injury in dimethyl sulfate poisoning. J Occup Med 1989;31:141–143.
5. Moeschlin S. Poisoning. Diagnosis and treatment. New York: Grune & Stratton 1965, pp. 1–707.
6. Kleinfeld M. Acute pulmonary edema of chemical origin. Arch Environ Health 1965;10:942–946.
7. Dimethyl sulfate. In: Encyclopedia of occupational health and Safety. Vol 1. International Labour Office. New York: McGraw-Hill, 1971, pp. 388–389.
8. Littler TR, McConnell RB. Dimethyl sulfate poisoning. Br J Ind Med 1955;12:54–56.
9. IARC (International Agency for Research or Cancer). Monograph on the evaluation of the carcinogenic risk of chemicals to humans. Supplement 4, 1987.
10. Ellgehausen D. Determination of volatile toxic substances in the air by means of a coupled gas chromatograph-mass spectrometer system. Anal Lett 1975;8:11–23.
11. Ellgehausen D. A gas chromatographic monitor for dimethyl sulfate in air. In: The monitoring of hazardous gases in the working environment. London, December 12–14, 1977. London: The Chemical Society, pp. 27–28.
12. Roux H, Gallet M, Vincent V, Frantz P. Poisoning by dimethyl sulfate (clinical aid bibliographic study). Acta Pharmacol Toxicol 1977;41(Suppl 2):428–433.

DIMETHYL SULFOXIDE

Dimethyl sulfoxide is a synthetic chemical capable of inducing renal, hepatic, hematopoietic, or central nervous system dysfunction when it is administered intravenously. Few controlled clinical studies have been performed in man. Treatment of overdose will be supportive and symptomatic. There are no known antidotes.

SYNONYMS

Rimso 50, Dermasorb dimethyl sulfoxide, DMS-70, DMS-90, Dromisol, Gamasol 90, Hyadur, Infiltrina, Somnipront, Syntexan, DMSO.[1]

USES

In industry DMSO is widely used as an industrial solvent for both organic and inorganic chemicals.[2] In the USA a 50% w/w aqueous solution is available clinically for intravesical instillation used for relief of symptoms of interstitial cystitis.[3] DMSO has been used as a vehicle for other drugs; it has been tried for cutaneous and musculoskeletal disorders, but has exhibited little evidence of beneficial effects.[2] DMSO has been used to protect living cells during cold storage.[4] In mice, DMSO has been shown to exert a protective effect against acetaminophen-induced hepatotoxicity.[5,6] No studies have been performed in humans. Clinical studies are under way on the intravenous administration of 10% DMSO or a treatment for intractable cerebral edema.[7,8]

PRODUCT FORMULATION

Each ml of the commercial preparation of DMSO contained 0.54 gm of DMSO for intravesical use.[3]

DOSE

Topical application of 80% DMSO daily for 12 weeks did not result in ocular toxicity.[9] Instillation of 7.5 to 60% DMSO in tetrahydrozoline for 1 to 15 months in patients with ocular problems did not induce ocular toxicity.[10] Daily injection of 10 to 40% DMSO in 5% dextrose or water for 3 days at a dose of 1 g/kg IV resulted in a dose-dependent hemolysis with hemoglobinuria.[11,12] There has been no lethal dose established in man.

TOXICOKINETICS

Absorption

Oral

Ingestion of 1 g/kg DMSO resulted in a peak serum concentration of about 1000 to 3000 μg/mL within 4 hours. The dimethyl sulfone ($DMSO_2$) concentration peaked 72 to 96 hours after administration with values of 300 to 600 μg/mL.[13]

Dermal

Dermal application of 1 g/kg of DMSO produced a maximum serum level of $DMSO_2$ of approximately 500 μg/mL within 4 to 8 hours. Serum levels of DMSO become maximal at concentrations of 300 to 500 μg/mL after 36 to 72 hours.[13]

Distribution (V_D)

Eight hours after the cutaneous application of 2 g of 90% DMSO, 20% remained at the application site. Within 24 hours, 10 to 15% of the total dose appeared in the urine.[14]

Elimination

Oral

The elimination half-life of oral DMSO is 20 hours; dimethylsulfone ($DMSO_2$) has an elimination half-life of 72 hours. At 120 hours 50% of an oral dose was excreted in the urine as DMSO and 9.6% as $DMSO_2$.[13]

Dermal

The elimination half-life of dermal DMSO is about 11 to 14 hours; the $DMSO_2$ half-life is approximately 60 to 70 hours.[13] DMSO is metabolized in man by oxidation to dimethyl sulfone ($DMSO_2$) or by reduction to dimethylsulfide. DMSO and $DMSO_2$ are excreted in the urine and feces. Dimethylsulfide is eliminated through the breath and skin and is responsible for the characteristic odor.[3] $DMSO_2$ can persist in the serum for over 2 weeks after a single intravesical installation.[3]

Drug Interactions

DMSO has been shown to enhance the absorption of heparin, insulin, sodium salicylate, Evans blue dye, sulfadiazine, aminophylline, and thio-TEPA in animals.[15] Other drugs include iron chloride, tertiary and quaternary ammonium compounds, glucocorticoids, local anesthetics, and antifungal, antibacterial, and anticholinesterase agents.[16]

Pregnancy/Lactation

DMSO has been placed in Pregnancy Category C by the U.S. Food and Drug Administration.[3] Teratogenic effects have been found in animals. There have been no adequate well-controlled studies in pregnant women. It is not known whether DMSO is excreted in human milk. Safety and effectiveness in children has not been established.

MECHANISM OF ACTION

DMSO appears to penetrate cell membranes due to its ability to form hydrogen bonds and to displace water.[17] It has also been reported to exhibit antiinflammatory activity, local analgesia, diuresis, vasodilation, and dissolution of collagen.[18]

CLINICAL PRESENTATION

Intravesical Administration

A garliclike taste may remain for 72 hours after its use intravesically. Transient chemical cystitis follows its use.

Dermal Application

In humans chronic dermal applications of DMSO have resulted in pruritus, urticaria, erythema, eosinophilia, a garlic odor to the breath, fatigue, headache, nausea, dizziness, eye irritation, exfoliation, and pigmentation at the site of application.[19] A 63-year-old arthritic patient applied 90% DMSO topically and experienced mixed sensorimotor peripheral neuropathy and segmental demyelination.[20]

Intravenous Use

Dose-dependent intravascular hemolysis with bilirubinemia and hemoglobinuria may follow intravenous use.[11,12] When used in a penetrating basis for other drugs, DMSO may enhance their toxic effects.[2] Abnormalities in renal function tests, hepatic enzymes, and coagulation parameters have been observed.[21,22] Transient encephalopathy, dysarthric speech, disorientation, hypoactive reflexes, and altered consciousness have been described.[21–24] Symptoms may not clear for 1 week. Acute tubular necrosis followed two IV infusions of 100 g of 20% DMSO.[21]

LABORATORY

Analytic Methods

DMSO and $DMSO_2$ have been measured by flame-ionization or electrocapture gas chromatography after solvent extraction or protein precipitation.[25]

Blood Levels

Intravenous administration of DMSO led to serum concentrations of DMSO (1600 μg/mL) and $DMSO_2$ (3000 μg/mL), which were associated with a severe garlic odor, disorientation, and dysarthric speech.[23]

Abnormalities

After dermal applications, infrequent elevations of renal function tests and hepatic enzymes may occur[24]; eosinophilia has been observed. Creatine kinase levels may rise.[21] Prothrombin and partial thromboplastin times may shorten.[21,22]

TREATMENT

Industrial Exposure

Use protective clothing, including gloves and head, foot, and body protection, to minimize skin contact. Use goggles and/or face shield when danger of splashing exists. Avoid breathing a spray or mist of DMSO or a high concentration of vapors. Use care in handling solutions of toxic materials in DMSO.

Intravesical Use

An overdose of DMSO in the course of intravesical use may result in symptoms of a chemical cystitis. Bladder antispasmodics and analgesic medication may be useful. The patient will require continued urologic care.

Intravenous Use

If DMSO is administered by the intravenous route, there may be an enhanced possibility of developing signs and symptoms of central nervous system, renal, hepatic, or hematopoietic dysfunction. Treatment will be supportive and symptomatic. There are no antidotes. Renal failure, unresponsive to conservative management, may respond to extracorporeal treatment measures. A paucity of toxicokinetic data does not provide a guide for the clinician. Clinical judgment based on severity of symptoms and laboratory parameters must form the basis for initiating hemodialysis or hemoperfusion.

Decontamination

Skin

Excess amounts of DMSO on the skin will require vigorous irrigation with water or saline.

Oral Ingestion

Ingestion of overdoses of DMSO have not been reported. An attempt should be made to empty the gastric contents with tracheal protection. Emetic agents have not been evaluated.

Antidote

There are no antidotes.

REFERENCES—DIMETHYL SULFOXIDE

1. Willhite CC, Katz PI. Dimethyl sulfoxide. J Appl Toxicol 1984; 4:155–160.
2. Reynolds JEF. *Martindale: The extra pharmacopoeia.* 29th ed. London: The Pharmaceutical Press, 1989; pp. 1426–1427.
3. Physicians Desk Reference. 46th ed. Montvale, New Jersey: Medical Economics Company, 1992, pp. 1836–1837.
4. McGann LE, Walterson ML. Cryoprotection by dimethyl sulfoxide and dimethyl sulfone. Cryobiology 1987;24:11–16.
5. Arndt K, Haschok WM, Jeffrey EH. Mechanism of dimethyl sulfoxide protection against acetaminophen hepatotoxicity. Drug Metab Rev 1989;20:261–269.
6. Park Y, Smith RD, Combs AB, Kehrer JP. Prevention of acetaminophen-induced hepatotoxicity by dimethyl sulfoxide. Toxicology 1988;52:165–175.
7. Waller FT, Tanabe CT, Paxton HD. Treatment of elevated intracranial pressure with dimethyl sulfoxide. Ann NY Acad Sci 1983;411:286–292.
8. Karaca M, Bilgin UY, Akar M, de la Torre JC. Dimethyl sulfoxide lowers ICP after closed head trauma. Eur J Clin Pharmacol 1991;40:113–114.
9. Hull FW, Wood DC, Brobyn RD. Eye effects of DMSO. Report of negative results. Northwest Med 1969;68:39–41.
10. Gordon DM. Dimethyl sulfoxide in ophthalmology with special reference to possible toxic effects. Ann NY Acad Sci 1967;141:392–401.
11. Bennett WM, Munther RS. Lack of nephrotoxicity in intravenous dimethyl sulfoxide. Clin Toxicol 1981;18:615–618.
12. Munther RS, Bennett WM. Effects of dimethyl sulfoxide on renal function in man. JAMA 1980;244:2081–2083.
13. Hucker HB, Miller JK, Hochberg A, Brobyn RD, Riordan FH, Calesnick B. Studies on the absorption, excretion and metabolism of dimethyl sulfoxide (DMSO) in man. J Pharm Exp Ther 1967;155:309–317.
14. Kolb KH, Janicke G, Kramer M, Schulze PE. Absorption, distribution and elimination of labeled dimethyl sulfoxide in man and animals. Ann NY Acad Sci 1967;141:85–95.
15. Jacob SW, Bischell M, Herschler RJ: Dimethyl sulfoxide (DMSO). A new concept in pharmacotherapy. Curr Ther Res 1964;6:134–135.
16. Rubin LF. Toxicity of dimethyl sulfoxide, alone and in combination. Ann NY Acad Sci 1975;243:98–103.
17. Szmant HH. Physical properties of dimethyl sulfoxide and its function in biological systems. Ann NY Acad Sci 1975;243: 20–23.
18. Wood DC, Wood J. Pharmacological and biochemical considerations of dimethyl sulfoxide. Ann NY Acad Sci 1975; 234:7–19.
19. Kligman AM. Topical pharmacology and toxicology of dimethyl sulfoxide—part II. JAMA 1965;193:923–928.
20. Reinstein L, Mahon R Jr, Russo GL. Peripheral neuropathy after concomitant dimethyl sulfoxide and sulindac therapy. Arch Phys Med Rehabil 1982;63:581–584.
21. Yellowlees P, Greenfield C, McIntyre N. Dimethyl sulfoxide induced toxicity. Lancet 1980;2:1004–1006.
22. Greenfield C. Dimethyl sulfoxide toxicity. Lancet 1981;1:276–277.
23. Bond GR, Curry SC, Dahl DW. Dimethyl sulfoxide-induced encephalopathy. Lancet 1989;1:1134–1135.
24. Boby RB. The human toxicology of dimethyl sulfoxide. Ann NY Acad Sci 1975;243:497–506.
25. Garretson SE, Aitchison P. Comparison of dimethyl sulfoxide levels in whole blood and serum using an auto sampler-equipped gas chromatography. Ann NY Acad Sci 1983;411:328–331.

GASOLINE[1–3]

Gasoline is a refined petroleum product that is used as a motor fuel. It is highly flammable and potentially explosive and contains more than 250 hydrocarbons and small quantities of additives and blending agents.

CHEMICAL COMPOSITION

The composition of gasoline varies depending on geographic region, season, performance requirements, and blending stocks. The typical hydrocarbon content of liquid gasoline (% volume) is as follows: approximately 60 to 70% alkanes (straight chain, branched chain, and cyclic), 5 to 10% alkenes (straight chain and branched chain), and 25 to 30% aromatics.

Benzene, a known hematotoxic agent, is present at an average concentration of approximately 1% in United States gasoline, but can be as high as 5% concentration in European formulations.

LEADED GASOLINE

Gasoline that contains more than 0.05 grams of lead per gram of gasoline is considered leaded gasoline. Organic lead is added to enhance a fuel's octane rating. In 1989 only 10% of the gasoline purchased in the United States was leaded gasoline. By 1997 the use of leaded gasoline in this country will have ceased. However, organic lead compounds are still added to gasoline in other parts of the world. Replacements for organic lead antiknock agents include ethanol, methanol, methyl tertiary butyl ether (MTBE), and tertiary butyl ether (TBE), which are typically added in concentrations of 5 to 15%.

EXPOSURE TO GASOLINE VAPOR

Self-service gasoline customers typically experience short-term exposures during refueling of approximately 200 parts per million (ppm) gasoline hydrocarbons and less than 1 ppm benzene for periods of about 2 minutes. The Occupational Safety and Health Administration (OSHA) short-term exposure limit (STEL) averaged over 15 minutes is 500 ppm for gasoline hydrocarbons and 5 ppm for benzene. Thus the exposure during self-service refueling of automobiles is not likely to be a significant hazard to the public.

EXPOSURE TO LIQUID GASOLINE

Exposure to liquid gasoline occurs by unintentional or intentional ingestion, accidental skin contact, or by misuse of the solvent. Misuse of gasoline, especially to clean and degrease floors, tools and machine parts, represents the single most important health risk from gasoline for the general public.

OCCUPATIONAL

Refinery workers and persons and workers involved in removal and maintenance of underground storage tanks are at greatest risk of exposure to gasoline. Persons who misuse gasoline to clean garage floors or use gasoline-soaked rags to clean hands or machinery parts risk toxicity from both inhalation and dermal absorption. Persons who unintentionally ingest gasoline while siphoning and those who intentionally inhale gasoline vapors to obtain euphoric effects risk serious health consequences.

TOXICOKINETICS

Absorption

Gasoline can be absorbed by inhalation, ingestion, and dermal exposure routes. The hydrocarbon components with higher blood/gas partition coefficients in the lungs (e.g., xylene, benzene, toluene) have a higher absorption rate during inhalation than components with lower coefficients (e.g., cyclohexane, ethane, ethylene). The rate of dermal absorption is low compared with absorption after ingestion, although the aromatic hydrocarbons such as benzene are expected to have higher skin penetration than the alkanes.

Distribution

After unintentional ingestion of gasoline, the highest gasoline concentrations are in the liver, gastric wall, and lungs. Service-station attendants who were exposed to gasoline, most likely by dermal contact, as well as inhalation, have elevated blood levels of hydrocarbons such as benzene, toluene, pentane, and hexane.

Metabolism

Mixed-function oxygenase activity is accelerated by gasoline. Some gasoline hydrocarbons are oxidized by liver microsomal-enzyme systems to products that are readily excreted in the urine. Alkanes are stable, saturated compounds that are not metabolized. Most of what is systemically absorbed is excreted unchanged through the lungs. Urinary phenol, a biologic indicator of benzene exposure, is elevated in gasoline-pump workers (average 40 mg/L) compared with persons with no occupational exposure to gasoline (less than 20 mg/L).

Gasoline Additives

Tetraethyl lead and tetramethyl lead can be rapidly absorbed through inhalation and skin contact. After absorption these organic lead compounds are rapidly dealkylated by the liver to trialkyl metabolites that are toxic. The trialkyl metabolites, which are water soluble, can accumulate in the brain and are slowly metabolized to inorganic lead.

Ingestion of large amounts of gasoline can result in absorption of methanol in a quantity sufficient to quickly overwhelm the folate-dependent metabolic pathway and produce severe toxicity. Ethanol toxicity in humans is rarely attributed to gasoline inhalation exposure. Depending on the dose and exposure route, 20 to 70% of the absorbed MTBE is rapidly exhaled. When metabolized, MTBE is oxidized to formaldehyde and demethylated to tertiary butyl alcohol, which may then be further oxidized to 2-methyl-1,2-propanediol and alpha-hydroxyisobutyric acid. These oxidation products are excreted in the urine.

CLINICAL PRESENTATION

Inhalation is the most common route of exposure. The major target organ of gasoline exposure is the central nervous system (CNS). Single oral doses of approximately 10 mL/kg body weight (or about 700 mL for an adult) may be fatal. Smaller amounts, if aspirated into the lungs, may lead to lipoid pneumonitis. Prolonged contact with liquid gasoline can defat the skin and cause irritation and dermatitis.

Chronic Abuse

Chronic intentional abuse (e.g., sniffing or "huffing") of gasoline can result in death. Chronic abuse of leaded gasoline may cause a range of neurologic effects, including encephalopathy, ataxia, and tremor. Chronic sniffers of leaded gasoline may show neurologic effects with elevated blood lead levels. Chronic abuse of gasoline through sniffing can cause cardiac dysrhythmias and tachycardia.

Respiratory Effects

At high concentrations, gasoline vapor is a respiratory-tract irritant. Pulmonary congestion, edema, acute exudative tracheobronchitis, and intrapulmonary hemorrhage have been observed after gasoline overexposure.

Hematopoietic Effects

Long-term exposure to gasoline vapor may lead to blood dyscrasias such as anemia, hypochromia, thrombocytopenia, and neutropenia thought to be due to the benzene in gasoline mixture.

Carcinogenic Effects

Epidemiologic studies have not substantiated the carcinogenic effects observed in experimental animals. In 1989 the International Agency for Research on Cancer (IARC) concluded that gasoline is possibly carcinogenic to humans.

Acute Exposure

High-concentration exposures by any route cause CNS depression, which results in confusion, tinnitus, disorientation, headache, drowsiness, weakness, seizures, and coma. Inhalation may produce respiratory-tract irritation, resulting in dyspnea, tachypnea, and rales that may progress rapidly to massive pulmonary edema; a burning sensation in the chest may be present. Ingestion may cause pain and irritation of the mucous membranes, resulting in nausea, vomiting, abdominal pain, and diarrhea. Irritation and dermatitis can occur after skin contact, and conjunctivitis can occur after eye contact.

Chronic Exposure Risks

Exposures to gasoline and its constituents, including benzene, *n*-hexane, and 1,3-butadiene during refueling of motor vehicles are not a serious health hazard for consumers. Organic lead compounds can produce chronic neurologic toxicity, but exposure to such compounds in gasoline is currently negligible in the United States. Ethanol, methanol, and other additives in gasoline pose potential exposure risks, particularly through unintentional ingestion or suicide attempts.

LABORATORY

Appropriate laboratory evaluation in the patient with neurologic signs and symptoms includes neurobehavioral testing and electroencephalography. After severe, acute overexposure to gasoline, degenerative changes may occur in the liver and kidneys; these effects should be evaluated through routine laboratory testing. Persons with suspected ingestion should also have a careful pulmonary evaluation, including a baseline chest radiograph to assess possible aspiration. A follow-up chest x-ray should be obtained in about 6 hours if pulmonary symptoms develop. Pulse oximetry or arterial blood-gas analyses may be needed to assess oxygenation.

TREATMENT

Acute Exposure

No specific antidotes exist for gasoline; medical management for exposed persons is supportive. Respiratory compromise may require intubation or surgical creation of an airway.

After ingestion, vomiting should not be induced because of the risk of pulmonary aspiration. Activated charcoal is of limited use. If skin or hair has been in contact with liquid gasoline, remove clothing and flush skin and hair with water (preferably under a shower) for 2 to 3 minutes. Wash with mild soap; rinse thoroughly with water. If eye contact has occurred, the eye should be flushed with water for at least 5 minutes or until pain resolves.

Chronic Exposure

In most cases, exposure cessation usually leads to complete recovery, even for patients who have evidence of CNS toxicity.

JET FUELS[4,5]

Aviation fuel consists primarily of straight-chain and branched-chain alkanes (paraffins), cyclic alkanes (naphthenes), alkenes (olefins), and aromatic hydrocarbons. JP-4 and JP-7 are grades of jet propulsion fuel. Components include benzene, xylene, and toluene. Acute exposure causes central nervous system depression, dizziness, nausea, and vomiting. Chronic exposure is associated with neuropsychiatric disorders and peripheral sensory neuropathy, as well as a dermatitis. Tests of liver function are usually normal. Inhalation may cause respiratory tract irritation. The carcinogenic effects are unknown. Ingestion may lead to coughing, dyspnea, tachypnea, rapidly developing pulmonary edema, and potentially fatal aspiration pneumonitis. Treatment is symptomatic and supportive. After dermal exposure, remove contaminated clothing and wash skin and hair thoroughly. Eyes should be irrigated with water or saline for at least 15 minutes. After ingestion, gastric emptying is not indicated. Induced emesis or lavage may increase the risk of aspiration. There is no specific treatment for chronic jet fuel toxicity. Recovery occurs within a few days after exposure.

STODDARD SOLVENT[6,7]

"Stoddard solvent" is the name adopted by the National Association of Dryers and Cleaners to honor W.J. Stoddard for his work with petroleum distillates used in the dry-cleaning industry. Stoddard solvent is a distillation fraction of crude petroleum (distilling between about 300°F (149°C) and 400°F (204°C) that contains at least 200 products, predominantly C_7 through C_{12} hydrocarbons. The mixture typically consists of 30 to 40% cycloalkanes (naphthenes) and 10 to 20% aromatic hydrocarbons. (Benzene, toluene, and xylene each represent less than 1% of the total mixture.) Although the toxicity of Stoddard solvent is not attributable to any one type of constituent, the aromatic components are considered to be more toxic than the paraffin or naphthene components. Stoddard solvent is a colorless, flammable liquid that is insoluble in water.

USES

Stoddard solvent is a solvent used in industry primarily as a dry-cleaning solvent, metal degreaser, and extractant. Consumers may be exposed to Stoddard solvent through inhalation or dermal contact with cleaning products, paints, paint thinners, furniture refinishers, pesticides, or residues on dry-cleaned products.

ODOR

The odor threshold for Stoddard solvent is less than 1 part per million (ppm). However, after about 6 minutes, the olfactory sense fatigues and Stoddard solvent is no longer detected by smell. Thus odor is not a reliable indicator of exposure and may not provide adequate warning of dangerously high concentrations.

TOXICOKINETICS

Stoddard solvent is metabolized in the liver, thus preexisting liver disease (e.g., hepatitis, cirrhosis) would likely decrease the rate of metabolism and increase the amount of Stoddard solvent circulating in the blood. Excretion occurs by the lungs and kidneys; persons with lung impairment (e.g., chronic obstructive pulmonary disease [COPD]) or renal insufficiency may retain Stoddard solvent or its metabolites, thereby increasing their risk of toxicity.

CLINICAL PRESENTATION

Acute Exposure

Acute exposure to Stoddard solvent at air concentrations below the odor threshold produces no adverse health effects. The major effect associated with inhalation of paraffin-like solvents is CNS excitation, followed rapidly by CNS depression. Reported symptoms of acute exposure to Stoddard solvent include lightheadedness, dizziness, visual disturbances, and drowsiness. Although case reports have been published of persons who were exposed to Stoddard solvent and subsequently suffered liver, kidney, or hematologic injury, a causal relationship has not been firmly established. However, cardiac dysrhythmias have not been reported in humans after exposure to Stoddard solvent.

Respiratory Effects

Acute exposure to high concentrations of Stoddard solvent can irritate mucous membranes and cause upper respiratory-tract irritation. Acute ingestion and attendant aspiration of hydrocarbon mixtures similar to Stoddard solvent have resulted in chemical pneumonitis that mimics adult respiratory distress syndrome (ARDS). Complications of severe overexposure by the aspiration route may also include pulmonary edema, pulmonary emphysema, pneumothorax, pleuritis, pleural effusion, empyema, and pneumatoceles.

Dermal Effects

Stoddard solvent is a skin irritant.

Carcinogenic Effects

Data from studies of Stoddard solvent exposure in experimental animals (dermal exposure) and in humans (inhalation exposure) have not conclusively demonstrated that Stoddard solvent is carcinogenic.

Reproductive and Developmental Effects

Stoddard solvent probably can cross the placenta and enter breast milk.

Chronic Exposure

Chronic exposure to Stoddard solvent has been associated with headaches, fatigue, intermittent episodes of inebriation, and memory deficits that generally resolve on discontinuation of exposure.

LABORATORY TESTS

No specific hydrocarbon in the plasma or tissues is a reproducible index of exposure.

Acute Exposure

1. The person should be removed immediately from the source of exposure.
2. Institute decontamination procedures. Remove contaminated clothing and wash exposed areas with mild soap and shampoo, then rinse thoroughly with water. Direct eye splashes should be treated by irrigation with saline or water for 15 minutes or until pain resolves.
3. Supplemental oxygen should be administered as needed. Blood gas analyses, chest radiography, ECG monitoring, and baseline liver and kidney function tests should be considered in serious overexposures.
4. Gastric decontamination (i.e., emesis, lavage, cathartic, activated charcoal) is not recommended in most cases. Corticosteroids and prophylactic antibiotics are not necessary. Patients who are asymptomatic after 6 hours of observation may be discharged from the hospital.

Chronic Exposure

In cases of persistent neurologic symptoms, neuropsychologic testing may be useful for diagnostic purposes and to establish baseline function.

REFERENCES—GASOLINE

1. Logan D, Dart R. Gasoline Toxicity. Case studies in environmental medicine. 31. Agency for Toxic Substances and Disease Registry, September 1993.
2. Edminster SC, Bayer MJ. Recreational gasoline sniffing. Acute gasoline intoxication and latent organolead poisoning. J Emerg Med 1985;3:365–370.
3. Weaver NH. The petroleum industry. State Art Rev Occup Med 1988;3(5).
4. Dabney BJ, Brent J. Jet fuel toxicity. Case studies in environmental medicine. 32. Agency for Toxic Substances and Disease Registry, September 1993.
5. Davies NE. Jet fuel intoxication. Aerospase Med 1964;35: 481–482.
6. Cocchiarella L, Hryhorczuk D, Garrettson LK. Stoddard solvent toxicity. Case studies in environmental medicine. 33. Agency for Toxic Substances and Disease Registry, September 1993.
7. McDermott HJ. Hygienic guide series: Stoddard solvent (mineral spirits, white spirits). Am Ind Hyg Assoc J 1975;36: 553–558.

METHANETHIOL

Methanethiol (CH_3SH) is derived predominantly from the breakdown of methionine or the methylation of H_2S. It is metabolized by oxidation to disulfides such as dimethyl disulfide ($CH_3S\text{-}SCH_3$) or to sulfate, methylation to dimethyl sulfide (Ch_3SCh_3), acetylation to thiolesters, and glucuronylation to thioglucuronides.[1] It may be one of the endogenous factors involved in the pathogenesis of hepatic encephalopathy.[2] Methanethiol and dimethyl sulfide have been found in the urine of patients with fulminant hepatic failure. The odor on the breath of patients with cirrhosis given methionine is caused by dimethyl sulfide.[3] Somnolence and disorientation in cirrhotic patients is probably caused by methanethiol from which dimethyl sulfide is derived.[1]

CLINICAL PRESENTATION

Occupational exposure to CH_3CH may induce headache, nausea, vomiting, eye irritation, chest tightness and wheezing, dizziness, diplopia, and a productive cough.[4]

LABORATORY

Analytic Methods

Methanethiol may be quantified by gas chromatography and mass spectrometry.[1]

REFERENCES—METHANETHIOL

1. Zreve L, Nagasawa HT. Methanethiol and derivatives in hepatic failure. J Lab Clin Med 1988;111:595–597.
2. Blom HJ, van den Elzen JPAM, Yap SH, Tangerman A. Methanethiol and methylsulfide formation for 3-methylthiopropionate in human and rat hepatocytes. Bioch Biophys Acta 1988;972:131–136.
3. Chen S, Zieve L, Mahadevan V. Mercaptans and dimethyl sulfide in the breath of patients with cirrhosis of the liver. J Lab Clin Med 1970;75:628–635.
4. Garrettson LK, Warren DA. Chronic methanethiol poisoning. Vet Hum Toxicol 1990;32:365.

MONOOCTANOIN

Monooctanoin has been used to dissolve cholesterol gallstones by intrabiliary perfusion. Rapid perfusion may result in respiratory compromise and cardiac arrest.

STRUCTURE AND CLASSIFICATION

Monooctanoin is a mixture of glycerol esters, principally glyceryl monoactanoate. The empirical formula is $C_{19}H_{22}O_4$; the molecular weight is 218.3 and the CAS No. is 26402-26-6.[1]

Synonyms and Proprietary Names

Capmine 8210; Moctanin (USA, UK).[2]

DOSES

Therapeutic

Monooctanoin has been used by continuous perfusion through a catheter inserted directly into the common bile duct at a rate of 3 to 5 mL per hour at a pressure of 10 cm of water for 7 to 21 days.[1]

Fatal

Cardiac arrest followed 0.4 mL injected through a central venous catheter.[3]

CLINICAL PRESENTATION

Abdominal pain, nausea, vomiting, and diarrhea occur frequently in patients treated with monooctanoin, especially with a rapid rate of perfusion. Two deaths have been reported and one patient died from blood loss from a duodenal ulcer. The second died from pancreatitis.[2–6] Episodes of dyspnea and hypoxemia and respiratory compromise have followed intrabiliary monooctanoin use.

A 57-year-old patient was accidentally given <1 mL of monooctanoin through a central venous catheter. The patient experienced respiratory, then cardiac arrest. Nine hours later the patient experienced ventricular fibrillation and died 9.5 hours after the inadvertent administration. Autopsy confirmed the cause of death as respiratory failure secondary to lung infiltration of monooctanoin.[3,7]

TREATMENT

Treatment is symptomatic and supportive. If symptoms develop, cease use of monooctanoin.

REFERENCES—MONOOCTANOIN

1. Reynolds JEF, ed. *Martindale: The extra pharmacopoeia.* 30th ed. London: The Pharmaceutical Press, 1993, p. 1390.
2. Monooctanoin for gallstones. Med Lett Drugs Ther 1987; p. 52.
3. Hejka AG, Poquett M, Wiebe DA, Huntington RW III. Fatal intravenous injection of monooctanoin. Am J Forensic Med Pathol 1990;11:165–170.
4. Minuk GY, Hoofnagle JH, Jones EA. Systemic site effects from the intrabiliary infusion of monooctanoin for the dissolution of gallstones. J Clin Gastroenterol 1982;4:133–135.
5. Shustak A, Noseworthy TW, Johnston RG et al. Noncardiogenic pulmonary edema during intrabiliary infusion of monooctanoin. Crit Care Med 1986;14:659–660.
6. Physicians desk reference. 41st ed. Oradell, NJ. Medical Economics, 1987;924–925.
7. Litovitz TL, Schmitz BF, Holm KC. 1988 Annual Report of the American Association of Poison Control Centers National Data Collection System. Case 436. Am J Emerg Med 1989;7:495–545.

TRIMELLITIC ANHYDRIDE (TMA)

PHYSICAL AND CHEMICAL CHARACTERISTICS

Trimellitic anhydride has the formula $C_9H_4O_5$ ($HOCOC_6H_3$ (CO_2) O) and a CAS number of 552-30-7. It is a white crystalline solid. Synonyms include anhidrotrimellitic acid, 1,2,4-benzenene tricarboxylic acid anhydrone; TMA; and 1,3-dihydro-1,3-dioxo-5-isobenzofuran carboylic acid. Molecular weight is 192.1.

USES

TMA is used as a curing agent for epoxy and other resins and as a vinyl plasticizer. It is also found in anticorrosive surface coatings, polymers, paints, dyes, and pharmaceuticals. These products find applications in high-temperature plastics, wire insulation, gaskets, and automobile upholstery.

CLINICAL PRESENTATION

TMA induces four clinical syndromes in humans,[1,2] three of which are thought to be immunologically related.[1–4] The first is an IgE-mediated allergic rhinitis; the second a late respiratory systemic syndrome (LRSS) characterized by cough, dyspnea, myalgias, fever, and chills that occur 4 to 12 hours after TMA inhalation. This is correlated with high levels of IgG, IgM, and IgA antibody to trimellityl substitute human proteins. The third is a pulmonary disease-anemia syndrome that is characterized by dyspnea, cough, hemoptysis, and symptoms related to anemia. This syndrome may lead to respiratory failure; associated clinical findings are restrictive lung disease, infiltrates on a chest roentgenogram, and hypoxemia. Pulmonary hemosiderosis may be found on biopsy. A fourth nonimmunologic, irritant syndrome reflects upper airway irritation in response to high concentrations of TMA dust or fumes. Treatment is symptomatic and supportive.[1–4] OSHA permissible limits in air for an 8-hour day are 0.005 ppm.

REFERENCES—TRIMELLITIC ANHYDRIDE

1. Zeiss CR, Wolkonsky P, Pruzansky JJ, Patterson R. Clinical and immunologic evaluation of trimellitic anhydride workers in multiple industrial settings. J Allergy Clin Immunol 1982;70:15–18.
2. Patterson R, Zeiss CR, Pruzansky JJ. Immunology and immunopathology of trimellitic anhydride pulmonary reactions. J Allergy Clin Immunol 1982;70:19–23.
3. Leach CL, Hatoum NS, Ratajczak HV, Zeiss CR, Garvin PJ. Evidence of immunologic control of lung injury induced by trimellitic anhydride. Am Rev Respir Dis 1988;137:186–191.
4. Zeiss CR, Leach CL, Smith LJ, Levitz D, Hatoum NS, Garvin PJ, Patterson R. A serial immunologic and histopathologic study of lung injury and histopathologic study of lung injury induced by trimellitic anhydride. Am Rev Respir Dis 1988;137:191–196.

TRIMETHYLAMINE (TMA)

CAS: 75-50-3. $(CH_3)_3n$. 1991 TLV-TWA: 10 ppm (24 mg/m^3).
TVL-STEL 15 ppm (36 mg/m^3)
Synonyms. *N-N*-Dimethylmethanamine; TMA.

TMA is a colorless gas used as an insect attractant, as a warming agent for natural gas, and in organic synthesis. It may be an irritant to the eyes, mucous membranes, and lungs.[1] The fish odor syndrome, recessively inherited, is probably due to trimethylamine in the sweat. Acid soaps and acid body lotions convert TMA to an odorless oxide.[2,3]

REFERENCES—TRIMETHYLAMINE (TMA)

1. Hathaway GJ, Proctor NH, Hughes JP, Fischman ML, eds. Proctor and Hughes' Chemical Hazards of the Workplace. 3rd ed. New York: Van Nostrand Reinhold, 1991; pp 568–569.
2. Wilcken B. Acid soaps in the fish odor syndrome. Br Med J 1993;307:1497.
3. Ayesh R, Mitchell SC, Zhang A, Smith RL. The fish odour syndrome: biochemical, familial and clinical aspects. Br Med J 1993;307:655–657.

AROMATIC HYDROCARBONS—*P*-DICHLOROBENZENE (SEE ALSO CHAPTER 53: HOUSEHOLD PRODUCTS)

USES

p-Dichlorobenzene is used as a moth killer and to make deodorant blocks used in restrooms. It is also used in the manufacture of certain resins, in the pharmaceutical industry, and as a general insecticide in farming.

TOXICITY LEVELS

The current OSHA permissible exposure limit (PEL) for para-dichlorobenzene (*p*-DCB) in the workplace as a time-weighted average (TWA) for 8 hours/day and 40 hours/week is 75 ppm (450 m/m^3) with a short-term (15 minute) exposure limit of 110 ppm (675 mg/m^3). *O*-dichlorobenzene (CAS 95-50-1) has a 50-ppm ceiling (300 mg/m^3). NIOSH guidelines for immediate danger to life and health are 1000 ppm for *p*-DCB.

TOXICOKINETICS

Absorption

p-DCB has been found in human blood, fatty tissue, and breast milk following inhalation exposure.

Elimination

The major route of elimination appears to be in the urine. 2,5-Dichlorophenol is the major urinary metabolite of *p*-DCBs.[1]

Laboratory

In a case of accidental ingestion of an unknown quanitity of *p*-DCB crystals by a 3-year-old boy, analysis of urine specimens yielded four unidentified phenols as well as 2,5-dichlorphenol. These were shown to be conjugated with glucuronic and sulfuric acid.[1] Methemóglobinemia, hyperchromic anemia, and acute hemolytic anemia have also been described.

TREATMENT

Treatment is mainly symptomatic and supportive.[2]

REFERENCES—*P*-DICHLOROBENZENE

1. Hallowell M. Acute haemolytic anemia following ingestion of paradichlorobenzene. Arch Dis Child 1959;34:74–75.
2. Agency for Toxic Substance Disease Registry. US Public Health Service. Toxicological profile for 1,4-dichlorobenzene. January 1989. ATSDR/TP-88/14.

HALOGENATED HYDROCARBONS—HALOGENATED SOLVENTS

Table 65–3 lists OSHA standards for halogenated hydrocarbons. Table 65–4 lists commercial uses of halogenated solvents.

STEL (short-term exposure limit) is the employees' 15-minute, time-weighted, average exposure that shall not be exceeded at any time during a workday.[1]

CHEMICAL PROPERTIES

Most halogenated hydrocarbons are clear and colorless liquids that are not inflammable and have chloroform-like odors. Most contain impurities such as other chlorinated hydrocarbons.

Table 65–3
Halogenated Hydrocarbons Occupational Health and Safety Standards (U.S.) Limits for Air Contaminants

	CAS #	TWA 8 hour	STEL (15 minutes unless otherwise noted)	Ceiling (15 minutes unless otherwise noted)	Acceptable Maximum Peak Above the Acceptable Ceiling Concentration for an 8-Hour Shift: Concentration	Acceptable Maximum Peak Above the Acceptable Ceiling Concentration for an 8-Hour Shift: Maximum Duration
1,2-Dichloroethane (Ethylene dichloride)	107-06-2	50 ppm	200 ppm	100 ppm	200 ppm	5 minutes in any 3 hours
1,2-Dichloroethane (1,2-Dichloroethylene)	540-59-0	200 ppm (790 ng/m³)				
Methylenechloride	75-09-7	500 ppm		1000 ppm	2000 ppm	5 minutes in any 2 hours
Propylene dichloride (1,2-Dichloropropane)	78-87-5	75 ppm (350 mg/m³)	110 ppm (510 mg/m³)			
1,2,2,2-Tetrabromoethane	79-27-6	1 ppm (14 mg/m³)				
1,1,2,2-Tetrachloroethane	79-34-5	1 ppm (7 mg/m³)				
Perchlorethylene	127-18-4	25 ppm (170 mg/m³)				
Carbon tetrachloride	56-23-5	2 ppm (12.6 mg/m³)		25 ppm	200 ppm	5 minutes in any 4 hours
1,1,1-Trichloroethane (Methyl chloroform)	71-55-6	350 (1900 mg/m³)		450 ppm (2450 mg/m³)		
Chloroform (Trichloromethane)	67-66-3	2 ppm (9.75 mg/m³)				Skin designation
1,1,2-Trichloroethylene (Trichloro-ethane)	79-01-6	50 ppm (270 mg/m³)	200 ppm (100 mg/m³)			
1,2,2-Trichloro-1,2,2-Trifluoroethane	76-13-1	1000 ppm (7600 mg/m³)	1250 ppm (9500 mg/m³)			
Betachloroprene	126-99-8	10 ppm (35 mg/m³)				
Ethylene dibromide	101-93-4	20 ppm		30 ppm	50 ppm	5 minutes
Methyl bromide	74-83-9	5 ppm (20 mg/m³)				
Methyl chloride	74-87-3	50 ppm (105 mg/m³)	100 ppm (210 mg/m³)			

Table 65–4
Uses of Halogenated Hydrocarbons

1,1-Dichloroethane	Cleansing agent; degreaser; solvent for plastics, oils, and fats; grain fumigant; chemical intermediate.
1,2-Dichloroethane	Manufacture of ethyl glycol, polyvinyl chloride, nylon, viscose rayon, styrene-butadeine, rubber; solvent; degreaser; extracting agents; fumigant.
1,2-Dichloroethylene	Solvent for waxes, resins, and ethylcellulose; extract of rubber; refrigerant; manufacture of pharmaceuticals.
Dichloromethane (Methylene dichloride)	Solvent, paint remover, manufacture of photographic fixant, aerosol propellants, urethane foam, degreaser.
Dichloropropane (Propylene dichloride)	Degreasing, dry cleaning, soil fumigant, manufacture of cellulose plastics, metal degreasing, stain remover, chemical intermediates.
Tetrabromoethane (Acetylene tetrabromide)	Gauge fluid, solvent, refractive index liquid in microscopy.
Tetrachloromethane (Carbon tetrachloride)	Manufacture of fluorocarbon propellants (Freon 2, Freon 11, Freon 12); solvent for oils, fats, lacquers, varnishes, and resins; degreasing and cleaning agents; grain fumigant. Synthesis of fluorocarbons, dry cleaning agents, fire extinguisher agents.
1,1,1-Trichloroethane	Solvent for adhesives (including food packaging adhesives, metal degreasing, pesticides, textile processing, vapor degreasing, aerosols, coating and inks. Used primarily for cold-cleaning, dip cleaning, bucket cleaning.
Trichloroethylene	Vapor degreasing of fabricated metal parts, chemical intermediates, general solvent, refrigerant, typewriter correction fluids, paint removers/stuffers, adhesives, rug cleaning fluids, spot removers.
Tetrachloroethylene	Solvent, chemical intermediate (for synthesis of fluorocarbon 113), dry cleaning and textile processing, industrial metal cleaning, vapor and liquid degreasing agent, anthelminthic, pesticide, intermediate.
1,1,2,2,Tetrachloroethane	Feed stock, in the production of trichloroethylene, tetrachloroethylene and 1,2-dichloroethylene solvent, cleaning and degreasing metals in paint removers.
1,1,2-Trichloro-1,2,2-trifluoroethane (Fluorocarbon 113, Freon 113)	Solvent for cleaning electronic equipment and degreasing of machinery, refrigerant, fire extinguishers, dry cleaning, polymer intermediates.

EXPOSURE

Case-control studies depend on the assumption that individuals in the "exposure occupations" have more hydrocarbon exposure than those in the control occupation. However, controls often include individuals with high solvent exposure, probable high solvent exposure, and uncertain status. Some factory workers have little chemical exposure, so workers listed under "Exposure Occupations" may not have more hydrocarbon exposure than several control groups.[2]

TOXICOKINETICS

Absorption

The pulmonary route is the primary source of toxic exposure to the halogenated hydrocarbons. Oral absorption is rapid but less complete than pulmonary absorption. Insignificant amounts are absorbed through the skin.

Distribution

Peak blood levels occur soon after inhalation, but peak levels of oral administration are usually found in 1 to 2 hours after ingestion. Distribution is highest in the fat, the brain, and the blood. Halogenated solvents cross the placenta and may be found in the fetus.

Metabolism

Halogenated hydrocarbons are metabolized in the liver by the cytochrome P450 oxidation. Partial glutathione conjugation may occur. Halogentated solvents are also excreted through the lungs.

CLINICAL PRESENTATION

Acute Toxicity

Neurologic

Inhalation induces central nervous system depression within minutes. Alterations in psychomotor performance occur. Cranial neuropathies have been observed.

Cherry and colleagues conducted a prospective, case-referred study and observed that occupational solvent exposure plus alcohol intake may be an important cause of organic brain damage.[3] An anecdotal study indicates that individuals with a history of 10 years or more of regular occupational exposure to solvents in confined space may present with a spectrum of neurologic disease resembling those seen in solvent abusers.[4,5]

Dermal

Insignificant penetration of human skin.

Oral

Hepatorenal failure, beginning a few days after exposure, and death.

Gastrointestinal

Hepatotoxicity and gastrointestinal irritation.

Chronic Toxicity

Study design flaws and inadequate neuropsychiatric testing procedures have not produced convincing evidence of chronic neurologic toxicity. Centrilobular hepatic necrosis may be observed. Degreaser's flush may result from ethanol-induced vasodilation of superficial skin vessels. This resolved in about 1½ hours.[6]

Painter's Syndrome

Although painter's syndrome (headaches, fatigue, difficulties in concentrating, problems with short-term memory, irritability, depression, and alcohol intolerance) has been classified as an occupational disease and is a cause of premature retirement in the Scandinavian countries, critical reviews of the literature[7,8] have reported that flawed methodology and inattention to compounding variables may have led to the erroneous conclusion that chronic solvent exposure causes organic damage to the central nervous system. Potential cofounders include age, sex, intelligence, alcohol ingestion, occupational exposure to other neurotoxins, and health status.[9]

Renal

Halogenated solvents are weakly nephrotoxic.

Several anecdotal studies have suggested that a relation may exist between exposure to occupational organic solvents and diseases of the kidney—particularly malignancy and glomerulonephritis.[10–12] Two case-referral studies on renal cancer and glomerulonephritis did not confirm any relation with exposure to solvents.[11] Indicators of renal dysfunction that might assert the integrity of the glomerulus (albuminuria, GBM antigens in blood and urine, circulating anti-GBM antibodies) and tubular function (low-molecular-weight proteinuria, hyperphosphatemia, acetyl glucoaminidase, tubular antigen excretion, prostaglandin excretion) have seen limited use in industrial studies.[13]

Cardiovascular

Hypotension, arrhythmias.

Lungs

Upper respiratory tract irritation. Little alveolar damage.

Pregnancy and Reproduction

No halogenated solvents have been definitively associated with teratogenicity.

Carcinogenicity

Suspected carcinogens include tetrachloromethane, 1-2, dichloroethane, dichloromethane, tetrachloroethylene, and trichloromethane.

LABORATORY

Ancillary Tests

Hepatotoxicity associated with hepatorenal failure may be indicated by elevated serum hepatic aminotransferase, bilirubin, alkaline phosphatase, ammonia, creatinine, and lactate lead. In addition, a prolonged prothrombin time and hypoglycemia may be seen. Tests usually return to normal in several weeks. Renal dysfunction may be associated with a rise in serum creatinine and reduced urine volume.

Analytic Methods

Gas chromatography with electron capture can be used to determine the concentration of halogenated solvents in biologic samples.

Abnormalities

Trichloroethylene, tetrachloroethylene, and trichloroethane metabolism may lead to the presence of trichloroacetone and (TCAA) in the urine. Other chemicals such as chloral hydrate may also be metabolized to TCAA. Trichloroethanol levels in exposed air, blood, and urine may be increased following trichloroethylene exposure.

Interpretation

Human data is inadequate to establish a dose-related tissue concentration effect.

TREATMENT

Stabilization

Treatment is largely supportive. Watch for respiratory depression and arrhythmias. Obtain arterial blood gases. Administer oxygen if there is evidence of altered mental status or dyspnea. Treat hypotension with volume expansion and vasopression. Use lidocaine or beta-blockers for ventricular arrhythmias.

Skin

Remove contaminated clothing. Wash affected area with soap and copious amounts of water.

Eye

Irrigate the eye for 15 to 20 minutes. Obtain a consultation if symptoms persist.

Oral

Most of the halogenated solvents ingested in quantities of one to two swallows may be partially removed by ipecac-induced emesis if administered within a few hours to a patient who has not lost the gag reflex, is not seizing, is not markedly lethargic, or is not in coma. Observe the patient in the upright position to lessen the possibility of aspiration. Activated charcoal is probably ineffective.[14]

Inhalation

Move from the contaminated area. Provide a source of oxygen and prepare for mechanical ventilation. If the patient is unconscious and the pulse is absent, initiate cardiopulmonary resuscitation measures.

Enhancement of Elimination

Maintain good ventilation. Hemodialysis or hemoperfusion are not likely to be useful because of the high lipophilic properties of these solvents. Hyperbaric oxygen is experimental.

Methyl Bromide

Methyl bromide intoxication is characterized by acute, resistant, myoclonic convulsions and severe and permanent mental and neurologic damage for which supportive treatment has been the mainstay of management. An anecdotal, uncontrolled report suggests the use of hemodialysis to remove the bromide from the blood.[15]

Antidote

N-acetylcysteine may restore depleated glutathione stores, but no adequate clinical studies are available to validate this possible treatment.

Supportive Care

Watch for cardiac dysrhythmias, aspiration pneumonitis, hepatotoxicity, and hypoxic encephalopathy. Monitor for arrhythmia for at least 24 hours and for hepatorenal failure for about 3 days. Obtain a chest x-ray, arterial blood gas, electrocardiogram, serum creatinine, and hepatic aminotransferase. Check electrolyte imbalance daily. Treat renal failure with dialysis and hepatic failure with fresh frozen plasma, vitamin K, a low-protein diet, neomycin, and lactulose. Watch fluid and electrolyte balance.

REFERENCES—HALOGENATED HYDROCARBONS

1. Part 1910. Occupational Safety and Health Standards. Subpart Z—Toxic and Hazardous Substances 695 to 702-0-30.
2. Ducatman AM, Prader-Willi. Syndrome and paternal hydrocarbon exposure. Lancet 1988;1:646.
3. Cherry NM, Labreche FP, McDonald JC. Organic brain damage and occupational solvent exposure. Br J Ind Med 1992;49:776–781.
4. Seaton A, Jellinek EH, Kennedy P. Major neurological disease and occupational exposure to organic solvents. Q J Med 1992;84:707–712.
5. Seedorff L, Olsen E. Exposure to organic solvents. I. A survey on the use of solvents. An Occup Hyg 1990;34:371–378.
6. Stewart RD, Hake CL, Peterson JE. "Degreaser's flush" dermal response to trichloroethylene and ethanol. Arch Environ Health 1974;29:1–5.
7. Grasso P, Sharra M, Davies DM, Irwin D. Neurophysiological and psychological disorders and occupational exposure to organic solvents. Ed Chem Toxicol 1984;22:819–852.
8. Errebo-Knudsen EO, Olsen F. Organic solvents and presenile dementia (The Painter's Syndrome). A critical review of the Danish literature. Sci Total Environ 1986;48:45–67.
9. Bolla KI, Schwartz BX, Agnew J, Ford PD, Blecker ML. Subclinical neuropsychiatric effects of chronic low-level solvent exposure in US pain manufacturers. J Occup Med 1990; 32:676–677.
10. Daniell WE, Couser WG, Rosenstock L. Occupational solvent exposure and glomerulonephritis. A case report and review of the literature. JAMA 1988;259:2280–2283.
11. Narvarte J, Saba SR, Ramirez G. Occupational exposure to organic solvents causing chronic tubulointerstitial nephritis. Arch Intern Med 1989;149:155–158.
12. Nelson NA, Robins TG, Port FK. Solvent nephrotoxicity in humans and experimental animals. Am J Nephrol 1990; 10:10–20.
13. Harrington JM, Whitby W, Gray CN, Reid FJ, Aw TC, Waterhouse JA. Renal disease and occupation exposure to organic solvents: a case report approach. Br J Ind Med 1989; 46:643–650.
14. Laass W. Therapy of acute oral poisonings by organic solvents. Treatment by activated charcoal in combination with laxatives. Arch Toxicol Suppl 1980;4:406–409.
15. Moosa MR, Jansen J, Edelstein CL. Treatment of methyl bromide proisoning with hemodialysis. Postgrad Med J 1994; 20:733–735.

POLYCHLORINATED BIPHENYLS (PCB) (FIG. 65–1)

OCCUPATIONAL EXPOSURE[1]

Because of their insulating and nonflammable properties, PCBs have been used as head exchange and dielectric fluids in transformers and capacitors, hydraulic and lubricating fluids, diffusion pump oils, plasticizers, extenders for pesticides, and as ingredients of caulking compounds, paints, adhesives, and flame retardants. PCBs have also been used in inks and carbonless paper. Trade names for PCBs include Aroclor, Askarel, Eucarel, Pyranol, Dykanol, Clorphen, Asbestol, Diaclor, Nepolin, and EEC-18.

Occupations entailing risk of PCB exposure include, but are not limited to, the following: electric cable repair, electroplating, emergency response, firefighting, hazardous waste hauling/site operating, heat exchange equipment

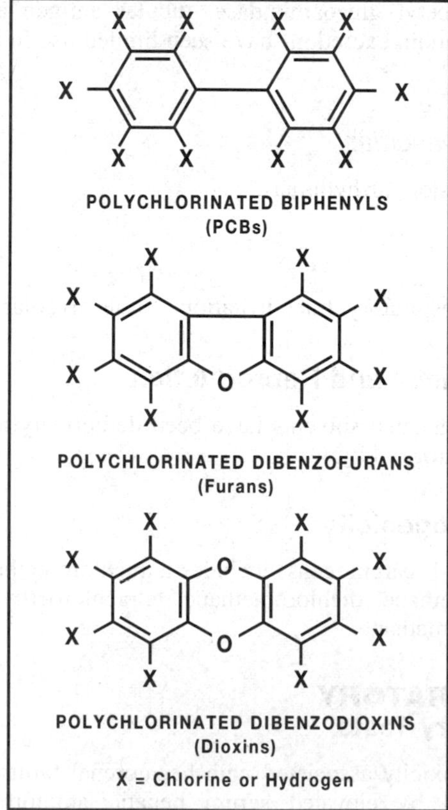

Figure 65–1 Polychlorinated biphenyls and related compounds.

repair, maintenance cleaning, metal finishing, paving and roofing, pipefitting/plumbing, timber products manufacturing, transformer/capacitor repair, and waste oil processing.[1]

FETUS AND NEONATES

Fetuses and neonates are potentially more sensitive to PCBs than adults because of transplacental distribution and physiologic differences. They lack the hepatic microsomal enzyme systems that facilitate metabolism and excretion of PCBs. Furthermore, PCBs accumulate in breast milk. Nursing infants are at additional risk because human milk contains a steroid that inhibits PCB glucuronidation and excretion.

Chloracne is the only overt effect of PCB exposure in humans, but absence of chloracne does not rule out exposure. Chloracne typically develops weeks or months after exposure. The lesions are often refractory to treatment and can last for years.

TREATMENT

Acute exposure

In the event of PCB splashes in the eyes, irrigate with tepid water immediately for at least 15 minutes and follow with ophthalmic evaluation. Remove contaminated clothing and discard properly. Gently wash affected skin with soap and warm water for at least 15 minutes.

If PCB-containing substances are ingested, induce vomiting if the patient is conscious. Activated charcoal has not been proven beneficial, but is not contraindicated.

Chronic Exposure

There is no specific treatment for PCB toxicity. Initial treatment of chloracne is based on cessation of exposure, good skin hygiene, and use of dermatologic measures commonly employed for acne vulgaris.

Since there are no known methods of reducing reserves of PCBs in lipid tissues, attempts to purge the body of PCBs should not be undertaken. Saunas and nutritional therapies have no proven efficacy. Crash diets risk mobilizing PCBs stored in fat. Patients should be encouraged to avoid exposure to other hepatotoxins such as antibiotics or medications with known hepatotoxicity, alcohol, and chlorinated solvents.

REFERENCE—POLYCHLORINATED BIPHENYLS

1. Wabeke R, Weinstein R, Letz G. Polychlorinated biphenyl toxicity. Case studies in Environmental Medicine. 12. Agency for Toxic Substances and Disease Registry, June 1990.

CHLORODIBENZOFURANS (CDFS)

SOURCE

Small amounts of CDFs can enter the environment from a number of sources. Accidental fires or breakdowns involving capacitors, transformers, and other electrical equipment (e.g., fluorescent light fixtures) that contain polychlorinated biphenyls (PCBs) are the main known sources of CDFs in the environment. A fire involving transformers containing PCBs contaminated the State Office Building in Binghamton, New York, with CDFs. Accidents of a different kind involving PCBs occurred in Japan and Taiwan. In Japan and Taiwan, where PCBs were used as a heat exchanger fluid for processing rice oil, PCBs contaminated with CDFs accidentally leaked into the oil causing "Yusho" or "Yu-Cheng" (oil disease) in about 4000 people. CDFs are also produced as unwanted compounds during the manufacture of several chemicals and consumer products such as wood-treatment chemicals, some metals, and paper products. When the waste water, sludge, or solids from these processes are released into waterways or soil in dumpsites, these locations become contaminated with CDFs. CDFs also enter into the environment from burning municipal and industrial waste in incinerators. The exhaust from cars that use leaded gasoline releases small amounts of CDFs in the environment. CDFs also enter into the environment from burning of coal, wood, or oil for home heating and production of electricity. Many of these chemicals or processes that produce CDFs in the environment are either being slowly phased out or strictly controlled.

CHEMICAL IDENTITY

Dibenzofuran is an organic compound that contains two benzene rings fused to a central furan ring. CDFs are a class of organic compounds in which one to eight chlorine atoms are attached to the benzene ring positions of a dibenzofuran structure. The general chemical structure for CDFs with the numbering system for the chlorine substituents is as follows:

Based on the number of chlorine substituents (one to eight) on the benzene rings, there are eight homologues of CDFs (monochlorinated through octachlorinated). Each homologous group contains one or more isomers. There are 135 possible CDF isomers, including 4 monoCDFs, 16 diCDFs, 28 triCDFs, and one octaCDF. Each one of these compounds is called a congener. Because of molecular asymmetry, CDFs have 135 congeners, compared with 75 for CDDs.[1]

REFERENCE—CHLORODIBENZOFURANS (CDFS)

1. Agency for Toxic Substances and Disease Registry. Toxicological Profile for Chlorinated Dibenzofurans Draft. US Department of Health and Human Services. October 1992.

POLYCYCLIC AROMATIC HYDROCARBONS

PHYSICAL AND CHEMICAL CHARACTERISTICS

Polycyclic aromatic hydrocarbons consist of three or more fused benzene rings in varying arrangements that contain only carbon and hydrogen. Naphthalene, which is a coal tar constituent used for mothballs, is not considered a polycyclic aromatic hydrocarbon because it contains only two fused benzene rings. The primary environmental sources of polycyclic aromatic hydrocarbons (PAHs) are forest fires and combustion of fossil fuel, where high temperatures convert organic substances to PAHs. Seafood and agricultural products contain PAHs because of their sedimentation from air and subsequent penetration into water systems. Crude coconut oil, heavily smoked ham, roasted coffee, tea, and charcoal-broiled meat contain PAHs in concentrations up to 20 to 40 μg/kg.

OCCUPATIONAL EXPOSURE

Occupational medicine began with Percival Pott's 1775 report[1] of an unusually high incidence in chimney sweeps of scrotal cancer, which, by the 1930s, was attributed to benzo-[*a*]pyrene and dibenz[*a,h*]anthracene in coal tar. Coke-oven, coal-tar, pitch, asphalt-fume, and carbon-black workers are all exposed to PAHs. The carcinogenic form of PAHs results from their oxidation by the mixed-function oxidase system to diol-epoxide derivatives. These compounds contain highly reactive "bay regions" that probably bind covalently to DNA.

PATHOPHYSIOLOGY

Direct covalent binding of a carcinogenic agent to DNA to produce carcinogen DNA adducts may be an essential step in the development of cancer. Polycyclic aromatic hydrocarbon (PAH) ONA adducts have been detected in lung tissue from patients with lung cancer. Benzo[*a*]pyrene (BP) is often measured as an indicator of PAH exposure and may be responsible for an increased risk of lung cancer among smokers, foundry workers, and coke-oven workers. Measurement of BP serum protein adduct concentrations appear to be a useful method by which groups exposed to BP may be biologically monitored.[2] Urinary 1-hydroxypyrene (1-OHPY) has promise as an environmental marker of exposures to PAH.[3] Following a meal high in PAHs, 1-OHPY appears in the urine with a half-life of 4.4 hours. Maximum concentrations are found in 6.3 hours.

OSHA permissible exposure limits in air over an 8-hour workday are 0.2 mg/m^3 measured as the benzene-soluble fraction of coal-tar pitch volatiles. The OSHA standard for coke-oven emissions is 0.15 mg/m^3.

CLINICAL PRESENTATION[4]

Acute toxicity is rarely reported. Exposure to high-risk PAHs via skin and lung absorption results in increased incidences of skin and lung cancer. Certain PAHs are considered carcinogenic, whereas others are not (e.g., anthracene and phenanthrene). Coke-oven emissions are complex mixtures of coal and coke material that include PAHs, and epidemiologic study of exposed workers indicated increased incidences of lung and urinary tract cancer. Soots, tars, and creosote contain a variety of by-products and contaminants that include PAHs, and epidemiologic study demonstrates increased incidences of skin, lung, bladder, and gastrointestinal cancer. Benzo[*a*]anthracene, benzo[*a*]pyrene, and dibenzo[*a,h*]pyrene are suspected carcinogens based on studies in animals that show increased incidences of skin, lung, and liver cancer.

Chronic Exposure[5]

Reported effects associated with chronic exposure to coal tar and its by-products include the following:

Skin

Erythema, burns, warts on sun-exposed areas with progression to cancer. Toxic effects of coal tar are enhanced by exposure to ultraviolet light.

Eyes

Irritation and photosensitivity.

Respiratory System

Cough, bronchitis, and bronchogenic cancer.

Gastrointestinal System

Leukoplakia, buccal-pharyngeal cancer, and cancer of the lip.

Hematopoietic System

Leukemia (inconclusive) and lymphoma.

Genitourinary

Hematuria, kidney and bladder cancers.

TREATMENT

Acute Exposure

Remove contaminated clothing as soon as possible. Decontaminate the skin by gently scrubbing with soap and water. Ocular exposure should be treated with irrigation and a complete eye examination. Ventilatory support should be available in the event of an acute inhalation exposure.

Chronic Exposure

Periodic evaluation of healthy patients who have been significantly exposed to PAHs, even in the absence of symptoms, is recommended to facilitate early diagnosis and intervention should a malignancy develop.[5]

REFERENCES—POLYCYCLIC AROMATIC HYDROCARBONS

1. Pott P. Chirurgical observations relative to the cataract, the polypus of the nose, the cancer of the scrotum, the different kinds of ruptures, and the mortification of the toes and feet. London: Hawkes, Clark and Collins, 1775.
2. Sherson D, Sabro P, Sigsgaard T, Johansen F, Acetrup H. Biological monitoring of foundry workers exposed to polycyclic aromatic hydrocarbons. Br J Ind Med 1990;47:448–453.
3. Buckley TJ, Lioy PJ. An examination of the time course from human dietary exposure to polycyclic aromatic hydrocarbons to urinary elimination of 1-hydroxypyrene. Br J Ind Med 1992;49:113–124.
4. Zedeck MS. Polycyclic aromatic hydrocarbons: a review. J Environ Pathol Toxicol 1980;3:537–567.

5. Brudzewski J, Shusterman D. Polynuclear aromatic hydrocarbons (PAH) toxicity. Agency for Toxic Substances and Disease Registry. Atlanta. US Department of Health and Human Services, June 1990.

CREOSOTES[1–4]

Creosote is a complex mixture of hydrocarbon compounds, including many polycyclic aromatic hydrocarbons. It has been used as a disinfectant and treatment for coughs. Creosote is a potent carcinogen. Skin cancer has been observed in workers exposed to creosote for long periods during timber treatment. The only products now routinely treated with creosotes are commercial wood products such as railroad ties and marine piers. Its use as a cough medicine can no longer be recommended.[1–3]

CLINICAL PRESENTATION

Creosotes cause irritation of the skin, mucous membranes, and conjunctiva. The skin may become red, papular, vesicular, or ulcerative. Photosensitization has been observed. Following ingestion of creosote, gastrointestinal irritation (nausea, vomiting, salivation, and abdominal discomfort) and cardiovascular instability (tachycardia, hypotension, respiratory distress, cyanosis, and pupillary changes) may occur. The fatal dose is about 0.1 g/kg body weight.

TREATMENT

Treatment is entirely symptomatic and supportive.

REFERENCES—CREOSOTES

1. Landrigan PJ. Health risks of creosotes. JAMA 1993;209: 1309.
2. Karlehagen S, Andersen A, Ohlson C-G. Cancer incidence among creosote exposed workers. Scand J Work Environ Health 1992;18:26–29.
3. Agency for Toxic Substances and Disease Registry. Toxicological Profile for Creosote. Atlanta, GA. Dept of Health and Human Services, Public Health Service, 1990; Publication TP 90-09.
4. Henson EV. Cresols, creosote and derivatives. In Parmeggiani L, ed. Encyclopaedia of occupational health and safety. 3rd (revised) ed. Geneva: International Labour Office, 1991; pp. 569–570.

CYCLIC ETHERS—TETRAHYDROFURAN

Tetrahydrofuran (THF) is a colorless organic solvent liquid belonging to a group of cyclic ethers with an odor similar to acetone.[1] It can dissolve many types of plastics (polyvinyl chloride, polyurethanes, epoxy compounds, and cellulosics) and a wide range of organic products. Its main applications include the manufacture of glues, paints, varnishes, inks, and wetting and dispersing agents in textile processing.

Synonyms

Cyclotetramethylene oxide, diethylene oxide, THF, tetramethylene oxide, 1,4-epoxybutane. Recently, it has been used as an iron oxide coating agent employed in the production of audio and video tapes. Tetrahydrofuran forms explosive peroxides when exposed to air.

The TWA NIOSH/OSHA standard in the United States is 590 mg/m^3 with a STEL of 735 mg/m^3. TWA standards in the United Kingdom are 200 ppm (590 mg/m^3); the STEL is 250 ppm (735 mg/m^3).[2] THF is readily absorbed across the alveolar membrane and from the digestive tract. It can cross the skin in toxic amounts.[3,4] THF has modest anesthetic properties in animals.[5]

TOXICOKINETICS

Metabolic products may include gamma-butyrolactone, which possesses convulsive properties.[4,5] Tetrahydrofuran is subject to oxidative metabolism.[6]

MECHANISM OF ACTION

THF is an inhibitor of a number of cytochrome P450 (P450)–dependent, mixed-function oxidase activities, with a particular affinity for the alcohol-induced enzyme P450 II E1.[7]

CLINICAL PRESENTATION

Symptoms after exposure may include nausea, headache, blurred vision, dizziness, fatigue, tinnitus, chest pain, and cough. Irritation of skin and mucous membranes may be experienced. THF may have contributed to the development of status epilepticus or awakening from an enflurane anesthesia in a patient occupationally exposed to solvent.[8] One patient developed a peripheral neuropathy after exposure.[8]

Tetrahydrofuran is an upper respiratory tract irritant. At high concentrations it is a central nervous system depressant. An adult ingested tetrahydrofuran and developed abdominal pain, nausea, and vomiting. The vomitus and breath had an unusual odor. The patient developed jaundice, oliguria, a high fever, and loss of consciousness. He died in 5 days. Lesions of the gastrointestinal tract and kidney (glomeruli) were observed.[9] The two primary signs of intoxication are narcosis and hepatocellular dysfunction, both occurring at doses of approximately half of the lethal doses in animals.

LABORATORY

Hepatic aminotransferases may be considerably elevated. The chest x-ray and electrocardiogram are normal. The blood count, renal function tests (serum creatinine, blood urea nitrogen) are usually normal. Muscle acetylcholinesterase appeared to be increased in animal studies.[6]

Analysis of the breath, blood, and urine is accomplished with the use of gas chromatography. The detection limit is 40 ppb. Measurement of THF concentration in the urine is a sensitive, specific method for monitoring of exposure.[10]

TREATMENT

Treatment is largely symptomatic and supportive.

REFERENCES—TETRAHYDROFURAN

1. Juntumen J, Kaste M, Markovan H. Cerebral convulsions after enflurane anaesthesia and occupational exposure to

tetrahydrofuran. J Neurol Neurosurg Psychiatry 1984;47: 1258–1259.
2. Occupational Exposure Limits for Airborne Toxic Substances. 3rd ed. Geneva: International Labour Office, 1991; pp. 382–383.
3. Garnier R, Rosenberg N, Puissant JM, Chauvet JP, Efthymiou ML. Tetrahydrofuran poisoning after occupational exposure. Br J Ind Med 1989;46:677–678.
4. Viader F, Lechevalier B, Morin P. Polynevrite toxique chez un travailleur du plastique. Role possible du methyl-ethyl-cetone. Presse Med 1975;4:1813–1815.
5. Stoughton RW, Robbins BH. The anesthetic properties of tetrahydrofuran. J Pharmacol Exp Ther 1936;58:171–173.
6. Klunk WE, McKeon AC, Covey DF, Farrendelli JA. Alpha substituted gamma-butyrolactones: new class of anticonvulsant drugs. Science 1982;217:1040–1042.
7. Moody DE. The effect of tetrahydrofuran on biological system: does a hepatotoxic potential exist? Drug Chem Toxicol 1991;14:319–342.
8. Elovaara E, Pfaffli P, Savolainen H. Burden and biochemical effects of extended tetrahydrofuran vapour inhalation of three concentration levels. Acta Pharmacol Toxicol 1984;54:221–226.
9. Nagata T, Hara M, Kageura M, Hara K, Kimura K. A fatal case of tetrahydrofuran poisoning. In Maes RAA, ed. Topics in forensic and analytic toxicology. Amsterdam: Elsevier, 1984; pp. 33–37.
10. Ong CN, Chia SE, Phoon WH, Tan KT. Biological monitoring of occupational exposure to tetrahydrofuran. Br J Ind Med 1991;48:616–621.

KETONES—CYCLOHEXANONE

Cyclohexanone (ketohexamethylene or pimelic ketone) is a cyclic 6-carbon ketone whose formula is CO $(CH_2)_4CH_2$. It is a colorless to slightly yellow liquid with an odor like peppermint. Molecular weight: 98.16. Cyclohexanone is slightly soluble in water. Synonyms: Anone, hexanon, ketohexamethylene, nadone, pimelic ketone, pimelin ketone.[1] Cyclohexanone will dissolve most plastics, resins, and rubber. It may react with oxidizing agents and nitric acid causing fires and explosions. Odor threshold: 0.88 ppm.

Urinary cyclohexanol concentrations correlate well with the time-weighted average concentration of cyclohexanone at the workplace. The detection limit for urinary cyclohexanol is 0.4 mg/L. It is specific enough to detect cyclohexanol in urine for those who are exposed to cyclohexanone below the current exposure limit of 25 ppm.

EXPOSURE LIMITS

The current Occupational Safety and Health Administration (OSHA) permissible exposure limit (PEL) is 50 ppm parts of air (200 mg/m^3) as a time-weight average (TWA) concentration over an 8-hour work shift. The NIOSH REL is 25 ppm (100 mg/m^3) as a TWA for up to a 10-hour work shift; 40-hour workweek. The ACGIH threshold limit value (TLV) is 25 ppm (100 mg/m^3) (skin) as a TWA for a normal 8-hour workday and a 40-hour workweek.[2]

USES

Cyclohexanone is a commonly used industrial solvent for cellulose acetate natural resins, vinyl resins, rubber, waxes, and fats. It is also used as a solvent sealer for polyvinyl chloride in many medical devices.[2] It has been found as a contaminant of intravenous dextrose and a parenteral feeding solution used in a newborn special care unit, where it was considered to be leached into infusion fluids from administration sets.[3]

TOXICOKINETICS

Metabolism

Cyclohexanone appears to be reduced to cyclohexanol at pH 7.0 by human liver alcohol dehydrogenase,[4] an enzyme demonstrated to be present in human fetal liver from as early as 2 months of gestation.[5] Cyclohexanol is metabolized further by hepatic and microsomal mixed-function oxidase and is excreted in human urine as *trans* 1,2 and *trans* 1,3-cyclohexanediol, the main metabolites, and *trans* 1,4-cyclohexandeliol with cyclohexane (excreted unchanged in small amounts (3.5%). Cyclohexanol disappears from the urine after 24 hours. Excretion of cyclohexanediol may continue for at least 10 days.[6] A 1-kg preterm newborn baby receiving 150 mL of dextrose pumped through an infusion set over 24 hours can receive up to 1 mg of cyclohexanone daily[6] (0.74 to 0.98 mg; 7.5 to 10.0 μmol, mean 9.1 μmol).

Cyclohexanone metabolites have been excreted by premature babies who were fed by the intravenous route.[7] Although cyclohexanone has been associated with central nervous system depression and hepatotoxicity in adults, its toxicity in neonates has not been evaluated. Foreign compounds that compete with bilirubin and drugs for transport proteins and glucuronosyltransferase in liver cells may increase the risk of kernicterus in the neonate or of drug toxicity. Further data is required to determine whether cyclohexanone might compete in this way. Ketamine hydrochloride is an anesthetic agent whose formula is (2-[*o*-chlorophenyl]-2-[methylamino] cyclohexanone hydrochloride.

Neonates

There is little information available on the toxicity of cyclohexanone in neonates. Foreign compounds that compete with bilirubin and drugs for blood transport proteins and with glucuronosyltransferase in liver cells may increase the risk of kernicterus or of drug toxicity. Further data is required to determine the extent of cyclohexanone effects in the liver.

Toxicity

In man exposure to 25 ppm of cyclohexanone vapor for 5 minutes did not cause side effects, but 75 ppm resulted in eye, nose, and throat irritation.[8] A 46-year-old man ingested 50 mL of a plastic catalyst containing methyl ethyl ketone and cyclohexanone peroxides in dimethyl phthalate. He collapsed, became comatose, and exhibited severe erosion of the mucosa of the posterior pharynx, oliguria, hepatotoxicity, and an erosive gastritis preceding death.[9]

A 55-year-old drank approximately 100 mL of a liquid cement for polyvinyl chloride resin containing acetone, methyl ethyl ketone, cyclohexanone, and polyvinyl chloride. He was lavaged, treated with plasma exchanges and hemoperfusions, developed a transient hyperglycemia and hepatotoxicity, and recovered. The largest component of the ingested liquid was cyclohexanone. Cyclohexanol was detected in the urine. The comatose state was considered to be caused mainly by cyclohexanol.[2]

ANALYTIC METHODS

A sensitive method for determining urinary cyclohexanol involves hydrolysis and gas chromatography with flame ionization detection.[10] Cyclohexanediol is assayed by gas chromatography and mass spectrometry.[4]

TREATMENT

Management is symptomatic and supportive.

REFERENCES—CYCLOHEXANONE

1. Cyclohexanone. Occupational Safety and Health Guidelines for Chemical Hazards. Cincinnati, OH: US Dept Health and Human Services. DHHS (NIOSH) Publication No. 89-104, Supplement II-OHG.
2. Sakata M, Kikuchi J, Haga M. Disposition of acetone, methyl ethyl ketone and cyclohexanone in acute poisoning. Clin Toxicol 1989;27:67–77.
3. Mills GA, Walker V. Urinary excretion of cyclohexanediol, a metabolite of solvent cyclohexanone, by infants in a special care unit. Clin Chem 1990;36:870–874.
4. Deetz JS, Luehr CA, Vallee BL. Human liver alcohol dehydrogenase isozymes: reduction of aldehydes and ketones. Biochemistry 1984;23:6822–6828.
5. Stave U. Liver enzymes. In: Stave U, Weech AA, eds. Perinatal physiology. New York: Plenum Medical, 1978; pp. 499–521.
6. Flek J, Sedivec V. Identification and determination of metabolites of cyclohexanone in human urine. Prac Lek 1989; 41:259–263.
7. Flek J, Sedivec V. Identification and determination of metabolites of cyclohexanone in human urine. Prac Lek 1989; 41.259–263.
8. Proctor NH, Hughes JP, Fischman ML. Chemical hazards of the workplace. 2nd ed. New York: Van Nostrand Reinhold, 1989, pp. 171–172.
9. Burger LM, Chandor SB. Fatal ingestion of plastic resin catalyst. Arch Environ Health 1971;23:402–404.
10. Ong CN, Sia GL, Chia SE, Phoon WH, Tan KT. Determination of cyclohexanol in urine and its use in environmental monitoring of cyclohexanone exposure. J Anal Toxicol 1991;15:13–16.

HYDROQUINONE

Hydroquinone ingestion in low doses (300 to 500 mg daily) may be relatively asymptomatic. In higher doses it can induce an acute gastroenteritis-like syndrome. When doses of 5 to 12 g are ingested, death ensues following hemolysis and renal and hepatic failure. Poisonings occur sporadically. Treatment is symptomatic and supportive.

STRUCTURE AND CLASSIFICATION

Synonyms

1,4 dihydroxybenzene; 1,4-benzendiol; alpha hydroquinone; beta-quinol, *p*-benzenediol, *p*-dihydroxybenzene, *p*-dioxobenzene, *p*-dioxybenzene, *p*-hydroquinone, *p*-hydroxyphenol, benzohydroquinone, benzoquinol, hydroquinol, hydroquinole, hydrochinon (Czech, Polish, German), idrochinone (Italian), pyrogentisic acid, quinol, 1-4 dihydroxybenzeen (Dutch), 1,4-dihydroxybenzol (German), 1-4 diidrobenzene (Italian), 4-hydroxyphenol (IARC).[1]

Odor and Warning Properties

Hydroquinone has a sweet taste.

USES

Hydroquinone is a reducing agent. It is used as a photographic developer in black-and-white photography; an antioxidant or stabilizer for certain materials that polymerize in the presence of oxidizing agents; a polymerization inhibitor for vinyl acetate and acrylic monomers; a stabilizer in paints, varnishes, motor fuels, and oils; an intermediate for rubber-processing chemicals; and a source of the productions of its mono- and dialkyl ethers.[1] Many of its derivatives are used as bacteriostatic agents, and others, especially 2,5-bi (ethyleneimino) hydroquinone, may be antimitotic and tumor-inhibiting agents.[2]

DOSES

Tolerable Dose

The daily ingestion of 300 to 500 mg of hydroquinone for 3 to 5 months by 19 volunteers caused no observable alterations in the blood and urine.[3]

Toxic Dose

"Health teas" prepared from the leaves of blueberry, red whortleberry, cranberry, or bearberry may contain hydroquinone in excess of 1% capable of causing irritation of the gastrointestinal mucosa and inducing systemic poisoning.[4] A 36-year-old man ingested 12 g of hydroquinone, developed cyanosis, and survived.[5]

Fatal Dose

Two other patients ingested 5 gm and 6 gm, respectively, of hydroquinone, developed cyanosis and icterus, and died.[5]

OCCUPATIONAL EXPOSURE

A partial list of occupations in which exposure may occur include:[2]

Antioxidant makers
Bacteriostatic-agent makers
Drug makers
Fur processors
Motor-fuel blenders
Organic-chemical synthesizers
Paint makers
Photographic-developer makers
Plastic-stabilizer workers
Stone-coating workers
Styrene-monomer workers

ENVIRONMENTAL EXPOSURE

Hydroquinone exists in a free state in pear leaves. Arbutin, a glucoside of hydroquinone, occurs widely in the leaves, bark, buds, and fruit of many plants, especially the Ericaceae.[1] Hydroquinone has been detected in cigarette smoke, and in the effluents from photoprocessing, coal-tar production, and the paper industry. The half-life of hydroquinone in the daylight environment is estimated from less than 5 weeks in June to over 240 weeks in January.[1]

TOXICOKINETICS

Elimination

Hydroquinone is readily absorbed from the gastrointestinal tract and is excreted in the urine as sulfate and glucuronide conjugates.[1,6]

Pregnancy/Lactation

No studies have been made to assess the teratogenic potential of hydroquinone.

MECHANISM OF ACTION

Oral Ingestion

In the few fatal cases described, death appeared to follow a massive hemolysis with renal and hepatic failure.[5]

Eye

In aqueous solutions, as in tears, hydroquinone is oxidized by air, especially rapidly in alkaline solutions in the presence of light, to form a brown color partly due to conversion to 1,4-benzoquinone.[7] Hydroquinone is known to be converted by human myeloperoxidase to 1,4-benzoquinone, a toxic compound.[8]

CLINICAL PRESENTATION

Oral

In July 1977 544 crewmen aboard a large U.S. Navy vessel developed an illness characterized by acute nausea, vomiting, abdominal cramps, and diarrhea all of which resolved within 12 to 36 hours. The white blood cell count was elevated. Drinking water had been contaminated with photographic developer.[9] Fatal cases have been reported after ingestion of between 5 to 12 g of hydroquinone.[5] These doses induced tinnitus, dyspnea, cyanosis, extreme somnolence, a dark color to the urine, icterus of the sclerae, and bile-stained urine. Two deaths were presumed to be due to extension hemolysis and renal and hepatic failure.[10]

Eye

Direct acute contamination of the eye with particles of hydroquinone (10 to 30 mg of vapor or dust of hydroquinone per cubic meter of air)[11,12] can cause immediate eye irritation; chronic, low-grade, and long-time exposure may result in ulcerations of the cornea with dark brown discoloration and distortion and opacification of the cornea.[7] The eye changes appear irreversible.

Skin

Skin-lightening preparations containing hydroquinone used by individuals with dark skin may produce severe and irreversible cutaneous damage.[13,14] The effects begin with a darkening and coarsening of the skin, followed by a hyperpigmented papular change, an exogenous ochronosis.[15]

LABORATORY

Analytic Methods

Liquid chromatographic analysis has been used to quantitate serum hydroquinone levels.[9] High-performance liquid chromatography can also be used for the detection (at 280 nm) of hydroquinone in water samples.[1]

Blood Levels

Acutely ill patients with gastrointestinal symptoms following hydroquinone ingestion had serum levels over 0.1 μg/mL.[9]

Abnormalities

Ingestion of 12 g of hydroquinone led to a black-colored urine that tested positive for phenol.[5]

Ancillary Tests

Hypoglycemia, hypercholesterolemia, leukocytosis, hemoglobinemia, and granular and hyaline casts in the urine have been observed after large oral ingestions (5 to 12 g).[5]

TREATMENT

Oral

The treatment of oral ingestions is symptomatic and supportive. Induction of emesis and gastric lavage have been employed.[16] On admission to the emergency department the patient should have access to a source of oxygen, to cardiac monitoring, and to an intravenous line. Blood should be drawn for a complete blood count, serum aminotransferases, alkaline phosphatase, bilirubin (total and indirect), glucose, creatinine, and blood urea nitrogen. Arterial blood gases and serum electrolytes should be obtained periodically.

Eye

Treatment of eye contamination consists of immediately flushing with water for 15 minutes; an ophthalmologic consultation should be obtained.[16]

Skin

Since contact with the skin may cause a dermatitis, the skin should be washed with soap and water.[16]

Antidotes

There are no antidotes.

Prevention

Contact with the eyes or inhalation of its dust or vapors must be avoided. Dust particles of hydroquinone may remain in the tears for a long period and in dissolving produce localized areas of high concentration.[4]

REFERENCES—HYDROQUINONE

1. Devillers J, Boule P, Vasseur P, Prevot P, Steinman R, Seigle-Murandi F et al. Environmental and health risks of hydroquinone. Ecotoxicol Environ Safety 1990;19:327–354.
2. Key MM, Henschel AF, Butler J, Ligo RN, Tabershaw IR, eds. Occupational diseases. A guide to their recognition. Revised edition. DHEW (NIOSH). Publication No. 77-181. Washington, DC: US Government Printing Office, 1977; pp. 249–250.
3. Carlson AJ, Brewer NR. Toxicity studies on hydroquinone. Proc Soc Exp Biol 1953;84:684–688.
4. Deichmann WB, Keplinger ML. Phenols and phenolic compounds. In: Patty FA, ed. Industrial hygiene and toxicology. 2nd revised ed. Vol II. New York: Interscience, pp. 1380–1383.
5. Zeidman I, Deutl R. Poisoning by hydroquinone and monomethyl-paraminophenol sulfate. Report of 2 cases with autopsy findings. Am J Med Sci 1945;210:328–333.
6. Harbison KG, Belly RT. The biodegradation of hydroquinone. Environ Toxicol Chem 1982;1:9–15.
7. Grant WM. Hydroquinone in toxicology of the eye. 2nd ed. Springfield, IL: Charles C Thomas, 1974; pp. 564–567.
8. Subrahmanyam UV, Kolachana P, Smith MT. Metabolism of hydroquinone by human myeloperoxidase: mechanisms of stimulation by other phenolic compounds. Arch Biochem Biophys 1991;286:76–84.
9. CDC. Hydroquinone poisoning aboard a navy ship. MMWR July 14, 1978; pp. 237–243.
10. Occupational Safety and Health Standards. Support Z-Toxic and Hazardous Substances. Code of Federal Regulations. Title 29, Section 1910.1000 air contaminants.
11. Anderson B. Corneal and conjunctival pigmentation among workers engaged in manufacture of hydroquinone. Arch Ophthalmol 1947;38:812–826.
12. Anderson B, Oglesby F. Corneal changes from quinone-hydroquinone exposure. Arch Ophthalmol 1958;59:495–501.
13. Scarpa A, Guerci A. Depigmenting procedures and drugs employed by melanoderm populations. J Ethnopharmacol 1987;19:17–66.
14. Schulz EJ, Summers B, Summers RS. Inappropriate treatment of cosmetic ochronosis with hydroquinone. S Afr Med J 1988;73:59–60.
15. Williams H. Skin lightening creams containing hydroquinone. The case for a temporary ban. Br Med J 1992;305:963.
16. Anonymous. Hydroquinone. Dangerous Properties of Industrial Materials. Report No. 3518820 000 8. 1988; pp. 51–60.

Chapter 66 Respiratory Toxicology

TOXICOLOGY OF THE LUNG

Metabolism

The major metabolic pathways can be divided into the phase I enzymes (cytochrome P-450 isoenzymes, flavin monoxygenases, prostaglandin synthetase, and epoxide hydrolase) and the phase II enzymes (glutathione-S-transferase, sulfotransferase, and glucuronyl transferase). Unlike the liver where damage is monitored by serum enzyme levels, the lung has no specific indicator of damage.[1]

Target Organ

The lung is a vulnerable target for chemicals due to the high exposure to air (approximately 10,000 L/day), the high blood cardiac output (about 7,000 L/day), and a large surface area.[2]

RESPIRATORY CELL TYPES (TABLE 66–1)

The five major cell populations of the lung include the type I and type II alveolar epithelial cells, capillary endothelial cells, alveolar macrophages, and interstitial cells (Table 66–1). These cells form the basic structures underlying gas exchange in the lung. The two other cell types (Clara cells and neuroendocrine cells) are of interest to the toxicologist because they appear to play important roles in xenobiotic metabolism and carcinogenesis.[3]

Alveolar Type I Epithelial Cells (Fig. 66–1)

These cells comprise 8% of the parenchymal cell population and cover over 90% of the alveolar surface. Possibly because of their relative lack of cytoplasmic organelles and the long distance between their cytoplasmic processes and cell nucleus, they are vulnerable to inhaled and bloodborne toxic agents. Type I cells expose the largest percentage of their epithelial surface to toxic agents. Type II cells may differentiate in vitro to type I cells.[4]

Alveolar Type II Epithelial Cells (Fig. 66–1)

The type II cell produces surfactant and may replace damaged type I cells. They cover 7% of the alveolar surface, but represent 16% of the total cell population.

Table 66–1
Some Specific Lung Cell Types and Their Function

Cell Types	Location and Function
Epithelium	
Clara cells	High metabolic activity; secretory; nonciliated; function not well-defined; may serve as precursor of goblet and ciliated cells
Ciliated cells	Most common epithelial cells in airways; may secrete mucus-like substances; controls perciliary fluid
Type II alveolar cells	Covers 3% of alveolar surface; secrete surfactant; replace injured Type 1 cells; high metabolic activity
Type I alveolar	Large and covers considerable surface area per cell; covers ≥95% of alveolar surface; forms the alveolar epithelium and facilitates gas exchange; low metabolic activity; incapable of self-reproduction
Mucus	Mucus-secreting
Serous	Mucus-secreting; perciliary fluid; stem cell
Brush cells	Chemoreceptor cells; preciliated
Globule leukocyte	Immunoglobulin transportation; releases inflammatory mediators
Endocrine	Secreto- and vaso-regulatory
Submucosal	
Goblet (mucus) cells	Epithelial linings; common in trachea and bronchioles; contribute to mucus production
Serous cells	Mucus-secreting; perciliary fluid; stem cell/proliferative
Endocrine cells	Secretes amines and neuropeptides
Lymphocytes	Immunoresponsive
Myoepithelial	Expulsion of mucus
Bronchoalveolar mast cells	Migratory cells located throughout respiratory tract; release mediators of bronchoconstriction when antigens bind to IgE antibodies on surface
Macrophage	Phagocytic; secrete mediators of inflammatory reactions; modulate lymphocytes and otherwise participate in immune response
Endothelial cells	Forty percent of lung parenchyma cells; metabolize blood-borne substances; proliferative
Fibroblasts (interstitial)	Predominant in alveolar wall and constitutes the basement membrane; become activated during disease states and produce elastin and collagen; proliferation leads to fibrosis, modulation of growth, bronchial tone, and mucosal secretion

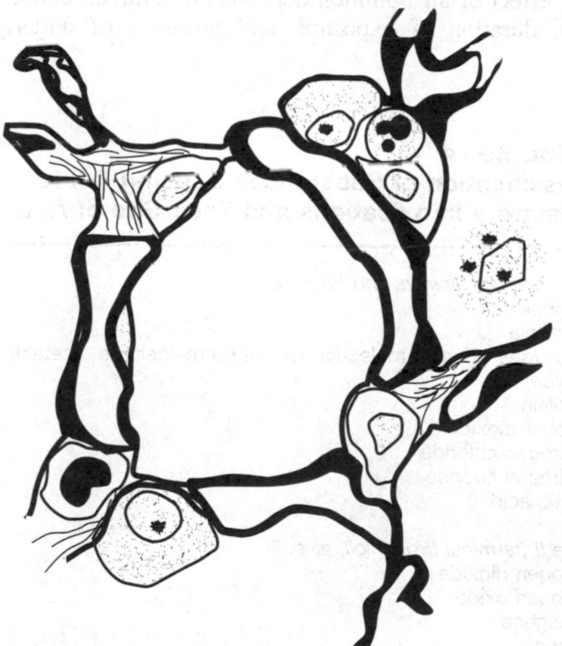

Figure 66–1 The pulmonary alveolar region. (Adapted from Finkelstein JN. Toxicology 1990;60:41–52 with permission.)

Interstitial Cells

Fibroblasts, lymphocytes, interstitial macrophages, mast cells, pericytes, and plasma cells constitute the lung cells that occupy the interstitial space and represent approximately 37% of all lung cells. When pulmonary epithelial cells react to toxic chemicals, there may be a subsequent increase in fibroblast number and an increase in collagen production, resulting in an interstitial pulmonary fibrosis. This may follow toxic lung damage induced by airborne substances, including oxidant gases, dusts, and fibers (silica, asbestos) or following bloodborne agents such as antineoplastic drugs.

Capillary Endothelial Cells

Capillary endothelial cells are the largest single cell population in the lung, comprising 30% of all human lung cells. They form the first line of defense against bloodborne toxic agents.

Alveolar Macrophages

Alveolar macrophages join in the defense against hostile pathogenic organisms. When they are compromised by toxic inhalants, they may increase susceptibility to infectious diseases. They are also involved in the development and pathogenesis of chronic lung disease such as silicosis and asbestosis.[5] They may work in collaboration with polymorphonuclear leucocytes.[6]

Clara Cells (Nonciliated Bronchiolar Cells)

Clara cells have a substantial agranular cytoplasmic reticulum. They function as the primary secretory cell type in the conducting airway of the centriacinar region (terminal bronchioles). The Clara cell replicates itself, or it may develop into a ciliated cell. It is the primary site of cytochrome P-450 monooxygenase activity within the lungs. Naphthalene, 4-ipomeanol, 3-methylfuran, methylindole, carbon tetrachloride, and trichloroethylene induce toxicity to the Clara cells following metabolic activation by the cytochrome P-450 monooxygenase system.[5]

Neuroendocrine Cells

Neuroendocrine cells are also known as APUD cells (aminoprecursor uptake and decarboxylase) or Kulchitsky cells. They are found in the mucosa lining the airways or in the pulmonary parenchyma.[7] These cells proliferate when exposed to hyperoxia.

Injury to the pulmonary epithelial cells by various toxic agents is summarized in Table 66–2.

Table 66-2
Injury to the Pulmonary Endothelial Cells[a]

	Primary Target
Inhalants	
Hyperoxia	Endothelium
Ozone	Endothelium
Nitrogen dioxide	Endothelium, type I epithelium
Chemotherapeutic agents	
Bleomycin	Type I and II epithelium
Doxorubicin	Type I and II epithelium
Nitrofurantoin	Type I and II epithelium
Amiodarone	Endothelium
Other drugs	
Beta-naphthylthiourea	Endothelium
Monocrotaline	Endothelium
Herbicides	
Paraquat	Type I and II epithelium
X-irradiation	Endothelium
Endotoxemia	Endothelium

[a]Adapted from Smith LL et al. Arch Toxicol 1986;58:214–218.

Table 66-3
A Preponderance of Certain Cells in Bronchoalveolar Fluid May be a Helpful Diagnostic Pointer [a]

Cell	Disorder
T4 helper	Sarcoidosis
	Beryllium disease
T8 suppressor	Extrinsic allergic alveolitis (Hypersensitivity pneumonitis)
	Talc
Neutrophil	Smoker
	Fibrosing alveolitis
	AIDS
	Mineral dust
	Collagen disease
Eosinophil	Drugs
	Eosinophilic pneumonia
	Bronchial asthma
Mast cell	Sarcoidosis
	Asthma
Multinucleate giant	Cobalt
Plasma	Multiple myelomatosis
Reed–Sternberg	Hodgkin's
Anaplastic	Lymphangitic carcinoma
OKT6 staining	Langerhans' histiocytosis

[a]Adapted from James DG. Postgrad Med J 1992;68:160–173.

Acute Inhalation Intoxication

Brochoalveolar lavage (Table 66–3) permits a wider perspective for the understanding of respiratory and multisystem disorders (e.g., asbestosis, cobalt lung, AIDS, pulmonary alveolar proteinosis, and other diseases).[8]

A classification of substances causing acute inhalatory intoxication with their sites of action is found in Table 66–4.[9] A schema for therapeutic consideration of three types of acute inhalatory intoxication is found in Table 66–5.[9]

AIR POLLUTION

A number of risk factors that predispose to the development of drug-induced pulmonary disease are found in Table 66–6. Drugs causing noncardiogenic pulmonary edema, hypersensitivity lung disease, and pneumonitis/fibrosis are found in Tables 66–7, 66–8, and 66–9, respectively.[10]

Typical indoor air pollution sources in the home, office, and transportation environment are summarized in Table 66–10. Concentrations of indoor air pollutants are depicted in Table 66–11.

HUMAN HEALTH EFFECTS

The effect of air pollution depends on pollutant concentration, duration of exposure, and presence of underlying

Table 66-4
Classification of Substances Causing Acute Inhalatory Intoxications and Their Site of Action[a,b]

Type I (upper airways and bronchi)
Chlorine
Ammonia
Aldehydes of lower molecular weight (formaldehyde, acetaldehyde)
Acrolein
Sulphur dioxide
Hydrogen chloride
Hydrogen fluoride
Acetic acid
Type II (terminal bronchioli, alveoli)
Nitrogen dioxide
Nitrogen oxide
Phosgene
Ozone
Type III absorption (without or with only slight pulmonary involvement)
Toluene
Xylene
Carbon dioxide
Carbon monoxide
Hydrogen cyanide
Propane
Carbon tetrachloride

[a]Adapted from Sangster B, Meulenbett J. Netherlands J Med 1988;33:91–100.
[b]This list is not a complete review, but it gives some examples of the substances belonging to one of the three types of acute inhalatory intoxication.

Table 66–5
A Schema for Therapeutic Consideration of Three Types of Acute Inhalatory Intoxication[a]

Inhalatory → Symptoms intoxication	*Type I* (bronchi)	*Type II* (alveoli, terminal bronchiol)	*Type III* (absorption)
	conjunctival irritation nasal discharge hemoptysis retrosternal pain laryngeal edema (stridor) bronchospasms	dyspnea cyanosis (bronchospasms)	no pulmonary damage
↓ No symptoms	↓ *Diagnostic procedures* blood gas analysis chest-X-ray	↓ *Diagnostic procedures* blood gas analysis chest x-ray	↓ frequently CNS involvement, infrequently other organs
→Type I → no observation needed	↓ *Therapy* bronchodilators[b] oxygen mechanical ventilation tracheostomy corticosteroid?[c]	↓ *Therapy* oxygen mechanical ventilation in an early stage bronchodilators[b] corticosteroid?[c]	↓ *Therapy* depends on which organ and which substance is involved
→Type II → observation 24 h →Type III → observation occasionally necessary			

[a]Adapted from Sangster B, Meulenblatt J. Netherlands J Med 1988;33:91–100.
[b]Bronchodilators (xanthine derivatives i.v., beta-1-adrenergic medications s.c.)
[c]The role of corticosteroids is doubtful. No double-blind, well-evaluated study is known to have been carried out on the effectivity of corticosteroids in inhalation toxicology.

Table 66–6
Risk Factors Predisposing to Development of Drug-Induced Pulmonary Disease[a]

Risk Factor	Drug(s) Implicated[b]
Cumulative dose	Bleomycin, carmustine (BCNU), amiodarone?
Unit dose	Amiodarone, heroin, propoxyphene methadone, ethchlorvynol, chlordiazepoxide, haloperidol colchicine, imipramine
Route of administration	Bleomycin
Frequency of administration	Methotrexate
Oxygen therapy	Bleomycin, mitomycin?, cyclophosphamide?, nitrofurantoin?
Radiotherapy	Bleomycin, busulfan?, mitomycin?
Other drug therapy	Bleomycin, camustine (BCNU), cyclophosphamide, mitomycin, methotrexate, vinca alkaloids
Age	Bleomycin
Previous pulmonary disease	Carmustine (BCNU), amiodarone
Blood component transfusions	Mitomycin, amphotericin
Renal failure	Bleomycin
Steroid tapering or adrenalectomy	Methotrexate
Pulmonary angiography	Amiodarone?

[a]Adapted from Cooper JA Jr, Matthay RA. Dis Mon 1987;33:61–120.
[b]? Indicates information is suggestive but not conclusive.

cardiopulmonary disease. Both acute symptoms and aggravation of chronic disease may result from exposure, but the complex variables involved in large epidemiologic studies make the detection of injury and the establishment of limits on exposure (threshold limit values) difficult. Ambient air quality standards have been proposed by 21 nations for

Table 66–7
Drugs That Cause Noncardiogenic Pulmonary Edema[a]

Cancer Chemotherapeutic Drugs	Other Drugs
Mitomycin	Amphotericin
Cyclophosphamide	Heroin
Methotrexate	Propoxyphene
Cytosine arabinoside	Methadone
VM-26	Ethchlorvynol
	Chlordiazepoxide
	Haloperidol
	Lidocaine
	Terbutaline
	Ritodrine
	Isoxsuprine
	Imipramine
	Colchicine

[a]Adapted from Cooper JA Jr, Matthay RA. Dis Mon 1987;32:61–120.

carbon monoxide, sulfur dioxide, nitrogen dioxide, and particulate matter (Table 66–12) and for ozone, fluorides, and asbestos (Table 66–13).

OZONE LAYER (SEE FLUOROCARBONS—THIS CHAPTER)

Background

In September 1987 24 nations signed the "Montreal Protocol on Substances that Deplete the Ozone Layer" (Montreal Protocol) (Table 66–14). The intent of the protocol was to control all substances that deplete the ozone layer.[12] A reduction schedule was set out:

1. A freeze in consumption at 1986 levels for Group I compounds:
   CFCs—Chlorofluorocarbons—starting on July 1, 1989:
   CFC 11—Trichlorofluoromethane (CCl_3F)
   CFC 12—Dichlorodifluoromethane (CCl_2F_2)
   CFC 113—Trichlorotrifluoroethane ($C_2Cl_3F_3$)
   CFC 114—Dichlorotetrafluoroethane ($C_2Cl_2F_4$)
   CFC 115—Chloropentafluoroethane (C_2ClF_5)
   Group II compounds:
   Halons (used in fire extinguishing equipment)—starting January 1, 1992:
   Halon 1211 Bromochlorodifluoromethane ($CBrClF_2$)
   Halon 1301 Bromotrifluoromethane ($CBrF_3$)
   Halon 2402 Dibromotetrafluoroethane ($C_2Br_2F_4$)
2. A reduction in consumption of CFCs:
   20% starting July 1, 1993
   50% starting July 1, 1998

As of January 1, 1990, about 50 nations had ratified the protocol. Since the signing of the Montreal Protocol studies have indicated that the scientific bases for the protocol understated the increasing levels of stratospheric bromine and chlorine.[13] In June 1990 phase 2 of the Montreal Protocol was agreed to in London,[14] committing signatory nations to a phase-out of CFCs, halons, and carbon tetrachloride by the year 2000 (Table 66–14). However, the phase-out date for methylchloroform has been put back to 2005; there is a 10-year derogation for nonindustrialized nations, and other ozone depleting chemicals are not included in the protocol. It is estimated that chlorine levels (normally 0.6 ppb) will not fall back to 1991 levels until the year 2050.

Chemical substitutes such as hydrochlorfluorocarbons (HCFCs) and hydrofluorocarbons (HFCs) have been proposed as a temporary solution by the chemical industry. These include the following[15]:

HCFC 123	CCl_2HCF_3
HCFC 141b	CCl_2FCH_3
HCFC 142b	$CClF_2CH_3$
HCFC 22	$CClF_2H$
HCFC 124	$CClFHCF_3$
HFC 134a	CF_3CFH_2
HFC 152a	CF_2HCH_3
HFC 125	CF_3CF_2H

These chemicals are more ozone friendly, but still have some ozone depleting potential. Additionally, evidence of an area of ozone loss in the Antarctic[16] and possibly the Arctic polar area,[17] together with the continued injection of some 75 tons of chlorine into the stratosphere from each rocket shuttle flight,[18] continue to exert pressure for more immediate ozone-saving measures.

Although the three main volatile anesthetic agents in present use, halothane ($CF_3CHBrCl$), enflurane (CHF_2-0-CF_2CHFCl), and isoflurane (CHF_2-0-$CHClCF_3$), resemble

Table 66–8
Drugs That Cause Hypersensitivity Lung Disease[a]

Bleomycin	Para-aminosalicylic acid
Methotrexate	Penicillin
Procarbazine	Cromolyn
Azathioprine	Dantrolene
Mercaptopurine	Methylphenidate
Sulfasalazine	Mephenesin carbamate
Nitrofurantoin	Hydralazine
Diphenylhydantoin	Mecamylamine
Carbamazepine	Ampicillin
Chlorpropamide	Febarbamate
Imipramine	Salazopyrin
Isoniazid	Naproxen
Sulfadimethoxine	

[a]Adapted from Cooper JA Jr, Matthay RA. Dis Mon 1987;32:61–120.

Table 66–9
Drugs That Cause Pneumonitis/Fibrosis[a]

Cancer Chemotherapeutic Agents	Other Drugs
Bleomycin	Nitrofurantoin
Mitomycin	Sulfasalazine
Neocarzinostatin	Amiodarone
Busulfan	Tocainide
Cyclophosphamide	Gold salts
Chlorambucil	Penicillamine
Melphalan	
Carmustine (BCNU)	
Semustine (methyl CCNU)	
Lomustine (CCNU)	
Chlorozotocin	
Methotrexate	

[a]Adapted from Cooper JA Jr, Matthay RA. Dis Mon 1987;32:61–120.

Table 66–10
Typical Sources of Indoor Air Pollution in the Home, Office, and Transportation Environment[a]

Environment	Source and Pollutants
Home	Tobacco smoking: respirable particles, CO, VOC[b]
	Gas stoves: NO_2, CO
	Woodstoves and fireplaces: respirable particles, CO, PAH[c]
	Building materials: formaldehyde, radon
	Earth underlying the home: radon
	Furnishings and household products: VOC, formaldehyde
	Gas-fueled space heaters: NO_2, CO
	Kerosene-fueled space heaters: NO_2, CO, SO_2
	Insulation: asbestos
	Moist materials and surfaces: biological agents
Office	Tobacco smoking: respirable particles, CO, VOC
	Building materials: VOC, formaldehyde
	Furnishings: VOC, formaldehyde
	Copying machines: VOC
	Air conditioning systems: biological agents, vehicle exhaust with combustion emissions containing particles, CO, and NO_2
Transportation	Tobacco smoking: respirable particles, CO, VOC
	Ambient air: ozone in jet aircraft, CO and lead in automobiles
	Auto air conditioners: biological agents

[a]Adapted from Samet JM, Marbury MC, Spengler JD. Am Rev Respir Dis 1987;136:1486–1508.
[b]Volatile organic compounds.
[c]Polycyclic aromatic hydrocarbons.

Table 66–11
The Principal Indoor Pollutants, Their Sources and Typical Concentrations[a]

Pollutant	Typical Sources	Pollutant Concentrations	Relevant Standards	Comments
Respirable particles	Tobacco smoke, unvented kerosene heaters, wood and coal stoves, fireplaces, outside air, attached facilities, occupant activities	>500 μg/m³ bars, meetings, waiting rooms with smoking 100 to 500 μg/m³ typical for smoking sections of planes 10 to 100 μg/m³ typical of homes 1,000 μg/m³ with burning food or fireplaces	265 μg/m³ EPA 24-h standard ambient air 75 μg/m³ EPA annual standard ambient air 150 μg/m³ Japanese indoor standard	Current EPA standards are for total and not only respirable suspended particles
NO, NO_2	Gas ranges and pilot lights, unvented kerosene and gas space heaters, gasoline engines, some gas floor furnaces, outside air	25 to 75 ppb typical range for homes with gas stoves 100 to 500 ppb peak values kitchens with gas stoves or kerosene gas heaters	160 ppb 1-h maximum, WHO guideline 50 ppb annual average EPA ambient standard	No current EPA short-term standard
CO	Gas ranges and pilot lights, unvented kerosene and gas space heaters, tobacco smoke, back drafting of water heater or furnace or woodstove, gasoline engines, camping lanterns and stoves Attached garages, street level intake vents, hockey rinks	>50 ppm when oven used for heating >50 ppm attached garages, air intakes, arenas 2 to 15 ppm cooking with gas stove 2 to 10 ppm heavy smoking in homes, bars, and other locations	35 ppm EPA 1-h standard 9 ppm EPA 8-h standard	
CO_2	People, unvented kerosene and gas space heaters, tobacco smoke, outside air	320 to 400 ppm outdoor air 2,000 to 5,000 ppm crowded indoor environment, inadequate ventilation	1,000 ppm Japanese indoor air standard	CO_2 concentrations below 1,000 ppm usually indicate adequate fresh air supply for buildings
Infectious, allergenic, irritating biological materials	Dust mites and cockroaches, animal dander, bacteria, fungi, viruses, pollens	Few systematic measurements of spores, bacteria, and viruses indoors Homes with mold problem, offices with water damage: >1,000 cfu/m³[b] Homes and offices without obvious problem: 500 ± 200 cfu/m³[b]	None	Interpretations of a level depend on the specific agent; cfu/m is only an indicator
Formaldehyde	Urea formaldehyde foam insulation (UFFI), glues, fiberboard, pressed board, plywood, particle board; carpet backing and fabrics	0.1 to 0.8 ppm homes with UFFI 0.5 ppm average in mobile homes >1 ppm in a few homes and mobile homes	0.2 to 0.5 ppm adopted by several states 0.1 ppm Sweden, new homes 0.7 ppm Sweden, maximum in old buildings 3 ppm U.S. OSHA 8-h time-weighted average	Formaldehyde concentrations in homes with UFFI decline by 50% every 2 to 3 yr.
Radon and radon daughters	Ground beneath a home, domestic water, and some utility natural gas	1.5 pCi/l estimated average in U.S. homes >8 pCi/l in 3% to 5% homes	8 pCi/l NCRP action level 4 pCi/l EPA limit for uranium processing site homes 2 pCi/l ASHRAE guidelines 5 pCi/l Sweden, maximum, existing buildings 3 pCi/l Sweden, maximum, new buildings	Radon or radon daughters can be measured. Standards are for radon. Lung cancer risk results from radon daughters.

[a]Adapted from Samet JM, Marbury MC, Spengler JD. Am Rev Respir Dis 1987;136:1486–1508.
[b]cfu/m³ = colony-forming units/m³.

(continued)

Table 66–11 *(Continued)*

Pollutant	Typical Sources	Pollutant Concentrations	Relevant Standards	Comments
Volatile organic compounds: benzene, styrene, tetrachloroethylene; dichlorobenzene; methylene chloride; chloroform	Outgassing from water, plasticizers, solvents, paints, cleaning compounds, mothballs, resins, glues, gasoline, oils, combustion, art materials, photocopiers, personal care products	Typical indoor concentrations of selected compounds: benzene—15 μg/m³; 1,1,1 trichloroethylene—20 μg/m³; chloroform—2 μg/m³; tetrachloroethylene—5 μm/m³; styrene—2 μg/m³; m,p-dichlorobenzene—4 μg/m³; m,p-xylene—15 μg/m³	No indoor standards for nonoccupational settings	EPA Carcinogenic Assessment Group potency factors available for many of the volatile organics
Semivolatile organics: chlorinated hydrocarbons, DDT, heptachlor, chlordane	Pesticides, transformer fluids, termicides, combustion of wood, tobacco, kerosene, and charcoal; wood preservatives, fungicides	Only limited data available	No indoor standards	
Semivolatile organics: polycyclic compounds, benzo(a)pyrene, polychlorinated biphenols	Herbicides, insecticides			
Asbestos	Insulation on building structural components; asbestos plaster around pipes and furnaces; tiles	No systematic measurements to determine typical fiber concentrations. >1,000 ng/m³ when friable asbestos	2 fibers/cc OSHA 8-h time-weighted average	EPA and state attention has been on schools and office buildings. Domestic problems not evaluated.

hydrochlorofluorocarbons, they appear to offer a minimal threat to the ozone layer.[19]

INDOOR AIR POLLUTANTS—SICK BUILDING SYNDROME

Problems associated with indoor air quality have been reported in newly constructed or remodeled buildings.[20] These are sealed and energy-efficient buildings with no opening windows, and outside air is provided only through a recirculated air-conditioning system. These buildings are known as "sick buildings." Perhaps 800,000 to 1,200,000 commercial buildings with 30 to 70 million occupants in the United States have problems that are manifested as the sick building syndrome.[21,22]

Clinical Presentation

"Sick Building Syndrome" (SBS) refers to symptoms frequently reported by those who work in these buildings and includes nasal, eye, and mucous membrane irritation; lethargy; dry skin; headaches; nausea; and sensitivity to odors.[21–23] No objective findings are diagnostic of SBS in symptomatic individuals.[24]

An outbreak of SBS is considered to be an excessive reporting of one or more such symptoms (work-related) by the occupants. Work-related refers to the occurrence of symptoms after coming to work, worsening of symptoms during work, and disappearance of symptoms after leaving work and especially on weekends and during holidays. In addition, there should be no evidence for a preexisting medical condition or exposure to occupational toxic materials.

Synonyms

Other terms for the Sick Building Syndrome (SBS) have included tight building syndrome, closed building problem, new building syndrome, indoor air pollution, and building-associated illness.[20]

No specific etiology has been discovered for SBS, although there have been associations studied with building ventilation systems and with a wide variety of indoor air pollutants,[23] including appliances, office equipment and supplies, animal and plant air allergens, bacteria, and fungi.[25] A number of other variants of clinical disease may be building related (Table 66–15).

A detailed protocol for the comprehensive evaluation of building-associated illness has been prepared.[24]

Management

Approaches to diminish the incidence of SBS include a complete history and physical examination, temporary

Table 66-12
Ambient Air Quality Standards Currently Applied in Twenty-One Nations for Carbon Monoxide, Sulfur Dioxide, Nitrogen Dioxide and Particulate Matter. All AAQS Values in μg/m³*

☐ **No receptor standards for some time scales** ⊟ **No receptor standards (emission standards may apply)**

	Substance											
	Carbon Monoxide CO			Sulphur Dioxide SO_2			Nitrogen Dioxide NO_2			Particulate Matter PM		
Country	Long Term	Medium Term	Short Term	Long Term	Medium Term	Short Term	Long Term	Medium Term	Short Term	Long Term	Medium Term	Short Term
WHO (1987)		10000^{e}	30000^{g} 60000^{h} 100000^{i}			350^{g} 500^{j}		150^{d}	400^{g}			
Australia												
Victoria (1981)		11400^{e}	34300^{g}		155^{d}	445^{g}		120^{d}	300^{g}	90^{a}		
Tasmania (1974)		12500^{e}	37500^{g}	50^{a}	160^{d}	450^{g}		120^{d}	310^{g}	90^{a}		
Austria (1987)		10000^{d}	40000^{g}		200^{d}	200^{h}			200^{h}		200^{d}	
Canada (1989)		6000^{e}	15000^{g}	30^{a}	150^{d}	450^{g}	60^{a}	200^{d}	400^{g}	60^{a}	120^{d}	
Finland (1982)		10000^{e}	30000^{g}	40^{a}	200^{d}	500^{g}		150^{d}	300^{g}	60^{a}	150^{d}	
Germany (1986)	10000^{a}		30000^{h}_{δ}	140^{a}		400^{h}_{δ}	80^{a}		200^{h}_{δ}	150^{a}		300^{h}_{δ}
Greece (1992)	—	—	—	—	—	—			200^{g}_{δ}	—	—	—
Hungary (1990)	2000^{a}	5000^{d}	10000^{h}	70^{a}	150^{d}	500^{h}	70^{a}	85^{d}	100^{h}	50^{a}	100^{d}	200^{h}
Israel (1992)		11000^{e}	60000^{h}	60^{a}	280^{d}	500^{h}		560^{d}	940^{h}	75^{a}	200^{d}	300^{g}
Italy (1989)	—	—	—	40^{a}	100^{d}		50^{g}_{ζ}		200^{g}_{δ}	40^{a}	100^{d}	
Japan (1990)		11400^{d} 22800^{e}			107^{d}	267^{g}		80^{d}			100^{d}	200^{g}
Kuwait (1989)		9100^{d} 11400^{e}	40000^{g}	80^{a}	160^{d}	453^{g}		100^{d}		90^{a}	350^{d}	
Mexico (1984)		14950^{e}			341^{d}				395^{g}		275^{d}	
Netherlands (1986)		6000^{g}_{δ}	40000^{g}_{α}		500^{d}	830^{g}			175^{g}		150^{d}	
New Zealand (1986)		10000^{e}	40000^{g}	50^{b}	125^{d}			100^{d}	200^{g}	60^{k}		
Poland (1990)	120^{a}	1000^{d}	5000^{h}	32^{a}	300^{d}	600^{h}	50^{a}	150^{d}	500^{h}	50^{a}	120^{d}	
Saudi Arabia (1991)		10000^{e}	40000^{g}	80^{a}	365^{d}	730^{g}	100^{a}		660^{g}	80^{a}	340^{d}	
South Africa (1965)	—	—	—	80^{a}	265^{d}	780^{g}	270^{a}	540^{d}	1080^{g}		150^{d}	350^{g}
Soviet Union			20000	—	—	—	85			4		
Switzerland (1985)		8000^{d}		30^{a}	100^{d}	100^{h}_{ϵ}	30^{a}	80^{d}	100^{h}_{ϵ}	70^{a}	150^{d}_{ϵ}	
Taiwan (1975)		11400^{d}	22900^{g}	133^{a}	267^{d}			100^{d}		240^{a} 210^{c}		
United States (1990)		10000^{e}	40000^{g}	80^{a}	365^{d}	1300^{f}	100^{a}			50^{a}	150^{d}	

*Adapted from Cochran LS et al. J Air Waste Manage Assoc 1992;42:1567–1572.
Remarks: *a:* annual mean; *b:* 3-month mean; *c:* 1-month mean; *d:* 24-hour mean; *e:* 8-hour mean; *f:* 3-hour mean; *g:* 1-hour mean; *h:* 30-minute mean; *i:* 15-minute mean; *j:* 10-minute mean; and *k:* 7-day mean.
α: 99.99 percentile; β: 99.5 percentile; γ: 99 percentile; δ: 98 percentile; ε: 95 percentile; and ζ: 50 percentile.

removal of an individual from the workplace, correction of building problems (switching to 100% outside air for a period of time), delaying occupancy of a new building for several weeks while ventilation is maintained at 100% outside air, repair of roof leaks, checking water contamination of central heating, ventilating, and air-conditioning systems (HVAC), use and frequent replacement of HVAC filters, recognition of an SBS outbreak, and banning of cigarette smoking.[26]

Psychosocial Factors—Mass Psychogenic Illness

The rapid spread of symptoms whose basis lies in psychosocial factors is not uncommon in the workplace. Mass psychogenic illness (MPI) may be similar to those symptoms typically reported in the sick building syndrome. Odors are the most common triggering event. The threshold for detection of chemical odor is often well below air concentrations associated with any toxicity. Workers may believe that the odors signal dangerous indoor air pollution.[22] Workers may be more alarmed if they believe that the environmental contaminants to which they are exposed may cause damaging long-term effects, particularly cancer or birth defects. Concerns are increased if the source, often an offensive odor, is unknown.

Office equipment sources may include laser printers, copiers, computers, visual display terminals (VDTs), duplicators, and microfiche and blueprint equipment. Carbonless copy paper and correction fluids and preprinted computer forms may be a source of contaminants.

Human Activities

Human respiration releases vapor, carbon dioxide, and microbes into the air. Heating, cooling, cooking, smoking, and pesticide applications may affect indoor air.[27]

Table 66-13
Ambient Air Quality Standards Currently Applied in Twenty-One Nations for Ozone, Lead, Fluorides and Asbestos. All AAQS values in $\mu g/m^3$*

[ ] **No receptor standards for some time scales** [—] **No receptor standards (emission standards may apply)**

	Substance											
	Ozone O_3			Lead Pb			Fluorides F			Asbestos		
Country	Long Term	Medium Term	Short Term	Long Term	Medium Term	Short Term	Long Term	Medium Term	Short Term	Long Term	Medium Term	Short Term
WHO (1987)		100[e]	150[g]	0.5[a]								
Australia												
Victoria (1981)		100[e]	240[g]	1.5[b]			0.5[b]	2.9[d]			33 fibre/l	
Tasmania (1974)				1.5[b]			0.5[b]	2.9[d]				
Austria (1987)		100[e]	120[h]	—	—	—	—	—	—	—	—	—
Canada (1989)	30[a]	30[d]	100[g]	—	—	—	0.2[b]	.085[d]		—	—	—
Finland (1982)	—	—	—	—	—	—	—	—	—	—	—	—
Germany (1986)	—	—	—	2.0[a]			1.0[a]		3.0[h][δ]	—	—	—
Greece (1992)	—	—	—	2.0[a]			—	—	—	—	—	—
Hungary (1990)		30[d]	60[h]		0.3[d]	0.3[h]	3.0[a]	5.0[d]	20.0[h]		5.0[d]	10[h]
Israel (1992)		160[e]	230[h]	0.5[a] 1.5[b]	5.0[d]		—	—	—		0.4[e] fibre/l	
Italy (1989)	—	—	—	—	—	—	—	—	—	—	—	—
Japan (1990)			118[g]			0.1	—	—	—		10 fibre/l	—
Kuwait (1989)			157[g]		2.0[d]		—	—	—	—	—	—
Mexico (1984)			216[g]	1.5[b]			—	—	—	—	—	—
Netherlands (1986)			120[g]	0.5[a]	2.0[d]		0.8[c]	2.8[d]		—	—	—
New Zealand (1986)		60[e]	120[g]	1.5[b]			0.5[b] 1.0[k]			—	—	—
Poland (1990)		30[d]	100[h]	0.2[a]	1.0[d]		1.6[a]	10.0[d]	30.0[h]	—	—	—
Saudi Arabia (1991)			295[g]	—	—	—		1.0[d]		—	—	—
South Africa (1965)		100[d]	240[g]	2.5[a]			—	—	—	—	—	—
Soviet Union			100	.01					20	2.0		
Switzerland (1985)			120[g] 100[h][δ]	1.0[a]			—	—	—	—	—	—
Taiwan (1975)	—	—	—	—	—	—	—	—	—	—	—	—
United States (1990)			240[g]	1.5[b]			—	—	—		10 fibre/l	

*Adapted from Cochran LS et al. J Air Waste Manage Assoc 1992;42:1567–1572.
Remarks: *a:* annual mean; *b:* 3-month mean; *c:* 1-month mean; *d:* 24-hour mean; *e:* 8-hour mean; *f:* 3-hour mean; *g:* 1-hour mean; *h:* 30-minute mean; *i:* 15-minute mean; *j:* 10-minute mean; and *k:* 7-day mean.
α: 99.99 percentile; β: 99.5 percentile; γ: 99 percentile; δ: 98 percentile; ε: 95 percentile; and ζ: 50 percentile.

Table 66-14
Montreal Protocol—Revised Control Measures[a]

Year	Fully[b] Halogenated CFCs	"Other" CFCs	Halons[c] (3)	CC14	Methyl[b] Chloroform	"Other" Halons "HCFCs"
Jan. 1 1992	(Freeze-in Protocol)		(Freeze-in Protocol)	—	—	(See Resolution-UNEP/ OzL. Pro.2/L.2)
1993	(20% step-in Protocol)	20%	—	—	Freeze	HCFCs:
1994	—	—	—	—	—	
1995	50%	—	50%	85%	30%	-confine to substitutes
1996	—	—	—	—	—	-phaseout by 2020–2040
1997	85%	85%	—	—	—	
1998	—	—	—	—	—	
1999	—	—	—	—	—	
2000	100%	100%	100%	100%	70% —	
2005	—	—	—	—	100%	
Base Year	1986	1989	1986	1989	1989	

[a]Adapted from Armstrong JA. Commercial Chemicals Branch. Conservation and Protection, Ottawa, Ontario, Canada, Environment Canada.
[b]Adopted on the understanding that the adequacy/feasibility of further control measures will be considered at 1992 meeting of the Parties.
[c]Decision to be taken by the Parties on essential uses if any, by January 1, 1993.

Table 66-15
Variants of Clinical Disease in Building-Related Illness[a]

Hypersensitivity pneumonitis or humidifier fever
Building-related asthma or allergic rhinitis
Infectious syndromes
Legionnaires' disease
Pontiac fever
Q fever
Building-related dermatitis
Annoyance and irritational syndromes
Intoxication syndromes
Mass hysteria

[a]Adapted from Bardana EJ Jr et al. Clin Rev Allergy 1988;6:61–89.

Biologic Agents

Appropriate humidity, appropriate temperature, and appropriate physical and nutritional substrates may enhance microbial growth.[28] Complex heating, ventilation, and air-conditioning systems; fiberglass insulation; fabrics; ceiling tiles; and carpets may be substrates for microbial growth.

Radon and Radon Daughters

HVAC—Heating, Ventilation, Air Conditioning

HVAC systems can be a source of indoor air contaminants such as combustion products, bioaerosols, fibers, and particulates.

Air Quality

Indoor air must satisfy three requirements: (a) thermal acceptability, (b) maintenance of normal concentrations of respiratory gases, and (c) removal of contaminants and pollutants to levels below health or odor thresholds.[24] Most IAQ (Indoor Air Quality) complaints in nonindustrial environments are triggered by chemical levels 100 to 1000-fold below published standards affecting performance and health. The increase in indoor air pollution is due to the following (Norback)[21]:

1. Increased use of synthetic building materials.
2. Building occupants are sealed in. They have little control over environmental factors such as temperature, humidity, lighting, and ventilation.
3. Over 90% of the United States population spends the majority of its time indoors.
4. Those most susceptible to indoor air pollutants (the very young, the very old, and the chronically ill) spend all of their time indoors.[29]
5. The office technology boom makes its contribution to IAQ problems.

Volatile Organic Compounds (VOCs)

VOCs such as formaldehyde,[27] airborne alcohols, aldehydes, aliphatic, and aromatic and halogenated hydrocarbons and ketones found in indoor air may be associated with irritation phenomena. Massive exposure to VOCs may result in reactive airway dysfunction syndrome, characterized by bronchial hyperresponsiveness.[30]

Many VOCs arise from building materials and interior furnishings. Common materials leading to problems in indoor air quality include paints, adhesives, caulks, carpeting, and other flooring products, glazing compounds, and insulation materials. Furnishings such as textiles and insulation materials provide a basis for microbial growth.

Particulates

Particulates and fibers from asbestos and fiberglass insulation may contribute to indoor air pollution problems.

Legionella Pneumophila[31]

Airborne exposure to this organism may lead to Legionnaires'[1] Disease (progressive pneumonia with confusion, vomiting, and diarrhea, and associated with low attack rates) and Pontiac fever (nonpneumonic febrile illness with dizziness,[27] sore throat, nausea and diarrhea, and high attack rates). Sources of this organism include air conditioning, cooling towers, evaporative condensers, shower heads, drinking water, and streams.

Toxins

Indoor fungi and mycotoxins may induce symptoms common to the sick building syndrome.[27]

Immunologic Disorders

Indoor air pollutants may contribute to allergies by both antibody-mediated (rhinitis and asthma) and cell-mediated (hypersensitivity pneumonitis) immune mechanisms. The contribution of microbial/plant products, irritant gases (NO_2, SO_2, O_3), and volatile organic compounds (VOCs) to these disorders has yet to be systematically studied.[24]

Human Health Effects

Persistent lung diseases such as cancer, emphysema, fibrosis, and chronic bronchitis may be due to inhaled gases or particulates. Nonindustrial environments, however, seldom harbor contaminants of sufficient concentration to be harmful.[32]

Respiratory Cancer[33]

Environmental tobacco smoke, radon, asbestos, organic particulates, and volatile organic compounds may exert individual and additive effects on the initiation of human cancer. The association between indoor air and induction of cancer has not been demonstrated by controlled studies.

Chronic Obstructive Pulmonary Disease (COPD)

Environmental tobacco smoke,[27] irritant gases, respirable fibers, dusts, particulates, and volatile organic compounds may contribute to the development or exacerbation of bronchiolitis, chronic bronchitis, and emphysema by direct effects on elastic fibers, connective tissue repair, and alteration of protease inhibitors. Further research is required to establish definite correlation between chronic indoor oxidant gas exposure (nitrogen dioxide, sulfur dioxide, ozone) and COPD development. Tobacco smoke and cleaning/renovation activities continue to be prominent sources of respirable particulates. Controlled studies of such contaminants and COPD have not been performed.

Humidifier Fever

Microbial contaminants of humidifiers, vaporizers, or saunas is often associated with a variant of hypersensitivity pneumonitis (HP) humidifier fever (HF). Symptoms of hypersensitivity pneumonitis and humidifier fever may be similar. HF is thought to be caused by microbial toxins. HP is linked to antigenic components of thermophilic actinomycetes, fungi, or organic dusts. Fever is observed more in HF than in HP. Symptoms of HF often begin in the first 4 to 6 hours after beginning the workweek and subside during the week. These may include headache, polyuria, weight loss, and joint pain. The etiologic agents of HF have not been defined.

Irritant Gases

Gases such as NO_2, SO_2, and O_3 are known irritants, but whether they cause irritation at concentrations commonly found in indoor air remains to be determined.

Fibers and Dusts

Most dusts and fibers are irritating to the eyes and mucous membranes. Man-made mineral fibers (MMMF), including fiberglass, glasswool, and rockwool, are extensively used in HVAC ducting. Any repair activities that disrupt the integrity of the duct-lining materials may introduce MMMF into indoor air.

Odors

Odors are more annoying to people who work in clean environments such as offices than to those who work in dirty environments such as print shops or garages. Odor-induced bronchospasm in asthmatics may follow exposure to tobacco smoke, perfumes, and colognes.

Investigation of IAQ problems requires a personal interview and clinical histories of the individuals involved,[25] walk-through environmental surveys,[25,34] environmental monitoring (if required), inspection of HVAC (heating, ventilation, and air conditioning) system, and communication of results.

ENVIRONMENTAL CONTROL MEASURES

Quinlan and colleagues have summarized environmental control measures[25]:

1. Isolating areas undergoing renovation from the rest of a building so that contaminants associated with the renovation do not mix with the air supplied to the occupied space.
2. Ensuring that contaminants from neighboring exhaust ducts do not enter a building. This may necessitate providing separate ventilation for garages or relocating outdoor air intakes.
3. Installing local exhaust systems to remove contaminants generated in specific areas such as blueprint copying machines.
4. Banning or restricting cigarette smoking. If cigarette smoking cannot be prohibited, then smoking areas should be designated. These rooms should have a separate exhaust system so that cigarette smoke is not recirculated to the rest of the building.
5. Ensuring that pesticide applications are done by well-trained personnel using only approved structural pesticides without organic hydrocarbon solvents. It is essential to restrict pesticide application to times that a building is unoccupied. Ensure that the building is well ventilated before reoccupation.
6. Replacing or thoroughly disinfecting water-damaged furnishings that have been contaminated with microorganisms.

PREVENTIVE MEASURES

Cone has provided the following suggestions for preventing SBS outbreaks[20,35]:

1. New or newly remodeled buildings should not be occupied until they are completely finished, including final touches. Ideally, occupancy should be delayed for several weeks after building completion, with ventilation maintained during that period at 100% outside air to allow solvents and other chemicals to dissipate adequately.
2. To prevent germination of fungal spores, roof leaks should be rapidly repaired, water contamination of HVAC units should be prevented, and relative humidity should be kept below 70%.
3. HVAC filters should be replaced regularly. Filters should have an efficiency rating of at least 50% as measured by the atmospheric dust spot test. Also, preventive maintenance on fans, ducts, and motors is essential to keep them at their designed efficiency over the life of the building.
4. Rapid recognition of a potential SBS outbreak by an alert clinician or building management can help reduce the severity of an outbreak and the complications that result when accurate diagnosis is delayed. Consultations by appropriate medical, epidemiologic, and industrial hygiene personnel is essential.
5. Cigarette smoking should be banned from all offices, public transportation (including airlines), and public buildings.

TREATMENT

Samet and associates have outlined some suggested control measures for specific pollutants (Table 66–16).[36]

Indoor air pollution concentrations can be kept below levels that produce illness by excluding or removing sources of contamination, diluting room air with "cleaner air"

Table 66–16
Control Measures for Pollutants[a]

Pollutant	Control Measures: Equipment and Materials	Control Measures: Ventilation and Design
Respirable particles	High efficiency filters	Zone and ventilate for smoking
	Tight sealing doors and grates	Supply outside combustion air to heater and fireplace
	Properly drafting chimney	Relocate air intakes
	Electrostatic precipitators	Maintain filter system
NO, NO_2	Remove gasoline engine	Effective hood vent over source
	Pilotless ignition	Isolate garage from indoor space
CO	Pilotless ignition	Supply outside combustion air
	Restrict heater use to uninhabited space	Vent emission outside
	Use catalytic converter	Kitchen/hood vent
	Replace indoor gasoline engines with electric	Relocate vents
		Provide smoking zones
		Isolate garage from indoor space
CO_2	Check static pressure in return air ducts to make sure return is not overriding fresh air intake	Isolate garage from indoor space
Agents from biological sources	Insulate to prevent condensation	Maintain inside relative humidities of 35–50%
	Damp-proof foundation, ducts	Exhaust bath and kitchen
	Proper drainage of drip pans under condenser coils	Vent crawl spaces
	Add bacteriocides to steam and water for humidifiers and cooling towers	
	Proper maintenance of filters and ducts	
	Routine cleaning	
	Discard water-damaged floor coverings	
	Do not use cool-mist humidifiers and vaporizers	
Formaldehyde	Substitute products such as phenolic resin plywood	Increase air exchange to house or office
	Seal sources	
	Removal of materials	
Radon and radon daughters	Vapor barrier around foundation	Vent crawl space
	Damp-proof basement and crawl space	Vent sumphole to exterior
	Seal cracks and holes in floor traps and drains	Subslab depressurization
	Install charcoal water scrubber for well water	Subslab depressurization
	Completely seal foundation	Vent bathroom and laundry to exterior
Volatile organic compounds	Substitute products	Use only with adequate ventilation
	Isolate storage area	Ventilate laundry, shop
	Apply only according to specifications	Provide separate ventilation to storage area
	Do not locate transformers indoors	
Asbestos	Removal	Ventilation does not provide adequate protection
	Injection sealant	
	Wrap pipes with plastic and duct tape	

[a]Adapted from Samet JM et al. Am Rev Respir Dis 1988;137:221–242.

(ventilation), removing contaminants from the air (filtration), and providing local exhausts.[24] Prevention of excessive indoor microbial contamination requires appropriate heating, ventilation, and air-conditioning installation, operation, and maintenance; outdoor air makeup that meets current ASHRAE (American Society of Heating, Refrigeration and Air Conditioning Engineers) standards[37]; appropriate humidity control, filtration to limit intrusion of outdoor bioaerosols, and adequate interior housekeeping and maintenance.[24] Irritant gases (NO_2, SO_2, O_3) are seldom controlled by filtration alone. Appropriate location of outdoor air intake and effective use of ventilation, including localized exhausts, may diminish indoor air pollution due to these contaminants. Filtration methods are also seldom effective in controlling VOCs. Prevention may be enhanced by using low-VOC-emitting materials, supplies, and equipment and assuring adequate ventilation. Unlike experience with gases and fumes, appropriate housekeeping and filtration of air are usually effective in reducing airborne concentrations of dusts, particulates, and fibers. Selection of materials with low odor levels plus adequate ventilation and housekeeping are usually effective in eliminating unacceptable odors.[38,39]

Increased Ventilation

Increased ventilation may paradoxically increase the risk of emissions from static surfaces such as the combinations of styrene, epoxy resins, phenol, and formaldehyde from pressed board; benzyl and benzol chlorides from plasticized vinyl tile; and sodium dodecyl sulfate detergent and mite allergens from carpets and bedding.[27] Removal, encasement, or other sealing-off of the source is required. Cleaning, sodium hypochlorite, ultraviolet treatment, and absolute dehydration of high-humidity sites can be effective in reducing mold growth.

Physical Factors

Temperature

Temperatures ranging from 20 to 26° C are usually felt to be acceptable. Above this range outgassing of volatile organic compounds may occur. Reduced alertness may be observed above 24° C.[40]

Humidity

In environments exceeding 70% relative humidity (RH) microbial growth and contamination may occur.[41] The EPA recommends a range of 40 to 50% RH. The American Society of Heating, Refrigerating, and Air Conditioning Engineers (ASHRAE) recommends RH be kept below 60%.

Other Factors

Lighting, vibrations, and noises can intensify indoor air pollution problems.

Sick Hospital Syndrome

Between 40 and 50% of operating room and recovery room personnel may have acute symptoms such as fatigue, headache, dizziness/light headedness, nausea, drowsiness, cough, and skin irritation[42,43] from exposure to nitrous oxide, ethylene oxide, and halogenated anesthetics. Germicidal agents, including isopropyl alcohol, glutaraldehyde, and parachlorphenol, have also been implicated. Airborne transmission of infectious organisms such as rubella, chickenpox, and *Legionella* contribute. Research laboratories may have an improper installation, operation, or design of the exhaust system.[43]

SMOG AND AIR POLLUTION DISASTERS

Photochemical Smog

Background

Air over areas such as Los Angeles and Houston contains primary and secondary pollutants, aerosols, and gases. In 1955, during a week-long heat wave, more than 247 deaths per day occurred as a result of the atmospheric and geographic conditions in the Los Angeles basin; high mountain ranges reduced the flow of free air through this area. A strong temperature inversion layer reduced the mixing height of pollutants and therefore increased pollutant concentration.

High temperatures and emission of hydrocarbons from automobile exhausts produce large amounts of photochemical smog. Minimal wind conditions produce stagnant air, which intensifies concentration of smog. Stable, warm weather increases concentrations of contaminants, which combine with sunlight to produce photochemical smog. Generally, these episodes are short-term and sporadic. Aesthetically, fine mists produced from hydrocarbons, sulfur dioxide, and nitrogen oxides cause obviously dirty air. Chemical oxidizing agents have a pungent odor; most people can detect nitrogen dioxide levels of 0.42 ppm.

Health Effects

Direct acute health effects of photochemical smog are difficult to establish. Eye irritation is frequent. Excess mortality is less easily demonstrated, because there are cyclical variations in various pollutant levels, and other factors (e.g., season, high temperatures, rapid temperature changes, holidays, day of week) have a stronger impact on death rates than pollution levels. At current air pollution levels, photochemical smog may increase the risk of asthmatic attacks in a small number of susceptible patients, reduce pulmonary function after long-term exposure, cause mucous membrane irritation and cough, and interfere with athletic performance; however, it probably causes no increased mortality or serious illness.[44]

Nonphotochemical Smog

High levels of carbon monoxide, sulfur oxides, and particulate matter with few secondary pollutants occur more frequently in the northeastern United States and parts of Europe. The high density of adjacent cities increases the background concentration of pollutants. Increasing the downwind length of the city (e.g., those situated in long and narrow valleys) increases the pollutant concentration.[45]

Meuse Valley, Belgium (1936)

High sulfur dioxide emissions from coal-burning plants combined with light winds to produce several thousand cases of pulmonary irritation and 65 deaths (primarily cardiac failure in elderly patients).

Donora, Pennsylvania (1948)

High concentrations of particulate matter and sulfur dioxide emissions from industrial smoke associated with poor environmental mixing of pollutants caused a severe pollution episode. Twenty excess deaths were recorded, and almost half of the city residents developed conjunctival and upper respiratory irritation along with gastrointestinal symptoms. These patients later had an increased prevalence of respiratory disease and increased mortality rates.

London (1952)

High particulate matter and sulfur dioxide concentrations in the absence of air movement produced over 4000 excess deaths.[46]

HUMAN HEALTH EFFECTS

The effect of air pollution depends on pollutant concentration, duration of exposure, and presence of underlying cardiopulmonary disease. Both acute symptoms and aggravation of chronic disease may result from exposure, but the complex variables involved in large epidemiologic studies make the detection of injury and the establishment of limits on exposure (threshold limit values) difficult.

Susceptibility to urban air pollution occurs in premature infants, the newborn, the elderly, those with chronic cardiac and pulmonary disease, some hypersensitive individuals, and heavy cigarette smokers. Suggested toxic effects of pollutants include impaired expiratory flow rate, airway inflammation, increased cough and sputum production, reduced resistance to pulmonary infections, decreased exercise tolerance in cardiac patients, unfavorable ECG changes, impaired oxygen transport, transient eye irritation, and excess death rates. Exercise performance is definitely reduced. Exposure to 0.5 ppm of ozone decreases athletic performance by 50%, which is greatest on the second day of exposure and minimal by the fifth day.[47] The use of antioxidants such as vitamin E does not ameliorate or prevent symptoms.[48]

The following summary lists individual pollutant effects at existing pollution levels. Refer to individual sections for high-dose effects.

Sulfur Dioxide

Both sulfates and sulfur dioxide together with particulate matter and photochemical pollutants aggravate chronic pulmonary disease and increase the risk of acute and chronic respiratory illness.[49] These compounds impair pulmonary mucociliary clearance, primarily in those patients with preexisting pulmonary disease, probably as a result of hydrogen ion deposition on the bronchial lining.[50] Sulfur dioxide has been responsible for the major air pollution disasters.[51] In high-exposure communities (community mean specific sulfur dioxide level of 45 μg/m^3 over 5 years), smokers and nonsmokers had a higher incidence of persistent cough and sputum production compared with controls in low-exposure communities.[52] Smoking remained the most important variable of the prevalence of persistent cough and sputum production.

Ozone

This chemical causes eye irritation and bronchitis, aggravates chronic obstructive pulmonary disease, and perhaps increases the risk of acute and chronic pulmonary disease, mutagenesis, and fetotoxicity. Ozone damages tissue by rapidly oxidizing thiol-containing compounds and unsaturated fatty acids. Symptoms of respiratory irritation and decreased forced expiratory volume occur at exposures above 0.3 ppm, but strenuous exercise causes these effects to develop at lower ozone levels.[53] In animals short-term exposure to ambient concentrations of ozone (below 1 ppm) indicates that ozone inhibits the capacity to kill intrapulmonary organisms and allows purulent bacteria to proliferate, but the applicability of these models to humans remains unclear.[54]

Nitrogen Oxides

Interstitial edema, epithelial proliferation, and, in high concentrations, fibrosis and emphysema develop after heavy nitrogen dioxide exposures. At current pollution levels nitrogen oxides are less toxic than ozone, and short-term exposures probably do not contribute to cardiorespiratory disease.[53]

Peroxyacetyl Nitrate

Lacrimation and pulmonary irritation are observed.

Aldehydes

Examples are acrolein and formaldehyde. Pulmonary irritation and bronchospasm are the health effects observed during exposure to concentrations present in the atmosphere.

Hydrocarbons

There are probably no adverse health effects at ambient air concentrations, but these compounds combine with primary pollutants and sunlight to form oxidants and mists.

Particulate Matter

Particulate matter alters lung function in children.

Carbon Monoxide

High concentrations impair oxygen transport; this may affect cardiac patients on smoggy days, but generally no effects occur in healthy individuals at existing levels.

AIR QUALITY STANDARDS

By legislation, the United States government sets ambient air quality standards at levels that provide an adequate margin of safety to protect health. These standards are based on threshold values established from animal experiments, experimental human exposures, and epidemiologic studies. Such threshold values do not represent no-effect values, because they are set to reduce detectable health effects to those levels "normally" seen in a general population. Hence, sensitive individuals (e.g., those with chronic cardiopulmonary disease) may sustain adverse effects even at these levels. The United States ambient air standards are as follows:

Sulfur dioxide	0.03 ppm Annual arithmetic mean
	0.14 ppm Maximum daily average
Suspended particulate matter	75 μg/m^3 Annual geometric mean
	260 μg/m^3 Maximum daily average
Ozone	0.12 ppm Maximal 1-hour average (Stage 2 smog alerts occur in Los Angeles at ozone levels of 0.20 ppm, Stage 3 alerts at 0.35 ppm)
Nitrogen dioxide	0.05 ppm Annual arithmetic mean
Carbon monoxide	9 ppm 8-hour average maximum
	35 ppm 1-hour average maximum
Lead	1.5 μg/m^3 Monthly average

CONTINUING AIR POLLUTION PROBLEMS

Acid Rain

In recent years the acidity of rain and snow has increased sharply over the northeastern United States and Canada, Western Europe, and Scandinavia. The normal pH of precipitation (5.6) is due to naturally occurring sulfur dioxide and hydrogen sulfide (e.g., from volcanoes), which are oxidized and hydrolyzed to sulfuric acid. Nitrogen oxides are similarly converted to nitric acid. The increasing release of sulfur and nitrogen oxide from burning fossil fuels has changed precipitation in certain areas from neutral solutions

200 years ago to dilute acidic solutions today. The most extreme case was the presence of rain at a pH of 2.4 (i.e., the pH equivalent of vinegar) in Scotland in 1974. Although human health effects have not been documented, damage to forests and lakes has been obvious. Potential human effects include the inhalation of nitrogen and sulfur oxides, as well as the mobilization of trace elements from the soil (e.g., lead, mercury, aluminum).[55,56] Efforts at control have been frustrated by the fact that damage occurs at great distances from the source of pollutants. Ironically, the building of large smokestacks has reduced local pollution but increased the transport of pollutants to distant areas where acid rain forms. Controlled studies suggest that the damage to vegetation by sulfur oxides is worse in the presence of nitrogen oxides and ozone. Thus programs that are designed to reduce the problem of acid rain must consider the effects of all air pollutants, including nitrogen oxides.[57]

REFERENCES—AIR POLLUTION

1. Smith AG. Toxicology of the lung. Hum Exper Toxicol 1993; 12:415–416.
2. Wheeldon EB. Mechanism of lung toxicity. Proc Br Toxicol Soc, September 1992. Hum Exper Toxicol 1993;12:419.
3. Witschi H, Oreffo V, Pinherton KE. Cell types and their importance in pulmonary toxicology. In: Volans GN, Sims J, Sullivan FM, Turner P, eds. Basic science In toxicology. London: Taylor & Francis, 1990.
4. Dobbs LG, Williams MC, Gonzalez C. Biochimica Biophysica Acta 1988;970:146–156.
5. Hansen K, Mossman B. Generation of superoxide from alveolar macrophages exposed to asbestiform and non fibrous particles. Cancer Research 1987;47:1681–1686.
6. Schoenberger CI, Hunninghake GW, Kawanami O, Ferrans VJ, Crystal RG. Role of alveolar macrophages in asbestosis: modulation of neutrophil migration to the lung after acute asbestos exposure. Thorax 1983;37:803–809.
7. Moldeus P, Cotgreave I. Mechanisms of endothelial lung damage. In: Volans GN, Sims J, Sullivan FM, Turner P, eds. Basis science in toxicology. London: Taylor & Francis, 1990, pp. 242–249.
8. James DG. Respiratory disease. Postgrad Med J 1992;68: 160–173.
9. Sangster B, Meulenbelt J. Acute pulmonary intoxications. Overview and practical guidelines. Netherlands J Med 1988; 33:91–100.
10. Cooper JAD Jr, Matthay RA. Drug-induced pulmonary disease. Dis Mon 1987;33:61–122 (Chicago: Year Book).
11. Smith LL, Cohen GM, Aldridge WN. Morphological and biochemical correlation of chemical-induced injury to the lung. Arch Toxicol 1986;58:214–218.
12. Technical Progress on Protecting the Ozone Layer Electronics, Degreasing and Dry Cleaning Solvents Technical Options Report. United Nations Environment Programme. June 30, 1989.
13. US EPA Future Concentrations of Stratospheric Chlorine and Bromine, July 1988.
14. Ozone depletion quickens. Lancet 1991;1:1132–1133 (editorial).
15. Scientific Assessment of Stratospheric Ozone, 1989. Volume II. Appendix: Alternative Fluorocarbon or Environmental Acceptability Study (AFEAS). World Meteorological Organization. Global Ozone Research and Monitoring Project. Report No 20. National Aeronautics and Space Administration, United Kingdom and United Nations.
16. Browne MW. Ozone hole reopens over Antarctica. New York Times, October 12, 1990.
17. Profitt MH, Martitan JJ, Kelly KK, Loewenstein M, Podolske JR, Chan KR. Ozone loss in the Arctic polar vertex inferred from high-altitude aircraft measurements. Nature 1990; 347:31–36.
18. Broad WJ. Some say the rocket's red glare is eating away at the ozone layer. New York Times, May 14, 1991.
19. Logan M, Farmer JG. Anaesthesia and the ozone layer. Br J Anaesth 1989;63:645–647.
20. Lyles WB, Greve KW, Bauer RM, Ware MC, Scharansmke CJ, Crouch J et al. Sick building syndrome. South Med J 1991;84:65–71.
21. Norback D, Michel I, Widstron J. Indoor air quality and personal factors related to the sick building syndrome. Scand J Work Environ Health 1990;16:121–128.
22. Boxer PA. Indoor air quality. A psychosocial perspective. J Occup Med 1990;32:425–428.
23. Hicks JB. Tight building syndrome: when work makes you sick. Occup Health Saf 1984;53:51–56.
24. Brooks BO, Utter GM, De Broy JA, Schinke RD. Indoor air pollution: an edifice complete. Clin Toxicol 1991;29:315–374.
25. Quinlan P, Macher JM, Alevantis LE, Cone JE. Protocol for the comprehensive evaluation of a building-associated illness. In: Occupational medicine: state of the art reviews. Philadelphia: Hanley & Belfus, 1989;4:771–797.
26. Woods JE. Cost avoidance and productivity in owning and operating buildings. In Cone JE, Hodgson MJ, eds. Problem buildings: building-associated illness and the sick building syndrome. Occup Med Soc Art Rev 1989;4:753–770.
27. Angle C. Indoor air pollutants. Adv Pediatr 1988;35:239–280.
28. Arundel A, Sterling E, Biggen J, Sterling T. Indirect health effects of relative humidity in indoor environments. Environ Health Perspect 1986;351–361.
29. Koenig JD, Pierson WE. Air pollutants and the respiratory system. Toxicity and pharmacologic interventions. Clin Toxicol 1991;29:40–41.
30. Boulet L. Increases in airway responsiveness following acute exposure to respiratory irritants. Reactive airway dysfunction syndrome or occupational asthma? Chest 1988;94:476–481.
31. Mahoney M, Lakhani A, Stephens A, Wallace JG, Youngs ER, Harper D. Legionnaire's disease and the sick building syndrome. Epidemiol Infect 1989;103:285–292.
32. Norback D, Edling C. Environmental, occupational and personal factors related to the prevalence of sick building syndrome in the general population. Br J Ind Med 1991;48: 451–462.
33. Samet JM, Marbury MC, Spengler JD. Health effects and sources of indoor air pollution. Part I. Am Rev Respir Dis 1987;136:1486–1508.
34. Building Air Quality. A Guide for Building Owners and Facility Managers. US Environmental Protection Agency, Indoor Air Division and National Institute for Occupational Safety and Health. Washington, DC: US Government Printing Office, December 1991.
35. Cone JE. Building associated illness and the tight building syndrome. San Francisco General Hospital, August 1982.
36. Samet JM, Marbury MC, Spengler JD. Health effects and sources of indoor air pollution. Part II. Am Rev Respir Dis 1988;137:221–242.
37. American Society of Heating, Refrigeration and Air Conditioning Engineers. Ventilation for Acceptable Indoor Air Quality. ASHRAE Standard 62, 1989; Atlanta, GA. ASHRAE, 1989.
38. Sim MR, Abramson MJ. Indoor air quality and sick buildings. Med J Aust 1991;155:651–652.
39. Samet JM, Spengler JD, eds. Indoor Air Pollution: a Health Perspective. Baltimore: Johns Hopkins University Press, 1991; p. 407.
40. Wyon D. The effects of moderate heat stress on typewriting performance. Ergonomics 1974;17:309–318.
41. Koren HS, Graham DE, Devlin RB. Exposure of humans to a volatile organic mixture. III. Inflammatory response. Arch Environ Health 1992;74:39–44.
42. Kreiss K. The epidemiology of building-related complaints and illness. Occup Med 1989;4:575–592.
43. Brandt-Rauf PW, Andrews LR, Schwarz-Miles J. Sick hospital syndrome. J Occup Med 1991;33:737–739.
44. Goldstein E, Hackney JD, Rokaw SN. Photochemical air pollution. Part 1. West J Med 1985;142:369–376.

45. De Nevers N. Community air pollution. In: Rom WN, ed. Environmental and occupational medicine. Boston: Little, Brown, 1983, pp. 797–810.
46. Logan WPD. Mortality in the London fog incident 1952. Lancet 1953;1:336–338.
47. Summer Olympics to be under ozone cloud. JAMA 1981; 246:202 (editorial).
48. Hackney JD, Linn WS, Buckley Rd et al. Vitamin E supplementation and repiratory effects of ozone in humans. J Toxicol Environ Health 1981;7:383–390.
49. French JG, Lowrimore G, Nelson WC et al. The effect of sulfur dioxide and suspended sulfates on acute respiratory disease. Arch Environ Health 1973;27:129–133.
50. Schlessinger RB. Comparative irritant potency of inhaled sulfate aerosols. Effects on bronchial mucociliary clearance. Environ Res 1984;34:268–279.
51. Buechley RW, Riggan WB, Hasselblad V. Sulfur dioxide levels and perturbations in mortality: a study of New York–New Jersey metropolis. Arch Environ Health 1973;27:134–137.
52. Chapman RS, Calafiore DC, Hasselblad V. Prevalence of persistent cough and phlegm in young adults in relation to long-term ambient sulfur dioxide exposure. Am Rev Respir Dis 1985;132:261–267.
53. McDonnel WF, Horstman DH, Hazucha MJ et al. Pulmonary effects of ozone exposure during exercise: dose-response characteristics. J Appl Physiol 1983;54:1345–1352.
54. Dungworth D, Goldstein E, Ricci PF. Photochemical air polution. Part II. West J Med 1985;142:523–531.
55. Acid rain: toxic metals. Lancet 1984;1:656–660 (editorial).
56. Acid-rain and human health. Lancet 1985;1:616–618 (editorial).
57. Abelson PH. Air pollution and acid rain. Science 1985;230:617.

CARBON DIOXIDE

The narcotic action of carbon dioxide in high concentration has been known since 1820.[1] Most people will lose consciousness after taking eight to twelve breaths of 30% carbon dioxide, and this exercise can cause a rise in arterial carbon dioxide tension (pCO_2) to more than 100 mm Hg with a lowering of the arterial pH to below 7.1. Numerous fatalities have occurred after individuals have entered fermentation vats, wells, and silos where air had been replaced by carbon dioxide.[2] Deaths and cerebral damage have been associated with accidental hypercapnia following the use of carbon dioxide in anesthesia.[3] Carbon dioxide embolism is a rare but potentially devastating complication of laparoscopy or hysteroscopy.[4] Carbon dioxide was blamed but not conclusively shown to be the cause for the deaths of approximately 1700 people in Cameroon, West Africa, in 1986 when a massive release of gas occurred from Lake Nyos, a volcanic crater lake.[5]

PHYSICAL PROPERTIES

Carbon dioxide is a colorless, odorless, noncombustible gas, soluble in water. It is commonly sold in the compressed liquid form, and the solid form (dry ice).[6]

SOURCES

Carbon dioxide is normally present in the atmosphere at a concentration of approximately 0.03% (300 ppm).[7] It is a normal body constituent arising from cellular respiration. Most commercially available carbon dioxide is recovered from industrial processes in which it is generated as a byproduct.[1] It is present in natural gas wells and is a product of fuel combustion and of fermentation. Carbon dioxide is a byproduct of ammonia production and lime kiln uses; carbon dioxide is used in the carbonation of beverages, as a propellant in aerosols, and as dry ice for refrigeration.[8]

ACUTE TOXIC LEVELS

Concentrations of 20 to 30% result in unconsciousness and convulsions within 1 minute of exposure.[1] Exposure to concentrations of 75,000 ppm (7.5%) for 15 minutes may result in headache, dizziness, restlessness, and/or dyspnea.[1] Neurologic signs, including eye flickering, myoclonic twitches, dilated pupils, and restlessness, have followed exposure to 100,000 to 150,000 ppm of carbon dioxide for 15 minutes.[1]

CHRONIC EXPOSURE

A 5-day exposure to 30,000 ppm (3%) of carbon dioxide has resulted in mild frontal headaches.[1] Chronic hypercapnia in patients suffering from pulmonary disease may include headache, somnolence, mental confusion, lassitude, irritability, and unconsciousness.[9]

PERMISSIBLE EXPOSURE LIMITS

The Federal OSHA Standard is 10,000 ppm (18,000 mg/m^3) as an 8-hour time-weighted average.

PATHOPHYSIOLOGY

Carbon dioxide exerts a key influence on the control of respiration and cerebral circulation. It acts peripherally, both as a vasodilator and as a vasoconstrictor, and is a powerful cerebral vasodilator. At high concentrations it exerts a stimulating effect on the central nervous system, while excessive levels exert depressant effects. It induces graded increases in respiratory minute volume and ventilatory rate. Increased carbon dioxide levels may result in respiratory acidosis. Blood pH values may decrease after 2 days' exposure to 3% (30,000 ppn) carbon dioxide.[1]

CLINICAL PRESENTATION

Acute Effects

Acute exposure to 6 to 10% of carbon dioxide may induce a decrease in vascular resistance, an increase in renal blood flow, increased cerebral blood flow, and an increase in systolic and diastolic blood pressure, pulse rate, and respiratory muscle volume with sweating and hyperpnea. Exposure to between 10 and 20% concentration may induce myoclonic twitching, dilated pupils, and restlessness; at 17% for 20 to 50 seconds throat irritation, increased rate of respiration, dimness of vision, dizziness, and unconsciousness may supervene.[1]

Chronic Effects

Exposures to concentrations of 1 to 1.5% for 30 to 42 days has led to increases in minute volume, respiratory rate, anatomic dead space, and tidal volume.

LABORATORY

Exposures to 7.5% carbon dioxide for 15 minutes may lead to a decrease in total eosinophils, increase in blood sugar, increase in arterial pCO_2 and H^+. After 7 to 14% carbon dioxide is inhaled for 10 to 20 minutes, there may be an increase in plasma catecholamines.

TREATMENT

Initial management of severe symptoms following carbon dioxide inhalation requires immediate removal from the source, establishment of an adequate oxygen supply, and careful attention to the airway, breathing, and circulation. Near fatal CO_2 embolism during laparoscopy and hysteroscopy has been successfully treated with cardiopulmonary bypass.[10] Symptomatic and supportive care should suffice. There are no antidotes.

REFERENCES—CARBON DIOXIDE

1. Westlake EK, Simpson T, Kaye M. Carbon dioxide narcosis in emphysema. Quart J Med 1955;24:155–172.
2. National Institute for Occupational Safety and Health. Criteria for a recommended standard. Occupational exposure to carbon dioxide. DHEW (NIOSH) Publication No. 76-194; pp. 67–72, 114–116. Washington, DC: US Government Printing Office, 1976.
3. Razis PA. Carbon dioxide—a survey of its use in anaesthesia in the UK. Anaesthesia 1989;44:348–351.
4. McGrath BJ, Zimmerman JE, Williams JF, Parmet J. Carbon dioxide embolism treated with hyperbaric oxygen. Can J Anaesth 1989;36:586–589.
5. Baxter PJ, Kapila M, Mfonfu D. Lake Nyos disaster, Cameroon, 1986: the medical effects of large scale emission of carbon dioxide. Br Med J 1989;298:1437–1441.
6. Key MM, Henschel AF, Butler J, Ligo RN, Tabershaw IR, eds. Occupational diseases. A guide to their Recognition. Rev. edition. June 1977. DHEW (NIOSH) Publication No. 77-181. Washington, DC: Superintendent of Documents USGPO, pp. 415–417.
7. Slonim NB, Hamilton LH. Respiratory physiology. 2nd ed. St. Louis: CV Mosby, 1971; pp. 16–25, 76–89, 207–210.
8. Proctor NH, Hughes JP, Fischman ML. Chemical hazards of the workplace. 2nd ed. New York: Van Nostrand Reinhold, 1989; pp. 119–120.
9. Johnston RF. The syndrome of carbon dioxide intoxication. Its etiology, diagnosis and treatment. Univ Mich Med Bull 1959;25:280–292.
10. Diakun TA. Carbon dioxide embolism: successful resuscitation with cardiopulmonary bypass. Anesthesiology 1991;74:1151–1157.

CARBON DISULFIDE

Although acute carbon disulfide toxicity is relatively rare, chronic carbon disulfide toxicity was well known in the French and German rubber industry by the late 1800s.[1] Early American industrial exposure resulted in severe debilitating CNS symptoms (e.g., irritability, mania, hallucinations, tremors, memory loss).[2] Recent concern centers on chronic industrial exposures, which may cause neuropsychiatric changes, peripheral neuropathies, and accelerated atherogenic changes.[3] Carbon disulfide is primarily a synthetic product that produces disturbances in trace mineral balance in humans. Minute amounts are found in coal and crude oil.

STRUCTURE/CHARACTERISTICS

The pure compound is a clear, colorless volatile liquid with the structural formula CS_2 and a sweet, aromatic odor resembling that of decaying cabbage. Carbon disulfide is an exceptional fat solvent. The highly flammable liquid releases sulfur dioxide on combustion. The density of the vapor is two and one-half times that of air.

SOURCES

Carbon disulfide is a man-made product. Most poisonings occur in the viscose rayon manufacturing industry. Commercial applications include use as a chemical intermediate for adhesives, a grain and soil fumigant, a solvent in the rubber and rayon industry, a grease remover, a corrosion inhibitor, and an insecticide.

TOXIC DOSAGE

The United States government (NIOSH)–recommended time-weighted average (TWA) exposure limit for a 40-hour workweek is 1 ppm. Exposure to a TWA of 11 ppm results in headache and dizziness. Exposure to a TWA of 20 ppm results in sleep disturbances, fatigue, nervousness, anorexia, and weight loss. Long-term exposure to levels in excess of 20 ppm may result in atherogenic and diabetogenic changes. Most acute carbon disulfide fatalities result from an ingestion of which 15 mL may be fatal to an adult.[1,4]

TOXICOKINETICS

Carbon disulfide is well absorbed through the lungs, and serious toxicity has resulted from ingestion. Peak blood concentrations appear 2 hours after inhalation. The plasma elimination half-life is about 1 hour. The liver and fat tissue store concentrated carbon disulfide. The body metabolizes between 80 and 90% of the absorbed dose; the lungs excrete all except a small fraction of the rest.[5] Disulfiram is metabolized by the body to carbon disulfide. Metabolic products seen in the urine include thiourea, 2-mercapto-2-thiazolin-5-one, and 2-thiazolidine-4-carboxylic acid. The iodine-azide test identifies these metabolites in the urine.

PATHOPHYSIOLOGY

Carbon disulfide reacts with a variety of nucleophilic compounds in the body, including pyridoxamine (one of the vitamin B_6 complex), cerebral monoamine oxidases, and dopamine decarboxylase, to block enzymatic processes. Carbon disulfide binds to microsomal enzymes, reducing activity; it also produces a centrilobular hepatic necrosis. In addition, carbon disulfide may interfere with copper and zinc metabolism by acting as a chelating agent.[6] Continued exposure to high levels of carbon disulfide results in a permanent axonal neuropathy.[1] Other causes (alcohol consumption, diabetes, dietary deficiencies, cancer, other chemicals) must be excluded by history, since histologic lesions are not pathognomonic.

CLINICAL PRESENTATION

Skin

Local contact results in erythema and pain since carbon disulfide is one of the most potent fat solvents. Prolonged contact produces vesiculation and chemical burns. Severe chemical burns of the cornea result from direct contact with the eyes.

Inhalation

Acute inhalation produces rapid onset of both local irritation and CNS symptoms ranging from pharyngitis, nausea, vomiting, dizziness, fatigue, headache, mood changes, lethargy, and blurred vision to agitation, delirium, hallucinations, convulsions, coma, and death.

Chronic Effects

Carbon disulfide is a potent nerve toxin; it also may accelerate coronary artery disease. Peripheral neuropathies, cranial nerve dysfunction, and neuropsychiatric changes are present in over 70% of chronic carbon sulfide poisoning victims.[1] Impaired psychomotor function (i.e., dexterity, speed) and higher cortical function (i.e., visuomotor skills, concentration), as well as neurasthenic symptoms (i.e., mood swings, irritability, headache, nausea, fatigue, malaise, memory loss), characterize the neurologic illness associated with excessive carbon disulfide exposures.[3] These neuropsychiatric symptoms may be irreversible.[7]

Chronic long-term exposures (e.g., in rayon workers) may result in elevated blood cholesterol, retinopathy (microaneurysms, optic neuropathy), peripheral neuropathy, decreased glucose tolerance, reduced serum thyroxine levels, and parkinsonism.[1,8] Increases in atherosclerosis, coronary artery disease, deaths, suicide rates, personality changes, and hypertensive disease have been suggested, but not confirmed, by epidemiologic studies.[9]

LABORATORY

The iodine-azide test for urinary metabolites of carbon disulfide is used to assess industrial exposure. Electromyography and nerve conduction studies are sensitive methods for the early detection of carbon disulfide peripheral neuropathy.

The Santa Ana Dexterity Test, tests of simple reaction time, and Wechsler Adult Intelligence Scale subtests on block design, digit symbols, and digit span have been suggested as accurate measures of carbon disulfide-induced neuropsychiatric dysfunction,[3] but the patients must be carefully matched to age-appropriate controls.

TREATMENT

Initial management of severe inhalation poisoning requires careful attention to airway, breathing, and circulation. Otherwise, treatment involves removal from source and symptomatic care.

REFERENCES—CARBON DISULFIDE

1. Davidon M, Feinleib M. Carbon disulfide poisoning: a review. Am Heart J 1972;83:100–114.
2. Goroy ST, Trumper M. Carbon disulfide poisoning. JAMA 1938;110:1543–1549.
3. Feldman RG, Ricks NL, Baker EL. Neuropsychological effects of industrial toxins: a review. Am J Ind Med 1980;1:211–227.
4. Foreman W. Notes of a fetal case of poisoning by bisulphide of carbon with post-mortem appearances and remarks. Lancet 1886;2:118–119.
5. Teisinger J, Soucek B. Absorption and elimination of carbon disulfide in man. J Ind Hyg Toxicol 1949;31:67–73.
6. Cohen AE, Scheel LD, Kopp JF et al. Biochemical mechanisms in chronic carbon disulfide poisoning. Am Ind Hyg Assoc J 1959;20:303–323.
7. Kleinfeld M, Tabershaw IR. Carbon disulfide poisoning. Report of two cases. JAMA 1955;159:677–679.
8. Corsi A, Maestrelli P, Picotti G et al. Chronic peripheral neuropathy in workers with previous exposure to carbon disulfide. Br J Ind Med 1983;40:209–211.
9. Partanen T. Coronary heart disease among workers exposed to carbon disulfide. Br J Ind Med 1970;27:313–325.

CARBON MONOXIDE

Sources

Sources of carbon monoxide include tobacco smoke, automobile exhaust, heating equipment, fire, and paint remover (methylene chloride).

METHYLENE CHLORIDE

Methylene chloride is a highly volatile liquid used as a degreaser, solvent, extraction medium, and paint remover. It has mild central nervous system depressant properties that are less pronounced than those of chloroform and carbon tetrachloride. Methylene chloride is a very weak hepatotoxic agent. Exposure to methylene chloride vapors for 2 to 3 hours produces arterial carboxyhemoglobin levels between 5 and 15%. Such carboxyhemoglobin levels may stress patients or workers with underlying cardiopulmonary disease or concomitant carbon monoxide exposure. The use of a paint remover in a poorly ventilated setting has been implicated in a fatal myocardial infarction.[1]

CARBON MONOXIDE PRODUCTION

An 8-hour exposure to 150 ppm methylene chloride produced carboxyhemoglobin levels similar to those produced by exposure to 35 ppm carbon monoxide. An 8-hour exposure to 250 ppm methylene chloride caused the carboxyhemoglobin level to exceed 8%.[2] Severe, acute methylene chloride exposures have resulted in carboxyhemoglobin levels as high as 50%.[3] Physical exercise and smoke produce an additive effect on the carboxyhemoglobin level.[4]

TOXICOKINETICS

Absorption

Methylene chloride is well absorbed by the lung (55% retention in rats, 35% in humans). Toxicity has resulted from oral ingestion. Methylene chloride can be absorbed by intact skin, but probably not in quantities sufficient to cause systemic toxicity.[5]

Elimination

The lungs exhale most of the absorbed dose of methylene chloride unchanged. The body metabolizes between one-quarter and one-third of the absorbed dose to carbon monoxide and the rest to carbon dioxide.[6,7] The carboxyhemoglobin elimination half-life after methylene chloride ingestion is longer than that after direct inhalation of carbon monoxide.

CLINICAL PRESENTATION

Acute Systemic Effects

Since methylene chloride inhalation elevates blood carboxyhemoglobin levels, symptoms of carbon monoxide poisoning may occur, especially in patients with cardiopulmonary disease or workers who are exposed to other carbon monoxide sources. Epidemiologic studies have not identified an increased mortality among methylene chloride workers,[8] but workers with cardiovascular disease may be more susceptible to methylene chloride vapor. Symptoms may persist longer than carboxyhemoglobin levels predict because of continuing in vivo carboxyhemoglobin production and the fact that carboxyhemoglobin affects more than oxygen transport.[9]

LABORATORY

Abnormalities

Laboratory workup of serious methylene chloride exposures should include complete blood count, hepatic aminotransferase levels, creatinine, urinalysis, urine myoglobin, and blood carboxyhemoglobin level. Exposure to about 1000 ppm methylene chloride for several hours resulted in carboxyhemoglobin levels as high as 15%. The carboxyhemoglobin level of the average worker exposed to 183 ppm (8-hour TWA) ranges from 4.5 to 9%.[10] Carboxyhemoglobin produced by methylene chloride metabolism has a half-life almost twice as long as equivalently inhaled carbon monoxide because of continuing carboxyhemoglobin formation after cessation of exposure. Methanol, exercise, and concomitant carbon monoxide exposures such as smoking elevate carboxyhemoglobin levels. Serious poisonings from methylene chloride exposure may occur without significant elevation of carboxyhemoglobin levels.[11]

Biologic Monitoring

Exposure measurements include blood methylene chloride and carboxyhemoglobin levels, as well as air sampling. For average, sedentary, nonsmoking workers maximum allowable exposures (200 ppm) produce methylene chloride levels of 80 ppm in expired air and 0.18 mg/100 mL in blood and carboxyhemoglobin levels of 6.8%.[6]

TREATMENT

Stabilization

As with inhalation or ingestion of other hydrocarbons, initial attention should be directed toward removal from exposure, support of respiration, and monitoring for dysrhythmias.

Elimination Enhancement

There are no measures to enhance elimination.

Antidotes

There are no antidotes.

Supportive Care

The usual measures suffice with primary attention given to the extent of hepatorenal toxicity and the carboxyhemoglobin level. Follow-up measurements of hepatic aminotransferase levels should be scheduled within 1 week of exposure.

BIOMASS FUELS

Most people in developing countries still depend on biomass fuels such as agricultural wastes, dried animal dung, wood, or charcoal that are burnt in traditional cook-stoves without a chimney.[12] It is estimated that at least 300 to 400 million people, mostly women, are exposed to such smoke. Data from India suggests that exposure to biomass smoke from cooking raises carboxyhemoglobin levels to about 13%.[13]

TOXIC AMBIENT LEVELS

At equilibration, atmospheric carbon monoxide levels of 50, 100, and 200 ppm produce average carboxyhemoglobin levels of 8, 16, and 30%, respectively.[14] Perceptible clinical effects occur with a 20-hour exposure to concentrations as low as 0.01% (100 ppm). Carbon monoxide toxicity is increased by numerous factors, including decreased barometric pressure (e.g., high altitude), increased alveolar ventilation (e.g., activity, high metabolic rate) (e.g., children, pets, birds), preexisting cardiovascular and cerebral vascular disease, reduced cardiac output, increased affinity of hemoglobin for CO (e.g., fetal hemoglobin has an oxygen dissociation curve to the left of adult hemoglobin so that fetal hypoxia may be greater for similar degrees of CO exposure), anemia, hypovolemia, pulmonary carbon monoxide diffusing capacity, and increased rate of endogenous CO production.

Industrial Exposure Limits

The TLV is 35 ppm for an 8-hour workday on a time-weighted average. This level allows for a maximum COHb level of 5% during an 8-hour period assuming normal activity. This TLV is based on an alveolar ventilation of 6L/min and a CO diffusing capacity of 30 mL/min/kg. The ceiling concentration to which a worker may be transiently exposed without altering COHb level is 200 ppm. This short-term exposure limit (STEL) implies that a worker would be asymptomatic 15 minutes after cessation of exposure.

TOXICOKINETICS

The lungs rapidly absorb carbon monoxide, which avidly combines with hemoglobin at 230 to 270 times greater affinity than oxygen. Elimination occurs exclusively through the lungs; the half-life of carboxyhemoglobin in room air is

3 to 4 hours depending on minute ventilation. Administration of 100% oxygen shortens the half-life to 30 to 40 minutes. Hyperbaric oxygen (100% oxygen at 2.5 atm) further reduces the half-life to as little as 15 to 20 minutes. The COHb half-life after methylene chloride exposure is more than two times longer because of continuing endogenous conversion to carbon monoxide. About 85% of absorbed CO combines with hemoglobin; the remainder attaches to myoglobin and blood proteins.

PREGNANCY/LACTATION

The fetus is particularly vulnerable to CO poisoning because of increased accumulation in fetal blood (10 to 15% higher than maternal levels) and lower initial fetal PO_2 levels (20 to 30 mm Hg compared with 100 mm Hg in adults.[15,16] Furthermore, the fetal hemoglobin dissociation curve lies to the left of the adult curve, resulting in greater tissue hypoxia at similar COHb levels. Animal studies suggest that maternal CO exposures as low as 125 ppm over 4 to 18 days may affect fetal growth.[17] Neonates are more susceptible, since fetal hemoglobin constitutes 20% of the total at 3 months.[18] Acute nonlethal maternal intoxication may result in fetal demise[19,20] or permanent neurologic sequelae (e.g., cerebral palsy).[21] A comatose woman delivered an apparently normal infant (4-month neurologic check-up was normal) despite an initial carboxyhemoglobin level of 58.2%.[22] Prolonged exposure to low doses (5 to 15% COHb in smoking mother) is associated with smaller babies and elevated neonatal mortality.[23] In addition to elevated carboxyhemoglobin levels, fetal cord blood from the smoking mother demonstrates a dose-related decreased pH and PO_2, as well as increased PCO_2 levels.[24]

PATHOPHYSIOLOGY

Physiology

CO toxicity results from impaired oxygen delivery and utilization, which lead to cellular hypoxia. Areas of poorly developed anastomotic vessels and high metabolic activity (e.g., brain, heart) are particularly susceptible. Carbon monoxide affects several different sites within the body, but the exact contribution of each pathophysiologic effect remains unclear.

1. Inhalation of carbon monoxide replaces oxygen on the hemoglobin molecule, leading to a relative anemia. The body requires 5 mL of oxygen per 100 mL of oxygen dissolves per 100 mL of blood; the remaining 3 mL of oxygen per 100 mL blood (3 vol%) comes from the release of oxygen from hemoglobin. Impairment of oxyhemoglobin formation by CO results in cellular hypoxia.
2. COHb impairs the release of oxygen from hemoglobin by increasing oxygen binding to hemoglobin. The result is a shift of the oxyhemoglobin dissociation curve to the left, which reduces unloading of oxygen in the tissues. Figure 66–2 demonstrates the altered oxyhemoglobin dissociation curve. Note that exercise (acidosis, hypoxia, hyperthermia) moves the curve to the right and toxins move it to the left.

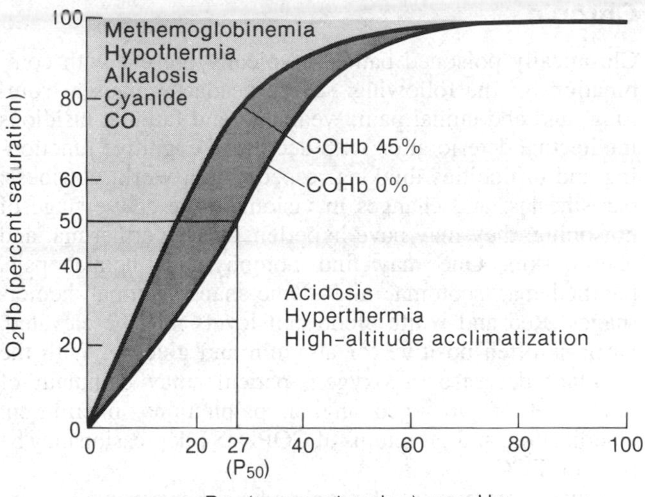

Figure 66–2 Factors that shift the oxygen-hemoglobin dissociation curve (shown at 37°C and pH 7.4). Note that exercise (acidosis and temperature elevation) moves the curve to the right, enhancing the oxygen delivery to the tissues. (Adapted from Goldfrank L, Lewin N, Kirstein R et al. Hosp Physician 1981;17(2):50.)

3. CO binds to cytochrome oxidase in vitro; however, the affinity of oxygen for cytochrome oxidase is so much greater than that of carbon monoxide that in vivo binding of carbon monoxide to cytochrome oxidase may be small.[25] Several authors used the inhibition of cellular respiration to explain the poor correlation of toxicity to carboxyhemoglobin blood levels and to justify the use of hyperbaric oxygen.[26]
4. CO saturates myoglobin in three times higher concentration than skeletal muscle. The resultant myocardial depression and hypotension cause ischemia and potentiate the hypoxia induced by impaired oxygen delivery.

Delayed Neurologic Deterioration

Delayed neurologic deterioration ususally becomes apparent within 2 to 3 weeks of the carbon monoxide exposure, but it may occur as early as 2 days later. Other precipitating causes of delayed neurologic deterioration include drug overdose, strangulation, and seizures.[27]

CLINICAL PRESENTATION

Thorpe[28] has summarized neurologic signs and symptoms in both acute and chronic carbon monoxide poisoning:

Acute

Patients presenting with acute poisoning may display weakness, fatigue, and "amnestic confabulatory state," apathy, impulsiveness, and distractibility. There may be fecal and urinary incontinence. There are often abnormal motor, sensory, and cerebellar findings, including abnormal reflexes. Three percent of those acutely poisoned develop permanent sequelae, including mental deterioration (98%), urinary and fecal incontinence (88%), and gait disturbance (81%).

Chronic

Chronically poisoned patients typically present with combinations of the following: severe headache, nausea, vomiting, and abdominal pain; weakness and fatigue; insidious intellectual deterioration with decreased cognitive functioning and difficulties thinking, especially at work; dizziness; paresthesias; and changes in vision. In the active stage of poisoning, they may have hypertension, hyperthermia, and cherry skin. One may find homonymous hemianopsia, papilledema, scotoma, and flame-shaped retinal hemorrhages. Red and white blood cell levels may be elevated. Urine is often positive for albumin and glucose. With the resultant decrease of oxygen, patients may complain of new-onset or worsened angina, palpitations, intermittent claudication, and symptoms of COPD. ST depression may be seen on ECG.

Forty-three percent of people who suffer chronic poisoning have neurologic sequelae at 3-year follow-up. Of these about 40% have memory impairment, including amnestic confabulatory states, and retro- and anterograde amnesias. Many have cerebral, cerebellar, and midbrain damage evidenced in findings of akinetic movements, agnosia, apraxia, rigidity, and brisk reflexes. Thirty-three percent have personality changes usually, including lethargy, apathy, and fatigue. They may show irritability, verbal aggression, violence, impulsiveness, moodiness, "affective incontinence," severe attention deficits, distractibility, and sexual outbursts. Eleven percent suffer gross neuropsychologic damage. Some are psychotic, disoriented, and blind. They may have vestibular dysfunction with poor hearing. One month after insult, I.Q. is usually normal except in the digit span test.

Criteria for mild, moderate, and severe carbon monoxide poisoning is presented in Table 66–17. Mistaken diagnoses often occur after poisoning with carbon monoxide (Table 66–18).[29]

Table 66–17
Severities of CO Poisoning[a]

Mild poisoning
- Criteria:
- COHb levels <30 percent
- No signs or symptoms of impaired cardiovascular or neurologic function
- May complain of headache, nausea, or vomiting
- Treatment:
- Admission of patients with COHb levels >25 percent
- Symptomatic medication
- 100 percent oxygen by nonrebreathing mask until COHb remains <5 percent
- Patients with underlying heart disease should be admitted and cardiac function be appropriately monitored regardless of COHb level.

Moderate poisoning
- Criteria:
- COHb levels from 30 to 40 percent
- No signs or symptoms of impaired cardiovascular or neurologic function
- Treatment:
- Admission
- Cardiovascular status should be followed closely even in absence of clear cardiac effects, especially in those patients with underlying heart disease.
- Determination of acid-base status (will be corrected by high-flow oxygen)
- 100 percent oxygen by nonrebreathing mask until COHb remains <5 percent

Severe poisoning
- Criteria:
- COHb levels >40 percent or
- Cardiovascular or neurologic functional impairment at any COHb
- Treatment:
- Admission
- Cardiovascular functioning monitoring
- Acid-base status monitoring
- 100 percent oxygen by nonrebreathing mask
- Transport to a hyperbaric oxygen facility, immediately if available, or if no improvement in cardiovascular or neurologic function is seen in within 4 h

[a]Adapted from Ilano AL, Raffin TA. Chest 1990;97:165–169.

Cardiovascular System (Table 66–19)

Patients with cardiovascular disease are particularly sensitive to carbon monoxide cardiotoxicity and develop in-

Table 66–18
Some Possible Mistaken Diagnoses in Patients With Carbon Monoxide Poisoning[a]

Misdiagnosis	Cause
Neurologic	
Cerebrovascular accident	cerebral ischemic accident due to CO poisoning
Migraine, tension headache	headache
Epilepsy	anoxic convulsions
Meningitis, encephalitis	vomiting, headache, bizarre neurologic symptoms
Parkinsonism	late-onset parkinsonian symptoms
Psychiatric	
Depression	lethargy, somatic symptoms
Anxiety state	hyperventilation, headache, malaise
Hyperventilation syndrome	hyperventilation
Acute confusional state	confusion, hallucinations
Cardiac	
Myocardial infarction	a critical coronary artery lesion decompensated through hypoxia
Cardiac arrhythmias	conduction system hypoxia
Pharmacologic and toxicologic	
Drug overdose	hypoxic coma, non-traumatic rhabdomyolysis
Ethylene glycol poisoning	coma and renal failure
Ethanol intoxication	vomiting, ataxia, slurred speech, coma
Drug abuse	agitation, confusion, hallucinations
Infections	
Influenza and other viral infections	muscle aches, tachypnea, headache, exhaustion
Post viral syndrome	lethargy, myalgia
Gastroenteritis and food poisoning	nausea, vomiting
Pneumonia	dyspnea, delirium
Sinusitis	headache, malaise
Others	
Cholecystitis and other acute abdominal conditions	abdominal pain, nausea, vomiting

[a]Adapted from Lowe-Ponsford FL, Henry JA. Adverse Drug React Acute Pois Rev 1989;8:217–240.

Table 66–19
Effects of CO Exposure on Human Cardiovascular System[a]

CO and/or COHb Level	Duration	Effects
5% CO 9% COHb	30–120 sec	Increase in coronary blood flow and oxygen extraction ratio and decrease in coronary sinus oxygen tension in subjects with normal hearts; no significant increase in coronary heart disease subjects at high COHb levels; oxygen extraction ratio increased and coronary sinus tension decreased in heart patients, altered lactate and pyruvate metabolism seen at high COHb levels
100 ppm 4.08% COHb	1 hr	Significant decrease in exercise time until marked dyspnea in subjects with chronic obstructive pulmonary disease
42–63 ppm 5.08% COHb	90 min	Exercise time until onset of angina decreased significantly in angina pectoris patients; systolic blood pressure and heart rate at angina also significantly decreased
50 and 100 ppm 2.9 and 4.5% COHb	4 hr	Exercise time until onset of angina in angina pectoris patients and reduced even at low COHb level; systolic blood pressure and heart rate also decreased at angina
7 and 20% COHb		Maximal exercise time for healthy subjects decreased with increasing COHb levels; no difference in blood lactate concentrations between exposed and control groups; maximum oxygen uptake decreased with increased COHb
100 ppm 3.95% COHb	1 hr	Mean exercise time until exhaustion decreased in middle-aged, healthy nonsmokers; reduced work time for exposed nonsmokers; no reduction in exposed smokers; respiratory pattern changes noted in smokers
50 ppm		Study of "admission case fatality rate" in hospitals divided into high- and low-pollution areas: significant difference found for fatality rates between high- and low-pollution area hospitals in 9 of 10 weeks when ambient CO levels were above a weekly mean of 9 ppm
		Significant low-level association observed between ambient CO levels and frequency of initial cardiorespiratory complaints at an emergency room of a hospital in Denver, Colorado, during high-pollution months.

[a]Adapted from Rylander R, Vesterlund J. Scand J Work Environ Health 1981;7(Suppl 1):17.

creased exertional angina at COHb levels as low as 5 to 10%. Sudden death has occurred in workers with severe arteriosclerotic heart disease when their carboxyhemoglobin levels exceeded 20%.[30] The presence of ischemic symptoms (chest pain, syncope, dyspnea, diaphoresis, nausea) depends on the existence of preexisting cardiovascular disease and COHb concentration. Occasionally, myocardial infarction occurs. Conduction defects, premature ventricular contractions, and atrial fibrillation also occur in these patients. Hypotension results from myocardial depression, even in healthy patients, when COHb levels exceed 60%. Chronic low-level exposure such as that seen with heavy cigarette smokers may accelerate atherosclerosis.

Warehouse Worker's Headache

Warehouse worker's headache follows use of propane-fueled forklifts in enclosed warehouses. Common complaints due to the carbon monoxide emissions include headache, nausea, and lightheadedness. Syncope and loss of consciousness may occur. Symptoms appear to resolve after breathing 100% oxygen at 2.45 atmospheres absolute (ATA) for 90 minutes.[31] No long-term sequelae were observed in one series of 17 patients.[7]

Gastrointestinal

Shock or left ventricular failure in severe carbon monoxide poisoning may lead to bowel ischemia.[32] Multiple family members may present with nausea, vomiting, and diarrhea.

The levels of carboxyhemoglobin can be dissimilar in individuals simultaneously exposed to the same source. The symptoms manifested by the individuals can be dissimilar despite similar carboxyhemoglobin levels. Levels of carboxyhemoglobin present in individuals riding in old vehicles can be as great or greater than those of individuals who are victims of house fires.[33]

A suggested overall estimate of the carboxyhemoglobin concentration at the time of removal from a carbon monoxide source follows[34]:

Calculation of $t_{1/2}$ from 2 values of [COHb] at different times.

Assumption:

The [COHb] decays exponentially.

$$t_{1/2} = \frac{\ln 2 \times t}{(\ln Col - \ln CO2)} \qquad \text{(Eq. 1)}$$

Where $t_{1/2}$ is in hours and appropriate to the PIO_2
ln = the natural logarithm
t = the time in hours between [COHb] determinations
CO1 = the 1st [COHb] in %
CO2 = the 2nd [COHb] in %

Calculation of administered O_2, "equivalent O_2 %" (Eq O_2).

Assumptions:

1. $t_{1/2}$ is inversely proportional to partial pressure of inspired O_2.
2. $t_{1/2}$ for air (approximately 20% O_2) at 1ATA = 5 hours

$$EqO_2 = \frac{100}{t_{1/2}} \qquad \text{(Eq. 2)}$$

Back calculation of the [COHb] at the time of patient removal from the CO source (the Max [COHb]).

Assumptions:

No additional ones are required.

$$Max[COHb] - [COHb] \times 2^{(T/t1/2} \quad \text{(Eq. 3)}$$

Where: t is hours from removal to [COHb] determination
[COHb] = the percent of hemoglobin combined with CO
Max[COHb] = [COHb] when patient is removed from CO source

Example: [COHb] 2.55 hours after removal = 6%. Find Max[COHb].

1. Assume air breathing since removal ($t_{1/2}$ = 5 hours). Max [COHb] = $6 \times 2^{(0.51)} = 7.5\%$
2. Assume ventilation with 100% 0_2 where $t_{1/2}$ = 1 hour. Max [COHb] = $6 \times 2^{(2.55)} = 35.1\%$

ABNORMALITIES

Arterial Blood Gases

P_{O2} is normal, but the oxygen saturation expressed as a percentage is decreased. Some laboratories calculate oxygen saturation rather than measure it with an oximeter. Therefore reliability depends on which laboratory method is used. A gap between the measured percentage HbO_2 and the calculated percentage HbO_2 indicates the necessity for measuring COHb. P_{CO2} may be normal or slightly reduced. Metabolic acidosis is a feature of CO poisoning and reflects both ischemia and hypoxia.

Electrocardiogram

The ECG is a sensitive test for the presence of myocardial damage in adults.[35] Ischemic changes range from ST depression and T-wave flattening or inversions to ST elevation indicative of myocardial infarction. Dysrhythmias range from frequent premature ventricular contractions to atrial fibrillation and ventricular tachyarrhythmias. Sinus tachycardia is the most common abnormality.

Electroencephalogram

Abnormal EEG findings are common (diffuse slow waves, low voltage) and parallel the progression of an hypoxic encephalopathy. The predictive value of the EEG is questionable, since a patient with a critically abnormal EEG may completely recover.

Radiography

Chest x-rays usually are normal on admission, but may display abnormalities such as ground-glass appearance, perihilar haze, peribronchial cuffing, and intraalveolar edema. The presence of x-ray abnormalities indicates a much worse prognosis.[36]

CAT Scan

Positive computerized axial tomography accurately predicts severe neurologic sequelae within 24 hours (e.g., low-density globus pallidus lesions), but not all patients with neurologic impairment have abnormal CAT scans.[37]

Magnetic Resonance Imaging (MRI)

Carbon monoxide causes cytotoxic edema and demyelination. White matter and basal ganglia are commonly damaged. These findings are nonspecific and may be associated with barbiturate intoxications; hypoglycemia; cyanide, disulfiram, and hydrogen sulfide poisoning. MRI may be more sensitive than CT scans in detecting tissue edema caused by demyelination.[38]

Ancillary Tests

Initial laboratory values should include complete blood count, glucose, creatinine, cardiac enzymes, urinalysis, carboxyhemoglobin, arterial blood gases, ECG, and chest x-ray. Clinical judgment determines the necessity of cyanide and methemoglobin levels. Muscle necrosis may result in elevated serum creatine kinase and lactate dehydrogenase levels and myoglobinemia. Elevated creatinine levels may result from either myoglobinuria- or ischemia-induced acute tubular necrosis. Patients with significant CO poisoning exhibit hypokalemia, hyperglycemia, and hemoconcentration that may be a result of elevated catecholamine levels as a response to acute cellular hypoxia. Elevated lactic acid levels despite a normal CO level reflect evidence of continued cellular hypoxia.[39]

Fetal hemoglobin interferes with carboxyhemoglobin (COHb) determinations by falsely elevating COHb in direct proportion to fetal hemoglobin. Interpretations of COHb level in infants younger than 90 days old should be considered in evaluating the clinical relevance of this observation. Further controlled studies are indicated.[40]

PULSE OXIMETRY

Pulse oximetry is a noninvasive method used to monitor oxygen saturation. It is relatively easy to perform, painless, rapid in its response, and accurate when arterial oxygen saturations are greater than 65%.[41,42] It requires no warm-up time, special skin preparation, or complex calibration.[13]

Accuracy[43–45]

The accuracy of pulse oximetry can be affected by patient movement, compression of the sensor, severe desaturation, low perfusion states, surgical electrocautery, hypothermia (<35°C), hypotension (<50 mm of mercury), severe vascular disease, vasopressor therapy,[46] infrared heating lamps, nail polish (other than red), black ink,[47] intravenous dyes,[48] and abnormal types of hemoglobins (carboxyhemoglobin, methemoglobin). Pulse oximetry (SaO_2) values are not affected by differences in skin pigmentation, total hemoglobin concentration, or thickness of the tissue at the site of monitoring.[49]

In carbon monoxide poisoning, pulse oximetry gives higher readings than the true HbO_2 (oxyhemoglobin) levels and fails to alert the physician to potentially lethal hypoxia.[50] COHb absorbs light almost identically to HbO_2 at 660 nm. The oximeter responds to COHb as if it were HbO_2.[51]

Similarly, the pulse oximeter progressively overestimates oxygen saturation with increasing methemoglobin concentrations and may not warn the physician that a dangerous hypoxic state is developing.[13] In fact, a disparity between the oxygen saturation calculated from PaO_2 values and pulse oximetry readings may offer a clue to the presence of methemoglobinemia.

Measurement

Oxygen saturation is measured by placing a special sensor on a patient's finger, toe, or nose. The sensor consists of a light-emitting diode that projects two discrete wavelengths of light corresponding to saturated and unsaturated hemoglobin (660 and 940 nm) together with a photodetector.

Smokers

In a smoker, the oximetry-measured oxygen saturation must be subtracted by the percent carboxyhemoglobin to find the true O_2 saturation.

Methylene Blue

Methylene Blue has a spectral absorption peak of 668 nm, and therefore it may absorb most of the 660-nm light emission causing the oximeter to interpret this as the presence of reduced hemoglobin and a fall in arterial oxygen saturation. If any doubt exists, an arterial blood sample should be obtained to confirm PaO_2 and hemoglobin saturation.[52]

Dangers

Pressure erosion or necrosis,[53] finger injuries due to overheating by a damaged probe,[54] and burns[55] have rarely followed use of pulse oximeters.

Co-oximeter

The co-oximeter measures light absorption at four wavelengths and uses the extinction coefficients at each wavelength to calculate the relative concentrations of HbO_2, reduced hemoglobin, carboxyhemoglobin, and methemoglobin.

Functional and Fractional Saturation[56]

Pulse oximeters measure the "functional saturation" defined as the percentage of oxyhemoglobin compared with the sum of oxyhemoglobin (oxyHB) and reduced hemoglobin (Hb) (Fig. 66–2).

$$\text{Functional saturation} = \frac{\text{OxyHb}}{\text{OxyHb} + \text{reduced Hb}}$$

Co-oximeters measure what is termed the "fractional saturation."

$$\text{Fractional saturation} = \frac{\text{OxyHb}}{\text{OxyHb} + \text{reduced Hb} + \text{COHb} + \text{MetHb}}$$

TREATMENT

Stabilization

Immediate removal from the contaminated environment, control of airway, support of breathing with ventilation, 100% O_2, and the institution of intravenous lines and cardiac monitoring are the initial priorities. Oxygen (100%) should be delivered through a tight-fitting mask or an endotracheal tube if the patient lacks adequate minute ventilation. Continue 100% O_2 until the COHb level falls below 15 to 20%. Fire victims should be evaluated for airway obstruction from thermal or chemical injury, pulmonary edema, trauma, concomitant toxin inhalation (e.g., cyanide and methemoglobin formers), and cerebral edema.

Elimination Enhancement

Oxygen

O_2 (100%) reduces the COHb half-life from 5 to 6 hours to ½ to 1 hour. It will increase dissolved oxygen from 0.3 mL O_2 per 100 mL blood to 2 mL O_2 per 100 mL blood. Hyperbaric oxygen (3 ATA) further reduces COHb half-life to 20 to 30 minutes.

Hyperbaric Oxygen

Hyperbaric oxygen (HBO) enhances the elimination of carboxyhemoglobin and increases the amount of dissolved oxygen in plasma, but its exact role in the treatment of carbon monoxide poisoning remains controversial. Some physicians feel strongly that victims of serious carbon monoxide poisoning should be transferred to HBO facilities, since published case reports attesting to the effectiveness of HBO and the threat of litigation exist.[57,58] In addition to decreased COHb elimination half-life, potential benefits may include increased tissue clearance of residual carbon monoxide, reduced cerebral edema, and reduced cytochrome oxidase inhibition. Other physicians indicate that the cost, complications, and difficulties in transport dictate caution and selective use of HBO.[59] The available literature does not contain enough information to guide therapy convincingly.[60] Individual responses to carbon monoxide levels vary, and predicting who will develop severe neurologic sequelae (e.g., demyelination) currently is inaccurate. Subtle neurologic/psychologic sequelae (e.g., personality changes, mood disturbances, headaches) may be a common long-term problem, but prior available tests have not been sensitive to these changes. Recent use of psychologic tests may improve detection of such sequelae.[61] No large, prospective, randomized study compares the long-term neurologic sequelae after 100% oxygen and HBO therapy. One study indicates that neurologic sequelae develop in 50% of patients with severe carbon monoxide poisoning despite intensive treatment with hyperbaric oxygen.[13] Other studies, which used more liberal criteria for hyperbaric oxygen therapy (any neurologic abnormality or history of unconsciousness), demonstrated a low incidence of delayed neurologic sequelae (0 to 4.5%).[62,63] In a series of 2967 patients hospitalized for acute carbon monoxide poisoning, 86 (2.7%) developed delayed neuropsychiatric symptoms.[64] Of these 86 patients, 32 patients (37%) received hyperbaric oxygen after the acute exposure.

Currently the decision to use HBO requires clinical judgment to evaluate the potential benefits and complications. Complications of HBO therapy include decompression sickness resulting from intravascular and intracellular expansion of dissolved nitrogen causing formation of bubbles, rupture of tympanic membranes, damaged sinuses, cerebral gas embolism, oxygen toxicity (convulsions and pulmonary edema), potentiation of pneumothorax, and complications of transport (e.g., cardiac dysrhythmias and hypotension may make transport hazardous). Seriously poisoned patients require a compression chamber large enough to support an intensive care setting with ventilators and cardiac monitoring. The Diving Accident Network at Duke University Medical Center provides a 24-hour hotline (919-684-8111) for the location of hyperbaric oxygen chambers. When readily available, HBO therapy should be considered for patients with serious carbon monoxide poisoning:

1. Symptomatic patients with COHb levels over 40%.
2. Comatose patients and those with significant neurologic impairment.
3. Pregnant patients when COHb levels exceed 20% or when fetal monitoring shows signs of distress.
4. Patients with a history of unconsciousness for more than a brief period, especially those who remain symptomatic in the hospital.

Supportive Care

1. The decision to admit must correlate symptoms, individual susceptibility, and peak carboxyhemoglobin levels. (Consider both room air elimination half-life [4 hours] and the 50 to 60% oxygen [3 hours] to estimate peak levels.) The following patients should be admitted:
   a. Pregnant patients with COHb levels over 10%.
   b. Patients with cardiovascular disease whose COHb levels exceed 15%.
   c. Symptomatic patients with COHb levels over 25%.
   d. Patients with a history of unconsciousness, abnormal neuropsychiatric examination, or ischemia-like chest pain.
   e. Patients with reduced body temperatures, metabolic acidosis, chest x-ray abnormalities, myoglobinuria, hypoxia, or abnormal ECG.
2. Monitor cardiac and respiratory status. Obtain baseline ECG and cardiac enzymes (creatine kinase—myocardial band, lactate dehydrogenase, aspartate aminotransferase) in all patients, as well as serial cardiac enzymes and ECGs in cardiac patients. Watch for suppression of hypoxic respiratory drive in chronic lung disease patients.
3. Consider other toxic inhalants (e.g., cyanide, methemoglobin formers, concomitant trauma, hypoxic encephalopathy) in patients who do not respond promptly to therapy.
4. Watch for the development of cerebral edema with serial neurologic exams, CAT scans, and fundoscopic examination. Obtain a neurologic consultation when the diagnosis of cerebral edema is suspected. Corticosteroids have been used, although their efficacy in preventing neurologic sequelae or improving CO-induced cerebral edema has not been proven. Hyperventilation (P_{CO2} 25 to 30 mm Hg), head elevation (35°), and mannitol (0.25 to 1 g/kg of a 20% solution over 30 minutes) constitute the initial treatment of elevated intracranial pressure.
5. Oxygen (100%) therapy may be stopped when the patient becomes asymptomatic or the COHb levels falls below 15 to 20%. No more than 4 hours of 100% oxygen should be necessary.
6. Metabolic acidosis should not be treated aggressively unless the acidosis itself contributes to toxicity (i.e., below 7.15). Acidosis increases the unloading of oxygen in tissues, and therapy has a theoretic advantage in carbon monoxide poisoning where the dissociation curve shifts leftward.
7. Physical activity should be minimized for 2 to 4 weeks after the exposure.[65]

Controversies in Treatment of Carbon Monoxide Poisoning[66]

Gorman and Runciman have provided a comprehensive outline of problems related to current therapeutic approaches.

A. Toxic Mechanisms—Pathophysiology
   1. CO toxicity is only due to Hgb binding and reduction in tissue oxygenation.
      But: a. CO has toxicity unrelated to tissue O_2 delivery.
      b. COHb itself is not toxic.
      c. Patient outcome does not correlate well with COHb levels in hospitals.
      d. Titration of treatment against COHb concentration is often unsuccessful.
      e. Body stores of CO remain elevated after COHb levels have returned to normal.
   2. CO binds to and inhibits other hemoproteins (myoglobin, reduced cytochrome C, reduced cytochromes of P_{450} type, and tryptophan dioxygenase).
      But: a. CO affinity for the mitochondrial enzymes is low compared with O_2.
      b. Severe intracellular hypoxia is a prerequisite for CO-cytochrome C binding.
      c. Patients who develop neuropsychiatric deficits after CO poisoning are often not acutely acidotic.
   3. CO causes lipid peroxidation
      a. Continues after removal of tissue from CO source.
      b. Dilates blood vessels in the absence of Hb.
   4. Pathologic change in severely poisoned patients (CT, MRI, postmortem) include necrosis of globus pallidus, cerebral cortex, hippocampus, cerebellum, and substantia nigra. MRI may be more sensitive than CT to early changes.[67]
      But: a. Changes in severe CO poisoning are not identical to those of hypoxic brain injury.
      b. Relevance to mild poisoning is uncertain.
   5. Poisoning with CO and CN in fires
      a. CO binds to Fe^{++}.
      b. CN binds to Fe^{+++}. Prevents reoxidation of reduced cytochrome A_3.
      c. In combined exposure toxicities of CO and CN are synergistic.
      But: Synergy cannot be explained by CO or CN concentrations.

B. Clinical Presentation—Course of CO poisoning
1. Neurologic dysfunction (reduced consciousness) dominates clinical presentation of CO poisoning.
2. Cardiovascular manifestations less common
   a. Asymptomatic ST-segment change
   b. Other infrequent presentation
      (1) Cardiac arrhythmias
      (2) Hypotension
      (3) Pulmonary edema
      (4) Cardiorespiratory arrest
   c. Cherry-red color rare, late, much less common than cyanosis.
3. Removal from CO source leads to recovery, accelerated by breathing O_2.
   But: a. Some recoveries are incomplete.
   b. Others continue after patient is discharged from the hospital (late recoveries).
   c. Patients who recover can also later relapse or deteriorate (late deteriorations).
      (1) In 1 day or up to 6 weeks.
      (2) Lipid peroxidation is inhibited by O_2, may occur after tissue removed from CO source.
      (3) HBO may be effective for these deteriorations.
4. 33% may be dying or dead on arrival; 2% have obvious neuropsychiatric deficits on discharge
   But: 3 years later 10.8%—gross NP deficits; 28%—personality deterioration; 36%—loss of memory functions.
5. Late deteriorations indicating morbidities (rates) at discharge must be restricted to those with measurements of long-term activities.

C. Assessment of severity of CO poisoning
1. COHb levels
   But: a. Outcomes correlate poorly with COHb levels in hospital. On this basis survivors cannot be distinguished from nonsurvivors.
   b. Due to CO toxicity that is not related to Hb, alternative body depots for CO other than Hb and rapid dissociation of COHb
      (1) Half-life COHb 320 to 480 minutes on room air
      (2) 60 to 80 minutes on normobaric O_2 (100% O_2 at atmospheric pressure)
      (3) 8 to 23 minutes (on HBO)
   c. Clinical assessment and ABG at time of admission do not identify which CO-poisoned patients will suffer a late deterioration. CT and psychometric testing not established.
   d. History of unconsciousness = severe CO poisoning? Not always.
   e. Increased COHb level only confirms exposure
   to CO.
2. Traditional patient selection criteria have little validity. Urgent need for a reliable marker of severe CO poisoning.
3. Treatment and follow-up should be pursued with all patients with a history of exposure to CO and intoxication (focal neurologic deficit, impaired consciousness, myocardial ischemia at time of exposure) regardless of condition on arrival at a hospital.

D. Treatment
1. Increased inspired O_2 tension—recommended treatment
   a. O_2 is competitive antagonist to CO for hemoprotein binding.
   b. Increased O_2 in solution in plasma offsets reduced tissue O_2 delivery dose to COHb formation.
   c. O_2 inhibits lipid peroxidation secondary to CO.
2. Optimal O_2 therapy (PiO_2, duration, frequency) is unknown.
3. Cyanide poisoning
   a. O_2 delivery to tissues is normal.
   b. O_2 does not antagonize CN^- binding to the cytochromes as CN binds to Fe^{+++} and not Fe^{++} iron.
   c. O_2-dependent increase in CN^- metabolism not yet demonstrated.
   d. Human data: only case reports.
   e. O_2 does not worsen outcome.
   f. O_2 reduces toxicity of amyl and sodium nitrate, profound vasodilators, produce Met Hb, reduce tissue O_2 delivery.
   g. Give O_2 to patients poisoned with CO, even if CN^- poisoning also suspected.
4. Ideal O_2 dose
   a. Cannot titrate against COHb level
   b. Normobaric O_2: mortality rate 30% not prevented by
      (1) Prolonged hyperventilation with O_2
      (2) Hypothermia
      (3) Moderate dehydration
      (4) Steroids
      (5) Barbiturate sedation
      (6) Neuromuscular blockade
   c. Long-term morbidity in survivors 12 to 66%. Despite initial recovery, late neurologic deterioration is 12%.
5. Single HBO treatment—similar poor outcome
   No impaired level of consciousness—32% long-term sequelae
   Impaired consciousness—45% long-term sequelae, 19 to 48% morbidity in other series
   (2ATA for 2 hours each) HBO on 1st day of admission
   15.4% died
   7.5% of survivors—long-term sequelae
   11% of survivors—minor sequelae
6. HBO on admission, repeated daily or by patient's condition
   Mortality—0 to 9.6%
   Long-term morbidity 0 to 4.4%
   None: late deterioration in brain function
   Exception: If unconscious for at least 6 hours and CT scan changes before HBO
7. HBO on admission (2 to 3 ATA for 1 to 2 hours) and daily thereafter as determined by patient's condition is the only adequate treatment of CO poisoning yet observed.
   a. May prevent late deteriorations.
   b. Permanent patient morbidity caused by HBO is low.
   c. Problem is not treatment regimen but patient selection.

8. Need prospective, randomized, controlled clinical studies with a wide range of O_2 therapies
9. Raphael[68] and colleagues compared normobaric oxygen and HBO and recommend that
   a. Patients who have sustained loss of consciousness: treat with NBO (normobaric oxygen), irrespective of initial COHb level
   b. Brief loss of consciousness—one session of HBO, irrespective of COHb level
   c. Coma—high risk. Two sessions of HBO not better than one.

GUIDELINES FOR CONSIDERING THE HYPERBARIC CHAMBER

1. Symptomatic patients with COHb levels over 40%.
2. Comatose patients and those with significant neurologic impairment.
3. COHb greater than 15% in a child, or a patient with cardiovascular disease. (This guideline has not been systematically evaluated.)
4. The pregnant female: COHb greater than 10% in a pregnant female at any time during exposure, neurologic signs regardless of COHb level, and signs of fetal distress. If distress 12 hours after initial treatment, additional HBO treatments may be considered. (This guideline has not been clinically evaluated.) Preliminary human data tend to suggest that the human fetus can tolerate the short duration of HBO therapy and its attendant hyperoxic exposure when HBO is used to treat the mother for CO poisoning.[60] Further observations are necessary to determine the long-term sequelae and effectiveness of treatment with HBO during pregnancy.
5. Ischemic chest pain or ECG abnormalities.
6. Abnormal neuropsychiatric examination (not universal agreement).
7. Patients with a history of unconsciousness for more than a brief period, especially those who remain symptomatic in the hospital.
8. Presence of hypoxia, myoglobinuria, or abnormal renal function. (This guideline has not been evaluated.)
9. Abnormal chest x-ray (controversial).

HBO Controversies

The controversy about the role and dose of oxygen in carbon monoxide poisoning can only be resolved by prospective, randomized, controlled clinical studies of a wide range of oxygen therapies. Problems with ethical consent underlie proposed studies comparing normobaric oxygen with repeated hyperbaric oxygen. A marker for the severity of poisoning is still needed.[70]

Only a few controlled studies with inconclusive results have compared HBO with 100% oxygen at 1 ATM.[71,72] In a prospective randomized study with patients diagnosed as mild to moderate carbon monoxide poisoning, Thom and associates observed that compared with 100% oxygen, HBO treatment decreased the incidence of delayed neurologic sequelae (DNS) but that the DNS cannot be predicted on the basis of the patient's clinical history or CO level.[73] The role of HBO therapy in recovery from carbon monoxide poisoning, while possibly significant, is still poorly understood.[74,75] Clarification of the mechanism of action of both carbon monoxide poisoning and the beneficial effects of oxygen therapy will aid in understanding the potential usefulness of HBO therapy.[76] There is, however, insufficient data to support the efficacy or safety for HBO therapy in wound healing, gas gangrene, carbon monoxide poisoning, radiation neurosis syndromes,[77] or multiple sclerosis.[78]

Sloan and colleagues conclude, after a 10-year retrospective study with HBO, that the transfer of CO-poisoned patients to a HBO therapy facility need not be deferred for fear of impending cardiac arrest, respiratory arrest, myocardial infarction, or worsening mental status if these complications have not occurred prior to or during the initial emergency department resuscitation. In contrast, dysrhythmias, hypotension, seizures, agitation, and emesis must be anticipated both during the initial resuscitation and later during transfer to a HBO facility.[79]

Risks

Patients who require chest compressions, intubation, positive pressure ventilation, or central venous catheterization during their emergency department resuscitation are at increased risk of a hyperbaric oxygen therapy–induced tension pneumothorax. Careful pulmonary examination and chest radiography of these high-risk patients immediately prior to and following hyperbaric oxygen therapy are recommended, and the need for emergency needle thoracotomy should be anticipated. Endotracheal and nasogastric tubes are indicated in obtunded patients to minimize their risk of aspiration. Otic barotrauma precludes prophylactic myringotomy prior to hyperbaric oxygen therapy.

Carbon Monoxide Detectors

Carbon monoxide (CO) detectors have been controversial. Krenzelok and colleagues in an initial unconfirmed study suggest that CO detectors with audible alarms used in a series of 101 possible CO exposures were effective in alerting the potential victims of CO poisoning of its presence and of reducing the potential development of symptomatic CO poisoning.[80] Further clinical studies will be required to validate the use of these detectors.

REFERENCES—CARBON MONOXIDE

1. Ratney RS, Wegman DH, Elkins HB. In vivo conversion of methylene chloride to carbon monoxide. Arch Environ Health 1974;28:223–236.
2. Lawwerys RR. Industrial chemical exposure: guidelines for biological monitoring. Davis, CA: Biomedical Publications, 1983, p. 83.
3. Fagin J, Bradley J, Williams D. Carbon monoxide poisoning secondary to inhaling methylene chloride. Br Med J 1980; 281:1461.
4. Di Vincenzo GD, Kaplan CJ. Effect of exercise or smoking on the uptake, metabolism and excretion of methylene chloride vapor. Toxicol Appl Pharmacol 1981;59:141–148.
5. Stewart RD, Dodd HC. Absorption of carbon tetrachloride, trichloroethylene, tetrachloroethylene, methylene chloride and 1,1,1-trichloroethane through the human skin. Am Ind Hyg Assoc J 1964;25:439–446.

6. Di Vincenzo GD, Kaplan CJ. Uptake, metabolism and elimination of methylene chloride vapors by humans. Toxicol Appl Pharmacol 1981;59:130–140.
7. Steward RD, Fisher TN, Hosko MJ et al. Carboxyhemoglobin elevation after exposure to dichloromethane. Science 1972; 176:295–296.
8. Friedlander BR, Hearne T, Hall S. Epidemiologic investigation of employees exposed to methylene chloride. Mortality analysis. J Occup Med 1973;20:657–666.
9. Langehennig PL, Seeler RA, Berman E. Paint removers and carboxyhemoglobin. N Engl J Med 1976;295:1137.
10. Stewart RD, Hake CC. Paint remover hazard. JAMA 1976; 235:398–401.
11. Hall AH, Mountain R, Kulig KW et al. Methylene chloride poisoning without significantly elevated carboxyhemoglobin level. Vet Hum Toxicol 1986;28:482–483 (abstract).
12. Mavalankar DV. Indoor air pollution in developing countries. Lancet 1991;1:358–359.
13. Behera D, Dash S, Malik SK. Blood carboxyhaemoglobin levels following acute exposure to smoke of biomass fuel. Indian J Med Res 1988;88:522–524.
14. Peterson JE, Steward RD. Absorption and elimination of carbon monoxide by inactive young men. Arch Environ Health 1970;21:165–171.
15. Longo LD. Carbon monoxide effects on oxygenation of the fetus in utero. Science 1976;194:523–525.
16. Longo LD. The biological effects of carbon monoxide on the pregnant woman, fetus, and newborn infant. Am J Obstet Gynecol 1977;129:69–103.
17. Singh J, Scott LJ. Threshold for carbon monoxide induced fetotoxicity. Teratology 1984;30:253–257.
18. Venning H, Robertson D, Milner AD. Carbon monoxide poisoning in an infant. Br Med J 1982;284:651.
19. Muller GL, Graham S. Intrauterine death of the fetus due to accidental carbon monoxide poisoning. N Engl J Med 1995;252:1075–1078.
20. Goldstein DP. Carbon monoxide poisoning in pregnancy. Am J Obstet Gyencol 1965;9:526–528.
21. Cramer CR. Fetal death due to accidental maternal carbon monoxide poisoning. J Toxicol Clin Toxicol 1982;19: 297–301.
22. Margulies JL. Acute carbon monoxide poisoning during pregnancy. Am J Emerg Med 1986;4:516–519.
23. De Haas JH. Parental smoking. Its effect on fetus and child health. Eur J Obstet Gynecol Reprod Biol 1975;5:283–296.
24. Harrison KL, Robinson AG. The effect of maternal smoking on carboxyhemoglobin levels and acid-base balance of fetus. Clin Toxicol 1981;18:165–168.
25. Coburn RF. Mechanisms of carbon monoxide toxicity. Prev Med 1979;8:310–322.
26. Meyers RAM, Lindberg SE, Crowley RA et al. Carbon monoxide poisoning. The injury and its treatment. JACEP 1979;8: 479–484.
27. Opeskin K, Drummer OA. Delayed death following carbon monoxide poisoning. A case report. Am J Forens Med Pathol 1994;15:36–39.
28. Thorpe T. Chronic carbon monoxide poisoning. Can J Psychiatry 1994;39:59–61.
29. Lowe-Ponsford FL, Henry JA. Clinical aspects of carbon monoxide. Adverse Drug React Acute Pois Rev 1989;8:212–220.
30. Atkins EH, Baker EL. Exacerbation of coronary artery disease by occupational carbon monoxide exposure: a report of two fatalities and a review of the literature. Am J Ind Med 1985;7:73–79.
31. Fawcett TA, Moon RE, Fracica PJ, Mebane GY, Theil DR, Piantadosi LA. Warehouse worker's headache. Carbon monoxide poisoning from propane-fueled forklifts. J Occup Med 1992;34:12–15.
32. Balzan M, Cacciottolo JM, Casha S. Intestinal infarction following carbon monoxide poisoning. Postgrad Med J 1993;69:302–303.
33. Sanchez R, Fosarelli P, Felt B, Greene M, Lacovara J, Hachett F. Carbon monoxide poisoning due to automobile exposure: disparity between carboxyhemoglobin levels and symptoms of victims. Pediatrics 1988;82:663–666.
34. Hyperbaric Center Advisory Committee Emergency Medical Service, City of New York. A registry for carbon monoxide poisoning in New York City. Clin Toxicol 1988;26:417–441.
35. Anderson R, Allensworth DC, De Groot WJ. Myocardial toxicity from carbon monoxide poisoning. Ann Intern Med 1967;67:1172–1182.
36. Sone S, Higoshihari T, Kotake T et al. Pulmonary manifestations in acute carbon monoxide poisoning. Am J Roentgenol 1974;120:865–871.
37. Sawada Y, Takahashi M, Ohashi N et al. Computerized tomography as an indication of long term outcome after acute carbon monoxide poisoning. Lancet 1980;1:783–784.
38. Kanaga N, Imaizumi H, Nakayana M, Nagai H, Yamaya K, Namiki A. The utility of MRI in acute stage of carbon monoxide poisoning. Intensive Care Med 1992;18:371–372.
39. Chiulli DA, Rivers EP, Kristal S, Smithline HA, Blake H, Reiser E et al. Metabolic abnormalities in patients with severe carbon monoxide poisoning: insights into pathophysiology. Ann Emerg Med 1992;22:180.
40. Perrone J, Hoffman RS. Fetal hemoglobin interference with carboxyhemoglobin determination. Clin Toxicol 1995;33:475–486 (abstract 163).
41. Watcha MF, Conner MT, Hing AV. Pulse oximetry in methemoglobinemia. AJDC 1989;143:845–847.
42. Yelderman M, New W. Evaluation of pulse oximetry. Anesthesiology 1983;59:349–352.
43. Ralston AC, Webb RK, Runciman WB. Potential errors in pulse oximetry. I. Pulse oximeter evaluation. Anaesthesia 1991;46:202–206.
44. Webb RK, Ralston AC, Runciman WB. Potential errors in pulse oximetry. II. Effects of changes in saturation and signal quality. Anaesthesia 1991;46:207–212.
45. Ralston AC, Webb RK, Runciman WB. Potential errors in pulse oximetry. III. Effects of interference dyes, dyshaemoglobins and other pigments. Anaesthesia 1991;46:291–295.
46. Gordon K III. Pulse oximetry in emergency medicine. West J Med 1989;151:67.
47. Battito MF. The effect of fingerprinting ink on pulse oximetry. Anesth Analg 1989;69:260–269.
48. Schiller MS, Unger RJ, Kelner MJ. Effects of intravenously administered dyes on pulse oximetry readings. Anesthesiology 1986;65:550–552.
49. Jennis MS, Peabody JL. Pulse oximetry: an alternative method for the assessment of oxygenation in newborn infants. Pediatrics 1987;79:524–528.
50. Barker SJ, Tremper KK. The effects of carbon monoxide inhalation on pulse oximetry and transcutaneous PO_2. Anesthesiology 1987;66:677–679.
51. Alexander CM, Teller LE, Gross JB. Principles of pulse oximetry: theoretical and practical considerations. Anesth Analg 1989;68:368–376.
52. Kessler MR, Side T, Humayun B, Poppers PJ. Spurious pulse oximeter desaturation with methylene blue injection. Anesthesiology 1986;65:435–436.
53. Miyasaka K, Ohata J. Burn erosion, and "sun" tan with the use of pulse oximetry in infants. Anesthesiology 1987;67: 1008–1009.
54. Sloan TB. Finger injury by an oxygen saturation monitor probe. Anesthesiology 1988;68:936–938.
55. Murphy KG, Secunda JA, Rockoff MA. Severe burns from a pulse oximeter. Anesthesiology 1990;73:350–352.
56. Schnapp LM, Cohen NH. Pulse oximetry. Uses and abuses. Chest 1990;98;1244–1250.
57. Myers RAM, Snyder SK, Linberg S et al. Value of hyperbaric oxygen in suspected carbon monoxide poisoning. JAMA 1981;246:2478–2480.
58. Neubauer RA. Carbon monoxide and hyperbaric oxygen. Arch Intern Med 1979;139:829.
59. Olson KR. Carbon monoxide poisoning: mechanism, presentation and controversies in management. J Emerg Med 1984;1:233–243.
60. Kumar S. Hyperbaric oxygen in treatment of carbon monoxide poisoning. Br Med J 1984;289:1315.
61. Myers RAM, Messier LD, Jones DW et al. New directions in the research and treatment of carbon monoxide exposure. Am J Emerg Med 1983;2:226–230.

62. Myers RAM, Snyder SK, Emhoff TA. Subacute sequelae of carbon monoxide poisoning. Ann Emerg Med 1985;14:1163–1167.
63. Matthieu D, Wolf M, Durocher A et al. Acute carbon monoxide poisoning. Risk of late sequelae and treatment by hyperbaric oxygen. Clin Toxicol 1985;23:315–324.
64. Min SK. A brain syndrome associated with delayed neuropsychiatric sequelae following acute carbon monoxide intoxication. Acta Psychiatr Scand 1986;73:80–86.
65. Ginsburg R, Pomano J. Carbon monoxide encephalopathy: need for appropriate treatment. Am J Psychiatry 1976; 133:317–320.
66. Gorman DF, Runciman WB. Carbon monoxide poisoning. Anaesth Intensive Care 1991;19:506–511.
67. Kanaya N, Imaizuni H, Nakayana M, Nagai H, Yamaya K, Niniki A. The utility of MRI in acute stage of carbon monoxide poisoning. Intensive Care Med 1992;18:371–372.
68. Raphael J-C, Elkharrat D, Jars-Guincertie M-C, Chastung C, Charles V, Verchen J-B, Gajdos P. Trial of normobaric and hyperbaric oxygen for acute carbon monoxide intoxication. Lancet 1989;2:414–419.
69. Van Hoesen KB, Camporesi EM, Moon RE, Hage ML, Piantadosi CA. Should hyperbaric oxygen be used to treat the pregnant patient for acute carbon monoxide poisoning? A case report and literature review. JAMA 1989;261: 1039–1043.
70. Gorman DF, Runciman WB. Carbon monoxide poisoning. Anaesth Intensive Care 1991;19:506–511.
71. Raphael J-C, Elharrat D, Jars-Guincestre M-C, Chastang C, Chasles V, Vercken J-P et al. Trial of normobaric and hyperbaric oxygen for acute carbon monoxide intoxication. Lancet 1989;2:414–419.
72. Goulon M, Barois A, Rapin M, Nouailhat F, Grosbuis S, Labrousse J. Carbon monoxide poisoning and acute anoxia. J Hyperbar Med 1986;1:23–41.
73. Thom SR, Tabe RI, Mendiguren II, Clark JM, Hardy KR, Fisher AR. Delayed neuropsychologic sequelae after carbon monoxide poisoning: prevention by treatment with hyperbaric oxygen. Ann Emerg Med 1995;25:474–480.
74. Broome JR, Sykes JJW, Francis TJR, Tighe SQM, Ertmonstone WM, Clark RJ. Hyperbaric oxygen for carbon monoxide poisoning. Lancet 1990;335:549–550.
75. Hamilton-Farrell MR, Hanson GC. Hyperbaric oxygen for carbon monoxide poisoning. Lancet 1990;335:550.
76. Grim PS, Gottlieb LJ, Boddie A, Batson E. Hyperbaric oxygen therapy. JAMA 1990;263:2216–2220.
77. Ingle R. Hyperbaric oxygen therapy. JAMA 1990;764: 1811.
78. Kindwall ER, McQuilen MP, Khatri BO, Gruchow HW, Kindwall ML. Treatment of multiple sclerosis with hyperbaric oxygen. Results of a National Registry. Arch Neurol 1991;48: 195–199.
79. Sloan EP, Murphy DG, Hast R, Crope MA, Turnbull T, Barrea RS, Ellerson B. Complications and protocol considerations in carbon monoxide poisoned patients who require hyperbaric oxygen therapy: report for a ten-year experience. Ann Emerg Med 1989;18:629–634.
80. Krenzelok EP, Full R, Roth R. Carbon monoxide. The silent killer with an audible slution. Clin Toxicol 1995;33:475–486 (abstract 132).

CYANIDE POISONING

Symptoms can occur within seconds of HCN inhalation, within minutes after ingestion of cyanide salts, and may be delayed up to 12 hours after ingestion of cyanogenic glycosides, nitriles, or thiocyanates.

Cyanide is one of the most rapidly acting lethal poisons and is well known to the public for such homicidal disasters as the Jonestown massacre and the cyanide-Tylenol deaths. Under normal conditions, cyanide appears in the blood of healthy individuals as a result of vitamin B_{12} metabolism and environmental factors such as food and smoking. Acute toxicity may result from medicinal uses (e.g., Laetrile), industrial exposures, genocide, and suicidal attempts (especially in chemists). Continuous nitroprusside infusions may produce a subacute cyanide toxicity after several days of therapy. Chronic cyanide exposure also presents a health hazard and is associated with tropical ataxic neuropathy from chronic cassava consumption, tobacco amblyopia from smoking, and Leber's optic atrophy from a congenital metabolic defect in cyanide metabolism.

STRUCTURE/CHARACTERISTICS

Cyanide exists as a gas or the liquid hydrogen cyanide (HCN), which is also known as prussic acid. Common salts of cyanide ion (CN^-) are potassium, sodium, and calcium. Cyanide appears in many forms, including cyanuric chloride, cyanoacetamide, cyanoacetonitrile, mercury compounds, cyanomethyl acetate, cyanoethyl acrylate, cyanamid, halogenated CN^- (Cl, Br, I, Fl), cyanates, phosphorous compounds, cobalticyanic acid, cyanuric acid, cyanoacetic acid, cyanodiethylamide, and cyanogenic glucosides (e.g., amygdalin); however, all of these compounds do not produce acute cyanide poisoning.

SOURCES

Industry

Commercial applications of cyanide include electroplating (HCN gas, CN^- particulates in air), extraction of ores (gold, silver), metal processing, photographic processes, production of synthetic rubber (acetonitrile, acrylonitrile, glyconitrile), chemical synthesis, manufacture of plastics, pesticide/rodenticide control (e.g., fumigant for rodents in ships and greenhouses, insecticides, oil sterilization), dehairing of hides, and laboratory processes. The most commonly employed method of illicit manufacture of phencyclidine (PCP) uses KCN, and an intermediate containing CN^- (cyclohexane carbonitrile) can contaminate improperly synthesized PCP.

Plants (Cyanogenic Glycosides)

Cyanogenic glucosides are present in significant concentrations in a wide variety of plants and plant parts (Table 66–20). Naturally occurring enzymes present in such plant parts as fruit pits hydrolyze the glycosides and release HCN. Hydrolysis of amygdalin (active ingredient of Laetrile) by the enzyme emulsin results in gentibiose (a sugar), benzaldehyde (an aldehyde), and HCN. Beta-glucosidase, which is present in the human gastrointestinal tract, nuts, seeds, fruit pits, and vegetables, will convert amygdalin to HCN in the human gut. Sources of common cyanogenic glycosides include the following:

Amygdalin

Bitter almonds and apricot seeds have high levels, whereas peach, plum, pear, and apple pits have smaller amounts.

Table 66-20
Cyanogenic Plants[a]

Christmas berry	Sudan grass
Velvet grass	Arrow grass
Linium species	Pear (seeds)
Prunus species (leaves, bark, seeds)	Apple (seeds)
	Crab apple (seeds)
Cherry laurel	Jetberry bush (jet bead)
Western chokeberry	Elderberry (leaves and shoots)
Mountain mahogany	Hydrangea (leaves and buds)
Pin cherry	Bamboo (sprouts)
Wild black cherry	Cassava (beans and roots)
Chokecherry	Cycad nut
Plum	Lima beans (black beans from Puerto Rico and tropical countries; not those grown in United States)
Bitter almond	
Peach	
Apricot	
Sorghum species	
Johnson grass	
Sorghum	

[a]Adapted from Kingsbury JM. Poisonous Plants of the United States and Canada. Englewood Cliffs, NJ: Prentice-Hall, 1964, p. 26.

Prunasin

Cherry laurel. Prunasin is the primary metabolite of orally administered amygdalin. It is produced at the mucosal absorption site by a true "first-pass" effect.

Dhurrin

Sorghum.

Linamarin

Cassava and certain lima beans (CN^- content varies between species with black Puerto Rican beans being the most lethal). Linase or acid hydrolysis yields hydrocyanic acid from linamarin.

Combustion

Polyurethane and polyacrylonitrile, which are commonly used in modern plastic furniture, release HCN on combustion. Natural products such as silk and wool also release cyanide during fires. Cyanide toxicity may be an important contributor to tissue hypoxia in some severe smoke inhalation injuries. Although carbon monoxide poisoning commonly accounts for most fire deaths, significantly elevated cyanide levels have been reported in survivors of severe smoke inhalation.[1] Each cigarette liberates between 150 and 200 μg of HCN, and smokers have high thiocyanate levels. Tobacco amblyopia may be secondary to cyanide in cigarette smoke.

MEDICINAL USES

Laetrile has been sanctioned for use in 22 states, including California, despite the fact that studies have disproven its usefulness in cancer treatment.[2] No FDA approval for Laetrile has been given. In the presence of gut beta-glucosidase or emulsin within the gastrointestinal tract, Laetrile releases cyanide. Intravenous Laetrile does not produce cyanide poisoning. Fatalities and near-fatalities have been reported from both suicidal ingestion in adults and accidental ingestion in children. Nitroprusside is an intravenous antihypertensive medication used for acute hypertensive crisis, aortic dissection, hypotensive anesthesia, and myocardial work reduction by the ischemic or infarcted heart. Cyanide is a metabolite of nitroprusside, and toxicity results from rapid infusion, prolonged use where tachyphylaxis requires high doses, or renal failure.

ACUTE TOXIC DOSAGE

Inhalation

Cyanide gas is a rapid-acting poison producing symptoms in seconds and death in minutes. Cyanide toxicity occurred in a man attempting mouth-to-nose ventilation on a dog who swallowed cyanide.[3] The threshold of bitter almond odor (genetically determined and absent in 20 to 40% of the population) is 0.2 to 5 ppm. The current United States exposure limit as an 8-hour TWA is 10 ppm, although reduction to 5 ppm has been recommended. Slight symptoms (e.g., headache) develop after several hours of exposure to 18 to 36 ppm. Animals tolerate exposure to 45 to 54 ppm for ½ to 1 hour without difficulty. Death probably occurs in 1 hour at 100 ppm; 300-ppm exposures prove fatal within several minutes.

Ingestion

Cyanide is a potent oral poison producing symptoms in minutes and death in minutes to hours. One teaspoon of 20% liquid HCN has been fatal. The lethal adult dose of HCN is 50 mg. The lethal oral adult dose of cyanide salts (e.g., KCN) is 200 to 300 mg, and the calculated lethal dose of KCN in children is 1.2 to 5 mg/kg. Survival has occurred after an adult ingested 300 g of CN^- salt.[4] A lethal dose for cyanogenic plant ingestions cannot be predicted because of variations in HCN content, extraction methods, and metabolism.

Laetrile is synthesized from amygdalin. One gram of Laetrile contains the equivalent of 60 mg of cyanide, and each Laetrile tablet may contain up to 100 mg of Laetrile. A 12- to 18-tablet Laetrile overdose produced severe metabolic acidosis and convulsions in an adult who responded to prompt administration of nitrites and thiosulfate.[5]

Nitroprusside Infusion

Higher-than-recommended doses and prolonged infusion produce symptoms of cyanide poisoning. Recommended limits are 1 to 1.5 mg/kg for 1 to 3 hours and 0.5 mg/kg/hr for treatment exceeding 48 hours.[6] Toxicity also results from rapid infusion and the presence of renal failure.

TOXICOKINETICS

Absorption

Usually, rapid absorption occurs. Inhalation of high cyanide gas concentrations results in symptoms within seconds. Hydrochloric acid in the stomach causes the release of HCN, which is rapidly absorbed as the cyanide ion (CN^-). Good absorption occurs across both mucous membranes and intact skin.

Distribution

Cyanide is concentrated in red blood cells at a RBC/plasma ratio of 100/1. The volume of distribution of cyanide ion is approximately 1.5 L/kg. About 60% of CN^- in plasma is protein bound.

Elimination

Cyanide is metabolized by at least four pathways. The enzyme rhodanese converts the majority of cyanide (80%) in the presence of thiosulfate to thiocyanate, which the kidney excretes. The rate-limiting step is the amount of thiosulfate:

$$CN^- + \text{thiosulfate } \textit{rhodanese} \rightarrow \text{thiocyanate} + \text{sulfite}$$

Rhodanese is present in high concentrations in the liver and kidney (especially mitochondria), but the supply of thiosulfate is limited. Alternate pathways include the conversion of hydroxocobalamin (vitamin B_{12a}) in the presence of HCN to the nontoxic cyanocobalamin (vitamin B_{12}). Only small amounts of cyanide are excreted in the lung and sweat, where they produce a bitter almond odor.

PATHOPHYSIOLOGY

Biochemistry

Cyanide binds to heme iron in the cytochrome a-a_3 complex with greatest affinity for oxidized iron (Fe^{3+}). This complex inhibits the final step of oxidative phosphorylation and halts aerobic metabolism. The patient essentially suffocates from an inability to use oxygen, since the tricarboxylic acid cycle requires cytochrome oxidase to produce 38 mol of ATP per mole of glucose. The diversion of carbohydrate metabolism from pyruvate to lactate production then results in a rapid accumulation of lactic acid. A number of enzymes are more sensitive to cyanide than cytochrome oxidase; therefore cyanide toxicity may be a complex biochemical lesion resulting from the inhibition of multiple enzyme systems involving Schiff-base intermediates and metalloenzymes.[7]

Acute Exposures

In minimal lethal doses, cyanide affects primarily the central nervous system. Cyanide initially stimulates the peripheral chemoreceptors, causing increased respirations. It also promotes slowing of the heart by stimulating the carotid body receptors. The electrical activity of the brain may stop while the heart is still beating. No specific pathologic changes characterize cyanide toxicity, although necrosis occurs more often than demyelination and lesions occur primarily in the white matter in monkeys.

Chronic Exposures

Visual abnormalities of tobacco amblyopia are associated with heavy smoking and vitamin B_{12} deficiency. Leber's hereditary optic atrophy probably results from inborn errors of metabolism that produce low urinary and plasma thiocyanate levels in the presence of normal liver rhodanese levels. The suspected inborn metabolic deficiency limits the ability of the patient to detoxify cyanide by conversion to thiocyanate. The signs and symptoms of tropical ataxic neuropathy have been linked with chronic cassava consumption and elevated thiocyanate levels.[8] These patients apparently are not deficient in vitamin B_{12}, and hydroxocobalamin is not as efficacious in treating tropical ataxic neuropathy as it is in treating Leber's hereditary optic atrophy.

Nitroprusside

Normal hepatic clearance of cyanide by conversion to thiocyanate corresponds to a nitroprusside infusion rate of less than 2 μg/kg/min. Nitroprusside infusions given at rates of over 4 μg/kg/min can produce toxic cyanide concentrations in 5 to 10 hours. Lactic acidosis and venous hyperoxemia may not be present for several hours after nitroprusside administration, making the diagnosis of nitroprusside-induced cyanide toxicity difficult. Patients with renal insufficiency are also at risk for developing thiocyanate toxicity, which may be manifested by confusion, hyperreflexia, seizures, coma, and death.[9,10]

Toxicity may result from the metabolism of the five cyanide groups of nitroprusside, $Na_2Fe(CN)_5NO$, although altered hemodynamic parameters also may play a role. One heme group on the hemoglobin molecule is oxidized to ferric form (Fe^{3+}) and, by trapping one of five cyanide groups, forms cyanomethemoglobin. The other four cyanide molecules diffuse into red blood cells and bind to cytochrome oxidase. CN in cyanomethemoglobin is inactive, although it is measured as part of the elevated blood cyanide levels seen during nitroprusside infusions. Simultaneous infusion of thiosulfate reduces toxicity.

CLINICAL PRESENTATION

Acute Toxicity

Signs and symptoms of acute cyanide poisoning reflect cellular hypoxia and often are nonspecific. Onset of symptoms depends on dose, route, and duration of exposure. Inhalation produces the most rapid and serious exposures, resulting in flushing, headache, tachypnea, and dizziness within 30 seconds and progressing to irregular stridorous breathing, coma, seizures, and death within 10 minutes. Oral exposures are less rapid because of slower entry into the circulation and passage of cyanide through the portal system, where the liver detoxifies some cyanide by the first-pass effect. Rapid onset of coma suggests toxins such as cyanide, hydrogen sulfide, carbon monoxide, nicotine, and rapidly acting narcotics or barbiturates. The absence of cyanosis despite respiratory depression suggests cyanide poisoning.

Nervous System

The central nervous system (CNS) is the most sensitive target organ of cyanide poisoning, with early stimulation followed by CNS depression. Early symptoms include lightheadedness, giddiness, tachypnea, nausea, vomiting, feeling of neck constriction and suffocation, confusion, restlessness, and anxiety. Initial tachypnea results from direct stimulation of carotid body chemoreceptors followed by respiratory depression. Severe cyanide poisonings progress to stupor, coma, opisthotonus, convulsions, fixed dilated pupils, and death.

Cardiovascular System

Depression of the cardiovascular system requires cyanide doses higher than those necessary for depression of the CNS. Initial tachycardia occurs followed by bradycardia. Dysrhythmias and hypotension often precede peripheral vascular collapse. The ECG may display striking ischemic changes; pulmonary edema may complicate severe intoxications.[4]

Skin/Ocular Signs

In serious poisonings, the skin is cold, clammy, and diaphoretic. Cyanosis may be a late finding, since poor tissue utilization of oxygen results in elevated venous oxygen levels. Retinal veins and arteries may appear similar in color because of the elevated venous oxygen level.

Differential Diagnosis

Diagnosis of cyanide toxicity is difficult because of the lack of pathognomonic signs. Classic signs of bright red venous blood, profound metabolic acidosis, and bitter almond breath often are absent. A hypertensive, bradycardiac, acyanotic, and tachypneic patient suggests cyanide poisoning, especially when the patient subsequently develops CNS and cardiovascular depression. Cyanide should be included in the differential diagnosis of rapid onset of coma and whenever coma and metabolic acidosis appear together.

Chronic and Subacute Exposures

Chronic Occupational Exposures

The most common symptoms of a long-term cyanide exposure that has exceeded current standards have been headache, dizziness, nausea or vomiting, and a bitter or almond taste.[11] Mild abnormalities of vitamin B_{12}, folate, and thyroid function have been noted, but symptoms did not correlate with these changes. Other excessive exposures to cyanide have resulted in psychosis and thyroid enlargement without symptoms of thyroid dysfunction.[12] Several clinical syndromes have been associated with chronic cyanide toxicity, although the American literature contains few studies confirming this link. These diseases may be due to high cyanide levels, impaired cyanide detoxification mechanisms, nutritional deficiencies, or some combination of these factors.[7]

Tobacco Amblyopia

This disease is similar to the retrobulbar neuritis associated with pernicious anemia. Central scotomata develop with occasional temporal pallor of the optic disk. Hydroxocobalamin (vitamin B_{12a}) improves visual acuity and field defects in some patients, despite the fact that saline loading in these patients reveals that vitamin B_{12} metabolism appears normal.

Leber's Hereditary Optic Atrophy

Depressed plasma thiocyanate levels occur. Hydroxocobalamin improves vision in some patients. Congenital susceptibility or metabolic defect may increase the sensitivity of the optic nerve to cyanide.

Nigerian Nutritional Ataxic Neuropathy

This disease is prevalent in populations consuming large portions of the cyanogenic glycoside–containing cassava *Manihot*, which constitutes the bulk of the south Nigerian diet. Segmental demyelination leads to a peripheral sensory neuropathy, optic atrophy, ataxia, and deafness. Glossitis, stomatitis, and scrotal dermatitis also may be present. Studies in these patients indicate elevated plasma thiocyanate levels and reduced concentrations of sulfur-containing amino acids, which suggests that nutritional factors are important in addition to cassava consumption.

Konzo

Individuals from the Central African Republic develop Konzo, an upper motor neuron disease associated with high dietary cyanide exposure from near-exclusive consumption of insufficiently processed bitter cassava containing cyanogenic glycosides plus a low protein intake. An isolated symmetric spastic paraparesis begins abruptly. The serum thiocyanate concentration is elevated.[13] This disorder is similar to Nigerian nutritional ataxic neuropathy.

Nitroprusside

Increasing tachyphylaxis requiring continuously higher nitroprusside doses to lower blood pressure, together with increasing metabolic acidosis, characterizes nitroprusside toxicity. Symptoms include tachycardia, dyspnea, vomiting, headache, ataxia, and altered mental status.[14]

LABORATORY

Blood Levels

Blood cyanide levels are useful in confirming toxicity, but therapeutic interventions usually must be made before the level is available. Although extensive data exist on cyanide blood levels in animals, documentation of human cyanide levels is sparse. (A 1977 case study cited only four cases with documented cyanide levels in the last 100 years.)[4]

The normal *plasma* cyanide level for nonsmoking patients is 0.004 μg/mL (1 μg/mL is equivalent to 1 ppm). Smoking elevates normal plasma levels to 0.006 μg/mL (smokers have both elevated cyanide and elevated thiocyanate levels in blood and urine), and concurrent nitroprusside therapy elevates them to between 0.01 and 0.06 μg/mL. Normal *whole blood* cyanide levels are higher than plasma cyanide levels because of the concentration of cyanide in the red blood cells (e.g., nonsmoking—0.016 μg/mL; smoking—0.041 μg/mL; concurrent nitroprusside therapy—0.05 to 0.5 μg/mL).

Correlation of symptoms to *whole blood* cyanide levels may be misleading, since the effect of cyanide depends on the *intracellular* concentration at the cytochrome oxidase binding sites, the duration of poisoning, and perhaps the route of toxicity. Levels lower than 0.2 μg/mL usually cause no symptoms. At concentrations between 0.5 and 1.0 μg/mL the patient is conscious and flushed with tachycardia. Stupor and agitation appear between 1.0 and 2.5 μg/mL. Levels over 2.5 μg/mL are associated with coma and are potentially fatal.

Assay

Although microdiffusion techniques using the Conway cell generally require 2 to 4 hours, a modification of the procedure involving pyridine-barbituric acid reagents allows a semiquantitative reading after 10 minutes of diffusion for the emergency situation.[15]

The Lee-Jones test is a quantitative cyanide rapid spot test performed on gastric aspirate.

1. Add a few crystals of ferrous sulfate to 5 mL of gastric aspirate.
2. Add 4 to 5 drops of 2% NaOH to precipitate iron.
3. Boil and then cool.
4. Acidify solution with 8 to 10 drops 10% HCl.
5. Interpret.

A greenish blue color or precipitate that intensifies on standing indicates cyanide. The presence of salicylate alone causes a purplish color. Presence of both salicylates and cyanide causes an immediate blue-green color, which may be masked by the purple color. No reaction occurs with barbiturates, phenothiazines, imipramine, benzodiazepines, or amitriptyline.

Rapid Tests

A paper test for cyanide in blood at blood cyanide concentrations of over 1.0 mg/liter is sensitive to a concentration of 0.2 mg/L of cyanide in whole blood. The paper (CYANTOSNO) is available in the United States from Fallard-Schlesinger, 584 Mineola Ave, Carle Place, NY 11514-1744). Preliminary studies suggest its potential usefulness in determination of the presence of over 0.5 mg/liter of cyanide after an acute cyanide poisoning or after exposure to fire.[16] Further clinical studies will no doubt determine its accuracy and clinical usefulness.

A rapid (about 20 minutes) specific and sensitive assay method for cyanide determination in whole blood has been developed by Laforge and colleagues.[17]

Surrogate Measure of Cyanide Intoxication[18]

Laboratory tests that suggest cyanide intoxication include:

1. A serum lactate level of more than 10 mmol/L may be highly predictive of "toxic" cyanide levels (more than 40 μmol/L or more than 1.00 μg/mL).
2. The serum anion gap, while less specific than a serum lactate level, also has been found to be elevated.
3. Whole blood cyanide levels are more closely related to pH than to anion gap.
4. Arterial blood gas determination (pH), while somewhat invasive, may be superior to the serum anion gap for the estimation of whole blood cyanide levels.
5. Even more specific may be the simultaneous determination of arterial and venous O_2 saturations with an eye toward so-called "arteriolization of venous blood" (decreased peripheral oxygen extraction).

Abnormalities

Changes noted on the ECG during cyanide intoxication are nonspecific and reflect cellular hypoxia. Tachycardia and nonspecific ST-T wave changes appear first. Atrioventricular block, a short Q-T interval, and an obliterated ST interval also can occur. Later, the ECG exhibits signs of progressive hypoxia with bradycardia and nodal or idioventricular rhythm, followed by atrioventricular block and a slow agonal rhythm. A striking ST elevation may be present, especially in patients with underlying cardiovascular disease.

Electrical activity in the basal ganglia, hypothalamus, and midbrain is depressed before similar depression in pons and medullary activity. Clinical parkinsonism due to cyanide exposure may be associated with bilateral lucencies in the putamen and external globus pallidus.[19–22] Arterial-venous oxygen difference often is diminished because of the decreased tissue utilization of oxygen. Severe metabolic acidosis occurs depending on the degree of cellular hypoxia.

TREATMENT

Stabilization

Rapid support of respiration and circulation is essential to successful treatment of cyanide intoxication. Massive cyanide overdoses have survived with only good supportive care.[4] Immediate attention should be directed toward assisted ventilation, administration of 100% oxygen, insertion of intravenous lines, and institution of cardiac monitoring. Obtain an arterial blood gas immediately and correct any severe metabolic acidosis (pH below 7.15). Oxygen (100%) should be used routinely in moderate or severely symptomatic patients even in the presence of a normal P_{O2}, since 100% O_2 increases O_2 delivery, may reactivate cyanide-inhibited mitochondrial enzymes, and potentiates the effect of thiosulfate.[23]

Decontamination

Remove contaminated clothing and rinse all cyanide-contaminated skin with green soap. Because of the rapid onset of cyanide toxicity, gut decontamination should follow antidote therapy. Gastric lavage, charcoal, and cathartics may be used after antidote therapy if less than 2 hours has passed since ingestion.

Elimination Enhancement

Hemodialysis and hemoperfusion are ineffective. Use of hyperbaric oxygen has been suggested, but few data on humans exist to recommend its use in cyanide toxicity. Hyperbaric oxygen therapy should be considered only in patients not responding to standard therapy, with the knowledge that its effectiveness is unproven.[24] Hyperbaric oxygen does not appear to add to the value of normobaric oxygen in the treatment of cyanide poisoning.[25]

ANTIDOTES

Although a variety of agents are effective antidotes in the experimental animal (nitrites, dimethylaminophenol, cobalt EDTA, hydroxocobalamin, stroma-free methemoglobin solutions, pyruvate, thiosulfate, sulfur sulfanes, mercaptopyruvate, oxygen), only the three-step Eli Lilly cyanide kit is approved in the United States.[26]

Nitrites

Mechanism of Action

These compounds induce methemoglobinemia, which was thought to attract cyanide off the heme group of cytochrome oxidase, allowing thiosulfate to detoxify the cyanide (Fig. 66–3). The antidotal effect of nitrite is very rapid, whereas the formation of methemoglobin by nitrites is relatively slow; however, nitrites and thiosulfates are equally effective either prophylactically or antidotally in animal models.[27] Hence, methemoglobinemia may not play a major role in cyanide detoxification.[7] Current research centers on the effect of nitrite-induced vasodilation on cyanide detoxification, although it remains unclear why nitrites work while other vasodilators do not. In some but not all animal studies chlorpromazine and phenoxybenzamine have been shown to potentiate the antidotal effect of thiosulfates, and alpha-agonist agents appear to abolish these positive effects.[28]

Indications

Because of the potentially adverse effects and the fact that patients have survived with supportive care only, nitrites should not be given indiscriminately. In all cases of moderate to severe cyanide poisoning, nitrites should be given along with thiosulfate. Mildly symptomatic patients who are alert may be given supportive care, unless their mental status deteriorates or they develop a metabolic acidosis.[29]

Dosage

Amyl nitrite perles are designed to produce 3 to 5% methemoglobinemia while an intravenous line is established for intravenous sodium nitrite. As a temporizing measure, the patient inhales the vapors until the sodium nitrite is ready. Because of the variability in methemoglobin production and the potential for cardiovascular collapse, this step may be omitted if sodium nitrite is readily available and the patient is not in extremis. Adequate ventilation and oxygenation are more important than administration of amyl nitrite. One perle (0.2 mL) is crushed and inhaled for 30 seconds every minute until intravenous nitrite is given. Sodium nitrite (3% solution), as 10 mL of a 3% solution (i.e., 300 mg), is administered IV slowly over 4 minutes to produce a 20% methemoglobin level in adults. Children should receive 0.33 mL of the 3% solution per kilogram initially at an infusion rate of 2.5 mL/min, up to a maximum of 10 mL. Administer sodium nitrite doses to children on the basis of body weight, since fatal methemoglobinemia has occurred in children. Time permitting, adjustments should also be made for hemoglobin concentrations, which can be estimated from

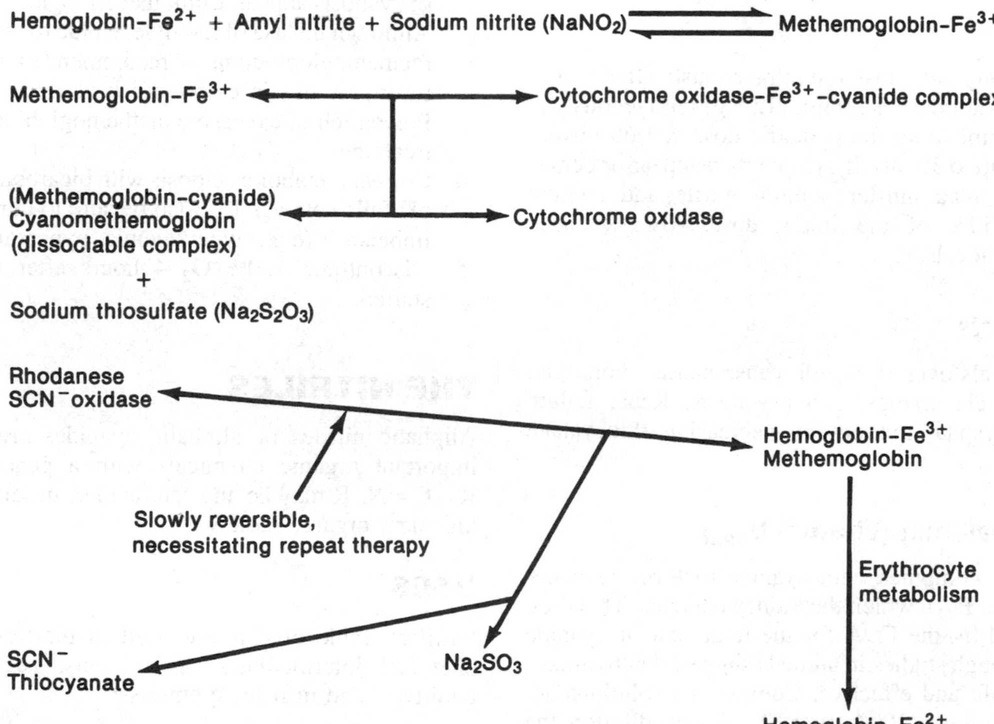

Figure 66–3 Mechanism of cyanide treatment. (Adapted from Goldfrank LR, Kirstein R: Cyanide (bitter almonds) in toxicologic emergencies. In: Goldfrank LR, Flomenbaum NE, Lewin NA et al, eds. A comprehensive handbook in problem solving. New York: Appleton-Century-Crofts, 1982, p. 99.)

centrifuged capillary tube blood specimens. The shelf life of amyl nitrite is 1 year, while that of sodium nitrite is 5 years.

Adverse Effects

Nitrites produce both hypotension and methemoglobinemia. Cyanosis appears at 15% methemoglobin levels, but symptoms usually do not appear until the level reaches 30 to 40%. The lethal methemoglobin level is 70%. Nitrites must be used with caution in patients with severe cardiovascular or cerebral vascular disease. Headache, nausea, vomiting, hypotension, and syncope can occur after nitrite administration.

Thiosulfates

Mechanism of Action

Rhodanese, a sulfur transferase enzyme located in the mitochondria, catalyzes the irreversible transfer of a sulfane donor from thiosulfate to cyanide, which produces the nontoxic thiocyanate. Since thiosulfate does not penetrate cells well, large doses are required and the detoxification rate is slow. Other sulfur transferase enzymes (e.g., mercaptopyruvate) may detoxify cyanide, provided adequate sulfur donors exist. A sulfur-sulfane serum albumin complex may provide the needed transport.[7] The kidney excretes thiocyanate.

Indications

Thiosulfates are given with nitrites for confirmed cyanide poisoning and are available in the Eli Lilly cyanide antidote kit.

Dosage

The 25% solution is administered intravenously after nitrites are given. The adult dose is 50 mL (12.5 g) intravenously at a rate of 3 to 5 mL/min; the pediatric dose is 1.65 mL/kg (412.5 mg/kg) up to 50 mL. If symptoms reappear or persist within 1 hour, readminister sodium nitrite and sodium thiosulfate at 50% of the initial dose. Always check methemoglobin levels.

Adverse Effects

Thiocyanate levels over 10 mg/dL cause nausea, vomiting, arthralgias, muscle cramps, and psychosis. Renal failure enhances thiocyanate toxicity by decreasing thiocyanate excretion.

Hydroxocobalamin (Vitamin B_{12a})

This compound combines with cyanide to form cyanocobalamin (vitamin B_{12}), which the kidney excretes. This drug is not approved by the FDA for the treatment of cyanide poisoning, although studies in animals suggest that hydroxocobalamin is safe and effective. Commercial solutions are expensive and dilute (1000 μg/mL). At this dilution the recommended dose (50 mg/kg) requires the administration of 3500 mL of fluid to a 70-kg adult. Limited human experience precludes a specific dosage recommendation for cyanide poisoning, although 50 times the ingested cyanide dose has been recommended. Continuous prophylactic use (25 mg hydroxocobalamin per hour) was suggested to prevent nitroprusside-induced cyanide toxicity,[30] but its current use in preference to thiosulfate cannot be recommended.

Cobalt EDTA

This compound is available in France (as Kelocyanor) but not in the United States. Cobalt compounds chelate cyanide and therefore cause no methemoglobinemia. Occasional vomiting and rare anaphylactic reactions occur. Patients have developed marked facial edema, retrosternal chest pain, diaphoresis, ventricular tachycardia, and laryngeal edema requiring intubation after intravenous administration of dicobalt edetate (Co_2EDTA) for cyanide poisoning.[31] Co_2EDTA acts more rapidly than nitrites and is used extensively in Britain and France. Concern about cobalt toxicity led to its recommended use as a second-line antidote after a lack of response to nitrites.[32]

Methylene Blue

Methylene blue is *not* an antidote. Its use increases cyanide release; clinical deterioration ensues when methylene blue is given to cyanide-intoxicated patients.

Supportive Care

1. Follow the patient for at least 24 to 48 hours.
2. Watch for development of pulmonary edema and aspiration pneumonia in comatose patients.
3. Follow methemoglobin levels during nitrite treatment beginning ½ to 1 hour after initial dose or when signs of cyanosis appear. Limit methemoglobin levels to 40%. Although the use of methylene blue to reverse excessive methemoglobinemia is recommended in the package insert, its use is extremely hazardous in this setting. Prevention of excessive methemoglobinemia is the best treatment.
4. Correct metabolic acidosis with bicarbonate when blood pH falls below 7.15. Also be sure to correct electrolyte imbalance (e.g., hyperkalemia, hypercalcemia).
5. Discontinue 100% O_2 4 hours after the antidote is started.

THE NITRILES

Aliphatic nitriles or aliphatic cyanides are commercially important organic chemicals with a general formula of $R-C\equiv N$. R may be any saturated or unsaturated aliphatic univalent organic moiety.[34]

USES

Nitriles (Table 66–21) are used in plastic production, as chemical intermediates, as solvents, as lubricating oil additives, and in resin synthesis.[33]

CLINICAL PRESENTATION

Human experience following exposure to nitriles is restricted to published data on exposure to acetonitrile,[35–40]

Table 66-21
The Nitriles

Acetonitrile	Solvent for removal of acrylic sculptured nails Chemical intermediate
Acrylonitrile	Plastic production fumigant
Adiponitrile	Nylon manufacture
Allylnitrile	
n-butyronitrile	Chemical intermediate
2-chlorobenzylidene malononitrile	Lacrimator (see Lacrimators)
Crotononotrile	
Glycolonitrile	Chemical intermediate
Isobutyronitrile	Gasoline additive Chemical intermediate
Malononitrile	Lubricating-oil additive Chemical intermediate
Methacrylonitrile	Plastic production
2-Methyllactonitrile	Resin synthesis intermediate
2-Pentenenitrile	
Propionitrile	Solvent, chemical intermediate
Succinonitrile	Chemical intermediate
Tetrachlorophthalonitrile	Agricultural chemical

methylactronitrile,[41] acrylonitrile,[42] ioxynil (4-hydroxy-3,5-di-iodobenzonitrile), and propionitrile.[43] Following acetonitrile exposure the earliest symptoms are nausea and vomiting. A latent period (hepatic production of cyanide) may last up to 12 hours. Other symptoms may include headache, lassitude, abdominal cramps, weakness, hyporeflexia, urinary frequency, stupor, shock, respiratory depression, hypothermia, and bradycardia.[44] There may be a rapid progression of coma, lactic acidosis, and respiratory arrest due to damage of brainstem neurons controlling respiratory drive. Other organs affected are the skin (painful blisters, sweating, rashes), eyes (conjunctivitis), gastrointestinal tract (nausea, vomiting), metabolism (metabolic acidosis with a decreased arteriovenous oxygen gradient), cardiovascular system (tachycardia, decreased cardiac output, hypotension, electrocardiographic evidence of depressed ST segments, varying degrees of AV block, erratic supraventricular rhythm or ventricular fibrillation), and respiratory tract (tachypnea, respiratory arrest).

CHRONIC EXPOSURE

Vertigo, mental deterioration, weakness, anorexia, and weight loss may be observed. Chronic cyanide poisoning may be associated with thyromegaly, altered B_{12} and folate metabolism, personality changes, extrapyramidal syndromes, optic atrophy, demyelinating syndromes, and psychosis.

LABORATORY

Confirmation of intoxication may be made by a blood cyanide concentration. These are not often available in time for clinical management decision.

0.5 to 1.0 mcg/mL: alert, flushed, tachycardic
1.0 to 2.5 mcg/mL: obtunded
Over 2.5 mcg/mL: coma, respiratory depression, death

Serial cyanide and thiocyanate levels are indicated because of the slow generation of cyanide after exposure to nitriles. Nitrile half-lives may be as long as 32 hours.[45]

TREATMENT

Remove victim to fresh air by a protected rescuer. Airway, breathing, and circulatory stability are confirmed (see Cyanide—Treatment of Overdose). Although the Lilly Antidote Kit is available in the United States, hydroxocobalamin (4 g) followed by sodium thiosulfate (80 g) IV is not. Decontamination of the gastrointestinal tract (include activated charcoal) has not been evaluated. Skin or eye exposure should be treated with active irrigation by water for at least 15 minutes. Patients should be repeatedly assessed for at least 24 hours.[46] Death may follow exposure to the acetonitriles.[2]

Although the metabolism of acetonitrile to inorganic cyanide usually requires 3 or more hours, (the parent compound is not toxic until converted to cyanide), acrylonitrile and methylactonitrile[47] may cause symptoms within 1 hour, and propionitrile may induce coma within minutes. Management follows the usual procedure for cyanide poisoning. (See Cyanide Treatment Protocol.)

REFERENCES—THE NITRILES

1. Clark CJ, Campbell D, Reid WH. Blood carboxyhemoglobin and cyanide levels in fire survivors. Lancet 1981;1:1332–1335.
2. Moertel CG, Fleming TR, Rubin J et al. A clinical trial of amygdalin (Laetrile) in the treatment of human cancer. N Engl J Med 1982;306:201–206.
3. Berumen U. Dog poisons man. JAMA 1983:249:353.
4. Graham DL, Laman D, Theodore J et al. Acute cyanide poisoning complicated by lactic acidosis and pulmonary edema. Arch Intern Med 1977;137:1051–1055.
5. Beamer WC, Shealy RM, Prough DS. Acute cyanide poisoning from Laetrile ingestion. Ann Emerg Med 1983;12:449–451.
6. Vesey CJ, Cole PV, Simpson PV. Cyanide and thiocyanate concentrations following sodium nitroprusside infusions in man. Br J Anaesth 1976;48:651–660.
7. Way JL. Cyanide intoxication and its mechanism of antagonism. Annu Rev Pharmacol Toxicol 1984;24:451–481.
8. Osintokun BD, Adenja AOG, Aladehoyinbo A. Free cyanide levels in tropical ataxic neuropathy. Lancet 1970;2:372–373.
9. Zerbe NF, Wagner BKJ. Use of vitamin B_{12} in the treatment and prevention of nitroprusside-induced cyanide toxicity. Crit Care Med 1993;21:465–467.
10. Rieves RD. Importance of symptoms in recognizing nitroprusside toxicity. South Med J 1984;77:1035–1037.
11. Blanc P, Hogan M, Mallin K et al. Cyanide intoxication among silver reclaiming workers. JAMA 1985;253:367–371.
12. Ghawabi SH, Gadfar MA, El-Saharti AA et al. Chronic cyanide exposure: a clinical radioisotope and laboratory study. Br J Ind Med 1975;32:215–219.
13. Tylleskar T, Legue FD, Peterson S, Kpizingui E, Stecker P. Konzo in the Central African Republic. Neurology 1994; 44:959–961.
14. Drew RH. The use of hydroxocobalamin in the prophylaxis and treatment of nitroprusside-induced cyanide toxicity. Vet Hum Toxicol 1983;25:342–345.
15. Holzbecher M, Ellenberger HA. An evaluation and modification of a microdiffusion method for the emergency determination of blood cyanide. J Anal Toxicol 1985;9:251–253.
16. Fligner CL, Luthi R, Linkaityte E, Raisys VA. Paper strip method for detection of cyanide in blood using CYANTESNO test paper. Am J Forensic Med Pathol 1992;13:81–84.

17. LaForge M, Buneaur F, Hoveto P, Bourgeois F, Bourdon R, Levillein P. A rapid spectrophotometric blood cyanide determination applicable to emergency toxicology. J Anal Toxicol 1994;18:173–175.
18. Shusterman D, Hargis C. Surrogate laboratory measures of cyanide intoxication. Ann Emerg Med 1994;74:527–538.
19. Rosenberg NL, Myers JA, Martin WRW. Cyanide-induced parkinsonism: clinical, MRI and 6-fluorodopa (FD) position emission tomography (PET) studies. Neurology 1988;38 (Suppl 1):203.
20. Kadushin FS, Bronstein AC, Riddle MW, Gilmore DA. Cyanide induced parkinsonism: Neuropsychology and radiological findings. Vet Hum Toxicol 1988;30:359.
21. Grandas F, Artieda J, Obeso JA. Clinical and CT scan findings in a case of cyanide intoxication. Movement Disorders 1989;4:188–193.
22. Rosenberg NL, Myers A, Martin WRW. Cyanide-induced parkinsonism: clinical, MRI and 6-fluorodopa PET studies. Neurology 1989;39:142–144.
23. Isom GE, Way JL. Effect of oxygen on cyanide intoxication. VI. Reactivation of cyanide-inhibited glucose metabolism. J Pharmacol Exp Ther 1974;189:235–243.
24. Litowitz TL, Larkin RF, Myers RAM. Cyanide poisoning treated with hyperbaric oxygen. Am J Emerg Med 1983;1:94–101.
25. Kizer KW. Hyperbaric oxygen and cyanide poisoning. Am J Emerg Med 1984;2:113.
26. Way JL. Cyanide antagonism. Fundam Appl Toxicol 1985;3:383–386.
27. Holmes RK, Way JL. Mechanism of cyanide antagonism by sodium nitrite. Pharmacologist 1982;24:182 (abstract 478).
28. Burrows GE, Way LJ. Antagonism of cyanide toxicity by phenoxybenzamine. Fed Proc 1976;35:533 (abstract 1805).
29. Vogel SN, Sultan TR. Cyanide poisoning. Clin Toxicol 1981;18:367–383.
30. Cotrell JE, Casthely P, Brodie JD et al. Prevention of nitroprusside induced cyanide toxicity with hydroxocobalamin. N Engl J Med 1978;298:809–811.
31. Dodds C, McKnight C. Cyanide toxicity after immersion and the hazards of dicobalt edetate. Br Med J 1985;291:785–786.
32. Nagler J, Provoost RA, Parizel G. Hydrogen cyanide poisoning. Treatment with cobalt EDTA. J Occup Med 1978;20:414–416.
33. Kunkel DB. Cyanide: looking for the source. Emerg Med 1987;19(9):115–125.
34. Willhite CC. Inhalation toxicology of acute exposure to aliphatic nitriles. Clin Toxicol 1981;18:991–1003.
35. Caravati EM, Litovitz TL. Pediatric cyanide intoxication and death from an acetonitrile-containing cosmetic. JAMA 1988;260:3470–3473.
36. Turchen SG, Managuera AS. Severe cyanide poisoning following suicidal ingestion of acetonitrile. Vet Hum Toxicol 1989;31:351.
37. Boggild MD, Peck RW, Tomson CRF. Acetonitrile ingestion delayed onset of cyanide poisoning due to concurrent ingestion of acetone. Postgrad Med J 1990;66:40–41.
38. Kirk MK, Voorhees SL, Kulig R, Rumack BH. Cyanide leverls after acetonitrile exposure. An in-vitro study. Ann Emerg Med 1990;19:628.
39. Geller RJ, Ekins BR, Iknoian RC. Cyanide toxicity from acetonitrile-containing false nail remover. Am J Emerg Med 1991;9:268–270.
40. Kurt T, Day LC, Reed WG, Gandy W. Cyanide poisoning from glue on nail remover. Am J Emerg Med 1991;9:271–272.
41. Bismuth C, Baud FJ, Djeghout H, Astier A, Aubriot D. Cyanide poisoning from propionitrile exposure. J Emerg Med 1987;5:191–195.
42. Vogel RA, Kirkendall KM. Acrylonitrile (vinyl cyanide) poisoning: a case report. Texas Med 1984;80:48–51.
43. Scolnick B, Hamel D, Woolf AD. Successful treatment of life-threatening propionitrile exposure with sodium nitrite/sodium thiosulfate followed by hyperbaric oxygen. J Occup Med 1993;35:577–580.
44. Hryhorczuk DO, Aks SE, Turk JW. Unusual occupational toxics. Occup Med State of the Art Reviews 1992;7:567–586.
45. Michaelis HC, Clemens C, Kijewski H, Newath H, Eggert A. Acetonitrile serum concentrations and cyanide blood levels in a case of suicidal oral acetonitrile ingestion. Clin Toxicol 1991;29:447–458.
46. Geller RJ, Ekins BR, Iknoian RC. Cyanide toxicity from acetonitrile-containing false nail remover. Am J Emerg Med 1991;9:268–270.
47. Winter ML, Nelson DA, Snodgrass WR. Industrial exposure to acetone cyanohydrine. Delayed onset cyanide toxicity. Vet Hum Toxicol 1989;31:354.

ACETONITRILE

Acetonitrile (methyl cyanide) is an organocyanide that is slowly metabolized to inorganic cyanide in a reaction forming hydrogen cyanide. The major toxicity of acetonitrile is due to the in vivo formation of cyanide as a metabolite.[1,2] The diagnosis of acetonitrile poisoning is difficult. It cannot be detected with conventional toxicology panels. The symptoms can mislead the clinician because the delayed onset of symptoms (3 to 12 hours) does not suggest typical cyanide intoxication. Initially the patient may be asymptomatic and sent home. Acetonitrile-induced poisoning must also be included in the differential diagnosis of anion gap and osmolar gap metabolic acidosis.[3,4]

Sufficient acetonitrile is contained in a typical 1-ounce sculptured nail glue removal bottle for severe fatal doses even in a child's single swallow.[5] The bottles do not have child-resistant lids.[6] Diagnosis of acetonitrile ingestion involves differentiating nail polish remover (acetone) from nail glue remover (acetonitrile). Initial symptoms of acetonitrile ingestion are indistinguishable from those of acetone and common alcohols.[4] Patients should be observed and repeatedly evaluated for at least 24 hours. In the absence of cyanide level determinations, lethargy, vomiting, seizures, and the lack of normal venous blood hemoglobin desaturation may be clues to cyanide toxicity.[7]

STRUCTURE AND CLASSIFICATION

Acetonitrile has a molecular formula of CH_3CN and a molecular weight of 41.05. Synonyms include methyl cyanide, ethanenitrile, cyanomethane, ethyl nitrite, and meobam carbonitrile.[1] It is a 2-carbone aliphatic nitrile.[1]

USES

Acetonitrile is used as a solvent remover of acrylic sculptured nails that are bonded to the natural nail with durable glues. The artificial nails are applied with cyanoacrylic glue. Glue-on nails remover should not be confused with regular nail polish removers that contain acetone.

PRODUCT FORMULATION

Acetonitrile is present in a number of products in the United States: Supernail Nailoff, Nailene Salon Quality Glue Remover (84% acetonitrile), Artificial Nail Tip and Glue Remover (95% or more acetonitrile), Super Nail Wrap Off Instant Glue Dissolver, Super Nail Tip Off, Ardell Instant Glue Remover (98 to 100% acetonitrile).[8]

These products are packaged in 0.75- to 2-fl-oz (22.5- to 60 mL) bottles with non–child resistant threaded closures.[8] Some of these products are marketed in supermarkets and drugstores, intended for the general public's use rather than for professional beauty operators. A potentially lethal amount of acetonitrile is present in a single container.[8]

SOURCES

Other alternative agents currently marketed by other manufacturers of acrylic or sculptured nail removers include acetone/ethyl ether, trichloroethylene/mineral oil, and dichloromethane/dimethylketone combinations.[8]

FATAL DOSE

A 16-month-old infant ingested 15 to 30 mL of Super Nail Nail Off (1.2 to 2.4 g/kg of acetonitrile), vomited in 20 minutes, and was found dead the next morning.[8] Ingestion of 5 mL may be fatal in a small child.[6] A 26-year-old who swallowed 40 g of acetonitrile experienced seizures, vomiting, acidosis (pH 6.4), shock, and coma following a 3-hour latency period. The patient recovered after treatment with dicobalt EDTA and hydroxocobalamin.[9]

ELIMINATION KINETICS

Elimination half-lives following an ingestion of 5 mL of 98% acetonitrile were 32 hours for acetonitrile and 15 hours for cyanide.[1]

CLINICAL PRESENTATION

Onset of symptoms are delayed 3 or more hours. Nausea and vomiting are the earliest symptoms. This latent period occurs because the parent molecule has no apparent intrinsic toxicity, but undergoes a two-step activation reaction mediated by cytochrome P450 enzymes (P-450IIE1). This reaction results in the formation of cyanohydrin, which undergoes peroxidation releasing hydrogen cyanide.[1,4,5] Cyanide is then eliminated by the rhodanese-mediated oxidation of endogenous thiosulfate to thiocyanate, that is, in turn, renally excreted. Symptoms do not appear until enough cyanide has been produced to exhaust endogenous stores of thiosulfate or to overwhelm the rhodanese pathway. Patients may exhibit signs and symptoms of cyanide intoxication, including lethargy, seizures, respiratory depression, and death.[4]

LABORATORY

Analytic Methods

Gas chromatography/mass spectrometry can confirm the identification of acetonitrile. A gas chromatography method using a flame-ionization detector has a lower limit of 1 μg/mL of acetonitrile in plasma.[1]

Blood Levels

Plasma cyanide may better correlate with symptoms than whole blood assays. Acetonitrile was present in the blood of a patient who died after an ingestion. The levels were 31 and 56 mg/dL in two samples.[10] Cyanide concentration in the blood was 4.4 μg/mL.[10] Acetonitrile serum levels in the first 25 hours can range from 40 to 80 μg/mL (0.97 to 1.95 mmol/L) and decrease with treatment over 120 hours.[1] Cyanide blood concentration will rapidly decrease after thiosulfate administration.[1,4] Very high serum acetonitrile and cyanide blood levels may be found in the absence of severe clinical symptoms.[1] A 30-year-old man ingested 5 mL of 95% acetonitrile. Five hours later the concentrations of acetonitrile and cyanide were 80 μg/mL and 7.1 μg/mL, respectively.

TREATMENT

Stabilization

Patients should be treated in an intensive care facility immediately after ingestion of acetonitrile where they may be administered antidotes before serious toxic effects occur. Fluid, electrolyte, and acid-base disturbance should be corrected. Supportive care and supplemental oxygen may be sufficient even without concomitant antidotes.[8]

Decontamination

Gastric lavage is advised, rather than syrup of ipecac, due to the anticipated onset of severe cardiovascular compromise and seizures. Activated charcoal may have limited efficacy in cases of inorganic cyanide poisoning due to the rapidity of cyanide's systemic absorption and the onset of severe manifestations of cyanide toxicity. Specific data on acetonitrile binding by activated charcoal is not available.[8]

Elimination Enhancement

Acetonitrile has a low volume of distribution and a low molecular weight. Hemodialysis and hemoperfusion may return thiocyanate concentrations to subtoxic levels. Hemodialysis may be considered for severely poisoned patients since severe symptoms can persist for several days and administration of antidotal therapy may be limited by the sodium content.[4]

Antidotes

Intravenous sodium thiosulfate is the drug of choice for treatment of acetonitrile poisoning. Its high sodium content (each 12.5 g ampule contains 103 meq sodium) and short half-life suggest that a continuous infusion, following an initial bolus, might maintain continuously high thiosulfate levels while minimizing total daily sodium dose. Low-sodium-content IV solutions should be used. Sodium nitrite may exacerbate the hypotension.[4] *P*-Methyl-aminophenol (250 mg) has also been used.[1] Its role in acetonitrile poisoning remains to be determined. Specific antidotes are recommended in seriously poisoned patients who fail to respond immediately to standard supportive measures.

Nitrites seem to be of dubious value. Sodium thiosulfate is probably the treatment of choice.[8] Animal data suggest that the specific cytochrome P-450 enzymes responsible for conversion of acetonitrile to cyanohydron are inducible by ethanol and 4-methylpyrazole.

Supportive Measures

Ethanol may be useful in acetonitrile toxicity. It may act by competing with acetonitrile for oxidation by P-450 IIE1, as well as by acting as a competitive substitute for the peroxidatic activity of catalase-H_2O_2.[5]

REFERENCES—ACETONITRILE

1. Michaelis HC, Clemens C, Kijewski H, Newath H, Eggert A. Acetonitrile serum concentrations and cyanide blood levels in a case of suicidal oral acetonitrile ingestion. Clin Toxicol 1991;29:447–458.
2. Pozzani UC, Carpenter CP, Palin PE, Weil CS, Nair JH III, Spracuse MS. Mammalian toxicity of acetonitrile. J Occup Med 1959;1:634–642.
3. Turchen SG, Manoguerra AS, Whitney C. Severe cyanide poisoning from the ingestion of an acetonitrile-containing cosmetic. Am J Emerg Med 1991;9:264–267.
4. Rainey PM, Roberts WL. Diagnosis and misdiagnosis of poisoning with the cyanide precursor acentonitrile: nail polish remover or nail glue remover? Am J Emerg Med 1993; 11:104–108.
5. Feierman DE, Cederbaum AI. Role of cytochrome P-450 IIE1 and catalase in the oxidation of acetonitrile to cyanide. Chem Res Toxicol 1989;2:359–366.
6. Kurt TL, Day LC, Reed WG, Gandy W. Cyanide poisoning from glue-on-nail remover. Am J Emerg Med 1991;9: 271–272.
7. Geller RJ, Ekins BR, Iknoian RC. Cyanide toxicity from acetonitrile-containing false nail remover. Am J Emerg Med 1991;9:268–270.
8. Caravati EM, Litovitz TL. Pediatric cyanide intoxication and death from an acetonitrile-containing cosmetic. JAMA 1988; 260:3470–3473.
9. Jaeger A, Temper JD, Porte AD, Stoeckel L, Mantz JM. Acute voluntary intoxication by acetonitrile. Acta Pharmacol Toxicol (Suppl):1977;41:340.
10. Swanson JR, Krasselt W. An acetonitrile related death. Proc Am Acad Forensic Sci, 44th Annual Meeting, New Orleans, February 17–22, 1992, p. 196.

ACRYLONITRILE

Acrylonitrile is the most commonly used aliphatic nitrile compound characterized by the structural formula $R-C=N$. Other commercially important nitriles include the relatively less toxic acetonitrile (CH_3CN, methyl cyanide) and the more toxic propionitrile (CH_3CH_2CN) and *n*-butyronitrile (CH_3CHCCH_2CN). Acute toxicity in this group resembles cyanide poisoning, with deaths reported from acute acetonitrile inhalation.[1,2] The use of sodium thiosulfate and sodium nitrite is effective in the mouse exposed to nitrile vapor when given prior to exposure,[3] and the use of conventional cyanide antidotes is suggested for severe exposures. Acrylonitrile has been listed as a substance that may reasonably be anticipated to be a carcinogen by the U.S. National Toxicology Program.

PHYSICAL AND CHEMICAL CHARACTERISTICS

Acrylonitrile is an explosive, flammable liquid with a boiling point of 77°C. The chemical structure is $CH_2=CHCN$, similar to the known chemical carcinogen vinyl chloride. Synonyms include acrylon, carbacryl, vinyl cyanide, cyanoethylene, and propene nitrile. Acrylonitrile decomposes to cyanide during pyrolysis and is heavier than air, which presents a significant hazard during fires.

USES

The major use of acrylonitrile is in the production of acrylic (e.g., blankets, carpets) and modacrylic (e.g., wigs, furs) fibers by copolymerization with agents such as vinyl chloride and methyl methacrylate. Other industrial applications include manufacture of the plastic acrylonitrile-butadiene-styrene (ABS) and the chemical production of acrylamide, adiponitrile, and a fumigant.

ESTIMATION OF ACUTE TOXICITY

Acrylonitrile is regulated as a suspected carcinogen with exposure levels set at 2 ppm as an 8-hour TWA.

TOXICOKINETICS

Absorption

Acrylonitrile is readily absorbed through stomach, skin, and lungs with most acute exposures resulting from inhalation. Cutaneous absorption (about 1%) does occur through contaminated leather and rubber because of excellent penetrating properties. After absorption most acrylontrile is converted to cyanide. This is then transformed to thiocyanate.

Elimination

Forty-seven percent of a single oral dose of acrylonitrile (30 mk/kg) was excreted as seven urinary metabolites.[4] The three major metabolites in order of excretion are thiocyanate, *N*-acetyl-*S*-(2-cyanoethyl)cysteine, and a thiazine. Eight-hour exposure to 4.2 ppm of acrylonitrile produced a mean urinary thiocyanate excretion of 11.4 mg/L.[5] However, the presence of hydrogen cyanide in smoke indicates that plasma levels of thiocyanate and cyanide are higher in smokers than in nonsmokers (e.g., 1.5 mg/mL versus 0.58 mg/mL, respectively).[6]

PATHOPHYSIOLOGY

Although cyanide is released from the hepatic biotransformation of acrylonitrile, acute toxicity results primarily from the whole molecule.[7,8] Detoxification of reactive vinyl groups and epoxide intermediaries can deplete glutathione stores,[4] which may lead to liver toxicity. Acute toxicity does not result from the in vivo release of cyanide.

CLINICAL PRESENTATION

Acute Effects

Acute inhalation may produce headache, sneezing, mucous membrane irritation, chest discomfort, nausea, vomiting, diarrhea, lightheadedness, weakness, and apprehension, with severe exposures resulting in asphyxia and cardiovascular collapse. The clinical syndrome resembles cyanide poisoning. Liver dysfunction may develop and is characterized by jaundice, malaise, anorexia, and leukocytosis.[9] Cutaneous exposure may produce a chemical burn that is exacerbated by prolonged contact with contaminated rubber or leather.

Cancer

Substantial evidence in animals incriminates acrylonitrile as a carcinogen, although evidence in humans is more limited. A retrospective cohort study of male workers exposed to acrylonitrile showed an excess cancer death rate, with the excess resulting primarily from increased respiratory cancer rates.[10] A small cohort of rubber workers exposed to acrylonitrile also showed an excess of lung cancer deaths.[11] At present, the size and design of these and British studies prevent a firm conclusion that exposure to acrylonitrile causes lung cancer, but animal studies and structural similarities to proven carcinogens strongly suggest that acrylonitrile is a carcinogen. Other epidemiologic studies have indicated increased incidences of stomach, brain, colon, and prostate cancer.[12]

Reproduction

Acrylonitrile may be weakly teratogenic in rats, but there is no evidence in humans to indicate that acrylonitrile is a reproductive risk.[13]

TREATMENT

Stabilization

Remove the patient from the source of the exposure. Severe acute inhalations should be treated like cyanide poisoning. The first priority is to establish adequate ventilation (100% oxygen) and circulation, since cyanide antidotes are theoretically useful but clinically unproven in acrylonitrile poisoning.

Decontamination

Contaminated clothing should be removed and placed in a sealed container. Attendants should use plastic gloves and should discard them after use since acrylonitrile may penetrate rubber, gloves, and leather. The usual decontamination measures (syrup of ipecac, lavage, charcoal) may be effective within the first 1 to 2 hours postingestion, but should not delay the use of nitrites and thiosulfate in significantly symptomatic patients.

Antidotes

Sodium nitrite and sodium thiosulfate have been recommended as antidotes, although their efficacy in human toxicity is unproven. Most exposures will not require an antidote, but the Lilly cyanide kit theoretically may be useful in severe exposures.

Supportive Care

Symptomatic management, especially of respiration, is the mainstay of treatment. Moderately to severely exposed patients should have an evaluation of liver function.

Toxicokinetics

Acrylonitrile is readily absorbed (about 95%) after oral ingestion or inhalation.[14] Dermal absorption is less than 1%. The major route of elimination is through the urine.

Mechanism of Action

Toxicity is based both on the release of cyanide and the degree of unsaturation.

DIMETHYLAMINE PROPIONITRILE (DMAPN)

USE

DMAPN is used as a catalyst in the polymerization process for the manufacture of polyurethane.

CLINICAL PRESENTATION

DMAPN is an aliphatic nitrile considered to be the causative agent in epidemics of urinary bladder dysfunction in workers exposed to the compound. Symptoms of bladder dysfunction include hesitancy, straining to void, decreased force of stream, and increased duration of urination.[15,16]

TREATMENT

Cessation of exposure. Supportive and symptomatic care.

ANTIDOTES

Nitrites

The hypotensive effects induced by sodium nitrite may be prevented by diluting the sodium nitrite dose in 50 to 100 mL of normal saline, beginning administration as a slow drip, with frequent blood pressure and methemoglobin monitoring, and then increasing the infusion rate to the most rapid tolerated.[17] The use of nitrites in victims of smoke inhalation should only be done with knowledge of both carboxyhemoglobin and methemoglobin levels. Kirk and colleagues, in a multicenter prospective study, concluded that administration of the cyanide antidote kit in the presence of concomitant carbon monoxide poisoning in smoke inhalation is a relatively safe procedure. Controlled clinical trials will be required to determine the effects of methemoglobin on oxygen delivery and on the extent of cyanomethemoglobin formation.[18]

4-Dimethylaminophenol

4-Dimethylaminophenol was introduced for the treatment of cyanide poisoning in Germany[19,20] after initial studies[21–23] indicated that it was able to generate a methemoglobin concentration of 30 to 50% within a few minutes.[21] A dose of 3.25 mg/kg IV results in a methemoglobin level of 15% within 1 minute and 30% within 10 minutes.[22] 4-Dimethylaminophenol is excreted largely as the glucuronide. Side effects observed after its use include an increase in bilirubin, a reticulocytosis, high levels of methemoglobin, and evidence of nephrotoxicity.[24,25] Hemolysis has been observed in overdose, as well as after therapeutic doses. Its use is contraindicated in patients with glucose 6-phosphate dehydrogenase deficiency.

Unexpectedly high levels of methemoglobin have followed an accidental overdose,[26,27] but the patient had also received sodium nitrite prior to this. Excess methemoglobinemia may be corrected with either methylene blue or toluidine blue. Caution is urged with the use of 4-dimethylaminophenol in cases of diagnostic uncertainty or in smoke inhalation victims who may have both cyanide toxicity and carbon monoxide poisoning; a further decrease in oxygen-carrying capacity by excess methemoglobin induction may be very dangerous to the patient.[17] 4-Dimethylaminophenol was deleted from the treatment guidelines for cyanide poisoning in Sweden in 1990, but is still available for use in severe hydrogen sulfide poisoning.[28]

Methylene Blue

Methylene blue is *not* an antidote. Its use increases cyanide release; clinical deterioration ensues when methylene blue is given to cyanide-intoxicated patients.

CYANIDE TREATMENT PROTOCOL

The following protocol summarizes the recommendations of a World Health Organization study[29]:

First Aid Measures[30]

These measures are to be undertaken only in cases of unequivocally severe poisonings.

Trained staff, wearing protective clothing and breathing apparatus if hydrogen cyanide or liquid cyanide preparations are involved, should do the following:

1. Stop further exposure.
2. Start artificial ventilation with 100% oxygen by a non-rebreathing system.
3. Give 0.2 to 0.4 mL amyl nitrite through an Ambu bag.

If a doctor is present immediately on the scene:

1. Start artificial ventilation with 100% oxygen by a non-rebreathing system.
2. Give 0.2 to 0.4 mL amyl nitrite through an Ambu bag.

Hospital Treatment

Hospital doctors must establish whether specific antidotal treatment was given at the time of the incident before further doses are given, especially in the case of agents that form methemoglobin.

In cases of severe poisoning when the patient is in deep coma with dilated, nonreactive pupils and deteriorating cardiorespiratory function (blood cyanide concentrations 115 to 154 μmol/L, 3 to 4 mg/L):

1. Start artificial ventilation with 100% oxygen.
2. Start cardiorespiratory support.

Then give either 10 mL of 3% sodium nitrite solution (300 mg) intravenously over 5 to 20 minutes or 5 mL 5% dimethylaminophenol solution (250 mg or 3 to 4 mg/kg) intravenously over 1 minute or 20 mL 1 to 5% dicobalt edetate solution (300 mg) intravenously over 1 minute or 10 mL 40% hydroxocobalamin solution (4 g) intravenously over 20 minutes and 50 mL 25% sodium thiosulphate solution (12.5 g) intravenously over 10 minutes (Fig. 66–3).

In cases of moderately severe poisoning when the patients have suffered a short period of unconsciousness, convulsions, vomiting, or cyanosis (blood cyanide concentrations 77 to 115 μmol/L (2 to 3 mg/L):

1. Give 100% oxygen but for no longer than 12 to 24 hours.
2. Observe in intensive care.
3. Give 50 mL 25% sodium thiosulphate solution (12.5 g) intravenously over 10 minutes.

In cases of mild poisoning when patients have nausea, dizziness, and drowsiness (blood cyanide concentrations <77 μmol/L (<2 mg/L):

1. Give oxygen.
2. Reassurance.
3. Prescribe bed rest.

See also Chapter 5—Antidotes.

SUGGESTED READINGS—CYANIDE IN SMOKE INHALATION

1. Becker CE. The role of cyanide in fires. Vet Hum Toxicol 1985;27:487–490.
2. Clark CJ, Campbell D, Reid WH. Blood carboxyhaemoglobin and cyanide levels in fire survivors. Lancet 1981;1 (8234): 1332–1335.
3. Hall AH, Rumack BH. Hydroxocobalamin/sodium thiosulfate as a cyanide antidote. J Emerg Med 1987;5:115–121.
4. Hall AH, Kulig KW, Rumack BH. Suspected cyanide poisoning in smoke inhalation: complications of sodium nitrite therapy. J Toxicol Clin Exp 1989;9:3–9.
5. Hart GB, Strauss MB, Lennon PA, Whitcraft DD III. Treatment of smoke inhalation by hyperbaric oxygen. J Emerg Med 1985;3:211–215.
6. Kizer KW. Hyperbaric oxygen and cyanide poisoning. Am J Emerg Med 1984;2:113 (letter).
7. Symington IS, Anderson RA, Thomson I, Oliver JS, Harland WA, Kerr JW. Cyanide exposure in fires. Lancet 1978;2(8080):91–92.

Government Documents

1. Agency for Toxic Substances and Disease Registry: Toxicological profile for cyanide. Oak Ridge, TN: Oak Ridge National Laboratory, 1989.
2. Environmental Protection Agency. Drinking water criteria document for cyanide. Cincinnati: Office of Health and Environmental Assessment, 1988.
3. Environmental Protection Agency. An exposure and risk assessment for cyanide. Washington, DC: Office of Water Regulations and Standards, 1981.

REFERENCES—ACRYLONITRILE

1. Amdur ML. Accidental group exposure to acetonitrile. J Occup Med 1959;1:627–633.
2. Garbois B. Fatal exposure to methyl cyanide. NY State Dept of Labor, Division of Industrial Hygiene Mon Rev 1955; 34(2):7–8.
3. Willhite CC. Inhalation toxicology of acute exposures to aliphatic nitriles. Clin Toxicol 1981;18:991–1003.

4. Langvardt PW, Potzig CL, Braun WH. Identification of the major urinary metabolites of acrylonitrile in the rat. J Toxicol Environ Health 1980;6:273–282.
5. Sakurai H, Onodera M, Utsunomiya T et al. Health effects of acrylonitrile in acrylic fibre factories. Br J Ind Med 1978;35: 219–222.
6. Butts WC, Kuehneman M, Widdowson GM. Automated method for determination of serum thiocyanate to distinguish smokers and non-smokers. Clin Chem 1974;20:1344–1348.
7. Tarkowski S. Studies in acrylonitrile effect on some properties of cytochrome oxidase. Med Pract 1968;19:525–530.
8. Magos L. A study of acrylonitrile poisoning in relation to methemoglobin—CN complex formation. Br J Ind Med 1962; 19:283–286.
9. Wilson RH, McCormick WF. Plastics and rubbers. Plastomers and monomers. Ind Med Surg 1954;23;479–486.
10. O'Berg MT. Epidemiologic study of workers exposed to acrylonitrile. J Occup Med 1980;22:245–252.
11. Delzell E, Monson RR. Mortality among rubber workers. VI. Man with potential exposure to acrylonitrile. J Occup Med 1982;24:767–769.
12. Fourth Annual Report on Carcinogens. Research Triangle Park, NC: National Toxicology Program, 1985, Publication 82-330.
13. Council on Scientific Affairs. Effects of toxic chemicals on the reproductive system. JAMA 1985;253:3431–3437.
14. Page NP, Cook B. Assessment of risk from exposure to acrylonitrile: the general approach used by a consultant. Sci Total Environ 1990;99:307–317.
15. Keough JP, Pestronek A, Wertheimer DS, Moreland R. An epidemic of urinary retention caused by dimethylaminopropionitrile. JAMA 1980;243:741–745.
16. Kreiss K, Wegman DH, Niles CA. Neurological dysfunction of the bladder in workers exposed to dimethylaminopropionitrile. JAMA 1980;243:741–745.
17. Hall AH, Rumack BH. Management of cyanide poisoning. Ann Emerg Med 1988;17:108–109.
18. Kirk MA, Gerace R, Kulig KW. Cyanide and methemoglobin kinetics in smoke inhalation victime treated with the cyanide antidote kit. Ann Emerg Med 1993;22:1413–1418.
19. Van Heijst ANP, Meredith TJ. Antidotes for cyanide poisoning. In: Volans GN, Sims J, Sullivan FM, Turner P, eds. Basic science in toxicology. London: Taylor & Francis, 1990; pp. 558–566.
20. Israeli A. Management of cyanide poisoning. Ann Emerg Med 1988;17:108.
21. Weger N. Aminophenole als Blausaure-antidote. Arch Toxikol 1968;14:49–50.
22. Kiese M, Weger N. Formation of ferrihaemoglobin with aminophenols in the human for treatment of cyanide poisoning. Eur J Pharmacol 1979;7:97–105.
23. Weger NP. Treatment of cyanide poisoning with 4-dimethylaminophenol (DMAP)—experimental and clinical overview. Fundam Appl Toxicol 1983;3:387–396.
24. Klimmek R, Krettek C, Szincicz L, Eyer P, Weger N. Effects and biotransformation of 4-dimethylaminophenol in man and dog. Arch Toxicol 1983;53:275–288.
25. Marrs TC. Antidotal treatment of acute cyanide poisoning. Adverse Drug React Acute Poisoning Rev 1988;4:179–206.
26. Van Dijk A, Glerum JH, Van Heijst ANP, Douze JMC. Clinical evaluation of the cyanide antagonist 4-DMAP in a lethal cyanide poisoning case. Vet Hum Toxicol 1987;39(Suppl 2): 38–39.
27. Van Heijst ANP, Douze JMC, Van Kesteren RG, Van Bergen JEAM, Van Dijk A. Therapeutic problems in cyanide poisoning. Clin Toxicol 1987;25:383–398.
28. Persson H. Swedish Poison Information Center. Personal communication. July 19, 1990.
29. Meredith TJ, Jacobsen D, Haines JA, Berger J-C, Van Heijst ANP, eds. Antidotes for poisoning by cyanide: International Program on Chemical Safety/Commission of the European Communities. Cambridge University Press, 1993.
30. Langford RM, Armstrong RF. Algorithm for managing injury from smoke inhalation. Br Med J 1989;299:902–905.

HYDROGEN SULFIDE

Hydrogen sulfide is the toxic gas commonly associated with the "rotten egg" smell of homemade "stink bombs," but in the workplace it is one of the leading causes of sudden death. Its excellent olfactory warning properties are lost at high concentrations, leading to insidious exposures and serious toxicity. Hydrogen sulfide is a by-product of organic decomposition (e.g., in sewers), the petroleum industry, tanning, rubber vulcanizing, and heavy water production. Serious toxicity and fatalities have been reported in poorly ventilated spaces after agitation of underground liquid manure tanks,[1] addition of sulfuric acid to a drain[2] and hydrochloric acid to a well,[3] cleaning of a propane tank,[4] and entry of both victims and rescuers into a sewer[5] and ship holds containing fish meal.[6] Occupations subject to exposure to hydrogen sulfide are listed in Table 66–22.

The most important determinants of clinical toxicity are gas concentration and duration of exposure. On exposure to levels exceeding 1000 ppm, victims rapidly develop coma,

Table 66–22
Occupations Having the Potential for Exposure to Hydrogen Sulphide (National Institute for Occupational Safety and Health, 1977)[a]

Animal fat and oil processors	Lithographers
Animal manure removers	Lithophone makers
Artificial-flavor makers	Livestock farmers
Asphalt storage workers	Manhole and trench workers
Barium carbonate makers	Metallurgists
Barium salt makers	Miners
Blast furnace workers	Natural gas production and processing workers
Brewery workers	Painters using polysulphide caulking compounds
Bromide-brine workers	Papermakers
Cable splicers	Petroleum production and refinery workers
Caisson workers	Phosphate purifiers
Carbon disulphide workers	Photoengravers
Cellophone makers	Pipeline maintenance workers
Chemical laboratory workers, teachers, students	Pyrite burners
Cistern cleaners	Rayon makers
Citrus root fumigators	Refrigerant makers
Coal gasification workers	Rubber and plastics processors
Coke oven workers	Septic tank cleaners
Copper-ore sulphidizers	Sewage treatment workers
Depilatory makers	Sewer workers
Dyemakers	Sheep dippers
Excavators	Silk makers
Felt makers	Slaughterhouse workers
Fermentation makers	Smelting workers
Fertilizer makers	Soapmakers
Fishing and fish-processing workers	Sugar beet and cane workers
Fur dressers	Sulphur spa workers
Geothermal-power drilling and production workers	Sulphur products processors
Gluemakers	Synthetic-fibre makers
Gold-ore workers	Tank gaugers
Heavy metal precipitators	Tannery workers
Heavy water manufacture	Textiles printers
Hydrochloric acid purifiers	Thiophene makers
Hydrogen sulphide production and sales staff	Tunnel workers
Landfill workers	Well diggers and cleaners
Lead ore sulphidizers	Wool pullers

[a]Adapted from Prior MG et al, eds. Proc Int Conf on Hydrogen Sulfide Toxicity. Banff, Alberta, Canada: June 18–21, 1989.

Table 66–23
Physiologic Effects of Human Exposure to Hydrogen Sulfide[a]

Concentration (ppm)	Physiologic Effect	Concentration (ppm)	Physiologic Effect
0.02	Odor threshold	100	Olfactory fatigue level
0.022	No odor	150	Olfactory nerve paralysis
0.025	Detectable odor	~200	Less intense odor; olfactory paralysis
~0.03	Olfactory threshold	200	Kills smell quickly, stings eyes and throat
0.13	Detectable, minimum perceptible odor	250	Prolonged exposure may cause pulmonary edema
0.15	Offensive odor		
0.2	Detectable odor	300–500	Pulmonary edema, imminent threat to life
0.3	Distinct odor	500	Systemic symptoms may occur in 0.5–1 h
0.77	Faint, weak odor, readily perceptible	500	In 0.5–1 h it will cause excitement, headache, dizziness, and staggering, followed by unconsciousness and respiratory failure
3–5	Offensive, moderately intense		
4.6	Fairly noticeable, moderate intensity		
10	Obvious and unpleasant odor	500	Dizziness, breathing ceases in a few minutes, needs prompt artificial respiration
10	Threshold limit value-time weighted average		
10	"Sore eyes"	500–1000	Acts primarily as a systemic poison causing unconsciousness and death through respiratory paralysis
20	Maximum allowable concentration for daily 8-h exposure		
20	Safe for 7-h exposure	700	Unconscious quickly, death will result if not rescued promptly
27	Strong, cogent, forceful, not intolerable odor		
20–30	Strong and intense odor, but not intolerable	700–900	Rapidly produces unconsciousness, cessation of respiraton, and death
50	Conjunctival irritation is first noticeable		
50	Marked irritant action on conjunctiva and respiratory tract	900+	Exposure to these concentrations may mean instant death
50/100	Mild irritation to the respiratory tract and especially to the eyes after 1 h of exposure	1000	Rapid collapse, respiratory paralysis, imminent coma, followed by death within minutes; nervous system paralysis
100	Loss of smell in 3 to 15 min, may sting eyes and throat	5000	Imminent death

[a]Adapted from Beauchamp RD Jr, Bus JS, Popp JA et al. CRC Crit Rev Toxicol 1984;13:40.

respiratory paralysis, and hypoxia. Death then occurs, unless the victim is quickly removed from the exposure and effective artificial ventilation is established. Although the exact mechanics of toxicity are unknown, hydrogen sulfide produces both local irritation and cellular asphyxia, probably by binding to the iron in cytochrome oxidase a_3. Pulmonary edema is a common complication of serious toxicity, whereas upper respiratory tract irritation, a keratoconjunctivitis, and nonspecific complaints (e.g., headache, nausea, dizziness) develop at lower exposure levels.

PHYSICAL PROPERTIES

Hydrogen sulfide is a colorless gas, heavier than air (1.19), with a strong "rotten eggs" odor detectable at 0.2 to 0.3 ppm. It burns with a blue flame, decomposing to water, sulfur dioxide, and elemental sulfur. At physiologic pH, approximately one-third of H_2S exists as the undissociated form (H_2S) and the remainder as hydrosulfide anion (HS^-). Very little of the H_2S exists as sulfide anion (S^{2-}).[7] Water solubility at 40°C is moderate (186 mL in 100 mL water). Blackened coins may be found in the pockets of victims poisoned by hydrogen sulfide.[8]

SOURCES

The addition of dilute sulfuric or hydrochloric acid to iron sulfide or the reaction of hydrogen with elemental sulfur produces hydrogen sulfide gas. Natural sources include subterranean emission (e.g., caves), volcanoes, and bacterial decomposition of sulfur in soil and the gastrointestinal tract (minor amounts). Decay of organic sulfur-containing products (e.g., fish, sewage, manure, septic tanks) and pouring of acid on sewage liberate hydrogen sulfide. Toxic gases released from the decomposing environment include hydrogen sulfide, carbon monoxide, sulfur dioxide, carbon dioxide, methane, ammonia, and amines (trimethylamine, diethylamine, *N*-butylamine). Common commercial exposures involve hydrogen disulfide as the manufacturing by-product of viscose rayon (along with carbon disulfide), silk, petroleum and tanning, paper mills, damp mines, geothermal energy and hot sulfur springs, roofing asphalt tanks, burning of wool, hair, meals, and hides, production of heavy water for nuclear reactors, metal refining, and vulcanization of sulfur-containing rubber.[9] Table 66–23 lists potential occupational exposures.

ACUTE TOXIC LEVELS

Most fatalities occur at the scene. Patients who have vital signs on arrival at the hospital usually survive, provided severe hypoxic encephalopathy is not present. Government regulations limit H_2S exposure (maximum allowable concentration) to less than 10 ppm over 10 minutes, and air levels over 50 ppm require evacuation. Table 66–23 lists exposure levels. An odor is detectable at 0.2 to 0.3 ppm, and a definite odor appears at 20 to 30 ppm, but olfactory paralysis develops between 100 and 150 ppm. Between 150 and 300 ppm, respiratory tract and eye irritation is prominent (blepharospasm, keratoconjunctivitis, blurred vision, colored halos around lights [gas eyes]), accompanied by mucous membrane irritation, bronchitis, and pulmonary edema. Severe systemic toxicity develops above 500 ppm (headache, nausea, vomiting, weakness, disorientation, coma within 30 minutes of exposure).

Above 700 ppm, cardiorespiratory arrest occurs and death is imminent. One reason for the insidious toxicity of hydrogen sulfide is the unpredictability of its presence and concentration, which leads to unexpected accidents. Agitation of solutions containing hydrogen sulfide may dramatically increase ambient air hydrogen sulfide levels.[4]

TOXICOKINETICS

Hydrogen sulfide is primarily a respiratory toxin, since cutaneous absorption is negligible. Inorganic sulfides are present in the body only in small quantities (0.05 mg/L). The toxicokinetics of hydrogen sulfide has not been studied in man. In animals, excretion of hydrogen sulfide by the lungs is minimal after parenteral administration.[7] Elimination occurs via oxidation to sulfate, methylation, and reaction with metalloproteins or disulfide-containing proteins. Detoxification of hydrogen sulfide occurs rapidly (85% of a lethal dose per hour in animals), with the red blood cell and liver mitochondria being the primary sites. Consequently, hydrogen sulfide is not a cumulative poison. Endogenous sulfide is mostly oxidized to thiosulfate, with a smaller portion excreted unchanged by the lungs and urine. Sulfhemoglobin is not produced by hydrogen sulfide poisoning.[10]

PATHOPHYSIOLOGY

Mechanism of Toxicity

Like cyanide, hydrogen sulfide probably is an intracellular toxin that inhibits cytochrome oxidase by disrupting electron transport. Hydrogen sulfide is a somewhat more potent inhibitor of the cytochrome oxidase system than cyanide.[11] The resulting switch to anaerobic metabolism causes lactate accumulation and metabolic acidosis. At lower doses, hydrogen sulfide is a mucous-membrane and respiratory irritant (200 ppm), but at high doses (1000 ppm) it causes direct respiratory depression. Death usually results from respiratory arrest and hypoxia.

Autopsy Findings

Autopsies demonstrate nonspecific findings such as visceral congestion, scattered petechiae, and hemorrhagic pulmonary edema. Greenish discoloration of gray matter, viscera, and bronchial secretions has been reported in documented hydrogen sulfide-related fatalities,[12] but may disappear after the injection of formalin.[5] The green discoloration may result from a denaturation product of sulfur and hemoglobin.[13] A sulfide smell may be present on the slicing of tissue, and autolysis of tissue may be accelerated.[14] Most but not all autopsy cases demonstrate pulmonary edema.

CLINICAL PRESENTATION

Acute Effects

In high doses the central nervous system is the primary target organ, with symptoms of irritation of the eyes and respiratory tract developing on prolonged exposure. Central nervous system depression may result in headache, lethargy, vertigo, horizontal or vertical nystagmus,[15] and coma; the combination of vomiting and CNS depression may lead to aspiration pneumonia. Symptoms of severe exposure in one large series were, in the order of frequency, loss of consciousness, dizziness, nausea, vomiting, headache, sore throat, conjunctivitis, weakness of extremities, dyspnea, convulsions, pulmonary edema, cyanosis, and hemoptysis.[16] Almost 5% of patients were dead on arrival at the hospital. Local irritant properties result in keratoconjunctivitis, rhinitis, pharyngitis, bronchitis, pneumonia, and pulmonary edema. Cardiac symptoms include dysrhythmias, myocardial depression, conduction defects, and abnormal ventricular repolarization.

Chronic Effects

Headache, weakness, nausea, vomiting, and weight loss occur in chronic exposures and may appear for several months after acute exposure. Long-term adverse effects are unusual in victims promptly resuscitated.[16] Spasticity, cerebellar ataxia, tremor, and exacerbation of exercise-induced angina have been reported in a patient rendered unconscious and cyanotic by a 30-minute hydrogen sulfide exposure.[8] Abrupt collapse strongly suggests hydrogen sulfide poisoning in the presence of a rotten-egg odor and may produce traumatic injuries (7% of cases in one series).[17]

Chronic exposure to at least 0.6 ppm of hydrogen sulfide for almost 1 year produced truncal ataxia, choreoathetosis, and dystonia with bilateral lucent areas in the basal ganglia in a 20-month-old child. Removal from the source of the gas resulted in clinical recovery with resolution of the basal ganglia abnormalities.[18]

LABORATORY

Ancillary Tests

All seriously poisoned patients should have chest x-rays and arterial blood gases to search for evidence of aspiration pneumonia and pulmonary edema. Early widening of the alveolar-arterial oxygen gradient suggests the development of pulmonary edema or pneumonia. A CAT scan revealed bilateral symmetric lucent areas within the cerebral hemispheres, which probably correspond to the lentiform nucleus.[19] Such lesions are consistent with focal brain lesions produced by hypoxia or hypotension.

Analytic Method

A specific ion electrode in combination with Conway microdiffusion cells has been developed to detect elevated sulfide ion in blood. Sulfide ion levels measured soon after hydrogen sulfide–induced death ranged from 1.70 to 3.75 mg/L.[20] Postmortem confirmation of toxic levels is complicated by the rapid endogenous destruction of the sulfide ion, formation of sulfide from protein degradation postmortem, and deterioration of the sulfide ion in storage.[13]

TREATMENT

A NIOSH alert addresses the dangers to farm workers entering manure pits where an anaerobic digestive fermentation process, which normally leads to the production of fertilizer, simultaneously generates four potentially dangerous gases: methane, hydrogen sulfide, carbon dioxide, and ammonia. Recommendations to avoid fatal exposure are detailed in the NIOSH document.[21]

Stabilization

Immediate supportive care is the most important phase of treatment, since most fatalities occur at the scene. Rescuers must very cautiously enter areas that potentially contain hydrogen sulfide. Such closed areas (e.g., inside storage tanks) require self-contained breathing apparatus, safety lines, and outside observation. Evacuate the immediate area and monitor hydrogen sulfide levels with Draeger tubes. Be sure to move the victim to an area without toxic hydrogen sulfide levels, since would-be rescuers have lost consciousness while applying mouth-to-mouth resuscitation.[9] After protection of the rescuer, the most important priority is the establishment of adequate ventilation and circulation. Supportive care and oxygen may be sufficient to treat the victim without the need to use nitrites.[22] Use MAXIMUM oxygen flow. Violent convulsive movements have required the use of muscle relaxants (i.e., succinylcholine) to complete intubation.[23]

Decontamination

Skin decontamination is not necessary due to poor cutaneous absorption.

Elimination Enhancement

Several anecdotal case studies suggest that HBO may be useful for severe hydrogen sulfide toxicity.[24,25] Although patients who continue to show symptoms after standard therapy may benefit from HBO therapy, the clinical efficacy of this modality remains to be determined.

Antidotes (Nitrites)

Mechanism of Action

Nitrites produce methemoglobin, which in turn attracts sulfide from the cytochrome oxidase and thus reactivates aerobic metabolism. Sulfmethemoglobin undergoes rapid spontaneous detoxification in the body. The use of nitrites in serious cases may be effective only at the exposure site, because data on animals indicate that the sulfmethemoglobin complex is short-lived and leads directly to the oxidation of sulfide by molecular oxygen.[26] The lifetime of sulfide in oxygenated blood is short, and induction of methemoglobin more than 10 to 15 minutes postexposure may not aid the victim.

Dosage

The use of an antidote must not delay the establishment of adequate ventilation and oxygenation. The dosages of nitrites are similar to those used in cyanide poisoning. An amyl nitrite perle is broken and inhaled for 30 seconds every minute until the intravenous line is established. This step should be omitted until good oxygenation is present. Adults should receive 300 mg (10 mL of 3% sodium nitrite solution) over 4 minutes intravenously similar to cyanide poisoning.[27] No absolute guidelines are available for the use of nitrites in hydrogen sulfide poisoning in the hospital setting, because most hospital inpatients survive with supportive care only and nitrites have inherent toxicity.[28] Thiosulfate is not required, because the body spontaneously detoxifies sulfmethemoglobin.

Supportive Care

1. Follow fluid and electrolyte balance carefully.
2. Watch for the development of aspiration pneumonia and pulmonary edema.
3. If nitrites are used, check methemoglobin levels.

REFERENCES—HYDROGEN SULFIDE

1. Morse DL, Woodbury MA, Rentmeester K et al. Death caused by fermenting manure. JAMA 1981;245:63–64.
2. Peters JW. Hydrogen sulfide poisoning in a hospital setting. JAMA 1981;246:1588–1589.
3. Thoman M. Sewer gas: hydrogen sulfide intoxication. Clin Toxicol 1969;2:383–386.
4. Vannatta JB. Hydrogen sulfide poisoning: report of four cases and brief review of the literature. J Okla Med Assoc 1982;75:29–32.
5. Adelson L, Sunshine I. Fatal hydrogen sulfide intoxication: Report of three cases occurring in a sewer. Arch Pathol 1966;81:375–380.
6. Dalgaard JB, Dencker F, Fallentin B et al. Fatal poisoning and other health hazards connected with industrial fishing. Br J Ind Med 1972;29:307–316.
7. Beauchamp RO Jr, Bus JS, Popp JA et al. A critical review of the literature on hydrogen sulfide toxicity. CRC Crit Rev Toxicol 1984;13:25–97.
8. Hurwitz LJ, Taylor GI. Poisoning by sewer gas with unusual sequelae. Lancet 1954;1:1110–1111.
9. Milby TH. Hydrogen sulfide intoxication: review of the literature and report of unusual accident resulting in two cases of nonfatal poisoning. J Occup Med 1962;4:431–437.
10. Smith RP, Gosselin RE. Hydrogen sulfide poisoning. J Occup Med 1979;21:93–97.
11. Nicholls P. The effect of sulphide on cytochrome a_3, isosteric and allosteric shifts of the reduced alpha peak. Biochim Biophys Acta 1975;396:24–35.
12. Winek CL, Collom WD, Wecht CH. Death from hydrogen sulphide fumes. Lancet 1968;1:1096.
13. Evans L. The toxicity of hydrogen sulphide and other sulphides. Q J Exp Physiol 1967;52:231–248.
14. Simson RE, Simpson GR. Fatal hydrogen sulphide poisoning associated with industrial waste exposure. Med J Aust 1971;1:331–334.
15. Stine RJ, Slosberg B, Beacham BE. Hydrogen sulfide intoxication. A case report and discussion of treatment. Ann Intern Med 1976;85:756–758.
16. Burnett WW, King EG, Grace M et al. Hydrogen sulfide poisoning: review of 5 years experience. CMA J 1977;117:1277–1280.
17. Arnold IMF, Dufresne RM, Alleyne BC et al. Health implication of occupational exposures to hydrogen sulfide. J Occup Med 1985;27:373–376.
18. Gaitonde VB, Sellar RJ, O'Hare AE. Long term exposure to hydrogen sulphide producing subacute encephalopathy in a child. Br Med J 1987;294:614.
19. Matsuo F, Cummins JW, Anderson RE. Neurological sequelae of massive hydrogen sulfide inhalation. Arch Neurol 1979;36:451–452.
20. McAnalley BH, Lowry WT, Oliver RD et al. Determination of inorganic sulfide and cyanide in blood using specific ion electrodes. Application to the investigation of hydrogen sulfide and cyanide poisoning. J Anal Toxicol 1979;3:111–114.

21. Millar JD. NIOSH alert. Request for assistance in preventing deaths of farm workers in manure pits. DHHS (NIOSH) Publication No. 90-103, May, 1990.
22. Ravizza AG, Carugo D, Cerchiari EL et al. The treatment of hydrogen sulfide intoxication: oxygen versus nitrites. Vet Hum Toxicol 1982;24:241–242.
23. Kemper FD. A near fatal case of hydrogen sulfide poisoning. CMA J 1966;94:1130–1131.
24. Whitcraft DD III, Bailey TD, Hart GB. Hydrogen sulfide poisoning treated with hyperbaric oxygen. J Emerg Med 1985;3:23–25.
25. Smilkstein MJ, Bronstein AC, Pickott HM et al. Hyperbaric oxygen therapy for severe hydrogen sulfide poisoning. J Emerg Med 1985;3:27–30.
26. Beck JF, Bradbury CM, Connors AJ et al. Nitrite as an antidote for acute hydrogen sulfide intoxication? Am Ind Hyg Assoc J 1981;42:805–809.
27. Hoidal CR, Hall AH, Robinson MD et al. Hydrogen sulfide poisoning from toxic inhalations of roofing asphalt fumes. Ann Emerg Med 1986;15:826–830.
28. Marcus SM. Hydrogen sulfide. Clin Toxicol Rev 1983;5(4):1–2.

Table 66–24
Some Products That May Be Abused by Inhalation[a]

Product	Major Volatile Components
Adhesives	
Balsa wood cement	Ethyl acetate
Contact adhesives	Toluene, hexane and esters
Cycle tire repair adhesive	Toluene and xylenes
PVC cement	Trichloroethylene
Aerosols	
Air freshener	Halons, butane and/or dimethyl ether
Deodorants, antiperspirants	Halons, butane and/or dimethyl ether
Fly spray	Halons, butane and/or dimethyl ether
Hair lacquer	Halons, butane and/or dimethyl ether
Paint	Halons, butane and esters
Anesthetics/analgesics	
Gaseous	Nitrous oxide, cyclopropane
Liquid	Diethyl ether, halothane, enflurane, isoflurane
Local	Halons 11 and 12, ethyl chloride
Commercial dry cleaning and degreasing agents	1,1,1-Trichloroethane, tetrachloroethylene, trichloroethylene (rarely carbon tetrachloride, 1,2-dichloropropane)
Domestic spot removers and dry cleaners	1,1,1-Trichloroethane, tetrachloroethylene, trichloroethylene
Fire extinguishers	Bromochlorodifluoromethane, halons 11 and 12
Fuel gases	
Cigarette lighter refills	*n*-Butane, isobutane and propane
Butane	*n*-Butane, Isobutane and propane
Propane	Propane and butanes
Nail varnish/nail varnish remover	Acetone and esters
Paints/paint thinners	Butanone, esters, hexane, toluene, xylene
Paint stripper	Dichloromethene and toluene
Surgical plaster/chewing gum remover	Trichloroethylene
Typewriter correction fluids/thinners	1,1,1-Trichloroethane

[a]Adapted from Flanagan RJ et al. Drug Safety 1990;5:359–383.

INHALANT ABUSE

SOURCES

Inhalation of fuel gases, especially lighter refills, accounted for 33% of 951 deaths due to abuse of volatile substances in the United Kingdom during the period from 1971 to 1989. The proportion due to fuel gases rose from 26% in 1971–1980 to 50% for 1989. Deaths due to inhalation of the contents of fire extinguishers may be rising sharply.[1,2] (See also Chapter 65—The Hydrocarbons.)

Products and volatiles compounds that may be abused by inhalation are summarized in Tables 66–24 and 66–25. A summary of clinical toxicities associated with inhalation is found in Table 66–26.[4]

Table 66–25
Volatile Compounds That May Be Abused by Inhalation[a]

Aliphatic hydrocarbons
Acetylene
n-Butane[b]
Isobutane (2-methylpropane)[b]
n-Hexane[c]
Propane[b]

Alicyclic/aromatic hydrocarbons
Cyclopropane (trimethylene)
Toluene (toluol, methylbenzene, phenylmethane)
Xylene (xylol, dimethylbenzene)[d]

Mixed hydrocarbons
Petrol (gasoline)[e]
Petroleum ethers[f]

Halogenated compounds
Bromochlorodifluoromethane (BCF)
Carbon tetrachloride (tetrachloromethane)
Chlorodifluoromethane (halon 22, propellant 22, 'Freon 22')
Chloroform (trichloromethane)
Dichlorodifluoromethane (halon 12, propellant 12, 'Freon 12')
Dichloromethane (methylene chloride)
1,2-Dichloropropane (propylene dichloride)
Enflurane (2-chloro-1,1,2-trifluoroethyl difluoromethyl ether)
Ethyl chloride (monochloroethane)
Halothane (2-bromo-2-chloro-1,1,1-trifluoroethane)
Isoflurane (1-chloro-2,2,2-trifluoroethyl difluoromethyl ether)
Methoxyflurane (2,2-dichloro-1,1-difluoroethyl methyl ether)
Tetrachloroethylene (perchloroethylene)
1,1,1-Trichloroethane (methylchloroform, 'Genklene')
Trichloroethylene ('trike,' 'Trilene')
Trichlorofluromethane (halon 11, propellant 11, 'Freon 11')
1,1,2-Trichlorotrifluoroethane (halon 113)

Oxygenated compounds
Acetone (dimethyl ketone)
butanone (butan-2-one, methyl ethyl ketone, MEK)
Diethyl ether (ethoxyethane)
Dimethyl ether (DME, methoxymethane)
Ethyl acetate
Methyl acetate
Methyl isobutyl ketone (MIBK, isopropyl acetone)
Methyl tert.-butyl ether (MTBE)
Nitrous oxide (dinitrogen monoxide, laughing gas)

[a]Adapted from Flanagan RJ et al Drug Safety 1990;5:359–383.
[b]Components of liquefied petroleum gas (LPG).
[c]Commercial 'hexane' is a mixture of *n*-hexane and *n*-heptane with small amounts of some higher aliphatic hydrocarbons.
[d]Mainly *o*-xylene (1,3-dimethylbenzene).
[e]Boiling range 40-200°C, atmospheric pressure.
[f]Mixtures of pentanes, hexanes, etc., with specified boiling ranges (for example 40-60°C).

Table 66-26
Toxicities from Inhalation[a]

Chemicals	Toxicities
Aliphatic Hydrocarbons	
Aliphatic nitrates (*n*-butyl, isobutyl, amyl nitrite)	Dizziness, syncope, giddiness, hypotension, cerebral ischemia, headache, tachycardia, increased intraocular pressure, confusion, sudden death, methemoglobinemia, convulsions, myocardial ischemia, coma, cardiovascular collapse, asphyxia, fatal overdose.
Petroleum distillates, naphtha, kerosene, gasoline	Irritation of mucous membranes, nausea, ataxia, dizziness, hallucinations, narcoses, cardiac arrhythmias (ventricular fibrillation), respiratory arrest, syncope, death. Myoclonia, chorea, encephalopathy and tremor, pulmonary hemorrhage and edema, pneumonitis, plumbism, anemia, lead encephalopathy, confusion, dementia, cerebral edema, peripheral and cranial neuropathies, paresthesias, proteinuria, hematuria, fatal overdose.
n-Hexane	Eye and nasopharynx irritation, dizziness, giddiness, nausea, headache, CNS depression, peripheral neuropathy, anemia, basophilic stippling, bone marrow depression, fatal overdose.
Aromatic Hydrocarbons	
Benzene	Irritation of conjunctiva and visual blurring, mucous membranes, dizziness, headache, unconsciousness, convulsions, tremors, ataxia, delirium, tightness in chest, irreversible brain damage with cerebral atrophy, fatigue, vertigo, dyspnea, respiratory arrest, cardiac failure and ventricular arrhythmias, leukopenia, anemia, thrombocytopenia, petechiae, blood dyscrasia, leukemia, bone marrow aplasia, fatty degeneration and necrosis of heart, liver, adrenal glands, fatal overdose.
Naphthalene	Irritation and injury of conjunctiva and cornea, perspiration, nausea, vomiting, headache, cataracts, hemolytic anemia (greater in glucose-6-phosphate dehydrogenase deficiency), hepatic necrosis, hematuria, jaundice, proteinuria, oliguria or anemia, excitement, confusion, convulsions and coma, dermatitis, fatal overdose.
Styrene	Irritation of mucous membranes, CNS depression and narcosis, fatal overdose.
Toluene	CNS depression, syncope, coma, cardiac arrhythmias and sudden death, ataxia, convulsions, rhabdomyolysis, increased creatine phosphokinase, abdominal pain, nausea, vomiting, hematemesis, peripheral neuropathy, paresthesias, encephalopathy, optic neuropathy, cerebellar ataxia, distal renal tubular acidosis, hyperchloremia, hypokalemia, azotemia, hypophosphatemia, hematuria, proteinuria, pyruria, hepatomegaly, lymphocytosis, macrocytosis, basophilic stippling, hypochromia, eosphinophil, EEG abnormalities, decreased cognitive function, fatal overdose.
Xylene	Irritation to eye and mucosa, CNS depression and narcoses, reversible corneal damage, death, pulmonary edema and hemorrhage, fatty degeneration of heart, liver, adrenals and increased LFTs, fatal overdose.
Esters	
(methy-, ethyl-, *n*-propyl- *n*-butyl acetate, methyl and ethyl formate)	Irritation of eyes, skin and mucous membranes, CNS depression, liver and kidney necrosis, fatal overdose.
Glycols	
(Ethylene glycol)	Oxalosis, impaired renal and liver function, stupor, coma, convulsions, irreversible brain damage, pulmonary edema, respiratory failure, nausea, vomiting, headache, tachycardia, hypotension, hypoglycemia, hypocalcemia, intravascular hemolysis, lymphocytosis, proteinuria, hematuria, fatal overdose.
Halogenated Inhalants Chlorinated Hydrocarbons	
Trichlorethane Trichoroethylene Methyl chloroform	Decreased myocardial contractility, arrhythmias, cardiac arrest and failure, myocarditis, hepatotoxia, renal failure, paresthesias, tinnitus, ataxia, headache, narcosis, CNS damage, sudden death, fatal overdose.
Carbon tetrachloride Ethylene dichloride	Nausea, vomiting, confusion, unconsciousness, coma, respiratory slowing, color blindness, blurred vision, memory loss, paresthesias, tremors, dermatitis, CNS edema, congestion and hemorrhage, edema and inflammation of lungs, kidneys, spleen, pancreas, fatty degeneration of liver, cardiac arrhythmias and sudden death, fatal overdose.
Methylene chloride	Cardiovascular death, liver and kidney abnormalities, fatal overdose.
Fluorinated Hydrocarbons	
Trichlorofluoromethane	Cardiac arrhythmia, decreased cardiac contractility and output, fatal overdose.
Alcohols	
Methyl alcohol	Abdominal discomfort, dizziness, fatigue, headache, nausea, vertigo, CNS depression, coma, vomiting, acidosis, mydriasis, retinal edema and ganglion cell destruction, philophobia, mydrasis, areflexia, hemorrhagic infiltration of basal ganglia, decreased vision and blindness, fatal overdose.
Ethyl alcohol	Irritation of mucous membranes, headache, excitability, narcosis, memory and cognitive impairment, cerebral and cerebellar atrophy, seizures, delirium, coma, peripheral neuropathy, myopathy, Wernicke-Korsakoff's optic neuropathy, ataxia, metabolic acidosis, fatty degeneration of liver, hepatitis, cirrhosis, hepatic splenomegaly, hepatoma, pancreatitis, pancreatic cancer, esophogeal ulcers and cancer, Mallory-Weiss syndrome, gastric ulcers and cancer, peptic ulcer, cardiac arrhythmias, cardiomegaly, cardiomyopathy, hypertension, microcytic and megaloblastic anemia, B6, B12/folate deficiency, bone marrow depression, leukopenia, thrombocytopenia, pulmonary and CNS infections, nasopharyngeal cancer, gonadal and adrenal insufficiency, fetal alcohol effects syndrome, fatal overdose.
Isopropyl alcohol and *n*-propyl alcohol	Irritation of eyes and mucous membranes, nausea, vomiting, abdominal pain, hematemesis, narcosis, coma, areflexia, depressed repression, oliguria and diuresis, fatal overdose.
Butyl alcohol	Irritation of eyes and mucous membranes, CNS depression, kidney and liver damage, fatal overdose.

[a]Adapted from Miller NS, Gold MS. Ann Clin Psychiatry 1990;2:85–92.

(continued)

Table 66–26 *(Continued)*

Chemicals	Toxicities
Ketones	
Acetone	Irritation of eyes and mucous membranes, dermatitis, dizziness, lacrimation, salivation, nausea, vomiting, dysuria, albuminuria, tachycardia, ataxia, stupor and coma, fatal overdose.
Methyl ethyl ketone	Irritation of mucous membranes, CNS depression, dermatitis, paresthesias, emphysema, liver and kidney congestion, fatal overdose.
Methyl-*n*-butyl ketone	Peripheral neuropathy.
Nitrous Oxide	Hallucinations, respiratory depression, paresthesias, seizures, respiratory arrest, brain hypoxia, coma, ataxia, impotence, leg weakness, fatal overdose.

RENAL DYSFUNCTION

Central nervous system depression, nausea, vomiting, shortness of breath, photophobia, and/or decreased visual acuity follows inhalation of methanol; blood methanol and formic acid levels are often elevated.[5]

CLINICAL PRESENTATION—GENERAL ACUTE EFFECTS

Typewriter Correction Fluid

Inhalation of typewriter correction fluid (1,1,1-trichloroethane and trichloroethylene) leads to nausea and vomiting, dizziness, coma, cerebral edema, and sudden death due to cardiac arrhythmias. Management is mainly supportive.[6,7]

Gasoline

Heavy abusers develop organic lead encephalopathy, arrhythmias, ataxia, delirium, tremor, and narcosis. Fifteen to 20 breaths of gasoline vapor produces a 5- to 6-hour intoxicated state (i.e., giddiness, dizziness, ataxia, excitement, confusion, restlessness, hallucinations), which resembles ethanol-induced CNS changes.[8] The most consistent neurologic signs are abnormal jaw jerk, gait abnormalities, hyperactive deep tendon reflexes, and intention tremor. Organic lead toxicity is primarily a neurologic problem, in contrast to inorganic lead toxicity, in which gastrointestinal and hematologic abnormalities also occur.[9]

Nitrites

Isobutyl, butyl, and amyl nitrites can cause mild methemoglobinemia, cyanosis, and hypotension.

Cyclohexane

Narcosis is observed.

Nitrous Oxide

Use of nitrous oxide cryosurgical probes produces a temporary decrease in psychomotor performance if ventilation is suboptimal. Nitrous oxide concentrations over 50 ppm reduce dexterity, cognition, and motor and audiovisual skills. Even occupational exposure to nitrous oxide may cause depression of vitamin B_{12} activity as measured by the impaired synthesis of deoxyribonucleic acid.[10] Evidence of disturbance in hematopoiesis usually requires approximately 5 hours of exposure to nitrous oxide in healthy patients and at least 1 hour in severely debilitated patients.[11,12]

LABORATORY

Visual evoked potentials, brainstem auditory evoked potentials, and somatosensory evoked potentials may be abnormal at an early stage of neurologic damage in inhalant abusers.[13] Confirmatory studies will ultimately indicate the clinical usefulness of these tests.

SUPPORTIVE CARE

1. Remove the offending agent that is producing the adverse consequences.
2. Perform a detailed physical and medical evaluation to assess the possible existence of additional toxicity.
3. The mainstay of the treatment is to confront the usual denial of the drug use and to establish a commitment to recovery. Involvement in 12-step programs such as Alcoholics Anonymous or Narcotics Anonymous may be useful to maintain abstinence from the solvents and other drugs.[4]

REFERENCES—INHALANT ABUSE

1. Wright SP, Pottier ACW, Taylor JC, Normal LL, Anderson HR, Ramsey JD. Trends in deaths associated with volatile substances 1971–1989. London: St. George's Hosp Med Sch 1991;337:548.
2. Breath of death. Lancet 1991;337:548 (editorial).
3. Flanagan RJ et al. Clinical toxicology of volatile substances. Drug Safety 1990;5:359–383.
4. Miller NS, Gold MS. Organic solvents and aerosols. An overview of abuse and dependence. Ann Clin Psych 1990;2: 85–92.
5. Frenia ML, Schauben JL. Methanol inhalation toxicity. Ann Emerg Med 1993;22:1919–1923.
6. Troutman WG. Additional deaths associated with the intentional inhalation of typewriter correction fluid. Vet Hum Toxicol 1987;29:479.
7. Wodka RM, Jeong EWS. Cardiac effects of inhaled typewriter correction fluid. Ann Intern Med 1989;110:91–92.
8. Poklis A, Burkett CD. Gasoline sniffing: A review. Clin Toxicol 1977;11:35–41.

9. Edminister SC, Bayer MJ. Recreational gasoline sniffing: acute gasoline intoxication and latent organolead poisoning. Case reports and literature review. J Emerg Med 1985;3: 365–370.
10. Sweeney B, Bingham RM, Amos RJ et al. Toxicity of bone marrow in dentists exposed to nitrous oxide. Br Med J 1985; 291:567–569.
11. Gillman MA. Analgesic nitrous oxide for addictive withdrawal states. S Afr Med J 1989;75:100–101.
12. Gillman MA. Haematological changes caused by nitrous oxide: cause for concern. Br J Anaesth 1987;59:143–146 (editorial).
13. Tenenbein M, Pillay N. Evoked potentials in clinically normal inhalant abusing adolescents. Vet Hum Toxicol 1990; 32:343.

NITRATES, NITRITES, AND METHEMOGLOBINEMIA

Congenital methemoglobinemia is rare. Acquired methemoglobinemia is caused by oxidizing agents (Table 66–27).[1] A comparison of methemoglobinemia cyanide and hydrogen sulfide poisoning is seen in Table 66–28.

ANILINE

This colorless oily liquid with a characteristic odor has the chemical structure $C_6H_5NH_2$. Commercial applications include use as an intermediate in dyestuff production and in the manufacture of pharmaceuticals, photographic developers, shoe polish, resins, varnish, perfumes, and organic chemicals.

Table 66–27
Reported Inducers of Methemoglobinemia[a]

Agent	Source
Inorganic nitrates/nitrites	Contaminated well water
	Meat preservatives
	Vegetables-carrot juice, spinach
	Silver nitrate burn therapy
	Industrial salts
	Contaminants of nitrous oxide canisters for anesthesia
Organic nitrites	
Butyl/isobutyl nitrite	Room deodorizer propellants
Amyl nitrite	Inhalant in cyanide antidote kit
Nitroglycerine	Oral, sublingual, or transdermal pharmaceuticals for treatment of angina
Others	
Amiline/aminophenols	Laundry ink
Nitrobenzene	Industrial solvents, gun-cleaning products
Local anesthetics	Benzocaine, lidocaine, propitocaine, prilocaine
Sulfonamides	Antibacterial drugs
Phenazopyridine	Pyridium
Antimalarials	Chloroquine, primaquine
Sulfones	Dapsone
p-Aminosalicylic acid	Bactericide (tuberculostatic)
Naphthalene	Mothballs
Copper sulfate	Fungicide for plants, seed treatment
Resorcinol	Antiseborrheic, antipruritic, antiseptic
Chlorates	Matches, explosives, pyrotechnics
Combustion products	Fires

[a]Adapted from Dabney BJ, Zelarny PT, Hall AH. Emerg Care Q 1990;6:65–80.

TOXIC DOSAGE
Nitrates

Sodium nitrate is a frequent cause of nitrate poisoning in China where at least 2 grams are ingested at each meal. Building workers appear to be more susceptible.[2] The ingestion of one hundred 0.4-mg nitroglycerin tablets over 2 days caused a fatal 7% methemoglobinemia in an elderly adult with severe cardiovascular disease.[3] Methemoglobin concentrations of 9% were associated with the extension of a recent myocardial infarction in a cardiac patient receiving high-dose intravenous nitroglycerin.[4]

A 15-year-old ingested 80 isosorbide-5 mononitrate (IS-5 MN) tablets (1.6 g) and 20 nitroglycerin tablets (20 mg). She developed severe headache, nausea, and vomiting. The skin was flushed and hot and dry. Symptoms disappeared in 24 hours.[5] IS-5-MN is the principal acetone metabolite of isosorbide dinitrate.

PATHOPHYSIOLOGY
Nitric Oxide—Nitrovasodilators

Nitric oxide now appears to be formed endogenously in man from L-arginine and has been found in macrophages, endothelial cells (EDRF—endothelium-derived relaxing factors), and in the central nervous system. Vasodilating

Table 66–28
Comparison of Methemoglobin, Cyanide, and Hydrogen Sulfide Poisoning

	Methemoglobinemia	Cyanide	Sulfide
Fe^{2+} (heme → Fe^{3+} in RBC	+	–	–
Binding to Fe^{3+} iron in cytochrome a_3 in tissues	–	+	+
Binding to Fe^{2+} in oxyhemoglobin	+	–	–
Arterial blood chocolate brown, does not become bright red when oxygen is bubbled through or shaken with air	+	–	–
Venous blood retains bright red color of oxyhemoglobin	–	+	+
Production of methemoglobin useful by nitrites	–	+	+
May respond to oxygen	–	+	±
Responds to methylene blue	+	–	–
Pa_{O_2}, Pa_{CO_2} normal	+	±	–
Pulses full, symmetric	+	–	–
Coma	+	+	+
Coma with metabolic acidosis	±	+	+
Bitter almond odor	–	+	–
ECG abnormal, responds to sodium nitrite	–	+	–
Rotten egg odor	–	–	+

Table 66–29
Contents of Common Ammonium Nitrate Cold Packs[a]

Brand Name	Manufacturer	Grams of Ammonium Nitrate			
		Small	Medium	Large Size	Other
American Instant Cold Pack	American Hospital Supply Co.	127	—	234	Binasol, water
Disposable Instant Cold Pack	Cramer	—	—	210	Water (plastic cover)
Reditemp-C Cold Pack	Wyeth Company	127	—	234	Water, modified starch
Zee Instant Ice Pack	Zee Medical Company	86	—	200[b]	Water
Kwick Kold Instant Ice Pack	American Pharmaceuticals	57	113	218[b]	Water
Instant Cold Pack	Jack Frost Company	50	150		Water

[a]Adapted from Challone KR, McCarron MM. J Emerg Med 1988;6:289–293.
[b]+/–5 to 10%.

organic nitrates are reduced to organic nitrite, which is then converted to nitric oxide. Nitric oxide is then converted to an S-nitrosothiol derivative by the addition of a sulfhydryl group. This activates guanylcyclase, thereby producing cyclic GMP, the mediator for relaxation of vascular smooth muscle. Hypotension, low systemic vascular resistance, and a reduced sensitivity to vasoconstrictors may follow.[6–8] Depletion of sulfhydryl group donors is considered to be the mechanism for tolerance to the organic nitrates in patients with angina pectoris. Such tolerance may be reversed by sulfhydryl group donors such as *N*-acetylcysteine.[9] Such tolerance reversal has not, however, been demonstrated in healthy patients following use of glyceryl trinitrate skin patches with concurrent administration of NAC.[10] Nitroglycerin, a vasodilator, is known to decompose to nitric oxide in biologic systems.[6] There is no evidence at present that nitrogen dioxide is endogenously formed from nitric oxide.

Acute Clinical Effects

Confusion between a tube of nitroglycerin ointment 2% and a look-alike tube of lanolin skin lubricant made by the same manufacturer resulted in episodes of flushing, headache, presyncope, and hypotension before the problem was clarified.[11] Another patient, unable to obtain a bandage, placed a nitroglycerin patch over a superficial laceration and developed headaches, dizziness, and weakness.[12]

A transient methemoglobinemia may be observed in infants (less than 3 months of age) who are cyanotic and have diarrhea and acidosis. The methemoglobinemia is responsive to methylene blue.[13]

Chronic Effects

A suggested hypothesis for the production of Kaposi's sarcoma in homosexuals is the formation of carcinogenic *N*-nitroso compounds by the use of the nitrosation agents amyl and butyl nitrite.

Ammonium Nitrate

Disposable ammonium nitrate cold packs are widely used in emergency departments instead of ice bags (Table 66–29).[14] Chronic ingestion of 6 to 12 g/day may cause gastritis, acidosis, isosmotic diuresis, and nitrite toxicity manifested by hemoglobinemia or vasodilitation. Five patients tore open the cold packs and ingested from 6 to 234 grams of ammonium nitrate in a single dose. None developed severe toxicity although three had symptoms of gastritis, three had slight methemoglobinemia, and two had mild hypotension. Prompt gastric lavage and supportive care appears to be sufficient for treatment. A decrease in anion gap was observed in one asymptomatic patient who ingested a commercial ice pack mixture containing ammonium nitrate. The decreased anion gap was due to an increase in CO_2 in the electrolyte. The instrument (Ektachem, Kodak) that measured the total CO_2 uses a method that crossreacts positively with nitrate. Nitrate may be considered in the list of toxins (e.g., lithium, bromide) that can decrease the anion gap,[3] using the mnemonic BLIND (Bromide, Lactate, Iodide, Nitrate, Diatrizoate sodium).[15]

LABORATORY

Analytic Methods

In nitrite/nitrate poisoning rapid tests may confirm the diagnosis. These include the diphenylamine blue test (DTA test), the sulfanilic acid—1 naphthylamine test (SA-INA test), and the "cooking test" (clotted blood sample placed in boiling water bath: after cooking and cooling, a blood sample containing nitrite will be salmon pink). A normal blood sample will be chocolate brown. Commercial urine reagent strips (used for detection of urinary tract infections due to nitrite-poisoning bacteria) may be more rapid and more sensitive.[16] An intense pink color develops in the presence of nitrites.

Because of similar absorption characteristics between methemoglobin and sulfhemoglobin, a cooximeter usually interprets sulfhemoglobin as methemoglobin. Hydrogen sulfide does not combine with hemoglobin to form sulfhemoglobin. Neither sulfhemoglobin nor any other abnormal pigments are found in significant concentration in the blood of patients poisoned by sulfide. Animal studies indicate that sulfhemoglobin levels are increased after sulfur dioxide inhalation.[17] Laboratory documentation of sulfhemoglobinemia is often inadequate, and it is probably underdiagnosed.[18]

Diagnosis

Evaluation of the child with "chocolate brown blood" should include a history (past history of same in infant/child or family member, drug exposure, source of drinking water, use of home remedies [including skin creams, ear drops], diarrhea, pica, specific foods and occupations or hobbies of child/parents); physical examination (cardiovascular disease, including clubbing), and laboratory tests (pH, PO_2, PCO_2, quantitative methemoglobin, G6PD screen, hemoglobin/hematocrit/reticulocyte count, quantitative hemoglobin electrophoresis in citrate agar and cellulose acetate, quantitative G6PD if deficient, quantitative NADH and DADPH methemoglobin reductase, stool culture, toxicology screen and/or quantitation of drugs, and others.

Blood Levels

Following an ingestion of isosorbide-5-mononitrate (1.6 g) plasma levels were 2993 (4 hours) and 3140 ng/mL (6 hours) as performed by gas chromatography.[5]

Methylene Blue Overdose

The recommended dose of methylene blue in infants has been reported as 2 mg/kg. At doses of 2 to 4 mg/kg, some infants develop hemolytic anemia and hyperbilirubinemia, Heinz body formation, and desquamation of the skin, which may terminate fatally.[19]

TREATMENT

Ensure airway. Use 100% oxygen and assisted ventilation as required. Administer methylene blue by the intravenous route.

Stabilization

Initial attention should be directed toward improving oxygen delivery with assisted ventilation, if necessary, and 100% oxygen while intravenous methylene blue is prepared. Institute cardiac monitoring, especially in patients with coronary artery or pulmonary disease. Hypotension should respond to Trendelenburg's position and intravenous fluids. Otherwise, dopamine may be needed. Naloxone, glucose, and thiamine should be given if a multiple ingestion is suspected.

Decontamination

Gut decontamination later than 4 hours may be effective if substances that delay gastric emptying or produce ileus are ingested. The administration of the usual doses of charcoal and cathartics after ipecac/lavage is theoretically beneficial. Be sure to remove clothes and wash contaminated skin.

Elimination Enhancement

Theoretically, hemodialysis, forced diuresis, and hemoperfusion are not effective for pure methemoglobinemia, but may be adjunctive treatment for aniline poisoning when supportive care is inadequate. Hyperbaric oxygen has not demonstrated conclusive benefits in animal models. Exchange transfusion and/or the transfusion of packed red blood cells may be useful for methylene blue failures or for patients with known G6PD or NADPH methemoglobin reductase deficiencies. The inherent risks of the large blood volumes required in adults limit the applicability of this method.

Antidotes

Methylene blue (tetramethylthionine chloride) is the antidote of choice for serious methemoglobinemia.

Mechanism of Action

Methylene blue acts as a cofactor to increase the erythrocyte reduction of methemoglobin in the presence of NADPH. The methylene blue is oxidized to leukomethylene blue, which is the electron donor molecule for the nonenzymatic reduction of methemoglobin to oxyhemoglobin.

Toxicokinetics

Methylene blue (blue, oxidized form) is poorly absorbed from the gastrointestinal tract and therefore must be given intravenously. Leukomethylene (colorless, reduced form) is excreted in the urine, although the urine may appear blue when the kidney also excretes sufficient quantities of methylene blue. At high levels of methemoglobin (over 70%), methylene blue reduces the methemoglobin half-life from an average of 15 to 20 hours to 40 to 90 minutes. Hence, improvement from methylene blue therapy should be observed within 1 hour of administration. Patients who ingest aniline may be less responsive to methylene blue, because the toxic intermediate, phenylhydroxylamine, may competitively block uptake of methylene blue by the erythrocytes.

Adverse Effects

High intravenous doses of methylene blue produce chest pain, dyspnea, anxiety, and tremor. Irritating effects on the urinary tract produce dysuria and frequency. High doses (over 7 mg/kg) have endogenous oxidizing properties. In animal models, doses as low as 5 mg/kg produce methemoglobinemia. Mild hemolysis, manifest by slight anemia, reticulocytosis, and hyperbilirubinemia, may appear as a result of the denaturation of hemoglobin by the oxidant. Severe hemolytic reactions are rare in normal patients but common in G6PD-deficient patients. Methylene blue may produce bluish skin discoloration similar to cyanosis.

Failure of Methylene Blue Therapy

1. G6PD deficiency due to low endogenous levels of NADPH.
2. Rare patients with NADPH methemoglobin reductase deficiencies who cannot activate the alternate pathway for methemoglobin reduction.

3. Presence of sulfhemoglobinemia for which methylene blue is ineffective.
4. Excessive methylene blue doses, which produce paradoxic formation of methemoglobin.
5. Continuing gastrointestinal absorption or methemoglobin formation (certain drugs such as aniline produce cyclic formation of methemoglobin).

Indications

Symptomatic patients with methemoglobin levels over 30% should receive methylene blue. Symptoms requiring treatment may appear below 30% in the presence of anemia, pulmonary disease, or processes that reduce coronary or cerebral perfusion. Cyanosis alone is not an indication for treatment without symptomatic evidence of hypoxia.

Contraindications

1. Hypersensitivity.
2. G6PD deficiency resulting from a propensity to precipitate severe hemolytic anemia and lack of efficacy in such patients.
3. NADPH methemoglobin reductase deficiency, a relative contraindication.

Dosage

The usual dose of methylene blue is 1 to 2 mg/kg (25 to 50 mg/m^2) of a 1% solution (10 mg/mL) intravenously over 5 minutes. The same dose may be repeated within 1 hour if symptoms of hypoxia fail to subside. Chemicals such as aniline that produce active metabolites may require repeat doses, but limit the total dose to 7 mg/kg. The administration of ascorbic acid (100 to 500 mg twice daily either orally or intravenously) is harmless, but probably has a minor effect on increasing methemoglobin reduction.

Supportive Care

1. Patients with preexisting pulmonary or cardiac disease require careful cardiac monitoring and evaluation for silent myocardial infarctions and congestive heart failure.
2. Repeat methemoglobin levels are required 1 to 2 hours after therapy to assess the effectiveness of methemoglobin reduction. Be sure to correlate symptoms to methemoglobin levels, and remember that large doses of methylene blue cause a bluish skin discoloration after methemoglobin levels return to normal. If the patient fails to improve within 1 hour after methylene blue therapy, reconsider the diagnosis and review the causes of treatment failure.
3. Follow with complete blood counts and reticulocyte counts for evidence of hemolysis. The need for blood transfusions to correct the anemia produced by hemolysis depends on the patient's ability to withstand decrements in oxygen-carrying capacity (e.g., underlying cardiovascular disease) and the degree of hemoglobin reduction.

REFERENCES—NITRITES, NITRATES, AND METHEMOGLOBINEMIA

1. Askew GL, Finell L, Genese CA, Sorhage FE, Sosin DH, Spitalney KC. Boilerbaisser. An outbreak of methemoglobinemia in New Jersey in 1992. Pediatrics 1994;94: 381–384.
2. Lu G, Yan-Sheng G. Acute nitrate poisoning. A report of 80 cases. Am J Emerg Med 1991;9:200–201.
3. Marshall JB, Eckland RE. Methemoglobinemia from overdose of nitroglycerin. JAMA 1980;244:330.
4. Gibson GR, Hunter JB, Raabe DS et al. Methemoglobinemia produced by high dose intravenous nitroglycerin. Ann Intern Med 1982;96:615–616.
5. Sobrino JM, Fernandez N, Martinez A, Pedrote A. Massive ingestion of isosorbid-5-mononitrate and nitroglycerin: suicide attempt by an adolescent girl without previous heart disease. Eur Heart J 1992;13:145.
6. Marletta MA: Nitric oxide, nitrovasodilators, and L-Arginine—An unusual relationship. West J Med 1991;154: 107–109.
7. Vallance P, Moncada S. Hypodynamic circulation in cirrhosis: a role for nitric oxide? Lancet 1991;337:776–778.
8. Griffith T, Randall M. Nitric oxide comes of age. Lancet 1989; 2:875–876.
9. Svendsen JH, Klarlund K, Aldershrile J, Waldorff S. *N*-Acetylcysteine modifies the acute effects of isosorbid-5-mononitrate in angina pectoris patients evaluated by exercise testing. J Cardiovasc Pharmacol 1989;13: 320–323.
10. Hogan JC, Lewis MJ, Henderson AH. N-acetylcysteine fails to attenuate haemodynamic tolerance to glyceryl trinitrate in healthy volunteers. Br J Clin Pharmac 1989;28: 421–426.
11. Ehrenpreis ED, Young MA, Loikin JD. Symptomatic nitroglycerin toxicity from erroneous use of topical nitroglycerine. Vet Hum Toxicol 1990;32:138–139.
12. Abrams J. Pharmacology of nitroglycerin and long-acting nitrates. Am J Cardiol 1985;56:12A–18A.
13. Yano SS, Danish EH, Hsia YE. Transient methemoglobinemia with acidosis in infants. J Pediatr 1982;100:415.
14. Challoner KR, McCarron MM. Ammonium nitrate cold pack ingestion. J Emerg Med 1988;6:200–201.
15. Senecal PD, Dyer JE, Osterloh JD. Nitrate as a cause of decreased anion gap. Vet Hum Toxicol 1991;33:375.
16. Rodriguez FS, Santiyan MPM, Zamorano JDP. Evaluation of reagent strips for the rapid diagnosis of nitrite poisoning. J Anal Toxicol 1992;16:63–64.
17. Baskurt OK. Acute hematologic and hemorheologic effects of sulfur dioxide inhalation. Arch Environ Health 1988;43: 345–348.
18. Park CM, Nagel RL. Sulfhemoglobinemia. Clinical and molecular aspects. N Engl J Med 1984;310:1579–1584.
19. Sills MR, Zinkhaim WA. Methylene blue-induced Heinz body hemolytic anemia. Arch Pediatr Adolesc Med 1994;148:306–310.

OCCUPATIONAL LUNG DISEASE[1–6] (PULMONARY RESPONSE TO INHALED TOXINS—OCCUPATIONAL ASTHMA)

Occupational asthma has become the most prevalent occupational lung disease in developed countries. About 250 agents can cause occupational asthma (Tables 66–30 and 66–31). Isocyanates are responsible for the most common form of the disease. The prevalence of isocyanate-induced

Table 66–30
Causes of Occupational Asthma: Allergic or Possibly Allergic Mechanism Low-Molecular-Weight Compounds[a]

Agents	Industries	Skin Test[b,c]	Specific IgE	Precipitin	Broncho-provocation Test
Diisocyanates					
Toluene diisocyanate	Polyurethane industry, plastics, varnish	±	±	–	+
Diphenylmethane diisocyanate	Foundries	–	+		+
Hexamethylene diisocyanate	Automobile spray painting		–	+	+
Anhydrides					
Phthalic anhydride	Epoxy resins, plastics	+	+		+
Trimellitic anhydride	Epoxy resins, plastics	+	+		+
Tetrachlorophthalic anhydride	Epoxy resins, plastics		–	–	+
Wood Dust					
Western red cedar *(Thuja plicata)*	Carpentry, construction, cabinet-making, sawmill	+	+	–	+
California redwood *(Sequoia sempervirens)*		–		–	+
Cedar of Lebanon *(Cedra libani)*		–		–	
Cocabolla *(Dalbergia retusa)*		–			
Iroko *(Chlorophora excelsa)*		+		+	+
Oak *(Quercus robur)*		–		+	–
Mahogany *(Shoreal spp)*		–		+	+
Abiruana *(Pouteria)*		+		–	+
African maple *(Triplochiton scleroxylon)*		+	+		+
Tanganyika aningre		+	–	–	+
Central American walnut *(Juglans olanchana)*		–	–	–	+
Kejaat *(Pterocarpus angolensis)*		+			
African zebra wood *(Microberlinia)*		+	+	–	+
Metals					
Platinus	Platinum refinery	+			+
Nickel	Metal plating	+	±	±	+
Chromium	Tanning	±	+		+
Cobalt	Hard metal industry	+		+	+
Vanadium	Hard metal industry				
Tungsten carbide	Hard metal industry				
Fluxes					
Aminoethyl ethanolamine	Aluminum soldering	–			+
Colophony	Electronic soldering				+
Drugs					
Penicillins	Pharmaceutical	–			+
Cephalosporins	Pharmaceutical	+			+
Phenylglycine acid chloride	Pharmaceutical	+	+		+
Piperazine hydrochloride	Chemical	+			+
Psyllium	Laxative manufacturer	+			+
Methyl dopa	Pharmaceutical	–			+
Spiramycin	Pharmaceutical	+			+
Salbutamol intermediate	Pharmaceutical				+
Amprolium HCl	Poultry feed mixer				+
Tetracycline	Pharmaceutical				+
Sulphone chloramides	Manufacturer, brewery	+			
Other Chemicals					
Dimethyl ethanolamine	Spray painting	–			+
Persulphate salts and henna	Hairdressing	+			+
Ethylene diamine	Photography	–			+
Azodicarbonamide	Plastics and rubber	–			
Hexachlorophene (sterilizing agent)	Hospital staff				+
Formalin	Hospital staff				+
Urea formaldehyde	Insulation, resin	–			+
Freon	Refrigeration	+			+
Paraphenylene diamine	Fur dyeing	+			+
Furfuryl alcohol (furan bases resin)	Foundry mold making				+

[a]Adapted from Chan-Yeung M, Lam S. Am Rev Respir Dis 1986;133:686–703.
[b]Skin test to specific antigen.
[c]± indicates both positive and negative results have been reported.

Table 66–31
Causes of Occupational Asthma: Allergic Mechanism High-Molecular-Weight Compounds[a]

Agents	Industries	Skin Test[b,c]	Specific IgE	Precipitin	Broncho-provocation Test
Animal Products, Insects, Other					
Laboratory animals					
Rats	Laboratory workers				
Mouse	Veterinarians	+			+
Rabbit	Animal handlers	+		−	
Guinea pig		+	+	−	+
Birds					
Pigeon	Pigeon breeders	+			+
Chicken	Poultry workers	+	+		+
Budgerigar	Bird fanciers				
Insects					
Grain mite	Grain workers	+		+	+
Locust	Research laboratory	+	+		
River fly	Power plants along rivers	+			
Screw worm fly	Flight crews	+			
Cockroach	Laboratory workers	+			
Cricket	Field contact	+	−	−	+
Bee moth	Fish bait breeder	+		−	+
Moth and butterfly	Entomologists	+			
Plants					
Grain dust	Grain handlers	±	−	±	+
Wheat/rye flour	Bakers, millers	±	±	±	+
Buckwheat	Bakers	+			
Coffee bean	Food processor	+	+		+
Castor bean	Oil industry	+	+		+
Tea	Tea worker	+			+
Tobacco leaf	Tobacco manufacturing	+	+		+
Hops *(Humulus lupulus)*	Brewery chemist	+			
Biologic Enzymes					
Bacillus subtilis	Detergent industry	+	+	+	+
Trypsin	Plastic, pharmaceutical	+	+	−	+
Pancreatin	Pharmaceutical				
Papain	Laboratory	+	+	+	
	Packaging	+	+	−	+
Pepsin	Pharmaceutical	+	+		+
Flaviastase	Pharmaceutical	+	+	+	
Bromelin	Pharmaceutical	+			+
Fungal amylase	Manufacturing, bakers	+			
Vegetables					
Gum acacia	Printers	+			+
Gum tragacanth	Gum manufacturing	+			
Other					
Crab	Crab processing	+			+
Prawn	Prawn processing	+	+	+	+
Hoya	Oyster farm	+	+		
Larva of silkworm	Sericulture	+	+		+

[a]Adapted from Chan-Yeung M, Lam S. Am Rev Respir Dis 1986;133:686–703.
[b]Skin test to specific antigens.
[c]± indicates both positive and negative results have been reported.

asthma in exposed workers is close to 10%.[7] Mechanisms of pathologic injury in occupational lung disease are summarized in Table 66–32.

CLASSIFICATION

The two categories of asthma in the workplace are occupational asthma and work-aggravated asthma. Occupational asthma is characterized by variable airflow limitation, bronchial hyperresponsiveness, or both, due to conditions in a particular work environment, not to stimuli outside the workplace. Work-aggravated asthma is preexisting or concurrent asthma that is aggravated by irritants or physical stimuli in the workplace. Occupational asthma may develop in a person with preexisting asthma or concurrent asthma after a workplace exposure.[7]

Two types of occupational asthma can be distinguished according to whether there is a latency period (Table 66–33). Occupational asthma with latency is the most common type. This develops after a period of exposure that may vary from a few weeks to several years. Occupational asthma with latency includes all instances of immunologic asthma, although the immunologic mechanism has not yet been identified for some agents (Table

66–34). Occupational asthma without a latency period follows exposure to high concentrations of irritant gases, fumes, or chemicals on one or several occasions.[7] A systematic approach to history taking and the diagnosis of occupational and environmental disease is depicted in Figure 66–4 (Table 66–35).

TREATMENT

The ideal treatment for patients with occupational asthma with a latency period is removal from exposure. Most people with occupational asthma have to be retrained for a job with another employer in a different field. Any patient with occupational asthma who returns to the same job should have close medical follow-up. Worsening of asthma should lead to immediate removal from exposure. Pharmacologic treatment is similar to the treatment of patients with other forms of asthma.[7]

Table 66–32
Mechanisms of Pathological Injury in Occupational Lung Diseases[a]

Mechanism	Tissue Reaction	Example
Irritant	Alveolitis	Phosgene
	Bronchiolitis obliterans	NO_2 inhalation
	Bronchitis	Coke workers
Immunologic		
Type I	Bronchial edema, plugging	Byssinosis
Type III	Interstitial infiltrate, granuloma	Farmer's lung
Type IV	Noncaseating granuloma	Berylliosis
Fibrogenesis	Dust macules (little scarring)	Iron, tin
	Dust nodules (marked scarring)	Silicosis
	With focal emphysema, "PMF"[b]	Coal dust
	With malignancy	Asbestosis

[a]Adapted from Hasan FM, Dodge RR. Occupational lung diseases—general principles and select topics. In: Occupational Safety and Health Administration Symposium, 1978. Washington, DC: National Institute of Occupational Safety and Health, 1979, p. 104.
[b]Progressive massive fibrosis.

RADS (TABLE 66–36)

RADS (Reactive Airway Disease Syndrome) differs from typical occupational asthma because of the absence of a preceding period for sensitization and the onset of illness after a single first-time exposure.[8] The subsequent inflammatory process may alter the threshold of receptors in the bronchial mucosa.[8] Viral respiratory infections may temporarily increase bronchial reactivity in healthy subjects.[9]

Reflex

Inert particles, noxious fumes, cold air, and exercise may cause direct bronchoconstriction by stimulating irritant receptors in the bronchial wall. Most subjects who develop reflex bronchospasm have preexisting asthma.

Causes

Polyethylene shrink wrapping (paper wrapper's asthma) may be due to the pyrolysis products of polyvinyl chloride produced by the shrink-wrapping processes. Bronchoprovocation tests exhibit a positive response.[10]

HYPERSENSITIVITY PNEUMONITIS (EXTRINSIC ALLERGIC ALVEOLITIS)[11,12]

Hypersensitivity pneumonitis (HSP) (Tables 66–37 and 66–38) is an immunologically induced inflammation of the lung parenchyma resulting from the repeated inhalation of a variety of etiologic agents, including organic dusts and simple chemicals.

Clinical Presentation

Both systemic and respiratory symptoms may occur. In the acute form, influenza-like symptoms often predominate, consisting of chills, fever, sweating, myalgias, lassitude, headache, and nausea that begin 2 to 9 hours after exposure, peak typically between 6 and 24 hours, and last from hours

Table 66–33
Types of Occupational Asthma

Characteristic	Asthma with Latency		
	IgE-dependent	IgE-independent	Asthma Without Latency
Clinical			
Interval between onset of exposure and symptoms	Longer	Shorter	Within hours
Pattern of asthmatic reaction on inhalation testing	Immediate, dual	Late, atypical	Testing not done
Epidemlologic			
Prevalence in exposed population	<5%	>5%	Unknown
Host predisposition	Atopy, smoking(?)	Unknown	Unknown
Pathologic*			
Eosinophil change	++	++	++
Lymphocyte change	++	++	+
Subepithelial fibrosis	+	+	++
Thickened basement membrane	++	++	++
Desquamation of epithelium	+	+	++

Chan-Yeung M and Malo J-C. N Engl J Med 1985;333:107–112.
*The symbol + denotes increased, and ++ markedly increased.

Table 66–34
Common Agents That Cause Occupational Asthma with Latency and Workers Who Are at Risk

Agent	Workers at Risk
High-molecular-weight agents	
Cereals	Bakers, millers
Animal-derived allergens	Animal handlers
Enzymes	Detergent users, pharmaceutical workers, bakers
Gums	Carpet makers, pharmaceutical workers
Latex	Health professionals
Seafoods	Seafood processors
Low-molecular-weight agents	
Isocyanates	Spray painters; insulation installers, manufacturers of plastics, rubbers, foam
Wood dusts	Forest workers, carpenters, cabinetmakers
Anhydrides	Users of plastics, epoxy resins
Amines	Shellac and lacquer handlers, solderers
Fluxes	Electronics workers
Chloramine-T	Janitors, cleaners
Dyes	Textile workers
Persulfate	Hairdressers
Formaldehyde, glutaraldehyde	Hospital staff
Acrylate	Adhesives handlers
Drugs	Pharmaceutical workers, health professionals
Metals	Solderers, refiners

Chan-Yeung M and Malo J-C. New Engl J Med 1995;333:107–112.

to days. Respiratory symptoms such as cough and dyspnea are common but not universal. The subacute form may appear gradually over several days to weeks, is marked by cough and dyspnea, and may progress to severe dyspnea with cyanosis, leading to urgent hospitalization. The chronic form has an insidious onset over a period of months, with increasing cough and exertion dyspnea. Fatigue and weight loss may be prominent symptoms.

Symptoms, signs, and other manifestations of hypersensitivity pneumonitis disappear within days, weeks, or months in most patients if the causative agent is no longer inhaled.

Differential Diagnosis

The diagnosis of HSP should be initially considered in any patient with a history of recurrent pneumonias or with interstitial lung disease, as well as in those with typical presentations of acute, subacute, or chronic HSP. Recurrent pneumonias also require that immunodeficiency syndromes, especially hypoimmunoglobulinemia, be ruled out. Common occupational lung diseases and occupational alveolar and airway disease are listed in Tables 66–39 and 66–40.

Pulmonary Myotoxicosis

Exposure to fresh silage. Fever, chills, and cough within a few hours.

Toxic Organic Dust Syndrome (Table 66–41)

Transient fever, muscle aches, with or without respiratory symptoms. Chest x-ray films usually appear normal.

Idiopathic Interstitial Fibrosis (Cryptogenic Fibrosing Alveolitis)

Autoimmune phenomena common, bronchopulmonary lavage helpful. Histopathology distinctive.

Cystic Fibrosis

Silo-Filler's Lung

Oxides of nitrogen from a freshly filled silo.

Psittacosis

In patients handling birds.

Eosinophilic Pneumonias

Striking eosinophilia; bronchial asthma.

Allergic Bronchopulmonary Aspergillosis

Precipitating antibodies to *Aspergillus fumigatus.*

Collagen Vascular Disease

Granuloma-vasculitis syndromes and sarcoidosis are multi system diseases. Hypersensitivity pneumonitis is confirmed to the lung.

Diagnostic Procedures

Radiologic Evaluation

The chest x-ray film sometimes appears normal, even in symptomatic patients. The acute phase may be associated with a small, poorly defined, uniform, rather discrete, and diffuse nodulation, occasionally symmetrically sparing the apices or bases. A diffuse, soft, stringy or patchy interstitial infiltrate may also be seen with or without nodulation. In the chronic fibrotic phase, the linear element becomes more distinct and the periphery may be more prominently involved. Abnormalities rarely seen in hypersensitivity pneumonitis include pleural effusion or thickening, hilar adenopathy, calcification, cavitation, atalectasis, and coin lesions.

Pulmonary Function Testing

Pulmonary function studies typically show a restrictive pattern, with decreased compliance and impaired gas exchange (DLco). After acute exposure, there is a decrease in forced vital capacity and 1-second forced expiratory volume (FEV_1) with maintenance of flow rates. If the chronic stage develops into progressive fibrosis, changes of airway obstruction, as well as restriction, may be increasingly prominent.

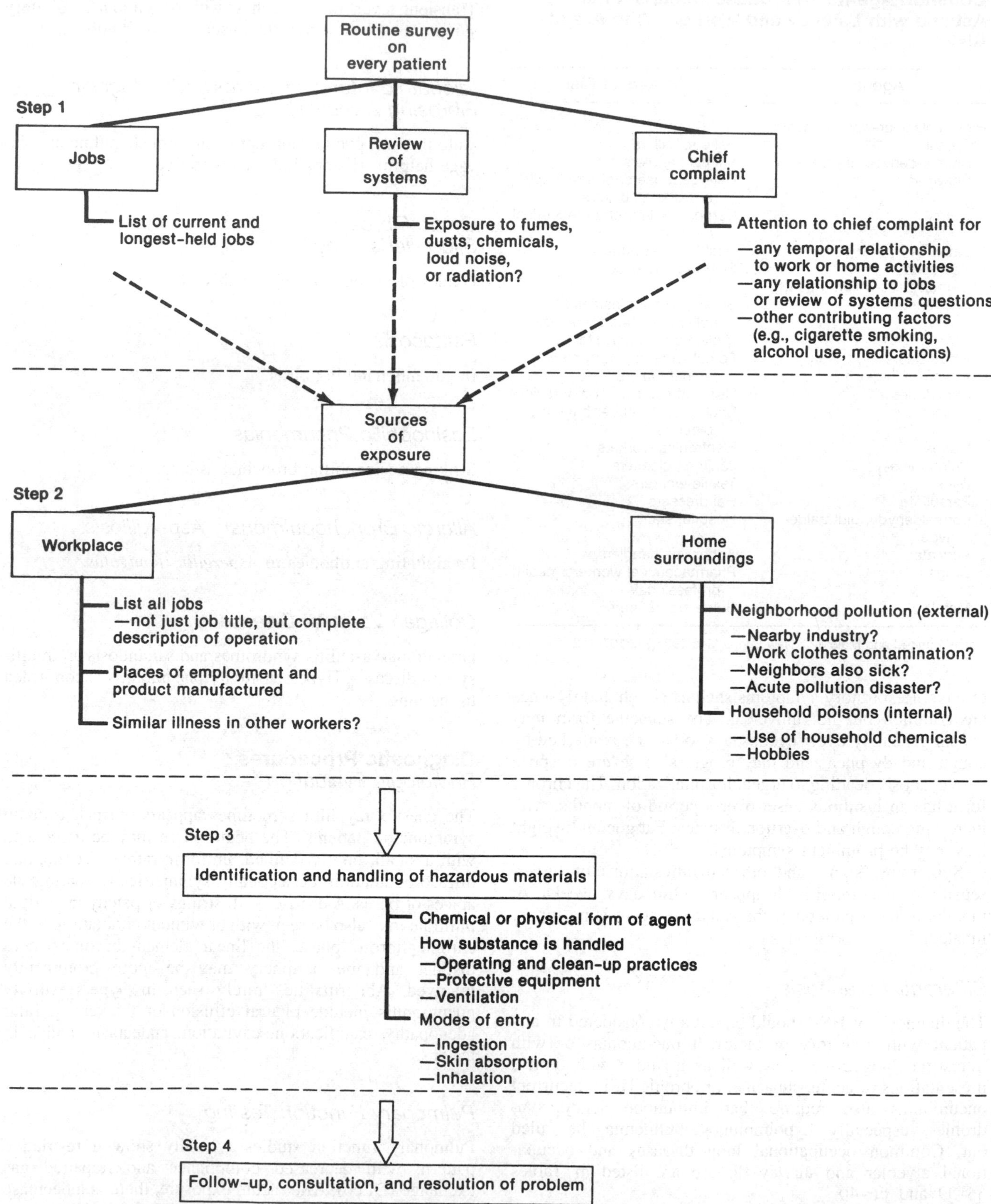

Figure 66–4 Systematic approach to history taking and diagnosis of occupational or environmental illness. (Adapted from Goldman RH, Peters JH. JAMA 1981;246:2832.)

Table 66–35
Advantages and Disadvantages of Diagnostic Methods for Occupational Asthma*

Method	Advantages	Disadvantages
Questionnaire	Simple, sensitive	Low specificity
Immunologic testing	Simple, sensitive	Only for high-molecular-weight and some low-molecular-weight agents; identifies sensitization, not disease; majority of allergens not available commercially
Bronchial responsiveness to methacholine or histamine	Simple, sensitive	Not specific for asthma or occupational asthma; occupational asthma not ruled out by a negative test
Measurement of FEV_1 before and after work	Simple, inexpensive	Low sensitivity and specificity
Peak expiratory flow monitoring	Relatively simple, inexpensive	Requires patient's cooperation and honesty; not as sensitive as FEV_1 in assessing airway caliber; no standardized method of interpreting graphs
Specific inhalation challenges in a hospital laboratory	If positive, confirmatory	Diagnosis not ruled out by a negative test (e.g., if wrong agent or subject no longer at work); expensive; few referral centers
Serial FEV_1 measurements at work under supervision	If negative, rules out diagnosis when patient tested under usual work conditions	A positive test may be due to irritation; requires collaboration of employer

Chan-Yeung M and Malo J-C. N Engl J Med 1995;333:107–112.
*FEV_1 denotes forced expiratory volume in one second.

Table 66–36
Clinical Criteria for the Diagnosis of Reactive Airways Dysfunction Syndrome (RADS)[a]

1. A documented absence of preceding respiratory complaints.
2. The onset of symptoms occurred after a single specific exposure incident or accident.
3. The exposure was to a gas, smoke, fume, or vapor that was present in very high concentrations and had irritant qualities to its nature.
4. The onset of symptoms occurred within 24 hours after the exposure and persisted for at least 3 months.
5. Symptoms simulated asthma with cough, wheezing, and dyspnea predominating.
6. Pulmonary function tests may show airflow obstruction.
7. Methacholine challenge testing was positive.
8. Other types of pulmonary diseases were ruled out.

[a]Adapted from Brooks SM et al. Chest 1985;88:376–384.

Serum Antibody

The attempted demonstration of antibody against suspected antigens by precipitin reactions in agar is an important part of the diagnostic workup. Precipitins are not demonstrable in all patients, and available antigens are not standardized.

General Laboratory Tests

After acute exposure, peripheral blood neutrophilia and lymphopenia are common. Eosinophilia is not expected. Mild elevations in erythrocyte sedimentation rate, C-reactive protein, rheumatoid factor, and in immunoglobulins of IgG, IgM, or IgA isotypes may be present occasionally, reflecting acute or chronic inflammatory changes. Antinuclear antibodies or other autoantibodies are seldom detected.[11]

In Vitro Tests for Cell-Mediated Immunity

There is no place in the routine diagnostic workup for measures of cell-mediated immune responses (e.g., antigen- or mitogen-induced blastogenesis or release of lymphokines such as macrophage migration inhibitory factor).[11]

Routine use of inhalational challenge is not recommended, especially in patients with forms of the disease other than simple, acute, recurrent, or transient attacks.[11]

Available information is insufficient to know to what extent bronchoalveolar lavage is useful in the routine diagnostic workup of patients with suspected HSP.

Lung Biopsy

To make a definitive diagnosis in patients without sufficient clinical criteria, lung biopsy may be indicated, especially to rule out other diseases requiring different treatment. Open lung biopsy will usually provide adequate material, whereas transbronchial biopsy may not.

Treatment
Therapeutic Trial

Removal of the causative agent from the patient's environment, or of the patient from the incriminated inhalant, should be followed by improvement in most acute cases within days, weeks, or months and will help confirm the diagnosis.[11]

ORGANIC DUST TOXIC SYNDROME (TABLE 66–41)

Organic Dust Toxic Syndrome (ODTS)[13] is a nonallergic, noninfectious, febrile respiratory illness caused by organic

Table 66–37
Hypersensitivity Pneumonitis (Extrinsic Allergic Alveolitis)—Reported Associations[a]

Disease	Antigen	Source of Particles
Farmer's lung	Thermophilic actinomycetes	"Moldy" hay, grain, silage
Bird fancier's, breeder's, or handler's lung	Parakeet, budgerigar, pigeon, chicken, turkey proteins	Avian droppings or feathers
Humidifier or air-conditioner lung (ventilation pneumonitis)	*Aureobasidium pullulans* or other microorganisms	Contaminated water in humidification and forced air air-conditioning systems
Chemical worker's lung	Isocyanates	Polyurethane foam, varnishes, lacquer, foundry casting
Bagassosis	Thermophilic actinomycetes	"Moldy" bagasse (sugar cane)
Malt worker's lung	*Aspergillus fumigatus* or *A. clavatus*	Moldy barley
Mushroom worker's lung	Thermophilic actinomycetes, other	Mushroom compost
Sequoiosis	*Aureobasidium, Graphium* sp.	Redwood sawdust
Maple bark disease	*Cryptostroma corticale*	Maple bark
Woodworker's lung	Wood dust; *Alternaria*	Oak, cedar, and mahogany dusts; pine and spruce pulp
Cheese washer's lung	*Penicillium casei*	Moldy cheese
Suberosis	Cork dust mold	Cork dust
Sauna taker's lung	*Aureobasidium* sp., other	Contaminated sauna water
Pituitary snuff taker's lung	Animal proteins	Heterologous pituitary snuff
Coffee worker's lung	Coffee bean dust	Coffee beans
Miller's lung	*Sitophilus granarius* (wheat weevil)	Infested wheat flour
Fish meal worker's lung	Fish meal dust	Fish meal
Furrier's lung	Animal fur dust	Animal pelts
Lycoperdonosis	Puffball spores	Lycoperdon puffballs
Familial HSP	*Bacillus subtilis*	Contaminated wood dust in walls
Compost lung	*Aspergillus*	Compost
Wood trimmer's disease	*Rhizopus* sp., *Mucor* sp.	Contaminated wood trimmings
Thatched roof disease	*Sacchoromonospora viridis*	Dried grasses and leaves
Streptomyces albus HSP	*Streptomyces albus*	Contaminated fertilizer
Cephalosporium HSP	*Cephalosporium*	Contaminated basement (sewage)
Detergent worker's disease	*Bacillus subtilis* enzymes	Detergent
Japanese summer house HSP	*Trichosporon cutaneum*	House dust? bird droppings
Potato riddler's lung	Thermophilic actinomycetes, *M. Faeni, T. Vulgaris, Aspergillus* sp.	"Moldy" hay around potatoes
Tobacco worker's disease	*Aspergillus* sp.	Mold on tobacco
Hot tub lung	*Cladosporium* sp.	Mold on ceiling
Winegrower's lung	*Botrytis cinerea*	Mold on grapes
Laboratory worker's HSP	Male rat urine	Laboratory rat
Tap water lung	Unknown	Contaminated tap water
Pauli's HSP	Pauli's reagent	Laboratory reagent
Woodman's disease	*Penicillium* sp.	Oak and maple trees

[a]Adapted from Richerson HB et al. J Allergy Clin Immunol 1989;84:839–844.
HSP, Hypersensitivity pneumonitis.

Table 66–38
Agents Inducing Hypersensitivity Pneumonitis[a]

Agent	Disease	Exposure
Thermophilic actinomycetes		
Micropolyspora faeni	Farmer's lung	Mold compost
Thermoactinomyces sacchari	Bagassosis	Moldy sugar cane
Thermoactinomyces vulgaris	Mushroom worker's lung	Moldy compost
Thermoactinomyces viridis	Mushroom worker's lung	Moldy compost
Thermoactinomyces candidus	Ventilation pneumonitis	Contaminated forced-air systems
Fungi		
Alternaria species	Wood worker's lung	Moldy wood chips
Pullularia pullulans	Sequoiosis	Moldy redwood dust
Aspergillus clavatus	Malt worker's lung	Moldy malt
Penicillium frequentans	Suberosis	Moldy work dust
Penicillium caseii	Cheese worker's lung	Moldy cheese
Penicillium roqueforti	Cheese worker's lung	Moldy cheese
Phoma species	Shower curtain	Moldy shower curtain
Mucor stolonifer	Paprika splitter's lung	Paprika dust
Cryptostroma corticale	Maple bark stripper's lung	Moldy maple bark

[a]Adapted from Levy MB, Fink JN. Ann Allergy 1985:54;168.

(continued)

Table 66-38 *(Continued)*

Agent	Disease	Exposure
Animal proteins		
Avian proteins	Bird breeder's lung	Avian droppings
Bovine and porcine	Pituitary snuff user's lung	Heterologous proteins
Rodent urinary proteins	Laboratory animal worker's lung	Rodent urine
Arthropods		
Sitophilus grainafius	Wheat weevil	Infested wheat
Chemicals		
Phthalic anhydride	Epoxy resin worker's lung	Expoxy resin
Toluene diisocyanate	Porcelain refinisher's lung	Paint catalyst
Trimellitic anhydride	Plastic worker's lung	Trimellitic anhydride
Other agents		
Ameba, various fungi	Ventilation pneumonitis	Contaminated air systems
Bacillus subtilis	Enzyme worker's lung	Detergent enzymes
Hair dust	Furrier's lung	Animal proteins

Table 66-39
Common Occupational Lung Diseases (Partial List)[a]

Inhalant	Disease	Exposure
Mineral (Inorganic Dusts)		
	Fibrosis and malignancy	
Free silica	Silicosis	Hard-rock or metal mining, foundry work, sand-blasting, pottery industry, slate industry
Asbestos	Asbestosis, lung cancer, mesothelioma	Mining and milling; manufacture of asbestos products; installation or removal of asbestos insulation
Coal dust	Progressive massive fibrosis	Coal mining
Diatomaceous earth, kaolin, talc, mica, tungsten carbide	Varying degrees of fibrosis	Mining, manufacturing
	Maculae	
Coal dust	Simple coal worker's pneumoconiosis	Coal mining
Iron oxide	Siderosis	Welding
Barium sulfate	Baritosis	Mining
Tin oxide	Stannosis	Mining
Organic Dusts		
Diffuse hypersensitivity pneumonia (extrinsic allergic alveolitis)		
Moldy hay	Farmer's lung	Farming
Bagasse	Bagassosis	Manufacture of wallboard, paper
Avian droppings or serum	Bird breeder's lung	Bird handling
Mushroom spores	Mushroom worker's lung	Mushroom farming
Variable airway obstruction (occupational asthma)		
Grain	Asthma	Grain elevator work
Castor or coffee beans	Asthma	Castor oil or coffee manufacturing
Proteolytic enzyme detergents	Asthma	Detergent manufacturing
Western red cedar dust	Asthma	Lumbering, woodworking
Cotton, flax, hemp	Byssinosis	Textile industry
Irritant Gases and Chemicals		
Acute heavy exposure	Diverse pathology	
Chlorine, phosgene, nitrogen oxide, ammonia	Tracheobronchitis, bronchiolitis, pulmonary edema	Transportation accidents, manufacturing accidents or malfunction
Chronic low level (continuous or intermittent)		
Toluene diisocyanate, phthalic anhydride, trimellitic anhydride	Occupational asthma	Plastics industry
Wide variety of irritants	Industrial bronchitis	Chemical industry
Chemical carcinogens	Lung cancer	
Chloromethyl ethers		Chemical industry
Uranium		Mining
Coke-oven emission		Steel industry
Metals (arsenic, chromates, nickel)		Mining or manufacturing

[a]Adapted from Weill H. Hosp Pract 1981;164:68.

Table 66–40
Origins of Occupational Alveolar and Airway Disease[a,b]

Source	Workers Affected	Airway Disease	Alveolar Disease
Microbes			
Bacteria			
Aerobacter cloacae	Air conditioner, humidifier		+
Phialophora sp.			
Escherichia coli endotoxin	Mill fever—textile workers	+	+
Pseudomonas sp.	Sewer workers	+	+
Fungi	Farmer's lung group		
Aspergillus sp., *Micropolyspora faeni*	Farmers	+	
Aspergillus clavatus	Malt workers	+	
Cladosporium sp.	Combine operators	+	+
Verticillium sp.			
Alternaria sp.			
Micropolyspora faeni	Mushroom workers	+	+
Penicillium casei	Cheese workers	+	
Penicillium frequentans	Suberosis (cork)	+	
Thermoactinomyces (vulgaris) sacchari	Bagassosis, sugar cane products	+	+
Amoeba			
Acathamoeba castellani	Air conditioning and humidifier	+	+
Acathamoeba polyphaga			
Naegleria gruberi			
Plants			
Castor bean—ricin	Oil mill	+	
Coffee bean	Roasters	+	
Cotton, hemp, flax, jute, kapok	Textile workers	+	
Flour dust	Millers	+	
Grain dust	Farmers	+	
Gum arabic, gum	Printers	+	
Papain	Preparation workers		+
Proteolytic enzymes, *Bacillus subtilus* (subtilisin, alcalase)	Detergent workers		+
Tamarind seed powder	Weavers	+	
Wood dust	Canadian red cedar, South African boxwood, rosewood (*Dalbergia* sp.)	+	
Animals			
Ascaris lumbricoides	Zoologists	+	
Ascidiacea	Oyster culture	+	
Dander	Farmers, fur workers, grooms	+	
Feathers	Turkey and chicken farmers	+	
Insect chitin			
Sitophilus granarius	Flour	+	
Mayfly	Outdoorsmen	+	
Screwfly	Screw-worm controllers	+	
Pancreatic enzymes	Preparation workers	+	+
Rat serum–urine	Laboratory workers	+	+
Chemicals			
Inorganic			
Calcium hydroxide/tricalcium silicate	Cement workers	+	
Chromium	Casters	+	
Vanadium pentoxide	Refinery workers	+	
Nickel sulfate	Platers	+	
Platinum chloroplatinate	Photographers	+	
Tungsten carbide (cobalt) hard metal	Hard metal workers	+	+
Zinc, copper, magnesium fumes	Welders, bronze (metal fume fever)	+	
Copper sulfate and lime	Vineyard sprayers		+
Organic			
Aminoethyl ethanolamine	Solderers	+	
Chlorinated biphenyls	Transformer manufacturers		+
Colophony (pine resin)	Solderers	+	
Diisocyanates—toluene, diphenylmethane	Production workers	+	
Formalin	Permapress, urethane foam	+	
Paraquat	Sprayers	+	+
Penicillin, ampicillin	Production workers, nurses	+	
Parathion	Sprayers	+	

[a]Adapted from Last JM, Maxcy-Roseman: Public health and preventive medicine. 11th ed. New York, Appleton-Century-Crofts, 1980, pp. 620–621.
[b]Reversible airway disease is occupational asthma, which occurs most often in atopic individuals. Alveolar disease is manifest as hypersensitive pneumonitis (British synonym is extrinsic allergic alveolitis).

(continued)

Table 66-40 *(Continued)*

Source	Workers Affected	Airway Disease	Alveolar Disease
Chemicals (continued)			
p-Phenylenediamine	Solderers	+	
Piperazine	Chemists	+	
Polymer fumes (polytetrafluoroethylene)	Teflon manufacture, use	+	+
Synthetic fibers—nylon, polysters, dacron	Textile workers		+
Vinyl chloride (phosgene) (hydrogen chloride)	Meat wrappers (asthma)	+	
	Firefighters		+
	Polymerization plant		+

Table 66-41
Environments in Which Reactions to Organic Dust Have Been Reported[a]

Environments with high or unknown endotoxin levels and probably low mold spore exposure
Cotton card room
Grain elevator
Swine confinement buildings
Plucking ducks
Offices with uncleaned humidifiers
Bath water
Sewage plants
Environments with high or unknown endotoxin levels but probably high mold spore concentrations in air
Moldy silo capping
Moldy grain
Moldy woodchips used as fuel
Partying in a room covered with hay
Work in storehouse with moldy oranges
Experimental exposures to dust causing ODTS in man
Grain dust
Cotton carding dust
Endotoxin

[a]Adapted from Malmberg P, Rask-Anderson A. Semin Respir Med 1993;14: 38–48.

dust from moldy silage, hay, or other agricultural products. It is also known as *pulmonary mycotoxicosis*[13] because the organic dust consists largely of microbial hyphae and spores. Exposure may occur when farm workers are involved in the dusty activity of transferring moldy silage. This condition has been referred to as *silo-unloader's syndrome.*[13,14]

The symptoms include chills, malaise, myalagia, a dry cough, dyspnea, headache, and nausea after a heavy organic dust exposure. ODTS is similar to acute farmer's lung and other forms of hypersensitivity pneumonitis in that both exhibit increased numbers of neutrophils in the bronchoalveolar lavage, both may be more common in nonsmokers, and both have a latency period of 4 hours or more. They differ in that the chest x-ray in ODTS does not show infiltrates, severe hypoxemia does not occur, prior sensitization to antigens in the organic dust toxic syndrome usually does not occur (serology-allergen panel is usually negative), and there are no known sequelae of physiologic significance.[13,15,16]

Table 66–42 differentiates ODTS from acute farmer's lung.[13–19] A tabulation of occupational hazards is presented in Table 66–43.

PNEUMOCONIOSIS (TABLE 66–44)

Silica

It is important to distinguish among the terms *silicon* (the element), *silica* (the minerals), *silicates* (the minerals), and *silicone* (a man-made synthetic polymer). Silica or silicon dioxide (SiO_2) exist in nature in amorphous and crystalline forms.[20] *Amorphous silica* includes natural glasses, such as are found in volcanic tuff; synthetic glasses of commerce, including the glasses in mineral wool; and fume silica. Amorphous silica is much less toxic than crystalline silica although it is not biologically inert. *Crystalline silica* forms in the earth's crust under conditions of increased heat and pressure. *Free silica* refers to pure crystalline silicon dioxide. It consists of silicon-oxygen tetrahedra in a number of polymorphic forms. The medically important crystalline phases of silicon dioxide are known as alpha quartz, cristobalite, and tridymite. Among these, alpha quartz is the most common mineral of commercial importance. It is a major constituent of igneous rocks such as granite and pegmatite, but it is also found in sandstone and sedimentary deposits such as slate and shale. Cristobalite and tridymite are formed from quartz at high temperatures and have a restricted geologic distribution. These crystalline types commonly form in refractories due to the high temperatures of the industrial process. Diatoms are composed of amorphous silica, but diatomaceous earth crystallizes at extreme temperatures and pressure, forming cristobalite and tridymite.

Silicates are less fibrogenic than silica when inhaled into the lungs, but cause characteristic lesions after heavy prolonged exposure.

Sandblasting is extremely hazardous and a notorious cause of silicosis. In Great Britain, sandblasting was banned in 1951, and the National Institute for Occupational Safety and Health recommended its prohibition in the United States in 1974.[21]

Sources

Silicosis results from the inhalation of crystalline or free silica, usually in the form of quartz. Workers at risk, in addition to sandblasters, include miners, tunnelers, silica millers, abrasives and flour workers, ceramics workers, glassmakers, and quarry and foundry workers.[21]

Table 66-42
Organic Dust Toxic Syndrome Versus Acute Farmer's Lung[a]

	Organic Dust Toxic Syndrome	Acute Farmer's Lung
Incidence	10–190/10,000	2–30/10,000
Clustering of cases	Yes	Uncommon
Season	Most common in summer, fall	Most common in winter, early spring
Sex	Most common in males (may be related to division of labor)	Male or female depending on division of labor
Age	Median = 30s, 40s	Median = 30–50s
Nonsmokers vs. smokers, former smokers	May be more common in nonsmokers	More common in nonsmokers
Exposure history	Heavy exposure to organic dust, commonly from "moldy" grain, silage "moldy" hay, or wood chips and others May occur with first exposure	Repeated exposure to causative agent, including spoiled hay, grain, poultry, and others
Causative agent	?Endotoxin ?Fungal toxins ?Others	Antigens in the thermophilic actinomycetes, *Aspergillus* spp. avian proteins, and others
Latency	4–12 hours	4–8 hours
Symptoms	Dry cough, chills, fever, malaise, dyspnea, myalgia, chest tightness, headache	Fever, chills, malaise, dry cough, dyspnea
Duration of acute symptoms	Usually less than 24 hours but may last 2–5 days	12–36 hours
Physical examination of the chest	Normal or scattered rales	End-inspiratory bibasilar rales
White blood count	Leukocytosis to 26,000 WBC/mm^3, neutrophilia	Leukocytosis to 25,000 WBC/mm^3, also mild to moderate eosinophilia may be seen
Arterial blood gases	Normal or mild respiratory alkalosis, mild hypoxemia, arterial-alveolar gradient	Hypoxemia, which may be severe Increased arterial-alveolar gradient
Serum allergic precipitins to farmer's lung	Usually negative	Usually positive
Chest x-ray	Normal or minimal interstitial infiltration	Patchy, ill-defined, parenchymal densities Interstitial strands
Pulmonary function tests	Normal or mild restriction and/or decreased DLCO	Moderate to severe restriction, decreased DLCO May also see evidence of obstruction
Brochoalveolar lavage findings	Elevated neutrophils	Elevated lymphocytes, neutrophils
Open lung biopsy results	Multifocal acute inflammation of terminal bronchioles, alveolar, interstitial area. Exudate consists of neutrophils, macrophages. Large numbers of fungal spores present	Acute granulomatous interstitial pneumonitis, with macrophages, foreign body giant cells, neutrophils, eosinophils
Treatment	O_2 if needed. Corticosteroids	O_2 if needed Corticosteroids
Prognosis	No sequelae known at this time	Recurrence with repeated exposure. May develop severe pulmonary fibrosis
Risk of recurrence	Recurs only with repeated heavy exposure to organic dust	Recurrence likely on any exposure to antigen
Prevention	Dust masks, avoidance of heavy exposure to organic dust	Absolute avoidance of exposure to causative antigen

[a]Adapted from Von Essen S et al. Clin Toxicol 1990;28:389–420.

Table 66-43
Occupational Hazards[a]

Occupation/Avocation	Toxins[b]
Acid dipper	*Arsine, cyanogens,* hydrochloric, nitric and sulfuric acid fumes
Acid finishing worker (glass)	*Hydrochloric* acid, sulfuric acid, lead
Agricultural worker	See Farmer
Aircraft mechanic	Alcohols, *chlorinated and other solvents,* gasoline and other fuels, zinc chromate
Aircraft pilot	See Aircraft mechanic
Crop duster	Pesticides and their solvents
Aircraft worker	Cyanides, chromates, fiberglass and resin plastics, *solvents* (especially chlorinated), hydrofluoric acid
Airplane hanger employee	As in other aircraft fields, *carbon monoxide*
Alcohol distiller	Alcohols (including methanol), *amyl acetate, benzene,* mercury, toluene, xylene
Aluminum extraction worker	Aluminum, *hydrofluoric acid,* manganese
Amber worker	*Formaldehyde* (artificial amber), lead

[a]Adapted from Done AK. Emerg Med 1986;14:196, 201, 205, 209, 213.
[b]The most important toxins, because of either severity or frequency of toxic effects, are italicized.

(continued)

Table 66–43
Occupational Hazards[a]

Occupation/Avocation	Toxins[b]
Art-glass worker	Amyl acetate, copper, *hydrofluoric acid, lead* methanol, volatile hydrocarbons (including benzine)
Asbestos products worker	*Asbestos,* benzene, formaldehyde, toluene, xylene
Automobile worker	Asbestos, chromates, *fiberglass and resin plastics,* gasoline, lead, *solvents*
Radiator cleaner	Borate, isopropanol, *oxalate,* sulfamic acid
Painter	Benzene, lead, *methanol,* zinc
Balloon operator	Arsine, *carbon monoxide*
Barber/beautician	Aliphatic solvents, alkyl sodium sulfates, borates, cadmium, cobalt, copper, detergents, *dyes,* essential oils, lead, oxalate (freckle remover), pyrogallol, resorcinol, salicylate, silver, *thioglycolate*
Barometer maker	Mercury
Battery worker	*Acids,* benzene, *mercury,* zinc
Blacksmith	*Carbon monoxide* and dioxide, cyanogens, lead
Blast furnace worker	*Carbon dioxide* and monoxide, *cyanogens,* hydrogen sulfide, *phosphine,* sulfur dioxide
Bleacher	Caustic alkali, *chlorine,* chromium, *hydrochloric acid,* hydrofluoric acid, *peroxides,* nitric acid, oxalic acid, phosgene, sulfur oxides
Bookbinder	Acetate, arsenic, *formalin,* lead, methanol, oxalate, polyvinyl, solvents
Brass worker (founder)	*Antimony, arsenic,* carbon dioxide and monoxide, copper, lead, phosphorus, sulfur oxides
Brazer	*Lead,* zinc
Brewer	*Amyl alcohol, carbon dioxide* or monoxide, cobalt, formaldehyde, hydrofluoric acid, phenol, sulfuric acid
Brick worker	Carbon monoxide and dioxide, epoxy resins, *hydrofluoric acid, lead, lime,* magnesium, manganese, *silica,* sulfur oxides
Bronzer	*Acetone,* ammonia amyl acetate, antimony, arsenic, benzene, benzine, cyanides, hydrochloric acid, hydrogen sulfide, lead, manganese mercury, methanol, sulfur oxides, *zinc*
Bullet reloader	See Cartridge maker
Burnisher	*Antimony, benzine,* carbon tetrachloride, sulfuric acid, trichloroethylene
Cabinetmaker (see also Painter)	Acetone, *benzine,* bleaches, *methanol, methylene chloride,* resins, solvents, turpentine
Ironwood	*Arsenic*
Candle maker	*Aniline,* borates, chromates, potassium nitrate, sodium hydroxide
Carpenter	See Cabinetmaker
Cartridge maker	*Lead,* mercury, nitrites
Case hardener	*Cyanogens,* sodium dichromate or nitrite
Caster	See specific occupation
Cementer (rubber, plastic, etc.)	*Benzene, benzine,* butyl alcohol, *carbon disulfide,* carbon tetrachloride, methanol, naphtha, tetrachloroethane, trichloroethylene
Cement (Portland) worker	Arsenic, chromates, cobalt, lime, pitch, *silica*
Ceramist	Arsenic, *barium,* carbon monoxide, *chromium,* cobalt, *feldspars,* hydrochloric or hydrofluoric acid, *lead,* manganese, mercury, selenium, *silica,* sulfur oxides, tellurium
Charcoal cook	*Carbon monoxide* or dioxide
Chrome plater (see also Electroplater)	*Chromium,* solvents, sulfuric acid
Coal miner	See Miner
Coal tar worker	*Aniline, creosote, cresol,* cyanogens, naphtha, phenol, pitch
Cobbler	Amyl acetate, aniline, *benzene and related solvents,* benzine, carbon tetrachloride, methanol, plastics
Coke oven worker (see also Coal tar worker)	*Ammonia, benzene, carbon monoxide,* hydrogen sulfide, sulfur oxides
Compositor	*Alkalis, aniline,* antimony, benzine, lead, *solvents*
Construction worker (see also Brick worker, Cabinetmaker, Cement worker, Ceramist, Painter)	*Arsenic, creosote,* gasoline, glass fibers, paint products, *pitch, silica,* solvent
Cosmetic worker	Aniline, *arsenic, mercury,* nitrobenzene, solvents
Dentist	Anesthetics, clove oil, disinfectants, *mercury*
Dockworker	See Longshoreman
Dry cleaner	*Amyl acetate, benzine,* carbon tetrachloride, dichloroethylene, methanol, *naphtha,* oxalate, tetrachloroethane, tetrachlorethylene, *trichloroethylene,* turpentine, waterproofing compounds
Dye maker	*Aniline,* antimony, arsenic, benzine, chlorates, chromates, coal tar products, cresol, *dimethyl sulfate,* ferrocyanides, formaldehyde, lead, manganese, mercury, methanol, nitrobenzene, phenol, titanium, *organotins*
Dyer	*Acetone, aniline,* other *aminobenzene derivatives,* bleaches, mercury, solvents, titanium, zinc
Electric apparatus maker	*Asbestos, epoxy and phenolic resins,* solvents
Electroplater	*Antimony, arsenic,* benzine, cadmium, *chromium,* copper, *cyanide,* gold, lead, lime, mercury, nickel, nitrous fumes, potassium hydroxide, silver, sulfuric acid, zinc
Enameler	*Amyl acetate,* antimony, arsenic, chromium, cobalt, lead, nickel, *silica*
Engraver	*Acids,* alkalis, *benzene, copper, cyanide,* solvents
Etcher	*Acids, alkalis, arsine, hydrofluoric acid,* nitrous fumes, picric acid
Explosives maker	Acetone, *ammonia amyl acetate,* mercury, nitrites, *nitroglycerin,* picric acid, TNT

(continued)

Table 66–43 *(Continued)*

Occupation/Avocation	Toxins[b]
Farmer	Carbon monoxide, *farmer's lung,* fertilizers, pesticides, plants with contact toxicity (poison ivy, sumac, oak, etc.), *silo filler's disease,* solvents
Felt hat worker	*Carbon monoxide,* hydrogen peroxide, hydrogen sulfide, *mercury,* methanol, nitrous fumes, *oxalic acid,* sulfuric acid
Fertilizer producer/user	*Ammonia,* arsenic, *calcium cyanamide,* carbon dioxide, castor bean pomace, cyanogens, fluoride, hydrogen sulfide, lime, magnesium, manganese, nitrates, nitric acid, phosphates, sulfur oxides, sulfuric acid
Fire extinguisher maker	Carbon dioxide, chlorobromomethane, *ethyl bromide, ethyl chloride,* ethylene dibromide, methyl bromide, sodium dichromate
Firearms maker	See Explosives maker, Gunsmith
Fireworks maker (see also Explosives maker)	*Antimony, arsenic,* barium, bismuth, mercury, phosphorus, picric acid, thallium
Fish-meal processor	*Hydrogen sulfide, triethylamine*
Foundry worker (see also particular occupation)	Acids, *carbon dioxide and monoxide, lime,* resins, silica
Furniture polisher	*Amyl acetate, benzine,* chromium, methanol, naphtha, petroleum hydrocarbons, pyridine, rosin, turpentine
Fur processor	*Alum, bleaches,* chromate, dyes, formaldehyde, hydrogen sulfide, lime, mercury, nitrous fumes
Galvanizer	Acids, *ammonia,* arsenic, *arsine,* benzine, nitrous fumes, sulfur oxides, trichloroethylene, *zinc*
Garage worker	*Benzine, carbon monoxide,* detergents, *epoxy resins,* gasoline, glass fibers, lead, paints, solvents
Gardener	Arsenic, calcium, cyanamide, *fertilizers, fungicides, herbicides, insecticides,* lead, *pesticides,* poisonous plants, venomous insects
Gem/lapidary/jewelry worker	*Arsenic,* asbestos, benzene, bisulfate, borates, cadmium, cyanide, epoxy resins, hydrochloric acid, *hydrofluoric acid,* lead, *mercury* (gold extraction), methanol, methyl salicylate, nitric acid, selenium, silica, sulfur oxides, sulfuric acid, trisodium phosphate, zinc
Glass worker (see also Art-glass worker)	Acids, *arsenic, borates,* carbon monoxide, chlorine, *glass fibers,* hydrofluoric acid, lead, nitrogen oxides, sulfur
Glazer (pottery)	See Ceramist
Gold and silver extractor	*Arsenic, arsine,* bromides, *cyanide,* formaldehyde, hydrofluoric acid, lead, *mercury*
Gunsmith/hunter/marksman (see also Explosives maker)	Cyanide, *kerosene, lead,* magnesium, mercury, nickel, *nitrites, nitrobenzene, solvents*
Bluing	*Chlorate, mercury,* methanol, nitrite, selenium
Browning	Benzine, *cyanide, lead,* petroleum hydrocarbons
Hairdresser	See Barber/beautician
Hunter	See Gunsmith
Ice cream maker	*Ammonia,* carbon dioxide
Ink maker	*Ammonia,* arsenic, benzene, benzine, *chromates, cobalt,* formaldehyde, lead, mercury, *nitrites,* other solvents, silver
Insecticide maker/applier	Solvents as well as specific insecticides
Insulation maker/applier	*Asbestos,* formaldehyde, glass fibers, *silica*
Iron/steel worker	*Arsenic,* cadmium, *carbon monoxide,* hydrofluoric acid, nitrogen oxides, sulfur oxides, *titanium*
Jeweler (see also Gem worker)	Acids, *amyl acetate,* chromates, *cyanide,* mercury, nickel, nitric acid, nitrous fumes, solder fluxes
Lacquer maker/applier	Acetaldehyde, *acetone,* alcohols, *amyl acetate,* benzine, butanone, cresyl phosphate, methylene chloride, solvents
Laundry worker	*Alkaline caustics, bleaches,* chloride, chlorine, detergents, formaldehyde, lime, ozone
Lead smelter	Antimony, *arsenic,* cadmium, carbon monoxide, *lead,* selenium, sulfur oxides, tellurium
Leather worker	Acids, *amyl acetate, barium,* carbon tetrachloride, methanol, trichloroethylene
Tanner	Acetates, acids, *aniline,* arsenic, benzene, carbon dioxide, chromates, cyanide, diethylamine, dyes, formaldehyde, hydrogen sulfide, mercury, *nitrites,* oxalate, picric acid, sodium sulfide, tannin
Linoleum worker	*Amyl acetate, asphalt,* benzene, benzine, carbon tetrachloride, chromates, *dyes,* methanol, resins, solvents
Linotyper	*Antimony,* carbon monoxide, lead
Lithographer	Acids, *aniline,* arsenic, benzene, benzine, chromates, lead, mercury, methanol, nitric acid, *nitrites,* oxalate, tetrachloroethane, turpentine
Longshoreman	Manganese, *various chemicals and fumigants* (depending on cargo), venomous insects and snakes
Match worker	Alkalis, antimony, carbon disulfide, *chlorates, chromates,* hydrogen sulfide, manganese, *phosphorus*
Metal polisher	Acids, *ammonia, benzine, cyanide,* methanol, *naphtha,* oxalates, solvents, trichloroethylene, triethanolamine
Miner (varies with type)	*Asbestos,* carbon dioxide and monoxide, hydrogen sulfide, manganese, nitrogen oxides, *silica, talc*
Mirror maker	*Acetaldehyde, ammonia,* benzene, cyanide, lead, mercury, silver, solvents
Painter	*Acetone, acids,* alkalis, aniline, arsenic, barium, *benzine,* carbon disulfide, carbon tetrachloride, chromates, *lead,* manganese, mercury, methanol, methylene chloride, nitrogen oxides, *solvents,* trichloroethylene, turpentine
Paint maker	Cadmium, *chlorinated diphenyls,* petroleum distillates, titanium, zinc
Paper maker	*Acids,* acrylamide, *alkalis,* ammonia, amyl acetate, bisulfide, calcium chloride, chromates, *DMSO,* formaldehyde, hydrofluoric acid, hydrogen sulfide, lead, resins, sulfur oxides, titanium
Petroleum refiner	Acetone, ammonia, arsenic, *benzene, benzine,* gasoline and other petroleum distillates, hydrofluoric acid, *hydrogen sulfide,* nitrites, solvents, sulfur oxides

(continued)

Table 66-43 *(Continued)*

Occupation/Avocation	Toxins[b]
Photoengraver	Acids, alkalis, *ammonia,* ammonium bichromate, *amyl acetate,* methanol, nitrous fumes, solvents
Photographer	*Acids, alkalis,* aminophenols, *amyl acetate,* benzene, borates, bromides, chromates, cyanide, ethylene glycol, formaldehyde, hydroquinone, iodine, lead, mercury, methanol, oxalate, pyrogallic acid, silver, *sodium bisulfite,* sodium hypochlorite, sodium sulfite, sodium thiosulfate, tellurium, trichloroethylene, uranium, vanadium
Plastics and resin maker/user	None with finished plastics but unreacted resins are toxic
Plumber	Acids, alkalis, *arsine, carbon monoxide, lead,* solvents, zinc
Pottery worker	See Ceramist
Printer	*Alkalis, aniline, benzine,* carbon tetrachloride, chromates, cyanide, lead, mercury, methanol, tetrachloroethylene, other solvents
Railroad shop/track worker	*Chromates,* contact plant poisons (poison ivy, etc.), *creosote,* detergents, dichlorobenzenes, diesel fuel oil, fungicides, herbicides, insecticides, paint, paint strippers, solvents
Rayon worker	*Acetic anhydride,* acids, ammonia, benzine, bleaches, butyl alcohol, *calcium bisulfite,* carbon disulfide, chlorinated diphenyls, cyanogens, *dioxane,* formaldehyde, hydrogen sulfide, methanol, nitrous fumes, solvents, sulfide, sodium sulfite, tetrachloroethane
Refrigeration worker	*Acrolein, ammonia,* carbon dioxide, carbon monoxide, *ethyl bromide, ethyl chloride,* glass fiber, *methyl bromide, methyl chloride,* methyl formate, ozone, sulfur oxides
Rubber worker	*Acetaldehyde, acetone,* amyl alcohol, aniline, antimony, arsenic, barium, benzene, benzine, carbon disulfide, carbon tetrachloride, *chloroprene,* chromates, cresol, ethylene dichloride, formaldehyde, lead, magnesium, methanol, nitrogen oxides, *plasticizers, pyridine,* silica, solvents, tellurium, zinc
Sewage worker	*Ammonia,* carbon dioxide, chlorine, *hydrogen sulfide,* methane
Shoemaker (see also Leather worker)	*Acetone, adhesives,* ammonia, amyl acetate, amyl alcohol, *aniline and dyes,* benzene, benzine, carbon tetrachloride, methanol, naphtha, plastics, tetrachloroethane, trichloroethylene, waxes
Solderer	*Acids,* antimony, arsenic, *arsine,* borates, cadmium, cyanide, *hydrazine salts, lead,* potassium bifluoride, rosin, zinc
Stone worker	*Lime, silica*
Sugar refiner	*Acids, ammonia, bagasse,* barium, burlap, carbon dioxide, hydrogen sulfide, sulfur oxides
Tannery worker	Acetic acid, acids, alum, ammonia, *amyl acetate, aniline and dyes,* arsenic, benzene, benzine, calcium hydrosulfide, chromates, cyanide, dimethylamine, dyes, formaldehyde, hydrogen sulfide, lead, lime, mercury, oxalate, sodium sulfide, solvents, sulfur oxides, tannin
Tar worker	*Arsenic, cresols,* pitch, tar
Taxidermist	*Arsenic,* calcined alum, *mercury,* solvents, tannin, zinc
Upholsterer (see also Lacquer maker)	*Glues, lacquer,* lacquer solvents, methanol
Waterproofer	*Alum,* benzene, *benzine,* carbon tetrachloride, chromates, formaldehyde, melamine, pitch, resins, solvents, tar
Welder	*Arsenic,* benzene, cadmium, chromates, fluoride, lead, manganese, mercury, nitrous fumes, ozone, phosphorus, selenium, zinc
Wood preserver	*Arsenic chlorophenols,* chromates, copper compounds, creosote, cresols, dinitrophenols, mercury, pitch, resins, tar, zinc
Woodworker	See Cabinetmaker

Clinical Presentation

Chronic silicosis, the most common form, results from low-to-moderate exposure for more than 20 years. Typical radiographic findings are nodular opacities, usually predominating in the upper lung zones. In simple silicosis the opacities are discrete and range from 1 to 10 mm in diameter. At first the nodules are usually 1 to 3 mm in diameter and limited to the upper lung fields; subsequently, the middle and lower zone tend to become involved. Typically, discrete silicotic nodules form, without interstitial fibrosis. In the early stages of simple silicosis there are usually no symptoms and signs. When findings are present, they are usually attributable to concomitant cigarette smoking or industrial bronchitis. As the disease progresses, however, decrements in pulmonary function become more apparent and are greater in smokers than nonsmokers. Enlargement of the hilar lymph nodes is common, with peripheral (eggshell) calcification in 5 to 10% of cases. This pattern is not pathognomonic for silicosis, but is highly suggestive if there is a history of exposure. Once silicosis begins, it continues to progress even in the absence of ongoing exposure. Complicated or conglomerate silicosis, caused by the coalescence of silicotic nodules, usually in the upper lung zones, is diagnosed when the radiographic opacities are greater than 1 cm in diameter. This condition, referred to as "progressive massive fibrosis," produces a restrictive pattern of pulmonary function, with decreased gas transfer, and may eventually result in cor pulmonale.[21]

Diagnosis

Three criteria are required: an appropriate history of exposure, radiologic findings consistent with silicosis, and the absence of a likely alternative explanation for the clinical and radiologic findings.[21]

Table 66–44
Pathologic and Physiologic Changes of Pneumoconiosis[a]

Agent	Type of Pathology	Type of Respiratory Impairment
Silica		
Simple	Nodular fibrosis	Restrictive, diffusion
Complicated	Conglomerate nodular fibrosis	Restrictive, obstructive, diffusion
Hematite	Nodular fibrosis	Restrictive, diffusion
Mixed dusts, iron and silica	Nodular fibrosis (Rarely, conglomerate nodular fibrosis)	Restrictive, diffusion
Silicates	Nodular fibrosis	Restrictive, obstructive
Talc	(Rarely, conglomerate nodular fibrosis)	
Kaolin		
Bentonite		
Diatomite		
Tripoli		
Fuller's earth		
Mica		
Sillimanite		
Cement	Nonspecific bronchitis	Obstructive
Coal		
Simple	Peribronchiolar macules, focal emphysema	Obstructive (small airways)
Complicated	Conglomerate nodular fibrosis	Obstructive, restrictive, diffusion
Graphite	Peribronchiolar macules, focal emphysema	Obstructive (small airways)
Aluminum	Interstitial fibrosis	Restrictive, diffusion
Asbestos	Interstitial fibrosis	Restrictive, diffusion
Beryllium	Interstitial fibrosis (granulomata)	Restrictive, diffusion
Tungsten carbide	Interstitial fibrosis	Restrictive, diffusion
Barium	Simple dust accumulation	None known
Cerium	Simple dust accumulation	None known
Iron	Simple dust accumulation	None known
Tin	Simple dust accumulation	None known
Titanium	Simple dust accumulation	None known

[a]Adapted from Key MM, Henschel AF, Butler J et al, eds. Occupational Diseases: A Guide to Their Recognition. Washington DC, US Department of Health, Education and Welfare, US Government Printing Office, 1977, p. 119.

Laboratory

The laboratory findings in patients with silicosis are nonspecific. A moderate elevation in the angiotensin-converting–enzyme concentration and various immunologic abnormalities are common. Positive antinuclear-antibody titers are found in 26 to 44% of patients. An increased prevalence of rheumatoid factor and elevated levels of immunoglobulins and immune complexes have also been found. In addition, scleroderma, rheumatoid arthritis, rheumatoid lung nodules, and glomerulonephritis have been reported.[21]

Acute Silicosis (Silicoproteinosis)

Acute silicosis or silicoproteinosis progresses rapidly, may develop after only a few years of very intense exposure to free silica, and may be seen in sandblasters. Acute silicosis resembles idiopathic alveolar proteinosis histologically, with the air spaces filled with material that is positive on periodic acid-Schiff staining. In patients with acute silicoproteinosis, x-ray films of the chest reveal diffuse air-space disease, and the findings may mimic those in pulmonary edema. Progressive restriction and impairment in gas transfer lead to extreme dyspnea, cor pulmonale, and death within several years.[21]

Accelerated Silicosis

Accelerated silicosis is a less well defined entity that is intermediate between chronic silicosis and acute silicoproteinosis. The features of accelerated disease are identical to those of chronic silicosis but more rapidly progressive, requiring only 4 to 8 years of exposure.[21]

Silicotuberculosis

Mycobacterial infection must also be ruled out whenever a patient with silicosis has radiographically evident progression or a deterioration in respiratory function. The increased risk of tuberculosis and atypical mycobacterial infections in patients with silicosis is well recognized. Before the introduction of effective therapy, tuberculosis was the most important cause of death in workers with silicosis. Aspergillus species may also colonize tuberculous or ischemic cavities in patients with silicosis. Superinfection with nocardia, sporothrix, and cryptococcus has been reported.[21]

Early in the course the patient may be asymptomatic and have no demonstrable radiographic changes other than those of preexisting silicosis.[21]

Treatment

All patients with silicosis should be tested annually with purified protein derivative (PPD), and any induration of 10 mm or more should be considered positive. A positive PPD test, symptoms, or radiographic changes suggesting tuberculosis require the examination of acid-fast smears and cultures for mycobacteria. Sputum cultures in patients with silicotuberculosis may not be consistently positive, and thus even a single positive result should be considered meaningful. Patients with positive smears or cultures should be treated initially with four drugs and for a year with at least two bactericidal agents.[21]

Radiographic Classification

Since 1950 the International Labour Office in Geneva, Switzerland, has periodically proposed classifications of the radiographic appearance of pneumoconiosis. The most recent classification was proposed in 1988.[22]

The ILO classification grades profusion from category 0 to category 3. Category 0 is normal or nearly normal, and categories 1 through 3 are abnormal. A category 3 pattern has a diffuse, "snowstorm" appearance.[23]

ASBESTOS-RELATED DISEASE (TABLE 66–45)

Exposure-response studies suggest a relationship between retained asbestos fiber size in the lung and specific disease predilection. Asbestos exposure indices have been summarized as follows[24]:

Asbestosis	Surface area of fibers with: Length >2 μm; diameters >0.15 μm.
Mesothelioma	Numbers of fibers with: Length >5 μm; diameter <0.1 μm.
Lung cancer	Number of fibers with Length >10 μm; diameter >0.15 μm

These findings require validation by further studies.

Radiographic findings in asbestosis are nonspecific. Small irregular opacities involving the lower lung field are commonly noted, but in the absence of an exposure history asbestosis may be difficult to distinguish clinically or radiographically from other pulmonary fibrotic disorders.

There is no evidence that smoking predisposes to the progression or development of asbestos-related disease, except that smoking greatly increases the risk of bronchogenic carcinoma in asbestos workers (5- to 50-fold). The incidence of esophageal cancer appears to be increased in asbestos workers, but elevation of the number of stomach cancers is questionable.[25] Further data suggest a probable causal association between asbestos exposure and kidney cancer.[26]

Several preliminary studies have indicated that there appears to be an increased number of deaths from colon cancer in asbestos workers.[27] Asbestos fibers frequently enter and reside in the wall of the colon and are often intimately associated with tumor tissue at the site of colon carcinoma in workers with asbestos exposure and colon carcinoma.[33] These data require validation to include confounding factors and selection and observer bias. A differential diagnosis of asbestosis is listed in Table 66–46.

The majority of lung tumors in asbestos-exposed patients arise from the lower lobes whereas upper-lobe tumors dominate in the general population. Such tumors can follow low-level exposure independent of pulmonary fibrosis.[28] Lung volume definitions are summarized in Figure 66–5. Severity of pulmonary function abnormalities is found in Table 66–47. Factors influencing the regional deposition of inhaled particles are depicted in Figure 66–6.

BYSSINOSIS

Byssinosis is an occupational lung disorder most commonly observed in textile workers and caused by the inhalation of cotton, flax, or hemp dust.[29] Initially, workers have chest tightness and shortness of breath on the first day of the workweek, "Monday chest tightness," and this is accompanied by a moderate and reversible decrease in ventilatory function. These symptoms subside as the week continues.[30] After many years of exposure, the symptoms worsen and may persist throughout the workweek, as well as in the absence of work exposure. Both obstructive and restrictive pulmonary dysfunction develops.[35,36] Endotoxin, a component of the cell walls of Gram-negative bacteria, known to colonize cotton plants grown in fields, is suspect as a possible causative agent of byssinosis.[31,35] Treatment is symptomatic.

MAN-MADE MINERAL FIBERS (MMMF)

Man-made mineral fibers, also known as man-made vitreous fibers (MMVF), are made by spraying or extruding molten glass, rock, or furnace slag.[32] The mortality from lung cancer appears, with limited evidence, to be increased in long-term follow-up studies of workers from the rock wool/slag wool industries. The mortality appears to be intermediate in the

Table 66–45
Radiographic Findings in Asbestosis[a]

Irregular opacities	75%
Honeycombing	35%
Kerley B lines	35%
Distribution	
Lower	35%
Lower & middle	30%
Pleural changes	50%
Shaggy heart or diaphragm	5%

[a]Adapted from Dunn MM. Chest 1989;95:1304–1308.

Table 66–46
Diseases To Be Considered in the Differential Diagnosis of Asbestosis[a]

- Congestive heart failure
- Chronic obstructive pulmonary disease
- Interstitial fibrosis
  - Progressive systemic sclerosis
  - Lupus
  - Hydralazine
  - Procainamide
  - Sarcoidosis
  - Polyarteritis nodosa
  - Eosinophilic granuloma
  - Miliary tuberculosis
  - Viral pneumonia
  - Rheumatoid disease
  - Idiopathic disease
- Interstitial fibrosis plus pleural thickening
  - Rheumatoid lung
  - Blastomycosis, other fungi
  - Drug induced
  - Other pneumoconioses (e.g., talc)
  - Silica

[a]Adapted from Murphy R. Comp Ther 1980;6(5):12.

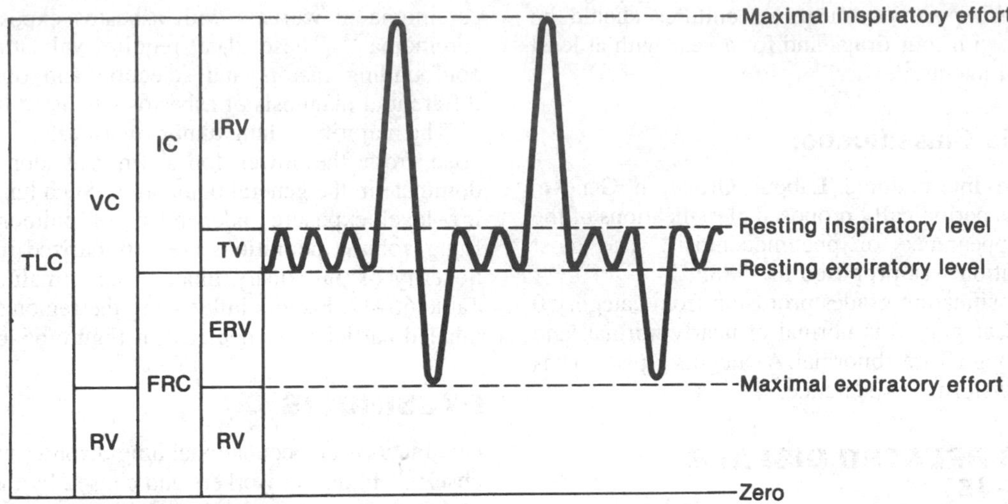

DEFINITIONS

Residual volume (RV): **amount of gas that cannot be exhaled after maximal expiratory effort**
Expiratory reserve volume (ERV): **difference between resting expiratory level and maximal expiratory effort**
Tidal volume (TV): **normal amount of gas exchanged during rest**
Inspiratory reserve volume (IRV): **difference between resting and maximal inspiratory effort**
Inspiratory capacity (IC): **TV + IRV**
Vital capacity (VC): **IRV + TV + ERV**
Functional residual capacity (FRC): **RV + ERV**
Total lung capacity (TLC): **RV + ERV + TV + IRV**

Figure 66–5 Lung volume definitions.

Table 66–47
Severity of Pulmonary Function Abnormalities[a,b]

Test	Normal	Mild	Moderate	Severe	Comment
	Degree of Abnormality				
Spirometry					
In restrictive disorders (FVC% of predicted)	>80	66–80	51–65	≤50	Presence of obstruction changes degree of abnormality
In obstructive disorders (FEV_1/FVC)	>0.69	0.61–0.69	0.45–0.60	<0.45	FVC considered normal; presence of restriction component changes degree of abnormality
Lung volume (TLC% of predicted)					
In restrictive disorders	≥81	66–80	51–65	≤50	
In hyperinflation	≤120	121–134	135–149	≥150	
Diffusing capacity (% of predicted)	81–140	61–80	41–60	≤40	

[a]Adapted from Rom WN, ed. Environmental and occupational medicine. Boston: Little, Brown, 1983, p. 101.
[b]Degree of pulmonary function abnormalities is based on percentage change from predicted values. Low FEV_1/FVC ratios and normal FVC volumes suggest obstruction, whereas low FVC volumes and normal FEV_1/FVC ratios suggest restrictive disease. Combined obstructive and restrictive defects alter the above severity classification.

glass wool sector and lowest in the continuous filament glass sector.[33,38] For both the glass wool and glass filament sectors the data are still considered as "inadequate evidence" in recent reviews.[34–36]

Risks for lung fibrosis, lung cancer, and mesothelioma from industrial exposure to most fibrous glass products are low, probably due to the mean glass fiber diameter of approximately 7.5 μm that results in mean aerodynamic diameters of over 22 μm.[38] Thus they do not penetrate into the lung to any great extent. The fraction that does penetrate breaks and is subject to dissolution. Rock wool and wool fibers appear to have increased hazards because of their smaller diameters and greater durability within the lungs.[38–41]

PRINCIPLES OF WORKPLACE CONTROL

The principles of workplace control in order of effectiveness include the following[37]:

1. Eliminating the harmful substances by substitution.
2. Enclosing the process so that workers are not exposed.

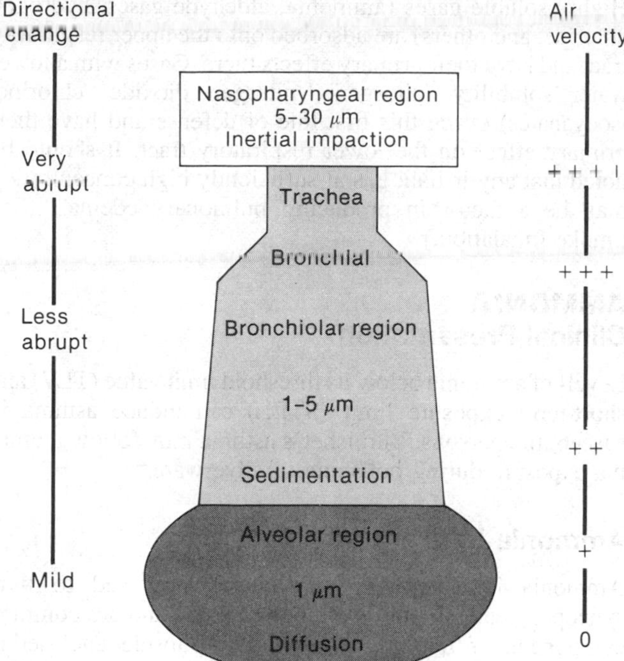

Figure 66–6 Factors influencing the regional deposition of inhaled particles. Submicron particles may be exhaled as well as deposited in the alveoli. (Adapted from Doull J, Klaassen CD, Amdun MO, eds. Casarett and Doull's Toxicology: the basic science of poisons. 2nd ed. New York: Macmillan, 1980, p. 258.)

3. Removing the substance by exhaust ventilation.
4. Diluting any fugitive emissions by improved general ventilation
5. Providing personal protection for workers by means of respirators.

REFERENCES—OCCUPATIONAL LUNG DISEASES

1. Rom WN, ed. Environmental and occupational medicine. Boston: Little, Brown, 1983.
2. Last JM. Maxcy-Roseman: public health and preventive medicine. 11th ed. New York: Appleton-Century-Crofts, 1980.
3. Klaassen CD, Amdun MO, Doull J, eds. Casarett and Doull's toxicology: basic science of poisons. 3rd ed. New York: Macmillan, 1986.
4. Finkel AJ, ed. Hamilton and Hardy's industrial toxicology, 4th ed. Boston: John Wright, 1983.
5. Key MM, Henschel AF, Butler J et al, eds. Occupational diseases. A guide to their recognition. Washington, DC: US Department of Health, Education and Welfare, US Government Printing Office, 1977.
6. Parkes WR. Occupational lung disorders. 2nd ed. London: Butterworth, 1982.
7. Chan-Yeung M, Malo J-C. Occupational asthma. N Engl J Med 1995;333:107–112.
8. Brooks SM, Weiss MA, Bernstein IL. Reactive airways dysfunction syndrome (RADS). Persistent asthma syndrome after high level irritant exposures. Chest 1985;88:376–384.
9. Empey DW, Laitinen LA, Jacobs L et al. Mechanisms of bronchial hyperreactivity in normal subjects after upper respiratory tract infections. Am Rev Respir Dis 1976;113:131–139.
10. Gannon PFG, Burge PS, Benfield GFA. Occupational asthma due to polyethylene shrink wrapping (paper wrapper's asthma). Thorax 1992;47:759.
11. Richerson HR, Bernstein L, Fink JN, Hunninghake GW, Novey HS, Reed CE, Salvaggio JE, Schuyler MR, Schwartz HJ, Stechschulte DJ. Guidelines for the clinical evaluation of hypersensitivity pneumonitis. J Allergy Clin Immunol 1989; 84:839–844.
12. Rose C, King TE Jr. Controversies in hypersensitivity pneumonitis. Am Rev Respir Dis 1992;145:1–2.
13. Brinton WT, Vastbinder EE, Greene JW, Marx JJ Jr, Hutcheson RH, Schaffner W. An outbreak of organic dust toxic syndrome in a college fraternity. JAMA 1987;258:1210–1212.
14. Emanual DA, Wenzel FJ, Lawton BP. Pulmonary mycotoxicosis. Chest 1975;67:293–297.
15. Van Essen S, Robins RA, Thompson AB, Rennard SI. Organic dust toxic syndrome: an acute febrile reaction to organic dust exposure distinct from hypersensitivity pneumonitis. Clin Toxicol 1990;128:389–426.
16. Yoshida K, Ando M, Araki S. Acute pulmonary edema in a storehouse of moldy oranges. A severe case of Organic Dust Toxic Syndrome. Arch Environ Health 1989;44:382–384.
17. Melinn M, McLaughlin H. Farmer's lung: a three year survey and comparison of ELISA and CIEP techniques in antibody detection. Irish J Med Sci 1989;158:173–174.
18. Muller-Wening D, Repp H. Investigation on the protective value of breathing masks in Farmer's Lung using an inhalation provocation test. Chest 1989;95:100–105.
19. Malmberg P, Rask-Anderson A. Organic dust toxic syndrome. Semin Respir Med 1993;14:38–48.
20. Silicosis and Silicate Disease Committee. Diseases associated with exposure to silica and nonfibrous silicate minerals. Arch Pathol Lab Med 1988;112:673–720.
21. Kales SN. Case 35-1995. Weekly clinicopathological exercises. Case records of the Massachusetts General Hospital. N Engl J Med 1993;333:1340–1346.
22. Classification of Radiographs of the Pneumoconioses. Med Radiogr Photogr 1981;57:3,4,7,17
23. Shepherd JD. Case 35-1995. Weekly clinicopathological exercises. Case records of the Massachusetts General Hospital. N Engl J Med 1993;333:1340–1346.
24. Lippmann M. Review. Asbestos exposure indices. Environ Res 1988;46:86–106.
25. Morgan RW, Foliart DE, Wong O. Asbestos and gastrointestinal cancer. A review of the literature. West J Med 1985;143: 60–65.
26. Smith AH, Shearn VI, Wood R. Asbestos and kidney cancer. The evidence supports a causal association. Am J Ind Med 1989;16:159–166.
27. Ehrlich A, Gordon RE, Dikman SH. Carcinoma of the colon in asbestos-exposed workers: Analysis of asbestos content in colon tissue. Am J Ind Med 1991;19:629–636.
28. Anttila S, Kajalainen A, Taikino-aho O, Kyrronen P, Vainio H. Lung cancer in the lower lobe is associated with pulmonary asbestos fiber count and fiber size. Environ Health Perspect 1993;101:166–170.
29. Castellan RM, Olenchock SA, Kinsley KB, Hankinson JL. Inhaled endotoxin and decreased spirometric values. An exposure-response relation for cotton dust. N Engl J Med 1987;317:605–610.
30. Schachter EN, Kapp MC, Beck GJ, Maunder LR, Witek TJ. Smoking and cotton dust effects in cotton textile workers. Chest 1989;95:997–1003.
31. Milton DK, Godleski JJ, Feldman HA, Greaves IA. Toxicity of intratracheally instilled cotton dust, cellulose and endotoxin. Am Rev Respir Dis 1990;142:184–192.
32. Lippmann M. Man-made mineral fibers (MMME): human exposures and health risk assessment. Toxicol Ind Health 1990; 6:225–246.
33. Marsh GM, Enterline PE, Stone RA, Henderson VL. Mortality among a cohort of US man made mineral fiber workers: 1985 follow-up. J Occup Med 1990;32:594–604.
34. Miettinen OS, Rossiter CE. Man-made mineral fibers and lung cancer. Epidemiologic evidence regarding the causal hypothesis. Scand J Work Environ Health 1990;16: 221–231.
35. Man-made mineral fibers. Environ Health Criteria No. 77; International Programme on Chemical Safety (IPCS), 1988.

36. Doll R. Symposium on MMMF Copenhagen, October 1986: Overview and conclusions. Am Occup Hyg 1987;31:805–819.
37. Seaton A. Management of the patient with occupational lung disease. Thorax 1994;49:627–628.

RESPIRATORY TRACT IRRITANTS

Weiss and Lakshminarayan[1] have surveyed the clinical manifestations associated with exposure to gaseous respiratory irritants, their mechanisms of injury (Table 66–48), and their physical properties (Table 66–49). Wald and Balmes have proposed hospital action criteria for toxic inhalations[2] (Table 66–50). Unusual effects of irritant gases relating to their water solubility are summarized in Table 66–51. Respiratory irritants are listed in Table 66–52.

Respiratory tract irritants may cause changes in the mucous membranes, upper and lower respiratory tract, and lung parenchyma (Table 66–53). Irritant gases can generally be divided into two categories based on water solubility.

Table 66–48
Categorization of Toxic Inhalants by Mechanism of Injury[a]

Toxic Inhalant	Mechanism of Injury
Irritants	
Ammonia (NH_3)	Direct mucosal injury from alkaline burn
Chlorine (CL_2)	Direct mucosal injury from acid burn and free radical formation
Sulfur dioxide (SO_2)	Low concentration exposure causes bronchoconstriction and increased mucous secretion. High concentration exposure causes acid burns
Asphyxiants	
Methane (CH_4)	Replaces atmospheric oxygen
Carbon monoxide (CO)	Competes for oxygen-binding sites on hemoglobin
Systemic toxins	
Benzene (C_6H_6)	Causes central nervous system toxicity and bone marrow suppression

[a]Adapted from Weiss SM, Lakshminarayan S. Clin Chest Med 1994;15: 103–116.

Highly soluble gases (ammonia, aldehyde gases, hydrogen chloride, and others) are adsorbed onto the upper respiratory tract and have their primary effects there. Gases with a lower water solubility (phosgene, nitrogen dioxide, chlorine, isocyanates) evade this first line of defense and have their primary effect on the lower respiratory tract. It should be noted that any irritant gas at sufficiently high concentration may be a factor in producing pulmonary edema.[3] (See Smoke Inhalation.)

AMMONIA

Clinical Presentation

Levels of ammonia below its threshold limit value (TLV) and short-term exposure limit (STEL) can induce asthma in susceptible persons. Burnisher's asthma may follow ammonia exposure during polishing of silverware.[4]

Ammonia Inhalants

Ammonia inhalants are mild stimulants used to treat syncope, weakness, or threatened collapse and are common components of first-aid kits. Each glass capsule, enclosed in a fiber mesh, may contain 0.33 mL of a mixture of 18% ammonia and 36% alcohol. When the aromatic ammonia "smelling salts" are bitten into by children, vomiting, drooling, dysphagia, cough, and oral pharyngeal burns may ensue. Endoscopy has usually not indicated any esophageal burns. Treatment is symptomatic. Endoscopy is reserved only for those children with clinical evidence suggestive of upper airway involvement such as stridor, dysphagia, or drooling.[5–7]

Ammonia Sprays

Ammonia sprays may be employed in cases of criminal assault during which victims are temporarily immobilized by ammonia solution squirted into their eyes. The preparation used may be household ammonia (9.5 to 35%). Ammonia causes an immediate and serious ocular chemical burn. Within a few seconds of injury it may diffuse through the cornea into the anterior chamber. Permanent impairment of vision and even blindness may follow. Treatment should

Table 66–49
Sources of Exposure, Physical Properties, and Mechanisms of Lung Injury of Gaseous Respiratory Irritants[a]

Irritant Gas	Sources of Exposure	Water Solubility	OSHA Standard Ceiling
Ammonia (NH_3)	Agriculture, mining, plastic and explosive manufacturing	High	50.0 ppm
Chlorine (Cl_2)	Paper and textile manufacturing, sewage treatment	Intermediate	1.0 ppm
Hydrogen chloride (HCl)	Dyes, fertilizers, textiles, rubber; thermal degradation of polyvinyl chloride	High	5.0 ppm
Oxides of nitrogen (NO, NO_2, N_2O_4)	Agriculture, mining, welding, and manufacturing of dyes and lacquers	Low	5.0 ppm
Ozone (O_3)	Welding, chemical industry, and high altitude transportation	Low	0.1 ppm
Phosgene ($COCl_2$)	Firefighters, welders, paint strippers; chemical intermediates (isocyanates, pesticides, dyes, and pharmaceuticals)	Low	0.1 ppm
Sulfur dioxide (SO_2)	Smelting, combustion of coal and oil, paper manufacturing, and food preparation	High	5.0 ppm

[a]Adapted from Weiss SM, Lakshminarayan S. Clin Chest Med 1994;15:103–116.
OSHA, Occupational Safety and Health Administration.

Table 66-50
Action Criteria for Toxic Inhalants[a]

- Criteria for transportation to the hospital
  - Trapped in an enclosed space
  - Burning of synthetic material
  - Altered mental status
  - Facial burns
  - Chest pain
  - Age greater than 60 years
- Criteria for admission to the hospital
  - Altered mental status
  - Any respiratory symptoms (e.g., cough, chest tightness, dyspnea)
  - Carbonaceous sputum
  - Hoarseness, wheezing
  - History of ischemic heart disease or chronic obstructive pulmonary disease
  - Elevated carboxyhemoglobin (greater than 20%)
- Criteria for admission to intensive care unit
  - Depressed consciousness
  - Abnormal levels of arterial blood gases
  - Abnormal electrocardiogram
  - Hoarseness, wheezing
  - Decreased peak flow or abnormal spirometry
- Criteria for intubation
  - Depressed consciousness
  - Laryngeal obstruction
  - Respiratory insufficiency on arterial blood gases

[a]Adapted from Wald PH, Balmes JR. J Intensive Care Med 1987;2:260–278.

Table 66-51
Water Solubility and Unusual Effects of Irritant Gases[a]

Agent	Water Solubility	Unusual Effects
Aldehyde gases	High	None
Ammonia	High	None
Chlorine	Moderate	None
Hydrogen chloride	High	None
Hydrogen fluoride	High	Hypocalcemia, hypomagnesemia
Nitrogen oxides	Low	Methemoglobinemia, delayed onset
Ozone	Low	None
Phosgene	Low	None
Sulfur dioxide	High	Bronchoconstriction

[a]Adapted from Wald PH, Balmes JR. J Intensive Care Med 1987;2:260–278.

Table 66-52
Respiratory Irritants[a]

Gas	Source	Pulmonary Effect	Systemic Effect
Acetylene	Welding operations	Irritant	Narcosis
Ammonia	Refrigerant, organic syntheses	Irritant, edema	
Butane	Cooking, heating	Asphyxia	
Carbon dioxide	Confined cargos of plant materials		Asphyxia
Carbon disulfide[b]	Solvent, disinfectant, fumigant	Irritant	CNS stimulant
Carbon monoxide	Incomplete burning of organic material	Dyspnea	Carboxyhemoglobinemia
Chloramine	Mixing ammonia and chlorine bleaches	Irritant	Slight narcosis
Chlorine[b]	Swimming pool treatment	Irritant, edema	
Chloroacetophenone[b]	Tear gas, Mace	Irritant	
Fluorine	Organic syntheses	Irritant, edema	
Formaldehyde	Disinfectant, fixative, wrinkle-proof fabrics	Irritant	
Gasoline vapor	Automotive, dry cleaning		Narcosis
Hydrogen chloride	Plastic (PVC) fires	Irritant, edema	Myocardial toxicity
Hydrogen cyanide	Industry, fruit pits and seeds	Asphyxia	
Hydrogen fluoride	Glass etching, petroleum industry	See Fluorine	
Hydrogen sulfide[b]	Sewer gas, shale oil industry, fertilizer manufacturing	Irritant, edema	Cellular asphyxia
Methane	Natural gas		Asphyxia
Methyl bromide, chloride, iodide[b]	Refrigerants, fumigants, herbicides, fire extinguishers	Irritant, edema	CNS depression, organ damage, acidosis
Natural gas	See Methane		
Nitric oxide or nitrogen dioxide	"Silo filler's disease," combustion of x-ray film	Edema, bronchiolitis obliterans	
Nitrogen tetroxide	Missile industry	Irritant	Narcosis, apnea
Nitrous fumes	(See Nitric Oxide and Nitrogen Tetroxide)		
Ozone	Smog, arc welding, electrical equipment, high-altitude flying	Irritant, edema, hemorrhage	CNS depression
Phosgene	Burning of chlorine compounds	Irritant, edema	
Polyvinyl chloride	See Hydrogen Chloride		
Propane	Cooking, heating		Narcosis, asphyxia
Sulfur dioxide	Illuminating, pulp and paper plants	Bronchospasm irritant, edema	

[a]Adapted from Done AK. Emerg Med 1976;8(5):306–307.
[b]Not attributable to hypoxia and/or shock or cardiac failure.

Table 66-53
Clinical Manifestations Associated With Exposure to Gaseous Respiratory Irritants

		Acute Respiratory Manifestations			Chronic Respiratory Sequelae		
Irritant Gas	Onset	Upper Airway Irritation	Pneumonia	Pulmonary Edema	Bronchitis	Bronchiolitis Obliterans	Obstructive Lung Disease
Ammonia	Minutes	Severe	+	+	+	–	+
Chlorine	Minutes to hours	Moderate	+	+	–	–	–
Hydrogen chloride	Minutes	Severe	–	–	?	?	?
Oxides of nitrogen	Hours	Mild	+	+	–	+	+
Ozone	Hours	Mild	–	–	?	?	?
Phosgene	Hours	Mild	+	+	?	?	?
Sulfur dioxide	Minutes	Severe	+	+	–	+	+

Weiss SM, Lakshminarayan S. Clin Chest Med 1994;15:103–116.
–, Exposure not reported to be associated with clinical entity.
+, Exposure reported to be associated with clinical entity.
?, Chronic respiratory sequelae not pursued in those with acute symptoms.

include prolonged (30 minutes or longer until the eye reaches neutral pH as tested in the conjunctival sac), immediate irrigation with water. Topical antibiotics and topical steroids may be required.[8]

SULFUR DIOXIDE
Clinical Presentation

Exposures of two miners to sulfur dioxide concentrations of at least 40 PPM resulted in severe airway obstruction, hypoxemia, markedly reduced exercise tolerance, ventilation perfusion mismatch, and evidence of active inflammation as documented by a positive gallium lung scan. Serial ventilation-perfusion scans over the first 12 months showed progressive improvement without returning to normal. This status has remained for 2 years.[9]

A 10-year follow-up study on workers exposed to mean sulfur dioxide concentrations ranging from 4 to 33 ppm did not reveal an increased prevalence of chronic respiratory disease or deteriorating pulmonary function as compared with a control group.

ACID AEROSOLS

Respirable sulfuric acid (H_2SO_4) aerosol studies have indicated no respiratory irritant effects in normal subjects exposed to H_2SO_4 concentrations <100 μg/m^3 or less.[10] In asthmatic subjects some studies with H_2SO_4 aerosol have found a decrease in lung function,[11] while others have found no decrease.[12,13] Respiratory disease has been reported from Japan with exposures of at least 159 μg/m^3 of H_2SO_4.[14,15] Further data are required to elucidate this possible relationship.

NITROGEN OXIDES
Sources

Combustion of gas during cooking and burning of pilot lights releases nitric oxide (NO), nitrogen dioxide, carbon monoxide, carbon dioxide, and water.[16] Normal use of an unvented gas cooking range may add 25 parts per billion (ppb) of nitrogen dioxide to the background concentration in a home.[17] These levels may reach 200 to 400 ppm.[18]

Nitrogen dioxide, a product of combustion in malfunctioning ice-resurfacing machines, can accumulate in indoor ice-skating arenas that are poorly ventilated. Inhalation of toxic gases in arenas has also been linked to carbon monoxide, which induces early symptoms compared with the latent period following nitrogen dioxide exposure.[19]

Pulmonary Injury

Inhalation of nitrogen dioxide results in pulmonary injury that is dose-dependent. The injury is characterized morphologically by loss of ciliated cells in the airways and degeneration of alveolar epithelial type I cells leaving the basement membrane denuded. The disappearance of type I cells, which normally cover 97% of the alveolar surface, will result in cellular hypertrophy of epithelial type II cells to replace the damaged type I cells. Within 72 hours the denuded basement membrane will be repopulated again, but with the rapidly proliferating type II cells.[20]

Nitric Acid Spills

Nitric acid spillage generates oxides of nitrogen, including nitrogen dioxide. Patients exposed to the fumes experience the familiar period of relative well-being lasting a few hours, followed by rapidly progressive and often fatal, noncardiogenic pulmonary edema. The structural lung injury is manifest mainly in the distal bronchioles and adjacent alveoli.[21]

ICE HOCKEY LUNG

Engine exhaust liberated in a confined space has been recognized as a cause of carbon monoxide poisoning. Less well known is the fact that nitrogen dioxide may also be released from malfunctioning ice resurfacers during ice hockey games.[22] Cough hemoptysis, chest pain, headache, and dyspnea may be experienced by ice hockey players, cheerleaders, and spectators during and within 48 hours of attending an ice hockey game.[23] This may be associated with mild evidences of abnormal pulmonary function tests.[24,25] No sequelae have been reported. Treatment is symptomatic. Proper ventilation of ice arenas and repair of faulty resurfacing equipment will assist in reducing exposure.

PULMONARY ALVEOLAR PROTEINOSIS

Pulmonary alveolar proteinosis (PAP) is an unusual disease marked by the accumulation of granular, eosinophilic, periodic-Schiff (PAS)-positive protein lipid material in the alveoli. It predominantly affects men in the second to fourth decade of life. No specific infectious agent or neoplastic process has been definitely implicated in its pathogenesis. It has been associated with silica and nitrogen dioxide. There may be a defect of type II cells and/or pulmonary surfactant that leads to an overproduction of surfactant. Treatment does not appear to alter the course of the disease. Aerolized acetylcysteine and whole-lung lavage may be possible therapeutic approaches.[26] Spontaneous remission may occur.[27]

PHOSGENE (SEE CYTOTOXIC AGENT CHAPTER)

CHLORINE (SEE CYTOTOXIC AGENT CHAPTER)

Household hypochlorite exposures are less massive than industrial or environmental releases, but can be lethal. The most frequent site of exposure is the bathroom (often the shower stall). Mixing hypochlorite with an acid (such as toilet bowl or tile cleaner) results in release of chlorine gas.[28] The combined use of calcium hypochlorite and trichloro-s-triazinetrione, both chlorinating agents, may induce an explosive release of chlorine gas.[29] When ammonia interacts with hypochlorite-containing products, a combination of monochloramine and dichloramine, fumes known as chloramine are produced.[30]

Summary

- Bleach (hypochlorite) + acidic cleaning agent (toilet bowl cleaners) → chlorine gas (moisture in mucous membrane).
- Hypochlorous acid + hydrochloric acid → hypochloric acid + O_2 free radicals.
- Bleach (hypochlorite) + ammonia → monochloramine + dichloraminne → fumes → chloramine gas → moisture (mucous membrane) → hypochloric acid + toxic nascent oxygen.[29,30]

Treatment

1. Pulmonary edema may occur up to 24 hours after exposure sometimes inducing severe hypoxemia in minutes. Patients who are well 24 hours after exposure may be discharged.[31] Persistent hypoxemia can be associated with a high mortality.[32]
2. Intravenous fluids should be given with great caution. Fluid overload is very dangerous in these patients; diuretics such as furosemide may be useful as indicated.[29]
3. Corticosteroids are controversial in the patient with pulmonary edema, and clinical studies evaluating their efficacy are lacking.[33]
4. Pulmonary edema may develop within the first 24 hours after exposure.
5. Acute hypoxemic respiratory failure includes the presence of severe hypoxemia despite oxygen therapy, radiographic evidence of diffuse pulmonary infiltrates, decreased lung compliance and intrapulmonary shunt, and normal cardiac function with a pulmonary artery occlusive pressure <17 mm Hg.[34] The patient with persistent hypoxemia may require positive end-expiratory airway pressure (PEEP), in addition to supplemental oxygen.
6. A complication of high PEEP is diminished cardiac output due to decreased venous return to the heart. Such low output is reflected in signs of peripheral vasoconstriction, decreased urine output, and tachycardia combined with an inadequate central venous pressure. In such cases intravascular fluid will be of assistance.
7. Nebulized sodium bicarbonate may ameliorate respiratory symptoms by neutralizing the acid found when chlorine gas comes into contact with water in the airways. This may result in an exothermic reaction. Patients should be carefully monitored before and after this procedure. Few clinical studies have confirmed this approach. It is not known if such therapy is safe or effective for severe toxicity (pulmonary edema, respiratory compromise).[35–37]

SULFUR TRIOXIDE

Sulfur trioxide is a clear, colorless, nonflammable liquid with a strong irritating odor used as a sulfating or sulfonating agent in the production of detergents, emulsifiers, and shampoo. Sulfur trioxide is strongly acidic (pHCl) and reacts violently with water in air or on the skin to form sulfuric acid. Direct exposure with the skin or by inhalation results in thermal burns and tissue destruction. Treatment includes the use of oxygen, decontamination with special attention to the eyes, and monitoring for hypoxic ischemia. Treatment should include use of beta-agonists for bronchospasm, repeat pulmonary function tests, and monitoring for delayed pulmonary edema. Steroids, antibiotics, and nebulized sodium bicarbonate have not been adequately studied.[38]

METAL FUME FEVER (TABLE 66–54) (SEE METALS CHAPTER)—ISOCYANATES

At Bhopal 500 persons died before receiving any medical treatment. Six thousand persons were severely injured with symptoms of respiratory, central nervous system, and circulatory system distress. Of these, 2000 persons died within the first week. Approximately 10,000 persons had severe respiratory tract symptoms, but were otherwise unaffected. It is estimated that 150,000 to 200,000 were affected to some extent.[39] Hydrogen cyanide does not appear to have been a definitive causative factor.[40–43]

Table 66–54
Metal Fumes and Metallic Compound Gases[a]

		Effects			
Agent	Mechanism	Tracheo-bronchitis	Pulmonary Edema	Systemic Effects	Specific Treatment
Fume fever chemicals[b]	?	+	–	+	. . .
Metal halides	Irritants	+	+	–	. . .
Cadmium	Irritant, systemic toxin	+	+	+	Dialysis?
Manganese	Systemic toxin	+	–	+	. . .
Mercury	Systemic toxin	+	+	+	Chelation?
Nickel carbonyl	Irritant	+	+	–	. . .
Osmium tetroxide	Irritant	+	–	–	. . .
Vanadium pentoxide	Irritant	+	–	–	. . .
Metal hydrides					
Arsine	Hemolytic agent	–	–	–	Hemodialysis, exchange transfusion
Diborane	Irritant, systemic toxin	+	+	+	CNS monitoring
Phosphine	Irritant, systemic toxin	+	+	+	CNS depression, monitoring of seizures
Silane	Asphyxiant	+	–	–	. . .

[a]Adapted from Wald PH, Balmes JR. J Intensive Care Med 1987;2:260–278.
[b]Includes zinc, copper, magnesium, aluminum, antimony, iron, manganese, nickel, selenium, gold, tin, and polytetrafluorethylene.
+ = present; – = absent; CNS = central nervous system.

These compounds are strong mucous membrane irritants and pulmonary sensitizers. The most common serious side effects of the methyl isocyanate exposure at Bhopal were pulmonary edema and corneal ulceration.

Clinical Presentation

Follow-up 3 years after exposure to methyl isocyanate at Bhopal showed an excess of eye irritation, eyelid infection, an apparent increase in cataracts, and a decrease in visual acuity among the exposed. Bhopal eye syndrome thus includes full resolution of the initial interpalpebral superficial erosion, a subsequent risk of eye infections, hyperresponsive phenomena (irritation, watering, and phlyctena), and possible cataracts. Fundoscopy has not revealed any abnormality, and there is no evidence of damage to color vision or afferent pupillary reflexes.[44]

Laboratory

It is possible to monitor exposure to toluene diisocyanate by monitoring plasma concentration of 2,2,4- and 2,6-toluenediamine.[45]

LACRIMATORS (TABLE 66–55) (SEE ALSO CYTOTOXIC DRUG CHAPTER)

Riot-control agents are aerosol-dispersed chemicals that produce eye, nose, mouth, skin, and respiratory tract irritation. Most of these symptoms resolve by 30 minutes postexposure. Both ocular and mucous membrane symptoms may persist for 24 hours. The three currently used agents are 1-chloroacetophenone (CN), 2-chlorobenzylidenemalononitrile (CS), and dibenz[*b,f*]-1,4-oxazepine (CR). In dilute concentrations, these agents cause profuse lacrimation and blepharospasm, as well as cutaneous erythema and pain.

Table 66–55
Riot-Control Agents[a]

Agent	
Most commonly used	
ortho-Chlorobenzylidene malononitrile	CS
w-Chloroacetophenone	CN
10-Chloro-5,10-dihydrophenarsazine	DM
Dibenz (b.f.)-1 : 4-oxazepine	CR
Other agents	
Brombenzyl cyanide	CA
Ethyliodo acetate	SK
Bromacetone	BA
Xylyl bromide	T-stoff
Benzyl iodide	
Ethyl bromo ethanoate	
Phenyl carbylamine chloride	
Benzyl bromide	
Acrolein	
Chloracetone	
Iodoacetone	
Oleoresin of capsicum	

[a]Adapted from Hu H. Toxicology of riot-control agents (lacrimators). In: Somani SM. Chemical warfare agents. San Diego: Academic Press, 1993, pp. 271–288.

Serious systemic toxicity is rare and occurs only when these agents are used in high concentrations within confined spaces. Delayed cutaneous sensitivity can develop after exposure to chloroacetophenone.[46]

Uses

The lacrimators (tear gases) such as CS (2-chlorobenzylidene malononitrile) and CN (chloroacetophenone) are used by many police forces in crowd control operations and for personal protection, by the general public for personal protection (CN), and under certain conditions by combat forces.[47] Some pulmonary irritants such as chloropicrin[48] and cyanogen chloride are also lacrimators.[44] Severe traumatic injury from exploding tear gas bombs, as well as lethal toxic injury, has been observed. A tear gas liquid spray made from cayenne peppers may produce serious respiratory problems.[49] CN may be a clastogenic and mutagenic agent.[50] The United Nations has initiated action to include tear gas agents among chemical weapons banned under the Geneva Protocol.[51]

Sources

Chemical mace is a 1% solution of tear gas (chloroacetophenone) in a solvent propellant mixture of 4% kerosene, 5% 1,1,1-trichloroethane, and Freon 113. A 1-second spray releases 25 mg of chloroacetophenone, but evaporation of the organic solvent may concentrate the mixture in the eyes and intensify damage.[51] Other aerosol protectants may contain capsicum (Guardian) or chlorobenzylidenemalononitrile (Paralyzer). Classically, tear gas powder (chloracetophenone) is combined with a pyrotechnic base that volatilizes and aerosolizes the compound on contact with cool air.

Structure

In their natural states, these lacrimators are solids that hydrolyze fairly rapidly in water. Both 1-chloroacetophenone and 2-chlorobenzylidenemalononitrile are alkylating agents. Dibenz[*b,f*]-1,4-oxazepine (CR) is the parent compound of the antipsychotic agent loxapine. The cyano groups of 2-chlorobenzylidenemalononitrile apparently do not cause systemic cyanide toxicity since a 1-minute exposure to an intolerable level (10 mg/m^3) produces less cyanide than two puffs of a cigarette.[52]

Acute Toxic Dosage

These lacrimators are relatively nontoxic except when dispersed in a confined, nonventilated space.

1-Chloroacetophenone

Tear gas is the most toxic lacrimator and has accounted for at least five deaths resulting from pulmonary injury and/or asphyxia.[53,54] Readily apparent irritation occurs at 40 mg/m^3. At higher concentrations, corneal epithelial damage and chemosis develop. The maximum safe dose for short-term inhalation is 500 mg/m^3.[51]

2-Chlorobenzylidenemalononitrile

This compound is a 10-times-more-potent lacrimator than 1-chloroacetophenone and is less toxic.

Dibenz[b,f]-1,4-oxazepine

This compound is the most potent lacrimator with the least systemic toxicity.

Toxicokinetics

2-Chlorobenzylidenemalononitrile reacts covalently with plasma proteins to form compounds some of which may be antigenic. On contact with water, it hydrolyzes into *o*-chlorobenzaldehyde and malononitrile. The kidney excretes *o*-chlorobenzaldehyde as the metabolites *o*-chlorohippuric acid (major) and *o*-chlorobenzoic acid (minor). Malononitrile is metabolized to thiocyanate. Significant amounts of free cyanide do not appear in the plasma.[55]

Pathophysiology

The lacrimators are strong mucous membrane irritants and chemical activators of the lacrimal glands. Both 1-chloroacetophenone and 2-chlorobenzylidenemalononitrile are alkylating agents that react with sulfhydryl groups and other nucleophilic sites. Tissue injury and necrosis probably result from the biochemical inhibition of important enzymes such as pyruvic decarboxylase. 2-Chlorobenzylidenemalononitrile has the ability to generate bradykin in both in vitro and in vivo.[55] Postmortem findings associated with 1-chloroacetophenone include acute tracheobronchitis with necrosis of the respiratory mucosa and pseudomembrane formation, focal intraalveolar hemorrhage, early bronchopneumonia, pulmonary edema, cerebral edema, and fatty metamorphosis of the liver.[53,54]

Clinical Presentation

Eyes

These compounds produce intense blepharospasm, pain, lacrimation, conjunctival erythema, periorbital edema, and a short-duration rise in intraocular pressure. Symptoms generally diminish within 30 minutes postexposure, but the persistence of symptoms depends on the concentration and duration of exposure. Ocular injuries range from conjunctival irritation, ecchymosis, corneal edema, and loss of epithelium to necrotizing keratitis, coagulative necrosis, iridocyclitis, and deformities of the anterior chamber angle.[56]

Upper Respiratory Tract

Rhinorrhea, nasal irritation and congestion, bronchorrhea, sore throat, cough, sneezing, unpleasant taste, and burning of the mouth occur immediately after exposure and rapidly resolve within minutes postexposure.

Lungs

Prolonged concentrated exposures (e.g., the gassing of a prison ward) can produce an acute laryngeotracheobronchitis.[57] An infant developed persistent wheezes, rales, cough, and bronchial secretions for 3 to 4 days after a 2- to 3-hour 2-chlorobenzylidenemalononitrile exposure in a house.[58] After 1 week of ampicillin and steroid therapy, the child developed a right upper lobe infiltrate that resolved over the next 10 days. In doses likely to occur during a riot (open space), pulmonary function tests in human volunteers indicate no adverse effects.[59]

Reactive airways dysfunction syndrome (RADS) may follow a high level exposure to CS and respiratory irritants similar to CS.[60–62] Cough and shortness of breath can continue for weeks after exposure.[51]

Concentrated exposure to CS may lead to acute changes (eyes, face, throat, nasal passages) with paroxysmal cough, a feeling of tightness and burning in the chest, and abnormal chest x-ray. Chronic changes may then ensue for many weeks (cough, shortness of breath) and lead to RADS.[54] In most exposures to CS gas, only short-term health effects are observed. Cough, shortness of breath, chest pain, sore throat, and fever generally resolve within 2 weeks.[63]

Gastrointestinal

Ingestion of CS will lead to repeated episodes of abdominal cramping pain and diarrhea. Two patients were treated with cathartics and antacids and recovered.[64]

Skin

Burning and sometimes erythema occur after exposure to lacrimators. Prolonged exposures, particularly those associated with wet clothing or the use of petroleum jelly, can cause second-degree chemical burns.[57] The development of skin effects depends on the thickness of the stratum corneum, as well as the extent of exposure. Skin previously exposed to dibenz[*b, f*]-1,4-oxazepine may become painful again for 24 to 48 hours on water contact.[65] Cutaneous erythema usually resolves within 3 hours, but 1-chloroacetophenone is a skin sensitizer and may produce an allergic contact dermatitis (pruritus, weeping, papulovesicular rash) within 72 hours of exposure.[46,57,66]

Laboratory

Analytic methods for lacrimators include gas chromatographic–mass spectrometric identification procedures.[67,68] Gas chromatography–mass spectrometry identification of tear gases provide a sensitivity level of 1 to 10 ng/mL.[69] Spectra data (ultraviolet, fluorescence, nuclear magnetic resonance, infrared and mass) and a capillary gas–liquid chromatography–mass spectrometric method that differentiate and identify CN and CS are available.[70] A significant leukocytosis (i.e., over 20,000 WBC/cm^3) may occur after exposure to 1-chloroacetophenone and can last for several days.[57,58]

Treatment

Stabilization

The immediate priority is removal from exposure and establishment of an airway. The development of laryngeal edema and/or spasm is a theoretical possibility. Patients with respiratory distress should receive oxygen, an evaluation of airway patency and ventilation, an intravenous line, and cardiac monitoring. Severe respiratory injuries can result from gassing in a confined space. Obtain arterial blood gases and chest x-rays in these patients. Bronchospasm may contribute to respiratory distress and may be treated with aminophylline and inhaled sympathomimetic drugs (salbutamol, metaproterenol).

Decontamination

Remove all contaminated clothing and seal it in a plastic bag. Medical personnel should use disposable rubber gloves when handling contaminated clothes. The eyes should be irrigated copiously with saline for 15 to 20 minutes. Contaminated skin should be washed thoroughly with mild liquid soap and water. Only a saline irrigation should be used over vesiculated skin.

If clothing is to be washed, cold water should be used because hot water will cause any residual CS gas to vaporize leading to symptons in attending staff.[71]

Supportive Care

The eyes should be examined for corneal abrasions and treated with oral analgesics, topical antibiotics (sulfacetamide), and mydriatics as needed. Vesiculated skin is treated like a second-degree chemical burn. Patients with respiratory distress should be admitted if symptoms persist several hours. These patients should be observed for the development of bronchospasm and pneumonia (e.g., serial chest x-rays, arterial blood gases). Prophylactic antibiotics and steroids probably are not effective. Humidified oxygen may provide symptomatic relief.

Irrigate ocular injuries with isotonic saline and remove the remaining powder with a cotton wool swab. Any remaining stromal particles should be removed with a needle tip with a slit lamp.[72]

REFERENCES—RESPIRATORY TRACT IRRITANTS

1. Weiss SM, Lakshminarayan S. Acute inhalation injury. Clin Chest Med 1994;15:103–116.
2. Wald PH, Balmes JR. Respiratory effects of short-term high intensity toxic inhalation: smoke, gases and fumes. J Intensive Care Med 1987;2:260–278.
3. Wald PH, Balmes JR. Respiratory effects of short-term, high-intensity toxic inhalations: smoke, gases, and fumes. J Intensive Care Med 1987;2:260–278.
4. Lee HS, Chan CC, Tan KT, Cheong TH, Chee CBE, Wang YT. Burnisher's asthma—a case due to ammonia from silverware polishing. Singapore Med J 1993;34:565–566.
5. Wason S, Stephan M, Breide C. Ingestion of aromatic ammonia "smelling salts" capsules. AJDC 1990;144:139–140.
6. Lopez GP, Dean BS, Krenzelok EP. Oral exposure to ammonia inhalants. A report of 8 cases. Vet Hum Toxicol 1988; 30:350.
7. Wallace DE. Consequence of exposure to aromatic ammonia solution in 15 patients. Vet Hum Toxicol 1989;31:399.
8. Beare JDL, Wilson RD, Marsh RJ. Ammonia burns of the eye: an old weapon in new hands. Br Med J 1990;296:590.
9. Rabinovitch S, Greyson ND, Weiser W, Hoffstein V. Clinical and laboratory features of acute sulfur dioxide inhalation poisoning: two-year follow-up. Am Rev Respir Dis 1989;239: 556–558.
10. Avol EL, Linn WS, Shamoo DA, Anderson KR, Peng R-C, Hochney JD. Respiratory responses of young asthmatic volunteers in controlled exposures to sulfuric acid aerosol. Am Rev Respir Dis 1990;142:343–348.
11. Koenig JQ, Covert DS, Pierson WE. Effects of inhalation of acidic compounds on pulmonary function in allergic adolescent subjects. Environ Health Perspect 1989;79:173–178.
12. Utell MJ. Effects of inhaled acid aerosols on lung mechanics. An analysis of human exposure studies. Environ Health Perspect 1985;63:39–44.
13. Folinsbee LJ. Human health effects of exposure to airborne acid. Environ Health Perspect 1989;79:195–199.

14. Kitagawa T. Cause analysis of the Yokkaichi asthma episode in Japan. J Air Pollution Control Assoc 1984;34:743–746.
15. Lippman M. Airborne acidity: estimates of exposure and human health effects. Environ Health Perspect 1985;63:63–70.
16. Samet JM, Marbury MC, Spengler JD. Health effects and sources of indoor air pollution. I. Am Rev Respir Dis 1987;136:1486–1508.
17. Spengler JD, Duffy CP, Letz R, Tibbitts TW, Ferris BG Jr. Nitrogen dioxide inside and outside 137 homes and implications for ambient air quality standards and health effects research. Environ Sci Technol 1983;17:164–168.
18. Spengler JD, Sexton K. Indoor air pollution: A public health perspective. Science 1983;221:9–17.
19. Soparkar G, Mayers I, Edouard L, Hoeppner VH. Toxic effects from nitrogen dioxide in ice skating arenas. Can Med Assoc J 1993;148:1181–1182.
20. Elsayed NM. Toxicity of nitrogen dioxide: an introduction. Toxicology 1994;89:161–174.
21. Hajela R, Janigan DT, Landrigan PL, Boudreau SF, Sebastian S. Fatal pulmonary edema due to nitric acid fume inhalation in three pulp-mill workers. Chest 1990;97:487–489.
22. Ice hockey lung: NO_2 poisoning. Lancet 1990;335:1191 (editorial).
23. Hedberg K, Hedberg CW, Iber C, White KE, Osterholic MT, Jones DBW et al. An outbreak of nitrogen dioxide-induced respiratory illness among ice hockey players. JAMA 1989;262:3014–3017.
24. Ford DP, Rothman N. Nitrogen dioxide-induced respiratory illness in ice hockey players. JAMA 1990;263:3024.
25. Hedberg K, MacDonald KL, Osterholm M, Hedberg C, White K. Nitrogen dioxide-induced respiratory illness in ice hockey players. JAMA 1990;263:3024–3025.
26. Dawkins SA, Gerhard H, Nevin M. Pulmonary alveolar proteinosis: a possible sequel of NO_2 experience. J Occup Med 1991;33:638–641.
27. Martinez-Lopez MA, Gomez-Cerazo G, Villasante C, Molina F, Diaz S, Cobo J, Medrano C. Pulmonary alveolar proteinosis: prolonged spontaneous remission in two patients. Eur Respir J 1991;4:377–379.
28. Blanc PD. Chlorine gas inhalation. AACT Update 1994;7(4): 1–2.
29. Martinez TT, Long C. Explosion risk from swimming pool chlorinators and review of chlorine toxicity. Clin Toxicol 1995; 33:349–359.
30. Krenzelok E, Mrvos R. Chlorine/chloramine. Clin Toxicol 1995;355–357.
31. Baxter PJ, Davies PC, Murray V. Medical planning for toxic releases into the community: the example of chlorine gas. Br J Ind Med 1989;46:277–285.
32. Heidemann SM, Goetting MG. Treatment of acute hypoxemic respiratory failure caused by chlorine exposure. Pediatr Emerg Care 1991;7:87–88.
33. Vinsel PJ. Treatment of acute chlorine gas inhalation with nebulized sodium bicarbonate. J Emerg Med 1990;8:327–329.
34. Zucker AR. Therapeutic strategies for acute hypoxemic respiratory failure. Crit Care Clin 1988;4:813–830.
35. Bosse M. Nebulized sodium bicarbonate in the treatment of chlorine gas inhalation. Vet Hum Toxicol 1993;35:357.
36. Vinsel PJ. Treatment of acute chlorine gas inhalation with nebulized sodium bicarbonate. J Emerg Med 1990;8: 327–329.
37. Chisholm CD, Singletary EM, Okerberg CV, Langlinais PL. Inhaled sodium bicarbonate therapy for chlorine inhalation injuries. Ann Emerg Med 1989;18:466.
38. Stueven HA, Coogan P, Vallery V. A hazardous material episode: sulfur trioxide. Vet Hum Toxicol 1993;35:37–38.
39. Lorin HG, Kulling PEJ. The Bhopal tragedy—what has Swedish disaster medicine planning learned from it? J Emerg Med 1986;4:311–316.
40. Mehta PS, Mehta AS, Mehta SJ, Makhijani AB. Bhopal tragedy's health effects. A review of methyl isocyanate toxicity. JAMA 1990;264:2781–2787.
41. Salmon AG. Bright red blood of Bhopal victims: cyanide or MIC? Br J Ind Med 1986;43:502–504.
42. Nemery B, Sparrow S, Dinsdale D. Methyl isocyanate. Thiosulphate does not protect. Lancet 1985;2:1245–1246.
43. Anderson N. Long-term effects of methyl isocyanate. Lancet 1989;1:1259.
44. Anderson N, Ajwani MK, Mahashabde S, Tiwari MK, Muir MK, Mehra V et al. Delayed eye and other consequences from exposure to methyl isocyanate. 93% follow-up of exposed and unexposed cohorts in Bhopal. Br J Ind Med 1990;47:553–558.
45. Persson P, Dalene M, Skarping G, Adensson M, Hagman L. Biological monitoring of occupational exposure to toluene diisocyanate: measurement of toluenediamine in hydrolysed urine and plasma by gas chromatography–mass spectrometry. Br J Ind Med 1993;50:1111–1118.
46. Frazier CA. Contact allergy to mace. JAMA 1976;236:2526.
47. Danto BL. Medical problems and criteria regarding the use of tear gas by police. Am J Forensic Med Path 1987;8:317–322.
48. Toxic gas in Tbilisi. Lancet 1989;1:1462–1663.
49. ACLU report calls pepper spray potentially deadly. New York Times, June 19, 1995.
50. Hu H, Fine J, Epstein P, Kelsey K, Reynolds P, Walker B. Tear gas-harrassing agent on toxic chemical weapon? JAMA 1989;262:660–663.
51. Beswick FW. Chemical agents used in riot control and warfare. Hum Toxicol 1983;2:247–256.
52. Verdict on CS. Br Med J 1971;2:721 (editorial).
53. Stein AA, Kirwan WE. Chloroacetophenone (tear gas) poisoning: a clinico-pathologic report. J Forensic Sci 1964;9: 374–382.
54. Chapman AJ, White C. Death resulting from lacrimatory agents. J Forensic Sci 1978;23:527–530.
55. Cucinell AA, Swentzel KC, Biskup R et al. Biochemical interactions and metabolic fate of riot control agents. Fed Proc 1971;30:86–91.
56. Leopold IH, Lieberman TW. Chemical injuries of the cornea. Fed Proc 1971;30:92–95.
57. Thorburn KM. Injuries after use of the lacrimatory agent chloroacetophenone in a confined space. Arch Environ Health 1982;37:182–186.
58. Park S, Giammonia ST. Toxic effects of tear gas on an infant following prolonged exposure. Am J Dis Child 1972;123: 245–246.
59. Beswick FW, Holland P, Kemp KH. Acute effects of exposure to o-chlorobenzylidenemalononitrile (CS) and the development of tolerance. Br J Ind Med 1972;29:298–306.
60. Brooks SM, Weiss MA, Bernstein IL. Reactive airways dysfunction syndrome (RADS). Chest 1985;88:376–384.
61. Brooks SM, Weiss MA, Bernstein IL. Reactive airways dysfunction syndrome. J Occup Med 1985;27:473–476.
62. Hu H, Christian D. Reactive airways dysfunction after exposure to tear gas. Lancet 1992;339:1535.
63. Wheeler H, Murray V. Poisons centre will monitor cases. Br Med J 1995;331:871.
64. Sidell FR. Civil emergencies involving chemical warfare agents: medical considerations. In: Somani SM, ed. Chemical warfare agents. San Diego: Academic Press, 1992; pp. 341–356.
65. Holland P. The cutaneous reactions produced by dibenzoxazepine (CR). Br J Dermatol 1974;90:657–659.
66. Penneys NS. Contact dermatitis to chloroacetophenone. Fed Proc 1971;30:96–99.
67. Wils ERJ, Hulst AG. Gas chromatographic-mass spectrometric identification of tear-gases in dilute solutions using large injection volumes. J Chromatogr 1985;330:379–382.
68. Ferslew KE, Orcutt RH, Hagardon AN. Spectral differentiation and gas chromatographic/mass spectrometric analysis of the lacrimators 2-chloroacetophenone and o-chlorobenzylidene malononitrile. J Forensic Sci 1986;31: 658–665.
69. Wils ERJ, Hulst AG. Gas chromatographic–mass spectrometric identification of tear gases in dilute solubions using large injection volumes. J Chromatogr 1985;330:379–382.
70. Ferslew KE, Orcutt RH, Hagardorn AN. Spectral differentiation and gas chromatographic/mass spectrometric analysis of the lacrimators 2-chloroacetophenone and o-chlorbenzylidene malononitrile. J Forensic Sci 1986;31: 658–665.

71. Gray PJ. Treating CS injuries to the eye. Br Med J 1995;311: 871.
72. Scott RAH. Illegal "Mace" contains more toxic CN particles. Br Med J 1995;311:871.

FLUOROCARBONS

Fluorocarbons are halogenated hydrocarbons; fluorocarbons that contain chlorine are called chlorofluorocarbons (CFCs). These colorless, noncombustible liquids are used as refrigerants, propellants, degreasers, fire extinguishers, deicers, and agents for cleaning electronic equipment and preparing frozen tissues for histopathology.

Of the more than 36 commercially available fluorocarbons, approximately 12 are produced and used in significant quantities. One of these, 1,1,2-trichloro-1,2,2-trifluoroethane, is more commonly known as CFC-113 or by such trade names as Freon 113, Genetron 113, Halocarbon, or Refrigerant 112. The National Occupational Hazard Survey (NOHS) estimates that 300,000 workers are potentially exposed to CFC-113 [NIOSH 1977].[1]

Fluorocarbons may be deposited on cigarettes from the air or from a worker's fingers. As the cigarette is smoked, fluorocarbons are then burned or "pyrolyzed" and the products of decomposition inhaled with the cigarette smoke.[2,3] The most common products of such pyrolysis include inorganic fluorides, hydrogen fluoride, carbonyl fluoride, and perfluoropropane.[4] A no-smoking rule should be in effect in areas where fluorocarbons are used.[5,6]

CHLOROFLUOROCARBONS (CFCs)

CFCs are being phased out to protect the ozone layer. Manufacturers will stop selling CFCs no later than year end 1995 in the United States and other developed countries. December 31, 1995, is the last day CFCs can be manufactured in the United States, but an international treaty permits American factories to produce 53,500 tons each year for export until the year 2005.[5] Odor thresholds for some CFCs are found in Table 66–56.[6]

1,1,2-Trichloro-1,2,2-trifluoroethane (Fluorocarbon 113-FC-113)

CAS 76-13-1

OSHA Exposure Limits:
8-hour time-weighted average 1000 ppm
7600 mg/m^3
Short-term exposure limit 1250 ppm
(15 minutes) 9500 mg/m^3

Table 66–56
Odor Thresholds—CFCs

Odor Thresholds	Odor Low (mg/m^3)	Odor High (mg/m^3)
Trichlorofluoromethane (Freon 1)	28.00	1170.40
Trichlorotrifluoroethane (Freon 113)	342.00	1026.00

Uses

FC-113 was introduced as a refrigerant (Freon 113). It is now used in the industrial setting as a refrigerant, degreaser, and dry-cleaning solvent.

Clinical Presentation

Fatalities attributed to cardiac arrhythmia, asphyxiation, or both have followed occupational exposure in confined spaces. Human health effects at various concentrations of CFC-113 are found in Table 66–57.

Several factors that contribute to the hazards of exposure to CFC-113 and that are applicable to other CFCs are as follows:

1. Use in confined spaces.
2. High vapor pressure, which results in hazardous vapor; concentrations, particularly in confined spaces.
3. Poor odor-warning properties and absence of irritation.
4. Relatively low toxicity up to approximately 2500 ppm, which leads workers to believe that the chemical is inherently safe.

These factors may work together to create situations in which workers may be exposed to CFC-113 or other CFCs at concentrations sufficient to cause death by cardiac arrhythmia or asphyxiation.

Risk factors

Medications that contain ingredients such as epinephrine, norepinephrine, dopamine, isoproterenol, and other sympathomimetic agents used by asthmatics and that induce a catecholamine response may be of concern. Another increased risk factor is the presence of preexisting cardiovascular disease.

Toxicokinetics

Following exposure to 1980, 4000, or 7630 mg/m^3 of FC-113, the average elimination half-life in the breath was 0.22 to 29 hours. About 2.6 to 4.3% of the dose is recovered unchanged in the breath.[7]

Table 66–57
Human Health Effects Related to Various Concentrations of CFC-113

Concentration (ppm)	Health Effect
1000	No adverse health effects (OSHAPEL)
2500	Impairs ability to perform simple tasks; induces mild lethargy and loss of ability to concentrate
4500[a]	Considered IDLH
7600 (measured 24 hr after exposure)	Death from cardiac arrhythmia (Case No. 1)
300,000 (estimated)	Death from asphyxiation and pulmonary edema (Case No. 2)

[a]The IDLH concentration can be reached in a confined, unventilated space by evaporating as little as 21 ounces of CPC-113 in an enclosed, 1000-cubic-ft area (10 by 10 by 10 ft) [AIHA 1982].

TABLE: Fluorocarbon in currently available metered-dose inhalers

	FC-11	FC-12	FC-14
Formula	Cl I Cl-C-F I Cl	Cl I F-C-F I Cl	F F I I F-C-C-F I I Cl Cl
Boiling point (C)	23.7	–29.8	4.1
Amount in dose (mg)			
Bricanyl	8.6	17.2	8.6
Berotec	17	37	15.5
Respolin 400	1.7	27	4.8
Respolin 200	3.4	54.2	9.6
Ventolin	23.7	61.2	0

Figure 66–7 Fluorocarbons in currently available metered-dose inhalers. (Adapted from Pierce RJ et al. Med J Aust 1991;154: 701–704.)

Laboratory

A 16-year-old collapsed fatally after exposure to FC-113. The blood FC-113 concentration was 2.3 μg/mL.[4]

Treatment

Minimize skin contact and absorption. Wear chemical protective clothing (CPC) such as gloves and aprons. CPC made from neoprene and nitrile rubber should provide adequate protection for at least 1 hour. If CFC-113 gets on the skin, promptly wash the contaminated area with soap or a mild detergent and water. Wear splash-proof safety goggles to prevent eye contact. If contact dose occur, wash eyes with copious amounts of water.

Trichlorotrifluoroethane

Three individuals suffered rapid fatal cardiac arrest when they were exposed to a compartment flooded with trichlorotrifluoroethane gas.[8]

Monochlorodifluoromethane (Freon-22)

Deaths have been reported following inhalation of Freon-22. Fatal blood concentrations in three fatal cases were 286 to 538 μg/mL.[9] Two children experienced severe central nervous system depression following accidental inhalation of Freon from toys inflated with the gas.[10]

Bromotrifluoromethane (Halon-1301)

Halon-1301 is a commonly used fire extinguisher. Changes in cognitive, psychomotor, and perceptual performance have been reported with exposures between 4 and 7%. Over 7% headache, dizziness, disorientation, and coma may occur. At higher levels cardiac arrhythmias have been observed.[11]

Bromodichlorodifluoromethane

Bromodichlorodifluoromethane is structurally similar to halothane. Rhabdomyolysis may be produced in individuals known to be susceptible to malignant hyperthermia.[12]

Bromochlorodifluoromethane (Halon-1211)

Halon-1211 is widely used as an extinguishing agent. Several cases of sudden death in teenagers associated with BCF abuse have been reported. In such cases, BCF sniffing has been followed by breathing difficulties, excitation, ventricular fibrillation, and loss of consciousness.[13]

A comparison of CFCs available in metered-dose inhalers is found in Figure 66–7.[14]

Trichlorofluoromethane (FC-11)
Dichlorodifluoromethane (FC-12)
Dichlorotetrafluoromethane (FC-114)

REFERENCES—FLUOROCARBONS

1. NIOSH Alert: Request for assistance in preventing death from excessive exposure to chlorofluorocarbon 113 (CFC-113). Washington, DC: US Government Printing Office. DHHS (NIOSH). Publication No. 89-109.
2. CDC-polymer-fume fever associated with cigarette smoking and the use of tetrafluoroethylene—Mississippi. MMWR 1987;36:515–522.
3. Albrecht WN, Bryant CJ. Polymer-fume fever associated with smoking and use of a mold-release spray containing polytetrafluoroethylene. J Occup Med 1987;29:817–819.
4. CDC. Criteria for a recommended standard: occupational exposure to decomposition products of fluorocarbon polymers. Cincinnati, OH: US Department of Health, Education and Welfare, Public Health Service, 1977; DHEW Publication No. (NIOSH) 77-193.
5. Begley S. Holes in the ozone treatment. Newsweek, September 25, 1995, p. 70.
6. Ruth JH. Odor thresholds and irritation levels of several chemical substances: a review. Am Ind Hyg Assoc J 1986; 47:A142–A151.
7. Woollen BH, Guest EA, Howe W, Marsh JR, Wilson HF, Auton TR et al. Human inhalation pharmacokinetics of 1,1,1,2-trichloro-1,2,2 trifluoromethane (FC-113). Int Arch Occup Environ Health 1990;62:73–78.
8. McGee MB, Meyer RF, Jejurikai SG. A death resulting from trichlorotrifluoromethane poisoning. J Forensic Sci 1990; 35:1453–1460.
9. Tsatsakis AM, Smialek J. A fatal case due to Freon-22 inhalation. Bull Int Assoc Forensic Toxicol 1991;21:33–36.
10. Thompson JD, Snodgrass WR. Inflatable toys—an unusual source of Freon toxicity. Vet Hum Toxicol 1991;33:363.
11. Holness DL, House RA. Health effects of Halon-1301 exposure. J Occup Med 1992;34:722–725.
12. Denborough MA, Hopkinsin KC, Banney DG. Firefighters and malignant hyperthermia. Br Med J 1988;296:1442–1443.
13. Lerman Y, Winkler E, Tirosh MS, Danon Y, Almog S. Fatal accidental inhalation of bromochlorodifluoromethane (Halon-1211). Hum Exper Toxicol 1991;10:125–128.
14. Pierce RJ, Seale JP, Ruffin RE. Inhaled respiratory medications and the use of chlorofluorocarbons (CFCs). Med J Aust 1991;154:701–704.

Table 66–58
Gradation of Individual Physiologic Response to Acute O_3 Exposure[a]

Gradation of Response	Mild	Moderate	Severe	Incapacitating
Change in spirometry $FEV_{1.0}$, FVC	5–10%	10–20%	20–40%	>40%
Duration of effect	Complete recovery in <30 min	Complete recovery in <6 hr.	Complete recovery in 24 hr	Recovery in >24 hr
Symptoms	Mild to moderate cough	Mild to moderate cough, pain on deep inspiration, shortness of breath	Repeated cough, moderate to severe pain on deep inspiration and shortness of breath; breathing distress	Severe cough, pain on deep inspiration and shortness of breath; obvious distress
Limitation of activity	None	Few individuals choose to discontinue activity	Some individuals choose to discontinue activity	Many individuals choose to discontinue activity

[a]Adapted from Lippman M. J Am Poll Control Assoc 1989;32:672–695.

OZONE

ACUTE TOXIC DOSAGE

Exposure to high concentrations of ozone produces damage to type I cells and replacement by a metaplastic cuboidal epithelium.[1]

Respiratory effects of ozone may be affected by the level of activity in most healthy adults exposed to ozone concentrations from 0.10 to 0.16 ppm.[2] Relationships between physiologic responses to various grades of severity of acute O_3 exposure are summarized in Table 66–58.[3]

Ambient exposures to ozone at levels below the National Ambient Air Quality Standard of 120 ppb may be associated with transient decreases in lung function.[4] The long-term significance of this is not certain. Airway hyperresponsiveness may also be a risk factor for ozone sensitivity even among healthy, asymptomatic athletes.[5]

TREATMENT

Treatment is supportive.

REFERENCES—OZONE

1. Rusznak C, Devalia JL, Davies RJ. A hole in our knowledge of ozone toxicity? Allergy 1994;49:21–27.
2. Paulo M, Gong H Jr. Respiratory effect of ozone: whom to protect, when and how? J Respir Dis 1991;12:482–499.
3. Lippman M. Health effects of ozone. A critical review. J Am Poll Control Assoc 1989;32:672–695.
4. Kinney PL, Ware JH, Spengler JD, Dockery DW, Speizer FE, Ferris BG Jr. Short-term pulmonary function change in association with ozone levels. Am Rev Respir Dis 1989; 139:56–61.
5. Aris R, Christian D, Sheppard D, Balmes JR. The effects of sequential exposure to acidic fog and ozone on pulmonary function in exercising subjects. Am Rev Respir Dis 1991;143:85–91.

SMOKE INHALATION—FIRE TOXICOLOGY

Toxicologic effects of fire gases are summarized in Table 66–59. Table 66–60 indicates common products of combustion. Pyrolysis products of building materials are listed in Table 66–61.

AIRBORNE TOXINS INCLUDED IN SMOKE INHALATION

Asphyxiants

Carbon Monoxide

CO results from incomplete combustion of hydrocarbons or the combustion of cellulose (wood, paper, cotton) and is the major gas in almost all fires. About 80% of all fire deaths are not due to burns, but are probably due to carbon monoxide.[1]

Cyanide

Cyanide contributes, with carbon monoxide, to a probably synergistic lethality, causing an augmented inhibitor of cytochrome oxidase in the central nervous system.[2] Few deaths after a fire occur in individuals in whom high blood cyanide concentrations are found with low or definitely sublethal carboxyhemoglobin concentrations.[3] Fire victims have exhibited sublethal concentrations of both carboxyhemoglobin and blood cyanide. Cyanide may exert a critical incapacitating effect exposing the victim to high concentrations of carbon dioxide.[4]

Methemoglobinemia

Small elevations in methemoglobin levels are found in some victims of smoke inhalation and may add to symptoms related to hypoxia, carbon monoxide exposure, and cyanide poisoning.[5]

Ancillary Tests

Pentetic acid (diethylenetriaminepentaacetic acid, DTPA) labeled with technetium Tc 99m (molecular weight 492 daltons) appears to reflect permeability of the epithelial layer of the alveolar-capillary barrier. 99m TC DTPA offers a possible means of rapidly detecting smoke-induced injury to the alveolar-capillary barrier. Lung clearance of 99m TcDTPA is a relatively fast (less than 20 minutes) test to

Table 66–59
Toxicologic Effects of Fire Gases[a]

Toxicant	Sources	Toxicologic Effects	Estimate of Short-term (10-min) Lethal Concentration (ppm)
Hydrogen cyanide (HCN)	From combustion of wool, silk, polyacrylonitrile, nylon, polyurethane and paper	A rapidly fatal asphyxiant poison.	350
Nitrogen dioxide (NO_2) and other oxides of nitrogen	Produced in small quantities from fabrics and in larger quantities from cellulose nitrate and celluloid	Strong pulmonary irritant capable of causing immediate death as well as delayed injury.	200
Ammonia (NH_3)	Produced in combustion of wool, silk, nylon and melamine, concentrations generally low in ordinary building fires.	Pungent, unbearable odor; irritant to eyes and nose.	1000
Hydrogen chloride (HCl)	From combustion of polyvinyl chloride (PVC), and some fire-retardant treated materials.	Respiratory irritant; potential toxicity of HCl coated on particulate may be greater than that for an equivalent amount of gaseous HCl.	500[b]
Other halogen acid gases (HF and HBr)	From combustion of fluorinated resins or films and some fire-retardant materials containing bromine.	Respiratory irritants.	HF ~400 HBr >500
Sulfur dioxide (SO_2)	From materials containing sulfur.	A strong irritant, intolerable well below lethal concentrations.	>500
Isocyanates	From urethane polymers; pyrolysis products, such as toluene-2,4-diisocyanate (TDI), have been reported in small-scale laboratory studies; their significance in actual fires is undefined.	Potent respiratory irritants; believed the major irritants in smoke of isocyanate-based urethanes.	~100 (TDI)
Acrolein	From pyrolysis of polyolefins and cellulosics at lower temperatures (~400°C).	Potent respiratory irritant.	30 to 100

[a]Adapted from Hartzell GE et al. Am Ind Hyg Assoc J 1983;44:248–255.
[b]If particulate is absent.

administer. Although its use in man is increasing, it is not yet a standard clinical procedure. Further data will be of interest before recommendations for routine use can be made.[6–9] Cyanide and carbon monoxide are important poisons affecting individuals suffering from smoke inhalation. Methemoglobinemia may also be observed, but its significance has not yet been evaluated.[5]

Plasma Lactate

Baud and associates studied victims of residential fires. Blood cyanide concentrations below 40 μmol/L (0.10 mg/dL) were defined as nontoxic, those greater than 40 to less than 100 μmol/L (0.26 mg/dL) as potentially toxic, and those over 100 μmol/L (0.26 mg/dL) as potentially lethal. In fire victims who survive, blood cyanide concentrations are elevated. Survival may occur despite a blood cyanide concentration in the lethal range. Plasma *lactate* concentrations at the time of hospital admission appear to correlate more closely with blood cyanide concentrations than with blood carbon monoxide concentrations. Metabolic acidosis occurs frequently in fire victims, and cyanide poisoning is a possible cause of the lactic acidosis. Plasma lactate concentrations above 10 mmol/L appear to be a sensitive indicator of cyanide intoxication, as defined by the presence of a blood cyanide concentration above 40 μmol/L. An elevated plasma lactate concentration may be a useful indicator of cyanide toxicity in fire victims who do not have severe burns.[10]

Treatment

After initial life-support measures, including oxygen therapy, have been administered, arterial blood samples should be collected for evaluation of blood gases, carboxyhemoglobin, cyanide, and lactate. A 12.5 g dose of sodium thiosulfate can then be given immediately. If the patient continues to exhibit findings suggestive of cyanide intoxication (coma, seizures, cardiac arrhythmias, acidemia, hypotension) and the plasma lactate level is over 10 mmol/L and is not due to other factors, then sodium nitrite can be administered while the blood pressure is carefully monitored. Plasma lactate levels and blood cyanide concentrations may take hours to perform.[11]

Hydroxocobalamin, which has been given orphan drug status in the United States, does not affect normal hemoglobin and is probably safer than sodium nitrite.[12] Its toxic effects include transient reddish discoloration of the skin, mucous membranes, and urine and, rarely, anaphylaxis.[13]

Samples used for the measurement of blood cyanide were obtained at the scenes of fires. Values reported were near the

Table 66-60
Common Toxic Combustion Products[a]

Product	Pulmonary Irritant	Systemic Toxin[b]
Acrylic	Hydrogen chloride	Carbon monoxide
Carbon tetrachloride extinguishers	Phosgene	
Cellulose nitrate	Nitrogen oxides	
Celluloid, cellulosic acid	Acrolein	Carbon monoxide
Chlorinated hydrocarbons	Phosgene	
Fabrics	Nitrogen oxides	
Cotton	Acetaldehyde, formaldehyde	Acetic acid, methane, formic acid
Nylon	Ammonia	Cyanide
Wool, silk	Ammonia, nitrogen oxides, carbon monoxide, carbon dioxide	Hydrogen sulfide and cyanide
Film		
Cellulose acetate	Acetaldehyde, formaldehyde	Carbon monoxide, acetic acid, methane
Nitrocellulose	Nitrogen oxides	Carbon monoxide, cyanide, hydrogen fluoride
Others		
Insulation wire	Hydrogen chloride	
Newsprint (resembles wood)		
Neoprene	?Pulmonary edema may result	
Paper		Cyanide
Photocopier paper		Nickel carbonyl
Polyacrylonitrile		Cyanide
Polyfluorocarbons	Octafluoroisobutylene	
Polyolefins	Acrolein	
Polystyrene	Styrene	
Polyurethane	Isocyanates	Cyanide, isocyanates
Polyvinyl acetate	Acetic acid and vapors	
Polyvinyl chloride (PVC)	Hydrogen chloride, phosgene, chlorine	Carbon monoxide, carbon dioxide
Polyvinyl methyl ether		Monomers, alcohols
Resins		
Melamine	Ammonia	Hydrogen cyanide
Phenolic	Ammonia, formaldehyde	Hydrogen cyanide
Retardant treatment	Hydrogen chloride	Bromine
Rubber		Hydrogen sulfide, sulfur dioxide
Urethane isocyanate polymers	Isocyanates	Isocyanates
Wood	Acetaldehyde, formaldehyde	Acetic acid, methane, formic acid, carbon monoxide
Xerox paper		Nickel carbonyl

[a]Adapted from Done AK. Emerg Med 1986;14:125.
[b]Carbon monoxide and carbon dioxide may be produced by all but are listed only when they are deemed exceptional contributors to toxicity.

Table 66-61
Pyrolytic Products of Building Materials[a]

Material Burned	Toxic Pyrolytic Products
Acrilan	Acrolein, hydrogen cyanide
Acrylic	Acrolein
Melamine resins	Ammonia, hydrogen cyanide
Nitrocellulose products	Acetic acid, formic acid, oxides of nitrogen
Nylon	Ammonia, hydrogen cyanide
Petroleum products	Acetic acid, acrolein, carbon monoxide, formic acid, sulfur dioxide
Polyfluorocarbons (PTFE)	Octafluoroisobutylene
Polystyrene	Carbon monoxide, styrene
Polyurethane	Hydrogen cyanide, isocyanates
Polyvinyl chloride	Carbon monoxide, hydrogen chloride, phosgene
Wallpaper	Acetaldehyde, acetic acid, formaldehyde, oxides of nitrogen
Wood, cotton, paper	Acetaldehyde, acetic acid, acrolein, carbon monoxide, formaldehyde, formic acid

[a]Adapted from Wald PH, Belmes JR. J Intensive Care Med 1987;2:260–278.
PTFE, Polytetrafluoroethylene.

peak blood cyanide concentrations. In some patients several blood samples were obtained that confirmed a rapid elimination half-life (1.2 hours) of cyanide.

The clinician in the United States has oxygen and the Lilly Cyanide Antidote Kit (two 300-mg ampules of sodium nitrite for IV use; two 12.5-g ampules of sodium thiosulfate; and for inhalation, 12 ampules of amyl nitrite). The sodium nitrite component presents a danger of hypotension due to vasodilatation and a risk of diminished peripheral oxygen delivery after methemoglobin induction in a patient who may already have a high concentration of carboxyhemoglobin. A dose of 300 mg of sodium nitrite will result in a peak hemoglobin concentration of about 10% 35 to 70 minutes later. By then, after oxygen administration is given (normobaric or hyperbaric), the carboxyhemoglobin concentration in a victim of smoke inhalation will be somewhat decreased from its peak. Hyperbaric oxygen administration has been recommended as adjunctive treatment of smoke inhalation to treat carbon monoxide poisoning, cyanide poisoning, chemical pneumonitis caused by smoke, and thermal burns.[11]

REFERENCES—SMOKE INHALATION

1. Beritic T. The challenge of fire effluents. Poisonous gases are potential killers. Br Med J 1990;300:696–698.
2. Norris JC, Moore SJ, Haine AS. Synergistic lethality induced by the combination of carbon monoxide and cyanide. Toxicology 1994;40:121–129.
3. Birky MM, Paabo M, Brown JF. Correlation of autopsy data and materials involved in the Tennessee jail fire. Fire Safety J 1979;80;2:17–22.
4. Birky MM, Clarke FB. Inhalation of toxic products from fire. Bull NY Acad Med 1981;57:997–1013.
5. Hoffman RS, Sauter P. Methemoglobinemia resulting from smoke inhalation. Vet Hum Toxicol 1989;31:168–170.
6. Witten ML, Quan SF, Sobonya RE, Lemen RJ. New developments in the pathogenesis of smoke inhalation-induced pulmonary edema. West J Med 1988;148:33–36.
7. Jones JG, Lawler P, Crawley JCW et al. Increased alveolar epithelial permeability in cigarette smokers. Lancet 1000; 1:66–68.
8. Minty BD, Rayston D, Jones JG et al. Changes in permeability of the alveolar-capillary barrier in fire fighters. Br J Ind Med 1985;42:631–634.
9. Sammut P, Cunnigham J, Witten M et al. Pulmonary epithelial permeability to 99m Tc DTPA in cystic fibrosis patients compared with normal subjects. Am Rev Respir Dis 1987;235:A464.
10. Baud FJ, Barriot P, Toffis V, Riou B, Vicaut E, Lecarpentier Y et al. Elevated blood cyanide concentrations in victims of smoke inhalation. N Engl J Med 1991;325:1761–1766.
11. Hart GB, Strauss MB, Lennon PA, Whitcraft DD III. Treatment of smoke inhalation by hyperbaric oxygen. J Emerg Med 1985;3:211–215.
12. Kulig K. Cyanide antidotes in fire toxicology. N Engl J Med 1991;325:1801–1802.
13. Hall AH, Rumack BH. Hydroxocobalamin/sodium thiosulfate as a cyanide antidote. J Emerg Med 1987;5:115–121.

Chapter 67

Metals and Related Compounds

ORGANOMETALS

Organometals are compounds of heavy metals and hydrocarbons. The valence sites on the metal are occupied with the attached hydrocarbon moiety, and the organometals may be more lipid soluble than the metal; hence, the possible development of encephalopathies after tetraethyl lead, organotin, and organomercury compounds. The use of chelating agents to extract organometals from the body remains an unresolved issue.

ALUMINUM

ABSORPTION

Normal ingestion of aluminum in the diet is about 3 to 5 mg/day. About 15 μg is absorbed through the wall of the gastrointestinal tract. This amount is usually excreted by the kidneys. The total body burden is maintained at about 30 mg.[1] Normal ingestion of aluminum in the diet from food and drinking water is about 3 to 5 mg/day of which only about 15 μg is absorbed through the wall of the gastrointestinal tract.[2] Patients on antacid or phosphate binding therapy ingest up to 5 g/dL/day.[3] Such individuals are in positive balance to the extent of 200 to 300 mg/day. Estimates of aluminum absorbed from various sources and representative values of A1 content in IV solutions and oral substances are found in Tables 67–1, 67–2 and 67–3.[4,5]

Most of the tissue aluminum stores (about 30 to 50 mg) reside in bone.[6] The mean plasma half-life of aluminum after intravenous administration in dogs is approximately 4.5 hours.[7] Current data indicate that biliary excretion is the major route of excretion,[7] but renal elimination appears more important after large aluminum loads.[8]

Aluminum concentrations in foods are low, usually less than 5 mg/kg. Vegetables and salads may contain 5 to 10 mg/kg aluminum, dried spices and particularly tea leaves tens or even hundreds mg/kg (brewed tea beverage—1 to 5 mg/L). Daily aluminum intake with food is 2 to 36 mg/d. Boiling of water in aluminum pans causes a marked increase in aluminum intake. The use of automatic coffee machines may also lead to increased aluminum intake.[9]

Table 67–1
Estimate of Aluminum (Al) Absorbed from Various Sources

At Risk Group	Al Intake	Al Absorbed	Estimated Retention
Normal adults	3–5 mg/day		
70 kg		0.04–0.07 μg/kg per day	0%
Individual ingesting	3,600 mg/day		
30 ml Al-containing antacid			
70-kg adult		42 μg/kg per day	Documented only in renal insufficiency
10-kg child		360 μg/kg per day	
Newborn ingesting cow's milk formula	160–320 μg/day		
4-kg infant		0.08 μg/kg per day	Unknown
Infants receiving i.v. therapy	10–20 μg/day		
0.75-kg infant		15–30 μg/kg per day	78%

Adapted from Sedman AB et al. Pediatr Nephrol 1992;6:383–393.

Table 67–2
Representative Values of Al Content in IV Solutions[a,b]

	Al/μg per l
Potassium phosphate	16,598
Sodium phosphate	5,977
Calcium gluconate	5,056
25% Albumin	1,822
5% Dextrose	72
TPN—high calcium and phosphate	306
Ringer's lactate	35

TPN, Total parenteral nutrition
[a]Adapted from references 1 and 18
[b]Measurements will vary from batch to batch
Adapted from Sedman A. Pediatr Nephrol 1992;6:383–393.

Table 67–3
Representative Values of Al Content in Oral Substances

	Al
Amphogel	636 mg/30 ml
Alternagel	966 mg/30 ml
Maalox	360 mg/30 ml
Sucralfate	207 mg/1,000 mg tablet
Kaopectate	100 mg/100 ml
Seawater	0.001 mg/1,000 ml
Tap water (Colorado)	0.012 mg/1,000 ml
Breast milk (Colorado) (n = 12)	0.009 ± 0.006 mg/1,000 ml
Cow's milk based formula	0.266 mg/1,000 ml
Soy formula	1.4 mg/1,000 ml
Spinach	87 mg/100 g
Rhubarb boiled in Al foil	1.62 mg/100 g

Adapted from Sedman AB. Pediatr Nephrol 1992;6:383–393.

The kidney can excrete up to 0.5 mg/24 hours.[10,11] The total body burden is maintained at about 30 mg.[10] Insoluble aluminum compounds such as aluminum hydroxide mixture, which contain varying amounts of the hydroxide, oxide, carbonate, or bicarbonate, are slowly but incompletely converted to aluminum chloride in the stomach.[1,4,12–14]

Encephalopathy, osteomalacia, and microcytic anemia secondary to aluminum toxicity are more likely to occur in individuals who take aluminum-containing phosphate binders or are exposed to high levels of parenteral aluminum.

CLINICAL PRESENTATION

Dialysis Exposure

Aluminum toxicity may be characterized by hypercalcemia, a reversible microcytic anemia, vitamin D refractory osteodystrophy, and a progressive encephalopathy (mixed dysarthria-apraxia of speech, asterixis, tremulousness, myoclonus, dementia, focal seizures, fracturing osteomalacia in children, bone pain, proximal myopathy, decline in visual memory, attention, and concentration, and arthropathy). In a study of hemodialysis, patients with higher serum levels of aluminum appeared to exhibit a decline in visual memory, lower vocabulary scores, and a decrease in attention concentration and frontal lobe functions.[15,16] Symptoms usually develop insidiously over months to years in chronic renal failure patients unless dietary aluminum loads are excessive. Even in the absence of severe anemia or microcytosis, aluminum contributes to anemia in dialysis patients, at least in part by impairing iron utilization. Hematopoietic toxicity from aluminum correlates with bone surface staining for aluminum but not with other measures of aluminum overload. [17,18]

Dialysis Encephalopathy

Classical dialysis encephalopathy[19] (Table 67–4) initially presents with a mild speech disturbance characterized by stuttering or stammering speech that most frequently occurs immediately following dialysis. This is associated with subtle mental changes such as directional disorientation and personality changes. As the disease progresses, the speech disorder is intensified accompanied by twitching, myoclonus, motor apraxia, seizures, visual and auditory hallucinations, and paranoid and suicidal behavior. Ultimately, the patients became immobile, mute, and obtunded. Death can follow in 6 to 9 months after the onset of symptoms. Electroencephalogram alterations are characterized by multifocal bursts of slow (delta) and sp/L activity. CT scans are either normal or show mild cortical atrophy. If begun early enough, chelation therapy with deferoxamine appears to be effective in treating dialysis encephalopathy.[20] Criteria for the diagnosis of aluminum encephalopathy are presented in Table 67–4.[21] Risk factors for aluminum intoxication in dialysis patients are presented in Table 67–6.[12]

Occupational Exposure

Pulmonary fibrosis is reported in some workers heavily exposed to fine aluminum dust (the Swedish term is aluminosis) (Table 67–5). A severe encephalopathy with incoordination, intention tremor, and cognitive deficits has been reported in aluminum workers with pulmonary fibrosis.[22] Three aluminum smelter workers developed spinocerebellar degeneration without peripheral nerve involvement.[23] These three workers were exposed to long-term, low-dose aluminum levels in the same environment.

A further study of 25 symptomatic workers from the same plant showed that 88% reported a frequent loss of balance, and 84% reported a memory loss. A neurologic syndrome is observed among workers in the pot room of aluminum smelting plants, previously termed "pot room palsy." The syndrome is characterized by incoordination, poor memory, impairment in abstract reasoning, and depression.[24]

Canadian and Soviet workers documented skin telangiectases at an aluminum plant.[25] Excesses of lung cancer[26] and bladder cancer[27] have been reported in epidemiologic studies of aluminum workers.

Table 67–4
Diagnostic Criteria for Dialysis Encephalopathy

I	On maintenance hemodialysis for at least 18 months, or having undergone at least 150 hemodialysis sessions
II	Other causes of neurological syndrome excluded
III	Two or more of: Speech difficulty Seizures Myoclonus Motor dyspraxia More than five pathological fractures and/or positive aluminum staining of bone
IV	Three or more of the following (in addition to one criterion from category III): Change in mood Change in behavior Intellectual deterioration Episodic confusion related to dialysis Asterixis Serum aluminum level >50 mcg/l Diffuse EEG abnormality Blood transfusions on 10 or more occasions over a 12-month period

Adapted from Garrett PJ et al. Quart J Med 1988;68:775–783.

Aluminum Potroom Asthma

The electrolyte production of aluminum is accompanied by emission of dust and gases inducing reversible asthmalike symptoms (potroom asthma). There is no immunologic or bronchial challenge test to confirm the diagnosis.[28,29] In sensitive individuals, aluminum may exacerbate asthma.[30]

Alzheimer's Disease

The differentiation of Alzheimer's disease from aluminum encephalopathy is found in Table 67–5.

Alum Irrigations

Continuous bladder irrigation with potassium aluminum sulfate (alum) induces an increase in the serum aluminum levels that can lead to a fatal encephalopathy.[31–33] The development of lethargy, confusion, seizures, or metabolic acidosis in a patient receiving intravesical alum mandates cessation of treatment, supportive measures, and the selection of an alternative modality to control the hematuria.[34]

Aluminum in Infants and Children

Plasma aluminum levels may become elevated in infants with normal renal function who are consuming high doses of aluminum-containing antacids.[35] Infants at particular risk of aluminum intoxication are those born prematurely and those with impaired renal function. Larger amounts of aluminum are absorbed during the first month after birth.[36] Sources of aluminum in infant formulas should be identified and wherever possible the amount of aluminum in these products should be reduced.

Amyotrophic Lateral Sclerosis (ALS)

Preliminary studies of high incidence foci of ALS in the Western Pacific strongly implicate low concentration of

Table 67–5
Distinguishing Characteristics of Alzheimer's Disease and Aluminum Encephalopathy

Brain atrophy	Grossly apparent	Microscopically normal
Senile plaques	Present	Absent
Neurofibrillary transfer	Abnormal neurofibrils	Normal neurofibrils
Tan protein	Bind to neurofibril tangles	Do not bind to neurofibril tangles
Lesions, cerebellar	Localized to cortical, subcortical, and hippocampal areas	Widespread, involving brain stem, spinal cord
Acetylcholine, serotonin, norepinephrine levels	Reduced	Reduced
Somatostatin levels	Reduced	Not reduced
Serum albumin levels	Not elevated	Elevated
Anemia, osteomalacia	Absent	Present
Chelation effect	No	Yes

calcium and magnesium combined with high levels of aluminum and manganese in drinking water in the pathogenesis of ALS.[37]

Bone

Transiliac bone biopsy remains the "gold standard" for the diagnosis of aluminum-related bone disease (ARBD) in patients on regular hemodialysis, but it is an invasive and at times painful procedure. A low-dose deferoxamine test (0.5 g in 200 mL of 0.9% sodium chloride given intravenously during the first 2 hours of a regular hemodialysis treatment) is performed with aluminum estimations before (T1) and 48 hours (T2) after the DFO challenge. This test may be considered positive if the T2 concentration is 150 μg/L or three times the amount of T1. The DFO test may be impaired in patients with hyperparathyroid or mixed uremic bone disease.[38] There is some suggestion that patients who have had a parathyroidectomy may be particularly prone to ARBD.[39,40]

There are little data to correlate plasma and bone aluminum levels. This suggests that plasma aluminum levels do not necessarily reflect the status of total body aluminum.[41]

Radiograph Detection

Soft tissues have a density of 1.08 to 1.5 g/cc, bone has a density of 2.5 to 5.9 g/cc, and aluminum has a density of 2.7 g/cc. Aluminum is radiopaque. Foreign bodies as small as 0.5 mm × 0.5 mm × 1 mm can be clearly visualized when projected away from underlying bone. Aluminum foreign bodies that are embedded in larger body parts or that have been swallowed or aspirated may not be detected radiographically. Swallowed aluminum pull tabs are difficult to detect radiographically. The United States government proposal to mint aluminum pennies was abandoned because of the frequency of coin ingestion in children and the difficulty in radiographically detecting aluminum in the respiratory and gastrointestinal tracts.[42]

Serum Levels and Mortality

A study of 10,646 patients undergoing long-term hemodialysis suggests that mortality was 18% higher in patients with serum aluminum levels between 1520 and 2220 mmol/L and increased to 60% higher for patients with aluminum levels above 7410 mmol/L. These data suggest that patients undergoing long-term hemodialysis should have periodic surveillance of the serum aluminum level, and that, in those with plasma levels of 1570 to 2220 mmol/L or higher, use of aluminum salts to control serum phosphorous levels should be reconsidered.[43]

Table 67–6
Risk Factors for Aluminum Intoxication in Dialysis Patients

Duration of dialysis	"Unsafe" aluminum level in water supply
High absorber	Parathyroidectomy
Enteropathy	Diabetic patients on hemodialysis
HLA–Fe?	Transplanted patients who returned to dialysis because of rejection
Drugs	Children
Aluminum-containing phosphate binders	
Aluminum-contaminated IV solutions	

Adapted from Van de Vyver FL et al. Contr Nephrol 1987;55:198–220.

TREATMENT (TABLE 67–7)

Czapla and colleagues suggest that coadministration of an H_2-receptor antagonist such as ranitidine (300 mg/day) can reduce absorption from aluminum-containing phosphate binders, resulting in lower plasma aluminum concentrations after 1 month together with a decrease in urinary aluminum excretion and a decrease in desferrioxamine-induced plasma aluminum.[44]

Deferoxamine has been used to treat dialysis encephalopathy[45] and osteomalacia[46] with symptomatic relief reported.[47] The use of deferoxamine for aluminum-toxic dialysis patients has been suggested for serum levels of aluminum between 100 and 200 μg/mL.[48,49] Deferoxamine also has been used to diagnose aluminum-related osteodystrophy. After a deferoxamine infusion of 40 mg/kg over 2 hours, an increment in plasma aluminum concentration of 200 μg/L identified 35 of 37 patients with biopsy-proven aluminum-related osteodystrophy (sensitivity, 94%; specificity, 50%).[50] Deferoxamine treatment for dialysis patients is adapted according to serum aluminum levels (Fig. 67–1).[12] Calcium disodium ethylenediaminetetraacetic acid does not appear as effective as deferoxamine in chelating aluminum.[51] Especially in dialysis patients, aluminum-containing medications should be reduced.

Dialysis Facilities

The FDA has recently recommended that dialysis facilities should be aware of the following precautions:

Routinely evaluate the dialysate delivery system, including the dialysate concentrate transfer and storage devices. The compatibility of all the various components used in the preparation and delivery of dialysate to the patient should be evaluated to ensure that leaching of trace elements does not occur.[52] Routinely monitor all dialysis patients' blood to determine serum aluminum levels. When elevated serum

Table 67–7
DFO Treatment

1 g desferrioxamine (in 250 ml glucose) during the last 30 min of a hemodialysis session (in the venous line)
Serum aluminum measurement before the subsequent dialysis (±44 hours later)
Adaptation of the DFO dose
- Serum aluminum above 400 μg/l: decrease DFO dose
- Serum aluminum less than double the serum aluminum before DFO administration and less than 400 μg/l: increase DFO dose

Evaluation (not earlier than 6 months after the start of DFO therapy)
- Second DFO test
- Second bone biopsy

Adapted from Van de Vyver FL et al. Contr Nephrol 1987;55:198–220.

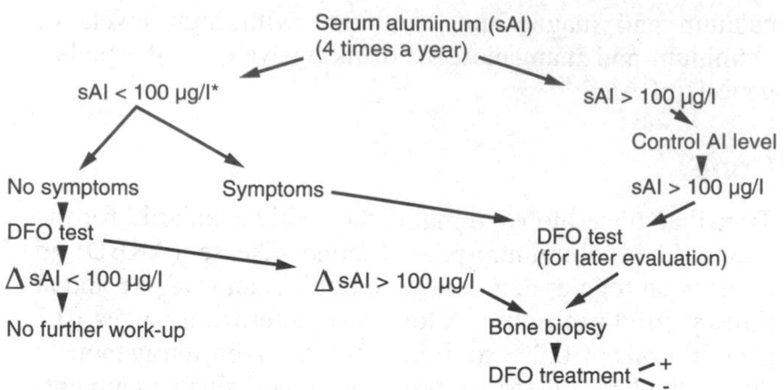

Figure 67–1 Tentative algorithm for the evaluation of the aluminum body burden and treatment. Serum A1 levels constantly below 30 µg/l without symptoms do not necessitate further workup. (Adapted from Van de Vyver FL et al. Contrib Nephrol 1987;55:198–220.)

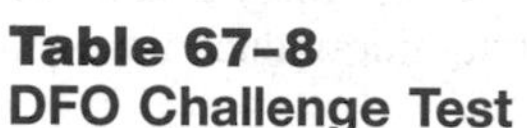

Table 67–8
DFO Challenge Test

1. Baseline serum aluminum measurement (Al_1)
2. 2 g DFO during the last 30 minutes of dialysis
3. Serum aluminum measurement (Al_2) before subsequent dialysis
4. Test is positive if $Al_2 - Al_1 > 100$ µg/L.

Table 67–9
Management of Aluminum Neurotoxicity

Acute intoxication
- Discontinue aluminum exposure
- Low-dose (1 g) DFO IM evening prior to dialysis
- Rapid removal of DFO-aluminum complex (high flux dialyzer or charcoal cartridge)
- Diazepam for seizures

Chronic intoxication
- Prolonged DFO treatment
- Treat until EEG normalized
- Relapse common after DFO stopped

Adapted from Coburn JW et al. Am J Kid Dis 1988;12:171–184.

aluminum levels are found, corrective actions such as avoiding aluminum-based phosphate binders and initiating chelation therapy should be taken. Elevated serum aluminum levels can cause anemia, bone irregularities, transient or permanent neurologic symptoms, and death.

Deferoxamine Challenge Test (Table 67–8)

Deferoxamine Toxicity

Side effects with deferoxamine mesylate may include posterior cataracts, hearing loss, audiovisual neurotoxicity, DFO-induced growth retardation, hypotension, anaphylactic reactions, and abdominal pain. Coadministration of isoniazid, a plasma MAO inhibitor, may ameliorate the side effects and permit continued DFO treatment.[53]

Anemia and Hemodialysis[54]

Hemoglobin levels, mean cell volume, and mean cell hemoglobin concentrations respond to a 3-month course of deferoxamine (30 mg/kg IV over the last 2 hours of dialysis, three times a week). Therapy with DFO significantly improved anemia in patients when sufficient levels of erythropoietin are present to stimulate erythropoiesis. Care must be taken to replete iron stores during therapy to avoid iron deficiency during treatment. Aluminum intoxication may cause resistance to erythropoietin by interference with heme synthesis with accumulation of protoporphyrin.

Aluminum Neurotoxicity

Table 67–9 summarizes management of aluminum neurotoxicity.[55]

Aluminum Bone Disease

Histologic features of aluminum bone disease may indicate an increase in bone aluminum (on foaming surface), a decrease in bone formation, and a decrease in cellularity of osteoblasts and osteoclasts.[12] If the increase in plasma aluminum is less than 150 µg/L, the probability of aluminum bone toxicity is low. If the increase in plasma aluminum exceeds 300 to 400 µg/L, the risk is substantial.[56]

REFERENCES—ALUMINUM

1. Winship KA. Toxicity of aluminum: a historical review. I. Adverse Drug React Toxicol Rev 1992;11:123–141.
2. Wilhelm M, Jager DE, Ohnesorge FK. Aluminum toxicokinetics. Pharmacol Toxicol 1990;66:4–9.
3. Nemery B. Metal toxicity and respiratory tract. Eur Respir J 1990;3:202–209.
4. Sedman A. Aluminum toxicity in childhood. Pediatr Nephrol 1992;6:383–393.
5. Committee on Nutrition. Finberg L, Dwech HS, Holmes F, Kretchmer N, Mauea AM, Reynolds JW et al. Aluminum toxicity in infants and children. Pediatrics 1986;78:1150–1153.
6. Henry PA, Goodman WO, Nudelman RK et al. Parenteral aluminum administration in the dog. I. Plasma kinetics, tissue levels, calcium metabolism and parathyroid hormones. Kidney Int 1984;25:362–369.
7. Williams JW, Santiago RV, Peters TG et al. Biliary excretion of aluminum in aluminum osteodystrophy with liver disease. Ann Intern Med 1986;104:782–785.
8. Lione A. Aluminum toxicology and the aluminum-containing medications. Pharmacol Ther 1986;29:255–285.
9. Liukkonen-Lija, Piepponen S. Leaching of aluminum from aluminum dishes and packages. Food Addit Contam 1992;9:213–223.
10. Fleming LW, Prescott A, Steward WK, Cargill RW. Bioavailability of aluminum. Lancet 1981;9:433.
11. Monteagudo FSE, Cassidy MJD, Fold PI. Recent developments in aluminum toxicology. Med Toxicol 1989;4:1–16.
12. Van de Vyver FL, Silva FJE, D'Haese PC, Verbucken AH, de Broe MI. Aluminum toxicity in dialysis patients. Contrib Nephrol 1987;55:198–220.
13. Federal Register 1990;55:No. 98:5/21; p. 20:799.

14. ASCN/Aspen Working Group on Standards for Aluminum Content of Parenteral Nutrition Solutions. Parenteral drug products containing aluminum as an ingredient or a contaminant: response to FDA. Notice of Intent. Am J Clin Nutr 1991;53:399–402.
15. Bolla KI, Briefel G, Spector D, Schwartz BS, Wieler L, Herron J et al. Neurocognitive effects of aluminum. Arch Neurol 1992;49:1021–1026.
16. Bartter T, Irwin RS, Abraham JL, Dascal A, Nash G, Himmelstein JS et al. Zirconium compound-induced pulmonary fibrosis. Arch Intern Med 1991;151:1197–1201.
17. Bia MJ, Cooper K, Schnell S, Daffy T, Henderl E, Malluche H, Solomon L. Aluminum induced anemia: pathogenesis and treatment in patients in chronic hemodialysis. Kidney Int 1989;36:852–853.
18. Rosenlof K, Fahrquist F, Tenhunen R. Erythropoietin, aluminum and anaemia in patients on haemodialysis. Lancet 1990; 335:247–249.
19. Alfrey AC, Mishell MM, Burks J, Contiguglia SR, Rudolph H, Lewin E et al. Syndrome of dyscrasia and multifocal seizures associated with chronic hemodialysis. Trans Am Soc Artif Intern Organs 1972;18:257–261.
20. Alfrey AC. Dialysis encephalopathy. Kidney Int 1986;29(Suppl 18):S53–S57.
21. Garrett RJ, Mulcahy D, Carmody M, O'Dwyer WS. Aluminum encephalopathy: clinical and immunological features. Q J Med 1988;69:775–783.
22. McLaughlin AIG, Kazantzis G, King E et al. Pulmonary fibrosis and encephalopathy associated with the inhalation of aluminum dust. Br J Ind Med 1962;16:123–125.
23. Longstretch WT, Rosenstock L, Heyer NJ. Potroom palsy? Neurologic disorder in three aluminum smelter workers. Arch Intern Med 1985;145:1972–1975.
24. White DM, Longstretch WT Jr, Rosenstock L, Claypoole KHJ, Brodkin CA, Townes BD. Neurologic syndrome in 25 workers from an aluminum smelting plant. Arch Intern Med 1992; 152:1443–1448.
25. Theriault G, Cordier S, Harvey R. Skin telangiectases in workers at an aluminum plant. N Engl J Med 1980;303:1278–1281.
26. Gibbs GW, Horowitz I. Lung cancer mortality in aluminum plant workers. J Occup Med 1979;21:347–353.
27. Theriault G, Tremblay C, Cordier S et al. Bladder cancer in the aluminum industry. Lancet 1984;1:947–950.
28. Kongerud J, Boe J, Soyseh V, et al. Aluminum potassium asthma: the Norwegian experience. Eur Respir J 1994; 7:165–172.
29. Desjardins A, Bergeron J-P, Ghezzo H, Cartier A, Malo J-C. Aluminum potassium asthma confirmed by monitoring of forced expiratory volume in one second. Am J Respir Crit Care Med 1994;150:1714–1717.
30. Musk AW, Greville HW, Tribe AE. Pulmonary disease from occupational exposure to an artificial aluminum silicate used for cat litter. Br J Ind Med 1980;37:367–372.
31. Seear MD, Dinmick JE, Rogers PC. Acute aluminum toxicity after continuous intravesical alum irrigation for hemorrhagic cystitis. Urology 1990;36:353–356.
32. Kavoussi LR, Gelstein GD, Andriole GL. Encephalopathy and an elevated serum aluminum level in a patient receiving intravesical alum irrigation for severe urinary hemorrhage. J Urol 1986;136:665–667.
33. Shoskes DA, Radzinski CA, Struthers NW, Honey RJ. Aluminum toxicity and death following intravesical alum irrigation in a patient with renal impairment. J Urol 1992;147:697–699.
34. Murphy CP, Cox RL, Harden EA, Stevens M, Heye M, Herzig RH. Encephalopathy and seizure induced by intravesical alum irrigations. Bone Marrow Transplant 1992;10:383–385.
35. Tsou WM, Young RM, Hart MH, Vanderhoof JA. Elevated plasma aluminum levels in normal infants receiving antacids containing aluminum. Pediatrics 1991;87:148–151.
36. Bishop N, McGraw M, Ward B. Aluminum in infant formulas. Lancet 1989;1:565.
37. Yasvi M, Yase Y, Oka K, Mukoyama M, Adachi K. High aluminum deposition in the central nervous system of patients with amyotrophic lateral sclerosis from Kae Kii peninsula, Japan. Two case reports. Neurotoxicology 1991;12:277–284.
38. Yaqoob M, Ahmad R, Roberts N, Helliwell T. Low-dose desferrioxamine test for the diagnosis of aluminum related bone disease in patients on regular hemodialysis. Nephrol Dial Transplant 1991;6:484–486.
39. Felsenthal AJ, Harrelson JM, Gutman RA, Wells SA, Drezner MK. Osteomalacia after parathyroidectomy in patients with uremia. Ann Intern Med 1982;97:34–39.
40. Pizzarelli F, Giordano R, Ballanti P, Costantin S, Mocetti P, Maggiore Q. Bone aluminum intoxication. An unpreventable sequel of parathyroidectomy? Nephron 1988;48:250–251.
41. Alfrey AC. Aluminum metabolism. Kidney Int 1986;29:(Suppl 18):S8–S11.
42. Ellio GL. Are aluminum foreign bodies detectable radiographically? Am J Emerg Med 1993;11:12–13.
43. Chazan JA, Lew NL, Lowrie EG. Increased serum aluminum. An independent risk factor for mortality in patients undergoing long-term hemodialysis. Arch Intern Med 1991; 151:319–320.
44. Czapla K, Rodger RSC, Halls DJ, Muralikrishna GS, MacDougall AI, Fell GS. Ranitidine reduced aluminum toxicity in patients with renal failure. Nephrol Dial Transplant 1992;7: 1246–1248.
45. Arze RS, Parkinson IS, Cartlidge NEF et al. Reversal of aluminum dialysis encephalopathy after desferrioxamine treatment. Lancet 1981;2:1116.
46. Brown DJ, Dawborn JK, Ham KN et al. Treatment of dialysis osteomalacia with desferrioxamine. Lancet 1982;2:343–345.
47. Freundlich M, Zilleruelo G, Faugere M-C et al. Treatment of aluminum toxicity in infantile uremia with deferoxamine. J Pediatr 1986;109:140–143.
48. Savory J, Berlin A, Courtoux C et al. Summary report of an international workshop on the role of biological monitoring of aluminum toxicity in man: Aluminum analysis in biological fluids. Ann Clin Lab Sci 1983;13:444–451.
49. Pogglitsch H, Knoff C, Wawschinek D et al. Aluminum intoxication in dialysis patients. Int J Artif Organs 1982;5:293–296.
50. Milliner DS, Nebeker HG, Ott SM et al. Use of deferoxamine infusion test in the diagnosis of aluminum related osteodystrophy. Ann Intern Med 1984;101:775–780.
51. Adhemar JP, Laederich J, Jaudon MC et al. Removal of aluminum from patients with dialysis encephalopathy. Lancet 1980;2:1311.
52. Dialysis patients face dangers from aluminum and other trace elements. FDA Med Bull 1992;22(2):8.
53. Kruch TPA, Fisher EA, McLachlan DRC. Suppression of deferoxamine mesylate treatment-induced side effect by coadministration of isoniazid in a patient with Alzheimer's disease subject to aluminum removal of ion-specific chelation. Clin Pharmacol Ther 1990;48:439–441.
54. Altman P, Plowman DH, Marsha F, Cunningham J. Aluminum chelation therapy in dialysis patients: evidence for inhibition of hemoglobin synthesis by low levels of aluminum. Lancet 1988;1:1012–1015.
55. Coburn JW, Norris KC, Sherrard DJ, Bia M, Llach F, Alfrey AC, Slatopolsky E. Toxic effects of aluminum in end stage renal disease. Discussion of a case. Am J Kidney Dis 1988;12:171–184.
56. Coburn JW, Norris KC, Sherrard DJ, Bia M, Llach F, Alfrey AC, Slatopolsky E. Toxic effects of aluminum in end stage renal disease. Discussion of a case. Am J Kidney Dis 1988;12:171–184.

ANTIMONY

Antimony is widely used in the production of alloys and is commonly found in ores associated with arsenic.[1,2] OSHA permissible exposure limits in air as a time-weighted average are 0.5 mg antimony/m^3.[1] The symptomatology in oral antimony intoxications derived from the medical literature and compared with patients who have ingested antimony potassium tartrate (tartar emetic) is found in Table 67–10.[2] Patients at risk from the adverse effects of antimony compounds include those treated with antileishmaniasis agents and workers occupationally exposed to dusts and fumes containing antimony.[3]

Table 67–10
Symptomatology in Oral Antimony Intoxications

System	Literature	Survivors	Nonsurvivors
Emesis	++++	++++	++++
Diarrhea	+++	++++	++++
Hematemesis	++	—	++++
Abdominal pain	+++	++	—
Cough	+	++	—
Hypoxia	—	++	++++
Liver failure	++	—	++++
Oliguria	—	+	++
Asthenia	++	++	—
EEG disturbances	—	+	+
Dermatitis	++	—	—
Thrombophlebitis	—	+++	+
Electrolyte disturbances	+++	++	+++

Adapted from Lauwers LF et al. Crit Care Med 1990;18:324–325.

Trivalent antimony compounds were used for the treatment of trypanosomiasis and leishmaniasis between 1908 and the 1920s. Because of their toxicity the trivalent antimony compounds were superseded by the less toxic pentavalent compounds in the 1920s. For the past 50 years the pentavalent antimonials, sodium stibogluconate (SSG) available as Pentostam and meglumine antimoniate (MA) available as Glucantime, have been the main drugs used for the management of visceral, cutaneous, and mucocutaneous leishmaniasis.[4] SSG is available in the United States from the Centers for Disease Control (CDC) under an investigational new drug protocol. CDC recommends a dose of 20 mg/kg/day with no upper limit on the daily dose.[5]

TOXICOKINETICS[6]

Absorption

In humans antimony compounds are only poorly absorbed from the gastrointestinal tract.

Distribution

Trivalent antimony compounds rapidly leave the plasma, but remain in the circulation bound to erythrocytes. They react with the red cell membrane and interfere with hemoglobin function. Pentavalent antimony is largely recovered from the plasma. Mean normal serum values for antimony are 0.05 to 0.5 μg per 100 mL.

Excretion

About 10% of the trivalent form is excreted by the kidney in 24 hours; 50 to 60% of the pentavalent form is found in the urine within 24 hours.

CLINICAL PRESENTATION (TABLE 67–10)

Stibine gas (SbH_3) exposure produces a clinical picture similar to that of arsine gas (AsH_3) exposure. Stibine gas appears when Sb alloys are treated with acids. Clinical features include hemolytic anemia, myoglobinuria, renal failure, weakness, profuse vomiting, nausea, headache, abdominal and low back pain, and hematuria.[7] Vomiting is usually prominent. Antimony levels may be determined by atomic absorption spectrophotometry.

Reversible side effects that are commonly associated with pentavalent antimonial therapy but seldom require discontinuing therapy include arthralgias, myalgias, increases in hepatocellular enzymes, and flattening or inversion of T-waves on electrocardiogram.[4] Occasional deaths that may have been due to cardiotoxicity have been reported, but they occurred in association with either high daily doses (30 to 60 mg/kg/day) or with underlying cardiac disease. Prolongation of the corrected QT interval (to >0.50s) and development of concave ST segments are considered to be ominous signs. A prospective study has shown an excess of lung cancer in exposed workers with a carcinogenic latency of 20 years.[8]

TREATMENT

Chelation with British Anti-Lewisite (BAL) for serious antimony exposures should be employed, as in arsenic intoxication. Dimercaptosuccinic acid (DMSA) and dimercaptopropane sulfonic acid (DMPS) have been proposed for the treatment of antimony intoxicants.[9] There is no evidence that BAL is useful for stibine gas exposure.[10] Dialyze as needed. The role of exchange transfusion is not clear. Be sure to monitor for dysrhythmias.

Treatment of an acute oral antimony intoxication includes gastric lavage, which, due to the slow absorption rate of antimony, can be used even several hours after ingestion. Repeated charcoal installations (1 g/kg body weight) may be useful. Fluid, electrolyte, and blood losses must be replaced. Chelation therapy (BAL, DMPS, DMSA) has been recommended.[2]

REFERENCES—ANTIMONY

1. Toxicological Profile for Antimony. Agency for Toxic Substances and Disease Registry. TP-91/02, September, 1992.
2. Lauwers LF, Roelants A, Rosseel PM, Heyndrickx B, Baute L. Oral antimony intoxications in man. Crit Care Med 1990;18:324–325.
3. de Wolff FA. Antimony and health incriminating stibine in the sudden infant death syndrome is difficult in current evidence. Br Med J 1995;310:1216–1217.
4. Berman JD. Chemotherapy for leishmaniasis: biochemical mechanisms, clinical efficacy and future strategies. Rev Infect Dis 1988;10:560–586.
5. Herwaldt BL, Berman JD. Recommendations for treating leishmaniasis with sodium stibogluconate (Pentostam) and review of pertinent clinical studies. Am J Trop Med Hyg 1992;46:296–306.
6. Winship KA. Toxicity of antimony and its compounds. Adverse Drug React Acute Pois Rev 1987;2:67–90.
7. Robbins A. Stibine, NIOSH Current Intelligence Bulletin 32. Vet Hum Toxicol 1980;22:108–109.
8. Jones PD. Survey of antimony workers: mortality 1961–1992. Occup Environ Med 1994;51:772–776.
9. Aaseth J. Recent advances in therapy of metal poisoning with chelating agents. Hum Toxicol 1983;2:257–272.
10. Teisinger J. BAL. In: Occupational Health and Safety. Vol. 1. Geneva: International Labour Office/New York: McGraw-Hill, 1976, p. 154.

ARSENIC

The treatment of inorganic and organic arsenic compounds is presented in Table 67–11.[1]

Table 67–11
Inorganic and Organic Arsenic Compounds Relevant to Human Health: Environmental Occurrence or Industrial Use

Chemical Name	Chemical Abstract Reg Serial No	Synonyms and Formula	Valence ( ), Physical Properties	Industrial Use or Biologioal Occurrence
Arsine	7784-42-1	**Arsine.** Arsenic trihydride, hydrogen arsenide AsH_3	(–3), colorless neutral gas, slightly w.s.	organic synthesis, solid state electronic components, by product of metal smelting
Arsenic (elemental)	7440-38-2	Grey arsenic, metallic arsenic, As	(0), gray shiny, brittle metallic-looking rhombohedra w.i.	alloys in order to increase the hardness and heat resistance
Arsenic trichloride	7784-34-1	Butter of arsenic, $AsCl_3$	(+3), a yellowish oily liquid, w.s., decomposes	pottery industry, manufacturing of chlorine-containing arsenicals
Arsenic trioxide	1327-53-3	**Arsenic Oxide, As_2O_3.** White arsenic, arsenic sesquioxide, arsenious anhydride As_2O_3	(+3), white amorphous or crystalline powder. Heated sublimes. Slowly w.s. Combines with water to form arsenious acid	manufacture of glass, insecticide, rodenticide
Sodium arsenite	7784-46-5	**Arsenious acid, sodium salt.** Arsenious acid sodium, meta-arsenite, $NaAsO_2$	(+3), white or grayish hygroscopic powder, very w.s.	veterinary use, insecticide, wood preservative. Used also in combination with other salts such as calcium-arsenite, lead arsenite, cupric acetoarsenite
Arsenic pentoxide	1303-28-2	**Arsenic oxide As_2O_5.** Arsenic acid, arsenic anhydride, As_2O_5	(+5), white amorphous deliquescent powder. Freely w.s. Combines with water to arsenic acid	manufacture of colored glass, insecticide, wood preservative
Lead arsenate	7784-40-9	**Arsenic acid, H_3AsO_4, lead (+2) salt, (1.1).** Acid lead arsenate, arsenate of lead approx. $PbHAsO_4$	(+5), heavy white powder, w.i. On heating emits toxic fumes	constituent of various insecticides also with other salts; calcium arsenate, sodium arsenate, potassium arsenate
Methylarsonic acid	2163-80-6	**Arsenic acid, methyl-mono-sodium salt.** Methanearsonic acid, monosodium salt, sodium methylarsonate, sodium methanearsonate $CH_3AsO(OH)ONa$	white powder, w.s.	constituent of various pesticides also as mixture with methylarsonic acid disodium salt. Excretion product of mammalian metabolism
Dimethylarsinic acid sodium salt	124-65-2	**Arsenic acid, dimethylsodium salt.** Cacodilic acid sodium salt, sodium cacodilate, sodium dimethylarsinate, arsine oxide, hydroxymethylsodium salt, $(CH_3)_2AsO(ONa)$	colorless crystals hygroscopic, w.s., slightly soluble in ethanol	constituent of various pesticides. Excretion product of mammalian metabolism
Trimethylarsine	593-88-4	Gosio gas, $As(CH_3)_3$	colorless neutral gas, slightly w.s., decomposes	produced after metabolic transformation of As compounds by bacteria and fungi especially in sewage
Arsanilic acid	98-50-0	4-aminobenzenearsonic acid, aminophenylarsine $NH_2C_6H_4–AsO(OH)_2$	white crystalline powder, w.s.	stimulator of growth of food-producing animals
Arsenobetaine		$(CH_3)_3As + CH_2COOH$	w.s.	organic arsenical compound in marine organisms
Arsenocholine		$(CH_3)_3As + CH_2CH_2OH$	w.s.	organic arsenical compound in marine organisms

Legenda: Chemical Abstracts services names are heavy typed.
w.s. = water soluble.
w.i. = water insoluble.

Epidemiologic studies of arsenic in drinking water suggest that arsenic can cause skin, liver, lung, kidney, and bladder cancer. Table 67–12 provides an estimate of risks of dying from cancer after arsenic exposure compared with environmental tobacco smoke and radon in homes.[2] Clinical findings in acute and chronic arsenic poisoning are summarized in Table 67–13.

TOXIC DOSAGE

The pentavalent form As^{5+} (arsenate or organic form) is less toxic than the trivalent form As^{3+} (arsenite or inorganic form) based on lower solubility. In general, the insoluble salts of arsenic (arsenic trioxide, lead arsenate) and organic alkane arsonates possess substantially fewer toxic properties than the soluble inorganic arsenic compounds (sodium arsenite, arsenic acid, arsenious acid).[3,4] The most toxic form is arsine gas (AsH_3). A wide range of toxicity occurs depending on the compound and form involved. Less than 1 mg/kg can cause serious illness in children; 2 mg/kg can cause death. The lethal range is 120 to 200 mg, although survival occurs at higher levels in adults. The ingestion of 9 to 14 mg of arsenic trioxide by a 16-month-old infant produced significant signs of poisoning, which required chelation therapy.[5]

Kingstrom and colleagues have observed that single, low-dose (less than 5 mL) pentavalent arsenate ingestions (less than 3%) of sodium arsenate–containing ant killers is associated with little toxicity and can be managed at home. The need for chelation following exposure to pentavalent compounds requires further study.[6] Even in cases of "trivial" exposure by careful history, patients exposed to sodium arsenate in an ant killer may present with significantly elevated levels of arsenic in 24-hour urine collections (range 3500 to 5300 µg/L, normal <50 µg/24 hours). The appearance of a "trivial" exposure in an asymptomatic child may represent a significant medical risk of arsenic poisoning.[7]

Arsine gas, a hazard from leaking cylinders and semiconductor factories, is a colorless, nonirritating gas that has poor olfactory warning properties and evolves from arsenic compounds on addition of an acid.[8] The TLV-TWA is 0.05 ppm. Immediate death occurs at 150 ppm. Fatalities with extensive hemolysis result in 30 minutes from exposure to 25 to 50 ppm, and in less than 30 minutes at 100 ppm.

Table 67–12
Estimated Lifetime Risks of Dying From Cancer Due to Exposure to Different Environmental Carcinogens in the United States

Carcinogen	Risk
Environmental tobacco smoke (passive smoking)	
Low exposure (not married to a smoker)	4/1000
High exposure (married to a smoker)	10/1000
Radon in homes	
Average exposure	3/1000
High exposure (1–3% of homes)	20/1000
Arsenic in drinking water (1.6 L/day)	
2.5 µg/L (U.S. estimated average)	1/1000
50 µg/L (U.S. water standard)	21/1000

Adapted from Smith AH et al. Envir Health Persp 1992;97:259–267.

TOXICOKINETICS

The half-life of inorganic arsenic in blood is about 2 hours; the half-life of the methylated metabolites range from 5 to 20 hours.

Absorption

Pentavalent arsenic is well absorbed through the gut, but the trivalent form is more lipid soluble. Toxicity results from the arsenite form (As^{3+}), especially by dermal absorption. Inhalation can result in symptomatic chronic exposure, particularly with arsine gas, which causes severe symptoms by inhalation. Arsenic compounds are well absorbed parenterally within 24 hours.

Distribution

Arsenic initially localizes in the blood bound to globulin. Redistribution occurs within 24 hours to the liver, lungs,

Table 67–13
Clinicopathologic Findings in Acute and Chronic Arsenic Poisoning

System	Acute	Chronic
Skin	Hair: delayed loss; nails: Mees's lines (2–3 weeks postingestion)	Melanosis, Bowen's disease, facial edema, hyperkeratosis, cutaneous cancers, hyperpigmentation
Neurologic	Hyperpyrexia, convulsions, tremor, coma	Encephalopathy, polyneuropathy, tremor, axonal degeneration
Gastrointestinal tract	Abdominal pain, dysphagia, vomiting, bloody or rice-water diarrhea, mucosal erosions	Nausea, vomiting, diarrhea; anorexia, weight loss
Liver	Fatty infiltration	Hepatomegaly, jaundice, cirrhosis
Kidney	Tubular and glomerular damage—oliguria, uremia	Nephritic findings
Hematologic		Bone marrow hypoplasia: anemia, leukopenia, thrombocytopenia; impaired folate metabolism; basophilic stippling and karyorrhexis
Cardiac	ST-T wave abnormalities, prolonged QT interval, ventricular fibrillation, atypical ventricular tachycardia	—

Adapted from Gorby MS. West J Med 1988;149:308–315.

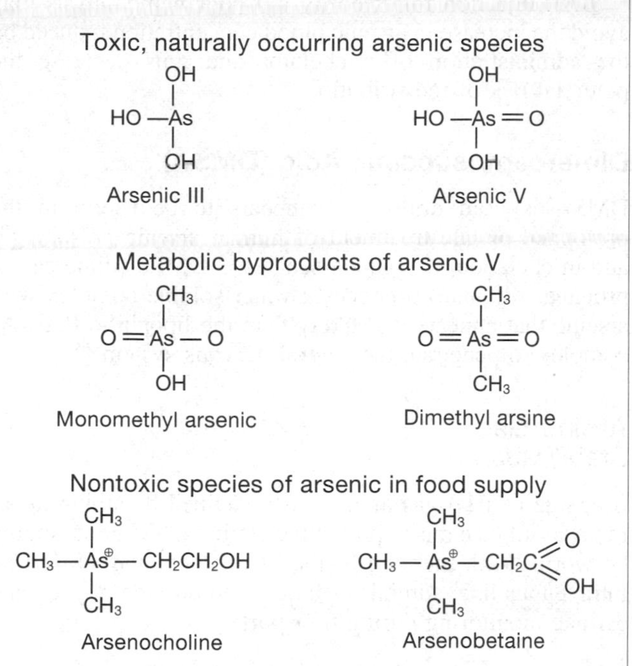

Figure 67–2 Chemical structures of common forms of arsenic found in biologic tissues. (Adapted from Moyer TP. Mayo Clin Proc 1993;68:1210–1211.)

intestinal wall, and spleen, where arsenic binds to the sulfhydryl groups of tissue proteins. Only small amounts of arsenic penetrate the blood–brain barrier. Arsenic replaces phosphorus in the bone where it may remain for years. Within 30 hours postingestion, arsenic deposits in the hair. Arsenic levels in hair sections may provide an indication of the time of exposure based on length from growth site. The hair of an individual who died 6 to 8 hours after ingestion of an arsenic overdose generally does not contain arsenic.

Organic Arsenic Sources

The two most commonly found organic, nontoxic variants of arsenic found in food regularly consumed by humans are arsenobetaine and arsenocholine. Considerable concentrations of organic acid are found in shellfish, cod, and haddock. After arsenobetaine and arsenocholine are ingested, they are rapidly cleared in the urine where they are completely excreted within 1 to 2 days (Fig. 67–2). No residual toxic metabolites are present. The half-life of organic arsenic is 4 to 6 hours.

Pregnancy

Inorganic arsenic crosses the placenta. A 22-year-old female at 20 weeks of gestation ingested 340 mg of sodium arsenate. The initial 24-hour urinary arsenic level was 3030 μg/L. Dimercaprol was administered. Fetal heart tones were normal. A healthy infant was delivered at 36 weeks. At birth 24-hour urinary arsenic levels were <50 μg/L in the infant and <100 μg/L in the mother. Another case of maternal arsenic ingestion at 30-week gestation resulted in infant death shortly after birth. Dimercaprol appears to be the agent of choice. D-penicillamine has been associated with teratogenicity.[9]

Gastrointestinal Tract

Dilation of splanchnic vessels causes submucosal vesicle formation. Rupture of these vesicles leads to rice-water stools and bleeding. Subsequently, a protein-losing enteropathy may develop.

Despite aggressive management of arsenic intoxication and a rapid decrease in blood and urine arsenic levels, neurologic defects may persist. It appears that distribution into neural tissue is rapid and may be irreversible even with chelation.[10,11]

Muscle

Fatal rhabdomyolysis dysfunction has been reported after an acute arsenic overdose.[12,13]

Metabolic/Hepatic

Negative nitrogen balance, hepatic fatty degeneration, central necrosis and cirrhosis, antagonism of thyroid hormone.

Skin Appendages

Alopecia (late), brittle fingernails, Mees's lines (horizontal white lines that appear after exposed nail bed area grows to exterior).

CLINICAL PRESENTATION (TABLE 67–13)[14]

Acute Arsine Gas Exposure

The classic presentation of arsine exposure involves a latent period up to 24 hours, followed by the onset of abdominal pain, hemolysis, and renal failure.[15,16] Sudden death resulting from overwhelming arsenic exposure may occur in the absence of pulmonary edema and hemolysis.

Blackfoot Disease

Blackfoot disease is a unique peripheral artery disease in an endemic area of chronic arsenicism on the southwest coast of Taiwan. Humic acid in well water may be the main cause of the disease.[17–19] Platelet activation and hypercoagulability may play a role in causing this disease.[20]

Lead Arsenate

Ingestion of lead arsenate may lead to nausea, vomiting, and abdominal pain. The vomitus may be milky due to lead chloride. There is a metallic taste in the mouth. Diarrhea or constipation may occur. The stools may be black due to lead sulfide. Paresthesias and muscle weakness may occur. Acute hemolytic crisis, oliguria, and shock occurs in severe cases. If the patient survives, the syndrome of chronic lead poisoning will develop. Treatment involves gastric lavage, followed by chelation therapy with both dimercaprol and calcium EDTA.[21]

LABORATORY

Analytic Methods

The current standard for arsenic analysis is atomic absorption spectroscopy, which measures total arsenic, does not distinguish between pentavalent, trivalent, or organic arsine.[6]

Blood Levels

The short half-life of arsenic in the blood means that blood arsenic levels are less useful than urine levels unless exposure occurred on the same day. Serum (or blood) arsenic levels are detectable only during the first 2 to 4 hours after ingestion, after which arsenic in any form is not readily detected in blood or serum.

Urine Levels

Inorganic AS^{+3} and AS^{+5}

AS^{+3} is more toxic than AS^{+5}. AS^{+3} and AS^{+5} are detected in the body shortly after ingestion. Monomethylarsine and dimethylarsine predominate more than 24 hours after ingestion. Urinary AS^{+3} and AS^{+5} levels present about 10 hours and return to normal in 20 hours. Urinary monomethylarsine and dimethylarsine levels peak at 40 to 60 hours and return to baseline in 6 to 20 days after ingestion. The half-life of inorganic arsenic in blood is 2 hours and that of the methylated metabolites 5 to 20 hours. Serum (or blood) arsenic levels are only detectable during the first 2 to 4 hours after ingestion.

Organic As (Fig. 67–2)[22]

Arsenobetaine and arsenochlorine have a half-life of about 4 hours and are completely excreted in 1 to 2 days.

Urine: No exposure—less than 25 µg/daily.
Toxic levels—50 to 50,000 µg daily.
After seafood—50 to 2,000 µg daily.

Hair Levels

Hair analysis for arsenic is a semireliable method for confirming chronic toxicity. It does not discriminate between externally deposited arsenic and arsenic found within the hair shaft.

Fingernails

Fingernail arsenic may provide an estimate of the air arsenic exposure for a worker.

TREATMENT

Mathieu and colleagues believe that hemodialysis can be considered in arsenic poisoning when the ingested dose is massive and signs of visceral involvement are present: hypotension in spite of fluid therapy, mental confusion or coma, oliguria, increased transferase, or lactic acidosis. BAL should be administered in combination with hemodialysis to avoid the possible deleterious effects of arsenic redistribution.[23]

BAL injection followed by a 4-hour hemodialysis may avoid the increase in arsenic blood concentration induced by the administration of a chelator and thus decrease the potential risk of redistribution.

Dimercaptosuccinic Acid (DMSA)

DMSA is used orally and appears to be useful in the prolonged or late treatment of human arsenic poisoning[24] and in chelation of organoarsenates.[25] DMPS (dimercaptopropane sulfonate) produces a water-soluble complex with arsenic that appears less likely than the lipophilic BAL-As complex to penetrate the central nervous system.[26]

Arsine Gas

Stabilization

In arsine (AsH_3) gas areas, self-contained breathing apparatus, a full face mask, protective clothing, and boots should be worn. Wash the skin of the victim copiously. Insert an intravenous line, administer fluids, and provide oxygen and cardiac monitoring during transport.

Supportive Care

Management in the Hospital[27]:

1. Evaluate and support ABCs (airway, breathing and circulation).
2. Provide O_2 by mask.
3. Monitor cardiac rhythm; obtain 12-lead EKG.
4. Laboratory Tests: Perform urine dipstick for occult blood and hemoglobin. Obtain a complete blood count, plasma free hemoglobin (PFHgb), urine hemoglobin, electrolytes, BUN and/or creatinine, bilirubin, blood type and screen, and other laboratory tests as appropriate. Urinary arsenic levels may be elevated for a few weeks after exposure.
5. If there is evidence of acute hemolysis, alkalinize the urine with sodium bicarbonate, 50 to 100 mEq in or added to 1 (one) liter of 5% dextrose administered IV at a rate to maintain urine output at 2 to 3 cc/kg/hr. Consider furosemide or mannitol. Follow electrolytes. Follow BUN, creatinine, and fluid status closely because renal failure may result in acute fluid overload.
6. If PFHgb exceed 1.5 g/dL, there has been a significant rapid drop in hematocrit (e.g., from 40 to 30 without other explanation), or there are other indications of intravascular hemolysis (severe abdominal pain, jaundice, shock), consider exchange transfusion after consultation with a medical toxicologist. Prepare for dialysis in the event of renal failure. Shock may occur and should be treated appropriately.

NOTE: BAL and other chelating agents are not effective for arsine exposure. Arsine does not produce the classical symptoms of arsenic poisoning.

REFERENCES—ARSENIC

1. Foa V, Colombi A, Maroni M, Buratti M. Arsenic. Biological Indicators for Assessment of Human Exposure to Indus-

trial Chemicals. Commission of the European Committee EUR 11135. 1987; pp. 25–46.
2. Smith PH, Hopenhayn-Rich C, Bates MN, Goeden HM, Hertz-Piccioto I, Duggan JM, Wood R et al. Cancer risks for arsenic in drinking water. Environ Health Perspect 1992; 97:256–267.
3. Done AK, Peart AJ. Acute toxicities of arsenical herbicides. Clin Toxicol 1971;1:343–355.
4. Boyd SD, Wasserman GS, Green VA et al. Lead arsenate ingestion in eight children. Clin Toxicol 1981;18:489–491.
5. Watson WA, Veltri JC, Metcalf TJ. Acute arsenic exposure treated with oral D-penicillamine. Vet Hum Toxicol 1981;23: 164–166.
6. Kingstrom RL, Hall S, Sioris L. Clinical observations and medical outcome in 149 cases of arsenate ant killer ingestion. Clin Toxicol 1993;31:581–591.
7. Scalzo AJ, Thompson MW, Peters DW. Asymptomatic presentation of pediatric arsenic ingestion from sodium arsenate ant killer. Vet Hum Toxicol 1989;31:340.
8. Parish GG, Glass R, Kimbrough R. Acute arsine poisoning in two workers cleaning a clogged drain. Arch Environ Health 1979;34:224–227.
9. Daya MR, Irwin R, Parshley MC, Handuy J, Burton BT. Arsenic ingestion in pregnancy. Vet Hum Toxicol 1989; 31:347.
10. Marcus SM. Survival after massive arsenic trioxide ingestion. Vet Hum Toxicol 1987;29:481.
11. Di Napoli J, Hall AH, Drake R, Rumack BH. Cyanide and arsenic poisoning by intravenous (IV) injection. Vet Hum Toxicol 1988;30:360.
12. Fernandez-Sola J, Nogue S, Grau JM, Casademont J, Munne P. Acute arsenic myopathy: morphological description. Clin Toxicol 1991;29:131–136.
13. Sanz P, Corbella J, Nogue S, Munne P, Rodriguez-Pazos M. Rhabdomyolysis in fatal arsenic trioxide poisoning. JAMA 1989;212:3271.
14. Gorby MS. Arsenic poisoning. West J Med 1988;149:308–315.
15. Pinto SS. Arsine poisoning: evaluation of the acute phase. J Occup Med 1976;18:633–635.
16. Kleinfeld MJ. Arsine poisoning. J Occup Med 1980;22:820–821.
17. Chen C-J. Blackfoot disease. Lancet 1990;2:442.
18. Lu FJ. Blackfoot disease: arsenic or humic acid? Lancet 1990;336:115–116.
19. Lu FJ, Shih SR, Liu TM, Shown SH. The effect of fluorescent humic substances existing in the well water of Blackfoot Disease in endemic areas in Taiwan on prothrombin time and activated partial thromboplastin time in vitro. Thromb Res 1990;57:747–752.
20. Shen M-C, Tsong W-P, Chen C-S. Increased circulating platelet aggregation and coagulation factors in patients with Blackfoot Disease. J Formosa Med Assoc 1983;82:816–821.
21. Tallis GA. Acute lead arsenate poisoning. Aust NZ J Med 1989;19:730–732.
22. Moyer TP. Testing from arsenic. Mayo Clin Proc 1993;68: 1210–1211.
23. Mathieu D, Mathieu-Nolf M, Germain-Alonso M, Neviere R, Furon D, Wattel F. Massive arsenic poisoning—effect of hemodialysis and dimercaprol or arsenic kinetics. Intensive Care Med 1992;18:47–50.
24. Kosnett MJ, Becker CE. Dimercaptosuccinic acid: utility in acute and chronic arsenic poisoning. Vet Hum Toxicol 1988; 30:369.
25. Shum S, Whitshead J, Vaughan L, Shum S, Hale T. Chelation of organoarsenate with dimercapton succinic acid. Vet Hum Toxicol 1995;37:239–242.
26. Moore DF, O'Callaghan CA, Berlyne G et al. Acute arsenic poisoning: absence of polyneuropathy and after treatment with 2,3-dimercaptopropanesulfonate (DMPS). J Neurol Neurosurg Psychiatry 1994;57:1133.
27. Hazardous Materials Medical Management Protocols. (California Emergency Medical Services Authority and Toxics Epidemiology Program, Los Angeles County Department of Health Services. March 26, 1989; p. 22.

BARIUM

Barium poisoning results in a rapid onset of gastrointestinal symptoms, paralysis, cardiac dysrhythmias, hypertension, and often severe hypokalemia. The acute syndrome can be fatal.[1]

Table 67–14
Toxicity of Barium Compounds to Humans[a]

Compound	Exposure Data	Effect
Barium carbonate	lowest lethal dose = 57 mg/kg	death
Barium carbonate	lowest toxic dose = 29 mg/kg	flaccid paralysis without anesthesia; paresthesia; muscle weakness
Barium chloride	lowest lethal dose = 11.4 mg/kg	death
Barium polysulfide	lowest toxic dose = 226 mg/kg	flaccid paralysis without anesthesia; muscle weakness; dyspnea

[a]Source; RTECS (1985).

Table 67–15
Drug Induced Hypokalemia

1. Barium salt poisoning
2. Theophylline overdose
3. Strychnine poisoning
4. Steroid use
5. Vitamin B 12 therapy
6. Toluene exposure, chronic
7. Salbutamol poisoning
8. Terbutaline administration

Adapted from Deng JF et al. Vet Hum Toxicol 1991;33:173–175.

Table 67–16
Clinical Toxicity of Barium Poisoning

Gastrointestinal
Salivation
Nausea, vomiting
Severe abdominal pain
Watery diarrhea
Increased peristalsis

Nervous System
Mydriasis
Anxiety
Circumoral and peripheral paresthesias
Diminished deep tendon reflexes
Headache
Confusion
Seizure

Respiratory
Respiratory failure
Pulmonary edema

Cardiac
Increased automaticity
Hypertension
Premature ventricular contractions
QT prolongation
Ventricular tachycardia
Ventricular fibrillation
Asystole

Muscle
Myoclonus
Myalgias
Rigidity
Cramps
Dysarthria
Flaccid paralysis

Adapted from Johnson CH et al. Ann Emerg Med 1991;20:1138–1142.

Table 67–17
Differential Diagnosis of Barium Poisoning

Condition	Hypertension	Hypokalemia	Numbness and/or Paresthesias	Weakness or Paralysis	Respiratory Paralysis	Cranial Nerve Involvement	Cardiac Dysrhythmia	Nausea, Vomiting, and Diarrhea
Barium poisoning	++	++	++	+	+	–	+	+++
Ciguatera fish poisoning	–	–	++	–	+	+	+¶	+++
Paralytic shellfish poisoning	–	–	++	++	+	–	–	++
Neurotoxic shellfish poisoning	–	–	++	–	–	–	–	++
Botulism	–	–	–	++	+	++	–	++††
Diphtheria	–	–	+	+§	+	+	+**	++‡‡
Familial hypokalemic periodic paralysis	–	+++†	–	+++	+	+	+	–
Thyrotoxic periodic paralysis	–	+++†	–	+++	+	+	+	–
Guillain-Barré syndrome	+*	–	++	+++	+	+	+	–
Gastroenteritis	–	+‡	–	+	+	–	+¶	+++

–, Absent or usually absent; +, occasionally present; ++, usually present; +++, always or almost always present
*Autonomic disturbances may cause hypertension, hypotension, and/or hyperthermia
†Potassium is usually normal or low-normal between episodes of paralysis
‡Other causes of hypokalemia, such as villous adenoma, diuretic use, licorice ingestion (glycyrrhiza extract), mineralocorticoid or glucocorticoid excess, renal tubular acidosis, hypomagnesemia, and alkalosis should also be considered.
§Paralysis occurs in up to 75% of severe cases, usually weeks after the acute syndrome is recognized
¶Correlates with degree of hypokalemia
*Sinus bradycardia
**Cardiac dysrhythmias occur in the setting of myocarditis
††Nausea and vomiting with abdominal pain and constipation are characteristic of food-borne botulism
‡‡This feature is seen mostly in children
Adapted from Johnson CH, Van Tassell VJ, Ann Emerg Med 1991;1138–1142.

DOSAGE

Oral ingestion of 0.8 to 1.5 g of absorbable barium chloride or barium carbonate (used for glazing pottery) may lead to hypokalemic paralysis and death.[2] A summary of lethal and toxic doses of barium salts is seen in Table 67–14.[3]

PATHOPHYSIOLOGY

Barium initially stimulates striated, cardiac, and smooth muscle and depresses serum potassium, which is forced intracellularly.[4] Subsequent muscle weakness may result from a direct depolarizing effect and neuromuscular blockade.[5] Some toxic causes of drug-induced hypokalemia are summarized in Table 67–15.[6]

Barium blocks the passive potassium conductance of muscle. The membrane potential remains normal at first, owing to the basal activity of the sodium-potassium pump. Since barium inhibits passive efflux and influx of potassium equally, basal sodium-potassium pumping results in a net uptake of potassium. Because the mass of skeletal muscle is very large (about 40 percent of body weight) the shift of extracellular potassium into muscle soon lowers the plasma potassium concentration. As the plasma potassium concentration falls, barium blockade of potassium permeability becomes more effective and the ionic diffusion potential is increasingly dominated by the sodium conductance, which exerts a depolarizing influence on the membrane potential. At the same time the falling concentration of plasma potassium rapidly shuts off the sodium-potassium pump, so that the membrane potential is now determined by the ionic diffusion potential, which has fallen to less than –60 mV. At this membrane potential the muscle is inexcitable and paralysis ensues.[7]

CLINICAL PRESENTATION

A survey of systemic reactions associated with barium poisoning is found in Table 67–16.[3,6]

Sequence of Symptoms

Within 1 or 2 hours after ingestion of the poison, patients experience tingling around the mouth, diarrhea, vomiting, and colicky abdominal pain. Arterial hypertension is usually observed. In 2 to 3 hours the tingling moves from the face to the hands, pupillary reactions are impaired, muscle stretch reflexes become depressed, muscle twitching is noticeable, and flaccid weakness begins to spread through the muscles of the upper and lower extremities. In some cases, complete flaccid quadriplegia develops within a few hours; in others, paralysis becomes severe on the second day of illness. Sensation is always preserved despite subjective paresthesias.[7] In most cases symptoms abate by 24 hours and patients can be ambulatory within 48 hours. In some patients muscle paralysis and weakness can persist for more than a week.[8] Table 67–17 depicts a differential diagnosis of barium poisoning.[9]

Long-term prognosis is favorable, but the acute syndrome, which can also include cardiac dysrhythmia, can be fatal and must be treated promptly.[9] Death may ensue in a few hours from cardiac arrest or respiratory paralysis, unless vigorous therapy is administered with intravenous potassium.[7]

LABORATORY

X-rays of the abdomen may indicate the presence of radiopaque concentrations in the small intestine and colon.[10]

An abdominal x-ray disclosed radiopaque material in the intestinal tract. Whole blood barium levels are elevated.

TREATMENT

1. Institute the usual measures of gastric decontamination.
2. Add 5 to 10 g of sodium sulfate to lavage solution or as fluid supplement to syrup of ipecac since sulfate salt is not absorbed.
3. Monitor cardiac rhythm and serum potassium closely to establish the trend over the first 24 hours.[4] In reported cases of barium poisoning, the serum potassium level remained low until a very large amount of potassium chloride had been administered. Barium and potassium appear to compete in their interaction with the potassium conductance channels. Presumably the administered potassium continues to enter muscle until the serum potassium level rises high enough to displace barium from the potassium channels. Moreover, raising the serum potassium level may allow the muscle membrane to repolarize by increasing electrogenic sodium-potassium pumping. Administration of a large volume of fluid also allows barium to be "flushed out" by the resulting diuresis.
4. Administer generous amounts of fluid replacement, but monitor the urine and serum for evidence of renal failure.
5. Magnesium sulfate (30 grams) administered through a nasogastric tube may prevent severe barium poisoning by precipitating insoluble barium sulfate.[11]
6. Barium is excreted in the feces. Therefore it is unlikely that diuresis, dialysis, or hemoperfusion will be effective.[12]
7. Hemodialysis shortens the half-life of barium and aids in the return to muscle strength.[13]
8. Hypokalemia is treated with potassium infusions.[13]

Pa Ping

A remarkable example of mass barium poisoning was experienced in 1943 in the Szechuan province of China where an endemic form of periodic paralysis known as Pa Ping was traced to massive contamination of table salt by barium chloride. Potassium citrate intravenously was followed by rapid and complete recovery of muscle strength.[7]

REFERENCES—BARIUM

1. Johnson CH, Van Tassell VJ. Acute barium poisoning with respiratory failure and rhabdomyolysis. Ann Emerg Med 1991;20:1138–1142.
2. Stedwell RE, Allen KM, Binder LS. Hypokalemic paralyses: a review of the etiologies, pathophysiology, presentation and therapy. Am J Emerg Med 1992;10:143–148.
3. Environmental Health Criteria 107. Barium. Geneva. World Health Organization, 1990; p. 89.

4. Wetherill SF, Guarino MJ, Cox RW. Acute renal failure associated with barium chloride poisoning. Ann Intern Med 1981; 95:187–188.
5. Phelan DM, Hagley SR, Guerin MD. Is hypokalemia the cause of paralysis in barium poisoning? Br Med J 1984;289: 882.
6. Deng JF, Jan IS, Cheng HS. The essential role of a poison center in handling an outbreak of barium carbonate poisoning. Vet Hum Toxicol 1991;33:173–175.
7. Layzer RB. Neuromuscular manifestations of systemic disease. Philadelphia: FA Davis, 1985; pp. 54–57.
8. Boehmert M, Shore N, Timperi R et al. Measurement of serum levels in acute barium chloride overdose. Vet Hum Toxicol 1985;28:291 (abstract).
9. Johnson CH, Van Tassell VJ. Acute barium poisoning with respiratory failure and rhabdomyolysis. Ann Emerg Med 1991;20:1138–1142.
10. Buylaert W, Vanhoe H, Van den Bogaerde J, Vogelaers D, Derom E, Versieck J, Verstraete A. Acute poisoning with barium carbonate. A case report. Proc Eur Assoc Pois Contr Cent Clin Toxicol 1988; p. 42.
11. Mills K, Kunkel D. Prevention of severe barium carbamate toxicity with oral magnesium sulfate. Vet Hum Toxicol 1993; 35:347.
12. Boehmert M. Soluble barium salts. Clin Toxicol Rev 1988; 10(5):1–2.
13. Scharn ThF, Olbricht CH, Schuler A, Franz A, Wittek K, Balks H-J et al. Barium carbonate intoxication. Intensive Care Med 1991;17:60–62.

BERYLLIUM

Uses and properties of some important beryllium compounds are found in Table 67–18.[1] Exposure to beryllium causes an acute chemical pneumonitis and chronic granulomatous disease similar to sarcoidosis and miliary tuberculosis.[2–4] A comparison of chronic beryllium disease, sarcoidosis, and extrinsic allergic alveolitis is found in Table 67–19.[5]

Table 67–18
Uses and Properties of Some Important Beryllium (Be) Compounds*

Compound	Total Be Consumption (%)	Formula	Density (g/cm³)	Melting Point (centigrade)	Uses
Beryllium (metallic)	33	Be	1.84	1290	Nuclear reactors and weapons, inertial guidance systems, aircraft brakes, x-ray tube windows, turbine rotor blades
Beryl	—	$3BeO\ A1_2C_36SiO_2$	2.70	1410	Principal beryllium ore
Bertrandite	—	$4BeO\ SiO_2\ H_2O$	2.60	—	Another beryllium ore
Beryllium oxide	5	BeO	3.01	2530	Spark plugs, laser tubes, electrical components, rocket engine liners, ceramic applications, intermediate in Be refining
Beryllium fluoride	†	BeF_2	1.99	‡	Intermediate in Be refining
Beryllium copper alloy (typically 2% beryllium in copper)	50				Springs, bellows, gears, aircraft engines, bearings, welding electrodes, electrical contacts

*From reference 5.
†Produced only as an intermediate.
‡Indefinite, softens at approximately 800°C.
Adapted from Kriebel D et al. Am Rev Resp Dis 1988;137:464–473.

Table 67–19
Comparison of Chronic Beryllium Disease, Sarcoidosis and Extrinsic Allergic Alveolitis

	Chronic Beryllium Disease	Sarcoidosis	Extrinsic Allergic Alveolitis
Occupational exposure	Yes	No	Yes
Beryllium in tissues	Yes	No	No
Erythema nodosum	No	Yes	No
Bilateral hilar/adenopathy	Uncommon	Common	No
Bone cysts	No	3%	No
Skin tests: tuberculin	Negative	Negative	Unaltered
Kveim Siltzbach	Negative	Positive	Negative
Beryllium patch	Positive	Negative	Negative
Beryllium lymphocyte transformation	Positive	Negative	Negative
Circulating precipitins	No	No	Yes
Elevated serum angiotensin converting enzyme	Uncommon	Common	Uncommon
Granulomas	Yes	Yes	Yes (acute)
Alveolitis	Prominent	Inconspicuous	Prominent
Prognosis	Poor	Good	Good

Adapted from Williams WJ. Postgrad Med J 1988;64:511–516.

Table 67-20
Occupations at Risk

1. Metal workers—pure beryllium, alloys, scrap metal, disposal.
2. Ceramic manufacturers—crucibles, cermats, jet engine blades, rocket covers, brake pads.
3. Electronic industry—transistors, heat sinks, X-ray windows.
4. Atomic energy industry—rocket fuels, heat shields.
5. Laboratory workers.
6. Beryllium extraction from ore.
7. Fluorescent lamp workers (ceased in 1951).

Adapted from Williams WJ. Postgrad Med J 1988;64:511–516.

CLINICAL PRESENTATION

Acute

The lung is the primary target organ, with a defect occurring in carbon monoxide diffusing capacity. In contrast to sarcoid, ocular involvement is absent. Multisystem involvement includes lymph nodes, spleen, liver, myocardium, kidney, and bone. Occasional hypercalcemia develops. Initially, nonspecific symptoms appear and are followed by dyspnea and cough. Symptoms are progressive, and steroids may help blunt the course of the disease. Occupations at risk for beryllium disease are listed in Table 67–20.[5]

Acute beryllium exposures produce chemical pneumonitis and pulmonary edema.[6] This metal is a cutaneous sensitizer and primary skin irritant that produces contact dermatitis, skin granulomas, and ulcers.[7] Aurin tricarboxylic acid effectively protected monkeys exposed to lethal quantities of beryllium, but no data on humans are available to substantiate its safety or effectiveness.[8] Acute beryllium disease with diffuse chemical pneumonitis has been virtually eliminated. In contrast, new occurrences of chronic beryllium disease (CBD) continue to be diagnosed each year. The treatment of choice for patients with CBD is corticosteroids.[9]

Chronic

Occupational exposure studies have shown an excess of lung cancer 15 years after the onset of exposure among patients with chronic berylliosis, and among some who had experienced acute berylliosis.[10,11]

Chronic low-level exposure to beryllium may cause chronic granulomatous lung disease. The blood beryllium lymphocyte transformation (BeLT) test is positive in most cases of chronic beryllium disease in which the lavaged BeLT is abnormal. Some persons with seemingly minor, incidental beryllium exposure should be considered to be at risk.[12]

Chronic Beryllium Disease (CBD)—Criteria

The criteria for the diagnosis of chronic beryllium disease adopted by the beryllium case registry at the Massachusetts General Hospital require at least four of the following six features and must include at least one of the first two:

1. Epidemiologic evidence of significant beryllium exposure.
2. Presence of beryllium in lung tissue, lymph nodes, or urine.
3. Evidence of lower respiratory tract disease and a clinical course consistent with beryllium disease.
4. Radiologic evidence of interstitial disease consistent with a fibronodular process.
5. Evidence of a restrictive or obstructive ventilatory defect or diminished carbon monoxide diffusing capacity.
6. Pathologic changes consistent with beryllium disease or examination of lung tissue and/or lymph nodes.[1,13]

Chronic beryllium disease (CBD) may develop decades after exposure has ended and is a progressive granulomatous disease that may lead to reduced lung volume, dyspnea, and diffuse irregular opacities on radiography. CBD involves a cell-mediated immune response.[14]

LABORATORY

Persons with chronic beryllium disease have cell-mediated immune responses to beryllium that can be detected by beryllium-specific blast transformation of lung lymphocytes obtained through bronchoalveolar lavage.[1] A beryllium-specific lymphocyte transformation blood test appears to be a sensitive screening test that may be useful in preventing chronic beryllium disease by early diagnosis in a subclinical phase. Not all individuals with a positive test may have beryllium disease at the time of their initial evaluation.[15,16] Bronchoalveolar cells of a patient with beryllium disease appear to be more reactive to in vitro stimulation by beryllium salts than peripheral blood cells. These findings are consistent with the concept that chronic berylliosis is a form of a hypersensitivity pneumonitis and that bronchoalveolar lavage may be helpful in establishing the diagnosis of this disease.[17,18]

In patients with chronic beryllium disease, beryllium acts as a class II restricted antigen, stimulating local proliferation and accumulation in the lung of beryllium-specific CD4+ (helper/inducer) T cells.[19] A laser microprobe mass spectrometry (LAMMS) may be able to detect beryllium in granulomas of chronic beryllium disease and distinguish such granulomas from those of sarcoidosis.[20]

The Kveim test is reported to be consistently negative in beryllium disease, but also has a high false-negative rate (20%) in sarcoidosis. Thus a negative result cannot be taken as compelling evidence of beryllium disease when signs and symptoms are consistent with either diagnosis.[1]

TREATMENT

Treatment of acute beryllium disease includes removal from exposure, bed rest, oxygen, mechanical ventilation as required, and corticosteroids. Chronic beryllium disease is treated symptomatically and supportively.[1]

REFERENCES—BERYLLIUM

1. Kriebel D, Brain JD, Sprince NL, et al. The pulmonary toxicity of beryllium. Am Rev Respir Dis 1988;137:464–473.
2. Cotes JE, Gilson JC, McKerrow CB et al. A long term follow up of workers exposed to beryllium. Br J Ind Med 1983; 40:13–21.
3. Hasan F, Kazemi H. Chronic beryllium disease: a continuing epidemiologic hazard. Chest 1974;65:289–293.
4. Sprince NL, Kanarek DJ, Weber AL et al. Reversible respiratory disease in beryllium workers. Am Rev Respir Dis 1978; 117:1011–1017.

5. Williams WJ. Beryllium disease. Postgrad Med J 1988;64: 511–516.
6. Hooper WF. Acute beryllium lung disease. NC Med J 1981; 42:551–553.
7. Rom WN, Lockey JE, Bank KM et al. Reversible beryllium sensitization in a prospective study of beryllium workers. Arch Environ Health 1983;38:302–307.
8. King ME, Shefner AM, Ehrlich R. Effectiveness of aurin tricarboxylic acid as an antidote for beryllium poisoning. Ind Med Surg 1964;33:566–569.
9. Aronchik JM. Chronic beryllium disease. Radiol Clin N Amer 1992;30:1209–1217.
10. Saracci R. Beryllium and lung cancer: adding another piece to the puzzle of epidemiologic evidence. J Natl Cancer Inst 1991;83:1362–1363.
11. Vainio H, Kleihues P. IARC Working Group on Carcinogenicity of Beryllium. J Occup Med 1994;36:1068–1069.
12. Newman LS, Kreiss K. Non-occupational beryllium disease masquerading as sarcoidosis: identification by blood lymphocyte proliferative response to beryllium. Am Rev Respir Dis 1992;145:1212–1214.
13. Sprince NL, Kazemi H. Beryllium disease. In: Rom W, ed. Environmental and occupational medicine. 1st ed. Boston: Little, Brown, 1983; pp. 481–490.
14. Steinland K, Ward E. Lung cancer incidence among patients with beryllium disease: a cohort mortality study. J Natl Cancer Inst 1991;83:1380–1385.
15. Kreiss K, Newman LS, Mroz MM, Campbell PA. Screening blood test identifies subclinical beryllium disease. J Occup Med 1989;31:603–608.
16. Newman LS, Kreiss K, King TE Jr, Seay S, Campbell PA. Pathologic and immunologic alterations in early stages of beryllium disease. Re-examination of disease definition and natural history. Am Rev Respir Dis 1989;139:1479–1489.
17. Epstein PE, Dauber JH, Rossman MD, Daniele PP. Bronchoalveolar lavage in a patient with chronic berylliosis: evidence for hypersensitivity pneumonitis. Ann Intern Med 1982;97:211–213.
18. Rossman MD, Kern JA, Elias JA, Cullen MP, Epstein PE, Preuss OP et al. Proliferative response of bronchoalveolar lymphocytes to Beryllium. A test for chronic beryllium disease. Ann Intern Med 1988;108:687–693.
19. Saltini C, Winstock K, Kirby M, Pinkston P, Crystal RG. Maintenance of alveolitis in patients with chronic beryllium disease by beryllium-specific helper T-cells. N Engl J Med 1989; 320:1103–1109.
20. Williams WJ, Wallach ER. Laser microprobe mass spectrometry (LAMMS) analysis of beryllium, sarcoidosis and other granulomatous disease. Sarcoidosis 1989;6:111–117.

BISMUTH

Between 1973 and 1980 approximately 1000 cases of bismuth-related neurotoxicity were reported in France; many cases were also reported in Australia, Belgium, Switzerland, and Spain. In Australia in 1974 this led to withdrawal from use of all preparations of bismuth subgallate for oral administration. In France the neurotoxicity was associated with the use of a bismuth substrate. All patients recovered within 2 to 12 weeks after ceasing bismuth administration. Bismuth salts were placed under prescription control, and other restrictions were initiated. In 1980 Austrian authorities withdrew pharmaceutical preparations containing bismuth. Canada has prohibited sale of all oral salts except the subgallate, which is available by prescription only. In Australia, Canada, France, and Austria the use of bismith preparations has been curtailed because of neurotoxicity. In the United States bismuth subsalicylate was considered safe in doses up to 4.8 g daily, but there was insufficient evidence to establish its effectiveness as an antinauseant/antiemetic. In the United Kingdom, bismuth products were limited to periods of 2 to 4 weeks, and dosage to less than 4 g daily.[1]

BISMUTH COMPOUND GROUPS

Pharmacologically active bismuth compounds have been subdivided by Serfontein and Mekel into the following four groups[2]:

Group 1: Simple inorganic salts and subsalts of bismuth such as bismuth subcarbonate, bismuth subnitrate, etc. These compounds are insoluble in water in the absence of complexing agents with minimal bismuth absorption and virtually no toxicity.
Typical example: bismuth subcarbonate.

Group 2: Predominantly lipid-soluble organic compounds and complexes of bismuth such as bismuth subgallate. They are absorbed as such leading to high bismuth blood levels and are mainly neurotoxic and possibly also hepatotoxic.
Typical example: bismuth subgallate.

Group 3: Predominantly water-soluble organic compounds and complexes of bismuth that are stable enough to be absorbed as such leading to high bismuth blood levels. Renal damage is a prominent feature of the toxicity syndrome in man of these compounds.
Typical example: bismuth triglycollamate.

Group 4: Water-soluble organic complexes of bismuth that decompose (hydrolyze) in the gastrointestinal system with the ultimate production of simple insoluble bismuth compounds such as bismuth subchloride and bismuth sulfide. Minimal absorption and practically no toxicity are characteristic features.
Typical example: Bicitropeptide.

CLINICAL PRESENTATION

Symptoms of systemic intoxication are similar to those of lead and mercury. Increased salivation, a bismuth line (bluish discoloration of the gums), pyorrhea, and loss of teeth have been observed. Permanent discoloration of the skin and ulcerative stomatitis with or without colitis are rarely seen. Methemoglobin may follow the reduction of bismuth substrate to nitrate. Diminished renal function with severe nephrosis and renal failure have been observed, in addition to hepatic degeneration and peripheral neuritis. Myoclonic encephalopathy has been described.[3,4]

Bone

Osteoarthropathy may complicate bismuth encephalopathy. Osteoporosis and osteomalacia may follow increased levels of bismuth stored in bone.

A 27-year-old man ingested 100 De-Nol (colloidal bismuth) tablets and later developed anorexia, nausea, vomiting, malaise, leg weakness, blurred vision, thirst, and poor urinary output. He was lucid. Bismuth blood levels were 260 μg/L. Renal function and neurologic signs resolved in 5 days.[5] Clinical studies in ulcer patients report a peak blood concentration at 2 to 3 hours postadministration of up to 100 μg/L.[6,7]

Encephalopathy

Despite the relative safety of oral bismuth preparations, encephalopathy (some fatal) has been reported after large or repetitive ingestions of water- or lipid-soluble salts.[1] The encephalopathy is characterized by altered mental status, ataxia, myoclonus, and a specific electroencephalographic abnormality.[8] Bismuth blood levels ranges from 1500 to 2000 μg/L (normal less than 20 μg/L).[9] Clinically, bismuth encephalopathy is separated into two clinical phases[1]:

1. A prodromal period lasting from a week to several months during which cognitive and affective disorders are predominant. The patients are asthenic, somnolent, depressed, and anxious, sometimes with visual hallucinations and even delusions of persecution (three cases). Jerky movements of varying severity are seen in this phase (15 patients), and disturbances of writing and speech occur more rarely.
2. A second phase of encephalopathy of rapid onset appears abruptly in 24 to 48 hours. Four symptoms are constant: confusion (progressing to coma or dementia), dysarthria, disturbances of walking and standing, and pseudotremor accompanied by myoclonic jerks. Myoclonic jerks are always present in this phase. Sometimes they predominate in the upper limbs and distally; at other times they are diffuse and involve the facial and axial muscles. They are increased by voluntary movements and by stimuli (change of position, noise).

These problems are usually reversible over several weeks or months when bismuth preparations are withheld.[10]

Chronic Toxicity

Chronic ingestion results in stomatitis, black spots in the mucosa and gums (bismuth lines), salivation, and pathologic fractures.[11] In animal models, bismuth alters the metabolism of certain heavy metals (copper, zinc) and induces the formation of low-molecular-weight metallothioneinlike proteins.[12] In mice models, *d*-penicillamine is a useful chelating agent.[13] The ingestion of over-the-counter mixtures containing bismuth subsalicylate (e.g., Pepto-Bismol) may result in serious symptoms (e.g., encephalopathy).[14] Chronic toxicity results in encephalopathy and acute nephrotoxicity following use of bismuth salts. Therapeutic doses lead to blood bismuth concentrations of 10 to 20 μg/L and urine levels of less than 5 μg/L, which are not toxic. An alerting level of 50 μg/L has been suggested. In the very early stages chelating agents (e.g., dimercaptopropanesulfonic acid) may be beneficial.[15] BAL is not advised because of its toxicity and the necessary intramuscular route of administration.[16]

Pepto-Bismol (see also Salicylate Chapter)

Doses of 5.2 to 9.4 grams of Pepto-Bismol daily led to an encephalopathy after 7 days. Blood bismuth levels were 200 μg/L (normal <5 μg/L). Urine levels were 2960 μg/L (normal <20 L). The patient died in 24 hours.[5]

LABORATORY

The method of choice for the quantification of bismuth in urine, blood, or serum is either electrothermal atomic absorption spectrophotometry (detectable limit 1 μg/L)[17,18] or MS with a hydride generator.[19] A reversed-phase high-performance liquid chromatography method (HPL) with on-column derivatization is available.[20]

Blood Levels

Confirmation of their validity should be obtained. Blood concentrations are not a reliable marker for neurotoxicity. No relationship is apparent between blood and urine bismuth concentration, or blood and cerebrospinal fluid bismuth concentration.

Abdominal X-ray

A radiopaque substance may be seen on a plain film of the abdomen in the large intestine of patients with bismuth encephalopathy.[1]

Electroencephalogram

Epileptic EEG patterns have appeared when the bismuth blood level was below 150 μg/L.[21] A characteristic EEG in bismuth toxicity displays low voltage and diffuse beta frequencies bilaterally, maximal in the frontal and central areas and accentuated by hyperventilation.[22]

CT Scans

On CT scan an increase in density may be present in the cortex of the cerebral hemisphere and in the basal ganglia. This increased density may be caused directly by the presence of bismuth, which is radiopaque. Hyperdensities in the basal ganglia, cerebellum, and cerebral cortex in one series were most marked when bismuth blood levels exceeded 2000 μg/L.

Pepto-Bismol

Bismuth subsalicylate (BSS), the active ingredient in Pepto-Bismol, is a highly insoluble salt of trivalent bismuth and salicylic acid. Each molecule contains 58% bismuth and 42% salicylate by weight. BSS is nearly completely hydrolyzed in the stomach to form bismuth oxychloride and salicylic acid. Bismuth is strongly associated with the mucosal surface of the stomach and may be responsible for the cytoprotective properties of Pepto-Bismol.[23] Dissociation of BSS occurs mostly in the stomach. Absorption of salicylate occurs in the small intestine. In the small intestine nondissociated BSS reacts with other anions (bicarbonate and phosphate) to form bismuth subcarbonate and bismuth phosphate salts, which are highly insoluble. In the colon nondissociated BSS and other bismuth salts react with hydrogen sulfide produced by anaerobic bacteria to produce bismuth sulfide, a highly insoluble black salt responsible for darkening of the stool. Unchewed and undissolved Pepto-Bismol tablets are radiopaque.[24]

TREATMENT

Treatment of overdose is largely symptomatic and supportive. Chelating agents may be effective early before tissue binding has occurred. D-penicillamine does not appear to facilitate excretion of bismuth.[25] Dimercaprol (BAL) enhanced bismuth clearance in two patients with myoclonic encephalopathy due to bismuth salts intoxication.[26] Dimercapto-1-propane sulfonic acid (DMPS) has led to a tenfold increase in urinary clearance of bismuth with clinical improvement of encephalopathy.[27] The role of hemodialysis has not been evaluated. Even after large overdoses, the prognosis is good.[5,15]

The main therapeutic measure in bismuth encephalopathy is to withdraw bismuth from the patient. Benzodiazepines or other anticonvulsants may be useful for myoclonic seizures, but few studies have been performed to support this.[17]

REFERENCES—BISMUTH

1. Winship KA. Toxicity of bismuth salts. Adverse Drug React Acute Pois Rev 1982;2:103–121.
2. Serfontein WJ, Mekel R. Bismuth toxicity in man. II. Review of bismuth blood and urine levels in patients after administration of therapeutic bismuth formulations in relation to the problem of bismuth toxicity in man. Res Commun Chem Pathol Pharmacol 1979;26:391–411.
3. Hoffman RS, Mendelowitz PC, Weber S. Bismuth absorption and myoclonic encephalopathy after bismuth subsalicylate therapy. Vet Hum Toxicol 1989;31:380.
4. Mendelowitz PC, Hoffman RS, Weber S. Bismuth absorption and myoclonic encephalopathy during bismuth subsalicylate therapy. Ann Intern Med 1990;112:140–141.
5. Hudson M, Ashley N, Mowat G. Reversible toxicity in poisoning with colloidal bismuth substrate. Br Med J 1989; 299:159.
6. Nwokolo CV, Gavy CJ, Smith JTL, Pounder RE. The absorption of bismuth from oral dose of tripotassium dicitrate bismuthate. Aliment Pharmacol Ther 1989;3:29–39.
7. Lauritsen K, Laursen LS, Rask-Madsen J. Clinical pharmacokinetics of drug used in the treatment of gastrointestinal diseases. I. Clin Pharmacokinet 1990;19:11–31.
8. Supino-Veterbo V, Sicard C, Risvegliato M, Rancurel G, Buge A. Toxic encephalopathy due to ingestion of bismuth salts: clinical and EEG studies of 45 patients. J Neurol Neurosurg Psychiatry 1977;40:748–752.
9. Buge A, Supino-Viterbo V, Rancirel G, Pontes C. Toxic epileptic phenomena in bismuth toxic encephalopathy. J Neurol Neurosurg Psychiatry 1982;44:62–67.
10. Gordon MF, Abrams RI, Rubin DB, Barr WB, Correa DD. Bismuth subsalicylate toxicity as a cause of prolonged encephalopathy with myoclonus. Movement Disorders 1995;10: 220–222.
11. Emil J, De Bray JM, Bernat M et al. Osteoarticular complications in bismuth encephalopathy. Clin Toxicol 1981;18: 1285–1290.
12. Szymanska JA, Zelazowski AJ, Kawiorski S. Some aspects of bismuth metabolism. Clin Toxicol 1981;18:1291–1298.
13. Basinger MA, Jones MM, McCroskey SA. Antidotes for acute bismuth intoxication. J Toxicol Clin Toxicol 1983;20:159–165.
14. Hasking G, Duggan J. Encephalopathy from bismuth subsalicylate. Med J Aust 1982;2:167.
15. Huwez F, Pall A, Lyons D, Stewart MJ. Acute renal failure after one dose of colloidal bismuth subcitrate. Lancet 1992; 340:1298.
16. Slikkerveer A, Helminth RB, Jong HB, de Wolff TA. Development of a therapeutic procedure for bismuth intoxication using chelating agents. Hum Exp Toxicol 1993;12:77–78.
17. Behrendt WA, Groger C, Kuhn D, Schulz H-V, Topfmeier P. A study relating to bioavailability and renal elimination of bismuth after oral administration of basic bismuth nitrate. Internat J Clin Pharmacol Ther Toxicol 1991;29:357–360.
18. Slikkerveer A. Bismuth: biokinetics, toxicity and experimental therapy of overdosage. PhD thesis. S. Gravenlage, Pasmans Opfset Drukerij 1992; pp. 1–185.
19. Slikkerveer A, de Wolff FA. Pharmacokinetics and toxicity of bismuth compounds. Med Toxicol Adverse Drug Dep 1989; 4:303–323.
20. Irth H, Brouwer E, de Jong GJ, Brinkman UA Th, Free RW. Trace enrichment and separation of AsIII, SbIII as diethyldithiophosphate complexes by reversed phase high performance liquid chromatography. J Chromatog 1988; 439:63–70.
21. Buge A, Supino-Viterbo V, Rancirel G, Pontes C. Toxic epileptic phenomena in bismuth toxic encephalopathy. J Neurol Neurosurg Psychiatry 1981;44:62–67.
22. Hasking GJ, Duggen JM. Encephalopathy for bismuth subsalicylate. Med J Aust 1982;2:167.
23. Bierer DW. Bismuth subsalicylate: history, chemistry and safety. Rev Infect Dis 1990;12(Suppl 1):S3–S8.
24. Woo OF, Jackson GM. Radiopacity of chewable Pepto-Bismol® tablets: report of two patients. Vet Hum Toxicol 1993;35:317.
25. Nwokolo CU, Pounder PE. D-penicillamine does not increase urinary bismuth excretion in patients treated with tripotassium dicitrato bismitate. Br J Clin Pharmacol 1990;30:648–650.
26. Molina JA, Calandre L, Bermajo F. Myoclonic encephalopathy due to bismuth salts: treatment with dimercaprol and analysis of CSF transmitters. Acta Neurol Scand 1989; 79:200–203.
27. Playford RJ, Matthews CH, Campbell MJ, Delves VT, Hla KK, Hodgson HJF et al. Bismuth induced encephalopathy caused by tripotassium dicitrato bismethate in a patient with chronic renal failure. GUT 1990;36:359–360.

CADMIUM

Cadmium poisoning is a rare type of heavy-metal poisoning associated with industrial exposures, ingestion of contaminated shellfish, or drinking of acidic beverages from contaminated vessels. It causes leg cramps, nausea, vomiting, and diarrhea.

EPIDEMIOLOGY

Acute exposures usually occur in the workplace via inhalation and initially affect the lungs. Chronic exposures produce renal dysfunction,[1] emphysema,[2] and osteomalacia.[3]

SOURCES

Environmental exposures involve zinc and lead smelters (cadmium is a common contaminant of metal ores), electroplated ice trays, as well as contaminated foodstuff (e.g., rice, cigarettes, soil).[4]

TOXICOKINETICS[5]

Pregnancy

There appears to be a maternal-fetal gradient of blood cadmium. Retention of cadmium in the placenta is related to the synthesis of metallothionein. The birth weight of offspring of mothers who smoke is decreased, but this has not definitely been attributed to cadmium exposure without smoking.[6]

CLINICAL PRESENTATION

Chronic Exposures

Cadmium-related symptoms and signs include "yellow teeth line," tubular or glomerular insufficiency (microhematuria, proteinuria, leukocyturia, hypertension), vertigo, fatigue, urinary calculus, osteopenia osteomalacia (musculoskeletal pain), rhinitis and anosmia (damage to the olfactory nerve, loss of sense of smell), anorexia, and dyspnea (lung damage).[8]

The most direct way to associate adverse health effects of Cd exposure is to correlate historical blood levels of Cd and other indicators of Cd exposure with symptoms and detection of renal damage by urinary *N*-acetylglucosaminidase excretion.

Itai-Itai disease is associated with impaired urine concentration ability. Animal data appear consistent with clinical observations on the contribution of nutritional deficiency to Itai-Itai disease and the benefit attributed to vitamin D_3 therapy.[9,10]

An IARC working group reported that there was sufficient evidence in experimental animals and limited evidence in humans for the carcinogenicity of cadmium and certain compounds. The overall IARC classification of cadmium was group 2A, probably carcinogenic to humans.[11]

LABORATORY

Analytic Methods

Quantitation of urine cadmium is accomplished with electrothermal atomic absorption spectrometry. The detection limit of urinary cadmium is 0.08 μg/L.[12]

Blood Levels

Concentration of cadmium in the blood in normal populations ranges from about 0.4 to 1.0 μg/L for nonsmokers and 1.4 to 4.0 μg/L for smokers. Values in occupationally exposed populations range from 10 to 100 μg/L.[13] Blood cadmium levels in workers involved in an outbreak of cadmium intoxication in a jewelry factory were higher (0.93 μg/100 mL) than those in unexposed workers (0.38 μg/100 mL). A dose-response relationship was observed between blood cadmium levels and symptoms of dyspnea, chest pain, dyscrasia, and dizziness. Segmental hair analysis revealed highest cadmium levels (up to 19 μg/g) in segments formed prior to cadmium exposure. Beta$_2$-microglobulin levels were within normal limits.[14]

Urine

When the urinary excretion of cadmium is less than 2 μg/24 hours, the risk of occurrence of renal effects remains low.[15] A urinary cadmium excretion of 2 μg/24 hours corresponds to a mean renal cortex concentration of 50 ppm (net weight). In nonsmokers this level is reached after 50 years of an oral daily cadmium intake of about 1 μg/kg of body weight.[15]

TREATMENT

Antidotes

$CaNa_2EDTA$ is the chelator of choice for acute cadmium exposures. Preliminary animal data suggest that dimercaptosuccinic acid (DMSA) may have a role in enhancing cadmium excretion and may be of clinical use in acute oral intoxication by cadmium compounds. Clinical studies confirming these observations remain to be done.[16,17] BAL increases nephrotoxicity and therefore is not indicated. Chronic exposures require no chelation, and treatment involves removal from contamination.

No chelation treatment presently available has been shown to reduce the cadmium body burden in human beings.[15]

REFERENCES—CADMIUM

1. Lerner S, Hong CD, Bozian RC et al. Cadmium nephropathy—a clinical evaluation. J Occup Med 1979;21:409–412.
2. Cadmium and the lung. Lancet 1973;2:1134–1135 (editorial).
3. Kressel J. Cadmium. Clin Toxicol Rev 1983;5:1–2.
4. Gloag D. Contamination of food: mycotoxin and metals. Br Med J 1981;282:879–882.
5. Perry HM, Thind CS, Perry AB. The biology of cadmium. Med Clin North Am 1976;60:759–768.
6. Goyer RA. Transplacental transfer of cadmium and fetal effects. Fundam Appl Toxicol 1991;16:22–23.
7. Buel G. Some biochemical aspects of cadmium toxicology. J Occup Med 1975;17:189–195.
8. Kahan E, Derazne E, Rosenboim J, Ashkenazi R, Ribak J. Adverse health effects in workers exposed to cadmium. Am J Ind Med 1992;21:527–537.
9. Nakada T, Furuta H, Koike H, Katayama T, Teranishi H. Impaired urine concentrating ability in Itai-Itai (ouch-ouch) disease. Int Urol Nephrol 1989;21:201–209.
10. Angle CR, Thomas DJ, Swanson SA. Cadmium and bone toxicity. Protective effect of 1,25 $(OH)_2$ vitamin D_3. Vet Hum Toxicol 1989;31:351.
11. Karakaya A, Yucesoy B, Sardas OS. An immunological study on workers occupationally exposed to cadmium. Hum Exp Toxicol 1991;13:73–75.
12. Ong CN, Chua LH, Lee BL, Ong HY, Chia KS. Electrothermal atomic absorption spectrometric determination of cadmium and nickel in urine. J Anal Toxicol 1990;14:29–31.
13. Agency for Toxic Substances and Disease Registry: Toxicological Profile for Cadmium. March, 1989;TSDR/TP-88/08.
14. Baker EL Jr, Coleman C, Peterson WA, Holtz JL, Landrigan PJ. Subacute cadmium intoxication in jewelry workers. An evaluation of diagnostic procedure. Arch Environ Health 1979;39:173–177.
15. Buchet JP, Lauwerys R, Roels H, Bernard A, Bruaux P, Claeys F et al. Renal effects of cadmium body burden of the general population. Lancet 1990;336:699–702.
16. Basinger MA, Jones MM, Holscher MA, Vaughan WK. Antagonists for acute oral cadmium chloride intoxication. J Toxicol Environ Health 1988;23:77–89.
17. Andersen O, Nielsen J. Chelation in acute oral cadmium intoxication. Fifth Int Congress of Toxicology July 16–21, 1989, Brighton, England. London: Taylor & Francis, 1990; p. 177.

CHROMIUM

A comparison of hexavalent and trivalent chromium is presented in Table 67–21.[1]

The OSHA permissible exposure limit (PEL) for chromic acid and chromates is 0.1 mg/m^3. For soluble Cr (VI) salts the PEL is an 8-hour time-weighted average (TWA) of 500 μg Cr/m^3. For chromic metal and for insoluble salts the TWA is 1000 μg Cr/m^3. The toxicity of chromium is due to the oxidizing properties of the hexavalent compounds and the pH (chromic acid has a pH of 5 and ammonia dichromate a pH of 13). Death has occurred after a 10% skin surface burn. The hexavalent form crosses the cell membrane and the

Table 67-21
Toxic Effects of Hexavalent and Trivalent Chromium

Cr^{6-}	Cr^{3-}
– excellent membrane penetration	– poor membrane penetration
– poor protein binding (poor tanning agent)	– excellent protein binding (good tanning agent)
– reduced to Cr^{3-} intracellularly } tissue damage, tanning	
– toxic	– said to have low toxicity
– Corrosive, causes tissue ulceration	– non-irritating
– Oral burns	– non-corrosive
– Nausea, vomiting, diarrhea	
– GI bleeding	
– GI necrosis	
– Renal failure—tubular damage	

GI, gastrointestinal.
Adapted from van Heerden PV et al. Intens Care Med 1994;20:145–147.

placenta and may be found in breast milk. The elimination half-life is 15 to 41 hours.[2]

DOSE

As little as 500 mg of ingested hexavalent chromium (such as chromic acid or chromium trioxide) may cause life-threatening toxicity in adults. Lethal doses of 1 to 2 g have been reported. 0.5 to 0.8 g of potassium dichromate may be lethal.[3,4]

TOXICOKINETICS

Hexavalent chromium compounds (sodium, potassium, ammonium, chromium trioxide, and chromic acid), which are more toxic, are readily absorbed by the lungs and gastrointestinal tract. Once absorbed, chromium is rapidly excreted mainly via the urinary tract, with a half-life estimated to range between 15 and 41 hours. Ingestion of hexavalent compounds usually leads to abdominal pains, vomiting, diarrhea, and intestinal bleeding. Death may ensue during the initial circulatory collapse. If the patient survives the initial phase, some renal tubular damage may occur. Hepatic failure, severe coagulopathy, or intravascular hemolysis have been observed. *N*-acetyl-beta-D-glucosaminidase (NAG) is a sensitive indicator of early renal injury.[5] The bivalent and trivalent (chromic oxide, chromic sulfate, and other salts) forms are relatively insoluble, poorly absorbed, and usually not of any clinical importance.

CLINICAL PRESENTATION

An adult who suffered full-thickness burns of the left calf (1% of body surface) from a concentrated chromic acid solution developed nausea and vomiting within 1 hour and complete anuria within 24 hours. Two weeks later the patient continued to receive hemodialysis three times each week.[6]

Survival in two cases of chromic acid ingestion has been achieved with vigorous hemodialysis.[7,8] Treatment of chromic acid burns by peritoneal dialysis is less successful.[9]

Intraperitoneal chromic phosphate is used as adjuvant therapy for early-stage ovarian carcinoma. The radiocolloid is a pure beta emitter with a mean depth of penetration of about 3 mm. Bowel perforations or obstruction may occur months to years after chromic phosphate therapy.[10]

Treatment is symptomatic. The efficacy of BAL, hemodialysis, and exchange transfusion has not been established.[11] Dimercapto-propane-sulfuric acid (DMPS) was given to a man who fell into a pool of chromic acid. The urine chromium level rose to 13,614 μg/mL. The patient recovered.[12]

LABORATORY

Hair chromium concentrations may be used as indices of industrial exposure to trivalent chromium.[13]

REFERENCES—CHROMIUM

1. van Heerden PV, Jenkins IR, Woods WPD, Rossi E, Cameron PD. Death by tanning—a case of fatal basic chromium sulphate poisoning. Intensive Care Med 1994;20:145–147.
2. Kapil V, Krogh J. Chronic toxicity. Case studies in environmental medicine. Agency for Toxic Substances and Disease Registry, June, 1990.
3. Sarayan LA, Reedy M. Chronic determinations in a case of chromic acid ingestion. J Anal Toxicol 1988;12:162–164.
4. Schonwald S. Chromium. Clin Toxicol Rev 1989;11(5):1–2.
5. Sanz P, Nogue S, Munne P, Torra R, Marques F. Acute potassium dichromate poisoning. Hum Exp Toxicol 1991;10: 228–229.
6. Stoner RS, Tong TG, Dart R, Sullivan JB, Saito G, Armstrong B. Acute chromium intoxication with renal failure after 1% body surface area burns from chromic acid. Vet Hum Toxicol 1988;30:361.
7. Fristedt B, Lindqvist B, Schutz A, Orrum P. Survival in a case of acute oral chromic acid poisoning with acute renal failure treated by hemodialysis. Acta Med Scand 1965;177:153–159.
8. Pedersen RS, Morch PT. Chromic acid poisoning treated with acute hemodialysis. Nephron 1978;22:592–595.
9. Wang X-W, Davies JWL, Sirvent Z, Robinsons WA. Chromic acid burns and acute chromic poisoning. Burns 1985;11: 181–184.
10. Proctor J, Doering D, Barnhill D, Park R. Bowel perforation associated with intraperitoneal chromic phosphate instillation. Gynecol Oncol 1990;39:125–127.
11. Langard S, Vigander T. Occurrence of lung cancer in workers producing chromium pigments. Br J Ind Med 1983; 40:71–74.
12. Donner A, Meisinger V, Scholtz I, Prick K, Hruby K. Dimercapto-propane-sulphuric acid (DMPS) in the treatment of an acid copper and an acid chromium poisoning. Toxicol Lett 1986;31(Suppl):154.
13. Randall JA, Gibson RS. Hair chromium as indices of chromium exposure of tannery workers. Br J Ind Med 1989;46:171–175.

DICHROMATE

PATHOPHYSIOLOGY

The hexavalent chromium in dichromate binds nonspecifically to proteins and nucleoproteins and is specifically taken up into red cells and platelets intracellularly. It is reduced to trivalent chromium, but this conversion, and perhaps the intermediate pentavalent chromium, combines to produce severe, free-radical damage to mitochondria, particularly in the kidney tubules and hepatocytes.[1]

CLINICAL PRESENTATION

Chronic Effects

Chromate dust causes conjunctivitis, chronic penetrating lesions of the skin, lacrimation, ulceration of the nasal septum, and respiratory cancer.[2]

Acute Effects

Vertigo, thirst, abdominal pain, vomiting, oliguria, anuria, shock, seizures, severe coagulopathy, intravascular hemolysis, and a hepatorenal syndrome can follow large doses.[2–6]

Case Studies

A 15-year-old girl ingested a few grains of potassium dichromate. She then vomited, became unconscious, and died in 12 hours. The blood contained 3.5 mg of chromium per 100 mL. High chromate concentrations were found in the liver, kidney, and stomach.[7]

LABORATORY

Elimination Enhancement

Following an ingestion of saturated solution of potassium dichromate by an adult hemodialysis removed about 5 mg of chromium after 5 hours. The patient was treated for 5 hours daily for 7 days. The serum chromium fell from initial values of 1.6 mg/L (normal 0.06 to 0.54 μg/L) to 0.86 mg/L. Urine chromium values fell from 2.4 mg/L (normal value 0.08 to 2.10 μg/L) to 0.88 mg/L. The patient recovered.[8]

BAL (dimercaprol), ascorbic acid, folic acid, and edetic acid have not been shown to have any effective role in treatment.[6]

Antidotes

Nasogastric lavage with an ascorbic acid solution and large IV doses of ascorbic acid may effectively reduce hexavalent chromium to the less toxic trivalent state.[9] IV *N*-acetylcysteine (140 mg/kg every 4 hours, continued for 48 hours) and hemodialysis was associated with hepatic and renal improvement in an adult who ingested sodium dichromate.[10]

Supportive Care

Monitor renal and hepatic function. Administer oxygen as required for respiratory compromise.

REFERENCES—DICHROMATE

1. Michie CA, Hayhurst M, Knobel GJ, Stokol JM, Hensley B. Poisoning with a traditional remedy containing potassium dichromate. Hum Exp Toxicol 1991;10:129–131.
2. Cooper P. Poisoning by drugs and chemicals. 3rd ed. London: Alchemist, 1974, pp. 180–181.
3. Castera J, Bourdais A, Bonsom R et al. Intoxication aigue par ingestion massive de bichromate de potassium. Guerison Bull Med Leg Toxic Med 1969;12:134–143.
4. Banner W, Frank J, Iserson K et al. Coagulopathy following ingestion of potassium dichromate. Vet Hum Toxicol 1982;24:288 (abstract).
5. Sharma BK, Singhal PC, Chugh KS. Intravascular hemolysis and acute renal failure following potassium dichromate poisoning. Postgrad Med J 1978;54:414–415.
6. Ellis EN, Brouhard BN, Lynch RE et al. Effects of hemodialysis and dimercaprol in acute dichromate poisoning. J Toxicol Clin Toxicol 1982;19:249–258.
7. Grusz-Harday E. Acute lethal potassium dichromate poisoning. Bull Int Assoc Forensic Toxicol 1974;10(1):7.
8. Sanz P, Nogue S, Munne P, Torra R, Marques F. Acute potassium dichromate poisoning. Hum Exp Toxicol 1990;10:228–229.
9. Meert KL, Ellis J, Aronow R, Perrin E. Acute ammonium dichromate poisoning. Ann Emerg Med 1994;24:748–750.
10. Vassallo S, Howland MA. Severe dichromate poisoning: survival after therapy with IV N-acetylcysteine and hemodialysis. Vet Hum Toxicol 1988;30:347.

COBALT—HARD METAL LUNG DISEASE

Hard metal is an alloy consisting of mainly tungsten carbide (75 to 95%) and cobalt (5 to 25%) as a matrix and others that may be added such as titanium, nickel, chromium, niobium, vanadium, and tantalum. Hard metal is 90 to 95% as hard as diamond. Tungsten carbide has been shown to be inert and cobalt is considered to be the cause of the lung damage.[1–3]

Hard metal interstitial lung disease (HMILD) was first described in 1940, and hard metal occupational asthma (HMOA) in 1967. Both disorders are considered to be idiopathic reactions to the cobalt component of hard metal, although nickel may play a part in HMOA. Workers with HMOA have had positive provocation inhalation tests with cobalt and may have immunoglobulin-E antibodies specific for cobalt.

CLINICAL PRESENTATION

Hard metal lung disease is an occupational pulmonary disease generally found in patients who work as grinders of material made from tungsten carbide.[4] It can occur as an interstitial lung disease with all the classical signs of pulmonary fibrosis and an obstructive airway syndrome.[4,5] Hard metal lung disease often starts as an allergic alveolitis that can progress to severe fibrosis if the exposure is not stopped. Hard metal asthma may be an IgE-antibody–mediated syndrome due to cobalt reactivity.[6] Nickel, as well as cobalt, sensitivity may play a role in hard metal asthma.[7] Review of occupational reports suggests that a woman can have a successful pregnancy despite severe pulmonary dysfunction secondary to hard metal lung disease.[8]

Pathology

Both the obstructive and the interstitial syndromes in hard metal disease are responses to the inhalation of cobalt.[6] Histologic abnormalities in subjects chronically exposed to inhalation of dust containing cobalt include an interstitial pneumonitis (fibrosing alveolitis) with infiltrates of lymphocytes, macrophages, plasma cell, and eosinophils. A more characteristic feature is the presence of many multinucleated giant cells of macrophage/monocyte origin within the alveoli and also in bronchoalveolar lavage flush

(Table 67–17). Cobalt induced by disease is more likely to occur when the threshold limit value for cobalt (0.05 mg/m^3) is exceeded.[6] Death may occur in cor pulmonale or respiratory failure.

Cobalt Lung

Interstitial lung disease attributed to cobalt not alloyed to carbides of hard metals may induce cough, chest tightness, dyspnea, weight loss, a severe restrictive defect, and a markedly decreased diffusing capacity and may be accompanied by the presence of multiple multinucleated giant cells in the bronchoalveolar lavage.[9] This condition may show a rapidly fatal progression.[10]

Cobalt Cardiomyopathy

Industrial cobalt exposure may cause fatal cardiomyopathy in adults employed in the hard metal industry.[11,12] Few causes of sudden onset cardiomyopathy in previously healthy young men exist. This was also observed during the 1960s after a large number of beer drinkers in three countries consumed beer to which cobalt chloride or cobalt sulfate had been added to enhance foaming. These cases had an abrupt onset of left and then right heart failure. Overall mortality approached 50%.[2] Similar findings leading to rapid fatalities were observed in young children who had swallowed cobalt chloride.[13]

Cancer

There are some data that suggest that metallic cobalt and certain cobalt compounds (e.g., cobalt oxide, sulfide, chloride, acetate and naphthenate) are probable chemical carcinogens and that such exposure has been associated with lung cancer.[14]

LABORATORY

Roentgenographic findings in the lung fields may reveal bilateral linear shadows, a reticulonodular pattern, or a nodular pattern. Respiratory function tests may show evidence of restrictive lung disease and a decrease in diffusion capacity of carbon monoxide D_2CO.[15]

An 11-year-old child swallowed two magnets consisting of 40% cobalt.[16] Vomiting, weight loss, polycythemia, thyromegaly, metabolic acidosis and cardiomyopathy (gallup rhythm), and an abdominal radiograph showing an opaque mass in the stomach were accompanied by a serum cobalt value of 4.1 mEq/dL (normal 0.35 to 1.7 mcg/dL) and a urine cobalt value of 1700 mcg/L (normal 1 to 7 mcg/L). Clinical improvement followed chelation with $CaNa_2EDTA$ 50 mg/kg/day for 5 days.[8] A cobalt concentrate of 0.5 mg/m^3 in air corresponds to 25 μg/liter of cobalt in whole blood and 300 μg/liter of cobalt in the urine.[17]

TREATMENT

Interruption of exposure usually leads to a rapid regression of complaints and a partial improvement of lung function.[9] Treatment is otherwise symptomatic and supportive.

REFERENCES—COBALT

1. Sjogren I, Hillerdal G, Andersson A, Zetterstron O. Hard metal lung disease importance of cobalt in coolants. Thorax 1980;35:653–659.
2. Coates EO, Watson JHL. Diffuse interstitial lung disease in tungsten carbide workers. Ann Intern Med 1971;75:706–711.
3. Harding H. Notes on the toxicology of cobalt metal. Br J Ind Med 1950;276:78.
4. Kusaka Y, Yokoyama K, Sera Y, Yamamoto S, Sone S, Kyono H et al. Respiratory disease in hard metal workers: an occupational hygiene study in a factor. Br J Ind Med 1986;43: 474–485.
5. Shirakawa T, Kugaka Y, Fujimura N, Goto S, Kato M, Heki S et al. Occupational asthma from cobalt sensitivity to workers exposed to hard metal dust. Chest 1989;95:29–37.
6. Cugell DW, Morgan WKC, Perkins DG, Rubin A. The respiratory effects of cobalt. Arch Intern Med 1990;150:177–183.
7. Shirakawa T, Kusaka Y, Fujimura N, Kato M, Heki S, Morimoto K. Hard metal asthma: cross immunological and respiratory reactivity between cobalt and nickel? Arch Intern Med 1990;150:177–183.
8. Ratto D, Balmes J, Boylen T, Sharma OP. Pregnancy in a woman with severe pulmonary fibrosis secondary to hard metal disease. Chest 1988;93:663–664.
9. Demedts M, Gheysens B, Nagels J, Verbeken E, Lawerryns J, Van den Eeckhout A et al. Am Rev Respir Dis 1984;130: 1330–1335.
10. Nemery B, Nagels J, Verbeken E, Dinsdale D, De Medis M. Rapidly fatal progression of cobalt lung in a diamond polisher. Am Rev Respir Dis 1990;141:1373–1378.
11. Barborik M, Duslek J. Cardiomyopathy accompanying industrial cobalt exposure. Br Heart J 1972;34:113–116.
12. Jarius JQ, Mammond E, Meier R, Robinson C. Cobalt cardiomyopathy. A report of two cases from mineral assay laboratories and a review of the literature. J Occup Med 1992; 34:620–626.
13. Jacobziner H, Raybin MW. Accidental cobalt poisoning. Arch Pediatr 1961;78:200–205.
14. Jensen AA, Tuchsen F. Cobalt exposure and cancer risk. Crit Rev Toxicol 1990;20(6):427–438.
15. Austenfeld JL, Colby TV. Recognizing lung diseases induced by hard metal exposure. J Respir Dis 1989;10:65–75.
16. Henretig F, Joffe M, Baffa G, Burns R, Bingham P, Burg F et al. Elemental cobalt toxicity and effects of chelation therapy. Vet Hum Toxicol 1988;30:372.
17. Beyersmann D, Hartwig A. The genetic toxicology of cobalt. Toxicol Appl Pharmacol 1992;115:132–145.

COPPER

Renal failure and death may follow ingestion of as little as 1 g of copper sulfate.[1] Fatal poisoning is rare. It may be a factor in the development of childhood cirrhosis.[2,3]

TOXICOKINETICS

Absorption

The current estimated safe and adequate daily dietary intake (ESADDI) range from copper is 2 to 3 mg/day.[4] The usual intake of copper in the United States population is considerably less than 2 mg/d and appear to average 1 mg/d.[5] A controlled study of copper balance suggests that 0.8 mg of copper/day may be close to the copper requirement for young adults.[6]

Metabolism

A review of copper metabolism is depicted in Fig. 67–3.[7,8] Copper is present in serum in two different forms: the copper

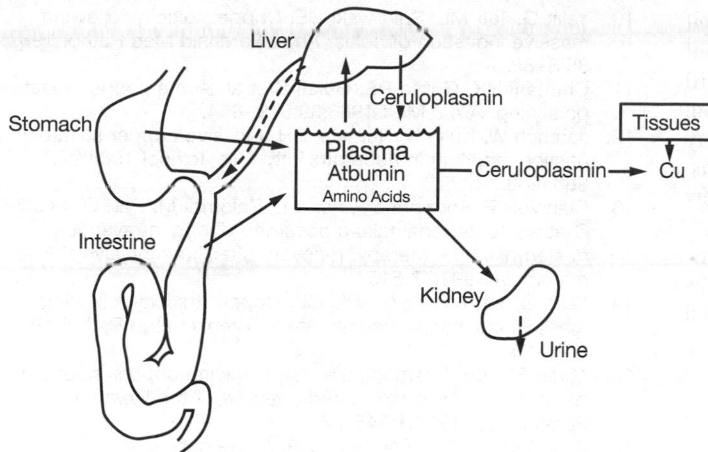

Figure 67–3 Basic aspects of mammalian copper metabolism. Dietary copper is absorbed from stomach and small intestine. In human adults the RDA is ~2.5 mg/day. Some copper in intestinal contents is biliary and serves as the major excretory route. Normally only small quantities of copper are lost in urine, but this increases during aminoaciduria. Copper is transported in portal plasma, bound principally to albumin and possibly as amino acid complexes. Hepatic uptake occurs via a saturable transport process. Systemic transport of copper from liver is primarily as ceruloplasmin, which appears to donate copper to tissues. Circulating level of ceruloplasmin increases in response to various stresses and disease-related processes. (Adapted from Cousins RJ. Physiol Rev 1985;65:238–309.)

that reacts directly with the copper colorimetric reagent, sodium diethyldithiocarbamate, is loosely bound to serum albumin. It is this function that is cytotoxic. This small fraction is concerned with the transportation of copper from the gastrointestinal tract to the tissues, and from one tissue to another. The larger fraction of serum copper is tightly bound to the serum copper enzyme ceruloplasmin. The copper in the enzyme does not react directly with carbonate.[8] About 7% of copper in the series is loosely bound to albumin, and 93% is bound to the ceruloplasmin enzyme. The mean value for total serum copper is 114 μg/100 mL, and for the direct-reacting copper, 7 μg/mL. The mean value of ceruloplasmin is 30 mg/100 mL. Erythrocytes contain 89 μg of copper per 100 mL of packed cells. The urine normally contains only traces of copper (5 to 25 μg/day).[8]

Total body copper content is 150 mg. The average serum copper level in an adult male is 17.31 μmol/L (1.1 mg/L). The half-life of copper in healthy individuals is about 26 days. System bioavailability of edible copper (5 mg/day) is 30%. The apparent volume of distribution of copper is 1.95 L/kg, and its clearance is 0.036 mL/min/kg. Copper (metallic and/or its azide salt) may be absorbed from the skin.[9] The copper content in a normal adult's liver is 18 to 45 ng/g dry weight. About 0.1 to 1.3 ng of copper is excreted through the bile daily and lost in the feces. When the concentration of hepatic copper is greater than 50 mg/d dry weight, liver cell necrosis, with release of copper into the serum, can occur. If a large amount of copper is suddenly released from the liver, it is taken up by erythrocytes. A hemolytic crisis may occur.[10] Massive ingestion of copper led to a fatality with a hepatic copper content of 1160 μg/g.[10] A 47-year-old man ingested 20 to 30 mL of a copper sulfate solution in 2½ days after profound vomiting, abdominal pain, diarrhea, and jaundice. The hepatic liver copper concentration was 61 μg/g unit weight.

CLINICAL PRESENTATION[11,12]

An inadvertent infusion in an adult of 33.7 g of deferoxamine in 18 hours (39 mg/kg/hour) led to headache, somnolence, nausea and vomiting, and an acute renal failure that responded to hemodialysis.[13]

Kidney

Copper causes a focal necrosis of the proximal tubule. The Fanconi syndrome–tubular proteinuria, generalized amino aciduria, phosphaturia, uricosuria, and hypercalciuria may result from the direct toxic effect of copper or the associated hemolysis.[14] Hemoglobinemia has been observed after ingestion of about 175 g of copper sulfate.[15]

Systemic Effects

The symptom complex of myalgia, abdominal pain, diarrhea, acidosis, pancreatitis, methemoglobin formation, and hemolysis is indicative of copper intoxication.[16]

Chronic Effects

When airborne the dusts of inorganic copper salts have low toxicity. Vineyard sprayer's lung disease has been associated with airborne copper sulfate. This is a histiocytic granulomatous lung and liver disease occurring in individuals exposed to copper sulfate spray for 2 to 15 years.[17] A syndrome of intravenous copper intoxication due to copper released from copper tubing during hemodialysis includes symptoms of nausea, vomiting, abdominal pain, diarrhea, anxiety, and depression. Plasma copper levels are over 150 μg/dL.[17]

Skin

Chronic copper poisoning has occurred after repeated application of a copper-containing topical cream to eczematous skin. The application of copper crystals to granulomatous tissue with burns has resulted in chronic poisoning with skin darkening.[18] Wounds sustained after copper azide explosions can propel metallic copper into the dermis. The most common form of skin contamination by copper is the production of green hair discoloration. The green hue is produced by an increased absorption of copper into the hair from copper algicidal chemicals used in swimming pools.[19]

Nigeria—"Spiritual Water"

Overdosage of copper salts is common in developing countries because of its wide use in various traditional preparations. Poisoning is due to the ingestion of "spiritual green water" following distribution to members of spiritual churches. The amount of copper sulfate ingested is about 10 to 20 g, a lethal dose. Within a few hours of ingestion, greenish vomiting and abdominal pain are seen. Anuria may supervene within 24 hours. Flapping tremor, toxic psychosis, hemolytic anemia, and jaundice may follow within a few days. Hepatic and renal failure precede death within 7 days. Patients appear to die within a few days of hemodialysis. Analysis of water has revealed copper sulfate concentrations of 100 to 150 g/L. Similar cases have occurred in the United States.[20]

LABORATORY

The serum concentration of copper ranges from 70 to 155 μg/dL. Patients with metal fume fever following exposure to the copper metal exhibit serum copper levels over 160 μg/dL.

Blood Levels

Ingestion of 20 to 30 mL of copper sulfate led to a blood copper level of 1.25 μg/mL in a patient who died.[21] Plasma copper concentration in a series of fatal cases involving copper poisoning ranged from 9.8 to 46 mg/L.[22] Ingestion of a copper sulfate solution led to death with a blood copper level of 25 μg/mL.[3,23]

TREATMENT

Removal of copper by dialysis may be useful in the early stages of poisoning when the metal is still present in the circulation as free copper.[24] The copper-chelating drug tetrathiomolybdate used in Wilson's disease has been associated with pancytopenia. Its use has not been reported in copper poisoning.[25] Ingestion of 10 to 20 g of copper sulfate is usually lethal. Hemodialysis has not prevented death in such cases.[20,26]

REFERENCES—COPPER

1. Lamont DL, Duflou JALC. Copper sulfate; not a harmless chemical. Am J Forensic Med Pathol 1988;9:226–227.
2. Muhlendahl K, Lange H. Copper and childhood cirrhosis. Lancet 1994;344:1515–1516.
3. Scheinberg IM, Sternlieb N. Is non-Indian childhood cirrhosis caused by excess dietary copper? Lancet 1994;344:1002–1004.
4. Committee on Dietary Allowances, Food and Nutrition Board, National Research Council. Recommended dietary allowances. 9th Ed. Washington, DC: National Academic Press, 1980.
5. Turnlund JR. Copper nutriture, bioavailability and the influence of dietary factors. J Am Diet Assoc 1988;88:303–310.
6. Turnlund JR, Keen CL, Smith RG. Copper status and urinary and salivary copper in young men at three levels of dietary copper. Am J Clin Nutr 1990;51:658–664.
7. Cousins RJ. Absorption, transport and hepatic metabolism of copper and zinc: Special reference to metallothionein and ceruloplasmin. Physiol Rev 1985;65:238–300.
8. Cartwright GE, Wintrobe MM. Copper metabolism in normal subjects. Am J Clin Nutr 1964;14:222–232.
9. Bentur Y, McGuigan M, Spielberg AP. An unusual skin exposure to copper: clinical and pharmacokinetic evaluation. Clin Toxicol 1988;26:371–380.
10. Yelin G, Taff ML, Sadowski GE. Copper toxicity following massive ingestion of coins. Am J Forensic Med Pathol 1987; 8:78–85.
11. Chuttani HK, Gupta PS, Gulati S et al. Acute copper sulfate poisoning. Am J Med 1965;39:849–854.
12. Jantsch W, Kulig K, Rumack BH. Massive copper sulfate ingestion resulting in hepatotoxicity. Clin Toxicol 1984;22: 585–588.
13. Cianciulli P, Sorrentino F, Forte L, Palombi M, Paili G, Meloni C et al. Acute renal failure occurring during intravenous desferrioxamine therapy: recovery after haemodialysis. Haematologia 1992;77:515.
14. Yelin G, Taff ML, Sadowski GE. Copper toxicity following massive ingestion of coins. Am J Forensic Med Pathol 1987; 8:78–85.
15. Mittal SR. Oxyhaemoglobinemia following copper sulphate poisoning. A case report and a review of the literature. Forensic Sci 1972;1:245–248.
16. Klein WJ Jr, Metz EN, Price AR. Acute copper intoxication. A hazard of hemodialysis. Arch Intern Med 1972;129: 580–582.
17. Bluhm RE, Welch L, Branch RA. Increased blood and urine copper after residential exposure to copper naphthenate. Clin Toxicol 1992;30:99–108.
18. Holgzman NA, Elliott DA, Heller PH. Copper intoxication: report of a case with observations on ceruloplasmin. N Engl J Med 1966;275:347–352.
19. Burnett JW. Copper. Cutis 189;43:322.
20. Akintonwa A, Mabadeje AFB, Odutola TA. Fatal poisonings by copper sulfate ingested from "spiritual water." Vet Hum Toxicol 1989;31:453–454.
21. Farmer JG. A fatality following copper sulphate ingestion. Bull Int Assoc Forensic Toxicol 1981;16(2):22–23.
22. Hla KK, House IM, Henry JA. Toxicity from ingestion of cupramonium carbonate. Proc Eur Assoc Pois Cont Centers Toxicol 1988; p. 94.
23. Gulliver GJM. A fatal copper sulphate poisoning. Bull Int Assoc Forensic Toxicol 1991;21(1):19–20.
24. Chugh KS, Sharma BK, Singhal PC, Das KC, Dotta BN. Acute renal failure following copper sulphate intoxication. Postgrad Med J 1977;53:18–23.
25. Harpe PL, Walshe JM. Reversible pancytopenia secondary to treatment with tetrathiomolybdate. Br J Haematol 1986;6: 851–853.
26. Dash SC. Copper sulphate poisoning and acute renal failure. Int J Artif Organs 1989;12:610.

GERMANIUM

Germanium is an element with chemical properties similar to those of silicon, tin, arsenic (to which it lies next in the periodic system), and antimony. The daily intake by man is about 1 mg, in foods such as oats and barley. It is rapidly absorbed in the gastrointestinal tract and excreted mainly through the kidneys. A 43-year-old female developed severe and fatal lactic acidosis in association with abuse of germanium.[1]

Germanium (atomic number 32; atomic weight 72.59) is a trace metal used industrially because of its semiconductive ratio.[2] Germanium-containing organic molecules are under investigation for their ability to modulate immune responses.[3]

Its role in man is unknown. In Japan,[2,4,5] the United Kingdom,[5] the United States,[6], and the Netherlands,[7] it has been used as a health food supplement. In Japan it has led to the death of two patients.[3] When used in doses of 50 to 250 mg/d for several months or longer, germanium dioxide has been associated with severe renal dysfunction.[2,4,7,8] Germanium may be found in the hair and nails.[4] A

43-year-old female ingested 2250 mg germanium lactate-citrate (40 mg germanium) per day and developed a fatal lactic acidosis with acute renal and hepatic failure.[1,8]

REFERENCES—GERMANIUM

1. Krapf R, Schaffner T, Hen PX. Abuse of germanium associated with lactic acidosis. Nephron 1992;62:351–356.
2. Sanai T, Okuda S, Onoyama K, Oochi N, Oh Y, Kobayashi K et al. Germanium dioxide-induced nephropathy: a new type of renal disease. Nephron 1990;54:56–60.
3. St. Georgieu V. New synthetic immunodilating agents. Trends Pharmaceut Sci 1988;9:446–451.
4. Okada K, Okagawa K, Kawakani K, Kuroda Y, Morizumi K, Sato H et al. Renal failure caused by long-term use of a germanium preparation as an elixir. Clin Nephrol 1989;31:219–224.
5. Germanium danger. Lancet 1989;2:755 (editorial).
6. Stopping toxic tablets. FDA Consumer 1989;23(10):34–35.
7. Van der Spoel JI, Stricker BHC, Esseveld MR, Schipper MEI. Dangers of dietary germanium supplements. Lancet 1990; 336:117.
8. Taleuchi A, Yoshizawa N, Oshina S, Kubata T, Oshikawa Y, Akashi Y et al. Nephrotoxicity of germanium compounds. Report of a case and review of the literature. Nephron 1992;60:436–442.

GOLD

All antirheumatic gold compounds contain gold in the gold (I) oxidation state. The adverse effect of gold-containing antirheumatics appear to be caused by gold III, an oxidation product of gold I.[1]

CLINICAL PRESENTATION

A 53-year-old male was accidentally injected with an intramuscular dose of 450 mg of sodium aurothiomalate. Palpebral edema and a rash were observed within 30 minutes. The gold blood levels reach 2970 μg/dL without significant toxicity. The patient was treated with BAL and recovered.[2]

Gold Lung

Gold lung is a rare toxic side effect of gold therapy that may begin after 300 to 1000 mg total gold dose has been administered. Dyspnea appears suddenly over a period of 2 to 10 days. The chest x-ray shows a diffuse bilateral pulmonary shading.[3] A moderate eosinophilia may be present. There is no clubbing of the fingers.[4] Lymphocyte transformation studies may suggest a hypersensitivity to gold.[5] The prognosis is good after simple withdrawal of gold.[4] Lung function tests show a restrictive defect with a reduced transfer factor for carbon monoxide. Impairment of lung function may be permanent.[6]

Nitritoid Reaction

The nitritoid reaction, a side effect of treatment with sodium aurothiomalate, consists of a brief episode of facial flushing, nausea, dizziness, and occasionally hypotension. It occurs several minutes after an intramuscular injection and appears unpredictably on the first week after gold treatments are begun. It is rarely seen. The nitritoid reaction may be more common if an angiotensin-converting-enzyme inhibitor is added to the regimen of gold therapy.[7]

Gastrointestinal

Gold-induced enterocolitis may follow treatment with either injected or orally administered gold and may involve any segment of the gastrointestinal tract.[8] Presenting symptoms may include fever, nausea, vomiting, and abdominal cramps with diarrhea. This condition may end fatally. Treatment consists of immediate discontinuation of gold. A trial of oral cromolyn may be useful.[9]

Hepatic

Intrahepatic cholestasis with eosinophilia may be observed after gold injections. The condition is self-limiting. On withdrawal of gold therapy, liver function tests returned to normal in about 3 months.[6,10]

Blood

Idiosyncratic agranulocytosis and aplastic anemia have been reported following gold therapy. Spontaneous neutrophil recovery may take 15 to 30 days after drug withdrawal. Filgastrin, 10 μcg/day (G-CSF) may enhance myeloid recovery.[11]

Lymphadenopathy

Enlarged regional lymph nodes following prolonged gold therapy may contain deposits of elemental gold.[12,13]

Renal

Proteinuria occurs in 2 to 20% of patients treated with injected gold and may be sufficiently severe to cause the nephrotic syndrome in 10 to 30% of those affected.[6] Renal biopsy may disclose a membranous glomerulonephritis.[14,15] The proteinuria usually resolves when the drug is stopped. Renal function does not deteriorate.[14,15] Corticosteroids are generally unnecessary.

Patients with an impaired sulfoxidation ability (decreased ability to oxidize sulfhydryl-containing compounds) may be predisposed to sodium aurothiomalate toxicity.[16]

REFERENCES—GOLD

1. Gleichman E, Kubicka-Murangi M, Kind P, Goldermann P, Goertz G et al. Insights into the mechanism of gold action provided by immunotoxicology: biooxidation of gold (I) to gold (III) detected from sensitized T-cells. Rheumatol Int 1991;11:219–220.
2. Barelli A, Calimici A, Pala F. Gold salts acute poisoning: a case report. Vet Hum Toxicol 1987;29(Suppl 2):108–110.
3. Gortenuti G, Parrinello A, Vicentini D. Diffuse pulmonary changes caused by gold salt therapy. Report of a case. Diagn Imag Clin Med 1985;54:298–303.
4. Richard AM. Gold lung. New Zeal Med J 1982;2:897–898.
5. McFadden RG, Traher LJ, Thompson JM. Gold-naproxen pneumonitis. A toxic drug interaction? Chest 1989;96:216–218.
6. Cohen MAH. Adverse reactions to gold compounds. Adverse Drug React Acute Poison Rev 1988;4:163–178.

7. Healey LA, Baches MB. Nitritoid reactions and angiotensin-converting-enzyme inhibitor. N Engl J Med 1989;326:763.
8. Jackson CW, Habouli NY, Whorwell PJ, Schofield PF. Gold-induced enterocolitis. Gut 1986;27:452–456.
9. Martin DM, Goldman JA, Gillian J, Nasrallah SM. Gold-induced eosinophilic enterocolitis: response to oral cromolyn sodium. Gastroenterology 1981;80:1567–1570.
10. Farre JM, Peree T, Hautefemille P, Tonnel F, Columbee JF et al. Cholestasis and pneumonitis induced by gold therapy. Clin Rheumatol 1989;8:538–540.
11. Brown SL, Hill ER. G-CSF in gold-induced aplastic anemia. Ann Rheum Dis 1994;53:213.
12. Rollins SO, Craig JP. Gold-associated lymphadenopathy in a patient with rheumatoid arthritis. Arch Pathol Lab Med 1991;115:175–177.
13. Spark RP. Cold-associated lymphadenopathy in a patient with rheumatoid arthritis. Arch Pathol Lab Med 1991;115: 861–862.
14. Hall CL. The natural coma of gold nephropathy. Br Med J 1988;296:293.
15. Hall CL, Fothergill NJ, Blackwell MM, Harrison PR, MacKenzie JC, Maciver AG. The natural course of gold nephropathy: long term study of 21 patients. Br Med J 1987;295:745–748.
16. Madhok P, Capell HA, Waring R. Does sulphoxidation state predict gold toxicity in rheumatoid arthritis? Br Med J 1987; 294:483.

IRON

Mills and Curry have comprehensively surveyed the current status of iron intoxication.[1] There has been an annual average of 22,000 reported exposures to medications containing iron over the last 3 years. Most exposures involve children less than 6 years of age who have ingested pediatric multivitamin preparations. Most of these patients remain asymptomatic or develop minimal toxicity. Concentrated iron supplement overdoses more often result in serious sequelae and may be fatal. Patients die at any stage of iron poisoning and can present to the emergency department at any stage. If a patient does not develop symptoms within 6 hours after ingestion, it is unlikely that iron toxicity will develop.

FORMULATIONS

Clinical toxicity is expected following an ingestion of at least 20 mg/kg of elemental iron. The amount of elemental iron in ferrous fumarate is 33%, in ferrous chloride 28%, ferrous sulfate (the most common source) 20%, ferrous chloride 20%, and ferrous gluconate 12%. Ingestion of as few as 5 or 6 tablets of a high-potency preparation could be fatal for a 10 kg (22 lb) child.[2]

CHEWABLE VITAMINS WITH IRON

The overdose of chewable vitamins with iron remains one of the most commonly encountered potential poisonings in children. Doses of 10 mg/kg of elemental iron in the form of children's chewable vitamins with iron, often considered to be a nontoxic dose, may produce serum iron concentrations close to baseline total iron-binding capacities (TIBCs).[3]

The kinetics of iron absorption after ingestion of chewable vitamins are not fully understood. However, one controlled study in human volunteers who were administered 6 mg elemental iron/kg body weight as chewable multivitamins with iron (MVI) showed that iron is very well absorbed from chewable MVI.[4] Chewable vitamins may enhance iron absorption so that "low" doses could cause systemic effects. There is little evidence to support the use of abdominal radiographs to identify iron remaining in the gastrointestinal tract following an overdose of chewable multivitamins with iron.[5]

Animal studies suggest four features of severe iron intoxication in dogs. First, there are decreases in cardiac output and mean arterial pressure that occur despite vigorous fluid resuscitation. Second, there is a fall in heart rate that is at least partially responsible for the fall in CO. Third, large quantities of IV fluid are required for maintenance of intravascular volume status. Fourth, metabolic acidosis occurs and persists in the face of unchanged oxygen consumption, suggesting that this acidosis is due to effects of iron intoxication that are separate from the hemodynamic alterations.[6]

CLINICAL PRESENTATION

Stages

I. Begins immediately postingestion. Vomiting, diarrhea, abdominal pain, hypotension, pallor, lethargy, metabolic acidosis, leukocytosis,and hyperglycemia may be observed.
II. Begins in 6 to 24 hours and lasts 12 to 24 hours. Signs of hypovolemia, lethargy, hypotension, and metabolic acidosis. Serum iron level may not have peaked.
III. Begins 12 to 24 hours after ingestion. Multiple organ failures (gastrointestinal, central nervous system, cardiovascular system, hepatorenal, metabolic coagulopathies, hypoglycemia). Fulminant hepatic failure is usually associated with a fatal outcome.
IV. Begins in 4 to 6 weeks. Gastric scarring, pyloric obstruction.

Gastrointestinal Tract

The corrosive effects of iron (mucosal irritation, hemorrhagic gastritis, ulceration, bleeding, ischemia, infarction, and perforation) can produce significant gastrointestinal symptoms even at doses far below those generally considered to cause systemic toxicity.

Coagulopathy

Depression of activities of factors V, VII, IX, and X and fibrinogen are typical abnormalities. The prothrombin time and partial thromboplastic time are increased. The coagulopathy may be biphasic with the initial phase occurring within hours of the overdose. It is reversible and serum iron dependent.[7,8] The second, a later phase, is characterized by hepatotoxicity with resultant coagulopathy and usually occurs at least 24 hours after ingestion. The coagulopathy is reversible and is dependent on the serum iron concentration.

LABORATORY

Serum Levels

Normal serum iron levels are 50 to 150 µg/dL. Peak serum iron levels are observed at about 4 hours after ingestion. Iron toxicity is not excluded by serum levels less than 350 μg/dL. The total iron-binding capacity (TIBC) (normal 300 to 435 μg/dL) becomes elevated in the presence of high serum iron concentrations or deferoxamine.[11] A serum iron level less than TIBC does not rule out acute iron poisoning. Fewer than 10% of patients with serum iron levels below 500 μg/dL will develop cardiovascular collapse or coma.

Deferoxamine, by providing iron binding sites, may cause falsely elevated measurements of TIBC.[9] The unreliability of the TIBC as a decision-making factor in the initiation of deferoxamine therapy may be due to a laboratory aberration in cases of iron poisoning.[10] Even though the serum iron may rise above 300 μg/dL, and there may be clinical toxicity, this level may not exceed the TIBC, which appears to rise by an unknown mechanism.[11]

A 22-month-old child poisoned with ferrous sulfate tablets was found to have a serum iron concentration of 16,700 μg/dL. Following DFO and intensive supportive therapy, the child survived.[12]

For chewable vitamins the 2-hour serum iron levels are too early to predict peak levels and to identify the potential for systemic toxicity.[13] The value of serum iron levels after chewable multivitamin ingestion remains to be established.

Abdominal X-rays

Abdominal x-rays can confirm the diagnosis of iron poisoning when positive, but cannot exclude it if negative. Although chewable vitamins with iron are radiopaque, visualization of these tablets clinically is unlikely (E. P. Krenzelok, personal communication).

Blood

Chyka and Butler[14] reviewed 128 cases of iron poisoning and were unable to confirm that vomiting, diarrhea, leukocytosis, hyperglycemia, and radiopacities alone indicated a serum iron concentration in excess of 300 μg/dL (54 μmol/L). At concentrations greater than 500 μg/dL (90 μmol/L) coma or the combination of leukocytosis, radiopacities, and an increased anion gap were commonly observed. Sole reliance on observations of vomiting, diarrhea, leukocytosis, hyperglycemia, and radiopacities may not be useful as screening tests to detect patients with iron poisoning. The absence of all these signs or symptoms is likely to be associated with serum concentrations less than 500 μg/dL. When coma, radiopacities, leukocytosis, and an elevated anion gap are present in suspected iron poisoning, further evaluation is warranted. The wide range of serum iron values from groups with and without cardiovascular symptoms make interpretation of individual values difficult. The presence of a serum iron level greater than the total iron-binding capacity was not associated with clinical symptoms or the occurrence of vin-rose urine after deferoxamine. Glucose levels over 150 mg/dL and white blood cell counts over 15,000 do not indicate iron levels over 300 mcg/dL.

TREATMENT

1. Do a complete history and physical examination.
2. Ensure adequate airway, ventilation, and circulation.
3. Perform a gastric lavage in patients after an intentional ingestion, a positive KUB radiography, and when the ingestion elemental iron content exceeds 20 mg/kg. Do not use sodium bicarbonate or phosphosoda.
4. Observation alone is usually sufficient when children have ingested multivitamins, the amount of elemental iron ingested is less than 20 mg/kg and the KUB radiograph is negative.
5. In symptomatic patients give a bolus of 20 mL/kg of isotonic normal saline.
6. Order serum iron levels, creatinine, electrolytes, blood hemoglobin concentration, blood prothrombin time, baseline liver function tests, and arterial blood gases in seriously poisoned patients.
7. Activated charcoal is ineffective.
8. Oral magnesium preparations may reduce serum iron absorption.

The treatment of a seriously ill patient (unexplained alteration of mental status, bleeding, or hypotension) with suspected iron toxicity should be prompt (deferoxamine) and not await the return of a serum iron level.

Decontamination—Elimination Enhancement

Extracorporeal Management

Whole-bowel irrigation in the treatment of acute iron poisoning appears to be a safe, effective means of gastrointestinal decontamination in iron poisoning, but there have been no controlled studies confirming this.[15] Because iron has a well known, direct corrosive effect on the gastrointestinal mucosa, late presentation after an acute iron ingestion may lead to significant gastrointestinal damage. Caution is therefore advised with the use of whole-bowel irrigation in a patient who may have sustained mucosal damage. Major gastrointestinal dysfunctions, including ileus, bowel obstruction, perforation, or significant gastrointestinal hemorrhage, are contraindications to whole-bowel irrigation.[16] Serial abdominal radiographs may be useful in documenting the elimination of large numbers of iron tablets from the intestine.[17] There is a suggestion based on an animal study that continuous arteriovenous hemofiltration may be useful to remove iron in severe iron intoxication, especially in the presence of renal failure.[18]

Deferoxamine (Desferal)[19]

Vin-rose urine is an insensitive marker for significantly elevated serum iron levels or serious iron poisoning. The absence of vin-rose urine after DFO use does not rule out acute iron toxicity or the need for DFO therapy. A DFO challenge test is therefore not useful. Intravenous DFO is the preferred route for characteristic acute iron poisoning. The recommended dose level of deferoxamine mesylate is 15 mg/kg/hour by continuous intravenous infusion, although there are few controlled clinical studies to support this dose. Cheney and colleagues have successfully administered infusions of 25 mg/kg/hour for 12 hours/day for 3 days in an infant with iron levels of 2687 μmol/L (over 15,000 μg/dL).[20] Oral deferoxamine does not decrease the absorption of low doses of iron in man.[21]

Uses

Chelation therapy with deferoxamine mesylate (DFO: Desferal) is indicated in any of the following four situations:

1. All symptomatic patients exhibiting more than transient minor symptoms (e.g., more than one episode of emesis or passage of one soft stool).
2. Patients with evidence of lethargy, significant abdominal pain, hypovolemia, or acidosis.
3. Patients with positive abdominal radiograph results demonstrating multiple radiopacities. The great majority of these patients will go on to develop symptomatic iron poisoning.
4. Any symptomatic patient with a serum iron level greater than 300 to 350 µg/dL regardless of TIBC. Bosse[22] suggests that a conservative approach without deferoxamine therapy or challenge should be considered when serum iron levels are in the 300 to 500 µ/dL range in asymptomatic patients, as well as in those with self-limited, nonbloody emesis or diarrhea without other symptoms.

Deferoxamine, by providing iron-binding sites, may cause falsely elevated measurements of TIBC, which can be assumed erroneously to reflect the level of iron-binding proteins (e.g., transferrin, lactoferrin). This may lead to a premature cessation of deferoxamine therapy in acute iron intoxication.[23]

Other Uses

Deferoxamine may have a potential usefulness as an antiproliferative, antiinflammatory, and immunosuppressive agent. Deferoxamine inhibits T-lymphocyte proliferation and blocks DNA synthesis by inhibition of ribonucleotide reductase.[24]

Toxicokinetics

In man total body clearance of deferoxamine is 0.296 L/hr/kg. Renal clearance accounts for about one-third of total body clearance. Its elimination half-life ranges between 10 and 30 minutes. Deferoxamine is rapidly metabolized mainly in the plasma, probably by an enzyme belonging to the alpha globulins.[25]

Ferrioxamine

The iron-deferoxamine complex, ferrioxamine, is poorly absorbed from the gastrointestinal tract. Its volume of distribution is about 20% of body weight, which corresponds to the extracellular space. It is not degraded to any appreciable extent and is rapidly excreted unchanged in the urine. Its elimination half-life is about 5.9 hours, and its renal clearance is 516 to 1766 L/kg/hr.

Adverse Effects

Anaphylactic/Anaphylactoid Reactions

IgE-mediated anaphylaxis following deferoxamine seldom occurs. Bolus administration/rapid infusion of over 15 mg/kg/hr causes histamine release and hypotension, especially in the presence of hypovolemia.

Infectious

Yersinia enterocolitica septicemia after an iron overdose treated with deferoxamine may be due to an iron enteritis or an iron/deferoxamine-induced growth promotion.[27,28] There appears to be a relationship between iron-overload states and bacterial infections when on dialysis, with or without deferoxamine. Mucormycosis and pneumocystic infection may occur in iron-overdose patients treated with deferoxamine.[29,30]

Ocular/Auditory

Retrobulbar optic neuropathy; mild, high-frequency, sensorineural hearing loss; and cataracts have been described.[31]

Renal/Other Toxic Effects

Acute renal failure, renal impairment, thrombocytopenia, and growth retardation may be seen.[32,33]

Pulmonary

Four patients treated with IV deferoxamine at a dose of 15 mg/kg/hour for 5 to 92 hours for acute iron poisoning developed a fatal adult respiratory distress syndrome.[34,35] The authors caution that deferoxamine should not be given by infusion for more than 24 hours. This observation has been challenged since iron poisoning itself may cause pulmonary injury; deaths may have been due to inadequate or late treatment, the daily use of deferoxamine use (57 to 120 g over 65 to 90 hours), and greatly exceeding the normally recommended dose (about 6 g/24 hours). High-dose deferoxamine-associated pulmonary injury has been reported previously in patients with thalassemia and advanced malignancy. Deferoxamine-induced pulmonary injury may occur following administration of high doses. The mechanism could involve either deferoxamine-induced free-radical production or impaired catalase and heme synthesis with iron-induced oxidant danger. The maximum safe rate of administration of DFO has not been determined.

Pregnancy

A 4-year study of iron overdose and deferoxamine treatment in pregnancy has been conducted in the United Kingdom.[36] The study concludes that (a) iron overdose does not appear to be markedly fetotoxic; (b) first-trimester overdose is so rarely reported that even a large poison center is unlikely even to estimate its consequences reliably; and (c) there is no evidence that deferoxamine adversely affects the outcome of pregnancy, so it should not be withheld. More vigorous teratologic studies of deferoxamine and ferriosamine are required. An assessment of the fetal effects of iron overload is also required to weigh the relative teratogenic risk of iron intoxication when compared with chelation therapy.[37] To summarize: in iron overdose during pregnancy with clinical evidence of moderate to severe iron intoxication, deferoxamine therapy should be instituted.[38] Whole-bowel irriga-

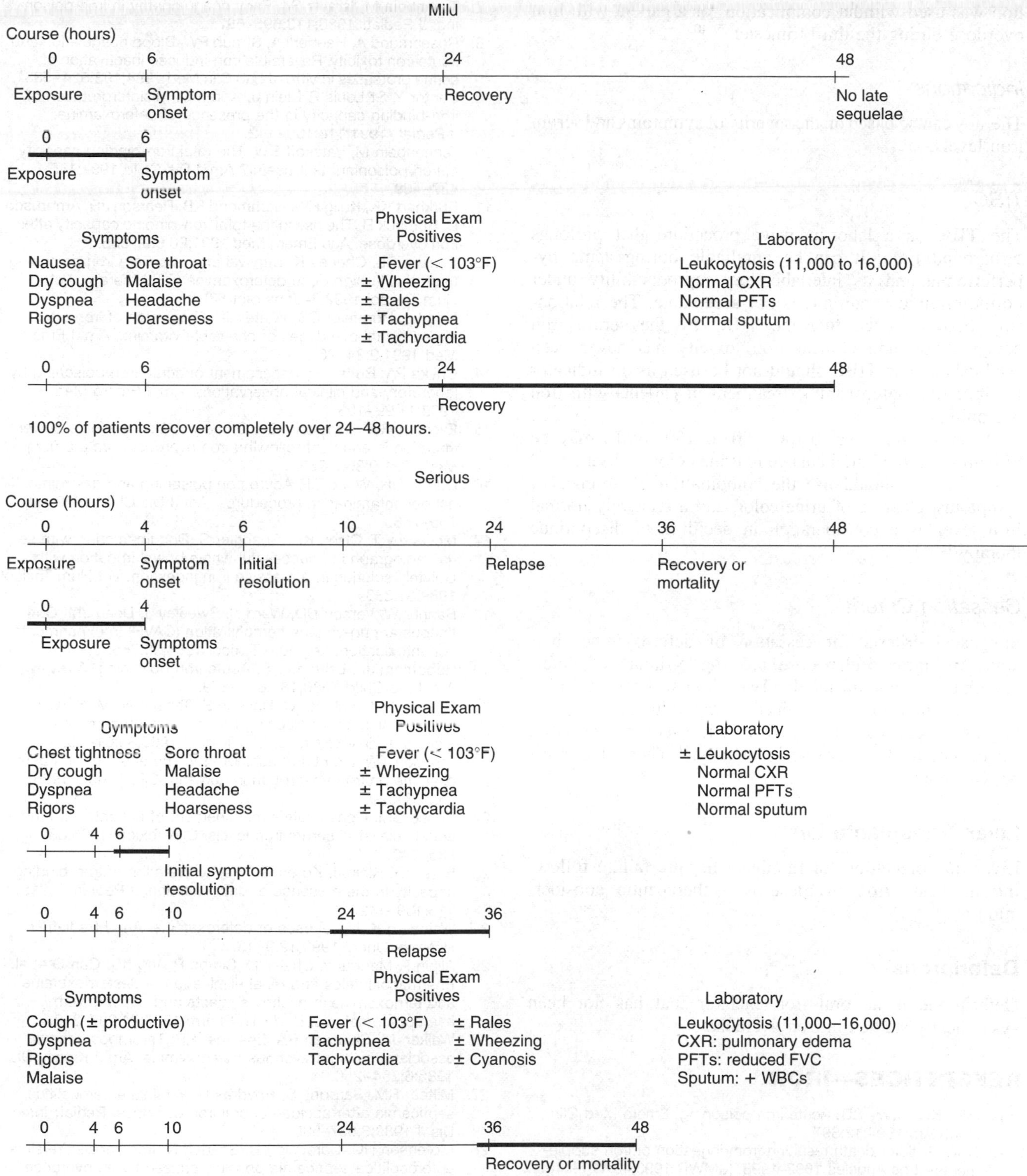

Patients usually recover symptomatically in 36–48 hours with CXR resolution over the next 14–45 days, but zinc chloride metal fume fever can progress to fatalities (usually in the first 5 days).

Diagnosis based on exposure history (HC smoke grenades or HC smoke pots, not smoke generators).

Treatment

Prevention-wear protective mask.

Careful observation-admit and observe for 36–48 hours in spite of mild symptoms.

Figure 67–4 Metal fume fever. (Adapted from Blount BW. Mil Med 1990;155:372–377.)

tion was used without complication for a patient with iron overdose during the third trimester.[39,40]

Indications

Therapy can be based on the severity of symptoms and serum iron levels.

TIBC

The TIBC is a labor-intensive procedure that prolongs turnaround time. It can be unreliable during acute hyperferremia and its interlaboratory reproducibility under normoferremic conditions is not acceptable. The relationship between exceeding the TIBC by the serum iron concentration and clinical iron toxicity has never been established. The TIBC should not be used as an indicator for initiating deferoxamine treatment in patients with iron poisoning.[10]

A serum iron level below 100 to 150 μg/dL may be of help when the initial change in urine color is absent.[41–43] The clinician should use the combination of absence of symptoms, clearing of urine color, and a relatively normal iron level as a consideration in deciding to discontinue therapy.[41–43]

Cessation Criteria

Suggested criteria for cessation of deferoxamine therapy: An intravascular dose (15 mg/kg/hour) of deferoxamine is administered. Two hours later a urine iron:creatinine ratio is obtained. If the value is over 12.5, the test is considered positive and is used as a criterion for cessation of deferoxamine therapy.[44] These data must be validated.

Liver Transplantation

Liver transplantation for fulminant hepatic failure following an acute iron overdose is a therapeutic consideration.[45]

Deferiprone

Deferiprone is an oral iron chelator that has not been systemically studied in iron overdose.

REFERENCES—IRON

1. Mills KC, Curry SC. Acute iron poisoning. Emerg Med Clin North Am 1994;12:397.
2. CDC. Toddler death resulting from ingestion of iron supplements—Los Angeles 1992–1993. MMWR 1993;42:111–113.
3. Ling LJ, Hornfeldt CS, Winter JP. Absorption of iron after experimental overdose of chewable vitamins. Am J Emerg Med 1991;9:24–26.
4. Linakis JG, Lacouture PG, Woolf AD. Iron absorption from chewable multivitamins with iron vs ferrous fumarate tablets. Vet Hum Toxicol 1989;21:342.
5. Everson GW, Oudjhane K, Young LW, Krenzelok EP. Effectiveness of abdominal radiographs in visualizing chewable iron supplements following overdose. Am J Emerg Med 1989;7:459–463.
6. Vernon DD, Banner W, Dean JM. Hemodynamic effects of experimental iron poisoning. Ann Emerg Med 1989;18: 863–866.
7. Tenenbein M, Israels SJ. Early coagulopathy in iron poisoning. J Pediatr 1988;113:695–697.
8. Rosenmund A, Haeberli A, Straub PW. Blood coagulation and acute iron toxicity. Reversible iron-induced inactivation of serine proteases in vitro. J Lab Clin Med 1984;103:524–533.
9. Bentur Y, St Louis P, Klein J, Koren G. Misinterpretation of iron-binding capacity in the presence of deferoxamine. J Pediatr 1991;118:139–142.
10. Tennenbein M, Yatskoff BW. The total iron-binding capacity in iron poisoning: Is it useful? Am J Dis Child 1991;145: 437–439.
11. Burkhart KK, Kulig KW, Hammond KB, Pearson JR, Ambrusco D, Rumack B. The rise in the total iron-binding capacity after iron overdose. Ann Emerg Med 1991;20:532–535.
12. Benson BL, Cheney K. Survival after a severe iron poisoning treated with high dose deferoxamine (DFL) therapy. Vet Hum Toxicol 1992;34:(abstract 53).
13. Ling LJ, Hornfeldt CS, Winter JP. Absorption of iron after experimental overdoses of chewable vitamins. Am J Emerg Med 1991;9:24–26.
14. Chyka PA, Butler AY. Assessment of acute iron poisoning by laboratory and clinical observations. Am J Emerg Med 1993;11:99–103.
15. Everson GW, Bertaccini EJ, O'Leary J. Use of whole bowel irrigation in an infant following iron overdose. Am J Emerg Med 1991;9:366–369.
16. Durbin DR, Wood BP. Acute iron poisoning and gastrointestinal decontamination procedures. Am J Dis Child 1992;146: 765–766.
17. McCarthy T, Olson KR, Spangler S. Documentation with serial radiographs of successful whole bowel irrigation with Golytely solution in a massive iron ingestion. Vet Hum Toxicol 1989;31:333.
18. Banner W, Vernon DD, Ward R, Sweeley J, Dean JM. Continuous arterio-venous hemofiltration (CAVH) in experimental iron intoxication. Vet Hum Toxicol 1988;30:755.
19. Robotham JL, Leitman PS. Acute iron poisoning. A review. Am J Dis Child 1980;134:875–879.
20. Cheney K, Gumbiner C, Benson B, Tenenbein M. Survival after a severe iron poisoning treated with intermittent infusions of deferoxamine. Clin Toxicol 1995;33:61–66.
21. Jackson TW, Ling LJ, Washington V. The effect of oral deferoxamine on iron absorption in humans. Clin Toxicol 1995; 33:325–329.
22. Bosse GM. Conservative management of patients with moderately elevated serum iron levels. Clin Toxicol 1995;33: 235–240.
23. Bentur Y, Klein J, Koren G. Misinterpretation of iron-binding capacity in the presence of deferoxamine. J Pediatr 1991; 118:139–142.
24. Weinberg K. Novel uses of deferoxamine. Am J Pediatr Heamtol Oncol 1990;12:9–13.
25. Allain P, Mauras Y, Chaleil D, Simon P, Ang KS, Can G et al. Pharmacokinetics and renal elimination of desferrioxamine and ferrioxamine in healthy subjects and patients with haemochromatosis. Br J Clin Pharm 1987;24:207–212.
26. Walker JA, Sherman RA, Ensinger RP: Thrombocytopenia associated with intravenous deferoxamine. Am J Kidney Dis 1985;6:254–256.
27. Milteer RM, Sarpony S, Poydras U. Yersinia enterocolitica septicemia after accidental oral iron overdose. Pediatr Infect Dis J 1989;8:537–538.
28. Mofenson HC, Caraccio TR, Sharieff N. Iron sepsis: Yersinia enterocolitica septicemia possibly caused by an overdose of iron. N Engl J Med 1987;316:1029–1093.
29. Bentur Y, McGuigan M, Koren G. Deferoxamine (desferrioxamine). New toxicities for an old drug. Drug Safety 1991; 6:37–46.
30. Ammon A, Rumpf KW, Homverich CP, Behrene-Bauman W, Ruchel R. Rhinocerebral incormyosis during deferoxamine treatment. Dtsch Med Wochenschr 1992;117:1434–1435.
31. Cohen A, Martin M, Mizanin J, Konkle DF, Schwartz E. Vision and hearing during deferoxamine therapy. J Pediatr 1990; 117:326–330.
32. Li Volti S, di Gregorio F, Schiliro G. Acute changes in renal function associated with deferoxamine therapy. Am J Dis Child 1990;144:1069–1070.

33. Koren G, Bentur Y, Strong D et al. Acute changes in renal function associated with deferoxamine therapy. Am J Dis Child 1989;143:1077–1080.
34. Tenenbein M, Kowalski S, Roberts D. Pulmonary toxicity in iron poisoning: deferoxamine induced? Vet Hum Toxicol 1990;32:343.
35. Tenenbein M, Kowalski S, Sienko A, Bowden DH, Adamson IYR. Pulmonary toxic effects of continuous desferrioxamine administration in acute iron poisoning. Lancet 1992;339: 669–701.
36. Roberts JC, McElhatton PR, Sullivan FM. Consequences of iron overdose and desferrioxamine treatment in pregnancy. Proc Lux-Tox '90 meeting, Luxembourg, 1990;OR518.
37. McElhatton PR, Roberts JC, Sullivan FM. The consequences of iron overdose and its treatment with desferrioxamine in pregnancy. Hum Exp Toxicol 1991;10:251–259.
38. Blanc P, Hryhorczuk D, Danol I. Deferoxamine treatment of acute iron intoxication in pregnancy. Obstet Gynecol 1984;64:125–145.
39. Van Ameyde KJ, Tenenbein M. Whole bowel irrigation during pregnancy. Am J Obstet Gynecol 1989;160:646–647.
40. Turk J, Aks S, Ampuero F, Hryhorezuk DO. Successful therapy of iron intoxication in pregnancy with intravenous deferoxamine and whole bowel irrigation. Vet Hum Toxicol 1993;35:441–443.
41. Schauben JL, Augenstein WL, Cox J, Sato R. Iron poisoning. Report of three cases and review of therapeutic intervention. J Emerg Med 1990;8:309–319.
42. Henretig FM, Temple AR. Acute iron poisoning in children. Emerg Med Clin North Am 1987;21:153–159.
43. Engle JP, Polink S, Stile IL. Acute iron intoxication: treatment controversies. Drug Intell Clin Pharm 1987;21:153–159.
44. Yatscoff RW, Wayne EA, Tenenbein M. An objective criterion for the cessation of deferoxamine therapy in the acutely iron poisoned patient. Clin Toxicol 1991;29:1–10.
45. Comes J, Walter FG, Kozaki K, Ekins BR, Lindsey J, Cox K et al. Liver transplantation for fulminant hepatic failure due to acute iron poisoning. Vet Hum Toxicol 1993;35:337.

LEAD

EPIDEMIOLOGY

Blood lead levels once thought to be safe have been shown to be associated with IQ deficits, behavior disorders, slowed growth, and impaired hearing. In fact, lead poisoning is, according to the Department of Health and Human Services, "the most important environmental health problem for young children."[1]

In the 1970s common effects in children of environmental contamination were encephalopathy and even death. In 1976 the estimated average blood lead level for the entire United States population was 16 µg/dL. Even for children of low socioeconomic class living in upper Manhattan, the average blood lead level that was 19 µg/dL just a few years ago, has now declined to 5 µg/dL. Clinically overt lead poisoning has essentially disappeared. An important reason for the nationwide decline of blood lead is the reduction of lead from many sources, and, most of all, the near-complete elimination of lead from gasoline.

LOW LEAD LEVELS

There is substantial epidemiologic evidence of adverse effects of lead at blood levels <20 µg/dL. Adverse effects of very low lead exposure are certainly minor. Consideration should be given to cost:benefit ratio. Parental anxiety, validity of intervention, and disruption of life should be weighed against potential benefits of screening. A recommendation was made to lower the threshold blood lead level for intervention to 10 µg/dL. Current technology cannot adequately measure with accuracy blood lead levels in the 10 to 15 µg/dL range. If the blood lead level were 10 to 15 µg/dL, its detection would accomplish no useful purpose for the individual child. In that range, the demonstration of minor effects of lead requires large numbers of children and sophisticated techniques of detection and analysis. The reduction in blood lead levels in the United States has resulted not from extensive screening, but from the removal of the most important sources of environmental lead. Screening is critical only in the high-risk areas, but is very inefficient in communities without lead exposure. It would be more logical today to test all the houses in which children live that were built before lead-based paint was eliminated. State legislatures, instead of decreeing mandatory screening of all children <6 years, should vote instead to establish mandatory inspection of all dwellings built before 1950 in which those children may live.[2]

Severe lead poisoning (BPb >55 µg/dL) can result in encephalopathy with permanent damage. Substantial data indicate that moderate lead poisoning (25 µg/dL through 55 µg/dL) causes neurobehavioral and intelligence deficits. Although lead is a toxin with no apparent threshold below which it is harmless, the question is how much harm does BPb <20 µg/dL cause to the developing nervous system of a child.[3]

OSHA (1985) has set an action level at air concentrations of 30 µg/m^3 in those exposed to this level over 30 days per year and a permissible exposure limit (PEL) of 50 µg/m^3, averaged over an 8-hour work period for employee exposure to airborne lead. For exposures over 8 hours, the maximum PEL is calculated by dividing 400 µg/m^3 by the hours of exposure. For exposures above the action level of 30 µg/m^3 OSHA mandates periodic determination of blood lead levels.[4]

SOURCES[5]

The three most common sources of lead in the home are paint, pottery (see Hobbies Chapter), and drinking water.[6–8]

Table 67–22 lists occupational, environmental, hobbies and related activities, and substance use as a source of lead exposure.

HAZARDS

Paint[9]

Paint used before 1950 may contain high levels of lead carbonate and lead oxide (up to 50%). Since 1950 allowable paint lead levels have dropped. Indoor and outdoor household paint manufactured since 1977 contains no more than 0.06% (600 parts per million) lead by dry weight. Industrial paints for cars, machinery, bridges, highway stripes, etc., still commonly contain 10 to 20% lead, and possibly up to 40%.

Flaking exterior paint that contains lead can cause problems by contaminating soil around the home. Children are at high risk of lead poisoning when they play with this contaminated soil or eat flaking lead-based paint chips. Old toys and furniture may also be painted with lead-based paint. Children who chew on these items regularly may develop

Table 67–22
Sources of Lead Exposure

Occupational	Environmental	Hobbies and Related Activities	Substance Use
Plumbers, pipe fitters	Lead containing paint	Glazed pottery making	Folk remedies
Lead miners	Soil/dust near lead industries, roadways, lead-painted homes	Target shooting at firing ranges	"Health foods"
Auto repairers	Plumbing leachate	Lead soldering (e.g., electronics)	Cosmetics
Glass manufacturers	Ceramicware	Painting	Moonshine whiskey
Shipbuilders	Leaded gasoline	Preparing lead shot, fishing sinkers	Gasoline "huffing"
Printers		Stained-glass making	
Plastic manufacturers		Car or boat repair	
Lead smelters and refiners		Home remodeling	
Policemen			
Steel welders or cutters			
Construction workers			
Rubber product manufacturers			
Gas station attendants			
Battery manufacturers			
Bridge reconstruction workers			

lead poisoning. In addition, deteriorating paint may release lead dust particles. People who live in homes with old deteriorating paint and inhale lead-containing dust are also at risk.

Exacerbation of lead poisoning may occur in children and adults following deleading of the home.[10,11]

ABATEMENT[12]

Lead in paint should always be considered a "potential" hazard. An immediate lead hazard exists when lead-based paint is (a) chipping, peeling, or flaking; (b) is chalking, thereby producing lead dust; (c) is on a part of a window that is abraded through the opening and closing of the window; (d) is on any surface that is walked on (like floors) or otherwise abraded; (e) can be mouthed by a child (for example, window sills); or (f) is disturbed by repainting or remodeling. A potential lead hazard can easily become an immediate hazard through natural aging, plumbing or roof leaks, or the paint being disturbed. All lead-based paint exceeding the action level should therefore be abated whenever possible. Otherwise, complicated records must be kept of unabated surfaces, and those surfaces must be inspected frequently to make certain that they have not become immediate hazards.

Proper abatement includes the following steps[19]:

1. Proper training of all workers involved in the abatement.
2. Protecting those workers whenever they are in the abatement area.
3. Containing lead-bearing dust and debris.
4. Replacing, encapsulating, or removing lead-based paint.
5. Cleaning the abatement area thoroughly.
6. Disposing of abatement debris properly.
7. Inspecting to make certain the property is ready for reoccupancy.

The three methods of abatement are replacement, encapsulation, and removal.[19]

Replacement is the process whereby the structures painted with lead-based paint are replaced. Doors, windows, and frames are particularly easy and cost-effective to remove. This is the best method for abating lead paint.[9]

Encapsulation involves securely covering or resurfacing painted surfaces with durable materials such as formica, paneling, tile, gypsum board, canvas backed vinyl, vinyl flooring, wood stone, plastic, or metal.

Removal of the lead paint from the structure is the most hazardous alternative and should only be considered if replacement and encapsulation are not feasible. If you have doors or woodwork that you wish to keep, they can be sent off-site for chemical stripping. Old toys and furniture can also be treated off-site. On-site removal is the most dangerous lead paint abatement method and requires careful attention to proper containment, disposal procedures, and worker safety.

Further detailed questions and answers on lead paint removal can be found in Pesce J, Pesce AJ: The Lead Paint Primer. Questions and Answers on Lead Paint Poisoning. Melrose McStone Industries, 1991.

In the United Kingdom significant amounts of lead have been found in beer. This is assumed to arise from contact with brass or bronze fittings containing lead.[13] Significant lead exposure and absorption can occur at outdoor firing ranges. The use of copper-jacketed ammunition may decrease air lead levels.[14,15]

DRINKING WATER

Lead in drinking water is probably absorbed more completely than lead in food. Adults absorb 35 to 50% of the lead they drink, and the absorption rate for children may be greater than 50%.[12,16]

Lead levels are typically low in ground and surface water, but may increase once the water enters the water distribution system. Contamination of drinking water can occur at five points in or near the residential, school public, or office plumbing, including (a) lead connectors (that is, goosenecks or pigtails), (b) lead service lines or pipes, (c) lead-soldered joints in copper plumbing throughout the building, (d) lead-containing water fountains and coolers, and (e) lead-containing brass faucets and other fixtures. The 1986 Safe Drinking Water Act Amendments banned the use of lead in public drinking water distribution systems and limited the lead content of brass used for plumbing to 8%.

Practical measures to reduce exposure to lead in drinking water include using fully-flushed water for drinking and cooking and always drawing water for ingestion from the cold water tap. The effectiveness of many point-of-use devices (treatment devices that are installed at the tap) in reducing lead in water varies and may be affected by the location of the device in relation to the lead source and by compliance with manufacturer's use and maintenance instructions. Some measures, like reverse osmosis and distillation units, may be effective. Carbon, sand, and cartridge filters do not remove lead.

The Environmental Protection Agency regulates the permissible lead content of water.

DRUG ABUSE

Lead contaminated heroin[17,18] or amphetamines[19–21] may produce concomitant lead poisoning. This may be suspected in a drug abuser who experiences abdominal pains, nausea, vomiting, lower back and leg pains, vomiting, weakness, weight loss, and anorexia. Laboratory studies may indicate an anemia and basophilic stippling of the red blood cells.

INFANTS

A review of a lead toxicology program in Massachusetts suggests that sources of plumbism in infants ranging from 1 through 12 months may include household renovation, direct ingestion of paint chips, infant formula preparations with lead-contaminated water, lead dust importation, and congenital exposure to an elevated maternal lead level. In children aged 18 through 30 months apparent sources of intoxication include mainly paint chip ingestion and, in a few instances, household renovation.[22]

GUNSHOT WOUNDS

Gunshot wounds in adults and children may lead to anorexia, abdominal pain, vomiting, anemia, encephalopathy, and seizures with blood lead levels up to 350 to 500 μg/dL. The surface area of retained lead particles (buckshot injuries with lead poisoning in about 8 months [23]; bullet—symptoms in 17 years; shrapnel—10 years), location of retained lead particles (near joint—chronic bath in synovial fluid dissolving lead), length of time one is exposed to lead (after years, unlikely to be seen in pediatric population), and type of activation (uncoated—greater surface area of lead for dissolution) are all factors that may lead to lead poisoning.

Treatment

The source of lead should be removed after a course of chelation therapy since surgery may cause mobilization of lead stores and result in acute postoperative poisoning.[23,24]

TOXICOKINETICS

Bone

Among adults, over 95% of lead is in the skeleton. For children, about 70% of total body lead is in osseous tissues. An L x-ray (x-ray fluorescence XRF) using an iodine-125 source and a K x-ray using either cadmium-109 or cobalt-57 sources is available for in vivo analysis of bone lead concentrations. These techniques analyze superficial bones near the skin, such as the tibia or calcaneus. The LXRF is limited to the top 1 or 2 mm of bone. The KXRF penetrates to about 20 to 40 mm of bone. The LXRF identifies a peak of lead that corresponds to recently deposited lead and correlates well with the EDTA-chelatable lead. The LXRF measurements of lead in cortical bone may have the potential to replace the more cumbersome $CaNa_2EDTA$ test. The KXRF appears to be more reflective of a chronic, cumulative exposure to lead. Lead has a long half-life in bone; over 10 years for many types of bones.[25–27] Until FDA approval is obtained, in vivo tibial XRF can be used only for investigational purposes.[28]

Significant amounts of skeletal lead may be mobilized under conditions of increased bone resorption, leading to significant blood lead level elevations. Multiple courses of chelation therapy may then be necessary to keep lead levels down.[29]

PREGNANCY AND REPRODUCTION[30,31]

Infants

A study of 260 infants prospectively followed from birth suggests that the expected stature of a child born to a mother with a prenatal blood lead concentration over 7.7 μg/dL is about 2 cm shorter at 15 months of age if, potentially, the infant also incurred a 10-μg/dL blood level increase during the 3- to 15-month interval of life.[32]

Male

There appears to be an association between blood lead concentrations of 40 to 70 μg/dL and adverse reproductive effects on sperm counts and hormonal parameters.[33,34] Moderate effects on follicle stimulating hormone and luteinizing hormone have been correlated with lead levels over about 50 μg/dL.[35,36] There is little information available covering reproductive impairment to males exposed to lead at the lower levels generally found in the nonoccupational environment.

Female

Blood lead levels are lower at delivery than they are 6 months postpartum possibly due to the rise in plasma volume during pregnancy.[37]

The U.S. Food and Drug Administration has warned that lead levels in table wine over 300 ppb may present an acute health hazard to pregnant and nursing women. Most urine contains less than this amount of lead.[38]

Lead is readily transferred from the mother to the developing infant during pregnancy. The cord blood lead concentration is approximately 85 to 90% as high as the mother's blood lead concentration.[39,40]

The relative risk of preterm delivery at exposure levels of 14 µg/dL or greater was 8.7 times the risk at levels of up to 8 µg/dL in one prospective study.[41] A Cincinnati study noted a half-week's reduction in gestation for every 10 µg/dL increment in blood lead.[42]

Malformations

A VACTERL (*v*ertebral anomalies, *a*nal atresia, *c*ardiac defect, *t*racheal, *e*sophageal fistula, *r*enal anomalies, and *l*imb abnormalities) association was present in an infant whose mother had high lead levels in the first trimester of pregnancy. Further studies are necessary to confirm this finding.[43] The infant's mother, who worked with leaded glass, had a blood lead level of 62 µg/dL (2.99 µmol/L) at 8 weeks of gestation and 15 µg/dL (0.73 µmol/L) at 12 weeks. (Normal levels are about 0 to 20 µg/dL or 0 to 0.97 µmol/L.) Whether lead exposure in utero results in an increased incidence of congenital malformation is unclear. Major malformations have rarely been reported.

Chromosomal Alterations

Lead is capable of producing chromosomal aberrations.[44] The contribution of these effects to reproductive toxicity is unclear.

Treatment

Treatment for pregnant women chronically exposed to lead is initially removal from continued exposure. Increasing iron and calcium intake and stopping or curtailing the use of alcohol and cigarettes may reduce lead absorption. Chelation therapy may be indicated in acute lead poisoning, but because neither calcium diodide edetate nor dimercaprol cross the placenta, chelation therapy does not decrease lead levels in the fetus.[45] Safe use of these agents during pregnancy has not been established.

PATHOPHYSIOLOGY

Kidney

In children no specific association of lead poisoning with nephropathy has been reported.[46] A slight impairment of renal function may lead to an increase in blood lead concentration.[47] This observation requires clinical confirmation.[48] *N*-acetyl-beta-glucosamidase (NAG) appears to be one of the most sensitive indicators for estimating renal dysfunction due to lead poisoning. Lead absorption associated with blood lead levels of over 80 µg/dL may cause renal tubular damage, and NAG is useful in indicating renal toxicity due to lead exposure.[49]

Cardiovascular System

There is some evidence to suggest that lead may play a primary role in hypertension through direct effects on arterioles and through metabolic processes related to calcium metabolism.[48,50] Individuals with hypertensive nephropathy do not have a greater body burden of lead than renal failure controls.[51]

Bone

More than 90% of the adult body lead burden occurs in bone, with a half-life in dense cortical bone of years to decades.[52]

Chronic Exposure—Biologic Marker

The blood lead level, a traditional index of absorption, reflects only recent exposure because the half-life of blood is only 36 days. In persons with chronic exposure, there is little correlation between a single randomly obtained blood level and either a cumulative index of absorption or the body lead burden.

CLINICAL PRESENTATION—TABLE 67-23

Neurologic—Adults

No relationship exists between maximal motor nerve conduction velocity (MMNCV) and blood lead concentrations of less than 20 µg/dL (Fig. 67-5).[53] Between 20 and 30 µg/dL the blood lead has a minor impact on nerve conduction velocity. Above that level there is a more substantial impact. Each increment of 10 µg/dL in blood lead level is associated with an approximately 20% slowing in MMNCV.[54] Though motor nerve conduction velocity in the ulnar and peroneal nerves may be intact in adults with blood lead levels in the range of 40 to 60 µg/dL, dysfunction in the central nervous system at those levels has been found. This suggests that the central nervous system is more vulnerable

Table 67-23
Continuum of Signs and Symptoms Associated with Lead Toxicity

Mild Toxicity	Moderate Toxicity	Severe Toxicity
Blood levels	Arthralgia	Blood levels
35–500 µg/dl–children	General fatigue	70 µg/dl or more–children
40–60 µg/dl–adult	Difficulty concentrating	100 µg/dl or more–adult
Myalgia or paresthesia	Muscular exhaustibility	Paresis or paralysis
Mild fatigue	Tremor	Encephalopathy—may abruptly lead to seizures, changes in consciousness, coma, and death
Irritability	Headache	Lead line (blue-black) on gingival tissue
Lethargy	Diffuse abdominal pain	Colic (intermittent, severe abdominal cramps)
Occasional abdominal discomfort	Vomiting	
	Weight loss	
	Constipation	

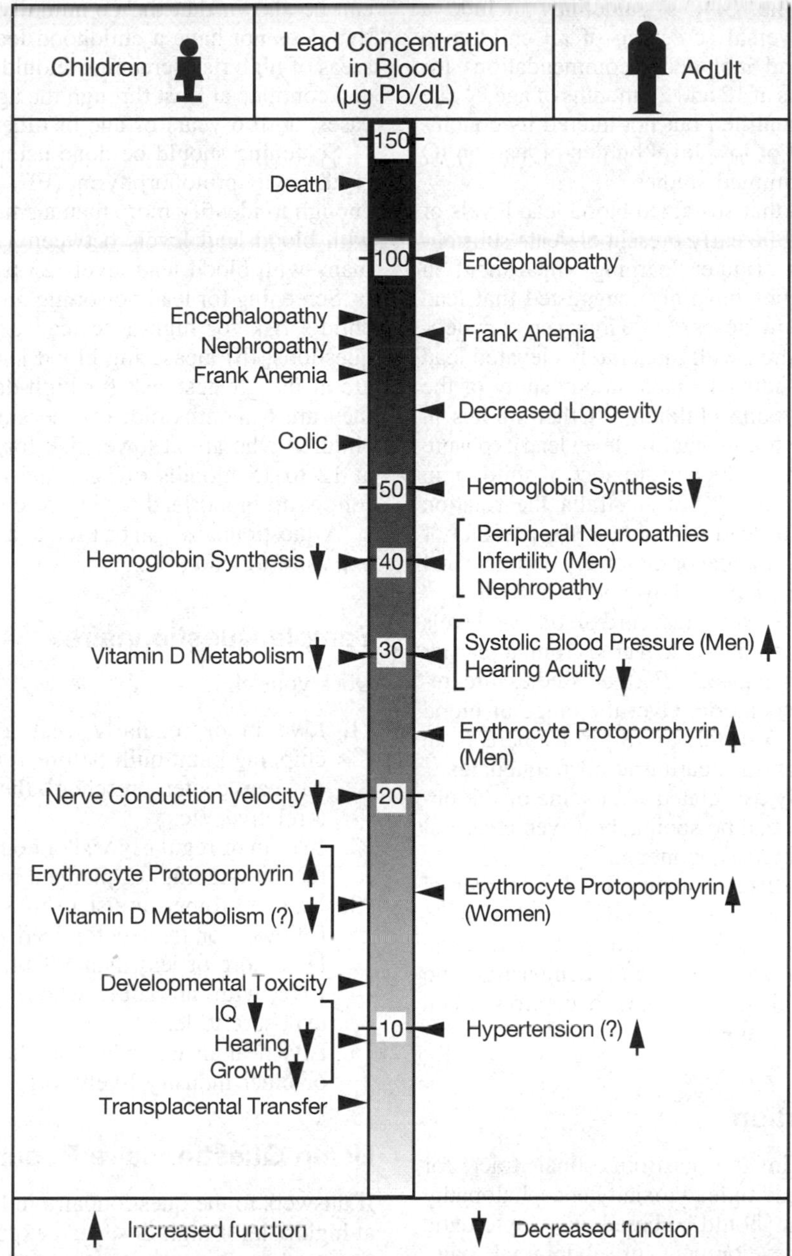

Figure 67–5 Effects of inorganic lead on children and adults—lowest observable adverse effect levels. (Adapted from Royce SE, Needleman HL. Case studies in environmental medicine. I. Lead Toxicity. June 1990. ATSDR. DHHS.)

to lead than is the peripheral nervous system.[54] Lead has not been shown to be an etiologic factor in the development of amyotrophic lateral sclerosis.[55,56]

Neurobehavioral Effects in Children

Chronic low-level lead exposure may cause neurologic impairment, including decreased intelligence, behavioral and learning disorders, and deficits in visuomotor function, perceptual integration, and verbal abstraction.[57]

Low-level lead exposure is related directly to neurobehavioral and cognitive deficits. Data from multiple studies tend to indicate that there is an average decrease of 0.25 IQ points for each 0.05 µmol/L (1.0 µg/dL) increase in blood lead levels. This relationship continued well below 0.48 µmol/L (10 µg/dL). Baghurst and colleagues estimate that, in the age range of 15 months to 4 years, an increase in blood lead concentration from 10 µg/dL (0.48 µmol/L) to 30 µg/dL (1.45 µmol/L) lead to an approximate deficit in IQ of 4 to 5%.[58] Based on these data, the Center for Disease Control has lowered the definition of childhood lead poisoning from 1.21 to 0.48 µmol/L (25 to 10 µg/dL).

Even if moderate increases in body lead burden adversely affect IQ, a threshold below which there is negligible influence cannot currently be determined. Because of these uncertainties, the degree of public health priority that should be devoted to detecting and reducing moderate increases in children's blood lead, compared with other important social detriments that impede children's development, needs careful consideration.[59]

Other initiatives in the CDC's guidelines include a recommendation for universal screening of all children 6 years of age or under and included recommendations for testing of blood lead levels at 12 and 24 months of age.[60] The CDC has subsequently qualified but not altered its conclusions regarding the effect of low-level burden of lead on IQ while recommending continued studies.[61]

Chisolm has indicated that sustained blood lead levels of 60 μg/dL or more during the early preschool years substantially increases the risk of later learning impairment in school.[62] Tooth lead studies have also suggested that lead impairs children's IQ at low doses.[63–65] However, iron deficiency, often seen in children with moderately elevated lead levels, may be a compounding variable in any study of the mental development of young children.[66] Other studies in the United Kingdom have found that low-level lead exposure has a small negative effect on the performance of children in ability and attainment tests.[67,68] In Australia the relation between low-level ambient lead exposure in the prenatal or early postnatal periods and mental or motor development at 4 years of age has not been supported by studies in Sydney.[69] By age 5 years children with umbilical cord blood lead levels of 10 to 25 μg/dL appear to have recovered from an earlier insult to cognitive performance.[70] Further studies are required to confirm this association. Over the range of blood lead concentrations from 6 μg/dL to 18 μg/dL there is an approximate 2 decibel loss of hearing at all frequencies.[71] Iron deficiency is strongly associated with some of the observed toxicities of lead. Lead poisoning, however, can exist without producing microcytosis or anemia.[72]

A significant predictor of subsequent neurodevelopmental outcome appears to be the blood lead concentration at 24 months of age. If a child's lead levels can be reduced to mean levels by 24 months of age, most will demonstrate no neurodevelopmental deficit compared with controls when tested at 5 and 10 years of age.[73]

Foreign Body Ingestion

Lead objects retained in the gastrointestinal tract for prolonged periods may lead to lead toxicity encephalopathy and death.[74–76] Treatment should be based on symptomatic care, observation for development of abdominal pain, vomiting, or fever, and an abdominal radiograph if the object does not pass within a few days. If the lead foreign body progresses through the GI tract, continued observation is warranted for 10 days. If the object has still not passed, than an abdominal radiograph and blood lead level should be obtained and repeated every 4 days. If the object does not appear to be progressing, if blood lead levels begin to rise, or if the patient develops abdominal signs or complications such as perforation, bleeding, or obstruction, surgical consultation will be necessary.

LABORATORY

Screening

Because almost all United States children are at risk for lead poisoning (although some children are at higher risk than others), all children should be screened at least at their first birthday, and if possible, at ages 18 to 24 months, unless it can be shown that the community in which these children live does not have a childhood lead-poisoning problem. In areas of high risk screening should begin at 6 months of age and continue at least through the age of 4 years and, in some cases, until 6 years of age or older.

Screening should be done using a blood lead test, since erythrocyte protoporphyrin (EF) levels are not sensitive enough to identify more than a small percentage of children with blood lead levels between 10 and 25 μg/L and miss many with blood lead levels 25 μg/L or more.[77]

Screening for lead poisoning requires (a) determining the child's risk for high-dose lead exposure by asking a few questions; (b) measuring blood lead levels in children who are at the greatest risk for high-dose lead poisoning when they are 6 months old; (c) measuring blood lead levels in children who are at lower risk for high-dose lead exposure at 12 to 15 months of age; and (d) conducting necessary follow-up blood lead testing of children.

A questionnaire can be used to assess the risk of high-dose exposure to lead.

Sample Questionnaire

Does your child—

1. Live in or regularly visit a house with peeling or chipping paint built before 1960? This could include a day care center, preschool, the home of a baby sitter or a relative, etc.
2. Live in or regularly visit a house built before 1960 with recent, ongoing, or planned renovation or remodeling?
3. Have a brother or sister, housemate or playmate being followed or treated for lead poisoning (that is, blood lead more or less than 15 μg/L)?
4. Live with an adult whose job or hobby involved exposure to lead?
5. Live near an active lead smelter, battery recycling plant, or other industry likely to release lead?

Using Questionnaire Results

If answers to the questionnaire indicate that the child is not at high risk for high-dose lead exposure, the child should be screened at 12 months of age, and, if resources allow, at 24 months of age.

If answers to the questionnaire indicate that the child is at risk for high-dose lead exposure, the child should be screened starting at 6 months of age.

For children previously at low risk, any history suggesting that exposure to lead has increased should be followed up with a blood lead test.

Screening Schedule

The following provides a minimum screening schedule for children aged 6 months up to 36 months and 36 to 72 months.

Children 6 Months and Up to 36 Months of Age

A questionnaire should be used at each routine office visit to assess the potential for high-dose lead exposure and therefore the appropriate frequency of screening.

Schedule if the child is at low risk for high-dose lead exposure by questionnaire:

1. A child at low risk for exposure to high-dose lead sources by questionnaire should have an initial blood lead test at 12 months of age.
2. If the 12-month blood lead result is <10 μg/L (0.50 μmol/L), the child should be retested at 24 months, if possible, since that is when blood lead levels peak.
3. If a blood lead test result is 10 to 14 μg/L (0.50 to 0.70 μmol/L), the child should be retested every 3 to 4 months. After two consecutive measurements are <10 μg/L or three are <15 μg/L (0.70 μmol/L), the child should be retested in a year.
4. If any blood lead test result is more than 15 μg/L (0.70 μmol/L), the child needs individual case management, which includes retesting the child at least every 3 to 4 months.

Schedule if the child is at high-risk for high-dose lead exposure by questionnaire:

1. A child at high risk for exposure to high-dose lead sources by questionnaire should have an initial blood lead test at 6 months of age.
2. If the initial blood lead result <10 μg/L, the child should be rescreened every 6 months. After 2 subsequent consecutive measurements are <10 μg/L or three are <15 μg/L, testing frequency can be decreased to once a year.
3. If a blood lead test result is 10 to 14 μg/L, the child should be screened every 3 to 4 months. Once two subsequent consecutive measurements are <10 μg/L or three are <15 μg/L, testing frequency can be decreased to once a year.
4. If any blood lead test result is 15 μg/L or over, the child needs individual case management, which includes retesting the child at least every 3 to 4 months.

Children 36 Months or Over and Less Than 72 Months of Age

As for younger children, a questionnaire should be used at each routine office visit of children from 36 to 72 months of age. Any child at high risk by questionnaire who has not previously had a blood lead test should be tested. All children who have had venous blood lead tests more than 15 μg/L or who are at high risk by questionnaire should be screened at least once a year until their sixth birthday (age 72 months) or later, if indicated (for example, a developmentally delayed child with pica). Children should also be rescreened any time history suggests exposure has increased. Children with blood lead levels 15 μg/L or more should receive follow-up as described below. In general, such children should receive blood lead tests every 3 to 4 months.

If the blood lead level is 15 to 19 μg/dL, the child should be screened every 3 to 4 months, the family should be given education and nutritional counseling, and a detailed environmental history should be taken to identify any obvious sources of pathways of lead exposure. When venous blood lead level is in this range in two consecutive tests 3 to 4 months apart, environmental investigation and abatement should be conducted, if resources permit.

If the blood lead level is 20 μg/dL or more, the child should be given a repeat test for confirmation. If the venous blood lead level is confirmed to be 20 μg/dL or over, the child should be referred for medical evaluation and follow-up. Such children should continue to receive blood lead tests every 3 to 4 months or more often if indicated. Children with blood lead levels 45 μg/dL or over (2.15 μmol/L) must receive urgent medical and environmental follow-up preferably at a clinic with a staff experienced in dealing with this disease. Symptomatic lead poisoning or a venous blood lead concentration 70 μg/dL or more is a medical emergency, requiring immediate inpatient chelation therapy.[12]

Free Erythrocyte Protoporphyrin

Recently, the Centers for Disease Control (CDC) recommended that all children between 9 months and 6 years of age should receive an FEP test. Although the FEP is a better measure of body lead burden (i.e., soft tissue levels) than blood lead, both tests should be used to estimate body lead burden since iron deficiency anemia causes an elevation of the FEP. The FEP may be elevated when blood lead is below 29 μg/dL. At lead levels of 30 μg/dL, 60% of females, but only 10% of males, have an elevated FEP level. The elevation of the FEP test persists long after cessation of lead exposure. An FEP level higher than 35 μg/dL and a blood lead level higher than 10 μg/dL indicate excess lead exposure and require further medical evaluation and environmental investigation. Table 67–24 correlates blood FEP with lead levels. The EP is not a sensitive test to identify children with blood lead levels below about 25 μg/dL and therefore it is no longer the screening test of choice. All elevated EP results should be followed by a venous blood lead test.

Iron Deficiency

An elevated EP level indicates impairment of the heme biosynthetic pathway. EP levels are sensitive screening tests for iron deficiency, and iron status should be assessed in any child with an elevated Ep level (that is, 35 μg/dL or more when standardized using 297 L cm-1 mmol-1, or 70 μmol/mol when measured in μmol/mol units).[78]

Some studies have suggested harmful effects at even lower levels, but the body of information accumulated so far is not adequate for effects below about 10 μg/dL to be evaluated definitely. As yet, no lowest threshold value has been identified for the harmful effects of lead.

Blood Lead

Table 67–24 provides an interpretation of blood lead results and recommended follow-up activities. Five classes of child-based blood lead concentrations are presented.[78,79]

Zinc protoporphyrin concentration may not be a sensitive indicator of lead levels in the absence of iron deficiency.[71]

Table 67–24
Interpretation of Blood Lead Test Results and Follow-up Activities: Class of Child Based on Blood Lead Concentration

Class	Blood Lead Concentration (µg/dL)	Comment
I	≤9	A child in Class I is not considered to be lead-poisoned.
IIA	10–14	Many children (or a large proportion of children) with blood lead levels in this range should trigger communitywide childhood lead poisoning prevention activities. Children in this range may need to be rescreened more frequently.
IIB	15–19	A child in Class IIB should receive nutritional and educational interventions and more frequent screening. If the blood lead level persists in this range, environmental investigation and intervention should be done.
III	20–44	A child in Class III should receive environmental evaluation and remediation and a medical evaluation. Such a child may need pharmacologic treatment of lead poisoning.
IV	45–69	A child in Class IV will need both medical and environmental interventions, including chelation therapy.
V	≥70	A child with Class V lead poisoning is a medical emergency. Medical and environmental management must begin immediately.

Source: CDC, *Preventing Lead Poisoning in Young Children,* October 1991, page 3.

Calcium Disodium EDTA Mobilization Test

Children

A $CaNa_2EDTA$ mobilization test is used to determine whether a child with an initial confirmatory blood lead level of 25 to 41 µg/dL will respond to chelation therapy with a brisk lead diuresis.[80,81] Because of the cost and staff time needed for quantitative urine collection, this test is used only in selected medical centers where large numbers of lead-poisoned children are treated. Children whose blood lead levels are 45 µg/dL or over should not receive a provocative chelation test; they should be referred for appropriate chelation therapy immediately.[82]

The outcome of the provocative chelation test is determined not by a decrease in the blood lead level but by the amount of lead excreted per dose of $CaNa_2EDTA$ given. This ratio correlates well with blood lead levels. In one study almost all children with blood lead levels of 45 µg/dL had positive provocative tests, 76% of the children with blood lead levels of 35 to 44 µg/dL had positive test results, and 35% of the children with blood lead levels of 25 to 34 µg/dL had positive test results.[81] This test should not be done until the child is iron repleted, since iron status may affect the outcome of the test.[83]

Conducting a $CaNa_2EDTA$ Provocative Chelation Test

First, a repeated baseline blood lead level must be obtained. The patient is asked to empty the bladder, and then $CaNa_2EDTA$ is administered at a dose of 500 mg/m^2 in 5% dextrose infused over 1 hour. (A somewhat painful but practical alternative is to administer intramuscularly the same dose mixed with procaine so that the final concentration of procaine is 0.5%.) All urine must be collected with lead-free equipment over the next 8 hours. (An 8-hour mobilization test has been shown to be as reliable as a 24-hour mobilization test.[84] An 8-hour test can be accomplished on an out-patient basis, but the patient should not leave the clinic during this test.) In the laboratory the urine volume should be carefully measured and stored at 20°C until the lead concentration is measured. Extreme care must be taken to ensure that lead-free equipment is used.

The use of lead-free apparatus for urine collection is mandatory. Special lead-free collection apparatus must be used if valid test results are to be obtained. The laboratory that will perform the analysis should supply the proper collection apparatus. Preferably, urine should be voided directly into polyethylene or polypropylene bottles that have been cleaned by the usual procedures, then washed in nitric acid, and thoroughly rinsed with deionized, distilled water. For children who are not toilet trained, plastic pediatric urine collectors can be used. Urine collected in this manner should be transferred directly to the urine collection bottles.

Interpretation of a $CaNa_2EDTA$ Provocative Chelation Test

To obtain the total lead excretion in micrograms, the concentration of lead in the urine (in micrograms per milliliter) is multiplied by the total urinary volume (in milliliters). The total urinary excretion of lead (micrograms) is divided by the amount of $CaNa_2EDTA$ given (milligrams) to obtain the lead excretion ratio:

$$\frac{\text{Lead excreted } (\mu g)}{CaNa_2EDTA \text{ given (mg)}}$$

An 8-hour $CaNa_2EDTA$ chelation provocative test is considered positive if the lead excretion ratio is >0.6.[3] Some clinicians use a cutoff of 0.5 for the lead excretion ratio.[85] Children with blood lead levels of 25 to 44 µg/dL and positive chelation test results should undergo a 5-day course of chelation.

Regardless of age, all children with elevated blood lead values and negative provocative chelation results should have blood lead levels measured monthly. If the elevation in blood lead value persists, the $CaNa_2EDTA$ provocative test can be repeated every 1 to 3 months and interpreted according to the above guidelines.

Data suggest (a) (UPb)/(UCr) >20 after an EDTA mobilization test can be used to identify a positive test in incomplete or (potentially) single-void urine specimens, and (b) (UCr) is decreased in children with larger lead burdens, suggesting subclinical renal injury.[86]

Lead poisoning and associated morbidity, such as renal failure, hypertension, and gout, appear to correlate with the body burden of lead estimated by the $CaNa_2EDTA$ mobilization test, direct measurement of lead in bone biopsy specimens, or x-ray fluorescence. Blood lead levels may be helpful in identifying trends in large populations. They are not very useful in studying selected populations such as patients with gouty nephropathy or hypertensive nephrosclerosis; only the EDTA lead mobilization test reveals unsuspected lead poisoning among these patients.[87]

TREATMENT—ANTIDOTES

D-Penicillamine

The Food and Drug Administration (FDA) has approved D-penicillamine for the treatment of Wilson's disease, cystinuria, and severe, active rheumatoid arthritis. Until the recent approval of succimer, it was the only commercially available oral chelating agent. It can be given over a long period (weeks to months). D-penicillamine has been used mainly for children with blood lead levels <45 μg/dL.[88]

Mechanism of Action

D-penicillamine enhances urinary excretion of lead, although not as effectively as $CaNa_2EDTA$. Its specific mechanism and site of action are not well understood.

Route of Administration and Dosage[89]

D-penicillamine is administered orally. It is available in capsules or tablets (125 mg and 250 mg). These capsules can be opened and suspended in liquid, if necessary. The usual dose is 25 to 35 mg/kg/day in divided doses. Side effects can be minimized, to an extent, by starting with a small dose and increasing it gradually, monitoring all the time for side effects. For example, 25% of the desired final dose could be given in week 1, 50% in week 2, and the full dose by week 3.

Precautions and Toxicity[90]

Toxic side effects (albeit minor in most cases) occur in as many as 33% of patients given the drug.[91] The main side effects of D-penicillamine are reactions resembling those of penicillin sensitivity, including rashes, leukopenia, thrombocytopenia, hematuria, proteinuria, hepatocellular enzyme elevations, and eosinophilia. Anorexia, nausea, and bloating are commonly seen. Vomiting is less frequent. Rarely, myasthenia gravis may follow D-penicillamine use.[92] Of most concern, however, are isolated reports of nephrotoxicity, possibly from hypersensitivity reactions. For these reasons, patients should be carefully and frequently monitored for clinically obvious side effects, and frequent blood counts, urinalyses, and renal function tests should be performed. In particular, blood counts and urinalyses should be done on day 1, day 14, day 28, and monthly thereafter. If the absolute neutrophil count falls to <1500 μL, the count should be rechecked immediately, and treatment should be stopped if it falls to <1200 μL. D-penicillamine should not be given on an outpatient basis if exposure to lead is continuing or the physician has doubts about compliance with the therapeutic regimen. D-penicillamine should not be administered to patients with known penicillin allergy. The drug should be continued until lead levels are less than 15 μg/dL. Rebound following cessation of therapy may raise the lead level to an additional 25% from its nadir.[93,94]

There is no evidence that penicillamine treatment or treatment with any chelating agent in children has any therapeutic value in preventing or reversing the effects of lead on cognitive development.[94,95] Penicillamine remains, however, of potential usefulness in children with low-level plumbism (whole blood lead levels 25 to 40 μg/dL).[94]

Termination of Treatment[96]

Treatment of D-penicillamine is terminated immediately if any of the following occur:

1. A rise in blood lead level—suggesting ongoing lead exposure.
2. Otherwise unexplained generalized urticarial rash.
3. Fall in platelet count below 100,000.
4. Fall in white blood cell count below 3000.
5. Appearance of abnormal urinalysis: proteinuria (>1+ on dipstick; hematuria (>10 red blood cells/high power field); or pyuria (>10 white blood cells/high power field).

ORAL BAL ANALOGS

DMPS (2,3 Dimercapto-1-Propane-Sulfonic Acid)

Although DMPS has shown promise in the treatment of lead poisoning,[89,97] Julian Chisolm and others have seen patients who have developed a Stevens-Johnson syndrome following its administration; therefore DMPS will probably not be a drug of choice for lead poisoning.[98] There is a need for further study of this product.

DMSA (Succimer)

The FDA approved succimer in January 1991 for treating children with blood lead levels >45 μg/dL. Liebelt and colleagues have recently shown that DMSA is effective in lowering BPb concentrations in children with BPb values from 0.97 to 2.17 μmol/L (20 to 45 μg/dL). Regardless of the BPb concentration, chelation therapy should never be used as a substitute for environmental assessment and abatement of lead hazards for lead-poisoned children.[99] Succimer appears to be an effective oral chelating agent. Its selectivity for lead is high, whereas its ability to chelate essential trace metals is low. Although its use to date has been limited, succimer appears to have promising potential, and a broader range of clinical research studies in children are being undertaken.[90,100]

Succimer is chemically similar to BAL, but is more water soluble, has a high therapeutic index, and is absorbed from the gastrointestinal tract. It is effective when given orally and produces a lead diuresis comparable to that produced by $CaNa_2EDTA$.[98] This diuresis lowers blood lead levels and reverses the biochemical toxicity of lead, as indicated by normalization of circulating aminolevulinic acid dehydrase levels.[100] Succimer is not indicated for prophylaxis of lead poisoning in a lead-containing environment. As with all chelating agents, succimer should only be given to children who reside in environments free of lead during and after treatment.

The efficacy of chelation therapy in lead poisoning cannot be judged by estimating blood lead concentrations alone. Determination of urine lead excretion must also be performed concomitantly. There are preliminary data to suggest that intravenous calcium disodium EDTA (75 mg/kg/day) is about four times more effective in promoting lead excretion than DMSA (30 mg/kg/day).[101]

Rosen and Markowitz have proposed guidelines for the use of DMSA in the treatment of childhood lead poisoning[102]:

1. As with all chelating agents, DMSA should be administered to children who are living only in thoroughly and definitively abated housing or living in transition housing, such as a Safe House.
2. It appears to be prudent to administer DMSA for the first 5 days either as a hospital in-patient or in a Safe House environment, where compliance, side effects, and the environment can be tightly and rigorously controlled.
3. The experience of using DMSA in children with a BPb value of 70 μg/dL or more is extremely limited; and at this time it is not recommended for use in high-level Pb poisoning. Accordingly, at present BAL and $CaNa_2EDTA$ are recommended to treat children with BPb levels equal to or greater than 70 μg/dL.
4. The potential capability of DMSA to ameliorate cognitive and neurobehavioral deficits produced by Pb must be carefully and systematically assessed and compared with $CaNa_2EDTA$ in a randomized, controlled study before the use of DMSA or $CaNa_2EDTA$ become uncritically accepted as the drug of choice to treat childhood Pb poisoning.

Mechanism of Action

Succimer is probably more specific for lead than the most commonly used chelating agent, $CaNa_2EDTA$; the urinary loss of essential trace elements (for example, zinc) appears to be considerably less with succimer than with $CaNa_2EDTA$.[103] The site of lead chelation by succimer is not known.

Route of Administration and Dosage[98]

Succimer is administered orally. It is available in 100-mg capsules. The recommended initial dose is 350 mg/m^2 (10 mg/kg) every 8 hours for 5 days, followed by 350 mg/m^2 (10 mg/kg) every 12 hours for 14 days. A course of treatment therefore lasts 19 days. If more courses are needed, a minimum of 2 weeks between courses is preferred, unless blood lead levels indicate the need for immediate retreatment. These doses may be modified as more experience is gained in using succimer.

Rebound

Multiple causes of DMSA may be required because of the rebound in blood lead levels after cessation of a course of treatment. Liebelt and Shannon use a postrebound blood lead level of <15 μg/dL as an endpoint of therapy.[96]

Patients who have received therapeutic courses of $CaNa_2EDTA$ with or without BAL may use succimer for subsequent treatment after an interval of 4 weeks. Data on the concomitant use of succimer and $CaNa_2EDTA$ with or without BAL are not available, and such use is not recommended.

If young children cannot swallow capsules, succimer can be administered by separating the capsule and sprinkling the medicated beads on a small amount of soft food or by putting them on a spoon and following with a fruit drink. Data are not available on how stable succimer is when it is suspended in soft foods for prolonged periods; succimer should be mixed with soft foods immediately before being given to the child.

Precautions and Toxicity[91]

To date, toxicity due to succimer (transient elevations in hepatic enzyme activities) appears to be minimal. The most common adverse effects reported in clinical trials in children and adults were primarily gastrointestinal and included nausea, vomiting, diarrhea, and appetite loss. A transient decrease in the whole blood cell count has been reported. Its clinical significance is not clear.[104] Rashes, some necessitating discontinuance of therapy, have been reported for about 4% of patients. Though succimer holds considerable promise for the outpatient management of lead poisoning, clinical experience with succimer is limited. Consequently, the full spectrum and incidence of adverse reactions, including the possibility of hypersensitivity or idiosyncratic reactions, have not been determined.

If succimer is used, the following precautions must be taken:

1. Monitor for side effects (especially effects on liver transaminases), the rapidity of the initial decrease in blood lead levels, and the course of the rebound in blood lead levels once treatment has ended.
2. Succimer, like other chelators, is not a substitute for effective and rapid environmental interventions. Use succimer as part of an integrated environmental and medical approach to treating patients with lead poisoning.
3. Do not give succimer (or any other chelating agent) in situations whose high-dose lead sources are available to the child. In rats gastrointestinal absorption of lead and whole-body lead retention were reduced by a single oral dose of succimer. The potential for enhancing human lead absorption from the gastrointestinal tract during the use of succimer is under study.
4. Children with blood lead levels >45 μg/dL who are being treated with succimer should, if possible, be

hospitalized until their blood lead levels fall below 45 μg/dL and the lead hazards in their homes are abated or alternative lead hazard-free housing has been identified.

5. Children with blood lead levels about 70 μg/dL should be immediately hospitalized. The decision to treat such children with succimer instead of $CaNa_2EDTA$ and BAL should be made with the understanding that experience with using succimer in children with these blood lead levels is limited.[90,93]
6. DMSA has been placed in pregnancy category C, indicating that animal studies have demonstrated adverse fetal effects, but controlled data in pregnant women do not exist. Transmission via breast milk is unknown.[93]

Rebound is common and may be as high as 70%[105] above the nadir. Initial trials are under way and appear to indicate a potential use of DMSA at levels under 45 μg/dL.[93,106,107] Vale and colleagues, however, indicate that the available literature does not support the view that DMSA is superior to calcium disodium EDTA in promoting urinary lead excretion.[101] Long-term clinical confirmation and correlation with this observation will be required. Both DMSA and DMPS effectively chelate arsenic, lead, organic and inorganic mercury, and other heavy metals, but cause minimal effects on iron, calcium, and magnesium. Small increases in urinary zinc and copper excretion may occur.[108]

Indications for Chelation Therapy

Symptomatic Children (Acute Symptomatic Plumbism)[78] (CDC Guidelines)

Start treatment with a dose of 75 mg/m^2 BAL only, given by deep intramuscular injection; administer BAL at a dose of 450 mg/m^2/day in divided doses of 75 mg/m^2 every 4 hours. Once this dose is given and an adequate urine flow is established, administer $CaNa_2EDTA$ at a dose of 1500 mg/m^2. Give $CaNa_2EDTA$ as a continuous intravenous infusion in dextrose and water or in a 0.9% saline solution. The concentration of $CaNa_2EDTA$ should not exceed 0.5% in the parenteral fluid. (When treating a child with encephalopathy, the physician may choose to give $CaNa_2EDTA$ intramuscularly to reduce the amount of fluid administered.) Treat with combined BAL-$CaNa_2EDTA$ therapy for a total of 5 days. During treatment, monitor renal and hepatic function and serum electrolyte levels daily.

A second course of chelation therapy with $CaNa_2EDTA$ alone (at blood lead levels of 45 to 69 μg/dL) or combined with BAL (at blood lead levels of 70 μg/dL) may be required once there is a rebound in the blood lead level after chelation. Wait at least 2 days before giving a second course of chelation. A third course is required only if the blood lead concentration rebounds to a value >45 μg/dL within 48 hours after the second course of treatment. Unless there are unusual and compelling clinical reasons, wait at least 5 to 7 days before beginning a third course of $CaNa_2EDTA$.

Asymptomatic Children (Subclinical Plumbism)

All patients with elevated blood lead levels should have repeat blood samples drawn to exclude the possibility of contamination or laboratory error and to measure FEP levels. Check blood iron levels before chelating because iron deficiency alone causes elevated FEP levels. FEP levels below 35 μg/dL are normal, whereas levels above 250 μg/dL are grossly abnormal.[96]

Blood lead level more than 70 μg/dL. Children with blood lead levels more than 70 μg/dL (with or without symptoms) represent an acute medical emergency. If the blood lead level is more than 70 μg/dL, give both BAL and $CaNa_2EDTA$ in the same doses and using the guidelines as for treatment of symptomatic lead poisoning. A second course of chelation therapy with $CaNa_2EDTA$ alone may be required if the blood lead concentration rebounds to a value of more than 45 μg/dL within 5 to 7 days after treatment. In general, allow at least 5 to 7 days before beginning a second course of $CaNa_2EDTA$. Some practitioners give a second course of chelation after a 3-day rest period if the immediate posttreatment blood lead level is >35 μg/dL.

Blood lead level 45 to 69 μg/dL. If the blood lead value is between 45 and 69 μg/dL, chelation treatment should be limited to $CaNa_2EDTA$ only. $CaNa_2EDTA$ is given for 5 days at a dose of 1000 mg/m^2/day intravenously by continuous infusion or in divided doses. During treatment evaluate renal and hepatic function and serum electrolyte levels regularly. Do not continue $CaNa_2EDTA$ treatment for more than 5 days.

A second course of chelation therapy with $CaNa_2EDTA$ alone may be required if the blood lead level rebounds to 45 μg/dL within 7 to 14 days after treatment. Allow 5 to 7 days before beginning a second course of $CaNa_2EDTA$.

Blood lead level 25 to 44 μg/dL. For this blood lead range, the effectiveness of chelation therapy in decreasing the adverse effect of lead on children's intelligence has not been shown. Treatment regimens vary from clinic to clinic. Some practitioners treat children with lead levels in this range pharmacologically. (Although it is not approved for this use, some use D-penicillamine for children in this blood lead range.) The minimum medical management for children with these blood lead levels is to decrease the children's exposure to all sources of lead to ensure that the child's blood lead levels are decreasing. Many experienced practitioners decide whether to use chelation therapy on the basis of the results of carefully performed $CaNa_2EDTA$ mobilization tests.

Blood lead level 20 to 24 μg/dL. Only very minimal data exist about chelating children with blood lead levels below 25 μg/dL, and such children should not be chelated except in the context of approved clinical trials. A child with a confirmed blood lead level of 20 to 24 μg/dL will require individual case management by a pediatric health-care provider. The child should have an evaluation with special attention to nutritional and iron status. The parents should be taught about (a) the causes and effects of lead poisoning, (b) the need for more routine blood lead testing, (c) possible sources of lead intake and how to reduce them, (d) the importance of adequate nutrition and of food high in iron and calcium, and (e) resources for further information. Sequential measurements of blood lead levels along with review of the child's clinical status should be done at least every 3 months. Iron deficiency should be treated promptly. Children with blood lead levels in this range should be referred for environmental investigation and management. Identifying and eradicating all sources of excessive lead exposure is the most important intervention for decreasing blood lead levels.

Studies of cognitive performance in untreated children with blood lead levels between 25 and 55 μg/dL (1.21 and 2.66 μmol/L) suggest that intelligence scores in such children increased 1 point for every decrease of 3 μg/dL (0.64 μmol/L) in blood lead levels after a full course of treatment with calcium disodium EDTA and/or orally administered iron supplement if iron deficient.[109]

Adults (See also DMSA)

Symptomatic patients should be chelated. Chelation based on specific blood levels for adults is controversial (Table 67–25). Asymptomatic patients with blood lead levels between 40 and 79 μg/dL and FEP levels of more than 60 μg/dL should have a provocation test and be chelated if positive.

Elimination Enhancement

Hemodialysis appeared to enhance the excretion of $CaNa_2EDTA$ chelated lead in one adult who ingested 40 g of lead oxide. Little confirmatory evidence of the usefulness of hemodialysis is available.[110] Whole-bowel irrigation has shown some usefulness in the prevention of lead toxicity by removal of a lead glaze preparation from the gastrointestinal tract.[111,112]

Thiamine

Animal studies suggest that thiamine 10 to 50 mg/kg body weight improves neurophysiologic changes related to lead poisoning.[113] In combination with zinc, this appears to reduce the lead-induced inhibition of Δ aminolevulinic dehydratase activity.[114] Clinical confirmatory studies demonstrating its usefulness are lacking.

Supportive Care

1. In an acute oral lead ceramic glaze ingestion, the potential for ongoing absorption of large amounts of lead from the gut makes GI contamination reasonable. No unanimity exists regarding optimal evacuation techniques.
2. Following gastric lavage, abdominal radiography should be obtained to gauge the efficacy of the procedure.
3. Whole-bowel irrigation can be of potential benefit in those situations in which cathartics should be avoided (e.g., renal failure, overload states, etc.).[115]

Graef[73,93,116,117] has proposed a therapeutic protocol for lead poisoning (Table 67–25).

Liebelt-Shannon Suggested Guidelines for DMSA Use[96]

1. DMSA was approved by the FDA for the treatment of lead poisoning in children with blood lead concentrations above 45 μg/dL.
2. For BPb <45 μg/dL DMSA was not approved in children, but the attending physician may use it if there is a determination of need.
3. Asymptomatic children with no clinical signs of lead encephalopathy and with BPb 35 to 70 μg/dL—DMSA potentially useful.
4. Consider hospitalization if BPb >50 μg/dL and there are ongoing lead exposures to ensure medication compliance and to obtain close monitoring for medical complication. Abatement of environmental lead hazards should be instituted prior to DMSA treatment on an outpatient basis.
5. If BPb in hospitalized children remains >35 μg/dL after chelation with $CaNa_2EDTA$, consider DMSA.
6. Children with BPb 35 to 50 μg/dL: outpatient DMSA therapy if (a) environment assessed to be safe; (b) abdominal radiograph does not contain radiopaque densities, and (c) they are likely to comply with medication administration and appropriate medical follow-up.
7. Children with BPb 20 to 35 μg/dL: use DMSA if (a) refractory elevated blood levels despite attempted chelation with D-penicillamine or $CaNa_2EDTA$, or (b) for children with complications from D-penicillamine.
8. DMSA: not for prophylaxis of lead poisoning in a lead-containing environment.

American Academy of Pediatrics Treatment Recommendations

The Committee on Drugs of the American Academy of Pediatrics in July 1995 presented the following treatment recommendations based on confirmed blood lead results[118]:

Venous blood samples should be used to determine treatment.

1. Chelation treatment is not indicated in patients with blood lead levels of less than 25 μg/dL, although environmental intervention should occur.
2. Patients with blood lead levels of 25 to 45 μg/dL need aggressive environmental intervention, but should not routinely receive chelation therapy because no evidence exists that chelation avoids or reverses neurotoxicity. If blood lead levels persist in this range despite repeated environmental study and abatement, some patients may benefit from (oral) chelation therapy by enhanced lead excretion.
3. Chelation therapy is indicated in patients with blood lead levels between 45 and 70 μg/dL. In the absence of clinical symptoms suggesting encephalopathy (e.g., obtundation, headache, and persistent vomiting), patients may be treated with succimer at 30 mg/kg per day for 5 days, followed by 20 mg/kg per day for 14 days. Children may need to be hospitalized for the initiation of therapy to monitor for adverse effects and institute environmental abatement. Discharge should be considered only if the safety of the environment after hospitalization can be guaranteed. An alternate regimen would be to use $CaNa_2EDTA$ as inpatient therapy at 25 mg/kg per day for 5 days. Before chelation with either agent is begun, if an abdominal radiograph shows that enteral lead is present, bowel decontamination may be considered as an adjunct to treatment.

Table 67-25
Therapeutic Protocol[116,117]

Acute Symptomatic Poisoning with Encephalopathy
A. Medical Emergency
B. Establish IV access
1. BAL 4 mg/kg (children) immediately
2. Cranial CT—rule out cerebral edema
3. KUB rule out lead chips in GI tract
4. Seizures—Rx: diazepam, phenobarbital
5. Cerebral edema: admit to ICU
after 1st dose of BAL give 10 cc/kg bolus of normal saline. (Establish urine flow). Follow with $CaNA_2$ EDTA 75 mg/kg/24 hr continuous infusion. Do not give oral DMSA in symptomatic lead poisoning.
6. Fluids to keep urine specific gravity under 1,020.
7. Foley catheter: monitor urinary specific gravity, sediment, lead content.
8. BAL 4 mg/kg q 4 hr until whole blood lead level is less than 40 ug/dL. Then reduce BAL to 12 mg/kg/day in 3 divided doses. $CaNa_2$EDTA can be reduced to 50 mg/kg/d as child's condition improves. BAL is discontinued when the blood lead is less than 40 µg/dL. Repeat courses of parenteral $CaNA_2$EDTA until asymptomatic and can tolerate oral chelation DMSA, d-penicillamine. Do not administer iron with BAL, but give with EDTA as required.

Severe Symptomatic Lead Poisoning (BPb >70 µg/dL).
1. Hospitalize immediately
2. BAL and $CaNa_2$EDTA both needed when blood lead level is >µg/d.
3. If child is asymptomatic
BAL 12 mg/kg/day; $CaNa_2$EDTA 50 mg/kg/day
begin with BAL; wait 4 hours for $CaNa_2$EDTA in continuous infusion.
4. 1 cc/kg bolus of normal saline. Encourage fluids (to 1½ times daily maintenance.)
5. Do KUB; if positive enhance elimination by catharsis with magnesium sulfate. Can begin chelation simultaneously.
6. Continue BAL until blood lead less than 40 µg/dL. Then continue EDTA alone.
7. Give 5 day course of $CaNa_2$EDTA
8. Change to oral DMSA dependent on condition of child, lead levels, ability to tolerate oral medication.
9. If the blood level is 45 to 70 µcg try DMSA
10. Discharge to lead-safe environment

Moderately severe asymptomatic Pb poisoning (BPb 45–70 µg/dL)
1. Hospitalize all children unless the lead source has been identified and the child removed from it.
2. Start therapy with parenteral $CaNa_2$EDTA
3. DMSA: stay in hospital until tolerance determined or lead safe environment found
4. No DMSA with a blood Pb <45 µg/dL if the child is not in a lead-safe environment
5. Correct iron deficiency
6. May need multiple chelations.

Moderate Symptomatic Lead Poisoning (BPb 35–45 µg/dL)
1. Lead mobilization test useful.

Mildly Asymptomatic Lead Poisoning (BPb 20–35 µg/dL)
1. D-Penicillamine useful. Monitor for side effects. 30 mg/kg/day in 2–3 divided doses. Therapy started with ¼ the calculated dose; doubled to ½ expected dose after 1 week
2. At 2 weeks—child to return to clinic for blood assays for white blood cells, differential, platelets, urinalysis, BUN, BPb, and EP double the dose of penicillamine to the full amount.
3. See child in 2 weeks.
4. Then monthly until BPb is less than 15 µg/dL or maximum of 3 months on full dose. If penicillamine is stopped, rebound can occur.

Graek J: Lead poisoning; Part I, II, III. in Clin Toxicol Rev 1992;14(8,9,12).
Graef JW: Lead Poisoning—Part III. Therapeutic Protocols, Clin Toxicol Rev 1992;14(12):1–2.

4. Patients with blood levels of greater than 70 µg/dL or with clinical symptoms suggesting encephalopathy require inpatient chelation therapy using the most efficacious parenteral agents available. Lead encephalopathy is a life-threatening emergency that should be treated using contemporary standards for intensive care treatment of increased intracranial pressure, including appropriate pressure monitoring, osmotic therapy, and drug therapy in addition to chelation therapy. Therapy is initiated with intramuscular dimercaprol (BAL) at 25 mg/kg per day divided into six doses. The second dose of BAL is given 4 hours later, followed immediately by intravenous $CaNa_2$EDTA at 50 mg/kg per day as a single dose infused during several hours or as a continuous infusion. Current labeling of $CaNa_2$EDTA does not support the intravenous route of administration, but clinical experience suggests that it is safe and more appropriate in the pediatric population. The hemodynamic stability of these patients, as well as changes in neurologic status that may herald encephalopathy, needs to be closely monitored. Adequate hydration should be maintained to ensure renal excretion.

Therapy needs to be continued for a minimum of 72 hours. After this initial treatment, two alternatives are possible: (a) the parenteral therapy with two drugs ($CaNa_2$EDTA and BAL) may be continued for a total of 5 days; or (b) therapy with $CaNa_2$EDTA alone may be continued for a total of 5 days. If BAL and $CaNa_2$EDTA are used for the full 5 days, a minimum of 2 days with no treatment should elapse before considering another 5-day course of treatment. In patients with lead encephalopathy, parenteral chelation should be continued with both drugs until they are clinically stable before therapy is changed.

Follow-Up

After chelation therapy, a period of reequilibration of 10 to 14 days should be allowed, and another blood lead concentration should be obtained. Subsequent treatment should be based on this determination, following the categories presented above.

LEAD-BASED PAINT

Central to the treatment of the lead-poisoned child is identification and removal of the lead source. A national health objective for the year 2000 is to reduce the prevalence in children aged 6 months through 5 years who have blood lead levels over 15 µg/dL to less than 500,000 and the prevalence of those with blood lead levels greater than 25 µg/dL to zero.

Deleading

The New Jersey Department of Health has developed a guide for the safe removal of lead paint.[119]

Lead-based paint should be removed only by professionals trained in hazardous material removal. Consumers should not attempt to remove lead-based paint. Any attempt to remove lead-based paint may create a serious hazard in the house.[120]

Homeowners should question contractors about their familiarity with the following procedures:

1. The room should be sealed from the rest of the house. All furniture, carpets, and drapes should be removed.
2. Workers should wear respirators designed to avoid inhaling lead.
3. No eating or drinking should be allowed in the work area. All food and eating utensils should be removed from the room. All cabinets, as well as food contact surfaces, should be covered and sealed.
4. Children and other occupants (especially infants, pregnant women, and adults with high blood pressure) should be kept out of the house until the job is completed.
5. Clothing worn in the room should be disposed of after working. The work clothing should not be worn in other areas of the house.
6. Debris should be cleaned up using special vacuum cleaners with HEPA (high-efficiency particle absorption) filters. A wet mop should be used after vacuuming.

Screening Strategies

The Centers for Disease Control and Prevention recommends decreasing exposure to lead through simple home-based intervention for children with blood levels between 0.50 µmol/L (10 µg/dL) and 0.70 µmol/L (14 µg/dL). More intensive home interventions and the identification of specific sources of lead in the child's environment are indicated when blood lead levels are between 0.75 µmol/L (15 µg/dL) and 0.96 µmol/L (19 µg/dL). Children whose blood lead levels are between 1.00 µmol/L (20 µg/dL) and 1.20 µmol/L (25 µg/dL) should have a detailed environmental and behavioral history, physical examination, and testing for iron deficiency, as well as a home inspection and lead abatement.[122]

SUGGESTED READING

1. Graef J. Lead poisoning. I, II, and III. Clin Toxicol Rev 1992; 14:8,9,12.
2. Commonwealth of Massachusetts: MGL Chapter III, SS190-199a. Childhood lead poisoning prevention act. Regulation for lead poisoning prevention and control. 105CMP560.000, 7/29/91.
3. Agency for Toxic Substances and Disease Registry. The nature and safety of lead poisoning in children in the United States: a report to Congress. Washington, DC: Superintendent of Documents, US Dept Health Human Services, July, 1988.
4. A new look at lead toxicity. Conference on Childhood Lead Toxicity. Comtact Corp CHE019, 1991.
5. Royce SE, Needleman HL. Case Studies in Environmental Medicine. Lead Toxicity. Atlanta: Agency for Toxic Substances and Disease Registry, June 1990.
6. The Lead Paint Primer. Questions and Answers on Lead Paint Poisoning. Melrose, MA: Star Industries.
7. Centers for Disease Control: Preventing Lead Poisoning in Young Children. Atlanta: US Dept Health Human Services. Public Health Service, October 1991.
8. Toxicological Profile for Lead. Agency for Toxic Substances and Disease Registry. ATSDR/TP-88/17, June 1990.

REFERENCES—LEAD

1. Committee on Environmental Health. Lead poisoning: from screening to primary prevention. Pediatrics 1993;92: 176–183.
2. Piomelli S, Wolff JA. Childhood lead poisoning in the '90s. Pediatrics 1994;93:508–510.
3. Harvey B. Should blood lead screening recommendations be revised? Pediatrics 1944;93:201–204.
4. Royce SE, Needleman HL. Case studies in environmental medicine. I. Lead toxicity. ATSDR, June 1990. Public Health Service.
5. Gloag D. Sources of lead pollution. Br Med J 1981;282: 41–44.
6. Public Health Service. Healthy People 2000: National Health Promotion and Disease Prevention Objectives. Washington, DC: US Department of Health and Human Services, Public Health Service 1990; DHHS Publication No (NHS) 90-50212.
7. New Jersey Department of Health. Accident Prevention and Poison Control Program. Manual for Safe Removal of Lead Paint, March 1992.
8. Consumer Product Safety Alert. CSSC warns about hazards of "do-it-yourself" removal of lead-based paint. Washington, DC: US Consumer Product Safety Commission, February 1989.
9. Smitherman J. Household lead exposure. Newscare Poison Prevention and Hazardous Materials Information, San Francisco Bay Area Regional Poison Center. 1989;5(1):1–2.
10. Amitai Y, Graef JW, Brown MJ, Gertler RS, Kahn N, Cochran PE. Hazards of "deleading" homes of children with lead poisoning. Am J Dis Child 1987;141:758–760.
11. Amitai Y, Brown MJ, Graef JW, Cograve E. Residential deleading: effects on the blood lead levels of lead-poisoned children. Pediatrics 1991;88:893–897.
12. CDC. Preventing lead poisoning in young children. USDHHS, October 1991; p. 71.

13. Newton D, Pickford CJ, Chamberlain AC, Sherlock JC, Hislop JS. Elevation of lead in urine blood from its controlled ingestion in beer. Hum Exp Toxicol 1992;11:3–9.
14. Goldberg RC, Hicks AM, O'Leary LM, London S. Lead exposure at uncovered outdoor firing ranges. J Occup Med 1991;33:718–719.
15. Tripathi RK, Sherertz PC, Llewellyn GC, Armstrong CW. Lead exposure in outdoor firearm instructors. Am J Public Health 1991;81:752–755.
16. ATSDR (Agency for Toxic Substances and Disease Registry). The nature and extent of lead poisoning in children in the United States: a report to Congress. Atlanta: ATSDR, 1988.
17. Parras F, Patier JL, Ezpeleta C. Lead-contaminated heroin as a source of inorganic lead intoxication. N Engl J Med 1987; 316:755.
18. Montefort S. Lead poisoning in heroin addicts. Br Med J 1987;299.
19. CDC. Lead poisoning associated with intravenous amphetamine use—Oregon 1988. MMWR 1989;38:830–831.
20. Norton RL, Kauffman KW, Chandler DB, Burton BT, Gordon J, Fostern LR. Intravenous lead poisoning associated with methamphetamine use. Vet Hum Toxicol 1989;31:379.
21. Allcott JV III, Barnhart RA, Mooney LA. Acute lead poisoning in two users of illicit methamphetamine. JAMA 1987;258: 510–511.
22. Shannon MW, Graef JW. Lead intoxication in infancy. Pediatrics 1992;89:87–90.
23. Selbst SM, Henretig F, Fee MA, Levy SE, Kitts AW. Lead poisoning in a child with a gunshot wound. Pediatrics 1986;77: 413–416.
24. Kikano GE, Stange KC. Lead poisoning in a child after a gunshot injury. J Fam Pract 1992;34:498–504.
25. Nordberg GF, Mahaffey KR, Fowler BA. Introduction and summary. International Workshop on lead in bone: implications for dosimetry and toxicology. Environ Health Perspect 1991;91:3–7.
26. Hu H, Milder FL, Burger DE. The use of x-ray fluorescence for measuring lead burden in epidemiological studies: high and low lead burdens and measurement uncertainty. Environ Health Perspect 1991;94:107–110.
27. Rosen JF, Markowitz ME, Baer PE, Jenks ST, Wielopolski L, Kalef-Ezra JF et al. Sequential measurements of bone lead content by x-ray fluorescence in $CaNa_2EDTA$-treated lead-toxic children. Environ Health Perspect 1991;91:57–62.
28. Wedeen RD. In vivo tibial XFR measurement of bone lead. Arch Environ Health 1990;45:69–70.
29. Shannon M, Lindy H, Anast C, Graef J. Recurrent lead poisoning in a child with immobilization osteoporosis. Vet Hum Toxicol 1988;30:586–588.
30. Sublet VH. Lead. A Reproductive Toxin in Humans. Fact or Fiction. Atlanta, GA: Agency for Toxic Substances and Disease Registry, US Department of Health and Human Services.
31. Needleman HL, Rabinowitz M, Leviton A et al. The relationship between prenatal exposure to lead and congenital anomalies. JAMA 1984;251:2956–2959.
32. Shukla R, Bornschein RL, Dietrich KV, Buncher CR, Berger OG, Hammond PB et al. Fetal and infant lead exposure: effect on growth in stature. Pediatrics 1989;84:604–612.
33. Winder C. Reproductive and chromosomal effects of occupational exposure to lead in the male. Reprod Toxicol 1989; 3:221–233.
34. Lancranjian I, Popescu HI, Gavanescu O, Klepsch I, Serbanescu M. Reproductive ability of workmen occupationally exposed to lead. Arch Environ Health 1975;30: 396–401.
35. McGregor AJ, Mason HJ. Chronic occupational lead exposure and testicular endocrine function. Hum Exp Toxicol 1990;9:371–376.
36. Mg TP, Goh HH, Ng LY, Ong HY, Ong C, Chia SE et al. Male endocrine function in workers with moderate exposure to lead. Br J Ind Med 1991;48:485–491.
37. Ernhart CB, Greene T. Postpartum changes in maternal blood lead concentrations. Br J Ind Med 1992;49:11–13.
38. Lead in table wines could pose hazards for pregnant and nursing women. FDA Med Bull 1991;21(3):6–7.
39. Mahaffey KR. Biokinetics of lead during pregnancy. Fundam Appl Toxicol 1991;16:15–16.
40. Goyer RA. Transplacental transport of lead. Environ Health Perspect 1990;89:101–105.
41. McMichael AJ, Vimpani GV, Robertson EF et al. The Port Pirie Cohort Study: maternal blood lead and pregnancy outcome. J Epidemiol Cancer Health 1986;40:18.
42. Bellinger DC, Leviton A, Needleman HL et al. Low level lead exposure and infant development in the first year. Neurobehav Toxicol Teratol 1986;8:151.
43. Levine F, Muenke M. Vacterl association with high prenatal lead exposure. Similarities to animal models of lead teratogenicity. Pediatrics 1991;87:390–392.
44. Farni A, Sciame A, Bertazzi PA, Alesio L. Chromosomal and biochemical studies in women occupationally exposed to lead. Arch Environ Health 1980;35:139–146.
45. Wong GP, Ng TL, Martin TR, Farquharson DF. Effects of low level lead exposure in utero. Obstet Gynecol Survey 1992;45: 285–289.
46. Bernard BP, Becker CE. Environmental lead poisoning and the kidney. Clin Toxicol 1988;26:1–34.
47. Staessen J, Yeoman WB, Fletcher AE, Markowe HLJ, Marmot MG, Rose G et al. Blood lead concentration, renal function and blood pressure in London civil servants. Br J Indust Med 1990 ;47:442–447.
48. Staessen JA, Lauwerys RR, Buchet J-P, Bulpitt CJ, Rondia D, Vanrenterghem Y et al. Impairment of renal function with increasing blood lead concentrations in the general population. N Engl J Med 1992;237:151–156.
49. Endo G, Horiguchi S, Kiyota I. Urinary *N*-acetyl-beta-D-glucosaminidase activity in lead-exposed workers. J Appl Toxicol 1990;10:235–238.
50. Pirkle JL, Schwartz J, Landis JR, Harlan WR. The relationship between blood lead levels and blood pressure and its cardiovascular risk implications. Am J Epidemiol 1985; 121:246–258.
51. Osterloh JD, Selvy JV, Bernard BP, Becker CE, Menke DJ, Tepper E et al. Body burdens of lead in hypertensive nephropathy. Arch Environ Health 1989;44:304–310.
52. Kosnett MJ, Becker CE, Osterloh JD, Kelly TJ, Pasta DJ. Factors influencing bone lead concentration in a suburban community assessed by noninvasive x-ray fluorescence. JAMA 1994;271:197–202.
53. Royce SE, Needleman HL. Case studies on environmental medicine. Lead toxicity. US Department of Health and Human Services, Agency for Toxic Substance and Disease Registry.
54. Schwartz J, Landrigan PJ, Feldman RG, Silbergeld EK, Baker EL, von Lindern IH. Threshold effect on lead-induced peripheral neuropathy. J Pediatr 1988;112:12–17.
55. Roelofs-Iverson PA, Mulder DW, Elvebach LR, Kurland LT, Molgoard CA. ALS and heavy metals: a pilot case-control study. Neurology 1984;34:393–395.
56. Boothby JA, de Jesus PV, Rowland LP. Reversible factor of motor neuron disease. Arch Neurol 1974;21:18–23.
57. Marecek J, Shapiro IM, Burke A et al. Low level exposure in childhood influences neuropsychological performance. Arch Environ Health 1983;38:355–359.
58. Baghurst PA, McMichael AJ, Wigg NP, Vimpani GV, Robertson EF, Roberts RJ et al. Environmental exposure to lead and children's intelligence at the age of seven years. The Post Pirie Cohort Study. N Engl J Med 1992;327:1275–1284.
59. Pocock SJ, Smith M, Baghurst P. Environmental lead and children's intelligence: a systematic review of the epidemiological evidence. Br Med J 1994;309:1189–1197.
60. Rosen JF. Health effects of lead at low exposure levels. Expert consensus and rationale for lowering the definition of childhood lead poisoning. Am J Dis Child 1992;146:1278–1281.
61. Thecker SB, Hoffman DA, Smith J, Steinberg K, Zall M. Effect of low-lead body burdens of lead on the mental development of children: limitations of meta-analysis in a review of longitudinal data. Arch Environ Health 1992;47:336–346.
62. Chisolm JJ Jr. The continuing hazard of lead exposure and its effects in children. Neurotoxicology 1984;5:23–42.

63. Needleman HL, Gatsonis CA. Low-level lead exposure and the IQ of children. A meta-analysis of modern studies. JAMA 1990;263:673–678.
64. Needleman HL, Schell A, Bellinger D, Leviton A, Allred EN. The long-term effects of exposure to low doses of lead in childhood. An 11-year follow-up report. N Engl J Med 1990;322:83–88.
65. Fergusson DM, Fergusson JE, Horwood LJ, Kinzett NG. A longitudinal study of dentine lead levels, intelligence study of school performance and behavior. I. Dentine lead levels and exposure to environmental risk factors. J Child Psychol Psychiatry 1988;29:781–792. II. Dentine lead and cognitive ability. J Child Psychol Psychiatry 1988;29:783–809.
66. Sargent JD, Meyers A, Weitzman M. Environmental exposure to lead and cognitive deficit in children. N Engl J Med 1989;320:595.
67. Smith M. The neuropsychological effects of lead in children. A review of the research 1984–1988. Report from the Medical Research Council (UK) Advisory Group on Lead and Neuropsychological Effects in Children. June 1988.
68. Ernhart CB. A critical review of low-level prenatal lead exposure in the human. II. Effects on the developing child. Reprod Toxicol 1992;6:21–40.
69. Cooney GH, Bell A, McBride W, Carter C. Low level exposure to lead: the Sydney lead study. Develop Med Child Neurol 1989;31:640–649.
70. Bellinger D, Leviton A, Sloman J. Antecedents and correlates of improved cognitive performance in children exposed in utero to low levels of lead. Environ Health Perspect 1990;89: 5–11.
71. Schwartz OD. Lead and minor hearing impairment. Arch Environ Health 1991;46:300–305.
72. Clark M, Royal J, Seeler R. Interaction of iron deficiency and lead and the hematologic findings in children with severe lead poisoning. Pediatrics 1988;81:247–254.
73. Graef J. Lead poisoning. I. Clin Toxicol Rev 1992;14(8):1–2.
74. Durbach LF, Wedin GP, Seidler DE. Management of lead foreign body ingestion. Clin Toxicol 1989;27:173–182.
75. Wiley JF II, Henretig FM, Selbst SM. Blood lead levels in children with foreign bodies. Pediatrics 1992;89:593–596.
76. Hugelmeyer CD, Morrhead JC, Horenblas L, Bayer MJ. Fatal lead encephalopathy following foreign body ingestion: case report. J Emerg Med 1988;6:397–400.
77. CDC. Preventing lead poisoning in young children. USDHHS, October 1991; p. 53.
78. CDC. Preventing lead poisoning in young children. USDHHS, October 1991; p. 46.
79. Hazardous Substances Public Health Agency for Toxic Substances and Disease Registry, 1992;2(1).
80. Piomelli S, Rosen JF, Chisolm JJ Jr, Graef JW. Management of childhood lead poisoning. J Pediatr 1984;105:523–532.
81. Markowitz ME, Rosen JF. Need for the lead mobilization test in children with lead poisoning. J Pediatr 1991;119:305–310.
82. CDC. Preventing lead poisoning in young children. USDHHS, October 1991; pp. 53–54.
83. Markowitz ME, Rosen JF, Bijur PE. Effects of iron deficiency on lead excretion in children with moderate lead intoxication. J Pediatr 1990;116:360–364.
84. Markowitz ME, Rosen JF. Assessment of lead stones in children: validation of an 8-hour $CaNa_2EDTA$ provocative test. J Pediatr 1984;104:337–342.
85. Weinberger HL, Post ER, Schneider T, Helu B, Friedman J. An analysis of 248 initial mobilization tests performed on an ambulatory basis. Am J Dis Child 1987;14:1266–1270.
86. Shannon MW, Kassner J, Garef J. Use of urinary creatinine in the interpretation of the lead mobilization test. Vet Hum Toxicol 1990;32:365.
87. Batuman V, Wedeen RR. Impairment of renal function with increasing blood lead concentrations. N Engl J Med 1992; 327:1394–1395.
88. CDC. Preventing Lead Poisoning in Young Children. US Department of Health and Human Services, October 1991, pp. 57.
89. Chisolm JJ Jr, Thomas DJ. Use of 2,3-dimercaptoprane-1-sulfonate in treatment of lead poisoning in children. J Pharmacol Exp Ther 1985;235:665–669.
90. CDC. Preventing Lead Poisoning in Young Children. US Department of Health and Human Services, October 1991, pp. 57–59.
91. Shannon M, Graef J, Lovejoy FH. Efficacy and toxicity of D-penicillamine in low-level lead poisoning. J Pediatr 1988; 12:799–804.
92. Adelman HM, Winters PR, Mahan CS, Wallach PM. D-penicillamine-induced myasthenia gravis: diagnosis observed by coexisting chronic obstructive pulmonary disease. Am J Med Sci 1995;309:191–193.
93. Graef J. Lead poisoning management. II. Clin Toxicol Rev 1992;14(9):1–2.
94. Shannon M, Grace A, Graef JW. Use of penicillamine in children with small lead burdens. N Engl J Med 1989;321: 979–980.
95. Graziano JH. Use of penicillamine in children with small lead burdens. N Engl J Med 1990;322:1888.
96. Liebelt EL, Shannon MW. Oral chelators for childhood lead poisoning. Pediatr Annals 1994;23:616–626.
97. Donner A, Hruby K, Pirich K, Kahls P, Schwarzacher K, Meisinger V. Dimercaptopropansulfonate (DMPS) in the treatment of acute lead poisoning. Vet Hum Toxicol 1987; 29(Suppl 2):37.
98. Chisolm JJ Jr. BAL, EDTA, DMSA and DMPS in the treatment of lead poisoning in children. Clin Toxicol 1992;30:493–504.
99. Liebelt EL, Shannon M, Graef JW. Efficacy of oral meso-2,3-dimercaptosuccinic acid therapy for low-level childhood plumbism. J Pediatr 1994;124:313–317.
100. Graziano JH, Lolacono NJ, Moulton T, Mitchell ME, Slavkovich V, Zarate C. Controlled study of meso 2,3-dimercaptosuccinic acid for the management of childhood lead intoxication. J Pediatr 1992;120:133–139.
101. Ching GWK, Rogers SM, Braithwaite RA, Vale JA. An oral treatment for lead toxicity. Postgrad Med J 1991;67: 953–956.
102. Rosen JF, Markowitz ME. Trends in the management of childhood lead poisonings. Neurotoxicology 1993;14:211–218.
103. Aposhian HV, Aposhian MM. Meso-2,3,dimercaptosuccinic acid: chemical, pharmacological and toxicological properties of an orally effective metal chelating agent. Ann Rev Pharmacol Toxicol 1990;30:279–306.
104. Hurlbut KM, Dart RC, Gercina RA, Brad GR, Philips S. Changes in white blood cell counts (WBC) associated with dimercaptosuccinic acid (DMSA) therapy. Vet Hum Toxicol 1993;35:353.
105. Chisolm JJ Jr. Evaluation of the potential role of chelation therapy in treatment of low to moderate lead exposure. Environ Health Perspect 1990;89:67–74.
106. Lovejoy FH, Shannon M, Woolf AD. Recent advances in clinical toxicology. Curr Probl Pediatr 1992 (March), pp. 119–129.
107. Liebelt E, Shannon M, Graef J. The efficacy of oral DMSA for lead childhood plumbism. Vet Hum Toxicol 1992;24:360.
108. Graziano JH. Role of 2,3-dimercaptosuccinic acid in the treatment of heavy metal poisoning. Med Toxicol 1986;1: 155–162.
109. Ruff HA, Bijur PE, Markowitz M, MA Y-C, Rosen JF. Declining blood lead levels and cognitive changes in moderately lead-poisoned children. JAMA 1993;269:1641–1646.
110. Pedersen RS. Lead poisoning treated with haemodialysis. Scand J Urol Nephrol 1978;12:189–190.
111. Roberge RJ, Martin T, Michelson EA. Whole bowel irrigation in acute lead ingestion. Vet Hum Toxicol 1991;33:353.
112. Murphy DG, Gerace RV, Peterson RG. The use of whole bowel irrigation in acute lead ingestion. Vet Hum Toxicol 1991;33:353.
113. Kim JS, Crichlow EC, Blakley BR. The effects of thiamine on the neurophysiological alterations induced by lead. Vet Hum Toxicol 1990;32:101–105.
114. Flora SJS, Singh S, Tandon SK. Thiamine and zinc in prevention therapy of lead intoxication. J Int Med Res 1989;17: 68–75.
115. Roberge RJ, Martin TG. Whole bowel irrigation in an acute oral lead intoxication. Am J Emerg Med 1992;10: 577–583.

116. Graef J. Lead poisoning. I, II, and III. Clin Toxicol Rev 1992; 14:8,9,12.
117. Graef JW. Lead poisoning. III. Therapeutic protocols. Clin Toxicol Rev 1992;14(12):1–2.
118. Committee on Drugs American Academy of Pediatrics. Treatment guidelines for lead exposure in children. Pediatrics 1995;96:155–160.
119. Waldron HA. Chasing the lead. Br Med J 1985;291:366–367.
120. Sawyer M, Kerny T, Spector S et al. Lead intoxication in children—Interdepartmental Conference, University of California, San Diego. (Specialty Conference) West J Med 1985;143:357–364.
121. Greeley A. Getting the lead out. FDA Consumer 1991;25(6): 26–31.
122. Centers for Disease Control. Preventing lead poisoning in young children. A statement by the Centers for Disease Control. Atlanta, GA: US Dept of Health and Human Services, 1991.

LITHIUM

Lithium is used as the drug of choice for manic-depressive affective disorders, adjunctive therapy of depressive disorders, mania control in children and adolescents, treatment of alcoholism, control of schizoaffective disorders, prophylaxis of cluster headaches, and amelioration of chemotherapy-induced neutropenia. This has also expanded the population at risk for toxicity.[1]

Although lithium is used industrially in nuclear reactor coolant, alkaline storage batteries, and alloys, occupational lithium toxicity is rare. Lithium has a narrow toxic therapeutic index, with most common poisonings resulting from altered drug kinetics during chronic therapeutic use. Side effects include thirst, polyuria, resting tremor, acne, hypothyroidism, and rarely dysarthria, ataxia, impaired cognition,[2] and pseudotumor cerebri,[3] alopecia,[4] keratoderma,[5] psoriasis of the fingernails,[6] restless legs syndrome,[7] and rhabdomyolysis associated with a hyperosmolar state followed by reduced renal tubular concentrating ability.[8–11]

TOXIC DOSAGE

A single ingestion of 40 mg of lithium salt per kilogram by a patient with a history of prior lithium use is capable of producing toxic lithium blood levels (>2 mEq/L).[12]

TOXICOKINETICS[12–19]

Bioavailability (%)	over 95%
Peak plasma levels	0.8 to 1.5 mmol/L
Peak plasma level time	30 minutes to 2 hours; in overdose: up to 72 hours
Volume of distribution	0.6 L/kg
Plasma protein binding	<10%
Elimination half-life	24 hours

DRUG INTERACTIONS

Table 67–26 lists many of the numerous drug interactions of lithium. Cisplatin effects on the glomeruli and tubules may either increase or decrease serum lithium concentration.[20] Lisinopril may induce elevations of lithium serum concentrations with CNS toxic effects.[21] Additional drug interactions are found in Table 67–27.

PREGNANCY[9,12,32–38]

Prospective controlled studies of pregnant women who have ingested lithium during the first trimester suggest that such ingestions do not lead to a significant increase in spontaneous or therapeutic abortions or to the incidence of major malformations.[32,33] If an association exists between Ebstein's anomaly and lithium, it is a weak one.[34,35] Lithium inhibits thyroid hormone release and stimulates thyroid-stimulating hormone production. Goiter in the newborn has been observed.[35]

The best estimate of the risk of major congenital anomalies among the children of women treated during early

Table 67–26
Lithium and Drug Interactions

Drug	Lithium Renal Clearance: Reduced	Lithium Renal Clearance: Increased	Toxic at Normal Therapeutic Lithium Levels	Other
Thiazide diuretics	+			
Ibuprofen	+			
Indomethacin	+			
Phenylbutazone	+			
Dictofenac	+			
Piroxicam	+			
Mazindol	+			
Phenytoin	+			
Tetracycline	+			
Acetazolamide		+		
Theophylline		+		
Verapamil		+		
Cisplatin		+		
Sodium bicarbonate		+		
Carbamazepine			+	Neurologic toxicity signs
Methyldopa	+		+	May exacerbate CNS response to lithium
Neuroleptics (high doses)			+	Neuroleptic syndrome, extrapyramidal symptoms

Adapted from Groleau G et al. Am J Emerg Med 1987;5:527–553.

Table 67–27
Conditions That May Increase the Risk of Lithium Toxicity

Chronic medical conditions
Increased age
Hypertension
Diabetes mellitus
Congestive heart failure
Chronic renal failure
Schizophrenia
Addison's disease
Acute medical conditions
Vomiting
Diarrhea
Low salt diet
Low food intake
Recent increase in lithium dosage
Intentional overdose

pregnancy is on the order of 4 to 12% in cohort studies. The prevalence of congenital anomalies in the untreated comparison groups was 2 to 4%. Patients who decide to conceive while taking lithium and who subsequently continue to take it should be counseled regarding the slightly increased risks of cardiovascular and other malformations in the fetus.[39] No difference with controls was observed in development milestones. Another study suggests a higher incidence of cardiac anomalies among newborn infants exposed to lithium carbonate in utero.[9]

Schou advises, as a general rule, that women of fertile age use contraceptive measures while receiving lithium treatment, that the treatment be discontinued before a planned pregnancy, and that it is stopped as soon as an unplanned pregnancy has been discovered. If the woman's past history indicates that the risk of manic-depressive relapse is high, one may consider starting treatment again after passage of the first half of the pregnancy when morphogenesis is finished. Pregnant women in lithium treatment should be referred to obstetric and gynecologic specialists for pregnancy or reproductive problems or questions. Lithium may need to be discontinued 2 to 3 days before the expected delivery date to lower the lithium concentration in the newborn and to prevent lithium accumulation caused by derangement of fluid and water balance during the delivery. Lithium treatment should be started again a few days after the delivery with an appropriately reduced dose. In infants blood lithium concentrations are about one-tenth to one-half the concentration in the mother's milk. There are little data to indicate that breast-feeding should be contraindicated.[35]

Lithium levels should be monitored throughout pregnancy and dosage adjusted as necessary. Sodium-restricted diets and diuretics should be used with caution. Lithium doses should be reduced with the onset of labor. Mothers who choose to breast-feed should watch for signs of toxicity in their babies.[38]

NEWBORNS

Lithium crosses the placenta readily. Fetal serum concentrations approximately equal maternal serum levels. Toxicity has been noted in newborns of mothers taking lithium and is manifested by hypotonicity, lethargy, and cyanosis. Lithium may be one of the causes of the "floppy baby" syndrome.[40] Lithium passes through breast milk.[41]

TARGET ORGANS

Central Nervous System

The major target organ of overdose is the central nervous system.[42]

Kidney

Up to 5% of patients treated with lithium for a long period develop renal insufficiency.[43] Both glomerular and tubular function are affected.[44] It remains undisputed that lithium is capable of causing a major disturbance in water balance, manifest as polyuria and secondary polydipsia (Fig. 67–6). A decreased urinary concentrating ability (nephrogenic diabetes insipidus) with a disturbed responsiveness of the distal nephron to the action of ADH (vasopressin) is demonstrable, and the symptoms are largely reversible on cessation of lithium or reduction of the dose. An acute histologic lesion of the distal nephron, corresponding to the site of lithium inhibition of the action of ADH and consisting of epithelial cellular swelling and glycogen deposition, also appears to be readily reversible.[45]

A single massive ingestion of lithium has no constant dose-dependent direct acute or chronic nephropathy.[46]

Cardiovascular System

Cardiac complications are common but rarely serious in chronic overdose.[42] Dysrhythmias are rare. Hypotension usually is secondary to coma.[47]

Repeat cardiac arrests may be observed during chronic lithium therapy.[48] Sinus arrests and asystole due to serum lithium intoxication may be seen in patients with preexisting conduction tissue disease.[49]

Lithium treatment, even with steady-state serum levels of less than 1.0 mEq, can result in sinus arrest and repolarization delay (prolonged QTc interval). Lithium may depress serum potassium concentrations. Oral supplementation of potassium may result in a reversing of the QTc interval toward prelithium levels while lithium levels remain unchanged. Sinus node dysfunction is the most common lithium-related conduction defect. Both the sinus node dysfunction and cardiac repolarization delays may be treated by oral potassium chloride.[50]

Respiratory

Severe lithium intoxication may be followed by a life-threatening acute respiratory distress syndrome.[1] It may be seen in a patient who is neurologically intact and has no infection. The diagnosis of noncardiogenic pulmonary edema with normal ventricular function will be confirmed by echocardiogram and a normal pulmonary capillary wedge pressure in the setting of normal systemic indices of perfusion.[1]

Rarely an acute respiratory distress syndrome (ARDS) confirmed by pulmonary artery catheterization has followed a lithium overdose. In one anecdotal report the patient

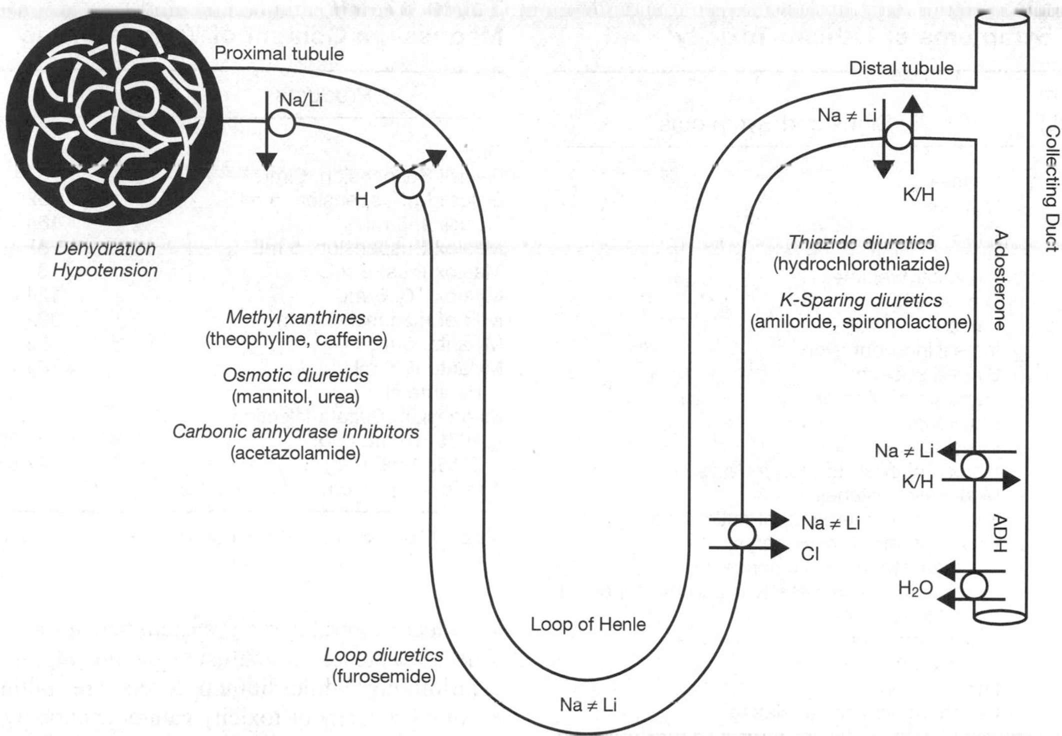

Figure 67–6 Renal handling of lithium. The lithium ion is freely filtered by the glomerulus. Clearance may, therefore, be influenced by various physiological factors which reduce renal blood flow and filtration rates (e.g., dehydration or hypotension). Reabsorption of lithium occurs in parallel with sodium in the proximal tubule and, to a lesser extent, the loop of Henle. In the distal tubule and collecting duct, antidiuretic hormone (ADH) and aldosterone facilitate the reabsorption of sodium and water but the tubular membrane appears to be impervious to lithium along the distal portion. As a result, the administration of distally acting diuretics (e.g., thiazides and spironolactone) will potentiate an increase in lithium reabsorption along the proximal tubule, while diuretics with more proximal activity [e.g., furosemide (frusemide)] are not associated with a compensatory increase in reabsorption rates. (Adapted from Finley PR et al. Clin Pharmacokinet 1995;29:172–191.)

survived after intubation and positive end-expiratory ventilation.[1]

Thyroid and Parathyroid

Lithium is concentrated in the thyroid gland and can reach levels 2.5 to 5 times those of its concentration in the serum.[51] Lithium inhibits thyroid hormone synthesis and metabolites at five different stages: (a) iodine uptake, (b) iodination of tyrosine, (c) release of thyroxine (T_4) and triiodothyronine T_3), (d) peripheral iodination of T_4 and T_3, and (e) modification of the effect of thyrotropin (TSH) on the thyroid gland.[51] Thyrotoxicosis has developed in the course of lithium therapy despite the general suppressive effect of lithium on thyroid hormone synthesis and release. Long-term lithium therapy may lead to laboratory evidence of hyperparathyroidism (elevated serum calcium, ionized calcium, and parathormone levels).[52] Lithium intoxication may exacerbate preexisting hypothyroidism to the point of respiratory arrest and myxedema coma.[53]

CLINICAL PRESENTATION

Jaeger and colleagues suggest three types of poisoning[54]:

1. Acute poisoning, voluntary or accidental, in patients not previously treated with lithium. This poisoning carries less risk and patients usually show only mild symptoms independent of the serum lithium concentration. However, more severe symptoms may appear after a delay if lithium elimination is impaired.
2. Acute on chronic poisoning, i.e., an acute overdose in patients who are under lithium treatment. In this type of poisoning, serum concentrations above 3 to 4 mmol/L are usually associated with severe symptoms.
3. Chronic or therapeutic poisoning that occurs in patients who are under lithium treatment. These patients develop progressive lithium toxicity following an increase in dosage, a decrease of lithium renal elimination, an intercurrent disease, or drug administration. Severity of symptoms usually correlates well with serum concentrations, although features of toxicity may also be present at concentrations below 1.5 mmol/L.

ACUTE AND CHRONIC TOXICITY

Table 67–28 compares acute and chronic lithium toxicity.

NEUROLOGIC EFFECTS

Lithium administered to patients with preexisting neurologic disease (e.g., stroke) may, at low to therapeutic plasma levels, enhance disabling neurologic symptoms.[55] Patients with lithium toxicity may present with a neurologic syndrome suggesting a diagnosis of Creutzfeldt-Jacob disease.[56]

Table 67–28
Signs and Symptoms of Lithium Toxicity*

Blood Lithium Level (mEq/L)	Signs and Symptoms
1.5	Nausea
	Diarrhea
2.0	Polyuria
	Blurred vision
	Muscular weakness
	Drowsiness
	Vertigo
	Increasing confusion
	Slurred speech
	Transient scotomas
	Blackouts
	Fasiculations
	Increased deep tendon reflexes
2.5	Myoclonic twitches
	Myoclonic movements of entire limbs
	Choreoathetoid movements
	Urinary or fecal incontinence
	Increasing restlessness followed by stupor, followed by coma
3.0	Epileptiform seizure
	Cardiac dysrhythmias
4.0	Hypotension
	Peripheral vascular collapse

WITHDRAWAL SYNDROME

If lithium and chlorpromazine are used in combination, the withdrawal of lithium may be potentially dangerous (prolonged QTc interval, low serum potassium, ventricular fibrillation). The dose of chlorpromazine may need to be reduced if lithium is to be discontinued.[57] Some components of the adenylate cyclase system that are sensitive to lithium inhibition may become supersensitive to stimulation after lithium withdrawal.[58] Withdrawal relapse after lithium treatment of patients with manic illness can begin 13 to 19 days after stopping the drug.[59]

LABORATORY

Serum Levels

Serum levels do not always correlate with symptoms in part because of drug interactions and coexisting disease processes. An approximate correlation is suggested by Groleau (Table 67–29).

In chronic lithium therapy in humans, red blood cell (RBC) lithium levels appear to correlate better than serum levels with clinical response and neurotoxicity. Early in an acute intoxication, RBC levels may be more useful than serum levels in predicting toxicity and the need for hemodialysis.[60] Rebound of lithium after hemodialysis may be due to a trichobezoar containing fragments of lithium tablets.[61] Seizures may occur in susceptible patients at therapeutic doses documented by normal serum lithium levels.[62]

Remember that in acute overdose lithium levels may be quite elevated without the patient exhibiting significant toxicity. Peak serum concentrations may occur much later after a large overdose than after a therapeutic dose. Severe toxicity may not occur after levels have peaked and significant central nervous system penetration has occurred. This may present a confusing picture of a patient who is deteriorating while lithium levels are falling. Thus the eventual severity of toxicity cannot accurately be predicted by either the presenting clinical status or the lithium levels. Patients can deteriorate late after presentation.[63]

Table 67–29
Magnesium Content of Various Drugs*

Products	mg	mEq
Oral		
Gelusil Suspension, 5 mL	82	6.8
Gelusil M Suspension, 5 mL	82	6.8
Gelusil II, 5 mL	164	13.7
Maalox Suspension, 5 mL	82	6.8
Maalox Plus, 5 mL	82	6.8
Maalox TC, 5 mL	124	10.3
Milk of magnesia, 10 mL	332	27
Mylanta, 5 mL	82	6.8
Mylanta II, 5 mL	164	13.7
Parenteral		
Magnesium Sulfate injection		
10%, 10 mL (1 g)	97.56	8.1
50%, 2 mL (1 g)	97.56	8.1
1 mEq magnesium ion weighs 12 mg		

Adapted from Mofenson HC and Caraccio TR. Clin Toxicol 1991;29:215–222.

Abnormalities

Lithium may impair renal-concentrating ability and can cause hypernatremia, as well as hypercalcemia and hypoparathyroidism. The effect on parathyroid secretion of parathyroid hormone (PTH) may be the initiating action. Periodic serum calcium measurements would appear to be indicated in chronic lithium use. If the hypercalcemia is mild (less than 2.8 mmol/L), no further action is indicated. If levels are higher, consider stopping lithium, if possible. If hypercalcemia persists, measure PTH levels. If these are elevated, consider neck exploration with a view to either subtotal parathyroidectomy or adenoma removal, depending on the findings.[64] Hyperbilirubinemia has been observed after therapeutic use. There were no abnormal liver function tests or evidence of hemolysis.[65]

CHRONIC INTOXICATION

Patients with chronic lithium intoxication experience a period of days to a few weeks with slight "nervous" symptoms. This will be accompanied by moderately elevated serum lithium, serum creatinine concentrations, and serum urea concentration.[66–68] Cerebrovascular deterioration, cerebellar dysfunction, and abnormal T waves are observed in patients with chronic lithium intoxication. T-wave abnormalities served to distinguish patients with acute versus chronic intoxication.[67] Patients with chronic lithium intoxication appear to be at greater risk of life-threatening events. Patients who have become chronically intoxicated from lithium have a delayed resolution of toxicity following return of lithium concentrations to therapeutic levels when compared with those with acute overdoses.

TREATMENT

Stabilization

In the obtunded patient, cumulative control of the airway, breathing, and circulation is a first priority. The patient should have access to a cardiac monitor and an IV line.[69]

Decontamination

Charcoal is not useful. No clinical data on humans are available to guide the administration of cathartics.

Sodium Polystyrene Sulfonate[70–74]

Hemodialysis is the treatment of choice for severe lithium intoxication, which presents a problem for facilities without dialysis equipment or in which there is a long delay before dialysis can be accomplished. Additional sustained-release lithium products are absorbed over a long period creating a need for repeat dialysis. Whole-bowel irrigation has reduced lithium absorption in healthy volunteers.[70] Sodium polystyrene sulfonate, which contains 4.1 mEq of sodium per gram of resin (danger for sodium overload in renal failure patients), administered to healthy volunteers after ingesting a 0.5-mEq/kg (18.5 mg/kg) lithium carbonate dose has decreased lithium absorption.[71] Another similar study used 30 g of polystyrene sulfonate followed by a similar delay in lithium absorption.

These studies were not performed in the presence of lithium overdose. They suggest that sodium polystyrene sulfonate may be given to patients immediately or soon after ingestion of a significant acute overdose of lithium when hemodialysis cannot be instituted promptly. Studies on repeat doses of sodium polystyrene sulfonate must be performed before repeated doses can be recommended to reduce absorption in lithium intoxication. Complications may include sodium overload and hypokalemia.[71,72]

Elimination Enhancement—Hemodialysis

Primary treatment should include measures such as artificial ventilation, use of anticonvulsants, and correction of hypotension, dehydration, and hypovolemia. Hemodialysis is not an emergency treatment in lithium poisoning.

Jaeger and colleagues suggest that hemodialysis may be indicated in patients satisfying several of the following clinical and kinetic criteria[16]:

Clinical Criteria

Severe intoxication (>grade 3) with coma, convulsions, or respiratory failure; progressive clinical deterioration; presence of an underlying disease that may favor the development of complications; patients with acute or chronic poisoning that increases the severity.

Kinetic Criteria

Impaired renal lithium excretion with increased serum concentration and half-life; continuing gastrointestinal absorption with rising serum concentrations or continuing cellular diffusion of lithium; amount of lithium expected to be removed by a 6 hour hemodialysis markedly higher than the 24-hour renal excretion.

Additional indications for hemodialysis include patients with serum levels over 4 mEq/L in those chronically taking lithium, those with levels between 2.5 and 4.0 mEq/L who develop serious central nervous system or cardiovascular symptoms, and those with serum lithium levels over 6 to 8 mEq/L in acute poisoning. Dialysis usually is unnecessary in patients with levels below 2.5 mEq/L. Repeat dialysis may be needed to compensate for rebound of serum levels.

The decision to undertake hemodialysis should be made some 8 to 12 hours after admission and should be based on the patient's clinical condition, the serum lithium level, and the spontaneous lithium kinetics. Hemodialysis significantly increases lithium clearance, with lithium extraction higher from serum than from whole blood or red blood cells.[75] In a chronic intoxication case, hemodialysis decreased the lithium serum half-life from 54 to 25 hours.[15]

On average, 4 hours of hemodialysis will reduce plasma lithium concentration by 1.0 mEq/L since rebound of lithium concentration may occur after dialysis. A dialysis time of 10 to 12 hours is suggested.[69]

Whole-Bowel Irrigation

Whole-bowel irrigation (WBI) with polyethylene glycol (PEG) electrolyte lavage solution at a rate of 2 L/hr for 5 hours, if begun within 1 hour after ingestion, has been shown in a crossover study to be effective for acute ingestions of sustained release lithium. Further studies will be required to confirm the use of WBI for large acute overdoses and acute on chronic overdoses.[70] Continuous arteriovenous hemodiafiltration (CAVH) can rapidly eliminate toxic quantities of lithium, does not require a hemodialysis trained staff, and is now available in an increasing number of intensive care units. The rebound increase in lithium concentrate after cessation of CAVH suggests that optimal therapy with this technique will require about 24 hours of treatment.[76]

Supportive Care

1. Patients with serum lithium levels less than 2.5 mEq/L can usually be treated with saline infusion unless they exhibit moderate or severe neurotoxicity or have significant underlying cardiac or renal disease. In the absence of these factors, physicians should first attempt a trial of rapid IV infusion of normal saline, giving 1 or 2 liters over 6 hours. Frequent monitoring of serum sodium levels is mandatory. Watch for hypernatremia. If the admitting serum levels are 2.5 to 4.0 mEq/L and there is no significant toxicity, hemodialyze the patient. Alternatively, a trial of saline infusion may be begun unless contraindicated by severe neurologic dysfunction, renal insufficiency, or congestive heart failure. Serum lithium levels above 4.0 mEq/L or patients with severe clinical symptoms require hemodialysis. Hemodialysis is also indicated if patients are asymptomatic and the serum lithium level is over 4.0 mEq/L at least 6 hours after ingestion.[77]
2. Neurologic signs with coma may require management with mechanical ventilation.

Admission Criteria

Admit symptomatic patients and asymptomatic patients with a lithium serum level exceeding 2.0 mEq/L. After serial serum levels at least 4 hours apart confirm a declining level, the asymptomatic patient may be discharged if the lithium level is below 2.0 mEq/L. Psychiatric counseling may be appropriate before discharge. Be sure to search for and correct factors contributing to toxicity (e.g., dehydration and loop diuretics).

REFERENCES—LITHIUM

1. Friedman PB, Bekes CE, Scott WE, Bartter T. ARDS following acute lithium carbonate intoxication. Intensive Care Med 1992;18:123–124.
2. Lewis DA. Unrecognized chronic lithium neurotoxic reactions. JAMA 1983;250:2029–2030.
3. Soul RF, Hamburger HA, Selhorst JB. Pseudotumor cerebri secondary to lithium carbonate. JAMA 1985;253:2869–2870.
4. Wagner KD, Teicher MH. Lithium and hair loss in childhood. Psychosomatics 1991;32:355–356.
5. Labelle A, La Pierre YD. Keratoderma: side effects of lithium. J Clin Psychopharmacol 1991;1:149–150.
6. Rudolph RI. Lithium induced psoriasis of the fingernails. J Am Acad Dermatol 1992;26:135–136.
7. Terao T, Terao M, Yoshimina R, Ave K. Restless legs syndrome induced by lithium. Biol Psychiatry 1991;30:1167–1170.
8. Bateman AMS, Larner AJ, McCartney SA, Rifkin IR. Rhabdomyolysis associated with lithium-induced hyperosmolar state. Nephrol Dial Transplant 1991;6:203–205.
9. Simard M, Gumbiner B, Lee A, Lewis H, Norman D. Lithium carbonate intoxication. A case report and review of the literature. Arch Intern Med 1989;149:36–46.
10. Amdisen A. Clinical features and management of lithium poisoning. Med Toxicol 1988;3:18–32.
11. Groleau G, Barch R, Tso E, Shye D, Brown B. Lithium intoxication: manifestations and management. Am J Emerg Med 1987;5:527–532.
12. Marcus S. Lithium. Clin Toxicol Rev 1980;2(5):1–2.
13. Friedberg RC, Spyker DA, Herold DA. Massive overdoses with sustained release lithium carbonate preparations: pharmacokinetic model based on two case studies. Clin Chem 1991;37:1205–1209.
14. Anton RF, Paladino JA, Morton A et al. Effect of acute alcohol consumption on lithium kinetics. Clin Pharmacol Ther 1985;38:52–55.
15. Jaeger A, Sander P, Kopferschmitt J et al. Toxicokinetics of lithium intoxication treated by hemodialysis. Clin Toxicol 1985;23:501–517.
16. Jaeger A, Sauder P, Kopferschmitt J, Tritsch L, Flesch I. When should dialysis be performed in lithium poisoning: A kinetic study in 14 cases of lithium poisoning. Clin Toxicol 1993;31:429–447.
17. Hunter R. Steady state pharmacokinetics of lithium carbonate in healthy subjects. Br J Clin Pharmacol 1988;25:375–380.
18. Jermain DM, Crismon ML, Martin ES III. Population pharmacokinetics of lithium. Clin Pharm 1991;10:376–381.
19. Chapron DJ. Comment on pharmacokinetics of lithium in the elderly. J Clin Psychopharmacol 1988;8:78.
20. Bijnen JH, Vlasveld LT, Wander J, Huinik WWB, Rodenhuis S. Effect of cisplatin-containing chemotherapy on lithium serum concentrations. Ann Pharmacother 1992;26:488–490.
21. Griffin JH, Halu SM. Lisinopril induced lithium toxicity. DICP Ann Pharmacother 1991;25:101.
22. Goodrich PJ, Schorr-Cain CB. Lithium pharmacokinetics. Psychopharmacol Bull 1991;27:475–491.
23. Binder EF, Cayabyab L, Ritchie DJ, Birge SJ. Diltiazed-induced psychosis in a possible diltiazem-lithium interaction. Arch Intern Med 1991;151:373–374.
24. Sacristan JA, Iglesias C, Arellano I, Leguesica J. Absence seizures induced by lithium: possible interaction with fluoxetine. Am J Psychiatry 1991;148:146–147.
25. Dinan TG, O'Keene V. Acute extrapyramidal reactions following lithium and sulpiride co-administration: two case reports. Hum Psychopharmacol Clin Exp 1991;6:67–69.
26. Helhmuth D, Ljaljevic Z, Ramirez L, Meltzer HY. Choreoathetosis induced by verapamil and lithium treatment. J Clin Psychopharmacol 1989;9:450–455.
27. Austin LS, Aran GW, Melvin JA. Toxicity resulting from lithium augmentation of antidepressant treatment in elderly patients. J Clin Psychiatry 1990;51:344–345.
28. Herbert V, Hirschman S, Jacobson J. Lithium for zidovudine-induced neutropenia in AIDS. JAMA 1988;260:3588.
29. Abou-Saleh MF. Reply. Br Med J 1987;294:1405.
30. Simon G. Combination angiotensive converting enzyme inhibitor/lithium therapy contraindicated in renal disease. Am J Med 1988;56:893–894.
31. D'Arcy PF. Nephrotoxic interaction: lithium and metronidazole. Int Pharm J 1988;2:44–45.
32. Jacobson SI, Jones KL, Johnson K, Ceolin L, Kaur P, Saber D et al. A prospective multicenter study of pregnancy outcome following lithium exposure during the first trimester of pregnancy. Pediatr Res 1992;31(4):691.
33. Jacobson SJ, Jones K, Johnson K, Ceolin L, Kaur P, Salm D et al. Prospective multicentre study of pregnancy outcome after lithium exposure during the first trimester. Lancet 1992;39:530–533.
34. Cunniff CM, Salm DJ, Johnson KA, Jones KJ. Pregnancy outcome in women treated with lithium. Clin Res 1988;36:217A.
35. Schou M. Lithium treatment during pregnancy, delivery, and lactation: an update. J Clin Psychiatry 1990;51:410–413.
36. Schou M, Goldfield MD, Weinstein MP, Elleneuve A. Lithium and pregnancy-I report from the Register of lithium babies. Br Med J 1973;2:135–136.
37. Schou M, Amdisen A, Steenstrup OR. Lithium and pregnancy. II. Hazards to women given lithium during pregnancy and delivery. Br Med J 1973;2:137–138.
38. Linden S, Rich CL. The use of lithium during pregnancy and lactation. J Clin Psychiatry 1983;44:358–361.
39. Cohen LS, Friedman JM, Jefferson JW, Johnson EM, Weiner ML. A reevaluation of risk of the in utero exposure to lithium. JAMA 1993;271:146–150.
40. Connoley G, Menahem S. A possible association between neonatal jaundice and long-term maternal lithium ingestion. Med J Aust 1990;157:272–273.
41. Ananth J. Lithium during pregnancy and lactation. Lithium 1993;4:231–237.
42. Hansen HE, Amdisen A. Lithium intoxication. Q J Med 1978;186:123–144.
43. Gitlin MJ. Lithium-induced renal insufficiency. J Clin Psychopharmacol 1993;13:276–279.
44. Bendz H, Aurell M, Balldin J et al. Kidney damage in long-term lithium patients: a cross-section study of patients with 15 years or more on lithium. Nephrol Dial Transplant 1994;9:1250–1254.
45. Walker RG. Lithium nephrotoxicity. Kidney Int 1993;44(Suppl 42):S93–S98.
46. Bismuth C, Baud FJ, Musczynski J, Galliot M. Renal function in lithium treatment. About 50 cases. Proc Eur Assoc Pois Cont Centers Toxicol 1988;83.
47. Tilkan AG, Schroeder JS, Kao JJ et al. The cardiovascular effects of lithium in man. A review of the literature. Am J Med 1976;61:665–670.
48. Kachel F, Boning JAL. Recurrent asystole due to arrhythmic changes during treatment with lithium. Pharmacopsychiatry 1991;24:104.
49. Ong ACM, Handler CE. Sinus arrest and asystole due to severe lithium intoxication. Int J Cardiol 1991;30:364–366.
50. Kast R. Reversal of lithium-related cardiac repolarization delay by potassium. J Clin Psychopharmacol 1990;10:304–305.
51. Chow CC, Cockram CS. Thyroid disorders induced by lithium and amiodarone: an overview. Adverse Drug React Acute Pois Rev 1990;9:207–222.

52. Stancer HC, Forbath N. Hyperparathyroidism, hypothyroidism and impaired renal function after 10 to 20 years of lithium treatment. Arch Intern Med 1989;149:1042–1045.
53. Santiago R, Rashkin MC. Lithium toxicity and myxedema coma in an elderly woman. J Emerg Med 1990; 8:63–66.
54. Jaeger A, Sauder P, Kopferschmitt J, Tritsch L, Flesch F. When should dialysis be performed in lithium poisoning? A kinetic study in 14 cases of lithium poisoning. Clin Toxicol 1993;31:429–447.
55. Moskowitz AS, Altschuler L. Increased sensitivity to lithium-induced neurotoxicity after stroke: a case report. J Clin Psychopharmacol 1991;1:272–273.
56. Smith SJM, Kocen RS. A Creutzfeldt-Jacob like syndrome due to lithium toxicity. J Neurol Neurosurg Psychiatry 1988; 51:120–123.
57. Stevenson RM, Blanshard C, Patterson DLH. Ventricular fibrillation due to lithium withdrawal—an interaction with chlorpromazine? Postgrad Med J 1989;65:936–938.
58. Risby E, Potter WZ, Moses F. Effects of lithium withdrawal on human platelets and lymphocyte adenylate cyclase activity. Clin Pharmacol Ther 1989;45:172.
59. Mander AJ, Loudon JB. Rapid recurrence of mania following abrupt discontinuation of lithium. Lancet 1988;2:15–17.
60. Martin TG, Mallinger AG, Michelson EA, Schneider SM. RBC lithium kinetics during an acute intoxication treated with hemodialysis. Vet Hum Toxicol 1991;33:363.
61. Thornley-Brown D, Galla JH, Williams PD, Kart S, Rashkin M. When toxicity is associated with a trichobezoar. Ann Intern Med 1992;116:739–740.
62. Massey EW, Folger WN. Seizures activated by therapeutic levels of lithium carbonate. South Med J 1984;77:1173–1174.
63. Kulig K. All lithium overdoses deserve respect. J Emerg Med 1992;10:757–758.
64. Larkens RG. Lithium and hypercalcemia. Aust NZ J Med 1991;21:675–677.
65. Cohen LS, Cohen DE. Lithium-induced hyperbilirubinemia in an adolescent. J Clin Psychopharmacol 1991;1: 274–275.
66. Arden A. Clinical features and management of lithium poisoning. Med Toxicol 1988;3:18–32.
67. Shannon MW, Eisen T, Linakus J, Woolf A. Clinical features of acute versus chronic lithium intoxication. Ann Emerg Med 1990;19:630.
68. Dyson EH, Simpson D, Prescott LF, Proudfoot AT. Self-poisoning and therapeutic intoxication with lithium. Hum Toxicol 1987;6:325–329.
69. Schonwald S. Lithium. Clin Toxicol Rev 1990;12(7):1–2.
70. Smith SW, Ling LJ, Halstenson CE. Whole bowel irrigation as a treatment for acute lithium overdose. Ann Emerg Med 1991;20:536–539.
71. Tomaszevski C, Musso C, Pearson JR, Kulig K, Marx JA. Lithium absorption prevented by sodium polystyrene sulfonate in volunteers. Ann Emerg Med 1992;21:130–131.
72. Belanger DR, Tierney MG, Dickinson G. Effect of sodium polystyrene sulfonate on lithium bioavailability. Ann Emerg Med 1992;21:1312–1315.
73. Linakis JG, Lacouture RG, Eisenberg MS et al. Administration of activated charcoal or sodium polystyrene sulfonate (Kayexalate) as gastric decontamination for lithium intoxication: an animal model. Pharmacol Toxicol 1989; 65:387–389.
74. Roberge RJ, Martin TG, Schneider SM. Use of sodium polystyrene sulfonate in lithium overdose. Ann Emerg Med 1993;22:1911–1915.
75. Clendeninn NJ, Pond SM, Kaysen G et al. Potential pitfalls in the evaluation of the usefulness of hemodialysis for the removal of lithium. J Toxicol Clin Toxicol 1982; 19:341–352.
76. Bellomo R, Kearly Y, Parkin G, Lowe J, Boyce N. Treatment of life-threatening lithium toxicity with continuous arteriovenous hemodiafiltration. Crit Care Med 1991;19:836–837.
77. Karkal SS, Mateer JR, Groleau G. Reducing the lethal potential of lithium intoxication. Emerg Med Rep 1989;10(18):141–148.

MAGNESIUM

Magnesium sulfate is a competitive antagonist of calcium. Magnesium serum levels of 9 to 12 mEq/L may cause respiratory arrest and cardiovascular collapse. Calcium charcoal blockers may potentiate the action of both substances.[1]

A profound neuromuscular blockade may be accompanied by preserved hearing, vision, and skin sensation. This has been observed with serum magnesium levels of 9.85 mmol/L (24 mg/dL) (normal range—0.75 to 1.5 mmol/L [9.5 to 14.8 mg/dL]). Coma has been reported with serum levels of 9.5 mmol/L (23 mg/dL). Extensive hypermagnesemia can cause parasympathetic blockade and fixed dilated pupils, in addition to neuromuscular blockade, mimicking a midbrain syndrome, and resulting in a pseudocomatose state.[2]

Hypertonic magnesium sulfate enemas administered to infants may result in absorption of Mg^{++} from the colon. Respiratory arrest, loss of consciousness, and depressed deep-tendon reflexes with electrocardiographic findings typical of magnesium intoxication may be observed. Serum magnesium levels have reached 5.87 mmol/L (normal 0.7 to 1.0 mmol/L) equal to 14.3 mg/100 mL (normal 1.7 to 2.4 mg/100 mL).[3–5] Calcium administration (10 mL 10% calcium gluconate IV) may reverse respiratory depression, improve consciousness, return deep-tendon reflexes to normal, and lead to reactive pupils.[4] Death may follow in spite of calcium administration.[5]

MAGNESIUM IN DRUGS (TABLE 67–29)

Magnesium-Containing Cathartics

Repeated magnesium citrate cathartics administered with activated charcoal may lead to magnesium intoxication with magnesium blood levels of up to or greater than 4.0 mcg/L.[6] Use of multiple doses of magnesium cathartics in patients with renal insufficiency resulting from chronic renal failure or dehydration is not advised.[7] Consider using non–magnesium-containing cathartics if multiple doses are indicated.[8] In patients who may receive frequent, repetitive doses of magnesium cathartics, frequent monitoring of deep-tendon reflexes, bowel motility, renal function, serum calcium, and magnesium levels is indicated.[9] Magnesium toxicity should also be anticipated when magnesium-containing agents are administered but catharsis does not occur due to decreased bowel function.[10]

Magnesium Hydroxide Laxatives[11]

Magnesium hydroxide laxatives administered to infants and neonates may induce symptoms of severe magnesium intoxication with elevated serum magnesium levels.[12,13] In adults iatrogenic magnesium toxicity rarely occurs in the absence of renal or intestinal disease.[12] In the infant or neonate renal immaturity may be a factor.[13]

An additional cause of hypermagnesemia may be the erroneous ordering of "one amp" of magnesium sulfate intravenously; a 50-mL vial of 50% magnesium sulfate may be erroneously given instead of a standard ampule containing 2 mL of 50% solution (4.03 mmol—1 g or 8.06 mEq) of magnesium. It may also be given instead of an order for 50 mL of 50% dextrose in water, which may have a similar size, shape, and label design to the 50% magnesium sulfate. Such

Table 67–30
Clinical Settings of Hypermagnesemia

Common
Acute renal failure
Chronic renal failure with exogenous Mg intake
Toxemia therapy

Less Common
Chronic renal failure without exogenous intake
Rectal administration of Mg-containing solutions

Uncommon
Parasitosis with exogenous Mg intake
Lithium therapy
Hypothyroidism
Certain neoplasms with skeletal involvement
Viral hepatitis
Hyperparathyroidism with renal disease
Pituitary dwarfism
Milk–alkali syndrome
Perforated viscus with exogenous Mg intake
Acute diabetic ketoacidosis
Addison's disease

Adapted from Graber TW, Yee AS, Baker TJ. Magnesium: Physiology, disorders and therapy. Ann Emerg Med 1982;10:53. Used with permission.

incidents may lead to severe magnesium intoxication and death. Removal and discontinuance of 50-mL vials of magnesium sulfate may be required.[14]

TOXICOKINETICS[15]

The gut absorbs about 30% of an orally administered dose. The glomerulus filters and the proximal tubule resorb 95% of the filtered load. Glomerular filtration rates below 30 mL/min predispose patients to hypermagnesemia. Both magnesium resorption and calcium resorption in the kidney are closely related. A common carrier exists for both calcium and magnesium, in addition to separate active processes. Hypercalcemia and high sodium intake increase magnesium excretion.

CLINICAL PRESENTATION

Cathartic Abuse

Hypermagnesemia (Table 67–30) impairs neuromuscular junction transmission by decreasing acetylcholine release from the presynaptic membrane, by diminishing the depolarizing action of acetylcholine at the postsynaptic junction, and by impairing postsynaptic junction sensitivity to acetylcholine.[16] Cardiovascular and neural effects of excess Mg are summarized in Tables 67–31 and 67–32.[17]

LABORATORY

Elimination Enhancement

Hemodialysis effectively removes magnesium and often is necessary to correct the associated renal dysfunction. Serum magnesium levels over 8 mEq/L suggest the need for dialysis.

Antidotes

Calcium is an antagonist of magnesium action. The exact mechanism of action is unknown, but calcium may displace magnesium from cell membranes. Treat with calcium when serum magnesium levels exceed 5 mEq/L and the patient exhibits symptoms. The adult dose of calcium gluconate is 10 mL of a 10% solution over several minutes. The dose may be repeated once; then the calcium level should be rechecked. Intravenous calcium gluconate is less irritating than calcium chloride.

Table 67–31
Common Cardiovascular Effects of Excess Mg

1. Hypotension
2. Transient tachycardia followed by bradycardia
3. Electrocardiographic changes
   a. Increased PR interval
   b. Increased QRS duration
   c. Increased QT interval
   d. Variable decrease in P-wave voltage
   e. Variable degree of T-wave peaking
4. Heart block at high concentration
5. Arrest in asystole at high concentration

Table 67–32
Neural Effects of Excess Mg

1. Impaired nerve conduction
2. Synaptic blockade
   a. Decreased transmitter release
   b. Diminished postsynaptic responsiveness
   c. Induction of acetylcholine esterase
   d. Increased reuptake of adrenergic transmitters
   e. Competition with calcium for common receptor sites
3. Primary central nervous system depression only if the blood-brain barrier is defective or if applied directly to central nervous tissue.
4. Secondary central nervous depression, in part due to hypotension and hypoxia.

Adapted from Mordes JP and Wacker WE. Pharmacolog Rev 1978;29:281.

REFERENCES—MAGNESIUM

1. Rabinerson D, Gruber A, Kaplan B, Roybürt M, Ovada J. Accidental cardiopulmonary arrest following magnesium sulphate overdose. Eur J Obstet Gynecol Reprod Biol 1994;55: 149–150.
2. Rizzo AM, Fisher M, Lock JP. Hypermagnesemia pseudocoma. Arch Intern Med 1993;153:1130–1136.
3. Ashton R, Sutton D, Nielson M. Severe magnesium toxicity after magnesium sulfate enema in a chronically constipated child. Br Med J 1990;300 :541.
4. Brown AT, Campbell WAB. Hazards of hypertonic magnesium enema therapy. Arch Dis Child 1978;53:920.
5. Outerbridge EW, Papageorgiou A, Stern L. Magnesium sulfate enema in a newborn. Fatal systemic magnesium absorption. JAMA 1973;224:1392–1393.
6. Green J, Woolf A. Hypermagnesemia associated with catharsis in a salicylate-intoxicated patient with anorexia nervosa. Ann Emerg Med 1989;18:200–203.
7. Woodard JA, Slauson M, Lacouture PG, Woolf A. Serum magnesium concentrations after repetitive magnesium cathartic administration. Am J Emerg Med 1990;8:297–300.
8. Smilkstein MJ, Steedle D, Kulig KW, Marx JA, Rumack BH. Magnesium levels after magnesium containing cathartics. J Toxicol Clin Toxicol 1988;26:51–65.
9. Jones J, Heiselman D, Dougherty J, Eddy A. Cathartic-induced magnesium toxicity during overdose management. Ann Emerg Med 1986;15:1214–1218.

10. Weber CA, Santiago RM. Hypermagnesemia. A potential complication during treatment of theophylline intoxication with oral activated charcoal and magnesium-containing cathartics. Chest 1989;95:56–59.
11. Brand JM, Greer FR. Hypermagnesemia and intestinal perforation following antadel administration in a premature infant. Pediatrics 1990;85:121–123.
12. Alison LH, Bulugahapitiya D. Laxative induced magnesium poisoning in a 6 week old infant. Br Med J 1990;300:125.
13. Mofenson HC, Caraccio TR. Magnesium intoxication in a neonate from oral magnesium hydroxide laxative. Clin Toxicol 1991;29:215–222.
14. Hoffman RS, Smilkstein MJ, Rubenstein F. An "amp" by any other name: the hazards of intravenous design. JAMA 1989; 261:557.
15. Graber TW, Yee AS, Baker FJ. Magnesium: Physiology, clinical disorders and therapy. Ann Emerg Med 1981;10:49–57.
16. Castelbaum AR, Donoforio PD, Walker FO, Troost BT. Laxative abuse causing hypermagnesemia, quadriparesis and neuromuscular junction defect. Neurology 1989;39: 746–747.
17. Mordes JP, Wacker WEC. Excess magnesium. Pharmacolog Rev 1978;29:274–286.

MANGANESE

CLINICAL PRESENTATION

Chronic Effects

The two main target organs affected by chronic exposure to manganese (Mn) dust are the lungs (increased incidence of pneumonia, bronchitis, and chronic nonspecific lung disease) and the central nervous system (neurobehavioral symptoms, Parkinson-like syndrome).[1]

"Locura manganica" or "manganese madness" is the insidious onset of psychiatric symptoms, including apathy, insomia, confusion, bizarre behavior, visual hallucinations, emotional lability, decreased libido, impotence, and anxiety. Neurologic manifestations include nystagmus, disequilibrium, paresthesia, memory impairment, a vocal pattern described as "whispering speech," problems with fine motor movement, lumbosacral pain, urgency, and incontinence. The neurologic syndrome is similar to Parkinson's disease with tremor, ataxia, loss of memory, flat affect, muscle rigidity, and gait disturbances. Unlike Parkinson's, however, pathologic lesions are found in the globus pallidus and the striatum rather than the globus pallidus and the substantia nigra.[2]

The most common respiratory symptom is dyspnea. Because of its low solubility in water, airborne manganese does not cause oral or dermal problems. Instead, it penetrates the lower respiratory tract toward the alveolar membrane, leading to the development of manifestations of pneumonitis, pneumonia, and bronchitis. This is true of most low-solubility airborne toxins.[2]

Patients with manganism have pathologic hepatic changes (increased golgi bodies and dilated biliary canaliculi), but rarely develop clinical hepatitis.[2]

If the physician does not ask for an occupational history, the patient may not volunteer one. A physician may not be able to figure out the problem without an awareness of the materials, processes, and hazards associated with the particular occupation. Standard heavy-metal screens only detect mercury, arsenic, bismuth, and antimony. If the physician suspects another heavy metal, it must be specifically requested. Most artists work in private studios not covered by occupational laws governing exposures.[2]

A number of islanders on the Australian island of Groote Eylandt where manganese is mined and cycads grown, have developed a neurologic disease complex with upper motor neuron and cerebellar signs and oculomotor symptoms, the "Angurugu Syndrome" associated with elevated blood manganese values.[3]

Acute Effects

Studies of neurologic and psychologic symptoms in workers exposed to manganese suggest that exposure to airborne dust below the current ACGIH TWA (5 mg/m^3) for 1 year or more may still lead to clinical signs of intoxication, especially respiratory symptoms, changes in lung ventilatory parameters, alteration of neurofunctional performances, and hypercalcemia.[1,4]

LABORATORY

Whole-blood manganese values are 0.4 to 2.0 µg/dL. Neurologic symptoms may be associated with blood manganese levels of 3.0 to 5.6 µg/dL.[5] Preliminary studies indicate that magnetic resonance imaging appears to be effective in visualizing manganese in the basal ganglia.[6] Serial MRI changes clearing in 5 to 7 months are characteristic of manganese encephalopathy.[7] MRI may add to the diagnosis of the presymptomatic stage.

TREATMENT

Treatment is supportive. A study from China suggests that symptoms of chronic manganese poisoning may be ameliorated by treatment with sodium para-aminosalicylic acid (PAS-Na, 6 g/day in 500 mL of 10% glucose solution by intravenous drip).[8] Further confirmatory studies will be required to evaluate this proposal.

Signs and symptoms of Parkinson's disease following chronic manganese poisoning appeared to improve after treatment with sodium para-aminosalicylic acid (PAS-Na 6 g/day in 500 mL of 10% glucose solution by intravenous drip given for 4 days, then off treatment 3 days, for 3 to 4 months). This study was uncontrolled and has not been validated by other observations. Other treatments have been used with limited success including L-dopa, 5-hydroxytryptophan, scopolamine, procyclidine (Kemadine), and trihexyphenidyl (Actane).[8] The role of DMSA has not been established.

REFERENCES—MANGANESE

1. Roels HA, Ghyselen P, Buchet JP, Ceulemans E, Lauwerys RR. Assessment of the permissible exposure level to manganese in workers exposed to manganese dioxide dust. Br J Ind Med 1992;49:25–34.
2. Lesser SH, Weiss SJ. Art hazards. Am J Emerg Med 1995; 13:451–458.
3. Angurugu syndrome. Lancet 1987;2:1537 (editorial).
4. Wennberg A, Iregren A, Struwe G, Cizinsky G, Hagman M, Johanssen L. Manganese exposure in steel smelters a health hazard to the nervous system. Scand J Work Environ Health 1991;17:255–262.

5. Ejima A, Imamura T, Nakamura S, Saito H, Matsumoto K, Momono S. Manganese intoxication during total parenteral nutrition. Lancet 1992;229:426.
6. Newland MC, Ceckler TL, Kordower JH, Weiss P. Visualizing manganese in the primate basal ganglia with magnetic resonance imaging. Exp Neurol 1989;106:251–258.
7. Angle C, Nelson K. Manganese encephalopathy. Utility of early magnetic resonance imaging. Vet Hum Toxicol 1992;34:350.
8. Shuqin K, Haishang D, Peiyi X, Wanda H. A report of two cases of chronic serious manganese poisoning treated with sodium para-aminosalicylic acid. Br J Ind Med 1992;49:66–69.

MERCURY POISONING—ELEMENTAL AND INORGANIC

SOURCES IN THE HOME

Potential sources of elemental mercury in the home include mercury switches and mercury-containing devices such as thermometers, thermostats, and barometers. Family members may also bring into the home elemental mercury obtained from laboratories, dental offices, or other industrial sources.[1,2]

CLINICAL PRESENTATION

Acute Inhalation

Patients may be asymptomatic during the first 1 to 4 hours following acute exposure to high air concentrations of mercury vapor.

Elemental mercury vapor is absorbed rapidly through the lungs reaching the blood and entering the brain.[3] A clinical picture evolves that may be divided into three phases. The initial phase (first few days after exposure) is manifested as metal fume fever or a flulike illness characterized by chills, fever, aching muscles, dryness in the mouth and throat, and headache. The intermediate phase (symptoms present 2 weeks after an accident) can be defined as the period during which severe multiorgan symptoms (central nervous system, respiratory tract, and gastrointestinal and urologic systems) may be involved. Severe cases progress to noncardiogenic pulmonary edema with dyspnea, cyanosis, and a chest x-ray exhibiting extensive bilateral infiltrates. Complications include subcutaneous emphysema, pneumomediastinum, pneumothorax, and death. Metallic mercury vapor toxicity may simulate mucocutaneous lymph node syndrome (Kawasaki disease). Rarely, acute renal failure, hepatocellular dysfunction, and seizures occur.[4] Subcutaneous injections cause local abscesses and pulmonary embolization, but systemic symptoms are unusual. The late phase involves the period when central nervous symptoms persist and other organ complaints resolve.[3] Thus acute exposure to elemental mercury and its vapor induce acute inorganic mercury toxicity and cause long-term, probably irreversible, neurologic sequelae.[5]

Chronic

Further exposure to mercury in an individual already suffering from coarse tremors of the hands and arms may lead to ataxia of the lower limbs, producing a characteristic reeling gait. There may be tremors of the lips and tongue, complaints of excessive salivation, and a dry metallic taste in the mouth. A blue line similar to that seen in poisoning by lead and bismuth develops in the alveolar margin of the gums. A urinary excretion of over 300 μg Hg/24 hours is confirmatory.[6]

The classic symptoms of metallic mercury vapor poisoning may include (a) intentional tremor; (b) erethism (loss of memory, lack of self control, irritability, excitability, loss of self confidence, drowsiness, and depression); and (c) gingivitis. In severe cases delirium with hallucinations, suicidal melancholia, or manic-depressive psychosis may occur. Shyness and loss of appetite may occur at exposures of less than 0.1 mg/m^3 time-weighted average (TWA) air concentration.

MERCURY ASPIRATION

Elemental mercury aspiration does not usually lead to signs of acute or chronic intoxication. Urine mercury concentrations may be elevated. Chest radiographs may display mercury opacities for 5 years after an aspiration. Treatment is symptomatic and supportive. The influence of chelating agents is minimal.[7]

CHILDREN-WORKER EXPOSURE

Mercury poisoning is often observed in the children of mercury workers. Symptoms include fever, irritability, tremor, and refusal to walk. Urine mercury concentrations can be increased. Chelating agents lead to a resolution of symptoms.[8] Clothing barriers need to be removed by the worker at the plant each day after work.

TOXICOKINETICS

After inhalation, elemental mercury is readily absorbed through the alveolar membrane and transported by blood to the brain and other tissues of the nervous system.

Mercury is rapidly converted by the blood to mercuric ions (Hg^{++}), which are then excreted in the urine and feces.

Elimination of elemental mercury occurs primarily in the urine with a half-life of about 60 days.

After oxidation, elemental mercury may act as mercuric or divalent mercury and thus be identical to the chemical form that occurs after dissociation of mercuric salts. The dissociated mercuric ion may then lead to renal tubular danger similar to that seen after ingestion of mercuric chloride or the mercurial diuretics.

The same areas of the brain are affected by both inorganic and organic mercury. The tremor, rigidity, and truncal unsteadiness impairing gait may produce a parkinsonian syndrome suggesting involvement of the basal ganglia and cerebellum. Involvement of the corpus callosum may be involved as indicated by performance on tests showing no improvement on switching to the preferred from the nonpreferred hand. Defects in memory suggest involvement of the temporal lobe.[9]

A urine excretion level of 300 mg/L probably represents mercury poisoning; 100 mg/L of mercury in urine usually requires treatment, and levels of 50 mg/L and lower are considered safe. However, urinalysis often yields unreliable results, and normal levels are not yet clearly established.

Careful behavioral and neurologic monitoring is recommended when urine levels are 100 μg/dL or greater.

GOLD MINING[10]

Symptoms of chronic mercury poisoning are prevalent in gold miners and in those involved in gold refining. Blood and urine mercury levels are better indicators of the miners' recent exposure than of past exposure, but do not correlate well with symptoms.[11] Whole-blood levels in residents in these areas have ranged from 0.4 to 13.0 μg/dL; spot urines ranged from 0 to 151 μg/L.[12]

Gold Ore Processing

The production of a mercury amalgam in home gold-ore processing has become a popular and widely used method. In a gold extraction factory a gold-mercury amalgam may be heated in a confined area. Home smelting of silver from dental amalgam containing mercury may lead to shortness of breath within 24 hours, an adult respiratory syndrome, and death.[13] Prompt treatment with penicillamine and corticosteroids may be useful. Radiologic pulmonary infiltrates may disappear within a week, but pulmonary function abnormalities (restriction and diffusion impairment) can persist for over 6 months.[14–16]

LAXATIVE ABUSE

In most types of inorganic mercury poisoning, toxicity results from absorption of the mercuric ion. Mercurous chloride laxative (calomel) ingested over a long period may produce toxic effects of mercury on the kidneys, gastrointestinal tract, and central nervous system. Small amounts of insoluble mercurous chloride are converted to mercuric ion in the bowel lumen. In addition, absorption of mercury ion or mercurous ion, which is subsequently oxidized to mercuric ion, may induce cellular toxicity when the mercuric ion binds to sulfhydryl groups. Melanosis coli is frequently observed.[15] Chronic mercury poisoning due to mercurous chloride–containing laxative preparations should be suspected in patients with a history of laxative abuse who present with unexplained renal failure, colitis, dementia, or tremor.[17]

INORGANIC MERCURY

Source

Inorganic mercury poisoning may be associated with the ingestion of pesticides, antiseptics, and germicides. Ingestion of a stool fixative (4.5% mercuric chloride [675 mg Hg], 5% glacial acetic acid, 10% formula) has resulted in immediate oropharyngeal burns, salivation, vomiting, abdominal pain and tenderness on palpation, and a guaiac-positive stool. The whole-blood and urine mercury levels are elevated. Treatment with BAL, *N*-acetylcysteine, and DMSA has been useful.[18]

Clinical Presentation

Following an ingestion of mercuric chloride some patients may remain asymptomatic, but the majority develop gastrointestinal symptoms. Of this latter group some may develop renal lesions that terminate fatally. Burning mouth, sore throat, nausea, and vomiting with severe gingivitis, stomatitis, and esophageal erosions may develop after inorganic mercury ingestion. Abdominal pain, weakness, fatigue, pallor, hematemesis, hematochezia, shock, and vascular collapse may follow.

The initial and frequently the only lesions are gastrointestinal sufficient to result in death in a few hours. Patients who develop renal involvement almost invariably have severe gastrointestinal symptoms.[19] Severe gastritis and colitis manifested by grossly bloody vomiting and diarrhea may vary from doses of less than 0.5 g to 4.0 g. The smallest lethal dose was 2.0 g in one series (1.0- to 4.0-g range).[19]

Toxicokinetics

About 10 minutes is required for a tablet of mercuric bichloride to be absorbed from the stomach. It is then widely distributed to the liver, kidney, blood, and muscle. Excretion begins soon after ingestion. The metal may be found in the urine within 2 hours. Excretion takes place through the large bowel, kidney, liver, gastric mucosa, salivary glands, and skin. Freedom from urinary findings for 48 hours tends to indicate a better prognosis.

Excretion

The loss of mercury from the lungs has a half-life of 1.7 days, from the kidney region 64 days, and from the head 21 days.[20] After the first week about 19% of a retained dose is eliminated through fecal excretion (50%), expired breath (37%), and urinary excretion (13%). The mean half-life for urinary mercury excretion is 59 to 64 days.[20] Blood mercury levels appear to be influenced by recent (1 to 2 days) exposure to mercury. Urinary mercury levels appear to relate more to the kidney content of mercury.

Air Exposure—Urine and Blood Correlations

The threshold limit value for mercury in air (50 μg/m^3) corresponds to blood mercury levels of 30 to 35 μg/L (150 to 175 nmol Hg/L).[21] (Normal blood mercury levels are 60 nmol/L; normal urine mercury levels are 60 nmol/L.) Signs of mercury poisoning are seldom observed in individuals with less than 750 to 1000 nmol (150 to 200 μg) per liter of urine. This may correspond to an air exposure of about 30 μg/m^3, a urine mercury excretion of about 195 nmol/L, and a blood level of mercury of about 100 nmol/L.[21]

Spot Urine

The air:urine ratio of mercury concentrations in occupationally exposed individuals is approximately one to one. The use of spot urine samples as an indicator to determine when an employee should be removed from further mercury exposure is highly variable and not necessarily indicative of the week's TWA exposure. A 16-hour composite urine sample appears to correlate well with measured TWA exposures.[22]

Blood

If airborne mercury concentration is less than 50 μg/m^3, elemental mercury in the blood is usually undetected. If airborne mercury levels are over 50 μg/m^3, blood elemental mercury levels are 0.08 to 1.22 nmol/L.[23]

Concentrations of mercury increase with increasing mercury exposure. The elemental blood mercury concentration is less than 0.2% of inorganic mercury concentration. In non–occupationally exposed individuals plasma mercury concentration is about 43 ng/mL (range 14 to 176) and the blood mercury concentration is about 61 ng/L. Both blood and plasma mercury levels increase according to age between ages 10 and 30 years. Mercury blood and plasma concentrations for ages 0.5 to 10 years are about 16 ng/mL and 17 ng/mL, respectively. Between 10 and 30 years levels rise to 50 and 44 ng/mL, respectively. Over 30 years of age levels are 77 and 62, respectively. The ratio of blood Hg/plasma Hg was less than 1 in the age group below 15 years and greater than 1 in the other.[24]

There may be significant correlations between neuropsychologic test performance and indices of mercury exposure. Seral mercury concentrations in the blood and urine verify the long half-life (45 to 56 days) and large volume of distribution (1.4 L/kg) of mercury.[5]

TREATMENT

Hemodialysis, peritoneal dialysis, hemofiltration, and hemodialysis with *N*-acetylcysteine infusions have all been tried in the patient with acute renal failure, but have had limited success in reducing the body load of mercury. Plasma exchange has shown some evidence in terms of removal of the mercury load[25] and may be useful in association with chelation therapy at the early phase of an intoxication.

INTRAVENOUS MERCURY INJECTIONS

Pulmonary embolism from metallic mercury is rare. It may occur after a deliberate intravenous injection of mercury as a suicide gesture, in the presence of drug abuse or severe psychiatric disturbance, with the hope of increasing athletic and sexual performance, and accidentally during right heart catheterization while sampling blood with mercury-containing syringes. The term "quicksilver" may be the origin of the misconception that mercury quickens a boxer's punches.[26] An injection of mercuric chloride led to nausea, vomiting, darkened gums, abdominal pain, and anemia. The patient survived even after dimercaprol and daily hemodialysis, which was not effective in removal of mercury.[27]

Injected mercury can pass through the pulmonary capillary bed and can be observed in systemic sites such as the liver, lungs,[28] kidney, brain, or heart[26] where it can then oxidize to mercuric ion and where it may produce toxic effects.

Clinical Presentation

Sequelae of intravenous mercury injections include local and embolic complications and the syndrome known as mercurialism. Local complications include thrombophlebitis and granuloma formation.[26] Mercurialism, which results from chronic inhalation of mercurial salts and vapor, is rarely described after intravenous administration.

The patient who has injected mercury intravenously may experience pleuritic pain, exertional dyspnea, and fatigue. There may be a low-grade fever and a low posterior pleural rub.[29] Repeated hemoptysis has been observed.[30] Multisystem toxicity (eye, kidney) may supervene.[31]

Treatment

Penicillamine therapy does not seem to be worth its adverse effects. Even with the use of chelating agents mercurialism may take months or years to recover and mental deterioration may be permanent. Local foci should probably be excised to preclude their role as a "reservoir" of mercury for continued slow absorption into the bloodstream.[26] Therapy with chelating agents may not be warranted since there is little evidence to suggest that intravascular mercury produces either acute or chronic toxicity.

Laboratory

After intravenous injection of mercury, urine levels of mercury have reached 1050 μg/L[28] and 640 μg/L.[32] There may be a moderate increase in the white blood cell count. The electrocardiogram will usually be normal.[30] Pelvic and abdominal x-rays may indicate mercury in the paraspinal and pelvic areas in addition to the injection site. Radionuclide images may indicate a right pleural effusion and multiple bilateral pulmonary emboli, while blood mercury levels may reach 2990 μg/dL (normal <59 μg/dL).[27] At a blood level of 500 μg/dL one patient was asymptomatic.[33]

Ancillary Tests

Neuropsychologic test results appear to offer a sensitive, quantitative assessment of heavy-metal toxicity.[32] Following an intravenous injection of mercury, neurologic examination may be within normal limits, demonstrating intact cranial nerves and reflexes, as well as no focal deficits. The cerebrospinal fluid results may also be noncontributory. On neuropsychologic testing severely impaired performance may be evident in memory, new problem solving, learning efficiency, and sustained attention/concentration. Psychologic symptoms may include depression, emotional lability, and anxiety.[34]

Differential Diagnosis[30]

Chest Radiograph

The chest radiograph may exhibit multiple fine, radiodense, spherical particles in the lungs[28] and a pooled metallic density in the right ventricle by echocardiography.[26] Despite its striking radiographic appearance, mercury that has embolized to the lung does not cause significant vascular obstruction as judged by angiography.

Accidental intrabronchial aspiration from rupture of the mercury-filled bag during the insertion or removal of an intestinal tube may produce the identical radiographic characteristics seen after pulmonary arterial mercury emboli.

Pulmonary Function

Respiratory symptoms are relatively uncommon. The patient may have mild dyspnea or transient chest pain. Mercury emboli have little or no effect on pulmonary function. They are like small "silent" thromboemboli. Spirometry may be normal or show a reversible restrictive pattern. The diffusing capacity may be low or normal. Metallic mercury causes a local chronic inflammation with progressive fibrosis with globules of metal still evident several years later.[28]

MERCURY SPILLS

A serious concern with broken thermometers lies in mercury in the home, not ingested mercury. When mercury is left in the home, it will volatilize and be inhaled.

A small vial (approximately 5 mL) of elemental mercury spilled on a rug can lead to the development of symptoms in a child (anorexia, irritability, insomnia, stomatitis, red, painful hands, and feet, BP 158/124). The child's increased susceptibility to the effects of mercury vapor are due to either (a) closer physical proximity to the source of mercury vapors, (b) increased respiratory rate resulting in increased absorption of mercury vapor, or (c) decreased body size.[3]

Attempts to remove the mercury often fail and may disperse the mercury over a larger surface area. The problem may require removal of the contaminated carpeting.[35] Elemental mercury should not be stored in residences and in particular those with carpeted surfaces. If mercury is spilled it should be removed before it can be dispersed. A contaminated carpet or rug should be vacuumed only with a specialized industrial mercury vacuum, or it should be removed completely.[36] If necessary, decontamination procedures should be undertaken to reduce the ambient mercury vapor concentration in a house to less than 1 $\mu g/m^3$.

Response Guidelines for Mercury Spills[37]

Clinical Thermometer

1. Verify that the broken thermometer contained a silver-colored (mercury) liquid, not a red (dibutyl phthalate) liquid.
2. Verify that the thermometer bulb is intact. If the bulb has been broken/crushed, the procedure for a larger device/unknown amount should be followed.
3. Before any work is performed, advise the caller not to use vacuum (or Dustbuster, etc.) in the spill area.
4. Determine the surface of the spill area. If the surface is porous (unfinished wood, carpet, etc.), recommend contacting the local environmental health department and/or a private company to assist with spill cleanup.
5. Remove gold jewelry prior to cleaning a spill. Turn off any sources of heat in the spill area. Do not sweep mercury with a broom; the bristles tend to break up the drops into small, harder-to-clean droplets. Minimize skin contact with the mercury droplets. Use index cards or other slightly stiff paper to gather droplets together into a jar with a lid or "ziplock" plastic baggie. Dispose of mercury through household hazardous waste program.
6. Recommend additional ventilation in the spill area for a few days to avoid distribution and buildup of vapors.

Larger device/unknown amount

1. Determine surface of spill area. If not porous (kitchen counter, linoleum floor, etc.), cleanup can proceed as above—pick up and contain—PLUS, recommend contacting a local environmental health department to perform air monitoring to verify completion (not necessary on clinical thermometer spills).
2. Spills on porous materials (furniture, carpets, unfinished wood, etc.) or on surfaces with many cracks/crevices require special attention and equipment to clean and to verify cleanup. Callers should contact their local environmental health department and/or a private consultant to assist with cleanup.

Even small amounts of mercury spilled in a small, possibly insufficiently aerated room can cause severe acrodynia.[38]

ACRODYNIA (PINK DISEASE)[39–43]

In 1948 Warkany and Hubbard made the connection between mercury and acrodynia.[39] As late as 1952 to 1953 and prior to the removal of calomel (mercuric oxide) from teething powders, acrodynia accounted for 3.6% of all admissions to a children's hospital in England.[42] Thousands of adults are exposed to mercury compounds that cause acrodynia in children, but they are not affected. Newborns are not affected.

Mercury Compounds Involved

Various forms of mercury can cause acrodynia, among them mercury vapor, phenylmercuric compounds, mercurous and mercuric salts, and ammoniated mercury ointment. More recently, cases involved school children who brought metallic mercury home with which to play. They inhaled the vapor for long periods.[42] Alkyl mercury compounds are rarely involved. Phenylmercuric compounds are now banned from paints in the United States. Children may still break thermometers in the home. Liquid mercury certainly remains an attractive hazard.

Clinical Presentation[42,43]

Acrodynia means painful extremities, one of the more interesting symptoms of this disorder.

Young Children

The onset of this illness is often insidious with anorexia, insomnia, and irritability. This is often attributed to teething. Sweating is usually profuse, often leading to miliaria type rashes. Photophobia is often experienced. Children bury their heads in pillows or blankets. The hands and feet become puffy, pink, painful, paresthetic, perspiring, and peeling. Children frequently rub their hands together resulting in shedding of skin, denudation, and secondary infection. In severe cases teeth are shed with ulceration of the gums. These children become dehydrated from perspiration in warm weather. The muscles are weak and the limbs can be hyperextended. Hypertension is usually present.

The Older Child

Clinical findings are less severe. The extremities are not as pink since the palms and soles are thicker. They are moist and cool. Asocial outbursts, fatigue, and insomnia are observed. Alopecia and hair loss are often present. Hypertension and hypotension are frequently observed.

Adults

In adults the presenting symptoms are insomnia, thirst, abdominal pain, aching extremities, and psychologic disturbance.

Catecholamine Effect

Mercury blocks catechol methyl transferase, the enzyme that converts catecholamines to metanephrine. Elevated levels of epinephrine and norepinephrine can be found in the urine. Vanillylmandelic acid and homovanillic acid in the urine are increased. Sweating, tachycardia, hypertension, and occasional glucosuria may be related to sympathetic overactivity.

Differential Diagnosis

Exposure to mercury vapor may be associated with the mucocutaneous lymph node syndrome or "Kawasaki disease," which has many similarities to pink disease. Kawasaki disease appears immunologically mediated with increased serum IgE and eosinophilia.[3]

Laboratory

Basal urinary excretion of mercury can be normal even in overt acrodynia.[38]

Treatment

Treatment of acrodynia requires careful monitoring of fluids and electrolyte balance. Avoid high ambient temperatures (profuse sweating). DMSA (dimercapto succinic acid) appears to increase the excretion of mercury to a greater extent than *N*-acetyl-D,L-penicillamine (NAP). During chelation little or no increase in blood mercury levels are observed.

INDUSTRIAL EXPOSURE

The National Institute of Occupational Safety and Health indicates that about 150,000 people in the United States are exposed annually to mercury at work.[44]

Industrial Sources

Industries that routinely use mercury or mercury-based compounds include chlor-alkali facilities; manufacturers of mercury-filled instruments (barometers, thermometers, manometers); lighting manufacturers (including neon, fluorescent lamps, and high-temperature mercury vapor lamps); and producers of batteries and electrical switches when mercury is used for thermostats and silent contacts. Mercury is also used to refine gold and other ores.[44]

Mercury Measurements in Industry

Mercury vapor detectors may determine the source of contamination. A dosimeter badge provides an immediate visual indication of mercury concentration.

Industrial Mercurialism

Three signs characterize the diagnosis of industrial mercurialism: gingivitis, tremor of the extremities, and emotional instability. The clinical course reflects an insidious onset and a slow and progressive evolution. Mercurialism, although a chronic intoxication most of the time, occasionally assumes the features of an acute overdose. Gingivitis, increased salivation, and a metallic taste are often present.

Micromercurialism

Preclinical evidence of impaired psychomotor function (micromercurialism) may become evident at urine mercury concentrations of over 500 μg/L.[18] Psychomotor measurements should include (a) tremor measurements, (b) bimanual coordination, (c) color determination, and (d) reaction time.[45]

Blood Mercury

Blood mercury levels of up to 50 to 70 nmol/L may be considered as "normal." When blood mercury concentrations do not exceed 150 nmol/L, no investigative or preventative measures are required other than continued routine checks of blood mercury levels. If the blood mercury levels exceed 150 nmol/L, control measures to reduce mercury exposure (blood, urine mercury levels) should be initiated. If the ratio of blood to urine mercury concentration is over 1, repeat the investigations in 2 to 4 weeks. If the mercury level in the blood still exceeds 150 nmol/L and the ratio still exceeds 1, special attention is recommended. At blood levels of over 300 nmol/L, exposure to mercury should stop.

Chest x-rays, pulmonary function tests, and electrocardiograms are usually not significantly abnormal in mercury exposed workers.[46]

Urine

Group average urine levels over 50 μg/L should arouse suspicion and levels above 100 μg/L call for correction of a faulty work situation. An individual with urine levels over 200 μg/L on two successive tests should be removed from exposure until the level has fallen below 50 μg/L. Clinical poisoning does not normally occur with levels below 300 μg/L unless kidney function is impaired.[47,48]

TWA (Time-Weighted Average) Correlations

A study of workers exposed to inorganic mercury in chloralkali plants suggests that a urine mercury level of 250 μg/L is a good "biological threshold limit value" and correlates with a blood mercury level of about 6 μg/100 mL. An air threshold limit value of 0.1 mg/m^3 corresponds to blood levels of 6 μg/100 mL and urine levels of 260 μg/L.

Few signs or symptoms are seen in persons exposed to mercury vapor at or below levels of 0.1 mg/m^3. The TWAs appear to be the best indicator of the probable appearance of symptoms.[49]

DENTAL EXPOSURE

In the United States over 100 tons of mercury are used by dentists annually. Individual dentists in private practice use an average of 2 to 3 pounds of mercury per year.[50] About 100 million fillings per year in the United States involve the use of amalgam.[51]

Dental Offices

About 14% of dental operating rooms exhibit levels of total mercury concentration (vapor and particulates) that exceed the threshold limit values of 0.1 mg/m^3. Particulates appear to be increased more than mercury vapor. Many dentists still knead the amalgam mass in the palms of their hands. In squeezing the mass to express excess mercury—also done by hand—mercury droplets sometimes fall to the floor where they are allowed to remain and vaporize. High levels may be found in a carpeted reception room.[18]

Dentists—Urinary Mercury Levels

Urine mercury levels are correlated with the number of hours of practice/week and with the number of amalgam restorations per week. In one study of dentists the mean urinary mercury levels were 14.2 μg Hg/liter urine; about 1.3% had levels greater than 100 μg/L, a level at which physiologic effects from mercury may first appear.[50]

Dentists—Tissue Mercury

A study of mercury levels in dentists using an x-ray fluorescence technique suggests that dentists with high tissue mercury levels may develop polyneuropathies, mild visuographic dysfunction, and some evidence of mild neuropsychopathy and distress.[52,53]

Dentists—Blood Levels of Mercury

Total and inorganic blood mercury levels appear to be elevated in dentists. Organomercurials are not similarly elevated. Significant enzymatic conversion of inorganic mercury compounds does not occur in vivo. The pathways postulated include

$$Hg^0 \xrightarrow{\text{Catalase}}_{\textit{Peroxidase}} Hg^{2+} \xrightarrow{\text{Methylase}}_{CH_3} CH_3Hg^+ \text{ or } (CH_3)_2Hg$$

do not appear to occur in vivo.[54]

Pregnancy in Dental Personnel

A Swedish study of 8157 infants born of dentists, dental assistants, or dental technicians suggests that there is no effect on spontaneous abortion rates, perinatal survival, or birthweight distribution that could be explained by occupational exposure in dentistry work.[55]

Table 67–33
Classification of Amalgams According to Metal Content

	Silver	Copper	Tin
1. Conventional amalgams:	65–70%	2–5%	25–30%
2. Non-gamma-2 amalgams:			
a) dispersion alloys, admix alloys:	65–70%	12%	18%
b) one-component alloys with 12–15% Cu:	55–60%	12–15%	25–30%
high-copper amalgams:	40–50%	20–30%	20–30%

Adapted from Stadtler P. Internat J Clin Pharmacol Therapy Toxicol 1991;29: 161–163.

DENTAL AMALGAMS (TABLE 67–33)

Conventional Composition—Transformation

Corrosion results in a release of about 30 μg mercury/day. *Abrasion* results in a release of 101 μg Hg/day. In Germany amalgams containing gamma-2 may be banned because of its instability and risk of releasing mercury during the filling procedure.[56]

The average life span of amalgam is about 10 years. Other alternatives to amalgam are (a) composites of plastic material (not always suitable for the back of the mouth where the bite is more forceful; shrink or set leaving gaps between fillings and teeth; not easy to use),[51] (b) porcelain (requires several visits), and (c) gold (requires several visits and is more expensive).[54]

Amalgam Fillings

Following placements of up to eight new amalgam restorations, urine mercury levels could not be detected at concentrations above the putative safe levels (<50 ng/mL mercury in blood; <30 ng/mL mercury in urine).[53] The release of mercury from an amalgam restoration is at its peak just after its placement in the cavity, declining to a lower steady-state level by 10 to 15 days.[57] The half-life for elimination of mercury from the blood after amalgam removal is about 30 days.[58] Removal of amalgams provides an additional exposure of about 1.5 ng Hg/mL that is rapidly cleared from the blood with a half-life of 2.9 days. The daily intake of mercury from removal of about 14 amalgam surfaces was estimated to be about 1.3 μg.[59] The blood level of mercury from amalgam sources is estimated as 1.12 ng Hg/mL, whereas toxic signs of mercury intoxication begin at blood levels of about 30 ng/mL.[60]

Human Exposure—Chewing Gum

The emission of mercury vapor after some minutes of intense chewing is normally increased three- to fivefold. An amalgam-free population occupationally unexposed to mercury indicates an average urinary excretion rate of 0.6 μg Hg/24 hours (0.5 μg Hg/L).

Although people with mercury amalgams may excrete more mercury than people without them, there is no evidence that this is sufficient to cause renal toxicity.[60]

Recommendations

The U.S. Food and Drug Administration Dental Devices Panel advises consumers that it is not necessary to have amalgam fillings removed. There is no valid data to demonstrate that the fillings are harmful in clinical use or that removing them would prevent adverse health effects or reverse the course of existing illness.[61–63] The only documented health problem associated with dental amalgam is an allergy to one of the metals—more often copper or silver than mercury. Composite plastic fillings are more likely to spark allergic reactions.[64]

REPRODUCTION AND PREGNANCY

Pregnancy Exposure

For mercury vapor the maximum allowable concentration of 50 μg/m^3 (ACGIH—8-hour TWA; OSHA ceiling standard for mercury is 100 μg/m^3) may not provide sufficient protection for the fetus since nervous excitability and enzyme concentration changes have been noted in adults exposed to 10 to 50 μg/m^3. Because of this, women of childbearing age should not be exposed to mercury vapor concentrations greater than 10 μg/m^3. Children born of mothers with a history of inorganic mercury exposure must be regularly evaluated by a neurologist who is aware of the occupational history.[65]

Male Fertility

A fertility study in male workers exposed to mercury vapor suggests that there is no difference in the reproductive experience (children born), but this study did not look specifically at the incidence of spontaneous abortion.[66]

Spontaneous Abortion

The rate of spontaneous abortion was higher than controls among the wives of 152 workers occupationally exposed to mercury vapor. This increase appeared to correlate with the urine mercury concentrations of the father during the months preceding pregnancy.[67] In Sweden a study of infants born to dentists, dental assistants, or dental technicians indicated no increase in stillborns, spontaneous abortions, or the malformation rate.[55]

Placental Function

The highest concentration of mercury is found in the placenta suggesting a barrier role.[68] In vitro studies of the human placenta suggest that the mercuric ion may interfere with placental amino acid transfer and with the placental oxygen consumption rate. This may indicate a role for the mercuric ion in impaired organogenesis in early pregnancy or deranged fetal growth during the last trimester.[69]

SYSTEMIC EFFECTS

Endocrine Effects—Pituitary Glands

Samples taken at necropsy from industrial workers exposed to elemental mercury (Hg^o) vapor and from dentists have shown high concentrations of mercury in the pituitary gland. Patients with several amalgam fillings may have increased concentrations of mercury in their pituitary glands. The clinical significance of this finding is not yet apparent.[70]

Although exposure to elemental mercury vapor results in an accumulation of mercury in the pituitary, the thyroid, and the testes, there is no change in basal serum concentrations of pituitary hormone (thyrotropin (TSH), prolactin (PRL), follicle stimulating hormone (FSH), and luteinizing hormone (LH).[71] There is no evidence that long-term low-level mercury exposure exerts a negative influence on the function of the pituitary hormones, thyroid stimulating hormone (TSH), and prolactin (PRL).[72]

The Eye[73]

The Brown Reflex

The brown reflex is evidence of protracted mercury exposure and persists unchanged for years after removal from mercury exposure. The brown reflex of the anterior lens capsule is bilateral and symmetrical and varies in intensity from light brown to coffee brown (mercurialentis).[74]

Lens Opacities

Fine punctate opacities are present bilaterally and are most evident in the anterior cortex of the lens.

Vascularity

Well-marked vascularity is observed at the corneoscleral junction.

Visual Fields

Visual fields are usually normal.

The Kidney

Renal Lesions

The nephrotoxicity associated with mercury may be manifested as either an acute tubular necrosis or as an immune complex glomerulonephritis. The nephrotic syndrome may develop secondary to a membranous glomerulonephritis (MGN). Complement (C_3, C_4, CH_{50}) tests are normal. The antinuclear antigen (ANA) titer and LE titers are normal. Renal venograms and intravenous pyelograms are normal. The urine contains occasional oval fat bodies, fatty casts, and hyaline casts.[75]

Etiology

MGN has been observed after the use of teething powders containing mercury given to pediatric patients, skin-lightening creams used by African black women, and use of ammoniated mercury ointment for psoriasis. Lesions have also been described after occupational mercury exposure.[76] In cases of the nephrotic syndrome associated with metal contaminants it is prudent to examine unstained material by electromicroscopy in all cases of idiopathic MGN and nephrotic syndrome associated with metal contaminants and to evaluate biopsy material with elemental analysis where indicated.

Renal Function[77]

The kidney has a remarkable capacity to concentrate mercury. It is a target organ following exposure to mercury.[33] The potential of mercuric salts (e.g., mercuric chloride) to produce overt renal tubular damage is well documented. The evidence that human exposure to metallic mercury vapor produces renal damage is less convincing.

In a study of chemical workers exposed to inorganic mercury, elevated urine mercury levels correlated with excessive neuropsychologic symptoms, elevated levels of urine *N*-acetyl-beta-D-glucosaminidase (a lysosomal enzyme present in renal tubular cells), and reduced mean motor-conduction velocities; no correlation was found between urine mercury levels and neurobehavioral tests, saccadic eye movements, or lenticular opacities.[78]

Proteinuria

There are two types of proteinuria associated with mercury toxicity: a glomerular proteinuria and a tubular proteinuria.[79] Glomerular proteinuria is characterized by the leakage of serum proteins (predominantly high molecular weight) through damaged glomeruli and is thought to represent an idiosyncratic immune-complex glomerulonephritis.[75] Tubular proteinuria consists of a variety of proteins and enzymes. Many of these markers are low-molecular-weight proteins (e.g., beta$_2$-microglobulin and retinol binding protein) normally filtered through the glomerulus and then reabsorbed in the proximal tubules. Others (enzymes such as NAG) are released directly into the urine from damaged proximal tubule cells. Tubular proteinuria may be a more sensitive marker for mercury toxicity. Elevated NAG levels may be more reflective of current activity of an injurious process than of acute toxicity. Elevated urinary beta$_2$-microglobulin (B_2 M) may be more representative of chronic than acute toxicity. Also since they are freely filtered, urinary B_2 M are more sensitive to serum levels. Serum B_2 M levels do not correlate well with measures of mercury exposures.[80]

Beta$_2$ Microglobulin

Following the ingestion of 1.5 g mercuric chloride by an 18-year-old B_2-microglobulins in the urine rose to 42,400 μg/d. An increased excretion of both albumin and B_2-microglobulin indicate the presence of both tubular and glomerular lesions.

Analytic Methods

Low-molecular-weight serum proteins are determined by acrylamide gel electrophoresis. B_2-microglobulin excretion is measured by specific radioimmunoassay.[73]

NAG (N-acetyl-beta-D-glucosaminidase)

Despite elevated blood and urine mercury levels, routine clinical testing such as physical examination, blood chemistries, and urinalysis are generally normal.[81] More sensitive indicators of toxicity may include evaluation of neuropsychologic symptoms, elevated urinary *N*-acetyl-beta-D-glucosaminidase (NAG) levels, decreased motor nerve conduction velocities, and the presence of lenticular opacities on slit-lamp examination.

Laboratory

A urinary mercury concentration of over 150 μg/L is a level associated with the earliest neurologic effects in adults. This may be associated with an 8-hour time-weighted average or concentration of elemental mercury vapor of 50 μg/m^3. The U.S. Environmental Protection Agency suggested ambient air concentration for mercury is less than 1 μg/m^3.[82]

Mercurous Chloride

Chronic ingestion of mercurous chloride laxative (e.g., 240 mg of mercurous chloride for 6 or more years) may lead to many of the classical signs and symptoms of inorganic mercury poisoning, including erethism (unusual timidity, loss of memory, lack of attention, decline of intellect) and fine tremors of the hand or face. In addition, intention tremors, myoclonic jerks, weakness, hyporeflexia, and deafness may occur in both mercurous and mercuric mercury poisoning.[83]

Central Nervous System

Repeated peak exposures may be more dangerous for the central nervous system than chronic low exposures because concentrations of free elemental mercury in the blood become much higher at peak exposures and the amount of mercury that passes the blood–brain barrier is dependent on the concentration of unoxidized elemental mercury in the blood.[84]

Tremor

Tremor is the most frequently reported sign of excessive mercury exposure.[85] It often occurs in workers exposed to mercury for more than 10 years.[86] Tremor has been described as evolving in progressive stages.[85]

1. Slight static tremor, evidenced with the arms outstretched and the fingers spread and often not manifest to the patient himself. It does not disturb to any extent a satisfactory muscular activity.
2. Static tremor of greater degree associated with early intention tremor, moderately affecting delicate muscular activity.
3. Static and intention tremor that prevents or seriously disturbs delicate muscular activities (writing, shaving, holding a glass).
4. Tremor inducing conspicuous difficulties in gross movements.
5. Generalized intense tremor, preventing daily living activities ("concussio mercurialis").

Mercury Levels

Tremor and electromyographic changes following chronic exposure to elemental mercury vapor are often associated with urine mercury levels over 500 μg/L during the prior year. Effects are reversible within 4 to 6 months on reduction of mercury exposure.[34,87,88] Mercury concentrations in blood and urine have generally failed to relate well to clinical neurologic findings, electrophysiologic measures, and neurobehavioral tests.[89] Tremor may present even many years after removal from exposure to mercury and even after ataxia, incoordination, dizziness, insomnia, and fatigue have long resolved.[90] Mercury half-life in the brain may exceed 1 year.[87] Measurement of tremor may show abnormalities of frequency on special testing apparatus even when finger tremor appears to be visibly normal.[89]

Toxicokinetics

Elemental mercury easily penetrates the blood–brain barrier and accumulates in brain tissue. Brain human mercury concentrations are highly correlated with total mercury concentrations in abdominal muscles.[91] Animals exposed to mercury vapor demonstrate a brain mercury content about ten times higher than animals injected with the same amount of mercury as mercuric salts.[5] Mercury vapor is taken up by the upper respiratory system (bronchi, larger bronchiolis) and alveolar wall and then passes into the blood. High levels accumulate in the cerebellum, brainstem (inferior olive nucleus, subthalamic nucleus), and choroid plexus.[5]

Pathophysiology

In man, mercury distributes to all parts of the body on absorption, reaching a peak over 1 to 2 days.[87] Elemental mercury is rapidly oxidized by the blood[5] to mercuric ion.[92] After a short exposure (14 to 24 minutes) the measured half-life in the head is about 21 days.[93,94] Eight days after elemental mercury vapor exposure to animals, studies show that the brain contains nearly as much mercury as the kidney.[92]

The "Mad Hatter"

Mercury was introduced during carrotting, the process of rubbing fur with mercuric nitrate to produce felt. Subsequent heating released mercury vapor that was inhaled during the later phases of felt-hat manufacturing: finishing, forming, and sizing. In 1860 J.A. Freeman of Orange, New Jersey, described Hatter's shakes. These characteristic tremors were sometimes called the Danbury Tremor in reference to Danbury, Connecticut, a former center for the hat-making industry. Common wisdom deemed hatters "mad" because of the curious jerking gait, extreme shyness, and stammering speech the hatters exhibited. Loss of teeth, salivation, and neurologic deficits were known to Ramazzine, the father of occupational medicine, in 1790. The notion that mercury accounted for the name of the "Mad Hatter" gained credibility as the popularity of Alice's Adventures in Wonderland, first published in 1865, spread.[95,96]

Psychologic Performance

Impaired mental efficiency, increased neurotic reactions, deficiencies in short-term memory, and decrements in psychomotor skill have followed exposure to mercury vapors.

Aging

Natural neuronal attrition may mask prior mercury exposure–related subclinical abnormalities. Disorders consistent with this hypothesis include late progression of prior poliomyelitis, trauma related to boxing with subsequent encephalopathy and parkinsonism, remote radiation-associated plexopathy or myelopathy, and the amyotrophic lateral sclerosis-demential complex of Guam linked to the cycad seed whose effects may be delayed up to 3 decades or more after exposure.[90]

The Skin

The skin is affected by mercury used in skin lightening creams, mercury used in soap, topical ammoniated mercury, mercuric oxide used in the treatment of eczema, topical metallic mercury, and by contact allergy.

Cutaneous Mercury Application

Mercury intoxication following the cutaneous application of inorganic mercury has been reported in the following conditions: (a) treatment of infected eczema or impetigo by application of different mercury salts; (b) cutaneous applications of calomel in syphilis; (c) topical use of ointment containing yellow mercuric oxide or ammoniated mercury in psoriasis; (d) use of skin lightening creams;[97] and (e) topical use of metallic mercury ointments.[98]

Pathophysiology

After exposure of the skin to mercury vapor the rate of uptake is approximately 2% of the rate of mercury reuptake by the lungs. About half of the mercury taken up is shed by desquamation of epidermal cells every several weeks. The remainder diffuses into the general circulation and can be measured as systemic mercury.[99] Mercury compounds are readily absorbed through the skin and cause depigmentation by the inhibition of melanin formation. By competing with copper, mercury inactivates the key melanin-forming enzyme, tyrosinase. The opposite effect, skin pigmentation, may occur rarely.

Skin Lightening Creams

Skin lightening creams are in high demand by Afrocaribbean women. Up to 50% of these women are not aware of the possible danger. Since the creams are cosmetics, they are not subject to stringent tests or regulations and the formulations used in them are not standardized.[100,101] Topical preparations based on mercury have been commonly used as freckle removers.

Proteinuria

Skin lightening creams, some of which contain 5 to 10% mercuric ammonium chloride (and others that contain mercuric iodide)[103] have been studied in Kenya.[104–106] Urine mercury levels over 100 μg/L were observed in the women studied. Serum proteins were normal. Seven (10%)

of 56 women studied had an unexplained but minimal proteinuria.

Nephrotic Syndrome

The nephrotic syndrome has been described in association with the use of ammoniated mercury ointments, the administration of mercurial diuretics, and exposure to other mercurial preparations.[104,105]

Mercury Contact Allergy

Mercury allergy in man may be either the anaphylactic type (e.g., allergy to thiomersalate, an organic mercury compound), or a delayed type hypersensitivity (contact dermatitis, lichenoid reactions in red tattoo areas or adjacent to amalgam fillings).

Blood Analytic Methods

Flameless atomic absorption spectrometry will detect as little as 1 ppb (1 ng/mL) of mercury.[107] High-performance liquid chromatography with indirectly coupled cold vapor plasma emission spectrometry can detect 35 ppb (ng/mL) of mercuric chloride simultaneously with methyl mercury chloride and ethyl mercury chloride with detection limits of 32 to 62 ppb (32 to 62 ng/mL).[108] An atomic absorption method has been described to determine total mercury and selectively inorganic mercury. Organic mercury is measured as the difference between total and inorganic mercury. Analyses of Alaskan communities indicate a mean red cell level of inorganic mercury of 2.4 ng/mL and mean inorganic mercury plasma levels of 1.0 mg/mL.[109]

Urine Mercury

The normal level of urine mercury is considered to be less than 1 mg/mL. This level may rise to 1000 ng/mL or more when individuals are exposed to a mercury-polluted environment.

Hair

Hair analysis may indicate past exposure resulting from concentration of mercury in sulfhydryl groups at a particular place on the hair. External contamination is a potential source of inaccurate analysis, particularly with methyl mercury compounds, which are more readily absorbed on the hair shaft than inorganic mercury. Hair analysis continues to require controlled clinical confirmatory studies.[110]

Analytic Methods

A study of mercury in human hair by cold vapor atomic absorption spectrometry indicated that the mean mercury concentration in the beards and hair of men was 2.13 µg/g and 1.62 µg/g, respectively.[111]

Hair grows at a rate of 0.4 mm/day. As the growing hair approaches the skin surface, it undergoes keratinization. Trace elements accumulated during hair formation are sealed into the protein structure of the hair.[110] Normal values for serum mercury are 2 to 6 µg/L, of urine 1 to 20 µg/L, and of hair 0.5 to 10 mg/kg.

Contamination of hair by external application of mercurials can be differentiated from mercury deposits in hair from the diet by means of special washing procedures that selectively remove the externally absorbed Hg^{o}, Hg^{2+}, and CH_3Hg^{+}. Even metallic mercury vapor is absorbed on the hair surface. Flameless atomic absorption can analyze total and inorganic hair mercury; gas chromatography can quantitate methyl mercury in hair.[112]

Blood, Urine, and Air Mercury Level Correlations

A rough correlation exists between airborne levels of exposure and biologic measurements of mercury.

Recent data suggest that renal neurobehavioral effects may appear with air mercury levels in the 50 to 100 µg/m^3 range, and there are reports of effects at even lower levels.[80] Urine mercury levels below 300 µg/L were thought to be safe, but recent reports suggest that neurobehavioral and subclinical renal effects may be detected in individuals with urinary levels as low as 50 to 100 µg/g creatinine. There are no established standards for urinary levels of inorganic mercury.[113]

Metallothionein

Metallothionein, which represents a group of low-molecular-weight proteins with a molecular weight of about 6000 to 7000 daltons, is an intracellular thiol that binds to zinc, copper, cadmium, silver, platinum, and mercuric ions. Metallothionein has not yet become a clinically useful measure of mercury toxicity.[114–116]

Somatosensory-Evoked Potential

Studies of evoked somatosensory potential have a potential use as an efficient early warning system for the prevention of mercury-induced clinical symptoms.[117] Visually evoked responses may indicate an effect on the nervous system many years after exposure to inorganic mercury has ceased.[118]

ANTIDOTES

BAL and BAL Analogues

Animal studies suggest that the less toxic hydrophilic BAL (dimercaprol) analogue DMPS is superior to other chelators, BAL and DMSA (dimercapto succinic acid), in preventing mortality after administration of oral mercuric chloride. Both DMSA and DMPS appear superior to BAL and NAPA (*N*-acetyl-D,L-penicillamine) in alleviating acute toxicity and in preventing the undesirable distribution of orally administered mercury, especially to the brain.[119]

Dimercaprol (BAL)

Dimercaprol is an option in the treatment of self-administered intravenous mercury poisoning even months after the original exposure, at which time patients often still continue to respond clinically and in addition exhibit positive effects in both the urine and blood mercury.[31] There are survivors of severe elemental mercury poisoning who have been treated only with supportive care.[4]

DMPS (Dimaval—Heyl and Co., Berlin)

2,3-Dimercaptopropane-1-sulfonate (DMPS) is less toxic than DMSA. In oral doses of 100 mg twice daily, DMPS significantly increased the urinary excretion of mercury, as well as copper and zinc. DMPS is an investigational drug used under U.S. Food and Drug Administration guidelines. The excretion half-life of mercury decreased from 33.1 days to 11.2 days in two workers who developed elevated mercury levels resulting from exposure to excessive elemental mercury vapors.[116]

Dosage

DMPS has been used intravenously in the treatment of mercury poisoning in a dose of 5 mg/kg (or six infusions of 250 mg IV/day)[120] followed by use orally in doses of 100 mg two to three times daily for 24 days.[115]

Adverse Effects

Maculopapular rashes, erythema multiforme, and mucous membrane reactions (mouth ulcers) can develop after a course of treatment.[121]

Toxicokinetics

The bioavailability of an oral dose is about 47%. The elimination half life of DMPS is about 10 hours, and the half-life of free DMPS is about 1½ hours. Approximately 10% and 8% is excreted unchanged in the urine after DMPS is given IV or orally, respectively. The apparent volume of distribution of free DMPS in the beta phase is about 4 L/kg; that of total DMPS is 1.8 L/kg.[122,123]

DMSA (Succimer)

DMSA (meso 2,3-dimercaptosuccinic acid) has been approved by the U.S. Food and Drug Administration for the treatment of lead poisoning in children with blood levels above 45 µg/dL.[142] It has been shown to be of possible use as an antidote in poisoning from mercury, arsenic, cadmium, antimony, tellurium, gold, zinc, nickel, platinum, silver, cobalt, and tin.[124]

Absorption

DMSA is rapidly but incompletely absorbed when administered orally to man.

Distribution

It is not known if DMSA passes through the human placental barrier or if it can affect reproductive capacity or cause fetal harm. DMSA in lactating females has not been studied.

Excretion

Approximately 8 to 12% of DMSA is excreted unchanged in the urine. The major DMSA metabolite in man has been identified as a mixed disulfide of L-cysteine. The elimination half-life of DMSA is 3.2 hours.[125]

Pregnancy

DMSA (Succimer) is classified as a Category C agent.

Dose

Doses of 30 mg/kg/day for 5 days followed by 20 mg/day for 14 days led to a threefold increase in urinary mercury excretion with a decrease in blood mercury concentration. Longer courses of therapy or sustained therapy may have a larger impact on total body mercury elimination following elemental mercury exposure.

Pathophysiology

Animal and clinical studies suggest that DMSA chiefly removes mercury from the main peripheral site of deposition, the kidney.[126]

Acetylcysteine

The principal target organs for mercuric chloride induced toxicity are the kidneys. Nonprotein sulfhydryl group may be directly involved in mercury entry into the tubular cells. Glutathione plays a role in this process. Its high concentration in renal tissue may explain the accumulation of the metal in the kidney. Animal studies suggest that the nephrotoxic effects of mercuric chloride (both functional and biochemical) are either enhanced by glutathione depletion or prevented by glutathione augmentation. A synergistic effect may exist between the direct effect of memory and renal glutathione deficiency. *N*-acetylcysteine promotes a significant increase in renal nonprotein sulfhydryl content.[127]

N-acetyl-D,L-Penicillamine (NAP)

N-acetyl-penicillamine is formed by the acetylation of the amine group of penicillamine. It is classified as a chemical and is not approved for clinical use in the United States.

This oral compound may be useful in the less severe symptomatic inorganic and elemental mercury inhalation exposures, but its actual value remains to be determined by clinical studies. D-Penicillamine reverses sulfhydryl binding in the blood and chelates both mercury and lead. The use of penicillamine is contraindicated in penicillin-sensitive patients. *N*-acetyl-D,L-penicillamine has been administered successfully to patients with inorganic mercury-induced neuropathies (tremor, ataxia) and chronic elemental mercury toxicity.

Although DMSA appears superior to NAP in enhancing urinary excretion of mercury, NAP remains of interest in the treatment of elemental mercury vapor poisoning. A further advantage of DMSA over NAP is that fewer adverse reactions appear to occur with DMSA and NAD. Reactions to NAP are predominantly allergic. There are rare reversible elevations in liver function tests with DMSA.[3] The role of DMPS (dimercaptopropane sulfonate) in inorganic or organic mercury poisoning has not been evaluated. Both the oral and IV forms increase mercury excretion in the urine.[128]

Other Chelators

Methicillin has been subject to early trials, but significant data are not available regarding its efficacy.[129] Animal data indicate that the thiol chelator alpha-mercapto-beta-(2-furyl) acrylic acid may be able to induce metallothionein biosynthesis capable of binding mercury and rendering it biologically inactive. Clinical data with this chemical are not yet available.

ELIMINATION ENHANCEMENT

Hemodialysis

Mercury is over 90% bound to red blood cells and plasma protein. At equilibrium the blood contains only 1% of total body mercury.[130] In man the elimination half-life of inorganic mercury is about 40 days. The kidneys retain mercury longer than other tissues in the body with reports of over 85% of the accumulated body burden present 15 days or more after absorption.[131]

Charcoal Hemoperfusion

Charcoal hemoperfusion and hemodialysis are ineffective in removing mercury even after the patient has been treated with dimercaprol (BAL).[130–149] Charcoal hemoperfusion does not offer a useful alternative to accelerate the elimination of mercury.[132]

Plasma Exchange

Plasma exchange may remove a small amount of the ingested mercury after an acute mercuric chloride poisoning. It appears to be most efficient for the elimination of inorganic mercury and may, together with chelation, be useful at an early phase of mercury intoxication and in acute renal failure.[132] These studies require confirmation.

ERCH (Extracorporeal Regional Coupling Hemodialysis)

DMSA-ERCH induces more than a tenfold greater removal of mercury into dialysate when compared with hemodialysis. This procedure may prove to be useful to enhance removal of mercury in mercuric chloride–induced renal failure.[136] Efficacy of the DMSA-ERCH procedure for inorganic mercury poisoning is likely to be improved as the interval between exposure and treatment is reduced.[137] ERCH has also appeared to be effective in reducing blood methyl mercury in two patients. If treatment is begun soon after exposure to methyl mercury and before the inception of signs and symptoms, the incidence and severity of methyl mercury poisoning may potentially decrease.[138]

N-acetylcysteine and In Vitro Equilibrium Dialysis

N-acetylcysteine may be clinically useful in the removal of mercury from the body during hemodialysis for acute mercury poisoning.[139,140] In vitro equilibrium dialysis may be a useful screening procedure for potential chelating agents to enhance mercury clearance in patients undergoing hemodialysis. With this method *N*-acetylcysteine and dimercaptosuccinic acid may significantly enhance transfer of mercury into the dialysate. Lesser effectiveness has followed use of diethyldithiocarbamate and dithiothreitol.[141]

CANCER

Mercury compounds are genotoxic mainly by inhibiting the mitotic spindle, but the direct mutagenic effect of the inorganic forms seems to be low.[20,142] The effect on the spindle mechanism is probably the high affinity of mercury for sulfhydryl groups in the spindle apparatus. Cytogenetic studies in subjects exposed to mercury vapor have in most cases shown no effect on human chromosomes. Chloralkali workers have a higher incidence of lymphocyte micronuclei, a sensitive cytogenetic procedure.[142] Sister chromatid exchange is a measure of the exchange of DNA material within the chromosome, is used as a screening test method for possibly carcinogenic compounds, and appears to correlate with mercury exposure from ingested food.[143]

ORGANIC MERCURY

In the 1950s an epidemic of methyl mercury poisoning developed in Minamata, Japan, affecting over 2500 individuals. MRIs showed residual brain damage in the calcarine cortices, parietal cortices, and cerebellum of the older children that accounted for many of their persistent clinical signs. Since methyl mercury primarily damages the cerebrum and cerebellum—areas of brain concerned with coordination, balance, and sensations—and relatively spares the vital areas of the brainstem, methyl mercury appears to be a more potent neurotoxin than a lethal agent. Some recovery does occur in older children. The prominence of choreoathetosis and ataxia slowly disappears, spasticity lessens, and seizures stop. However, the cortical blindness and the constricted visual fields do not improve. MRIs demonstrated focal cortical atrophy in the calcarine and somatomotor cortices. Methyl mercury easily crosses the blood–brain barrier, while inorganic mercury crosses the blood–brain barrier poorly.[144]

REFERENCES—MERCURY

1. Taueg C, Sanfilippo DJ, Rowens B, Szejde J, Hesse JL. Acute and chronic poisoning from residential exposure to elemental mercury—Michigan 1989–1990. Clin Toxicol 1992; 30:63–67.
2. Campbell JS. Acute mercurial poisoning by inhalation of metallic vapour in an infant. Can Med Assoc J 1948;58:72–75.
3. Bluhm RE, Bobbitt RG, Welch LW, Wood AJJ, Bonfiglio JF, Sarzen C, Heath AJ, Branch RA. Elemental mercury vapour toxicity, treatment and prognosis after acute intensive exposure in chloralkali plant workers. I. History, neuropsychological findings and chelator effects. Hum Exp Toxicol 1992;11:201–210.

4. Jaffe KM, Shurtleff DB, Robertson WO. Survival after acute mercury vapor poisoning. Role of intensive supportive care. Am J Dis Child 1983;137:749–751.
5. Berlin M, Fazackerley J, Nordberg G. The uptake of mercury in the brains of mammals exposed to mercury vapor and to mercuric salts. Arch Environ Health 1969;18:719–729.
6. Bidstrup PL, Bonnell JA, Harvey DG, Locket S. Chronic mercury poisoning in men repairing direct-current meters. Lancet 1951;2:856–861.
7. McLauchlan GA. Acute mercury poisoning. Anesthesia 1991; 46:110–112.
8. Swineheart LT. Elemental mercury exposure. Pediatrics 1988; 81:743–744.
9. Vroom FQ, Greer M. Mercury vapour intoxication. Brain 1972;95:305–318.
10. Levin M, Jacobs J, Polos PG. Acute mercury poisoning and mercurial pneumonitis from gold ore purification. Chest 1988; 94:554–556.
11. Erickson T, Aks S, Branches FJ, Naleway C, Chou H-N, Hryhorszuk DO. Fractional mercury levels in Brazilian gold refiners and miners. Vet Hum Toxicol 1992;34:354.
12. Branches F, Erickson T, Aks S, Hryhorczuk DO. The price of gold: mercury poisoning in the Amazonian rain forest. Vet Hum Toxicol 1992;34:354.
13. Kanluen S, Gottlieb CA. A clinical pathologic study of four adult cases of acute mercury inhalation toxicity. Arch Pathol Lab Med 1991;115:56–60.
14. Tennant R, Johnston HJ, Wells JB. Acute bilateral pneumonitis associated with the inhalation of mercury vapor. Report of five cases. Connecticut Med 1961;25:106–109.
15. Weiss SW, Wands JR, Yardley JH. Demonstration by electron diffraction of black mercuric sulfide: (beta-HgS) in a case of "melanosis coli and black kidneys" caused by chronic inorganic mercury poisoning. Lab Invest 1973;28:401–402.
16. Snodgrass W, Sullivan JB, Rumack BH, Hashimoto C. Mercury poisoning from home gold ore processing. Use of penicillamine and dimercaprol. JAMA 1981;246:1929–1931.
17. Wands JR, Weiss SW, Yardley JH, Maddrey WC. Chronic inorganic mercury poisoning due to laxative abuse. Am J Med 1974;57:92–101.
18. Williamson AM, Teo RKC, Sanderson J. Occupational mercury exposure and its consequence for behaviour. Int Arch Occup Environ Health 1982;50:273–286.
19. Troen P, Kaufman SA, Katz KH. Mercuric bichloride poisoning. N Engl J Med 1951;244:59–71.
20. Barregard L, Sallsten G, Jarvholm B. Mortality and cancer incidence in chloralkali workers exposed to inorganic mercury. Br J Ind Med 1990;47:99–104.
21. Lindstedt G, Gottberg I, Holmgren B, Jonsson T, Karlsson G. Individual mercury exposure of chloralkali workers and its relation to blood and urinary mercury levels. Scand J Work Environ Health 1979;5:59–69.
22. Bell ZG, Lovejoy HB, Vizena TR. Mercury exposure evaluations and their correlation with urine mercury excretions. III. Time-weighted average (TWA) mercury exposures and urine mercury levels. J Occup Med 1973;15:501–508.
23. Yoshida M. Relation of mercury exposure to elemental mercury levels in the urine and blood. Scand J Work Environ Health 1985;11:33–37.
24. Jaeger A, Livardjani F, Dahlet M, Flexch F. Plasma and blood mercury concentrations in a non-occupationally exposed population. 1990;LuxTox'90, Luxembourg.
25. Arnold W. Elimination of mercury in urine after aspiration into the lungs. TIAFT, Proceedings of the 25th International Meeting, The International Association of Forensic Toxicologists. Groningen, June 27–30, 1988.
26. Manoukian SV, Wenger NK. Mercury in the heart. Am J Cardiol 1991;67:317–318.
27. Will VK, Burton BT, Magnusson AR, Solter J. Mercuric chloride: intravenous (IV) injection resulting in transient anuric renal failure. Vet Hum Toxicol 1991;33:388.
28. Stahl MG, Bonekat HW, Shigeoka JW. Concomitant pulmonary thromboembolism and metallic mercury embolism. A diagnostic dilemma. Chest 1985;88:787–789.
29. Clague JR, Gray HH, Kay PH. Self injection with mercury. BMJ 1989;299:1567.
30. Cassar-Pullicino VN, Taylor DN, Fitz-Patrick JD. Multiple metallic mercury emboli. Br J Radiol 1985;58:470–474.
31. Murray KM, Hedgpeth JC. Intravenous self-administration of elemental mercury: efficacy of dimercaprol therapy. Drug Intell Clin Pharm 1988;22:972–975.
32. Zillmer EA, Lucci K-A, Barth JT, Peake TH, Spyker DA. Neurobehavioral sequelae of subcutaneous injection with metallic mercury. Clin Toxicol 1986;24(2):91–110.
33. Friberg L, Hammarstrom S, Nystrom A. Kidney injury after chronic exposure to inorganic mercury. Arch Ind Hyg Occup Med 1953;8:149–153.
34. Langolf GD, Chaffin DB, Henderson R, Whittle HP. Evaluation of workers exposed to elemental mercury using quantitative tests of tremor and neuromuscular functions. Am Ind Hyg Assoc J 1978;39:976–984.
35. Sexton DJ, Powell KE, Liddle J, Smrek A, Smith JC, Clarkson TW. A nonoccupational outbreak of inorganic mercury vapor poisoning. Arch Environ Health 1978;33:186–191.
36. Blair E, Cross RE, Stave GM et al. Elemental mercury vapor poisoning. MMWR 1989;38:770–772.
37. Toxic Information Center Case Rounds. What is the proper technique for cleaning a mercury spill in a home? San Francisco Regional Poison Center, February 11, 1991.
38. Muhlendahl KEV. Intoxication from mercury spilled on carpets. Lancet 1990;336:1578.
39. Warkany J, Hubbard DM. Mercury in the urine of children with acrodynia. Lancet 1948;May 29:829–830.
40. Mellick C. Mercury poisoning from paint exposure. Rocky Mountain Poison Center Bulletin 1991;10(1):1–4.
41. Warkany J. Acrodynia. Postmortem of a disease. Am J Dis Child 1966;112:147–156.
42. Dathan JG. Acrodynia associated with excessive intake of mercury. Br Med J 1954;1:247–249.
43. Tunnessen WW, McMahon KJ, Baser M. Acrodynia from exposure to mercury in fluorescent light bulbs. Pediatrics 1987; 79:786–789.
44. Rapaport DS. Exposure to mercury vapor endangers workers' mental, physical health. Occup Health Saf 1989;58(10): 47–50.
45. Schuckmann F. Study of preclinical changes in workers exposed to inorganic mercury in chloralkali plants. Int Arch Occup Environ Health 1979;44:193–200.
46. Smith RG, Vorwald AJ, Patil LS, Mooney TF Jr. Effects of exposure to mercury in the manufacture of chlorine. Am Ind Hyg Assoc J 1970;3:687–700.
47. Ladd AC, Zuskin E, Valic F, Almonte JB, Gonzales TV. Absorption and excretion of mercury in miners. J Occup Med 1966;8:122–137.
48. Danziger SJ, Possick PA. Metallic mercury exposure in scientific glassware manufacturing plants. J Occup Med 1973; 15:15–20.
49. Stonard MD, Chater BV, Duffield DP, Nevitt AL, O'Sullivan JJ, Steel GT. An evaluation of renal function in workers occupationally exposed to mercury vapor. Int Arch Occup Environ Health 1983;52:177–189.
50. Naleway C, Sakaguchi R, Mitchell E, Muller T, Ayer WA, Hefferren JJ. Urinary mercury levels in US dentists, 1975–1983: review of Health Assessment Program. JADA 1985; 222:37–42.
51. Hancocks S. Is dental amalgam bad for you? Br Med J 1991;302:488.
52. Litovitz TL, Schmitz BF, Bailey KM. 1989 Annual Report of the American Association of Poison Control Centers National Data Collection System: 433. Case 124.
53. Fung YK, Molvar MP. Toxicity of mercury from dental environment and from amalgam restorations. Clin Toxicol 1992; 30(1):59–61.
54. Bergman M. Side-effects of amalgam and its alternatives: local, systemic and environmental. Int Dental J 1990;40:4–10.
55. Ericson A, Kallen B. Pregnancy outcome in women working as dentists, dental assistants or dental technicians. Int Arch Occup Environ Health 1989;61:329–333.
56. Tuffs A. Germany: amalgam fillings. Lancet 1992;339:419.
57. Olstad ML, Holland RI, Pettersen AH. Effect of placement of amalgam restorations on urinary mercury concentration. J Dent Res 1990;69(9):1607–1609.

58. Molin M, Bergman B, Marklund SL, Schutz A, Skerfving S. Mercury, selenium and glutathione peroxidase before and after amalgam removal in man. Acta Odontol Scand 1990;48: 189–202.
59. Snapp KR, Boyer DB, Peterson LC, Svare CW. The contribution of dental amalgam to mercury in blood. J Dent Res 1989;68(5):780–785.
60. Eti S, Weisman RS, Hoffman RS. Lack of renal toxic effect of mercury amalgam fillings. Vet Hum Toxicol 1992;34:354.
61. Panel advises further research on dental amalgam. FDA Consumer 1991;25(5):4–5.
62. Friedman PK. Safety of dental amalgam. JAMA 1988;260: 2295.
63. Nightingale SL. Safety of dental amalgam. JAMA 1991;215: 2934.
64. Baratz R. Dental amalgam. Heavy metal. Harvard Health Letter. 1991;16(11):4–5.
65. Melkonian R, Baker D. Risks of industrial mercury exposure in pregnancy. Obstet Gynecol Survey. 1988;43(112): 637–641.
66. Lauwerys R, Roels H, Genet P, Toussaint G, Bouckaert A, De Cooman S. Fertility of male workers exposed to mercury vapor or to manganese dust: a questionnaire study. Am J Ind Med 1985;7:171–176.
67. Cordier S, Deplan F, Mandereau L, Hemon D. Paternal exposure to mercury and spontaneous abortions. Br J Ind Med 1991;48:375–381.
68. Kuhnert PM, Kuhnert BR, Erhard P. Comparison of mercury levels in maternal blood, fetal cord blood and placental tissues. Am J Obstet Gynecol 1981;139:209–213.
69. Urbach J, Boadi W, Brandes JM, Kerner H, Yannai S. Effect of inorganic mercury on in vitro placental nutrient transfer and oxygen consumption. Reprod Toxicol 1992;6:69–75.
70. Takahata N, Hayashi H, Watanabe S, Anso T. Accumulation of mercury in the brains of two autopsy cases with chronic inorganic mercury poisoning. Folia Psychiatrica et Neurologica Japonica 1970;24:59–69.
71. Erfurth EM, Schutz A, Nilsson A, Barregard L, Skerfving S. Normal pituitary hormone response to thyrotropin and gonadotrophin releasing hormones in subjects exposed to elemental mercury vapour. Br J Ind Med 1990;47:639–644.
72. McGregor AJ, Mason HJ. Occupational mercury vapour exposure and testicular, pituitary and thyroid endocrine function. Hum Exp Toxicol 1991;10:199–203.
73. Pesce AJ, Hanenson I, Sethi K. Beta$_2$ microglobulinuria in a patient with nephrotoxicity secondary to mercuric chloride ingestion. Clin Toxicol 1977;11:390–395.
74. Hunter D, Lister A. Mercurialentis. Br J Ophthalmol 1953;37: 234–235.
75. Tubbs RR, Gephardt GN, McMahon JT, Polh MC, Vidt DG, Barenberg SA, Valenzuela R. Membranous glomerulonephritis associated with industrial mercury exposure. Study of pathogenetic mechanisms. Am J Clin Pathol 1982;77:409–413.
76. Buchet JP, Roels H, Bernard A, Lauwerys R. Assessment of renal function of workers exposed to inorganic lead, cadmium or mercury vapor. J Occup Med 1980;22:741–750.
77. Clarkson TW. The pharmacology of mercury compounds. Annu Rev Pharmacol Toxicol 1972;12:375–406.
78. Rosenman KD, Valciukas JA, Glickman L, Meyers BR, Cinotti A. Sensitive indicators of inorganic mercury toxicity. Arch Environ Health 1989;41:208–215.
79. Winek CL, Fochtman FW, Bricker JD et al. Fatal mercuric chloride ingestion. Clin Toxicol 1981;18:261–262.
80. Ehrenberg RL, Vogt RL, Smith AB et al. Effects of elemental mercury exposure at a thermometer plant. Am J Ind Med 1991;19:495–507.
81. Leaback DE, Walker DG. The fluorometric assay of *N*-acetyl-beta-glucosaminadase. Biochem J 1981;78:151–156.
82. Elemental mercury vapor poisoning—North Carolina 1988. MMWR 38:770–777.
83. Fahn S. Differential diagnosis of tremors. Med Clin North Am 1972;56:1363–1375.
84. Langworth S, Almkvist O, Soderman E, Wikstrom B-A. Effects of occupational exposure to mercury vapor on the central nervous system. Br J Ind Med 1992;49:545–555.
85. Battigelli MC. Mercury toxicity from industrial exposure. A critical review of the literature. II. J Occup Med 1960;Aug: 394–399.
86. Verberk MM,Salle HJA, Kemper CH. Tremor in workers with low exposure to metallic mercury. Am Ind Hyg Assoc J 1987; 47(8):559–562.
87. Cavanaugh JB. Long-term persistence of mercury in the brain. Br J Ind Med 1988;15:619–651.
88. Miller JM, Chaffin DB, Smith RG. Subclinical psychomotor and neuromuscular changes in workers exposed to inorganic mercury. Am Ind Hyg Assoc J 1975;Oct:725–733.
89. Chapman LJ, Sauter SL, Henning RA, Dodson VN, Reddan WG, Matthews CG. Differences in frequency of finger tremor in otherwise asymptomatic mercury workers. Br J Ind Med 1990;47:838–843.
90. Albers JW, Kallenbach LR, Fine LJ et al. Mercury Workers Study Group. Neurological abnormalities associated with remote occupational elemental mercury exposure. Ann Neurol 1988;24:651–659.
91. Nylander M, Friberg L, Weiner J. Muscle biopsy as an indicator for predicting mercury concentrations in the brain. Br J Ind Med 1990;47:575–576.
92. Magos L. Mercury-blood interaction and mercury uptake by the brain after vapor exposure. Environ Res 1967; 323–337.
93. King GW. Acute pneumonitis due to accidental exposure to mercury vapor. Ariz Med 1954;11:335.
94. Bluhm RE, Breyer J, Bobbitt RG, Welch LW, Wood AJJ, Bonfiglio JF, Branch RA. Hyperchloremia as a manifestation of elemental mercury vapor toxicity in chloralkali workers. Vet Hum Toxicol 1991;33:373.
95. Freeman JR. Mercurial disease among hatters. Trans Med Soc NJ, 1960; pp. 61–64.
96. Wedeen RP. Were the hatters of New Jersey "mad"? Am J Ind Med 1989;16:225–233.
97. De Bont B, Lauwerys R, Govaerts H, Moulin D. Yellow mercuric oxide ointment and mercury intoxication. Eur J Pediatr 1986;145:217–218.
98. Bourgeois M, Dooms-Goossens A, Knockaert D, Sprengers D, Van Boven M, Van Tittelboom T. Mercury intoxication after topical application of a metallic mercury ointment. Dermatologica 1986;172:48–51.
99. Hursh JB, Clarkson TW, Miles EF, Goldsmith LA. Percutaneous absorption of mercury vapor by man. Arch Environ Health 1989;44:120–127.
100. Godlee F. Skin lighteners cause permanent damage. BMJ 1992;305:333.
101. Barr RD, Woodger BA, Rees PH. Levels of mercury in urine correlated with the use of skin lightening creams. Am J Clin Pathol 1973;59:36–40.
102. Dyall-Smith DJ, Scurry JP. Mercury pigmentation and high mercury levels from the use of a cosmetic cream. Med J Aust 1990;153:409–415.
103. Moria A. Health hazards from mercury soap. Lancet 1989; 1:448.
104. Becker CG, Becker EL, Maher JF. Nephrotic syndrome after contact with mercury. Arch Intern Med 1962;110:178–186.
105. Silverberg DS, McCall JT, Heut JC. Nephrotic syndrome with use of ammoniated mercury. Arch Intern Med 1967;170: 581–586.
106. Schrallhammer-Benkler K, Ring J, Przybilla B, Meurer M, Landthaler M. Acute mercury intoxication with lichenoid drug eruption followed by mercury contact allergy and development of antinuclear antibodies. Acta Derm Venereol (Stockh) 1992;72:294–296.
107. Gaffin SL, Hornung H. Rapid determination of mercury in urine by flameless atomic absorption spectrometry. Clin Toxicol 1977;10:345–351.
108. Krull IS, Bushee DS, Schleicher RG, Smith SB Jr. Determination of inorganic and organomercury compounds by high-performance liquid chromatography-inductively coupled plasma emission spectrometry with cold vapour generation. Analyst 1986;111:345–349.
109. Magos L, Clarkson TW. Atomic absorption determination of total, inorganic and organic mercury in blood. J Assoc Off Anal Chem 1972;55:966–971.

110. Landrigan PJ. Occupational and community exposure to toxic metals: lead, cadmium, mercury and arsenic. West J Med 1982;137:531–539.
111. Pineau A, Piron M, Boiteau H-L, Etourneau M-J, Guillard O. Determination of total mercury in human hair samples by cold vapor atomic absorption spectrometry. J Analyt Toxicol 1990;14:235–238.
112. Giovanoli-Jakubczak, Greenwood MR, Smith JC, Clarkson TW. Determination of total and inorganic mercury in hair by flameless atomic absorption and of methylmercury by gas chromatography. Clin Chem 1974;20:222–229.
113. Kazantzis G, Schiller KFR, Asscher AW, Drew RG. Albuminuria and the nephrotic syndrome following exposure to mercury and its compounds. Q J Med 1962;31: 403–419.
114. Zalups RK, Cherian MG. Renal metallothionein metabolism after a reduction of renal mass. I. Effect of unilateral nephrectomy and compensatory renal growth on basal and metal-induced renal metallothionein metabolism. Toxicology 1992;71:83–102.
115. Mant TGK. Clinical studies with dimercaptopropane sulphonate in mercury poisoning. Hum Toxicol 1985;4:346.
116. Campbell JR, Clarkson TW, Omar MI. Therapeutic use of 2,3-dimercaptopropane-1-sulfonate in two cases of inorganic mercury poisoning. JAMA 1986;256:3127–3130.
117. Lamm O, Pratt H. Subclinical effects of exposure to inorganic mercury revealed by somatosensory-evoked potentials. Eur Neurol 1985;24:237-243.
118. Ellingsen D, Morland T, Anderson A, Kjuus H. Nervous system effects associated with previous exposure to inorganic mercury. Neurotoxicology 1991;12(4):808.
119. Nielsen JB, Andersen O. Effect of four thiol-containing chelators on disposition of orally administered mercuric chloride. Hum Exp Toxicol 1991;10:423–430.
120. Toet AC, van Dijk A, Savelkoul TJF, Meulenbelt J. A case of severe mercury chloride poisoning treatment with dimercapto-1-propane sulfonate (DMPS). Proc Eur Assoc Pois Cont Centers Clin Toxicol, Istanbul, May 24–27, 1992.
121. Hla KK, Ashton CE, Henry JA, Volans GN, Mant TGK. Adverse effects of 2,3 dimercapto-1-propane sulfonate (DMPS). Proc Eur Assoc Pois Cont Centers Clin Toxicol, Istanbul, May 24–27, 1992; p. 13.
122. Aposhlan HV, Maiorino RM, Hurlbut KM, Dart RC, Bruce DS, Aposhlan MM. Pharmacokinetics of DMPS and DMSA in humans. Proc Eur Assoc Pois Cont Centers Clin Toxicol, Istanbul, May 24–27, 1992; p. 12.
123. Product literature: (Succimer®). McNeil Consumer Products, 1991.
124. Ding G-S, Liang Y-Y. Antidotal effects of dimercaptosuccinic acid. J Appl Toxicol 1991;11:7–14.
125. Maiorino MM, Bruce DC, Aposhian HV. Determination of dithiol chelating agents. VI. Isolation and identification of the mixed sulfides of meso-2,3 dimercaptosuccinic acid with L-cysteine in human urine. Toxicol Appl Pharmacol 1989;97: 338–349.
126. Roels HA, Boeckx M, Ceulemans E, Lauwerys RR. Urinary excretion of mercury after occupational exposure to mercury vapour and influence of the chelating agent meso-2,3-dimercaptosuccinic acid (DMSA). Br J Ind Med 1991;48: 247–253.
127. Girardi G, Elias MM. Effectiveness of N-acetylcysteine in protecting against mercuric chloride-induced nephrotoxicity. Toxicol 1991;67:155–164.
128. Feychting K, Kulling P, Skold H, Sjerstrom H, Furuland H, Bennis J. DMPS and DMSA in mercury poisoning. Presentation at Eur Assoc Pois Cent Clin Toxicol 1994, Krakow.
129. Lyle WH. Evaluation of the chelating action of methicillin in prolonged experimental metallic mercury poisoning. Br J Ind Med 1987;44:71.
130. Keller F, Koeffer C, Von Keyserling HJ, Schutze G. Hemoperfusion for organic mercury detoxication. Klin Wochenschr 1981;59:865–866.
131. Clarkson TW. Recent advances in the toxicology of mercury with emphasis on the alklymercurials. Crit Rev Toxicol 1972; 1:203–234.
132. Leumann EP, Brandenberger H. Hemodialysis in a patient with acute mercuric cyanide intoxication. Concentrations of mercury in blood, dialysate, urine, vomitus and feces. Clin Toxicol 1977;11:301–308.
133. Worth DP, Lewins AM, Davison AM, Ledgerwood MJ, Taylor A. Haemodialysis and charcoal haemoperfusion in acute inorganic mercury poisoning. Postgrad Med J 1984;60: 636–638.
134. Lowenthal DT, Chardo F, Reidenberg MM. Removal of mercury by peritoneal dialysis. Arch Intern Med 1974;134: 139–141.
135. Pellonen TJ, Karjalainer K, Haaparen JE. Hemoperfusion in mercury poisoning. J Toxicol Clin Toxicol 1983;120: 187–189.
136. Kostyniak PJ, Greizerstein HB, Goldstein J et al. Extracorporeal regional complexing haemodialysis treatment of acute inorganic mercury intoxication. Hum Toxicol 1990;9: 137–141.
137. Cunningham LE, Kostyniak PJ, Goldstein J, Greizerstein HB, Lachaal M, Reddy P et al: Extracorporeal regional complexing hemodialysis. Treatment of acute inorganic mercury intoxication. Kidney Int 1990;37:292.
138. Al-Abbasi AH, Kostyniak PJ, Clarkson TW. An extracorporeal complexing hemodialysis system for the treatment of methylmercury poisoning. III. Clinical applications. J Pharmacol Exp Ther 1978;207:249–254.
139. Ferguson CL, Cantilena LR Jr. Enhanced mercury clearance during hemodialysis with chelating agents. Clin Pharmacol Ther 1991;49:131.
140. Ferguson CL, Cantilena LR. Mercury clearance from human plasma during in vitro dialysis: screening systems for chelating agents. Clin Toxicol 1992;30:423–441.
141. Ferguson CL, Cantilena LR Jr. In vitro equilibrium dialysis as a screening procedure for chelating agents effective in enhancing mercury clearance from human plasma. Am Soc Clin Pharmacol Ther 1992;Feb:186.
142. Barregard L, Sallstein G, Schutz A, Attewell R, Skerfving S, Jarvholm B. Kinetics of mercury in blood and urine after brief occupational exposure. Arch Environ Health 1992;46: 176–184.
143. Wulf HC, Kromann N, Kousgaard N, Jansen J, Niebuhr E, Alboge K. Sister chromatid exchange (SCE) in Greenlandic Eskimos. Dose-response relationship between SCE and seal diet, smoking and blood cadmium and mercury concentrations. Sci Total Environ 1986;48:81–94.
144. Davis LE, Kornfeld M, Mooney HS et al. Methylmercury poisoning: long-term clinical, radiological, toxicological and pathological studies of an affected family. Ann Neurol 1994;35:680–688.

MOLYBDENUM

Lesser and Weiss have detailed effects of exposure to molybdenum.[1] The fumes from molybdenum, an additive in some welding rods or in the steel itself, produce a unique clinical picture. The symptoms of molybdenum exposure are decreased appetite, listlessness, weakness, fatigue, anorexia, headache, arthralgias, myalgias, chest pain, nonproductive cough, and diarrhea. Molybdenum increases production of xanthine oxidase and is a cofactor required for transferases to bind iron. Therefore patients with high molybdenum levels develop gouty attacks and a hypochromic microcytic anemia. The patient may develop an x-ray pattern that looks like a pneumoconiosis. Chronic molybdenism causes testicular atrophy.

REFERENCES—MOLYBDENUM

1. Lesser SH, Weiss SJ. Art hazards. Am J Emerg Med 1995;13:451–458.

NICKEL

NICKEL SULFATE

Nickel sulfate may be fatal[1] or may produce evidence of respiratory, circulatory, and neurologic distress.[2,3]

NICKEL CARBONYL

This product is considered to be one of the most toxic chemicals used in industry. The magnitude of its morbidity and mortality has been compared to that of hydrogen cyanide.[4]

Types of nickel poisoning are summarized in Table 67–34.[3] Spyker has comprehensively reviewed nickel exposure categories.[5]

STRUCTURE AND CLASSIFICATION

Nickel is found in metallic nickel, as nickel oxide (green), nickel oxide (black), nickel chloride hexahydrate, nickel sulfate hexahydrate, and nickel nitrate hexahydrate. Nickel may exist in many oxidation states, the most prevalent being Ni^{2+}.

SOURCES

The largest nickel source found in the atmosphere is from fuel oil combustion.[1] Other sources of atmospheric emissions include mining and refining operations, municipal waste incinerators, and windblown dust. Nickel sources in water soil include stormwater runoff and wastewater from municipal sewage treatment plants. Consumer products contribute little to exposure. Nickel occurs in most food items. The highest level of exposure to nickel comes from dietary intake.[1]

THERAPEUTIC DOSES

Foods with nickel concentrations over 1 mg/kg include oatmeal, wheat bran, fried beans, soya products, hazelnuts, peanuts, sunflower seeds, licorice, cocoa, and dark chocolate.[1] Consumption of such foods in large amount could raise the nickel intake to 900 μg/d.[7,3] Ingestion of 0.5 to 2.5 g of nickel sulfate led to transient symptoms and full recovery in 32 workers who drank water contaminated with both nickel sulfate and chloride (1.63 g Ni/liter).[2]

Table 67–34
Types of Nickel Poisoning

Inhalation ($Ni(CO)_4$, Ni, Ni_3S_2, NiO, Ni_2O_3)
- *Acute*
  - Pneumonitis with adrenal cortical insufficiency; hyaline membrane formation; pulmonary edema and hemorrhage; hepatic degeneration; brain and renal congestion
- *Chronic*
  - Cancer of respiratory tract; pulmonary eosinophilia (Loeffler's syndrome); asthma

Skin Contact
- Primary irritant dermatitis; allergic dermatitis; eczema

Parenteral (Prosthetic Implantations)
- Allergenic reactions; osteomyelitis; osteonecrosis; malignant tumors

Oral
- Food and beverage; drugs

FATAL DOSE

A fatal case of nickel poisoning by the oral route occurred in a 2½-year-old girl who ingested 15 g of nickel sulfate crystals (3.3 g Ni)[6] (3.3 g of nickel is equivalent to 220 mg/kg body weight).

OCCUPATIONAL EXPOSURE

Occupations in which nickel exposure may occur include the following: Battery makers, ceramic makers, coal gasification workers, dyers, electroformers, electroplaters, enamellers, glassworkers, ink makers, jewelers, magnet makers, metalworkers, nickel miners, nickel refiners, nickel smelters, oil dehydrogenators, paint makers, sandblasters, spark plug makers, spray painters, stainless steel makers, textile dyers, varnish makers, and welders.[1]

CARCINOGENICITY

Occupational exposure to nickel refinery dust, which contains nickel subsulfide, has been associated with an increased risk of lung and nasal cancers, and possibly cancer of the larynx.[7] Nickel subsulfide is considered to be a known human carcinogen. Nickel carbonyl is a probable human carcinogen.[7,8] Metallic nickel, nickel oxide, and soluble nickel salts may be associated with lung and nasal sinus cancer.[9]

ENVIRONMENTAL EXPOSURE

The OSHA permissible exposure limit for nickel and soluble nickel compounds is 1 mg/m^3.[10] Based on studies of stainless steel workers a future limit volume for nickel concentration in the urine should be between 20 and 50 μg/L corresponding to an exposure of 500 μg Ni/m^3.[11]

BLOOD

Normal levels of nickel have been reported to be less than 0.1 mg/kg body weight in tissues, 3 to 7 μg/L in whole blood, 1 to 5 μg/L in blood serum, and 2.5 μg/L (2 to 4 μg/L) in urine.[7] After absorption, concentrations are highest in the kidneys, lungs, liver, and pituitary gland.[5] The fatal nickel burden in man is about 10 mg. After exposure to nickel in the air at a concentration of 39 $\mu g/m^3$, the plasma nickel concentration was 93 μg/L, and the concentration in the urine 18.5 μg.[1]

ELIMINATION

Absorbed nickel is excreted predominantly in the urine. It is also excreted in perspiration and is deposited in the hair. The half-life of nickel in the serum is 11 hours.[1] Nickel appears to have a short half-life in the body of several days with little tissue accumulation.

Table 67–35
Symptoms of Acute Nickel Carbonyl Poisoning

Immediate	Latent	Delayed
Mild, non-specific Symptoms disappear when subject removed to uncontaminated air Headache; dizziness Sternal and epigastric pains Nausea and vomiting occasionally	1 to 5 days May be essentially asymptomatic	Constriction in chest Chills, sweating Shortness of breath Unproductive cough Muscle pains Weakness, fatigue Gastrointestinal symptoms occasionally Convulsions and delirium—sometimes terminally

PREGNANCY/LACTATION

No human studies are available relative to effects of nickel on pregnancy or lactation. Nickel crosses the placental barrier in animals and may do so in man.[8]

MECHANISM OF ACTION

Nickel readily crosses the cell membrane via Ca^{2+} channels and competes with Ca^{2+} for specific receptors.[3]

CLINICAL PRESENTATION

Nickel Carbonyl (Table 67–35)[3]

Nickel carbonyl is the most toxic form of nickel. The immediate symptoms following exposure include nausea, vertigo, headache, dyspnea, and chest pain followed in 1 to 5 days by severe pulmonary symptoms and possibly death.[12] Acute toxic effects usually occur in two stages, immediate and delayed. Following an exposure to an air concentration of nickel over 50 mg/m^3 symptoms referable to the respiratory and nervous system may appear within 30 minutes to 1 hour[13] followed within 24 hours by more serious life-threatening events. Fatalities usually occur after 4 to 11 days and are attributed to neurologic and respiratory toxicity.[3,4]

Nickel Hypersensitivity

Asthma, urticaria, erythema multiforme, contact dermatitis, and hand eczema may follow use of objects made with nickel. Stainless steel sutures may induce a hypersensitivity reaction in a patient allergic to nickel.[14] Patch tests may be useful. Nickel disposable surgical skin clips may be contraindicated in patients with nickel allergy.[14,15]

Dimethylglyoxine Test[14,16]

A spot test kit contains 1% dimethylglyoxine in alcohol solution (1 fluid ounce) and 10% ammonium hydroxide solution (1 fluid ounce). Add a few drops of each solution to the metallic object, solution, or skin to be tested. A positive reaction is indicated by a red precipitate, denoting the presence of available nickel in sufficient concentration (at least 1:10,000) to produce dermatitis in nickel-sensitive persons. Stainless steel objects may give a negative reaction and should be safe for use by those who are sensitive to nickel.[16] Dimethylglyoxine test kits may be obtained from Alloderm Laboratories, P.O. Box 931, Mill Valley, CA 94941.[14]

LABORATORY

Analytic Methods

Electrothermal atomic absorption spectrometry is useful for determinations of nickel concentration in the urine. The limit of detection of nickel is 0.1 μg/L.[17]

Abnormalities

Exposure to nickel carbonyl fumes may induce a leukocytosis that may parallel the severity of intoxication. Eosinophilia is usually not found. The electrocardiogram may show a sinus tachycardia or bradycardia with or without heart block and a toxic myocarditis (changes in ST, T-waves, QT interval prolongation).[13] Irregular linear shadows may be seen on a chest x-ray.

Ancillary Tests

Transient elevations of blood reticulocytes, urine albumin, and serum bilirubin may follow a nickel sulfate ingestion.[2]

The lymphocyte proliferation test appears to be useful in assessing the relevance of nickel contact in occupational hand eczema.[18]

TREATMENT

Nickel Carbonyl Inhalation

Mild cases can be treated with bed rest after removal from exposure. Bronchodilators and symptomatic drugs may be useful. In moderate cases oxygen, glucose, ascorbic acid, and corticosteroids may be useful. Dithiocarb, antibiotics, and other drugs may help resolve the pulmonary edema, pneumonia, and toxic myocarditis.[13] Most patients recover without severe sequelae. Symptoms may persist for 3 to 6 months. Disulfiram may be used because it is metabolized to two molecules of dithiocarb (diethyldithiocarbamate).[4] Dithiocarb is investigational in the United States. Data on dithiocarb and disulfiram have not been subjected to controlled clinical studies.

Nickel Sulfate, Nickel Chloride

Individuals who have ingested either nickel sulfate or nickel chloride should be treated with symptomatic and supportive care.[2,3] No evidence exists to support the efficacy of topical dithiocarb or disulfiram in treatment of nickel dermatitis.

REFERENCES—NICKEL

1. Cormish H, Kniep TJ, Sunderman FW Jr. Toxicological profile for nickel. Agency for Toxic Substances and Disease Registry and EPA ATSDR/TP-88/19, December 1988.
2. Sunderman FW Jr, Dingle B, Hopfer SM, Surft T. Acute nickel toxicity in electroplating workers who accidentally ingested a solution of nickel sulfate and nickel chloride. Am J Ind Med 1988;14:257–266.

3. Sunderman FW Jr. A pilgrimage into the archives of nickel toxicology. Ann Clin Lab Sci 1989;19:1–16.
4. Kurta DL, Dean BS, Krenzelok EP. Acute occupational nickel carbonyl poisoning. Vet Hum Toxicol 1991;33:372.
5. Spyker DA. Nickel toxicokinetics. A white paper. Pharmaceutical Research Association, Inc., Charlottesville, VA 22901.
6. Daldrup T, Haarhoff K, Szathmary SC. Toedliche nickel sulfate—intoxikation. Bericht Gericht Med 1986;141: 141–144.
7. National Research Council, Canada. Effects of nickel in the Canadian environment, 1981; citation 18568.
8. Sunderman FW Jr. Mechanisms of nickel carcinogenesis. Scand J Work Environ Health 1989;15:1–2.
9. US EPA, CEC, Energy, mines and Resources, Canada, National Health and Welfare, Canada, Ontario Ministry of Labour, Nickel Producers Environmental Research Association. Report of the International Committee on Nickel Carcinogenesis in Man. Scand J Work Environ Health 1990;16: 1–82.
10. OSHA (Occupational Safety and Health Administration). Occupational Standards Permissible Exposure Limits. 29 Code of Federal Regulations 1910.10000.
11. Angerer J, Lehnert G. Occupational chronic exposure to metals. II. Nickel exposure of stainless steel welders—biological monitoring. Int Arch Occup Environ Health 1990;62:7–10.
12. Webster JD, Parker TF, Alfrey AC, Smythe WR, Kubo H, Neal G et al. Acute nickel intoxication by dialysis. Ann Intern Med 1980;92:631–633.
13. Zhicheng S. Acute nickel carbonyl poisoning: a report of 179 cases. Br J Ind Med 1986;43:422–424.
14. Fisher AA. Medico-legal aspects of the use of stainless steel sutures in nickel-sensitive persons. Cutis 1988;45:25–26.
15. US EPA. Project Survey, Health Assessment Document for Nickel. EPA/600/58-3/012, July 1990.
16. Fisher AA. The dimethylglyoxamine test in the prevention and management of nickel dermatitis. Cutis 1990;46: 467–468.
17. Ong CN, Chua LH, Lee BL, Ong HY, Chia KS. Electrothermal atomic absorption spectrometric determination of cadmium and nickel in urine. J Anal Toxicol 1990;14:29–33.
18. Rasanen L, Tuomi M-L. Diagnostic value to the lymphocyte proliferation test on nickel contact allergy and provocation in occupational coin dermatitis. Contact Dermatitis 1992;27:250–254.

PALLADIUM

Palladium occurs in nature with platinum or gold. It is found in nickel sulfide ores. Palladium compounds include palladium chloride ($PdCl_2.2H_2O$), palladium iodide (PdI_2), palladium oxide (PlO), palladium nitrate ($Pd(NO_3)_2$) and palladium trifluoride (PdF_3).[1] No cases of occupational poisoning from palladium or its compounds have been reported. In Austria palladium has begun to replace amalgam in dental fillings because of concerns about mercury toxicity.[2] Contact dermatitis has been reported.[3]

REFERENCES—PALLADIUM

1. Mastromatteo E. Palladium alloys and compounds. In: Parmeggiani L, ed. Encyclopaedia of occupational health and safety. 3rd ed. Geneva: International Labour Office 1991; pp. 1587–1588.
2. Aberer W, Holub H, Strobal R, Slavick R. Palladium in dental alloys—the dermatologist's responsibility to warn? Contact Dermatitis 1993;28:163–165.
3. Olivarius F de F, Menne T. Contact dermatitis from metallic palladium in patients reacting to palladium chloride. Contact Dermatitis 1992;27:71–77.

PHOSPHORUS

A preliminary case study of nonsmoking men who live in the central Florida phosphate mining section suggests that they experience an increased risk of lung cancer.[1] This has not yet been confirmed.

A low-birth-weight infant of 28 weeks was inadvertently administered 460 mg of phosphorus daily instead of 46 mg as a preventive measure for metabolic bone disease. The infant developed apneic attacks with cyanosis, a distended abdomen, generalized muscle spasms in both arms and legs, an extreme hypocalcemia, and a hyperphosphatemia. Calcium supplements led to the child's recovery.[2]

CLINICAL PRESENTATION

Phosphine Gas

Exposures to phosphine gas cause gastrointestinal tract symptoms, as well as respiratory, cardiovascular, and central nervous system changes resulting from metabolic changes. Prominent clinical manifestations of acute phosphine gas exposure include headache, fatigue, nausea, vomiting, cough, dyspnea, paresthesias, jaundice, ataxia, intention tremor, weakness, and diplopia.[3] On autopsy fatal cases revealed centrilobulbar necrosis of the liver,[4] congestive heart failure with pulmonary edema, and focal myocardial necrosis.[3]

REFERENCES—PHOSPHORUS

1. Stockwell HG, Lyman GH, Waltz J, Peters JT. Risks associated with residence in the central Florida phosphate mining region. Am J Epidemiol 1988;128:78–84.
2. Van den Anker JN, Fetter WPF, Sauer PJJ. Acute phosphorous intoxication in very low birthweight infant. Eur J Pediatr 1992;151:619–620.
3. Wilson R, Lovejoy FH, Jaeger RJ et al. Acute phosphine poisoning aboard a grain freighter. JAMA 1980;244:148–150.
4. Singh S, Dilawandi JB, Vashist R et al. Aluminum phosphide ingestion. Br Med J 1985;290:1110–1111.

PLATINUM[1,2]

CLINICAL PRESENTATION

Potassium Chloropalatinite

Potassium chloropalatinite (K_2PtC16; CAS# 10025-99-7) is a soluble, nonorganic salt of platinum used in photography, in the chemical and electrical industries, in electroplating, and in the manufacture of catalysts. A 31-year-old man ingested 10 mL of a photographic tonic solution containing 600 mg of potassium chloropalatinite and subsequently developed an acute oliguric renal failure, metabolic acidosis, fever, muscle cramps, gastroenteritis, and rhabdomyolysis. Laboratory studies indicated mildly elevated liver enzymes and an elevated peripheral blood neutrophil and eosinophil count. A spot serum platinum concentration was 245 μg/dL, and a spot urine platinum concentration was 4200 μcg/L. The patient recovered within 6 days after supportive treatment. The blood and urine platinum levels were obtained by atomic absorption spectrophotometry using a graphite furnace. Sensitivity of this method is 1 to 2 μg/dL.[3] The nephrotoxicity appeared similar to that seen after the use of *cis*-platinum.

REFERENCES—PLATINUM

1. Vaisrub S. Humble therapeutic beginnings for a noble metal. JAMA 1979;241:2738.
2. Krakoff IH. Nephrotoxicity of cis-dichlorodiamine platinum (II). Cancer Treat Rep 1979;63:1523–1525.
3. Woolf AD, Ebert TH. Toxicity after self-poisoning by ingestion of potassium chloropalatinite. Clin Toxicol 1991;29:467–472.

POTASSIUM

CLINICAL PRESENTATION

Slow-release potassium tablets in overdose may lead to serious arrhythmias and death.[1,2] One patient ingested 100 slow-release potassium tablets, developed ventricular tachycardia, and survived.[3] A 27-year-old ingested 60 tablets of slow-K (sustained-release potassium chloride, 600 mg, 8 mmol each of K^+ and Cl^-), developed a first-degree heart block, wide QRS complexes, and tall T-waves. The plasma potassium concentration was 91 mmol/L.[4] The patient survived.

A 53-year-old male ingested 1 tablespoonful (21 grams) of a salt substitute containing 52.8% potassium, an ingestion representing 283 mmol of potassium. The patient developed a hyperkalemia that led to asystole and death.[5]

Oral ingestion of saltpeter (K^+NO_3) should be added to the differential diagnosis of hyperkalemia with a spuriously elevated Co_2 and a negative anion gap in patients with normal renal function.[6]

Dialysis effectively removes potassium. Patients who cannot tolerate fluid loads or those with severe renal dysfunction benefit from early hemodialysis. Treatment of hyperkalemia is summarized in Table 67–36.

Table 67-36
Treatment of Hyperkalemia

	Dose	Onset/Duration of Action	Mechanism of Action	Comments
Calcium gluconate (10%) or calcium chloride (10%)	10 cc IV (May repeat × 2 prn q 5–10 min)	1–5 min/~1 h	Antagonizes membrane effects of K+	ECG monitoring required Do not mix with HCO_{3-} Beware: Hypercalcemia
Sodium bicarbonate	50 mg IV (May repeat × 1 prn)	~10–15 min/1–2 h	Intracellular movement of K+	Beware: Volume overload Hypertonicity Alkalosis (Seizures)
Glucose/insulin	10–20 units regular insulin per 100 g glucose	30 min/while infusion continued	Intracellular movement of K+	Beware: Hyperglycemia Hypoglycemia Infused volume may be decreased by using D10, D20 or D50
Kayexalate	25 g in 25 mL 70% sorbitol po q6h ± 50 g in 50 mL 70% sorbitol by retention enema q6h	Hours/while cont'd	Exchange of K+ for Na+	Beware: Na+ overload Enema must be retained × 30–45 min.
Dialysis	Hemodialysis Peritoneal dialysis	Minutes/while cont'd	Removal of K+ from blood	May remove 50 mEq/h (HD) Beware: K+ rebound May remove 15 mEq/h (PD)
Intravenous diuretics (volume if hypovolemic)	(Depending on renal function)	Minutes/while diuresis continued	Urinary K+ excretion	Only in patients with residual renal function

Adapted from Wolfson AB and Singer I. J Emerg Med 1988;6:61–70.

REFERENCES—POTASSIUM

1. Illingworth RN, Proudfoot AT. Rapid poisoning with slow-release potassium. Br Med J 1980;28:485–486.
2. Saxena K. Clinical features and management of poisoning due to potassium chloride. Med Toxicol Adverse Drug Exp 1989;4:429–443.
3. Survival after massive overdose of slow release potassium. Scott Med J 1988;33:279.
4. Steedman DJ. Poisoning with sustained release potassium. Arch Emerg Med 1988;5:206–211.
5. Restuccio A. Fatal hyperkalemia from a salt substitute. Am J Emerg Med 1992;10:171–173.
6. Sporer KA, Mayer AP. Saltpeter ingestion. Am J Emerg Med 1991;9:165.

POTASSIUM BICHROMATE

Ingestion of match heads may lead to acute renal failure.[1]

REFERENCES—POTASSIUM BICHROMATE

1. Picaud JC, Cochat P, Parchoux JC, Berthier JC, Gilly J, Careyre S et al. Acute renal failure in a child after chewing of match heads. Nephron 1995;57:225–226.

POTASSIUM PERMANGANATE

CLINICAL PRESENTATION

Acute hemorrhagic pancreatitis, which can terminate fatally, may be the underlying disorder in patients who develop widespread visceral damage after potassium permanganate poisoning.[1] Solutions over 1:5000 concentrations are irritating to tissues. Potassium permanganate solutions are deep purple, but they leave a deep brown stain of manganese dioxide.

REFERENCES—POTASSIUM PERMANGANATE

1. Middleton SJ, Jacyna M, McClaren D, Robinson R, Thomas HC. Hemorrhagic pancreatitis—a cause of death in severe potassium permanganate poisoning. Postgrad Med J 1990;66:657–658.

SELENIUM

USE

The effectiveness of dietary selenium repletion on human diseases linked to selenium deficiency (e.g., the familial cerebral degenerative cases known as Batten's disease) remains unproven.[1]

Selenium is widely used in industry (e.g., electronics, glass, ceramics, steel, pigment manufacturing). Solutions contain lethal amounts of selenious acid, in addition to lesser amounts of copper nitrate and nitric acid. Medicinal uses of selenium include antidandruff shampoos, dietary supplements, and the treatment of cystic fibrosis (controversial). Human toxicity is rare. Chronic elemental selenium exposure can cause dental caries, but adverse effects are unusual.[2] Selenious acid is the most toxic form of selenium and usually causes fatalities.[3]

ACUTE TOXIC DOSAGE

Elemental Selenium

This form is nontoxic in therapeutic doses (50 to 200 μg/d),[4] with a normal daily intake in one study of 81 μg.[5] The estimated ingested dose of superpotent selenium in a series of toxic cases ranged from 27 to 2310 mg, with nausea, vomiting, nail changes, fatigue, and irritability as the most common manifestations.[6] Selenium dusts produce respiratory tract irritation manifested by nasal discharge, loss of smell, epistaxis, and cough.

Selenium Salts

The ingestion of 22 mg of sodium selenate per kilogram produced minimal toxicity despite a substantial rise in the blood level.[7] Consumption of 1 to 5 mg of sodium selenite per kilogram by five adults caused nausea, vomiting, abdominal pain, and tremor, which resolved in 24 hours.

Selenate is the least toxic inorganic selenium form; selenite is more toxic. Vitamin C reduces selenite to the elemental form.

Selenious Acid

This compound is the most toxic inorganic selenium compound. A 15-mL ingestion of gun blue (2% selenious acid) by a 2-year-old[8] and a 30- and 60-mL ingestion by an adult[3] resulted in death.

Selenium Oxide

Selenium dioxide is a white crystalline solid that decomposes in water to selenious acid. An estimated 10-g oral dose produced apnea and asystole within 8 hours of ingestion.[9]

TOXICOKINETICS

In animals after 4 hours, selenious acid is well absorbed from the lungs (97%) and gastrointestinal tract (87%). Absorption of elemental selenium was slightly less from the lungs and gastrointestinal tract (57% and 50%, respectively).[10] About 50% of systemically absorbed selenium was eliminated (mostly in the urine) with a biologic half-life of 1.2 days.[11] The terminal half-life (roughly 20% of the absorbed dose) was 34 days.

CLINICAL PRESENTATION

Chronic Selenium Toxicity

This syndrome resembles arsenic toxicity.[6] Hair loss, white horizontal streaking on fingernails, paronychia, fatigue, irritability, hyperreflexia, nausea, vomiting, garlic odor on breath, and metallic taste characterized toxicity.[12] Muscle tenderness, tremor, lightheadedness, and facial flushing are observed in selenite poisoning. Serum selenium levels are elevated, but do not correlate well with symptoms. Blood chemistries, hematology, and liver and renal function tests are usually normal. Fatal cardiomyopathy has been reported in long-term parenteral nutrition patients who developed low selenium levels (5 to 12%).[13]

Acute Selenious Acids Toxicity

These ingestions are almost invariably fatal. Stupor, respiratory depression, hypotension, and death can result several hours postingestion.[14,15] Severe hypotension develops secondary both to decreased contractility from a toxic cardiomyopathy and to inappropriately low peripheral vascular resistance.[16] Terminal respiratory failure developed after a selenious acid ingestion (15 mL gun bluing solution) despite the use of an extracorporeal membrane oxygenator. Death occurred on the 18th hospital day. The postmortem examination demonstrated myocardial and pulmonary infarction, ascites, obstructive mucous plugs in the bronchi, interstitial pulmonary emphysema, bronchopulmonary dysplasia, barotrauma, and *Hemophilus legionella* infection.[8]

LABORATORY

A fluorometric assay of total selenium in plasma and urine has a limit of detection of 10 μg/L (0.126 μmol/L).[17] Stable isotope dilution gas chromatography–mass spectrometry using any of the three derivatizing reagents NPD (4-nitro-o-phenylenediamine), DBPD (c,5-dibro-o-phenylenediamine), and TFMPD (4-trifluoromethyl-phenylenediamine) can be used for the determination of Se in urine samples.[18]

Laboratory abnormalities include thrombocytopenia, moderate hepatorenal dysfunction, and elevated serum creatine kinase levels. The electrocardiogram may demonstrate ST elevations and T-wave changes characteristic of myocardial infarction. The urinary excretion of selenium is rapid. In a fatal case the plasma selenium level reached 285 µg/mL on the first hospital day and returned to normal levels by day 4.[8]

ACUTE HYDROGEN SELENIDE INHALATION[19]

Accidental inhalation of hydrogen selenide gas produced initial upper respiratory tract irritation and wheezing followed in 18 hours by progressive dyspnea, pneumomediastinum, and markedly reduced expiratory flow rates. Improvement occurred over 5 days, but some restrictive and obstructive changes remained on pulmonary function testing 3 years later.

TREATMENT

Management of chronic intoxication is supportive with elimination of the selenium source. BAL and $CaNa_2EDTA$ may enhance toxicity. The treatment of ingestions of compounds containing selenious acid (i.e., gun bluing solutions) is not well studied. Even small amounts of this chemical are potentially lethal. All patients who ingest selenious acid should be evaluated by a physician and should usually be hospitalized for observation. Gun bluing compound containing selenious acid is corrosive and will produce esophageal burns; however, since this acid is a serious systemic poison, the decision to use decontamination measures is based on clinical judgment. Factors to consider in the decision to use these measures include the time since exposure, the amount of spontaneous emesis, the clinical condition of the patient, and the amount ingested. There are no antidotes to selenious acid toxicity; treatment is expectant (cardiopulmonary monitoring in an intensive care setting) and supportive (intravenous infusion, supplemental oxygen, and ventilation as needed).

REFERENCES—SELENIUM

1. Katz MA. The expanding role of oxygen free radicals in clinical medicine. West J Med 1986;144:441–446.
2. Hadjimarkos DM. Selenium in relation to dental caries. Food Cosmet Toxicol 1973;11:1083–1095.
3. Pentel P, Fletcher D, Jentzen J. Fatal acute selenium toxicity. J Forensic Sci 1985;30:556–562.
4. Committee on Dietary Allowances Food and Nutrition Board Recommended Dietary Allowances, 9th rev ed. Washington, DC: National Academy of Sciences, 1980, p. 162.
5. Welsh SO, Holden JM, Wolf WR et al. Selenium in self-restricted diets of Maryland residents. J Am Diet Assoc 1981;79:277–285.
6. Selenium intoxication—New York. MMWRT 1984;33:157–158.
7. Civil IDS, McDonald MJA. Acute selenium poisoning. Case report. NZ Med J 1978;87:354–356.
8. Natal AJ, Brown M, Dery P et al. Acute poisoning by selenious acid. Vet Hum Toxicol 1985;27:531–533.
9. Koppel C, Baudisch H, Beyer KH et al. Fatal poisoning with selenium dioxide. Clin Toxicol 1986;24:21–35.
10. Medinsky MA, Cuddihy RG, McClellan RO. Systemic absorption of selenious acid and elemental selenium aerosols in rats. J Toxicol Environ Health 1981;8:917–928.
11. Weissman SH, Cuddihy RG, Medinsky MA. Absorption, distribution and retention of inhaled selenious acid and selenium metal aerosols in beagle dogs. Toxicol Appl Pharmacol 1983;67:331–337.
12. Yang G, Wang S, Zhou R et al. Endemic selenium intoxication of humans in China. Am J Clin Nutr 1983;37:972–981.
13. Quercia RA, Korn S, O'Neill D et al. Selenium deficiency and fatal cardiomyopathy in a patient receiving long-term home parenteral nutrition. Clin Pharm 1984;3:531–535.
14. Carter RF. Acute selenium poisoning. Med J Aust 1966;1:525–528.
15. Normann SA, Nisbet K, Manoguerra AS. Acute selenious acid poisoning—case report. Vet Hum Toxicol 1984;26 (Suppl 2):48 (abstract A-40).
16. Sioris LJ, Guthrie K, Pentel PR. Acute selenium poisoning. Vet Hum Toxicol 1980;22:364.
17. Sheehan TMT, Gao M. Simplified fluorometric assay of total selenium plasma and urine. Clin Chem 1990;36:2124–2126.
18. Aggarwal SK, Kinter M, Herold DA. Determination of selenium in urine by isotope dilution gas chromatography mass spectrometry using 4-nitro-o-phenylenediamine, 3,5-dibromo-o-phenylenediamine, and 4-trifluoromethyl-o-phenylenediamine as derivatizing reagents. Anal Biochem 1992;202:367–374.
19. Schecter A, Shanske W, Stenzler A et al. Acute hydrogen selenide inhalation. Chest 1980;77:554–555.

SILVER

Silver is still available in several forms: sulfadiazine silver (Silvadene), colloidal silver iodide (e.g., Neo-silvol), and mild silver protein (e.g., Argynol eye drops). Silver nitrate ointment and solution have well-established roles in the prophylaxis of perinatal gonococcal conjunctivitis. Argyria is an irreversible generalized blue-grey pigmentation of the skin found in patients who have ingested silver compounds for prolonged periods.[1] It is commonly caused by mechanical impregnation of the skin by small silver particles in workers involved in silver mining, refining of silver, and in the manufacture of silverware and metal alloys, metallic films on glass and china, electroplating solutions, and photographic processing.[2] Silver nitrate may be locally corrosive. Ingestion of concentrated silver nitrate did not produce any serious complaints in two children.[3]

Advertising materials in health food stores promote colloidal silver protein (CSP) use in more than 650 different diseases. Colloidal silver proteins are being touted as powerful antimicrobials against viruses, bacteria, parasites, and fungi, including human immunodeficiency virus (HIV), herpes, *Candida,* and tuberculosis. The CSPs have also been advertised as "an immune system stimulant and antiinflammatory agent" for use in such conditions as diabetes, chronic fatigue syndrome, allergies, and cancer.[4]

Silver is not an essential mineral supplement and has no known physiologic function. The use of silver products as germicidals has chiefly been replaced. Efficacy claims for the treatment of infectious diseases such as tuberculosis, malaria, and systemic fungal infections or for the prevention of cancer, acquired immunodeficiency syndrome (AIDS), and diabetes remain unproven. Neurologic deficits and diffuse silver deposition in visceral organs have been reported with long-term use of oral silver products. Renal damage and metal fume fever have been reported with high silver exposures.[4]

REFERENCES—SILVER

1. Karakashian GV, Burnett JW. Argyria. Cutis 1989;43:209.
2. Shall L, Stevens A, Millard LG. An unusual case of acquired localized argyria. Br J Dermatol 1990;123:403–407.
3. Raiber A, Bruner B. Ingestion of concentrated silver nitrate. A report of two cases. Vet Hum Toxicol 1987;29:321–322.
4. Fung MC, Weintraub M, Bowen DL. Colloidal silver proteins marketed as health supplements. JAMA 1995;274:1196–1197.

TELLURIUM

Tellurium is a white elemental metal chemical related in behavior and in the periodic table to selenium.[1]

USE

Tellurium is used as a component of many alloys of the base metals. It is a powerful carbide stabilizer. It is used in the synthetic rubber, glass, and steel production industries.

TOXICOKINETICS

Tellurium is absorbed by ingestion, by inhalation, and through the skin. Tellurium compounds are reduced to the relatively harmless elemental tellurium and methyl telluride. Ninety percent of the body stores of tellurium are in bone. The normal background levels in urine and serum are 0.6 μg/mL and 1.0 μg/mL, respectively.[2]

CLINICAL PRESENTATION

About 15 mg of tellurium in humans can cause a garlic odor lasting over 200 days.[3] Workers exposed to tellurium fumes may experience a garlic odor of the breath and sweat, dryness of the mouth, metallic taste, nausea, anorexia, weight loss, decreased sweating, dry itchy skin, gastrointestinal disturbances, and somnolence.[4] Loss of consciousness and death following inadvertent ingestion of sodium tellurium have been reported. Tellurium is teratogenic in a rat model.[5] Blue-black discoloration in the finger webs have followed exposure to tellurium hexafluoride gas.[6]

TREATMENT

There has been no effective treatment reported for tellurium poisoning. Only supportive and symptomatic care can be recommended. There are no specific antidotes.

REFERENCES—TELLURIUM

1. Finkel AJ, Hamilton A, Hardy HL. Tellurium. In: Finkel AJ, ed. Hamilton and Hardy's industrial toxicology. 4th ed. Bristol, UK: John Wright, 1983; pp. 128–130.
2. Schroeder HA, Buckman J, Belasse JJ. Abnormal trace elements in man. J Chron Dis 1967;20:147–161.
3. De Meio RH. Tellurium: effect of ascorbic acid on the tellurium breath. J Ind Hyg Toxicol 1947;29:393–395.
4. Shie MD, Deeds FE. The importance of tellurium as a health hazard in industry. Public Health Perspect 1970;35:939–954.
5. Duckett S. Teratogenesis caused by tellurium. Ann NY Acad Sci 1972;192:220–221.
6. Blackadder ES, Manderson WG. Occupational absorption of tellurium. A report of two cases. Br J Ind Med 1975;32: 59–61.

THALLIUM

Tabandeh and colleagues have provided a concise description of the clinical features of thallium intoxication.[1]

The clinical picture of thallium intoxication is variable; however, the diagnosis is often suspected in the presence of the triad of symptoms: (a) alopecia and skin rash, (b) painful peripheral neuropathy, and (c) confusion and lethargy.

The lethal dose for humans is 15 to 20 mg/kg of body weight; nonfatal intoxication occurs below this dose. The first symptoms of poisoning are abdominal pain, gastroenteritis, tachycardia, and headache, which usually occur within 12 hours.[2] A characteristic dark, pigmented band appears in the scalp hair within 4 days. Neurologic symptoms appear in 2 to 5 days and include confusion, hallucinations, and convulsions. In severe cases coma, respiratory paralysis, and death occur within 1 week. When smaller doses are taken painful peripheral sensorimotor neuropathy and ataxia are the outstanding symptoms. Other neurologic features include cranial nerve palsies, optic neuropathy, choreoathetosis, tremor, and encephalopathy. Scalp alopecia is the best known symptom of chronic thallium poisoning, which begins 10 days after the ingestion and is completed within 1 month. Skin may be involved by acneiform eruptions, a papulomacular rash, and dystrophy of the nails (Mees's stripes). Autonomic dysfunction, hypertension, cardiomyopathy, electrocardiographic changes, testicular toxicity, hypokalemia, renal failure, abnormal liver function, leukocytosis, and thrombocytopenia have been reported. Electroencephalopathy shows nonspecific slow wave activity and electromyography is suggestive of distal axonopathy.

Ophthalmologic manifestations include loss of the lateral half of the eyebrows, eyelid skin lesions, blepharoptosis, facial nerve palsy, internal and external ophthalmoplegia, and nystagmus. Noninflammatory keratitis and lens opacities have also been described. Optic atrophy as a sequel to thallium-induced toxic optic neuropathy is well reported. Functional changes include impairment of contrast sensitivity, abnormal color vision (tritanomaly), impaired visual acuity, and central or cecocentral scotomas. There is also electroretinographic abnormality and a delayed visual-evoked response. Optic neuropathy and cranial nerve palsies are the most marked features.

Thallium does cross the placental barrier, and produced alopecia and nail abnormalities in a fetus exposed in the last trimester.[3]

Because of the rarity of this type of poisoning and the paucity of toxicology laboratories that perform an assay for thallium, suspicions of this agent in any case of unexplained acute neuropathy, especially with sudden alopecia, is important.[4] Hair regrowth usually occurs. Thallium poisoning may be reported in groups of patients.[5]

DIFFERENTIAL DIAGNOSIS

The differential diagnosis of thallium poisoning includes other heavy-metal intoxication such as those by mercury, lead, arsenic, and selenium; Guillain-Barré syndrome; acute porphyria; acute psychosis; botulism; polio; medications such as isoniazid, hydralazine, and phenytoin; and thiamine deficiency.[6]

LABORATORY

Tests of contrast sensitivity and color vision are useful in the early detection of optic neuropathy in thallium intoxication.[7]

SUPPORTIVE TREATMENT

Gastric lavage, activated charcoal, and use of Prussian blue have been suggested by Herrero and colleagues.[8] Thallium concentrations in the blood and urine should probably be measured initially three times per week. Pay special attention to mouth hygiene since a severe stomatitis may occur. Shaving the patient's head may reduce the stress of tractional hair loss and may improve the patient's morale. Physical therapy prevents muscle contractures. Reassure the patient that recovery from the acute episode is the rule once the diagnosis has been made and medical care started. Recovery may take a long time.[9]

REFERENCES—THALLIUM

1. Tabandeh H, Crowston JG, Thompson FM. Ophthalmological features of thallium poisoning. Am J Ophthalmol 1994;112: 243–248.
2. Wax PM. Tortilla the votoxicosis. Clin Toxicol 1995;33:265.
3. Moeschlin S. Thallium poisoning. Clin Toxicol 1980;17: 133–146.
4. Schwartz JG, Stuchey JH, Kunkel SP, Dowd DC, Kagen-Hallet. Poisoning from thallium. Texas Med J 1988;84: 46–48.
5. Villanueva E, Hernandez-Cueto C, Lachica E, Rodrigo MD, Ramos V. Poisoning by thallium. A study of five cases. Drug Safety 1990;5:384–389.
6. Stack AM. Thallium. Clin Toxicol Rev 1992;14(4):1–2.
7. Tabandeh H, Thompson GM. Visual function in thallium toxicity. Br Med J 1993;307:324.
8. Herrero F, Fernandez E, Gomez J, Pretel L, Canizares F, Frias J et al. Thallium poisoning presenting with abdominal colic paresthesia and irritability. Clin Toxicol 1995;33:261–264.
9. Moore D, House I, Dixon A. Thallium poisoning. Grand Rounds, Guy's Hospital., Br Med J 1993;306:1527–1529.

TIN

Tributyl tin oxide may induce an occupational asthma.[1] Its addition to indoor paint can induce eye and throat irritation, loss of appetite, nausea and vomiting, and a burning sensation in the nose.[2] The Occupational Safety and Health Administration's permissible exposure limit for organic tin compounds is 0.1 mg/m^3 as an 8-hour, time-weighted exposure for workers.[3]

PHYSICAL CHARACTERISTICS

OSHA permissible exposure limits for inorganic compounds are 2 mg/m^3 in air and for organic tin compounds 0.1 mg/m^3 in air.[4,5]

PATHOPHYSIOLOGY

Morphologic changes after TMT intoxication are confined to the nervous system. All neurons are almost equally affected with central chromatolysis and accumulation of lysosomal disease bodies.[6]

Table 67–37
Common Tin Compounds and Their Toxicity

Substance	Use	Toxicity
Metallic Tin	Metal plating, alloy production	
Inorganic Tin	Ceramics, toothpaste additive	Metal fume fever, stannosis GI and dermal irritant
Organotin		
Alkyltin		
Monoalkyltin	Stabilizer	Hepatotoxicity in animals
Dialkyltin	Stabilizer, catalyst	Irritant, immunotoxicity in animals
Trialkyltin		
Trimethyltin	Byproduct of dimethyltin	Neurotoxicity
Triethyltin	Contaminant	Neurotoxicity
Tributyltin	Fungicide	Irritant
Tetraalkyltin	Converted to trialkyltin	Neurotoxicity
Aryltin		
Triaryltin		
Triphenyltin	Molluscicide	Neuro-, hepato-, renal-, dermal toxicity

Adapted from Wax PM and Dockstader. Clin Toxicol 1995;33:239–241.

CLINICAL PRESENTATION

Besser and colleagues describe an acute limbic-cerebellar syndrome following inhalation of trimethyl tin (TMT), which resembles prior reports but is additionally characterized by hearing loss, confabulation, hyperphagia, disturbed sexual behavior, nystagmus, partial and tonic–clonic seizures, and a sensory neuropathy. Severity appeared to parallel maximal urinary organ tin levels, which occurred between day 1 and 10.[7]

Oral triethyl tin, a contaminant in the production of a diethyl tin-containing bactericidal drug against *Staphylococcus* (Stalinon) was characterized by symptoms of increased intracranial pressure paralysis and generalized tonic–clonic seizures. More than 100 people died.[8] Wax and Dockstader have tabulated tin toxicity (Table 67–37).[9]

REFERENCES—TIN

1. Shelton D, Urch B, Tarlo SM. Occupational asthma induced by a carpet fungicide-tributyl tin oxide. J Allergy Clin Immunol 1992;90:274–275.
2. MMWR. Acute effect of indoor exposure to paint containing bis(tributyrin) oxide. 1991;40:280–281.
3. Office of the Federal Register 1989;29:CFR:1910.1000.
4. Barnes JM, Stoner HB. The toxicology of tin compounds. Pharmacol Rev 1959;11:211–231.
5. Toxicological Profile for Tin and Compounds. Life System Inc. Agency for Toxic Substances and Disease Registry. ATSDR/TP 91/26. September 1992.
6. Kreyberg S, Torvik A, Bjorneboe A, Wiik-Larsen W, Jacobsen D. Trimethyl tin poisoning: report of a case with postmortem examination. Clin Neuropathol 1992;11:256–259.
7. Besser R, Kramer G, Thumler R, Bohl J, Gutmann L, Hopf HC. Acute trimethyl tin limbic cerebellar syndrome. Neurology 1987;37:945–950.
8. Alajouanine T, Derobest L, Theffry S. Etude clinique d'encemble de 210 cas d'intoxication par les sels organique d'etain. Rev Neurol (Paris) 1958;98:85–96.

9. Wax PM, Dockstader L. Tributyl tin use in interior paints: a continuing health hazard. Clin Toxicol 1995;33:239–241.

TITANIUM

Titanium dioxide (TiO_2) is a white pigment used in paints, linoleum lacquers, leather, inks, rubber, soaps, textiles, ceramics, and plastics. It is approved by the U.S. Food and Drug Administration for use in adhesives, cellophane, cosmetics, paper products, poultry products, and to whiten salads and spreads. The most common finding associated with TiO_2 exposure is increased pulmonary dust disposition, which may lead to alveolar cell hyperplasia and fibrosis. There was no evidence of an association of TiO_2 and risk of lung cancer, chronic respiratory disease, and chest roentgenogram abnormalities in one study of workers exposed to TiO_2.[1]

There are relatively few cases of pulmonary disease reported in association with exposure to titanium dust. In some subjects there may be evidence of a hypersensitivity to titanium.[2]

REFERENCES—TITANIUM

1. Chen JL, Fayerweather WE. Epidemiologic study of workers exposed to titanium dioxide. J Occup Med 1988;30:937–942.
2. Redline S, Barna BP, Tomashefski JF Jr, Abraham JC. Granulomatous disease associated with pulmonary deposition of titanium. Br J Ind Med 1986;43:652–656.

URANIUM

Although gamma radiation is present in all uranium mines, levels rarely exceed the acceptable standard of 5 rads per year. Adverse effects from uranium mining result from the inhalation of radon daughters. The decay of radium produces radon, which in turn forms short-life radon daughters (isotopes of lead, bismuth, and polonium). These products attach to dust particles that are inhaled by workers. Alpha radiation delivers 95% of the radiation dose to the tracheobronchial epithelium. Mortality of uranium miners from lung cancer and chronic lung disease strongly depends on radon exposure, cigarette smoking, and height.[1] Although both squamous and oat cell tumor types display a dose-response effect, there is some difference in the strength of the association.[2]

REFERENCES—URANIUM

1. Archer VE. Health concerns in uranium mining and milling. J Occup Med 1981;23:502–505.
2. Chavil A. The epidemiology of primary lung cancer in uranium miners in Ontario. J Occup Med 1981;23:417–421.

ZINC

Inhalation of zinc oxide is the most common cause of metal fume fever.

SOURCES[1]

CLINICAL PRESENTATION

Metal Fume Fever

This syndrome resembles a flulike illness. Onset occurs in 4 to 6 hours, generally on the evening after exposure to fumes. Fatigue, chills, fever, myalgias, cough, dyspnea, leukocytosis, thirst, metallic taste, and salivation characterize this self limited illness, with resolution of symptoms appearing in 36 hours. The chest x-ray usually is clear. Tolerance develops in workers, but may be lost over the weekend ("Monday Morning Fever"). Metal fume fever can also follow exposure to fumes of copper, magnesium, aluminum, antimony, iron, manganese, and nickel in welding, galvanizing, or smelting operations.

Synonyms

Other names have been used for metal fume fever including Monday fever, brass chills, zinc ague, welder's ague, spelter shakes, foundry fever, the smothers, and brass founders' ague.[2]

Metals

Various metals that have been associated with metal fume fever include cadmium, aluminum, magnesium, nickel, copper, manganese, antimony, and tin. Exposure to zinc oxide fumes occurs mainly during welding or the galvanization of steel.

Occupations

Other occupations at risk include smelters, shipyard workers, junk metal refiners, electroplaters, metallic pigment makers, metal polishers, and alloy makers.

Diagnosis

The diagnosis of metal fume fever is usually made when the clinical picture is combined with history of metal fume exposure. The disorder is usually of short duration, lasting no more than 24 to 48 hours. The complaints of metallic taste in the mouth, fever, chills, malaise, fatigue, headache, myalgias, and cough usually occur within 3 to 10 hours after exposure.

Laboratory

The symptoms may start when the employee is at home. Laboratory studies include leukocytosis (15,000 to 20,000 cells/mL) with excess of polymorphonuclear cells. Lactate dehydrogenase may be elevated with the pulmonary fraction showing the greatest increase. Zinc levels may be elevated in the serum and urine, but the absence of zinc does not rule out exposure of the diagnosis.

Physical

Physical findings may vary from person to person. Fever, sweating, tachycardia, chills, pleural friction rub, and pulmonary rales have been described. Pulmonary function study results may be normal or may show acute changes consistent with reduced lung volumes (forced vital capacity and forced expiratory volume in 1 second) and decreased carbon monoxide diffusing capacity. Over time the pulmonary function abnormalities revert to normal.

The abrupt onset of symptoms on the job or within 3 to 10 hours after work and a history of welding of galvanization of steel should make the diagnosis. Cadmium exposure from solder and welding fumes presents a similar initial presentation, but may lead to a toxic pneumonitis with pulmonary infiltrates and a picture consistent with acute respiratory distress syndrome. Exposure to pyrolysis products of fluorine-containing plastics has been associated with a clinical syndrome similar to metal fume fever.

Acute high concentrations of ozone generated during gas metal arc welding of aluminum with argon gas for shielding have been associated with an acute chemical pneumonitis. Phosgene and nitrogen dioxide in high concentrations are associated with coughing, shortness of breath, and noncardiac pulmonary edema.

Exposure to high concentrations of organic dusts (contaminated with thermophilic bacteria and fungal spores) has produced symptoms similar to metal fume fever. This has been described mostly in the summer and fall season and associated with shoveling damp wood chips, leaves, or silage. Massive grain dust exposure has also been associated with a febrile reaction similar to the organic dust toxic syndrome. New mill workers' exposure to cotton dust also is associated with a clinical picture similar to that of metal fume fever. Tolerance develops with continued exposures. The treatment of metal fume fever is symptomatic and nonspecific.

Prevention of metal fume fever includes implementation of engineering controls, general room ventilation, local exhaust ventilation, process enclosure, down-draft or cross-draft tables, and use of fume extractors built into welding equipment.

Blount has described two forms of metal fume fever, a mild form (Table 67–38)[3] caused by numerous metal fumes (Table 67–39) and a serious form (Table 67–40) associated with zinc chloride fume–generated military smoke. Figure 67–4 summarizes the mild and serious forms.[3]

Table 67–38
Metals Causing Mild Metal Fume Fever[a]

Zinc	Nickel	Selenium
Copper	Manganese	Beryllium
Magnesium	Mercury	Vanadium
Iron	Cobalt	Silver
Chromium	Lead	Aluminum
Cadmium	Antimony	

Zinc Chloride Inhalation[4]

Two autopsies revealed severe inflammation of the upper respiratory tract mucosa and pulmonary edema. No toxic changes appeared in the kidney or liver.

Two soldiers who were not wearing gas masks during inhalation of hexite smoke ($ZnCl_2$) while on military training developed a severe adult respiratory distress syndrome accompanied by an increased plasma zinc concentration. Both soldiers died.[5]

Patients who receive zinc supplementation may develop hypocupremia and hyperceruloplasminemia.[6] Sideroblastic anemia has been associated with copper deficiency, and copper excretion is enhanced by the ingestion of zinc.[7] Zinc concentrates in the pancreas, and this organ should be considered a potential target in zinc poisoning. Hyperamylasemia has been reported in human beings with oral or parenteral zinc toxicity. Monitor pancreatic amylase. Later development of chronic pancreatic exocrine deficiency should also be considered.[8]

Intravenous

Hypotension, diarrhea, vomiting, pulmonary edema, jaundice, hyperamylasemia, oliguria, anemia, and thrombocytopenia occurred after a suicidal zinc injection.[4]

Table 67–39
Mild MFF Manifestations[a]

Symptoms	Signs
Headache	Leukocytosis
Sweet metallic taste	Granulocytosis
Myalgias	Fever
Malaise	High Sed Rate
Cough	Hypoxemia[b]
Thirst[b]	Reduced pulmonary function tests
Chest tightness	Rales
Nausea	High lactate dehydrogenase
Chills	Wheezing
Dyspnea	Tachypnea
Diaphoresis	Tachycardia

[a]Listed in order of decreasing frequency.
[b]Manifestations below this point are seen in less than one half of the patients.
Adapted from Blount BW. Milit Med 1990;155:372–377.

Table 67–40
Serious MFF Manifestations[a]

Symptoms	Signs
Dyspnea	Abnormal CXR
Cough	Reduced pulmonary function tests
Sore throat	Tachypnea
Chest tightness	Conjunctivitis
Nausea[b]	Leukocytosis
Metallic taste	Cyanosis (gray)
Malaise	Tachycardia
Hoarseness	Granulocytosis
Chills	Hypoxemia[b]
	Fever
	Rales
	Wheezing

Adapted from Blount BW. Two Types of Metal Fume Fever. Mild vs Serious. Milit Med 1990;155:372–377.

LABORATORY

Normal values for plasma zinc are 60 to 100 μg/dL, and for 24 hours with zinc. Plasma zinc may decrease after chelation (CaN_2EDTA) with improvement of lethargy and hypertension.[9]

Kidney, ureter, and bladder studies will demonstrate the radiopaque tablets in the bowel.[10] Serum zinc levels may be elevated (normal 68 to 136 μg/dL).[11]

TREATMENT

The usual measures for decontamination (ipecac or lavage, charcoal, cathartics) may be administered, although patients usually have sufficient vomiting not to require them. $CaNa_2EDTA$ has been used successfully to normalize zinc levels[12,13] and is considered the agent of choice.

D-penicillamine has increased mortality in animal models.[13] Recently, *N*-acetylcysteine has been found to increase urinary zinc excretion in rats.[14]

Whole-bowel irrigation was useful in improving rectal elimination in one patient who had ingested 50 zinc sulfate tablets.[10]

REFERENCES—ZINC

1. Key MM, Henschel AF, Butler J, eds. Occupational diseases: a guide to their recognition. Rev ed. Washington, DC: US Department of Health, Education and Welfare, 1977, pp. 406–408.
2. Perry GF. Occupational medicine forum. J Occ Med 1994; 36(10):1061–1063.
3. Blount BW. Two types of metal fume fever: mild vs serious. Mil Med 1990;115:372–377.
4. Evans EH. Casualties following exposure to zinc chloride smoke. Lancet 1945;2:368–370.
5. Hjortso E, Zvist J, Bud MI, Thomsen JL, Andersen JB, Wiberg-Jorgenson F et al. ARDS after accidental inhalation of zinc chloride smoke. Intensive Care Med 1988;14:17–24.
6. Prasad AS, Brewer GJ, Schoomaker ER, Rabbani P. Hypocupremia induced by zinc therapy in adults. JAMA 1978;240: 2166–2168.
7. Brown ER, Greist A, Tricet G, Hoffman R. Excessive zinc ingestion. A reversible cause of sideroblastic anemia and bone marrow depression. JAMA 1990;164:1441–1443.
8. McKinney PE, Brent J, Kulig K. Zinc chloride ingestion in a child: Exocrine pancreatic insufficiency. Ann Emerg Med 1995;25:562.
9. McKinney P, Brent J, Kulig K, Rumack B. Zinc chloride soldering flux ingestion in a child. Vet Hum Toxicol 1991; 33:366.
10. Burkhart KK, Kulig KW, Rumack B. Whole bowel irrigation as treatment for zinc sulfate overdoses. Ann Emerg Med 1990; 119:1167–1170.
11. Hedtker J, Daja MR, Neac G, Burton BT. Local and systemic toxicity following zinc chloride ($ZnCl_2$) ingestion. Vet Hum Toxicol 1989;31:342.
12. Potter JL. Acute zinc chloride ingestion in a young child. Ann Emerg Med 1981;10:267–269.
13. Chobasanian SJ. Accidental ingestion of liquid zinc chloride: local and systemic effects. Ann Emerg Med 1981;10: 91–93.
14. Banner W, Koch M, Hopf S et al. *N*-acetylcysteine in the chelation of zinc sulfate. Vet Hum Toxicol 1985;28:293 (abstract).

ZIRCONIUM

Subcutaneous granulomas develop from the use of deodorant sticks and poison ivy lotions, probably as a result of hypersensitivity reactions. Minimal industrial toxicity apparently occurs, and a study of occupational zirconium inhalation failed to detect pulmonary abnormalities.[1]

However, a sarcoid granulomatous type of chronic pulmonary hypersensitivity reaction may follow long-term exposure to zirconium. Zirconium can also cause an acute and fulminant allergic alveolitis-like hypersensitivity reaction.[2]

REFERENCES—ZIRCONIUM

1. Hadjimichael OC, Brubaker RE. Evaluation of an occupational respiratory exposure to zirconium-containing dust. J Occup Med 1981;23:543–547.
2. Liippo KK, Anttila SL, Taikina-Aho O, Ruokonen E-L, Toivonen ST, Tuomi T. Hypersensitivity pneumonitis and exposure to zirconium silicate in a young ceramic tile worker. Am Rev Respir Dis 1993;148:1089–1092.

Chapter 68
Pesticides

Acute pesticide poisoning is an important cause of worldwide morbidity and mortality. It has been estimated that there are three million severe cases of acute pesticide poisoning each year with some 220,000 deaths. Ninety-five percent of fatal pesticide poisonings occur in developing countries. Serious cases of pesticide poisoning are more likely to occur in adults than in children. Rodenticides remain the most common cause of suspected pediatric pesticide poisoning in the United Kingdom (42%), while other animal poisons are the second most common cause (33%). In declining order of incidence, herbicides and fungicides (13%), creosote (7%), and mothballs (5%) were responsible for the remaining cases. In the United Kingdom pesticides are responsible for only 1.1% of deaths from poisoning. No deaths from acute pesticide poisoning in children under 10 years of age were reported by Casey and colleagues in the United Kingdom survey in more than 2 decades. About three-quarters of the pesticide fatalities were due to suicide. Paraquat was the most common cause of fatal pesticide poisoning.[1–3]

Brender and colleagues have summarized characteristics of pesticide poisonings (Table 68–1). In an effort to control occupational pesticide poisoning in the United States, reentry intervals have been proposed for workers exposed to organophosphate pesticides (Table 68–2). A comprehensive and clinically useful guide to the recognition and treatment of pesticide poisonings has been prepared by Morgan.[4]

DEFINITION OF AGENTS

On the basis of current agricultural practices, chemicals used to alter our environment are defined by their intended target:

Pesticides

Compounds that are used to kill pests.

Insecticides

Compounds that are used to kill insects and related species (e.g., organophosphates, organochlorines, carbamates).

Table 68–1
Characteristics of Acute Pesticide Poisoning[a]

Chemical Basis (Examples of Compounds)[b]	Pharmacologic Action or Site of Toxicity	Routes of Absorption	Major Acute Signs and Symptoms	Laboratory Tests
Chlorinated hydrocarbons [chlorobenzilate, Kelthane, Thiodan, methoxychlor, lindane, heptachlor, toxaphene, chlordane]	Neurotoxin; CNS, kidney, liver	Ingestion, dermal, inhalation	Apprehension, excitability, dizziness, headache, disorientation, weakness, paresthesia, convulsions	Pesticides and/or metabolites measured in blood; concentration more important than mere presence
Organophosphates [diazinon, malathion, methyl parathion, parathion, Guthion, chlorpyrifos (Dursban), Di-Syston, dichlorvos, S-Seven]	Irreversible inhibition of acetylcholinesterase enzyme	Ingestion, dermal, inhalation	*Mild:* fatigue, headache, blurred vision, dizziness, numbness of extremities, nausea, vomiting, excessive sweating and salivation, tightness in chest *Moderate:* weakness, difficulty talking, muscular fasciculations, miosis *Severe:* unconsciousness, flaccid paralysis, moist rales, respiratory difficulty, and cyanosis *Other:* cardiac arrhythmias	Red blood cell cholinesterase, plasma cholinesterase
Carbamates [aldicarb (Temik), methomyl, oxamyl, carbaryl (Sevin), carbofuran, Baygon]	Reversible inhibition of acetylcholinesterase enzyme	Ingestion, dermal, inhalation	Diarrhea, nausea, vomiting, abdominal pain, excessive sweating and salivation, blurred vision, difficulty breathing, headache, muscular fasciculations	Red blood cell and plasma cholinesterase may be normal and thus not reliable detectors of poisoning; carbamate metabolites in urine
Halocarbon and sulfuryl fumigants [methyl bromide, carbon disulfide, chloropicrin, ethylene dibromide, dibromochloropropane]	CNS, enzyme systems, liver, kidney, lungs	Ingestion, dermal, inhalation	Dizziness, headache, nausea, vomiting, abdominal pain, mental confusion, tremor, convulsions, pulmonary edema	Methyl bromide—blood bromide concentrations; carbon disulfides in urine
Phosphine fumigants [aluminum phosphide (Phostoxin)]	Lungs, CNS, liver kidney	Inhalation, dermal, ingestion	Dizziness, headache, nausea, vomiting, dyspnea, pulmonary edema	None known; victim's breath may smell like garlic or acetylene
Cyanide fumigants [Cyclon]	Inactivates the cytochrome oxidase of cells in critical tissues, primarily the heart and brain	Ingestion, inhalation, dermal (rare)	*Large dose:* collapse and cessation of respiration *Smaller dose:* headache, weakness, confusion, nausea, vomiting, dizziness, hyperpnea, apprehension, convulsions *Other:* breath may smell like bitter almonds	Cyanide in blood and tissues; thiocyanate metabolite in urine and saliva
Nitrophenolic and nitrocresolic herbicides [dinitrocresol, dinoseb (Dinitro-3), dinitrophenol]	Liver, kidney, and nervous system; stimulation of oxidative metabolism in cell mitochondria	Ingestion, inhalation, dermal	Yellow staining of skin and hair; profuse sweating, headache, thirst, malaise, warm flushed skin, tachycardia, fever	Nitrophenols and nitrocresols in urine and serum
Chlorophenoxy compounds [2,4-D, Silvex, 2,4,5-T, Dicamba]	Skin, eyes, respiratory and gastrointestinal linings	Ingestion, dermal, inhalation	*Inhalation:* burning sensations in the nasopharynx and chest, dizziness *Ingestion:* vomiting, esophagitis, abdominal pain, diarrhea, fibrillary muscle twitching, stiffness of muscles of extremities, metabolic acidosis in large doses	Chlorophenoxy compounds in blood and urine
Dipyridyls [diquat (Aquacide), paraquat (Dextrone X)]	Injury of epithelial tissue: skin, nails, cornea, liver, kidney, and linings of gastrointestinal and respiratory tracts	Ingestion, dermal, inhalation	*Ingestion early:* nausea, vomiting, diarrhea, melena, pain (oral, substernal, abdominal) *48–72 hours after exposure:* oliguria, jaundice, cough, dyspnea, tachypnea, pulmonary edema, convulsions, coma	Paraquat and diquat in blood and urine

[a]Adapted from Brender JD et al. Tex Med 1988;84:29–35.
[b]Use of trade names is for identification only and does not imply endorsement by the Texas Department of Health or the National Institute for Occupational Safety and Health, Centers for Disease Control.

Table 68–2
Reentry Intervals for Pesticides Used on Crops Requiring Workers To Perform Labor-Intensive Activities in Texas[a,b]

Re-entry Level	Pesticide
24 hours	Any pesticide with registered agricultural uses when used on crops requiring workers to perform labor-intensive activities, unless the pesticide has been granted an exemption. (As of April 4, 1986, six formulations of Dipel are exempt).
48 hours	azinphos-methyl (Guthion)
	carbophenothion
	demeton
	dicrotophos
	disulfoton
	endosulfan
	endrin
	ethion
	methidathion
	methyl parathion
	mevinphos
	monocrotophos
	oxydemeton-methyl
	phorate
	phosphamidon
7 days	ethyl parathion

[a]Adapted from Brender JD et al. Tex Med 1988;84:29–35.
[b]Texas Department of Agriculture. Reentry Intervals [Texas Register, Jan 1, 1985 (10 Tex Reg 39-401).] Notice of Exemption from Interim 24-hour Reentry Interval established for Agricultural Pesticides [Texas Register, Apr 4, 1986 (II Tex Reg 1164).]

Rodenticides

Compounds that are used to kill rats, mice, moles, and other rodents (e.g., anticoagulants, thallium, Vacor).

Herbicides

Compounds that are used to kill weeds (e.g., paraquat, diquat, [2,4-dichlorophenoxy]acetic acid [2,4-D]).

Fungicides

Compounds that are used to kill fungi and molds (e.g., dithiocarbamates, Captan).

Fumigants

Gases that are used to sterilize products (e.g., ethylene dibromide, methyl bromide).

PESTICIDES THAT CAUSE POISONING IN MAN

The following compounds may cause toxicity whether or not they are used as pesticides.[5] Cases of ingestion or other exposure without subsequent illness are omitted.

Inorganic and Organometallic Pesticides

Arsenic trioxide, barium carbonate, copper sulfate, lead arsenate, mercuric chloride, phosphorus, sodium arsenate, sodium chlorate, sodium fluoride, thallium sulfate, zinc phosphide, several methyl and ethyl mercury compounds.

Pesticides Derived From Plants and Other Organisms

Anabasine, nicotine, pyrethrum, rotenone, sabadilla, strychnine.

Solvents, Propellants, and Oil Insecticides

Dichlorodifluoromethane, kerosene, Tetralin, xylene.

Fumigants and Nematocides

Acrylonitrile, aluminum phosphide, carbon tetrachloride, chloropicrin, 1,2-dibromethane, *p*-dichlorobenzene, 1,2-dichloroethane, hydrogen cyanide, hydrogen phosphide, Lethane 384, methyl bromide, methylene chloride, naphthalene, Nemagon, sulfuryl fluoride, tetrachloroethylene, trichloroethane.

Chlorinated Hydrocarbon Insecticides

Aldrin, chlordane, DDT, dieldrin, *p,p*-dichlordiphenylmethyl carbinol (DMC), endosulfan, endrin, isobenzan, hexachlorocyclohexane (all isomers are toxic: the gamma-isomer [lindane] has the highest acute toxicity), methoxychlor, tetrachlorodiphenylethane (TDE), toxaphene.

Organophosphate Insecticides

Azinphosmethyl, carbophenothion, demton-*O*-methyl, demeton-methyl, diazinon, dichlorvos, dicrotophos, dimethoate, endothion, EPN, fensulfothion, fenthion, Hinosan, methyl demeton, methyl parathion, mevinphos, mipafox, mononcrotophos, naled, parathion, phorate, phosphamidon, Phostex, tetraethyl pyrophosphate (TEPP), thiometon, trichlorfon.

Carbamates and Related Pesticides

Aldicarb, 4-benzothienyl-*N*-methyl carbamate, bufencarb (BUX), carbaryl, carbofuran, isolan, 2-isopropyl phenyl-*N*-methyl carbamate, 3-isopropyl phenylmethyl carbamate, maneb, propoxur, thiram, Zectran, zineb, ziram.

Phenolic and Nitrophenolic Pesticides

Dinitrobutylphenol, 2,4-dinitrophenol, dinocap, dinitrocresol (DNOC), pentachlorophenol.

Miscellaneous Pesticides

Chlorfenson.

Synthetic Organic Rodenticides

Coumafuryl, fluoroacetamide, sodium fluoroacetate, warfarin.

Molluscicides

Metaldehyde.

Herbicides and Related Compounds

Acrolein, 2,4-D, dalaphon, dicamba, diquat, dichlorprop, (4-chloro-2-methyl-phenoxy)acetic acid (MCPA), paraquat, propazine, simazine, (2,4,5-trichlorophenoxy)acetic acid (2,4,5-T), trichloroacetic acid (TCA).

Fungicides and Related Compounds

Captafol, diphehyl, hexachlorobenzene, sodium azide, thiabendazole.

Repellents and Attractants

Chloralose, diethyltoluamide (DEET)

Evidence of carcinogenicity of many pesticides is listed in Table 68–3. No pesticides except arsenic and vinyl chloride have definitely been proved to be carcinogenic in man.

TOXIC EXPOSURES

The National Human Adipose Tissue Survey has tabulated the pesticide, semivolatiles, polychlorinated phenyls, volatiles, and polychlorinated dibenzo-*p*-dioxins and polychlorinated dibenzofuranes found in the adipose tissue of individuals residing in different areas in the United States. When pesticide ranks for all age groups were combined, the East South Central and West South Central States of the United States were the highest ranked regions. A general trend of increasing pesticide concentrations with increasing age appears to exist, indicating that continued exposure results in higher levels of toxins in human adipose tissue because of bioaccumulation. The ultimate correlation of this data with scientific proof that toxic chemicals in the environment pose significant threats to humans has not yet been defined.

Note: Many metabolites have not been correlated with exposure or with treatment. Methodology is frequently not available in clinical laboratories.[6]

Additional useful guides include Work Safety—With Farm Chemicals, National Agricultural Chemical Association, 1155 Fifteenth Street, Washington, DC 20005, July 1985 (English and Spanish); US EPA Citizen's Guide to Pesticides. Office of Pesticides and Toxic Substances, Washington, DC 20460, September 1987.

INSECTICIDES—THE ANTICHOLINESTERASES—ORGANOPHOSPHATE COMPOUNDS (SEE ALSO CHEMICAL WARFARE CHAPTER)

PREGNANCY

Patients who ingest organophosphorus insecticides during the second or third trimesters of pregnancy have been treated successfully with atropine and pralidoxime and later delivered healthy newborns with no significant abnormalities.[7]

DRUG INTERACTIONS

Patients who may develop low plasma cholinesterase activity after exposure to an organophosphate may subsequently develop a prolonged apnea after administration of succinylcholine.[8,9]

MECHANISM OF ACTION

Muscle

Karalliede and Henry[10] have studied the effects of the organophosphates on skeletal muscle. Organophosphate compounds produce muscle weakness by three different mechanisms. The first occurs during the cholinergic phase. Fasciculations progress to paralysis due to depolarization and desensitization blocks at the neuromuscular junction.

The Intermediate Syndrome (Table 68–4)

During the second or intermediate phase excessive entry of calcium ions into the muscle due to prolonged transmitter receptor interaction probably produces muscle necrosis, although the intermediate syndrome is probably due to long-lasting cholinesterase inhibition.[11] This necrosis and the subsequent muscle weakness and paralysis begins 48 to 96 hours after intoxication. In both the cholinergic and intermediate phases the muscle of respiration may be affected and lead to death from respiratory failure. The cholinergic phase weakness often recovers within 48 hours. The weakness due to muscle necrosis may last up to 4 weeks. Early administration of cholinesterase reactivators (oximes) and rest may reduce the severity of paralysis of intermediate onset, but this has not been demonstrated in controlled clinical studies. Finally, muscle weakness may be due to demyelination of nerves. This begins 2 to 3 weeks after intoxication and spares the muscle of respiration. Recovery may not be complete. The intermediate syndrome requires clinical validation. It does not appear to differ from that which would be expected with prolonged acetylcholinesterase inhibition.

de Bleecker and colleagues have studied patients with the intermediate syndrome and observed that such patients exhibited a prolonged red blood cell acetylcholinesterase inhibition and prolonged excretion of metabolites in the urine.[12] This syndrome exhibits clinical and electromyographic hallmarks of combined pre- and postsynaptic impairment of neuromuscular transmission.[12,13] The intermediate syndrome may result from inadequate treatment of the acute episode (e.g., inadequate amount and time of administration of oximes, inadequate assisted ventilation).

Structure-Activity Relationships

Oximes are useful only if the acetylcholinesterase (AChE) is an "unaged" form. Efficacy of the oximes depends on the chemical form of the acetylcholinesterase inhibitor, the plasma oxime concentration, the duration of oxime treatment, and the plasma cholinesterase concentration. Spontaneous reactivation of the alkyl-phosphorylated cholinester-

Table 68–3
Evidence for Carcinogenicity[a]

Compound	Evidence				
	Animal	Human	In Vitro	IARC[b]	EPA[c]
Aldrin	Limited	Inadequate	Inadequate	3	C
Amitrole	Sufficient	Inadequate	Inadequate	2B	B2
	Sufficient	Inadequate	Inadequate	3	C
α-Naphthylthiourea	Inadequate	Inadequate	. . .	3	C
Aramite	Sufficient	. . .	. . .	. . .	. . .
Arsenicals	Inadequate	Sufficient	Limited	1	A
Benzal chloride	Limited	Inadequate	Limited	3	C
Benzotrichloride	Sufficient	Inadequate	Limited	2B	B2
Benzoyl chloride	Inadequate	Inadequate	Inadequate	3	C
Benzyl chloride	Limited	Inadequate	Sufficient	3	C
Captan	Limited	Insufficient	. . .	. . .	. . .
Carbon tetrachloride	Sufficient	Inadequate	Inadequate	2B	B2
Chlordane	Limited	Inadequate	Inadequate	3	C
Chlordimeform (metabolite)	No data	Insufficient	. . .	. . .	. . .
	Sufficient	. . .	. . .	. . .	. . .
Chlorobenzilate	Limited	Insufficient	. . .	. . .	. . .
Chlorophenols	. . .	Limited	. . .	2B	B2
Chlorothalonil	Limited	Insufficient	. . .	. . .	. . .
Diallate	Limited	Insufficient	. . .	. . .	. . .
1,2-Dibromochloropropane	Sufficient	. . .	. . .	. . .	. . .
p-Dichlorobenzene	Sufficient	No data	. . .	2B	B2
2-Dichloroethane	Sufficient	. . .	. . .	. . .	. . .
2,4-Dichlorophenoxyacetic acid esters	Inadequate	Inadequate	Inadequate	3	C
p,p′-Dichlorodiphenyltrichloroethane	Sufficient	Inadequate	Inadequate	2B	B2
Dicofol (Kelthane)	Limited	Insufficient	. . .	. . .	. . .
Dieldrin	Limited	Inadequate	Inadequate	3	C
Ethylene dibromide	Sufficient	Inadequate	Sufficient	2B	B2
Ethylene oxide	Limited	Inadequate	Sufficient	2B	B2
	Sufficient	Inadequate	. . .	. . .	. . .
Ethylene thiourea	Sufficient	Inadequate	Limited	2B	B2
Fluometuron	Inadequate	No evaluation	. . .	. . .	. . .
Formaldehyde	Sufficient	Inadequate	Sufficient	2B	B2
Heptachlor	Limited	Inadequate	Inadequate	3	C
Hexachlorobenzene	Sufficient	. . .	. . .	. . .	. . .
Kepone (chlordecone)	Sufficient	. . .	. . .	. . .	. . .
Lindane (γ-hexachlorocyclohexane)	Limited	Inadequate	Inadequate	3	C
Malathion	No evidence	No data	. . .	. . .	. . .
(4-chloro-2-methylphenoxy) acetic acid	Inadequate	Inadequate	. . .	3	C
Methyl parathion	No evidence	No evidence	. . .	3	C
Mirex	Sufficient	. . .	. . .	. . .	. . .
Nitrofen	Sufficient	No data	. . .	. . .	. . .
Parathion	Inadequate	Insufficient	. . .	. . .	. . .
Pentachlorophenol	Inadequate	Inadequate	Inadequate	3	C
Phenoxy acids	. . .	Limited	. . .	2B	B2
α-Phenylphenol	Limited	Insufficient	. . .	. . .	. . .
Piperonyl butoxide	No evidence	No evidence	. . .	. . .	. . .
Sulfallate	Sufficient	No data	. . .	. . .	. . .
2,3,7,8-Tetrachlorodibenzo-*p*-dioxin	Sufficient	Inadequate	Inadequate	2B	B2
Tetrachlorovinphos	Limited	Insufficient	. . .	. . .	. . .
Thiourea	Sufficient	. . .	. . .	. . .	. . .
Toxaphene	Sufficient	. . .	. . .	. . .	. . .
Trichlorfon	Inadequate	Insufficient	. . .	. . .	. . .
2,4,5-Trichlorophenol	Inadequate	Inadequate	No data	3	C
2,4,6-Trichlorophenol	Sufficient	Inadequate	No data	2B	B2
2,4,5-Trichlorophenoxyacetic acid	Inadequate	Inadequate	Inadequate	3	C
Vinyl chloride	Sufficient	Sufficient	Sufficient	1	A

[a]Adapted from Council on Scientific Affairs. American Medical Association. JAMA 1988;260:959–966.

[b]IARC indicates International Agency for Research on Cancer. Evidence is divided into the following categories: 1, evidence is sufficient to establish a causal relationship between the agent and human cancer; 2, agent, or process, is probably carcinogenic to humans; 2A, limited, almost sufficient evidence for carcinogenicity in humans; 2B, combination of sufficient evidence in animals and inadequate human data; and 3, cannot be classified according to carcinogenicity in humans.

[c]EPA indicates Environmental Protection Agency. Evidence is divided into the following groups: A, carcinogenic to humans (epidemiologic evidence supports a causal relationship); B, probably carcinogenic to humans (B1, epidemiologic evidence is limited or the weight of evidence from animal studies is sufficient or B2, evidence is sufficient from animal studies but epidemiologic studies provide inadequate evidence or no data); and C, possibly carcinogenic to humans (limited evidence from animal studies and no human data).

Table 68–4
Organophosphate Neurotoxicity[a]

Type	Neuropathy	Treatment
Acute cholinergic crisis	Muscarinic, nicotinic, central nervous system effects, acetylcholinesterase inhibition	Atropine, oximes
Intermediate (usually associated with fenthion, dimethiate) (begins 1 to 4 days after acute poisoning)	Appears in interval between acute cholinergic crises and onset of delayed neuropathy. No muscle fasciculations. Acute respiratory paresis, weakness in area of motor cranial nerves, weakness of neck flexor and proximal limb muscles. Depressed tendon reflexes. Death from respiratory failure. Pre- and postsynaptic impairment of neuromuscular transmission. Acetylcholinesterase inhibition.	Not responsive to atropine, oximes
Delayed sensorimotor polyneuropathy[b] exposure (nerve demyelination?)	Not related to acetylcholinesterase inhibition. Neuropathy target esterase inhibition. Flaccid weakness and atrophy in distal limb muscles, spasticity, ataxia. Spares muscles of respiration.	Not responsive to anticholinergics or oximes

[a]Adapted from de Bleecker JL, van den Neuck K, Colardyn F. Crit Care Med 1993;21:1706–1711.
[b]Driskell WJ, Groce DF, Hill RH Jr. J Anal Toxicol 1991;15:339–340.

Table 68–5
Cholinergic Manifestations of Organophosphate Poisoning

Muscarinic Effects (Parasympathetic)	
Bronchial tree	Tightness in chest, wheezing, suggestive of bronchoconstriction, rhinitis, dyspnea, increased bronchial secretion, cough, pulmonary edema, cyanosis
Gastrointestinal system	Nausea, vomiting, abdominal tightness and cramps, diarrhea, tenesmus, fecal incontinence
Sweat glands	Increased sweating
Salivary glands	Increased salivation
Lacrimal glands	Increased lacrimation
Cardiovascular system	Bradycardia, fall in blood pressure, rare atrial fibrillation, ventricular tachycardia
Pupils	Miosis, occasionally unequal
Ciliary body	Blurring of vision
Bladder	Freqeuncy, urinary incontinence
Nicotinic Effects (Sympathetic and Somatic Motor)	
Striated muscle	Muscular twitching, fasciculation, weakness, cramps, weakness including muscles of respiration
Sympathetic ganglia	Pallor, tachycardia, elevation of blood pressure, hyperglycemia

ase is dependent on whether the organophosphate insecticide carries either two methyl (e.g., demeton-5-methyl, dichlorvos, dimethoate, malathion) or two ethyl (e.g., chlorpyrifos, diazinon, parathion) ester groups attached to the phosphorus atom. From either group the dimethyl phosphorylated AChE or diethyl phosphorylated AChE, respectively, will be generated. Dimethyl phosphorylated AChE is spontaneously reactivated rapidly. Patients may improve even without oxime therapy. Patients poisoned with diethyl phosphorylated insecticides will more likely benefit from oxime therapy.

CLINICAL PRESENTATION

Acute Effects

Cholinergic Features

The cholinergic effects of organophosphate poisoning depend on the balance between muscarinic and nicotinic receptors (Table 68–5). Patients may have elevated blood pressure and tachycardia (nicotinic), rather than bradycardia or hypotension (muscarinic). Miosis is the most constant sign, but its absence does not exclude organophosphate poisoning. The differential diagnosis of miosis includes opiates (except for meperidine), pilocarpine, bromides, phenothiazines, parasympathomimetics, propoxyphene, and phencyclidine. Muscle fasciculations are a highly reliable sign. The presence of excessive secretions (lacrimation, salivation, bronchorrhea, diaphoresis) is helpful in confirming the diagnosis. The mnemonic DUMBELS describes signs of cholinergic excess.

*D*iarrhea
*U*rination
*M*iosis
*B*ronchospasm
*E*mesis
*L*acrimation
*S*alivation

Pancreas

Pancreatitis after ingestion of organophosphates may be painless and terminate fatally,[14] although all children in one study had a complete recovery.[15] Pancreatic enzyme estimation in serum or urine, as well as imaging procedures such as ultrasound or computed tomography, should be performed in cases of parathion ingestions. Serum hemoperfusion is a useful therapy in acute pancreatitis. Overlooking the possibility of a diagnosis of acute pancreatitis may incur the risk of hemorrhages or hemorrhagic pancreatitis.[13]

Chronic Effects

Suggested diagnostic criteria for the organophosphate-induced delayed syndrome include the following[16]:

1. A history of severe acute organophosphate poisoning about 1 to 6 weeks prior to the onset.
2. Symptoms and signs of polyneuropathy and later with or without concurrent pyramidal signs.

3. Denervation changes shown by electromyography.
4. Slow recovery.
5. Reasonable exclusion of other nervous disease.

Sheep Farmers' Disease

Sheep farmers involved in long-term sheep-dip operations and organophosphates appear to develop subtle psychiatric changes.[17]

Plasma Levels

During the 51 days of hospitalization following a methylparathion ingestion, the parathion level measured peak concentrations of 0.46 mg/L for methylparathion (MPT) and 5.8 mg/L for parathion (P). Plasma PT and MPT concentrations fell during charcoal hemoperfusion (on day one) but rebounded again. Plasma PT levels were detectable for 27 days and fell with a terminal half-life of 2.1 days. RBC and plasma cholinesterase levels did not begin to rise until day 32.[18]

In the delayed neuropathy syndromes the electromyogram may display evidence of denervation. The cerebrospinal fluid is usually normal with the exception of a slight rise in protein.[19] Early inhibition of a lymphocytic neurotoxic esterase may be a useful predictor of the later (2 to 3 weeks) development of organophosphate induced delayed neuropathy.[20,21]

Blood Levels

A fatal ingestion of malathion by an 80-year-old was associated with a delayed polyneuropathy and a blood malathion concentration of 23.9 μg/L.[22]

ANTIDOTES

Atropine

Atropine noncompetitively antagonizes both muscarinic and CNS effects of organophosphate poisoning by alleviating excessive bronchial secretions, salivation, sweating, anorexia, nausea, epigastric and chest "tightness", abdominal cramps, vomiting, and bradycardia. Atropine has no effect on muscle weakness or respiratory failure in severe poisoning, since this drug does not reactivate the cholinesterase enzymes. For diagnosis, use an intravenous dose of 1 mg (adult) or 0.015 mg/kg (child) and watch for signs of atropinization (dilated pupils, dry or red skin, confusion, tachycardia, fever, ileus) within 10 minutes of administration. For a therapeutic intravenous dose in symptomatic patients, use 2 to 4 mg in adults or 0.015 to 0.05 mg/kg in children every 15 minutes as needed. Mild atropinization may be needed for up to 48 hours in cases of moderate toxicity. The administration of atropine as an antidote does not require confirmation by acetylcholinesterase levels. Atropine is rapidly metabolized, and large doses often are needed within the first 24 hours. Seriously poisoned patients develop marked resistance to the usual doses of atropine. A severe parathion ingestion required 20 g of atropine over 24 days,[23] and an intentional Cygon ingestion necessitated the use of an atropine drip of 0.5 to 2.4 mg/kg over 6 weeks.[24] The drying of secretions or full atropinization, rather than dilated pupils, is the effective endpoint of atropine titration. Do not wait for the return of cholinesterase levels before treating significantly symptomatic patients with atropine. Prophylactic use of atropine is not recommended.

TREATMENT

Decontamination Procedures

1. Stand victim in shower (or sit in chair) and supervise washing.
2. Three different washes are recommended. Sequence of water temperatures changes is important since absorption conceivably could be enhanced if hot-water wash were administered first.
   a. Cold water for 5 minutes. Wash from head to toe with tincture of green soap or any nongermicidal soap.
      (1) Wash hair each time
      (2) Wash under nails
      (3) Remove contact lenses/glasses
      (4) Rinse with cold water
   b. Repeat wash and rinse procedure with warm water.
   c. Repeat wash and rinse procedure with hot water.

Elimination Enhancement

A study of the use of charcoal hemoperfusion in malathion poisoning indicated that its effectiveness was limited by the short duration of effective removal (120 minutes) afforded by the column and the wide distribution of malathion in the body. Over a prolonged time in severe, acute malathion poisoning the column must be changed when it becomes saturated with the pesticide.[25]

Alternate routes for atropine administration (when rapid intravenous access cannot be achieved) may induce the intraosseous route in children,[26] and nebulized atropine by inhalation in adults.[27]

Pralidoxime (2PAM)

In children pralidoxime (2PAM) administration may be instituted with a 25-mg/kg intravenous dose given for 15 to 30 minutes, followed by a continuous infusion of 10 to 20 mg/kg/hour. Therapy with 2PAM should be continued for at least 18 hours or longer, depending on the patient's clinical status and the properties of the suspected toxin.[28]

In a severely poisoned adult the dosage of pralidoxime (e.g., 500 mg/hour) should be continuously maintained until clear and irreversible clinical improvement is achieved. This may take days until residual insecticide is cleared from body stores.[29,30] To achieve the recommended plasma pralidoxime concentration of 4 mg/L pralidoxime should be administered in doses of 30 mg/kg body weight by bolus dose intravenously over 4 to 6 hours or 8 to 10 mg/kg/hour intravenously until full recovery occurs[29] and atropine is no longer required to treat cholinergic signs and symptoms. Professor Eyer of Munich prefers obidoxime 250 mg intravenously, then 750 mg for 24 hours IV. The red blood cell acetylcholinesterase level provides an indication of reversibility of the AChE.

Obidoxime

Obidoxime [N,N^1-oxidimethylene *bis* (pyridinium-4-aldoxime) dichloride] is an antidote for organophosphate intoxication used in Israel, the Netherlands, Scandinavian countries, Germany, Belgium, and Portugal. An anecdotal study in a 20-year-old with methamidophos intoxication revealed the elimination half-life of obidoxime to be 6.9 hours, volume of distribution 0.845 L/kg, total body clearance 85.4 mL/min, and renal clearance 69 mL/min (creatinine clearance 54 mL/min). Eighty percent of the dose was excreted in the urine over 5 hours. The relationship between obidoxime blood levels and therapeutic efficacy has not been established. Based on a rat study, obidoxime plasma levels of 1 to 4 µg/mL have been proposed as possibly effective therapeutic levels. Further studies are required to establish the therapeutic window for obidoxime and its disposition in organophosphate intoxicated patients. Its dose should meanwhile be adjusted to renal function. Bentur and colleagues suggest that special attention should also be given to suspected toxicity, which includes QT prolongation, ventricular tachyarrhythmias, and liver enzyme abnormalities.[31] There have been no controlled clinical studies that suggest the superiority of pralidoxime over obidoxime or other oximes in the treatment of anticholinesterase poisonings.

Cautions

1. Use for all symptomatic patients after a nerve gas exposure.
2. If severely dyspneic give 4 to 6 mg atropine plus 2PAMCl 1 g IV. Watch heart rate, blood pressure.
3. If moderate exposure to vapor (respiratory distress, gastrointestinal signs and symptoms, muscle twitching): give 6 mg atropine and 2PAMCl. Always give diazepam (10 mg IM).
4. Seizures often respond to atropine and 2PAMCl. If they do not, give diazepam (5 to 10 mg IV) over 3 to 5 minutes in adults; 0.24 to 0.4 mg/kg IV (up to 10 mg) over 2 to 3 minutes in children. Watch for worsening of respiratory depression (after diazepam is used) caused by nerve agents.

Observe for recurrence of nicotinic symptoms. If they do not recur for the next 24 hours, discontinue therapy. If they recur, record time of breakthrough, estimate level of pralidoxime (MEC = minimum effective concentration) in patient at that moment. Reload immediately with 1 g of pralidoxime when breakthrough symptoms occur. Give a continuous IV infusion of pralidoxime to maintain a level approximately 10% above the estimated MEC. Weaning the patient off should be performed by set increments (e.g., 25% every 8 hours). Watch the patient for at least 1 hour after each adjustment. These guidelines may not be applicable to fat-soluble organophosphate pesticides; they may be affected by organophosphate agent properties such as "aging," redistribution, and delayed absorption; the patient may alter the toxicokinetics of pralidoxime (renal function, serum pH); interactions with atropine effect must be considered.[31]

Doses For Organophosphate Insecticide Poisoning—Other Methods

The usual adult dose of pralidoxime consists of 1 to 2 g for a 70-kg person (14 to 28 mg/kg) IV in 100 to 150 mL of saline given slowly over 15 to 30 minutes. A suggested initial dose for children is 15 to 25 mg/kg. Sidell recommends an initial dose of 15 mg/kg for infants.

Child Dose

Seven children were poisoned with organophosphate insecticides and received a loading dose of 2PAMCl: 15 to 50 mg/kg in 0.9% saline to yield a blood concentration of 10 to 20 mg/mL, given IV over a 30-minute period. A maintenance IV infusion of 9 to 19 mg/kg/hr was then administered. Using the toxicokinetics of 2PAMCl ($T_{1/2}$ 1.14 hours; V_D 0.73 L/kg) a continuous infusion of 18 mg/kg/hr would lead to a steady-state 2PAM serum concentration of about 40 µg/mL. Therefore in children a continuous infusion of 10 to 20 mg/kg/hr should provide >4-µg/mL levels.

This data suggest initiation of treatment with 25-mg/kg IV 2PAMCl doses for 15 to 30 minutes, then continuous infusion 10 to 20 mg/kg/hr. Continue for 18 hours or longer depending on the patient's clinical status and the properties of the suspected toxin.[28]

Supportive Care

1. Avoid parasympathomimetic agents (physostigmine, succinylcholine) because they may potentiate anticholinesterase activity. Apnea for 3½ hours followed the administration of succinylcholine to an infant suffering from organophosphate poisoning.[32]
2. Phenothiazines and antihistamines have anticholinesterase activity and may potentiate organophosphate toxicity.
3. Central nervous system depressants (e.g., opiates) may increase the likelihood of respiratory arrest.
4. During antidote administration, the patient should be followed closely for signs of respiratory failure and atropinization in an intensive care setting. The patient should be observed at least 48 hours after the last dose of atropine.
5. Administer fluids only to replace losses.

Prognosis

Full recovery generally occurs within 10 days when optimum treatment is quickly instituted. Fatality usually occurs in untreated, severely intoxicated patients within 24 hours. Persistent CNS effects (irritability, nervousness, fatigue, lethargy, impaired memory, depression, and schizophrenic reactions) and peripheral neuropathies similar to those in Jamaican ginger paralysis (TOCP) have been reported in a few survivors. No prolonged effect on liver function, coagulation, skin, or respiratory tract has been documented. The patient must avoid reexposure until cholinesterase activity is over 75% of normal.

TRICRESYLPHOSPHATES (TOCP)

Childhood presentation of acute tricresylphosphate intoxication is similar to adult cases.[33] Typical findings of gastrointestinal complaints are followed by the resolution of symptoms, and then by delayed neuropathic change often with permanent sequellae. Mass intoxication occurred in the southern United States during the 1930s when TOCP was employed as an adulterant of Jamaica Ginger ("Jake"), a popular alcohol-containing medicament of the Prohibition Era. The resulting neurologic syndrome was known as Ginger Paralysis or Jack-Leg because of its predilection for paralysis of the lower extremity.

CHLORMEQUAT (CHLOROCHOLINE) [2-CHLOROETHYL) TRIMETHYL AMMONIUM CHLORIDE]

Chlormequat (chlorocholine) [(2-chloroethyl) trimethyl ammonium chloride] is an anticholinesterase chemical that is used as a plant growth regulant marketed as Cycockl (11.8% chloroquat). Dizziness, profuse perspiration, visual disturbances, excessive salivation, T-wave inversions, seizures, bradycardia, ventricular fibrillation, and asystole have been observed after ingestion. Chlormequat is not detected in the blood, liver, or kidney by thin-layer chromatography.[34]

DIMETHOATE

Dimethoate is an organothiophosphate widely used as a pesticide.[4] The clinical presentation of dimethoate poisoning includes all the signs of cholinergic intoxication:

1. Muscarinic effects: miosis, lacrimation, hypersalivation, diarrhea, bradycardia, and bronchial hypersecretion.
2. Nicotinic effects: muscular fibrillations and fasciculations.
3. Effects on CNS: nausea, vomiting, ataxia, tonic–clonic convulsions, respiratory insufficiency, and coma.[35]

Severe poisoning with dimethoate is associated with an unfavorable prognosis. Ingestion in man may be fatal.[36]

STRUCTURE AND CLASSIFICATION

Dimethoate (Cygon, Defend, Ethim, Roxlon, Rogor L20, Sistemin 40) is an organophosphate insecticide that is considered to be moderately toxic by the U.S. Environmental Protection Agency.[4] It is a phosphorodithioate.

TOXIC DOSE—120 G

A 52-year-old patient ingested 20 g of dimethoate, was treated with atropine and hemoperfusions and recovered.[35] A 20-year-old injected 4 g of dimethoate subcutaneously. He received atropine and an oxime (H1-6) and was discharged in good health on day 24.[37]

FATAL DOSE

Ingestions of about 10 to 12 g of dimethoate have been fatal.[38,39]

DISTRIBUTION (V_D)

The apparent volume of distribution is about 30 L/kg.[35]

ELIMINATION

The plasma half-life in one patient[40] is 5 hours. In humans and rats 76 to 90% of a dose of radioactive dimethoate is excreted in the urine within 24 hours.[35] Dimethoate is oxidized by the liver to omethoate and to three further metabolites, all inhibitors of acetylcholinesterase.

MECHANISM OF ACTION

The toxic action of dimethoate is located in the tissue compartments where it binds reversibly and, after some time, irreversibly to the nerve endings.[41] Only the reversibly bound dimethoate in the tissues is in equilibrium with the dimethoate in the blood. Therefore the effect of hemoperfusion is restricted to this reversibly bound fraction.[35]

CLINICAL PRESENTATION

A 52-year-old male was admitted 2 hours after ingesting 20 g of dimethoate. On admission he was comatose and exhibited muscular fasciculation, extreme miosis, hypersalivation, and respiratory insufficiency. Pseudocholinesterase was unmeasurable. After treatment with gastric lavage, atropine, and hemoperfusions (activated charcoal, and amberlite XAD4) he recovered and was discharged in 25 days.[35] Dimethoate, as well as dichlorvos and methylparathion, does not appear to produce organophosphate-induced peripheral neuropathy.[42]

LABORATORY

Analytic Methods

Dimethoate in plasma urine and gastric lavage fluid may be determined by gas chromatography.[35]

Blood Levels

Plasma dimethoate levels after ingestion of dimethoate may reach concentrations of 50 μg/mL.[35] The half-times for reactivation of serum cholinesterase was 10.3 days and for red cell cholinesterase, 36.8 days, even though an oxime cholinesterase reactivator (HI-6) was used.[38] The patient clinically improved even though cholinesterase reactivation by the oxime was relatively ineffective and slow.[38] Injection of 4 g of dimethoate was followed by blood levels of 1.7 μg/mL and urine levels of 94 μg/mL.[38]

Abnormalities

The electrocardiogram may exhibit a sinus tachycardia.[38] A metabolic acidosis, leukocytosis, hypokalemia, and moderate rise in liver enzymes may follow dimethoate poisoning.[38]

TREATMENT

Stabilization

Treatment includes administration of high doses of atropine and supportive measures. Reactivation of cholinesterase has been recommended for the early state.[38] Koppel and colleagues administered bolus injections of 20 mg of atropine every 20 minutes, the dosage based on peristalsis of the gut and pupillary size.[35]

Decontamination

After ingestion of 20 g of dimethoate, gastric lavage fluid removed about 10 mg.[30]

Elimination Enhancement

Extracorporeal detoxication and hemoperfusion (HP) and combined hemoperfusion/hemodialysis (HP/HD) have been reported. The efficacy of these procedures has been preliminarily studied.[42]

Dimethoate has a dialysance of 59 mL/min (blood flow 100 mL/min, dialysate flow 600 mL/min, ultraflow 200 membrane) and a HP clearance of 88 mL/min (flow 100 mL/min, activated charcoal). Two cases of using HP and HD/HP in severe dimethoate poisoning have been published:

1. Fifteen hours after suicidal ingestion of 12 g dimethoate (plasma level before HP 5 μg/mL) HP with activated charcoal was performed. A dimethoate clearance of 87 mL/min (flow 162 mL/min) was calculated. A considerable rebound effect was observed on day 6 after ingestion. The patient died on day 11 from adult respiratory distress syndrome after prolonged pneumonia.
2. Two hours after suicidal ingestion of 10 g dimethoate (plasma level 2.34 μg/mL 30 min after ingestion), HP/HD was performed using activated charcoal for HP. A HP clearance of 95 mL/min and a dialysate of 85 mL/min (flow 200 mL/min, C-DAK hollow fiber dialyzer Cordis Dow) was determined; 55.3 mg dimethoate was eliminated by HP, 25.3 mg by HD. No rebound effect was observed. During extracorporeal detoxication the dimethoate plasma half-life was 1.8 hour.[39,42]

After an ingestion of about 20 g of dimethoate by an adult 142 mg and 72 mg were removed by HP with activated charcoal and amberlite XAD4, respectively. Clinically, HP did not markedly change the condition of the patient. HP may be more effective at an early stage of intoxication when the distribution of dimethoate in tissues is not complete and the fraction irreversibly bound is low.[35] Ten mg of the unchanged pesticide (after an ingestion of 20 g) was excreted in the urine during the first 4 days.[35]

Antidotes

An infusion of H1-6 (an oxime) in doses of 4 g/day was accompanied by a very slow rise in serum and red cell cholinesterase (10 to 36 days in one patient).[38]

Supportive Measures

Supportive measures should be employed similar to those administered after an organophosphate insecticide poisoning (intubation, oxygen, positive end-expiratory pressure, treatment of metabolic acidosis, daily monitoring of serum and red cell cholinesterase levels, vital signs).

CARBAMATES

Carbamate pesticides cause a decrease in cholinesterase activity. These poisonings are less severe because they bind reversibly to the active site on the cholinesterase enzyme, in contrast to the organophosphate pesticides that, over time, bind irreversibly. Carbamates cause the same excess in muscarinic stimulation and nicotinic stimulation followed by weakness seen in organophosphate poisonings, but for a relatively shorter duration.

An adult ingested 7.5 g of carbaryl and became nauseated, flushed, salivated, and diaphoretic. No antidotes were given. Symptoms subsided in 3 hours.[43]

LABORATORY

Three hours following ingestion of 7.5 g of carbaryl the blood carbaryl and alpha naphthol were analyzed by HPLC. Carbaryl and alpha naphthol concentrations were 833 and 516 ng/mL, respectively. Following first-order kinetics the half-life of carbaryl was 1.30 hours; the half-life of alpha naphthol was 1.13. The volume of distribution of carbaryl was 32.9 L/kg and clearance 3080 m/min.[43]

TREATMENT

Oximes do not appear to provide any additional benefit compared with atropine alone in carbaryl poisoning. Oxime therapy in carbaryl poisoning may lead to the production of a carbamylated oxime that may be a more potent acetylcholinesterase inhibitor than carbaryl itself.[44–46] With other carbamate insecticides (e.g., aldicarb) oximes may be a useful adjunct to atropine therapy[47,48] but the use of pralidoxime for carbamate pesticide poisoning continues to be controversial. Most carbamate poisonings resolve within several hours without treatment other than atropine. In an aldicarb poisoning, muscle weakness and clonus appeared to slowly improve after bolus IV doses of pralidoxime (1 g) were followed by an infusion of 0.5 g/hour over 40 hours. Cholinesterase inhibition continued for 52 hours. This anecdotal report must be validated by further controlled studies.[44]

The use of 2PAM is indicated as an adjunct to atropine (a) in serious, potentially fatal poisonings with unknown cholinesterase inhibitors; (b) in a serious poisoning with a mixture of organophosphorus and carbamate compounds together, and (c) if a patient known to have carbamate poisoning does not respond to full atropinization.[49,50]

METHOMYL

Methomyl (a synthetic carbamate) was introduced in 1966 in the United States. It is now available throughout the world.

Exposure to the spray may induce typical manifestations of cholinesterase inhibition.[51] Ingestion may lead to similar symptoms and can be fatal.[52–54] Treatment of poisoning is largely symptomatic and supportive. Atropine has been useful to diminish cholinergic activity. Oximes may form a toxic complex with the carbamate and may diminish atropine effectiveness.[55] and, in many cases, are not necessary to revert the intoxication.[56]

USES

Methomyl is a broad-spectrum carbamate insecticide used on various vegetable crops (e.g., cabbage, cauliflower, broccoli, lettuce).[52]

PRODUCT FORMULATION

Methomyl is usually marketed as an aqueous solution, but may also be sold in solid form.[52]

SOURCES

Methomyl is a synthetic carbamate.

TOXIC DOSE

A 39-year-old female ingested 4.5 mg/kg, lost consciousness, and exhibited a diminished respiratory rate and blood pressure. The patient recovered.[57] Eleven adult patients were exposed (ingestion, skin) to from 2 to 16 g of methomyl (30 to 200 mg/kg), developed symptoms of a cholinesterase inhibitor, and survived.[57]

FATAL DOSE

A lethal dose is approximately 12 to 15 mg/kg.[52,54]

MECHANISM OF ACTION

Methomyl may induce profound clinical signs and symptoms reflective of cholinesterase inhibition.

CLINICAL PRESENTATION

Clinical symptoms after exposure to methomyl are similar to those produced by organophosphates, although of lesser intensity and duration.[56] There is often an absence of bradycardia. Typical manifestations of cholinesterase inhibition include nausea, miosis, headache, lacrimation, salivation, vomiting, and abdominal pain. Diminished respirations, hypotension, and muscle fasciculations have been observed. Frothing from the mouth has been seen.[54] Tachycardia is often observed.[52] Fatalities have followed ingestions of methomyl.[52–54,58] Acute methomyl poisoning depresses the nervous system. Symptoms may include headache, dizziness, weakness, ataxia, tremor, nausea, and death. Workers at pesticide plants manufacturing methomyl often require hospitalization for illness related to methomyl exposure in packaging production and maintenance functions.[59]

LABORATORY

Analytic Methods

High-pressure liquid chromatography, gas chromatography, and gas chromatography/mass spectrometry methods are available.[54] The lower limit of detectability of the oxamyl oxime is 0.5 mg.[60]

Blood Levels

A 73-year-old female who ingested about 30 mg/kg of methomyl had a blood level of 44 μg/mL and then died. Her husband, who also ingested 30 mg/kg of methomyl, had a blood level of 0.01 to 0.1 μg/mL. He survived.[54] A 39-year-old female ingested about 4.5 mg/kg, developed methomyl blood levels of 1.6 μg/mL, and survived.[57] Blood methomyl concentrations from nine individuals who died after methomyl ingestion ranged from 8 to 56 μg/mL.[51] These individuals who were found unresponsive had methomyl blood levels of 8 to 57 μg/mL.[57] Blood concentrations of 700 and 1400 ng/mL were reported in suicides after ingestion.[61] After ingesting 2.25 g of methomyl one person developed a blood concentration of 1600 ng/mL within 6 hours.[57] An aerial spray pilot who died when his aircraft crashed while he was spraying methomyl had a whole blood methomyl concentration of 570 ng/mL.[61] Methomyl blood concentrations are dependent on the difference between the time of methomyl administration and the time of blood sampling.[62]

Abnormalities

The electrocardiogram after methomyl exposure may exhibit a sinus tachycardia or T-wave changes (decrease in height, inversion). Such changes may revert to preexposure status within 1 week.[51] No changes in the P-wave, PR interval, or QRS complex were observed. Premature beats were not seen. One patient exhibited an atrioventricular block.[56]

Ancillary Tests

There may be a decrease in plasma cholinesterase concentrations but no decrease in red blood cell cholinesterase levels. The lactic and dehydrogenase levels may be elevated after methomyl exposure. The aspartate aminotransferase levels were unchanged in one series of patients.[51] Leukocytosis (15,000 white cells/mm^3 with an increase in bands) was observed in 11 patients after methomyl exposures.[56] Determination of plasma cholinesterase may be useful even 20 hours after exposure. If plasma cholinesterase values have returned to normal, red blood cell cholinesterase values may be useful. Cholinesterase determination should be within 4 hours of exposure.[56]

TREATMENT

Stabilization

Patients should be admitted to an intensive care facility where access to a central line, oxygen, and cardiac monitoring will be available. Exposure after spraying will require careful washing of the entire (nails, intertriginous areas) body with tincture of green soap (contains alcohol, useful to remove fat-soluble compounds). Remove all contaminated clothing. Immediate life-threatening symptoms usually result from weakness of the respiratory muscles, central respiratory depression, bronchospasm, bronchial secretions, and pulmonary edema, all of which may result in hypoxemia. Frequent suctioning, endotracheal intubation, and ventilatory assistance may be required. Monitor the PO_2 with repeat arterial blood gases. Excessive secretions and bronchospasm should respond to adequate doses of atropine.

Decontamination

Gastric lavage and activated charcoal should be used if the patient presents within 4 hours after exposure. Health personnel should use rubber gloves and avoid direct contact with contaminated material.

Elimination Enhancement

Methods for elimination are not recommended in view of the short action of the carbamates and the effectiveness of atropine.

Antidote

Atropine (IV 0.6 mg for adults; 0.007 mg/kg for children) may be useful without reaching complete atropinization (dilated pupils, dry or red skin, confusion, tachycardia, fever ileus). It can be administered every 15 minutes as needed. Pralidoxime is usually unnecessary and may reduce the effectiveness of atropine, although it may reduce fasciculations.[63] Patients may require 6 to 8 hours of atropine treatment. Significant poisoning may require at least 24 hours of observation after the last atropine dose.

Supportive Measures

Follow the patient for any signs of respiratory failure for at least 24 hours after the last atropine dose. Administer fluids to replace losses. Avoid central nervous system depressants (e.g., opiates); they may increase the possibility of respiratory arrest.

GLUFOSINATE

Glufosinate, a herbicide used in Japan as Basta, is a phosphorus-containing amino acid with a molecular weight of 198.2. Human poisonings have been characterized by diminished consciousness, nausea, vomiting, pyrexia to 38 to 40°C, generalized seizures, disturbances of eye movements, generalized edema, elevation of leukocyte counts and serum aminotransferase, gastric mucosal erosion, and retrograde partial amnesia. Death may follow due to hemodynamic failure.[64]

ORGANOCHLORINES

EPIDEMIOLOGY

As a result of positive findings in carcinogenicity assays the U.S. Environmental Protection Agency suspended all uses of products containing heptachlor in 1976, except for treatment of seeds, control of ants in Hawaiian pineapple plants, and control of termites and the narcissus bulbs. In August 1987, the EPA and the manufacturers agreed to halt all sales of the products.[65]

STRUCTURE/PRODUCT FORMULATIONS

Acute Toxic Dosage

Dieldrin

The acute adult lethal dose of dieldrin is approximately 1.5 to 5 g.[66] Endrin, a stereoisomer of dieldrin, has a similar toxicity, producing death after a 6-g ingestion.[67]

Lindane

The fatal dose in adults is approximately 10 to 30 g; doses of 1.6 and 45 g are capable of producing seizures in young children and adults, respectively. A 16-year-old boy survived a 392-g ingestion after treatment of apnea and status epilepticus.[68] A single application of lindane to adults may lead to seizures.[69] Ingestion of 250 mg of lindane led to seizures within 30 minutes.[70] A 43-year-old female ingested 8 oz of a 20% lindane solution (about 48 g) and died.[71] Pseudotumor cerebri has also been reported after exposure to lindane.[72]

TOXICOKINETICS

In breast milk heptachlor poses a special risk because the body absorbs it rapidly and can store it in fatty tissue for a year or more. Breast milk may be considered a main route for the elimination of heptachlor from the mother's body.[73]

Lindane crosses the placenta. Lindane levels in human blood and placental and fetal tissues are higher in cases of spontaneous abortion and prematurity than in normal-term pregnancies. Tissues from stillborn babies show the same range of lindane values as adult tissues.[74]

CLINICAL PRESENTATION

Pregnancy

An anecdotal report describes a 16-week-pregnant woman who ingested an organochlorine insecticide in an attempt to commit suicide. This resulted in the death of twin fetuses and vaginal bleeding. Respiratory arrest followed termination of the pregnancy. The patient survived with symptomatic care.[75]

Ingestion of 5 g of lindane by an 18-week-pregnant woman led to hypotension, episodes of respiratory arrest, and intrauterine death. The mother recovered after supportive therapy and an induced abortion.[76]

LABORATORY
Lindane

Blood levels as low as 0.21 μg/mL have been measured following seizure.[70] Ingestion of about 250 mg of lindane led to blood lindane levels of 0.13 μg/mL associated with seizure.[70] Geriatric patients who seized after a single application of lindane had serum lindane levels of 1.9 to 9.3 mg/mL. After an ingestion of about 48 g of lindane a 43-year-old adult had a serum lindane concentration of 1.3 μg/mL.[69]

TREATMENT

Daily oral mineral oil appeared to reduce the amount of lindane in the fat (biopsy) and plasma of a 30-year-old patient who had applied lindane lotion to the total body twice weekly for 6 months. Further clinical trials will be indicated to confirm this approach to treatment.[76]

Antidotes

There is no antidote.

ENDOSULFAN

Endosulfan (Thiodan, Malix, Thionax) is a cyclic sulfurous ester organochlorine and is registered in Italy for use as an insecticide.[77] It is moderately soluble in organic solvent and insoluble in water.[78]

CLINICAL PRESENTATION

Ten patients ingested 50 to 500 mL of the 35% concentrate (17.5 to 175 g endosulfan). Patients experienced vomiting within ½ hour, hypotension, tonic–clonic seizures, fever, metabolic acidosis, and elevation in liver function enzymes. The acute toxidrome of endosulfan poisoning includes GI irritation, CNS irritability, respiratory depression, cardiovascular collapse,[79] and death within 2 hours.[78] Five out of 10 patients died in 4 to 60 hours.

Five patients developed severe gastrointestinal disorders. One died. Six patients ingested an undetermined quantity of endosulfan and within 3 hours developed nausea, vomiting, headache, dizziness, convulsions, and metabolic acidosis. Three developed aspiration bronchopneumonia and thrombocytopenia; one died with disseminated intravascular coagulation, acute renal failure, acute respiratory distress syndrome, and massive pulmonary thromboembolism.[80,81]

The clinical course of a patient who survived after ingestion 200 mL of 30% thionax (60 grams) may be divided into 3 stages:

1. Convulsive and hemodynamic instability stage lasting 16 hours with alveolar hypoventilation, pulmonary edema, and hemodynamic instability. Episodes of tachycardia, hypertension, and mydriasis followed by cardiogenic shock were observed.
2. The next phase lasted 2 weeks and may be characterized by convulsions, recurrent aspiration pneumonias, and the need for mechanical ventilation.
3. This is followed by a slow recovery of psychosomatic function.[78]

LABORATORY

A 55-year-old female was found dead. The blood endosulfan concentration was 30 μg/mL.[77] Analysis was made by using a gas chromatography with a flame photometric detector. Four of five patients who ingested endosulfan had blood levels of 0.29 to 2.85 μg/mL. One who died had a blood level of 0.57 μg/mL. Urine levels ranged from 0.09 to 3.00 μg/mL.[82]

TREATMENT

Treatment is symptomatic and supportive. Seizures are treated with diazepam.

PYRETHRUM AND SYNTHETIC PYRETHROIDS

CLINICAL PRESENTATION
Synthetic Pyrethroids

The clinical manifestations of inhalation exposure to pyrethrins can be local or systemic. Localized reactors confined to the upper respiratory tract include rhinitis, sneezing, scratchy throat, oral mucosal edema, and even laryngeal mucosal edema. Localized reaction of the lower respiratory tract include cough, shortness of breath, wheezing, and chest pain. An asthmalike reaction occurs with acute exposures in sensitized patients. Hypersensitivity pneumonitis characterized by chest pain, cough, dyspnea, and bronchospasm may occur in an individual chronically exposed. About 50% of persons sensitive to ragweed exhibit cross-sensitivity to pyrethrum (ragweed and chrysanthemum are in the same botanical group). Hypersensitivity to pyrethroids has not been reported.[83]

The diagnosis of acute pyrethroid poisoning should be made on the basis of verified exposure to pyrethroids within 2 days before onset, of corresponding symptoms and signs, and of reasonable exclusion of other diseases.

A 36-year-old woman with a history of asthma developed severe shortness of breath 5 minutes after she began to wash her dog with an insecticide shampoo containing 0.05% pyrethrin. She soon developed gasping respiration. In 5 minutes she was in cardiopulmonary arrest. Despite resuscitative efforts she died. Postmortem findings were considered to be compatible with asthma.

LABORATORY
Pyrethrums[84–90]

No common laboratory tests are available to the emergency physician that have diagnostic or prognostic values. A color test with 2-2(2-amino ethylamine) ethanol produces a red to violet color in the presence of pyrethroidal substances, but is not suitable for analysis of these agents in body fluids. Plasma levels are not clinically useful.[88] The radioallergosorbent test (RAST) or wheal-and-flare skin testing can detect the presence of antigen-specific immunoglobulin antibodies.[89]

Pyrethroids

Blood cholinesterase levels are normal. Cerebrospinal fluid is usually normal. The electrocardiogram may indicate ST-T changes, sinus tachycardia, and verticular premature beats.[85]

TREATMENT

Pyrethrum Exposure

The additives (e.g., petroleum distillate), when present, represent a greater toxic threat to the patient than the active ingredient itself. There are no specific antidotes regardless of route of toxicity. Atropine and pralidoxime are not indicated. Emesis should not be induced when petroleum distillate additives are present unless the product ingested is estimated to contain a near lethal dose (1 g/kg) of pyrethrum or pyrethrins. The alert person with an intact gag reflex and a sublethal pyrethrum ingestion without other toxic constituents may have emesis induced by ipecac, followed by a saline cathartic and slurry of activated charcoal. Oils and fats, including milk, promote the intestinal absorption of pyrethrums and should be avoided. Pulmonary and allergic sequelae are treated symptomatically with airway maintenance, oxygen, and ventilatory assistance as required. Standard drugs and management protocols may be used for treatment of bronchospasm and anaphylaxis. Seizures are treated with diazepam.[88]

CROTAMITON

Crotamiton is used topically as an antipruritic and scabicide.[91,92] It is a derivative of ortho-toluidine, a compound that may induce methemoglobinemia.[93] Several cases of ingestion of the product have been reported and, in one case, ended fatally.[94]

STRUCTURE AND CLASSIFICATION

Crotamiton is *N*-ethyl-crotono-*o*-toluidide (crotonyl-*N*-ethyl-*O*-toluidine), an antipruritic and scabicide.

USES

Crotamiton is used as a sarcoptocide and antipruritic.[91,92]

PRODUCT FORMULATION

Crotamiton is available as a cream or lotion continuing 10% crotamiton with water, petrolatum, propylene glycol, steareth-2, cetyl alcohol, dimethicone, laureth-23, fragrance, magnesium aluminum silicate, carbomer-934, sodium hydroxide, diazolidinyl urea, methyl chloroisothiazolinone, methylisothiazolinone, and magnesium nitrate. In addition, the cream contains glyceryl stearate.[90] It is available commercially as Eurax, Crotamitex, and Euraxil.[95]

SOURCES

Crotamiton is a synthetic chemical.

DOSES

Therapeutic Doses

Crotamiton is usually applied to the whole body twice in 24 hours, using a 60-gm tube.

Toxic Dose

The highest known doses ingested have been 2 g of cream by a child age 1½ years, and 1 ounce of lotion by a 2-year-old child.[91] The 2-year-old may have died following this ingestion.[93] One patient drank approximately 10 mL of Eurax lotion; clinical details are not available.[96] An adult drank an unknown amount of Eurax emulsion. She survived.[94]

Fatal Dose

An undetermined amount of crotamiton may have been ingested by a 2-year-old. The child died.[93]

TOXICOKINETICS

Absorption

After oral ingestion crotamiton may be found in the serum.[94]

Distribution

Crotamiton probably is metabolized in the liver to two metabolites.

Elimination

Crotamiton appears to be eliminated in the urine as the parent drug and as desethyl and hydroxy derivatives.[94]

MECHANISM OF ACTION

The mechanism of action of crotamiton is not known. It may induce methemoglobinemia.[92] Mechanisms of central nervous system toxicity have not been elucidated.

CLINICAL PRESENTATION

A 2-year-old is reported to have ingested 1 ounce of Eurax lotion, and subsequently developed abdominal pain and purpura of the ankles and feet; the condition was diagnosed as an interstitial glomerulonephritis or acute tubular necrosis and the child died.[93] A 2½-month-old child was treated topically with three applications of crotamiton in 1 day for scabies and presented with pallor and cyanosis of the lips and extremities. The patient was treated for methemoglobinemia and survived.[93] A 23-year-old woman who ingested an unknown amount of Eurax emulsion was treated with a salt-water emetic, gastric lavage, activated charcoal, and metoclopramide, following which she suffered from grand mal convulsions, developing coma, hyperreflexia, ankle clonus, and hypotension that responded to a plasma substitute. She recovered.[96]

LABORATORY

Analytic Methods

Gas chromatography/mass spectrometry has been used to detect crotamiton in the serum and both crotamiton and metabolites in the urine.[96]

Blood Levels

Following an ingestion by an adult, serum crotamiton levels were 34 μg/mL.[96]

Abnormalities

Methemoglobin levels may be elevated.[93] Renal dysfunction may be present.[93]

TREATMENT

Treatment is supportive and symptomatic. An intravenous line, cardiac monitoring, and oxygen should be available. Hypotension may require position change, intravenous fluids, and pressor amines. Patients may experience seizures soon after ingestion. Repeat seizures may be treated with diazepam or phenytoin as indicated. Use of syrup of ipecac to induce emesis would therefore not be advised. If methemoglobinemia supervenes, use of methylene blue or other antimethemoglobin measures may be indicated, depending on clinical judgment. Follow-up serial determinations of methemoglobin levels and renal function (serum creatinine, urinalyses) may be indicated.

LABORATORY

Analytic Method

Gas chromatographic techniques (electron capture, flame ionization) can detect warfarin blood levels that range from 0.6 to 3.1 mg/L in patients on long-term therapy.

SODIUM MONOFLUOROACETATE ("1080")

EPIDEMIOLOGY

Sodium monofluoroacetate is a rodenticide. Fluoracetic acid is the major isolate of the poisonous South African gifblaar plant *(Dichapetalum cymosum).* Monofluoroacetic acid produces toxicity when livestock consume plants from the South American genus *Palicourea* and the Australian genera *Gastrolobium, Oxylobium,* and *Acacia.* Toxicity varies 10,000-fold among experimental animals, but the extremely high toxicity among mammals has resulted in severe restrictions on the use of this compound.[97] Sodium monofluoroacetate is a white, odorless, tasteless substance that is mixed with black dye and added to grain baits.

ACUTE TOXIC DOSAGE

Estimates of the mean lethal human dose range from 2 to 10 mg/kg with a mean of 5 mg/kg, similar to values for strychnine.[98] Survival despite renal failure was reported after a 400-mg adult suicidal ingestion.[99]

A 20-year-old attempted suicide by ingesting 50 mL of 1% of monofluoroacetate (approximately 500 mg). He survived.[100]

TOXICOKINETICS

Sodium monofluoroacetate is absorbed from the gastrointestinal tract, lungs, and mucous membranes but probably not from intact skin.

CLINICAL PRESENTATION

A latent period of 30 to 150 minutes precedes the onset of gastrointestinal symptoms. Initially, nausea, vomiting, and abdominal pain occur, followed by anxiety, agitation, muscle spasm, stupor, seizures, and coma.[101] Sinus tachycardia and hypotension are the common cardiovascular signs, and the cardiac rhythm may deteriorate into ventricular tachycardia or fibrillation. Renal failure may occur within 3 to 4 days. Late cerebellar degeneration and cerebral atrophy have been associated with suicidal ingestions.[102]

Two weeks after an ingestion of about 500 mg of monofluoroacetate an adult male developed paresthesias and weakness. Nerve conduction velocity studies, an electromyogram, and nerve biopsy suggested polyneuropathy, mainly of the axonal type. Four weeks later the patient exhibited marked motor weakness, muscle atrophy and tenderness, impaired position/vibratory sense, and an inability to stand.[100]

LABORATORY

Abnormalities

Hyperglycemia, hyperuricemia, and elevated serum hepatic aminotransferases and creatinine levels associated with metabolic acidosis are observed.

Analytic Method

Normal human body fluids and tissues contain fluoride and citrate but no fluoroacetate. Both gas-liquid and high-performance liquid chromatographic techniques are available to detect fluoroacetate in biologic specimens.

TREATMENT

The approach to sodium monofluoroacetate-poisoned patients is primarily supportive. Pay careful attention to respiratory status, pH, and cardiac rhythm in moderate to severe poisonings.

Animal studies suggest that calcium gluconate in combination with sodium succinate may offer a promising therapy modality in sodium fluoroacetate intoxication.[103] Clinical studies with these chemicals have not been performed.

ALPHA-CHLORALOSE

Alpha-chloralose, formed by the condensation of glucose with chloral, is metabolized to chlorine, then to trichlorethanol and trichloracetic acid. In England it is sold as "Alphakill" containing 4% alpha-chloralose. A toxic dose of chloralose is about 1 g in adults and 20 mg/kg in infants, although recovery has occurred after an alleged ingestion of 6 g. Clinical features in poisoning include hyperreflexia and hypersensitivity followed by flaccid paralysis and respiratory depression that may require artificial ventilation. Coma may be rapid (within 1 hour) in onset. Management is supportive. Gastric lavage is the preferred method of removal of unabsorbed chloralose. Chloralose may inhibit vomiting. Therefore emetics are ineffective. Keep the patient in a quiet darkened room. Seizure may respond to diazepam. Endotracheal intubation will assist ventilation and also remove excess secretion.[104]

REFERENCES—INSECTICIDES

1. Casey P, Vale JA. Deaths from pesticide poisoning in England and Wales: 1945–1989. Hum Exper Toxicol 1994;13: 95–101.
2. Thompson JP, Casey PB, Vale JA. Suspected paediatric pesticide poisoning in the UK. II. Home accident surveillance system, 1989–1991. Hum Exp Toxicol 1994;13:534–536.
3. Casey PB, Thompson JP, Vale JA. Suspected paediatric poisoning in the UK. I. Home accident surveillance system, 1982–1988. Hum Exper Toxicol 1994;13:529–533.
4. Morgan DR. Recognition and management of pesticide poisonings. 4th ed. Washington, DC: US Environmental Protection Agency EPA-540/9-88-001, 1989.
5. Hayes WJ Jr. Toxicology of pesticides. Baltimore, MD. Williams & Wilkins, 1975, p. 317.
6. Brewster MA, Hulka BS, Lavy TL. Biomarkers of pesticide exposure. Rev Environ Contam Toxicol 1992;128:17–42.
7. Karalliedde L, Senanayake N, Ariaratnam A. Acute organophosphorus insecticide poisoning during pregnancy. Hum Toxicol 1988;7:363–364.
8. Guillermo FP, Pretel CMM, Roya FT, Macias MJP, Ossorio RA, Gomez JAA, Vidal CJ. Prolonged suxamethonium-induced neuromuscular blockade associated with organophosphate poisoning. Br J Anaesth 1988;61:233–236.
9. Weeks DB, Ford D. Prolonged suxamethonium-induced neuromuscular block associated with organophosphate poisoning. Br J Anaesth 1989;62:237.
10. Karalliedde L, Henry JA. Effects of organophosphates on skeletal muscle. Hum Exp Toxicol 1993;12:289–296.
11. de Bleecker JL, Van den Neucker K, Colardyn F. Intermediate syndrome in organophosphorus poisoning: a prospective study. Crit Care Med 1993;21:1706–1711.
12. de Bleecker J, Van den Neucker K, Willems J. The intermediate syndrome in organophosphate poisoning. Presentation of a case and review of the literature. Clin Toxicol 1992; 30:321–329.
13. de Bleecker J, Willems J, Van der Neucker K, De Reuck J, Vogelaers D. Prolonged toxicity with intermediate syndrome after combined parathion and methyl parathion poisoning. Clin Toxicol 1992;30:333–345.
14. Lankisch PG, Muller C-H, Niederstadt H, Brand A. Painless acute pancreatitis subsequent to anticholinesterase insecticide (Parathion) intoxication. Am J Gastroenterol 1990; 85:872–875.
15. Weizman Z, Sofen S. Acute pancreatitis in children with anticholinesterase insecticide intoxication. Pediatrics 1992;90: 204–206.
16. Haddad LM. Organophosphate poisoning—intermediate syndrome? Clin Toxicol 1992;30:331–332.
17. Stephens R, Spurgeon A, Calvert IA, Beach J, Levy LS, Berry H et al. Neuropsychological effects of long-term exposure to organophosphates in sheep dip. Lancet 1995;345: 1135–1149.
18. Gerkin R, Cury S. Persistently elevated plasma insecticide levels in severe methylparathion poisoning. Vet Hum Toxicol 1987;29:483–484.
19. He F. Organophosphates and delayed neuropathy—is NTE alive and well? Toxicol Appl Pharmacol 1990;102:395–399.
20. Lotti M. Scientific basis of risk assessment and biological monitoring for organophosphorus induced polyneuropathy. In: Volans GN, Smith J, Sullivan FM, Turner P, eds. Basic science in toxicology. London: Taylor & Frances, 1990; 133–142.
21. Mandel JS, Berlinger NT, Kay N, Conwett J, Reape M III. Organophosphate exposure inhibits nonspecific esterase staining in human blood monocytes. Am J Indust Med 1989; 15:207–212.
22. Zovot U, Castorena JJ, Garriott JC. A case of fatal ingestion of malathion. Am J Forensic Med Pathol 1993;14:51–53.
23. Golsousidis H, Kokkas V. Use of 19,590 mg of atropine during 24 days of treatment after a case of unusually severe parathion poisoning. Hum Toxicol 1985;4:339–340.
24. Le Blanc FN, Benson BE, Gilg AD. A severe organophosphate poisoning requiring the use of an atropine drip. Clin Toxicol 1986;24:69–76.
25. Burgess ED, Audette RJ. Limited effectiveness of charcoal hemoperfusion in malathion poisoning. Pharmacotherapy 1990;10:410–412.
26. Haley KJ, Mortensen ME. Intraosseous infusion of antidote in an organophosphate poisoned child. Vet Hum Toxicol 1990; 32:370.
27. Shockley LW. The use of inhaled nebulized atropine for the treatment of malathion poisoning. Clin Toxicol 1989;27: 183–192.
28. Farrar HC, Wells TG, Kearns GL. Use of continuous infusion of pralidoxime for treatment of organophosphate poisoning in children. J Pediatr 1990;116:648–661.
29. Johnson MK, Vale JA, Marrs TC, Meredith TJ. Pralidoxime for organophosphorus poisoning. Lancet 1992;340:6.
30. Vale JA, Meredith TJ, Heath A. High dose atropine in organophosphorus poisoning. Postgrad Med J 1990;66:878–881.
31. Bentur Y, Nutenko I, Tsipinicek A, Raichlin-Eisenkraft B, Teitelman U. Pharmacokinetics of obidoxime in organophosphate poisoning associated with renal failure. Clin Toxicol 1993;31:315–322.
32. Selden BS, Curry SC. Prolonged succinylcholine-induced paralysis in organophosphate insecticide poisoning. Ann Emerg Med 1987;16:215–217
33. Goldstein DA, McGuigan MA, Ripley BD. Acute tricresylphosphate intoxication in childhood. Hum Toxicol 1988;7:179–182.
34. Winek CL, Whaba WW, Edelstein J. Sudden death following accidental ingestion of chlormequat. J Anal Toxicol 1990; 14:257–258.
35. Koppel C, Forycki Z, Ibe K. Hemoperfusion in severe dimethoate poisoning. Intensive Care Med 1986;12:110–112.
36. Lie B, Breder O, Rygnestad T, Stromme JH, Wickstrom E, Jacobson D. Dimethoate self-poisoning in three cases. Proc Eur Assoc Pois Cont Centers Clin Toxicol, 1988; p. 16.
37. Javanovic D, Randjelovic S, Joksovic D. A case of unusual suicide poisoning by organophosphorus insecticide methoate. Hum Exp Toxicol 1990;9:99–151.
38. Magler J, Braekmann PA, Willems JL, Verpooten GA, De Broe ME. Combined hemoperfusion-hemodialysis in organophosphate poisoning. J Appl Toxicol 1981;1:199.
39. Okonek S, Henningsen B, Bork R, Kusche P, Maintz J, Schuster CJ. Hemoperfusion zar behandling von intoxikatimen durch die insektizide demeton-S-methylsulfoxide und dimethoate. In: Mengler S, Kleber B, Seiffert B, eds. Moglichkeiten und Granzen der Hemoperfusion. Fresenices, Wetzlar, 1978; pp 66.
40. Jackson RJ. Pesticides as a public health concern in California. West J Med 1983;139:363–364.
41. Desi I, Nagymajtenyi L. Acute and subacute neurotoxicity and cardiotoxicity of anticholinesterases. In: Ballantyne B, Marrs TL, eds. Clinical and experimental toxicology of organophosphates and carbamates. Oxford: Butterworth-Heinemann, 1992, pp. 84–89.
42. Okonek S, Boelcke G, Hollmann N. Therapeutic properties of hemodialysis and blood exchange transfusion in organophosphate poisoning. Eur J Intensive Care Med 1976;2:13.
43. Heath A, May DG, Naukam RJ, Kamban JR, Branch RA. Insecticide overdose. A case study on carbaryl kinetics. Proc Euro Assoc Pois Cont Center Toxicol, 1988; p. 65.

44. Burgess JL, Bernstein JN, Hurlbut K. Aldicarb poisoning. A case report with prolonged cholinesterase inhibition and improvement after pralidoxime therapy. Arch Intern Med 1994;154:221–224.
45. Lifshitz M, Rotenberg M, Sofer S, Tamiri T, Shahak E, Almog S. Carbamate poisoning and oxime treatment in children: a clinical and laboratory study. Pediatrics 1984;93:652–655.
46. Sterr SH, Rognerud B, Fiskum SE, Lyngaas S. Effect of toxogonin and P25 on the toxicity of carbamates and organophosphates. Acta Pharmacol Toxicol 1979;45:9–15.
47. Natoff IL, Reiff B. Effects of oximes on the acute toxicity of anticholinesterase carbamates. Toxicol Appl Pharmacol 1973;25:569–573.
48. Casey P. Should we recommend the use of pralidoxime in carbamate insecticide poisoning. Personal communication. Birmingham, UK: First European Training Course for Poisons Information Specialists and Clinical Toxicologists, November 1992.
49. Garber M. Carbamate poisoning. The "other" insecticide. Pediatrics 1987;79:734–738.
50. Kurtz PH. Pralidoxime in the treatment of carbamate intoxication. Am J Emerg Med 1990;8:68–70.
51. Saiyed HN, Sadhu HG, Bhatnagar VK, Dewan A, Venkaiah K, Kahyap SK. Cardiac toxicity following short-term exposure to methomyl in spraymen and rabbits. Hum Exper Toxicol 1992;11:93–97.
52. Liddle JA, Kimbrough RD, Needham LL, Cline RE, Smrek AL, Yert LV et al. A fatal episode of accidental methomyl poisoning. Clin Toxicol 1979;15:159–167.
53. Michalodimitrakis EN, Tsatsakis AM. Fatal methomyl poisoning in Crete. Abstract K20. Proc Am Acad Forensic Sci, New Orleans, February 17–22, 1992.
54. Miyazaki T, Yashiki M, Kojuma T, Chikasue F, Ochiai A, Hidam Y. Fatal and non-fatal methomyl intoxication in an attempted double suicide. Forensic Sci Int 1989;42:263–270.
55. Natoff I, Reiff B. Effects of oximes on the acute toxicity of anticholinesterase carbamates. Toxicol Appl Pharmacol 1973;25:469–473.
56. Martinez-Chuecos J, Molinero-Somolino F, Sole-Violan J, Rubio-Sanz R. Management of methomyl poisoning. Hum Exp Toxicol 1990;9:251–254.
57. Kojima T, Noda J, Yashiki M, Chikasue F, Miyazaki T. Methomyl poisoning: an intoxication case and an animal experiment. Proc 24th Meeting Int Assoc Forensic Toxicol. Banff, Canada, July 28–31, 1987; pp. 505–511.
58. Tsatsakis AM, Michalodimitrakis EN, Tsakalof AK. Three lethal cases of poisoning involving lannate (methomyl). Bull Int Assoc Forensic Toxicol 1992;22:23–26.
59. Morse DL, Baker EL Jr, Kimbrough Rd, Wisseman CL. Propanil-chloracne and methomyl toxicity in workers of a pesticide manufacturing plant. Clin Toxicol 1979;15:13–21.
60. Chapman RA, Harris CR. Determination of residues of methomyl and oxamyl and their oximes in crops by gas-liquid chromatography of oxime trimethylsilyl ethers. J Chromatogr 1979;171:249–262.
61. Driskell WJ, Groce DF, Hill RH Jr. Methomyl in the blood of a pilot who crashed during aerial spraying. J Anal Toxicol 1991;15:339–340.
62. Tsakalof AK, Tsatsakis AM, Mixadodimetratis. Two fatal poisonings due to methomyl. Bull Int Assoc Forensic Toxicol 1993;23:24–27.
63. Ekins BR, Geller RJ, Khasigian PA, Carlson TS. Severe carbamate poisoning caused by methomyl with clinical improvement produced by pralidoxime. Vet Hum Toxicol 1993;35:358.
64. Koyama K, Andou Y, Saruki K, Matsuo H. Delayed and severe toxicities of a herbicide containing glufosinate and a surfactant. Vet Hum Toxicol 1994;36:17–18.
65. Stehr-Green PA, Wohlleb JC, Royce W, Head SL. An evaluation of serum pesticide residue levels and liver function in persons exposed to dairy products contaminated with heptachlor. JAMA 1988;259:374–377.
66. Steentoft A. A case of fatal dieldrin poisoning. Med Sci Law 1979;19:268–269.
67. Reddy DB, Edward VD, Abrahams GJS et al. Fatal endrin poisoning: a detailed autopsy, histopathological and experimental study. J Ind Med Assoc 1966;46:121–124.
68. Davies JE, Dedhia HV, Morgade C et al. Lindane poisonings. Arch Dermatol 1983;119:142–144.
69. Tenenbein M. Seizures after lindane therapy in adults. Vet Hum Toxicol 1990;32:363.
70. Burton BT, Will UK, Brunett PH, Chandler DB, Wagner S, Giffin S. Seizure following lindane ingestion in a patient pretreated with phenytoin. Vet Hum Toxicol 1991;33:391.
71. Rao CVSR, Shreenivas R, Singh V, Perez-Atayde A, Woolf A. Disseminated intravascular coagulation in a case of fatal lindane poisoning. Vet Hum Toxicol 1988;30:132–134.
72. Verderber L, Lavin P, Wesley R. Pseudotumor cerebri and chronic benzene hexachloride (lindane) exposure. Thorax 1991;454:1123.
73. Farley D. From tainted feed to mother's milk. A pesticide's devastating journey through the food chain. FDA Consumer 1987;21:38–40.
74. Curley A, Copeland MF, Kimbrough RD. Chlorinated hydrocarbon insecticides in organs of stillborn and blood of newborn babies. Arch Environ Health 1969;19:628.
75. Konje JC, Otolorin EO, Sotunmbi PT, Ladipo OA. Insecticide poisoning in pregnancy. A case report. J Reprod Med 1992;37:992–994.
76. Hadrzynski CL, Morgan DR, Winsett O, Roy D, Snodgrass WR. Mobilization of a halogenated hydrocarbon pesticide from body fat in man: lindane. Vet Hum Toxicol 1986;28: 471.
77. Bernardelli BC, Gennari MC. Death caused by ingestion of endosulfan. J Forensic Sci 1987;32:1109–1112.
78. Shemesh Y, Bourvine A, Gold D, Bracha P. Survival after acute endosulfan intoxication. Clin Toxicol 1988;26:265–268.
79. Tsai WJ, Yang GY, Ger J, Chung HM, Deng JF. Acute massive endosulfan poisoning. A study of 14 cases. Vet Hum Toxicol 1988;30:370.
80. Coronado JLB, Gomez RJG, Rubi JCM, Rull JRV, Martinez AMS, Martinez MP. Acute intoxication by endosulfan. Proc 5th World Congress on Intensive and Critical Care Medicine. Kyoto, Japan, September 3–8, 1989, p. 225.
81. Blanco-Coronago JL, Repetto M, Ginestal RJ, Vincente JR, Yelamis F, Lardelli A. Acute intoxication by endosulfan. Clin Toxicol 1992;30:575–583.
82. Menendez M, Martinez D, Gimenez P, Jurado C, Repetto M. Five cases (one of them fatal) of endosulfan poisoning. Bull Int Assoc Forensic Toxicol 1988;20(1):28–29.
83. Wax PM, Hoffman RS, Goldfrank LR. Fatality associated with inhalation of a pyrethrum insecticide. Vet Hum Toxicol 1991; 33:363.
84. Tucker SB, Flannigan SA. Cutaneous effects from occupational exposure to fenvalerate. Arch Toxicol 1983;54:195–202.
85. He F, Wang S, Liu L, Chen S, Zhang Z, Sun J. Clinical manifestations and diagnosis of acute pyrethroid poisoning. Arch Toxicol 1989;63:54–58.
86. Chen S, Zhang Z, He F, Yao P, Wu Y, Sun J et al. An epidemiological study on occupational acute pyrethroid poisoning in cotton farmers. Br J Ind Med 1991;48:77–81.
87. Taplin D, Meinking FL. Pyrethrins and pyrethroids in dermatology. Arch Dermatol 1990;126:213–221.
88. Paton DL, Walker JS. Pyrethrin poisoning from commercial shampoo. Flee and tick spray. Am J Emerg Med 1988;6:232–235.
89. Culver CA, Malina JJ, Talbert RL. Probable anaphylactoid reaction to a pyrethrin pediculicide shampoo. Clin Pharm 1988;7:846–849.
90. Fumigants. In: Morgan DR, ed. Recognition and management of pesticide poisonings. Washington, DC. US Environmental Protection Agency. EPA-540/9-88-001. 1989, pp. 131–145.
91. Reynolds JEF. Martindale: The extra pharmacopoeia. London: The Pharmaceutical Press, 1989, p. 918.
92. Physicians desk reference. 45th ed. Oradell, NJ: Medical Economics, 1991, p. 2294.
93. Arditti J, Jouglard J. Surdosage percutane de crotaminon et suspission de methemoglobinemie. Bull Med Leg Toxicol 1978;21:661–662.
94. Green RC. Westwood Squibb. Buffalo, NY: Personal Communication, March 20, 1991.

95. De Wilde A-R, Heyndrickx A, Carton D. A case of fatal rotenone poisoning in a child. J Forensic Sci 1986;31:1492–1498.
96. Meredith TJ, Dawling S, McMicol MW. Crotamiton overdose. Hum Exp Toxicol 1990;9:57.
97. Egekeze JO, Oehme FW. Sodium monofluoroacetate (SMFA, Compound 1080): a literature review. Vet Hum Toxicol 1979;21:411–416.
98. Gajdusek DC, Luther G. Fluoroacetate poisoning: a review and report of a case. Am J Dis Child 1950;79:310–320.
99. Chung HM. Acute renal failure caused by acute monofluoroacetate poisoning. Vet Hum Toxicol 1984;26(Suppl 2):29–32.
100. Yang GY, Tominack RL, Kaok P, Deng JF. Toxic neuropathy following rodenticide poisoning. Vet Hum Toxicol 1987; 29:480.
101. Reigart JR, Brueggeman L, Keil JE. Sodium fluoroacetate poisoning. Am J Dis Child 1975;129:1224–1226.
102. Trabes J, Rason N, Abrahami E. Computed tomography demonstration of brain damage due to acute sodium monofluoroacetate poisoning. Clin Toxicol 1982;20:85–92.
103. Omara F, Sisodia CS. Evaluation of potential antidotes for sodium fluoroacetate in mice. Vet Hum Toxicol 1990;32:407–431.
104. Thomas HM, Sumpan D, Prescott LF. The toxic effects of alpha-chloralose. Hum Toxicol 1988;7:285–287.

HERBICIDES

PARAQUAT

Paraquat (1,1-dimethyl-4,4'-bipyridylium chloride), a para-substituted quaternary bipyridyl cation, is the most important bipyridyl herbicide in the group of five: paraquat, diquat, chlormequat, difenzoquat, and morfamquat.[1]

Although deaths are reported from accidental paraquat exposure by inhalation and transdermal absorption, the method for suicide is nearly always oral ingestion. Ingestion of concentrated liquid solutions invariably proves fatal, whereas dilute solid formulations rarely cause death. Self-injections (intramuscularly of 2.5% and 20% paraquat solution) led to death in 72 hours and 8 days in 2 patients, respectively. Serum paraquat levels were 1300 μg/L in one patient 9 hours after injection and 3200 μg/L 6 hours after injection in the other.[2] One patient died of paraquat poisoning following insertion per vagina of a tampon inadvertently soaked in paraquat.[3] Chronic occupational exposure to paraquat does not appear to cause pulmonary toxicity.[4]

A nonswallowable formulation—paraquat water-dispersible granule (WRD) contains a natural thickening agent that makes it more difficult to swallow.[5]

STRUCTURE AND CLASSIFICATION

Chemically, paraquat is 1,1'-dimethyl-4,4'-bipyridylium ion. It is present in commercial preparations as the dichloride or dimethyl sulfate salt.[6] 4,4'-Bipyridyl as an impurity is permitted in paraquat at a maximum concentration of 0.25%.[7] When paraquat is thermally decomposed, it may release toxic degradation products such as carbon monoxide, hydrogen chloride, and oxides of sulfur and nitrogen.[7]

USES

Paraquat is used as a desiccant, contact herbicide, defoliant, and plant growth regulator. Paraquat is classified for restricted use under the U.S. Federal Insecticide, Fungicide, and Rodenticide Act (FIFRA) and is limited to use by or under the supervision of a certified pesticides applicator.

PRODUCT FORMULATION

Paraquat is formulated as a water-dilutable liquid concentration (20 to 44%), a medium concentration (7 to 10%), as granules (2.5%) to be dissolved in water, or as an aerosol (0.44%). It is sold commercially under the trade names Cekuquat, Dextron X, Dextrone, Gramoxone, Herbaxon, Herboxone, Pillarxone, Pillarquat, Total, and Toxer and was previously available under the trade names Esgram, Goldquat, Dexuron, Sweep, and Weedol.[6,8]

Paraquat is commonly combined with diquat in commercial herbicides.[9] It is available in trade name combination products such as Actor, Herbaxon, Preglone, Priglone, and Weedol (with diquat); and Terraklene and Pathclear (with simazine).[6,7,10]

Common commercial preparations are a 5% powder for domestic use and a 10 to 30% aqueous concentrate for agricultural usage.[11–13] The liquid technical product is of 20 to 50% concentration.[14] A stenching agent, a blue-colored dye, and an emetic have been added to liquid formulations manufactured by Imperial Chemical Industries (ICI) in an attempt to reduce the likelihood of fatal ingestion poisoning.[11,15]

Concentrated solutions (12 to 20%) are more dangerous than dilute solutions because they are more caustic, and also because they contain a greater amount of paraquat per unit volume. Solid (granular) preparations are available commercially in several countries. These usually cause benign poisonings because their paraquat concentrations are low.

ACUTE TOXIC DOSAGE

Vale and colleagues have distinguished three degrees of paraquat intoxication that appear dose related[16]:

Group 1

Mild poisoning follows the ingestion or injection of <20 mg of paraquat ion/kg body weight (i.e., <1 sachet of 2.5% [w/v] Weedol). Patients are asymptomatic or develop vomiting and diarrhea. Full recovery occurs, but there may be a transient fall in the gas transfer factor (TLCO) and vital capacity.

Group 2

Moderate to severe poisoning follows the ingestion or injection of 20 to 40 mg of paraquat ion/kg body weight (i.e., >1 sachet of 2.5% [w/v] Weedol or <15 mL of 20% [w/v] concentrate). Patients suffer vomiting and diarrhea and develop generalized symptoms indicative of systemic toxicity. Pulmonary fibrosis develops in all cases, but recovery may occur. In addition, renal failure and sometimes hepatic dysfunction may supervene. Death occurs in the majority of cases, but can be delayed for 2 or 3 weeks.

Group 3

Acute fulminant poisoning follows the ingestion of more than (usually considerably in excess of) 40 mg of paraquat ion/kg body weight (i.e., >15 mL of 20% [w/v] concentrate). In addition to nausea and vomiting, there is marked ulceration of the oropharynx with multiple organ (cardiac, respiratory, hepatic, renal, adrenal, pancreatic, neurologic) failure. In this group the mortality is 100%. Death may occur within 24 hours of the overdose, but is never delayed for more than 1 week.

Marijuana

No cases of paraquat pulmonary toxicity have every been documented among smokers of paraquat-treated marijuana, and it has been shown that the temperatures generated by smoking inactivate the paraquat.[17]

OCCUPATIONAL EXPOSURE

Several cases of ocular damage were reported in workers who accidentally splashed paraquat in their eyes during preparation or application. Initial irritation has been followed by conjunctival loss and anterior uveitis,[18] corneal lesions,[19] severe ocular surface destruction,[20] severe eye injury,[21] or variable degrees of conjunctivitis. Healing of such ocular lesions has been relatively slow, taking between 2 and 10 weeks,[22,23] but recovery has always been complete as long as secondary infections were controlled and palpebral adhesions prevented.

Long-term

Long-term use of paraquat has been found to be safe under appropriate conditions of hygiene, with protective equipment, and avoidance of aerosol inhalation.[24]

TOXICOKINETICS

Absorption

Pulmonary Absorption

Following inhalation, paraquat is poorly absorbed because most aerosolized particles have a diameter greater than 5 μm and cannot reach the alveolar barrier. Only a few cases of systemic paraquat poisoning by the inhalational route have been described.[25]

Dermal Absorption

Paraquat cannot be absorbed significantly through intact human skin. However, damage to the skin, either by paraquat itself or by other means, allows greater systemic absorption and, possibly, poisoning.

A single exposure of healthy skin to paraquat solution induced paraquat levels in the plasma and urine less than 50 mg/mL.[26] Prolonged contact with paraquat solutions at concentrations as low as 5 g/L paraquat cation can cause systemic poisoning that may be fatal.

Subcutaneous Absorption

Daniel and Gage[27] have reported systemic absorption of paraquat following subcutaneous administration as being about 10% of the administered dose.

Ingestion

Absorption after ingestion is considered to be small, ranging from 1 to 5% of the quantity ingested.[28] Under these conditions, very low lethal plasma paraquat concentrations may be observed (2 mg/L after 4 h, 0.16 mg/L after 16 h, and 0.1 mg/L after 24 h, respectively) following paraquat ingestion (35 mg/kg).[29] Absorption is relatively rapid, with the peak plasma level occurring 2 to 4 hours after ingestion.

Distribution (V_D)

Lungs

The lungs are the principal target organ for paraquat toxicity.[30] The kinetics of paraquat in the lungs show a rapid decline with an elimination half-life of 20 minutes, followed by a slower decline with a half-life of about 50 hours.[31] Peak paraquat concentrations in this tissue are reached 4 to 5 hours after intravenous administration and 5 to 7 hours after ingestion, provided that renal function is normal.

Volume of Distribution

The apparent volume of distribution (V_D) ranges from 1.2 to 1.6 L/kg.

The uptake of paraquat by lung tissue in the human is an early process that is essentially complete at the time of presentation to medical facilities.[32]

Plasma paraquat concentration (Figs. 68–1 and 68–2) exhibits a mean distribution half-life ($T_{1/2}$) of 5 hours and a mean elimination half-life ($T_{1/2}$ beta) of 8 hours. Cardiovascular collapse appears early in intoxication and is associated with the distribution phase. Death related to pulmonary fibrosis is late and is associated with the elimination phase. Muscle may represent an important reservoir, explaining the long persistence of paraquat in plasma and urine for several weeks or months after poisoning.[33]

Elimination

Renal elimination is rapid, with 80 to 90% being excreted in the first 6 hours and urinary recovery being almost 100% complete by 24 hours.[34] Paraquat is not metabolized, but is reduced to an unstable free radical that is then reoxidized to produce a superoxide radical.

INTERACTIONS

Ethanol

Three chronic rum drinkers who drank 80 g ethanol per day survived after each had drunk more than 20 mL "Gramoxone" (20% w/v paraquat). The exact mechanism of interaction remains to be elucidated.[35]

Pregnancy

Paraquat levels in one case of paraquat exposure during pregnancy disclosed paraquat levels five times higher in cord blood and the baby than in the mother. Paraquat may be detected in the amniotic fluid. The value of emergency cesarean operation in these patients is unclear. No fetus has survived.[36]

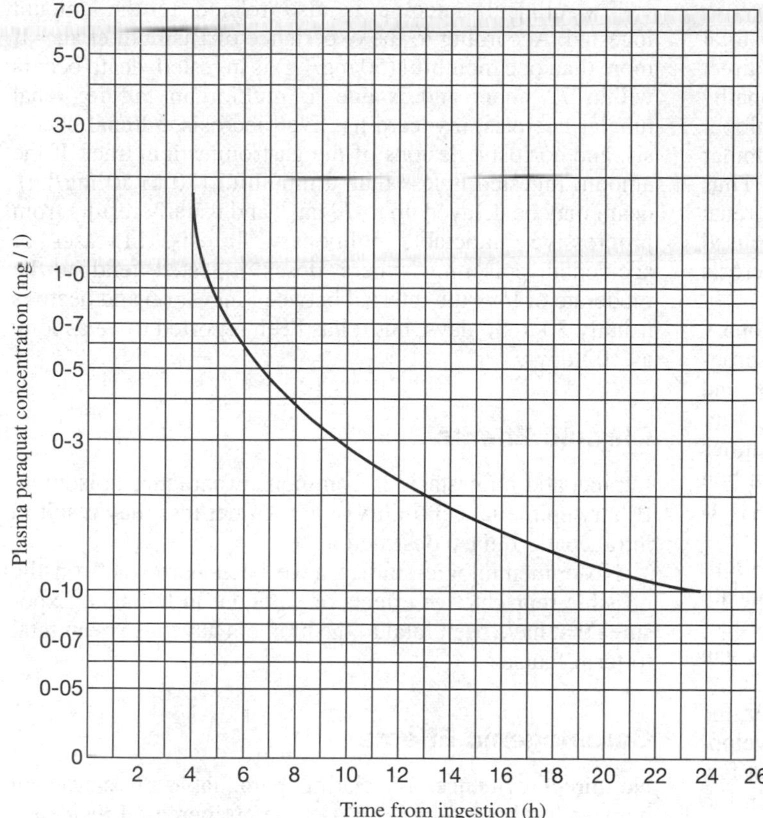

Figure 68–1 Patients whose plasma paraquat concentrations related to time from ingestion are above the line are likely to die, and those below survive. There are insufficient data to interpret concentrations measured within 4 hours. (Adapted from Proudfoot AT. Acute poisoning. 2nd ed. Oxford: Butterworth-Heinemann, 1993.)

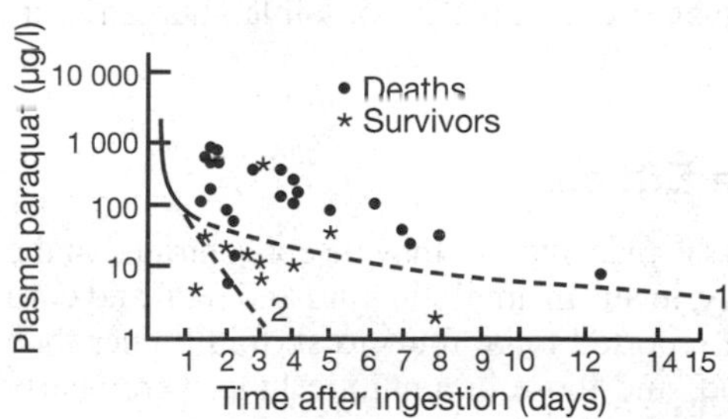

Figure 68–2 Plasma paraquat concentrations for 30 patients admitted after 24 h. The dashed lines represent the prolongation of Proudfoot's line using the hyperbolic equation (curve 1) and the triexponential equation (curve 2). (Adapted from Scherrmann JM et al. Hum Toxicol 1987;6:91–93.)

A woman of 28 weeks gestation died of paraquat poisoning 20 days after ingestion.[37] A 20-week-pregnant female drank a few sips of "Weedol" containing paraquat. One hour afterwards she had a gastric lavage and 30% Fuller's Earth orally every 2 hours for 24 hours, then 4 hourly for 24 hours. She also received 40 mg furosemide intramuscularly with her first dose. Blood paraquat levels were: 1 hour 18 µg/L, 3 hour 8 µg/L, 8 hour <1 µg/L. The baby was born at term and did well.[38]

CLINICAL PRESENTATION

Ingestion

Bismuth, Wong, and Hall[39] describe several forms of acute poisoning:

1. The Typical Form[40]
   This form is noted following ingestion of 30 to 50 mg/kg of paraquat, equivalent to a single swallow of 12 to 20% concentrated commercial products.

   a. Initial phase. The initial phase is characterized by the appearance of lesions due to the herbicide's causticity. Ingestion is immediately followed by buccopharyngeal, esophageal, epigastric, and gastric pain. Vomiting almost always ensues, even in the absence of emetic additives in the commercial preparation. Secondarily, abdominal colic and diarrhea are noted occasionally. Caustic lesions of the lips, oral cavity, and gastrointestinal tract are established over the first few hours following ingestion.[40] Patients with such lesions can be completely aphonic and aphasic and may thus require total parenteral nutrition (TPN). Fibroptic esophagogastroscopy frequently shows mucosal lesions. These are usually superficial, although several cases of gastric perforation and massive gastrointestinal hemorrhage have been reported.[41–43]
   b. Second phase. Between the second and fifth days following ingestion, renal failure[44,45] and hepatocellular necrosis develop. Functional insufficiency is

often noted, due to hypovolemia secondary to gastrointestinal fluid losses and a decreased or total lack of oral fluid intake. Paraquat itself has direct renal toxicity. It generally causes a pure tubulopathy with proximal predominance. Such renal tubulopathies usually evolve—as with all causes of tubular necrosis—to full recovery without sequelae. Thus paraquat-poisoned patients frequently recover renal function by the time of death. The liver lesion caused by paraquat is centrilobular hepatocellular necrosis and is most often moderate.[16]

c. Third phase. Delayed development of pulmonary fibrosis is responsible for the generally poor prognosis in acute paraquat poisoning. Clinically and radiographically, this appears several days after ingestion. However, alveolar-capillary abnormalities are present much earlier. A decrease in the carbon monoxide diffusing capacity (DL_{CO} or TL_{CO}) is noted from the first day.[46]

   Pulmonary fibrosis leads rapidly to the development of refractory hypoxemia, resulting in death over a period of 5 days to several weeks. Neither spontaneous nor assisted artificial ventilation can delay the fatal outcome.

   Pulmonary changes are shown to depend on the quantity of paraquat ingested, with fibrosis developing only in those patients who survived the first few days after ingestion. Death usually occurs within 1 to 2 weeks, but progressive pulmonary fibrosis and respiratory failure can occur even up to 6 weeks after paraquat ingestion.

d. Destructive Phase. Irrespective of the route of administration, the earliest observed pulmonary changes caused by paraquat occur in the type I alveolar epithelial cells. The alveolar type II cell represents the only other cell type to show overt damage during this early phase of paraquat toxicity.[47]

e. Proliferative Phase. The onset of the proliferative phase occurs several days after paraquat ingestion and is characterized by a rapidly forming, extensive fibrosis.

2. The Hyperacute Form
   In cases of massive ingestion (greater than 55 mg/kg of paraquat), patients usually survive for less than 4 days and die in a setting of cardiogenic shock.[48,49] Renal and hepatic lesions are common in such cases.
3. The Subacute Form
   Ingestion of doses less than 30 mg/kg results in benign intoxication. The initial gastrointestinal insult is usually moderate. Renal and hepatic lesions are either minimal or absent.

Mortality

Mortality is related to the circumstances of the poisoning and also the type of paraquat formulation. Mortality is very high in patients poisoned with a 20% concentrate and lower with less concentrated solutions.[50] This relationship between mortality and paraquat formulation was demonstrated by Proudfoot et al[51]: mortality was 65% in patients who ingested the concentrated formulation and only 4% in those who ingested dilute solutions of the herbicide (2.5% w/v).

The clinical outcome is also related to the amount ingested. According to the experience of Bismuth et al,[52] if more than one mouthful (50 mg/kg) is ingested, death occurs within 72 hours and is due to multiorgan failure, renal tubular necrosis, myocarditis, liver necrosis, adrenal necrosis, and corrosive lesions of the gastrointestinal tract. If the amount ingested is less than a mouthful (20 to 50 mg/kg), death may be delayed up to 70 days and usually results from progressive intractable pulmonary fibrosis. In cases of accidental poisoning where doses ingested tend to be moderate or low, the interval between ingestion and death is usually 20 to 30 days, but it has been reported to be as long as 102 days.[53]

Chronic Effects

Intrahepatic cholestasis is common in paraquat poisoning. Biliary epithelial cell injury and bile duct loss may result in intrahepatic biliary obstruction.[54]

No epidemiologic studies have been performed on the possible reproductive effects of paraquat in humans. Exposures that have been fatal to the mothers have also been fatal to term fetuses.

Carcinogenic Effects

No direct evidence associating paraquat with cancer in humans has been found.[55] Based on an increased incidence of squamous cell carcinoma in the head region of Fischer 344 rats, the US Environmental Protection Agency (EPA) has classified paraquat in group C (possible human carcinogen).[56]

Reproductive Effects

Paraquat crosses the placenta and may be concentrated in the fetus. In one study, levels in amniotic fluid and fetal and cord blood have been reported to be four- to sixfold higher than in maternal blood, and those in amniotic fluid were nearly twice the maternal level.[57] Previous exposure to paraquat may not be hazardous to future pregnancies.

LABORATORY

Analytic Methods

The dithionite test does not require sophisticated equipment as for RIA procedures, uses single reagents and 1 to 2 mL of urine, and is not time-consuming. Samples giving no color or a very light blue color come from patients who have a good prognosis. Blue colors are generally associated with a fatal prognosis. For "out of hours" emergency use the direct qualitative dithionite colorimetric urine paraquat test is useful.[58] The color intensity is well correlatcd to the prognosis with the first urine sample following paraquat ingestion (analysis time, 5 minutes).[59] Use an immunoassay for quantitative analysis of paraquat in plasma and compare the paraquat level with those given by prognosis scales (analysis time, 60 minutes). Plasma paraquat concentrations have a higher predictive role, but the use of urine data may assist the clinician in making therapeutic decisions more rapidly.[60]

Paraquat and diquat in serum and urine may be assayed simultaneously using second-derivative spectroscopy. The method is less sensitive than a HPLC method; however, all serum analyses are complete within about 10 minutes and urine samples within 5 minutes.[60] A high-performance liquid chromatography is available for the determination of 4-4′-bipyridine (a major product in paraquat manufacturing) in water and air. The limit of detection is 2 ng of 4-4′-bipyridine.[61] A radioimmunoassay proposed for paraquat has a sensitivity to at least 0.5 ng paraquat.[62]

Urine Paraquat

The preferred method to measure paraquat in urine due to favorable sensitivity, analysis time, and cost is spectrophotometry. Many potentially interfering components in human urine make the direct use of dithionite reagent difficult. A method has been proposed for pretreating the urine specimen with an anion exchange resin. It requires 8 mL of urine and takes 20 minutes for the full procedure. The urinary paraquat in most patients who survive is below 1 μg/mL. Detection limits are 100, 0.05, and 0.005 μg/L by spot test, zero-order, and second-derivative spectrophotometry, respectively.

Plasma Levels

Limited anecdotal evidence suggests that survivors of paraquat poisoning may be left with a restrictive type of pulmonary dysfunction.[63]

Blood Levels

Serum levels greater than 0.2 μg/mL at 24 hours and 0.1 μg/mL at 48 hours are usually associated with a fatal outcome.[29,64,65]

In 1979 Proudfoot et al[29] first demonstrated prognostic value of paraquat plasma levels. All patients whose plasma levels were less than those on a plot joining 2 mg/L at 4 hours after ingestion and 0.1 mg/L at 24 hours after ingestion survived; those whose plasma levels were above this line at comparable times died (Fig. 68–1). Scherrmann et al[58] expanded the above plot beyond 24 hours after ingestion while retaining its prognostic value (Fig. 68–2).

Paraquat plasma levels allow prediction of the circumstances of death: plasma paraquat concentrations greater than 10 mg/L suggest that death will occur from cardiogenic shock during the first 2 days after ingestion, while plasma concentrations less than 10 mg/L suggest a late death from pulmonary fibrosis. However, patients whose initial plasma paraquat concentrations exceed 3 mg/L do not survive, regardless of the time after ingestion when the levels are measured and despite treatment with such therapeutic modalities as hemoperfusion.[66]

Proudfoot et al[29] reported on plasma paraquat concentrations (measured by three different techniques) in 79 poisoned patients.[67] After plotting the admission plasma concentrations (on a semilogarithmic scale) from the 71 patients who presented within 24 hours, an arbitrary line was drawn joining 2.0, 0.6, 0.3, 0.16, and 0.10 mg/L at 4, 6, 10, 16 and 24 hours after ingestion, respectively, to separate fatal cases (above the line) from survivors (below the line). This line has come to be known as the *predictive* line (Fig. 68–1).

Urine Screens

All patients who die rapidly in less than 24 hours appear to show urine paraquat levels of up to 10 μg/mL. When paraquat concentrations are less than 1 μg/mL, all patients survive. Patients who died from pulmonary fibrosis had urine paraquat levels between 1 and 1000 μg/mL in a study of 30 patients.[58] When urine concentrations of less than 500 μg/L are present, no color is observed with the dithionite colorimetric test. Patients who died with pulmonary fibrosis had urine paraquat levels between 1 and 1000 mg/L.[58] This observation indicates that urine determinations may offer a rapid predictive test, but plasma paraquat concentrations have higher prognostic value.[58] If the qualitative test for urinary paraquat remains negative over the first 24 hours after an exposure, serious toxicity would not be expected.[12]

Abnormalities

Electrolytes

Hypokalemia is reported to be induced by paraquat itself and/or the additive and may be a good prognostic indicator.[68] The interval of time from ingestion to admission, serum creatinine concentration, serum potassium concentration, and arterial blood HCO_3 may bear a significant relationship to the prognosis of acute paraquat poisoning.

Radiology

Radiologic changes do not always parallel the severity of clinical symptoms. Thus the chest x-ray may be normal, particularly in those patients who die soon after ingestion from multiorgan failure. More often, patchy infiltration develops, which may progress to opacification of one or both lung fields.[16] The fibrosis can also be demonstrated on lung scans, where multiple reticulated areas adjoin cystic and tubular lucencies.[69]

Ancillary Tests

Severity Index

Sawada et al[70] developed a severity index of paraquat poisoning (SIPP) based on a study of serum paraquat concentrations in 30 patients, 20 of whom died and 10 of whom survived. Concentrations were plotted against the time from ingestion for the predictive line, and the boundary between death and survival was defined—SIPP being the time to treatment multiplied by the serum paraquat level on admission. A SIPP value of 10 separated fatal from nonfatal cases and described a line that lay above the predictive line proposed by Proudfoot et al.[29]

Plasma Concentrations and the Mode of Death

Cardiogenic shock is the usual cause of death in patients with very high plasma concentrations, while death from lower levels is due to pulmonary fibrosis and respiratory failure.

TREATMENT

Patients who ingest paraquat should be treated as medical emergencies even if asymptomatic. Ensure that ingestion has not occurred even if the patient claims to have had only dermal, inhalational, or ocular contact.[12]

Information

Specific information should be obtained including the following:

1. Delay between ingestion and admission.
2. Circumstances of poisoning (accidental or suicidal.
3. Name and concentration of the paraquat formulation and other compounds it may contain.
4. Whether the formulation ingested was diluted beforehand.
5. Amount ingested.
6. Timing and extent of vomiting after ingestion.
7. Delay between the last meal and ingestion.[71]

First 2 Hours

Perform upper gastrointestinal endoscopy to identify the extent and severity of any mucosal lesions in the esophagus or stomach. Perform rapid qualitative analysis for paraquat on urine and gastric fluid. If the qualitative test for urinary paraquat remains negative over the first 24 hours after the exposure serious toxicity will be unlikely.[12]

Priorities

Initial management has four priorities. First, fluid loss should be replaced; second, the prognosis should be determined; third, symptoms due to ulceration of the oropharynx must be relieved; fourth, appropriate supportive care for patients and relatives must be provided. In addition, it may be appropriate to consider referral to a specialist treatment center.[16]

Decontamination

Gastric Lavage

There is no definite evidence that gastric lavage is of any value in the treatment of paraquat poisoning in humans. If this procedure is used, any possible benefit is likely to be confined to the first hour following ingestion.[72]

Syrup of Ipecac

No clinical or experimental studies involving the use of ipecac syrup in paraquat poisoning have been reported. Syrup of Ipecac is no longer recommended for any ingestion, for patients who are in the hospital.

Cathartics

Whole-gut lavage has not improved outcome to date and may produce pulmonary edema in compromised patients.

Bentonite and Fuller's Earth

There is no evidence to demonstrate an improved prognosis associated with the administration of Fuller's Earth.

Activated Charcoal

Activated charcoal has not been shown to reduce systemic absorption significantly enough to affect either the morbidity or mortality in cases of paraquat poisoning.

Elimination Enhancement

Hemoperfusion

Plasma paraquat levels peak early in the course of the poisoning. Intervention with hemodialysis-hemoperfusion should thus be attempted early, probably within 10 to 12 hours after ingestion, before the absorbed paraquat is distributed extensively to the tissues.[73,74] No patients whose initial plasma paraquat concentration was greater than 3 mg/L have survived, regardless of the time after ingestion when plasma levels were measured and despite treatment with hemoperfusion.[75] Therefore patients with plasma levels of 3 mg/L or greater should probably not be considered for hemoperfusion treatment because of the uniformly poor prognosis and a lack of demonstrated efficacy of the procedure.[76]

Because of the relative ease with which continuous arteriovenous hemofiltration (CAVH) can be performed, its low cost compared with that of hemoperfusion or hemodialysis, and the continuous nature of the procedure, CAVH may still be worth considering in paraquat poisoning. It may be used in those patients who have developed renal failure or while patients are being prepared for hemoperfusion.[77] Prospective studies are indicated.

Nevertheless, even if delays incurred in measuring plasma paraquat concentration and in setting up hemodialysis or hemoperfusion could be reduced to a minimum, elimination by these procedures would achieve little because paraquat disappears rapidly from the plasma in the first few hours after ingestion as it is taken up by the tissue and excreted into the urine.[78,79]

Antidotes

Paraquat-specific antibodies have reduced the uptake of a toxic concentration of paraquat by type II cells in vitro, but no clinical studies have validated the usefulness of this procedure.[80] No antidote can be recommended currently on the basis of convincing evidence obtained in patients.[81–83]

Supportive Care

Meticulous attention to supportive care has improved the prognosis of poisoned patients and remains the mainstay of treatment for paraquat poisoning. Management includes protection of the airway, maintenance of the circulation, frequent monitoring of vital signs and blood gases, treatment of secondary infection, adequate pain relief, prevention or treatment of renal failure, replacement of blood losses, treatment of complications such as arrhythmias and seizures, and counseling of the patient and family.

The patient should be washed thoroughly with soap and water. Do not use scrubbing brushes (skin abrasion, percutaneous absorption).

Pain and distress should be reduced to a minimum. It is difficult to abolish the severe pain produced by local ulceration. Mouthwashes, ice cold fluids (e.g., ice cream, lemon mucilage), local anesthetic sprays, and lozenges have all been employed with varying degrees of success. Opiates will be required eventually in most patients to relieve general, as well as local, pain and distress. Above all, inappropriate treatment should be avoided. Thus, for example, the repeated use of cathartics when the outlook is hopeless is therapeutically irrelevant and clinically harmful.

Radiotherapy for pulmonary damage may be useful.[84] The cation resin, Kayexalate, may ultimately be useful to adsorb paraquat.[85]

Lung Transplantation

Lung transplantation would appear to be useful in a patient with extensive irreversible pulmonary fibrosis from paraquat toxicity, but with reversible damage to all other organs. Unfortunately, in the few situations where this has been attempted, there was new uptake by the transplanted lung of paraquat sequestered in other organs and the subsequent development of paraquat toxicity.[86] Lung transplantations have not reduced mortality because either the transplanted lung developed toxicity or technical complications have led to death.[77] High-dose cyclophosphamide and dexamethasone appear unlikely to improve the prognosis of paraquat poisoning.[87]

DIQUAT (TABLE 68–6)

Diquat is a dipyridyl herbicide used less frequently than paraquat. Although diquat is less toxic in animal models than paraquat, seven deaths were reported by 1983 in the English-language medical literature. Mortality in reported cases approaches 50% despite a lower LD_{50} (400 mg/kg) than for paraquat (25 to 50 mg/kg). Survival has been reported after ingestion of 300 mL of 20% diquat.[88]

TOXICOKINETICS

Humans are poisoned by oral and, rarely, pulmonary routes.[89] In animal models, only multiple large dermal applications produce toxic effects.[90] In rats, 90% of an oral dose remains in the feces. The majority (90%) of an absorbed dose is excreted unchanged by the kidneys within 24 hours.[91] No metabolites are known. Deaths have occurred after ingestion of 20 to 50 mL of Reglone (diquat 20 g/100 mL).[92]

PATHOPHYSIOLOGY

The mechanism of toxicity is similar to that of paraquat, in which superoxide radicals destroy lipid membranes; however, diquat does not cause pulmonary lesions, because of its lower affinity for lung tissue.

The activity of diquat, as well as paraquat, may be based on the liberation of hydrogen peroxide, leading to tissue destruction.[92]

CLINICAL PRESENTATION

Parkinsonism may develop within days after exposure to a diquat solution.[93] Acute and persistent parkinsonism has followed exposure of the hand to an aqueous solution of 10%

Table 68–6
Current Diquat Formulations[a]

Trade Name	Country	Formulation Type	Active Ingredients
Professional Formulations			
Reglone	UK	Aqueous solution	140 g/liter diquat ion
Reglone	Europe	Aqueous solution	200 g/liter diquat ion
Aquacide	UK	Aqueous solution	140 g/liter diquat ion
Preeglone	Spain	Aqueous solution	80 g/liter diquat ion 120 g/liter paraquat ion
Priglone	France Switzerland	Aqueous solution	80 g/liter diquat ion 120 g/liter paraquat ion
Ortho diquat Herbicide concentrate	USA	Aqueous solution	200 g/liter diquat ion
Ortho diquat Water weed killer	USA	Aqueous solution	200 g/liter diquat ion
Nonprofessional Formulations[b]			
Weedol	Various	Soluble granules	2.5 diquat ion 2.5 paraquat ion
Preeglone	Denmark Norway	Soluble granules	2.5 diquat ion 2.5 paraquat ion
Duanti	West Germany	Soluble granules	2.5 diquat ion 2.5 paraquat ion
Pathclear	UK	Soluble granules	2.5 diquat ion 2.5 paraquat ion 5.0 simazine
Gesal Super herbicide	Switzerland	Soluble granules	2.5 diquat ion 10.0 terbutylazine

[a]Adapted from Vanholder R et al. Am J Med 1981;70:1268.
[b]Active ingredients expressed as percents.

diquat dibromide. This may relate to the chemical similarity between diquat and MPTP (1-methyl-4-phenyl-1,2,3,6-tetrahydropyridine) known to elicit chronic parkinsonism in humans.[93]

LABORATORY

An enzyme-linked immunosorbent assay (ELISA) is available to determine the diquat level in human tissues.

A pyrolysis gas chromatography method is available for determination of diquat serum levels. Diquat serum levels of 0.45 μg/mL and 4.5 μg/mL have been associated with fatalities.[92]

TREATMENT

Gastric lavage should be considered early in treatment, but care must be exercised because of the expected occurrence of extensive tissue necrosis in the esophagus and stomach.[94] Prompt aggressive therapy as soon after the ingestion of diquat as possible remains the hallmark of effective therapy, even in those who have a relatively symptom-free initial interval.

MONOLINURON

Monolinuron [3-(4-chlorophenyl)-1-methoxy-1-methylurea] is a substituted urea herbicide effective against annual grasses and broad-leaved weeds. Products containing monolinuron and marketed in Europe include Arresin (monolinuron 200 g/L), Gramonol (monolinuron 140 g/L + paraquat 110 g/L), Gramonol 5 (monolinuron 154 g/L + paraquat 100 g/L), and Sonalan M (monolinuron 200 g/kg + ethalfluralin 300 g/kg).[95]

Methemoglobinemia is probably caused by the metabolites of monolinuron, which may include a hydroxychloraniline derivative. Methemoglobinemia may exacerbate the effects of a paraquat-induced hypoxia. Treat with intravenous methylene blue 1 to 2 mg/kg.

Table 68–7
Pesticide, Polychlorinated Biphenyl, Semivolatile, Volatile, and Polychlorinated Dibenzo-*p*-dioxin and Polychlorinated Dibenzofuran Data Selected from the 1982 National Human Adipose Tissue Survey for Analysis[a]

Pesticides	*Polychlorinated biphenyls*
Beta benzene hexachloride	Total PCBs
*p-p′*DDE	Trichlorobiphenyls
*p-p′*DDT	Tetrachlorobiphenyls
Mirex	Pentachlorobiphenyls
Dieldrin	Hexachlorobiphenyls
Hexachlorobenzene	Heptachlorobiphenyls
Trans nonachlor	Octachlorobiphenyls
	Nonachlorobiphenyls
	Decachlorobiphenyls
Semivolatiles	*Volatiles*
1,2,4-Trichlorobenzene	Chloroform
Triphenyl phosphate	1,1,1-Trichlorethane
Tributyl phosphate	Bromodichloromethane
Tris(2-chloroethyl)phosphate	Benzene
Diethyl phthalate	Tetrachloroethene
Di-*n*-butyl phthalate	Dibromochloromethane
Di-*n*-octyl phthalate	1,1,2-Trichloroethane
Butyl benzyl phthalate	Toluene
Naphthalene	Chlorobenzene
Phenanthrene	Ethyl benzene
	Bromoform
	Styrene
	1,1,2,2-Tetrachloroethane
	1,2-Dichlorobenzene
	1,4-Dichlorobenzene
	Ethyl phenol
	Xylene
*Polychlorinated dibenzo-*p*-dioxins and polychlorinated dibenzofurans*	
Tetrachlorodibenzo-*p*-dioxin	
1,2,3,7,8-Pentachlorodibenzo-*p*-dioxin	
Hexachlorodibenzo-*p*-dioxin	
1,2,3,4,7,8,9-Heptachlorodibenzo-*p*-dioxin	
Octachlorodibenzo-*p*-dioxin	
2,3,7,8-Tetrachlorodibenzofuran	
2,3,4,7,8-Pentachlorodibenzofuran	
Hexachlorodibenzofuran	
1,2,3,4,6,7,8-Heptachlorodibenzofuran	
Octachlorodibenzofuran	

[a]Adapted from Phillips LJ, Birchard GF. Arch Environ Contam Toxicol 1991;21:159–168.

DIOXINS[96,97] (TABLE 68–7)

EPIDEMIOLOGY

Dioxins and furans are terms applied to polychlorinated dibenzo-*p*-dioxins and polychlorinated dibenzofurans. Because 2,3,7,8-tetrachlorodibenzo-*p*-dioxin (TCDD) is the most thoroughly studied and most toxic of the 75 dioxin isomers, the term TCDD is used interchangeably with dioxins throughout.

Some Vietnam veterans were potentially exposed to dioxins through the military use of the defoliant Agent Orange (a mixture of 2,4,5-trichlorphenoxyacetic acid [2,4,5-T] and 2,4-dichlorophenoxyacetic acid [2,4-D] contaminated with TCDD).

The largest known dioxin contamination occurred between 1962 and 1970, when 12 million gallons of Agent Orange, a defoliant mixture contaminated with a form of the most toxic dioxin, were sprayed over southern and central Vietnam.[98] Tests on the Vietnamese population as recently as 1992 found that those living in the former South Vietnam had 10 times as much dioxin in blood and tissue samples as did the North Vietnamese. Now that relations between the United States and Vietnam have improved, further studies are planned of the health effects of the spraying.

Several areas of the United States have been contaminated as a result of industrial discharges or spraying of dirt roads with dioxin-contaminated waste oils. Three areas that have received notoriety are Love Canal in Niagara Falls, New York; Times Beach, Missouri; and Newark, New Jersey. The most highly publicized accident affecting a residential population was an explosion at a chemical plant that resulted in an airborne discharge of dioxins over Seveso, Italy, in 1976. More than 37,000 people lived in an area that may have been contaminated by dioxins. There were no deaths from acute poisoning.

STRUCTURE/PRODUCT FORMULATION

Dioxins are formed during the production of many chlorinated organic solvents, hexachlorophene, and the herbicide 2,4,5-T. Emission from coal-burning power plants, exhaust from diesel engines, and the incomplete burning of wastes containing chlorine, such as PVC plastic, form both dioxins and furans.

TOXICOKINETICS

Dioxins enter the body by ingestion, inhalation, and dermal absorption. The metabolic pathway of TCDD for humans has not been established. Metabolism is primarily by hepatic detoxification, with the major metabolites consisting of hydroxylated or methoxylated TCDD derivatives. These are excreted as glucuronide and sulfate conjugates. Because of the lipophilic nature of milk, nursing females decrease their body burden of TCDD through lactation. Dioxins distribute to organs according to lipid content and readily accumulate in body fat.

The half-life of TCDD ranges from several hours (on the surface of plants) to 7.1 years (in human serum and adipose tissue).

EFFECTS

No deaths due to systemic dioxin toxicity in humans have been reported. Only two clinical effects have been repeatedly observed in exposed populations: chloracne and transient hepatic effects. Soft-tissue sarcomas, lymphomas, peripheral neuropathy, birth defects, and reproductive effects have been studied but remain unconfirmed.

Dermatologic Effects (Chloracne)

Acneform lesions may appear as early as 1 to 3 weeks after dioxin exposure. The lesions are small, pale yellow cysts that arise from altered differentiation of acinar sebaceous basal cells in keratinocytes. The acne primarily involves the face, especially the periorbital, temporal, and malar areas, as well as the upper body. Most cases of chloracne resolve in 1 to 3 years. Chloracne can also be caused by chloro- and bromonaphthalenes, polychlorinated and polybrominated biphenyls (PCBs, PBBs), pentachlorophenol, and tetrachlorobenzene.

Chloracne is the only overt effect of dioxin exposure in human populations; the absence of this effect does not rule out dioxin exposure. It may develop weeks or months after exposure and may be dependent on individual predisposition. It can result from inhalation, ingestion, or dermal contact and may indicate systemic toxicity.

Other reported dermal effects include hyperpigmentation, hirsutism, increased skin fragility, and vesicular eruptions on exposed areas of the skin.

Neurologic Effects

Data from human studies have been inconsistent and inconclusive. No case of peripheral neuropathy was found after the Seveso accident.

Hepatic Effects

There is no evidence that TCDD causes long-term hepatotoxicity in humans. Some studies have shown a transient increase in liver enzymes without clinical disease. Epidemiologic studies of TCDD-exposed workers have shown no difference in serum levels of hepatic enzymes compared with those of matched controls.

Reproductive and Developmental Effects

Studies of Vietnam servicemen possibly exposed to Agent Orange revealed no overall increase of debilitating birth defects in progeny. Studies of the Seveso area have failed to demonstrate increased risk of birth defects due to dioxin exposure.

Carcinogenic Effects

EPA and the National Institute of Occupational Safety and Health (NIOSH) consider TCDD to be a "cancer promoter" in conjunction with certain other chemicals. NIOSH classifies TCDD as a "potential occupational carcinogen." EPA considers TCDD to be a probable human carcinogen.

CLINICAL PRESENTATION

The onset of symptoms after acute exposure to TCDD-containing substances can take days to weeks and may include skin, eye, and respiratory tract irritation; headache; dizziness; and nausea. Many signs and symptoms are nonspecific.

LABORATORY TESTS

Some researchers believe that serum levels correlate with adipose tissue levels in persons with long-term exposure. Analyses of serum or fat TCDD levels by GC-MC are expensive and time-consuming and are not recommended. Levels of 20 ppt in adipose tissue have been measured in persons with no known exposure to TCDD. People in the Seveso, Italy, accident had TCDD levels a thousand times greater than the average found in the general unexposed population and did not experience illness.

TREATMENT

Treatment of chronic exposure to dioxin-containing agents is primarily supportive. It is most important to remove the patient from the source of exposure. Chloracne is often refractory and unresponsive to common acne treatments. Long-term topical treatment with dilute retinoic acid and administration of tetracycline to treat secondary pustular follicles have been used. In severe cases acne surgery or dermabrasion may be effective.

Contaminated fish such as those from the Baltic Sea are an important source of exposure to polychlorinated dibenzofurans and dibenzodioxins in persons who eat fish regularly. The clinical consequence of such exposure remains uncertain.[99]

In the United Kingdom the Committee on the Toxicity of Chemicals in Food, Consumer Products, and the Environ-

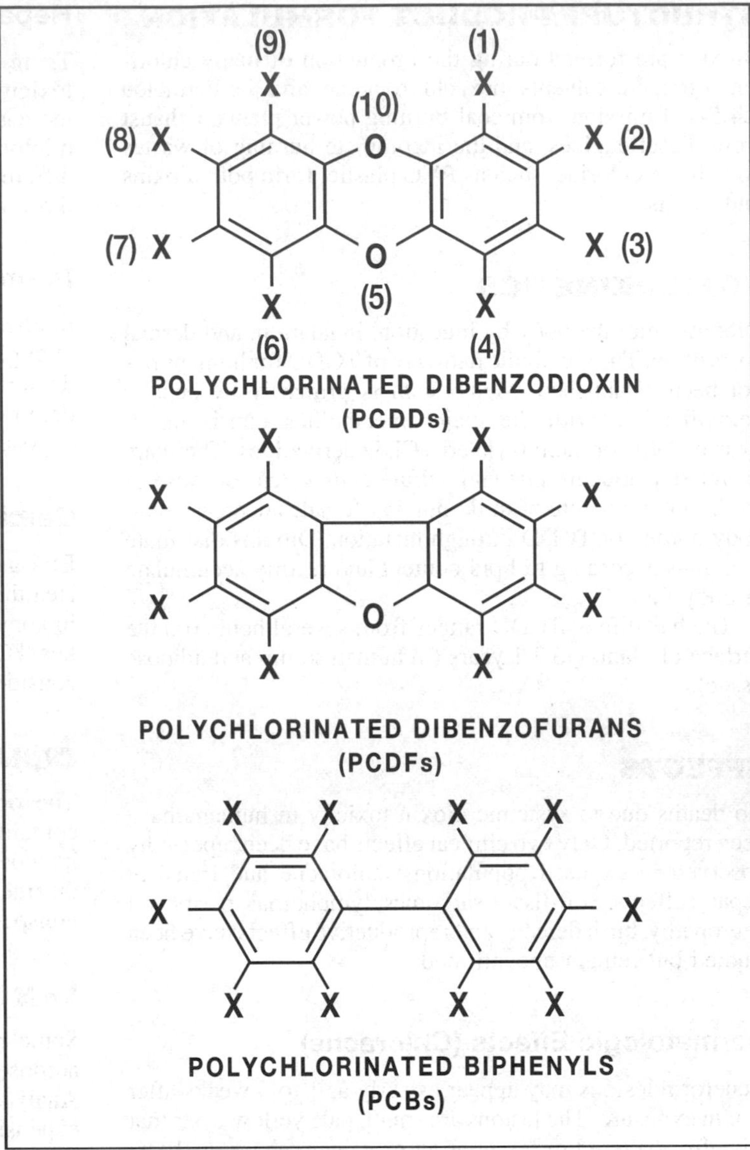

Figure 68–3 Chemical structure of dioxins and related compounds.

ment suggests a maximum advised intake for all dioxins equivalent to pg/kg body weight per day of TCDD. In West Germany an adult on an average diet may have a daily intake of 1.3 pg dioxin/kg body weight per day.[100]

The sources of dioxin are listed below.[101] The structure of dioxins and furans is found in Figure 68–3.

An ingestion of 199.5 g of MCPP together with ioxynil and a hormonal weedkiller produced a toxic effect that led to fatality.[102] An ingestion of 41 g of MCPP with 2,D-D and chlorpyrofos was followed by death in 30 hours.[103]

DIOXIN SOURCES[101]

The main environmental sources of 1,2,7,8-TCDD are as follows:

1. Use of herbicides containing 2,4,5-trichlorophenoxy acids (2,4,5-T).
2. Production and use of 2,4,5-trichlorophenol in wood preservatives.
3. Production and use of hexachlorophene as a germicide.
4. Pulp and paper manufacturing plants.
5. Incineration of municipal and certain industrial wastes.
6. Small amounts formed during the burning of wood in the presence of chlorine.
7. Accidental transformer/capacitor fires involving chlorinated benzenes and biphenyls.
8. Exhaust from automobiles powered with leaded gasoline.
9. Improper disposal of certain chlorinated chemical wastes.

Consumer sources are as follows:

1. Skin contact with surfaces such as soil or vegetation contaminated by the chemical.
2. Skin contact and inhalation of wood dusts from use of pentachlorophenol-treated woods.
3. Inhalation of air near improperly maintained dump sites or municipal incinerators.

4. Consumption of fish and cow's milk from contaminated areas.
5. Consumption of breast milk containing 2,3,7,8-TCDD by babies.
6. Minute exposure from the use of paper towels, napkins, coffee filters, computer papers, and other contaminated paper products.

Workers at risk of contacting 2,3,7,8-TCDD are as follows:

1. Workers who have been involved in the production or use of trichlorophenol and salts, hexachlorophene, and 2,4,5-T or other herbicides containing this chemical. The production of 2,4,5-T and 2,4,5-trichlorophenol, however, has been discontinued in the United States.
2. Workers in the pulp and paper industry.
3. Workers at certain municipal and industrial incinerators.
4. Workers involved in the high-temperature/pressure treatment of woods with pentachlorophenol.
5. Workers at certain hazardous waste sites.
6. Workers involved in the cleanup of certain accidental capacitor/transformer fires and in the salvaging of transformers.
7. Workers who have been involved in spraying of phenoxy herbicides such as Agent Orange.

TOXIC DOSAGE—CHLOROPHENOXY ACIDS

Death has followed absorption of 2,4-dichlorphenol through the skin.[104]

MCPP

Two adults about 70 years of age ingested an unknown quantity of MCPP (2-methyl-4 chlorphenoxypropionic acid). Both developed coma, muscle cramps, arterial hypotension, hyperkalemia, transient thrombocytopenia, and renal failure. They did not have seizures. The renal failure was secondary to the rhabdomyolysis (increased serum myoglobin, increased serum aldolase) that may have resulted from the muscle cramps or a direct toxic action of the chemical on the muscles. The hyperkalemia was due to the renal failure, muscle cell damage, and metabolic acidosis. Both patients recovered.[105]

Vietnam

A study of enlisted men who entered the U.S. Army from 1965 to 1971 indicated that Vietnam veterans experienced an increase in depression, anxiety, and alcohol abuse or dependence.[106] Study of Air Force veterans of Operation Ranch Hat, the unit responsible for aerial spraying of herbicides in Vietnam, indicates that these veterans experienced an increase in basal cell carcinomas, but not melanoma or systemic cancer in comparison with veterans not exposed to herbicides.[107] No other increase was noted in hepatic or cardiovascular profiles. There was no increased risk of mortality from accidental malignant neoplasm or circulatory deaths.[108]

Carcinogenesis

A National Academy of Sciences' Institute of Medicine panel found sufficient evidence for a statistical association between exposure to herbicides and soft-tissue sarcomas, Hodgkin's disease, non-Hodgkin's lymphoma, chloracne, and porphyria tarda; limited or suggestive evidence of an association between herbicide exposure and respiratory cancers, prostate cancer, and multiple myeloma, inadequate evidence to demonstrate an association for most other cancers and disorders; and for a small group cancers—those of the skin, gastrointestinal system, bladder, and brain—a sufficient number of well-designed studies provide suggestive evidence that no association between the disease and herbicide exposure existed.[109]

Most of the studies reviewed looked at the health of industrial and agricultural workers who were exposed to much higher levels of herbicides for much longer periods than the average soldier in Vietnam. Hence, the committee recommended that an independent agency be established to determine the amount of herbicide exposure experienced by United States servicemen by reconstructing the history of herbicide use during the war.[110]

Studies of mortality in United States chemical workers who had been exposed to substances contaminated with TCDD suggest that the medical history of a patient with a soft-tissue sarcoma should include a search for dioxin exposure. The diagnostic workup of exposed persons should include a search for soft-tissue sarcoma.[111,112] The probability at present points to results that are consistent with TCDD being a carcinogen.[112–114]

Teratogenesis

Although TCDD is teratogenic in animal models, studies of both Australian and American servicemen exposed to Agent Orange did not reveal an increased incidence of congenital malformations in their children.[115] Veterans with greater exposure did not seem to be at greater overall risk for fathering babies with birth defects, although a few specific types of defect were more common than expected.[116] Spontaneous abortion rates in exposed mothers did increase after the 1976 Seveso dioxin accident, but no difference was observed between women from areas of low, moderate, and high contamination.[117] Data collected after the Seveso incident failed to demonstrate any increased risk of birth defects associated with TCDD.[118]

LABORATORY

Analytic Methods

A high-performance liquid chromatographic assay useful as an aid in the diagnosis of acute poisoning by 2,4-D and related components has a limit of detection of 20 μg/mL.[119]

Moderately to severely 2,4-D-poisoned patients should receive the following tests: serum aldolase, creatinine, electrolytes, hepatic aminotransferase, and urinalysis.

Vietnam veterans who were heavily exposed to Agent Orange exhibited an increase in both blood and adipose tissue levels of TCDD.[120] The high correlation of blood and adipose tissue levels suggests that there may be a mobile equilibrium between them and that blood measurement could replace adipose tissue measurements of TCDD levels.[120]

During 1986 CDC's Division of Environmental Health Laboratory Science developed a method for measuring TCDD in human serum that is highly correlated with measurements of TCDD in adipose tissue. The half-life of TDD body burden in man is estimated as approximately 6 to 10 years. Only about 2 to 2.5 TCDD half-lives have elapsed since potential exposure in Vietnam. TCDD medians for Vietnam veterans (3 ppt) and non-Vietnam veterans (3.9 ppt) are almost the same.[121,122] Human serum in the general population with no known exposure to TCDD contains a mean of 47.9 ppg (and 7.5 pptr on a life weight basis). The results are in agreement with levels in human adipose tissue of 6.4 to 7.1 pptn.[123,124] Human adipose tissue from Vietnam veterans contained 13.4 ppt, similar to civilians (1.5 ppt) and non-Vietnam veterans (12.5 ppt).[122]

Seveso

At least 1.3 kg of TCDD contaminated a populated area of about 2 km^2 near Seveso, Italy. All who developed a severe chloracne had TCDD levels over 12,000 ppt. The results were 3000 to 4000 times higher than background human levels. These data suggest that chloracne is not the most sensitive marker of overt exposure to TCDD but that the actual measurement of TCDD in human samples is.[125]

Workers exposed to dioxin had adipose tissue levels with a mean of 246 ppt. Unexposed workers had levels of 8.6 ppt.[124] Nine workers with a history of exposure to PCDDs and chloracne in 1971 to 1973 had TCDD serum levels of 340 pg per gram blood lipid in 1990. This was higher than blood levels in workers without chloracne (18 pg).[126]

Tissue concentrations of phenoxy herbicides were determined in a patient who died 30 hours after ingesting MCPP, 2,4-D, and chlorpyrifos. After ingesting about 44 g of MCPP, tissue concentration of MCPP ranged from 161 to 277 μg/g. In the brain there was a striking difference between the grey matter concentration of MCPP (75 μg/g) and white matter concentration of MCPP (178 μg/g). The patient had ingested about 39 g of 2,4-D. Tissue concentrations of 2,4-D ranged from 180 to 301 μg/L. Concentration in the grey matter was 186 μg/g and the white matter 298 μg/g.[103] Four hours after an ingestion of 5 mg/kg of 2,4-D a plasma peak level of about 25 μg/mL was obtained.[127]

TBrDD

Thirty-five years after an exposure to 2,3,8-tetrabromodibenzo dioxin (TBrDD) or TCDD and the subsequent development of chloracne, the whole blood lipid level of 2,3,7-TBrDD was 625 ppt and the TCDD level 18 ppt compared with TCDD levels of 5 ppt in the United States population.[128]

TREATMENT

Four patients who had ingested from 40 to 160 g of 2,4-D were treated with hemodialysis. Three were admitted in coma within 2 to 3 hours after ingestion. Recovery followed hemodialysis in three patients and hemodialysis and resin hemoperfusion in the fourth. They survived after high 2,4-D serum concentrations (177 m/100 mL and 37 mg/100 mL).[129]

After MCPP ingestion, a tracheostomy, mechanical ventilation, gastric lavage, activated charcoal, cathartics, supplemental oxygen, plasma infusions, and hemodialysis were employed in two patients who survived.[105]

A study of 38 patients with herbicide poisoning suggests that alkaline diuresis should be used to treat acute poisoning with chlorphenoxy herbicides in the presence of coma or other poor prognostic indicators, such as acidemia or if plasma total chlorophenoxy concentrations are 0.5 g/L or more.[130] There is one report in the literature to support the use of extracorporeal methods for removal of 2,4-D.[129]

CHLORATE SALTS (SODIUM, POTASSIUM)

Sodium chlorate is a powerful oxidizing agent that causes methemoglobinemia, hemolytic anemia, and direct nephrotoxic effects. Coma and death within a few hours can result from either tissue hypoxia (severe methemoglobinemia), hyperkalemia from massive hemolysis, or acute renal failure compounded by hemoglobinuria.

ACUTE TOXIC DOSAGE

A 34-year-old adult ingested 50 g of sodium chlorate. In spite of a methemoglobinemia of 32% and impaired renal and respiratory dysfunction, she recovered after IV fluids, toludine blue IV, hemodialysis, and plasmapheresis.[131]

CLINICAL PRESENTATION

Within 2 to 24 hours gastrointestinal symptoms develop, including nausea, vomiting, diarrhea, and abdominal pain. After absorption, hemoglobin rapidly oxidizes to methemoglobin, leading to cyanosis, dyspnea, and coma in severe cases. Intravascular hemolysis also can occur.[132] Seven of 14 patients in the largest published chlorate poisoning series developed acute renal failure within 48 hours of hospital admission.[133]

LABORATORY

Blood abnormalities include normocytic normochromic anemia, thrombocytopenia, free plasma haptoglobin, polymorphonuclear leukocytosis, Heinz bodies, ghost cells, dark brown "chocolate" serum, methemoglobin levels exceeding 10%, mildly elevated hepatic aminotransferases, hyperkalemia, and elevated serum creatinine. Proteinuria and hemoglobinuria also may be present.

TREATMENT

Stabilization

Obviously ill patients should be evaluated for the adequacy of airway, ventilation, and circulation. Methemoglobin levels, complete blood count, serum electrolytes, and creatinine should be drawn immediately after the establishment of adequate ventilation and an intravenous line. The patient should receive cardiac monitoring and supplemental oxygen. Watch carefully for signs of hyperkalemia (e.g., widening of the QRS and PR prolongation) on the ECG.

Decontamination

The usual measures of gut decontamination (lavage, activated charcoal, cathartics) may be useful within the first several hours after exposure. The effectiveness of charcoal, however, has not been established.[134]

Elimination Enhancement

Sodium chlorate is freely dialyzable, and hemodialysis or early exchange transfusion is recommended, particularly when renal failure is present. Such procedures may prevent the ensuing hemolysis, which may be fatal.[134]

Antidotes

Sodium thiosulfate either orally or intravenously (2 to 5 g in 200 mL of 5% sodium bicarbonate) inactivates chlorate ion and is a potentially useful antidote on the basis of anecdotal reports.[135]

Methemoglobin can be reduced to hemoglobin by intravenous methylene blue; however, methylene blue may have minimal effect in the treatment of chlorate intoxication. The clinical course of chlorate poisoning appears to be determined by hemolysis, disseminated intravascular coagulation, and renal failure.[134]

ATRAZINE

This herbicide (2-chloro-4-ethylamino-6-isopropylamino-5-triazine) is widely used in agriculture. Oral doses of atrazine, 400 mg/kg, produce diffuse subcutaneous hemorrhage, liver necrosis, ataxia, black stool, and death in cattle.[136] Reports of human toxicity are rare. Atrazine is an irritant capable of causing local eye and skin inflammation.

CLINICAL PRESENTATION

Ingestion of 100 g of atrazine may lead to coma, circulatory collapse, metabolic acidosis, and gastric bleeding, which can be followed by renal failure, hepatic necrosis, and a disseminated intravascular coagulopathy that may be fatal. This compound was implicated in the development of sensorimotor polyneuropathy in a farmer who sustained a cutaneous exposure over several days.[137]

Following an ingestion of atrazine 100 g together with aminotriazole, ethylene glycol, and formaldehyde, a 38-year-old man developed coma, circulatory collapse, metabolic acidosis, and gastric bleeding, which led to death in 3 days. Plasma atrazine concentrations were determined by high-performance liquid chromatography and reached 2.0 μg/mL within 1 hour of ingestion. Within 1 hour after hemodialysis the plasma atrazine levels dropped to undetectable levels.[138] Overexposure to triazinic herbicides (atrazine, simazine, propazine) may induce fatigue, dizziness, nausea, irritation of the skin, eyes and respiratory tract, allergic eczema, or asthma.[139] Ingestion of 100 g leads to a plasma concentration of 2 μg/mL. Hemodialysis induces the atrazine clearance of 250 mL/min.[138] A high-performance liquid chromatography method is available for measurement of atrazine in human plasma.[140]

LABORATORY

Enzyme-limited immunosorbent assays (ELISAs) detect atrazine and its principal metabolites in the urine (mercapturic acid conjugate) with a minimum detectable level of 0.02 μg/L.[141]

AMITROLE

Amitrole-containing herbicides are commonly used by home and cottage owners for spraying grass. They are manufactured and distributed under names such as Amitrole-T, Amizol, Azolan, Cytrol, and Weedizol. Amitrole is a water-soluble compound whose chemical formula is $C_2H_4N_4$ (3-amino, 1,2,4-triazole). It is also known as aminotriazole. First introduced in 1954, its mechanism of herbicidal action is due to inhibition of chlorophyll formation and herb regrowth. Human toxicity appears to be limited to cutaneous allergies. A 74-year-old healthy ex-smoker sprayed an amitrole-containing herbicide for 2 hours without wearing a protective mask. He developed a dry cough. Pulmonary function tests indicated lung restriction; x-ray disclosed a right-sided patchy infiltrate and bilateral pleural effusions. Transbronchial lung biopsy disclosed a toxic alveolitis. Partial relief followed IV corticosteroids.[142]

ENDOTHALL

Endothall (Acuchrate, Endothall Weed Killer, Aquathol, Des-i-cate, Endothal Turf Herbicide, Hydrothol, Herbicide 273) is a phthalate (Fig. 68–4). As the free acid or as sodium, potassium, or amine salts, endothall is used as a contact herbicide, defoliant, aquatic herbicide, and algicide. It is formulated in aqueous solutions and granules at various strengths.[143]

MECHANISM OF ACTION

Systemic toxic mechanism are (a) corrosive effect on the gastrointestinal tract (especially with high concentrations of the free acid); (b) myocardiopathy and vascular injury leading to shock; (c) central nervous system injury causing seizures and respiratory depression.[144]

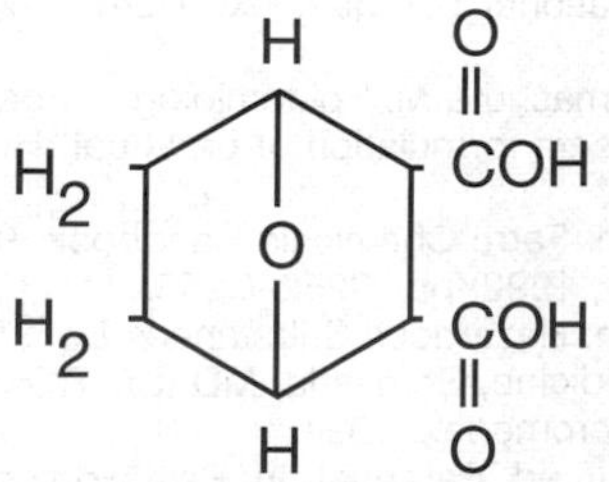

Figure 68–4 Chemical structure of endothall.

CLINICAL PRESENTATION

Endothall is irritating to the skin, eyes, and mucous membranes. It is well absorbed across abraded skin and from the gastrointestinal tract.[143] A 23-year-old adult ingested 40 mL of endothall. He vomited spontaneously four times. In an hour he developed abdominal pain and vomited again. Within 6 hours he complained of abdominal pain and dyspnea. In the next several hours he vomited bright red blood and developed hypotension, acidosis, anuria, DIC, and cardiovascular collapse. He expired in 12 hours after the ingestion.[144]

TREATMENT

1. Wash endothall from the skin with soap and water. Flush contamination from the eyes with copious amounts of clean water.
2. If endothall has been ingested, activated charcoal may limit toxicant concentration in the gastrointestinal tract. Repeat the charcoal administration every 2 to 4 hours at half or more of the original dosage.
3. If there is no evidence of corrosive effect on pharyngeal tissue, or on the esophagus, the stomach may be carefully lavaged with a slurry of activated charcoal after all measures are taken to protect the airway from aspiration of vomitus.
4. If there are indications of corrosive effect in the pharynx, do not attempt gastric intubation because of the risk of esophageal perforation.
5. Oxygen may be administered by mask. Assisted ventilation may be required.
6. Monitor blood pressure closely. Give IV fluids to correct dehydration, stabilize electrolytes, provide sugar, and support mechanisms for toxicant disposition.
7. In view of the myocardiopathy use vasopressor amines only with caution.
8. Seizures may require diazepam.
9. It is not known whether hemodialysis or hemoperfusion would be effective in removing endothall from the blood. This option may be necessary if the patient's condition deteriorates despite supportive care.

REFERENCES

1. Winchester JF. History of paraquat intoxication. In: Bismuth C, Hall AH, eds. Paraquat poisoning: mechanisms—prevention—treatment. New York: Marcel Dekker, 1995.
2. Dawling S, Braithwaite RA. Fatal poisoning by paraquat injection. Bull Int Assoc Forensic Toxic 1991;21:33–35.
3. Ong ML, Glew S. Paraquat poisoning per vagina. Postgrad Med J 65:835–836.
4. Kline JN, Darden IL, Lohne E, Larson RK. Pulmonary function of San Joaquin Valley agricultural laborers with occupational paraquat exposure. Chest 1990;98 (Suppl):65S.
5. Naito H, Yamashute M. Epidemiology of paraquat in Japan and a new safe formulation of paraquat. Hum Toxicol 1987;6: 87–88.
6. Paraquat. In: Farm Chemicals Handbook '92. Willoughby, OH: Meister, 1992; pp. C252–C253.
7. Paraquat. In: Hazardous Substances Data Bank. National Library of Medicine, Bethesda, MD (CD-ROM version). Denver, CO. Micromedex, 1994.
8. Hayes WJ Jr, ed. Paraquat. In: Pesticides studied in man. Baltimore: Williams & Wilkins, 1982; pp 543–558.
9. Hall AH. Paraquat usage. Environmental fate and effects. In: Bismuth C, Hall AH, eds. Paraquat poisoning: mechanisms—prevention—treatment. New York: Marcel Dekker, 1995.
10. Hayes WJ Jr, Laws ER Jr. Quaternary nitrogen compounds. In: Handbook of pesticide toxicology. Vol 3. Classes of pesticides. San Diego, CA: Academic Press, 1991; pp 1356–1408.
11. Baselt RC. Paraquat. In: Biological monitoring methods for industrial chemicals. 2nd ed. Littleton, MA: PSG Publishing Company, 1988; pp 240–243.
12. Pond SM. Manifestations and management of paraquat poisoning. Med J Aust 1990;152:356–359.
13. Hall AH, Becker CE. Occupational health and safety considerations in paraquat handling. In: Bismuth C, Hall AH, eds. Paraquat poisoning: mechanisms—prevention—treatment. New York: Marcel Dekker, 1995.
14. Morgan DP. Paraquat. In: Recognition and management of pesticide poisonings. 4th ed. Washington, DC: U.S. Environmental Protection Agency, EPA-540/9-88-0015, Government Printing Office, 1989; pp. 76–82.
15. Onyon LJ, Volans GN. The epidemiology and prevention of paraquat poisoning. Hum Toxicol 1987;6:19.
16. Vale JA, Meredith TJ, Buckley BM. Paraquat poisoning: clinical features and immediate general management. Hum Toxicol 1987;6:41–47.
17. Selden BS, Clark RF, Curry SC. Marijuana. Emerg Med Clin North Am 1990;8:527.
18. Cant JS, Lewis DRH. Ocular damage due to paraquat and diquat. Br Med J 1978;2:224.
19. Joyce M. Ocular damage caused by paraquat. Br J Ophthalmol 1968;53:688.
20. Vlahos K, Goggin M, Coster D. Paraquat causes chronic ocular surface toxicity. Aust NZ J Ophthalmol 1993; 32(3):187.
21. Watanabe I, Sakai H, Toyama K, Veno M, Watanabe M. Ocular impairment due to paraquat dichloride. Jpn Rev Clin Ophthalmol 1979;73:660.
22. Guardascione V, Mazella di Bosco M. Contribution to the knowledge of occupational intoxication with paraquat, dipyridilium herbicide. Folia Med (Naples) 1969;52:728.
23. Oishi S. A cause of ocular injury by paraquat dichloride. Jpn J Ind Health 1975;17:522.
24. Howard JK, Sabapathy NN, Whitehead PA. A study of the health of Malaysian plantation workers with particular reference to paraquat spraymen. Br J Ind Med 1981; 38:110.
25. Houze P, Scherrman JM, Baud FJ. Toxicokinetics of paraquat. In: Bismuth C, Hall AH, eds. Paraquat poisoning: mechanisms—prevention—treatment. New York: Marcel Dekker, 1995.
26. Hoffer E, Taitelman U. Exposure to paraquat through skin absorption. Clinical and laboratory observations of accidental splashing in healthy skin of agricultural workers. Hum Toxicol 1989;8:483–484.
27. Daniel JW, Gage JC. Absorption and excretion of diquat and paraquat. Br J Ind Med 1966;23:133.
28. Reference Deleted
29. Proudfoot AT, Stewart MS, Levitt T, Widdop B. Paraquat poisoning. Significance of plasma paraquat concentrations. Lancet 1979;1:330.
30. Clark DG, McElligott TF, Westonhurst E. The toxicity of paraquat. Br J Ind Med 1966;23:126.
31. Sharp CWM, Ottolenghi A, Posner HS. Correlation of paraquat toxicity with tissue concentrations and weight loss of the rat. Toxicol Appl Pharmacol 1972;22:241.
32. Baud FJ, Houze P, Bismuth C, Scherrmann J-M, Jaeger A, Keyers C. Toxicokinetics of paraquat through the heart-lung block. Six cases of acute human poisoning. Clin Toxicol 1988;26:35–50.
33. Houze P, Baud FJ, Mouy R, Bismuth C, Bourdon R, Scherrmann JM. Toxicokinetics of paraquat in humans. Human Exp Toxicol 1990;9:5–12.
34. Hawksworth GM, Bennett PN, Davies DS. Kinetics of paraquat elimination in the dog. Toxicol Appl Pharmacol 1981;57:139.

35. Ragouoy Gengler O, Pileire D, Daijardin JB. Survival from severe paraquat intoxication in heavy drinkers. Lancet 1991; 380:1461.
36. Talbot AR, Fuh CC, Hsieh MF, Shaw HJ. Paraquat intoxication during pregnancy. A report of 9 cases. Vet Hum Toxicol 1988;30:12–17.
37. Fennelly JJ, Gallagher JT, Carroll RJ. Paraquat poisoning in a pregnant woman. Br Med J 1968;3:722.
38. Musson FA, Porter CA. Effect of ingestion of paraquat on a 20 week gestation fetus. Postgrad Med J 1982;58:732.
39. Bismuth C, Wong A, Hall AH. Paraquat ingestion exposure. In: Bismuth C, Hall AH, eds. Paraquat poisoning: mechanisms—prevention—treatment. New York: Marcel Dekker, 1995.
40. Pasi A. The Toxicology of paraquat, diquat and morfamquat. Bern, Switzerland: Hans Humber, 1978.
41. Ackrill P, Haselton PS, Ralston AJ. Oesophageal perforation due to paraquat. Br Med J 1978;1:6122, 1252.
42. Frelon JH, Merigot P, Garnier R, Bismuth C, Efthymiou ML. Facteurs prognostiques de l'intoxication aigue par le paraquat. Etude retrospective des cas enrigistres au Centre Anti-Poisons de Paris en 1981. Toxicol Eur Res 1983;5:163.
43. Malone JDG, Carmody M, Keogh B, O'Dwyer WF. Paraquat poisoning. A review of nineteen cases. J Irish Med Assoc 1971;64:59.
44. Kodagoda N, Jayewardene RP, Attygalle D. Poisoning with paraquat. Forensic Sci 1973;2:107.
45. Vaziri ND, Ness RL, Fairshter RD, Smigh WR, Rosen SM. Nephrotoxicity of paraquat in man. Arch Intern Med 1979;139:172.
46. Baguley E, Iles PB, Wright N. Serial lung function tests in paraquat poisoning. Hum Toxicol 1983;2:418.
47. Lewis CPL, Nemery B. Pathophysiology and biochemical mechanisms of the pulmonary toxicity of paraquat. In: Bismuth C, Hall AH, eds. Paraquat poisoning: mechanisms—prevention—treatment. New York: Marcel Dekker, 1995.
48. Bismuth C, Garnier R, Dally S, Fournier PE, Scherrmann JM. Prognosis and treatment of paraquat poisoning: a review of 20 cases. J Toxicol Clin Toxicol 1982;19:461.
49. Reif RM, Lewinsohn G. Paraquat myocarditis and adrenal cortical necrosis. J Forensic Sci 1983;28:505.
50. Pronczuk de Garbino J. Epidemiology of paraquat poisoning in Bismuth C, Hall AH, eds. Paraquat poisoning: mechanisms—prevention—treatment. New York: Marcel Dekker, 1995.
51. Proudfoot AT, Prescott LF, Jarvie DR. Hemodialysis for paraquat poisoning. Hum Toxicol 1987;6:63.
52. Bismuth C, Baud FJ, Garnier R, Muszinski J, Houze P. Paraquat poisoning: biological presentation. J Toxicol Clin Exp 1988;8:211.
53. Ohkubo T, Takeda K, Okano T, Shigeizumi Y, Oikawa M, Toyohara T, Hayashi S et al. A case of death due to paraquat intoxication. J Jpn Soc Rural Med 1979;28:472.
54. Takagoshi K, Nakanuma Y, Ohta M, Thoyanna T, Okuda K, Kono N. Light and electron microscopic study of the liver in paraquat poisoning. Liver 1988;8:330–336.
55. Dabney BJ. Genetic, carcinogenic and reproductive effects of paraquat. In: Bismuth C, Hall AH, eds. Paraquat poisoning: mechanisms—prevention—treatment. New York: Marcel Dekker, 1995.
56. IRIS, Integrated Risk Information System, U.S. Environmental Protection Agency (CD-ROM version). Denver, CO. Micromedex, edition expires 7/31/94.
57. Talbot AR, Fu CC, Hsieh MF. Paraquat intoxication during pregnancy: a report of 9 cases. Vet Hum Toxicol 1988;30:12.
58. Scherrmann JM, Houze P, Bismuth C, Bourdon R. Prognostic value of plasma and urine paraquat concentrations. Hum Toxicol 1987;6:91–93.
59. Fuke C, Amero K, Arneno S, Kiriu T, Shinohara T, Sogo K, Ijiri I. A rapid simultaneous determination of paraquat and diquat in serum and urine using second-derivative spectroscopy. J Anal Toxicol 1992;16:214–216.
60. Scherrmann JM. Analytical procedures and predictive value of late plasma and urine paraquat concentrations. Personal communication. Jan 7, 1993. To be published.
61. Kuo H-W, Wang J-D, Lin J-M. Determination of 4,-4'-bipyridine vapor. Am Ind Hyg Assoc J 1992;53:514–518.
62. Nagao M, Takatori T, Terazawa K, Wu R, Wakasugi C, Masui PM, Ikeda N. Development and application of immunoassay for paraquat radioimmunoassay. J Forensic Sci 1989;34: 547–552.
63. Bismuth C, Hall AH. Pulmonary dysfunction in paraquat poisoning survivors. In: Bismuth C, Hall AH, eds. Paraquat poisoning: mechanisms—prevention—treatment. New York: Marcel Dekker, 1995, pp 349–355.
64. Hart TB, Nevitt A, Whitehead A. A new statistical approach to the prognostic significance of plasma paraquat concentrations. Lancet 1984;2:1222.
65. Scherrmann JM, Galliot M, Garnier R, Bismuth C. Acute paraquat poisoning: prognostic significance and therapeutical interest of blood assay. Toxicol Eur Res 1983;3:141.
66. Hampson ECGM, Pond SM. Failure of haemoperfusion and haemodialysis to prevent death in paraquat poisoning. Med Toxicol 1988;6:91.
67. Proudfoot AT. Predictive value of early plasma paraquat concentrations. In: Bismuth C, Hall AH, eds. Paraquat poisoning: mechanisms—prevention—treatment. New York: Marcel Dekker, 1995.
68. Yamaguchi H, Sato S, Watanabe S, Naito H. Pre-embarkment prognostication for acute paraquat poisoning. Hum Exper Toxicol 1990;9:1384.
69. Im JG, Lee KS, Han MC, Kim SJ, Kim IO. Paraquat poisoning: findings on chest radiography and CT in 42 patients. Am J Roentgenol 1991;4:697.
70. Sawada Y, Yamamoto I, Hirokane T, Nagai Y, Satoh Y, Ueyama M. Severity index of paraquat poisoning. Lancet 1988;1:1333.
71. Duke SO. Overview of herbicide mechanism of action. Environ Health Perspect 1990;87:263–271.
72. Meredith T, Vale JA. Treatment of paraquat poisoning. Gastrointestinal decontamination. In: Bismuth C, Hall AH, eds. Paraquat poisoning: mechanisms—prevention—treatment. New York: Marcel Dekker, 1995.
73. Widdop B, Medd RK, Braithwaite RA. Charcoal haemoperfusion in the treatment of paraquat poisoning. Eur Soc Toxicol 1977;18:156.
74. Smith LL. Mechanism of paraquat toxicity in lung and its relevance to treatment. Hum Toxicol 1987;6:31.
75. Bismuth C. Treatment of paraquat poisoning. Modification of toxicokinetics in Bismuth C, Hall AH, eds. Paraquat poisoning: mechanisms—prevention—treatment. New York: Marcel Dekker, 1995.
76. Hampson ECGM, Pond SM. Failure of haemoperfusion and haemodialysis to prevent death in paraquat poisoning: a retrospective review of 42 patients. Med Toxicol 1988;3:64.
77. Pond SM, Johnston SC, Schoof DD, Hampson ED, Boules M, Wright DM, Petrie JJ. Repeated hemoperfusion and continuous arteriovenous hemofiltration in a paraquat poisoned patient. Clin Toxicol 1987;25:305–316.
78. Proudfoot AT, Prescott LF, Jarvie DR. Haemodialysis in paraquat poisoning. Hum Toxicol 1987;6:69–74.
79. Bismuth C, Scherrmann JM, Barnier R, Baud FJ, Pontal PG. Elimination of paraquat. Hum Toxicol 1987;6:63–67.
80. Pond SM, Chen N, Bowles MR. Prevention of paraquat toxicity in alveolar type II cells by paraquat-specific antibodies. Vet Hum Toxicol 1993;35:337.
81. Paraquat poisoning. Lancet 1986;1:333.
82. Bateman DN. Pharmacological treatments of paraquat poisoning. Hum Toxicol 1987;6:57.
83. Pond SM. Treatment of paraquat poisoning. In: Bismuth C, Hall AH, eds. Paraquat poisoning: mechanisms—prevention—treatment. New York: Marcel Dekker, 1995.
84. Talbot AR, Barnes AAR. Radiotherapy for the treatment of pulmonary complications of paraquat poisoning. Hum Toxicol 1988;7:325–332.
85. Yamashita M, Maito H, Takagi S. The effectiveness of a cation resin (Kayexalate) as an adsorbent of paraquat. Experimental and clinical studies. Hum Toxicol 1987;6:89–90.
86. Blain PG. Aspects of pesticide toxicology. Adverse Drug React Acute Pois Rev 1990;9:37–68.

87. Perriens JH, Benimadho S, Kiauw IL, Wisse J, Chee H. High-dose cyclophosphamide and dexamethasone in paraquat poisoning: a prospective study. Hum Exper Toxicol 1992;11: 129–134.
88. Mahieu P, Bonduelle Y, Bernard A et al. Acute diquat intoxication: Interest of its repeated determination in urine and the evaluation of renal proximal tubule integrity. Clin Toxicol 1984;22:363–369.
89. Wood TE, Edgar H, Salcedo J. Recovery from inhalation of diquat aerosol. Chest 1976;70:774–775.
90. Clark DG, Hurst EW. The toxicity of diquat. Br J Ind Med 1970;27:51–55.
91. Daniel JW, Gage JC. Absorption and excretion of diquat and paraquat in rats. Br J Ind Med 1966;23:133–136.
92. Vanholder R, Colardyn F, De Reuck J, Praet M, Lameire N, Ringoir S. Diquat intoxication. Report of two cases and review of the literature. Am J Med 1981;70:1267–1271.
93. Sechi GP, Agnetti V, Piredda M, Canu M, Deserra F, Omar HA et al. Acute and persistent parkinsonism after use of diquat. Neurology 1992;42:261–263.
94. McCarthy LG, Speth CR. Diquat intoxication. Ann Emerg Med 1983;12:394–396.
95. Casey PB, Buckley BM, Vale JA. Methemoglobinemia following ingestion of a monolinuron/paraquat herbicide (Gramonol®). Clin Toxicol 1994;32:185–189.
96. Demers R, Perrin E. Dioxin toxicity. Case studies in environmental medicine. 7. Agency for Toxic Substances and Disease Registry, June 1990.
97. Skene SA, Dewhurst IC, Greenberg M. Polychlorinated dibenzo-*p*-dioxins and polychlorinated dibenzofurans: the risks to human health. A review. Hum Toxicol 1989;8: 172–204.
98. Schecter A, Dai LC, Bich LT, Quynh HT, Minyh DQ, Cau HD, Phiet PH et al. Agent Orange and the Vietnamese: the persistence of elevated dioxin levels in human tissues. Am J Public Health 1995;85:516–522.
99. Svensson B-G, Nilsson A, Hansson M, Rappe C, Akesson B, Skerfung S. Exposure to dioxins and dibenzofurans through the consumption of fish. N Engl J Med 1991;324:8–12.
100. A daily dose of dioxin. Lancet 1989;2:59 (editorial).
101. Dickson LC, Buzik SC. Health risks of "dioxins": a review of environmental and toxicological considerations. Vet Hum Toxicol 1993;35:68–77.
102. Dickey W, McAleer JJA, Callender ME. Delayed sudden death after ingestion of MCPP and ioxynil. An unusual presentation of hormonal weedkiller intoxication. Postgrad Med J 1988;64:681–682.
103. Osterloh J, Lotti M, Pond SM. Toxicologic studies in a fatal overdose of 2,4D, MCPP and chlorpyrifos. J Anal Toxicol 1983;7:125–129.
104. Kintz P, Tracqui A, Mangin P. Accidental death caused by the absorption of 2,4-dichlorphenol through the skin. 1992;66: 298–299.
105. Meulenbelt J, Zwaveling JH, van Zooner P, Notermans NC. Acute MCPP intoxication. Report of two cases. Hum Toxicol 1988;7:289–292.
106. Centers for Disease Control Vietnam Experience Study. Health status of Vietnam veterans. I. Psychosocial characteristics. JAMA 1998;259:2701–2707.
107. Wolfe WH, Michalek JE, Miner JC, Rake A, Silva J, Thomas WF et al. Health status of air force veterans occupationally exposed to herbicides in Vietnam. I. Physical health. JAMA 1990;264:1824–1831.
108. Michalek JE, Wolfe WH, Miner JC. Health status of air force veterans occupational exposed to herbicides in Vietnam. II. Mortality. JAMA 1990;264:1832–1836.
109. McCarthy M. Agent Orange. Lancet 1993;342:367.
110. Veterans and Agent Orange: health effects of herbicides used in Vietnam. Washington, DC: National Academy Press, 1993.
111. Baiker JCH. How dangerous is dioxin? N Engl J Med 1991; 324:260–262.
112. Fingerhut MA, Halperin WE, Marlow DA, Piactelli LA, Hanchar PA. Cancer mortality in workers exposed to 2,3,7,8-tetrachloro dibenzo-*p*-dioxin. N Engl J Med 1991;324: 212–218.
113. Fingerhut MA, Steanland K, Sweeney MH, Halperin WE, Piactelli LA, Marlow DA. Old and new reflections on dioxin. Epidemiology 1992;3:69–72.
114. Eriksson M, Hardell L, Adani HO. Exposure to dioxins as a risk factor for soft tissue sarcoma. A population based case-control study. J Natl Cancer Inst 1990;82:486–496.
115. Donovan JW, MacLennan R, Adena M. Vietnam service and the risk of congenital abnormalities: a case control study. Med J Aust 1984;140:394–397.
116. Erickson JD, Mulinare J, McClain PW et al. Vietnam veterans' risks for fathering babies with birth defects. JAMA 1984; 252:903–912.
117. Reggiani G. Anatomy of a TCDD spill: the Seveso accident. Hazard Assess Chem Curr Dev 1983;2:269–342.
118. Mastroiacovo P, Spagnola A, Marni E, Meazzo L, Bertollini R, Segni G. Birth defects in the Seveso area after TCDD contamination. JAMA 1988;259:1668–1672.
119. Flanagan RJ, Ruprah M. HPLC measurement of chlorphenoxyherbicides, bromoxynil and ioxynil in biological specimens to aid diagnosis of acute poisoning. Clin Chem 1989;35:1342–1347.
120. Kahn PC, Gochfeld M, Nygren M, Hansson M, Rappe C, Velez H et al. Dioxins and dibenzofurans in blood and adipose tissue of Agent Orange-exposed Vietnam veterans and matched controls. JAMA 1988;259:1661–1667.
121. CDC Serum dioxin in Vietnam-era veterans. Preliminary report. MMWR 1987;36:470–475.
122. Kang HK, Watanabe KK, Breen J, Renuvers J, Conomos MG, Stanley J et al. Dioxins and dibenzofurans in adipose tissue of US Vietnam veterans and controls. Am J Public Health 1991;81:344–349.
123. Patterson DG, Hampton L, Lapeza CR Jr, Belser WT, Green V, Alexander L et al. High resolution gas chromatographic/high resolution mass spectrometric analysis of human serum on a whole-weight and lipid basis for 2,3,7,8-tetrachlorodibenzo-*p*-dioxin. Anal Chem 1987;59: 2000–2005.
124. Patterson DG, Fingerhut MA, Roberts DW, Needham LL, Sweeney MH, Marlow DA et al. Levels of polychlorinated dibenzo-*p*-dioxin and dibenzofurans in workers exposed to 2,3,7,8-tetrachlorbenzo-*p*-dioxin. Am J Ind Med 1989;16:135–146.
125. Mocarelli P, Needham LL, Marocchi A, Patterson DG Jr, Branbille P, Gerthoux PM et al. Serum concentration of 2,3,7,8-tetrachloro dibenzo-*p*-dioxin and test results for selected residents of Seveso, Italy. J Toxicol Environ Health 1991;32:357–366.
126. Neuberger M, Landvoight W, Derntl F. Blood levels of 2,3,7,8-tetrachlordibenzo-*p*-dioxin chemical workers after chloracne and in comparison groups. Inst Arch Occup Environ Health 1991;63:325–327.
127. Sauerhoff MW, Braun WH, Blau GE, Gehring PJ. The fate of 2,4-dichlorophenoxy acetic acid (2,4-D) following oral administration to man. Toxicology 1977;8:3111.
128. Schecter A, Ryan JJ. Persistent brominated and chlorinated dioxin blood levels in a chemist 35 years after dioxin exposure. J Occup Med 1992;32:702–707.
129. Durakovic Z, Durakovic A, Durakovic S, Ivanovic D. Poisoning with 2,4-dichlorophenoxy acetic acid treated by hemodialysis. Arch Toxicol 1992;66:518–521.
130. Flanagan RJ, Meredith TJ, Ruprah M, Onyon LJ, Liddle A. Alkaline diuresis for acute poisoning with chlorophenoxy herbicides and ioxynil. Lancet 1990;335:454–458.
131. Donner A, Lenz K, Wagner L, Walgran M, Hruby K. Survival after massive self-poisoning with sodium chlorate. Proc Eur Assoc Pois Cont Cent Clin Toxicol, 1988; p. 80.
132. Lee DBN, Brown DL, Baker LRI et al. Haematological complications of chlorate poisoning. Br Med J 1970;2:31–32.
133. Sanger B, Wegman RCC, Hofstee AWM. Nonoccupational exposure to pentachlorophenol: clinical findings and plasma PCP concentrations in three families. Hum Toxicol 1982;1: 123–133.
134. Steffen C, Wetzel E. Pathologic aspects of chlorate poisoning. Hum Toxicol 1985;4:541–542 (abstract).
135. Helliwell M, Nunn J. Mortality in sodium chlorate poisoning. Br Med J 1979;1:1119.

136. Kobel W, Sumnor DD, Campbell JD et al. Protective effect of activated charcoal in cattle poisoned with atrazine. Vet Hum Toxicol 1985;27:185–188.
137. Castano P, Ferrario VF, Vizzotto L. Sciatic nerve fibres in albino rats after atrazine treatment: a morpho-quantitative study. Int J Tissue React 1982;4:269–275.
138. Pommery J, Mathieu M, Mathieu D, Lhermitte M. Atrazine in plasma and tissue following atrazine-aminotriazole-ethylene glycol-formaldehyde poisoning. Clin Toxicol 1993;31:323–331.
139. Scott AR. Questions. Br Med J 1989;299:615.
140. Pommery J, Mathieu M, Mathieu D, Lhermitte M. High performance liquid chromatographic determination of atrazine in human plasma. J Chromatogr 1990;526:569–574.
141. Lucas AD, Jones AD, Goodrow MH, Saiz SG, Blewett G, Seiber JN et al. Determination of atrazine metabolites in human urine: development of a biomarker of exposure. Chem Res Toxicol 1993;6:107–116.
142. Balkisson R, Murray D, Hoffstein V. Alveolar damage due to inhalation of amitrole-containing herbicide. Chest 1992; 101:1174–1175.
143. Morgan DP. Recognition and management of pesticide poisonings. 4th ed. Washington, DC. US Env Prot Agency. EPA-540/9-88-001. 1989, pp. 154–155.
144. Day LC. Delayed death by endothall, a herbicide. Vet Hum Toxicol 1988;30:366.

BENZONITRILES—IOXYNIL AND BROMOXYNIL

Ioxynil (4-hydroxy-3,5,diiodo benzonitrile) and bromoxynil (3,5-dibromo-4-hydroxbenzonitrile)[1] have herbicidal properties similar to those of the chlorophenoxy and herbicides such as 2,4-D (2,4-dichloro-phenoxyacetic acid) and 2,4,5-T (2,4,5-trichlorophenoxyacetic acid).[2] Fatalities have been reported[3–6] with cardiac arrests occurring 5 to 8 hours after admission.[3]

STRUCTURE/PRODUCT FORMULATIONS

Ioxynil may be ingested as potassium, sodium, dimethylamine, or triethanolamine salts alone or with chlorophenoxy compounds.[4]

TOXIC DOSE

Ingestion of 18 g of ioxynil by an adult resulted in coma, shock, and death with acute pulmonary edema.[5]

TOXICOKINETICS

In one patient with plasma levels of 10 μg/mL ioxynil was cleared from the plasma with a half-life of approximately 112 hours.[4]

PATHOPHYSIOLOGY

The principal action of the benzonitriles (ioxynil and bromoxynil) is to uncouple oxidative phosphorylation.

CLINICAL PRESENTATION

The symptoms of acute poisoning with these two products are similar to those produced by other uncouplers such as pentachlorophenol and dinitrophenol. These include fatigue, excessive sweating, thirst, pyrexia, anxiety, tachycardia, and hyperventilation. Symptoms may resolve on cessation of exposure. This course was observed in four patients studied in France.[5]

A fatality occurred in a 54-year-old man who ingested an unknown quantity of ioxynil and died 45 minutes after admission to a hospital. Autopsy indicated brain, liver, and gut edema with upper gastrointestinal erosions.[6]

LABORATORY

A high-performance liquid chromatographic assay has been used to determine plasma levels of ioxynil and bromoxynil.[7] This method is able to separate these products from phenoxyacetic acids, which can then be analyzed concurrently. Chlorophenoxy and benzonitrile herbicides are often formulated together with other herbicides or other pesticides.[2] Urinary ioxynil has been assayed by gas-liquid chromatography with electron-capture detection of the acetylated derivative.[2] The limit of sensitivity was 0.2 μg/mL.[7]

Blood Levels

Total blood ioxynil concentrations performed on patients ranged from 10 to 320 μg/mL.[4] In that series ioxynil was encountered in seven fatalities, three of whom died in the hospital. Ioxynil levels in the serum were 300 μg/mL in a patient who died and 450 μg/mL in a patient who survived.[5]

Ioxynil blood levels 8 hours after ingestion of approximately 7 grams of ioxynil were 317 μg/mL. At postmortem 17 hours after ingestion the ioxynil level was 299 μg/mL. A serum ioxynil level of 300 μg/mL was observed 90 minutes after ingestion of 18 g of the product. Serum levels decreased to only 285 μg/mL 6 hours after hemoperfusion.[3] Two patients who died in a hospital had initial plasma ioxynil values of 290 μg/mL and 230 μg/mL. One patient died with a plasma ioxynil level of 40 μg/mL.[7]

Ancillary Tests

Thiocyanate urinary excretion was elevated in three of the four patients studied. One patient with severe muscular pain exhibited an elevation in the creatine kinase, lactic acid dehydrogenase, aldolase, and aminotransferases.[5]

Serum cyanide levels following a suicide attempt by an adult were 1.2 μg/mL and following administration of a cobalt compound remained in the range of 0.12 to 0.28 μg/mL for 48 hours. Urinary cyanide excretion rose following the cobalt compound (cobalt tetracemate) with a peak of 0.2 μg%.[4] Plasma thiocyanate levels were 2.5 to 4.8 μg/mL in one patient followed for 31 days.

TREATMENT

Stabilization

Benzonitrile ingestions require immediate care in an intensive care unit where intravenous lines, oxygen, and cardiac monitoring will be available. Arterial blood gases and oxygen status should be determined. For hyperpyrexic patients (rectal temperature over 39°C) the temperature should be reduced rapidly with cooling measures and the body temperature monitored with a rectal probe. Muscle rigidity may be associated with respiratory depression. Increase in muscular rigidity and a deteriorating acid-base balance may require neuromuscular paralysis.

Decontamination

Within the first few hours the usual methods of gastrointestinal decontamination (lavage, activated charcoal, cathartics) may diminish the amount of the benzonitriles absorbed. If there has been occupational exposure remove contaminated clothing and wash underlying skin with soap and water.

Elimination Enhancement

Charcoal hemoperfusion does not appear to affect either the clinical course or the serum ioxynil levels.[3,5] Alkaline diuresis did not influence ioxynil clearance in one series of cases.[7] However, alkaline diuresis may ameliorate the toxicity of ioxynil without influencing clearance.[7] Alkaline diuresis was used to treat three patients with initial plasma ioxynil concentrations of 70 to 320 mg/mL and all survived.[7] More data will be required before firm recommendations can be made.[7]

Antidotes

Although cobalt compounds have been used,[8] there are no antidotes that have been subjected to controlled clinical studies.

Supportive Care

Similarity of the clinical picture to that seen in malignant hyperthermia suggests possible use of dantrolene. No studies have used this drug.

REFERENCES—IOXYNIL AND BROMOXYNIL

1. Carpenter K, Cottrell HJ, De Silva WH, Hewyood BJ, Leeds WG, Rivett KF et al. Clinical and biological properties of two new herbicides—ioxynil and bromoxynil. Weed Res 1964;4:175–195.
2. Flanagan RJ, Ruprah M. HPLC measurement of chlorphenoxyherbicides, bromoxynil and ioxynil in biological specimens to aid diagnosis of acute poisoning. Clin Chem 1989;35:1342–1347.
3. Abi Khalil F, Alvoet C, Ectors M, Molle L. Acute fatal ioxynil intoxication. The International Association of Forensic Toxicologists: Proceedings of the 24th International Meeting, Banff. 1988; pp. 512–515.
4. Dickey W, McAleer JJA, Callender ME. Delayed sudden death after ingestion of MCPP and ioxynil. An unusual presentation of hormonal weedkiller intoxication. Postgrad Med J 1988;64:681–682.
5. Vogelaers D, Ectors M, de Wilde V, Klostin M, Khalil A, de Wispelaere I, Heyndrickx A. Ionxynil intoxication. Proc Eur Assoc Pois Control Cent. Edinburgh, September 1988. Newsletter Europ Assoc Pois Control Cent, March, 1989.
6. Smysl B, Smyslova O, Kosatik A. Akute todliche ioxynil vergiftung. Arch Toxicol 1977;37:241–245.
7. Conso F, Neel P, Pouzoulet C, Efthymiou ML, Gervais P, Gaultier M. Toxicite aigue chez l'homme des derives halogenes de l'hydroxybenzonitrile (ioxynil, bromoxynil). Arch Mal Prof 1977;38:674–677.

PROPIONITRILE

Propionitrile exposure in a chemical plant resulted in cyanide poisoning with coma and blood cyanide level of 220 mmol/L (57 μg/mL) 2 hours after exposure. The toxic effects responded to hydroxocobalamin (4 g) and sodium thiosulfate (8 g IV over less than 30 minutes).[1,2] Hydroxocobalamin has not been approved for general use in the United States.

Hydroxocobalamin administered with sodium thiosulfate in experimental poisoning results in excretion of thiocyanate as a primary urinary detoxification product. When hydroxocobalamin is administered alone, the primary elimination product is cyanocobalamin. Although up to 50% of hydroxocobalamin is excreted unchanged in the urine, it may be effective in cyanide detoxification by binding cyanide (forming cyanocobalamin), which is later given up to rhodanese for complexing with sulfone (producing thiocyanate and regenerating hydroxocobalamin).[1]

REFERENCES—PROPIONITRILE

1. Bismuth C, Baud FJ, Djeghout H, Astier A, Rubriot D. Cyanide poisoning from propionitrile exposure. J Emerg Med 1989;5:191–195.
2. Bismuth C, Baud FJ, Djeghout H, Astier A. Blood cyanide and thiocyanate kinetics after propionitrile exposure: effects of hydroxocobalamin and thiosulfate. Vet Hum Toxicol 1987;29(Suppl 2):41.

GLYPHOSATE SURFACTANT HERBICIDE

Glyphosate-surfactant herbicide concentrate (Roundup) (Gly SH) has often been ingested in an attempted suicide. The toxic syndrome produced consists of mucosal and gastrointestinal irritation, hypotension, metabolic acidosis, pulmonary insufficiency, and oliguria. Extensive clinical data suggest that individuals over 40 years of age who have ingested amounts of the concentrate varying from over 100 to 150 ml are at highest risk of death. Patients may appear to do well for many hours and then slowly lapse into a hypotensive, apparently nonhypovolemic shock that can be refractory to fluids and pressor amines and often ends fatally. Few deaths have followed accidental ingestion (usually children).[1] Most deaths have followed a suicidal attempt. About one in three patients do not develop systemic symptoms.

STRUCTURE AND CLASSIFICATION

Glyphosate is *N*-(phosphonomethyl) glycine. Its structural formula is $HOC\text{-}CH_2\text{-}NH\text{-}CH_2\text{-}P(OH)_2$. The molecular formula of glyphosate is $C_3H_8NO_5P$ and its isopropylamine salt, $C6H_{17}N_2O_4P$. Glyphosate has a molecular weight of 169.1. The isopropylamine salt has a molecular weight of 228.20. Glyphosate is a nonvolatile, white solid with a melting point of 230°C (decomposition). It is soluble to the extent of 12 g/liter in water at 25°C and is insoluble in common organic solvents.[2] Glyphosate is a broad-spectrum herbicide.

Synonyms in Taiwan

Nien nien chun, Hao Ni Chun, Lan Da, Fukwei Chun, Mien Tswu Tsao.[3]

Other Synonyms for Roundup

Glyphosate-surfactant herbicide (GlySH).

USES

Glyphosate is a herbicide useful in crop, noncrop, and aquatic weed control.[4]

PRODUCT FORMULATION

Roundup is a clear, yellowish brown liquid with a pH of 4.8[5] and has no distinctive odor. Its constituents include Glyphosate (the isopropylamine salt of *N*-(phosphonomethyl) glycine)—41%; polyoxyethyleneamine (POEA), a surfactant—15%; and water—44%. The product in use may be diluted 40 times to a concentration of glyphosate 1% and POEA 0.4%.[3] The diluted product produces little or no irritation of the skin or eyes.[6] Other products with glyphosate include Accord (for forestry), Honcho Herbicide, Ranger (for quackgrass), Rodeo (for aquatic use), Bronco (with alachlor), Fallow Master (with dicamba), Landmaster (with 2,4 D), Landmaster II (with 2,4 D), Landmaster BW (with 2,4 D), and Vision (for forestry use in Canada).[4]

SOURCES

Glyphosate is a synthetic chemical.

DOSAGE

Asymptomatic patients (Table 68–8) in one series appeared to ingest about 5 to 50 mL; mild symptoms were observed with ingestions of 5 to 150 mL. Moderate symptoms followed 20 to 500 mL, and severe symptoms, 85 to 200 mL.[7]

Toxic Dose

Ingestions of 30 to 60 mL of the concentrate may lead within 15 minutes to emesis, pharyngeal pain, and nausea. Within 6 to 8 minutes diarrhea supervenes, which may last 1 week. Such patients usually recover.[5] Survivors have usually ingested no more than 100 to 120 mL of the concentrate. These patients will develop gastrointestinal symptoms and pharyngeal inflammation. The symptoms may be due to the surfactant POEA.[5] Individuals have survived ingestion of up to 500 mL of the Roundup concentrate with mild to moderate symptomatology.[7,8] In general, adults swallowing 0.5 mL/kg or more of Roundup herbicide are at risk for serious symptoms.[3]

Fatal Dose

Fatalities have followed ingestions of over 100 mL of the concentrate.[3,5] The average dose of the concentrate in nonsurvivors ranged from 85 to 200 mL in one series,[7] to 263 more or less than 100 mL in another.[3] A minimal lethal dose of 150 mL has been suggested.[3] The LD_{50} of polyoxyethylene amine (the surfactant) is 1 to 2 g/kg; it is approximately three times more toxic than glyphosate.[9] Similar surfactants may cause gastrointestinal bleeding, sedation, hemolysis, and renal dysfunction.[10,11]

TOXICOKINETICS

There is little data available on the toxicokinetics of glyphosate in man. In animals 15 to 35% of glyphosate appears to be absorbed.[3] In dogs the apparent volume of distribution is 0.28 L/kg.[12] Its major metabolite is (aminomethyl) phosphonic acid (AMPA), which appeared in the plasma in man 3.5 hours after glyphosate ingestion in some nonsurvivors.[13] Both glyphosate and its metabolite (AMPA) are excreted in the urine.[14]

PATHOPHYSIOLOGY

Glyphosate is a useful herbicide because it effectively inhibits plant aromatic amino acid biosynthesis by inhibiting the enzyme 5-enol-pyruvyl shikimate-3-phosphate synthase. The shikimic acid pathway does not exist in animals.[15] Glyphosate does not act as an acetylcholinesterase inhibitor in man. Some data indicate that glyphosate may interfere with mitochondrial oxidative phosphorylation,[16] but tachypnea, tachycardia, and significant hyperpyrexia are not usually observed clinically.[3] The profound hypotensive shock observed in many of the nonsurvivors combined with a relative absence of hypovolemia suggests a direct cardiotoxic effect.[7] Death may be associated with severe hypotension, shock, renal failure, or a respiratory distress syndrome.[12]

CLINICAL PRESENTATION (TABLE 68–8)

Summary: A toxic syndrome follows the ingestion of a large volume of glyphosate-surfactant herbicide (Roundup) and

Table 68–8
Classification of Severity in Acute Poisoning with Roundup Herbicide[a]

Classification	Description
Asymptomatic	No complaints, and no abnormalities on physical or laboratory examination.
Mild	Mainly GI symptoms (nausea, vomiting, diarrhea, abdominal pain, mouth and throat pain) that resolved within 24 h. Vital signs were stable, and there was no renal, pulmonary or cardiovascular involvement.
Moderate	GI symptoms lasting longer than 24 h, GI hemorrhage, endoscopically verified esophagitis or gastritis, oral ulceration, hypotension responsive to intravenous fluids, pulmonary dysfunction not requiring intubation, acid–base disturbance, evidence of transient hepatic or renal damage, or temporary oliguria.
Severe	Pulmonary dysfunction requiring intubation, renal failure requiring dialysis, hypotension requiring treatment with pressor amines, cardiac arrest, coma, repeated seizures, or death.

[a]Adapted from Talbot AR et al. Hum Exp Toxicol 1991;10:1–8.

consists of oral-pharyngeal, mucosal, and gastrointestinal irritation, hypotension, pulmonary insufficiency, metabolic acidosis, and oliguria.[17] Effects on organs other than the gastrointestinal tract tend to occur with increasing amounts ingested. Adults over 40 years of age who have ingested over 100 to 150 mL of the GlySH appear to be at the highest risk of a fatal outcome.[3,7,8] There may be a low-grade fever after 6 to 24 hours.[18] Symptoms may reflect toxicity representing an interaction between glyphosate and POEA.

Mental Status

Initial mental status is usually abnormal when other substances have been coingested. In severe poisoning mental status alteration may develop after up to 6 hours, often attributable to hypoxia or hypotension.

Oral Mucosa

Sore throat, burning sensation in the mouth and throat, salivation, erythema, and oral ulcerations have been observed.

Gastrointestinal Tract

Spontaneous vomiting, nausea, epigastric and abdominal pain, diarrhea, and dysphagia are seen. Hematemesis and bloody stool have been observed. Paralytic ileus is rarely seen.[19] Acute pancreatitis has been observed.[19,20]

Endoscopy

Erosions of the pharynx and larynx were described in one series.[7] The esophagus was involved in 39% of cases with development of esophageal ulcers, superficial or corrosive esophagitis with mucosal edema, erosions, and hemorrhage.[7] Transmural injury or perforation has not been observed. The stomach is often involved (up to 96%) with gastritis and ulceration; the duodenum is involved in about 26% of patients with duodenitis or infrequently duodenal ulcer. Colitis has been observed rarely.[7] Gastric and esophageal abnormalities may follow ingestion of as little as 25 mL of GlySH.[8]

Pulmonary

Asymptomatic mild hypoxemia may be detected by arterial blood gas analysis. More serious involvement ranges from alveolar or interstitial infiltrates seen on a chest x-ray, tachypnea, dyspnea, cough, and bronchospasm to cyanosis, aspiration pneumonia, frank pulmonary edema, and respiratory failure. Lung injury may be due to toxic effects of both glyphosate and the surfactant.[21,22]

Cardiovascular

Hypotensive shock is often observed within hours after GlySH ingestion. In survivors this may be transient. In one series hypotensive shock occurred in all nonsurvivors. The hypotension may respond initially to position change, hydration, and pressor amines, but later becomes refractory to these measures. Hypovolemia does not appear to be the cause since hematocrit and blood urea nitrogen have been normal and there was no response to fluid resuscitation or vasopressors.[7,8]

Renal

Renal abnormalities may include oliguria, anuria, and infrequently gross or microscopic hematuria. Blood urea nitrogen and serum creatinine tend to be normal or slightly elevated initially.

Hepatic

Aminotransferases (AST, ALT) may be mildly elevated. Jaundice is not seen.

Central Nervous System

Confusion and coma may appear. Glasgow Coma Scale scores have ranged from 9 to 13 and can improve rapidly without treatment.[7]

Hematologic

GlySH does not appear to exert a primary toxic effect on bone marrow. Hemolysis has not been documented. No platelet or coagulation abnormalities have been reported.

Metabolic

A metabolic acidosis has been observed in most seriously poisoned patients. Initial blood pH measurements in one series were 7.18 more or less than 0.13 compared with 7.25 more or less than 0.20 in nonfatal cases. The metabolic acidosis is more often seen in those with serious poisoning, hypoxemia, or anuria. Lactate production may be a factor. In some fatal cases the metabolic acidosis has not responded to bicarbonate therapy.

Eyes

Temporary conjunctival irritation can occur from ocular exposure.

Skin

No significant absorption occurs through the skin. Prolonged contact can lead to a "detergent dermatitis."[8] Glyphosate does not appear to induce skin irritations, photo irritation, skin sensitizations, or photosensitization.[23,24] Table 68–8 presents a severity classification after acute poisoning with Roundup.[13]

POEA

The role of the surfactant POEA on symptom production has not been defined.

LABORATORY

Analytic Methods

Glyphosate and AMPA (aminomethyl) phosphonic acid can be quantitated by gas chromatography,[25] high-performance liquid chromatography,[24,26,27] gas chromatography/mass spectrometry,[28] and nuclear magnetic resonance spectroscopy.[29] Air samples of glyphosate can be measured by GC/MS to levels of 0.1 ng/mL (0.3 μg/m^3). Urine samples of glyphosate can be detected to a level of 0.1 ng/μL; AMPA can be detected to a level of 0.05 ng/μL (0.5 μmol/L).[14] Urine can be used as an indicator of glyphosate exposure. There is no clinical assay available to measure the surfactant. A high-performance chromatography method using ultraviolet detection can be performed rapidly for serum glyphosate (detection limits 0.3 μg/mL) and serum AMPA (detection limit 0.2 μg/mL) determinations.[30]

Blood Levels

Glyphosate and AMPA concentrations appear to be decreased after hemodialysis.[19] Levels diminish 50% by day 3 after an ingestion.[31] Following 100 mL of GlySH (Roundup), equivalent to 48 g of glyphosate, blood levels of glyphosate were 497 μg/mL and the urine concentration was 15,100 μg/mL. By day 3 less than 2.5 μg/mL was present in the blood. On the ninth day urine levels had fallen to 7.9 μg/mL.[5] Blood levels are not a good prognostic indicator of severity of poisoning. In one study survivors had glyphosate plasma levels of 0 to 725 μg/mL. Two nonsurvivors had plasma glyphosate levels of 918 μg/mL and 1515 μg/mL, respectively, with plasma AMPA levels of 88 and 32 μg/mL, respectively.[13]

Abnormalities

The serum amylase is frequently elevated, usually due to a salivary gland isoenzyme.[8] The electrocardiogram may exhibit sinus tachycardia or sinus bradycardia.[7] Atrioventricular block and ventricular ectopy has been observed.[10–12] Slight elevations in serum aminotransferases and bilirubin may be seen.[3,7,8] Serum acetylcholinesterase values are normal.[8] Between 10 and 20 hours after a 200- to 250-mL ingestion of GlySH concentrate the serum potassium level rose from 5.4 to 7.0.[18]

Ancillary Tests

About one-half of patients exhibit a leukocytosis; this appears more frequently in the more severely affected patients (see Table 68–1). Hyperglycemia has been observed in 30% of patients in one series.[32]

TREATMENT

Stabilization

Treatment of glyphosate surfactant herbicide (GlySH or Roundup) ingestion is based on aggressive symptomatic and supportive care. Patients who have ingested more than 0.5 mL of Roundup herbicide per kilogram of body weight should be admitted to an intensive care facility for evaluation and monitoring. Ensure patency of the airway and respiration. Careful monitoring of the status of pulmonary, cardiovascular, and renal functions is essential. Administer 100% oxygen initially. Respiratory distress may require cricothyroidotomy if endotracheal intubation is contraindicated by excessive swelling. Intravenous lines should be immediately established to aid in precluding the possibility of circulatory compromise. Do not administer buffering agents (e.g., antacids) since they may induce a exothermic reaction without altering the pH. Attempt to avoid further emesis by limiting the oral fluid intake.

Decontamination

If emesis has not occurred, the patient presents within 4 hours of ingestion, and about 0.5 mL/kg body weight of concentrate has been ingested, gastric lavage may be indicated. Protect against aspiration by frequent oral suctioning, placing the patient in the left lateral decubitus position, and inserting a cuffed endotracheal tube during lavage as required. Activated charcoal (50 to 100 g in water) may absorb the surfactant. There is no clinical evidence to support the use of multiple doses of activated charcoal or a cathartic. If the patient is oliguric or anuric, magnesium blood levels should be monitored before using magnesium sulfate as a cathartic.

Elimination Enhancement

There is no evidence to support the use of forced diuresis. Care must be taken to monitor fluid balance and prevent either fluid depletion or fluid overload. Hemodialysis or hemoperfusion have not been systematically studied, but may be useful in view of the low molecular (169) and the low volume of distribution (0.28 L/kg) seen in dogs.[12] The surfactant (POEA) may be metabolized, but little is known of its toxicokinetics. Hemodialysis is indicated for renal failure and intractable metabolic acidosis.[33]

Antidote

There is no antidote for the treatment of glyphosate surfactant herbicide toxicity.

Supportive Measures

1. Confusion may exist that glyphosate surfactant herbicide (Roundup) is an organophosphate compound. It is not. Do not give atropine or 2-pralidoxime (2PAM).
2. Gastrointestinal—Rinse the mouth with water. Topical anesthetics such as viscous lidocaine may be useful for oral pain in a conscious, alert patient. Patients should not be fed orally until endoscopy has confirmed the extent of injury.
3. Histamine-2 antagonists such as cimetidine, ranitidine, and other similar drugs may be considered.
4. Serial abdominal examinations, and, if indicated, radiography and water-soluble contrast studies may aid in management of gastric or duodenal ulcers.
5. Steroids have not been systematically evaluated in this ingestion. Antibiotics should be reserved for documented infections.

6. Cardiovascular—Hypotension may develop hours after ingestion. Cardiac monitoring should be available. If hypotension develops, treat initially with IV fluids and place the patient in the Trendelenburg position. If the patient is unresponsive to fluid challenges, use pressor amines. A central venous pressure line or Swan-Ganz catheter should be used to guide fluid therapy where clinically required. An arterial line for constant blood pressure monitoring is advisable. Fluid overload may lead to pulmonary edema.
7. Pulmonary—Respiratory function should be evaluated by serial chest x-rays, arterial blood gas determination, and clinical evidence of signs of respiratory distress (dyspnea, cyanosis, tachypnea). Adequate oxygenation may require intubation, assisted ventilation, high inspiratory oxygen flow rates, and positive end-expiratory pressure (PEEP). Use antibiotics for documented infection. When fluid overload or left ventricular failure is evident, furosemide may be useful. Morphine may compromise blood pressure, depress cardiac output, or impair the central respiratory drive.
8. Renal—Urine output should be monitored hourly. Adequate circulating volume and systolic blood pressure should be ensured. Do not use diuretics for volume depletion or hypotension. Mannitol may precipitate pulmonary edema. It should not be used in an anuric patient. Dialysis is indicated for renal failure.
9. Metabolic acidosis—Monitor blood pH and serum bicarbonate. Treat significant acidosis with bicarbonate infusion. Failure to reverse acidosis may be an indication for hemodialysis to correct the acid-base balance.
10. Laboratory—Monitor white cell count, hematocrit, hemoglobin, electrolytes, blood urea nitrogen, creatinine, bilirubin, amylase (isoenzyme), hepatic aminotransferases, acid-base status, arterial blood gas, chest x-ray, central venous pressure, pulmonary capillary wedge pressure, pulmonary capillary wedge pressure, and cardiac output as indicated clinically.
11. Inhalation exposure—Remove from aerosol exposure; use drinking water to wash the throat; nasal irrigation as required.
12. Dermal exposure—Wash contaminated skin with mild soap and water; bland ointments for rashes.
13. Eye exposure—Irrigate eyes with normal saline or water for at least 15 to 20 minutes. Artificial tears may relieve residual irritation. If irritation persists, call an ophthalmologist.

Occupational Precautions[29,31]

1. Wear chemical-resistant gloves, head covering, long-sleeved shirt, long pants, and shoes with socks.
2. Avoid getting glyphosate surfactant herbicide concentrate on the skin or eyes.
3. Launder clothing worn during application of the herbicide separately from the family laundry.
4. Children and pets should be kept from close contact with an area sprayed for 24 hours after use.
5. Store in its original container, in a secure place, away from children and pets.
6. Do not pour unused product down sinks or into showers.

Glyphosate may be contaminated with *N*-nitrosoglyphosate. The State of California classifies glyphosate as a mouse oncogen.[34–36]

BIALOPHOS[37,38]

Bialophos (CAS 35597-43-4) is a sodium salt of L-2-amino-4-[(hydroxy) (methyl)phosphinoyl]butyryl-L-alanyl-L-alanine, with a molecular weight of 345.26. It is one of the glyphosate herbicides fermented from *Streptomyces hygroscopicus.* In plants, bialophos is metabolized to glufosinate, an irreversible inhibitor of the binding of glutamine to glutamine synthetase. This causes a toxic accumulation of ammonia. Ingestion of 100 mL (32% w/v%) of bialophos by an adult led to vomiting in 30 minutes, cyanosis, a metabolic acidosis, nystagmus, respiratory arrest 36 hours later, seizures 44 hours following ingestion, and fever. The patient recovered. Bialophos is detected in human serum as its metabolite, L-AMPB, by aminometric analysis.[38] Respiratory support, intravenous fluid, orogastric intubation, gastric lavage, sodium bicarbonate, and furosemide have been used in management.

An anecdotal study indicates that bialophos may induce respiratory arrest, seizures, nystagmus, reversible hepatic dysfunction, and a metabolic acidosis. Bialophos is measured in serum by aminometric analysis. Treatment is symptomatic and supportive.[38]

GLUFOSINATE (BASTA)

Basta contains glufosinate ammonium 18.5%. Acute poisoning with over 1 to 9 mL/kg of herbicides containing glufosinate may lead to delayed (several hours) central nervous system disorders such as coma, convulsions, and respiratory arrest. Deaths from circulatory failure have occurred after ingestion of 5.5 mg/kg. Hemodialysis may be useful.[39,40]

REFERENCES

1. Jackson JR. Toxicity of herbicide containing glyphosate. Lancet 1988;1:414.
2. Glyphosate. WHO Monograph. Food and Agriculture Organization, United Nations Pesticide Residue in Food Evaluation. Part 2. Toxicology. Rome, 1986. Paper 78/2.
3. Tominack RL, Yang G-Y, Tsai W-J, Chung H-M, Deng J-F. Taiwan National Poison Center Survey of glyphosate-surfactant herbicide ingestions. Clin Toxicol 1991;29:91–109.
4. Glyphosate. In: [Humburg, NE, Chairman] Chicago, IL: Herbicide Handbook of the Weed Science Society of America. 6th ed. Weed Science Society of America, 1989.
5. Kawamura K, Nobuhara H, Tsuda K, Tanaka A, Matsubara Y, Yamauchi N. Two cases of glyphosate (Roundup) poisoning. Pharmaceuticals Monthly 1987;29:163 (Japanese, translated).
6. Tominack RL. Acute human exposure to glyphosate-surfactant herbicide. Proc Internat Cong Clin Toxicol, Poison Control, Anal Toxicol. LuxTox'90, May 2–5, 1990, Luxembourg.
7. Talbot AR, Sahw MH, Huang J-S, Yang S-F, Goo T-S, Wang S-H, Chen C-L, Sanford TR. Acute poisoning with a glyphosate-surfactant herbicide ("Roundup"): a review of 93 cases. Hum Exp Toxicol 1991;10:1–8.
8. Tominack R, Conner P, Yamashita M. Clinical management of Roundup herbicide exposure. Jpn J Toxicol 1989;2:187–192.

9. Kubota T, Hamada K, Nika H, Konoe A, Ikeda K, Hisaaki I et al. A case of glyphosate poisoning. Gekkan Yakuji 1986; 28(8):7 (abstract) (Japanese, translated by Dr. Alan Talbot).
10. Sawada Y, Nagai Y: Roundup poisoning—its clinical observation. Possible involvement of surfactant. J Clin Exp Med (Igaku No Ayumi) 1987;143(1):25–27 (Japanese, translated).
11. Sawada Y, Nagai Y, Veyama M, Yamamoto I. Probable toxicity of surface-active agent in commercial herbicide containing glyphosate. Lancet 1988;1:299.
12. Deng J-F, Chung H-M, Yang Y-G, Tsai W-J, Ger J. The treatment of Nien Nien Chun ingestion poisoning. Clinical Medicine (Taiwan) 1988;22:469–473 (Translation).
13. Talbot AR, Chen ZL, Goo TS, Huang JS, Wang SH, Sahw MH, Yang SF. Plasma levels and hemodynamics in acute glyphosate poisonings. Vet Hum Toxicol 1990;32:370.
14. Jauhiainen A, Rasanen K, Sarantila R, Nuutinen J, Kangas J. Occupational exposure of forest workers to glyphosate during brush saw spraying work. Am Ind Hyg Assoc J 1991; 52:61–64.
15. Duke SO. Overview of herbicide mechanism of action. Environ Health Perspect 1990;87:263–271.
16. Orlorunsogo OO, Bababunmi EA, Bassir O. Effect of glyphosate on rat liver mitochondria in vivo. Bull Environ Cont Toxicol 1979;22:357–364.
17. Yamashita M, Mizutani T, Nakamura K, Koike J, Tsuchiya Y, Yamamoto S. Four cases of Roundup poisoning. ICU to CCU 1987;11(Autumn Suppl):156–157 (abstract) (Japanese, translated by Dr. Alan Talbot).
18. Menkes DB, Temple WA, Edwards IR. Intentional self poisoning with glyphosate-containing herbicides. Hum Exp Toxicol 1991;10:103–107.
19. Nonaka J, Niki H, Aizawa K, Ikeda K, Makino Y, Itoo M, Isshiki J. A case of glyphosate poisoning. Tokyo Idai Shi 1986; 44(3):575 (abstract) (Japanese, translated by Dr. Alan Talbot).
20. Nishimoto K. Pesticide poisoning in our hospital - especially in regard to poisoning with glyphosate (Roundup). Masui to Sosei 1987;23(2):149 (abstract) (Japanese, translated by Dr. Alan Talbot).
21. Martinez TT, Long WC, Hiller R. Comparison of the toxicology of the herbicide Roundup by oral and pulmonary routes of exposure. Proc West Pharmacol Soc 1990;33:193–197.
22. Martinez TT, Brown K. Oral and pulmonary toxicology of the surfactant used in Roundup herbicide. Proc West Pharmacol Soc 1991;34:43–46.
23. Maibach H. Irritation, sensitization, photoirritation and photosensitization assays with a glyphosate herbicide. Contact Dermatitis 1986;15:152–156.
24. Hoogheem TJ. The safety of Roundup pesticide. JAMA 1989;262:2679.
25. Deyrup CL, Chang SM, Weintraub RA, Moye HA. Simultaneous esterification and acetylation of pesticides for analysis by gas chromatography. I. Derivatization of glyphosate and (aminomethyl) phosphoric acid with fluorinated alcholos-perfluorinated anhydrides. J Ag Food Chem 1985;33:944–947.
26. Moye HA, Miles CJ, Scherer SJ. A simplified high-performance liquid chromatographic residue procedure for the determination of glyphosate herbicide and (aminomethyl) phosphoric acid in fruits and vegetables employing postcolumnar fluorogenic labelling. J Ag Food Chem 1983;31:69–76.
27. Cowell JE, Kumstman J, Nord PJ, Steinmetz JR, Wilson GR. Validation of an analytical method for analysis of glyphosate and metabolite: an interlaboratory study. J Ag Food Chem 1986;34:955–960.
28. Kageura M, Hara K, Heida Y, Kashimura S. A derivatization of glyphosate and aminomethylphosphoric acid for GC/MS analysis. Bull Int Assoc Forensic Toxicol 1988;20(1):43.
29. Dickson SJ, Meinhold RH, Beer ID, Koelmeyer TD: Rapid determination of glyphosate in post-mortem specimens using 31P NMR. J Anal Toxicol 1988;12:284–286.
30. Tomita M, Okuyama T, Watanabe S, Uno B, Kawai S. High performance liquid chromatographic determination of glyphosate and (amino methyl) phosphoric acid in human serum after conversion into p toluenesulphonyl derivatives. J Chromatogr Biomed Appl 1991;566:239–243.
31. Hara Y, Hiraoka H, Morimoto T, Sasaki H, Ishikawa K, Kirimoto K et al. Three cases of pesticide poisoning focusing on fatalities due to glyphosate. Iryo 1985;39(Suppl 2): 310 (abstract) (Japanese, translated by Dr. Alan Talbot).
32. Ong HC, Tsai WJ, Deng JF. An analysis of the clinical findings observed in the case of glyphosate ingestion. Poisonings XIVth International Congress of European Association of Poison Control Centres. Milan, Italy, September 25–28, 1990, p. 160.
33. Harry P, Tirot P, Maigret P, Bouachour G. Haemodialysis in glyphosate poisoning. Toxicol Lett 1992;5 (Suppl):319.
34. Moses M. Glyphosate herbicide toxicity. JAMA 1989;261: 2549.
35. Moses M. The safety of Roundup pesticide. JAMA 1989;262: 2679.
36. Medical Toxicology Branch. Summary of Toxicology Data: Glyphosate, Isopropylamine Salt. Sacramento. State of California Dept of Food and Agriculture, 1988, Publication SB950-241.
37. Wada S, Ushlimaru H, Nozawa K et al. A case of acute intoxication of bialophos. Jpn J Acute Med 1988;12:245–247.
38. Matsukawa Y, Hachisuka H, Sawada S, Horie T, Kitamini Y, Nishijima S. Bialophos poisoning with apena and metabolic acidosis. Clin Toxicol 1991;29:141–146.
39. Koyama K, Matsuo H, Saraki H, Andou Y. The acute oral toxic dose of herbicide containing glufosinate. Clin Toxicol 1995;33:475–486 (abstract 85).

FUNGICIDES—PENTACHLOROPHENOL

EPIDEMIOLOGY

Acute poisoning has occurred in workers exposed while dipping wood in liquid formulations, immersion of their hands in the solutions, spraying pentachlorophenol (PCP) solutions as a molluscicide, by hobbyists after brushing PCP onto logs intended for a recreational log cabin, and by the use of insecticides containing PCP to clean wood furniture.[1]

CONTAMINANTS

The content of PCP in commercially available PCP solutions is about 80 to 90%, with tetrachlorophenol 4 to 12% trichlorophenol less than 0.1 to 10%, and hydroxychlorodiphenylether 1 to 5%. The 5% of "inert" ingredients contain varying quantities of dioxins and furans.[1]

TOXIC DOSAGE

In groups of individuals not specifically exposed to PCP, net daily intake varied from 5 μg (Nigeria) to 37 μg (the Netherlands). Net intake was 51 μg/day to 57 μg/day in residents of homes made of PCP-treated logs. In individuals occupationally exposed to PCP, net daily intake varied from 35 μg to about 24,000 μg.[2]

TOXICOKINETICS

Absorption

Significant amounts of pentachlorophenol have been reported in human serum, adipose tissue, and urine. PCP is even found in people not occupationally exposed to this toxin or not living in PCP-treated log houses.[3]

Acute Effects

Within several hours of exposure fever, perspiration, headache, malaise, abdominal pain, anorexia, nausea, vomiting, weakness, myalgias, and thirst develop; in severe cases these symptoms progress to coma, convulsions, cerebral edema, and vascular collapse.

CLINICAL PRESENTATION

Chronic Effects

Chronic poisoning is often difficult to detect because symptoms can often be vague and include anorexia, weight loss, general weakness, dizziness, headache, personality changes, anxiety, urticaria, pemphigus vulgaris, and chloracne. Fever is seen in chronic, as well as acute, intoxication. Upper respiratory complaints, conjunctivitis, and chronic sinusitis have been seen.[1]

Gerhard and colleagues suggest that prolonged exposure to pentachlorophenol may be a factor in hirsutism, alopecia, unexplained infertility, repeated abortions, and other endocrine and immunologic disorders in women. Further observations will be required to validate these findings.[4]

Workers with a documented episode of direct skin contact with PCP appear to have a significant increased risk of chloracne. Such chloracne is associated with exposure to PCP contaminated with hexachlorinated, heptachlorinated, and octochlorinated dibenzo-*p*-dioxins and dibenzofurans.[5]

A case-referent preliminary study on occupational risk factors among patients with gliomas suggests a raised risk among wood workers.[6]

Carcinogenicity

Pentachlorophenol is considered as possibly carcinogenic to humans (Group 2B) by the International Agency for Research on Cancer (IARC). There is an inconclusive series of studies suggesting an increase in risk for nasal and nasopharyngeal cancer in wood nodes.[1]

LABORATORY

PCP reduces both glomerular filtration rates and tubular function. An increased anion gap and a metabolic acidosis has been observed in acute PCP poisoning. A typical odor of PCP can be noted in the urine after a massive acute poisoning in addition to proteinuria, acetone, and an aminoacidosis. Chronic exposure may be associated with decreased high-density lipoprotein cholesterol and increased triglyceride levels. Two studies have observed a decrease in serum bilirubin levels.[1]

In nonoccupationally exposed individuals, blood pentachlorophenol concentrations range up to 1 mg/L, whereas pentachlorophenol-exposed workers have levels up to 10 mg/L. Obvious intoxication occurs with blood pentachlorophenol levels exceeding 40 mg/L.[7] One postmortem blood study of an occupational exposure revealed a level of 162 ppm.[8] Electron-capture gas chromatography of a methyl or ethyl derivative is the preferred method of analysis.[9]

One study of occupational exposure of workers exposed to pentachlorophenol (PCP) in a wood factory indicated that plasma PCP concentrations varied from 50 to 200 μg/L in workers without direct exposure and from 500 to 600 μg/L in workers handling and applying PCP on the wood. Urine PCP concentration ranged from 5 to 12 μg/L except for subjects having home exposure from indoor wooden surfaces who showed urinary values up to 100 μg/L.[10]

Pentachlorophenol has been observed in the cerebrospinal fluid (0.24 to 2.03 μg/L [ppb]). The CSF level did not correlate with the serum PCP concentration nor with the protein level of the cerebrospinal fluid.[1]

Antidotes

There is no antidote.

TREATMENT

Supportive Care

1. Solutions spilled on the skin should be removed promptly by thorough washing with soap and water.
2. Eyes should be flushed to remove all chemicals.
3. The use of antipyretics are not recommended to control fever since antipyretics such as aspirin produce salicylate in the body. Salicylate is also an uncoupler of oxidative phosphorylation and could add to toxicity.[1]

FUNGICIDES—ALAR (DAMINOZIDE)

Studies in the 1970s suggested that daminozide was carcinogenic in animals. This effect appears largely due to its hydrolysis product 1,1-demethylhydrazine.[11]

In February 1989 the Environmental Protection Agency stated that alar posed a significant risk of cancer in humans.[12] Strong disagreement to this view was voiced by Bruce Ames in May 1989.[13] A month later the EPA reversed its advice. The manufacturer, Uniroyal, voluntarily withdrew the chemical from the United States market, but is still selling it to the United Kingdom, where at least 7% of the apple crop is sprayed with the substances. Friends of the Earth has called for a ban on the chemical in the United Kingdom.[14]

Some apple juice brands were tested by Consumers Union and no detectable levels of alar were found in 1988 or 1989.[15] The laboratory process was able to detect to 0.02 ppm.[15] By 1990 the FDA and Consumers Union found little detectable alar on apples in the United States.[16] There have been no confirmed cases of acute poisoning from ingesting legally applied pesticides on food in California. There have been no epidemiologic studies indicating an actual human cancer incidence following the use of alar on apples.

CHLORTHALONIL

Chlorthalonil (Bravo, Clotocaffaro, Clortosip, Daconil 2787, Exotherm Terinil, Tuffcide), CAS Registry number 1897-45-6, is used as a fungicide in the culture of many vegetables, fruits, and ornamental plants.[17]

CLINICAL PRESENTATION

Chlorthalonil has caused irritation of skin and mucous membranes of the eyes and respiratory tract on contact. It is poorly absorbed across the skin and the gastrointestinal mucosa. Few cases of systemic poisoning have been reported.[18]

LABORATORY

Chlorthalonil can be measured in blood by gas chromatography.[19]

TREATMENT

Toxicity for chlorthalonil is similar to that after hexachlorthiazine. Treatment is primarily supportive.

METALDEHYDE

During 1990 there were 292 exposures to metaldehyde reported to the American Association of Poison Control Centers National Data Collection System.[20] Most reports concerned children under age 6 years. Almost all were accidental. They exhibited moderate to life-threatening symptomatology. There were no deaths.

STRUCTURE/PRODUCT FORMULATIONS

Metaldehyde is a tetramer composed of an eight-member ring containing aldehyde (CH_3CHO) molecules. In the United States, metaldehyde formulations are limited to concentrations less than 4% by weight and occasionally contain other toxic components (e.g., carbaryl, arsenate, organophosphates). European uses for metaldehyde include Meta-fuel tablets, which are portable energy products and equally common sources of poisoning. European metaldehyde concentrations in commercial molluscicides may reach 50%.

TOXIC DOSAGE

Although serious metaldehyde poisonings are extremely rare in the United States, several accidental and suicidal deaths resulting from ingestion of Meta-fuel tablets have been reported in Europe.[21] American children exposed to metaldehyde almost always are asymptomatic.[22]

LABORATORY

Ingestion of about 100 to 150 mg/kg of metaldehyde led to peak serum levels of metaldehyde (120 µg/mL) 35 hours after ingestion and urine levels of 53 µg/mL in 14 hours. Acetaldehyde levels in the serum were less than 1.0 µg/mL.[23] A gas chromatographic assay for use with plasma or urine has a sensitivity of 1 µg/mL for urine and 2 µg/mL for plasma.[24]

A 44-year-old alcoholic individual consumed vodka with 1 cupful of Deadline (containing 4% metaldehyde). The patient presented in 10 hours with vomiting, seizures, a Glasgow coma scale of 6, heart rate 140 bpm, blood pressure 222/117, and respirations 44 to 48/minute. Despite phenytoin and phenobarbital IV intermittent seizures continued. By 12 hours his temperature had risen to 39.8°C. He remained unresponsive, flushed, and diaphoretic. At 16 hours his serum contained 1 mg/dL of acetaldehyde derived from metaldehyde and his urine contained 3 mg/dL of acetaldehyde. On day 8 he was discharged without sequelae.[25]

INSECT REPELLENTS—DIETHYLTOLUAMIDE

The American military finds 75% diethyltoluamide (DEET) useful to protect its forces in jungles infested with disease-carrying mosquitos. Yet preparations containing 100% DEET are available in the United States, some of which may be used in children (Table 68–9).

FORMULATIONS

DEET is a colorless to amber liquid found in "Muskol" (spray 25%, lotion 100%), "Deep Woods Off" (liquid 100%, aerosol 40%), "Jungle Plus" (100%), "Jungle Formul" (75%), "Repel" (20%), "Off" (aerosol 15%, Towelettes 31%), Cutter (spray 17.9%), "6-12 plus" (5%). Because of its water insolubility it is usually prepared in an ethyl or 0.5 propyl alcohol vehicle.

TOXICOKINETICS[26–28]

DEET is absorbed by the oral and dermal routes. About 9 to 56% of a topically applied dose is absorbed within 6 hours. Peak plasma concentration for gastrointestinal and dermal absorption sites is usually reached within 1 hour. About 10 to 15% of each dose can be recovered unchanged from the urine. Volume of distribution is 2.1 L/kg. Plasma half-life is 2.5 hours. DEET is eliminated by hepatic oxidative metabolism through the P450 enzyme system. About 10 to 14% is excreted in the urine unchanged. Urinary half-life is 4 hours. DEET and its metabolites can be detected in the urine for 2 weeks and from the skin and adipose tissues for 1 to 3 months after dermal application. It exhibits an enterohepatic recirculation.[29]

Table 68–9
Selected Insect Repellents Containing Diethyltoluamide[a]

Product	Manufacturer (Location)	Form	% Diethyltoluamide[b]
6-12 Plus	Sterling Drug (Montvale, NJ 07645)	Aerosol	5
		Stick	9.1
Off!	S.C. Johnson and Son (Racine, WI 53403)	Aerosol	15
		Towelettes	32.31
Deep Woods Off!	S.C. Johnson and Son	Aerosol	20
		Pump spray	20
		Lotion	30
Deep Woods Off! Maximum Strength	S.C. Johnson and Son	Liquid	100
Cutter Insect Repellent	Cutter Division of Miles Laboratories (Chicago, IL 60638)	Spray	17.9
		Stick	33
		Cream	51.75
Muskol	Plough, Inc. (Memphis, TN 38151)	Spray	40
		Lotion	100
		Liquid	100

[a]Adapted from Edwards DL, Johnson CE. Clin Pharm 1987;6:496–498.
[b]All of the products also contain isomers of diethyltoluamide. Percentages reflect total diethyltoluamide content.

The optimal concentration of DEET for prevention of tick bites is unknown. Repellents containing 20 to 30% DEET applied to clothing are approximately 90% effective in preventing tick attachment.[30] Use of 10% DEET in small children may be especially dangerous.[31,32] Repeated cutaneous application of varying concentrations of DEET in children can lead to behavioral, ataxia, encephalopathy, seizures, coma, and death.[33] Ingestion of DEET has resulted in hypotension, seizures, coma, and death.

CLINICAL PRESENTATION

Skin

Immediate-contact urticaria[34,35] and a general pruritus that led to a generalized angioedema (after spraying with a 52% solution of DEET)[36] have been described.

LABORATORY

Analytic Method

A procedure for monitoring *N,N'*-diethyl-*m*-toluamide in urine and serum by high-performance liquid chromatography has been described. Limit of detection is 0.09 μg/mL in urine and 0.09 μg/g for serum.[33]

Blood level

Applications of 0.14 to 1.86 g over wide skin areas led to serum values of 0.15 μg/g to 1.17 μg/g with the peak serum concentrations occurring 1 to 2 hours after DEET application.[33] Only 2 of 9 subjects had measurable quantities of DEET in their urine though levels of 0.3 μg/mL were found 22 hours after application. A routine cutaneous application of DEET in man (133 mg/kg) led to serum levels of 0.31 mg/dL (3.10 μg/mL) (0.16 mmol/L).[37] Application of 10 to 12 g of DEET to 75% of the body surface led to maximum DEET blood concentrations of 0.087 mg/L (0.0045 mmol/L) and 0.092 mg/dL (0.0048 mmol/L) in 2 volunteers, respectively.

Blood levels were obtained for 4.1 and 5.5 hours, respectively. Ingestion of about 50 g of DEET led to blood levels of 16.8 mg/dL (0.88 mmol/L) in one patient who died and 24 mg/dL (1.25 mmol/L) in another patient who was found dead.

Two of five patients who ingested insect repellents containing DEET developed coma, seizures, and hypotension within 1 hour of ingestion. Two died. Three had no sequelae.[33,38–40] Ingestion of a 25% solution of DEET resulted in a concentration of 0.32 mg/L in 1 hour. Fatalities have been associated with blood concentrations of 240 mg/L.[41] Seizures may begin from 8 to 48 hours after last using DEET. Ataxic psychosis developed in a 30-year-old adult after daily applications of a 70% solution of DEET.[31,42–46]

Seizures may begin from 8 to 48 hours after last using DEET. A toxic psychosis developed in a 30-year-old adult after daily application of a 70% solution of DEET.

TREATMENT

Treatment is supportive. To minimize the possibility of adverse reactions to DEET, the following precautions are suggested[33]:

1. Apply repellent sparingly only to exposed skin or clothing.
2. Avoid applying high-concentration products to the skin, particularly of children.
3. Do not inhale or ingest repellents or get them into the eyes.
4. Wear long sleeves and long pants, when possible, and apply repellent to clothing to reduce exposure to DEET.
5. Avoid applying repellents to portions of the children's hands that are likely to have contact with eyes or mouth.
6. Never use repellents on wounds or irritated skin.
7. Use repellent sparingly; one application will last 4 to 8 hours. Saturation does not increase efficacy.
8. Wash repellent-treated skin after coming indoors.
9. If a suspected reaction to insect repellents occurs, wash treated skin, and call a physician. Take the repellent can to the physician.

Specific medical information about the active ingredients in insect repellents is available from the National Pesticide Telecommunications Network, Telephone (800) 858-7378.

Establish and maintain vital function. Seizures are treated with diazepam and phenytoin. Decontaminate with gastric lavage after ingestion. Do not use emetics because of the rapid onset of seizures. Administer activated charcoal initially with a cathartic. Repetitive doses of activated charcoal may be useful because of the possible enterohepatic recirculations. For dermal exposure, remove the clothing and wash the skin thoroughly with tepid water and soap. Cerebral edema is treated with hyperventilation, fluid restriction, head elevation, and mannitol. Consider intracranial pressure monitoring. Monitor for inappropriate secretion of the antidiuretic hormone.[29]

Phthalates are also insect repellents. They can cause skin irritation and, if ingested, may lead to coma.

FUMIGANTS

Chemicals used as fumigants[47] include halocarbons (methylene chloride, methyl bromide, chloroform, carbon tetrachloride, chloropicrin, ethylene dichloride, dibromochloropropane, ethylene dibromide, dichloropropene, dibromochloropropene, paradichlorobenzene), oxides, and aldehydes (ethylene oxide, propylene oxide, formaldehyde, paraformaldehyde, acrolein).

Commercial products under study include the following:

Hydrocarbon

Naphthalene (naphthene).

Halocarbons

Methylene chloride, methyl bromide (bromomethane, Brom-O-Gas, Brom-O-Sol, Meth-O-Gas, Terr-O-Gas, Brom-O-Gaz, Celfume, Kayafume, MeBr), chloroform (trichloromethane), carbon tetrachloride, chloropicrine (nitrochloroform, Chlor-O-Pic, Aquinite, Dojyopicrine, Dolochlor, Laracide, Pic-Clor, Tri-Clor), ethylene dichloride (dichloroethane, EDC), ethylene dibromide (dibromoethane, Bromofume, Celmide, E-D-Bee, EdB, Kopfume, Nephis), dichloropropene (Telone II Soil Fumigant, D-D92), dichloropropene plus dichloropropane (D-D), dibromochloropropane (Nemafume, Nomanax, Nemaset, DBCP, Nematocide), paradichlorobenzene (PDB, Paracide).

Oxides and Aldehydes

Ethylene oxide (epoxyethane, ETO, Oxirane), propylene oxide, formaldehyde (formalin is a 40% aqueous solution), paraformaldehyde, acrolein (propenal, acrylaldehyde, Aqualin).

Sulfur Compounds

Sulfur dioxide, sulfuryl fluoride (Vikane), carbon disulfide.

Phosphorus Compounds

Phosphine (liberated from aluminum phosphide: phostoxin, AIP, Fumitoxin).

Nitrogen Compounds

Hydrogen cyanide (hydrocyanic acid, prussic acid, Cyclon), acrylonitrile (Acritet, Carbacryl, Acrylofume—all mixtures with carbon tetrachloride).

Naphthalene, methylene chloride, methylbromide, chloroform, carbon tetrachloride, ethylene dichloride, ethylene dibromide, dibromochlorpropane, dichloropropane, paradichlorobenzene, ethylene oxide, formaldehyde, acrolein, sulfur dioxide, carbon disulfide, hydrogen cyanide, and acrylonitrile are discussed in other chapters.

TREATMENT

Flush contaminating fumigants from the skin and rinse with copious amounts of water for at least 15 minutes. Remove victims to fresh air immediately. Watch for corrosive damage to the cornea, pulmonary edema, shock, and seizures. Treat supportively and symptomatically.

ALUMINUM PHOSPHIDE

Aluminum phosphide orally is rapidly becoming a very commonly used agent for self-poisoning in India.[48–50] It is highly lethal due to the fact that, in the presence of moisture, aluminum phosphide releases phosphine, which can cause severe pulmonary edema in humans. Taken orally phosphine is liberated in the stomach causing gastrointestinal irritation and intractable peripheral circulatory failure. The number of people killed by phosphine every year in India may be greater than the methyl isocyanate deaths in the Union Carbide tragedy at Bhopal in 1984.[50] Occupational phosphine exposure has occurred in Indian workers.[51]

STRUCTURE AND CLASSIFICATION

Aluminum phosphide, $Al \equiv P$, in the presence of moisture liberates phosphine, PH_3.

USES

Aluminum phosphide is used as a grain preservative. Fumigation depends on the release of phosphine gas from the aluminum phosphide when it comes into contact with the moisture in the grain.

PRODUCT FORMULATION

It is marketed in India as Cephos, Quickphas, Synfume, and Phosphine tablets of 3 g each containing 57% aluminum phosphide.[48]

TOXIC DOSE

Phosphine concentrations in the work environment ranged from 0.17 to 2.11 ppm when workers involved in fumigation became ill.[52] Clinical effects from phosphine may occur at levels below the olfactory threshold of 1.5 to 3 ppm.[53]

FATAL DOSE

Less than 500 mg is a usual lethal dose of aluminum phosphide in India.[49]

MECHANISM OF ACTION

The exact mechanism of action of aluminum phosphide is not known. In animals it induces a noncompetitive inhibition of mitochondrial cytochrome oxidase.[48]

CLINICAL PRESENTATION

Aluminum Phosphide

Following an ingestion of aluminum phosphide patients will present with profuse vomiting and pain in the upper abdomen. Clinical presentation may also be characterized by a marked tachycardia, altered sensorium, anemia, and pulmonary edema.[48,54] Intractable shock is usually present, and death occurs within half an hour to 3 days of admission.[52]

Aluminum phosphide tablets mistakenly placed in a home for rodent control released phosphine gas. A 6-year-old experienced a heavy inhalation exposure. She also ingested one or more aluminum phosphide tablets. She presented to the hospital in profound shock 36 hours later and developed multisystem failure with asystole 16 hours after admission.[55] After resuscitation, peritoneal dialysis, and vitamin B she recovered. If patients survive the initial 6 to 24 hours, the adult respiratory distress syndrome may supervene. Patients with mild toxicity recover. If the patient reaches the hospital with significant hypotension, death is a probable outcome. Workers engaged in fumigation of stored grains reported minor symptoms, including cough, dyspnea, tightness around the chest, headache, giddiness, numbness, lethargy, anorexia, and epigastric pain. They exhibited diffuse bilateral rhonchi and absent ankle reflex. Motor nerve conduction velocities of the median and peripheral nerves and sensory conduction velocity of the median and sural nerves were normal.[51]

Phosphine

Symptoms from acute exposure are generally transient and findings are often absent on physical examination and laboratory tests.

LABORATORY
Abnormalities

Minor increases in blood aminotransferase and serum bilirubin have been observed.[48] The electrocardiogram has revealed a subendocardial infarction in a few patients and occasional transient atrial fibrillation. ST elevation or depression, a wandering pacemaker, and heart block has been observed.[56] Clinical diagnosis can be confirmed by analysis of gastric aspirate or breath, both of which blacken a paper impregnated with silver nitrate.[57]

Ancillary Tests

The leukocyte count may be increased. Hypermagnesemia (over 2.5 mEq/L) and hypokalemia (less than 0.7 mEq/h) may be observed.[58]

TREATMENT
Stabilization

Supportive treatment with fluids, bicarbonate, oxygen, and vasopressors have been unsuccessful in many patients with severe poisoning. Corticosteroids appear to be ineffective.[49] Pulmonary edema and shock should be treated symptomatically. Intravenous magnesium sulfate has been attempted without clear therapeutic results.[48]

Decontamination

If fumigant liquid or solid has been ingested less than several hours prior to treatment, quantities remaining in the stomach should be removed as effectively as possible by gastric intubation, aspiration, and lavage after all possible precautions have been taken to protect the respiratory tract from aspirated gastric contents.[59]

Antidotes

There are no antidotes.

Supportive Measures

Patients will be treated symptomatically and supportively. Renal failure may require dialysis. Vitamin E may prevent liver damage from phosphorus-induced lipoperoxidation.[55]

ZINC PHOSPHIDE

Zinc phosphide produces its immediate toxicity by the production of phosphine gas. Signs and symptoms of toxicity include nausea, vomiting, dyspnea, and changes in mental status.[60] Immediate death results from pulmonary edema. Delayed effects follow the absorption of phosphide affecting primarily the liver, heart, and kidneys. Delayed death is due to a direct cardiotoxicity. Treatment is symptomatic and supportive. Aggressive airway management and circulatory support are critical.[61–63]

CHLOROPICRIN

Chloropicrin was initially synthesized in 1848. It was used as a tear gas during World War I because of its irritant properties. Since 1917 it has been used as an insecticidal fumigant. The water solubility of chloropicrin is very low and its toxicity appears to be intermediate between chlorine and phosgene.[64] Less water soluble agents such as chloropicrin tend to damage the lower respiratory tract.

STRUCTURE AND CLASSIFICATION

Chloropicrin (CAS No. 76-06-2) has an empirical formula of $CC1_3NO_2$.[65]

Synonyms

Trichloronitromethane, nitrochloropen.

198 TLV = al ppm
The structural formula is

$$\begin{array}{c} C1 \\ C1 - C - NO_2 \\ C1 \end{array}$$

USES

Chloropicrin is used as a fumigant for cereals and grains; as a soil insecticide; and as a war gas. It is also used as a deterrent to reentry after residential fumigation. Chloropicrin is used in most control agents. A small amount of chloropicrin is added to other toxic, odorless fumigants or utilized as a prewarning gas in ship fumigation before introducing cyanogen gas.[66]

PRODUCT FORMULATION

The product is a colorless, slightly oily liquid.

TOXIC DOSES

A concentration of 15 ppm could not be tolerated longer than 1 minute; exposure to 4 ppm for a few seconds is temporarily disabling because of its irritant effects.[67] Concentrations of 0.3 to 0.37 ppm can lead to painful eye irritation in 3 to 30 seconds.[68] Exposure to air containing 4 mg/L chloropicrin for a few seconds renders a soldier unfit for fighting;[69] 15 mg/L results in respiratory tract injury.[65,66]

FATAL DOSE

A lethal exposure in humans is approximately 119 ppm for 30 minutes,[65] or 0.8 mL/L,[66] death usually resulting from pulmonary edema.[65]

CLINICAL PRESENTATION

Human exposure results in lacrimation, cough, nausea, vomiting, and skin irritation.[65] Aspiration causes vomiting and choking.[66] An 18-year-old girl was sprayed with chloropicrin and died of pulmonary edema 3 hours later. A friend similarly exposed recovered after 30 days.[66]

LABORATORY
Analytic Methods

Gas chromatography (GC) and gas chromatography–mass spectrometry has been used to identify chloropicrin.[66]

TREATMENT

Treatment will be largely symptomatic and supportive and includes flushing contaminating fumigants from the skin and eyes with copious amounts of water or saliva for at least 15 minutes, removal to fresh air immediately, resuscitation with positive pressure oxygen apparatus, intravenous fluids, pressors (with caution), position change, controlling seizures, and using morphine or aminophylline as indicated.

PHOSPHINE GAS

Industrial exposures occur after the use of PH_3 in the production of acetylene gas or when it is used as a doping agent for the manufacture of silicon crystals. Aluminum phosphide grain fumigants and zinc phosphide rodenticides release phosphine gas on contact with moisture, leading to fatalities.[70] This gas has a garlic odor and causes severe gastrointestinal symptoms. In severe cases coma, convulsions, hypotension, and pulmonary edema develop. Unlike arsine gas, phosphine gas does not produce hemolytic anemia.

CLINICAL PRESENTATION

Exposures to phosphine gas cause gastrointestinal tract symptoms, as well as respiratory, cardiovascular, and central nervous system changes resulting from metabolic changes. Prominent clinical manifestations of acute phosphine gas exposure include headache, fatigue, nausea, vomiting, cough, dyspnea, paresthesias, jaundice, ataxia, intention tremor, weakness, and diplopia.[71] On autopsy fatal cases revealed centrilobular necrosis of the liver,[72] congestive heart failure with pulmonary edema, and focal myocardial necrosis.[71]

TREATMENT
Prehospital Management in the Hot Zone/ Decon Area[73]

Very small amounts of phosphine can be trapped in a victim's clothing after an overwhelming exposure, but are not usually sufficient to create a hazard for health care personnel away from the scene.

1. Rescuers should wear fully self-contained breathing apparatus and agent-specific protective clothing and gloves.
2. Quickly evaluate ABCs, spine stabilization (if trauma suspected), establish airway and breathing, and administer supplemental oxygen.
3. Flush the victim with water spray, and if gas is likely to be trapped in clothing (i.e., significant exposure in an enclosed area), remove and double-bag clothing.

Management in the Hospital

1. Evaluate and support ABCs (airway, breathing, and circulation).
2. Administer O_2 by mask, if the patient has respiratory distress.
3. Monitor cardiac rhythm; obtain 12-lead EKG. Following severe exposures, rule out myocardial infarction.
4. Laboratory tests: HCT, electrolytes, BUN and/or creatinine, liver enzymes, Ca, Mg, and blood gases. Other laboratory tests should be requested.
5. Treat pulmonary edema. Symptoms may not develop for 72 hours.
6. Liver damage may become evident 2 to 3 days later.

1,3-DICHLOROPROPENE

In 1985 2,3-dichloropropene (DCP) was the most widely applied active ingredient of the soil fumigants in a flower-bulb area in the Netherlands.[74]

PHYSICAL AND CHEMICAL CHARACTERISTICS

1,3-dichloropropene: CAS: 542-75-6. Structural formula: 1 ppm (5 mg/m^3). Synonyms: Propene; 1-3-dichloro; dichloro 2,3-propane. Telone—Telone II, DD fumigants. Physical form: white to amber-colored liquid. Molecular weight III.

USES

Soil fumigant for nematodes.

TOXICOKINETICS

1,3-dichloropropene mercapturic acid metabolites have urinary elimination half-lives of about 5 hours. About 45 and 15% of Z- and E-DCP are excreted as their respective mercapturic acid metabolites.[74,75]

CLINICAL PRESENTATION

Applicants of 1,3-dichloropropene are potentially exposed orally, dermally, or through the respiratory tract to Z- and E,1,3-dichloropropene. Exposure to DCP results in headache, mucous membrane irritation, dizziness, and chest discomfort.[76]

LABORATORY

Slight elevation of aminotransferases may be observed.[76]

SULFURYL FLUORIDE

Sulfuryl fluoride (Vikane) has been used extensively for structural fumigation and is currently a popular tent fumigant for insect extermination, used in approximately 100,000 homes each year since 1957.[77]

Sulfuryl fluoride (SO_2F_2), also known as sulfuric oxyfluoride, was first introduced in 1957. It is a colorless, odorless, nonflammable compound with a boiling point of −52°C and a molecular weight of 102.07. It is shipped and stored as a compressed gas. When heated it gives off toxic fumes such as hydrofluoric acid.[78] The TLV is 5 ppm.

DOSE

One death followed exposure to an apartment fumigated and charged with 22.5 kg (50 lb) of sulfuryl fluoride. Another individual was found dead next to an empty tank that normally held 31.5 kg (70 lb) of material.[78] Normally, a fumigation tent is charged or filled with 0.675 kg (1½ lb) per 30 m^3 (1000 ft^3) calculated to treat the volume of the structure to a peak of 16 to 24 ppm.[78]

CLINICAL PRESENTATION

A healthy elderly couple were given permission to reenter their home 20 hours after fumigation with Vikane. That evening they experienced extreme weakness, nausea, and shortness of breath. Next day the husband had a seizure and died. The wife developed a severe interstitial pulmonary edema and developed a fatal cardiorespiratory arrest.[77] Two adults were found dead after sulfuryl fluoride exposure. Another adult died 12 hours after exposure to sulfuryl fluoride.[78] Symptoms 6 hours after the exposure included cough, chest discomfort, hyperexcitability, and hyperventilation leading to a supraventricular tachycardia, productive cough, pulmonary edema, carpal/pedal tetany, cardiac dysrhythmias, and death.[78] Renal injury has induced proteinuria and azotemia.[79]

LABORATORY

Analytic Method

Serum or plasma fluoride concentrate is determined by a modification of a method that uses a Conway diffusion cell and spectrophotometrically measures the fluoride and sodium salt.[80]

Blood Levels

A fatal fluoride concentration has not been defined, but up to 3 mg/L has been proposed.[80] Blood fluoride concentrations were 50.42 mg/L and 20 mg/L in two patients who died.[78] Serum fluoride levels in one patient who died were 0.5 ng/L 4 days after exposure.[77] Serum fluoride in persons not exceptionally exposed rarely exceed 0.1 mg/L.

TREATMENT

Patients should be immediately removed to fresh air. Pulmonary edema, shock, and seizures should be managed symptomatically and supportively.

Precautions[81]

Both methyl bromide (MeBr) and sulfuryl fluoride (Vikane) are safe to be used for structural termite control when properly applied and when the precautions are observed.

STRYCHNINE

Strychnine poisoning was once considered to be the most serious form of accidental drug poisoning in children under 5 years of age. Reported deaths averaged over three per week in the late 1920s, but more recent national statistics report 190 cases and only one death due to strychnine in the year 1989.[82–84] This decrease is largely due to the removal of strychnine from various over-the-counter tonics and laxatives. Strychnine use is restricted to veterinary preparations and nonmedicinal preparations such as rodenticides. Strychnine has been found in adulterated street drugs. Accidental, suicidal, or homicidal cases of strychnine poisoning still occur.[82]

Fatal doses of strychnine are reported to be as low as 5 to 10 mg but, more significantly, survival can follow ingestion of very high doses (over 3500 mg). Strychnine ingestion should be considered in all cases of convulsion of obscure etiology, especially if the person is an agricultural worker or is known to have access to the poison.[85]

FORMULATION

Strychnine, a basic alkaloid, is an odorless, bitter-tasting white crystalline material derived from the ripe seeds of the Strychnos plant, *S. nux-vomica,* a tree native to India. It was introduced in the sixteenth century in Germany for use as a rodenticide. It was first used medically in 1540 and was used as recently as the 1960s in many cathartics, stimulants, and tonics. Many tablets had brightly colored sugar or sweet-chocolate coatings making them attractive to children. Strychnine-containing medications are no longer routinely found in American pharmacies, but it is still found in some veterinary preparations, rodenticides, avicides, and sometimes in adulterated street drugs such as cocaine.[82]

Most preparations sold for household use contain 0.25% to 0.35% strychnine, although more concentrated forms are available. Currently, poisoning usually occurs under three circumstances:

1. Accidental ingestion of proprietary "tonics" or vermicides by children.
2. Suicide attempts using vermicides.
3. Use of adulterated illicit drugs (especially cocaine).[86]

FATAL DOSE

Fatal doses of strychnine are reported to be as low as 5 to 10 mg, but, more significantly, survival can follow ingestion of very high doses (over 3500 mg).[85] Ingestion of 75 one-grain tablets (4.8 grams) was fatal.[83]

OCCUPATIONAL EXPOSURE

Strychnine poisoning is seen more often in veterinarians or in those associated with agricultural activities.

TOXICOKINETICS

Absorption

Strychnine is rapidly absorbed from the gastrointestinal tract or nasal mucosa. There is little protein binding.[83]

Distribution (V_D)

The apparent volume of distribution in one patient was 13 L/kg.[83]

Elimination

The half life of absorption is about 15 minutes.[83] Metabolism is by first-order kinetics primarily by enzymatic degradation involving the liver microsomal system. The half-life is about 10 hours.[83] Less than 1% of the product is excreted unchanged in the urine.[83]

MECHANISM OF ACTION

Strychnine prevents the uptake of glycine at inhibitory synapses, especially in the ventral horns of the spinal cord (Fig. 68–5). This results in a net excitatory effect, with minimal sensory stimulation, resulting in diffuse muscle contractions. This causes the classical clinical picture of convulsive activity in an awake patient with no postictal phase.[87]

CLINICAL PRESENTATION

Onset of symptoms usually begins within 15 to 30 minutes following ingestion and as soon as 5 minutes after inhalation. Initial symptoms include apprehension, a heightened sense of awareness, and muscle spasms. Generalized hyperreflexia and hypersensitivity to stimuli are usually present. This is followed by overwhelming convulsions, typically lasting 30 seconds to 2 minutes, often precipitated by minimal external stimuli. Opisthotonic posturing develops with the back arched, extremities hyperextended, and the jaw tightly clamped. Facial muscle spasm may be so violent as to produce the sardonic smile (risus sardonicus). Muscle relaxation usually occurs between convulsions. The patient generally maintains a clear sensorium during and after the convulsions. This is of major diagnostic importance.[86] Most patients do not tolerate more than five convulsive episodes, and death commonly occurs within several hours after ingestion. Respiratory arrest secondary to spasm of the respiratory muscles is the usual fatal event. Prognosis for survival is good if the patient survives beyond 5 hours.[86]

Complications from strychnine-induced muscle spasms include hypoxia, hyperthermia, cardiac arrest, rhabdomyolysis, and acute renal failure. Chest muscle and diaphragm spasm results in hypoxia and hypercarbia. The excessive muscle activity, if not controlled, results in hyperthermia and rhabdomyolysis. Severe metabolic acidosis is often present and may be out of proportion to the degree of lactic acidosis. Acute renal failure has resulted from rhabdomyolysis.[83]

Differential Diagnosis[82]

The differential diagnosis includes tetanus, rabies, meningitis, hysteria, and ingestions of phenothiazines, cocaine, PCP, chlorinated hydrocarbons, isoniazid, or other substances that may cause myoclonus or seizures.

LABORATORY

Analytic Methods

Strychnine may be detected in the gastric aspirate, urine, blood, and tissues through a variety of methods. Rapid spot tests relying on color changes exist, but lack specificity. Thin-layer chromatography (TLC) gives reliable qualitative information, while high-performance liquid chromatography (HPLC) provides quantitative data. For most purposes it is adequate to confirm strychnine poisoning with a qualitative test such as TLC. The urine and gastric aspirate are the most useful specimens for confirming the diagnosis. Blood levels are not reliable.

Blood Levels

Blood levels may reach up to 11 mg/L.[83]

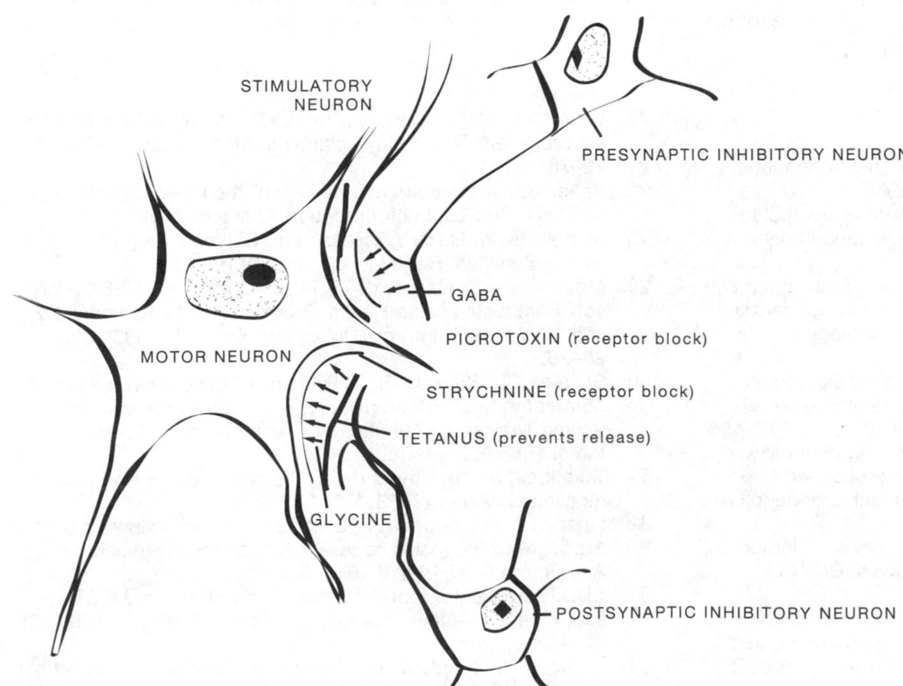

Figure 68–5 Motor neuron. Strychnine provides disinhibition by blocking glycine uptake at the motor neuron. Tetanus toxin exerts a similar effect by blocking glycine release and picrotoxin by competing with gamma-aminobutyric acid (GABA) for presynaptic inhibitory neurons. (Adapted from Heiser JM et al. Clin Toxicol 1992;30: 269–283.)

TREATMENT

Stabilization

Treatment is directed at preventing absorption, reversing hypoxia and acidosis, minimizing muscle spasm, and maintaining an adequate urine output. Early aggressive airway management is the priority. Ipecac is contraindicated since the onset of convulsions is rapid and vomiting may actually elicit muscle spasms or at least complicate their management. Gastric lavage should always follow protection of the airway since pharyngeal stimulation may result in uncontrolled convulsions. Activated charcoal should be administered both prior to and following gastric lavage. Since 1 g of activated charcoal binds 950 mg of strychnine, early use of charcoal can reduce the amount of toxin absorbed.[83]

Elimination Enhancement

Intravenous fluid sufficient to maintain a brisk urine output is indicated pending assessment of myoglobinuria. Serial physical examinations and appropriate surgical consultation should be done to assess for compartment syndromes. Measures to enhance elimination, such as forced diuresis and peritoneal dialysis, have not been studied adequately enough to be recommended.[86]

Antidotes

There are no antidotes.

Supportive Measures

Aggressive control of convulsions is the key to successful management. Diazepam is considered to be the first-line drug and large total doses may be required (e.g., more than 1 mg/kg of diazepam). Lorazepam is another intravenous benzodiazepine that should be effective. If control of convulsions is unsuccessful following intravenous benzodiazepines and barbiturates, neuromuscular blockade with an agent such as pancuronium (0.04 to 0.1 mg/kg) is necessary.[86] The clinical course is rapid. Complete recovery generally occurs with successful management.[86]

REFERENCES

1. Jorens PG, Schepens PJC. Human pentachlorophenol poisoning. Hum Exp Toxicol 1993;12:479–495.
2. Reigner BG, Bois FY, Tozer TN. Assessment of pentachlorophenol exposure in humans using the clearance concept. Hum Exp Toxicol 1992;11:17–21.
3. Jorens PG, Janssens JJ, Van Tichelen WI, Van Paesschen W, De Deyn PB, Schepens PJC. Pentachlorophenol concentrations in human cerebrospinal fluid. Neurotoxicology 1991;12:1–8.
4. Gerhard I, Derner M, Runnebaum B. Prolonged exposure to wood preservatives induces endocrine and immunological disorders in women. Am J Obstet Gynecol 1991;165:487–488.
5. O'Malley MA, Carpenter AV, Sweeney MH, Fingerhut MA, Marlow DA, Halperin WE et al. Chloracne associated with employment in the production of pentachlorophenol. Am J Indust Med 1990;17:411–421.
6. Cordier S, Poisson M, Gerin M, Vaum J, Conso F, Hemon D. Gliomas and exposure to wood preservatives. Br J Ind Med 1988;45:705–709.
7. Sanger B, Wegman RCC, Hofstee AWM. Nonoccupational exposure to pentachlorophenol: clinical findings and plasma PCP concentrations in three families. Hum Toxicol 1982;1: 123–133.
8. Gray RE, Gilliland RD, Smith EE et al. Pentachlorophenol intoxication: Report of a fatal case with comments on the clinical course and pathologic anatomy. Arch Environ Health 1985;40:161–164.
9. Benvenue A, Emerson ML, Casarette LJ et al. A sensitive gas chromatographic method for the determination of pentachlorophenol in human blood. J Chromatogr 1968;38:467–472.
10. Colosio C, Maroni M, Garratini S, Knoffel H. Abstract 223. V Internat Congress of Toxicology, July 16–21, 1989, Brighton, England. London: Taylor & Frances, p. 75.
11. Jackson RJ, Faw AM. Pesticides in food. West J Med 1990; 152:286–287.
12. Shabecoff P. 100 chemicals for apples add up to enigma on safety. New York Times, February 5, 1989.
13. Ames BN, Gold LS. Pesticides, risk and applesauce. Science 1989;224:755–756.
14. Alar withdrawn in US. Lancet 1989;1:145 (editorial).
15. Consumers Union. Alar free juice. Wall Street Journal, March 20, 1989.
16. Alar vanishing. FDA Consumer 1990;24(7):4–5.
17. Spencer JR, Bissell SR, Sanborn JR, Schneider FA, Maytich SS, Kriger MI. Chlorthalonil exposure of workers on mechanical tomato harvesters. Toxicol Lett 1991;55: 99–107.
18. Chlorthonil. In: Morgan D, ed. Recognition and management of pesticide poisonings. 4th ed. Washington, DC. US Environmental Protection Agency (EPA-540/9-88-001), 1989; p. 95.
19. Jongen MJ, Engel R, Leenheers LH. Determination of the pesticide chlorthalonil by HPLC and UV detection for occupational exposure assessment in Greenhouse Carnation Culture. J Anal Toxicol 1991;15:30–34.
20. Litovitz TL, Bailey KM, Schmitz BF, Holm KC, Klein-Schwartz W. 1990 Annual Report of the American Association of Poison Control National Data Collection System. Am J Emerg Med 1991;9:461–499.
21. Lewis DR, Madel GA, Drury J. Fatal poisoning by "Meta" fuel tablets. Br Med J 1939;1;1283–1284.
22. Longstreet WT, Pierson DJ. Metaldehyde poisoning from slug bait ingestion. West J Med 1982;137:134–137.
23. Moody JP, Inglis FG. Persistence of metaldehyde during acute molluscicide poisoning. Hum Exp Toxicol 1992;11:361–362.
24. Booze TF, Oehme FW. Gas chromatographic analysis of metaldehyde in urine and plasma. J Anal Toxicol 1985;9:172–177.
25. Keller KH, Shimizu G, Walter FG, Olson KR. Acetaldehyde analysis in severe metaldehyde poisoning. Vet Hum Toxicol 1991;33:374.
26. Anderson A. *N, N*-diethyl-*m*-toluamide (DEET). Clin Toxicol Rev 1989;11(7):1–4.
27. Laurie AA, Gleiberman SE, Tsizin YS. Pharmacokinetics of insect repellent *D,N*-diethyltoluamine. Med Parazitol 1979;47: 72–76.
28. Knaak JB. A Toxicological Review of the Insect Repellent DEET. Hazard Evaluation Section, Office of Environmental Health Hazard Assessment. California Department of Health Services, Berkeley, CA, March 1987;1–12.
29. Mofenson HC, Caraccio TR et al. Update on DEET. Poison Perspectives for Health Professional. LI Regional Poison Center at Winthrop University Hospital. 1993;12(6): 23–26.
30. Schreek CE, Snoddy EL, Spielman A. Pressurized sprays of permethrin or DEET on military clothing for personal protection against *Ixodes dammini* (Acari: Ixodidae). J Med Entomol 1986;23:396–399.
31. Tenenbein M. Toxicity of diethyltoluamide-containing insect repellents. JAMA 19088;259:2339–2340.
32. Lipscomb JW, Kramer JE, Leikin JB. Seizure following brief exposure to the insect repellent *N,N*-diethyl-*M*-toluamide. Ann Emerg Med 1992;21:315–317.
33. CDC. Seizures temporally associated with use of DEET insect repellent—New York and Connecticut. MMWR 1989;38: 678–680.
34. Maibach HI, Johnson HL. Contact urticaria syndrome. Arch Dermatol 1975;111:726–730.

35. Von Mayenburg J, Rakoski J. Contact urticaria to diethyltoluamide. Contact Dermatitis 1983;9:171.
36. Miller JD. Anaphylaxis associated with insect repellent. N Engl J Med 1982;307:1341–1342.
37. Smallwood AW, De Bord KE, Lowry LK. *N,N'*Odiethyl-*m*-toluamide (*m*-DEET): analysis of an insect repellent in human urine and serum by high performance liquid chromatography. J Anal Toxicol 1992;16:10–13.
38. Leikin JB, Kramer J, Lipscomb JW, Stewart MD. Seizure following brief exposure to the insect repellent *N,N*-diethyl-m-toluamide. Vet Hum Toxicol 1990;32:363.
39. Insect Repellents. Med Lett Drugs Ther 1989;31(792):45–48.
40. Edwards DL, Johnson CE. Insect repellent induced toxic encephalopathy in a child. Clin Pharm 1987;6:496–498.
41. Singer PP, Jones GR. Distribution of diethyltoluene (DEET) after fatal overdosage. Bull Int Assoc Forensic Toxicol 1993; 23(2):23–25.
42. Wu A, Pearson NH, Shekoski LL, Sato RJ, Steward DR. High resolution gas chromatography/mass spectrometric characterization of urinary metabolites of *N,N*-diethyl-*n*-toluamide (DEET) in man. J High Resolution Chromatogr Commission 1979;2:558–562.
43. Davies MH, Soto RJ, Stewart RD. Toxicity of diethlytoluamide-containing insect repellents. JAMA 1988; 259:2329.
44. Tenenbein M. Severe toxic reactions and death following the ingestion of diethyltoluamide-containing insect repellents. JAMA 1987;258:1509–1511.
45. Crowley RJ, Geyer R, Muir SG. Analysis of *N, N*-diethyl-*m*-toluamide (DEET) in human post mortem specimens. J Forensic Sci 1986;31:280–282.
46. Heick HMC, Peterson RG, Dalpe-Scott M, Quresli IA. Insect repellent, *N,N*-diethyl-*m*-toluamide, effect on ammonia metabolism. Pediatrics 1988;82:373–376.
47. Morgan DR. Recognition and management of pesticide poisonings. 4th ed. US Environmental Protection Agency. EPA-540/9-88-001. March 1989, p. 132.
48. Chopra JS, Kabra OP, Malik WS, Sharma R, Chandra A. Aluminum phosphide poisoning: a prospective study of 16 cases in one year. Postgrad Med J 1986;62: 113–115.
49. Banjaj R, Wasir HS. Epidemic aluminum phosphide poisoning in Northern India. Lancet 1988;1:820–821.
50. Kabra SG, Narayanan R. Aluminum phosphide: worse than Bhopal. Lancet 1988;1:1333.
51. Misera VK, Bhargava SK, Nag D, Kidwai MM, Lol MM. Occupational phosphine exposure in Indian workers. Toxicol Letters 1988;41:257–263.
52. Chugh SN, Dyhyant SR, Arora B, Malhotra KC. Incidence and outcome of aluminum phosphide poisoning in a hospital setting. Indian J Med Res 1991;[B]94:232–235.
53. Feldstein A, Heumann M, Barnett M. Fumigant intoxication during transport of grain by railroad. J Occup Med 1991;33: 64–65.
54. Misera VK, Tripathi AK, Pandey R, Bhargwa B. Acute phosphine poisoning following ingestion of aluminum phosphide. Hum Toxicol 1988;7:343–345.
55. Augenstein WL, Sokol R, Kulig K, Rumach BH. Phosphine poisoning: a report of six cases. Vet Hum Toxicol 1988; 30:344.
56. Khosla SM, Nand M, Kumar P. Cardiovascular complications of aluminum phosphide poisoning. Angiology April 1988, pp. 355–357.
57. Mital HS, Mehrotra TN, Dwivedi KK, Gera M. A study of sluminum phosphide poisoning with special reference to its spot diagnosis by silver nitrate test. J Assoc Physicians India 1992;40:473–474.
58. Singh RB, Singh RG, Singh U. Hypermagnesemia following aluminum phosphide poisoning. Int J Clin Pharmacol Ther Toxicol 1991;29:82–85.
59. Gupta S, Ahlawat SK. Aluminum phosphide poisoning—a review. Clin Toxicol 1995;33:19–24.
60. Rosenberg HD, Chang CC, Watson WA. Zinc phosphide ingestion. A case report and review. Vet Hum Toxicol 1989; 33:359–360.
61. Casteel SW, Bailey EM Jr. A review of zinc phosphide poisoning. Vet Hum Toxicol 1986;28:151–154.
62. Mack RD. A hard day's knight. Zinc phosphide poisoning. NC Med J 1989;50:17–18.
63. Stephenson JBP. Zinc phosphide poisoning. Arch Environ Health 1967;15:83–88.
64. Buckley LA, Jiang XZ, James RA, Morgan KT, Burrow CS. Respiratory tract lesions induced by sensory irritants at the RD50 concentration. Toxicol Appl Pharmacol 1974;30:408.
65. Proctor NH, Hughes JP, Fischman ML, eds. Chemical hazards of the workplace. 2nd ed. New York. Van Nostrand Reinhold, 1989, p. 149.
66. Gonmonri K, Muto H, Yamamoto T, Takahashi K. A case of homicidal intoxication by chloropicrin. Am J Forensic Med Pathol 1987;8:135–138.
67. Chloropicrin. Documentation of TLVs and BEs. 5th ed. Cincinnati: American Conference of Governmental Industrial Hygienists (ACGIH), 1986 p. 134.
68. Stokuyer HE. Aliphatic nitro compounds, nitrates, nitrites. In: Clayton GD, Clayton FE, eds. Patty's industrial hygiene and toxicology. 3rd ed. Vol 2C. Toxicology. New York: Wiley-Interscience, 1982; pp. 464–466.
69. Flury F, Zernik F. Schadliche gas. Berlin. Springer, 1931, p. 418.
70. Heyndrickx A, Van Peteghem C, Van den Heede M et al. A double fatality with children due to fumigated wheat. Eur J Toxicol 1976;9:113–118.
71. Wilson R, Lovejoy FH, Jaeger RJ et al. Acute phosphine poisoning aboard a grain freighter. JAMA 1980;244:148–150.
72. Singh S, Dilawandi JB, Vashist R et al. Aluminum phosphide ingestion. Br Med J 1985;290:1110–1111.
73. Phosphine: Hazardous Materials Medical Management Protocols. Calif Emerg Med Services Authority and Toxins Epidemiology Program, Los Angeles County Department of Health Services, March 26, 1989.
74. Brouwer DH, Brouwer EJ, de Vreede JAF, von Welia PTH, Vermeulen NPE, van Hemnen JJ. Inhalation exposure to 1,3-dichloropropene with Dutch flower-bulb culture. I. Environmental monitoring. Arch Environ Contam Toxicol 1991; 20:1–5.
75. van Wehe RTH, van Duyn P, Brouwer DH, van Hemnen JJ, Brouwer EJ, Vermeulen NPE. Inhalation exposure to 1,3 dichloropropene in the Dutch flower bulb culture. II. Biological monitoring by measurement of urinary excretion of two mercapturic acid metabolites. Arch Environ Contam Toxicol 1991;20:6–12.
76. Flessel P, Goldsmith JR, Kahn E, Weslolowski JJ. Acute and possible long-term effects of 1,3-dichloropropene. MMWR 1978;27:50.
77. Dammann KZ, Nuchols J, Wiley SH, Spyler DA. Delayed deaths following Vikane exposure. Vet Hum Toxicol 1987;29: 464.
78. Scheuerman EH. Suicide by exposure to sulfuryl fluoride. J Forensic Sci 1986;31:1154–1158.
79. Morgan DP. Recognition and management of pesticide poisonings. 4th ed. Washington, DC. US Environmental Protection Agency, 1989, pp. 135, 138.
80. Sunshine I, Finkle BS. Fluoride type B procedure. In: Methodology for analytical toxicology, Cleveland: CRC Press, 1975.
81. Toxic Information Center Case Recors. San Francisco Poison Information Center, September 18, 1989.
82. Yamarick W, Walson P, DiTraglia J. Strychnine poisoning in an adolescent. Clin Toxicol 1992;30(1):141–148.
83. Heiser JM, Daya MR, Magnussen AR, Norton RL, Spyker DA, Allen DW, Krasselt W. Massive strychnine intoxication: serial blood levels in a fatal case. Clin Toxicol 1992;30(2): 269–283.
84. Litovitz TL, Schmitz BF, Bailey KM. Annual Report of the American Association of Poison Control Centers. National Data Collection System. J Emerg Med 1990;8:394–442.
85. Burn DJ, Tomson CRV, Seviour J, Dale G. Strychnine poisoning as an unusual cause of convulsions. Postgrad Med J 1989;65:563–564.
86. Smith BA. Strychnine poisoning. J Emerg Med 1990;8:321–325.
87. Van Heerden PV, Edibaum C, Augustson B, Thompson WR, Power BM. Strychnine poisoning—alive and well in Australia. Anaesth Intensive Care 1993;21:876–878.

Chapter 69

Plastics, Plasticizers, and Epoxy Resins

THE ACRYLATES

Methylmethacrylate monomers and polymers, especially those used in orthopedics and by dental technicians, may induce a severe contact dermatitis, peripheral neuropathy, occupational asthma, hypotension, atrioventricular block, and cardiac arrest.

STRUCTURE AND CLASSIFICATION

The basic structure of acrylic monomers is the ester of acrylic acid:

$$\mathrm{CH = \underset{H}{C} - COOR}$$

The nature of the R group determines the properties of each ester and the polymer it forms.[1] If R is a methyl group, the monomer, methyl acrylate, is produced. Replacement of the hydrogen with a methyl group forms the ester of methacrylic acid, and if R is again a methyl group, the most used monomer in the acrylic series results: methyl methacrylate. The lower molecular weight acrylic monomers are liquid and have a characteristic, often unpleasant odor.

A typical self-curing acrylic may have the following formula:

Component A

Methyl methacrylate monomer with 2% dimethyl-*p*-toluidine (initiator).

Component B

Polymerized methyl methacrylate in granular form and 2 to 3% benzoyl peroxide (activator).

Combining these two components mixes the activator and the initiator, bringing about polymerization of the monomer, which, in turn, binds the powder particles together forming a solid mass. Within 3 to 5 minutes the mass has hardened into its desired state. A residual quantity of monomer, less than 2%, remains in the final acrylic resin.[2]

Methyl methacrylate (e.g., Surgical Simplex P Radiopaque bone cement) is similar as a liquid and a powder mixed shortly before use. The liquid consists of methylmethacrylate monomer (the "monomer") and small quantities of dimethyl-*p*-toluidine and hydroquinone. Hydroquinone prevents premature polymerization. Dimethyl-*p*-toluidine promotes cold curing of the finished compound. The powder consists basically of methylmethacrylate powder. The mixture forms a dough that sets hard (in 5 to 10 minutes) in a marked exothermic reaction to produce a cementlike complex.[3,4]

USES

The largest use for polymethacrylate is as a glazing, lighting, or decorative material. Polymethacrylates are used in the manufacture of dentures, denture bases, and filling materials. In the orthodontics market, methacrylates have found acceptance as sealants or pit-and-fissure resin sealants painted over teeth, which act as barriers to tooth decay. Polymethacrylates are also used as bone cement masses[5,6] and for preparation of both soft and hard contact lenses.[7] Other uses are in the manufacture of artificial nails[8–10] (Table 69–1).[9]

Table 69–1
Acrylic Monomers in Various Nail Preparations[a]

Brand Name	Contains
Mona Sculptured Nails Liquid	Ethyl methacrylate monomer Ethylene glycol dimethacrylate
Audette Artificial Nail Set	Ethyl methacrylate monomer Butyl methacrylate monomer Trimethylolpropane trimethacrylate monomer
Polynail Artificial Nail Set	Ethyl methacrylate monomer Isobutyl methacrylate monomer
Magic Sculptura Nails	Methacrylic acid monomer Ethyl methacrylate monomer Isobutyl methacrylate monomer
Pattinail Nail Extender	Ethyl methacrylate monomer Isobutyl methacrylate monomer
House of Nails Nail Extender	Ethyl methacrylate monomer Butyl methacrylate monomer
Super Nail Artificial Fingernail	Ethyl methacrylate monomer Isobutyl methacrylate monomer
Lee Nails Nail Extender	Ethyl methacrylate monomer Tetrahydrofurfuryl methacrylate monomer Diethylene glycol dimethacrylate monomer

[a]Adapted from Fisher AA. Cutis 1989;43:404–405.

OCCUPATIONAL EXPOSURE (TABLE 69–2)

The levels of methylmethacrylate (MMA) and formaldehyde in the workroom air of a dental laboratory following work with a denture base resin do not usually exceed the respective threshold limit values in air.[11] The maximum exposure limit to MMA mandated by OSHA for workplaces is 100 ppm or 410 mg/m^3 averaged over an 8-hour shift.[12] Its odor is noticeable at 0.2 to 0.3 ppm.[4] Levels of MMA in the operating room during total hip replacement at the time of mixing reach 225 ppm, decreasing to about 50 ppm 2 minutes after mixing, to 4 ppm in 6 minutes, and to zero at the time of curing.[13]

Suggested occupational exposures (ACGIH) for *n*-butyl acrylate in the United States is 55 mg/m^3 TWA.[14] Exposure limits for ethylacrylate in the United States (ACGH) are 20 mg/m^3 (TWA) and 100 mg/m^3 (short-term exposure—skin).

ENVIRONMENTAL EXPOSURE

Most of the health and safety aspects of acrylic polymers are involved with their manufacture, such as in violent polymerizations.[1,7] Acrylics are involved as thermal decomposition products of synthetic polymers[15] (Table 69–3).

Table 69–2
Acrylates—OSHA Standards[a,b]

	Molecular Weight	OSHA TWA	IDLH	Physical Description
Ethyl acrylate $CH_2 = CHCOOCH_2CH_3$	100.1	5 ppm (20 mg/m^3) Short term 25 ppm (100 mg/m^3) (skin)	Ca 2000 ppm	Colorless liquid with an acrid odor
Methyl acrylate $CH_2 = CHCOOCN_3$	86.1	NIOSH/OSHA 10 ppm (35 mg/m^3) (skin)	1000 ppm	Colorless liquid with an acrid, sharp, fruity odor
Methylmethacrylate (methacrylate monomer) $CH_2 = C(CH_3)COOCH_3$		NIOSH/OSHA 100 ppm (410 mg/m^3)	4000 ppm	Odorless liquid with an acrid, fruity odor
Butyl methacrylate (Sweden)		TWA 50 ppm (300 mg/m^3) STEL 75 ppm (450 mg/m^3)		
Methacrylic Acid $CH_2 = C(CH_3COOH)$	86.1	70 mg/m^3 (skin)		
Ethyl-2 cyanacrylate (Sweden)		TWA 2 ppm (10 mg/m^3) STEL 4 ppm (20 mg/m^3)		
Acrylic Acid ($CH_2 = CHCOOH$)	72	Maximum allowable concentration USSR 5 mg/m^3 USI 30 mg/m^3 (skin)		Colorless liquid with a sharp odor

[a]Occupational Exposure Limits for Airborne Toxic Substances. 3rd ed. Geneva: International Labour Office, 1991.
[b]NIOSH Pocket Guide to Chemical Hazards. DHHS (NIOSH). Publication No. 90-117. Washington, DC: Superintendent of Documents. June 1990.

Table 69–3
Thermal Decomposition Products of Synthetic Polymers[a]

Type of Polymer	Degradation Condition	Products
HYDROCARBON		
Polyethylene	Pyrolysis	Mainly shorter chain alkene and alkene-type hydrocarbons, ethylene monomer, toluene, ethylbenzene, and polycyclic aromatic hydrocarbons
	Combustion	Principal combustion products were CO, CO_2, carboxylic acids, formaldehyde, acetaldehyde, acrolein, and complex mixtures of oxygen-containing organic compounds
Polypropylene	Pyrolysis	Pentane is the major aliphatic saturated hydrocarbon and propylene the main unsaturated hydrocarbon produced
	Combustion	CO, CO_2, H_2O, other low-molecular-weight oxygenated compounds, aromatic hydrocarbons such as benzene, toluene and xylene, and aliphatic compounds in 1–6 carbon range
Polystyrene	Pyrolysis	Principal product is styrene: lesser amounts of benzene, toluene, and ethylbenzene
	Combustion	Large amounts of styrene and CO, CO_2, acetophenone, benzaldehyde, phenylethanol, methane, ethylene, and acetylene
OXYGEN-CONTAINING		
Acrylics		
Simple methacrylate homopolymers (e.g. primary esters)	Pyrolysis	Mainly monomer and small amounts of CO, CO_2, olefins corresponding to the ester group, methane, ethane, ethylene, acetylene, formaldehyde, and alcohols
	Combustion	CO and small quantiites of formaldehyde and acrolein
Complex methacrylate homopolymers (e.g., secondary or tertiary esters)	Pyrolysis	Mainly olefin corresponding to the ester group, small amounts of monomer
	Combustion	No data
Methacrylate copolymers	Pyrolysis	Monomer or olefin corresponding to ester group depending on complexity of polymer
	Combustion	No data
Simple acrylate homopolymers	Pyrolysis	Chain fragments and alcohols corresponding to the ester group; also substantial quantities of corresponding olefin and CO_2; minor compounds include corresponding monomers, alkyl methacrylate, and alkanes, and CO, H_2, methane, ethane, ethylene, and oxygenated compounds
	Combustion	No data
Complex acrylate homopolymers	Pyrolysis	Olefin corresponding to the ester group and CO_2, very small quantities of corresponding alcohol and CO
	Combustion	No data
Acrylate copolymers	Pyrolysis	Alcohol corresponding to ester group and monomers
	Combustion	No data
Acrylate-methacrylate copolymer	Pyrolysis	Acrylate and methacrylate monomer
	Combustion	Monomer and alcohol
Epoxy	Pyrolysis	CO, CO_2, H_2, methane, acetaldehyde, H_2O, phenol, formaldehyde, benzene, acetone, and toluene
	Combustion	HCl and smaller amounts of CO, CO_2, O_2, acetylene, ethylene, chlorine, and ethane
Phenolics	Pyrolysis	CO, CO_2, H_2O, H_2, methane, formaldehyde, C_2 and C_1 compounds, aromatic hydrocarbons, and tarry substances
	Combustion	Aromatic hydrocarbons (phenol methyl phenol), CO, CO_2, and methane
Polycarbonate	Pyrolysis	No data
	Combustion	CO, CO_2, and methane, smaller amounts of low-molecular-weight aliphatic and oxygenated hydrocarbons and benzene-related compounds
Polyester	Pyrolysis	CO, CO_2, and H_2O aromatic polyesters produced fewer saturated and unsaturated hydrocarbons than aliphatic polyesters and moderate amounts of benzene
	Combustion	CO, CO_2, methane, acetaldehyde ethane, benzene, and a wide variety of benzene-related compounds
Metamine formaldehyde	Specific conditions unknown	CO, CO_2, HCN, formaldehyde, and NH_3

[a]Adapted from Orzel RA. Occup Med 1983;8:422–423.

(continued)

Table 69–3 *(Continued)*

Type of Polymer	Degradation Condition	Products
OXYGEN/NITROGEN-CONTAINING		
Rigid polyurethane foam	Pyrolysis and combustion	Major products are CO and HCN in addition to great number of different compounds
Flexible polyurethane foam	Pyrolysis and combustion	CO, CO_2, HCN, other nitrogen-contailing compounds such as acetonitrile, acrylonitrile, pyridine, benzonitrile, and low-molecular-weight hydrocarbons
Urea-formaldehyde	Pyrolysis	No data
	Combustion	CO, CO_2, HCN, and NH_1
HALOGENATED		
Polytetrafluoroethylene (PIFF)	Pyrolysis	Main products are carbonyl fluoride and carbon tetrafluoride; hexafluoroethane, octafluorocyclobutane, decafluoro-*n*-butane, tetrafluoroethylene, hexafluoropropylene, and octafluoro-*n*-propane are also produced
	Combustion	Similar to above plus CO and CO_2
Polyvinyl chloride (PVC)	Pyrolysis and combustion	CO, CO_2, HCl, benzene, and saturated aromatic hydrocarbons, and benzene- and chloride-related compounds and particulate matter; phosgene (particularly with electric arc heat source)

TOXICOKINETICS

Absorption

Kim and Ritter[16] demonstrated methacrylate in the venous blood of patients after cement insertion into the femur and the acetabulum. A peak blood level was noted at 3 minutes after insertion. After 5 and 10 minutes methylmethacrylate (MMA) was not detected. They found no correlation between methyl methacrylate blood levels and the degree of hypotension.[3] Crout and colleagues[5] found maximum blood concentrations of methylmethacrylate of 0.24 to 8.05 µg/mL in the first 5 minutes after insertion of cement into the acetabulum cavity. Maximum levels of 3.10 µg/mL were observed in the first 5 minutes after inserting cement into the femoral cavity. Methacrylic acid (MA) was also observed in concentrations of 1.10 and 2.40 µg/mL during these two periods, respectively.[5]

Methyl methacrylate, the monomeric component of the polymethyl methacrylate cement used in orthopedic surgery, undergoes hydrolysis to methacrylic acid during hip replacement operations. No correlations have been observed between changes in the concentration of MMA and MA and changes in blood pressure.[5]

Distribution (V_D)

Methylmethacrylate is present in blood cells in concentrations twice as large as plasma. It disappears from plasma at a rate at least 10 times faster than from the cells. Methyl methacrylate appears to be broken down exclusively in the plasma phase. The cells act as a storage place from which the monomer is released into the plasma.[17]

Elimination

The half-life of methylmethacrylate in whole blood at 20°C is 3 hours. Methacrylate is not found in the urine of healthy controls. Dental technicians exposed to methylmethacrylate may develop urine concentrations as high as 373 nmol/mmol creatinine.[18]

Pregnancy/Lactation

There is one report of an increase in spontaneous abortion in women employed in polystyrene manufacture but not in polyolefine or polyvinyl processing.[19]

CLINICAL PRESENTATION—METHYL METHACRYLATE

Systemic Reaction

An operating room nurse developed a sensitivity reaction to the odor of orthopedic cement characterized by hypertension, dyspnea, and generalized erythroderma. She recovered. Methylmethacrylate air concentrations were 0.4 ppm, 1.0 ppm, and 1.5 ppm monitored over 15-minute periods.[4] Operating room personnel are exposed for about 30 minutes for each orthopedic procedure. When averaged over an 8-hour period such exposures rarely exceed the OSHA limits of 100 ppm.[11,12] Increased complaints of respiratory, cutaneous, and genitourinary problems have been observed in workers exposed to MMA at concentrations of 4 to 49 ppm over an 8-hour time-weighted average.[4]

Dermal

The acrylic bone cement used in orthopedic surgery leaves some residual monomer unpolymerized. These monomers penetrate practically all rubber and polyvinyl gloves, but butyl rubber gloves (0.48 mm thick) may prevent the development of contact dermatitis.[20] Many orthopedic surgeons have acquired allergic contact dermatitis from the acrylic monomers and have shown strongly positive patch-test reactions to methylmethacrylate. Patients very rarely become sensitized.[21]

Patients Sensitive to Methylmethacrylate

Loss of fingernails may be due to an allergic reaction to an acrylic nail preparation (Table 69–1).[9]

N-butyl and ethylmonomers do not appear to crossreact in patients sensitive to methyl methacrylate. Patients who acquire an allergic contact dermatitis to ethyl methacrylate and butyl methacrylate may also have a positive patch-test reaction to methyl methacrylate monomer.[9] A history of skin disease during childhood or allergic conjunctivitis or rhinitis may predispose an individual to the dermatologic effects caused by methyl methacrylate.[22] Paresthesias and tenderness in areas of contact dermatitis frequently outlast the eruption.[4]

Cardiac

Several cases of intraoperative cardiac arrest have been reported in patients undergoing hip replacements, although the occurrence is rare.[3,23] Hypotension occurs during 50 to 80% of total hip replacements. The drop in blood pressure rarely exceeds 15 mm Hg, reaches its maximum 30 to 60 seconds following insertion of the prosthesis, and usually returns to normal in 90 seconds.[24] The contributing role of fat emboli,[25] micropulmonary emboli, or free MMA in causing these cardiovascular effects is unclear. A second-degree atrioventricular block and a bradycardia that progressed to a fatal third-degree heart block has been reported during hip arthroplasty using MMA cement.[26] Graham reports four deaths with fat embolism.[25]

Nervous System

Peripheral Nervous System

An adult had a 40-year career as a dental technician. During this work he had extensive and repeated skin and inhalational exposure to methyl methacrylate monomer. This led to a generalized sensorimotor peripheral neuropathy of the axonal degeneration type confirmed by a sural nerve biopsy.[6] Between 3 to 5% of methylmethacrylate is unreacted monomer, posing an occupational hazard among dental technicians who experience feelings of numbness, coldness, and pain in the dominantly exposed hand.[22] Sensory conduction velocities in finger nerves are slowed in conjunction with the numbness.[27,28] Urine output of methylmethacrylate in such dental technicians reflects a percutaneous absorption.[22]

Central Nervous System

Irritability, rapid fatigue, and headache have been observed in workers engaged in pouring methylmethacrylate (MMA) into forms. Such workers were exposed to 25 to 146 ppm of MMA.[29] These findings have not been evaluated in controlled studies.

Gastrointestinal

Dental students have observed nausea while working with MMA and have experienced a lack of appetite that lasts several hours.[4] Plastic particles from a polypropylene syringe induced a fatal bowel necrosis in a neonate.[30]

Respiratory

At high concentrations MMA causes irritation to the respiratory tract. A transient decrease in PaO_2 occurs within seconds after application of MMA and is reversed within minutes.[4] The transient hypoxia may be due to fat and bone marrow emboli resulting from the high intramedullary pressure during insertion of the prosthesis.[4,25,31] In one study two cases of intraoperative death occurred during insertion of the hip prosthesis with use of MMA polymer as bone cement. Widespread marrow emboli were found.[31]

Plastics and Cancer

The International Agency for Research on Cancer has labeled three plastic compounds as carcinogenic with varying degrees of certainty: vinyl chloride (definite); acrylonitrile (probable), and chloroprene (under suspicion).[14]

In the early 1940s workers in jobs entailing highest exposures to vapor-phase ethyl methacrylate and methyl methacrylate monomer appeared to be subject to excess mortality from cancer of the colon 2 decades after the equivalent of 3 year's employment in jobs with the most intense exposures.[32] These observations were not corroborated in a subsequent cohort study of 2671 men that concluded that there was no evidence to support the hypothesis that methyl methacrylate is a human carcinogen.[33]

Ethyl Acrylate, Butyl Acrylate

Drowsiness, headache and nausea have followed exposure. No electroencephalographic changes have been observed.[14]

LABORATORY

Analytic Methods

Gas chromatography (GC) with a flame ionization detector is used to detect monomer in blood and can detect concentrations as low as 1 ppm. GC measures methyl methacrylate only and, unlike ^{14}C-labeled methyl methacrylate, it does not measure radioactive metabolites.[17]

TREATMENT

Stabilization

Treatment of adverse reactions to methyl methacrylate monomer or polymer is largely symptomatic and supportive.

Prevention

Cardiac

Measures that can be taken prior to application of the cement have been suggested.[3,16] The prophylactic administration of blood and fluids, such as 500 mL of blood and 2000 mL of balanced salt solution, before cement insertion may be helpful in limiting the hypotensive response.

Dermal

To prevent dermatitis the orthopedic cement can be mixed mechanically and applied with a spatula. Two pairs of cotton gloves over them can be worn and removed as soon as possible and discarded. Skin contamination can be cleaned with alcohol or methylethylketone and the hands washed with ample soap and water.[21]

Antidote

There are no antidotes.

CYANOACRYLATES

Cyanoacrylates are used as adhesives. Occupational exposure may lead to an allergic type asthma. Accidental exposure in the eye may lead to corneal damage. On the skin these compounds lead to a bonding that can often be treated conservatively by simple manipulation. Chronic dermatitis may follow their use on fingernails.[34]

STRUCTURE AND CLASSIFICATION

Three cyanoacrylates available for medical use are bucrylate (isobutyl 2-cyanoacrylate, $C_8H_{11}NO_2$ m.w. 153.2), *n* butyl cyanoacrylate (butyl-2-cyanoacrylate $C_8H_{11}NO_2$ m.w. 1532), and mecrylate (methyl 2-cyanoacrylate $C_5H_5NO_2$ m.w. 11.1).[35,36] Butyl cyanoacrylate adhesive is sold commercially as Histoacryl-blue (Melsungen, Germany). Ethyl cyanoacrylate is sold as Krazy Glue.

USES

Primary uses for cyanoacrylates include skin closure, particularly during reconstructive surgery of the eyelids and the nose; immobilization of grafts for hair transplants; local hemostasis; closure of gingival flaps in periodontal surgery; and restorative procedures on teeth or on fixed dental prostheses. Cosmetic applications, such as "gluing" of nail overlays, synthetic eyelashes, eyebrows, small hairpieces, and facial prostheses, also seem to be common.[36]

In addition, cyanoacrylate adhesives have been used to treat corneal leaks, to seal aqueous leaks following trauma, and for spontaneous corneal melting.[37] Other uses have included temporary tarsorrhaphy for seventh-nerve palsy (37) and facial lacerations[38] (Table 69–4).[39]

PRODUCT FORMULATION

Industrial and consumer grades of adhesives include Crazy Glue, Durabond, Eastman 910, and Loctite 12.[36] Blais and Campbell[36] described the modifications of cyanoacrylate requiring improved handling characteristics and mechanical properties.[36]

Commercial preparations are often modified by the addition of substances of high molecular weight such as prepolymerized cyanoacrylates, methylmethacrylate, and polystyrene, as well as fillers such as talc, powdered glass, alumina, and fumed silica, most of which are not resorbable and can act as embedded foreign bodies in tissue. In addition, these preparations incorporate strong desiccating agents and stabilizers to prevent premature curing in the reopenable container. Frequently used compounds include phosphoric anhydride, sulfur dioxide, and sulfur trioxide, sometimes at levels as high as 15% of the total preparation. These are potent irritants; thermal and chemical burns from the additives or incidental to the exothermic reaction that may take place during the curing step are other possible side effects.[36]

Eastman 910 consists of methyl 2-cyanoacrylate monomer modified with a plasticizer (a sebacate), a thickening agent (methyl methacrylate), and an inhibitor (SO_2).[36] Aron Alpha consists of monomeric alkyl cyanoacrylate.[40]

SOURCES

Cyanoacrylate monomers are usually synthesized by base-catalyzed condensation of formaldehyde and a cyanoacetate. This produces a polycyanoacrylate that is then depolymerized to yield the monomer, decomposing to formaldehyde and a cyanoacetate. This degradation mechanism is probably the major cause of the tissue toxicity of cyanoacrylate adhesives.[39] Methyl, butyl, and alkyl cyanoacrylates have been used as adhesives.[40]

Table 69–4
Use of Cyanoacrylate Adhesives in Ocular Surgery[a]

Type of Cyanoacrylate	Ocular Application or Surgery	Experimental (E) or Clinical (C)
Methyl- or Eastman 910	Skin, lid, conjunctiva, corneal or intracorneal, scleral, muscle, intraocular injection, evisceration, exenteration, glaucoma, corneal and limbal incisions	E
	Plastic lid procedures—tarsorrhaphy	C
Isobutyl-, n-heptyl-, n-octyl	Corneal perforations and lacerations	E
Methyl-[21]	Glued-on contact lens (artificial epithelium or epikeratoprosthesis)	E
Isobutyl- n-heptyl-[21] n-octyl-		C
n-heptyl-	Artificial endothelium	E
		C
Isobutyl-	Keratoprosthesis	C
	Cataract wound closure	E
	Lamellar corneal transplantation	E
	Scleral and macular buckling without sutures	E
	Choroidal perforations	
	Postoperative (glaucoma, cataract, keratoplasty	C

[a]Adapted from Refojo MF et al. Surv Ophthalmol 1971;15:217–236.

OCCUPATIONAL EXPOSURE

A suggested threshold limit value for methyl 2-cyanoacrylate is 2 ppm (8 mg/m^3).[41]

CLINICAL PRESENTATION

Eastman 910 applied superficially to the cornea of animals produces a mild corneal haze and mild inflammatory reaction that together with the corneal haze clears in 1 week.

Alkyl cyanoacrylates (ethyl cyanoacrylate, methyl cyanoacrylate) appear to act as allergens, including an immunologic reaction (type I) leading to the development of asthma with sneezing, nasal discharge, coughing stridor, and dyspnea beginning several hours after (42) work and not recurring on days off work.[40] A 2-year-old child bit into a tube of Super Glue 3. The glue adhered to the lower lip and lower incisors and remained firm after 12 hours.[43] A chronic dermatitis similar to small plaque parapsoriasis may follow use of the adhesive on fingernails.[34]

TREATMENT

Stabilization

Asthma is treated symptomatically. Bonding of the lips together with sealing of the nostrils may require a tracheotomy.[43] Adherence to the corneal conjunctiva and/or eyelid may require (a) copious irrigation of the exposed eye with tepid tap water for at least 15 minutes, (b) application of mineral oil to the external eyelid surface after irrigation, and (c) referral to an appropriate health care facility for an ophthalmologic evaluation.[44] Acetone has been used to remove the adhesive from the fingernails.[34]

MULTIFUNCTIONAL ACRYLATES (MFA)

Multifunctional acrylates and methacrylates (MFAs) are used in photocurable coatings: UV curing inks, paints, dental sealants, resins, and varnishes.

TOXICITY

MFAs have been mainly studied in animals. Few clinical reports are available. They are severe eye and skin irritants. Repeated dermal application may lead to seizures, tremors, or ataxia. Sensitization leads to a delayed contact dermatitis. MFAs do not appear to be potent fetotoxins or teratogens. They are not strong skin carcinogens, but may be potentially absorbed leading to tumors of the viscera.[4]

FOOD PACKAGING

The U.S. Food and Drug Administration has approved plastic for use on food. Many tests have been performed at temperatures up to 250 to 300°F. The use of polymer materials in microwaves that are capable of heating foods to 500°F may ultimately lead to an increased rate of polymer (and monomer) transfer to food, in addition to other thermal degradation products.[46]

PLASTICS

Some plastics currently used in the food packaging business include the following (1):

Polyethylene; polypropylene; ethylene-vinyl acetate copolymer; vinyl plastics and vinyl copolymers: (PVC—resists fat absorption, used in trays, inserts, and shrinkwrap), vinyl chloride (used to wrap cheese and as an over-wrap for paper-wrapped products), polystyrene (used for yogurt, cottage cheese containers), styrene-acrylonitrile (used for measuring cups, juice squeezers), ABS (acrylonitrile-butadiene-styrene), used for margarine tubs; acrylics: XT polymer = acrylic acid + ?—used for peanut butter; nylons (used to vacuum seal—bacon, cheese), polyethylene terephthalate (Terylene), used for boil-in-the-bag foods; polycarbonates (used for nondisposable plates, cups).

Additives: antioxidants, brighteners, colorants, and lubricants may be used in plastics intended for food use.

To minimize any possible exposure and, therefore, risk, the FDA U.S. Department of Agriculture recommends[1]:

1. Follow package directions. Remember that the FDA approves packaging only for use under specific conditions.
2. Use only cookware labeled for microwave use in the microwave.
3. Wrap plastic wrap tightly over container openings rather than letting it touch food directly.

FLUOROPOLYMERS (FIG. 69–1)

Polytetrafluoroethylene ("Polytef")

Polytetrafluoroethylene ("Polytef") (Fig. 69–1) is used in the treatment of vocal cord disorders and urinary incontinence. Toxic respiratory tract effects have been observed during manufacture. There are no controlled studies that indicate carcinogenicity.[47,48]

Polymer fume fever (an influenza-like syndrome starting 2 to 3 hours after exposure and clearing up spontaneously within 36 to 48 hours) has been observed in the home after unattended utensils have been heated to more than 340°C (Fig. 69–2). There is no known association of polymer fume fever and an increased risk of development of cancer.[49]

$$\left[-CF_2 - CF_2 - \right]_n$$ Polytetrafluoroethylene (Teflon®)

$$\left[-CH_2 - CF_2 - \right]_n$$ Polyvinylidine fluoride (Kynar®)

$$\left[-CH_2 - CHF_2 - \right]_n$$ Polyvinyl fluoride (Tedlar®)

Figure 69–1 Chemical structures of some common fluoropolymers. Teflon and Tedlar are tradenames of E.I. duPont; Kynar is a tradename of Elf Atochem North America, Inc. (Adapted from Shusterman DJ. Occup Med 1993;8:519–531.)

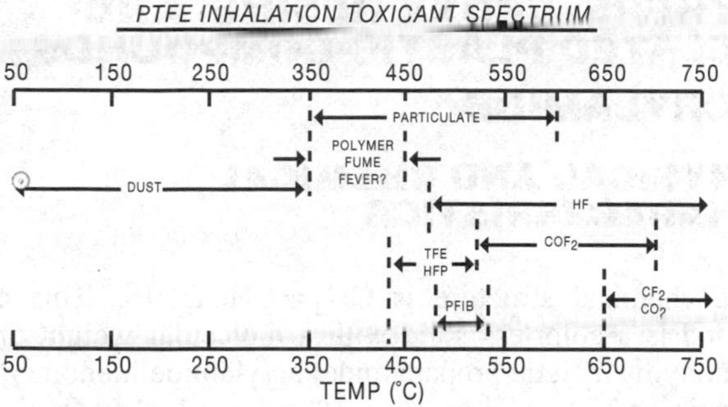

Figure 69–2 PTFE inhalation toxicant spectrum as a function of temperature (heated in air). *TFE,* Tetrafluoroethylene; *PFIB,* Octafluoroisobutene; *HPF,* hexafluoropropylene; and CF_4, carbonylfluoride. (Adapted from Waritz RS. Environ Health Perspect 1975;11:197–203.)

In comparison to metal fume fever, exposures producing polymer fume fever are more likely to result in pulmonary consolidation, including radiologic abnormalities possibly due to the liberation of hydrogen fluoride deep in the lungs at PTFE pyrolysis product inhalation. Unlike metal fume fever, polymer fume fever episodes appear to have little or no tendency to diminish in intensity after serial daily exposure. These patients should be observed for 24 to 48 hours for signs of lung consolidation. Treatment is supportive, including oxygen and intubation with positive end-expiratory pressure if respiratory distress is severe.[50] Chemical structure of common synthetic polymers are found in Table 69–4.[15] Fluoropolymers are found in Figure 69–2.[50]

MEAT WRAPPERS' ASTHMA

Inhalation of thermal degradation products of plastic fumes from heated polyvinyl chloride (PVC) or polyethylene meat-wrapping film or heated price labels may cause bronchospasm or "meat wrappers" asthma. Patients may have a history of preexisting bronchospastic disease. Treatment is symptomatic and supportive. Patients may require removal from work exposure.[51,52]

POLYPROPYLENE

Initial studies suggest an elevated colorectal cancer incidence has been observed in workers employed in the production of polypropylene.[53] Polyp prevalence rates also appear elevated in such workers.[54] These studies require epidemiologic confirmation.[55,56]

REFERENCES—PLASTICS

1. Kine BB, Novak RW. Acrylic ester polymers. In: Kirk-Othmer encyclopedia of chemical Technology. 3rd ed. Vol 1, New York: John Wiley, 1978; pp. 386–408.
2. Autian J. Structure-toxicity relationship of acrylic monomers. Environ Health Perspect 1975;11:141–152.
3. Hyderally H, Miller R. Hypotension and cardiac arrest during prosthetic hip surgery with acrylic bone cement. Orthop Rev 1976;5:55–61.
4. Scolnick B, Collins J. Systemic reaction to methylmethacrylate in an operating room nurse. J Occup Health 1986;28: 196–198.
5. Crout DHG, Corkill JA, Jones ML, Ling RSM. Methylmethacrylate metabolism in men. The hydrolysis of methylmethacrylate to methacrylic acid during total hip replacement. Clin Orthop 1978;141:90–95.
6. Donaghy M, Rushworth G, Jacobs JM. Generalized peripheral neuropathy in a dental technician exposed to methyl methacrylate monomer. Neurology 1991,41: 1112–1116.
7. Kine BB, Novak RW. Methacrylic polymers. In: Kirk-Othmer encyclopedia of chemical technology. 3rd ed. Vol 1, New York: John Wiley, 1978; pp. 377–398.
8. Kechijian P. Dangers of acrylic fingernails. JAMA 1990; 236:458.
9. Fisher AA. Permanent loss of fingernails due to allergic reaction to an acrylic nail preparation. A sixteen-year follow-up study. Cutis 1989;43:404–405.
10. Hecht A. Artificial fingernails: apply with caution. FDA Consumer 1988;22.(1):18–21.
11. Brune E, Beltesbrekke H. Levels of methylmethacrylate, formaldehyde and asbestos in dental workroom air. Scand J Dent Res 1981;89:113–116.
12. Guidelines for Protecting the Safety and Health of Health Care Workers. 5.1.9. Methyl Methacrylate. Centers for Disease Control. US Department of Health and Human Services. September 1988, pp. 5-30–5-31. DHHS (NIOSH) Publication No. 88-119.
13. McLaughlin RE, Barkalow JA, Allen MS. Pulmonary toxicity of methyl methacrylate vapors: an environmental study. Arch Environ Health 1979;34:336–338.
14. Reference Deleted
15. Orzel PA. Toxicological aspects of firesmoke: polymer pyrolysis and combustion. In: Shusterman DJ, Peterson JE, eds. De nova toxicants: combustion toxicology mixing incompatibilities and environmental activation of toxic agents. State of the Art Reviews 1993;8:415–429, Philadelphia: Hanley & Belfus, 1993.
16. Kim KC, Ritter MA. Hypotension associated with methylmethacrylate in total hip arthroplasty. Clin Orthop 1972;88: 154–160.
17. Rijke AM, Johnson RA. On the fate of methyl methacrylate in blood. J Biomed Mater Res 1977;11:211–221.
18. Rajaniemi R, Pfaffli P, Savolainen H. Percutaneous absorption of methyl methacrylate by dental technicians. Br J Ind Med 1989;46:356–357.
19. McDonald AD, Lavoie J, Cote R, McDonald JC. Spontaneous abortion in women employed in plastics manufacture. Am J Ind Med 1988;14:9–14.
20. Kassis W, Videl P, Darre E. Contact dermatitis to methyl methacrylate. Contact Dermatitis 1984;11:26–28.
21. Fisher AA. Reactions to acrylic bone cement in orthopedic surgeons and patients. Cutis 1986;32(6):425–426.
22. Rajaniemi R, Tola S. Subjective symptoms among dental technicians exposed to the monomer methyl methacrylate. Scand J Work Environ Health 1985;11:281–286.
23. Durbin FC, Jeffery CC, Jones CB, Ling RSM, Scott PJ, Woodyard JE et al. Cardiac arrest and bone cement. Br Med J 1970;2:176–177.
24. Schuh FT, Schuh SM, Viguera MG, Terry RN. Circulatory changes following implantation of methylmethacrylate bone cement. Anesthesiology 1973;39:455–459.
25. Gresham GA, Kuczynski A. Cardiac arrest and bone cement. Br Med J 1970;2:465.
26. Learned DW, Hantler CB. Lethal progression of heart block after prosthesis cementing with methylmethacrylate. Anesthesiology 1992;77:1044–1046.
27. Rajanieni R. Clinical evaluation of occupational toxicity of methylmethacrylate monomer in dental technicians. J Soc Occup Med 1986;36:56–59.
28. Seppalainen AM, Rajanieni R. Local neurotoxicity of methyl methacrylate among dental technicians. Am J Ind Med 1984; 5:471–477.
29. Innes DL, Tansy MF. Central nervous system effects of methyl methacrylate vapor. Neurotoxicology 1981;2:515–522.

30. Cant AJ, Lenney W, Kirkham N. Plastic material from a syringe causing fatal bowel necrosis in a neonate. Br Med J 1988;296:968–969.
31. Kepes ER, Underwood PS, Becsey L. Intraoperative death associated with acrylic bone cement. Report of two cases. JAMA 1972;22:576–577.
32. Walker AM, Cohen AJ, Loughlin JE, Rothman KJ, de Fonso LR. Mortality from cancer of the colon or rectum among workers exposed to ethyl acrylate and methyl methacrylate. Scand J Work Environ Health 1991;17:7–19.
33. Collins JJ, Page LC, Caporossi JC, Utidjian HM, Saipher JM. Mortality patterns among men exposed to methyl methacrylate. J Occup Med 1989;31:41–46.
34. Shelley ED, Shelley WB. Chronic dermatitis-simulating small-plaque parapsoriasis due to cyanoacrylate adhesive used on fingernails. JAMA 1984;252:2455–2456.
35. Reynolds JEF. Martindale: *The extra pharmacopoeia.* 29th ed. London: The Pharmaceutical Press, pp. 1561–1562.
36. Blais P, Campbell RW. Cyanoacrylates in medicine. Can Med Assoc J 1982;126:227–228.
37. Diamond JP. Temporary tarsorrhaphy with cyanoacrylate adhesive for seventh-nerve palsy. Lancet 1990;335:1039.
38. Watson DP. Use of cyanoacrylate tissue adhesive for closing facial lacerations in children. Br Med J 1989;299:1014.
39. Refojo MF, Dohlman CH, Koliopoulos J. Adhesives in ophthalmology: a review. Surv Ophthalmol 1971;15:217–236.
40. Nakazawa T. Occupational asthma due to alkyl cyanoacrylate. J Occup Med 1990;32:709–710.
41. Coover HW Jr, McIntire JM. Two cyanoacrylic ester polymers. In: Kirk-Othemer encyclopedia of chemical technology. 3rd ed. Vol 1. New York: John Wiley, 1978, pp. 408–413.
42. Lozewicz S, Davison AG, Hopkirk A, Burge PS, Boldy D, Riordan IF et al. Occupational asthma due to methylmethacrylate and cyanoacrylates. Thorax 1985;40: 836–839.
43. De Fonsek ACP. Danger of instant adhesives. Br Med J 1976;2:234.
44. Dean BS, Krenzelok EP. Cyanoacrylates and corneal abrasions. Clin Toxicol 1989;27:169–172.
45. Andrews LS, Clary JJ. Review of the toxicity of multifunctional acrylates. J Toxicol Environ Health 1986;19: 149–164.
46. Hiatt P. Toxic Information Center Case Rounds. Tox Info Center, San Francisco General Hospital Medical Center, January 16, 1990.
47. Dewan PA. Is injected polytetrafluoroethylene (Polytef) carcinogenic? Br J Urol 1992;69:29–33.
48. International Agency for Research on Cancer. Tetrofluoroethylene and polytetrafluoroethylene. IARC Monogr Eval Carcinog Risks Hum 1979;19:285–301.
49. Roe FJC. Br Med J 1988;297:783 (letter).
50. Shusterman DJ. Polymer fume fever and other fluorocarbon pyrolysis-related syndromes. In: Shusterman DJ, Peterson JE, eds. De nova toxicants: combustion toxicology mixing incompatibilities and environmental activation of toxic agents. State of the Art Reviews 1993;8:415–429, Philadelphia: Hanley & Belfus, 1993.
51. Sokol WN, Aelony Y, Beall GH. Meat-wrappers' asthma: a new syndrome? JAMA 1973;226:639–641.
52. Skevfving S, Akesson B, Simonsson BG. "Meat wrappers" asthma caused by thermal degradation products of polyethylene. Lancet 1980;1:211.
53. Acquavella JF, Douglass TS, Phillips SC. Evaluation of excess colorectal cancer incidence among workers involved in the manufacture of polypropylene. J Occup Med 1988;30: 438–440.
54. Acquavella JF, Douglass TS, Vernon S, Hughes JI, Thar WE. Assessment of colorectal cancer screening outcomes among workers involved in polypropylene manufacture. J Occup Med 1989;31:785–791.
55. Dougherty J. Polypropylene and colorectal adenomas: searching for prevalence. J Occup Med 1990;32:1141–1142.
56. Gibbs GW. Colorectal cancer and polypropylene exposure: how good is the evidence? J Occup Med 1990;32:1143.

ETHERS, EPOXY RESINS, AND RELATED PLASTIC COMPOUNDS

ACRYLAMIDE

PHYSICAL AND CHEMICAL CHARACTERISTICS

The chemical structure is $CH_2=CHCONH_2$. This compound is a colorless solid with a molecular weight of 71. Synonyms include propanamide, acrylamide monomer, and acrylic amide.

USES

Most toxic exposures occur during its use as a soil waterproofing agent in mining and tunneling operations as a result of pyrolysis during fires. Other industrial applications include the use of vinyl monomer in production of special monomers for grout and dyes and the use of acrylamide as a sizing agent in the paper and permanent press fabric industries.

ESTIMATION OF ACUTE TOXICITY

The United States exposure limit is 0.03 mg/m^3 as an 8-hour TWA for acrylamide, but the polymer is nontoxic. Toxicity can result from handling the crystalline powder, primarily through cumulative skin absorption.[1]

PATHOPHYSIOLOGY

Acrylamide neurotoxicity resembles the "dying back" peripheral neuropathy of tri-*o*-cresyl phosphate in which the distal regions of the longest and largest axons are affected. Acrylamide may inhibit energy production of distal nerves through progressive inhibition of glycolytic enzymes involved with rapid axonal transport.[2] Recent studies in rats indicate that in vivo activities of glycolytic enzymes remain intact, casting doubt on the hypothesis that acrylamide neuropathy begins with a reduction in metabolic energy.[3] Other routes that may result in the secondary loss of metabolic energy involve glutathione conjugation and nicotinamide antagonism.[4,5]

CLINICAL PRESENTATION

Chronic Effects

Long-term acrylamide exposure produces a motor and sensory polyneuropathy that is insidious and distal in onset. The presence of ataxia and, occasionally, dysarthria and tremor suggests central midbrain involvement.[1] Signs and symptoms include weakness, paresthesias, fatigue, lethargy, decreased pinprick sensation, vibratory loss, decreased reflexes, and positive Romberg sign. Severity is worse in distal portions of the extremities. Desquamation of the palms and soles, sweating, and peripheral vasoconstriction are more prominent in acrylamide peripheral neuropathy compared with other industrial neuropathies.[6] Recovery typically occurs within several months to a year of cessation of exposure, although severe exposures may result in permanent sequelae.[1]

Acute Effects

Severe exposure may produce central nervous system symptoms. In severe acute intoxication confusion and hallucinations may be observed; in moderate subacute intoxication drowsiness, loss of concentration, and ataxia are seen.[7]

Midbrain and cerebellar signs such as dysarthria, tremor, positive Romberg sign, and gait disturbances are most common. Visual changes (reduction of red and green discrimination) and a hypertensive retinopathy were associated with one severe case of acrylamide peripheral neuropathy.[8]

Ingestion by an adult of 18 grams of acrylamide crystals was followed within 5 hours by hallucinations, hypotension, seizures, gastrointestinal bleeding, and adult respiratory distress syndrome. Symptoms of peripheral neuropathy and hepatotoxicity appeared 3 days after ingestion.[9]

TREATMENT

Management involves the cessation of exposure and symptomatic treatment.

REFERENCES—ACRYLAMIDE

1. Garland TO, Patterson MWH. Six cases of acrylamide poisoning. Br Med J 1967;4:134–138.
2. Spencer PS, Sabri MI, Schaumberg HH et al. Does a defect of energy metabolism in the nerve fiber underly axonal degeneration in polyneuropathies? Ann Neurol 1979; 5:501–507.
3. Brimijoin SW, Hammond PI. Acrylamide neuropathy in the rat: Effects on energy metabolism in sciatic nerve. Mayo Clin Proc 1985;60:3–8.
4. Kaplan ML, Murphy SD, Gilles FH. Modification of acrylamide neuropathy produced by selected factors. Toxicol Appl Pharmacol 1973;24:564–579.
5. Sharma RP, Obersteiner EJ. Acrylamide cytotoxicity in chick ganglia cultures. Toxicol Appl Pharmacol 1977;42:149–156.
6. Auld RB, Bedwell SF. Peripheral neuropathy with sympathetic overactivity from industrial contact with acrylamide. Can Med Assoc J 1967;96:652–654.
7. Le Quesne PM. Clinical and morphological findings in acrylamide toxicity. Neurotoxicology 1985;6:17–24.
8. Mapp C, Mazzotta M, Bartolucci GB et al. Five cases of acrylamide intoxication. Med Lav 1977;68:1–12.
9. Donovan JW, Pearson T. Ingestion of acrylamide with severe encephalopathy, neurotoxicity and hepatotoxicity. Vet Hum Toxicol 1987;29:462.

DIMETHYLACETAMIDE

Dimethylacetamide (DMAC), like dimethylformamide, can induce liver damage in man. A relationship exists between the amount of DMAC absorbed and the amount of its metabolite monomethylacetamide excreted in the urine. High doses induce mental changes that are reversible. Skin exposure should be avoided.

STRUCTURE AND CLASSIFICATION

Dimethylacetamide (DMAC) is a colorless liquid whose chemical formal is $CH_3CON(CH_3)_2$. It exhibits wide organic and inorganic solubility, water miscibility, a high boiling point (329°F), low freezing point (–4°F), and good stability.[1] DMAC has a weak ammonia or fishlike odor.[2] Its molecular weight is 87.1. One part per million (ppm) = 3.62 mg/m^3 DMAC is a substituted amide.

Synonyms

Acetyldimethylamine; *N,N*-dimethylacetamide; DMAC.[3]

USES

Dimethylacetamide has excellent solvent properties. Because of this it is widely used in the production of plastics, resins, synthetic fibers and gums, and as a booster solvent in coatings and adhesive formulations.[4] DMAC is useful for dissolving polyacrylonitrile, polyvinylchloride (PVC), polyamides, polyimides, cellulose derivatives, styrenes, and linear polyester.[1]

OCCUPATIONAL EXPOSURE

DMAC can be perceived by some humans at 21 ppm, and by all at 47 ppm.[5] Most countries have established acceptable exposure levels for the workplace at 10 ppm. In the United States permissible exposure limits (time-weighted average) is 10 ppm (35 mg/m^3) (skin).[4]

TOXICOKINETICS

Absorption

DMAC is readily absorbed in man after oral, dermal, or inhalation exposure. After absorption it undergoes sequential demethylation to the monomethyl derivative (*N*-methylacetamide MMAC) and the demethylated product, acetamide.[1]

Elimination

About 2% of a dose of dimethylacetamide is recovered in the urine as MMAC after inhalation; 10% is recovered after inhalation plus skin exposure. Exposure to 10 ppm of DMAC results in complete excretion of MMAC within 30 hours.[6] Maximal concentrations of 45 and 100 ppm (mg/L) of MMAC in the urine are found in subjects exposed both by inhalation and skin. In workers continuously exposed to DMAC vapor (inhalation plus skin) and subjected to DMAC airborne levels of 6 to 22 ppm (8-hour TWA from 0.7 to 50 ppm DMAC), about 13.5% of the estimated dose is excreted as MMAC in the urine. Some workers may excrete about 30% of a dose as MMAC.[4]

Mean DMAC air concentrations studied on each day of the workweek ranged from 0.79 to 1.08 ppm in one study.[7] The MMAC urine concentration varied from 10 to 14 ppm, rising toward the end of the week.[8] Urinary MMAC reflected the amount of DMAC in the air. At measured exposures of 0.5 ppm DMAC in air, urinary MMAC levels had a mean of 6 ppm (range 4 to 11 ppm). At measured exposure of 1.5 ppm DMAC in air, mean MMAC values were 14 ppm (range 7 to 20 ppm). The data suggest that for each part per million of DMAC in air, approximately 10 ppm MMAC appear in the end of shift urine sample. A buildup of urine MMAC during the week may be due to dermal contact. For biologic monitoring in situations where air levels approach 10 ppm, urinary levels of 100 ppm MMAC might be expected.[6]

Pregnancy/Lactation

Teratogenic effects have been observed in rats at DMAC doses of 2400 mg/kg.[5]

Carcinogenicity

DMAC appears to be noncarcinogenic. Long-term feeding of relatively high levels of acetamide produces liver cancer in rats.[6]

CLINICAL PRESENTATION

Jaundice has been observed in workers exposed to 20 to 25 ppm with skin penetration contributing to this effect.[9] Workers exposed to DMAC from 2 to 10 years exhibited varying evidence of hepatotoxicity.[10] There were no data to link these changes to either dermal contact or specific air levels. Hepatomegaly was diagnosed in 14 of 41 workers studied. When DMAC was used as the solvent for injection of a triazine antifolate anticancer drug, three to four injections for 9 consecutive days did not result in any measurable toxicity.[11] Doses of DMAC of 400 mg/kg for 3 or more days in 13 of 15 patients with advanced malignancies induced depression, lethargy, and occasional confusion and disorientation. All patients (after the fourth or fifth dose) developed hallucinations (primarily visual), perceptual distortions, and delusions. All patients were judged to be normal several days after discontinuing DMAC treatment.[12,13] Repeated exposures of healthy males to DMAC have not induced an increase in epidermal mitosis or skin irritation.[14] The concentration considered to be an immediate danger to life and health is 400 ppm.[2]

LABORATORY

Analytic Methods

DMAC in air is measured by gas chromatography with a flame ionization detector.[15] Urine level of MMAC is measured by gas chromatography.[16]

Abnormalities

Bromosulphthalein (BS) retention was increased in 9 of 10 workers exposed to DMAC for 7 to 10 years and in 10 of 20 exposed for 2 to 7 years.[10] Liver function tests were altered also (serum aminotransferases, alkaline phosphatase, bilirubin). Workers exposed to DMAC in the production of heat-resistant enamel wire showed increases in hemoglobin and leukocytes with sporadic serum aminotransferase increase following long-term exposure.[1]

TREATMENT

DMAC is not an irritant to human skin,[14] but can enter the body through the skin. Control of DMAC workplace air levels may not be totally effective in cases where dermal contact may occur. A relationship exists between the amount of DMAC absorbed and the amount of MMAC excreted in the urine so that biomonitoring of urinary metabolites may indicate situations in which total exposure, both dermal and inhalation, are excessive. Workers exposed to DMAC should be informed about its adverse health effects and trained to avoid skin contact. Appropriate protective equipment and work practices should be emphasized. Employers should institute adequate engineering controls to ensure that DMAC exposures do not exceed the NIOSH recommended exposure limit/OSHA permissible exposure limit of 10 ppm.

Skin exposures should be followed by prompt water flushing. Eye exposure should be followed by immediate saline irrigation and an ophthalmology review. Oral ingestions of DMAC should be treated symptomatically and supportively in a hospital. Liver function tests should be obtained periodically as indicated.

REFERENCES—DIMETHYLACETAMIDE

1. Kennedy GL Jr. Biological effects of acetamide, formamide and their monomethyl and dimethyl derivatives. CRC Crit Rev Toxicol 1986;17:129–182.
2. NIOSH Pocket Guide to Chemical Hazard. DHHS (NIOSH) Publication No 90-117. Washington, DC: US Government Printing Office, p. 94.
3. Proctor NH, Hughes JP, Fischman ML, Hathaway GW. The chemical hazards. In: Proctor NH, Hughes JP, Fischman ML, eds. Chemical hazards of the work place, 2nd ed. New York: Van Nostrand Reinhold, 1989; pp. 206–207.
4. Borm PJA, de Jong L, Vliegen A. Environmental and biological monitoring of workers occupationally exposed to dimethylacetamide. J Occup Med 1987;29:898–903.
5. Leonardous G, Kendall D, Barnard N. Odor threshold determinations of 53 odorant chemicals. J Air Pollut Control Assoc 1965;19:91–95.
6. Maxfield ME, Barnes JR, Azar A, Trochimowicz HT. Urinary excretion of metabolite following experimental human exposures to DMF or to DMAC. J Occup Med 1975;17:506–511.
7. Kennedy GL Jr, Pruett JW. Biologic monitoring for dimethylacetamide: measurement for 4 consecutive weeks in a work place. J Occup Med 1989;31:47–50.
8. Stula EF, Karuss WC. Embryotoxicity in rats and rabbits from cutaneous application of amide-type solvents and substituted ureas. Toxicol Appl Pharmacol 1977;41:35–55.
9. Threshold limit values for chemical substances and physical agents in the work environment. Cincinnati: American Conference of Governmental Industrial Hygienists, 1982, p. 17.
10. Corsi GC. Dimethylacetamide-induced occupational disease; with particular attention to hepatic functions. Med Lav 1971;62:28–42.
11. Corbett TH, Leopold WR, Dykes DJ, Roberts BJ, Griswold DP, Schabel FM. Toxicity and anticancer activity of a new triazine antifolate (NSC 127755). Cancer Res 1982;42:1707.
12. Weiss AJ, Mancall EL, Koltes JA, White JC, Jackson LG. Dimethylacetamide: a hitherto unrecognized hallucinogenic agent. Science 1962;136:151–152.
13. Weiss AJ, Jackson LG, Carabasi RA, Mancall EL, White JC. A phase 1 study of dimethylacetamide. Cancer Chemother Rep No. 16; February 1972, p. 477.
14. Fisher LB, Maibach HI. Effect of some irritants on human epidermal mitosis. Contact Dermatitis 1975;1:273–276.
15. National Institute for Occupational Safety and Health. Manual of Sampling Data Sheets. Washington, DC: US Department of Health, Education and Welfare, 1977, Publication No. 254-1-3.
16. Barnes JR, Henry NW III. The determination of *N*-methylformamide and *N*-methylacetamide in urine. Ind Hyg Assoc J 1974;35:84–87.

DIMETHYLFORMAMIDE

Approximately 94,000 United States workers are potentially exposed to dimethylformamide (DMF).[1] Clinical studies suggest a probable association between exposure to DMF and the production of liver damage,[2–12] and a role as a "possible" carcinogen in view of its putative association with testicular cancer,[13–17] prostate cancer, buccal cavity and pharynx cancer, and malignant melanomas.[18,19] DMF has been postulated as the probable cause of hepatic damage in poisoning due to ingestion of T61, a veterinary euthanasia drug[12] (see Veterinary Drug Section).

Synonyms

DMF, DMFA.

USES

Dimethylformamide is a versatile and widely used laboratory and industrial chemical and is an excellent solvent. It is used primarily in the manufacture of polyurethane products and acrylic fibers, as well as in the production of pharmaceuticals, pesticides, and other products.[4] It is also present in textile dyes and pigments, paint stripping solvents, and coating, printing, and adhesive formulations.[20] In veterinary medicine it is used as a vehicle for drug administration.

TOXIC EXPOSURE

Dimethylformamide exposure to air concentrations of 3500 ppm is considered immediately dangerous to life or health (IDLH).[21]

TOXICOKINETICS

Absorption

Dimethylformamide is readily absorbed through the skin, respiratory system, and gastrointestinal tract.[4] It reaches an average level of 2.8 μg/ml in the blood when subjects have been exposed to 21 ppm of the vapor for 4 hours; it is not detected in the blood after 4 hours.[22–24] Exposure to 87 ppm of the DMF vapor for 4 hours results in peak blood levels of about 14 μg/mL and 8 μg/mL, for dimethylformamide and methylformamide, respectively, measured at 0 and 3 hours after exposure.[23]

Elimination

A metabolite of DMF, methylformamide, maintains a blood level of 1 to 2 μg/mL for 4 hours after exposure.[24] DMF is metabolized by *N*-demethylation to methylformamide and formamide, which are largely excreted in the urine. The amount of *N*-methylformamide recovered in the urine represents only 2 to 6% of the dose of dimethylformamide inhaled.[25,26] A substantial portion of an absorbed dose of DMF is excreted unchanged in the expired breath. The urinary concentration of *N*-methylformamide is probably the best index of worker exponent dimethylformamide.[22–25]

Dimethylformamide →	Methylformamide →	formamide
$HCON(CH_3)_2$	$HCONHCH_3$	$HCONH_2$

Concentrations of *N*-methylformamide above 50 mg/24 hour urine indicates exposure exceeding 20 ppm.[23]

Concentrations of *N*-methylformamide in the urine collected at the end of a work shift that do not exceed 40 to 50 mg/g of creatinine suggests an exposure that is possibly safe with regard to the acute and possibly also with regard to the long-term (5 years) effects of DMF on liver function. The long-term data must still be corroborated by prospective studies with consecutive measurements of DMF air and urine concentrations and of its metabolites, together with periodic liver function studies. However, if skin absorption can be ruled out, this concentration of *N*-methylformamide in the postshift sample corresponds to an average concentration of DMF vapor of 14 mg/m³ (45 ppm) during a 6-hour period, higher than the NIOSH/OSHA permissible limits of 10 ppm.[26]

Drug Interactions

Ingestion of alcohol during or after an exposure to dimethylformamide can produce a disulfiram-like reaction, with facial flushing, dizziness, sweating, nausea, palpitation, breathlessness, and loss of consciousness. This is probably due to the inhibition of acetaldehyde dehydrogenase by methylformamide.[8]

No studies in human pregnancy or lactation are available.

CLINICAL PRESENTATION

A NIOSH Alert Fact Sheet is available.[27]

Complaints of abdominal pain, nausea, vomiting, dizziness, headaches, loss of appetite, and alcohol intolerance have been reported in workers exposed to dimethylformamide.[5–10]

Liver

Dimethylformamide hepatotoxicity is believed to be dose-dependent. Hepatic necrosis and steatosis have been observed on liver biopsy specimens from exposed workers[5–16] (see Laboratory). The long-term hepatic effects of dimethylformamide exposure are not known.[4]

Testicular Cancer

Several studies[13–15] of workers exposed to DMF indicate a possible role for this chemical in the development of testicular concerns. Animal studies have not demonstrated that DMF is mutagenic or carcinogenic.[14] A DMF manufacturers' study of potentially exposed employees found no excess of testicular cancer, but did find significant excesses of buccal and pharyngeal cancer and malignant melanoma. The International Agency for Research on Cancer has classified DMF as a "possible" carcinogen.

LABORATORY

Analytic Methods

Dimethylformamide and methylformamide in blood may be measured after extraction into ethanol by nitrogen-selective gas chromatography.[22,23] Methylformamide determinations in the urine may be quantified by flame-ionization gas

NIOSH Fact Sheet on DMF

Dimethylformamide (DMF) WARNING!

Avoid skin contact with dimethylformamide (DMF)! This chemical is easily absorbed through the skin and can cause liver damage and other adverse health effects.

Dimethylformamide is associated with the following health effects:

- Liver damage
- Alcohol intolerance
- Skin problems

Exposed workers have also reported the following symptoms:

- Weakness
- Nausea and vomiting
- Abdominal pain
- Dizziness
- Headache
- Constipation

Some reports suggest an increase in cancer among workers exposed to DMF, but the evidence is not conclusive at this time. The excess cancer observed could have resulted from exposure to other chemicals or tobacco, or from chance alone.

Take the following precautions if you are exposed to DMF on the job:

1. Obtain and read the material safety data sheet (MSDS) for DMF and the NIOSH Alert on DMF (see ordering information at right).
2. Avoid skin contact with DMF: Use chemical protective clothing such as gloves and aprons made from butyl rubber, Teflon(R), or polyethylene/ethylene (for example, 4H(R) or Silvershield(R)).
3. Use respiratory protection when concentrations of DMF in workplace air may exceed 10 ppm as a 8-hour time weighted average (for example, during emergencies or maintenance operation).
4. Participate in your company's medical screening program if you qualify.

Figure 69–3 NIOSH Fact Sheet on DMF. (Adapted from NIOSH Health Alert, 1981.)

chromatography. The method is sensitive from 5 to 500 μg/liter.[28]

Abnormalities

Elevation of serum aminotransferase concentrations (aspartate-AST and alanine-ALT) have been observed following occupational exposure to DMF. A finding of the ratio of AST to ALT levels less than one may be useful in differentiating toxic from alcoholic hepatitis.[4] Resolution of the abnormal liver enzymes may take up to 1 to 7 months. Elevation of liver enzyme levels has been found in 76% of production workers exposed routinely to DMF without accidental overexposure or unusual circumstances.[4] The long-term effects of DMF exposure are not known.

Ancillary Tests

Elevations of blood creatine phosphokinase (CPK) may follow a high exposure to DMF.[10] Dermal and respiratory exposure to DMF sufficient to induce abdominal pain, hypertension, leukocytosis and hepatic damage may be associated with a positive urine porphobilinogen.[3] Sister chromatic exchange rates appear related to the intensity of DMF exposure.[29]

TREATMENT (FIG. 69-3)

Workers exposed to DMF should be informed about its adverse health effects and trained to avoid skin contact and to use appropriate protective equipment and work practices. Employees should institute engineering controls to ensure that DMF exposure does not exceed the NIOSH recommended exposure limit/OSHA permissible exposure limit of 10 ppm as an 8-hour time-weighted average.[20] NIOSH/OSHA recommend maximum concentrations for various respirator uses at 100 ppm and above.

Eye exposure should be followed by immediate saline irrigations and an ophthalmology review. Skin exposure is followed by prompt water flushing. Oral ingestion of DMF should be treated supportively in a hospital. Liver function tests should be obtained within 24 hours and followed weekly.

Antidote

There are no antidotes to DMF overexposure.

REFERENCES—DIMETHYLFORMAMIDE

1. CDC. NIOSH alerts on work place hazards: falls through skylights and roof openings, death of farm workers in manure pits and exposure to dimethylformamide. MMWR 1991; 40:142–143.
2. Fleming LE, Shalat SL, Redlich CA. Liver injury in workers exposed to dimethylformamide. Scand J Work Environ Health 1990;16:289–292.
3. Potter HP. Dimethylformamide-induced abdominal pain and liver injury. Arch Environ Health 1973;27:340–341.
4. Redlich CA, Beckett WS, Sparer J, Barwich KW, Riely CA, Miller H et al. Liver disease associated with occupational exposure to the solvent dimethylformamide. Ann Intern Med 1988;108:680–686.
5. Tolot F, Arcadio F, Lenglet JP, Roche L. Intoxication par la dimethylformamide. Arch Mal Prof 1968;29:714–717.
6. Tolot F, Droin M, Generois M. Intoxication par la dimethylformamide. Arch Mal Prof 1958;19:602–606.
7. Reinl W, Urban HJ. Erkrankungen durch dimethylformamide. Int Arch V Gewerbepathol Gewerbehyg 1965;21: 333–346.
8. Lyle WH, Spence TW, McKinneley WM, Duckers K. Dimethylformamide and alcohol intolerance. Br J Ind Med 1979;36: 63–66.
9. Chivers CP. Disulfiram effect from inhalation of dimethylformamide. Lancet 1978;1:331 (letter).
10. Wang J-D, Lai M-Y, Chen J-S, Lin J-M, Chiang J-R, Shiau S-J, Chang W-S. Dimethylformamide-induced liver damage among synthetic leather workers. Arch Environ Health 1991;46:161–166.
11. Scailteur V, Lauwerys RR: Dimethylformamide (DMF) hepatotoxicity. Toxicology 1987;43:231–238.
12. Nicolas F, Rodineau P, Rouzioux J-M, Tack I, Chabac S, Merain D. Fulminant hepatic failure in poisoning due to ingestion of T61, a veterinary euthanasia drug. Crit Care Med 1990;18:573–574.
13. Levin SM, Baker DB, Landrigan PJ et al. Testicular cancer in leather tanners exposed to dimethylformamide. Lancet 1987;2:1153 (letter).
14. CDC. Testicular cancer in leather workers—Fulton County, New York. MMWR 1989;38:105–114.
15. Calvert GM, Fajen JM, Hills BW, Halperin WE. Testicular cancer, dimethylformamide and leather tanneries. Lancet 1990; 336:1253–1254.
16. Ducatman AM. Dimethylformamide, metal dyes, and testicular cancer. Lancet 1989;1:911.
17. Gollins WJF. Dimethylformamide and testicular cancer. Lancet 1991;337:306–307.
18. Chen JL, Kennedy GL Jr. Dimethylformamide and testicular cancer. Lancet 1988;1:55.
19. Chen JL, Fayerweather WE, Pell S. Cancer incidence of workers exposed to dimethylformamide and/or acrylonitrile. J Occup Med 1988;30:813–818.
20. Office of the Federal Register. Code of Federal Regulations: occupational Safety and Health Standards. Subpart Z: Air contaminants—permissible exposure limits. Table Z-1-A. Washington, DC: Office of the Federal Register. National Archives and Records Administration, 1989 (29CFR1910.1000).
21. NIOSH pocket guide to chemical hazards. DHHS (NIOSH) Publication No. 90-117. NIOSH. US Government Printing Office, Washington, DC: June 1990.
22. Kimmerle G, Eben A. Metabolism of *N,N*-dimethylformamide. I. Studies in rats and dogs. Int Arch Arbeitsmed 1975;34: 109–126.
23. Kimmerle G, Eben A. Metabolism studies of *N,N*-dimethylformamide. Int Arch Arbeitsmed 1975;34:127–136.
24. Baselt RC, Cravey RH. Disposition of toxic drugs and chemicals in man. 3rd ed. Chicago: Year Book, 1989; pp. 280–282.
25. Yonemoto J, Suzuki S. Relation of exposure to dimethylformamide vapor and the metabolite, methylformamide, in urine of workers. Int Arch Occup Environ Health 1980;46: 159–165.
26. Lauwerys RR, Kivits A, Lhoir M, Rigolet P, Houbeau D, Beucket JP, Roels HA. Biological surveillance of workers exposed to dimethylformamide and the influence of skin protection on its percutaneous absorption. Int Arch Occup Environ Health 1980;45:189–203.
27. NIOSH alert on dimethylformamide. [DHHS (NIOSH) 90-105].
28. Barnes JR, Henry NW III. The determination of *N*-methylformamide and *N*-methylacetamide in urine. Am Ind Hyg Assoc J 1974;35:84–87.
29. Seij K, Inoue O, Cai S-K, Kowai T, Watane T, Ikeda M. Increase in sister chromatid exchange rates in association with occupational exposure to *N-N*-dimethylformamide. Int Arch Occup Environ Health 1992;64:65–67.

PLASTICIZERS—PHTHALATE ESTERS

USE

Vinyl plastic is used in the manufacture of blood bags and associated medical devices used in the collection, processing, storing, and dispensing of human blood and blood components.[1] It is also used in consumer products such as imitation leather, rainwear, footwear, upholstery, flooring, tablecloths, shower curtains, food packaging materials, and children's toys.[2] To be pliable vinyl plastic must have added to it a chemical, referred to as a "plasticizer," at levels up to 30 to 40% of the final weight.

DEHP

The most widely used plasticizer worldwide, particularly for medical devices, is a phthalic acid ester (Fig. 6–4) known as di (2-ethyl hexyl) phthalate.[3] DEHP is not bound chemically to the vinyl plastic, but is dissolved physically in it. DEHP is leached from polyvinyl chloride containers by cyclosporin, miconazole, teniposide, etoposide, chlordiazepoxide, the surfactants polysorbate 80 and polyoxyethylated castor oil, and the vehicles used in paclitoxel and docetanel formulation.[4,5] The possibility therefore exists for migration of the plasticizer from the plastic film. It is practically insoluble in water but soluble in fat and can migrate into food containing

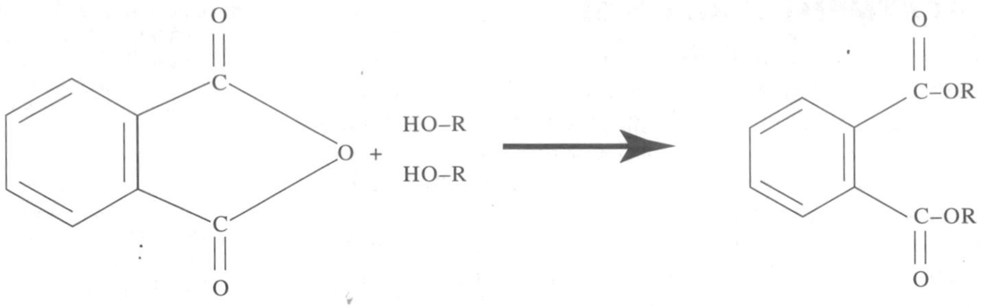

Figure 69–4 Structures of several common phthalate esters. (Adapted from Kluwe W. Environ Health Perspect 1988;45:3–10.)

lipophilic material such as fats and oils.[6] The OSHA PEL-TWA skin designation is 5.0 mg/m^3.

TOXICOKINETICS

Absorption

DEHP may enter the body through the lungs, skin, or gastrointestinal tract, as well as through direct injection.[7] It readily forms aerosols. It is absorbed rapidly and extensively following oral administration. DEHP is absorbed primarily as its non-deesterified metabolite, MEHP.[8] The hydrolysis occurs in intestinal cells, mucosa cells, blood, and tissues. Little DEHP is detected in the body after oral exposure, except after massive doses have saturated the capacity of the body to hydrolyze it. MEHP undergoes oxidative metabolism to yield 13 or more metabolites excreted in the urine.[9]

Distribution

A whole-body exchange transfusion in a 70-kg man with 21-day-old blood was estimated to result in the intravenous administration of 300 mg of DEHP, a dose of 4 to 5 mg/kg body weight.[10] In newborn infants undergoing a single exchange transfusion, DEHP (0.8 to 3.3 mg/kg) and MEHP (0.05 to 0.20 mg/kg) were infused.[11] The plasma levels ranged between 5.8 and 19.6 μg/ml, but declined rapidly. DEHP disappeared from the blood with a half-life of 28 minutes. The clearance of DEHP was approximately 78 mL/min/m^2. Maximal plasma levels of MEHP were about 5 μg/ml. The elimination half-life was approximately 10 hours. Patients undergoing maintenance hemodialysis for renal failure were exposed to about 105 mg of DEHP in a single dialysis session (23.8 to 360 mg).[12] Blood levels of DEHP averaged 1.9 μg/mL and of MEHP 1.3 μg/mL. Blood concentrations of phthalic acid averaged 5.2 μg/mL. The apparent volume of distribution is 2.8 L/m^2 (approximately 0.06 L/kg).

Excretion

Approximately 4.5 to 15% of a single oral dose of 10 g to 30 g of DEHP was excreted as metabolites in the urine of human volunteers.[13,14] These oxidized metabolites (2 ethyhexanoic acid [EAH] and 2-ethyl-5-hydroxyhexanoic acid [5-OH-EHA])[15] are excreted in humans as glucuronides.[16]

Toxicity

Based on animal data DEHP may have potential toxicity in the heart, lungs, liver, and reproductive organs in man. There have been no specific defined lesions in humans associated with its use. However, most male patients receiving hemodialysis treatment have been observed to be sterile, with testicular atrophy,[17] and polycystic kidney disease is prevalent in long-term hemodialysis patients.[18,19] Limited data, in man seem to suggest that humans exposed to "normal" amounts of phthalates are not susceptible to the possible cytogenic effects. Patients repeatedly exposed to phthalate esters in infusion fluids have not yet been adequately studied sufficiently to prove a causal relationship between exposure and renal pathology.[1]

The inhalation of DEHP has been associated with pulmonary dysfunction and bronchial asthma.[20] Exposure of workers to high levels of mixed phthalates in the workplace area may produce transient irritation of the nose and throat. MEHP causes bronchial hyperactivity in rats.[21] A necrotizing dermatitis[22] and a plasticizer-induced hepatitis-like syndrome[23] have been described following extensive use of blood tubing. Polyneuropathies have been described in one series of patients[24] but not in another.[25]

A 59-year-old patient developed repeated bouts of cutaneous necrotizing dermatitis, which showed a clear temporal relation to the use of polyvinyl chloride tubing during dialysis.[26]

OTHER USES

"Cling films," the thin, clear, flexible plastic films used for packaging foods, are made from polyvinyl chloride (PVC) or vinylidine chloride (VDC) copolymers. Plasticizers are required to provide flexibility to the PVC and VDC.[27] Plasticizers used most widely in PVC cling films are di-2-ethyl hexyl adipate (DEHA) and polymeric species (polyesters of dicarboxylic acids and di hydric alcohols); acetyl tributyl citrate (ATBC) is used with VDC copolymer films. PVC films have been recently reformulated, with DEHA replaced largely by polymeric species; DEHA dietary intake has fallen, but is still approximately 8 mg per day. No adverse health effects have been observed at this level of intake. ATBC intake has risen from 0.05 to 1.5 mg/day since 1987.[28]

A United Kingdom government report recommends that cling films not be used in conventional ovens or for wrapping food or lining dishes for cooking in a microwave oven. Because plasticizers are fat soluble, cling films should not be used to wrap food with a high fat content.[29] The metabolism of DEHA in man indicates that acidic urinary metabolites are eliminated within 24 hours.[30]

DI-*N*-BUTYLPHTHALATE

Limited data exist on exposure to di-*n*-butylphthalate, a liquid used to make soft plastics, paints, glue, insect repellents, hair spray, nail polish, and rocket fuel.[31] Workers were observed to develop hypertension, pain, numbness, spasm, reflex disturbances, depression of vestibular function, and hyperbilirubinemia at a frequency that increased with length of employment.[32] They were also exposed to other plasticizers.

Glo sticks and other glow products are very popular with children, especially in the summer months. They provide a heatless chemical luminescence in an array of vivid colors. Contact of any body parts with the liquid contents induces a burning sensation. Little or no morbidity is observed. Eye irrigation, gut dilution, and washing with soap are adequate treatment in most cases. Referral to a health care facility is usually unnecessary.[33]

DIMETHYL PHTHALATE

A 34-year-old male consumed a liquid plastic catalyst containing methyl ethyl ketone peroxide and dimethyl phthalate. He was initially stuporous and later developed an esophageal stricture that responded to treatment.[34]

TRIBUTOXYETHYL PHOSPHATE

This chemical has been used as a plasticizer for rubber stoppers in blood specimen containers and has been identified in postmortem blood samples.[35]

N-BUTYL BENZENE SULFONAMIDE (NBBS)

NBBS, a sulfonamide plasticizer, is used for the polymerization of polyamide compounds in the production of plastic resins and as a starting agent in the synthesis of an agricultural herbicide.[36,37]

Toxicity

A container-derived contaminant from plastic ware (NBBS) induced a progressive spastic myelopathy in rabbits.[36] Human exposure to NBBS may occur from agricultural fungicides and waste-water effluents.[38] Workers engaged in the production of plastics seem to be at an increased risk for the development of amyotrophic lateral sclerosis.[39] The levels of NBBS required to induce human neurodegenerative disease, the conditions most likely to result in leaching of NBBS, and the human bioavailability of NBBS have not yet been determined.[36] Leaching of plasticizers from plastic products depends not only on pH, temperature, and duration of storage but also on the chemical composition of foods or biologic products stored in them.[40]

Analytic Method

Liquid-liquid extraction followed by capillary gas chromatography has been developed to screen solutions leached from packaging material. This procedure screens cyclohexanone, 2-ethyl-l-hexanol, phthalide, 2,6-di-tet-butyl-*p*-cresol, dibutyl phthalate and di (2-ethyl hexyl) phthalate (DEHP).[41] Plasma concentrations of DEHP- and MEHP-derived metabolites were determined by gas chromatography–chemical ionization spectrometry and gas chromatography–electron impact mass spectrometry, respectively.[12] The structure of DEHP can also be determined by NMR spectroscopy, mass spectrometry, and microanalysis.[42] DEHP metabolites in urine samples may be of use in monitoring the occupational exposure to DEHP.[43]

BENZOTHIAZOLES (FIG. 69–5)

Sources

A contaminant found to leach into the contents of disposable syringes was identified as 2-(2-hydroxyethylthio) benzothiazole (HEB) formed during manufacture of the syringes as a result of a reaction between 2-mercaptobenzothiazole, a rubber vulcanization accelerator, and ethylene oxide, used for sterilization. The contaminant was isolated from the rubber plunger seal.[44]

HEB has also been found in certain rubber components of intravenous administration sets.[45]

Toxicity—Metabolism

2-Mercaptobenzothiazole (2-MB) may cause dermatologic reactions in man[46–48] and has been assumed in animals.[49] In mice 2-MB resulted in central nervous system stimulation, peripheral vasodilatation, salivation, and a severe liver toxicity. This was also produced by 2-(2-hydroxyethylmercapto) benzothiazole (HEB).

2-(carboxymethylthio) benzothiazole (CMB) is a product that may, by a simple oxidation process, be derived from HEB (Fig. 69–5). Neonates have been observed to have serum levels of CMB in proportion to the duration of intravenous therapy (35-595 µmol/L).[45] The half-life of CMB is 9 days; it passes the blood–brain barrier (found in cerebrospinal fluid) and is 99% protein bound to albumin binding sites.[45] It appears possible that CMB could displace bilirubin from albumin and hence increase the risk of kernicterus.

Analytic Method

High-performance liquid chromatography and mass spectrometry were used to determine serum levels of CMB.[45]

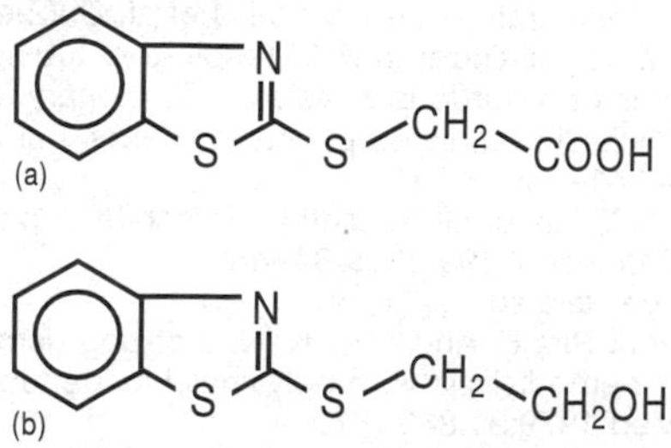

Figure 69–5 Chemical structure of the two benzothiazoles. (a) 2-(carboxymethylthio)benzothiazole (CMB). (b) 2-(hydroxyethylthio)-benzothiazole (HEB). Conversion factors: CMB 1 µmol = 225 µg; HEB 1 µmol = 211 µg. (Adapted from Meek JH, Pettit BR. Lancet 1985;2:1090.)

REFERENCES—PHTHALATE ESTERS

1. Rubin RJ, Ness PM. What price progress? An update on vinyl plastic blood bags. Transfusion 1989;29:358–361.
2. Toxicological profile for di (2-ethyl hexyl) phthalate. Agency for Toxic Substances and Disease Registry, US Public Health Service. ATSDR/TP-88/15, 1989.
3. Kluwe WM. Overview of phthalate ester pharmacokinetics in mammalian species. Environ Health Perspect 1988;45: 3–10.
4. Pearson SD. Leaching of diethylhexylphthalate from polyvinyl chloride containers by selected drugs and formulation components. Am J Hosp Pharm 1993;50:1405–1409.
5. Alexander M, Matsumura F, Lech J (Peer review panel). ATSDR. Toxicological profile for diethyl phthalate draft. May 1993.
6. Dickson SJ, Missen AW, Down GJ. The investigation of plasticizer contaminants in post-mortem blood samples. J Forensic Sci 1974;4:155–159.
7. Albro PW, Lavenhar SR. Metabolism of di (2-ethyl hexyl) phthalate. Drug Metab Rev 1989;21:13–34.
8. White RD, Carter DE, Earnest O, Mueller J. Absorption and metabolism of three phthalate diesters by the rat small intestine. Food Cosmet Toxicol 1980;18:383–386.
9. Albro PW, Thomas R, Fishbein L. Metabolites of dietary diethylhexyl phthalate by rats. Isolation and characterization of the urinary metabolites. J Chromatogr 1983;76:321–330.
10. Jaeger RJ, Rubin RJ. Migration of phthalate ester plasticizer from polyvinyl chloride blood bags into stored human blood and its localization in human tissues. N Engl J Med 1972; 287:1114–1118.
11. Sjoberg POJ, Bondesson VG, Sedin EG, Gustaffson JP. Exposure of newborn infants to plasticizers. Plasma levels of DEHP and MEHP during exchange transfusion. Transfusion 1985;25:424–428.
12. Pollack GM, Buchanan JF, Slaughter RL, Kohli RK, Shen DD. Circulating concentrations of DEHP and its de-esterified phthalic acid products following plasticizer exposure in patients receiving hemodialysis. Toxicol Appl Pharmacol 1985; 79:257–267.
13. Shaffer CB, Carpenter CB, Smyth HF. Acute and subacute toxicity of DEHP with note upon its metabolism. J Ind Hyg Toxicol 1945;27:130–135.
14. Schmid P, Schlatter C. Excretion and metabolism of DEHP in man. Xenobiotica 1985;15:251–256.
15. Steel GT, Woollen BH, Loftus NJ, Laird WJD, Wilks MF, Olver GJA. Biological monitoring of exposure to plasticizers. Hum Exp Toxicol 1992;11:287–288.
16. Albro PW, Corbett JT, Schroeder JL, Jordan S, Matthews HB. Pharmacokinetics, interactions with macromolecules and species differences in metabolism of DEHP. Environ Health Perspect 1982;14:19–25.
17. Reference Deleted
18. Woodward KN. Phthalate esters, cystic kidney disease in animals and possible effects on human health: a review. Hum Exp Toxicol 1990;9:297–301.
19. Dunnill MS, Millare PR, Oliver D. Acquired cystic disease of the kidney. A hazard of long-term intermittent hemodialysis. J Clin Pathol 1977;30:868–877.
20. Roth B, Herkenrath P, Lehmann HJ et al. Di-(2-ethyl hexyl) phthalate as plasticizer in PVC respiratory tubing systems: indications of hazardous effects on pulmonary function in mechanically ventilated pre-term infants. Eur J Pediatr 1988;147:41–46.
21. Kamrin MA, Mayor GHY. Diethyl phthalate: A perspective. J Clin Pharmacol 1991;31:484–489.
22. Reference Deleted
23. Bommer J, Ritz E, Andrassy K. Necrotizing dermatitis resulting from hemodialysis with polyvinylchloride tubing. Ann Intern Med 1979;91:869–870.
24. Gilioli R, Bulgheroni C, Terrana T, Filippini G, Masselto N, Bocri R. A neurological, electromyographic and electroneurographic study in subjects working at the production of phthalate plasticizers: preliminary results. Med Lavoro 1978; 69:620–622.
25. Nielsen J, Akesson B, Skerfring S. Phthalate ester exposure—air levels and health of workers processing polyvinyl chloride. Am Ind Hyg Assoc J 1985;46:643–647.
26. Bommer J, Ritz E, Andrassy K. Necrotizing dermatitis resulting from hemodialysis with polyvinyl chloride tubing. Ann Intern Med 1979;91:869–870.
27. Neergaard J, Nielsen B, Faubry V, Christensen DH, Nielson OF. Plasticizers in P.V.C. and the occurrence of hepatitis in a haemodialysis unit. Scand J Urol Nephrol 1971;5:141–145.
28. Plasticizers in food. Lancet 1990;336:1309 (editorial).
29. Plasticizers: continuing surveillance. MAFF Food Surveillance Paper 30. London: HM Stationery Office, 1990, ISBNO-11-242905-X. p. 52.
30. Loftus N-J, Laird WJD, Leeser JE, Steel GT, Woolen BH. The metabolism and pharmacokinetics of Deuterium labelled di-(2-ethyl hexyl) adepate (DEHA) in human volunteers following oral administration. Hum Exper Toxicol 1990;9:326.
31. Di-*n*-butyl phthalate. Toxicological profile. Agency for Toxic Substances and Disease Registry. TP-90-10. 1990.
32. Milkov LE, Aldryeva MV, Poporia TB et al. Health status of workers exposed to phthalate plasticizers in the manufacture of artificial leather and films based on PVC resins. Environ Health Perspect 1973;3:175–178.
33. Keys N, Erickson T, Lipscomb J. Glow compound exposure. Clin Toxicol 1995;33:475–486 (abstract 5).
34. Deisher JB. Poisoning with a liquid plastic catalyst. Northwest Medicine 1958;57:46.
35. Snell RB, Capillary GC. Analysis of compounds leach into parenteral solutions packaged in plastic bags. J Chromatogr Sci 1989;27:524–528.
36. Strong MJ, Garruto RM, Wolff AV, Yanagahira R, Chou SM, Fox SD. *N*-butyl benzene sulphonamide, a novel neurotoxic plasticizing agent. Lancet 1990;336:640.
37. Strong MJ, Wolff AV, Yanagahira R, Garruto RM, Chou SM. *N*-butyl benzene sulfonamide: a plasticizing agent inducing a chronic neurofilamentous degenerative neurology. 1990; 40(Suppl 1):430.
38. Sheldon LS, Hites RA. Sources and movement of organic chemicals in the Delaware River. Environ Sci Technol 1979; 13:574–579.
39. Deaper DM, Henderson BE. A case-control study of amyotrophic lateral sclerosis. Am J Epidemiol 1986;123:790–797.
40. Rubin RJ, Ness PM. What price progress? An update on vinyl blood bags. Transfusion 1989;29:358–361.
41. Snell RB. Capillary GC analysis of compounds leach into parenteral solutions packaged in plastic bags. J Chromatogr Sci 1989;27:524–528.
42. Cohen H, Charrier C, Sarfaty J. Extraction and identification of a plasticizer, di(2-ethylhexyl) phthalate from a plastic bag containing contaminated cor n. Arch Environ Contam Toxicol 1991;210:437–444.
43. Dirven HAAM, Van den Broek PHH, Arends AM, Nordkamp HH, de Lepper AJGM, Henderson PT et al. Metabolites of the plasticizer di (2-ethyl hexyl) phthalate in urine samples of workers in polyvinylchloride processing industries. Int Arch Occup Environ Health 1993;64:549–554.
44. Peterson MC, Vine J, Ashley JJ, National RL. Leaching of 2-(2-hydroxyethylmercapto) benzothiazole into contents of disposable syringes. J Pharmaceut Sci 1981;70:1139–1143.
45. Meek JH, Pettit BR. Avoidable accumulation of potentially toxic levels of benzothiazoles in babies receiving intravenous therapy. Lancet 1985;2:1090–1092.
46. Bonnevie P, Marcussen PV. Rubber products as a widespread cause of eczema. Report of 80 cases. Acta Dermatovener 1945;25:163–178.
47. Cronin E. Shoe dermatitis. Br J Dermatol 1966;78:617–625.
48. Wilson HTH: Rubber dermatitis. An investigation of 106 cases of contact dermatitis caused by rubber. Br Med J 1969;81:175–180.
49. Salmone G, Assaf A, Bayte-Sorbier A, Airauda ChB. Mass spectral identification of benzothiazole derivatives leached into injections by disposable syringes. Biomed Mass Spectrom 1984;9:450–454.

EPICHLORHYDRIN (ECH)

Epichlorhydrin (ECH) or 1-chloro-2,3-epoxy propane (CH_2 - CH - CH_2 - Cl) is a colorless liquid at room temperature with an odor comparable to chloroform. Its molecular weight is 92.53. The CAS no. is 106-89-5. OSHA permissible exposure limits are 2 ppm for an 8-hour time-weighted average. It is used as a basic material for the manufacture of epoxy resins, glycerin, insecticides, solvents, and other chemicals. ECH is an alkylating agent.

An epidemiologic study of workers followed for 20 years after probable exposure to ECH suggested a moderate increase in heart disease. Evidence for the relation between exposure to ECH and both respiratory cancer and leukemia is not strong.[1–3] A study of exposed workers from four European plants did not indicate an increase in cancer mortality.[3] Two of the three studies were performed by individuals associated with manufacturers.[2,3] Further validation of these observations appears to be required.

REFERENCES—EPICHLORHYDRIN

1. Enterline PE, Henderson V, Marsh G. Mortality of workers potentially exposed to epichlorhydrin. Br J Ind Med 1990;47: 269–276.
2. Tsai SP, Cowles SR, Tackett DL, Barclay MT, Ross CE. Morbidity prevalence study of workers with potential exposure to epichlorhydrin. Br J Ind Med 1990;47:392–399.
3. Tassignon JP, Bas GD, Craigen AA, Jacquet B, Kueng HL, Lanouziere-Simon C, Pierre C. Mortality in an European cohort occupationally exposed to epichlorhydrin (ECH). Int Arch Occup Environ Health 1983;51:325–333.

Chapter 70
Radiation Poisoning

TYPES OF RADIATION

Radiation is characterized as either ionizing or nonionizing (Tables 70–1 and 70–2). Ionizing radiation is capable of physically disrupting neutral atoms by dislodging orbital electrons, thus forming an ion pair consisting of the dislodged electron and the residual atom. Ion pairs are chemically reactive and may produce toxic agents in the cell (e.g., free radicals from water), which can interfere with normal life processes. Nonionizing radiation, on the other hand, does not dislodge orbital electrons or destroy the physical integrity of an impacted atom.[1]

IONIZING RADIATION[2]

SOURCES

Ionizing radiation is part of the natural environment, and since the discovery of x-rays and radioactivity, it has become part of the work environment as well.

BACKGROUND RADIATION (TABLES 70–3 AND 70–4)

1. Varies between 1 and 10 mGy (100 and 1000 mrad) per year.
2. Maximum annual permissible total body dose by radiation standard for the general public is 5 mGy (500 mrad). On an annual basis, radiation workers are permitted to receive a dose ten times higher (e.g., 50 mGy [5000 mrad]).
3. Radiation exposure from television sets, luminous dials on watches and clocks, and reactors are several orders of magnitude below background.

DEFINITIONS (TABLE 70–5)

Radiation is measured and defined as follows (SI units are given in the definitions):

Curie — A measure of a substance's radioactivity. 1 curie (Ci) = 3.7×10^{10} disintegrations per second.

Table 70–1
Ionizing Radiation

Acute radiation syndrome
Cancer—secondary
Chernobyl
Diagnostic radiology
Low-dose radiation
Nuclear reactor accidents
Radiation therapy
Radionuclides
Radon
Short-wavelength electromagnetic radiation
  Gamma radiation
  Irradiation
Particulate radiation
  Alpha
  Beta
  Neutron
  Proton

Table 70–2
Nonionizing Radiation

Electromagnetic field
  Microwave
  Radio frequency
  Low frequency
Optical fields
  Ultraviolet
  Visible
  Infrared
Lasers
MRI
Ultrasound
Ultraviolet
Video display units

Absorbed dose	The amount of radiation that the body absorbs.
Exposure	The amount of radiation to which the body is exposed.
Radioactive half-life	The time required for the radioactivity of an isotope to decrease by 50%.
Rem (rem)	Acronym for roentgen equivalent man—the dosage of any ionizing radiation that will cause biologic injury to human tissue equal to the injury caused by 1 roentgen of x-ray or gamma-ray dosage. 1 rem = 0.01 sievert (SV).
Millirem (mrem)	10^{-3} rem. 1 mrem = 0.01 mSV.
Rad	Acronym for radiation absorbed dose—a unit that measures the absorbed dose of ionizing radiation. 1 Rad = 100 ergs/gm = 0.01 Gray (Gy).
Roentgen	Unit of measure for quantity of ionization produced by x-radiation or gamma radiation. 1 Roentgen (R) = 2.58×10^{-4} coulomb/kg.

The relationship between old and new radiation units is shown in Table 70–6.

Table 70–3
Typical Average Annual Exposures to Individuals from Background Radiation in the United States[a]

	Radiation Dose in Millirems (prorated over total population)
Natural Sources	
External	
From cosmic radiation	28
From the earth	26
From building materials	3
Internal Sources (elements found naturally in human tissues)	28
Total, Natural Sources	85
Man-made Sources	
Medical Procedures	
Diagnostic x-rays	79
Radiopharmaceuticals	14
Nuclear industry	<1
Consumer products	3–4
Radioactive fallout	4–5
Total, Man-made Sources	103
Total, Natural and Man-made Sources	**188**

[a]Data from *The Effects on Populations of Exposure to Low Levels of Ionizing Radiation*, typescript edition (Washington, DC: National Academy of Sciences, 1980), table III-23.

Table 70–4
Radiation Doses in Perspective[a]

Background radiation (average)
  Natural: 240 mrem (2.4 mSv)/year
  Man-made: 35 mrem (0.35 mSv)/year
    Total: 275 mrem (2.75 mSv)/year
Transatlantic flight; <38,000 feet: 5 mrem (0.05 mSv)
Occupational limit; >18 years old: 5,000 mrem (50 mSv)
Astronaut, 35 years old: 250,000 mrem (2,500 mSv)/career
Chest x-ray; 1 film: 10 mrem (0.10 mSv)
Upper GI series: 450 mrem (4.5 mSv)
Lumbosacral spine series: 300 mrem (3.0 mSv)
Nausea, vomiting: 100,000 mrem (1,000 mSv)
Lethal dose, 50%, 60 days: 325,000 mrem (3,250 mSv)
Cancer treatment series: 6,000,000 mrem (60,000 mSv)
  100 rad/rem = 1 Gy/Sv

[a]Sources: BEIR III (1980), UNSCEAR (1988), NCRP REPORTS 98 (1989), 100 (1989)

TYPES

The different types of ionizing radiation vary in their penetrative powers, as well as in the number of ions they produce while traversing matter. Ionizing radiation is produced naturally by the decay of radioactive elements or artificially by such devices as x-ray machines. A radioactive element is one that spontaneously changes to a lower-energy state, emitting particles and gamma rays from the nucleus in the process. The particles commonly emitted are alpha or beta particles. X-rays are produced when high-energy electrons strike the nuclei of a suitable target such as tungsten. When these fast-moving electrons approach the electrical field around the nuclei of the target material, the electrons are deflected from their path and release energy in the form of high-energy electromagnetic radiation (x-rays).

Alpha particles usually have energies of 4 to 8 million electron volts (MeV). They travel a few centimeters in air and up to 60 microns into tissue. The high energy and short path result in a dense track of ionization along the tissues with which the particles interact. Alpha particles will not penetrate the stratum corneum of the skin, and thus they are not an external hazard. However, if alpha-emitting elements are taken into the body by inhalation or ingestion or from open wounds, serious problems such as cancer may develop. Radium implants (radium-226 and radium-222) are examples of alpha particle emitters that may be used in hospitals.

Beta particles interact much less readily with matter than do alpha particles and will travel up to a few centimeters into tissue or many meters through air. Exposure to external sources of beta particles is potentially hazardous, but internal exposure is more hazardous. Examples of beta-particle emitters are the isotopes carbon-14, gold-198, iodine-131, radium-226, cobalt-60, selenium-75, and chromium-51.

Gamma rays are electromagnetic energy (like x-rays) emitted from the nucleus. They have a range of many meters in air and many centimeters in tissue and, like beta particles, constitute a biologic hazard both internally and externally.

Beta and *gamma* emitters are most likely to be encountered by emergency medicine personnel. *Alpha* emitters are primarily transuranic isotopes and are generally found in nuclear chemistry laboratories and isotope production facilities. Examples of gamma emitters are cobalt-60, cesium-137, iridium-192, and radium-226. When checking a patient for radioactivity, however, one must monitor for alpha, as well as beta and gamma, radiation.[3]

Protons with energies of a few MeV are produced by high-energy accelerators and are quite effective in producing tissue ionization. The path length of a proton is somewhat longer than that of an alpha particle of equivalent energy.

X-rays generally have longer wavelengths, lower frequencies, and thus lower energies than gamma rays. The biologic effects of x-rays and gamma rays are better known than those of any of the other forms of ionizing radiation. X-rays may be encountered during the use of electronic tubes and electron microscopes.

USES

Ionizing radiation is used in the hospital for (a) diagnostic radiology, including diagnostic x-ray, fluoroscopy and angiography, dental radiography, and computerized axial tomography scanners (CAT scanners); (b) therapeutic radiology; (c) dermatology; (d) nuclear medicine in diagnostic and therapeutic procedures; and (e) radiopharmaceutical laboratories. A radiation hazard may exist in areas where radioactive materials are stored or discarded. Radiation safety is usually well managed in diagnostic and therapeutic radiology units by the radiation protection officer. Staff in departments where portable x-rays are taken (operating rooms, emergency rooms, and intensive care units) are often inadvertently exposed and inadequately monitored for the effects of radiation exposure.[2]

Table 70–5
Units of Radiation Measurement [a]

Characteristic	Unit	Description
Energy	Electron volt (eV) (also ergs, joule)	Kinetic energy of an electron as it moves through a potential difference of 1 volt.
Rate of radioactive decay	Curie (Ci)	Radioactivity emitted per unit of time (1 Ci = 3.7×10^{10} disintegrations per second).
Air exposure	Roentgen (R)	Amount of X and gamma radiation that causes ionization in air. One roentgen of exposure will produce about 2 billion ion pairs per cubic centimeter of air.
Absorbed dose	Rad	Dose resulting from one roentgen of ionizing radiation deposited in any medium, typically water or tissue. One rad results in the absorption of 100 ergs of ionizing radiation per gram of medium.
Biologic effectiveness	Rem	Dose of any form of ionizing radiation that produces the same biological effect as 1 roentgen; 1 rem = 1 rad × Radiation Weighting Factor (RWF), where the value of RWF depends on the type of radiation as follows: X radiation = 1.0 gamma radiation = 1.0 beta = 1.0 alpha = 20 neutrons = 5 to 20, depending on their energy

[a]Adapted from Wald N. Ionizing radiation. ATS DR. October 1993.

Table 70–6
Relationship Between Old and New Radiation Units

Quantity	Old Unit	Symbol	New Unit	Symbol	Relationship
Activity	curie	Ci	becquerel	Bq	1 Ci = 3.7×10^{10} Bq
Absorbed dose	rad	rad	gray	Gy	1 rad = 0.01 Gy
Dose equivalent	rem	rem	sievert	Sv	1 rem = 0.01 Sv

Table 70–7
Summary of Recommendations for Ionizing Radiation[a]

Dose Limits for Workers[b]	**ICRP, 1991[c]**	**NCRP, 1993[d]**
Based on stochastic effects[e] (e.g., cancer and genetic damage)	5 rem (50 mSv) annual effective dose limit and 10 rem (100 mSv) as 5-year cumulative effective dose limit	5 rem (50 mSv) annual effective dose limit and 1 rem (10 mSv) times age in years cumulative effective dose limit
Based on nonstochastic effects[e] (e.g., lens cataracts and fertility impairment)	15 rem (150 mSv) equivalent dose limit to lens of eye and 50 rem (500 mSv) annual equivalent dose limit to skin, hands, and feet	15 rem (150 mSv) annual equivalent dose limit to lens of eye and 50 rem (500 mSv) annual equivalent dose limit to skin, hands, and feet
Dose Limits for the Public[b]	**ICRP, 1991**	**NCRP, 1993**
Based on stochastic effects	0.1 rem (1 mSv) annual effective dose limit, and, if needed, higher values provided that the annual average over 5 years does not exceed 0.1 rem	0.1 rem (1 mSv) annual effective dose limit for continuous exposure and 0.5 rem (5 mSv) annual dose limit for infrequent exposure
Based on nonstochastic effects	1.5 rem (15 mSv) annual equivalent to lens of eye and 5 rem (50 mSv) annual equivalent dose limit to skin, hands, and feet	5 rem (50 mSv) annual equivalent dose limit to lens of eye, skin, and extremities
Embryo-fetus	0.2 rem (2 mSv) equivalent dose to the woman's abdomen once pregnancy has been declared	0.05 rem (0.5 mSv) equivalent dose limit in a month once pregnancy is known

[a]Adapted from Wald N. Ionizing radiation. ATSDR. October 1993.
[b]The dose limits for both workers and the public exclude medical and natural background exposures. Note that the dose limits for the public are lower, in general, than those for workers. Workers, by virtue of the ability to work, tend to be a healthier population than the public, which includes susceptible populations, the elderly, and children.
[c]International Commission on Radiological Protection. 1990 Recommendations of the International Commission on Radiological Protection, ICRP Publication 60, Annals of the ICRP 21. Elmsford, New York: Pergamon Press, 1991.
[d]National Council on Radiation Protection and Measurements (NCRP). Limitation of exposure to ionizing radiation. Bethesda, Maryland: NCRP, 1993. NCRP Report No. 116.
[e]Stochastic effects are those effects for which the probability of occurrence, rather than the magnitude of the effect, is proportional to dose. Not all irradiated persons show such effects; however, the probability that they will can be described by a dose response curve that extends to zero with no threshold. Nonstochastic effects are proportional in severity to the magnitude of the absorbed dose; they probably have a threshold below which no effect will be observed because simultaneous injury to many cells is required.

DOSE LIMITS

Recommendations for ionization radiation exposure for workers and the public is summarized in Table 70–7.[4]

DIAGNOSTIC RADIOLOGY

Radiation doses seen in perspective are summarized in Tables 70–8. and 70–9. Radiation exposures and maximal lifetime risks from selected radiographic examinations are depicted in Table 70–10.

PREGNANCY

All medical exposures should be kept as low as reasonably achievable. The possibility of pregnancy should be considered in deciding whether to examine a woman of reproductive ability. In the first 10 days after menstruation it is unlikely that there is a conceptus and therefore unlikely to be additional risk. During the rest of the first month any risk is likely to be so small that no special limitation on diagnostic exposures is required. During the second month of gestation malformation of specific organs has occurred in experimental animals exposed to irradiation. Between 8 and 15 weeks after conception irradiation of the forebrain may result in mental retardation, but no evidence of this has been shown in the first 8 weeks. The risk of cancer may be increased by doses as low as few tenths of mGy to an extent comparable with, or perhaps rather higher than, that in adults. The ovum is sensitive to irradiation during at least the 7 weeks before ovulation.[5]

PRACTICAL GUIDELINES

1. Assume a woman in the reproductive years is pregnant unless proved otherwise. Acceptable proofs that she is not pregnant are the following: onset of menses in the last 10 days, taking oral contraceptives, having an intrauterine device, or having had surgical sterilization.
2. If a woman may be in the first trimester of pregnancy, avoid inclusion of the pelvis in the primary x-ray beam if at all possible.
3. Where feasible, always shield the pelvis and abdomen of women when performing diagnostic roentgenographic studies.
4. If there is a valid medical indication to perform a diagnostic study using radiation on a pregnant woman, this will generally outweigh the remote possibility of harm to the patient or her fetus.
5. If a woman receives a relatively large amount of radiation (5 to 15 rads) to the pelvis in the first trimester

Table 70–8
Radiation Exposure[a]

Technique	Site	Number of Views	Whole Body Dose (mRad)	Marrow Dose (mRad)	Gonadal Dose (mRad) Males	Gonadal Dose (mRad) Females
Roentgenogram	Chest	2	++	++	0	0
Roentgenogram	Upper GI	4	++++	++++	0	+++
Roentgenogram	Ba enema	4	++++	++++	+++	+++++
Roentgenogram	IVP	5	++++	++++	+++	+++++
Roentgenogram	Both hands	1	0	0	0	0
Roentgenogram	Shoulder	2	++	++	0	0
Roentgenogram	Hip	2	+++	++	++++	+++
Roentgenogram	C-spine	3	++	++	0	0
Roentgenogram	T-spine	2	+++	+++	0	0
Roentgenogram	LS-spine	3	++++	++++	+++	+++++
Roentgenogram	Pelvis	1	+++	++	+++	++++
Scintigram (15 mCi ^{99m}Tc)	Any		++++	++++	++++	++++
Scintigram (4mCi ^{67}Ga)	Any		+++++	+++++	+++++	+++++
CT Scan	SI joints		NA	+++++	+++++	+++++

Legend: 0 less than 1.0 mRad
+ = 1.0–4.9 mRad
++ = 5.0–24.9 mRad
+++ = 25.0–99.9 mRad
++++ = 100.0–499.0 mRad
+++++ = 500.0 mRad or more
NA = not applicable
[a]Adapted from Whalen JP, Balter S. Dis Mon 1982;28:1–96.

Table 70–9
Gross Comparison of Relative Radiation Levels[a,b]

	Relative Levels[c]
NATURAL BACKGROUND	50–100 chest examinations/year
Diagnostic radiology	0.1–500 chest examinations/study [d]
Nuclear imaging	50–1,000 chest examinations/study
Start of acute radiation syndrome	30,000 chest examinations in *one* day
Lethal dose ($LD50_{30}$)	300,000 chest examinations in *one* day
Radiation therapy (small volumes of tissue)	100,000–1,000,000 chest examinations in a few weeks
Ultrasound	This scale does not apply

[a]Adapted from Whalen JP, Balter S. Dis Mon 1982;28:1–96.
[b]Due to differential tissue distributions and sensitivities, such estimates are intended to be rough comparisons (50–100 chest examinations will not have exactly the same biologic impact as 100–200 mrads of natural background).
[c]One PA chest examination ≅ 5 millirad average tissue dose in thorax, which corresponds to a whole-body equivalent dose of 2 millirads.
[d]Dependent on examination types and techniques.

Table 70–10
Estimated Maximal Lifetime Risks from Selected Radiographic Examinations[a]

Radiograph	Fatal Leukemias per Million Examinations	Genetic Disease per Million Examinations
Cervical spine	1	<0.5
Thoracic spine	10	6
Lumbar spine	20	400
Pelvis	4	200
Hip	3	300
Chest	2	<0.5
Intravenous pyelogram	20	300
Barium enema	40	500
Spontaneous incidence	9800[b]	107,000[c]

[a]Adapted from Whalen JP, Balter S. Dis Mon 1982;28:1–96.
[b]Per million population.
[c]Per million live births.

of pregnancy, the increased risk of a congenital anomaly of the fetus is from 1 to 3%. Such a risk may justify therapeutic abortion. On the other hand, if the parents are psychologically able to handle the slightly increased risk of a malformed child, one can recommend that the pregnancy continue.[6]

RADON[7]

Radon (^{222}Rn) is an odorless, colorless, inert, gaseous element produced during the decay of uranium (^{238}U), specifically from radium (^{226}Ra). It has been postulated that radon, as the source of most background environmental radiation, accounts for between 1000 to 20,000 cases of lung cancer in the United States annually.[8]

SOURCES

Radon gas is derived from the radioactive decay of radium, a ubiquitous element found in rock and soil. The decay series begins with uranium-238 and goes through four intermediates to form radium-226, which has a half-life of 1600 years.

Radium-226 then decays to form radon-222 gas. Radon's half life, 3.8 days, provides sufficient time for it to diffuse through soil and into homes, where further disintegration produces the more chemically and radiologically active radon progeny ("radon daughters"). These radon progeny, which include four isotopes with half-lives of less than 30 minutes, are the major source of human exposure to alpha radiation (high-energy, high-mass particles, each consisting of two protons and two neutrons). This alpha radiation is responsible for cellular transformation in the respiratory tract, which results in radon-induced lung cancer.

Underground uranium mines found throughout the world, including the western United States and Canada, pose the greatest risk because of their high concentration of radon. Iron ore, potash, tin, fluorspar, gold, zinc, and lead mines also have been found to have significant levels of radon, often due to radium in the surrounding rock. In the past it was not uncommon to use the tailings from these mines as fill on which to build homes, schools, and other structures.

DEFINITIONS

Almost all measurements of radon levels in the home or outdoors are expressed as the concentration of radon in units of picocuries per liter of air (pCi/liter), or in SI units as becquerels per cubic meter (Bq/m^3), and radon daughters are expressed in working levels (WL). A working level month (WLM) is defined as 170 hr (21.25 working days/month × 8 hrs/day) in a workplace at one WL. Thus a 12 hr/day exposure in the home at one WL corresponds to about 26 working level months per year, that is, 2.1 × the occupational exposure, assuming equal radon levels at home and in the workplace, other things being equal. Exposure rate is typically given in working level months per year (WLM/yr). Dosimetrically, it corresponds to the dose delivered in 1 liter of air that results in the emission of 1.3×10^5 MeV of potential alpha energy. Typical outdoor levels in the United States are given by NCRP No. 78 as 0.2 pCi/liter.[9]

The recommended safe radon exposure limits for the general public (<0.02 WL or <4 pCi/L) are much lower than those for occupationally exposed individuals (4.0 WLM per year in the United States). The average national exposure to radon indoors is estimated to be 0.005 WL (1.0 pCi/L). It is estimated that being exposed to a radon concentration of 2 pCi/L annually is a lung cancer risk equivalent to having 100 chest x-rays; an exposure to radon at 4 pCi/L/year is a lung cancer risk equivalent to smoking half a pack of cigarettes per day. If those same 100 people were exposed to an average 1.0 WL (200 pCi/L) for 70 years, between 14 to 42 out of 100 would develop a lung cancer due to the effects of radon.[8]

MECHANISM OF ACTION

The external dose from ^{222}Rn and its airborne progeny is a very small fraction of the natural external radiation dose received by individuals. Inhalation of radon and its daughters may be followed by deposition of potentially large amounts of energy, that is, absorbed dose in the tracheobronchial epithelium (TBE) from the short-lived alpha and beta particle-emitting decay products (primarily ^{218}Po, ^{214}Pb, ^{214}Bi, and ^{214}Po).[9]

Dose to the TBE from radon per se is negligible, since its intrapulmonary residence time is short with respect to its half-life. The high absorbed dose is from the decay of radon daughters attached to the TBE. Alpha particles contribute more than 85% of the TBE dose, which will be deposited within 30 μm of the decay site.[9]

RISK FACTORS

Factors that may intensify human exposure risks from radon include cigarette smoking (Table 70–11), job-related radiation exposures, high ambient radon levels, a long duration of exposure, and a high average minute ventilation (e.g., children).[8]

HOMES

Radon may be carried into some homes via the water supply. With municipal water or surface reservoirs, most of the radon volatilizes to air or decays before the water reaches homes. However, water from private wells may be another matter. Groundwater that comes from deep subterranean sources and passes over rock rich in radium, such as that found in northern New England, may dissolve some of the radon gas produced from radium decay. As the water splashes during showering, toilet flushing, dishwashing, and laundering, radon is released into the air and may result in inhalation exposure. Radon may also be present in natural gas supplies.

The amount of radon emanating from the earth and concentrating inside homes varies considerably by region and locality. Nearly every state in the United States has dwellings with measured radon levels above acceptable limits. The EPA estimates that 6% of American homes (approximately 6 million) have concentrations of radon above 4pCi/L. In Clinton, New Jersey, near a geologic formation high in radium, called the Reading Prong, all 105 homes tested were above the recommended guidelines; 40 had levels exceeding 200 pCi/L.

Areas of the country that are likely to have homes with elevated radon levels are those with significant deposits of granite, uranium, shale, and phosphate—all high in radium content and therefore potential sources of radon gas. Some homes in these areas, however, may not have elevated levels of radon. Due to the many determinants of indoor radon levels, local geology alone is an inadequate predictor of risk.

CANCER

Even conservative estimates based on current knowledge suggest that radon is one of the most important environmental causes of death. The EPA estimates that approximately 14,000 deaths annually in the United States are due to lung cancer caused by indoor radon exposure. It has also been estimated that approximately 14% of all current cases of lung cancer are attributable to radon. For a lifetime exposure to radon at 4 pCi/L, the EPA estimates that the risk of developing lung cancer is 1 to 5%. The National Research Council estimates the risk at 0.8 to 1.4%.

Table 70–11
Radon Risk Evaluation Chart[a]

Radon Risk If You Smoke			
Radon Level	If 1000 People Who Smoked Were Exposed to This Level Over a Lifetime . . .	The Risk of Cancer From Radon Exposure Compares to . . .	What To Do: Stop Smoking and . . .
20 pCi/L	About 135 people could get lung cancer	← 100 times the risk of drowning	Fix your home
10 pCi/L	About 71 people could get lung cancer	← 100 times the risk of dying in a home fire	Fix your home
8 pCi/L	About 57 people could get lung cancer		Fix your home
4 pCi/L	About 29 people could get lung cancer	← 100 times the risk of dying in an airplane crash	Fix your home
2 pCi/L	About 15 people could get lung cancer	← 2 times the risk of dying in a car crash	Consider fixing between 2 and 4 pCi/L
1.3 pCi/L	About 9 people could get lung cancer	(Average indoor radon level)	(Reducing radon levels below 2 pCi/L is difficult)
0.4 pCi/L	About 3 people could get lung cancer	(Average outdoor radon level)	

Note: If you are a former smoker, your risk may be lower.

Radon Risk If You've Never Smoked			
Radon Level	If 1000 People Who Never Smoked Were Exposed to This Level Over a Lifetime . . .	The Risk of Cancer From Radon Exposure Compares to . . .	What To Do:
20 pCi/L	About 8 people could get lung cancer	← The risk of being killed in a violent crime	Fix your home
10 pCi/L	About 4 people could get lung cancer		Fix your home
8 pCi/L	About 3 people could get lung cancer	← 10 times the risk of dying in an airplane crash	Fix your home
4 pCi/L	About 2 people could get lung cancer	← The risk of drowning	Fix your home
2 pCi/L	About 1 person could get lung cancer	← The risk of dying in a home fire	Consider fixing between 2 and 4 pCi/L
1.3 pCi/L	Less than 1 person could get lung cancer	(Average indoor radon level)	(Reducing radon levels below 2 pCi/L is difficult)
0.4 pCi/L	Less than 1 person could get lung cancer	(Average outdoor radon level)	

Note: If you are a former smoker, your risk may be higher.
[a]Adapted from EPA. ATSDR September 1992.

CLINICAL PRESENTATION

Radon exposure causes no acute or subacute health effects, no irritating effects, and has no warning signs at levels normally encountered in the environment. The only established human health effect currently associated with residential radon exposure is lung cancer. Epidemiologic studies of miner cohorts have reported an increased frequency of chronic, nonmalignant lung diseases such as emphysema, pulmonary fibrosis, and chronic interstitial pneumonia, all of which increased with increasing cumulative exposure to radiation and with cigarette smoking.

Epidemiologic studies and a recent study of groundwater radon and cancer mortality have found no association with extrapulmonary cancers such as leukemias and gastrointestinal cancers. There is also no evidence that environmental radon exposure is causally associated with adverse reproductive effects.[7]

Some studies have not found a significant cause-effect relationship between very low radon exposure in the home (1.25 pCi/L) and lung cancer.[10] An association remains at indoor levels of 4 pCi/L and above.

DIMINISHING HOME EXPOSURE[11] (TABLE 70–12)

The U.S. Environmental Protection Agency suggests that homes should be tested for radon. Construction changes may be indicated if the radon level is 4 pCi/L or higher. Radon levels less than 4 pCi/L still pose a risk and in many cases may be reduced. Radon passes into the home through cracks in solid floors, construction joints, cracks in walls, gaps in suspended floors, gaps around service pipes, cavities inside walls, and the water supply.

SHORT-TERM TESTING

The quickest test is a short-term test. Short-term tests remain in the home for 2 days to 90 days, depending on the device. "Charcoal canister," "alpha track," "electret ion chamber," "continuous monitor," and "charcoal liquid scintillation" detectors are most commonly used for short-term testing. Because radon levels tend to vary from day to day and season to season, a short-term test is less likely than a long-term test to indicate year-round average radon level. If results are needed quickly, a short-term test followed by a second short-term test may be used to decide whether to fix the home.

LONG-TERM TESTING

Long-term tests remain in the home for more than 90 days. "Alpha track" and "electret" detectors are commonly used for this type of testing. A long-term test will provide a reading that is more likely than a short-term test to indicate the year-round average home radon level.[11]

RADON ABATEMENT

If excessive levels of indoor radon are found in a structure, low-cost, quick-fix methods should be implemented first. These include limiting the amount of time spent in contaminated areas and increasing ventilation. It is wise to consult with the state radiation protection office before implementing major abatement projects. Reduction can be obtained from several sources listed in the Suggested Reading list and in the Sources of Information section prepared by Upfal.[7]

Besides increasing ventilation, radon control measures include sealing the foundation, subslab depressurization (creating negative pressure in the soil), pressurizing the home, and using air-cleaning devices. Methods of increasing ventilation include opening windows, ventilating basements and crawl spaces, ventilating sumpholes and floor drains to the outside of the house, and increasing air movement with ceiling fans. Ventilation must be modified properly, however, since increased ventilation can depressurize the house in some cases, causing an increase of soil gas entry to the home. Heat exchangers provide a way of bringing fresh air indoors without major heat loss, but these must be properly balanced or they can make the problem worse.[7]

RADIATION EXPOSURES

PARENTAL RADIATION

It is highly unlikely that there is a direct causal relation between paternal exposure to radiation before conception and childhood leukemia.[12,13]

NUCLEAR ACCIDENTS

Between 1944 and 1988 3005 nuclear misadventures occurred (Table 70–13). About 4000 people were potentially exposed in Juarez in 1984, but none required immediate medical assistance. In contrast, until the 1987 accident in Goiania, Brazil, about 250 persons were irradiated to more than clinically significant levels (four fatally; 36 required medical surveillance and 20 were hospitalized).[14]

Of the radionuclides potentially available for release in a nuclear reactor accident in the short-term, radioiodines, particularly iodine-131, are by far the most significant in view of their huge quantities in the reactor core and their volatility, which contributes to their wide, although nonuniform, dispersion. In addition, they are readily absorbed by the body and rapidly and highly concentrated by the thyroid gland.[15]

PHYSIOLOGY OF IODINE

Iodine is rapidly and completely absorbed by the gastrointestinal tract within 30 to 60 minutes of ingestion. Inhaled radioiodines reach equilibrium in the blood within about 30 minutes. Iodide is rapidly concentrated by the thyroid, reaching its maximum euthyroid uptake in 48 hours. It is almost instantaneously synthesized into thyroid hormones, primarily thyroxine, which is only slowly (biologic half-life = 89 days) released. The radiation dose the thyroid receives is directly proportional to the uptake because of its long thyroidal retention.

Table 70–12
EPA Recommendations[a]

How quickly should action be taken?
In considering whether and how quickly to take action based on test results, the following guidelines may prove to be useful. The EPA believes that radon levels should try to be permanently reduced as much as possible. Based on currently available information, the EPA believes that levels in most homes can be reduced to about 0.02 WL (4 pCi/liter).

If results are about 1.0 WL or higher *or* about 200 pCl/liter or higher:
Exposures in this range are among the highest observed in homes. Residents should undertake action to reduce levels as far below 1.0 WL (200 pCi/liter) as possible. It is recommended that action should be taken within several weeks. If this is not possible, consultation with appropriate state or local health or radiation protection officials can determine if temporary relocation is appropriate until the levels can be reduced.

If results are about 0.1 to about 1.0 WL *or* about 20 to about 200 pCl/liter:
Exposures in this range are considered greatly above average for residential structures. Action should be undertaken to reduce levels as far below 0.1 WL (20 pCl/liter) as possible within several months.

If results are about 0.02 to about 0.1 WL, *or* about 4 pCl/liter to about 20 pCl/liter:
Exposures in this range are considered above average for residential structures. Action should be undertaken to lower levels to about 0.02 WL (4 pCl/liter) or below within a few years, sooner if levels are at the upper end of this range.

If results are about 0.02 WL *or* lower, *or* about 4 pCl/liter or lower:
Exposures in this range are considered average or slightly above average for residential structures. Although exposures in this range do present some risk of lung cancer, reductions of levels this low may be difficult, and sometimes impossible, to achieve.

NOTE: There is increasing urgency for action at higher concentrations of radon. The higher the radon level in a home, the faster action should be taken to reduce exposure.

[a]Adapted from Brill AB et al. J Nucl Med 1994;35:368–385.

Table 70–13
Summary of Military Nuclear Weapon Accidents[a]

Date	Vehicle	Location
Feb. 13, 1950	B-36	Off coast British Columbia [b]
April 11, 1950	B-29	Monzano Base, New Mexico [b]
July 13, 1950	B-50	Lebanon, Ohio [b]
August 5, 1950	B=29	Fairfield, California [b]
Nov. 10, 1950	B-50	Over water, outside U.S.[d]
March 10, 1956	B-47	Mediterranean Sea [d]
July 27, 1956	B-47	Overseas base
May 22, 1957	B-36	Kirtland AFB, New Mexico[b]
July 28, 1957	C-124	Atlantic Ocean [d]
October 11, 1957	B-47	Homestead AFB, Florida[b]
January 31, 1958	B-47	Overseas base
February 5, 1958	B-47	Savannah River, Georgia[d]
March 11, 1958	B-47	Florence, South Carolina[b]
November 4, 1958	B-47	Dyess AFB, Texas[b]
November 26, 1958	B-47	Chennault AFB, Louisiana [b]
January 18, 1959	F-100	Pacific base
July 6, 1959	C-124	Barksdale AFB, Louisiana
September 25, 1959	P-5M	Off Whidbey Island, Washington [d]
October 15, 1959	B-52/ KC-135	Hardinsburg, Kentucky
June 7, 1960	BOMARC missile	McGuire AFB, New Jersey
January 24, 1961	B-52	Goldsboro, North Carolina
March 14, 1961	B-52	Yuba City, California
November 13, 1963	Storage Igloo	Medina Base, Texas[b]
January 13, 1964	B-52	Cumberland, Maryland
December 5, 1964	Minutemen ICBM	Ellsworth AFB, South Dakota
December 8, 1964	B-58	Grissom AFB, Indiana
October 11, 1965	C-124	Wright-Patterson AFB, Ohio
December 5, 1965	A-4	Pacific Ocean[d]
January 17, 1966	B-52/ KC-135	Palomares, Spain[c]
January 21, 1968	B-52	Thule, Greenland[c]
Spring 1968	Classified	Classified
September 19, 1980	Titan II ICBM	Damascus, Arkansas

[a]Adapted from Mettler FA et al, eds. Medical management of radiation accidents. Boca Raton, FL: CRC Press, 1990.
[b]Detonation of high explosive portion without significant plutonium dispersal.
[c]Extensive plutonium dispersal.
[d]One or more weapons not recovered.

If 100 mg of KI is administered at the same time or shortly before exposure to radioiodine, thyroid blockade is almost 97% complete, and the thyroid takes up only 3% of the administered radioiodine. If the KI is given 12 hours before exposure to ^{131}I, there will still be a 90% protective effect; even 24 hours before exposure, KI will produce a 70% blockade of thyroid uptake.

Potassium iodide given 3 hours later reduces the uptake to only 50% of control value, and after 6 hours KI no longer has a significant protective effect. If there is no new exposure to fallout, KI administration should be continued for 2 or 3 additional days; if exposure persists, then administration of KI should be continued.

NONTHYROIDAL EFFECT

The major nonthyroidal effects are dose-dependent, and the most common reactions such as sialadenitis and some skin reactions (dermatitis and ioderma) usually occur only after taking large iodine doses. Of most concern are reactions due to iodide sensitivity. Edema of the face and glottis and such dermatologic reactions as eczema and exacerbation of pustular psoriasis have been reported.[15]

NUCLEAR FACILITIES

There is no convincing evidence of a cause-effect relationship between nuclear facilities and cancer occurrence in nearby populations (e.g., Three Mile Island).[16,17]

INFORMATION SOURCES

Draft toxicologic profiles for plutonium, thorium, uranium, and radium were disseminated by the Agency for Toxic Substances and Disease Registry in February 16, 1990.

THE ATOM BOMB

Classic papers on the pathology of atomic bomb casualties were presented by Liebow and colleagues.[18,19] These studies formed the basis for subsequent studies on the acute radiation syndrome.[20]

NEUTRONS

In clinical trials until now, neutron therapy has demonstrated significant advantages in the treatments of salivary and prostate cancers, despite the relatively low-energy neutron beam used in the early stages of these trials.[21]

Neutrons deposit 20 to 100 times more energy per unit path length than do high-energy photons from either a linear accelerator or a gamma source. This property provides neutron radiation with two important biologic advantages:

First, neutrons are less dependent on the oxygen status of cells than photons and are thus better able to kill hypoxic cells. This is important for rapidly growing tumors that tend to outstrip their blood supply such as melanomas, sarcomas, and renal cell carcinomas.

Secondly, the cell-killing properties of neutrons are less sensitive to where the cell is in its growth cycle. There is less ability for noncycling cells to repair radiation damage. This can be important for tumors that are slowly growing such as those of prostate cancer.[21]

TREATMENT[22]

Procedures in Case of Significant Overexposure

1. Escort evacuees from the scene of the accident to a convenient area in which radiation levels are low enough to permit contamination and activation measurements. Inquire if any of them saw a flash of light at the time of the accident.
2. Identify persons with external contamination, and initiate appropriate decontamination procedures.
3. Check contamination-free persons for neutron exposure by gamma-ray measurements of body midsection or by indium foil monitor. Record readings.
4. Interview exposed persons to ascertain position, orientation, and movement relative to the radiation source. Complete retention of all information is facilitated by

use of a tape recorder. Record information about positions, orientation, and movement on a drawing of the building or the area in which the accident occurred. Try to determine the time of the accident and obtain photographs of the scene of the accident.

5. Collect all monitoring devices worn by exposed persons. Record position of the device on the body.
6. Obtain blood samples from exposed persons prior to any oral or intravenous administration of inactive sodium. Secure hair samples, recording the exact location (e.g., position on head or body) from which hair is taken. Samples should be preserved by freezing.
7. Collect personal items likely to contain induced radioactivity; for example, pens and pencils, coins (Cu, Ni, Ag), keys, match folders (Cl in match heads, P on striking surface), jewelry, metal buttons, buckles, garters, eyeglasses (Si, Na, Ba in lenses), dental appliances, etc. Record position on body.
8. Forward well-labeled blood and hair samples, monitoring devices, and personal items to a radioactivity laboratory, together with all recorded data and information.
9. If facilities are available, and with the consent of the attending physician, arrange for whole-body counting of exposed persons.
10. The following procedures *should* be carried out at the accident scene.[23]
    a. As soon as it is safe to do so, recover monitors and dosimeters installed in the vicinity of the accident.
    b. Search for small objects that may possess induced radioactivity; for example, tools, components of experimental apparatus, scrap materials solder (Sn), semiconductor devices (Ge, Si), dry batteries (Mn, Zn), thermometers (Hg), etc. Without disturbing the existing arrangement of furniture and equipment, collect such objects in sufficient number to supplement the installed monitors in their function of defining the neutron field. Label each item and record its location (and elevation) on a drawing of the area.
    c. Forward monitoring devices and miscellaneous objects to the dosimetry laboratory, together with pertinent recorded information and an indication of the contamination status of each item. Use protective coverings to prevent spread of contamination.
    d. Check all operating radiation detection of equipment in the area for recorder charts that may indicate the time and/or intensity of a radiation burst. Note both the time at which a chart record is terminated and the identification numbers of the recorder (so that chart speed may be established). Send labeled charts to the dosimetry laboratory.
    e. If the accident involved a criticality, arrange for radiochemical analysis of reaction material to determine total number of fissions.
    f. Interview persons familiar with operations related to the accident to obtain additional information of possible value in evaluating exposure; for example, normal position and movement-sequence of an equipment operator.

ACUTE RADIATION SYNDROME[24]

CLINICAL SUMMARY (FIG. 70–1)

1. Early prodromal phase—Few hours to 1–2 days
   Nausea
   Vomiting
2. Latent stage—Days to several weeks
   Feels well
3. Third stage—Begins 3rd to 5th week
   Abrupt onset of severe gastrointestinal tract disturbances
   Bleeding
   Infection
   Epilation
4. Fourth stage—Weeks to months
   Recovery

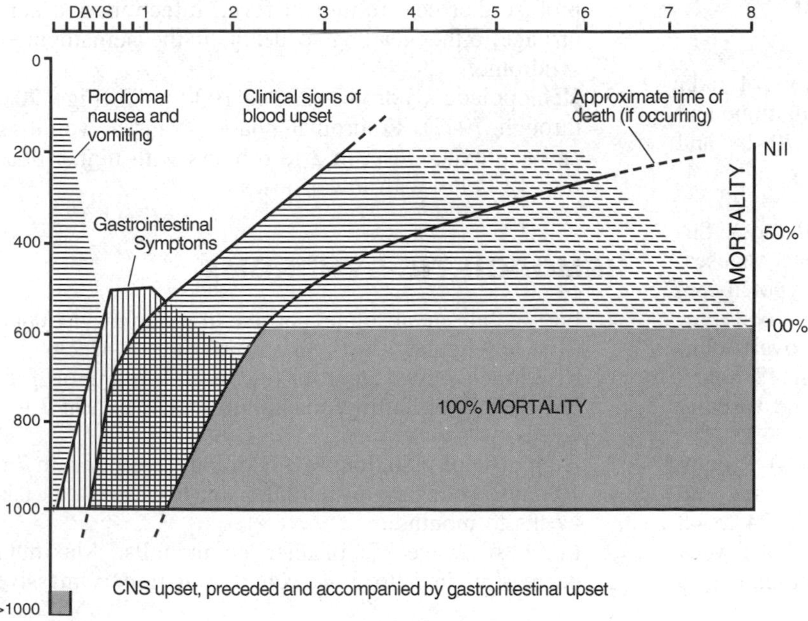

Figure 70–1 The acute radiation syndrome: time sequence of the main events according to dose. (Adapted from Llewellyn C. In: Reis MD, Dolve E, eds. Manual of disaster medicine. Berlin: Springer-Verlag, 1989.)

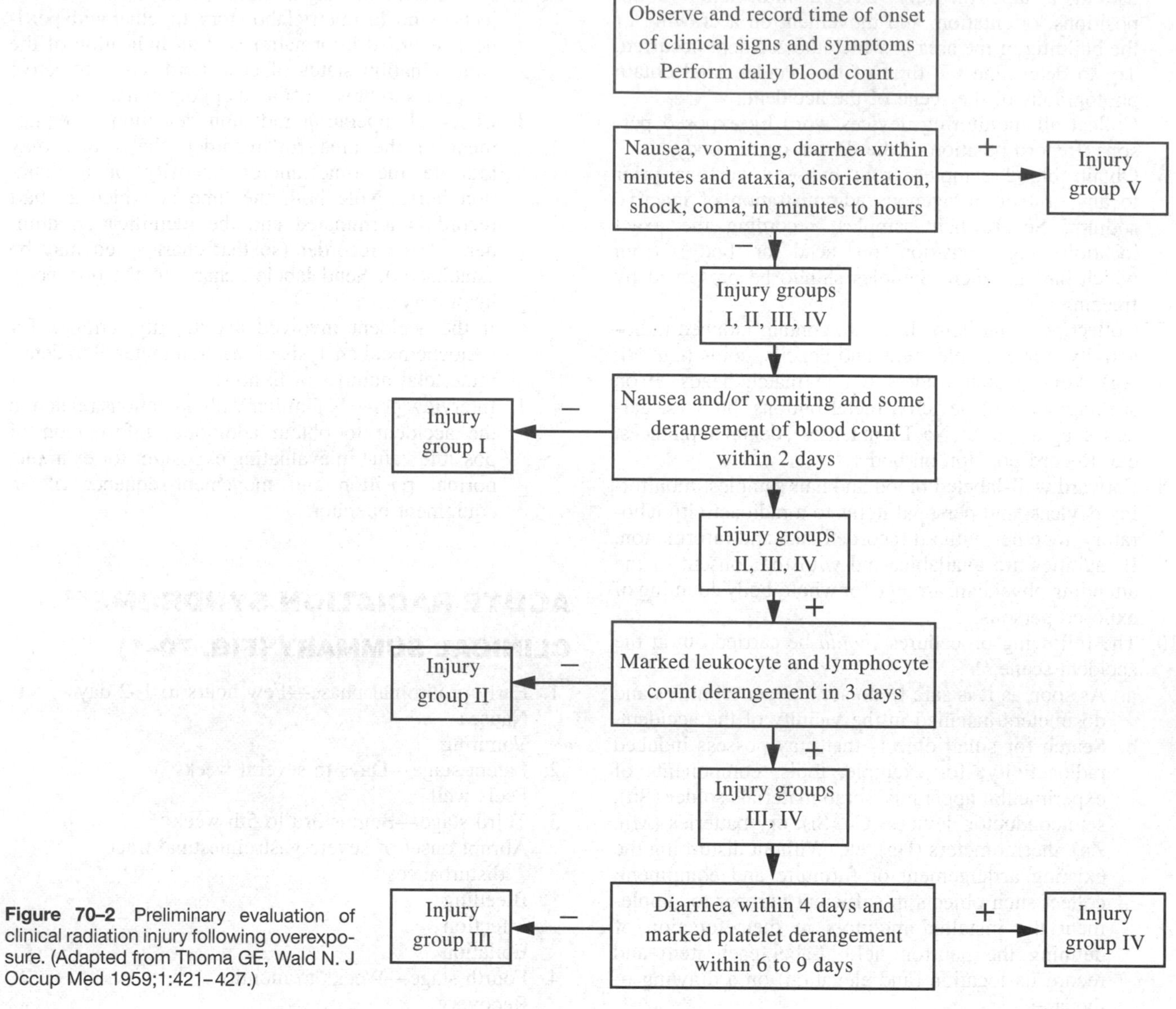

Figure 70–2 Preliminary evaluation of clinical radiation injury following overexposure. (Adapted from Thoma GE, Wald N. J Occup Med 1959;1:421–427.)

INJURY SUBGROUPS (FIG. 70–2)

Syndromes

Three major organ systems with different levels of radiation sensitivity respond to penetrating radiation and thereby contribute to the syndrome (Tables 70–14 and 70–15)

1. Cardiovascular/CNS syndrome (over 2000 rads). Supralethal dose, always fatal. Immediate nausea, vomiting, blood diarrhea, irreversible hypotension, apathy, ataxia, convulsions, and coma. No prodrome or latent phase. Progression to overt clinical illness in 3 to 6 hours. Death within 48 hours. Lesion involves endothelial radionecrosis and vascular collapse.
2. Gastrointestinal syndrome (1000 to 3000 rads). Prompt onset (3 to 12 hours) of profuse diarrhea, nausea, and vomiting. Patient becomes asymptomatic in 24 to 48 hours. Lymphocyte depression. Latent period of 1 week or less followed by denuding of the GI tract leading to profuse diarrhea, fulminant fever, infection, and hemorrhage, either leading to death or the hematopoietic syndrome.
3. Hemopoietic syndrome (200 to 1000 rads) (Figs. 70–3 through 70–7). Prodromal phase—Nausea, vomiting, and anorexia. Onset in 2 to 6 hours with higher dose; 6 to 12 hours with lower doses.

HEMOPOIETIC SYNDROME

1. Early—fall in absolute peripheral lymphocyte count (first few hours)—lasts for several days to weeks.
2. Rise in leukocyte count for few days, leveling off for a few days, then falling: maximum leukopenia in 2 to 5 weeks.
3. High dose of radiation: severe granulocytopenia in 7 to 10 days. Poor prognostic indicator. Recovery can take weeks to months.
4. In 1 to 2 weeks, platelet count falls. Maximum depression in 4 to 5 weeks. If radiation is massive,

Table 70–14
The Acute Radiation Syndrome[a]

Dose (rems)	1 h	2–6 h	6–8 h	24–48 h		1 2 3 4	Presenting type of illness	Treatment required from	Outcome	
50–150		?	Symptoms reach maximum	Prodromal symptoms subside	LATENT PERIOD		Little clinical upset Perhaps only laboratory evidence of blood upset	?	Recovery likely	50–150
200–400		□ Nausea, vomiting				← Latent period 2–3 weeks →	Clinical and laboratory evidence of blood upset	3rd–4th week	50% or more recover	200–400
* 400–600	□ Nausea, vomiting			Symptoms may continue for several days . . .		← L.P. → 1–2 weeks	Severe clinical evidence of blood upset. Gastrointestinal upset at higher doses.	2nd week	50% or more die	400–600
600–1400	□ Nausea, vomiting, diarrhea			. . . and may merge into manifest illness →		← L.P. → 0–7 days	Severe gastrointestinal upset. At lower doses patient may survive long enough to show severe blood upset later.	1st week	Death likely	600–1400
>1400	□ Vomiting, diarrhea, shock, CNS impairment. Death within hours.					Patient already dead				>1400

[a]Adapted from Llewellyn C. In: Reis MD, Dolve E, eds. Manual of disaster medicine. Berlin: Springer-Verlag, 1989.
The prodromal phase, onset and duration of symptoms according to dose received.
* Thick horizontal line is drawn at the LD_{50} level.
□ Onset of symptoms.

Duration of the latent period and presenting type of the manifest illness according to dose received.

Table 70–15
Acute Effects of Whole-Body Doses of Ionizing Radiation[a]

rem[b]	
0–25	No detectable clinical effects; small increase in risk of delayed cancer and genetic effects
25–100	Temporary reductions in lymphocytes and neutrophils; sickness not common; long-term effects possible
100–200	Minimal symptoms; nausea/vomiting/diarrhea/fatigue in a few hours; reduction in lymphocytes and neutrophils, with delayed recovery; possible bone growth retardation in children
200–300	Nausea and vomiting on first day; following latent period of up to 2 weeks, symptoms (loss of appetite and general malaise) appear but are not severe; hematopoietic subsyndrome; recovery likely in about 3 months unless complicated by previous poor health
300–600	Nausea, vomiting, and diarrhea in first few hours, followed by latent period as long as 1 week with no definite symptoms; loss of appetite, general malaise, and fever during second week, followed by hemorrhage, purpura, inflammation of mouth and throat, diarrhea, and intestine destruction in third week; some deaths in 2–6 weeks; possible eventual death to 50% of those exposed
600–1000	Vomiting in 100% of victims within first few hours; diarrhea, hemorrhage, and fever toward end of first week; rapid emaciation; almost certain death
1000–5000	Vomiting within 5–30 minutes; 100% incidence of death within 2–4 days
>5000	Vomiting immediately; 100% incidence of death within a few hours to 2 days
Also	
>15	In men yields temporary sterility
>300	In women yields permanent sterility

[a]Adapted from Goldman M. Ionizing radiation and its risks. In: Occupational disease—new vistas for medicine. West J Med 1982;137:540–547.
[b]rem = rad equivalent in man or mammal.

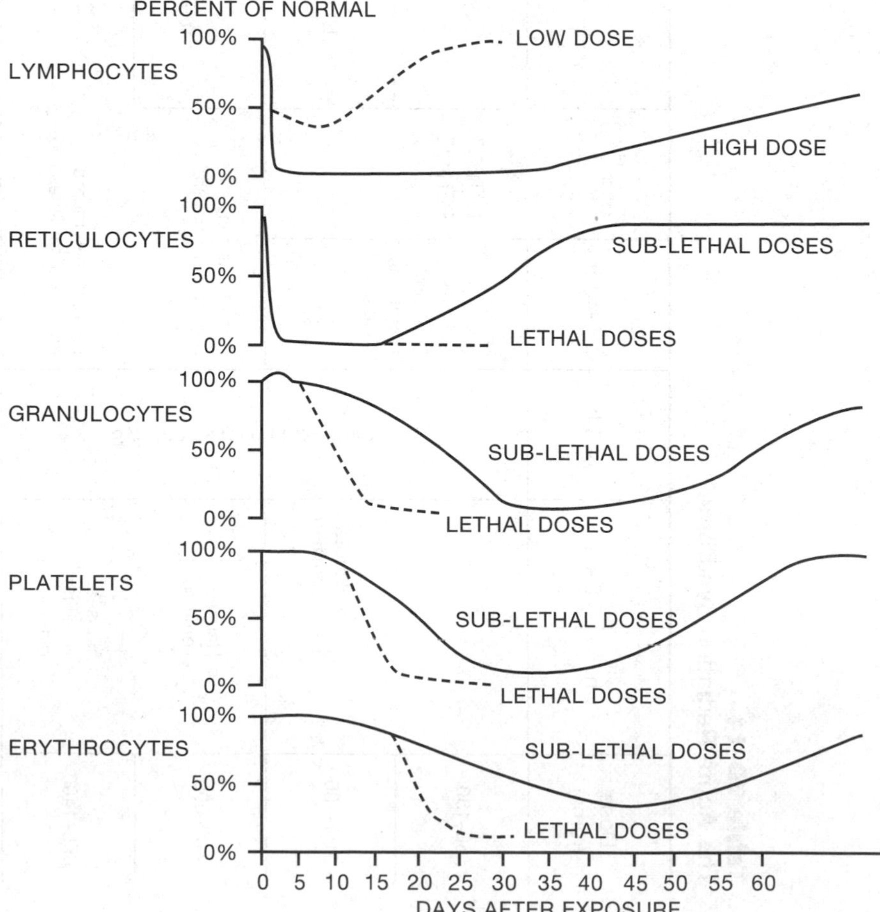

Figure 70–3 The blood element response to acute whole body radiation is shown. (Adapted from Milroy WC. Emerg Med Clin North Am 1984;2:667–686.)

severe platelet drop occurs earlier. Return to normal may take several months.

5. RBC: slow decline with reticulocytopenia. Extent depends on amount of radiation exposure and severity of acute radiation syndrome. Blood loss from gastrointestinal tract or into tissues may lead to earlier anemia.

Signs and Symptoms During the Prodromal Period

Nausea and Vomiting

Onset within the first hour with explosive, bloody diarrhea signals a fatal outcome. Appearance during the first 2 to 3 hours indicates a high dose. Onset between 6 to 12 hours and termination within 24 hours suggests a sublethal (100 to 200 rads) dose. This must be documented at the initial and each subsequent examination and differentiated from a normal stress/anxiety response.

Hyperthermia

Significant rise in body temperature in the first hours after exposure is associated with a fatal outcome. Fever and chills in the first 24 hours indicate a similar prognosis.

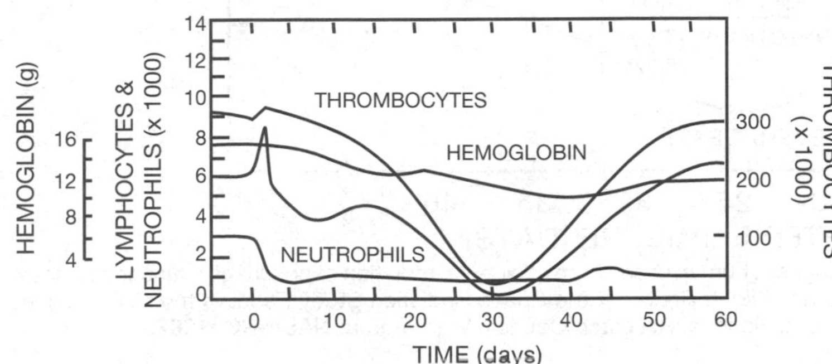

Figure 70–4 Hematologic response to 300 rads whole-body exposure. (Adapted from Llewellyn C. In: Reis MD, Dolve E, eds. Manual of disaster medicine. Berlin: Springer-Verlag, 1989.)

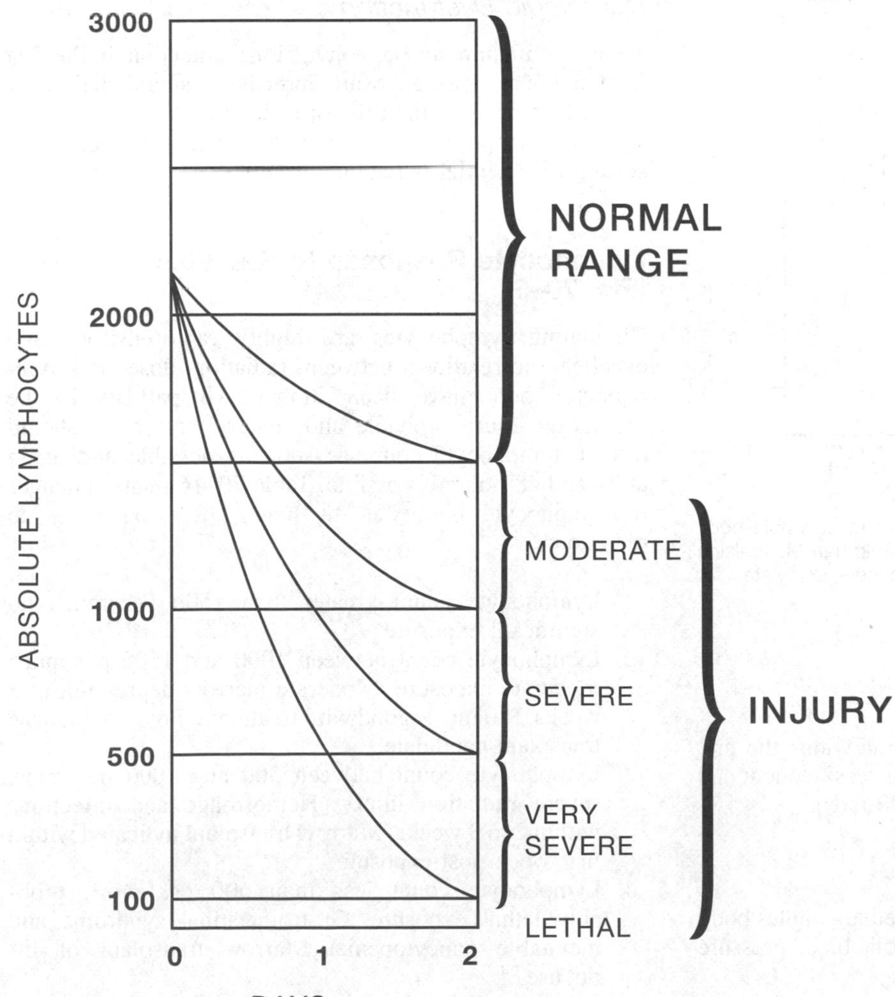

Figure 70–5 Schematic relationships between absolute lymphocyte level and clinical injury as estimated in the first 2 days after exposure. (From Andrews GA, Auxier JA, Lushbaugh CC. The importance of dosimetry to the medical management of persons accidentally exposed to high levels of radiation. In: Personnel Dosimetry for Radiation Accidents. Vienna: International Atomic Energy Agency, 1965.)

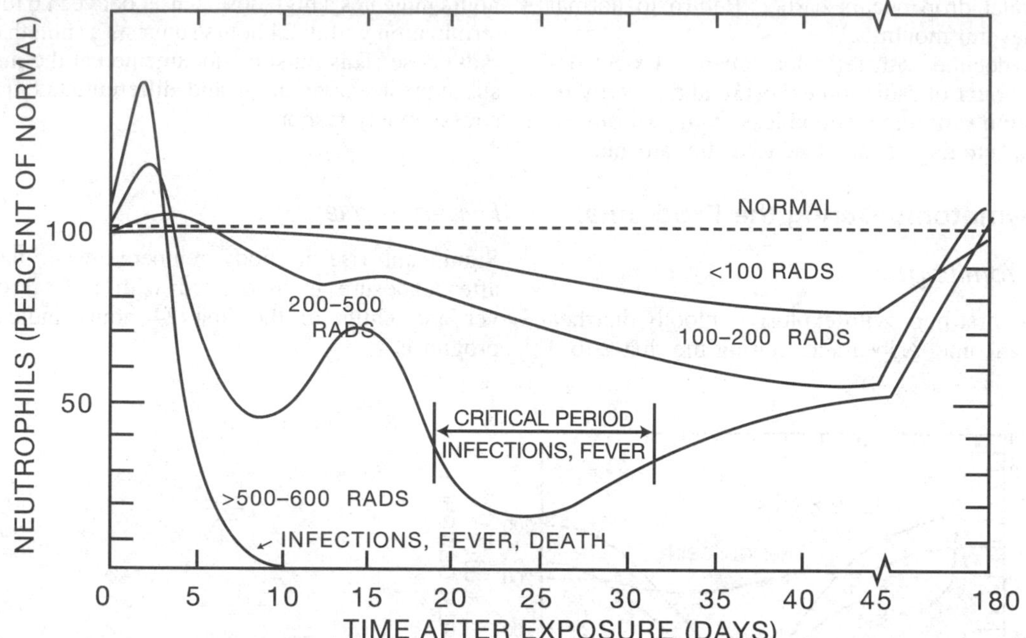

Figure 70–6 Smoothed average time-course of neutrophil changes in human cases from accidental radiation exposure as a function of dose. (From Langham WL, ed. Radiobiological Factors in Manned Space Flight: Report of the Space Radiation Study Panel of the Life Sciences Committee, Space Science Board, National Academy of Sciences, National Research Council. Washington: NAS/NRC, 1967.)

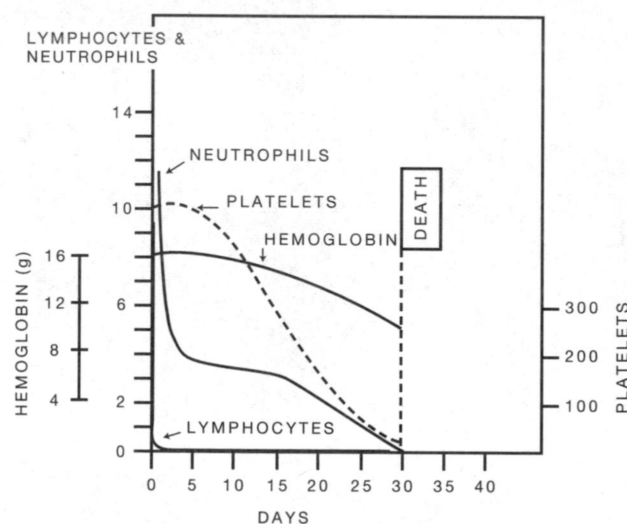

Figure 70–7 Typical hematologic response* to a whole-body radiation dose of 450 rads. (Adapted from Goldman M. Ionizing radiation and its risks. In: Occupational disease—new vistas for medicine. West J Med 1982;137:540–547.)

Erythema

Doses of 1000 to 2000 rads cause erythema within the first 24 hours of exposed body surfaces. This is less frequent and later in appearance with lower doses (400 rads).

Hypotension

Hypotension is associated with supralethal whole body irradiation. More than a 10% drop in systolic blood pressure is significant.

Neurologic Dysfunction

Mental confusion, ataxia, convulsions, and coma in the first 2 to 6 hours after exposure indicate a supralethal dose. Careful attention to the time of onset and duration of these signs and symptoms enables the physician to do rapid early sorting of potential radiation casualties.

Lymphocyte Response to Radiation (Fig. 70–5)

Circulating lymphocytes are highly radiosensitive, and excellent correlations between radiation dose and lymphocyte count have been shown. All patients in the "radiation injury probable and severe" categories should have a lymphocyte count as soon as possible and again at 24 and 48 hours if possible. Table 70–16 relates changes in lymphocyte count at 48 hours after exposures to radiation:

1. Lymphocyte count greater than 1500 per mm^3: no significant exposure.
2. Lymphocyte count between 1000 and 1500 per mm^3: moderate exposure. Moderate marrow depression in 3 weeks. Prognosis good with treatment. Possible marrow transplant candidate.
3. Lymphocyte count between 500 and 1000 per mm^3: severe radiation injury. Hemorrhage and infections within 2 to 3 weeks. Marrow transplant indicated within first week post exposure.
4. Lymphocyte count less than 500 per mm^3: probably lethal exposure. Gastrointestinal syndrome and inevitable pancytopenia. Marrow transplant of little use.[24]

Table 70–10
Absolute Lymphocyte Count at 48 Hours[a]

Lymphocyte Count	Significance
Above 2000/cubic mm	No life-threatening dose of radiation.
1200–2000/cubic mm	Significant, but probably nonlethal injury has occurred.
Less than 1200/cubic mm	Serious injury.
Below 500/cubic mm	Possible lethal injury.
Below 100/cubic mm	Lethal radiation injury.

[a]Adapted from Berger ME et al. Am J Med Technol 1981;47:831–834.

TREATMENT (FIG. 70–8)

Triage (Fig. 70–9)

Rather than a definitive diagnosis of radiation injury, attention should be focused early on sorting into three categories: radiation injury unlikely; radiation injury probable; and radiation injury severe.

Radiation Injury Unlikely

No signs or symptoms of radiation sickness. Return to duty unless other injuries or medical problems exist.

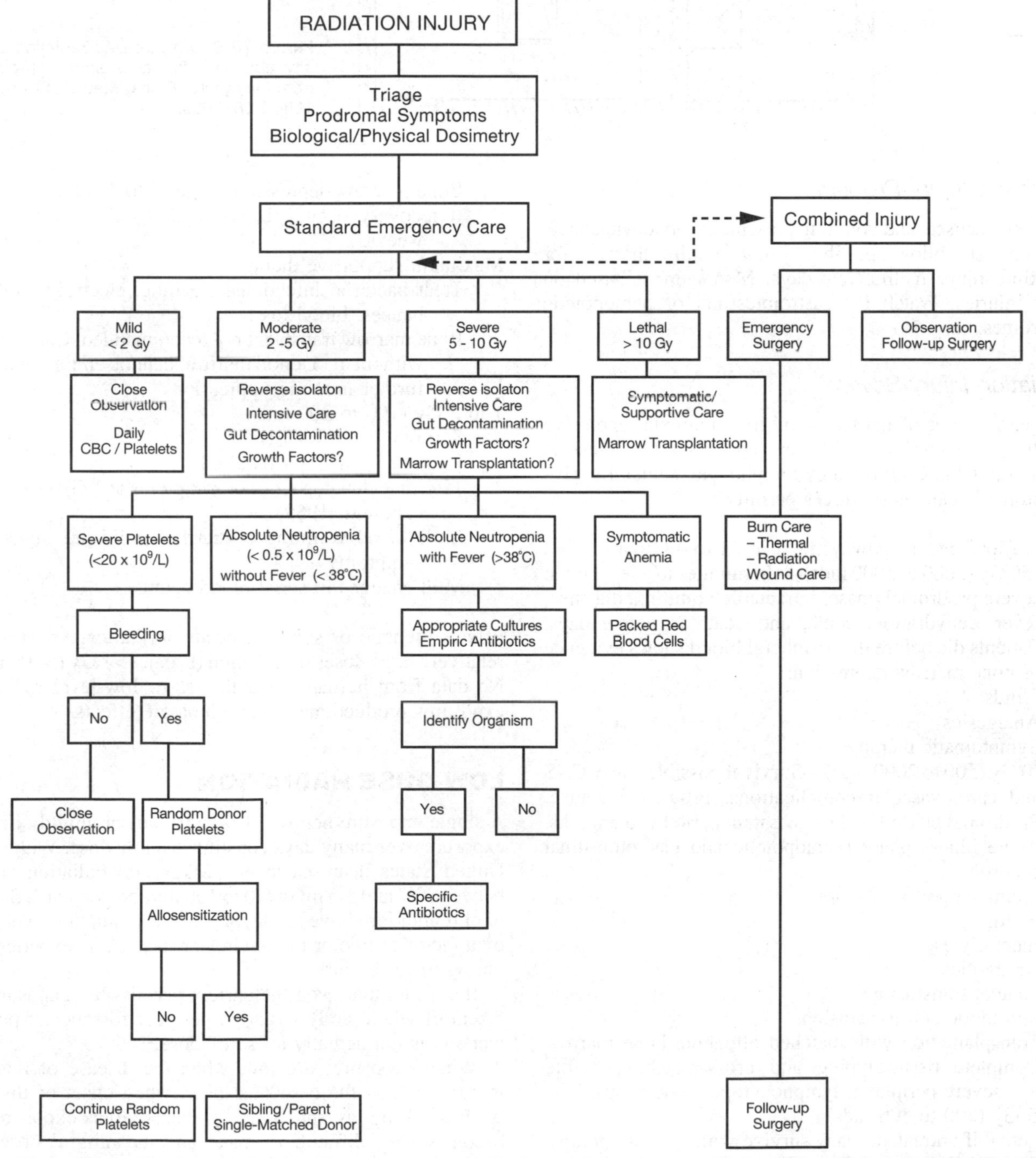

Figure 70–8 Treatment scheme for patients receiving an acute high-dose radiation exposure. (Adapted from Browne D, Weiss JF, MacVitlie TJ, Pillai MV. Treatment of radiation injuries. New York: Plenum Press, 1990.)

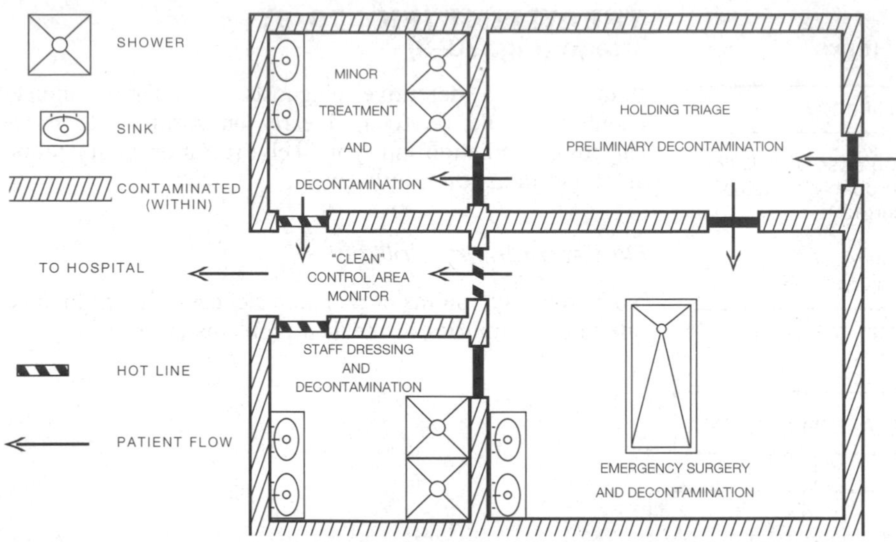

Figure 70–9 An idealized radiation casualty treatment facility is shown. (Adapted from Milroy WC. Emerg Med Clin North Am 1984;2:667–686.)

Radiation Injury Probable

Anorexia, nausea, and vomiting present. Lymphocyte counts indicated as follow-up. Should not require therapy for radiation injury in first few days. Management based on other injuries. Watch for gastrointestinal or hemopoietic syndromes.

Radiation Injury Severe

Very early onset of nausea, vomiting, anorexia, explosive diarrhea, hypotension, and neurologic disability. Dose is potentially fatal. Confirmed by lymphocyte counts. Receive symptomatic care as resources permit.[24]

50 Gy (5000 rads)—Always fatal in 24 to 48 hours.
30 to 50 Gy (3000 to 5000 rads)—(In minutes to a few hours: severe prodromal phase: intractable vomiting, diarrhea, fever, dehydration, coma, and death in a few days. Patients die before the peripheral blood shows evidence of bone marrow depression.)
- Fluids
- Analgesics
- Symptomatic therapy

5 to 20 Gy (500 to 2000 rads)—Survival possible; early CNS and cardiovascular complications. Protracted course. Prodromal phase 1 to 2 days. Latent period 1 to 2 weeks. Acute illness phase (hemopoietic and gastrointestinal syndrome).
Maximum supportive therapy
- Fluids
- Electrolytes
- Antibiotics
- Platelet transfusions
- Red blood cell transfusions
- Transplantation with matched allogenic bone marrow
- Complete tissue typing and cross-matching before severe peripheral lymphocytopenia develops.

2 to 5 Gy (200 to 500 rads)
- Lethal if untreated; many survive with optimal therapy.
- Signs and symptoms similar to above group; more delayed, less severe.
- Bone marrow depression phase: 3 to 4 weeks.
- If recovery occurs: begins at 6th week, over 2 to 3 weeks.

Maximum supportive therapy
- Treat bacterial infections, bleeding, electrolyte disturbances, blood loss.
- Bone marrow transplant not recommended: Can survive without it. Donor marrow cannot engraft without further immunosuppression.

1 to 2 Gy (100 to 200 rads)
- Survive
- Little or no therapy required.
- 15% may develop signs or symptoms at 1 Gy (100 rads) (Thomas, 1959)
- Little or no vomiting or diarrhea, mild late signs and symptoms
- Mild changes in serial blood counts.

Effects (genetic or somatic) occur only after exposures to relatively large doses of radiation (usually >1 Gy (>100 rad). No data from humans exist that show low-level radiation exposures produce measurable biologic effects.

LOW-DOSE RADIATION

A single exposure below 0.1 Gy (10 rad) or slightly higher exposure over many days constitutes a low dose. Within the United States near sea level, background radiation varies between 0.7 and 1.5 mGy (70 to 150 mmrad per year). Skiing or climbing far above sea level increases radiation exposure by a factor of two or three. Greater increase is experienced during travel by air.

It appears that even the current permissible exposure of 5 rem of whole-body radiation per year for nuclear-power workers is not actually a "safe" dose.[25]

When exposures are low, when the disease of interest is rare, and, in the case of cancer, when onset of disease is delayed by as much as 30 years after exposure, it becomes very difficult to make any meaningful observations on cause and effect.[26,27] There is as yet no way to determine precisely the cancer risks of low-level ionizing radiation exposure, and it is unlikely that this question will be resolved soon.[28]

RADIONUCLIDES (TABLE 70–17)

SOURCES

Most patients given radioactive substances present only a small risk to others, but guidance needs to be followed carefully to ensure that the risk is kept to a minimum—particularly in the case of those given radiolabeled iodine (iodine-131) therapeutically.

HAZARDS

Radiotherapy with sealed radioactive sources is carried out in designated centers on inpatients under controlled conditions of isolation, and the patients are not discharged until the treatment has been completed and the sources have been removed. On the other hand, unsealed radioactive sources are used more commonly in more hospitals for diagnosis, as well as for treatment, and in outpatients, as well as inpatients. These procedures present two distinct types of hazard. First, radiation is emitted from the patient so that members of the public, porters, nurses, and other hospital staff are exposed. Second, specimens of the patient's tissue and body fluids such as blood and urine may become radioactive, presenting a risk to family members and other people at home and to people in hospital wards, operating theaters, and the mortuary.

By far the greatest hazard comes from giving iodine-131 therapeutically. Radioiodide is secreted in body fluids such as sweat and saliva, and more stringent precautions must be taken against both contamination and close contact. Conventional doses for treating thyrotoxicosis are normally given to outpatients, but the higher doses given for thyroid carcinoma mean that patients have to remain in the hospital nursed under conditions of isolation similar to those that apply to treatments from sealed sources.

Staff with infrequent contact with radioactive patients should be reassured that most staff in departments of nuclear medicine, who may be subject to almost continual exposure, receive annual whole body radiation doses that are less than the current legal limit for members of the public.[29]

TREATMENT—INTERNAL CONTAMINATION (TABLE 70–18)

Following internal contamination there is usually a period of time before the radionuclide has been absorbed, transported, and taken up by tissue cells. The absorption from the lung, gut, or wound can sometimes be reduced by chemical manipulation in the GI tract, or by hastening the passage of the material through the body. Alkalizing the stomach may cause the formation of relatively insoluble hydroxides or will at least keep the pH high enough to reduce solubility of some metal salts. Metals such as copper, iron, or plutonium are generally more available for later absorption after spending some time in the acid milieu of the stomach. With chromium, the opposite is true. Acid gastric juice reduces hexavalent chromium to the poorly absorbed trivalent ion. The administration of a cathartic such as magnesium sulfate will shorten the intestinal transit time, thereby reducing absorption and radiation exposure to the gut wall and nearby tissues. Once absorbed, uptake can be reduced by the use of blocking agents, isotopic dilution, or chelating agents.

A *blocking agent* is a chemical that saturates a tissue with a nonradioactive element, thereby reducing the uptake of the radionuclide. *Isotopic dilution* refers to the administration of large quantities of the stable isotope of the radionuclide so that, on a statistical basis alone, the opportunity for incorporation of atoms of the radionuclide is lessened.

Chelating agents (Table 70–19) bind metals into complexes, preventing tissue uptake and allowing urinary excretion. If given promptly, diethylenetriaminepentaacetic acid (DTPA) will greatly reduce the uptake of absorbed ^{239}Pu into the skeleton. Chelating agents such as EDTA, DTPA, BAL, penicillamine, or deferoxamine are sometimes useful after uptake has occurred, but their effectiveness is greatly reduced.

BREAST MILK (TABLE 70–20)

It is considered advisable to separate radiopharmaceuticals crudely into the following three categories according to their physical properties and according to their magnitude and effective half-life of excretion in breast milk:

1. Breast-feeding must be discontinued.
2. Breast-feeding must be interrupted for a short period during which milk should be expressed at normal feeding times and discarded.
3. Breast-feeding need not be interrupted.

Table 70–20 lists recommended minimum periods of interruption to breast-feeding.[30]

RADIATION ACCIDENTS AND RADIOTHERAPY

A radiation accident is defined as an uncontrolled exposure to radiation or radioactive materials causing injury or contamination. Radiation accidents have been rare in the past, but with the increasing use of ionizing radiation in industry, research, power production, and defense and in the diagnosis and treatment of disease, the possibility of an increased number of injuries associated with radiation exists. Selected examples of radiation accidents include the misadministration/mishandling of therapeutic or diagnostic radionuclides; careless use/loss of radiography sources; failure of safety-interlock systems in high-flux x-ray-or gamma ray–producing devices; and, in very rare instances, release of radioactive materials in transportation accidents.

There are four general types of radiation accidents involving humans: (a) those in which the victim has been irradiated by penetrating radiation to the whole body or some part of the body; (b) those in which the victim has received surface contamination with radionuclides; (c) those in which victims have been contaminated internally with radionuclides such as by inhalation, ingestion, injection, or absorption through skin or wounds; and (d) those with combina-

Table 70–17
Radionuclides Listed Alphabetically

Radionuclide	Physical Half-Life*	Effective Half-Life	Radiation
Americium 241	458 yrs	139 yrs	α, e⁻, γ
Americium 243	7950 yrs	194 yrs	α, γ
Antimony 122	67 hrs	—	β⁻, β⁺, γ
Antimony 124	60 days	—	β⁻, γ
Antimony 125	2.7 yrs	—	β⁻, e⁻, γ
Argon 37	35 days	—	γ
Arsenic 74	18 days	17 days	β⁻, β⁺, γ
Arsenic 76	26.5 hrs	—	β⁻, γ
Arsenic 77	39 hrs	24 hrs	β⁻, γ
Barium 131	12 days	—	γ, e⁻
Barium 133	7.2 yrs	—	γ, e⁺
Barium 137m	2.55 min	—	γ, e⁻
Barium 140	13 days	11 days	β⁻, e⁻, γ
Beryllium 7	53 days	—	γ
Bismuth 207	30 yrs	—	e⁻, γ
Bismuth 210	5.01 days	—	α, β⁻, γ
Bromine 82	35.34 hrs	—	β⁻, γ
Cadmium 109	453 days	140 days	e⁻, γ
Cadmium 115	53.5 hrs	—	β⁻, γ
Cadmium 115	43 days	—	β⁻, γ
Calcium 45	165 days	162 days	β⁻
Calcium 47	4.5 days	4.5 days	β⁻, γ
Californium 243	2.6 yrs	2.2 yrs	γ, α, N
Carbon 11	20.3 min	—	β⁺, γ
Carbon 14	5730 yrs	12 days	β⁻
Cerium 141	33 days	30 days	β⁻, e⁻, γ
Cerium 144	284 days	280 days	β⁻, e⁻, γ
Cesium 131	9.70 days	—	γ
Cesium 134	2.05 yrs	—	β⁻, γ
Cesium 137	30.0 yrs	70 days	β⁻, e⁻, γ
Chlorine 36	3.1 × 10⁵ yrs	—	β⁻, γ
Chromium 51	27.8 days	27 days	e⁻, γ
Cobalt 57	270 days	9 days	e⁻, γ
Cobalt 58	71.3 days	8 days	β⁺, γ
Cobalt 60	5.26 yrs	10 days	β⁻, γ
Copper 64	12.8 hrs	—	β⁻, e⁻, β⁺, γ
Curium 242	163 days	155 days	α, N, γ
Curium 243	32 yrs	27.5 days	α, γ
Curium 244	17.6 yrs	16.7 yrs	α, N, γ
Dysprosium 159	144 days	—	e⁻, γ
Erbium 169	9.4 days	—	β⁻, e⁻, γ
Europium 152	13 yrs	3 yrs	β⁻, β⁺, e⁻, γ
Europium 154	16 yrs	3 yrs	β⁻, e⁻, γ
Europium 155	2 yrs	1.3 yrs	β⁻, e⁻, γ
Fluorine 18	2 hrs	2 hrs	β, γ
Gadolinium 153	242 days	—	e⁻, γ
Gallium 67	78.1 hrs	—	γ
Gallium 68	68.3 min	—	β⁺, γ
Gallium 72	14.1 hrs	12 hrs	β, γ
Germanium 71	11.4 days	—	γ
Gold 195	183 days	—	e⁻, γ
Gold 198	2.7 days	2.6 days	β⁻, e⁻, γ
Gold 199	75.6 hrs	—	β⁻, e⁻, γ
Hafnium 181	42.5 days	—	β⁻, e⁻, γ
Holmium 166	26.9 hrs	—	β⁻, e⁻, γ
Hydrogen 3	12 yrs	12 days	β⁻
Indium 111	2.8 days	—	γ
Indium 113m	100 min	—	e⁻, γ
Indium 114	72 sec	—	β⁻, β⁺, γ
Indium 114m	49 days	27 days	e⁻, γ (DR)
Iodine 123	13 hrs	—	γ
Iodine 125	60 days	42	e⁻, γ
Iodine 129	1.7 × 10⁷ yrs	—	β⁻, e⁻, γ
Iodine 130	12.4 hrs	—	β⁻, γ
Iodine 131	8.05 days	8 days	β⁻, e⁻, γ
Iridium 192	74 days	—	β⁻, e⁻, γ
Iridium 194	17.4 hrs	—	β, χ, γ

**sec*, second; *min*, minute; *hrs*, hours; *yrs*, years; *DR*, daughter radiation; *N*, neutron.

(continued)

Table 70–17 *(Continued)*

Radionuclide	Physical Half-Life*	Effective Half-Life	Radiation
Iron 52	8.3 hrs	—	β^-, γ
Iron 55	2.6 yrs	1 yr	γ
Iron 59	45 days	42 days	β^-, γ
Krypton 81m	13.0 sec	—	γ
Krypton 85	10.76 yrs	—	β^-, γ
Lanthanum 140	40.22 hrs	—	β^-, γ
Lead 210	2 yrs	1.3 yrs	α, β^-, e^-, γ
Lutetium 177	6.7 days	—	β^-, e^-, γ
Magnesium 28	21 hrs	—	β^-, e^-, γ
Manganese 54	303 days	—	e^-, γ
Mercury 197	2.7 days	2.3 days	e^-, γ
Mercury 197m	24 hrs	—	e^-, γ
Mercury 203	4 days	11 days	β^-, e^-, γ
Molybdenum 99	67 hrs	1.5 days	β^-, γ
Neodymium 147	11.1 days	—	β^-, e^-, γ
Neptunium 237	2×10^6 yrs	200 yrs	α, γ (DR)
Neptunium 239	2.3 days	2.3 days	β, γ
Nickel 63	92 yrs	—	β^-
Niobium 95	35 days	—	β^-, γ
Nitrogen 13	10 min	—	β^+, γ
Osmium 191	15 days	—	β^-, e^-, γ
Oxygen 15	124 sec	—	β^+, γ
Palladium 103	17 days	—	γ
Palladium 109	13.47 hrs	—	β^-, e^-, γ
Phosphorus 32	14 days	14 days	β^-
Plutonium 238	88 yrs	63 yrs	γ, α
Plutonium 239	2.4×10^4 yrs	197 yrs	γ, α
Polonium 210	138 days	46 days	α, γ
Potassium 42	12 hrs	12 hrs	β^-, γ
Praseodymium 142	19.2 hrs	—	β^-, γ
Praseodymium 143	13.6 days	—	β^-
Praseodymium 144	17.3 min	—	β^-, γ
Promethium 147	2.6 yrs	1.6 yrs	β^-
Promethium 149	2.2 days	2.2 days	β^-, γ
Protactinium 233	27.0 days	—	β^-, e^-, γ
Protactinium 234	6.75 hrs	—	β^-, e^-, γ
Radium 224	3.6 days	3.6 days	γ, α (DR)
Radium 226	160 yrs	44 yrs	α, e^-, γ (DR)
Rhenium 186	90 hrs	—	β^-, e^-, γ
Rhodium 106	30 sec	—	β^-, γ
Rubidium 82	1.3 min	—	β^+, γ
Rubidium 86	19.0 days	13.2 days	β^-, γ
Ruthenium 97	2.9 days	—	e^-, γ
Ruthenium 103	39.6 days	—	β^-, γ
Ruthenium 106	367 days	2.5 days	β^- (DR)
Samarium 151	87 yrs	—	β^-, e^-, γ
Samarium 153	47 hrs	—	β^-, e^-, γ
Scandium 46	84 days	40 days	β^-, γ
Selenium 75	120.4 days	—	e^-, γ
Selenium 77m	17.5 sec	—	γ
Silver 110	24.4 sec	—	β^-, γ
Silver 110m	253 days	5 days	β^-, e^-, γ
Silver 111	7.5 days	—	β^-, γ
Sodium 22	2.60 yrs	11 days	β^+, γ
Sodium 24	15 hrs	14 hrs	β^-, γ
Strontium 85	64 days	64 days	e^-, γ
Strontium 87m	2.83 hrs	—	e^-, γ
Strontium 89	52 days	—	β^-, γ
Strontium 90	28 yrs	15 yrs	β^- (DR)
Sulfur 35	88 days	44 days	β^-
Tantalum 182	115 days	—	β^-, e^-, γ
Technetium 99	2.12×10^5 yrs	20 days	β^-
Technetium 99m	6.0 hrs	—	e^-, γ
Tellurium 132	78 hrs	—	β^-, e^-, γ
Terbium 160	72.1 days	—	β^-, e^-, γ
Thallium 201	73 hrs	—	γ (DR)
Thallium 204	3.8 yrs	—	β^-, γ
Thorium 230	8×10^4 yrs	200 yrs	α, γ

(continued)

Table 70–17 *(Continued)*

Radionuclide	Physical Half-Life*	Effective Half-Life	Radiation
Thorium 232	1.4×10^{10} yrs	200 yrs	α, γ (DR)
Thulium 170	130 days	—	β^-, e^-, γ
Tin 113	115 days	—	γ
Tin 119m	250 days	—	e^-, γ
Titanium 44	48 hrs	—	e^-, γ (DR)
Tungsten 185	75 days	—	β^-
Tungsten 187	23.9 hrs	—	β^-, e^-, γ
Uranium 235	7.1×10^8 yrs	15 days	α, γ (DR)
Uranium 238	4.51×10^9 yrs	—	α, e^-, γ (DR)
Xenon 127	36.4 days	—	e^-, γ
Xenon 133	5.27 days	—	β^-, e^-, γ
Ytterbium 169	32 days	—	e^-, γ
Yttrium 90	64 hrs	64 hrs	β^-
Yttrium 91	58.8 days	—	β^-, γ
Zinc 65	245 days	194 days	β^+, e^-, γ
Zinc 69	57 min	—	β^-
Zirconium 95	66 days	56 days	β^-, γ (DR)

Table 70–18
Treatment Summary for Internal Contamination, by Selected Radioactive Elements[a]

The benefit from therapy recommendations in the Immediate Actions to Consider (column 2) and Drugs to Consider (column 3) will be influenced by the route of exposure: ingestion, inhalation, skin absorption, injection, or contaminated wounds. The chemical form and solubility of the radionuclide will also change markedly the efficacy of the recommended treatment. The table below lists therapeutic procedures or drug therapy that may be helpful for the listed elements in favorable circumstances.

Element	Immediate Actions to Consider	Drugs to Consider	Information and Comment
Americium (Am)	DTPA*	DTPA	Chelation should be started as soon as treatment decision can be made. CaEDTA† may be used if CaDTPA¶ is not immediately available.
Arsenic (As)	Lavage	Dimercaprol	Short-lived isotopes. Use of dimercaprol is not indicated except in massive exposures.
Barium (Ba)	Lavage, purgatives	See column 4	Use of sodium or magnesium sulfate with and after stomach lavage will precipitate insoluble barium sulfate.
Calcium (Ca)	Lavage, purgatives, calcium	Calcium, furosemide	Massive exposure may warrant use of the sodium salt of EDTA§, but with caution over a 3- to 4-hour period to avoid tetany. Furosemide enhances urinary excretion.
Californium (Cf)	DTPA, lavage, purgatives	DTPA	Same as for Americium.
Carbon (C)	(None listed)	No treatment available	Low-energy beta rays of carbon-14 are not detected by survey instruments; collect samples and smears for special low-energy beta counting in laboratory.
Cerium (Ce)	DTPA, lavage purgatives	DTPA	Same as for Americium.
Cesium (Cs)	Prussian blue, lavage, purgatives	Prussian blue	Ion exchange resins should be as effective as Prussian blue, but have not been used in humans.
Chromium (Cr)	Lavage, purgatives	No treatment available for anionic forms; DTPA or DFOA** for cationic forms	Antacids are contraindicated. Adsorbents, such as charcoal, may reduce intestinal tract absorption.
Cobalt (Co)	Lavage, purgatives	See column 4	Penicillamine may be considered for therapeutic trial in large exposures.
Curium (Cm)	DTPA, lavage, purgatives	DTPA	Same as for Americium.
Europium (Eu)	Lavage, purgatives	DTPA	None.

[a]Adapted from Wald N. Ionizing radiation. ATSDR. October 1993.
*DTPA = diethylenetriaminepentaacetic acid.
†CaEDTA = calcium salt of ethylenediaminetetraacetic acid.
¶CaDTPA = calcium diethylenetriaminepentaacetic acid.
§EDTA = ethylenediaminetetraacetic acid.
**DFOA = deferoxamine or desferrioxamine.
††Depends on major isotope(s) in mixture, which varies with age of the isotope mixture.

(continued)

Table 70–18 *(Continued)*

Element	Immediate Actions to Consider	Drugs to Consider	Information and Comment
Fission Products	Lavage, purgatives	††	Gamma-ray spectroscopy of air or swipe samples may identify prominent radionuclides (mixed). Check also for possible alpha emitters.
Fluorine (F)	Aluminum hydroxide gel	See column 4	Very short half-life. Oral aluminum hydroxide gel will reduce absorption in the gastrointestinal (GI) tract.
Gallium (Ga)	See column 4	See column 4	Short half-life. Penicillamine can be considered for therapeutic trial.
Gold (Au)	None	Dimercaprol and penicillamine are possible therapeutic agents.	No known therapy for colloidal gold.
Iodine (I)	Potassium iodide, lavage	Potassium iodide	Success of stable iodine depends on early administration.
Iron (Fe)	Lavage	DFOA	Materials that reduce GI absorption include egg yolk or adsorbents. Oral penicillamine also chelates iron.
Lanthanum (La)	Lavage, purgatives	DTPA	CaEDTA may be used if CaDTPA is not immediately available.
Lead (Pb)	Lavage	EDTA	Dimercaprol and penicillamine are less satisfactory alternative drugs.
Mercury (Hg)	Lavage	Pencillamine	Dimercaprol may be considered for alternative therapy. Gastric lavage with egg white solution or 5% sodium formaldehyde sulfoxide; if unavailable, use a 2% to 5% solution of sodium bicarbonate.
Phosphorus (P)	Lavage, aluminum hydroxide	Phosphates	Severe overdosage may be treated with parathyroid extract (intramuscular) in addition to oral phosphates.
Plutonium (Pu)	DTPA	DTPA	DFOA may be used initially if DTPA is not available. CaEDTA may also be used, but is less effective.
Polonium (Po)	Lavage, purgatives	Dimercaprol	Consider toxicity of dimercaprol before using in cases of low-level exposure. Penicillamine is an alternative treatment.
Potassium (K)	Purgatives, diuretics, aluminum hydroxide	Diuretics	Use aluminum hydroxide antacids first to reduce GI tract absorption. Use oral liquid potassium supplements for dilution.
Promethium (Pm)	DTPA	DTPA	Chelation treatment should be started as soon as possible.
Radium (Ra)	Magnesium sulfate, lavage, purgatives	See column 4	Use 10% magnesium sulfate solution for gastric lavage and as saline cathartic. Oral sulfates reduce intestinal absorption. No effective therapy after absorption.
Rubidium (Rb)	Prussian blue	Prussian blue	Chemical properties are similar to potassium, but efficacy of similar treatments is unknown.
Ruthenium (Ru)	Lavage, purgatives	See column 4	Chlorthalidone causes enhanced urinary excretion. DTPA has variable effectiveness.
Scandium (Sc)	Lavage, purgatives	DTPA	EDTA may be used in place of DTPA.
Sodium (Na)	Lavage	Diuretic	Isotopic dilution (1 liter of 0.9% sodium chloride) by intravenous route, followed by furosemide or other diuretic agent.
Strontium (Sr)	Aluminum phosphate, lavage	Strontium or calcium intravenously	Corticosteroid may be considered, but adverse reactions should be balanced against probable limited effectiveness.
Technetium (Tc)	(None listed)	(None listed)	Potassium perchlorate has been used effectively to reduce thyroid dose.
Thorium (Th)	(None listed)	DTPA or DFOA for soluble compounds	Treatment not effective for thorotrast (ThO_2).
Tritium (^3H)	Forced water	Forced water	Low-energy beta rays of ^3H are not detectable by survey instruments; requires samples for special low-energy beta counting in laboratory.
Uranium (U)	DTPA	(None listed)	DTPA must be given within 4 hours to be effective. Sodium bicarbonate protects the kidneys from damage.
Yttrium (Y)	(None listed)	DTPA	CaEDTA may be used if CaDTPA is not immediately available.
Zinc (Zn)	Lavage	DTPA	Zinc sulfate or CaEDTA may be used as a diluting agent if CaDTPA is not immediately available. Penicillamine is another alternative.

tions of these problems. These patients may also have complicating medical and surgical problems.

Irradiation

The irradiated patient may have been exposed to electromagnetic radiation from an x-ray machine, an accelerator, or from a sealed source containing a gamma emitter. Sources of high-energy electrons (betatrons) can also produce this type of injury. Exposure may be to a part of the body or to the whole body.

Contamination

The victim who has been contaminated by radionuclides in an accident may, depending on the degree of contam-

Table 70–19
Medications and Mechanisms of Decorporation. (Modified from Safety Series 47, IAEA)

Radionuclide	Medication	Applications In: Ingestion/Inhalation	Applications In: Wound	Principle of Action
Iodine	KI	130 mg (tabl) stat, followed by 130 mg q.d. × 7 if indicated	Same	Blocking
Rare earths Plutonium Transplutonics Yttrium	DTPA	1 g Ca-DTPA in 500 ml 5% D/W IV over 60 min; or 1 g (4 ml) in 6 ml 5% D/W by slow IV injection (1 min)	Irrigate wound with 1 g of Ca-DTPA in 250 ml D5W	Chelation
Polonium Mercury Arsenic Bismuth Gold	BAL	One ampule (= 300 mg) i.m. q4h for 3 days—(first test for sensitivity with ¼ amp.)	Same	Promotes excretion
Uranium	Bicarbonate	Slow IV infusion of bicarbonated physiologic solution (250 ml at 14%)	Slow IV infusion of bicarbonated physiologic solution (250 ml at 14 percent) and wash with bicarbonate	Alkalinization of urine; reduces chance of ATN
Cesium Rubidium Thallium	Prussian Blue* [Ferrihexacyano-Ferrate (II)]	1 g in 100–200 ml water p.o. t.i.d. for several days	Same	Mobilization from organs and tissues—reduction and absorption
Radium	Ca-gluconate	May be tried; 20% Ca-gluconate 10 ml IV once or twice daily	Same	Displacement
Strontium	Ammonium chloride	3 g t.i.d. p.o.	Same	Demineralizing agent
Tritium	Water	Have patient drink 6–12 liters of water per day	Same	Isotopic dilution
Strontium Radium	$BaSO_4$	100 g $BaSO_4$ in 250 ml of water	Same	Reduces absorption
Calcium Barium	Sodium alginate	10 g in a large glass of water	Same	Inhibits absorption
Copper Polonium Lead Mercury Gold	D-penicillamine	1 g IV q.d. or 0.9 g p.o. q4–6 hr	Same	Chelation

*Not FDA approved as of publication date.

Table 70–20
Recommended Minimum Periods of Interruption to Breast-Feeding[a]

Radiopharmaceutical	Period (h)
^{131}I-MAA	Discontinue
^{125}I-HSA	Discontinue
^{125}I-Fibrinogen	Discontinue
Na-^{131}I	Discontinue
^{67}Ga-citrate	Discontinue
^{75}Se-methionine	Discontinue
Sodium ^{32}P phosphate	Discontinue
Chromic ^{32}P phosphate	Discontinue
^{131}I-hippuran	24
^{125}I-hippuran	24
^{99}Tc^{m}-pertechnetate	12
^{99}Tc^{m}-MAA	6
^{99}Tc^{m}-DTPA	Not essential
^{99}Tc^{m}-EDTA	Not essential
^{99}Tc^{m}-MDP	Not essential
^{99}Tc^{m}-erythrocytes	Not essential
^{51}Cr-EDTA	Not essential
^{111}In-leukocytes	Not essential

[a]Adapted from Mountford PJ, Coakley AJ. Nucl Med Commun 1986;7: 399–401.

ination, be cared for with strict isolation precautions to prevent the transfer of radionuclides to other personnel or other areas of the hospital. The contaminant can be in the form of liquids or particulate matter. The latter may range from powdery, invisible substances to large particles. The contaminant can consist of radionuclides that emit particulate radiation (alpha or beta radiation), or electromagnetic radiation (x-rays, gamma rays), or combinations of these.

Internal Contamination

Radiation accident victims with internal contamination present no special hazard to medical laboratory personnel. Only two situations exist in which precautions in the clinical laboratory might be necessary. These occur (a) in the extremely unlikely situation where the patient has been exposed to a very high level of neutron radiation, and (b) if the victim of internal contamination is undergoing therapy that facilitates excretion of radionuclides and prevents their incorporation into body tissues.[31]

CLINICAL PRESENTATION[23-31]

Acute

Normal tissues typically involved in acute radiation reactions include the bone marrow, gut, skin, and epithelium of the upper digestive tract and bladder. Bone marrow depression, mucositis, epithelitis, epilation, and gastrointestinal upset are ultimately the result of failure to maintain the integrity of the proliferative compartments of the corresponding cell-renewal systems.

Treatment of acute mucosal and epithelial reactions should be symptomatic. Antispasmodics, opiates, and analgesics are useful for gastrointestinal and urologic symptoms. Local anesthetics can alleviate symptoms in the mouth, pharynx, and esophagus.[35]

Intermediate Effects

Intermediate effects result from injury to cells of a slowly proliferating cell-renewal system, possibly endothelium or connective tissue. Radiation pneumonitis and pericarditis are particularly important intermediate effects. They occur shortly after irradiation and are usually transient, mild in severity, and not associated with permanent sequelae.

Late Effects

Late radiation sequelae are directly related to the total effective dose received by the limiting normal tissue within a treatment portal. Although it is assumed to be endothelium or connective tissue, the nature of this critical target tissue is by no means certain. The development of tissue necroses, fistulas, and dense fibrosis is clearly related to the total effective radiation dose. Late complications may occur as early as a few months to as long as several years after irradiation. Unlike acute and intermediate radiation reactions, however, these complications are chronic and not always amenable to surgical correction. Moreover, they do not necessarily bear any relation to prior acute or intermediate reactions. It is the development of these late effects that limits the total effective dose delivered to a tumor.

An initial prospective clinical study suggests that hyperbaric oxygen (20 sessions of 100% oxygen inhalation at 3 bar for 90 minutes) should be considered in patients with severe radiation-induced hematuria.[36]

There appears to be an association between low-dose x-irradiation for lymphoid hyperplasia and the development of thyroid nodules later in life.[37] Breast cancer incidence in women includes radiation treatment for fibroadenomatosis and mastitis.[38]

Eye[35]

The lacrimal-corneal complex is most sensitive to radiation damage.

Cerebral Necrosis[39,40]

Delayed radiation necrosis of the brain should be considered whenever a patient who has received cranial irradiation develops neurologic symptoms.

Lungs[41]

Radiation pneumonitis is characterized by the insidious onset of cough, dyspnea, and fever, usually occurring between 6 and 12 weeks after radiotherapy. The chest roentgenogram and computed tomographic scan of the thorax show changes that vary from an ill-defined, nonhomogeneous opacification to a dense alveolar infiltrate associated with air bronchograms. A characteristic feature of the roentgenographic infiltrate is that is has a sharply defined border that corresponds to the edge of the radiation field. Radiation pneumonitis probably represents a form of immunologically mediated hypersensitivity pneumonitis.

Local Radiation Injury (See Tables 70–21 and 70–22)[42]

Radiation Accident Management (Tables 70–23 and 70–24) (Fig. 70–8)

Training sources and training aids are found in Table 70–25.

Drugs and Radiation

Increased mucosal and cutaneous radiation toxicity is observed in patients receiving amiodarone, aminoglutethimide, benoxaprofen,[43–45] trimethoprim-sulfamethoxazole, cocaine,[46] doxorubicin, cyclophosphamide, vincristine, methotrexate, and actinomycin D.

Second Cancers

The induction of second cancers is a particularly important late side effect of cancer treatment. Several epidemiologic studies demonstrated increased risks of leukemia and solid tumors in patients exposed to radiotherapy. Large increases in leukemia risk have also been observed after chemotherapy with alkylating agents.

The BEIR report indicated that almost all types of cancer can be caused by exposure to ionizing radiation. However, certain organs such as the thyroid gland and the female breast appear to be more radiosensitive than others.[47,48]

THOROTRAST

Thorotrast (25% thorium dioxide), a radiologic contrast agent used between 1928 and 1955, was abandoned following a report of hepatic angiosarcoma attributed to Thorotrast exposure. Thorium dioxide has radioactive properties due to the emission of alpha-, beta-, and gamma-rays with a biologic half-life of 400 years. Its use has been

Table 70–21
Clinical Manifestations of Local Radiation Injury [a]

Finding	Time of Onset
Irritation, tenderness, itching	Within 1–2 wks
Restriction of motion, stiffness	Within 1–2 wks
Erythema, edema, decreased sensation	Within 1–3 wks
Bullae, ulceration	Within 1–4 wks

[a]These findings and times of onset may vary.

Table 70–22
Organ Damage, Dysfunction, Treatment, and Prognosis After Local Irradiation[a]

Organ	Acute Lesion	Delayed Lesion	Clinical Signs	Treatment	Prognosis
Bone marrow	Pancytopenia	Vascular occlusion Myelofibrosis	Infection Hemorrhage	Antibiotics Transfusion	Good if % of total marrow irradiation small
Intestine	Flattened villi	Fibrosis, obstruction	Diarrhea	Fluid, electrolyte acute Resection for obstruction	Good for acute Obstruction can be fatal
CNS	Edema	Necrosis	Headache Focal neurologic	 Resection	Poor Fair
Skin	Desquamation	Ulcer, necrosis	Pain, oozing	Cleansing, ointments, graft	Good
Lung	Pneumonitis	Fibrosis	Cough, fever, cyanosis Dyspnea	Corticosteroids	Good at low dose Good if small volume
Heart	Pericarditis	Carditis	Fever, dyspnea	Anti-inflammatory, pericardiocentesis	Fair
Liver	Central venous thrombosis	Fibrosis	Ascites	Diuretics	Fair
Kidney	Tubular degeneration	Fibrosis	Protenuria Hypertension, renal failure	Dialysis Transplant	Fair

[a]Adapted from Phillips TL. In: Wyngaarden JB, Smith LH Jr, eds. Cecil textbook of medicine. Philadelphia: WB Saunders, 1988.

Table 70–23
Field Operation Protocols for Radiation Accidents[a]

1. Approach site with caution—look for evidence of hazardous materials.
2. If radiation hazard is suspected, position personnel, vehicles, and command post at a *safe distance* (200–300 feet) upwind of the site.
3. Notify proper authorities and hospital (see inside back cover for call list).
4. Put on protective gear and use dosimeters and survey meters if immediately available.
5. Determine the presence of injured victims.
6. Assess and treat life-threatening injuries immediately. Do not delay advanced life support if victims cannot be moved or to assess contamination status. Perform routine emergency care during extrication procedures.
7. Move victims away from the radiation hazard area, using proper patient transfer techniques to prevent further injury. Stay within the controlled zone if contamination is suspected.
8. Expose wounds and cover with sterile dressings.
9. Victims should be monitored at the control line for possible contamination only after they are medically stable. Radiation levels above background indicate the presence of contamination. Remove the contaminated accident victims' clothing.
10. Move the ambulance cot to the clean side of the control line and unfold a clean sheet or blanket over it. Place the victim on the covered cot and package for transport. Do not remove the victim from the backboard if one was used.
11. Package the victim by folding the stretcher sheet or blanket over and securing them in the appropriate manner.
12. Before leaving the controlled area, rescuers should remove protective gear at the control line. If possible, the victim should be transported by personnel who have not entered the controlled area. Ambulance personnel attending victims should wear gloves.
13. Transport the victims to the hospital emergency department. The hospital should be given additional, appropriate information, and the ambulance crew should ask for any special instructions the hosptal may have.
14. Follow the hospital's radiological protocol upon arrival.
15. The ambulance and crew should not return to *regular* service until the crew, vehicle, and equipment have undergone monitoring and necessary decontamination by the radiation safety officer.
16. Personnel should not eat, drink, smoke, etc., at the accident site, in the ambulance, or at the hospital until they have been released by the radiation safety officer.

[a]Adapted from Ricks RC. Oak Ridge, February 1987 Hospital Management of Radiation Incidents PRAV-223.

associated with the development of a wide range of malignancies, mainly of hepatic origin.[49]

USE

Thorotrast is used for cerebral arteriography and ventriculography, hepatoportosplenography, instillation for visualizing body cavities, and pyelography.[49]

DIAGNOSIS

The diagnosis of Thorotrast exposure is made on the basis of metallic hyperdensities in the liver, spleen, and lymph nodes, detected by a plain film of the abdomen that shows the pathognomonic increased density of liver, spleen, and lymph nodes. Such a finding should alert the clinician to the possibility of radiation-induced malignancy. CT will confirm this, while MRI and ultrasound do not provide any further information. A liver biopsy will confirm the malignancy, while the presence of Thorotrast can be confirmed by autoradiography.[49]

The risk of developing malignancies as a result of Thorotrast exposure continues throughout the patient's life as the radiation is continuous and linked with the long half-life of Thorotrast. This historical pathology obviously will disappear with time, but must be kept in mind for at least 2 decades when confronted with atypical abdominal pain in elderly patients.[49]

CHERNOBYL

The explosion and fire at the Chernobyl number 4 nuclear power plant on April 16, 1986, was the most significant nuclear event—in terms of acute injuries and deaths, the amount of radioactivity released into the environment, the size of the affected area, and the probable magnitude of long-term consequences—since the bombings of Hiroshima and Nagasaki. It was the worst commercial nuclear power plant disaster in history and the second to involve a meltdown of nuclear fuel—7 years after the first such instance at Three Mile Island in 1979.[50]

DOSE

It is now estimated that approximately 50 individuals were irradiated with doses greater than 500 rad (5 Gy), approximately 100 received doses of between 300 rad (3 Gy) and 500 rad, and perhaps another 100 received doses of between 100 rad (1 Gy) and 300 rad (R.P. Gale, MD, statement to Moscow press, June 6, 1986).[50]

Table 70–24
Some Ideas for Use in Planning for Multiple Casualties in Radiation Accidents

A. Designate:
  (1) Treatment area (emergency treatment and surgery) for both *contaminated* and *non contaminated* patients.
  (2) Morgue areas for contaminated and uncontaminated bodies.
  (3) Storage areas for (a) contaminated clothing and personal items, (b) waste.
  (4) Showers for ambulatory patients and staff.

B. Plan for efficient use of *all* personnel.
  (1) Rotate personnel if possible.
  (2) Do not use pregnant personnel in contaminated areas.
  (3) Security personnel will be needed in the triage area.
  (4) Housekeeping personnel will need to supply linen (large quantities) to *both* contaminated and noncontaminated areas.
  (5) Central supply and pharmacy will also need to supply two areas.

C. Plan to have a triage area that is big enough to allow movement of patients on stretchers and to allow presence of medical, nursing, and other personnel for monitoring, recordkeeping, etc.

D. Plan to have necessary equipment and supplies available for use: protective clothing for staff, towels, soap, shampoo, gowns, slippers, etc. for shower use, plastic bags, survey instruments and probes, dosimetry, etc.

E. *Plan to control contamination*
  1. Assume the triage area is contaminated.
  2. Assume contamination when in doubt.
  3. Ambulance personnel should not cross the control line to enter a clean area.
  4. Keep ambulance stretchers in the triage area—do not move them across a control line. Transfer patients from stretcher to stretcher at the control line.
  5. Use the radiology department to x-ray patients. Use portable x-ray equipment in the contaminated area. (Put all films in separate bags *before* taking them into the contaminated area.) A radiology technician shuld remain in the controlled area.
  6. If hallways must be shared, use rope/dividers and floor coverings for contaminated areas.
  7. Have *(at least)* booties, gloves, and assorted sizes of plastic bags available at *all* control points.
  8. *Change gloves between patients.*
  9. Have plenty of hampers/boxes etc. (lined with plastic) readily available in the controlled area.

F. Plan to facilitate communication, to keep patients and staff informed, and to minimize anxiety.
  1. Use signs, posters (even hastily made) to direct patients and to give instructions. Make use of copy machines to mass-produce information.
  2. Keep patients, families, etc. busy. Have them fill out their own history, if possible. *Encourage self-help.*
  3. Use intercom as a means of providing information to staff, patients, and families.
  4. Expect phone systems to be tied up.

G. Plan for recordkeeping.
  1. Expect and plan for computer systems failure (and hope for the best).
  2. Have clerks available in controlled and uncontrolled areas.

H. Plan to adapt medical care:
  1. What diagnostic procedures should be performed on patients who may have been:
     -internally contaminated
     -irradiated
     Where will tests be done and who will do them?
  2. Will uninjured but irradiated patients be admitted or sent home?
  3. Are references, phone numbers of consultants, state radiologic health depts., etc. available?
  4. What adaptations are necessary in trauma management?
     Some considerations:
     -transfusions
     -immediate or delayed closure of wounds
     -timing of surgical intervention

Table 70–25
Training Sources and Training Aids[a]

1. American Occupational Medical Association
   2340 S. Arlington Heights Road
   Arlington Heights, Illinois 60005
Periodically sponsors post-graduate training seminars. May also serve as a source of speakers for locally sponsored programs.
2. Radiation Accident Preparedness
   Medical and Managerial Aspects
   Eugene L. Saenger, M.D.; Gould A. Andrews, M.D.; Roger E. Linnemann, M.D., and Neil Wald, M.D.
   Sponsored by Edison Electric Institute
   Produced and distributed by Science-Thru-Media, Inc.
   305 Fifth Avenue, Suite 803
   New York, New York, 10016
A series of taped lectures with text and self-assessment examination providing CME/I credit.
3. Radiation Emergency Assistance Center/Training Site (REAC/TS)
   Oak Ridge Associated Universities
   Post Office Box 117
   Oak Ridge, Tennessee 37830
REAC/TS provides a series of excellent courses in handling radiation accidents for physicians, nurses, health physicists and EMTs. REAC/TS has recently completed a set of videotapes for the Federal Emergency Management Agency (FEMA) for use in training packages currently in preparation. These packages should be ready for distribution in the very near future.
4. Training Resources, a division of Nuclear Support Services, Inc.
   Suite B-3, 9150 Rumsey Center
   Columbia, Maryland 21045
Excellent slide programs for use in in-house training.

[a]Adapted from Milroy WC. Emerg Med Clin North Am 1984;2:669–686.

The vast majority of children received relatively small amounts of radiation due to the accident. Some preliminary data indicate that 80,000 children received thyroid doses from radioactive iodine of less than 200 rem (2 Sv), while 12,000 received doses between 200 and 500 rem (2 and 5 Sv), and 4000 received doses greater than 500 rem (5 Sv).[51]

RADIONUCLIDES

The major contiminants identified were as follows: iodine-131 and -132; cesium-134 and -137; niobium-95; cerium-144; ruthenium-103 and -106; and plutonium-239. Of these, cesium and iodine isotopes predominated and accounted for 90% of the absorbed dose contributed by internal radionuclides.[52]

TREATMENT

Those with estimated exposure of 500 rad or more were the first candidates for bone marrow transplantation. In general, treatment consisted of specific therapy for burns, platelet and red blood cell transfusions, prophylactic antibiotics and specific antibiotic therapy when infections developed, and fluid maintenance and parenteral hyperalimentation. Patients were placed in single rooms with sterile precautions and laminar air flow facilities. All of the fatalities had received doses of more than 600 rad (6 Gy) to bone marrow plus severe beta-radiation burns of the skin, and in many cases also thermal burns.[50] Potassium iodide was administered to much of the population near the accident site.

The 31 deaths resulting from the Chernobyl nuclear reactor accident approximately equaled the total number of accidental radiation deaths occurring in the world during the previous 42 years. About half of the Chernobyl victims had moderate to severe thermal or radiation burns of the skin; 203 persons were said to have had some level of radiation sickness that eventually required hospitalization. The 29 persons in the highest illness category were estimated to have received 6 Gy (600 rad) or more of radiation exposure.

THYROID CANCER

These children, who received unknown amounts of radiation through ingestion and inhalation, may develop hypothyroidism or cancer of the thyroid. The full incidence of thyroid cancers may not be expressed for 30 years.[53]

Early in the summer of 1989 plutonium was found in the underground waters of the Red Forest. However, as it decays to americium, plutonium, a health hazard, becomes even more medically dangerous and more likely to migrate in water. Americium-241, moreover, has a long half-life (433 years). By the year 2060, the alpha-particle emission rate of americium-241 in the affected area will be twice that of plutonium.[54]

EUROPE—CANCER AND FETAL EFFECTS

Childhood leukemia in Finland or Sweden was not increased between 1976 and 1992. No significant increase in birth defects or abortion rate was observed in Austria. No association was observed between the exposure and small head circumference, congenital cataracts, anencephaly, spina bifida, and low birth weight in Norway or Finland.[55] The incidence of thyroid cancer in children in parts of the Soviet Union affected by fallout from the Chernobyl reaction continues to rise.[56,57]

NONIONIZING RADIATION (TABLE 70–26)

ELECTROMAGNETIC FIELDS

Most of the recent research on possible biologic effects of 60-hertz EMFs suggests that the magnetic, rather than the electric, fields are more likely to produce significant effects. Electric charges create electric fields. Electric charges that move (i.e., electric current) create magnetic fields. An appliance that is plugged in, and therefore connected to a source of electricity, has an electric field even when the appliance is turned off. To produce a magnetic field, however, the appliance must be not only plugged in, but also operating, so that the current is flowing. These fields can be characterized by either their wavelength or their frequency, which are related. The amount of energy an electric or magnetic field can carry depends on the frequency and wavelength of the field. The wavelength describes how far it is between one peak on the wave and the next peak. The frequency, measured in hertz, describes how many wave peaks pass by in one second of time.[58]

The Electromagnetic Spectrum

The low end of the spectrum includes electric and magnetic fields produced by everyday electrical appliances. At the top of the spectrum are x-rays and gamma rays (Figs. 70–10 and 70–11). "EMFs" usually refers to electric and magnetic fields at the extremely low frequency (or ELF) end of the spectrum, such as those associated with the use of electric power. Electric fields from most appliances primarily create charges of current on or near the surface of the body and not in the internal organs. Magnetic fields, however, pass through the body and actually induce electric currents within the body. Individuals can be easily shielded from the higher-frequency microwaves' magnetic fields, but not from the 60-hertz magnetic fields. This is because even though the microwaves' frequency is higher, its length is much, shorter (about 1 cm) then the wavelength of a 60-hertz field (about 5000 kilometers). The shorter wave can be blocked by materials such as thin metal sheets, whereas the much longer wave cannot. The term "radiation" simply means energy transmitted by waves. "Ionizing" radiation has enough energy to strip electrons from atoms. (X-rays are a form of ionizing radiation.) Higher frequency nonionizing radiation such as microwaves can heat up biologic tissue by vibrating molecules. The lower-frequency, 60-hertz EMFs cannot. Because of their relatively lower energy, 60-hertz EMFs were not, until recently, thought to be connected with any potential health problems.[59]

Magnetic Field Strength

The strength of the magnetic field is measured in units of gauss (G) or milligauss (mG). A milligauss is 1/1000th of a gauss. (The international standard unit is microtesla, which is the same as 10 milligauss.) It is important to keep in mind that a typical American home has a background magnetic field level (away from any appliances) ranging from 0.5 mG to 4 mG.[59–61]

ELECTROMAGNETIC WAVES

The term "electromagnetic field" applies to a type of energy that is beamed through the air. These fields have two components, as the name implies: an electric charge and a magnetic attraction. Light, radio waves, radar, x-rays, and gamma rays are all forms of electromagnetic radiation. Physically, they differ from one another only in frequency (the back-and-forth oscillation of the field's force); the higher the frequency, the more energy contained in the field.[62] Both the electric and magnetic components of the 60-hertz field act on charged particles, but too weakly to disrupt the bonds in molecules. The strongest 60-hertz field produced by high-voltage power lines and generators does not damage DNA, even in someone standing very close, and it would contribute less than a millionth the amount of heating that results from normal metabolism.[62]

The electric component influences primarily those particles at the surface of a nearby object, whereas the magnetic field penetrates to the interior. Ambient levels of the two components vary from place to place. Someone walking directly underneath a high-voltage power line has relatively high exposure to both. But if he or she enters a building or a grove of trees, only the magnetic component continues to have much influence, because electric fields are easily shielded by trees or walls.[62]

Sources

Bathroom sources include hair dryers and electric shavers. Kitchen sources include blenders, can openers, coffee makers, crock pots, dishwashers, food processors, garbage disposals, microwave ovens, mixers, electric ovens, electric ranges, refrigerators, and toasters. Living/family room sources include ceiling fans, window air conditioners, tuners/tape players, and color and black-and-white TVs. Laundry/utility room sources include electric clothes dryers, washing machines, irons, portable heaters, and vacuum cleaners. Bedroom sources include digital clocks, analog (conventional clock-face) clocks, and baby monitors. Office sources include air cleaners, copy machines, FAX machines,

Table 70–26
Comparative Aspects of Various Forms of "Radiation"[a]

Type	Physical Characteristics	Biologic Effects
X-rays Gamma rays	Short wavelength. Electromagnetic waves, highly penetrating, with the capability of producing ionization within tissues and subsequent electrochemical reactions.	Electrochemical reactions. Can result in tissue damage at high exposures that result in cell death, mutation, cancer, and developmental defects. These effects are dose-related.
Microwaves Radar Diathermy	Longer-wave electromagnetic waves with variable ability to penetrate but no ability to produce ionization within tissues.	The primary biologic effect is hyperthermia, although the existence of nonthermal effects of these electromagnetic waves is still being investigated. Cataract development is the most widely known complication of extensive microwave or radar exposure.
Ultrasound	Sound waves with a frequency above the audible range; they produce mechanical compressions and variations in matter with no capability of producing ionization.	Sound waves can cause tissue disruption if the energy is high enough by producing cavitation and streaming as well as hyperthermia. None of these effects occur with the energies utilized in diagnostic ultrasonography.

[a]Adapted from Brent RL. Pediatr Ann 1980;9:469–473.

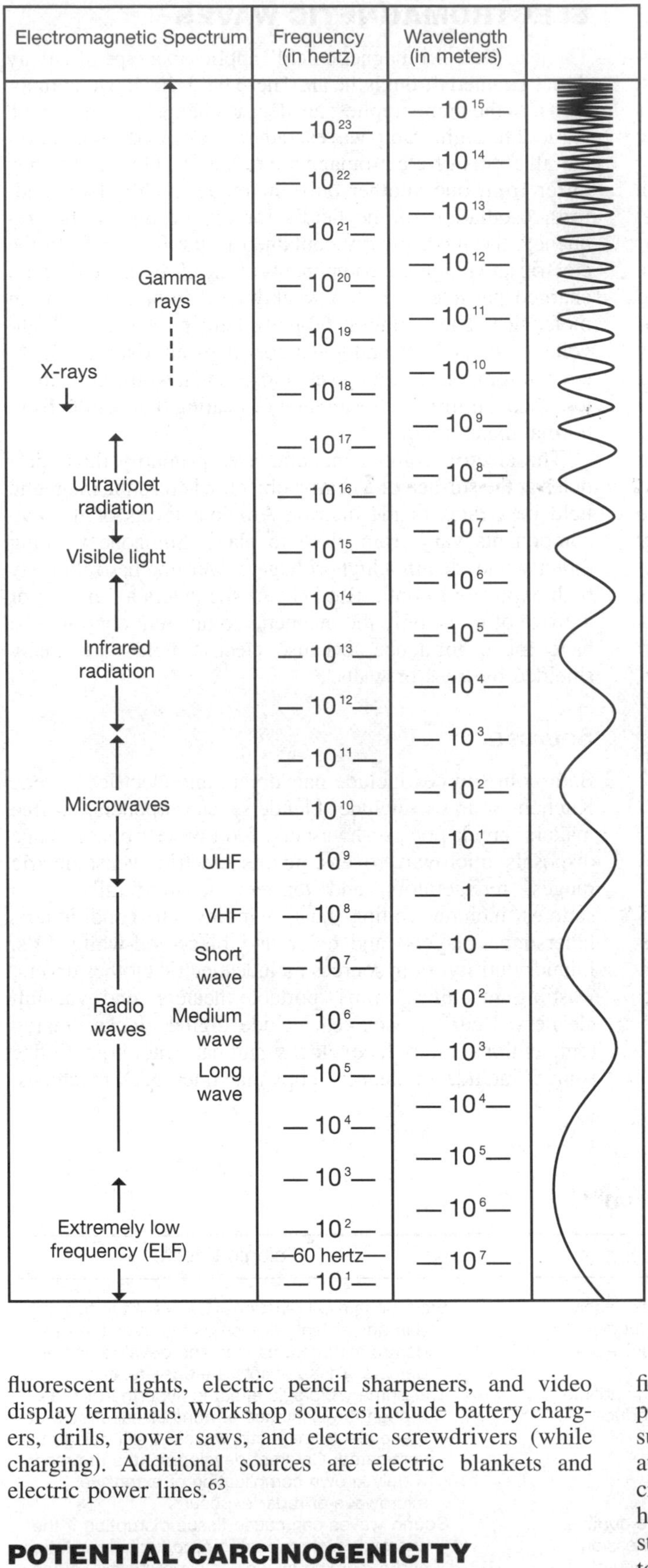

Electromagnetic Spectrum | Frequency (in hertz) | Wavelength (in meters)

Gamma rays
X-rays
Ultraviolet radiation
Visible light
Infrared radiation
Microwaves
UHF
VHF
Short wave
Radio waves
Medium wave
Long wave
Extremely low frequency (ELF)

— 10^{23} —
— 10^{22} —
— 10^{21} —
— 10^{20} —
— 10^{19} —
— 10^{18} —
— 10^{17} —
— 10^{16} —
— 10^{15} —
— 10^{14} —
— 10^{13} —
— 10^{12} —
— 10^{11} —
— 10^{10} —
— 10^{9} —
— 10^{8} —
— 10^{7} —
— 10^{6} —
— 10^{5} —
— 10^{4} —
— 10^{3} —
— 10^{2} —
—60 hertz—
— 10^{1} —

— 10^{15} —
— 10^{14} —
— 10^{13} —
— 10^{12} —
— 10^{11} —
— 10^{10} —
— 10^{9} —
— 10^{8} —
— 10^{7} —
— 10^{6} —
— 10^{5} —
— 10^{4} —
— 10^{3} —
— 10^{2} —
— 10^{1} —
— 1 —
— 10 —
— 10^{2} —
— 10^{3} —
— 10^{4} —
— 10^{5} —
— 10^{6} —
— 10^{7} —

Figure 70–10 This illustrates the point that the higher the frequency, the shorter the wavelength. The wavelengths are infinitely long at the bottom and infinitesimally short at the top of the spectrum so, obviously, the drawing cannot be done to scale.

fluorescent lights, electric pencil sharpeners, and video display terminals. Workshop sources include battery chargers, drills, power saws, and electric screwdrivers (while charging). Additional sources are electric blankets and electric power lines.[63]

POTENTIAL CARCINOGENICITY

Current Status

During the past 20 years a number of studies have suggested an increased risk of cancer induced by electromagnetic fields.[64–66] A news report on nonionizing irradiation is published in the United Kingdom.[67] Potential confounders of such studies include socioeconomic status, benzene associated with traffic density, ionizing radiation, trauma (brain), cigarette smoking, solvent exposures, sun rays, and household exposure to pesticides, herbicides, and other substances. Parental occupational confounders include exposure to polychlorinated biphenyls, naphthalene, epoxy resins, rubber, solder fumes, varnishes, solvents, machine oil, platinum, and tellurium. Other problems with these studies have been addressed.[68]

Reviews of cancer studies and electromagnetic fields (overhead power lines) indicate that there is no firm evidence of the existence of a carcinogenic hazard from exposure of paternal gonads, the fetus, children, or adults to the extremely low frequency electromagnetic fields that might be associated with residences near major sources of electricity supply, the use of electrical appliances, or work in the electronic and telecommunication industries.[69–71]

INFRARED RADIATION

Infrared radiation (IR) falls between microwaves and visible light in the electromagnetic spectrum. The biologic effects associated with IR exposure revolve around its ability to heat tissue at relatively high field intensity levels (>100 mW/cm^2). The eye is particularly sensitive to IR, especially at wavelengths between 750 and 1500 nm. Corneal, iritic, and lenticular lesions have been observed in experimental studies. The prevalence rates of subcapsular, cuneiform, and nuclear cataracts were found to be elevated among glassworkers exposed to IR when compared with rates in an unexposed group. This condition, also known as "glassblower's cataract," has been recognized for some time as an effect of occupational IR exposure. Most accidents involving the eyes occur during setup or alignment procedures when appropriate eye goggles are not worn. The threshold limit value for occupational exposure to IR has been set at 10 mW/cm^2 at wavelengths of more than 770 nm.[72]

LASERS

The term of "laser" is an acronym. It stands for "Light Amplification by Stimulated Emission of Radiation." Thus the laser is a device that produces and amplifies light. The mechanism by which this is accomplished, stimulated emission, was postulated by Einstein in 1917. Lasers vary greatly in output power, from a few milliwatts in the helium-neon gas laser, to thousands of watts in the carbon dioxide gas laser. Lasers are capable of operating continuously or in pulses with millions of watts of power in each pulse.[59]

Properties of Laser Light

1. Divergence: When light emerges from the laser, it does not diverge (spread) very much at all. Thus the energy

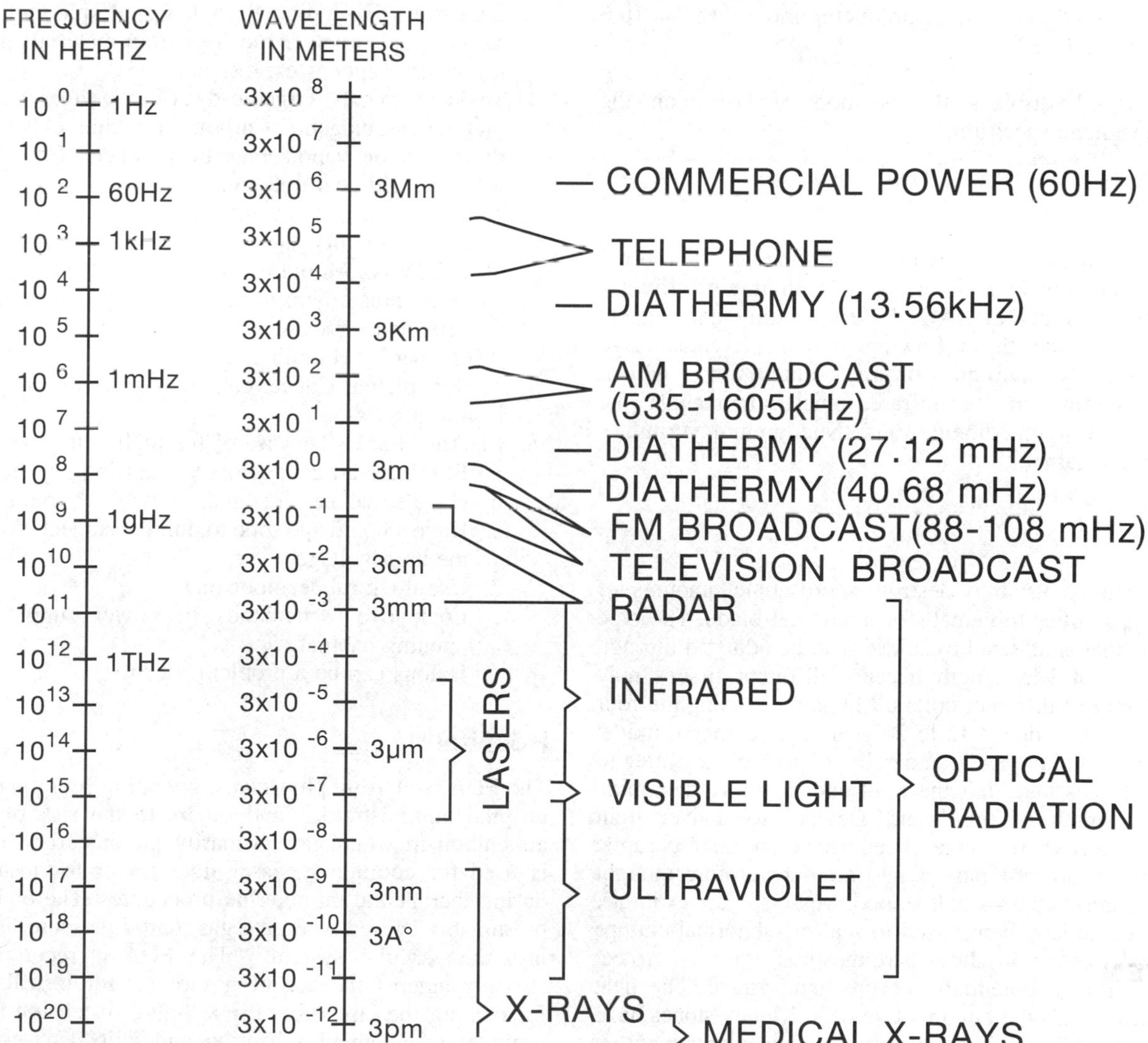

Figure 70–11 The electromagnetic spectrum. (Adapted from Hughes R. University of Southern California.)

is not greatly dissipated as the beam travels. Laser beam divergence is measured in milliradians or 1×10^{-3} radians. There are two radians in a circle, so one milliradian equals about 3 minutes of arc. A typical He-Ne laser has a rated divergence of 0.5 to 1.5 milliradians.

2. Monochromaticity: Laser light is very close to being monochromatic. The term "monochromatic" means one color, or one wavelength, of light. Actually, very few lasers produce only one wavelength of light. A typical He-Ne laser emits light at 632-638 nm, which is orange-red, and at 1150 nm and 3390 nm in the near and middle infrared regions. The He-Ne laser is usually designed to emit only one of the three wavelengths of light, and the variation in this wavelength is slight.
3. Coherence: Coherence is a term used to describe particular relationships between two waveforms. Two waves with the same frequency, phase, amplitude, and direction are termed spatially coherent. No source of perfectly spatial coherent light is yet known; however, laser light comes so close that for most practical purposes it can be considered perfectly coherent.
4. High Intensity: Laser light can be very intense. The sun emits about 7×10^3 W/cm^2/Sr/um at its surface. Lasers are presently capable of producing more than 1×10^{10} W/cm^2/Sr/um.[59]

Figure 70–11 displays the position of lasers on the electromagnetic spectrum.[73]

Types[74]

Lasers emitting in the ultraviolet region include the following: excimer (excited dimer), and Neodymium:yttrium - aluminum - garnet (Nd:YAG). Lasers emitting in the visible spectrum include the following: Argon, Krypton, Dye Lasers, and Neodymium:yttrium - aluminum - garnet. Lasers emitting in the infrared spectrum include the following: Carbon dioxide and Neodymium:yttrium - aluminum - garnet.[74]

Uses[75]

Lasers can be used to destroy microscopic amounts of tissue—quantities too small for a surgical blade. The type of tissue that is affected by a laser can be adjusted through the choice of wavelength because different tissues may absorb light of different colors. Medicine is using the four basic lasers introduced 15 to 20 years ago: carbon dioxide, argon, neodymium/YAG, and ruby. (These names refer to the substances that emit the light and therefore determine the wavelength of the laser.) Devices to deliver light virtually anywhere have been developed. Fiberoptic bundles can now be passed into areas heretofore thought of as unreachable—small blood vessels, for example. Lasers are already being used to seal off abnormal clumps of blood vessels in the gastrointestinal tract to protect patients from a potentially severe hemorrhage. The heat of the laser seals the abnormal vessels. Kidney stones have also been disintegrated with lasers. Laser treatment is cheaper than the shock-wave procedure and can be used to reach some stones on which shock waves cannot be used. Abnormal growth of blood vessels in the retina, a common complication of diabetes, can be treated by laser beams, which can also be used to create channels for the drainage of fluid from an eye with glaucoma. The newest target for lasers is the arterial plaque of atherosclerosis. The hope is to cut away an area of plaque by threading a fiberoptic tube into the artery and then firing a laser through it. Passing a catheter complete with fiberoptics and a laser channel into a coronary artery is feasible. The difficulty has been in how to hit a moving target. By sending out pulsed energy thousands of times a second and monitoring the reflection and fluorescence of each pulse, the laser should be able to distinguish between normal and abnormal tissue. The process can be repeated many times a second until the entire plaque is gone.[75]

Hazards

1. Radiation. Most lasers have high voltage power supply exceeding 15,000 volts.
2. Fire. Exploding flash lamps may ignite alcohol in the dye. CO_2 lasers ignite materials in the sheet covering the patient.
3. Explosion. Exploding flash lamps. Exploding energy storage capacitors. Explosions from materials processing where vapor is explosive.
4. Toxic chemicals. Organic dyes can be toxic; IR dyes may be carcinogenic. Carbon monoxide, chloride, and fluorine toxic vapors may be produced from cutting, welding, and heat treating.
5. Nonlaser optical radiations (e.g., a fluorescence out of side walls of tube and b argon ion laser—significant ultraviolet comes out of the side) can lead to sunburn.
6. Acoustic noise: Nuisance. Some lasers are loud when they fire and some are named after the noise they make: "Thumper," "Humdinger."
7. Tumor splatter: Cancer cells may spread during vaporization process.
8. Electric shock—because of the high voltage
   a. Eliminate all conductors worn, (dog tags etc.).
   b. Have someone on standby with CPR training.
   c. Have a board and rope to pull the subject away from the high voltage.
   d. Use thick rubber floor mats.
   e. Look over schematics of power supply before opening cabinet.
   f. Halons can be a problem for fires.

Hospital

The FDA is alerting physicians, operating room personnel, hospital administrators, and others to the risk of gas or air embolism when gas, primarily air or carbon dioxide, is used for cooling the laser fiber tip or for insufflation during therapeutic intrauterine procedures. The emboli are presumably caused when the gas, under pressure, is forced into the vascular system.[76] The FDA is recommending strongly against the use of gas or air for insufflation or for cooling the laser fiber tip. A liquid distension medium provides adequate visualization and will also serve as a cooling agent for the tip.[77]

Clinical Presentation

Most accidents occur during setup or alignment procedures when goggles are not worn. Laser radiation may be either absorbed, scattered, or reflected from biologic tissues. In most cases a combination of all of these effects occurs. However, the biologic effect is caused only by absorption. From approximately 280 nm to 3.0 μm in the infrared, reflection may exceed 10%, and significant penetration will also occur, such that scattering may play an important role in determining the final exposure to the target tissue.[66]

The Eye

For visible and IR-A radiation, the eye is generally the most critical organ in terms of vulnerability to laser radiation. A retinal injury that occurs in the macula, the most central sensitive area of the retina, is serious and will be immediately apparent to the victim. Injury to the paramacula or peripheral retinal region may have only a minimal effect on vision and in many cases may go undetected by the victim. In some instances limited visual recovery can be observed after limited macular injury, but such recovery may not occur for many months following exposure.

Infrared radiation of wavelengths greater than 1.4 μm can cause thermal injury to the cornea and conjunctiva. The biologic response to ultraviolet laser radiation is similar to that produced by noncoherent UVR (ultraviolet radiation) sources. Photophobia, tearing, conjunctival discharge, surface exfoliation, and stromal haze are the expected consequences of exposure to these lasers. Damage to the corneal epithelium probably results from the photochemical denaturation of proteins. In the UVC (100 nm to 280 nm) and UVB (280 nm to 315 nm) regions, photokeratitis may be produced. Photokeratitis usually has a latency period varying from 80 minutes to as long as 20 hours depending inversely on the severity of the exposure. A sensation of sand in the eyes accompanied by various degrees of photophobia, lacrimation, and blepharospasm is the usual result. In the UVA region (315 nm to 400 nm) photokeratitis may be produced only by chronic high-level exposure.

Skin

The biologic consequences of irradiating the skin with laser radiation are considered to be less than those to the eye, since skin damage is often repairable or reversible. On the other hand, exposure of the skin to high levels of optical radiation can cause depigmentation, severe burns, and possible damage to underlying organs. The aperture assumed for skin exposure measurements is 1 mm with the purpose of limiting the exposed areas.

The effects of UVR laser radiation on the skin are the same as for UVR from conventional sources: erythema from acute exposure and accelerated skin aging and skin cancer from chronic exposure. Our knowledge of UVR dose-effect relationships in man is insufficient and further studies are necessary, especially epidemiologic studies of UVR carcinogenesis.

THE ANTIPERSONNEL LASER

Antipersonnel lasers have been promoted as "dazzle guns," producing temporary visual loss through dazzle or bleaching of photopigments without permanent injury. Under daylight conditions it is questionable whether reversible blinding can occur without risk of permanent injury. However, it is on this basis that antipersonnel lasers have been introduced into the armed forces. Examples are the Royal Navy Laser Dazzle Gun and antipersonnel rifles developed by the U.S. Department of Defense under the Dazer and Cobra programs.[78]

Laser Safety Equipment Suppliers

Laser Safety Eyewear

Fish-Schurman Corp, Inc.
P.O. Box 319
New Rochelle, NY 10802-0319
(914) 636-1300

Fred Reed Optical Co.
P.O. Box 1336
Bryn Mawr SE
Albuquerque, NM 87103
(505) 265-3531

Glendale Optical Co., Inc.
130 Crossways Park Drive
Woodbury, NY 11797
(516) 921-5800

Phase -R
Old Bay Road
P.O. Box G-2
New Durham, NH 03855
(603) 859-3800

Spectra Optics
12317 Gladstone Avenue
Sylmar, CA 91342
(213) 361-0949

(Single or multiple frequency)

Uvex Winter Optical, Inc.
10 Thurber Blvd
Smithfield, RI 02917-1896
(401) 232-1200

(Filter and frame guaranteed to withstand 10 sec or 100 pulses)

Laser Safety and Interlock Systems

Molectron Corporation
177 North Wolfe Road
Sunnyvale, CA 94086
(408) 738-2661

Safety Equipment and Screens for Work Area

Glendale Optical Co., Inc.
130 Crossways Park Drive
Woodbury, NY 11797
(516) 921-5800

Warning Signs and Labels

Rockwell Associates, Inc.
P.O. Box 43018
Cincinnati, OH 45243
(513) 271-1568

Laser Safety Software

High-Rez Diagnostics, Inc.
260 Clark Way
Angwin, CA 94508
(707) 965-3574

Suggested Reading

1. Thompson C. Laser tackles bone. Lancet 1995;345:1001.
2. Healing with light. Harvard Medical School Letter 1988; 13:3–5.

3. Sliney DH, Bosnjakovic B, Court LA, McKinlay AF, Szabo LD, Coppee GH. The Use of Lasers in the Workplace. Occupational Safety and Health Series No. 68. International Non-ionizing Radiation Committee of the International Radiation Protection Association and the International Labour Organization, 1993, Geneva.
4. Gelb AF. Lasers in pulmonary treatment. West J Med 1990; 153:70–71.
5. Nightingale SL. Warning about gas/air embolism during intrauterine laser surgery. JAMA 1990;264:168.
6. Edmunds D. Laser protective eyewear: determining the correct lens. Occup Health Safety, July/August 1994;31–34.
7. Patlak M. Light for sight. Lasers beginning to solve vision problems. FDA Consumer 1990;24:15–17.
8. Lewis R. Erasing skin marks with lasers. FDA Consumer 1992;26:23–26.
9. Excimer laser 1991. Lancet 1991;338:730–731 (editorial).
10. Tanner M. Increasing use, power of lasers make eye protection essential. Occup Health Safety, July 1990;44–45.
11. American National Standards Institute. May 23, 1989. 3rd printing. September 1989. AN SI Z136.1-1986. The Laser Institute of America, 12424 Research Parkway, Orlando, FL 32826.

MAGNETIC RESONANCE IMAGING

In 1946 Felix Block and Edward Purcell first demonstrated the nuclear magnetic resonance principle, and they jointly received the Nobel Prize for Physics in 1952 for their discoveries. The device consists of a main magnet system, magnetic gradient coil assemblies, radio frequency coil assemblies, associated power supplies, filters, amplifiers, signal analysis, display, recording, storage and communication equipment, and patient support and positioning equipment, as well as physiologic motion gating and compensating devices and accessories. The main (static) magnetic field is generated by either a permanent magnet, a resistive magnet, or a superconducting magnet.

USES

Electromagnetic signals are acquired from the body using nuclear magnetic resonance phenomena with a static magnetic field, gradient magnetic fields, and radiofrequency magnetic fields. Computers process this information and present an image, a spectrum, or localized nuclear magnetic resonance parameter data. Various imaging techniques and spectroscopy acquisition protocols are used.

CLINICAL PRESENTATION[65,79]

Risks

Risks to health include the following:

1. Adverse effects of whole or partial body exposure to the static magnetic field.
2. Adverse effects of exposure to time-varying magnetic fields.
3. Adverse effects of absorption of energy from radiofrequency magnetic fields.
4. Hazards from high acoustic noise levels.
5. Hazards from laser beams.
6. Electrical and mechanical hazards.
7. Insufficient image or spectral quality resulting in reduced clinical utility.

STATIC MAGNETIC FIELDS

The static magnetic field produced by the main magnet determines the resonant radiofrequency of the nuclei of interest. No adverse effects are expected from whole-body exposure or exposure of the head to magnetic fields with strength of 2 tesla or less for a period of 1 hour or less.

TIME-VARYING MAGNETIC FIELDS

Time-varying magnetic fields (dB/dt) occur during switching of the magnetic gradients used for spatial localization of the acquired NMR signal. Many thousands of patients have been exposed to such limited strength time-varying magnetic fields without exhibiting deleterious effects attributable to these fields.

RADIOFREQUENCY MAGNETIC FIELDS

Radiofrequency magnetic fields occur at the resonant frequency of the nuclei of interest. Radiofrequency energy absorption in the patient may cause systemic thermal overload and local thermal injury. Radiofrequency power deposition may cause heating around metallic implants, tattoos, or permanent eyeliner. These risks can be controlled by placing appropriate warnings in the labeling.

HIGH ACOUSTIC NOISE LEVELS

High acoustic noise levels may be generated on pulsing of the electrical current energizing the gradient coils. Acoustic noise may be annoying, cause discomfort, or beyond certain levels be hazardous. These risks can be reduced by following a standard that limits acoustic noise to levels below the occupational limits recommended by the American Conference of Governmental Industrial Hygienists for exposures of up to 1 hour per day or below the permissible time-averaged and peak noise exposure given by the Occupational Safety and Health Association.

LASER SYSTEM

A laser system may be used in patient positioning. A laser has the potential for causing permanent eye injury, although no such injury has been reported.

ELECTRICAL AND MECHANICAL HAZARDS

Potential electrical and mechanical hazards can be controlled by a standard that requires that devices have adequate design specifications and adherence to good design practices.

OTHER POTENTIAL HAZARDS

The field near the magnet, that is, the fringe field, may be strong enough to attract ferromagnetic objects such as tools with great force, causing a collision. This potentially hazardous situation can be controlled by placing warning statements in the labeling such as warnings to restrict access to only authorized personnel and to require in-place procedures for emergency services of patients in areas where the fringe field is weaker. The field in or near the magnet may fatally interfere with the operation of devices such as cardiac pacemakers. The static magnetic field may move or dislodge ferromagnetic materials within the patient's body such as intracranial aneurysm clips, shrapnel fragments, and prostheses constructed of ferromagnetic material, each of which could cause life-threatening situations. Prompted by a recent magnetic resonance (MR) imaging-related death of a patient with an intracranial aneurysm clip, the U.S. Food and Drug Administration (FDA) is urging physicians to be especially cautions in ordering or performing MR imaging in patients who have these implants.[80] There is no way to be certain that a patient with one of these clips can be safely imaged. The physician and the patient should be aware that there is still a risk of serious complications from magnetic interactions with the aneurysm clip. Because there is no established method for testing the magnetic properties of aneurysm clips, manufacturers cannot positively ensure that clips will not be affected by the MR field.[80]

FETUSES AND INFANTS

Special concerns arise when scanning fetuses or infants who are particularly susceptible to thermal overload and require careful monitoring for signs of cardiocirculatory and respiratory distress.

LIQUID HELIUM, NITROGEN CRYOGENS

Liquid helium and nitrogen cryogens are used to cool the superconducting wire in a superconducting magnet. Some boil-off of the gases occurs during normal operation. If the magnet quenches, the boil-off rate of the cryogens will increase and gas could suddenly be released into the room causing asphyxiation of site personnel or patients.

CLAUSTROPHOBIA

Due to the configuration of the system and the length of the examination, some patients become claustrophobic.[67]

CONTRAINDICATIONS

Magnetic resonance imaging entails a strong static magnetic field and changing magnetic and radiofrequency fields. Problems arise from any metal objects present in the body. With magnetic resonance imaging, the whole body is in the magnetic field, and sensitive organs cannot be "screened" as they can in most techniques that use ionizing radiation.[81] Cleaners, engineers, and anyone accompanying the patient during imaging are subject to the same risks: nobody known or suspected of harboring any hazardous object should come near the imager.

A cardiac pacemaker, the best known contraindication to entry to a magnetic resonance imaging suite, may be moved in the tissues by the electromagnetic fields or be irreversibly switched from demand to fixed rate operation. The intracardiac wires of even a nonfunctioning pacemaker could cause arrhythmias. Some devices with magnetically or electronically operated switches such as cochlear implants, neurostimulators, implanted infusion pumps, and ventricular shunt valves, whose opening pressure can be changed transcutaneously, are also contraindications to magnetic resonance imaging. Detachable objects such as magnetic stoma plugs and dental implants should be removed before imaging. Ocular prostheses may, however, have permanently implanted magnets, which, like those used with some radiotherapeutic implants, may be moved or demagnetized.

Static hardware, including most of that used for orthopedic and spinal work (with the exception of halo fixation devices), does not contraindicate magnetic resonance imaging; the procedure should, however, be stopped if patients experience pain in the region of large implants. Ventricular shunts used to treat hydrocephalus and most hemostatic clips do not pose problems. Magnet imaging should be deferred for at least 6 weeks after metal clips are applied to the fallopian tubes and in patients with the intravascular coils, stents, and filters that are increasingly used by interventional radiologists to allow their firm incorporation into the vessel. Nonmagnetic dental implants are harmless as are intrauterine and diaphragm contraceptive devices. Some penile and inflatable breast implants may, however, be hazardous. Prosthetic heart valves are compatible with magnetic resonance imaging, although they were originally believed not to be so. Metal fragments introduced accidentally, including pellets, bullets, or shrapnel, may be a contraindication, particularly soon after introduction.[81] Shellock and colleagues have provided a comprehensive list of metallic implants, material, devices, or objects and their movement or deflection during exposure to static magnetic fields.[82]

ULTRASOUND

Ultrasound is the mechanical vibration of an elastic medium that is produced in the form of alternating compressions and expansions. The vibration may be produced by continuous or impulse sound in the form of a sequel of interrupted vibrations. The medical uses of ultrasound include therapeutic, surgical, and diagnostic procedures.

A comparison of x-rays or gamma rays, microwaves, radar and diathermy, and ultrasound is summarized in Table 70.26. Ultrasound does not produce tissue ionization.[83] No epidemiologic studies up to the present time indicate that diagnostic ultrasound results in any measurable or significant biologic effects.

MICROWAVE RADAR

PHYSICS

Microwave field intensity is described by both electric field strengths (volts per minute) and power density (milliwatts per square centimeter). Microwaves encompass a range of electromagnetic nonionizing radiation whose energy levels and tissue penetration depend on wavelength. All radar systems, microwave ovens, diathermy machines, and a variety of industrial heat sources produce specific wavelengths of microwave energy to achieve their effects.

CLINICAL PRESENTATION

Although exposure to ultrasound does not appear to pose a human health risk, exposure to audible high-frequency

Table 70–27
Ultraviolet Spectrum[a]

Radiation Band[b]	Description	Spectrum	Comments
UV-A	Long-wave, near UV, blacklight	Short-wave UV-A, 320 to 340 nm Long-wave UV-A, 340 to 400 nm	Virtually no UV-A absorbed by ozone layer; biologic effects of short- and long-wave UV-A differ in both animals and humans
UV-B	Middle UV, "sunburn" radiation	290 to 320 nm	Substantial portion absorbed in the ozone layer
UV-C	Short-wave, far UV, germicidal radiation	Below 290 nm	Absorbed by ozone layer in atmosphere; has no role in photobiology of natural sunlight.

[a]Adapted from Council on Scientific Affairs. JAMA 1989;262:380–384.
[b]UV indicates ultraviolet; UV-A, ultraviolet A radiation; UV-B, ultraviolet B radiation; and UV-C, ultraviolet C radiation.

radiation above 10 kHz can result in a syndrome involving nausea, headaches, tinnitus, pain, dizziness, and fatigue. Temporary hearing loss and threshold shifts are also possible from high-frequency ultrasound radiation.

Low-frequency ultrasound radiation may produce local effects when a person touches parts of materials being processed by ultrasound. The hands are often involved in the area where ultrasound acts most strongly. Exposure to powerful sources of ultrasound may result in damage to peripheral nervous and vascular structures at the points of contact. Airborne ultrasound vibration may produce effects on the central nervous system and on other systems and organs through the ear and through extra-auditory routes.[2]

Microwave interference with cardiac pacemakers has resulted in shielding of current devices. Hypogonadism occurred in a man exposed to a very high level of microwaves. Lenticular opacities have been associated with short- and long-term exposures.[84]

ULTRAVIOLET (TABLES 70–27 AND 70–28)

ERYTHEMA AND SUNBURN

A personal history of sunburning, peeling, and the ability to tan may be useful to help classify people of different ethnic backgrounds into six sun-reactive types, although a recent study concludes that self-reported burning-tanning histories may be unreliable as a means of skin typing. Ultraviolet B radiation (UV-B), particularly the shorter wavelengths, is most efficient in causing erythema and sunburn. All ultraviolet A radiation (UV-A) also can cause erythema, but levels 800 to 1000 times higher than those of UV-B are required.

TANNING

Two different types of tanning occur in response to UVR exposure: so-called immediate tanning, which is more correctly termed *immediate pigment darkening,* and delayed tanning. Immediate pigment darkening is a transient grayish brown discoloration of the skin induced by UV-A and exposure to certain visible light wavelengths. It begins during exposure and is maximal at the end of the radiation period. Persistence of the effect depends on the duration of

Table 70–28
Classification of Sun-Reactive Skin Types[a]

Skin Type	History of Sunburning or Tanning[b]
I	Always burns easily, never tans
II	Always burns easily, tans minimally
III	Burns moderately, tans gradually and uniformly (light brown)
IV	Burns minimally, always tans well (moderate brown)
V	Rarely burns, tans profusely (dark brown)
VI	Never burns, deeply pigmented (black)

[a]Adapted from Council on Scientific Affairs. JAMA 1989;262:380–384.
[b]Based on first 45 to 60 minutes of sun exposure after winter with no sun exposure.

exposure; immediate pigment darkening will begin fading within minutes following a short exposure, but will last more than 36 hours after prolonged exposure to high-intensity UV-A. The darker the natural skin and previously acquired tan, the more pronounced the response.[85]

Delayed tanning occurs 48 to 72 hours following UVR exposure, peaks in 7 to 10 days, and persists for several weeks to months. It can be maintained by repeated exposure to UVR.[85] Both UV-A and UV-B induce delayed tanning, but the levels of radiation needed are quite different. Considerably larger doses of UV-A than UV-B are required.[86]

Ultraviolet A radiation is not uniformly effective in producing a tan. Ultraviolet A sunbeds generally produce a tan in people who tan well in sunlight (sun-reactive skin types III and over), but those who tan poorly or not at all or who are burnt easily by the sun (skin types I and II) are likely to be disappointed with the cosmetic results.

SUNBEDS[87]

People taking drugs or applying cosmetics with photosensitizing potential and who then use ultraviolet A sunbeds may develop a photosensitivity reaction. Sunbeds can also cause the common photodermatosis polymorphous light eruption—a transient, irritating, papular reaction—and they exacerbate light-aggravated dermatoses such as systemic lupus erythematosus. Immunologic changes, both cutaneous and systemic, have been seen after exposure to ultraviolet radiation from a sunbed. Excessive use of ultraviolet A sunbeds produces increased skin fragility and blistering. It may also cause melanocytic lesions with malignant potential.

PHOTODAMAGE (PHOTOAGING)

Although UV-B is responsible for much of the dermal connective-tissue destruction in the photoaging process, high-intensity UV-A (315-400 nm) can cause vasodilation accompanied by endothelial cell enlargement, mast cell hypogranulation, and fibrin deposition; intercellular and intracellular edema with a decrease in the number of Langerhans cells; and elastosis. However, although UV-A penetrates deeper into the dermis than UV-B, the elastosis caused by UV-A is less dense than that produced by UV-B; also, at wavelengths of 340 to 400 nm (peak emission, 365 nm), only mild elastic fiber hyperplasia occurs. Other effects related to photoaging include the development of actinic keratoses (solar keratoses). Actinic keratoses are most common in older people, but may be seen in younger individuals exposed to sunlight over a prolonged period (e.g., beach lifeguards, outdoor laborers, farmers, and sailors). Blacks are seldom affected.[86]

Other solar-induced skin changes include cutis rhomboidalis nuchae, a severe form of skin wrinkling that occurs on the posterior portion of the neck; visible facial telangiectasias, especially on the cheeks, nose, and ears; and increased vascular fragility of the skin.[86]

CARCINOGENS

Ultraviolet radiation (UVR) is a complete carcinogen, acting at all three of the major recognized stages of carcinogenesis—initiation, promotion, and progression.[88]

PHOTOCARCINOGENESIS

The most common skin cancer in the United States is basal cell carcinoma. It occurs with greatest frequency in men who spend much time outdoors and who may posses other high-risk characteristics such as type I skin.[86] Another common skin cancer in whites is squamous cell carcinoma. Some forms of human squamous cell carcinoma may be related to skin exposure. The incidence of cutaneous malignant melanoma (CMM) has markedly increased. A history of sunburn is significantly more common in individuals with CMM. There is a markedly lower incidence of CMM in races with deeply pigmented skin than in whites.

There are essentially no data in humans to suggest that even shorter wavelength UV-A causes carcinoma; an exception is that UV-A combined with oral psoralen (psoralen-UV-A therapy) significantly increases the risk of squamous cell carcinoma and keratoacanthoma, particularly in those individuals with type I skin. Likewise, there is little or no evidence that UV-A alone causes actinic keratosis, basal cell epithelioma, or contributes to the development of malignant melanoma in humans. Nevertheless, there is increasing evidence that the occurrence of skin cancer in humans may be related to changes in the immune system in the skin, and all UVR, including UV-A, affects the immune system.

MELANOMA[89]

In 1990 it was predicted that 27,600 people in the United States would develop melanoma and 6300 die from it. One in 120 Americans can expect to develop this cancer during his or her lifetime—a twelvefold increase since the 1930s, when the figure was only 1 in 1500. Although depletion of the ozone in the stratosphere will increase the rate of squamous- and basal-cell skin cancers, its effect on melanoma is unclear.

Data suggest that the use of ultraviolet A sunbeds is a weak risk factor in inducing melanoma. The British Photodermatology Group has therefore recommended that the use of ultraviolet A sunbeds for cosmetic tanning should be discouraged. In particular, several groups should not use them at all: children under 16; people who burn easily, do not tan, or tan poorly; those taking drugs or using cosmetics thought to be photoactive; those suffering from a skin disorder induced or aggravated by exposure to sunlight; those with a history of skin cancer; and those with risk factors for cutaneous melanoma. The risk factors include more than 20 benign pigmented nevi above 2 mm in diameter; a tendency to freckle; clinically atypical nevi; a history of severe sunburn, particularly in childhood or adolescence; and a family history of cutaneous melanoma.

People with fair skin, blond or red hair, or marked freckling in the upper back are more likely to get melanoma. Also at increased risk are people who have actinic keratoses, usually developing after age 40. Merely living closer to the equator, which increases exposure to ultraviolet light, may be a predisposing factor. Total sun exposure over one's lifetime should be factored into the overall estimate of risk.

FLUORESCENT LIGHTS[90]

Compared with natural ultraviolet B radiation, fluorescent lighting is unlikely to be a significant factor in the induction of skin cancer by ultraviolet B radiation.[91]

PHOTOEFFECTS ON THE EYE

Excessive exposure to UVR may result in erythema and sunburn of the eyelids. In conditions such as aphakia or pseudoaphakia, in which ultraviolet absorption does not occur in the lens, retinal damage is more likely. The UV-A spectrum at which retinal damage may occur is between 325 and 441 nm.

PHOTOIMMUNOLOGY

There is indirect evidence in humans that the immune system is involved in cutaneous carcinogenesis, since organ transplant recipients undergoing immunosuppressive therapy appear to be at much greater risk of skin cancer than the normal population.[86]

PHOTOTOXICITY AND PHOTOALLERGY (TABLE 70–29)

One form of chemical photosensitivity, referred to as "phototoxicity," does not depend on an immunologic response in that the reaction can occur on first exposure to the offending material. Most phototoxic agents are activated in the range of 320 to 400 nm.[86]

Another type of chemical photosensitivity, photoallergy, differs from phototoxicity in that it is an acquired altered reactivity of the skin that is dependent on antigen-,

Table 70–29
Phototoxicity and Photoallergy[a]

Characteristic	Phototoxic	Photoallergic
Incidence	Potentially a high proportion of those exposed	Generally a low proportion
Dose dependency (of both drug and light)	+	–
Reaction on first exposure	+	–
Latency after exposure	Minutes to several hours	One to a few days
Cross reaction with structurally related sensitizers	–	++
Clinical features	Resembles sunburn with tingling and burning proceeding to erythema ± edema ± vesiculation. Well localized to sun-exposed areas	More variable morphology. May be eczematous or papular or, rarely, lichenoid. Less well localized
Subsequent pigmentation	++	+
Persistent light reaction	–	++
Histology	Epidermal necrosis Dermo-epidermal junctional separation Sparse superficial lymphohistiocytic infiltrate	Epidermal spongiosis Edema of papillary dermis Deep and superficial lymphocytic infiltrate

[a]Adapted from Smith AG. Adverse Drug React Bull 1989, No. 136, p. 509.

antibody-, or cell-mediated hypersensitivity. It is manifested clinically as urticaria (hives) or dermatitis.

Individuals using medications or using topical agents known to be sensitizing should avoid sun exposure altogether, if possible, and absolutely shun any form of UV-A from artificial sources.

PHOTOPROTECTIVE MEASURES

Skin

Sunscreens

In addition to wearing protective clothing or staying out of the sun and not using tanning devices, the primary method of mitigating the harmful effects of UVR is the use of sunscreens. There are two types of topical sunscreens: (a) chemical sunscreens that provide protection by absorbing UVR, and (b) physical sunscreens that block UVR from reaching the skin. Ultraviolet-absorbing preparations may contain one or more chemical entities in a carrier base; these are formulated as clear or milky lotions, gels, creams, or ointments and are intended to be applied as a thin film to exposed skin. Depending on the chemicals used, a sun protective factor of 2 to 50 can be achieved.[86]

The physical sunscreens contain materials such as zinc oxide, talc, or titanium dioxide in an ointment base. These preparations scatter both ultraviolet and visible radiation and thus are opaque to all wavelengths of light. They are effective and useful in protecting selected areas of the body (e.g., nose, cheeks, and shoulders) if applied thickly, but they may be cosmetically unappealing.

Sunscreens should be used daily on sun-exposed skin by individuals habitually exposed to the sun, by people with skin types I and II, and by those who are hypersensitive to sunlight. Frequent use of sunscreens should become a standard procedure for children. Bald-headed men should apply sunscreens to the exposed area regularly. Additional applications should be made following swimming, after exercise that has caused profuse sweating, or when clothing or beach towels have rubbed off part of the original application. One application a day usually is not sufficient.

Prevention of Severe Burning and Eye Damage

Minimize Exposure to UVR

The effects of the sun are greatest between 10 AM and 2 PM; therefore plan outdoor activities in the morning or late afternoon. Wear a hat and protective clothing while outdoors.

Beware of Reflective Surfaces

Sand, snow, ice, and concrete reflect from 10% to more than 50% of the sun's rays.

Use a Sunscreen

For individuals with skin types I to III, sunscreens with a sun protection factor of 15 and light-screening lipsticks are usually adequate to prevent burning. Preparations with a higher sun protection factor can be used, if indicated, particularly at high elevations. Use a sunscreen on cloudy, overcast, or hazy days, as well as on sunny days. People at high risk (fair-skinned individuals, outdoor workers, and persons who have had skin cancer) should use sunscreen more liberally than the average population.

Protecting Infants and Children

Keep infants out of the sun as much as possible and apply a sunscreen when children are to be outdoors for prolonged periods (the U.S. Food and Drug Administration recommends that use of sunscreens containing aminobenzoic acid be avoided in infants younger than 6 months). Begin teaching children sun protection early in life, since damage begins with the first exposure and accumulates over a lifetime.

Avoid Tanning Machines

Exposure to UVR in a tanning booth may increase the risk of skin cancer. If individuals tan poorly and burn easily in sunlight, they also will not tan and may burn in a tanning booth. People with type I skin and those who already have solar keratoses, severe reactions to sunlight, or a history of skin cancer should never use tanning devices. Such devices are especially hazardous if photosensitizing medications are being used.

If tanning equipment is used, those who tan moderately well should limit their exposure to 30 to 50 half-hour sessions per year or less (30 minimal erythemic doses). The device must be properly calibrated and have a timer that has not been tampered with by the owner or the client. Ideally, one should keep a record of the total number of joules of exposure just as those individuals who work with ionizing radiation keep a record of the dose-equivalent in sieverts they receive over a given period. Protective goggles containing yellow glass lenses that absorb all UV-A, UV-B, and visible light up to 500 nm should be worn; simply closing the eyes, using regular sunglasses, or putting cotton balls over the eyes may not protect against eye damage. Finally, when using a tanning machine, an attendant should always be nearby to help in any emergency.[86]

EYE (TABLE 70–30)

Cataracts

Most of the ultraviolet radiation is filtered out by the cornea, and only wavelengths of 295 nm or greater pass through, but the lens absorbs nearly all the ultraviolet from 295 nm to 400 nm, and the high prevalence of cataracts in countries with hot climates has meant that the harmful effect of ultraviolet radiation has long been suspected. Absorbing ultraviolet radiation from sunlight is an important risk factor in forming cataracts.[92]

Ocular exposure to ultraviolet B can be reduced by half by wearing a hat with a brim and wearing ordinary glasses with plastic lenses may reduce it to about 5%. Thus to minimize ocular exposure to ultraviolet B, people should be advised to wear a hat with a brim and close-fitting sunglasses with ultraviolet B–absorbing lenses at times of maximal exposure to sunlight.[93]

ULTRAVIOLET

Sun Protection[94,95]

1. Apply an effective sunscreen generously to exposed skin. Remember to use the sunscreen consistently.
2. Reapply the sunscreen after swimming, bathing, or heavy sweating.
3. Wear sunglasses that block out ultraviolet rays (wrap-around sunglasses are the best). A broad-brimmed hat can decrease eye exposure to sunlight up to 50%.
4. Use sunscreens when sitting under a beach umbrella or protective awning. White sand can reflect up to 20 to 25% of the sun's rays, while fresh snow, aluminum, or white surfaces may reflect 70 to 85%.
5. Sunlight can penetrate water up to several feet, so swimmers and snorkelers can get a sunburn even while swimming in cool water. When the sun is directly overhead, water can act like a mirror, reflecting up to 95% of the sun's rays.
6. For every 1000 feet of elevation above sea level, there is a 4% increase in ultraviolet light exposure since there is less atmosphere to absorb the sun's rays.
7. The ozone layer over the equator is thinner and more UV-B rays reach the earth's surface.
8. Try to avoid going out in the sun between the hours of 10:00 AM and 2:00 PM (11:00 AM to 3:00 PM daylight savings time).
9. Do not forget that ultraviolet rays are invisible.
10. When driving a truck or car, keep the driver's window closed, since window glass will block out most of the UV-B rays contained in sunlight.
11. Wear tightly-woven, light-colored clothing to shield your skin from the sun.
12. Avoid tanning booths, sunbeds, and sunlamps, since they produce ultraviolet rays that damage your skin.
13. Keep infants under 6 months of age out of the sun. Teach your children to protect their skin and eyes from the sun's rays.

Table 70–30
Eye Effects of Ultraviolet

Keratitis solaris
Cataract—cortical cataract
Keratitis photoelectrics
Macular degeneration
Photokeratitis
Erythropsin
Actinic keratitis
Cystic macular edema after cataract surgery
Aging of receptors
Loss of photoreception sensitivity (after chronic exposure to UV)

OZONE

The absorption of ultraviolet radiation by stratospheric ozone (O_2) is crucial to the protection of living organisms. About 3% of the sun's electromagnetic output is emitted as UV radiation, but only a fraction reaches the surface of the earth. UV-C in the 240 to 290 nm range is virtually eliminated by ozone, and only a proportion of UV-B (290 to 320 nm) penetrates the terrestrial environment. Because UV-B and UV-C span the photoabsorption spectrum of DNA, ozone is crucial to the viability of primitive life forms, particularly in aquatic ecosystems, and in human beings it greatly limits the carcinogenic impact of solar radiation. Plant photosynthesis, too, is intimately linked to ambient levels of O_2, O_3, and solar radiation.[96]

SUNGLASSES[86]

The New Ratings[97,98]

The Sunglass Association of America, in cooperation with the U.S. FDA, adopted a voluntary program in 1990 to provide information about light absorption of sunglass lenses. The rating system was developed in 1986 by the American National Standards Institute (ANSI). The tag on any pair of nonprescription sunglasses distributed under the new program states that it meets or exceeds "ANSI Z80.3" requirements for one of three categories: cosmetic, general purpose, or special purpose. The new labels also state the percentage of UV-A and UV-B light absorbed by lenses. UV-A light is closest to the visible spectrum. UV-B has a shorter wavelength, is more energetic, and has the greatest potential to cause injury. Protection from sun damage depends mainly on the absorption of UV-B.

Cosmetic lenses absorb at least 70% of UV-B and 20% of UV-A, and they absorb less than 60% of visible light. Such lenses are appropriately worn for comfort rather than protection in really bright sunlight.

General-purpose lenses absorb at least 95% of UV-B and 60% of UV-A, and they absorb 60 to 92% of visible light. They are recommended for most outdoor activities in temperate regions.

Special purpose lenses block at least 99% of UV-B, 60% of UV-A, and 20 to 97% of visible light. They are advisable for activity in highly reflective environments—bright sun combined with sand, snow, or water.

Sunglasses that absorb "UV up to 400 nm" block all ultraviolet light. Purchasers of prescription lenses can ask for information about ultraviolet absorption.

VISUAL DISPLAY TERMINAL (VDT)

CLINICAL PRESENTATION

In the late 1970s to early 1980s, it was suggested that three types of adverse health effects were caused by working with a visual display terminal (VDT): cataracts, adverse pregnancy outcomes, and skin rashes. Initial concerns were primarily focused on radiation such as x-rays or UVR. These were dismissed because of the very low or nonexistent exposure levels of these radiations. The majority of epidemiologic studies have failed to demonstrate an increased occurrence of spontaneous abortion and malformed children in relation to VDT use.

Visual display terminals do not cause permanent ocular damage, but the use of these terminals, often combined with a change in work routine, may be associated with ocular and general musculoskeletal discomfort. These can be alleviated by having the worker's reading glasses checked for proper working distance; by paying adequate attention to ergonomic factors such as having seating and angle of the VDT adjustable to each worker's comfort needs; by adjusting the lighting to minimize glare; by using high-quality monitors whose contrast and brightness can be controlled by the operator; and by making provisions for periodic rest breaks.

Any individual with eye symptoms related to VDT use should have a complete eye examination by an ophthalmologist.[99]

Discomfort with use of visual display terminals such as aches, smarting, gritty feeling, itching, sensitivity to light, teariness, and dryness may be caused by older age, use of glasses, and low relative humidity.

SEIZURES

Seizures have been induced by playing video games. This appears to be similar to television-induced seizures, which have been well recognized in epileptic patients who are sensitive to flickering lights or geometric patterns.[100] Photosensitive epilepsy occurs in approximately 1 to 3% of patients with epilepsy (1 in 10,000 of the general population) and is commonly manifested by generalized tonic–clonic seizures that occur while the patient is watching television.[101,102]

PHYSICS

A survey of the literature suggests that computer monitors do not emit microwaves. Some companies have done a brisk business selling lead-lined aprons to worried computer operators who believe that the radiation given off by monitors is the same as that given off by dental and medical x-rays. Fear of possible radiation effects has sometimes caused VDT operators to consider protective devices such as special aprons or radiation shields. These are of no value because they are designed either to shield radiographers from x-rays, which VDTs do not emit, or to minimize low-level electromagnetic fields, which are not regarded as hazardous in any case.

The magnetic fields cannot be stopped by lead aprons, concrete walls, so-called radiation shields or glare guards that fit over the screen of the monitor, or other barriers. The best precaution against high levels of exposure to these fields is simply to sit at least an arm's length from the front of a computer monitor and at least 3 or 4 feet away from the sides and backs of nearby monitors.

Radiation and fields emitted from the VDT include optical radiations: ultraviolet radiation (UVR), visible radiation, and infrared (IR) radiation. Inside the cathode ray tube, soft x-rays are produced, but the glass prevents any emission of x-rays from VDTs.

Ultraviolet Radiation (UVR)

UV-A (long-wavelength UVR) radiation can be detected from certain VDTs. The levels are, however, insignificant compared with the present general population and occupational standards, and also insignificant compared with emission from other sources (e.g., sunlight through windows).

Light

Visible radiation is emitted and is necessary to perform the intended function of the VDTs—to provide a visual display. Luminance levels are adjustable to the comfort of the operators and are far below current exposure limits.

Infrared Radiation (IR)

IR is emitted from all bodies. Since all surfaces of the VDT are at room temperature or slightly above, IR can be detected, although at levels far below any limits of concern for health.

Low-Frequency Electromagnetic Fields

In the radiofrequency (very low frequency, VLF) range and extremely low frequency (ELF) field range, electric and magnetic fields can be measured. The dominant sources are the power supply (at 50/60 Hz) and the horizontal and vertical sweep generators (at frequencies of 15 to 35 kHz and 50 to 80 Hz, respectively). These fields do not represent any risk factor when compared with current IRPA/INIRC general population or occupational guidelines. Epidemiologic studies have generally failed to show an association between the use of VDTs emitting those fields and various health problems that have been suggested as due to those fields. Attempts to relate health hazards to explicitly measured fields emanating from VDTs have also been unsuccessful.

Electrostatic Fields, Air Ions

Electrostatic fields at VDT workplaces have been suggested as a possible cause of skin disorders. The magnitudes of electrostatic fields are greater in the environment of VDT operators than for office workers without VDT work. This may, in turn, cause changes in light air ion concentrations. No correlations between electrostatic fields from the VDTs or air ions at operator positions and skin problems have, however, been found.

Ultrasound

Airborne ultrasonic (acoustic) radiation is produced in CRTs as a result of mechanical vibrations generated in the core of the flyback transformer (responsible for the horizontal sweep of 15 to 35 kHz). The sound pressure levels found are considerably below existing general public and occupational limits of exposure levels. Some individuals may detect this or a subharmonic in the higher noise frequency region as an annoying factor.[103]

RADON PROGENY

Recent reports indicate that VDTs can collect radon progeny from the air. Although some radioactivity may be released during the cycle, room air currents redistribute it into the room with no detectable levels being inhaled by users.[104]

CONCLUSIONS

No association has been found between radiation emissions from VDTs and reported spontaneous abortions, birth defects, cataracts, or other injuries.[103,105–110] Representative equipment has been monitored for all forms of electromagnetic and other emissions, and the levels have been below presently accepted standards of exposure.[111] The levels of most radiations and electromagnetic fields emitted from VDTs are much less than those from natural sources such as the sun or even the human body, and all are well below levels considered harmful by expert bodies such as the International Radiation Protection Association and the World Health Organization. Radiation emissions from VDTs are not considered to be harmful to health.

GUIDELINES FOR HEALTH CARE WORKERS[112]

NIOSH studies have resulted in a report titled *Potential Health Effects of Video Display Terminals* (NIOSH 1981h), which contains specific recommendations for the installation, maintenance, and use of VDTs.

1. Workstation design: VDT units, supporting tables, and operator chairs should be designed with maximum flexibility. VDTs should have detachable keyboards, and work tables should be adjustable for height. Chairs should be adjustable for height and should provide proper back support.
2. Illumination: Sources of glare should be controlled through VDT placement (i.e., parallel to windows, and parallel to and between lights), proper lighting, and the use of glare-control devices on the VDT screen surface. For VDT tasks requiring screen-intensive work, illumination levels should be lower than those needed when working with hard copy, which may require local lighting in addition to normal office lighting.
3. Work regimens: Continuous work with VDTs should be interrupted periodically by rest breaks or other work activities that do not produce visual fatigue or muscular tension. As a minimum, a break should be taken after 2 hours of continuous VDT work. Breaks should be more frequent as visual, mental, and muscular burdens increase.
4. Vision testing: VDT workers should have visual testing before beginning VDT work and periodically thereafter to ensure that they have adequately corrected vision to handle such work.[15]

REFERENCES—RADIATION POISONING

1. Wald N. Ionizing radiation. ATSDR October 1993.
2. Guidelines for protecting the safety and health of health care workers. US Dept of Health and Human Services. September 1988; DHHS (NIOSH) Publication No. 88-119. pp. 5–71.
3. Leonard RB, Ricks RC. Emergency department radiation accident protocol. Ann Emerg Med 1980;9:462–470.
4. Whalen JP, Balter S. Radiation risks associated with diagnostic radiology. Disease-A-Works, Yearbook, 1982; pp. 1–92.
5. Pearson R. Radiography in women of childbearing ability. Br Med J 1989;299:1175–1176.
6. Swartz HM, Reichling BA. Hazards of radiation exposure for pregnant women. JAMA 1978;239:1907–1908.
7. Upfal M, Sanat JM. Radon toxicity. ATSDR Case Studies in Environmental Medicine 14. September 1992.
8. Woolf AD. Radon. Clin Toxicol Rev 1991;43:1–2.
9. Brill AB, Becker DV, Donahoe K, Goldsmith SJ, Greenspan B, Kase K et al. Radon update: facts concerning environmental radon: levels, mitigation strategies, dosimetry, effects and guidelines. J Nucl Med 1994;35:368–385.
10. Leary WE. Studies raise doubts about need to lower home radon levels. New York Times, September 6, 1994;27, B7.
11. A Citizen's Guide to Radon. 2nd ed. The Guide to Protecting Yourself and Your Family From Radon. United States Environmental Protection Agency. Air and Radiation (ANR-464), May, 1994. NCRP Report No 103. Control of Radon in Houses. Bethesda, MD: National Council on Radiation Protection and Measurements.
12. McLaughlin JR, King WD, Anderson TW, Clarke EA, Ashmore JP. Paternal radiation exposure and leukaemia in offspring. The Ontario case-control study. Br Med J 1993; 307:959–966.
13. Godlee F. Sellafield cancer link "fragile" says HSE. Br Med J 1993;307:1096.
14. Lushbaugh CC. Keynote address: radiation accidents worldwide. An additional decade of experience. In: Ricks RC, Fry SA, eds. The medical basis for radiation accident preparedness II. New York: Elsevier, pp. xxxv-xxxix.
15. Becker DV. Reactor accidents. Public health strategies and their medical implications. JAMA 1987;258;649–654.
16. Hatch MC, Beyena J, Nieves JW, Susser M. Cancer near the Three Mile Island nuclear plant: radiation emissions. Am J Epidemiol 1990;132:397–412.

17. Jablon S, Hrubec Z, Boice JD Jr, Stone BJ. Cancer in populations living near nuclear facilities. Volume for Report and Survey. National Cancer Institutes NIH Publication No. 90-874, July 1990; pp. 1–96.
18. Liebow AA, Warren S, DeCoursey E. Pathology of atomic bomb casualties. Am J Pathol 1947;25:853–1028.
19. Liebow AA. Encounter with disaster—a medical diary of Hiroshima, 1945. Yale J Biol Med 1965;38:61–239.
20. Keller PD. A clinical syndrome following exposure to atomic bomb explosions. JAMA 1946;131:504–506.
21. Randall T. A lean mean cyclotron revs up neutron therapy. JAMA 1992;267:614–616.
22. NRCP Report No. 38. Protection Against Neutron Radiation. Washington, DC: January 4, 1971.
23. Henshaw DL, Eatough JP, Richardson RB. Radon as a causative factor in induction of myeloid leukemias and other cancers. Lancet 1990;335:1008–1012.
24. Llewellyn C. Medical aspects of thermonuclear disasters. In: Reis MD, Dolve E, eds. Manual of disaster medicine. Civilian and military. Berlin: Springer-Verlag, 1989; pp. 124–148.
25. Gofman JW. Radiation-induced cancer from low-dose exposure: an independent analysis. San Francisco Committee for Nuclear Responsibility, 1990.
26. Marwick C. More studies pending of low-dose radiation. JAMA 1990;264:944.
27. Marwick C. Low-dose radiation: latent data renew questions of "safe" level. JAMA 1990;264:553–554.
28. Yalow RS. Concerns with low-level ionizing radiation. Mayo Clin Proc 1994;69:436–440.
29. Mountford PJ, Coakley AJ. Radioactive patients. Patients given radioactive substances represent a small risk to others. Br Med J 1989;298:1538–1539.
30. Mountford PJ, Coakley AJ. Guidelines for breast feeding following maternal pharmaceutical administration. Nuclear Med Comm 1986;7:399–401.
31. Berger ME, Thompson DW, Ricks RC, Kaufmann D. The medical technologist and the radiation-accident victim. Am J Med Technol 1981;47:831–834.
32. Bloomer WD, Hellman S. Normal tissue responses to radiation therapy. N Engl J Med 1975;293:80–83.
33. Brahan D. Radiotherapy overdose. Lancet 1988;2:975.
34. Polish RA. Prediction of radiation-related small bowel damage. Radiology 1980;135:219–221.
35. Jiang GL, Tucker SL, Guttenberger R, Peters LJ, Morrison WH, Garden AS et al. Radiation-induced injury to the visual pathway. Radiotherap Oncol 1994;30:17–25.
36. Bevers RFM, Bakker DJ, Kurth KH. Hyperbaric oxygen treatment for hemorrhagic radiation cystitis. Lancet 1995;346: 803–805.
37. Pottern LM, Kaplan MM, Larsen PR, Silva JE, Koenig RJ, Lubin JH et al. Thyroid nodularity after childhood irradiatin for lymphoid hyperplasia: a comparison of questionnaire and clinical findings. J Clin Epidemiol 1990;43:449–460.
38. Leith JT, Hercbergs AA. Radiation-induced breast cancer: long-term follow-up of radiation therapy for benign breast disease. J Natl Cancer Inst 1994;86:393–394.
39. Morris JGL, Grattan-Smith P, Panegyres PK, O'Neill P, Soo YG, Langlands AO. Delayed cerebral radiation necrosis. Q J Med 1994;87:119–129.
40. Malapert D, Brugieres P, Degos JD. Motor neurone syndrome in the arms after radiation treatment. Thorax 1991;54
41. Gibson PG, Bryant DH, Morgan GW, Yeates M, Fernandez V, Penny R et al. Radiation-induced lung injury: A hypersensitivity pneumonitis? Ann Intern Med 1988;109:288–291.
42. Phillips TL. Radiation injury. In: Wyngaarden JB, Smith LH Jr, eds. Cecil textbook of medicine. 18th ed. Philadelphia: WB Saunders, 1988; pp. 2375–2378.
43. De Neve W, Fortan L, Storme G. Increased mucosal and cutaneous epus radiation toxicity in two patients taking amiodarone. Int J Radiat Oncol Biol Phys 1992;22:224.
44. Vanek N, Horotobagyi GN, Buzden AV. Radiotherapy enhances the toxicity of aminoglutethimide. Med Pediatr Oncol 1990;18:162–164.
45. Ramakrishnas S, Macleod P, Tyrrell CJ. Acute radiation skin reaction and persistent photosensitivity after benoxapropon. Lancet 1988;2:913.
46. Shelley WB, Shelley ED, Campbell EAC, Weigensberg IJ. drug eruptions presenting at sites of prior radiation damage (sunlight and electronic beam). J Am Acad Dermatol 1984; 11:53–57.
47. Boivin J-T. Second cancers and other late side effects of cancer treatment. A review. Cancer 1990;65:770–775.
48. Curtis RE, Boise JD Jr, Stovall M, Bernstein L, Greenberg RS, Flannery JT et al. Risk of leukemia after chemotherapy and radiation treatment for breast cancer. N Engl J Med 1992;326:1745–1751.
49. Weber E, Laarbai F, Michel L, Donckier J. Abdominal pain: do not forget Thorotrast! Postgrad Med J 1995;7: 367–369.
50. Geiger HJ. The accident at Chernobyl and the medical response. JAMA 1986;256:609–612.
51. US and IAEA Chernobyl delegations assess radiation effects. J Nuclear Med 1991;32:11N–13N.
52. Linnemann RE. Soviet medical response to the Chernobyl nuclear accident. JAMA 1987;258:637–643.
53. Finch SC. Acute radiation syndrome. JAMA 1987;258: 164–167.
54. Rich V. New hazard at Chernobyl. Lancet 1994;343:108.
55. Boice J, Linet M. Chernobyl, childhood cancer, chromosome 21. Probably nothing to worry about. Br Med J 1994;309: 139–140.
56. Kingman S. Thyroid cancer increases around Chernobyl. Br Med J 1993;307:1230.
57. Furmanchuk AW, Averkin JI, Egloff B, Ruchti C, Abelin T, Schappi W. Korotkevich EA. Pathomorphological findings in thyroid cancers of children from the Republic of Belarus: a study of 86 cases occurring between 1986 ("post-Chernobyl") and 1991. Histopathology 1992;21: 401–408.
58. EMF in your environment. Magnetic field measurements of everyday electrical devices. US Environmental Protection Agency. 402-R-92008, December 1992.
59. Hughes RS. Laser safety. Principles of laser action. University of Southern California Institute of Safety and Systems Management Professional Program, 1990.
60. Extremely low frequency (ELF) fields. Environmental Health Criteria 35. Geneva: World Health Organization, 1984.
61. Magnetic Fields. Environmental Health Criteria 69. Geneva: World Health Organization, 1987.
62. Harvard Medical School Health Letter 1990;15(8):1–4.
63. Saritz DA, Pearce NE, Pook C. Methodological issues in the epidemiology of electromagnetic fields and cancer. Epidemiol Rev 1989;11:59–78.
64. Savitz DA, Calle EZ. Leukemia and occupational exposure to electromagnetic fields: review of epidemiologic surveys. J Occup Med 1987;20:47–51.
65. Herring A. Hazards of magnetic resonance imaging. Lancet 1991;337:1477.
66. The Use of Lasers in the Workplace. A Practical Guide. Occupational Safety and Health Series No. 68. Geneva: International Labour Office, 1993; pp. 49–56.
67. Magnetic Resonance Diagnostic Panel. Panel recommendations and report on petitions for MR reclassification. Fed Reg 1988;53:7575–7579.
68. Jauchem JR. Potential confounders in epidemiologic studies of electric and magnetic fields and childhood leukemia. Environ Carino Ectox Revs 1993;11:163–183.
69. Connor S. No risk of cancer from electromagnetic fields. Br Med J 1992;304:938–939.
70. Draper G. Electromagnetic fields and childhood cancer. No causal relation has been established. Br Med J 1993;307: 884–885.
71. Feychting M, Ahlbom A. Magnetic fields and cancer in children residing near Swedish high-voltage power lines. Am J Epidemiol 1993;138:467–481.
72. Hoffman DA. Biologic effects of infrared radiation. JAMA 1988;260:703.
73. Performance Standards for Light-emitting Products. Code of Federal Regulations. H1. Part 1040.10 (Laser Products), April 1, 1995; pp. 344–360.
74. Council on Scientific Affairs. Lasers in medicine and surgery. JAMA 1986;256:900–907.

75. Healing with light. Harvard Medical School Health Letter, February 1988;13(4):3–5.
76. Nightingale SL. Warning about gas/air embolism during intrauterine laser surgery. JAMA 1990;264:168.
77. Pathak MA, Fitzpatrick TB, Greiter FJ, Kraus EW. Principles of photoprotection in sunburn and suntanning and topical and systemic photoprotection in health and diseases. J Dermatol Surg Oncol 1985;1:575–579.
78. Gillow JT. Another weapon too far: the anti-personnel laser. J R Soc Med 1995;88:347P–340P.
79. Chalmers JWT, Maclean IH, Breen DA. Hazards of magnetic resonance imaging. Lancet 1991;237:1477.
80. Johnson GC. Need for caution during MRI imaging of patients with aneurysm clips. Radiology 1993;188:287–288.
81. Moseley I. Safety and magnetic resonance imaging. Avoid imaging patients with metal objects in their body. Br Med J 1994;308:1181–1182.
82. Shellock FG, Morisoli S, Kanal E. MR procedures and biomedical implants, materials and devices: 1993 update. Radiology 1993;189:587–599.
83. Brent RL: X-ray, microwave and ultrasound: the real and the unreal hazards. Pediatr Ann 1989;9:43–47.
84. Forman SA. Sublethal exposure to microwave radar. JAMA 1988;259:3129.
85. Council on Scientific Affairs. Harmful effects of ultraviolet radiation. JAMA 1989;262:380–384.
86. Harvard Medical School Health Letter 1990;15(9):3
87. Diffey BL. Tanning with ultraviolet A sunbeds. Should be discouraged. Br Med J 1990;301:773–774.
88. Choo V. Ultraviolet radiation and carcinogenesis. Lancet 1994;344:1499.
89. The melanoma epidemic. Harvard Medical School Health Letter 1990;15:1–3.
90. Walter SD, Manrett LD, Shannon HS. From Hertzman C: The association of cutaneous malignant melanoma and fluorescent light fixtures. Am J Epidemiol 1992;135:749–762.
91. Griffiths AP, Fairney A. Fluorescent lights, ultraviolet lamps and cutaneous melanoma. Br Med J 1988;297:1041.
92. Cheng H: Causes of cataract. Age, sugars and probably ultraviolet B radiation. Br Med J 1989;298:1470–1471.
93. Taylor HR, West SK, Rosenthal FS, Munoz B, Newland HS, Abbey H, Emmett EA. Effect of ultraviolet radiation on cataract formation. N Engl J Med 1988;319:1429–1433.
94. Hendricks WM. Sun protection. NCMJ 1989;50:435–440.
95. Hendricks WM. How much sun is enough? NCMJ 1989;50:272–273.
96. Jones PR. Ozone depletion and cancer risk. Lancet 1987;2:443–446.
97. Pitts DG. Threat of ultraviolet radiation to the eye—how to protect against it. J Am Optom Assoc 1981;52:949–957.
98. McDonagh AF, Nguyen ML. Spectacles, ultraviolet radiation and formation of cataracts. N Engl J Med 1989;321:1478–1479.
99. Secretariat for Governmental Relations and Public Information Committee. American Academy of Ophthalmology. Video display terminals (VDTs) and the eye, July 1984.
100. Dahlquist NR, Mellinger JF, Klass DW. Hazard of video games in patients with light-sensitive epilepsy. JAMA 1983;249:776–777.
101. Hart EJ. Nintendo epilepsy. N Engl J Med 1990;322:1473.
102. Harding GFA. Video-game epilepsy. Lancet 1994;344:1710.
103. Knave B, Repacholi M, Stolwijk J, Stuchly M, Bergqvist U. Visual Display Units: Radiation Protection Guidance. Occupational Safety and Health Series 70. Geneva: International Labour Office, 1994.
104. Ziegler JF, Zabel TH, Curtis HW. Video display terminals and radon. Health Phys 1993;65:252–264.
105. Schnorr TM, Grajewski BA, Murray WE, Hornung RW. Magnetic fields of video display terminals and spontaneous abortion. Am J Epidemiol 1993;138:902–903.
106. Bentur Y. Ionizing and nonionization radiation in pregnancy. In: Koren G, ed. Maternal-fetal toxicology. New York: Marcel Dekker, 1990; pp. 205–251.
107. Perry G, Weissenberger DI, Milroy WC, Clever LH, Ducatman AM, Anstadt GW et al. VDT exposure and pregnant workers. J Occup Med 1991;33:675–676.
108. Schnorr TM, Grajewski BA, Hornung RW, Thun MJ, Egeland GM, Murray WE et al. Video display terminals and the risk of spontaneous abortion. N Engl J Med 1991;324:727–733.
109. Schnorr TM. The NIOSH study of reproductive outcomes among video display terminal operators. Reprod Toxicol 1990;4:61–65.
110. Bergqvist UO, Knave BG. Eye discomfort and work with visual display terminals. Scand J Work Environ Health 1994;20:27–33.
111. Council on Scientific Affairs. Health effects of video display terminals. JAMA 1987;257:1508–1510.
112. Guidelines for Protecting the Safety and Health of Health Care Workers. US Department of Health and Human Services. DHHS (NIOSH) Publication No. 88-119, pp. 5-72, 5-73.

Chapter 71
Veterinary Product Poisonings in Man

PHARMACEUTICAL PRODUCTS

Veterinary pharmaceutical products have been used by man to induce suicide,[1–5] in suicide attempts,[5–8] and for pain treatment.[9–12] Many who attempt suicide with veterinary euthanasia agents are employed in the veterinary profession. There have also been occasional reports of ingestions of antibiotics in cat food,[13] of antiprotozoal products mixed with flour (some fatal),[14] of dog heart tablets with a theophylline analog,[7] and of a beta-blocker added to animal feed.[15] Finally, accidental human exposures occur with organophosphorus insecticides used for veterinary purposes.[16–19] An increase in spontaneous abortions appears to follow exposure by female veterinarians to radiographic examinations.[20] Most states do not require child-resistant packaging for prescription veterinary medicines.

STRUCTURE AND CLASSIFICATION

Veterinary pharmaceutical products that have been involved in induction of human poisoning include those commonly used for veterinary euthanasia (Table 71–1),[5] nonsteroidal antiinflammatory drugs (equine phenylbutazone,[9–11] flunixin meglumine),[12] antibiotics (penicillin),[13] antiprotozoans (monensin sodium),[14] etamphylline,[7] and clenbuterol (added to animal feed).[15] Frequent exposure to radiographic examinations appears to be a risk factor in the induction of spontaneous abortions in female veterinarians.[20] Organophosphorus insecticides are a frequent toxic exposure source for the veterinarian.[16,17]

DOSAGE
Barbiturates (Table 71–1)

A veterinarian was found dead after ingesting about 1500 mg of a veterinary euthanasia preparation (Toxital) containing pentobarbital (178 mg/mL) in a 50% propylene glycol base, in addition to ethanol.[1] A veterinary assistant was found dead clutching a 50-mL syringe with an intravenous line from the syringe that entered the left antecubital fossa. Approximately 40 mL of the drug, twice the recommended lethal dose for animals, had been injected.[2] A 17-year-old was found with a partially emptied syringe still inserted in his right antecubital fossa. The

Table 71–1
Products Commonly Used for Veterinary Euthanasia[a]

Brand Name	Manufacturer	Ingredients
Beuthanasia-D Special	Burns-Biotec	390 mg/mL Na pentobarbital 50 mg/mL phenytoin 18% propylene glycol 10% alcohol
Euthanasia Solution	Med-Tech	325 mg/mL Na pentobarbital Propylene/glycol Alcohol
Fatal	North American Pharmacal	325 mg/mL Na pentobarbital Propylene glycol Alcohol
Lethal	Eli Lilly	260 mg/mL Na pentobarbital Isopropanol 20% polyethylene glycol-200
Repose	Diamond	400 mg/mL secobarbital 50 mg mephenesin 10% propylene glycol
Sleepaway	Fort Dodge	260 mg/mL Na pentobarbital 10% isopropanol 20% propylene glycol
Socumb	The Butler Company	360 mg/mL Na pentobarbital 31.2% isopropanol 2.38% propylene glycol
T-61	American Hoechst	200 mg/mL embutramide [b] 50 mg/mL mebezonium[c] 5 mg/mL tetracaine 0.6 mL dimethylformamide/ mL T-61

[a]Adapted from Cordell WH et al. Ann Emerg Med 1986;15:939–943.
[b]*N*-[2-(m-methoxy phenyl)-2-ethyl-butyl-(1)]-gamma-hydroxy-butyramide.
[c]4,4,-methylene-*bis* (cyclohexyl-trimethyl-ammonium iodide).

veterinary euthanasia used was a multidose vial of Socumb (Table 71–1) containing pentobarbital, 360 mg/mL. The patient later died. [5] A suicide was attempted by a 29-year-old woman who ingested another veterinary euthanasia drug, Sleepaway, containing pentobarbital, isopropanol, and propylene glycol (Table 71–1) in addition to drinking wine. She survived.[5] Fifty milliliters of sodium pentobarbital (65 mg/L) was ingested together with 15 mL of T-61 (see T-61). She survived.[5]

Phenylbutazone

Phenylbutazone is probably the most frequently used nonsteroidal antiinflammatory agent in equine medicine. It is often referred to as "bute" by racetrack personnel such as jockeys, grooms, and trainers who take it for muscle aches and bruises.[9] An adult race horse track worker ingested equine phenylbutazone (1 g/tablet) for 3 months. He survived.[9] A jockey ingested 2 g of equine phenylbutazone (1 g/tablet) for 3 days and died.[10] A greyhound racing dog handler ingested 17 g of equine phenylbutazone over a period of 24 hours and survived.[11]

Flunixin meglumine (Banamine)

An adult ingested 250 mg of flunixin meglumine was found in coma, regained consciousness in 24 hours, and survived.[12]

VETERINARY FOOD POISONING

Penicillin

An 11-month-old child with a prior history of eating cat food ate cat food with a high penicillin content and died with a hypersensitivity type myocarditis.[13]

Ingestion of an antiprotozoal, anticoccidian chicken food additive, sodium monensin (a complex ester of butyric acid—$C_{36}H_{62}OI_{11}$), by seven people following its mistaken addition to wheat flour led to severe abdominal pain, nausea and vomiting, weakness, muscle cramps, and joint pains in five of the seven and death within 15 days of the other two patients.[14]

Clenbuterol

Clenbuterol, a veterinary and human beta-agonist, is used illicitly in animal feeding where it may induce regression of body lipids, muscle growth, and weight gain. Much of it accumulates in the liver where it may subsequently poison humans who ingest it.[15,21] In the United Kingdom, clenbuterol is licensed for use in respiratory disease in horses and cattle and to relax the uterus in cows at parturition. Some farmers have added clenbuterol to animal feed and several may have died after inhaling it.[21]

Detomidine

Detomidine hydrochloride is an $alpha_2$ adrenergic agonist similar to clonidine and xylazine used as a veterinary sedative. It has a plasma half-life of about 2.5 to 4 hours. The dose of detomidine required for anesthesia in horses is 40 to 80 μg/kg either IM or IV (5 to 6 mg IM/70 kg). An intramuscular injection of 50 mg in a 36-year-old man together with butorphanol led to sedation and signs of opiate poisoning that responded to naloxone.[22]

T-61

T-61 has been used for veterinary euthanasia in Germany since 1962 and in the United States since 1963.[5] T-61 (Table 71–1), a veterinary euthanasia product, contains embutramide (a general anesthetic), mebezonium iodide (a neuromuscular blocker), and tetracaine (a local anesthetic) in a dimethylformamide solvent (see Hydrocarbon section). In one suicide attempt a 20-year-old female injected 12 mL intramuscularly and survived.[6] Murder of a 7-year-old, a murder attempt of a 6-year-old, and a suicide attempt by a young mother occurred after injection of about 50 mL of T-61. The mother and 6-year-old survived.[8] A 37-year-old was found dead approximately 20 to 30 minutes after ingesting about 100 mL of T-61.[3] Ingestion of 5 mg (1 mL/kg) of T-61 together with clorazepate potassium 500 mg by an adult terminated fatally.[4] An adult ingested 15 mL of T-61 together with about 3250 mg of sodium pentobarbital. The patient survived.[5]

Tilmicosin (Micotil)

Tilmicosin is a veterinary antibiotic. Each milliliter of preconstituted solution contains 300 mg tilmicosin phosphate and 70% propylene glycol w/v. The Ontario Regional

Poison Information Centre in Toronto has collected 36 reports of accidental human exposure, most of whom were exposed to less than 1 mL mostly from needle punctures. Local symptoms (pain at site) predominate. Patients who may experience nausea or vomiting or respiratory difficulty within 30 minutes should be evaluated in a hospital. Treatment is supportive and symptomatic. Consider epinephrine for anaphylactic reactions, although epinephrine-tilmicosin interactions have not been evaluated.[23]

Etamphylline

A 15-year-old, in a suicide attempt, ingested her dog's heart tablets, containing approximately 12,100 mg of etamphylline camsylate, a xanthine compound similar in action to theophylline. Etamphylline is a bronchodilator estimated to have about one-fifth the strength of theophylline.[24,25] She survived.[7]

Radiation

Epidemiologic data suggest that female veterinarians who perform five or more radiographic examinations per week may be at an increased risk for spontaneous abortion.[20]

Organophosphorus Insecticides

A veterinarian technician was accidentally exposed (face, bare parts of body, clothes) to a commercial, canned product formulation containing an organophosphorus and carbamate insecticide, dichloromethane, 1,1-difluoroethane, and 1,1,1 trichloroethane as solvents. He survived.[17] In 1991 the Veterinary Medicine Directorate of the United Kingdom received 135 reports of adverse reactions following exposure to organophosphorus compounds in veterinary medicines (veterinary sheep dips). Accidental self-injection was the most frequently reported history.[26,27]

CLINICAL PRESENTATION

Acepromazine

Acepromazine maleate, an aliphatic phenothiazine structurally similar to chlorpromazine, is used as an aid in controlling intractable animals. It is available in 10 and 25 mg tablets. Overdose in humans presents with central nervous system dysfunction ranging from coma and sedation to extrapyramidal symptoms and seizures. Cardiovascular effects may include a sinus tachycardia, ventricular arrhythmias, intraventricular conduction delays, hypotension, miosis, hypothermia, hyperthermia, and pulmonary edema. Treatment is largely symptomatic and supportive.[28,29]

A 19-year-old veterinary assistant attempted suicide by ingestion of acepromazine 1.25 g. She became lethargic and deeply sedated. Pupils were normal; she was normotensive and exhibited a sinus tachycardia on the electrocardiogram. She was treated with ipecac, charcoal, and a cathartic and discharged in 36 hours.[30] A 2½-year-old ingested 75 to 100 mg of acepromazine used to calm a dog. The child developed marked sedation, tachycardia, and evidence of poor perfusion. Following supportive care the child recovered within 6 hours.[31]

Azaperone

Azaperone is a butyrophenone used as a sedative for animal handling. An adult ingested about 2 g of azaperone. Following identification by thin-layer chromatography and mass spectrometry the patient recovered in 2 days.[32]

Barbiturates

Three of the four patients who ingested or injected veterinary euthanasia preparations of pentobarbital were found dead.[1,2,5] The fourth became lethargic and then recovered.[5] Barbiturate solutions used in veterinary euthanasia frequently contain glycols such as propylene glycol. Toxic doses of propylene glycol can cause hyperosmolarity, acidosis, and CNS depression and may contribute to the toxicity of these solutions.

Equine Phenylbutazone

Signs of equine phenylbutazone intoxication in one patient included melena and a gastric bleeding ulcer with recovery in 4 weeks.[9] Pallor and ecchymosis were observed in a patient who ingested equine phenylbutazone and subsequently died of aplastic anemia.[10] Hypertension, grand mal seizures, renal and hepatic dysfunction, respiratory failure, and coma were seen in a patient who recovered after 6 weeks.[11]

Flunixin Meglumine (See Banamine)

Ingestion of Banamine granules for the relief of arthritic pain led to Cheyne-Stokes respiration, response only to deep pain, and hypertension. The patient was fully alert and neurologically intact 24 hours after ingestion and was discharged on day 3.[12]

VETERINARY FOOD POISONING

Penicillin

Consumption by an 11-month-old child of cat food with high levels of penicillin led to nausea, vomiting, fever (to 40°C), and death.[13]

Sodium Monensin

Seven people ate flour contaminated by sodium monensin used as an additive in chicken feed. They developed severe abdominal pain, nausea and vomiting, weakness, muscle cramps, and joint pains. Within 15 days two patients died.[14]

Clenbuterol

Ingestion by 195 patients of bovine liver contaminated by clenbuterol led to the onset of symptoms, following a period of between 30 minutes and 6 hours, consisting of muscle tremors, palpitations/tachycardia, nervousness, asphalgia, and myalgia lasting about 60 hours.[15] Symptoms have also included dizziness, nausea, vomiting, fever, and seizures and have appeared to cease spontaneously after about 48 hours.[33]

Closantel

Eleven Lithuanian women lost their eyesight after closantel, a veterinary antihelminthic supplied to Lithuania by donor agencies, was inadvertently prescribed for a gynecologic condition. The eyesight later returned, but eye pain persisted. The half-life of closantel in animals ranges from 3 to 28 days. The drug is 99% bound to plasma albumin.[34] Vacuolation of the optic nerve has been described. Plasmapheresis and activated charcoal may enhance elimination. The syndrome in animals has an inflammatory component. High-dose corticosteroids (up to 500 mg methylprednisolone IV for 5 days) may also be considered.[35]

T-61

Injections of T-61 have led to seizures, coma, respiratory arrest,[5,6,8] cyanosis of the mucous membranes, decreased deep tendon reflexes,[3,8] sinus bradycardia, hypotension, and constricted and nonreactive pupils. Pulmonary infiltrates and fever were observed in one patient who subsequently recovered.[5] Three of five patients who have been reported have died.[2,4,8] After regaining consciousness on the second day after ingesting T-61, a patient developed dizziness, epigastric pain, and vomiting on the fourth day. Jaundice, a flapping tremor, and hepatic fetor were observed on the sixth day. Coma and renal failure ensued before death occurred 9 days after the T-61 ingestion.[4]

Methimazole

Methimazole illicitly used in animal feeding as a weight enhancer has been associated with congenital scalp aplasia.[36]

Etamphylline

Etamphylline camsylate overdose led, within 45 minutes, to nausea, weakness of the lower limbs, a generalized coarse tremor, restlessness, hyperventilation, hypertension, olfactory hallucinations, seizures, cyanosis, and a sinus tachycardia. In 15 hours the patient was sufficiently recovered to await a psychiatric interview.[7]

Organophosphorus/carbamate Exposure

A veterinary technician who was splashed with an organophosphorus carbamate mixture developed headache, nausea, vomiting, diarrhea, and difficulty in breathing. These signs and symptoms remained for 4 days. Following a chemical pneumonia the patient was released on the thirteenth day.[17]

Hypersensitivity to Veterinary Drugs

Hypersensitivity in humans to products used in veterinary medicine includes reactions to penicillin (anaphylaxis), chloramphenicol (aplastic anemia), and levamisole (agranulocytosis).[33]

Bayo-N-Ox-1

This quinoline derivative (2-[*N*-2′hydroxyethyl-carbamoyl] 3-methyl-quinoxaline-1,4 dioxide) is used as a feed additive for the prevention of bacterial enteritis in pigs. Allergic contact dermatitis and photocontact dermatitis have been experienced by pig breeders using the product.[37,38]

Mail-Order Drugs—Carisoprodol

A 46-year-old adult became dependent on a veterinary carisoprodol product that she ordered over the counter through a veterinary mail-order outlet. Federal law does not restrict such sales from states that permit them.[39] Carlsoprodol is not legally classified as a drug of abuse.[40]

Spiramycin

Spiramycin, a macrolide antibiotic used by chick breeders, induced bronchial asthma and dermatitis in a nonatopic woman. Patch test showed a vigorous delayed reaction to the drug.[41] Asthma following exposure to this veterinary product was observed in an adult male employee of a pharmaceutical company.[42]

LABORATORY

A gas chromatography/mass spectrometry method is available for the quantification of embutramide in biologic material.[43]

Barbiturates

Following an ingestion of 1500 mg of pentobarbital, blood pentobarbital levels reached 15 mg/100 mL (fatal levels over 2 mg/100 mL) when the patient died.[1] Intravenous injection of pentobarbital and amobarbital product led to pentobarbital postmortem blood levels of 4.5 mg/100 mL.[2]

Phenylbutazone

Ingestion of equine phenylbutazone led to hematocrits of 18% following gastric ulcer bleeding,[9] bone marrow biopsy findings of a fatty marrow with nearly complete aplasia,[10] and serum phenylbutazone concentrations of 900 μg/mL (normal steady state 25 to 75 μg/mL).[11] Electrocardiogram findings have been generally restricted to a sinus tachycardia.

T-61

Increased values of liver function tests followed an injection of T-61 in a patient who survived.[6] Another patient who ingested T-61 with clorazepate potassium developed abnormal hepatic aminotransferase concentrations, abnormal coagulation parameters (prothrombin complex activity, Factor II, V, VII, and X, fibrinogen), and an elevation in serum creatinine with oliguria prior to death.[4] Embutramide blood levels taken postmortem have revealed levels of 31 ppm, with 17 ppm in the liver.[3]

Etamphylline

Overdose of etamphylline was accompanied by hypokalemia, sinus tachycardia, and an etamphylline concentration of 43 μg/mL (by an enzyme immunoassay technique—Syva, Palo Alto, CA).[7] The patient survived.

Organophosphorus Insecticides

Toxicity with organophosphorus insecticides is often accompanied by a sharp decrease in red blood cell acetylcholinesterase and plasma pseudocholinesterase values (see pesticide chapter).

TREATMENT

Barbiturates

Patients who have overdosed on veterinary euthanasia products should be hospitalized in an intensive care facility after emergency evaluation to ascertain adequate respiratory, airway, and circulatory status. Oxygen and cardiac monitoring should be available. Endotracheal intubation with mechanical ventilation may be required. The treatment of pentobarbital poisoning consists mainly of symptomatic and supportive care. If pentobarbital solution has been ingested, gastric lavage with endotracheal protection and administration of activated charcoal may be useful.

Elimination Enhancement

After massive overdoses of pentobarbital, and following continued deterioration despite supportive care, charcoal hemoperfusion may be effective, although this procedure is usually more effective for elimination of the longer acting barbiturates.

T-61

Supportive care would appear to be the mainstay of therapy. Seizures may be controlled with adequate oxygenation and diazepam. Musculoskeletal paralysis can be reversed with anticholinesterase agents such as pyridostigmine. Embutramide may produce a respiratory arrest from its CNS depressive actions. Decontamination of the gastrointestinal tract with gastric lavage, under tracheal protection, and activated charcoal may be useful. There is no evidence of hepatic glutathione depletion that could encourage use of acetylcysteine in patients with T-61–induced hepatotoxicity.

Phenylbutazone

Overdoses of equine phenylbutazone require symptomatic and supportive treatment. Gastric dysfunction may be ameliorated with H_2 receptor antagonists (cimetidine, ranitidine). Aplastic anemia will frequently require bone marrow transplants. Hemodialysis is probably ineffective (high protein binding, low water solubility). The value of hemoperfusion remains controversial, although it has been recommended for severe phenylbutazone poisoning.[28,29]

Organophosphorus—Solvents

Prompt showers and removal of contaminated clothing should be performed while preparations are made for specific therapy. Safety information should be printed on product containers. A toll-free telephone number to the product manufacturer's medical department should also be clearly printed on the product containers and on the package.

Antidotes

There are no antidotes for barbiturate, phenylbutazone, penicillin, or etamphyllin overdosages. Organophosphorus exposure may be ameliorated by atropine and oxime injection.

SELF-INOCULATION

Self-inoculations (autoinoculation) of veterinary vaccines may induce injury to biologic aides, veterinarians, animal caretakers, and biologic technicians[44] by physical tissue injury, direct toxicity, stimulation of host immune response, or infection.[45] Such self-inoculations usually occur when an inadequately restrained animal gives a sudden jerk during a vaccination procedure.[46]

Hazard Classes

The National Animal Disease Center (NADC), a U.S. Department of Agriculture Agricultural Research Service Laboratory, has classified etiologic agents according to risk assessment for laboratory and professional workers:

Class 1

Agents of no or minimal hazards under ordinary conditions of handling.

Class 2

Agents of ordinary potential hazard, which may produce disease of varying degrees of severity from accidental inoculation or injection or other means of cutaneous penetration, but which are contained by ordinary laboratory techniques.

Class 3

Agents involving special hazards that require special conditions for containment.

Class 4

Agents that require the most stringent conditions for containment because they are extremely hazardous to laboratory personnel or may cause serious epidemic disease in animals.[44]

Physical Injury

Physical injury by the entry of a needle to the tissues may penetrate nerves, blood vessels, or tendons, or if the needle has previously passed through animal tissue or another nonsterile field, it may introduce foreign bodies, infectious material, or both. Oil adjuvants in veterinary vaccines may induce vasospasm and ischemia, which can lead to loss of a finger.[44,47,48] The Veterinary Products Committee in the United Kingdom has advised that a warning should appear on all containers of oil-based injectable products to emphasize immediate care of accidental self-injections at an accident and emergency department.[49]

Direct Toxicity

Veterinary medications are usually prepared in conformity with strict governmental guidelines before they are approved for sale. Toxic effects are infrequent.

Immune Response

If a veterinary vaccine is accidentally self-inoculated to an individual previously exposed to the same organism, a hypersensitivity reaction may develop within a few hours characterized by local pain, redness, swelling, chills, and fever. Recovery occurs within several days.[50] The local area of irritation may undergo necrosis for some months. Antibiotics and steroids will usually be effective. Similar self-inoculation in a nonpreviously sensitized individual will produce a transient mild elevation of temperature after a latent period of a few days.[46]

Infection

Autoinoculations of 38 individuals were recorded during a 25-year-period by the NADC; three patients became infected. The organisms at highest exposure risk included *Brucella* sp., *Mycorbacteria* sp., and *Leptospira* sp. Of 419 cases of brucellosis reported to the Communicable Disease Center of the Public Health Laboratory Service between 1975 and 1979, veterinarians (37 cases) formed a highly susceptible group since they were at risk not only from a diseased animal but from exposure to live *B. abortus* strain 19 vaccine, the manufacture of which ceased by 1982.[51]

Veterinary Antiinfective Products Ingested Orally

A 14-year-old drank two glasses of milk from a gallon inoculated with 21 vials of live Newcastle Virus Vaccine intended to immunize baby chicks. The patient was asymptomatic for the next 28 days. Treatment was restricted to cathartics and observation. The patient survived.[52]

LABORATORY

Laboratory studies useful after self-inoculation of auto-infective biologic products should include repeated blood cultures, cultures of the wound site, an initial agglutination titer, and serial titers. Serum aminotransferases, creatine kinase, and lactic acid dehydrogenase levels should be obtained to follow hepatic function and muscle status.

TREATMENT

Treatment of hypersensitivity reactions will usually include an antibiotic and a steroid (e.g., prednisone). Non-hypersensitivity reactions should respond to symptomatic and supportive therapy and antibiotics (e.g., tetracycline for *Brucella* sp.). There are no antidotes. Veterinary surgeons who handle vaccines and are self-inoculated by strains of bacteria or virus vaccine should be screened by periodic skin tests and agglutination titers where applicable.[53] Accidental self-inoculations, especially into the hand, require immediate attention at an accident or emergency health care facility where early incision and irrigation of the injected area may be required.[49]

National Animal Poison Control Center [54]

The National Animal Poison Control Center (NAPCC) is at 2001 South Lincoln Avenue, Urbana, IL 61801. The hotline to the center is 800-548-2423, administrative telephone: 217-333-2053, FAX: 217-333-4628. Harold L. Trammel, Pharm D is Operation Director. The NAPCC has collected information on human exposures to veterinary medication since 1987.[55] Prof. Guy Lorgue at the Lyon Animal Poison Control Center in France has additional information on human cases.

AMITRAZ

Amitraz is a component of veterinary acaricides and insecticides. It is usually formulated in a xylene preparation. When humans are exposed to amitraz they manifest symptoms and signs of both xylene and amitraz exposure. Treatment is largely symptomatic and supportive. Fatalities have been reported.

STRUCTURE AND CLASSIFICATION

Amitraz is a formamidine pesticide.[56]

USES

Amitraz is active against mites on fruit trees and kills mange mites on livestock and ticks on cattle.[57] It is an acaricide and insecticide intended for use on animals and plants. In Turkey amitraz is widely used for agricultural and public health purposes.[57]

PRODUCT FORMULATION

Formulations include the following: METABAN liquid concentration—amitraz, xylene, propylene oxide, blend of alkyl benzene sulfonates, and ethoxylated polyethers.[58] MITAC 20 EC[1]—Amitraz in 75% xylene. In Turkey some amitraz formulations contain 20% amitraz, and some veterinary formulations may contain 12.5 to 13.6% amitraz. The amount of xylene as a solvent varies between 30 and 70%.[57]

SOURCES

Amitraz is a synthetic chemical compound.

DOSAGE

Toxic Dose

In about one-half of the cases observed in Turkey 2.5 to 10 mL (0.3 to 1.25 g of the 12.5% formulation or 0.5 to 2 g of the 20% formulation) were ingested. In the remaining patients up to 10 g were ingested.[57]

Fatal Dose

Death followed ingestion of 30 mL of a product with 6 g of amitraz.[51] MITAC 20ED led to a suicide, following a survival for 6 days, in Japan.[55]

ELIMINATION

The hydrolyzed metabolic products of amitraz include 2,4-dimethylanaline, and *N*-(2,4-dimethylphenyl)-N^1-methylformamidine. These metabolites are further metabolized to 2,4-dimethylaniline and ultimately to 4-amino-3-methylbenzoic acid, the principal amitraz metabolite found in the urine and liver.[58] Xylene is excreted in the urine largely as methylhippuric acid with about 2% appearing in the urine as xylenol. From 3 to 6% of an absorbed dose of xylene is excreted through the lungs unchanged (see Hydrocarbon Products).

PREGNANCY/LACTATION

There are no adequate or controlled studies available of either amitraz or xylene during pregnancy or lactation. A 25-year-old mother who abused xylene during the 3rd to 16th week of pregnancy delivered a stillborn baby with multiple deformities.[59]

MECHANISM OF ACTION

Amitraz exhibits monoamine oxidase–inhibiting properties in vitro,[60] but only at high doses does it or its main metabolite (*n*-2,4 dimethylphenyl-*N*-methyl-formamide—BTS 27-271) exhibit central monoamine oxidase–inhibiting properties in animals in vivo.[61] The hydrolyzed metabolic product 2,4-dimethylaniline is a relatively weak methemoglobin formed in dog and presumably man.[58] Topical application of high doses of amitraz in the dog increases plasma glucose and suppresses insulin.[61] Amitraz appears to be a central $alpha_2$-adrenoceptor agonist whose action results in diminished peripheral sympathetic tone with a lowering of blood pressure and heart rate. Peripherally, it exhibits both $alpha_1$ and $alpha_2$ adrenoceptor agonist activity resulting in some elevation of blood pressure. The xylene present in amitraz formulations is more likely to induce central nervous system depression.

CLINICAL PRESENTATION

Animals

In animals amitraz by mouth induces bradycardia and hypotension within 1 to 5 hours; this later reverses. The hypotensive action may be mediated by the action of the metabolite BTS 27-271 on presynaptic adrenergic receptors. Common signs and symptoms in animals include CNS depression with episodes of hyperexcitability, hypotension, bradycardia, hypothermia, hypoglycemia, and in some cases hemoconcentration.[55] Recovery may be slow, requiring 7 to 10 days.

Xylene

Xylene in man may, after acute exposure, induce central nervous system depression with ataxia, impaired motor coordination, nystagmus, stupor, and coma. Ingestion may cause a burning sensation of the mouth, possibly blistering of the mucosa, substernal and abdominal pain, nausea, vomiting, diarrhea, headache, dizziness, sedation, and incoordination. Studies with a commercial product (MITACC20EC) in animals indicate that the early toxic effects of amitraz formulations are probably due to the xylene.

Amitraz Overdoses in Man

Clinical signs and symptoms after human exposure to an amitraz formulation initially include drowsiness, loss of consciousness, confused mental state, or agitation, with weakness, headache, vomiting, and malaise. Absent bowel sounds, miosis or mydriasis, abdominal pain and tenderness, and hyperactive deep tendon reflexes have been observed in children.[55,57] Exposure to amitraz formulations in man may terminate fatally.[55,57] In Turkey during 1989 about 17% of cases (seven patients) were suicidal and 84.4% accidental. In 37 cases poisoning followed ingestion, and in eight cases it followed dermal application.[57] In China a 61-year-old woman drank a swallow of a product containing Amitraz and developed CNS depression, respiratory depression, and bradycardia. This disappeared 36 hours later.[62]

LABORATORY

Analytic Method

A sensitive and rapid quantitation of Amitraz in plasma has been proposed using gas chromatography with nitrogen-phosphorous detection. The detection limit is 0.5 mg/mL.[63]

Abnormalities

Glycosuria, ketonuria, increased serum aminotransferases and alkaline phosphatase, and a neutrophil leukocytosis have been observed.[55,57]

TREATMENT

Stabilization

Initial attention should be directed toward evaluation and support of ventilation, with oxygen and endotracheal intubation provided as required. Cardiac monitoring is advisable because of the possibility of cardiac arrhythmias. Unconscious patients should be hospitalized, monitored, and treated as a coma emergency.

Decontamination

In the first 4 hours following an oral ingestion of an amitraz formulation gastric lavage, with tracheal protection, may be useful. A baseline chest x-ray and later follow-up films within the first 6 to 24 hours may provide an indication of aspiration pneumonitis (probably from xylene) if it develops. Activated charcoal and cathartics in this setting have not been studied and may not be useful. Following skin contact immediately remove contaminated clothing and wash with copious amounts of soap and water.

Elimination Enhancement

There are no clinical studies indicating that measures to enhance elimination (charcoal, whole bowel irrigation, extracorporeal approaches) would be useful.

Antidote

There are no antidotes. Yohimbine, an alpha-2-adrenergic agonist, reversed central nervous system depression and bradycardia in dogs, in addition to improving gastrointestinal signs following Amitraz toxicity.[64]

Supportive Measures

Patients should be admitted to a hospital where a complete blood count, liver function tests, blood and urine glucose and ketone levels, and a serum creatinine concentration can be obtained. Symptomatic and supportive care should be useful for amelioration of the hypotension (intravenous fluids) and bradycardia (atropine). Patients should be monitored for hypothermia. Patients may not be fully conscious for several days after an ingestion. Oral symptoms can be treated supportively.

BERENIL

Berenil is used in veterinary medicine for the treatment of trypanosomiasis and babesiosis.[65] Because of its toxic effects in animals (brain damage in dogs and asses, pyelonephritis in horses and camels), its use in human treatment has not been recommended by the manufacturers. When it has been used in man, it has induced toxic reactions, including fever, numbness, pain in the feet (plantar surface), paralysis, and nausea and vomiting. Such effects appear to be reversible. Guillain-Barré syndrome has been reported.[66]

STRUCTURE AND CLASSIFICATION

Diminazene accturate is an aromatic diamidine derivative related to pentamidine. Its proprietary name is Berenil.[65]

USES

Berenil has been used in veterinary medicine for the treatment of trypanosomiasis and babesiosis.

CLINICAL

Three doses of berenil 5 mg/kg body weight at 1- to 2-day intervals were administered to 99 patients. Toxic effects following treatment included paralysis, coma, and numbness of the legs all of which were reversible. Use of berenil in two pregnant patients at the sixteenth week of pregnancy was followed by an uneventful antenatal period and full-term normal deliveries. Laboratory examinations, including blood, urine, and cerebrospinal fluid, were normal except for parasites.[66]

XYLAZINE

Xylazine (5,6-dihydro-2-[2,6 xylidino]-FH-1,3 thiazine) is a sedative, analgesic, and skeletal muscle relaxant veterinary drug effective in a wide range of domestic and wild animals. In the United States the drug is marked under the trade name Rompun and is available in a 50-mL vial of 100 mg/L xylazine hydrochloride intended for either intravenous or intramuscular injection in animals.[67] Xylazine, a 1,3 thorazine, shares certain pharmacologic properties with a number of structurally related drugs: phenothiazines (1,4-thiazines), tricyclic antidepressants, and the imidazole derivative clonidine.[68]

TOXICOKINETICS

The relative concentration of the drug in tissues compared with blood is consistent with second-order toxicokinetics in which the drug is rapidly biotransformed and distributed to visceral organs and skeletal muscle. The half-life of xylazine is 2 to 3 hours; 70% is excreted by the kidneys; 8% is excreted unchanged.[69]

MECHANISM OF ACTION

Xylazine acts on the alpha$_2$ adrenoceptor that controls central neuronal dopamine and narconephrine storage and/or rales.

CLINICAL PRESENTATION

Reports of human overdose are summarized in Table 71–2.[68] Pronounced initial bradycardia, significant CNS and respiratory depression, electrocardiographic abnormalities, including possibly ventricular arrhythmia, and transient hyperglycemia have been observed in reported cases. Phenothiazines, tricyclic antidepressants, and clonidine may also produce bradycardia, CNS depression, and ECG abnormalities (Table 71–3).[68] Transient hypoglycemia may be associated with clonidine overdose. Nitroprusside may be useful for paradoxical hypertension and atropine or dopamine for hypotension and bradycardia.[69] Pulmonary edema may be fatal.

LABORATORY

Analytic methods

A gas chromatography method is useful for quantitative analysis of body fluids and is sensitive to about 20 ng/mL.[67]

TREATMENT

Sinus tachycardia and ventricular premature beats may be treated with lidocaine. Supportive measures must be used for the comatose patient. Yohimbine (0.125 mg/kg) and tolazoline, both alpha$_2$ adrenoceptor blockers, reverse xylazine sedative in animals.[70] Supportive measures include endotracheal intubation, ventilatory assistance, control of hypotension with intravenous fluids, position change, bladder catheterization, central venous pressure monitoring,[71] and cautious use of vasopressors (dopamine), maintenance of acid-base and electrolyte pathways, extended clinical observations and cardiac monitoring for possible myocardial infarction and ventricular arrhythmias, use of lidocaine for

Table 71–2
Xylazine Poisonings

	Age (yr)	Sex	Dose (mg)	Clinical	Blood Level (ng/mL)	History	Died
Veterinarian	36	M	3800	Found dead	0.2	1 month	yes
	34	M	1000	Found comatose, apneic, areflexic; hyperglycemic. Elevated cardiac enzyme; ECG and sinus tachycardia, flattened T-wave. Ventricular premature beats Respiratory depression Extubated in 60 hours.	IM injection of xylazine		no
	39	F		Sinus bradycardia drowsiness, slurred speech	30	Abused xylazine, alcohol. Prior attack of tiredness, faintness, blurred vision	no
Horse trainer	20	F	400	Drowsy, incontinent	Unknown	Prior injection of xylazine	no
				Dizzy, weak			
				CNS depression (drowsiness, disorientation, hyporeflexia). Bradycardia, hyperglycemia. Apneic spells, hypotensive episodes, premature ventricular beats. Extubated in 24 hours			
		M		Unconscious 13 hours	30		no
(volunteer)				Anesthesia, bradycardia 44 min.	7 IV		no
	19	F		Difficult to rouse, cyanosed, hyporeflexia, small pupils, sinus bradycardia; hyperglycemia Extubated in 8 hours	200 IV		no
	37	F		#1 mild hypotension, respiratory depression	0.73 ng/kg #1 no subcutaneous		no
				severe bradycardia	23 ng/kg #2		
				mild apnea	24		
	59	F		Pulmonary edema	16 mg/L		yes

Table 71–3
Comparison of Pharmacologic and Toxicologic Effects of Xylazine, Clonidine, Phenothiazines, and Tricyclic Antidepressants[a,b]

Effects	Animals	Xylazine	Clonidine	Phenothiazines	TCA
Hypotension	+	+	+	+	+
Hypertension	+	N.A.	+	–	+
Sedation	+	+	+	+	+
Respiratory depression	+	+	+	+	+
Bradycardia	+	+	+	–	–
Tachycardia	–	+?	–	+	+
Quinidine-like effects	+?	N.A.	+?	+	+
Alpha-adrenergic effect (central or peripheral)	+	N.A.	+	–	–
Alpha-adrenergic blocking	+	N.A.	+	+	+
Hyperglycemia	+	+	+	N.A.	N.A.
Temperature disturbance	N.A.	N.A.	+	+	+
EKG abnormalities	+	+	+	+	+

[a]Adapted from Gallanosa AG et al. Clin Toxicol 1981;18:663–678.
[b]+ = present, – = absent, +? = data suggestive but not established, N.A. = no data available.

ventricular arrhythmia, and control of hyperglycemia in susceptible patients.[68]

REFERENCES—VETERINARY PRODUCT POISONINGS IN MAN

1. Poklis A, Hameli AZ. Two unusual barbiturate deaths. Arch Toxicol 1975;34:77–80.
2. Clark MA, Jones JW. Suicide by intravenous injection of a veterinary euthanasia agent: report of a case and toxicologic studies. J Forensic Sci 1979;24:762–767.
3. Smith RA, Lewis D. Suicide by ingestion of T-61. Vet Hum Toxicol 1989;31:319–320.
4. Nicolas F, Rodineau P, Rovzioux J-M, Tack I, Chabac S, Meram D. Fulminant hepatic failure in poisoning due to ingestion of T-61, a veterinary euthanasia drug. Crit Care Med 1990;18:573–575.

5. Cordell WH, Curry SC, Furbee RB, Mitchell-Flynn DL. Veterinary euthanasia drugs as suicidal agents. Ann Emerg Med 1986;15:939–943.
6. Kingston RL, Saxena K. Intentional poisoning by injection of veterinary euthanasia drug. Clin Toxicol 1979;15:492 (abstract).
7. Brown M. An overdose of dog's heart tablets. Hum Exp Toxicol 1990;9:201.
8. Cavaliere U, Andreano C, Raducci G, Andreioni C, Iacovella A. Intossicazione da T-61 (Tanax[R]). Min Anest 1982;48: 001–004.
9. Cohen ML, Ming RH, Gogel HK, Davis M, Pitcher JL. Horse pill ("bute") hemorrhage. J Clin Gastroenterol 1988;10: 210–212.
10. Ramsey R, Golde DW. Aplastic anemia from veterinary phenylbutazone. JAMA 1976;236:1049.
11. Newton TA, Rose SR. Poisoning with equine phenylbutazone in a racetrack worker. Ann Emerg Med 1991;20: 204–207.
12. Thompson JD. Human intoxication with banamine. Vet Hum Toxicol 1990;32:352.
13. Markus CK, Chow LH, Wycoff DM, McManus BM. Pet food derived penicillin residue as a potential cause of hypersensitivity myocarditis and sudden death. Am J Cardiol 1989;63:1155–1156.
14. Boutelba K, Belmati E, Merad R, Drif M. Talking of a strange intoxication by an anti-coccidian of veterinary use. Proc Intern Cong Clin Toxicol Pois Cont Anal Toxicol. Lux Tox '90, Luxembourg, May 2–5, 1990, p. 499.
15. Martinez-Navarro JF. Food poisoning related to consumption of illicit beta-agonist in liver. Lancet 1990; 336:1311.
16. Woodward KN, Gray AK. Adverse reactions in humans following occupational exposure to veterinary drugs. Hum Exp Toxicol 1990;9:326.
17. Sidhu KS, Collisi MB. A case of an accidental exposure to a veterinary insecticide product formulation. Vet Hum Toxicol 1989;31:63–64.
18. Woodward KN, Gray AK. Adverse reactions in humans arising from the use of veterinary drugs. Abstract 000. Brighton, England: Fifth International Congress of Toxicology, July 16–21, 1989.
19. Woodward KN. Veterinary Medicines Directorate, UK. Personal communication, August 6, 1990.
20. Schenker MB, Samuels SJ, Green RS, Wiggins P. Adverse reproductive outcomes among female veterinarians. Am J Epidemiol 1990;132: 96–106.
21. Reference Deleted.
22. Reid FM, Tracey JA. Parenteral exposure to detomidine and butorphanol. Clin Toxicol 1994;32:465–469.
23. McGuigan MA. Human exposures to tilmocosin (Micotil[R]). Vet Hum Toxicol 1994;36:306–398.
24. Vazquez C, Labayru T, Rodriguez-Soriano J. Poor bronchodilator effect of oral etamphylline in asthmatic children. Lancet 1984;1:914.
25. Addis GJ. Absence of bronchodilator effect from etamphylline. Lancet 1984;1:1083.
26. Gray AK. Suspected adverse reaction surveillance scheme 1991: summary of results. Vet Rec 1993;132:4–6.
27. Murray VSG, Wiseman HM, Dawling S, Morgan I, Hosue IM. Health effects of organophosphate sheep dips. Br Med J 1992;305:1090.
28. Strong JE, Wilson J, Douglas JF et al. Phenylbutazone self-poisoning treated by charcoal haemoperfusion. Anaesthesia 1979;34:1038–1040.
29. Berlinger WC, Spector R, Flanigan MJ et al. Hemoperfusion for phenylbutazone poisoning. Ann Intern Med 1982;96: 334–335.
30. Clutton RE. Attempted suicide with acepromazine maleate: a case report. Vet Hum Toxicol 1985;27:391.
31. Berns SD, Wright JL. Pediatric acepromazine poisoning. The importance of child-resistant packaging for veterinary drugs. Am J Emerg Med 1993;11:247–248.
32. Van Boren M, Daenens P. Analysis and identification of azaperone and its metabolites in humans. J Anal Toxicol 1992; 16:33–35.
33. Woodward KN. Hypersensitivity in humans and exposure to veterinary drugs. Vet Hum Toxicol 1991;33:168–171.
34. Hoen E, Hodgkin C, Mikevicious D. Harmful human use of donated veterinary drugs. Lancet 1993;342:308–309.
35. Amery WF, Veys P, Gheuens J. Beerse, Belgium, Janssen Research Foundation. Personal communications, March 2, 1993.
36. Martinez-Frias ML, Cereijo A, Rodriguez-Pinilla E, Uriose M. Methimazole in animal feed and congenital aplasia. Lancet 1992;339:742–743.
37. Bedello PG, Goitre M, Cane D, Roncarolo G. Allergic contact dermatitis to Bayo-N-Ox-1. Contact Dermatitis 1985;12:284.
38. Francalanci S, Gola M, Giorgini S, Muccinelli A, Sertoli A. Occupational photocontact dermatitis from olaquindox. Contact Dermatitis 1986;15:112–114.
39. Luehr JG, Meyerle KA, Larson EW. Mail-order (veterinary) drug dependence. JAMA 1990;263:657.
40. Reference Deleted.
41. Paggiaro PL, Loi AM, Toma G. Bronchial asthma and dermatitis due to spiramycin in a chick breeder. Clinical Allergy 1979;9:571–574.
42. Davies RJ, Pepys J. Asthma due to inhaled chemical agents—the macrolide antibiotic spiramycin. Clinical Allergy 1975;1:99–107.
43. Braselton WE Jr, Ray JS, Slanker MR, Rumler PC. Determination of embutramide in mammalian tissues. Vet Hum Toxicol 1988;30:536–539.
44. Miller CD, Songer JR, Sullivan JF. A twenty-five year review of laboratory-acquired human infections at the National Animal Disease Center. Am Ind Hyg Assoc J 1987;48:271–275.
45. Geller RJ. Human effects of veterinary biological products. Vet Hum Toxicol 1990;32:479–480.
46. Gulasekharan J. Illness following accidental self-inoculation of *Brucella abortus* strain 19 vaccine. Med J Aust 1970:2: 642–643.
47. Committee on Safety of Medicines. Accidental self-injection of oil-based veterinary vaccines. London Committee on Safety of Medicines 1981;20:3–4.
48. Woodward KN. Veterinary Medicines Directorate. Weybridge, Surrey, UK: Personal communication. August 6, 1990.
49. Warning about veterinary vaccines. Br Med J 1987;7:294–352.
50. Joffe B, Diamond MT. Brucellosis due to self-inoculation. Ann Intern Med 1966;65:564–565.
51. Constable PJ, Harrington JM. Risks of zoonosis in a veterinary service. Br Med J 1982;284:146–148.
52. Crosby AD, Geller RJ. Human effects of veterinary biological products. Vet Hum Toxicol 1986;28:569–571.
53. McCaullugh NB. Medical care following accidental injection of *Brucella abortus,* strain 19 in man. J Am Vet Med Assoc 1963;143:617.
54. Trammel HL. National Animal Poison Control Center. Urbana, IL: Personal communication, December 3, 1990.
55. Bonsall JL, Turnbull GJ. Extrapolation from safety data to management of poisoning with reference to amitraz (a formamide pesticide) and xylene. Hum Toxicol 1983;2:587–592.
56. Hollingworth RM. Chemistry, biological activity, and uses of formamidine pesticides. Environ Health Perspect 1976;14: 57–62.
57. Besbelli N, Oto N, Yalcinlar O, Ikinciogullari A. Poisoning cases with amitraz, 1990. Proc XIV Int Congress Eur Assoc Poison Control Centres. Milan, Italy: September 25–29, 1990.
58. Jones RD. Xylene/amitraz: a pharmacologic review. Vet Hum Toxicol 1990;32:446–448.
59. Kucera J. Exposure to fat solvents, a possible cause of sacralagenesis in man. J Pediatr 1968;72:857–859.
60. Azia SA, Knowles CO. Inhibition of monoamine oxidase by the pesticide chlordimeform and related compounds. Nature 1973;242:417–418.
61. Hsu WH, Schaffer DD. Effects of topical application of amitraz on plasma glucose and insulin concentrations in dogs. Am J Vet Res 1988;49:130–131.
62. Yamaguchi Y, Shirakawa Y, Ogura S, Ameno K, Fuke C, Ogli K. A case of Amitraz poisoning. Jpn J Toxicol 1989;2:289–292.
63. Ameno K, Fuke C, Ameno S, Kiriu T, Shinohara T, Ijiri I. A rapid and sensitive quantitation of Amitraz in plasma by gas chromatography with nitrogen-phosphorus detection and

its application for pharmacokinetics. J Anal Toxicol 1991;15: 116–118.

64. Hovda LR, McManus AC. Yohimbine for treatment of Amitraz poisoning in dogs. Vet Hum Toxicol 1993;35:329.
65. Reynolds JEF. Martindale: The extra pharmacopoeia. 29th ed. London: The Pharmaceutical Press, 1989, p. 663.
66. Abaru DE, Lewo DA, Isakina D, Okori EE. Retrospective long-term study of effects of berenil by follow-up of patients treated since 1965. Trop Med Parasitol 1984;35:148–150.
67. Poklis A, Machell MA, Case MES. Xylazine in human tissues and fluids in a case of fatal drug abuse. J Anal Toxicol 1985;9:234–236.
68. Gallanosa G, Spyker DA, Shipe JR, Morris LD. Human xylazine overdose: a comparative review with clonidine, phenothiazines and tricyclic antidepressants. Clin Toxicol 1981; 18:663–678.
69. Spoerke DG, Hall AH, Grimes, MJ, Honea BN, Rumack BH. Human overdose with the veterinary tranquilizer xylazine. Vet Hum Toxicol 1985;28:190.
70. Mackintosh C. Potential antidote for Rompun (xylazine) in humans. New Zeal Med J 1985;9:714–715.
71. Carruthers SG, Nelson M, Wexler HR, Stiller CR. Xylazine hydrochloride (Rompun) overdose in man. Clin Toxicol 1979;15:281–285.

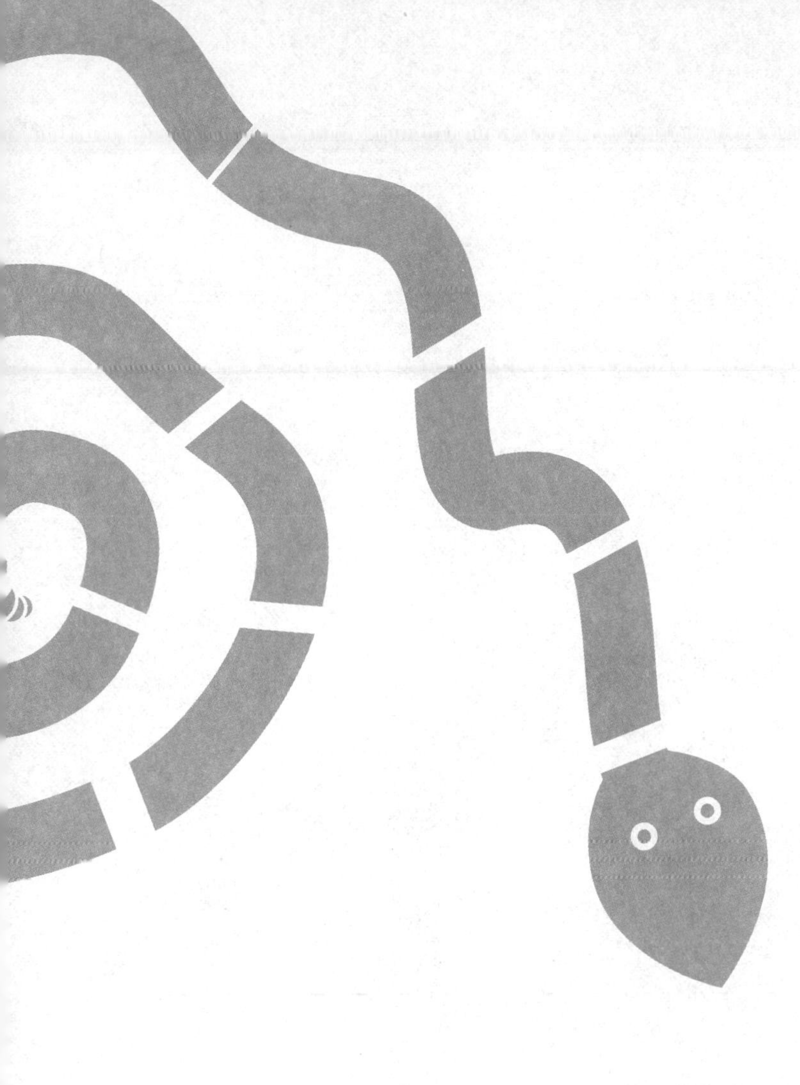

Section V
NATURAL TOXINS

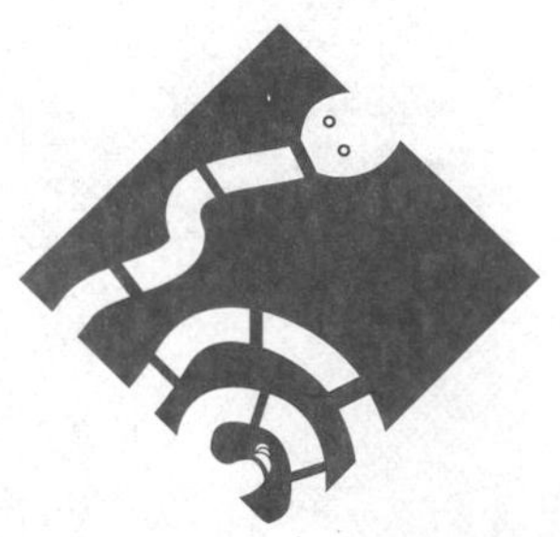

Chapter 72

Envenomations—Bites and Stings

SNAKES—INTERNATIONAL

VENOMOUS SNAKES[1]

There are five families of venomous snakes:

1. Colubridae—back-fanged, arboreal snakes such as the African boomslang and twig snakes
2. Elapidae—cobras, kraits, mambas, coral snakes, and the terrestrial Australasian venomous snakes; rattlesnakes (Crotalidae)
3. Hydrophiidae—sea snakes
4. Viperidae—vipers, adders, pit vipers, and rattlesnakes
5. Atractaspididae—burrowing asps or stiletto snakes, formerly known as burrowing or mole vipers and adders

EPIDEMIOLOGY

Injuries and death due to snakes occur in most parts of the world (Table 72-1),[2] especially in the tropics where they may represent a major health problem.[3] Guidelines to snakebite management discussed in this chapter are derived from experience with snakebites throughout the world and can be considered for envenomations in the United States.

In Costa Rica hospital admissions for snakebites have been estimated as high as 22.4 per 100,000 population per year, with five deaths per 100,000 (mostly due to bites by *Bothrops atrox asper).* In South America 90% of snakebites are caused by *Bothrops* species. Mortality has been estimated as high as 2.4%, but may be as high as 8% when no antivenom is given. After rattlesnake envenomation *(Crotalus durissus terrificus)* about 75% of the untreated victims die; in those who receive antivenom, mortality falls to 12%.[2]

In North Africa scorpion stings are medically more important than snakebites. In the savanna regions of West Africa, the carpet viper *(Echis carinatus)* is the most important cause of snakebite morbidity and mortality.

In Europe snakebite is relatively rare. Only 14 deaths due to adder bites *(Vipera berus)* have occurred in Britain during the last 100 years.[4] In England and Wales only one death from adder bite was recorded from 1950 to 1972, but there were 61 deaths from bee or wasp stings. The last adder bite death in Germany was in 1959. In Europe bites by imported venomous snakes are sometimes fatal. In France about 1000

Table 72–1
Medically Important Snake Species[a]

Definition

Species are considered to be of medical importance if (from published medical reports of bites by identified species) they fall into one of three categories:
(1) Commonly cause death or serious disability.
(2) Uncommonly cause bites but are recorded to cause serious effects (death or local necrosis).
(3) Commonly cause bites but serious effects are very uncommon.

Geographical Areas

Area	Category 1	Category 2	Category 3
North America	*Agkistrodon piscivorus* *Crotalus adamenteus* *C. atrox* *C. viridis*	*Crotalus scutulatus* *Micrurus fulvius*	*Agkistrodon contortrix* *Crotalus horridus* *Sistrurus miliarius*
Mexico and Central America	*Bothrops atrox asper* *Crotalus atrox* *C. basiliscus* *C. durissus*	*Agkistrodon bilineatus* *Crotalus molossus* *C. triseriatus* *C. polystictus* *C. scutulatus* *Lachesis muta* *Micrurus nigrocinctus*	*Bothrops schlegeli* *B. lateralis*
South America	*Bothrops atrox atrox* *B. jararaca* *B. neuwiedi* *Crotalus durissus* *C. durissus terrificus*	*Bothrops alternatus* *B. jararacussu* *Lachesis muta* *Micrurus corallinus* *M. lemniscatus* *M. mipartitus*	*Bothrops bilineatus* *B. schlegeli*
North Africa	*Bitis arietans* *Echis carinatus* *Naja nigricollis*	*Atractaspis* sp. *Naja haje*	*Cerastes* sp.
Mid-Africa	*Bitis arietans* *Echis carinatus* *Naja mossambica* *N. nigricollis*	*Atractaspis* sp. *Bitis gabonica* *Dendroaspis* sp. (mainly *D. polylepis*) *Dispholidus typus* *Naja haje* *Thelotornis kirtlandii*	*Causus* sp.
Southern Africa	*Bitis arietans* *Naja nigricollis*	*Atractaspis* sp. *Dendroaspis* sp. *Dispholidus typus* *Naja haje* *N. nivea* *Thelotornis kirtlandii*	*Causus* sp.
Europe		*Vipera lebetina*	*Vipera ammodytes* *V. aspis* *V. berus*
Near and Middle East	*Bitis arietans* *Echis carinatus* *Naja naja* *Vipera lebetina* *V. xanthina*	*Atractaspis* sp. *Echis coloratus* *Naja haje*	*Agkistrodon halys* *Cerastes* sp. *Vipera ammodytes*
Southeastern Asia (Pakistan to Sulawesi)	*Agkistrodon rhodostoma* *Echis carinatus* *Enhydrina schistosa* *Naja naja* *Vipera russelli*	*Bungarus caeruleus* *Hydrophis cyanocinctus* *Lapemis hardwicki* *Ophiophagus hannah* *Trimeresurus purpureomaculatus*	*Trimeresurus albolabris* *T. wagleri*
Far East	*Naja naja* *Trimeresurus flavoviridis* (Ryukyu) *T. mucrosquamatus*	*Agkistrodon acutus* *Bungarus multicinctus* (China, Province of Taiwan) *Hydrophis cyanocinctus* *Lapemis hardwicki* *Ophiophagus hannah*	*Agkistrodon blomhoffi* *A. caliginosus* *A. halys* group *Trimeresurus albolabris* *T. stejnegeri* (China, Province of Taiwan) *Pseudechis porphyriacus*
Australia and Pacific Islands	*Acanthopis antarcticus* *Notechis scutatus* *Pseudonaja textilis*	*Austrelaps superba* *Oxyuranus scutellatus* *Pseudechis australis* *Pseudechis papuanus* *Tropidechis carinatus*	

[a]Adapted from Progress in the Characterization of Venoms and Standardization of Antivenoms. WHO Offset Publication No. 58, Geneva, World Health Organization, 1981.

Table 72-2
Snakebite Mortality in Southeastern Asia[a]

Country or Area	Average No. of Bites per Year	Average No. of Deaths per Year	Yearly Mortality per 100,000 Population
Burma	8,508	75.9	2.700
China (Province of Taiwan)		36	0.270
Hong Kong	203	1.3	0.090
India (Maharashtra State)		1,093	2.100
Japan	610	5.6	0.570
Malaysia	2,480	16	0.180
Philippines		294	0.770
Sri Lanka		104	0.820
Thailand	3,989	302	0.860

[a]Adapted from Progress in the Characterization of Venoms and Standardization of Antivenoms. WHO Offset Publication No. 58, Geneva, World Health Organization, 1981.

to 2000 bites mostly due to *Vipera aspis* and *Vibera berus* are reported each year, with a mortality of about 0.5%.[5]

In Southeastern Asia over 2500 deaths due to snakebite are reported annually. Mortality is high in Myanmar (Burma), India, the Philippines, Sri Lanka, and Thailand (Table 72-2). In the Maharashtra State of India, more than 1000 deaths per year due to snakebite have been recorded. In Australia about 3000 suspected cases of snakebite are reported each year, and 600 victims are treated with antivenom. Few now die.

There is a high incidence of disability from local necrosis. Older concepts of cytotoxic and hemotoxic viperid venoms, neurotoxic elapid venoms, and mycotoxic sea snake venoms are no longer relevant. Clinical syndromes of envenomation are rarely diagnostic. There remains a need for rapid diagnostic tests of venom origin. Enzyme-refined equine antivenoms are clinically effective against hemostasis disorders, hypotension, and postsynaptic neurotoxicity, but much less effective against presynaptic neurotoxicity, nephrotoxicity, and local necrosis.[6] Poisonous toxins and environmental neurotoxins are summarized in Tables 72-3 and 72-4.

Table 72-3
Poisonous Toxins

Toxin	Source	Action	Locale
Myotoxins	*Crotalus viridis*		Southwestern U.S.A.
	Crotalus atrox		
Cardiotoxin	Mojave rattlesnake *(Crotalus scatulatus)*		
	Southern Pacific rattlesnake *(Crotalus viridishelleri)*		Southwestern U.S.A.
Bufotoxin	Colorado river toad *(Bufo alvarious)*		
Batrachotoxin	*Phyllobates terribilis*	Activates sodium channel	Central America
Pumiliotoxin B	*Phyllobates bicolor*	Increases sodium conduct range	
Isodihydrohistrionicotoxin	*Phyllobates aurptaemoa*	Stabilizes sodium channel	
		Swelling of nerve axon	
Pumilotoxin C	(Colombian poison-dart frogs)		
Gephyrotoxin			
Tetrodotoxin	Newt	Sodium channel blocker	
	Taricha granulosa		West Coast, U.S.A.
	Notophthalmus		Carolines, Eastern U.S.A.
Saxitoxin		Sodium channel blocker	
Hemorrhagin	King cobra		
Ciguatoxin (CTX)			
CTX-1	Spanish mackerel *(Scomberomorus commersoni)*		
CTX-2	Moray Eel		South Pacific
CTX-3	Barracuda *(Sphjyraena jello)*		
Maitotoxin	Lipid-soluble toxin (from *Gambierdiscus toxicus)*		South Pacific
	Water-soluble toxin (from *Gambierdiscus toxicus)* (not accumulated in flesh of fishes)		
Gambiertoxins	*Gambierdiscus toxicus* (oxidized to ciguatoxins)		
Apamin	*Hymenoptera*		
	Bee venoms		
	Yellow jacket		
	White-faced hornet		
	Yellow hornet		
	Fire ant		
	Wasp		
Postsynaptic	King cobra *(Ophiophagus hannah)*		India through Burma Thailand Malaysia Indochina Southern China Indonesia Philippines

Table 72–4
Envenomation Neurotoxins[a]

Toxin	Source	Chemistry	Mode of Action
Na^+ channel			
Polypeptide toxins			
Alpha-scorpion toxins	Scorpions: Toxin I; *Androctonus australis; Buthus occitanus*	Peptides, approx. 64 amino acids	Hyperexcitability, repetitive firing in motor units, accelerated respiration, convulsions, spastic paralysis; eventual respiratory failure
Sea anemone toxins (Toxin I, II, III; ATX I, II, III)	Sea anemone: *Anemonia sulcata*	Peptide	Action similar to alpha-scorpion toxins
Beta-scorpion toxins	Scorpions: (*Centruroides suffusus suffusus; Centruroides sculpturatus*	Peptide	Similar to alpha-scorpion toxins, except that hyperexcitability less pronounced; heavy perspiration, tremor
u-conotoxins (GIIIA, GIIIB, GIIIC geographutoxin)	Piscivorous snails: *Conus geographus*	Peptides, 22 amino acids	Flaccid paralysis caused by block of action potentials in skeletal muscle, but not in cardiac muscle or neurons
u-agatoxins (I-VI)	Funnel web spider: *Agelenopsis aperta*	Peptides, 36–37 amino acids	Paralysis in insects characterized by excitation, tremor; associated with repetitive action potentials in motor axons and increase in frequency of spontaneous transmitter release; apparently insect-specific
Lipophilic toxins			
Batrachotoxin	Poison dart frogs: *Phyllobates aurotaenia;* Hooded pitohui bird: *Pitohui dichrous*	Alkaloid	Hyperexcitability, resulting from long-lasting membrane depolarization
Pyrethroids	Synthetic analogs of pyrethrins; two groups (Type I and Type II)	Organic ester	Lethal paralysis in insects; Type I is generally excitatory, Type II induces flaccid paralysis; also paralytic to vertebrates
Pumiliotoxins (Pumiliotoxin A, pumiliotoxin B)	Skin of neotropical frogs: *Dendrobates pumilio* (Dendrobatidae)	Alkaloid	Cardiotonic myotonic activity; increases Na^+ influx into guinea-pig synaptosomes
K^+ channels			
Apamin	Bee venom: *Apis mellifera*	Peptide, 18 amino acids	Clonic convulsions, respiratory failure
Tityus toxins	Scorpion: *Tityus serrulatus*	Peptides	Not determined
Scyllatoxin (Leiurotoxin I)	Scorpion venom: *Leiurus quinquestriatus hebraeus*	Peptide, 31 amino acids	Blocks the adrenaline-induced relaxation of guinea-pig taenia coli, while having no effect on the rate or force of contraction of guinea-pig atria or rabbit portal vein
Mast cell–degranulating peptide (MCDP)	Bee venom: *Apis mellifera*	Peptide, 22 amino acids	Convulsions, hyperactivity
Charybdotoxin	Scorpion: *Leiurus quinquestriatus hebraeus*	Peptide, 37 amino acids	Transient increase in blood pressure after intravenous injection
Dendrotoxin (Alpha, $beta_1$, $beta_2$, gamma, delta forms)	Mamba snake venom: *Dendroaspis polylepis; Dendroaspis angusticeps*	Peptide, 59 amino acids; sequence similar to that of bovine pancreatic trypsin inhibitor, but no enzymatic activity observed.	Convulsant; facilitates release of transmitter
Ca^{2+} channels			
Polypeptide toxins			
Omega-conotoxins			
Omega-conotoxin GVIA	Piscivorous cone snail: *Conus geographus*	Peptide, 27 amino acids	Long-lasting block of neuromuscular transmission in vertebrates (except for mammals); produces "shaker" symptoms when injected intracranially into young mice
Omega-agatoxins			
Omega-Aga-IA	Funnel-web spider: *Agelenopsis aperta*	Heterodimeric peptide, major chain contains 66 amino acids, minor chain, connected by disulphide bridge, contains 3 amino acids	Paralytic to injected insects; no effect after intracranial injection in mice

[a]Adapted from Adams ME, Swanson G. Neurotoxins. Trends Neurosci Suppl April 1994.

(continued)

Table 72–4 *(Continued)*

Toxin	Source	Chemistry	Mode of Action
Presynaptic toxins			
Snake toxins			
Beta bungarotoxin	Snake venom: *Naja, Bungarus, Laticauda* spp.	Dimeric polypeptide toxin; A chain in basic phospholipase A_2, B chain is similar to proteinase inhibitors such as bovine pancreatic trypsin inhibitor	Inhibition of elicited transmitter release
Crotoxin	Snake venom: *Crotalus durrisus terrificus*	Dimeric polypeptide; component A probably involved in specific binding, component B involved in biologic effect	Inhibition of elicited transmitter release; three phases—initial transient inhibition, facilitation of ACh release, irreversible inhibition resulting from transmitter depletion
Notexin	Australian tiger snake: *Notechis scutatus scutatus*	Single-chain polypeptide toxin (seven disulphide bridges)	Lethal paralysis associated with inhibition of transmitter release
Mojave toxin	Rattlesnake: *Crotalus s. scutatus*	Heterodimeric polypeptide	Inhibition of neurotransmitter release; can cause fusion of myoblasts
Textilotoxin	Australian common brown snake venom: *Pseudonaja textilis*	Multimeric polypeptide (four chains, 133 amino acids each)	Inhibition of elicited transmitter release; no known myotoxic activity
Taipoxin	Australian taipan snake venom: *Oxyuranus s. scutellatus*	Trimeric polypeptide; toxin	Triphasic effect on nerve terminals: transient inhibition, facilitation of ACh release; irreversible depression; depletion of presynaptic vesicles
Spider toxins			
Alpha-latrotoxin	Black widow spider: *Latrodectus mactans*	Peptide, 1401 amino acids	Causes massive exocytotic transmitter release followed by depletion and irreversible block; selective for vertebrate presynaptic terminals
Alpha-latroinsectotoxin	Black widow spider: *Latrodectus mactans*	Peptide, 1411 amino acids	Apparently similar to alpha-latrotoxin, but specific for spider neuromuscular junction
Wasp toxins			
Mandaratoxin	Wasp: *Vespa mandarinia*	Polypeptide, 20 kDa	Blocks neuromuscular transmission in lobster
Acetylcholine receptors nicotinic (antagonist):			
Alpha-bungarotoxin (alpha-Btx)	Banded krait: *Bungarus multicinctus*	Peptides: Type I: 61-62 amino acids	Flaccid paralysis
Cobra alpha-neurotoxin	Cobra: *Naja naja*	Type II: 71-74 amino acids	
Erabutoxin	Sea snake: *Laticauda semifasciata*		
Transmitter re-uptake			
Glutamate			
Delta-philanthotoxin	Solitary wasp venom: *Philanthus triangulum*	Acylpolyamine	Paralytic; block glutamatergic neuromuscular transmission in insects

Table 72–5
World's Most Venomous Snakes in Order of Lethal Potency [a]

Small-scaled snake	Death adder	King cobra[b]
Brown snake	Gwardar	Blue-bellied black snake
Taipan	Australian copperhead	Collet's snake
Tiger snake	Indian cobra[b]	King brown snake
Reevesby Island tiger snake	Dugite	Red-bellied black snake
Beaked sea snake	Papuan black snake	Small-eyed snake
Western Australian tiger snake	Yellow banded snake	Eastern diamondback rattlesnake
Chappell Island tiger snake	Rough-scaled snake	

[a]Adapted from Sutherland SK. Aust Fam Physician 1990;19:24–42.
[b]Not Australian snakes.

Table 72-6
Scientific and Common Names for North American Pit Vipers[a]

Scientific Name	Common Name	Scientific Name	Common Name
C. mitchellii angelensis	Angel de la Guarda Island speckled	*A. contortrix mokeson*	Northern copperhead
C. viridis cerberus	Arizona black	*C. viridis oreganus*	Northern Pacific
C. willardi willardi	Arizona ridge-nosed	*C. durissus culminatus*	Northwestern Neotropical
C. unicolor	Aruba Island	*C. basiliscus oaxacus*	Oaxacan
C. lannomi	Autlan	*C. intermedius gloydi*	Oaxacan small-headed
C. lepidus klauberi	Banded rock	*C. intermedius omiltemanus*	Omilteman small-headed
C. mollossus subspecies	Black-tailed	*A. contortrix phaeogaster*	Osage copperhead
A. contortrix laticinctus	Broad-banded copperhead	*C. v. oreganus* or *C. v. helleri*	Pacific
C. horridus atricaudatus	Canebrake	*C. mitchellii stephensi*	Panamint
S. miliarius miliarius	Carolina pigmy	*S. miliarius* subspecies and *S. ravus*	Pigmy
C. exsul	Cedros Island diamond	*C. viridis viridis*	Prairie
C. durissus durissus	Central American	*C. triseriatus aquilus*	Queretaran dusky
C. triseriatus triseriatus	Central-plateau dusky	*C. catalinensis*	Rattleless
C. enyo cerralvensis	Cerralvo Island	*C. ruber ruber*	Red diamond
C. cerastes laterorepens	Colorado Desert sidewinder	*C. willardi* subspecies	Ridge-nosed
A. bilineatus bilineatus	Common cantil	*C. lepidus* subspecies	Rock
C. viridis caliginis	Coronado Island	*C. enyo furvus*	Rosario
C. transversus	Cross-banded mountain	*C. molossus estebanensis*	San Esteban Island
C. willardi amabilis	Del Nido ridge-nosed	*C. ruber lucasensis*	San Lucan diamond
S. catenatus edwardsii	Desert massasauga	*C. mitchellii mitchellii*	San Lucan speckled
C. adamanteus, C, atroix, C. rubber, etc.	Diamond or diamond back	*C. catalinensis*	Santa Catalina Island
		C. cerastes subspecies	Sidewinder
C. triseriatus subspecies and *c. pussilus*	Dusky	*C. intermedius* subspecies	Small-headed
		C. cerastes cercobombus	Sonoran Desert sidewinner
S. m. barbouri	Dusky pigmy	*C. durissus terrificus*	South American
A. piscivorus piscivorus	Eastern cottonmouth	*A. contortrix contortrix*	Southern copperhead
C. adamanteus	Eastern diamondback	*C. viridis helleri*	Southern Pacific
S. catenatus catenatus	Eastern massasauga	*C. willardi meridionalis*	Southern ridge-nosed
C. pricei miquihuanus	Eastern twin-spotted	*C. mitchellii pyrrhus*	Southwestern speckled
C. m. muertensis	El Muerto Island speckled	*C. mitchellii* subspecies	Speckled
A. piscivorus conanti	Florida cottonmouth	*C. lepidus morulus*	Tamaulipan rock
C. viridis abyssus	Grand Canyon	*C. pusillus*	Tancitaran dusky
C. viridis lutosus	Great Basin	*A. bilineatus taylori*	Taylor's cantil
C. viridis nuntius	Hopi	*C. tigris*	Tiger
C. scutulatus salvini	Huamantlan	*C. horridus horridus*	Timber
C. polystictus	Lance-headed	*C. tortugensis*	Tortuga Island diamond
C. stejnegeri	Long-tailed	*C. intermedius intermedius*	Totalcan small-headed
C. enyo	Lower California	*C. durissus totanacus*	Totonacan
C. catenatus subspecies	Massasauga	*A. contortrix pictigaster*	Trans-Pecos copperhead
C. molossus nigrescens	Mexican black-tailed	*C. pricei* subspecies	Twin-spotted
C. polystictus	Mexican lance-headed	*C. vegrandis*	Uracoan
S. ravus	Mexican pigmy	*C. willardi silus*	West Chihuahua ridge-nosed
C. basiliscus basiliscus	Mexican west-coast	*C. viridis* subspecies	Western
C. viridis concolor	Midget faded	*A. piscivorus leucostoma*	Western cottonmouth
C. scutulatus scutulatus	Mojave	*C. atrox*	Western diamondback
C. cerastes cerastes	Mojave Desert sidewinder	*S. catenatus tergeminus*	Western massasauga
C. lepidus lepidus	Mottled rock	*S. miliarius streckeri*	Western pigmy
C. durissus subspecies	Neotropical	*C. pricei pricei*	Western twin-spotted
C. molossus molossus	Northern black-tailed	*C. durissus tzabcan*	Yucatan Neotropical

[a]Adapted from Davidson TM. J Wilderness Med 1992;3:397–421.

Australian elapids induce a coagulopathy characterized by defibrination and normal platelet counts. Factors V and VIII, protein C, and plasminogen are significantly depleted. Specific antivenom therapy reverses these findings. Venom from the brown snakes, *Pseudonaja* spp., tiger snakes, *Notechis* spp., and the taipan, *Oxyuranus* spp., all exhibit a coagulopathy, and all have a powerful procoagulant that converts prothrombin to thrombin.[7] Tables 72-3 and 72-4 compares poisonous toxins associated with snakes, marine envenomations, and some arthropods. Sutherland has ranked the world's most venomous snakes in order of lethal potency[8,9] (Table 72-5).

About 120 species of snakes reside in the United States, 26 of which are considered poisonous. Approximately 8000 people are bitten annually by poisonous snakes in the United States, resulting in 14 to 20 deaths.[10]

Scientific and common names for North American pit vipers are listed in Table 72-6.[11] Distribution of snake by state in the United States is found in Table 72-7.

VENOMS

In elapid venoms, polypeptide neurotoxins may predominate. These cause respiratory paralysis by blocking the

Table 72–7
Some Medically Important Snakes of the United States[a,b]

Snakes	WA, OR, ID	CA, NE	AZ, NM	TX	MT, MI, WI, MN, SD, ND, NE, IA, WY, UT, CO	KS, OK, AR, MO	TN, KY, IL, IN, OH	NC, SC, GA, AL, MS, LA	FL	PA, NJ, MD, DE, VA, WV, NY, New England
Pit vipers (Crotalidae)										
Cottonmouths and copperheads *(Agkistrodon)*										
Cottonmouths *(A. piscivorus)*				X	NE, IA	X	TN, KY, IL	X	X	VA
Copperheads *(A. contortrix)*				X	NE, IA	X	X	X	X	X
Rattlesnakes *(Crotalus)*										
Eastern diamondback *(C. adamanteus)*								X	X	
Western diamondback *(C. atrox)*		X	X	X		OK, AR				
Sidewinder *(C. cerastes)*		X	AZ		UT					
Timber *(C. horridus)*				X	MN, WI, NE, IA	X	X	X	X	X
Rock *(C. lepidus)*			X	X						
Speckled *(C. mitchellii)*		X	AZ							
Black-tailed *(C. molossus)*			X	X						
Twin-spotted *(C. pricei)*			AZ							
Red diamond *(C. ruber)*		CA								
Mojave *(C. scutulatus)*		X	X	X						
Tiger *(C. tigris)*			AZ							
Prairie *(C. viridis viridis)*	ID	X	X		KS, OK Not MI, W, MN					
Grand Canyon *(C. v. oreganus)*			AZ							
Southern Pacific *(C. v. helleri)*		CA								
Great Basin *(C v. lutosus)*	OR, ID	X	AZ		UT					
Northern Pacific *(C v. oreganus)*	X	X								
Ridge-nosed *(C. willardi)*			AZ							
Massasauga and pigmy *(Sistrurus)*										
Massasauga *(S. ratenatus)*			X	X	MI, WI, MN, NE, IA, CO	Not AR	IL, IN, OH			NY, PA
Pigmy *(S miliarius)*						OK, AR, MO	TN	X	X	
Coral Snakes (Elapidae)										
Western coral snakes *(Micruroides euryxanthus)*			X							
Eastern coral snake *(Micrurus fulvius)*				X		AR		X	X	

[a]Adapted from Russell FE. Vet Hum Toxicol 1991;33:584–586.
[b]Certain groups of adjoining states are treated as units. The symbol "X" indicates that distribution of the species is widespread within the unit. Restriction of a species to a part of a unit is indicated appropriately.

Table 72-8
Effects of Envenoming by Snakes on the Hemostatic System[a]

Clinical Features	Venom Component	Species Commonly Responsible
Nonclotting blood Bleeding from sites of trauma (fang marks, venepuncture sites, recent wounds)	Procoagulants Anticoagulants Fibrinolytics	Many Viperidae, some Australasian elapids and some colubrids
Thrombocytopenia, petechiae, poor clot retraction	Platelet aggregation inducers/inhibitors	Many Viperidae, some Australasian elapids and some colubrids
Spontaneous systemic bleeding (gums, nose, gastrointestinal tract, local bruising, discord ecchymoses)	Hemorrhagins	Many Viperidae, some Australasian elapids and some colubrids
Macroangiopathic hemolysis Ischemia, infarction of kidney, anterior pituitary, lung, etc. DIC with fibrin deposition in microcirculation	Factor X and prothrombin activators	*D. russelli, Bothrops* spp. *Echis* sp., *O. scutellatus*

[a]Adapted from Hutton RA, Warrell DA. Blood Rev 1993;7:176–189.

nicotinic acetylcholine receptors at the postsynaptic motor endplates and/or they affect the mode of neurotransmitter release at the presynaptic motor nerve endings. Postsynaptically acting neurotoxins are small molecules with a single chain cross-linked by four or five invariant disulfide bonds. Presynaptically acting neurotoxins found in elapid and some viperid snake venoms have a basic phospholipase A_2 in common that may be complexed with acidic basic or neutral protein units.[12]

Crotalid or viperid venoms in animals usually produce a precipitous fall in systemic blood pressure, terminating in cardiac arrest.[2] Circulatory shock with internal hemorrhage is a main cause of death following viper and pit viper bites. Viper venoms may also activate the coagulation system leading to sudden death due to disseminated intravascular coagulation. Elapid snakebites very occasionally induce hematologic disturbances.[12] Table 72-8 summarizes effects of envenomation by snakes on the hemostatic system.[13] Antivenom sources worldwide are found in the comprehensive compilation of Theakston and Warrell.[14]

ASIA PACIFIC SNAKEBITES

TREATMENT

There is little substantive clinical evidence (prospective, controlled, randomized studies) on which to base recommendations for treatment of the Asia Pacific snakebites. David Warrell has delineated some of his personal experiences, and these are summarized below.[15]

First Aid Treatment

The aims of first aid are (a) to deliver patients as quickly as possible to a place where they can be seen by medical staff; (b) to delay the evolution of life-threatening envenomation at least until patients reach a place where they can receive medical care; and (c) to alleviate early symptoms of envenomation.

General Recommendations for First Aid:

1. Reassure the patient.
2. Do not tamper with the bite wound: wipe it once with a damp cloth to remove the surface venom.
3. Immobilize the bitten limb.
4. Transport the patient to a place where they can be seen by a medically trained person.
5. Take along the dead snake for identification. Be sure it is dead. Severed snake heads, both fresh and preserved, have inflicted severe and even fatal bites.
6. Do not apply tourniquets, ligatures, or constricting bands unless the snake is a neurotoxic envenomating species: elapids (cobras, kraits); Australasian "elapids" (genera *Acanthopis, Micropechis, Oxyuranus, Pseudechis,* and *Pseudonaja*); sea snakes.
7. Avoid potentially harmful traditional first-aid measures such as cauterization, incision, excision, or amputation of the bite site; suction by mouth, vacuum pump, or syringe; combined incision and suction by "Venomex" apparatus; injection or instillation of compounds such as potassium permanganate, phenol (carbolic soap), and trypsin; application of electric shocks or ice (cryotherapy); herbal, folk, and ayurvedic remedies such as emetic plant products and parts of the snake; multiple incisions and tattooing; insufflation of oily substances into the trachea; and application of irritants to the conjunctivae.

Dangers of Tourniquets, Compression Bandages, and Other Occlusive Methods

1. Ischemia and gangrene.
2. Damage to superficial peripheral nerves, especially the lateral popliteal (common peroneal) nerve at the neck of the fibula.
3. Increased fibrinolytic activity in the occluded limb.
4. Congestion, swelling, and increased bleeding from the occluded limb.
5. Shock on releasing a tight tourniquet.
6. Intensification of local effects of venom in the occluded limb.

A firmly applied crepe bandage exerting a compression of approximately 55 mm Hg may be used after bites by neurotoxic elapids and sea snakes and may be left in place for several hours. Tourniquets tight enough to obliterate the arterial pulse are painful and must be released for about 1 minute after an hour. If reapplied, they can be finally removed after 2 hours in a hospital or dispensary after an intravenous infusion of antivenom is begun and drugs and resuscitation equipment is ready for immediate use.

Treatment of Early Manifestations of Envenomation (Before the Patient Reaches the Hospital)

1. Fear: reassurance, sedation (chlorpromazine or other tranquilizing drug).
2. Pain: oral acetaminophen.
3. Vomiting (seen early after bites by elapids, Australasian snakes, sea snakes, vipers): lay on side, head down position; chlorpromazine 25 to 50 mg (adults), 1 mg/kg (children) by mouth, injection, or suppositories.
4. Anaphylaxis (within a few minutes by some species of *Vipera* and Australian "elapids"): adrenaline; if hypotensive tip head downwards; bronchospasm, dyspnea, cyanosis: give oxygen. H_1 blockers are used to treat severe allergic reactions.
5. Vasovagal syncope: head down tilt.
6. Bulbar, respiratory paralysis (may begin within 1 to 2 hours: first, difficulty in focusing, eyelids feel heavy; later, external ophthalmoplegia, inability to open the mouth, protrude the tongue, speak, and swallow. Paralysis of the jaw and tongue may lead to upper airway obstruction and aspiration. Respiratory muscle paralysis may lead to respiratory failure: Lay the patient on the side, elevate jaw, insert oral airway if available; if cyanosed, give oxygen; artificial ventilation may be required; mouth-to-mouth or mouth-to-nose ventilation may be life saving; if the patient is unconscious and no femoral or carotid pulse can be felt, external cardiac massage and mouth-to-mouth ventilation should be started immediately.

Medical Treatment in Health Stations, Dispensaries, Hospitals, Etc.

Preliminary questions

1. In which part of your body were you bitten?
2. How long ago were you bitten?
3. Have you brought the snake, or can anyone describe it? Circumstances of bite can provide a clue. Bitten while asleep in a hut in Southern Asia—*Bungarus species* (krait); biting fresh-water fishermen—cobras; plantation workers in Southeast Asia—*Calloselasma rhodostoma;* rice farmers—*Vipera russelli.*

History of Evolution of Symptoms

Symptoms of systemic envenomation: vomiting, fainting, muscular pain and weakness, abdominal pain, and bleeding.

Examination

Local swelling, tenderness, lymph node involvement seen early: Viperidae, Asian cobras. However, 9 to 18% of systemic envenomation by *Vipera russelli* in Sri Lanka and Burma exhibit: no local swelling. Neurotoxic venomous snakes (sea snakes, kraits, Australian elapids). almost no swelling. Gingival bleeding; shock; ptosis; respiratory muscle weakness (measure peak expiratory flow, vital capacity, or expiratory pressure using mercury manometer of a sphygmomanometer); coma; muscle tenderness, resistance to passive muscle stretching; trismus-rhabdomyolysis due to venoms of sea snakes, some Australasian elapids, Sri Lankan/South Indian *Vipera russelli.* Oliguria after bite by *Vipera russelli.* Massive intravascular hemolysis (black urine): Sri Lankan and Indian *Vipera russelli.* Urine: myoglobin. Severe hypofibrinogenemia: blood runs out of tube after sitting for 20 minutes.

Check every hour:

1. Level of consciousness.
2. Presence or absence of ptosis.
3. Pulse rate and rhythm.
4. Blood pressure.
5. Respiratory rate.
6. Extent of local swelling.
7. New symptoms or signs.

Antivenom Treatment

Do not use routinely and indiscriminately because of the following:

1. All commercial antivenoms carry a risk of potentially serous serum reactions.
2. Antivenom is not always necessary; many patients are bitten by nonvenomous snakes, and a large proportion of those bitten by venomous snakes are not envenomated.
3. Antivenoms have a range of specific and paraspecific neutralizing activity and are useless for venoms outside that range. Specific antivenoms are not available for treatment of envenomation by some species (e.g., *Bungarus candidus* in Southeast Asia).
4. Antivenom is expensive, always in short supply, and has a limited shelf life.

Indications for Antivenom

A. Systemic envenomation
   1. Hemostatic disturbances: spontaneous systemic bleeding (e.g., gums, epistaxis), coagulopathy (e.g., incoagulable blood, prolonged clotting time, elevated FDR, or thrombocytopenia).
   2. Cardiovascular abnormalities: shock, hypotension, abnormal electrocardiogram, arrhythmia, cardiac failure, pulmonary edema.
   3. Neurotoxicity.
   4. Generalized rhabdomyolysis.
   5. Impaired consciousness of any cause.

6. In patients with definite signs of local envenomation, the following indicate significant systemic envenomation: neutrophil leukocytosis, elevated creatine phosphokinase and aminotransferases, hemoconcentration, uremia, hypercreatinemia, oliguria, hypoxemia, acidosis, and vomiting.

B. Severe local envenoming
Local swelling involving more than half the bitten limb, or associated with extensive blistering or bruising, especially in patients bitten by species whose venoms are known to cause local necrosis (e.g., many Viperidae, Asian cobras). Bites on digits carry a high risk of necrosis.

Contraindications to Antivenom

There is no absolute contraindication to antivenom in patients with life-threatening systemic envenomation. However, patients with an atopic history (asthma, hay fever, vernal conjunctivitis, eczema, food and drug allergies) and those who have had reactions to equine antiserum on previous occasions have an increased risk of severe reactions. In these cases pretreatment with subcutaneous adrenaline and intravenous antihistamine and corticosteroids may prevent or diminish the reaction. Rapid desensitization is not recommended.

Timing of Antivenom

Give as soon as signs of systemic or severe local envenomation are evidenced. Average time between bite and death:

Asian cobras—8 hours (12 minutes to 120 hours)
Bungarus caeruleus—18 hours (3 to 63 hours)
Vipera russelli—3 days (15 minutes to 264 hours)
Echis carinatus—5 days (25 hours to 41 days)

It is almost never too late to try antivenom treatment: it has been effective up to 2 days after sea snake bites and 10 days or more after *Echis carinatus* bites.

Antivenom Specificity

Optimal treatment consists of monospecific antivenom. If no dead snake is brought in for identification, a polyspecific antivenom may be useful.

Administration

Give intravenously: 5 mL/minute, or diluted in isotonic fluid, infused over 30 to 60 minutes. Dress venipuncture sites with a pressure bandage. Injection of antivenom into the fang marks is probably ineffective and is painful.

Dosage

Children must be given the same dose of antivenom as adults.

Response to Antivenom: Time to Possible Response

Neurotoxicity—slowly
Cardiovascular effects (hypotension, bradycardia)—10 to 20 minutes
Stopping spontaneous systemic bleeding—15 to 30 minutes
Blood coagulability restored—1 to 6 hours

Repeat the initial dose of antivenom if severe cardiovascular or neurotoxic symptoms persist for more than 30 minutes and incoagulable blood persists for more than 6 hours after the first dose.

Antivenom Reactions

1. Early reactions
10 to 60 minutes after starting IV antivenom. Cough, tachycardia, itching (especially of scalp), urticaria, fever, palpitations, nausea, vomiting, headache. Over 5% with early reactions develop manifestations of severe systemic anaphylaxis: hypotension, bronchospasm, angioedema. Few die. Treatment: Adrenaline (epinephrine) subcutaneously: 0.5 to 1.0 mL 0.1% (1 in 1000) for adults; 0.01 mg/kg for children. In severe cases, give same dose by intramuscular injections, or during cardiac resuscitation, by slow IV or even intracardiac injection. Follow with an antihistamine (e.g., chlorpheniramine maleate—10 mg (adults); 0.2 mg/kg (children).
2. Pyrogenic reactions
Develop 1 to 2 hours after treatment. Chills, cutaneous vasoconstriction, goose flesh, shivering. Drop in temperature. Sweating, vomiting, diarrhea. Treatment: Lie flat; reduce temperature by fanning, tepid sponging, hypothermia blankets, or antipyretic drugs such as acetaminophen (5 mg/kg by mouth, suppository, or via nasogastric tube).
3. Late reactions (serum sickness type)
About 7 days after treatment (5 to 24 days).Treatment: Antihistamines may contain a milder attack. Steroids may be useful in more severe cases.

Ancillary Treatment

Local Envenomation

1. Secondary infection: Prevent with penicillin or erythromycin and booster dose of tetanus toxoid.
2. Clean wound with antiseptic.
3. Bullae can be aspirated to dryness with a fine sterile needle.
4. Nurse limbs in most comfortable position.
5. Examine wound frequently for evidence of necrosis.

Intracompartmental Syndromes

Excessive pain, weakness of muscles contained by the compartment, pain when muscles are passively stretched, hyperesthesia of the skin supplied by nerves running through the compartment, and obvious tension of the compartment. Palpable distal arterial pulses do not exclude intracompartmental ischemia. Intracompartmental pressure above 45 mm Hg (60 cm of water) are associated with a high risk of ischemic necrosis and may be regarded as an indication for fasciotomy. However, this procedure may not save envenomated muscles. Fasciotomy should not be performed before blood coagulability has been restored by antivenom.

Hemostatic Abnormalities

After specific antivenom is administered, fresh whole blood, fresh frozen plasma, cryoprecipitates (containing fibrinogen, factor VII, fibronectin, and some factors V and XIII), or platelet concentrates may be used. Because of attendant risks Burgess and Dart[16] recommend use of blood products in pit viper envenomation only if antivenom is not effective for active bleeding or for specific coagulation abnormalities. Heparin and epsilon aminocaproic acid have not yet been shown to accelerate recovery.

Neurotoxic Envenomation—Bulbar, Respiratory Paralysis

Keep airway clear; head down, lie on side, jaw elevated, oral airway, tracheostomy if required, cuffed endotracheal intubation if necessary. Manual or mechanical ventilation may be required for many weeks.

Anticholinesterases

Prostigmine has not reversed the paralytic effects of South American venoms. Clinical response is more likely if postsynaptic neurotoxin (see later) predominate in the venoms. All patients with neurotoxic symptoms should be given the benefit of a "Tensilon" (Edrophonium) test as in the case of patients with suspected myasthenia gravis (see Philippines).

1. Atropine sulfate (0.6 mg adults; 50 µg/kg children) IV to block unpleasant muscarinic effects of acetylcholine-increased secretion, abdominal colic.
2. Edrophonium chloride (10 mg adults; 0.25 mg/kg children) IV 2 mg at first, then 8 mg after 45 seconds to evaluate effect.
3. Measure duration of lid retraction on upward gaze, maximum interdental distance on mouth opening, forced expiratory pressure, or vital capacity.
4. If patients respond convincingly, maintain on neostigmine methylsulfate (50 to 100 µg/kg) and atropine sulfate (15 µg/kg) by subcutaneous injection every 4 hours or by continuous IV infusion. If patient can swallow tablets, give neostigmine (initial adult dose 15 mg four times daily) or pyridostigmine (initial adult dose 60 mg four times daily) with atropine (0.6 mg twice daily) or propantheline hydrochloride (15 mg twice daily).

Generalized Rhabdomyolysis or Myonecrosis

Some venoms contain phospholipase A_2 with presynaptic neurotoxic activity and can induce a generalized breakdown of skeletal muscle resulting in myoglobinemia, myoglobinuria, hyperkalemia, hyperphosphatemia, and hypocalcemia. Creatine phosphokinase and aspartate aminotransferase enzymes may be greatly elevated. Generalized muscle tenderness, pain on passive stretching of muscle, generalized weakness, and trismus associated with dark reddish brownish or black urine may be seen. To prevent myoglobinuric nephropathy: Adults—mannitol 25 g and sodium bicarbonate, 100 mEq, are added to 1 liter 5% dextrose infused over 4 hours: monitored central venous pressure and urine output. If no diuresis, follow with furosemide 240 mg IV over 15 minutes. Potential dangers of mannitol are hyponatremia, fluid overload, and hyperkalemia; bicarbonate may exacerbate hypocalcemia.

Hypotension and Shock

Specific antivenom; plasma expander; raise foot of bed; monitor central venous pressure or pulmonary arterial pressure (Swan-Ganz catheter); systemic blood pressure measured frequently. If patients do not respond, give dopamine.

Renal Failure

Record urine output, fluid balance. If urine output falls below 400 mL/24 hours, insert urethral catheter and monitor central venous pressure (CVP). Cautious rehydration with isotonic fluid to increase CVP to 3 cm H_2O followed by up to 100 mg of furosemide IV and finally dopamine (2.5 µg/kg/minute) by continuous infusion into a central vein may be used. If these measures fail to increase urine output, consider dialysis.

Snake Venom Ophthalmia

"Spitting cobras" *(N.n. sputatrix, N.n. philippinensis, N.n. sumatrana, N.n. sumarensis)* occur in Thailand, Malaysia, Indonesia, and the Philippines. Wash venom from the eye with large volumes of water. Treat as if patient has a corneal injury. Topical antimicrobial tetracycline or chloramphenicol and dressing pad to a closed eye can be useful.

Clinical Effects

Clinical effects of envenomation by Australian elapid snakes are summarized in Table 72-9.

Envenomation[20]

Early signs of systemic envenomation include headache, nausea, vomiting, blurred vision, abdominal pain, collapse, and convulsions (especially in children) beginning within 5 to 10 minutes to several hours. Blood may become hypocoagulable within 15 to 30 minutes. A persistent ooze from the bite is more common. Renal effects are unlikely in the first few hours, other than oliguria or anuria. Myolysis is first evidenced by dark urine (myoglobinuria), muscle weakness, and muscle movement pain usually beginning within 1 to several hours. Neurotoxic paralysis also may begin within the first hour and is seen first as ptosis, then blurred vision and diplopia, followed by ophthalmoplegia, facial weakness, loss of expression, tongue weakness, and dysarthria. In severe cases limb weakness, paralysis of

Table 72–9
Summary of Clinical Effects of Envenomation by Australian Elapid Snakes[a]

	Local Problems at the Bite Site			Systemic Problems			
Snake/Venom Group	Pain	Swelling	Bruising (Mild Necrosis)	Unconsciousness	Paralysis	Coagulopathy	Muscle Destruction (Muscle Movement Pain/Myoglobinuria)
Brown snakes (*Pseudonaja* spp.)	Absent or minimal	Nil	Nil	Usual (convulsions)	Uncommon	Usual, severe	Nil
Tiger snakes (*Notechis* spp.)	Frequent	Frequent but mild	Often present	Usual (convulsions)	Usual and sometimes severe	Usual, severe	Frequently present
Mulga snake (*Pseudechis australis*)	Often minor	Usually severe	Usually absent or minimal but necrosis may occur	Usual	True paralysis not seen	Frequent, but often mild	Usual and sometimes severe
Red-bellied black snake (*Pseudechis porphyriacus*)	Often minor	Usual	Variable	Occasionally	Not seen	Unlikely	Frequently present, though often minor
Death adders (*Acanthophis* spp.)	Frequent	Minimal or absent	Absent	Unusual	Usual and sometimes severe	Unlikely	Not seen
Taipans (*Oxyuranus* spp.)	Variable, sometimes absent	Often minimal	Unusual	Usual (convulsions)	Usual and sometimes severe	Usual, severe	Probably frequently present

[a]Adapted from White J. J Wilderness Med 1991;2:219–244.

Table 72-10
Laboratory Evaluation for Rattlesnake Envenomation[a]

Complete blood cell count with differential and platelet count
Coagulation parameters
Prothrombin time
Partial thromboplastin time
Fibrinogen levels
Fibrin degradation products
Serum levels of electrolytes, urea nitrogen, creatinine, calcium, phosphorus, alanine aminotransferase, lactate dehydrogenase, and bilirubin
Urinalysis (macroscopic and microscopic)[b]
Free protein
Hemoglobin
Myoglobin
Electrocardiogram
Additional tests as needed or indicated by patient's hospital course

[a]Adapted from Davidson TM, Schafer SF. Postgrad Med 1991;96:107–114.
[b]Intermittent catheterization or an indwelling Foley catheter is often useful.

respiration (requiring mechanical ventilation), and fixed, dilated pupils may be observed.

Management of Complications of Envenomation[20]

Coagulopathy—Antivenom therapy; replacement therapy (e.g., fresh frozen plasma only if life-threatening hemorrhage). Heparin therapy is hazardous.

Paralysis—Presynaptic neurotoxins (e.g., brown snakes, tiger snakes, taipans, rough-scaled snake, copperheads). Given antivenom early before severe paralysis; antivenom is unlikely to reverse established paralysis. Postsynaptic neurotoxins (e.g., death adder): antivenom may induce some reversal of paralysis; anticholinesterases possibly useful.

Renal failure—follow urine output, fluid therapy, central venous pressure.

Myolysis—Watch for myoglobinuria, hyperkalemia; physiotherapy for early contractures.

LABORATORY

Suggested laboratory investigations in cases of snakebite injuries are outlined in Table 72-10.[21]

TREATMENT

Principles of treatment of snakebite in the South Pacific and Asian areas have been comprehensively summarized by Dr. D.A. Warrell (see Asia Pacific Snakebite Summary) and are summarized here. An overall plan for treatment of snakebite injuries is presented in Figure 72-1. Use of adrenaline prior to antivenom administration is controversial. Adrenaline is probably best reserved for treatment of a severe reaction should it occur. If there is a history of previous exposure to antivenom, or allergy to horse serum, or a history of severe allergic reactions or asthma, consideration should be given to prior treatment with subcutaneous adrenaline, intravenous antihistamine, and, in addition, intravenous hydrocortisone. Failure to show resolution of coagulopathy or worsening coagulopathy 2 hours after administration of antivenom is evidence of continuing circulating venom and is an indication for further antivenom therapy. Antivenoms may not reverse any paralysis due to a venom containing neurotoxin. The antivenom will not prevent the early signs of paralysis such as ptosis and double vision, but may prevent further more severe and life-threatening paralysis.[22] Recommended doses of antivenom (intravenous) for Australian snakes are presented in Table 72-11[21] where snake identity is known.

Most venoms produce the death of poisoned creatures by paralysis of the muscles of respiration. The action occurs on nerve membranes on or about the motor cord plate region. Sutherland has delineated presynaptic and postsynaptic toxins.[21]

Presynaptic Venoms

Snake neurotoxins usually have a high molecular weight (13,000 to 85,000). Botulinus toxin (MW 140,000) is the most neurotoxic substance known. Presynaptic venoms (except for Bungarotoxin [from the Asian banded krait] and Botulinus toxin [MW 140,000]) produce detectable ultrastructural changes and a paralysis that is difficult to reverse with antivenoms. Examples include lathrotoxin (red-black spider venom—MW 130,000), notexin (tiger snake venom—MW 13,500), taipoxin (Taipan venom—MW 45,000), and textilar (common brown snake venom—MW 88,000).

Postsynaptic Venoms

Smaller neurotoxins from snake venoms block acetylcholine receptors. No ultrastructural changes are observed. Paralysis is more easily reversed by antivenom. Examples include Australian snake venoms (MW 6000), alpha-Bungarotoxin (MW 7400), and conotoxins.[21]

Use of Antivenoms[17]

The decision to use antivenom must be an absolute one, not a "try-and-see" decision. If the decision to use antivenom is not made a priori in an absolute sense, an impossible dilemma occurs if a severe reaction develops. Under these (uncommon) latter circumstances, if a patient is envenomated after a life-threatening bite, one still must press on with antivenom albeit with a modified pharmacologic technique with supplementary drugs and a slower infusion rate.

The patient should receive the antivenom in an intensive-care unit of a referral hospital, if at all possible.

The administration technique is straightforward and of proved efficacy in practice.

Dilute the antivenom 1 in 10 in an appropriate fluid carrier, such as normal saline, or glucose saline. In small children it may be necessary to dilute the antivenom 1 in 5, because of potential fluid overload.

Give an intravenous injection of an antihistamine agent.

Give a subcutaneous injection of adrenaline (1 in 100 solution). The suggested dose is 0.3 mL for an adult and 0.1 mL for a child. Warn the patient that the effects of the adrenaline will develop over the next few minutes, and that these are not a result of the snake venom itself.

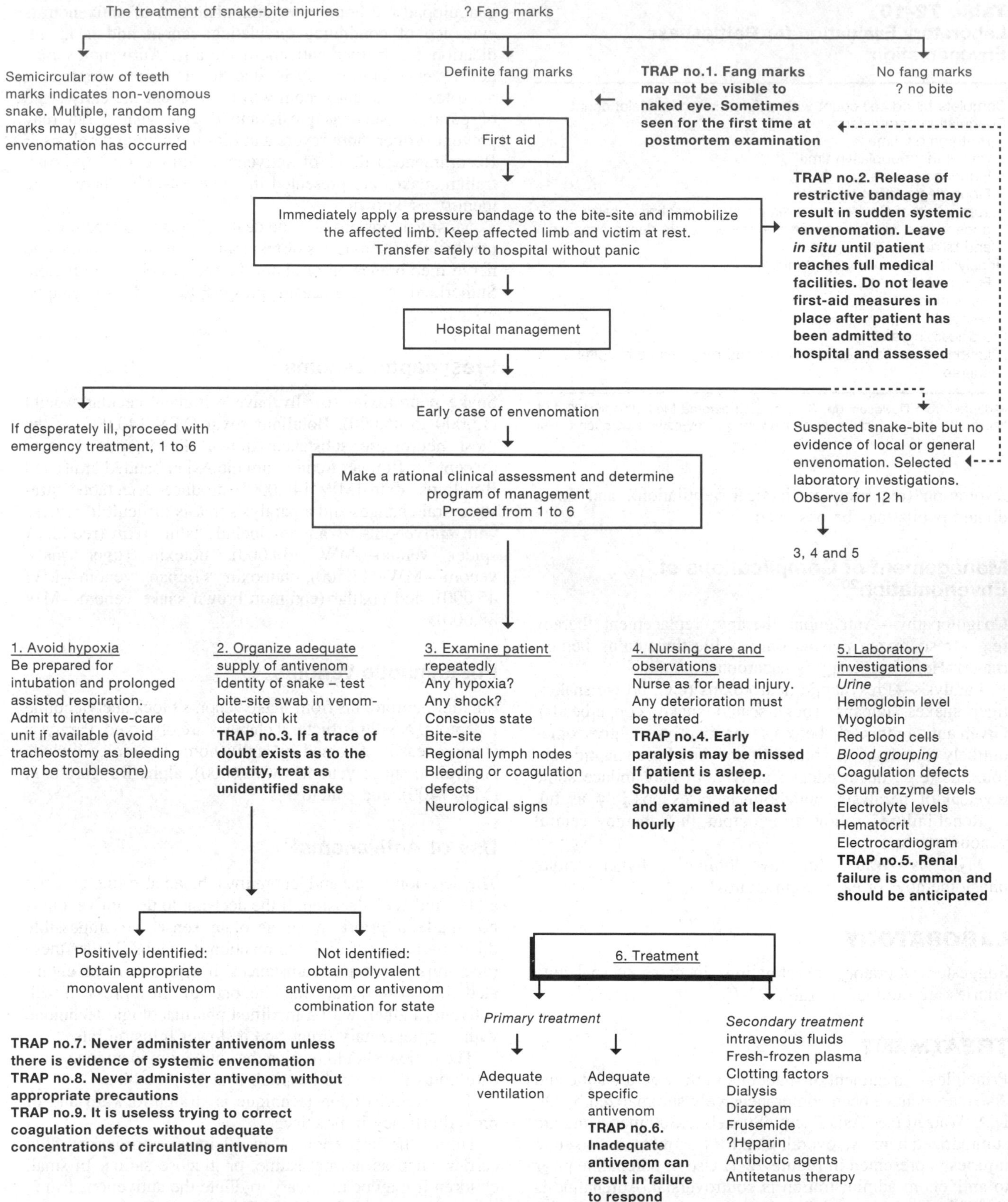

Figure 72-1 The treatment of snake-bite injuries. (Adapted from Sutherland SK, King K. Management of snake bite injuries. Monograph Series Number One. Royal Flying Doctor Service of Australia, 43 Bridge Street, Hurstville NSW 2220, 1991.)

In some circumstances, administer hydrocortisone by the intravenous route (the dose is empirical; 100 mg is used currently as the initial dose). Hydrocortisone is used to reduce the incidence of subacute and chronic reactions such as serum sickness. The circumstances in which it is recommended specifically include children; those who will be receiving a large volume of antivenom, for example, polyvalent antivenom, or when it is anticipated that multiple vials of monovalent antivenom will be required; and those with a history of previous allergic reactions to equine protein.

Commence the intravenous infusions of antivenom, running the infusion slowly at first (not faster than 1 mL/min for 3 to 5 minutes). Plan to give the infusion over 30 to 40 minutes, unless allergic reactions are encountered.

Monitor the patient in an intensive care unit for at least 6 hours after the antivenom is given.

Table 72–11
Amount of Monovalent Antivenom Where Snake Identity Is Known[a]

Snake	Appropriate Monovalent Antivenom	Initial Dose
Common Tiger Snake *Notechis scutatus*	Tiger Snake	3,000 units
Western Tiger Snake *N. ater occidentalis*	Tiger Snake	6,000 units
Kreffts Tiger Snake *N. ater ater*	Tiger Snake	6,000 units
Peninsular Tiger Snake *N. ater niger*	Tiger Snake	6,000 units
Tasmanian Tiger Snake		
King Island Tiger Snake *N. ater humphreysi*	Tiger Snake	6,000 units
Chappell Island Tiger Snake *N. ater serventyi*	Tiger Snake	9,000 units
Taipan *Oxyuranus scutellatus*	Taipan	12,000 units
Inland Taipan *Oxyuranus microlepidotus*	Taipan	12,000 units
Copperhead *Austrelaps superbus*	Tiger Snake	3,000 units 6,000 units (in Tasmania)
Common Brown Snake *Pseudomaja textilis*	Brown Snake	1,000 units
Dugite *Pseudomaja affinis*	Brown Snake	1,000 units
Western Brown Snake *Pseudomaja nuchalis*	Brown Snake	1,000 units
Peninsula Brown Snake *Pseudomaja inframacula*	Brown Snake	1,000 units
Ingrams Brown Snake *Pseudomaja ingrami*	Brown Snake	1,000 units
Speckled Brown Snake *Pseudomaja guttata*	Brown Snake	1,000 units
Death Adder *Acanthophis antarcticus*	Death Adder	6,000 units
Desert Death Adder *Acanthophis pyrrhus*	Death Adder	6,000 units
Northern Death Adder *Acanthophis praelongus*	Death Adder	6,000 units

[a]Adapted from Mirtschin PJ, Crowe GR, Davis R. In: Gopalakrishnakone P, Chou LM, eds. Snakes of medical importance (Asia Pacific region). Singapore: Venom and Toxin Research Group. National University of Singapore. 1990, pp. 1–173.

Failure of Antivenom Therapy[20]

If the antivenom fails to give the expected response, there may be several problems:

1. The wrong monovalent antivenom was chosen; use polyvalent antivenom if there is a problem in identifying the snake.
2. Insufficient antivenom was used.
3. Inactive venom—check expiration date.
4. Wrong route of administration (e.g., intramuscular route).
5. Too great a delay, but antivenom therapy has been useful up to 60 hours after envenomation.

Reptile Handlers

Experience in South Australia indicates that about 25% or less of all presentations for snakebite treatment occur in reptile handlers. In this group most bites are glancing and minor and alcohol is not a universal, but is a frequent association. Problems with keepers include a history of repeated bites, an increased risk of antivenom and venom allergy, a tendency to late presentation for medical care, and usually an increase in medical costs that may need to be paid by the community.[18]

PAPUA, NEW GUINEA, AUSTRALIAN OUTBACK

The Papuan black snake, *Pseudechis papuanus,* is a main cause of serious snakebites in Southern Papua. The introduction of the cane or marine toad *Bufomarinus* from South America during the 1930s and 1940s has, because of its powerful bufotoxin, caused the death of many frog-eating snakes. About 155 admissions per year to Papuan hospitals follow snakebites, or suspected snakebites. The New Guinea death adder *(Acanthrophis antarcticus)* produces a venom that appears to act postsynaptically by blocking cholinergic receptors causing a severe flaccid paralysis and death due to respiratory failure. Early signs of Australasian elapid envenomation include vomiting, headaches, localized pain of the lymph nodes, abdominal pain, loss of consciousness, shortness of breath, cyanosis of the lips and gums, and heaviness of limbs. Bleeding from the gums and gingival sulci are not observed following death adder envenomation. Antivenom for Papua New Guinea are produced by the Commonwealth Serum Laboratories in Victoria, Australia. A polyspecific Papuan antivenom is available. Nonspecific death adder, taipan, black snake, or brown snake antivenoms are available. Anticholinesterases administered together with atropine may be useful during the initial critical stage of envenomation and allow the bite victim to gain valuable time needed to reach a hospital. However, anticholinesterase therapy alone may not adequately prevent progression of neurotoxicity in severe envenomation.[19–21]

AUSTRALIA

There are over 120 species of snake in Australia—these represent 6% of the world's snakes. About 60% of these are from the Elapidae (or cobralike) family. Australia possesses

40% of the world's elapid snakes, and about 23% of all venomous snakes of the world. Twenty-seven of these species are capable of causing death. Nevertheless, the mortality due to snakebite is only two to three per year.[22] Much of this is due to the work of the Commonwealth Serum Laboratories (CSL) and to Dr. Struan Sutherland who has produced antivenoms for all of Australia's dangerous snakes, as well as a Venom Detection Kit and specific monovalent antivenom. A second group based in Brisbane is headed by Dr. J. Pearn of the University of Queensland. Dr. Julian White, who leads a third group at Adelaide Children's Hospital, has also been active in emphasizing the clinical aspects of diagnosis and treatment of snakebite. Sutherland estimates up to 500 cases of envenomation occur requiring antivenom per year, and about 3000 cases of bite remain asymptomatic and require no treatment.[23] The inland taipan *(Oxyuranus microlepidotus)* may be Australia's most dangerous snake.

Snake Venom[18,22,24–26]

The most important systemic effects of Australian snake venom in man are as follows:

1. Neurotoxicity (N)
   Postsynaptic neurotoxins: more common, rapidly acting, less toxic.
   Presynaptic neurotoxins: more potent, all have a phospholipase A2 as a principal component and are either single chain (e.g., notexin from *Notechis suitatus*), or multichain (e.g., taipoxin from *Oxyuranus scutellatus*).
2. Myotoxins (M)—watch for rhabdomyolysis.
3. Hemotoxins (C)—affecting platelets (less important); clotting pathway; fibrinolytic pathway; possibly resulting in intravascular hemolysis.
4. Renal damage (R)—possibly secondary in many cases.
5. Local tissue destruction—not usually seen in Australia.
6. Local edema (E)

Identification

Identification may require handling the snakes (may be very dangerous for the untrained layman), comparing color photographs for a similar color, and comparing the scalation count and head scales. Common Australian snakes include the brown snakes (genus *Pseudonaja*) the tiger snakes (*Notechis* spp.), the taipans (genus *Oxyuranus*), the death adders (genus *Acanthopus*), the black or Mulga snakes (genus *Pseudechis*), the copperheads (genus *Austrelaps*), the broad-headed snakes (genus *Hoplocephalus*), and other snakes. Monovalent antivenoms are employed to neutralize the five major groups of Australian snake venom.

Venom Detection Kits

CSL has developed snakebite venom detection kits that can detect venom levels as low as 5 to 10 nanograms of venom and can be performed in about 30 minutes. Although a positive result may be obtained from the kit, antivenom should be withheld if no symptoms develop in the patient. If a negative result is obtained, and symptoms develop, antivenom treatment should be started.

BURMA[27]

Each year 10,000 snakebites, from 144 species, occur in Burma with 1000 lives lost. Russell's viper and the common cobra are deadly. Ten percent of bites are fatal annually. Farmers are usually the victims. Cobra bites are responsible for 5% of deaths due to venomous snakebites in Burma. Russell's viper is perhaps the most venomous snake and is responsible for 85% of poisonous snake bites; significant envenomation in 70% of bites and 95% of the fatalities due to venomous snakebites in Burma. In minimal envenomation there are mild symptoms and slight local swelling. If severe, in a few hours, hemorrhagic effects (bleeding gums, epistaxis, hemoptysis, hematemesis, hematuria, orbital edema, and subconjunctival hemorrhages) may be observed. Shock may be seen. The patients may experience a burning sensation in the epigastrium. Blood does not coagulate. The prothrombin time is much prolonged and the plasma fibrinogen extremely low. After antivenom therapy the coagulation time comes back to normal within 2 to 3 hours. The platelet count remains low for 7 to 10 days. Acute renal failure may supervene.[28] Pituitary failure has been observed—Sheehan's syndrome-like.[29,30] Treatment: 20 mL specific antivenom IV; usually 60 mL is sufficient, but up to 160 mL have been given. Follow clotting times every hour for 6 hours, then every 2 hours. Shock may respond to massive doses of hydrocortisone. Polyvalent cobra venom is available. Both antivenoms are prepared by the Burma Pharmaceutical Industry, Rangoon.

CHINA

In China there are 200 species, 62 genera, and 8 families; 57 species are venomous. In recent years at least a million snakes were captured and killed on mainland China; all parts of the snake are sold and used—venoms, skin (arts and crafts), bile (traditional medicine), and meat (food). Antivenoms are produced by the Shanghai Institute of Biological Products of the Ministry of Public Health for the whole country. No statistical data on snakebites are available. Antivenom against *Agkistrodon blomhoffi brevicaudus* can be used for snakebite of all species of Agkistrodons. That against *A. acutus* and *brevicaudus* can be used for genus *Trimeresurus* (cross-immunization). The antivenoms of Elapidae and Viperidae are very specific. Therefore it is

Table 72–12
Initial Antivenom ([Crotalidae] Polyvalent [Wyeth]) Dose According to Grade of Severity [a]

Envenomation	Amount Administered
No envenomation	None
Minimal	0 to 5 vials
Moderate	10 to 20 vials
Severe	20 or more

Place 5 vials (50 mL) in 200 mL of 0.5 normal saline; infuse at 1 mL/min for first 10 minutes.
[a]Adapted from Blackman JR, Dillon S. J A Board Fam Pract 1992;5:399–405.

important to have accurate identification of species before using these antivenoms. Potency and dosage of antivenoms are found in Table 72-12.[31,32] *Bungarus multicinctus* (banded krait) often induces respiratory arrest and multisystem organ failure. Antivenom and respiratory support are essential for survival.[33]

HONG KONG

Snakebites in Hong Kong are most commonly due to *Trimeresurus albolabris* (the white-lipped pit viper, bamboo snake).[34] Most induce a coagulopathy, probably resulting from the presence of a thrombinlike substance that induces defibrination and secondary fibrinolysis. Increased blood concentration of fibrin degradation products is the most sensitive test for detecting the abnormality, although a decrease in fibrinogen concentration and thrombocytopenia are also seen. Problems remain with the purification of the antivenom. Its use should probably be restricted to high-risk patients such as children and pregnant women and other patients with systemic envenomation (nonclotting blood) associated with spontaneous systemic bleeding. In the remaining patients appropriate use of replacement therapy should remain the mainstay of treatment. Fatalities have rarely occurred.[34] A bedside whole blood clotting time in excess of 20 minutes appears indicative of serious envenomation. Green pit viper antivenom (Thai Red Cross) is specific for use in the treatment of white-lipped viper bites.

INDIA

There are four medically important venomous land snakes in India—the Indian krait *(Bungarus caeruleus);* the common cobra *(Naja naja);* the saw-scaled viper *(Echis carinatus);* and Russell's viper *(Vipera russelli).* Only Russell's viper has been locally reported as a cause of renal failure. Peritoneal dialysis appears to be an adequate form of treatment for most of these patients.[35] Nevertheless, 10,000 to 15,000 deaths from snakebite are reported annually.[36] The frequency of snakebite peaks in the rainy season, which coincides with increased agricultural operations. During this season the eggs of cobras and kraits hatch. Farmers and their families are the main victims.[36] Vasculotoxic and neuroparalytic signs predominate. In addition to general supportive care, polyvalent antivenom is the mainstay of treatment. Neostigmine with atropine is used to reverse the neuroparalysis. Ventilatory support is essential. Whole blood transfusions and transfusions of fibrinogen with heparin are used to correct the bleeding diathesis. The polyvalent snake venom is equine (horse) in origin and is a mixture of venoms of the four snakes detailed above.[37]

JAPAN

Rhabdophis tigrinus (family Natricidae) is one of the most common venomous snakes in Japan.[38] *Agkistrodon blomhoffi blomhoffi* (family Crotalidae) is the other major venomous snake found in Japan. Others are found in the Ryuku archipelago: *Calliophis* sp. (family Elapidae) and *Trimeresurus (habu)* sp. (family Crotalidae). Antivenoms against habu *(Trimeresurus),* mamushi *(A. b. blomhoffi),* and yamakagashi *(Rhabdophis tigrinus)* are commercially produced by the Laboratory of Chemotherapy and Serotherapy, Kumamoto, Japan. Antimamushi antivenom is also available commercially at China Prefectural Serum Laboratory, Konodai, Chiba, Japan. A toxoid has been developed that may decrease the severe local necrosis of habu.[39]

MALAYSIA

In Malaysia 17 of 105 strictly land snakes are venomous and dangerous to man.[40] These snakes belong to two families: Elapidae and Viperidae. All 14 species of freshwater snakes are harmless, but all of the 22 species of sea snakes are venomous. The family Viperidae has a distinctive triangular shaped head with a pit situated between the eye and the nostril, and it has long poison fangs. Two genera are involved: *Agkistrodon* with a single species, and *Trimeresurus* with seven species. The family Elapidae has enlarged poison fangs at the front of each upper jaw. All the really dangerous land snakes found in Malaysia belong to the Elapidae family: cobras, kraits, and the coral snakes. Most snake species are forest dwellers. The elapid snakes are mainly terrestrials; the viperid snakes are semiarboreal. Cannibalism is common among the elapid, but not viperid snakes. The genus *Agkistrodon* (family Viperidae) is represented by one species—*Calloselasma rhodostoma,* which is probably the most common cause of snakebite in Malaysia.[41] It produces either local swelling or systemic poisoning with varying effects on blood clotting leading, in its severe form, to a hemorrhagic syndrome and in some instances, shock. Antivenom treatment may not prevent hemorrhage.[42]

Neurotoxic symptoms or signs are seldom seen. Hemoptysis is the earliest sign of generalized poisoning and may precede the coagulation defects observed. *Trimeresurus,* the other genus of the Viperidae family, is represented by seven species, one of which is the temple or speckled pit viper *(Trimeresurus wagleri).* Its bite results in pain and swelling. Although most clinically significant land snakebites in Malaysia are due to the common black cobra *(Naja naja)* and the Malayan pit viper *(Calloselasma rhodostona),* only 11 out of 83 snakebites in one series resulted in systemic poisoning and required antivenom.[43] Fatality rate is about 2%.

MIDDLE EAST

Echis coloratus (family Viperidae) inhabits the arid zones of the Middle East, including the Jordan valley, Judean desert, and northern Negev. *Echis carinatus* is the other major snake causing envenomation in this area. The venom of all species of *Echis* causes hemostatic failure, with disseminated intravascular coagulation and occasional thrombocytopenia. Unlike *E. coloratus,* untreated envenomation by *E. carinatus* is associated with overt bleeding in up to 57% of victims and a 10 to 20% mortality mostly due to cerebral hemorrhage. The most remarkable feature of envenomation by *E. coloratus* is the discrepancy between the severe hemostatic failure and its benign clinical course. Antivenom treatment is recommended for all victims of *E. coloratus* with past exposure to antivenom who are judged to be at an average risk of a second envenomation in the future, and who present with any of the following: any bleeding, anemia, azotemia, thrombocytopenia, or proteinemia.[44]

ISRAEL

Of the 35 or more snake species of Israel eight are venomous and belong to three families: Viperidae (six species)—*Vipera palestinae, Vipera bornmuelleri, Echis coloratus, Pseudocerastes fieldi, Cerastes cerastes, Cerastes vipera;* Elapidae (one species)—*Walterinnesia aegyptia;* and Atractaspididae (one species)—*Atractaspis engaddensis. Vipera palestinae* is the clinically most important snake of Israel: 100 to 300 bites/year, 0 to 2 fatalities. About 20% of the bites may carry no envenomation. Within 15 to 20 minutes after a bite weakness, restlessness, vomiting, profuse perspiration, and abdominal pain are experienced. Diarrhea, hypotension, unmeasurable blood pressure and pulse, rapid heart beat, angioneurotic edema of the upper lip, and swelling of the bitten extremity may follow. Major bleeding, anemia, and azotemia may be seen after an *Echis coloratus* envenomation.[45,46] A monospecific antivenom is available and effective (50 to 60 mL IV) for *V. palestinae* bites and for *Echis coloratus* (Rogoff Wellcome Institute) and against *Walterinnesia aegypti* (Department of Zoology, Tel Aviv University).[47]

PERSIAN GULF[48–50]

The Arabian Peninsula and the waters that surround it harbor at least 51 species of snake, of which 18 are poisonous.[48] Of the land snakes nine must be considered dangerous: Innes' cobra *(Walterinnesia aegypti)* very aggressive, seen in arid desert areas; Arabian cobra *(Naja naja arabicus)* fast, aggressive; horned viper, sand viper *(Ceristes cerastes gasperittii)* triangular head, found from sea level to altitudes of 5000 feet; Levant viper *(Vipera lebitina)* seen only in Yemen; *Pseudocerastes persica fieldi,* found in rocky, dry, and mountainous areas; puff adder *(Bitis lactesis)* found in southern mountains; burrowing adder *(Atractaspis microlepidota andersonii);* carpet viper *(Echis carinatus),* a fast, aggressive and very dangerous snake; unnamed viper *(Echis coloratus).*[51] Sea snakes (family Hydrophidae) are found throughout the tropical seas, usually in shallow coastal water. The bite is rarely painful, but the venom is neurotoxic and more potent than that of a cobra. These snakes are often found resting in underwater pipes and ledges. There are nine types of sea snakes in the area, and all are dangerous.[48] Venomous sea snake antivenom can be obtained from Commonwealth Serum Laboratories, 45 Poplar Road, Parkville 3052, Melbourne, Australia, 061-3389-1911.

PHILIPPINES

The snake fauna of the Philippines is related to those in Malaysia and Western Indonesia, but it lacks the genera *Bungarus* and *Agkistrodon.*[52] Out of more than 60 species, seven are venomous. Three are *Trimeresurus* (family Crotalidae) and four are elapids (family Elapidae). Probably the most important snake in the Philippines is the Philippine cobra, *Naja naja phillippinensis.* Cobras are the leading cause of snakebite death in the Philippines.

N.n. philippinensis produces a clinical syndrome significantly different from other Asian cobras in which local swelling and necrosis but not paralysis are the most distinctive features.[53] Neurotoxicity dominates the clinical picture and can be severe in the absence of any swelling or necrosis at the bite site. Vomiting is an early sign, but is seen in only one out of every three patients. Neurotoxic signs may not occur until 24 hours after a bite. Neurotoxicity is often rapid in onset: ptosis may occur within 5 minutes, but usually begins 1 hour after a bite. Respiratory dysfunction and apnea may begin in 10 minutes, but usually take 30 to 78 minutes.[54] No primary cardiotoxicity is observed. Arrhythmias and hypotension may occur in some patients with severe respiratory paralysis and may be related to hypoxemia.

Since the neurotoxins are considered to bind to acetylcholine receptor sites on the motor end plate, they may produce effects similar to those of curare and myasthenia gravis. It was the use of krait and cobra toxins that permitted the identification of the acetylcholine-receptor abnormality in myasthenia.[55] The number of acetylcholine receptor sites on the motor end plates is also decreased.

Anticholinesterase Use

Neurotoxic venoms differ in the site of action and the avidity with which they are bound. The presynaptic blockage produced by the krait beta-bungarotoxin is completely resistant to anticholinesterases. Anticholinesterases have benefitted patients envenomated by Russell's viper *(Vipera russelli pulchella),* the green mamba *(Dendroaspis viridis),* cobras (*N. naja* and *N. melanaleuca*),[53] and as a supplement to antivenom death adder bites *(A. antarcticus).*[25,26]

Patients with neurotoxic envenomation by bites of the Philippine cobra *(N.n. phillipinensis)* were given an anticholinesterase drug (edrophonium chloride, 10 mg I.V.) administered after an atropine injection (0.6 mg slow IV), which resulted in an improvement in ptosis and endurance of upward gaze. The expiratory and inspiratory pressures, forced vital capacity, and ability to cough, speak, and swallow also improved after edrophonium.[56]

Edrophonium

A test dose of edrophonium is given to patients with neurologic signs who have been bitten by any species of snake, especially cobras. Atropine sulfate (0.6 mg for adults, 50 μg/kg body weight for children) is given by intravenous injection and is followed by edrophonium chloride (Tensilon) (10 mg for adults; 0.25 mg/kg body weight for children). If improvement occurs, the patient can be maintained on a longer-acting anticholinesterase preparation such as neostigmine methylsulfate (by intravenous injection or by continuous intravenous or subcutaneous infusion).[56]

Precautions should be exercised with edrophonium use. Bronchoconstriction may be precipitated or exacerbated. Cardiac arrest has followed edrophonium use. Neostigmine's safety may be a serious problem. Elderly patients may not tolerate these agents well.[57,58] However, most victims of neurotoxic snakebite in Australasia are young rural farmers who have few cardiac risk factors and are not taking medications. Neurotoxic snakebite is a medical emergency; the effects of edrophonium can be life saving.[56]

Cobra antivenom (monovalent) is produced by the National Serum Vaccine Laboratories in the Philippines.[52]

SRI LANKA

The snakes of Sri Lanka include all the known families of venomous or medically important snakes such as the kraits and cobra (family Elapidae); sea snakes (family Hydrophiidae); and Russell's viper, saw-scaled viper, hump-nosed viper, and green pit viper (family Viperidae).[59] The common krait *(Bungarus caeruleus),* cobra *(Naja naja naja),* and Russell's viper *(Vipera russelli pulchella)*[60] account for 97% of deaths due to snakebite envenomation in Sri Lanka. The victims of the common krait *(Bungarus caeruleus)* run a greater risk of death than from any other snake in Sri Lanka. Sri Lanka has one of the highest incidences of death from snakebite in the world (5.3/100,000 population). Most of these deaths occur without receiving antivenom. The Elapidae family are the most important group of snakes in Sri Lanka. Their venom is mainly neurotoxic.

Venomous snakes of Sri Lanka include the following[59]:

1. Highly venomous snakes where a significant proportion of bites produce systemic envenomation possibly culminating in death (e.g., sea snakes, kraits, cobra, Russell's viper, saw-scaled viper).
2. Moderately venomous snakes where there are occasional reports of systemic envenomation and death (e.g., hump-nosed vipers) or severe local reactions (e.g., hump-nosed vipers and green pit viper).
3. Mildly venomous snakes where there are no reported deaths or systemic or severe local reactions, but where the venom gland, or Duverney's Gland, and fangs that are canalized or grooved are present with reports of mild local envenomation by some species (e.g., cat snakes and green vine snakes).

The cobra bite *(Naja naja naja)* may induce the following clinical picture:

1. Immediate burning pain that spreads up the limb.
2. Maximum swelling reached about 24 hours after the bite.
3. Dark discoloration around the site of the bite and tenderness.
4. Necrosis may be observed.
5. Hematemesis occasionally.[59]

Envenomations with *Vipera russelli pulchella* (Russell's viper) are followed by symptoms of local pain, blurred or double vision, difficulty in swallowing, bleeding, black urine, and generalized muscle aching. Signs include external ophthalmoplegia, ptosis, restriction of mouth opening, incoagulable blood, and generalized muscle tenderness.[60]

Snakebites are treated in Sri Lanka by the indigenous (Ayurvedic) system of traditional medicine and by the allopathic or western system. Lyophilized polyvalent antisnake venom serum effective against the venoms of Indian, *Naja naja, Bungarus caeruleus, Vipera russelli,* and *Echis carinatus* are imported from the Haffkine Institute in Bombay, India.

THAILAND [61]

There are 160 species and 9 families; 46 species or 2 families are deadly venomous. Twenty-four are land snakes; the rest, sea snakes. Each year 10,000 individuals are bitten; 600 die. The Siamese cobra *(Naja kaouthia)* induces the highest mortality rate. The spitting cobra *(Naja sputatrix)* can spit venom several feet toward the head or face of an enemy. Permanent blindness may result. The king cobra *(Ophiophagus hannah)* is perhaps the longest venomous snake in the world. Bites may be fatal in 3 minutes. The banded krait *(Bungarus fasciatus)* is the least aggressive venomous snake in Thailand, but produces a potent neurotoxin. Kraits are nocturnal. The Malayan krait *(Bungarus candidus)* is more aggressive. Russell's viper *(Vipera russelli siamensis)* makes a hissing sound when disturbed, feeds at night on rodents, birds, and frogs and induces varying degrees of acute renal failure in man.[62,63]

The main systemic targets of Russell's viper venom are hemodynamics (hypotension); coagulation system (activation of factor X, classical disseminated intravascular clotting); red blood cells (hemolysis); and kidneys (acute renal failure). Multiple bleeding sites are often observed.[64] Few fatalities follow bites of the green pit vipers (*Trimeresurus* sp.). The Malayan pit viper (*Agkistrodon rhodostoma* or *Calloselasma rhodostoma*) is not aggressive; although it bites often, the mortality rate is low. Twenty-two of Thailand's 23 varieties of sea snakes are venomous. Sea snakebite poisoning is least commonly observed. Neuromuscular symptoms are caused by bites of the Elapinae (cobras and kraits) and Hydrophinae (see snakes). Ptosis of the eyelids, blurred vision, paresthesias, headache, increased salivation, trismus, and paralysis of the muscles of deglutition, tongue, and vocal cord are seen. Myoglobinuria and renal failure may follow.

Antivenoms (from the Queen Saovapha Memorial Institute) are administered in a dose of 40 to 100 mL IV followed by 20 to 30 mL every 10 to 15 minutes as required. An average of 200 mL is used in a patient. The dosage is the same for the bite of the cobra, king cobra, or krait. Skin tests have been recommended prior to antivenom administration, but their value is questioned since they do not appear useful in predicting early anaphylactic reactions.[65] Prostigmine and edrophonium chloride have a variable therapeutic history. Cobra bites often leave a tissue necrosis for which a skin graft may be required.

Viper bite treatment aims at prevention of the venom from reaching the systemic circulation, neutralization of circulating venom, correction of venom-induced abnormalities, and general supportive care. Specific antivenom is used when the nonclotted blood or venous clotting time lasts longer than 30 minutes.[61] Monovalent antivenom, 4 to 6 vials, is administered in 5% dextrose in ½ N saline, 250 mL IV over 30 minutes, repeated in 6 hours if indicated. Heparin infusion may be considered in Russell's viper bite.

In Thailand, when cobra antivenom was not available, some neurotoxic snakebites (*N.n. kaouthia* and other Elapidae) were treated symptomatically (assisted ventilation) and locally (early cleaning of wounds and antibiotics) without antivenom. About 46% of patients developed local necrosis and 87.5% required skin grafting.[66]

A reverse latex agglutination test (RLA) has been developed for the detection of the six medically important snake venoms of Thailand: *Naja naja siamensis, Bungarus fascatus, Ophiophagus hannah, Vipera russelli, Calloselasma rhodostoma,* and *Trimeresurus albolabris.* Sensitivity of serum samples is 52.5%, the positive detection of venom in wound swabs is 38.5%. The test time is about 40 minutes. ELISA, an immunoassay currently in use, still lacks required specificity, is too slow for treatment needs, may be too expensive for use in developing countries, and is often not sufficiently stable for storage and transportation conditions in tropical areas.[67] The RLA test will require further clinical trials.

EUROPE

Vipera berus, Vipera aspis, Vipera ammodytes, and *Vipera ursini* are found in Europe.

HABITAT

Vipera berus (common European adder)—the whole of Europe below the Arctic circle except for the most southern area, the major Mediterranean islands and Ireland; *Vipera aspis*—southern Europe, the Pyrenees, the Alps, Southern Germany; *Vipera latasti*—the Iberian peninsula; *Vipera ursini*—central and eastern Europe; *Vipera ammodytes*—southeast of Europe, Northern Italy, Austria; *Vipera labetina*—Cyprus. The common European adder, *Vipera berus,* is the only naturally occurring venomous snake in Sweden and Britain.[68]

CLINICAL

Edema, local swelling, relatively little local pain, vomiting, abdominal pain, diarrhea, leukocytosis, shock (weakness, sweating, peripheral coolness, pallor, thirst, tachycardia, hypotension), confusion, somnolence, and occasional loss of consciousness. Bronchospasm, renal dysfunction, fever, exanthem, coagulopathy, and hemolysis may be observed. About 10 to 12% suffer a severe poisoning. No fatalities were observed in 136 patients recently treated in Sweden, but 44 died from 1911 to 1978.[69] Children recover quickly, but adults recover over weeks to months.[70] In most cases symptomatic treatment is enough, but all patients should be carefully monitored. Zagreb antivenom is available (Table 72-13).

In France *Vipera aspis* venom levels in the blood (or urine) can be quantitated by ELISA testing (sensitivity 7 ng/mL and 2 ng/mL, respectively) and correlated with signs of envenomation graded according to the extent of the edema:

- GO (no envenomation), fang marks or edema or local reaction.
- G1 (minimal envenomation), local edema, no systemic symptoms.
- G2 (moderate envenomation), regional edema, moderate systemic symptoms.[71]
- G3 (severe envenomation), extensive edema, severe systemic symptoms.

In the United Kingdom the European adder *(Vipera berus)* was not reported by poison centers in Cardiff and London to have caused a human fatality for the years 1983 to 1991.[72] The serum venom level is maximal in less than 2 hours after a bite. The elimination half-life varies from 6 to 16 hours.[73]

Table 72-13
Reid's Criteria for Antivenom Therapy [a] Modified by Persson [b]

Prolonged or recurring hypotension
Persistent or recurring shock in spite of symptomatic treatment
Pronounced leukocytosis (more than 20 × 10/L)
Protracted gastrointestinal symptoms
Acidosis
ECG changes
Raised serum creatine phosphokinase levels
Early extensive swelling in adults
Hemolysis
Small children, pregnant females

[a]Reid HA. Br Med J 1976;2:153–156.
[b]Persson H, Irestedt B. Acta Med Scand 1981;210:433–439.

Venom[74–78]

The *Vipera* venoms contain hyaluronidase and proteolytic enzymes—cause local damage to subcutaneous structures and capillary endothelium; phospholipase—hemolysis, coagulopathies, toxic polypeptides, amino acids, and carbohydrates. Direct neurotoxic activity has been associated with *V. ammodytes,* and cardiotoxicity has followed bites with *V. berus* and *V. aspis.* Histamine, bradykinin, prostaglandins, and serotonin may be released during reaction to a *Vipera* bite.

LABORATORY

An enzyme-linked immunosorbent assay (ELISA) appears to indicate a correlation between clinical signs of envenomation and the level of venom antigens in blood or urine.[71]

TREATMENT

Supportive care has been the mainstay of treatment in symptomatic cases. The Zagreb antivenom has been favorably received. Reassurance, immobilization of the bitten limb, tetanus protection, low-dose heparin as required, volume substitution (crystalloids, colloids), and correction of acid base balance and electrolyte abnormalities will suffice in most cases. An affinity purified specific Fab ovine antivenom has been developed that may become useful in the treatment of *Vipera berus* envenomation.[79,80]

Following severe reactions high-dose steroids and inotropic drugs may be required. Anaphylactic reactions may require epinephrine, antihistamines, and corticosteroids. Mild cases may be observed for 6 to 8 hours, moderate to severe cases with progressive symptomatology will require observation for at least 24 hours. All children should be observed in a hospital following a bite.

SOUTH AMERICA (TABLE 72-14)

Brazil experiences about 70,000 snakebites annually with a morality of treated cases of 1.7 to 2.4%. Snakebites are

Table 72–14
Members of the Genus *Bothrops*[a]

Species	Common Name	Distribution
B. alternatus	Urutu	Brazil, Paraguay, Argentina
B. ammodytoides	Patagonian lance-head	Argentina
B. andianus	Andean lance-head	Peru
B. asper	Terciopelo	Southern Mexico, Central America, North South America
B. atrox	Common lance-head	South America except Chile, Paraguay, Uruguay and Argentina
B. barnetti	Barnett's lance-head	Peru
B. brazili	Brazil's lance-head	Northern and Central South America
B. carribbaeus	Saint Lucia lance-head	Saint Lucia Island, Lesser Antilles
B. cotiara	Cotiara	Argentina, Brazil
B. erythromelas	Caatinga lance-head	Northeast Brazil
B. fonsecai	Fonseca's lance-head	Southeast Brazil
B. iglesiasi	Sertao lance-head	Piaui, Brazil
B. insularis	Golden lance-head	Ilha Queimada Grande Brazil
B. itapetiningae	Sao Paulo lance-head	South central Brazil
B. jararaca	Jararaca	Brazil, Paraguay, Argentina
B. jararacussu	Jararacussu	Brazil, Paraguay, Southern Bolivia, Northeast Argentina
B. lanceolatus	Martinique lance-head	Martinique, West Indies
B. leucurus	White-tailed lance-head	Bahia, Brazil
B. lojanus	Logan lance-head	Southern Ecuador
B. marajoensis	Marajo lance-head	Extreme Northern Brazil
B. microphthalmus	Small-eyed lance-head	Colombia, Ecuador, Peru
B. moojeni	Brazilian lance-head	Brazil, Paraguay
B. neuwiedi	Neuwied's lance-head	Brazil, Paraguay, Bolivia, Uruguay, Argentina
B. pictus	Desert lance-head	Costal peru
B. pirajai	Piraja's lance-head	Bahia, Brazil
B. pradoi	Prado's lance-head	Espirito Santo, Brazil
B. pulcher	Dusky lance-head	Coastal Northwestern South America
B. roedingeri	Roedinger's lance-head	Ica, Peru
B. sanctaecrucis	Bolivian lance-head	Central Bolivia
B. venezuelensis	Venezuelan lance-head	Northern Venezuela
B. xanthogrammus	Cope's lance-head	Southern Ecuador

[a]Adapted from Davidson TM et al. J Wilderness Med 1992;3:397–421.

usually due to various species of *Bothrops* (about 94%); *Crotalus* (4%); *Micrurus* (1%); and *Lachesis* (1.1%). Intravascular disseminated coagulation by *Bothrops* and blood incoagulability and mydriasis by *Crotalus* carry a serious prognosis.[81] Acute interstitial nephritis may follow *Crotalus* bites.[82] Hemorrhagic, myonecrotic, and edema-inducing toxins have been isolated from some species of *Bothrops.*[83] An enzyme-linked immunosorbent assay may be useful for detection of *Bothrops jararaca* venom in fluids.[84] The lethal toxicity of *Crotalus durissus terrificus* (Crotalidae, Viperidae) can be attributed mainly to the presence of a neurotoxic protein, crotoxin, which also shows phospholipase A_2 activity.[85] The venom also has hemolytic, nephrotoxic, and anticoagulant activity. An antivenom factor present in the alpha$_1$-globulin fraction of blood may be able to neutralize the lethal and phospholipase activities of the crotoxin.[85] This may be a factor in the recovery of the patient envenomated by *Crotalus durissus terrificus* who survived after receiving only supportive and symptomatic treatment without the use of antivenom.[86]

In Brazil, snakes of genus *Bothrops* (lance-headed vipers) are responsible for more than 80% of bites in which the snake is identified (Table 72-14).[87] These pit vipers are also the most common cause of envenomation in other parts of Latin America. Since the introduction of antivenom, case fatality has decreased from about 25 to 0.60% in 1986 to 1989. Acute renal failure is the major cause of death. Shock, intracranial hemorrhage, and blood incoagulability have also been reported with *Bothrops* envenomation.[88,89]

The 20-minute whole blood clotting time test (WBCT20) is correlated with plasma fibrinogen concentrations and has been used in assessing the effectiveness of antivenom therapy in relation to the restoration of blood coagulability after South American snake envenomations.[90]

Bothrops insularis, a Brazilian snake found only on Queimada Grande Island (Sao Paulo), produces a venom that induces a myonecrosis and is more toxic than *B. jararaca* venom.[91]

Systemic envenomation with *Bothrops jararaca* may result in incoagulable blood due to fibrinogen consumption, with elevated levels of FDP and thrombin; antithrombin III complex; and decreased levels of factors V and VIII and platelets. Bleeding appears to be associated with the presence of thrombocytopenia.[92] These phenomena have also been studied with *Bothrops atrox.*

A polyvalent antiserum is produced by the Instituto Butartan (Brazil) to neutralize the activity of *Bothrops neuwiedi pauloensis.*[93]

In Bahia, Brazil, *Bothrops jararaca* or "jararacussu" or "patrona" is responsible for the major percentage of phidian (snakebite) accidents. Snakebites by Colubridae are next in frequency with rare *Crotalus, Micrurus,* and *Lachesis* bites.[94]

The jararaca *(Bothrops jararaca)* is responsible for 90% of all snakebite cases in southeastern Brazil. Swelling, ecchymosis, necrosis, coagulopathy, and spontaneous systemic bleeding may follow envenomation. The bleeding is often correlated with the presence of thrombocytopenia.[95]

CENTRAL AMERICA (TABLE 72-14)

Bothrops asper is responsible for the majority of snakebites in Central America. Venoms from the adult *B. asper* induce local myonecrosis, hemorrhage, edema, defibrination, systemic hemorrhage, cardiovascular shock, and acute renal failure. Many bites in Central America are caused by newborn and juvenile species of *B. asper.*[96] The newborn *B. asper* exhibits higher lethal, hemorrhagic, edema-forming, and proteolytic activities than the adult. Polyvalent antivenom is used in Central America for the treatment of envenomation induced by Crotalidae snakes.

AFRICA

The viper *Echis carinatus* is probably responsible for more deaths and injuries caused by snakebite than any other species.[97] It may cause thousands of deaths a year in the savannah region of Nigeria alone.[98,99]

GABOUN VIPER *(BITIS GABONICA)*[100]

Envenomations

Neurologic, respiratory, cardiac, and hematologic symptoms appear.

Treatment

Identify snake. Administer antivenom. Zoos may have a small amount of antivenom, but can provide information on how to obtain more.

NORTH AMERICA

CROTALIDAE

Incidence

Of the approximately 45,000 snakebites reported annually in the United States, about 18%, or 8000 per annum, are inflicted by poisonous snakes. Although annually an estimated 12 to 15 deaths result from snake venom toxicity,[101,102] only one death was reported in the English-language medical literature between 1965 and 1985.[103] Not all bites by poisonous snakes result in envenomation. Rattlesnakes fail to inject venom in up to 20% of bites. The highest rates of venomous snakebite (i.e., reported bites per 100,000 population) occur in the southern United States[104]; the top five states in order are North Carolina, Texas, Arkansas, Mississippi, and Louisiana. The typical victim of a pit viper (Crotalidae family) is a young male (11 to 35 years of age, with highest incidence between 11 and 19 years) who is bitten on the hand while trying to handle the snake.[104]

About two-thirds of bites involve the upper extremity, one-third involve the lower extremity, and less than 1% occur on other body parts. Life-threatening airway obstruction may develop when the soft-tissue structures of the mouth (e.g., tongue) are directly envenomated.[105] Since snakes either hibernate or are inactive during winter, the peak snakebite season is April through October.

The vast majority (95%) of poisonous snakebites are inflicted by members of the Crotalidae (pit viper) family. The three main genera in this family are *Crotalus* (rattlesnake), *Agkistrodon* (copperhead, cottonmouth), and *Sistrurus* (pigmy rattler, massasauga). Eastern and western diamondback rattlesnakes are the most dangerous species, accounting for 95% of fatalities but only 10% of bites.[106] Rarely, envenomation results from foreign snakes imported to private or public collections (about 2% of poisonous snakebites).

CLASSIFICATION OF AMERICAN VENOMOUS SNAKES

Crotalidae

Four characteristics (listed below) separate poisonous pit vipers (Crotalidae family) from most of the other nonpoisonous snake species (Figs. 72-2 and 72-3). Coloration and diamondback patterns do not exclusively identify rattlesnakes because nonpoisonous snakes mimic these markings as defensive mechanisms:

1. Triangular or arrow-shaped head, compared with smooth tapered body and narrow head of nonpoisonous snakes.
2. Facial pits located between the nostril and eye; this organ functions as a heat and vibration sensor.
3. Vertical, elliptical pupils similar to the eyes of cats, in contrast to the round pupil of nonpoisonous varieties; however, poisonous coral snakes have round pupils.
4. Single row of subcaudal scales, compared with the double row in nonpoisonous snakes.

The poisonous Elapidae (cobra) genera is not distinguished from nonpoisonous snakes on the basis of the above criteria for pit viper (Crotalidae) identification. All pit vipers have movable fangs that inject a voluntarily controlled amount of venom, compared with the fixed fangs of the *Elapidae.*

True Rattlesnakes

Although all pit vipers share the four characteristics, variations in coloration and body features separate the genera. Most, but not all, rattlesnakes (genus *Crotalus*) have a set of interlocking, terminal horny segments known as rattles. An exception is *Crotalus catalinensis,* which is found only off Santa Catalina Island near Los Angeles. A characteristic buzzing similar to the sound of escaping steam usually, but not always, occurs before a strike. Each molting (average of three to four times per year) adds a rattle, but trauma or congenital abnormalities may lead to their absence.

Elapidae (Coral)

Two genera of poisonous coral snakes *(Micrurus, Micruroides)* represent this family in the United States. Coral snakes are slender snakes ranging from 2 to 4 feet; brightly colored

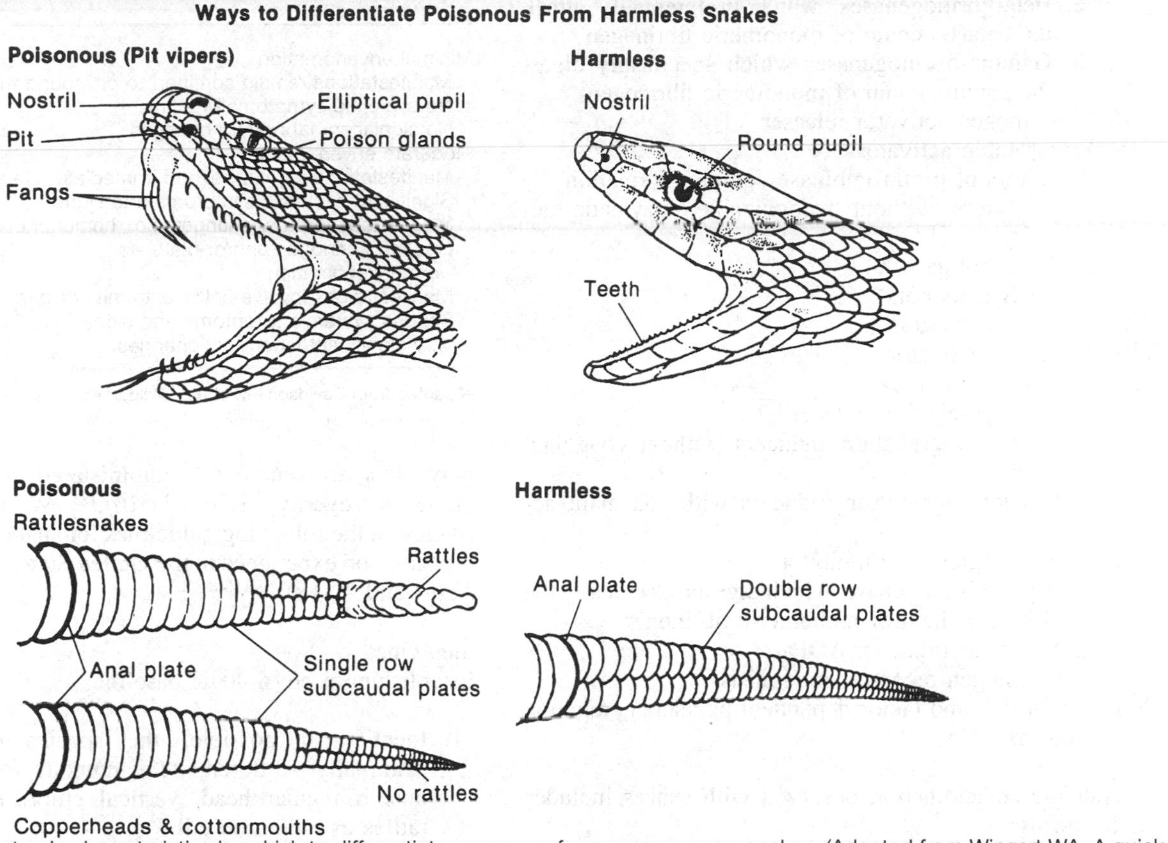

Ways to Differentiate Poisonous From Harmless Snakes

Poisonous (Pit vipers)
Nostril
Pit
Fangs
Elliptical pupil
Poison glands
Harmless
Nostril
Round pupil
Teeth
Poisonous
Rattlesnakes
Rattles
Anal plate
Single row subcaudal plates
No rattles
Copperheads & cottonmouths
Harmless
Anal plate
Double row subcaudal plates

Figure 72-2 Anatomic characteristics by which to differentiate venomous from nonvenomous snakes. (Adapted from Wingert WA. A quick handbook on snake bites. Res Staff Physician 1977;23(5):59.)

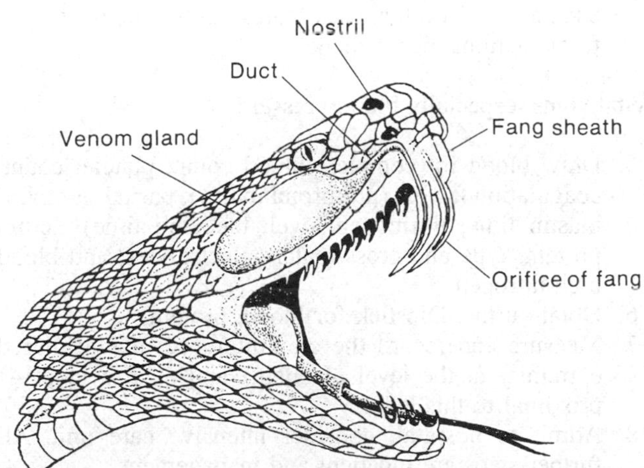

Figure 72-3 Venom apparatus of snakes. (Adapated from Russell FE, Picchioni AL. Snake venom poisoning. Clin Toxicol Consult 1983;5:75.)

rings circle the body but not the head or tail. In North America the coral snake's red and yellow rings are contiguous, whereas nonvenomous snakes that mimic coral snakes have a black ring separating the red and yellow rings. The following mnemonic helps differentiate the coral snake from nonpoisonous snakes: "Red on yellow, kill a fellow; red on black, good for Jack."[107]

Coral snakes have round pupils, fixed fangs, small heads, and no facial pits, in contrast to pit vipers. Generally, coral snakes are docile, preferring to chew rather than bite, since their fangs are fixed. The eastern coral snake *(Micrurus fulvius fulvius)* inhabits the southern United States from Arkansas to Florida; the Texas coral snake subspecies *(Micrurus fulvius tenere)* extends to west Texas. The Arizona or Sonoran coral snake *(Micruroides euryxanthus)* is found in the southwestern United States (Arizona, New Mexico).

True Rattlesnake *(Crotalus)*

Approximately 8000 people in the United States are bitten by venomous snakes each year, resulting in fewer than 12 deaths. Only six species of crotalids are known to inhabit southern California: the red diamond rattlesnake *(Crotalus ruber),* southern Pacific rattlesnake *(C. viridis helleri),* speckled rattlesnake *(C. mitchelli),* western diamondback rattlesnake *(C. atrox),* sidewinder *(C. cerastes),* and Mojave rattlesnake *(C. scutulatus).*[108]

MECHANISM OF ACTION

Blood

Snake venom components affecting blood coagulation and platelet function can be classified into the following groups[109]:

I. Components coagulating fibrinogen
II. Fibrino(geno)lytic enzymes
   1. Alpha-fibrinogenases, which digest specifically the alpha(A)-chain of monomeric fibrinogen

2. Beta-fibrinogenases, which preferentially attack the beta(B)-chain of monomeric fibrinogen
3. Gamma-fibrinogenases which specifically digest the gamma-chain of monomeric fibrinogen

III. Plasminogen activator releaser
IV. Prothrombin activators
V. Inhibitors of prothrombinase complex formation
   1. Inhibitors without recognizable enzymatic activity
   2. Phospholipase A_2
VI. Factor X activators
VII. Factor V activators
VIII. Factor XI activator
IX. Protein C activators
X. Platelet aggregation inducers
   1. Platelet aggregation inducers without coagulant activity
   2. Platelet aggregation inducers with coagulant activity
XI. Platelet aggregation inhibitors
   1. Alpha-fibrinogenase, which digests specifically the alpha(A)-chain of monomeric fibrinogen
   2. 5′-Nucleotidase or ADPase
   3. Fibrinogen receptor antagonists
XII. von Willebrand factor-dependent platelet aggregation inducers

Systemic envenomation observed with snakes includes the following:

Crotalid:

Hypotension, shock bleeding, blood cell changes, sometimes neurologic effects.

Vipers:

Spontaneous hemorrhage; nonclotting blood; defibrinogenation.

Elapids:

Neuromuscular junction principally; other organs also.

Sea Snakes:

Myotoxic, especially to skeletal muscles.

Local Envenomation:

Local necrosis: vipers, African spitting cobras *(e.g., Naja nigricollis),* Asian cobras.

A classification system for grading the clinical severity of crotalid envenomation has been suggested as a possible guide to the administration of antivenom[110] (Table 72-15).

Table 72–15
Grade of Envenomation [a]

Minimal envenomation
- Manifestations remain confined to or around the bite area.
- No systemic symptoms or signs.
- No significant laboratory changes.

Moderate envenomation
- Manifestations extend beyond immediate bite area.
- Significant systemic symptoms and signs.
- Moderate laboratory changes; i.e., hemoconcentraton, decreased fibrinogen and/or platelets.

Severe envenomation
- Manifestations involve entire extremity or part.
- Serious systemic symptoms and signs.
- Very significant laboratory changes.

[a]Adapted from Davidson TM et al. J Wilderness Med 1992;3:397–421.

TREATMENT (FIG. 72-4)

Algorithms applicable to the evaluation and treatment of North American pit viper envenomation have been prepared by Davidson and colleagues and by Sutherland and are shown as Figs. 72-1 and 72-4.[8,11] Initial doses of crotalid polyvalent antivenom are administered according to the grade of severity (Table 72-16).[111] Willis Wingert has suggested the following guidelines for snake venom poisoning based on experience in the United States (see also Tables 72-17 and 72-18)[112,113]:

Step One:
Establishing a physiologic baseline

1. Identify, if possible, the species of the snake. Minimally—differentiate venomous from nonvenomous: triangular head, vertical elliptical pupil, fangs, rattles or button on tail.
2. Note size of offending snake.
3. Note circumstances of bite.
4. Evaluate rapidly signs and symptoms: Fangs, local edema, local ecchymoses, paresthesia (mouth, scalp), fasciculations, hemorrhage.

Vital signs, especially blood pressure

5. Draw blood for complete blood count, platelet count, coagulation factors (prothrombin time, partial thromboplastin time, fibrinogen level, bleeding time), serum protein, type and cross-match, electrolytes, and blood urea nitrogen.
6. Obtain urine. Dipstick for blood, protein.
7. Measure and record the circumference of the injured extremity at the level of edema and at a level of 4″ proximal to this level.
8. Admit to hospital; consider intensive care unit. All further steps are inpatient and management.

Step Two:
Determine severity of envenomation.

Grade 0:	No local or systemic reactions (occurs in approximately 20%).
Minimal:	Local swelling at bite site, no systemic reactions.
Moderate:	Swelling progressing beyond site of bite with some systemic reaction and/or laboratory changes. History of large-sized snake.
Severe:	Marked local reaction with rapidly progressing edema, severe symptoms, falling blood pressure, hemorrhage, and markedly abnormal changes.

Step Three:
Perform skin tests for horse serum sensitivity following instructions in antivenom brochure. **(Note: This test is not completely reliable.)**

Step Four:
Reconstitute antivenom (quantity below) and add to 300 mL ½ N.S. If patient is severely envenomated, start infusions in two extremities, one for antivenom and one for life support. (Note: Antivenom is difficult to dissolve. Warm the diluent and shake hard.)
Note: If patient is hypotensive, administer a plasma expander, *not* crystalloid solution.

Step Five:
Administer adequate amount of antivenom intravenously over 2 hours. Grade 0: None; Minimal: 5 vials; Moderate: 10 vials; Severe: 15 vials; *increase* dose by 50% for children. Bites by *C. scutulatus* (Mojave green): 10 vials.

Step Six:
Monitor the progress of envenomation:

1. Measure the level of progression of swelling every 30 minutes.
2. Vital signs as indicated but at least q 30 minutes in moderate or severe envenomations.
3. Repeat laboratory work as indicated, especially serum protein (10'Yo decrease is significant) hematocrit, and platelet count.

If the swelling continues to progress 2 hours after the initial antivenom dose, repeat antivenom in increments of 5 vials every hour until signs and symptoms are controlled.

Step Seven:
Support vital functions, oxygen, assisted respiration. Transfusion or plasma expander (*not* crystalloid solutions) for shock.

Step Eight:
Administer a broad-spectrum antibiotic such as ampicillin, amoxicillin, or cephalcor if the bite has been incised and/or suctioned.

Step Nine:
Administer tetanus toxoid or human antitoxin, if indicated.

Step Ten:
Splint the injured extremity in position of function and maintain at level of heart.

Step Eleven:
Consultation is available.

Step Twelve:
Avoid the following drugs or procedures:

1. Incisions *anywhere.*
   (Bite marks, edematous extremities, etc.)
2. Steroids
3. Antihistamines
4. Tourniquets
5. Narcotics
6. Cryotherapy of any sort.

Note: Many snakebite victims could have significant serum levels of alcohol and other drugs complicating their management.

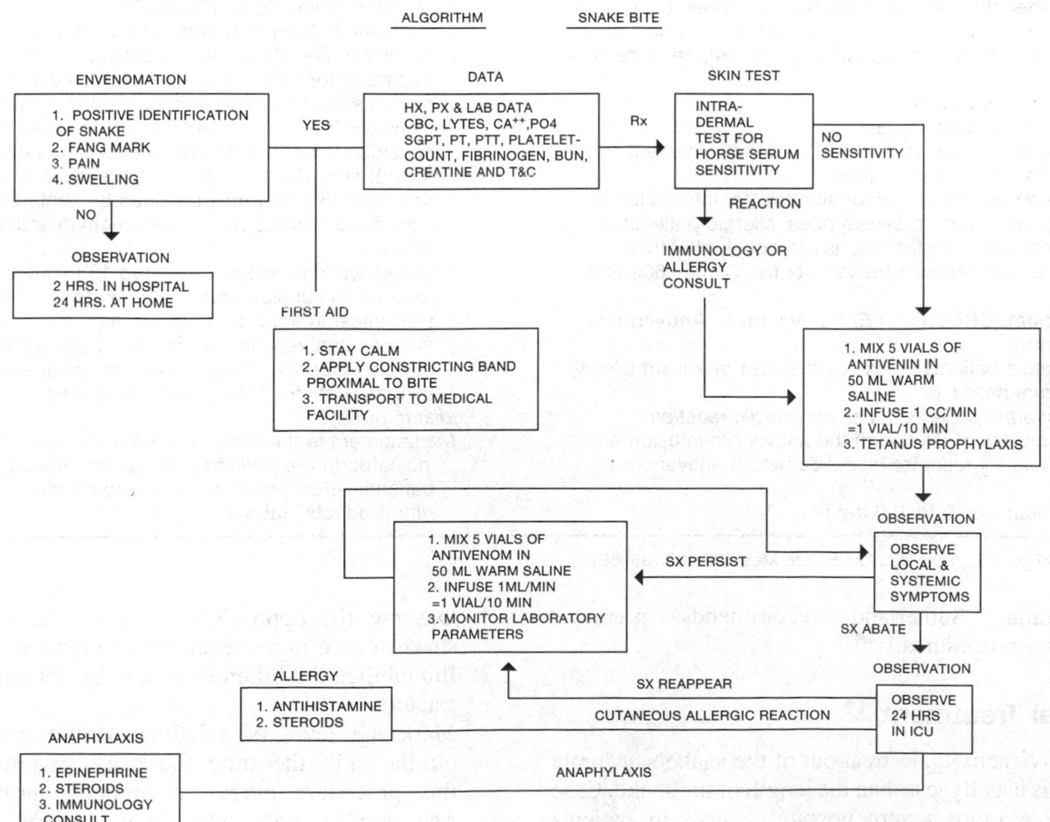

Figure 72-4 Algorithmic display of the evaluation and treatment for North American pit viper envenomation. (Adapted from Davidson TM et al. J Wilderness Med 1992;3:397–421.)

Table 72–16
Guidelines for Use of Antivenom (CROTALIDAE) Polyvalent and Management of Allergic Reactions[a]

Standard Administration of Antivenom (CROTALIDAE) Polyvalent
1. Read package insert.
2. Check allergy history, especially to horse serum products.
3. Perform skin test if antivenom is indicated using the skin test material included with the antivenom.
   - Never perform a skin test unless you are sure antivenom will be administered.
   - If skin test is positive (wheal and flare within 20 to 30 minutes) and antivenom is necessary, request consultation through regional poison center. Antivenom may be administered in many cases despite a positive skin test.
4. Dosage and administration of antivenom (CROTALIDAE) polyvalent
   - Dosage
     - Minimal or trivial envenomation: no antivenom
     - Moderate envenomation: five to ten vials
     - Severe or rapidly progressive envenomation: ten to 30 vials, or more
   - Mixing and infusion
     - Add 10 mL of the diluent provided or normal saline to each vial. Mix by rolling between hands. Do not shake.
     - Then, dilute by injecting into normal saline IV bag (eg, five to ten vials in 250 mL). Give intravenously at a slow rate initially and then at a faster rate (about five to ten minutes per vial) if no reaction occurs. Reduce volume of diluent in pediatric patients.
     - Attempt to give total dose during first one to two hours.
   - Use after 24 hours is currently limited to reversal of coagulopathy.
5. Guide to subsequent administration of antivenom should include response to the first dose and evidence of continuing injury. If swelling, coagulopathy, or any other problem is worsening after the initial administration, further antivenom is probably warranted. Consultation with a physician experienced in the treatment of complicated snakebite is recommended.

General Recommendations
1. Do not leave patient unattended.
2. Do not delay immediate or vigorous treatment if patient has a moderate or severe envenomation.
3. Consult poison control center for all bites (for informational purposes). In moderate-to-severe bites, allergic patients, or cases with complicating factors, ask to speak directly to toxicologist on call (Arizona Poison Control Center, 602/626-6016).

Use of Antivenom (CROTALIDAE) Polyvalent in Antivenom-Allergic Patients
1. Possible allergic patients—Positive skin test or known allergy to horse serum products
   - *Treatment of adult patients at risk for allergic reaction*
   - Treatment consists of dilution of the antivenom infusion and **both** H_1- and H_2-receptor blockade before antivenom infusion
     - Diphenhydramine 50 to 100 mg/IV
     - Cimetidine 300 mg IV or ranitidine 50 mg/IV
     - Dilute antivenom to half or normal concentration—about one vial/100 mL.
     - Start infusion at a rate of 25 to 50 mL/hr, and double the rate every ten to 15 minutes until a rate is reached that will infuse the volume in two hours.
     - In case a severe allergic reaction develops, the patient should be cardiac monitored, and equipment for airway control and epinephrine should be available at the bedside.
   - *Pediatric patients*
     - Diphenhydramine 1.25 mg/kg IV
     - Cimetidine 5 to 10 mg/kg or ranitidine 1 to 2 mg/kg IV
     - Dilute antivenom to half of normal concentration—about one vial/100 mL (1:10 dilution). However, it is recommended that total volume not exceed 20 mL/kg.
     - Start infusion at a slow rate (about 25 to 50 mL/hr); double the rate every ten to 15 minutes until a rate is reached that will infuse the total volume in two hours.
     - Keep epinephrine 1:1,000 available at the bedside for possible reactions.
2. Patients currently having a reaction
   - Diagnosis—Any of the following signs or symptoms developing during antivenom infusion: anxiety, chills, weakness, nausea, pruritis, sneezing, feeling of throat constriction, hypotension, stridor, urticaria, wheezing, emesis, dyspnea, diaphoresis, fever, or erythematous streaking from injection site.
   - Treatment of patients having an allergic reaction
   - Treatment consists of dilution and slowing of antivenom infusion
     - and **both** H_1- and H_2-receptor blockade
     - Stop antivenom infusion.
     - Epinephrine 1:1000, 0.3 to 0.5 mg SQ; may be repeated every 15 minutes
     - Diphenhydramine 50 to 100 mg IV
     - Cimetidine 300 mg IV or ranitidine 50 mg IV
     - A second IV line should be established. First line of treatment for hypotension is isotonic fluid infusion. Vasopressors may be needed in particularly severe cases.
     - Reconsider the need for antivenom. The primary considerations include the severity of the envenomation (life- or limb-threatening) and the seriousness of the reaction. This decision may be aided by contacting a physician experienced in the use of antivenom in antivenom-allergic patients.
     - If antivenom is needed, wait ten to 15 minutes for initial reaction to subside and for patient to stabilize. Then, restart infusion at 25 to 50 mL/hr. Increase the rate every 15 minutes until reaching a rate that is 25 mL/hr below the rate at which the allergic response occurred. Continue at this rate until the total volume is infused.
   - *Pediatric patients*
     - Management is the same, except that doses are reduced as indicated in the pediatric section of "Possibly allergic patients—Positive skin test or known allergy to horse serum products" (above)

[a]Adapted from Burgess JL, Dart RC. Ann Emerg Med 1991;20:795–801.

In Australia, Sutherland recommends pressure/immobilization procedures.[114,115]

Prehospital Treatment[112]

Avoid excessive activity. Retreat out of the snake's accurate range, which is usually less than the length of the snake. Case studies show a more severe hospital course in patients extremely active after envenomation compared with patients immobilized early:

1. Observe the approximate size of the snake. Larger snakes cause more severe envenomation.
2. Immobilize the bitten extremity by splinting as if for a fracture.
3. Mark the level of swelling with a pen, and write on the skin the time the mark was made. Repeat this procedure every 15 minutes during transport. The rapidity with which the swelling appears and progresses is an important factor in assessing severity.

Table 72-17
Indications for Antivenin Treatment of Snakebite [a]

Systemic envenoming
- Hypotension, shock, ECG abnormalities, cardiac arrhythmias
- Neurotoxic signs: ptosis, ophthalmoplegia, bulbar or respiratory paralysis
- Impaired consciousness of any cause (eg, respiratory or circulatory failure)
- Spontaneous systemic bleeding or excessive bleeding from new and old wounds
- Incoagulable blood
- Rhabdomyolysis: dark urine, tender stiff muscles

Local envenoming
- Venom known to be necrotic (eg, vipers, African spitting cobras, Asian cobras)
- Swelling spreading to involve more than half of the bitten limb
- Rapidly progressive local swelling
- Bites involving digits and into other tight fascial compartments (for example anterior tibial compartment)

[a]Adapted from Warrell DA, Fenner PJ. Br Med Bull 1993;49:423–439.

4. Transport the victim at a safe speed to the nearest medical facility that is equipped and staffed to care for envenomation—that is, one that has an adequate supply of antivenom available and a knowledgeable professional staff.

A summary of current recommendations includes the following:

1. Make an incision across the bite? No.
2. Use mouth suction to try and remove venom? No.
3. Use a commercially available suction venom extractor? Mild difference of opinion.
4. Use a venous constricting tourniquet above the wrist? No.
5. Pack the arm in snow? No.
6. Immobilize the arm in a splint? OK.
7. Hold the hand above the head during transport? No–at *heart level.*
8. Inject antivenom intravenously? Yes, *but only in hospital.*
9. Kill the snake for identification? No.

Unintended effects of an extractor can include spreading the venom if the device is used incorrectly, exacerbating tissue damage, and possibly infecting wounds made by nonvenomous bites.[116]

Antivenins

There has been a paucity of research on antivenoms, but efficacy against hemostatic abnormalities and shock has been established. Conventional antivenoms may reverse predominantly postsynaptic neurotoxicity. They usually fail to prevent nephropathy and local necrosis. Further critical assessment of antivenoms is necessary. Anticholinesterases (e.g., edrophonium chloride—Tensilon) have been reported to be useful in the treatment of postsynaptic neurotoxic envenomation. Mechanical ventilation, dialysis, and surgical intervention may be indicated.[1] Table 72-17 summarizes some indications for antivenom treatment of snakebite.[1] Table 72-16 depicts use of polyvalent antivenom (Crotalidae).

Table 72-18
How Not to Treat a Snakebite[a]

Though United States medical professionals may not agree on every aspect of what to do for snakebite first aid, they are nearly unanimous in their views of what *not* to do. Among their recommendations are the following:
1. *No* ice or any other type of cooling on the bite. Research has shown this to be potentially harmful.
2. *No* tourniquets. This cuts blood flow completely and may result in loss of the affected limb.
3. *No* electric shock. This method is under study and has yet to be proven effective. It could harm the victim.
4. *No* incisions in the wound. Such measures have not been proven useful and may cause further injury.

[a]Adapted from Henkel J. FDA Consumer 1995;29:23–27.

Sutherland suggests the use of subcutaneous adrenaline 10 minutes before antivenom administration to lessen the possibility and severity of an immediate adverse reaction to snake antivenom.[117] Antihistamine use as a preventative has been questioned.[118]

Snake Venom Allergy

Snake venom allergy is uncommon.[119] The individual becomes sensitized to the protein in the venom from recurrent exposure through bites. Snake handlers are at particular risk. The allergy is similar in severity to bee venom allergy, and fatalities have occurred. Management is to avoid all contact with snakes or any species since the venoms of different species often share common proteins. Desensitization cannot be done at present because of the complexity and toxicity of the venoms. Treat anaphylaxis with snake antivenom and parenteral adrenaline. The antivenom should be administered by rapid infusion and should be able to neutralize the allergenic protein of the venom.[18,118] Steroids and oral antihistamines may additionally be effective.[120]

Use of electric shocks for treatment of venomous bites and stings is not supported by adequate controlled clinical studies.[121] The U.S. Food and Drug Administration banned the use of such devices on April 9, 1990.[122] In one patient who was envenomated, electric shock induced loss of consciousness and incontinence.[122]

Experimental studies are under way with purified immunoglobulin G and possibly F(ab) fragments.[123] Hyperbaric oxygen therapy has been studied in animals as a possible means of treating rattlesnake venom–induced tissue damage and myonecrosis.[124] Studies in rabbits suggest that muscle necrosis secondary to *Crotalus atrox* venom poisoning is not ameliorated by hyperbaric oxygen when added to the antivenom.[125] No controlled data in humans are available.

Laboratory

An enzyme-linked immunosorbent assay (ELISA) has been developed for antigens of European vipers and is sensitive to limits of 7 to 2 ng/mL for *Vipera aspis* venom in serum and urine.[126]

NEUROTOXINS[127] (TABLE 72-4)

Neurotoxins are found in the venoms of vipers, elapids, and hydrophids. Kraits and cobras are a major cause of snakebite mortality in Asia. Textilotoxin, from the Australian brown snake *(Pseudomya textilis)* is the most potent snake venom toxin known. In Africa neurotoxic venoms occur in both elapids (cobras and mambas) and vipers (horned puff adder). In North and South America the elapids are the coral snake (genus *Micrurus*), and the vipers are rattlesnakes *(Crotalus scutulatus)* in the United States and *(Crotalus durissus terrificus)* in South America. Neurotoxic sea snakes are found not only in the sea but also in rivers and fresh-water lakes. Venoms may be predominantly postsynaptic (e.g., Philippine cobra venom, *Naja naja phillipinesis),* predominantly presynaptic (e.g., most sea snake venoms), or have components acting both pre- and postsynaptically (e.g., beta- and alpha-bungarotoxins from the venoms of the Chinese krait, *Bungarus multicinctus*).

Mechanism of Action

Neurotoxins acting presynaptically are thought to bind almost irreversibly at acetylcholine-releasing sites on the nerve ending. The resultant neuromuscular blockade is considered not to be amenable to therapeutic intervention.

Clinical Presentation

Death occurs very rapidly after envenomation by a neurotoxin species. Respiratory failure occurs within hours after the bite of a neurotoxic elapid, whereas death from bleeding or renal failure after envenomation by a viper occurs several days after the bite. Respiratory paralysis has developed within 10 minutes after bites by cobras *(Naja naja phillipinensis),* and deaths have occurred within 15 minutes of bites by mambas (genus *Dendroaspis*). Antivenins can rarely be relied on to promptly reverse paralysis. Respiratory compromise after bites by both the tropical rattlesnake *(Crotalus durissus terrificus)* and coral snakes (genus *Micrurus*) also responds poorly to antivenom therapy.

Treatment

Supportive treatment underlies effective management. Patients with paralysis of the muscles of the jaw and tongue, as well as paralysis of the muscle of coughing and swallowing, are at high risk for aspiration pneumonia. Place patients on their sides and provide frequent suctioning. Insert an oral airway and hyperextend the neck. Maintain ventilation. Recovery may follow respiratory paralysis after manual ventilation by relatives and nurses for up to 30 days.

All effects of neurotoxins are eventually reversible if adequate oxygenation can be maintained. Predominantly postsynaptic venoms can benefit from the use of edrophonium chloride (Tensilon).[23] The Tensilon test should be given to all patients with severe paralytic envenomation and anticholinesterase administered to those with a positive response. Atropine sulfate (0.6 mg for adults; 50 µg/mg for children) is given by IV injection followed by Tensilon (10 mg for adults; 0.25 mg/kg for children). If improvement occurs, the patient can be maintained on a longer-acting anticholinesterase preparation such as neostigmine methyl sulfate (initial dose is 25 µg/kg/hour given by constant IV infusion). The amount given is titrated to the patient's clinical response. One member of this aminopyridine family of drugs, 3,4-diaminopyridine, has been found to be effective in botulism and Lambert-Eaton myasthenia, which also affect acetylcholine-releasing sites. This compound merits further investigation. Prophylactic steroids given over a period of 4 to 5 days may diminish serum sickness.[128]

Intracompartmental Pressure

Intracompartmental pressure measurements can be performed by either using a simple syringe, tubing, needle, and saline or with a commercially available solid-state transducer device (Styker, Kalamazoo, MI). Normal intracompartmental pressure ranges from 0 mm Hg to 9 mm Hg. Normal pressure at the arterial end of the capillary is 30 to 35 mm Hg. Capillary blood flow may be severely compromised at compartment pressures of 30 to 40 mm Hg. The arterial capillary pressure is dependent on mean arterial pressure. It is suggested that the capillary microcirculation is compromised at compartment pressures within 30 mm Hg of the patient's mean arterial pressure. Compartment syndromes may develop at relatively low compartment pressures in a hypotensive individual. The compartment pressures required to compromise the microcirculation are well below the pressures of the patients' palpable arterial pulses.[129]

Prevention[130]

1. Do not place any part of your body where you have not first looked.
2. Do not use your hands to lift anything a snake could be under.
3. Gather firewood in the daylight.
4. Do not place your camp, boots, or clothes near brush, rubbish, rock piles, cave entrances, or swampy areas.
5. Do not disturb, capture, or attempt to kill snakes unless you are experienced in handling them.
6. Do not move suddenly when you hear a rattlesnake sound; locate the snake and carefully move away. Remember, there could be others nearby.
7. Take along a friend when traveling in snake habitat.
8. Stay on paths and avoid tall grass and heavy undergrowth.
9. Wear adequate protective clothing, including tall boots with pant legs worn on the outside.
10. Do not handle freshly killed snakes or the heads of decapitated snakes, which have been known to bite reflexively up to one-half hour after death.
11. Carry a flashlight at night.
12. Watch for snakes at altitudes of up to 9500 feet in warm climates, up to 11,000 feet in California and up to 14,500 feet in central Mexico.
13. Do not avoid snake habitats out of fear, but be careful.
14. Do not keep poisonous snakes as pets or consume alcohol when handling them.

Suggested laboratory studies for rattlesnake envenomations are found in Table 72-10. Administration of crotalid polyvalent antivenoms is presented in Table 72-16.

Dart, Horowitz, and Gomez have provided a guide to the management of poisonous snakebites in the United States.[131] Distribution of the Mojave rattlesnake in the United States is seen in Figure 72-5.

MASSASAUGA *(SISTRURUS)*

Members of the genus *Sistrurus* in the United States are divided into the pigmy rattlesnakes *(Sistrurus miliarius)* and the massasaugas *(Sistrurus catenatus)*. The massasaugas are comprised of three subspecies: the desert (subspecies *edwardsi*) located in the southwest, the western (subspecies *(tergeminus)* located in the middle midwest, and the eastern (subspecies *catenatus*). The latter is one of the few members of the Crotalidae family indigenous to the Great Lakes region (Fig. 72-6).

Characteristics

In contrast to *Sistrurus, Crotalus* species have small crown scales. In body build the eastern massasauga is similar to other small rattlesnakes such as the twin-spotted or ridge-nosed. Following rainstorms, with flooding of the marshland habitat, the eastern massasauga or swamp rattler will often seek higher ground, thereby increasing its chance for human encounter. Although this snake will bite if cornered or provoked, it remains more reclusive and docile than other types of rattlesnakes. This snake is found primarily in prairie marshes or fields with heavy grass cover. The venom of *S. catenatus* reportedly has an LD_{50} of 2.91 mg/kg^{-1} when given intravenously to mice. This toxicity is greater than that of copperheads (*Agkistrodon contortrix,* 10.92 mg/kg^{-1}) or cottonmouths (*A. piscivorus,* 4.17 mg/kg^{-1}) [132]

Clinical Presentation

Envenomations involve the same organ systems as *Crotalus* bites, but the clinical picture usually is much less severe. Often bites occur without envenomation. The clinical picture of *Sistrurus* envenomation more closely resembles copperhead than *Crotalus* bites. Edema is much less severe, but hemorrhagic blebs frequently occur after massasauga envenomation. Some nausea develops, but vomiting, paresthesias, and fasciculations are uncommon. Laboratory abnormalities and fatalities are rare.

Treatment

Management of *Sistrurus* envenomation follows *Crotalus* protocols, with gradation of clinical symptoms and administration of Antivenin (Crotalidae) Polyvalent as needed. Often, antivenom is not necessary.

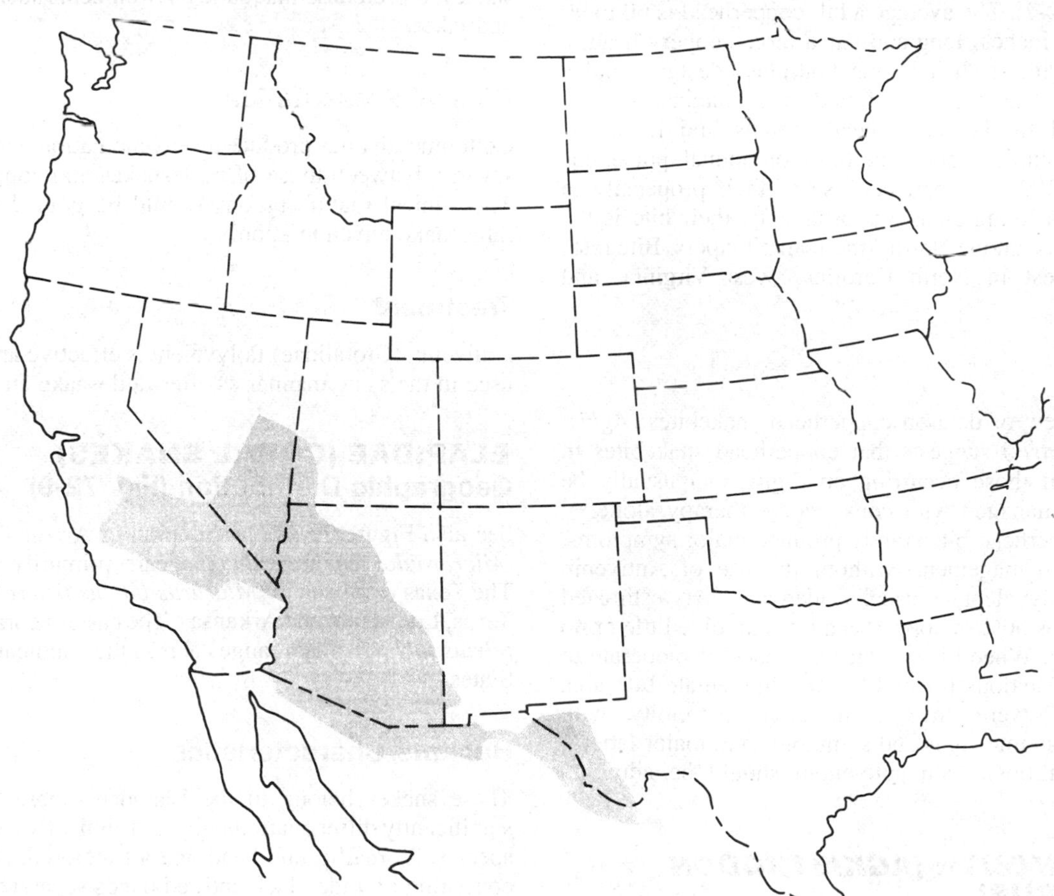

Figure 72-5 United States distribution of Mojave rattlesnake *(Crotalus scutulatus scutulatus)*. (Adapted from Russell FE. Snake venom poisoning. Great Neck, NY: Scholium International, 1983, p. 60.)

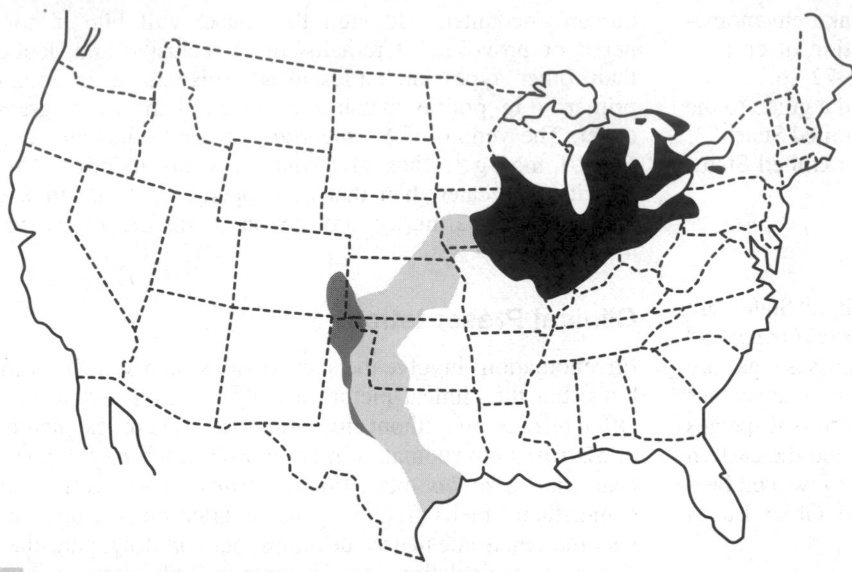

Figure 72-6 United States distribution of massasauga species. (Adapted from Russell FE. Snake venom poisoning. Great Neck, NY: Scholium International, 1983, p. 63.)

COPPERHEAD *(AGKISTRODON CONTORTRIX)*

Five species range from the eastern United States to southern Texas (Fig. 72-7). The average adult copperhead is 60 to 90 cm (24 to 30 inches) long and has a large coppery head, a thick body with reddish brown hourglass designs, and a rattleless tail. This species is found in mountains, wooded hillsides, and in the south near streams and lowlands. Copperheads inflict about one-third of annual poisonous bites (about 3000), in part because of their propensity to invade human living areas[133]; fortunately, their bite is the least venomous among North American pit vipers. Bite rates are the highest in North Carolina, West Virginia, and Arkansas.

Treatment

A recent review of data on copperhead snakebites *(Agkistrodon contortrix)* suggests that copperhead snakebites in children, even those occurring on digits, can usually be successfully managed with conservative therapy alone.[134]

Since copperhead bites rarely produce major symptoms, conservative management, without the use of Antivenin Crotalidae Polyvalent, is usually adequate. It is estimated that as many as 50% of copperhead bites involve little or no envenomation. When bites induce evidence of moderate to severe manifestations (extend beyond immediate bite area and may, if severe, involve the entire extremity, with significant systemic signs and symptoms and major laboratory abnormalities), then antivenom should be administered.[135]

COTTONMOUTH *(AGKISTRODON PISCIVORUS)*

Three species are distributed across the semiaquatic environments of the southeastern United States (Fig. 72-8). A unique white buccal mucosa on a dark head, a broad heavy body, and a rattleless tail characterize this species. The cottonmouth shares pit viper characteristics with rattlesnakes. It prefers semiaquatic environments such as swamps and lakes.

Clinical Presentation

Cottonmouth bites produce an envenomation intermediate in severity between those of rattlesnakes and copperheads.[136] The clinical manifestations should be graded similarly to rattlesnake envenomation.

Treatment

Antivenin (Crotalidae) Polyvalent is effective and should be used in the same manner as after rattlesnake envenomation.

ELAPIDAE (CORAL SNAKES)

Geographic Distribution (Fig. 72-9)

See also Figure 72-7. The Sonoran or Arizona coral snake *(Micruroides euryxanthus)* appears primarily in Arizona. The Texas coral snake *(Micrurus fulvius tenere)* is found in Texas, Louisiana, and Arkansas. The eastern coral *(Micrurus fulvius fulvius)* snake ranges across the southeastern United States.

Habitats/Characteristics

These snakes belong to the Elapidae (cobra) family and significantly differ anatomically and clinically from *Crotalus* species. A small round head and a tricolored, slender body consisting of wide black and red bands separated by yellow or white stripes characterize this genus. Their eyes are round, and their fangs are fixed. Bites leave a row of teeth marks rather than fang marks, because the coral snake needs prolonged contact (about 30 seconds) to work the venom into the skin. This secretive snake avoids human contact; most bites result from molestation of the snake. Coral snakes account for only 1 to 2% of annual poisonous snakebites in the United States.

Venom

Coral snake venom is primarily a neurotoxin and causes little local tissue reaction. Systemic reactions (i.e., neurologic) are common. The rate of fatalities from bites of the eastern coral snake (but not the Arizona coral snake) is about 9% compared with 0.2% for pit viper bites.

Clinical Presentation

Some pain may be present at the bite site, but usually edema, erythema, and pain are minimal. Typically, several hours after envenomation, neurologic signs and symptoms develop. Euphoria, lightheadedness, or drowsiness appears first. Fasciculations, tremor, weakness, increased salivation, and nausea and vomiting then occur. Symptoms may progress to bulbar palsy, paralysis, and respiratory depression after 5 to 10 hours manifested by diplopia, slurred speech, ptosis, dysphagia, and dyspnea. Convulsions can develop in small children. After coral snake bites, symptoms may be delayed 7 to 10 hours and no local reaction may be present to confirm envenomation.[137] Death usually occurs within 24 hours as a result of respiratory depression, although hypotension and cardiovascular collapse may contribute to mortality. The Arizona coral snake causes headache, blurred vision, abdominal pain, and gait disturbances, but usually not the serious CNS symptoms noted above for the Texas and eastern coral snakes.[138]

Treatment

First Aid

Transport the patient to an emergency medical facility as soon as possible (i.e., the keys to your car or the telephone is the best first-aid device you have). Capture of the snake is an important measure to help identify the species if it can be done promptly, safely, and with minimal hazard to both victim and rescuer.

Do not give alcohol to the victim. Tourniquets probably are not effective, although one study in an animal model suggested that pressure wrapping and immobilization decrease the spread of venom.

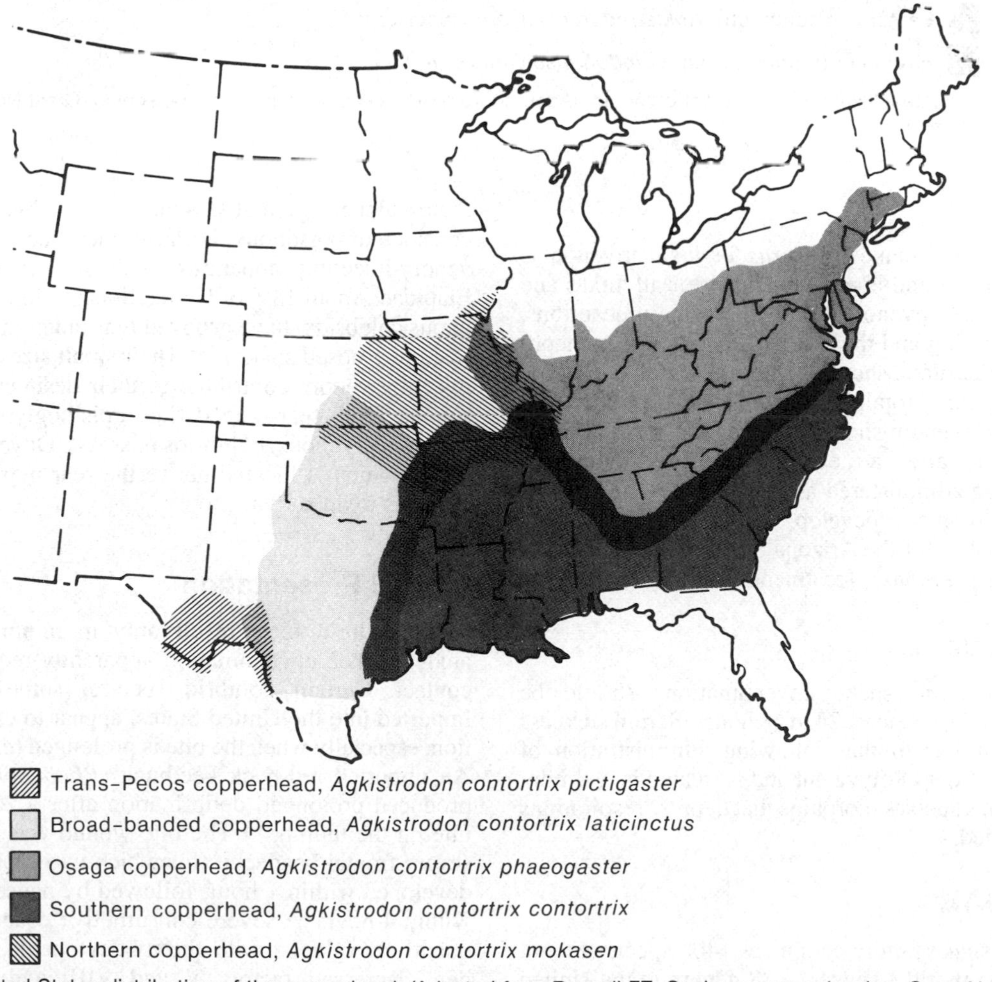

Figure 72-7 United States distribution of the copperhead. (Adapted from Russell FE. Snake venom poisoning. Great Neck, NY: Scholium International, 183, p. 64.)

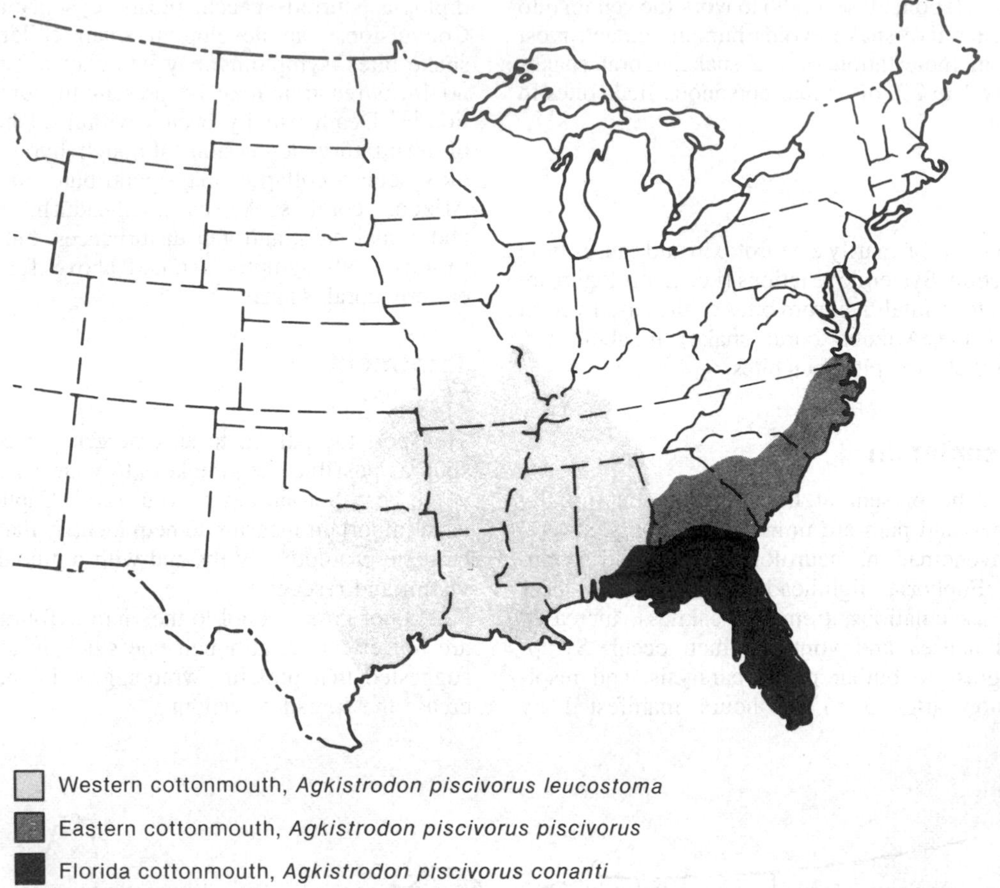

Figure 72-8 United States distribution of the cottonmouth. (Adapted from Russell FE. Snake venom poisoning. Great Neck, NY: Scholium International, 1983, p. 64.)

Antivenom

North American coral snake *(Micrurus fulvius)* antivenom is an effective antidote and is recommended for all Texas and eastern coral snake envenomations. The same precautions, including skin testing and the quick availability of epinephrine and other measures, should be used as for the administration of Antivenin (Crotalidae) Polyvalent. Approximately 3 to 5 vials of antivenom should be given in 250 to 500 mL of normal saline after a negative skin test. The antivenom should be administered as soon as possible without waiting for symptoms to develop. There is no commercial antivenom available for the Arizona or Sonoran coral snake *(Micruroides euryxanthus)*. Treatment is usually supportive.

Supportive Care

All victims of coral snake envenomations should be carefully observed for at least 24 to 48 hours. Serum sickness may develop similar to that following administration of Antivenin (Crotalidae) Polyvalent and is treated in a similar fashion. Narcotics such as morphine that depress respirations should be avoided.

COLUBRIDAE

This enormous snake family comprises 1400 species (about two-thirds of the world's snakes)—38 genera in the United States alone. Generally, snakes from this family are not considered poisonous because they lack the specialized venom-injecting apparatus seen in the Crotalidae and Elapidae. About 13% of United States colubrids (opisthoglyphous colubrids) have grooved rear fangs and venom glands (e.g., hog-nosed snake).[139] Their small size and difficulty in injecting venom contribute to their designation as nonpoisonous. Both rear-fanged (i.e., opisthoglyphous) and nonfanged (aglyphous) colubrids possess a Duvernoy's (parotid) gland, which is located above the rear maxillary teeth and contains toxic saliva.[140]

Clinical Presentation

Most colubrid bites result only in minor abrasions and anxiety, since envenomation apparently requires continued contact. Certain colubrid species, some of which are imported into the United States, appear to cause envenomation, especially when the bite is prolonged (e.g., 30 seconds). An imported red-neck keelbuck *(Rhabdophis subminatus)* produced prolonged defibrination after a 20- to 30-second bite on the thumb.[141] The bite wound was not painful, but severe frontal headache (for which two aspirin were taken) developed within 1 hour, followed by nausea and vomiting within 4 hours. A severe consumptive coagulopathy subsequently developed with thrombocytopenia, absent fibrinogen, depressed factors V and VIII, and elevated fibrin degradation products. Hemostasis did not begin returning toward normal until the seventh hospital day. Hematemesis and hematuria required cryoprecipitate, packed red blood cells, and fresh-frozen plasma transfusions. Bites by the Japanese colubrid snake known as yamakagashi *(Rhabdophis trigrinus),* a close relative of the American garter snake, produce nausea, vomiting, headache, and coagulation disorders that have resulted in massive local ecchymosis[140] and hematuria.[142] A prolonged bite by a large wandering garter snake *(Thamnophis elegans vagrans)* produced pain, edema, and localized hemorrhage that involved the hand, but no systemic symptoms.[143] Two nonindigenous African colubrid species are considered venomous and have caused fatalities (e.g., African twig snake and boomslang). Evidence of toxic saliva exists for five colubrid genera (*Coniophanes, Hypsiglena, Leptodria, Oxybelis,* and *Triniorphodon*), but these snakes are not as poisonous as the tropical colubrids.[141]

Treatment

Management is mainly supportive, since experience with treatment procedures is very limited. First aid involves primarily limiting the duration of bite to minimize the possibility of envenomation by placing the body of the snake on the nearest surface and striking its head. Hemorrhage appears to be the most serious threat to life. Supportive care (e.g., cryoprecipitate, fresh-frozen plasma, RBC transfusions) appears to be the best therapy. Heparin and aminocaproic acid are not recommended.[142] The effectiveness of colubrid antivenoms is not known, and their use should probably be avoided except in severe envenomations.

Nonvenomous Snakebites

Of the approximately 50,000 people bitten by snakes in the United States each year, more than 80% are not envenomated. Patients bitten by a nonvenomous snake (e.g., garden snakes—genus: *Thermophilis;* little brown snakes-genus: *Storeria*) can usually be discharged on completion of tetanus toxoid inoculation and local wound care. If the snake cannot be identified, the patient should be closely observed for 4 to 6 hours for symptoms and signs of envenomation. Prophylactic antibiotic therapy is usually unnecessary. Persistently tender snakebite wounds may contain an embedded tooth fragment that can be detected radiographically.[144]

Snake Database

A worldwide database on venomous snakes is being established in Switzerland (Azemiops, Herpetological Data Center, 8, Route de Ravieres, 1258 Perly, Geneva, Switzerland). Its aim is to cover all publications on venomous snakes since 1758.

It will also contain an international listing of sources of antivenom, as well as amino acid sequences of venomous snake proteins and DNA sequences.[145] It should shortly be available in CD-ROM.

GILA MONSTER

Helothermine has been isolated from *Heloderma horridum horridum* (Mexican beaded lizard) venom. It has an apparent molecular weight of 25,500, is composed of approximately

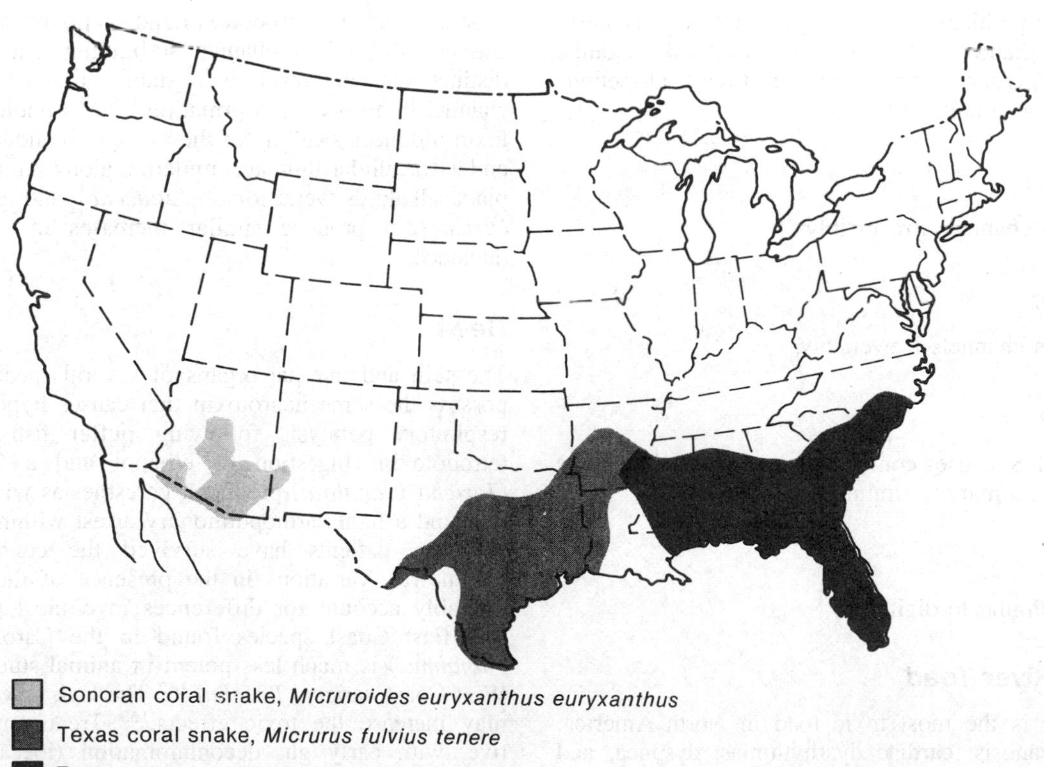

Figure 72-9 United States distribution of the coral snake. (Adapted from Russell FE. Snake venom poisoning. Great Neck, NY: Scholium International, 1983, p. 65.)

220 amino-acid residues, has an isoelectric point of 6.8, and has a unique *N*-terminal amino-acid sequence. Helothermine does not appear to affect Na^+, K^+, or Ca^{++} ion channels. In mice it induces lethargy, partial paralysis of the limbs, and a lowering of the body temperature.[146]

Clinical Presentation

Symtpoms and signs may include pain (begins immediately, peaks at 15 to 45 minutes), hypotension, tachycardia, generalized weakness, edema, nausea, and vomiting. The teeth of the Gila monster are easily dislodged and may remain in the wound. They do not show up on x-rays.

Laboratory

In one patient who developed an acute anterolateral infarction following a *H. suspectum cinctum* bite, a right bundle branch block and left posterior fascicular block were also observed on the electrocardiogram. The conduction abnormalities disappeared after 3 days, but the ST-segment changes persisted.[147,148]

Treatment

Hypotension responds to fluids. Broad-spectrum antibiotics and tetanus antitoxin are used as needed. Observe for at least 6 hours after exposure. Pliers may be necessary to pry open the jaws. Holding a flame under the Gila monster's jaws may effect release in a few seconds.[149]

AMPHIBIAN VENOMS[150]

The skin of amphibians (toads, frogs, newts, salamanders) contains small glands used for protection of the skin against infection by microorganisms. Many are toxins. *O*-methylbufotenin acts as a hallucinogen.

Batrachotoxin

Opens sodium channels irreversibly.

Tetrodotoxin

Blocks sodium channels irreversibly.

Samandarin

Acts on the CNS, causes convulsions and paralysis, affects Na^+ channel in a manner similar to batrachotoxin.

Bufotalin

Cardiotoxin, similar to digitalis.[151]

Colorado River Toad

Bufo alvarius is the most toxic toad in North America. Salivation, cyanosis, cardiac dysrhythmias, dyspnea, and seizures are common complications of the ingestion of *B. alvarius* by domestic animals.[152] A 5-year-old boy developed drooling and generalized tonic–clonic seizures within 15 minutes of placing a toad in his mouth.[153] Seizures lasted 1 hour until controlled by diazepam and phenobarbital in the emergency department. Physical examination revealed a total left-sided hemiparesis, Babinski sign, slurred speech, tachypnea, tachycardia, and systolic hypertension. The serum potassium level was 2.5 mEq/L. The neurologic deficit resolved over 1 week on high-dose hydrocortisone sodium succinate.

Colombian Poison-Dart Frogs

On the basis of LD_{50} experiments in mice, the amphibian group contains some of the most toxic substances known to man.[154] The skin secretions of the Colombian poison-dart frogs contain the steroidal alkaloid, batrachotoxin (molecular weight 538), pumiliotoxin B, isodihydrohistrionicotoxin, pumiliotoxin C, and gephyrotoxin.[155] In guinea pig atria, batrachotoxin demonstrates positive chronotropic and inotropic properties; dysrhythmias and atrial arrest develop after the application of batrachotoxin to isolated cardiac muscle preparations. At least three species of frogs *(Phyllobates terribilis, Phyllobates bicolor, Phyllobates aurotaenia)* from lower Central America and northwestern South America possess the powerful poison batrachotoxin.[156] The mouse LD_{50} for this toxin is 2 μg/kg compared with 8 μg/kg for tetrodotoxin and 500 μg/kg for curare.[157]

One freshly caught *P. terribilis* frog (the most dangerous species) contains up to 1.9 mg of batrachotoxin; the lethal dose in humans ranges from 0.02 to 0.2 mg.[158] This toxin depolarizes electrical membranes by increasing the permeability to sodium ions; fast axonal transport also is blocked at high concentrations. In contrast with the sodium channel blockers, tetrodotoxin and saxitoxin, batrachotoxin activates the sodium channel by binding to a separate and distinct site; the result is a stabilization of the sodium channel in an open conformation.[159] Morphologically, this toxin produces swelling of the axon at the node of Ranvier and extracellular fluid accumulation along the axon.[160] The plant alkaloids veratridine *(Liliaceae)* and grayanotoxin *(Ericaceae)* produce similar increases in sodium conductance.

Newt

The skin and internal organs of several species of newts possess the same neurotoxin that causes hypotension and respiratory paralysis following puffer fish ingestion—tetrodotoxin. Ingestion of ethanol and a 20-cm newt *(Taricha granulosa)* produced paresthesias within 15 minutes and a fatal cardiopulmonary arrest within 2 hours[161]; however, patients have survived the consumption of five newts. Variations in the presence of the neurotoxin probably account for differences in clinical presentation. The East Coast species found in the Carolinas *(Notophthalmus)* is much less potent in animal studies than the West Coast variety *(Taricha)*.[162] The lack of vomiting also may increase the toxic effects.[163] Treatment is supportive, with early gut decontamination (ipecac, charcoal, cathartics) recommended. Patients should be observed for 24 hours for signs of respiratory depression and hypotension.

SUGGESTED READINGS

1. Harvey AL, ed. International encyclopedia of pharmacology and therapeutics. Sct 134, Snake toxins. Elmsford, NY: Pergamon Press, 1991.
2. Tu AT, ed. Reptile venoms and toxins. In: Handbook of natural toxins, vol. 5. New York: Marcel Dekker, 1991.
3. Covacevich J, Davie P, Pearn J, eds. Toxic plants and animals. A guide for Australia. Queensland Museum, 1987.
4. Sutherland SK. Australian animal toxins. The creatures, their toxins and care of poisoned patient. Melbourne: Oxford University Press, 1983.
5. Edmunds C. Dangerous marine creatures. Reed Books Pty Ltd. 2 Aquatic Drive, Frenchs Forest, NSW 2086, 1989.
6. Edmunds C. A diving medical centre monograph. Biomedical Marine Services Pty Ltd., 25 Battle Blvd, Seaforth 2092, Australia, 1984.
7. Sutherland SK. Venomous creatures of Australia. A field guide with notes on first aid. Melbourne: Oxford University Press, 1988.
8. Pearn J, Covacevich J. Venoms and victims. South Brisbane: The Queensland Museum and Amphion Press, 1988.
9. Sutherland SK. First aid for snake bites and stings in Australia, with notes on first aid for bites and stings by other animals including spiders. CSL, April 1991.
10. Gopalakrishnakone P, Chou LM, eds. Snakes of medical importance (Asia-Pacific region). Singapore: Venom and Toxin Research Group, National University of Singapore, 1990.
11. White J, Snake bite: an Australian perspective. J Wilderness Med 1991;2:219–244.
12. Iyaniwura TT. Snake venom constituents: biochemistry and toxicology. I and II. Vet Hum Toxicol 1991;33:468–480.
13. Phelps T. Poisonous Snakes. Revised editions. London: Blandford Press, 1990.
14. Russell FE. Snake venom immunology. Historical and practical considerations. J Toxicol Toxin Reviews 1988;7:1–82.
15. Theakston RDG, Warrell DA. Antivenoms: a list of hyperimmune sera currently available for the treatment of envenoming by bites and stings. Toxicon 1991;29(12):1419–1470.
16. Kochva E. The origin of snakes and evaluation of the venom apparatus. Toxicon 1987;25:65–106.
17. Gopalakrishnakone P, Chou LM, eds. Snakes of medical importance (Asia-Pacific region). Singapore: Venom and Toxin Research Group, National University of Signapore, 1990, p. 670.
18. The International Society of Toxinology newsletter: IST Bite, Sting, and Poison Newsletter. Editors: Prof. Dr. G. Habermehl, Dept of Chemistry, Veterinary University, D-3000 Hanover, Germany. Prof. Dr. D Mebs. Zentrum der Rechtsmedizine, University of Frankfurt, D-6000 Frankfurt, Germany.
19. Sutherland SK. Treatment of snake bite. Aust Fam Physician 1990;19:21–41.
20. White J. Snake bite: an Australian perspective. J Wilderness Med 1991;2:219–244.
21. Sutherland SK. Deaths from snake bites in Australia, 1981–1991. Med J Aust 1992;157:740–746.

Middle East

1. Gilon D, Shalev O, Benbassat J. Treatment of envenomation by Echis coloratus (Mid-East Saw Sealed Viper): a decision tree. Toxicon 1989;27:1105–1112.
2. Russell FE. Venomous snakes of the Middle East. Vet Hum Toxicol 1991;33:68.
3. Kirchberg JS, Davidson TM. Envenomation by the colubrid snake Atarctaspis bibronii: a case report. Toxicon 1991;29:379–381.

Australia

1. Mirtschin PJ, Crowe GR, Davis R. Dangerous snakes of Australia. In: Gopalakrishnakone P, Chou LM, eds. Snakes of medical importance (Asia Pacific Region). Singapore: Venom and Toxin Research Group. National University of Singapore, 1990, pp. 1–174.
2. White J. Venomous snakes of medical importance in Australia. Clinical toxinology. In: Gopalakrishnakone P, Chou LM, eds. Snakes of medical importance (Asia Pacific region). Singapore: Venom and Toxin Research Group. National University of Singapore, 1990.
3. White J. Snakebite: an Australian perspective. J Wilderness Med 1991;2:219–244.
4. Sutherland SK. Treatment of snakebite. Aust Fam Physician 1990;19:1–13.
5. Covacevich J. Australia's dangerous snakes. In: Pearn J, Covacevich J, eds. Venoms and victims. South Brisbane: The Queensland Museum and Amphion Press, 1988, pp. 73–86.
6. Pearn J. Snakebite victims. In: Pearn J, Covacevich J, eds. Venoms and victims. South Brisbane: The Queensland Museum and Amphion Press, 1988, pp. 87–96.
7. Pearn J. Human snakebite—effects and first aid. In: Pearn J, Covacevich J, eds. Venoms and victims. South Brisbane: The Queensland Museum and Amphion Press, 1988, pp. 97–110.
8. Sutherland SK. First aid for snakebite in Australia. CSL Commonwealth Serum Laboratories, April 1991.
9. White J. Management of snakebite in South Australia. A management plan. South Australian Health Commission. Country Health Services Division, August 1991, pp. 1–36.
10. Sutherland SK, King K. Management of snakebite injuries. Monograph Series Number One. Royal Flying Doctor Service of Australia, 43 Bridge Street, Hurstville NSW 2220, 1991.
11. Jamieson R, Pearn J. An epidemiological and clinical study of snakebites in childhood. Med J Aust 1989;150:698–702.
12. Sutherland SK, Coulter AR, Harris RD. Rationalization of first-aid measures for elapid snakebite. Lancet 1979;1:183–186.

REFERENCES—REPTILES/AMPHIBIANS

1. Warrell DA, Fenner PJ, Venomous bites and stings. Br Med Bull 1993;49:423–439.
2. Phelps T. Poisonous snakes. Revised edition. London: Blandford Press, 1989.
3. Progress in the characterization of venoms and standardization of antivenoms. WHO Offset Publication No. 58. Geneva: World Health Organization, 1981.
4. Harborne DJ. Emergency treatment of adder bites: case reports and literature review. Arch Emerg Med 1993;10:223–243.
5. Audebert F, Grosselet O, Sabouraud A, Bone C. Quantitation of venom antigens from European vipers in human serum or urine by ELISA. J Anal Toxicol 1993;17:236–240.
6. Warrell DA. The global problems of snake bites: its prevention and treatment. In: Proc 10th World Congress on Animal Plant and Microbial Toxins, National University of Singapore, November 3–8, 1991. Abstract #004, p. 56.
7. White J, Duncan B, Wilson C, Williams V, Lloyd J. Coagulopathy following Australian elapid snakebite: a review of 20 cases. In: Proc 10th World Congress on Animal Plant and Microbial Toxins, National University of Singapore, November 3–8, 1991. Abstract #022, p. 84.
8. Sutherland SK. Treatment of snake bite. Aust Fam Physician 1990;19:26.
9. Sutherland SK. Treatment of snake bite. Aust Fam Physician 1990;19:1–13.
10. Ryan KC, Caravati EM. Life-threatening anaphylaxis following envenomation by two different species of Crotalidae. J Wilderness Med 1994;5:263–268.
11. Davidson TM, Schafer SF, Jones J. North American pit vipers. J Wilderness Med 1992;3:397–421.
12. Meier J. Effects of snake venoms on hemostasis. CRC Cnst Rev Toxicol 1991;21:171–182.
13. Hutton RA, Warrell DA. Action of snake venom components in the haemostatic system. Blood Rev 1993;7:176–189.
14. Theakston RDG, Warrell DA. Antivenoms: a list of hyperimmune sera currently available for the treatment of envenomation by bites and stings. Toxicon 1991;29(12):1419–1470.

15. Warrell DA. Treatment of snake bite in the Asia-Pacific Region: a personal view. In: Gopalakrishnakone P, Chou LM, eds. Snakes of medical importance (Asia Pacific region). Singapore: Venom and Toxin Research Group. National University of Singapore, 1990, pp. 641–670.
16. Burgess JL, Dart RC. Snake venom coagulopathy use and abuse of blood products in the treatment of pit viper envenomation. Ann Emerg Med 1991;20:795–801.
17. Jamieson R, Pearn J. An epidemiological and clinical study of snake bites in childhood. Med J Aust 1989;150:608–702.
18. White J. A review of snake bites and suspected snake bites treated in South Australia with particular reference to reptile handlers. In: Proc 10th World Congress on Animal Plant and Microbial Toxins, National University of Singapore, November 3–8, 1991. Abstract 181. p. 33.
19. O'Shea MT. The highly and potentially dangerous elapids of Papua, New Guinea. In: Gopalakrishnakone P, Chou LM, eds. Snakes of medical importance (Asia Pacific region). Singapore: Venom and Toxin Research Group. National University of Singapore, 1990, pp. 585–640.
20. Hudson BJ. Positive response to edrophonium in death adder *(Acanthophis antarcticus)* envenomation. Aust NZ J Med 1988;18:792–794.
21. Currie BJ, Richens J, Korinihona A, Worthington J. Anticholinesterase therapy for death adder envenomation. Aust NZ J Med 1990;20:190.
22. Mirtschin PJ, Crowe GR, Davis R. Dangerous snakes of Australia. In: Gopalakrishnakone P, Chou LM, eds. Snakes of medical importance (Asia Pacific region). Singapore. Venom and Toxin Research Group. National University of Singapore, 1990, pp. 1–173.
23. Sutherland SK. Australian animal toxins. The creatures, their toxins and care of the poisoned patient. Melbourne: Oxford University Press, 1983.
24. White J. Venomous snakes of medical importance in Australia: clinical toxinology. In: Gopalakrishnakone P, Chou LM, eds. Snakes of medical importance (Asia Pacific region). Singapore. Venom and Toxin Research Group. National University of Singapore, 1990, pp. 175–210.
25. Sutherland SK, King K. Management of snakebite injuries. Monograph Series Number One. Royal Flying Doctor Service of Australia, 43 Bridge Street, Hurstville, NSW 2220, 1991.
26. White J. Snakebite: an Australian perspective. J Wilderness Med 1991;2:219–244.
27. Aye MM. Venomous snakes of medical importance in Burma. In: Gopalakrishnakone P, Chou LM, eds. Snakes of medical importance (Asia Pacific region). Singapore. Venom and Toxin Research Group. National University of Singapore, 1990, pp. 211–241.
28. Soe-Soe, Than-than, Khin-Ei-Han. The nephrotoxic action of Russell's viper (Vipera russelli) venom. Toxicon 1990;28: 461–467.
29. Tun-Pe, Warrell DA, Tra-Nu-Swe, Phillips RE, Moore RA, Myint-Lwm. Acute and chronic pituitary failure resembling Sheehan's syndrome following bites by Russell's viper in Burma. Lancet 1987;2:763–767.
30. Proby C, Tha-Aung, Thet-Win, Hla-Mon, Burrin JM, Joplin GF. Immediate and long-term effects in hormone levels following bites by the Burmese Russell's viper. Q J Med 1989;276:399–411.
31. Zhao E. Venomous snakes of China. In: Gopalakrishnakone P, Chou LM, eds. Snakes of medical importance (Asia Pacific region). Singapore. Venom and Toxin Research Group. National University of Singapore, 1990, pp. 243–268.
32. Chen Yuan-Cong. Venomous snake bites and snake venom research in China. In: Gopalakrishnakone P, Chou LM, eds. Snakes of medical importance (Asia Pacific region). Singapore. Venom and Toxin Research Group. National University of Singapore, 1990, pp. 269–279.
33. Yu P-N, Lian Z-J, Lu Z-Y. Emergency treatment of respiratory arrest due to Chinese banded krait bite (33 case reports). Int Symp Natural Toxins (ISNt-89), Builin, China. J Toxicol Tox Rev 1990;9(1):134.
34. Cockram CS, Chan JCN, Chow KY. Bites by the white lipped pit viper *(Trimeresurus albolabris)* and other species in Hong Kong. A survey of 4 years' experience at the Prince of Wales Hospital. J Trop Med Hyg 1990;93:69–86.
35. Shastry JCM, Date A, Carman RH, Johny KV. Renal failure following snake bite. A clinicopathological study of nineteen patients. Am J Trop Med Hyg 1977;26:1032–1038.
36. Murthy TSN. Venomous snakes of medical importance in India (part A). In: Gopalakrishnakone P, Chou LM, eds. Snakes of medical importance (Asia Pacific region). Singapore. Venom and Toxin Research Group. National University of Singapore, 1990, pp. 281–297.
37. Khaire A, Khaire N, Joshi DN. Venomous snakes of medical importance in India (Part B)—clinical aspects. In: Gopalakrishnakone P, Chou LM, eds. Snakes of medical importance (Asia Pacific region). Singapore. Venom and Toxin Research Group. National University of Singapore, 1990, pp. 299–309.
38. Toriba M, Sawai Y. Venomous snakes of medical importance in Japan. In: Gopalakrishnakone P, Chou LM, eds. Snakes of medical importance (Asia Pacific region). Singapore. Venom and Toxin Research Group. National University of Singapore, 1990, pp. 323–347.
39. Murata R, Fukishima H. Immune response of man to habu venom toxoid. Jpn J Med Sci Biol 1981;34:197–212.
40. Liat LB. Venomous land snakes of Malaysia. In: Gopalakrishnakone P, Chou LM, eds. Snakes of medical importance (Asia Pacific region). Singapore. Venom and Toxin Research Group. National University of Singapore, 1990, pp. 387–417.
41. Reid HA, Thean PC, Chan KE et al. Clinical effects of bites by Malayan viper *(Ancistrodom rhodostoma).* Lancet 1963;1: 617–621.
42. Tau KK, Choo KE, Ariffin WA. Snake bite in Kelantanese children: a five-year experience. Toxicon 1990;28:225–230.
43. Tau NH, Saifuddin MN. Isolation and characterization of a hemorrhagin from the venom of *Ophiophagus hannah* (king cobra). Toxicon 1990;28:285–292.
44. Benbassat J, Shalev O. Envenomation by Echis coloratus (Mideast saw-scaled viper): a review of the literature and indications for treatment. Isr J Med Sci 1993;29:239–250.
45. Porath A, Gilon D, Schulchynska-Castel H, Shalev O, Keynan A, Benbasset J. Risk indications after envenomation in humans by Echis coloratus (Mideast saw-scaled viper). Toxin 1992;30:35–42.
46. Schulchynska-Castel H, Dvilansky A, Keynan A. Echis colorata bites: clinical evaluation of 42 patients. A retrospective study. Isr J Med Sci 1986;22:880–883.
47. Kochva E. Venomous snakes of Israel. In: Gopalakrishnakone P, Chou LM, eds. Snakes of medical importance (Asia Pacific region). Singapore. Venom and Toxin Research Group. National University of Singapore, 1990, pp. 311–326.
48. Strunk HK. Guidebook of infections and communicable diseases and other health hazards of the Arabian Peninsula. Pearl Harbor, HI: US Naval Forces Central Command, 1984.
49. Baker MS, Strunk HK. Medical aspects of Person Gulf operations: environmental hazards. Mil Med 1991;156:381–385.
50. Vick JA. Medical studies of the poisonous land and sea snakes found in and around Saudi Arabia. Mil Med 1992; 157:159–162.
51. Coppola M, Hogan DE. Venomous snakes of Southwest Asia. Am J Emerg Med 1992;10:230–236.
52. Toriba M. Venomous snakes of medical importance in the Philippines. In: Gopalakrishnakone P, Chou LM, eds. Snakes of medical importance (Asia Pacific region). Singapore. Venom and Toxin Research Group. National University of Singapore, 1990, pp. 463–469.
53. Watt G, Padre L, Tuazon L, Theakston RDG, Laughlin L. Bite by the Philippine cobra *(Naja naja philippinensis):* prominent neurotoxicity with minimal local signs. Am J Trop Med Hyg 1988;39:306–311.
54. Watt G, Theakston RDG, Hayes CG, Yamboa ML, Sangalang R, Ranoa CP, Alquizalas E, Warrell DA. Positive response to edrophonium in patients with neurotoxic envenomation by cobras *(Naja naja philippinensis).* A placebo-controlled study. N Engl J Med 1986;315:1444–1448.
55. Drachman DB. Myasthenia gravis. N Engl J Med 1978;298: 136–142, 186–193.

56. Watt G, Hayes CG. Edrophonium for cobra bite. N Engl J Med 1987;316:1609.
57. Riding JE, Robinson JS. The safety of neostigmine. Anaesthesia 1961;16:346–354.
58. Arsura EL. Edrophonium for cobra bite. N Engl J Med 1987; 316:1608–1609.
59. de Silva A. Venomous snakes, their bites and treatment in Sri Lanka. In: Gopalakrishnakone P, Chou LM, eds. Snakes of medical importance (Asia Pacific region). Singapore. Venom and Toxin Research Group. National University of Singapore, 1990, pp. 479–556.
60. Phillips RE, Theakston RDG, Warrell DA, Galigedara Y, Abeysekera DTDJ, Dissanayaka P et al. Paralysis, rhabdomyolysis and haemolysis caused by bites of Russell's viper (Vipera russelli pulchella) in Sri Lanka. Failure of Indian (Haffkine) antivenom. Q J Med 1988;68:691–716.
61. Jintakune P, Limthongkul S, Mahasandana S, Meemano K, Pochanugool C, Sitprija V. Venomous snakes and snake bite in Thailand. In: Gopalakrishnakone P, Chou LM, eds. Snakes of medical importance (Asia Pacific region). Singapore. Venom and Toxin Research Group. National University of Singapore, 1990, pp. 557–579.
62. Sanguanvungsirikul S, Chomdej B, Suivanprasert K, Wattanavah P. Acute effect of Russell's viper (Vipera russelli siamensis) on renal hemodynamics and antiregulation of blood flow in dogs. Toxicon 1989;27:1199–1207.
63. Sitprija V, Suvanpha R, Pochanugool C, Chusil S, Tungsanga K. Acute interstitial nephritis in snake bite. Am J Trop Med Hyg 1982;31:408–410.
64. Mitrakul C, Juzi V. Pongrujikorn W. Antivenom therapy in Russell's viper bite. Am J Clin Pathol 1991;95:412–417.
65. Malasit P, Warrell DA, Chanthavanich P, Viravan C, Mongkolsapaya J, Singhthong B, Supich C. Prediction, prevention, and mechanism of each (anaphylactic) antivenom reactions in victims of snake bites. Br Med J 1986;292:17–20.
66. Pochamgool C, Limthogkul S, Mecmano K. Clinical features of non-antivenom treated neurotoxic snake bite patients. In: Gopalakrishnakone P, Tan CK. Progress in Venom and Toxin Research. Proc First Asia-Pacific Congress on Animal, Plant and Microbial Toxins. Singapore: June 24–27, 1987, pp. 46–51.
67. Chinonavanig L, Karnchaachetanee C, Pongsettakul P, Ratanabanangkoon K. Diagnosis of snake venoms by a reverse latex agglutination test. Clin Toxicol 1991;29: 493–503.
68. Persson H. Features of viper bites in Europe. Management and indications for antivenom immune therapy. Proc Eur Assoc Pois Cont Cent Toxicol Technical Meeting. Lyon, France: May 22–24, 1991.
69. Persşon H, Irestedt B. A study of 136 cases of adder bite treated in Swedish Hospitals during one year. Acta Med Scand 1981;210:433–439.
70. Reid HA. Adder bites in Britain. Br Med J 1976;2:153–156.
71. Audebert F, Sorkine M, Bon C. Clinical gradation and ELISA quantification of envenomations following viper bites in France. In: Proc. 10th World Congress on Animal Plant and Microbial Toxins, National University of Singapore, November 3–8, 1991. Abstract 127, p. 179. (Also see Toxicon 1992;30: 599–609.)
72. Alldridge G, Campbell A, Routledge PA, Volans GN. Survey of enquiries concerning *Vipera berus* bites received by United Kingdom Poison Center 1983–1991. In: 10th World Congress on Animal Plant and Microbial Toxins, National University of Singapore, November 3–8, 1991. Abstract 128, p. 180.
73. Audebert F, Grosselet O, Sabourand A, Bon C. Quantification of venom antigens from European vipers in human serum or urine by ELISA. Personal communication, June 18, 1993.
74. Stahel E, Wellauer R, Freyvogel TA. Vergiftungen durch einheimische Vipera (*Vipera berus* and *Vipera aspis*). Schweiz Med Wochenschr 1985;115:890–896.
75. Pozio E. Venomous snake bites in Italy: epidemiological and clinical aspects. Trop Med Parasitol 1988;39:62–66.
76. Theakston RDG, Reid HA. Effectiveness of Zagreb antivenom against envenomation by the adder, *Vipera berus.* Lancet 1976;2:121–123.
77. Antonini G, Rasura M, Conti G, Mattia C. Neuromuscular paralysis in *Vipera aspis* envenomation: pathogenetic mechanisms. J Neurol Neurosurg Psych 1991.
78. Hawley A. Adder bites in the British Army 1979–1988: a decade of experience. J R Army Med Corps 1990;136:114–118.
79. Smith DC, Reddi KR, Laing G, Theakston RGD, Landon J. An affinity purified ovine antivenom for the treatment of *Vipera Berus* envenomation. Toxicon 1992;30:865–871.
80. Persson H. Initial experience with *Vipera berus* specific Fab antivenom. Proc Eur Assoc Pois Centers Clin Toxicol, Istanbul, May 1991, p. 3.
81. Rodrigues D, Machado MA. Poisonous animals: a study of human accidents in the State of Bahia, Brazil. II. Ophidian accidents. Vet Hum Toxicol 1987;29(Suppl 2):76–78.
82. Burdmann E, Barcellos MA Cardoso JL, Malheiros R, Abdulkader R, Dakes E et al. Acute interstitial nephritis after snake bite. Ren Fail 1989;11:51–52.
83. Selistre HS, Queiroz LS, Cunha OAB, De Souza GEP, Giglio JR. Isolation and characterization of hemorrhagic, myonecrotic and edema inducing toxins from *Bothrops insularis* (Jararaca Ilhoa) snake venom. Toxicon 1990;28:261–273.
84. Barral-Netto M, Schreifer A, Vinhas V, Almeida AR. Enzyme linked immunosorbent assay for the detection of *Bothrops jararaca* venom. Toxicon 1990;28:1053–1061.
85. Fortes-Dias CL, Fonseca BCB, Kochva E, Diniz CR. Purification and properties of an antivenom factor from the plasma of the South American rattlesnake *(Crotalus durissus terrificus).* Toxicon 1991;29:997–1008.
86. Jaeger A, Sander PH, Kopferschmitt J, Flesch F. Afibrinogenemia and rhabdomyolysis following rattlesnake bite *(Crotalus durissus terrificus).* XIII Int Cong Eur Assoc Pois Control Centers, Edinburgh. September 12–14, 1988.
87. Davidson TM, Schafer SF, Moseman J. Central and South American vipers. J Wilderness Med 1993;4:416–440.
88. Cardosa JLC, Fan HW, Franco FOS, Jorge MT, Leite RP, Nichioka SA et al. Randomized comparative trial of three antivenoms in the treatment of envenoming by lance-headed vipers *(Bothrops jaruaca)* in Sao Paulo, Brazil. Q J Med 1993;86:312–325.
89. Bratt DE, Boos HEA. *Bothrops atrox* snakebite in a six-year-old child. West Ind Med J 1993;41:130.
90. Sano-Martins IS, Fan HW, Castro SCP, Tomy SC, Franca FOS, Jorge MT et al. Reliability of the simple 20 minute whole blood clotting test (WBCT20) as an indicator of low plasma fibrinogen concentration in patients envenomated by *Bothrops* snakes. Toxicon 1994;32:1045–1050.
91. Cogo JC, Prado-Franceschi J, Rodrigues, Simioni L. Effect of *Bothrops insularis* on the neuromuscular junction. In: Proc 10th World Congress on Animal Plant and Microbial Toxins, National University of Singapore, November 3–8, 1991. Abstract 135, p. 187.
92. Kamiguti AS. Coagulopathy induced by *Bothrops jararaca* envenomations. In: Proc 10th World Congress on Animal Plant and Microbial Toxins, National University of Singapore, November 3–8, 1991. Abstract 152, p. 204.
93. Moreno RA, Gutierrez JM, Prado-Franceschi J. The neutralization by commercial antiserum (AS) of the systemic and local effects induced by *Bothrops neuwiedi pauloensis* venom. In: Proc 10th World Congress on Animal Plant and Microbial Toxins, National University of Singapore, November 3–8, 1991. Abstract 159, p. 211.
94. Nunes TB, Rodrigues DS. Poisonous animals. A study of human accidents in the State of Bahia, Brazil. Vet Hum Toxicol 1987;29(Suppl 2):73–75.
95. Kamiguti AS, Cardoso JLC, Theakston RDG, Sano-Martins IS, Hutton RA, Rugman RF et al. Coagulopathy and haemorrhage in human victim of *Bothrops jararaca* envenoming in Brazil. Toxicon 1991;29:961–972.
96. Chaves F, Gutierrez JM, Brenes F. Pathological and biochemical changes induced in mice after intramuscular injection of venom from newborn specimens of the snake *Bothrops asper* (Terciopelo). Toxicon 1992;2:1099–1109.
97. Desmond HP, Crampton JM, Theakston RDG. Rapid isolation and partial characterization of two phospholipases from Kenyan *Echis carinatus leakeyi* (Leakey's saw-scaled viper) venom. Toxicon 1991;29:536–539.

98. Pugh RNH, Theakston RDG. The incidence and mortality of snake bite in savanna Nigeria. Lancet 1980;2:1181–1183.
99. Warrell DA, Davidson N McD, Greenwood BM, Ormerod LD, Pope HM, Watkins J, Prentice CRM. Poisoning by bites of the saw-scaled or carpet viper *(Echis carinatus)* in Nigeria. Q J Med 1977;46:33–62.
100. Brown R, Brasch L, Leichter D, Canfield D. Gabon viper envenomation: An unexpected big city emergency. Pediatr Emerg Care 1989;5:248–249.
101. Russell FE, Carlson RW, Wainschel J et al. Snake venom poisoning in the United States: experience with 550 cases. JAMA 1975;233:341–344.
102. Watt CH. Poisonous snake bite treatment in the United States. JAMA 1978;240:654–656.
103. Curry SC, Kunkel DB. Death from a rattlesnake bite. Am J Emerg Med 1985;3:227–235.
104. Wingert WA. Poisoning by animal venoms. Top Emerg Med 1980;2(3):89–118.
105. Gerkin R, Curry S, Vance M et al. Life-threatening airway obstruction from rattlesnake bite to the tongue. Vet Hum Toxicol 1986;28:487 (abstract).
106. Clement JE, Pietrusko RG. Pit viper snakebite envenomation in the United States. Clin Toxicol 1979;14:515–538.
107. Russell FE. Snake venom poisoning. Great Neck, NY: Scholium International, 1983.
108. Bush SP, Jansen PW. Severe rattlesnake envenomation with anaphylaxis and rhabdomyolysis. Ann Emerg Med 1995; 25:845–848.
109. Ouyang C, Teng C-M, Huang T-F. Characterization of snake venom components acting on blood coagulation and platelet function. Toxicon 1992;30(9):945–966.
110. Swindle GM, Seaman KG, Arthen DC, Almquist TD. The six-hour observation rule for grade I crotalid envenomation: is it sufficient? Case report of delayed envenomation. J Wilderness Med 1992;3:168–172.
111. Blackman JR, Dollon S. Venomous snakebite: past, present and future treatment options. J Am Board Fam Pract 1992;53:399–405.
112. Wingert WA, Chan L. Rattlesnake bites in Southern California and rationale for recommended treatment. West J Med 1988;148:37–44.
113. Walter FG, Olson KR. First aid for snakebite. AACT Clinical Toxicology Update 1995;8:1.
114. Sutherland SK. First aid for snakebite in Australia with notes on first aid for bites and stings by other animals including spiders. Fourth Revision. April 1991. Commonwealth Serum Laboratories, pp. 4–5.
115. Sutherland SK, Coulter R, Harris RD. Rationalisation of first aid measures for Elapid snake bite. Lancet 1979;1:183–186.
116. Gellert GA. Snake venom and insect venom extractors: an unproved therapy. N Engl J Med 1992;327:1322.
117. Sutherland SK. Premedication before antivenom therapy. Med J Aust 1991;155:722.
118. Fatovich DM, Turner VF, Hirsch RL. Premedication before antivenom therapy. Med J Aust 1992;156:510.
119. Kirkland G. Snake venom allergy. Med J Aust 1990;153:570–571.
120. Caravati EM, Wallace DE. Anaphylactic reaction to snake venom. Vet Hum Toxicol 1990;21:66.
121. Bucknall NC. Electrical treatment of venomous bites and stings. Toxicon 1991;29:397–400.
122. Dart RC, Gustafson RA. Failure of electric shock treatment for rattlesnake envenomation. Ann Emerg Med 1991;20:659–661.
123. Sullivan JB Jr. Past, present, and future immunotherapy of snake venom poisoning. Ann Emerg Med 1987;16:938–944.
124. Kelly JJ, Sadeghani K, Gottlieb SF, Ownly CL, Van Meter KW, Torbati D. Reduction of rattlesnake venom–induced myonecrosis in mice by hyperbaric oxygen therapy. J Emerg Med 1991;9:1–7.
125. Stolpe MR, Norrus RL, Chisholm CD, Hartshorne MF, Okerberg C, Ehler WJ, Posch J. Preliminary observation on the effects of hyperbaric oxygen therapy on western diamondback rattlesnake *(Crotalus atrox)* venom poisoning in the rabbit model. Ann Emerg Med 1989;18:871–874.
126. Audebert F, Gorsselet O, Sabourand A, Bond C. Quantitation of venom antigens from European vipers in human serum or urine by ELISA. J Anal Toxicol 1993;17:236–240.
127. Watt G. Ancillary treatments of neurotoxic envenomation. Toxicon 1993;31:932–933.
128. Sutherland SK. Commonwealth Serum Laboratories, Melbourne, Australia: Personal communication. May 4, 1992.
129. Mars M, Hadley GP, Aitchison JM. Direct intracompartmental pressure measurement in the management of snakebites in children. S Afr Med J 1991;80:227–228.
130. Blackman JR, Dillon S. Venomous snakebite: past, present and future treatment options. J Am Board Fam Pract 1992;5: 399–405.
131. Dart RC, Horowitz R, Gomez H. Management of poisonous snakebite in the United States. Rocky Mountain Poison and Drug Center and University of Colorado, Denver, CO. Revised September 18, 1994.
132. Sing K, Erickson T, Aks S, Rothenberg H, Lipscomb J. Eastern massasauga rattlesnake envenomations in an urban wilderness. J Wilderness Med 1994;5:77–87.
133. Parrish HM, Carr C. Bites by copperheads *(Agkistrodon contortrix)* in the United States. JAMA 1967;201:107–112.
134. Rodgers GC, Roe D, Matyunas NJ. Copperhead *(Agkistrodon contortrix)* envenomations in children. Report of thirty-two cases. In: Proc 10th World Congress in Animal Plant and Microbial Toxins, National University of Singapore, November 3–8, 1991. Abstract 166. p. 218.
135. White BD, Rodgers GC, Matyunas NJ, Allen F. Copperhead snake bites reported to the Kentucky Regional Poison Center 1986: epidemiology and treatment suggestions. J Kentucky Med Assoc 1988;86:61–66.
136. Watt CH. Poisonous snake bite treatment in the United States. JAMA 1978;240:654–656.
137. Treatment of snakebites in the USA. Med Lett 1982;24:87–89.
138. Russell FE. Bites by the Sonoran coral snake, *Micruroides euryxanthus.* Toxicon 1967;5:39–42.
139. Mandell F, Bates J, Mittleman MS et al. Major coagulopathy and "non-poisonous" snake bites. Pediatrics 1980;65: 314–317.
140. MckKinstry DM. Evidence of toxic saliva in some colubrid snakes of the United States. Toxicon 1978;16:523–534.
141. Cable D, McGehee W, Wingert WA et al. Prolonged defibrination after a bite from a "nonvenomous" snake. JAMA 1984;251:925–926.
142. Minton SA. Beware: nonpoisonous snakes. Clin Toxicol 1978; 15:259–265.
143. Vest DK. Envenomation following the bite of a wandering garter snake *(Thamnophis elegans vagrans).* Clin Toxicol 1981;18:573–579.
144. Weed HG. Nonvenomous snakebite in Massachusetts: prophylactic antibiotics are unnecessary. Can Emerg Med 1993; 22:220–224.
145. Golay P, Stocklin R. Azemiops: a worldwide database on venomous snakes. In: Proc 10th World Congress on Animal Plant and Microbial Toxins, National University of Singapore, November 3–8, 1991. Abstract 102, p. 154.
146. Mochca-Morales J, Martin BM, Possani LD. Isolation and characterization of helothermine, a novel toxin from *Heloderma horridum horridum* (Mexican beaded lizard) venom. Toxicon 1990;28:299–309.
147. Bou-Abboud CF, Karassakis DG. Acute myocardial infarction following a Gila monster *(Heloderma suspectum cinctum)* bite. West J Med 1988;148:577–579.
148. Preston CA. Hypotension, myocardial infarction and coagulopathy following Gila monster bite. J Emerg Med 1989;7:37–40.
149. Hooker KR, Caravati EM. Gila monster envenomation. Ann Emerg Med 1994;24:731.
150. Fletcher JE, Jodokowsky M, Tripolitis L. Calcium release induced by *Naja naja kaouthia* cardiotoxin in skeletal muscle sarcoplasmic reticulum exhibits a species-dependent association with the threshold of cardiotoxin-induced calcium release. In: Proc 10th World Congress on Animal Plant and Microbial Toxins, National University of Singapore, November 3–8, 1991. Abstract 021, p. 73.
151. Habermehl G. Chemistry and pharmacology of amphibian venoms. In: Proc 10th World Congress on Animal Plant and Microbial Toxins, National University of Singapore, November 3–8, 1991. Abstract 113, p. 165.

152. Palumbo NE, Perri S, Read G. Experimental induction and treatment of toad poisoning in the dog. J Am Vet Med Assoc 1975;167:1000–1005.
153. Hitt M, Ettinger DD. Toad toxicity. N Engl J Med 1986;314: 1517.
154. Daly JW. Biologically active alkaloids from poison frogs *(Dendrobatidae).* J Toxicol Toxin Rev 1982;1:33–86.
155. Mensah-Dwumah M, Daly JW. Pharmaclotical activity of alkaloids from poison-dart frogs *(Dendrobatidae).* Toxicon 1968;16:189–194.
156. Myers CW, Daly JW, Malkin B. A dangerously toxic new frog *(Phyllobates)* used by Enbera Indians of western Colombia with discussion of blowgun fabrication and dart poisoning. Bull Am Mus Nat Hist 1978;101:311–365.
157. Daly J, Witkop B. Batrachotoxin, an extremely active cardio- and neurotoxin from the Colombian arrow poison frog *(Phyllobates aurotaenia).* Clin Toxicol 1971;4:331–342.
158. Daly JW, Myers CW, Warnick JE et al. Levels of batrachotoxin and lack of sensitivity to its action in poison-dart frogs *(Phyllobates).* Science 1980;208:1383–1385.
159. Brown GB. ^{3}H-Batrachotoxin—a benzoate binding to voltage-sensitive sodium channels: inhibition by the channel blockers tetrodotoxin and saxitoxin. J Neurosci 1986;6:2064–2070.
160. Wayne Moore GR, Boegman RJ, Robertson DM et al. Acute stages of batrachotoxin-induced neuropathy: a morphologic study of a sodium channel toxin. J Neurocytol 1986;15: 573–583.
161. Bradley SG, Klika LJ. A fatal poisoning from the Oregon roughskinned newt *(Taricha granulosa).* JAMA 1981;246: 247.
162. Brodie ED Jr. Investigations of the skin toxins of the adult rough-skinned newt, *Taricha granulosa.* Copeia 1974; 68(1):306–313.
163. Brodie ED Jr, Hansel JL, Johnson JA. Toxicity of the urodele amphibians *Taricha notophthalmus cynops* and *Paramesotriton salamandridae.* Copeia 1974(2):506–511.

ARTHROPODS

Some general characteristics of arthropods are summarized in Table 72-19. Available antivenoms are summarized in Table 72-20. The wasp, hornet, and yellow jacket are depicted in Figures 72-10, 72-11, and 72-12.

Table 72–19
Habits and Effects of Various Arthropods [a]

			Method of Attack		Time of Activity				Local Reaction					Distribution of Lesions			
									Onset		Duration						
Insect	Average Length[b] (mm)	Usual Location	Bite	Sting	Day	Night	Dusk	Dawn	Immediate	Delayed	Hours	Days	Weeks	Single	Scattered	Grouped	Residua
Bumblebee	20–25	Flowers		X	X				X	X	X	X		X			None
Honeybee	10–15	Flowers		X	X				X	X	X	X		X			None
Mud-dauber wasp	20–25	Orchards, garbage pails		X	X				X			X		X			None
Yellow jacket	10–15	Orchards, garbage pails		X	X				X		X			X			None
Hornet	20–30	Woods, flowers		X	X				X		X			X			None
Harvester ant	7–9	Vegetation, kitchen		X	X							X		X			None
Fire ant	6–7	Fields		X	X				X			X				X	Pigmented macules, occasionally nodules
Stable fly	6–7	Barns	X		X				X		X			X			None
Horse fly	10–20	Barns	X		X				X		X			X			None
Deer fly	7–9	Cattle	X		X				X		X			X	X		None
Black fly	1–5	Woodlands, running water	X		X			X		X			X		X		Nodules, scars
Sand fly	1–4	Woodlands	X			X			X			X			X		Bluish spots
Biting midges	0.6–5	Marshlands	X				X		X		X				X		None
Chigger mite	0.2–1	Vegetation	X		X					X		X				X	Hyperpigmentation
Ticks	5–15	Vegetation	X								X	X		X	X		Granulomas
Brown Recluse Spider	10–15	Closets, attics	X						X		X	X		X			Scar
Black Widow Spider	10	Basements, outhouses	X						X		X	X		X			None
Tarantula	15–20	Vegetation	X											X			None
Scorpion	15–200	Stones and sand		X		X			X		X			X			None
Wheel bug	20+	Vegetation	X		X				X		X			X			None
Kissing bug	20+	Bedroom	X			X				X		X				X	None

[a]Adapted from Frazier CA. Clin Symp (Ciba) 1968;20(3):101.
[b]10 mm = ⅜ in.

Table 72–20
Table of Poisonous Animals and Available Antivenins[a]

Producer or Distributor	Venoms Used in Preparation	Trade or Common Name	Common Name of Arthropod	Additional Venoms Neutralized	Comments
Merck, Sharp and Dome, Westpoint, Pennsylvania 19486, USA	*Latrodectus mactans*	Black widow	Black widow (spider)		
Instituto Nacional de Higiene, Av. M. Escobedo No. 20, Mexico City D.F., Mexico	*Centruroides noxius*	Antialacrás polyvalent			
Laboratorio Zapata, Mexico City D.F., Mexico	*Centruroides suffusus* *Centruroides noxius*	Antialacrás polyvalent			
Laboratorios "MYN," S.A. Av. Coyoacan 1707, Mexico City, 12, D.F. Mexico	*Centruroides suffusus* *Centruroides noxius* or *C. limidus*	Antialacras polyvalent			
Institutio Nacional de Higiene, Lima, Peru	*Loxosceles* sp.	Anti-Loxoscelico			Ammonium sulfate precipitation. Supplied as liquid.
Instituto Butantan, Caixa Postal 65, 05504 São Paulo, Brazil	*Phoneutria* *Loxosceles* *Lycosa*	Antiarachnidico polivalente			
Institute of Immunology, Rockefellerova, 2, Zagreb, Yugoslavia	*Scorpaena porcus*	Scorpion fish antivenom	Scorpion fish		
Institut d'Etat des serums et Vaccins Razi, P.O. Box 656, Teheran, Iran	*Androctonus crassicauda* *Buthotus saulcyi* *Hemiscorpius lepturus* *Mesobuthus eupeus* *Odontobuthus doriae* *Scorpio maurus*	Polyvalent scorpion serum	Scorpions		Ammonium sulfate precipitation. Supplied in liquid form.
Commonwealth Serum Laboratories, 45 Poplar Road, Parkville, Victoria 3052, Australia	*Latrodectus mactans hasselti*	Red-black spider antivenom	Red-back spider		Pepsin digestion and ammonium sulfate precipitation.
	Chironex fleckeri	Sea-wasp	Sea-wasp	*Chiropsalmus quadrigatus*	
	Synanceja trachynis	Stonefish	Stonefish		
Institut Pasteur d'Algérie, rue Docteur Laveran, Algiers, Algeria	*Androctonus australis*	Scorpion antivenin			
Lister Institute of Preventive Medicine, Elstree, Herts WD6 3AX, England	*Androctonus australis* *Buthus occitanus* *Leiurus quinquestriatus*	Scorpion			
South African Institute for Medical Research, Hospital Street, Johannesburg, South Africa	*Latrodectus* *Parabuthus*	Black widow Scorpion			

[a]Adapted from Theakston RDG, Warrell DA. Toxicon 1991;29(12):1419–1470.

BEHAVIOR AND STINGING APPARATUS

Killer Bees (Africanized Honey Bees *[Apis mellifera scutellata]*)

Swarms of killer bees have gradually moved from Latin America to the United States (Fig. 72-13). They attack in large numbers and have led to the development of hypersensitivity with the risk of fatal anaphylaxis. Multiple stings are necessary to cause death by direct toxicity, but as few as 30 to 50 stings have proved fatal in children.

Venoms of European honey bees *(Apis mellifera),* the common honey bees of Europe and their descendants brought to North America, include mellitin, phospholipase A_2 (PLA_2), and hyaluronidase. These components appear to be present in similar concentrations in European and Africanized bee venom.[1–3]

African Bees

Once Africanized honey bee colonies are established in a state, there will probably be two or three more deaths per year than usual from bee stings in the area.[4]

Hospital admission should be considered in all patients who have received more than 50 bee stings or who have an anaphylactic reaction. Maintain airway patency and blood pressure.

Treatment of Envenomation

Schumacher and Egen[2] have provided a synopsis of treatment of Africanized bee stings.

Stabilization

Epinephrine (0.3 to 0.5 mL of 1:1000 epinephrine, intramuscularly) and an antihistamine (e.g., 50 mg of diphenhydramine orally or parenterally) should be given immediately because it may be difficult to distinguish systemic toxic effects from anaphylaxis when relatively small numbers of stings are sustained and because anaphylaxis and toxic effects could occur simultaneously in the venom-allergic patient. When large numbers of stings are sustained, transportation to an emergency department and treatment for the toxic effects of venom must be started immediately, even if the initial presentation is suggestive of an allergic reaction.

Supportive Therapy

Supportive therapy must be started immediately. Airway management and assurance of adequate ventilation and oxygenation are the first priorities. Aggressive fluid resuscitation may be necessary if shock is present, and increased fluid requirement will be obvious in the many patients who exhibit vomiting and diarrhea. Maintenance of adequate cardiac output and blood pressure is clearly important. Both histamine$_1$ and histamine$_2$ antagonists should be given intravenously to treat the vascular effects of histamine in bee venom, since the combination of the two types of antihistamine is more effective than either one alone.

Over the following 2 days, acute renal failure may occur due to rhabdomyolysis and myoglobinuria, hemoglobinuria, renal ischemia, or immune mechanisms. Monitoring urine output, hemoglobinuria, levels of serum electrolytes and creatinine, and urea concentration is indicated, as well as repeated urinalysis. The patient should also be tested for the presence of intravascular hemolysis and rhabdomyolysis. Maintenance of blood pressure, renal perfusion, urine output, and urine alkalinization is recommended to minimize pigment nephropathy.

Continuous electrocardiographic monitoring should be done routinely because of the possiblity of myocardial damage, arrhythmia, and hyperkalemia. Monitoring to detect disseminated intravascular coagulation and the acute respiratory distress syndrome is indicated for the early management of these complications.

If only a few stings are sustained, the stingers should be removed within 1 minute of the attack. Studies have shown that the entire contents of domestic bee venom sacs are empty within 2 minutes of the time when the stinger is embedded in the skin.

Antivenom

No specific antivenom is currently available. Persistence of circulating venom in fatal and near-fatal victims of multiple stings for many hours or days suggests that even some delay in antivenom administration would not necessarily contraindicate its potential use. The Fab or (Fab′)$_2$ digestion

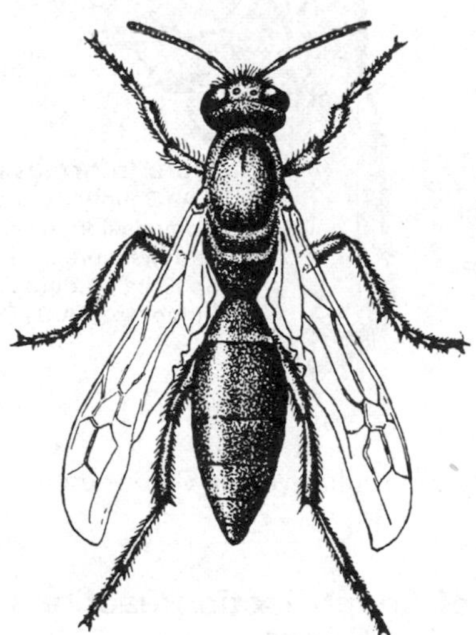

Figure 72-10 Wasp (Vespoidea). (Adapted from Frazier CA. Anaphylactic response to insect stings. Comp Ther 1976;2:68.)

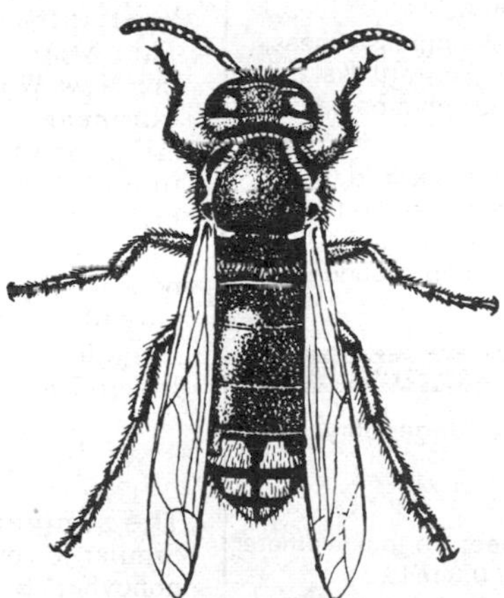

Figure 72-11 Hornet (Vespoidea). (Adapted from Frazier CA. Anaphylactic response to insect stings. Comp Ther 1976;2:68.)

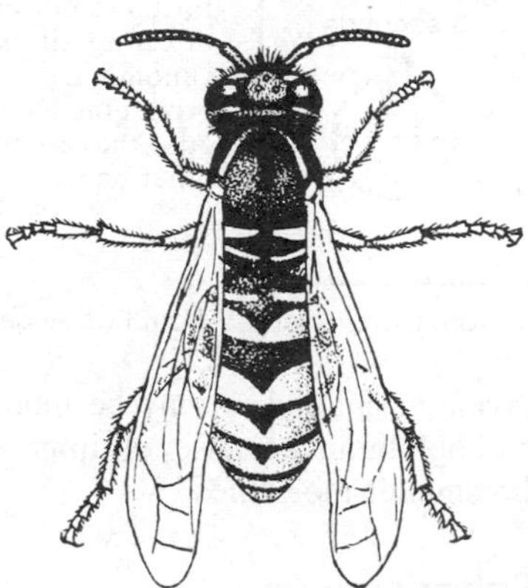

Figure 72-12 Yellow jacket (Vespoidea). (Adapted from Frazier CA. Anaphylactic response to insect stings. Comp Ther 1976;2:69.)

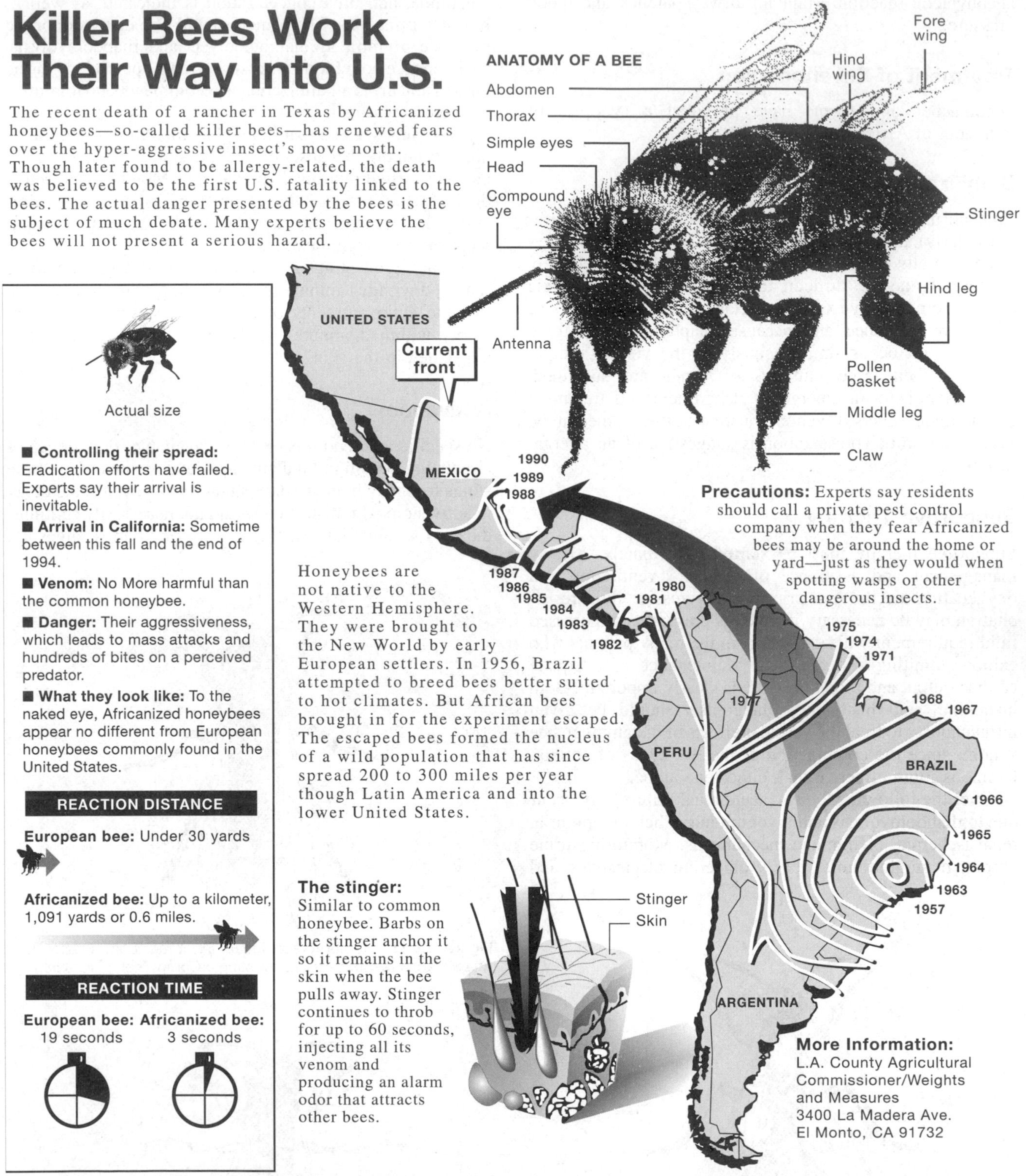

Killer Bees Work Their Way Into U.S.

The recent death of a rancher in Texas by Africanized honeybees—so-called killer bees—has renewed fears over the hyper-aggressive insect's move north. Though later found to be allergy-related, the death was believed to be the first U.S. fatality linked to the bees. The actual danger presented by the bees is the subject of much debate. Many experts believe the bees will not present a serious hazard.

Actual size

- **Controlling their spread:** Eradication efforts have failed. Experts say their arrival is inevitable.
- **Arrival in California:** Sometime between this fall and the end of 1994.
- **Venom:** No More harmful than the common honeybee.
- **Danger:** Their aggressiveness, which leads to mass attacks and hundreds of bites on a perceived predator.
- **What they look like:** To the naked eye, Africanized honeybees appear no different from European honeybees commonly found in the United States.

REACTION DISTANCE

European bee: Under 30 yards

Africanized bee: Up to a kilometer, 1,091 yards or 0.6 miles.

REACTION TIME

European bee: 19 seconds

Africanized bee: 3 seconds

ANATOMY OF A BEE

Abdomen
Thorax
Simple eyes
Head
Compound eye
Antenna
Fore wing
Hind wing
Stinger
Hind leg
Pollen basket
Middle leg
Claw

UNITED STATES
Current front
MEXICO
PERU
BRAZIL
ARGENTINA
1990 1989 1988 1987 1986 1985 1984 1983 1982 1981 1980 1977 1975 1974 1971 1968 1967 1966 1965 1964 1963 1957

Honeybees are not native to the Western Hemisphere. They were brought to the New World by early European settlers. In 1956, Brazil attempted to breed bees better suited to hot climates. But African bees brought in for the experiment escaped. The escaped bees formed the nucleus of a wild population that has since spread 200 to 300 miles per year though Latin America and into the lower United States.

Precautions: Experts say residents should call a private pest control company when they fear Africanized bees may be around the home or yard—just as they would when spotting wasps or other dangerous insects.

The stinger: Similar to common honeybee. Barbs on the stinger anchor it so it remains in the skin when the bee pulls away. Stinger continues to throb for up to 60 seconds, injecting all its venom and producing an alarm odor that attracts other bees.

Stinger
Skin

More Information:
L.A. County Agricultural Commissioner/Weights and Measures
3400 La Madera Ave.
El Monto, CA 91732

Figure 72-13 Envenomation. (Adapted from Los Angeles Times, August 11, 1993.)

fragments of antivenom antibodies may be more effective than whole immunoglobulin because of improved tissue distribution of the smaller molecules.

Elimination Enhancement

In severe cases hemodialysis should be considered not only for the treatment of renal failure but also for removal of circulating low-molecular-weight venom components such as mellitin.

Treatment of Anaphylactic Reactions to Africanized Bee Stings

If the victim of multiple stings is known to be allergic to bee stings or if severe manifestations follow a small number of stings (fewer than 50), rapid transportation to an emergency department and additional treatment for anaphylaxis is indicated. This includes the administration of one or more additional doses of epinephrine (0.01 mg/kg intramuscularly, or the same dose of epinephrine given intravenously over a 10-minute period) and the following medications given intravenously: a $histamine_1$ antagonist (e.g., diphenhydramine, 1.5 mg/kg, or chlorpheniramine, 0.3 mg/kg), a $histamine_2$ antagonist (e.g., cimetidine, 7.5 mg/kg), and corticosteroids (e.g., methylprednisolone, 50 mg, or hydrocortisone, 200 mg). Oxygen should be administered to all patients, and most will require intravenous fluids beginning with a 10- to 20-mL/kg bolus of saline. Bronchodilator aerosol therapy and/or endotracheal intubation may be necessary.

Prevention of Multiple Stings

Since Africanized bees are known to establish their colonies in wall cavities and other protected sites close to homes, it is necessary to ensure that all holes and defects in exterior walls where pipes and conduit enter above ground are properly caulked, and to maintain garages and sheds similarly. Discarded boxes, junk automobiles, and unused equipment such as old water heaters should be removed from yards, or, if possible, sealed.

A healthy adult can usually outrun attacking bees because they do not pursue for distances more than 0.25 mile. If possible, the victim should cover the mouth and nose to try to prevent airway stings. Bees continuing to attack may be killed by spraying them with soapy water.

Prevention of Anaphylaxis Caused by Africanized Bee Stings

All individuals with a history of systemic reactions to bee stings should carry an anaphylaxis emergency treatment kit that allows for two doses of epinephrine (one Ana-Kit, Miles Inc, West Haven, Conn, or two Epipen injectors, Center Laboratories, Port Washington, NY) whenever engaged in outdoor activities. Such persons should consult an allergist for venom skin testing and venom immunotherapy, even though it is unclear as to whether current bee venom immunotherapy schedules are effective in preventing toxic reactions to multiple bee stings.

For 4 to 6 weeks after an episode of multiple stings, allergic skin-test reactivity to bee venom may be found because of sensitization by the episode or from preexisting sensitivity. In the case of positive skin tests, venom immunotherapy should be considered. Although venom immunotherapy is known to reduce the risk of systemic reactions to single stings from more than 50% to less than 100%, it is not known if conventional venom immunotherapy given for 3 to 4 years would be similarly effective in preventing anaphylaxis from multiple stings.

Hornets

Multiple organ failure may terminate fatally.[5]

CLINICAL PRESENTATION

Intravascular hemolysis, respiratory distress with acute respiratory distress syndrome, hepatic dysfunction, rhabdomyolysis (with myoglobulinemia and myoglobinuria), hypertension, myocardial damage (perhaps explained by release of endogenous catecholamines by venom phospholipa A_2 and mellitin), shock, coma, acute renal failure, and bleeding have been observed. Death may intervene. Laboratory findings include gross neutrophil leukocytosis and elevated serum enzymes (AST, ALT, LDH, CPK, predominantly CPK-MM) and creatinines. There is no specific antivenoms.[6,7] Treatment is supportive and symptomatic.

JUMPER ANTS (AUSTRALIA)

Jumper ants *(Myrmecia pilosula)* are among the most primitive living ants. They display aggressive behavior and may jump 10 cm to attack victims. About 5% of humans stung by jumper ants exhibit a generalized allergic reaction, with symptoms such as swelling of the larynx, vomiting, bronchoconstriction, rash, faintness, unconsciousness, and even death.[8] Local reactions may include intense sharp pain, swelling, and severe itching. Pharmacologic studies suggest that jumper ant venom contains histamine, appears to be able to stimulate release of cyclo-oxygenase products, and includes a hemolytic heat-labile factor.[9]

Immunotherapy—Venoms

Guidelines for indications for venom immunotherapy have been proposed[10–12] (Tables 72-21 and 72-22).

Table 72-21
Indications for Venom Immunotherapy in Patients with Positive Venom Skin Tests [a,b]

Reaction to Insect Sting	Venom Immunotherapy
Anaphylaxis	
Severe	Yes
Moderate	Yes
Mild, dermal only	
Children	No
Adults	Yes
Serum sickness	Probably
Toxic reaction	Possibly
Extensive local swelling	No
Normal reaction (transient pain, swelling)	No

[a]Adapted from Reisman RE. N Engl J Med 1994;331:523–527.
[b]Venom immunotherapy is not indicated for people with negative venom skin tests.

Table 72-22
Venom Immunotherapy

1. Purified venom should be used for diagnosis and treatment of Hymenoptera hypersensitivity.
2. Only persons with a history of a severe systemic reaction to Hymenoptera and demonstrated venom-specific IgE should be treated with venom immunotherapy.
3. Children who experience only cutaneous sting reactions are not candidates for venom immunotherapy.
4. Venom immunotherapy is not indicated for the treatment of large local reactions or non-IgE-mediated reactions.

FIRE ANTS *(SOLENOPSIS INVECTA)*

Anaphylaxis occurs in about 4% of bites. The bites may be fatal. Almost all persons stung by imported fire ants have a wheal-and-flare reaction at the site of the sting. This resolves in 30 minutes to an hour and evolves into a sterile pustule at the site of the sting within 24 hours.[13] Life-threatening systemic reactions may occur (apnea, asystole, shock, metabolic acidosis, coagulopathy, no evidence of cerebral function).

Fire ants are abundant in the southern United States and are increasingly found on corpses in both urban and rural settings making determination of postmortem intervals difficult.[14] An enzyme-linked immunosorbent assay (ELISA) has been developed for in vitro measurement of IgE specific for *Solenopsis invecta* venom.[15]

Imported fire ant–whole body extract (IFA-WBE) in one controlled study appeared effective in decreasing the incidence of anaphylaxis during subsequent field stings, reducing specific immunoglobulin E as demonstrated by skin testing, and protecting against systemic reactions provoked by a sting challenge with a single IFA.[16] Chemicals used to control fire ants around homes are listed in Table 72-23.[17]

Administration

Venom immunotherapy is probably unnecessary for children whose reaction to insect stings has been limited to the skin.[18]

Large local reactions that may develop in individuals stung by bees, wasps, hornets, yellow jackets, and fire ants may not require immunotherapy since such responses have not been proven to predispose patients to systemic allergic reactions.[19]

Pregnancy

Venom immunotherapy in the Hymenoptera-allergic pregnant patient receiving immunotherapy to venoms has not been associated with any significant increase in abortions and malformations.[20] The number of venoms administered did not appear to affect the outcome.[18]

Preventive Measures

1. First-aid kits containing epinephrine should be prescribed to patients who have sustained prior systemic reactions and perhaps to those with large local reactions.[21] EpiPen and EpiPen JR are designed for self-administration of 0.3 and 0.15 mg, respectively, of epinephrine subcutaneously and may be kept in the home, car, or personal belongings.
2. A warning bracelet or tag should be worn.
3. Hymenoptera nests in areas around the living space of the sensitized patient should be destroyed.
4. Sensitized individuals should keep their feet covered outdoors.
5. Bright, flowered clothing and attractive scents, soaps, and shampoos should be avoided.
6. Tight rather than floppy clothing should be worn.
7. Light-colored, long-sleeved clothing should be worn, especially for working with plants.
8. Materials or plants that attract Hymenoptera (e.g., clover, dandelions, uncovered sweet drinks) should be reduced.
9. Hymenoptera should not be swatted when encountered. Slow retreat or standing still is recommended. If the hymenopteran lands on skin, it should be quickly brushed off.

Table 72–23
Spider Bites

	Loxosceles	*Latrodectus*
Marking	Violin	Hourglass
Pairs of eyes of face	3	4
Bite symptoms lag period	2–8 hours	10–20 minutes
Necrotic	+	–
Laboratory tests diagnostic	–	– Oliguria, high specific gravity, albuminuria, Increased CPK, blood sugar, eosinophils
Lymphocyte blast transformation	+	–
Signs and symptoms	Confined to bite site Erythema –> violaceous –> blue macula –> eschar –> ulcer	Systemic: chest, abdomen, lumbar region, lower extremities, BP elevated
Eschar—ulcer	+	–
Systemic effects	24–72 hours after bite	Early, within hours
Hematuria	+	–
Hemoglobinuria	+	–
Hemolysis	+	–
WBC elevation	+	+
Fibrin degradation products	+	+
Corticosteroids/ antibiotics	–	–
for skin lesions	–	–
Steroids for hemolysis	+	–
Antivenin	–	+
Dapsone	+	–

LEPIDOPTERA

The most common stinging caterpillar is the puss caterpillar *Megalopyge opercularis),* also the "woolly slug." In various regions of the United States and Mexico it is also known as the "tree asp," "Italian asp," "nasty worm," "opossum bug," "el perrito" (little dog), and "Bicho peludo negro" (black hairy bug).[22]

Clinical Presentation

Hairs act as primary skin irritants and produce a characteristic pruritic erythematous lesion at the contact site. The chitinous spines are capable of penetrating the human epidermis and causing contact urticaria.[23] The term erucism refers to urtication by Lepidoptera larvae.[24]

Responses may include muscle spasms, paresthesias and dizziness, diaphoresis, nausea, abdominal pain, radiating pain to an extremity, joint stiffness, and lymphadenopathy.[25,26]

Treatment

Supportive care includes immobilization and elevation of the involved extremity, tetanus prophylaxis, inspection for broken off spines, early application of ice, morphine sulfate, meperidine or codeine for pain, and IV calcium gluconate (10 milliliters of 10% solution). Epinephrine 1 : 1000 administered subcutaneously may be useful if the patient presents with a shocklike syndrome.[20]

CHILOPODA (CENTIPEDES)

Clinical Presentation

An Australian 6-month-old apparently ingested a centipede identified as the species *Scutigera morpha,* following which he became pale and lethargic with a marked generalized hypotonia. Reflexes and tests of sensation were normal. He vomited a few times and slowly improved over the next 48 hours with no specific treatment.[27]

ARACHNIDA—SPIDERS (TABLES 72-23 AND 72-24)

HABITATS/CHARACTERISTICS

All except two of 20,000 American spider species are venomous, but only about 50 species have fangs capable of penetrating the human skin. Spiders are ubiquitous and are found in concentrations of up to two million per acre of grassland. They generally live for 1 to 2 years. Anatomically, the spider consists of cephalothorax (fused head and chest) and an abdomen, with four pairs of legs protruding from the thorax as opposed to Hymenoptera (i.e., ants, bees, wasps), which have six legs. Spiders depend primarily on a sense of touch, since they are extremely shortsighted. Two clawlike fangs, the celicerea, protrude from the head and are connected to venomous glands believed to be under voluntary control. Spiders molt 5 to 10 times before maturity. During this period they shed their hard shells and may change coloration or markings. Although their venom is more potent than pit viper venom, small quantities and weak injection mechanisms limit seriously venomous spiders to two genera (*Latrodectus* and *Loxosceles*).

LOXOSCELES (BROWN RECLUSE) (FIG. 72-14)

Classification

Loxosceles (Brown Recluse Spiders)

Clinical problems range from mild local necrosis to rare hemolysis, coagulopathy, and death.

Latrodectus (Widow Spiders)

The venom is primarily neurotoxic, producing little local tissue reaction.

Table 72-25 lists the genera and distribution of spiders known to inflict clinically significant bites on humans.

Necrosis-Inducing Spiders

At least four species, excluding *Loxosceles* species, indigenous to the United States are capable of producing necrotic lesions.[28] Other species (e.g., *Atrax, Pamphobeteus*) not indigenous to the United States are capable of causing local necrosis and may enter by ship or airplane cargo.[29]

Phidippus

The jumping spider is probably the most common cause of necrotic arachnidism and is characterized by short legs, white stripes, and fluorescent green mouth parts. A bite produces a sharp, painful site that may develop into urticarial swelling and pruritus lasting several days.[30]

Golden Orb Weaver or Running Spider *(Chiracanthium)*[31]

Envenomation produces urticarial and necrotic lesions; in one reported case envenomation caused pain without inflammation.[32]

Black and Yellow Garden Spider *(Argiope)* and Wolf Spider *(Lycosa)*[31]

These can inflict noticeable skin lesions on humans.

Geographic Distribution of *Loxosceles* (Brown Recluse, Fiddleback, Violin, or Brown Spider)

This rapidly expanding group currently includes 54 species and is found throughout the world. Thirteen species are indigenous to the United States.

Loxosceles reclusa

This spider is the most widely reported species and is found from the East Coast to California with the highest concentrations in the Southeast. The term brown recluse technically applies only to this species.

Loxosceles laeta

This spider is the most dangerous species. Native to South America, this species has immigrated to the United States (a colony was established in the Sierra Madre section of Los Angeles in 1969).[33] No bites from *L. laeta* have as yet been reported in the United States.

Loxosceles deserta

This less potent species, residing in the western deserts, is appropriately named the desert recluse.

Loxosceles unicolor

This species is found in California, Arizona, Nevada, Utah, and Texas.

Table 72–24
Spiders Known to Envenomate Humans[a]

Genus	Family	Common Name	Distribution
Aganippe species	Idiopidae (formerly Ctenizidae)	Trap-door spider	Australia
Araneus species	Araneidae	Orbweaver	Worldwide
Arbanitis species	Idiopidae (formerly Ctenizidae)	Trap-door spider	Australia, East Indies
Argiope species	Araneidae	Orbweaver	Worldwide
Atrax species	Hexathelidea (formerly Macrothelinae)	Funnel-web spider	Australia, Tasmania
Bothriocyrtum species	Ctenizidae	Trap-door spider	California
Chiracanthium species	Clubionidae	Running spider or sac spider	Europe, North Africa, Orient, North America
Cupiennius species	Ctenidae	Banana spider	Central and South America, West Indies
Diallomus species (formerly *Elassoctenus*)	Zoridae (formerly Ctenidae)	Zorid (formerly ctenid)	Australia
Drassodes species	Gnaphosidae	Running spider	Worldwide
Dysdera species	Dysderidae	Dysderid	Eastern Hemisphere, Americas
Filistata species	Filistatidae	Hackled-band spider	Temperate and tropical zones worldwide
Harpactirella species	Theraphosidae	Trap-door spider	South Africa
Hermeas species (formerly *Dyarcyops*)	Idiopidae (formerly Ctenizidae)	Trap-door spider	Australia, New Zealand
Heteropoda species	Sparassidae	Giant crab spider	Tropical zones worldwide
Isopoda species	Sparassidae	Giant crab spider	Australia, New Guinea, East Indies
Ixeuticus species	Desidae (formerly Amaurobiidae)	Desid (formerly amaurobiid)	New Zealand, Southern California
Lampona species	Gnaphosidae	Running spider	Australia, New Zealand
Latrodectus species	Theridiidae	Widow spider	Temperate and tropical regions worldwide
Liocranoides species	Clubionidae	Running spider	Appalachia and California
Loxosceles species	Loxoscelidae	Brown or violin spider	Americas, Africa, Europe, Australia, Pacific Islands
Lycosa species	Lycosidae	Wolf spider	Worldwide
Missulena species	Actinopodidae	Trap-door spider	Australia
Misumenoides species	Thomisidae	Crab spider	North and South America
Miturga species	Miturgidae	Running spider	Australia
Mopsus species	Salticidae	Jumping spider	Australia
Neoscona species	Araneidae	Orbweaver	Worldwide
Olios species	Sparassidae	Giant crab spider	North and South America
Pamphobeteus species	Theraphosidae	Tarantula	South America
Peucetia species	Oxyopidae	Lynx spider	Worldwide
Phidippus species	Salticidae	Jumping spider	Worldwide
Phoneutria species	Ctenidae	Hunting spider	Central and South America (has been transported to other areas)
Rheostica species (formerly *Aphonopelma*)	Theraphosidae	Tarantula	North America
Selenocosmia species	Theraphosidae	Tarantula	East Indies, India, Australia
Steatoda species (*Teutana, Asagena,* and *Lithyphantes* are now *Steatoda*)	Theridiidae	Tangleweb weaver, false black widow	Worldwide
Thiodina species	Salticidae	Jumping spider	Americas
Trechona species	Dipluridae	Funnel-web spider	Central and South America
Ummidia species	Ctenizidae	Trap-door spider	North and Central America

[a]Adapted from Russell F. Emerg Med 1986;18(11):9, 13.

Loxosceles arizonica

Arizona is home to this species.

Loxosceles rufescens

Found in the eastern United States and Texas, *L. rufescens* is a Mediterranean species.

A differential diagnosis of *Loxosceles* bites is seen in Table 72-25. Systemic loxoscelism with hemolytic anemia is a rare but potentially fatal complication of envenomation by the brown recluse spider.

Systemic Reactions

Systemic reactions occur uncommonly and do not correlate with the severity of cutaneous lesions.[34] Typically, systemic symptoms develop within 24 to 48 hours of envenomation and are characterized by fever, chills, malaise, nausea, vomiting, myalgias, hemolysis, and consumptive coagulopathy (DIC).[35–37] Coma, convulsions, and renal dysfunction are probably secondary effects. Hemolytic anemia may be insidious, often requiring 2 to 3 days to develop.

It occurs with greatest frequency in children. The evolution of cutaneous loxoscelism is depicted in Figure 72-15.[38] Dapsone, which has been advocated in the management of the local dermatonecrotic lesions associated with brown recluse spider bite, may itself cause a dose-dependent hemolytic anemia that is mild, does not appear until after 14 days of treatment, and stabilizes by the sixth week. Systemic steroids are of unproven benefit. The use of dapsone in the management of the local lesion has not been validated in a controlled clinical study and cannot be recommended for use in children.[39]

No routine laboratory tests are available to diagnose necrotic arachnidism. The white blood cell count may rise to 20,000 to 30,000 cells per cubic millimeter in the absence of secondary infection. Rarely, a consumptive coagulopathy appears with depressed levels of fibrinogen, clotting factors, and platelets, as well as increased fibrin degradation products. Renal and liver dysfunction may be seen in severe cases. Patients with systemic symptoms should receive a complete blood count, including platelets, coagulation profile (prothrombin time, partial thromboplastin time, fibrinogen level, fibrin degradation products), urinalysis, blood electrolytes, liver function tests, and serum creatinine.

A passive hemagglutinated inhibition test to diagnose brown recluse spider bite envenomation has been proposed by Barrett and colleagues.[40]

LATRODECTUS (WIDOW SPIDERS) (TABLE 72-26)

Geographic Distribution

These cosmopolitan spiders are found in all parts of the world except at ecologic extremes (highest mountains,

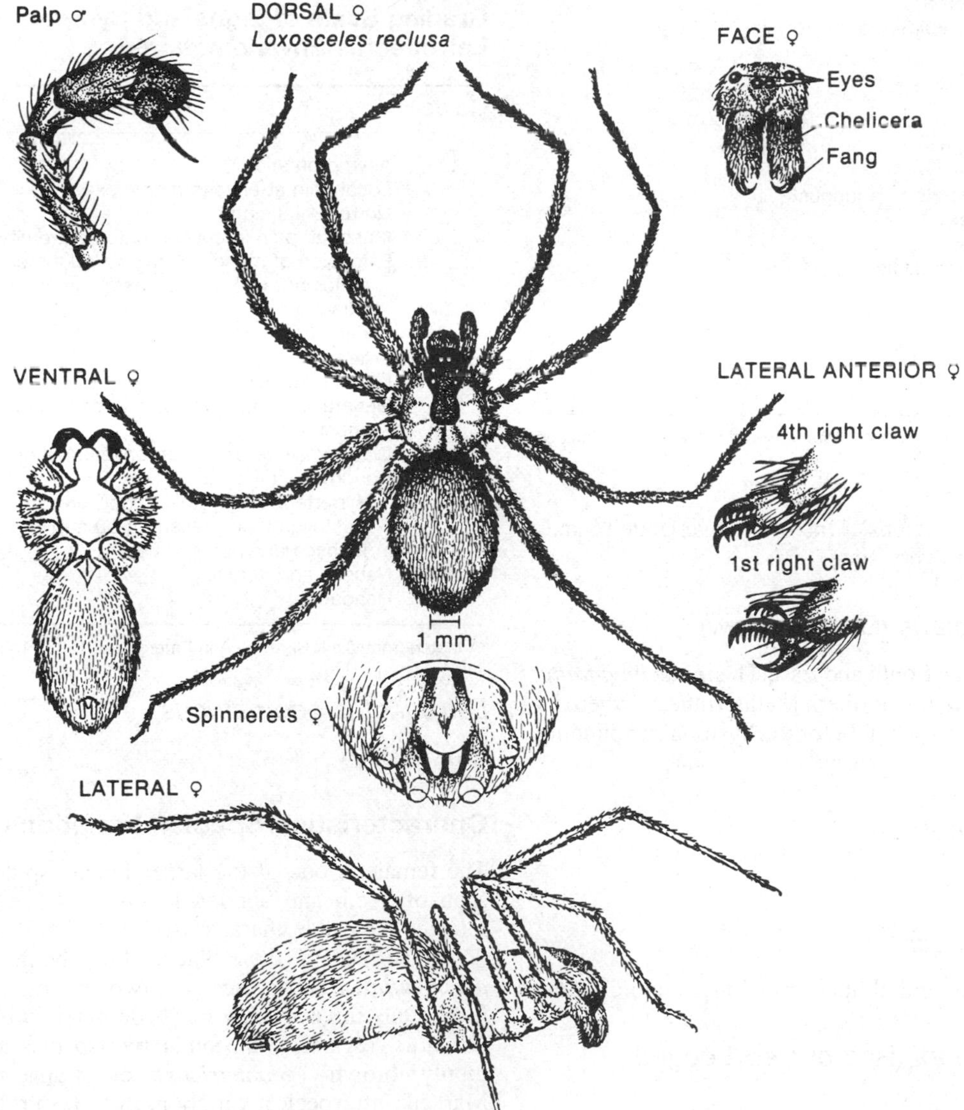

Figure 72-14 Anatomy of brown recluse spider (Loxosceles reclusa). (Adapted from Anderson PC. Necrotizing spider bites. Am Fam Physician 1982;26:199.)

Table 72-25
Differential Diagnosis of *Loxosceles* (Brown Recluse) Bites[a]

Bites of Spiders From Other Genera	Other Insects Brought in as "Spiders"/Other Lesions
Aphonopehna	Solpugids
Steatoda	Ticks (esp. *Ornithodoros coraceus*)
Araneus	Assassin bugs
Argiope	Jerusalem crickets
Heteropoda	Grasshoppers
Misumenoides	Other orthopterans
Chiracanthium	Kissing bug *(Triatoma protracta)*
Drassodes	Infected flea bites
Lycosa	Imbedded tick mouth parts
Phidippus	Mite
	Bed bug
	Fly bite
	Hymenoptera stings

Admitted Misdiagnosis of "Brown Recluse Bite"
Erythema chronicum migrans
Stevens–Johnson syndrome
Lyell's syndrome (toxic epidermal necrolysis)
Erythema nodosum
Erythema multiforme
Periarteritis nodosa
Lymphoid papulosis
Pyoderma gangrenosum
Sprotrichosis
Keratin-mediated response to a fungus
Chronic herpes simplex
Infected herpes simplex
Gonococcal arthritis–dermatitis
Purpura fulminans
Diabetic ulcer
Bed sore
Poison oak
Poison ivy

[a]Adapted from Russell FE, Gertsch WJ. Letter to the Editor. Toxicon 1983;21(3):337–339.

hottest deserts, polar regions). One of the five United States species is present in every state.

Latrodectus mactans (Black Widow)

Generally found in the South and East. The *tredecimguttatus* subspecies is native to the northern Mediterranean, where its bites probably were responsible for the hysteria surrounding the tarantula in the 17th century.[41]

Latrodectus hesperus

Western black widow.

Latrodectus variolus

Found in the eastern United States ranging up into Canada.

Latrodectus bishopi (Red or Red-Legged Widow)

Confined to small area of scrub pines in central Florida.

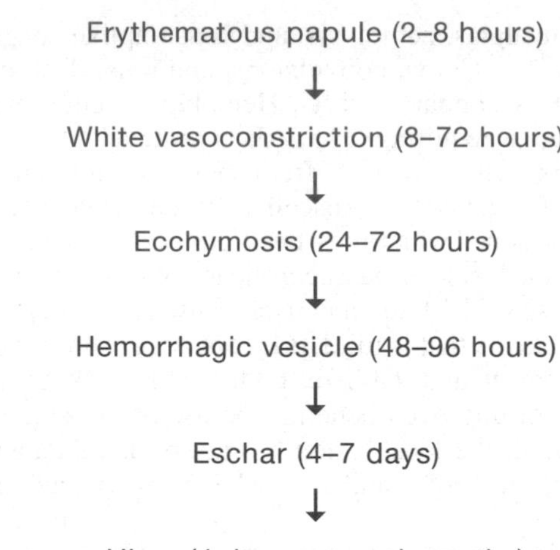

Figure 72-15 Flow diagram showing the sequential evolution of cutaneous loxoscelism. (Adapted from Walker JS, Hogan DE. Acad Emerg Med 1995;2:223–237.)

Table 72-26
Grading Scale of Signs and Symptoms Following Latrodectus Envenomations[a]

Grade	Description
1	Asymptomatic
	Local pain at envenomation site
	Normal vital signs
2	Muscular pain in envenomated extremity
	Extension of muscular pain to abdomen if envenomated on lower extremity or chest if envenomated on upper extremity
	Local diaphoresis of envenomation site or involved extremity
	Normal vital signs
3	Generalized muscular pain in back, abdomen, and chest
	Diaphoresis remote from envenomation site
	Abnormal vital signs:
	Hypertension (systolic blood pressure >140 mm Hg or diastolic blood pressure >90 mm Hg)
	Tachycardia (pulse >100)
	Nausea and vomiting
	Headache

[a]Adapted from Clark RF et al. Ann Emerg Med 1992;21:782–787.

Latrodectus geometricus

Brown widow.

Characteristics/Species Variations

The female is one of the larger female spiders, with a leg span of 5 cm and a body length of 1.5 cm. *L. mactans* females have the characteristic red hourglass spot on the dorsal surface of their black, shiny bodies, but the *tredecimguttatus* subspecies has two red marks that do not meet. Only three species are predominantly black *(mactans, hesperus, variolus);* the other two species are more commonly brown *(geometricus)* or orange-red *(bishopi)*. Marked intraspecies variation may occur as a result of molting. The black spiders become darker with less prominent red spots on each of nine moltings. In fact, black widow spiders can turn brown and then revert to the original color.[47] The male has more colorful white markings and is smaller than the female at maturity. Its smaller venom apparatus and less aggressive nature make it clinically insignificant to humans. Female widows are venomous from birth, but their venom toxicity is seasonal and is greatest in the warmer months.

Habitats

These shy, trapping spiders use their venom to paralyze entrapped prey and then suck the hemolymph. They form irregular, untidy, three-dimensional webs in dark, hidden, protected places such as crevices, ground cover, stone walls, woodpiles, barns, stables, or outdoor toilets. A period of lassitude postcopulation allows the male spider to escape unless the female has a voracious appetite. Contrary to popular belief, both females and males may be found living together. Although earlier encounters involved bites to the buttocks and genitalia during outdoor toilet use, the body part most commonly bitten now is the hand.

Clinical Presentation

Envenomation from *Latrodectus* is rarely fatal. Clark and colleagues have used a grading scale of signs and symptoms following *Latrodectus* envenomation[43] (Table 72-27). Its correlation with clinical outcome remains to be determined.

Laboratory

Leukocytosis and mildly elevated creatine kinase (CK) are common in more severe cases.[42] Albuminuria may appear, but renal dysfunction resulting from factors other than prerenal causes is uncommon.

Table 72–27
Usefulness of Scorpion Antivenins

Benefit	No Benefit	Country
	–	Israel[1]
+		Brazil[2]
+		USA[3]
		USA, Mexico[4]
	–	Israel[5]
+		Saudi Arabia[6]
+		Mexico[7]

1. Sofer S, Shaht Z, Gueron M. Scorpion envenomation and antivenom therapy. J Pediatr 1994;124:973–978.
2. Nishikawa AK, Caricat CP, Lima MLSR, Dos Santis MC, Kipnis TL, Eikstedt VRD et al. Antigenic cross-reactivity among the venoms for several species of Brazilian scorpions. Toxicon 1994;32:989–998.
3. Bond GR. Antivenin administration for Centruroides scorpion sting: risks and benefits. Ann Emerg Med 1992;21:788–791.
4. Gateau T, Bloom M, Clark R. Response to specific *Centruroides sculpturatus* antivenom in 151 cases of scorpion stings. Clin Toxicol 1994;21:165–171.
5. Gueron M, Sofer S. The role of the intensivist in the treatment of the cardiovascular manifestations of scorpion envenomation. Toxicon 1994; 32:1027–1029.
6. Ismail M. The treatment of the scorpion envenoming syndrome: The Saudi experience with serotherapy. Toxicon 1994;32:1019–1025.
7. Dehesa-Davila M, Possani LD. Scorpionism and serotherapy in Mexico. Toxicon 1994;32:1015–1016.

Treatment

Although calcium gluconate usually has been considered as first-line treatment of severe envenomation by black widow spiders, Clark and colleagues in a review of 163 cases found it ineffective for pain relief compared with a combination of IV opioids and benzodiazepines. Antivenin use may shorten the duration of symptoms in severe envenomation.[29]

Antivenin

Because of concern about anaphylaxis the use of *Latrodectus*-specific antivenom should be restricted to patients who have the most severe envenomation (small children, the elderly) and no allergic contraindications and in whom IV or IM analgesics were unsuccessful for pain relief.[29] The usual dosage is one or two vials diluted in 50 to 100 mL of saline and infused over 1 hour. Symptoms usually resolve within an hour. Antivenins have been effective as late as 30 hours after envenomation.[44] The antivenom has been used successfully in pregnant women.[45] Delayed hypersensitivity or serum sickness is infrequently observed. Death has followed its use in a patient with bronchial asthma. Symptomatic treatment with opiates and benzodiazepines should be the mainstays of therapy.[29]

Muscle spasms, pain, and elevated blood pressure may be refractory to treatment with calcium gluconate, diazepam, and methocarbamol and only temporarily decreased with meperidine. All symptoms can resolve following use of specific equine-derived *L. mactans* antivenom (Merck, Sharp and Dohme), which blocks the ability of the venom to bind to presynaptic membrane and has been useful as late as 46 hours postenvenomation.[46]

Cutaneous

Local treatment has been controversial. Some advocate early excision[47,48]; others suggest that such therapy is ineffective, expensive, and disfiguring.[49] Surgical intervention may be necessary for cosmetic purposes, especially when the lesion exceeds 4 cm at 12 hours after envenomation,[48] but successful surgical management results from allowing the necrosis to delineate and then excising it with wide margins.[50] General wound care (cleansing with bactericidal agents, tetanus prophylaxis as indicated, immobilization, elevation), serial observation, and antipruritic agents (e.g., hydroxyzine, diphenhydramine) are the mainstays of treatment. Infections are uncommon but do occur. Anecdotally, the application of heat to *Loxosceles* bites appears to worsen cutaneous symptoms.[51]

Steroids

Experiments in animals do not support a role for steroids in local treatment.

Dapsone

The use of polymorphonuclear leukocyte inhibitors such as dapsone (4,4′-diaminodiphenylsulfone) has been suggested for large violaceous lesions on the basis of laboratory data and a human case.[52]

A prospective clinical trial of dapsone treatment involving *Loxosceles* bites in 17 patients revealed that objectionable scarring developed in one patient; wound infections complicated the treatment of 5 patients.[53] Methemoglobinemia has complicated dapsone use for *Loxosceles* envenomations.[54] At this point, serious adverse effects, small scale of studies in humans, and the fact that leukocyte migration may be a secondary phenomenon limit human use of dapsone for *Loxosceles* envenomations.[55] Inadequately controlled and documented human cases, as well as the difficulty in predicting the course of the cutaneous lesions, make incisional therapy contraindicated.[29] For patients with signs of necrotic lesions, baseline hemoglobin, urinalysis, and platelet count should be followed daily together with wound observation for at least 3 days. The development of fever or dark urine should prompt an immediate follow-up by a physician.

Systemic

All patients with systemic reactions should be followed in the hospital for evidence of increasing hemolysis, coagulopathy, and renal failure. Systemic corticosteroids have not been proven effective in controlled studies (there are too few cases), but given early in doses of 1 to 2 mg/kg/d over 4 days, they may be useful. Treatment for hemolysis and coagulopathy is supportive (i.e., RBC transfusions, platelets, cryoprecipitate, fresh-frozen plasma). Urine alkalinization promotes hemoglobin excretion and may prevent renal failure. Follow fluid and electrolyte status closely and hemodialyze for renal failure. (Neither hemoglobin nor spider venom is removed by artificial means.) Effective *Loxosceles* antivenom currently is not available in the United States.

TARANTULAS (MYGALOMORPHAE)

Beginning in the 17th century, panic spread from the southern Italian city of Taranto throughout Europe concerning spider bites that caused muscle contractions and pain. The spider involved was believed to be the largest European spider, the wolf spider *Lycosa tarantula*. The name *tarantula* has limited zoologic meaning, since the term has been applied to any big spider. Such hysteria led to the development of a special dance called the tarantella, designed to protect the envenomated victim. Such concern over the tarantula persists today despite the fact that the widow spider *(Latrodectus),* not the wolf spider,[38] probably was responsible for the envenomations. The mild-mannered North American tarantula species produces a bite similar to that of a Hymenoptera sting except that systemic toxicity does not occur. Local therapy (i.e., ice packs, cleansing) is usually all the treatment necessary. Urticarial hairs on the abdomen of the tarantula may cause dermatitis and conjunctivitis on contact.

Dapsone has been used, but may result in a hemolytic anemia or methemoglobinemia. Systemic steroid use is controversial.[56]

AUSTRALIA

All deaths in Australia due to arachnids have been attributed to one of three species—the red-back spider, the Sydney funnel-web spider, and the common bush tick. In many cases the bite produces no superficial illness.

Red Back Spider *(Latrodectus mactans hasselti)*[57]

Geographic Distribution

This spider is found in all states of Australia. It is related to the black widow spider of America (the male is supposedly eaten after mating) and to the katipo of New Zealand.

Habitats/Characteristics

The male is very small, too small to bite man effectively; it is considered harmless. The red-back spider is not aggressive. If disturbed, it will usually fall to the ground, curl up, and feign death. If disturbed while guarding her eggs or if cornered, a female red-back will bite the intruder with her minute but effective fangs.

Venoms

The main toxin in red-back spider venom is a protein of molecular weight 130,000 that acts at nerve endings to deplete either acetylcholine or catecholamines.

Clinical Presentation (Fig. 72-16)

Most cases of human envenomation occur in summer. At least 300 cases annually in Australia warrant use of the specific antivenom. Bites are usually on the extremities. The bite is immediately painful, and the spider is often identified. Perspiration is observed at the bite site initially and then becomes generalized. Later nausea, vomiting, and headaches occur. In very severe cases, muscle paralysis develops. Migrating joint pains are common. Abdominal pain may be a dominant feature, especially in children. Some hypertension may be seen. If untreated, the signs and symptoms may increase in severity for up to 24 hours, then, in nonfatal cases, slowly resolve over the next week. Without specific treatment, resolution of muscle weakness and spasm may require months.

Antivenom

The antivenom available from the Commonwealth Serum Laboratories (CSL) is a purified equine immunoglobulin that contains 500 units in a volume of 0.75 mL, including preservative, per ampule. This is given intramuscularly, usually within 24 hours of the bite, if definite or distressing evidence of envenomation is present. CSL recommends pretreatment with an appropriate dose of a parenteral antihistamine with full resuscitation facilities available. Adrenaline (e.g., 0.5 mg subcutaneous) is given to a patient with a known allergy to equine protein or who has received antivenom before. Some withhold the adrenaline unless the antivenom is being administered intravenously for severe envenomation, when it is diluted tenfold in Hartmann's sodium lactate solution as recommended by CSL.[58]

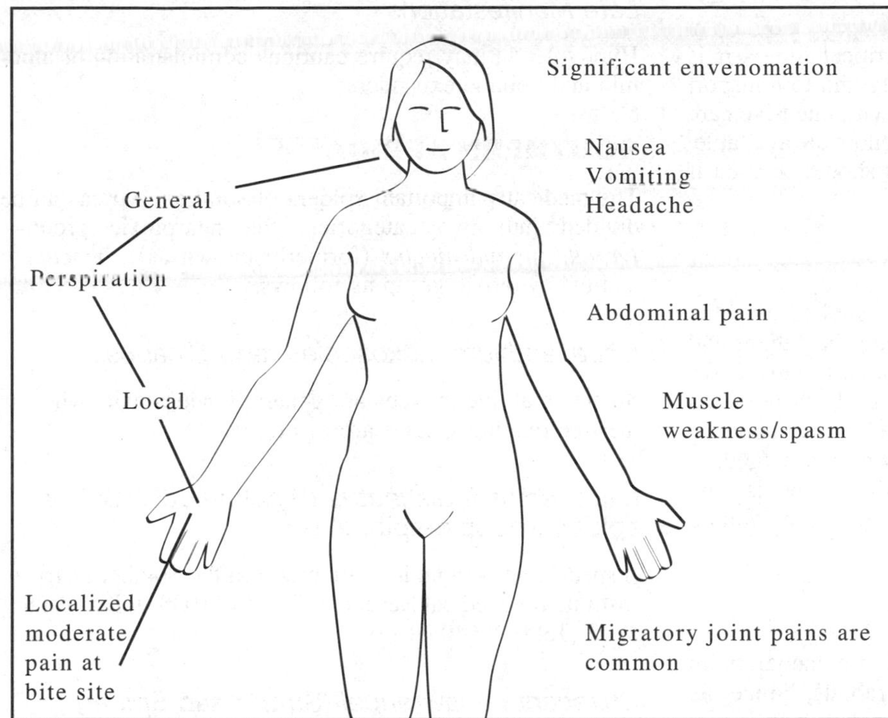

Figure 72-16 Symptoms of red-back spider bite. (Adapted from Sutherland SK. Aust Fam Physician 1990;19:1–10.)

Treatment

Envenomation is far more serious in the young, the frail, and the elderly. If the victim develops only a local reaction with no evidence of systemic envenomation after a 24-hour observation period, antivenom should not be used. All other victims should be given antivenom as directed by the leaflet enclosed with the antivenom. The antivenom is given intramuscularly. If patients have a severe envenomation, the intravenous route may be used. Patients may present up to a week after a bite with persistent symptoms and still rapidly respond to antivenom. The last death in Australia occurred in 1955. Almost 2000 bites are reported in Australia annually.[59]

Funnel-web Spiders[34,60,61]

Geographic Distribution

The funnel-web spider is found mainly in Australia, in Southern Queensland, and eastern parts of New South Wales, Victoria, and Tasmania, as well as near Adelaide.

Atrax robustus (the Sydney funnel-web spider).
Appears to be limited to an area with a radius of about 160 kilometers from Sydney.
Hadronyche formidabilis (Northern or tree-dwelling funnel-web spider).
Hadronyche versata (Blue Mountains funnel-web spider)
Hadronyche cerebera (Southern tree-dwelling funnel-web spider)

Habitats/Characteristics

Both sexes are very aggressive. When approached, they usually rear up in a position ready to strike with their massive fangs. Males tend to roam and often enter houses, particularly in summer after heavy rains.

Venom

The venom of the male spider is more toxic to animals than that of the female. Man and monkeys appear to have a special apparent effect following exposure to the venom. All recorded human deaths by funnel-webs have involved a male spider. The main component of the venom is atraxotoxin, which acts on nerve fibers, causing a release of acetylcholine at the motor endplates and of acetylcholine, adrenaline, and noradrenaline throughout the autonomic nervous system.

Clinical Presentation

There are two critical stages at which death may occur in monkeys and humans. Within 20 minutes of an injection in a limb, generalized piloerection and widespread muscle fasciculation may be seen. The fasciculations are usually seen first in the facial, tongue, or intercostal muscles. In five minutes tachycardia, severe hypertension, and coma may occur. Intracranial pressure may rise and pupils become nonreactive. Within 30 minutes muscle writhing begins and excessive sweating, salivation, and lacrimation are then evident. Apnea, hyperthermia, and cardiac arrhythmia may occur. Spasm of the jaw and laryngeal muscles may be severe. Pulmonary edema may follow. Several hours later, the hypertension, muscle twitching, salivation, and sweating subside. If the venom dose is small, consciousness may return; if the dose is large, death ensues. The last deaths due to funnel-web spider bites occurred in January 1979 and January 1980.[13] No deaths have occurred since introduction of the funnel-web spider antivenom in December 1980.

Laboratory

An elevation of plasma creatine phosphokinase and metabolic acidosis may be observed.

Treatment

Because of the rapidity of onset of a critical illness it is important to provide first aid immediately and to transport the patient to a center where monitoring with intensive care resuscitation facilities and stocks of antivenom are available. Intensive care ambulances or helicopters should be used if available.

First Aid

Firm pressure with a bandage should be applied over the bitten area. The limb is kept immobilized. The patient and the spider are transported safely the hospital. In most cases effective envenomation has not occurred. If there is no evidence after 4 hours of local muscle fasciculation or systemic envenomations, the patient can be discharged. If local muscle fasciculation is present or there is any suggestion of central movement of the venom, antivenom may be required.

Antivenom

The antivenom preparation consists of immunoglobulin (IgG) isolated from hyperimmunized rabbits. Since its release in 1980, it has been given to at least 40 patients, all of whom have rapidly recovered with no adverse reactions.

Indications for Antivenom

Urgent use should be considered if an effective bite has been made by a male specimen of *Atrax robustus* and there is clear evidence of systemic envenomation. Any of the following signs or symptoms after a bite of a male *Atrax robustus* indicates that significant envenomation has occurred: muscle fasciculation in the limb involved or remote from the bite, usually first seen in the tongue or lips when systemic spread of venom has occurred; marked salivation or lacrimation; piloerection; significant tachycardia; hypertension in a previously normotensive patient (late in the syndrome, the patient may become hypotensive); dyspnea; disorientation; confusion or depressed level of consciousness.

Administration of the Antivenin

Skin testing is not recommended. Pretreatment is usually with a nonsedating antihistamine. Minimum initial dose for a mild case is two ampules of antivenom repeated in 15 minutes if there is no improvement. Give the antivenom slowly by the intravenous route.

General Management

Additional measures that may be indicated include oxygen; atropine 0.6 mg for an adult to curtail salivation and bronchorrhea; a secure intravenous line; muscle relaxants and sedatives to facilitate mechanical ventilation and control intracranial pressure; intermittent positive-pressure ventilation (IPPV) and positive end-expiratory pressure (PEEP) for respiratory failure and intracranial hypertension; sympathetic blockage for hypertension and severe tachycardia; and maintenance of adequate mechanical respiration to correct and prevent respiratory acidosis. Vomiting is an airway and aspiration hazard.

Late Manifestations

Hypovolemia may require cautious administration of albumin and volume expanders.

SOUTHERN AFRICA[62,63]

The medically important spiders of southern Africa can be divided into two categories: the neurotoxic group—*Latrodectus indistinctus* (formerly known as *L. mactans*); and the cytotoxic group as follows:

Chiracanthium, Loxosceles, and *Sicarius*

Spiders that live in webs are generally neurotoxic, whereas the free-ranging species are cytotoxic.

Latrodectus indistinctus (Black widow, Button spider, Knoppie-spinnekop)

A specific antivenom is available from the Southern African Institute for Medical Research, PO Box 1038, Johannesburg 2000 (Tel 011 640 7130).

Chiracantum lawrencei (Strand-sac Spider)

Most victims are bitten while asleep in bed or when dressing in garments harboring the spiders. The bite is not particularly painful. The area surrounding the bite becomes edematous and painful. After 4 to 5 days the lesion ulcerates leaving a necrotic area about 10 mm across. The lesion should heal in 2 weeks. The lesion is self limiting and usually heals provided secondary infections are prevented. No antivenom is available.

Loxosceles species

Similar to *L. reclusa*. No antivenom is available in South Africa.

Sicarius species (Six-eye Crab Spider)

Found in arid and semi-arid areas. Massive tissue necrosis and a disseminated intravascular coagulation (DIC) syndrome follow its envenomation. There is no antivenom. Treatment is directed at combating secondary infections and DIC.

SOUTH AMERICA

There were 1863 spider bites reported in 1988 in Brazil. Some of the bites caused a local inflammation at the bite site followed by local necrosis. This may follow a bite by the wolf spider (*Lycosa raptoria* or *Scaptocosa raptoria*), which appear to produce a necrotizing venom. Bites usually occur on the feet and hands. Common signs and symptoms include pain, local swelling, and local erythema. Most patients have not required medical care. Antivenin administration is rarely used. Since 1985 the Butantan Institute antivenom against spider bites has not included the anti-Lycosid fraction. Adequate documentation of bites by this group of spiders is scarce.[64]

Reports of wolf spider bites in the United States *(Lycosidae)* suggest the immediate presence of sharp pain or a burning sensation and erythema. Necrosis is not described in contrast to the South American wolf spider species *(L. raptoria)*. Local applications of ice, tetanus immunization, and oral antibiotics have been recommended.[65]

Brazil

The spider *Loxosceles gaucho* is the most common species of this genus in the state of Sao Paulo, Brazil, and is responsible for the majority of accidents in that region. IgG antibodies are detected as early as 9 days and as late as 120 days after a bite.[66] Antivenin serum administered IV in a clinical study ranged from 2 to 10 vials. The diagnosis of loxascelism was supported by clinical signs such as swelling, infiltration area, erythema, ecchymosis, blister, ischemia, exanthema, and necrosis. Table 72-20 summarizes arthropod antivenom sources.[67]

SCORPIONS (FIG. 72-17)

BUTHUS TAMULUS (INDIA)

Signs of autonomic stimulation following *Buthus tamulus* envenomation in India include mild to severe pain at the sting site, local edema, cool extremities, urticaria, vomiting, profuse and diffuse sweating, priapism, parasternal lift, excessive salivation, hypertension, brady- and tachyarrhythmias, and ventricular premature contractions. Early electrocardiographic changes include peaked T waves in leads V_2 to V_6, Q waves, ST-segment elevation in leads I and AVL, and left anterior hemiblock. Pulmonary edema may develop within 2 to 3 hours after a sting with death within 3 to 4 hours.[68,69]

LEIURUS QUINQUESTRIATUS

Scorpion stings in tropical and subtropical areas with *Leiurus quinquestriatus* have been reported to induce bradycardia, tachycardia, and hypertension in children; heart failure and pulmonary edema are less frequent.[70,71] Abdominal pain, nausea, and vomiting due to an acute pancreatitis may be seen more often in older children and adults.[72] Perioral paresthesias have been described after envenomation by *Leiurus quinquestriatus.*[70]

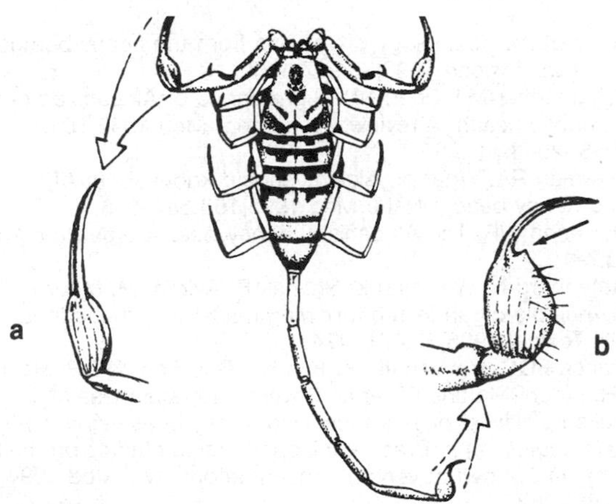

Figure 72-17 Bark scorpion *(Centruroides sculpturatus):* **(a)** enlarged chela; **(b)** enlarged vesicle showing a tubercle below the stinger. The body length, including telson, is 55 mm. (Adapted from Curry SC, Vance MV, Ryan PS et al. J Toxicol Clin Toxicol 1983–1984;21:420.)

TREATMENT

An intensive care of scorpion envenomation has been suggested by Gueron and Sofer in Israel[74]:

1. Fluid loss due to vomiting, perspiration, and increased salivation commonly complicates the clinical course. Every effort should be directed toward correcting the fluid balance; if left uncorrected such fluid loss may complicate the hemodynamic abnormalities and lead to death.
2. The presence of respiratory failure with or without CNS disturbances in the presence of hypertension or complicating those patients with pulmonary edema should be aggressively treated with early ventilation, afterload reduction, careful sedation, and acid-base balance correction.
3. Rhythm disturbances and conduction abnormalities may be observed during the initial hours after the sting, sometimes in the presence of pulmonary edema. These abnormalities are of short duration, are rarely sustained, and usually do not need a specific treatment except on the rare occasions that tachyrhythmias contribute to the hemodynamic failure.
4. The mechanism of the shock syndrome or severe hypotension has not been elucidated, as hemodynamic or noninvasive evaluations are not available. Antivenin is not effective, and every effort should be directed in supportive treatment, correction of hypovolemia, and possible invasive monitoring in the presence of pulmonary edema, CNS, or respiratory disturbances, in addition to severe hypotension.
5. In patients with pulmonary edema with or without hypertension the management should be directed to relieve the afterload without compromising the preload. Inotropic drugs such as digitalis are ineffective and the routine use of diuretics without control may be dangerous in the presence of hypovolemia.
6. Occasionally, parasympathetic effects of the venom may be present, rarely dominating the clinical picture. In these unusual situations, one should avoid the complete abolition of the parasympathetic effects, thus permitting the domination of the overstimulated sympathetic system.
7. Frequent noninvasive monitoring of the left ventricular function (systolic and diastolic) is extremely helpful in the management of scorpion envenomations.

Management of severe human scorpion envenomation should be directed toward neutralizing the overstimulated autonomic nervous system. All patients with systemic manifestations such as severe hypertension, hypovolemia, and pulmonary edema or patients in shock should be admitted to a critical care unit under close electrocardiographic, echocardiographic, and, if necessary, invasive hemodynamic monitoring. Management should include sedation, fluid replacement, and afterload reduction. Patients with respiratory failure or with CNS disturbances should be mechanically ventilated. Acid-base imbalance should be corrected. Avoid atropine, calcium antiinflammatory drugs, and steroids. Antivenin is not effective.[75] Controversy exists relating to its value.[76]

CARDIOVASCULAR MANIFESTATIONS

Scorpion venom appears to stimulate the central and autonomic nervous systems, increase circulatory catecholamines, and elevate renin-aldosterone blood levels. Treatment of the cardiovascular manifestation should include careful cardiac monitoring, correction of hypovolemia and abnormal gas exchange, and the rational use of calcium-channel blockers, angiotensin-converting enzyme inhibitors, and vasodilators. Anticholinergic drugs such as atropine are justified where required. Experience suggests that treatment should be directed against the overstimulated sympathetic nervous system, rather than specifically against the venom.[77]

AGITATION

Intravenous use of phenobarbital (5 to 10 mg/kg intravenously) in this setting may improve neurologic symptoms such as agitation or hyperactivity, but probably does not decrease the duration of symptoms. Large phenobarbital doses may depress respirations and may have contributed to the mortality and morbidity seen in earlier studies. No rational basis exists for the use of antihistamines, corticosteroids, or calcium in the treatment of nonhypersensitivity reactions to scorpion stings. Propranolol has effectively and rapidly reversed tachydysrhythmias, but has not improved other hemodynamic or neurologic parameters.[78]

BUTHUS TAMULUS

Suggested treatments in India include treatment in an intensive care unit, oral nifedipine for reduction of hypertension, and an alpha blocker (prazosin hydrocholoride) to block peripheral effects of the venom. Digoxin, aminophylline, oxygen, diuretics, and sodium nitroprusside are used as indicated. Antivenin is not used by some groups.[47] Continuous cardiopulmonary monitoring is essential.

LEIURUS QUINQUESTRIATUS

Cardiac monitoring is required as long as the patient is symptomatic. Respiratory failure may require mechanical ventilation. Excessive fluids should be avoided due to the risk of pulmonary edema. Calcium blocking agents and vasodilators may be useful in the treatment of hypertension. Hydralazine and nifedipine have been useful.[79]

A retrospective review of *Centruroides* scorpion envenomation in young children indicates a rapid resolution of symptoms in 12 patients treated with antivenom. The use of antivenom for the less severe envenomation common in older children and adults may subject them to an unjustified risk.[80]

Specific antivenom for *Centruroides sculpturatus* (not FDA approved) is available through seven laboratories worldwide (Antivenin Production Laboratory, Arizona State University, Tempe, Arizona, USA; Laboratorio "Myn," S.A., Mexico City, Mexico; Institudio Butantan, Sao Paulo, Brazil; Central Institute of Hygiene, Ankara, Turkey; Institute d'Pasteur, Algiers, Algeria; State Scientific and Vaccine Institute, Cairo, Egypt; South African Institute for Medical Research, Johannesburg, South Africa).[81]

SCORPION ANTIVENIN

Most patients who benefit from the use of scorpion antivenom (resolution of neurologic, respiratory, and cardiovascular symptoms within 1 to 3 hours) may develop rash, urticaria, or serum sickness within 2 weeks of antivenom administration. Antivenin appears to shorten the duration of respiratory failure and may prevent rhabdomyolysis. Its use carries a potential for anaphylaxis and an increased risk for a delayed reaction; therefore it should be restricted for those with more severe symptoms.[82] Usefulness of scorpion antivenoms varies between countries (Table 72-27).

PREVENTIVE MEASURES

1. Avoid contact with scorpions in an infested area, if possible.
2. As a rule, if you find one scorpion, there are others about. Females give birth to as many as 60 young and they remain close to where they are born. In the interest of safety, kill them all if you are to remain in the area.
3. Inspect boots, clothing, and bedding for scorpions.
4. Do not reach into places you cannot see.
5. Clear debris and trash from any areas you may inhabit.
6. Spraying is effective. Use a mixture of 2% chlorine, 10% DDT, and 0.2% pyrethrins in an oil base. Spray building foundations and roof complexes. Although less effective, a mix of fuel oil, kerosene, and small amounts of creosote can be used for a spray.[83]

SUGGESTED READINGS

1. Blum MS. Antivenoms: chemical and pharmacological properties. J Toxicol Toxin Rev 1992;11:115–164.
2. Sutherland SK. Antivenom use in Australia. Premedication, adverse reactions and the use of venom detection kits. Med J Aust 1992;157:734–739.
3. Warrell DA, Fenner PJ. Venomous bites and stings. Br Med Bull 1993;49:423–439.

REFERENCES—ARTHROPODS

1. Schmidt JA. Toxinology of venoms from the honey bee genus *apis*. Toxicon 1995;33:917–927.
2. Schumacher MJ, Egen NB. Significance of Africanized bees for public health. A review. Arch Intern Med 1995;155: 2038–2043.
3. Sherman RA. What physicians should know about Africanized honey bees. West J Med 1995;163:541–546.
4. McKenna WR. The Africanized honey bee. Allergy Proc 1992; 13:7–10.
5. Watenberg N, Weizman Z, Shahak E, Aviram M, Maor E. Fatal multiple organ failure following massive hornet stings. Clin Toxicol 1995;33:471–474.
6. Franca FOC, Benvenuti LA, Fan HV, Dos Santos DR, Hain SH, Picchi-Martins FR et al. Severe and fatal mass attacks by "killer" bees (Africanized honey bees—*Apis mellifera scutellata*) in Brazil: clinicopathologic studies on measurement of serum venom concentrations. Q J Med 1994; 8:269–282.
7. Tunget CL, Clark RF. Invasion of the "killer" bees. Separating fact from fiction. Postgrad Med 1993;94:92–102.
8. Sutherland SK. Venomous arthropods of medical importance, other than spiders and ichs in Australian Animal Toxins. The

Creatures, Their Toxins and Care of Poisoned Patient. Melbourne: Oxford University Press, 1983, pp. 316–326.
9. Maluszek MA, Hodgson WC, Sutherland SK, King RG. Pharmacological studies of jumper ant *(Myrmecia pilosula)* venom: evidence for the presence of histamine and haemolytic anc cicoanoid-releasing factors. Toxicon 1992;30: 1081–1091.
10. Golden DBK, Schwartz HJ. Guidelines for venom immunotherapy. J Allergy Clin Immunol 1986;77:727.
11. Warpinski JR, Buck RK. Stinging insect allergy. J Wilderness Med 1990;1:249–257.
12. Reisman RE. Insect stings. N Engl J Med 1994;331:523–527.
13. De Shazo RD, Butcher BT, Banks WA. Reactions to the stings of the imported fire ant. N Engl J Med 1990;323:462–466.
14. Hayes J. Fire ants—forensic implication and potential impact upon determination of post mortem interval. Abs G88. Proc American Academy Forensic Sci, February 14–19, 1994.
15. Ponder RD, Stafford CF, Kiefer CR, Ford JL, Thompson WO, Hoffman DR. Development of an enzyme-like immunosorbent assay for measurement of fire and venom-specific IgE. Ann Allergy 72:329–332.
16. Freeman TM, Hylander R, Ortiz A, Martin ME. Imported fire ant immunotherapy: effectiveness of whole body extracts. J Allergy Clin Immunol 1992;90:210–215.
17. De Shazo RD, Williams DF. Multiple fire ant stings indoors. South Med J 1995;88:712–715.
18. Valentine MD, Schuberth KC, Kagey-Sobotka A, Graft DF, Kurterovich KA, Szklo M, Lichtenstein LM. The value of immunotherapy with venom in children with allergy to insect stings. N Engl J Med 1990;323:1601–1603.
19. Lockey RF. Immunotherapy for allergy to insect stings. N Engl J Med 1990;323:1627–1628.
20. Herrera AM. Review of Schwartz HJ, Golden DB, Lockey RF: J Allergy Clin Immunol 1990;85:709–712. Pediatrics 1991; 87(Suppl):990.
21. Frazier CA. Emergency first aid for allergic reactions to insect bites or stings. Cutis 1977;19:770–772.
22. Pinson RT, Morgan JA. Envenomation by the pass caterpillar *(Megalopyge Opercularis)*. Ann Emerg Med 1991;20:562–564.
23. Edwards EK Jr, Edwards EK, Kowalczyk AP. Contact urticaria and allergic contact dermatitis to the saddleback caterpillar with histologic correlation. Int J Dermatol 1986;25:467.
24. Finkelstein Y, Raikhlin-Eisenkraft B, Taitelman U. Systemic manifestation of erucism: A case report. Vet Hum Toxicol 1988;30:573–574.
25. Everson GW, Chapin JB, Normann SA. Caterpillar envenomations: a prospective study of 112 cases. Vet Hum Toxicol 1988;30:368 (abstract).
26. Everson GW, Chapin JB, Normann SA. Caterpillar envenomations: a prospective study of 112 cases. Vet Hum Toxicol 1990;32:114–119.
27. Barnett PLJ. Centipede ingestion by a six-month-old infant: Toxic side effects. Pediatr Emerg Care 1991;7:229–230.
28. Anderson PC. Necrotizing spider bites. Am J Fam Pract 1982;26:198–203.
29. Wasserman GS, Anderson PC. Loxoscelism and necrotic arachnidism. J Toxicol Clin Toxicol 1983–1984;21:451–472.
30. Russell FE. Bite of the spider *Phidippus formosus:* case history. Toxicon 1970;8:193–194.
31. Gorham JR, Rheney TB. Envenomation by the spiders *Chiracanthium inclusum* and *Argiope aurantia.* JAMA 1968;206: 1958–1962.
32. Furman DP, Reeves WC. Toxic bite of a spider: *Chiracanthium inclusum* Hentz. Calif Med 1947;87:114.
33. Russell FE, Madon NB. New names for the brown recluse and the black widow. Postgrad Med 1981;70(6):31.
34. Wasserman GS, Siegel C. Loxascelism (brown recluse spider bite): a review of the literature. Clin Toxicol 1979;14:353–358.
35. Chu JY, Rush CT, O'Connor DM. Hemolytic anemia following brown spider *(Loxosceles reclusa)* bite. Clin Toxicol 1978; 12:531–534.
36. Vorse IT, Seccareccio P, Woodruff K et al. Disseminated intravascular coagulopathy following fatal brown spider bite (necrotic arachnidism). J Pediatr 1972;80:1035–1037.
37. Madrigal GC, Ercolani RL, Wenzl JE. Toxicity from a bite of the brown spider *(Loxosceles reclusus):* skin necrosis, hemolytic anemia and hemoglobinuria in a nine year old child. Clin Pediatr 1972;11:641–644.
38. Walker JS, Hogan DE. Bite to the left leg. Acad Emerg Med 1995;2:223–237.
39. Murray LM, Seger DL. Hemolytic anemia following a presumptive brown recluse spider bite. Clin Toxicol 1994; 32:451–456.
40. Barrett SM, Romine-Jenkins M, Blick KE. Passive hemoglutination inhibition test for diagnosis of brown recluse spider bite envenomation. Clin Chem 1993;3:2104–2107.
41. Rauber A. Black widow spider bites. J Toxicol Clin Toxicol 1983-1984;21:473–485.
42. Rauber AP. The case of the red widow: a review of latrodectism. Vet Hum Toxicol 1980;22(Suppl 2):39–41.
43. Clark RF, Wethern-Kestner S, Vance MV, Gerkin R. Clinical presentation and treatment of black widow spider envenomation: a review of 163 cases. Ann Emerg Med 1992; 21:782–787.
44. Schtorntham S, Roberts JR, Nilsen GJ. Dramatic clinical response to the delayed administration of black widow spider antivenom. Ann Emerg Med 1994;24:1198–1199.
45. Russell FE. Black widow spider envenomation during pregnancy: report of a case. Toxicon 1979;17:188–189.
46. Allen RC, Norris RL. Delayed use of antivenom in black widow spider *(Latrodectus mactans)* envenomation. J Wilderness Med 1991;2:181–192.
47. Arnold RE. Brown recluse spider bites: five cases with a review of the literature. JACEP 1976;5:262–264.
48. Auer AI, Hershey B. Surgery for necrotic bites of the brown spider. Arch Surg 1974;108:612–618.
49. Anderson PC. What's new in locoscelism—1978. Mo Med 1977;74(7):549–552, 556.
50. Rees R, Shack B, Withers E et al. Managment of the brown recluse spider bite. Plast Reconstruct Surg 1981;68:768–773.
51. King LE Jr. Brown recluse spider bites: Stay cool. JAMA 1985;254:2895–2896.
52. King LE, Rees RS. Dapsone treatment of a brown recluse spider. JAMA 1983;250:648.
53. Rees RS, Altenbern DP, Lynch JB et al. Brown recluse spider bites: a comparison of early surgical excision versus dapsone and delayed surgical excision. Ann Surg 1985;202:659–663.
54. Iserson KV. Methemoglobinemia from dapsone therapy for a suspected brown spider bite. J Emerg Med 1985;3:285–288.
55. Berger RS. Management of brown recluse spider bite. JAMA 1984;251:889.
56. Murray LM, Seger DC. Hemolytic anemia following a presumptive brown recluse spider bite. Clin Toxicol 1994; 32:451–456.
57. Sutherland SK. Treatment of arachnid poisoning in Australia. Aust Fam Physician 1990;19:1–10.
58. Brown AFT. Delayed diagnosis of red-back spider envenomation; a timely reminder. Med J Aust 1989;151:705–706.
59. Jelinek GA, Banham NDG, Dunjey SJ. Red-back spider bites at Freemantle Hospital, 1982–1987. Med J Aust 1989;150: 693–695.
60. Sutherland SK. Australia animal toxins. Melbourne: Oxford University Press, 1983, p. 276.
61. Duncan AW, Tibbales J, Sutherland SK. Effects of Sydney funnel-web spider envenomation in monkeys and their clinical implications. Med J Aust 1980;2:429–435.
62. Newland G, Atkinson P. Review of Southern African spiders of medical importance with notes on the signs and symptoms of envenomation. S Afr Med J 1988;73:235–239.
63. Newland G, Atkinson P. Behavioural and epidemiological considerations pertaining to necrotic arachnidism in Southern Africa. S Afr Med J 1990;77:92–95.
64. Ribeiro LA, Jorge MT, Presco PV, Nishioka SdA. Wolf spider bites in Sao Paulo, Brazil: a clinical and epidemiological study of 515 cases. Toxicon 1990;28:715–717.
65. Campbell DS, Rees RS, King LE. Wolf spider bites. Cutis 1987;39:113–114.

66. Barbaro KC, Cardoso JLC, Eikstedt VRD, Mota I. IgG antibodies to *Loxosceles* sp. spider venom in human envenomation. Toxicon 1992;30:1117–1121.
67. Theakston RDG, Warrell DA. Antivenoms: a list of hyperimmune sera currently available for the treatment of envenoming by bites and stings. Toxicon 1991;29(12):1419–1470.
68. Bawaskar HS, Bawaskar PH. Scorpion sting: a review of 121 cases. J Wilderness Med 1991;2:164–174.
69. Krishna Murthy KR, Zolfagharian H, Medh JD, Kadalkar JA, Yeolekar ME, Sandit SP et al. Disseminated intravascular coagulation and disturbances in carbohydrate and at metabolism in acute myocarditis produced by scorpion *(Buthotus tamulus)* venom. Indian J Med Res 1988;87:318–325.
70. Sofer S, Shahak E, Slonim A, Gueron M. Myocardial injury without heart failure following envenomation by the scorpion *Leiurus quinquestriatus* in children. Toxicon 1991;29:382–385.
71. Sofer S, Gueron M. Respiratory failure in children following envenomation by the scorpion *Leiurus quinquestriatus:* Hemodynamic and neurological aspects. Toxicon 1988;26: 931–939.
72. Sofer S, Shaler H, Weizman Z, Shahak E, Gueron M. Acute pancreatitis in children following envenomation by the yellow scorpion *Leiurus quinquestriatus.* Toxicon 1991;29:125–128.
73. Bogomolksi-Yahalom V, Amitai Y, Stalnikowicz R. Paresthesia in envenomation by the scorpion *Leiurus quinquestriatus.* Clin Toxicol 1995;33:79–82.
74. Gueron M, Sofer S. The role of the intensivist in the treatment of the cardiovascular manifestations of scorpion envenomation. Toxicon 1994;32:1027–1029.
75. Gueron M, Margulic G, Ilia R, Sofen S. The management of scorpion envenomation. Toxicon 1993;31:1071–1083.
76. Ismail M. Serotherapy of the scorpion envenoming syndrome is irrationally convicted without trial. Toxicon 1993;31:1077–1083.
77. Gueron M, Sofer S. Scorpion envenomation and the heart. J Wilderness Med 1991;2:175–177.
78. Rachesky IJ, Banner W, Dansky J et al. Treatments for *Centruroides exilicauda* envenomation. Am J Dis Child 1984; 138:1136–1139.
79. Sofer S. Gueron M. Vasodilators and hypertensive encephalopathy following scorpion envenomation in children. Chest 1991;97:118–120.
80. Bond GR. Antivenin administration for *Centruroides* scorpion sting: risks and benefits. Ann Emerg Med 1992;21:788–791.
81. Binder LS. Acute arthropod envenomation. Incidence, clinical features and management. Med Toxicol Adverse Drug Exp 1989;4:163–173.
82. Bond GR. Antivenin administration for *Centruroides* scorpion sting—risks, benefits. Vet Hum Toxicol 1990;32:367.
83. Baker MS, Strunk HK. Medical aspects of Persian Gulf operations. Environmental hazards. Mil Med 1991;156:381–385.

MARINE ANIMALS

An approach to the emergency management of a marine envenomation has been suggested by Auerbach[1] (Fig. 72-18). Treatment of marine vertebrates and invertebrates has been summarized by McGoldrick and Marx (Tables 72-28 and 72-29).[2,3] Table 72-30 summarizes some antivenoms available for marine venoms.

COELENTERATES

Contact with coelenterates accounts for most marine envenomations. Coelenterates, a group of invertebrates, compromise more than 9000 species, of which approximately 100, belonging to the phylum Cnidaria, are recognized as venomous. The Cnidaria are subdivided into three classes: Hydrozoa, for example, Portuguese man-of-war; Schiphozoa, for example, jellyfish and sea nettle; and Anthozoa, for example, sea anemone and corals. Cnidaria inflict their stings with organelles, called nematocysts, located in their epithelial tissues.

SEA BATHERS' ERUPTION

Sea bathers' eruption ("sea lice") has been reported predominantly in the Florida Keys. It is an intensely pruritic, vesicular or maculopapular eruption primarily affecting skin surfaces covered by swimwear.[14] Symptoms begin within 24 hours of ocean exposure, last for 3 to 5 days, and usually resolve spontaneously. Outbreaks occur intermittently between March and August, but peak during early April through early July.[2,5] The eruption is probably caused by the larvae of *Linuche unguiculata* ("thimble jellyfish"). Treatment has included antihistamines and antipruritic agents. Topical steroids may be used. All treatment may be disappointing in severe cases. Topical agents (isopropyl alcohol, vinegar, papain, baking soda, aluminum sulfate/surfactant) are unlikely to be effective in neutralizing venoms after a sting has occurred. Changing swimwear and showering are probably effective in preventing stings.[6]

Documented fatalities have occurred from the Atlantic species, but death after a Pacific *Physalia* sting is not yet known. A scuba diver was a victim in one of the fatalities when stung by the multitentacled Atlantic *Physalia.* By contrast, the single-tantacled *Physalia*—typified by the familiar Australian bluebottle—inflicts what may be the world's most common, nonserious jellyfish sting, a painful, "beaded" urticarial cutaneous eruption.[7]

ATLANTIC PORTUGUESE MAN-OF-WAR *(PHYSALIA PHYSALIA)*

Its habitat includes the Atlantic Ocean and Caribbean Sea. The gastric cavity is 5 to 10 cm in diameter, similar to the Pacific variety, but the tentacles are longer and more numerous.

PACIFIC PORTUGUESE MAN-OF-WAR *(PHYSALIA URTRICULUS)*

This smaller version of the Atlantic variety is distributed across the Pacific and Indian oceans. Another common name is the bluebottle. The body rarely grows larger than 8 to 10 cm in diameter, and the tentacles seldom reach 30 m.

A woman emerged from the ocean with a Portuguese man-of-war wrapped about both arms. She became comatose, developed electrocardiographic evidence of myocardial ischemia, and died after 5 days of ventilator support.[8]

SCYPHOZOA—BOX JELLYFISH *(CHIRONEX FLECKERI)*

The box jellyfish is also known as "box jelly," "cubomedusan," "cubo," "fire medusa," "indringa," "sea-stinger."[9] It is the only known stinging coelenterate that is lethal to humans. It can be very difficult to see a box jellyfish in the water under natural conditions. Their relative transparency makes them almost invisible, except to trained spotters, even in clear sunlit seawater.[8,10]

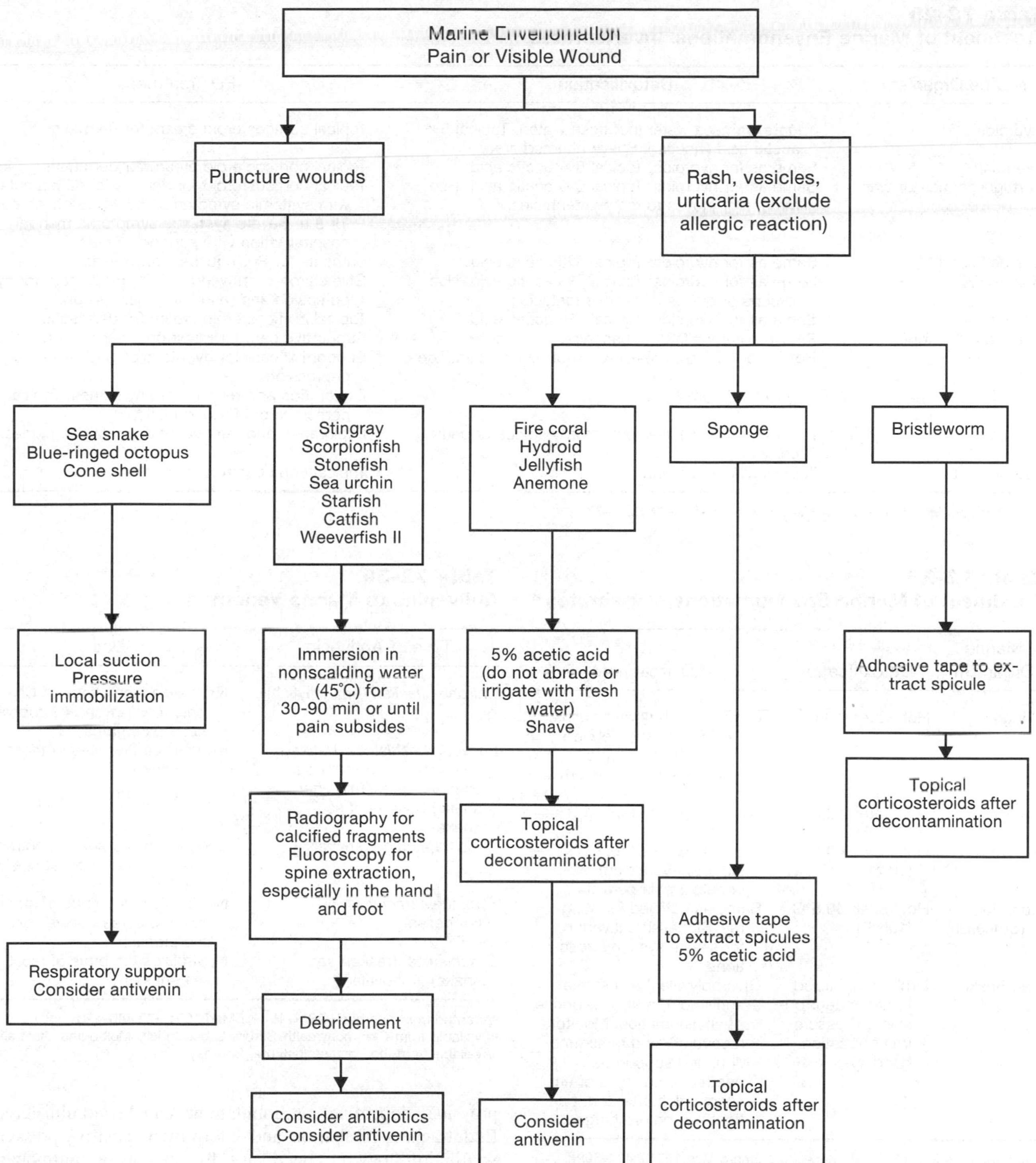

Figure 72-18 Approach to emergency management of marine envenomation. (Adapted from Auerbach PS. N Engl J Med 1991;325:486–493.)

HABITATS/CHARACTERISTICS

Species are ubiquitous throughout United States coastal waters (e.g., *Chrysaora cyanae).* The sea nettle *(Chrysaora quinquecirrha)* found near Chesapeake Bay and North Carolina sounds, especially in late summer, is one of the most common and best studied species. An estimated 500,000 annual jellyfish envenomations occur in the Chesapeake Bay and 60 to 200,000 in Florida. The presence of *Physalia physalia* (Portuguese man-of-war) is very unusual in Maryland waters.[11]

CLINICAL PRESENTATION (TABLE 72-31)

Rapidly developing acute pulmonary edema in previously healthy adults may follow envenomation by a jellyfish,

Table 72–28
Treatment of Marine Envenomations: Invertebrates [a]

Marine Organism	Detoxification	ED Treatment
Hydroids	Irrigate with sea water (not fresh water). Topical 5% acetic acid (vinegar). Shave affected area.	Topical corticosteroid cream for dermatitis.
Fire coral	Same as for hydroids. Topical 5% acetic acid.	Topical corticosteroid cream for dermatitis.
Portuguese man-of-war	Same as for hydroids. Topical 5% acetic acid. Use forceps or gloves to remove tentacles.	Topical corticosteroid for dermatitis. All patients with systemic symptoms should be observed for 8 h. Severe systemic symptoms mandate hospitalization with supportive care.
Sea nettles	Same as for hydroids. Topical 5% acetic acid.	Same as for Portuguese man-of-war.
Box jellyfish	Same as for hydroids. Topical 5% acetic acid. Use forceps or gloves to remove tentacles.	Give chironex antivenom. Supportive care for hypotension and respiratory depression.
Anenomes	Same as for hydroids. Topical 5% acetic acid.	Topical corticosteroid cream for dermatitis.
Blue-ringed octopus	Pressure immobilization bandage.	Supportive care for respiratory depression.
Cone shell	Hot water (105°F). Pressure immobilization bandage.	Supportive care for hypotension and respiratory depression.
Starfish	Irrigation with fresh water.	Exploration and removal of any spines. Topical corticosteroid for dermatitis.
Sea urchin	Hot water (105°F). Removal of any spines or pedicellariae.	Exploration and removal of any retained spines.
Sea cucumber	Topical 5% acetic acid.	Topical corticosteroid for dermatitis.

[a]Adapted from McGoldrick J, Marx JA. J Emerg Med 1992;10:71–77.

Table 72–29
Treatment of Marine Envenomations: Vertebrates [a]

Marine Organism	Detoxification	ED Treatment
Stingray	Hot water (105°F)	Irrigation with normal saline. Exploration and debridement. Observation for 3–4 h to rule out systemic envenomation.
Catfish	Hot water, 40.5°C (105°F)	Same as outlined for stingray.
Weeverfish	Hot water, 40.5°C (105°F)	Same as outlined for stingray. IV calcium gluconate if pain persists.
Scorpionfish (Stonefish)	Hot water, 40.5°C (105°F)	Same as outlined for stingray. Stonefish antivenom for severe systemic reactions.
Sea Snake	Limb immobilized in dependent position. Pressure immobilization bandage.	Give polyvalent sea snake antivenom for any evidence of envenomation. Monitor respiratory and renal function, and support as needed. If no signs of envenomation after 8 h, patient can be discharged.

[a]Adapted from McGoldrick J, Marx JA. J Emerg Med 1991;9:497–502.

Table 72–30
Antivenins to Marine Venoms [a]

Type of Antivenin	Use
Chironex fleckeri (box-jellyfish)[b]	Neutralizes the stings of *Chironex fleckeri* and *Chiropsalmus quadrigatus*
Enhydrina schistosa (beaked sea snake) and *Notechis scutatus* (terrestrial tiger snake) polyvalent sea snake[b]	Neutralizes the bites of most sea snakes
N. scutatus (tiger snake)[b]	Second-choice agent; neutralizes the bites of most sea snakes
Synanceja trachynis (stonefish) [b]	Neutralizes the stings of stonefish and some species of scorpionfish
E. schistosa (beaked sea snake) monovalent[c]	Neutralizes the bites of most sea snakes

[a]Adapted from Auerbach PS. N Engl J Med 1991;325:486–493.
[b]Available from Commonwealth Serum Laboratories, Melbourne, Australia.
[c]Available from the Haffkine Institute, Bombay, India.

probably *Carukia barnesi.* This has been referred to as the "Irukandji syndrome." The clinical picture presents many features of unchecked catecholamine release. Treatment may require large doses of meperidine or morphine for pain, phentolamine 5 mg slowly IV followed by 10 mg IV repeated when necessary for treatment of hypertension, shaking, and sweating and symptomatic management of pulmonary edema or cardiopulmonary complications with IV diuretics, opiates, or sublingual nitrites; Swan-Ganz right heart catheterization to monitor pressure so that IV nitroprusside, dopamine, or dobutamine can be administered. Endotracheal intubation and intermittent positive-pressure ventilation may be necessary for increasing pulmonary edema not responding to the above therapy, or if the pulmonary edema is noncardiogenic.[12]

TREATMENT (TABLE 72-32)[13]

Measures similar to those described for the Portuguese man-of-war are effective. A sheep antivenom is available (from Commonwealth Serum Laboratories, Melbourne, Australia) and should be given intravenously as one vial (20,000 units) in all serous envenomations. Fluids, vasopressors, and antidysrhythmic agents may be required in severe envenomations.

Anaphylaxis from jellyfish envenomations should be treated by maintaining the airway and cardiovascular system. Insert an intravenous line. Give epinephrine as required. Verapamil may be useful for arrhythmias.[14]

Use of verapamil in mice after intravenous challenge with box jellyfish venom suggests that calcium antagonists may be useful in the acute treatment of box jellyfish stings.[13,15] Analgesics may be required. Current first-aid advice is to douse the sting area with at least 2 liters of vinegar. When vinegar is not available, the rescuers should pick off any adherent tentacles with their fingers (there is little danger of significant stinging through the thicker keratin of the rescuers' fingers) before the application of compression, immobilizing bandages. Vinegar saturation of the bandage-covered sting area should be carried out at the earliest opportunity. A specific box jellyfish antivenom directed against box jellyfish envenomations (Commonwealth Serum Laboratories, Melbourne, Australia), e.g., in doses of 3 ampules (60,000 units with a total volume of 8.2 mL), is injected intramuscularly into the anterior thigh of the patient above the compression bandages. Beneficial effects appear maximal when the antivenom is given within 4 to 6 hours after a serious *Chironex* envenomation.[16]

Chiropsalmus quadrumanus envenomation has rarely led to fatalities with cardiac shock, hypotension, and acute pulmonary edema.[17] Studies of peripheral monocytes from a patient exposed to crude sea nettle venom suggest evidence of induced immunosuppressive activity.[18]

Solutions of 3% to 10% acetic acid (in vinegar) have been shown to rapidly inactivate the penetrating nematocysts of *Chironex fleckeri*.[19] Willis Wingert[20] suggests that many local agents have been recommended in treatment of cnidarian stings. Some remedies have a theoretical effectiveness. The following procedure appears to be most beneficial:

1. Remove any adhering tentacles *carefully*. Tactile pressure may cause additional nematocyst discharge.
2. Inactivate the unexploded nematocysts by topical application for at least 30 minutes of any of the following solutions:
   a. Vinegar (3 to 5% acetic acid). Altering pH below 6.0 may inactivate the venom.
   b. A slurry (50% w/u) of baking soda. This chemical raises local pH above 8 and dissolves tentacular material.
   c. Aluminum subacetate 10 to 20% solution (Burow's solution). The aluminum ion denatures protein components of the venom. The solution is highly effective when combined with 5% detergent (2 tsps liquid detergent per pint of Stingase).
   d. Meat tenderizer contains papain. This may be beneficial because of the protein-denaturing trypsin-like activity, but the results are inconsistent and high concentrations cause skin peeling.
3. Apply dry baking soda, flour, sand, or shaving soap to the area.

Table 72–31
Jellyfish Envenomations[a]

Local reactions
- Toxin-induced
- Exaggerated local reaction (angioedema)
- Recurrent reactions up to four episodes
- Delayed persistent reactions up to several months
- Distant site reactions
- Contact dermatitis
- Papular urticaria up to one month

Long-term reactions
- Keloids
- Pigmentation
- Fatty atrophy
- Contractions
- Gangrene
- Vascular spasm
- Mercuritis
- Autonomic nerve paralysis
- Ataxia

Postepisode dermatitis
- Herpes simplex
- Granuloma annulare

Reactions from jellyfish ingestion
- Gastrointestinal symptoms
- Urticaria

Systemic reactions
- Toxin-induced
- Irukanji syndrome
- Respiratory acidosis

Fatal reactions
- Toxin-induced
  - Immediate cardiac arrest
  - Rapid respiratory arrest
  - Delayed renal failure
- Anaphylaxis

[a]Adapted from Burnett JW, Calton GJ. Ann Emerg Med 1987;16:1000–1005.

Table 72–32
Treatment of *Chironex* Stings[a]

First aid

Retrieve the victim from the water if necessary (children) or restrain if necessary (adults)

Send others for an ambulance/medical help and antivenom

Assess the conscious state and treat airway, breathing, and circulation if necessary

Liberally pour vinegar over the stung area for a minimum of 30 seconds to inactivate remaining stinging cells on any adherent tentacles

Apply compression bandages to major stings (one covering an area greater than 50% of one limb or one causing impairment of conscious state)

Remain with the victim, treating with cardiopulmonary resuscitation if necessary

Hospital treatment

Continue treating airway, breathing, and circulation if necessary. Add oxygen if available

Secure an intravenous line with a crystalloid solution running, and administer a minimum of one ampoule of antivenom (20,000 units slowly by the intravenous route) if none has been given. Up to three ampoules may be used if the sting is severe, or if the response to a lesser amount of antivenom is not sufficient clinically

Monitor breathing and circulation, and give verapamil (5 mg) by the intravenous route for any cardiac abnormality (arrhythmia and/or hypotension) which persists in spite of antivenom therapy

Intravenously administered analgesia (1–2 mg/kg of pethidine [50 mg for an adult patient]) whenever necessary in conscious patients

[a]Adapted from Fenner PJ et al. Med J Aust 1989;151:708–710.

4. Scrape remaining nematocysts from the wound with a sharp instrument such as a knife. Do not use a razor.
5. Wash the area with sea (salt) water.
6. Apply a steroid cream or lotion (i.e., triamcinolone 0.1%).
7. If ulcerating lesions develop, clean the area daily with Burow's solution and cover with dry dressings.
8. Administer appropriate tetanus prophylaxis.
9. If severe systemic symptoms develop, oxygen and intravenous fluids may be required. Severe pain should be controlled with intramuscular codeine or meperidine (Demerol). Calcium gluconate (10%) intravenously may relieve painful muscle spasms.

ECHINODERMATA[20]

Animals:

This phylum includes sea urchins, starfish, and sea cucumbers. Of 6000 species, 80 are venomous to man. The toxins vary in chemistry and modes of action. Actions in experimental animals include erythrocyte hemolysis, heart block, hypotension, neuromuscular blockage, and release of histamine.

The globular body of sea urchins is covered with calcareous spines of many sizes and shapes, some of which contain poison glands. Between the spines are small pincerlike organs called pedicellariae, which also serve as venom organs. Traumatic injury by penetration of the spines may occur without envenomation.

Symptoms

Stepping on a sea urchin may result in a puncture wound, and the brittle spine may break and remain embedded in the wound. A foreign-body reaction, pain, and secondary infection may follow. If the spine is left in situ, a granuloma forms or the spine may be absorbed within 48 hours. Surgical removal may be required. Hot candle wax applied to the affected area can lead to diminution of pain.[21]

Treatment (Method of Willis Wingert)[20]

Mild echinoderm stings may be treated by washing the area and applying steroid ointment. The spines may be demonstrated on x-ray. Therefore the extremity should be examined radiologically and broken spines removed surgically as soon as possible before there is migration into deeper tissues. Severe poisoning may require cardiopulmonary support as indicated until the venom is metabolized. No antidotes are currently available.

ANTHOZOA

Sea Anemones

Contact with coelenterates accounts for most marine envenomations. Coelenterates are a group of invertebrates comprising more than 9000 species of which about 100, belonging to the phylum Cnidaria are venomous. The Cnidaria are divided into three classes: Hydrozoa (e.g., Portuguese man-of-war); Schiphozoa (e.g., jellyfish and sea nettle); and Anthozoa (e.g., sea anemone and corals). Sea anemone sting may induce fulminant hepatic failure.[22]

Irukandji Reaction

An irukandji reaction follows envenomation from several carybdeid jellyfish *(Carukia barnesi)* in northeastern Australia. The reaction follows a minor painful sting.[23] After 5 to 40 minutes, a boring pain begins in the trunk spreading quickly to the chest and thigh. Waves of numb pain intensify over a few minutes.[24] There may be increased sighing respiration, restlessness, tremor, anxiety, headache, localized or general piloeruption, sweating, pallor, cyanosis, oliguria, tachycardia, nausea, hypertension, pulmonary edema with left ventricular dilatation, cardiac failure,[25] and feelings of imminent death that last 1 to 2 days. Some symptoms may be reversed with phentolamine and IV narcotics.[11]

The Commonwealth Serum Laboratories specific box jellyfish *(Chironex fleckeri)* antivenom is largely ineffective in the "Irukandji syndrome."[26]

VENOMOUS FISH[20]

Animals:

Stingray, scorpion, zebra, stonefish, weevers, toadfish, stargazers, ratfish, catfish, surgeonfish, and several species of sharks.

Venomous fish have a defensive apparatus, usually spines or stings, containing specialized tissue that secretes a pain-producing toxin. Over 200 species, including stingray, scorpion fish, zebra fish, stonefish, weevers, toadfish, stargazers, ratfish, catfish, surgeon fish, and several species of sharks, are known to be venomous. Generally, these fish are found in shallow water, reefs, kelp beds, around coral, or inshore mostly in tropical waters in the South Pacific. They are nonmigratory, slow swimming, and often found buried in the sand on the ocean floor.

All fish venoms are characterized by instability due to small temperature changes. Toxicity is lost by drying, and the substance is unstable even at room temperature.

Stingrays (elasmobranches) range in size from several inches in diameter to over 14 feet. They usually lie quietly, half buried in mud or sand, in shallow water, although a few species are found in deep water. Rays do not attack humans; wounds occur when a swimmer runs into the surf and accidentally steps on the fish. Pressure causes the tail to thrust up and forward usually into the victim's leg or foot.

Symptoms

Stings cause severe lacerations from 5 to 20 cm long, usually on a lower extremity. The edges of the wound tend to become necrotic. Intense pain occurs immediately and spreads rapidly up the extremity. Paresthesias, cardiac arrhythmias, and convulsions have been reported. Nausea, vomiting, and abdominal pain may be due either to some component of the toxin or to the extreme anguish of the victim. If untreated, the pain subsides over 6 to 48 hours.

Treatment

First aid for stings includes immediate irrigation of the wound with salt water to remove as much venom as possible. If any portion of the integumentary sheath is visible in the laceration, it should be removed. The extremity then should be submerged in very hot water until the pain has completely subsided, usually 30 to 90 minutes. After the toxin has been inactivated by the heat, the wound should be explored for fragments of the sheath, debrided, and sutured. Secondary infection is rare if the wound is thoroughly cleansed. The patient should be immunized appropriately for tetanus.

SCULPIN[20]

Animals:

Stonefish, zebra, and lionfish.

The sculpin is a common fish found on the Pacific Coast and is considered highly edible. Stings are common on the hands of fishermen who encounter sculpin that are caught in nets with other fish. Stonefish are well camouflaged and sluggish and usually lie buried in sand or mud in shallow water; they are usually 10 to 15 inches in length, but may reach 24 inches and may weigh 3 pounds. The zebra fish is a bright-colored tropical fish with large, fanlike but highly venomous fins.

Symptoms

All envenomations cause excruciating, often incapacitating, pain radiating through the entire extremity. Numbness and paresthesias occur around the wound with swollen. Respiratory depression, cyanosis, primary shock, and cardiac arrhythmias may follow. Stonefish stings are especially dangerous; in addition to extensive necrosis at the site of the wound, deaths have been reported.

Treatment

Immersion in very hot water until the angonizing pain is relieved, usually a minimum of 30 minutes. Injection of emetine hydrochloride directly into the wound may be of value if it can be done within 30 mintues after the sting. Meperidine hydrochloride may be required for pain. Patients stung by stonefish and lionfish must be monitored carefully for cardiotoxic effects and respiratory depression.

Antivenin is available for stonefish stings and usually may be obtained from local zoos or aquariums. It should be used in all serious cases.

CATFISH STINGS

The stinging apparatuses of the catfish are the bony dorsal and pectoral fins, each of which contains a spine attached to venom glands in its leading edge. The spines have a series of razor-sharp teeth that act as barbs, and extraction of these brittle structures is difficult. The spines normally lie flat against the side of the fish, but they extend when the fish is frightened or excited.[27]

There are over 1000 species of fresh- and saltwater catfish worldwide, many of them venomous. Toxicity results from both the classically described venom, delivered when a spine punctures the victim, and a more recently elucidated skin toxin found over the entire surface of the catfish. Death has been reported, but symptoms are usually limited to the involved extremity and respond within hours to supportive therapy.[28]

The major groups of persons at risk for catfish envenomation are fishermen and water-sports participants. Worldwide, saltwater fishermen have sustained many serious envenomations from the Arabian Gulf catfish *(Aurius thalasinus)* and the potentially lethal Oriental catfish *(Plotosus lineatus),* which possesses one of the most potent known marine toxins. In North America, the Carolina madtom *(Noturus furiosus)* and the Ictalurids (genus *Ictalurus*) are most commonly responsible for dangerous catfish envenomations. This group includes the brown bullhead (sp. *nebulosus*), channel catfish (sp. *punctatus*), blue catfish (sp. *furcatus*), and white catfish (sp. *catus*).[28]

The Stinging Apparatus

The classically known mechanism of catfish envenomation involves spinous puncture of the victim. Penetration of the spine into the victim is coincident with rupture of the venom glands located in the tissues surrounding the fins, thus allowing venom to trickle into the wound.[28]

A second mechanism of catfish toxicity, crinotoxicity, has been found in some catfish species (*A. thalasinus* and *P. lineatus*). Crinotoxins are proteinaceous toxins found in catfish epidermal secretions that coat the entire body, including the fins. Agitation of the catfish causes locked extension of the fins and also causes secretion of the crinotoxins.[28]

Clinical Presentation

Severe pain, paresthesias, and numbness are described. Other localized symptoms commonly found with catfish envenomation are erythema, cyanosis, edema, sweating, lymphangitis, and muscle fibrillation. Any of these may progress to involve the entire extremity. Wounds inflected by catfish spines often bleed more freely than expected for their size. Systemic findings occur less frequently in catfish envenomation and may include fever, convulsive muscular contractions, coagulopathy, palpitations, nausea, hypotension, weakness, and altered level of consciousness.[28]

There are no specific antitoxins for catfish envenomations. Treatment is directed toward pain control and prevention of wound complications. Tetanus prophylaxis is given when indicated. Initially, the wound should be inspected and all foreign material removed, with x-rays taken to confirm absence of radiopaque foreign material. Catfish spines usually do not break off when skin is punctured, but radiographs may reveal the spines when they are present.[28]

Treatment

The affected body part should then be immersed in hot water (~110°F/43°C) for at least 30 minutes. Hot water immersion, originally thought to provide relief through toxin inactivation, may result in at least partial symptomatic improvement through reversal of painful vascular and muscular spasm.

Opiate analgesics may be required to control pain, but local anesthesia with bupivacaine may reduce the need for systemic analgesics.[28]

Optimal wound outcome depends not only on removal of foreign material but also on consideration of secondary bacterial infection. Deep wounds should be cultured. Bacteremia resulting from wound infection with *Aeromonas* or *Vibrio* is relatively more likely in patients with diabetes, cirrhosis, or arthritis or the immunocompromised. Tetracycline, beta-lactamase–stable beta-lactams, and aminoglycosides may all be necessary to eradicate serious *Aeromonas* or *Vibrio* infections. Oral tetracycline or cotrimoxazole should be adequate. Empiric intravenous antibiotics should be started pending culture results. Inpatient therapy may also be required in health patients with deep wounds, long delays in wound care, wounds with retained foreign material or with spine penetration of sterile body cavities, and wounds with inflammatory changes persisting beyond 12 hours after envenomation.[28]

REFERENCES—MARINE ENVENOMATION

1. Auerbach PS. Marine envenomations. N Engl J Med 1991;325:486–493.
2. McGoldrick J, Marx JA. Marine envenomations. II. Invertebrates. J Emerg Med 1992;10:71–77.
3. McGoldrick J, Marx JA. Marine envenomations. I. Vertebrates. J Emerg Med 1991;9:497–502.
4. Russell MT, Tomchik RS. Sea bather's eruption or "sea lice": New findings and clinical implications. J Emerg Nurse 1993;19:197–201.
5. Freundentel AR, Joseph PR. Sea bather's eruption. N Engl J Med 1993;329:542–544.
6. Tomchik RS, Russell MT, Szmant AM, Black NA. Clinical perspectives on seabathers' eruption also known as "sea lice." JAMA 1993;269:1169–1172.
7. Burnett JW, Fenner PJ, Kokelj F, Williamson JA. Serious *Physalia* (Portuguese man o'war) stings: implications for scuba divers. J Wilderness Med 1994;5:71–76.
8. Stein MR, Marraccini JV, Rothschild NE, Burnett JW. Fatal Portuguese Man-O-War *(Physalia physalis)* envenomation. Ann Emerg Med 1989;18:312–315.
9. Williamson JA, Callanan VI, Hartwick RF. Serious envenomation by the northern Australian box jellyfish: the continuing search for lethal mechanisms. Med J Aust 1980;1:13–15.
10. Williamson J. Current challenges in marine envenomation: an overview. J Wilderness Med 1992;3:422–431.
11. Burnett JW. Human injuries following jellyfish stings. Maryland Med J 1992;41:506–513.
12. Fenner PJ. Irukandji—a "new" danger. In: Pearn J, Covacevich J, eds. Vemons and victims. South Brisbane: The Queensland Museum and Amphion Press, 1988.
13. Fenner PJ, Williamson JA, Blenkin JA. Successful use of *Chironex* antivenom by members of the Queensland Ambulance Transport Brigade. Med J Aust 1989;151:708–710.
14. Burnett JW, Calton GJ. Response of the box jellyfish *(Chironex fleckeri)* cardiotoxin to intravenous administration of verapamil. Med J Aust 1983;2:192–194.
15. Burnett JW, Othman IB, Endean R, Fenner PJ, Callanan VI, Williams JA. Verapamil potentiation of *Chironex* (box jellyfish) antivenom. Toxicon 1990;28:242–244.
16. Beadnell CE, Rider TA, Williamson JA, Fenner PJ. Management of a major box jellyfish *(Chironex fleckeri)* sting. Lessons from the first minutes and hours. Med J Aust 1992;156:655–658.
17. Bengston K, Nichols MM, Schnadig V, Ellis MD. Sudden death in a child following jellyfish envenomation by *Chiropsalmus quadrumanus.* Case report and autopsy findings. JAMA 1991;266:1404–1406.
18. Wachsman M, Aurelian L, Burnett JW. Human immunosuppression induced by sea nettle *(Chrysavra Quinquecirrha)* venom. Toxicon 1991;29:386–390.
19. Hartwick R, Callanan V, Williamson J. Disarming the box jellyfish. Nematocyst inhibition in *Chironex fleckeri.* Med J Aust 1980;1:15–20.
20. Wingert W. Poisoning by marine animals. Personal communication.
21. Laird P. Sea-urchin injuries. Lancet 1995;346:1240.
22. Garcia PJ, Shein MH, Burnett JW. Fulminant hepatic failure from a sea anemone sting. Ann Intern Med 1994;120:665–666.
23. Burnett JW. Human injuries following jellyfish stings. Maryland Med J 1992;41:506–513.
24. Fenner PJ, Williamson J, Callanan VI, Audly I. Further understanding of and a new treatment for "Irukandju" *(Carukia barnesi)* stings. Med J Aust 1986;145:569–574.
25. Martin JC, Audley I. Cardiac failure following irukandji envenomation. Med J Aust 1990;153:166–168.
26. Fenner PJ, Williamson JA, Burnett JW, Colquhoun DM, Godfrey S, Gunawardane K, Murtha W. The "Irukandji Syndrome" and acute pulmonary edema. Med J Aust 1988;149:150–156.
27. Das SK, Johnson MB, Cohly HHP. Catfish stings in Mississippi. South Med J 1995;88:809–812.
28. Shepherd S, Thomas SH, Stone CK. Catfish envenomation. J Wilderness Med 1994;5:67–70.

Chapter 73
Indigenous Toxicology—Folk Medicine

It is not unusual for patients who used traditional medicines to seek advice and treatment with traditional ethnic practitioners before resorting to more conventional medical advice. Physicians must be alert to the possibility of unusual heavy metal poisonings in such patients. Often patients may complain of a progressive general malaise, anorexia, vague abdominal discomfort, and impaired taste. In the United States, Canada, France, Great Britain, Germany, and other nations immigrant neighborhoods may have local ethnic stores that carry familiar products often imported from home, including traditional foods, utensils, medicines, and cosmetics. Importation of these items appears to be unregulated in part because many of these items have never been tested for possible health hazards. Table 73–1 lists potential side effects and toxicity from traditional remedies. Some liliiflorae (see Table 73–2) known to have caused fatal human or animal poisoning are summarized in Table 73–2.

INFORMATION SOURCES

Information sources are available that are related to traditional medicine, herbal and magical medicine, food supplements, and alternative medicine.[1–3]

CLINICAL PRESENTATION

Joubert and Mathibe have summarized acute poisoning in developing countries.[4]

In general, acute poisoning with traditional medicines presents with one of three major clinical syndromes. The most common is a varying degree of gastrointestinal irritation affecting either the upper or lower, or the whole, gastrointestinal tract. Upper gastrointestinal symptoms may vary from mild epigastric discomfort and nausea to severe vomiting with dehydration. Diarrheas of varying severity and even frank bleeding from the gastrointestinal tract may occur. Many traditional medicines are purgatives used to "clean out" the body, and many herbal remedies are administered as enemas.

The second syndrome is that of hepatic or renal toxicity or both. The latter may be accompanied by hematuria.

Table 73–1
Potential Side Effects and Toxicity From Traditional Remedies [a]

Substance or Therapy	Other Names	Possible Toxicity or Side Effects
Various Asian patent medicines	Many—mainly herbal	Heavy-metal toxicity
Toad secretions		Neurotoxicity
Dried insects, scorpions		Convulsions, shock
Various Hispanic patent medicines	Many	Mercury, lead toxicity
Vietnamese coin rubbing cupping	Caogio	Ecchymoses
Mexican rattlesnake		*Salmonella,* other Gram-negative bacteria
Aloe	Carrisyn, Huang-chi	Catharsis, hypotension, hypoglycemia
Black tree fungus	Mo-Ehr	Anticoagulation
Burdock		Atropinic, diuretic, hypoglycemic, estrogenic effects
Chaparrel	Creosote	Nausea, vomiting, diarrhea, abdominal cramps
Comfrey tea		Veno-occlusive liver disease
Dandelion		Nausea, vomiting, increased gastric secretions, dermatitis
Garlic	Dasuan	Gastroenteritis, nausea, diarrhea, platelet inhibition, inhibition of iodine uptake by thyroid
Ginseng	Wuchaseng, Wujia, Ren-shen	Diarrhea, CNS stimulation, hypertension, MAO-inhibitor interaction
Hypercicin	St. John's wort, Sho-ren-gyo	Photosensitivity, MAO-inhibitor interaction
Iscador	Mistletoe	Hepatitis, gastroenteritis, seizures, shock
Kelp	Kombu	Goiters, jodbasedow (iodine-induced hyperthyroidism)
Licorice	Gan-cao	Hyperaldosterone state
Lycium fruit	Kuo-chi-tzu, Gouquizi, wolfberry	Atropinic, hypoglycemic effects
Peony	Mountain bark, Chi-shao, Bai-shao, Mudan-pi	Nausea, diarrhea, CNS depression, hypotension
Prunella	Xia-ku-cao, woundwort, allheal	Catharsis, uterine hypotension
Red clover		Anticoagulation (warfarin-like)
Salvia	Tan-shen	Platelet inhibition, sedation, hypotension, diuresis, hypoglycemia
Yarrow	Milfoil	Anticoagulation, photosensitivity, dermatitis

[a]Goldman L, ed. Cross cultural medicine in MKSAP 10: General Internal Medicine. American College of Physicians, 1994; p. 142.
CNS, Central nervous system; *MAO,* monoamine oxidase.

Table 73–2
Some Liliiflorae Known to Have Caused Fatal Human or Animal Poisoning [a]

Botanical Name, Family, Local Names	Indicated Active Principle	Features of Poisoning	Deaths, Postmortem Indications	Traditional Medicinal Usage
Gloriosa superba Colchicaceae *iHlamu* (X, Z) *uHlamvu* (Z)	Cholchicine, superbine [2]	Mucous membrane irritation, severe vomiting and diarrhea, abdominal pain, hypotension, respiratory failure [21]	Recorded human and stock deaths due to exhaustion or respiratory failure [2]	Barrenness (X, Z), sterility (Z), sex determination (Z), ascites (Z), aphrodisiac (Z)
Eriospermum sp. Eriospermaceae *isiDagwa* (Z)	Colchicine-like alkaloid[2]		Recorded human death following medication[1]	Emetic to clear liver (Z), given to wife and husband after miscarriage (Z)
Albuca sp. Hyacinthaceae	Haemolytic sapogenin (in *Albuca setosa*)[2]	Effects on experimental rabbit: listlessness, anorexia and diarrhea, death within 36 h[2]	Death in experimental rabbit: hyperemia of lungs, acute catarrhal gastritis, patchy hyperemia of intestinal mucosa [2]	Purge (Z), venereal disease (X, Z)
Bowiea volubilis Hyacinthaceae *uGibisisila* (Z) *uMgaqaqana* (X)	3 cardiac glucosides, bovosides A, B, and C[2]	Hemolysis, digitalis action, vomiting and purging[2]	Recorded human death following medication,[22] death due to heart failure in experimental frog[2]	Ascites, dropsy, purge (X), barrenness, headaches (X), pregnancy (X, Z), love-charm emetic (Z)

[a]Adapted from Hutchings A, Terblanche SE. S Afr Med J 1989;75:62–69.
X, Xhosa; *Z,* Zulu.

(continued)

Table 73–2 *(Continued)*

Botanical Name, Family, Local Names	Indicated Active Principle	Features of Poisoning	Deaths, Postmortem Indications	Traditional Medicinal Usage
Eucomis autumnalis (= *E. undulata*) Hyacinthaceae *uMakhadakantsele* (Z) *uMathunga* (Z) *ubuHlungu becanti* (X)	Hemolytic saponin [2]	In human case: diarrhea for 1 d, blood in urine and stool, oliguria followed by anuria.[2] In experimental sheep: listlessness, anorexia, inactivity of the rumen, tympanites, foaming at the mouth, dyspnea, strong pulse terminating in death[2]	Death in experimental sheep: general cyanosis, ascites, hydrothorax, hydropericardium, hyperemia of the tracheal mucosa, hyperemia, edema and emphysema of the lungs, degenerative changes in myocardium and liver, tympanites of the rumen[2]	Urinary disease (Z), emetic and enema in fever (Z), ingredient in infusion taken during pregnancy (Z)
Scilla natalensis Hyacinthaceae *I(li)chitha* (Z) *inGuduza* (Z) *uBulika* (Z)		Toxic to experimental sheep with dyspnea, weak quickened pulse [2]	Death of experimental sheep within 12 h[2]	Used as an enema for children (Z), ingredient in infusion taken regularly during pregnancy (Z), dried leaves given to child late in walking (Z)
Scilla nervosa (= *Schizocarpus nervosus* = *S. rigidifolius*) *inGcino* (Z) *inGcolo* (Z) *Magaqana* (X)	Digitalis glycosides[18]	Toxic to sheep with tympanites, dyspnea, quickening of pulse, apathy and anorexia in experimental sheep [2]	Recorded human and stock deaths;[18] death in experimental sheep: generalized cyanosis, fluid in serous sacs, subendocardial and subpericardial petechiae, hyperemia, and edema of lungs[2]	Dysentery remedy (X), small doses given for rheumatic fever (Z)
Urginea altissima Hyacinthaceae *Skanama* (Z)	Altoside, scillitoxin, scillipain[1]	Causes "slangkop" poisoning in cattle with severe gastric intestinal tract inflammation, diarrhea, tremors/paralysis, heart failure,[22] frequency of urination[2]	Human deaths recorded.[2] Stock deaths by cardiac arrest show general cyanosis, dilation of the ventricles, degeneration of myocardium, hyperemia and edema of lungs and mediastinal lymph nodes, hemorrhage at trachea bifurcation and mediastinal lymph nodes[2]	Emetic for stomach troubles and high blood pressure (Z), diuretic (X), catarrh, asthma (X), bronchitis (X)
Boophane disticha Amaryllidaceae *inCwadi* (X, Z) *iBadi* (Z) *iswadi* (Z)	Ipuranol (glucoside), buphanine (alkaloid), narcissine, hemanthine (convulsant alkaloid[2])	Dizziness, visual disturbance, excitation or depression, stupor, coma[21]	Recorded human death following medication: engorgement of mucous membranes of stomach and intestines[19]	Hysteria (X, Z), headaches (Z), chest pain (Z), narcotic (X), boils, wounds (X)
Scadoxcus puniceus Amaryllidaceae *i(li) dumbilikha* *Nhloyile* (Z) *umPhompo* (Z)	Patalensine (= hemanthine)[2]	Dizziness, visual disturbance, excitation or depression, stupor, coma[21]	Recorded human death[18]	Ingredient in infusion taken during pregnancy (Z), emetic for coughs (Z)
Clivia nobilis Amaryllidaceae *um Gulufu* (Z)	Cliviine, clivianine, glucoside of low toxicity[2]	Feeble emetic [2]	Suspected human death[18]	Protective charm

Patients can develop hepatic or renal failure with severe metabolic disturbances.[4]

The third syndrome is that of central nervous system involvement. The picture usually reflects cerebral irritation, and patients can be confused or may even hallucinate. Psychoactive and nonpsychoactive substances used in herbal preparations are listed in Tables 73–3 and 73–4.[5]

ADVERSE REACTIONS

De Smet has classified adverse reactions to herbal remedies[6]:

Type A Reactions

These are pharmacologically predictable and usually dose-dependent, for example, the induction of hypertension and anxiety by yohimbine, the major alkaloid in yohimbe bark preparations.

Type B Reactions

These are idiosyncratic reactions that occur in only a minority of patients, but which can be serious and potentially fatal; for example, normal doses of yohimbine were associated with bronchospasm and increased mucus production in a patient with severe allergic dermatitis, and with progressive renal failure and a lupuslike syndrome in another patient.

Type C Reactions

These may develop during long-term therapy, for example, muscular weakness due to hypokalemia in long-term users of herbal anthranoid laxatives (Tables 73–5 and 73–6).

Type D Reactions

These consist of delayed effects such as carcinogenicity and teratogenicity. Some herbs are known to have carcinogenic and teratogenic potential.

HERBAL PRODUCTS

Members of the Long Island Regional Poison Control Center[7] at Winthrop-University Hospital have classified herbs as the following:

1. Volatile oils—which are odorous plant ingredients that evaporate at room temperature.

Table 73–3
Psychoactive Substances Used in Herbal Preparations[a]

Labeled Ingredient	Botanical Source	Pharmacologic Agent	Suggested Use	Effects
African yohimbine bark; yohimbe	*Corynanthe yohimbe*	Yohimbe	Smoke or tea as stimulant	Mild hallucinogen
Broom; Scotch broom	*Cytisus* spp.	Sparteine	Smoke for relaxation	Questionable sedative—hypnotic
California poppy	*Eschscholtzia californica*	Coptisine, sanguinarine	Smoke as marijuana substitute	Probably none
Catnip	*Nepeta cataria*	Nepetalactone	Smoke or tea as marijuana substitute	Mild hallucinogen
Cinnamon	*Cinnamomum camphora*	?	Smoke with marijuana	Mild stimulant
Damiana	*Turnera diffusa*	?	Smoke as marijuana substitute	Mild stimulant
Hops	*Humulus lupulus*	Lupuline	Smoke or tea as sedative and marijuana substitute	None
Hydrangea	*Hydrangea paniculata*	Cyanogenic glycosides	Smoke as marijuana substitue	Cyanide toxicity
Juniper	*Juniper macropoda*	?	Smoke as hallucinogen	Strong hallucinogen
Kavakava	*Piper methysticum*	Yangonin, pyrones	Smoke or tea as marijuana subsitute	Mild hallucinogen
Khat	*Catha edulis*	Cathine, cathinone	Tea, chew	Strong stimulant
Kola nut, gotu kola	*Cola* spp.	Caffeine, theobromine, kolanin	Smoke, tea, or capsules as stimulant	Stimulant
Lobelia	*Lobelia inflata*	Lobeline	Smoke or tea as marijuana substitute	Mild euphoriant
Mandrake	*Mandragora officinarum*	Scopolamine, hyoscyamine	Tea as hallucinogen	Anticholinergic toxicity
Mate	*Ilex paraguayensis*	Caffeine	Tea as stimulant	Stimulant
Mormon tea	*Ephedra nevadensis*	Ephedrine	Tea as stimulant	Stimulant
Nutmeg	*Myristica fragrans*	Myristicin	Tea as hallucinogen	Hallucinogen
Passion flower	*Passiflora incarnata*	Harmine alkaloids	Smoke, tea, or capsules as marijuana substitute	Mild stimulant, convulsions, tremors in excess
Periwinkle	*Catharanthus roseus*	Indole alkaloids	Smoke or tea as euphoriant	Hallucinogen
Prickly poppy	*Argemone mexicana*	Protopine, bergerine isoquinilines	Smoke as euphoriant	Narcotic–analgesic
Snakeroot	*Rauwolfia serpentina*	Reserpine	Smoke or tea as tobacco substitute	Tranquilizer
Thorn apple	*Datura stramonium*	Atropine, scopolamine	Smoke or tea as tobacco substitute or hallucinogen	Anticholinergic toxicity
Tobacco	*Nicotiana* spp.	Nicotine	Smoke as tobacco	Strong stimulant
Valerian	*Valeriana officinalis*	Chatinine, velerine alkaloids	Tea or capsules as tranquilizer	Tranquilizer
Wild lettuce	*Lactuca sativa*	Lactucarine	Smoke as opium subsititute	Qeustionable Narcotic–analgesic
Wormwood	*Artemisia absinthium*	Absinthine	Smoke or tea as relaxant	Narcotic–analgesic

[a]Adapted from Siegel RK. Herbal intoxication. JAMA 1976;236:474.

Table 73–4
Nonpsychoactive Toxic Effects of Herbal Preparations [a]

Herb Name	Botanical Source	Pharmacologic Principle	Herbalist's Use	Clinical Effects	Toxicity	Miscellaneous
Cardiovascular System						
Buchu	*Barosma betulina*	Diosphenol (volatile oil)	Diuretic Also GU uses	Diuretic	Nausea, vomiting	Abandoned by the medical profession
Cayenne pepper	*Capsicum frutescens*	Capsaicin	Improve circulation GI irritant Counterirritant		Nausea, vomiting Diarrhea, local irritation	
Elder	(See GI System)			Diuretic		
Foxglove	*Digitalis purpurea*	Digitoxin Gitalin Gitoxin	Heart stimulant	Cardioactive	Vomiting Bradycardia Arrhythmias	
Garlic	*Allium sativum*	Allyl disulfides	Hypertension Colic Hyperlipemia Antineoplastic		Hypotension Rashes Leukocytosis	Fatalities have been reported in children after massive ingestion
Hellebore	*Veratrum viride*	Steroidal glycoalkaloids (germidine, germutine)	Decreases blood pressure Toxemia of pregnancy		Vomiting Bradycardia Hypotension	*Veratrum* alkaloids produce reflexive decreases in blood pressure and heart rate
Juniper	*Juniperus communis* Oil of sabural *Juniperus depressa*		Diuretic (See CNS System, Rheumatological System)		Renal and CNS toxicity GI irritation Psychiatric changes	
Lily of the Valley	*Convallaria majalis*	Convallarin (glycosides) Convallotoxin	Heart stimulant Diuretic	Cardioactive Diuretic	Nausea, vomiting Purgative Arrhythmias Dermatitis with contact	Similar to digitalis Little cumulative tendency, unlike digitalis more of a diuretic Convallotoxin is 10 times more cardioactive than digitoxin
Jalap	*Exagonium purga* Conquer root	Jalapin glycoside (resin), or convolvulin	Cathartic	Watery diarrhea	Profuse fluid and electrolyte imbalances secondary to hypercatharsis	Can cause GI symptoms if applied to open wound
Olive oil	*Olea europaea*	Olein (fixed oil)	Laxative	Emollient	Diarrhea	
Peanut oil	*Arachis hypogaea*	Olein	Laxative Herb vehicle	Demulcent	Diarrhea	
Rheumatologic System						
Guaiac	*Guaiacum officinale*	Guaiaconic acid	Laxative Diuretic (Rheumatism: no longer recommended)		GI irritant Nausea, vomiting	Used as a test for oxidizing enzymes for occult blood Blood + H_2O_2 + guaiac = blue
Juniper	*Juniperus communis*	Oil of sabinol	Gout Diuretic GI dyspepsia		Catharsis Personality changes Renal toxicity Seizures	
Respiratory System						
Grindelia	*Grindelia camporum* *Grindelia humilis* *Grindelia squarrosa*	Balsamic resin	Expectorant Asthma Bronchitis Mild sedative	Drowsiness Decreases heart rate Mydriasis Increases blood pressure Stimulates expectoration	Renal toxicity ?Selenium Cardiotoxicity	

[a]Adapted from Goldfrank L, Lewin N, Flomenbaum N et al. Hosp Physician 1982;18(10):66–69, 73.

(continued)

Table 73–4 *(Continued)*

Herb Name	Botanical Source	Pharmacologic Principle	Herbalist's Use	Clinical Effects	Toxicity	Miscellaneous
Respiratory System *(continued)*						
Jimsonweed	(See CNS System)		Asthma	Bronchodilatation	(See CNS System)	
Lobelia	(See CNS System)		Asthma Expectorant			
Integumentary System						
Aloe	*Aloe vera* *Aloe barbadensis* *Aloe officinalis*	Aloe—emodins Resinol—tannol	Burns Laxative	Soothes burn	Irritation to skin Nausea, vomiting Diarrhea Red urine	Clears lower bowel Stimulates peristalsis Works in concert with bile in gut
Horse chestnut	*Aesculus hippocastanum*	Aesculin (coumarin glycoside)	Absorbs UV light (sunscreen) Antithrombin agent	Sunscreen	Nausea, vomiting Increases temperature Hemolysis	
Metabolic and Others						
Galega	*Galega officinalis*	Galegine (alkaloid) Tannins	Diabetes	Hypoglycemia	May decrease blood sugar	Replaced by more effective hypoglycemic agents Claim that galega increases breast milk is not substantiated in literature
Oleander	*Nerium oleander*	Oleandrin, other cardioactive glycosides	Heart stimulant	Cardioactive	Similar to digitalis Vomiting and diarrhea	Dried root and rhizomes used in tea or made into tincture
Gastrointestinal System						
Aloe	(See Integumentary System)					
Black cohosh	*Climicifuga* spp.	Climicifugin (resin)	Dyspepsia	Dyspepsia Cathartic Emetic	Nausea, vomiting	
Caraway	*Carum carvi*	Carvone (ketone) Terpene (volatile oil) Calcium oxalate	Colic	Carminative Flavoring agent	Nausea, vomiting CNS depression	
Cardamom	*Ellettaria cardamonum* *Amonum cardamonum*	Cardamom	Condiment	Carminative Purgative	Nausea, vomiting, diarrhea	
Castor bean	*Ricinus communis*	Castor oil (fixed oil) Ricin	Laxative Cathartic		Nausea, vomiting Bleeding	Phytotoxin General protoplasmic poison Toxalbumin
Catnip	*Nepeta cataria*	Citral Limonene Geraniol (volatile oil)	Carminative CNS effects	CNS stimulant Antispasmodic		
Chamomile	*Anthemis flores*	Tiglic (volatile oil)	Carminative	Antispasmodic	Anaphylaxis reported in patients with allergy to ragweed pollens (Compositae family)	
Coconut	*Cocos nucifera*	Trilaurin	Anthelmintic	Cathartic	Diarrhea	
Dandelion	*Taraxacum officinale*	Taraxacerin (resin)	Dyspepsia Diuretic	May stimulate gastric secretion	Vomiting	High vitamin A, C, and niacin; protein, fat, iron

(continued)

Table 73–4 *(Continued)*

Herb Name	Botanical Source	Pharmacologic Principle	Herbalist's Use	Clinical Effects	Toxicity	Miscellaneous
Gastrointestinal System *(continued)*						
Elder	*Sambucus* spp.	Sambucine	Laxative Diuretic	Laxative	Stems used by children as blow guns leading to cyanide poisoning (main toxicity is stem) Inner bark is purgative, emetic	
Garlic	*Allium sativum*	Allyl disulfides	Colic	(See Cardiovascular System)		
Gentian	*Gentiana lutea*	Gentiopicrin (glycoside)	Stomachic	Stimulates gastric secretion	Nausea, vomiting	Questionable use in malaria
Golden seal	*Hydrastis* spp.	Hydrastine	Dyspepsia Aid to stop postpartum bleeding	Nausea, vomiting	Nausea, vomiting Paresthesia CNS stimulant Respiratory failure Paralysis	Fatalities have occurred
Guaiac	See Rheumatologic System					
Ipecac	*Cephaelis acuminata* *Cephaelis ipecacuanha*	Emetine Cephaelin		Emetic		
Ginseng	*Panax quinquefolium* *Panax ginseng*	Saponin glycosides	Impotence Anemia Depression Diabetes Edema Hypertension	Decreases serum glucose Increases cortisol	Ginseng abuse syndrome	"Adaptogen" "Biocatalyzer" Native to Georgia *(Panax quinquefolium)*
Heliotrope	*Heliotropium europaeum*	Pyrrolizidine			Hepatotoxicity	Heliotrope is a common weed—"not garden heliotrope"
Ipecac	*Cephaelis* *Cephaelis ipecacuanha*	Cephaelin Emetine	?Edema ?Stress	Emetic	Myotoxicity	
Periwinkle	(See CNS System)		Hypoglycemia	(See CNS System)		

Table 73–5
Examples of Increased Toxicity Due To Interactions Between Herbal Preparations and Conventional Medicines [a]

Drug	Herbal Compound	Comment
Increased toxicity of the herbal compound		
Pipemidic acid Ciprofloxacin Enoxacin	Caffeine in *Cola, Ilex,* and *Paullinia* preparations	The antibacterial quinolones pipemidic acid, ciprofloxacin and enoxacin inhibit the hepatic metabolism of caffeine.[39–42] As a result, users of caffeine-containing *Cola, Ilex,* and *Paullinia* preparations may have an increased risk of adverse effects, such as tremors or tachycardia
Quinidine Haloperidol Moclobemide	Sparteine in *Cytisus scoparius*	The antiarrhythmic drug quinidine is a potent inhibitor of the oxidative metabolism of sparteine,[43] and a similar effect has been observed with haloperidol[44] and moclobemide.[45] Sparteine is a quinolizidine alkaloid from *Cytisus scoparius* which was recently found in a herbal slimming remedy on the UK market. Substantial doses in slow metabolizers could be expected to be associated with various adverse reactions, such as circulatory collapse[46]
Increased toxicity of the conventional medicine		
Theophylline Phenytoin	Piperine in *Piper* spp.	Piperine, a major alkaloid of *Piper longum* and *Piper nigrum* (both of which occur in Ayurvedic formulations), can enhance the bioavailability of conventional drugs, such as theophylline and phenytoin[47–51]
Calcium antagonists	Grapefruit juice	Grapefruit juice increases the bioavailability of certain calcium antagonists and might interact in a similar way with certain other conventional drugs[52]

[a] Adapted from De Smet PAGM. Drug Safety 1995;13:81–93.

Table 73–6
Examples of Teratogenic and/or Carcinogenic Herbs [a]

Herbs	Comments
Acorus calamus	The Jammu variety of calamus oil has been shown to be carcinogenic in rats; as studies on the calamus constituent β-asarone have revealed similar activities, this compound is considered to be the causative agent
Aristolochia species	Many *Aristolochia* species contain carcinogenic aristolochic acids
Blighia sapida	The unripe fruit of this tree has high levels of a potent hyoglycemic amino acid, known as hypoglycin A, which is teratogenic in animal experiments
Conium maculatum	Contains the poisonous piperidine alkaloid conine and related alkaloids. It has well established teratogenic activity in certain animal species
Croton tiglium	Croton oil contains tumor-promoting phorbol diesters
Genista tinctoria	Contains toxic quinolizidine alkaloids, such as anagyrine, cytisine and *N*-methylcytisine. Anagyrine is a suspected animal teratogen, whereas cytisine has been shown to have teratogenic activity in rabbits
Sassafras albidum	The wood of sassafras root contains 1 to 2% of volatile oil, which in turn consists largely of safrole. This constituent is hepatocarcinogenic in laboratory animals. Experiments in mice suggest the possibility of transplacental carcinogenesis
Symphytum officinale and other herbs containing pyrrolizidine alkaloids	Hepatocarcinogenic pyrrolizidine alkaloids occur in a large number of medicinal plants, which occur notably in the genera of *Crotalaria, Cynoglossum, Heliotropium, Petasites, Senecio* and *Symphytum.* Animal studies have also shown that transplacental passage is possible, and there is a human case of fatal neonatal liver injury in which the mother had used a herbal cough tea containing pyrrolizidine alkaloids throughout her pregnancy

[a]Adapted from De Smet PAGM. Drug Safety 1995;13:81–93.

2. Resins—which are complex mixtures or alcohols, resinol, esters, and resenes.
3. Alkaloids—which are alkaline, organic compounds.
4. Glycosides—such as sugar esters containing glycol and aglone. Hydrolysis yields one or more sugars.
5. Fixed oils—which are esters of long-chain fatty acids and alcohols.

Popular herb products include the following:

Absinthe or wormwood *(Artemisia absinthe)* is a toxic liquor. It contains a volatile oil, alpha and beta thujone. It is now banned in the United States. It caused "absinthism," which includes psychosis, hallucinations, and intellectual deterioration. It is rumored to have produced effects in Van Gogh. Its CNS effects are similar to camphor. Absinthe was a flavoring and coloring agent in alcoholic drinks. It produces ataxia, vertigo, headache, vomiting, diarrhea, and diaphoresis.

Aconite *(Aconitum napellus)* is known as monkshood or wolfsbane. (See Chu an wu.) Fatal doses are 5 mL of aconite tincture, 2 mg of pure aconite, and 1 gram of the plant.

Aloe *(Aloe vera, barbadensis, officinalis)* soothes skin burns and rashes. May cause hypersensitivity, skin irritation, diarrhea, vomiting, and red urine.

Birch bark (bark leaves) (*Betula* sp.) contains methylsalicylate.

Black balls or Tung Shueh pills. They contain diazepam, heavy metals and steroids.[8]

Black cohosh *(Cimicifuga racemosa)* has estrogenic effect and has been used for "female complaints" and other disorders. Adverse effects of this plant include nausea, vomiting, dizziness, and weakness. Tannin has also been present and has the potential for liver damage.

Black snake root (*Zigadenus* spp.), similar to veratamine, produces hypotension and bradycardia.

Buckthorn types (Hipothae momnoides) is suspected to contain **anthroquinones** which can produce severe watery diarrhea. **Buckthorn** (*Rhammus* spp.) bark yields a toxin that causes spinal cord demyelination and paralysis. It has been used as a cathartic.

Burdock root *(Articum minus)* has anticholinergic actions.

Bush tea *(Crotalaria spp.)* contains pyrrolizidine alkaloids, which are hepatotoxic.

Capsicum (*Capsicum* peppers) contains capsaicin, an alkaloid contained in various capsaicin red peppers (used as a herbal remedy for pain for centuries) and exhibits widespread pharmacologic properties, notably on type C nociceptive afferent nerve fibers. It is believed to deplete substance P, a neurotransmitter of pain. The application of capsaicin produces desensitization to thermal, chemical, and mechanical stimuli in a dose-dependent manner.

Cassia spp. **(Senna), cascara sagrada** *(Rhamnus purshiana)* contain strong botanical laxatives and diuretics and produce symptoms of laxative abuse syndromes, including severe electrolyte disturbances leading to cardiac dysrhythmias.

Catnip *(Nepeta cataria)* is a mild central nervous system (CNS) stimulant and hallucinogen. It is used by insufflation.

Chamomile teas are members of the Composita family. One type *(Anthemis cotula)* is found in the western United States; another species *(Matricaria recutita)* is found in Germany. It has been recommended for its antispasmodic and carminative actions. It is made from the fragrant pollen-laden flowering heads that have a cross-allergic reaction with other members of the Composita family, which includes ragweed, asters, and chrysanthemums. A single cup can cause allergic reactions such as anaphylactoid reactions, hives, and respiratory distress. In Mexico it is called manzanilla.

However, a double-blind study on the efficacy of herbal tea preparations (Calma-Bebi, Bonomelli, Dalzago [Italy]) containing the following extracts of natural herbs, chamomile (*Matricaria chamomilla*), vervain (*Verbena officinalis*), licorice (*Glycyrrhiza glabra*) fennel (*Foeniculum vulgare*), and balm mint (*Melissa officinalis*) eliminated colic in 19 of 33 infants (57%), whereas a placebo was helpful in nine (26%). There were no adverse reactions in this group of patients.

Chaparral from the leaves of the creosote bush (*Larres tridentas*) is recommended as an antioxidant or free-radical scavenger to retard aging and treat a variety of skin disorders. It has been a traditional Indian medicine. It contains nordihydroguaiaretic acid (NDGA), a potent antioxidant that can act as a cyclooxygenase and lipoxygenase pathway inhibitor.

Chromium III chelated to picolinate is not a truly herbal product but a heavy metal. It is an isomer of niacin that is claimed to have lowered cholesterol and enhanced absorption of the usually poorly soluble chromium III. It has been used by body builders to enhance glucose utilization and increase lean body mass. Toxicity is unlikely with a single acute dose. The gastrointestinal absorption is estimated to be less than 1%. The minimum daily dose of chromium has not been established; however, 50 to 200 μg appear to be safe, but long-term exposure to other chromium salts is a possible carcinogen.

The differential diagnosis is with licorice (*Glycyrrhiza glabra*), which can cause weakness from hypokalemia, especially in individuals predisposed to hypokalemic paralysis (exclude by finding normal potassium).

Chu an wu may also be made from toad venom (*Bufo melanosticus*), which contains bufotoxins structurally and pharmacologically similar to digoxin. Patients may present with symptoms of digoxin poisoning.

Chuifong fokwan made in Asia and sold illegally in the United States as Miracle Herb contains cadmium, a probable carcinogen and on long-term exposure has caused osteomalacia.

Chuen Lin (Coptis chinensis/japonicum) is a tonic used in infants and has displaced the bilirubin from its serum protein binding causing hyperbilirubinemia.

Clove cigarettes contain an essential oil, eugenol 60% and tobacco 40%. Smoking has been known to cause epistaxis, respiratory problems, hemoptysis, and death, in addition to the hazards of tobacco.

Cocoa bean contains theobromine, which is dangerous to dogs if ingested. Sixty milliliters caused death in a 30-pound dog.

Comfrey or **Russian comfrey** (*Heliatropium, Crotolaria, Scencio,* and *Symphytum officinale* (common type), *asperium* (prickly type), and *uplandicum* (Russian) are used as herbal teas and digestive aids, which have been linked to pyrrolidine poisoning and liver damage (venoocclusive disease, hepatic failure, hepatic carcinogen). It causes hepatic carcinoma in rats. In South Africa they had produced Scencio disease characterized by abdominal pain, vomiting, and ascites. Epidemics have occurred in India, Afghanistan, and Jamaica due to contamination of grain and bush tea. Nature's Herb manufacturers in Utah has discontinued its production in 1991, but some are still on the shelves of Health Food Stores.

The mechanism of toxic action is the formation of pyrroles, which are highly reactive molecules capable of alkylating neurophilic groups on macromolecules of DNA and result in cell necrosis venous occlusive disease similar to Budd-Chiari syndrome. They are capable of mutagenesis and carcinogenesis. They are available in comfrey-pepsin capsules of 2.9 mg pyrrolizidine. Liver damage has been produced by 2 capsules for 4 months. Severe liver disease is found in animals with LD50 30 to 40 μg/kg/day.

The differential diagnosis for comfrey is encephalitis, Reye syndrome, salicylism, chlordane, and antabuse intoxication. Management consists of gastrointestinal decontamination in acute ingestions. In chronic intoxication treatment is supportive therapy. Portal shunts may be necessary.

Eucalyptus oil contains 38 to 68% eucalyptol. Toxic dose is 3.5 to 5 mL of 100%. As little as 1 mL is fatal in a child. It causes GI upset, seizures, and coma. The toxin is eucalyptol. The onset of symptoms may occur within 10 to 20 minutes. Ingestion can cause rapid onset of convulsions and apnea, aspiration pneumonia, bronchospasm, and permanent neurologic sequelae.

European mistletoe (*Viscum album*) is cardiotoxic and produces vasoconstriction. The American mistletoe (*Phoradendron flavescens*) is also cardiotoxic and has potential vasopressor effects.

Garlic (*Allium sativum*) and **onions** (*Allium cepa)* are members of the Lilliaceae or lily family. They have been used as traditional culinary adjuncts since ancient times.

In 1944 allicin (diallyl disulfide), the antibacterial agent in garlic, was isolated. Fresh garlic has a broad spectrum for Gram-positive and Gram-negative organisms, including strains that are resistant to other antimicrobials. Garlic has been found useful against experimental shigellosis in rabbits. Recently garlic's fibrinolytic activities, prophylactic activities against hypercholesterolemia, hyperlipidemia, and atherosclerotic plaque formation have been recognized. It is claimed to retard aging.

However, garlic can induce nausea, vomiting, diarrhea, bronchospasm, hypoglycemia, contact dermatitis, and garlic burns when applied to the skin for a prolonged time. The contact dermatitis has been attributed to the sulfides in garlic, especially diallyl disulfide, which has bactericidal activities against bacteria, fungi, and larva.

Gan mao tong pian contains phenylbutazone and has been reported to induce aplastic anemia.[9]

Ginseng (*Panax quinquefolium* native to North America or *P. ginseng* native to Korea) is recommended for many ailments. It was used in China for treatment of impotence, fatigue, ulcers, and stress. It is a composite of many active compounds. There are two types of ginseng, and both contain 17 beta-hydroxylated steroidal saponin glycosides that are reported to produce direct CNS stimulation and arousal. It increases GI motility.

Ginseng metabolically can affect the glucose metabolism and lowers blood glucose, increases erythropoiesis, increases iron absorption, lowers cholesterol, and increases blood pressure. Some varieties produce paradoxical hypotension due to the presence of damarenetriol glycosides.

Chronic or excessive use can produce the ginseng-abuse syndrome (TAS) characterized by diarrhea, nervousness, insomnia, hypertension, tachycardia, and increased motor and cognitive activity. An eruptive dermatitis has occurred in 33 of 133 users. Both ginseng species cause fluid and electrolyte imbalance, gynecomastia, and can produce hemolysis. Treatment is to discontinue use and monitor blood pressure and blood glucose.

Germander, wild germander, wall germander, or **tealine** in the United Kingdom (*Teucruium chamaedrys*) comes in the form of a tea or capsule used for weight loss and anal pruritus. It has produced hepatitis and hepatotoxic death. In April 1992 it was prohibited from sale in France after it was believed to have produced 26 cases of hepatitis.

Golden seal (*Hydrastis canadensis* and other *Hydrastis* spp.) is a natural laxative. Golden seal in overdose has produced nausea, vomiting, diarrhea, and paresthesias. In very large amounts hypotension, respiratory depression, and seizures can occur.

Gordolobo yerba. Jamaicans and Mexicans consume a product called gordolobo yerba (*Senecio longilobus*), which contains pyrrolizidine alkaloids and can produce fulminant liver disease.

Groundsel (*Senecio vulgaris, S. spartoides*) contains pyrrolizidine, which is hepatotoxic and has produced cirrhosis in children fed a tea containing this product.

Heliotripium used as an anticonvulsant produced two deaths in American Indians because of pyrrolizidine.

Herbal balls are aromatic, malleable, earth-toned, roughly spherical, hand-rolled mixtures of primarily herbs and honey. They are 1.5 to 2.5 cm in diameter and weigh 2.5 to 9.0 g. These balls are factory produced, patented medicinal agents manufactured in mainland China. The recommended adult dose of the preparation is two herbal balls daily, which can provide up to 73 mg of arsenic and over 1200 mg of mercury, both doses of which can induce either chronic arsenic sulfide poisoning or chronic mercury sulfide poisoning (Table 73–7).[8]

Hops (*Humulus lupulus*) may contain lupuline, which may produce intravascular hemolysis and paroxysmal nocturnal hemoglobinuria.

Kava-kava (*Piper methysticum*) contains methysticine, which causes ataxia, blurred vision, CNS intoxication, deafness, skin yellowing, and dermatosis.

Khat, chat (*Catha edulis*). It is a hallucinogen and stimulant from a plant grown in East Africa and the Arabian Peninsula. The active ingredient is norpseudoephedrine. Methcathinone, the designer stimulant from Russia, is a derivative of cathinone, a potent amphetamine-like constituent occurring naturally in the fresh evergreen leaves of khat. It belongs to the class of phenylalkylamine alkaloids. A medieval Arabic medical treatise recommends chewing khat leaves to avoid hunger and fatigue. Khat use has mainly occurred in North Yemen, Ethiopia, Kenya, adjacent Djibouti, and Somalia. In the United States, Switzerland, and several other countries its use is prohibited. It has been recommended by the World Health Organization that cathinone, the active principle of khat, should be a Schedule I drug of the United Nations and be put under international control. It may produce hypertension, cerebral hemorrhage, myocardial infarction, and pulmonary edema.

It became a Schedule I drug under the Federal Controlled Substances Act in May 1992. Wisconsin has designated it a Schedule I drug. It is also a white, yellowish white, or off-white powder made from the oxidation of over-the-counter ephedrine. It is now being abused in Michigan, Wisconsin, and Ohio. The *l*-isomer of methcathinone parallels the physiologic parameters of *d*-amphetamine. Methcathinone is more potent than cathinone and amphetamine. Methcathinone produces amphetamine-like CNS stimulation. In Russia it is used by IV injection in a cycle binge of 4 days, followed by abstinence for 1 week.

Kelp has high sodium and potassium content.

Kola nut (*Cola nitida*) contains caffeine and theobromine, which act as stimulants.

Ibogaine (*Tabernathe ibogafrom*) is a hallucinogen classified since 1967 as a drug similar to LSD. It is an extract obtained from the roots of the flowering shrub native to the West African nation of Gabon. Ibogaine is classified by the United States government as a Schedule I drug, which indicates no medical value and a high potential for abuse. Its alkaloid, ibogaine, is being promoted for Food and Drug Administration studies and is claimed to be nonaddictive and to make it easier for addicts to curb cocaine and heroin addiction with as little as one dose. Heroin and cocaine ordinarily trigger dopamine release in the brain's "reward center." Ibogaine interrupts this mechanism, and in rats it kills the brain cells that are associated with repetitive obsessive behavior. It is under investigation at the University of Miami.

Table 73–7
Ranges of Arsenic and Mercury Concentrations in Herbal Balls[a,b]

Herbal-Ball Preparation	Chinese Manufacturer	No. Analyzed	Arsenic (mg)	Mercury (mg)
An Gong Niu Huang Wan	Tung Jen Tang Pharmaceutical Factory, Nanjing	3	3.21–36.6	80.7–621.3
Da Huo Luo Wan	Guangzhou Chen Li Ji Pharmaceutical Factory, Guangzhou	6	ND–0.1	12.9–23.3
Dendrobium Moniliforme Night Sight Pills	Tientsin Drug Manufactory, Tientsin	3	ND–0.6	18.9–28.1
Niu Huang Chiang Ya Wan	Tianjiin Drug Manufactory, Tianjin	3	6.9–8.4	42.5–45.4
Niu Huang Chiang Ya Wan	Tianjiin Drug Manufactory, Tianjin	3	8.5–9.5	ND
Niu Huang Ching Hsin Wan	Peking Tung Jen Tang, Beijing	3	1.3–2.7	22.3–181.8
Niu Huang Ching Hsin Wan	Tientsin Drug Manufactory, Tientsin	5	3.4–9.9	24.5–70.5
Ta Huo Lo Tan	Beijing Tung Jen Tang, Beijing	3	14.9–22.1	41.6–99.0
Tsai Tsao Wan	Peking Tung Jen Tang, Beijing	3	ND–0.6	7.8–15.9

[a]Adapted from Espinoza EO, Mann M-J, Bleasdell B. N Engl J Med 1995;333:803–804.
[b]The herbal balls were dissolved in concentrated hydrochloric acid and nitric acid, and the resulting solutions were analyzed with flame atomic absorption spectroscopy.
ND denotes not determined.

Juniper (*Juniperus macropodia*) is a hallucinogen, but renal toxicity and gastrointestinal irritation may occur.

Licorice (*Glycyrrhiza glabra*) produces mineralocorticoid effects, sodium retention, edema, hypertension, and hypokalemia.

Lobelia (*Lobelia inflata*) contains lobeline, atropine, and scopolamine and pyridine alkaloids, which can produce anticholinergic actions and may be a potential hepatotoxin.

Mandrake (*Mandragon officinarum*) or "satan's apple" contains scopolamine and hyoscyamine and can produce anticholinergic effects. **Mandrake** (*Podophyllum peltatrum*) resins also produce keratolytic effects, hypotension, and seizures after ingestion. The ripe fruit is nontoxic.

Ma Hwang (*Ephedra sinica*) or Chinese ephedra is an ephedra herb that has been banned. It contains ephedrine and pseudoephedrine in the Asiatic species. North American varieties are high in tannins and 10 species native to North America contain no useful alkaloids. Symptoms are palpitations, vomiting, tingling, and numbness of the extremities.

Manzanilla. See Chamomile tea.

Mate (*Ileus partaguayensis*) may contain caffeine and pyrrolizidine alkaloids, which may be hepatotoxic and hallucinogenic.

Miracle herb. See *Chuifong fokwan*.

Melaleuca oil from leaves of *Melateuca alternifolia* contains 50 to 60% terpenes and related alcohols and produces CNS depression. It is used for skin conditions.

Mescal bean is from *Sophora secundiflora* that grows on an evergreen shrub native to the southwestern United States and northern Mexico. Used as a hallucinogen, half of a seed has produced toxicity. A suicidal attempt using this shrub resulted in myoclonic jerking, seizures, hypertension, agitation, and hypotension.

Mistletoe berry tea (*Phoradendron flavescens*) is a cardiotoxin with vasopressor effects.

Moon seed *(Menispermacae)* contains toxin with convulsant properties.

Mormon tea (*Ephedra nevadensis*) contains ephedrine and can result in the symptoms of sympathomimetic overdose.

Morning glory seeds (*Ipomea purpora* or *violacea* or *Rivea corymbosa*) is used as a hallucinogen. One seed can contain up to 25 μg of lysergic acid. It may produce nausea, vomiting, confusion, and coma.

Nutmeg (*Myristica fragrans*) is used to treat dyspepsia (carminative), musculoskeletal disorders, and arthritis and as an abortifacient. It has weak monoamine oxidase inhibitor properties and myristicin. It is metabolized into an amphetamine-like metabolite. Nutmeg is the dried ripe fruit of *Myristica fragrans,* a tree native to the South Pacific islands. Ground nutmeg is a cooking spice. Nutmeg contains volatile terpenes and aromatic ethers. The perceptible dose is 5 to 15 grams (1 to 3 ground nutmeg seeds) of myristica oil or nutmeg oil. It is a carminative in a dose of 0.03 mL. It is used as a hallucinogen in doses of 2 to 4 teaspoonfuls. It causes GI upset, agitation, coma, miosis, hypertension, and dry mouth.

Myristicin and **alamecin**, which resemble endogenous catecholamine neurotransmitters, are believed to be responsible for CNS effects. Myristica may also produce cardiovascular effects, including palpitations and mild hypertension. One fatality in an 8-year-old boy who ingested 14 grams was reported in 1908. It can produce miosis to differentiate it from anticholinergic agents. Effects begin 3 to 6 hours after ingestion, and the duration is up to 60 hours. Effects are similar to LSD and include tachycardia, tachypnea, mild hypertension, and mydriasis. Severe reactions with shock, hypotension, cyanosis, and hypothermia have been reported.

Onions (*Allium cepa*) have been used with garlic in traditional culinary fare since ancient times. See Garlic.

Oleander tea (*Nerium oleander*) contains cardiac glycosides, which could produce malignant, dysrhythmias and cardiac arrest.

Paraguay tea (*Ilex paraguayensis*) contains caffeine, theophylline, and essential oils. It is used medicinally as a bowel antispasmodic. It also contains belladonna alkaloids (atropine, scopolamine, hyoscyamine), which produced toxic anticholinergic symptoms and sent five people to the hospital in Queens in March 1994.

Panagamate. See Vitamin B-15.

Passion flower may produce convulsions and hypotension.

Pennyroyal (*Mentha pulegium* and *Hedeoma pulegiodes*) has oxytocic properties and has been used as an abortifacient. It has also been used for the regulation of menstruation. It contains *pulegone,* an aromatic ketone as its main toxin, which is bioactivated to a hepatotoxin by cytochrome P-450 (depletes the glutathione stores), and the mechanism of toxicity may also be due to an epoxide metabolite. Pennyroyal oil has produced GI bleeding, seizures, hematuria, shock, hepatotoxicity, and death. *N*-acetylcysteine has successfully treated one human case, but was unsuccessful in an animal model at doses used to treat acetaminophen.

Periwinkle vinca gives vinca alkaloids for cancer treatment.

Periwinkle rose (*Cathararhus rosus*) is a hallucinogen, but has produced seizures, GI upset, hepatotoxicity, and alopecia.

Pokeweed (*Phytolocca americana, P. decandra*) is called inkberry and Jerusalem artichoke. It contains saponins, triterpenes, and glycoproteins. Pokeweed may produce decreased vision, respiratory depression, seizures, and cardiac dysrhythmias. It has a mitogen action and may produce fulminant bloody diarrhea. It has produced possible mitogen aberrations. It is tolerated when rinsed twice in boiling water.

Royal jelly (queen bee jelly) is a milky white viscid secretion from the salivary glands of the worker hive bee *Apis mellifera* (Apidae). It is essential for the development of the queen bees. Royal jelly has been used as a "general tonic" and has been incorporated in some cosmetic preparations for its supposed beneficial effect on skin tissue. Consumption of royal jelly (about 2 capsules) by man has been followed by severe respiratory distress, asthma, anaphylaxis, and death.[10–12]

Sassafras (*Sassafras albidum*) contains safrole and derivatives that are carcinogenic in animals. It may be associated with hepatic tumors. The FDA has banned safrole-containing products. Safrole inhibits microsomal enzymes. In animals ataxia, hypothermia, CNS depression, hepatotoxic, and hepatic tumors have occurred.

Senna (*Cassia acutifolia* or *C. angustifolia*) is a natural laxative; however, too large a dose will cause diarrhea. Senna in very large doses may produce liver toxicity, electrolyte disturbances, and cardiac dysrhythmias.

Skullcap. See Geramander.

Simplex plus is mainly 200 mg/2 mL of a bitter alkaloid of the plant *Menispermum condense* and has been promoted as a muscle-building and testosterone-increasing agent. Plant steroids are used in the manufacture of steroidal drugs, but there is no scientific evidence that natural steroids are converted into testosterone in the human body.

Slang nut in Thailand and Southeast Asia is called *Salang chai nut,* which contains strychnine from *Strychnos nux vomica.*

Snake root (*Rauwolfia serpentina*) contains reserpine, which can produce hypotension, bradycardia, and CNS intoxication.

Tansy ragwort (*Senecio jacobea*) contains hepatotoxic pyrrolizidine alkaloids.

Tonka bean (*Dipteryx odoratum* and *Doumarouna oppositofilia*) contains coumarin and produces prolonged prothrombin time and bleeding.

Tung Shueh pills (see Black balls) contain mefenamic acid and diazepam, neither of which is listed on the label. Acute renal failure has followed the use of mefenamic acid, phenylbutazone, and aristolochic acid in these preparations.[13]

Tu-san-chi (*Gynura segetum*) contains hepatotoxic pyrrolizidine.

Valerian (*Valerian officianalis*) has been used as an antispasmodic and sedative since the Middle Ages. It can produce ataxia and hypotension.

Vitamin B-15 or **Panagamate** is not a B vitamin and is obtained from apricot seeds. It is similar to laetrile. It has the potential to cause cyanide poisoning if ingested.

Woodruff (*Galium segetum*) contains coumarin, which can cause prolonged prothrombin time and bleeding.

Wormwood. See Absinthe.

Yellow root. See Golden seal.

Yohimbe, YoYo (*Crynanthe yohimbine*) is used as an aphrodisiac and hallucinogen. In overdose it may cause hypertension, weakness, and paralysis.

Tuba-tuba from the black Jatropha seed is a Philippine remedy. It produces vomiting, abdominal pain, nausea, muscle twitching, salivation, and weakness.

DRUG-HERBAL INTERACTIONS

Increased toxicity may follow the use of herbal compounds and conventional medications (Table 73–5). Herbs may be associated with teratogenic and carcinogenic properties.[6]

DRUG COMBINATIONS

The use of unapproved imported drug combinations is common among recent immigrants to the United States, particularly those from Asia and Latin America. These products are frequently perceived as relatively harmless "folk remedies." They often contain corticosteroids or anabolic steroids; nonsteroidal, antiinflammatory drugs; prescription antibiotics such as tetracycline and chloramphenicol; and controlled substances such as diazepam and narcotics.

AFRICA, MIDDLE EAST[14–26]

IDENTIFICATION OF HERBS

There are four ways to name a herb: the English common name, transliteration of the herb name, the latinized pharmaceutical name, and the scientific name. For example, the corresponding names for ginseng are ginseng, ren-shen, vadix ginseng, and *Parax ginseng.* Common names are usually very loose: the name ginseng is also applied to *P. ginseng* (oriental ginseng), *P. Quinquefolium* (American ginseng), and *Eleutherococus senticosus* (Siberian ginseng). The Chinese Medicinal Material Research Centre at the Chinese University of Hong Kong can be of considerable assistance in identifying the true identity of herbs.[27]

TRADITIONAL MEDICINES

Chinese traditional medicines are used as first-line medication by the majority of Chinese people in Hong Kong for the common cold, a sore throat, cough, or general health.[28] Few adverse effects have been observed. Some of these medications may be obtained in the United States from health food stores, Chinese markets, or by mail order. These preparations may contain such toxic chemicals as aminopyrine, lead,[29] phenylbutazone,[30] and cardiac glycosides. Additional drugs found in Chinese herbal medicine include betamethasone, chlordiazepoxide, dexamethasone, diazepam, hydrocortisone, indomethacin, mefanamic acid, methyltestosterone, prednisolone, prednisone, aminopyrine, caffeine, chlorpheniramine, chlorzoxazone, ethaverine, hydrochlorothiazide, paracetamol, phenylbutazone, and thiamine.[31] Herbal medicine obtained in Korea induced both lead and arsenic poisoning.[32]

LEAD POISONING

Lead poisoning due to traditional ethnic remedies has been reported in a number of countries.[19] Asian preparations are often "tonics" and aphrodisiacs, which appear to be a particular hazard. Analysis of such remedies may disclose the presence of lead oxide, lead sulfate, and lead nitrate.[24]

KOHL

Kohl is a cosmetic predominantly used as an eye makeup by women and men and on children and babies and has been purchased in Morocco, Mauritania, Great Britain, and the United States.[16–18] When tested, samples have contained in excess of 50% lead, often as galena, or lead sulfide, in addition to ground antimony.[14]

SURMA[15,19]

The substance known as kohl in the Middle East and Africa is identical to surma, a commonly used eye makeup in India, Iran, Pakistan, Bangladesh, Nepal, and southern regions of the former Soviet Union.[6] Frequently, mothers or relatives apply this product to infants and children as a traditional measure to beautify and to protect the child from the "evil eye." Such patients may present with plumbism, which can end fatally.[23] Lead absorption is alimentary following wiping of the irritant compound from the eyes followed by subsequent finger sucking. Great Britain outlawed the importation and sale of surma under the Cosmetics Products Safety Regulation in 1984. This has been marginally successful in curtailing its use. Laboratory confirmation of the lead content of some surmas is available.[15]

KHAT

(See Amphetamine chapter.)[33]

TRADITIONAL HERBAL MEDICINES

Acute renal failure has followed use of traditional herbal remedies in Kenya. Herbal plants associated with renal damage include *Euphorbia matabelensis* and *Cotalaria laburnifolia*.[34] Traditional medicinal plants used by Zulu and Xhosa residents of South Africa include various families of the superorder *Liliiflorae sona*. Some fatalities are summarized in Table 1C.[35]

In Cameroon tetracycline capsules are extremely popular and have been given the local (Bulu) name of Fokolo, which means wound healer.[24,25]

TURKEY

About 69 medicinal plants have been used as part of folk medicine. Yesilada and colleagues have identified the plants, parts used, methods of preparation, and traditional users.[36]

"SPIRITUAL WATER"

Overdosage of copper salts is common in developing countries because of its wide use in various traditional preparations. Poisoning due to the ingestion of "spiritual green water" follows distribution to members of spiritual churches. The amount of copper sulfate ingested is about 10 to 20 g, a lethal dose. Within a few hours of ingestion, greenish vomiting and abdominal pain are seen. Anuria may supervene within 24 hours. Flapping tremor, toxic psychosis, hemolytic anemia, and jaundice may follow within a few days. Hepatic and renal failure precede death within 7 days. Patients appear to die within a few days of hemodialysis. Analysis of water has revealed copper sulfate concentrations of 100 to 150 g/L. Similar cases have occurred in the United States.[37]

PARAPHENYLENEDIAMINE (PPD)

Paraphenylenediamine (PPD), an aromatic diamine, is a hair dye used as a cosmetic in Africa, the Middle East, and the countries of the Indian subcontinent where it is commonly mixed with henna (leaves of *Lausonia alba*) and applied to color the palms of the hands and soles of the feet and to dye hair a dark red shade.[38] Ingestion produces a characteristic clinical sequence of events that is often fatal. In the Sudan it is a frequent cause of suicidal poisoning.[38,39] Intensive supportive care may lead to recovery.[40]

STRUCTURE AND CLASSIFICATION

p-Phenylenediamine (1,4-diaminobenzene) is an aromatic diamine. The dyeing action of PPD depends on its oxidation by the addition of hydrogen peroxide. Its molecular weight is 108.2. PPD is a pale crystalline solid.[40]

USES

PPD is mainly used as an oxidizable hair dye, in dyeing furs, and in the photochemical and tire vulcanizing industries.[39]

PRODUCT FORMULATION

PPD is sold in local markets as a powder or as small stony lumps.

SOURCES

PPD is a synthetic chemical.

TOXIC DOSE

An oral dose of about 7 g may be followed by serious side effects.[39] The lethal dose in man is estimated to be 10 g.

CLINICAL PRESENTATION

Symptoms usually appear within 4 to 6 hours after ingestion.[40]

1. Initially local irritation of the mucous membranes and skin results in intense edema often requiring a tracheostomy. Yogi describes the acute PPD poisoning phase: edema of the head and neck and a wooden, hard, swollen, protruding tongue. The clinical picture may resemble a Ludwig's angina.[41]
2. Upper respiratory tract obstruction. Endotracheal intubation may be difficult.
3. Drowsiness, tremors, seizures, and disturbance of consciousness.[42]
4. Vomiting and dysphagia.
5. Rigid painful limbs.
6. Rhabdomyolysis, acute renal failure, and sudden cardiac death have been observed.
7. Acute renal failure may be due to methemoglobin formation and hemolysis.[39,42] The metabolic products of PPD are quinones, which may be nephrotoxic.
8. Rare permanent blindness and exophthalmia have been described.[39,42]
9. Hypotensive shock is associated with a poor prognosis.
10. Death is usually due to acute respiratory distress.[38]

LABORATORY

Analytic Methods

Urine PPD may be detected by thin-layer chromatography plates sprayed with 0.2% aqueous potassium permanganate. This method is sensitive to 1 μg of PPD.[39]

Blood Levels

No dye has been detected in the blood.

Abnormalities

The urine is usually chocolate brown in color and clears to a normal color within 48 to 72 hours.[39]

Ancillary Tests

Anemia, leukocytosis, hemoglobinemia, and hemoglobinuria have been observed.

TREATMENT

Stabilization

Patients should be hospitalized. Treatment is mainly supportive and symptomatic. The major early challenge to life is asphyxia followed by renal failure. Early tracheostomy is advisable. Renal dialysis may be lifesaving when oliguria develops. Hydrocortisone 100 mg to 300 mg intravenously and 100 mg every 3 to 6 hours, together with an intravenous antihistamine (e.g., chlorpheniramine maleate 4 to 6 mg intravenously)[39] have been used empirically. Treatment following prompt diagnosis or suspicion of acute hair dye poisoning is usually successful. There are no antidotes.

IBOGAINE

Ibogaine, an alkaloid, is an investigational drug being developed as a possible addiction interrupter for heroin, cocaine, amphetamine, nicotine, and alcohol. The product is used in Gabonese villages to induce visions during initiation rites. It has not been approved for general use by the U.S. Food and Drug Administration. The concept of a hallucinogen disrupting addictive behavior has not been clinically tested. Ibogaine exerts stimulatory, hallucinogenic, and tremorigenic properties. Its major effects appear to be (a) inhibition of cholinesterase resulting in hypotension; (b) central nervous system stimulation leading to seizures, paralysis, and respiratory arrest at high doses in animals, and (c) visual and other hallucinations often associated clinically with severe anxiety and apprehension.

STRUCTURE AND CLASSIFICATION

The ibogaine molecular formula is $C_{20}H_{26}N_2O$. Ibogaine hydrochloride is an indole alkaloid.[43]

Synonym

Endabuse.

Ibogaine is a Schedule I controlled substance in the United States similar to other hallucinogenic substances such as LSD and mescaline like heroin.

SOURCES

One of the main alkaloids extracted from the roots of *Tabernanthe iboga,* a shrub indigenous in French equatorial Africa, is ibogaine. It may also be synthesized. The plant belongs to the Apocynaceae family. The powdered bark is cultivated by West Africans.

DOSES

Therapeutic Doses

Doses of 500 mg (7.7 mg/kg) to 1000 mg have been used in clinical investigation. The usual regimen by individuals who choose to use this chemical involves one or two test doses (50 to 100 mg orally) followed the next day by a therapeutic doses (9 to 25 mg/kg). Data in humans is limited.[44]

Toxic Doses

At doses of 150 mg some difficulty in sleeping and perception of colored lights may be experienced. Doses of 20 mg or higher lead to dilation of the pupils and an increase in systolic blood pressure but no effects on temperature, pulse rate, or respiratory rate.[45] At 300 mg of the dried root bark powder slight nausea, dizziness, and a lack of muscular control or coordination may be experienced. Visual imagery and heightened empathy are experienced. At doses 1 gram ibogaine is a type of hallucinogen. In humans single oral doses of 5 to 25 mg/kg lead to an onset of CNS and cardiovascular effects in 15 to 40 minutes.

TOXICOKINETICS

Many of the toxicokinetic studies have been performed on animals.

Distribution

The volume of distribution is estimated at about 5 L/kg.

Elimination

The 24-hour recovery of unchanged ibogaine in the urine is less than 5% of the dose. An indole metabolite accounts for about 15% of the dose.[46] The elimination half-life is about 38 hours.

Drug Interactions

Ibogaine prevents the rise in brain dopamine levels usually observed after a morphine injection.[47] Ibogaine antagonizes adrenaline, acetylcholine, yohimbine, and atropine.[44] Ibogaine in animals enhances amphetamine- and cocaine-induced increases in brain dopamine levels.

MECHANISM OF ACTION

In animal studies a negative chronotropic effect on the heart has been observed. Both a blood pressure fall (vasodilatory) and rise have been seen. This is caused by an excitatory action of ibogaine on the reticular activating system.[43] Negative chronotropic and inotropic effects are seen.[48] This alkaloid has distinct central stimulating properties. Ibogaine is a central stimulant that exhibits weak but definite anticonvulsant properties.[44] Ibogaine itself is nonaddictive. Ibogaine inhibits the oxidation of serotonin and catalyzes that of catecholamines by a monoamine oxidase, ceruloplasmin. Ibogaine does not possess opiate-like pharmacologic properties. It does not produce physical dependence. It is not a substitute for morphine, and it has no analgesic properties. Ibogaine does not modulate the effects of norepinephrine, serotonin, acetylcholine, and histamine in the heart. Ibogaine produces a selective degeneration of Purkinje cells in the cerebellum.[49] This may be related to its putative antiaddictive effects, suggesting that the cerebellum may be involved in addictive behavior.[50]

CLINICAL PRESENTATION

Crude extracts of *Tabernanthe iboga* have been associated with a feeling of excitement, drunkenness, mental confusion, and hallucinations in high doses.[43] The effect of ibogaine lasts about 30 hours during which time ibogaine exerts a stimulant effect. Effects are noticed in 15 to 20 minutes after oral administration. Initially, a numbing of the skin is accompanied by an auditory buzzing and oscillating sounds. In 25 to 30 minutes objects appear to vibrate. Nausea may follow. The visions end abruptly, and the numbness of the skin begins to abate followed by 6 to 8 hours of a high energy state with "lighting" or flashes of light dancing about the subjects. Between 26 and 36 hours stimulation diminishes and the subject falls asleep. Ibogaine results in the complete elimination of narcotic withdrawal sequelae.[44] Postural tremor, vertigo, and nystagmus have been observed clinically. There is little controlled clinical data to support its use in treating opiate addiction.[50]

Acute

Acute effects have included photophobia, ataxia, oscillating vision, dizziness, out-of-body experiences, vertigo, nystagmus, nausea, and hallucinations. Peak cardiovascular and CNS effects occur in 1.5 to 2 hours after ingestion of about 20 mg/kg. Most patients recover from tremor and ataxia in 4 to 8 hours. Animal studies indicate that clinical signs of toxicity include tremors, abnormal breathing, spasticity of the legs, and seizures. Parasympathomimetic findings include diarrhea, lacrimation, salivation, and nasal discharge. Body temperature rise is dose related.

ASIAN CONTINENT

CHUIFONG TOKUMAN

Chuifong tokuman, a pharmaceutical product manufactured in Hong Kong, is a combination product containing diazepam, hydrochlorothiazide, mefenamic acid, dexamethasone, lead, and cadmium. It is not approved by the U.S. Food and Drug Administration and not legal for sale in or importation into the United States. It is available in Texas. The drug is distributed illegally in the United States. Chuifong tokuman may increase the body burden of cadmium. Renal tubular cell damage has been reported in such patients.[51]

KUSHTAY

Preparations called "kushtay," used especially as tonics and aphrodisiacs, contain oxidized heavy metals such as arsenic, mercury, tin, zinc, and lead. A typical kushtay may contain 10 to 12% of each of several of these metals. (See China.)

PAYLOOAH

Paylooah is used in Southeast Asia for rash or fever. It is an orange-red powder and may contain lead.[51]

CANTHARIDIN

One of the best known traditional medicines responsible for acute poisoning is the cantharidin beetle. There are over 300 species producing cantharidin belonging to the Meloidae family in South Africa. It is ground to a powder and used in a medicine called seletsa by the Tswanas as an aphrodisiac, abortifacient, and for purifying the blood. Seletsa poisoning produces severe gastrointestinal irritation and ulceration. Nephrotoxicity occurs with hematuria and dysuria, and fatalities are relatively common. It is a common cause of death associated with traditional medicine poisoning.

Cantharidin is a toxic terpenoid produced by beetles.[52,53] The dried and powdered blister beetle is termed cantharides. Cantharidin was for many years wrongly believed to be an aphrodisiac and an abortifacient based on its tendency to cause marked irritation to the genitourinary system leading to priapism in men and pelvic congestion in women. In overdose it may lead to death.[53–57]

STRUCTURE

Cantharidin (hexahydro-2 alpha, 7 alpha-dimethyl-4 beta, 7 beta-epoxyisobenzofura-1,3,dione) is the anhydride of cantharidic acid derived from beetles.[53]

USES

Cantharidin has been used as an aphrodisiac, abortifacient, wart remover (topically), and as a diuretic agent in veterinary medicine.

PRODUCT FORMULATION

Crystals of cantharides are colorless, odorless, and glistening, and are very water insoluble (1 : 30,000 cold), slightly soluble in alcohols, and soluble in acetone at 1 : 40 dilutions.[58,59] It is soluble in oils, which help dissolve the toxin and increase intestinal absorption.

SOURCES

Insects producing cantharidin are beetles belonging to the order *Coleoptera*, family Meloidae, and are commonly known as "blister beetles" or the "Spanish fly" (*Lytta vesicatoria*,[60] *Cantharis vesicatoria*). There are perhaps more than 1500 species of cantharidin-yielding beetles with several species in the United States.[59] The ovaries, soft tissues, and blood of blister beetles have the highest concentrations of cantharidin.[59] *Epicauta vittata* and *E.*

pennsylvanica are found in the south and southwestern parts of the United States and propagate in alfalfa, along fence rails, and in flower beds. They range up to 1 inch in size and are variable in color.[61,62] Cantharidin poisoning is relatively common in South Africa because of the widespread use of cantharides by local herbalists.[60,63]

TOXIC DOSE

Patients have survived after ingestions of 75 mg and 175 mg, respectively,[53] and after ingestion of 20 mg.[64]

FATAL DOSE

The fatal dose has varied between approximately 10 mg[59] and 65 mg.[56]

MECHANISM OF ACTION

Cantharidin is a severe irritant to epithelial linings (gastrointestinal tract, urinary tract, skin). It leads to a separation of cells in the skin and liver similar to acantholysis. Details of the mechanism of its toxicity are unknown.[65,66]

CLINICAL PRESENTATION[53–57,59,60,64–72]

Skin—Topical use

Symptoms after application of a toxic quantity of cantharidin to the skin can result in a full spectrum of toxicity ranging from inflammation followed by blistering within 4 to 5 hours to death within 12 hours.[59] Handling the beetles, crushing them on the skin, or applying their vesiculating fluid to the genitals can result in blisters on the skin of the penis, scrotum, and labia.[62] Cantharidin liquor was painted on an area of the abdomen measuring 7 × 2¾ inches. Within 1 hour there were signs of urgency, hematuria, tachycardia, profuse sweating, pain at the distal end of the penis, and dysuria, followed by oliguria. The patient survived.[68]

Mouth

Within 10 minutes after ingestion of cantharidin burning of the lips, mouth, and pharynx begin. Ulcerations and excoriations of the lips and buccal mucosa develop with perilabial encrustations of blood. The tongue becomes swollen.

Gastrointestinal

Nausea, vomiting, and diarrhea may begin within 5 minutes to 1 hour, accompanied by midline abdominal pain and tenderness and by hematemesis.

Genitourinary

Frequency, dysuria, hematuria, and flank pain are early signs developing within the first hour and progressing over the first 12 hours. This may progress to oliguria for up to 15 days.[68] Pathology of the kidney frequently reveals an acute tubular necrosis. Priapism may be painful.[57] Death may follow renal failure.[53]

Cardiac

Sinus tachycardia with a normal blood pressure may be observed within the first hour. Arrhythmias commonly observed have included ventricular fibrillation and asystole. Multiple punctate hemorrhages have been observed in the pericardium and subendocardium.[59,67,69,72]

Hematologic

Leukocytosis and a pseudopolycythemia have been described, which revert to normal after dehydration is corrected.[67]

Neurologic

Several days after ingestion patients may develop dilated pupils that are nonreactive to light, numbness of the hands and feet, and a "glove and stocking" type peripheral neuropathy that may be associated with diminished deep tendon reflexes (ankle jerk, knee jerk). Within 10 days bilateral lower motor neuron lesions of the facial nerves with weakness of the upper limbs may be seen. After 3 weeks these signs begin to improve.[60]

Pulmonary

Pulmonary edema, coma, and death may follow cantharidin use.[62]

LABORATORY

Analytic Methods

Identification of cantharidin is based on its x-ray diffraction, its melting point, its ability to cause a skin reaction of pain and blistering when applied cutaneously,[59] and by a gas chromatography/mass spectrometry (GC/MS) method using clofibrate as an internal standard. The GC/MS detection limit is 26 nM/L (5 ng/ml).[52,57]

Blood Levels

Blood levels of cantharidin have ranged from 72.3 ng/mL to 110 ng/mL[57] in patients who died.

Abnormalities

Hypokalemia, hypocalcemia, and moderate elevations of serum bilirubin and serum aminotransferase levels have been observed.[62,67] Hematuria (gross and microscopic) and proteinuria may be associated with elevations in blood urea concentration and serum creatinine levels. Serum amylase levels may be elevated.[53]

Ancillary Tests

The electrocardiogram may show elevations of the ST segments in lead II, III, AVF, V_1 to V_3 with T-wave inversion in V_2 and V_3.[67] Elevations of the hematocrit, red blood cell counts, and hemoglobin levels have been noted, with increased red blood cells in the cerebrospinal fluid.[60]

TREATMENT

Stabilization

Patients should be admitted to a hospital where fluids (intake and output) and electrolytes may be monitored. Immediate symptomatic and supportive care to mouth lesions will provide some relief. Cardiac monitoring, intravenous fluids, and oxygen should be available. Intravenous fluids will be required to correct a dehydration. Arterial blood gases, hematologic studies (hemoglobin, packed red cell volume, red blood cell, and leukocyte counts), serum amylase, serum creatinine, liver function studies (aminotransferases), serum electrolytes, and urinalysis should be closely followed. Diarrhea will be treated supportively and symptomatically. Tracheostomy may be required. Esophagoscopy will delineate damage to the esophagus.

Decontamination

Hemorrhagic excoriations in the mouth, esophagus, and stomach will preclude vigorous attempts at removal of the toxic substance. A nasogastric tube carefully inserted may provide a vehicle through which careful gastric lavage may be performed and into which antacids may be inserted. There is no evidence that activated charcoal or cathartics will be useful. Cathartics may compromise an already inflamed bowel.

Elimination Enhancement

There is no evidence to support the usefulness or safety of activated charcoal or cathartics. Where required to ameliorate anuria, hemodialysis may be required. Diuresis in the face of oliguria or anuria may predispose the patient to fluid overload, acute pulmonary edema, and, in view of the cardiac pathology that has been observed, possible heart failure.

Antidote

There are no antidotes.

Supportive Measures

Patients should be admitted to an intensive care unit for follow-up care of pain control, cardiologic changes, diarrhea, hematemesis, and neurologic abnormalities. Intravenous hydrocortisone and antibiotics have been administered, but further work remains to confirm their usefulness.[72]

Skin lesions should be cleansed with acetone, ether, fatty soap, or alcohol, since these substances dissolve or dilute the cantharidin.[62] Lesions then should be thoroughly and repeatedly washed with soap and water. Calamine lotion containing a steroid may be useful. Treatment is largely symptomatic and supportive.[73]

PLANTS (TABLES 73–8 AND 73–9)

Several plants containing oils that are irritant laxatives are used as traditional medicines. These include the castor oil plant *(Ricinus communis),* which is used as a laxative, and *Jatropha curcas*, known as mohlapametsi. The latter contains curcanoleic acid and is used as a laxative, or the oil from the seeds is applied to painful joints. Poisoning presents with watery diarrhea. Dehydration in these cases may need intravenous fluid replacement.

Another well-known plant used as a traditional medicine is *Datura stramonium*, which contains belladonna alkaloids. It is known as mokhura to the Tswanas, and the features of

Table 73–8
Some Poisonous Plants Commonly Used in Traditional Practice in Zimbabwe [a]

Plant	Local Name	Part Used	Medicinal Use
Aloe	Chikowa (C)	Leaves	Constipation, Abortion
chabaudii Schonl.	Chinyangami (T)		
christianii Reynolds	Chinyangami (T)	Leaves	Poisons to pregnant women, abortion, gynecological problems
globuligema Pole-Evans	Chinyangami (T)	Leaves	Abdominal pains, venereal diseases
Boophane disticha	Mumhandwe (C)	Bulb	To arouse spirits (ancestral)
(L.f) Herb	Ingcotho (N)		
Capparis Tomentosa	Mukorongwe (T)	Root	Illness due to miscarriage
Lam	Gondashindi (H)		
Chenopodium ambresioides L.	Dungurachirombo (C)	Leaves	Convulsions, psychosis
		Whole plant	Snake repellent
Croton megalobotrys	Mutonga (T)	Root or Bark	Purgative, malaria
Muell. Arg.	Mubvuguta		Dropsy, abortion
Dalbergia nitidula	Murima (C)	Bark	Ulcers washed with infusion
Bak.	Linvani (H)		
Datura stramonium L.	Chowa (C)	Leaves	Asthma, aid in divination
Euphorbia ingens	Umhlonhlo (N)	Latex	Emetic, purgative
Boiss	Mukonde (C)		
Gnidia, kraussiana	Chitupatupa (C)	Tuber	Emetic?
Meisn.	Isidikili (N)		Constipation
Securidaca longepedunculata	Mufufu (C)	Root	Epilepsy, headache
Fresen	Umfumfu (N)		Emetic, purgative, rheumatism

[a] Adapted from Nyazema NZ. Cent Afr J Med 1984;30:80–83.
C, Central Shona; *T*, Tonga; *N*, Ndebele; *H*, Hlengwe.

Table 73–9
Medicinal Plants and Their Chemical Constituent(s) [a]

Plant	Constituent(s)
Aloe spp.	Oxymethylanthraquinone derivatives
Boophane disticha	Buphanine, buphanitine, caranine, buphanamine
Capparis tomentosa	1-Stachydine, alkaloids, sulphur oil
Chenopodium ambrosioides	Nitrates
Croton megalobotrys	Opium? 4-hydroxyhygric acid
Datura stramonium	Hyocynamine, hyoscine, atropine
Euphorbia ingens	Polycyclic ketone
Gnidia kraussiana	Mezareine, phytosterol
Securidaca longe-pedunculata	Methyl salicylate, steroid glycoside, saporia

[a]Adapted from Nyazema NZ. Cent Afr J Med 1984;30:80–83.

acute poisoning are due to its anticholinergic effects and include dilatation of the pupils, tachycardia, and central nervous system irritation and even hallucinations.

Poisoning due to the plant *Callilepis laureola* is a well-described entity in Natal. It is known as "impela" to the Zulus and poisoning results in severe hepatotoxicity associated with hypoglycemia. *Urginea burkei* is known as sekanama to Tswana traditional healers who use the bulb for purifying the blood. It contains a cardiac glycoside, and poisoning manifests with nausea and vomiting. In severe cases cardiac depression may occur.[4]

Reports to the National Poisons Unit in London have included heavy metal poisoning associated with Asian medicines, drowsiness, and severe liver damage from herbal tranquilizers, and thyrotoxicosis from exposure to kelp.[74]

CHINA[75,80]

The Ministry of Public Health is trying to combat the trade in bogus and inferior pharmaceuticals. Special telephone lines have been set up to give the public information about the production and sale of bogus medicine, which in the past 6 years has included 90 products with over 45,000 reports of the production and sale of such materials.[81]

The Chinese Medicinal Material Research Center in 1992 identified the following issues as high priority: education in the proper use of traditional Chinese medicine, the drawing up of "potent herbs" list to facilitate control, and the introduction of registration and regulation of practitioners of traditional Chinese medicine.[82]

CHINESE PATENT MEDICINE (TABLE 73–10)

Chinese patent medicines (CPM) in North America have become more significant to the clinician because of a number of contributory factors, including the increasing number of immigrants from Asia; the increasing quantity, sources, and availability of CPM in the open market; increasing non-Asian users (particularly patients with serious chronic diseases); inadequate regulation by the U.S. Food and Drug Administration and manufacturers (or distributors); lack of communication between consumer and "prescriber"; limited improvisation available on CPM for health care, professional, and the general public; and finally, the inadequate reporting of adverse drug reactions and toxic experiences.[83]

INFORMATION SOURCES

Herbal medicine deriving from traditional Chinese medicine has been reviewed by several authors.[84–86]

MERCURY (TABLE 73–10)[80]

Chinese patent medicines may commonly contain cinnabar (mercuric sulfide) and calomel (mercurous chloride).[80] The influx of new immigrants to North America has resulted in an increase in the availability and use of CPM orally. There is also an increase in the number of non-Chinese CPM users due to the impact of the "back-to-nature" movement.

LEAD

Lead poisoning from ingestion of a herbal medication of Chinese origin, in the form of orange and red pills, has been reported. These were found to contain lead at a concentration of 0.5 mg per pill.[76]

PLANTS FOR SNAKEBITE

In China plant products are used for the treatment of snakebite as an interim measure until qualified support is available. There have been no systematic investigations to indicate any efficacy for these products.[87]

THALLIUM

Thallium intoxication has been observed following ingestion of a Chinese herbal medication/nutritional supplement purchased in the United States.[88]

Chinese herbal remedies have served as a basis for the development of useful therapeutic products (Table 73–11).[84]

ACONITE

Herb-induced aconite poisoning is great in Chinese communities worldwide. In China alone there were over 600 reported cases in the past 30 years. The genus *Aconitum* belongs to the Ranunculaceae family and is widely distributed throughout the Northern Hemisphere. There are over 350 species worldwide and approximately 170 in China alone. Aconite tubers are among the most toxic plants known, but have been used in Eastern and Western therapeutics for centuries. The raw tuber is usually processed by drying, soaking, or boiling, which significantly reduces its toxicity. In Europe aconite is derived from the species *Aconitum napellus*, also known as Monkshood or Wolfsbane. Aconite last appeared in the British Pharmacopoeia in 1953 and is now only used in Western countries as a proarrhythmic agent in animal studies to test the efficacy of antiarrhythmic agents.[89]

In Hong Kong at present there are no regulatory controls, and it is estimated that 75% of Chinese herbal medicine–related admissions to hospitals are due to aconite toxicity.[82] The alkaloids are sodium channel activators, which affect all excitable tissues. Cardiotoxicity is due to an indirect effect (via stimulation of the vagal medullary center) resulting in bradycardia, sinus node arrest, and hypotension, and due to a direct effect on the myocardium in which prolonged repolarization results in triggered automaticity and a variety of tachyarrhythmias. Symptoms of poisoning usually occur within an hour of ingestion.[89]

DOSES

Therapeutic Doses

The recommended dose of cured Caowu and Chaanwu in China is 1.5 to 3 g.[90]

Toxic Dose

Severe poisoning occurs with as little as 0.2 mg of aconite or the consumption of concoctions prepared for prescriptions containing 6 g of cured aconite.[90]

The aconites are among the most toxic plants known. Severe poisoning can occur after ingestion of as little as 5 mL of aconite tincture, 0.2 mg of aconitine, or 1 g of cured plant.[88]

Fatal Dose

Fatalities have followed ingestions of 9 to 18 g.[90]

MECHANISM OF ACTION

The diterpene alkaloids, aconitine, mesaconitine, and hypaconitine, are known neurotoxins that can cause conduction block and paralysis through their action on the voltage-sensitive sodium channels in the axons.[92]

Symptoms generally begin within 0.5 to 1.5 hours after drinking the broth and last up to 30 hours. Patients generally present with features that are typical of aconitine poisoning, namely, cardiovascular (palpitations, hypotension, ventricular ectopics/arrhythmias), gastrointestinal (nausea, vomiting, diarrhea), and neurologic (numbness, paresthesia, and weakness of extremities) signs and symptoms.[93] The conscious state may be reduced. Hypotensive, sustained, ventricular tachyarrhythmias are the direct cause of death. Acidosis and hypokalemia are seen.[82]

CLINICAL PRESENTATION

Most cases of serious poisoning by Chinese herbal medicines (CHM) are related to the use of the aconites Chaowi, the root of *Aconitum kusrezoffii,* and Chuanwu, the root of *Aconitum carmichaeli.* The alkaloids are sodium channel activators. Presenting signs and symptoms may be neurologic (paresthesia and numbness in the mouth, lips, and limbs and/or seizures). Deep tendon reflexes may be absent. Cardiac arrhythmias or gastrointestinal (nausea, vomiting, diarrhea) symptoms of poisoning usually occur within an hour of ingestion. Aconite cardiotoxicity usually resolves within 24 hours. The main causes of death are cardiovascular collapse and ventricular arrhythmias.

TREATMENT

Stabilization

1. Symptoms begin within 1 hour after ingestion. Induced emesis with syrup of ipecac is therefore contraindicated because of the damage of pulmonary aspiration.
2. Refer the patient to health care facility immediately.
3. If patients are seen within 1 to 2 hours, gastric lavage may be attempted.
4. Activated charcoal may assist in decreasing absorption of the alkaloid.
5. Perform an arterial blood gas, serum electrolytes, creatine phosphokinase (fractionated), and an electrocardiogram.
6. Serum levels of aconites are not of value.
7. Aggressive supportive care is the mainstay of therapy.

Elimination Enhancement

Serial activated charcoal, forced diuresis, hemodialysis, and hemoperfusion have not been studied and cannot be recommended.

Antidote

There is no antidote.

Supportive Measures

1. Provide airway support as required.
2. Establish vascular access.
3. Treat seizures with a benzodiazepine (diazepam) followed by phenytoin as required.
4. Treat metabolic acidosis and hypokalemia.
5. Atropine is administered for bradycardia and hypersalivation, but data for its use in tachyarrhythmias are inconclusive.[89]

Cardiotoxicity

1. The ideal drug therapy for aconite-induced tachyarrhythmias is not known.
2. No single antiarrhythmic agent is uniformly effective.[82,89]
3. DC cardioversion is ineffective in controlling tachyarrhythmias.[89]
4. Cardiopulmonary bypass and a left ventricular assist device were useful in treatment of one patient with severe aconite-induced cardiotoxicity.[89]

Anticholinergic Poisoning

Most cases of anticholinergic poisoning after ingestion of CHM are probably due to yangjinhua or naoyanghua, flowers of *Datura metel L* and *Flos rhododendri mollis,* respectively. These herbs may contain scopolamine, hyoscyamine, and atropine. Intoxication may result in confusion, coma, flushed dry skin, dilated pupils, tachycardia, fever, and urinary retention.

Table 73–10
Chinese Patent Medicine[a]

	English	Chinese	Source	Form	Total Weight	% HgS	% Hg2Cl2	Normal Dosage	Route	Claimed Common Disease Applications
1	She Dan Chen Pi San	蛇膽陳皮散	Guang Zhou United Pharm.	Powder	0.6 g	12.33% (.074 g)		A—1 vial BID C—½ vial BID	PO w/warm water	1. Acute pneumonia 2. Acute bronchitis 3. Whooping cough
2	Xi Gua Shuang (Water Melon Frost)	西瓜霜	Kweilin Drug Manu	Powder	2 g/vial	2% (0.04 g)		Int—1 vial BID–TID Ext—1 vial Q2–3hrs	PO/Ext	1. Disease of the mouth: ulcers, stomatitis 2. Burns on the skin
3	An Gong Niu Huang Wan	安宮牛黃丸	Beijing Tung Jen Tan Pharm.	Pill	3 g/pill	11.11% (0.033 g)		A—1 QD–TID	PO	1. Spasm due to high fever in epidemic diseases 2. Stroke, seizure
4	Ci Zhu Wan	磁朱丸	Guang Zhou Pharm. Industry Co.	Pill		14.40%		A—5–6 pills BID	PO	1. Kidney/heart disharmony 2. Epileptic seizures
5	An Shen Bu Nao Pian (Ansenpunaw Tablets)	安神補腦丸	Chung Lian Drug Works, Hang Zhou	Pill		6.90%		A—4 pills TID	PO	1. Neurasthenia 2. Meniere's syndrome 3. Hyperthyroidism
6	Bai Zi Yang Xin Wan (Pai Tze Yang Hsin Wan)	柏子養心丸	Lanzhou Chinese Medicine Works	Pill		3.80%		A—8–10 pills BID	PO	1. Neurasthenia w/chills, palpitations, etc.
7	Zhu Sha An Shen Wan (Cinnabar Sedative Pill)	硃砂安神丸	Lanzhou Chinese Medicine Works	Pill		17.40%		A—6 pills TID PC w/warm water	PO	1. Neurasthenia w/poor memory and depression 2. Hysteria
8	Jian Nao Wan (Healthy Brain Pills)	健腦丸	Tsingtao Medicine Works	Pill		4%		A—10 pills TID		1. Meniere's syndrome (tinnitus, vertigo)
9	Qi Li San	七厘散	Tung Jen Tang Pharmacy, Beijing	Powder	1.5 g/vial	7% (0.105 g)		Int—0.2–0.9 g TID Ext—apply QD		1. Sport, traumatic injuries w/open wound 2. Skin infection and sores 3. Pain due to chronic hepatitis

10	San Li Hui Chun Dan	三粒回春丹	Hong Kong	Wax ball		Coating only		C (>1yo)—1 BID–TID C(1–2 yo)—2 BID–TID C (8–12 yo)—5 BID–TID	PO	1. Pediatric: acute bronchitis, pneumonia, acute encephalitis, meningitis, gastroenteritis
11	Zi Jin Ding	紫金定		Powder	0.3 g or 3 g	6.25%		Int—0.6 g–1.5 g BID Ext—Apply as paste	PO/Ext	1. Pediatric: pneumonia, bronchitis 2. Summer heat stroke 3. Early stages of skin infection
12	Bao Ying Dan	保嬰丹	Guangzhou United Pharm. Manuf.	Powder Pill	0.3 g/vial 0.5 g/pill	4.98%		<1 mon—0.1 g BID–TID 1 yo—0.3 g BID–TID	PO	1. High-grade fever 2. Acute pneumonia, bronchitis
13	Hu Po Bao Long Wan (Po Lung Yuen Med. Pills)	琥珀抱龍丸	Hong Kong	Pill		4.70%		<1 mon—⅓ pill BID >1 yo—1 pill BID–TID	PO	1. Acute bronchitis, pneumonia 2. Epidemic encephalitis 3. High-grade fever assoc. w/measles
14	Wan Shi Niu Huang Qing Xin Wan	方氏牛黃清心丸	Beijing Tung Jen Tang Pharm.	Pill	3 g/pill	60 g/box?		A—1 pill BID C (<1 yo)—½ pill BID	PO	1. Acute stroke 2. Infantile convulsions, pneumonia 3. High-grade fever w/infection
15	Zi Xue Dan (Tzuh-sueh Tan)		Guangzhou United Drug Manuf.	Powder	0.8 g/via	not spec.		A—2 vials BID C (<1 yo)—½ vial BID	PO	1. Epidemic encephalitis, meningitis 2. Childhood measles
16	Tse Koo Choy	宏興鷓鴣菜	Wang Hing Co. H.K.	Powder	Powder paper		0.0096 g		PO	1. Pediatric: gastroenteritis
17	Su He Xiang Pills		Not available			not spec.				
18	Peaceful		Turtle Mount, USA			0.10%				1. Hypertension 2. Mental agitation, poor memory 3. Reduces blood cholesterol

[a]Adapted from Kang Yum E. Nyack NY: Hudson Valley Regional Poison Center.

Table 73–11
Drugs From Ancient Chinese Therapeutics[a]

		Use
Artemisin (quinghaosu)	Arterisia annua	Malaria
Henbane drug	Atropa belladonna Hyocyamus niger	Septic shock
Tetrahydro-palmitine	Corydalis yan husuo (Chinese famenot)	Sedative, tranquilizer
Yanhua (lilac daphne)	Daphne genkwa	Abortifacient
Trichesantin	Trichosanthese kilowii M	Abortifacient Hydotial mole
Indirubin	Indigo naturals	Cytotoxic
Triptonygium	Tripterygium spells	Antiinflammatory

[a]Adapted from Guang-Sheng D. Clin Ther 1987;9:345–357.

Table 73–12
Pharmacokinetics of *Ginkgo Biloba* Extract[a,b]

	Ginkgo-flavone glycosides	Ginkgolides (A or B)	Bilobalide
Oral bioavailability (%)	>60	>98 (A) >80 (B)	70
Time to peak concentration (h)	1.5–3	1–2	1–2
Volume of distribution (liters)	?	40–60 (A) 60–100 (B)	170
Protein binding	Unknown	Unknown	Unknown
Elimination half-life (h)	2–4	4–6	3
Clearance (ml/min)	?	130–200 (A) 140–250 (B)	600

[a]Adapted from Kleijnen J, Knipschild P. Lancet 1992;340:1136–1139.
[b]Preliminary data, partly from unpublished results.

ARTEMISIN

Artemisin compounds are effective antimalarials. Artemisin derivatives have been developed in China from the traditional remedy quinghamosu.[94,95]

BOUI-OUGI-TOU

Boui-ougi-tou is a mixture of Chinese crude drugs containing glycyrrhizin, which has been associated with a Fanconi syndrome in an anecdotal report of a patient who survived.[96]

DAIDZIN

The root of kudzu vine has been used by traditional Chinese healers to treat alcohol abuse. An extract of the herb *Radix puerariae* contains daidzinane daidzin and may reduce the craving for alcohol. Controlled clinical studies have not yet been performed.[97]

EPHEDRAS

Six different ephedrine alkaloids have been isolated from Chinese ephedras. Of these, ephedrine, pseudoephedrine, and norephedrine (phenylpropanolamine) are commonly used in the United States as decongestants or bronchodilators, and the other three—methylephedrine, methylpseudoephedrine, and norpseudoephedrine—are not available in the United States in pharmaceutical dosage form. Most species of Chinese ephedras contain methylephedrine, methylpseudoephedrine, ephedrine, pseudoephedrine, norephedrine, and norpseudoephedrine. Erythroderma has followed ingestion.[95] In the United States ephedrine is legal and can be obtained in over-the-counter diet and pep pills.[99] Activated charcoal may be useful in the overdose patient. Gastric lavage may increase the associated hypertension. Nifedipine and phentolamine or nitroprusside may be required.

FANG-JI

Fang-ji is dereived from *Aristolocha fangchi,* and contains aristolochic acid, which is nephrotoxic.[100–102] This has been the probable cause of an epidemic of Chinese herb nephropathy in over 80 women who ingested slimming remedies containing the Chinese herbs *Magnolia officinalis* and *Stephania tetrandra,* both containing the mutagenic *Aristolochia fangchi.* Chinese herb nephropathy may be associated with an increased risk for developing urothelial tumors.[103]

GINKGO BILOBA

Extracts from the dried leaves of Ginkgo biloba (maidenhair tree) are used by the Chinese to make tea for the treatment of asthma, bronchitis, peripheral vascular disease, and a number of central nervous system problems. Ingredients of ginkgo include flavonoids (ginkgo-flavone glycosides) and terpenoids (ginkgolides and bilobalide). Toxicokinetics of Ginkgo biloba extract are found in Table 73–12. Doses of 120 to 160 mg/day have been associated with headache, allergic skin reactions, and mild gastrointestinal complaints.[104]

HAI GE FEN

Hai Ge Fen (clamshell powder) may be contaminated with copper, chromium, arsenic, or lead.[105,106]

LICORICE

Glycyrrhiza uralensis (licorice) is a common component of traditional Chinese formulations. It contains glycyrrhetinic acid, which also has antiinflammatory properties, and it has been shown to potentiate the effect of topically applied hydrocortisone.[107]

JIN BU HUAN-LEVO: TETRAHYDROPALIMITINE (L-THP)

Jin Bu Huan is a Chinese herbal medication derived from plants of the genera *Stephania* and *Corydalis* and is used for relieving pain. Following ingestion of between 7 and 60 tablets, each containing 28.8 mg of L-THP, rapid-onset, life-threatening bradycardia and central nervous system and respiratory depression develop, which appears to respond to symptomatic and supportive therapy (activated charcoal, gastric lavage). There are no permanent sequelae. Hepatotoxicity (hepatitis) has been observed.[108,109] Analysis of L-THP in tablets may be performed using nuclear magnetic resonance and gas chromatography/mass spectroscopy. This is an example of a Chinese herbal product available in the United States.[110,111] Botanical ingredients may be incorrectly identified on the labeling.[112] Clinical studies suggest that the biochemical action of THP is similar to that of reserpine-like drugs. Brain dopamine, noradrenaline, and serotonin (%HT) concentrations are depleted.[113]

HERBAL MEDICINE

Naoyanghua (*Flos rhododenilipollis*)

This Chinese herbal medicine contains hyosena and atropine. Ingestion may lead to symptoms of anticholinergic poisoning.[114]

Yixin Wan (Toad Venom)

Yixin Wan is a nonprescription Chinese medication that contains toad venom (Ch'an Su), ginseng, pearl (Chem Chu), and musk (She Hsiang). The product is sold in the United States in ethnic grocery stores and pharmacies. Toad venom contains a digitalis-like immunoreactive cardiotrophic substance (bufotoxin). Bufotalin, a major bufotoxin in toad venom, has a chemical structure similar to digitalis.[115] Anecdotal reports indicate that ingestion of Yixin Wan has been followed by therapeutic levels of serum digoxin and atrioventricular node conduction dysfunction.[115]

Undeclared Synthetic Drugs

There have been reports that some traditional Chinese medicines contain potent synthetic drugs without disclosure of their presence (e.g., acetaminophen, prednisolone)[116] and other steroids.[117]

Yangjinhua

Yangjinhua, the dried flowers of *Datura metel L*, are used in southern Asia and southern China for treating bronchial asthma and chronic bronchitis. This preparation contains scopolamine, hyoscyamine, and atropine, which account for the anticholinergic symptoms of poisoning (dry mouth, dilated pupils, agitation, tachycardia, tachypnea, unsteady gait, hallucinations, coma, and death).[118]

Quinghaosu

Quinghaosu (artemisinin) is a sesquiterpene lactone peroxide derived from the leaves of the Chinese medicinal herb quinghao (*Artemisiana annua L*), a traditional Chinese medication used for the treatment of febrile illnesses. Artemisinin and its derivatives (e.g., dihydroartemisinin) appear to have antimalarial activity. Toxic effects reported have included a rare first-degree heart block, dose-related decrease in reticulocyte and neutrophil counts, increases in serum aspartate aminotransferase, abdominal pain, and diarrhea. Significant toxicity has been infrequent.[119,120]

EAST INDIES

East Indian herbal medicines often contain lead, mercury, arsenic, or cadmium. These may be used locally and by immigrants to the United States and elsewhere who have obtained such preparations from local practitioners unlicensed in the United States.[121]

SOUTHEAST ASIA

Acute hepatitis and renal failure following ingestion of raw carp gallbladders have been recognized in persons in Taiwan, Hong Kong, and South Korea. This syndrome includes acute gastrointestinal symptoms followed several days later by jaundice and oliguria. Bile components responsible for this syndrome have not been characterized. Cyprinol, a C_{27} alcohol, may have a direct toxic effect on the kidneys. No specific treatment has been identified; renal and hepatic impairment generally resolve within 3 weeks with supportive care.[122]

HONG KONG

At least 7000 species of medicinal plants are used in China. Of the 150 species most commonly used, about 10 are toxic. In Hong Kong the use of herbal remedies is widespread among the local Chinese.

Infants

About half of Chinese infants in Hong Kong are given chuenlin by their mother to clear various products of pregnancy. The chief alkaloid of chuenlin, berberine, can displace bilirubin from its serum binding proteins, which can result in a rise in the free bilirubin concentration. Southern Chinese have a high prevalence of glucose-6-phosphate dehydrogenase deficiency. Hence, kernicterus is common in Chinese infants even when they do not have clinically defined hemolysis.

Adulteration and Inadvertent Dispensing

Serious poisonings by CHM (Chinese herbal medicine) can occur when an importer or retailer mistakes one herb for another. Adulteration of CHM by cheaper and often more toxic substrates is common. Ingestion of ginseng (Panaxginseng) bought in China has occasionally led to symptoms of anticholinergic poisoning. Inadvertent dispensing has led to patients being given guijiu, which contains podophylline, instead of the intended longdancao (*Gentiana* species).

CHINESE PROPRIETARY MEDICINES (CPM)

CPM may contain Western drugs such as acetaminophen (paracetamol), aspirin, antihistamines, or steroids. The manufacturer's information leaflet may not warn of their side effects. CPM may contain heavy metals such as cadmium, lead, and arsenic. Many overseas Chinese obtain Chinese herbal medicine from visiting friends or by postal delivery.[123]

HMONG

Arsenic Poisoning[124–130]

Adult Hmong Southeast Asian refugees in Minnesota have presented with manifestations of arsenic poisoning, including anorexia, weight loss, paresthesias, depression, hyperkeratosis, blood dyscrasias, electrolyte disturbance, and a prolonged QT interval. Arsenic levels in the urine have been elevated. Patients have responded to treatment with BAL and penicillamine.[126]

LEAD POISONING

Medications such as Pay-Loo-Ah, a red and orange powder, are fed to children as a cure for fever and rash. Two samples confirmed lead at concentrations of 1 and 80%.[128]

INDIA[121,127,132,133]

METAL TOXICITY

Metal intoxication (arsenic, lead, and mercury) has been observed after ingestion of Indian ethnic remedies dispensed by Indian ethnic practitioners or hakin.[134]

Lead—Ghasard, Bola Goli, Kandu, Moha Yogran Guggulu

A fatal case of lead poisoning from medications originating in India was reported in 1984.[127] The highest of the three suspected materials, of East Indian origin, contained 1.6% lead by weight. This was a brown powder known as Ghasard administered as a tonic once daily to a 9-month-old child who later developed a blood lead concentration of 214 μg/dL and died from acute encephalopathy.[127] Two other medications from India used for stomachache have been Bola Goli (a round, flat, black bean) and Kandu (a red powder) containing 25 ppm and 7 ppm lead, respectively.[133] Moha Yogran Guggulu is taken for back pain and has a lead content of 6.47%.

Bal jivan chamcho is recommended for children with bronchitis, diarrhea, rickets, croup, and convulsions. It contains lead.

AYURVEDIC MEDICINES (BHASMAS)

In India a widely practiced type of traditional medicine is known as Ayurveda, which employs preparations such as vegetable products, animal products, and metals and minerals, most often lead and mercury.[121,133] Modern pharmaceuticals are even prescribed by traditional healers. Ayurvedic healers frequently administer penicillin. Other indigenized drugs are analgesics, antipyretics, and corticosteroids.[20]

Ayurvedic traditional medicinal preparations, commonly known as bhasmas and commonly used in Asia, are administered orally for systemic use or are applied locally. In Ayurvedic medicine, lead is regarded as an aphrodisiac and its reputed role may have been to counter the impotence associated with autonomic neuropathy in the diabetic male.[135] Bhasmas are fine ashes of metals and metallic salts (iron, copper, etc.) and a variety of natural products (oyster shells, conches). The ingredients are subjected to several cycles of heating, cooling, and grinding until the preparation turns to a fine ash. All contain polycyclic aromatic hydrocarbons. They may be significantly contaminated with benzo(a)pyrene, a chemical carcinogen.[136] Putative therapeutic uses of Ayurvedic bhasmas are summarized in Table 73–13.[113]

Gymnema (*Gymnema sylvestre*) has been used by Ayurvedic practitioners in India for centuries either alone or as a compound of Tribang shia, a mixture of tin, lead, zinc, *G. Sylvestre* leaves, neom (*Melia azadirachta*) leaves, *Enicostenna littorale,* and janbul (*Eugena jambolana*) seeds. It has also been used in traditional African medicines. It appears to have hypoglycemic properties, approximately that of tolbutamide.[137]

Table 73–13
Therapeutic Uses of Ayurvedic Bhasmas [a]

Common Name	Ingredient	Major Use
Made from iron		
1. Lauha	Iron	Anemia, weakness, cough
2. Kashees	Iron sulfate	Anemia, weakness, cough, leprosy
3. Mandoor	Filth of Iron	Anemia, jaundice, infection
Made from copper		
1. Tamra	Copper	Asthma, cough, piles
2. Swarnmakshik	Copper pyrite	Angina pectoris, antiseptic
3. Mayurchandrika	Copper sulfate	Spleen enlargement, cough, indigestion, paralysis, leprosy
Made from lead		
1. Nag	Lead	Paralysis and leprosy
Made from natural products		
1. Abarakh	Mica	T.B., cough, anemia
2. Panna	Beryl	Anemia, cough, weakness
3. Muktashukti	Oyster shell	Diabetes, respiratory disease
4. Shankh	Conches	Vomiting, asthma, liver and spleen disorders
5. Varatika	Kawrie	T.B., leprosy
6. Mrigashringa	Horn	Asthma, joint pain, chest pain, cough

[a] Adapted from Jani JP et al. Hum Exp Toxicol 1991;10:347–350.

AFLATOXIN

High levels of aflatoxin B_1, B_2, and G_1 used for the treatment of liver disorders have been found in herbal plant material sold in India.[138]

BETEL NUT

Betel nut is also known as supari in India. The Indian Ministry of Information has issued a health warning on the chewing of supari and has banned all advertisements for supari because of its association with oral cancer.[139]

The areca nut, commonly known as betel nut, grows on an Areca palm tree (*Areca catechu*) Thought to have originated on the Malay Peninsula, it is the oldest known masticatory used by Asians. Many older Cambodian refugee women in the United States chew betel nut quid, a combination of areca nut, betal leaf (from Piper beetle), lime paste, and leaf tobacco. The women are easily identified because the quid causes the teeth to turn black-brown and stains the tongue and oral mucosa. Arecoline, a cholinomimetic alkaloid, is a major constituent of the betel nut. It is a potent diaphoretic; it stimulates the salivary, lacrimal, gastric, pancreatic, and intestinal glands and the mucosal cells of the respiratory tract; increases muscle tonus and plan muscle movement throughout the body; slows the heart rate; constricts the pupils of the eyes; and mimics the action of acetylcholine in the body. The lime that is part of the betel quid hydrolizes the arecoline into arecaidine, a central nervous system stimulant that, in combination with the essential oil of the betel pepper (a mixture of phenols and terpenelike constituents), accounts for the euphoric properties of the betel quid when absorbed from the buccal mucosa.[140]

Arecoline, the main constituent of betel nut, produces widespread cortical arousal similar to the action of acetylcholine. This arousal from arecoline administration is associated with an elevation of acetylcholine concentrations in the central nervous system.[141]

JAPAN

KAMPO

Traditional Chinese herbal medicines imported from China into Japan are referred to as Kampo medicines containing magnolol, an inhibitor of 11-beta-hydroxysteroid dehydrogenase. Magnolol can be isolated from the urine.[142]

Herbal medicines are used for treatment of anxiety and depression (Saiko-Ka-Ryukotu-Borei-To), agitated depression and nightmare (Yokukan-San-Ka-Chinpi-Hange), headache (Choto-San), and exhausted depression (Hochu-Ekki-To). These products are generally a mixture of herbs. For example, Saiko-Ka-Ryukotu-Borei-To is composed of a number of constituents.[143]

KYUSHIN

Kyushin, a popular Chinese medicine used in Japan, exhibits immunoreactive digoxin-like activity. The major component is Chan-su, the dried venom of the Chinese Toad (*Bufo bufo gargarizans Cantor),* which contains several cardiotoxic steroids such as cinobufagin, bufotalin, and bufalin. The chemical structures of these chemicals are similar to that of digoxin.[144]

SHO-SAIKO-TO

This herbal medicine has been used in the treatment of cirrhosis of the liver and is associated with an increase in cytokine (IL-beta, GM-CSF) production. Controlled clinical studies have yet to be performed.[145]

ITALY

Herbal tea mixtures that contain extracts of licorice, fennel, anise, and *Galega officinalis* are used to stimulate lactation and have induced hypotonia, lethargy, emesis, weak cry, and poor sucking in nursing infants.[146]

KOREA[147,148]

Chronic lead and arsenic poisoning has been described in a 33-year-old Korean woman following consumption of a Korean herbal medicine prescribed for hemorrhoids. The material contained 26.4 mg/g of lead and 9.65 mg/g of arsenic. She developed elevated blood lead and arsenic levels and responded to DMSA.

MALAYSIA

Jamu is a form of traditional medicine widely known in Malaysia, Indonesia, and Brunei. Jamu may contain traces of toxic metals such as arsenic and copper.[149]

Minyak is used for external application, but traditional healers (bomohs) may contain methylsalicylate, which can induce an acute salicylism after ingestion.[150]

MEXICO[151,152]

Lead compounds are used to treat "empacho," which is believed to be caused by a block in the digestive tract, resulting in diarrhea and/or vomiting.[153] These include greta, azarcon, and albayalde.

Greta

Lead oxide is incorporated with a mustard-colored powder called "greta" in Spanish, generally used as a glaze for low-priced pottery.[154]

Azarcon[155–158]

Lead tetroxide is a bright orange-colored powder called "azarcon" in Spanish. Both greta and azarcon are over 90% lead by weight.

Albayalde

Albayalde is lead carbonate, used commonly to make paint. Azarcon and greta are also known as Liga, Maria Luisa, Alarcon, Coral, and Rueda.[158]

HERBAL MEDICATIONS

Herbal medications derived from pyrollizidine-containing plants (see Plant chapter) are commonly sold under the name of Gordolobo, a *Senecio longilobus* species. Common local names include Manzanilla del Rio, Mullein, Punchon, candelaria, and verbasco.[159] These plant ingestions may lead to severe liver damage and death.

Ingestion of *Packera candidissima,* known as chucaca, lechuguilla de la sierra, te de milagras, and hierba de milagro, is associated with pyrrolizidine alkaloid poisoning (veno occlusive disease of the liver, arterial hypertension, and right ventricular hypertrophy).[160]

Medications may be obtained from a local curandera—folk healer.[159]

RATTLESNAKE CAPSULES[161–166]

Rattlesnake capsule ingestion is a common practice among Mexican-Americans in the Los Angeles Area. It is a Mexican folk remedy used to treat cancer, diabetes, arthritis, and skin disorders. The reptile is decapitated, skinned, dried in the sun, pulverized, placed in capsules, and sold under various names—*vibora de cascabel, polvo de vibora,* and *carne de vibora*—without prescription in farmacias: *Salmonella arizonae* infections may follow its use.

MEXICAN BORDER PURCHASES[167]

Purchases by Americans traveling to Mexico and by local Mexicans have included many drugs and other products sold over the counter[168] (Table 73–14),[169] including corticosteroids[170–172]; dipyrone (dipirona, metamizol)[173–175]; oxyphenbutazone[176]; dapsone[177]; diet medications[172] containing various combinations of stimulants, sympathomimetics, anticholinergics, thyroid preparations, digitalis, and tranquilizers (e.g., REDOTEX—pseudoephedrine, liothyronine, atropine, and diazepam and also ASENLIX—clobenzorex, PONDEREX—fenfluramine)[178–180]; and fruit drinks that have contained lead, amygdalin, ergot alkaloid, indomethacin, chlorpheniramine, trifluoperazine, and tranylcypromine.[181] Prescriptions of such products is not followed by many reputable Mexican physicians.[171]

Table 73–14
Potentially Dangerous Medications Readily Available Over the Counter in Cuidad Juarez [a]

Drug Name	Approximate Cost (US Currency)	Common Use in Mexico and Adverse Reactions
Prodolina and Neo-Melubrina (dipyrone salts)	$0.08 per tablet	Powerful analgesics used to relieve headaches, sore throats, joint pain, toothaches, etc. Banned in US by FDA; associated with agranulocytosis.
Senociclin Balsamico (chloramphenicol & tetracycline)	$2.41 per ampule	Most frequently used to treat common cold. This combined antibiotic has been banned by US FDA. Chloramphenicol is used in US only for serious infections and can cause aplastic anemia.
Artridol (indomethacin, methocarbamol, betamethasone)	$0.18 per tablet	Widely used to reduce inflammation. Betamethasone can lead to many serious problems characteristic of corticosteroids.
Entero Vioformo (iodochlorhydroxyquin)	$0.09 per tablet	Commonly used to relieve upset stomach and diarrhea. No longer available in US because of an epidemic of subacute myelo-optic neuropathy in Japan.
Lincocin (lincomycin)	$1.02 per ampule	Used to treat laryngitis. Currently available in US for limited uses. Can cause diarrhea, colitis, and pseudomembranous colitis.
Espasmo Cibalgina (adiphenine hydrochloride)	$0.12 per tablet	Used mainly to relieve muscle spasms. Not sold in US. Can cause agranulocytosis.

FDA, Food and Drug Administration.
[a]Adapted from Tabet SR, Wiese WH. South Med J 1990;83:271–273.

THIAZOLIDINE CARBOXYLIC ACID

In Mexico, Europe, and Central and South America, thiazolidine carboxylic acid is available as a "hepatoprotector" under a variety of trade names, including Celepat, Hepalidine, Heparagene, and Thiobiline. The *Diccionaro de Especialidades Farmaceuticas,* 24th Edition, claims that the drug "reactivates the enzymatic processes of the liver . . . normalizes the transaminases and shortens the icteric and recuperation periods." Ingestion of 4 or 5 to 30 100-mg tablets have resulted in coma, seizures, acidosis, and hypoglycemia. Many patients have also exhibited fever, tachycardia, respiratory distress, and miosis.[182] Death in cardiorespiratory arrest has followed in one of five children who ingested an overdose.[183,184] Management should be directed to supportive care, correction of acidosis, and control of seizures.[185]

PHILIPPINES

Indigenized pharmaceuticals include "Diatabs," "Polymagma" (antidiarrheals), and penicillin tablets. Diatabs (sulfaguanidine, charcoal, bismuth bicarbonate, pectin, dicyclonic HC1) and Polymagma (streptomycin, polymyxin pectin) are inexpensive and are sold in small shops known as "sari sari stores" and are known to everybody.[24]

GREECE

Ecbalium (Echallium) elaterium (EE), known as the wild or squirting cucumber, is a hairy perennial herbaceous vine of the Cucurbitaceae family endemic to the Mediterranean region. All parts of the plant are toxic, particularly the gherkinlike fruits. In Greece the juice of the squirting cucumber is used as a folk medication for multiple diseases, including constipation, rheumatic diseases, and malignancies. In some areas of Crete it is used for the treatment of sinusitis by nasal aspiration. The juice of EE can cause severe skin irritation, inflammation, and edema. Large doses can cause severe vomiting, diarrhea, neurotoxicity, anuria, uremia, and cardiorespiratory failure and may be fatal. EE poisoning begins with local irritation, erythema, and edema and is followed by systemic toxicity with renal, cardiac, and respiratory insufficiency.[186]

URGINEA MARTIMA (SQUILL)[187]

The most important plant sources of cardiac glycosides are digitalis (foxglove), strophanthus, and squill. Squill is *Urginea martima,* the sea onion that grows near the Mediterranean shore and in the southwest region of Turkey. The bulb, but possibly the whole plant, contains several related steroidal cardioactive glycosides, including scillaren A, Glucoscillaren A, Scillaridin A, and scilliroside that exert digitalis-like toxicity. Ingestion of squill as a folk remedy may result in fatal toxicity. The toxic effects of squill are reportedly similar to those of digitalis glycosides. In patients presenting with gastrointestinal symptoms and bradyarrhythmias due to presumed poisoning by herbal medicines, cardiac glycoside poisoning should be suspected.

NIGERIA

In Nigeria, Tiro, similar to kohl and surma, has been used as a cosmetic, leading to elevated blood lead levels in children.[188]

SOUTHERN AFRICA[189–192]

Analysis of chemicals that may be present in traditional medicine in South Africa has been systematized by a screening method using an HPLC Diode Array Detection.[193] Poisonous plants commonly used in traditional practice in Zimbabwe are found in Tables 73–8 and 73–9.[194] Deaths in South Africa presumed to have been caused by herbal medicine have been subjected to chemical investigation. Cardiac glycosides have been found in about half of the cases.[195] *Callilepsis laureola* is known to the Zulu tribe as *Impila* (Zulu for health).[35] Toxic plants are used for medicinal purposes by the Zulu population of southern Africa.[193] Clinical symptoms of *Impila* intoxication are abdominal pain, jaundice, hypoglycemia, and disturbed hepatic and renal function. The hepatotoxin has not been identified, but the nephrotoxin and hypoglycemia inducing agents is a diterpene glycoside, atractyloside.[197,198]

POTASSIUM DICHROMATE

Traditional remedies in South Africa urban areas include potassium dichromate, used primarily for its coloring rather than disinfectant action. This resulted in death of a 48-year-old Xhosa man.[196,197]

AMIDOPYRINE

Drugs such as amidopyrine, withdrawn in the West, have produced toxic effects when used by indigenous populations in some Third World countries.[191,192]

ZIMBABWE

In Zimbabwe, indigenous and naturalized plants are known to be used medically.[199] Poisonings may due to berries or other plants (muti-traditional).[199] Poisoning due to traditional medicines (muti) represent the largest single cause of poisoning admissions in Zimbabwe. Most poisonings are accidental and may result in death. Active ingredients, in most cases, are not known. Management consists mainly of supportive and symptomatic treatment. Some cases of traditional medicine poisoning have been caused by orthodox medicines.[190,200] There is a need to standardize traditional medicines.[201] In Zimbabwe the most common toxic agents involved in poisoning of children were household products.[200]

OVERDOSES

Overdoses of therapeutic drugs have included analgesics, sedatives, hypnotics, antipsychotics, antimalarials, antidepressants, antimicrobials, and alcohol. The mortality rate is 3.9%. Most of these deaths are suicides.[202]

DEATH

In South Africa, Joubert reports that the major cause of death among black South Africans were traditional medicines (about 50% of deaths) followed by kerosine (about 25% of deaths). The traditional healer is the main source of traditional medicine in addition to African medicine.[203,204] Considerable secrecy still surrounds traditional medicine, hampering rational therapy. Venter and Joubert are currently building up a library of traditional medicines that includes a picture of the particular substance, the colloquial name(s), traditional uses, botanical information, and toxicologic profile.[200]

Traditional medicines (or mutis) are usually administered orally or as an enema by a traditional healer. Cardiac glycosides are often found in autopsies where death was presumed to have been caused by herbal medicine.[205]

TRADITIONAL HEALER PRACTITIONERS

From published reports and interviews with a traditional healer (personal communication), there appear to be different categories of traditional healer practitioners: (a) diviners, who receive a strong "calling" from ancestors by way of dreams; (b) *inyangas,* the majority of whom are men, who diagnose and prescribe medicine, but not always through visions or dreams; *sangomas,* predominantly women, who usually diagnose and then send the patient to an *inyanga;* (c) herbalists, men or women, who usually sell or prescribe herbal remedies; (d) members of the family (e.g., grandmothers) whose knowledge is passed down through the generations, who collect plants for medicinal purposes to administer to their children and grandchildren; and (e) it is suspected there also exist "traditional healers" who practice without any formal training or "calling" and have a low success rate—this appears to represent the negative aspect of traditional healing.

NYANGAS

Nyangas (traditional township healers) are consulted for a wide range of problems and are more likely to dispense enemas or emetics than any other form of treatment. Such enemas may contain chloroxylenol, vinegar, battery acid, potassium permanganate, copper sulfate, or potassium dichromate. Renal failure may occur.[189]

SOUTH AMERICA[24,206,207]

Villagers in the Andean region of Peru believe in popular and traditional medicine (magical plants) such as Ilanten *(Plantago major)* as compresses for inflammation, or alfalfa *(Medicago sativa)* in juice or tea for nasal hemorrhage.[3] In western South America, Susto (known as the "fright illness") is treated with arsenic in a home remedy.[206] Western pharmaceuticals are increasingly "indigenized," that is, incorporated into the local culture.[24] Terramicina (oxytetracycline) and "Ambra-Sinto" (tetracycline HC1) are taken for intestinal disturbances. The contents of a capsule are mashed together with pork fat after the fashion of certain herbal treatments. A herbal medicine used in this way has acquired the name Terramicina do Matto (herbal terramicina).[24]

PERU

"Sapo" is obtained from the skin of the frog *Phyllomedusa bicolor* and is used by the Peruvian Matses Indians in shamanic limiting practices. Active peptides induce severe gastrointestinal and cardiovascular toxicity in man.[207,208]

TAIWAN

TUNG SHUEH

Tung Shueh pills containing diazepam and mefanamic acid have been associated with an acute interstitial nephritis.[209]

UNITED KINGDOM

Five cases of lead poisoning due to traditional remedies in the West Midlands were reported. All patients developed typical clinical features, although in two cases the diagnosis was first suspected because the blood film showed basophilic stippling of red cells. Two patients were given chelation therapy, one with penicillamine and one with calcium edetate. One patient was left with a permanent neurologic deficit.[210]

UNITED STATES

HAWAII

A Hawaiian materia medica or medicinal plants known to Hawaiian Kahunas for asthma has been compiled by B.E. Hope. Polynesian Herbal Medicine has been written by A.W. Whistler of the National Tropical Garden at Lauwaii on Kawaii.[211]

ELEMENTAL SULFUR[212]

Elemental sulfur is widely used as a folk remedy. It is usually combined with a sweet syrup or molasses. It has internal uses that include intestinal "spring-cleaning," treatment for dyspnea, and as a "tonic." Its usefulness for these indications is subject to doubt, but it has been generally held to be harmless. Sulfur is used widely in the treatment of dermatologic disease.[213] The lethal oral dose in humans is estimated to be between 0.5 and 5 mg/kilogram body weight. There is no evidence that sulfur ingestion by man leads to hydrogen sulfide toxicity.

CLINICAL TOXICOKINETICS

In man, elemental sulfur is probably converted first to sulfide by colonic bacteria and then to sulfate. Ferritin, abundant in the gut, may be important in detoxifying hydrogen sulfide produced by colonic bacteria. Excess sulfate ion is rapidly excreted by the kidneys by filtration, with little subsequent tubular resorption.

CLINICAL PRESENTATION

An ingestion of 250 g by an adult over 2 days led to lethargy, confusion, a serum sulfate concentration of 2.3 mEq/liter (normal 0.16 to 0.38), hyperchloremia, and a metabolic acidosis with a normal anion gap. The patient survived following intravenous hydration, modest doses of sodium bicarbonate, and enemas to remove sulfur from the colon. In 1 week the serum sulfide was 0.27 mEq/liter.

THE LUMBEE

The Lumbee Indians are the largest group of Indians residing east of the Mississippi River. Most live in Robeson County in North Carolina. They do not have a distinct language and religion. Their unique body of folklore and tradition appear to identify them. They live in rural areas with access to a number of plant communities. Medical care is rendered by physicians and herbalists. Plant medicines are made into teas, poultices, and salves. Many acute symptoms of poisoning are easily noted by patients and practitioners.[214]

Avon "Skin So Soft" is a concentrated bath oil used as a "folk medicine" insect repellent. It may offer protection for over 30 minutes. Controlled clinical studies have not been performed.[215]

COLLOIDAL SILVER PROTEINS (CSP) (SEE ALSO SILVER, CHAPTER 67)

In the 19th century, colloidal silver proteins (CSPs) were promoted as cure-alls to prevent and treat diseases such as tetanus and rheumatism. In this century up until World War II, CSPs were widely used to treat colds and gonorrhea. However, in recent decades, the medicinal use of silver has been largely replaced by safer and more effective therapies.

Since 1990 interest has resurged in promoting CSP products as "essential" mineral supplements with multiple health claims. For example, advertising materials in health food stores promote CSP use in more than 650 different diseases. Colloidal silver proteins are being touted as powerful antimicrobials against viruses, bacteria, parasites, and fungi, including human immunodeficiency virus (HIV), herpes, *Candida,* and tuberculosis. The CSPs also have been advertised as "an immune system stimulant and antiinflammatory agent" for use in conditions such as diabetes, chronic fatigue syndrome, allergies, and cancer.[216]

CSPs are now widely available throughout the United States because of aggressive marketing by distributors. Efficacy claims for the treatment of infectious diseases such as tuberculosis, malaria, and systemic fungal infections or for the prevention of cancer, acquired immunodeficiency syndrome (AIDS), and diabetes remain unproven.[216]

Silver is not without toxicity. Silver accumulates in the body and may result in bluish skin discoloration (argyria). Argyria is irreversible and has no effective treatment. In addition, neurologic deficits and diffuse silver deposition in visceral organs have been reported with long-term use of oral silver products. Renal damage and metal fume fever have been reported with high silver exposures. The Food and Drug Administration's Nontraditional Drug Compliance Branch is currently evaluating the legitimacy of marketing these products.[213]

CHEN-SU ("ROCKHARD")

From February 1993 to May 1995 the New York City Poison Control Center (NYCPCC) was informed about onset of illness in five previously healthy men after they ingested a substance marketed as a topical aphrodisiac; four of the men died.[217] The decedents died from cardiac dysrhythmias, and all five patients had measurable levels of digoxin detected in their serum. The purported aphrodisiac contains bufadienolides, naturally occurring cardioactive steroids that have digoxin-like effects.

Chan Su, a traditional Chinese medication, is used as a topical anesthetic and cardiac medication and also contains bufadienolides. Cardioactive steroids, including bufadienolides, have a narrow therapeutic index, and unintentional therapeutic intoxication is well documented. These steroids can adversely affect the myocardium, and the most life-threatening manifestations of toxicity include arrhythmias, ventricular ectopy, sinus bradycardia, atrial arrhythmias, and hyperkalemia. Cardiac steroids are found in other nontraditional therapies such as teas made from oleander *(Nerium oleander)* and foxglove *(Digitalis purpurea).*

In New York City the product, marketed as an aphrodisiac, is sold under names such as "Stone," "LoveStone," "BlackStone," and "RockHard" and is available in grocery stores and smoke shops and from street vendors.

Physicians and the public should report adverse reactions to purported aphrodisiacs to FDA's MedWatch Program, telephone (800) 332-1088 or (301) 738-7553.

KOMBUCHA "MUSHROOM"[218,219]

Kombucha tea is a popular health beverage made by incubating the Kombucha mushroom in sweet black tea. Although advocates of Kombucha tea have attributed many therapeutic effects to the drink, its beneficial and/or adverse effects have not been determined scientifically.

Composition

The Kombucha "mushroom" is a symbiotic colony of several species of yeast and bacteria that are bound together by a surrounding thin membrane. Although the composition of the Kombucha colony varies, some of the species reportedly found in the mushroom include *S. ludwigii, S. pombe, Bacterium xylinum, B. gluconicum, B. xylinoides, B. katogenium, Pichia fermentans,* and *Torula* sp. Kombucha tea can contain up to 1.5% alcohol and a variety of other metabolites (e.g., ethyl acetate, acetic acid, and lactate). There are at least two commercial producers of Kombucha mushrooms in the United States. Sharing of the mushrooms is believed to have helped to promote its popularity in the United States.

Possible Beneficial Effects

Beneficial effects attributed to consumption of Kombucha tea have included prevention of cancer, relief of arthritis, treatment of insomnia, and stimulation of regrowth of hair. Because the tea is believed to stimulate the immune system, it has become popular among persons with human immunodeficiency virus infection. In addition the tea has become popular among the elderly (who are less likely to try alternative therapies).

Contamination

The FDA has evaluated the practices of the commercial producers of the Kombucha mushroom and has found no pathogenic organisms or hygiene violations. However, because the tea is produced under varying conditions in individual homes, contamination with pathogenic organisms such as *Aspergillus* is possible.

Clinical

Because folk medicines and herbal remedies, including Kombucha tea, are considered neither a food nor a drug, they are not routinely evaluated by the FDA or the U.S. Department of Agriculture. Drinking this tea in quantities typically consumed (approximately 4 oz. daily) may not cause adverse effects in healthy persons. The potential health risks are unknown for those with preexisting health problems or those who drink excessive quantities of the tea.

Because of the acidity of Kombucha tea, it should not be prepared or stored in containers made from materials such as ceramic or lead crystal, which both contain toxic elements that can leach into the tea. Because of the increasing use of this tea (even in groups that usually do not use alternative therapies), health-care professionals should consider consumption of Kombucha tea in the differential diagnosis of persons with unexplained lactic acidosis. Consumption of Kombucha tea has been associated with hepatotoxicity. Physicians and the public should report adverse health effects associated with the consumption of Kombucha tea to FDA Med/Watch program, telephone (800) 332-1088 or (301) 738-7553.

SUGGESTED READINGS

1. D'Arcy PF. Adverse reactions and interactions with herbal medicines. I. Adverse reactions. Adverse Drug React Toxicol Rev 1991;10:189–208.
2. D'Arcy PF. Adverse reactions and interactions with herbal medicine. II. Drug interactions. Adverse Drug React Toxicol Rev 1993;12:147–162.

REFERENCES—INDIGENOUS TOXICOLOGY—FOLK MEDICINE

1. Murray V, Perharic-Walton L. Toxicological problems resulting from exposure to traditional medicines and food supplements. National Poisons Unit, Guy's Hospital, St. Thomas Street, London, SE1, 9RT (Tel. 071-639-9653) and Simpson G, Edwards N. National Poisons Information Service, Avonley Road, London SE1, 45ER (Tel 071-635-9191).
2. Kirkland J, Matthews HF, Sullivan CW III, Baldwin K, eds. Herbal and magical medicine. Traditional healing today. Durham, NC: Duke University Press, 1992; pp. 235.
3. Perharic L, Shaw D, Murray V. Toxic effects of herbal medicines and food supplements. Lancet 1993;342:180–181.
4. Joubert PH, Mathibe L. Acute poisoning in developing countries. Adverse Drug React Acute Poisoning Rev 1989;8(3): 165–178.
5. Goldman L, ed. Cross cultural medicine in MKSAP 10: General Internal Medicine. American College of Physicians, 1994; p. 142.
6. De Smet PAGM. Health risks of herbal remedies. Drug Safety 1995;13:81–93.
7. Mofenson HC, Caraccio TR, Brody G, Greensher J, Leggiadro R, Mancini R, Sherman J. Herbal products. Poison Perspective for Health Professionals 1994;13:54–62.
8. Espinoza EO, Mann M-J, Bleasdell B. Arsenic and mercury in traditional Chinese herbal balls. N Engl J Med 1995;333: 804–805.
9. Nelson L, Shih R, Hoffman R. Aplastic anemia induced by an adulterated herbal preparation. Clin Toxicol 1995;33:467–470.
10. Martindale: The extra pharmacopoeia. 30th ed. London: The Pharmaceutical Press, 1993, p. 1410.
11. Peacock S, Murray V, Turton C. Respiratory distress and royal jelly. Br Med J 1995;310:1472.
12. Bullock RJ, Rohan A, Straatmans JA: Fatal royal jelly–induced asthma. Med J Aust 1994;160:44.
13. Abt AB, Oh JY, Huntington RA. Chinese herbal medicine-induced acute renal failure. Arch Intern Med 1995;155:211.
14. Parry C, Easton J. Kohl: a lead-hazardous eye make-up from the Third World to the First World. Environ Health Perspect 1991;94:121–123.
15. Ali A, Smales O, Aslam M. Surma and lead poisoning. Br Med J 1978;2:915–916.
16. Snodgrass G, Ziderman D, Gulati V, Richards J. Cosmetic plumbism. Br Med J 1973;27:230.
17. Pontifex AH, Gary AK. Lead poisoning from an Asian Indian folk remedy. Can Med Assoc J 1985;133:1227–1228.
18. Zaloga CP, Deal J, Spurling T, Richter J, Chernow B. Unusual manifestations of arsenic intoxication. Am J Med Sci 1985; 289:210–214.
19. Aslam M, Healy MA, Daris SS, Ali AR. Surma and blood lead in children. Lancet 1980;1:568–569.
20. Dolan G, Jones AP, Blumsohn A, Reilly JT, Brown MJ. Lead poisoning due to Asian ethnic treatment for impotence. J R Soc Med 1991;84:630–631.
21. Lead poisoning with the use of Asian medicine. Pharmacy J 1991;5:248.
22. CDC. Cadmium and lead exposure associated with pharmaceuticals imported from Asia—Texas. MMWR 1989;38: 612–614.
23. Fernando A, Healy M, Aslam M, Davis S, Hussein A. Lead poisoning and traditional practices: the consequences for world health. A study in Kuwait. Public Health 1981;95: 250–260.
24. Haak H, Hardon AP. Indigenized pharmaceuticals in developing countries: widely used, widely neglected. Lancet 1988; 2:620–621.
25. Abdullah MA. Lead poisoning among children in Saudi Arabia. J Trop Med Hyg 1984;87:67–70.
26. Van der Gusti S. Tetracycline against children's diarrhea. A note from South Asia, Africa, Middle East. Cameroon, Amsterdam (CASA) 1985.
27. But PP-H. Need for correct identifying of herbs in herbal poisoning. Lancet 1993;341:637.
28. Tomlinson B, Leung SKF, Chan TYK, Critchley JAJH. Adverse effects and usage of Chinese traditional medicine in Hong Kong. Br J Clin Pharmacol 1991;31:6115.
29. Goldman JA. Chinese herbal medicine: Camouflaged prescription antiinflammatory drugs, corticosteroids and lead. Arthritis Rheum 1991;31:1207.
30. Segasothy M, Samad S. Illicit herbal preparation containing phenylbutazone causing analgesic nephropathy. Nephron 1991;59:166–167.
31. Gertner E, Marshall PS, Filandrinos D, Potek AS, Smith TM. Complications resulting from the use of Chinese herbal medications containing undeclared prescription drugs. Arthritis Rheum 1995;38:614–617.
32. Mitchell-Higgs CAV, Conway M, Cassar J. Herbal medicine as a cause of combined lead and arsenic poisoning. Hum Exp Toxicol 1990;9:1994–195.
33. Balint GA, Balint EE. On the medico-social aspects of khat *Catha edulus:* chewing habit. Hum Psychopharmacol 1994;9: 125–128.
34. Otieno LS, McLigeyo SO, Luta M. Acute renal failure following the use of herbal remedies. East Afr Med J 1991;61: 993–998.
35. Hutchings A, Terblanche SE. Observations on the use of some known and suspected toxic *Liliiflore* in Zulu and Xhosa medicine. S Afr Med J 1989;75:62–69.
36. Yesilada E, Honda G, Sezik E, Tabata M, Goto K, Ikeshino Y. Traditional medicine in Turkey. IV. Folk medicine in the Mediterranean subdivision. J Ethnopharmacol 1993;39:31–38.
37. Akintonwa A, Mabadeje AFB, Odutola TA. Fatal poisonings by copper sulfate ingested from "spiritual water." Vet Hum Toxicol 1989;31:453–454.
38. El-Ansary EH, Ahmed MEK, Clague HW. Systemic toxicity of para-phenylenediamine. Lancet 1983;1:1341.
39. Ashraf W, Dawling S, Farrow J. Systemic para-phenylenediamine (PPD) poisoning: a case report and review. Hum Exp Toxicol 1994;13:167–170.
40. Yagi H, El Hind AM, Khalil SI. Acute poisoning from hair dye. East Afr Med J 1991;68:404–411.
41. Lifshits M, Yagupsky P, Sofen S. Fatal paraphenylenediamine (hair dye) intoxication in a child resembling Ludwig's angina. Clin Toxicol 1993;31:653–656.
42. Sullman SM, Homeida M, Aboud OI. Paraphenylenediamine induced acute tubular necrosis following hair dye ingestion. Hum Toxicol 1983;2:633–635.
43. Schneider JA, Sigg EB. Neuropharmacological studies on ibogaine, an indole alkaloid with central stimulant properties. Ann NY Acad Sci 1956;66:766–776.
44. Endabuse[R] (Ibogaine hydrochloride). NDA International Inc, 46 Oxford Place, Staten Island, NY 10301.
45. Isbell H. USPHS Hospital, Addiction Research Center, Lexington, KY. Preliminary trials with ibogaine, November 1956. Personal communication to Ciba.

46. Dhahir HI. A comparative study on the toxicity and serotonin. Doctoral Dissertation. University Microfilm International 71-25-34. Ann Arbor, MI. Indiana University, PhD. 1971. Pharmacology, p. 151.
47. Maissoneuve IM, Keller RW, Glick SD. Interactions between ibogaine, a potential anti-addictive agent and morphine: an in vivo microdialysis study. Eur J Pharmacol 1991;199:35–42.
48. Schneider JA, Rinhart RR. Analysis of the cardiovascular action of ibogaine hydrochloride. Arch Int Pharmacodyn 1957;110:92–102.
49. Reference Deleted.
50. O'Hearn EO, Molliver ME. Degeneration of Purkinje cells in parasagittal zones of cerebellar vermis after treatment with ibogaine or harmaline. Neuroscience 1993;55:363–370.
51. CDC. Lead poisoning associated with use of traditional ethnic remedies—California, 1991–1992. MMWR 1993;24: 521–524.
52. Steyn JM, Hundt HKL. GC/MS identification and quantitation of cantharidin in post-mortem serum. Uges DRQ, deZeeuw RA, eds. Proc. 25th International Meeting, Int Assoc Forensic Toxicol. Groningen, June 27, 1988.
53. Hundt HLK, Steyn JM, Wagner L. Post-mortem serum concentration of cantharidin in a fatal case of cantharides poisoning. Hum Exp Toxicol 1990;9:35–40.
54. Lecritier MA. A case of cantharidin poisoning. Br Med J 1954;2:1399–1400.
55. Craven JD, Polak A. Cantharidin poisoning. Br Med J 1954; 2:1386–1388.
56. Nickolls LC, Teare D. Poisoning by cantharidin. Br Med J 1954;2:1384–1386.
57. Kok-Choi C, Hee-Ming L, Bobby SSF, David YCP. A fatality due to the use of cantharides from *Mylabris Phalerata* as an abortifacient. Med Sci Lau 1990;30:336–340.
58. Cantharidin. The Merck Index. 9th ed. Rahway, NJ: Merck and Co., p. 222.
59. Till JS, Majmuder BN. Cantharidin poisoning. South Med J 1981;74:444–447.
60. Harrisberg J, Deseta JCH, Cohen L, Temlett J, Milne FJ. Cantharidin poisoning with neurological complications. So Afr Med J 1984;65:614–615.
61. Edwards WO, Edwards RM, Ogden L, Whaley M. Cantharidin—Content of two species of Oklahoma blister beetles associated with toxicosis in horses. Vet Hum Toxicol 1989; 31:442–444.
62. Burnett JW, Calton GJ, Morgan RJ. Blister beetles: "Spanish fly." Cutis 1987;40(1):22.
63. Andrews CH. A case of poisoning by cantharidin. Lancet 1921;2:654–655.
64. Rosin RD. Cantharides intoxication. Br Med J 1967;4:33.
65. Graziano MJ, Waterhouse AL, Casida JE. Cantharidin poisoning associated with specific binding site in liver. Biochem Biophys Res Commun 1987;149:79–85.
66. Weakley DR, Eikenbinder JM. The mechanics of cantharidin acantholysis. J Invest Dermatol 1962;39–45.
67. Oaks WB, DiTunno JF, Magnani T, Levy HA, Mills LC. Cantharidin poisoning. Arch Intern Med 1960;105:574–582.
68. Avery JS. A case of acute cantharides poisoning. Lancet 1908;2:800.
69. Tenschert W, Behrenbeck T, Rolf N, Ahlmann J, Winterberg B, Heepe J et al. Kantharidin-Intoxikation. Fortschr Med 1987;105:686–688.
70. Villadsen AB, Hansen HE. Akut nyreinsuficiens efter indtagelse af "spank flue." Ugeskr Laeger 1984;146:1436–1437.
71. Fisch HP, Reutter FW, Gloor F. Schadigung der nieren und der ableitenden harnwege durch kantharidin. Schweiz Med Wochenschr 1978;108:1664–1667.
72. Ewart WB, Rabkin SW, Mitenko PA. Poisoning by cantharides. Can Med Assoc J 1978;118:1199.
73. Presto AJ, Muecke EC. A dose of Spanish fly. JAMA 1970; 214:591–592.
74. Perhark L, Shaw D, Murray V. Toxic effects of herbal medicines and food supplements. Lancet 1993;342:180–181.
75. China: attack on bogus drugs. Lancet 1992;340:1243 (editorial).
76. Winship KA. Toxicity of lead: a review. Adverse Drug React Acute Pois Rev 1989;8:117–152.
77. Lightfoote J, Blair HJ, Cohen JP. Lead intoxication in an adult caused by Chinese herbal medication. JAMA 1977;238:1539.
78. Levitt C, Paulson D, Duvall K et al. Folk remedy-associated lead poisoning in Hmong children. JAMA 1983;250:3149–3150.
79. Chan H, Yeh Y-Y, Billmeier GJ, Evans WE, Chan H. Lead poisoning from ingestion of Chinese herbal medicine. Clin Toxicol 1977;10:273–281.
80. Kang-Yum E, Oransky SH. Chinese patent medicine as a potential source of mercury poisoning. Vet Hum Toxicol 1992; 34:235–238.
81. Gorey JD, Wahlqvist ML, Boyce NW. Adverse reaction to a Chinese herbal remedy. Med J Aust 1992;157:484–486.
82. Tai Y-T, But PP, Young K, Lau CP. Adverse effects from traditional Chinese medicine. Lancet 1993;341:892–893.
83. Kang-Yum E. Personal communication. Nyack, NY: Hudson Valley Regional Poison Center, Tel. 915-348-2615.
84. Huang KC. The pharmacology of Chinese herbs. Boca Raton, FL: CRC Press, 1993, pp. 388.
85. Guang-Sheng D. Important Chinese herbal remedies. Clin Ther 1987;9:345–357.
86. Zhen-Gang W, Gan-Zhong L. Advances in natural products in China. Trends Pharmacol Sci 1985;6:423–426.
87. Martz W. Plants with a reputation against snakebite. Toxicon 1992;30:1131–1142.
88. Schaumburg NH, Berger A. Alopecia and sensory polyneuropathy from thallium in a Chinese herbal medication. JAMA 1992;268:3430–3431.
89. Fitzpatrick AJ, Crawford M, Allan RM, Wolfenden H. Aconite poisoning managed with a ventricular assist device. Anaesth Intensive Care 1994;22:714–717.
90. But PP H, Tai Y-T, Young K. Three fatal cases of herbal aconite poisoning. Vet Hum Toxicol 1994;36(3):212–215.
91. Shannon M. Herbal medicine—the aconites. Clin Toxicol Rev 1995;17(4):1–2.
92. Chan TYK, Tomlinson B, Critchley JAJH, Cockram CS. Herb-induced aconitine poisoning presenting as tetraplegia. Vet Hum Toxicol 1994;36:133–134.
93. Chan TYK, Critchley JAJH. The spectrum of poisonings in Hong Kong: An overview. Vet Hum Toxicol 1994;36(2); 135–137.
94. Taylor TE, Wilk BA, Kazembe P, Chisak M, Wirima JJ, Ratsma EYEG, Molyneux ME. Rapid coma resolution with artemether in Malawian children with cerebral malaria. Lancet 1993;341:661–662.
95. Van Thiel PPAM, van Gool T, Buma APCCH, Tendeloo CH, Leentraar-Kuijpers A, Kager PA. Artemisinin compounds in treatment of malaria. Lancet 1993;34:1034–1035.
96. Izumotani T, Ishimura E, Tsumura K, Goto K, Nishizawa Y, Morii H. An adult case of Fanconi syndrome due to a mixture of Chinese crude drugs. Nephron 1993;65:137–140.
97. Dicke W. Ancient Chinese herbal remedy found to curb desire for alcohol. New York Times, November 2, 1993.
98. Catlin DH, Sekera M, Adelman DC. Erythroderma associated with ingestion of an herbal product. West J Med 1993;159: 491–492.
99. Bullock C. Herbal diet causes one death and other attacks. Emerg Med News, August, 1994; p. 8.
100. Atherton DJ, Rustin MN, Brostoff J. Need for correct identification of herbs in herbal poisoning. Lancet 1993;341:637–638.
101. Van der Weghem J-L, Depierreux M, Tielemans C, Abramowicz D, Dratwa M, Jadoul M et al. Rapidly progressing interstitial renal fibrosis in young women: association with slimming regimen including Chinese herbs. Lancet 1993;341: 387–391.
102. Cosyns J-P, Jadol M, Squifflet J-P, de Plaen J-F, Ferluga N, de Strihou CW. Chinese herbs nephropathy: A clue to Balkan endemic nephropathy. Kidney Int 1994;45:1680–1685.
103. Van Ypersele de Strihou C, Vanherweghen JL. The tragic paradigm of Chinese herbs nephropathy. Nephrol Dial Transplant 1995;10:157–160.
104. Kleijnen J, Knipschild P. Ginkgo biloba. Lancet 1992;340: 1136–1139.
105. Hill GJ. Lead poisoning due to Hai Ge Fen. JAMA 1995;273: 24–25.

106. Markowitz SB, Nunez CM, Klitzman S, Munshi AA, Kim WS, Eisinger J, Landrigan PJ. Lead poisoning due to Hai Ge Fen. The porphyric content of individual erythrocytes. JAMA 1994;271:932–934.
107. Harper J. Traditional Chinese medicine for eczema. Br Med J 1994;308:489–490.
108. CDC. Jin Buttauan toxicity in adults—Los Angeles, 1993. MMWR 1993;42:920–922.
109. Woolf GM, Petrovic LM, Rojter SE, Wainwright S, Villamil FG, Katkov WN et al. Acute hepatitis associated with the Chinese herbal product Jin Bu Huan. Intern Med 1994;121:229–235.
110. CDC. Jin Bu Huan toxicity in children—Colorado 1993. MMWR 1993;42:633–636.
111. Feldhaus KM, Horowitz RS, Dart RC, Brent J, Gomez H, Moore L et al. Life-threatening toxicity from tetrahydropalmitine (THP) in an herbal medicine product. Vet Hum Toxicol 1993;35:329.
112. Jin Bu Huan toxicity in children—Colorado 1993. JAMA 1993;270:1298–1302.
113. Liu G-Q, Algeri S, Garattini S. D-L-Tetrahydropalmitine as monoamine depletor. Arch Int Pharmacodyn 1982;258:39–50.
114. Chan JCN, Chan TYK, Chum KL, Leung NWY, Tomlinson B, Critchley JAJH. Anticholinergic poisoning from Chinese herbal medicines. Aust N Zeal Med J 1994;24:317–318.
115. Kwan T, Paiusco AD, Kohl L. Digitalis toxicity caused by toad venom. Chest 1992;102:949–950.
116. Karuranithy R, Smita KP. Undeclared drugs in traditional Chinese antirheumatoid medicine. Intern J Pharm Pract 1991; 1:117–119.
117. Hughes JR, Higgins EM, Pembroke AC. Oral dexamethasone masquerading as a Chinese herbal remedy. Br J Dermatol 1994;130:261.
118. Chan TYH. Anticholinergic poisoning due to Chinese herbal medicine. Vet Hum Toxicol 1995;32:156–157.
119. Hien TT, White NJ. Quinghaosu. Lancet 1993;341:603–608.
120. Fernando A. Medicinal plants. Ceylon Med J 1992;37:90–95.
121. McElvaine MD, Harder EM, Johnson L, Baer RD, Satzger ND. Lead poisoning from the use of Indian folk medicine. JAMA 1990;264:2212–2213.
122. CDC. Acute hepatitis and renal failure following ingestion of raw carp gallbladders—Maryland and Pennsylvania, 1991 and 1994. MMWR 1995;44:565–566.
123. Chan TYP, Chan JCN, Tomlinson B, Critchey JAJH. Chinese herbal medicines revisited: a Hong Kong perspective. Lancet 1993;342:1532–1534.
124. CDC. Folk remedy associated lead poisoning in Hmong children—Minnesota. MMWR 1983;32:555–556.
125. CDC. Folk remedy associated lead poisoning in Hmong children. JAMA 1983;250:3149–3150.
126. Hall SW, Night FE, Holtan NR, Eberhardt MS. Arsenic poisoning in Hmong adults. Vet Hum Toxicol 1989;31:351.
127. CDC. Non-fatal arsenic poisoning in three Hmong patients—Minnesota. MMWR. 1984;33:347–349.
128. Rubio EL, Ekins BR, Singh PD, Docus J. Hmong opiate folk remedy toxicity in three infants. Vet Hum Tox 1987;29: 323–325.
129. Tay C-H. Arsenic poisoning from anti-asthmatic herbal preparations. Med J Aust 1975;2:424–428.
130. Tay CH. Cutaneous manifestations of arsenic poisoning due to certain Chinese herbal medicines. Aust J Dermatol 1974;15:121–131.
131. CDC. Lead poisoning associated death from Asian Indian folk remedies—Florida. MMWR 1984;33:638–645.
132. Smitherman J, Harber P. A case of mistaken identity: herbal medicine as a cause of lead toxicity. Am J Ind Med 1991; 20:795–798.
133. Saryan LA. Surreptitious lead exposure from an Asian Indian medication. J Anal Toxicol 1991;15:336–338.
134. Kew J, Morris C, Aihie A, Fysh R, Jones S, Brooks D. Arsenic and mercury intoxication due to Indian ethnic remedies. Br Med J 1993;305:506–507.
135. Keen RW, Deacon AC, Delues HT, Moreton JA, Frost PG. Indian herbal remedies for diabetes as a cause of lead poisoning. Postgrad Med J 1994;70:113–114.
136. Jani JP, Raiyani CV, Mistry JS, Kashyap SK. Polycyclic aromatic hydrocarbons or traditional medicinal preparations. Hum Exp Toxicol 1991;10:347–350.
137. Gymnema. Lawrence Review of Natural Products. St. Louis: Facts and Comparisons, August 1993.
138. Kuman S, Roy AK. Occurrence of aflatoxin in some liver curative herbal medicine. Lett Appl Microbial 1993;17: 112–114.
139. Mangla betel nut warning. Lancet 1993;341:810–819.
140. Pickwell SM, Schimelpfening S, Palinkas LA. "Betelmania." Betel quid chewing by Cambodian women in the United States and its potential health effects. West J Med 1994;160: 326–330.
141. Chu N-S. Effects of betel chewing on electroencephalographic activity: spectral analysis and topographic mapping. J Formosa Med Assoc 1994;93:167–169.
142. Homma M, Oka K, Niitsuna T, Itah H: Pharmacokinetic evaluation of traditional Chinese herbal remedies. Lancet 1993; 341:1595.
143. Sarai K. Oriental medicine as therapy for resistant depression: use of some herbal drugs in the Far East (Japan). Prog Neuropsychopharmacol Biol Psychiatry 1992;16:171–180.
144. Fushimi R, Kohn T, Iyama S, Yasuhara M, Tachi J, Kohda K et al. Digoxin-like immunoreactivity in Chinese Medicine. Ther Drug Monit 1990;12:242–245.
145. Yamashiki M, Kosaka Y, Nishimura A, Okuta Y, Hamaguchi K et al. The herbal medicine sho-saiko-to improves cytokine production of peripheral blood mononuclear cells in patients with liver cirrhosis. Curr Ther Res 1993;54:86–97.
146. Rosti L, Nardini A, Bettinalli ME, Rosti D. Toxic effects of a herbal tea mixture in two newborns. Acta Paediatr 1995; 83:683.
147. Mitchell-Heggs CAW, Conway M, Cassar J. Herbal medicine as a cause of combined lead and arsenic poisoning. Hum Exp Toxicol 1990;9:195–196.
148. Chung JG, Yoon YB, Kim CY. A case of lead poisoning by herbal medicine. J Korean Med Assoc 1980;23:517–522.
149. Ibrahim N. Trace element analysis of the tradition medicine, Jamu. Bull Environ Contam Toxicol 1993;51:199–202.
150. Malik AS, Zabidi MH, Noor AP. Acute salicylism due to accidental ingestion of a traditional medicine. Singapore Med J 1994;35:215–216.
151. Anderson PA. Hazardous Mexican drug alert: metamizol. Vet Hum Toxicol 1992;34:555.
152. Foulke JE. Toddler's blood test leads to FDA recall. FDA Consumer 1992;41.
153. Sankury T, Cooper D, Bradley R et al. Lead poisoning from Mexican folk remedies—California. JAMA 1983;250:3149.
154. Trotter RT III. The cultural parameters of lead poisoning: a medical anthropologist's view of intervention in environmental lead exposure. Environ Health Perspect 1990;89:79–84.
155. Bose A, Vashishta K, O'Loughlin BJ. Azarcon por empacho—another cause of lead toxicity. Pediatrics 1983;72:106–110.
156. Levitt C, Godes J, Eberhardt M, Ing R, Simpson JM. Sources of lead poisoning. JAMA 1984;252:3127–3128.
157. CDC. Use of lead tetroxides as a folk remedy for gastrointestinal illness. MMWR 30:546–547.
158. Corchado A. Folk healers stay popular with poor in rural southwest. Wall Street Journal, January 4, 1989.
159. Huxtable RJ. The harmful potential of herbal and other plant products. Drug Safety 1990;5(Suppl 1):126–136.
160. Bah M, Bye R, Pereda-Miranda P. Hepatotoxic pyrrolizidine alkaloids in the Mexican medicinal plant *Packera candidissima (Asteraceae Senecioneae).* J Ethnopharmacol 1994;43:19–30.
161. Cone LA, Boughton WH, Cone LA, Lehr LH. Rattlesnake capsule-induced Salmonella arizonae bacteremia. West J Med 1990;153:315–316.
162. Waterman SH, Juarez G, Carr SJ, Kilman L. Salmonella arizonae infections in Latinos associated with rattlesnake folk medicine. Am J Public Health 190;80:286–289.
163. Babu K, Sonnenberg M, Kathpalia S, Ortega P, Suriatlo AL, Kocka FE. Isolation of Salmonella from dried rattlesnake preparations. J Clin Microbiol 1990;28:361–362.
164. Riley KB, Antoniskis D, Maris R, Leedon JM. Rattlesnake capsule-associated Salmonella arizonae infections. Arch Intern Med 1988;148:1207–1210.
165. Bhatt BD, Zuckerman MJ, Foland JA, Guerra LG, Polly SM. Rattlesnake meat ingestion—a common Hispanic folk remedy. West J Med 1988;149:605.

166. Noskin GA, Clarke JT. Salmonella arizonae bacteremia as the presenting manifestation of human immunodeficiency virus infection following rattlesnake meat ingestion. Rev Infect Dis 1990;12:514–517.
167. Casner PR, Guerra GG. Prescription medications on the U.S.–Mexican border. J Clin Pharmacol 1990; 30;831–862.
168. Casner PR, Guerra LG. Purchasing prescription medication in Mexico without a prescription. The experience at the border. West J Med 1992;156:512–516.
169. Tabet SR, Wiese WH. Medications obtained in Mexico by patients in southern New Mexico. South Med J 1990;83:271–270.
170. Rubin FK, Le Gatt DF, Audette RJ. The Mexican asthma cure. Systemic steroids for gullible gringos. Chest 1990;97: 959–961.
171. Chavaje N. The Mexican asthma "cure." Chest 1991;99:1052.
172. Blackburn JL, Hindmarsh KW. Corticosteroids contained in Mexican cures for arthritis and asthma. Can Med Assoc J 1976;1114:299–300.
173. Ruiz-Arguelles GJ, Alarcon-Segovia. Letter to the Editor: Mexican aspirin—a derogatory term. Am J Hematol 1990;34: 159.
174. Hargis JB, Redmond J, Wright DG. Author's reply. Am J Hematol 1990;34:160.
175. Hargis JB, La Russa VF, Redmond J, Kessler SW, Wright DG. Agranulocytosis associated with "Mexican aspirin" (dipyrone): evidence for an autoimmune mechanism affected multi-potential hematopoietic progenitors. Am J Hematol 1989;31:213–215.
176. Jachnowitz AI, Walker BK. Agranulocytosis and hepatitis as a result of Mexican drug therapy. Drug Intell Clin Pharm 1984;18:66–68.
177. Ifediba T, Haynes JF, Nelson B. Management of severe methemoglobinemia from dapsone ingestion in a binational community. Vet Hum Toxicol 1988;30:362.
178. Marti R. Description and incidence of Mexican diet medications at the Texas State Poison Center. Vet Hum Toxicol 1988;30:358–359.
179. Thompson RC. Dangerous diet drugs from south of the border. FDA Consumer 1987;21(4):29.
180. Maesner JE, Reynolds MS, St. Peter WL. Mexican diet clinical and drugs. Drug Intell Clin Pharm 1987;21.
181. Hindmarsh KW, Le Gatt DF. Mexican drug therapy. Clin Toxicol 1980;17:85–99.
182. Iarlori R, Foppiano M, Gimenez ER. Intoxicaciones agudas por acido tiazolidin carboxilico (ATC). Rev Hosp Ninix (Buenos Aires) 1977;19:125–126.
183. Kahn RS, Managuerra AS. Acute poisoning with thiazolidine carboxylic acid. Clin Toxicol 1981;18:527–530.
184. Sandler B, Bouchet H. Intoxication grave par l'acide thiazolidine carboxylique. Pediatrie 1972;27:76.
185. Baer RD, Ackerman A. Toxic Mexican folk remedies for the treatment of empacho. The case of azarcon, greta and albayalde. J Ethnopharmacol 1988;24:31–39.
186. Vlachos P, Kanitsakis NN. Fatal cardiac and renal failure due to *Ecbalium Elaterium* (squirting cucumber). Clin Toxicol 1994;32:737–738.
187. Tuncok Y, Kozan O, Cavdar C, Guven H, Fowler J. *Urginea maritima* (Squill) toxicity. Clin Toxicol 1995;33:83–86.
188. Healy MA, Aslam M, Bamgboye DA. Traditional medicine and lead containing preparations in Nigeria. Public Health (London) 1984;98:26–32.
189. Michie CA, Hayhurst M, Knobel GJ, Stokol JM, Hensley B. Poisoning with a traditional remedy containing potassium dichromate. Hum Exp Toxicol 1991;10:129–131.
190. Wood R, Mills PB, Knobel GJ, Hurlow WE, Stokol JM. Acute dichromate poisoning after use of traditional purgatives. A report of 7 cases. So Afr Med J 1990;77:640–642.
191. Epstein P, Yudkin JS. Agranulocytosis in Mozambique due to amidopyrine, a drug withdrawn in the West. Lancet 1980;2: 254–255.
192. Yudkin JS. Ciba-Geigy, amidopyrine and the Third World. Lancet 1981;2:114.
193. Foukaridis GN, Joubert PH, Forte M. A computerized library search routine using an HPLC diode array detector for the identification of poisoning by traditional medicines. Clin Toxicol 1992;30:149–151.
194. Nyazema NZ. Poisoning due to traditional remedies. Cent Afr J Med 1984;30:80–83.
195. McVann A, Havlik I, Joubert PH, Monteagudo FST. Cardiac glycoside poisoning involved in deaths from traditional medicines. So Afr Med J 1992;81:139–141.
196. Bye SN, Dutton MF. Poisonings from the incorrect use of traditional medicaments—an introduction. Proc Int Assoc Forensic Toxicol. Edinburgh: Scottish Academic Press, 1992; pp. 120–122.
197. Bye SM, Dutton MF. Development of an Elisa and immunochemistry for atractyloside, a toxin from *Callilepsis laureola*. In: Oliver JS, ed. Forensic Toxciology. Edinburgh: Scottish Academic Press, 1992; pp. 123–127.
198. Savage A, Hutchings A. Poisoned by herbs. Br Med J 1987; 295:1650–1651.
199. Nyazema NZ. Poisoning due to traditional remedies. Cent Afr J Med 1984;30:80–83.
200. Kasilo OMJ, Nhachi CFB. The pattern of poisoning from traditional medicine in urban Zimbabwe. S Afr Med J 1992; 82:187–188.
201. Kasilo OMJ, Nhachi CFB. A pattern of acute poisoning in children in urban Zimbabwe: ten years experience. Hum Exp Toxicol 1992;11:335–340.
202. Nhachi CFB, Habane T, Saturba P, Kasilo OMJ. Aspects of orthodox medicines (therapeutic drugs) poisoning in urban Zimbabwe. Hum Exp Toxicol 1992;11:329–333.
203. Joubert PH. Poisoning admission of black South Africans. Clin Toxicol 1990;28:85–94.
204. Venter CP, Joubert PH. Aspects of poisoning with traditional medicines in southern Africa. Biomed Environ Sci 1988;1: 388–391.
205. McVann A, Havlik I, Joubert PH, Monteagudo FSE. Cardiac glycoside poisoning involved in deaths from traditional medicines. S Afr Med J 1992;81:139–141.
206. Baer RD, Ackerman A. Arsenic as a home remedy. Treatment of Susto in Western South America. Social Pharmacol 1988;2: 37–49.
207. Santa-Maria SF. Health mission at 5000 m. J Wilderness Med 1992;3:460–461.
208. Erspamer V, Erspamer GF, Severini C, Potenza RL, Barra D, Mignogna G, Bianchi A. Pharmacological studies of "Sapo" from the frog *Phyllomedus bicolor* skin: a drug used by the Peruvian Matses Indians in Shamanic limiting practices. Toxicon 1993;31:1099–1111.
209. Diamond JR, Pallone PL. Acute interstitial nephritis following use of Tung Shueh pills. Am J Kidney Dis 1994;24:219–221.
210. Bayly GR, Braithwaite R, Sheehan TMT, Ferner RE. Lead poisoning from traditional Asian remedies in the West Midlands. Hum Exp Toxicol 1994;13:626.
211. Editor: Native Hawaiian medical lore. Hawaii Med J 1993;52: 156.
212. Blum JE, Coe FL. Metabolic acidosis after sulfur ingestion. N Engl J Med 1977;297:869–870.
213. Lin AN, Reimer RJ, Carter DM. Sulfur revisited. J Am Acad Dermatol 1988;18:553–558.
214. Croom EM Jr. Herbal medicine among the Lumbee Indians. In: Kirkland J, Mathews HF, Sullivan CW III, Baldwin K, eds. Herbal magical medicine. Traditional healing today. Durham, NC: Duke University Press, 1992; pp. 137–169.
215. Meier B. New York Times, April 8, 1990; p. 50.
216. Fung MC, Weintraub M, Bowen DL. Colloidal silver proteins marketed as health supplements. JAMA 1995;274:1196–1197.
217. CDC. Deaths associated with a purported aphrodisiac—New York City, February 1993–May 1995. MMWR 1995;44:853–855; also JAMA 1995;274:1828–1829.
218. CDC. Unexplained severe illness possibly associated with consumption of Kombucha tea—Iowa 1995. MMWR 1995;44:892–900.
219. Perron AD, Patterson JA, Yanofsky NN. Kombucha "mushroom" hepatotoxicity. Ann Emerg Med 1995;26:660–661.

Chapter 74 Plants—Mycotoxins—Mushrooms

PLANTS

A few plant species in certain localities can produce serious toxicity, including oleander *(Nerium oleander),* foxglove *(Digitalis purpurea),* jequirity pea *(Abrus precatorius),* castor beans *(Ricinus communis),* water hemlock *(Cicuta maculata),* Jerusalem cherry *(Solanum pseudocapsicum),* tree tobacco *(Nicotiana glauca),* jimsonweed *(Datura stramonium),* false hellebore *(Veratrum* spp.), plants containing pyrrolizidine alkaloids (e.g., *Senecio longilobus* teas), autumn crocus *(Colchicum autumnale),* and hepatotoxic mushrooms *(Amanita phalloides, Amanita virosa).* Each year a few deaths from plant poisonings occur in the United States.

PLANT IDENTIFICATION

A working relationship with a botanist or the local poison control center represents a valuable resource to optimize therapy in an emergency. As soon as a toxic ingestion is recognized, a portion of the plant, including reproductive parts, should be taken to the appropriate place (e.g., nursery, botanist, emergency department) for identification.

PHYSICAL EXAMINATION

Gastrointestinal Irritants (Table 74–1)

Pokeweed *(Phytolacca americana)* and holly bush (*Ilex* spp.) are common causes of gastroenteritis. The toxalbumin-containing plants, castor bean *(Ricinus communis)* and jequirity bean *(Abrus precatorius),* produce a severe gastroenteritis and, rarely, multiorgan failure.

Cardiovascular Abnormalities

Common oleander *(Nerium oleander),* lily of the valley *(Convallaria majalis),* foxglove *(Digitalis purpurea),* and yellow oleander *(Thevetia peruviana)* contain cardiac glycosides resembling digitalis.

Convulsions

Water hemlock (*Cicuta* spp.) ingestions produce convulsions within 30 to 60 minutes of exposure. Chinaberry *(Melia*

Table 74–1
Some Primary Gastrointestinal Irritants

Aloe spp.	All parts
Amaryllis (*Hippeastrum equestre*)	Bulb
Baneberry (*Actaea* spp.)	All parts, especially berries
Barberry (*Berberis vulgaris*)	Root, root bark
Bellyache bush (*Jatropha gossypifolia*)	Fruit
Bittersweet, American (*Celastrus scandens*)	All parts
Boxwood (*Buxus* spp.)	Leaves, stems
Buttercup (*Ranunculus* spp.)	All parts
Chinaberry (*Melia azedarach*)[a]	Fruits, leaves
Christmas rose (*Helleborus niger*)	All parts, especially rootstocks, leaves
Coral plant (*Jatropha multifida*)	Fruit
Crown of thorns (*Euphorbia milii*)	All parts
Daffodil (*narcissus pseudonarcissus*)	All parts, especially bulb
Daphne (*Daphne*)[a]	All parts, especially bark, fruit
Desert potato (*Jatropha macrorhiza*)	Root
English ivy (*Hedera helix*)	All parts
Euonymus (*Euonymus* spp.)	All parts
Four o'clocks (*Mirabilis jalapa*)	Roots, seeds
Holly (*Ilex* spp.)	Berries; leaves less toxic
Hyacinth (*Hyacinthus orientalis*)	Bulb
Iris (*Iris*)	Bulb leaves
Marsh marigold (*Caltha palustris*)	All parts
Mayapple (*Podophyllum peltatum*)[a]	Green fruit, roots, foliage
Mistletoe (*Phoradendron flavescens*)[a]	All parts, especially berries
Pokewood (*Phytolacca americana*)[a]	All parts
Privet (*Ligustrum* spp.)	Berries, leaves
Purging nut (*Jatropha curcas*)	Seeds, perhaps leaves
Purple rattlebox (*Daubentonia longifolia*)	Seeds
Pyracantha (*Pyracantha* spp.)	Berries (mild)
Tung nut (*Aleurites fordii*)	Nut
Yew (*Taxus* spp.)[a]	All parts, except fleshy red aril
Wisteria (*Wisteria sinensis*)	Pods

[a]Anecdotally, fatalities have been associated with large ingestions.

azedarach), moonseed *(Menispermum canadense),* and *Coriaria myrtifolia* contain potential convulsants. Occasionally, convulsions have resulted from serious ingestions of *Aconitum* (monkshood), *Taxus* (yew), and *Veratrum* plant species.

Nicotine and Nicotine-like Toxicity

Several plant species contain nicotine-like toxins, including the golden chain tree *(Laburnum anagyroides),* tree tobacco *(Nicotiana glauca),* Indian tobacco *(Lobelia inflata),* and poison hemlock *(Conium maculatum).* Nausea, vomiting, salivation, and abdominal cramps begins soon after exposure and are followed by headache, confusion, tachycardia, mydriasis, fever, and ataxia.

Atropine Poisoning (Table 74–2)

Atropine, scopolamine, and hyoscyamine appear in a variety of plants, the most common of which are jimsonweed *(Datura stramonium),* deadly nightshade *(Atropa belladonna),* henbane *(Hyoscyamus niger),* angel's trumpet (*Brugmansia* spp., formerly *Datura sauveolens*), and matrimony vine *(Lycium halimifolium).* Clinical manifestations of toxicity are similar to those of classic atropine poisoning with headache, nausea, dry skin and mouth, tachycardia, mydriasis, and urinary retention.

Hallucinations (Table 74–3)

Nutmeg *(Myristica frangans),* the ergot fungus *(Claviceps purpurea),* morning glory seeds *(Ipomoea violacea),* peyote *(Lophophora williamsii), Mimosa* spp., psilocybin-containing mushrooms (e.g., *Psilocybe* or *Paneolus*), ibotenic acid–containing mushrooms (e.g., *Amanita muscaria*), and marijuana (*Cannabis* spp.) possess mind-altering properties.

Kidney

Rhubarb plants contain soluble oxalate crystals, which can produce renal failure after chronic consumption. Decreased renal function also occurs secondary to the hepatorenal syndrome seen after *Amanita phalloides* poisoning. Autumn crocus *(Colchicum autumnale)*, podophyllum resin, and *Cortinarius* mushrooms can produce primary renal dysfunction.

Liver

Hepatotoxic mushrooms are well described. Less well known are the pyrrolizidine alkaloids, which produce hepatic failure both sporadically (e.g., when ingested as teas from *Senecio longilobus*) and epidemically (e.g., consumption of cereals contaminated by *Crotolaria* or *Heliotropmum* seeds). Akee fruit, a South African tuber *(Callilepis laureola),* and sassafras root also cause hepatic dysfunction in severe cases.

DISTRIBUTION

Willis has tabulated common poisonous plants in North America according to their site of toxic action (Table 74–4).[1] Plants of abuse are listed in Table 74–5.[2] Nonpoisonous plants that do not generally causes symptoms are listed in Table 74–6.[3] John Henry has compiled a review of the possibly fatal amount of some plants (Table 74–7).[4] Nephrotoxic plants are listed in Table 74–8.[5] The frequency of plant exposures in the United States in 1993 are listed in Table 74–9.[6] The most important potentially serious exposures follow ingestion of cardiac glycosides (e.g., oleander), anticholinergics (e.g., jimsonweed), cyanogenic glycosides (amygdalin, *Prunus* spp. pits, bean, jequirity peas), solanine (e.g., green potato, nightshade), and water hemlock. Visual recognition of oleander, foxglove, jimson seed pod, castor bean, and jequirity bean is important.

Table 74–2
Hyoscyamine- and Hyoscine-Containing Plants (Alkaloids With a Tropane Nucleus)[a]

Scientific Name	Common Name	Description	Distribution	Poisonous Component
(a) *Datura stramonium*	Tolguacha Apple of Peru Jimsonweed Jamestown weed Devil's apple Thorn apple Devil's trumpet Stinkweed Loco seeds or locoweed	Large erect plant; funnel-shaped white or purple flowers; spreading branches; hard prickly ovate; many-seeded fruit	Cultivated or noncultivated fields; widespread in United States	Hyoscyamine (leaves, roots, seeds) Hyoscine (roots)
(b) *Hyoscyamus niger*	Henbane Black henbane	Tall erect stem; multibranched stem having fetid odor; yellowish flowers; encapsulated seeds	Common in United States	Hyoscyamine Hyoscine
(c) *Atropa belladonna*	Belladonna Deadly nightshade	Fleshy erect stem; hairy leaves; purple flowers; purple-black many-seeded berry when ripe	Cultivated in Eastern states; rarely survives in wild form	Hyoscyamine (throughout plants)
(d) *Lycium halimifolium*	Matrimony vine	Vine or shrub; bell-shaped flowers; ovoid orange-red berry	Northern United States	Hyoscyamine
(e) *Cestrum nactornum* *Cestrum diurnum*	Night-blooming jessamine	Large, attractive shrubs; fragrant trumpet flowers; small berry	Coastal plains in South and Southwest	Atropine (?), gastroenterotoxin
(f) *Mandragora officinarum*	Mandrake	Native Mediterranean plant whose leaves resemble lettuce	Greece and Mediterranean countries	Roots, fruit, and leaves contain hyoscyamine, scopolamine, pseudohyoscyamine, and mandragorine

[a]Adapted from Goldfrank L, Melinek M. Hosp Physician 1979;15(8):40.

TOXIC PLANT SUBSTANCES (TABLE 74–10)

Toxic plant substances belong to a relatively few broad categories of compounds. Major groupings of these compounds include alkaloids, glycosides, proteinaceous compounds, organic acids, alcohols, resins and resinoids (including phenolics), mineral toxins, and nonorganic compounds.[7]

Alkaloids

1. The belladonna type (tropane or atropine alkaloids) such as belladonna *(Atropa)*, jimsonweed *(Datura)*, henbane *(Hyoscyamus)*, mandrake *(Mandragora)*, and coca tree *(Erythroxylum)*.
2. The groundsel type (pyrrolizidine alkaloids) such as groundsel *(Senecio)*, blue devil *(Echium)*, and heliotrope *(Heliotropium)*.
3. Hemlock type (pyridine or piperidine alkaloids) such as poison hemlock *(Conium)* and Indian tobacco *(Lobelia)*.
4. Nicotine or tobacco type (pyridine alkaloids) such as tobacco *(Nicotiana)* and horsetail *(Equisetum)*.
5. Caffeine or caffeine type (purine alkaloids) such as coffee *(Coffea)*; chocolate, "cola," cocoa *(Theobroma)*, and tea *(Camellia)*.
6. Quinine type (quinoline alkaloids) such as the quinone tree *(Cinchona)* and globe thistle *(Echinops)*.

Table 74–3
Major Hallucinogenic Plants and Their Active Principles[a]

Plant	Family	Active Principle
Cannabis sativa	Cannabinaceae	Δ^1-Tetrahydrocannabinol
Lophophora williamsii	Cactaceae	Mescaline
Piptadenia species	Leguminosae	Substituted tryptamines
Mimosa species	Leguminosae	Substituted tryptamines
Virola species	Myristacaceae	Substituted tryptamines
Banistereopsis species	Malpighiaceae	Harmaline, harmine
Peganum harmala	Zygophyllaceae	Harmaline, harmine
Tabernanthe iboga	Apocynaceae	Ibogaine
Ipomoea violacea	Convolvulaceae	*d*-Lysergic acid amide *d*-Isolysergic acid amide
Turbina corymbosa	Convolvulaceae	*d*-Lysergic acid amide *d*-Isolysergic acid amide
Datura species	Solanaceae	Scopolamine
Methysticodendron amesianum	Solanaceae	Scopolamine
Amanita muscaria	Agaricaceae	Pantherine, ibotenic acid
Psilocybe mexicana	Agaricaceae	Psilocybine

[a]Adapted from Farnsworth NR. Science 1986;162:1090.

Table 74–4
Common Poisonous Plants Native to and Cultivated in North America[a]

Name	Toxic Parts	Toxic Compounds
Anticholinergics		
• Deadly nightshade *Atropa belladonna*	All	Atropine and related compounds
• Henbane *Hyoscyamus niger*	All	Hyoscyamine, hyoscine, atropine
• Jimsonweed (Angel's trumpet, thorn apple) *Datura stramonium*	All	Hyoscyamine, hyoscine, atropine
• Lantana (bunchberry) *Lantana* spp.	Berries, leaves	Lantadene
Cardiac toxins		
• Azalea *Rhododendron* spp.	All	Grayanotoxins
• Death camass (black snakeroot) *Zigadenus* spp.	All	Zygadenine, veratrine
• False hellebore (corn lily) *Veratrum californicum*	All	Veratrum alkaloids
• Foxglove *Digitalis purpurea*	Leaves, seeds	Digitalis glycosides
• Green hellebore (American white hellebore) *Veratrum viride*	All	Veratrum alkaloids
• Japanese pieris *Pieris japonica*	All	Grayanotoxins
• Larkspur *Delphinium ambiguum*	All	Delphinin and other alkaloids
• Lily of the valley *Convallaria majalis*	All	Convallarin, convallamarin
• Monkshood (aconite) *Aconitum* spp.	Leaves, roots, seeds	Aconitine, aconine
• Mountain laurel *Kalmia latifolia*	All	Grayanotoxins
• Oleander *Nerium oleander*	All	Oleandrin, oleandrosine
• Yew *Taxus* spp.	All parts except flesh of berry	Taxine
CNS stimulants		
• Chinaberry *Melia azedarach*	All	A resinoid
• Water hemlock *Cicuta maculata*	All parts, especially roots	Cicutoxin
• Western water hemlock *Cicuta douglasii*	All parts, especially roots	Cicutoxin
Cyanogenic glycosides		
• Cherry laurel *Prunus laurocerasus*	Foliage, pits	Amygdalin
• Choke cherry *Prunus virginiana*	Foliage, pits	Amygdalin
• Elderberry *Sambucus nigra*	Foliage, pits	Amygdalin
• *Hydrangea* spp.	All	Hydrangin
Dermatitis-producing		
• Poinsettia *Euphorbia pulcherrima*	All	Vesicant sap
• Poison ivy *Rhus toxicodendron*	All	Oleoresin
• Poison oak *Toxicodendron* spp.	All	Oleoresin
Gastrointestinal irritants		
• Amaryllis *Hippeastrum puniceum*	Bulb	Lycorine
• Autumn crocus *Colchicum autumnale*	All	Colchicine
• Daffodil, narcissus, jonquil *Narcissus* spp.	All parts	Lycorine, narcissine

[a]Adapted from Willis GA. Medicine North America. December 14, 1990, pp. 1753–1759.

(continued)

Table 74–4 *(Continued)*

Name	Toxic Parts	Toxic Compounds
Gastrointestinal irritants *(continued)*		
• Daphne *Daphne* spp.	All	Daphnin, narcissine
• Holly *Ilex* spp.	Berries	Ilicin
• Horsechestnut (buckeye) *Aesculus hippocastanum*	Nut	Esculin
• Hyacinth *Hyacinthus orientalis*	Bulb	Narcissine
• Iris (blue flag) *Iris* spp.	Bulb, leaves	Irritant resins
• Mistletoe *Phoradendron flavescens*	All parts, especially berries	Sympathetic amines
• Oak *Quercus* spp.	Acorns	Tannins
• Poinsettia *Euphorbia pulcherrima*	Sap	Irritant
• Pokeweed (inkberry) *Phytolacca americana*	All	Resins, saponins, alkaloids
• Privet *Ligustrum* spp.	All	Not known
• Snowberry (waxberry) *Symphoricarpus albus*	Berries	Loturidine
• Snowdrop *Galanthus nivalis*	Bulb	Narcissine, lycorine
• Wisteria *Wisteria* spp.	Seeds, pods	Wisterin, resin
Nicotinics		
• Laburnum (golden chain) *Laburnum anagyroides*	All	Cystisine
• Lobelia (cardinal flower) *Lobelia* spp.	All	Lobeline
• Poison hemlock *Conium maculatum*	All	Coniine
• Tobacco *Nicotiana* spp.	All	Nicotine
Oxalates		
• Caladium *Caladium* spp.	All	Calcium oxalate
• Dumb-cane *Dieffenbachia* spp.	All	Calcium oxalate
• Elephant's ear *Colocasia* spp.	All	Calcium oxalate
• Jack-in-the-pulpit *Arisaema triphyllum*	All parts, except rhizome	Calcium oxalate
• Philodendron	All	Calcium oxalate
• Pothos *Scindapsus aureus*	All	Calcium oxalate
• Rhubarb *Rheum rhaponticum*	Leaves	Oxalic acid and soluble oxalates
• Skunk cabbage *Symplocarpus aureus*	All	Calcium oxalate
Solanine		
• Black nightshade *Solanum nigrum*	Leaves, fruit	Solanine, alkaloids
• Jerusalem cherry *Solanum pseudocapsicum*	Leaves, fruit	Solanine, alkaloids
• Potato *Solanum tuberosum*	Sprouts, sun-greened tuber	Solanine, alkaloids
Toxalbumins		
• Black locust (black acacia) *Robinia pseudoacacia*	All parts, except flowers	Robin, robitin
• Castor bean *Ricinus communis*	All parts (mainly)	Ricin
• Jequirity bean (rosary pea) *Abrus precatorius*	Seeds	Abrin

Table 74–5
Miscellaneous Plants of Abuse[a]

Plant	Part Used	Toxic Agent
Argyreia nervosa	Seed	Ergoline hallucinogens
Atropa belladonna	Seed	Tropane alkaloids
Banisteriopsis species	Various	Harmaline (hallucinogen)
Cola nitida	Seed	Caffeine
Datura speciosa	Seed	Tropane alkaloids
Hyoscyamus niger	Whole plant	Tropine alkaloids
Ilex paraguarensis	Leaf	Caffeine
Lophophora		
Mandragora officinarum	Whole plant	Tropane alkaloids
Methysticodendron amesianum	Stems/Leaf	Tropane alkaloids
Mimosa hostilis	Root	Phenylamine hallucinogens
Olmedioperebea sclerophylla	Fruit	Unknown hallucinogen
Passiflora incarnata	Stem/Leaf	Harmaline (hallucinogen)
Pelganum harmala	Seed	Harmaline (hallucinogen)
Piper methysticum	Root	Methysticin/Kawain
Piptadenia colubrina	Seed	Phenylamine hallucinogens
Piptadenia excelsa	Seed	Phenylamine hallucinogens
Piptadenia macrocarpa	Seed	Phenylamine hallucinogens
Piptadenia peregrina	Seed/Bark	Phenylamine hallucinogens
Salvia divinorum	Leaf	Unknown hallucinogen
Sophora secundiflora	Seed	Cytisine (stimulant)
Tabernanthe iboga	Root	Ibogaine (hallucinogen)
Trichocereus pachanoi	Cactus	Mescaline
Virola calophylla	Bark	Phenylamine hallucinogens

[a]Adapted from Spoerke DG, Hall AH. Emerg Clin North Am 1990;8:579–593.

Table 74–6
Nonpoisonous Houseplants That Generally Do Not Cause Symptoms

Common Name	Botanical Name
African violet	*Episcia reptans*
Aluminum plant	*Pilea cadierei*
Aralia	*Fatsia japonica*
Baby tears	*Helxine soleirolli*
Bird's nest fern	*Asplenium nidus*
Bridal veil	*Tradescantia*
Coleus X hydrus	*Coleus*
Corn plant	*Dracaena fragrans*
Creeping Charlie[a]	*Lysimachia nummularia*
Creeping Charlie[a]	*Pilea nummularifolia*
Creeping Jenny	*Lysimachia*
Dracaena indivisa	*Cordyline indivisa*
Dwarf Schefflera	*Schefflera arboricola*
Emerald ripple	*Peperomia caperata*
Fiddleleaf fig	*Ficus lyrata*
Gardenia	*Gardenia jasminoides*
Grape ivy	*Cissus rhombifolia*
Jade plant	*Crassula argentea*
Wandering Jew	*Tradescantia albiflora*
Wandering Jew (red and green)	*Zebrina pendula*
Parlor palm	*Chamaedorea elegans*
Peacock plant	*Calathea*
Piggyback begonia	*Begonia hispida var. Cuculifera*
Piggyback plant	*Tolmiea menziesii*
Prayer plant	*Maranta leuconeura*
Rubber tree	*Ficus elastica Decora*
Schefflera, umbrella plant	*Brassaia actinophylla*
Snake plant	*Sansvieria trifasclata*
Spider plant	*Chlorophytum comosum*
String of hearts	*Ceropegia woodii*
Swedish ivy	*Plectranthus verticallatus*
Velvet plant	*Gynura aurantiaca*
Wax plant	*Hoya carnosa*
Zebra plant	*Aphelandra squarrosa*

[a]There are species in this group that are poisonous.

Table 74–7
Common Fatal Plants[a]

Plant	Toxic Principle	Possibly Fatal Amount (in an adult)
Ackee *(Blighia sapida)*	Hypoglycin	One fruit
Apple or pear seeds (*Pyrus* spp.)	Amygdalin (cyanogenic glycoside)	50 seeds
Castor oil plant *(Ricinus communis)*	Ricin	One bean
Death cap *(Amanita phalloides)*	Amanitin, phalloidin (cyclopeptides)	One mushroom
Galerina spp. mushrooms	Amanitin-type cyclopeptide	One mushroom
Gyromitra spp. mushrooms	Monomethylhydrazine	One mushroom
Holly *(Ilex aquifolium)*	Ilicin	30 berries
Jequirity *(Abrus precatorius)*	Abrin	One bean
Oleander *(Nerium oleander)*	Oleandrin (cardiac glycoside)	One leaf
Stone fruid kernels (*Prunus* spp.)	Amygdalin (cyanogenic glycoside)	30 kernels
Hemlock water dropwort *(Oenanthe crocata)*	Oenanthetoxin	One root
Yew *(Taxus baccata)*	Taxine A and B (cardiac glycosides)	50 needles

[a]Adapted from Henry JA. Eur Assoc Pois Cont Center Newsletter, May 1985.

Table 74–8
Nephrotoxic Plants[a]

Plant	Scientific Name	Toxic Compounds
Autumn crocus	*Colchicum autumnaie*	Colchicine
Castor bean	*Ricinus communis*	Ricin and recinine
Daphne	*Daphne mezereum*	Daphnin, vesicant resin, and mezerenic acid anhydride
Herbal remedies	Exact plants unknown	Unknown
Impila	*Callilepsis laureola*	Atractyloside
Marking-nut tree	*Semecarpus anacardium*	Phenolic constituents
Poison mushrooms	*Amanita phalloides* and *Cortinarius* species	Amatoxin cyclopeptides
Rosary pea	*Abrus precatorius*	Abrin and abric acid
?	*Securidaca longipedunculata*	Methyl salicylate, saponius, tanins, and gaultherin
Water hemlock	*Cicuta maculata*	Cicutoxin

[a]Adapted from Abuelo JG. Arch Intern Med 1990;150:505–510.

Table 74–9
Frequency of Plant Exposures by Plant Type[a]

Botanical Name	Common Name	Frequency
Philodendron species	Philodendron	4,726
Capsicum annuum	Pepper	3,912
Dieffenbachia species	Dumbcane	2,837
Euphorbia pulcherrima	Poinsettia	2,798
Ilex species	Holly	2,651
Phytolacca americana	Pokeweed, inkberry	2,231
Spathiphyllum species	Peace lily	2,086
Crassula species	Jade plant	1,658
Epipremnum aureum	Pothos, devil's ivy	1,401
Toxidodendron/Rhus radicans	Poison ivy	1,306
Brassaia actinophylla	Umbrella tree	1,141
Saintpaulia ionantha	African violet	1,137
Rhododendron species	Rhododendron, azalea	1,029
Taxus species	Yew	969
Eucalyptus Globulus	Eucalyptus	945
Pyracantha species	Pyracantha	894
Chlorophytum comusum	Spider plant	787
Schlumbergera bridgesii	Christmas cactus	781
Hedera helix	English ivy	765
Solanum dulcamara	Climbing nightshade	754

[a]Adapted from Litovitz TL et al. Am J Emerg Med 1994;12:546–584.

Table 74–10
Plant Toxins[a]

Toxin	Source	Chemistry	Mode of Action
Na^+ channel			
Lipophilic toxins			
Veratridine	Plant rhizome Veratrum album (Lilaceae) or seeds of *Schoenocauon officinale*	Alklaoid	Hyperexcitability resulting from reversible membrane depolarization
Aconitine	Monk's hood: *Aconitum napellus* (Ranunculaceae)	Alkaloid	Cardiac arrhythmia, repetitive firing of nerve
Grayanotoxins (GTX)	Leaves of *Rhodendendron, Kalmia, Leucothoe* (Ericaceae)	Diterpenoid	Membrane depolarization
Pyrethrins	Chrysanthemum flower *Chrysanthemum cinaerofolium*	Organic ester	Insecticidal; lethal convulsive paralysis in insects; also used historically in humans as stimulant, aphrodisiac
Ca^+ channels			
Ryanodine	Plant: *Ryania speciosa* (Flacourticeae)	Alkaloid	Insecticidal; causes muscle contracture
Glutamate-gated channels			
Ibotenic acid	Fly agaric mushroom: *Amanita muscaria*	Amino acid	Depolarization of cells possessing glutamate receptors
Kainic acid	Red alga: *Digenea simplex*	Cyclic amino acid	Depolarization of crayfish and insect muscle
Domoic acid	Alga: *Nitzschia Pungens* found in blue mussel, *Mytilus edulis*; Seaweed: *Chondria armata*	Cyclic amino	Excitotoxic; causes amnesia
Acromelic acid	Mushroom: *Clitocybe* spp.	Cyclic amino acid	Following systemic administration in rats causes forced hindlimb extension; seizures; wet-dog shakes; degeneration of spinal interneurons

[a]Adapted from Adams ME, Swanson G. Trends Neurosci Suppl, April 1994.

(continued)

Table 74–10 *(Continued)*

Toxin	Source	Chemistry	Mode of Action
Acetylcholine receptors			
Nicotine	Tobacco: *Nicotiana tabacum*	Alkaloid	CNS stimulant: decreases skeletal muscle tone; nausea and vomiting at high doses
Anatoxin-A	Freshwater cyanobacterium: *Anabaena flos-aquae*	Bicyclic alkaloid	Flaccid paralysis
Muscarinic (agonist):			
Muscarine	Fly agaric mushroom: *Amanita muscaria*	Quaternary ammonium-substituted alkaloid	Stimulates parasympathetic system, smooth muscle; slows heart rate; CNS arousal
Arecoline	Betel nut: *Areca catechu*	Tertiary amine-substituted alkaloid	Stimulates parasympathetic system, smooth muscle; slows heart rate; CNS arousal
Pilocarpine	Leaves of plant: *Pilocarpus* spp.	Tertiary amine-substituted alkaloid	Stimulates parasympathetic system, smooth muscle; slows heart rate; CNS arousal
Muscarinic (antagonist):			
Scopolamine (Hyoscine)	Henbane: *Hyoscyamus niger* or *Scopolia carniolica*	Alkaloid	Depression of salivary and bronchial secretion and sweating; pupil dilation; increases heart rate at higher doses
Atropine	Deadly nightshade: *Atropa belladonna* *Jimson weed:* *Datura stramonium*	Alkaloid	Depression of salivary and bronchial secretion and sweating; pupil dilation; increases heart rate at higher doses
GABA receptors agonist			
Muscimol	Fly agaric mushroom: *Amanita muscaria*	Alkaloid; cyclic GABA analogue	Hallucinogenic; potentiates morphine-induced analgesia
Glycine receptor			
Strychnine	Seed: *Strychnos nux-vomica*	Heterocyclic alkaloid	CNS convulsant; acts primarily on spinal cord and brainstem
Transmitter re-uptake			
GABA			
Guvacine	Seeds of betel nut: *Areca catechu* (Palmae)	Nicotinic acid analogues	Anticonvulsant
Catecholamines			
Cocaine	Leaves of coca plant: *Erythroxylon coca*	Benzoylmethyl-ecgonine	Stimulates CNS, vasoconstrictor
ATPase			
Digitoxin	Foxglove: *Digitalis purpurea*	Glycoside	Cardiac acceleration
Ouabain (Strophanthin G)	Seeds: *Strophanthus gratus*	Glycoside	Ataxia, rapid breathing, cardioacceleration, tremor, convulsions
Toxins with unknown targets			
Capsaicin	Peppers: *Capsicum* spp. (Solenaceae)	Diterpene	Irritant of mucous membranes; prolonged exposure reduces pain sensation; can cause selective degeneration of primary sensory afferents in newborn rats
Cycasin	Seeds of cycad: *Cycas revoluta*	b-D-glucopyranoside	Neurotoxic; might be causal agent in slow neurodegenerative disease; western Pacific ALS and parkinsonism; dementia complex

7. Opium or morphine type (isoquinoline alkaloids) such as opium poppy *(Papaver),* blood root *(Sanguinaria),* squirrel corn *(Dicentra),* golden seal *(Hydrastis),* and fumatory *(Corydalis).*
8. Ergot type (indole or indolizidine alkaloids) such as ergot *(Claviceps),* magic mushroom *(Psilocybe),* locoweed *(Astragalus),* Carolina jessamine *(Gelsemium),* and strychnine *(Strychnos).*
9. Lupine type (quinolizidine alkaloids—cytisine type) such as lupines *(Lupinus),* golden chain *(Laburnum),* false indigo *(Baptisia),* Scotch broom *(Cytisus),* and Kentucky coffee tree *(Gymnocladus).*

10. Tomato or solanine type (steroidal, glycoalkaloids) such as tomato *(Lycopersicon),* Irish potato *(Solanum),* and nightshades *(Solanum).*
11. Veratrum type (steroid alkaloids) such as false hellebore *(veratrum)* and death camus *(Zigadenus).*
12. Larkspur type (diterpenoid alkaloids) such as larkspur *(Delphinium)* and monkshood *(Aconitum).*
13. Mescaline type (phenylalanine alkaloids) such as peyote *(Lophophora)* and ephedra *(Ephedra).*

Glycosides

1. Cyanogenic (cyanogenic glycoside) aglycone is hydrocyanic acid (e.g., amygdalin in seeds or pits of wild cherry, peach, apricot, apple, and almond), which on hydrolysis yields sugar, cyanide, and benzaldehyde. Amygdalin from ground up apricot pits is laetrile.
2. Steroid glycosides: sugar is joined to a steroid molecule. (a) Cardiac glycosides (see Chapter 32—Antiarrhythmic Drugs), e.g., foxglove (digoxin, *Digitalis purpurea),* lily of the valley *(Convallaria),* ouabain *(Strophanthus),* dogbane *(Apocynum),* milkweed *(Asclepias),* and oleander *(Nerium).* (b) Saponin (sapogenic) glycosides: pokeweed *(Phytolacca),* English ivy *(Hedera).* Cause gastric irritation; aglycones are hemolytic.
3. Coumarin glycosides: sugar attached to a coumain aglycone, e.g., Ohio buckeye *(Aesculus glabra),* yellow and white sweet clover (*Melilotus* spp.): anticoagulants.
4. Anthraquinone and mustard oil glycosides: cathartics, GI irritants.

Proteinaceous Compounds

1. Proteins: phytotoxins (toxalbumins), e.g., abrin—seeds of rosary bean *(Abrus precatorius);* ricin (castor bean—*Ricinus communis* seeds).
2. Polypeptides: amatoxins, phallotoxins, phalloides in *Amanita phalloides.*
3. Amines: e.g., *Lathyrus*—aminopropionitrile, degeneration of motor tracts of spinal cord—lathrism, mistletoe berries (tyramine, phenylethylamine): acute gastroenteritis, cardiovascular collapse.

Oxalates

The leaves, stems, and roots of many plants contain oxalates. Rhubarb leaves contain up to 1% soluble sodium and potassium oxalates. Other plants containing high amounts of insoluble calcium oxalates in their leaves include dieffenbachia, philodendron, and sorrel. Insoluble calcium oxalate crystal needles are contained in raphides, then bundled into elongated idioblasts that fire the needles as projectiles where force such as chewing is applied (Fig. 74–1). Highest levels are found in the families Polygonaceae *(Rheum, Rumex),* Chenopodiaceae *(Halogetin, Glomeratus),* Spinaciae, Oxalidaceae *(Oxalis cirnua),* Portulacaceae *(Portulaca),* and Ficoidaceae *(Tetragonia).* Ingestion of a small amount of plant parts with high oxalate concentrations usually causes only mild irritation of the mouth and esophageal mucosa. More pronounced gastrointestinal effects may follow ingestion of large amounts of soluble oxalate: spinach, rhubarb, and dieffenbachia.[8]

Alcohols

Cicutoxin from *Cicuta maculata*—water hemlock is a convulsant, and tremetol from white snakeroot *(Eupatorium nyosum)* produces trembling in cattle.

Resins and Resinoids

Phenolic Resins

Tetrahydrocannabinol (THC) from *Cannabis sativa.*

Resinoids

Urushiol (from poison ivy, poison oak, and poison sumac) and hypericin (from *Hypericum perforatum,* St. John's wort).

Phenolics

Gossypol (seed oil of Gossypium). Male contraceptive.

Mineral Toxins

Weed species (goosefoot, *Chenopodium album,* and pigweed, *Amaranthus* spp.) accumulate potassium nitrate.

DATABASES

A microcomputer-based database on dangerous animals and plants with capabilities of displaying color pictures plus textual information has been developed by the National University of Singapore.[9] A database has been completed for Poison Control Center inquiries for 103 common houseplants described in lay terms.[10] The Colorado Group has developed a berry identification approach.[11] Additional approaches to plant information systems are available.[12–14] An image-based computerized identification system for poisonous plants and fungi in the United Kingdom has been initiated by the National Poisons Unit at Guy's Hospital in London and the Royal Botanic Gardens in Kew.[15]

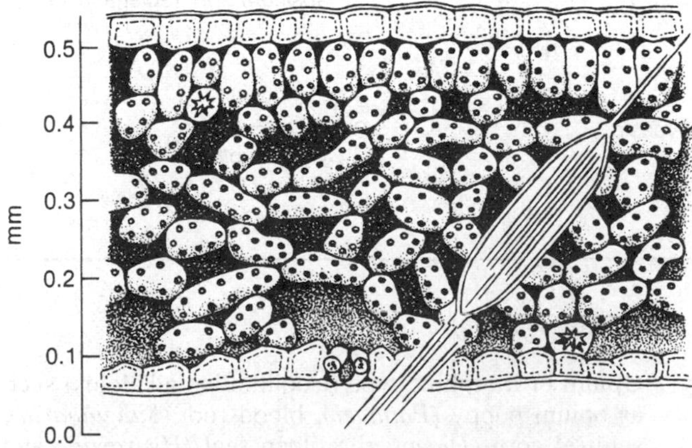

Figure 74–1 Diagrammatic section of leaf of *Dieffenbachia,* showing needlelike crystals of calcium oxalate inside the specialized bivented idioblast situated in the spongy mesophyll. Two druses are also shown. (Adapted from Dore WC. JAMA 1963;185:1045.)

Table 74–11
Some Herbs That Should Not Be Used in Foods, Beverages or Drugs[a]

Botanical Name of Plant Source	Common Names	Remarks
Arnica montana L.	Arnica. Arnica Flowers. Wolf's-bane. Leopard's Bane. Mountain Tobacco. Flores Arnicae.	Aqueous and alcoholic extracts of the plant contain choline, plus two unidentified substances that affect the heart and vascular systems. Arnica, an active irritant, can produce violent toxic gastroenteritis, nervous disturbances, change in pulse rate, intense muscular weakness, collapse, and death.
Atropa belladonna L.	Belladonna. Deadly Nightshade.	Poisonous plant that contains the toxic solanaceous alkaloids hyoscyamine, atropine and hyoscine.
Solanum dulcamara L.	Bittersweet twigs. Dulcamara. Bittersweet. Woody Nightshade. Climbing Nightshade.	Poisonous. Contains the toxic glycoalkaloid solanine; also solanidine and dulcamarin.
Sanguinaris canadensis L.	Bloodroot. Sanguinaria. Red Puccoon.	Contains the poisonous alkaloid sanguinarine and other alkaloids.
Cytisus scoparius (L) Link.	Broom-tops. Scoparius. Spartium. Scotch Broom. Irish Broom. Broom.	Contains toxic sparteine, isosparteine, and other alkaloids; also hydroxytyramine.
Aesculus hippocastanum L.	Buckeyes. Aesculus. Horse Chestnut.	Contains a toxic coumarin glycoside, aesculin (esculin). A poisonous plant.
Acorus calamus L.	Calamus. Sweet Flag. Sweet Root. Sweet Cane. Sweet Cinnamon.	Oil of calamus, Jammu variety, is a carcinogen. FDA regulations prohibit marketing of calamus as a food or food additive.
Heliotropium europaeum L.	Heliotrope.	A poisonous plant. It contains alkaloids that produce liver damage. Not to be confused with garden heliotrope (*Valeriana officinalis* L.).
Conium maculatum L.	Hemlock. Conium. Poison Hemlock. Spotted Hemlock. Spotted Parsley. St. Bennet's Herb. Spotted Cowbane. Fool's Parsley.	Contains the poisonous alkaloid coniine and four other closely related alkaloids. Often confused with water hemlock (*Cicuta maculata* L.). Not to be confused with hemlock, hemlock spruce, etc. (*Tsuga canadensis* (L). Carr.).
Hyoscyamus niger L.	Henbane. Hyoscyamus. Black Henbane. Hog's Bean. Poison Tobacco. Devil's Eye.	Contains the alkaloids hyoscyamine, hyoscine (scopolamine) and atropine. A poisonous plant.
Exogonium purga (Wenderoth) Bentham. *Ipomoea jalapa* Nutt, and Coxe. *Ipomoea purga* (Wenderoth) *Hayne. Exagonium jalapa* (Wenderoth) Baillon.	Jalap Root. Jalap. True Jalap. Jalapa. Vera Cruz Jalap. High John Root. (Possibly also known as High John the Conqueror, John Conqueror. St. John the Conqueror Root. Hi John Conqueror.)	A large twining vine of Mexico, this plant has undergone many name changes. The drug is a powerful, drastic cathartic. Purgative powers of jalap reside in its resin. In overdoses, jalap may produce dangerous hypercatharsis.
Datura stramonium L.	Jimson Weed. Datura. Stramonium. Apple of Peru. Jamestown Weed. Thornapple. Tolguacha.	Contains the alkaloids atropine, hyoscyamine and scopolamine. Illegal drug for nonprescription use. A poisonous plant.
Convallaria majalis L.	Lily of the Valley. Convallaria. May Lily.	Contains the toxic cardiac glycosides convallatoxin, convallarin and convallamarin. Poisonous plant.
Lobelia inflata L.	Lobelia. Indian Tobacco. Wild Tobacco. Asthma Weed. Emetic Weed.	A poisonous plant that contains the alkaloid lobeline plus a number of other pyridine alkaloids. Overdoses of the plant or extracts of the leaves or fruits produce vomiting, sweating, pain, paralysis, depressed temperatures, rapid but feeble pulse, collapse, coma, and death.
Mandragora officinarum L.	Mandrake. Mandragora. European Mandrake.	The plant is a poisonous narcotic similar in its properties to belladonna. Contains the alkaloids hyoscyamine, scopolamine, and mandragorine.
Podophyllum peltatum L.	Mandrake. May Apple. Podophyllum. American Mandrake. Devil's Apple. Umbrella Plant. Vegetable Calomel. Wild Lemon. Vegetable Mercury.	A poisonous plant, it contains podophyllotoxin, a complex polycyclic substance, and other constituents.
Phorandendron flavescens (Pursh.) Nutt. *Viscum flavescens* (Pursh.)	Mistletoe. Viscum. American Mistletoe.	Poisonous. Contains the toxic pressor amines β-phenylethylamine and tyramine.

[a]Adapted from Larkin T. FDA Consumer, 1983;14:5–10.

(continued)

Table 74–11 *(Continued)*

Botanical Name of Plant Source	Common Names	Remarks
Phoradendron juniperinum Engelm.	Mistletoe. Viscum. Juniper. Mistletoe.	May be poisonous. Little is known about its properties.
Viscum album L.	Mistletoe. Viscum. European Mistletoe.	Poisonous. Contains the toxic pressor amines β-phenylethylamine and tyramine.
Ipomoea purpura (L) Roth	Morning Glory.	Contains a purgative resin. In addition, morning glory seeds contain amides of lysergic acid but with a potency much less than that of LSD.
Vinca major L. and *Vinca minor* L.	Periwinkle. Vinca. Greater Periwinkle. Lesser Periwinkle.	Contains pharmacologically active, toxic alkaloids such as vinblastine and vincristine that have cytotoxic and neurological actions and can injure the liver and kidneys.
Hypericum perforatum L.	St. Johnswort. Hypericum. Klamath Weed. Goatweed.	A primary photosensitizer for cattle, sheep, horses and goats. Contains hypericin, a fluorescent pigment, as a photosensitizing substance.
Euonymus europaeus L.	Spindle-tree.	Violent purgative.
Dipteryx odorata (Aubl.) Willd. *Coumarouna odorata* (Aubl.) and *Dipteryx oppositifolia* (Aubl.) Willd. *Coumarouna oppositifolia* (Aubl.)	Tonka Bean. Tonco Bean. Tonquin Bean.	Active constituent of seed is coumarin. Dietary feeding of coumarin to rats and dogs causes extensive liver damage, growth retardation, and testicular atrophy. FDA regulations prohibit marketing of coumarin as a food or food additive.
Euonymus atropurpureus Jacq.	Wahoo Bark. Euonymus. Burning Bush. Wahoo.	The poisonous principle has not been completely identified. Laxative.
Eupatorium rugosum Houtt. *E. ogeratoides* L.f. and *E. urticaefolium*	White Snakeroot. (Also called Snake-root, Richweed.)	Poisonous plant. Contains a toxic, unsaturated alcohol called *tremetol* combined with a resin acid. Causes "trembles" in cattle and other livestock. Milk sickness is produced in humans by ingestion of milk, butter, and possibly meat from animals poisoned by this plant.
Artemisia absinthium Linné	Wormwood. Absinthium. Absinth. Absinthe. Madderwort. Wermuth. Mugwort. Mingwort. Warmot. Magenkraut. Herba Absinthii.	Contains a volatile oil (oil of wormwood) that is an active narcotic poison. Oil of wormwood is used to flavor *absinthe,* an alcoholic liqueur illegal in this country because its use can damage the nervous sytem and cause mental deterioration.
Corynanthe yohimbi Schum. *Pausinystalia yohimbe* (Schum.) Pierre	Yohimbe. Yohimbi.	Contains the toxic alkaloid yohimbine (quebrachine) and other alkaloids.

HERBS

The FDA has compiled a list of some herbs that should not be used in foods, beverages, or drugs (Table 74–11)[16] (see also Chapter 73—Indigenous Toxicology). Potential toxicity of herbal teas is found in Table 74–12.[17] Medicinal herbs are frequently used by AIDS patients[18] (Table 74–13). D'Arcy has written a comprehensive review of the adverse reactions encountered with herbal medicines.[19]

Huxtable[20] indicates that herbal poisoning may be due to misidentified or unknown plant species or toxicity of a correctly identified plant. He has suggested some commonsense guidelines for the public:

If ill, see a doctor.
Do not take herbs if pregnant or attempting to become pregnant.
Do not take herbs if you are nursing.
Do not give herbs to your baby.
Do not take a large quantity of any one preparation.
Do not take any herb on a daily basis.
Buy only preparations on which the plants are listed on the packet (no guarantee of safety or correctness, but better than nothing).
Do not take anything containing comfrey.

Information on traditional Chinese medicines derived from herbs may be obtained from the Chinese Medicinal Material Research Centre, Chinese University of Hong Kong, Shatin, New Territories, Hong Kong[21] (see Indigenous Toxicology Chapter). Herbs that may induce hepatic toxicity are listed in Table 74–14.[22–24] Useful cautions relative to safe use of plants and mushrooms are listed in Table 74–15.[25]

PLANT IDENTIFICATION REFERENCES

A number of suggested reference books include the following (see also Appendix—Plants and Mushrooms):

Table 74–12
Potential Toxicity of Herbal Teas[a]

Tea Constituent	Botanical Source	Commercially Available	Suspected Toxin	Clinical Toxicity
Buckthorn	*Hippophae rhamnoides*	Yes	Anthraquinones	Cathartic toxin
				Severe watery diarrhea
Burdock root	*Arctium minus*	Yes	Atropine	Anticholinergic blockade
Chamomile	*Chamomilla recutita*	Yes	Antigens of Compositae family	Anaphylactic shock
	Chamaemelum nobile			Contact dermatitis (in patients sensitive to ragweed, asters, chrysanthemum)
Comfrey	*Symphytum officinale*	Yes	Pyrrolizidine alkaloids	Veno-occlusive disease
				Hepatic failure
				?Hepatocarcinogen
Foxglove tea	*Digitalis purpurea*		Digitalis	Malignant arrhythmias
				Cardiac arrest
Gordolobo	*Senecio longilobus*	Yes	Pyrrolizidine alkaloids	Veno-occlusive disease
Groundsel	*Senecio vulgaris*			Hepatic failure
	Senecio spartoids			
Hops	*Humulus lupulus*	Yes	?Lupuline	?Intravascular hemolysis
				?PNH-like defect
Jimson tea	*Datura stramonium*		Atropine	Anticholinergic blockade
			Scopolamine	
			Hyoscyamine	CNS intoxication, hallucinations
			Stramonium	Ataxia, blurred vision
Kavakava tea	*Piper methysicum*		Methysticin	CNS intoxication, ataxia, deafness
				Skin yellowing, dermatosis
Lobelia	*Lobelia inflata*	Yes	Lobeline	Anticholinergic blockade
			Atropine	
			Scopolamine	
			Pyridine alkaloids	?Potential hepatotoxin
Mandrake	*Mandragora officinarum*		Scopolamine	Anticholinergic blockade
			Hyoscyamine	
Mate	*Ilex paraguariensis*	Yes	?Pyrrolizidine alkaloids	?Veno-occlusive disease
				?Hepatic failure
Melilot	*Melilotus officinalis*		Coumarin	Hemorrhagic diathesis
				Prolonged prothrombin time
Mormon tea	*Ephedra nevadensis*		Ephedrine	Sympathomimetic overdose
Nutmeg tea	*Myristica fragrans*	Yes	Monoamine oxidase inhibitors	CNS intoxication, hallucination
				Visual disturbances
			Myristicin	?Hepatic damage
Oleander	*Nerium oleander*		Cardiac glycosides	Malignant arrhythmias
			Digitoxigenin	Cardiac arrest
			Nerioside	
			Oleandroside	
Poke root	*Phytolacca americana*	Yes	Saponins	Gastroenteritis, bloody diarrhea
	Phytolacca decandra		Poke weed mitogen	?Respiratory depression
				?Mitogenic alterations
Sassafras	*Sassafras albidum*	Yes	Safrole	Hepatocarcinogen
Senna	*Cassia acutifolia*	Yes	Anthraquinones	Cathartic toxin
	Cassia angustifolia			Severe watery diarrhea
Snakeroot	*Rauwolfia serpentina*		Reserpine	Potential CNS intoxication
Tansy ragwort	*Senecio jacobea*	Yes	Pyrrolizidine alkaloids	?Veno-occlusive disease
				?Hepatic failure
Thornapple	*Datura species*		Atropine	Anticholinergic blockade
			Scopolamine	
			Hyoscyamine	
Tonka bean	*Dipteryx odoratum*		Coumarin	Hemorrhagic diathesis
	Coumarouna oppositofilia			Prolonged prothrombin time
T'u-san-chi	*Gynura segetum*		Pyrrolizidine alkaloids	Veno-occlusive disease
				Hepatic failure
Woodruff	*Galium odoratum*	Yes	Coumarin	Hemorrhagic diathesis
				Prolonged prothrombin time
Yohimbe bark	*Corynanthe yohimbe*		Yohimbine	Alpha-2 (pre-synaptic) sympathetic blockade

[a]Adapted from Ridker PM. Arch Environ Health 1987;42:133–136.

Table 74–13
Medicinal Herbs Used by Human Immunodeficiency Virus-Infected Patients, Their Pharmacologic Principle, and Potential Adverse Effects Including Gastrointestinal (GI), Hematologic (Heme), Central Nervous System (CNS), Allergic/Dermatologic (Allergic), and Systemic (Other) Toxicities[a]

Common Name	Botanical Name(s)	Other Names	Pharmacologic Principle(s)	Potential Effects
Aloe	*Aloe vera*	Carrisyn	Anthraquinones	GI: cathartic
Astragalus	*Astragalus membranaceus*	Huang-chi	?	Other: hypotension, diuretic, hypoglycemic
Atractylodes	*Atractylodes ovata, Atractylodes macrocephali*	Bai-zhu, pai-chu	Atractylone, sequesterpene furfural, atractyloside	GI: hepatotoxicity CNS: sedative action; Other: diuretic, hypoglycemia
Burdock	*Arctium lappa*	. . .	Atropinelike alkaloid	CNS: anticholinergic effects; Other: diuretic, hypoglycemic, estrogen activity
Chaparrel	*Larrea divaricata, Larrea tridentata*	Creosote bush	Nordihydroguaiaretic acid	GI: nausea, vomiting, diarrhea, abdominal cramps; Allergic: dermatitis; Other: stomatitis, possible stimulation of tumor growth
Codonopsis	*Codonopsis pilosula*	Tang-shen	Alkaloids	Other: hypotension
Comfrey	*Symphytum officinale*	. . .	Pyrrolizidine alkaloids	GI: hepatic veno-occlusive disease
Compound Q	*Trichosanthes kirilowii*	Gualougen, GLQ-223, Chinese cucumber root	Trichosanthin	GI: cathartic; CNS: severe neurologic toxicity (parenteral); Other: hypoglycemia, abortifacient
Dandelion	*Taraxacum officinale*	. . .	Taraxacin, compositae antigens (sesqueterpene lactones)	GI: increased gastric secretion, nausea, and vomiting; Allergic: dermatitis, anaphylaxis; Other: diuretic
Echinacea	*Echinacea angustifolio, echinacea pallida, echinacea purpurea*	Coneflower	Caffeic acid glycoside, compositae antigens (sesqueterpene lactones)	CNS: stimulant; Allergic: dermatitis, anaphylaxis
Ganoderma	*Ganoderma lucidum, Ganoderma japonicum*	Ling-zhi, reishi	Adenosine, coumarin, ergosterol	Heme: inhibition of platelet aggregation, anticoagulation
Garlic	*Allium sativum*	Dasuan	Allicin	GI: gastroenteritis, nausea, vomiting, diarrhea, weight loss, anorexia; Allergic: contact dermatitis; Heme: inhibition of platelet aggregation; Other: inhibition of iodine uptake by thyroid
Ginseng	*Eleutherococcus senticosus, Panax ginseng* (50 other species)	Wuchaseng, siberian ginseng, wujia, ren-shen	Saponin glycocides, estrogens	GI: diarrhea; CNS: stimulant, nervousness, insomnia, depression, confusion; Allergic: histamine release, dermatitis; Other: hypertension, estrogen activity, interaction with monoamine oxidase inhibitor
Hypericin	*Hypericum perforatum*	St John's wort, klamath weed, sho-ren-gyo	Hypericin	Other: photosensitivity, monoamine oxidase inhibitor
Isatis	*Isatis tinctoria*	Pan-lan-ken, dyers' wood root	Hypoxanthine, uracil, uridine, salicylic acid indigo	Heme: inhibits platelet aggregation
Iscador	*Viscum album*	Mistletoe	Sympathomimetic-amines, lectins, viscotoxin	GI: gastroenteritis, hepatitis; CNS: seizures; Other: vasoconstriction, shock (parenteral)
Kelp	*Laminara japonica*	Kombu	Iodide	Other: inhibition of thyroid hormone synthesis; goiters from seaweed consumption in Japan
Licorice	*Glycyrrhiza lepidata, Glycyrrhiza glabra, Glycyrrhiza uralensis*	Gan-cao	Glycyrrhizinic acid	Other: mineralocorticoid effects (sodium retention, edema, hypertension, hypokalemia)

[a]Adapted from Kassler WJ et al. Arch Intern Med 1991;151:2281–2288.

(continued)

Table 74–13 *(Continued)*

Common Name	Botanical Name(s)	Other Names	Pharmacologic Principle(s)	Potential Effects
Lycium fruit	*Lycium chinensis, Lycium barbarum (haliminifolium)*	Kuo-chi-tzu, gouqizi, wolfberry, false jessamine	Atropinelike alkaloids	Other: hypoglycemia, anitcholinergic effects
Paud' arco	*Tabebuia altissima, Tabebuia impetiginosa*	Taheebo	Lapachol	GI: nausea and vomiting, weight loss; Heme: anticoagulation
Peony	*Paeonia suffruticosa, Paeonia lactiflora, Paeonia officinale*	Moutan bark, chi-shao, bai-shao, mudan-pi	Paeonol, paeoniflorin	GI: gastroenteritis, nausea, diarrhea; CNS: depressant; Other: hypotension, diuretic
Privet	*Ligustrum lucidum, Ligustrum vulgare*	Nuzhenzi	Ligustrone, fatty acids	GI: cathartic; Other: hypotension, renal failure
Propolis	. . .	. . .	Resins, balsams, waxes, oils	Allergic: contact dermatitis
Prunella	*Prunella vulgaris*	Xia-ku-cao, woundwort, allheal	Ursolic acid, triterpenoid saponins	GI: cathartic; Other: hypotension, diuretic, uterine contraction
Red clover	*Trifolium pratense*	. . .	Coumarin, salicylic acid	Heme: anticoagulation
Rehmennia	*Rehmannia glutinosa*	Sheng-ti-huang	?	Other: hypoglycemia
Salvia	*Salvia miltiorrhizia*	Tan-shen	Ursolic acid, volatile oils	Heme: inhibition of platelet aggregation; CNS: sedative; Other: hypotension, diuretic, hypoglycemia
Schizandra	*Schizandra chinensis, Schizandra sphenanthea*	Gomishi	?	CNS: stimulant, ether extract is depressant; Other: hypotension, uterine contractions
Shiitake	*Lentinus edodes*	Xiangling	Lentinan, adenosine	Heme: inhibition of platelet aggregation; Allergic: dermatitis; Other: hypotension
Tang-kuei	*Angelica sinensis, Angelica pubecens, Angelica polymophia, Angelica dahurica*	Du-huo, bai-zhi	Psoralens, coumarins, angelicin, osthole	Heme: inhibition of platelet aggregation, anticoagulation; depressant; Other: photosensitivity
Tremella	*Auriculariaceae* species	Bai-muer, white tree ear	?	Heme: inhibition of platelet aggregation
Sweet wormwood	*Artemisa anna, Artemisa apiacea, Artemisa vulgaris*	Quinghaosu, mugwort	Compositae antigens (sesqueterpene lactones), endoperoxide, thujone	Allergic: dermatitis, anaphylaxis; CNS: altered mental status
Yarrow	*Achillea millefolium*	Milfoil	Psoralens, compositae antigens (sesqueterpene lactones), furanocoumadin	Heme: anticoagulation; Allergic: dermatitis, anaphylaxis; Other: photosensitivity

[a]Adapted from Kassler WJ et al. Arch Intern Med 1991;151:2281–2288.

Table 74–14
Herb-Induced Hepatotoxicity

Herb	Active Ingredient
Scutellaria laterifolia (skullcap)	
Senecio longilobus (groundsel)	
Symphytum spp. (comfrey)	Pyrollizidine alkaloids
Heliotropium spp.	
Crotalaria spp.	
Phoradendron and *Viscum* spp. (mistletoe)	
Cassia acutifolia (senna)	
Larrea tridentata (chapparal leaf, creosote bush)	Nondihydroguaiaretic acid
Teucrium chamaedrys (germander)	

Table 74–15
Do's and Don'ts

1. Never eat any part of an unknown plant or mushroom. Teach your children never to put leaves, stems, bark, seeds, nuts, or berries from any plant into their mouths.
2. Store poisonous house plants, bulbs, and seeds out of sight and out of reach.
3. Learn the names of the plants in your home and yards.
4. Do not think a plant is not poisonous just because birds or other wildlife eat it.
5. Do not rely on cooking to destroy poisons in plants.
6. Never use anything prepared from nature as medicine or "tea" unless the plant is nonpoisonous.

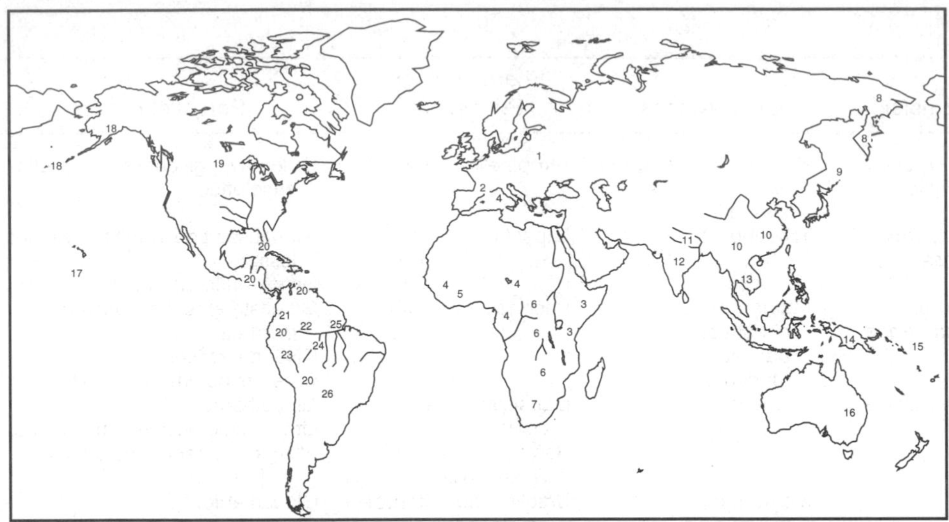

Figure 74–2 The distribution of the principal known arrow and dart poisons. (Adapted from Bisset NG. Ethnopharmacology 1989;25: 1–41.)

1. Gibbons W, Haynes RR, Thomas JL. Poisonous plants and venomous animals of Alabama and adjoining states. Tuscaloosa: University of Alabama Press, 1990.
2. Stary F. Poisonous Plants. London: Hamlyn, 1983. (color pictures—brief description of poisonous principle).
3. Blackwell WH. Poisonous and medicinal plants. Englewood Cliffs, NJ: Prentice-Hall, 1990. (Drawings. Chapter with formulas on major toxic plant alkaloid. Structure and forms of leaf.)
4. Thompson CJS. Poisons and poisoners. New York: Macmillan, 1931.
5. Wiltens J. Thistle greens and mistletoe. Edible and poisonous plants of northern California. Berkeley: Wilderness Press, 1988. (Drawings.)
6. Frohne D, Pfander HJ. A colour atlas of poisonous plants. London: Wolfe Publishing, 1984.

A central and very extensive repository for plant information in the United States is found in the Lloyd Library, Plum Street, Cincinnati, Ohio.

General Review Article

Ogzewalla, Bonfiglio, and Sigell have presented a comprehensive review of common plants and their toxicity with characteristics of poisonous and edible plants relating to the toxic parts of such plants.[26]

LABORATORY

If the patient is symptomatic, obtain blood for electrolytes and complete blood count and perform renal and hepatic function tests and urinalysis. Toxic analyses should be done on samples of emesis or lavage fluid, blood, and urine. Electrocardiographic monitoring is indicated in cardiac glycoside poisonings *(Digitalis purpurea, Nerium oleander)* and anticholinergic or cholinergic ingestions.

TREATMENT

Decontamination

The majority of casual ingestions require no specific therapy. Emesis is preferred to lavage because plant particles are difficult to remove by gastric tube from children. Activated charcoal absorbs most alkaloids well and should be administered in almost all symptomatic cases.

Elimination Enhancement

Most plant poisonings respond to supportive care. Hemoperfusion has been used after *Amanita phalloides* and *Podophyllum* poisonings, but its precise role remains controversial.

Antidotes

Few antidotes to plant poisonings are available. Laetrile toxicity has been successfully treated with use of the Lilly Cyanide Kit. Digoxin-specific Fab fragments have been administered to symptomatic patients who ingested digitalis-containing plants.

ARROW AND DART POISONING

Besset, in a series of papers in the Journal of Ethnopharmacology, has systematized the study of arrow and dart poisoning in both plants and animals throughout the world[27,28] (Fig. 74–2). (See also Moffett MW. Poison-dart frogs. Lurid and lethal. National Geographic 1995;187:98–111.)

REFERENCES—GENERAL PLANT TOXICOLOGY

1. Willis GA. Common poisoning by plants. Medicine. North America. December 14, 1990; pp. 1753–1759.
2. Spoerke DG, Hall AH. Plants and mushrooms of abuse. Emerg Med Clin North Am 1990;8:579–593.
3. Reference Deleted
4. Henry JA. Eur Assoc Pois Cont Centers Newsletter. May 1985.
5. Abuelo JG. Renal failure. Arch Intern Med 1990;150:505–510.
6. CDC. MMWR 1995;44:42–44.

7. Toxic plant substances. The chemistry of poisonous and medicinal plants. In: Blackwell WH, ed. Poisonous and medicinal plants. Englewood Cliffs, NJ: Prentice-Hall, 1990; pp. 34–52.
8. Fassett DW, Chap IC. Oxalates in toxicants occurring naturally in foods. 2nd ed. Washington, DC: National Academy of Sciences, 1973.
9. Gopalakrishnakone P. A computer based colour-photo database system for dangerous animals and plants. Academic and public information networks. Toxicon 1990;28:1285–1292.
10. Metsger DA. Microcomputer-assisted telephone identification of plants in response to Poison Control calls. Clin Toxicol 1990;28:135–157.
11. Spoerke DG, Spoerke SE, Rumack BH. Berry identification using a modified botanic key. Vet Hum Toxicol 1988;30:260–264.
12. Wagstaff DJ, Raisbeck M, Wagstaff AT. Poisonous plant information system (PPIS). Vet Hum Toxicol 1989;31:237–238.
13. Wisepelaere C. Identification of berries with a microcomputer. Vet Hum Toxicol 1987;29(Suppl 2):149.
14. Wagstaff DJ, Wagstaff AT, Goshorn JC. A poisonous plant file in Toxline. Toxicon 1989;27:259–263.
15. Murray V, Knott C (National Poisons Unit, Guy's Hospital, London) and Leon C (Royal Botanic Gardens, Kew). An image-based computerized identification system for poisonous plants and fungi. (A pilot study in the United Kingdom.)
16. Larkin T. Unsafe herbs. FDA Consumer 1993;14:5–10.
17. Ridker PM. Potential toxicity of herbal teas. Arch Environ Health 1987;42:133–136.
18. Kassler WJ, Blanc P, Greenblatt P. Use of medicinal herbs by human immunodeficiency virus infected patients. Arch Intern Med 1991;151:2281–2289.
19. D'Arcy PF. Adverse reactions and interactions with herbal medicines. I. Adverse reactions. Adverse Drug React Toxicol Rev 1992;10:189–208.
20. Huxtable RJ. The harmful potential of herbal and other plant products. Drug Safety 1990;5(Suppl 1):126–136.
21. But P P-H. Need for correct identification of herbs in herbal poisoning. Lancet 1993;341:637.
22. Chapparal-induced toxic hepatitis in California and Texas 1992. MMWR 1992;41:812–814.
23. Katz M, Salbil F. Herbal hepatitis: subacute hepatic necrosis secondary to chapparal leaf. J Clin Gastroenterol 1990;12: 203–206.
24. Larrey D, Vial T, Pauwels A, Castot A, Biour M, David M et al. Hepatitis after Germander *(Teucrium chamaedrys)* administration: another instance of herbal medicine hepatotoxicity. Ann Intern Med 1992;117:129–132.
25. Reference Deleted
26. Ogzewalla CD, Bonfiglio JF, Sigell LT. Common plants and their toxicity. Pediatr Clin North Am 1987;34:1557–1598.
27. Bisset NG. Arrow and dart poisons. J Ethnopharmacol 1989; 25:1–41.
28. Bisset NG. Arrow poisons in China. II. Aconitum—botany, chemistry and pharmacology. J Ethnopharmacol 1981;4:247–336.

ORNAMENTAL "BEANS" AND SEEDS

CASTOR BEANS (*RICINUS COMMUNIS L*)

A study of 424 cases of castor bean intoxication revealed symptoms including acute gastroenteritis, fluid and electrolyte depletion, gastrointestinal bleeding, hemolysis, and hypoglycemia. Fourteen patients died due to hypovolemic shock.[1] The clinical severity of the intoxication cannot be predicted on the basis of the number of beans ingested.

Castor oil increases peristalsis of the small intestine by the action of ricinoleic acid on the small intestine. The oil extract of the castor bean contains the ricinoleic acid; the fibrous portion contains the toxic protein ricin.

TOXIN

Structure

The toxicity of this plant (Fig. 74–3) results from the effects of ricin, which is one of the most toxic parenteral substances in the plant kingdom. Ricin contains two polypeptide chains, held together by a single disulfide bond; the total molecular weight is 66,000. Chain B is a lectin that binds to the surface of the cell to facilitate toxin entry into the cell. Chain A disrupts protein synthesis by activating the 60 S ribosomal subunit (Fig. 74–4). Hence, its toxic effects are delayed and widespread. The pulp of the seed contains allergenic glycoproteins, which cause allergic dermatitis, rhinitis, and asthma in sensitized industrial workers. In addition, the leaves, stem, and seeds contain potassium nitrate and hydrocyanic acid.

LETHAL DOSE

The lethal dose of ricin in man has been estimated to be 1 mg/kg body weight; this corresponds to eight seeds. An ingestion should be considered dangerous, especially in children. Because of the potential of anaphylaxis, one seed may be fatal.

CLINICAL PRESENTATION

Signs/Symptoms

Toxic effects from ricin usually require several hours to develop. Allergic reactions in sensitized individuals may occur immediately after exposure. The most common initial symptoms result from gastrointestinal irritation and include burning in the alimentary tract, nausea, vomiting, diarrhea, and colicky abdominal pain. In severe poisoning, these symptoms progress to hemorrhagic gastritis and dehydration. There is a latent period for nonallergenic reactions, which has been reported to vary between 2 and 24 hours. The primary target organs are the kidney, liver, and pancreas.

Fatalities

Ricin is several hundred times more toxic when administered parenterally than by ingestion.

TREATMENT

Decontamination

Every patient should receive the usual measures to prevent absorption (syrup of ipecac, charcoal, cathartics) after the usual precautions and contraindications are observed.

If either syrup of ipecac or activated charcoal is available at home, it should be given promptly. Recommended treatment for asymptomatic patients who have chewed one or more beans includes emergency department evaluation, gastric decontamination, administration of activated charcoal, observation until 4 to 6 hours after ingestion, and discharge with instructions to return if symptoms develop. After decontamination and activated charcoal symptomatic patients require hospitalization for treatment with IV fluids,

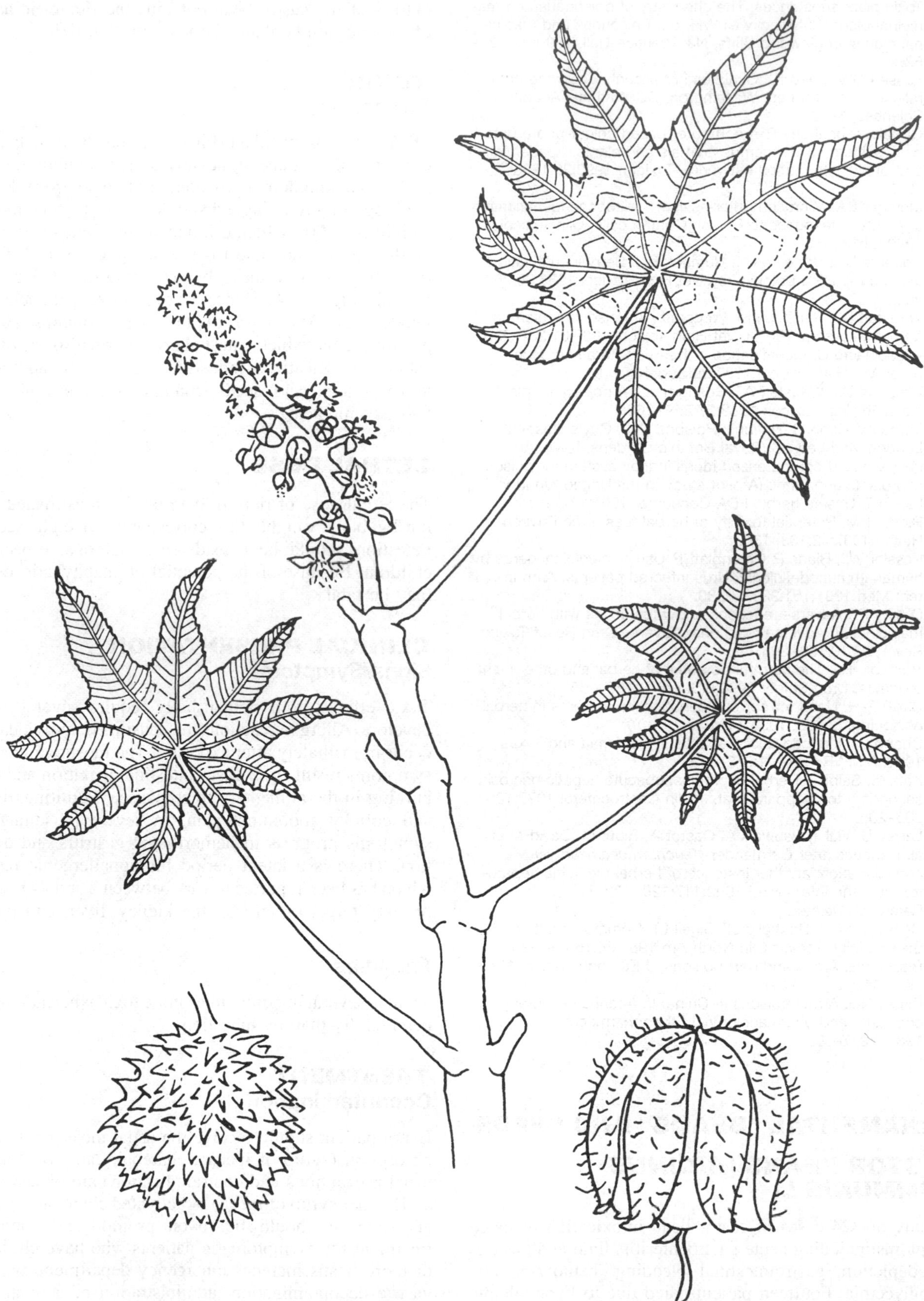

Figure 74–3 Castor bean (*Ricinus communis*). (Adapted from Lampe KF, Fagerström R. Plant toxicity and dermatitis. Baltimore: Williams & Wilkins, 1968.)

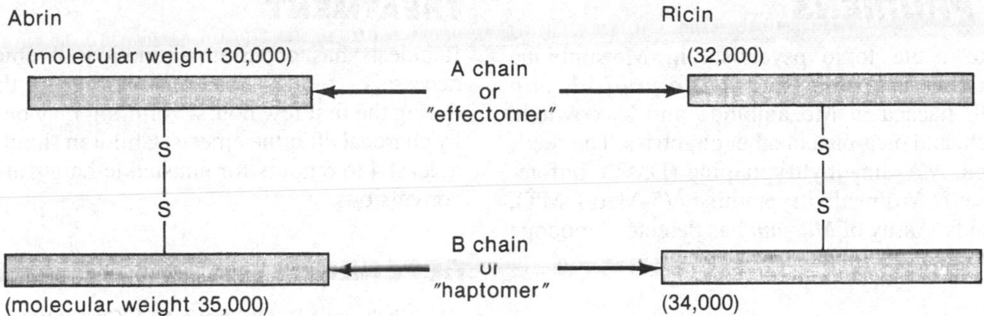

Figure 74-4 Schematic structures of abrin and ricin. (Adapted from Olsnes S. Refsnes K, Pihl A. Nature 1974;249:627.)

supportive care, and monitoring for hypoglycemia, hemolysis, and complications of hypovolemia.

Castor beans and their dusts are highly allergenic and may cause anaphylaxis.[2] Ricin (water-soluble) is not dialyzable, and little is excreted in the urine. Therefore hemodialysis or forced diuresis is not indicated. Most patients respond well to IV fluid and electrolyte replacement and recover without permanent sequelae.

Antidotes

There are no postingestion antidotes to ricin.

Supportive Care

Attempt to identify the plant and seed. The maintenance of fluid and electrolyte balance is the most important aspect of supportive care.

Admission Criteria

Symptomatic patients should be hospitalized. Asymptomatic patients may be discharged with instructions to return immediately should symptoms develop. Asymptomatic pediatric patients who have ingested more than several beans should be observed for at least 4 to 6 hours postingestion. Initial daily outpatient follow-up for several days is important to identify target organ toxicity for those patients released.

JEQUIRITY BEANS

IDENTIFICATION

Scientific Name. *Abrus precatorius.*

Common Name. Jequirity bean, rosary pea, Buddhist rosary bead, Indian bead, Seminole bead, prayer head, crab's eye, weather plant, lucky bean, ojo de pajaro.

TOXIN

The jequirity bean contains *N*-methyltryptophan, abric acid, glycyrrhizin (the active principle of licorice), a lipolytic enzyme, and abrin. Structurally, abrin has the same two-subunit configuration as ricin.

POISONOUS PARTS

Most ingestions to date involve children attracted to the bright colors of the seed.

CLINICAL PRESENTATION

Symptoms/Signs

Serious abrin ingestion produces a severe gastroenteritis several hours after consumption and is followed by the development of diarrhea that may become bloody. Symptoms may last as long as 10 days.

Deaths

Reported fatalities associated with abrin consumption occur after a 3- to 4-day course characterized by persistent gastroenteritis.

TREATMENT

Decontamination

All patients who ingest the seeds and are seen within 4 hours of ingestion should receive the usual measures of decontamination (lavage, charcoal, and cathartics). The presence of spontaneous diarrhea may obviate the need for cathartics.

Elimination Enhancement

There is no effective method.

Antidotes

There is no antidote.

JATROPHA SEEDS

The black seeds of unripe Jatropha fruit are known in the Philippines as "tuba-tuba." They are commonly ingested by children. A prospective study describes vomiting, abdominal pain, nausea, muscle twitching, weakness, salivation, and sweating following their ingestion. Most patients were discharged in 24 to 48 hours with only supportive therapy. The toxicity may be due to the ricin (a toxalbumin) and tannic acid content.[3]

MUCUNA PRURIENS

An outbreak of acute toxic psychosis in Mozambique followed ingestion of the seeds of *Mucuna pruriens,* also known as feijao nacaca in Mozambique and as cowitch, cowhage, kaunch, and pica-pica in other countries. The seeds contain levodopa, *N,N*-dimethyltryptamine (DMT), bufotenine, 5-methoxy-*N,N*-dimethyltryptamine (5-Meo-DMT), and other alkaloids. Assay of *Mucuna* has detected levodopa yields of 3.1 to 6.1% of the mature seed.[4]

TREATMENT

If emesis has occurred, induction of emesis may not be necessary. If emesis has not occurred or the patient is seen during the first few hours, vomiting may be helpful followed by charcoal after the emesis. Children should be observed for at least 4 to 6 hours for unusual lethargy, ataxia, delirium, or convulsions.

REFERENCES—ORNAMENTAL "BEANS"

1. Challoner KR, McCarron MM. Castor bean intoxication. Ann Emerg Med 1990;19:1177–1183.
2. Steingrub JS, Lopez T, Teres D, Steingart R. Amniotic fluid embolism associated with castor oil ingestion. Crit Care Med 1988;16:642–643.
3. Makalinao IP. A descriptive study on the clinical profile of Jatropha seed poisoning. Vet Hum Toxicol 1993;35:330.
4. Infante ME, Perez AM, Simoo MR, Manda F, Baguette EF, Fernandes AM, Cliff JL. Outbreak of acute toxic psychosis attributed to *Mucuna pruriens.* Lancet 1992;336:1129.
5. Spoerke DG, Murphy MA, Wruk KM, Rumack BH. Five cases of *Thermopsis* poisoning. Clin Toxicol 1988;26:397–406.

QUINOLIZIDINE ALKALOIDS

THERMOPSIS IDENTIFICATION

Scientific Name

Thermopsis spp.

Common Name

Golden banner, false lupine, buck bean, buffalo pea, yellow bean, mountain thermopsis.

Family

Leguminosae.

Botanical Description

Occurrence

Various *Thermopsis* species are found in the foothills and plains of the Rocky Mountains. These plants are herbaceous with leaves containing three leaflets; bright yellow, peaklike flowers; and a flat, pealike pod (legume). They bloom from May to July and soon after 2 to 3 weeks develop long pods.

TOXIN

The seeds contain the highest plant concentration of quinolizidine alkaloids. Symptoms may follow ingestion of the flowers or blossoms. *Thermopsis rhombifolia* contains anagyrine, thermopsine, rhombfoline, cytisine, *N*-methylcytisine, 5-6-dehydrolupanine, and lupanine. The two principal alkaloids of the group are anagyrine and thermopsine. The most studied of the group are cytosine, the primary toxin of *Laburnum anagyroides,* which exerts a nicotine-like activity (see *Laburnum*), and anagyrine, which is a teratogen in cattle.[6] No specific toxic dose is known for humans, but a "handful" of seeds produce symptoms.

CLINICAL PRESENTATION

Symptoms seen in quinolizidine alkaloid poisoning include abdominal pain, cramping, vomiting, convulsions, and death through respiratory paralysis. A serious cytisine case could exhibit nausea, abdominal pain, vomiting, stupor, giddiness, muscular weakness, incoordination, and ataxia followed by respiratory paralysis. Headaches occur within 4 to 6 hours postingestion and usually clear within 12 to 24 hours.

LUPIN BEANS

Lupins are legumes cultivated extensively in Australia, South America, eastern Europe, and the Mediterranean as supplemental feed for livestock. Humans ingest lupins as bean dishes, appetizers or in high-fiber breads, pastas, and biscuits containing lupin flour.[1]

CLINICAL PRESENTATION

There are two forms of lupin toxicity: an alkaloid-induced syndrome and a mycotoxin (phomopsin)–induced hepatoxicosis (Lupinosis). Quinolizidine alkaloids are present in lupin plants, and the beans are responsible for acute lipin toxicity. Fatalities among children and four moderately severe acute anticholinergic reactions have been reported. A motor neuron disease–like presentation associated with chronic and excessive consumption of lupin beans containing high levels of alkaloids have been observed.[1]

REFERENCE—LUPIN BEANS

1. Lowen RJ, Alam FKA, Edgar JA. Lupin bean toxicity. Med J Aust 1995;162:256–257.

GUAR GUM[1]

IDENTIFICATION

Scientific Name

Cyamopsis tetragonolobus Taub.

Common Name

Indian cluster bean, guar plant.

Family

Leguminosae.

Botanical Description

The guar plant is a nitrogen-fixing annual that bears pods, each containing a number of seeds.

Occurrence/Use

Native to tropical Asia, the plants grow throughout India and Pakistan and have been growing in the United States since the early 1900s. It has been used in the management of hypercholesterolemia and as an over-the-counter diet pill.

TOXIN

Guar gum contains about 80% guaran (a galacto composed of D-mannose and D-galactose unit) with a molecular weight of about 220,000. The viscosity of guar gum varies in proportion to the degree of galacto cross-linking. The guar gum is isolated from the endosperm of the Indian cluster bean.

CLINICAL PRESENTATION

Esophageal and small bowel obstruction have been reported following use of Cal-Ban 3000, guar gum "diet pills" in tablet and capsule formulations. Of 18 individuals reported to the FDA who developed esophageal obstruction, preexisting esophageal or gastric disorders were present in nine (50%).

TREATMENT

Management has included endoscopic removal from the esophagus or stomach. This is difficult because of its tenacious sticky consistency. Surgery has been required for small bowel obstruction. In Australia the galacto diet pills were banned in 1985. The U.S. FDA has taken similar measures. An unknown number of individuals may still be using the diet pills.[2]

REFERENCE—GUAR GUM

1. Guar gum. The Lawrence review of natural products. St. Louis: Facts and Comparisons, November 1990.
2. Lewis JH. Esophageal and small bowel obstruction from guar gum-containing "diet pills." Analysis of 26 cases reported to the Food and Drug Administration. Am J Gastroenterol 1992;87:1424–1428.

SUNFLOWER SEED SYNDROME

CLINICAL PRESENTATION

The clinical features of obstipation, rectal pain with defecation, and a "crunchy" sensation on rectal examination subsequent to ingestion of unhusked sunflower seeds appear due to undigested shards impinging on the delicate anoderm. Attempts to defecate enhance the symptoms.[1]

TREATMENT

Disimpact under general anesthesia or enemas requiring nitrous oxide anesthesia. Insert the lavage tube through the anoscope to relieve the obstruction.[2,3]

REFERENCES

1. Phillips RW, Moses FR. Sunflower seed syndrome: a prickly proctological problem. Ann Emerg Med 1991;20: 1049–1050.
2. Melchreit R, McGowan G, Hyams IS. "Colonic crunch" sign in sunflower-seed bezoar. N Engl J Med 1984;310:1748–1749.
3. Cloonan CC, Kleinschmidt K, Gatrell C. Rectal bezoar from sunflower seeds. Ann Emerg Med 1988;17:161–162.

COLCHICINE

CLINICAL PRESENTATION

Folpini and Furfori have provided a summary of the phases of colchicine toxicity[1] (Table 74–16).

Antidotes

Investigators at the Hospital Fernand Widal in Paris have produced IgG colchicine antibodies in goats, which have been beneficial to mice given an LD_{50} dose of colchicine. The steady-state volume of distribution decreased significantly in the treated mice. There was sequestration of free colchicine in the intravascular space (low free plasma toxins) and a decrease in colchicine concentration in most tissues.[2] Even after the distribution phase the IgG antidote decreased the mortality rate.[3]

A 25-year-old female ingested colchicine 1 mg/kg and was admitted 24 hours later with vomiting, diarrhea, hypotension, disseminated intravascular coagulation, oliguria, ARDS, and cardiogenic shock refractory to dobutamine. On admission the plasma colchicine concentration was 24 ng/mL. Specific goat colchicine Fab fragments (480 mg) were administered. There was a sixfold increase in total colchicine 10 minutes after starting the Fab infusion. Free colchicine became undetectable in 7 hours. Urinary excretion rate of colchicine increased sixfold. The cardiogenic shock improved. She survived even after a bacteremia, neutropenia, total hair loss, and transient polyneuritis.[4] A 4.4-fold decrease of colchicine distribution volume

Table 74–16
Phases of Colchicine Toxicity[a]

0–24 h
Abdominal pain, nausea and vomiting, diarrhea, leukocytosis
Electrolyte balance disorders, hypovolemia
Excessive fibrinolytic activity
Coagulation factors consumption
Massive cytolysis
Days 2, 3, 4, 5, 6, 7
Bone marrow hypoplasia, leukopenia, thrombocytopenia
Spontaneous hemorrhages, anemia
Cardiac arrhythmias
Hepatic insufficiency
Confusion, delirium, convulsions, coma
Possible MOF[b] and ARDS
From the 7th day on
Beginning of alopecia
Rebound of leukocytosis

[a]Adapted from Folpini A, Furfori P. Clin Toxicol 1995;33:71–77.
[b]Multiple organic failure.

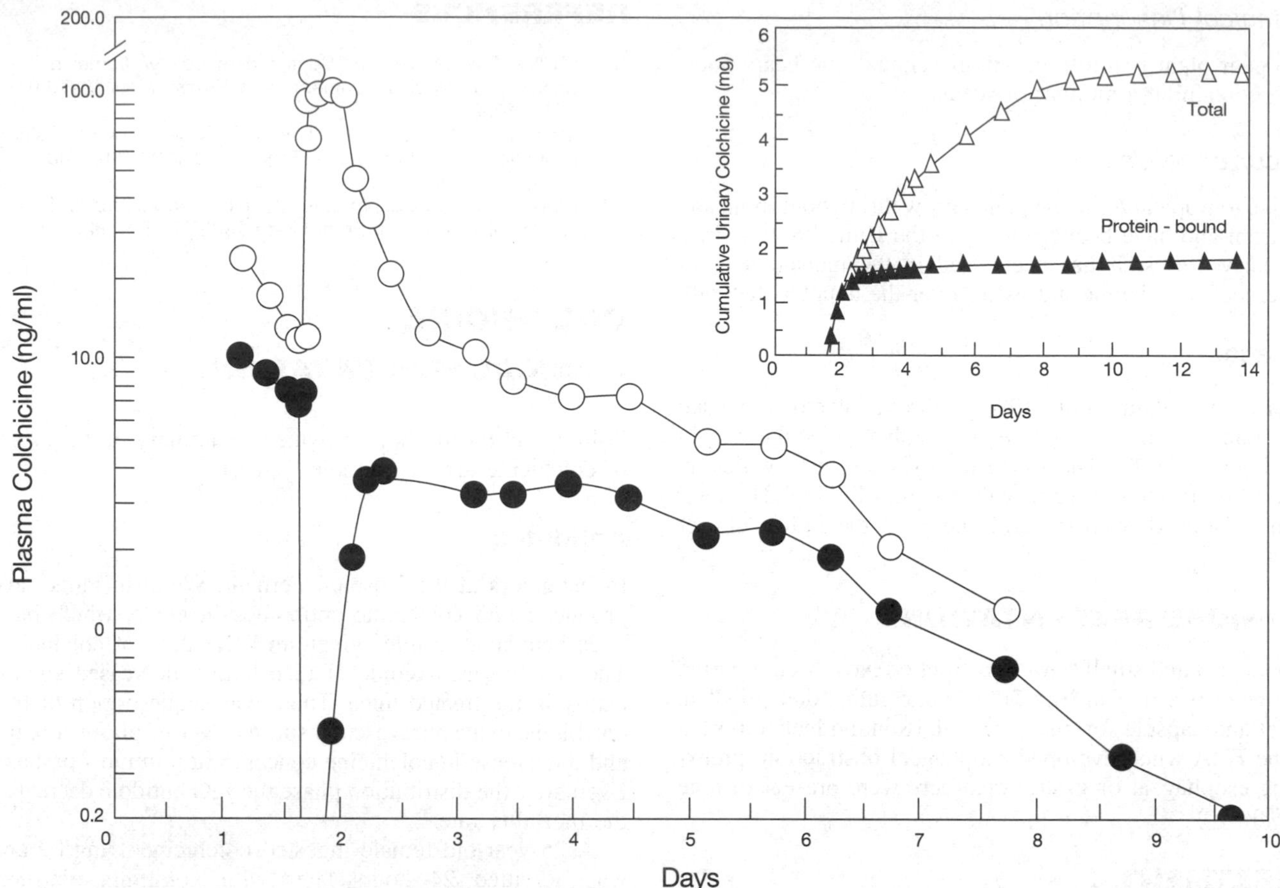

Figure 74–5 Concentrations of colchicine in the plasma and urine of the study patient. The colchicine overdose occurred on day 0, and the infusion of colchicine-specific Fab fragments began on day 1.66. For plasma colchicine, concentrations of total and unbound colchicine are shown. The inset shows the cumulative urinary excretion of total and protein-bound colchicine. (Adapted from Baud FJ et al. N Engl J Med 1995;332:642–645.)

(29 L/kg) under Fab treatment indicated that substantive amounts of colchicine were being removed from peripheral sites and redistributed into the extracellular space. Neutralization yield of Fab fragments was near 100%. The amount of neutralized colchicine was estimated at 3.7 ng of the 9 mg of colchicine present in the body prior to Fab dosing[5,6] (Fig. 74–5).

Supportive Care

Granulocyte colony stimulating factor (filgrastim) is useful in alleviating pancytopenia after a colchicine overdose. It is commercially available as Neupogen. A 19-year-old received a single dose (300 μg) of G-CSF. The pancytopenia resolved and the patient recovered.[7]

PLANTS CULTIVATED AS FOOD SOURCES AND BULBS

Atractylis gummifera Indentification

Scientific Name

Atractylis gummifera.

Common Name

White chameleon.

Family

Compositae.

Botanical Description

Tuber with long serrated leaves (thistle).

Occurrence/Use

Located especially around the Mediterranean Sea (Greece, Italy, Sicily, Spain, Portugal, North Africa). It is also used to prepare an extract from the root as a traditional medicine for oxyuriasis.

Toxin

The leaves secrete a gum that is used by children as chewing gum. All the intoxication duc to *Atractylis gummifera* has been due to ingestion of the root where the toxins are found. *Atractylis gummifera* contains two toxic glucosides, atractyloside and 4-carboxy-atractyloside. These norditerpenes have structural similarities to the aconitine-delphinidine alkaloids.[8] Both are inhibitors of mitochondrial adenosine nucleotide translocation, resulting in inhibition of oxidative phosphorylation and disturbance of the Krebs cycle oxidative reactions.[8]

CLINICAL PRESENTATION

Patients may appear a few days after ingestion in coma, with epigastric pain and vomiting. The liver is palpable. The patient then proceeds into respiratory arrest and renal insufficiency and develops hypoglycemia; jaundice deepens prior to death in a few hours to days. Postmortem examination of the liver reveals a diffuse necrosis of the hepatic parenchyma with collapse of the interstitial connective tissue.[9,10]

TREATMENT

Treatment of the intoxicated patient is largely symptomatic and supportive. There are no antidotes.

REFERENCES—COLCHICINE

1. Folpini A, Furfori P. Colchicine toxicity—clinical features and treatment. Massive overdose case report. Clin Toxicol 1995;33:71–77.
2. Terrier N, Urtizberrea M, Scherrmann JM. Influence of goat colchicine-specific antibodies on murine colchicine disposition. Toxicology 1989;59:11–22.
3. Terrier N, Urtizberrea M, Scherrmann JM. Reversal of advanced colchicine toxicity in mice with goat colchicine-specific antibodies. Toxicol Appl Pharmacol 1990;104:504–510.
4. Baud FJ, Sabouraud A, Vicaut E, Taboulet P, Lang J, Bismuth C, Rouzioux JM, Scherrmann J-M. Brief report. Treatment of severe colchicine overdose with colchicine-specific Fab fragments. N Engl J Med 1995;332:642–645.
5. Sabouraud A, Urtizberrea M, Scherrmann JM, Caraux J, Baud FJ, Bismuth C. First pharmacokinetic investigation of colchicine-specific FAB fragments in one case of human colchicine poisoning. Eur Assoc Pois Cent Clin Toxicol XIV Congress, Istanbul, May 24–27, 1992 (abstract P11).
6. Scherrmann JM, Sabouraud A, Urtizberea M, Rouzioux J, Lang J, Baud F, Bismuth C. Clinical use of colchicine-specific Fab fragments in colchicine poisoning. Vet Hum Toxicol 1992;34:334.
7. Katz R, Chuang LC, Sutton JD. Use of granulocyte colony-stimulating factor in the treatment of pancytopenia secondary to colchicine overdose. Ann Pharmacother 1992;26:1087–1088.
8. Frohme D, Pfander HJ. A colour atlas of poisonous plants. Stuttgart Wolfe Publishing, 1984; p 64.
9. Georgiou M, Siandidou L, Hatzis T, Papadatos J, Koutselinis A. Hepatotoxicity due to *Atractylis gummifera* L. Clin Toxicol 1988;26:487–493.
10. Nogue S, Sanz P, Botey A, Esforzado N, Blanche C, Alvarez L. Insuffisance renale aigue due a une intoxication par le chardona glu *(Atractlyis gummifera).* Presse Medicale 1992;21:130.

HOUSEPLANTS

POINSETTIA

Botanical Description

A popular indoor Christmas ornamental plant with large (3 to 7 in.) alternating leaves and prominent red, pink, yellow, or cream bracts clustered at the tops of the stems.

Clinical Presentation

Poinsettia toxicity is limited to its ability to produce local irritation, contact dermatitis, mucosal burns, and keratoconjunctivitis.

Treatment

Treatment is supportive (as in *Dieffenbachia* exposure).

DIEFFENBACHIA

Botanical Description

A popular ornamental plant that has broad, shiny leaves and grows to 6 ft. This tropical American native has leaves that may be spotted or variegated; it grows well indoors.

Clinical Presentation

Dieffenbachia species cause salivation and severe swelling of the lips, mouth, and tongue, which may lead to interference with swallowing and breathing.

Treatment

Most encounters involve casual contact. Usually demulcents (milk, water) and cold packs are all that is required. The most severe sequela appears to be the potential for respiratory obstruction, which progresses over the first 6 hours. Only those patients with significant edema require direct medical observation. Otherwise, only symptomatic care with topical agents (e.g., Cepacol, Orabase Plain) is necessary. Severe cases require more potent analgesics. Admission criteria should be based on the presence of respiratory obstruction and the ability to maintain fluid balance. Antihistamines are of questionable value since the role of histamine-induced edema is unclear. Diphenhydramine may be used as a topical anesthetic.

MISTLETOE

Botanical Description

A semiparasitic perennial that grows chiefly on oak trees. It grows as a 1- and 4-ft bush in the oak branches and is distinguished from the oak by light green leaves and hairy stems. Small white berries grow in grapelike clusters. Several species are present in the United States, including the familiar Christmas mistletoe *(Phoradendron flavescens).* The dominant European mistletoe species is *Viscum album,* which has been studied extensively for its cardiotoxin.

Poisonous Parts

All parts of the plants are poisonous. The berries have been a common source of gastrointestinal poisoning.

Clinical Presentation

Ingestion of large quantities of berries causes gastroenteritis. Although anecdotal reports support the cardiac toxicity of these agents, the severity of their human cardiotoxicity remains to be documented. Symptoms begin in less than 6 hours after ingestion. Seizures have been observed. Most mistletoe exposure involves children.[1,2] In the Krenzelok series, symptoms were rare.

Treatment

There are no specific antidotes to mistletoe toxicity. Patients who manifest dysrhythmias or electrolyte imbalance should be hospitalized for observation overnight. "Mistletoe hepatitis" remains a curiosity and should be considered in serious or chronic ingestions. Asymptomatic patients may be discharged after several hours of observation.

HOLLY

The genus *Ilex* contains 300 to 350 species found throughout regions with temperate and tropical climates, where they grow as deciduous and evergreen shrubs and trees. They have bright green leaves, often with hard teeth on the leaf margins, which discourage leaf consumption. The red or black berries (Christmas holly) are attractive ornaments, especially to curious children.

Clinical Presentation

Ilex species produce gastrointestinal distress in some but not all ingestions.

Treatment

Treatment is supportive.

PLANTS CULTIVATED AS FOOD SOURCES AND BULBS

RHUBARB

Botanical Description

A garden vegetable plant with large, leathery, heart-shaped leaves and a reddish color.

Toxin

The leaf blade is the toxic part of the plant, containing somewhat less than 1% soluble oxalates. The stalks have much lower oxalate levels and therefore are edible. Cooking does not make rhubarb leaves edible. The soluble oxalates are readily absorbed from the gastrointestinal tract. Systemic formation of calcium oxalate may produce hypocalcemia; precipitation of insoluble salts in the renal system may lead to kidney dysfunction and electrolyte imbalance.

Clinical Presentation

Early symptoms result from the mucosal irritant effect of oxalate on the gastrointestinal tract and include sore throat, nausea, vomiting, anorexia, diarrhea, and abdominal pain. Gastrointestinal symptoms are not always present in rhubarb poisoning. Kidney dysfunction and electrolyte imbalance are the major causes of death and appear after signs of gastrointestinal distress develop. Anuria, oliguria, proteinuria, hematuria, and oxaluria are present in severe cases.

Paresthesias, tetany, hyperreflexia, muscle twitches, and muscle cramps reflect hypocalcemia.

Treatment

Decontamination

Patients who ingest rhubarb leaves and are seen early in their clinical course (4 to 6 hours postingestion) should receive the usual measures of decontamination (syrup of ipecac, cathartics, charcoal) after the usual precautions have been observed. Lavage with 0.15% calcium hydroxide (lime water) to precipitate insoluble calcium oxalate in the gastrointestinal tract has been suggested for serious ingestions, but no clinical substantiation of its effectiveness exists. Magnesium cathartics are the preferable cathartics.

Elimination Enhancement

Generous fluid replacement should be given to promote the excretion of calcium oxalate crystals from the kidney tubules.

Supportive Care

Symptomatic patients should receive a complete blood count and serum electrolytes, including calcium and kidney function tests (creatinine, urinalysis). Kidney function may deteriorate over the first week; careful management of fluid and electrolyte balance may be necessary. Intravenous calcium may be necessary to reverse the oxalate-induced hypocalcemia. To an adult, 10 mL of 10% calcium gluconate may be given intravenously with cardiac monitoring over a 10-minute period and repeated if symptoms, signs, and ECG evidence (e.g., shortened QT interval) persist.

POTATOES, TOMATOES, AND SOLANINE TOXICITY (FIG. 74–6)

TOXIN

Structure

Species of *Solanum* contain the toxic glycoalkaloid solanine. Since solanidine is structurally similar to steroids, its proposed biosynthetic pathway is from acetate through cholesterol.

POISONOUS PARTS

Ripe fruit contain the least amount of solanine. Solanine occurs in highest concentrations in areas of high metabolic rate such as the sprouts, green skin, and stems.

CLINICAL PRESENTATION

Gastrointestinal and neurologic symptoms predominate in cases of solanine poisoning depending on the amount ingested. Vomiting, headache, and flushing are the most common symptoms reported in children ingesting plant parts.

Deaths have been associated with consumption of toxic potatoes, but those reports involved malnourished patients who may not have received adequate care. Headache, abdominal pain, vomiting, thirst, restlessness, and

SCIENTIFIC NAME	COMMON NAME	DESCRIPTION	DISTRIBUTION	POISONOUS COMPONENT
Solanum dulcamara	European bittersweet, blue nightshade, woody nightshade, climbing nightshade	Shrub or slender vine, purple flowers, bright red berry, various seeds	Along fences, streams, ditches. Most common in the east and north central states	Solanine
Solanum nigrum (or) *S. americanum*	Black nightshade, poison berry, common nightshade	Multibranched vines or bushes, white flowers, purple-black berries	In fields, woods, waste places. Widespread in United States	Solanine Other glycoalkaloids
Solanum tuberosum	Irish potato, common potato	Vines, "eyes" and sprouts, peelings or tubers exposed to light turning green	Mainly in Northeast, Northwest	Solanine Solanidine
Solanum pseudocapsicum	Jerusalem cherry, natal cherry	Ornamental plant, orange, cherrylike berries	Various species throughout United States	Solanine Solanidine Solanocapsine
S. villosum	Hairy nightshade			
S. aculeatissimum	Devil's apple, bull nettle			
S. triflorum	Three-flowered nightshade, cut-leafed nightshade			
S. melongena	Eggplant			
S. carolinense	Horse nettle			
S. gracile	Bull nettle, wild tomato			
S. eleagnifolium	White horse nettle, silver leaf nightshade, tropillo			
S. sodomeum	Apple of Sodom, popalo			
S. rostratum	Buffalo burr, sandburr, Colorado burr, Texas thistle			
S. intrusum soria	Garden huckleberry, wonderberry			
Lycopersicon esculentum	Tomato	Vines and suckers of tomato plant	Worldwide	Glycoalkaloids of solanine type
Solandra species	Trumpet flower, chalice vine	Large showy yellow or white flowers	Greenhouse or warmest parts of United States	Solanine type
Physalis heterophylla	Ground cherry	Perennial, solitary flowers, many-seeded	Eastern North America	
P. longifolia	Husk tomato	Yellow berry	Weed meadows, pastures	

[a]Solanines and solanidine are gastroenterotoxins as well as being toxic to the central nervous system.

Figure 74-6 Solanine and solanidine-containing plants[a]. (Adapted from Goldfrank L, Melinek M. Hosp Physician 1979;15(8):25.)

apathy preceded death, but no convulsions or fever developed.

TREATMENT

General supportive care is the key to treatment. Fluid status should be evaluated in every patient by means of orthostatic pulse and blood pressures. Electrolytes should be checked on those patients who exhibit profound changes or who take medications that alter fluid or electrolyte balance. An intravenous line should be established on those patients who exhibit orthostatic hypotension or neurologic signs. For those seriously ill patients who do not respond to fluid replacement, cardiac monitoring and vasopressors may be needed. Seizures should respond to diazepam. Those patients with neurologic signs or orthostatic changes should be admitted for at least 24 hours of observation.

REFERENCES

1. Spiller HA, Willias DB, Gorman SE, Sanftleban J. Retrospective study of mistletoe ingestion. Clin Toxicol 1995;33:475–486 (abstract 156).
2. Krenzelok EP, Jacobsen TD, Aronic JM. Mistletoe exposures—the kiss of death? Clin Toxicol 1995;33:475–486 (abstract 150).

CYANOGENIC PLANTS

CASSAVA

Cassava *(Manihot esculenta)* has been estimated as the second largest carbohydrate crop in the world. It forms a majority of the diet for millions of people.[1]

Toxin

The main toxin, which occurs in varying amounts in all parts of the cassava plant, is a compound called linamarin, a cyanogenic glycoside. Cassava is often eaten without processing during the dry season when the diet is completely dominated by cassava due to a lack of other food items. Dietary cyanide exposure from cassava will result from consumption of insufficiently processed (to remove cyanide) roots, probably from liberation of cyanide in the gut from ingested linamavin. The detoxification mechanism for cyanide in the body converts cyanide into the far less toxic thiocyanate. The substrate for this reaction is sulfur originating from proteins in the diet.

Clinical Presentation

Cyanide intake from a cassava-dominated diet has been proposed as a contributing factor to two forms of nutritional neuropathies: tropical ataxic neuropathy (TAN)—Nigeria, and epidemic spastic paraperesis (ESP) described from Mozambique, Tanzania, and Zaire. TAN has occurred in Nigeria, was found among adult males, and resulted in ataxia. A low dietary protein intake resulting in sulfur deficiency was proposed as a contributing factor.[2] ESP mainly affected women and children in Mozambique (1102 cases in 1981) and Zaire during droughts and resulted in a spastic paralysis of both legs (Table 74–17). A list of cyanogenic plants is found in Chapter 66.

Treatment

Treatment for the neuropathies is supportive and symptomatic.[2]

AMYGDALIN

Distribution

Amygdalin is minimally protein bound and distributed in the extracellular department.

Elimination

Rapidly filtered by the kidney with small hepatic clearance,[3] amygdalin is eliminated with a half-life of about one-half hour. Of an orally administered "therapeutic" amygdalin dose, 62 to 96% is excreted within the first 24 hours.[4]

Clinical Presentation

The clinical picture of amygdalin poisoning mimics cyanide poisoning. The rapid onset of dyspnea, cyanosis, vomiting, diaphoresis, weakness, lightheadedness, and excitement followed by convulsions, stupor, disorientation, paralysis, weakness, coma, and cardiovascular collapse characterizes cyanide toxicity. Symptoms typically start within one-half hour of consumption and progress quickly.

Ingestion of 45 mL (10.5 g) laetrile caused severe headache, dizziness, coma, and convulsions within 8 minutes.[5] An estimated ingestion of 500 to 2500 mg of amygdalin by an 11-month-old child caused vomiting and listlessness within one-half hour followed quickly by obtundation, depressed respirations, and shock.[6] Consumption of 48 apricot kernels as a milkshake caused vomiting, headache, flushing, diaphoresis, and lightheadedness after 1 hour, which rapidly subsided after ipecac-induced emesis at an emergency department.[7] Ingestion of 20 to 40 apricot kernels resulted in similar symptoms plus disorientation, reversal of which required sodium nitrite and thiosulfate.[8] Ingestion of 12 bitter almonds produced vomiting, abdominal pain, coma, lactic acidosis, and transient pulmonary

Table 74–17
Environmental Neurotoxins[1]

Clinical	Source	Site	Chemical
Lathyrism[1]	Chickling pea seed *(Lathyrus sativa)*	Africa, Asia	Beta-*N*-oxalylamino-L-alanine
ALS parkinsonism Dementia complex[2–4]	Seeds of false Sago plant *(Cycas circinalis)*	Guam	Beta-*N*-methylamino-L-alanine
Parkinsonism[5]	Synthetic opiate contaminate		MPTP
Spastic paralysis[6]	Cassava (inadequate preparation) *(Manihot esculenta)*	Mozambique	Cyanogenic glycoside
Motoneuron disease[7]		Leather workers+	Solvents?
Motoneuron disease[8]			Lead, mercury, aluminum, manganese[9]
Neurodegenerative disease[10]	Mussels	Canada	Domoic acid
Sporadic motoneuron disease[11]		UK	Glycine[9]

1. Martyn CN. Br Med J 1987;295:346–347.
2. Spencer PS et al. Science 1987;237:517–522.
3. Garruto RM, Yanagihara R, Gajdusek DC. Lancet 1988;2:1079.
4. Duncan MW et al. Neurology 1990;40:767–772.
5. Mitchell JD. Arch Toxicol 1991;15:130–139.
6. Tylleskar T et al. Lancet 1992;339:208–211.
7. Hawkes CH, Cavanagh JB, Fox AJ. Lancet 1989;1:73–75.
8. Boothby JA, de Jesus PV, Rowland LP. Arch Neurol 1974;31:18–23.
9. Williams DB, Windebank AJ. Mayo Clin Proc 1991;66:54–82.
10. Teitlebaum JC et al. N Engl J Med 1990;322:1781–1787.
11. Lane RJM, Dick JPR, de Balleroche J. Lancet 1991;337:732–733.

edema starting within 15 minutes.[9] Wild apricot seed ingestion commonly causes the sudden onset of vomiting and crying, followed by fainting, lethargy, or coma in children in Turkey.[10] Skin eruptions, hepatosplenomegaly, and progressive neuromuscular weakness have been associated with laetrile treatment.[11]

Treatment

Treatment is identical to that for cyanide poisoning. When the cyanide antidote is administered to children, appropriate adjustments for weight and hemoglobin content must be made in the nitrite dose to avoid a fatal methemoglobinemia. Mild to moderate ingestions may require only decontamination and supportive care. Alteration in mental status, severe acidosis, continuous seizures, or refractory hypotension indicates the need for the antidote. Clinical features that suggest an appropriate response to the antidote include the following: normalization of blood pressure, pulse, and mentation; cessation of seizure activity; and return of spontaneous respirations.[12]

PEPPER

The pungency of peppers is the sum of the concentration and potencies of five compounds.[13] Topical capsaicin has been used for the treatment of neuralgia associated with herpes zoster infection,[14] psoriasis,[15] (substance P (SP) is released from cutaneous sensory nerve endings and is increased in the regional skin in psoriasis). Capsaicin depletes SP through inducing degeneration of primary sensory neurons, (thus relieving itching),[15] diabetic neuropathy,[16–18] pruritus related to hemodialysis,[19] and posttraumatic amputation stump pain.[20] In diabetics receiving ACE inhibitors, topical capsaicin may enhance the ACE inhibitor cough.[21] Workers exposed to hot chili cayenne peppers *(Capsicum annum)* may experience an increase in cough ("chili workers' cough").[22] Capsaicin, the active principle of the hot peppers (genus *Capsicum),* has been a subject of child abuse when a split jalapeno pepper was placed in the child's mouth resulting in burning of the mouth, throat, and stomach and burning at the anus.[23]

CLINICAL PRESENTATION

Peeling of chili peppers in New Mexico is performed manually causing burning pain, irritation, and erythema. Such "chili burns" are improved after immersion into cool tap water and vegetable oils.[24] "Hunan hand" is a contact dermatitis resulting from the direct handling of chili peppers containing capsaicin.[25]

Eight patients died due to aspiration of pepper. Seven deaths involved homicides. These deaths occurred in different states.[26] A 4-year-old boy with a history of pica aspirated table pepper with subsequent respiratory arrest, severe anoxia, and death.[27] Black pepper (*Piper nigrum* [Piperaceae]) contains terpinoids (*d*-limonene, *L*-pinene, linalool, and philadendrone), which are reported to be potential carcinogens.[28] Black pepper force fed to Egyptian toads primarily induced tumors in the liver.[28] Intragastric administration of red or black pepper is associated with a significant increase in gastric acid and pepsin secretion, mucosal exfoliation, and potassium loss.[29]

GARLIC

Sith Garliche then hath power to save from death,
Bear with it though it make unsavoury breathe,
And scorne not Garliche like some that thinke
It only makes men winke and drinke and stinke.[30]

IDENTIFICATION

Scientific Name

Allium sativum.

Common Names

Garlic, stinking rose, rustic treacle, nectar of the gods, camphor of the poor.[31]

Family

Liliaceae.

Botanical Description

A perennial bulb with a tall erect flowering stem. The plant produces pink to purple flowers that bloom from July to September. The bulb is odoriferous.

OCCURRENCE/USE

Garlic has been used as a medicine in many cultures as reported in folk medicine literature. It has been utilized as an antipyretic, antibiotic, antifungal, and antiviral agent.[32] Preliminary data indicate that it may affect antifibrinolytic activity in humans, decrease atherosclerotic plaque formation, and decrease lipid and cholesterol levels in man.[33–39] Most of these claims have not been subjected to controlled clinical studies.

TOXIN

Garlic contains about 0.5% of a volatile oil composed of sulfur-containing compounds (diallyl disulfide, diallyl trisulfide, and methylallyl trisulfide. The enzyme allicinase converts alliin (5-allyl-L-cysteine sulfoxide) to 2-propenesulfene acid, which dimerizes to form allicin. Allicin gives the pungent characteristic odor to crushed garlic and probably is the cause of skin reactions.[30]

CLINICAL PRESENTATION

Adverse effects have included arrhythmias, asthma,[40] contact dermatitis, and partial-thickness second-degree burns.[30]

MANAGEMENT

Management is supportive and symptomatic. Topical burns will respond to sterile dressings. "Wel loved he garlek, oynons, and eek rekes, and for to drinken strong wyn, reed as blood." Chaucer, The Canterbury Tales.[41]

ACKEE FRUIT AND JAMAICAN VOMITING SICKNESS

Potential risk behaviors for ackee poisoning include the following[42]:

1. Selection and cooking of unripe ackee.
2. Purchase of tampered, forcibly opened ackee.
3. Reuse of the water in which unripe ackee has been cooked.

Undernutrition is also thought to be associated with both susceptibility to and severity of THS (toxic hypoglycemic syndrome), particularly among children in Jamaica.

PREGNANCY

Hypoglycin A has been associated with a high incidence of fetal resorption and malformations (encephalocele syndactyly and stunted growth) in animals (rats). These teratogenic effects may be due to the metabolite of hypoglycin, methylene cyclopropane acetic acid.[43] This may have been a factor in the production of 33 neonatal human stillborn and neonatal deaths with anencephaly, spina bifida, and hydrocephalus observed out of an estimated 54,400 total births in Jamaica between September 1986 and August 1987.[44]

KAVA

IDENTIFICATION

Scientific Name

Piper methysticum.

Common Name

Kava-kava, kew, tonga, awa.

Family

Piperaceae.

Botanical Description

The plant is indigenous to the islands of the South Pacific. It has been imported into aboriginal communities in Arnhem Land in Australia in commercial quantities since the early 1980s.

TOXIN

Kava is an intoxicating drink prepared from the rhizome of *P. methysticum.* The pulverized roots are steeped in water. Lactones (kawain, dihydrokawain, methysticin, dihydromethysticine, desmethoxyyanogonin, and yanogonin are the major constituents present in kava resin. This extract may induce sedation, protection from electric shock, local anesthetic action, smooth muscle relaxation, and potentiation of barbiturate narcosis.[45]

The plasma elimination half-life of kavain is 2.8 to 6.7 hours.[46] Time to peak plasma concentration of 277 ng/mL is 1.8 to 3.0 hours.[47]

A gas chromatography–mass spectrometry method to determine urinary metabolites of L-kavain is available.[48]

CLINICAL PRESENTATION

Kava drinkers generally appear to suffer from ill health, shortness of breath, malnutrition, and loss of body fat.[49,50] A scaly ichthyotoxic skin rash may be present.[51] Its main effect appears to be on the liver, kidneys, blood, and lungs where it induces biochemical and functional evidence of damage. Signs suggestive of central dopaminergic antagonism, including dystonic reactions and dyskinesias, have been observed.[52]

Albumin and plasma proteins are decreased. High-density lipoprotein cholesterol levels are increased. Red-cell volume is increased. Platelet and lymphocyte counts are decreased. There is decrease in lung volume.[46]

TREATMENT

Reduction of consumption of kava and improvement of nutrition appear to be reasonable approaches to lessening the problems induced by this drink.

GINKGO (SEE ALSO CHAPTER 73)

IDENTIFICATION

Scientific name

Ginkgo biloba.

Common names

Ginkgo, maidenhair tree, kew tree.

Family

Ginkgoaceae.

Occurrence/Use

The ginkgo is the world's oldest living tree species. The extract of its fruit has been used for peripheral arterial disease and organic brain syndromes in the elderly. There is little controlled clinical evidence to support its use.[53–55]

TOXIN

The ginkgo contains a number of terpenes, proarthocyanidines, heterosides, and bioflavones. Its terpenoids include ginkgolides and bilobalides.[54]

CLINICAL PRESENTATION

Ingestion of ginkgo extract has been associated with mild gastrointestinal disturbance and headache. The whole ginkgo plant has been associated with severe allergic reactions. Ginkgolides and bilobalides are structurally similar to the allergens of poison ivy, mango rind, and cashew nut shell oil. Contact with the fruit pulp causes erythema, edema, vesicles, and itching, which may last 7 to 10 days.[54]

TREATMENT

Treatment is symptomatic and supportive. There are no desensitization preparations in clinical use.

MATE

Scientific Name

Ilex paraguariensis.

Common names

Mate, yerba mate, Paraguay tea, St. Bartholomero's tea, Jesuit's tea.

Botanical Description

Mate is a beverage, not a plant, and is prepared from the leathery leaves of *Ilex paraguariensis,* a species of holly that is found in South America. In areas where mate is drunk it largely replaces coffee and tea. The leaves are plunged into hot water.

TOXIN

Yerba mate contains phenylpropanoids, including caffetannin, yielding caffeic acid when hydrolyzed, chlorogenic acid, neochlorogenic acid, and isochlorogenic acid. The beverage contains caffeine (about 2%), theobromine, and theophylline.[56]

Heavy use of yerba mate has been associated with a high risk of esophageal cancer. This may be due to the hot drinks, rather than the alkaloids.[57]

THUJONE AND ABSINTHE[56–58]

IDENTIFICATION

Scientific Name

Artemisia absinthium.

Common Name

Wormwood, absinthium, armoise, wermut, absinthe, absinthites, ajenjo.

Family

Compositae.

Botanical Description

Wormwood is a perennial shrub native to Europe, but also grown in the northeast and north central United States. The leaves and stems are covered with fine silky hairs, and the plant grows to a height of about 3 feet. The small flowers are green-yellow, and the indented leaves have a silver-gray color.

OCCURRENCE/USE

In the first century a wine fortified with extract of wormwood *(Artemisia absinthium)* was described as "absinthites" by Pliny the Elder. A stronger drink, with 70 to 80% alcohol by volume, was developed by a Frenchman who sold the recipe to M. Pernod in 1797.[58]

TOXIN

The deleterious compound in absinthe that appeared to produce hallucinations and psychosis was thujone. Thujone is a terpene. Thujone occurs in a variety of plants, including tansy *(Tanacetum vulgare)* and sage *(Salvia officinalis),* as well as in all trees of the arborvitae group of which the thuja *(Thuja occidentalis),* or white cedar, is one. Wormwood is a bitter plant. The bitterness is due to a compound called absinthin ($C_{30}H_{40}O_6$).

CLINICAL PRESENTATION

Ingestion of absinthe may lead to a group of neurologic symptoms described as "absinthism" and characterized by digestive disorders, thirst, restlessness, vertigo, tremor, numbness of extremities, diminished intellect, delirium, paralysis, and death. Fifteen grams of the volatile oil can cause convulsions and coma in humans. Van Gogh was known to repeatedly drink absinthe and painted a still life with absinthe. Edouard Manet painted the Absinthe Drinker (1859), and Edgar Degas painted "L'Absinthe" in 1876.

TREATMENT

Treatment is symptomatic and supportive. Some countries have banned absinthe.[58–60]

BETEL NUT

Scientific Name

Areca catechu L.

Common Name

Betel nut.

Family

Palmae (Arecaceae).

TOXIN

About six reduced pyridine alkaloids are present in these nuts. Arecaidine may have carcinogenic effects and may be a factor in the associated increased incidence of oral cancer.[61] Arecoline, a major component of the *Areca* (betel nut), is a cholinergic agent of similar structure to methacholine. Asthmatic patients challenged with inhaled arecoline respond with bronchoconstriction.[62]

The Ministry of Health and Family Welfare for India has included betel nut or *supari* as a food item "injurious to health" because of its causal association with oral cancer.

Supari is chewed alone or as pan, a mixture of *supari,* lime, and other ingredients with or without tobacco wrapped in a betel leaf *(Piper betal). Pan masala* is a concentrated powdered form of the preparation used in pan.[63]

REFERENCES—PLANTS CULTIVATED AS FOOD SOURCES AND BULBS

1. Rosling H. Cassava toxicity and food security. 2nd ed. UNICEF, 1988, pp. 1–40.
2. Osuntokun RO, Durooju JE, McFarlane WJ. Plasma aminoacids in the Nigeria nutritional ataxic neuropathy. Br Med J 1968;3:647–649.
3. Rauws AG, Olling M, Timmerman A. The pharmacokinetics of amygdalin. Arch Toxicol 1982;49:311–319.
4. Moertel CG, Ames MM, Kovach JS et al. A pharmacologic and toxicological study of amygdalin. JAMA 1981;245: 591–594.
5. Sadoff L, Fuchs K, Hollander J. Rapid death associated with laetrile ingestion. JAMA 1978;239:1582.
6. Humbert JR, Tress JH, Braico KT. Fatal cyanide poisoning. Accidental ingestion of amygdalin. JAMA 1977; 238:482.
7. Townsend WA, Boni B. Cyanide poisoning from ingestion of apricot kernels. Morbid Mortal Week Rep 1975;24:427.
8. Rubino MJ, Davidoff F. Cyanide poisoning from apricot seeds. JAMA 1979;241:359.
9. Shragg TA, Albertson TE, Fisher CJ. Cyanide poisoning after bitter almond ingestion. West J Med 1982;136:65–69.
10. Sayre JW, Kaymakcalan S. Cyanide poisoning of apricot seeds among children in central Turkey. N Engl J Med 1964; 270:1113–1115.
11. Smith FP, Butler TP, Cohan S et al. Laetrile toxicity: a report of two cases. JAMA 1977;238:1361.
12. Hall AH, Linden CH, Kulig KW et al. Cyanide poisoning from laetrile ingestion: role of nitrite therapy. Pediatrics 1986;78: 269–272.
13. Cordell GA, Araujo DE. Capsaicin: identification, nomenclature and pharmacotherapy. Ann Pharmacother 1993;27:330–331.
14. Don PC. Topical capsaicin for treatment of neuralgia associated with herpes zoster infection. J Am Acad Dermatol 1988;18:1135–1136.
15. Kurkcuoglu N, Alaybeyi F. Topical capsaicin for psoriasis. Br J Dermatol 1990;123:549–550.
16. Tandan R, Lewis G, Fried T, Kallal J. Safety of topical capsaicin in diabetic neuropathy. Neurology 1990;40(Suppl 1):160.
17. Ross DR, Varepapa RJ. Treatment of painful diabetic neuropathy with topical capsaicin. N Engl J Med 1989;321:474–475.
18. Levy DM, Abraham RR, Tomkinson DR. Topical capsaicin in the treatment of painful diabetic neuropathy. N Engl J Med 1991;324:776.
19. Breneman DL, Cardose JS, Kaufmann PS, Lather RM. Topical capsaicin for treatment of pruritus related to hemodialysis. Clin Pharmacol Ther 1989;45:188.
20. Weintraub M, Golik A, Rubio A. Capsicum for treatment of post-traumatic amputation stump pain. Lancet 1990;336: 1003–1004.
21. Kakas JF Jr. Topical capsaicin induces cough in patients receiving ACE inhibitors. Ann Allergy 1990;65:322.
22. Blanc P, Liu D, Juarez C, Boushey HA. Cough in hot pepper workers. Chest 1991;99:27–32.
23. Tominack RL, Spyker DA. Capsicum and capsaicin—review: case report of the use of hot peppers in child abuse. Clin Toxicol 1987;25:591–601.
24. Jones LA, Tandberg D, Troutman WG. Household treatment for "chili burns" of the hand. Clin Toxicol 1987; 25:483–491.
25. Williams SR, Clark RF, Dunford JW. Contact dermatitis associated with capsaicin. Hunan hand syndrome. Ann Emerg Med 1995;25:713–715.
26. Cohle SD, Trestrail JD III, Graham MA, et al. Fatal pepper aspiration. Amer J Dis Child 1988;1242:633–636.
27. Sheahan K, Page DV, Kemper T, Suarez R. Childhood sudden death secondary to accidental aspiration of black pepper. Am J Forensic Med Pathol 1988;9:51–57.
28. El-Mofty MM, Soliman AA, Abdel-Gawad AF, Sakr SA, Schwairlb MA. Carcinogenicity testing of black pepper *(Piper nigrum)* using the Egyptian toad *(Bufo regularis)* as a quick biological test animal. Oncology 1988;45:247–252.
29. Myers BM, Smith JL, Graham DY. Effect of red pepper and black pepper on the stomach. Am J Gastroenterol 1987; 82:211–214.
30. Sir John Harrington: The Englishman's Doctor. 1609.
31. Olin BR, ed. The Lawrence review of natural products. St. Louis; Facts and Comparisons. Garlic. January 1988, pp. 1–2.
32. Garlic Therapy Symposium. Br J Clin Pract 1988;44(Suppl 69).
33. Roser D. Garlic. Lancet 1990;335:114–115.
34. Parish RA, McIntire S, Heimbach DM. Garlic burns: a naturopathic remedy gone awry. Pediatr Emerg Care 1987;3:258–260.
35. Kleijnen J, Knipschild P, Ter Piet G. Garlic, onions and cardiovascular risk factors. A review of the evidence for human experiments with emphasis on commercially available preparations. Br J Clin Pharmacol 1989;28:535–544.
36. Caporaso N, Smith SM, Eng RHK. Antifungal activity in human urine and serum after ingestion of garlic *(Allium sativum).* Antimicrobial Agents Chemother 1983;23:700–702.
37. Bordia A. Effect of garlic on blood lipids in patients with coronary heart disease. Am J Clin Nutr 1991;34:2100–2103.
38. Ariga T, Oshiba S, Tamad T. Platelet aggregation inhibition in garlic. Lancet 1981;1:150–151.
39. Aier W, Eiher A, Hertkorn E, Hoehfeld E, Koehnle U, Lorenz A, Mader FV. Garlic therapy: hypertension and hyperlipidemia: garlic helps in mild cases. Br J Clin Pract 1988;44(Suppl 69).
40. Lybarger JA, Gallagher JS, Pulver DW, Litwin A, Brooks S, Bernstein IL. Occupational asthma induced by inhalation and ingestion of garlic. J Allergy Clin Immunol 1982;69:948–957.
41. Editor. Well loved he garleek, oynons. Lancet 1989;2:1409–1410.
42. CDC. Toxic hypoglycemic syndrome—Jamaica 1989–1991. MMWR 1992;41:53–55.
43. Persaud TVN. Foetal abnormalities caused by the active principle of the fruit of Blighia sapida (Ackee). West Indian Med J 1967;16:193–197.
44. Golding J, Foster-Williams K, Coard K, Ashley D. A cluster of central nervous system defects in Jamaica. Hum Exp Toxicol 1990;9:13–16.
45. Duffield AM, Lidgard RO. Analysis of Kava resin by gas chromatography and electron impact and negative ion chemical ionization mass spectrometry. New trace constituents of Kava resin. Biomed Environ Mass Spectrom 1986;13:621–626.
46. Droege H, Walter K, Huber HD, Knoch A, Gay S, Stanislaus F. Preliminary results of Kavain on pharmacokinetics and bioavailability from Neuronika in man. Eur J Drug Metab Pharmacokin 1990;15:26.
47. Droege H, Walter K, Huber HJ, Jank P, Schmoll H, Stanislaus F. Metabolic profile of Kavain in human plasma. Eur J Drug Metab Pharmacokin 1990;15:28.
48. Koppel C, Tenczer J. Mass spectral characterization of urinary metabolites of D,L-Kawain. J Chromatography (Biomed Appl) 1991;562:207–210.
49. Editor. Kava. Lancet 1988;1:258–259.
50. Mathews JD, Riley MD, Fejo L, Munoz E, Milns MR, Gardner ID et al. Effects of the heavy usage of kava on physical health: summary of a pilot survey in an aboriginal community. Med J Aust 1988;148:548–555.
51. Ruze P. Kava-induced dermopathy: a niacin deficiency? Lancet 1990;335:1442–1445.
52. Schelovsky L, Raffauf C, Jendroska K, Poewe W. Kava and dopamine antagonism. J Neurol Neurosurg Psychiatry 1995;58:639–640.
53. Olin BR, ed. The Lawrence review of natural products. St. Louis: Facts and Comparisons. Ginkgo. February 1988.

54. *Gingko biloba* extract: over 5 million prescriptions a year. (West Germany). Lancet 1080;2:1510–1514.
55. Hofferberth B. Effect of *Ginkgo biloba* extract on neurophysiological and psychomatic measurement results in patients with cerebro-organic syndrome. A double-blind study versus placebo. Arzneimittel-forsch/Drug Res 1989;39:918–919.
56. Mate. Lawrence review of natural products. St. Louis: Facts and Comparisons, April 1988.
57. de Stefani E, Munoz N, Esteve J, Vasallo A, Victora CG, Teuchmann S. Mate drinking, alcohol, tobacco, diet and esophageal cancer in Uruguay. Cancer Res 1990;5:426–431.
58. Arnold WN. Vincent van Gogh and the thujone connection. JAMA 1988;260:3042–3044.
59. Arnold WN. Absinthe. Sci Am 1989;260(6):112–117.
60. Wormwood. Lawrence review of natural products. St. Louis: Facts and Comparisons, April 1991.
61. Ashby J, Styles JA, Boyland E. Betel nuts, arecaidine, and oral cancer. Lancet 1979;1:112.
62. Betel nuts and asthma. Lancet 1992;339:1134.
63. Editor. India: Betel nut warning. Lancet 1993;341:819.

PLANT ESTROGENS

Some foods contain potential estrogenic analogues such as the isoflavonoids, lignins, and resorcylic acid lactones, which may be activated or inactivated. Plant estrogens may include soy flour, sprouts, and linseed. Such foods can modulate the severity of the menopause.[1,2]

FAVA BEANS AND FAVISM

Scientific Name

Vicia faba.

Common Name

Broadbean.

Family

Fabaceae (Papilionaceae).

Botanical Description

A coarse erect annual vine without tendrils.[3] Fruit up to 14 inches long, a thick many-seeded legume, the large seeds compressed or globular, and variously colored from green to purple or blue.

Occurrence/Use

Vicia faba is widely cultivated in Canada and often grown as an ornamental vine in the United States. It is of European origin and often cultivated there.[3,4]

GLUCOSE-6-PHOSPHATE DEHYDROGENASE DEFICIENCY

The hemolytic syndrome associated with favism has been recognized since antiquity. Glucose-6-phosphate dehydrogenase deficiency (G6PD) is the most common disease-producing enzyme disorder of humans with an estimated 7% of the world's population carrying the gene. The G6PD gene is located in the X chromosome. It is inherited in a sex-linked manner and is fully expressed in homizygote males and homozygous females. A high incidence of low activity G6PD variants is typical of the Mediterranean area and the Middle East in addition to Taiwan and South China. About 12% of black American men are reported to have the deficiency.[5–7]

Mechanism of Action

G6PD catalyzes the first step in the hexosemonophosphate pathway. (See Methemoglobin discussion in Airborne Toxic chapter.) This results in reduction of the cofactor nicotinamide phosphate (NADP) to NADPH. NADPH is necessary to protect the -SH groups of enzymes and of the beta-chain of hemoglobin from oxidation. This protection is mediated by glutathione, which is present in red blood cells almost entirely in the reduced form (GSH). GSH becomes oxidized to GSSG as it restores oxidized -SH groups. NADPH in turn regenerates GSH through the enzyme glutathione reductase. Red blood cells do not have alternative enzyme systems capable of generating NADPH. In the absence of adequate G6PD activity, hemolysis is the primary effect of an oxidative stress. Sensitivity to favism is a poorly understood phenomenon that appears to be determined by a separate gene.[5,7]

Clinical Presentation

About 10 to 20% of G6PD-deficient individuals who consume fava beans experience fava crises. The first symptoms of favism are malaise, generalized weakness to severe lethargy, nausea and vomiting, headache, and lumbar or abdominal pain. Chills, tremors, and fever are often present. After a delay of up to 48 hours, jaundice appears accompanied by enlargement of the spleen and liver. A few hours after fava bean intake hemoglobinuria begins and may continue for several days. Anemia and reticulocytosis follow. In most cases the hemolysis is self-limited. During an acute episode the measured G6PD levels may be normal.[5]

Treatment

The disorder induces a self-limited to low-grade hemolytic anemia, light or no hemoglobinuria, and slight jaundice. It may require no treatment or only supportive therapy (intravenous hydration to maintain urine output and diuresis to prevent precipitation of hemoglobin in the kidneys). If anemia is life-threatening, transfusion is required.

REFERENCES—PLANT ESTROGENS

1. Wilcox G, Wahlqvist ML, Burger HG, Medley G. Oestrogen effects of plant foods in postmenopausal women. Br Med J 1990;301:905–906.
2. Farnsworth NR, Bingel AS, Cordell GA, Crane FA, Fong HHS. Potential value of plants as sources of new antifertility agents. II. J Pharm Sci 1975;64:714.
3. Lewis WH, Elvin-Lewis MPF. Medical botany. Plants affecting man's health. New York: John Wiley, 1977.
4. Frohne D, Pfander HJ. A colour atlas of poisonous plants. London: Wolfe, 1983; pp. 129–130.
5. Hasler J, Lee S. Acute hemolytic anemia after ingestion of fava beans. Am J Emerg Med 1992;11:560–561.

6. O'Connell JT, Henderson AR. Glucose-6-phosphate dehydrogenase revisited. J Natl Med Assoc 1984;76:1135–1136, 1139, 1143.
7. Cooper RA, Bunn HF. Hemolytic anemias. In: Wilson JD, Braunwald E, Isselbacher KJ, Petersdorp RG, Martin JB, Fauci AS, Root RK, eds. Harrison's principles ofi nternal medicine. 12th ed. New York: McGraw-Hill, 1991; p. 1542.

CYCADS

Scientific Name

Cycas circinalis.

Common Name

False sago palm.

Family

Cycadaceae.

Botanical Description

A tropical plant with palmlike leaves that grow outward encircling a central trunk.[1]

Occurrence/Use

The seeds of the false sago palm have been used as a dietary staple for the Chamorro indigenous population of the Mariana Islands in the Western Pacific.[2]

TOXIN

The leaves and seeds of the false sago palm contain a glycoside, cycasin, and an unusual nonprotein amino acid, alpha-amino-beta-methyl aminopropionic acid or BMAA, chemically similar to BOAA (beta-*N*-oxalyl-amino-alanine), a toxin found in the pea, *Lathyrus sativus* (see above, Sweet Pea and Lathyrism), associated with a motor or neuron disease in India[3] (Table 74–17).[1]

CLINICAL PRESENTATION

Much evidence links motor neuron disease parkinsonism in Guam to BMAA. Cycad was the main source of edible starch among the Chamorros before and during the 1939–1945 war. Motor neuron disease accompanied by parkinsonism and dementia was common among Chamorrs in this area.[4] Now more than 80% of the total BMAA content is lost from seeds during processing.[4] Therefore, even when cycad flour is eaten regularly, it is unlikely at present that it causes the ALS (amyotrophic lateral sclerosis) and parkinsonism dementia (PD) complex of Guam.[4,5]

A gas chromatographic/mass spectrometric method for quantitation of BMAA in cycad seeds is available.[6] Cycad ingestion by sheep and cattle in Australia produces ataxia and liver necrosis.[7]

TREATMENT

Treatment of the ALS-PD syndrome is symptomatic and supportive. If children ingest the seeds, syrup of ipecac or gastric emptying reduces exposure.

REFERENCES—CYCADS

1. Spoerke D, Evans B, Linaburg B. The hidden hazards in house and garden plants. Missoula, MT: Pictorial Histories, 1991; p. 75.
2. Spencer PS. Guam ALS/parkinsonism—dementia. A long-lasting neurotoxic disorder caused by "slow toxin(s)" in food? Can J Neurol Sci 1987;14:347–357.
3. Editorial. A poison tree. Lancet 1987;2:947–948.
4. Duncan MW, Kopin IJ, Garruto MM, Lavine L, Markey SP. 2-amino-3-(methylamino) propionic acid in cycad-derived form is an unlikely cause of amyotrophic lateral sclerosis/parkinsonism. Lancet 1988;2:631–632.
5. Duncan MW, Steele JC, Kapin IJ, Markey SR. 2-amino-3-(methylamino) propionic acid (BMAA) in cycad flour: an unlikely cause of amyotrophic lateral sclerosis and parkinsonism—dementia (ALS-PD) of Guam. Neurology 1990;40: 767–772.
6. Duncan MW, Kopin IJ, Crowley JS, Jones SM, Markey SP. Quantification of the putative neurotoxin 2-amino-3-(methylamino) propionic acid (BMAA) in Cycadales: analysis of the seeds of some members of the family Cycadaceae. J Anal Toxicol 1989;13:169-175.
7. Hall WTK. Cycad (*Zamia*) poisoning in Australia. Aust Vet J 1987;64:149–150.

ORNAMENTAL SHRUBS AND TREES

RHODODENDRON

Clinical Presentation

A 33-year-old woman ingested tea made from fresh rhododendron leaves and complained of weakness, dizziness, blurred vision, nausea, and vomiting. She was hypotensive and bradycardic and experienced a transient episode of complete A-V dissociation. Her hypotension improved with IV fluids alone. She was asymptomatic the following day when she was discharged.[1]

Symptoms following honey ingestions (between 2 and 5 teaspoonfuls) by 23 people in Turkey began within 30 minutes and up to 2 hours after ingestion and included nausea, vomiting, sweating, dizziness, hypotension, bradycardia, and impairment of consciousness. Electrocardiographic changes included bradycardia, junctional rhythm, complete atrioventricular blocks, and Wolff-Parkinson-White syndrome with sinus bradycardia. Patients regained consciousness or felt better in 30 minutes to 6 hours, and recovered completely in 1 or 2 days. ECGs were normal in 24 hours.[2] The intoxication is rarely fatal.[3]

A group of 30 patients with food poisoning due to honey were seen in Turkey from 1983 to 1986. Symptoms included hypotension, bradycardia, nausea, vomiting, sweating, dizziness, impaired consciousness, exhaustion, fainting, blurred vision or diplopia, cyanosis, and chills. Ages varied from 7 months to 61 years. The amount of toxic honey ingested ranged between 2 teaspoonfuls and 5 tablespoonfuls. Symptoms began within 30 minutes to 2 hours. An electrocardiographic bradycardia, junctional rhythm, complete atrioventricular block, and Wolff-Parkinson-White syndrome with sinus bradycardia were often observed.

Patients regained consciousness in ½ hour to 6 hours and recovered in 1 to 2 days. ECGs were normal in 24 hours.[2]

REFERENCES—ORNAMENTAL PLANTS AND SHRUBS

1. Meier KH, Hemmich RS. Bradycardia and complete heart block after ingestion of rhododendron tea. Vet Hum Toxicol 1992;34:351.
2. Yavuz H, Ozel A, Akkus I, Erkul I. Honey poisoning in Turkey. Lancet 1991;337:789–790.
3. Biberoglu K, Komsuoglu B, Biberoglu S. Transient Wolff-Parkinson-White syndrome during honey intoxication. Isr J Med Sci 1988;24:253–254.

COMMON OLEANDER (FIG. 74–7)

CLINICAL PRESENTATION

Oleander poisoning closely resembles digitoxin poisoning with predominantly gastrointestinal and cardiac symptoms. Nausea and vomiting usually occur within several hours. Serious toxic effects result from cardiotoxicity and specifically from ventricular ectopy and cardiovascular collapse. Conduction delays may persist 3 to 6 days, displaying classical digitalis toxicity as characterized by increased ectopy and conduction delay (e.g., supraventricular tachycardia with atrioventricular block).[1,2] In a fatal suicidal ingestion, a 40-kg 96-year-old woman developed a cardiac arrest shortly after arrival in the emergency department.[3] Cardiac monitoring displayed ventricular ectopy, including ventricular tachycardia and ventricular fibrillation, both of which were unresponsive to the standard therapies of the American Heart Association's Advanced Cardiac Life Support guidelines. Her admission potassium level was 8.6 mEq/L. A 30-year-old woman presented in cardiogenic shock with an idioventricular rhythm 10 hours after ingesting an oleander tea. She died after 1 hour of resuscitation with a potassium level of 6.6 mEq/L.[4]

LABORATORY

The Abbott TDx Digoxin II assay is a rapid method useful for confirming the ingestion of glycosides from the plants *Nerium oleander, Thevetia peruviana*, and *Adonis microcarpa,* as well as from the toad, *Bufo marinus*.[5] Serum from a 17-year-old boy suspected of ingesting a leaf from an oleander tree (clinically normal, normal electrocardiogram) had an apparent digoxin concentration of 0.45 μg/L and 0.14 μg/L measured by radioimmunoassay and TDx methods, respectively. Many asymptomatic patients suspected of *Thevetia peruviana* ingestion have apparent digoxin concentrations in the serum of 0.5 to 1.2 μg/L. A 5-year-old was asymptomatic for 24 hours after swallowing *Thevetia* seeds before developing severe vomiting, bradycardia, and electrocardiographic changes that persisted for 4 days. The patient recovered. The apparent digoxin concentration in the serum 50 hours after ingestion was 1.5 μg/L. A 2½-year-old child died 16 hours after ingestion of *Thevetia peruviana* seeds. A postmortem apparent digoxin level was 11.0 μg/L. The patient had been asymptomatic for 4 to 5 hours after the *Thevetia* ingestion.

A 37-year-old man ingested a "handful" of oleander leaves (probably *Nerium oleander*). He developed bradycardia, a sinotrial nodal arrest, and junctional escape. He was treated with a single dose of 5 vials (200 mg) of digoxin-specific FAB antibody fragments. Prior to treatment the digoxin level was 1.5 ng/mL. After treatment the rhythm stabilized with residual bradycardia. The patient recovered.[6]

TREATMENT

Treatment is mainly supportive. Gastric lavage, fluid administration, atropine, isoproterenol, antiarrhythmics, and early administration of activated charcoal may be useful. Hemodynamic decompensation may require the temporary use of a cardiac pacemaker and digoxin-specific Fab antidote fragments. Doses of 200 mg and 480 mg intravenously have improved life-threatening oleander intoxication.[7]

REFERENCES—COMMON OLEANDER

1. Chin D, Wei-liang C. Auricular tachycardia with auriculo-ventricular block in oleander leaf poisoning. Chin Med J 1957;75:74–77.
2. Spevak L. Dva slucaja trovanja cajem od oleanderovog lisca. Arh Hig Rada 1975;26:147–150.
3. Osterloh J, Harold S, Pond S. Oleander interference in the digoxin radioimmunoassay in a fatal ingestion. JAMA 1982;247:1596–1597.
4. Haynes BE, Bessen HA, Wrightman WD. Oleander tea: herbal draught of death. Ann Emerg Med 1985;14:350–353.
5. Cheung K, Hinds JA, Duffy P. Detection of poisoning by plant origin cardiac glycoside with the Abbott TDx analyzer. Clin Chem 1989;35:295–296.
6. Shumaik GM, Wu AW, Pine AC. Oleander poisoning: treatment with digoxin-specific FAB antibody fragments. Ann Emerg Med 1988;17:732–735.
7. Safadi R, Ley I, Amitai Y, Caraco Y. Beneficial effect of digoxin-specific Fab antibody fragments in oleander intoxication. Arch Intern Med 1995;155:2121–2125.

WISTERIA

Scientific Name

Wisteria spp.

Common Name

Wisteria.

Botanical Description

The 12.5- to 15-cm pods contain three to five seeds, which are flat, nearly circular, and brown.[1]

TOXINS

The known toxins are wistarin, alectin, and a glycoside.

CLINICAL PRESENTATION

About 3 hours following ingestion of two to ten seeds, headache, nausea, vomiting, diarrhea, dizziness, abdominal pain, and drowsiness may ensue. There have been no fatalities reported. A leukocytosis may be present.

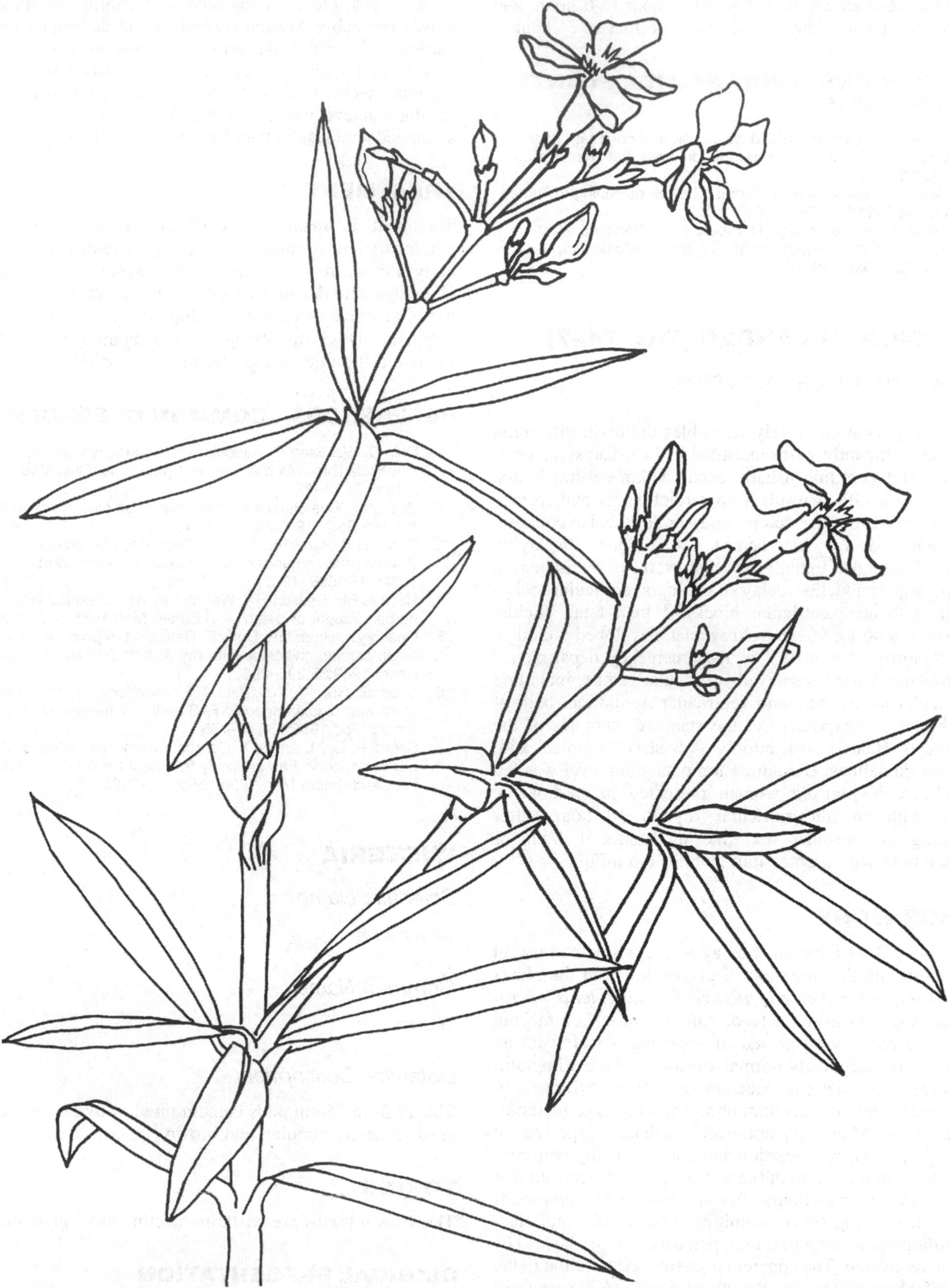

Figure 74–7 Oleander (*Nerium oleander*). (Adapted from Lampe KF, Fagerström R. Baltimore; Williams & Wilkins, 1968.)

TREATMENT

Treatment is largely symptomatic and supportive.

BRACKEN

Scientific Name

Pteridium aquilinum.

Common Name

Bracken.

Family

Polypodiaceae.

Occurrence/Use

Found in mountainous areas. Occasionally, the fronds are put into floral displays and are used in table decorations.

Botanical Description

A dark brown, coarse fern with stiff fronds (leaves) that are somewhat fan shaped.

TOXIN

Bracken contains thiaminase, which destroys thiamine and results in a vitamin B deficiency poisoning horses and cattle. It has not been reported to be toxic to children when ingested. Bracken is carcinogenic in animal species perhaps due to shimic, a possible carcinogen in animals.[2] Further data are required to establish a human carcinogenic association with bracken.[3]

REFERENCES—MOIST WOODLAND PLANTS AND TREES

1. Rondeau ES. Wisteria toxicity. Clin Toxicol 1993;31:107–112.
2. Trotter WR. Is bracken a health hazard? Lancet 1990;336: 1563–1564.
3. Spoerke D, Evans R, Linaburg B. Tho hidden hazards in house and garden plants, Missoula, MT: Pictorial Histories, 1991, p. 142.

JIMSONWEED (FIG. 74–8)

D. stramonium grows throughout the United States and, historically, was used by American Indians for medicinal and religious purposes. All parts of the jimsonweed plant are poisonous, containing the alkaloids atropine, hyoscyamine, and scopolamine. Jimsonweed—also known as thorn apple, angel's trumpet, and Jamestown weed (because the first record of physical symptoms following ingestion occurred in Jamestown, Virginia, in 1676)—is a member of the nightshade family. Although all parts of the plant are toxic, the highest concentrations of anticholinergic occur in the seeds (equivalent to 0.1 mg of atropine per seed). The estimated lethal doses of atropine and scopolamine in adults are more or less than 10 mg and >2 to 4 mg, respectively.

CLINICAL PRESENTATION

Symptoms of jimsonweed toxicity usually occur within 30 to 60 minutes after ingestion and may continue for 24 to 48 hours because the alkaloids delay gastrointestinal motility. Ingestion of jimsonweed manifests as classic atropine

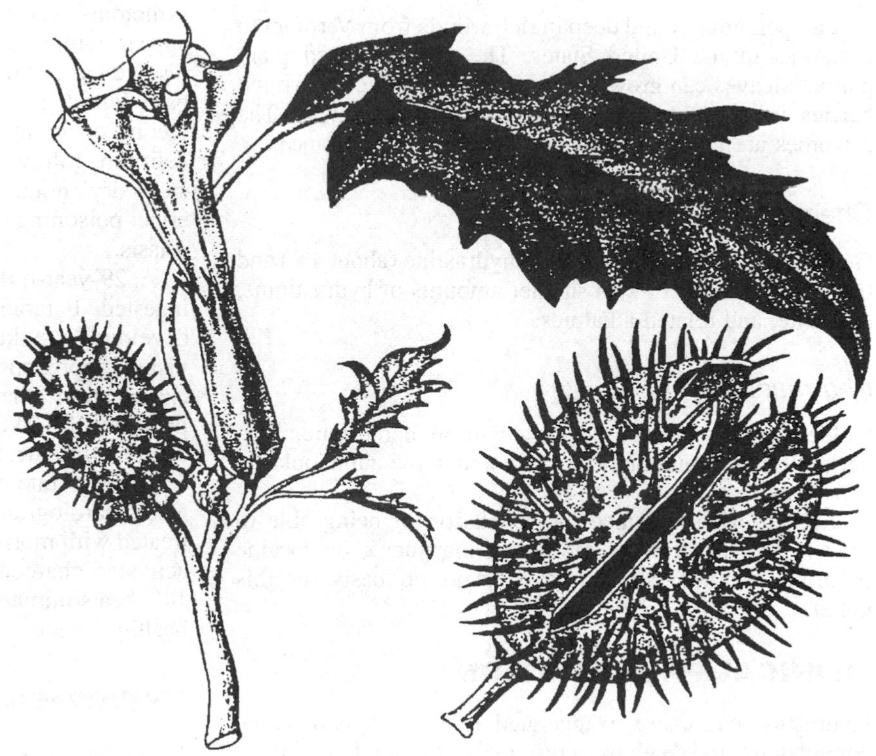

Figure 74–8 Drawing of jimsonweed. (Adapted from Rosen CS, Lechner M. N Engl J Med 1967;267:449.)

poisoning. Initial manifestations include dry mucous membranes, thirst, difficulty swallowing and speaking, blurred vision, and photophobia and may be followed by hyperthermia, confusion, agitation, combative behavior, and hallucinations typically involving insects, urinary retention, seizures, and coma.

TREATMENT

Treatment consists of supportive care, gastrointestinal decontamination (i.e., lavage and/or activated charcoal), and physostigmine in severe cases.[1]

REFERENCES—JIMSONWEED

1. CDC. Jimson weed poisoning—Texas, New York and California, 1994. MMWR 1995;44:41–44.

GOLDENSEAL

Scientific Name

Hydrasis canadensis L.

Family

Ranunculaceae.

Common Names

Eye balm, eye root, goldenseal, ground raspberry, Indian dye, jaundice root, orange root, turmeric root, yellow Indian paint, yellow puccoon, yellow root.

Botany

A stout perennial found deep in rich woods from Vermont to Arkansas in the United States. The 5- to 9-lobed plant palmate leaves can grow to 10 inches. It produces dark red berries in April and May from green-white flowers. The rhizomes are golden yellow and knotted in appearance.

Chemistry

Goldenseal contains the alkaloids hydrastine (about 4%) and berberine (up to 6%) with smaller amounts of hydrastinine, canadine, and related alkaloids.

Pharmacology

Goldenseal has been used as a uterine hemostatic. Berberine has weak antibiotic activity and some antineoplastic activity.

Goldenseal had gained the reputation of being able to prevent the detection of morphine, marijuana, or cocaine in urine samples. Studies have found no basis for this belief.

CLINICAL PRESENTATION

Hydrastine can cause exaggerated reflexes, hypertension, convulsions, and death from respiratory failure. Large doses of the plant irritate the mouth and throat and cause nausea, vomiting, diarrhea, and paresthesias. Central nervous system stimulation and respiratory failure induced by the plant can be fatal.[1]

REFERENCE

1. Dombek C, ed. Lawrence review of natural products. St. Louis: Facts and Comparisons, May 1994.

PSYCHOACTIVE AND HALLUCINOGENIC PLANTS (TABLE 74–3)

The hallucinogenic plants can be subdivided into two groups based on the presence of nitrogen in the active principle. Marijuana (*Cannabis sativa*) and nutmeg (*Myristica fragrans*) are two representatives of the nonnitrogen group. The nitrogenous group includes peyote (*Lophophora williamsii*), South American *Piptadenia* and *Mimosa* spp., hallucinogenic mushrooms (*Psilocybe, Clitocybe, Amanita muscaria*), Indian spice (*Peganum harmala*), morning glory seeds, and tropanes of the Solanaceae family. Table 74–3 lists the major plant hallucinogens. Many more plants are used as herb teas for their psychoactive properties. The increased popularity of these teas has led to increased cases of clinical toxicity.

NUTMEG

CLINICAL PRESENTATION

Approximately 10 to 50 g of nutmeg is required to produce symptoms. (One nutmeg weighs about 6 g.) Symptoms appear within 3 to 6 hours of ingestion and generally resolve by 24 hours. Initially, nausea, vomiting, abdominal pain, chest pain, restlessness, agitation, tremor, and a feeling of doom occur; alternating periods of lethargy and delirium follow. Facial flushing, tachycardia, hypertension, dry mouth, and delirium may stimulate anticholinergic poisoning, but miosis is more common than mydriasis.

A 29-year-old 30-week pregnant female inadvertently ingested 1 tablespoon of nutmeg (equal to 7 g). She developed a sudden onset of palpitations, agitation, blurred vision, apprehension, chest tightening, and dry mouth. On examination she presented with flushed facies, blood pressure of 170/80 mm Hg, and regular pulse rate of 170 beats per minute. She had no delusions or hallucinations. The fetal heart rate was 160 to 170 beats per minute. The electrocardiogram showed a sinus tachycardia. She was treated with morphine sulfate IV and magnesium citrate and activated charcoal orally. The fetal beat returned to 120 to 140 beats/minute within 24 hours. She later delivered a healthy infant.[1]

TREATMENT

Management is supportive.

ARGYREIA NERVOSA

Scientific Name

Argyreia nervosa.

Common Name

Hawaiian baby woodrose.

Family

Convolaceae.

BOTANICAL DESCRIPTION/ OCCURRENCE/USE[2]

Argyreia nervosa is characterized by heart-shaped leaves with dense, white, silky hairs beneath. This member of the morning-glory group is available in southern California, Florida, and Hawaii. Its seeds are ingested by juveniles who seek hallucinating experiences.

TOXIN

Each grain of seed contains 3 mg of alkaloids, of which 0.36 mg is represented by one of the psychoactive constituents, ergine. Ergine (lysergic acid amide) and isoergine (isolysergic acid amide) have been identified in *A. nervosa* by TLC.

CLINICAL PRESENTATION

Ingestion of about 100 *A. nervosa* seeds leads to nausea and vomiting in 30 minutes. Feelings of paranoia may follow. The experience is similar to ingestion of LSD. Agitation, tachycardia, hypertension, and dilated pupils may be seen. Bowel sounds are present. The skin is not flushed.[3]

TREATMENT

Management is largely supportive (activated charcoal, diazepam, cardiac monitoring). Within 24 hours the tachycardia and hypertension returns to normal.[3]

PEYOTE AND CACTUS HALLUCINOGENS

Scientific Name

Lophophora williamsii.

Common Name

Peyote, mescal button, mescal.

TOXIN

Mescaline is the major hallucinogenic agent among at least 16 active beta-phenylethylamine and isoquinoline alkaloids. An average mescaline dose of 5 mg/kg produces psychic effects and visual hallucinations. Peyote buttons are round fleshy tops from the cactus that are sliced and dried for prolonged storage. Each button contains the equivalent of 45 mg of mescaline.

CLINICAL PRESENTATION

Mescaline is rapidly absorbed and produces a phase of mild gastrointestinal distress (nausea, vomiting, rarely diarrhea) within 30 to 60 minutes followed by a phase of sympathomimetic effects (mydriasis, mild tachycardia and hypertension, diaphoresis, tremor). Nystagmus, ataxia, and hyperreflexia also may occur. The sensory phase begins after the nausea and vomiting subside and peaks between 4 and 6 hours postingestion. The phase is similar to LSD intoxication and is characterized by vivid visual hallucinations. Although the sensorium remains clear, emotional lability, anxiety, and panic reactions predispose such patients to self-inflicted or accidental trauma. Mescaline doses over 20 mg/kg can be associated with hypertension, bradycardia, and respiratory depression, but death from the drug is less common than traumatic fatalities resulting from altered perception. Symptoms usually resolve about 12 hours after ingestion.

TREATMENT

A quiet dark environment and calm reassurance provide the best setting. Decontamination usually is not necessary unless a more toxic drug has also been consumed. Diazepam is the sedative of choice (orally or intravenously) if a reassuring environment does not calm the patient.

MORNING-GLORY FAMILY (CONVOLVULACEAE)

IDENTIFICATION

The seeds of certain members of the morning-glory family contain psychotomimetic indole compounds that are structurally related to LSD.

CLINICAL PRESENTATION

Clinical effects are dose dependent and similar to those caused by the sympathomimetic and hallucinogenic properties of LSD. Ingestion of 250 *I. violacea* seeds produce dilated pupils, hyperreflexia, facial erythema, a dissociative state, and emotional lability within 3 hours. Other reported adverse effects include nausea, vomiting, numbness, cool extremities, lethargy, uterine stimulation (*I. violacea* seeds only), and hypotension (intravenous injection). Like LSD, morning-glory seeds can cause panic reactions, marked paranoia, violent behavior, and persistent changes in perception and sensation when ingested.

TREATMENT

Management involves reassurance to calm the patient and a protective environment to prevent self-harm, similar to LSD treatment. Diazepam is the sedative of choice. Normally, symptoms resolve within 8 hours.

KHAT (SEE DRUG ABUSE—AMPHETAMINES)

REFERENCES—PSYCHOACTIVE AND HALLUCINOGENIC PLANTS

1. Levy G. Nutmeg intoxication in pregnancy. A case report. J Reprod Med 1987;32:63–64.
2. Chao J-W, Der Marderosian AH. Ergoline alkaloidal constituents of Hawaiian Baby Woodrose, *Argyreia nervosa* (Burm. f.) Bojer J Pharmaceutical Sci 1973;62:588–591.
3. Furbee RB, Curry SC, Kunkle DB: Ingestion of *Argyreia nervosa* (Hawaiian Baby Woodrose) seeds. Vet Hum Toxicol 1991;33

GOSSYPOL (FIG. 74–9)

IDENTIFICATION

Scientific Name

Gossypium spp.

Common Name

Cotton seed.

Family

Malvaceae.

OCCURRENCE/USE

Gossypol has potential use as a male contraceptive, but it may not be effective as a vaginal spermicide.[1] It also has antineoplastic activity.[2] There are about 15 gossypol pigments in extracts of cottonseed or cottonseed oil. The predominant naturally occurring gossypol pigment is the yellow pigment gossypol with a molecular weight of 518.5. It is soluble in organic solvents and insoluble in water.[3]

TOXIN

Gossypol (3,2'-*bis*-(8-formyl-1,6,7-trihydroxy-5-isopropyl-3-methyl naphthalene) is present as the racemate. Its two enantiomers, (+) and (-) gossypol, have been separated.[4] Gossypol is a binaphthalaldehyde with polyphenolic hydroxy groups.[4,5] Racemic gossypol tablets, each containing 20 mg gossypol acetate, have been used in man. An analytic method to quantitate plasma concentrations of gossypol with high-performance liquid chromatography and electrochemical detector has been described.[6]

After a 20-mg oral dose of racemic gossypol peak plasma concentrations of 996 ng/mL are reached in about 5 hours.[4] The beta $T_{1/2}$ (elimination half-life) averaged 286 hours. Gossypol, (both (+) and (-), may act as an antifertility agent by inhibiting prostaglandin synthesis at the level of arachidonic acid release.[7]

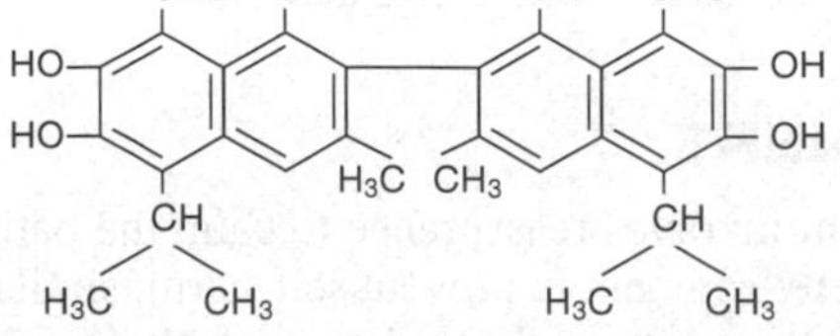

Figure 74–9 Chemical structure of gossypol. (Adapted from Wu D. Drugs 1989;38:333–341.)

CLINICAL PRESENTATION

Gossypol is a pigment present in various parts of the cotton plant. In the 1960s attention began to be paid to the antifertility activity of gossypol when farmers in some rural areas of China developed fatigue and a burning sensation on the face, hands, and other exposed parts of the body. This was given the name "Hanchuan fever" because it was first recognized in Hanchuan County. The farmers called it "burning fever." Epidemiologists showed that patients with this burning fever had consumed homemade unheated cottonseed oil containing gossypol. Many couples from these areas were found to be infertile. The women had amenorrhea and the men had oligospermia or azoospermia. Gossypol has since been considered as a possible male contraceptive or a therapeutic agent for some gynecologic diseases.[5]

The use of gossypol 50 mg/week results in abrupt decreases in sperm counts after 3 months that are sometimes recoverable. A hyperkalemia due to renal potassium loss has been seen.[5]

TREATMENT

Treatment is mainly symptomatic and supportive. Sperm morphology and count often return to normal values in about 3 months after gossypol use is discontinued.[5]

REFERENCES—GOSSYPOL

1. Hong CY, Huang JJ, Wu O. The inhibitory effect of gossypol on human sperm motility: relationship with time, temperature and concentration. Hum Toxicol 1989; 8:49–51.
2. Reidenberg MM, Flack MR, Pyle RG, Mullens NM, Lorenzo B, Wu YW et al. Gossypol treatment of metastatic adrenal cancer. Clin Pharmacol Ther 1992;51:145.
3. Bernardi LC, Goldblatt LA, Liener IE, ed. In: Toxic constituents of plant foodstuffs. 2nd ed. New York: Academic Press, 1980; pp. 184–230.
4. Wu D-F, Yu Y-W, Tang Z-M, Wang M-Z. Pharmacokinetics of (+-)-, (+)-, and (-)- gossypol in humans and dogs. Clin Pharmacol Ther 1986;30:613–618.
5. Wu D. An overview of the clinical pharmacology and therapeutic potential of gossypol as a male contraceptive agent and in gynaecological disease. Drugs 1989;38:333–341.
6. Wang MZ, Wu DF, Yu YW. High-performance liquid chromatography with electrochemical detection of gossypol in human plasma. J Chromatogr (Biomed Appl) 1985;343:387–391.
7. Diammo X, Xiao-Lu W, Jun-bao Z, Hua-Cu C. Effects of gossypol on phorbol ester-calcimycin-induced prostaglandin synthesis by macrophages. Chinese Med J 1991;104: 321–325.

HERBAL MEDICINE (SEE ALSO INDIGENOUS TOXICOLOGY CHAPTER)

HERBAL TEAS (TABLE 74–11)

GERMANDER AND HERBAL HEPATOTOXICITY

Scientific Name

Teucrium chamaedrys.

Common Name

Wall germander.

Family

Lamiaceae.

Botanical Description/Occurrence/Use

The blossoms of wall germander may be used in preparations of herbal teas (1 gram per bag), a medicinal liquor in which germander is mixed with various other herbs (70 to 150 mg germander per 100 mL), and capsules containing germander powder either alone (200 or 270 mg per capsule) or mixed with green tea (150 mg germander and 250 mg tea per capsule).[1]

Hepatotoxicity of Herbs[2]

Hepatitis may occur after the ingestion of preparations containing valerian, asafetida, skullcap, and gentian, as well as after senna fruit extracts, Chinese herbs, mistletoe, and chaparral leaf.[3] Veno-occlusive disease of the liver is reported after exposure to pyrollizidine alkaloids (see section). Germander may induce hepatitis.

Treatment

Treatment is supportive.

CHAPARRAL

Identification

Scientific Name

Larrea tridentata (Larrea divaricata Cav.).

Common Name

Chaparral, creosote bush, greasewood, hediondillo.[4]

Family

Zygophyllaceae.

Botanical Description/Occurrence/Use

The chaparrals are a group of closely related wild shrubs found in the deserts of the American Southwest and Mexico. Chaparral is derived from the ground leaves of the creosote bush. It is found in health food stores as leaflets and twigs. Chaparral has been used by Native Americans in teas, capsules, and tablet form for a variety of disorders.[5]

Toxins

Nordihydroguaianetic acid (NDGA) and related lignans appear to be antioxidants at the cellular levels. NDGA also inhibits collagen- and ADP-induced platelet aggregation and platelet adhesiveness in aspirin treated patients.[4]

Clinical Presentation

Chronic ingestion of chaparral may be associated with acute or chronic hepatotoxicity.[5–7] In December 1992 the United States issued a public warning following four cases of hepatitis.[7]

Treatment

Cessation of use may lead to improvement in liver function. The U.S. FDA has an information service for chaparral toxicity. Telephone: 202-205-4198 (Lori A. Love, M.D., Ph.D.).

PYRROLIZIDINE ALKALOIDS

Comfrey

The pyrrolizidine alkaloids compose 180 compounds that occur in at least eight plant families, but four genera—*Heliotropium, Crotalaria, Senecio,* and *Symphytum*—have accounted for most toxic ingestions. The last genus includes common comfrey (*Symphytum officinale*), prickly comfrey (*S. asperus*), and Russian comfrey (*S. uplandicen*).[8,9]

Uses

Comfrey has been employed by herbalists as a demulcent, an antihemorrhagic, an antirheumatic, and an antiinflammatory agent. The dried roots and also the dried or fresh leaves are used, taken orally or applied topically. Comfrey may be the most widely recognized source of dietary pyrrolizidine alkaloids in developed countries.[9]

Mechanism of Toxicity

An essential structural requirement for toxicity is the presence of the unsaturated pyrrolizidine ring structure.[10] The hepatotoxic alkaloids have a 1,2-double bond in the pyrrolizidine ring. The pyrrolizidine alkaloids (PAs) occur as free bases and *N*-oxides. The latter are reduced to the free bases in the gastrointestinal tract and have a similar toxicity when ingested orally. Saturated PAs do not exhibit toxicity. The pyrrolizidine nucleus is dehydrogenated in the liver to the corresponding pyrrole, which is chemically reactive and which serves as a biologic alkylating agent. Pyrroles cause a similar toxic picture in animals to that seen with the parent pyrrolizidines.[10,11] The PAs in themselves are not toxic and are largely cleared from the body in 24 hours.[10] They are activated in the liver where they are metabolized by mixed-function oxidase to pyrrolic dehydroalkaloids, which are the reactive alkylating agents. These metabolites induce the liver cell necrosis and vascular lesions characterized by primary pulmonary hypertension.[10]

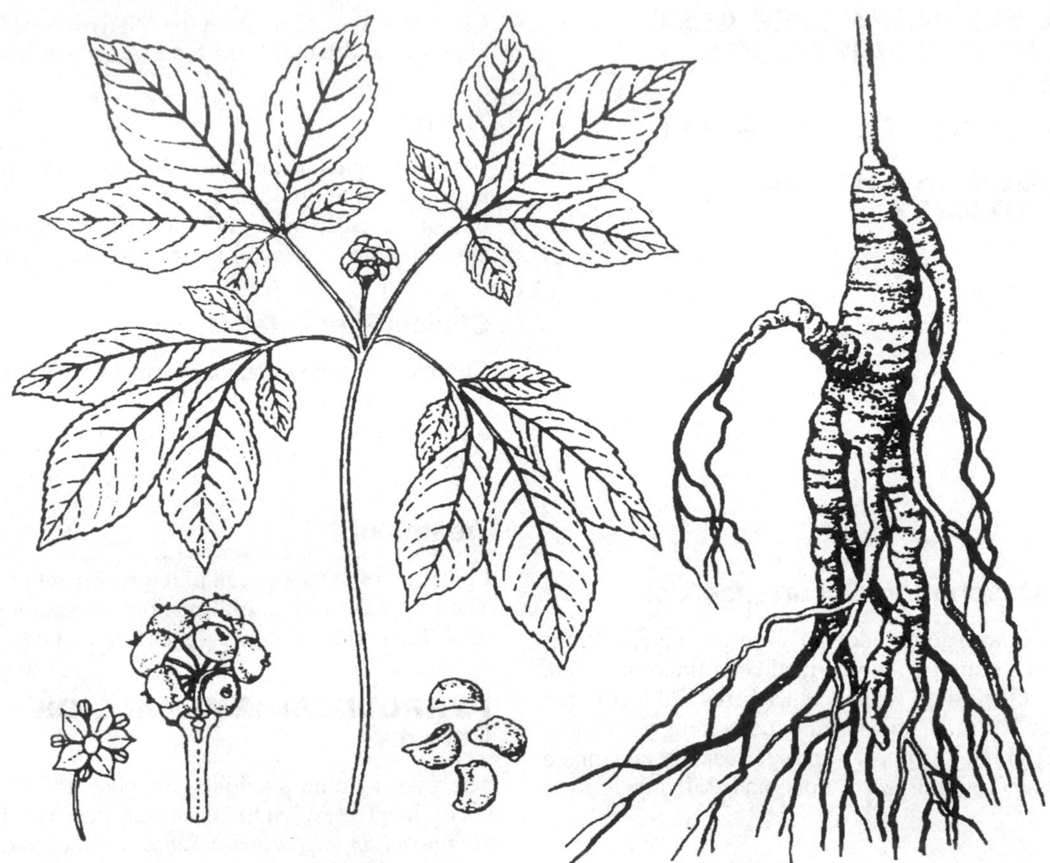

Figure 74–10 American ginseng: branch, root, flower, berries, and seeds. (Adapted from Minor JR. Hosp Formul 1979;14(2):188.)

Reproductive Effects and Fetotoxicity

Use of herbal tea/medicines by mouth throughout pregnancy (one cup of tea per day; total exposure of 0.125 mg of senecionine per kg) has led to birth of an infant with fatal hepatic veno-occlusive disease. No studies are available on the presence of PA in the milk of the lactating woman.

Toxicity

The characteristic hepatic veno-occlusive lesion and the endothelial proliferation, arterial medial hypertrophy pulmonary arterial hypertension, right ventricular hypertrophy, and cor pulmonale are probably due to the release of pyrrole metabolites by the liver.[12]

Levels of Intake

Liver toxicity follows consumption of herbal teas for up to several years. A high level of comfrey consumption as salad is about 5 to 6 leaves daily. Intake from comfrey tea is at the same level. The average alkaloidal content of the leaves are 1 mg per leaf. Alkaloid intake may vary from 1 to 6 mg/day. In fatal cases the total intake ranged from 6 to 167 mg/kg body weight; in nonfatal cases of veno-occlusive disease, it was 2 to 27 mg/kg body weight. Comfrey-root tea can yield as much as 26 mg of PA per day. Comfrey-papain capsules can contain as much as 2.9 ng/d total pyrrolizidines.[13]

Diagnosis

The diagnosis of PA poisoning can only be made by exclusion of veno-occlusive disease in all patients with hepatic failure, recognition of the pathognomonic histopathologic changes in hepatic biopsy specimen, and analysis for PA in herbal preparations to which the patient has been exposed.[11]

GINSENG (FIG. 74–10)

During the past three decades, consumption of ginseng has greatly increased in Western countries. It is one of the most popular and best known herbal remedies in Oriental medicine. The recommended daily dose for dried ginseng root is 0.5 to 2.0 g.[14] In general, commercial ginseng preparations are not well defined, and they are known to contain a large number of substances. The most characteristic compounds in the ginseng roots are the ginsenosides, and most biologic effects have been ascribed to these compounds. Ginsenosides, being glycosylated steroids, are very difficult to analyze and quantify in small amounts.[15]

Pregnancy

No reproductive studies are available that address the safety of ginseng use during pregnancy. A 30-year-old female ingested ginseng throughout pregnancy and early lactation. She experienced repeated premature uterine contractions during late pregnancy and noted increased and thicker hair growth on her head, face, and pubic area. Her full-term baby had thick, black pubic hair, hair over the entire forehead, and swollen red nipples.[16] The mother had undetectable testosterone levels when ingesting the ginseng and normal levels when ingesting placebo.[17] The ginseng may contain a compound that acts like and suppresses endogenous testosterone.[18]

Clinical Presentation

A patient developed cerebral arteritis after ingestion of a large quantity of ginseng extract (about 25 grams drug weight).[17]

Siegel[19] described ginseng abuse syndrome consisting of hypertension, nervousness, sleeplessness, skin eruptions, and morning diarrhea. The subjects took an average of 3 grams of ginseng root per day, and the symptoms usually occurred 1 to 3 weeks after daily ingestion.

Treatment

Treatment is supportive.

POISON HEMLOCK (*CONIUM MACULATUM*)

Scientific Name

Conium maculatum.

Botanical Description

Conium maculatum is a poisonous biennial herb that grows erect to an average height of 1 to 3 m (3¼ to 9¾ ft). The larger stems of maturing plants contain numerous purple spots that are an identifying characteristic. First-year-growth plants have fine, light-green, fernlike leaves and usually grow no taller than 46 cm (18 in). Poison hemlock has a long white taproot that is solid and parsniplike. Plants generally persist in localized stands because the seeds drop near the parent plant. Occasionally, seeds are spread by water, birds, or rodents.[20]

Toxins

The toxins in poison hemlock are simple piperidine alkaloids. Coniine and gamma-coniceine are the predominant toxicants that have been implicated in overt toxicity in animals and humans. The oral median lethal dose in mice for gamma-coniceine, the most toxic and most plentiful of the alkaloids, is 12 mg per kg.

Mechanism of Action

The mechanism of action of these alkaloids is twofold. The most serious effect occurs at the neuromuscular junction where they act as nondepolarizing blockers, similar to curare. Death, when it occurs, is usually caused by respiratory failure. As a result of their action at the autonomic ganglia, the toxins produce biphasic nicotinic effects, including salivation, mydriasis, and tachycardia followed by bradycardia. Less commonly, rhabdomyolysis and acute tubular necrosis have occurred.

Poison hemlock is often confused with water hemlock (*Cicuta* species) because the two are similar in appearance and belong to the same family. The toxin in water hemlock, cicutoxin, has primarily central nervous system effects, including seizures.

Clinical Presentation

Poison hemlock poisoning may be suspected in patients with an altered level of consciousness, myalgias, fasciculations, or flaccid paralysis following the ingestion of a plant substance. Supportive laboratory data include elevated muscle enzyme levels and myoglobinuria.

Laboratory

A method for a multiresidue chemical screen for alkaloids in plant material was recently described that provides the basis of confirming a case of poison hemlock or water hemlock toxicosis.[21]

Management

Because no antidote exists for coniine poisoning, treatment is supportive. Respiratory support and gastric decontamination should be instituted immediately. Anticonvulsants should be administered as needed. Forced diuresis may be useful in preventing renal failure from rhabdomyolysis and myoglobinuria.

OIL OF MELALEUCA (TEA TREE OIL)

Oil of melaleuca is promoted as a remedy for certain skin conditions. Melaleuca oil is extracted from the leaves of the Australian native tree *Melaleuca alternifolia* (where it is also known as tea tree oil) and contains 50 to 60% terpenes and related alcohols.[22] It has been used as an antiseptic and antifungal agent. Cineol, a skin irritant, is a major component of eucalyptus oil. Terpine-4-ol is a hydrocarbon of the terpene class with possible antimicrobial properties. Ingestion of 100% melaleuca oil has led to confusion, inability to walk, disorientation, ataxia, and a eucalyptus-like odor on the breath. Recovery follows treatment with activated charcoal.[21]

Both substances are capable of producing central nervous system depression, gastrointestinal and dermal irritation, vomiting, and diarrhea. Treatment is symptomatic and supportive.[23–25]

EUCALYPTUS OIL[26]

Adults and children may develop symptoms (vomiting, CNS depression, premature ventricular contractions, and apnea [in one child]) with as little as a swallow of eucalyptus oil.[27] Ingestion of "taste" amounts seem to be relatively harmless. This observation should be confirmed. Survival has been reported with ingestion of 21 to 30 mL in an 8-year-old, 23 mL in an adult, and 120 mL to 240 mL in a treated adult.[28] A child ingested 10 mL and survived. The child was seen within 30 minutes of ingestion and was deeply comatose with miosis, absent deep tendon reflexes, and shallow, irregular respiration. His breath had a strong odor of eucalyptus.[29]

SASSAFRAS[30]

An adult ingested 5 mL of sassafras oil. Within 1 hour vomiting, "shakiness," flushing, and tachycardia were observed. The patient recovered.[31] A 72-year-old patient drank 10 cups of sassafras teas daily. She developed diaphoresis and hot flashes that resolved on cessation of drinking the tea.[32]

CINNAMON OIL

A 7½-year-old boy ingested 2 ounces (about 6 mL) of oil of cinnamon and immediately felt a burning sensation in his mouth, chest, and stomach lasting for about 15 minutes. He then developed double vision, dizziness, vomiting, and collapse. Following ipecac and activated charcoal he developed diarrhea, more vomiting, dizziness, abdominal cramps, and burning in the rectal area. The white blood count was 29,800/mm^3. Gastrointestinal symptoms and sleepiness persisted for 5 hours.[33]

Abuse

Cinnamon oil is easily obtained from pharmacies in 5 to 10 mL amounts for use as a flavoring agent and in craft items. Cinnamon oil abuse in young adolescents follows sucking on toothpicks or fingers dipped in cinnamon oil. A rush or sensation of warmth, facial flushing, and oral burning may be experienced. No residual symptoms have been observed.[34]

OIL OF CITRONELLA

Oil of citronella is a fragrant, volatile oil obtained by distillation from fresh grass of *Cymbopogon nardus* Rendle or *C. winterianus* Jowitt (family Gramineae). The main constituents are geraniol and citronellol. Countries producing this oil include Sri Lanka, Indonesia, and Taiwan. Ceylon oil has 10% citronellol and 18% geraniol, and Java oil has 35% citronellol and 21% geraniol. Citronella oil is used in perfumery, in insect repellents, and other veterinary products.

Clinical Presentation

A child of 21 months drank 3 teaspoons of a preparation containing oil of citronella. The child became cyanosed, had seizures, vomited, and died in 5 hours. The child had been given an emetic of salt and water that may have contributed to the clinical course.[35] Five cases of oil of citronella poisoning were reviewed in New Zealand.[36] The doses were not specified. Mild cough or vomiting appear benign.

Treatment

Treatment is symptomatic.

OIL OF CLOVES

Use

Clove oil is obtained without prescription for the treatment of toothaches.

Origin

Clove oil is obtained from the dried flower buds or leaves of the *Syzygium aromaticum (Eugenia caryophyllus)* tree of the myrtle family (Myrtaceae) and contains about 70 to 90% of eugenol with a number of impurities.[37,38]

Clinical Presentation

Consumption of 5 to 15 mL of oil of cloves may induce a high anion gap acidosis, seizures, coagulopathy, acute liver damage, behavioral changes, and coma. A clove oil spill may lead to a stinging erythematous reaction with diminished sweating and reduced sensation in the affected areas.[37,38]

Treatment

Treatment is symptomatic and supportive. Gastric lavage was used safely in one patient.[38]

Seizures, central nervous system depression, acidosis, and disseminated intravascular coagulation was observed after an ingestion of 5 to 10 mL of oil of cloves containing 70 to 90% eugenol.[37] Symptomatic and supportive therapy led to recovery.

Clove oil contains 84 to 88% eugenol used as an anesthetic for dental procedures, a flavoring agent in foods and pharmaceuticals, in the manufacture of textiles, and in herbal medicines. Ingestion can lead to central nervous system depression, seizures, a coagulopathy, a lactic acidosis,[37,38] and hepatic dysfunction. Like acetaminophen it is metabolized by glucuronide and sulfate conjugates in the liver. Animal studies suggest that the hepatic damage is reversed by *N*-acetylcysteine. Evidence for this in man is not available.[37] Topically, one report indicates a stinging and erythematous reaction followed by diminished sensation.

PENNYROYAL OIL

Identification

Scientific Name

Mentha pulegium, Hedeoma pulegioides.

Common Name

Pennyroyal, squaw mint, mosquito plant.

Botanical Description/Occurrence/Use

Pennyroyal oil is a volatile oil derived from *M. pulegium* and *H. pulegioides,* which are indigenous plants present from Canada to Florida and west to Nebraska. Herbalists use pennyroyal oil as an abortifacient and to induce menses. Toxic effects usually result from the misuse of the herb in folk medicine.

Toxin

Pulegone is the ketone, cyclohexanone, which constitutes 85% of pennyroyal oil and produces direct hepatic damage. Ten milliliters of this compound produced gastrointestinal distress; 30 mL resulted in a fatal hepatic necrosis.

Clinical Presentation

Pennyroyal oil consumption produces direct toxic effects on the gastrointestinal tract and the liver. Depending on the dose, the clinical presentation includes nausea, vomiting, abdominal pain, burning of the throat, and dizziness within 2 hours of ingestion followed by liver dysfunction. In fatal cases, hepatomegaly, coagulation abnormalities, and renal failure, as well as shock, consumptive coagulopathy, massive hepatic necrosis, and hepatorenal failure, developed. Multiple grand mal seizures occurred within a 24-hour period after the ingestion of 40 pennyroyal tablets over 4 days.

Treatment

Decontamination

The usual measures of decontamination (syrup of ipecac/lavage, charcoal, cathartics) should be administered to all patients who have ingested significant amounts of pennyroyal oil (i.e., more than a taste) and who present within the first several hours. Asymptomatic patients or those whose symptoms subside within 4 hours postingestion may be discharged. Symptomatic patients should be admitted.

Elimination Enhancement

No methods are available.

Antidotes

No antidotes are available.

Supportive Care

Patients who are admitted should have a complete blood count, electrolytes, creatinine, liver function tests, urinalysis, and coagulation profiles. Hepatic necrosis usually occurs within 24 hours. Such patients should be observed for development of bleeding secondary to coagulation abnormalities and treated with platelet packs, fresh-frozen plasma, and blood transfusions as necessary. Seizures are self-limited and should respond to diazepam.

FEVERFEW

Identification

Scientific Name

Tanacetum parthenium (syn. *Chrysanthemum parthenium), Leucanthemum parthenium, Pyrethrum parthenium.*

Common Name

Feverfew, featherfew, midsummer daisy, nosebleed, Santa Maria.

Family

Compositae.

Botanical Description

A short bushy perennial that grows 15 to 60 cm tall along fields and roadsides. Its yellow-green leaves and yellow flowers resemble those of chamomile. The flowers bloom from July to October.[39]

Use

Feverfew has been used for the treatment of disorders often controlled by aspirin such as fever, rheumatic inflammations, and headache (migraine). Feverfew is taken orally either as fresh leaves or in tablets.[40–42]

Toxin

The plant is rich in sesquiterpene lactones, principally parthenolide. It appears to inhibit platelet aggregation, histamine release from mast cells, and the production of prostaglandins, thromboxanes, and leukotrienes.[40]

Clinical Presentation

Symptoms such as mouth ulcers, swollen lips, and abdominal pain have been experienced.[40] It does not appear to be mutagenic.[43]

Treatment

Management is supportive. There are no controlled studies on its use during pregnancy or lactation.

KUDZU

Identification

Scientific Name

Pueraria lobata (Willd) Ohuri.

Common Name

Japanese arrowroot, kudzu vine.

Family

Leguminosae.

Botanical Description/Occurrence/Use

Kudzu is a fast-growing vine native to the tropics, China, and Japan. It is used as fodder, as a ground cover crop, and to control soil erosion. It has taken hold in the moist southern regions of the United States.

Chemistry

Several isoflavones have been identified in an extract of kudzu root (radix puerariae). The isoflavones may be reversible inhibitors of alcohol dehydrogenase and may enhance the management of alcoholism.[44,45]

LICORICE ROOT[46]

Scientific Name

Glycyrrhiza glabra.

Common Name

Licorice root.

Family

Leguminosae.

Botanical Description/Occurrence/Use

Licorice root has been claimed to have many medicinal properties (e.g., laxative, gastritis, peptic ulcer disease).

Chemistry/Toxin

The principal toxic component is 10 to 20% glycyrrhizic acid. Consumption of 100 grams of commercial licorice (0.3% glycyrrhizic acid) is equivalent to a dose of 300 mg glycyrrhetic acid. Glycyrrhetic acid inhibits both the hepatic and renal 11-beta hydroxysteroid dehydrogenase enzyme, which converts active cortisol to the inactive 11-dehydro product, cortisone, and is present in the kidneys, gonads, placenta, lungs, and intestinal mucosa. A daily dose of 10 mg glycyrrhizic acid is probably safe in healthy adults.

Clinical Presentation

Chronic excess consumption of licorice leads to weakness, edema, weight loss, hypertension, hypokalemia, and confusion. Licorice candy, licorice flavored soft drinks, medicinals, chewing tobacco, and chewing gum may be toxic when excessive amounts are consumed chronically. About 2 to 4 licorice twist candies can contain about 100 grams of licorice—enough, when ingested daily for weeks to months, to be toxic.

Laboratory

Glycyrrhetic acid may be detected in the blood by enzyme-linked immunosorbent assay (ELISA) techniques. After 2 to 4 licorice twists daily for 2 to 4 weeks plasma glycyrrhetic acid concentrations may reach 480 ng/mL.

Treatment

Obtain a careful history of dietary sources of licorice in patients with hypertension and hypokalemia, with or without muscle weakness. Stop all licorice intake. Monitor serum electrolytes, fluid balance, acid/base status, electrocardiograph and cardiac monitoring; if necessary, in patients with electrolyte imbalances. Advise patients with hypertension or circulatory disorders to avoid licorice intake. Many confections are made with artificial flavorings that taste like licorice but contain no licorice root extract. In the patient with hypomagnesemia and hypokalemia intravenous potassium chloride and/or magnesium sulfate may be useful.

REFERENCES—HERBAL MEDICINE

1. Larrey D, Vial T, Pauwels A, Castot A, Biour M, David M et al. Hepatitis after germander (*Teucrium chamaedrys*) administration: another instance of herbal medicine hepatotoxicity. Ann Intern Med 1992;117:129–132.
2. De Smet PAGM. Health Risks of herbal remedies. Drug Safety 1995;13:81–93.
3. Huxtable RJ: The myth of beneficent nature. The risks of herbal preparations. Ann Intern Med 1992;117:165–166.
4. MacGregor FB, Abernethy VE, Dahabras S, Cobden I, Hayes PC. Hepatotoxicity of herbal remedies. Br Med J 1989;299: 1150–1157.
5. Chaparral. Lawrence Review of Natural Products. St. Louis: Facts and Comparisons, August 1993, pp. 1-2.
6. Nightingale SL. Public warning about herbal product "chaparral." JAMA 1993;269:328.
7. CDC. Chapparal-induced toxic hepatitis in California and Texas 1992. MMWR 1992;41:812–814.
8. Katz M, Saibil F. Herbal hepatitis: subacute hepatic necrosis secondary to chapparal leaf. J Clin Gastroenterol 1990;12: 203–206.
9. Ridker PM, McDermott WW. Comfrey herb tea and hepatic occlusive disease. Lancet 1989;1:657–658.
10. Abbott PJ. Comfrey: assessing the low-dose health risk. Med J Aust 1988;149:678–682.
11. Winship KA. Toxicity of comfrey. Adverse Drug React Toxicol Rev 1991;10:47–59.
12. Huxtable RJ. Activation and pulmonary toxicity of pyrrolizidine alkaloids. Pharmacol Ther 1990;47:371–389.
13. Roulet M, Laurini R, Rivier L, Calane A. Hepatic veno-occlusive disease in newborn infant of a woman drinking herbal tea. J Pediatr 1988;112:433–436.
14. Bach N, Thung SN, Schaffner F. Comfrey herb tea-induced hepatic veno-occlusive disease. Am J Med 1989;87:97–99.
15. Ryu S-J, Shien Y-Y. Ginseng-associated cerebral arteritis. Neurology 1995;45:829–830.
16. Cui J, Garle M, Eneroth P, Bjorkhem I. What do commercial ginseng preparations contain? The Lancet 1994;344:134.
17. Koren G, Randor S, Martin S, Danneman D. Maternal ginseng use associated with neonatal androgenization. JAMA 1990;264:2866.
18. Basett IB, Pannowitz DL, Barnetson RS-C. A comparative study of tea-tree oil versus benzoyl peroxide in the treatment of acne. Med J Aust 1990;153:455–458.
19. Koren G. Maternal use of ginseng and neonatal androgenization. JAMA 1991;265:1828.
20. Frank BS, Michelson WB, Panter KE, Gardner DR. Ingestion of poison hemlock (*Conium maculatum*). West J Med 1995;163:573–574.
21. Holstege DM, Seiber JN, Galey FD. Rapid multiresidue screen for alkaloids in plant material and biological samples. J Agricult Food Chem 1995;43:691–699.
22. Siegel RK. Ginseng abuse syndrome: problems with the panacea. JAMA 1070;241:1614–1615.
23. Hornfeldt CS. Malaleuca oil poisoning. A case report. Vet Hum Toxicol 1993;35:329.
24. Jacobs MR, Hornfeldt CS. Melalueca oil poisoning. Clin Toxicol 1994;32:461–464.
25. Knight TE, Hansen BM. Melaleuca oil (tea tree oil) dermatitis. J Am Acad Dermatol 1994;30:423–427.
26. Courtemanche NJ, Li M, Peterson RG. Coma following acute ingestion of eucalyptus oil in a child. Vet Hum Toxicol 1983;25 (Suppl):46.
27. Spoerke DG, Vandenberg S, Smolinske S, Kulig K, Rumack B. Eucalyptus oil. 14 cases of exposure. Vet Hum Toxicol 1989;31:166–168.
28. Mack RD. Fair dinkum roala kruisine—eucalyptus oil poisoning. NCMJ 1988;49:599–600.
29. Patel S, Wiggins J. Eucalyptus oil poisoning. Arch Dis Child 1980;55:405.
30. Segelman AB, Segelman FP, Karliner J et al. Sassafras and herb tea. Potential health hazards. JAMA 1976;236:477.
31. Grande GA, Dannewitz SR. Symptomatic sassafras oil ingestion. Vet Hum Toxicol 1987;29:463.

32. Haines JD Jr. Sassafras tea and diaphoresis. Postgrad Med 1991;9:75–76.
33. Pilapil VR. Toxic manifestations of cinnamon oil ingestion in a child. Clin Pediatr 1989;28:276.
34. Perry PA, Dean BS, Krenzelok EP. Cinnamon oil abuse by adolescents. Vet Hum Toxicol 1990;32:162–163.
35. Mant AK. Association proceedings. VI. A case of poisoning by oil of citronella. Med Sci Law 1961;112:170–171.
36. Temple WA, Smith NA, Beasley M. Management of oil of citronella poisoning. Clin Toxicol 1991;29:257–262.
37. Hartnoll G, Moore D, Douek D. Near fatal ingestion of oil of cloves. Arch Dis Child 1993;69:392–393.
38. Lane BW, Ellenhorn MJ, Vulbert TV, McCarron M. Clove oil ingestion in an infant. Hum Exp Toxicol 1991;10:291–294.
39. Olin BD, ed. Feverfew. The Lawrence review of natural products. St. Louis: Facts and Comparisons, June 1990.
40. Baldwin CA, Anderson LP, Phillipson JD. What pharmacists should know about feverfew. Pharm J 1987;239: 237–238.
41. Heptinstall S. Feverfew—an ancient remedy for modern times. J R Soc Med 1988;81:373–374.
42. Murphy JJ, Heptinstall S, Mitchell JRA. Randomized double-blind placebo-controlled trial of feverfew in migraine prevention. Lancet 1988;2:189–192.
43. Johnson ES, Kadam MP, Anderson D, Jenkinson PC, Dewdrey RB, Blowers SD. Investigation of possible genotoxic effects of feverfew in migrans patients. Hum Toxicol 1987;6: 5333–5334.
44. Kudzu: Lawrence review of natural products. St. Louis: Facts and Comparisons, June 1994.
45. Anonymous. Kudzu extract shows potential for moderating alcohol abuse. Am J Hosp Pharm 1994;51:750.
46. Woolf A. Licorice root poisoning. Clin Toxicol Rev 1994; 16(9):1–2.

VALERIAN

Valerian (*Valeriana officinalis*) is a herbaceous perennial widely distributed in the temperate regions of North America, Europe, and Asia and used since the Middle Ages as a sedative and antispasmodic. Valerian is much used in traditional Chinese and Indian medicines. In the United States valerian is sold in natural food stores, either alone as a sleep-promoting herbal preparation or combined with other herbal products. In Europe valerian is used as a homeopathic remedy.[1]

PLANT TOXINS

Dried valerian root has a characteristic malodorous aroma. The plant consists of three distinctive types of compounds: essential oils (valerenic acid and valenol), valepotriates (nonglycosidic iridoid esters), and a small number of alkaloids. The valepotriates appear the most active of these chemicals.

CLINICAL PRESENTATION

Valerian increases the quality of sleep and decreases sleep latency. Valerian has relaxant effects on gastrointestinal smooth muscle, as well as coronary dilating and antiarrhythmic properties. An intravenous injection of raw valerian root with tap water was followed by drowsiness, dilated pupils, chest pain, hypotension, hypocalcemia, hypophosphatemia, and hyperkalemia. The patient recovered in 12 hours with supportive therapy.[2] Adverse reactions that have been reported from chronic use of valerian include headaches, excitability, uneasiness, cardiac disturbances, and hepatotoxicity. A 20-g valerian overdose in an adult appeared benign, supporting previous reports that valerian has a low order of toxicity.[1]

REFERENCES—VALERIAN

1. Willey LB, Mady SP, Cogaugh DJ, Wax PM. Valerian overdose: a case report. Vet Hum Toxicol 1995;37(4):364–365.
2. Wells SR. Intentional intravenous administration of a crude valerian root extract. Clin Toxicol 1995;33:475–486 (abstract 148).

SENNA

Scientific Name

Cassia senna L. Caesalpiniaceae *(Cassia acutifolia)* known as Alexandrian senna and *Cassia angustifolia* Vahl, Caesalpiniaceae, commonly known as Tinnevelly senna.

Common Name

Senna.

Family

Leguminosae.

Botanical Description

Senna is an annual herbaceous subshrub. The leaves are alternated originating from zigzag bromides. Originating from the flowers are the fruits, "seed pods" each containing five to seven seeds. Both leaves and seeds are used in preparation of the commercial product.[1]

ORIGIN/OCCURRENCE

Alexandrian senna is cultivated along the upper Nile, whereas Tinnevelly senna is native to Somalia and southern Arabia and is cultivated in northwest Pakistan and southern India. It is also grown in California.

TOXICOKINETICS

Anthranoids

Anthranoids with a laxative activity can be divided into three classes: anthraquinone O-glycosides, anthrone C-glycosides, and dianthrine O-glycosides, which release anthraquinones, anthrone, and dianthrones in the intestinal tract, respectively.[2]

TOXIN

Anthranoid derivatives are present in several drugs of plant origin, especially as O- or C-glycosides. The best characterized compounds are sennoside, a dianthrone O-glycoside present in senna leaves and senna pods, and its aglycone (rhein anthrone).[2]

CLINICAL PRESENTATION

(See Laxative Abuse in Gastrointestinal chapter.)

PRIMARILY PLANT IRRITANTS

A large number of plants produce substances that cause direct irritation of exposed skin. In contrast to direct contact allergic dermatitis, almost all exposed patients develop lesions on exposure. Reaction occurs soon after exposure and the clinical response depends on both the concentration of the irritant and the susceptibility of the victim's skin. Treatment consists of skin cleansing, cool soaks, and topical corticosteroid treatment. Antihistamines may be given for symptomatic relief.

HONEYSUCKLE

Honeysuckle derives from the genus *Lonicera* and family Caprifoliaceae. Many varieties include bushes or twining climbers. They are distinct from Toxicodendroids. *Lonicera japonica* Halliana (Hall's Japanese honeysuckle) produces a sap that induces a Gell and Coombs type 4 reaction within 24 hours after contact consisting of pruritus, edema, and blisters at the contact site. Recovery follows immediate washing and use of topical steroids.[3]

REFERENCES—PLANT DERMATITIS

1. Granz G. The senna drug and its chemistry. Pharmacology 1993;47(Suppl 1):2–6.
2. de Witte P. Metabolism and pharmacokinetics of anthronoids. Pharmacology 1993; 47(Suppl 1):86–97.
3. Webster RM. Honeysuckle contact dermatitis. Cutis 1993;55:424.

MYCOTOXINS (TABLES 74–18, 74–19, 74–20, AND 74–21)

The natural occurrence of mycotoxins is presented in Table 74–18. Pohland[1] has summarized mutagenic, teratogenic, and carcinogenic effects of mycotoxins (Table 74–19), has listed postulated human mycotoxicoses (Table 74–20), and has tabulated the regulatory limits of mycotoxicosis in venous commodities (Table 74–21).

Five major mycotoxin groups occur in North America. Aflatoxin is common under warm humid conditions; zearalenone is most commonly reported in the north central cornbelt; trichothecene mycotoxins, especially deoxnivalenol, are common in cool damp regions; orchratoxin is reported in the Carolinas and Canada; and ergot infects small grains such as barley, rye, and wheat in the northern Great Plains.[2]

AFLATOXINS

AFB_1 may be present in corn to levels of 10 to 900 μg/kg.[1] The FDA has found that 6% of field corn in problem areas may contain more than 20 μg/g of ARB_1.[3]

Aflatoxins have been incriminated, mainly on weak evidence, in hepatocellular carcinoma, acute hepatic failure, and Reye's syndrome. Kwashiorkor, a widespread and serious disorder of children in the tropics, may be associated with ingestion of aflatoxins by infants. Exposure to aflatoxins may begin prenatally,[1,4] persist during breast-feeding,[5,6] and continue into adult life. Aflatoxins may (a) play a role in the etiology of kwashiorkor; (b) increase neonatal susceptibility to infection and jaundice; (c) increase childhood susceptibility to infections and malignant disease; (d) compromise normal response in prophylactic envenomations, and (e) play a role in the pathogenesis of diseases in heroin addicts.[7,8] Acute fatal aflatoxin poisoning may appear as "hepatitis."[9] The subject demands further serious exploration.

Table 74–18
Natural Occurrence of Mycotoxins[a]

Toxin	Producing Fungus	Occurrence
Alfatoxin	*Aspergillus flavus, A. paraciticus*	Corn, peanuts, cotton seed, rye, barley, etc.
Citrinin	*Penicillium citrinum, P. veridicatum*	Wheat, barley, peanuts
Ochratoxin A	*Aspergillus ochraceus, P. veridicatum, P. cyclopium*	Wheat, oats, rice
Sterigmatocystin	*Aspergillus versicolor, A. flavus, A. ruber, P. luteum*	Wheat, rice, peanuts
Zearalenone	*Fusarium roseum, F. moniliforme, F. nivale, F. oxysporum*	Corn, sorghum, wheat
Trichothecenes	*Fusarium roseum, F. tricinctum, F. nivale*	Corn, barley
Patulin	*Aspergillus clavatus, Penicillium patuluns*	Silage, apples
Penicillic acid	*Aspergillus clavatus, Penicillium puberulum*	Corn, beans
Alternariol, alternariol monomethyl ether	*Alternaria tenuis, A. dauci*	Weathered grain, sorghum, pecan pickouts
Tenuazonic acid	*Alternaria tenuis, A. tamarii, Sphaeropsidales sp, Pyricularia oryzae, Phoma sorghina*	Diseased rice plants
Ergot alkaloids (ergotamine, etc.)	*Claviceps spp, Aspergillus spp, Penicillium spp*	Ergots, ergot-infected pasture grass
Sporidesmin	*Pithomyces chartarum*	0.1% in spores on dead pasture grass
PR toxin	*Penicillium roqueforti*	Silage
Kojic acid	*Aspergillus flavus, A. oryzae*	Moldy corn

[a]Adapted from Hayes AW. Clin Toxicol 1980;17:48.

Table 74–19
Toxicologic Effects of Mycotoxins[a]

Mycotoxin	M	T	C
Aflatoxin	+++	+++	+++
Citrinin	−+	−	+
Cyclochlorotine			+
Fumonisin B_1			+
Fusarenone X		+	+
Griseofulvin			++
Luteoskyrin	−		+
Ochratoxin A	−	+	+
Patulin	+	+	+
Penicillic acid	+	−	+
Rugulosin	−+		+
Sterigmatocystin	+		+++
T-2 toxin	−	+	+
Zearalenone	+	−	+

[a]Adapted from Pohland AE. Food Addit Contam 1993;10:17–28.
M, Mutagenic; *T*, teratogenic; *C*, carcinogenic.

Table 74–20
Postulated Human Mycotoxicoses[a]

Aflatoxicosis	Aflatoxin
AIDS	Cyclosporins Gliotoxin
Akakabi-byo disease	*Fusarium* metabolites
Alimentary toxic aleukia	Trichothecenes
Balkan nephropathy, renal tumors	Ochratoxin
Cardiac beriberi	Citreoviridin
Cervical cancer	Zearalenone
Encephalopathy, fatty degeneration of the liver	Aflatoxin
Ergotism	Ergot alkaloids
Hepatocarcinogenesis	Aflatoxin
Immunosuppression	Aflatoxin
Indian childhood cirrhosis	Aflatoxin
Kashin-Beck disease	*F. equiseti* metabolites
Kodua poisoning	Cyclopiazonic acid
Kwashiorkor	Aflatoxin
Mushroom poisoning	Amatoxins, agaritine, amanitins, phallotoxins
Eoesophageal cancer	*F. moniliforme* metabolites
Onyalai disease	Moniliformin Tenuazonic acid
Pellagra	T-2 toxin
Premature thelarche	Zearalenone
Reye's syndrome	Aflatoxin
Tremors	Penitrem(?)

[a]Adapted from Pholand AE. Food Addit Contam 1993;10:17–28.

Consumption of aflatoxin in many parts of the world varies from 0 to 30,000 ng/kg/day. In most areas consumption varies from 10 to 200 ng/kg/day.[10] Aflatoxin may be secreted in breast milk up to 3 to 84 ng/L.[5,9] If a 5-kg baby were to drink half a liter of contaminated breast milk in 24 hours, the child's consumption could be as high as 8 ng/kg/24 hr.[3,6,9,11–19] The measured serum level of AFB_1 in one study rose from 33.6 to 218 pg per mL after a meal.[9]

Table 74–21
Regulations[a]

Mycotoxin	Reg. Limit (ng/kg)	Commodities	Country
Aflatoxins	0–50	All foods	53 countries
B_1, B_2, G_1, G_2, P_1, aflatoxicol, M_1	0–0.5	Milk, dairy	15 countries
B_1, B_2, G_1, G_2	10–1000	Feeds	43 countries
Chetomin	0	All foods	Romania
Deoxynivalenol	1000–4000	Wheat	5 countries
Diacetoxyscirpenol	100	Grain	Israel
Ochratoxin A	1–300	Rice, barley, beans, corn, pork kidney	6 countries
Patulin	20–50	Apple juice	10 countries
Phomopsin	5	Lupin products	Australia
Stachybotryotoxin	0	All goods	Romania
T-2 toxin	100	Grains	2 countries
Zearalenone	30–1000	All foods	4 countries

[a]Adapted from Pohland AE. Food Addit Contam 1993;10:17–28.

Metabolism

AFB_1 is converted in the adult liver by the cytochrome P450 enzyme P450 IIIAY, and in the fetal liver with P450 IIIA6,[4] to AFQ_1, the major metabolite of AFB_1.[9] Other major metabolites in the human include AFM_1, Aflatoxicol (AFL), $AFLH_1$, AFP_1, AFB_2alpha, and AFB_1-2.2-dihydriol.[9] About 80% of a total dose of AFB_1 is excreted in 1 week. The plasma half-life is 36.5 minutes, volume of distribution 14% of body weight, and body clearance is 1.25 L/kg/hour.[9] AFM_1 is mostly excreted within 48 hours of ingestion and compresses 1 to 4% of ingested AFB_1. It is possible that its measurement gives a reasonable estimate of recent aflatoxin ingestion.[9]

AFM probably comprises 1 to 4% of consumed AFB_1. Since it is conjugated and is easily detectable in urine, it may be useful in assessing aflatoxin conjugation.[9] The route of activation is to the reactive hydrophilic AFB_1-2-3-epoxide. This may be the most important product from the carcinogenic point of view. This highly reactive substance can combine with DNA bases such as guanine to produce alterations in DNA.[9]

Placental Transfer

A study of the Chinese population in Taiwan with a high mortality from primary hepatocellular carcinoma indicates that aflatoxin B_1-DNA adducts are present in human umbilical cord sera, suggesting that transplacental transfer of AFB_1 may play a biologic role in the initiation of primary hepatocellular carcinoma in the progeny.[20]

Heroin Contamination

Aflatoxin has oncogenic and immunosuppressive effects that may influence the pattern of infection with the human immunodeficiency virus (HIV). Heroin may be contaminated with aflatoxin. Two samples contained 507 and 1346 pg/g of aflatoxin B_1 in heroin. Intravenous heroin users are probably injecting aflatoxin B_1 into their systemic circulation and thereby suppress cell-mediated immunity.[6,7]

An outbreak of food poisoning resulting in 13 deaths in children occurred in Malaysia during the Chinese festival of the Nine Emperor Gods in 1988. The food poisoning was attributable to aflatoxins and boric acid. Clinical features included an initial Reye-like syndrome with vomiting, fever, diarrhea, abdominal pain, anorexia, seizures, and coma. Patients died in acute hepatic and renal failure. High levels of aflatoxins B_1, B_2, G_1, M_1, M_2, and aflatoxicol were found in various organs.[21]

Laboratory

Radioimmunoassays and the ELISA method are the most sensitive indices of exposure.[22] The enzyme immunoassay of ARB_1 is sensitive to 10 pg/mL in a range of 10 to 1650 pg/mL.[23] The ELISA method of breast milk analysis is sensitive to 2 pg of AFM_1/mL milk.[4] Levels of serum aflatoxin are usually not over 20 ng/mL (4 pmol/L).[18] Levels of AFM_1 in breast milk may react 20 to 1816 pg/mL; AFM_2 164 to 1075 pg/mL; AFB_1 130 to 8218 pg/mL; AFB_2 49 to 50 pg/mL; and aflatoxicol 614 to 270 pg/mL.[5] Assays of p53 codon 249Ser mutations may provide information on the probability of hepatocellular carcinoma after aflatoxin exposure.[10,11] Aflatoxin-guanine adduct concentration in the urine may provide a marker for liver cancer risk.[24]

TRICHOTHECENES (TABLE 74–22)

There is no evidence in long-term animal studies to indicate that T-2 toxin, fuarenon-x (a derivative), and nivalenol are tumorigenic.[25]

One disease outbreak from China was associated with the consumption of scabby wheat containing 1.0 to 40.0 ng DON (deoxyonivalenol)/kg. Zearalenone was also detected (0.25 to 0.5 mg/kg). The latency period for onset of symptoms was 5 to 30 min. The disease was characterized by gastrointestinal symptoms, abdominal pain, dizziness, and headache. No deaths occurred in humans. An analogous outbreak was reported from India and was associated with consumption of baked bread made from contaminated wheat.[26] Mycotoxin in samples of the refined wheat flour included DON, acetyl deoxyonivalenol, NIV, and T-2 toxin. The disease was characterized by gastrointestinal symptoms and throat irritation that developed within 15 minutes to 1 hour following ingestion of the bread.[24] DON has been shown to be teratogenic in animals.

Safe limits of trichothecenes in wheat for human consumption have been prescribed for DON (but not for the other trichothecenes) in Canada (2000 μg/kg in unclean soft wheat, 100 μg/kg for unclean soft wheat for infant foods, and 1200 μg/kg for imported nonstaple food), the former USSR (1000 μg/kg for durum wheat and 500 μg/kg for other wheat), and Romma (5 μg/kg in all feeds). The U.S. FDA suggests a limit of 2000 μg/kg in wheat intended for milling and 1000 μg/kg for finished products meant for human consumption.

Activated charcoal appears to be an effective antidote for treatment of T-2 toxicosis in mice.[27]

MILDEWED SUGAR CANE POISONING[28,29] (3-NITROPROPIONIC ACID)

Acute mildewed sugar cane poisoning is an acute intoxication resulting from ingestion of mildewed sugar cane. It is characterized by a toxic encephalopathy following initial gastrointestinal symptoms and by a delayed dystonia in most severe cases. There have been 217 outbreaks of acute mildewed sugar cane poisoning between 1972 and 1989 in China resulting in 884 patients and 88 deaths. Epidemiologic and experimental studies have found that 3-nitropropionic acid, a mycotoxin produced by *Arthrinium*-contaminated sugar canes, is the probable etiologic factor of the disease.

Clinical Presentation

The onset was abrupt with latent periods ranging from 2 to 3 hours after the ingestion of mildewed sugar cane. Initial symptoms were nausea, vomiting, abdominal pain without diarrhea, and anorexia that followed headache and dizziness. Coma and convulsions develop within 3 to 18 hours after onset. Coma lasted 20 days in one case. Following the coma motor aphasia, inability of voluntary movement, and urinary and fecal incontinence appeared. There was no fever. The focal cerebral impairments were reversible. Dystonia began 11 to 60 days after the coma. CT scans indicated bilateral lenticular lesions in the putanes and pallidum. The content of nitropropionic acid in a mildewed sugar cane sample that caused a fatality was 6600 ppn.

Table 74–22
Clinical Symptoms and Signs of Tricothecene Toxicosis[a]

Stage	Duration	Clinical Findings
I	3–9 d	Burning sensation of skin and mucous membranes Headache, dizziness, and weakness Vomiting, diarrhea, and abdominal pain Fever and sweating Tachycardia and cyanosis
I	2–4 wk	Leukopenia, granulocytopenia, and lymphocytosis Thrombocytopenia Anemia Headache, fatigue, vertigo Petechiae
III	Indeterminate; may result in death or progress to convalescence	Petechiae and focal necrotic lesions of skin and mucosa; ulcerative pharyngitis Hemorrhages of mucous membranes Gastrolntestinal hemorrhage Lymphadenopathy Progression of hematologic abnormalities complicated by sepsis
IV	3 wk to 2 mo	Resolution of necrotic lesions and hemorrhages Gradual improvement in hematologic findings Continuing risk of complication by infection

[a]Adapted from Stahl CJ, Green CC, Famum JB. J Forensic Sci 1985;30:329.

Table 74–23
Ergot Alkaloids[a]

Pharmacologic Effect	Amine (Ergonovine, Methysergide, Methyl Ergonovine)	Amino Acid (Ergotamine)	Dihydrogenated (Hydergine)	Bromocriptine (Parlodel)
Vasoconstriction	+	+++	++	0
Myometrial stimulation	+++	+++	+	0
α-Adrenergic blockade	0	++	+++	+
Emesis	+	+++	++	++

[a]Adapted from McGuigan MA. Clin Toxicol Rev 1984;6(6):1.

Treatment

Treatment is symptomatic and supportive. Clonazepam has led to improvement in involuntary movements in one patient.

ERGOT ALKALOIDS (TABLE 74–23)

The natural source of ergot alkaloids are fungi of the genus *Claviceps,* which infect cereal grains.

BROMOCRIPTINE

Interactions

The addition of a therapeutic sympathomimetic agent to therapy of severe headache treated by bromocriptine may result in a severe worsening of symptoms with life-threatening complications (e.g., ventricular tachycardia, seizures, cerebral vasospasm).[30]

Dosage—Toxic

Reports to the manufacturer indicate that doses of 2.5 to 25 mg were ingested by 18 children aged 2 weeks to 3 years. All survived.[31] A 19-year-old woman may have ingested as much as 225 mg of bromocriptine, developed dizziness, nausea, and transient hallucinations. She survived.[32,33]

Bromocriptine has induced postpartum psychosis at low doses of 2.5 mg every 24 hours.[34] It can potentially induce or exacerbate psychosis in psychiatric patients, mostly in those not receiving neuroleptic medication. This effect is usually seen at higher doses (over 10 mg/day).[35] Postpartum bromocriptine has been associated with myocardial infarction,[36] hypertension and pulmonary edema (in cocaine user),[37] cerebrovascular accident disorders (with antecedent cocaine use),[38] and brainstem thrombosis. Cocaine used with bromocriptine may predispose to cerebrovascular and cardiovascular sequela when bromocriptine is used postpartum.[39]

Bromocriptine in about 2 to 3% of males over 55 years of age, given in Parkinson's disease in doses of 22.5 or 50 mg/d, has appeared to produce pleuropulmonary fibrosis after treatment ranging from 9 months to 4 years.[40,41] Retroperitoneal fibrosis has also been noted in patients with Parkinson's disease treated with bromocriptine for 18 months to 5 years at doses of 20 to 22.5 mg/L.[40]

Pathophysiology—Chronic Ergotism

Rarely valvular heart disease has been associated with chronic ergotamine toxicity.[42] The structural similarity of ergotamine and methysergide may induce fibroblastic valvular stimulation after ergotamine similar to that found with methysergide.

A number of patients using ergot alkaloids for prolonged periods (e.g., one or more ergotamine suppositories daily for 6 to 20 years; methysergide 1 to 6 mg/d for 6 years) develop mitral and/or aortic valve disease, both regurgitant and stenotic. Echocardiographic findings are indistinguishable from those seen in patients with chronic rheumatic valvular disease. Such valvular lesions have been sufficiently symptomatic to necessitate valve replacement in all patients.[43] Ergotism is a vasospastic condition resulting from the use of ergot alkaloids (St. Anthony's fire).

Laboratory—Analytic Studies

An HPLC system is able to separate ergot alkaloids.[44] A gas chromatography–mass spectrometry method identifies and quantifies ergotamine in plasma or serum with linearity in the range of 50 pg/mL to 50 ng/mL in plasma.[45]

A 35-year-old female with ergotamine toxicity following an overdose of about 40 mg of ergotamine tartrate presented with severe ischemia of both legs. She responded within 5 hours to intravenous administration of prostacyclin (epoprostenol, prostaglandin$_2$) given up to a dose of 20 mg/kg/minute.[46]

REFERENCES—MYCOTOXINS

1. Pohland AE. Mycotoxin in review. Food Addit Contam 1993; 10:17–28.
2. De Vries HR, Maxwell SM, Hendrickse RG. Foetal and neonatal exposure to aflatoxins. Acta Paediatr Scand 1989; 78:373–378.
3. Sabino M, Prado G, Inomata EI, Pedroso MO, Gardia RV. Natural occurrence of aflatoxins and zearalenone in maize in Brad. II. Food Addit Contam 1989;6:327–331.
4. Wild CP, Rasheed FM, Jawla MFB, Hall AJ, Jansen LAM, Montesano R. In-utero exposure to aflatoxin in West Africa. Lancet 1991;337:1602.
5. Wild CP, Pionneau FA, Montesano R, Mutino CF, Chetscaga CJ. Aflatoxin detected in human breast milk by immunoassay. Trop Dis Bull 1988;85:908.
6. Lamplugh SM, Hendrickse RG, Apeagyei F, Muanmut DD. Aflatoxins in breast milk, neonatal cord blood and serum of pregnant women. Br Med J 1988;296:968.
7. Hendrickse RG, Maxwell SM. Heroin addicts, AIDS and aflatoxins. Br Med J 1988;296:1257.
8. Hendrickse RG, Maxwell SM, Young R. Aflatoxins and heroin. Br Med J 1989;299:492–493.
9. Hendrickse RG. Clinical implication of food contaminated by aflatoxins. Ann Acad Med Surg 1991;20:84–90.

10. Denning DW. Aflatoxin and human disease. Adverse Drug React Acute Pois Rev 1987;4:175–209.
11. Patel P, Stephenson J, Scheuer RJ, Francis GJ. p 53 codon 249 set mutations in hepatocellular carcinoma patients with low aflatoxin exposure. Lancet 1992;339:881.
12. Reference Deleted
13. Autrup JL, Schmidt J, Seremet T, Autrup H. Determination of exposure to aflatoxins among Danish workers in animal feed production through the analysis of aflatoxin B_1 adducts to serum albumin. Scand J Work Environ Health 1991;17: 436–440.
14. Campbell TC, Junshi C, Brun TA, Liu C, Geissler CA. Aflatoxin and liver cancer. Lancet 1990;335:1165.
15. Denning DW, Sykes JA, Wilkinson AP, Morgan MRA. High serum concentrations of aflatoxin in Nepal as measured by enzyme-labeled immunosorbent serum assay. Hum Exp Toxicol 1990;9:143–146.
16. Scott PM. Methods for determination of aflatoxin N_1 in milk and milk products—a review of performance characteristics. Food Addit Contam 1989;6:283–305.
17. Aflatoxin in corn. FDA Consumer 1989;23 (4):2–3.
18. Degan P, Montagnoli G, Wild CR. Time-resolved fluoroimmunoassay of aflatoxins. Clin Chem 1989;32:2308–2310.
19. Wilkinson AP, Denning DW, Morgan MRA. Analysis of UK sera for aflatoxin by enzyme-linked immunosorbent assay. Hum Toxicol 1988;7:353–356.
20. Hsieh L-L, Hsieh T-T. Detection of aflatoxin B_1-DNA adducts on human placenta and cord blood. Cancer Res 1993;53: 1278–1280.
21. Chao T-C, Maxwell SM, Wong S-T. An outbreak of aflatoxicosis and boric acid poisoning in Malaysia: a clinicopathological study. J Pathol 1991;164:225–233.
22. Okoye ZSC, Neal GE, Judah DJ. The detection of exposure to aflatoxins using EUSA. Hum Toxicol 1985;5:400–401.
23. Cheschan J, Neal GE, Woods H. A rapid enzyme immunoassay for extracted aflatoxin. Hum Toxicol 1986;5:405.
24. Ros RK, Yu MC, Henderson BE, Yuan J-M, Qian G-S, Tu J-T, Guo TT, Wogan GN, Groopman JD. Aflatoxin biomarkers. Lancet 1992;340:119.
25. Selected mycotoxins: ochratoxins, trichothecenes, ergot. Environmental Health Criteria 105. Geneva: World Health Organization, 1990.
26. Bhat RV, Beedu SR, Ramakrishna Y, Munshi KL. Outbreak of trichothecene mycotoxicosis associated with consumption of mould. Danish wheat products in Kashmir Valley, India. Lancet 1982;1:35–37.
27. Friche RF, Jorge J. Assessment of efficacy of activated charcoal for treatment of acute T-2 toxin poisoning. Clin Toxicol 1990;28:421–431.
28. He F, Zhand S, Li C, Qia F, Liu X, L X. Mycotoxin induced encephalopathy and dystonia in children. Fifth World Congress in Intensive and Critical Care Medicine, Kyoto, Japan, September 3–8, 1989.
29. He F, Quan F, Zhang S, Liu X, Zhang C, Lo X. Mycotoxin induced encephalopathy and dystonia in children. In: Volans GN, Sims J, Sullivan FM, Turne P, eds. Basic science in toxicology. London: Taylor and Francis, 1990; pp. 596–604.
30. Kulig K, Moore LL, Kirk M, Smith D, Stallworth J, Rumack B. Bromocriptine-associated headache. Possible life-threatening sympathomimetic interaction. Obstet Gynecol 1991;78:941–943.
31. Vermund SH, Goldstein RG, Romano AA, Atwood SJ. Accidental bromocriptine ingestion in childhood. J Pediatr 1984;105:839–840.
32. Warren DE, Nakfoor E. Acute overdose of bromocriptine. Drug Intell Clin Pharm 1983;17:374.
33. Mack RB. Mairzy doats and dozy doats and a kiddle eat almost anything. Bromocriptine (Parlodel) overdose. NC Med J 1988;49:17–18.
34. Canterbury RJ, Haskins B, Kahu N, Saathoff G, Yazel JJ. Postpartum psychosis induced by bromocriptine. South Med J 1987;81:1463–1464.
35. Perovich RM, Lieberman JA, Fleischhacker WW, Alvir J. The behavioral toxicity of bromocriptine in patients with psychiatric illness. J Clin Psychopharmacol 1989;9:417–477.
36. Iffy L, Tentlone W, Frisole G. Acute myocardial infarction on the puerperium in patients receiving bromocriptine. Am J Obstet Gynecol 1986;155:371–372.
37. Bakht FR, Kirshon B, Baker T, Cotton DB. Postpartum cardiovascular complications after bromocriptine and cocaine use. Am J Obstet Gynecol 1990;162:1065–1066.
38. Maurel C, Abhay K, Schaeffer A, Lange F, Castot A, Melon E. Acute thrombotic accidents in the postpartum period in a patient receiving bromocriptine. Crit Care Med 1990; 118:1180–1181.
39. Ruch A, Duhring JL. Postpartum myocardial infarction in a patient receiving bromocriptine. Obstet Gynecol 1989;74: 448–451.
40. McElvaney NG, Wilcox PG, Chung A, Fleetham JA. Phenopulmonary disease during bromocriptine treatment of Parkinson's disease. Arch Intern Med 1988;148:2231–2236.
41. Kains J-PD, Hardy J-C, Chevalier C, Collier A. Retroperitoneal fibrosis in two patients with Parkinson's disease treated with bromocriptine. Acta Clin Belg 1990;45:306–310.
42. Auster SM, El-Hayek A, Comianos M, Tamulonis DJ. Mitral valve disease associated with long-term ergotamine use. South Med J 1993;86:1179–1181.
43. Redfield MM, Nicholson WJ, Edward WD, Tajik AJ. Valve disease associated with ergot alkaloid use. Echocardiographic and pathologic correlations. Ann Intern Med 1992;117:50–52.
44. Gill R, Key JA. High-performance liquid chromatography system for the separation of ergot alkaloids with applicability to the analysis of illicit lysergide (LSD). J Chromatogr 1985; 346:423–427.
45. Feng N, Minder EI, Grampp T, Vonderschmitt DJ. Identification and quantification of ergotamine in human plasma by gas chromatography-mass spectrometry. J Chromatog 1992; 575:289–294.
46. Edwards RJ, Fulde GWO, McGrath MA. Successful limb salvage with prostaglandin infusion: a review of ergotamine toxicity. Med J Aust 1991;155:825–827.

MUSHROOMS

INCIDENCE/EPIDEMIOLOGY

John Trestrail, Chairman, Toxicology Committee, North American Mycological Association, (Telephone: 616-774-7851) has analyzed mushroom case exposure reported in 1989 to the American Association of Poison Control Centers National Data Collection System. The data suggest an incidence of five mushroom exposures per 100,000 population per year.[1] In 1989 five species involved included *Chlorophyllum molybdites, Lycoperdon candidum, Morchella angusticeps, Omphalotus olearium,* and *Coprinus atramentarius.* Mushroom exposures by toxin group were cyclopeptides 0.7%, orellanine (1 case), ibotenic acid/muscinol 6.2%, monoethylhydrazine 0.6%, muscarine (3 cases), coprine 0.3%, hallucinogenics 3 to 6%, GI irritants 2.2%, and nontoxics 1.9%.[1]

An on-line program for computer identification of poisonous and hallucinogenic mushrooms has been developed by Dr. P. Margot and colleagues at the Forensic Science Unit, Strathclyde University, Glasgow GllXW, UK.[2] The database is biased toward European species, although a fair number of American species are included. (See Fig. 74–11.)

MYTHS[3]

1. A mushroom is safe to eat if it does not turn a silver spoon black when boiled together.
2. A mushroom is safe to eat if the cap has been peeled.

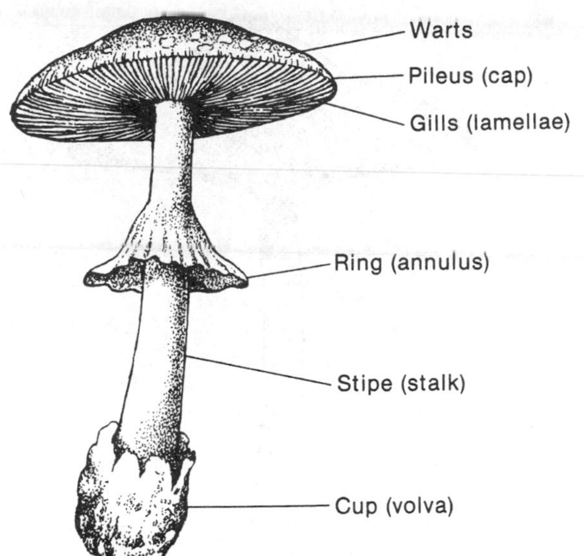

Figure 74–11A Composite of the mushroom. Basic structure of an *Amanita* mushroom.

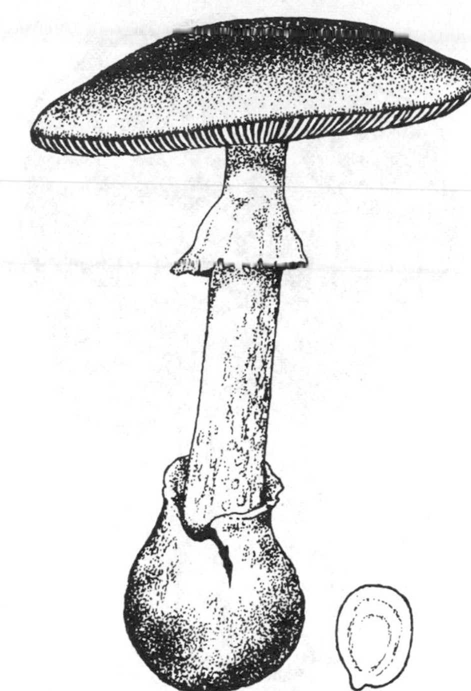

Figure 74–11C Death cap, *Amanita phalloides.* (Adapted from Lincoff G. The Audubon Society Field Guide to North American Mushrooms. New York: Alfred A. Knopf, 1981.)

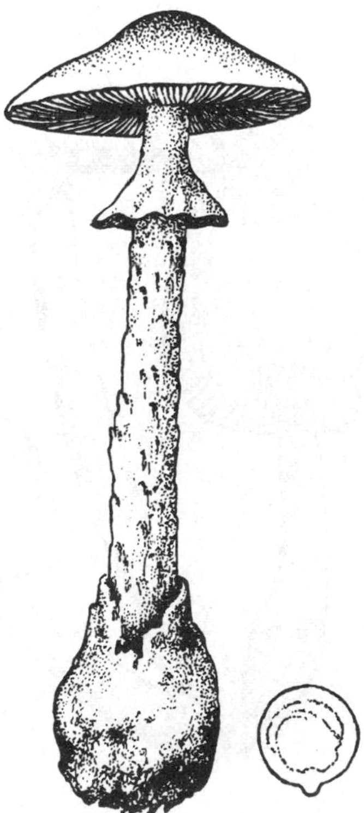

Figure 74–11B Destroying angel, *Amanita virosa.* (Adapted from Lincoff G. The Audubon Society Field Guide to North American Mushrooms. New York: Alfred A. Knopf, 1981.)

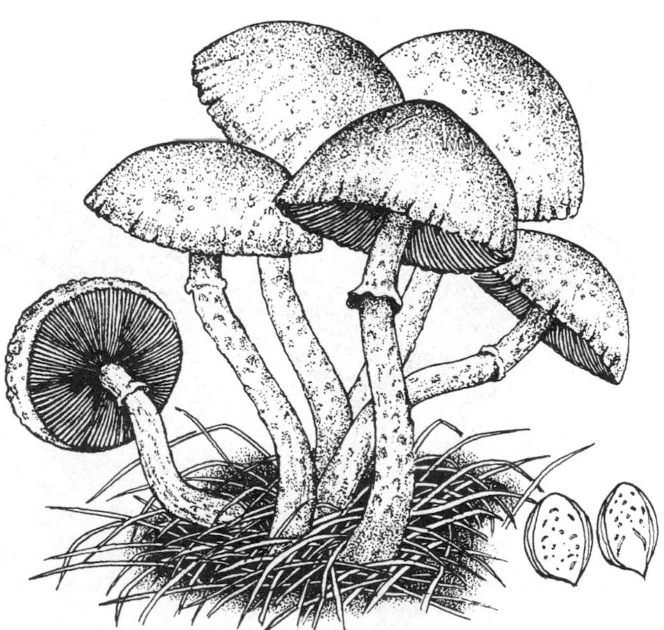

Figure 74–11D *Galerina marginata.* (Adapted from Lincoff G. The Audubon Society Field Guide to North American Mushrooms. New York: Alfred A. Knopf, 1981.)

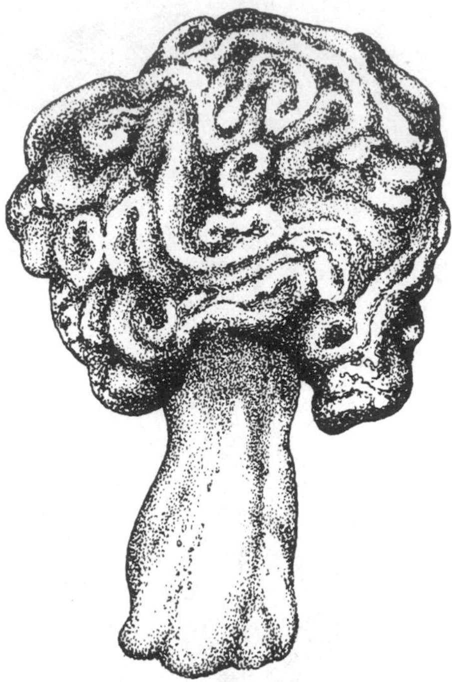

Figure 74–11E False morel (*Gyromitra esculenta*). (Adapted from Lincoff G. The Audubon Society Field Guide to North American Mushrooms. New York: Alfred A. Knopf, 1981.)

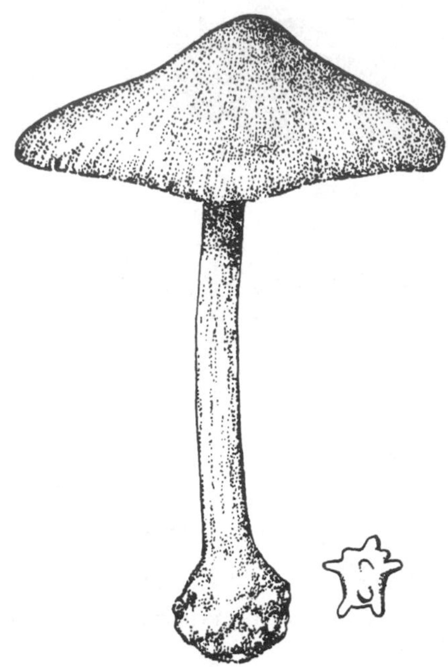

Figure 74–11G Turnip-bulb inocybe, *Inocybe napipes.* (Adapted from Lincoff G. The Audubon Society Field Guide to North American Mushrooms. New York: Alfred A. Knopf, 1981.)

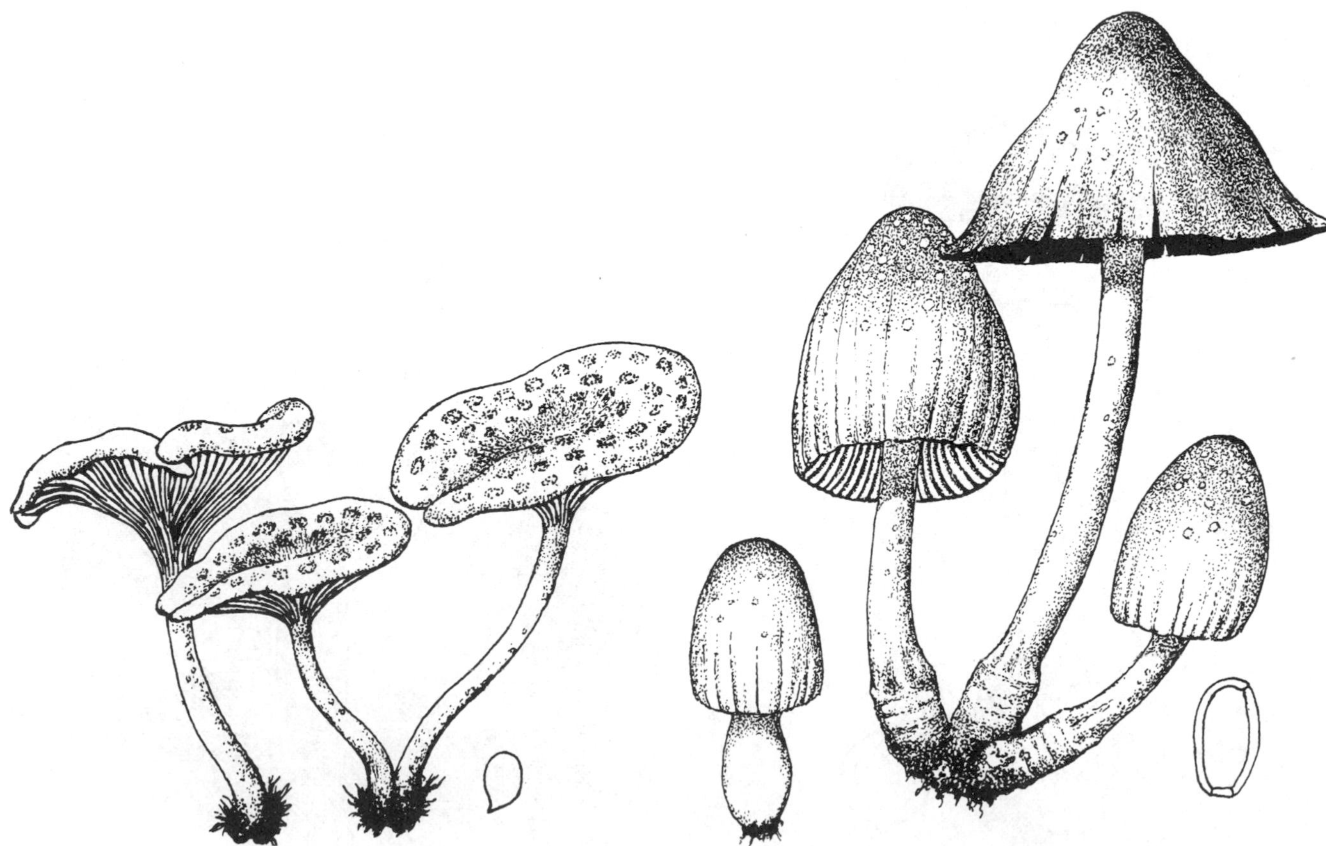

Figure 74–11F *Clitocybe dealbata.* (Adapted from Lincoff G. The Audubon Society Field Guide to North American Mushrooms. New York: Alfred A. Knopf, 1981.)

Figure 74–11H Inky cap, *Coprinus atramentarius.* (Adapted from Lincoff G. The Audubon Society Field Guide to North American Mushrooms. New York: Alfred A. Knopf, 1981.)

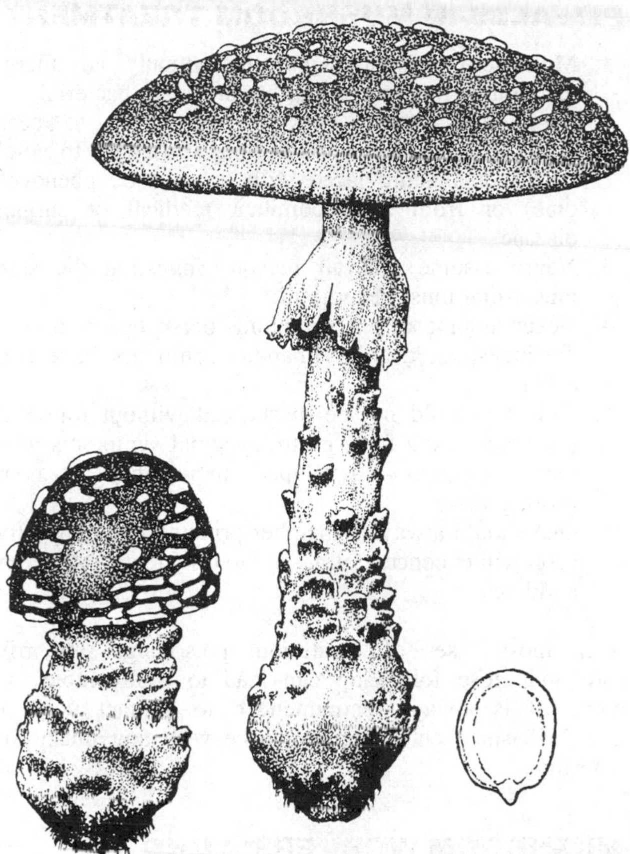

Figure 74–11I Fly agaric, *Amanita muscaria.* (Adapted from Lincoff G. The Audubon Society Field Guide to North American Mushrooms. New York: Alfred A. Knopf, 1981.)

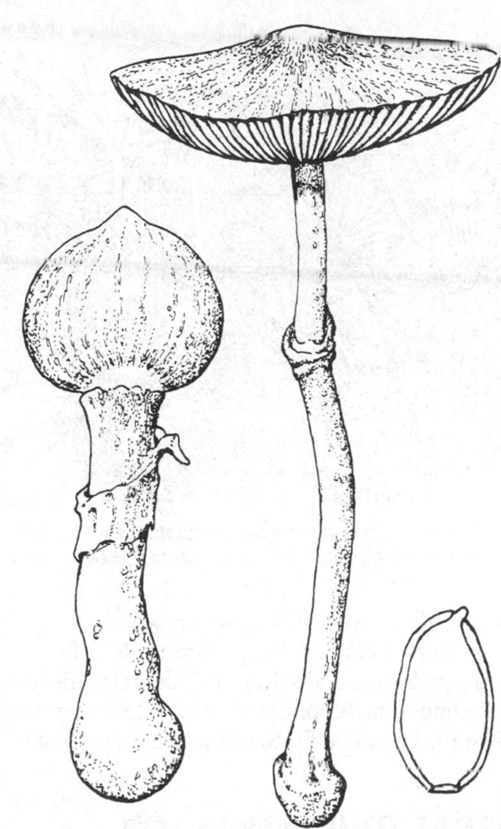

Figure 74–11K *Psilocybe cubensis.* (Adapted from Lincoff G. The Audubon Society Field Guide to North American Mushrooms. New York Alfred A. Knopf, 1981.)

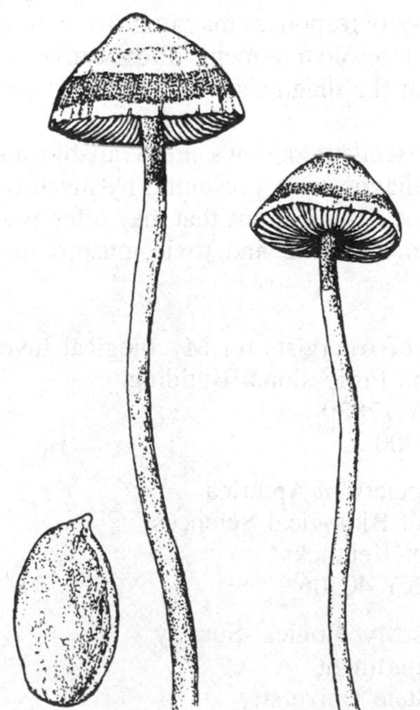

Figure 74–11J Mower's mushroom, *Panaeolus foenisecii.* (Adapted from Lincoff G. The Audubon Society Field Guide to North American Mushrooms. New York: Alfred A. Knopf, 1981.)

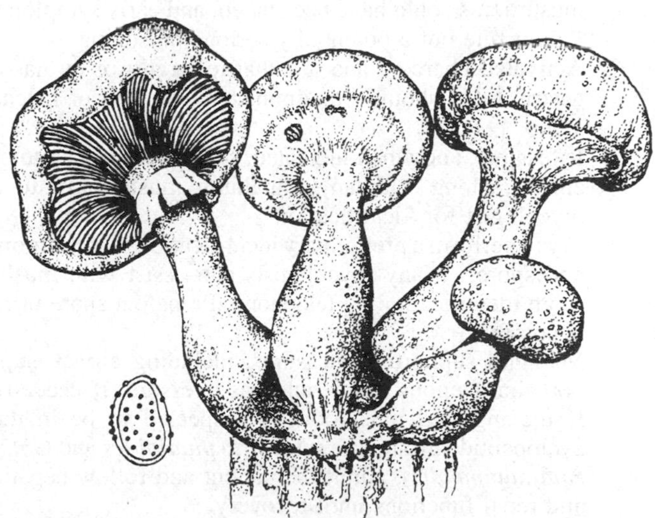

Figure 74–11L *Gymnopilus spectabilis* (66% actual size). (Adapted from Lincoff G. The Audubon Society Field Guide to North American Mushrooms. New York: Alfred A. Knopf, 1981.)

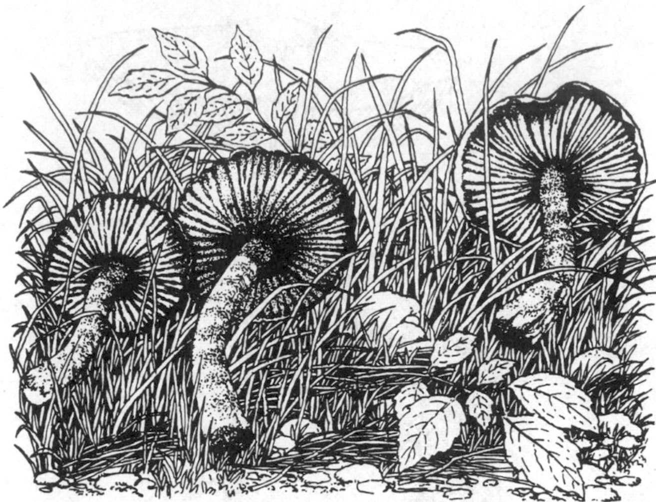

Figure 74–11M *Cortinarius speciosissimus.* (Adapted from Short AIK, Watling R, MacDonald MK et al. Lancet 1980;2:942.)

3. No deadly mushrooms grow on wood.
4. If an animal eats it, the mushroom is safe.
5. Boiling, drying, and salting will detoxify the mushroom.
6. Poisonous mushrooms will turn rice-water red.
7. Mushrooms are safe; toadstools are poisonous.

GENERAL GUIDELINES FOR MANAGEMENT

The following are some general guidelines for management of mushroom poisoning:

1. Determine the history of ingestion: how many types of mushrooms ingested; time of ingestion; if anyone else ate them; and what the current symptoms are.
2. Obtain a history of symptom presentation with emphasis on chronology. Usually, potentially lethal mushrooms produce symptoms 6 hours or longer after ingestion, whereas nonlethal mushrooms produce symptoms within 6 hours. However, keep in mind a variety of mushrooms could have been eaten, and early symptoms *do not* rule out a potentially serious poisoning.
3. Activated charcoal and a cathartic, orally or by nasogastric tube, should be administered in lieu of ipecac syrup.
4. If feasible, and when indicated, send gastric aspirate or emesis, along with any remaining mushrooms, to a mycologist for identification.
5. Try to perform a preliminary identification of mushroom and spores. Many mycologists can assist with mushroom identification by telephone. Prepare a spore print if possible.
6. Maintain supportive measures, including airway support, intravenous fluids, and vasopressors (if needed).
7. If the ingested mushroom is suspected to be in the cyclopeptide group, (i.e., *Amanita phalloides* and *Galerina autumnalis*), admit the patient and follow hepatic and renal functions until recovery.
8. Avoid antispasmodics for gastrointestinal symptoms.
9. Consider the use of specific antidotes when indicated.

PITFALLS IN MUSHROOM TREATMENT

1. Mushroom poisoning may be actually an allergic reaction or food poisoning secondary to bacteria.
2. Symptoms actually may be secondary to pesticides sprayed on the mushroom, secondary to edible mushrooms being laced with drugs (i.e., phencyclidine) or from a concomitant medical or surgical disease.
3. Never assume that all persons ingesting the same mushroom must become ill.
4. Never assume that if symptoms occur before 6 hours postingestion, deadly Amanitas could not have been eaten.
5. Patients should not be discharged without follow-up after recovering from gastrointestinal symptoms when those symptoms developed more than 6 hours postingestion.
6. One should always remember principles of supportive care while concentrating on toxin identification and antidotes.

In most cases of mushroom poisoning, supportive care and close follow-up can lead to a favorable outcome. It is always recommended to contact your regional Poison Center for assistance with any mushroom ingestion.

MUSHROOM WORKERS' LUNG

Respiratory disease may arise at various stages of the commercial production of mushrooms: during the preparation of the compost, mushroom spawning, mushroom growing, in the picking and sorting of the mushrooms, during the disposal of spent mushroom compost, and during the preparation of a mushroom food product.[4–6] Disease may affect both the airways and the lung parenchyma. Hypersensitivity responses may improve with removal from exposure and steroid treatment.[7] Provocative inhalation tests may assist in the diagnosis.[8] Pulmonary reactions may be fatal.

Several excellent reviews are available addressing the differential diagnosis of poisoning by mushrooms[9,10] (Fig. 74–12). Some organizations that may offer assistance in the identification of edible and toxic mushrooms include the following:

Association of Allergists for Mycological Investigations
444 Hermann Professional Building
Houston, TX 77030
(713) 797-0900

Botanical Society of America
c/o School of Biological Sciences
University of Kentucky
Lexington, KY 40506

Los Angeles Mycological Society
Biology Department
California State University
5151 State University Drive
Los Angeles, CA 90032
(publishes The Spore Print Journal)

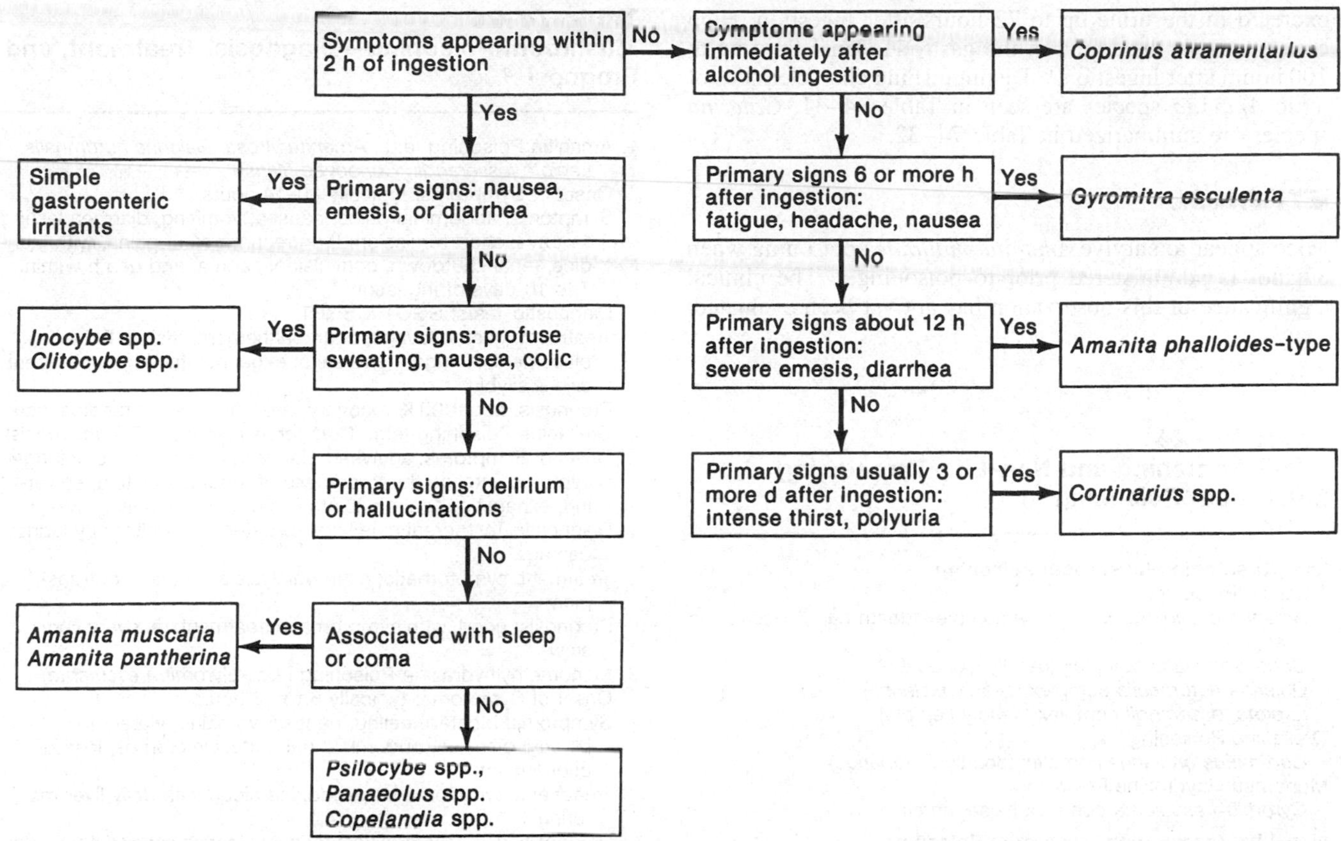

Figure 74–12 Differential diagnosis of mushroom intoxications by symptoms. (Adapted from Lampe KF. Paediatrician 1977;6:290.)

Infectious Disease Section
Centers for Disease Control
U.S. Dept HHS/Public Health Service
Atlanta, GA 30333
(404) 329-3311

International Society for Human and Animal Mycology
Animal Mycology
c/o Prof. W. Loeffler
Gellerstrasse 11A
Ch-4052 Basel, Switzerland

International Society for Mushroom Science
Institut fur Bodenbiologie
Landwirtschaft
D-3300 Braunschweig-Bundesalle 50
Germany

Mycology Society of America
c/o Department of Botany
University of Rhode Island
Kingston, RI 02881
(401) 792-2161

National Clearinghouse for Poison Control Centers
FDA Bureau of Drugs/Div of Poison Control
5600 Fishers Lane, Rm. 1345
Rockville, MD 20857
(301) 443-6260

North American Mycological Association
3556 Oakwood
Ann Arbor, MI 48104-5213

(Newsletter Editor Jay Justice
16055 Michale Dr.
Alexander, AR 22002)

Dr. Gary Lincoff
New York Botanical Gardens
(212) 662-2651

Lincoff has presented a summation of life-threatening and non–life-threatening mushroom poisoning[11] (Table 74–24). A summary of diagnostic features, treatment, and prognosis for mushroom poisoning prepared by Lincoff is found in Table 74–25.

Koppel has reviewed mushroom target organs and the latent periods after ingestion for each group[12] (Table 74–26).

A differential diagnosis of mushroom-induced gastritis is summarized in Table 74–27. Structural characteristics for toxic North American mushroom species are listed in Table 74–28. Poisonous mushrooms and their structurally similar edible species are summarized in Table 74–29. Table 74–30 summarizes mushroom toxicity by clinical classification.

AMATOXINS (*AMANITA PHALLOIDES*)

TOXICOKINETICS

Amatoxins are found in the serum as late as 30 hours after ingestion in concentrations of 0.5 to 24 ng/mL. They are excreted in the urine up to 72 hours after ingestion. High concentrations are found in the gastroduodenal fluid up to 100 hours after ingestion.[13] Distinguishing characteristics of toxic *Amanita* species are seen in Table 74–31. *Galerina* species are summarized in Table 74–32.

ETHANOL

Mice appear to survive *Amanita phalloides* poisoning when ethanol is administered prior to poisoning.[14] The clinical significance of this observation has not yet been evaluated.

Table 74–24
Life-Threatening and Non–Life-Threatening Mushroom Poisoning[a]

Life-Threatening Mushroom Poisoning
Amanitin Poisoning
- *Amanita phalloides* & *A. virosa* complex (death cap & destroying angels)
- *Conocybe filaris* complex (deadly *Conocybe*)
- *Galerina autumnalis* complex (deadly *Galerina*)
- *Lepiota josserandii* complex (deadly *Lepiota*)

Orellanine Poisoning
- *Cortinarius orellanus* complex (deadly *Cortinarius*)

Monomethylhydrazine Poisoning
- *Gyromitra esculenta* complex (false morel)

Non–Life-Threatening Mushroom Poisoning
Muscarine Poisoning
- *Inocybe* spp. (fiber caps)
- *Clitocybe dealbata* complex (the sweater)

Muscimol-Ibotenic Acid Poisoning
- *Amanita muscaria* complex (fly agaric)
- *Amanita pantherina* complex (the panther)

Hallucinogenic Mushroom Poisoning
- *Conocybe cyanopus* complex (psychoactive *Conocybe*)
- *(Cortinarius infractus)* (reported in Europe)
- *Gymnopilus spectabilis* complex (big laughing gym)
- *(Inocybe aeruginascens)* (reported in Europe)
- *Panaeolus* spp.
- *Pluteus salicinus*
- *Psilocybe* spp. (blue staining complex) (magic mushrooms)

Coprine Poisoning
- *Coprinus atramentarius* (alcohol inky cap)
- *Clitocybe clavipes* (fat-footed *Clitocybe*)

Miscellaneous Mushroom Poisoning
- A. Serious and potentially fatal (at least in Europe)
  - *Paxillus involutus* complex (poison pax)
- B. Serious but rarely fatal, if at all
  - *Chlorophyllum molybdites* (green-spored *Lepiota*)
  - *Omphalotus olearius* (jack o'lantern)
- C. Not usually requiring medical care
  1. Gilled mushrooms
     - *Agaricus xanthodermus* complex (malodorous, yellow foot fleshed *Agaricus*)
     - *Armillaria mellea* complex (honey mushroom)
     - *Entoloma* spp.
     - *Hebeloma* spp. (poison pie complex)
     - *Tricholoma pardinum* complex (dirty trich)
  2. Nongilled mushrooms
     - *Marchella* (black morels)
     - *Ramaria* spp. (some coral mushrooms)
     - *Polyporus* s.l. spp. (some tyramine-rich polypores)
     - *Boletus* spp. (red-pored, blue-staining)
     - *Suillus* spp. (slippery jack complex)
     - *Scleroderma citrinum* (pigskin false puffball)

[a]Adapted from Lincoff G. International Congress of Clinical Toxicology: Mushroom Workshop. September 9, 1993.

Table 74–25
Mushroom Poisoning—Diagnosis, Treatment, and Prognosis[a]

1. Amanitin Poisoning (e.g., *Amanita virosa, Galerina autumnalis, Lepiota josserandii, Conocybe filaris*)
   Onset of Symptoms: typically 10–14 hours
   Symptoms: abdominal pains, nausea, vomiting, diarrhea lasting 1+ days; short remission; then recurrence of pains, with jaundice, renal shutdown, convulsions, coma, and death within 7 to 10 days of ingestion.
   Diagnostic Tests: SGOT & SGPT.
   Treatment: gastric lavage, charcoal hemoperfusion; IV replacement of sugars and salts; experimental: high dose penicilin & silybin
   Prognosis: about 90% recovery rate with modern medical care
2. Orellanine Poisoning (e.g., *Cortinarius orellanus, C. rainierensis*)
   Onset of Symptoms: anywhere between 2 and 17 days or longer
   Symptoms: intense thirst, dryness of mouth, vomiting, shivering, exhaustion, pain in joints & muscles, oliguria
   Diagnostic Test: creatinine level to detect & monitor any kidney damage
   Treatment: symptomatic; haemodialysis as required or transplant
   Prognosis: good, with symptomatic treatment; recovery very slow
3. Monomethylhydrazine Poisoning (e.g., *Gyromitra esculenta*)
   Onset of Symptoms: typically 6 to 12 hours
   Symptoms: bloated feeling, nausea, vomiting, watery (or bloody) diarrhea, abdominal pain, muscle cramps, loss of coordination
   Treatment: symptomatic; pyridoxine along with daily liver monitoring
   Prognosis: very few fatalities; recovery in mild cases within a day
4. Muscarine Poisoning (e.g., *Inocybe* spp., *Clitocybe dealbata*)
   Onset of Symptoms: 30 minutes to 2 hours
   Symptoms: perspiration, lacrimation, salivation syndrome, blurred vision, constriction of pupils, fall in blood pressure
   Treatment: atropine if symptoms justify use
   Prognosis: good; symptoms often subside within 6 to 24 hours
5. Muscimol Poisoning (e.g., *Amanita muscaria, A. pantherina*)
   Onset of Symptoms: 30 minutes to 2 hours
   Symptoms: staggering, hyperactivity, muscle spasms, deep sleep, visions
   Treatment: symptomatic; atropine only for cholinergic symptoms
   Prognosis: good; recovery typically within 24 hours
6. Psilocybin Poisoning (e.g., *Psilocybe cubensis, Gymnopilus spectabilis*)
   Onset of Symptoms: 30 minutes to 2 hours
   Symptoms: mood change, muscle weakness, hilarity, panic, visions
   Treatment: symptomatic; reassurance
   Prognosis: good; recovery usually complete within 6 hours
7. Coprine Poisoning (e.g., *Coprinus atramentarius, Clitocybe clavipes*)
   Onset of Symptoms: about 30 minutes after drinking something alcoholic as long as 5 days (typically about a day) after eating mushroom
   Symptoms: flushing of face & neck; tingling of fingers & toes; headache
   Treatment: symptomatic, if violent vomiting occurs
   Prognosis: good; recovery typically spontaneous within 2 to 4 hours
8. Miscellaneous Mushroom Poisoning (e.g., *Agaricus xanthodermus, Boletus satanus, Chlorophyllum molybdites, Entoloma* spp., *Omphalotus* spp.)
   Onset of Symptoms: 30 minutes to 3 hours
   Symptoms: usually nausea, vomiting, diarrhea; severe in some species
   Treatment: symptomatic
   Prognosis: good; recovery usually within a day or two

[a]Adapted from Lincoff G. International Congress of Clinical Toxicology: Mushroom Poisoning Workshop. September 9, 1993.

Table 74–26
Mushroom Target Organs[a]

Syndromes	Target	Latent Period
Phalloides	Liver	6–24 hours
Gyromitra	Liver	6–12 hours
Orellanus (*Cortinarius*)	Kidney	30 hours–14 days
Muscarinic	Autonomic nervous system	0.5–2 hours
Coprine	Autonomic nervous system	0.5 hours after ethanol
Pantherina	Central nervous system	0.5–3 hours
Psilocybin		0.5–3 hours
Gastrointestinal	Intestine	0.5–3 hours

[a]Adapted from Koppel C. Toxicon 1993;31:1513–1540.

Table 74–27
Differential Diagnosis of Mushroom-Induced Gastritis

Drugs		
Digitoxin	Pilocarpine	Cocaine
Ergot	Ethanol	Procaine
Cathartics	Nicotine	Colchicine
Boric acid	Salicylate	
Infections		
Viral gastroenteritis	*Vibrio cholerae*	
	Clostridium botulinum A and B (home-canned foods)	
Food poisoning	*Vibrio parahaemolyticus* (seafood)	
	Staphylococcus aureus (unrefrigerated dairy products)	
	Salmonella enteritis (wild and domestic animals)	
	Bacillus cereus (meat, pudding, rice)	
Chemicals		
Heavy metals	Corrosives	Halogens
Cholinesterase inhibitors	DDT	Creosol
Phenols	Phosphorus	
Toxins		
Botulinum toxin	Muscarine	Methanol

Table 74–28
Distribution and Structural Characteristics of Toxic North American Mushroom Species[a]

Genus and Species	Distribution[b]	Season[b]	Pileus	Spore Print	Amyloid Reaction[b]
Group I. Cyclopeptide Poisoning					
Amanita					
A. bisporigera	E NA, Pac Coast (rare)	Sp, S, F	White	White	Positive
A. virosa (destroying angel)	E NA, Pac Coast (rare)	Sp, S, F	White	White	Positive
A. verna (death angel)	E NA, Pac Coast (rare)	Sp, S, F	White	White	Positive
A. phalloides (death cap)	Rare—E NA, PNW, Pac Coast	S, F	Pale yellow green to green	White	Positive
A. brunnescens	E NA	S, F	Brown with white margin	White	Positive
A. pantherina (see also Group V)	Common; widely, esp. RM, PNW	Sp, S, F	Light brown to brown with buff or yellowish margin	White	Negative
Galerina					
G. autumnalis	Common, widely	Late F, early Sp	Dark brown to leathery light tan	Rust brown	Negative
G. venenata	Rare—PNW	Late F, W	Cinnamon brown	Rust brown	Negative
Group II. Monomethylhydrazine Poisoning					
Gyromitra					
G. californica	Common, RM, PNW, PSW	Early Sp	Tan to red-brown	Brown	Negative
G. brunnea	Common, E NA	Early Sp	Chocolate brown, white beneath	Brown	Negative
G. esculenta	Common, widely, esp. RM, PNW	Late Sp	Brown to red-brown	Brown	Negative
Group III. Disulfiram-like Poisoning					
Coprinus					
C. atramentarius	Common, widely	S, F	Light gray-brown (exhibits deliquescence)	Black	Negative

[a]Adapted from Geehr EC. Toxic plant ingestions. In: Auerbach PS, Geehr EC, eds. Management of wilderness and environmental emergencies. New York: Macmillan, 1983.
[b]Key: E NA, Eastern North America; Mid W, Middle Western States; N Eng, New England; NE, Northeastern States; Pac Coast, Pacific Coast; PNW, Pacific Northwest; RM, Rocky Mountain States; SE, Southeastern States; widely, distributed throughout North America; common, found in abundance during the fruiting season; Sp, spring; S, summer; F, fall; W, winter; positive, spores turn blue in Melzer's reagent; negative, spores do not turn blue in Melzer's reagent.
[c]The stalks of hallucinogenic *Psilocybe* species stain blue with bruising.
[d]Beware of all *Lactarius* species that stain lilac when bruised and emit latex from the gills.

(continued)

Table 74–28 *(Continued)*

Genus and Species	Distribution[b]	Season[b]	Pileus	Spore Print	Amyloid Reaction[b]
Group IV. Muscarine Poisoning					
Inocybe	Common, widely, woodlands	S, F	Brown to dark brown	Brown	Negative
I. napipes					
I. fastigiata					
I. patouillardii					
I. interaria					
I. lanuginose					
I. geophylla			White to lilac	Clay brown	Negative
Clitocybe					
C. dealbata	Common, widely	S, F	Dull white	White	Negative
C. rivulosa					
C. trunicola					
Paneolus					
P. separatus	Common, widely	Sp, S, F	Light gray to dull gray-white	Black	Negative
Gymnopilus					
G. spectabilis also:	Common, widely	Sp, S, F, early W	Buff yellow to yellow-orange	Rusty orange	Negative
G. luteus					
G. decurrens					
G. valipides					
G. aeruginosus					
G. viridans					
Also reported					
G. stropharia					
G. copelandia					
G. conocyte					
G. pholiotina					
Group V. Isoxazole Derivatives: Ibotenic Acid and Muscimol Poisoning					
Amanita					
A. muscaria	Common, widely, esp. N Eng, Pac Coast, RM	Sp, S, F	Orange or straw yellow (N Eng) to bright red (Pac Coast) (often with pileal warts)	White	Negative
A. pantherina	Common, widely, esp. RM, PNW	Sp, S, F	Light brown to brown with buff or yellowish-white margin	White	Negative
Group VI. Hallucinogens					
Psilocybe[c]					
P. cubensis	Rare, Florida	Late W to F	Whitish to pale yellow	Purple-brown	Negative
P. balocystis	Oregon, Washington	W to F		Purple-brown	Negative
P. semilanceata	PNW, Britain	F, W	Buff-gray to gray-green	Purple-brown	Negative
P. stuntzii also:	PNW	F, W	Brown to ochre	Dark-purple	Negative
P. venenosus					
P. mexicana					
P. quebecensis					
Paneolus					
P. campanulatus	Common, widely	Sp, S, F	Gray, speckled dark purple-brown	Black	Negative
P. foenisecii	Common, widely	Sp, S, F	Dark brown or reddish brown to tan or light gray-brown	Purple-brown	Negative
Group VII. Gastrointestinal Irritants					
Agaricus					
A. hondensis	Common, widely	S, F	White-brown, gray-brown	Chocolate brown	Negative
Boletus					
B. luridus	Rare, NE, SE, Mid W	S, F	Mixed, many colors	Olive-brown	Negative
B. eastwoodiae	Rare, Pac Coast	F	Dark to red-brown	Olive-brown	Negative
B. satanas	Rare, Pac Coast		Olive, buff	Olive-brown	Negative
B. sensibilis				Olive-brown	Negative
Chlorophyllum					
C. molybdites	Common, widely	Sp, S, F	White with buff scales	Green	Negative

(continued)

Table 74–20 *(Continued)*

Genus and Species	Distribution[b]	Season[b]	Pileus	Spore Print	Amyloid Reaction[b]
Group VII. Gastrointestinal Irritants *(continued)*					
Entoloma					
E. lividum	Common, widely	S, F	Tan	Salmon-pink	Negative
Gomphus					
G. floccosus	Common, widely			Smoky gray to black	Negative
Hebeloma					
H. crustuliniforme	Rare, widely	F	Brown to cream at margin	Yellow to olive-brown	Negative
H. mesophaeum	Common, widely	Sp, S, F	Brown	Yellow to olive-brown	Negative
Lactarius species[d]	Common, widely	Sp, S, F	Variable	White to yellow	Positive
Marasmius					
M. ureus	Common, widely	S, F		White	Negative
Naematoloma					
N. fasciculare	Common, esp. PNW, SE	Sp, F, W	Yellow to orange-yellow	Purple-brown	Negative
Omphalatus					
O. olearius	E NA, S, US, Pac Coast	S, F	Yellow-orange to bright orange	White	Negative
Paxillus					
P. involutus	Common, widely	S, F	Red-brown	Clay-brown, yellow-brown	Negative
Ramaria (coral fungus)					
R. formosa	Common, widely	F, W	Pink to light orange (coral branches)	Red-brown	Negative
Rhodophyllus (R. sinuatus; see *Entoloma lividum*—same species)					
Russula					
R. emetica	Common, widely	S, F	Bright red	White	Negative
R. densifolia	Common, widely, esp. E NA	S, F	White to gray	White	Positive
Scleroderma (puffball fungi) species	Common, esp. E NA	S, F	Gleba (spore mass) purple to purple-brown; surface tan to white	Brown	Negative
Tricholoma species	Common, widely, esp. NE, RM, PNW, and Mid W	F	Gray-brown	White	Negative

PREGNANCY

A 21-year-old woman with *A. phalloides* intoxication had symptoms of nausea, vomiting, abdominal pain, and diarrhea within 10 hours of mushroom ingestion. The diagnosis was confirmed by blood and amniotic fluid alpha-amanitin levels. The serum level was 18.5 ng/mL by HPLC; no level was detected in the amniotic fluid. Alpha amanitin, with a molecular weight of 900, does not appear to cross the placental barrier even 24 hours after ingestion of *A. phalloides.*[15] Fourteen of 77 individuals poisoned with amatoxin containing *Lepiota* species (*Lepiota helveola* and *Lepiota castanea*) died of liver failure in Turkey. There were no deaths from renal failure.[16]

LABORATORY

Alpha and beta amanitins in plasma, urine, gastroduodenal fluid, feces, and tissues may be analyzed by high-performance liquid chromatography with separations of the alpha and beta amanitin performed on a reversible-phase analytic column under isocratic conditions with UV detection at 280 nm.[17] The detection limit is 5 ng/mL for both toxins. Detection in plasma at concentrations of 2 ng/mL may be performed using high-performance liquid chromatography with amperometric detection.

High-performance liquid chromatography allows the quantitation of alpha and beta amanitin separately. The detection limit is 5 ng/mL for both toxins.[13]

Blood and Urine and Gastroduodenal Fluid Levels

Plasma amatoxins have been detected by Jaeger and colleagues in *Amanita phalloides* poisoning at levels of 8 to 190 ng/mL for alpha and 23.5 to 162 ng/mL for beta. Urine amatoxins were detected with an hourly excretion of 32.18 μg for alpha and 80.15 μg for beta. Amatoxins were usually detectable in plasma before 36 hours, but were present in the urine until day 4. There was no correlation between amatoxin plasma concentrations and the clinical severity or outcome. Maximal urine excretion occurred during the 72 hours following ingestion. High concentrations were found in the gastroduodenal aspiration fluid from 48 to 110 hours.[13] A suggested high-performance liquid chromatography assay of alpha-amanitin and beta-amanitin in human serum, urine, or stomach washings has been described. The tests are sensitive to 20 μg/mL.[18] In animal studies no correlation has been observed between the plasma amatoxin concentration and the clinical outcome.[19]

Ancillary Tests

Routine laboratory tests for symptomatic cases include a complete blood count, electrolytes, blood urea nitrogen, creatinine, prothrombin time, bilirubin urinalysis, and blood glucose. Determinations should be repeated daily until clinical improvement occurs.

TREATMENT

Stabilization

Initial treatment requires the restoration of fluid and electrolyte balance. Obtunded patients should receive intravenous glucose immediately because of the common complication of hypoglycemia. Patients have presented to an emergency department in cardiac arrest resulting from fluid loss and massive gastrointestinal hemorrhage. Fresh-frozen plasma and vitamin K may be needed in addition to packed red blood cell transfusions and balanced electrolyte infusions.

Hemoperfusion

Patients who present prior to 24 hours after ingestion should receive charcoal hemoperfusion if a lethal dose (>50 g of mushroom) has been eaten.[20]

Decontamination

Forced Diuresis

Since most of the toxin is eliminated during the initial 24 to 48 hours, it is necessary to start this treatment as soon as possible. There are, however, no data to indicate that this treatment can decrease the amount of amatoxins found in the liver. Forced diuresis (6 to 9 L/day) has not been shown to be more efficient than maintenance of a normal or slightly enhanced urine volume.[13]

Plasma Exchange

In two series plasma exchange was attempted in 42 patients poisoned by *Amanita phalloides* mushrooms. Three patients

Table 74–29
Poisonous Mushrooms and Their Structurally Similar Edible Species[a]

Poisonous Mushrooms	Edible Mushrooms
Group I: Cyclopeptide Poisoning	
Amanita phalloides	*Amanita fulva*
	Agaricus spp.
	Lepiota procera
	Tricholoma flavovirens
	Tricholoma portentosum
Amanita verna-virosa group	*Amanita vaginata*
	Lepiota naucina[b]
	Agaricus spp (buttons)
Amanita buttons	*Lycoperdon perlatum*
Galerina (Pholiota) autumnalis	*Pholiota mutabilis*
Galerina (Pholiota) marginata	*Armillariella mellea*
	Flammulina (Collybia) velutipes
Group II: Monomethylhydrazine (MMH) Poisoning	
Gyromitra esculenta and spp.	*Morchella esculenta* and spp.
	Gyromitra gigas[b]
Group III: Coprine Poisoning	
Coprinus atramentarius	*Coprinus micaceus*[b]
Group IV: Muscarine Poisoning	
Clitocybe dealbata	*Marasmius oreades*
Inocybe spp.	*Marasmius oreades*
Omphalotus olearius	*Cantharellus cibarius*
	Clitocybe aurantiaca[b]
	Armillariella mellea
Group V: Ibotenic Acid–Muscimol Poisoning	
Amanita muscaria	*Amanita caesarea*
	Amanita rubescens
	Armillariella mellea
Amanita pantherina	*Amanita rubescens*
Amanita gemmata	*Russula* spp.
Amanita cothurnata	*Lepiota* spp.
Amanita "solitaria" group	*Agaricus* spp.
Group VI: Psilocybin–Psilocin Poisoning	
Panaeolus foenisecii	*Psathyrella candolleana*
	Agrocybe pediades
	Marasmius oreades
Panaeolus spp.	*Coprinus* spp.
Gymnopilus spectabilis	*Armillariella mellea*
Group VII: Gastrointestinal Irritants	
Agaricus spp.	*Agaricus augustus*
	A. arvensis
	A. campestris
Amanita brunnescens	*Amanita rubescens*
	Amanita inaurata
Boletus sensibilis	*Boletus* spp.
Chlorophyllum molybdites	*Lepiota* spp.
Entoloma spp.	*Pluteus cervinus*
	Entoloma (Clitopilus) abortivum, unaborted
Hebeloma crustuliniforme	*Rozites caperata*
Naematoloma fasciculare	*Armillariella mellea*
	Naematoloma sublateritium
	Naematoloma capnoides
Paxillus involutus	*Lactarius* spp.
Ramaria formosa	*Ramaria* spp.
Ramaria gelatinosa	
Scleroderma aurantium and spp.	*Lycoperdon perlatum* and spp.
Tricholoma pessundatum var. *montanum*	*Tricholoma pessundatum* var. *populinum* (*Tricholoma populinum*)

[a]Adapted from Lincoff O, Mitchel DH. Toxic and hallucinogenic mushroom poisoning. A handbook for physicians and mushroom hunters. New York: Van Nostrand Reinhold, 1977.
[b]Reportedly poisonous to some.

Table 74–30
Clinical Classification of Mushroom Toxicity[a]

Group	Toxins	Principal Mushrooms	Onset of Symptoms	Symptoms
Toxins Causing Cellular Destruction—Delayed Onset				
I	Cyclopeptides (amanitins)	*Amanita bisporigera* *A. ocreata* *A. phalloides* *A. verna* *A. virosa* *Galerina autumnalis* *G. marginata* *G. venenata* *Lepiota* sp.	6–24 h (typically 10–14 h)	Abdominal pains, nausea, vomiting, and diarrhea lasting 1+ days; short remission of symptoms; then recurrence of pains with jaundice, renal shutdown, convulsions, coma, and death
II	Gyromitrin Monomethylhydrazine (MMH)	*Gyromitra esculenta* and others	6–12 h	Bloated feeling, nausea, vomiting, watery (or bloody) diarrhea, abdominal pains, muscle cramps, faintness, loss of coordination and, in severe cases, convulsions, coma, and death
Toxins Affecting the Autonomic Nervous System—Rapid Onset				
III	Muscarine and other muscarinic compounds	*Clitocybe dealbata, C. cerusata,* and perhaps *C. illudens* (*Omphalotus olearius* and others; *Inocybe*—most spp.)	0.5–2 h	Cholinergic-like syndrome (perspiration, salivation, lacrimation), blurred vision, abdominal cramps, watery diarrhea, constriction of pupils, fall in blood pressure, slow pulse
IV	Coprine (Antabuse-like)	*Coprinus atramentarius, Clitocybe clavipes*	About 30 min after drinking alcohol; as long as 5 days after eating mushrooms	Flushing of face and neck, distension of neck veins, swelling and tingling of hands, metallic taste, tachycardia and hypotension; later, nausea, vomiting, and sweating
Toxins Affecting the Central Nervous System—Rapid Onset				
V	Ibotenic acid, muscimol (isoxazoles)	*Amanita muscaria, A. pantherina,* and others	0.5–2 h	Dizziness, incoordination, staggering (intoxication); muscular jerking and spasms; hyperkinetic activity; comalike deep sleep and "visions"
VI	Psilocybin and psilocin (indoles)	*Psilocybe cubensi, P. baeocystis,* and many others	30–60 (180) min	Pleasant or apprehensive mood; unmotivated laughter; hilarity; compulsive movements; muscle weakness; drowsiness; "visions" while awake, then sleep
Toxins Affecting the Gastrointestinal Tract—Rapid Onset				
VII	Diverse, mostly unknown	Many species from diverse genera	0.5–2 h	Principally nausea, vomiting, diarrhea, and abdominal pain
Toxins Affecting Renal Function—Delayed Onset				
VIII	*Cortinarius* sp.	Mainly European but toxic species present in United States	30 h 3–14 d	Gastritis Renal failure

[a]Adapted from Mitchel DH. Annu Rev Med 1980;31:52–53.

died.[21,22] Further data will be needed to support this interesting approach to treatment.

Antidotes

Penicillin

Penicillin appears to displace amatoxin from plasma protein-binding sites allowing for increased renal excretion. It also may inhibit the penetration of amatoxin into hepatocytes. In one retrospective clinical study of 205 patients, doses of 300,000 to 1,000,000 units of benzyl penicillin daily tended to be more often associated with survival than below 300,000 U/d.[14] Despite experimental data, the overall survival of patients treated with penicillin is not impressively higher than that of the total population.[23] Animal data suggest that cephalosporin may be similarly useful, but clinical studies have not yet been performed.[24]

Treatment of Acute Liver Failure[25] (See also Chapter 10 —Acetaminophen)

A. General Principles

1. Individuals with ALF require hospital admission in a specialized unit designed to manage such patients.

2. The availability of an established liver transplant program is highly recommended.
3. Invasive monitoring is necessary to detect complications before they become clinically evident and while they are still treatable.
4. A central venous pressure monitor, arterial line, urinary catheter, and nasogastric tube should be placed in all cases.
5. If the patient is in grade 3 or 4 coma, endotracheal intubation is essential to prevent aspiration.
6. Patients should also be monitored with continuous pulse oximetry.
7. Mechanical ventilation should be instituted when hypercapnia ($PaCO_2$ greater than 6.5 kPa) or hypoxia (PaO_2 less than 10 kPa) develops. Ascitic fluid and wounds, if present, should be cultured at regular intervals and whenever clinically indicated.
8. Sites of catheter insertion should be examined regularly; catheters should be replaced and their tips cultured at 3 to 5-day intervals.
9. Hypoglycemia should be prevented by a continuous infusion of 5 or 10% dextrose. Hypoglycemia may be undetected unless blood glucose determinations are made every 2 to 3 hours in comatose patients.
10. When blood glucose concentrations fall below 60 mg/dL, these must be corrected immediately with the infusion of a 50% dextrose solution given with an appropriate upward adjustment of the existing infusion rate.

Table 74–31
Distinguishing Characteristics of Toxic *Amanita* Species[a]

	A. verna	*A. virosa*	*A. bisporigera*	*A. tenuifolia*	*A. ocreata*	*A. phalloides*
Cap						
Size	2–5 in. across	2–5 in. across	1½–3 in. across	2½–3¼ in. across	2–5 in.? across	2½–6 in. across
Shape and color	Convex, viscid, smooth, no warts, white, at times discoloring in age to cream on disc; no color change when touched with 3%–10% KOH (or NaOH) solution	Convex to broadly umbonate, viscid, smooth, no warts, white, discoloring in age to pinkish cream or pale gray-brown (in some cases); staining yellow in KOH (or NaOH)	Convex, viscid, smooth, no warts, white, discoloring in age to pinkish cream; staining yellow in KOH (or NaOH)	Convex, viscid, smooth, shining when dry, no warts, white, becoming yellowish on disc with age or on drying; no data with KOH	Convex, viscid, smooth, no warts, white, discoloring in age to buff, pinkish or pale brownish; staining yellow in KOH (or NaOH)	Convex, viscid, smooth, no warts, yellowish green to greenish brown, paler toward margin, with flattened radiating hairs
Gills	Free or attached to stalk by a line; white	Free or attached to stalk by a line; white	Free or attached to stalk by a line; white	Adnate; white	Free or attached to stalk by a line; white	Free or attached to stalk by a line; white
Stalk	3–8 × ¼–¾ in. enlarging downward to basal bulb; smooth to floccose; white	3–8 × ¼–¾ in. enlarging downward to basal bulb; floccose; white	3–5 × ¼–¾ in. enlarging downward to basal bulb; smooth to finely floccose; white	3 × ¼–½ in. enlarging downward to basal bulb; smooth and shining white	3–8 × ¼–¾ in. ? enlarging downward to basal bulb; floccose?; white	3–5 × ½–⅘ in. enlarging downward to basal bulb; smooth; off-white to gray or greenish yellow
Annulus	Superior, pendant, membranous, persistent, white	Superior, pendant, membranous, lacerated to partly free, white	Superior, pendant, membranous, persistent, white	Superior, pendant, membranous, persistent, white	Superior, pendant, membranous, persistent, white	Superior, pendant, membranous, persistent, white
Volva	1+ in. high, membranous, persistent, saclike, white	1+ in. high, membranous, persistent, saclike, white	1+ in. high, membranous, persistent, saclike, white	1+ in. high, membranous, persistent, saclike, white	1+ in. high, membranous, persistent, saclike, white	1+ in. high, membranous, persistent, saclike, white
Spores	White spore print 8–11 × 7–9 µm (L/W ratio > 1.35), elliptical with distinct apiculus, thin-walled, amyloid (turns blue in Melzer's reagent)	White spore print 8–10 µm, (L/W ratio < 1.25), typically subglobose with distinct apiculus, thin-walled, amyoid	White spore print 7–10 µm, globose, with distinct apiculus, thin-walled, amyloid; two per basidium (all others in chart have four-spored basidia)	White spore print 12 × 5 µm, cylindrical, with distinct apiculus, thin-walled, amyloid	White spore print 9–14 µm, ovoid to subellipsoid, with distinct apiculus, thin-walled, amyloid	White spore print 8–11 × 7–9 µm, with distinct apiculus, subglobose, thin-walled, amyloid

[a]Adapted from Lincoff G, Mitchel DH. Toxic and hallucinogenic mushroom poisoning. A handbook for physicians and mushroom hunters. New York: Van Nostrand Reinhold, 1977.

Table 74–32
Characteristics of Toxic *Galerina* Species[a]

	G. autumnalis	*G. marginata*	*G. venenata*
Cap			
Size	1–2½ in. across	⅔–1½(3) in. across	½–1½ in. across
Shape and color	Convex becoming plane or with slightly obtuse umbo; smooth; viscid, with separable pellicle; margin striate when moist; dark brown (when moist) to ochre tawny fading to buff or pale yellow on drying and in age, disc at times remaining darker	Obtuse to convex becoming broadly convex, plane, or slightly umbonate; smooth; moist but not viscid; margin striate when moist; margin extending somewhat beyond gills; dark brown when moist fading to yellowish or dull tan, disc at times remaining darker	Convex to broadly convex; smooth; moist but not viscid; margin wavy and split in age; pale bay-brown to reddish cinnamon-brown
Gills	Adnate or with slight decurrent tooth, close, light brown at first, becoming rusty brown at maturity	Adnate to subdecurrent, close, yellowish to pallid brown when young, becoming tawny or darker at maturity	Attached, subdistant, golden brown to dull cinnamon
Stalk			
Size	(1¼)2–3½ × ⅛–⅓ in.	(⅘)1¼–2½ × ⅛–⅓ in.	1¼–1½ × ⅛–¼ in.
Shape and color	Equal to subclavate, hollow; dry; brown streaked with white fibrils; white mycelial covering about base	Equal to slightly enlarged downward; hollow; dry; brown to reddish brown or darker; white mycelial covering about base	Equal; dry; hairless; brownish; white mycelium just at base
Annulus (ring) (partial veil)	Almost fibrillose, superior, evanescent, thin, white, hairy ring	Submembranous to fibrillose, median to superior, often evanescent, becoming brown from spores	Hairy bandlike ring above middle of stalk
Spores	Brown to rusty brown spore print 8.5–10.5 × 5–6.5 μm ovate—elliptical, with apiculus, wrinkled to rough depression near base (by apiculus) and wrinkled exosporium	Brown to rusty brown spore print 8–10 × 5–6 μm ovate—elliptical, with apiculus, warty-wrinkled with base and wrinkled exosporium	Rusty brown spore print 8–11 × 6–6.5 μm ovate—elliptical, with apiculus, roughened, near base of spore

[a]Adapted from Lincoff G, Mitchel DH. Toxic and hallucinogenic mushroom poisoning. A handbook for physicians and mushroom hunters. New York: Van Nostrand Reinhold, 1977.

11. When crystalloid or colloid solutions fail to maintain blood pressure, dopamine or, in cases with very low vascular resistance, dopamine and noradrenaline can be given.
12. Renal failure is managed with careful volume monitoring. The continuous infusion of dopamine (2 to 4 μg/kg per hour) may reverse or slow renal deterioration by increasing renal blood flow.
13. Dialysis or arteriovenous ultrafiltration is required when the serum creatinine exceeds 400 μmol/L (4.5 mg/dL), in addition to the conventional indications such as severe metabolic acidosis, hyperkalemia, and fluid overload.
14. Gastroduodenal bleeding can be prevented by regular doses of H_2-antagonists or omeprazole to maintain intragastric pH above 5.

B. Hepatic encephalopathy
Lactulose and dietary protein withdrawal are used commonly to treat acute hepatic encephalopathy. Other agents include metronidazole and neomycin.

C. Cerebral edema
ICP monitoring seems to be helpful in directing therapy toward the prevention of brainstem herniation, in the selection of patients for liver transplantation, and in guiding anesthetic management during the transplant procedure.

Osmotic diuretics
Mannitol at a dose of 1 g/kg body weight is given as a rapid intravenous infusion of a 20% solution whenever ICP rises above 30 mm Hg for more than 5 minutes or, in the absence of ICP monitoring, clinical signs suggestive of cerebral edema are recorded. Mannitol infusions may be repeated provided the plasma osmolarity does not exceed 320 mOsm. In patients with renal failure, mannitol should be used only in combination with hemofiltration or ultrafiltration to prevent hyperosmolarity and fluid overload.

Barbiturates
Thiopental (3 to 5 mg/kg) is infused slowly over 15 minutes until signs of intracranial hypertension resolve or a maximum of 500 mg of drug is given. Subsequently, a continuous infusion of thiopentone at the lowest rate required to maintain an ICP <20 mm Hg was administered. Whenever clinical signs of ICP have resolved for more than 4 hours, the infusion is discontinued.

Positioning
In the absence of ICP monitoring, patients with ALF should be positioned in a head-upright position with the head no higher than 30° above horizontal.

Charcoal hemoperfusion
Charcoal hemoperfusion does not confer an additional benefit in survival over and above that obtained with intensive liver care.

Corticosteroids
Corticosteroids are not beneficial either as prophylaxis or as active treatment of cerebral edema in ALF.

D. Infection
Aggressive daily microbiologic surveillance is mandatory in patients with ALF if early detection and appropriate treatment of bacterial and fungal infections are to take place. Prophylactic antimicrobial treatments are useful to prevent infection in patients with ALF.

E. Coagulopathy
Fresh-frozen plasma (FFP)
The use of FFP is limited to patients who are bleeding or before an invasive procedure.

F. Hemodynamic abnormalities and tissue hypoxia
The addition of circulatory vasodilator agents, such as prostacyclin and *N*-acetylcysteine, may prevent the development of tissue hypoxia in patients with ALF who are given vasopressor therapy.

G. Artificial liver support devices
Extracorporeal liver assist device (ELAD) needs further testing in controlled trials to determine its real efficacy as a hepatic support device.

H. Orthotopic liver transplantation (OLT)
Every patient with ALF should be evaluated and listed for OLT as early as possible, generally at admission, even when the need for liver transplantation is still controversial.

Transplantation

Once hepatic coma develops in a patient who ingests *Amanita* mushrooms the chances of survival with medical therapy alone is remote.[26] Candidates for orthotopic liver transplantation will include the following:

1. Patients who experience progression to state II encephalopathy or beyond;
2. Prologation of prothrombin time greater than 2 times normal despite vigorous replacement with fresh-frozen plasma; and
3. Serum bilirubin levels greater than 25 mg/dL.[26]

Other patients with findings such as acidosis, hypoglycemia, gastrointestinal hemorrhage, and hypofibrinogenemia following marked serum aminotransferase elevation should be considered for urgent liver transplantation without waiting for progression to advanced hepatic encephalopathy, azotemia, or jaundice.[27]

Additional suggested criteria for orthotopic liver transplantation (OLT) following Amanita poisoning include peak prothrombin time less than 10% (>100 sec), factor V concentration less than 10%, lactic acidosis, gastrointestinal bleeding, and age less than 12 years. When OLT may be indicated, there does not appear to be a risk of intoxication from the transplanted liver, because, after day 4, no further circulating amatoxins are detected.[28] Guidelines for surveillance of patients who may need OLT should include repeated clinical examinations, prothrombin times, factor V, pH, blood lactose, EEG, and liver echography.[26,27,29]

A 4-year-old child in a coma after ingesting *Amanita phalloides* received an orthotopic liver transplant 70 hours after ingestion and regained consciousness in 24 hours.[30]

GYROMITRIN (GROUP II)
Clinical Presentation (Fig. 74–13)

Two patients who ate about 10 *Gyromitra esculenta* mushrooms developed moderate liver damage with the signs of hemolysis. One patient was treated with combined hemodialysis and hemoperfusion, together with pyridoxine 25 mg/kg and symptomatic therapy.[31] *Lycoperdon* are mushroom species belonging to the Basidiomycete family.[32,33] Puff balls are usually safe, but may produce nausea and vomiting within 6 to 12 hours after exposure and respiratory symptoms (e.g., shortness of breath), fever (up to

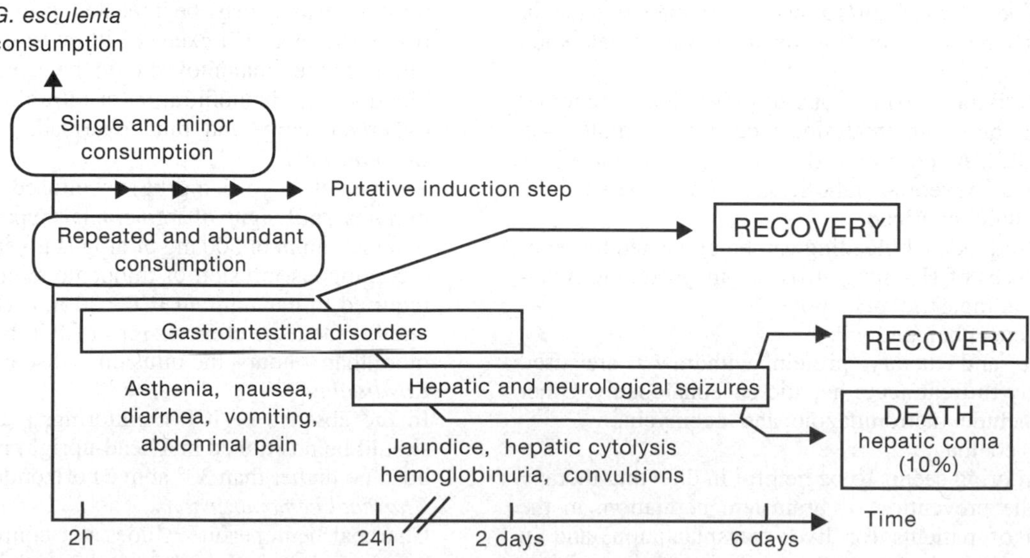

Figure 74–13 Chronology and development of *Gyromitra esculenta* poisoning. (Adapted from Michelot D, Toth B. J Appl Toxicol 1991;11:235–243.)

103°F), myalgia, and fatigue within 3 to 7 days following inhalation and ingestion.[34] The respiratory symptoms (lycoperdonosis) may include symptoms of pneumonia and widespread nodular densities on an x-ray of the lungs. One puff ball species (*L. marginatum*) can produce psychoactive effects.[35] Biopsy specimens of the lung reveal an inflammatory process and the presence of yeastlike structures consistent with *Lycoperdon* spores. Patients recover within 1 to 4 weeks with no apparent sequela.[32,36,37]

Laboratory

Methemoglobin may be detected early in the course of the poisoning and is an indicator of MMH exposure. Free hemoglobin may be detected early in the poisoning. There are few clinical studies that have evaluated methemoglobinemia in *Gyromitra esculenta* poisoning.[38]

MUSCARINIC POISONING (GROUP IV)

Elevated levels of liver function tests and hypokalemia have been observed after jack o'lantern mushroom poisoning (*Omphalotus illudens).*[39] Ingestions of nine jack o'lantern mushrooms *(Omphalotus illudens)* by 14 people led to vomiting in eight, diarrhea in five, weakness in two; tiredness and the feeling of being cold occurred in eight. Recovery was complete within 18 hours.[40] Seven adults who ingested jack o'lantern mushrooms experienced nausea, vomiting, abdominal cramping, diarrhea, weakness, dizziness, and diaphoresis. All symptoms began within 15 to 90 minutes after ingestion. Three had mildly elevated liver function tests; one had hypokalemia requiring potassium supplementation. All were given IV fluids and oral activated charcoal. They were discharged the following day.[39]

GROUP V

Amanita pantherina often contains compounds, in addition to ibotenic acid and miscimol (found also in *A. muscarina*), such as stizolobic and stizolobinic acid in concentrations that may be clinically significant. These compounds are related to L-dopa oxidation products and can produce anticholinergic effects.[41–43]

HALLUCINOGENIC MUSHROOMS (GROUP VI)

The adolescent substance abuser when seen in a state of panic may have ingested hallucinogenic mushrooms possibly with simultaneous LSD, alcohol, PCP, and marijuana.[44]

A number of other plants can be considered to be agents of abuse and are often taken in combination with other pharmacologically active substances. This group includes jimsonweed (*Datura stramonium*); nutmeg *(Myristica fragrans)*—active ingredients myristica, elemicine, eugenol, safrole, and botrenol; morning glory *(Ipomoea tricolori*—active ingredients, various amides of lysergic acid; ololiuqui *(Rivea corymbosa)*—active ingredient 0.5% total indole alkaloids in the seeds; khat (*Catha edulis*—active ingredients phenylethylamines; peyote *(Lophophora williamsii)*—active ingredient mescaline. Other plants of abuse are listed in Table 74–3.[45]

GASTROENTERITIS-PRODUCING MUSHROOMS (GROUP VII)

Clinical Presentation

A 6-year-old presented with hypotension, lethargy, and shallow respirations. This followed an episode of abdominal pain and diarrhea which began 1.5 hours after ingestion of *Chlorophyllum molybdites (Lepiota morgani*). She was treated symptomatically with IV fluids, pressor amines, activated charcoal, IV ranitidine, and penicillin G. She recovered in 3 days.[46] Gastrointestinal hemorrhage with disseminated intravascular coagulation has followed ingestion of *Chlorophyllum molybdites.*[47]

CORTINARIUS (GROUP VIII)

Toxin

The chronology and development of poisoning by *Cortinarius* mushrooms is depicted in Figure 74–12.[48]

Twenty-six young men ingested mushroom soup made only with *Cortinarius orellanus.* They were hospitalized 10 to 12 days after the incident: 12 presented with acute tubulointerstitial nephritis with acute renal failure; eight required hemodialysis; nine were given corticosteroids. Of these 12, eight patients recovered rapidly; four suffered from chronic renal failure for several months.[49]

The presence of normal liver function together with the delayed acute renal failure (up to 20 days after ingestion), abdominal pain, and burning thirst characterize the symptom complex. Orellanine, the toxin thought to cause tubulointerstitial nephritis, and orelline may be isolated from urine, serum, and feces.[50]

Orellanine can be detected by fluorometry after thin-layer chromatography.[51] The assay sensitivity for orellanine and orelline is 10 ng.[52]

SUGGESTED READING

1. Koppel C. Clinical symptomatology and management of mushroom poisoning. Toxicon 1993;31:1513–1540.

REFERENCES—MUSHROOMS

1. Trestrail JH. Mushroom poisoning in the United States. An analysis of 1989. United States Poison Center data. Clin Toxicol 1991;29:459–465.
2. Margot P, Farquhar G, Watling R. Identification of toxic mushrooms and toadstools (Agarics). An on-line identification program. In: Allkin R, Bisby FA, eds. Databases in systematics. London: Academic Press, 1984.
3. Hogue K. Another look at mushrooms. Rocky Mountain Poison Center Bulletin. 1988;7(2):6–7.
4. Pickering CAC. Mushrooms and the lungs. J R Soc Med 1987;80:667.
5. Tarvainmen K, Salonen J-P, Kanerva L, Estlander T, Keskinen H, Rantanen P. Allergic and toxicoderma from shitake mushrooms. J Am Acad Dermatol 1991;24:64–66.
6. Satre J, Ibanez MD, Lopez M, Lehrer SB. Respiratory and immunological reactions among shitake *(Lentinus edodes)* mushroom workers. Clin Exp Allergy 1990;20:13–19.
7. Phillips MS, Robinson AA, Higenbottom TW, Calder IM. Mushroom compost workers' lung. J R Soc Med 1987;80: 674–677.
8. Nakazawa T, Tochigi T. Hypersensitivity pneumonitis due to mushroom *(Pholiata mameko)* spores. Chest 1989;95: 149–151.

9. Lampe KF, McCann MA. Differential diagnosis of poisoning by North American mushrooms with particular emphasis on *Amanita phalloides*-like intoxication. Ann Emerg Med 1987;16:956–962.
10. Hall AH, Spoerke DG, Rumack BH. Mushroom poisoning. Identification, diagnosis and treatment. Pediatr 1987;8:291–298.
11. Lincoff G. Presentation. Mushroom workshop. International Congress of Clinical Toxicology. September 9, 1993.
12. Koppel C. Clinical symptomatology and management of mushroom poisoning. Toxicon 1993;31:1513–1540.
13. Jaeger A, Jehl F, Flesch F, Sauder P, Kopferschmitt J. Kinetics of amatoxins in human poisoning: therapeutic complications. Clin Toxicol 1993;31:63–80.
14. Floerscheim GL. Influence of ethanol on toxicity of paraquat and *Amanita phalloides.* Lancet 1992;339:437.
15. Belliardo F, Massano G, Accomo S. Amatoxins do not cross the placental barrier. Lancet 1982;1:11387.
16. Paydras S, Kocak R, Erturk F, Erken E, Zaksu KS, Gurcay A. Poisoning due to amatoxin-containing *Lepiota* species. Br J Clin Pract 1990;4:450–453.
17. Jehl F, Gallion C, Birchel P, Jaeger A, Flesch F, Minck R. Determination of alpha-amantin and beta-amantin in human biological fluids by high performance liquid chromatographic determination with amperometric detection of alpha-amantin in human plasma based on its voltametric study. J Chromatogr Biomed Appl 1991;563:299–311.
18. Jehl F, Gallion C, Birckel P, Jaeger A, Flesch F, Minck R. Determination of alpha-amanitin and beta-amanitin in human biological fluids by high performance liquid chromatography. Anal Biochem 1985;149:35–42.
19. Becker CE, Tong TG, Boerner V et al. Diagnosis and treatment of *Amanita phalloides*-type mushroom poisoning. West J Med 1976;125:100–109.
20. Feinfeld DA, Mofenson HC, Caraccio T, Kee M. Poisoning by amatoxin-containing mushrooms in suburban New York—report of four cases. Clin Toxicol 1994;31(6):715–721.
21. Ponikvar R, Drinovec J, Kandus A, Varl J, Gucek A, Malovich M. Plasma exchange in management of severe acute poisoning with *Amanita phalloides.* Prog Clin Biol Res 1990;337: 327–329.
22. Mecuriali F, Sirchia G. Plasma exchange for mushroom poisoning. Transfusion 1977;17:644–646.
23. Floerscheim GL. Treatment of human amatoxin mushroom poisoning: myths and advances in therapy. Med Toxicol 1987;2:1–9.
24. Neftel K, Keusch G, Cottagnoud P, Widner U, Hany M et al. Sind cephalosporine bei der intoxikation mit knollenblatterplilz besser winksam als penicillin-G? Schweiz Med Wochenschr 1988:118:49–51.
25. Caraceni P, Van Thiel DH. Acute liver failure. Lancet 1995; 345:163–169.
26. Klein AS, Hart J, Brens JJ, Goldstein L, Lewin K, Busuttil RW. Amanita poisoning: treatment and the role of liver transplantation. Am J Med 1989;66:187–193.
27. Pinson CW, Daya MR, Benner KG, Norton RL, Deveney KE, Aschen ML, Roberts PL et al. Liver transplantation for severe *Amanita phalloides* mushroom poisoning. Am J Surg 1990; 159:493–499.
28. Jaeger A, Jehl F, Flesch F, Sander P, Kopferschmitt J, Minck R, Mantz JM. Amatoxin kinetics in *Amanita phalloides* poisoning. Vet Hum Toxicol 1989;31:360.
29. Jaeger A, Kopferschmitt J, Flesch F, Berton C, Leveres H, Sander P. Liver transplantation for *Amanita* poisoning. Proc Eur Assoc Pois Cont Cent Toxicol XV Congress, Istanbul, May 24-27, 1992; p. 103.
30. Kern C, Zilker T, Clarmann M. Successful liver transplantation in a child after *Amanita* poisoning. Proc Eur Assoc Pois Cont Centers Toxicol XV congress, Istanbul, Turkey, May 24–27, 1992; p. 126.
31. Zilker T, v Clarmann M, Felgenhaser N, Hibler A. A rarity in Western Europe: a mushroom poisoning with *Gyromitra esculenta.* Proc XIV Internat Congress Eur Assoc Pois Control Centers. Milan, Italy, Sept. 25–29, 1990; p. 98.
32. Lincoff G, Mitchel DH. Toxic and hallucinogenic mushroom poisoning. A handbook for physicians and mushroom hunters. New York: Van Nostrand Reinhold, 1977; pp. 156–157.
33. Lewis WH, Elvin-Lewis MPF. Medical botany. Plants affecting man's health. New York: John Wiley, 1977; p. 398.
34. Vachuska C, Vachuska P. "Puff ball madness" or "How low can you go to get high." The spore print. J Los Angeles Mycolog Soc. #201, December 1994 (Biology Department, California State University, 5151 State University Drive, Los Angeles, CA).
35. Henriksen NT. Lycoperdonosis. Acta Paediatr Scand 1976; 65:643–645.
36. CDC. MMWR. Respiratory illness associated with inhalation of mushroom spores—Wisconsin, 1994. JAMA 1994;272: 508.
37. Strand RD, Neuhausen EBD, Sornberger CF. Lycoperdonosis. N Engl J Med 1967;277:89–91.
38. Lincoff G, Mitchell DH. Toxic and hallucinogenic mushroom poisoning. A handbook for physicians and mushroom hunters. New York: Van Nostrand Reinhold, 1977; pp. 19; 190–191; 49–61.
39. Vanden Hoek LL, Erickson T, Hryhorczuk D, Narasimhan K. Jack O'Lantern mushroom poisoning. Ann Emerg Med 1991; 20:559–561.
40. Cochran KW. Mushroom poisoning case registry. JAMA 1984;252:1685.
41. Chilton WS, Ott J. Toxic metabolites of *Amanita pantherina, A. cothurnata, A. muscarina* and other *Amanita* species. Lloydia 1976;39:150–157.
42. Clitton WS, Hsu CP, Zdybak WT. Stizolobic and Stizolobinic acid: L-dopa oxidation products of *A. pantherina.* Phytochemistry 1974;13:1179–1181.
43. Benjamin DR. Mushroom poisoning in infants and children. The *Amanita pantherina/muscarina* group. Clin Toxicol 1992; 30:13–22.
44. Schwartz PH, Smith DE. Hallucinogenic mushrooms. Clin Pediatr 1888;27:70–73.
45. Spoerke DG, Hall AH. Plants and mushrooms of abuse. Emerg Clin North Am 1990;8:579–593.
46. Stenklyft PH, Augenstein WL. *Chlorophyllum molybdites*-severe mushroom poisoning in a child. Clin Toxicol 1990;28: 159–168.
47. Levitan D, Macy JI, Weissman J. Mechanism of gastrointestinal hemorrhage in a case of mushroom poisoning by *Chlorophyllum molybdites.* Toxicon 1981;19:179–180.
48. Michelot D, Tebbett I. Poisoning by member of the genus *Cortinarius*—a review. Mycol Res 1990;94:289–298.
49. Bouget J, Bousser J, Pats B, Ramee M-P, Chevet D, Rifle G et al. Acute renal failure following collective intoxication by *Cortinarius orellanus.* Intensive Care Med 1990;16:506–510.
50. Moore B, Burton BT, Lindgren J, Rieders F, Kuehnel E, Fisher P. *Cortinarius* mushroom poisoning resulting in anuric renal failure. Vet Hum Toxicol 1991;33:360.
51. Andar C, Rapior S, Delpech N, Huchard G. Laboratory confirmation of *Cortinarius* poisoning. Lancet 1989;1:213.
52. Lampe KF, Ammirati JF. Human poisoning by mushrooms in the genus *Cortinarius.* Mellrainea 1990;9:225.

Appendix A
Poison Information Sources

GENERAL

Local and Regional Poison Information Centers
Poison Information Center Newsletters
POISINDEX—MICROMEDEX INC.
660 Bannock Street, Suite 350
Denver, CO 80204
(800) 525-9083
TOXIFILE—Chicago Micro Corporation
3525 West Petersen Avenue
Chicago, IL 60659
(312) 583-8150, (800) 572-1239
VIEW DATA SYSTEM—Scottish Poisons
Information Bureau
Royal Infirmary
Edinburgh
EH3 9YW, Scotland

INFORMATION RESOURCE AGENCIES

Agency for Toxic Substances and Disease Registry (ATSDR)
Emergency Response Coordinators—24 hours
(404) 452-4100 days
(404) 329-2888 nights, weekends
Cancer Information Service
(National Cancer Institute)
Office of Cancer Communication
NCI Building 31, Room 10A18
Bethesda, MD 20205
(800) 4-CANCER
5:00 am to 9:00 pm (California time)
Center for Occupational Hazards
(Art Hazards Information Center)
5 Beekman Street
New York, NY 10038
(212) 227-6220
10:00 am to 5:00 pm, Monday-Friday
Chemical Transportation Emergency Center (CHEMTREC)
2501 M Street, NW
Washington, DC 20037
(800) 424-9300, (202) 887-1100
24 hours
Chevron/Ortho Emergency Information Center
(415) 233-3737 (collect)
24 hours
Drug Abuse Warning Network (DAWN)
Division of Epidemiology and Statistical Analysis
National Institute on Drug Abuse
Rockville, MD 20857
(301) 443-6504, (301) 443-6543
National Center for Drugs and Biologics, HFN-310
Food and Drug Administration
5600 Fishers Lane, Rockville, MD 20857
(301) 443-2895
National Institute for Environmental Health Sciences (NIEHS)
Dr. Edward Gardner, Jr., Program Director
Research Grants Programs
Extramural Program
NIEHS
PO Box 12233
Research Triangle Park, NC 27709
(919) 541-3345
8:30 am to 5:00 pm
National Pesticide Telecommunications Network
Department of Preventive Medicine
School of Medicine
Texas Technical University Health Sciences Center
Lubbock, TX 79430
(800) 858-7378 (toll-free in US)
(806) 743-3091 (outside of US, non-toll free)
24 hours
National Response Center
(Oil and Chemical Spills)
US Coast Guard Headquarters
2100 2nd Street, SW, Room 2611
Washington, DC 20590
(800) 424-8802, (202) 426-2675
24 hours
Office of Toxic Substances
(Environmental Protection Agency)
401 M Street, SW
Washington, DC 20460
(202) 382-3813

Office of Consumer Affairs, HFE-88
Food and Drug Administration
5600 Fishers Lane, Rockville, MD 20857
US Agency for Toxic Substances and Disease Registry
Atlanta, GA 30333
Emergency Response
(404) 452-4100, (404) 329-2888 (24 hours)
(415) 974-8927 (California)

GOVERNMENT AGENCIES

Washington Area
Food and Drug Administration
Office of Consumer Affairs (HFE-88)
5600 Fishers Lane
Rockville, MD 20857
(301) 443-3170
Food and Safety Inspection Service
US Department of Agriculture
Meat and Poultry Hotline
Room 1163S
Washington, DC 20250
(800) 535-4555
Animal and Plant Health Inspection Service (Animal Vaccines)
US Department of Agriculture
Washington, DC 20250
(202) 436-8633
Federal Trade Commission
6th Street and Pennsylvania Avenue, NE
Washington, DC 20580
(202) 523-3598
Bureau of Alcohol, Tobacco, and Firearms
Room 4402
Ariel Rios Federal Building
1200 Pennsylvania Avenue, NW
Washington, DC 20226
(202) 566-7135
Consumer Product Safety Commission
Washington, DC 20207
(800) 638-CPSC
Drug Enforcement Administration
US Department of Justice
1405 Eye Street, NW
Washington, DC 20537
(202) 633-1000
National Institute on Drug Abuse
5600 Fishers Lane, Room 10A43
Rockville, MD 20857
(301) 443-6500
Environmental Protection Agency
401 M Street, SW
Washington, DC 20460
(202) 829-3535
Nuclear Regulatory Commission
Office of Public Affairs
Washington, DC 20555
(202) 492-7715
National Marine Fisheries Service
US Department of Commerce
Washington, DC 20235
(202) 634-7111
National Institute for Occupational Safety and Health
NIOSH Regional Offices
(513) 533-8236
Boston
HHS, PHS, CDC, NIOSH, Region I
JFK Federal Building, Room 1401
Boston, MA 02203
(617) 223-4045
Atlanta
HHS, PHS, CDC, NIOSH
101 Marietta Tower, Suite 1007
Atlanta, GA 30323
(404) 221-2396
Denver
HHS, PHS, CDC, NIOSH, Region VIII
1194 Federal Office Building
Denver, CO 80294
(303) 837-6382
1994 Annual Report of American Association of Poison Control Centers
Litovitz TL, Felberg L, Soloway RA, Ford M, Geller R
Toxic Exposure Surveillance System
American Journal of Emergency Medicine 1995; 13: 551-597.
European Association of Poison Centres and Clinical Toxicologists
Vale JA
National Poisons Information Service
West Midlands Poison Unit
Dudley Road Hospital
Birmingham B18 7QH, United Kingdom

Appendix B Guidelines for Disposition of the Poisoned Patient in the Emergency Department

Admissions Criteria for the Hospitalization of a Poisoned Patient to a Monitored Bed[1,2]:

1. All suicide attempts—obtain psychiatric consultation.
2. Life-threatening signs and symptoms, e.g., hypotension, seizures, arrhythmias, increased respiratory rate or temperature, altered mental status, visual complaints, coma, intubation, significant fluid losses, electrolyte imbalance, rhabdomyolysis.
3. Manifestations of allergy or hypersensitivity: immediate threat of anaphylaxis or angioneurotic edema.
4. Any ingestion of unknown amounts of a potentially dangerous poison in a child.
5. Child who requires antidotal therapy.
6. Child who comes from a home environment not considered to be safe.
7. The patient who has received *physostigmine.*
8. History of ingestion of an *extended release preparation.*
9. Any patient requiring hyperbaric oxygen who exhibits an acidosis, carboxyhemoglobin level greater than 20% after *carbon monoxide* exposure.
10. Body stuffers of *cocaine* until all packets are passed.
11. Ingestion of *acetonitrile-containing* compounds.
12. *Paralytic shellfish poisoning* or *tetrodotoxin* exposure with respiratory depression.
13. *Hydrocarbons:* Symptoms during first 6 hours of observation after a hydrocarbon ingestion.
14. *Iron:* Child requiring intravenous chelation for iron poisoning.
15. *Isoniazid:* Symptomatic patients.
16. Symptomatic *methemoglobinemia* in children (levels over 20% in patients requiring methylene blue administration).
17. Symptomatic child with acute *neuroleptic poisoning.*
18. *Snakebites* requiring antivenom.

Emergency Department Observation for About 6 to 8 Hours Followed by Discharge:

1. No overt signs of toxicity after decontamination and administration of activated charcoal.
2. Toxic agent ingested is not a sustained-release product.
3. *Methanol:* no evidence of acidosis, blood levels below 10 mg/dL.
4. *Cyclic antidepressant poisoning* with no tachycardia, QRS widening, anticholinergic symptoms or drowsiness.

Note: See test for more specific recommendations relating to poisoning.

REFERENCES

1. Tintinalli JE, Ruiz E, Krome RL, eds. Emergency medicine. A comprehensive study guide. 4th ed. New York: McGraw-Hill, 1996.
2. Strange GR, Ahrens W, Lelyveld S, Schafermeyer R, eds. Pediatric emergency medicine. A comprehensive study guide. New York: McGraw-Hill, 1996.

Appendix C
Toxicological Profiles: ATSDR

Table C–1
Toxicologic Profiles (as of May 1994)[a]

Acetone	May, 1994
Carbon tetrachloride (update)	May, 1994
Chlordane (update)	May, 1994
Chlorodibenzofurans	May, 1994
4,4′DDT-4,4′-DDE,4,4′DDD (update)	May, 1994
Hexchlorobutadiene	May, 1994
Alpha-, beta-, gamma- and delta-hexachlorocyclo-hexane (update)	May, 1994
Methoxychlor	May, 1994
4-4′-Methylenebis-(2-chloraniline) (MBOCA)	May, 1994

[a]Adapted from US Department of Health and Human Services. Agency for Toxic Substances and Disease Registry. Division of Toxicology/Toxicology Information Branch, 1600 Clifton Road NE, E29, Atlanta, GA 30333.

Table C–2
Toxicologic Profiles (as of June 1995)[a]

Automotive gasoline	June, 1995
Diethyl phthalate	June, 1995
Fuel oils	June, 1995
Jet fuels (JP4 and JPT)	June, 1995
Otto fuels II	June, 1995
RDX	June, 1995
Stoddard Solvent	June, 1995
Tetryl	June, 1995
1,3-Dinitrobenzene/1,3,5-trinitrobenzene	June, 1995
2,4,6-Trinitrotoluene	June, 1995

[a]Adapted from US Department of Health and Human Services. Agency for Toxic Substances and Disease Registry. Division of Toxicology/Toxicology Information Branch, 1600 Clifton Road NE, E29, Atlanta, GA 30333.

Table C–3
Toxicologic Profiles (as of August 1995)[a]

Asbestos
Benzidine (update)
Dinitrocresols
Dinitrophenols
Disulfoton
Mirex and chlordecone
Naphthalene (update)
Polycyclic aromatic hydrocarbons (PAHS) (update)
Polybrominated biphenyls (PBBS)
1,1,1-Trichloroethane (update)
Xylenes (update)

[a]Adapted from US Department of Health and Human Services. Agency for Toxic Substances and Disease Registry. Division of Toxicology/Toxicology Information Branch, 1600 Clifton Road NE, E29, Atlanta, GA 30333.

Appendix D General References/ Additional Suggested Readings

Listed below are some useful references in addition to those cited in each chapter:

Reynolds JEF, ed: Martindale. The extra pharmacopoeia. 13th ed. London: The Pharmaceutical Press, 1993.

Dollery C, ed. Therapeutic drugs. Edinburgh: Churchill Livingstone, 1991 (2 vol: Supplement one 1992, Supplement two 1994).

Feely J, ed. New drugs. 3rd ed. London: BMJ Publishing Group, 1994. ISBN 0 7279-0821-9.

Proceedings. 4th International Symposium on Protection Against Chemical Warfare Agents. Stockholm, Sweden, June 8–12, 1992. ISSN 0281-0220.

Baselt RC, Crayey RH, eds. Disposition of toxic drugs and chemicals in man. 3rd ed. Chicago: Yearbook, 1989. ISBN 0-8151-0547-9.

Hoffman RS, Goldfrank LP, eds. Contemporary management in critical care. Critical care toxicology. New York: Churchill Livingstone, 1991. ISBN 0-443-00830-6. ISSN 1050-9623.

Clinical pharmacokinetics. Drug data handbook. 2nd ed. Auckland: ADIS Press, 1990.

British National Formulary, 1994. London: John Feely, Smith, BMJ Publishing Group, 1994. ISBN 0-7279-08219.

Last JM, Wallace RB, eds. Maxey-Rosenau-Last. Public health and preventive medicine. 13th ed. Norwalk: Appleton and Lange, 1992. ISBN 0-8385-6188-8.

Gopalakrishnakone P, Chou LM, eds. Snakes of medical importance (Asia Pacific region). Venom and Toxin Research Group. National University of Singapore, 1990. ISBN 9971-62-217-3.

Sullivan JB Jr, Krieger GR, eds. Hazardous materials toxicology. Baltimore: Williams & Wilkins, 1992. ISBN 0-683-08025-3.

Goldfrank's toxicologic emergency. 5th ed. Norwalk: Appleton-Lange, 1994. ISBN 0-8384-3146-6.

Reisdorff EJ, Roberts MR, Wiegenstein JG, eds. Pediatric emergency medicine. Philadelphia: WB Saunders, 1993. ISBN 0-7216-3281-5.

Melmon and Morellis clinical pharmacology. Basic principles in therapeutics. 3rd ed. New York: McGraw-Hill, 1992. ISBN 0-07-105385-9.

Reproductive health hazards in the workplace. Office of Technology Assessment Task Force. London: JB Lippincott, 1988. ISBN 0-397-53003-4.

Levine DP, Sobel JD, eds. Infections in intravenous drug abusers. New York: Oxford University Press, 1991. ISBN 0-19-506223-X.

Koren G (ed). Maternal-fetal toxicology. A clinician's guide. New York: Marcel Dekker, 1990. ISBN 0-8247-8173-9.

Long JW. Clinical management of prescription drugs. Philadelphia: Harper and Row, 1984. ISBN 0-016-141555-3.

Zollo AJ Jr. Medical secrets. Philadelphia: Hanley & Belfus, 1991. ISBN 1-56053-011-1 (paper).

Gopalakrishnakone P, Tam CK, eds. Recent advances in toxicology research. Vol 1, 2, 3. Singapore: Venom and Toxin Research Group, National University of Singapore, 1992.

Leikin JB, Paloucek FB. Poisoning and toxicology handbook 1995–96. Hudson, OH: Leni-Comp, 1995.

Ford MD, Olshaker JC. Concepts and controversies in toxicology. Emerg Med Clin North Am 1994; 12:285–570.

Bismuth C, Hall AH, eds. Paraquat poisoning. Mechanism, prevention, treatment. New York: Marcel Dekker, 1995.

Proudfoot AT. Acute poisoning. Diagnosis and management. 2nd ed. Oxford: Butterworth Heinemann, 1993.

Rodgers GC Jr, Matyunas NU, eds. Handbook of common poisonings in children. 3rd ed. Elk Grove, Il.: American Academy of Pediatrics, 1994.

Viccellio P, eds. Handbook of medical toxicology. Boston: Little, Brown, 1993.

Olson KR, eds. Poisoning and drug overdose. 2nd ed. Prentice-Hall International, 1994.

Johnson KB, ed. The Harriett Lave handbook. A manual for pediatric house officers. 13th ed. St. Louis: Mosby, 1993.

Benitz WE, Tatro DS. The pediatric drug handbook. 2nd ed. Chicago: Year Book, 1988.

Cooper MR, Johnson AW. Poisonous plants and fungi. An illustrated guide. Ministry of Agricultural Fisheries and Food. London: Her Majesty's Stationery Office, 1988.

Spoerke DJ Jr, Smolinske SC: Toxicity of houseplants. Boca Raton, FL: CRC Press, 1990.

Phelps T. Poisonous snakes. Revised ed. London: Blandford Press, 1989.

Sutherland SK. Australian animal toxins. Oxford: Oxford University Press, 1983.

Wilson JD et al, eds. Harrison's principles of internal medicine. 12th ed. New York: McGraw-Hill, 1991.

Humphreys DJ. Veterinary toxicology. 3rd ed. London: Baillière Tindall, 1988.

McEvoy GK, ed. AHFS drug information 94. Bethesda: American Society of Hospital Pharmacists, 1994.

Occupational safety and health guidelines for chemical hazards DHHS (NIOSH). Publication No. 89-104, Supplement II-OHG. Cincinnati: US Department of Health and Human Services, National Institute for Occupational Safety and Health, 1988.

Chemical data guide for bulk shipment by water. US Department of Transportation. United States Coast Guard. Marine Technical and Hazardous Materials Division. Commandant Instruction No. 16616.68. Washington: Superintendent of Documents, 1990.

Meredith TJ, Jacobsen D, Haines JA, Berger J-C, Van Heijst ANP, eds. IPCS/CED Evaluation of Antidotes Series. 1. Naloxone, flumazenil and dantrolene as antidotes, 1993; 2. Antidotes for poisoning by cyanide, 1993; Antidotes for poisoning by paracetamol, 1995. Cambridge: Cambridge University Press.

Barash PG, Cullen BF, Stoelting: Handbook of clinical anesthesia. New York: JB Lippincott, 1991.
Gopalakrishnakone P, Tan CK, eds. Progress in venom and toxin research. Venom and Toxin Research Group. National University of Singapore, 1987.
Blumer JL, Bond GR, ed. Toxic effects of drugs used in the ICU. Crit Care Clin 1991;7:489–762.
Yinon J. Toxicity and metabolism of explosives. Boca Raton, FL: CRC Press, 1990.
Notten WRF, Herber RFM, Hunter WJ, Monster AC, Zielhuis RL, eds. Health surveillance of individual workers exposed to chemical agents. Berlin: Springer-Verlag, 1986. ISBN 3-540-19016-3; ISBN 0-387-19016-3.
Plunkett EF. Handbook of industrial toxicology. New York: Chemical Publisher, 1976. ISBN 085501-214-5.
Ballantyne B, Marrs TC. Clinical and experimental toxicology of organophosphates and carbamates. Oxford: Butterworth-Heinemann, 1992.
Clinical Toxicology Reviews. Coordinators: McGuigan MA, Gaudreault P, Woolf A. Boston: Massachusetts Poison Control System (published monthly).
Wexler P. Information resources in toxicology. 2nd ed. New York: Elsevier Science, 1988.
Hathaway GL, Proctor NH, Hughes JP, Fischman ML, eds. Proctor and Hughes chemical hazards of the workplace. 3rd ed. New York: Van Nostrand Reinhold, 1991.
Hall JB, Schmidt GA, Wood LD, eds. Principles of critical care. New York: McGraw-Hill, 1992.
Mandell GL, Douglas RG, Bennett JE, eds. Antiinfective therapy. New York: John Wiley, 1985. ISBN 0-47-80442-8.
Barsan WG, Jastremski MS, Syverud SA, eds. Emergency drug therapy. Philadelphia: WB Saunders, 1991. ISBN 0-7216-2584-3.
Powis G, Hacker MP, eds. The toxicity of anticancer drugs. New York: Pergamon Press, 1991. ISBN 0-08-040302-6 (hardcover).
Matossian MK. Poisons of the past. Molds, epidemics and history. New Haven: Yale University Press, 1989. ISBN 0-300-03942-9 (paper).
Gunther FA, ed. Residue reviews. Vol 89. New York: Springer-Verlag, 1983. ISBN 0-387-90884-6; ISBN 3-540-90884-6.
Noji EK, Kelen GD, eds. Manual of toxicologic emergencies. Chicago: Year Book, 1989. ISBN 0-8151-6450-5.
Dawood R. Travellers' health. How to stay healthy abroad. Oxford: Oxford University Press, 1989. ISBN 0-19-261831-8.
Organochlorine solvents. Health risks to workers. Brussels, Belgium: Royal Society of Chemistry, 1986. ISBN 0-8586-078-8.
Solvents in common use. Health risks and worker. Brussels, Belgium: 1988. ISBN 0-85186-088-5.
Woolf AD, Shannon MW. Clinical toxicology for the pediatrician. Pediatr Clin North Am 1995; 42:317–333.
Fine JS, Goldfrank LR. Update in medical toxicology. Pediatr Clin North Am 1992; 39:1031–1051.
Litovitz TL, Felberg L, Soloway RA, Ford M, Geller R. Annual report of the American Association of Poison Control Centers, 1994. Toxic exposure surveillance system. Am J Emerg Med 1995;13:551–597.
Vale JA. Clinical toxicology. Postgrad Med J 1993;69:19–32.
Liebelt EL, Shannon MW. Small doses, big problems: a selected review of highly toxic common medications. Pediatr Emerg Care 1993;9:292–297.
Bjorn Ekwall. MEIC monographs on time-related, high survival and lethal blood concentrations of chemicals from acute human poisonings. Uppsala, Sweden: Dept of Pharmaceutical Biosciences. Division of Toxicology, Uppsala University, BMC, Box 594, 1995.
Mofenson HC et al, eds. Poison perspectives for health professionals. LI Regional Poison Control Centers at Winthrop-University Hospital.
Tintinalli JE, Ruiz E, Krome RL, eds. Emergency medicine. A comprehensive study guide. 4th ed. New York: McGraw-Hill, 1996.
Strange GR, Ahrens W, Lelyveld S, Schafermeyer R, eds. Pediatric emergency medicine. A comprehensive study guide. New York: McGraw-Hill, 1996.
Mettler FA Jr, Kelsey CA, Ricks RD. Medical management of pediatric accidents. Boca Raton, FL: CRC Press, 1990.
Ricks RC, Fry SA, eds. The medical basis for radiation accident preparedness II. New York: Elsevier, 1990.
National Research Council. Health effects of exposure to low levels of ionizing radiation. BEIR V. Washington, DC: National Academy Press, 1990.
United Nations Scientific Committee on the Effects of Atomic Radiation. Sources, effects and risks of ionizing radiation. New York: United Nations, 1988.
Guidelines for protecting the safety and health of health care workers. National Institute for Occupational Safety and Health. Washington: Superintendent of Documents, 1988.
Bourdeau P, Green G, eds. Methods for assessing and reducing injury for chemical accidents. Scope 40. Chichester: John Wiley, 1989.
Chemical warfare agents. Fourth International Symposium on Protection Proceedings. National Defence Research Establishment Department of NBC Defence. S-900 82, Umea, Sweden: June 1992.
Medical manual of defence against chemical agents. JSP 312. Ministry of Defence. London: Her Majesty's Stationery Office, 1987.
Morgan DR. Recognition and management of pesticide poisonings. 4th ed. Washington, DC: US Environmental Protection Agency, 1989. EA-540/9-88-001.
Somani SM. Chemical warfare agents. San Diego: Academic Press, 1992.
Treatment of chemical agent casualties and conventional military chemical injuries. Army FM 8-285, Navy NaVMed P-5041, Air Force AFM 160-11, Field Manual, Washington, DC: February 1990.

Chapter 1

Fine JS, Goldfrank LR: Update in medical toxicology. Pediatr Clin North Am 1992;39:1031–1051.
Joyce DA, Ilett KF. Therapeutics. What's new? Med J Aust 1994; 161:622–626.
Vale JA. Clinical toxicology. Postgrad Med J 1993;69:19–32.
Liebelt EL, Shannon MW. Small doses, big problems: a selected review of highly toxic common medications. Pediatr Emerg Care 1993;9:292–297.

The Pediatric Patient

Woolf AD, Shannon MW: Clinical toxicology for the pediatrician. Ped Clin North Am 1995;42:317–353.
Jopreiatro JA. Pediatric toxixology: new poisons—new perils. J US Army Med Dept 1993;11–15. PB8-93-9/10, September/October.
Mofenson HC, Caraccio PR. Pediatric medications. NCMC Regional Poison Control Center PP/T News 1990;6:207–217; Update on pediatric poisoning 1995;14:1–17; Update on pediatric poisonings (continued) 1995;14:15–36; 1989;8:128–138; 1993;12:27–46; 1989;8:139–147.

Chapter 2

Binder L, Frederickson L. Poisonings in laboratory personnel and health care professionals. Am J Emerg Med 1991;9:11–15.
Flanagan RJ. The poisoned patients: the role of the laboratory. Br J Biomed Sci 1995;52:202–213.

Chapter 5

Hoffman RS, Goldfrank LP. Poisoned patients with altered consciousness. JAMA 1995;274:562–569.

Chapter 6

Working Group on Status Epilepticus. Treatment of convulsive status epilepticus. Recommendations of the Epilepsy Foundation of America's Working Group on Status Epilepticus. JAMA 1993;270:854–859.
Tunik MG, Young GM. Status epilepticus in children. The acute management. Pediatr Clin North Am 1992;39:1007–1030.

Chapter 7

Slaughter RL, Edwards DJ. Recent advances: the cytochrome P450 enzymes. Ann Pharmacother 1995;29: 619–624.

Chapter 10

Vale JA, Proudfoot AT. Paracetamol (acetaminophen) poisoning. Lancet 1995;346:547–552.

Wendon JA, Ellis A, Williams R. Management of paracetamol poisoning. Lancet 1995;346:1236.

Ward SJ, Connor P, Matthey F. Management of paracetamol poisoning. Lancet 1995;346:1236–1237.

Chapter 15

Drugs for AIDS and associated infections. Med Lett Drugs Ther 1995;37(Issue 959):87–94.

Chapter 19

Braithwaite RA, Jarvie DR, Mintoy PSB, Simpson D, Widdop B. Screening for drugs of abuse. I. Opiates, amphetamines and cocaine. Ann Clin Biochem 1995;32:123–153.

Shesser R, Jotte R, Olshaker J. The contribution of impurities to the acute morbidity of illegal drug use. Am J Emerg Med 1991;9:336–344.

Chapter 21

McCance EF, Price LH, Kosten TR, Jatlow PI. Cocaethylene: pharmacology, physiology and behavioral effects in humans. J Pharmacol Exp Ther 1995;274:215–223.

Cone EJ. Pharmacokinetics and pharmacodynamics of cocaine. J Anal Toxicol 1995;19:459–478.

Chapter 39

Power DM, Hackett LP, Dusci LJ, Ilett KF. Antidepressant toxicity and the need for identification and concentration monitoring in overdose. Clin Pharmacokinet 1995;29:154–171.

Chapter 64

Lesser SH, Weiss SJ. Art hazards. Am J Emerg Med 1995;13: 451–458.

Chapter 66

Chan-Yeung M, Malo J-L. Occupational asthma. N Engl J Med 1995;333:107–112.

Chapter 72

Strong PN. Potassium channel toxins. Pharmacol Ther 1990;46: 137–162.

Appendix E
Pediatric Emergency Drugs

Table E–1
Use of Emergency Drugs in Pediatrics

Drug Generic (Brand)	Preparation	Dose & Route of Administration	Toxicity or Adverse Effects	Contraindications
		Analgesia		
Acetaminophen (Tylenol, Panadol, Tempra, APAP)	Drops: 80 mg/0.8 mL Elixir: 80, 120, 160, 325 mg/5 mL Liquid: 160 mg/5 mL Suppository: 120, 125, 325, 600, 650 mg Tabs: 325, 500, 650 mg	10–15 mg/kg/dose PO q 4 h. Maximum 5 doses in 24 h	Hepatic toxicity in overdose situations; nausea, vomiting, diaphoresis, malaise	Recent (4h) acetaminophen dose, liver disease
Acetylsalicylic acid (ASA, aspirin)	Tabs: 65, 75, 200, 300, 325, 500, 600, 650 mg Suppository: 60, 65, 130, 150, 195, 200, 300, 325, 600 mg	10–15 mg/kg PO q 4 h; maximum 60–80 mg/kg in 24 h or 3.6 g in 24 h	Anaphylactic shock, rash, bleeding, Reye syndrome, salicylism—nausea, vomiting, tinnitus, hearing impairment, headache, dizziness, drowsiness, hyperpnea, hyperventilation, tachycardia, sweating, thirst	Contact with varicella or influenza illnesses, known hypersensitivity, severe bleeding disorder, coagulopathy, severe liver damage, concomitant anticoagulation therapy, peptic ulcer disease
Fentanyl (Sublimaze)	Injection: 50 μg/mL	1–5 μg/kg IV q 30–60 min	Respiratory depression, apnea, muscle rigidity, circulatory depression, bradycardia, nausea, vomiting, cardiopulmonary arrest	Known intolerance; use in monitored setting only
Ibuprofen (Advil, Motrin, Nuprin)	Liquid: 100 mg/5 mL Tabs: 200, 300, 400, 600, 800 mg	10–15 mg/kg/dose PO q 4–6 h	GI hemorrhage, ulcer formation with chronic use, dizziness, nervousness, rash, tinnitus, decreased appetite, edema, bleeding	Known hypersensitivity, syndrome of nasal polyps, angioedema, bronchospasm with ASA or other NSAID, GI hemorrhage or ulcer disease
Ketorolac (Toradol)	Injection: 30, 60 mg	1 mg/kg/dose IM; maximum 60 mg	GI hemorrhage, ulcer formation with chronic use, edema, nausea, dyspepsia, diarrhea, nervousness, dizziness, headache, sweating	Known hypersensitivity, syndrome of nasal polyps, angioedema, bronchospasm with ASA or other NSAID use; not officially approved for use in children
Meperdine (Demerol)	Injection: 10, 25, 50, 75, 100 mg/mL Syrup: 50 mg/5 mL Tabs: 50, 100 mg	1–2 mg/kg IM or IV q 3–4 h	Vomiting, dystonic reactions, paradoxical crying, constipation, hypotension, seizures from toxic intermediary metabolites, respiratory depression	Known hypersensitivity, concomitant use of monoamine oxidase inhibitors

[a]Adapted from Baren JM, Seidel JS. Pediatr Rev 1995;16:229–238.

(continued)

Table E–1 *(Continued)*

Drug Generic (Brand)	Preparation	Dose & Route of Administration	Toxicity or Adverse Effects	Contraindications
		Analgesia *(Continued)*		
Morphine	Injection: 2, 4, 5, 8, 10, 15 mg/mL	0.1–0.2 mg/kg IM, SC, IV, q 2–4 h; maximum 15 mg/dose	Central nervous system and respiratory depression, nausea, vomiting, hypotension, bradycardia, increased intracranial pressure, miosis, biliary or urinary spasm, stiff chest syndrome, histamine release	Altered mental status, hypotension, bradycardia, apnea, or respiratory depression; use in monitored setting only
		Anaphylaxis/Allergic Reaction		
Cimetidine (Tagamet)	Injection: 150 mg/mL	20–40 mg/kg IV divided q 6 h	Diarrhea, dizziness, somnolence, headache, confusion, cardiac arrhythmias with rapid IV bolus	Known hypersensitivity
Methylprednisolone (Solu-Medrol) Hydrocortisone (Solu-Cortef)	Injection: 20, 40, 62.5, 80, 125 mg/mL Single-dose vials of 100, 250, 500, 1000 mg	2 mg/kg IV q 6–8 h 4–8 mg/kg IV q 6 h; maximum dose 250 mg	Sodium and fluid retention, peptic ulcer formation, myopathy, adrenocortical insufficiency, impaired mineralocorticoid secretion, mood lability, suppression of growth and development (full range of effects beyond the scope of this text)	Do not use in preterm infants when preparation contains benzyl alcohol; systemic fungal or other infections; known hypersensitivity; caution in immunosuppressed patients
Diphenydramine (Benadryl, Genahist)	Injection: 10, 50 mg/mL Caps: 25, 50 mg Elixir/Syrup: 12.5 mg/5 mL Tabs: 25, 50 mg	5 mg/kg per 24 h PO, IM divided q 6 h For anaphylaxis: 1–2 mg/kg slow IV push; maximum 300 mg in 24 h	Central nervous system depression, incoordination, hallucinations, coma, urticaria, hypotension, tachycardia, headache, epigastric distress, thickening of bronchial secretions	Altered mental status, newborn or preterm infants, known hypersensitivity
Epinephrine	Injection 1:1000 (1 mg/mL)	Infusion: 0.1–0.4 µg/kg/min, 0.01 mg/kg SC; maximum 0.3 mL = 0.3 mg	Palpitations, tachycardia, sweating, nausea, vomiting, cardiac arrhythmias	No contraindications in life-threatening situations; tachyarrhythmias
Hydroxyzine (Vistaril, Atarax)	Injection: 25, 50 mg/mL	0.5–1 mg/kg q 4–6 h IV	Dizziness, dry mouth, tremor, blurred vision	Concurrent barbiturate use
		Cyanosis		
Morphine	(See under Analgesia)			
Oxygen	100% concentration	Deliver by nasal cannula (16 L/min), face mask (10 L/min), or ETT (100%)	Dry mucous membranes	Caution: F_{IO_2} level may need to be adjusted for patients who have COPD
		Dehydration		
Fluids	Normal saline	20 mg/kg boluses IV as needed	Pulmonary edema, IV infiltration, fluid overload	Use judiciously in congestive heart failure and renal failure

(continued)

Table E–1 *(Continued)*

Drug Generic (Brand)	Preparation	Dose & Route of Administration	Toxicity or Adverse Effects	Contraindications
		Fever		
Acetaminophen; acetylsalicylic acid; ibuprofen	(See under Analgesia)			
		Hyperglycemia		
Insulin	Regular 100 U/mL	0.1 U/kg IV bolus then 0.1 U/kg/h IV infusion	Sweating, syncope, altered mental status, hypoglycemia	Hypoglycemia
		Hypertension		
Furosemide (Lasix)	Injection: 10 mg/mL Oral: 10 mg/mL, 40 mg/5 mL Tabs: 20, 40, 80 mg	1 mg/kg IM, IV q 6–12 h prn; maximum dose 600 mg in 24 h; 2 mg/kg PO	Electrolyte depletion, alkalosis, hyperuricemia, hypotension, dehydration, tinnitus, hearing loss	Anuria, known hypersensitivity, caution in hepatic disease
Hydralazine (Apresoline)	Injection: 20 mg/mL Tabs: 10, 25, 50, 100 mg	0.1–0.5 mg/kg IM, IV q 4–6 h (hypertensive crisis)	Lupus-like illness (rare), headache, anorexia, nausea, vomiting, diarrhea, palpitations, tachycardia, angina, hypotension, skin flushing, rash, abdominal pain	Known hypersensitivity, coronary artery disease, mitral valve disease, caution in renal disease
Nifedipine (Adalat, Procardia)	Capsules: 10, 20 mg Sustained release: 30, 60, 90 mg	0.25–0.5 mg/kg PO q 6–8 h; maximum 30 mg/dose or 180 mg/d	Hypotension, dizziness, flushing, headache, nausea, peripheral edema, tachycardia, syncope	Known hypersensitivity; not officially approved for use in children
Nitroprusside (Nipride)	50-mg vials; mix only with 5% dextrose in water (D5W)	0.5–10 μg/kg/min; not to exceed 6 μg/kg/min in neonates. Mix in D5W and cover with aluminum foil	Cyanide toxicity with prolonged use, methemoglobinemia, tachyphylaxis, profound hypotension, nausea, vomiting, headache, anxiety, arrhythmias, metabolic acidosis, altered mental status	Compensatory hypertension secondary to AV shunt or coarctation of the aorta; use in monitored setting only
		Hypoglycemia		
Glucagon	Injection: 1-, 10-mg vials (1 U/mg)	Neonates: 0.3 mg/kg IM, IV q 4 h prn Children: 0.03–0.1 mg/kg IM, IV, SC q 20 min; maximum 1 mg	Nausea and vomiting	Known hypersensitivity, pheochromocytoma, suspected insulinoma
Glucose	25% dextrose in water	0.5 mg/kg (2–4 mL/kg) IV as needed	Hyperglycemia	Bedside determination of normoglycemia
		Hypotension		
Dobutamine	Injection: 12.5 mg/mL; do not add to alkaline solutions	2.5–15 μg/kg/min; maximum 40 μg/kg/min Infusion preparation: 0.6 × patient's weight = mg of drug added to 100 mL of IV fluid; desired dose (μg/kg/min) = IV infusion rate (mL/h)	Increased heart rate, increasd blood pressure, ventricular ectopic activity, hypotension, phlebitis, nausea, angina, palpitations, headache, dyspnea	Idiopathic hypertrophic subaortic stenosis, known hypersensitivity use in monitored setting only

(continued)

Table E–1 *(Continued)*

Drug Generic (Brand)	Preparation	Dose & Route of Administration	Toxicity or Adverse Effects	Contraindications
		Hypotension *(Continued)*		
Dopamino	Injection: 40, 80, 160 mg/mL; inactivated if added to alkaline solution	2–20 µg/kg/min, depending on desired effect Infusion preparation: 0.6 × patient's weight = mg of drug added to 100 mL IV fluid; desired dose (µg/kg/min) = IV infusion rate (mL/h)	Ectopic beats, nausea, vomiting, tachycardia, angina, palpitations, dyspnea, headache, hypotension, vasoconstriction, aberrant conduction, bradycardia, widened QRS	Pheochromocytoma, uncorrected tachyarrhythmias or V fib, uncorrected hypovolemia; use in monitored setting only
Epinephrine	Injection: 1:1000 (1 mg/mL)	Infusion 0.1–0.4 µg/kg/min Infusion preparation: 0.6 × patient's weight = mg of drug added to 100 mL IV fluid to give an infusion rate of 0.1 µg/kg/min or 1 mL/h	Palpitations, tachycardia, sweating, nausea, vomiting, cardiac arrhythmias, rebound hypertension	No contraindications in life-threatening situations; tachyarrhythmias; use in monitored setting only
Norepinephrine (Levarterenol, Levophed)	Injection: 1 mg/mL	0.1 µg/kg/min initially; titrate to desired effect	Severe peripheral and visceral vasoconstriction, decreased renal perfusion and urine output, tissue hypoxia, lactic acidosis, skin necrosis with extravasation, cardiac arrhythmias (V tach and V fib)	Hypotension secondary to blood volume deficits, mesenteric or peripheral thromboses; use in monitored setting only
		Narcotic Overdose		
Naloxone (Narcan)	Injection: 0.4 mg/mL, 1 mg/mL.	0.05–0.1 mg/kg SC, IM, IV	Nausea, vomiting, sweating, tachycardia, hypertension, tremulousness, seizure, cardiopulmonary arrest	Known hypersensitivity
		Poisoning		
Cathartic (magnesium citrate)	300-mL bottle	4 mg/kg PO once following administration of charcoal	Hypotension	Renal failure
Cathartic (sorbitol combined with activated charcoal)	75% solution: 25 g/120 mL, 50 g/240 mL	15–30 g in 75% solution PO	Diarrhea, thirst, fluid shifts	Avoid in very young children
Charcoal	Powder: 15, 30, 40, 120, 240 g Suspension: 12.5 g/60 mL, 15 g/75 mL, 25 g/120 mL	1–2 g/kg PO; maximum dose 50 g in 24 h	Constipation, aspiration	None
Ipecac	1.5%, 2% syrup	6–12 mo: 10 mL PO 1–12 y: 15–30 mL PO >12 y: 30–60 mL Po Repeat once in 20 min if no emesis	Aspiration, failure to prevent drug absorption	Children <6 mo, caustic ingestions, hydrocarbon ingestion, gypsum weed ingestion, coma or seizures

(continued)

Table E–1 *(Continued)*

Drug Generic (Brand)	Preparation	Dose & Route of Administration	Toxicity or Adverse Effects	Contraindications
		Pulmonary Edema		
Digoxin	Injection: 100, 250 μg/mL	20–40 μg/kg IV (complex dosing schedule—consult cardiology text)	Conduction disturbances, arrhythmias, anorexia, nausea, vomiting, diarrhea, blurred or yellow vision, sweating	V fib, bradycardia, high-grade AV block, bypass tract present
Furosemide (Lasix)	Injection: 10 mg/mL	1–2 mg/kg/dose IV, IM q 6–24 h; maximum 6 mg/kg/dose	Dehydration, electrolyte depletion, alkalosis, hypotension, hyperuricemia, tinnitus, hearing loss	Anuria, known hypersensitivity; caution in hepatic disease
Nitroglycerin (Nitrostat, Nitro-Bid)	Injection: 0.5, 0.8, 5, 10 mg/mL Must be diluted in D5W or normal saline for infusion	0.5–20 μg/kg/min continuous IV infusion; maximum 5 μg/kg/min for children; no fixed optimum dose, titrate to response	Headache, hypotension, tachycardia, nausea, vomiting, palpitations	Known hypersensitivity, hypotension, uncorrected hypovolemia, increased intracranial pressure, constrictive pericarditis, cardiac tamponade, inadequate cerebral circulation
Oxygen	100% concentration	Deliver by nasal cannula (16 L/min), face mask (10 L/min), or ETT (100%)	Dry mucous membranes	Caution: F_{IO_2} level may need to be adjusted for patients who have COPD
		Rhythm Disturbances		
Adenosine (Adenocard)	Injection: 6 mg/2 mL	0.1 mg/kg rapid IV bolus; may increase by 0.05 mg/kg increments to maximum of 0.25 mg/kg or 12 mg/dose; repeat with careful monitoring.	Hypotension, chest pain or pressure, dyspnea, tingling, heart block, arrhythmias	Second- or third-degree AV block, sick sinus syndrome, hypersensitivity
Atropine	Injection 0.05, 0.1, 0.3, 0.4, 0.5, 0.8, 1.0 mg/mL	0.01–0.03 mg/kg IV q 2–5 min to a maximum of 1–2 mg; minimum dose 0.1 mg	Paradoxical bradycardia, tachyarrhythmias	Tachyarrhythmias
Digoxin (Lanoxin)	Injection: 100, 250 μg/mL Liquid: 50 μg/mL Tabs: 0.125, 0.25, 0.5 mg	20–40 μg/kg IM or IV (complex dosing schedule—consult cardiology text)	Conduction disturbances, arrhythmias, anorexia, nausea, vomiting, diarrhea, blurred or yellow vision, sweating	V fib, bradycardia, high-grade AV block, bypass tract present
Epinephrine	Injection: 1:10,000, 1:1000	0.01 mg/kg/dose IV q 5 min; second dose or via ETT increase to 0.1 mg/kg	Palpitations, tachycardia, sweating, nausea, vomiting, cardiac arrhythmias	None in life-threatening situations; tachyarrhythmias; use in a monitored setting only
Fluids	Normal saline	20 mL/kg IV bolus as needed	IV infiltration, fluid overload	Pulmonary edema, congestive heart failure, renal failure
Lidocaine	Injection (in D5W): 2, 4, 8, 10, 20 mg/mL Drip: 40, 100, 200 mg/mL	Loading dose: 1 mg/kg IV q 5–10 min until arrhythmia controlled or maximum dose 5 mg Maintenance: 20–50 μg/kg/min IV	Central nervous system excitation, seizures, vomiting, bradycardia, hypotension	Hypersensitivity to amide-based local anesthetics, WPW or severe AV block, seizures; use in a monitored setting only

(continued)

Table E–1 *(Continued)*

Drug Generic (Brand)	Preparation	Dose & Route of Administration	Toxicity or Adverse Effects	Contraindications
		Rhythm Disturbances *(Continued)*		
Verapamil (Calan, Isoptin)	Injection: 2.5 mg/mL	0.1–0.3 mg/kg IV q 15 min × 2 doses; maximum 5 mg	Constipation, dizziness, hypotension, bradycardia, AV block	Children <1 y, severe left ventricular dysfunction, hypotension, sick sinus syndrome, second- or third-degree AV block, A fib or A flutter with a bypass tract; use in a monitored setting only
		Sedation		
Chloral hydrate	Syrup: 250, 500 mg/5 cc Suppository: 324, 500, 648 mg	25–75 mg/kg PO, PR depending on desired effect; maximum dose 2 g in 24 h	Prolonged sedation	Hepatic failure
Ketamine	Injection: 10, 50, 100 mg/mL	1–2 mg/kg IV, 2–4 mg/kg IM	Emergence reactions, vivid imagery, hallucinations, delirium, confusion, hypertension, tachycardia, hypotension, arrhythmias, apnea with rapid IV bolus, laryngospasm, diplopia, nystagmus, muscle twitching	Any patient in whom blood pressure elevation or increased intracranial pressure would be hazardous, known hypersensitivity; use in a monitored setting only
Methohexital (Brevital)	Injection: 0.5-, 2.5-, 5.0-g vials	10 mg/kg IM; 25–30 mg/dose PR	Circulatory depression, respiratory depression, cardiopulmonary arrest, thrombophlebitis, laryngospasm, bronchospasm, nausea, emesis, abdominal pain, skeletal muscle hyperactivity	Porphyria, known hypersensitivity to barbiturates, if general anesthesia is contraindicated; use in a monitored setting only
Midazolam (Versed)	Injection: 1, 5 mg/mL	0.1 mg/kg IM, IV; 0.3 mg/kg PR; 0.5 mg/kg PO; 0.4–0.6 mg/kg intranasal	Respiratory depression, hypotension, bradycardia	Caution when used with benzodiazepines; use in a monitored setting only
		Seizures/Status Epilepticus		
Diazepam (Valium)	Injection: 5 mg/mL	Neonates: 0.1–0.3 mg/kg IV q 15–30 min Children: 0.2–0.5 mg/kg IV q 15–30 min; maximum dose 10 mg; administer slowly over 5–10 min; 0.3–0.5 mg/kg PR	Drowsiness, fatigue, ataxia, apnea, bradycardia, hypotension, venous thrombosis or phlebitis, pain at injection site	Known hypersensitivity to diazepam, acute narrow-angle glaucoma; use in a monitored setting only
Glucose	25% dextrose in water	0.5 g/kg (2–4 mL/kg) IV	Hyperglycemia	Bedside glucose determination normal
Lorazepam (Ativan)	Injection: 2, 4 mg/mL; refrigeration suggested	0.05–0.1 mg/kg IM or IV; may repeat q 15–20 min; maximum 1 mg/dose to total of 4 mg	Central nervous system depression, pain at injection site, hypotension, hypertension, partial airway obstruction, arterial spasm if injected intraarterially	Known hypersensitivity to lorazepam or propylene glycol, acute narrow-angle glaucoma; use in a monitored setting only

(continued)

Table E–1 *(Continued)*

Drug Generic (Brand)	Preparation	Dose & Route of Administration	Toxicity or Adverse Effects	Contraindications
		Seizures/Status Epilepticus *(Continued)*		
Phenobarbital	Injection: 30-, 60-, 65-, 75-, 120-, 130-mg/mL; 120-mg vials	10–20 mg/kg IV initially, no faster than 1 mg/kg/min, then 5–10 mg/kg IV q 20 min until seizure controlled or maximum dose 40 mg/kg; 10 mg/kg IM	Central nervous system depression, particularly somnolence; hypoventilation, apnea	Known hypersensitivity, marked impairment of liver function, porphyria, respiratory disease with dyspnea or obstruction
Phenytoin (Dilantin)	Injection: 50 mg/mL	15–20 mg/kg IV initially, not faster than 1 mg/kg/min, maximum 50 mg/min; successive doses 5–10 mg/kg IV q 30 min until seizure controlled or maximum dose 25 mg/kg or 1000 mg in 24 h	Local tissue irritation, hypotension with rapid administration, cardiovascular collapse, central nervous system depression, crystallizaton of drug in IV tubing	Known hypersensitivity, sinus bradycardias, AV block, signs of toxicity—ataxia, nystagmus
Pyridoxine	Injection: 100 mg/mL	100 mg IV	Chronic administration associated with neurologic abnormalities	No documented pyridoxine deficiency
		Stridor		
Racemic epinephrine (Vaponefrin)	2.25% solution	0.05 mL/kg diluted to 3 cc with normal saline nebulized q 1–4 h; maximum 0.5 mL/dose	Palpitations, tachycardia, sweating, nausea, vomiting, cardiac arrhythmias, rebound stridor	Tachyarrhythmias, no contraindications in life-threatening situations; use in a monitored setting only
Dexamethasone (Decadron)	Injection: 4, 10, 20, 24 mg/mL	0.25–0.5 mg/kg IV q 6 h for airway edema; 0.6 mg/kg IM once for croup	Multiple effects with long-term use (see prednisone)	Systemic fungal infections, known hypersensitivity, caution in immunosuppressed individuals
Oxygen	100% concentration	Delivery by nasal cannula (16 L/min), face mask (10 L/min), or ETT (100%)	Dry mucous membranes	Caution: F_{IO_2} level may need to be adjusted for patients who have COPD
		Wheezing		
Albuterol (Proventil, Ventolin)	Metered dose inhaler (MDI): 90 µg/puff Inhalation solution: 5 mg/mL (0.5%) or unit dose 2.5 mg/3 mL normal saline	MDI: 1–2 puffs q 5 min to maximum of 12 puffs Nebulization: 0.15–0.3 mg/kg/dose q 15–20 min	Tremor, dizziness, headache, nausea, tachycardia, hypertension, paradoxical bronchospasm	Hypersensitivity, tachycardia >180–200 beats/min
Epinephrine (Adrenalin)	Injection: 1:1000 (1 mg/mL)	0.01 mg/kg SC, maximum 0.3 mL = 0.3 mg; repeat q 15 min × 3–4 doses	Palpitations, tachycardia, sweating, nausea, vomiting, cardiac arrhythmias, rebound wheezing	No contraindications in life-threatening situations; tachyarrhythmias; use in a monitored setting only
Ipratropium bromide (Atrovent)	Inhalation solution: 250, 500 µg/dose MDI: 18 µg/dose	250–500 µg q 4 h nebulized or 2 puffs via MDI q 4–6 h; maximum 12 doses in 24 h	Palpitations, nervousness, dizziness, headache, nausea, vomiting, tremor, blurred vision, dry mouth	Hypersensitivity, narrow-angle glaucoma, bladder neck obstruction

(continued)

Table E–1 *(Continued)*

Drug Generic (Brand)	Preparation	Dose & Route of Administration	Toxicity or Adverse Effects	Contraindications
		Wheezing *(Continued)*		
Long acting epinephrine (SusPhrine)	Injection: 1:2000 (5 mg/mL)	0.005 mL/kg SC; maximum 0.15 mL q 8–12 h	Palpitations, tachycardia, sweating, nausea, vomiting, cardiac arrhythmias	Tachycardia, rhythm disturbances, vomiting
Methylprednisolone (Solu-Medrol) Hydrocortisone (Solu Cortef)	(See under Anaphylaxis)			
Oxygen	100% concentration	Deliver by nasal cannula (16 L/min), face mask (10 L/min), or ETT (100%)	Dry mucous membranes	Caution: FIO_2 level may need to be adusted for patients who have COPD
Prednisone (Pediapred, Prelone)	Oral solution: 1, 3, 5 mg/mL Tabs: 1, 2.5, 5, 10, 20, 25, 50 mg	1–2 mg/kg PO bid or q d	See methylprednisolone	See methylprednisolone

Appendix F
Chapter XVII—Occupational Safety and Health Administration Department of Labor (Continued)

EDITORIAL NOTE: Chapter XVII is continued in the volumes containing 29 CFR Parts 1911 to 1925, Part 1926 and Part 1927 to End.

PART 1910—OCCUPATIONAL SAFETY AND HEALTH STANDARDS (CONTINUED)

Subpart Z—Toxic and Hazardous Substances

Subpart Z—Toxic and Hazardous Substances

AUTHORITY: Sections 6 and 8 Occupational Safety and Health Act, 29 U.S.C. 655, 657: Secretary of Labor's Order 12071 (36 FR 8754), 9–76 (41 FR 25059), 9–83 (48 FR 35736) or 1–90 (55 FR 9033), as applicable; and 29 CFR part 1911.

All of subpart Z issued under section 6(b) of the Occupational Safety and Health Act, except those substances which have exposure limits listed in Tables Z–1, Z–2, and Z–3 of 29 CFR 1910.1000. The latter were issued under section 6(a) [29 U.S.C. 655(a)].

Section 1910.1000, Tables Z–1, Z–2, and Z–3 also issued under 5 U.S.C. 553. Section 1910.1000, Tables Z–1, Z–2, and Z–3 not issued under 29 CFR part 1911 except for the arsenic (organic compounds), benzene, and cotton dust listings.

Section 1910.1001 also issued under section 107 of Contract Work Hours and Safety and Standards Act, 40 U.S.C. 333 and 5 U.S.C. 553.

Section 1910.1002 not issued under 29 U.S.C. or 29 CFR part 1911; also issued under 5 U.S.C. 553.

Section 1910.1003 through 1910.1018 also isued under 29 CFR 653.

Section 1910.1025 also issued under 29 U.S.C. 653 and 5 U.S.C. 553.

Section 1910.1028 also issued under 29 U.S.C. 653.

Section 1910.1030 also issued under 29 U.S.C. 653.

Section 1910.1043 also issued under 5 U.S.C. 551 et seq.

Section 1910.1045 and 1910.1047 also issued under 29 U.S.C. 653.

Section 1910.1048 also issued under 29 U.S.C. 653.

Sections 1910.1200, 1910.1499, and 1910.1500 also issued under 5 U.S.C. 553.

Section 1910.1450 is also issued under sec. 6(b), 8(c) and 8(g)(2), Pub. L. 91–596, 84 Stat. 1593, 1599, 1600; U.S.C. 655, 657.

SOURCE: 39 FR 23502, June 27, 1974, unless otherwise noted. Redesignated at 40 FR 23072, May 28, 1975.

§1910.1000 Air contaminants.

An employee's exposure to any substance listed in Tables Z–1, Z–2, or Z–3 of this section shall be limited in accordance with the requirements of the following paragraphs of this section.

(a) *Table Z–1.* (1) *Substances with limits preceded by "C"—Ceiling Values.* An employee's exposure to any substance in Table Z–1, the exposure limit of which is preceded by a "C," shall at no time exceed the exposure limit given for that substance. If instantaneous monitoring is not feasible, then the ceiling shall be assessed as a 15-minute time weighted average exposure which shall not be exceeded at any time during the working day.

(2) *Other substances—8-hour Time Weighted Averages.* An employee's exposure to any substance in Table Z–1, the exposure limit of which is not preceded by a "C," shall not exceed the 8-hour Time Weighted Average given for that substance in any 8-hour work shift of a 40-hour work week.

(b) *Table Z–2.* An employee's exposure to any substance listed in Table Z–2 shall not exceed the exposure limits specified as follows:

(1) *8-hour time weighted averages.* An employee's exposure to any substance listed in Table Z–2, in any 8-hour work shift of a 40-hour work week, shall not exceed the 8-hour time weighted average limit given for that substance in Table Z–2.

(2) *Acceptable ceiling concentrations.* An employee's exposure to a substance listed in Table Z–2 shall not exceed at any time during an 8-hour shift the acceptable ceiling concentration limit given for the substance in the table, except for a time period, and up to a concentration not exceeding the maximum duration and concentration allowed in the column under "acceptable maximum peak above the acceptable ceiling concentration for an 8-hour shift."

(3) *Example.* During an 8-hour work shift, an employee may be exposed to a concentration of Substance A (with a 10 ppm TWA, 25 ppm ceiling and 50 ppm peak) above 25 ppm (but never above 50 ppm) only for a maximum period of 10 minutes. Such exposure must be compensated by exposures to concentrations less than 10 ppm so that the cumulative exposure for the entire 8-hour work shift does not exceed a weighted average of 10 ppm.

(c) *Table Z–3.* An employee's exposure to any substance listed in Table Z–3, in any 8-hour work shift of a 40-hour work week, shall not exceed the 8-hour time weighted average limit given for that substance in the table.

(d) *Computation formulae.* The computation formula which shall apply to employee exposure to more than one substance for which 8-hour time weighted averages are listed in subpart Z of 29 CFR part 1910 in order to determine whether an employee is exposed over the regulatory limit is as follows:

(1)(i) The cumulative exposure for an 8-hour work shift shall be computed as follows:

$$E = C_aT_a + C_bT_b + \ldots C_nT_n) + 8$$

Where:

E is the equivalent exposure for the working shift.

C is the concentration during any period of time T where the concentration remains constant.

T is the duration in hours of the exposure at the concentration C.

The value of E shall not exceed the 8-hour time weighted average specified in subpart Z of 29 CFR part 1910 for the substance involved.

(ii) To illustrate the formula prescribed in paragraph (d)(1)(i) of this section, assume that Substance A has an 8-hour time weighted average limit of 100 ppm noted in Table Z–1. Assume that an employee is subject to the following exposure:

Two hours exposure at 150 ppm
Two hours exposure at 75 ppm
Four hours exposure at 50 ppm

Substituting this information in the formula, we have

$$(2 \times 150 + 2 \times 75 + 4 \times 50) \div 8 = 81.25 \text{ ppm}$$

Since 81.25 ppm is less than 100 ppm, the 8-hour time weighted average limit, the exposure is acceptable.

(2)(i) In case of a mixture of air contaminants an employer shall compute the equivalent exposure as follows:

$$E_m = (C_1 \div L_1 + C_2 \div L_2) + \ldots (C_n \div L_n)$$

Where:

E_m is the equivalent exposure for the mixture.

C is the concentration of a particular contaminant.

L is the exposure limit for that substance specified in subpart Z of 29 CFR part 1910.

The value of E_m shall not exceed unity (1).

(ii) To illustrate the formula prescribed in paragraph (d)(2)(i) of this section, consider the following exposures:

Substance	Actual concentration of 8-hour exposure (ppm)	8-hour TWA PEL (ppm)
B................	500	1,000
C................	45	200
D................	40	200

Substituting in the formula, we have:

$$E_m = 500 + 1{,}000 + 45 + 200 + 40 + 200$$
$$E_m = 0.500 + 0.225 + 0.200$$
$$E_m = 0.925$$

Since E_m is less than unity (1), the exposure combination is within acceptable limits.

(e) To achieve compliance with paragraphs (a) through (d) of this section, administrative or engineering controls must first be determined and implemented whenever feasible. When such controls are not feasible to achieve full compliance, protective equipment or any other protective measures shall be used to keep the exposure of employees to air contaminants within the limits prescribed in this section. Any equipment and/or technical measures used for this purpose must be approved for each particular use by a competent industrial hygienist or other technically qualified person. Whenever respirators are used, their use shall comply with 1910.134.

(f) *Effective dates.* The exposure limits specified have been in effect with the method of compliance specified in paragraph (e) of this section since May 29, 1971.

Table Z-1
Limits for Air Contaminants

Substance	CAS No. (c)	ppm (a)[1]	mg/m³ (b)[1]	Skin designation
Acetaldehyde	75–07–0	200	360	
Acetic acid	64–19–7	10	25	
Acetic anhydride	108–24–7	5	20	
Acetone	67–64–1	1000	2400	
Acetonitrile	75–05–8	40	70	
2-Acetylaminofluorine; see 1910.1014	53–96–3			
Acetylene dichloride; see 1,2-Dichloroethylene.				
Acetylene tetrabromide	79–27–6	1	14	
Acrolein	107–02–8	0.1	0.25	
Acrylamide	79–06–1	....	0.3	X
Acrylonitrile; see 1910.1045	107–13–1			
Aldrin	309–00–2	....	0.25	X
Allyl alcohol	107–18–6	2	5	X
Allyl chloride	107–05–1	1	3	
Allyl glycidyl ether (AGE)	106–92–3	(C)10	(c)45	
Allyl propyl disulfide	2179–59–1	2	12	
alpha-Alumina	1344–28–1			
Total dust		....	15	
Respirable fraction		....	5	
Aluminum, metal (as Al)	7429–90–5			
Total dust		....	15	
Respirable fraction		....	5	
4-Aminodiphenyl; see 1910.1011	92–67–1			
2-Aminoethanol; see Ethanolamine.				
2-Aminopyridine	504–29–0	0.5	2	
Ammonia	7664–41–7	50	35	
Ammonium sulfamate	7773–06–0			
Total dust		....	15	
Respirable fraction		....	5	
n-Amyl acetate	628–63–7	100	525	
sec-Amyl acetate	626–38–0	125	650	

[1] The PELs are 8-hour TWAs unless otherwise noted; a (C) designation denotes a ceiling limit. They are to be determined from breathing-zone air samples.
(a) Parts of vapor or as per million parts of contaminated air by volume at 25°C and 760 torr.
(b) Milligrams of substance per cubic meter of air. When entry is in this column only, the value is exact; when listed with a ppm entry, it is approximate.
(c) The CAS number is for information only. Enforcement is based on the substance name. For an entry covering more than one metal compound, measured as the metal, the CAS number for the metal is given—not CAS numbers for the individual compounds.
(d) The final benzene standard in 1910.1028 applies to all occupational exposures to benzene except in some circumstances the distribution and sale of fuels, sealed containers and pipelines, coke production, oil and gas drilling and production, natural gas processing, and the percentage exclusion for liquid mixtures; for the excepted subsegments, the benzene limits in Table Z–2 apply. See 1910.1028 for specific circumstances.
(e) This 8-hour TWA applies to respirable dust as measured by a vertical elutriator cotton dust sampler or equivalent instrument. The time-weighted average applies to the cotton waste processing operations of waste recycling (sorting, blending, cleaning and willowing) and gameting. See also 1910.1043 for cotton dust limits applicable to other sectors.
(f) All inert or nuisance dusts, whether mineral, inorganic, or organic, not listed specifically by substance name are covered by the Particulates Not Otherwise Regulated (PNOR) limit which is the same as the inert or nuisance dust limit of Table Z–3.
[2] See Table Z–2.
[3] See Table Z–3.
[4] Varies with compound.

(continued)

Table Z–1 *(Continued)*

Substance	CAS No. (c)	ppm (a)[1]	mg/m³ (b)[1]	Skin designation
Aniline and homologs	62–53–3	5	19	X
Anisidine (o-, p-isomers)	29191–52–4	....	0.5	X
Antimony and compounds (as Sb)	7440–36–0	....	0.5	
ANTU (alpha Naphthylthiourea)	86–88–4	....	0.3	
Arsenic, inorganic compounds (as As); see 1910.1018	7440–38–2			
Arsenic, organic compounds (as As)	7440–38–2	....	0.5	
Arsine	7784–42–1	0.05	0.2	
Asbestos; see 1910.1001	(4)			
Azinphos-methyl	86–50–0	....	0.2	X
Barium, soluble compounds (as Ba)	7440–39–3	....	0.5	
Barium sulfate	7727–43–7			
Total dust		....	15	
Respirable fraction		....	5	
Benomyl	17804–35–2			
Total dust		....	15	
Respirable fraction		....	5	
Benzene; see 1910.1028	71–43–2			
See Table Z-2 for the limits applicable in the operations or sectors excluded in 1910.1028[d]				
Benzidine; see 1910.1010	92–87–5			
p-Benzoquinone; see Quinone.				
Benzo(a)pyrene; see Coal tar pitch volatiles.				
Benzoyl peroxide	94–36–0	....	5	
Benzyl chloride	100–44–7	1	5	
Beryllium and beryllium compounds (as Be).	7440–41–7		(2)	
Biphenyl; see Diphenyl.				
Bismuth telluride, Undoped	1304–82–1			
Total dust		....	15	
Respirable fraction		....	5	
Boron oxide	1303–86–2			
Total dust		....	15	
Boron trifluoride	7637–07–2	(C)1	(C)3	
Bromine	7726–95–6	0.1	0.7	
Bromoform	75–25–2	0.5	5	X
Butadiene (1,3-Butadiene)	106–99–0	1000	2200	
Butanethiol; see Butyl mercaptan.				
2-Butanone (Methyl ethyl ketone)	78–93–3	200	590	
2-Butoxyethanol	111–76–2	50	240	X
n-Butyl-acetate	123–86–4	150	710	
sec-Butyl acetate	105–46–4	200	950	
tert-Butyl acetate	540–88–5	200	950	
n-Butyl alcohol	71–36–3	100	300	
sec-Butyl alcohol	78–92–2	150	450	
tert-Butyl alcohol	75–65–0	100	300	
Butylamine	109–73–9	(C)5	(C)15	X
tert-Butyl chromate (as CrO_3)	1189–85–1	....	(C)0.1	X
n-Butyl glycidyl ether (BGE)	2426–08–6	50	270	
Butyl-mercaptan	109–79–5	10	35	
p-tert-Butyltoluene	96–51–1	10	60	
Cadmium (as Cd); see 1910.1027	7440–43–9			
Calcium carbonate	1317–65–3			
Total dust		....	15	
Respirable fraction		....	5	
Calcium hydroxide	1305–62–0			
Total dust		....	15	
Respirable fraction		....	5	
Calcium oxide	1305–78–8	....	5	
Calcium silicate	1344–95–2			
Total dust		....	15	
Respirable fraction		....	5	
Calcium sulfate	7778–18–9			
Total dust		....	15	
Respirable fraction		....	5	
Camphor, synthetic	76–22–2	....	2	
Carbaryl (Sevin)	63–25–2	....	5	
Carbon black	1333–86–4	....	3.5	
Carbon dioxide	124–38–9	5000	9000	
Carbon disulfide	75–15–0		(2)	
Carbon monoxide	630–08–0	50	55	

(continued)

Table Z-1 *(Continued)*

Substance	CAS No. (c)	ppm (a)[1]	mg/m³ (b)[1]	Skin designation
Carbon tetrachloride	56–23–5		(2)	
Cellulose	9004–34–6			
Total dust		....	15	
Respirable fraction		....	5	
Chlordane	57–74–9	....	0.5	X
Chlorinated camphene	8001–35–2	....	0.5	X
Chlorinated diphenyl oxide	55720–99–5	....	0.5	
Chlorine	7782–50–5	(C)1	(C)3	
Chlorine dioxide	10049–04–4	0.1	0.3	
Chlorine trifluoride	7790–91–2	(C)0.1	(C)0.4	
Chloroacetaldehyde	107–20–0	(C)1	(C)3	
a-Chloroacetophenone (Phenacyl chloride)	532–27–4	0.05	0.3	
Chlorobenzene	108–90–7	75	350	
o-Chlorobenzylidene malononitrile	2698–41–1	0.05	0.4	
Chlorobromamethane	74–97–5	200	1050	
2-Chloro-1,3-butadiene; see beta-Choroprene.				
Chlorodiphenyl (42% Chlorine) (PCB)	53469–21–9	....	1	X
Chlorodiphenyl (54% Chlorine) (PCB)	11097–69–1	....	0.5	X
1-Chloro-2,3-epoxypropane; see Epichlorohydrin.				
2-Chloroethanol; see Ethylene chlorohydrin.				
Chloroethylene; see Vinyl chloride.				
Chloroform (Trichloromethane)	67–66–3	(C)50	(C)240	
bix(Chioromethyl) ether; see 1910.1008.	542–88–1			
Chloromethyl methyl ether; see 1910.1006.	107–30–2			
1-Chloro-1-nitropropane	600–25–9	20	100	
Chloropicrin	76–06–2	0.1	0.7	
beta-Chloroprene	126–99–8	25	90	X
2-Chloro-6-(trichloromethyl) pyridine	1929–82–4			
Total dust		....	15	
Respirable fraction		....	5	
Chromic acid and chromates (as CrO_3)	(4)		(2)	
Chromium (II) compounds. (as Cr)	7440–47–3	....	0.5	
Chromium (III) compounds. (as Cr)	7440–47–3	....	0.5	
Chromium metal and insol. salts (as Cr).	7440–47–3	....	1	
Chrysene; see Coal tar pitch volatiles.				
Clopidol	2971–90–6			
Total dust		....	15	
Respirable fraction		....	5	
Coal dust (less than 5% SiO_2), respirable fraction.			(3)	
Coal dust (greater than or equal to 5% SiO_2), respirable fraction.			(3)	
Coal tar pitch volatiles (benzene soluble fraction), anthracene, BaP, phenanthrene, acridine, chrysene, pyrene	65966–93–2	....	0.2	
Cobalt metal, dust, and fume (as Co)	7440–48–4	....	0.1	
Coke oven emissions; see 1910.1029.				
Copper	7440–50–8			
Fume (as Cu)		....	0.1	
Dusts and mists (as Cu)		....	1	
Cotton dust[e]; see 1910.1043		....	1	
Crag herbicide (Sesone)	136–78–7			
Total dust		....	15	
Respirable fraction		....	5	
Cresol, all isomers	1319–77–3	5	22	X
Crotonaldehyde	123–73–9; 4170–30–3	2	6	
Cumene	98–82–8	50	245	X
Cyanides (as CN)	(4)	....	5	
Cyclohexane	110–82–7	300	1050	
Cyclohexanol	108–93–0	50	200	
Cyclohexanone	108–94–1	50	200	
Cyclohexene	110–83–8	300	1015	
Cyclopentadiene	542–92–7	75	200	
2,4-D (Dichlorophenoxyacetic acid)	94–75–7	....	10	
Decaborane	17702–41–9	0.05	0.3	X
Demeton (Systox)	8065–48–3	....	0.1	X
Diacetone alcohol (4-Hydroxy-4-methyl-2-pentanone).	123–42–2	50	240	
1,2-Diaminoethane; see Ethylenediamine.				
Diazomethane	334–88–3	0.2	0.4	
Diborane	19287–45–7	0.1	0.1	
1,2-Dibromo-3-chloropropane (CBCP); see 1910.1044.	96–12–8			

(continued)

Table Z-1 *(Continued)*

Substance	CAS No. (c)	ppm (a)[1]	mg/m³ (b)[1]	Skin designation
1,2-Dibromoethane; see Ethylene dibromide.				
Dibutyl phosphate	107–66–4	1	5	
Dibutyl phthalate	84–74–2	....	5	
o-Dichlorobenzene	95–50–1	(C)50	(C)300	
p-Dichlorobenzene	106–46–7	75	450	
3,3′-Dichlorobenzidine; see 1910.1007	91–94–1			
Dichlorodifluoromethane	75–71–8	1000	4950	
1,3-Dichloro-5,5-dimethyl hydantoin	118–52–5	....	0.2	
Dichlorodiphenyltrichloroethane (DDT)	50–29–3	....	1	X
1,1-Dichloroethane	75–34–3	100	400	
1,2-Dichloroethane; see Ethylene dichloride.				
1,2-Dichloroethylene	540–59–0	200	790	
Dichloroethyl ether	111–44–4	(C)15	(C)90	X
Dichloromethane; see Methylene chloride.				
Dichloromonofluoromethane	75–43–4	1000	4200	
1,1-Dichloro-1-nitroethane	594–72–9	(C)10	(C)60	
1,2-Dichloropropane; see Propylene dichloride.				
Dichlorotetrafluoroethane	76–14–2	1000	7000	
Dichlorvos (DDVP)	62–73–7	....	1	X
Dicyclopentadienyl iron	102–54–5			
Total dust		....	15	
Respirable fraction		....	5	
Dieldrin	60–57–1	....	0.25	X
Diethylamine	109–89–7	25	75	
2-Diethylaminoethanol	100–37–8	10	50	X
Diethyl ether; see Ethyl ether.				
Difluorodibromomethane	75–61–0	100	860	
Diglycidyl ether (DGE)	2238–07–5	(C)0.5	(C)2.8	
Dihydroxybenzene; see Hydroquinone.				
Diisobutyl ketone	108–83–8	50	290	
Diisopropylamine	108–18–9	5	20	X
4-Dimethylaminoazobenzene; see 1910.1015.	60–11–7			
Dimethoxymethane; see Methylal.				
Dimethyl acetamide	127–19–5	10	35	X
Dimethylamine	124–40–3	10	18	
Dimethylaminobenzene; see Xylidine.				
Dimethylaniline (N,N-Dimethylaniline)	121–69–7	5	25	X
Dimethylbenzene; see Xylene.				
Dimethyl-1,2-dibromo-2,2-dichloroethyl phosphate.	300–76–5	....	3	
Dimethylformamide	68–12–2	10	30	X
2,6-Dimethyl-4-heptanone; see Diisobutyl ketone.				
1,1-Dimethylhydrazine	57–14–7	0.5	1	X
Dimethylphthalate	131–11–3	....	5	
Dimethyl sulfate	77–78–1	1	5	X
Dinitrobenzene (all isomers)			1	X
(ortho)	528–29–0			
(meta)	99–65–0			
(para)	100–25–4			
Dinitro-o-cresol	534–52–1	....	0.2	X
Dinitrotoluene	25321–14–6	....	1.5	X
Dioxane (Diethylene dioxide)	123–91–1	100	360	X
Diphenyl (Biphenyl)	92–52–4	0.2	1	
Diphenylmethane diisocyanate; see Methylene bisphenyl isocyanate.				
Dipropylene glycol methyl ether	34590–94–8	100	600	X
Di-sec octyl phthalate (Di-(2-ethylhexyl) phthalate).	117–81–7	....	5	
Emery	12415–34–8			
Total dust		....	15	
Respirable fraction		....	5	
Endosulfan	115–29–7	....	0.1	X
Endrin	72–20–8	....	0.1	X
Epichlorohydrin	106–89–8	5	19	X
EPN	2104–64–5	....	0.5	X
1,2-Epoxy-1-propanol; see Glycidol.				
Ethanethiol; see Ethyl mercaptan.				
Ethanolamine	141–43–5	3	6	
2-Ethoxyethanol (Cellosolve)	110–80–5	200	740	X
2-Ethoxyethyl acetate (Cellosolve acetate)	111–15–9	100	540	X
Ethyl acetate	141–78–6	400	1400	
Ethyl acrylate	140–88–5	25	100	X

(continued)

Table Z-1 *(Continued)*

Substance	CAS No. (c)	ppm (a)[1]	mg/m³ (b)[1]	Skin designation
Ethyl alcohol (Ethanol)	64–17–5	1000	1900	
Ethylamine	75–04–7	10	18	
Ethyl amyl ketone (5-Methyl-3-heptanone).	541–85–5	25	130	
Ethyl benzene	100–41–4	100	435	
Ethyl bromide	74–96–4	200	890	
Ethyl butyl ketone (3-Heptanone)	106–35–4	50	230	
Ethyl chloride	75–00–3	1000	2600	
Ethyl ether	60–29–7	400	1200	
Ethyl formate	109–94–4	100	300	
Ethyl mercaptan	75–08–1	(C)10	(C)25	
Ethyl silicate	78–10–4	100	850	
Ethylene chlorohydrin	107–07–3	5	16	X
Ethylenediamine	107–15–3	10	25	
Ethylene dibromide	106–93–4		(2)	
Ethylene dichloride (1,2-Dichloroethane).	107–06–2		(2)	
Ethylene glycol dinitrate	628–96–6	(C)0.2	(C)1	X
Ethylene glycol methyl acetate; see Methyl cellosolve acetate.				
Ethyleneimine; see 1910.1012	151–56–4			
Ethylene oxide; see 1910.1047	75–21–8			
Ethylidene chloride; see 1,1-Dichloroethane.				
N-Ethylmorpholine	100–74–3	20	94	X
Ferbam	14484–64–1			
Total dust		....	15	
Ferrovanadium dust	12604–58–9	....	1	
Fluorides (as F)	(4)	....	2.5	
Fluorine	7782–41–4	0.1	0.2	
Fluorotrichloromethane (Trichlorofluoromethane).	75–69–4	1000	5600	
Formaldehyde; see 1910.1048	50–00–0			
Formic acid	64–18–6	5	9	
Furfural	98–01–1	5	20	X
Furfuryl alcohol	98–00–0	50	200	
Grain dust (oat, wheat, barley)	....	....	10	
Glycerin (mist)	56–81–5			
Total dust		....	15	
Respirable fraction		....	5	
Glycidol	556–52–5	50	150	
Glycol monoethyl ether; see 2-Ethoxyethanol.				
Graphite, natural, respirable dust	7782–42–5		(3)	
Graphite, synthetic				
Total dust		....	15	
Respirable fraction		....	5	
Guthion; see Azinphos methyl.				
Gypsum	13397–24–5			
Total dust		....	15	
Rspirable fraction		....	5	
Hafnium	7440–58–6	....	0.5	
Heptachlor	76–44–8	....	0.5	X
Heptane (n-Heptane)	142–82–5	500	2000	
Hexachloroethane	67–72–1	1	10	X
Hexachloronaphthalene	1335–87–1	....	0.2	X
n-Hexane	110–54–3	500	1800	
2-Hexanone (Methyl n-butyl ketone)	591–78–6	100	410	
Hexone (Methyl isobutyl ketone)	108–10–1	100	410	
sec-Hexyl acetate	108–84–9	50	300	
Hydrazine	302–01–2	1	1.3	X
Hydrogen bromide	10035–10–6	3	10	
Hydrogen chloride	7647–01–0	(C)5	(C)7	
Hydrogen cyanide	74–90–8	10	11	X
Hydrogen fluoride (as F)	7664–39–3		(2)	
Hydrogen peroxide	7722–84–1	1	1.4	
Hydrogen selenide (as Se)	7783–07–5	0.05	0.2	
Hydrogen sulfide	7783–06–4		(2)	
Hydroquinone	123–31–9	....	2	
Iodine	7553–56–2	(C)0.1	(C)1	
Iron oxide fume	1309–37–1	....	10	
Isoamyl acetate	123–92–2	100	525	
Isoamyl alcohol (primary and secondary).	123–51–3	100	360	
Isobutyl acetate	110–19–0	150	700	
Isobutyl alcohol	78–83–1	100	300	

(continued)

Table Z–1 *(Continued)*

Substance	CAS No. (c)	ppm (a)[1]	mg/m³ (b)[1]	Skin designation
Isophorone	78–59–1	25	140	
Isopropyl acetate	108–21–4	250	950	
Isopropyl alcohol	67–63–0	400	980	
Isopropylamine	75–31–0	5	12	
Isopropyl ether	108–20–3	500	2100	
Isopropyl glycidyl ether (IGE)	4016–14–2	50	240	
Kaolin	1332–58–7			
Total dust		....	15	
Respirable fraction		....	5	
Ketene	463–51–4	0.5	0.9	
Lead, inorganic (as Pb); see 1910.1025.	7439–92–1			
Limestone	1317–65–3			
Total dust		....	15	
Respirable fraction		....	5	
Lindane	58–89–9	....	0.5	X
Lithium hydride	7580–67–8	....	0.025	
L.P.G. (Liquefied petroleum gas)	68476–85–7	1000	1800	
Magnesite	546–93–0			
Total dust		....	15	
Respirable fraction		....	5	
Magnesium oxide fume	1309–48–4			
Total particulate		....	15	
Malathion	121–75–5			
Total dust		....	15	X
Maleic anhydride	108–31–6	0.25	1	
Manganese compounds (as Mn)	7439–96–5	....	(C)5	
Manganese fume (as Mn)	7439–96–5	....	(C)5	
Marble	1317–65–3			
Total dust		....	15	
Respirable fraction		....	5	
Mercury (aryl and inorganic) (as Hg)	7439–97–6		([2])	
Mercury (organo) alkyl compounds (as Hg).	7439–97–6		([2])	
Mercury (vapor) (as Hg)	7439–97–6		([2])	
Mesityl oxide	141–79–7	25	100	
Methanethiol; see Methyl mercaptan.				
Methoxychlor	72–43–5			
Total dust		....	15	
2-Methoxyethanol (Methyl cellosolve)	109–86–4	25	80	X
2-Methoxyethyl acetate (Methyl cellosolve acetate).	110–49–6	25	120	X
Methyl acetate	79–20–9	200	610	
Methyl acetylene (Propyne)	74–99–7	1000	1650	
Methyl acetylene-propadiene mixture (MAPP).		1000	1800	
Methyl acrylate	96–33–3	10	35	X
Methylal (Dimethoxy-methane)	109–87–5	1000	3100	
Methyl alcohol	67–56–1	200	260	
Methylamine	74–89–5	10	12	
Methyl amyl alcohol; see Methyl isobutyl carbinol.				
Methyl n-amyl ketone	110–43–0	100	465	
Methyl bromide	74–83–9	(C)20	(C)80	X
Methyl butyl ketone; see 2-Hexanone.				
Methyl cellosolve; see 2-Methoxyethanol.				
Methyl cellosolve acetate; see 2-Methoxyethyl acetate.				
Methyl chloride	74–87–3		([2])	
Methyl chloroform (1,1,1-Trichloroethane).	71–55–6	350	1900	
Methylcyclohexane	108–87–2	500	2000	
Methylcyclohexanol	25639–42–3	100	470	
o-Methylcyclohexanone	583–60–8	100	460	X
Methylene chloride	75–09–2		([2])	
Methyl ethyl ketone (MEK); see 2-Butanone.				
Methyl formate	107–31–3	100	250	
Methyl hydrazine (Monomethyl hydrazine).	60–34–4	(C)0.2	(C)0.35	X
Methyl iodide	74–88–4	5	28	X
Methyl isoamyl ketone	110–12–3	100	475	
Methyl isobutyl carbinol	108–11–2	25	100	X
Methyl isobutyl ketone; see Hexone.				
Methyl isocyanate	624–83–9	0.02	0.05	X
Methyl mercaptan	74–93–1	(C)10	(C)20	
Methyl methacrylate	80–62–6	100	410	
Methyl propyl ketone; see 2-Pentanone.				

(continued)

Table Z–1 *(Continued)*

Substance	CAS No. (c)	ppm (a)[1]	mg/m³ (b)[1]	Skin designation
alpha-Methyl styrene	98–83–9	(C)100	(C)480	
Methylene bisphenyl isocyanate (MDI)	101–68–8	(C)0.02	(C)0.2	
Mica; see Silicates.				
Molybdenum (as Mo)	7439–98–7			
Soluble compounds		....	5	
Insoluble compounds.				
Total dust		....	15	
Monomethyl aniline	100–61–8	2	9	X
Monomethyl hydrazine; see Methyl hydrazine.				
Morpholine	110–91–8	20	70	X
Naphtha (Coal tar)	8030–30–6	100	400	
Naphthalene	91–20–3	10	50	
alpha-Naphthylamine; see 1910.1004.	134–32–7			
beta-Naphthylamine; see 1910.1009	91–59–8			
Nickel carbonyl (as Ni)	13463–39–3	0.001	0.007	
Nickel, metal and insoluble compounds (as Ni).	7440–02–0	....	1	
Nickel, soluble compounds (as Ni)	7440–02–0	....	1	
Nicotine	54–11–5	....	0.5	X
Nitric acid	7697–37–2	2	5	
Nitric oxide	10102–43–9	25	30	
p-Nitroaniline	100–01–6	1	6	X
Nitrobenzene	98–95–3	1	5	X
p-Nitrochlorobenzene	100–00–5	....	1	X
4-Nitrodiphenyl; see 1910.1003	92–93–3			
Nitroethane	79–24–3	100	310	
Nitrogen dioxide	10102–44–0	(C)5	(C)9	
Nitrogen trifluoride	7783–54–2	10	29	
Nitroglycerin	55–63–0	(C)0.2	(C)2	X
Nitromethane	75–52–5	100	50	
1-Nitropropane	108–03–2	25	90	
2-Nitropropane	79–46–9	25	90	
N-Nitrosodimethylamine; see 1910.1016.				
Nitrotoluene (all isomers)		5	30	X
o-isomer	88–72–2			
m-ismer	99–08–1			
p-isomer	99–99–0			
Nitrotrichloromethane; see Chloropicrin.				
Octachloronaphthalene	2234–13–1	....	0.1	X
Octane	111–65–9	500	2350	
Oil mist, mineral	8012–95–1	....	5	
Osmium tetroxide (as Os)	20816–12–0	....	0.002	
Oxalic acid	144–62–7	....	1	
Oxygen difluoride	7783–41–7	0.05	0.1	
Ozone	10028–15–6	0.1	0.2	
Paraquat, respirable dust	4685–14–7; 1910–42–5; 2074–50–2	....	0.5	X
Parathion	56–38–2	....	0.1	X
Particulates not otherwise regulated (PNOR)[f].				
Total dust		....	15	
Respirable fraction		....	5	
PCB; see Chlorodiphenyl (42% and 54% chlorine)				
Pentaborane	19624–22–7	0.005	0.01	
Pentachloronaphthalene	1321–64–8	....	0.5	X
Pentachlorophenol	87–86–5	....	0.5	X
Pentaerythritol	115–77–5			
Total dust		....	15	
Respirable fraction		....	5	
Pentane	109–66–0	1000	2950	
2-Pentanone (Methyl propyl ketone)	107–87–9	200	700	
Perchloroethylene (Tetrachloroethylene).	127–18–4		(2)	
Perchloromethyl mercaptan	594–42–3	0.1	0.8	
Perchloryl fluoride	7616–94–6	3	13.5	
Perlite	93763–70–3			
Total dust		....	15	
Respirable fraction		....	5	
Petroleum distillates (Naphtha) (Rubber Solvent).		500	2000	
Phenol	108–95–2	5	19	X
p-Phenylene diamine	106–50–3	....	0.1	X

(continued)

Table Z-1 *(Continued)*

Substance	CAS No. (c)	ppm (a)[1]	mg/m³ (b)[1]	Skin designation
Phenyl ether, vapor	101–84–8	1	7	
Phenyl ether-biphenyl mixture, vapor		1	7	
Phenylethylene; see Styrene.				
Phenyl glycidyl ether (PGE)	122–60–1	10	60	
Phenhydrazine	100–63–0	5	22	X
Phosdrin (Mevinphos)	7786–34–7	....	0.1	X
Phosgene (Carbonyl chloride)	75–44–5	0.1	0.4	
Phosphine	7803–51–2	0.3	0.4	
Phosphoric acid	7664–38–2	....	1	
Phosphorus (yellow)	7723–14–0	....	0.1	
Phosphorus pentachloride	10026–13–8	....	1	
Phosphorus pentasulfide	1314–80–3	....	1	
Phosphorus trichloride	7719–12–2	0.5	3	
Phthalic anhydride	85–44–9	2	12	
Picloram	1918–02–1			
Total dust		....	15	
Respirable fraction		....	5	
Picric acid	88–89–1	....	0.1	X
Pindone (2-Pivalyl-1,3-indandione)	83–26–1	....	0.1	
Plaster of Paris	26499–65–0			
Total dust		....	15	
Respirable fraction		....	5	
Platinum (as Pt)	7440–06–4			
Metal		....	....	
Soluble salts	....		0.002	
Portland cement	65997–15–1			
Total dust		....	15	
Respirable fraction		....	5	
Propane	74–98–6	1000	1800	
beta-Propriolactone; see 1910.1013	57–57–8			
n-Propyl acetate	109–60–4	200	840	
n-Propyl alcohol	71–23–8	200	500	
n-Propyl nitrate	627–13–4	25	110	
Propylene dichloride	78–87–5	75	350	
Propylene imine	75–55–8	2	5	X
Propylene oxide	75–56–9	100	240	
Propyne; see Methyl acetylene.				
Pyrethrum	8003–34–7	....	5	
Pyridine	110–86–1	5	15	
Quinone	106–51–4	0.1	0.4	
RDX; see Cyclonite.				
Rhodium (as Rh), metal fume and insoluble compounds.	7440–16–6	....	0.1	
Rhodium (as Rh), soluble compounds	7440–16–6	....	0.001	
Ronnel	299–84–3	....	15	
Rotenone	83–79–4	....	5	
Rouge				
Total dust		....	15	
Respirable fraction		....	5	
Selenium compounds (as Se)	7782–49–2	....	0.2	
Selenium hexafluoride (as Se)	7783–79–1	0.05	0.4	
Silica, amorphous, precipitated and gel	112926–00–8		(3)	
Silica, amorphous, diatomaceous earth, containing less than 1% crystalline silica.	61790–53–2		(3)	
Silica, crystalline cristobalite, respirable dust.	14464–46–1		(3)	
Silica, crystalline quartz, respirable dust.	14808–60–7		(3)	
Silica, crystalline tripoli (as quartz), respirable dust.	1317–95–9		(3)	
Silica, crystalline tridymite, respirable dust.	15468–32–3		(3)	
Silica, fused, respirable dust	60676–86–0		(3)	
Silicates (less than 1% crystalline silica)				
Mica (respirable dust)	12001–26–2		(3)	
Soapstone, total dust	....		(3)	
Soapstone, respirable dust	....		(3)	
Talc (containing asbestos); use asbestos limit; see 29 CFR 1910.1001.	....		(3)	
Talc (containing no asbestos), respirable dust.	14807–96–6		(3)	
Tremolite, asbestiform; see 1910.1001.				
Silicon	7440–21–3			
Total dust		....	15	
Respirable fraction		....	5	

(continued)

Table Z–1 *(Continued)*

Substance	CAS No. (c)	ppm (a)[1]	mg/m³ (b)[1]	Skin designation
Silicon carbide	409–21–2			
Total dust		....	15	
Respirable fraction		....	5	
Silver, metal and soluble compounds (as Ag).	7440–22–4	....	0.01	
Soapstone; see Silicates.				
Sodium fluoroacetate	62–74–8	....	0.05	X
Sodium hydroxide	1310–73–2	....	2	
Starch	9005–25–8			
Total dust		....	15	
Respirable fraction		....	5	
Stibine	7803–52–3	0.1	0.5	
Stoddard solvent	8052–41–3	500	2900	
Strychnine	57–24–9	....	0.15	
Styrene	100–42–5		([2])	
Sucrose	57–50–1			
Total dust		....	15	
Respirable fraction		....	5	
Sulfur dioxide	7446–09–5	5	13	
Sulfur hexafluoride	2551–62–4	1000	6000	
Sulfuric acid	7664–93–9	....	1	
Sulfur monochloride	10025–67–9	1	6	
Sulfur pentafluoride	5714–22–7	0.025	0.25	
Sulfuryl fluoride	2699–79–8	5	20	
Systox; see Demetron.				
2,4,5-T (2,4,5-trichlorophenoxyacetic acid).	93–76–5	....	10	
Talc; see Silicates.				
Tantalum, metal and oxide dust	7440–25–7	....	5	
TEDP (Sulfotep)	3689–24–5	....	0.2	X
Tellurium and compounds (as Te)	13494–80–9	....	0.1	
Tellurium hexafluoride (as Te)	7783–80–4	0.02	0.2	
Temephos	3383–96–8			
Total dust		....	15	
Respirable fraction		....	5	
TEPP (Tetraethyl pyrophosphate)	107–49–3	....	0.05	X
Terphenyls	26140–60–3	(C)1	(C)9	
1,1,1,2-Tetrachloro-2,2-difluoroethane	76–11–9	500	4170	
1,1,2,2-Tetrachloro-1,2-difluoroethane	76–12–0	500	4170	
1,1,2,2-Tetrachloroethane	79–34–5	5	35	X
Tetrachloroethylene; see Perchloroethylene.				
Tetrachloromethane; see Carbon tetrachloride.				
Tetrachloronaphthalene	1335–88–2	....	2	X
Tetraethyl lead (as Pb)	78–00–2	....	0.075	X
Tetrahydrofuran	109–99–9	200	590	
Tetramethyl lead (as Pb)	75–74–1	....	0.075	X
Tetramethyl succinonitrile	3333–52–6	0.5	3	X
Tetranitromethane	509–14–8	1	8	
Tetryl (2,4,6-Trinitrophenylmethylnitramine).	479–45–8	....	1.5	X
Thallium, soluble compounds (as T1)	7440–28–0	....	0.1	X
4,4′-Thiobis (6-tert, Butyl-m-cresol)	96–69–5			
Total dust		....	15	
Respirable fraction		....	5	
Thiram	137–26–8	....	5	
Tin, inorganic compounds (except oxides) (as Sn).	7440–31–5	....	2	
Tin, organic compounds (as Sn)	7440–31–5	....	0.1	
Titanium dioxide	13463–67–7			
Total dust		....	15	
Toluene	108–88–3		([2])	
Toluene-2,4-diisocyanate (TDI)	584–84–9	(C)0.02	(C)0.14	
o-Toluidine	95–53–4	5	22	X
Toxaphene; see Chlorinated camphene.				
Tremolite; see Silicates.				
Tributyl phosphate	126–73–8	....	5	
1,1,1-Trichloroethane; see Methyl chloroform.				
1,1,2-Trichloroethane	79–00–5	10	45	X
Trichloroethylene	79–01–6		([2])	
Trichloromethane; see Chloroform.				
Trichloronaphthalene	1321–65–9	....	5	X
1,2,3-Trichloropropane	96–18–4	50	300	
1,1,2-Trichloro-1,2,2-trifluoroethane	76–13–1	1000	7600	
Triethylamine	121–44–8	25	100	

(continued)

Table Z–1 *(Continued)*

Substance	CAS No. (c)	ppm (a)[1]	mg/m³ (b)[1]	Skin designation
Trifluorobromomethane	75–63–8	1000	6100	
2,4,6-Trinitrophenyl; see Picric acid.				
2,4,6-Trinitrophenylmethylnitramine; see Tetryl.				
2,4,6-Trinitrotoluene (TNT)	118–96–7	....	1.5	X
Triorthocresyl phosphate	78–30–8	....	0.1	
Triphenyl phosphate	115–86–5	....	3	
Turpentine	8006–64–2	100	560	
Uranium (as U)	7440–61–1			
Soluble compounds		....	0.05	
Insoluble compounds		....	0.05	
Vanadium	1314–62–1			
Respirable dust (as V_2O_5)		....	(C)0.5	
Fume (as V_2O_5)		....	(C)0.1	
Vegetable oil mist				
Total dust		....	15	
Respirable fraction		....	5	
Vinyl benzene; see Styrene.				
Vinyl chloride; see 1910.1017	75–01–4			
Vinyl cyanide; see Acrylonitrile.				
Vinyl toluene	25013–15–4	100	480	
Warfarin	81–81–2	....	0.1	
Xylenes (o-, m-, p-isomers)	1330–20–7	100	435	
Xylidine	1300–73–8	5	25	X
Yttrium	7440–65–5	....	1	
Zinc chloride fume	1314–13–2	....	5	
Zinc oxide	1314–13–2			
Total dust		....	15	
Respirable fraction		....	5	
Zinc stearate	557–05–1			
Total dust		....	15	
Respirable fraction		....	5	
Zirconium compounds (as Zr)	7440–67–7	....	5	

Table Z–2

Substance	8-Hour Time Weighted Average	Acceptable Ceiling Concentration	Acceptable Maximum Peak Above the Acceptable Ceiling Concentration for an 8-hr Shift	
			Concentration	Maximum Duration
Benzene[a] (Z37.40–1969)	10 ppm	25 ppm	50 ppm	10 minutes.
Beryllium and beryllium compounds (Z37.29–1970)	2 μg/m³	5 μg/m³	25 μg/m³	30 minutes.
Cadmium fume[b] (Z37.5–1970)	0.1 mg/m³	0.3 mg/m³	....	
Cadmium dust[b] (Z37.5–1970)	0.2 mg/m³	0.6 mg/m³		
Carbon disulfide (Z37.3–1968)	20 ppm	30 ppm	100 ppm	30 minutes.
Carbon tetrachloride (Z37.17–1967)	10 ppm	25 ppm	200 ppm	5 min. in any 4 hrs.
Chromic acid and chromates (Z37.7–1971)	....	1 mg/10m³	P	
Ethylene dibromide (Z37.31–1970)	20 ppm	30 ppm	50 pm	5 minutes.
Ethylene dichloride (Z37.21–1969)	50 ppm	100 ppm	200 ppm	5 min. in any 3 hrs.
Fluoride as dust (Z37.28–1969)	2.5 mg/m³	....	....	
Formaldehyde; see 1910.1048	....	....	....	
Hydrogen fluoride (Z37.28–1969)	3 ppm	....	....	
Hydrogen sulfide (Z37.2–1966)	....	20 ppm	50 ppm	10 mins. once, only if no other meas. exp. occurs.
Mercury (Z37.8–1971)	....	1 mg/10 m³	....	
Methyl chloride (Z37.18–1969)	100 ppm	200 ppm	300 ppm	5 mins. in any 3 hrs.
Methylene chloride (Z37.23–1969)	500 ppm	1,000 ppm	2,000 ppm	5 mins. in any 2 hrs.
Organo (alkyl) mercury (Z37.30–1969)	0.01 mg/m³	0.04 mg/m³	....	
Styrene (Z37.15–1969)	100 ppm	200 ppm	600 ppm	5 mins. in any 3 hrs.
Tetrachloroethylene (Z37.22–1967)	100 ppm	200 ppm	300 ppm	5 mins. in any 3 hrs.
Toluene (Z37.12–1967)	200 ppm	300 ppm	500 ppm	10 minutes.
Trichloroethylene (Z37.19–1967)	100 ppm	200 ppm	300 ppm	5 mins. in any 2 hrs.

[a]This standard applies to the industry segments exempt from the 1 ppm 8-hour TWA and 5 ppm STEL of the benzene standard at 1910.1028.
[b]This standard applies to any operations or sectors for which the Cadmium standard, 1910.1027, is stayed or otherwise not in effect.

Table Z-3
Mineral Dusts

Substance	mmpcf[a]	mg/m³
Silica:		
Crystalline		
Quartz (Respirable)	$\frac{250^{b}}{\%SiO_2 + 5}$	$\frac{10\ mg/m^{3e}}{\%SiO_2 + 2}$
Quartz (Total Dust)	....	$\frac{30\ mg/m^{3}}{\%SiO_2 + 2}$
Cristobalite: Use ½ the value calculated from the count or mass formulae for quartz		
Tridymite: Use ½ the value calculated from the formulae for quartz		
Amorphous, including natural diatomaceous earth	20	$\frac{80\ mg/m^{3}}{\%SiO_2}$
Silicates (less than 1% crystalline silica):		
Mica	20	
Soapstone	20	
Talc (not containing asbestos)	20[c]	
Talc (containing asbestos) Use asbestos limit.		
Tremolite, asbestiform (see 29 CFR 1910.1001).		
Portland cement	50	
Graphite (Natural)	15	
Coal Dust:		
Respirable fraction less than 5% SiO_2	....	$\frac{2.4\ mg/m^{3e}}{\%SiO_2 + 2}$
Respirable fraction greater than 5% SiO_2	....	$\frac{10\ mg/m^{3e}}{\%SiO_2 + 2}$
Inert or Nuisance Dust:[d]		
Respirable fraction	15	5 mg/m³
Total dust	50	15 mg/m³

Note—Conversion factors – mppcf × 35.3 = million particles per cubic meter = particles per c.c.

[a]Millions of particles per cubic foot of air, based on impinger samples counted by light-field techniques.

[b]The percentage of crystalline silica in the formula is the amount determined from airborne samples, except in those instances in which other methods have been shown to be applicable.

[c]Containing less than 1% quartz; if 1% quartz or more, use quartz limit.

[d]All inert or nuisance dusts, whether mineral, inorganic, or organic, not listed specifically by substance name are covered by this limit, which is the same as the Particulates Not Otherwise Regulated (PNOR) limit in Table Z–1.

[e]Both concentration and percent quartz for the application of this limit are to be determined from the fraction passing a size-selector with the following characteristics:

Aerodynamic Diameter (Unit Density Sphere)	Percent Passing Selector
2	90
2.5	75
3.5	50
5.0	25
10	0

The measurements under this note refer to the use of an AEC (now NRC) instrument. The respirable fraction of coal dust is determined with an MRE; the figure corresponding to that of 24 mg/m³ in the table for coal dust is 4.5 mg/m³K.
[58 FR 35340, June 30, 1993; 58 FR 40191, July 27, 1993]

§1910.1001 Asbestos.

(a) Scope and application. (1) This section applies to all occupational exposures to asbestos in all industries covered by the Occupational Safety and Health Act, except as provided in paragraph (a)(2) and (3) of this section.

(2) This section does not apply to construction work as defined in 29 CFR 1910.12(b). (Exposure to asbestos in construction work is covered by 29 CFR 1926.1101).

(3) This section does not apply to ship repairing, shipbuilding and shipbreaking employments and related employments as defined in 29 CFR 1915.4. (Exposure to asbestos in these employments is covered by 29 CFR 1915.1001).

(b) Definitions.

Asbestos includes chrystotile, amosite, crocidolite, tremolite asbestos, anthophyllite asbestos, actinolite asbestos, and any of these minerals that have been chemically treated and/or altered.

Asbestos-containing material (ACM) means any material containing more than 1% asbestos.

Assistant Secretary means the Assistant Secretary of Labor for Occupational Safety and Health, U.S. Department of Labor, or designee.

Authorized person means any person authorized by the employer and required by work duties to be present in regulated areas.

Building/facility owner is the legal entity, including a lessee, which exercises control over management and record keeping functions relating to a building and/or facility in which activities covered by this standard take place.

Certified industrial hygienist (CIH) means one certified in the practice of industrial hygiene by the American Board of Industrial Hygiene.

Director means the Director of the National Institute for Occupational Safety and Health, U.S. Department of Health and Human Services, or designee.

Employee exposure means that exposure to airborne asbestos that would occur if the employee were not using respiratory protective equipment.

Fiber means a particulate form of asbestos 5 micrometers or longer, with a length-to-diameter ratio of at least 3 to 1.

High-efficiency particulate air (HEPA) filter means a filter capable of trapping and retaining at least 99.97 percent of 0.3 micrometer diameter mono-disperse particles.

Homogeneous area means an area of surfacing material or thermal system insulation that is uniform in color and texture.

Industrial hygienist means a professional qualified by education, training, and experience to anticipate, recognize, evaluate and develop controls for occupational health hazards.

PACM means "presumed asbestos containing material."

Presumed asbestos containing material means thermal system insulation and surfacing material found in buildings constructed no later than 1980. The designation of a material as "PACM" may be rebutted pursuant to paragraph (j)(8) of this section.

Regulated area means an area established by the employer to demarcate areas where airborne concentrations of asbestos exceed, or there is a reasonable possibility they may exceed, the permissible exposure limits.

Surfacing ACM means surfacing material which contains more than 1% asbestos.

Surfacing material means material that is sprayed, troweled-on or otherwise applied to surfaces (such as acoustical plaster on ceiling and fireproofing materials on structural members, or other materials on surfaces for acoustical, fireproofing, and other purposes).

Thermal System Insulation (TSI) means ACM applied to pipes, fittings, boilers, breeching, tanks, ducts or other structural components to prevent heat loss or gain.

Thermal System Insulation ACM means thermal system insulation which contains more than 1% asbestos.

(c) Permissible exposure limit (PELS)—(1) Time-weighted average limit (TWA). The employer shall ensure that no employee is exposed to an airborne concentration of asbestos in excess of 0.1 fiber per cubic centimeter of air as an eight (8)-hour time-weighted average (TWA) as determined by the method prescribed in Appendix A to this section, or by an equivalent method.

(2) Excursion limit. The employer shall ensure that no employee is exposed to an airborne concentration of asbestos in excess of 1.0 fiber per cubic centimeter of air (1 f/cc) as averaged over a sampling period of thirty (30) minutes as determined by the method prescribed in Appendix A to this section, or by an equivalent method.

(3) Exposure monitoring.—(1) General. (i) Determinations of employee exposure shall be made from breathing zone air samples that are representative of the 8-hour TWA and 30-minute short-term exposures of each employee.

Appendix G Laboratories Acceptable for Urine Testing (Federal)

Substance Abuse and Mental Health Services Administration

Current List of Laboratories Which Meet Minimum Standards To Engage in Urine Drug Testing for Federal Agencies and Laboratories That Have Withdrawn From the Program

AGENCY: Substance Abuse and Mental Health Services Administration, HHS. (Formerly: National Institute on Drug Abuse, ADAMHA, HHS).

ACTION: Notice

SUMMARY: The Department of Health and Human Services notifies Federal agencies of the laboratories currently certified to meet standards of Subpart C of Mandatory Guidelines for Federal Workplace Drug Testing Programs (59 FR 29916, 29925). A similar notice listing all currently certified laboratories will be published during the first week of each month, and updated to include laboratories which subsequently apply for and complete the certification process. If any listed laboratory's certification is totally suspended or revoked, the laboratory will be omitted from updated lists until such time as it is restored to full certification under the Guidelines.

If any laboratory has withdrawn from the National Laboratory Certification Program during the past month, it will be identified as such at the end of the current list of certified laboratories, and will be omitted from the monthly listing thereafter.

FOR FURTHER INFORMATION CONTACT: Mrs. Giselle Hersh, Division of Workplace Programs, Room 13A-54, 5600 Fishers Lane, Rockville, Maryland 20857; Tel.: (301) 443-6014.

SUPPLEMENTARY INFORMATION:
Mandatory Guidelines for Federal Workplace Drug Testing were developed in accordance with Executive Order 12564 and section 503 of Pub. L. 100-71. Subpart C of the Guidelines, "Certification of Laboratories Engaged in Urine Drug Testing for Federal Agencies," sets strict standards which laboratories must meet in order to conduct urine drug testing for Federal agencies. To become certified an applicant laboratory must undergo three rounds of performance testing plus an on-site inspection. To maintain that certification a laboratory must participate in a quarterly performance testing program plus periodic, on-site inspections.

Laboratories which claim to be in the applicant stage of certification are *not* to be considered as meeting the minimum requirements expressed in the HHS Guidelines. A laboratory must have its letter of certification from SAMHSA, HHS (formerly: HHS/NIDA) which attests that it has met minimum standards.

In accordance with Subpart C of the Guidelines, the following laboratories meet the minimum standards set forth in the Guidelines:

ACCU-LAB, Inc., 405 Alderson St., Schofield, WI 54476, 800-627-8200 (formerly: Alpha Medical Laboratory, Inc. Employee Health Assurance Group, ExpressLab, Inc.).

Aegis Analytical Laboratories, Inc., 624 Grassmere Park Rd., Suite 21, Nashville, TN 37211, 615-331-5300.

Alabama Reference Laboratories, Inc., 543 South Hull St., Montgomery, AL 36103, 800-541-4931/205-263-5745.

American Medical Laboratories, Inc., 14225 Newbrook Dr., Chantilly, VA 22021, 703-802-6900.

Associated Pathologists Laboratories, Inc., 4230 South Burnham Ave., Suite 250, Las Vegas, NV 89119-5412, 702-733-7866.

Associated Regional and University Pathologists, Inc. (ARUP), 500 Chipeta Way, Salt Lake City, UT 84108, 801-583-2787.

Baptist Medical Center—Toxicology Laboratory, 9601 I-630, Exit 7, Little Rock, AR 72205-7299, 501-227-2783 (formerly: Forensic Toxicology Laboratory Baptist Medical Center).

Bayshore Clinical Laboratory, 4555 W. Schroeder Dr., Brown Deer, WI 53223, 414-355-4444/800-877-7016.

Cedars Medical Center, Department of Pathology, 1400 Northwest 12th Ave., Miami, FL 33136, 305-325-5810.

Centinela Hospital Airport Toxicology Laboratory, 9601 S. Sepulveda Blvd., Los Angeles, CA 90045, 310-215-6020.

Clinical Reference Lab, 11850 West 85th St., Lenexa, KS 66214, 800-445-6917.

CORNING Clinical Laboratories, South Central Division, 2320 Schuetz Rd., St. Louis, MO 63146, 800-288-7293 (formerly: Metropolitan Reference Laboratories, Inc.).

CORNING Clinical Laboratories, 8300 Esters Blvd., Suite 900, Irving, TX 75063, 800-526-0947 (formerly: Damon Clinical Laboratories, Damon/MetPath).

CORNING MetPath Clinical Laboratories, 1355 Mittel Blvd., Wood Dale, IL 60191, 708-595-3888 (formerly: MetPath, Inc.).

CORNING MetPath Clinical Laboratories, One Malcolm Ave., Teterboro, NJ 07608, 201-393-5000 (formerly: MetPath, Inc.).

CORNING National Center for Forensic Science, 1901 Sulphur Spring Rd., Baltimore, MD 21227, 410-536-1485 (formerly: Maryland Medical Laboratory, Inc., National Center for Forensic Science).

CORNING Nichols Institute, 7470-A Mission Valley Rd., San Diego, CA 92108-4406, 800-446-4728/619-686-3200 (formerly: Nichols Institute, Nichols Institute Substance Abuse Testing (NISAT)).

Cox Medical Centers, Department of Toxicology, 1423 North Jefferson Ave., Springfield, MO 65802, 800-876-3652/417-836-3093.

Dept. of the Navy, Navy Drug Screening Laboratory, Great Lakes, IL., Building 38-H, Great Lakes, IL 60088-5223, 708-688-2045/708-688-4171.

Diagnostic Services Inc., dba DSI. 4048 Evans Ave., Suite 301. Fort Myers, FL 33901, 813-936-5446/800-735-5416.

Doctors Laboratory, Inc., P.O. Box 2658, 2906 Julia Dr., Valdosta, GA 31604 912-244-4468.

Drug Labs of Texas, 15201 I-10 East, Suite 125, Channelview, TX 77530, 713-457-3784.

DrugProof, Division of Dynacare/Laboratory of Pathology, LLC, 1229 Madison St., Suite 500, Nordstrom Medical Tower, Seattle, WA 98104, 800-898-0180/206-386-2672 (formerly: Laboratory of Pathology of Seattle, Inc., DrugProof, Division of Laboratory of Pathology of Seattle, Inc.).

DrugScan, Inc. P.O. Box 2969, 1119 Mearns Rd., Warminster, PA 18974, 215-674-9310.

Eagle Forensic Laboratory, Inc., 950 N. Federal Highway, Suite 308, Pompano Beach, FL 33062, 305-946-4324.

ElSohly Laboratories, Inc., 5 Industrial Park Dr., Oxford, MS 38655, 601-236-2609.

General Medical Laboratories, 36 South Brooks St., Madison, WI 53715, 608-267-6267.

Harrison Laboratories, Inc., 9930 W. Highway 80, Midland, TX 79706, 800-725-3784/915-563-3300 (formerly: Harrison & Associates Forensic Laboratories).

HealthCare/MetPath, 24451 Telegraph Rd., Southfield, MI 48034, 800-444-0106 ext. 650 (formerly: HealthCare/Preferred Laboratories).

Holmes Regional Medical Center Toxicology Laboratory, 5200 Babcock St., NE., Suite 107, Palm Bay, FL 32905, 407-726-9920.

Jewish Hospital of Cincinnati, Inc., 3200 Burnet Ave., Cincinnati, OH 45229, 513-569-2051.

LabOne, Inc., 8915 Lenexa Dr., Overland Park, Kansas 66214, 913-888-3927 (formerly: Center for Laboratory Services, a Division of LabOne, Inc.).

Laboratory Specialists, Inc., 113 Jarrell Dr., Belle Chasse, LA 70037, 504-392-7961.

Marshfield Laboratories, 1000 North Oak Ave., Marshfield, WI 54449, 715-389-3734/800-222-5835.

MedExpress/National Laboratory Center, 4022 Willow Lake Blvd., Memphis, TN 38175, 901-795-1515.

Medical College Hospitals Toxicology Laboratory, Department of Pathology, 3000 Arlington Ave., Toledo, OH 43699-0008, 419-381-5213.

Medlab Clinical Testing, Inc., 212 Cherry Lane, New Castle, DE 19720, 302-655-5227.

MedTox Laboratories, Inc., 402 W. County Rd. D, St. Paul, MN 55112, 800-832-3244/612-636-7466.

Methodist Hospital of Indiana, Inc., Department of Pathology and Laboratory Medicine, 1701 N. Senate Blvd., Indianapolis, IN 46202, 317-929-3587.

Methodist Medical Center Toxicology Laboratory, 221 N.E. Glen Oak Ave., Peoria, IL 61636, 800-752-1835/309-671-5199.

MetPath Laboratories, 875 Greentree Rd., 4 Parkway Ctr., Pittsburgh, PA 15220-3610, 412-931-7200 (formerly: Med-Chek Laboratories, Inc., MedChek/Damon).

MetroLab-Legacy Laboratory Services, 235 N. Graham St., Portland, OR 97227, 503-413-4512, 800-237-7808 (x4512).

National Health Laboratories Incorporated, 2540 Empire Dr., Winston-Salem, NC 27103-6710, Outside NC: 919-760-4620/800-334-8627/Inside NC: 800-642-0894.

National Health Laboratories Incorporated, d.b.a. National Reference Laboratory, Substance Abuse Division, 1400 Donelson Pike, Suite A-15, Nashville, TN 37217.

National Health Laboratories Incorporated, 13900 Park Center Rd., Herndon, VA 22071, 703-742-3100.

National Psychopharmacology Laboratory, Inc., 9320 Park W. Blvd., Knoxville, TN 37923, 800-251-9492.

National Toxicology Laboratories, Inc., 1100 California Ave., Bakersfield, CA 93304, 805-322-4250.

Northwest Toxicology, Inc., 1141 E. 3900 South, Salt Lake City, UT 84124, 800-322-3361.

Oregon Medical Laboratories, P.O. Box 972, 722 East 11th Ave., Eugene, OR 97440-0972, 503-687-2134.

Pathology Associates Medical Laboratories, East 11604 Indiana, Spokane, WA 99206, 509-926-2400.

PDLA, Inc. (Princeton), 100 Corporate Court, So. Plainfield, NJ 07080, 908-769-8500/800-237-7352.

PharmChem Laboratories, Inc., 1505-A O'Brien Dr., Menlo Park, CA 94025, 415-328-6200/800-446-5177.

PharmChem Laboratories, Inc., Texas Division, 7606 Pebble Dr., Fort Worth, TX 76118, 817-595-0294 (formerly: Harris Medical Laboratory).

Physicians Reference Laboratory, 7800 West 110th St., Overland Park, KS 66210, 913-338-4070/800-821-3627 (formerly: Physicians Reference Laboratory Toxicology Laboratory).

Poisonlab, Inc., 7272 Clairemont Mesa Rd., San Diego, CA 92111, 619-279-2600/800-882-7272.

Puckett Laboratory, 4200 Mamie St., Hattiesburg, MS 39402, 601-264-3856/800-844-8378.

Regional Toxicology Services, 15305 N.E. 40th St., Redmond, WA 98052, 206-882-3400.

Roche Biomedical Laboratories, Inc., 1120 Stateline Rd., Southaven, MS 38671, 601-342-1286.

Roche Biomedical Laboratories, Inc., 69 First Ave., Raritan, NJ 08869, 800-437-4986.

Roche CompuChem Laboratories, Inc., A Member of the Roche Group, 3308 Chapel Hill/Nelson Hwy., Research Triangle Park, NC 27709, 919-549-8263/800-833-3984 (formerly: CompuChem Laboratories, Inc.—Special Division).

Scientific Testing Laboratories, Inc., 463 Southlake Blvd., Richmond, VA 23236, 804-378-9130.

Scott & White Drug Testing Laboratory, 600 S. 25th St., Temple, TX 76504, 800-749-3788.

S.E.D. Medical Laboratories, 500 Walter NE, Suite 500, Albuquerque, NM 87102, 505-848-8800.

Sierra Nevada Laboratories, Inc., 888 Willow St., Reno, NV 89502, 800-648-5472.

SmithKline Beecham Clinical Laboratories, 7600 Tyrone Ave., Van Nuys, CA 91045, 818-376-2520.

SmithKline Beecham Clinical Laboratories, 801 East Dixie Ave., Leesburg, FL 34748, 904-787-9006 (formerly: Doctors & Physicians Laboratory).

SmithKline Beecham Clinical Laboratories, 3175 Presidential Dr., Atlanta, GA 30340, 404-934-9205 (formerly: SmithKline Bio-Science Laboratories).

SmithKline Beecham Clinical Laboratories, 506 E. State Pkwy., Schaumburg, IL 60173, 708-885-2010 (formerly: International Toxicology Laboratories).

SmithKline Beecham Clinical Laboratories, 400 Egypt Rd., Norristown, PA 19403, 800-523-5447 (formerly: SmithKline BioScience Laboratories).

SmithKline Beecham Clinical Laboratories, 8000 Sovereign Row, Dallas, TX 75247, 214-638-1301 (formerly: SmithKline Bio-Science Laboratories).

South Bend Medical Foundation, Inc., 530 N. Lafayette Blvd., South Bend, IN 46601, 219-234-4176.

Southwest Laboratories, 2727 W. Baseline Rd., Suite 6, Tempe, AZ 85283, 602-438-8507.

St. Anthony Hospital (Toxicology Laboratory), P.O. Box 205, 1000 N. Lee St., Oklahoma City, OK 73102, 405-272-7052.

Toxicology & Drug Monitoring Laboratory, University of Missouri Hospital & Clinics, 301 Business Loop 70 West, Suite 208, Columbia, MO 65203, 314-882-1273.

Toxicology Testing Service, Inc., 5426 N.W. 79th Ave., Miami, FL 33166, 305-593-2260.

TOXWORX Laboratories, Inc., 6160 Variel Ave., Woodland Hills, CA 91367, 818-226-4373 (formerly: Laboratory Specialists, Inc.; Abused Drug Laboratories; MedTox BioAnalytical, a Division of MedTox Laboratories, Inc.).

UNILAB, 18408 Oxnard St., Tarzana, CA 91356, 800-492-0800/818-343-8191 (formerly: MetWest-BPL Toxicology Laboratory).

No laboratories withdrew from the Program in March.

Richard Kopanda,

Acting Executive Officer Substance Abuse and Mental Health Services Administration.

(FR Doc. 95-8015 Filed 3-31-95; 8:45 am)

BILLING CODE 4160-20-U

Appendix H
The Poisoned Patients and the Laboratory—"The Flanagan Tables"

THE FLANAGAN TABLES

Flanagan (Poisons Unit of Guy's and St. Thomas Hospital Trust, London, UK) has summarized laboratory use in a series of tables.[1] Sample requirements for general analytic toxicology and for metals and trace elements analysis are summarized in Tables H-1 and H-2. A summary of drugs and other common poisons detected in blood and in urine by commonly available methods is found in Table H-3. Emergency toxicologic analyses that may affect active treatment are listed in Table H-4. Factors affecting the interpretation of toxicology results are listed in table H-5. Drugs, metabolites, and other poisons unstable in whole blood or plasma are presented in Table H-6. Spot tests are reviewed in Table H-7.

SPECIMEN COLLECTION, TRANSPORT, AND STORAGE

If possible, all specimens should be stored at 4°C for 4 to 6 weeks. If there are medicolegal implications, then any specimen remaining should be kept at –20° or below until investigation of the incidence is concluded. All specimens should be clearly labeled with the patient's family or last name and any forenames, the date and time of collection, and the nature of the specimen if this is not self-evident. Hospital and/or casualty numbers should also be recorded.

CHAIN OF CUSTODY

If the analyses clearly have medicolegal implications, for example, if a serious medication error is suspected, then strict chain-of-custody procedures should be implemented. The physician or nurse taking the sample should seal the sample bag with a tamper-proof device, and sign and date the seal. A chain-of-custody form should also accompany the specimen. Each person taking possession of the sample should sign and date the form. The sample should be secured in a locked container or refrigerator if left unattended before arrival at the laboratory.

SPECIMEN SOURCES

Urine is useful for "screening" since it is often available in large volumes and usually contains higher concentrations of drugs and some other poisons than blood.

Stomach contents may be the best sample on which to perform certain tests. If obtained soon after an ingestion, large amounts of poison may be present. It may also be possible to identify tablets or capsules simply by inspection. Emetine from syrup of ipecacuanha may be present, especially in children.

Plasma or serum is normally used for quantitative assays, but some poisons are best measured in whole blood. EDTA tubes are preferred for aminoglycoside antibiotics (gentamicine, kanamycin, tobramycin, vancomycin), carboxyhemoglobin, and lead and some other metals (Table H-2). A fluoride/oxalate tube should be used if ethanol, cocaine, nitrazepam, or clonazepam is suspected. The use of disinfectant swabs containing alcohols (ethanol, 2-propanol) prior to venipuncture should be avoided, as should heparin, which contains phenolic preservatives (chlorbutol, cresol). The blood collection site should be remote from any infusion site. Vigorous discharge of blood through a syringe needle can cause sufficient hemolysis to invalidate a serum iron assay. Use plastic tubes if paraquat is to be measured, and (ideally) glass if volatiles are suspected.

CONTAINERS

Evacuated blood tubes and containers containing gel separators or soft rubber stoppers are not recommended if a toxicologic analysis is to be performed. Phosphate and phthalate plasticizers used in many such tubes may interfere in chromatographic methods.

PLASMA VERSUS SERUM

There are no significant differences in the concentrations of poisons between plasma and serum. Poisons such as carbon monoxide, cyanide, and lead are found primarily in erythrocytes, and thus whole blood is needed for such measurements. The space above the blood in the tube ("headspace")

Table H–1
Sample Requirements for General Analytic Toxicology

Sample	Notes*
Whole blood	10 mL (lithium heparin or EDTA tube—use fluoride/oxalate if ethanol suspected; plastic tube if paraquat suspected; glass or plastic tube with minimal headspace if carbon monoxide or other volatiles suspected)
[*or* Plasma/serum	5 mL (send whole blood of volatiles, metals and some other compounds suspected—see text)]
Urine†	20–50 mL (plain bottle, no preservative‡)
Gastric contents§	25–50 mL (plain bottle, no preservative)
Scene residues∞	As appropriate
Other samples	Vitreous humor, bile or liver (about 5 g) can substitute for urine in postmortem work. Other tissues (brain, liver, kidney, lung, subcutaneous fat—5 g) may also be valuable, especially if organic solvents or other volatile poisons are suspected

*Smaller volumes may often be acceptable, for example in the case of children.
†All that is normally required for drugs of abuse screening.
‡Sodium fluoride (1% w/v) should be added if ethanol is suspected and blood is not available.
§Includes vomit, gastric lavage (stomach washout, first sample), *etc.*
∞Tablet bottles, drinks containers, aerosol canisters, *etc.*—pack entirely separately from biological samples, especially if poisoning with volatiles is a possibility.

Table H–2
Sample Requirements for Metals/Trace Elements Analysis

Element	Sample Requirements
Aluminum	10 mL whole blood in plastic (not glass) tube—no anticoagulant/separating beads*, 20 mL dialysate/supply water in plastic bottle rinsed several times with portions of the intended sample*
Antimony	5 mL heparinized whole blood, 20 mL urine
Arsenic†	5 mL heparinized whole blood, 20 mL urine
Bismuth	5 mL heparinized whole blood
Cadmium	2 mL EDTA whole blood*, 10 mL urine*
Chromium	2 mL heparinized whole blood*‡, 20 mL urine (hard plastic bottle)*
Copper	2 mL heparinized or clotted whole blood, or 1 mL plasma/serum, 10 mL urine
Iron	5 mL clotted blood or 2 mL serum (no hemolysis)
Lead	2 mL EDTA whole blood (no clots)
Lithium	5 mL clotted blood or 2 mL serum (not lithium heparin tube)
Manganese	1 mL heparinized whole blood, or 0.5 mL plasma*‡
Mercury	5 mL heparinized whole blood§, 20 mL urine (hard plastic bottle)§
Selenium	2 mL heparinized whole blood or 1 mL plasma/serum
Silver	2 mL heparinized whole blood or 1 mL plasma
Strontium	2 mL heparinized whole blood or 1 mL plasma
Thallium	5 mL heparinized whole blood, 20 mL urine
Zinc	2 mL whole blood (heparinized or clotted but not EDTA) or 1 mL plasma/serum

*Send unused sample container from the same batch as used for sample collection to check for possible contamination.
†To diagnose chronic poisoning exclude seafood (shellfish, *etc.*) from diet for 15 days before sample collection.
‡Use of a plastic cannula to collect blood is advisable.
§Send samples promptly to avoid loss of mercury on storage.

Table H–3
Summary of Drugs and Other Common Poisons Detected in Blood and in Urine by Commonly Available Methods

1. Acidic and neutral drugs
   (a) Anticonvulsants, barbiturates, nonbarbiturate hypnotics and some hypoglycemics (blood, GLC)
   (b) Anticonvulsants and barbiturates (urine, TLC)
   (c) Paracetamol, salicylates* (blood/urine, various methods)
   (d) Nonsteroidal antiinflammatory drugs (blood, HPLC)
   (e) Caffeine, theophylline (blood, HPLC)
2. Basic drugs
   (a) *Detectable in blood after overdose (GLC).* Induces amphetamine and analogues, some antiarrhythmics, some antihistamines, some antimalarials, cocaine, dextropropoxyphene†, some opioids, some phenothiazines, tricyclic and related antidepressants
   (b) *Detectable in urine/gastric contents (GLC).* Most of those in 2(a) including:
      β-Adrenoceptor blockers (but not atenolol, sotalol)
      Amphetamines [includes MDA (methylenedioxyamphetamine), MDEA (methylenedioxyethylamphetamine) and MDMA (methylenedioxymethamphetamine)]
      Antiarrhythmics (includes disopyramide, flecainide, mexiletine)
      Antibiotics (includes chloramphenicol, metronidazole, trimethoprim)
      Anticholinergics (includes dicyclomine, benzhexol, procyclidine)
      Antihistamines (includes chlorpheniramine, cyclizine, diphenhydramine, terfenadine)
      Local anesthetics (includes bupivacaine, lignocaine, mepivacaine, prilocaine)
      Narcotic analgesics (but not heroin/morphine)
      Pesticides (includes some chlorinated pesticides, and some organophsophates and carbamates)
      Phenothiazines (but not flupenthixol and some other low-dose compounds)
      Tricyclic and related antidepressants (includes amitriptyline, clomipramine, desipramine, dothiepin, imipramine, nortriptyline)
   (c) *Detectable in urine gastric contents (TLC).* Those in Group 2(b) plus β-adrenoceptor blockers, cimetidine, heroin, mefenamic acid, morphine, phenothiazines, ranitidine

*May include aminosalicylate, aspirin, methyl salicylate and salicylamide if Trinder's test used.
†Quantitation by HPLC recommended.
‡From chloral hydrate, dichloralphenazone, trichloroethylene, or triclofos.

(continued)

Table H–3 *(Continued)*

3. Hypnotics/anxiolytics
   - (a) Ethchlorvynol, chlormethiazole, 2,2,2-trichloroethanol‡ (blood, GLC)
   - (b) Benzodiazepines (blood, GLC-ECD)
   - (c) Benzodiazepines (urine, immunoassay). Group identification only
4. Solvents and related compounds
   - (a) Anesthetics, fuel gases, solvents and other volatile substances (blood/urine, GC) (acetone, ethanol, 2-propanol and methanol commonly measured separately by direct injection GC; others measured by headspace GC)
   - (b) Ethylene glycol, 1,2-propanediol (blood/urine, GLC)
5. Substance abuse (various methods depending on circumstances; immuoassays group specific for amphetamines and opiates)
   - (a) Amphetamines (urine). Includes MDA, MDEA, MDMA
   - (b) Cannabis (urine, as cannabinoids)
   - (c) Cocaine (urine, as benzoylecgonine)
   - (d) Lysergic acid diethylamide (LSD) (urine)
   - (e) Opioids (urine). Includes codeine, dihydrocodeine, heroin, morphine
   - (f) Diuretics (urine, TLC). Includes thiazides, spironolactone
   - (g) Laxatives (urine, TLC). Includes bisacodyl, danthron, phenolphthalein, rhein (*e.g.* from *Senna*)
6. Pesticides
   - (a) Chlorphenoxy and hydroxybenzonitrile herbicides (blood/urine, HPLC). Includes 2,4-D (2,4-dichlorophenoxyacetic acid), DCPP (2,4-dichlorophenoxypropionic acid), ioxynil, MCPA (4-chloro-2-methylphenoxyacetic acid), MCPP (4-chloro-2-methylphenoxy-propionic acid), 2,4,5-T (2,4,5-trichlorophenoxyacetic acid)
   - (b) Diquat, paraquat (blood/urine, HPLC)
   - (c) Chlorinated pesticides (blood, GLC). Includes chlordane, DDT (1,1,1-trichloro-di-(4-chlorophenyl)ethane), dieldrin, lindane, pentachlorophenol
   - (d) Organophosphate and carbamate insecticides (blood/urine, GLC)
7. Toxic metals (separate assays, mostly atomic absorption spectrophotometry)
8. Miscellaneous poisons. Includes bromide, carbon monoxide (as carboxyhemoglobin), cyanide, lithium, digoxin

Table H–4
Emergency Toxicologic Analyses That May Influence Active Treatment

Treatment	Poison	Plasma Concentration Associated With Serious Toxicity*
1. Protective therapy		
N-Acetylcysteine or methionine	Paracetamol	200 mg/L at 4 h, 30 mg/L at 15 h
Ethanol	Ethylene glycol	0.5 g/L
2. Chelation therapy	Methanol	0.5 g/L
	Aluminum	50–250μg/L (serum
Deferroxamine	Iron	8 mg/L (serum
EDTA†/DMSA‡	Antimony	200 μg/L (whole blood)
	Cadmium	20 μg/L (whole blood)
	Lead	800 μg/L (whole blood)
DMSA‡/DMPS§	Arsenic	200 μg/L (whole blood)
	Bismuth	200 μg/L (whole blood)
	Mercury	100 μg/L (whole blood)
3. Active elimination therapy		
Oral Prussian Blue∞	Thallium	0.1 mg/L (whole blood)
Alkaline diuresis	Chlorophenoxy herbicides	500 mg/L
	Barbitone	300 mg/L
	Phenobarbitone	100 mg/L
	Salicylates	500 mg/L
Hemodialysis/peritoneal dialysis	Barbitone	300 mg/L
	Ethanol	5 g/L
	Ethylene glycol	0.5 g/L
	Lithium	10 mg/L
	Methanol	0.5 g/L
	Phenobarbitone	200 mg/L
	2-Propanol	4 g/L
	Salicylates	750 mg/L

*Many factors may modify response in a given patient.
†Calcium disodium ethylenediamine tetra-acetate.
‡Dimercaptosuccinic acid.
§Dimercaptopropane sulfonate.
∞Potassium ferrihexacyanoferrate.

Table H–5
Some Factors That May Affect Interpretation of Toxicology Results

Acidosis/alkalosis (water-soluble ionizable poisons)
Age
Burns (state of hydration)
Disease
Drug therapy (long-term and recent)
Duration of exposure
Ethanol consumption (short- and long-term)
Formulation (sustained release, racemate, *etc.*)
Genetics
Hemolysis
Idiosyncrasy
Infection
More than one poison present
Nutrition
Occupation
Pregnancy
Route of exposure (especially if intravenous or inhalational rather than oral)
Shock
Site of sampling (especially important if patient undergoing an infusion and in post-mortem cases)
Surgery
Time of sampling relative to exposure and/or death
Tolerance
Trauma

Table H–6
Some Drugs, Metabolites, and Other Poisons Unstable in Whole Blood or Plasma

Compound/Group of Compounds (Examples)
(i) Volatile compounds
All (aerosol propellants, anesthetic gases, carbon monoxide, ethanol, mercury, organic solvents, paraldehyde)
(ii) Nonvolatile compounds
Alkyl nitrites (glyceryl trinitrate)
Aspirin
Cocaine
Cyanide ion
Cyclosporin*
1,4-Dihydropyridines (nifedipine)
Insulin
N-Glucuronide metabolites (nomifensine)
7-Nitrobenzodiazepines (clonazepam, nitrazepam)
N-Oxide metabolites (nomifensine)
N-Sulfate metabolites (minoxidil)
Peroxides and other strong oxidizing agents
Paracetamol
Phenelzine
Phenothiazines†
Physostigmine
Quinol metabolites (4-hydroxypropranolol)
S-Oxide metabolites
Thiol (sulfydryl-containing) drugs (captopril)
Thiopentone

*Redistributes between plasma and red cells on standing—use whole blood
†Particularly those without an electron-withdrawing substituent at the 2-position.

Table H–7
Some Commonly Used Spot Tests

Test	Analyte(s)	Fluid	Limit of Sensitivity (mg/L)	Additional Compounds Detected
ortho-Cresol/ammonia	Paracetamol	Urine	1*	Aniline† Benorylate Nitrobenzene† Phenacetin† Ethylenediamine‡
Diphenylamine	Oxidizing agents	Gastric contents§	10	Bromates Chlorates Iodates Nitrates Nitrites Peroxides
Dithionite	Paraquat (blue) Diquat (yellow-green)	Urine∞	1 5	—
Ethchlorvynol/ diphenylamine	Ethchlorvynol	Urine	1	—
Forrest	Imipramine	Urine	25	Clomipramine Desipramine Trimipramine
FPN**	Phenothiazines	Urine	25††	—
Fujiwara	Trichloro compounds	Urine	1‡‡	Chloral hydrate Chloroform Dichloralphenazone Trichloroethylene Triclofos
Trinder's§§	Salicylates	Plasma Urine Gastric contents§	10	Aloxiprin† Aminosalicylate Aspirin† Benorylate† Methyl salicylate† Salicylamide†

*As 4-aminophenol.
†After metabolism or hydrolysis.
‡From aminophylline, for example.
§Includes vomit, stomach wash out, scene residues and similar samples.
∞Can be used on plasma in severe cases.
**Ferric chloride/perchloric acid/nitric acid.
††As chlorpromazine.
‡‡As trichloroacetate.
§§Ketones interfere.

should be minimized if carbon monoxide or other volatiles are suspected.

SCREENING

In clinical poisons screening, the main aim is to detect central nervous system (CNS)–depressant drugs and those where active treatment may be indicated. Normally, such analyses will be performed to help diagnose the cause of serious, often life-threatening conditions such as coma or convulsions.

Many difficulties may be encountered when performing qualitative and quantitative analyses for poisons. The substances that may be present include gases such as carbon monoxide, drugs, solvents, pesticides, metal salts, and naturally occurring toxins. Plasma concentrations associated with serious toxicity range from µg/L in the case of drugs such as digoxin to g/L in the case of ethanol. All relevant information about a patient gathered from a clinician, nurse, or poisons information specialist should be recorded in the laboratory using a suitably designed form. A note of a patient's occupation or hobbies can be valuable as this may indicate access to particular poisons.

General toxicologic analyses (poisons "screens") must use reasonable amounts of commonly available samples (see Table I-1). If any tests are to influence immediate patient management, the (preliminary) results should be available within 2 to 3 hours of receiving the specimens (1 hour in the case of paracetamol). A quantitative analysis carried out on whole blood or plasma is usually needed to confirm poisoning unequivocally, but this may not be possible. A "positive" result on a poisons screen does not of itself confirm poisoning, since such a result may arise from incidental or occupational exposure to the poison in question or the use of drugs in treatment.

Benzodiazepines, tricyclic and related antidepressants, anticonvulsants, narcotic and other analgesics, nonsteroidal antiinflammatory drugs (NSAIDs), and, of course, ethanol are all encountered regularly; multiple overdosage is frequent. Poisoning with certain compounds is not infrequently misdiagnosed, especially if the patient presents in the later stages of an episode. Examples include cardiorespiratory arrest (cyanide), hepatitis (paracetamol), diabetes (hypoglycemics, including ethanol in young children), paresthesias (thallium), progressive pneumonitis (paraquat), and renal failure (ethylene glycol). Quantitative measurements in urine are generally of little use except when assessing occupational exposure to certain compounds.

REFERENCES

1. Flanagan RJ. The poisoned patient: the role of the laboratory. Br J Biomed Sci 1995;52:202–213.

Appendix I
Drugs Discontinued 1974–1993

Table I–1
New Chemical Entities (NCEs) and New Biologic Entities (NBEs) Approved and Subsequently Discontinued in Light of a Safety Question in the United Kingdom, the United States, or Spain, 1974 Through 1993[a]

Drug	Trade Name(s)*	Country	Therapeutic Class	Safety Issue
Azaribine	Triazure	U.S.	Antipsoriatic	Thromboembolism
Bendazac	Bendalina	Spain	Antiinflammatory, for prevention of cataracts	Liver damage
Benoxaprofen	Opren, Oraflex, Bexopron	U.K., U.S., Spain	Antiinflammatory	Liver damage, serious skin reactions
Cianidanol	Catergen	Spain	Hepatoprotector	Hemolytic anemia
Cinepazide	Vasolande, Arteripax	Spain	Vasodilator	Agranulocytosis
Dilevalol	Unicarde	U.K.	β-Blocker, vasodilator	Liver damage
Encainide	Enkaid	U.K., U.S.	Antiarrhythmic	Proarrhythmic effect
Fenclofenac	Flenac	U.K.	Antiinflammatory	Serious skin reactions, carcinogenicity in animals
Feprazone	Methrazone	U.K.†	Antiinflammatory	Serious skin reactions, multiple problems
Flosequinan	Manoplax	U.K., U.S.	Vasodilator	Increased mortality
Gangliosides	Nevrotal	Spain	"Neurotrophic," treatment of neuritis, etc.	Acute polyneuropathy
Indoprofen	Flosint, Flosin	U.K., Spain	Antiinflammatory	Carcinogenicity in animals, multiple problems
Isoxicam	Pacyl	Spain	Antiinflammatory	Serious skin reactions
Nebacumab	Centoxin	U.K., Spain	Monoclonal antibody for treatment of septic shock	Increased mortality in patient subgroup
Nomifensine	Merital, Alival	U.K., U.S., Spain	Antidepressant	Hemolytic anemia
Perhexiline	Pexid	U.K., Spain	Vasodilator, antianginal	Peripheral neuropathy, liver damage
Pirprofen	Rengasil	Spain	Antiinflammatory	Gastrointestinal toxicity, liver damage
Polidexide	Secholex	U.K.	Hypolipidemic	Toxic impurities
Remoxipride	Roxiam	U.K.	Antipsychotic	Aplastic anemia
Somatropin	Crescormone, Asellacrin	U.K., U.S., Spain	Natural growth hormone	Creutzfeldt-Jacob disease
Suloctidyl	Loctidon	Spain	Vasodilator	Liver damage
Suprofen	Suprol, Supranol	U.K., U.S., Spain	Antiinflammatory	Renal toxicity, lumbar pain
Temafloxin	Teflox	U.K., U.S.	Antibiotic	Multiorgan reactions
Terodiline	Terolin, Micturin, Uromictrol	U.K., Spain	Anticholinergic, calcium antagonist for urinary incontinence	Cardiac arrhythmias
Ticrynafen (tienilic acid)	Selacryn	U.S.	Diuretic	Liver damage
Triazolam	Halcion	U.K.‡	Hypnotic, anxiolytic	Amnesia, various psychiatric reactions
L-Tryptophan	Optimax, Pacitron	U.K.	Antidepressant	Eosinophilia-myalgia syndrome
Zimeldine	Zelmid	U.K.	Antidepressant	Neuropathy, convulsions, liver damage
Zomepirac	Zomax	U.K., U.S., Spain	Analgesic, antiinflammatory	Anaphylactic shock, renal failure

[a]Adapted from Bakke OM et al. Cln Pharmacol Ther 1995;58:108–117.
*Only originator's and/or principal licensee's trade name shown.
†Still marketed in Spain; not approved in the United States.
‡Still marketed in the United States and Spain.

A number of new drugs have been discontinued from the market because of severe toxicity (Table I–1).[1]

REFERENCE

1. Bakke OM, Monocchia M, de Abajo F, Kaitinsk I, Lasagna L. Drug safety discontinuations in the United Kingdom, the United States, and Spain from 1974 through 1993: a regulatory perspective. Clin Pharmacol Ther 1995;58:108–117.

Appendix J
Conversion Formula

Readers who wish to convert drug concentrations to or from SI units may apply the following formulas:

To determine the conversion factor (CF): $CF = \frac{1000}{\text{mol wt}}$

To convert to SI units: (μg/mL) × CF = (μmol/liter)
To convert from SI units: (μmol/liter divided by CF = (μg/mL)

Example: Phenytoin conversion

Conversion factor: $CF = \frac{1000}{\text{mol wt}} = \frac{1000}{252.3} = 3.96$

Conversion: (μg/mL) × 3.96 = (10 μg/mL) × 3.96 = 39.6 μmol/liter (39.6 μmol/liter divided by 3.96 = 10 μg/mL)

Table J–1
SI Unit Conversions

Substance in Blood					
Old unit × factor = new (SI unit) × factor = old unit					
Calcium	mg/dL	0.250	mmol/L	4.00	mg/dL
Copper	μg/dL	0.1574	μmol/L	6.353	μg/dL
Sodium	mEq/L	1.0	mmol/L	1.0	mEq/L
Lead	μg/dL	0.0483	μmol/L	20.70	μg/dL
Zinc	μg/dL	0.1530	μmol/L	6.536	μg/dL
Magnesium	mEq/L	0.500	mmol/L	2.00	mEq/L
Potassium	mEq/L	1.00	mmol/L	1.00	mEq/L
Substance in Urine					
Mercury	μg/24 hr	4.985	nmol/d	2.00	μg/24 hr.

Appendix K
Système International Conversion Factors for Frequently Used Laboratory Components

Table K–1
Système International Conversion Factors for Frequently Used Laboratory Components[a]

System*	Component	Traditional Reference Interval†	Traditional Unit‡	Conversion Factor	Reference SI Interval†	SI Unit	Significant Digits§	Suggested Minimum Increment
S	Copper	70–140	µg/dL	0.1574	11.0–22.0	µmol/L	XX.X	0.2 µmol/L
U	Copper	<40	µg/24 hr	0.0574	<0.6	µmol/d	X.X	0.2 µmol/d
P	Corticotropin (ACTH)	20–100	pg/mL	0.2202	4–22	pmol/L	XX	1 pmol/L
S	Creatine Male	0.17–0.50	mg/dL	76.25	10–40	µmol/L	X0	10 µmol/L
	Female	0.35–0.93	mg/dL	76.25	30–70	µmol/L	X0	10 µmol/L
U	Creatine Male	0–40	mg/24 hr	7.625	0–300	µmol/d	XX0	10 µmol/L
	Female	0–80	mg/24 hr	7.625	0–600	µmol/d	XX0	10 µmol/d
S	Creatine kinase (CK)	0–130 (37°C)	Units/L	1.00	0–130	U/L	XXX	1 U/L
S	Creatine kinase isoenzymes, MB fraction	>5 in myocardial infarction	%	0.01	>0.05	1	X.XX	0.01
S	Creatinine	0.6–1.2	mg/dl **(Dual report)**	88.40	50–110	µmol/L	XX0	10 µmol/L
U	Creatinine	Variable	g/24 hr **(Dual report)**	8.840	Variable	mmol/d	XX.X	0.1 mmol/d
S, U	Creatinine clearance	75–125	mL/min **(Dual report)**	0.01667	1.24–2.08	mL/s	X.XX	0.02 mL/s
U	Cystine	10–100	mg/24 hr	4.161	40–420	µmol/d	XX0	10 µmol/d
P	Digoxin, therapeutic	0.5–2.2	ng/mL **(Dual report)**	1.281	0.6–2.8	nmol/L	X.X	0.1 nmol/L
		0.5–2.2	µg/L **(Dual report)**	1.281	0.6–2.8	nmol/L	X.X	0.1 nmol/L
S	Estradiol, male >18 y	15–40	pg/mL **(Dual report)**	3.671	55–150	pmol/L	XXX	1 pmol/L
P	Ethyl alcohol	>100	mg/dL	0.2171	>22	mmol/L	XX	1 mmol/L
P	Fibrinogen	200–400	mg/dL	0.01	2.0–4.0	g/L	X.X	0.1 g/L
P	Follicle-stimulating hormone (FSH) Female	2.0–15.0	mIU/mL	1.00	2–15	IU/L	XX	1 IU/L
	Peak production	20–50	mIU/mL	1.00	20–50	IU/L	XX	1 IU/L
	Male	1.0–10.0	mIU/mL	1.00	1–10	IU/L	XX	1 IU/L
U	Follicle-stimulating hormone (FSH) Follicular phase	2–15	IU/24 hr	1.00	2–15	IU/d	XXX	1 IU/d

[a]Adapted from JAMA 1995;274:97–98.
*P represents plasma; B, blood; S, serum; U, urine; CSF, cerebrospinal fluid; RBCs, red blood cells; and WBCs, white blood cells.
†These reference values are not intended to be definitive since each laboratory determines its own values. They are provided for illustration only.
‡Traditional units should be reported parenthetically after the SI units *only* for those units marked "Dual report."
§"Significant digits" refers to the number of digits used to describe the reported results. XX implies that results expressed to the nearest whole number are meaningful; XX0, that results are only meaningful when rounded to the nearest 10, and that results reported to lower numbers or decimal points are beyond the sensitivity of the procedure.

(continued)

Table K–1 *(Continued)*

System*	Component	Traditional Reference Interval†	Traditional Unit‡	Conversion Factor	SI Reference Interval†	SI Unit	Significant Digits§	Suggested Minimum Increment
	Midcycle	8–40	IU/24 hr	1.00	8–40	IU/d	XXX	1 IU/d
	Luteal phase	2–10	IU/24 hr	1.00	2–10	IU/d	XXX	1 IU/d
	Menopausal women	35–100	IU/24 hr	1.00	35–100	IU/d	XXX	1 IU/d
	Male	2–15	IU/24 hr	1.00	2–15	IU/d	XXX	1 IU/d
S	γ-Glutamyltransferase (GGT)	0–30 (30°C)	Units/L	1.00	0–30	U/L	XX	1 U/L
P	Glucose	70–110	mg/dL **(Dual report)**	0.05551	3.9–6.1	mmol/L	XX.X	0.1 mmol/L
B	Hemoglobin Male	14.0–18.0	g/dL	10.0	140–180	g/L	XXX	1 g/L
	Female	11.5–15.5	g/dL	10.0	115–155	g/L	XXX	1 g/L
S	Immunoglobulins IgG	500–1200	mg/dL	0.01	5.00–12.00	g/L	XX.XX	0.01 g/L
	IgA	50–350	mg/dL	0.01	0.50–3.50	g/L	XX.XX	0.01 g/L
	IgM	30–230	mg/dL	0.01	0.30–2.30	g/L	XX.XX	0.01 g/L
	IgD	<6	mg/dL	10	<60	mg/L	XX0	10 mg/L
	IgE 0–3 y	0.5–1.0	U/mL	2.4	1–24	μg/L	XX	1 μg/L
	3–80 y	5–100	U/mL	2.4	12–240	μg/L	XX	1 μg/L
S	Iron Male	80–180	μg/dL **(Dual report)**	0.1791	14–32	μmol/L	XX	1 μmol/L
	Female	60–160	μg/dL **(Dual report)**	0.1791	11–29	μmol/L	XX	1 μmol/L
S	Iron-binding capacity	250–460	μg/dL **(Dual report)**	0.1791	45–82	μmol/L	XX	1 μmol/L
S	Lactate dehydrogenase (L → P)	50–150 (37°C)	Units/L	1.00	50–150	U/L	XXX	1 U/L
			Wroblewski units/mL	0.482	. . .	U/L	XXX	1 U/L
S	Lactate dehydrogenase isoenzymes LD_1	15–40	%	0.01	0.15–0.40	1	X.XX	0.01
	LD_2	20–45	%	0.01	0.20–0.45	1	X.XX	0.01
	LD_3	15–30	%	0.01	0.15–0.30	1	X.XX	0.01
	LD_4 and LD_5	5–20	%	0.01	0.05–0.20	1	X.XX	0.01
	LD_1	10–60	Units/L	1	10–60	U/L	XX	1 U/L
	LD_2	20–70	Units/L	1	20–70	U/L	XX	1 U/L

(continued)

Table K–1 *(Continued)*

System*	Component	Traditional Reference Interval†	Traditional Unit‡	Conversion Factor	SI Reference Interval†	SI Unit	Significant Digits§	Suggested Minimum Increment
	LD_3	10–45	Units/L	1	10–45	U/L	XX	1 U/L
	LD_4 and LD_5	5–30	Units/L	1	5–30	U/L	XX	1 U/L
B	Lead, toxic	>60	µg/dL **(Dual report)**	0.04826	>2.90	µmol/L	X.XX	0.05 µmol/L
			mg/dL **(Dual report)**	48.26	. . .	µmol/L	X.XX	0.05 µmol/L
U	Lead, toxic	>80	µg/24 hr **(Dual report)**	0.004826	>0.40	µmol/d	X.XX	0.05 µmol/d
P	Lipids, total	400–850	mg/dL **(Dual report)**	0.01	4.0–8.5	g/L	X.X	0.1 g/L
P	Lipoproteins Low-density (LDL), as cholesterol	50–190	mg/dL **(Dual report)**	0.02586	1.30–4.90	mmol/L	X.XX	0.05 mmol/L
	High-density (HDL), as cholesterol Male	30–70	mg/dL **(Dual report)**	0.02586	0.80–1.80	mmol/L	X.XX	0.05 mmol/L
	Female	30–90	mg/dL **(Dual report)**	0.02586	0.80–2.35	mmol/L	X.XX	0.05 mmol/L
S	Magnesium	1.8–3.0	mg/dL **(Dual report)**	0.4114	0.80–1.20	mmol/L	X.XX	0.02 mmol/L
P	Phenytoin, therapeutic	10–20	mg/L	3.964	40–80	µmol/L	XX	5 µmol/L
P	Phosphatase, acid (prostatic)	0–3	King-Armstrong units/dL	1.77	0–5.5	U/L	X.X	0.05 U/L
			Bodansky units/dL	5.37	0–16.1	U/L	X.X	0.5 U/L
S	Phosphatase, alkaline	30–120	Units/L	1.00	30–120	U/L	XXX	1U/L
			Bodansky units/dL	5.37	161–644	U/L	XXX	1 U/L
			King-Armstrong units/dL	7.1	213–852	U/L	XXX	1 U/L
S	Phosphate (as phosphorus)	2.5–5.0	mg/dL **(Dual report)**	0.3229	0.80–1.60	mmol/L	X.XX	0.05 mmol/L
S	Potassium	3.5–5.0	MEq/L	1.00	3.5–5.0	mmol/L	X.X	0.1 mmol/L
P	Progesterone Follicular phase	<2	ng/mL	3.180	<6	nmol/L	XX	2 nmol/L
	Luteal phase	2–20	ng/mL	3.180	6–64	nmol/L	XX	2 nmol/L
S	Protein, total	6–8	g/dL	10.0	60–80	g/L	XX	1 g/L
CSF	Protein, total	<40	mg/dL	0.01	<0.40	g/L	X.XX	0.01 g/L
U	Protein, total	<150	mg/24 hr	0.001	<0.15	g/d	X.XX	0.01 g/d
S	Sodium	135–147	mEq/L	1.00	135–147	mmol/L	XXX	1 mmol/L
S	Sodium ion	135–147	mEq/L	1.00	135–147	mmol/L	XXX	1 mmol/L
U	Sodium ion	Diet dependent	mEq/24 hr	1.00	Diet dependent	mmol/d	XXX	1 mmol/d

(continued)

Table K–1 *(Continued)*

System*	Component	Traditional Reference Interval†	Traditional Unit‡	Conversion Factor	SI Reference Interval†	SI Unit	Significant Digits§	Suggested Minimum Increment
U	Steroids							
	Hydroxycorticosteroids (as cortisol)							
	Female	2–8	mg/24 hr	2.759	5–25	µmol/d	XX	1 µmol/d
	Male	3–10	mg/24 hr	2.759	10–30	µmol/d	XX	1 µmol/d
U	17-Ketogenic steroids (as dehydro-epiandrosterone)							
	Female	7–12	mg/24 hr	3.467	25–40	µmol/d	XX	1 µmol/d
	Male	9–17	mg/24 hr	3.467	30–60	µmol/d	XX	1 µmol/d
U	17-Ketosteroids (as dehydroepian-drosterone)							
	Female	6–17	mg/24 hr	3.467	20–60	µmol/d	XX	1 µmol/d
	Male	6–20	mg/24 hr	3.467	20–70	µmol/d	XX	1 µmol/d
U	Ketosteroid fractions							
	Androsterone							
	Female	0.5–3.0	mg/24 hr	3.443	1–10	µmol/d	XX	1 µmol/d
	Male	2.0–5.0	mg/24 hr	3.443	7–17	µmol/d	XX	1 µmol/d
	Dehydroepiandrosterone							
	Female	0.2–1.8	mg/24 hr	3.467	1–6	µmol/d	XX	1 µmol/d
	Male	0.2–2.0	mg/24 hr	3.467	1–7	µmol/d	XX	1 µmol/d
	Etiocholanolone							
	Female	0.8–4.0	mg/24 hr	3.443	2–14	µmol/d	XX	1 µmol/d
	Male	1.4–5.0	mg/24 hr	3.443	4–17	µmol/d	XX	1 µmol/d
				58.07	580–870	µmol/L	XX0	10 µmol/L
P	Testosterone							
	Female	<0.6	ng/mL **(Dual report)**	3.467	<2 0	nmol/L	XX.X	0.5 nmol/L
	Male	4.0–8.0	ng/mL **(Dual report)**	3.467	14.0–28.0	nmol/L	XX.X	0.5 nmol/L
S	Thyroxine (T_4)	4–11	µg/cL **(Dual report)**	12.87	51–142	nmol/L	XXX	1 nmol/L
S	Thyroxine-binding globulin (TBG), as thyroxine	12–28	µg/cL **(Dual report)**	12.87	150–360	nmol/L	XX0	10 nmol/L
S	Thyroxine, free	0.8–2.8	ng/cL **(Dual report)**	12.87	10–36	pmol/L	XX	1 pmol/L

(continued)

Table K–1 *(Continued)*

System*	Component	Traditional Reference Interval†	Traditional Unit‡	Conversion Factor	SI Reference Interval†	SI Unit	Significant Digits§	Suggested Minimum Increment
S	Triiodothyronine (T_3)	75–220	ng/dL	0.01536	1.2–3.4	nmol/L	X.X	0.1 nmol/L
S	Urate (as uric acid)	2.0–7.0	mg/dL	59.48	120–420	μmol/L	XX0	10 μmol/L
U	Urate (as uric acid)	Diet dependent	g/24 hr	5.948	Diet dependent	mmol/d	XX	1 mmol/d
S	Urea nitrogen	8–18	mg/dL **(Dual report)**	0.3570	3.0–6.5	mmol/L of urea	X.X	0.5 mmol/L
U	Urea nitrogen	12–20 (diet dependent)	g/24 hr **(Dual report)**	35.70	430–700	mmol/L of urea	XX0	10 mmol/d
U	Urobilinogen	0–4.0	mg/24 hr	1.693	0.0–6.8	μmol/d	X.X	0.1 μmol/d
S	Zinc	75–120	μg/dL	0.1530	11.5–18.5	μmol/L	XX.X	0.1 μmol/L
U	Zinc	150–1200	μg/24 hr	0.0153	2.3–18.3	μmol/d	XX.X	0.1 μmol/d

Appendix L
Odor Threshold Values, 1985–1991

Table L-1
Odor Threshold Values and 1985–1986 Threshold Limit Values

Substance	Odor Threshold (ppm)[a]	1985–1986 TLV-TWA (ppm)[a–d]
Acetaldehyde	0.031	100
Acetic acid	24	10
Acetone	1.5 and 0.20	750
Acetophenone	0.17	—
Acrolein	1.5 and 0.20	0.1
Acrylonitrile	19	2 (skin)
Allyl alcohol	1.4	2 (skin)
Allylamine	6.3	—
Allyl chloride	15,000 and 0.21	1
Allyl disulfide	0.00010 and 0.0012	—
Allyl isocyanide	0.018	—
Allyl isothiocyanate	0.0074 and 0.15	—
Allyl mercaptan	5.0×10^{-5}	—
Allyl sulfide	0.00014	—
Ammonia	0.019 and 55	25
n-Amyl acetate	0.080	100
Amyl alcohol	35	—
Amylene	0.0022	—
i-Amyl mercaptan	0.0043	—
Amyl sulfide	0.0030	—
Anethol	0.0033	—
Aniline	70	2
Apiol	0.0063	—
Arsenic hydride	1	0.2 mg/M³
Benzaldehyde	0.0060 and 0.042	—
Benzene	31	10
Benzyl chloride	0.040	1
Benzyl mercaptan	0.00035 and 2.6×10^{-3}	—
Benzyl sulfide	0.0060	—
Bornyl acetate	0.0078	—
Bromine	1	0.1
Bromoacetone	0.090	—
Butadiene	0.16	1,000 (1,3-Butadiene)
i-Butane	1.2	—
n-Butane	5.5	800
i-Butanol	40	—
n-Butanol	11	—
s-Butanol	43	—
t-Butanol	73	—
2-Butanone	4.8	200
Butyl acetate	20	150
i-Butyl acetate	4	—
n-Butyl acetate	7	150
i-Butylene	0.07	—
trans-2-Butylene	0.57	—
n-Butyl formate	17	—
Butyl mercaptan	0.0060	0.5
i-Butyl mercaptan	0.00054	—
n-Butyl mercaptan	0.0008	0.5
Butyl sulfide	0.00020 and 0.015	—
Butyric acid	0.00028 and 0.00056	—
Camphor	0.018 and 1.6	2 (Synthetic)
Carbon disulfide	0.0011 and 0.0081	10 (Skin)
Carbon tetrachloride	200	5 (Skin)
Carvacrol	0.0023	—
Chlorine	0.010	1
Chlorine dioxide	0.10	0.1
Chloroacetic acid	0.0–5	—
Chloroacetophenone	0.016	0.15 (Phenacylchloride) (α-Chloroacetophenone)
Chlorobenzene	0.21 and 0.94	75 (Monochlorobenzene)
Chloroform	200	10 (Trichloromethane)
o-Chlorophenol	0.0036	—
p-Chlorophenol	1.2	—
Chlorovinylarsine	1.6	—
Cinnamaldehyde	0.0026	—

[a]Oelert HH, Florian TH. Detection and evaluation of odor nuisance from diesel exhaust gases. Appendix. Odor Threshold Values. Staub 1972;32:20–31.
[b]TLV's: Threshold Limit Values for Chemical Substances in the Work Environment. Adopted by ACGIH with Intended Changes for 1985–1986. Cincinnati, Ohio, American Conference of Governmental Industrial Hygienists, 1985, pp 9–33.
[c]TLV—threshold limit value—refers to the airborne concentrations of a substance and represents conditions under which it is believed that nearly all workers may be repeatedly exposed day after day without adverse effects. See footnote *b*.
[d]TLV-TWA—threshold limit value time-weighted average—is the time-weighted average concentration for a normal 8-hour work day and a 40-hour work week to which nearly all workers may be repeatedly exposed, day after day, without adverse effect.

(continued)

Table L–1 *(Continued)*

Substance	Odor Threshold (ppm)[a]	1985–1986 TLV-TWA (ppm)[a–d]
Coumarin	0.00032 and 0.0033	—
m-Cresol	0.0076 and 0.68	5
o-Cresol	0.00068 and 0.68	5
p-Cresol	0.00047	5
Crotonaldehyde	0.035	2
Crotyl mercaptan	5.6×10^{-5} and 1.6×10^{-4}	—
Cyclohexane	0.41	300
Decanoic acid	0.0020	—
Decanol	0.0064	—
1-Decylene	0.12	—
Diacetyl	0.025	—
Diallyl ketone	9.0	—
O-Dichlorobenzene	50	50
Dichlorodiethyl sulfide	0.19	—
Dichloroethane	120	200 (1,1-Dichloroethane) 50 (1,2-Dichloroethane)
Dichloroethylene	0.085	200 (1,2-Dichloroethylene)
Bis-α-dichloroethyl sulfide	0.0023	—
Dichloroisopropyl ether	0.32	—
2,4-Dichlorophenol	0.21	—
1,2-Dichloropropane	50	75 (Propylene dichloride)
Diethyl selenide	0.00014	—
Diethyl succinate	0.016	—
Dimethylamine	0.021	10
1,1-Dimethylhydrazine	6	—
Dimethyl sulfide	0.0010 and 0.020	—
Dimethyl trithiocarbonate	0.0058	—
Dioxane	2.7 and 170	25 (Diethylene dioxide [skin])
Diphenylchloroarsine	0.030	—
Diphenylcyanoarsine	0.30	—
Diphenyl ether	0.10 and 0.0010	—
Diphenyl sulfide	0.00034 and 0.0021	—
Diphosgene	1.2	—
Dithioethylene glycol	0.031	—
Dodecanol	0.0064	—
Ethane	150	—
1,2-Ethanedithiol	0.0042	—
Ethanol	5100	1,000
Ethyl acetate	0.056	400
Ethyl butyrate	0.0082	—
Ethyl decanoate	0.00017	—
Ethyldichloroarsine	1.4	—
Ethyl disulfide	5.4×10^{-5} and 2.8×10^{-3}	—
Ethyl ether	0.33	400
Ethyl glycol	25	—
Ethyl hexanoate	0.0016 and 0.0056	—
Ethyl isothiocyanate	1.6	—
Ethyl mercaptan	1.6×10^{-5} and 5.1×10^{-4}	0.5
Ethyl methacrylate	9.8×10^{-5} and 0.0067	—
Ethyl pelargonate	0.0014	—
Ethyl selenide	6.4×10^{-5} and 1.2×10^{-3}	—
Ethyl selenomercaptan	1.8×10^{-6} and 3.0×10^{-4}	—
Ethyl sulfide	3, 0.00025, and 0.00060	—
Ethyl undecanoate	0.00054	—
Ethyl i-valerate	0.12	—
Ethyl n-valerate	0.060	—
Ethylene bromide	25	—
Ethylene glycol	0.080	50 ppm (Vapor)
Ethylene oxide	700	1
Eugenol	0.0046	—
Formaldehyde	0.98	1
Formic acid	21	5
n-Heptal chloride	0.060	—
Heptaldehyde	0.050	—
n-Heptane	50 and 200	400
Heptanol	0.057	—
Hexanoic acid	0.0061	—
Hexanol	0.0050	—
Hydrazine	3	0.1 (Skin)
Hydrocinnamyl alcohol	0.00027	—
Hydrocyanic acid	0.070	—
Hydrogen selenide	0.30	0.05
Hydrogen sulfide	0.0011 and 0.0081	10
Ionone	5.9×10^{-9} and 1.2×10^{-5}	—
Indoform	0.00050	—
Isocyanochloride	0.98	—
Lauric acid	0.0034	—
Light gasoline	800	—
Linoleyl acetate	0.0016	—
Menthol	1.5	—
2-Mercaptoethanol	0.64	—
Mesitylene	0.027	—
Methanol	5,900	200
Methoxynaphthalene	0.00012	—
Methyl acetate	0.21 and 200	200
Methylamine	3.3	10
Methyl anthranilate	0.00066	—
2-Methyl-2-butanol	2.3	—
Methyl n-butyrate	0.0026	—
Methyl chloride	10	50
Methyldichloroarsine	0.11	—
Methyl ethyl ketone	25	200 (2-Butanone)
Methylethylpyridine	0.050	—
Methyl formate	2000	100
Methyl glycol	60	—
Methyl isobutyl ketone	8.0	50 (Hexone)
Methyl mercaptan	0.041 and 0.0010	0.5
Methyl methacrylate	0.21	—

(continued)

Table L–1 *(Continued)*

Substance	Odor Threshold (ppm)[a]	1985–1986 TLV-TWA (ppm)[a–d]
2-Methylpropene	0.57	—
Methyl salicylate	0.00060 and 0.096	—
Methyl sulfide	0.0015	—
Methyl thiocyanate	0.25	—
Methylene chloride	150	100 (Dichloromethane)
Methylvinylpyridine	0.040	—
Mineral spirits	30	—
Monostyrene	25	—
Musk (synthetic)	4.0×10^{-7}	
Naphthalene	0.027	10
Nitric oxide	0.3 and 1	25
Nitrobenzene	1.9	1
n-Octane	150 and 0.19	300 (Octane)
Octanoic acid	0.0014	—
1-Octanol	0.0021	—
2-Octanol	0.0026	—
Oenanthic acid	0.015	—
Ozone	0.020	0.1
Pelargonic acid	0.00086	—
n-Pentane	2.2	600 (Pentane)
Pentanone	8.0	200 (Methylpropyl ketone)
Pentanol	0.0065	—
i-Pentyl acetate	0.0028	—
n-Pentyl acetate	0.00090	—
i-Pentyl mercaptan	0.00021	—
i-Pentyl sulfide	0.00041	—
n-Pentyl sulfide	2.8×10^{-5}	—
i-Pentyl i-valerate	0.0010 and 0.0066	
n-Pentyl i-valerate	0.00041	—
Phenol	0.05 and 5	5 (Skin)
Phenyl isocyanide	0.0010	—
Phenyl isothiocyanate	0.094	—
Phosgene	0.50	0.1 (Carbonyl chloride)
Phosphine	2.7	0.3
α-Pinene	0.010	—
Piperonal	0.0044	—
i-Propanol	45	—
n-Propanol	30	—
Propargyl aldehyde	0.015 and 0.16	
Propionic acid	0.018	—
i-Propyl acetate	30 and 400	—
n-Propyl acetate	20	200
Propyl mercaptan	7.5×10^{-5} and 1.6×10^{-3}	—
Propyl sulfide	0.0016 and 0.011	—
Pyridine	0.013 and 0.82	5
Quinoline	0.71	—
Safrole	0.0032	—
Skatole	7.5×10^{-8} and 0.019	—
Styrene	0.080 and 0.73	50 (Monomer) (Phenyl ethylene)
Sulfur dioxide	2 and 3	2
Tetrachloroethylene	50	50 (Perchloroethylene)
Tetrahydrofuran	30	200
Tetramethylbenzene	0.0029	0.0029
Thiocresol	0.00028 and 0.0027	—
Thiophenol	0.00026 and 14	—
Thymol	0.00086	—
Toluene	40	100 (Toluol)
1,1,1,-Trichloroethane	400	350 (Methyl chloroform)
Trimethylamine	1.7	—
2,4,6,-Trinitro-tert-butylxylene	6.5×10^{-6}	—
n-Undecane	0.12	—
Valeric acid	0.00060	—
i-Valeric acid	0.0018	—
Vanillin	3.2×10^{-8}	—
Xylene	2.2 and 20	100 (Xylol)
m-Xylene	3.7	100
p-Xylene	0.49	100
Xylidine	0.0048	2 (Skin)

Appendix M
SI Conversion Factors for Common Serum Drug Concentrations

Table M–1
Conversion Factors for Common Serum Drug Concentrations[a]

Drug	Molecular Weight (g/mol)	Present Unit	Conversion Factor (μg/mL to μmol/L)	Therapeutic Range μg/mL	Therapeutic Range μmol/L
Acetaminophen (P)	151.16	mg/dL	6.616	>5.0 mg/dL toxic	>330 toxic
Amitriptyline (P,S)	277.39	ng/mL	3.605	50–200 ng/mL	180–720 nmol/L
Carbamazepine (P)	236.27	mg/L	4.233	4–12	17–51
Chlordiazepoxide (P)	299.76	mg/L	3.336	0.5–5	2–17
Chlorpromazine (P)	318.88	ng/mL	3.136	50–300 ng/mL	150–950 nmol/L
Chlorpropamide (P)	276.74	mg/L	3.613	75–250	270–900
Desipramine (P)	266.37	ng/mL	3.754	50–200 ng/mL	170–700 nmol/L
Diazepam (P)	284.75	mg/L	3.512	100–250 ng/mL	350–900 nmol/L
Dicumarol (P)	336.30	mg/L	2.974	8–30	25–90
Digoxin (P)	780.95	ng/mL	1.281	0.5–2.2 ng/mL	0.6–2.8 nmol/L
Disopyramide (P)	339.48	mg/L	2.946	2–6	6–18
Doxepin (P)	279.37	ng/mL	3.579	50–200 ng/mL	180–720 nmol/L
Ethchlorvynol (P)	144.60	mg/L	6.915	>40 toxic	>280 toxic
Ethosuximide (P)	141.17	mg/L	7.084	40–110	280–780
Glutethimide (P)	217.27	mg/L	4.603	>20 toxic	>92 toxic
Gold (S)	196.96	μg/dL	0.051	300–800 μg/dL	15–40
Imipramine (P)	280.40	ng/mL	3.566	50–200 ng/mL	180–710 nmol/L
Isoniazid (P)	137.14	mg/L	7.291	>3.0 toxic	>22 toxic
Lidocaine (P)	234.34	mg/L	4.267	1.0–5.0	4.5–21.5
Lithium ion (S)	6.94	mEq/L	1.00	0.5–1.5 mEq/L	0.5–1.5
Maprotiline (P)	277.41	ng/mL	3.605	50–200 ng/mL	180–720 nmol/L
Meprobamate (P)	218.25	mg/L	4.582	>40 toxic	>180 toxic
Methaqualone (P)	250.29	mg/L	3.995	>30 toxic	>120 toxic
Methotrexate (S)	454.44	mg/L	2.200	>2.3 toxic	>5.0 toxic
Methsuximide (P) (as desmethylsuximide)	188.18	mg/L	5.285	10–40	50–210
Methyprylon (P)	183.25	mg/L	5.457	>40 toxic	>220 toxic
Nortriptyline (P)	263.37	ng/mL	3.797	25–200 ng/mL	90–760 nmol/L
Pentobarbital (P)	226.27	mg/L	4.419	20–40	90–170
Phenobarbital (P)	232.23	mg/dL	43.06	2–5 mg/dL	85–215
Phensuximide (P)	189.21	mg/L	5.285	4–8	20–40
Phenylbutazone (P)	308.37	mg/L	3.243	<100	<320
Phenytoin (P)	252.27	mg/L	3.964	10–20	40–80
Primidone (P)	218.26	mg/L	4.582	6–10	25–46
Procainamide (P)	235.33	mg/L	4.249	4–8	17–34
N-Acetylprocainamide† (P)	314.81	mg/L	3.606	4–8	14–29
Propoxyphene (P)	339.48	mg/L	2.946	>2.0 toxic	>5.9 toxic
Propranolol (P)	259.34	ng/mL	3.856	50–200 ng/mL	190–770 nmol/L
Protriptyline (P)	263.38	ng/mL	3.797	100–300 ng/mL	380–1140 nmol/L
Quinidine (P)	324.41	mg/L	3.082	1.5–3.0	4.6–9.2

[a]Adapted from Drug Intel Clin Pharm 1988;22:992.
†A metabolite of procainamide.
P = plasma; S = serum.

(continued)

Table M–1 *(Continued)*

Drug	Molecular Weight (g/mol)	Present Unit	Conversion Factor (µg/mL to µmol/L)	Therapeutic Range	
				µg/mL	µmol/L
Salicylic acid (S)	138.12	mg/dl	0.0724	>20 mg/dl toxic	1.45 toxic
Theophylline (P)	180.17	mg/L	5.550	10–20	55–110
Thiocyanate (P) (nitroprusside toxicity)	59.09	mg/dL	0.1722	10 mg/dL	1.7
Thiopental (P)	241.33	mg/L	4.126		
Tolbutamide (P)	270.35	mg/L	3.699	50–120	180–450
Trimethadione (P)	143.14	mg/L	6.986	<50	<350
Trimipramine (P)	294.42	ng/mL	3.397	50–200 ng/mL	170–680 nmol/L
Valproic acid (P)	144.21	mg/L	6.934	50–100	350–700
Warfarin (P)	308.32	mg/L	3.243	1.0–3.0	3.3–9.8

Appendix N
Reduce the Risk!

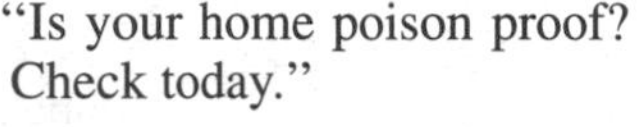

"Is your home poison proof?
Check today."

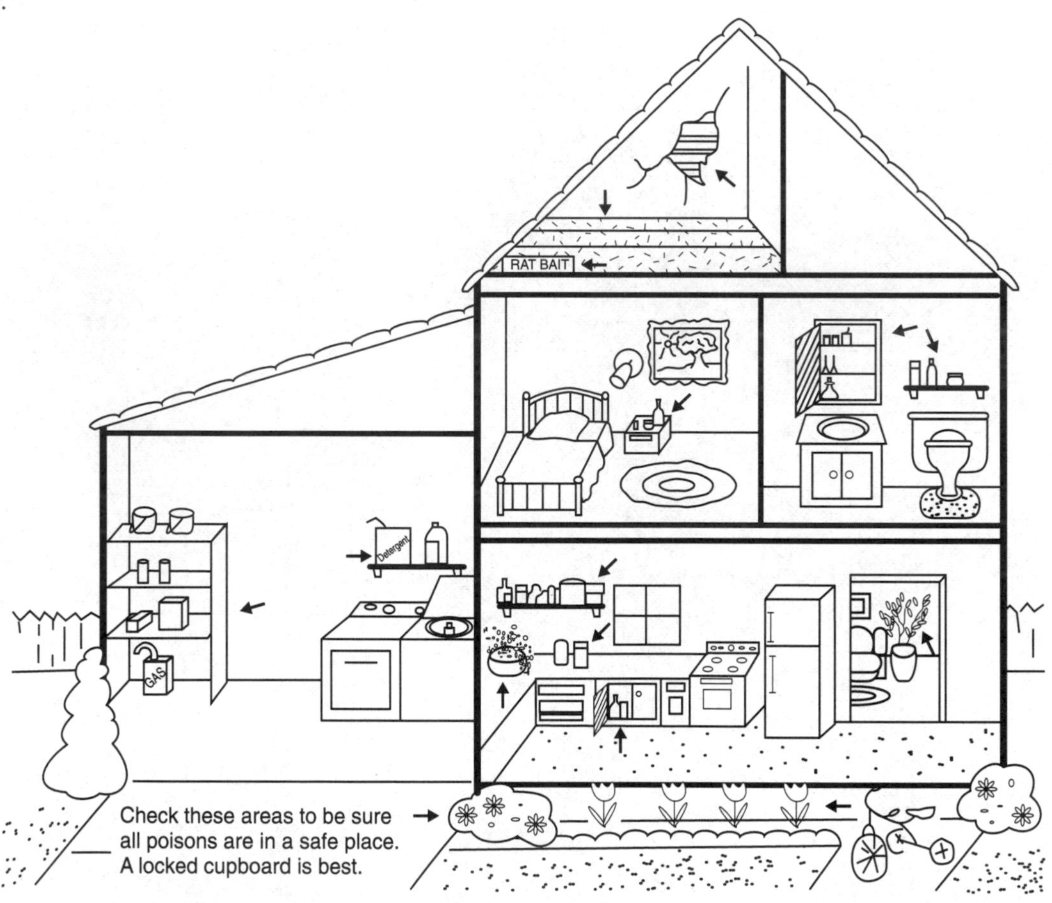

Kitchen	Garage	Bedroom	Bathroom	Attic	Yard
*Detergents	*Insect Spray	Medications	*Medications	*Insulation	*Flowers
*Drain Cleaner	*Fertilizer	*Perfume	*Vitamins	*Poison Bait	*Berries
*Old Food	*Weed Killer	*False Teeth Cleaners	*Sprays	*Broken Plaster	*Seeds
*Cleaners	*Laundry Aids	*Lotions	*Fluoride	*Peeling Paint	*Mushrooms
*Waxes/Polish	*Gas/Car Products	*House Plants	*Rubbing Alcohol		*Leaves
*Liquor	*Paint		*Shampoo		
*Undissolved Soap in Dishwasher	*Turpentine		*Polish Remover		
	*Lighter Fluid		*Mouthwash		

Printed as a Courtesy of the Rocketdyne Division/Rockwell International.

Appendix O
How to Poison-Proof Your Home[a]

Detergents, disinfectants, drain cleaners. . . .

To adults, these products are common household helpers. To young children, they can be lethal weapons.

You can avoid potential tragedy by poison-proofing your home:

- Store household cleaners, cosmetics, medicines, insecticides, and garage products out of children's sight and reach—in locked cabinets or cabinets secured with safety latches.
- Ask your pharmacist to put all prescription drugs in child-resistant packaging. However, be aware that children can open these containers.
- NEVER reuse empty household containers.
- DON'T follow antidote instructions on product labels without first contacting the Poison Control Center.
- NEVER call medicine candy.
- NEVER allow children to play with medicine bottles.
- DON'T take medicines in front of children who tend to imitate adults.
- Discard all old and unlabeled medicines by flushing them down the toilet.
- Store food away from household cleaners.

[a]Adapted from L.I. Regional Poison Control Center at Winthrop-University Hospital, 259 First Street, Mineola, NY 11501.

Appendix P U.S. Consumer Product Safety Commission Poison Lookout Checklist

This checklist should be completed by an adult.

Is your home poison-proof? If it's not, someone may get hurt—and soon. But it's easy to poison-proof your home. Help your parents use this checklist. Whatever you answer "no" should be fixed quickly.

Poison-Proofing the Kitchen	YES	NO
1. Do all harmful products in the cabinets have child-resistant caps? Products like furniture polishes, drain cleaners, and some oven cleaners should have safety packaging to keep small children from accidentally opening the packages.	☐	☐
2. Are all potentially harmful products in their original containers? There are two dangers if products aren't stored in their original containers. Labels on the original containers often give first-aid information if someone should swallow the product. And if products are stored in containers like drinking glasses or pop bottles, someone may think it is food and swallow it.	☐	☐
3. Are harmful products stored away from food? If harmful products are placed next to food, someone may accidentally get a food or a poison mixed up and swallow the poison.	☐	☐
4. Have all potentially harmful products been put up high and out of reach of children? The best way to prevent poisoning is making sure that it's impossible to find and get at the poisons. Locking all cabinets that hold dangerous products is the best poison prevention.	☐	☐

Poison-Proofing the Bathroom	YES	NO
1. Did you ever stop to think that medicines could poison if used improperly? Many children are poisoned each year by overdoses of aspirin. If aspirin can poison, just think of how many other poisons might be in your medicine cabinet.	☐	☐
2. Do your aspirins and other potentially harmful products have child-resistant closures? Aspirins and most prescription drugs come with child-resistant caps. Check to see yours have them.	☐	☐
3. Have you thrown out all out-of-date prescriptions? As medicines get older, the chemicals inside them can change. So what was once a good medicine may now be a dangerous poison. Flush all old drugs down the toilet. Rinse the container well, then discard it.	☐	☐
4. Do you always give medicine only to the person the doctor prescribed it for? The medicine that worked wonders on one person may harm the next. Give drugs only to the person the doctor told you to give them to.	☐	☐

Poison-Proofing the Bathroom—cont'd

	YES	NO
5. Are all medicines in their original containers with the original labels? Prescription medicines may or may not list ingredients. The prescription number on the label will, however, allow rapid identification by the pharmacist of the ingredients should they not be listed. Without the original label and container, you can't be sure of what you're taking. After all, aspirin looks a lot like poisonous roach tablets.	☐	☐

Poison-Proofing the Garage or Storage Area

	YES	NO
1. Did you know that almost everything in your garage or storage area that can be swallowed is a terrible poison? Violent, horrible reactions occur to people who swallow such everyday substances as charcoal lighter, paint thinner and remover, antifreeze, and turpentine.	☐	☐
2. Do all these poisons have child-resistant caps?	☐	☐
3. Are they stored in the original containers?	☐	☐
4. Are the original labels on the containers?	☐	☐
5. Have you made sure that no poisons are stored in drinking glasses or pop bottles?	☐	☐
6. Are all these harmful products locked up and out of sight and reach?	☐	☐

When you can answer all the questions with a "yes," your house is poison-proofed. Then, to make sure your house stays poison-proof, when you buy potentially harmful products make sure they have child-resistant closures and keep these products out of sight and reach.

Appendix Q
American Association of Poison Control Centers

CERTIFIED REGIONAL POISON CENTERS, NOVEMBER 1995

ALABAMA

Alabama Poison Center, Tuscaloosa
408-A Paul Bryant Drive
Tuscaloosa AL 35401
Emergency Phone: (800) 462-0800 (AL only) or (205) 345-0600
E-mail address: fisher 3@aol.com

Regional Poison Control Center
The Children's Hospital of Alabama
1600-7th Ave. South
Birmingham AL 35233-1711
Emergency Phone: (205) 939-9201, (800) 292-6678 (AL only) or (205) 933-4050
E-mail address: N/A

ARIZONA

Arizona Poison and Drug Information Center
Arizona Health Sciences Center, Rm. #1156
1501 N. Campbell Ave.
Tucson AZ 85724
Emergency Phone: (800) 362-0101 (AZ only), (520) 626-6016
E-mail address: mcnally@tonic.pharm.arizona.edu

Samaritan Regional Poison Center
Good Samaritan Regional Medical Center
Ancillary-1
1111 E. McDowell Road
Phoenix AZ 85006
Emergency Phone: (602) 253-3334
E-mail address: richardt@samaritan.edu

CALIFORNIA

Central California Regional Poison Control Center
Valley Children's Hospital
3151 N. Millbrook, IN31
Fresno CA 93703
Emergency Phone: (800) 346-5922 (Central CA only) or (209) 445-1222
E-mail address: N/A

San Diego Regional Poison Center
UCSD Medical Center
200 West Arbor Drive
San Diego CA 92103-8925
Emergency Phone: (619) 543-6000, (800) 876-4766 (in 619 area code only)
E-mail address: amanoguerra@ucsd.edu

San Francisco Bay Area Regional Poison Control Center
San Francisco General Hospital
1001 Potrero Ave., Building 80, Room 230
San Francisco CA 94110
Emergency Phone: (800) 523-2222
E-mail address: N/A

Santa Clara Valley Regional Poison Center
Valley Health Center-Suite 310
750 South Bascom Ave.
San Jose CA 95128
Emergency Phone: (408) 885-6000, (800) 662-9886 (CA only)
E-mail address: wielanmic@wpgate.hhs.co.santa-clara.ca.us

University of California, Davis, Medical Center Regional Poison Control Center
2315 Stockton Blvd
Sacramento CA 95817
Emergency Phone: (916) 734-3692; (800) 342-9293 (Northern California only)
E-mail address: N/A

COLORADO

Rocky Mountain Poison and Drug Center
8802 E. 9th Avenue
Denver CO 80220-6800
Emergency Phone: (303) 629-1123
E-mail address: N/A

CONNECTICUT

Connecticut Regional Poison Center
University of Connecticut Health Center
263 Farmington Avenue
Farmington CT 06030
Emergency Phone: (800) 343-2722 (CT only); (203) 679-3056
E-mail address: N/A

DISTRICT OF COLUMBIA

National Capital Poison Center
3201 New Mexico Avenue, NW, Suite 310
Washington, DC 20016
Emergency Numbers: (202) 625-3333; (202) 362-8563 (TTY)
E-mail address: N/A

FLORIDA

Florida Poison Information Center-Jacksonville
University Medical Center
University of Florida Health Science Center-Jacksonville
655 West 8th Street
Jacksonville, FL 32209
Emergency Numbers: (904) 549-4480; (800) 282-3171 (FL only)
E-mail address: schauben.pcc@mail.health.ufl.edu

The Florida Poison Information Center and Toxicology Resource Center
Tampa General Hospital
Post Office Box 1289
Tampa FL 33601
Emergency Phone: (813) 253-4444 (Tampa) (800) 282-3171 (Florida)
E-mail address: sven.normann@ashp.com

GEORGIA

Georgia Poison Center
Grady Memorial Hospital
80 Butler Street S.E.
P.O. Box 26066
Atlanta GA 30335-3801
Emergency Phone: (800) 282-5846 GA only; (404) 616-9000
E-mail address:lopez_g@L1.mercer.peachnet.edu

INDIANA

Indiana Poison Center
Methodist Hospital of Indiana
1701 N. Senate Boulevard
P.O. Box 1367
Indianapolis IN 46206-1367
Emergency Phone: (800) 382-9097 (IN only), (317) 929-2323
E-mail address: jmowry@mhi.com

KENTUCKY

Kentucky Regional Poison Center of Kosair Children's Hospital
Medical Towers South, Suite 572
P.O. Box 35070
Louisville, KY 40232-5070
Emergency Phone: (502) 629-7275 or (800) 722-5725 (KY only)
E-mail address: N/A

MARYLAND

Maryland Poison Center
20 N. Pine St.
Baltimore MD 21201
Emergency Phone: (410) 528-7701, (800) 492-2414 (MD only)
E-mail address: N/A

National Capital Poison Center (D.C. suburbs only)
3201 New Mexico Avenue, NW, Suite 310
Washington, DC 20016
Emergency Numbers: (202) 625-3333; (202) 362-8563 (TTY)
E-mail address: N/A

MASSACHUSETTS

Massachusetts Poison Control System
300 Longwood Ave.
Boston MA 02115
Emergency Phone: (617) 232-2120, (800) 682-9211
E-mail address: N/A

MICHIGAN

Poison Control Center
Children's Hospital of Michigan
4160 John R., Suite 425
Detroit MI 48201
Emergency Phone: (313) 745-5711, (800) 764-7661
E-mail address: Scsmoli@CMS.CC.Wayne.edu

MINNESOTA

Hennepin Regional Poison Center
Hennepin County Medical Center
701 Park Ave.
Minneapolis MN 55415
Emergency Phone: (612) 347-3141, Petline: (612) 337-7387, TDD (612) 337-7474
E-mail address: N/A

Minnesota Regional Poison Center
8100 34th Avenue S.
PO Box 1309
Minneapolis MN 55440-1309
Emergency Phone: (612) 221-2113
E-mail address: Lsioris@poison1.sprmc.healthpartners.com

MISSOURI

Cardinal Glennon Children's Hospital Regional Poison Center
1465 S. Grand Blvd.
St. Louis MO 63104
Emergency Phone: (314) 772-5200, (800) 366-8888
E-mail address: mike@pcc.slu.edu

MONTANA

Rocky Mountain Poison and Drug Center
8802 E. 9th Avenue
Denver CO 80220
Emergency Phone: (303) 629-1123
E-mail address: N/A

NEBRASKA

The Poison Center
8301 Dodge St.
Omaha NE 68114
Emergency Phone: (402) 390-5555 (Omaha), (800) 955-9119 (NE & WY)
E-mail address: N/A

NEW JERSEY

New Jersey Poison Information and Education System
201 Lyons Ave.
Newark NJ 07112
Emergency Phone: (800) POISON-1 (800-764-7661)
E-mail address: toxdoc@IBM.net

NEW MEXICO

New Mexico Poison and Drug Information Center
University of New Mexico
Health Sciences Library, Room 125
Albuquerque NM 87131-1076
Emergency Phone: (505) 843-2551, (800) 432-6866 (NM only)
E-mail address: troutman@medusa.unm.edu

NEW YORK

Hudson Valley Regional Poison Center
Phelps Memorial Hospital Center
701 North Broadway
North Tarrytown, NY 10591
Emergency Phone: (800) 336-6997, (914) 366-3030
E-mail address: N/A

Long Island Regional Poison Control Center
Winthrop University Hospital
259 First Street
Mineola NY 11501
Emergency Phone: (516) 542-2323, 2324, 2325, 3813
E-mail address: N/A

New York City Poison Control Center
N.Y.C. Department of Health
455 First Ave., Room 123
New York NY 10016
Emergency Phone: (212) 340-4494, (212) P-O-I-S-O-N-S, TDD (212) 689-9014
E-mail address: N/A

NORTH CAROLINA

Carolinas Poison Center
1000 Blythe Boulevard
PO Box 32861
Charlotte, NC 28232-2861
Emergency Phone: (704) 355-4000, (800) 84-TOXIN (1-800-848-6946)
E-mail address: wahoo@med.unc.edu

OHIO

Central Ohio Poison Center
700 Children's Drive
Columbus OH 43205-2696
Emergency Phone: (614) 228-1323, (800) 682-7625, (614) 228-2272 (TTY), (614) 461-2012
E-mail address: N/A

Cincinnati Drug & Poison Information Center
and Regional Poison Control System
PO Box 670144
Cincinnati OH 45267-0144
Emergency Phone: (513) 558-5111, 800-872-5111 (OH only)
E-mail address: N/A

OREGON

Oregon Poison Center
Oregon Health Sciences University
3181 S.W. Sam Jackson Park Road, CB550
Portland OR 97201
Emergency Phone: (503) 494-8968, (800) 452-7165 (OR only)
E-mail address: 'lastname'@ohsu.edu

PENNSYLVANIA

Central Pennsylvania Poison Center
University Hospital
Milton S. Hershey Medical Center
Hershey PA 17033
Emergency Phone: (800) 521-6110
E-mail address: N/A

The Poison Control Center
3600 Sciences Center, Suite 220
Philadelphia PA 19104-2641
Emergency Phone: (215) 386-2100
E-mail address: N/A

Pittsburgh Poison Center
3705 Fifth Avenue
Pittsburgh PA 15213
Emergency Phone: (412) 681-6669
E-mail address: krenzee@chplink.edu

RHODE ISLAND

Rhode Island Poison Center
593 Eddy St.
Providence RI 02903
Emergency Phone: (401) 277-5727
E-mail address: N/A

TEXAS

North Texas Poison Center
5201 Harry Hines Blvd.
P.O. Box 35926
Dallas TX 75235
Emergency Phone: (214) 590-5000, (800) 764-7661 (800-POISON-1)
E-mail address: N/A

Southeast Texas Poison Center
The University of Texas Medical Branch
301 University Avenue
Galveston TX 77550-2780
Emergency Phone: (409) 747-1460, (800) 764-7661 (800-POISON-1)
E-mail address: mellis@mspo1.med.utmb.edu

UTAH

Utah Poison Control Center
410 Chipeta Way, Suite 230
Salt Lake City UT 84108
Emergency Phone: (801) 581-2151, (800) 456-7707 (UT only)
E-mail address: barbara.crouch@hsc.utah.edu

VIRGINIA

Blue Ridge Poison Center
Box 67
Blue Ridge Hospital
Charlottesville VA 22901
Emergency Phone: (804) 924-5543, (800) 451-1428
E-mail address: N/A

National Capital Poison Center (Northern VA only)
3201 New Mexico Avenue, NW, Suite 310
Washington, DC 20016
Emergency Numbers: (202) 625-3333; (202) 362-8563 (TTY)
E-mail address: N/A

WASHINGTON

Washington Poison Center
155 N.E. 100th Street, Suite #400
Seattle, WA 98125
Emergency Numbers: (206) 526-2121; (800) 732-6985; (800) 572-0638 (TDD only); (206) 517-2394
E-mail address: N/A

WEST VIRGINIA

West Virginia Poison Center
3110 MacCorkle Ave. S.E.
Charleston WV 25304
Emergency Phone: (800) 642-3625 (WV only), (304) 348-4211
E-mail address: N/A

WYOMING

The Poison Center
8301 Dodge St.
Omaha NE 68114
Emergency Phone: (402) 390-5555 (Omaha), (800) 955-9119 (NE & WY)
E-mail address: N/A

Index

Note: Page numbers in *italics* indicate illustrations; those followed by t indicate tables.

C

E

G

H

I

M

N

O

P

Q

R

S

T

U

W

X

Y

Z